clinical evidence

The international source of the best available evidence for effective health care

13
JUNE 2005

Editorial Office
BMJ Publishing Group, BMA House, Tavistock Square, London, WC1H 9JR, United Kingdom. Tel: +44 (0)20 7387 4499 • Fax: +44 (0)20 7383 6242 • www.bmjpg.com

Subscription prices for *Clinical Evidence*
Clinical Evidence and *Clinical Evidence Concise* are both published six monthly (June/December) by the BMJ Publishing Group. The annual subscription rates (for December, Issue 12 and June, Issue 13) are:

Concise edition
Personal: £95 • €140 • US$170
Institutional: £200 • €295 • US$365
Student/nurse: £42 • €62 • US$76

Full edition
Personal: £105 • €155 • US$190
Institutional: £220 • €325 • US$400
Student/nurse: £48 • €71 • US$87

There are special combined rates if you wish to purchase both editions.

All individual subscriptions (personal, student, nurse) include online access at no additional cost. Institutional subscriptions are for print editions only. Institutions may purchase online site licences separately. For information on site licences and individual electronic subscriptions please visit the subscription pages of our website www.clinicalevidence.com or email us at CEsubscriptions@bmjgroup.com (UK and ROW) or clinevid@pmds.com (Americas). You may also telephone us or fax us on the following numbers:

UK and ROW Tel: +44 (0)20 7383 6270 • Fax: +44 (0)20 7383 6402
Americas Tel: +1 800 373 2897/240 646 7000 • Fax: +1 240 646 7005

Bulk subscriptions for societies and organisations
The Publishers offer discounts for any society or organisation buying bulk quantities for their members/specific groups. Please contact Miranda Lonsdale, Sales Manager at mlonsdale@bmjgroup.com.

Rights and permission to reproduce
For information on translation rights, please contact Kate McPartlin at KMcPartlin@bmjgroup.com. To request permission to reprint all or part of any contribution in *Clinical Evidence* please contact Michelle McNeely at mmcneely@bmjgroup.com.

British Library Cataloguing in Publication Data. A catalogue record for this book is available from the British Library. ISSN 1462-3846, ISBN 0-9548965-3-X.

Legal Disclaimer
The information contained in this publication, is intended for medical professionals. Categories presented in *Clinical Evidence* indicate a judgement about the strength of the evidence available to our authors prior to publication and the relative importance of benefits and harms.

We rely on our authors to confirm the accuracy of the information presented, and to describe generally accepted practices, and therefore we as the publisher, and our editors, cannot warrant its accuracy. Readers should be aware that professionals in the field may have different opinions. Because of this fact and also because of regular advances in medical research, we strongly recommend that readers independently verify specified treatments and drugs, including manufacturers' guidance. Also, the categories do not indicate whether a particular treatment is generally appropriate or whether it is suitable for a particular individual. Ultimately it is the readers' responsibility to make their own professional judgements, so to appropriately advise and treat their patients.

Description or reference to a product or publication does not imply endorsement of that product or publication, unless it is owned by the BMJ Publishing Group Limited.

To the fullest extent permitted by law, BMJ Publishing Group Limited and its editors, are not responsible for any losses, injury or damage caused to any person or property, (including under contract, by negligence, products liability or otherwise), whether they be direct or indirect, special, incidental or consequential, resulting from the application of the information in this publication.

Printed in Great Britain by William Clowes Ltd, Beccles, Suffolk, UK.

Designed by Pete Wilder, The Designers Collective, London, UK.

Team and Advisors

Editor David Tovey **Clinical Editors** Mike Bedford, Klara Brunnhuber, Luis Gabriel Cuervo Amore, Richmal Oates-Whitehead, Anjana Patel, Bazian Ltd **Senior Editor** Karen Pettersen **Assistant Editors** Claire Castle, Alan Thomas **Quality Assurance Editor** James Woodcock **North American Editor** David Goldmann **Publishing Manager** Polly Brown **Production Editor** Michelle McNeely **Editorial Assistant** Marie Traisneau **Production Assistant** Julia Stimpson **Technical Editors** Andy Baker, Jemma Carter, Maysoon Delahunty, Anne Lawson, Sean McNamara, Adrienne Penfield **Indexer** Angela Cottingham **Technology Manager** Jonathan Peterson **Technology Team** Michael Blake, Alex Hooper, Jeremy Gillies, Kourosh Mojar, James Freeman **Webmaster/Product Manager** David Ansley **Typesetting** BMJ Journal Production **Print Production** Catherine Harding-Wiltshire **Information Specialist Manager** Andrea Lane **Information Specialists** Mick Arber, Olwen Beaven, Sarah Greenley, Jane McHugh, Alex McNeil, Tamara Rader, Judith van Berkom **Information Specialist Administrator** Varsha Mistry **Business Manager** Rachel Armitage **Business Development Manager** Charlotte Pestridge **Department Administrator** Hannah Lawrence **Marketing and Sales Manager** Diane Harris **Marketing and Sales Team** Jaspal Chaggar, Miranda Lonsdale, Kate McPartlin, Nisha Patel

SECTION ADVISORS

Blood and lymph disorders Mark Best, Cayman Islands **Cardiovascular disorders** Nick Hicks, UK **Child health** Mary Rudolf, UK and Virginia Moyer, USA **Digestive system disorders** David Cave, USA, John McDonald, Canada, and David Metz, USA **Ear, nose, and throat disorders** George Browning, UK **Endocrine disorders** Shereen Ezzat, Canada and Victor Montori, USA **Eye disorders** Andrew Dick, UK **HIV and AIDS** Nandi Siegfried, South Africa **Infectious diseases** Paul Garner, UK **Kidney disorders** Fred Coe, USA and Michael Conlin, USA **Men's health** Peter Schlegal, USA and Robyn Webber, UK **Mental health** John Geddes, UK **Musculoskeletal disorders** Troels Mork Hansen, Denmark and John Stothard, UK **Neurological disorders** Tony Marson, UK **Oral health** Aubrey Sheiham, UK **Perioperative care** Andrew Smith, UK and Valerie Palda, Canada **Poisoning** Robin Ferner, UK and Allister Vale, UK **Pregnancy and childbirth** Metin Gulmezoglu, Switzerland **Respiratory disorders** Satyendra Sharma, Canada and Chris del Mar, Australia **Sexual health** George Schmid, USA **Skin disorders** Hywel Williams, UK and Jane McGregor, UK **Sleep disorders** Michael Hensley, Australia **Women's health** Mike Dixon, UK **Wounds** Nicky Cullum, UK

EDITORIAL BOARD

Don Berwick, USA • Jonathan Burton, UK • Enrico Coiera, Australia • Nicky Cullum, UK • Chris Del Mar, Australia • Paul Glasziou, UK • Peter Götzche, Denmark • Andrew Haines, UK • Brian Haynes, Canada • Ryuki Kassai, Japan • Christian Koeck, Austria • Alessandro Liberati, Italy • Ruaridh Milne, UK • Elizabeth Mullen, USA • Cynthia Mulrow, USA • Andrew Oxman, Norway • Eleanor Wallace, USA

Acknowledgements

The BMJ Publishing Group thanks the following people and organisations for their advice and support: The Cochrane Collaboration, and especially Iain Chalmers, Mike Clarke, Phil Alderson, and Carol Lefebvre; the National Health Service (NHS) Centre for Reviews and Dissemination, and especially Jos Kleijnen and Julie Glanville; the NHS, and especially Tom Mann, Ron Stamp, Ben Toth, Veronica Fraser, Muir Gray, and Nick Rosen; the British National Formulary, and especially Dinesh Mehta, Eric Connor, and John Martin; Martindale: The Complete Drug Reference, and especially Sean Sweetman; the Health Information Research Unit at McMaster University, and especially Brian Haynes and Ann McKibbon; the United Health Foundation (UHF), and especially Reed Tuckson and Yvette Krantz; Bazian Ltd, and especially Anna Donald and Vivek Muthu; Paul Dieppe, Tonya Fancher, and Richard Kravitz who are working with *Clinical Evidence* to explore ways of presenting evidence on the usefulness of diagnostic test; previous staff who have contributed to this issue; the clinicians, epidemiologists, and members of patient groups who have acted as contributors, advisors, and peer reviewers; and members of our user panels: Liz Hawthorne and colleagues at Didcot Health Centre; Murray Lough and colleagues at Airdrie Health Centre; Alex Potter and colleagues at Clydebank Health Centre; and Aimee Brame, Chris Clark, Gloria Daly, Hilary Durrant, Sarah Gwynne, James Harper, Diane Hickford, Sarosh Irani, Alison Kedward, Denise Knight, Sarah Lourenco, Michael Murphy, Ross Overshott, Deborah Rigby, and Catherine Tighe.

The BMJ Publishing Group values the ongoing support it has received from the global medical community for *Clinical Evidence*. In addition to others, we wish to acknowledge the efforts of the UHF and the NHS who have provided educational funding to support wide dissemination to health professionals in the USA (UHF) and UK (NHS). We are grateful to the clinicians and patients who have taken part in focus groups, which are crucial to the development of *Clinical Evidence*. Finally, we would like to acknowledge the readers who have taken the time to send us their comments and suggestions.

Contents

Some topics listed here are not printed in this issue but are available on the website while awaiting update (www.clinicalevidence.com).

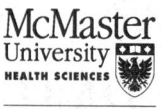

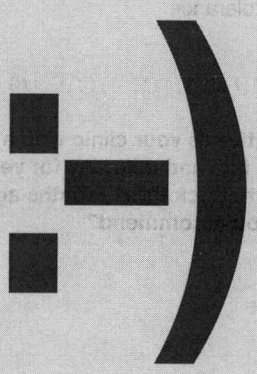

Welcome to Issue 13

Welcome to Issue 13 of *Clinical Evidence*, the international source of the best available evidence on the effects of common clinical interventions. *Clinical Evidence* summarises the current state of knowledge and uncertainty about the prevention and treatment of clinical conditions, based on thorough searches and appraisal of the literature. It is neither a text book of medicine, nor a set of guidelines. It describes the best available evidence from systematic reviews, RCTs, and observational studies where appropriate, and if there is no good evidence it says so.

DEALING WITH UNCERTAINTY

Clinical Evidence and its sister product for patients, Best Treatments, aim to help people make informed decisions about which treatments to use. For clinicians and patients we wish to highlight treatments that work and for which the benefits outweigh the harms, especially those treatments that may currently be underused. We also wish to highlight treatments that do not work or for which the harms outweigh the benefits. Crucially, *Clinical Evidence* and Best Treatments can help people to distinguish between uncertainty due to gaps in the evidence or due to gaps in their own knowledge.

For the research community, *Clinical Evidence* and Best Treatments show where more research is needed—where there are currently no good RCTs or no RCTs that look at certain groups of people or important patient outcomes. We are pleased to be working closely with the James Lind Alliance, which is establishing partnerships between patients and clinicians to identify and prioritise current uncertainties about the effects of treatments. One important product of this initiative will be the free access Database of Uncertainties about the Effects of Treatments (DUET).

HOW MUCH DO WE KNOW?

So what can *Clinical Evidence* tell us about the state of our current knowledge? What proportion of commonly used treatments are supported by good evidence, what proportion should not be used or used only with caution, and how big are the gaps in our knowledge? Of the 2404 treatments covered in this issue, 360 (15%) are rated as beneficial, 538 (22%) likely to be beneficial, 180 (7%) as trade off between benefits and harms, 115 (5%) unlikely to be beneficial, 89 (4%) likely to be ineffective or harmful, and 1122 (47%), the largest proportion, as unknown effectiveness (see figure 1). Dividing treatments into categories is never easy. It always involves a degree of subjective judgement and is sometimes controversial. We do it because users tell us it is helpful, but judged by its own rules the categorisation is certainly of unknown effectiveness and may well have trade offs between benefits and harms. However, the figures above suggest that the research community has a large task ahead and that most decisions about treatments still rest on the individual judgements of clinicians and patients.

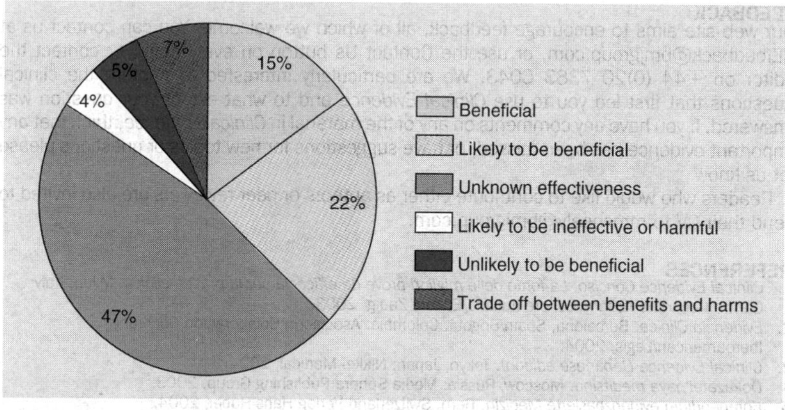

Figure 1

WHAT'S NEW

Clinical Evidence is continuously updated, with full literature searches on each topic every 12 months. Print copies containing the latest version of each topic are published every six months, and the website is refreshed, with new and updated content, every month. Before each topic is updated, we thoroughly review the structure of the topic, including the questions and the treatments covered, with the help of our expert authors and advisors in the field, to ensure maximum clinical relevance.

The content of *Clinical Evidence* Issue 13 is a snapshot of all content that was ready for publication in February 2005. Ten new topics have been added since Issue 12: Common cold, Angina (stable), Acne, Cervical cancer, Carbon monoxide poisoning, Non-Hodgkin's lymphoma, Glycaemic control in type 1 diabetes, End stage renal disease, Uncomplicated malaria and Kidney stones. In addition, 67 chapters have been updated, and by the time this reaches you more new and updated topics will have been posted on the website (www.clinicalevidence.com).

The regular updating of *Clinical Evidence* is now supplemented by BMJ Updates (www.bmjupdates.com), which provides readable summaries of the best and most relevant clinical research articles as they are published. You can ask the service to alert you to valid research in the areas that most interest you. BMJ Updates is a collaboration between the BMJ Publishing Group and McMaster University and can be accessed free via the *Clinical Evidence* website.

INTERNATIONAL REACH

Clinical Evidence has an international circulation, reaching more than a million clinicians worldwide in seven languages. In the USA, 500 000 clinicians receive copies of the concise edition thanks to the United Health Foundation. In the UK, the National Health Service distributes 50 000 copies of the concise edition to clinical staff in England, with free online access to everyone in England and Wales, and the BMA sends the concise edition to 10 500 UK medical students once a year. The governments of Norway and New Zealand now provide everyone in their countries with free online access, and thanks to the Italian Ministry of Health and the work of the Italian Cochrane Centre, 300 000 doctors in Italy receive a copy of the concise edition in Italian.[1]

Clinical Evidence is available in other non-English language editions. The Spanish translation (published in collaboration with the Iberoamerican Cochrane Centre and Legis) now comes in all formats: full, concise and online.[2] The full text is available in Japanese[3] and Russian[4] (seven broad speciality editions). The concise edition is also available in German[5] and French[6].

Finally, *Clinical Evidence* continues to be available free online to people in developing countries as part of the HINARI initiative spearheaded by the World Health Organization and the BMJ Publishing Group. Details of those countries that qualify are available from the *Clinical Evidence* website (www.clinicalevidence.com).

FEEDBACK

Our web-site aims to encourage feedback, all of which we welcome. You can contact us at CEfeedback@bmjgroup.com, or use the Contact Us button on every page, or contact the editor on +44 (0)20 7383 6043. We are particularly interested to capture the clinical questions that first led you to use *Clinical Evidence* and to what extent your question was answered. If you have any comments on any of the material in *Clinical Evidence*, think that any important evidence has been missed, or have suggestions for new topics or questions please let us know.

Readers who would like to contribute either as authors or peer reviewers are also invited to send their CV to mmcneely@bmjgroup.com.

REFERENCES

1. *Clinical Evidence Conciso: La fonte delle migliori prove de efficacia per la pratica clinica*. Milan, Italy: Centro Cochrane Italiano/Editore Italiano/Editore Zadig, 2003.
2. *Evidencia Clinica*. Barcelona, Spain/Bogotá, Colombia: Asociacón Colaboración Cochrane Iberoamerican/Legis, 2004.
3. *Clinical Evidence (Japanese edition)*. Tokyo, Japan: Nikkei Medical, 2004.
4. *Dokazatel'naya meditsina*. Moscow, Russia: Media Sphera Publishing Group, 2003.
5. *Kompendium evidenzbasierte Medizin*. Bern, Switzerland Verlag Hans Huber, 2004.
6. *Décider pour traiter abrégé*. Meudon, France: RanD, 2004.

About Clinical Evidence

The inspiration for *Clinical Evidence* came in a phone call in 1995. Tom Mann and his colleagues at the NHS Executive asked the BMJ Publishing Group to explore the possibility of developing an evidence "formulary" along the lines of the British National Formulary. They recognised that clinicians were under increasing pressure to keep up to date and to base their practice more firmly on evidence, but that few had the necessary time or skills to do this. Their idea was to provide a pocketbook containing concise and regularly updated summaries of the best available evidence on clinical interventions. However, they didn't think that the NHS could develop such a formulary itself. "It would be marvellous", said Tom Mann, "if somebody would just do it." A small team at the BMJ set to work to produce a pilot version of what was then called the Clinical Effectiveness Directory.

Since that pilot, a great deal has changed. In collaboration with the American College of Physicians–American Society of Internal Medicine, we convened an international advisory board, held focus groups of clinicians, talked to patient support groups, and adopted countless good ideas from early drafts by our contributors. Throughout we kept in mind an equation set out by Slawson et al.[1] This states that the usefulness of any source of information is equal to its relevance, multiplied by its validity, divided by the work required to extract the information. In order to be as useful as possible, we aimed for high relevance, high validity, and low work in terms of the reader's time and effort. We also kept in mind principles of transparency and explicitness. Readers needed to understand where our information came from and how it was assembled.

A UNIQUE RESOURCE

Clinical Evidence is one of a growing number of sources of evidence-based information for clinicians. But it has several features that make it unique.

- Its contents are driven by questions rather than by the availability of research evidence. Rather than start with the evidence and summarise what is there, we identify important clinical questions, and then search for and summarise the best available evidence to answer them.
- It identifies but does not try to fill important gaps in the evidence. In a phrase used by Jerry Osheroff, who has led much of the research on clinicians' information needs,[2] *Clinical Evidence* presents the dark as well as the light side of the moon. We feel that it is helpful for clinicians to know when their uncertainty stems from gaps in the evidence rather than gaps in their own knowledge.
- It is continuously updated, with full literature searches in each topic every twelve months. Print copies containing the latest version of each topic are published every six months and the website is refreshed, with new and updated content, every month.

COMPLEMENTARY BUT DIFFERENT

We are often asked how *Clinical Evidence* differs from two other high quality sources of evidence-based information: The *Cochrane Library*; and the evidence-based journals *ACP Journal Club*, *Evidence-Based Medicine*, *Evidence-Based Mental Health*, and *Evidence-Based Nursing*.

Clinical Evidence is complementary to but different from the work of the Cochrane Collaboration (www.cochrane.org), which produces and publishes high quality systematic reviews of controlled trials. *Clinical Evidence* has been called the friendly front end of the Cochrane Library, because it takes this and other high quality information and pulls it together in one place in a concise format. Many of our advisors and contributors are active members of the Cochrane Collaboration, and we are exploring closer ties between *Clinical Evidence* and the Collaboration in the way the evidence is searched for, summarised, and accessed by users.

Clinical Evidence is also complementary to but different from the evidence-based journals, which select and abstract the best and most clinically relevant articles as they appear in the world's medical literature. Together these journals form a growing archive of high quality abstracts of individual articles. *Clinical Evidence* takes a different approach. It begins not with the journals but with clinical questions. It is able to answer some. For others it simply reports that no good evidence was found.

A WORK IN PROGRESS

Clinical Evidence continues to evolve. We knew when we started that we were undertaking an enormous task, and the more we work on it, the more we realise its enormity. Although we have made every effort to ensure that the searches are thorough and that the appraisals of studies are objective (see How Clinical Evidence is put together), we will inevitably have missed some important studies. In order not to make unjustified claims about the accuracy of the information, we use phrases such as 'we found no systematic review' rather than 'there is no systematic review'. In order to be as explicit as possible about the methods used for each contribution, we have asked each set of contributors to provide a brief methods section, describing the searches that were performed and how individual studies were selected.

Clinical Evidence is now a family of products, appearing in different formats and languages for different audiences. Our expectation is that *Clinical Evidence* will evolve further over the years, in response to the needs of clinicians and patients.

REFERENCES

1. Slawson DC, Shaughnessy AF, Bennett JH. Becoming a medical information master: feeling good about not knowing everything. *J Fam Pract* 1994;38:505–513.
2. Ely JW, Osheroff JA, Ebell MJ, et al. Analysis of questions asked by family doctors regarding patient care. *BMJ* 1999;319:358–361.

A guide to the text

SUMMARY PAGE

The summary page for each topic presents the questions addressed, key messages, and a list of the interventions covered (in alphabetical order), categorised according to whether we have found evidence that they are effective or not. We have developed categories of treatment effects based on the Cochrane Collaboration's *A guide to effective care in pregnancy and childbirth*.[1] These categories are explained in the table below:

TABLE Categorisation of treatment effects in *Clinical Evidence*

Beneficial	Interventions for which effectiveness has been demonstrated by clear evidence from RCTs, and for which expectation of harms is small compared with the benefits.
Likely to be beneficial	Interventions for which effectiveness is less well established than for those listed under 'beneficial'.
Trade off between benefits and harms	Interventions for which clinicians and patients should weigh up the beneficial and harmful effects according to individual circumstances and priorities.
Unknown effectiveness	Interventions for which there are currently insufficient data or data of inadequate quality.
Unlikely to be beneficial	Interventions for which lack of effectiveness is less well established than for those listed under 'likely to be ineffective or harmful'.
Likely to be ineffective or harmful	Interventions for which ineffectiveness or harmfulness has been demonstrated by clear evidence.

Fitting interventions into these categories is not always straightforward. For one thing, the categories represent a mix of several hierarchies: the size of benefit (or harm), the strength of evidence (RCT or observational data), and the degree of certainty around the finding (represented by the confidence interval). Another problem is that much of the evidence that is most relevant to clinical decisions relates to comparisons between different interventions rather than to comparison with placebo or no intervention. Where necessary, we have indicated the comparisons. A third problem is that interventions may have been tested, or found to be effective, in only one group of people, such as those at high risk of an outcome. Again, we have indicated this where possible. But perhaps most difficult of all has been trying to maintain consistency across different topics. We continue to work on refining the criteria for putting interventions under each category. Interventions that cannot be tested in an RCT for ethical or practical reasons are sometimes included in the categorisation table and are identified with an asterisk.

NEGATIVE FINDINGS

A surprisingly hard aspect to get right is the reporting of negative findings. Saying that there is no good evidence that a treatment works is not, of course, the same as saying that the treatment doesn't work. We recognise that to get this right, we need a better handle on the power of individual systematic reviews and trials to demonstrate statistically significant differences between groups, and better information on what constitute clinically important differences in the major outcomes for each intervention. In the meantime, we hope that the text makes a clear distinction between lack of benefit and lack of evidence of benefit.

OUTCOMES

Clinical Evidence focuses on outcomes that matter to patients, meaning those that patients themselves are aware of, such as symptom severity, quality of life, survival, disability, walking distance, and live birth rate. We are less interested in proxy outcomes such as blood lipid concentrations, blood pressure, or ovulation rates. Each topic includes a list of the main patient oriented outcomes, and where possible describes how these are measured. We have for the moment decided not to address the vexed question of what constitutes a clinically important change in an outcome, but we would welcome suggestions on how to do this.

EFFECTS, NOT EFFECTIVENESS

A key aim of *Clinical Evidence* is to emphasise the important trade offs between advantages and disadvantages of different treatment options. We therefore talk about the effects of interventions, both positive and negative, rather than the effectiveness, and for each question or intervention option we present data on benefits and harms under separate headings.

HARMS

Good information about harms is often more difficult to find than information about benefits.[2] Most controlled trials are designed to investigate benefits. Many either fail to document harms or present the information in a form that is difficult to analyse or interpret. When drugs are licensed they may have been used clinically in only a few thousand people; the absence of documented harms is not strong evidence that harms will not be discovered in the years after licensing.

Clinical Evidence recognises that the evidence about harms is often weaker than that about benefits. In an attempt to correct for this bias, *Clinical Evidence* has lowered the threshold for evidence to be included in the harms sections. Much of the evidence for harms comes from observational studies ranging from prospective cohort studies to case reports, and these are included when the harm is serious or when there is good corroborating evidence that the harm can be attributed to the treatment.

DRUG NAMES

Clinical Evidence has an international audience. Difficulties can arise when different names for the same drug are used in different parts of the world. We state the recommended or proposed International Name where possible and give only the generic or non-proprietary names of drugs rather than the brand names. Where an international name for a drug is not available we use the most common name (e.g. aspirin). A regularly updated table of equivalent drug names, put together by *Martindale: The Complete Drug Reference*,[3] is available on the *Clinical Evidence* website (www.clinicalevidence.com).

INFORMATION ON COST

In previous issues we did not include information on the cost or cost effectiveness of interventions. This was not because we believed cost to be unimportant, but because the question of what constitutes good evidence on cost is much disputed and because costs vary greatly both within and between countries. In response to feedback from users and customers we have decided to relax this restriction. In future issues we will allow authors to add cost information and comparisons where they are both important and generally applicable.

NUMERICAL DATA

Whenever possible, data are presented in the same form as in the original studies. However, sometimes we have changed the units or type of information in an attempt to present the results in a systematic and easily interpretable form.

AN INTERNATIONAL APPROACH

Clinical Evidence takes an international approach to the evidence. This means including drugs that are not licensed in some countries. It also means keeping in mind the practicalities of treating people in poorer countries, by covering some interventions even if they have been superseded (for example, single drug treatment for HIV infection as opposed to three drug treatment).

COMPETING INTERESTS

In line with the BMJ's policy,[4] our aim is not to try to eliminate conflicts of interest but to make them explicit so that readers can judge for themselves what influence, if any, these may have had on the contributors' interpretation of the evidence. We therefore ask all contributors (and peer reviewers) to let us know about any potential competing interests, and we append any that are declared to the end of the contribution. Where the contributor gives no competing interests, we record 'none declared'.

CHANGES SINCE THE LAST UPDATE

Substantive changes since the last update are listed at the end of each topic. These are defined as:

- Presentation of additional evidence that either confirms or alters the conclusions
- Re-evaluation of the evidence
- Correction of an important error

WEB ONLY TOPICS

Some topics appear only on the website and not in the paper edition. These include topics whose search date is more than 20 months before an editorial deadline for the paper edition (February for the June edition and August for the December edition each year) and a few topics that we are no longer updating.

REFERENCE LINKS TO FULL TEXT

Clinical Evidence references link to the full text on PubMed.

EMAIL ALERTING SERVICE

If you wish to be notified by email about new topics, updates, or corrections, you can register for our alerting service at www.clinicalevidence.com.

HOW TO USE THE INFORMATION IN *CLINICAL EVIDENCE*

The type of information contained in *Clinical Evidence* is necessary but not sufficient for the provision of effective, high quality health care. It is intended as an aid to clinical decision making, to be used in conjunction with other important sources of information. These other sources include estimates of people's baseline risk of a condition or outcome based on history, physical examination and clinical investigations; individual preferences; economic arguments; availability of treatments; and local expertise. Some guidance on how to apply research evidence in practice is available on our website (www.clinicalevidence.com) and in appendix 3.

REFERENCES

1. Enkin M, Keirse M, Renfrew M, et al. *A guide to effective care in pregnancy and childbirth*. Oxford: Oxford University Press, 1998.
2. Derry S, Loke YK, Aronson JK. Incomplete evidence: the inadequacy of databases in tracing published adverse drug reactions in clinical trials. BMC Medical Research Methodology 2001;1:7. http://www.biomedcentral.com/1471-2288/1/7 (last accessed 13 October 2003).
3. Sweetman SC (Ed). *Martindale: The Complete Drug Reference*. 33rd ed. London: Pharmaceutical Press, 2002. http://www.pharmpress.com (last accessed 13 October 2003) or contact martindale@rpsgb.org.uk.
4. Smith R. Beyond conflict of interest. *BMJ* 1998;317:219-292.

How Clinical Evidence is put together

The summaries in *Clinical Evidence* result from a rigorous process aimed at ensuring that they are both reliable and relevant to clinical practice.

SELECTING TOPICS
Clinical Evidence aims to cover common or important clinical conditions seen in primary and hospital care. To decide which conditions to cover we review national data on consultation rates, morbidity and mortality, we take account of national priorities for health care such as those outlined in the UK National Service Frameworks and in the US Institute of Medicine reports, and we take advice from generalist clinicians and patient groups. Our website (www.clinicalevidence.com) provides a list of conditions that we are planning to cover in future issues. Further suggestions are welcome.

SELECTING THE QUESTIONS
The questions in *Clinical Evidence* concern the benefits and harms of preventative and therapeutic interventions, with emphasis on outcomes that matter to patients. Questions are selected for their relevance to clinical practice by section advisors and contributors, in collaboration with clinicians and patient groups. Each new issue of *Clinical Evidence* includes new questions as well as updates of existing questions. We invite readers to suggest new clinical questions using the feedback slips to be found at the back of the book and on clinicalevidence.com, or by writing directly to *Clinical Evidence*.

SEARCHING AND APPRAISING THE LITERATURE
For each question, the literature is searched using the Cochrane Library, Medline, Embase and other electronic databases as required, looking first for good systematic reviews of RCTs; then for good RCTs published since the search date of the review. Where we find no good recent systematic reviews, we search for individual RCTs back to 1966. The date of the search is recorded in the methods section for each topic. Of the studies that are identified in the search, we select and summarise only a small proportion. The selection is done by critically appraising the abstracts of the studies identified in the search, a task performed independently by information scientists using validated criteria similar to those of Sackett et al[1] and Jadad.[2,3] Where the search identifies more than one or two good reviews or trials, we select those we judge to be the most robust and relevant. Where we identify few or no good reviews or trials, we include other studies but highlight their limitations. Contributors, chosen for their clinical expertise in the field and their skills in epidemiology, are asked to review our selection of studies and to justify any additions or exclusions they wish to make.

Our search strategy and critical appraisal criteria are available on clinicalevidence.com.

SUMMARISING THE EVIDENCE, PEER REVIEW, AND EDITING
Our external contributors summarise the evidence relating to each question. Each topic is then peer reviewed by at least two external expert clinicians, and by an editorial committee including external expert clinicians and epidemiologists. The revised text is then extensively edited by editors with clinical and epidemiological training, and data are checked against the original study reports. Bazian Ltd edits a proportion of topics and provides additional content and support.

FEEDBACK AND ERROR CORRECTIONS
Despite the extensive peer review and editorial quality checks, we expect that a text of this size will contain some errors and inconsistencies. Please let us know if you find any errors, either by returning the comment page at the back of this book, emailing us at CEfeedback@bmjgroup.com, or going to 'Contact us' on clinicalevidence.com.

Any errors considered to be major will be corrected immediately on clinicalevidence.com; minor errors will be corrected as part of our monthly updating of the website. All errors will be corrected in the next printed issue. Errors that have been corrected will be marked as a substantive change on the website (the text in benefits, harms, or comment will be highlighted light blue, and an 'i' in a circle will link through to the substantive change text).

If you are using the information in *Clinical Evidence* to guide your clinical practice we advise that you (regularly) check our website in order to remain as up to date as possible.

REFERENCES

1. Sackett DL, Haynes RB, Guyatt GH, et al. Clinical Epidemiology: A basic science for clinical medicine. 2nd ed. Boston: Little Brown, 1991.
2. Jadad A. Assessing the quality of RCTs: Why, what, how and by whom? In: Jadad A, ed. Randomised Controlled Trials. London: BMJ Books, 1998:45–60.
3. Jadad AR, Moore RA, Carroll D, et al. Assessing the quality of reports of randomized clinical trials: is blinding necessary? *Control Clin Trials* 1996;17:1–12.

Glossary

Absolute risk (AR) The probability that an individual will experience the specified outcome during a specified period. It lies in the range 0 to 1, or is expressed as a percentage. In contrast to common usage, the word "risk" may refer to adverse events (such as myocardial infarction) or desirable events (such as cure).

Absolute risk increase (ARI) The absolute difference in risk between the experimental and control groups in a trial. It is used when the risk in the experimental group exceeds the risk in the control group, and is calculated by subtracting the AR in the control group from the AR in the experimental group. This figure does not give any idea of the proportional increase between the two groups: for this, relative risk (RR) is needed (see below).

Absolute risk reduction (ARR) The absolute difference in risk between the experimental and control groups in a trial. It is used when the risk in the control group exceeds the risk in the experimental group, and is calculated by subtracting the AR in the experimental group from the AR in the control group. This figure does not give any idea of the proportional reduction between the two groups: for this, relative risk (RR) is needed (see below).

Allocation concealment A method used to prevent selection bias by concealing the allocation sequence from those assigning participants to intervention groups. Allocation concealment prevents researchers from (unconsciously or otherwise) influencing which intervention group each participant is assigned to.

Applicability The application of the results from clinical trials to individual people. A randomised trial only provides direct evidence of causality within that specific trial. It takes an additional logical step to apply this result to a specific individual. Individual characteristics will affect the outcome for this person.

Baseline risk The risk of the event occurring without the active treatment. Estimated by the baseline risk in the control group.

Best evidence Systematic reviews of RCTs are the best method for revealing the effects of a therapeutic intervention.

Bias Systematic deviation of study results from the true results, because of the way(s) in which the study is conducted.

Blinding/blinded A trial is fully blinded if all the people involved are unaware of the treatment group to which trial participants are allocated until after the interpretation of results. This includes trial participants and everyone involved in administering treatment or recording trial results.

Block randomisation Randomisation by a pattern to produce the required number of people in each group.

Case control study A study design that examines a group of people who have experienced an event (usually an adverse event) and a group of people who have not experienced the same event, and looks at how exposure to suspect (usually noxious) agents differed between the two groups. This type of study design is most useful for trying to ascertain the cause of rare events, such as rare cancers.

Case series Analysis of series of people with the disease (there is no comparison group in case series).

Cluster randomisation A cluster randomised study is one in which a group of participants are randomised to the same intervention together. Examples of cluster randomisation include allocating together people in the same village, hospital, or school. If the results are then analysed by individuals rather than the group as a whole bias can occur.

Cohort study A non-experimental study design that follows a group of people (a cohort), and then looks at how events differ among people within the group. A study that examines a cohort, which differs in respect to exposure to some suspected risk factor (e.g. smoking), is useful for trying to ascertain whether exposure is likely to cause specified events (e.g. lung cancer). Prospective cohort studies (which track participants forward in time) are more reliable than retrospective cohort studies.

Completer analysis Analysis of data from only those participants who remained at the end of the study. Compare with intention to treat analysis, which uses data from all participants who enrolled (see below).

Confidence interval (CI) The 95% confidence interval (or 95% confidence limits) would include 95% of results from studies of the same size and design in the same population. This is close but not identical to saying that the true size of the effect (never exactly known) has a 95% chance of falling within the confidence interval. If the 95% confidence interval for a relative risk (RR) or an odds ratio (OR) crosses 1, then this is taken as no evidence of an effect. The practical advantages of a confidence interval (rather than a P value) is that they present the range of likely effects.

Controlled clinical trial (CCT) A trial in which participants are assigned to two or more different treatment groups. In Clinical Evidence, we use the term to refer to controlled trials in which treatment is assigned by a method other than random allocation. When the method of allocation is by random selection, the study is referred to as a randomised controlled trial (RCT; see below). Non-randomised controlled trials are more likely to suffer from bias than RCTs.

Controls In a controlled trial, controls refer to the participants in the comparison group, who may be allocated to placebo, no treatment, or a standard treatment.

Correlation coefficient A measure of association that indicates the degree to which two variables change together in a linear relationship. It is represented by r, and varies between -1 and $+1$. When r is $+1$, there is a perfect positive relationship (when one variable increases, so does the other, and the proportionate difference remains constant). When r is -1 there is a perfect negative relationship (when one variable increases the other decreases, or vice versa, and the proportionate difference remains constant). This, however, does not rule out a relationship—it just excludes a linear relationship.

Crossover randomised trial A trial in which participants receive one treatment and have outcomes measured, and then receive an alternative treatment and have outcomes measured again. The order of treatments is randomly assigned. Sometimes a period of no treatment is used before the trial starts and in between the treatments (washout periods) to minimise interference between the treatments (carry over effects). Interpretation of the results from crossover randomised controlled trials (RCTs) can be complex.

Cross sectional study A study design that involves surveying a population about an exposure, or condition, or both, at one point in time. It can be used for assessing prevalence of a condition in the population.

Disability Adjusted Life Year (DALY) A method for measuring disease burden, which aims to quantify in a single figure both the quantity and quality of life lost or gained by a disease, risk factor, or treatment. The DALYs lost or gained are a function of the expected number of years spent in a particular state of health, multiplied by a coefficient determined by the disability experienced in that state (ranging from 0 [optimal health] to 1 [deaths]). Later years are discounted at a rate of 3 per year, and childhood and old age are weighted to count for less.

Effect size (standardised mean differences) In the medical literature, effect size is used to refer to a variety of measures of treatment effect. In *Clinical Evidence* it refers to a standardised mean difference: a statistic for combining continuous variables (such as pain scores or height), from different scales, by dividing the difference between two means by an estimate of the within group standard deviation.

Event The occurrence of a dichotomous outcome that is being sought in the study (such as myocardial infarction, death, or a four-point improvement in pain score).

Experimental study A study in which the investigator studies the effect of intentionally altering one or more factors under controlled conditions.

Factorial design A factorial design attempts to evaluate more than one intervention compared with control in a single trial, by means of multiple randomisations.

False negative A person with the target condition (defined by the gold standard) who has a negative test result.

False positive A person without the target condition (defined by the gold standard) who has a positive test result.

Fixed effects The 'fixed effects' model of meta-analysis assumes, often unreasonably, that the variability between the studies is exclusively because of a random sampling variation around a fixed effect (see random effects below).

Hazard ratio (HR) Broadly equivalent to relative risk (RR); useful when the risk is not constant with respect to time. It uses information collected at different times. The term is typically used in the context of survival over time. If the HR is 0.5 then the relative risk of dying in one group is half the risk of dying in the other group.

Heterogeneity In the context of meta-analysis, heterogeneity means dissimilarity between studies. It can be because of the use of different statistical methods (statistical heterogeneity), or evaluation of people with different characteristics, treatments or outcomes (clinical heterogeneity). Heterogeneity may render pooling of data in meta-analysis unreliable or inappropriate.

Homogeneity Similarity (see heterogeneity above).

Incidence The number of new cases of a condition occurring in a population over a specified period of time.

Intention to treat (ITT) analysis Analysis of data for all participants based on the group to which they were randomised and not based on the actual treatment they received.

Likelihood ratio The ratio of the probability that an individual with the target condition has a specified test result to the probability that an individual without the target condition has the same specified test result.

Meta-analysis A statistical technique that summarises the results of several studies in a single weighted estimate, in which more weight is given to results of studies with more events and sometimes to studies of higher quality.

Morbidity Rate of illness but not death.

Mortality Rate of death.

Negative likelihood ratio (NLR) The ratio of the probability that an individual with the target condition has a negative test result to the probability that an individual without the target condition has a negative test result. This is the same as the ratio (1-sensitivity/specificity).

Negative predictive value (NPV) The chance of not having a disease given a negative test result (not to be confused with specificity, which is the other way round; see below).

Non-systematic review A review or meta-analysis that either did not perform a comprehensive search of the literature and contains only a selection of studies on a clinical question, or did not state its methods for searching and appraising the studies it contains.

Not significant/non-significant (NS) In *Clinical Evidence*, not significant means that the observed difference, or a larger difference, could have arisen by chance with a probability of more than 1/20 (i.e. 5%), assuming that there is no underlying difference. This is not the same as saying there is no effect, just that this experiment does not provide convincing evidence of an effect. This could be because the trial was not powered to detect an effect that does exist, because there was no effect, or because of the play of chance. If there is a potentially clinically important difference that is not statistically significant then do not say there was a non-significant trend. Alternative phrases to describe this type of uncertainty include, 'Fewer people died after taking treatment x but the difference was not significant' or 'The difference was not significant but the confidence intervals covered the possibility of a large beneficial effect' or even, 'The difference did not quite reach significance.'

Number needed to harm (NNH) One measure of treatment harm. It is the average number of people from a defined population you would need to treat with a specific intervention for a given period of time to cause one additional adverse outcome. NNH can be calculated as 1/ARI. In *Clinical Evidence*, these are usually rounded downwards.

Number needed to treat (NNT) One measure of treatment effectiveness. It is the average number of people who need to be treated with a specific intervention for a given period of time to prevent one additional adverse outcome or achieve one additional beneficial outcome. NNT can be calculated as 1/ARR (see appendix 2). In *Clinical Evidence*, NNTs are usually rounded upwards.

NNT for a meta-analysis Absolute measures are useful at describing the effort required to obtain a benefit, but are limited because they are influenced by both the treatment and also by the baseline risk of the individual. If a meta-analysis includes individuals with a range of baseline risks, then no single NNT will be applicable to the people in that meta-analysis, but a single relative measure (odds ratio or relative risk) may be applicable if there is no heterogeneity. In *Clinical Evidence*, an NNT is provided for meta-analysis, based on a combination of the summary odds ratio (OR) and the mean baseline risk observed in average of the control groups.

Odds The odds of an event happening is defined as the probability that an event will occur, expressed as a proportion of the probability that the event will not occur.

Odds ratio (OR) One measure of treatment effectiveness. It is the odds of an event happening in the experimental group expressed as a proportion of the odds of an event happening in the control group. The closer the OR is to one, the smaller the difference in effect between the experimental intervention and the control intervention. If the OR is greater (or less) than one, then the effects of the treatment are more (or less) than those of the control treatment. Note that the effects being measured may be adverse (e.g. death or disability) or desirable (e.g. survival). When events are rare the OR is analagous to the relative risk (RR), but as event rates increase the OR and RR diverge.

Odds reduction The complement of odds ratio (1-OR), similar to the relative risk reduction (RRR) when events are rare.

Open label trial A trial in which both participant and assessor are aware of the intervention allocated.

Placebo A substance given in the control group of a clinical trial, which is ideally identical in appearance and taste or feel to the experimental treatment and believed to lack any disease specific effects. In the context of non-pharmacological interventions, placebo is usually referred to as sham treatment (see sham treatment below).

Positive likelihood ratio (LR+) The ratio of the probability that an individual with the target condition has a positive test result to the probability that an individual without the target condition has a positive test result. This is the same as the ratio (sensitivity/1-specificity).

Positive predictive value (PPV) The chance of having a disease given a positive test result (not to be confused with sensitivity, which is the other way round; see below).

Power A study has adequate power if it can reliably detect a clinically important difference (i.e. between two treatments) if one actually exists. The power of a study is increased when it includes more events or when its measurement of outcomes is more precise.

Pragmatic study An RCT designed to provide results that are directly applicable to normal practice (compared with explanatory trials that are intended to clarify efficacy under ideal conditions). Pragmatic RCTs recruit a population that is representative of those who are normally treated, allow normal compliance with instructions (by avoiding incentives and by using oral instructions with advice to follow manufacturers instructions), and analyse results by 'intention to treat' rather than by 'on treatment' methods.

Prevalence The proportion of people with a finding or disease in a given population at a given time.

Publication bias Occurs when the likelihood of a study being published varies with the results it finds. Usually, this occurs when studies that find a significant effect are more likely to be published than studies that do not find a significant effect, so making it appear from surveys of the published literature that treatments are more effective than is truly the case.

P value The probability that an observed or greater difference occurred by chance, if it is assumed that there is in fact no real difference between the effects of the interventions. If this probability is less than 1/20 (which is when the P value is less than 0.05), then the result is conventionally regarded as being 'statistically significant'.

Quality Adjusted Life Year (QALY) A method for comparing health outcomes, which assigns to each year of life a weight from 1 (perfect health) to 0 (state judged equivalent to death) dependent on the individual's health related quality of life during that year. A total score of years multiplied by weight can then be compared across different interventions. There is disagreement about the best methods for measuring health-related quality of life.

Quasi randomised A trial using a method of allocating participants to different forms of care that is not truly random; for example, allocation by date of birth, day of the week, medical record number, month of the year, or the order in which participants are included in the study (e.g. alternation).

Random effects The 'random effects' model assumes a different underlying effect for each study and takes this into consideration as an additional source of variation, which leads to somewhat wider confidence intervals than the fixed effects model. Effects are assumed to be randomly distributed, and the central point of this distribution is the focus of the combined effect estimate (see fixed effects above).

Randomised controlled trial (RCT) A trial in which participants are randomly assigned to two or more groups: at least one (the experimental group) receiving an intervention that is being tested and an other (the comparison or control group) receiving an alternative treatment or placebo. This design allows assessment of the relative effects of interventions.

Regression analysis Given data on a dependent variable and one or more independent variables, regression analysis involves finding the 'best' mathematical model to describe or predict the dependent variable as a function of the independent variable(s). There are several regression models that suit different needs. Common forms are linear, logistic, and proportional hazards.

Relative risk (RR) The number of times more likely (RR > 1) or less likely (RR < 1) an event is to happen in one group compared with another. It is the ratio of the absolute risk (AR) for each group. It is analogous to the odds ratio (OR) when events are rare.

Relative risk increase (RRI) The proportional increase in risk between experimental and control participants in a trial.

Relative risk reduction (RRR) The proportional reduction in risk between experimental and control participants in a trial. It is the complement of the relative risk (1-RR).

Sensitivity The chance of having a positive test result given that you have a disease (not to be confused with positive predictive value [PPV], which is the other way around; see above).

Sensitivity analysis Analysis to test if results from meta-analysis are sensitive to restrictions on the data included. Common examples are large trials only, higher quality trials only, and more recent trials only. If results are consistent this provides stronger evidence of an effect and of generalisability.

Sham treatment An intervention given in the control group of a clinical trial, which is ideally identical in appearance and feel to the experimental treatment and believed to lack any disease specific effects (e.g. detuned ultrasound or random biofeedback).

Significant By convention, taken to mean statistically significant at the 5% level (see statistically significant below). This is the same as a 95% confidence interval not including the value corresponding to no effect.

Specificity The chance of having a negative test result given that you do not have a disease (not to be confused with negative predictive value [NPV], which is the other way around; see above).

Standardised mean difference (SMD) A measure of effect size used when outcomes are continuous (such as height, weight, or symptom scores) rather than dichotomous (such as death or myocardial infarction). The mean differences in outcome between the groups being studied are standardised to account for differences in scoring methods (such as pain scores). The measure is a ratio; therefore, it has no units.

Statistically significant Means that the findings of a study are unlikely to have arisen because of chance. Significance at the commonly cited 5% level ($P < 0.05$) means that the observed difference or greater difference would occur by chance in only 1/20 similar cases. Where the word 'significant' or 'significance' is used without qualification in the text, it is being used in this statistical sense.

Subgroup analysis Analysis of a part of the trial/meta-analysis population in which it is thought the effect may differ from the mean effect.

Systematic review A review in which specified and appropriate methods have been used to identify, appraise, and summarise studies addressing a defined question. It can, but need not, involve meta-analysis (see meta-analysis). In *Clinical Evidence*, the term systematic review refers to a systematic review of RCTs unless specified otherwise.

True positive A person with the target condition (defined by a gold standard) who also has a positive test result.

Validity The soundness or rigour of a study. A study is internally valid if the way it is designed and carried out means that the results are unbiased and it gives you an accurate estimate of the effect that is being measured. A study is externally valid if its results are applicable to people encountered in regular clinical practice.

Weighted mean difference (WMD) A measure of effect size used when outcomes are continuous (such as symptom scores or height) rather than dichotomous (such as death or myocardial infarction). The mean differences in outcome between the groups being studied are weighted to account for different sample sizes and differing precision between studies. The WMD is an absolute figure and so takes the units of the original outcome measure.

Non-Hodgkin's lymphoma (diffuse large B cell lymphoma)

Search date February 2004

Ellen Roxane Copson

QUESTIONS

INTERVENTIONS

*Based on consensus

See glossary G

Key Messages

First line treatment

- **CHOP 21*** CHOP 21 is the standard treatment for aggressive non-Hodgkin's lymphoma (not including Burkitt's lymphoma) and placebo or no treatment controlled trials would be considered unethical. Six RCTs identified by two systematic reviews found that no alternative regimen (MACOP-B, m-BACOD, ProMACE-CytaBOM, or PACEBOM) was shown to be consistently superior to CHOP 21 in terms of overall survival. Toxicity was generally similar with the different regimens.
- **CHOP 14** We found one RCT comparing CHOP 21 with CHOP 14 in people aged 18–60 years with good prognosis aggressive lymphoma and a second RCT comparing CHOP 21 with CHOP 14 in people aged 61–75 years with aggressive lymphoma. The RCT in younger people found no significant difference between CHOP 14 and CHOP 21 in complete response rates or 5 year event free survival. However, overall 5 year survival was higher with CHOP 14. The RCT in older people found that CHOP 14 improved complete response rate, 5 year event free survival, and overall survival compared with CHOP 21. Toxicity was similar with CHOP 14 and CHOP 21 in both studies.
- **CHOP 21 plus rituximab (increased survival compared with CHOP 21 alone)** One RCT found that in people aged 60–80 years with stage II–IV disease, CHOP 21 plus rituximab reduced events and death compared with CHOP 21 alone at 2 years.

Non-Hodgkin's lymphoma (diffuse large B cell lymphoma)

- **Short schedule CHOP 21 plus adjuvant radiotherapy (increased survival compared with longer schedule CHOP 21 alone)** One RCT found that short schedule CHOP 21 plus adjuvant radiotherapy improved 5 year progression free survival and overall survival compared with longer schedule CHOP 21 alone. Longer schedule CHOP 21 alone increased the risk of congestive heart failure, and slightly increased the risk of myelosuppression, although this increase was not significant.

Treatment for relapsed disease

- **Conventional dose salvage chemotherapy (consensus that treatment should be given but relative benefits of different regimens unclear)*** We found no RCTs comparing different conventional dose salvage chemotherapy regimens (PACEBOM, ESHAP, RICE, IVAC) in people with relapsed aggressive non-Hodgkin's lymphoma. Consensus is that people with relapsed disease should be treated with salvage chemotherapy. One systematic review identified 22 phase II trials of various conventional dose salvage chemotherapy regimens. All regimens reported similar response rates and no single superior regimen could be identified.
- **High dose chemotherapy plus autologous transplant stem cell support (increased survival compared with conventional dose chemotherapy in people with chemosensitive disease)** One systematic review identified one RCT comparing high dose chemotherapy plus autologous bone marrow transplantation with conventional dose chemotherapy in people with a chemosensitive relapse of aggressive non-Hodgkin's lymphoma. It found that high dose chemotherapy plus autologous bone marrow transplantation improved 5 year event free survival and overall survival compared with conventional chemotherapy. We found no RCTs in people in people with chemotherapy resistant disease.

*Based on consensus

DEFINITION Non-Hodgkin's lymphoma (NHL) consists of a complex group of cancers arising mainly from B lymphocytes (85% of cases) and occasionally from T lymphocytes. NHL usually develops in lymph nodes (nodal lymphoma) but can arise in other tissues almost anywhere in the body (extranodal lymphoma). NHL is categorised according to its appearance under the microscope (histology) and the extent of the disease (stage). **Histology:** Since 1966, four major different methods of classifying NHLs according to their histological appearance have been published (see table 1, p 12); see table 2, p 12; see table 3, p 13; see table 4, p 13). At present, the World Health Organization (WHO**G**)[1] system is accepted as the gold standard of classification. The WHO system is based on the underlying principles of the REAL**G** classification system.[2] Historically, NHLs have been divided into slow growing "low grade" lymphomas and fast growing "aggressive**G**" lymphomas. This chapter deals only with the most common aggressive NHL – diffuse B cell lymphoma (WHO classification; see table 1, p 12). Interpretation of older studies is complicated by the fact that histological methods have changed and there is no direct correlation between lymphoma types in the WHO and other classification systems. Attempts to generalise results must therefore be treated with caution. We have however included some older studies referring to alternative classification methods if they included people with the following types of aggressive lymphomas, which overlap substantially with the WHO classification of interest: Working Formulation Classification – primarily intermediate grades (grades E–H; see table 2, p 12);[3] Kiel classification – centroblastic, Immunoblastic, and anaplastic (see table 3, p 13)[4] Rappaport classification – diffuse histiocytic, diffuse lymphocytic poorly differentiated, and diffuse mixed (lymphocytic and histiocytic; see table 4, p 13).[5] **Stage:** NHL has traditionally been staged according to extent of disease spread using the Ann Arbor**G** system (see table 5, p 14).[6] The term "early disease"**G** is used to describe disease that falls within Ann Arbor stage I or II while "advanced disease"**G** refers to Ann Arbor stage III or IV disease. However, all people with bulky disease, usually defined as having a disease site larger than 10 cm in diameter, are treated as having advanced disease regardless of their Ann Arbor staging. **Relapsed disease:** Relapsed disease refers to the recurrence of active disease in a person who had previously achieved a complete response**G** to initial treatment for NHL. Most studies of treatments in relapsed disease require a minimum duration of complete response of 1 month before relapse.

Non-Hodgkin's lymphoma (diffuse large B cell lymphoma)

INCIDENCE/ PREVALENCE Non-Hodgkin's lymphoma occurs more commonly in males than females, and is increasing in incidence in the Western world by 4% a year. It is the seventh most common cancer in the UK with 9189 new cases per 100 000 population diagnosed in 2000 and causing 4654 deaths per 100 000 population in 2002.[7]

AETIOLOGY/ RISK FACTORS The aetiology of most Non-Hodgkin's lymphomas (NHLs) is unknown. Incidence is higher in individuals who are immunosuppressed (congenital or acquired). Other risk factors include viral infection (human T cell leukaemia virus type-1, Epstein Barr virus, human immunodeficiency virus), bacterial infection (e.g. *Helicobacter pylori*), previous treatment with diphenylhydantoin or antineoplastic drugs, and exposure to pesticides or organic solvents.[8]

PROGNOSIS **Overall survival:** Untreated aggressive🅖 Non-Hodgkin's lymphomas (NHLs) would generally result in death in a matter of months. High grade lymphomas, particularly diffuse large B cell lymphomas and Burkitt's lymphomas, have a high cure rate, with both initial and salvage chemotherapy.[9] The 5 year relative age standardised survival for people diagnosed with and treated for NHL between 2000 and 2001 was 55% for men and 56% for women.[7] **Relapse:** About 50% of people with NHL will be cured by initial treatment. Of the rest, about 30% will fail to respond to initial treatment (so called "chemotherapy refractory disease"), and about 20–30% will relapse. Most relapses occur within 2 years of completion of initial treatment. Up to 50% of these have chemosensitive disease; the remainder tend to have chemotherapy resistant disease. **Prognostic indicators:** Prognosis depends on histological type, stage, age, performance status🅖, and lactate dehydrogenase levels. Prognosis varies substantially within each Ann Arbor🅖 stage, and further information regarding prognosis can be obtained from applying the International Prognostic Index (IPI).[8] The IPI model stratifies prognosis according to the presence or absence of five risk factors: age (< 60 years *v* > 60 years), serum lactate dehydrogenase (normal *v* elevated), performance status (0 or 1 *v* 2–4), Ann Arbor stage (I or II *v* III or IV), and number of extranodal sites involved (0 or 1 *v* 2–4). People with two or more high risk factors have a less than 50% chance of relapse free and overall survival at 5 years. IPI staging is currently the most important system used to define disease stage and treatment options. However, most studies identified by our search pre-date the IPI staging system.

AIMS OF INTERVENTION To increase disease free survival, achieving cure if possible. Additionally, to palliate by achieving remission and prolonging survival, to minimise harmful effects of treatment and to maximise quality of life.

OUTCOMES **Benefits:** Overall survival (median and 5 year survival), disease free survival, chemotherapy response rates (complete response🅖 and partial response🅖; variously defined in different studies but usually measured at 1–2 months), quality of life. **Harms:** treatment related deaths, other adverse effects of treatment.

METHODS *Clinical Evidence* search and appraisal February 2004. Only studies from 1990 onwards have been included. This chapter applies to all stages of diffuse large B cell lymphomas (and other similar aggressive🅖 NHL (see definition, p 2). This chapter includes all stages (early and advanced🅖) unless otherwise specified at the option level. This chapter looks at all adults, but excludes those with HIV. CHOP 21🅖 chemotherapy is the standard treatment for aggressive NHL (not including Burkitt's lymphoma) and placebo controlled trials would be considered unethical.

QUESTION What are the effects of first line treatments for aggressive non-Hodgkin's lymphoma (diffuse large B cell lymphoma)? New

OPTION CHOP 21 New

CHOP 21 is the standard treatment for aggressive non-Hodgkin's lymphoma (not including Burkitt's lymphoma) and placebo or no treatment controlled trials would be considered unethical. Six RCTs identified by two systematic reviews found that no alternative regimen (MACOP-B, m-BACOD, ProMACE-CytaBOM, or PACEBOM) was shown to be consistently superior to CHOP 21 in terms of overall survival. Toxicity was generally similar with the different regimens.

Non-Hodgkin's lymphoma (diffuse large B cell lymphoma)

Benefits: **Versus other regimens (MACOP-B, m-BACOD, ProMACE-CytaBOM, PACEBOM, BCOP, HOP):** We found two systemic reviews (search date not reported,[10] and 2000;[11] 6 RCTs reported in 9 publications;[12–20] 3241 people) comparing CHOP 21Ⓖ versus MACOP-BⒼ, m-BACODⒼ, ProMACE-CytaBOMⒼ, and PACEBOMⒼ. No alternative regimen was consistently shown to be significantly superior to CHOP 21 in terms of overall survival (see table 6, p 15). The review did not find any RCTs comparing CHOP 21 versus BCOPⒼ or HOPⒼ that met inclusion criteria for this chapter.

Harms: No alternative regimen was shown to be superior to CHOP 21Ⓖ in terms of adverse effects (see table 6, p 15).

Comment: CHOP 21Ⓖ is the standard treatment for aggressiveⒼ non-Hodgkin's lymphoma (not including Burkitt's lymphoma) and placebo controlled trials would be considered unethical. **Older people:** We found a third systematic review (search date 2000) which assessed different chemotherapy regimens in people aged at least 60 years old with previously untreated advancedⒼ stage aggressive non-Hodgkin's lymphoma.[21] Twelve RCTs were reviewed, three of which compared CHOP 21 versus alternative regimens covered by our search (all of which were identified by the two included reviews[10,11]). The authors confirmed that the use of anthracycline containing regimens such as CHOP 21 resulted in superior outcomes compared with other regimens in this age group. However, all trials except one excluded people with significant co-morbidity.

OPTION — CHOP 21 PLUS ADJUVANT RADIOTHERAPY — New

One RCT found that short schedule CHOP 21 plus adjuvant radiotherapy improved 5 year progression free survival and overall survival compared with longer schedule CHOP 21 alone. Longer schedule CHOP 21 alone increased the risk of congestive heart failure, and slightly increased the risk of myelosuppression, although this increase was not significant.

Benefits: We found one systematic review (initial search date 1993,[22] updated in 2001;[23] 1 RCT[24]). The RCT identified by the review (401 people with stage I or II Working Formulation grades D–J lymphoma, excluding lymphoblastic lymphoma; 75% grades G and H; 49% ≥60 years) comparing CHOP 21Ⓖ alone (8 cycles) versus CHOP 21 plus adjuvant radiotherapy (3 cycles plus a total dose of radiotherapy of 40–55 Gy).[24] It found that short schedule CHOP 21 plus adjuvant radiotherapy significantly improved progression free survival and overall survival at 5 years compared with long schedule CHOP 21 (estimated progression free survival: 77% with CHOP 21 plus radiotherapy *v* 64% longer with CHOP 21 alone; estimated HR 1.5, 95% CI 1.0 to 2.2; estimated overall survival: 82% with CHOP 21 plus radiotherapy *v* 72% longer with CHOP 21 alone; estimated HR 1.7, 95% CI 1.1 to 2.7).

Harms: The RCT identified by the review found that two people died as a result of treatment.[24] One person treated with longer schedule CHOP 21Ⓖ alone died of sepsis associated with neutropenia and one person treated with short schedule CHOP 21 plus adjuvant radiotherapy died of liver failure, consistent with radiation induced hepatitis. Life threatening toxic events were more common in people treated with longer schedule CHOP 21 alone but the difference was not significant (61/200 [31%] with CHOP 21 plus radiotherapy *v* 80/201 [40%] with longer CHOP 21 alone; $P = 0.06$). The most common life threatening adverse event was myelosuppression, which caused grade 4 neutropenia (absolute neutrophil count $< 500/mm^3$: 71/201 (35%) with longer schedule CHOP 21 *v* 54/200 (27%) with short schedule CHOP 21 plus radiotherapy; $P = 0.09$). The RCT also found that significantly more people with longer schedule CHOP 21 alone experienced symptoms or signs of congestive heart failure or more than a 20% decrease from baseline in the left ventricular ejection fraction (0/201 [0%] with CHOP 21 plus radiotherapy v 7/201 [3.5%] with longer CHOP 21; P = 0.02).

Comment: None.

OPTION **CHOP 21 PLUS RITUXIMAB** New

One RCT found that in people aged 60–80 years with stage II–IV disease, CHOP 21 plus rituximab reduced events and death compared with CHOP 21 alone at 2 years.

Benefits: We found one systematic review (search date 2002),[25] which identified one RCT[26] comparing CHOP 21**G** alone versus CHOP 21 plus rituximab. The RCT included 399 people aged 60–80 years with previously untreated stage II–IV diffuse large B cell lymphoma. Participants were randomised to receive either eight cycles of CHOP 21 (197 people) or eight cycles of CHOP 21 plus rituximab (375 mg/m^2; 202 people) given on day 1 of each CHOP 21 cycle. The complete response**G** rate was significantly higher with CHOP 21 plus rituximab than with CHOP 21 alone (76% with CHOP 21 plus rituximab v 63% with CHOP 21 alone; P = 0.0005). CHOP 21 plus rituximab significantly reduced events and death compared with CHOP 21 alone at 2 years (AR for event: 43% with CHOP 21 plus rituximab v 61% with CHOP 21 alone; adjusted RR 0.58, 95% CI 0.44 to 0.77; AR for death: 29% with CHOP 21 plus rituximab v 41% with CHOP 21 alone; adjusted RR 0.64, 95% CI 0.45 to 0.89).

Harms: The RCT found that the incidence of grade 3 and 4 adverse events occurred with similar frequency in people taking CHOP 21 alone or CHOP 21 plus rituximab (overall figures not reported).[26] There was a higher incidence of cardiac events with CHOP 21**G** plus rituximab, which was due to an increase in grade 1 events (AR for cardiac events: 47% with CHOP 21 plus rituximab v 35% with CHOP 21 alone; AR for grade 1 cardiac events: 24% with CHOP 21 plus rituximab v 13% with CHOP 21 alone; significance of either comparison not reported). This difference was thought to be due to mild to moderate infusion reactions associated with rituximab, as predicted by Phase II studies. Grade 3 or 4 infusion related events were observed in 19 people (9%) treated with CHOP 21 plus rituximab, the most frequent of these being respiratory symptoms, chills, fever, and hypotension. In all cases the symptoms resolved on slowing of the infusion and all participants were able to receive subsequent infusions of rituximab without recurrence of grade 3 or 4 infusion related reaction. No participants died as a result of a rituximab infusion related event. In total 23 participants in both groups died during the treatment period (16 [4%] from infection, 4 [1%] from cachexia, and 3 [0.8%] from cardiovascular events). There was no significant difference in non-lymphoma mortality between treatment groups (absolute figures and P values not reported).

Comment: We found no RCTs comparing CHOP 21**G** versus CHOP 21 plus rituximab in people under 60 years of age. The systematic review[25] identified one small uncontrolled Phase II study (33 people) of CHOP 21 plus rituximab in people with newly diagnosed aggressive**G** non-Hodgkin's lymphoma (stage I–IV).[27] The Phase II study found that response rate was at least as good in people aged less than 60 years as in people aged over 60 years.

Non-Hodgkin's lymphoma (diffuse large B cell lymphoma)

OPTION **CHOP 14** New

We found one RCT comparing CHOP 21 with CHOP 14 in people aged 18–60 years with good prognosis aggressive lymphoma and a second RCT comparing CHOP 21 with CHOP 14 in people aged 61–75 years with aggressive lymphoma. The RCT in younger people found no significant difference between CHOP 14 and CHOP 21 in complete response rates or 5 year event free survival. However, overall 5 year survival was higher with CHOP 14. The RCT in older people found that CHOP 14 improved complete response rate, 5 year event free survival, and overall survival compared with CHOP 21. Toxicity was similar with CHOP 14 and CHOP 21 in both studies.

Benefits: We found no systemic review. We found two RCTs that compared CHOP 21Ⓖ versus CHOP 14Ⓖ.[28,29] The first RCT included 710 people aged 18–60 years with previously untreated aggressiveⒼ non-Hodgkin's lymphoma (NHL) according to the REALⒼ classification (see comment below) with good prognosis (defined as normal lactate dehydrogenase level).[28] The study compared four six cycle treatments in a 2 x 2 factorial design: CHOP 14 (172 people), CHOP 21 (176 people), CHOP 14 plus etoposide (177 people), and CHOP 21 plus etoposide (185 people).[28] Participants in the CHOP 14 regimens also received granulocyte colony stimulating factor (G-CSF; filgrastim) support between days 4 and 13 (inclusive). Radiotherapy (36 Gy) was given to sites of initial bulky disease and extranodal disease at completion of chemotherapy. The RCT found no significant difference between CHOP 14 and CHOP 21 in complete remissionⒼ rates or estimated 5 year event free survival (AR for no complete remission: 21.5% with CHOP 14 *v* 19.9% with CHOP 21; adjusted OR 1.10, 95% CI 0.66 to 1.86; AR for event: 39.2% with CHOP 14 *v* 45.3% with CHOP 21; adjusted RR 0.93, 95% CI 0.66 to 1.29). However, CHOP 14 significantly increased estimated overall 5 year survival compared with CHOP 21 (AR for death: 15% with CHOP 14 *v* 25.1% with CHOP 21; adjusted RR 0.61, 95% CI 0.37 to 0.96). The second RCT included people aged 61–75 years with previously untreated, aggressive NHL according to the REAL classification (see comment below).[29] The study compared four six cycle treatments in a 2 x 2 factorial design: CHOP 14 (172 people), CHOP 21 (178 people), CHOP 14 plus etoposide (169 people), and CHOP 21 plus etoposide (170 people).[29] G-CSF (filgrastim) and radiotherapy were given as in the first RCT. CHOP 14 significantly improved complete remission rates (AR for no complete remission: 23.9% with CHOP 14 *v* 39.9% with CHOP 21; adjusted OR 0.45, 95% CI 0.28 to 0.73). CHOP 14 significantly improved estimated 5 year event free survival and overall survival compared with CHOP 21 (AR for event: 56.2% with CHOP 14 *v* 67.5% with CHOP 21; adjusted RR 0.66, 95% CI 0.50 to 0.87; AR for death: 46.7% with CHOP 14 *v* 59.4% with CHOP 21; adjusted RR 0.58, 95% CI 0.43 to 0.79).

Harms: In both RCTs, toxicity in the CHOP 21Ⓖ and CHOP 14Ⓖ arms was similar.[28,29] Due to the use of filgrastim in the biweekly regimen, grade 3 and 4 leucopenia occurred less frequently with CHOP 14 than with CHOP 21 (first RCT: 33.6% with CHOP 14 *v* 34.1% with CHOP 21;[28] second RCT: 70.1% with CHOP 14 *v* 72.1% with CHOP 21;[29] significance not reported). Grade 3 and 4 anaemia occurred more frequently with CHOP 14 than with CHOP 21 (first RCT: 5.6% with CHOP 14 *v* 3.6% with CHOP 21;[28] second RCT: 19.5% with CHOP 14 *v* 4.7% with CHOP 21[29]). Grade 3 and 4 thrombocytopenia was more frequent with CHOP 14 than CHOP 21 in the second RCT, in older participants, but not in the first RCT (first RCT: 1.2% with CHOP 14 *v* 2.4% with CHOP 21;[28] second RCT: 15.1% with CHOP 14 *v* 4.7% with CHOP 21[29]). Infection occurred in 4.2% (first RCT[28]) and 10.6% (second RCT[29]) with CHOP 14 and

1.8% (first RCT[28]) and 8.0% (second RCT[29]) with CHOP 21. Other toxicities were alopecia (64.8 %[28] and 58.3%[29] with CHOP 14 *v* 63.6%[28] and 62.5%[29] with CHOP 21), nausea and vomiting (6.5%[28] and 13.5%[29] with CHOP 14 *v* 11.7%[28] and 8.0%[29] with CHOP 21) and mucositis (3.0%[28] and 7.1%[29] with CHOP 14 *v* 2.9%[28] and 0%[29] with CHOP 21). There was no increase in the incidence of neurological toxicity with the bi-weekly regimen (0.6%[28] and 3.6%[29] with CHOP 14 *v* 3.5%[28] and 3.4%[29] with CHOP 21). There were no treatment related deaths in either study.[28,29]

Comment: Both RCTs included people with very aggressive**G** lymphomas, namely Burkitt's lymphomas (first RCT: 1.4% of people;[28] second RCT: 3.7% of people[29]) and lymphoblastic lymphomas. In the second study there was an imbalance in the frequency of diffuse large B cell lymphoma in the treatment arms (74.4% in CHOP 14**G** group *v* 63.5% in CHOP 21**G** group; significance not reported).[29] Adjustment for diffuse large B cell lymphoma in the second RCT did not significantly affect the comparison of CHOP 14 and CHOP 21 (RR for an event remained at 0.66).[29] The first RCT included only people with "good prognosis", defined by having a lactate dehydrogenase level within normal limits.[28]

QUESTION What are the effects of treatments for relapsed aggressive non-Hodgkin's lymphoma (diffuse large B cell lymphoma)?

New

OPTION CONVENTIONAL DOSE SALVAGE CHEMOTHERAPY (PACEBOM, ESHAP, RICE, IVAC)

New

We found no RCTs comparing different conventional dose salvage chemotherapy regimens (PACEBOM, ESHAP, RICE, IVAC) in people with relapsed aggressive non-Hodgkin's lymphoma. Consensus is that people with relapsed disease should be treated with salvage chemotherapy. One systematic review identified 22 phase II trials of various conventional dose salvage chemotherapy regimens. All regimens reported similar response rates and no single superior regimen could be identified.

Benefits: **Versus each other:** We found one systematic review (search date not reported)[10] which identified no RCTs (see comment below) comparing conventional dose**G** salvage chemotherapy (PACEBOM**G**, ESHAP, RICE**G**, IVAC) in people with relapsed aggressive**G** non-Hodgkin's lymphoma.

Harms: The systematic review did not discuss harms.[10]

Comment: The consensus is that people with relapsed disease should be treated with salvage chemotherapy. The systematic review identified 22 phase II studies (1210 people overall; individual trials from 20–208 people) using 15 different combinations of cytotoxic drugs for conventional dose**G** second line (salvage) chemotherapy. The most common included drugs were etoposide (20 studies), ifosfamide (14 studies), and methotrexate (11 studies). Other drugs included cisplatin (6 studies), cytarabine (4 studies), mitoxantrone (3 studies), bleomycin (3 studies), and methylGAG (methylglyoxal-bis(guanylhydrazone); 3 studies). All 22 studies revealed similar results, with second line combination chemotherapy frequently inducing remission in people with relapsed or refractory aggressive**G** non-Hodgkin's lymphoma. The review found that overall 60–70% of people with relapsed disease showed objective tumour responses. Complete remission**G** was seen in

20–40% of people. However, these remissions were frequently short lived, with a maximum of 10% of responders remaining disease free after 3–5 years. The authors of the review were unable to conclude that any particular salvage chemotherapy regimen was superior to any of the others from the literature reviewed.

OPTION HIGH DOSE CHEMOTHERAPY PLUS AUTOLOGOUS STEM CELL SUPPORT New

One systematic review identified one RCT comparing high dose chemotherapy plus autologous bone marrow transplantation with conventional dose chemotherapy in people with a chemosensitive relapse of aggressive non-Hodgkin's lymphoma. It found that high dose chemotherapy plus autologous bone marrow transplantation improved 5 year event free survival and overall survival compared with conventional chemotherapy. We found no RCTs in people in people with chemotherapy resistant disease.

Benefits: **In people with chemotherapy sensitive disease:** We found one systematic review (search date 2000),[30] which identified one RCT[31] (see comment below). The multicentre RCT identified by the review enrolled 215 people aged 18–60 years, with a first or second relapse of intermediate grade or high grade NHL.[31] Participants had achieved a complete response**G** to previous treatment with a doxorubicin containing regimen, maintained for at least 4 weeks. All participants were initially treated with two cycles of DHAP**G** chemotherapy. Participants who responded to DHAP (109 people) were considered to have chemotherapy sensitive lymphoma, and were randomised to receive either conventional chemotherapy (a further 4 courses of DHAP plus involved field radiotherapy to bulky disease sites; 54 people) or high dose BEAC**G** chemotherapy with autologous bone marrow transplantation plus involved field radiotherapy (55 people). Among the 109 randomised participants, five (4.6%) had International Working Formulation Classification grade I or J lymphoma, and six (5.5%) had grade D lymphoma. The RCT found that the response rate was higher with autologous transplantation than with conventional chemotherapy**G** (84% with transplantation *v* 44% with conventional chemotherapy; significance not reported). Autologous transplantation significantly improved 5 year event free survival and overall survival compared with conventional chemotherapy (median follow up 63 months; 5 year event free survival: 46% with transplantation *v* 12% with conventional chemotherapy; P = 0.001; 5 year overall survival: 53% with transplantation *v* 32% with conventional chemotherapy; P = 0.038).[31] **In people with chemotherapy resistant disease:** We found no RCTs comparing high dose chemotherapy plus autologous bone marrow transplantation or peripheral blood stem cell transplant in people with chemotherapy resistant relapses.

Harms: **In people with chemotherapy sensitive disease:** The RCT found that toxicity was greater in the group receiving high dose chemotherapy plus autologous bone marrow transplantation than the group receiving conventional chemotherapy**G**.[31] In the high dose chemotherapy plus autologous bone marrow transplantation group, four people (6%) died from treatment related complications (2 from sepsis, 1 from cardiac toxicity, and 1 from a late pulmonary infection). There were no treatment related deaths in the conventional chemotherapy group. Autologous transplant was associated with increased incidences of bacterial infection (30 episodes with autologous transplant *v* 6 episodes with conventional chemotherapy; 1 case of septic shock in each group), viral infection (8 *v* 2 episodes), fungal infection (6 *v* 1 episodes), hepatic toxicity (4 *v* 1 episode), mucositis (27 *v* 4 episodes), and diarrhoea (16 *v* 3 episodes; significance not reported for any comparison). Three people in each treatment arm had pneumonitis and one person in the autologous transplant group developed grade 4 cardiac toxicity compared with two people with grade 1 cardiac toxicity in the conventional chemotherapy group. Only renal toxicity was more common in the conventional chemotherapy group than the autologous transplant group (14 cases with conventional chemotherapy *v* 5 with autologous transplantation; significance not reported).

Comment: The systematic review also identified seven retrospective studies involving 460 people treated for chemosensitive relapse of aggressive**G** NHL with high dose chemotherapy plus stem cell support.[30] No comparisons were made with conventional dose**G** salvage chemotherapy in these studies. The RCT identified by the review excluded 90 people who failed to respond to treatment with DHAP**G** before randomisation.[31] An additional 16 responders were also excluded from randomisation for unspecified protocol violations. Of the 55 people randomised to autologous transplant (and analyzed with this group), six people were not treated according to the trial protocol. This was because of early disease**G** progression in four cases, the development of new cardiac problems in one case and failure to harvest adequate stem cells from bone marrow in the final case. Twenty two of 55 people (40%) in the autologous transplant group received radiotherapy compared with only 12/54 people (22%) in the conventional chemotherapy group (significance not reported). Eighteen of the 45 people (40%) in the conventional chemotherapy group who had further relapses were subsequently treated with high dose chemotherapy plus autologous bone marrow transplantation. Since publication of this RCT,[31] the standard procedure for high dose chemotherapy has changed from transplantation of stem cells harvested from bone marrow to peripheral blood stem cell transplantation.[32] This change is based on European Bone Marrow Transplant registry data, retrospective studies, and clinical experience, including experience in all sub-types of NHL. Although there have been no direct comparisons of peripheral blood stem cell transplantation with autologous bone marrow transplantation in aggressive NHLs, peripheral blood stem cell transplantation seems to be more effective than transplantation of autologous bone marrow stem cells in several other diseases.[33]

GLOSSARY

Aggressive disease Diffuse large B cell lymphoma has been classified variously as diffuse histiocytic lymphoma, and occasionally as grades E–H); Kiel[4] classification: centroblastic, immunoblastic, and anaplastic; Rappaport[5] classification: diffuse histiocytic, diffuse lymphocytic poorly differentiated, and diffuse mixed (lymphocytic and histiocytic).

Ann Arbor See table 5, p 14.

BCOP BCNU, cyclophosphamide, vincristine, prednisone.

BEAC Carmustine, etoposide, cytarabine, cyclophosphamide.

CHOP 14 Cyclophosphamide, doxorubicin, vincristine, prednisolone given at 14 day intervals.

CHOP 21 Cyclophosphamide, doxorubicin, vincristine, prednisolone given at 21 day intervals (standard CHOP cycle).

Complete response/remission Complete disappearance of all lymph node masses to < 1.5 cm in transverse diameter as well as the normalisation of any biochemical abnormalities and a negative bone marrow result (if the bone marrow had previously been shown to have been involved). These criteria were recommended by the International Workshop on Non-Hodgkin's Lymphoma in 1999, before 1999 there were no consensus criteria for defining response to treatment in non-Hodgkin's lymphoma.[33]

Conventional dose chemotherapy Chemotherapy delivered at a dose that does not suppress bone marrow to such an extent that stem cell support is required.

DHAP Dexamethasone, cisplatin, cytarabine.

Non-Hodgkin's lymphoma (diffuse large B cell lymphoma)

Early and Advanced Disease Staging is historically done by the Ann Arbor system (See table 5, p 14). We have treated people with stage I or stage II non-bulky disease as having early disease, whereas stage III or IV, or bulky disease are included as advanced disease. It is recognised that there will be substantial variation even within these groups and that more recent trials participant's stage will be assessed by use of the International Prognostic Index (IPI).
HOP Doxorubicin, vincristine, prednisolone.
MACOP-B Methotrexate, leucoverin rescue, doxorubicin, cyclophosphamide, vincristine, prednisone, bleomycin.
m-BACOD Low dose methotrexate, leucoverin rescue, doxorubicin, cyclophosphamide, vincristine, prednisone, bleomycin.
PACEBOM Prednisolone, doxorubicin, cyclophosphamide, etoposide, bleomycin, vincristine, methotrexate.
Partial response A minimum decrease of 50% in the sum of the products of the greatest diameters of the six largest nodes or nodal masses. This criterion was recommended by the International Workshop on NHL in 1999, before 1999 there were no consensus criteria for defining response to treatment in NHL.[33]
Performance status Scale grading the level of normal activity a person with aggressive non-Hodgkin's lymphoma is capable of, where a minimum score of 0 represents normal activity and a maximum score of 4 represents being constantly bedridden.
ProMACE-CytaBOM Prednisone, methotrexate, doxorubicin, cyclophosphamide, etoposide, cytarabine, bleomycin, vincristine, methotrexate, with leucoverin rescue.
REAL A precursor to the present WHO classification system.[2]
RICE Rituximab, ifosfamide, cytarabine, etoposide.
WHO The World Health Organization classifies lymphomas on the basis of standard stains (e.g. H and E, and reticulin) supplemented by immunophenotyping using an increasing battery of monoclonal antibodies. Where possible fresh tissue is also obtained for cytogenetic analysis. The classification then consists of an amalgamation of the above data with clinical information, ideally in a multidisciplinary team setting (see table 1, p 12).

REFERENCES

1. Harris NL, Jaffe ES, Diebold J, et al. The World Health Organization classification of neoplastic diseases of the haematopoietic and lymphoid tissues. Report of the Clinical Advisory Committee meeting, Airlie House, Virginia, November, 1997. *Ann Oncol* 1999;10:1419–1432.
2. Harris NL, Jaffe ES, Stein H, et al. A revised European-American classification of lymphoid neoplasms: a proposal from the International Lymphoma Study Group. *Blood* 1994;84:1361–1392.
3. The Non-Hodgkin's Lymphoma Pathologic Classification Project. National Cancer Institute sponsored study of classification of non-Hodgkin's lymphomas. Summary and description of a working formulation for clinical usage. *Cancer* 1982;49:2112–2135.
4. Stansfeld AG, Diebold J, Noel H, et al. Updated Kiel classification for lymphomas. *Lancet* 1988;8580:292–293. [Erratum in: *Lancet* 1988;8581:372]
5. Rappaport H. Tumours of the Haemapoietic System. In: Atlas of Tumour Pathology, Section 3, fascicle 8. Washington DC: Armed Forces Institute of Pathology, 1966.
6. Carbone PP, Kaplan HS, Musshof K, et al. Report of the Committee on Hodgkin's Disease Staging Classification. *Cancer Res* 1971;31:1860–1861.
7. <EXTREFLtp://info.cancerresearchuk.org/cancerstats/nhl/survival/>
8. Ferris Tortajada J, Garcia Castell J, Berbel Tornero O, et al. Risk factors for non-Hodgkin's lymphomas. *An Esp Pediatr* 2001;55:230–238. [In Spanish]
9. The International Non-Hodgkin's Lymphoma Prognostic Factors Project. A predictive model of aggressive non-Hodgkin's lymphoma. *New Engl J Med* 1993;329:987–994.
10. Kimby E, Brandt L, Nygren P, et al. A systematic review of chemotherapy effects in aggressive non-Hodgkin's lymphoma. *Acta Oncol* 2001;40:198–212.
11. Messori A, Vaiani M, Trippoli S, et al. Survival in patients with intermediate or high grade non-Hodgkin's lymphoma: meta-analysis of randomized studies comparing third generation regimens with CHOP. *Br J Cancer* 2001;84:303–307.
12. Fisher RI, Gaynor ER, Dahlberg S, et al. Comparison of a standard regimen (CHOP) with three intensive chemotherapy regimens for advanced non-Hodgkin's lymphoma. *New Engl J Med* 1993;328:1002–1006.
13. Fisher RI, Gaynor ER, Dahlberg S, et al. A Phase III comparison of CHOP vs. m-BACOD vs. ProMACE-CytaBOM vs. MACOP-B in patients with intermediate- or high-grade non-Hodgkin's lymphoma: results of SWOG-8516 (Intergroup 0067), the National High Priority Lymphoma Study. *Ann Oncol* 1994;5(Suppl 2):91–95.
14. Cooper IA, Wolf MM, Robertson TI, et al. Randomized comparison of MACOP-B with CHOP in intermediate-grade non-Hodgkin's lymphoma. The Australian and New Zealand Lymphoma Group. *J Clin Oncol* 1994;12:769–778.
15. Wolf M, Matthews JP, Stone J, et al. Long-term survival advantage of MCOP-B over CHOP in intermediate-grade non-Hodgkin's lymphoma. The Australian and New Zealand Lymphoma Group. Ann Oncol 1997;8(S1):71–75.
16. Jerkeman M, Anderson H, Cavallin-Stahl E, et al. CHOP versus MACOP-B in aggressive lymphoma – a Nordic Lymphoma Group randomised trial. *Ann Oncol* 1999;10:1079–1086.
17. Gordon LI, Harrington D, Andersen J, et al. Comparison of a second-generation combination chemotherapeutic regimen (m-BACOD) with a

standard regimen (CHOP) for advanced diffuse non-Hodgkin's lymphoma. *N Engl J Med* 1992:327:1342–1349.
18. Montserrat E, Garcia-Conde J, Vinolas N, et al. CHOP vs. ProMACE-CytaBOM in the treatment of aggressive non-Hodgkin's lymphomas: long-term results of a multicenter randomized trial (PETHAMA: Spanish Cooperative Group for the Study of Hematological Malignancies Treatment, Spanish Society of Hematology). *Eur J Haematol* 1996;57:377–383.
19. Linch DC, Vaghan Hudson B, Hancock BW, et al. A randomised comparison of a third-generation regimen (PACEBOM) with a standard regimen (CHOP) in patients with histologically aggressive non-Hodgkin's lymphoma: a British National Lymphoma Investigation report. *Br J Cancer* 1996;74:318–322.
20. Linch DC, Smith P, Hancock BW, et al. A randomized British National Lymphoma Investigation trial of CHOP vs. a weekly multi-agent regimen (PACEBOM) in patients with histologically aggressive non-Hodgkin's lymphoma. *Ann Oncol* 2000;11(Suppl 1):87–90.
21. Kouroukis T, Browman GP, Esmail R, et al. Chemotherapy for older patients with newly diagnosed, advanced stage, aggressive-histology non-Hodgkin lymphoma: a systematic review. *Ann Intern Med* 2002;136:144–152.
22. Gustafsson A. Non-Hodgkin's lymphomas. *Acta Oncol* 1996;35(Suppl 7):102–116.
23. Gustavsson A, Osterman B and Cavallin-Stahl E. A systematic overview of radiation therapy effects in non-Hodgkin's lymphoma. *Acta Oncol* 2003;42:605–619.
24. Miller TP, Dahlberg S, Cassady JR, et al. Chemotherapy alone compared with chemotherapy plus radiotherapy for localized intermediate- and high-grade non-Hodgkin's lymphoma. *New Engl J Med* 1998;339:21–26.
25. UK NHS. National Coordinating Centre for Health Technology Assessment 3AD. Rituximab (Mabthera) for aggressive non-Hodgkin's lymphoma – NICE Technology Assessment Report (project). 2002.
26. Coiffier B, Lepage E, Briere J, et al. CHOP chemotherapy plus rituximab compared with CHOP alone in elderly patients with diffuse large-B-cell lymphoma. *N Engl J Med* 2002;346:235–242.
27. Vose JM, Link BK, Grossbard ML, et al. Phase II study of rituximab in combination with CHOP chemotherapy in patients with previously untreated, aggressive non-Hodgkin's lymphoma. *J Clin Oncol* 2001;19:389–397.
28. Pfreundschuh M, Trumper L, Kloess M, et al. Two-weekly or 3-weekly CHOP chemotherapy with or without etoposide for the treatment of young patients with good-prognosis (normal LDH) aggressive lymphomas: results of the NHL-B1 trial of the DSHNHL. *Blood* 2004;104;626–633.
29. Pfreundschuh M, Trumper L, Kloess M, et al. Two-weekly or 3-weekly CHOP chemotherapy with or without etoposide for the treatment of elderly patients with aggressive lymphomas: results of the NHL-B2 trial of the DSHNHL. *Blood* 2004;104;634–641.
30. Hahn T, Wolff SN, Czuczman M, et al. The role of cytotoxic therapy with hematopoietic stem cell transplantation in the therapy of diffuse large cell B-cell non-Hodgkin's lymphoma: an evidence-based review. *Biol Blood Marrow Transplant* 2001;7:308–331.
31. Philip T, Guglielmi C, Hagenbeek A, et al. Autologous bone marrow transplantation as compared with salvage chemotherapy in relapses of chemotherapy-sensitive non-Hodgkin's lymphoma. *New Engl J Med* 1995;333:1540–1545.
32. Cheson BD, Horning SJ, Coiffier B, et al. Report of an international workshop to standardize response criteria for non-Hodgkin's lymphomas. *J Clin Oncol* 1999;17:1244–1253. [Erratum in: *J Clin Oncol* 2000;18:2351]
33. Molineux G, Pojda Z, Hampson IN, et al. Transplantation potential of peripheral blood stem cells induced by granulocyte colony-stimulating factor. *Blood* 1990;76:2153–2158.

Ellen Copson
CRC Wessex Medical Oncology Unit, Center Care Dorectorate, Southampton General Hospital
Southampton
UK

Competing interests: none declared.

Non-Hodgkin's lymphoma (diffuse large B cell lymphoma)

TABLE 1 **WHO Classification 2001 (see text, p 2).[1]**

Precursor B-cell neoplasm
Precursor B-lymphoblastic leukemia/lymphoma (precursor B-cell acute lymphoblastic leukemia)

Mature (peripheral) B-cell neoplasms
B-cell chronic lymphocytic leukemia/small cell lymphocytic lymphoma
Lymphoplasmacytic lymphoma
Splenic marginal zone B-cell lymphoma (± villous lymphocytes)
Hairy cell leukemia
Plasma cell myeloma/plasmacytoma
Extranodal marginal zone B-cell lymphoma of MALT type
Nodal marginal zone B-cell lymphoma (± monocytoid B cells)
Follicular lymphoma
Mantle cell lymphoma
Diffuse large B-cell lymphoma
- Mediastinal large B-cell lymphoma
- Primary effusion lymphoma
Burkitt's lymphoma/Burkitt's cell leukemia

MALT, mucosa-associated lymphoid tissue; WHO, World Health Organization. Reproduced with permission of the copyright holder. Harris N, Jaffe E, Diebold J, et al. The World Health Organization Classification of Neoplastic Diseases of the Hematopoietic and Lymphoid Tissues. *Ann Oncol* 1999; 10:1419–1432.

TABLE 2 **International Working Formulation Classification (see text, p 2).[2]**

Grade	Working formulation	Classification
Low grade		
A	Small lymphocytic, consistent with chronic lymphocytic leukaemia	SL
B	Follicular, predominantly small cleaved cell	FSC
C	Follicular, mixed small cleaved and large cell	FM
Intermediate grade		
D	Follicular, predominately large cell	FL
E	Diffuse, small cleaved cell	DSC
F	Diffuse mixed, small and large cell	DM
G	Diffuse, large cell cleaved or non cleaved cell	DL
High grade		
H	Immunoblastic, large cell	BL
I	Lymphoblastic, convoluted or non-convoluted cell	LL
J	Small non-cleaved cell, Burkitt's or non-Burkitt's	SNC

TABLE 3 Updated Kiel classification (see text, p 2).[4]

B Cell lymphoma	T cell lymphoma
Low grade	
Lymphocytic, chronic lymphocytic, and prolymphocytic leukaemia; hairy cell leukaemia	Lymphocytic, chronic lymphocytic, and prolymphocytic leukaemia
Lymphoplasmacytic/cytoid	Small, cerebriform cell mycosis fungoides, Sezary's syndrome
Plasmacytic	Lymphoepithedloid (Lennert's syndrome)
Centroblastic/centrocytic, follicular, and diffuse	Angioimmunioblastic T zone
High grade	
Centrocytic	Pleomorphic, small cell
Immunoblastic	Immunoblastic
Large cell anaplastic	Large cell anaplastic
Burkitt's lymphoma	
Lymphoblastic	Lymphoblastic

TABLE 4 Rappaport classification (see text, p 2).[5]

Description	Classification
Diffuse lymphocytic, well differentiated	DLWD
Nodular lymphocytic poorly differentiated	NLPD
Nodular mixed, lympocytic and histiocytic	NM
Nodular histiocytic	NH
Diffuse lymphocytic poorly differentiated	DLDP
Diffuse mixed, lymphocytic and histiocytic	DM
Diffuse histiocytic	DH
Diffuse lymphoblastic	DL
Diffuse undifferentiated, Burkitt's or non-Burkitt's	DU

Non-Hodgkin's lymphoma (diffuse large B cell lymphoma)

TABLE 5 **Ann Arbor classification (see text, p 2).[6]**

Stage	Description
I	Involvement of a single lymph node region or of a single extralymphatic organ or site.
II	Involvement of two or more lymph node regions on the same side of diaphragm or localised involvement of extralymphatic organ or site of one or more lymph node regions on the same side of the diaphragm.
III	Involvement of lymph node regions on both sides of the diaphragm, which may also be accompanied by localised involvement extralymphatic organ or site or by involvement of the spleen of both.
IV	Diffuse or disseminated involvement of one or more extralymphatic organs of tissues with or without associated lymph node involvement.

Reproduced with permission of American Association of Cancer Research (Cancer Research, 31: 1860–1861, 1971).

TABLE 6 **Comparison of CHOP 21 versus alternative chemotherapy regimens for first line treatment.**

Comparison	Population	Benefits	Harms
CHOP *v* MACOP-B[14,15]	304 people aged 16–72 years (67% < 60 years) with Working Formulation intermediate (D–G; 6% grade D) or high (H) grade lymphoma; stage I (bulky) to stage IV disease (64% stage III or IV); median follow up 6.5 years (65 people excluded on histological or other grounds)	**Complete response rate:** 65/111 [59%] with CHOP *v* 64/125 [51%] with MACOP-B; P = 0.3 **Overall survival estimated at:** *4 years:* 51% with CHOP *v* 56% with MACOP-B; P = 0.7 *5 years:* 41% with CHOP *v* 54% with MACOP-B; P = 0.035 *8 years:* 36% with CHOP v 45% with MACOP-B; P = 0.16 **Disease free survival estimated at:** *4 years:* 32% with CHOP v 44% with MACOP-B; P = 0.47 *5 years:* 30% with CHOP *v* 42% with MACOP-B; P = 0.045 *8 years:* 25% with CHOP *v* 37% with MACOP-B; P = 0.057	**Stomatitis:** 9% with CHOP *v* 45% with MACOP-B; P < 0.0001 **Cutaneous toxicity:** 0% with CHOP *v* 11% with MACOP-B; P = 0.0001 **Gastrointestinal ulceration:** 4% with CHOP *v* 12% with MACOP-B; P = 0.0001 **Grade 3–4 haematological toxicity:** Significantly lower with CHOP; P = 0.04 (no further data reported) **Alopecia:** 71% with CHOP *v* 48% with MACOP-B; P = 0.0006 **Tolerance:** MACOP-B was poorly tolerated in older people (> 60 years) with 43% completing treatment compared with 83% of younger people

TABLE 6 continued

Comparison	Population	Benefits	Harms
CHOP *v* MACOP-B[16]	405 people aged 18–67 years with aggressive lymphomas according to the Kiel classification (centroblastic, immunoblastic, anaplastic large cell and peripheral T cell), stage I–IV disease (51.6% stage III or IV); median follow up 57 months (31 people excluded on histological or other grounds)	**Complete response rate:** 37% with CHOP *v* 41% with MACOP-B; P = NS **Overall survival estimated at 5 years:** 59% with CHOP *v* 60% with MACOP-B; P = NS **Disease free survival estimated at 5 years:** 44% with CHOP *v* 47% with MACOP-B; P = NS **QoL:** QoL was assessed by 1 centre in 92/106 (87%) people. It found significantly lower QoL with MACOP-B at 12 weeks (P = 0.04; European Organisation for Research into Treatment of Cancer 30, modified QoL score) and worse physical function. However, at 56 weeks the difference was no longer significant	**Treatment related mortality:** 1.9% with CHOP *v* 1.7% with MACOP-B; P = NS Less appetite loss with MACOP-B but more fatigue *After 12 weeks (MACOP-B course completed, CHOP still ongoing):* constipation, diarrhoea, fatigue, dry mouth, nausea/vomiting dizziness, hair loss, and mucositis were higher in the CHOP arm *At 56 weeks:* neuropathic symptoms and mucositis more common in the MACOP-B arm. (Absolute figures not reported; results presented graphically)
CHOP *v* MACOP-B *v* m-BACOD *v* Pro-MACE-Cyta-BOM[12,13]	1138 people aged 15–81 years (75% < 65 years old), with Working Formulation intermediate or high grade lymphomas D–H, and J (15% grade D or E; 4% grade J); stage II (bulky) to stage IV disease; median follow up 49 months (239 people excluded after histology revealed low grade lymphoma)	**Complete response rate:** 44% with CHOP *v* 51% with MACOP-B *v* 48% with m-BACOD *v* 56% with ProMACE-CytaBOM; P = NS **Overall survival estimated at 3 years:** 55% with CHOP *v* 49% with MACOP-B *v* 51% with m-BACOD *v* 53% with ProMACE-CytaBOM; overall P = 0.68 **Disease free survival estimated at 3 years:** 43% with CHOP *v* 40% with MACOP-B *v* 43% with m-BACOD *v* 44% with ProMACE-CytaBOM; overall P = 0.40	**Fatal toxicity:** 1% with CHOP *v* 6% with MACOP-B *v* 5% with m-BACOD *v* 3% with ProMACE-CytaBOM **Life threatening toxicity:** 31% with CHOP *v* 43% with MACOP-B *v* 29% with m-BACOD *v* 54% with ProMACE-CytaBOM **Overall toxicity:** significantly lower with CHOP and ProMACE-CytaBOM than m-BACOD and MACOP-B (P = 0.001)

TABLE 6 continued

Comparison	Population	Benefits	Harms
CHOP *v* m-BACOD[17]	392 people (51% aged ≥ 60 years) with Working Formulation lymphoma grades F–H; stage III or IV; median follow up 4 years (67 people excluded due to incorrect pathological assessment)	**Complete response rate:** 51% with CHOP *v* 56% with m-BACOD; P = 0.32 **Overall survival estimated at 5 years:** 48% with CHOP *v* 49% with m-BACOD; P = 0.54 **Disease free survival:** Results shown graphically; P = NS	**Grades 2–4 pulmonary toxicity:** 3% with CHOP *v* 23% with m-BACOD; P < 0.001 **Grades 3 and 4 infection:** 13% with CHOP *v* 35% with m-BACOD; P < 0.001 **Grades 3 and 4 thrombocytopaenia:** 2% with CHOP *v* 13% with m-BACOD; P = 0.003 **Grades 3 and 4 stomatitis:** 2% with CHOP *v* 37% with m-BACOD; P = 0.001 **Treatment related mortality:** 8/174 [4.6%] with CHOP *v* 9/151 [6.0%] with m-BACOD; P = NS
CHOP v Pro-MACE-CytaBOM[18]	175 people aged 21–82 years (47% < 60 years) with Working Formulation intermediate or high grades D–H (7% with grade D); stages II–IV disease (75% stages III and IV); median follow up 52 months (27 people excluded from study; further 14 people excluded from analysis due to early death or treatment refusal)	**Complete response rate:** 57.5% with CHOP *v* 62.3% with ProMACE-CytaBOM; P = NS **Overall survival estimated at 5 years:** 42% for both CHOP and ProMACE-CytaBOM; P = NS Median survival: 45 months with CHOP *v* 27 months with ProMACE-CytaBOM; significance not reported	Grade 3 and 4 toxicity: P = NS (absolute figures not reported) Treatment related mortality: 1/72 [1.4%] with CHOP *v* 6/76 [7.9%] with ProMACE-CytaBOM; P = 0.126

TABLE 6 continued

Comparison	Population	Benefits	Harms
CHOP *v* PACEBOM[19,20]	459 people aged 16–69 years, with Working Formulation lymphoma grades F and G, stages II–IV disease (67% stage III or IV)	**Complete response rate:** 57% with CHOP *v* 64% with PACEBOM; P = 0.14 (Criteria for complete response stricter than for most RCTs, required normal results 3 months after treatment) **Overall survival estimated at:** *5 years:* 50% with CHOP *v* 60% with PACE-BOM; P = 0.18 *8 years:* 41% with CHOP *v* 51% with PACE-BOM; P = 0.11 **Disease free survival estimated at:** *5 years:* 59% CHOP *v* 67% PACEBOM; P = 0.9 *8 years:* 60% with CHOP *v* 65% with PACE-BOM; P = 0.65	**Treatment related mortality:** 3/226 [1.3%] with CHOP *v* 4/233 [1.7%] with PACEBOM; significance not reported **WHO grade 3 or 4 haematological toxicity:** 34% with CHOP *v* 50% with PACEBOM; P = 0.02

CHOP – cyclophosphamide, doxorubicin, vincristine, prednisolone; m-BACOD – low dose methotrexate, leucoverin rescue, doxorubicin, cyclophosphamide, vincristine, prednisone, bleomycin; MACOP-B – methotrexate, leucoverin rescue, doxorubicin, cyclophosphamide, vincristine, prednisone, bleomycin; NS, not significant; PACEBOM – prednisolone, doxorubicin, cyclophosphamide, etoposide, bleomycin, vincristine, methotrexate; ProMACE-CytaBOM – prednisone, methotrexate, doxorubicin, cyclophosphamide, etoposide, cytarabine, bleomycin, vincristine, methotrexate, with leucoverin rescue; QoL – quality of life.

Sickle cell disease

Search date September 2003

Martin M Meremikwu

QUESTIONS

INTERVENTIONS

See glossary G

Key Messages

Prevention

- **Penicillin prophylaxis in children under 5 years of age** One systematic review found that penicillin prophylaxis in children younger than 5 years reduced invasive pneumococcal infections and related deaths compared with no penicillin or placebo, irrespective of pneumococcal immunisation status.

- **Hydroxyurea** One RCT in adults identified by a systematic review found that hydroxyurea reduced the incidence of painful sickle cell crisis over a mean 21 months compared with placebo. Another RCT in children identified by a systematic review found that hydroxyurea reduced the duration of hospital stay compared with placebo. The RCT in adults also found that hydroxyurea reduced acute chest syndrome and the need for blood transfusion in people with sickle cell disease over a mean 21 months. It found no significant difference in stroke, hepatic sequestration, and mortality related to sickle cell disease between hydroxyurea and placebo, but it may have lacked power and fewer people taking hydroxyurea than taking placebo had these outcomes. Hydroxyurea has been associated with neutropenia, hair loss, skin rash, and gastrointestinal disturbances. We found no RCTs assessing the long term effects of hydroxyurea.
- **Piracetam** One RCT identified by a systematic review found that piracetam reduced the incidence of sickle cell crisis in children compared with placebo.
- **Zinc sulfate** One RCT identified by a systematic review found that zinc sulfate reduced the incidence of sickle cell crisis compared with placebo.
- **Malaria chemoprophylaxis** *Falciparum* malaria is believed to precipitate sickle cell crisis and to increase the risk of death in children with sickle cell anaemia, therefore regular chemoprophylaxis with anti-malarial drugs is advocated by consensus. However, one quasi randomised trial identified by a systematic review provided insufficient evidence to assess routine malaria chemoprophylaxis in people with sickle cell disease.
- **Pneumococcal vaccines** We found no RCTs evaluating the clinical benefits of pneumococcal vaccines in sickle cell disease. Three RCTs found that pneumococcal vaccines caused local reaction and fever but no severe adverse effects.
- **Avoidance of cold environment; limiting physical exercise** We found no RCTs or observational studies of sufficient quality evaluating these interventions in preventing sickle cell crisis and other life threatening complications.

Treatment

- **Controlled release oral morphine given after an initial intravenous bolus dose of morphine (as effective as repeated doses of intravenous morphine)** We found no RCTs comparing morphine versus placebo in people with sickle cell crisis. One RCT in children with painful crisis found that, after an intravenous loading dose of morphine at onset of treatment, controlled release oral morphine was as effective for reducing pain as intravenous morphine.
- **Patient controlled analgesia** Two small RCTs in adults with sickle cell crisis found no significant difference in pain between patient controlled analgesia using either meperidine or morphine and intermittent parenteral treatment. The incidence of adverse effects was also similar in both regimens.
- **Corticosteroid as adjunct to narcotic analgesics** One RCT found that adding high dose intravenous methylprednisolone to intravenous morphine reduced the duration of inpatient analgesia compared with placebo in people with acute severe painful sickle cell crisis. It found no significant difference between adding methylprednisolone and placebo in the proportion of people readmitted to hospital for recurrent pain within two weeks of stopping treatment, although more people taking methylprednisolone were readmitted. Another RCT found that adding dexamethasone to intravenous morphine reduced the number of doses and duration of intravenous analgesia compared with placebo in people with acute sickle cell chest syndrome. Some of the known adverse effects of corticosteroids are increased risk of infections, weight gain, hypertension, poor glucose metabolism, cataracts, and poor growth in children.
- **Acupuncture** We found no RCTs of acupuncture in people with sickle cell crisis.
- **Diflunisal** One RCT in adults with vaso-occlusive sickle cell crisis found no significant difference between adding diflunisal to intramuscular meperidine and adding placebo in pain or in dose of meperidine administered, but it is likely to have been underpowered to detect a clinically important difference.

- **Hydration** We found no RCTs on the effects of routinely giving extra fluids to treat people with sickle cell crisis.
- **Ketorolac** Four RCTs provided insufficient evidence to assess ketorolac in people with vaso-occlusive sickle cell crisis.
- **Oxygen** One RCT in children provided insufficient evidence to assess oxygen therapy in people with sickle cell crisis.
- **Aspirin; codeine; ibuprofen; paracetamol** We found no RCTs evaluating these analgesics in people with sickle cell crisis.

DEFINITION **Sickle cell disease** refers to a group of disorders caused by inheritance of a pair of abnormal haemoglobin genes, including the sickle cell gene. It is characterised by chronic haemolytic anaemia, dactylitis, and acute episodic clinical events called "crises".[1] Vaso-occlusive (painful) crisis is the most common and occurs when abnormal red cells clog small vessels causing tissue ischaemia. The others are hyper-haemolytic crisis (excessive haemolysis), acute chest syndrome, sequestration crisis, and aplastic crisis**G**. A common variant of sickle cell disease, also characterised by haemolytic anaemia, occurs in people with one sickle and one thalassaemia gene. **Sickle cell trait** occurs in people with one sickle gene and one normal gene. People with sickle cell trait do not have any clinical manifestation of illness. This topic covers people with sickle cell disease with or without thalassaemia.

INCIDENCE/ PREVALENCE Sickle cell disease is most common among people living in or originating from sub-Saharan Africa.[2] The disorder also affects people of Mediterranean, Caribbean, Middle Eastern, and Asian origin. The sickle cell gene is most common in areas where malaria is endemic: sickle cell trait affects about 10–30% of Africa's tropical populations.[3] Sickle cell disease affects an estimated 1–2% (120 000) of newborns in Africa annually. Approximately 178 babies (0.28 per 1000 conceptions) are affected by sickle cell disease in England annually.[4] About 60 000 people in the USA[4] and 10 000 in the UK suffer from the disease.[5]

AETIOLOGY/ RISK FACTORS Sickle cell disease is inherited as an autosomal recessive disorder. For a baby to be affected, both parents must have the sickle cell gene. In parents with sickle cell trait, the risk of having of an affected baby is one in four for each pregnancy. Painful (vaso-occlusive) crisis is the most common and most distressing feature of the disease, and these episodes start in infancy and early childhood.[6] Factors that precipitate or modulate the occurrence of sickle cell crisis are not fully understood, but infections, hypoxia, dehydration, acidosis, stress (such as major surgery or childbirth), and cold are believed to play some role. In tropical Africa, malaria is the most common cause of anaemic and vaso-occlusive crisis.[3] High levels of fetal haemoglobin are known to ameliorate the severity and incidence of sickle cell crisis and other complications of the disease.

PROGNOSIS People affected by sickle cell disease are predisposed to bacterial infections, especially to those caused by encapsulated organisms such as *Pneumococcus*, *Haemophilus influenzae*, *Meningococcus*, and *Salmonella* species. Severe bacterial infections such as pneumonia, meningitis, and septicaemia are common causes of morbidity and mortality, especially among young children.[7] About 10% of children with sickle cell anaemia may develop a stroke, and more than half of these may suffer recurrent strokes.[8] Abnormal features of cerebral blood vessels shown by transcranial Doppler scan predict a high risk of stroke in children with sickle cell disease.[9] Frequent episodes of crisis, infections, and organ damage reduce the quality of life of people with sickle cell disease. High rate of vaso-occlusive (painful) crisis is an index of clinical severity that correlates with early death. Life expectancy remains low, especially in communities with poor access to health services. In some parts of Africa, about 50% of children with sickle cell disease die before their first birthday.[3] The average life expectancy for men and women with sickle cell disease in the USA is about 42 and 48 years, respectively.[10] Frequent blood transfusions could increase the risk of immune reactions and infections, such as HIV and hepatitis B or C viruses, and Chagas' disease. The need for repeated blood transfusions in people with sickle cell disease predisposes them to the risk of iron overload.[11]

AIMS OF INTERVENTION To reduce mortality, the incidence and severity of sickle cell crises and other acute complications; to prevent organ damage; to improve quality of life and increase life expectancy; to achieve effective pain relief during crises, with minimal adverse effects.

OUTCOMES Mortality; dactylitis, incidence of crisis; severity of crisis; incidence of other acute complications (e.g. malaria, stroke, infectious complications [invasive pneumococcal infection or acute osteomyelitis]); quality of life; adverse effects of treatment (e.g. gastrointestinal bleeding due to non-steroidal anti-inflammatory drugs, addiction to narcotic analgesics, immune reactions and infections due to blood transfusions [e.g. HIV, viral hepatitis, and Chagas' disease]). Secondary outcomes include duration of crisis, days out of school or work, requirement for blood transfusion for severe anaemia. Fetal and total haemoglobin levels are considered proxy outcomes and are not addressed in this chapter.

METHODS *Clinical Evidence* search and appraisal September 2003; this included a search for observational studies on limiting physical exercise and avoidance of cold environment.

QUESTION What are the effects of interventions to prevent sickle cell crisis and other acute complications in people with sickle cell disease?

OPTION ANTIBIOTIC PROPHYLAXIS

One systematic review found that penicillin prophylaxis in children younger than 5 years reduced invasive pneumococcal infections and related deaths compared with no penicillin or placebo, irrespective of pneumococcal immunisation status.

Benefits: We found one systematic review (search date 2001, 3 RCTs, 857 children with sickle cell anaemia).[12] Two RCTs identified by the review compared penicillin versus no penicillin or placebo and the third assessed stopping penicillin prophylaxis after the age of 5 years. The review found that penicillin prophylaxis significantly reduced the risk of pneumococcal infections regardless of vaccination status compared with no penicillin or placebo (2 RCTs, 9/248 [3.6%] with penicillin prophylaxis *v* 19/209 [9.1%] without penicillin prophylaxis; RR 0.39, 95% CI 0.17 to 0.88). It found no significant difference in mortality between penicillin and no penicillin (0/105 [0.0%] with penicillin *v* 4/110 [3.6%] without penicillin; RR 0.12, 95% CI 0.01 to 2.14).[12] The wide confidence interval in the assessment of mortality suggest that the RCTs may have been underpowered to detect a difference in mortality. The first RCT (242 children in Jamaica, aged 6–36 months) had a factorial design**G** and compared monthly intramuscular penicillin injection (dose not specified) versus no injection. Half of the children receiving penicillin and half of those not receiving penicillin also received either polysaccharide pneumococcal vaccine or *H influenzae* vaccine. The second RCT (215 children in the USA, aged 3–36 months) compared oral penicillin 125 mg twice daily versus placebo. All children received polysaccharide pneumococcal vaccine**G** at the ages of 1 and 2 years. The RCT was discontinued earlier than planned because of a significant reduction in the risk of pneumococcal infection in the penicillin group compared with no penicillin (RR 0.16, 95% CI 0.04 to 0.70), which made it unethical to continue recruitment.[13] The third RCT (400 children aged 5 years) identified by the review[12] compared continuing penicillin prophylaxis after the age of 5 years versus placebo.[14] All of the children had received prophylactic penicillin for ≥2 years and polysaccharide pneumococcal vaccine at age 2–3 years. The RCT found no significant difference between continuing penicillin 125 mg twice daily and placebo in the risk of pneumococcal infections (RR 0.47, 95% CI 0.09 to 2.56), or in mortality (RR 0.99, 95% CI 0.14 to 7.08) [14]

Harms: One RCT identified by the review found minor adverse effects, including localised reactions to vaccine and nausea and vomiting (3 cases); the difference in nausea and vomiting between penicillin prophylaxis and placebo was not significant (2/210 [0.95%] v 1/199 [0.50%]; RR 1.90, 95% CI 0.17 to 20.74).

Comment: Antibiotic prophylaxis and pneumococcal vaccines are recommended to reduce morbidity and mortality from pneumococcal infections in vulnerable groups, including children with sickle cell disease.[15] The effectiveness of antibiotic prophylaxis could be diminished by high incidence of *S pneumoniae* resistance. Allergy to penicillin is a contraindication. Erythromycin is usually the recommended alternative to penicillin but its value in sickle cell disease has not been evaluated in an RCT.

OPTION MALARIA CHEMOPROPHYLAXIS

***Falciparum* malaria is believed to precipitate sickle cell crisis and to increase the risk of death in children with sickle cell anaemia, therefore regular chemoprophylaxis with anti-malarial drugs is advocated by consensus. However, one quasi randomised trial identified by a systematic review provided insufficient evidence to assess routine malaria chemoprophylaxis in people with sickle cell disease.**

Benefits: We found one systematic review (search date 2003, 1 quasi randomised trial, 126 children with sickle cell disease) comparing weekly malaria chemoprophylaxis using chloroquine plus antibiotic prophylaxis using monthly injection of long acting benzathine penicillin versus sterile water.[16] The review found that malaria chemoprophylaxis plus antibiotics significantly reduced the incidence of malaria compared with sterile water (5/73 [7%] with chemoprophylaxis *v* 36/84 [43%] with sterile water; RR 0.16; 95% CI 0.07 to 0.39). It found no significant difference in dactylitis**G** between malaria chemoprophylaxis plus antibiotics and sterile water ($P < 0.1$; no further data reported).

Harms: The trial identified by the review gave no information on adverse effects.[16] Adverse effects of drugs commonly used for malaria prophylaxis (chloroquine, proguanil, doxycycline, mefloquine and atovaquone–proguanil) are described elsewhere (see malaria: prevention in travellers, p 956).

Comment: Inadequate allocation concealment and poor randomisation technique limit the validity of the results of the RCT identified by the review.[16] The RCT was performed between 1962 and 1964, at a time when chloroquine resistant *Plasmodium falciparum* was not as widespread as it is today. Using chloroquine for malaria chemoprophylaxis in areas where chloroquine resistance is known to be high is unlikely to be effective. Because *Falciparum* malaria is believed to precipitate sickle cell crisis and to increase the risk of death in children with sickle cell anaemia, regular chemoprophylaxis with anti-malarial drugs is advocated by consensus.[3] The evidence presented in the review is insufficient to support or refute this practice.

OPTION PNEUMOCOCCAL VACCINES

We found no systematic review or RCTs evaluating the clinical benefits of pneumococcal vaccines in sickle cell disease. Three RCTs found that pneumococcal vaccines caused local reaction and fever but no severe adverse effects.

Benefits: We found no systematic review. **Polysaccharide pneumococcal vaccine:** We found one RCT (123 Zambian residents with sickle cell anaemia, 106 aged 2–15 years).[17] It compared polyvalent polysaccharide pneumococcal vaccine**G** versus placebo for a period of 2 years, but reported no data on clinical benefits. **Pneumococcal conjugate vaccine:** We found no systematic reviews or RCTs of pneumococcal conjugate vaccine**G** that assessed clinical benefits (see comment below).

Harms: **Polyvalent polysaccharide vaccine:** The RCT found that pneumococcal polysaccharide vaccine increased adverse effects (sore arm, induration at the site of injection, and fever) compared with no vaccine, although the difference was not significant (3/61 [5%] with vaccine *v* 0/62 [0%] with no vaccine; ARI +4.9%, 95% CI –3.7% to +11.6%).[17] Another RCT (32 children with sickle cell disease aged < 5 years who had been immunised with the same vaccine 2 or more years before, crossover design) compared the incidence of reactions following booster immunisation versus placebo.[18] It found no significant difference in post-vaccination reactions (muscle pain, fever, headache, or rash) after crossover between booster immunisation and placebo (16/32 [50%] with booster vaccine *v* 7/32 [22%] with placebo; RR 2.29, 95% CI 1.09 to 4.79). **Pneumococcal conjugate vaccine:** We found one RCT (22 children, 11 allocated to each intervention) comparing a combined schedule of 7 valent pneumococcal conjugate vaccine followed by 23 valent polysaccharide pneumococcal vaccine versus 23 valent vaccine alone.[19] It found no significant difference between groups in the incidence of post-vaccination fever (27.3% with combined schedule *v* 18.1% with single; RR 1.50, 95% CI 0.31 to 7.30).[19]

Comment: The RCTs assessed antibody levels rather than incidence of pneumococcal infections.[17,19] Antibiotic prophylaxis and pneumococcal vaccines are recommended to reduce morbidity and mortality from pneumococcal infections in vulnerable groups, including children with sickle cell disease.[15] An increase in penicillin resistant strains of *Streptococcus pneumoniae* has highlighted the potential for pneumococcal vaccination as an alternative. Polyvalent polysaccharide pneumococcal vaccine offers no protective immunity to children younger than 2 years, who have the highest rates of invasive pneumococcal infections.[15] Newly developed pneumococcal conjugate vaccines show protective efficacy in children younger than 2 years and are recommended for routine use in young infants,[20] but this has not been demonstrated in infants with sickle cell disease.

OPTION HYDROXYUREA

One RCT in adults identified by a systematic review found that hydroxyurea reduced the incidence of painful crisis over a mean 21 months compared with placebo. Another RCT in children identified by a systematic review found that hydroxyurea reduced the duration of hospital stay compared with placebo. The RCT in adults also found that hydroxyurea reduced acute chest syndrome and the need for blood transfusion in people with sickle cell disease over a mean 21 months. It found no significant difference in stroke, hepatic sequestration, and mortality related to sickle cell disease between hydroxyurea and placebo, but it may have lacked power and fewer people taking hydroxyurea than taking placebo had these outcomes. Hydroxyurea has been associated with neutropenia, hair loss, skin rash, and gastrointestinal disturbances. We found no RCTs assessing the long term effects of hydroxyurea.

Benefits: We found one systematic review (search date 2001, 2 RCTs).[21] Both of the included RCTs compared hydroxyurea versus placebo (25 children, crossover design;[22] 299 adults, parallel group design[23]). **Painful crisis:**

The review found that, in adults, hydroxyurea reduced the number of painful crises compared with placebo after a mean follow up of 21 months (1 RCT, 299 adults, mean number of episodes during follow up 5.1 with hydroxyurea *v* 7.9 with placebo; WMD –2.8, 95% CI –4.74 to –0.86).[21] It also found that, children taking hydroxyurea had shorter hospital stay over 6 months before crossover than children taking placebo (1 RCT, 25 children, mean duration of hospital stay 5.3 days with hydroxyurea *v* 15.2 days with placebo; CI not reported).[22] **Other crises and mortality:** The RCT in adults identified by the review found that hydroxyurea significantly reduced the risk of acute chest syndrome**G** (RR 0.44, 95% CI 0.28 to 0.68) and the need for blood transfusion compared with placebo (RR 0.67, 95% CI 0.52 to 0.87).[21] It found no significant difference between hydroxyurea and placebo in stroke (RR 0.64, 95% CI 0.11 to 3.80), hepatic sequestration (RR 0.32, 95% CI 0.03 to 3.06), or mortality related to sickle cell disease (RR 0.48, 95% CI 0.09 to 2.60), although fewer people taking hydroxyurea had these outcomes, and the RCT was too small to rule out a clinically important difference. **Quality of life:** The RCT in adults identified by the review reported data on quality of life collected at 6 monthly intervals using the Health Status Survey, Profile of Mood States, and the Ladder of Life.[21] Lower scores reflect lower quality of life in all scales. It found no significant difference between hydroxyurea and placebo in quality of life, although changes from baseline on all the quality of life scales at 12 months were higher with hydroxyurea than placebo (general health perception: WMD +0.60, 95% CI –0.18 to +1.38; social function: WMD +0.20, 95% CI –0.36 to +0.76; pain recall: WMD +0.40, 95% CI –0.18 to +0.98; and Ladder of Life: WMD +0.40, 95% CI –0.15 to +0.95).

Harms: Neutropenia (neutrophil count ≤ 2500 x 10^9/L) was reported in 79% of the people in the hydroxyurea group compared with 37% of the people allocated to placebo, but no case of infection was related to neutropenia. Some participants suffered hair loss, skin rash, and gastrointestinal disturbances, but these did not differ significantly between groups.[21] The long term safety of hydroxyurea in sickle cell disease remains uncertain.

Comment: In the RCT in adults, hydroxyurea in adults was given at 15 mg/kg daily, and the dose increased at 12 weekly intervals by 2.5 mg/kg daily until mild bone marrow suppression was detected (indicated by a neutrophil count below 2000/mm^3, a reticulocyte or platelet count < 80 000/mm^3, or a haemoglobin level <4.5 g/dL).[23] Dose in children was 20 mg/kg daily and increased to a maximum of 25 mg/kg daily.[22]

OPTION PIRACETAM

One RCT identified by a systematic review found that piracetam reduced the incidence of sickle cell crisis in children compared with placebo.

Benefits: We found one systematic review (search date 2003, 1 RCT, 103 children aged 3–12 years) comparing piracetam versus placebo.[24] The RCT found that piracetam 160 mg/kg daily significantly reduced the incidence of crisis compared with placebo (mean 2.4 with piracetam *v* 4.3 with placebo; WMD –1.9, 95% CI: –3.01 to –0.79). No deaths occurred in either group.

Harms: The RCT identified by the review stated that "no toxic effects" associated with piracetam were observed.[24]

Comment: It is likely that this RCT was not adequately powered to provide reliable information on adverse effects. It is necessary to obtain more reliable data on the safety of piracetam.

OPTION ZINC SULFATE

One RCT identified by a systematic review found that zinc sulfate reduced the incidence of sickle cell crisis compared with placebo.

Benefits: We found one systematic review (search date 2003, 1 RCT, 145 people aged 12–27 years) comparing zinc sulfate versus placebo.[24] The RCT identified by the review found that zinc sulfate significantly reduced the mean number of sickle cell crises (including vaso-occlusive, haemolytic, sequestration and aplastic crisis) compared with placebo (mean 2.46 with zinc sulfate *v* 5.29 with placebo (WMD –2.83; 95% CI –3.51 to –2.15). No deaths occurred in either group.

Harms: The RCT identified by the review stated that "no significant toxicity" associated with zinc sulfate was observed, although it was unclear which adverse effects were monitored.[24]

Comment: None.

OPTION LIMITING PHYSICAL EXERCISE

We found no RCTs or observational studies of sufficient quality evaluating limiting exercise to prevent sickle cell crisis and other life threatening complications of sickle cell disease.

Benefits: We found no systematic review, RCTs, or observational studies of sufficient quality.

Harms: We found no RCTs or observational studies of sufficient quality.

Comment: Moderate exercise is generally accepted to be beneficial, especially in reducing risk of cardiovascular disease. Moderate exercise is therefore unlikely to cause harm in people with sickle cell disease. Strenuous exercise is suspected to lead to factors that may precipitate sickle cell crisis, such as low tissue oxygen saturation, dehydration, and stress.

OPTION AVOIDANCE OF COLD ENVIRONMENT

We found no RCTs or observational studies of sufficient quality evaluating avoiding exposure to cold environment to prevent crisis and other life threatening complications of sickle cell disease.

Benefits: We found no systematic review, RCTs, or observational studies of sufficient quality.

Harms: We found no RCTs or observational studies of sufficient quality.

Comment: A 10 year retrospective study found a close correlation between cold weather and admissions for sickle cell painful crisis.[25] One observational study in 60 men with sickle cell disease and 30 adults with normal haemoglobin genotype found that vasoconstriction induced by skin cooling was significantly more likely to occur in people with sickle cell disease than in those with normal haemoglobin genotype (83% *v* 60%; P = 0.03).[26] Among people with sickle cell disease, the frequency of painful crises was significantly greater in those prone to cooling induced vasoconstriction than those less prone (0.36 crises per year *v* 0.12 crises per year; P = 0.04).[26]

QUESTION What are the effects of interventions to treat pain and reduce complications in people with sickle cell crisis?

OPTION ASPIRIN

We found no RCTs of aspirin in people with sickle cell crisis.

Benefits: We found no systematic review or RCTs.

Harms: We found no RCTs.

Comment: Aspirin is widely used by clinicians to relieve mild pain and fever, although there is concern about using it in children because it has been associated with Reye's syndrome. The adverse effects of aspirin in different populations are discussed in other *Clinical Evidence* topics. (see primary prevention [web only]; stroke prevention, p 167; and non-steroidal anti-inflammatory drugs, p 1525) Studies on long term aspirin prophylaxis address a different question to that addressed here on treating acute pain in sickle cell crisis.

OPTION CODEINE

We found no RCTs of codeine in people with sickle cell crisis.

Benefits: We found no systematic reviews or RCTs.

Harms: Codeine is widely used by clinicians to relieve moderate pain. Prolonged use of narcotic analgesics may lead to addiction. Codeine is known to be less addictive than other narcotic analgesics like morphine and meperidine.

Comment: None.

OPTION IBUPROFEN

We found no RCTs of ibuprofen in people with sickle cell crisis.

Benefits: We found no systematic review or RCTs.

Harms: Ibuprofen is widely used by clinicians to relieve mild pain and fever. The adverse affects of ibuprofen in other populations are discussed in other *Clinical Evidence* topics (see acute otitis media, p 227; carpal tunnel syndrome, p 1388; and migraine headache, p 1622).

Comment: Adverse events associated with non-steroidal anti-inflammatory drugs have been reviewed elsewhere in *Clinical Evidence* (see non-steroidal anti-inflammatory drugs, p 1525; low back pain [acute, p 1465 and chronic, p 1479]; osteoarthritis, [Web only]; tennis elbow, p 1572; and dysmenorrhoea, p 2303).

OPTION PARACETAMOL

We found no RCTs of paracetamol (acetaminophen) in people with sickle cell crisis.

Benefits: We found no systematic review or RCTs.

Harms: We found no RCTs.

Comment: Paracetamol is widely used by clinicians to relieve mild pain and fever. Standard clinical dosage of paracetamol is well tolerated and unlikely to cause harm, but overdose is known to cause liver toxicity. See paracetamol (acetaminophen) poisoning, p 1756.

OPTION DIFLUNISAL

One RCT in adults with vaso-occlusive sickle cell crisis found no significant difference between adding diflunisal to intramuscular meperidine and adding placebo in pain or in dose of meperidine administered, but it is likely to have been underpowered to detect a clinically important difference.

Benefits: We found no systematic review. We found one RCT (32 adults, 46 episodes of vaso-occlusive crisis), which compared oral diflunisal (1000 mg loading dose followed by 500 mg 12 hourly for 5 days) versus placebo.[27] Pain episodes were the basis for randomisation. Intravenous meperidine (1.0–1.5 mg/kg) and hydroxyzine (0.5 1.0 mg/kg) were given every 3–4 hours as necessary for pain relief in all people. A categorical pain scale ranging from 0–5 was used to assess response to treatment. The RCT found no significant difference in pain intensity scores between diflunisal and placebo (P reported as non-significant, CI not reported). It also found no significant difference in the mean total dose of meperidine administered (1400 mg with diflunisal *v* 1000 mg with placebo; WMD +400.0, 95% CI –28.6 to +828.6). The RCT is likely to have been underpowered to detect a clinically important difference between treatments.

Harms: The RCT found that diflunisal significantly increased nausea compared with placebo (6/22 [27%] *v* 2/15 [13%]; $P < 0.05$).[27] One person discontinued diflunisal because of a facial rash. Adverse events associated with non-steroidal anti-inflammatory drugs have been reviewed elsewhere in *Clinical Evidence* (see non-steroidal anti-inflammatory drugs, p 1525; low back pain [acute, p 1465 and chronic, p 1479]; osteoarthritis, [Web only]; tennis elbow, p 1572; and dysmenorrhoea, p 2303).

Comment: None.

OPTION KETOROLAC

Four RCTs provided insufficient evidence to assess ketorolac in people with vaso-occlusive sickle cell crisis.

Benefits: We found no systematic review but found four small RCTs.[28–31] **Versus meperidine:** One crossover RCT (20 adolescents aged 11–19 years) compared parenteral ketorolac (1.0 mg/kg) versus parenteral meperidine (1.5 mg/kg) in sickle cell vaso-occlusive crisis in the first phase (150 minutes) before crossover.[28] Pain was measured in a visual analogue scale (VAS) ranging from 0–80 mm where 0 mm denotes "no pain" and 80 mm denotes "the worst pain I've ever had". Measurements were taken at 30 minutes and 150 minutes. It found that ketorolac significantly reduced pain compared with meperidine at 30 minutes (mean VAS 39 mm with ketorolac *v* 54 mm with meperidine; $P < 0.01$) and at 150 minutes (mean VAS 33 mm with ketorolac *v* 56 mm with meperidine; $P < 0.01$). It found no significant difference between ketorolac and meperidine in the proportion of people who were pain free at 150 minutes (4/10 [40%] with ketorolac *v* 2/10 [20%] with meperidine; RR 2.0, 95% CI 0.47 to 8.56), but the RCT was too small to rule out clinically important differences. Data obtained after crossover were not included because it is deemed unsuitable to confirm the effect of either drug. **Ketorolac plus meperidine versus placebo plus meperidine:**

We found two RCTs.[29,30] The first RCT (18 adults with vaso-occlusive sickle cell crisis) found no significant difference in pain between a single dose of intramuscular ketorolac (60 mg) and placebo given as a supplement to repeated doses of intravenous meperidine (mean pain score assessed by VAS: 44 with ketorolac *v* 37 with placebo; P = 0.49).[29] The second RCT (21 people with sickle cell crisis, aged > 14 years) compared intravenous infusion of ketorolac (150 mg first day, 120 mg subsequent days for total of 5 days) versus placebo as a supplement to intermittent intramuscular meperidine (100 mg every 3 hours if pain level is moderate or severe).[30] It found that people taking intravenous ketorolac required a significantly lower amount of meperidine to control pain compared with placebo (WMD –937.8 mg of meperidine, 95% CI –1803.2 mg to –72.4 mg). **Ketorolac plus morphine sulfate versus placebo plus morphine sulfate:** One RCT (29 people, 41 episodes of vaso-occlusive sickle cell crisis, aged 5–17 years) compared intravenous ketorolac (0.9 mg/kg) versus placebo as a supplement to simultaneous treatment with parenteral morphine sulfate (0.1 mg/kg).[31] Morphine was repeated every 2 hours based on pain intensity rated on the VAS. Pain episodes were the basis for randomisation. The RCT found no significant difference in the need for morphine between ketorolac and placebo (0.28 mg/kg with ketorolac *v* 0.32 mg/kg with placebo; WMD –0.04 mg/kg, 95% CI –0.09 mg/kg to +0.01 mg/kg). It also found no significant difference between ketorolac and placebo in the proportion of people requiring admission for further management of severe pain (9/22 [41%] with ketorolac *v* 10/19 [53%] with placebo; RR 0.78, 95% CI 0.40 to 1.50).

Harms: No severe adverse events were reported in the RCTs apart from one case of epistaxis in a person that received ketorolac.[30] Other adverse events (mostly gastrointestinal disturbances) were similar between treatment groups.

Comment: None.

OPTION MORPHINE

We found no RCTs comparing morphine versus placebo in people with sickle cell crisis. One RCT in children with painful crisis found that, after an intravenous loading dose of morphine at onset of treatment, controlled release oral morphine was as effective for reducing pain as intravenous morphine.

Benefits: We found no systematic review. **Versus placebo:** We found no RCTs comparing morphine versus placebo. **Oral versus intravenous morphine:** We found one double blind placebo controlled RCT (56 children aged 5–17 years with painful crisis) comparing controlled release morphine given orally (1.9 mg/kg every 12 hours) plus intravenous placebo (saline) versus intravenous morphine (0.04 mg/kg) plus placebo tablets for sickle cell vaso-occlusive crisis.[32] All children were given an intravenous loading dose of morphine (0.15 mg/kg) at onset of treatment. The RCT found no significant difference in pain assessed by the Children's Hospital of Eastern Ontario Pain Scale(G) (WMD +0.10 units, 95% CI –0.09 units to +0.70 units) or other clinical pain scales (Oucher, faces or clinical pain scales: –0.20 units, 95% CI –0.54 units to +0.14 units) throughout the observation period (at 0900, 1300, 1700, and 2100 every day). It also found no significant difference between oral and intravenous morphine in the mean frequency of rescue analgesia (WMD –0.12 doses/day, 95% CI –0.30 doses/day to +0.06 doses/day) and the mean duration of pain (WMD +1.20 days, 95% CI –0.01 days to +2.41 days).

Harms: The RCT found no significant difference in the frequency of spontaneously reported adverse events between oral and intravenous morphine (62 for oral *v* 52 for intravenous; 16 *v* 19 for severe intensity events). Common adverse events were fever, pruritus, nausea, vomiting, and constipation; these did not differ significantly between study groups.

Comment: None.

OPTION PATIENT CONTROLLED ANALGESIA

Two small RCTs in adults with sickle cell crisis found no significant difference in pain between patient controlled analgesia using either meperidine or morphine and intermittent parenteral treatment using either meperidine or morphine. The incidence of adverse effects was also similar in both regimens.

Benefits: We found no systematic review. **Meperidine:** One RCT (20 adults, age range 17–39 years) compared patient controlled analgesia (infusion of meperidine 25–30 mg/hour plus oral hydroxyzine 50 mg every 6 hours) versus intermittent intravenous analgesia (intramuscular meperidine 75–100 mg plus intramuscular hydroxyzine 50–75 mg given as necessary every 3–4 hours).[33] It found no significant difference between patient controlled and intermittent analgesia in pain over 3 days as measured by categorical and analogue pain scales (categorical scores on day 2: WMD +4.0 mm, 95% CI –1.09 mm to +9.09 mm; analogue scores: WMD +68.0 mm, 95% CI –25.35 mm to +161.35 mm). It also found no significant difference in the amount of meperidine used each day after 3 days (WMD +451 mg, 95% CI –70 mg to +972 mg). The units being measured in the pain scales were not defined. **Morphine:** One RCT compared patient controlled analgesia with morphine versus intermittent intravenous injections of morphine in two phases of high and low dose regimen, respectively, in adult patients with sickle cell crisis pain.[34] In the first phase (20 people), the intermittent therapy group received either 4 mg intravenous bolus of morphine sulfate every 30–60 minutes as needed to achieve a linear analogue pain intensity score < 50 mm. The patient controlled analgesia group received 2 mg bolus of intravenous morphine sulfate followed by 1 mg intravenous controlled by the patient with 6 minute lock out. The dose of morphine was increased to 6 mg for the intermittent therapy group, and 1.5 mg for the patient controlled analgesia group if pain control by the end of the first 30 minutes was inadequate (pain score > 50 mm). The second phase (25 people) was similar but used higher doses of morphine for the PCA (2.7 mg with 10 minutes' lock out) and the intermittent intravenous group (8 mg every 30–60 minutes). The RCT found a reduction in pain scores on the linear analogue scale in both groups, with no significant difference between treatment groups in both the first phase (WMD –0.10 mm, 95% CI –27.03 mm to +26.83 mm) and the second phase (WMD +9.0 mm, 95% CI –18.25 mm to +36.25 mm). It found no significant difference in the total amount of morphine administered between patient controlled analgesia and intermittent intravenous analgesia in the first phase (WMD –6.70 mg, 95% CI –23.35 mg to +9.95 mg) or the second phase of the study (WMD +6.40 mg, 95% CI –8.71 mg to +12.51 mg).

Harms: **Meperidine:** The RCT gave no information on adverse effects.[33] Severe adverse effects such as seizures and respiratory depression have been associated with meperidine.[35] There are concerns of possible addiction to narcotic analgesics, but some studies show a relatively low rate of addiction (0–11%) in people with sickle cell disease.[36] **Morphine:** The RCT found that nausea, vomiting, and pruritus were common events observed with both high and low dose morphine, with 44% and 31%

requiring antiemetic therapy (prochlorperazine) in the intermittent intravenous and PCA groups, respectively.[34] It found a no significant difference in the proportion of people who had adverse effects (53% with patient controlled *v* 47% with intermittent; P = 0.715), but no details were given about the types of adverse effects or their severity. Respiratory depression or clinically significant hypotension was not observed during the RCT. Respiratory depression is a well known adverse effect of narcotic drugs.

Comment: None.

OPTION ACUPUNCTURE

We found no RCTs of acupuncture in people with sickle cell crisis.

Benefits: We found no systematic reviews or RCTs.

Harms: Acupuncture is widely used to relieve pain. Adverse effects of acupuncture in different populations are discussed in other *Clinical Evidence* topics (see low back pain [acute, p 1465 and chronic, p 1479]; and nausea and vomiting in early pregnancy, p 1769).

Comment: None.

OPTION OXYGEN

One RCT in children provided insufficient evidence to assess oxygen therapy in people with sickle cell crisis.

Benefits: We found no systematic review. One RCT (25 children and adolescents aged 3–18 years with vaso-occlusive crisis) compared 50% oxygen versus air as an adjunct to continuous intravenous morphine infusion.[37] It found no significant difference between 50% oxygen and air in the duration of severe pain (0.94 days with 50% oxygen *v* 0.95 days with air; WMD –0.19, 95% CI –0.91 to +0.89), amount of narcotic analgesic administered, or further hospitalisation for pain (reported as non-significant for all outcomes, CI not reported). It also found no significant difference in the proportion of people with progression of crisis indicated by appearance of new pain sites (5/14 [36%] with 50% oxygen *v* 4/11 [36%] with air; reported as non-significant, CI not reported). The RCT may have been underpowered to detect a clinically important difference between interventions.

Harms: The RCT gave no information about adverse effects associated with oxygen therapy.[37]

Comment: The RCT was reported in two publications.[37,38] Low tissue oxygen saturation is a dominant factor in the mechanism that results in sickling. Given that increased sickling is a key component of the pathophysiology of vaso-occlusive crisis and acute chest syndrome**G**, oxygen therapy is expected to ameliorate these conditions. Oxygen therapy is recommended routinely for treatment of sickle cell acute chest syndrome, but people with acute chest syndrome were excluded from the RCT.[37]

OPTION HYDRATION

We found no RCTs on the effects of routinely giving extra fluids to treat people with sickle cell crisis.

Benefits: We found no systematic review or RCTs (see comment below).

Harms: We found no RCTs.

Comment: It is standard practice to give extra intravenous or oral fluids to dehydrated patients. This widely accepted clinical practice also applies to people with sickle cell who are dehydrated. However it is unclear whether giving extra fluids routinely to people with sickle cell painful crisis without dehydration will be beneficial or harmful.

OPTION CORTICOSTEROIDS

One RCT found that adding high dose intravenous methylprednisolone to intravenous morphine reduced the duration of inpatient analgesia compared with placebo in people with acute severe sickle cell crisis. It found no significant difference between adding methylprednisolone and placebo in the proportion of people readmitted to hospital for recurrent pain within two weeks of stopping treatment, although more people taking methylprednisolone were readmitted. Another RCT found that adding dexamethasone to intravenous morphine reduced the number of doses and duration of intravenous analgesia compared with placebo in people with acute sickle cell chest syndrome. Some of the known adverse effects of corticosteroids are increased risk of infections, weight gain, hypertension, poor glucose metabolism, cataracts, and poor growth in children.

Benefits: We found no systematic review but found two RCTs.[39,40] The first RCT compared high dose intravenous methylprednisolone versus placebo, given as an adjunct to narcotic analgesia (intravenous morphine followed by oral codeine plus paracetamol) in 56 acute episodes of severe sickle cell painful crisis in 34 people aged 2–19 years. Pain episodes were the basis for randomisation.[39] It found that methylprednisolone significantly reduced the duration of inpatient analgesia (intravenous or oral) compared with placebo (41.3 hours with methylprednisolone *v* 71.3 hours with placebo; $P = 0.01$). It found no significant difference between methylprednisolone and placebo in readmissions to hospital for recurrent pain within 2 weeks, although more people taking methylprednisolone were readmitted (4/26 [15%] with methylprednisolone *v* 1/30 [3%] with placebo; RR 4.62, 95% CI 0.55 to 38.74). The RCT may have lacked power to rule out a clinically important difference between groups. The second RCT compared intravenous dexamethasone versus placebo, given as an adjunct to narcotic analgesia (intravenous morphine followed by oral codeine plus paracetamol) in 43 acute episodes of acute sickle cell chest syndrome in 34 children aged 1–13 years. It found that dexamethasone significantly reduced the mean number of doses and duration of intravenous analgesia compared with placebo (mean number of doses: 2.5 with dexamethasone *v* 20.0 with placebo; $P < 0.001$; duration: 16.8 hours with dexamethasone *v* 76.8 hours with placebo; $P < 0.001$).[40]

Harms: The first RCT found no adverse effects associated with methylprednisolone.[39] The second RCT found no adverse effects associated with dexamethasone, but may have been underpowered to detect clinically important adverse effects.[40] Some of the known adverse effects of corticosteroids are increased risk of infections, weight gain, hypertension, poor glucose metabolism, cataracts, and poor growth in children.

Comment: None.

GLOSSARY

Acute chest syndrome Acute chest syndrome is a life-threatening complication of sickle cell disease characterised by fever, cough, chest pain, difficult breathing, worsening anaemia, and new pulmonary infiltrates on radiography. It is difficult to differentiate acute chest syndrome clinically from pneumonia and pulmonary infarctions.

Aplastic crisis Sudden cessation of the bone marrow from making new blood cells.

CHEOPS scale (Children's Hospital of Eastern Ontario Pain scale) A behavioural scale used to evaluate postoperative pain. It was initially validated in children aged 1–5 years, and subsequently validated in children from other populations and ages.[41] CHEOPS scale is used to monitor the effectiveness of interventions for reducing the pain and discomfort. Scores obtained from adding points from six different parameters range from 4–13.

Dactylitis Inflammation of the bones of the hands and feet resulting in swelling, redness, and pain in the affected parts. It is common in young infants with sickle cell disease, and is precipitated by the sickle process that characterises sickle cell disease. Because it tends to occur bilaterally in the hands and feet with swelling of the dorsum, it is commonly described as sickle cell "hand and foot syndrome".

Factorial design An RCT design which attempts to evaluate more than one intervention compared with control in a single trial, by means of multiple randomisations.

Fetal haemoglobin (Hb F) This is the predominant type of normal haemoglobin (i.e. the oxygen carrying molecule in the human red blood cell) in the unborn child. Following birth, another type of normal haemoglobin (Hb A) replaces Hb F and remains predominant throughout life. Hb F binds oxygen stronger than HbA and maintains higher tissue oxygen tension than Hb A.

Haemoglobin S (Hb S) This is an inherited type of abnormal haemoglobin that has a tendency to form crystals when oxygen saturation is low. Under such conditions, red blood cells become deformed (many shaped like "sickle"), more rigid, and easily breakable. This is the main disorder responsible for the clinical syndrome experienced by people with sickle cell anaemia. People affected by sickle cell anaemia who also have high levels of fetal haemoglobin tend to have fewer episodes of crisis because fetal haemoglobin maintains a higher level of tissue oxygen saturation.

Pneumococcal conjugate vaccines These are polysaccharide pneumococcal vaccines linked with proteins such as those of the outer membrane meningococcus, tetanus, or diphtheria toxoids. The conjugate pneumococcal vaccines have been shown to be immunogenic in children younger than 2 years, and is recommended for routine use in infants beginning from the age of 2 months.[19,42]

Polyvalent polysaccharide pneumococcal vaccine (PPV) This type of vaccine contains the purified capsular polysaccharides of several *S pneumoniae* serotypes. Many of the polysaccharides contained in the vaccines do not induce protective immunity in children younger than 2 years. This type of pneumococcal vaccine is recommended for children aged 2 years and older affected by conditions that predispose them to increased risk of invasive pneumococcal infection.[42]

Sequestration crisis Sudden pooling of blood in spleen and liver, with the result that the patient becomes very anaemic and hypotensive, with the affected organ becoming remarkably enlarged and painful.

REFERENCES

1. Akinyanju OO. A profile of sickle cell disease in Nigeria. *Ann N Y Acad Sci* 1989;565:126–136.
2. Serjeant GR. *Sickle cell disease*, 2nd revised ed. Oxford: Oxford University Press, 1992.
3. Ohene-Frempong K, Nkrumah FK. Sickle cell disease in Africa. In: Embury SH, Hebbel RP, Mohandas N, Steinberg MH, eds. *Sickle cell disease: basic principles and clinical practice*. 1994; New York: Raven Press Ltd.
4. Hickman M, Modell B, Greengross P, et al. Mapping the prevalence of sickle cell and beta thalassaemia in England: estimating and validating ethnic-specific rates. *Br J Haematol* 1999;104:860–867.
5. Davies SC, Oni L. The management of patients with sickle cell disease. *BMJ* 1997;315:656–660.
6. Effiong CE. Sickle cell disease in childhood. In: Fleming AF (Ed) Sickle cell disease: A handbook for general clinicians. Edinburgh: Churchill Livingstone, 1982: 57–72.
7. Overtuff GD, Powars D, Baraff LJ. Bacterial meningitis and septicemia in sickle cell disease. *Am J Dis Child* 1977;131:784–787.
8. Cohen AR, Norris CF, Smith-Whitley K. Transfusion therapy for sickle cell disease. In: Capon SM, Chambers LA, eds. *New directions in pediatric hematology*. Bethesda MD: American Association of Blood Banks, 1996:39–85.
9. Adams R, McKie V, Nichols F, et al. The use of transcranial Ultrasonography to predict stroke in sickle cell disease. *N Engl J Med* 1992;326(9):605–610.
10. Platt OS, Brambilla DJ, Rosse WF, et al. Mortality in sickle cell disease: life expectancy and risk factors for early death. *N Engl J Med* 1994;330:1639–1643.
11. Harmatz P, Butensky E, Quirolo K, et al. Severity of iron overload in patients with sickle cell disease receiving chronic red blood cell transfusion therapy. *Blood* 2000;96:76–79.
12. Riddington C, Owusu-Ofori S. Prophylactic antibiotics for preventing pneumococcal infection in children with sickle cell disease. In: The Cochrane Library, Issue 4, 2002. Oxford: Update Software. Search date 2001; primary sources Cochrane Cystic Fibrosis and Genetic Disorders Group specialised trials register on haemoglobinopathies and hand searches of bibliographic references of all retrived literature.

13. Gaston MH, Verter JI, Woods G, et al. Prophylaxis with oral penicillin in children with sickle cell anemia: a randomized trial. *N Engl J Med* 1986;314:1593–1599.
14. Falletta JM, Woods GM, Verter JI, et al. Discontinuing penicillin prophylaxis in children with sickle cell anemia. *J Pediatr* 1995;127:685–690.
15. Overturf GD. Pneumococcal vaccination in children. *Semin Pediatr Infect Dis* 2002;13:155–164.
16. Oniyangi O, Omari AAA. Malaria chemoprophylaxis in sickle cell disease (Cochrane Review). In: The Cochrane Library, Issue 3, 2003. Oxford: Update Software. Search date 2003; primary sources Cochrane Infectious Diseases Group trials register, Cochrane Central Register of Controlled Trials, Medline, Embase , Lilacs, plus hand searches of reference lists of articles and contact with individual researchers working in sickle cell disease research to identify any unpublished trials.
17. Chintu C, Gupta K, Osborne C, et al. Clinical trial of the protective role of polyvalent pneumococcal vaccine in sickle cell anaemia patients in Zambia. *Med J Zambia* 1983;17:73–76.
18. Rigau-Perez JG, Overtuff GD, Chan LS, et al. Reactions to booster pneumococcal vaccination in patients with sickle cell disease. *Pediatr Infect Dis* 1983;2:199–202.
19. Vernacchio L, Neufeld EJ, MacDonald K, et al. Combined schedule of 7-valent pneumococcal conjugate vaccine followed by 23-valent pneumococcal vaccine in children and young adults with sickle cell disease. *J Pediatr* 1998;133:275–278.
20. Pai VB, Heyman CA, Erramouspe J, et al. Conjugated heptavalent pneumococcal vaccine. *Ann Pharmacother* 2002;36:1403–1413.
21. Davies S, Olujohungbe A. Hydroxyurea for sickle cell disease. In: The Cochrane Library, Issue 4, 2002. Oxford: Update Software. Search date 2001; primary sources Cochrane Cystic Fibrosis and Genetic Disorders Group specialised trials register on haemoglobinopathies and hand searches of bibliographic references of all retrieved studies and reviews and personal contact with the pharmaceutical manufacturer.
22. Ferster A, Vermylen C, Cornu G, et al. Hydroxyurea for treatment of severe sickle cell anemia: a pediatric clinical trial. *Blood* 1996;88:1960–1964.
23. Charache S, Terrin M, Moore RD, et al. Effect of hydroxyurea on the frequency of painful crisis in sickle cell anemia. *N Engl J Med* 1995;332:1317–1322.
24. Riddington C, De Franceschi L. Drugs for preventing red blood cell dehydration in people with sickle cell disease (Cochrane Review). In: The Cochrane Library, Issue 3, 2003. Oxford: Update Software. Search date July 2003, primary sources Cochrane Cystic Fibrosis and Genetic Disorders Group trials register which comprises of references identified from comprehensive electronic database searches and handsearching of relevant journals and abstract books of conference proceedings.
25. Redwood AM, Williams EM, Desal P, et al. Climate and painful crisis of sickle-cell disease in Jamaica. *BMJ* 1976;1:66–68.
26. Mohan J, Marshall JM, Reid HL, et al. Peripheral vascular response to mild indirect cooling in patients with homozygous sickle cell (SS) disease and the frequency of painful crisis. *Clin Sci* 1998;94:111–120.
27. Perlin E, Finke H, Castro O, et al. Treatment of sickle cell pain crisis: a clinical trial of diflunisal (Dolobid). *Clin Trials J* 1988;25:254–264.
28. Grisham JE, Vichinsky EP. Ketorolac versus meperidine in vaso-occlusive crisis: a study of safety and efficacy. *Int J Pediatr Hematol Oncol* 1996;3:239–247.
29. Wright SW, Norris RL, Mitchell TR. Ketorolac for sickle cell vaso-occlusive crisis pain in the emergency department: lack of a narcotic-sparing effect. *Ann Emerg Med* 1992;21:925–928.
30. Perlin E, Finke H, Castro O, et al. Enhancement of pain control with ketorolac tromethamine in patients with sickle cell vaso-occlusive crisis. *Am J Hematol* 1994;46:43–47.
31. Hardwick WE, Givens TG, Monroe KW, et al. Effect of ketorolac in pediatric sickle cell vaso-occlusive pain crisis. *Pediatr Emerg Care* 1999;15:179–182.
32. Jacobson SJ, Kopecky EA, Joshi P, Babul N. Randomised trial of oral morphine for painful episodes of sickle-cell disease in children. *Lancet* 1997;350:1358–1361.
33. Perlin E, Finke H, Castro O, et al. Infusional/patient-controlled analgesia in sickle-cell vaso-occlusive crises. *Pain Clinic* 1993;6:113–119.
34. Gonzalez ER, Bahal N, Hansen LA, et al. Intermittent injection vs patient-controlled analgesia for sickle cell crises pain: comparison in patients in the emergency department. *Arch Intern Med* 1991;151:1373–1378.
35. Hagmeyer KO, Mauro LS, Mauro VF. Meperidine-related seizures associated with patient-controlled analgesia pumps. *Annals of Pharmacotherapy* 1993;27:29–33.
36. Shapiro BS, Ballas SK. The acute painful episode. In: Embury SH, Hebbel RP, Mohandas N, Steinberg MH, eds. *Sickle cell disease: principles and clinical practice*. New York: Raven Press Ltd.
37. Robieux IC, Kellner JD, Coppes MJ, et al. Analgesia in children with sickle cell crisis: comparison of intermittent opioids vs. continuous intravenous infusion of morphine and placebo-controlled study of oxygen inhalation. *Pediatr Hematol Oncol* 1992;9:317–326.
38. Zipursky A, Robieux IC, Brown EJ, et al. Oxygen therapy in sickle cell disease. *Am J Pediatr Hematol Oncol* 1992;14:222–228.
39. Griffin TC, McIntire D, Buchanan GR. High-dose intravenous methylprednisolone therapy for pain in children and adolescents with sickle cell disease. *N Engl J Med* 1994;330:733–737.
40. Bernini JC, Rogers ZR, Sandler ES, et al. Beneficial effect of intravenous dexamethasone in children with mild to moderately severe acute chest syndrome complicating sickle cell disease. *Blood* 1998;92:3082–3089.
41. Suraseranivongse S, Santawat U, Kraiprasit K, et al. Cross-validation of a composite pain scale for preschool children within 24 hours of surgery. *Br J Anaesth* 2001;87:400–405 [link: http://bja.oupjournals.org/cgi/content/full/87/3/400]
42. American Academy of Pediatrics. Technical report: Prevention of pneumococcal infections, including the use of pneumococcal conjugate and polysaccharide vaccines and antibiotics prophylaxis. *Pediatrics* 2000;106;(Pt 1/3):367–376.

Martin Meremikwu
Dr
Department of Paediatrics College of Medical Sciences University of Calabar
Calabar
Nigeria

Competing interests: None declared.

Acute myocardial infarction

Search date October 2003

Nicolas Danchin, Edoardo De Benedetti, and Philip Urban

QUESTIONS

INTERVENTIONS

See glossary G

Key Messages

Improving outcomes in acute myocardial infarction

- **Angiotensin converting enzyme inhibitors** One systematic review in people treated within 14 days of acute myocardial infarction has found that angiotensin converting enzyme inhibitors reduce mortality after 6 weeks compared with placebo. However, a non-systematic review found that angiotensin converting enzyme inhibitors increase persistent hypotension and renal dysfunction at 6 weeks compared with placebo.
- **Aspirin** One systematic review in people with acute myocardial infarction has found that aspirin reduces mortality, reinfarction, and stroke at 1 month compared with placebo.

Acute myocardial infarction

- **β Blockers** Two systematic reviews and one subsequent RCT found that β blockers reduced mortality compared with no β blockers. One RCT in people receiving thrombolytic treatment found that immediate treatment with metoprolol reduced rates of reinfarction and chest pain at 6 days compared with delayed treatment, but had no significant effect on mortality at 6 days or at 1 year.
- **Primary percutaneous transluminal coronary angioplasty versus thrombolysis (performed in specialist centres)** One systematic review found that primary percutaneous transluminal coronary angioplasty reduced a combined outcome of death, non-fatal reinfarction, and stroke compared with thrombolysis.
- **Thrombolysis** One non-systematic review in people with acute myocardial infarction and ST segment elevation or bundle branch block on their initial electrocardiogram found that prompt thrombolytic treatment (within 6 hours and perhaps up to 12 hours and longer after the onset of symptoms) reduced mortality compared with placebo. RCTs comparing different types of thrombolytic agents versus each other found no significant difference in mortality. One non-systematic review found that thrombolytic treatment increased the risk of stroke or major bleeding compared with control. The review also found that intracranial haemorrhage was more common in people of advanced age and low body weight, those with hypertension on admission, and those given tissue plasminogen activator rather than another thrombolytic agent. One non-systematic review found conflicting results for intracerebral haemorrhage with bolus treatment compared with infusion of thrombolytic agents. One systematic review found that thrombolysis was less effective at reducing a combined outcome of death, non-fatal reinfarction, and stroke compared with primary percutaneous transluminal coronary angioplasty.
- **Adding low molecular weight heparin (enoxaparin) to thrombolytics (reduces acute myocardial infarction rates)** One RCT found that adding enoxaparin (a low molecular weight heparin) to streptokinase reduced acute myocardial infarction rates compared with adding placebo in people with early evidence of a developing infarction. One systematic review identified five RCTs comparing enoxaparin (a low molecular weight heparin) plus thrombolytic treatment versus unfractionated heparin plus thrombolytic treatment. Two of the RCTs identified by the review found that enoxaparin plus thrombolytics reduced acute myocardial infarction rates compared with unfractionated heparin plus thrombolytics, while three RCTs found no significant difference between treatments. The review found no significant difference in mortality between enoxaparin and unfractionated heparin when added to thrombolytic treatment and no significant difference between added enoxaparin and added unfractionated heparin in the risk of intracranial or other major bleeding.
- **Nitrates (in the absence of thrombolysis)** One systematic review of the trials conducted in the prethrombolytic era found that nitrates reduced mortality in people with acute myocardial infarction compared with placebo.
- **Glycoprotein IIb/IIIa inhibitors** Two large RCTs found that combined treatment with half dose thrombolysis plus abciximab did not reduce mortality at 1 month in people with acute myocardial infarction compared with full dose thrombolysis, but found limited evidence that combined treatment reduced non-fatal cardiovascular events. However, the RCTs found that combined treatment with abciximab increased bleeding complications, particularly extracranial haemorrhage. Three RCTs found conflicting evidence about the benefits of adding abciximab to primary coronary angioplasty or stenting in people with acute myocardial infarction, although all found that adding abciximab increased bleeding risk. One RCT found no difference in survival or morbidity outcomes between early or late tirofiban administration in people undergoing primary coronary angioplasty. It also found no difference in minor or major bleeding complications between early and late tirofiban administration, although the study may have been too small to detect clinically important differences.
- **Adding unfractionated heparin to thrombolytics** Two RCTs found no significant difference in mortality or acute myocardial infarction rates between unfractionated heparin plus thrombolytics and thrombolytics alone. One systematic review identified five RCTs comparing enoxaparin (a low molecular weight heparin) plus thrombolytic treatment versus unfractionated heparin plus thrombolytic treatment. Two of

the RCTs identified by the review found that enoxaparin plus thrombolytics reduced acute myocardial infarction rates compared with unfractionated heparin plus thrombolytics, while three RCTs found no significant difference between treatments. The review found no significant difference in mortality between enoxaparin and unfractionated heparin when added to thrombolytic treatment. The systematic review found no significant difference between added enoxaparin and added unfractionated heparin in the risk of intracranial or other major bleeding.

- **Nitrates (in addition to thrombolysis)** Two RCTs in people with acute myocardial infarction (after thrombolysis was introduced) found no significant difference in mortality between nitrates and placebo.
- **Calcium channel blockers** We found evidence that neither dihydropyridines nor verapamil reduce mortality compared with placebo. One RCT found limited evidence that, in people with left ventricular dysfunction, nifedipine given in the first few days after myocardial infarction may increase mortality compared with placebo.

Treating cardiogenic shock after acute myocardial infarction

- **Early invasive cardiac revascularisation** One large RCT found that early invasive cardiac revascularisation reduced mortality after 6 and 12 months compared with medical treatment alone in people with cardiogenic shock within 48 hours of acute myocardial infarction. A second, smaller RCT found similar results, although the difference was not significant.
- **Intra-aortic balloon counterpulsation** An RCT presented only in abstract form found limited evidence of no significant difference in mortality at 6 months between intra-aortic balloon counterpulsation plus thrombolysis versus thrombolysis alone in people with cardiogenic shock.
- **Early cardiac surgery; positive inotropes; vasodilators; pulmonary artery catheterisation; ventricular assistance devices and cardiac transplantation** We found no evidence from RCTs about the effects of these interventions.
- **Thrombolysis** Subgroup analysis of one RCT found no significant difference in mortality after 21 days between thrombolysis and no thrombolysis in people with cardiogenic shock.

DEFINITION **Acute myocardial infarction (AMI):** The sudden occlusion of a coronary artery leading to myocardial cell death. **Cardiogenic shock:** Defined clinically as a poor cardiac output plus evidence of tissue hypoxia that is not improved by correcting reduced intravascular volume.[1] When a pulmonary artery catheter is used, cardiogenic shock may be defined as a cardiac index**G** below 2.2 L/minute/m^2 despite an elevated pulmonary capillary wedge pressure (≥ 15 mm Hg).[1–3]

INCIDENCE/ PREVALENCE **AMI:** Acute myocardial infarction is one of the most common causes of mortality worldwide. In 1990, ischaemic heart disease was the world's leading cause of death, accounting for about 6.3 million deaths. The age standardised incidence varies among and within countries.[4] Each year, about 900 000 people in the USA experience AMI, about 225 000 of whom die. About half of these people die within 1 hour of symptoms and before reaching a hospital emergency room.[5] Event rates increase with age for both sexes and are higher in men than in women and in poorer than richer people at all ages. The incidence of death from AMI has fallen in many Western countries over the past 20 years. **Cardiogenic shock:** Cardiogenic shock occurs in about 7% of people admitted to hospital with AMI.[6] Of these, about half have established cardiogenic shock at the time of admission to hospital, and most of the others develop it during the first 24–48 hours after their admission.[7]

AETIOLOGY/ RISK FACTORS **AMI:** The immediate mechanism of AMI is rupture or erosion of an atheromatous plaque causing thrombosis and occlusion of coronary arteries and myocardial cell death. Factors that may convert a stable plaque into an unstable plaque (the "active plaque") have yet to be fully elucidated. Shear stresses, inflammation, and autoimmunity have been proposed. The changing rates of coronary heart disease in different populations are only partly explained by changes in the standard risk factors for ischaemic heart disease (particularly a fall in blood pressure and smoking). **Cardiogenic shock:** Cardiogenic shock after AMI usually follows a reduction in functional ventricular myocardium, and is caused by left ventricular infarction (79% of people with cardiogenic shock) more often than by right ventricular infarction (3% of people with cardiogenic shock).[8] Cardiogenic shock after AMI may also be caused by cardiac structural defects, such as mitral valve regurgitation due to papillary muscle dysfunction (7% of people with cardiogenic shock), ventricular septal rupture (4% of people with cardiogenic shock), or cardiac tamponade after free cardiac wall rupture (1% of people with cardiogenic shock). Major risk factors for cardiogenic shock after AMI are previous myocardial infarction, diabetes mellitus, advanced age, hypotension, tachycardia or bradycardia, congestive heart failure with Killip class II–III**G**, and low left ventricular ejection fraction (ejection fraction < 35%).[7,8]

PROGNOSIS **AMI:** May lead to a host of mechanical and cardiac electrical complications, including death, ventricular dysfunction, congestive heart failure, fatal and non-fatal arrhythmias, valvular dysfunction, myocardial rupture, and cardiogenic shock. **Cardiogenic shock:** Mortality rates for people in hospital with cardiogenic shock after AMI vary between 50–80%.[2,3,6,7] Most deaths occur within 48 hours of the onset of shock (see figure 1, p 59). People surviving until discharge from hospital have a reasonable long term prognosis (88% survival at 1 year).[10]

AIMS OF INTERVENTION To relieve pain; to restore blood supply to heart muscle; to reduce incidence of complications (such as congestive heart failure, myocardial rupture, valvular dysfunction, and fatal and non-fatal arrhythmia); to prevent recurrent ischaemia and infarction; to decrease mortality, with minimal adverse effects of treatments.

OUTCOMES **Efficacy outcomes:** Rates of major cardiovascular events, including death, recurrent acute myocardial infarction, refractory ischaemia, and stroke. **Safety outcomes:** Rates of major bleeding and intracranial haemorrhage.

METHODS *Clinical Evidence* search and appraisal October 2003.

QUESTION Which treatments improve outcomes in acute myocardial infarction?

Nicolas Danchin

OPTION ASPIRIN

One systematic review in people with acute myocardial infarction has found that aspirin reduces mortality, reinfarction, and stroke at 1 month compared with placebo.

Benefits: **Versus placebo:** We found one systematic review (search date 1990, 9 RCTs, 18 773 people), which compared antiplatelet agents begun soon after the onset of acute myocardial infarction (AMI) and for at least 1 month afterwards versus placebo.[11] Almost all (> 95%) of the people in these studies were randomised to either aspirin or placebo. The absolute and relative benefits found in the systematic review are shown in figure 2, p 60. The largest of the RCTs identified by the review (17 187 people with suspected AMI) compared aspirin 162.6 mg versus placebo chewed and swallowed on the day of AMI and continued daily for 1 month.[12] There was a 2.4% absolute reduction in vascular death at 35 days. The survival benefit was maintained for up to 4 years.[13] In the systematic review, the most widely tested aspirin regimens were 75–325 mg daily.[11] Doses throughout this range seemed similarly effective, with no evidence that "higher" doses were more effective (500–1500 mg/day aspirin *v* placebo; OR for all vascular events 21%, 95% CI 14% to 27%) than "medium" doses (160–325 mg/day aspirin *v* placebo; OR for all vascular events 28%, 95% CI 22% to 33%), or "lower" doses (75–160 mg/day aspirin *v* placebo; OR 26%, 95% CI 5% to 42%). The review found insufficient evidence for efficacy of doses below 75 mg daily. One RCT identified by the review found that a loading dose of 160–325 mg daily achieved a prompt antiplatelet effect.[14]

Harms: The largest RCT identified by the review found no significant difference between aspirin and placebo in rates of cerebral haemorrhage or bleeds requiring transfusion (AR: 0.4% with aspirin and placebo).[12] It also found a small absolute excess of "minor" bleeding (ARI 0.6%, CI not reported; $P < 0.01$).

Comment: None.

OPTION THROMBOLYSIS

One non-systematic review of large RCTs in people with acute myocardial infarction and ST segment elevation or bundle branch block on their initial electrocardiogram found that prompt thrombolytic treatment (within 6 hours and perhaps up to 12 hours and longer after the onset of symptoms) reduced mortality compared with placebo. RCTs comparing different types of thrombolytic agents with each other found no significant difference in mortality. One non-systematic review found that thrombolytic treatment increased the risk of stroke or major bleeding compared with control. The review also found that intracranial haemorrhage was more common in people of advanced age and low body weight, those with hypertension on admission, and those given tissue plasminogen activator rather than another thrombolytic agent. One non-systematic review found conflicting results for intracerebral haemorrhage with bolus treatment compared with infusion of thrombolytic agents. One systematic review found that thrombolysis was less effective at reducing a combined outcome of death, non-fatal reinfarction, and stroke compared with primary percutaneous transluminal coronary angioplasty.

Benefits: **Versus placebo:** We found one non-systematic review of high quality RCTs (9 RCTs, 58 600 people with suspected acute myocardial infarction [AMI]) comparing thrombolysis versus placebo.[15] Baseline electrocardiograms showed ST segment elevation in 68% of people and ST segment depression, T wave abnormalities, or no abnormality in the rest. The review found that thrombolysis significantly reduced short term mortality compared with placebo (9.6% with thrombolysis *v* 11.5% with placebo; RR 0.82, 95% CI 0.77 to 0.87). The greatest benefit was found in the large subgroup of people presenting with ST elevation (RR 0.79, CI not reported) or bundle branch block (RR 0.75, CI not reported). Reduced death rates were seen in people with all types of infarction, but the benefit was several times greater in those with anterior infarction (ARR 3.7%) compared with those with inferior infarction (ARR 0.8%) or infarctions in other zones (ARR 2.7%). One of the RCTs included in the overview found that thrombolysis significantly reduced mortality after 12 years compared with placebo (36/107 [34%] died with thrombolysis *v* 55/112 [49%] with placebo; ARR 15.0%, 95% CI 2.4% to 29.0%; RR 0.69, 95% CI 0.49 to 0.95; NNT 7, 95% CI 4 to 41).[16] **Timing of treatment:** The non-systematic review found that the earlier thrombolytic treatment was given after the onset of symptoms, the greater the absolute benefit of treatment (see figure 3, p 61).[15] For each hour of delay in thrombolytic treatment, the absolute risk reduction for death decreased by 0.16% (ARR for death if given within 6 hours of symptoms 3%; ARR for death if given 7–12 hours after onset of symptoms 2%).[15] Too few people in the review received treatment more than 12 hours after the onset of symptoms to determine whether the benefits of thrombolytic treatment given after 12 hours would outweigh the risks (see comment below). **Streptokinase versus tissue plasminogen activator (tPA):** We found one non-systematic review,[17] which found three RCTs[18–20] (see table 1, p 56) comparing streptokinase versus tPA. The first RCT, in people with ST segment elevation and symptoms of AMI for less than 6 hours, was unblinded.[18] People were first randomised to intravenous tPA 100 mg over 3 hours or streptokinase 1.5 MU over 1 hour and then further randomised to subcutaneous heparin 12 500 U twice daily beginning 12 hours later, or no heparin. There was no significant difference in mortality between tPA 100 mg and streptokinase (9.0% with tPA 100 mg *v* 8.6% with streptokinase; RR 1.05, 95% CI 0.95 to 1.16). In the second RCT, people with suspected AMI presenting within 24 hours of symptoms were first randomised to receive either streptokinase 1.5 MU over 1 hour, tPA 0.6 MU/kg every 4 hours, or anisoylated plasminogen streptokinase activator complex 30 U every 3 minutes, and then further randomised to subcutaneous heparin 12 500 U starting at 7 hours and continued for 7 days, or no heparin.[19] All people received aspirin on admission. The RCT found no significant difference between thrombolytic agents in mortality (AR of death: 10.6% with streptokinase *v* 10.5% with anisoylated plasminogen streptokinase activator complex *v* 10.3% with tPA). The third RCT was unblinded and included people with ST segment elevation presenting within 6 hours of symptom onset.[20] People were randomised to one of four regimens: streptokinase 1.5 MU over 1 hour plus subcutaneous heparin 12 500 U twice daily starting 4 hours after thrombolytic treatment; streptokinase 1.5 MU over 1 hour plus intravenous heparin 5000 U bolus followed by 1000 U every hour; accelerated tPA 15 mg bolus then 0.75 mg/kg over 30 minutes followed by 0.50 mg/kg over 60 minutes, plus intravenous heparin 5000 U bolus then 1000 U every hour; or tPA 1.0 mg/kg over 60 minutes, 10% given as a bolus, plus streptokinase 1.0 MU over 60 minutes.[20] Meta-analysis of the three trials, weighted by sample size, found no significant difference between treatments in the combined outcome of any stroke or death (AR 9.4% for streptokinase only regimens *v* 9.2% for tPA based regimens, including the combined tPA and streptokinase arm in the third trial; ARR for tPA *v* streptokinase +0.2%, 95% CI –0.2% to +0.5%).[17]

tPA versus other thrombolytics: We found two RCTs that compared tPA versus other thrombolytic agents in people with AMI (participants also received aspirin and heparin).[21,22] The first RCT (15 059 people from 20 different countries with AMI evolving for < 6 hours, with ST segment elevation or with the appearance of a new left bundle branch block on their electrocardiogram) compared tPA (accelerated iv administration according to the study regimen) versus reteplase (recombinant plasminogen activator; two 10 MU iv boluses, 30 minutes apart).[21] It found no significant difference in mortality after 30 days (OR 1.03, 95% CI 0.91 to 1.18). The second RCT (16 949 people; see comment below) compared tPA (accelerated iv administration) versus tenecteplase (a genetically engineered variant of tPA; 30–50 mg iv according to body weight as a single bolus).[22] It found no significant difference between treatments in total mortality after 30 days (6% with tenecteplase *v* 6% with tPA; RR 1.0, 95% CI 0.91 to 1.10).

Harms: **Stroke/intracerebral haemorrhage:** The overview found that thrombolytic treatment significantly increased the risk of stroke compared with control (ARI 0.4%, 95% CI 0.2% to 0.5%; NNH 250, 95% CI 200 to 500).[15] In the third RCT comparing streptokinase versus tPA, the overall incidence of stroke was 0.7%, of which 31% were severely disabling and 50% were intracerebral haemorrhages.[20] The RCT also found that tPA significantly increased the risk of haemorrhagic stroke compared with streptokinase plus subcutaneous heparin or streptokinase plus intravenous heparin (AR for combined streptokinase arms 0.52% *v* 0.72% with tPA; P = 0.03 for tPA compared with combined streptokinase arms). The RCT comparing reteplase versus tPA found that the incidence of stroke was similar with both treatments, and the odds ratio for the incidence of death or disabling stroke was 1.0.[21] The RCT comparing tenecteplase versus tPA found no significant difference between treatments in the rate of stroke or death (7% with tenecteplase *v* 7% with tPA; RR 1.01, 95% CI 0.91 to 1.13).[22] We found one non-systematic review that compared bolus thrombolytic treatment versus infusion treatment.[23] Meta-analysis of nine small phase II trials (3956 people) found no significant difference between bolus and standard infusion thrombolysis for intracerebral haemorrhage (bolus *v* infusion: OR 0.53, 95% CI 0.27 to 1.01). However, meta-analysis of six larger phase III trials (62 673 people) found that bolus treatment significantly increased the risk of intracerebral haemorrhage (OR 1.25, 95% CI 1.06 to 1.49). **Predictive factors for stroke/intracranial haemorrhage:** Multivariate analysis of data from a large database of people who experienced intracerebral haemorrhage after thrombolytic treatment identified four independent predictors of increased risk of intracerebral haemorrhage: age 65 years or older (OR 2.2, 95% CI 1.4 to 3.5); weight less than 70 kg (OR 2.1, 95% CI 1.3 to 3.2); hypertension on admission (OR 2.0, 95% CI 1.2 to 3.2); and use of tPA rather than another thrombolytic agent (OR 1.6, 95% CI 1.0 to 2.5).[21] Absolute risk of intracranial haemorrhage was 0.26% on streptokinase in the absence of risk factors and 0.96%, 1.32%, and 2.17% in people with one, two, and three risk factors, respectively.[24] Analysis of 592 strokes in 41 021 people from the trials found seven factors to be predictors of intracerebral haemorrhage: advanced age, lower weight, history of cerebrovascular disease, history of hypertension, higher systolic or diastolic pressure on presentation, and use of tPA rather than streptokinase.[25,26] **Major bleeding:** The overview also found that thrombolytic treatment significantly increased the risk of major bleeding compared with placebo (ARI 0.7%, 95% CI 0.6% to 0.9%; NNH 143, 95% CI 111 to 166).[15] Bleeding was most common in people undergoing procedures (coronary artery bypass grafting or percutaneous transluminal coronary angioplasty). Spontaneous bleeds were observed most often in the gastrointestinal tract.[20]

Comment: Extrapolation of the data from the overview (see figure 3, p 61) suggests that, at least for people suspected of having an AMI and with ST segment elevation on their electrocardiogram, there may be some net benefit of treatment between 12–18 hours after symptom onset (ARR for death 1%).[15] The evidence from the RCT comparing reteplase versus tPA is consistent with a similar efficacy for both treatments, although formal equivalence cannot be established because the trial was designed as a superiority trial.[21] The evidence suggests that it is far more important to give prompt thrombolytic treatment than to debate which thrombolytic agent should be used. A strategy of rapid thrombolysis in a broad population is likely to lead to the greatest impact on mortality. When the results of RCTs are taken together, tPA based regimens do not seem to confer a significant advantage over streptokinase in the combined outcome of any stroke and death (unrelated to stroke). The legitimacy of combining the results of the three trials can be questioned, as the selection criteria and protocols differed in important aspects (see review for arguments to justify combining the results of these trials despite their apparent differences).[17]

OPTION ADDING ANTICOAGULANTS TO THROMBOLYTICS

Two RCTs found no significant difference in mortality or acute myocardial infarction rates between unfractionated heparin plus thrombolytics and thrombolytics alone in people with early evidence of a developing infarction. One RCT found that adding enoxaparin (a low molecular weight heparin) to streptokinase reduced acute myocardial infarction rates compared with adding placebo. One systematic review identified five RCTs comparing adding enoxaparin (a low molecular weight heparin) to thrombolytic treatment versus adding unfractionated heparin to thrombolytic treatment. Two of the RCTs identified by the review found that enoxaparin plus thrombolytics reduced acute myocardial infarction rates compared with unfractionated heparin plus thrombolytics, while three RCTs found no significant difference between treatments. The review found no significant difference in mortality between

enoxaparin and unfractionated heparin when added to thrombolytic treatment and no significant difference between added enoxaparin and added unfractionated heparin in the risk of intracranial or other major bleeding.

Benefits: **Versus thrombolytics alone:** We found three RCTs.[18,19,27] The first RCT (20 768 people with ST segment elevation and symptoms of acute myocardial infarction [AMI] for < 6 hours) was unblinded and compared streptokinase versus tissue plasminogen activator (tPA) with or without heparin.[18] People were first randomised to intravenous tPA 100 mg over 3 hours or streptokinase 1.5 MU over 1 hour and then further randomised to subcutaneous heparin 12 500 U twice daily beginning 12 hours later, or no heparin. It found no significant difference in mortality or AMI rate between thrombolytic plus heparin compared with thrombolytic alone (AR of death in hospital 8.5% with thrombolytic plus heparin *v* 8.9% with thrombolytic alone; RR 0.95, 95% CI 0.86 to 1.04; AR of AMI 1.9% with thrombolytic plus heparin *v* 2.3% with thrombolytic alone; P reported as not significant). In the second RCT (about 27 000 people), people with suspected AMI presenting within 24 hours of symptoms were first randomised to receive either streptokinase 1.5 MU over 1 hour, tPA 0.6 MU/kg every 4 hours, or anisoylated plasminogen streptokinase activator complex 30 U every 3 minutes, and then further randomised to subcutaneous heparin 12 500 U starting at 7 hours and continued for 7 days, or no heparin.[19] All participants received aspirin on admission. The RCT found no significant difference in mortality or AMI rate between thrombolytic plus heparin and thrombolytic alone (AR of death within 35 days: 10.3% with thrombolytic plus heparin *v* 10.6% with thrombolytic alone, P reported as not significant; AR of AMI: 3.16% with thrombolytic plus heparin *v* 3.47% with thrombolytic alone, P = 0.09). The third RCT (496 people) compared streptokinase (1.5 MU over 1 hour) plus enoxaparin (a low molecular weight heparin; 30 mg iv bolus then subcutaneously every 12 hours) versus streptokinase plus placebo.[27] It found that streptokinase plus enoxaparin significantly reduced AMI rates compared with streptokinase plus placebo after 30 days, although it found no significant difference in mortality rates between treatments (AR of AMI: 6/253 [2.4%] with enoxaparin *v* 18/243 [7.4%] with placebo; OR 0.30, 95% CI 0.12 to 0.78; AR of death: 17/253 [6.7%] with enoxaparin *v* 17/243 [7.0%] with placebo; OR 0.96, 95% CI 0.48 to 1.92). Thrombolytics plus low molecular weight heparins versus thrombolytics plus unfractionated heparins: We found one systematic review (search date 2002; 5 RCTs, 5757 people) comparing thrombolytics plus enoxaparin (a low molecular weight heparin) or plus unfractionated heparin (see comment below).[28] Adjunctive thrombolytic treatment was tPA in one RCT, tenecteplase in two RCTs, streptokinase in one RCT, and either streptokinase, anistreptase, or tPA in one RCT. The first RCT (312 people) identified by the review found no significant difference between added enoxaparin and added heparin in mortality rates or combined mortality and AMI rates after 30 days (AR for death: 13/154 [8.4%] with added heparin *v* 11/158 [7.0%] with added enoxaparin; OR 0.86, 95% CI 0.36 to 1.98; AR for death or AMI: 23/154 [14.9%] with unfractionated heparin *v* 15/158 [9.5%] with enoxaparin; OR 0.63, 95% CI 0.32 to 1.23). The second RCT identified by the review[28] (6095 people treated within 6 hours of ST segment elevation AMI) compared three treatments: full dose tenecteplase (30–50 mg according to body weight) plus unfractionated heparin (60 U/kg bolus plus 12 U/kg/hour); full dose tenecteplase plus enoxaparin (30 mg immediately then 1 mg/kg every 12 hours); or half dose tenecteplase plus full dose abciximab (0.25 mg/kg bolus plus 0.125 μg/kg/minute for 12 hours).[29] It found that added enoxaparin significantly reduced AMI rates compared with added unfractionated heparin plus tenecteplase after 30 days, although mortality rates were similar between treatments (AR for AMI: 86/2038

[4.2%] with added heparin *v* 54/2040 [2.7%] with added enoxaparin; OR 0.62, 95% CI 0.44 to 0.87; AR for death: 122/2038 [6.0%] with added heparin *v* 109/2040 [5.4%] with added enoxaparin; OR 0.89, 95% CI 0.68 to 1.16).[28] The third RCT identified by the review[28] (300 people) compared thrombolytics (streptokinase anistreptase or t-PA; see comment below) plus enoxaparin or heparin. It found no significant difference between added enoxaparin and added heparin in mortality rates or AMI rates after 90 days (AR for death: 16/151 [10.6%] with unfractionated heparin *v* 9/149 [6.0%] with enoxaparin; OR 0.54, 95% CI 0.23 to 1.27; AR for AMI: 30/151 [19.9%] with unfractionated heparin *v* 22/149 [14.8%] with enoxaparin; OR 0.70, 95% CI 0.38 to 1.28). The fourth RCT (483 people) identified by the review[28] compared enoxaparin versus heparin when added to either full dose tenecteplase (0.53 mg/kg) or half dose tenecteplase plus full dose abciximab (0.25 mg/kg bolus plus 0.125 µg/kg/minute for 12 hours).[30] It found that added enoxaparin significantly reduced AMI rates compared with added heparin after 30 days, although mortality rates were similar between treatments (see comment below; AR for AMI: 6/324 [1.9%] with enoxaparin *v* 12/159 [7.5%] with unfractionated heparin; OR 0.23, 95% CI 0.09 to 0.63; AR for death: 10/324 [3.1%] with enoxaparin *v* 5/159 [3.1%] with unfractionated heparin; OR 0.98, 95% CI 0.33 to 2.92). The fifth RCT identified by the review[28] (400 people) found no significant difference between tPA plus enoxaparin and tPA plus unfractionated heparin in mortality rates or AMI rates (AR for death: 10/200 [5.0%] with unfractionated heparin *v* 9/200 [4.5%] with enoxaparin; OR 0.90, 95% CI 0.36 to 2.5; AR for AMI: 8/200 [4%] with unfractionated heparin *v* 8/200 [4%] with enoxaparin; OR 1.0, 95% CI 0.37 to 2.72).

Harms: **Thrombolytics plus low molecular weight heparins versus thrombolytics plus unfractionated heparins:** The systematic review comparing enoxaparin plus thrombolytic treatment versus unfractionated heparin plus thrombolytic treatment found no significant difference in the risk of intracranial bleeding between treatments (5 RCTs; OR 1.0, 95% CI not reported; P = 0.99).[28] It found no significant difference in the risk of major bleeding between treatments (5 RCTs; OR 1.34, 95% CI 0.97 to 1.87).[28]

Comment: **Thrombolytics plus low molecular weight heparins versus thrombolytics plus unfractionated heparins:** There were methodological problems with the systematic review comparing enoxaparin plus thrombolytic treatment versus unfractionated heparin plus thrombolytic treatment.[28] Firstly, the review presented meta-analytic results for six RCTs, including a comparison of thrombolytic plus enoxaparin versus thrombolytic plus placebo, resulting in an unreliable comparison of enoxaparin versus unfractionated heparin. We have, therefore, presented the results for each relevant RCT separately. Secondly, in the third RCT identified by the review,[28] 66% of people had received streptokinase, 28% had received anistreptase, and 6% had received tPA, although treatment groups were balanced at baseline. Finally, in the presentation of the results for the fourth RCT, the systematic review pooled results that included a comparison of heparins added to tenecteplase alone and to tenecteplase plus abciximab. The results, therefore, do not strictly reflect the comparison of enoxaparin versus heparin added to a "pure" thrombolytic regimen.

OPTION GLYCOPROTEIN IIB/IIIA INHIBITORS

Two large RCTs found that combined treatment with half dose thrombolysis plus abciximab did not reduce mortality at 1 month in people with acute myocardial infarction compared with full dose thrombolysis, but found limited

evidence that the combined treatment reduced non-fatal cardiovascular events. However, the RCTs found that combined treatment with abciximab increased bleeding complications, particularly extracranial haemorrhage. Three RCTs found conflicting evidence about the benefits of adding abciximab to primary coronary angioplasty or stenting in people with acute myocardial infarction, although all found that adding abciximab increased bleeding risk. One RCT found no difference in survival or morbidity outcomes between early and late tirofiban administration in people undergoing primary coronary angioplasty. It also found no difference in minor or major bleeding complications between early or late tirofiban administration, although the study may have been too small to detect clinically important differences.

Benefits: **Added to thrombolytic:** We found two RCTs.[29,31] The first RCT (16 588 people treated within 6 hours of ST segment elevation myocardial infarction; unblinded design) compared half dose reteplase plus abciximab (0.25 mg/kg bolus plus 0.125 μg/kg/minute for 12 hours) versus standard dose reteplase (total dose 20 U).[31] It found no significant difference in all cause mortality or stroke at 30 days between combined treatment and standard dose reteplase alone (mortality: AR 5.9% for reteplase alone *v* 5.6% for combined treatment; OR 0.95, 95% CI 0.83 to 1.08; any stroke: AR 0.9% for reteplase *v* 1.0% for combined treatment; OR 1.10, 95% CI 0.80 to 1.51). It found that combined treatment reduced the composite end point of mortality or non-fatal reinfarction at 30 days (AR 8.8% for thrombolysis alone *v* 7.4% for combined treatment; OR 0.83, 95% CI 0.74 to 0.93). At 1 year, there was no significant difference in mortality between combination treatment and standard dose reteplase (692/8260 [8.4%] with standard reteplase *v* 698/8328 [8.4%] with combined therapy; HR 1.00, 95% CI 0.90 to 1.11).[32] The second RCT (6095 people treated within 6 hours of ST segment elevation myocardial infarction; unblinded design) compared three treatments: full dose tenecteplase (30–50 mg according to body weight) plus unfractionated heparin (60 U/kg bolus plus 12 U/kg/hour); full dose tenecteplase plus enoxaparin (30 mg immediately then 1 mg/kg every 12 hours); or half dose tenecteplase plus full dose abciximab (0.25 mg/kg bolus plus 0.125 μg/kg/minute for 12 hours).[28] It found no significant difference among groups in mortality at 30 days (AR 6.0% with unfractionated heparin *v* 5.4% with enoxaparin *v* 6.6% with abciximab; P = 0.25). It found that added abciximab increased composite risk of death, non-fatal cardiovascular events, or haemorrhage at 30 days compared with added enoxaparin but reduced risk compared with added unfractionated heparin (AR 13.8% with enoxaparin, 14.2% with abciximab, and 17.0% with unfractionated heparin). **Primary percutaneous transluminal coronary angioplasty with or without glycoprotein IIb/IIIa inhibitors:** We found four RCTs.[33–36] The first RCT (483 people with ST segment elevation myocardial infarction in the past 12 hours referred for primary angioplasty) compared abciximab (bolus + 12 hour infusion) versus placebo, given before the procedure. It found no significant difference between abciximab and placebo in the composite end point of death, reinfarction, or need for revascularisation of the target vessel at 6 months (AR 28% in both groups; OR 1.01, 95% CI 0.68 to 1.50; P = 0.90).[33] The second RCT (300 people with acute myocardial infarction [AMI] in the past 12 hours referred for primary coronary angioplasty) found that abciximab significantly reduced the composite end point of death, reinfarction, or urgent revascularisation of the target vessel at 30 days compared with placebo (AR 6.0% with abciximab *v* 14.6% with placebo; RR 0.41, 95% CI 0.18 to 0.93).[34] The third RCT (2082 people with AMI) compared percutaneous transluminal coronary angioplasty with or without stenting and with or without abciximab given during the procedure (2 x 2 unblinded factorial design).[35] At 6 months, it found that adding abciximab to angioplasty or stenting significantly reduced the risk of the composite end point of death, reinfarction, disabling stroke, or ischaemia driven revascularisation of the target vessel compared with either procedure alone (AR 20.0% after angioplasty alone *v* 16.5% after angioplasty plus abciximab; CI and P values not reported; AR 11.5% after stenting alone *v* 10.2% after stenting plus abciximab; CI and P values not reported). The fourth RCT (100 people with AMI in the past 12 hours referred for primary coronary angioplasty) compared tirofiban administered in the emergency room (early administration) versus tirofiban administered in the catheterisation laboratory after diagnostic angiography (late administration).[36] It found no significant difference between early or late tirofiban administration in death, reinfarction, or rehospitalisation, although the study may have been too small to detect clinically significant differences (death rate: 2% with early *v* 2% with late; recurrent myocardial infarction: 0% with early *v* 2% with late; rehospitalisation: 4% with early *v* 6% with late; P > 0.05 for each outcome).

Harms: **Glycoprotein IIb/IIIa inhibitors plus thrombolysis versus thrombolysis alone:** The first RCT found that abciximab plus half dose thrombolysis significantly increased severe or moderate extracranial bleeding at 30 days compared with full dose thrombolysis (AR 4.6% with combined treatment *v* 2.3% with full dose thrombolysis; OR 2.03, 95% CI 1.70 to 2.42).[31] However, it found no significant difference in rates of intracranial haemorrhage (AR 1.0% with combined treatment *v* 0.9% with thrombolysis alone; OR 1.10, 95% CI 0.80 to 1.81). The second RCT found that rates of any stroke and of intracranial haemorrhage were similar for thrombolysis plus abciximab, enoxaparin, or unfractionated heparin (AR for any stroke about 1.5%; AR for intracranial haemorrhage about 0.9%).[28] **Primary percutaneous transluminal coronary angioplasty with or without glycoprotein IIb/IIIa inhibitors:** The largest RCT found that abciximab given during percutaneous angioplasty or stenting increased the need for transfusion compared with no abciximab (AR for needing transfusion: 5.4% *v* 3.4%; P = 0.02; RR and CI not reported).[35] The remaining two RCTs found that giving abciximab before percutaneous angioplasty increased minor bleeding[34] and major bleeding[33] compared with no abciximab (minor bleeding: AR 12% *v* 3%; RR 3.7, 95% CI 1.3 to 10.1;[34] major bleeding: 16.6% *v* 9.5%; P = 0.02; CI not reported[33]). The fourth RCT comparing early versus late tirofiban administration before primary coronary angioplasty found similar rates of minor or major bleeding complications, although the study may have been too small to detect clinically important differences (AR for minor bleeding: 10% with early *v* 6% with late; P > 0.05; AR for major bleeding 2% with early *v* 2% with late; P > 0.05).[36]

Comment: None.

OPTION β BLOCKERS

Two systematic reviews and one subsequent RCT found that β blockers reduced mortality compared with no β blockers. One RCT in people receiving thrombolytic treatment found that immediate treatment with metoprolol reduced rates of reinfarction and chest pain at 6 days compared with delayed treatment, but had no significant effect on mortality at 6 days or at 1 year.

Benefits: **Versus no β blocker:** We found two systematic reviews (search dates 1997[37] and not reported[38]) and one subsequent RCT[39] of β blockers in people with acute myocardial infarction (AMI). The first review (27 RCTs) found that, within 1 week of treatment, β blockers significantly reduced the risk of death and major vascular events (for the combined outcome of death, non-fatal cardiac arrest, or non-fatal reinfarction: 1110 events with β blockers *v* 1298 events with no β blockers; RR 0.84, CI not reported; P < 0.001).[38] The more recent review (82 RCTs, 54 234 people) separately analysed 51 short term RCTs (people within 6 weeks after the onset of pain) and 31 long term RCTs (people treated for up to 48 months after AMI).[37] In most of the RCTs, the participants did not receive thrombolysis. In the short term studies, seven RCTs reported no deaths and many reported only a few. The short term RCTs reporting at least one death found no significant difference in mortality between β blockers and no β blockers (ARR 0.4%; OR 0.96, 95% CI 0.85 to 1.08). In the longer term RCTs, β blockers significantly reduced mortality over 6 months to 4 years compared with no β blockers (OR 0.77, 95% CI 0.69 to 0.85). No significant difference in effectiveness was found between different types of β blocker (based on cardioselectivity or intrinsic sympathomimetic activity). Most evidence was obtained with propranolol, timolol, and metoprolol. The subsequent RCT (1959 people within 3–21 days of AMI and with left ventricular dysfunction, of whom 46% had received thrombolysis or percutaneous transluminal coronary angioplasty at the acute stage of their infarction and 97% had received angiotensin converting enzyme inhibitors) compared carvedilol (6.25 mg increased to a maximum of 25 mg over 4–6 weeks) versus placebo.[39] It found that carvedilol significantly reduced mortality and non-fatal AMI compared with placebo (AR for death: 12% with carvedilol *v* 15% with placebo; HR 0.77, 95% CI 0.60 to 0.98; for non-fatal AMI: HR 0.59, 95% CI 0.39 to 0.90), but found no difference between treatments in the combined end point of total mortality and hospital admission for any cardiovascular event after a median of 1.3 years (HR 0.92, 95% CI 0.80 to 1.07). **Early versus delayed treatment:** We found one RCT (1434 people with AMI who had received tissue plasminogen activator thrombolysis), which compared early versus delayed metoprolol treatment.[40] Early treatment began on day 1 (iv then oral) and delayed treatment on day 6 (oral). It found that early treatment significantly reduced rates of reinfarction and recurrent chest pain after 6 days (AR for reinfarction: 2.7% with early treatment *v* 5.1% with delayed treatment; CI not reported; $P = 0.02$; AR for chest pain: 18.8% with early treatment *v* 24.1% with delayed treatment; $P < 0.02$). There were no significant differences in mortality or left ventricular ejection fraction between the two groups at 6 days or 1 year.

Harms: People with asthma or severe congestive cardiac failure were excluded from most trials. One RCT found that people given immediate versus delayed β blockers after tissue plasminogen activator experienced increased frequency of heart failure during the initial admission to hospital, although the result was not statistically significant (15.3% with immediate *v* 12.2% with delayed; $P = 0.10$).[40] The presence of first degree heart block and bundle branch block was associated with more adverse events.

Comment: Until recently, trials involving the use of β blockers in AMI were conducted mostly in people considered to be at low risk of heart failure (because of the supposed deleterious effect of β blockers on left ventricular function), and many of these trials took place in the prethrombolytic era. β Blockers may reduce rates of cardiac rupture and ventricular fibrillation. This may explain why people older than 65 years and those with large infarcts benefited most, as they have higher rates of these complications. The trial comparing early versus delayed β blockade after thrombolysis was too small to rule out an effect on mortality of β blockers when added to thrombolysis.[40]

OPTION **ANGIOTENSIN CONVERTING ENZYME INHIBITORS**

One systematic review in people treated within 14 days of acute myocardial infarction found that angiotensin converting enzyme inhibitors reduce mortality after 6 weeks compared with placebo. However, a non-systematic review found that angiotensin converting enzyme inhibitors increase persistent hypotension and renal dysfunction at 6 weeks compared with placebo.

Benefits: We found one systematic review (search date 1997, 15 RCTs with ≥ 6 weeks' follow up, 15 104 people), which compared angiotensin converting enzyme (ACE) inhibitors started within 14 days of acute myocardial infarction (AMI) versus placebo.[41] It found that ACE inhibitors decreased overall mortality and sudden cardiac death compared with placebo after 2–42 months (overall mortality: 1105/7658 [14.4%] with ACE inhibitors *v* 1251/7446 [16.8%] with placebo; OR 0.83, 95% CI 0.71 to 0.97; sudden cardiac death: OR 0.80, 95% CI 0.70 to 0.92).[41]

Harms: One non-systematic review of RCTs (search date not reported, 4 RCTs, 98 496 people within 36 hours of AMI) found that ACE inhibitors significantly increased persistent hypotension and renal dysfunction at 6 weeks compared with placebo (hypotension: AR 17.6% with ACE inhibitor *v* 9.3% with control; CI for difference not reported; P < 0.01; renal dysfunction: AR 1.3% *v* 0.6%; P < 0.01).[42] The relative and absolute risks of these adverse effects were uniformly distributed across both the high and lower cardiovascular risk groups. The systematic review did not report on harms.[41]

Comment: ACE inhibitors in people with AMI work best when treatment is started within 24 hours. The evidence does not answer the question of which people with an AMI should be offered ACE inhibitors, nor for how long after AMI it remains beneficial to start treatment. We found one systematic review (search date not reported; based on individual data from about 100 000 people in RCTs of ACE inhibitors), which found that people receiving both aspirin and ACE inhibitors had the same relative risk reduction as those receiving ACE inhibitors alone.[43] Of the 12 RCTs in the systematic review that reported on left ventricular function among participants, all reported a mean left ventricular ejection fraction of 54% or less. Six of these RCTs reported a mean left ventricular ejection fraction of 40% or less. However, there is debate over whether the benefits of ACE inhibitors also benefit people with normal left ventricular function after AMI.

OPTION **NITRATES**

One systematic review in people with acute myocardial infarction in the prethrombolytic era found that nitrates reduce mortality compared with placebo. Two RCTs in people with acute myocardial infarction (after thrombolysis was introduced) found no significant difference in mortality between nitrates and placebo.

Benefits: **Without thrombolysis:** We found one systematic review (search date not reported, 10 RCTs, 2000 people with acute myocardial infarction [AMI] who did not receive thrombolysis), which compared intravenous glyceryl trinitrate or sodium nitroprusside versus placebo.[44] The review found that nitrates significantly reduced mortality compared with placebo (RR 0.65, 95% CI 0.45 to 0.84). **With aspirin/thrombolysis:** We found two RCTs, which compared nitrates (given acutely) versus placebo in people with AMI, of whom 90% received aspirin and about 70% received thrombolytic treatment.[45,46] The first RCT (58 050 people with

AMI) compared oral controlled release isosorbide mononitrate 30–60 mg daily versus placebo.[45] It found no significant difference in mortality between isosorbide mononitrate and placebo (ARR nitrates *v* placebo 0.20%; OR 0.97, 95% CI 0.91 to 1.03). The second RCT (17 817 people with AMI) compared intravenous glyceryl trinitrate for 24 hours, followed by transdermal glyceryl trinitrate, versus placebo. It found no significant difference in mortality between nitrates and placebo (ARR nitrates *v* placebo 0.4%; OR 0.94, 95% CI 0.84 to 1.05). Neither RCT found significant differences in mortality in subgroups of people with different risks of dying.

Harms: The systematic review and the large RCTs found no significant harm associated with routine use of nitrates.[44–46]

Comment: Results for the two large RCTs were limited because a large proportion of people took nitrates outside the study, there was a high rate of concurrent use of other hypotensive agents, people were relatively low risk, and nitrates were not titrated to blood pressure and heart rate.[45,46] The RCTs found that nitrates were a useful adjunctive treatment to help control symptoms in people with AMI.

OPTION CALCIUM CHANNEL BLOCKERS

We found evidence that neither dihydropyridines nor verapamil reduce mortality compared with placebo. One RCT found limited evidence that, in people with left ventricular dysfunction, nifedipine given in the first few days after acute myocardial infarction may increase mortality compared with placebo.

Benefits: **Dihydropyridine calcium channel blockers:** We found two RCTs, which compared short acting nifedipine versus placebo within the first few days of acute myocardial infarction (AMI).[47,48] The first RCT (4491 people) was terminated prematurely because of concerns about safety.[47] It found that nifedipine increased mortality by 33% compared with placebo, although the increase did not reach statistical significance. The second RCT (1006 people) found no significant difference in mortality between nifedipine and placebo (18.7% with nifedipine *v* 15.6% with placebo; OR 1.60, 95% CI 0.86 to 3.00).[48] We found no RCTs of sustained release nifedipine, amlodipine, or felodipine in this setting. **Verapamil:** We found one systematic review (search date 1997, 7 RCTs, 6527 people with AMI).[49] It found no significant difference in mortality between verapamil and placebo (RR 0.86, 95% CI 0.71 to 1.04).

Harms: Two systematic reviews (search dates not reported; including both randomised and observational trials) investigating the use of calcium channel blockers in people with AMI found non-significant increases in mortality of about 4% and 6%.[50,51] One RCT (2466 people with AMI) compared diltiazem (60 mg orally 4 times daily starting 3–15 days after AMI) versus placebo.[52] It found no significant difference in total mortality or reinfarction between diltiazem and placebo. Subgroup analysis in people with congestive heart failure found that diltiazem significantly increased death and reinfarction (RRI 1.41, 95% CI 1.01 to 1.96).

Comment: None.

OPTION PRIMARY PERCUTANEOUS TRANSLUMINAL CORONARY ANGIOPLASTY VERSUS THROMBOLYSIS

One systematic review found that primary percutaneous transluminal coronary angioplasty reduced a combined outcome of death, non-fatal reinfarction, and stroke compared with thrombolysis.

Benefits: We found one systematic review (search date not reported, 23 RCTs, 7739 people with or without cardiogenic shock), which compared primary percutaneous transluminal coronary angioplasty (PTCA) versus thrombolysis (streptokinase and fibrin specific agents) in people with acute ST segment myocardial infarction.[53] It found that PTCA significantly reduced the combined end point of death, non-fatal reinfarction, and stroke at 4–6 weeks compared with thrombolysis (253/3089 [8%] with PTCA *v* 442/3085 [14%] with thrombolysis; OR 0.53, 95% CI 0.45 to 0.63; no significant heterogeneity was detected; P = 0.35). It also found that PTCA significantly reduced the combined outcome at 6–18 months (approximately 11% *v* 20%, results presented graphically; P < 0.0001). Results were similar for PTCA compared with streptokinase and for PTCA compared with fibrin specific agents (PTCA *v* streptokinase, 8 RCTs, 1837 people: OR 0.40, 95% CI 0.28 to 0.58; PTCA *v* fibrin specific agents, 15 RCTs, 5902 people: OR 0.57, 95% CI 0.48 to 0.63). The review also found that emergency hospital transfer for primary PTCA (average delay 39 minutes) significantly reduced the combined outcome compared with on-site thrombolysis (5 RCTs, 2909 people: 8% with PTCA *v* 15% with thrombolysis, results presented graphically; P < 0.0001).

Harms: **Stroke:** The review found that PTCA reduced the risk of all types of stroke compared with thrombolysis (all stroke: 1.0% with PTCA *v* 2.0% with thrombolysis; P < 0.001; haemorrhagic stroke: 0.05% with PTCA *v* 1.1 % with thrombolysis; P = 0.03).[53] **Major bleeding:** The review also found that PTCA increased major bleeding at 4–6 weeks compared with thrombolysis (7% with PTCA *v* 5% with thrombolysis; OR 1.30, 95% CI 1.02 to 1.56).[53]

Comment: Although collectively the trials found an overall short term and long term reduction in deaths with PTCA compared with thrombolysis, there were several pitfalls common to individual RCTs, most of which may have inflated the benefit of PTCA.[54] RCTs comparing PTCA versus thrombolysis could not be easily blinded, and ascertainment of end points that required some judgement, such as reinfarction or stroke, may have been influenced by the investigators' knowledge of the treatment allocation (the vast majority of the earlier trials did not have blinded adjudication events committees). In addition, the RCTs conducted before the GUSTO RCT (published 1997)[55] should be viewed as hypothesis generating, in that the composite outcome (death, reinfarction, and stroke) was not prospectively defined, and attention was only placed on these end points after there seemed to be some benefit on *post hoc* analysis. The lower mortality and reinfarction rates reported with primary PTCA are promising but not conclusive, and the real benefits may well be smaller. Only in a minority of centres (such as those who participated in the randomised trials) that perform a high volume of PTCA, and in the hands of experienced interventionists, may primary PTCA be clearly superior to thrombolytic treatment. Elsewhere, primary PTCA may be of greatest benefit in people with contraindications to thrombolysis, in people in cardiogenic shock, or in people in whom the mortality reduction with thrombolysis is modest and the risk of intracranial haemorrhage is increased, for example elderly people.[56] The value of PTCA over thrombolysis in people presenting to hospital more than 12 hours after onset of chest pain remains to be tested. In one large RCT, the collective rate of haemorrhagic stroke in people given thrombolysis was 1.1%, substantially higher than that observed in trials comparing thrombolysis versus placebo.[55] This may have been because the trials summarised above were in older people and used tissue plasminogen activator. However, the lower rates of haemorrhagic stroke with primary PTCA were consistent across almost all trials, and this may be the major advantage of PTCA over thrombolysis.

QUESTION **Which treatments improve outcomes for cardiogenic shock after acute myocardial infarction?**

Edoardo De Benedetti and Philip Urban

OPTION **EARLY INVASIVE CARDIAC REVASCULARISATION**

One large RCT found that early invasive cardiac revascularisation reduced mortality after 6 and 12 months compared with medical treatment alone in people with cardiogenic shock within 48 hours of acute myocardial infarction. A second, smaller RCT found similar results, although the difference was not significant.

Benefits: We found no systematic review. We found two RCTs in people with cardiogenic shock within 48 hours of acute myocardial infarction comparing early invasive cardiac revascularisation**G** versus initial medical treatment alone (see comment below).[2,3,57] The first RCT (302 people) found that early invasive cardiac revascularisation significantly reduced mortality after 6 and 12 months (see table 2, p 58).[2,57] The second RCT (55 people) found that early invasive cardiac revascularisation reduced mortality after 30 days and at 12 months, although the difference was not significant (see table 2, p 58).[3] **Percutaneous transluminal coronary angioplasty versus coronary artery bypass graft:** We found no RCTs in people with cardiogenic shock after acute myocardial infarction comparing percutaneous transluminal coronary angioplasty versus coronary artery bypass grafting.

Harms: Pre-specified subgroup analysis in the first RCT found that there was a non-significant increase in 30 day mortality in people aged 75 years or more with early invasive cardiac revascularisation compared with initial medical treatment alone (56 people in subgroup; 18/24 [75%] with early invasive cardiac revascularisation *v* 17/32 [53%] with medical treatment alone; RR 1.41, 95% CI 0.95 to 2.11).[2,57] The first RCT also found that acute renal failure (defined as a serum creatinine level > 265 μmol/L) was significantly more common in the medical treatment alone group than the early cardiac revascularisation group (36/150 [24%] *v* 20/152 [13%]; RR 1.82, 95% CI 1.1 to 3.0; NNH 9, 95% CI 5 to 48). Other harms reported by the RCT included major haemorrhage, sepsis, and peripheral vascular occlusion, although comparative data between groups for these harms were not reported. The second RCT did not report harms.[3]

Comment: In the first RCT, medical treatment included intra-aortic balloon counterpulsation**G** and thrombolytic treatment.[2,57] In the second RCT, medical treatment was not defined.[3] The second RCT was stopped prematurely because of difficulties with recruitment. Both RCTs were conducted in centres with expertise in early invasive cardiac revascularisation. Their results may not necessarily be reproducible in other settings.[2,3,57]

OPTION **THROMBOLYSIS**

Subgroup analysis of one RCT found no significant difference in mortality after 21 days between thrombolysis and no thrombolysis in people with cardiogenic shock.

Benefits: We found no systematic review. We found one RCT (11 806 people with acute myocardial infarction), which compared streptokinase versus no thrombolysis and performed a subgroup analysis on people with cardiogenic shock (see comment below).[58] The subgroup analysis found no significant difference in inpatient mortality after 21 days (280 people; 102/146 [70%] with thrombolysis *v* 94/134 [70%] with no thrombolysis; RR 1.0, 95% CI 0.85 to 1.16).

Harms: The RCT did not specifically report harms in the subgroup of people with cardiogenic shock.[58] Overall, adverse reactions attributed to streptokinase were found in 705/5860 (12%) people either during or after streptokinase infusion. These adverse reactions included minor and major bleeding (3.7%), allergic reactions (2.4%), hypotension (3.0%), anaphylactic shock (0.1%), shivering/fever (1.0%), ventricular arrhythmias (1.2%), and stroke (0.2%). See harms of thrombolysis in acute myocardial infarction, p 40.

Comment: The RCT was not blinded.[58] Data presented are from a retrospective subgroup analysis. Randomisation was not stratified by the presence of cardiogenic shock.

OPTION POSITIVE INOTROPES (DOBUTAMINE, DOPAMINE, ADRENALINE [EPINEPHRINE], NORADRENALINE [NOREPINEPHRINE], AMRINONE)

We found no RCTs comparing inotropes versus placebo.

Benefits: We found no systematic review or RCTs. We found three non-systematic reviews, which did not include RCTs evaluating positive inotropes specifically in people with cardiogenic shock after acute myocardial infarction (AMI).[1,59,60]

Harms: Positive inotropes may worsen cardiac ischaemia and induce ventricular arrhythmias.[1,59,60] We found no studies of harms specifically in people with cardiogenic shock after AMI (see harms of positive inotropic drugs under heart failure, p 115).

Comment: There is consensus that positive inotropes are beneficial in cardiogenic shock after AMI. We found no evidence to confirm or reject this view.

OPTION VASODILATORS (ANGIOTENSIN CONVERTING ENZYME INHIBITORS, NITRATES)

We found no RCTs comparing vasodilators versus placebo.

Benefits: We found no systematic review or RCTs.

Harms: We found no systematic review or RCTs.

Comment: The risk of worsening hypotension has led to concern about treating acute cardiogenic shock with any vasodilator.[60]

OPTION PULMONARY ARTERY CATHETERISATION

We found no RCTs comparing pulmonary artery catheterisation versus no catheterisation.

Benefits: We found no systematic review and no RCTs.

Harms: Observational studies have found an association between pulmonary artery catheterisation and increased morbidity and mortality, but it is unclear whether this arises from an adverse effect of the catheterisation or because people with a poor prognosis were selected for catheterisation.[61] Harms such as major arrhythmias, injury to the lung, thromboembolism (see thromboembolism, p 194), and sepsis occur in 0.1–0.5% of people undergoing pulmonary artery catheterisation.[61]

Comment: Pulmonary artery catheterisation helps to diagnose cardiogenic shock, guide correction of hypovolaemia, optimise filling pressures for both the left and right sides of the heart, and adjust doses of inotropic drugs.[1] There is consensus that pulmonary artery catheterisation benefits people with cardiogenic shock after acute myocardial infarction,[62,63] although we found no evidence to confirm or reject this view.

OPTION INTRA-AORTIC BALLOON COUNTERPULSATION

An RCT presented only in abstract form found limited evidence of no significant difference in mortality at 6 months between intra-aortic balloon counterpulsation plus thrombolysis and thrombolysis alone in people with cardiogenic shock.

Benefits: We found no systematic review. We found one abstract of an RCT (57 people), which compared intra-aortic balloon counterpulsation❻ plus thrombolysis versus thrombolysis alone in people with cardiogenic shock after acute myocardial infarction (AMI; see comment below).[64] The RCT found no significant difference in mortality after 6 months (22/57 [39%] with thrombolysis plus balloon counterpulsation *v* 25/57 [43%] with thrombolysis alone; RR 0.90, 95% CI 0.57 to 1.37; P = 0.3).

Harms: Harms were not reported in the abstract of the RCT.[64]

Comment: The abstract did not describe detailed methods for the trial, making interpretation of results difficult.[60] We also found two additional small RCTs (30 people[65] and 20 people[66]), which compared intra-aortic balloon counterpulsation versus standard treatment in people after AMI. Neither RCT specifically recruited or identified data from people with cardiogenic shock after AMI. Neither RCT found a reduction in mortality with intra-aortic balloon counterpulsation. There is consensus that intra-aortic balloon counterpulsation is beneficial in people with cardiogenic shock after AMI. We found no evidence to confirm or reject this view.

OPTION VENTRICULAR ASSISTANCE DEVICES AND CARDIAC TRANSPLANTATION

We found no RCTs evaluating either ventricular assistance devices or cardiac transplantation.

Benefits: We found no systematic review and no RCTs.

Harms: We found no evidence of harms specifically associated with ventricular assistance devices❻ or cardiac transplantation in people with cardiogenic shock after acute myocardial infarction.

Comment: Reviews of observational studies[1,60,67] and retrospective reports[68,69] have suggested that ventricular assistance devices may improve outcomes in selected people when used alone or as a bridge to cardiac transplantation. The availability of ventricular assistance devices and cardiac transplantation is limited to a few specialised centres. Results may not be applicable to other settings.

OPTION EARLY CARDIAC SURGERY

We found no RCTs evaluating early surgical intervention for ventricular septal rupture, free wall rupture, or mitral valve regurgitation complicated by cardiogenic shock after acute myocardial infarction.

Benefits: We found no systematic review and no RCTs.

Harms: We found no evidence about the harms of surgery in people with cardiogenic shock caused by cardiac structural defects after acute myocardial infarction.

Comment: Non-systematic reviews of observational studies have suggested that death is inevitable after free wall rupture without early surgical intervention and that surgery for both mitral valve regurgitation and ventricular septal rupture is more effective when carried out within 24–48 hours.[1,60]

GLOSSARY

Cardiac index A measure of cardiac output derived from the formula: cardiac output/unit time divided by body surface area (L/minute/m^2).

Intra-aortic balloon counterpulsation A technique in which a balloon is placed in the aorta and inflated during diastole and deflated just before systole.

Invasive cardiac revascularisation A term used to describe either percutaneous transluminal coronary angioplasty or coronary artery bypass grafting.

Killip class A categorisation of the severity of heart failure based on easily obtained clinical signs. The main clinical features are Class I: no heart failure; Class II: crackles audible half way up the chest; Class III: crackles heard in all the lung fields; Class IV: cardiogenic shock.

Ventricular assistance device A mechanical device placed in parallel to a failing cardiac ventricle that pumps blood in an attempt to maintain cardiac output. Because of the risk of mechanical failure, thrombosis, and haemolysis, ventricular assistance devices are normally used for short term support while preparing for a heart transplant.

REFERENCES

1. Califf RM, Bengtson JR. Cardiogenic shock. *N Engl J Med* 1994;330:1724–1730.
2. Hochman JS, Sleeper LA, Webb JG, et al, for the SHOCK investigators. Early revascularization in acute myocardial infarction complicated by cardiogenic shock. *N Engl J Med* 1999;341:625–634.
3. Urban P, Stauffer JC, Khatchatrian N, et al. A randomized evaluation of early revascularization to treat shock complicating acute myocardial infarction. The (Swiss) Multicenter Trial of Angioplasty for Shock — (S)MASH. *Eur Heart J* 1999;20:1030–1038.
4. Murray C, Lopez A. Mortality by cause for eight regions of the world: global burden of disease study. *Lancet* 1997;349:1269–1276.
5. National Heart, Lung, and Blood Institute. *Morbidity and mortality: chartbook on cardiovascular, lung, and blood diseases*. Bethesda, MD: US Department of Health and Human Services, Public Health Service, National Institutes of Health; May 1992.
6. Goldberg RJ, Samad NA, Yarzebski J, et al. Temporal trends in cardiogenic shock complicating acute myocardial infarction. *N Engl J Med* 1999;340:1162–1168.
7. Hasdai D, Califf RM, Thompson TD, et al. Predictors of cardiogenic shock after thrombolytic therapy for acute myocardial infarction. *J Am Coll Cardiol* 2000;35:136–143.
8. Hochman JS, Buller CE, Sleeper LA, et al. Cardiogenic shock complicating acute myocardial infarction — etiology, management and outcome: a report from the SHOCK trial registry. *J Am Coll Cardiol* 2000;36(3 suppl A):1063–1070.
9. Urban P, Bernstein M, Costanza M, et al. An internet-based registry of acute myocardial infarction in Switzerland. *Kardiovasc Med* 2000;3:430–441.
10. Berger PB, Tuttle RH, Holmes DR, et al. One year survival among patients with acute myocardial infarction complicated by cardiogenic shock, and its relation to early revascularisation: results of the GUSTO-1 trial. *Circulation* 1999;99:873–878.
11. Antiplatelet Trialists' Collaboration. Collaborative overview of randomised trials of antiplatelet therapy I: prevention of death, myocardial infarction, and stroke by prolonged antiplatelet therapy in various categories of people. *BMJ* 1994;308:81–106. Search date 1990; primary sources Medline and Current Contents.
12. Second International Study of Infarct Survival (ISIS-2) Collaborative Group. Randomized trial of intravenous streptokinase, oral aspirin, both or neither among 17 187 cases of suspected acute myocardial infarction. *Lancet* 1988;ii:349–360.
13. Baigent BM, Collins R. ISIS-2: four year mortality of 17 187 patients after fibrinolytic and antiplatelet therapy in suspected acute myocardial infarction study [abstract]. *Circulation* 1993;88(suppl I):I-291–I-292.
14. Patrignani P, Filabozzi P, Patrono C. Selective cumulative inhibition of platelet thromboxane production by low-dose aspirin in healthy subjects. *J Clin Invest* 1982;69:1366–1372.
15. Fibrinolytic Therapy Trialists' (FTT) Collaborative Group. Indications for fibrinolytic therapy in suspected acute myocardial infarction: collaborative overview of early mortality and major morbidity results of all randomized trials of more than 1000 patients. *Lancet* 1994;343:311–322.

16. French JK, Hyde TA, Patel H, et al. Survival 12 years after randomization to streptokinase: the influence of thrombolysis in myocardial infarction flow at three to four weeks. *J Am Coll Cardiol* 1999;34:62–69.
17. Collins R, Peto R, Baigent BM, et al. Aspirin, heparin and fibrinolytic therapy in suspected acute myocardial infarction. *N Engl J Med* 1997;336:847–860.
18. Gruppo Italiano per lo studio della streptochinasi nell'infarto miocardico (GISSI). GISSI-2: a factorial randomised trial of alteplase versus streptokinase and heparin versus no heparin among 12 490 patients with acute myocardial infarction. *Lancet* 1990;336:65–71.
19. Third International Study of Infarct Survival (ISIS-3) Collaborative Group. ISIS-3: a randomised comparison of streptokinase vs tissue plasminogen activator vs anistreplase and of aspirin plus heparin vs aspirin alone among 41 299 cases of suspected acute myocardial infarction. *Lancet* 1992;339:753–770.
20. The GUSTO Investigators. An international randomized trial comparing four thrombolytic strategies for acute myocardial infarction. *N Engl J Med* 1993;329:673–682.
21. The Global Use of Strategies to Open Occluded Coronary Arteries (GUSTO III) investigators. A comparison of reteplase with alteplase for acute myocardial infarction. *N Engl J Med* 1997;337:1118–1123.
22. Assessment of the Safety and Efficacy of a New Thrombolytic (ASSENT-2) investigators. Single bolus tenecteplase compared to front-loaded alteplase in acute myocardial infarction: the ASSENT-2 double-blind randomised trial. *Lancet* 1999;354:716–722.
23. Eikelboom JW, Mehta SR, Pogue J, et al. Safety outcomes in meta-analyses of Phase 2 vs Phase 3 randomized trials: intracranial hemorrhage in trials of bolus fibrinolytic therapy. *JAMA* 2001;285:444–450.
24. Simoons MI, Maggioni AP, Knatterud G, et al. Individual risk assessment for intracranial hemorrhage during thrombolytic therapy. *Lancet* 1993;342:523–528.
25. Gore JM, Granger CB, Simoons MI, et al. Stroke after thrombolysis: mortality and functional outcomes in the GUSTO-1 trial. *Circulation* 1995;92:2811–2818.
26. Berkowitz SD, Granger CB, Pieper KS, et al. Incidence and predictors of bleeding after contemporary thrombolytic therapy for myocardial infarction. *Circulation* 1997;95:2508–2516.
27. Simoons M, Krzeminska-Pakula M, Alonso A, et al. for the AMI-SK Investigators. Improved reperfusion and clinical outcome with enoxaparin as an adjunct to streptokinase thrombolysis in acute myocardial infarction. The AMI-SK study. *Eur Heart J* 2002;23:1282–1290.
28. Théroux P, Welsh RC. Meta-analysis of randomized trials comparing enoxaparin versus unfractionated heparin as adjunctive therapy to fibrinolysis in ST-elevation acute myocardial infarction. *Am J Cardiol* 2003;91:860–864.
29. The Assessment of the Safety and Efficacy of a New Thrombolytic regimen (ASSENT) 3 investigators. Efficacy and safety of tenecteplase in combination with enoxaparin, abciximab, or unfractionated heparin: the ASSENT-3 randomised trial in acute myocardial infarction. *Lancet* 2001;358:605–613.
30. Antman EM, Louwerenburg HW, Baars HF, et al. Enoxaparin as adjunctive antithrombin therapy for ST-elevation myocardial infarction: results of the ENTIRE-Thrombolysis in Myocardial Infarction (TIMI) 23 Trial. *Circulation* 2002;105:1642–1649.
31. The GUSTO V investigators. Reperfusion therapy for acute myocardial infarction with fibrinolytic therapy or combination reduced fibrinolytic therapy and platelet glycoprotein IIb/IIIa inhibition: the GUSTO V randomised trial. *Lancet* 2001;357:1905–1914.
32. Lincoff AM, Califf RM, Van de Werf F, et al. Mortality at 1 year with combination platelet glycoprotein IIb/IIIa inhibition and reduced-dose fibrinolytic therapy vs conventional fibrinolytic therapy for acute myocardial infarction: GUSTO V randomized trial. *JAMA* 2002;288:2130–2135.
33. Brener SJ, Barr LA, Burchenal JEB, et al. Randomized, placebo-controlled trial of platelet glycoprotein IIb/IIIa blockade with primary angioplasty for acute myocardial infarction. *Circulation* 1998;98:734–741.
34. Montalescot G, Barragan P, Wittenberg O, et al. for the ADMIRAL investigators. Platelet glycoprotein IIb/IIIa inhibition with coronary stenting for acute myocardial infarction. *N Engl J Med* 2001;344:1895–1903.
35. Stone GW, Grines CL, Cox DA, et al. Comparison of angioplasty with stenting, with or without abciximab, in acute myocardial infarction. *N Engl J Med* 2002;346:957–966.
36. Lee DP, Herity NA, Hiatt BL, et al. Adjunctive platelet glycoprotein IIb/IIIa receptor inhibition with tirofiban before primary angioplasty improves angiographic outcomes: results of the TIrofiban Given in the Emergency Room before Primary Angioplasty TIGER-PA) pilot trial. *Circulation* 2003;107:1497–1501.
37. Freemantle N, Cleland J, Young P, et al. Beta blockade after myocardial infarction: systematic review and meta regression analysis. *BMJ* 1999;318:1730–1737. Search date 1997; primary sources Medline, Embase, Biosis, Healthstar, Sigle, IHTA, Derwent drug file, dissertation abstracts, Pascal, international pharmaceutical abstracts, Science Citation Index, and hand searches of reference lists.
38. Yusuf S, Peto R, Lewis S, et al. Beta-blockade during and after myocardial infarction: an overview of the randomized trials. *Prog Cardiovasc Dis* 1985;27:335–371. Search date not stated; primary sources computer-aided search of the literature, manual search of reference lists, and enquiries to colleagues about relevant papers.
39. The CAPRICORN investigators. Effect of carvedilol on outcome after myocardial infarction in patients with left-ventricular dysfunction: the CAPRICORN randomized trial. *Lancet* 2001;357:1385–1390.
40. Roberts R, Rogers WJ, Mueller HS, et al. Immediate versus deferred beta-blockade following thrombolytic therapy in patients with acute myocardial infarction: results of the thrombolysis in myocardial infarction (TIMI) II-B study. *Circulation* 1991;83:422–437.
41. Domanski MJ, Exner DV, Borkowf CB, et al. Effect of angiotensin converting enzyme inhibition on sudden cardiac death in patients following acute myocardial infarction. A meta-analysis of randomized clinical trials. *J Am Coll Cardiol* 1999;33:598–604. Search date 1997; primary sources Medline and hand searches of reference lists.
42. ACE Inhibitor Myocardial Infarction Collaborative Group. Indications for ACE inhibitors in the early treatment of acute myocardial infarction: systematic overview of individual data from 100 000 patients in randomised trials. *Circulation* 1998;97:2202–2212. Search date not stated; primary source collaboration group of principal investigators of all randomised trials who collated individual patient data.
43. Latini R, Tognoni G, Maggioni AP, et al. Clinical effects of early angiotensin-converting enzyme inhibitor treatment for acute myocardial infarction are similar in the presence and absence of aspirin. Systematic overview of individual data from 96 712 randomized patients. *J Am Coll Cardiol* 2000;35:1801–1807. Search date not stated; primary source individual patient data on all trials involving more than 1000 patients.
44. Yusuf S, Collins R, MacMahon S, et al. Effect of intravenous nitrates on mortality in acute myocardial infarction: an overview of the randomised trials. *Lancet* 1988;1:1088–1092. Search date not stated; primary sources literature, colleagues, investigators, and pharmaceutical companies.
45. Fourth International Study of Infarct Survival (ISIS-4) Collaborative Group. ISIS-4: a randomised factorial trial assessing early oral captopril, oral mononitrate,

and intravenous magnesium sulphate in 58 050 patients with suspected acute myocardial infarction. *Lancet* 1995;345:669–685.
46. Gruppo Italiano per lo studio della streptochinasi nell'infarto miocardico (GISSI). GISSI-3: effects of lisinopril and transdermal glyceryl trinitrate singly and together on 6-week mortality and ventricular function after acute myocardial infarction. *Lancet* 1994;343:1115–1122.
47. Wilcox RG, Hampton JR, Banks DC, et al. Early nifedipine in acute myocardial infarction: the TRENT study. *BMJ* 1986;293:1204–1208.
48. Goldbourt U, Behar S, Reicher-Reiss H, et al. Early administration of nifedipine in suspected acute myocardial infarction: the Secondary Prevention Reinfarction Israel Nifedipine Trial 2 Study. *Arch Intern Med* 1993;153:345–353.
49. Pepine CJ, Faich G, Makuch R. Verapamil use in patients with cardiovascular disease: an overview of randomized trials. *Clin Cardiol* 1998;21:633–641. Search date 1997; primary sources Medline, Science Citation Index, Current Contents, and hand searches of reference lists.
50. Yusuf S, Furberg CD. Effects of calcium channel blockers on survival after myocardial infarction. *Cardiovasc Drugs Ther* 1987;1:343–344. Search dates and primary sources not reported.
51. Teo KK, Yusuf S, Furberg CD. Effects of prophylactic antiarrhythmic drug therapy in acute myocardial infarction: an overview of results from randomized controlled trials. *JAMA* 1993;270:1589–1595. Search date not stated; primary sources Medline and correspondence with investigators and pharmaceutical companies.
52. The Multicenter Diltiazem Post Infarction Trial Research Group. The effect of diltiazem on mortality and reinfarction after myocardial infarction. *N Engl J Med* 1988;319:385–392.
53. Keeley EC, Boura JA, Grines CL. Primary angioplasty versus intravenous thrombolytic therapy for acute myocardial infarction: a quantitative review of 23 randomised trials. *Lancet* 2003;361:13–20.
54. Yusuf S, Pogue J. Primary angioplasty compared to thrombolytic therapy for acute myocardial infarction [editorial]. *JAMA* 1997;278:2110–2111.
55. The GUSTO IIb Angioplasty Substudy Investigators. A clinical trial comparing primary coronary angioplasty with tissue plasminogen activator for acute myocardial infarction. *N Engl J Med* 1997;336:1621–1628.
56. Van de Werf F, Topol EJ, Lee KL, et al. Variations in patient management and outcomes for acute myocardial infarction in the United States and other countries: results from the GUSTO trial. *JAMA* 1995;273:1586–1591.
57. Hochman JS, Sleeper LA, White HD, et al. One year survival following early revascularization for cardiogenic shock. *JAMA* 2001;285:190–192.
58. GISSI-1. Effectiveness of intravenous thrombolytic treatment in acute myocardial infarction. *Lancet* 1986;1:397–401.
59. Herbert P, Tinker J. Inotropic drugs in acute circulatory failure. *Intensive Care Med* 1980;6:101–111.
60. Hollenberg SM, Kavinsky CJ, Parrillo JE. Cardiogenic shock. *Ann Int Med* 1999;131:47–59. Search date 1998; primary sources Medline and hand searches of bibliographies of relevant papers.
61. Bernard GR, Sopko G, Cerra F, et al. Pulmonary artery catheterization and clinical outcomes. *JAMA* 2000;283:2568–2572.
62. Hollenberg SM, Hoyt J. Pulmonary artery catheters in cardiovascular disease. *New Horiz* 1977;5:207–213. Search date 1996; primary sources not stated.
63. Participants. Pulmonary artery catheter consensus conference: consensus statement. *Crit Care Med* 1997;25:910–925.
64. Ohman EM, Nanas J, Stomel R, et al. Thrombolysis and counterpulsation to improve cardiogenic shock survival (TACTICS): results of a prospective randomized trial [abstract]. *Circulation* 2000;102(suppl II):II-600.
65. O'Rourke MF, Norris RM, Campbell TJ, et al. Randomized controlled trial of intraaortic balloon counterpulsation in early myocardial infarction with acute heart failure. *Am J Cardiol* 1981;47:815–820.
66. Flaherty JT, Becker LC, Weiss JL, et al. Results of a randomized prospective trial of intraaortic balloon counterpulsation and intravenous nitroglycerin in patients with acute myocardial infarction. *J Am Coll Cardiol* 1985;6:434–446.
67. Frazier OH. Future directions of cardiac assistance. *Semin Thorac Cardiovasc Surg* 2000;12:251–258.
68. Pagani FD, Lynch W, Swaniker F, et al. Extracorporeal life support to left ventricular assist device bridge to cardiac transplantation. *Circulation* 1999;100(suppl 19):II-206–210.
69. Mavroidis D, Sun BC, Pae WE. Bridge to transplantation: the Penn State experience. *Ann Thorac Surg* 1999;68:684–687.

Nicolas Danchin
Professor of Medicine Université Paris VI
H pital Européen Georges Pompidou, Paris, France

Philip Urban
Director, Interventional Cardiology
H pital de la Tour, Meyrin-Geneva, Switzerland

Edoardo De Benedetti
Cardiologist
C.H.U.V., Lausanne, Switzerland

Competing interests: PU has received funds for research and public speaking from a variety of pharmaceutical and device companies, both related and unrelated to products discussed here. EDB and ND none declared. *We would like to acknowledge the previous contributors to this chapter, including Shamir Mehta and Salim Yusuf.*

TABLE 1 Direct randomised comparisons of the standard streptokinase regimen with various tissue plasminogen activator based fibrinolytic regimens in people with suspected acute myocardial infarction in the GISSI-2, ISIS-3, and GUSTO-1 trials (see text, p 39).[18–20]

Trial and treatment	Number of people randomised	Any stroke Absolute number (%)	Any death Absolute number (%)	Death not related to stroke Absolute number (%)	Stroke or death Absolute number (%)
GISSI-2†[18]					
Streptokinase	10 396	98 (0.9)	958 (9.2)	916 (8.8)	1014 (9.8)
tPA	10 372	136 (1.3)	993 (9.6)	931 (9.0)	1067 (10.3)
Effect/1000 people treated with tPA instead of streptokinase		3.7 ± 1.5 more	3.6 ± 4.0 more	1.7 ± 4.0 more	5.3 ± 4.2 more
ISIS-3‡[19]					
Streptokinase	13 780	141 (1.0)	1455 (10.6)	1389 (10.1)	1530 (11.1)
tPA	13 746	188 (1.4)	1418 (10.3)	1325 (9.6)	1513 (11.0)
Effect/1000 people treated with tPA instead of streptokinase		3.5 ± 1.3 more	2.4 ± 3.7 fewer	4.4 ± 3.6 fewer	1.0 ± 3.8 fewer
GUSTO-1§[20]					
Streptokinase (sc heparin)	9841	117 (1.2)	712 (7.3)	666 (6.8)	783 (8.0)
Streptokinase (iv heparin)	10 410	144 (1.4)	763 (7.4)	709 (6.8)	853 (8.2)
tPA alone	10 396	161 (1.6)	653 (6.3)	585 (5.6)	746 (7.2)
tPA plus streptokinase	10 374	170 (1.6)	723 (7.0)	647 (6.2)	817 (7.9)
Effect/1000 people treated with tPA-based regimens instead of streptinokinase		3.0 ± 1.2 more	6.6 ± 2.5 fewer	8.6 ± 2.4 fewer	5.5 ± 2.6 fewer
$chi^2/2$ heterogeneity of effects between 3 trials		0.7	5.6	7.0	5.4
P value		0.3	0.06	0.03	0.07

TABLE 1 continued

Trial and treatment	Number of people randomised	Any stroke Absolute number (%)	Any death Absolute number (%)	Death not related to stroke* Absolute number (%)	Stroke or death Absolute number (%)
Weighted average of all 3 trials¶					
Effect/1000 people treated with tPA-based regimens instead of streptokinase		3.3 ± 0.8 more	2.9 ± 1.9 fewer	4.9 ± 1.8 fewer	1.6 ± 1.9 fewer
P value		< 0.001	> 0.1	0.01	0.4

Values are numbers (%). This table should not be used to make direct non-randomised comparisons between the absolute event rates in different trials, because the patient populations may have differed substantially in age and other characteristics. Deaths recorded throughout the first 35 days are included for GISSI-2 and ISIS-3 and throughout the first 30 days for GUSTO-1. Numbers randomised and numbers with follow up are from the ISIS-3 report[19] and GUSTO-1[20] (supplemented with revised GUSTO-1 data from the National Auxiliary Publications Service), and numbers with events and the percentages (based on participants with follow up) are from the ISIS-3 report[19] and Van de Werf, et al.[59] Plus-minus values are ± standard deviation. In all three trials, streptokinase was given in intravenous infusions of 1.5 MU over a period of 1 hour.

AMI, acute myocardial infarction; iv, intravenous; tPA, tissue plasminogen activator; sc, subcutaneous.

*Death not related to stroke was defined as death without recorded stroke.

†In the GISSI-2 trial, the tPA regimen involved an initial bolus of 10 mg, followed by 50 mg in the first hour and 20 mg in each of the second and third hours.

‡In the ISIS-3 trial, the tPA regimen involved 40 000 clot-lysis U/kg of body weight as an initial bolus, followed by 360 000 U/kg in the first hour and 67 000 U/kg in each of the next 3 hours.

§In the GUSTO-1 trial, the tPA alone regimen involved an initial bolus of 15 mg, followed by 0.75 mg/kg (up to 50 mg) in the first 30 minutes and 0.5 mg/kg (up to 35 mg) in the next hour; in the GUSTO-1 trial the other tPA based regimen involved 0.1 mg/kg of tPA (up to 9 mg) as an initial bolus and 0.9 mg/kg (up to 81 mg) in the remainder of the first hour, plus 1 MU of streptokinase in the first hour.

¶The weights are proportional to the sample sizes of the trials, so this average gives most weight to the GUSTO-1 trial and least to the GISSI-2 trials.[17] Reproduced with permission from Collins R, Peto R, Baigent BM, et al. Aspirin, heparin and fibrinolytic therapy in suspected AMI. *N Engl J Med*

TABLE 2 **Comparison of early invasive cardiac revascularisation versus initial medical treatment on mortality at 30 days, 6 months, and 12 months (see text, p 50).[2,3,57]**

Time after AMI	Mortality in early invasive cardiac revascularisation group Number dead/total number (%)	Mortality in medical treatment alone group Number dead/total number (%)	ARR (95% CI)	RR (95% CI)	NNT (95% CI)
SHOCK study[2,57]					
30 days	71/152 (47)	84/150 (56)	9.3% (–2 to +20.2)	0.83 (0.67 to 1.04)	NA
6 months	76/152 (50)	94/150 (63)	12.7% (1.5 to 23.4)	0.80 (0.65 to 0.98)	8 (5 to 68)
12 months	81/152 (53)	99/150 (66)	12.7% (1.6 to 23.3)	0.80 (0.67 to 0.97)	8 (5 to 61)
SMASH study[3]					
30 days	22/32 (69)	18/23 (78)	9.5% (–14.6 to +30.6)	0.88 (0.64 to 1.2)	NA
12 months	23/32 (74)	19/23 (83)	10.7% (–12.7 to +30.9)	0.87 (0.65 to 1.16)	NA

AMI, acute myocardial infarction; NA, not applicable.

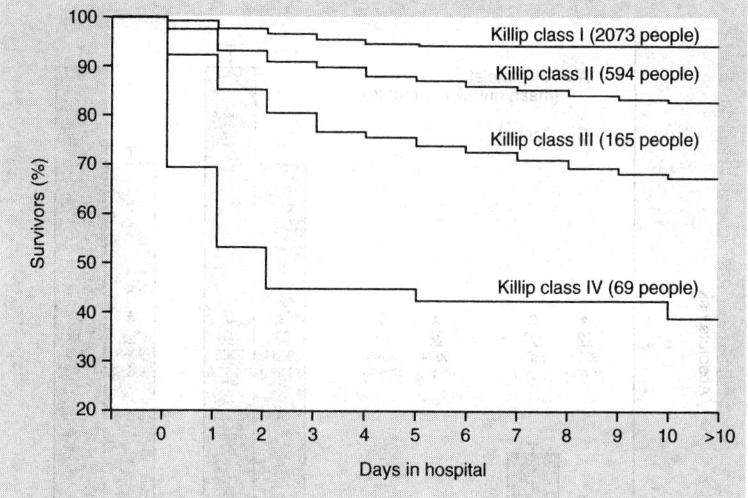

FIGURE 1 **The AMIS registry Kaplan–Meier survival curves as a function of Killip class⊕ at hospital admission for 3138 people (2901 evaluable) admitted in 50 Swiss hospitals between 1977 and 1998. Published with permission: Urban P, Bernstein MS, Costanza MC, et al, for the AMIS investigators. An internet-based registry of acute myocardial infarction in Switzerland. *Kardiovasc Med* 2000;3:430–441 (see text, p 38).[9]**

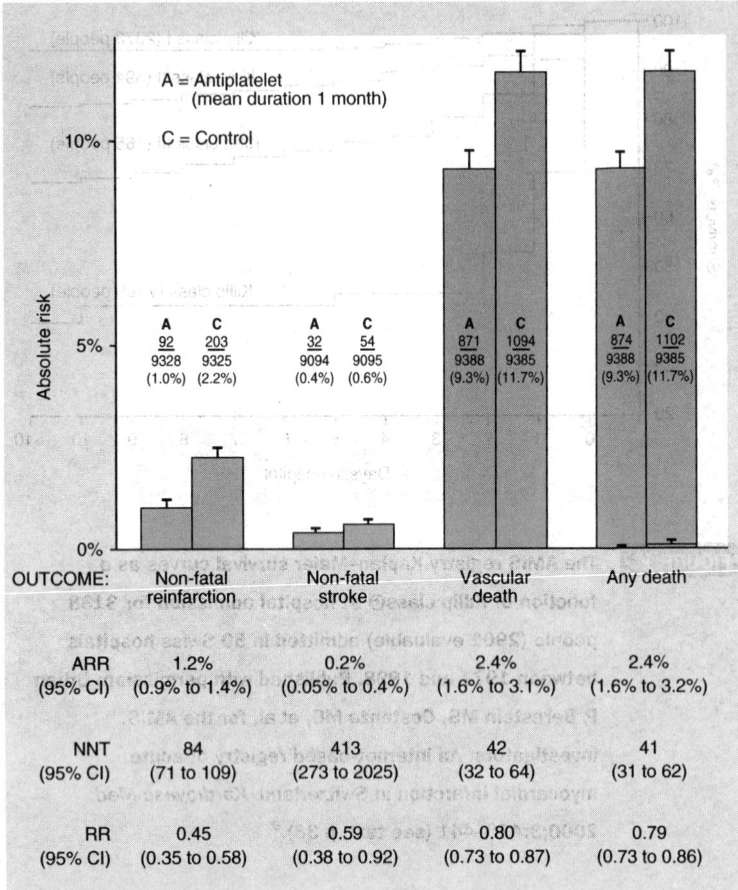

	Non-fatal reinfarction	Non-fatal stroke	Vascular death	Any death
ARR (95% CI)	1.2% (0.9% to 1.4%)	0.2% (0.05% to 0.4%)	2.4% (1.6% to 3.1%)	2.4% (1.6% to 3.2%)
NNT (95% CI)	84 (71 to 109)	413 (273 to 2025)	42 (32 to 64)	41 (31 to 62)
RR (95% CI)	0.45 (0.35 to 0.58)	0.59 (0.38 to 0.92)	0.80 (0.73 to 0.87)	0.79 (0.73 to 0.86)

FIGURE 2 **Absolute effects of antiplatelet treatment on outcomes in people with a prior suspected or definite acute myocardial infarction (AMI).[11] The columns show the absolute risks over 1 month for each category; the error bars are the upper 95% confidence interval (CI). In the "any death" column, non-vascular deaths are represented by lower horizontal lines. The table displays for each outcome the absolute risk reduction (ARR), the number of people needing treatment for 1 month to avoid one additional event (NNT), and the risk reduction (RR), with their 95% CI values (see text, p 38). Published with permission.[11]**

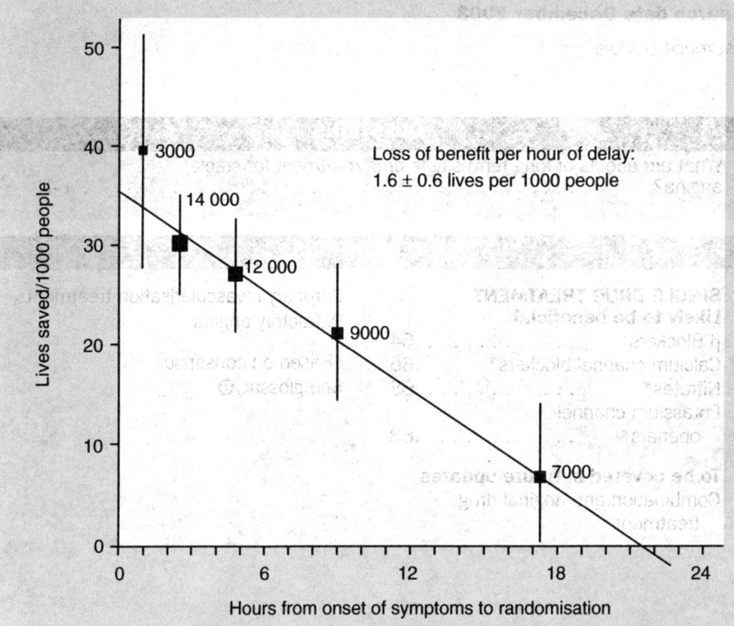

FIGURE 3 **Absolute number of lives saved at 1 month/1000 people receiving thrombolytic treatment plotted against the time from the onset of symptoms to randomisation among 45 000 people with ST segment elevation or bundle branch block.[15] Numbers along the curve are the number of people treated at different times (see text, p 39). Published with permission: Collins R, Peto R, Baigent BM, et al. Aspirin, heparin and fibrinolytic therapy in suspected AMI. *N Engl J Med* 1997;336:847–860. Copyright © 1997 Massachusetts Medical Society. All rights reserved.[17]**

Angina (stable)

Search date December 2003

Laurence O'Toole

QUESTIONS

INTERVENTIONS

*Based on consensus
See glossary G

Key Messages

Single drug treatment

- **β Blockers*** One small RCT found no significant difference between a β blocker (propranolol) and placebo in angina frequency or exercise duration after 6 months. However, this trial may have lacked power to detect a clinically important difference between groups. There is consensus that β blockers are effective for treating the symptoms of stable angina. RCTs found no significant difference between β blockers and calcium channel blockers in the frequency of angina attacks, exercise duration, mortality, or non-fatal cardiovascular events at 6 months to 3 years. However, these RCTs may have lacked power to detect clinically important differences between groups. One RCT also found no significant difference between β blockers and calcium channel blockers in quality of life.
- **Calcium channel blockers*** One small RCT found no significant difference between bepridil and placebo in the frequency of angina attacks. It found that bepridil increased exercise duration compared with placebo at 6 months. There is consensus that calcium channel blockers are effective for treating the symptoms of stable angina. RCTs found no significant difference between calcium channel blockers and β blockers in the frequency of angina attacks, exercise duration, mortality, or non-fatal cardiovascular events at between 6 months and 3 years. However, these RCTs may have lacked power to detect clinically important differences between groups. One RCT also found no significant difference between calcium channel blockers and β blockers in quality of life. One RCT found no significant difference between amlodipine and isosorbide mononitrate in the frequency of angina attacks or in quality of life. It found that amlodipine increased exercise duration compared with isosorbide mononitrate at 6 months. The RCT found that peripheral oedema was more common with amlodipine than with isosorbide mononitrate, whereas headache was more common with isosorbide mononitrate.

- **Nitrates*** We found no RCTs comparing long term single drug treatment with nitrates versus placebo for stable angina. However, there is consensus that nitrates are effective for treating the symptoms of stable angina. One RCT found no significant difference between amlodipine and isosorbide mononitrate in the frequency of angina attacks or in quality of life. It found that amlodipine increased exercise duration compared with isosorbide mononitrate at 6 months. The RCT found that peripheral oedema was more common with amlodipine than with isosorbide mononitrate, whereas headache was more common with isosorbide mononitrate.
- **Potassium channel openers*** We found no RCTs on the effects of long term single drug treatment with potassium channel openers for stable angina. However, there is consensus that potassium channel openers are effective for treating the symptoms of stable angina.

  *Based on consensus

DEFINITION Angina pectoris, often simply known as angina, is a clinical syndrome characterised by discomfort in the chest, shoulder, back, arm, or jaw.[1] Angina is usually caused by coronary artery atherosclerotic disease. Rarer causes include valvular heart disease, hypertrophic cardiomyopathy, uncontrolled hypertension, or vasospasm or endothelial dysfunction not related to atherosclerosis. The differential diagnosis of angina includes non-cardiac conditions affecting the chest wall, oesophagus, and lungs. Angina may be classified as stable or unstable. **Stable angina** is defined as regular or predictable angina symptoms that have been occurring for over 2 months. Symptoms are transient and are typically provoked by exertion, and alleviated by rest or nitroglycerin. Other precipitants include cold weather, eating, or emotional distress. This chapter deals specifically with stable angina caused by coronary artery atherosclerotic disease. **Unstable angina** is diagnosed if there is a rapid decline in exercise capacity or if there are episodes of pain at rest. This is usually associated with atherosclerotic plaque instability and, as myocardial infarction and death may ensue, should be treated as a medical emergency, usually requiring hospital admission (see chapter on unstable angina, [Web only]).

INCIDENCE/ PREVALENCE The prevalence of stable angina remains unclear.[1,2] Epidemiological studies in the UK estimate that 6–16% of men and 3–10% of women aged 65–74 years have experienced angina.[3–5] Annually, about 1% of the population visits their general practitioner with symptoms of angina[4] and 23 000 people with new anginal symptoms present to their general practitioner each year in the UK.[6] These studies did not distinguish between stable and unstable angina.[3–6]

AETIOLOGY/ RISK FACTORS Stable angina resulting from coronary artery disease is characterised by focal atherosclerotic plaques in the intimal layer of the epicardial coronary artery. The plaques encroach on the coronary lumen and may limit blood flow to the myocardium, especially during periods of increased myocardial oxygen demand. The major risk factors that lead to the development of stable angina are similar to those that predispose to coronary heart disease. These risk factors include increasing age, male sex, overweight, hypertension, elevated serum cholesterol level, smoking, and relative physical inactivity.[7]

PROGNOSIS Stable angina is a marker of underlying coronary heart disease, which accounts for 1 in 4 deaths in the UK.[8] People with angina are 2–5 times more likely to develop other manifestations of coronary heart disease than people that do not have angina.[7,9] One population based study (7100 men aged 51–59 years at entry) found that people with angina had higher mortality than people with no history of coronary artery disease at baseline (16 year survival rate: 53% with angina *v* 72% without coronary artery disease *v* 34% with a history of myocardial infarction).[10] Clinical trials in people with stable angina have tended to recruit participants who were not felt to be in need of coronary revascularisation and in these people prognosis is better, with an annual mortality of 1–2% and annual rate of non-fatal myocardial infarction of 2–3%.[11–14] Features that indicate a poorer prognosis include: more severe symptoms, male sex,[15] abnormal resting electrocardiogram[16] (present in about 50% of people with angina[17]), previous myocardial infarction,[10,18] left ventricular dysfunction,[19] easily provoked or widespread coronary ischaemia on stress testing (present in about one third of people referred to hospital with stable angina), and significant stenosis of all three major coronary arteries or the left main coronary artery.[6,19] In addition, the standard coronary risk factors continue to exert a detrimental and additive effect on prognosis in people with stable angina.[9,20,21] Control of these risk factors is dealt with in the *Clinical Evidence* chapter on secondary prevention of ischaemic cardiac events, (Web only).

AIMS OF INTERVENTION	To prevent death and future cardiovascular events, and to improve symptoms, exercise capacity, and quality of life.
OUTCOMES	**Primary outcomes:** mortality, non-fatal myocardial infarction, and unstable angina. **Secondary outcomes:** anti-anginal efficacy (as determined by symptom frequency and total exercise time on treadmill testing), quality of life (assessed by questionnaire), and adverse effects of treatment.
METHODS	*Clinical Evidence* search and appraisal December 2003. The search was limited to RCTs with at least 6 months of follow up, that compared single drug anti-anginal treatment versus placebo or another single drug anti-anginal treatment, in people with stable angina believed to be caused by coronary artery atherosclerotic disease. The anti-anginal drug classes covered by the search were β blockers, calcium channel blockers, long acting nitrate preparations, and potassium channel openers. We excluded RCTs where participants received combinations of anti-anginal drugs. Combination anti-anginal treatment will be dealt with in future updates.

QUESTION What are effects of long term single drug treatment for stable angina? New

OPTION β BLOCKERS New

One small RCT found no significant difference between a β blocker (propranolol) and placebo in angina frequency or exercise duration after 6 months. However, this trial may have lacked power to detect a clinically important difference between groups. There is consensus that β blockers are effective for treating the symptoms of stable angina. RCTs found no significant difference between β blockers and calcium channel blockers in the frequency of angina attacks, exercise duration, mortality, or non-fatal cardiovascular events at 6 months to 3 years. However, these RCTs may have lacked power to detect clinically important differences between groups. One RCT also found no significant difference between β blockers and calcium channel blockers in quality of life.

Benefits: We found one systematic review (search date 1996).[22] **Versus placebo:** The review[22] identified one RCT[23] (191 people of < 70 years of age with abnormal exercise stress test**G** or previous myocardial infarction). It compared three treatments: β blocker (propranolol; 78 people), calcium channel blocker (bepridil; 78 people), and placebo (35 people). It found no significant difference between propranolol and placebo in the reduction in frequency of angina attacks or improvement in duration of exercise at 6 months (mean reduction in weekly angina attacks from baseline: 71% with propranolol *v* 77% with placebo; P reported as not significant; increase in exercise duration from baseline: 24% with propranolol *v* 8% with placebo; P = 0.09). Serious cardiac events (cardiac death, myocardial infarction, or angina deterioration) were more common with propranolol than placebo, but the significance of this difference was not reported (AR for serious cardiac events: 8/78 [10.3%] with propranolol *v* 2/35 [5.7%] with placebo; P value not reported). **Versus calcium channel blockers:** The systematic review[22] identified five RCTs that met our inclusion criteria (1818 people). The first RCT (191 people of < 70 years of age, with abnormal exercise stress test or previous myocardial infarction),[23] compared three treatments: β blocker (propranolol 60–240 mg/day; 78 people), calcium channel blocker (bepridil 100–400 mg/day; 78 people), and placebo (35 people). It found no significant difference between propranolol and bepridil in the reduction in the frequency of angina attacks or improvement in duration of exercise at 6 months (reduction in weekly angina attacks from baseline: 69% with bepridil *v* 71% with propranolol; P reported as not significant; increase in exercise duration from baseline: 24% with propranolol *v* 31% with bepridil; P = 0.26). The incidence of serious cardiac events (cardiac death, myocardial infarction, or angina deterioration) was similar with propranolol and bepridil (AR for serious cardiac events: 8/78 [10.3%] with propranolol *v* 6/78 [7.7%] for bepridil; P value not reported). The second RCT (80 people aged ≤ 80 years with abnormal exercise stress test)[24] compared a β blocker (nadolol 40–160 mg once daily) with a calcium channel blocker (amlodipine 2.5–10 mg once daily) in people with stable angina. It found no significant difference in the reduction in frequency of angina attacks or change in exercise duration at 6 months (change in median number of angina attacks a week from baseline to 6 months: from 3.0 to 0.3 with nadolol *v* from 4.0 to 0.3 with amlodipine; P reported as not significant; change in total exercise treadmill time from baseline to 6 months: 490 seconds to 475 seconds [–3%] with nadolol *v* 454 seconds to 462 seconds [+2%] with amlodipine; P reported as not significant). The third RCT (56 people < 80 years of age with abnormal exercise stress test) compared a β blocker (metoprolol 100 mg twice daily; 26 people) with a calcium channel blocker (diltiazem 120 mg twice daily; 30 people) in people with stable angina.[25] It found no significant difference in the change in exercise capacity between groups at 32 weeks (39 people evaluable: 19 people with metoprolol *v* 20 people with diltiazem; analysis not by intention to treat; mean change in duration of exercise from baseline to 32 weeks: +0.2 minutes with metoprolol *v* +0.3 minutes with diltiazem; P reported as not significant). The effect of treatments on the frequency of angina symptoms was not reported. The fourth RCT (809 people aged < 70 years selected on the basis of typical clinical history and response to nitroglycerin or, if history was not typical, an abnormal stress test) compared a β blocker (metoprolol 200 mg once daily) with a calcium channel blocker (verapamil 240 mg twice daily).[26] It found no significant difference in either mortality or the combined outcome of mortality or non-fatal cardiovascular event between metoprolol and verapamil after a median follow up of 3.4 years (AR for mortality: 22/406 [5.4%] with metoprolol *v* 25/403 [6.2%] with verapamil; OR 0.87, 95% CI 0.48 to 1.56; AR for mortality or non-fatal cardiovascular event: 128/406 [31.5%] with metoprolol *v* 123/403 [30.5%] with verapamil; OR 1.03, 95% CI 0.84 to 1.30. It also found no significant difference in three quality of life variables between metoprolol and verapamil (Cornell Medical Index psychomatic symptom index, score range 39–195: mean score change –1.1 with metoprolol *v* –2.2 with verapamil; P = 0.34; overall life satisfaction, score range 0–120: mean score change –3.0 with metoprolol *v* –2.5 with verapamil; P = 0.85; sleep disturbances, score range 9–36: mean score change –0.7 with both treatments: P = 0.97). The fifth RCT (682 people with stable angina who were not immediately being considered for coronary revascularisation) compared three treatments: atenolol (50 mg twice daily), nifedipine (20 or 40 mg twice daily as tolerated), and atenolol plus nifedipine.[13] It found no significant difference between atenolol alone and nifedipine alone in the combined outcome of mortality, myocardial infarction, or unstable angina, after a mean follow up of 2 years (AR for combined death, myocardial infarction, or unstable angina: 29/226 [12.8%] with atenolol *v* 25/232 [10.8%] with nifedipine; log rank P = 0.32). **Versus nitrates or potassium channel openers:** We found no RCTs.

Harms: **Versus placebo:** The RCT identified by the review found no significant difference between propranolol and placebo in the proportion of people experiencing at least one non-cardiac adverse effect (AR 23/78 [29.5%] with propranolol *v* 6/35 [17.1%] with placebo; P = 0.08).[23]

There was no significant difference between groups in treatment withdrawal owing to lack of efficacy or severe adverse effects (17/78 [21.8%] with propranolol *v* 6/35 [17.1%] with placebo; P = 0.58). **Versus calcium channel blockers:** The first RCT identified by the review found that the proportion of people experiencing at least one non-cardiac adverse event was significantly higher with propranolol than with bepridil (AR for at least one non-cardiac adverse event: 23/78 [29.5%] with propranolol *v* 9/78 [11.5%] with bepridil; P = 0.003).[23] This was mostly due to an increased incidence of fatigue in the propranolol group (14/78 [17.9%] with propranolol *v* 6/78 [7.7%] with bepridil; P = 0.05). However, there was no significant difference between groups in treatment withdrawal owing to lack of efficacy or severe adverse effects (17/78 [21.8%] with propranolol *v* 15/78 [19.2%] with bepridil; P = 0.69). The second RCT found that significantly more people taking nadolol experienced adverse effects than people taking amlodipine (AR 33/40 [82.5%] with nadolol *v* 17/40 [42.5%] with amlodipine; P < 0.0001).[24] However, similar numbers of people were withdrawn owing to adverse effects in both groups (4/40 [10.0%] with nadolol *v* 3/40 [7.5%] with amlodipine; P value not reported). The third RCT reported that most adverse events were mild, and that there was no significant difference in the incidence of adverse events with metoprolol and diltiazem (figures not reported, P reported as non-significant).[25] The fourth RCT (809 people) found that significantly more people withdrew from the study because of gastrointestinal upset with verapamil than with metoprolol (AR 22/403 [5.5%] with verapamil *v* 10/406 [2.5%] with metoprolol; P = 0.029). However, it found no significant difference in overall withdrawal owing to adverse effects between the two treatments (AR 59/403 [14.6%] with verapamil *v* 45/406 [11.1%] with metoprolol; P = 0.13). The fifth RCT (682 people) found that, over an average of 2 years' follow up, significantly more people discontinued treatment because of adverse effects in the nifedipine group than in the atenolol group (AR 93/232 [40.0%] with nifedipine *v* 60/226 [26.5%] with atenolol; log rank P = 0.001).[13] **Versus nitrates or potassium channel openers:** We found no RCTs.

Comment: There is consensus that β blockers are effective for treating the symptoms of stable angina. Many of the RCTs included in the review were unlikely to have been sufficiently powered to detect a clinically important difference between groups.[22]

OPTION CALCIUM CHANNEL BLOCKERS New

One small RCT found no significant difference between bepridil and placebo in the frequency of angina attacks. It found that bepridil increased exercise duration compared with placebo at 6 months. There is consensus that calcium channel blockers are effective for treating the symptoms of stable angina. RCTs found no significant difference between calcium channel blockers and β blockers in the frequency of angina attacks, exercise duration, mortality, or non-fatal cardiovascular events at between 6 months and 3 years. However, these RCTs may have lacked power to detect clinically important differences between groups. One RCT also found no significant difference between calcium channel blockers and β blockers in quality of life. One RCT found no significant difference between amlodipine and isosorbide mononitrate in the frequency of angina attacks or in quality of life. It found that amlodipine increased exercise duration compared with isosorbide mononitrate at 6 months. The RCT found that peripheral oedema was more common with amlodipine than with isosorbide mononitrate, whereas headache was more common with isosorbide mononitrate.

Benefits: We found one systematic review (search date 1996).[22] **Versus placebo:** The review[22] identified one RCT (191 people of < 70 years of age with abnormal exercise stress test**G** or previous myocardial infarction).[23] It compared three treatments: calcium channel blocker (bepridil; 78 people), β blocker (propranolol; 78 people), and placebo (35 people). It found no significant difference between bepridil and placebo in the reduction in frequency of angina attacks at 6 months (mean reduction in weekly angina attacks from baseline: 69% with bepridil *v* 77% with placebo; P reported as not significant). It found that bepridil significantly increased duration of exercise compared with placebo at 6 months (increase in exercise duration from baseline: 31% with bepridil *v* 8% with placebo; P = 0.03). It found that the rate of serious cardiac events (defined as death, myocardial infarction, or unstable angina) was higher with bepridil than placebo, but the significance of this difference was not reported (AR for major cardiac events: 6/78 [7.7%] with bepridil *v* 2/35 [5.7%] with placebo; P value not reported). **Versus β blockers:** See benefits of beta blockers versus calcium channel blockers, p 64. **Versus nitrates:** The systematic review did not find any RCTs.[22] We found one subsequent RCT (196 people, aged ≥65 years with an abnormal exercise stress test) comparing amlodipine (5–10 mg once daily) versus isosorbide mononitrate (25–50 mg once daily).[27] It found no significant difference either in the number of weekly anginal attacks or in quality of life (assessed using the short form 36 [SF-36] questionnaire) between amlodipine and isosorbide mononitrate at 6 months (median weekly number of angina attacks: 0 for both groups; P reported as not significant; mean improvement in SF-36 bodily pains scale score from baseline: about 5 for both groups; P reported as not significant; mean improvement in SF-36 health transition score from baseline: about 11 for both groups; P reported as not significant). It found a significant improvement in exercise duration with amlodipine compared with isosorbide mononitrate at 6 months (mean change in exercise duration from baseline to 6 months: from 436 seconds to 548 seconds [+112 seconds] with amlodipine *v* from 462 seconds to 494 seconds [+32 seconds] with isosorbide mononitrate; P = 0.016). **Versus potassium channel openers:** We found no RCTs.

Harms: **Versus placebo:** The RCT[23] found no significant difference between bepridil and placebo in the proportion of people experiencing at least one non-cardiac adverse effect at 6 months (AR 9/78 [11.5%] with bepridil *v* 6/35 [17.1%] with placebo; P = 0.22). **Versus β blockers:** See harms of β blockers versus calcium channel blockers, p 65. **Versus nitrates:** The RCT found no significant difference between amlodipine and isosorbide mononitrate in the proportion of people reporting any adverse event at 6 months, the proportion of people with serious adverse effects was also similar in both groups (AR for any adverse event: 58% with amlodipine *v* 53% with isosorbide mononitrate; P value reported as not significant; AR for a serious adverse event: reported as about 7% in both groups; P value not reported).[27] About 8% of people in the amlodipine group and 18% of people in the isosorbide mononitrate group discontinued the study because of adverse events (significance not reported). Only two withdrawals (2%; both oedema) in the amlodipine group and seven withdrawals (7.3%; all headache) in the isosorbide mononitrate group were considered to be treatment related (significance not reported). The RCT found that peripheral oedema was more common with amlodipine than with isosorbide mononitrate, whereas headache was more common with isosorbide mononitrate than with amlodipine (AR for peripheral oedema: 14% with amlodipine *v* 0% with isosorbide mononitrate; AR for headache: 13% with isosorbide mononitrate *v* 2% with amlodipine; P value not reported for either comparison). **Versus potassium channel openers:** We found no RCTs.

Comment: There is consensus that calcium channel blockers are effective for treating the symptoms of stable angina.

OPTION NITRATES New

We found no RCTs comparing long term single drug treatment with nitrates versus placebo for stable angina. However, there is consensus that nitrates are effective for treating the symptoms of stable angina. One RCT found no significant difference between amlodipine and isosorbide mononitrate in the frequency of angina attacks or in quality of life. It found that amlodipine increased exercise duration compared with isosorbide mononitrate at 6 months. The RCT found that peripheral oedema was more common with amlodipine than with isosorbide mononitrate, whereas headache was more common with isosorbide mononitrate.

Benefits: **Versus placebo, β blockers, or potassium channel openers:** We found no systematic review or RCTs (see comment below). **Versus calcium channel blockers:** See benefits of calcium channel blockers versus nitrates, p 67.

Harms: **Versus placebo, β blockers, or potassium channel openers:** We found no systematic review or RCTs. **Versus calcium channel blockers:** See harms of calcium channel blockers versus nitrates, p 67.

Comment: There is consensus that nitrates are effective for treating the symptoms of stable angina.

OPTION POTASSIUM CHANNEL OPENERS New

We found no RCTs on the effects of long term single drug treatment with potassium channel openers for stable angina. However, there is consensus that potassium channel openers are effective for treating the symptoms of stable angina.

Benefits: **Versus placebo, β blockers, calcium channel blockers, or nitrates:** We found no systematic review or RCTs (see comment below).

Harms: **Versus placebo, β blockers, calcium channel blockers, or nitrates:** We found no systematic review or RCTs.

Comment: There is consensus that potassium channel openers are effective for treating the symptoms of stable angina.

GLOSSARY

Exercise stress testing is widely used in the evaluation of people with chest pain. The person walks on a treadmill, the speed and slope of which is varied according to protocol, while being monitored by electrocardiogram. Exercise induced horizontal or down-sloping ST segment depression is strongly suggestive of myocardial ischaemia, particularly when associated with typical chest pain. ST segment depression at a low workload usually indicates severe coronary artery disease, as may exercise induced ventricular arrhythmia or a fall in blood pressure.

REFERENCES

1. Gibbons RJ, Abrams J, Chatterjee K, et al. ACC/AHA 2002 guideline update for the management of patients with chronic stable angina: a report of the American College of Cardiology/American Heart Association Task Force on Practice Guidelines (Committee to Update the 1999 Guidelines for the management of Patients with Chronic Stable Angina). 2002. Available at http://www.acc.org/clinical/guidelines/stable/stable.pdf (last accessed 12 January 2005).
2. Martin RM, Hemingway H, Gunnell D, et al. Population need for coronary revascularisation: are national targets for England credible? *Heart* 2002;88:627–633.
3. Joint Health Surveys Unit. *Health survey for England 1998*. The Stationery Office: London, 1999.
4. Royal College of General Practitioners, the Office of Population Censuses and Surveys and the Department of Health. *Morbidity statistics from general practice: fourth national study 1991–1992*. HMSO: London, 1995.

5. Gill D, Mayou R, Dawes M, et al. Presentation, management and course of angina and suspected angina in primary care. *J Psychosom Res* 1999;46:349–358.
6. Gandhi MM, Lampe FC, Wood DA. Incidence, clinical characteristics, and short-term prognosis of angina pectoris. *Br Heart J* 1995;73:193–198.
7. Dawber TR. *The Framingham study. The epidemiology of atherosclerotic disease.* Cambridge, MA: Harvard University Press, 1980.
8. Office for National Statistics. *Social trends 27.* The Stationery Office: London, 1997.
9. Sigurdsson E, Sigfusson N, Agnarsson U, et al. Long-term prognosis of different forms of coronary heart disease: the Reykjavik Study. *Int J Epidemiol* 1995;24:58–68.
10. Rosengren A, Wilhelmsen L, Hagman M, et al. Natural history of myocardial infarction and angina pectoris in a general population sample of middle aged men: a 16-year follow-up of the Primary Prevention Study, Goteborg, Sweden. *J Intern Med* 1998;244:495–505.
11. CASS Principle Investigators and their Associates. Coronary Artery Surgery Study (CASS): a randomised trial of coronary artery bypass surgery. Survival data. *Circulation* 1983;68:939–950.
12. Brunelli C, Cristofani R, L'Abbate A. Long-term survival in medically treated patients with ischaemic heart disease and prognostic importance of clinical and echocardiographic data. *Eur Heart J* 1989;10:292–303.
13. Dargie HJ, Ford I, Fox KM. Total Ischaemic Burden European Trial (TIBET). Effects of ischaemia and treatment with atenolol, nifedipine SR and their combination on outcome in patients with chronic stable angina. *Eur Heart J* 1996;17:104–112.
14. The IONA study group. Effect of nicorandil on coronary events in patients with stable angina: the Impact Of Nicorandil in Angina (IONA) randomised trial. *Lancet* 2002;359:1269–1275. [Erratum in: *Lancet* 2002;360:806]
15. Murabito JM, Evans JC, Larson MG, et al. Prognosis after the onset of coronary heart disease. An investigation of differences in outcome between sexes according to initial coronary disease presentation. *Circulation* 1993;88:2548–2555.
16. Hammermeister KE, DeRouen TA, Dodge HT. Variable predictors of survival in patients with coronary artery disease. Selection by univariate and multivariate analyses from clinical, electrocardiographic, exercise, arteriographic, and quantitative evaluation. *Circulation* 1979;59:421–430.
17. Connolly DC, Elveback LR, Oxman HA. Coronary heart disease in Residents of Rochester, Minnesota. IV. Prognostic value of the resting electrocardiogram at the time of diagnosis of angina pectoris. *Mayo Clin Proc* 1984;59:247–250.
18. Bluck WJ Jr, Crumpacker EL, Dry TJ, et al. Prognosis of angina pectoris: observations in 6882 cases. *JAMA* 1952;150(4):259–264.
19. Mock MB, Ringqvist I, Fisher LD, et al. Survival of medically treated patients in the Coronary Artery Surgery Study (CASS) registry. *Circulation* 1982;66:562–568.
20. Hagman M, Wilhelmsen L, Pennert K, et al. Factors of importance for prognosis in men with stable angina pectoris derived from a random population sample. The Multifactor Primary Prevention Trial, Gothenburg, Sweden. *Am J Cardiol* 1988;61:530–535.
21. Rosengren A, Hagman M, Wedel H, et al. Serum cholesterol and long-term prognosis in middle-aged men with myocardial infarction and angina pectoris. A 16-year follow-up of the Primary Prevention Study in Goteborg, Sweden. *Eur Heart J* 1997;18:754–761.
22. Schulpher M, Petticrew M, Kelland JL, et al. Resource allocation in chronic stable angina: a systematic review of the effectiveness, costs and cost-effectiveness of alternative interventions. *Health Technol Assess* 1998;2:i–iv,1–176.
23. Destors JM, Boissel JP, Philippon AM, et al. Controlled clinical trial of bepridil, propranolol and placebo in the treatment of exercise induced angina pectoris. *Fundam Clin Pharmacol* 1989;3:597–611.
24. Singh S. Long-term double-blind evaluation of amlodipine and nadolol in patients with stable exertional angina pectoris. *Clin Cardiol* 1993;16:54–58.
25. Vliegen HW, van der Wall EE, Niemeyer MG, et al. Long-term efficacy of diltiazem controlled release versus metoprolol in patients with stable angina pectoris. *J Cardiovasc Pharmacol* 1991;18(suppl 9):S55–S60.
26. Rehnqvist N, Hjemdahl P, Billing E, et al. Effects of metoprolol vs verapamil in patients with stable angina pectoris: the Angina Prognosis Study in Stockholm (APSIS). *Eur Heart J* 1996;17:76–81. [Erratum in: *Eur Heart J* 1996;17:483]
27. Hall R, Chong C. A double-blind parallel-group study of amlodipine versus long-acting nitrate in the management of elderly patients with stable angina. *Cardiology* 2001;96:72–77.

Laurence O'Toole
Consultant Cardiologist and Honorary Senior Clinical Lecturer
Dept of Cardiology
Royal Hallamshire Hospital
Sheffield
UK

Competing interests: LOT has attended international cardiological conferences as a guest of a number of pharmaceutical companies. He has been paid by Novartis and Pfizer for running educational programmes and has received research funds from Sanofi-Synthelabo.

Atrial fibrillation (acute)

Search date October 2003

Gregory Y H Lip and Bethan Freestone

QUESTIONS

INTERVENTIONS

See glossary G

Key Messages

Prevention of embolism

- **Antithrombotic treatment before cardioversion** We found no RCTs on use of aspirin, heparin, or warfarin as thromboprophylaxis before attempted cardioversion in acute atrial fibrillation.

Conversion to sinus rhythm

- **Flecainide** One RCT found that intravenous flecainide increased the proportion of people who reverted to sinus rhythm within 1 hour and in whom the sinus rhythm was maintained after 6 hours compared with placebo. Flecainide has been associated with serious adverse events such as severe hypotension and torsades de point. Two RCTs found that oral flecainide increased the proportion of people who reverted to sinus rhythm within 8 hours compared with intravenous amiodarone. We found insufficient evidence to draw any conclusions about comparisons between intravenous flecainide and intravenous amiodarone and between flecainide and quinidine. Three RCTs found no significant difference in rates of conversion to sinus rhythm between flecainide and propafenone. Flecainide and propafenone are not used in people with known or suspected ischaemic heart disease because they may cause arrhythmias.

- **Propafenone** One systematic review and subsequent RCTs have found that propafenone increased the proportion of people converting to sinus rhythm within 1–4 hours compared with placebo. One RCT in people with onset of atrial fibrillation of less than 48 hours found no significant difference between intravenous propafenone and amiodarone in the proportion of people who converted to sinus rhythm within 1 hour. Another RCT in people with onset of atrial fibrillation of less than 2 weeks found that a higher proportion of people converted to sinus rhythm with oral propafenone within 2.5 hours compared with amiodarone but the difference did not remain significant at 24 hours. Three RCTs found insufficient evidence to compare rates of conversion to sinus rhythm between propafenone and flecqinide. Propafenone and flecainide are not used in people with known or suspected ischaemic heart disease.
- **Amiodarone** We found insufficient evidence from three RCTs about the effects of amiodarone as a single agent compared with placebo for conversion to sinus rhythm in people with acute atrial fibrillation in people who are haemodynamically stable. Four small RCTs found no significant difference in rate of conversion to sinus rhythm at 24–48 hours for amiodarone compared with digoxin, although the studies may have lacked power to exclude clinically important differences. One small RCT found that amiodarone increased rate of cardioversion compared with verapamil at 3 hours. One RCT in people with onset of atrial fibrillation of less than 48 hours found no significant difference between intravenous propafenone and amiodarone in conversion to sinus rhythm within 1 hour. Another RCT in people with onset of atrial fibrillation of less than 2 weeks found that a higher proportion of people converted to sinus rhythm with oral propafenone within 2.5 hours compared with amiodarone but the difference did not remain significant at 24 hours. Two RCTs found that intravenous amiodarone reduced the proportion of people who reverted to sinus rhythm within 8 hours compared with oral flecainide. We found insufficient evidence to draw any conclusion between intravenous flecainide compared with intravenous amiodarone. We found no RCTs comparing amiodarone with either DC cardioversion or diltiazem.
- **DC cardioversion** We found no RCTs of DC cardioversion in acute atrial fibrillation in people who are haemodynamically stable.
- **Quinidine** We found no RCTs of DC cardioversion that compared quinidine versus placebo. One small RCT in people with onset of atrial fibrillation of less than 48 hours found that quinidine plus digoxin increased the proportion of people converting to sinus rhythm within 12 hours compared with sotalol. We found insufficient evidence to draw any conclusions about comparisons between flecainide and quinidine.
- **Sotalol** We found no RCTs comparing sotalol versus placebo. One small RCT in people with onset of atrial fibrillation of less than 48 hours found that quinidine plus digoxin increased the proportion of people who converted to sinus rhythm within 12 hours compared with sotalol.
- **Digoxin** We found no placebo controlled RCTs limited to people with acute atrial fibrillation. Three RCTs in people with atrial fibrillation of up to 7 days' duration found no significant difference between digoxin and placebo in conversion to sinus rhythm. Four RCTs found no significant difference between amiodarone and digoxin in conversion to sinus rhythm at 24–48 hours, although these trials may have lacked power to detect clinically important differences.

Heart rate control

- **Digoxin** We found no placebo controlled RCTs limited to people with acute atrial fibrillation. Two RCTs found that compared with placebo, digoxin reduced ventricular rate after 30 minutes and after 2 hours in people with atrial fibrillation of up to 7 days' duration. One RCT found that compared with digoxin, intravenous diltiazem reduced heart rate within 5 minutes in people with acute atrial fibrillation and atrial flutter.

Atrial fibrillation (acute)

- **Diltiazem** One RCT in people with atrial fibrillation (of unspecified duration) or atrial flutter found that intravenous diltiazem reduced heart rate in people within 15 minutes compared with placebo. One RCT found that in people with acute atrial fibrillation and atrial flutter, intravenous diltiazem reduced heart rate within 5 minutes compared with intravenous digoxin. One RCT found no significant difference between intravenous verapamil and intravenous diltiazem in rate control or measures of systolic function in people with acute atrial fibrillation or atrial flutter, but verapamil caused hypotension in some people.
- **Timolol** We found no RCTs limited to people with acute atrial fibrillation. One small RCT in people with atrial fibrillation of unspecified duration found that intravenous timolol (a β blocker) reduced ventricular rate within 20 minutes compared with placebo.
- **Verapamil** Two RCTs found that intravenous verapamil reduced heart rate at 10 or 30 minutes compared with placebo in people with atrial fibrillation or atrial flutter. One RCT in people with atrial fibrillation or acute atrial flutter found no significant difference between intravenous verapamil and intravenous diltiazem in rate control or measures of systolic function, but verapamil caused hypotension in some people. The RCT found that amiodarone increased the rate of cardioversion compared with verapamil at 3 hours.
- **Amiodarone** We found no RCTs examining effects of amiodarone alone on heart rate in people with acute atrial fibrillation.
- **Sotalol** We found no RCTs comparing sotalol versus placebo.

DEFINITION **Acute atrial fibrillation** is rapid, irregular, and chaotic atrial activity of less than 48 hours' duration. It includes both the first symptomatic onset of chronic, or persistent, atrial fibrillation and episodes of paroxysmal atrial fibrillationⒼ. It is sometimes difficult to distinguish new onset of atrial fibrillation from long standing atrial fibrillation that was previously undiagnosed. Atrial fibrillation within 72 hours of onset is sometimes called recent onset atrial fibrillation. By contrast, **chronic atrial fibrillation** is more sustained and can be described as paroxysmal (with spontaneous termination and sinus rhythm between recurrences), persistent, or permanent atrial fibrillationⒼ. This review deals only with people with acute atrial fibrillation who are haemodynamically stable. The consensus is that people who are not haemodynamically stable should be treated with immediate DC cardiversion. We have excluded studies in people with atrial fibrillation arising during or soon after cardiac surgery.

INCIDENCE/ PREVALENCE We found limited evidence of the incidence or prevalence of acute atrial fibrillation. Extrapolation from the Framingham study suggests an incidence in men of 3/1000 person years at age 55 years, rising to 38/1000 person years at 94 years.[1] In women, the incidence was 2/1000 person years at age 55 years and 32.5/1000 person years at 94 years. The prevalence of atrial fibrillation ranged from 0.5% for people aged 50–59 years to 9% in people aged 80–89 years. Among acute emergency medical admissions in the UK, 3–6% had atrial fibrillation, and about 40% were newly diagnosed.[2,3] Among acute hospital admissions in New Zealand, 10% (95% CI 9% to 12%) had documented atrial fibrillation.[4]

AETIOLOGY/ RISK FACTORS Common precipitants of acute atrial fibrillation are acute myocardial infarction and the acute effects of alcohol. Age increases the risk of developing acute atrial fibrillation. Men are more likely to develop atrial fibrillation than women (38 years' follow up from the Framingham Study, RR after adjustment for age and known predisposing conditions 1.5).[5] Atrial fibrillation can occur in association with underlying disease (both cardiac and non-cardiac) or can arise in the absence of any other condition. Epidemiological surveys have found that risk factors for the development of acute atrial fibrillation include ischaemic heart disease, hypertension, heart failure, valve disease, diabetes, alcohol abuse, thyroid disorders, and disorders of the lung and pleura.[1] In a British survey of acute hospital admissions of patients with atrial fibrillation, a history of ischaemic heart disease was present in 33%, heart failure in 24%, hypertension in 26%, and rheumatic heart disease in 7%.[3] In some populations, the acute effects of alcohol explain a large proportion of the incidence of acute atrial fibrillation. Paroxysms of atrial fibrillation are more common in athletes.[6]

PROGNOSIS **Spontaneous reversion:** Observational studies and placebo arms of RCTs have found that more than 50% of people with acute atrial fibrillation revert spontaneously within 24–48 hours, especially if atrial fibrillation is associated with an identifiable precipitant such as alcohol or myocardial infarction. **Progression to chronic atrial fibrillation:** We found no evidence about the proportion of people with acute atrial fibrillation who develop more chronic forms of atrial fibrillation (e.g. paroxysmal, persistent, or permanent atrial fibrillation). **Mortality:** We found little evidence about the effects on mortality and morbidity of acute atrial fibrillation where no underlying cause is found. Acute atrial fibrillation during myocardial infarction is an independent predictor of both short term and long term mortality.[7] **Heart failure:** Onset of atrial fibrillation reduces cardiac output by 10–20% irrespective of the underlying ventricular rate[8,9] and can contribute to heart failure. People with acute atrial fibrillation who present with heart failure have worse prognoses. **Stroke:** Acute atrial fibrillation is associated with a risk of imminent stroke.[10–13] One case series used transoesophageal echocardiography in people who had developed acute atrial fibrillation within the preceding 48 hours; 15% had atrial thrombi.[14] An ischaemic stroke associated with atrial fibrillation is more likely to be fatal, have a recurrence, and leave a serious functional deficit among survivors than a stroke not associated with atrial fibrillation.[15]

AIMS OF INTERVENTION To reduce symptoms, morbidity, and mortality, with minimum adverse effects.

OUTCOMES Major outcomes include measures of symptoms, recurrent strokes, or transient ischaemic attacks; thromboembolism; mortality; and major bleeding. Proxy measures include heart rhythm, ventricular rate, and time to restoration of sinus rhythm. Frequent spontaneous reversion to sinus rhythm makes it difficult to interpret short term studies of rhythm; treatments may accelerate restoration of sinus rhythm without increasing the proportion of people who eventually convert. The clinical importance of changes in mean heart rate is also unclear.

METHODS *Clinical Evidence* search and appraisal October 2003. Current contents, textbooks, review articles, and recent abstracts were reviewed. Many studies were not solely in people with acute atrial fibrillation. The text indicates where results have been extrapolated from studies of paroxysmal, persistent, or permanent atrial fibrillation. Atrial fibrillation that follows coronary surgery was excluded. We found no RCTs that reported on quality of life, functional capacity, or mortality.

QUESTION **What are the effects of interventions to prevent embolism in people with acute atrial fibrillation who are haemodynamically stable?**

OPTION **ANTITHROMBOTIC TREATMENT BEFORE CARDIOVERSION**

We found no RCTs on use of aspirin, heparin, or warfarin as thromboprophylaxis before attempted cardioversion in acute atrial fibrillation.

Benefits: We found no RCTs on use of aspirin, heparin, or warfarin as thromboprophylaxis before cardioversion in acute atrial fibrillation.

Harms: We found no RCTs.

Comment: There is consensus to give heparin to people who undergo cardioversion within 48 hours of the onset of arrhythmia, but we found insufficient evidence from trials. The decision to give anticoagulation both in the short term and after cardioversion is usually based on an individual's intrinsic risk of thromboembolism.[16] Warfarin is not used as an anticoagulant in acute atrial fibrillation because of its slow onset of action. One transoesophageal echocardiography study in people with a recent embolic event found left atrial thrombus in 15% of people with acute atrial fibrillation of less than 3 days' duration.[14] This would suggest that such people may benefit from formal anticoagulation or need to be evaluated by transoesophageal echocardiography before safe cardioversion. One ongoing trial is assessing the feasibility and effects of such a strategy by comparing low molecular weight and unfractionated heparin in people with atrial fibrillation of more than 2 days' duration who undergo transoesophageal echocardiographically guided early electrical or chemical cardioversion.[17]

QUESTION **What are the effects of interventions for conversion to sinus rhythm and for controlling heart rate in people with acute atrial fibrillation who are haemodynamically stable?**

OPTION DC CARDIOVERSION

We found no RCTs of DC cardioversion in acute atrial fibrillation in people who are haemodynamically stable.

Benefits: We found no systematic review. **Versus no cardioversion:** We found no RCTs. **Versus chemical conversion:** We found no RCTs.

Harms: Adverse events from synchronised DC cardioversion include those associated with a general anaesthetic, generation of a more serious arrhythmia, superficial burns, and thromboembolism.

Comment: It might be unethical to conduct RCTs of DC cardioversion in people with acute atrial fibrillation and haemodynamic compromise. The only evidence for DC cardioversion in acute atrial fibrillation is extrapolated from its use in chronic atrial fibrillationⒼ. DC cardioversion has been used for the treatment of atrial fibrillation since the 1960s.[18] Consensus is that immediate DC cardioversion for acute atrial fibrillation should be attempted only if there are signs of haemodynamic compromise.[16] Otherwise, full anticoagulation is recommended (warfarin for 3 weeks before and 4 weeks after cardioversion) to reduce the risk of thromboembolism in people with acute atrial fibrillation of more than 48 hours' duration.[16] We found insufficient evidence on whether cardioversion or rate control is superior for the treatment of acute atrial fibrillation.

OPTION AMIODARONE

We found insufficient evidence from three RCTs about the effects of amiodarone as a single agent compared with placebo for conversion to sinus rhythm in people with acute atrial fibrillation who are haemodynamically stable. Four small RCTs found no significant difference in rate of conversion to sinus rhythm at 24–48 hours for amiodarone compared with digoxin, although the studies may have lacked power to exclude clinically important differences. One small RCT found that amiodarone increased rate of cardioversion compared with verapamil at 3 hours. One RCT in people with onset of atrial fibrillation of less than 48 hours found no significant difference between intravenous amiodarone and propafenone in conversion to sinus rhythm within 1 hour. Another RCT in people with onset of atrial fibrillation of less than 2 weeks found that a higher proportion of people converted to sinus rhythm with oral propafenone within 2.5 hours compared with amiodarone but the difference did not remain significant at 24 hours. Two RCTs found that intravenous amiodarone reduced the proportion of people who reverted to sinus rhythm within 8 hours compared with oral flecainide. We found insufficient evidence to draw any conclusions between intravenous flacainide. We found insufficient evidence to draw any conclusions between intravenous flacainide and intravenous amiodarone. We found no RCTs comparing amiodarone with either DC cardioversion or diltiazem.

Benefits: **Versus placebo:** We found two systematic reviews (search dates 2001, 2 RCTs that compared amiodarone as a single agent with placebo, 104 people with acute onset atrial fibrillation)[19,20] and one subsequent RCT.[21] Both RCTs included in the reviews found no significant difference in rates of conversion from atrial fibrillation to sinus rhythm between intravenous amiodarone and placebo at 8 hours (first RCT: 40 people; cardioversion rate 37% with amiodarone 5 mg/kg bolus plus 1800 mg/day *v* 48% with placebo; P value reported as not significant, CI not reported; second RCT: 64 people; cardioversion rate 59% with amiodarone 7 mg/kg bolus *v* 56% with placebo; P value reported as not significant, CI not reported).[22,23] The subsequent RCT (72 people) found higher cardioversion rates with oral amiodarone compared with placebo at 8 hours (50% cardioverted with amiodarone 30 mg/kg/day *v* 20% with placebo; $P < 0.0001$).[21] **Versus digoxin:** We found two systematic reviews (search date 2001, 3 RCTs, 148 people with acute onset atrial fibrillation;[19] search date 2001, 3 RCTs, 114 people, no statistical pooling of results[20]). Together, the reviews identified four small RCTs (34, 45, 50, and 30 people). None found any statistically significant difference in rates of conversion to sinus between amiodarone and digoxin at 24–48 hours. **Versus diltiazem:** We found no systematic review or RCTs in people with acute atrial fibrillation. **Versus verapamil:** We found two systematic reviews (both search dates 2001, 1 RCT, 24 people).[19,20] The RCT found that amiodarone increased conversion to sinus rhythm compared with verapamil at 3 hours (AR for cardioversion 77% with amiodarone *v* 0% with intravenous verapamil; $P < 0.05$).[24] **Versus propafenone:** See benefits of propafenone, p 80. **Versus DC cardioversion:** We found no systematic review or RCTs.

Harms: **Versus placebo:** One systematic review found that the most common adverse effects of intravenous amiodarone were phlebitis, hypotension, and bradycardia.[20] Pooled adverse event rates were higher with amiodarone than placebo (AR for any adverse effect 17% with amiodarone *v* 11% with placebo). Other reported adverse effects of amiodarone in the acute setting include heart failure and arrhythmia. **Versus propafenone:** One RCT that compared amiodarone versus propafenone found no serious adverse events.[25]

Comment: The RCTs were small. Those that found no significant difference between treatments may have lacked power to detect clinically important effects.

OPTION DIGOXIN

We found no placebo controlled RCTs limited to people with acute atrial fibrillation. Three RCTs in people with atrial fibrillation of up to 7 days' duration found no significant difference between digoxin and placebo in conversion to sinus rhythm but two of the RCTs found that digoxin reduced ventricular rate after 30 minutes and after 2 hours. Four RCTs found no significant difference between amiodarone and digoxin in conversion to sinus rhythm at 24–48 hours, although these trials may have lacked power to detect clinically important differences. One RCT found that compared with digoxin, intravenous diltiazem reduced heart rate within 5 minutes in people with acute atrial fibrillation and atrial flutter.

Benefits: We found no systematic review. We found no RCTs limited to people with acute atrial fibrillation **Versus placebo:** We found three RCTs in people with atrial fibrillation of up to 7 days' duration.[26–28] One RCT (239 people within 7 days of onset of atrial fibrillation, mean age 66 years, mean ventricular rate 122 beats/minute) found that intravenous digoxin (mean 0.88 mg) did not increase the restoration of sinus rhythm at 16 hours compared with placebo (51% with digoxin *v* 46% with placebo).[26] It found a rapid and clinically important reduction in ventricular rate at 2 hours (to 105 beats/minute with digoxin *v* 117 beats/minute with placebo; P = 0.0001). The second RCT (40 people within 7 days of the onset of atrial fibrillation, mean age 64 years, 23 men) compared high dose intravenous digoxin 1.25 mg versus placebo.[27] Restoration to sinus rhythm was not significantly different (9/19 [47%] with digoxin *v* 8/20 [40%] with placebo; P = 0.6). The ventricular rate after 30 minutes was significantly lower with digoxin versus placebo (P < 0.02). The third RCT (36 people within 7 days of the onset of atrial fibrillation) compared oral digoxin (doses of 0.6, 0.4, 0.2, and 0.2 mg at 0, 4, 8, and 14 hours, or until conversion to sinus rhythm, whichever occurred first) versus placebo. Conversion to sinus rhythm at 18 hours was not significantly different (50% with digoxin *v* 44% with placebo; ARR +6%, 95% CI −11% to +22%).[28] **Versus amiodarone:** See benefits of amiodarone, p 75. **Versus diltiazem:** See benefits of diltiazem, p 76.

Harms: **Versus placebo:** In one RCT, some people developed asymptomatic bradycardia and one person with previously undiagnosed hypertrophic cardiomyopathy suffered circulatory distress.[26] In the second RCT, two people developed bradyarrhythmias.[27] No adverse effects were stated in the third RCT.[28] Digoxin at toxic doses could result in visual, gastrointestinal, and neurological symptoms; heart block; and arrhythmias. **Versus amiodarone:** Two RCTs did not report adverse events.[29,30] One RCT reported episodes of bradycardia occurring in two patients (4%) in the control group on digoxin after conversion to sinus rhythm, but this was not significantly greater than in the amiodarone group (P = 0.24).[31] The final RCT reported hypotension developing in four patients, vomiting in two patients, one episode of atrial flutter, and one episode of a transient junctional rhythm in the group given digoxin.[32] **Versus diltiazem:** The RCT was not large enough to report adverse effects adequately.

Comment: The evidence suggests that digoxin is no better than placebo for restoring sinus rhythm in people with recent onset atrial fibrillation. The peak action of digoxin is delayed for up to 6–12 hours. We found one systematic review (search date 1998)[33] and RCTs of digoxin versus placebo in people with chronic atrial fibrillation**G**, which found that control of the ventricular rate during exercise was poor unless a β blocker or rate limiting calcium channel blocker (verapamil or diltiazem) was used in combination.[34,35]

OPTION DILTIAZEM

One RCT in people with atrial fibrillation of unspecified duration or atrial flutter found that intravenous diltiazem reduced heart rate in people within 15 minutes compared with placebo. One RCT found that in people with acute atrial fibrillation and atrial flutter, intravenous diltiazem reduced heart rate within 5 minutes compared with intravenous digoxin. One RCT found no significant difference between intravenous verapamil and intravenous diltiazem (both calcium channel blockers) in rate control or measures of systolic function in people with acute atrial fibrillation or atrial flutter, but verapamil caused hypotension in some people.

Benefits: We found no systematic review but found three RCTs.[36–38] **Versus placebo:** One RCT (113 people; 89 with atrial fibrillation of unspecified duration and 24 with atrial flutter**G**; ventricular rate > 120 beats/minute; systolic blood pressure ≥ 90 mm Hg without severe heart failure; 108 people with at least one underlying condition that may explain atrial arrhythmia; mean age 64 years) compared intravenous diltiazem versus placebo.[36] After randomisation, a dose of intravenous diltiazem (or equivalent placebo) 0.25 mg/kg every 2 minutes was given; if the first dose had no effect after 15 minutes, then the code was broken and diltiazem 0.35 mg/kg every 2 minutes was given regardless of randomisation. The RCT found that intravenous diltiazem significantly decreased heart rate during a 15 minute observation period compared with placebo (ventricular rate below 100 beats/minute 42/56 [75%] with diltiazem v 4/57 [7%] with placebo; $P < 0.001$; average decrease in heart rate, 22% with diltiazem v 3% with placebo; median time from start of drug infusion to maximal decrease in heart rate 4.3 minutes; mean rate decreased from 139 beats/minute to 114 beats/minute with diltiazem).[36] The RCT found no difference in response rate to diltiazem in people with atrial fibrillation compared with those with atrial flutter. **Versus digoxin:** One RCT (30 consecutive people, 10 men, mean age 72 years, 26 with acute atrial fibrillation, four with atrial flutter, unspecified duration) compared intravenous diltiazem versus intravenous digoxin versus both drugs given on admission to the emergency department.[37] Heart rate control was defined as a ventricular rate of < 100 beats/minute. Intravenous digoxin (25 mg as a bolus at 0 and 30 minutes) and intravenous diltiazem (initially 0.25 mg/kg over the first 2 minutes, followed by 0.35 mg/kg at 15 minutes and then a titratable infusion at a rate of 10–20 mg/hour) were given to maintain heart rate control. The dosing regimens were the same whether the drugs were given alone or in combination. The RCT found that diltiazem significantly decreased ventricular heart rate within 5 minutes compared with digoxin ($P = 0.0006$; mean rates 111 beats/minute with diltiazem v 144 beats/minute with digoxin). The decrease in heart rate achieved with digoxin did not reach statistical significance until 180 minutes ($P = 0.01$; mean rates 90 beats/minute with diltiazem v 117 beats/minute with digoxin). No additional benefit was found with the combination of digoxin and diltiazem. **Versus verapamil:** See benefits of verapamil, p 83.[38]

Harms: **Versus placebo:** In one RCT, in the diltiazem treated group, seven people developed asymptomatic hypotension (systolic blood pressure < 90 mm Hg), three developed flushing, three developed itching, and one developed nausea and vomiting; these were not significantly different from placebo.[36] **Versus digoxin:** The RCT was not large enough to adequately assess adverse effects, and none were apparent.[37] **Versus verapamil:** See harms of verapamil, p 83. Rate limiting calcium channel blockers may exacerbate heart failure and hypotension.

Comment: The evidence suggests that calcium channel blockers such as verapamil and diltiazem reduce ventricular rate in acute or recent onset atrial fibrillation, but they are probably no better than placebo for restoring sinus rhythm. We found no studies of the effect of rate limiting calcium channel blockers on exercise tolerance in people with acute or recent onset atrial fibrillation, but studies in people with chronic atrial fibrillation(G) have found improved exercise tolerance.

OPTION FLECAINIDE

One RCT found that intravenous flecainide increased the proportion of people who reverted to sinus rhythm within 1 hour and in whom sinus rhythm was maintained after 6 hours compared with placebo. Flecainide has been associated with serious adverse events such as severe hypotension and torsades de pointes. Two RCTs found that oral flecainide increased the proportion of people who reverted to sinus rhythm within 8 hours compared with intravenous amiodarone. We found insufficient evidence to draw any conclusions about comparisons between intravenous flecainide and intravenous amiodarone and between flecainide and quinidine. Three RCTs

found no significant difference in rates of cardioversion to sinus rhythm between flecainide and propafenone. Flecainide and propafenone are not used in people with known or suspected ischaemic heart disease because they may cause arrhythmias.

Benefits: We found no systematic review. **Versus placebo:** We found three RCTs.[22,23,39] One single-blind RCT (62 patients, recent onset atrial fibrillation [< 1 week], found that flecainide increased the rate of conversion to sinus rhythm compared with placebo at 8 hours (20/22 patients [91%] with flecainide *v* 10/21 [48%] with placebo; P < 0.01).[22] In the second RCT (98 patients, duration of atrial fibrillation AF < 72 hours, included postsurgical patients) flecainide increased the rate of conversion to sinus rhythm by 2 hours compared with placebo (20/34 [58%] with intravenous flecainide *v* 7/32 [22%] with placebo; P = 0.007), but this difference was no longer significant at 8 hours.[23] The third RCT (102 people with recent onset atrial fibrillation [< 72 hours]) also found that intravenous flecainide significantly increased the proportion of people who reverted to sinus rhythm within 1 hour and in whom the sinus rhythm was maintained after 6 hours (reversion to sinus rhythm within 1 hour of starting treatment compared with placebo; 29/51 [57%] with flecainide *v* 7/51 [14%] with placebo; OR 8.3, 95% CI 2.9 to 24.8; maintenance of sinus rhythm after 6 hours: 34/51 [67%] *v* 18/51 [35%]; OR 3.67, 95% CI 1.50 to 9.10). Participants were randomised to receive flecainide 2 mg/kg over 30 minutes (maximum dose 150 mg) or placebo and were monitored in intensive care or coronary care units. Intravenous digoxin 500 µg over 30 minutes was given to all people who had not previously received digoxin.[39] **Versus amiodarone or propafenone:** We found five RCTs.[40–44] The first RCT (five arm study, 417 people, onset of atrial fibrillation ≤ 7 days) found no significant difference between oral flecainide and intravenous amiodarone in the proportion of people who converted to sinus rhythm at 1 and 3 hours but found a higher rate of conversion to sinus rhythm with oral flecainide at 8 hours (conversion to sinus rhythm at 1 hour: 9/69 [13%] with oral flecainide *v* 3/51 [6%] with intravenous amiodarone; RR 2.2, 95% CI 0.6 to 7.8; at 3 hours, 39/69 [57%] with oral flecainide *v* 13/51 [25%] with intravenous amiodarone; RR 2.20, 95% CI 0.96 to 1.51; and at 8 hours: 52/69 [75%] with oral flecainide *v* 29/51 [57%] with intravenous amiodarone; RR 1.30, 95% CI 1.01 to 1.74).[40] The other groups in the RCT were placebo, intravenous propafenone, and oral propafenone. The RCT found no significant difference between oral flecainide and oral propafenone in the proportion of people who converted to sinus rhythm at 1, 3, or 12 hours (at 1 hour: 9/69 [13%] with oral flecainide *v* 10/119 [8%] with oral propafenone; RR 1.55, 95% CI 0.66 to 3.63; at 3 hours: 39/69 [57%] with oral flecainide *v* 54/119 [45%] with oral propafenone; RR 1.25, 95% CI 0.94 to 1.66; at 8 hours: 52/69 [75%] with oral flecainide *v* 91/119 [76%] with oral propafenone; RR 0.99, 95% CI 0.83 to 1.17).[40] The second RCT (three arm study, 62 people aged > 75 years, onset of atrial fibrillation ≤ 7 days) found that oral flecainide significantly increased the proportion of people who converted to sinus rhythm at 8 hours compared with intravenous amiodarone (20/22 [91%] with flecainide *v* 7/19 [37%] with amiodarone; RR 2.47, 95% CI 1.35 to 4.51).[41] The RCT also found that significantly higher proportion of people converted to sinus rhythm with flecainide compared with placebo (P < 0.01).[41] The third RCT (three arm study, 150 people, onset of atrial fibrillation ≤ 48 hours) found that intravenous flecainide significantly increased the proportion of people who converted to sinus rhythm at 1, 8, and 12 hours compared with intravenous amiodarone (at 1 hour: 29/50 [58%] with flecainide *v* 7/50 [14%] with amiodarone; RR 4.14, 95% CI 2.00 to 8.57; at 8 hours: 41/50 [82%] with flecainide *v* 21/50 [42%] with amiodarone; RR 1.95, 95% CI 1.38 to 2.77; at 12 hours:

45/50 [90%] with flecainide v 32/50 [64%] with amiodarone; RR 1.41, 95% CI 1.12 to 1.77).[44] The RCT found no significant difference between intravenous flecainide and intravenous propafenone in the proportion of people who converted to sinus rhythm at 1 and 8 hours. It found a significantly higher conversion rate at 12 hours with flecainide compared with propafenone (at 1 hour, 29/50 [58%] with flecainide v 30/50 [60%] with propafenone; RR 0.97, 95% CI 0.70 to 1.34; at 8 hours: 41/50 [82%] with flecainide v 34/50 [68%] with propafenone; RR 1.21, 95% CI 0.96 to 1.51; and at 12 hours: 45/50 [90%] with flecainide v 36/50 [72%] with propafenone; RR 1.25, 95% CI 1.03 to 1.52).[39] The fourth RCT (three arm study, 98 people, onset of atrial fibrillation ≤ 72 hours) found no significant difference between intravenous flecainide and intravenous amiodarone in the proportion of people who converted to sinus rhythm within 2 hours (20/34 [59%] with flecainide v 11/32 [34%] with amiodarone; RR 1.71, 95% CI 0.98 to 2.98). The RCT also found that significantly higher proportion of people converted to sinus rhythm with flecainide compared with placebo within 2 hours (20/34 [59%] with flecainide v 7/32 [22%] with placebo; RR 2.69, 95% CI 1.32 to 5.48).[42] The fifth RCT (three arm study, 352 people) found significantly faster conversion to sinus rhythm with intravenous flecainide within 1 hour after treatment compared with propafenone (72.5% with flecainide v 54.3% with propafenone; P = 0.05; absolute numbers not given).[43] **Versus quinidine:** One small RCT found insufficient evidence to draw any conclusions about the effectiveness of flecainide versus quinidine for conversion to sinus rhythm (60 people aged 16–92 years, of whom 36 people had atrial fibrillation < 10 days; conversion to sinus rhythm [time period not given], 18/21 [86%] with flecainide v 12/15 [80%] with quinidine; RR 1.07, 95% CI 0.79 to 1.46).[45]

Harms: **Versus placebo:** One RCT reported an asymptomatic pause of 9.3 seconds in a patient who took flecainide.[22] The second RCT reported hypotension during the study period but this was not significantly different between flecainide and placebo (8/34 [24%] of patients in the flecainide group versus 8/32 [25%] with placebo).[23] However, another RCT found that a higher proportion of people developed severe hypotension (a decrease in systolic arterial pressure by ≥ 33%) with flecainide compared with placebo (11/51 [22%] with flecainide v 3/51 [6%] with placebo; OR 4.40, 95% CI 1.03 to 18.60). One person in the flecainide group with no history of ventricular arrhythmia and a normal QT interval developed torsades de pointes.[39]

Comment: Following the increased mortality observed in post-myocardial infarction patients randomised to flecainide or ecainide in the Cardiac Arrhythmia Suppression Trial, flecainide is not used for the treatment of atrial fibrillation in patients with known ischaemic heart disease because of the risk of proarrhythmia.[46]

OPTION PROPAFENONE

One systematic review and subsequent RCTs have found that propafenone increased the proportion of people converting to sinus rhythm within 1–4 hours compared with placebo. One RCT in people with onset of atrial fibrillation of less than 48 hours found no significant difference between intravenous propafenone and amiodarone in the proportion of people who converted to sinus rhythm within 1 hour. Another RCT in people with onset of atrial fibrillation of less than 2 weeks found that a higher proportion of people converted to sinus rhythm with oral propafenone within 2.5 hours compared with amiodarone but the difference did not remain significant at 24 hours. Propafenone and flecainide are not used in people with known or suspected ischaemic heart disease because they may cause arrhythmias.

Benefits: **Versus placebo:** We found one systematic review (search date 1997, 27 controlled clinical trials including some non-randomised trials, 1843 people),[47] one additional RCT,[48] and five subsequent RCTs (see table 1, p 88).[49–53] The systematic review found that people treated with propafenone were more likely to convert to sinus rhythm at 4 and 8 hours after initial treatment compared with placebo but the difference between the groups did not remain significant after 24 hours (at 4 hours: ARR 31.5%, 95% CI 24.5% to 38.5%; at 8 hours: ARR 32.9%, 95% CI 24.3% to 41.5%; P < 0.01 for both time points; at 24 hours: ARR +11.0%, 95% CI −0.6% to +22.4%; absolute numbers not given).[47] In the trials included in the systematic review, propafenone was given either intravenously (2 mg/kg as initial bolus followed by infusion) or orally (450–600 mg).[47] The systematic review included people with either acute or chronic fibrillation❻, but it did not stratify the data. The number of RCTs was not stated clearly. All of the five subsequent RCTs found propafenone to be more effective than placebo in terms of conversion to sinus rhythm within 6 hours (see table 1). The additional RCT (75 people aged 18–75 years, onset of atrial fibrillation < 72 hours) found that intravenous propafenone significantly increased the proportion of people who converted to sinus rhythm within 3 hours compared with placebo (24/41 [58.5%] with propafenone *v* 10/34 [29.4%] with placebo; OR 3.2, 95% CI 1.3 to 7.9; see table 1, p 88).[48] The first subsequent multicentre RCT (240 people, mean age 59 years with atrial fibrillation duration < 7 days) found that propafenone significantly increased the proportion of people in sinus rhythm at 3 and 8 hours after treatment compared with placebo (at 3 hours: 54/119 [45%] with propafenone *v* 22/121 [18%] with placebo; ARR 27%, 95% CI 17% to 39%; RR 2.5, 95% CI 1.6 to 3.8; at 8 hours: 91/119 [76%] with propafenone *v* 45/121 [37%] with placebo; ARR 39%, 95% CI 29% to 52%; RR 2.1, 95% CI 1.6 to 2.6; see table 1, p 88).[49] After stratification by age (≤ 60 years or > 60 years of age), the RCT found that conversion to sinus rhythm with propafenone was more likely in people aged under 60 years old compared with older people (in people ≤ 60 years of age: OR 3.78, 95% CI 1.80 to 7.92 at 3 hours *v* OR 4.74, 95% CI 2.12 to 10.54 at 8 hours; in people aged > 60 years of age: OR 5.03, 95% CI 2.08 to 12.12 at 3 hours *v* OR 6.75, 95% CI 3.38 to 73.86 at 8 hours).[54] The second subsequent RCT (55 people, mean age 59 years, duration of atrial fibrillation < 7 days) found that a significantly higher proportion of people converted to sinus rhythm within 2 hours with propafenone compared with placebo, and the significant difference was maintained up to 6 hours but not at 12 or 24 hours (at 2 hours: 12/29 [41%] with propafenone *v* 2/26 [8%] with placebo, P = 0.005; at 6 hours: 65% with propafenone *v* 31% with placebo, P = 0.015; at 12 hours: 69% with propafenone *v* 31% with placebo, P = 0.06; and at 24 hours: 79% with propafenone *v* 73% with placebo, P = 0.75; see table 1, p 88).[50] The third subsequent RCT (156 people aged 18–80 years, onset of atrial fibrillation < 72 hours) found that intravenous propafenone significantly increased the proportion of people who converted to sinus rhythm within 2 hours compared with placebo: 57/81 [70.3%] with propafenone *v* 13/75 [17.3%] with placebo; ARR 53%, 95% CI 42% to 68%; RR 4.06, 95% CI 2.43 to 6.79; (see table 1, p 88).[51] The fourth subsequent RCT (123 people, onset of atrial fibrillation < 72 hours) found that intravenous or oral propafenone significantly increased the proportion of people who converted to sinus rhythm within 1 and 4 hours but not at 8 hours after initial treatment compared with placebo (within 1 hour: 25/81 [31%] with propafenone *v* 7/42 with placebo [17%]; RR 1.85, 95% CI 0.87 to 3.92; within 4 hours, 49/81 [61%] with propafenone *v* 14/42 [33%] with placebo; RR 1.82, 95% CI 1.14 to 2.88; and within 8 hours: 53/81 [65%] *v* 20/42 [48%]; RR 1.37, 95% CI 0.96 to 1.96; see table 1, p 88).[52] The RCT also found that the time to conversion to sinus rhythm was significantly shorter with intravenous propafenone compared with oral propafenone (1 hour: 19/40 [48%] with intravenous propafenone *v* 6/41 [15%] with oral propafenone; RR 3.25, 95% CI 1.45 to 7.28; within 4 hours: 20/40 [50%] with intravenous propafenone *v* 29/41 [71%] with oral propafenone; RR 0.71, 95% CI 0.49 to 1.02; see table 1, p 88).[52] The fifth subsequent RCT (three arm study, 123 people aged 18–75 years, onset of atrial fibrillation < 72 hours) found that a significantly higher proportion of people converted to sinus rhythm with propafenone compared with placebo but found no significant difference between digoxin and placebo conversion to sinus rhythm with 1 hour (20/41 [49%] with propafenone *v* 6/42 [14%] with placebo; RR 3.42, 95% CI 1.53 to 7.63; 13/40 [33%] with digoxin *v* 6/42 [14%] with placebo; RR 2.28, 95% CI 0.96 to 5.40; see table 1, p 88).[53] After 1 hour, people who had not converted to sinus rhythm were switched to the alternative drug (see table 1, p 88).[53] **Versus amiodarone:** We found no systematic review. We found two RCTs.[25,55] The first RCT (three arm study, 143 people, onset of atrial fibrillation < 48 hours) found no significant difference between intravenous propafenone and amiodarone in the proportion of people who converted to sinus rhythm within 1 hour (36/46 [78.2%] with propafenone *v* 40/48 [83.3%] with amiodarone; RR 0.94, 95% CI 0.77 to 1.15).[55] The RCT also found that a significantly higher proportion of people converted to sinus rhythm within 1 hour with propafenone and amiodarone than with placebo; (36/46 [78.2%] with propafenone *v* 27/49 [55.1%] with placebo; RR 1.42, 95% CI 1.06 to 1.91; 40/48 [83.3%] with amiodarone *v* 27/49 [55.0%] with placebo; RR 1.51, 95% CI 1.14 to 2.01). Intravenous propafenone was given as 2 mg/kg in 15 minutes then 10 mg/kg in 24 hours. Amiodarone was given as 300 mg in 1 hour then 20 mg/kg over 24 hours plus 1800 mg daily in three oral doses.[55] The second RCT (86 people, onset of atrial fibrillation < 2 weeks) found a faster rate of conversion to sinus rhythm with oral propafenone compared with amiodarone but no significant difference in the proportion of people who converted to sinus rhythm at 24 and 48 hours (median time to sinus rhythm; 2.4 hours with propafenone *v* 6.9 hours with amiodarone; P = 0.05; conversion to sinus rhythm at 24 hours, 56% with propafenone *v* 47% with amiodarone; NS, results presented graphically).[25] **Versus flecainide:** See benefits of flecainide, p 78.

Harms: **Versus placebo:** The systematic review did not comment on adverse events.[47] One RCT that included people with structural heart disease and hypertension found no significant difference between propafenone and placebo in terms of adverse events (sustained atrial flutter**G** or tachycardia lasting > 1 minute: 8/119 [7%] with propafenone *v* 7/121 [6%] with placebo, P > 0.2; pauses of > 2 seconds: 1/119 [1%] with propafenone *v* 3/121 [2%] with placebo, P > 0.2). No cases of ventricular proarrhythmia were reported.[49] Five other RCTs that compared propafenone versus placebo reported no serious adverse events.[48,50–52,54] **Other comparisons:** We found one RCT (246 people with onset of atrial fibrillation < 48 hours) that evaluated the safety of an oral loading dose of propafenone (600 mg for > 60 kg body weight, then 300 mg if persistent) compared with that of digoxin plus propafenone, digoxin plus quinidine, or placebo.[56] The RCT found no serious adverse events. The RCT found transient atrial flutter (13/66 [20%] with propafenone *v* 12/70 [17%] with digoxin plus propafenone *v* 9/70 [13%] with digoxin plus quinidine *v* 3/40 [8%] with placebo), asymptomatic salvos of up to four ventricular beats (4/70 [6%] with digoxin plus propafenone *v* 1/70 [1%] with digoxin plus quinidine), transient left bundle branch block (3/66 [5%] with propafenone *v* 2/70 [3%] with digoxin plus propafenone *v* 2/70 [3%] digoxin plus quinidine), transient Wenkebach 2 : 1 heart block (2/66 [3%] with propafenone *v* 2/70 [3%]

with digoxin plus quinidine), and transient mild hypotension (5/66 [8%] propafenone *v* 1/70 [1%] digoxin plus quinidine). The RCT found no significant difference between groups for non-cardiac adverse events such as nausea, headache, gastrointestinal disturbance, dizziness, and paraesthesia.[56]

Comment: Extrapolation of the results of the cardiac arrhythmia suppression trial mean that other class 1c antiarrhythmic agents including propafenone tend not to be used in patients with ischaemic heart disease because of concerns over a possible increase in proarrhythmic effects in this group of people.[46] In addition, the increased frequency of cardiac adverse events with long term propafenone noted in people with structural heart disease means that trials in acute atrial fibrillation have, for the main part, excluded people with significant heart disease.[57]

OPTION QUINIDINE

We found no RCTs that compared quinidine versus placebo. One small RCT in people with onset of atrial fibrillation of less than 48 hours found that quinidine plus digoxin increased the proportion of people converting to sinus rhythm within 12 hours compared with sotalol. We found insufficient evidence to draw any conclusions about comparisons between flecainide and quinidine.

Benefits: We found no systematic review. **Versus placebo:** We found no RCTs that compared quinidine versus placebo. **Quinidine plus digoxin versus sotalol:** One small RCT (61 people aged 18–75 years, mean age about 54 years, with recent onset atrial fibrillation of < 48 hours) found that quinidine plus digoxin significantly increased the proportion of people who converted to sinus rhythm within 12 hours compared with sotalol (24/28 [85.7%] with quinidine plus digoxin *v* 17/33 [51.5%] with sotalol; ARR 34%, 95% CI 16% to 58%; RR 1.66, 95% CI 1.16 to 2.39; NNT 3, 95% CI 2 to 6).[58] Quinidine was given as 200 mg orally up to three times with 2 hour intervals, and up to 0.75 mg of digoxin was given intravenously if the initial heart rate was greater than 100 beats/minute. Sotalol 80 mg was given orally, and the dose was repeated at 2, 6, and 10 hours after the initial dose if sinus rhythm was not achieved.[58] **Versus flecainide:** See benefits of flecainide, p 78.

Harms: One RCT reported broad complex tachycardia in 7/28 (27%) people with quinidine plus digoxin compared with 4/33 (13%) people with sotalol. Electrocardiogram R-R interval prolongation was also reported in both groups (total three people, longest R–R 3.8 seconds with digoxin plus quinidine *v* 6.4 seconds with sotalol).[58]

Comment: None.

OPTION SOTALOL

We found no RCTs comparing sotalol versus placebo. One small RCT in people with onset of atrial fibrillation of less than 48 hours found that quinidine plus digoxin increased the proportion of people converting to sinus rhythm within 12 hours compared with sotalol.

Benefits: **Versus placebo:** We found no systematic review or RCTs that compared sotalol versus placebo in people with acute atrial fibrillation for conversion to sinus rhythm or heart rate control. **Versus quinidine plus digoxin:** See benefits of quinidine, p 82.

Harms: We found no RCTs that compared sotalol versus placebo.

Comment: We found one systematic review (search date 1996) that identified one open label RCT in people with acute atrial fibrillation.[59] The RCT compared oral sotalol 80 mg versus quinidine, but digoxin was also given to people with a heart rate of less than 100 beats/minute in the quinidine group. The RCT found insufficient evidence to draw any conclusions.[59] We also found another systematic review that compared β blockers with placebo in people with acute or chronic atrial fibrillation**G**.[33] See comment on timolol, p 83.

OPTION TIMOLOL

We found no RCTs limited to people with acute atrial fibrillation. One small RCT found that timolol (a β blocker) reduced ventricular rate within 20 minutes compared with placebo.

Benefits: We found no systematic review. **Versus placebo:** We found no RCTs limited to people with acute atrial fibrillation. We found one RCT (61 people with atrial fibrillation of unspecified duration, ventricular rate > 120 beats/minute) that compared intravenous timolol 1 mg (a β blocker) versus intravenous placebo given immediately and repeated twice at 20 minute intervals if sinus rhythm was not achieved.[60] It found that 20 minutes after the last injection, intravenous timolol significantly increased the proportion of people who had a ventricular rate below 100 beats/minute compared with placebo (41% with timolol *v* 3% with placebo; $P < 0.01$).

Harms: In the RCT, the most common adverse effects were bradycardia (2%) and hypotension (9%).[60] β Blockers may exacerbate heart failure and hypotension in acute atrial fibrillation. β Blockers plus rate limiting calcium channel blockers (diltiazem and verapamil) may increase the risk of asystole and sinus arrest.[61–63] β Blockers can precipitate bronchospasm.[64]

Comment: We found one systematic review of β blockers versus placebo in people with acute or chronic atrial fibrillation**G**.[33] It found that in 7/12 (58%) comparisons at rest and in all during exercise, β blockers reduced ventricular rate compared with placebo.

OPTION VERAPAMIL

Two RCTs found that intravenous verapamil reduced heart rate at 10 or 30 minutes compared with placebo in people with atrial fibrillation or atrial flutter. One RCT found no significant difference between intravenous verapamil and intravenous diltiazem in rate control or measures of systolic function in people with acute atrial fibrillation or atrial flutter, but verapamil caused hypotension in some people. One small RCT found that amiodarone increased cardioversion rate compared with verapamil at 3 hours.

Benefits: We found no systematic review in people with acute atrial fibrillation. **Versus placebo:** We found two RCTs.[65,66] Both found that that intravenous verapamil reduced heart rate at 10 or 30 minutes compared with placebo in people with atrial fibrillation or atrial flutter. The first RCT (21 men with atrial fibrillation and a rapid ventricular rate, age 37–70 years) was a crossover comparison of intravenous verapamil versus placebo (saline).[65] It found that intravenous verapamil reduced ventricular rate within 10 minutes compared with placebo (reduction > 15% of the initial rate: 17/20 [85%] with verapamil *v* 2/14 [14%] with saline; $P < 0.001$). The second RCT (double blind, crossover study of 20 people with atrial fibrillation or atrial flutter**G** for 2 hours to 2 years) compared intravenous low dose verapamil 0.075 mg/kg versus placebo.[66] A positive response was defined as conversion to sinus rhythm or a decrease of the ventricular response to less than 100 beats a minute or by more than 20% of the initial rate. If a positive response did not occur within 10 minutes, then a second bolus injection was given (placebo for people who initially received verapamil, and verapamil for people who initially received placebo). With the first bolus injection, verapamil versus placebo significantly reduced ventricular rate (mean heart rate 118 beats/minute with verapamil *v* 138 with placebo), and more people converted to sinus rhythm within 30 minutes but the difference was not significant (3/20 [15%] with verapamil *v* 0/15 [0%] with placebo; P = 0.12). **Versus diltiazem:** We found one small double blind, crossover RCT (17 men, five with acute atrial fibrillation, 10 with atrial flutter, and two with a combination of atrial fibrillation and atrial flutter; ventricular rate ≥ 120 beats/minute, systolic blood pressure > 100 mm Hg) compared intravenous verapamil versus intravenous diltiazem.[38] It found no significant differences in rate control or measures of systolic function. **Versus amiodarone:** See benefits of amiodarone, p 74.

Harms: **Versus placebo:** One RCT reported that intravenous verapamil caused a transient drop in systolic and diastolic blood pressure greater than with placebo (saline), which did not require treatment, but it did not state the number of people affected.[65] The second RCT reported development of 1:1 flutter in one person with previous Wolff Parkinson White syndrome**G** and 2:1 flutter.[66] **Versus diltiazem:** In the third RCT, which compared verapamil versus diltiazem, 3/17 (18%) people who received verapamil as the first drug developed symptomatic hypotension and were withdrawn from the study before crossover.[38] Two people recovered, but the episode in the third person was considered to be life threatening. In people with Wolff Parkinson White syndrome, verapamil may increase ventricular rate and can cause ventricular arrhythmias.[67] Rate limiting calcium channel blockers may exacerbate heart failure and hypotension.

Comment: See comment on diltiazem, p 77.

GLOSSARY

Atrial flutter A similar arrhythmia to atrial fibrillation but the atrial electrical activity is less chaotic and has a characteristic saw tooth appearance on an electrocardiogram.

Chronic atrial fibrillation Refers to more sustained or recurrent forms of atrial fibrillation, which can be subdivided into paroxysmal, persistent, or permanent atrial fibrillation.

Paroxysmal atrial fibrillation If the atrial fibrillation recurs intermittently with sinus rhythm, with spontaneous recurrences or termination, it is designated as "paroxysmal", and the objective of management is suppression of paroxysms and maintenance of sinus rhythm.

Permanent atrial fibrillation If cardioversion is inappropriate, and has not been indicated or attempted, atrial fibrillation is designated as "permanent", where the objective of management is rate control and antithrombotic treatment.

Persistent atrial fibrillation When atrial fibrillation is more sustained than paroxysmal, atrial fibrillation is designated "persistent" and needs termination with pharmacological treatment or electrical cardioversion.

Torsades de pointes A form of ventricular tachycardia with atypical QRS complexes ECG pattern.

Wolff Parkinson White syndrome Occurs when an additional electrical pathway exists between the atria and ventricles as a result of anomalous embryonic development. The extra pathway may cause rapid arrhythmias. Worldwide it affects about 0.2% of the general population. In people with Wolff Parkinson White syndrome, β blockers, calcium channel blockers, and digoxin can increase the ventricular rate and cause ventricular arrhythmias.

REFERENCES

1. Benjamin EJ, Wolf PA, Kannel WA. The epidemiology of atrial fibrillation. In: Falk RH, Podrid P, eds. *Atrial fibrillation: mechanisms and management.* 2nd ed. Philadelphia: Lippincott-Raven Publishers, 1997:1–22.
2. Lip GYH, Tean KN, Dunn FG. Treatment of atrial fibrillation in a district general hospital. *Br Heart J* 1994;71:92–95.
3. Zarifis J, Beevers DG, Lip GYH. Acute admissions with atrial fibrillation in a British multiracial hospital population. *Br J Clin Pract* 1997;51:91–96.
4. Stewart FM, Singh Y, Persson S, et al. Atrial fibrillation: prevalence and management in an acute general medical unit. *Aust N Z J Med* 1999;29:51–58.
5. Kannel WB, Wolf PA, Benjamin EJ, et al. Prevalence, incidence, prognosis, and predisposing conditions for atrial fibrillation: population-based estimates. *Am J Cardiol* 1998;82:2N–9N.
6. Furlanello F, Bertoldi A, Dallago M, et al. Atrial fibrillation in elite athletes. *J Cardiovasc Electrophysiol* 1998;9(8 suppl):63–68.
7. Pedersen OD, Bagger H, Kober L, et al. The occurrence and prognostic significance of atrial fibrillation/flutter following acute myocardial infarction. TRACE Study group. TRAndolapril Cardiac Evaluation. *Eur Heart J* 1999;20:748–754.
8. Clark DM, Plumb VJ, Epstein AE, et al. Hemodynamic effects of an irregular sequence of ventricular cycle lengths during atrial fibrillation. *J Am Coll Cardiol* 1997;30:1039–1045.
9. Schumacher B, Luderitz B. Rate issues in atrial fibrillation: consequences of tachycardia and therapy for rate control. *Am J Cardiol* 1998;82:29N–36N.
10. Peterson P, Godfredson J, Embolic complications in paroxysmal atrial fibrillation. *Stroke* 1986;17:622–626.
11. Sherman DG, Goldman L, Whiting RB, et al. Thromboembolism in patients with atrial fibrillation. *Arch Neurol* 1984;41:708–710.
12. Wolf PA, Kannel WB, McGee DL, et al. Duration of atrial fibrillation and imminence of stroke: the Framingham study. *Stroke* 1983;14:664–667.
13. Corbalan R, Arriagada D, Braun S, et al. Risk factors for systemic embolism in patients with paroxysmal atrial fibrillation. *Am Heart J* 1992;124:149–153.
14. Stoddard ME, Dawkins PR, Prince CR, et al. Left atrial appendage thrombus is not uncommon in patients with acute atrial fibrillation and a recent embolic event: a transesophageal echocardiographic study. *J Am Coll Cardiol* 1995;25:452–459.
15. Lin HJ, Wolf PA, Kelly-Hayes M, et al. Stroke severity in atrial fibrillation. The Framingham Study. *Stroke* 1996;27:1760–1764.
16. Fuster V, Ryden LE, Asinger RW, et al. ACC/AHA/ESC guidelines for the management of patients with atrial fibrillation: executive summary. *Circulation* 2001;104:2118–2150.
17. Murray RD, Shah A, Jasper SE, et al. Transoesophageal echocardiography guided enoxaparin antithrombotic strategy for cardioversion of atrial fibrillation: the ACUTE II pilot study. *Am Heart J* 2000;139:1–7.
18. Lown B, Amarasingham R, Neuman J. Landmark article Nov 3, 1962: new method for terminating cardiac arrhythmias. Use of synchronised capacitator discharge. *JAMA* 1986:256;621–627.
19. Slavik RS, Tisdale JE, Borzak S. Pharmacological conversion of atrial fibrillation: a systematic review of available evidence. *Prog Cardiovasc Dis* 2001;44:121–152. Search date 2001; primary sources Medline, Embase, Current Contents, reference lists, recent review articles, personal files, experts in the field, and manual searching.
20. Hilleman DE, Spinler SA. Conversion of recent onset atrial fibrillation with intravenous amiodarone: a meta-analysis of randomised control trials. *Pharmacotherapy* 2002;22:66–74. Search date 2001; primary sources Medline, pertinent reviews, and references.
21. Peuhkurinen K, Niemela M, Ylitalo A, et al. Effectiveness of amiodarone as a single oral dose for recent onset atrial fibrillation. *Am J Cardiol* 2000;85:462–465.
22. Capucci A, Lenzi T, Boriani G, et al. Effectiveness of loading oral flecainide for converting recent onset atrial fibrillation to sinus rhythm in patients without organic heart disease or with only systemic hypertension. *Am J Cardiol* 1992;70:69–72.
23. Donovan KD, Power BM, Hockings BE, et al. Intravenous flecainide versus amiodarone for recent onset atrial fibrillation. *Am J Cardiol* 1995;75:693–697.
24. Noc M, Stager D, Horrat M. Intravenous amiodarone versus verapamil for acute cardioversion of paroxysmal atrial fibrillation to sinus rhythm. *Am J Cardiol* 1990;65:679–680.
25. Blanc JJ, Voinov C, Maarek M. Comparison of oral loading dose of propafenone and amiodarone for converting recent-onset atrial fibrillation. PARSIFAL Study Group. *Am J Cardiol* 1999;84:1029–1032.
26. Digitalis in Acute AF (DAAF) Trial Group. Intravenous digoxin in acute atrial fibrillation. Results of a randomized, placebo-controlled multicentre trial in 239 patients. *Eur Heart J* 1997;18:649–654.
27. Jordaens L, Trouerbach J, Calle P, et al. Conversion of atrial fibrillation to sinus rhythm and rate control by digoxin in comparison to placebo. *Eur Heart J* 1997;18:643–648.
28. Falk RH, Knowlton AA, Bernard SA, et al. Digoxin for converting recent-onset atrial fibrillation to sinus rhythm. *Ann Intern Med* 1987;106:503–506.
29. Hou ZY, Chang MS, Chen CY, et al. Acute treatment of recent-onset atrial fibrillation and flutter with a tailored dosing regimen of intravenous amiodarone. A randomised, digoxin controlled study. *Eur Heart J* 1995;16:521–528.
30. Vardas PE, Kochiadakis GE, Igoumendis NE, et al. Amiodarone as a first choice drug for restoring sinus rhythm in patients with atrial fibrillation: a randomised controlled trial. *Chest* 2000; 117: 1538–1545.
31. Cotter G, Blatt A, Metzkor-Cotter E, et al. Conversion of recent onset paroxysmal atrial fibrilation to normal sinus rhythm: the effect of no treatment and high-dose amiodarone. A randomised placebo-controlled study. *Eur Heart J* 1999;20:1833–1842
32. Galve E, Rius T, Ballester R, et al. Intravenous amiodarone in treatment of recent onset atrial fibrillation: results of a randomised controlled study. *J Am Coll Cardiol* 1996;27:1079–1082.
33. McNamara RL, Bass EB, Miller MR, et al. Management of new onset atrial fibrillation. Evidence Report/Technology Assessment No. 12 (prepared by the John Hopkins University Evidence-based Practice Center in Baltimore, MD, under contract no. 290–97–0006). AHRQ publication number 01-E026. Rockville, MD: Agency for Healthcare Research and Quality. January 2001. Search date 1998; primary sources The Cochrane Library, Medline, Pubmed's "related links" feature, reviews of Cochrane hand search results, hand searches of reference lists, and scanning of tables of contents from relevant journals.
34. Farshi R, Kistner D, Sarma JS, et al. Ventricular rate control in chronic atrial fibrillation during daily activity and programmed exercise: a crossover open-label study of five drug regimens. *J Am Coll Cardiol* 1999;33:304–310.

35. Klein HO, Pauzner H, Di Segni E, et al. The beneficial effects of verapamil in chronic atrial fibrillation. *Arch Intern Med* 1979;139:747–749.

36. Salerno DM, Dias VC, Kleiger RE, et al. Efficacy and safety of intravenous diltiazem for treatment of atrial fibrillation and atrial flutter: the Diltiazem-Atrial Fibrillation/Flutter Study Group. *Am J Cardiol* 1989;63:1046–1051.

37. Schreck DM, Rivera AR, Tricarico VJ. Emergency management of atrial fibrillation and flutter: intravenous diltiazem versus intravenous digoxin *Ann Emerg Med* 1997;29:135–140.

38. Phillips BG, Gandhi AJ, Sanoski CA, et al. Comparison of intravenous diltiazem and verapamil for the acute treatment of atrial fibrillation and atrial flutter. *Pharmacotherapy* 1997;17:1238–1245.

39. Donovan KD, Dobb GJ, Coombs LJ, et al. Efficacy of flecainide for the reversion of acute onset atrial fibrillation. *Am J Cardiol* 1992;70:50A–55A.

40. Boriani G, Biffa M, Cappuci A, et al. Conversion of recent-onset atrial fibrillation to sinus rhythm: effects of different drug protocols. *Pacing Clin Electrophysiol* 1998;21:2470–2474.

41. Capucci A, Lenzi T, Boriani G, et al. Effectiveness of loading oral flecainide for converting recent-onset atrial fibrillation to sinus rhythm in patients without organic heart disease or with only systemic hypertension. *Am J Cardiol* 1992;70:69–72.

42. Donovan KD, Power BM, Hockings BE, et al. Intravenous flecainide versus amiodarone for recent-onset atrial fibrillation. *Am J Cardiol* 1995;75:693–697.

43. Romano S, Fattore L, Toscano G, et al. Effectiveness and side effects of the treatment with propafenone and flecainide for recent-onset atrial fibrillation. *Ital Heart J* 2001;2(suppl):41–45. [Italian]

44. Martinez-Marcos FJ, Garcia-Garmendia JL, Ortega-Carpio A, et al. Comparison of intravenous flecainide, propafenone, and amiodarone for conversion of acute atrial fibrillation to sinus rhythm. *Am J Cardiol* 2000;86:950–953.

45. Borgeat A, Goy JJ, Maendley R, et al. Flecainide versus quinidine for the conversion of atrial fibrillation to sinus rhythm. *Am J Cardiol* 1986;58:496–498.

46. Akiyama T, Pawitan Y, Greenberg H, et al. Increased risk of death and cardiac arrest from encainide and flecainide in patients after non-Q-wave acute myocardial infarction in the Cardiac Arrhythmia Suppression Trial. CAST Investigators. *Am J Cardiol* 1991;68:1551–1555.

47. Reimold SC, Maisel WH, Antman EM, et al. Propafenone for the treatment of supraventricular tachycardia and atrial fibrillation: a meta-analysis. *Am J Cardiol* 1998;82:66N–71N. Search date 1997; primary sources Medline and Paperchase.

48. Fresco P, Proclemer A, Pavan A, et al. Intravenous propafenone in paroxysmal atrial fibrillation: a randomized, placebo-controlled, double-blind multicenter clinical trial. Paroxysmal Atrial Fibrillation Italian Trial (PAFIT)-2 Investigators. *Clin Cardiol* 1996;19:409–412.

49. Boriani G, Biffi M, Capucci A, et al. Oral propafenone to convert recent-onset atrial fibrillation in patients with and without underlying heart disease. A randomized, controlled trial. *Ann Intern Med* 1997;126:621–625.

50. Azpitarte J, Alverez M, Baun O, et al. Value of a single oral loading dose of propafenone in converting recent-onset atrial fibrillation. Results of a randomized, double-blind controlled study. *Eur Heart J* 1997;18:1649–1654.

51. Ganau G, Lenzi T. Intravenous propafenone for converting recent onset atrial fibrillation in emergency departments: a randomized placebo-controlled multicentre trial. FAPS Investigators Study Group. *J Emerg Med* 1998;16:383–387.

52. Botto GL, Bonini W, Broffoni T, et al. Randomized, crossover comparison of oral loading versus intravenous infusion of propafenone in recent-onset atrial fibrillation. *Pacing Clin Electrophysiol* 1998;21:2480–2484.

53. Bianconi L, Mennuni M. Comparison between propafenone and digoxin administered intravenously to patients with acute atrial fibrillation. PAFIT-3 Investigators. The Propafenone in Atrial Fibrillation Italian Trial. *Am J Cardiol* 1998;82:584–588.

54. Boriani G, Biffi M, Capucci A, et al. Oral loading with propafenone: a placebo-controlled study in elderly and nonelderly patients with recent onset atrial fibrillation. *Pacing Clin Electrophysiol* 1998;21:2465–2469.

55. Kochiadakis GE, Igoumenidis NE, Simantirakis EN, et al. Intravenous propafenone versus intravenous amiodarone in the management of atrial fibrillation of recent onset: a placebo-controlled study. *Pacing Clin Electrophysiol* 1998;21:2475–2479.

56. Capucci A, Villani GQ, Aschieri D, et al. Safety of oral propafenone in the conversion of recent onset atrial fibrillation to sinus rhythm: a prospective parallel placebo-controlled multicentre study. *Int J Cardiol* 1999;68:187–196.

57. Podrid PJ, Anderson JL, for the Propafenone Multicenter Study Group. Safety and tolerability of long term propafenone therapy for supraventricular tachyarrhythmias. *Am J Cardiol* 1996;78:430–434.

58. Halinen MO, Huttunen M, Paakinen S, et al. Comparison of sotalol with digoxin–quinidine for conversion of acute atrial fibrillation to sinus rhythm (the Sotalol-Digoxin-Quinidine Trial). *Am J Cardiol* 1995;76:495–498.

59. Ferreira E, Sunderji R, Gin K. Is oral sotalol effective in converting atrial fibrillation to sinus rhythm. *Pharmacotherapy* 1997;17:1233–1237. Search date 1996; primary sources Medline and hand searches of reference lists.

60. Sweany AE, Moncloa F, Vickers FF, et al. Antiarrhythmic effects of intravenous timolol in supraventricular arrhythmias. *Clin Pharmacol Ther* 1985;37:124–127.

61. Lee TH, Salomon DR, Rayment CM, et al. Hypotension and sinus arrest with exercise-induced hyperkalemia and combined verapamil/propranolol therapy. *Am J Med* 1986;80:1203–1204.

62. Misra M, Thakur R, Bhandari K. Sinus arrest caused by atenolol–verapamil combination. *Clin Cardiol* 1987;10:365–367.

63. Yeh SJ, Yamamoto T, Lin FC, et al. Repetitive sinoatrial exit block as the major mechanism of drug-provoked long sinus or atrial pause. *J Am Coll Cardiol* 1991;18:587–595.

64. Doshan HD, Rosenthal RR, Brown R, et al. Celiprolol, atenolol and propranolol: a comparison of pulmonary effects in asthmatic patients. *J Cardiovasc Pharmacol* 1986;8(suppl 4):105–108.

65. Aronow WS, Ferlinz J. Verapamil versus placebo in atrial fibrillation and atrial flutter. *Clin Invest Med* 1980;3:35–39.

66. Waxman HL, Myerburg RJ, Appel R, et al. Verapamil for control of ventricular rate in paroxysmal supraventricular tachycardia and atrial fibrillation or flutter: a double-blind randomized cross-over study. *Ann Intern Med* 1981;94:1–6.

67. Strasberg B, Sagie A, Rechavia E, et al. Deleterious effects of intravenous verapamil in Wolff-Parkinson-White patients and atrial fibrillation. *Cardiovasc Drugs Ther* 1989;2:801–806.

Atrial fibrillation (acute)

Bethan Freestone
Research Fellow

Gregory Y H Lip
Professor of Cardiovascular Medicine
Haemostasis Thrombosis and Vascular
Biology Unit University Department of
Medicine City Hospital
Birmingham
UK

Competing interests: GYHL has been reimbursed by various pharmaceutical companies for attending several conferences, and running educational programmes and research projects. BF none declared.

TABLE 1 **RCTs comparing propafenone versus placebo in conversion to sinus rhythm in people with acute atrial fibrillation (see text, p 79).**

RCT	Population	Intervention	Control	Outcome	Time	Result
48	75 people aged 18–75 years, onset of atrial fibrillation < 72 hours	Propafenone intravenous	Placebo	Conversion to sinus rhythm	3 hours	24/41 (58.5%) with propafenone *v* 10/34 (29.4%) with placebo (OR 3.2, 95% CI 1.3 to 7.9)
49	240 people, mean age 59 years, duration of atrial fibrillation < 7 days	Propafenone	Placebo	Conversion to sinus rhythm	3 hours	54/119 (45%) with propafenone *v* 22/121 (18%) with placebo (ARR 27%, 95% CI, 17% to 39%)
					8 hours	91/119 (76%) with propafenone *v* 45/121 (37%) with placebo (ARR 39%, 95%, 29% to 52%)
50	55 people, mean age 59 years, duration of atrial fibrillation < 7 days	Propafenone	Placebo	Conversion to sinus rhythm	2 hours	12/29 (41%) with propafenone *v* 2/26 (8%) with placebo (P = 0.005)
					6 hours	65% with propafenone *v* 31% with placebo (P = 0.015)
					12 hours	69% with propafenone *v* 31% with placebo (P = 0.06)
					24 hours	79% with propafenone *v* 73% with placebo (P = 0.75)
51	156 people aged 18–80 years, onset of atrial fibrillation < 72 hours	Propafenone	Placebo	Conversion to sinus rhythm	2 hour	57/81 (70.3%) with propafenone *v* 13/75 (17.3%) with placebo (ARR 53% 95% CI, 42% to 68%, 95% CI; RR 4.06, 95% CI, 2.43 to 6.79)

TABLE 1 continued

RCT	Population	Intervention	Control	Outcome	Time	Result
52	123 people, onset of atrial fibrillation < 72 hours	Propafenone intravenous or oral	Placebo	Conversion to sinus rhythm	1 hour	25/81 (31%) with propafenone *v* 7/42 with placebo (17%) (RR 1.85, 95% CI, 0.87 to 3.92)
					4 hours	49/81 (61%) with propafenone *v* 14/42 (33%) with placebo (RR 1.82, 95% CI, 1.14 to 2.88)
					8 hours	53/81 (65%) *v* 20/42 (48%) (RR 1.37, 95% CI, 0.96 to 1.96)
					1 hour	19/40 (48%) with intravenous propafenone *v* 6/41 (15%) with oral propafenone (RR 3.25, 95% CI, 1.45 to 7.28)
		Propafenone intravenous	Propafenone oral		4 hours	20/40 (50%) with intravenous propafenone *v* 29/41 (71%) with oral propafenone (RR 0.71, 95% CI, 0.49 to 1.02)
53	Three arm study, 123 people aged 18–75 years, onset of atrial fibrillation < 72 hours	Propafenone	Placebo	Conversion to sinus rhythm	1 hour	20/41 (49%) with propafenone *v* 6/42 (14%) with placebo (RR 3.42, 95% CI, 1.53 to 7.63)

Changing behaviour

Search date September 2003

Margaret Thorogood, Melvyn Hillsdon, and Carolyn Summerbell

QUESTIONS

INTERVENTIONS

See glossary Ⓖ

Key Messages

- **Advice from physicians and trained counsellors to quit smoking** Systematic reviews have found that simple, one off advice from a physician during a routine consultation increased the proportion of smokers quitting smoking and not relapsing for 1 year. One systematic review found that advice from trained counsellors also increased quit rates compared with minimal intervention.
- **Advice on cholesterol lowering diet** Systematic reviews have found that advice on cholesterol lowering diet (i.e. advice to lower total fat intake or increase the ratio of polyunsaturated : saturated fatty acid) leads to a small reduction in blood cholesterol concentrations in the long term (≥6 months).
- **Advice on reducing sodium intake to reduce blood pressure** One systematic review found that, compared with usual care, intensive interventions to reduce sodium intake provided small reductions in blood pressure, however effects on deaths and cardiovascular events are unclear.

Clin Evid 2005;13:90–114.

- **Antidepressants (bupropion or nortriptyline) as part of a smoking cessation programme (but no evidence of benefit for selective serotonin reuptake inhibitors or moclobemide)** Systematic reviews have found that quit rates are increased by bupropion and nortriptyline given as part of a smoking cessation programme, but not by moclobemide or selective serotonin reuptake inhibitors.
- **Antismoking interventions in people at high risk of disease** (evidence that counselling or bupropion are effective in this group) Systematic reviews and four subsequent RCTs have found that antismoking advice improves smoking cessation in people at high risk of smoking related disease. We found no evidence that high intensity advice is more effective than low intensity advice in high risk people. One RCT found that bupropion increased cessation rates in smokers with cardiovascular disease.
- **Antismoking interventions for pregnant women** Two systematic reviews have found that antismoking interventions in pregnant women increase abstinence rates during pregnancy. One RCT found that nicotine patches did not significantly increase quit rates in pregnant women compared with placebo.
- **Exercise advice to women over 80 years of age** One RCT found that exercise advice delivered in the home by physiotherapists increased physical activity and reduced the risk of falling in women over 80 years.
- **Lifestyle interventions for sustained weight loss** Two large RCTs found that weight loss advice resulted in greater weight loss than no advice. One RCT found that cognitive behavioural therapy was more effective than usual care in promoting weight loss. Systematic reviews have found that using behavioural therapy to support advice on diet and exercise is probably more effective in achieving weight loss than diet advice alone. One systematic review found limited evidence that partial meal replacement plans reduced weight loss at 1 year compared with reduced calorie diet in people who completed the treatment.
- **Nicotine replacement in smokers who smoke at least 10 cigarettes daily** One systematic review found that nicotine replacement is an effective additional component of cessation strategies in smokers who smoke at least 10 cigarettes daily. We found no evidence of any particular method of nicotine delivery having superior efficacy. We found limited evidence from five RCTs (follow up 2–8 years) that the benefit of nicotine replacement treatment on quit rates decreased with time.
- **Advice from nurses to quit smoking** One systematic review found limited evidence that advice from nurses to quit smoking increased quitting at 1 year compared with no advice.
- **Counselling sedentary people to increase physical activity** We found limited evidence from systematic reviews and subsequent RCTs that counselling sedentary people increased physical activity compared with no intervention. Limited evidence from RCTs suggests that consultation with an exercise specialist rather than or in addition to a physician may increase physical activity at 1 year. We found limited evidence that interventions delivered by new media can lead to short term changes in physical activity.
- **Lifestyle interventions to maintain weight loss** One systematic review and additional RCTs have found that most types of maintenance strategy result in smaller weight gains or greater weight losses compared with no contact. Strategies that involve personal contact with a therapist, family support, walking training programmes, or multiple interventions, or are weight focused, seem most effective.
- **Self help materials for people who want to stop smoking** One systematic review found that self help materials slightly improved smoking cessation compared with no intervention. It found that individually tailored materials were more effective than standard or stage based materials. One subsequent RCT found no significant difference in abstinence rates at 6 months between self help materials based on the stages of change model and standard self help literature.
- **Telephone advice to quit smoking** One systematic review found limited evidence that telephone counselling improved quit rates compared with interventions with no personal contact.

- **Lifestyle advice to prevent weight gain** One small RCT found that low intensity education plus a financial incentive increased weight loss compared with no treatment. A second RCT found no significant effect on prevention of weight gain from a postal newsletter with or without a linked financial incentive compared with no contact. One RCT found that lifestyle advice prevented weight gain in perimenopausal women compared with assessment alone. One small RCT comparing a nutrition course for female students with no nutrition course found no significant increase in weight from baseline in either group at 1 year.
- **Physical exercise to aid smoking cessation** One systematic review found limited evidence that exercise may increase smoking cessation.
- **Training health professionals in promoting weight loss** One systematic review of poor quality RCTs provided insufficient evidence on the sustained effect of interventions to improve health professionals' management of obesity. One subsequent cluster RCT found limited evidence that training for primary care doctors in nutrition counselling plus a support programme reduced body weight of the people in their care over 1 year compared with usual care.
- **Training health professionals to give advice on smoking cessation (increases frequency of antismoking interventions, but may not improve effectiveness)** One systematic review found that training health professionals increased the frequency of antismoking interventions being offered. It found no good evidence that antismoking interventions are more effective if the health professionals delivering the interventions received training. One RCT found that a structured intervention delivered by trained community pharmacists increased smoking cessation rates compared with usual care delivered by untrained community pharmacists.
- **Acupuncture for smoking cessation** One systematic review found no significant difference between acupuncture and control in smoking cessation rates at 1 year.
- **Anxiolytics for smoking cessation** One systematic review found no significant difference in quit rates between anxiolytics and control.

DEFINITION	Cigarette smoking, diet, and level of physical activity are important in the aetiology of many chronic diseases. Individual change in behaviour has the potential to decrease the burden of chronic disease, particularly cardiovascular disease. This chapter focuses on the evidence that specific interventions lead to changed behaviour.
INCIDENCE/ PREVALENCE	In the developed world, the decline in smoking has slowed and the prevalence of regular smoking is increasing in young people. A sedentary lifestyle is becoming increasingly common and the prevalence of obesity is increasing rapidly.
AIMS OF INTERVENTION	To encourage individuals to reduce or abandon unhealthy behaviours and to take up healthy behaviours; to support the maintenance of these changes in the long term.
OUTCOMES	Ideal outcomes are clinical, and relate to the underlying conditions (longevity, quality of life, and rate of stroke or myocardial infarction). However, the focus of this chapter, and the outcomes reported by most studies, are proxy outcomes, such as the proportion of people changing behaviour (e.g. stopping smoking) in a specified period.
METHODS	*Clinical Evidence* search and appraisal September 2003.

QUESTION **What are the effects of interventions aimed at changing people's behaviour?**

OPTION ADVICE TO QUIT SMOKING

Systematic reviews have found that simple, one off advice from a physician during a routine consultation increased the proportion of smokers quitting smoking and not relapsing for 1 year. One systematic review found that advice from trained counsellors also increases quit rates compared with minimal intervention. One systematic review found limited evidence that advice to quit smoking from nurses increased quitting at 1 year compared with no advice.

One systematic review provided limited evidence that telephone counselling improved quit rates compared with interventions with no personal contact. One systematic review found that self help materials slightly improved smoking cessation compared with no intervention. It found that individually tailored materials were more effective than standard or stage based materials. One subsequent RCT found no significant difference in abstinence rates at 6 months between self help materials based on the stages of change model and standard self help literature.

Benefits: We found five systematic reviews[1–5] and two subsequent RCTs.[6,7] **Physicians:** The first review (search date 2000, 34 RCTs, 28 000 smokers) considered advice given by physicians, most often in the primary care setting, but also in hospitals and other clinics.[1] It found that brief advice improved quit rates compared with no advice (16 trials, 12 with follow up for at least 1 year; 451/7705 [5.9%] with brief advice *v* 241/5870 [4.1%] with no advice; meta-analysis OR 1.69, 95% CI 1.45 to 1.98). Intensive advice slightly improved quit rates compared with minimal advice among smokers not at high risk of disease (10 trials, 7 with follow up for at least 1 year; OR with intensive *v* minimal advice 1.23, 95% CI 1.02 to 1.49). The first subsequent RCT tested a brief (10 minute) intervention given by general practitioners who had received 2 hours of training.[6] The intervention increased the abstinence rate at 12 months (7.3% with control *v* 13.4% with intervention; $P < 0.05$). **Counsellors:** The second systematic review (search date 2002, 15 RCTs) examined individual counselling of at least 10 minutes by professionals trained in smoking cessation (social work, psychology, psychiatry, health education, and nursing).[2] Follow up was at 6–12 months. The review found that counselling increased the rate of quitting (340/2590 [13%] with counselling *v* 232/2592 [9%] with control; OR of quitting 1.64, 95% CI 1.33 to 2.01).[2] The authors did not find a greater effect of intensive counselling compared with brief counselling (3 RCTs; OR 0.98, 95% CI 0.61 to 1.56). **Nurses:** The third review (search date 2001, 22 RCTs, 5 with follow up for < 1 year) considered the effectiveness of smoking interventions delivered by a nurse. It found that advice from a nurse increased the rate of quitting by the end of follow up (meta-analysis of 18 studies: 646/4836 [13.4%] with advice *v* 405/3356 [12.1%] with control; OR 1.50, 95% CI 1.29 to 1.73).[3] However, this review did have methodological weaknesses (see comment below). **Telephone advice:** The fourth systematic review (search date 2000, 23 RCTs) considered counselling delivered by telephone.[4] Ten of the included trials (9 with follow up for at least 12 months) compared proactive telephone counselling versus minimum intervention (involving no person to person contact). Pooled analysis was not possible because of statistical heterogeneity among trials. However, three trials found that telephone counselling was significantly more effective than minimum intervention, four trials found a non-significant benefit, and none of the trials found significant harms of telephone counselling. **Self help materials:** We found one systematic review (search date 2002, 51 RCTs)[5] that examined effects of providing materials giving advice and information to smokers attempting to give up on their own and one subsequent RCT.[7] The review found that self help materials without face to face contact slightly improved smoking cessation compared with no intervention (11 RCTs, including 8 RCTs with at least 12 months' follow up; OR 1.24, 95% CI 1.07 to 1.49). Individually tailored materials were more effective than standard or stage based materials (10 RCTs; OR for cessation 1.36, 95% CI 1.13 to 1.64). The subsequent RCT (2471 smokers) found no significant difference in abstinence rates at 6 months between self help materials based on the stages of change model and standard self help literature (abstinence: OR for stage of change materials *v* standard self help material 1.53, 95% CI 0.76 to 3.10).[7]

Harms: We found no evidence of harm.

Comment: The effects of advice may seem small, but a year on year reduction of 2% in the proportion of smokers would represent a significant public health gain (see smoking cessation under primary prevention, [Web only]). In the systematic review of advice provided by nurses,[3] there was significant heterogeneity of the study results and many studies may not have been adequately randomised (7/18 [39%] studies did not specify the randomisation method and 3/18 [17%] used an inadequate form of randomisation).

OPTION NICOTINE REPLACEMENT FOR SMOKING CESSATION

One systematic review found that nicotine replacement is an effective additional component of cessation strategies. We found no evidence of any particular method of nicotine delivery having superior efficacy. We found limited evidence from five RCTs (follow up 2–8 years) that the benefit of nicotine replacement treatment on quit rates decreased with time.

Benefits: **Abstinence at 12 months:** We found one systematic review (search date 2002)[8] that identified 51 trials of nicotine chewing gum, 34 of nicotine transdermal patches, four of nicotine intranasal spray, four of inhaled nicotine, and three of sublingual tablets. All forms of nicotine replacement were more effective than placebo. When the abstinence rates for all trials were pooled according to the longest duration of follow up available, nicotine replacement increased the odds of abstinence compared with placebo (3335/19 783 [16.8%] with nicotine replacement *v* 1835/17 977 [10.2%] with placebo; OR 1.74, 95% CI 1.64 to 1.86). The review found no significant difference in abstinence with different forms of nicotine replacement in indirect comparisons (OR 1.66 for nicotine chewing gum *v* 2.27 for nicotine nasal spray) or direct comparisons (1 RCT, inhaler *v* patch; OR 0.57, 95% CI 0.19 to 1.65). In trials that directly compared 4 mg with 2 mg nicotine chewing gum, the higher dose improved abstinence in highly dependent smokers (OR 2.18, 95% CI 1.49 to 3.17). High dose patches slightly increased abstinence compared with standard dose patches (6 RCTs; OR 1.21, 95% CI 1.03 to 1.42). The review found no significant difference in effectiveness for 16 hour compared with 24 hour patches, and no difference in effect in trials where the dose was tapered compared with those where the patches were withdrawn abruptly. Use of the patch for 12 weeks was as effective as longer use and there was limited evidence that repeated use of nicotine replacement treatment in people who have relapsed after an initial course may produce further quitters, though the absolute effect was small. One included RCT (3585 people) found that abstinence at 1 week was a strong predictor of 12 month abstinence (25% of those abstinent at 1 week were abstinent at 12 months *v* 2.7% of those not abstinent at 1 week).[9] One meta-analysis of relapse rates in nicotine replacement trials found that nicotine replacement increased abstinence at 12 months, but that continued nicotine replacement did not significantly affect relapse rates between 6 weeks and 12 months.[10] **Longer term abstinence:** We found five RCTs[11–15] that found nicotine replacement did not affect long term abstinence. In one RCT that compared nicotine spray with placebo, 47 people abstinent at 1 year were followed for up to a further 2 years and 5 months, after which there was still a significant, although smaller, difference in abstinence (abstinence in the longer term 15.4% with nicotine spray *v* 9.3% with placebo; NNT [for 1 extra person to abstain] 7 at 1 year *v* 11 at 3.5 years).[11] The second RCT compared 5 months of nicotine patches plus nicotine spray versus the same patches plus a placebo spray. It found no significant difference between treatments after 6 years (16.2% abstinent with nicotine spray *v* 8.5% with placebo spray; P = 0.08).[12] The third RCT compared patches delivering different nicotine doses versus placebo patches. The trial followed everyone that quit at 6 weeks for a further 4–5 years and found no significant difference in relapse between the groups. Overall, 73% of people who quit at 6 weeks relapsed.[13] The fourth RCT followed up 840 of 1686 people, 8 years after they participated in a trial of nicotine replacement therapy.[14] It found similar rates of relapse in the active and placebo groups, with no significant difference between the groups in 8 year continuous abstinence rates (OR 1.39, 95% CI 0.89 to 2.17).[14] The fifth RCT followed 107 of 311 health care workers 5 years after they participated in a trial comparing nicotine replacement therapy versus placebo patch.[15] It found no significant difference in abstinence rates at 5 years (18% with nicotine *v* 14% with placebo; P = 0.797).

Harms: Nicotine chewing gum has been associated with hiccups, gastrointestinal disturbances, jaw pain, and orodental problems. Nicotine transdermal patches have been associated with skin sensitivity and irritation. Nicotine inhalers and nasal spray have been associated with local irritation at the site of administration. Nicotine sublingual tablets have been reported to cause hiccups, burning, smarting sensations in the mouth, sore throat, coughing, dry lips, and mouth ulcers.[16]

Comment: Nicotine replacement may not represent an "easy cure" for nicotine addiction, but it does improve the cessation rate. The evidence suggests that the most of smokers attempting cessation fail at any one attempt or relapse over the next 5 years. Multiple attempts may be needed.

OPTION ACUPUNCTURE FOR SMOKING CESSATION

One systematic review found no significant difference between acupuncture and control in smoking cessation rates at 1 year.

Benefits: We found one systematic review (search date 2002, 22 RCTs, 4158 adults, 330 young people aged 12–18 years) comparing acupuncture with sham acupuncture, other treatment, or no treatment.[17] Seven RCTs (2701 people) reported abstinence after at least 12 months. The review found no significant difference in smoking cessation with acupuncture compared with control at 12 months (OR 1.08, 95% CI 0.77 to 1.52).

Harms: None reported.

Comment: None.

OPTION PHYSICAL EXERCISE FOR SMOKING CESSATION

One systematic review found limited evidence that physical exercise may increase smoking cessation.

Benefits: We found one systematic review (search date 2002, 8 RCTs)[18] comparing exercise versus control interventions. Only one of the eight trials found evidence for exercise aiding smoking cessation. However, the trials which did not show a significant effect of exercise on smoking abstinence were too small to exclude reliably an effect of intervention and had numerous methodological limitations. One RCT (281 women) found that three exercise sessions a week for 12 weeks plus a cognitive behavioural programme**G** improved continuous abstinence from smoking at 12 months compared with the cognitive behavioural programme alone (11.9% with programme plus exercise *v* 5.4% with programme alone; OR 2.36, 95% CI 0.97 to 5.70).[19]

Harms: None reported.

Comment: None.

OPTION **ANTIDEPRESSANT AND ANXIOLYTIC TREATMENT FOR SMOKING CESSATION**

Systematic reviews have found that quit rates are increased by bupropion and nortriptyline given as part of a smoking cessation programme, but not by moclobemide, selective serotonin reuptake inhibitors, or anxiolytics.

Benefits: **Antidepressants:** We found one systematic review of antidepressants given as part of a smoking cessation programme (search date 2002, 30 RCTs).[20] Sixteen of the RCTs (7397 people) reported 12 month cessation rates. The review found that bupropion significantly increased quit rates compared with placebo at 6–12 months (data from 10 RCTs with 12 months' follow up plus 6 RCTs with 6 months' follow up; OR of quitting 1.97, 95% CI 1.67 to 2.34).[20] Two RCTs identified by the review compared bupropion plus a nicotine patch versus patch alone and found different results. One RCT (893 people) found that combined treatment improved cessation compared with patch alone (OR 2.65, 95% CI 1.58 to 4.45). The second RCT (244 people) found no significant difference (OR 0.75, 95% CI 0.59 to 3.00). Five other included RCTs (3 with 6 months' and 2 with 12 months' follow up) found that nortriptyline improved long term (6–12 month) abstinence rates compared with placebo (OR 2.80, 95% CI 1.81 to 4.32). One RCT of moclobemide found no significant difference in abstinence at 12 months. Four included RCTs of selective serotonin reuptake inhibitors found no significant effect (OR 0.97, 95% CI 0.71 to 1.32). **Anxiolytics:** We found one systematic review of anxiolytics (search date 2000, 6 RCTs).[21] Four of the RCTs (626 people) reporting 12 month cessation rates found no significant increase in abstinence between anxiolytics and control treatment.[21]

Harms: **Antidepressants:** Headache, insomnia, and dry mouth were reported in people using bupropion.[21] Nortriptyline can cause sedation and urinary retention, and can be dangerous in overdose. One large RCT found that discontinuation rates caused by adverse events were 3.8% with placebo, 6.6% for nicotine replacement treatment, 11.9% for bupropion, and 11.4% for bupropion plus nicotine replacement treatment.[22] Allergic reactions to bupropion have been reported in about 1/1000 people. **Anxiolytics:** Anxiolytics may cause dependence and withdrawal problems, tolerance, paradoxical effects, and impair driving ability.

Comment: None.

OPTION **ANTISMOKING INTERVENTIONS FOR PREGNANT WOMEN**

Two systematic reviews found that antismoking interventions in pregnant women increased abstinence rates during pregnancy. One RCT found that nicotine patches did not significantly increase quit rates in pregnant women compared with placebo.

Benefits: We found two systematic reviews[23,24] and three additional RCTs.[25–27] The most recent review (search date 1998, 44 RCTs) assessed smoking cessation interventions in pregnancy. It found that smoking cessation programmes improved abstinence (OR of continued smoking in late pregnancy with antismoking programmes *v* no programmes 0.53, 95% CI 0.47 to 0.60).[23] The findings were similar if the analysis was restricted to trials in which abstinence was confirmed by means other than self reporting. The review calculated that of 100 smokers attending a first antenatal visit, 10 stopped spontaneously and a further six or seven stopped as the result of a smoking cessation programme. Five included trials examined the effects of interventions to prevent relapse in 800 women who had quit smoking. Collectively, these trials found no evidence that the interventions reduced relapse rate.[23] One earlier systematic review (search date not reported, 10 RCTs, 4815 pregnant women)[24] of antismoking interventions included one trial of physician advice, one trial of advice by a health educator, one trial of group sessions, and seven trials of behavioural therapy based on self help manuals. Cessation rates among trials ranged from 1.9–16.7% in the control groups and from 7.1–36.1% in the intervention groups. The review found that antismoking interventions significantly increased the rate of quitting (ARI with intervention *v* no intervention 7.6%, 95% CI 4.3% to 10.8%).[24] One additional RCT found that nicotine patches did not significantly alter quit rates in pregnant women compared with placebo.[25] The second additional RCT (1120 pregnant women) compared a brief (10–15 minute) smoking intervention delivered by trained midwives at booking interviews versus usual care.[26] It found no significant difference in smoking behaviour between women receiving intervention compared with usual care (abstinence in final 12 weeks of pregnancy until birth 17% in each group; abstinence for 6 months after birth 7% with intervention *v* 8% with control). The intervention was difficult to implement (see comment below). The third additional RCT compared motivational interviewing**G** with usual care in 269 women in their 28th week of pregnancy who had smoked in the past month.[27] It found no significant differences in cessation rate between intervention and control group at 34th week or at 6 months post partum.

Harms: None reported.

Comment: The recent review found that some women quit smoking before their first antenatal visit, and most of these will remain abstinent.[23] Recruitment to the RCT comparing midwife delivered intervention versus usual care was slow. Midwives reported that the intervention was difficult to implement because of a lack of time to deliver the intervention at the booking appointment.[26]

OPTION ANTISMOKING INTERVENTIONS FOR PEOPLE AT HIGH RISK OF DISEASE

Systematic reviews and four subsequent RCTs have found that antismoking advice improves smoking cessation in people at high risk of smoking related disease. We found no evidence that high intensity advice is more effective than low intensity advice in high risk people. One RCT found that bupropion increased cessation rates in smokers with cardiovascular disease.

Benefits: We found no trials in which the same intervention was used in high and low risk people. We found one systematic review (search date not reported, 4 RCTs, 13 208 healthy men at high risk of heart disease),[24] one systematic review among people admitted to hospital (search date 2002, 17 RCTs),[28] one systematic review among people with chronic obstructive pulmonary disease (search date 2002, 5 RCTs),[29] and five subsequent RCTs.[30–34] The first review found that antismoking advice improved smoking cessation rates compared with control interventions among healthy men at high risk of heart disease (ARI of smoking cessation 21%, 95% CI 10% to 31%; NNT 5, 95% CI 4 to 10).[24] One early trial (223 men) that was included in the review used non-random allocation after myocardial infarction. The intervention group was given intensive advice by the therapeutic team while in the coronary care unit. The trial found that the self reported cessation rate at 1 year or more was higher in the intervention group than the control group (63% quit in the intervention group *v* 28% in the control group; ARI of quitting 36%,

95% CI 23% to 48%).[35] The second review included seven trials (6 of them with at least 12 months' duration) of high intensity behavioural interventions (defined as contact in hospital plus active follow up for at least 1 month) among smokers admitted to hospital. The review found that active intervention increased quit rates compared with usual care (OR 1.82, 95% CI 1.49 to 2.22).[28] The third review (search date 2002, 2 RCTs reporting cessation rate at ≥12 months) concentrated on smoking cessation among people with chronic obstructive pulmonary disease.[29] It found that psychosocial interventions plus nicotine replacement therapy plus a bronchodilator significantly increased cessation rates at 5 years compared with no treatment (RR 4.00, 95% CI 3.25 to 4.93). The first subsequent RCT compared postal advice on smoking cessation versus no intervention in men aged 30–45 years with either a history of asbestos exposure, or forced expiratory volume in 1 second in the lowest quartile for their age. Postal advice increased the self reported sustained cessation rate at 1 year compared with no intervention (5.6% with postal advice *v* 3.5% with no intervention; $P < 0.05$).[30] The second subsequent RCT (254 smokers admitted to hospital with coronary artery disease) compared a stepped care approach where people who did not quit by the end of each stage received successively more intense interventions (consisting of counselling plus nicotine patch) versus a brief cessation intervention.[31] It found no significant difference in cessation rates at 1 year (39% with more intensive intervention *v* 36% with brief intervention; $P = 0.36$). The third subsequent RCT (223 smokers admitted to hospital) compared intensive counselling plus outpatient follow up plus nicotine patches versus minimal counselling plus nicotine patches.[32] It found no significant difference in cessation rate between intensive and minimal intervention at 12 months (16% with intensive counselling *v* 9% with minimal counselling; $P = 0.21$). The fourth subsequent RCT (432 people with cancer) compared a brief structured intervention from a physician versus usual care.[33] It found no significant difference between interventions in cessation rates at 1 year (13.3% with intervention *v* 13.6% with usual care; $P = 0.52$). The fifth subsequent RCT (629 people with cardiovascular disease) compared sustained release bupropion (150 mg/day increasing to 150 mg twice daily) therapy versus placebo for 7 weeks.[34] It found that bupropion significantly increased cessation rates at 12 months compared with placebo (22% with bupropion *v* 9% with placebo; $P < 0.001$).

Harms: The fifth subsequent RCT found that bupropion increased insomnia, dry mouth, and cardiovascular events compared with placebo (insomnia: 24% with bupropion *v* 12% with placebo; dry mouth: 18% with bupropion *v* 10% with placebo; cardiovascular events: 7.7% with bupropion *v* 4.5% with placebo; P value not reported).[34] The systematic reviews and other RCTs did not report harms.

Comment: There was heterogeneity in the four trials included in the review among healthy men at high risk of heart disease, partly because of a less intense intervention in one trial and the recording of a change from cigarettes to other forms of tobacco as success in another.[24] One of the included trials was weakened by use of self reported smoking cessation as an outcome and non-random allocation to the intervention.[35]

OPTION — TRAINING HEALTH PROFESSIONALS TO ENCOURAGE SMOKING CESSATION

One systematic review found that training health professionals increases the frequency of antismoking interventions being offered. It found no good evidence that antismoking interventions are more effective if the health

professionals delivering the interventions received training. One RCT found that a structured intervention delivered by trained community pharmacists increased smoking cessation rates compared with usual care delivered by untrained community pharmacists.

Benefits: We found one systematic review[36] and one subsequent RCT.[37] The review (search date 2000, 9 RCTs) included eight RCTs of training medical practitioners and one RCT of training dental practitioners to give antismoking advice.[36] All the trials took place in the USA. The training was provided on a group basis, and variously included lectures, videotapes, role play, and discussion. The importance of setting quit dates and offering follow up was emphasised in most of the training programmes. The review found no good evidence that training health professionals leads to higher quit rates in people receiving antismoking interventions from those professionals, although training increased the frequency with which such interventions were offered. Three of the trials used prompts and reminders to practitioners to deploy smoking cessation techniques, and found that prompts increased the frequency of health professional interventions.[36] The subsequent RCT compared a structured smoking cessation intervention delivered by community pharmacists, who had received 3 hours of training versus no specific training or antismoking intervention.[37] Intervention delivered by trained pharmacists improved abstinence compared with usual care (AR of abstinence at 12 months: 14.3% with intervention *v* 2.7% with usual care; RR 5.3; NNT 9; CI values not reported; $P < 0.001$).

Harms: None reported.

Comment: The results of the systematic review should be interpreted with caution because there were variations in the way the analysis allowed for the unit of randomisation.

OPTION COUNSELLING FOR INCREASING PHYSICAL ACTIVITY IN SEDENTARY PEOPLE

We found limited evidence from systematic reviews and subsequent RCTs that counselling sedentary people increased physical activity compared with no intervention. Limited evidence from RCTs suggests that consultation with an exercise specialist rather than or in addition to a physician may increase physical activity at 1 year. We found limited evidence that interventions delivered by new media can lead to short term changes in physical activity.

Benefits: We found three systematic reviews that focused on different types of interventions[38–40] and nine subsequent RCTs.[41–49] The first review (search date 1996, 11 RCTs based in the USA, 1699 people) assessed the effect of single factor physical activity promotion on exercise behaviour.[38] Seven trials evaluated advice to undertake exercise from home (mainly walking, but including jogging and swimming), and six evaluated advice to undertake facility based exercise (including jogging and walking on sports tracks, endurance exercise, games, swimming, and exercise to music classes). An increase in activity in the intervention groups was seen in trials in which home based moderate exercise was encouraged and regular brief follow up of participants was provided. In most of the trials, participants were self selected volunteers, so the effects of the interventions may have been exaggerated. The second systematic review (search date not reported, 3 RCTs, 420 people) compared "lifestyle" physical activity interventions with either standard exercise treatment or a control group.[39] Lifestyle interventions were defined as those concerned with the daily accumulation of moderate or vigorous exercise as part of everyday life. The first RCT in the review (60 adults, 65–85 years old) found significantly more self reported physical activity in the lifestyle group than a standard exercise group. The second RCT in the review (235 people, 35–60 years old) found no significant difference in physical activity between the groups. The third RCT in the review (125 women, 23–54 years old) of encouraging walking found no significant difference in walking levels at 30 months' follow up between people receiving an 8 week behavioural intervention and those receiving a 5 minute telephone call and written information about the benefits of exercise, although both groups increased walking. The third review (search date 2002, 7 RCTs and 1 quasi-randomised trial, 9054 people) examined the efficacy of exercise counselling from a primary care clinician compared with a control or comparison group.[40] Counselling was delivered using advice only, the promotion of self efficacy, posted educational materials, referral to community resources, and written exercise prescriptions. The review found equivocal results and at least one methodological limitation in most studies. There was limited evidence that the interventions in these studies led to short term (< 3 months) improvements in physical activity. There were insufficient studies to consider the relationship between the components of the interventions and the reported efficacy. Only two RCTs identified by the review[40] were rated as good quality.[50,51] The first good quality RCT identified by the review (874 people) compared 3 minutes of physician advice plus educational materials, all the above plus behavioural counselling plus interactive mail, and all the above plus telephone counselling plus classes.[50] It found no significant difference in self reported activity between interventions at 24 months. The second good quality RCT identified by the review (355 sedentary people) compared a brief 5 minute message, a prescription for exercise, and a follow up visit with usual care.[51] It found no significant difference in the proportion of people meeting the Healthy People 2010 goal after 8 months (28% with advice or prescription *v* 23% with usual care; difference +5%, 95% CI –6% to +14%). All but two of the subsequent trials[47,49] involved primary care delivered interventions, although they were not restricted to clinician led interventions.[41–46] Two of the three trials in which advice was delivered by an exercise specialist rather than a physician found significant improvement in self reported physical activity at long term (> 6 months) follow up compared with controls.[43,44] A third RCT (1658 people in a primary care setting), which compared a client centred, negotiating style to direct advice and a no intervention control group, did not find any significant difference in changes in physical activity.[46] One cluster RCT (878 people from 42 rural and urban general practices) compared clinician advice plus a written "green" exercise prescription and up to three 10–20 minute telephone calls from an exercise specialist over 3 months versus usual care.[48] Clinicians in the intervention practices were offered training in motivational interviewing**G** and interviews averaged 7 minutes of general practitioner time or 13 minutes of nurse time. The physical activity goals in the "green" exercise prescription were tailored to the individual but typically involved home based physical activity or walking. It found that the intervention significantly increased physical activity at 12 months compared with usual care (leisure exercise per week: 55 minutes with intervention *v* 17 minutes with usual care; difference: 33.6 minutes, 95% CI 2.4 minutes to 64.2 minutes). Short term improvement was found in two further trials, but not maintained at 9 months or 1 year.[41,42] One RCT (298 people) compared physical activity counselling with nutrition counselling, both delivered with automated telephone conversations using digitised human speech.[47] The system used information about current behaviour and some known determinants to counsel people on either physical activity or nutrition. The percentage of individuals meeting current physical activity recommendations at 3 months' follow up was significantly greater in the physical activity group compared with the nutrition group at 3 months. However, there was no significant difference at 6 months (3 months: 26% with activity counselling *v* 19.6% with dietary counselling; P = 0.04). One RCT (229 women) of encouraging women to increase walking found significantly increased walking in the intervention group at 10 years' follow up (86% of women available for follow up, median estimated calorie expenditure from self reported amount of walking 1344 kcal/week with encouragement *v* 924 kcal/week with no encouragement; P = 0.01).[52] A further RCT (260 people in a primary care setting) compared the additional offer of community walks (led by lay people) versus advice alone.[45] It found no significant difference in physical activity at 12 months' follow up (ARR for achieving at least 120 minutes of moderate intensity activity a week +6%, 95% CI −5% to +16.4%). One RCT (299 office based civil servants) in a workplace setting compared individual counselling tailored according to the workers' stage of change (7 sessions of 20 minutes each) versus written information on lifestyle.[49] It found that the intervention significantly increased energy expenditure and cardiorespiratory fitness at 9 months compared with information only (difference in energy expenditure: 176.2 kcal/day, 95% CI 60.6 kcal/day to 291.8 kcal/day; difference in submaximal heart rate: −4.7 beats/minute, 95% CI −7.4 beats/minute to −2.05 beats/minute).[14] It found no significant difference in the proportion of people meeting criteria for moderate intensity physical activity (OR 1.46, 95% CI 0.76 to 2.79).

Harms: Insufficient detail is available from these studies to judge the potential harm of exercise counselling. In the RCT comparing behavioural counselling with brief advice identified by the third systematic review,[40] 60% of participants experienced a musculoskeletal event during the 2 years of the study.[50] About half of these required a visit to the physician. About 5% of all participants were admitted to hospital for a suspected cardiovascular event. The trial lacked a non-intervention control group. We found no evidence that counselling people to increase activity levels increased adverse events compared with no counselling.

Comment: Self reporting of effects by people in a trial, especially where blinding to interventions is not possible (as is the case with advice or encouragement), is a potential source of bias. Few studies conduct intention to treat analyses, which may lead to an exaggeration of the true effect of interventions. Methodological problems in RCTs included in the third review included only moderate follow up rates, highly motivated providers, differences in physical activity levels at baseline between intervention groups, uncertain or low provided adherence, inclusion of some counselling advice in usual care control groups, and inadequate power to detect a clinically important difference.[40]

OPTION EXERCISE ADVICE IN WOMEN AGED OVER 80 YEARS

One RCT found that exercise advice increased physical activity in women aged over 80 years and decreased the risk of falling.

Benefits: We found no systematic review. One RCT (233 women > 80 years old, conducted in New Zealand) compared four visits from a physiotherapist who advised a course of 30 minutes of home based exercises three times a week that was appropriate for the individual versus a similar number of social visits.[53] After 1 year, women who had received physiotherapist visits were significantly more active than women in the control group, and 42% were still completing the recommended exercise programme at least three times a week. The mean annual rate of falls in the intervention group was 0.87 compared with 1.34 in the control group, a difference of 0.47 falls a year (95% CI 0.04 falls/year to 0.90 falls/year).

Harms: No additional harms in the intervention group were reported.

Comment: None.

OPTION ADVICE ON A CHOLESTEROL LOWERING DIET

Systematic reviews have found that advice on eating a cholesterol lowering diet (i.e. advice to reduce fat intake or increase the polyunsaturated : saturated fatty acid ratio in the diet) leads to a small reduction in blood cholesterol concentrations in the long term (≥ 6 months).

Benefits: **Effects on blood cholesterol:** We found three systematic reviews[16,54,55] and two subsequent RCTs[56,57] that reported biochemical rather than clinical end points. None of the reviews included evidence after 1996. One review (search date 1993) identified five trials of cholesterol lowering dietary advice (principally advice from nutritionists or specially trained counsellors) with follow up for 9–18 months.[54] It found a mean reduction in blood cholesterol concentration in the intervention group of 0.22 mmol/L (95% CI 0.05 mmol/L to 0.39 mmol/L) compared with the control group. There was significant heterogeneity ($P < 0.02$), with two outlying studies — one showing no effect and one showing a larger effect. This review excluded trials in people at high risk of heart disease. Another systematic review (search date 1994) identified 13 trials of more than 6 months' duration and included people at high risk of heart disease.[16] It found that dietary advice reduced blood cholesterol (mean reduction in blood cholesterol concentration with advice 4.5%, 95% CI 3.9% to 5.1%; given a mean baseline cholesterol of 6.3 mmol/L, mean AR about 0.3 mmol/L). The third systematic review (search date 1996, 1 trial,[58] 76 people) found no significant difference between brief versus intensive advice from a general practitioner and dietician on blood cholesterol at 1 year.[55] The first subsequent RCT (186 men and women at high risk of coronary heart disease) compared advice on healthy eating versus no intervention. At 1 year it found no significant differences between groups in total and low density lipoprotein cholesterol concentrations for either sex, even though the reported percentage of energy from fat consumed by both women and men in the advice group decreased significantly compared with that reported by the women and men in the control group.[56] These results may reflect bias caused by self reporting of dietary intake. The second RCT, in 531 men with hypercholesterolaemia (with and without other hyperlipidaemias) and fat intake of about 35%, compared dietary advice aimed at reducing fat intake to 30% versus 26% versus 22%. All interventions were similarly effective for reducing fat intake (total fat intake after intervention about 26% in all groups).[57]
Effects on clinical outcomes: We found two systematic reviews that reported on morbidity and mortality.[16,59] The first review (search date 1994) compared 13 separate and single dietary interventions.[16] It found no significant effect of dietary interventions on total mortality or coronary heart disease mortality (total mortality: OR 0.93, 95% CI 0.84 to 1.03; coronary heart disease mortality: OR 0.93, 95% CI 0.82 to 1.06). However, it found a reduction in non-fatal myocardial infarction (OR 0.77, 95% CI 0.67 to 0.90). The second review (search date 1999, 27 studies including 40 intervention arms, 30 901 person years) found dietary advice to reduce or modify dietary fat had no significant effect on total mortality or cardiovascular disease mortality compared with no dietary advice (total mortality: HR 0.98, 95% CI 0.86 to 1.12; cardiovascular disease mortality: HR 0.98, 95% CI 0.77 to 1.07). However, dietary advice significantly reduced cardiovascular disease events

(HR 0.84, 95% CI 0.72 to 0.99).[59] RCTs in which people were followed for more than 2 years showed significant reductions in the rate of cardiovascular disease events. The relative protection from cardiovascular disease events was similar in both high and low risk groups, but was significant only in high risk groups.

Harms: We found no evidence about harms.

Comment: The finding of a 0.2–0.3 mmol/L reduction in blood cholesterol in the two systematic reviews accords with the findings of a meta-analysis of the plasma lipid response to changes in dietary fat and cholesterol.[60] The analysis included data from 244 published studies (trial duration 1 day to 6 years), and concluded that adherence to dietary recommendations (30% energy from fat, < 10% saturated fat, and < 300 mg cholesterol/day) compared with average US dietary intake would reduce blood cholesterol by about 5%.

OPTION ADVICE ON REDUCING SODIUM INTAKE

One systematic review found that, compared with usual care, intensive interventions to reduce sodium intake provided small reductions in blood pressure, however effects on deaths and cardiovascular events are unclear.

Benefits: We found one systematic review (search date not reported).[61] The review identified three RCTs in 2326 normotensive people, five RCTs in 387 people with untreated hypertension, and three RCTs in 801 people with treated hypertension.[61] Follow up ranged from 6 months to 7 years. The large, high quality RCTs compared intensive behavioural interventions aimed at reducing salt intake (including comprehensive dietary and behaviour change programmes, group counselling sessions, newsletters, self assessment, goal setting, food tasting, and recipes) versus control interventions that did not promote salt reduction. In the included RCTs, outcomes were inconsistently defined and reported. Overall, the RCTs reported no significant difference in mortality between low salt and usual diet (4 RCTs; AR 8/1151 [0.69%] with low sodium *v* 9/1242 [0.72%] with control; P = 0.8). The review found no significant difference in cardiovascular events between low sodium diet and usual diet (2 RCTs; AR 42/374 [11.2%] with low sodium *v* 51/374 [13.6%] with usual diet; P = 0.3). It found that advice to reduce salt intake significantly reduced systolic blood pressure and reduced diastolic blood pressure at 13–60 months compared with control, although the reduction in diastolic pressure was not statistically significant (4 RCTs, 2347 people; reduction in systolic blood pressure: 1.1 mm Hg, 95% CI 1.8 mm Hg to 0.4 mm Hg; reduction in diastolic blood pressure: +0.6 mm Hg, 95% CI +1.5 mm Hg to –0.3 mm Hg). The degree of reduction in sodium intake was not related to change in blood pressure. The review found no significant difference between treatments for systolic or diastolic blood pressure at 7 years but may have lacked power to detect a clinically important difference (1 RCT, 128 normotensive people, change in systolic blood pressure: –1.6 mm Hg with low salt diet *v* +2.20 mm Hg with usual diet; P = 0.07; change in diastolic blood pressure: –7.5 mm Hg with low salt diet *v* –5.3 mm Hg with usual diet; P = 0.1). One large RCT identified by the review found that low salt diet advice significantly improved maintenance of blood pressure control after antihypertensive treatment medications were stopped compared with usual diet (1 RCT, 975 people, combined outcome of high blood pressure or restarting treatment or clinical cardiovascular event: RR 0.83, 95% CI 0.75 to 0.92).

Harms: None reported.

Comment: None.

OPTION **LIFESTYLE INTERVENTIONS FOR SUSTAINED WEIGHT LOSS**

Two large RCTs found that weight loss advice resulted in greater weight loss than no advice. One RCT found that cognitive behavioural therapy was more effective than usual care in promoting weight loss. Systematic reviews found that using behavioural therapy to support advice on diet and exercise is probably more effective in achieving weight loss than diet advice alone. One systematic review found limited evidence that partial meal replacement plans reduced weight loss at 1 year compared with reduced calorie diet in people who completed the treatment.

Benefits: We found four systematic reviews[62–65] and 21 additional RCTs (see table 1, p 111).[66–86] The first systematic review (search date 1995) identified one relevant RCT that found that the combination of diet and exercise in conjunction with behavioural therapy produced significantly greater weight loss than diet alone at 1 year (mean weight loss: 7.9 kg with diet plus exercise plus behavioural therapy *v* 3.8 kg with diet alone; significance result not reported).[62] The second systematic review (search date 1997, 3 RCTs) found that diet supported by behavioural therapy was more effective than diet alone at 1 year.[63] The third systematic review of the detection, prevention, and treatment of obesity (search date 1999) included eight RCTs comparing dietary prescriptions versus exercise, counselling, or behavioural therapy for the treatment of obesity, and three RCTs comparing dietary counselling alone versus no intervention. In both comparisons, initial weight loss was followed by gradual weight regain once treatment had stopped (mean difference in weight change at least 2 years after baseline, 2–6 kg with dietary prescription *v* 2–4 kg with dietary counselling).[64] The fourth systematic review (search date 2001, 6 RCTs, 487 people, 75% women, 24% with diabetes) found that partial meal replacement plans**G** significantly increased weight loss at 1 year compared with a reduced calorie diet (weight loss for 219 completers, fixed effects model: 7.31 kg with partial meal *v* 2.61 kg with reduced calorie; $P = 0.001$).[66] However, results should be interpreted with caution, because of the high rate of withdrawal (47% with partial meal *v* 64 % with reduced calorie; P for difference = 0.001) and significant heterogeneity among RCTs ($P \leq 0.005$). The additional RCTs are summarised in table 1, p 111. Two large RCTs found that weight loss advice resulted in greater weight loss than no advice.[66,79] One RCT found that cognitive behavioural therapy significantly increased weight loss compared with usual care at 1 year.[85] The heterogeneity of interventions used in the additional RCTs makes comparison of trials difficult, but no major differences were found among the various weight loss programmes.

Harms: The systematic reviews and RCTs provided no evidence about harms.

Comment: In one RCT (78 obese women), the withdrawal rate for a diet programme was 41% compared with 8% in a non-diet control.[73]

OPTION **LIFESTYLE INTERVENTIONS FOR MAINTAINING WEIGHT LOSS**

One systematic review and additional RCTs found that most types of maintenance strategy result in smaller weight gains or greater weight losses compared with no contact. Strategies that involve personal contact with a therapist, family support, walking training programmes, or multiple interventions, or are weight focused, seem most effective.

Benefits: We found one systematic review[63] and nine additional RCTs.[87–95] The systematic review (search date 1995, 21 studies) compared different types and combinations of interventions. It found that increased contact with a therapist in the long term produced smaller weight gain or greater weight loss, and that additional self help peer groups, self management techniques, or involvement of the family or spouse may increase weight loss. The largest weight loss was seen in programmes using multiple strategies. Two additional small RCTs (102 people[87] and 100 people in two trials[91]) assessed simple strategies without face to face contact with a therapist. Frequent telephone contacts, optional food provision, continued self monitoring, urge control, or relapse prevention did not reduce the rate of weight regain. One small RCT (117 people) found that telephone contacts plus house visits did reduce the rate of weight regain compared with no intervention (3.65 kg with telephone contacts plus house visits *v* 6.42 kg with no intervention; $P = 0.048$).[88] One further small RCT (80 obese women) found no difference in weight change at 1 year between participants offered relapse prevention training or problem solving compared with no further contact.[93] One RCT (82 women) compared two walking programmes (4.2 or 8.4 MJ/week) plus diet counselling versus diet counselling alone after a 12 week intensive weight reduction programme.[92] Both walking programmes reduced weight regain at 1 year (reduction in weight gain compared with dietary counselling alone 2.7 kg, 95% CI 0.2 kg to 5.2 kg with low intensity programme and 2.6 kg, 95% CI 0 kg to 5.1 kg with high intensity programme). At 2 years, weight regain was not significantly different between high intensity programme and control, but was reduced in the low intensity group (reduction in weight gain 3.5 kg, 95% CI 0.2 kg to 6.8 kg with low intensity programme and +0.2 kg, 95% CI –3.1 kg to +3.6 kg with high intensity programme). One additional small RCT (67 people) found that people on a weight focused programme maintained weight loss better than those on an exercise focused programme (weight gain 0.8 kg with weight focused programme *v* 4.4 kg with exercise focused programme; $P < 0.01$).[89] One 5 year RCT (489 menopausal women) compared behavioural intervention in two phases aimed at lifestyle changes in diet and physical activity with lifestyle assessment. People in the intervention group were encouraged to lose weight during the first 6 months (phase I), and thereafter maintain this weight loss for a further 12 months (phase II). The intervention resulted in weight loss compared with control during the first 6 months (–8.9 lb [–4.0 kg] with intervention *v* –0.8 lb [–0.4 kg] with control; $P < 0.05$), most of which was sustained over phase II (–6.7 lb [–3.0 kg] with intervention *v* –0.6 lb [–0.3 kg] with control; $P < 0.05$).[90] One RCT (90 obese men) compared the effects of walking, resistance training of moderate dose at 6 months, and no increase in exercise control after a 2 month weight loss programme with a very low energy diet.[95] It found no significant difference in long term weight maintenance between walking and resistance training programmes and control at 23 months (adjusted mean difference in weight compared with control: +0.8 kg with walking, 95% CI –4.0 kg to +5.6 kg *v* –0.5 kg with resistance, 95% CI –5.0 kg to +4.0 kg; P between interventions = 0.8). There was poor adherence to prescribed exercise (82% with walking *v* 66% with resistance).[95] One RCT (122 overweight men and women, 101 analyzed) compared the effects of a weight maintenance programme conducted in person (frequent support or minimal support) or over the Internet for 1 year, after a 6 month weight loss programme.[94] It found significantly less weight loss with Internet support compared with in person support (weight loss: –5.7 kg with Internet support *v* –10.4 kg with minimal in person support *v* –10.4 kg with frequent in person support; $P < 0.05$).[94]

Harms: We found no direct evidence that interventions designed to maintain weight loss are harmful.

Comment: Weight regain is common. The resource implication of providing long term maintenance of any weight loss may be a barrier to the routine implementation of maintenance programmes. One RCT (122 obese people) comparing in person and Internet support for weight maintenance, found attrition rates of 18% after 6 months and 24% after 18 months.[94]

OPTION LIFESTYLE ADVICE TO PREVENT WEIGHT GAIN

One small RCT found that low intensity education plus a financial incentive increased weight loss compared with no treatment. A second RCT found no significant effect on prevention of weight gain from a postal newsletter with or without a linked financial incentive compared with no contact. One RCT found that lifestyle advice prevented weight gain in perimenopausal women compared with assessment alone. One small RCT comparing a nutrition course for female students with no nutrition course found no significant increase in weight from baseline in either group at 1 year.

Benefits: We found three systematic reviews (search dates 1995,[62] 1999,[63] and not reported[96]) that included the same two RCTs[97,98] and two subsequent RCTs.[99,100] The first RCT (219 people) compared low intensity education with a financial incentive to maintain weight versus an untreated control group. It found significantly greater average weight loss in the intervention group than in the control group (–0.95 kg with intervention *v* –0.14 kg with control; P = 0.03).[97] The second RCT (228 men and 998 women) compared a monthly newsletter versus the newsletter plus a lottery incentive versus no contact. There was no significant difference in weight gain after 3 years between the groups (1.6 kg with newsletter *v* 1.5 kg with newsletter plus lottery incentive *v* 1.8 kg with no contact).[98] The first subsequent RCT (535 perimenopausal women) found that lifestyle advice reduced weight gain over 2 years compared with assessment alone (weight gain 0.5 kg with advice *v* 11.5 kg with assessment alone).[99] The second small subsequent RCT (40 female students, 33 analyzed) compared the effects of a one semester nutrition course (4 months) with no such course.[100] It found no significant change from mean baseline weight in either group 1 year after the end of intervention (66.7 kg at baseline to 67.7 kg at 1 year with course *v* 65.7 kg at baseline to 68.9 kg at 1 year with no course).

Harms: None reported.

Comment: None.

OPTION TRAINING HEALTH PROFESSIONALS IN PROMOTING WEIGHT LOSS

One systematic review of poor quality RCTs provided insufficient evidence on the sustained effect of interventions to improve health professionals' management of obesity. One subsequent cluster RCT found limited evidence that training for primary care doctors in nutrition counselling plus a support programme reduced body weight of the people in their care over 1 year compared with usual care.

Benefits: We found one systematic review (search date 2000, 18 RCTs, 8 with follow up > 1 year)[101] and one subsequent cluster RCT.[102] The studies in the review were heterogeneous and poor quality.[101] The subsequent cluster RCT (1162 people registered with 45 primary care doctors) compared nutrition counselling training plus a support programme for primary care doctors versus usual care (see comment below).[102] The nutrition supported intervention compared with usual care increased weight loss at 1 year (additional weight loss 2.3 kg; P < 0.001).

Harms: None reported.

Comment: In the subsequent RCT, the doctors were randomly allocated to training but the analysis of results was based on the people in the care of those doctors.[102] No allowance was made for cluster bias. This increases the likelihood that the additional weight loss could have occurred by chance.

GLOSSARY

Behavioural choice therapy A cognitive behavioural intervention based on a decision making model of women's food choice. This relates situation specific eating behaviour to outcomes and goals using decision theory. The outcomes and goals governing food choice extend beyond food related factors to include self esteem and social acceptance.
Cognitive behavioural programme Traditional cognitive behavioural topics (e.g. self monitoring, stimulus control, coping with cravings and high risk situations, stress management, and relaxation techniques) along with topics of particular importance to women (e.g. healthy eating, weight management, mood management, and managing work and family).
Motivational interviewing A goal directed counselling style that helps participants to understand and resolve areas of ambivalence that impede behavioural change.
Partial meal replacement plan A programme that prescribes a low energy (between 800–1600 kcal/day) diet, where one or two daily meals are replaced by commercially available, energy reduced products that are fortified with vitamins and minerals, and remaining meals consist of normal food.
Standard behavioural therapy A behavioural weight management programme that incorporates moderate calorie restriction to promote weight loss.

REFERENCES

1. Silagy C, Stead LF. Physician advice for smoking cessation. In: The Cochrane Library, Issue 3, 2004. Oxford: Update Software. Search date 2000; primary sources Cochrane Tobacco Addiction Group Trials Register and the Cochrane Controlled Trials Register.
2. Lancaster T, Stead LF. Individual behavioural counselling for smoking cessation. In: The Cochrane Library, Issue 3, 2004. Oxford: Update Software. Search date 2002; primary source Cochrane Tobacco Addiction Group Trials Register.
3. Rice VH, Stead LF. Nursing interventions for smoking cessation. In: The Cochrane Library, Issue 3, 2004. Oxford: Update Software. Search date 2003; primary sources Cochrane Tobacco Addiction Group Trials Register and Cinahl.
4. Stead LF, Lancaster T. Telephone counselling for smoking cessation. In: The Cochrane Library Issue 3, 2004. Oxford: Update Software. Search date 2002; primary source Cochrane Tobacco Addiction Group Trials Register.
5. Lancaster T, Stead LF. Self-help interventions for smoking cessation (Cochrane review). In: The Cochrane Library Issue 3, 2004. Oxford: Update Software. Search date 2002; primary sources previous reviews and meta-analyses, the Tobacco Addiction Review Group register of controlled trials identified from Medline Express (Silverplatter) to March 2002 and Science Citation Index to 7 March 2002.
6. Pieterse ME, Seydel ER, de Vries H, et al. Effectiveness of a minimal contact smoking cessation program for Dutch general practitioners: a randomized controlled trial. *Prev Med* 2001;32:182–190.
7. Aveyard P, Griffin C, Lawrence T, et al. A controlled trial of an expert system and self-help manual intervention based on the stages of change versus standard self-help materials in smoking cessation. *Addiction* 2003;98:345–354.
8. Silagy C, Mant D, Fowler G, et al. Nicotine replacement therapy for smoking cessation. In: The Cochrane Library, Issue 3, 2004. Oxford: Update Software. Search date 2004; primary source Cochrane Tobacco Addiction Group Trials Register.
9. Tonneson P, Paoletti P, Gustavsson G, et al. Higher dose nicotine patches increase one year smoking cessation rates: results from the European CEASE trial. *Eur Respir J* 1999;13:238–246.
10. Stapleton J. Cigarette smoking prevalence, cessation and relapse. *Stat Methods Med Res* 1998;7:187–203.
11. Stapleton JA, Sutherland G, Russell MA. How much does relapse after one year erode effectiveness of smoking cessation treatments? Long term follow up of a randomised trial of nicotine nasal spray. *BMJ* 1998;316:830–831.
12. Blondal T, Gudmundsson J, Olafsdottir I, et al. Nicotine nasal spray with nicotine patch for smoking cessation: randomised trial with six years follow up. *BMJ* 1999;318:285–289.
13. Daughton DM, Fortmann SP, Glover ED, et al. The smoking cessation efficacy of varying doses of nicotine patch delivery systems 4 to 5 years post-quit day. *Prev Med* 1999;28:113–118.
14. Yudkin P, Hey K, Roberts S, et al. Abstinence from smoking eight years after participation in randomised controlled trial of nicotine patch. *BMJ* 2003;327:28–29.
15. Glavas D, Rumboldt M, Rumboldt Z. Smoking cessation with nicotine replacement therapy among health care workers: randomized double-blind study. *Croat Med J* 2003;44:219–224.
16. Ebrahim S, Davey Smith G. Health promotion in older people for the prevention of coronary heart disease and stroke. *Health promotion effectiveness reviews series*, No 1. London: Health Education Authority, 1996. Search date 1994; primary sources Medline, hand searches of reference lists, and citation search on Bids for Eastern European trials.
17. White AR, Rampes H, Ernst E. Acupuncture for smoking cessation (Cochrane review) In: The Cochrane Library Issue 3, 2004. Oxford: Update Software. Search date 2002; primary sources Cochrane Tobacco Addiction Group Register, Medline, Psychlit, Dissertation Abstracts, Health Planning and Administration, Social SciSearch, Smoking and Health, Embase, Biological Abstracts, and Drug.

18. Ussher MH, West R, Taylor AH, et al. Exercise interventions for smoking cessation (Cochrane review). In: The Cochrane Library, Issue 3, 2004. Chichester, UK: John Wiley & Sons, Ltd. Search date 2002; primary source Cochrane Tobacco Addiction Group Register.
19. Marcus BH, Albrecht AE, King TK, et al. The efficacy of exercise as an aid for smoking cessation in women. *Arch Intern Med* 1999;159:1229–1234.
20. Hughes JR, Stead LF, Lancaster T. Antidepressants for smoking cessation (Cochrane review). In: The Cochrane Library, Issue 3, 2004. Chichester, UK: John Wiley & Sons, Ltd. Search date 2002; primary source Cochrane Tobacco Addiction Group Trials Register.
21. Hughes JR, Stead LF, Lancaster T. Anxiolytics for smoking cessation. In: The Cochrane Library, Issue 3, 2004. Oxford: Update Software. Search date 2003; primary source Cochrane Tobacco Addiction Group Trials Register.
22. Jorenby DE, Leischow SJ, Nides MA, et al. A controlled trial of sustained-release bupropion, a nicotine patch, or both for smoking cessation. *N Engl J Med* 1999;340:685–691.
23. Lumley J, Oliver S, Waters E. Interventions for promoting smoking cessation during pregnancy. In: The Cochrane Library, Issue 3, 2004. Oxford: Update Software. Search date 1998; primary source Cochrane Tobacco Addiction Group Trials Register.
24. Law M, Tang JL. An analysis of the effectiveness of interventions intended to help people stop smoking. *Arch Intern Med* 1995;155:1933–1941. Search date not reported; primary sources Medline and Index Medicus.
25. Wisborg K, Henriksen TB, Jespersen LB, et al. Nicotine patches for pregnant smokers: a randomized controlled study. *Obstet Gynecol* 2000;96:967–971.
26. Hajek P, West R, Lee A, et al. Randomized trial of a midwife-delivered brief smoking cessation intervention in pregnancy. *Addiction* 2001;96:485–494.
27. Stotts A, DiClemente CC, Dolan-Mullen P. One-to-one. A motivational intervention for resistant pregnant smokers *Addict Behav* 2002;27:275–292.
28. Rigotti NA, Munafro MR, Murphy MFG, et al. Interventions for smoking cessation in hospitalised patients. In: The Cochrane Library, Issue 3, 2004. Oxford: Update Software. Search date 2002; primary sources Cochrane Controlled Trials Register, Centre for Disease Control Smoking and Health database, Cinahl, and experts.
29. van der Meer RM, Wagena EJ, Ostelo RW, et al. Smoking cessation for chronic obstructive pulmonary disease (Cochrane Review). In: The Cochrane Library, Issue 3, 2004. Chichester, UK: John Wiley & Sons, Ltd. Search date 2002; primary sources Medline, Embase, Psychlit, and Centrale.
30. Humerfelt S, Eide GE, Kvale G, et al. Effectiveness of postal smoking cessation advice: a randomized controlled trial in young men with reduced FEV_1 and asbestos exposure. *Eur Respir J* 1998;11:284–290.
31. Reid R, Pipe A, Higginson L, et al. Stepped care approach to smoking cessation in patients hospitalized for coronary artery disease. *J Cardiopulm Rehabil* 2003;23:176–182.
32. Simon JA, Carmody TP, Hudes ES, et al. Intensive smoking cessation versus minimal counseling among hospitalized smokers treated with transdermal nicotine replacement: a randomized trial. *Am J Med* 2003;114:555–562.
33. Schnoll RA, Zhang B, Rue M, et al. Brief physician-initiated quit-smoking strategies for clinical oncology settings: a trial coordinated by the Eastern Cooperative Oncology Group. *J Clin Oncol* 2003;21:355–365.
34. Tonstad S, Farsang C, Klaene G, et al. Bupropion SR for smoking cessation in smokers with cardiovascular disease: a multicentre, randomised trial. *Eur Heart J* 2003;24:946–955.
35. Burt A, Thornley P, Illingworth D, et al. Stopping smoking after myocardial infarction. *Lancet* 1974;1:304–306.
36. Lancaster T, Silagy C, Fowler G. Training health professionals in smoking cessation. In: The Cochrane Library, Issue 3, 2004. Oxford: Update Software. Search date 2000; primary source Cochrane Tobacco Addiction Group Trials Register.
37. Maguire TA, McElnay JC, Drummond A. A randomized controlled trial of a smoking cessation intervention based in community pharmacies. *Addiction* 2001;96:325–331.
38. Hillsdon M, Thorogood M. A systematic review of physical activity promotion strategies. *Br J Sports Med* 1996;30:84–89. Search date 1996; primary sources Medline, Excerpta Medica, Sport Sciesarch, and hand searches of reference lists.
39. Dunn AL, Anderson RE, Jakicic JM. Lifestyle physical activity interventions. History, short- and long-term effects and recommendations. *Am J Prev Med* 1998;15:398–412. Search date not reported; primary sources Medline, Current Contents, Biological Abstracts, The Johns Hopkins Medical Institutions Catalog, Sport Discus, and Grateful Med.
40. Eden KB, Orleans CT, Mulrow CD, et al. Does counseling by clinicians improve physical activity? A summary of the evidence for the U.S. Preventive Services Task Force. *Ann Intern Med* 2002;137:208–215. Search date 2002; primary sources: the Cochrane Database of Systematic Reviews, Cochrane Controlled Trials Register, Medline, Healthstar, contact with experts, and hand searches of reference lists.
41. Harland J, White M, Drinkwater C, et al. The Newcastle exercise project: a randomised controlled trial of methods to promote physical activity in primary care. *BMJ* 1999;319:828–832.
42. Taylor A, Doust J, Webborn N. Randomised controlled trial to examine the effects of a GP exercise referral programme in Hailsham, East Sussex, on modifiable coronary heart disease risk factors. *J Epidemiol Community Health* 1998;52:595–601.
43. Stevens W, Hillsdon M, Thorogood M, et al. Cost-effectiveness of a primary care based physical activity intervention in 45–74 year old men and women; a randomised controlled trial. *Br J Sports Med* 1998;32:236–241.
44. Halbert JA, Silagy CA, Finucane PM, et al. Physical activity and cardiovascular risk factors: effect of advice from an exercise specialist in Australian general practice. *Med J Aust* 2000;173:84–87.
45. Lamb SE, Bartlett HP, Ashley A, et al. Can lay-led walking programmes increase physical activity in middle aged adults? A randomised controlled trial. *J Epidemiol Community Health* 2002;56:246–252.
46. Hillsdon M, Thorogood M, White I, et al. Advising people to take more exercise is ineffective: a randomized controlled trial of physical activity promotion in primary care. *Int J Epidemiol* 2002;31:808–815.
47. Pinto BM, Friedman R, Marcus BH, et al. Effects of a computer-based, telephone-counseling system on physical activity. *Am J Prev Med* 2002;23:113–120.
48. Elley CR, Kerse N, Arroll B, et al. Effectiveness of counselling patients on physical activity in general practice: cluster randomised controlled trial. BMJ 2003;326:793–796.
49. Proper KI, Hildebrandt VH, Van der Beek AJ, et al. Effect of individual counseling on physical activity fitness and health: a randomized controlled trial in a workplace setting. *Am J Prev Med* 2003;24:218–226.
50. The Writing Group for the Activity Counseling Trial Research Group. Effects of physical activity counseling in primary care: the Activity Counseling Trial: a randomised controlled trial. *JAMA* 2001;286:677–687.
51. Norris SL, Grothaus LC, Buchner DM, et al. Effectiveness of physician-based assessment and counseling for exercise in a staff model HMO. *Prev Med* 2000;30:513–523.
52. Pereira MA, Kriska AN, Day RD, et al. A randomized walking trial in postmenopausal women: effects on physical activity and health 10 years later. *Arch Intern Med* 1998;158:1695–1701.

53. Campbell AJ, Robertson MC, Gardner MM, et al. Randomised controlled trial of a general practice programme of home based exercise to prevent falls in elderly women. *BMJ* 1997;315:1065–1069.
54. Brunner E, White I, Thorogood M, et al. Can dietary interventions change diet and cardiovascular risk factors? A meta-analysis of randomised controlled trials. *Am J Public Health* 1997;87:1415–1422. Search date 1993; primary sources computer and manual searches of databases and journals.
55. Tang JL, Armitage JM, Lancaster T, et al. Systematic review of dietary intervention trials to lower blood total cholesterol in free living subjects. *BMJ* 1998;316:1213–1220. Search date 1996; primary sources Medline, Human Nutrition, Embase, Allied and Alternative Health, and hand searches of *Am J Clin Nutr* and reference lists.
56. Stefanick ML, Mackey S, Sheehan M, et al. Effects of diet and exercise in men and postmenopausal women with low levels of HDL cholesterol and high levels of LDL cholesterol. *N Engl J Med* 1998;339:12–20.
57. Knopp RH, Retzlaff B, Walden C, et al. One year effects of increasingly fat-restricted, carbohydrate-enriched diets in lipoprotein levels in free living subjects. *Proc Soc Exp Biol Med* 2000;225:191–199.
58. Tomson Y, Johannesson M, Aberg H. The costs and effects of two different lipid intervention programmes in primary health care. *J Intern Med* 1995;237:13–17.
59. Hooper L, Summerbell CD, Higgins JPT, et al. Reduced or modified dietary fat for preventing cardiovascular disease. In: The Cochrane Library, Issue 3, 2004. Oxford: Update Software. Search date 1999; primary sources Cochrane Library, Medline, Embase, CAB Abstracts, CVRCT registry, related Cochrane Groups' Trial Registers, trials known to experts in the field, and biographies.
60. Howell WH, McNamara DJ, Tosca MA, et al. Plasma lipid and lipoprotein responses to dietary fat and cholesterol: a meta-analysis. *Am J Clin Nutr* 1997;65:1747–1764. Search date 1994; primary sources Medline, hand search of selected review publications, and bibliographies.
61. Hooper L, Bartlett C, Davey Smith G, Ebrahim S. Reduced dietary salt for prevention of cardiovascular disease (Cochrane Review). In: The Cochrane Library, Issue 3, 2004. Chichester, UK: John Wiley & Sons, Ltd. Search date not reported; primary sources The Cochrane Library, Medline, Embase, CAB Abstracts, CVRCT registry, Sigle, and bibliographies of identified studies and reviews.
62. Glenny AM, O'Meara S, Melville A, et al. The treatment and prevention of obesity: a systematic review of the literature. *Int J Obesity* 887:21;715–737. Published in full as NHS CRD report 1997, No 10. A systematic review of interventions in the treatment and prevention of obesity. http://www.york.ac.uk/inst/crd/obesity.htm (last accessed 7 June 2004). Search date 1995; primary sources Medline, Embase, DHSS data, Current Research in UK, Science Citation Index, Social Science Citation Index, Conference Proceedings index, Sigle, Dissertation Abstracts, Sport, Drug Info, AMED (Allied and alternative medicine), ASSI (abstracts and indexes), CAB, NTIS (national technical information dB), Directory of Published Proceedings (Interdoc), Purchasing Innovations database, Health promotion database, S.S.R.U., DARE (CRD, database of systematic reviews, NEED, CRD, database of health economic reviews), and all databases searched from starting date to the end of 1995.
63. The National Heart, Lung, and Blood Institute. Clinical guidelines on the identification, evaluation, and treatment of overweight and obesity in adults. Bethesda, Maryland: National Institutes of Health, 1998; http://www.nhlbi.nih.gov/guidelines/obesity/ob_home.htm (last accessed 7 June 2004). Search date 1997; primary sources Medline, and hand searches of reference lists.
64. Douketis JD, Feightner JW, Attia J, et al. Periodic health examination, 1999 update. Detection, prevention and treatment of obesity. Canadian Task Force on Preventive Health Care. *Can Med Assoc J* 1999;160:513–525. Search date 1999; primary sources Medline, Current Contents, and hand searches of reference lists.
65. Heymsfield SB, van Mierlo CA, van der Knaap HC, et al. Weight management using a meal replacement strategy: meta and pooling analysis from six studies. *Int J Obes Relat Metab Disord* 2003;27:537–549.
66. Whelton PK, Appel LJ, Espeland MA, et al. Sodium reduction and weight loss in the treatment of hypertension in older persons. A randomized controlled Trial of Nonpharmacologic Interventions in the Elderly (TONE). *JAMA* 1998;279:839–846.
67. Wing RR, Venditti E, Jakicic JM, et al. Lifestyle intervention in overweight individuals with a family history of diabetes. *Diabetes Care* 1998;21:350–359.
68. Anderson RE, Wadden TA, Barlett SJ, et al. Effects of lifestyle activity v structured aerobic exercise in obese women. *JAMA* 1999;281:335–340.
69. Jakicic JM, Winters C, Lang W, et al. Effects of intermittent exercise and use of home exercise equipment on adherence, weight loss, and fitness in overweight women. *JAMA* 1999;282:1554–1560.
70. Sbrocco T, Nedegaard RC, Stone JM, et al. Behavioural choice treatment promotes continuing weight loss. *J Consult Clin Psychol* 1999;67:260–266.
71. Harvey-Berino J. Calorie restriction is more effective for obesity treatment than dietary fat restriction. *Ann Behav Med* 1999;21:35–39.
72. Wing RR, Jeffery RW. Benefits of recruiting participants with friends and increasing social support for weight loss and maintenance. *J Consult Clin Psychol* 1999;67:132–138.
73. Jeffery RW, Wing RR, Thorson C, et al. Use of personal trainers and financial incentives to increase exercise in a behavioural weight loss program. *J Consult Clin Psychol* 1998;66:777–783.
74. Craighead LW, Blum MD. Supervised exercise in behavioural treatment for moderate obesity. *Behav Ther* 1989;20:49–59.
75. Donnelly JE, Jacobsen DJ, Heelan KS, et al. The effects of 18 months of intermittent vs. continuous exercise on aerobic capacity, body weight and composition, and metabolic fitness in previously sedentary, moderately obese females. *Int J Obesity* 2000;24:566–572.
76. Rapoport L, Clark M, Wardle J. Evaluation of a modified cognitive-behavioural programme for weight management. *Int J Obesity* 2000;24:1726–1737.
77. Wing R, Epstein LH, Paternostro-Bayles M, et al. Exercise in a behavioural weight control program for obese patients with type 2 (non insulin dependent) diabetes. *Diabetologica* 1988;31:902–909.
78. Ramirez EM, Rosen JC. A comparison of weight control and weight control plus body image therapy for obese men and women. *J Consult Clin Psychol* 2001;69:444–446.
79. Stevens VJ, Obarzanek E, Cook NR, et al. for the Trials of Hypertension Prevention Research Group. Long term weight loss and changes in blood pressure: results of the Trials of Hypertension Prevention, Phase II. *Ann Intern Med* 2001;134:1–11.
80. Wylie-Rosett J, Swencionis C, Ginsberg M, et al. Computerized weight loss intervention optimises staff time: the clinical and cost results of a controlled clinical trial conducted in a managed care setting. *J Am Dietetic Assoc* 2001;101:1155–1162.
81. Bacon L, Keim NL, Van Loan MD, et al. Evaluating a 'non-diet' wellness intervention for improvements of metabolic fitness, psychological well-being and eating and activity behaviours. *Int J Obes Relat Metab Disord* 2002;26:854–865.
82. McManus K, Antinoro L, Sacks F. A randomized controlled trial of a moderate-fat, low-energy diet compared with a low-fat, low-energy diet for weight loss in overweight adults. *Int J Obes Relat Metab Disord* 2001;25:1503–1511.

83. Esposito K, Pontillo A, DiPalo C, et al. Effect of weight loss and lifestyle changes on vascular inflammatory markers in obese women: a randomized trial. *JAMA* 2003;289:1799–1804.
84. Heshka S, Anderson JW, Atkinson RL, et al. Weight loss with self-help compared with a structured commercial program: a randomized trial. *JAMA* 2003:289:1792–1798.
85. Munsch S, Biedert E, Keller U. Evaluation of a lifestyle change programme for the treatment of obesity in general practice. *Swiss Med Wkly* 2003;133:148–154.
86. Tate DF, Jackvony EH, Wing RR. Effects of Internet behavioral counseling on weight loss in adults at risk for type 2 diabetes: a randomized trial. *JAMA* 2003;289:1833–1836.
87. Bonato DP, Boland FJ. A comparison of specific strategies for long-term maintenance following a behavioural treatment program for obese women. *Int J Eat Disord* 1986;5:949–958.
88. Hillebrand TH, Wirth A. Evaluation of an outpatient care program for obese patients after an inpatient treatment. *Prev Rehabil* 1996;8:83–87.
89. Leermakers EA, Perri MG, Shigaki CL, et al. Effects of exercise-focused versus weight-focused maintenance programs on the management of obesity. *Addict Behav* 1999;24:219–227.
90. Simkin-Silverman LR, Wing RR, Boraz MA, et al. Maintenance of cardiovascular risk factor changes among middle-aged women in a lifestyle intervention trial. *Women's Health* 1998;4:255–271.
91. Wing RR, Jeffery RW, Hellerstedt WL, et al. Effect of frequent phone contacts and optional food provision on maintenance of weight loss. *Ann Behav Med* 1996;18:172–176.
92. Fogelholm M, Kukkonen-Harjula K, Nenonen A, et al. Effects of walking training on weight maintenance after a very-low-energy diet in premenopausal obese women: a randomized controlled trial. *Arch Intern Med* 2000;160:2177–2184.
93. Perri MG, Nezu AM, McKelvey WF, et al. Relapse prevention training and problem-solving therapy in the long-term management of obesity. *J Consult Clin Psychol* 2001;69:722–726.
94. Harvey-Berino J, Pintauro S, Buzzell P, et al. Does using the Internet facilitate the maintenance of weight loss? *Int J Obes Relat Metab Disord* 2002;26:1254–1260.
95. Borg P, Kukkonen-Harjula K, Fogelholm M, et al. Effects of walking or resistance training on weight loss maintenance in obese, middle-aged men: a randomized trial. *Int J Obes Relat Metab Disord* 2002;26:676–683.
96. Hardeman W, Griffin S, Johnston M, et al. Interventions to prevent weight gain: a systematic review of psychological models and behaviour change methods. *Int J Obesity* 2000;4:131–143. Search date not reported; primary sources Medline, Embase, Psychlit, The Cochrane Library, Current Contents, ERIC, Healthstar, Social Science Citation Index, and hand searches of reference lists.
97. Forster JL, Jeffery RW, Schmid TL, et al. Preventing weight gain in adults: a pound of prevention. *Health Psychol* 1988;7:515–525.
98. Jeffery RW, French SA. Preventing weight gain in adults: the pound of prevention study. *Am J Public Health* 1999;89:747–751.
99. Kuller LH, Simkin-Silverman LR, Wing RR, et al. Women's health lifestyle project: a randomized clinical trial. *Circulation* 2001;103:32–37.
100. Matvienko O, Lewis DS, Schafer E. A college science nutrition course as an intervention to prevent weight gain in female college freshmen. *J Nutr Educ* 2001;33:95–101.
101. Harvey EL, Glenny A, Kirk SFL, et al. Improving health professionals' management and the organisation of care for overweight and obese people. In: The Cochrane Library, Issue 3, 2004. Oxford: Update Software. Search date 2000; primary sources Specialised Registers of the Cochrane Effective Practice and Organisation of Care Group; the Cochrane Depression, Anxiety and Neurosis Group; the Cochrane Diabetes Group; the Cochrane Controlled Trials Register; Medline; Embase; Cinahl; Psychlit; Sigle; Sociofile; Dissertation Abstracts; Resource Database in Continuing Medical Education; and Conference Papers Index.
102. Ockene IS, Hebert JR, Ockene JK, et al. Effect of physician-delivered nutrition counseling training and an office-support program on saturated fat intake, weight, and serum lipid measurements in a hyperlipidemic population: Worcester area trial for counseling in hyperlipidemia (WATCH). *Arch Intern Med* 1999;159:725–731.

Margaret Thorogood
Professor of Epidemiology
Warwick Medical School University of Warwick, Coventry, UK

Melvyn Hillsdon
Lecturer in Health Promotion
London School of Hygiene and Tropical Medicine University of London, London, UK

Carolyn Summerbell
Reader in Human Nutrition
School of Health University of Teesside, Middlesbrough, UK

Competing interests: None declared.

TABLE 1 **RCTs examining lifestyle interventions to achieve sustained weight loss.**

Reference	Participants	Interventions	Results
66	585 overweight and hypertensive elderly people (subgroup analysis)	Weight loss advice *v* no weight loss advice	Weight loss advice reduced body weight more than no weight loss advice, but significance not reported (weight change at 30 months: –4.7 kg with weight loss programme *v* –0.9 kg with no weight loss programme)
67	154 non-diabetic people who were 30–100% overweight, with family history of diabetes	Compared 4 treatments for 2 years: diet (reduced calories and fat), exercise, diet + exercise, and no treatment	No significant difference between treatments at 2 years for weight change (–2.1 kg with diet *v* +1.0 kg with exercise *v* –2.5 kg with diet + exercise *v* –0.3 kg with no treatment; P value not reported)
68	40 obese women aged 21–60 years, BMI 32.9 kg/m2	16 week treatment programme: diet + lifestyle advice (advice to increase activity) *v* diet + aerobics (3 classes/week)	83% completed; no significant difference in weight regain 1 year after treatment (1.6 kg with aerobic *v* 0.08 kg with lifestyle; $P = 0.06$)
69	148 sedentary overweight women	Compared 3 behavioural weight control programmes: LB exercise, SB exercise, and SBEQ programme	78% completed 18 month programme; SBEQ significantly increased weight loss compared with SB (7.4 kg with SBEQ *v* 3.7 kg with SB; $P < 0.05$). No significant difference between weight loss with LB (5.8 kg) and either SB or SBEQ
70	24 obese women	Behavioural choice therapy *v* SBT	Behavioural choice therapy increased weight loss at 12 months compared with OFF (10.1 kg with behavioural choice therapy *v* 4.3 kg with SBT; $P < 0.01$)
71	80 obese non-smoking people aged 25–45 years, 120–140% ideal body weight	Energy restricted diet *v* fat restricted diet	Energy restricted diet significantly increased weight loss compared with fat restricted diet at 6 and 18 months (at 6 months: 11.2 kg with energy restricted diet *v* 6.1 kg with fat restricted diet; $P < 0.001$; at 18 months: 7.5 kg with energy restricted diet *v* 1.8 kg with fat restricted diet; $P < 0.001$)
72	166 people	SBT + support from friends *v* SBT without support	No additional weight loss at 16 months with social support from friends (4.7 kg with behavioural therapy + support *v* 3.0 kg with behavioural therapy without support; $P > 0.05$)

TABLE 1 continued

Reference	Participants	Interventions	Results
73	193 obese men and women	5 treatments compared: SBT, SW, SBT + SW, SBT + SW + PT, SBT + SW + PT + I	No significant difference between treatments in weight loss at 18 months (7.6 kg with SBT *v* 3.8 kg with SW *v* 2.9 kg with SBT + SW *v* 4.5 kg with SBT + SW + PT *v* 5.1 kg with SBT + SW + PT + I)
74	42 moderately obese young women, age 18–30 years, 6.8–20.5 kg overweight	3 12 week treatments compared: standard behaviour intervention (weekly meetings + exercise contracting), intensive intervention (weekly meetings + supervised exercise sessions 3 times/week), minimal contact intervention (written lessons with feedback)	38 completers analyzed. Intensive intervention significantly increased weight loss at 1 year compared with standard behaviour intervention or minimal contact (4.6 kg with supervised exercise *v* 4.3 kg with contracted exercise *v* 4.2 kg with minimal contact; $P < 0.05$)
75	22 sedentary moderately obese women	Continuous exercise (supervised exercise 30 minutes 3 times/week) *v* intermittent exercise (advice to walk briskly, twice daily for 15 minutes/session)	Continuous exercise reduced weight at 16 months but the reduction was not significant (from 81.4 kg to 79.7 kg with continuous *v* from 85.6 kg to 85 kg with intermittent; P value not reported)
76	76 women, 58 analyzed	Cognitive behavioural programme (10 weeks) *v* modified cognitive behavioural programme (10 weeks)	No significant difference between programmes after 1 year follow up (weight loss: 2.1 kg with modified programme *v* 3.8 kg with standard programme; P value not reported)
77 (Study 1)	25 people with type 2 diabetes	Diet + moderate exercise for 10 weeks *v* diet alone	19 people analyzed. No significant difference in weight loss at year (7.8 kg with diet + exercise *v* 4.0 kg with diet alone; $P > 0.10$)
77 (Study 2)	30 people with type 2 diabetes	Diet + more intensive exercise for 10 weeks *v* diet alone	Diet + intensive exercise significantly increased weight loss compared with diet alone at 1 year (from 104 kg to 96.2 kg with intensive exercise *v* from 102 kg to 98.2 kg with diet alone; $P = 0.01$)
78	65 obese men and women	Body image treatment + dietician led treatment *v* dietician led treatment alone	No significant difference in weight loss between treatments at 1 year (4.96% with body image + dietician led *v* 5.90% with dietician led alone; P value not reported)

TABLE 1 continued

Reference	Participants	Interventions	Results
79	1191 overweight and hypertensive people	Weight loss advice *v* no weight loss advice	Weight loss advice significantly reduced weight and hypertension more than no weight loss advice at 3 years (weight change at 3 years: –0.2 kg with advice *v* +1.8 kg with control; RR for hypertension with advice *v* control 0.81, 95% CI 0.70 to 0.95)
79	588 overweight people	Compared 3 different cognitive behavioural approaches for tailoring lifestyle modification goals to the individual: workbook alone (no tailoring), workbook + computerised tailoring (using computer kiosks with touch screen monitors), workbook + computerised tailoring + personal tailoring (staff consultation)	After 12 months, mean weight loss from baseline was significant in all groups. Combined computerised + personal tailoring significantly improved weight loss compared with workbook alone (mean weight loss: 1 kg with workbook *v* 2.1 kg with computerised tailoring *v* 3.3 kg with personal + computerised tailoring; P = 0.02 for workbook *v* combined group)
81	78 obese women, described as 'chronic dieters'	24 week 'non-diet' wellness programme *v* traditional 'weight loss' programme	Weight loss programme significantly increased weight loss compared with non-diet programme at 1 year (from 101.1 kg to 95.2 kg with diet *v* from 99.6 kg to 99.9 kg with non-diet; P < 0.001)
82	101 obese men and women	Moderate fat (based on the Mediterranean diet), low energy diet *v* low fat, low energy diet	Moderate fat diet increased weight loss compared with low fat diet after 18 months (mean weight change: –4.1 kg with moderate fat/low energy diet *v* +2.9 kg with low energy/low fat diet; difference in weight change 7.0 kg, 95% CI 5.3 kg to 8.7 kg)
83	120 premenopausal obese women	Advice to eat a low energy Mediterranean style diet *v* advice on healthy food choices. Both groups advised to increase their levels of physical activity	Low energy Mediterranean style diet advice increased weight loss compared with healthy food choice advice at 2 years (difference –11 kg, 95% CI –14 kg to –8 kg, intention to treat analysis)

TABLE 1 continued

Reference	Participants	Interventions	Results
84	423 moderately overweight people	Commercial weight loss programme *v* self help group	Commercial weight loss programme significantly reduced weight compared with self help at 2 years (weight change: −2.9 kg with commercial programme *v* + 0.2 kg with self help; $P < 0.001$, intention to treat analysis). Withdrawal rate was similar between groups (29% with commercial programme *v* 25% with self help)
85	122 people treated in general practice	CBT (16 sessions of about 90 minutes each) *v* usual care	CBT group significantly increased weight loss compared with usual care at 1 year (1.8 kg with CBT *v* 0.2 kg with usual care; $P < 0.001$). Withdrawal rate was similar with both treatments (23% with CBT *v* 29% with usual care)
86	92 obese people	Internet based weight loss programme + email based behavioural counselling *v* Internet-based weight loss programme alone	Combined intervention significantly increased weight loss compared with Internet-based programme alone at 1 year (4.4 kg with combined *v* 2.0 kg with Internet programme alone; $P = 0.04$, intention to treat analysis)

BMI, body mass index; CBT, cognitive behavioural therapy; I, monetary incentives; LB, long bout; PT, personal trainer; SB, short bout; SBEQ, short bout exercise plus home exercise equipment; SBT, standard behavioural therapy; SW, supervised walks

Heart failure

Search date February 2004

Robert McKelvie

QUESTIONS

INTERVENTIONS

See glossary Ⓖ

Key Messages

Non-drug treatments

- **Exercise** One systematic review found that exercise training reduced death rates and hospital admissions compared with usual care Ⓖ.
- **Multidisciplinary interventions** One systematic review found that multidisciplinary programmes reduced admissions to hospital compared with conventional care, but found no significant difference in mortality. The review found that telephone contact plus improved coordination of primary care had no significant effect on admission rate. Two RCTs included in the review found that home based support reduced

cardiovascular events at 3–6 years compared with usual care. Subsequent RCTs found that education, nurse led support, and multidisciplinary programmes reduced death and hospital readmission and improved quality of life at 12 weeks to 1 year compared with usual care.

Drug treatments

- **Angiotensin II receptor blockers** One systematic review and one subsequent RCT provided evidence that angiotensin II receptor blockers reduced mortality and admission for heart failure compared with placebo in people with New York Heart Association class II–IV heart failure, and were an effective alternative in people who were intolerant to angiotensin converting enzyme inhibitors. One systematic review found no significant difference between angiotensin II receptor blockers and angiotensin converting enzyme inhibitors in all cause mortality or hospital admission. One systematic review and one subsequent RCT found that angiotensin II receptor blockers plus angiotensin converting enzyme inhibitors reduced cardiovascular mortality and admission for heart failure compared with angiotensin converting enzyme inhibitors alone. Effects on all cause mortality remained uncertain.
- **Angiotensin converting enzyme inhibitors** Systematic reviews and RCTs found that angiotensin converting enzyme inhibitors reduced ischaemic events, mortality, and hospital admission for heart failure compared with placebo. Relative benefits were similar in different groups of people, but absolute benefits were greater in people with severe heart failure.
- **Digoxin (improves morbidity in people already receiving diuretics and angiotensin converting enzyme inhibitors)** One systematic review found that, in people in sinus rhythm with heart failure, digoxin reduced clinical worsening of heart failure compared with placebo. One large RCT in people already receiving diuretics and angiotensin converting enzyme inhibitors found that digoxin reduced the proportion of people admitted to hospital for worsening heart failure at 37 months compared with placebo, but found no significant difference between groups in mortality.
- **β Blockers** Systematic reviews found strong evidence that adding a β blocker to an angiotensin converting enzyme inhibitor decreased mortality and hospital admission in symptomatic people with heart failure of any severity. Limited evidence from a subgroup analysis of one RCT found no significant effect on mortality in black people.
- **Eplerenone (in people with myocardial infarction complicated by left ventricular dysfunction and heart failure already on medical treatment)** One large RCT in people with recent myocardial infarction complicated by left ventricular dysfunction and clinical heart failure already on medical treatment (which could include angiotensin converting enzyme inhibitors, angiotensin receptor blockers, diuretics, β blockers, or coronary reperfusion therapy) found that adding eplerenone (an aldosterone receptor antagonist) reduced mortality compared with adding placebo.
- **Implantable cardiac defibrillators in people at high risk of arrhythmia** One RCT found good evidence that an implantable cardiac defibrillator reduced mortality in people with heart failure who had experienced a near fatal ventricular arrhythmia. Two RCTs found that implantable cardiac defibrillators reduced mortality compared with medical treatment in people with heart failure and at high risk of arrhythmia.
- **Spironolactone in people with severe heart failure** One large RCT in people with severe heart failure taking diuretics, angiotensin converting enzyme inhibitors, and digoxin found that adding spironolactone reduced mortality after 2 years compared with adding placebo.
- **Amiodarone** Systematic reviews found weak evidence that amiodarone may reduce mortality compared with placebo. However, we were not able to draw firm conclusions about the effects of amiodarone in people with heart failure.
- **Anticoagulation** A preliminary report from one RCT found no significant difference between warfarin and no antithrombotic treatment or between warfarin and aspirin in the combined outcome of death, myocardial infarction, and stroke after 27 months. However, the RCT may have lacked power to detect a clinically important difference.

- **Antiplatelet agents** A preliminary report from one RCT found no significant difference between aspirin and no antithrombotic treatment or between aspirin and warfarin in the combined outcome of death, myocardial infarction, and stroke after 27 months. However, the RCT may have lacked power to detect a clinically important difference.
- **Calcium channel blockers** One systematic review found no significant difference in mortality between second generation dihydropyridine calcium channel blockers and placebo. RCTs comparing other calcium channel blockers versus placebo also found no evidence of benefit.
- **Non-amiodarone antiarrhythmic drugs** Evidence extrapolated from one systematic review in people treated after a myocardial infarction suggested that other antiarrhythmic drugs (apart from β blockers) may have increased mortality in people with heart failure.
- **Positive inotropes (other than digoxin)** RCTs in people with heart failure found that positive inotropic drugs other than digoxin (ibopamine, milrinone, and vesnarinone) increased mortality over 6–11 months compared with placebo. One systematic review in people with heart failure found a non-significant increase in mortality with intravenous inotropic drugs that act through the adrenergic pathway compared with placebo or control, and insufficient data to determine whether symptoms improved. It suggested that their use may not be safe.

High risk people: ACE inhibitors

- **Angiotensin converting enzyme inhibitors in people with asymptomatic left ventricular dysfunction or other risk factors** RCTs in people with asymptomatic left ventricular systolic dysfunction and in people with other risk factors found that angiotensin converting enzyme inhibitors delayed the onset of symptomatic heart failure, reduced cardiovascular events, and improved long term survival compared with placebo.

Diastolic heart failure

- **Angiotensin II receptor blockers** One RCT found that candesartan, an angiotensin II receptor blocker, reduced the combined outcome of cardiovascular death or hospital admission for heart failure compared with placebo, although the difference was not significant. It found no significant difference in cardiovascular death between the two groups, but found that candesartan reduced hospital admission compared with placebo.
- **Other treatments** We found no RCTs examining effects of other treatments in people with diastolic heart failure.

DEFINITION Heart failure occurs when abnormality of cardiac function causes failure of the heart to pump blood at a rate sufficient for metabolic requirements under normal filling pressure. It is characterised clinically by breathlessness, effort intolerance, fluid retention, and poor survival. It can be caused by systolic or diastolic dysfunction and is associated with neurohormonal changes.[1] Left ventricular systolic dysfunction (LVSD) is defined as a left ventricular ejection fraction below 0.40. It may be symptomatic or asymptomatic. Defining and diagnosing diastolic heart failure can be difficult. Recently proposed criteria include: (1) clinical evidence of heart failure; (2) normal or mildly abnormal left ventricular systolic function; and (3) evidence of abnormal left ventricular relaxation, filling, diastolic distensibility, or diastolic stiffness.[2] However, assessment of some of these criteria is not standardised.

INCIDENCE/ PREVALENCE Both the incidence and prevalence of heart failure increase with age. Studies of heart failure in the USA and Europe found that under 65 years of age the incidence is 1/1000 men a year and 0.4/1000 women a year. Over 65 years, incidence is 11/1000 men a year and 5/1000 women a year. Under 65 years the prevalence of heart failure is 1/1000 men and 1/1000 women; over 65 years the prevalence is 40/1000 men and 30/1000 women.[3] The prevalence of asymptomatic LVSD is 3% in the general population.[4–6] The mean age of people with asymptomatic LVSD is lower than that for symptomatic individuals. Both heart failure and asymptomatic LVSD are more common in men.[4–6] The prevalence of diastolic heart failure in the community is unknown. The prevalence of heart failure with preserved systolic function in people in hospital with clinical heart failure varies from 13–74%.[7,8] Fewer than 15% of people with heart failure under 65 years have normal systolic function, whereas the prevalence is about 40% in people over 65 years.[7]

AETIOLOGY/ RISK FACTORS Coronary artery disease is the most common cause of heart failure.[3] Other common causes include hypertension and idiopathic dilated congestive cardiomyopathy. After adjustment for hypertension, the presence of left ventricular hypertrophy remains a risk factor for the development of heart failure. Other risk factors include cigarette smoking, hyperlipidaemia, and diabetes mellitus.[4] The common causes of left ventricular diastolic dysfunction are coronary artery disease and systemic hypertension. Other causes are hypertrophic cardiomyopathy, restrictive or infiltrative cardiomyopathies, and valvular heart disease.[8]

PROGNOSIS The prognosis of heart failure is poor, with 5 year mortality ranging from 26–75%.[3] Up to 16% of people are readmitted with heart failure within 6 months of first admission. In the USA, heart failure is the leading cause of hospital admission among people over 65 years of age.[3] In people with heart failure, a new myocardial infarction increases the risk of death (RR 7.8, 95% CI 6.9 to 8.8). About a third of all deaths in people with heart failure are preceded by a major ischaemic event.[9] Sudden death, mainly caused by ventricular arrhythmia, is responsible for 25–50% of all deaths, and is the most common cause of death in people with heart failure.[10] The presence of asymptomatic LVSD increases an individual's risk of having a cardiovascular event. One large prevention trial found that, for a 5% reduction in ejection fraction, the risk ratio for mortality was 1.20 (95% CI 1.13 to 1.29). For hospital admission for heart failure, the risk ratio was 1.28 (95% CI 1.18 to 1.38) and the risk ratio for heart failure was 1.20 (95% CI 1.13 to 1.26).[4] The annual mortality for people with diastolic heart failure varies in observational studies (1.3–17.5%).[7] Reasons for this variation include age, the presence of coronary artery disease, and variation in the partition value used to define abnormal ventricular systolic function. The annual mortality for left ventricular diastolic dysfunction is lower than that found in people with systolic dysfunction.[11]

AIMS OF INTERVENTION To relieve symptoms; to improve quality of life; to reduce morbidity and mortality; with minimum adverse effects.

OUTCOMES Functional capacity (assessed by the New York Heart Association Ⓖ functional classification or more objectively by using standardised exercise testing or the 6 minute walk test);[12] quality of life (assessed with questionnaires);[13] mortality; adverse effects of treatment. Proxy measures of clinical outcome (e.g. left ventricular ejection fraction and hospital readmission rates) are used only when clinical outcomes are unavailable.

METHODS *Clinical Evidence* search and appraisal February 2004. Generally, RCTs with fewer than 500 people have been excluded because of the number of large RCTs available. If for any comparison very large RCTs exist then much smaller RCTs have been excluded, even if they have more than 500 people.

QUESTION What are the effects of non-drug treatments?

OPTION MULTIDISCIPLINARY INTERVENTIONS

One systematic review found that multidisciplinary programmes reduced admissions to hospital compared with conventional care, but found no significant difference in mortality. The review found that telephone contact plus improved coordination of primary care had no significant effect on admission rate. Two RCTs included in the review found that home based support reduced cardiovascular events at 3–6 years compared with usual care. Subsequent RCTs found that education, nurse led support, and multidisciplinary programmes reduced death and hospital readmission and improved quality of life at 12 weeks to 1 year compared with usual care.

Benefits: We found one systematic review (search date 1999, 11 RCTs, 2067 people with heart failure)[14] and eight subsequent RCTs.[15–22] Multidisciplinary programmes in the review included treatments such as nutrition advice, counselling, patient education, and exercise training. The review found that multidisciplinary interventions significantly reduced hospital admission compared with conventional care (11 RCTs; 406/1001 [40.6%] with multidisciplinary programme *v* 474/1011 [46.9%] with conventional care; RR 0.87, 95% CI 0.79 to 0.96), but found no significant difference in mortality (7 RCTs; 104/534 [19.5%] with multidisciplinary programme *v* 121/572 [21.2%] with conventional care; RR 0.94, 95% CI 0.75 to 1.19). However, the hospital admission results were heterogeneous by intervention. Specialised follow up by a multidisciplinary team significantly reduced admissions to hospital (9 RCTs, 1366 people with heart failure; RR 0.77, 95% CI 0.68 to 0.86), but there was no benefit from telephone contact plus improved coordination of primary care services (2 RCTs, 646 people with heart failure; RR 1.15, 95% CI 0.96 to 1.37). One subsequent report of two RCTs included in the review (297 people living at home with at least 1 hospital admission for heart failure) found that home based support significantly increased event free survival at 3–6 years compared with usual care (median event free survival: 7 months with support *v* 3 months with usual care; $P < 0.01$).[23] However, it found no significant difference in mortality between support and usual care at 5 years (83/149 [56%] with support *v* 96/148 [65%] with usual care; $P = 0.06$). The first subsequent RCT (88 people recently discharged after admission for heart failure) found that, compared with usual care, nurse led education and support significantly reduced the proportion of people who either died or had at least one readmission at 1 year (25/44 [57%] with support *v* 36/44 [82%] with usual care; RR 0.69, 95% CI 0.52 to 0.92).[15] The second subsequent RCT (200 people admitted with chronic heart failure) found no significant difference between protocol driven support plus management by nurses and usual care in mortality at 6 months (7/102 [7%] with support *v* 13/98 [13%] with usual care; $P = 0.14$).[16] It found that support significantly improved quality of life compared with usual care at 6 months (Minnesota Living with Heart Failure Questionnaire: final score 35.7 with support *v* 45.3 with usual care; $P = 0.01$). The third subsequent RCT (98 people) found that nurse led education plus specialist dietician advice significantly reduced readmission rate for heart failure compared with usual care at 12 weeks (readmission for heart failure: 1/51 [2%] with support *v* 11/47 [23%] with usual care; $P < 0.01$; OR 0.07, 95% CI 0.01 to 0.53).[17] The fourth subsequent RCT (216 people with heart failure) compared home nurse visit management (3 visits during the first week, 2 visits during the second and third weeks, 1 visit during the fourth and fifth week, then as needed) versus a nurse telemanagement programme (home monitoring device to measure weight, blood pressure, heart rate, and oxygen saturation, which transmitted data daily to a secure internet site to be reviewed by an advanced practice nurse and cardiologist) after hospital discharge.[18] It found that the nurse telemanagement programme significantly reduced heart failure readmissions after 3 months compared with the home nurse visit programme (13 with nurse telemanagement *v* 24 with home nurse visit; $P < 0.001$) and significantly reduced length of hospital stay (49.5 days with nurse telemanagement *v* 105 days with home nurse visit; $P < 0.001$). The fifth subsequent cluster RCT (197 people with heart failure) compared an integrated primary and secondary care programme (involving review at a hospital based heart failure clinic, individual and group education sessions, personal diary to record medication and body weight, booklets, and follow up alternating between the hospital and general practitioner) versus usual care after hospital discharge.[19] The unit of randomisation was the person's general practitioner. The RCT found no significant difference between the integrated programme and usual care in the combined end point of death or readmission after 1 year. It found that the integrated programme significantly reduced multiple admissions after 1 year compared with usual care (56 with integrated programme *v* 95 with usual care; P = 0.015). The sixth subsequent cluster RCT (358 people with heart failure) compared a telephone case management programme (including a registered nurse using a decision support software programme, printed educational material, reports sent to the person's physician, guidelines for treatment of heart failure) versus usual care after hospital discharge.[20] The unit of randomisation was the person's general practitioner. The RCT found that the telephone programme significantly reduced heart failure hospitalisation rate after 3 and 6 months compared with usual care (3 months: 45.7% lower, P = 0.03; 6 months: 47.8% lower, P = 0.01). It found that, compared with usual care, the telephone programme significantly reduced heart failure hospital days (P = 0.03) and multiple readmission (P = 0.03) after 6 months. The seventh subsequent RCT (234 people with heart failure) compared a heart failure management programme delivered by a day hospital (staff included a cardiologist, nurses, physiotherapist, with a plan of care structured for each person) versus usual care after hospital discharge.[21] It found that the programme significantly reduced readmissions to hospital after 12 months compared with usual care (13 with programme *v* 78 with usual care; P < 0.00001). It also found that the programme significantly reduced cardiac death after 1 year compared with usual care (3/112 [3%] with programme *v* 21/112 [17%] with usual care; P < 0.0007). The eighth subsequent RCT (106 people with New York Heart Association**G** II–IV heart failure) compared a multidisciplinary nurse led heart failure clinic versus usual care for 12 months after discharge from hospital.[22] It found that multidisciplinary care significantly reduced death rates and significantly improved self care compared with usual care at 12 months (death: 7 with multidisciplinary care *v* 20 with usual care; P = 0.005; self care score: P = 0.01; results presented graphically). However, it found no significant difference in admission rate between multidisciplinary care and usual care (82 with multidisciplinary care *v* 92 with usual care; P = 0.31).

Harms: The review and subsequent RCTs did not report on harms (see comment below).

Comment: The RCTs were small, involved highly selected patient populations, many lasted less than 6 months, and were usually carried out in academic centres, and so the results may not generalise to longer term outcomes based in smaller community centres. The review suggested that disease management programmes may fragment care such that peoples' other conditions are overlooked.[14] However, it did not provide evidence to support this.

OPTION EXERCISE

One systematic review found that exercise training reduced death rates and hospital admissions compared with usual care.

Benefits: We found one systematic review (search date not reported; 9 RCTs; 801 people; mean New York Heart Association class**G** about 2.5), which compared exercise training (to 60–80% of peak heart rate or peak oxygen consumption) versus usual care.[24] It found that exercise training significantly reduced death rate and the combined outcome of death or hospital admission compared with usual care (death: HR 0.65, 95% CI 0.46 to 0.92; death or admission: HR 0.72, 95%CI 0.56 to 0.93).

Harms: The systematic review did not report on adverse effects of exercise training.[24]

Comment: The studies were small, involved highly selected patient populations, and were carried out in well resourced academic centres. The results may not generalise to smaller community centres. The specific form of exercise training varied among studies, and the relative merits of each strategy are unknown. The studies generally lasted less than 1 year, and long term effects are unknown. A large RCT over a longer period of time is required to assess further the clinical benefits of exercise training.

QUESTION What are the effects of drug and invasive treatments in heart failure?

OPTION ANGIOTENSIN CONVERTING ENZYME INHIBITORS

Systematic reviews and RCTs found that angiotensin converting enzyme inhibitors reduced ischaemic events, mortality, and hospital admission for heart failure compared with placebo. Relative benefits were similar in different groups of people, but absolute benefits were greater in people with severe heart failure.

Benefits: **Versus placebo:** We found two systematic reviews (search dates 1994[25] and not reported[26]) of angiotensin converting enzyme (ACE) inhibitors versus placebo in heart failure. The first review (search date 1994, 32 RCTs, duration 3–42 months, 7105 people, New York Heart Association class**G** III or IV) found that ACE inhibitors significantly reduced mortality compared with placebo (611/3870 [16%] with ACE inhibitors *v* 709/3235 [22%] with placebo; ARR 6%, 95% CI 4% to 8%; OR 0.77, 95% CI 0.67 to 0.88).[25] Relative reductions in mortality were similar in different subgroups (stratified by age, sex, cause of heart failure, and New York Heart Association class). The second review (search date not reported, 5 RCTs, 12 763 people with left ventricular dysfunction or heart failure of mean duration 35 months) analysed long term results from large RCTs that compared ACE inhibitors versus placebo.[26] Three RCTs examined effects of ACE inhibitors in people for 1 year after myocardial infarction. In these three postinfarction trials (5966 people), ACE inhibitors significantly reduced mortality compared with placebo (702/2995 [23.4%] with ACE inhibitors *v* 866/2971 [29.1%] with placebo; OR 0.74, 95% CI 0.66 to 0.83), readmission for heart failure (355/2995 [11.9%] with ACE inhibitors *v* 460/2971 [15.5%] with placebo; OR 0.73, 95% CI 0.63 to 0.85), and reinfarction (324/2995 [10.8%] with ACE inhibitors *v* 391/2971 [13.2%] with placebo; OR 0.80, 95% CI 0.69 to 0.94). For all five trials, ACE inhibitors significantly reduced mortality compared with placebo (1467/6391 [23.0%] with ACE inhibitors *v* 1710/6372 [26.8%] with placebo; OR 0.80, 95% CI 0.74 to 0.87), reinfarction (571/6391 [8.9%] with ACE inhibitors *v* 703/6372 [11.0%] with placebo; OR 0.79, 95% CI 0.70 to 0.89), and readmission for heart failure (876/6391 [13.7%] with ACE inhibitors *v* 1202/6372 [18.9%] with placebo; OR 0.67, 95% CI 0.61 to 0.74). The relative benefits began soon after the start of treatment, persisted in the long term, and were independent of age, sex, and baseline use of diuretics, aspirin, and β blockers. Although there was a trend towards greater relative reduction in mortality or readmission for heart failure in people with lower ejection fraction, benefit was apparent over the range examined. **Dose:** We found one large RCT (3164 people with New York Heart Association class II–IV heart failure), which compared low dose lisinopril (2.5 or 5.0 mg/day) versus high dose lisinopril (32.5 or 35.0 mg/day).[27] It found no significant difference in mortality (717/1596 [44.9%] with low dose *v* 666/1568 [42.5%] with high dose; ARR 2.4%; CI not reported; HR 0.92, 95% CI 0.80 to 1.03; P = 0.128), but found that high dose lisinopril reduced the combined outcome of death or hospital admission for any reason (events: 1338/1596 [83.8%] with low dose *v* 1250/1568 [79.7%] with high dose; ARR 4.1%; CI not reported; HR 0.88, 95% CI 0.82 to 0.96) and reduced admissions for heart failure (admissions: 1576/1596 [98.7%] with low dose *v* 1199/1568 [76.5%] with high dose; ARR 22.2%; CI not reported; P = 0.002). **Comparison of different ACE inhibitors:** The first systematic review found similar benefits with different ACE inhibitors.[25]

Harms: The main adverse effects in large RCTs were cough, hypotension, hyperkalaemia, and renal dysfunction. Compared with placebo, ACE inhibitors increased cough (37% with ACE inhibitor *v* 31% with placebo; ARI 7%, 95% CI 3% to 11%; RR 1.23, 95% CI 1.11 to 1.35), dizziness or fainting (57% with ACE inhibitor *v* 50% with placebo; ARI 7%, 95% CI 3% to 11%; RR 1.14, 95% CI 1.06 to 1.21), increased creatinine concentrations above 177 μmol/L (10.7% with ACE inhibitor *v* 7.7% with placebo; ARI 3.0%, 95% CI 0.6% to 6.0%; RR 1.38, 95% CI 1.09 to 1.67), and increased potassium concentrations above 5.5 mmol/L (AR 6.4% with ACE inhibitor *v* 2.5% with placebo; ARI 4%, 95% CI 2% to 7%; RR 2.56, 95% CI 1.92 to 3.20).[28] Risk of angio-oedema was similar with ACE inhibitors and placebo (3.8% with enalapril *v* 4.1% with placebo; ARI +0.3%, 95% CI –1.4% to +1.5%).[28] The trial comparing low versus high doses of lisinopril found that most adverse effects were more common with high dose (dizziness: 12% with low dose *v* 19% with high dose; hypotension: 7% with low dose *v* 11% with high dose; worsening renal function: 7% with low dose *v* 10% with high dose; significant change in serum potassium concentration: 7% with low dose *v* 7% with high dose; P values not reported), although there was no difference in withdrawal rates between groups (18% discontinued with low dose *v* 17% with high dose). The trial found that cough was less commonly experienced with high dose compared with low dose lisinopril (cough: 13% with low dose *v* 11% with high dose). We found one systematic review (search date 1999), which specifically examined adverse effects of ACE inhibitors in people with heart failure. It found that ACE inhibitors significantly increased withdrawal because of adverse effects compared with control (placebo or non-ACE inhibitor treatments) after about 2 years (22 RCTs, 9668 people; AR 13.8% with ACE inhibitor *v* 9.4% with control; RR 1.54, 95% CI 1.30 to 1.83).[29] ACE inhibitors significantly increased cough, hypotension, renal dysfunction, dizziness, and impotence compared with control treatments (cough: RR 3.19, 95% CI 2.22 to 4.57; hypotension: RR 1.95, 95% CI 1.39 to 2.74; renal dysfunction: RR 1.84, 95% CI 1.20 to 2.81; dizziness: RR 1.60, 95% CI 1.15 to 2.23; impotence: RR 6.46, 95% CI 1.14 to 36.58).[29]

Comment: The relative benefits of ACE inhibitors were similar in different subgroups of people with heart failure. Most RCTs evaluated left ventricular function by assessing left ventricular ejection fraction, but some studies defined heart failure clinically, without measurement of left ventricular function in people at high risk of developing heart failure (soon after myocardial infarction). It is unclear whether there are additional benefits from adding ACE inhibitor to antiplatelet treatment in people with heart failure (see antiplatelet agents, p 133).

OPTION ANGIOTENSIN II RECEPTOR BLOCKERS

One systematic review and one subsequent RCT provided evidence that angiotensin II receptor blockers reduced mortality and admission for heart failure compared with placebo in people with New York Heart Association class II–IV heart failure, and were an effective alternative in people who were intolerant to angiotensin converting enzyme inhibitors. One systematic review found no significant difference between angiotensin II receptor blockers and

angiotensin converting enzyme inhibitors in all cause mortality or hospital admission. One systematic review and one subsequent RCT found that angiotensin II receptor blockers plus angiotensin converting enzyme inhibitors reduced cardiovascular mortality and admission for heart failure compared with angiotensin converting enzyme inhibitors alone. Effects on all cause mortality remained uncertain.

Benefits: **Versus placebo:** We found one systematic review (search date 2001, 11 RCTs, 2259 people with New York Heart Association class**G** II–IV, follow up 4 weeks to 2 years)[30] and one subsequent RCT.[31] The systematic review found no significant difference between angiotensin II receptor blockers and placebo in all cause mortality and admission for heart failure, although a smaller proportion of people died or were admitted with heart failure with angiotensin II receptor blockers (all cause mortality: 7 RCTs; AR 2% with angiotensin II receptor blockers *v* 3% with placebo; OR 0.68, 95% CI 0.38 to 1.22; admission for heart failure: 1 RCT; 8% with angiotensin II receptor blockers *v* 12% with placebo; OR 0.67, 95% CI 0.29 to 1.51). The numbers of deaths and admissions were small, which may explain why the difference did not reach significance. The subsequent RCT (2028 people with New York Heart Association class II–IV heart failure, left ventricular ejection fraction 40% or less, and intolerance to angiotensin converting enzyme inhibitors) compared candesartan (started at 4 or 8 mg daily with target dose 32 mg once daily from 6 weeks onwards) versus placebo.[31] It found that, during a median follow up of 33.7 months, candesartan significantly reduced the combined outcome of cardiovascular death or hospital admission for chronic heart failure, as well as each individual component, compared with placebo (cardiovascular death: 21.6% with candesartan *v* 24.8% with placebo; adjusted HR 0.80, 95% CI 0.66 to 0.96; hospital admission for heart failure: 20.4% with candesartan *v* 28.2% with placebo; adjusted HR 0.61, 95% CI 0.51 to 0.73; combined outcome of cardiovascular death and hospital admission for heart failure: 33% with candesartan *v* 40% with placebo; adjusted HR 0.70, 95% CI 0.60 to 0.81). **Versus angiotensin converting enzyme inhibitors:** We found one systematic review (search date 2001, 6 RCTs, 4682 people with New York Heart Association class II–IV, follow up 4 weeks to 1.5 years) comparing angiotensin II receptor blockers versus angiotensin converting enzyme inhibitors.[30] It found no significant difference between treatments for all cause mortality or rate of admission for heart failure (all cause mortality: 6 RCTs; OR 1.09, 95% CI 0.92 to 1.29; admission for heart failure: 3 RCTs; OR 0.95, 95% CI 0.8 to 1.13). **Plus angiotensin converting enzyme inhibitors versus angiotensin converting enzyme inhibitors alone:** We found one systematic review (search date 2001, 6 RCTs, 5712 people with New York Heart Association class II–IV heart failure)[30] and one subsequent RCT comparing angiotensin II receptor blockers plus angiotensin converting enzyme inhibitors versus angiotensin converting enzyme inhibitors alone.[32] The review found that combined treatment significantly reduced hospital admission for heart failure (3 RCTs; OR 0.74, 95% CI 0.64 to 0.86). However, it found no significant difference between treatments for all cause mortality (6 RCTs; OR 1.04, 95% CI 0.91 to 1.20). The subsequent RCT (2548 people with New York Heart Association class II–IV heart failure, left ventricular ejection fraction 40% or less) compared candesartan (started at 4 or 8 mg daily with target dose 32 mg once daily from 6 weeks onwards) plus angiotensin converting enzyme inhibitors versus placebo plus angiotensin converting enzyme inhibitors.[32] It found that, during a median follow up of 41 months, adding candesartan to angiotensin converting enzyme inhibitors significantly reduced the combined outcome of cardiovascular death or hospital admission for heart failure, as well as each individual component, compared with placebo (cardiovascular death: 23.7% with candesartan v 27.3% with placebo; adjusted HR 0.83, 95% CI 0.71 to 0.97; hospital admission for heart failure: 24.2% with candesartan v 28% with placebo; adjusted HR 0.83, 95% CI 0.71 to 0.97; combined outcome of cardiovascular death and hospital admission for heart failure: 37.9% with candesartan v 42.3% with placebo; adjusted HR 0.85, 95% CI 0.75 to 0.96).

Harms: **Versus placebo:** The systematic review did not report on harms.[30] The subsequent RCT found that candesartan non-significantly increased permanent discontinuation of treatment because of an adverse event or an abnormal laboratory value compared with placebo (main adverse effects were hypotension, hyperkalaemia, and increased serum creatinine; AR 21.5% with candesartan v 19.3% with placebo; P = 0.23).[31] **Versus angiotensin converting enzyme inhibitors:** The systematic review did not report on harms.[30] **Plus angiotensin converting enzyme inhibitors versus angiotensin converting enzyme inhibitors alone:** The systematic review did not report on harms.[30] The subsequent RCT found that candesartan plus angiotensin converting enzyme inhibitors significantly increased permanent discontinuation of treatment because of an adverse event or an abnormal laboratory value compared with angiotensin converting enzyme inhibitors plus placebo (main adverse effects were hypotension, hyperkalaemia, and increased serum creatinine; AR 24.2% with addtional candesartan v 18.3% with additional placebo; P = 0.0003).[32]

Comment: None.

OPTION POSITIVE INOTROPIC AGENTS

One systematic review found that, in people in sinus rhythm with heart failure, digoxin reduced clinical worsening of heart failure compared with placebo. One large RCT in people already receiving diuretics and angiotensin converting enzyme inhibitors found that digoxin reduced the proportion of people admitted to hospital for worsening heart failure at 37 months compared with placebo, but found no significant difference between groups in mortality. RCTs in people with heart failure found that positive inotropic drugs other than digoxin (ibopamine, milrinone, and vesnarinone) increased mortality over 6–11 months compared with placebo. One systematic review in people with heart failure found a non-significant increase in mortality with intravenous inotropic drugs that act through the adrenergic pathway compared with placebo or control, and insufficient data to determine whether symptoms improved. It suggested that their use may not be safe.

Benefits: **Digoxin:** We found one systematic review (search date 1992, 13 RCTs, duration 3–24 weeks, 1138 people with heart failure and sinus rhythm)[33] and one subsequent large RCT.[34] The systematic review found that six of the 13 RCTs enrolled people without assessment of ventricular function and may have included some people with mild or no heart failure. Other limitations of the older trials included crossover designs and small sample sizes. In people who were in sinus rhythm with heart failure, the review found significantly fewer people with clinical worsening of heart failure (52/628 [8.3%] with digoxin v 131/631 [20.8%] with placebo; ARR 12.5%, 95% CI 9.5% to 14.7%; RR 0.40, 95% CI 0.29 to 0.54), but found no significant difference in mortality (16/628 [2.5%] with digoxin v 15/631 [2.4%] with placebo; ARR –0.2%, 95% CI –2.6% to +1.1%; RR 1.07, 95% CI 0.53 to 2.23). The subsequent large RCT (6800 people, 88% male, mean age 64 years, New York Heart Association class Ⓖ I–III, 94% already taking angiotensin converting enzyme inhibitors, 82% taking diuretics) compared blinded additional treatment with either digoxin or placebo for a mean of 37 months.[34] It found no significant difference between digoxin and placebo in all cause mortality (1181/3397 [34.8%] with digoxin v 1194/3403 [35.1%] with placebo; ARR +0.3%, 95% CI −2.0% to +2.6%; RR 0.99, 95% CI 0.93 to 1.06). It found that digoxin significantly reduced admission rates for heart failure over 37 months compared with placebo (910/3397 [27%] with digoxin v 1180/3403 [35%] with placebo; ARR 8%, 95% CI 6% to 10%; RR 0.77, 95% CI 0.72 to 0.83; NNT 13, 95% CI 10 to 17) and reduced the combined outcome of death or hospital admission caused by worsening heart failure (1041/3397 [31%] with digoxin v 1291/3403 [38%] for placebo; ARR 7.3%, 95% CI 5.1% to 9.4%; RR 0.81, 95% CI 0.75 to 0.87). **Other inotropic agents:** One non-systematic review (6 RCTs, 8006 people) of RCTs found that non-digitalis inotropes increased mortality compared with placebo.[10] The largest RCT in the review (3833 people with heart failure) found significantly increased mortality with vesnarinone (60 mg/day) compared with placebo over 9 months (292/1275 [23%] with vesnarinone v 242/1280 [19%] with placebo; ARI 4%, 95% CI 1% to 8%; RR 1.21, 95% CI 1.04 to 1.40).[10,35] Another large RCT (1088 people with heart failure) found that milrinone significantly increased mortality over 6 months compared with placebo (168/561 [30%] with milrinone v 127/527 [24%] with placebo; ARI 6.0%, 95% CI 0.5% to 12.0%; RR 1.24, 95% CI 1.02 to 1.49).[36] A third large RCT (1906 people with heart failure) compared ibopamine versus placebo over 11 months.[37] It found that ibopamine significantly increased mortality compared with placebo (232/953 [25%] with ibopamine v 193/953 [20%] with placebo; RR 1.26, 95% CI 1.04 to 1.53). The review found that some RCTs reported improved functional capacity and quality of life, but this was not consistent across all RCTs. One systematic review (search date 2000, 21 RCTs, 632 people) examined the use of intravenous inotropic agents that act through the adrenergic pathway in people with heart failure.[38] Sixteen RCTs (474 people) contributed data from acute invasive haemodynamic studies of symptomatically severe heart failure, and five RCTs (158 people) were based on intermittent inotropic treatment in an outpatient context. Included RCTs were often small. It found 11 RCTs comparing inotropic agents (including dobutamine, dopexamine, toborinone, and milrinone) versus placebo or control. The review found that, compared with placebo or control, intravenous inotropes that act through the adrenergic pathway tended to increase mortality, although this did not reach significance (11 RCTs; OR 1.50, 95% CI 0.51 to 3.92; absolute numbers not reported). It reported that there were insufficient data to determine whether symptoms improved (see comment below).[38]

Harms: We found no systematic review. **Digoxin:** The RCT (6800 people) found that significantly more people had suspected digoxin toxicity in the digoxin group compared with placebo (11.9% with digoxin v 7.9% with placebo; ARI 4.0%, 95% CI 2.4% to 5.8%; RR 1.50, 95% CI 1.30 to 1.73).[34] The RCT found no significant difference between digoxin and placebo in the risk of ventricular fibrillation or tachycardia (37/3397 [1.1%] with digoxin v 27/3403 [0.8%] with placebo; ARI +0.3%, 95% CI −0.1% to +1.0%; RR 1.37, 95% CI 0.84 to 2.24). It found that, compared with placebo, digoxin significantly increased rates of supraventricular arrhythmia (2.5% with digoxin v 1.2% with placebo; ARI 1.3%, 95% CI 0.5% to 2.4%; RR 2.08, 95% CI 1.44 to 2.99) and second or third degree atrioventricular block (1.2% with digoxin v 0.4% with placebo; ARI 0.8%, 95% CI 0.2% to 1.8%; RR 2.93, 95% CI 1.61 to 5.34). **Other inotropic agents:** Most RCTs found that inotropic agents other than digoxin increased risk of death (see benefits above).

Comment: The systematic review on intravenous inotropic agents in people with heart failure concluded that "intravenous inotropic agents acting through the adrenergic pathway are often used in patients with worsening heart failure to achieve arbitrary haemodynamic targets. Our analyses show that there is very little evidence that such treatment improves symptoms or patient outcomes and may not be safe."[38]

OPTION β BLOCKERS

Systematic reviews found strong evidence that adding a β blocker to an angiotensin converting enzyme inhibitor decreased mortality and hospital admission in symptomatic people with heart failure of any severity. Limited evidence from a subgroup analysis of one RCT found no significant effect on mortality in black people.

Benefits: We found two systematic reviews (search dates 2000[39] and not reported[40]) and two subsequent RCTs[41,42] of the effects of β blockers in heart failure. **In people with any severity of heart failure:** The first systematic review (search date 2000, 22 RCTs, 10 315 people with heart failure, most people receiving triple therapy, in particular angiotensin converting enzyme inhibitors) found that β blockers significantly reduced the risk of death and hospital admission compared with placebo (death: 444/5273 [8.4%] with β blockers *v* 624/4862 [12.8%] with placebo; OR 0.65, 95% CI 0.53 to 0.80; hospital admissions: 540/5244 [10.3%] with β blockers *v* 754/4832 [15.6%] with placebo; OR 0.64, 95% CI 0.53 to 0.79).[39] This is equivalent to three fewer deaths and four fewer hospital admissions per 100 people treated for 1 year. The results were consistent for selective and non-selective β blockers. Sensitivity analysis and funnel plots found that publication bias was unlikely. **In people with severe heart failure:** The second systematic review (search date not reported, 4 RCTs, 635 people with class IV heart failure, on angiotensin converting enzyme inhibitors and diuretic with or without digitalis) found that β blockers significantly reduced the risk of death compared with placebo (56/313 [17.9%] with β blockers *v* 81/322 [25.1%] with placebo; RR 0.71, 95% CI 0.52 to 0.96).[40] The two subsequent RCTs compared β blockers versus placebo in people with New York Heart Association class**G** III or IV heart failure.[41,42] The first RCT (2289 people with class IV heart failure, who were euvolaemic [defined as the absence of rales and ascites and the presence of no more than minimal peripheral oedema] and who had an ejection fraction of < 25%, but were not receiving intensive care, iv vasodilators, or positive inotropic drugs) compared carvedilol versus placebo over 10.4 months.[41] It was stopped early because of a significant beneficial effect on survival that exceeded the pre-specified interim monitoring boundaries. It found that β blockers significantly reduced mortality compared with placebo (130/1156 [11.2%] with β blockers *v* 190/1133 [16.8%] with placebo; RR 0.65, 95% CI 0.52 to 0.81) and the combined outcome of death or hospital admission (425/1156 [36.8%] with β blockers *v* 507/1133 [44.7%] with placebo; RR 0.76, 95% CI 0.67 to 0.87). One subsequent report from this RCT found that, compared with placebo, carvedilol significantly reduced days in hospital for any reason or for heart failure compared with placebo (mean days in hospital for any reason: 6.2 per person with carvedilol *v* 8.5 per person with placebo; $P = 0.0005$; mean days in hospital for heart failure: 2.9 per person with carvedilol *v* 4.9 per person with placebo; $P < 0.0001$).[43] Another report from this RCT examined the short term risks of initiating carvedilol in severe heart failure.[44] During the first 8 weeks of treatment it found that, compared with placebo, carvedilol non-significantly reduced mortality and the combined outcome of death or hospitalisation compared with placebo (mortality: HR 0.75, 95% CI 0.41 to 1.35; death or hospitalisation for any reason:

HR 0.85, 95% CI 0.67 to 1.07).[44] The second RCT compared bucindolol versus placebo in people with severe heart failure (2708 people with class III or IV heart failure and ejection fraction ≤ 35%; about 70% of the people were white and 24% were black).[42] The RCT was stopped early because of accumulated evidence from other studies. It found that death was more common with placebo, but the difference did not reach significance (411/1354 [30.4%] with bucindolol *v* 449/1354 [33.1%] with placebo; HR 0.90, 95% CI 0.78 to 1.02). The RCT found a significant interaction of treatment effect with race (black *v* non-black people). There was no evidence of benefit in black people (HR 1.17, 95% CI 0.89 to 1.53), although there was a significant effect for non-black people (HR 0.82, 95% CI 0.70 to 0.96).[42]

Harms: The first subsequent RCT found that fewer people with carvedilol required permanent discontinuation of treatment because of adverse events other than death compared with placebo (P = 0.02).[41] Cumulative withdrawals at 1 year were 14.8% with carvedilol compared with 18.5% with placebo. For the subgroup of people with recent or recurrent cardiac decompensation or severely depressed cardiac function, the difference in withdrawal rates was greater (17.5% with carvedilol *v* 24.2% with placebo).[41] After 6 months of maintenance treatment it found that significantly more people felt improved and fewer felt worse with carvedilol than with placebo (P = 0.0009). It also found that a significantly smaller proportion of people with carvedilol experienced a serious adverse event compared with placebo (39% with carvedilol v 45.5% with placebo; P = 0.002). Another subsequent report of this RCT examined the short term risks of initiating carvedilol in severe heart failure.[44] The second subsequent RCT found that 23% of people in the bucindolol group and 25% of people in the placebo group permanently discontinued the medication.[42]

Comment: Fears that β blockers may cause excessive problems with worsening heart failure, bradyarrhythmia, or hypotension have not been confirmed. Good evidence was found for β blockers in people with moderate symptoms (New York Heart Association class**G** II or III) receiving standard treatment, including angiotensin converting enzyme inhibitors. The value of β blockers is uncertain in heart failure with preserved ejection fraction and in asymptomatic left ventricular systolic dysfunction. One recent RCT (1959 people) has found that carvedilol reduced all cause mortality compared with placebo (AR for death: 12% with carvedilol *v* 15% with placebo; HR 0.77, 95% CI 0.60 to 0.98) in people with acute myocardial infarction and left ventricular ejection fraction 40% or less.[45] The RCTs of β blockers have consistently found a mortality benefit, but it is not clear whether this is a class effect. One recent small RCT (150 people) of metoprolol versus carvedilol found some differences in surrogate outcomes, but both drugs produced similar improvements in symptoms, submaximal exercise tolerance, and quality of life.[46] Another recent RCT (3029 people) compared carvedilol versus metoprolol tartrate in people with heart failure.[47] It found that carvedilol significantly reduced all cause mortality compared with metoprolol (512/1511 [34%] with carvedilol *v* 600/1518 [40%] with metoprolol; HR 0.83, 95% CI 0.74 to 0.93). It found no significant difference between groups for the composite outcome of mortality or all cause admission (P = 0.122). The results of this RCT suggest that carvedilol extends survival compared with metoprolol. However, potential limitations to this RCT were that the target dose of metoprolol was less than usually suggested, and metoprolol was not the long acting formulation used in a previous RCT[39] that had shown significant clinical benefit. The results for non-black people were consistent between bucindolol and carvedilol. The lack of observed benefit for black people in one RCT[42] raises the possibility that there may be race specific responses to pharmacological treatment for cardiovascular disease.

OPTION CALCIUM CHANNEL BLOCKERS

One systematic review found no significant difference in mortality between second generation dihydropyridine calcium channel blockers and placebo. RCTs comparing other calcium channel blockers versus placebo also found no evidence of benefit.

Benefits: **After myocardial infarction:** See calcium channel blockers under acute myocardial infarction, p 035. **Other heart failure:** We found one systematic review (search date not reported, 18 RCTs, 3128 people with moderate to advanced heart failure for > 2 months) of second generation dihydropyridine calcium channel blockers,[48] one non-systematic review of all calcium channel blockers (3 RCTs, 1790 people with heart failure),[10] and one subsequent RCT.[49] The systematic review found no significant difference in mortality (2 RCTs, 1603 people; OR 0.94, 95% CI 0.79 to 1.12; significant heterogeneity was found; P = 0.48).[48] The largest RCT in the non-systematic review (1153 people with New York Heart Association class🅖 III or IV, left ventricular ejection fraction < 0.30, using diuretics, digoxin, and angiotensin converting enzyme inhibitors) found no significant difference between amlodipine and placebo on the primary combined end point of all cause mortality and hospital admission for cardiovascular events over 14 months (222/571 [39%] with amlodipine *v* 246/582 [42%] with placebo; ARR +3.4%, 95% CI –2.3% to +8.8%; RR 0.92, 95% CI 0.79 to 1.06).[10,50] Subgroup analysis of people with primary cardiomyopathy found a significant reduction in mortality with amlodipine (45/209 [22%] with amlodipine *v* 74/212 [35%] with placebo; ARR 13%, 95% CI 5% to 20%; RR 0.62, 95% CI 0.43 to 0.85). There was no significant difference in the group with heart failure caused by coronary artery disease. The second RCT (186 people, idiopathic dilated cardiomyopathy, New York Heart Association class I–III) compared diltiazem versus placebo.[10] It found no evidence of a difference in survival between diltiazem and placebo in people who did not have a heart transplant, although people on diltiazem had improved cardiac function, exercise capacity, and subjective quality of life. The third RCT (451 people with mild heart failure, New York Heart Association class II or III) compared felodipine versus placebo.[10] It found no significant effect. The subsequent RCT (2590 people with New York Heart Association class II–IV heart failure, mean follow up of 1.5 years with mibefradil and 1.6 years with placebo) found no significant difference in death rates between mibefradil and placebo (350/1295 [27.0%] with mibefradil *v* 319/1295 [24.6%] with placebo; RR 1.10, 95% CI 0.96 to 1.25).[49]

Harms: Calcium channel blockers have been found to exacerbate symptoms of heart failure or increase mortality in people with pulmonary congestion after myocardial infarction or where ejection fraction was less than 0.40 (see calcium channel blockers under acute myocardial infarction, p 035).[10] One RCT found mibefradil increased risk of death in people taking digoxin, class I or II antiarrhythmics, amiodarone, or drugs associated with torsade de pointes compared with placebo.[49] The review found that second generation dihydropyridine calcium channel blockers did not cause significant adverse effects.[48]

Comment: Many of the RCTs were underpowered and had wide confidence intervals. One RCT of amlodipine in people with primary dilated cardiomyopathy is in progress.

OPTION ALDOSTERONE RECEPTOR ANTAGONISTS

One large RCT in people with severe heart failure taking diuretics, angiotensin converting enzyme inhibitors, and digoxin found that adding spironolactone reduced mortality after 2 years compared with adding placebo. One large RCT in people with recent myocardial infarction complicated by left ventricular dysfunction and clinical heart failure already on medical treatment (which could include angiotensin converting enzyme inhibitors, angiotensin receptor blockers, diuretics, β blockers, or coronary reperfusion therapy) found that adding eplerenone reduced mortality compared with adding placebo.

Benefits: We found no systematic review but found two RCTs.[51,52] The first RCT (1663 people with heart failure, New York Heart Association class**G** III or IV, left ventricular ejection fraction < 0.35, all taking angiotensin converting enzyme inhibitors and loop diuretics, and most taking digoxin) compared spironolactone (25 mg/day) versus placebo.[51] The trial was stopped early because spironolactone significantly reduced all cause mortality compared with placebo after 2 years (mortality: 284/822 [35%] with spironolactone *v* 386/841 [46%] with placebo; ARR 11%, 95% CI 7% to 16%; RR 0.75, 95% CI 0.66 to 0.85; NNT 9, 95% CI 6 to 15).[51] The second RCT compared eplerenone (a selective aldosterone receptor antagonist) versus placebo in people found to have left ventricular dysfunction (ejection fraction of ≤ 40%) and clinical symptoms of heart failure after an acute myocardial infarction within the previous 3–14 days.[52] People were already receiving "optimal" medical treatment, which could include angiotensin converting enzyme inhibitors, angiotensin receptor blockers, diuretics, β blockers, or coronary reperfusion therapy, but excluded potassium sparing diuretics. The RCT found that eplerenone significantly reduced death from any cause after 16 months compared with placebo (478/3319 [14%] with eplerenone *v* 554/3313 [17%] with placebo; RR 0.85, 95% CI 0.75 to 0.96). It found that, compared with placebo, eplerenone significantly reduced death from cardiovascular causes (407/3319 [12%] with eplerenone *v* 483/3313 [15%] with placebo; RR 0.83, 95% CI 0.72 to 0.94) and significantly reduced the composite end point of death from cardiovascular causes or hospitalisation for cardiovascular events (885/3319 [27%] with eplerenone *v* 993/3313 [30%] with placebo; RR 0.87, 95% CI 0.79 to 0.95).[52]

Harms: The first RCT found no evidence that adding spironolactone to an angiotensin converting enzyme inhibitor increased risk of clinically important hyperkalaemia. Gynaecomastia or breast pain were reported in 10% of men given spironolactone and 1% of men given placebo.[51] In the RCT comparing eplerenone versus placebo, the rate of serious hyperkalaemia was significantly higher in the eplerenone group (180/3307 [5.5%] with eplerenone *v* 126/3301 [3.9%] with placebo; P = 0.002).[52]

Comment: The first RCT was large and well designed. As only people with New York Heart Association**G** functional class III or IV were included, these results cannot necessarily be generalised to people with milder heart failure.

OPTION ANTIARRHYTHMIC DRUG TREATMENT

Systematic reviews found weak evidence that amiodarone may reduce mortality compared with placebo. However, we were not able to draw firm conclusions about the effects of amiodarone in people with heart failure. Evidence extrapolated from one systematic review in people treated after a myocardial infarction suggested that other antiarrhythmic agents (apart from β blockers) may have increased mortality in people with heart failure.

Benefits: **Amiodarone:** We found two systematic reviews comparing amiodarone versus placebo in heart failure.[53,54] The most recent review (search date 1997, 10 RCTs, 4766 people) included people with a wide range of conditions (symptomatic and asymptomatic heart failure, ventricular arrhythmia, recent myocardial infarction, and recent cardiac arrest).[53] Eight of these RCTs reported the number of deaths. The review found that treatment with amiodarone over 3–24 months significantly reduced the risk of death from any cause compared with placebo or conventional treatment (436/2262 [19%] with amiodarone *v* 507/2263 [22%] with control; ARR 3.0%, 95% CI 0.8% to 5.3%; RR 0.86, 95% CI 0.76 to 0.96). This review did not perform any subgroup analyses in people with heart failure. The earlier systematic review (search date not reported) found eight RCTs (5101 people after myocardial infarction) comparing prophylactic amiodarone versus placebo or usual care, and five RCTs (1452 people) in people with heart failure.[54] Mean follow up was 16 months. Analysis of results from all 13 RCTs found a lower total mortality with amiodarone than control (annual mortality: 10.9% with amiodarone *v* 12.3% with control). The effect was significant with some methods of calculation (fixed effects model: OR 0.87, 95% CI 0.78 to 0.99) but not with others (random effects model: OR 0.85, 95% CI 0.71 to 1.02). The effect of amiodarone was significantly greater in RCTs that compared amiodarone versus usual care than in placebo controlled RCTs. It found that amiodarone significantly reduced arrhythmic death or sudden death compared with placebo (OR 0.71, 95% CI 0.59 to 0.85). Subgroup analysis found that amiodarone significantly reduced mortality in the five heart failure RCTs compared with placebo (annual mortality: 19.9% with amiodarone *v* 24.3% with placebo; OR 0.83, 95% CI 0.70 to 0.99). **Other antiarrhythmics:** Apart from β blockers, other antiarrhythmic drugs increase mortality in people at high risk (see class I antiarrhythmic agents under secondary prevention of ischaemic cardiac events, [Web only]).

Harms: **Amiodarone:** Amiodarone did not significantly increase non-arrhythmic death rate (OR 1.02, 95% CI 0.87 to 1.19).[54] In placebo controlled RCTs, after 2 years 41% of people in the amiodarone group and 27% in the placebo group had permanently discontinued study medication.[54] In 10 RCTs comparing amiodarone versus placebo, amiodarone increased the odds of reporting adverse drug reactions compared with placebo (OR 2.22, 95% CI 1.83 to 2.68). Nausea was the most common adverse effect. Hypothyroidism was the most common serious adverse effect (7.0% with amiodarone *v* 1.1% with placebo). Hyperthyroidism (1.4% with amiodarone *v* 0.5% with placebo), peripheral neuropathy (0.5% with amiodarone *v* 0.2% with placebo), lung infiltrates (1.6% with amiodarone *v* 0.5% with placebo), bradycardia (2.4% with amiodarone *v* 0.8% with placebo), and liver dysfunction (1.0% with amiodarone *v* 0.4% with placebo) were all more common in the amiodarone group.[54] **Other antiarrhythmics:** These agents (particularly class I antiarrhythmics) may increase mortality (see class I antiarrhythmic agents under secondary prevention of ischaemic cardiac events, [Web only]).

Comment: **Amiodarone:** RCTs of amiodarone versus usual treatment found larger effects than placebo controlled trials.[54] These findings suggest bias; unblinded follow up may be associated with reduced usual care or improved adherence with amiodarone. Further studies are required to assess the effects of amiodarone treatment on mortality and morbidity in people with heart failure.

OPTION IMPLANTABLE CARDIAC DEFIBRILLATORS

One RCT found good evidence that an implantable cardiac defibrillator reduced mortality in people with heart failure who had experienced a near fatal ventricular arrhythmia. Two RCTs found that implantable cardiac defibrillators reduced mortality compared with medical treatment in people with heart failure and at high risk of arrhythmia.

Benefits: We found no systematic review. We found three RCTs examining the effects of implantable cardiac defibrillators (ICDs) in people with left ventricular dysfunction.[55–57] The first RCT (1016 people resuscitated after ventricular arrhythmia and either syncope or other serious cardiac symptom and left ventricular ejection fraction ≤ 0.40) compared an ICD versus an antiarrhythmic drug (mainly amiodarone).[55] It found that ICDs improved survival at 1, 2, and 3 years (1 year survival: 89.3% with ICD *v* 82.3% with antiarrhythmic; 2 year survival: 81.6% with ICD *v* 73.7% with antiarrhythmic; 3 year survival: 75.4% with ICD *v* 64.1% with antiarrhythmic; P < 0.02). The second RCT included 196 people with New York Heart Association class Ⓖ I–III heart failure and previous myocardial infarction, a left ventricular ejection fraction 0.35 or less, a documented episode of asymptomatic unsustained ventricular tachycardia, and inducible non-suppressible ventricular tachyarrhythmia on electrophysiological study.[56] The RCT found that ICDs significantly reduced mortality over a mean of 27 months compared with conventional treatment (deaths: 15/95 [16%] with ICD [11 from cardiac cause] *v* 39/101 [39%] with conventional treatment [27 from cardiac cause]; HR 0.46, 95% CI 0.26 to 0.82). The third RCT (1232 people with prior myocardial infarction and left ventricular ejection fraction < 0.30) compared an ICD (742 people) versus conventional medical treatment (490 people).[57] It found that ICD reduced all cause mortality after 20 months' mean follow up compared with conventional treatment (AR 14.2% with ICD *v* 19.8% with conventional treatment; HR 0.69, 95% CI 0.51 to 0.93).

Harms: The RCTs found that the main adverse effects of ICDs were infection (about 5%), pneumothorax (about 2%), bleeding requiring further operation (about 1%), serious haematomas (about 3%), cardiac perforation (about 0.2%), problems with defibrillator lead (about 7%), and malfunction of defibrillator generator (about 3%).[55–58]

Comment: The RCTs were in people with reduced left ventricular function, and included people with and without previous cardiac arrest or inducible arrhythmia. It is uncertain whether asymptomatic ventricular arrhythmia is in itself a predictor of sudden death in people with moderate or severe heart failure.[59] Several RCTs of prophylactic ICD treatment in people with heart failure and in survivors of acute myocardial infarction are ongoing.[60]

OPTION ANTICOAGULATION

A preliminary report from one RCT found no significant difference between warfarin and no antithrombotic treatment or between warfarin and aspirin in the combined outcome of death, myocardial infarction, and stroke after 27 months. However, the RCT may have lacked power to detect a clinically important difference

Benefits: **Versus placebo:** We found one systematic review (search date 2000, 1 RCT, 279 people, 70% with New York Heart Association class Ⓖ III).[61] The RCT identified by the review was a pilot study comparing warfarin (international normalised ratio 2.5), aspirin (300 mg/day), and no antithrombotic treatment.[62] The RCT found no significant difference between warfarin and no antithrombotic treatment in the combined outcome of death, myocardial infarction, and stroke after mean follow up of 27 months (combined outcome: 26% with warfarin *v* 27% with no antithrombotic treatment; P value not reported).[62] **Versus antiplatelet agents:** See benefits of antiplatelet agents, p 133.

Harms: **Versus placebo:** The RCT found four haemorrhagic events with warfarin versus none with no antithrombotic treatment (total number of people in each group not reported).[62]

Comment: The systematic review (search date 2000)[61] found three additional non-randomised trials. Meta-analysis of these trials and the RCT[62] found that anticoagulant significantly reduced death from all causes and cardiovascular event rates compared with control (death from all causes in 1087 people: OR 0.64, 95% CI 0.45 to 0.90; cardiovascular event rates in 1130 people: OR 0.26, 95% CI 0.16 to 0.43).[61] Meta-analysis of two non-randomised trials (645 people) found no significant difference in bleeding complications between warfarin and no warfarin (OR 1.52, 95% CI 0.56 to 4.10).[61] The non-randomised controlled studies were performed in the early 1950s in hospitalised people with a high prevalence of rheumatic heart disease and atrial fibrillation, and the methods used may be considered unreliable today. One retrospective analysis assessed the effect of anticoagulants used at the discretion of individual investigators in RCTs on the incidence of stroke, peripheral arterial embolism, and pulmonary embolism.[63] The first cohort was from one RCT (642 men with chronic heart failure) comparing hydralazine plus isosorbide dinitrate versus prazosin versus placebo. The second cohort was from another RCT (804 men with chronic heart failure) comparing enalapril versus hydralazine plus isosorbide dinitrate. All people were given digoxin and diuretics. The retrospective analysis found that, without treatment, the incidence of all thromboembolic events was low (2.7/100 patient years in the first RCT; 2.1/100 patient years in the second RCT) and that anticoagulation did not reduce the incidence of thromboembolic events (2.9/100 patient years in the first RCT; 4.8/100 patient years in the second RCT). In this group of people, atrial fibrillation was not found to be associated with a higher risk of thromboembolic events. The second retrospective analysis was from two large RCTs (2569 people with symptomatic and asymptomatic left ventricular dysfunction), which compared enalapril versus placebo.[64] The analysis found that people treated with warfarin at baseline had significantly lower risk of death during follow up (HR adjusted for baseline differences 0.76, 95% CI 0.65 to 0.89). Warfarin use was associated with a reduction in the combined outcome of death plus hospital admission for heart failure (adjusted HR 0.82, 95% CI 0.72 to 0.93). The benefit with warfarin use was not significantly influenced by the presence of symptoms, randomisation to enalapril or placebo, sex, presence of atrial fibrillation, age, ejection fraction, New York Heart Association classification**G**, or cause of heart failure. Warfarin reduced cardiac mortality, specifically deaths that were sudden, or associated with either heart failure or myocardial infarction. Neither of the retrospective studies was designed to determine the incidence of thromboembolic events in heart failure or the effects of treatment. Neither study included information about the intensity of anticoagulation or warfarin use. We found several additional cohort studies that showed a reduction in thromboembolic events with anticoagulation, but they all reported results for too few people to provide useful results. An RCT is needed to compare anticoagulation versus no anticoagulation in people with heart failure.

OPTION ANTIPLATELET AGENTS

A preliminary report from one RCT found no significant difference between aspirin and no antithrombotic treatment or between aspirin and warfarin in the combined outcome of death, myocardial infarction, and stroke after 27 months. However, the RCT may have lacked power to detect a clinically important difference.

Benefits: We found one systematic review (search date 2000, 1 RCT, 279 people, 70% with New York Heart Association class Ⓖ III).[61] The RCT identified by the review was a pilot study comparing aspirin (300 mg/day) versus warfarin (international normalised ratio 2.5) versus no antithrombotic treatment.[62] **Versus placebo:** The RCT found no significant difference between aspirin and no antithrombotic treatment for the combined outcome of death, myocardial infarction, and stroke after mean follow up of 27 months (combined outcome: 32% with aspirin *v* 27% with no antithrombotic treatment; P value reported as not significant).[62] It found that aspirin significantly increased all cause hospital admission compared with placebo (P < 0.05; no data reported). **Versus warfarin:** The RCT found no significant difference between aspirin and warfarin for the combined outcome of death, myocardial infarction, and stroke after mean follow up of 27 months (combined outcome: 32% with aspirin *v* 26% with warfarin; P value reported as not significant).[62] It found that all cause hospital admissions were significantly higher for aspirin compared with warfarin (P = 0.05; no data reported).

Harms: Preliminary information on one RCT reported five haemorrhagic events with aspirin compared with four with warfarin (total number of people in each group not reported).[62] The total number of serious adverse reactions were similar in all groups (198 with aspirin *v* 173 with warfarin *v* 178 with no antithrombotic treatment).[65]

Comment: **In people not taking angiotensin converting enzyme inhibitors:** We found no systematic review and no RCTs. We found one retrospective cohort analysis within one RCT in 642 men with heart failure.[63] The RCT compared hydralazine plus isosorbide dinitrate versus prazosin versus placebo in men receiving digoxin and diuretics. Aspirin or dipyridamole, or both, were used at the discretion of the investigators. The number of thromboembolic events was low in both groups (1 stroke, 0 peripheral, and 0 pulmonary emboli in 184 people years of treatment with antiplatelet agents *v* 21 strokes, 4 peripheral, and 4 pulmonary emboli in 1068 people years of treatment without antiplatelet agents; 0.5 events/100 people years with antiplatelet agents *v* 2.0 events/100 patient years without antiplatelet agents; P = 0.07). **In people taking angiotensin converting enzyme inhibitors:** We found no RCTs. We found two large retrospective cohort studies.[63,66] The first retrospective analysis assessed the effect of antiplatelet agents used at the discretion of individual investigators on the incidence of stroke, peripheral arterial embolism, and pulmonary embolism within one RCT.[63] The RCT (804 men with chronic heart failure) compared enalapril versus hydralazine plus isosorbide dinitrate. It found that the incidence of all thromboembolic events was low without antiplatelet treatment and found no significant difference between groups (1.6 events/100 patient years with antiplatelet treatment *v* 2.1 events/100 people years with no antiplatelet treatment; P = 0.48). The second cohort analysis was from two large RCTs, which compared enalapril versus placebo (2569 people with symptomatic and asymptomatic left ventricular dysfunction). It found that people treated with antiplatelet agents at baseline had a significantly lower risk of death (HR adjusted for baseline differences 0.82, 95% CI 0.73 to 0.92).[66] Subgroup analysis suggested that antiplatelet agents might have an effect in people randomised to placebo (mortality HR for antiplatelet treatment at baseline *v* no antiplatelet treatment at baseline 0.68, 95% CI 0.58 to 0.80), but not in people randomised to enalapril (mortality HR for antiplatelet treatment *v* no antiplatelet treatment 1.00, 95% CI 0.85 to 1.17). Both retrospective studies have important limitations common to studies with a retrospective cohort design. One study did not report on the proportions of people taking aspirin and other antiplatelet agents.[63] The other study noted that more than 95% of people took aspirin, but the dosage and consistency of antiplatelet use was not recorded.[66] One retrospective non-systematic review (4 RCTs, 96 712 people) provided additional evidence about the effect of aspirin on the benefits of early angiotensin converting enzyme inhibitors in heart failure.[67] It found a similar reduction in 30 day mortality with angiotensin converting enzyme inhibitor versus control for those people not taking aspirin compared with those taking aspirin (aspirin: OR 0.94, 95% CI 0.89 to 0.99; no aspirin: OR 0.90, 95% CI 0.81 to 1.01). However, the analysis may not be valid because the people who did not receive aspirin were older and had a worse baseline prognosis than those taking aspirin. The effects of antiplatelet treatment in combination with angiotensin converting enzyme inhibitors in people with heart failure requires further research.

QUESTION What are the effects of angiotensin converting enzyme inhibitors in people at high risk of heart failure?

OPTION ANGIOTENSIN CONVERTING ENZYME INHIBITORS IN PEOPLE AT HIGH RISK OF HEART FAILURE

RCTs in people with asymptomatic left ventricular systolic dysfunction and in people with other risk factors found that angiotensin converting enzyme inhibitors delayed the onset of symptomatic heart failure, reduced cardiovascular events, and improved long term survival compared with placebo.

Benefits: **In people with asymptomatic left ventricular systolic dysfunction:** We found no systematic review but found three RCTs, one of which reported 12 year follow up of the first RCT.[68–70] The first large RCT (4228 people) compared an angiotensin converting enzyme (ACE) inhibitor (enalapril) versus placebo over 40 months in people with asymptomatic left ventricular systolic dysfunction (ejection fraction < 0.35).[68] It found no significant difference between enalapril and placebo in total mortality and cardiovascular mortality (all cause mortality: 313/2111 [14.8%] with ACE inhibitor *v* 334/2117 [15.8%] with placebo; ARR +0.9%, 95% CI –1.3% to +2.9%; RR 0.94, 95% CI 0.81 to 1.08; cardiovascular mortality: 265/2111 [12.6%] with ACE inhibitor *v* 298/2117 [14.1%] with placebo; ARR +1.5%, 95% CI –0.6% to +3.3%; RR 0.89, 95% CI 0.76 to 1.04). During the study, more people assigned to the placebo received digoxin, diuretics, or ACE inhibitors that were not part of the study protocol, which may have contributed to the lack of significant difference in mortality between the two groups. The RCT found that, compared with placebo, enalapril significantly reduced symptomatic heart failure, hospital admission for heart failure, and fatal or non-fatal myocardial infarction (symptomatic heart failure: 438/2111 [21%] with ACE inhibitor *v* 640/2117 [30%] with placebo; ARR 9.5%, 95% CI 7.0% to 12.0%; RR 0.69, 95% CI 0.61 to 0.77; admission for heart failure: 306/2111 [15%] with ACE inhibitor *v* 454/2117 [21%] with placebo; ARR 7%, 95% CI 5% to 9%; RR 0.68, 95% CI 0.59 to 0.77; fatal or non-fatal myocardial infarction: 7.6% with ACE inhibitor *v* 9.6% with placebo; ARR 2%, 95% CI 0.4% to 3.4%; RR 0.79, 95% CI 0.65 to 0.96).[9,68] Twelve year follow up of this RCT found that enalapril given for

3–4 years significantly reduced death from all causes and cardiac deaths compared with placebo (all cause mortality: HR 0.86, 95% CI 0.79 to 0.93; cardiac death: HR 0.85, 95% CI 0.77 to 0.94).[70] The second RCT in asymptomatic people after myocardial infarction with documented left ventricular systolic dysfunction found that an ACE inhibitor (captopril) reduced the risk of all ischaemic events, all myocardial infarctions, and fatal myocardial infarctions compared with placebo (all ischaemic events: 29% with captopril *v* 33% with placebo; RR 0.86, 95% CI 0.74 to 1.0; total myocardial infarctions: 12% with captopril *v* 15% with placebo; RR 0.75, 95% CI 0.60 to 0.95; fatal myocardial infarctions: 5% with captopril *v* 7% with placebo; RR 0.68, 95% CI 0.49 to 0.96).[69] **In people with other risk factors:** We found one large RCT comparing ramipril 10 mg daily versus placebo, for a mean of 5 years, in 9297 high risk people (people with vascular disease or diabetes plus one other cardiovascular risk factor) who were not known to have left ventricular systolic dysfunction or heart failure.[71] It found that ramipril significantly reduced the risk of heart failure compared with placebo (9.0% with ramipril *v* 11.5% with placebo; RR 0.77, 95% CI 0.67 to 0.87; $P < 0.001$). Ramipril also reduced the combined risk of myocardial infarction or stroke or cardiovascular death, the risk of these outcomes separately, and all cause mortality (see ACE inhibitors under secondary prevention of ischaemic cardiac events, p 000). During the trial, 496 people had an echocardiography; 2.6% of these people were found to have ejection fraction less than 0.4. Retrospective review of charts found that left ventricular function had been documented in 5193 people; 8.1% had a reduced ejection fraction.

Harms: **In people with asymptomatic left ventricular systolic dysfunction:** The first RCT over 40 months found that a high proportion of people in both groups reported adverse effects (76% with enalapril *v* 72% with placebo).[68] Dizziness or fainting (46% with enalapril *v* 33% with placebo) and cough (34% with enalapril *v* 27% with placebo) were reported more often in the enalapril group (P value not reported). The incidence of angio-oedema was the same in both groups (1.4%). Study medication was permanently discontinued by 8% of the people in the enalapril group versus 5% in the placebo group (P value not reported). The 12 year follow up of this RCT did not report on adverse effects.

Comment: Asymptomatic left ventricular systolic dysfunction is prognostically important, but we found no prospective studies that have evaluated screening to detect its presence.

QUESTION What are the effects of treatments for diastolic heart failure?

OPTION TREATMENTS FOR DIASTOLIC HEART FAILURE

One RCT found that candesartan, an angiotensin II receptor blocker, reduced the combined outcome of cardiovascular death or hospital admission for heart failure compared with placebo, although the difference was not significant. It found no significant difference in cardiovascular death between the two groups, but found that candesartan reduced hospital admission compared with placebo. We found no RCTs examining effects of other treatments in people with diastolic heart failure.

Benefits: **Angiotensin II receptor blockers:** We found one RCT (3023 patients with New York Heart Association class G II–IV heart failure and left ventricular ejection fraction > 40%), which compared candesartan (started at 4 or 8 mg daily with target dose 32 mg once daily from 6 weeks onwards) versus placebo.[72] It found that, during a median follow up of 36.6 months, candesartan reduced the combined outcome of cardiovascular death or hospital admission for chronic heart failure compared with placebo (22% with candesartan *v* 24.3% with placebo; adjusted HR 0.86, 95% CI 0.74 to 1.00). It found no significant difference in cardiovascular death between the two groups, but found that candesartan significantly reduced hospital admission for heart failure compared with the placebo group (cardiovascular death: 11.2% with candesartan *v* 11.3% with placebo; adjusted HR 0.95, 95% CI 0.76 to 1.18; hospital admission for congestive heart failure: 15.9% with candesartan *v* 18.3% with placebo; adjusted HR 0.84, 95% CI 0.70 to 1.00). **Other treatments:** We found no RCTs.

Harms: **Angiotensin II receptor blockers:** The RCT found that candesartan significantly increased permanent discontinuation of therapy because of an adverse event or an abnormal laboratory value compared with placebo (adverse events were hypotension, hyperkalemia, and increase in plasma creatinine; 17.8% with candesartan *v* 13.5% with placebo; P = 0.001).[72]

Comment: The causes of diastolic dysfunction vary among people with diastolic heart failure. Current treatment is largely based on the results of small clinical studies and consists of treating the underlying cause and coexistent conditions with interventions optimised for individuals.[6,73,74] Further RCTs with clinically relevant outcome measures are needed to determine the benefits and harms of treatments other than angiotensin II receptor blockers in diastolic heart failure.

GLOSSARY

New York Heart Association classification Classification of severity by symptoms. Class I: no limitation of physical activity; ordinary physical activity does not cause undue fatigue or dyspnoea. Class II: slight limitation of physical activity; comfortable at rest, but ordinary physical activity results in fatigue or dyspnoea. Class III: limitation of physical activity; comfortable at rest, but less than ordinary activity causes fatigue or dyspnoea. Class IV: unable to carry out any physical activity without symptoms; symptoms are present even at rest; if any physical activity is undertaken, symptoms are increased.

Usual or conventional care describes the comparator arm of some controlled trials. It refers to appropriate drug and non-drug treatment, in the absence of the intervention being examined in the active treatment arm of the trial.

REFERENCES

1. Poole-Wilson PA. History, definition, and classification of heart failure. In: Poole-Wilson PA, Colucci WS, Massie BM, et al, eds. *Heart failure. Scientific principles and clinical practice*. London: Churchill Livingston, 1997:269–277.
2. Working Group Report. How to diagnose diastolic heart failure: European Study Group on Diastolic Heart Failure. *Eur Heart J* 1998;19:990–1003.
3. Cowie MR, Mosterd A, Wood DA, et al. The epidemiology of heart failure. *Eur Heart J* 1997;18:208–225.
4. McKelvie RS, Benedict CR, Yusuf S. Prevention of congestive heart failure and management of asymptomatic left ventricular dysfunction. *BMJ* 1999;318:1400–1402.
5. Bröckel U, Hense HW, Museholl M. Prevalence of left ventricular dysfunction in the general population [abstract]. *J Am Coll Cardiol* 1996;27(suppl A):25.
6. Mosterd A, deBruijne MC, Hoes A. Usefulness of echocardiography in detecting left ventricular dysfunction in population-based studies (the Rotterdam study). *Am J Cardiol* 1997;79;103–104.
7. Vasan RS, Benjamin EJ, Levy D. Congestive heart failure with normal left ventricular systolic function. *Arch Intern Med* 1996;156:146–157.
8. Davie AP, Francis CM, Caruana L, et al. The prevalence of left ventricular diastolic filling abnormalities in patients with suspected heart failure. *Eur Heart J* 1997;18:981–984.
9. Yusuf S, Pepine CJ, Garces C, et al. Effect of enalapril on myocardial infarction and unstable angina in patients with low ejection fractions. *Lancet* 1992;340:1173–1178.
10. Gheorghiade M, Benatar D, Konstam MA, et al. Pharmacotherapy for systolic dysfunction: a review of randomized clinical trials. *Am J Cardiol* 1997;80(8B):14H–27H.
11. Gaasch WH. Diagnosis and treatment of heart failure based on LV systolic or diastolic dysfunction. *JAMA* 1994;271:1276–1280.
12. Bittner V, Weiner DH, Yusuf S, et al, for the SOLVD Investigators. Prediction of mortality and morbidity with a 6-minute walk test in patients with left ventricular dysfunction. *JAMA* 1993;270:1702–1707.
13. Rogers WJ, Johnstone DE, Yusuf S, et al, for the SOLVD Investigators. Quality of life among 5025 patients with left ventricular dysfunction randomized between placebo and enalapril. The studies of left ventricular dysfunction. *J Am Coll Cardiol* 1994;23:393–400.
14. McAlister FA, Lawson FME, Teo KK, et al. A systematic review of randomized trials of disease management programs in heart failure. *Am J Med* 2001;110:378–384. Search date 1999; primary sources Medline, Embase, Cinahl, Sigle, Cochrane Controlled Trials Register, the Cochrane Effective Practice and Organization of Care Study Register, hand searches of bibliographies of identified studies, and personal contact with content experts.

15. Krumholz HM, Amatruda J, Smith GL, et al. Randomized trial of an education and support intervention to prevent readmission of patients with heart failure. *J Am Coll Cardiol* 2002;39:83–89.
16. Kasper EK, Gerstenblith G, Hefter G, et al. A randomized trial of the efficacy of multidisciplinary care in heart failure outpatients at high risk of hospital readmission. *J Am Coll Cardiol* 2002;39:471–480.
17. McDonald K, Ledwidge M, Cahill J, et al. Heart failure management: multidisciplinary care has intrinsic benefit above the optimization of medical care. *J Card Fail* 2002;8:142–148.
18. Benatar D, Bondmass M, Ghitelman J, et al. Outcomes of chronic heart failure. *Arch Intern Med* 2003;163:347–352.
19. Doughty RN, Wright SP, Pearl A, et al. Randomized, controlled trial of integrated heart failure management: The Auckland Heart Failure Management Study. *Eur Heart J* 2002;23:139–146.
20. Riegel B, Carlson B, Kopp Z, et al. Effect of a standardized nurse case-management telephone intervention on resource use in patients with chronic heart failure. *Arch Intern Med* 2002;162:705–712.
21. Capomolla S, Febo O, Ceresa M, et al. Cost/utility ratio in chronic heart failure: comparison between heart failure management program delivered by day-hospital and usual care. *J Am Coll Cardiol* 2002;40:1259–1266.
22. Stomberg A, Martensson J, Fridlund B, et al. Nurse-led heart failure clinics improve survival and self-care behaviour in patients with heart failure: results from a prospective, randomized trial. *Eur Heart J* 2003;24:1014–1023.
23. Stewart S, Horowitz JD. Home-based intervention in congestive heart failure: long-term implications on readmission and survival. *Circulation* 2002;105:2861–2866.
24. ExTraMATCH Collaborative. Exercise training meta-analysis of trials in patients with chronic heart failure (ExTraMATCH). *BMJ* 2004;328:189–192. Search date not reported; primary sources Medline, Cochrane Reviews database, consulting with researchers in exercise physiology and heart failure, scrutinising reference lists from review articles, and abstracts presented at scientific sessions and published in *Circulation*, the *Journal of the American College of Cardiology*, and the *European Heart Journal*.
25. Garg R, Yusuf S, for the Collaborative Group on ACE Inhibitor Trials. Overview of randomized trials of angiotensin-converting enzyme inhibitors on mortality and morbidity in patients with heart failure. *JAMA* 1995;273:1450–1456. Search date 1994; primary sources Medline and correspondence with investigators and pharmaceutical companies.
26. Flather M, Yusuf S, Kober L, et al, for the ACE-Inhibitor Myocardial Infarction Collaborative Group. Long-term ACE-inhibitor therapy in patients with heart failure or left-ventricular dysfunction: a systematic overview of data from individual patients. *Lancet* 2000;355:1575–1581. Search date not reported; primary sources Medline, Ovid, hand searches of reference lists, and personal contact with researchers, colleagues, and principal investigators of the trials identified.
27. Packer M, Poole-Wilson PA, Armstrong PW, et al, on behalf of the ATLAS Study Group. Comparative effects of low and high doses of the angiotensin-converting enzyme inhibitor, lisinopril, on morbidity and mortality in chronic heart failure. *Circulation* 1999;100:2312–2318.
28. SOLVD Investigators. Effect of enalapril on survival in patients with reduced left ventricular ejection fractions and congestive heart failure. *N Engl J Med* 1991;325:293–302.
29. Agusti A, Bonet S, Arnau JM, et al. Adverse effects of ACE inhibitors in patients with chronic heart failure and/or ventricular dysfunction: meta-analysis of randomized clinical trials. *Drug Saf* 2003;26:895–908.
30. Jong P, Demers C, McKelvie RS, et al. Angiotensin receptor blockers in heart failure: meta-analysis of randomized controlled trials. *J Am Coll Cardiol* 2002;39:463–470. Search date 2001; primary sources Medline, Embase, Biological Abstracts, International Pharmaceutical Abstracts, Cochrane Controlled Trials Database, McMaster Cardiovascular Randomized Clinical Trial Registry, and Science Citation Index.
31. Granger CB, McMurray JJ, Yusuf S, et al. (CHARM Investigators and Committees). Effects of candesartan in patients with chronic heart failure and reduced left-ventricular systolic function intolerant to angiotensin-converting-enzyme inhibitors: the CHARM-Alternative trial. *Lancet* 2003;362:772–776.
32. McMurray JJ, Ostergren J, Swedberg K, et al. (CHARM Investigators and Committees). Effects of candesartan in patients with chronic heart failure and reduced left ventricular systolic function taking angiotensin-converting-enzyme inhibitors: the CHARM-Added trial. *Lancet* 2003;362:767–771.
33. Kraus F, Rudolph C, Rudolph W. Effectiveness of digitalis in patients with chronic heart failure and sinus rhythm. Review of randomized, double-blind and placebo controlled studies. [German]. *Herz* 1993;18:95–117. Search date 1992; primary source Medline.
34. Digitalis Investigation Group. The effect of digoxin on mortality and morbidity in patients with heart failure. *N Engl J Med* 1997;336:525–533.
35. Cohn J, Goldstein S, Greenberg B, et al. A dose-dependent increase in mortality with vesnarinone among patients with severe heart failure. *N Engl J Med* 1998;339:1810–1816.
36. Packer M, Carver JR, Rodeheffer RJ, et al, for the PROMISE Study Research Group. Effect of oral milrinone on mortality in severe chronic heart failure. *N Engl J Med* 1991;325:1468–1475.
37. Hampton JR, van Veldhuisen DJ, Kleber FX, et al. Randomised study of effect of ibopamine on survival in patients with advanced severe heart failure. *Lancet* 1997;349:971–977.
38. Thackray S, Easthaugh J, Freemantle N, et al. The effectiveness and relative effectiveness of intravenous inotropic drugs acting through the adrenergic pathway in patients with heart failure – a meta-regression analysis. *Eur J Heart Fail* 2002;4:515–529. Search date 2000; primary sources Medline, Embase, Cochrane Database of Trials, hand searches of reference lists, existing bibliographies, and reviews.
39. Brophy JM, Joseph L, Rouleau JL. β-blockers in congestive heart failure: a Bayesian meta-analysis. *Ann Intern Med* 2001;134:550–560. Search date 2000; primary sources Medline, Cochrane Library, Web of Science, and hand searches of reference lists from relevant articles.
40. Whorlow SL, Krum H. Meta-analysis of effect of β-blocker therapy on mortality in patients with New York Heart Association class IV chronic congestive heart failure. *Am J Cardiol* 2000;86:886–889. Search date not reported; primary sources Medline and hand searches of reference lists from relevant reviews.
41. Packer M, Coats A, Fowler MB. Effect of carvedilol on survival in severe chronic heart failure. *N Engl J Med* 2001;344:1651–1658.
42. The Beta-Blocker Evaluation of Survival Trial Investigators. A trial of the β-blocker bucindolol in patients with advanced chronic heart failure. *N Engl J Med* 2001;344:1659–1667.
43. Packer M, Fowler MB, Roecker EB, et al. Effect of carvedilol on the morbidity of patients with severe chronic heart failure: results of the carvedilol prospective randomized cumulative survival (COPERNICUS) study. *Circulation* 2002;106:2194–2199.
44. Krum H, Roecker EB, Mohacsi P, et al. Effects of initiating carvedilol in patients with severe chronic heart failure: results from the COPERNICUS Study. *JAMA* 2003;289:712–718.
45. The CAPRICORN Investigators. Effect of carvedilol on outcome after myocardial infarction in patients with

left ventricular dysfunction: the CAPRICORN randomized trial. *Lancet* 2001;357:1385–1390.
46. Metra M, Giubbini R, Nodari S, et al. Differential effects of β-blockers in patients with heart failure: a prospective, randomized, double-blind comparison of the long-term effects of metoprolol versus carvedilol. *Circulation* 2000;102:546–551.
47. Poole-Wilson PA, Swedberg K, Cleland JG, et al. Comparison of carvedilol and metoprolol on clinical outcomes in patients with chronic heart failure in the Carvedilol Or Metoprolol European Trial (COMET): randomised controlled trial. *Lancet* 2003;362:7–13.
48. Cleophas T, van Marum R. Meta-analysis of efficacy and safety of second-generation dihydropyridine calcium channel blockers in heart failure. *Am J Cardiol* 2001;87:487–490. Search date not reported; primary source Medline.
49. Levine TB, Bernink P, Caspi A, et al. Effect of mibefradil, a T-type calcium channel blocker, on morbidity and mortality in moderate to severe congestive heart failure. The MACH-1 study. *Circulation* 2000;101:758–764.
50. Packer M, O'Connor CM, Ghali JK, et al, for the Prospective Randomized Amlodipine Survival Evaluation Study Group. Effect of amlodipine on morbidity and mortality in severe chronic heart failure. *N Engl J Med* 1996;335:1107–1114.
51. Pitt B, Zannad F, Remme WJ, et al, for the Randomized Aldactone Evaluation Study Investigators. The effects of spironolactone on morbidity and mortality in patients with severe heart failure. *N Engl J Med* 1999;341:709–717.
52. Pitt B, Willem R, Zannad F, et al. Eplerenone, a selective aldosterone blocker, in patients with left ventricular dysfunction after myocardial infarction. *N Engl J Med* 2003;348:1309–1321. [Erratum in: *N Engl J Med* 2003;348:2271].
53. Piepoli M, Villani GQ, Ponikowski P, et al. Overview and meta-analysis of randomised trials of amiodarone in chronic heart failure. *Int J Cardiol* 1998;66:1–10. Search date 1997; primary source unspecified computerised literature database.
54. Amiodarone Trials Meta-analysis Investigators. Effect of prophylactic amiodarone on mortality after acute myocardial infarction and in congestive heart failure: meta-analysis of individual data from 6500 patients in randomised trials. *Lancet* 1997;350:1417–1424. Search date not reported; primary sources literature reviews, computerised literature reviews, and discussion with colleagues.
55. The Antiarrhythmic versus Implantable Defibrillators (AVID) Investigators. A comparison of antiarrhythmic-drug therapy with implantable defibrillators I patients resuscitated from near-fatal ventricular arrhythmias. *N Engl J Med* 1997;337:1576–1583.
56. Moss AJ, Hall WJ, Cannom DS, et al. Improved survival with an implanted defibrillator in patients with coronary disease at high risk for ventricular arrhythmia. *N Engl J Med* 1996;335:1933–1940.
57. Moss AJ, Zoreba W, Hall J, et al, for the Multicenter Automatic Defibrillator Implantation Trial II Investigators. Prophylactic implantation of a defibrillator in patients with myocardial infarction and reduced ejection fraction. *N Engl J Med* 2002;346:877–883.
58. Bigger JT for The Coronary Artery Bypass Graft (CABG) Patch Trial Investigators. Prophylactic use of implanted cardiac defibrillators in patients at high risk for ventricular arrhythmias after coronary-artery bypass graft surgery. *N Engl J Med* 1997;337:1569–1575.
59. Teerlink JR, Jalaluddin M, Anderson S, et al. Ambulatory ventricular arrhythmias in patients with heart failure do not specifically predict an increased risk of sudden death. *Circulation* 2000;101:40–46.
60. Connolly SJ. Prophylactic antiarrhythmic therapy for the prevention of sudden death in high-risk patients: drugs and devices. *Eur Heart J* 1999;(suppl C):31–35.
61. Lip GYH, Gibbs CR. Anticoagulation for heart failure in sinus rhythm (Cochrane Review). In: The Cochrane Library, Issue 3, 2004. Chichester, UK: John Wiley & Sons, Ltd. Search date 2001; primary sources Cochrane Controlled Trials Register, Medline, Embase, NHS Database of Abstracts of Reviews of Effectiveness, abstracts from national and international cardiology meetings, authors of identified studies, and reference lists.
62. Jones CG, Cleland JGF. Meeting report: the LIDO, HOPE, MOXCON, and WASH studies. *Eur J Heart Fail* 1999;1:425–431.
63. Dunkman WB, Johnson GR, Carson PE, et al, for the V-HeFT Cooperative Studies Group. Incidence of thromboembolic events in congestive heart failure. *Circulation* 1993;87:94–101.
64. Al-Khadra AS, Salem DN, Rand WM, et al. Warfarin anticoagulation and survival: a cohort analysis from the studies of left ventricular dysfunction. *J Am Coll Cardiol* 1998;31:749–753.
65. Lip GYH, Gibbs CR. Antiplatelet agents versus control or anticoagulation for heart failure in sinus rhythm (Cochrane Review). In: The Cochrane Library, Issue 2, 2003. Oxford: Update Software. Search date 2000; primary sources Medline, Embase, Dare, abstracts from national and international meetings, and contact with relevant authors.
66. Al-Khadra AS, Salem DN, Rand WM, et al. Antiplatelet agents and survival: a cohort analysis from the Studies of Left Ventricular Dysfunction (SOLVD) Trial. *J Am Coll Cardiol* 1998;31:419–425.
67. Latini R, Tognoni G, Maggioni AP, et al, on behalf of the Angiotensin-converting Enzyme Inhibitor Myocardial Infarction Collaborative Group. Clinical effects of early angiotensin-converting enzyme inhibitor treatment for acute myocardial infarction are similar in the presence and absence of aspirin. Systematic overview of individual data from 96 712 randomized patients. *J Am Coll Cardiol* 2000;35:1801–1807.
68. SOLVD Investigators. Effect of enalapril on mortality and the development of heart failure in asymptomatic patients with reduced left ventricular ejection fractions. *N Engl J Med* 1992;327:685–691.
69. Rutherford JD, Pfeffer MA, Moyé LA, et al. Effects of captopril on ischaemic events after myocardial infarction. *Circulation* 1994;90:1731–1738.
70. Jong P, Yusuf S, Rousseau MF, et al. Effect of enalapril on 12-year survival and life expectancy in patients with left ventricular systolic dysfunction: a follow-up study. *Lancet* 2003;361:1843–1848.
71. The Heart Outcome Prevention Evaluation Study Investigators. Effects of an angiotensin-converting-enzyme inhibitor, ramipril, on cardiovascular events in high-risk patients. *N Engl J Med* 2000;342:145–153.
72. Yusuf S, Pfeffer MA, Swedberg K, et al. (CHARM Investigators and Committees). Effects of candesartan in patients with chronic heart failure and preserved left-ventricular ejection fraction: the CHARM-Preserved Trial. *Lancet* 2003;362:777–781.
73. The Task Force of the Working Group on Heart Failure of the European Society of Cardiology. The treatment of heart failure. *Eur Heart J* 1997;18:736–753.
74. Tendera M. Ageing and heart failure: the place of ACE inhibitors in heart failure with preserved systolic function. *Eur Heart J* 2000;2(suppl I):I8–I14.

Robert McKelvie
Professor of Medicine
McMaster University, Hamilton, ON, Canada

Competing interests: RM has been paid by AstraZeneca and Bristol-Myers Squibb to serve on steering committees and has been paid by AstraZeneca and Merck Frosst to give presentations.

Peripheral arterial disease

Search date December 2003

Paul Bachoo

QUESTIONS

INTERVENTIONS

See glossary Ⓖ
*Based on observational evidence and consensus

Key Messages

- **Antiplatelet treatment** Systematic reviews have found strong evidence that antiplatelet agents reduce major cardiovascular events over an average of about 2 years compared with control treatment. Systematic reviews have found that antiplatelet agents reduce the risk of arterial occlusion and revascularisation procedures compared with placebo or no treatment. The balance of benefits and harms is in favour of treatment for most people with symptomatic peripheral arterial disease, because as a group they are at much greater risk of cardiovascular events.
- **Exercise** Systematic reviews and subsequent RCTs in people with chronic stable claudication have found that regular exercise at least three times weekly for between 3 and 6 months improves total walking distance and maximal exercise time after 3–12 months compared with no exercise. One RCT found that a "stop smoking and keep walking" intervention increased the maximal walking distance compared with usual care at 12 months. One RCT found that vitamin E plus regular exercise increased walking duration compared with placebo at 6 months.
- **Bypass surgery (compared with thrombolysis in people with acute limb ischaemia)** One systematic review in people with acute limb ischaemia found that surgery reduced amputation rate and pain compared with thrombolysis, but found no significant difference in mortality after 1 year.
- **Percutaneous transluminal angioplasty (transient benefit only)** Two small RCTs in people with mild to moderate intermittent claudication found limited evidence that percutaneous angioplasty improved walking distance after 6 months compared with no angioplasty but found no significant difference after 2 or 6 years. Two small RCTs identified by a systematic review and four additional RCTs in people with femoro-popliteal or aorto-iliac artery stenoses found no significant difference between angioplasty alone and angioplasty plus stent placement in patency rates, occlusion

rates, or clinical improvement. The RCTs may lack power to rule out an important clinical effect. One systematic review found that in people with chronic progressive peripheral arterial disease percutaneous transluminal angioplasty was less effective in improving patency compared with surgery after 12–24 months but found no significant difference after 4 years. The review found no difference in mortality after 12–24 months.

- **Smoking cessation** RCTs of advice to stop smoking would be considered unethical. The consensus view is that smoking cessation improves symptoms in people with intermittent claudication. One systematic review of observational studies found inconclusive results from stopping smoking, both in terms of increasing absolute claudication distance and reducing the risk of symptom progression compared with people who continue to smoke.
- **Cilostazol** Six RCTs found that cilostazol improved claudication distance at 12–24 weeks compared with placebo. However, adverse effects of cilostazol were common in the RCTs, and included headache, diarrhoea, and palpitations. One RCT found limited evidence that cilostazol increased initial and absolute claudication distance compared with pentoxifylline.
- **Bypass surgery (compared with percutaneous transluminal angioplasty)** One systematic review found that surgery improved primary blood vessel patency after 12–24 months compared with percutaneous transluminal angioplasty, but found no significant difference after 4 years. The review found no significant difference in mortality after 12–24 months. Although the consensus view is that bypass surgery is the most effective treatment for people with debilitating symptomatic peripheral arterial disease, RCTs provided inadequate evidence on long term clinical outcomes to confirm this view.
- **Pentoxifylline** One systematic review and one subsequent RCT found insufficient evidence to compare pentoxifylline with placebo. One RCT found limited evidence that pentoxifylline was less effective at improving initial and absolute claudication distance compared with cilostazol.

DEFINITION Peripheral arterial disease arises when there is significant narrowing of arteries distal to the arch of the aorta. Narrowing can arise from atheroma, arteritis, local thrombus formation, or embolisation from the heart or more central arteries. This topic includes treatment options for people with symptoms of reduced blood flow to the leg that are likely to arise from atheroma. These symptoms range from calf pain on exercise (intermittent claudication Ⓖ) to rest pain, skin ulceration, or symptoms of ischaemic necrosis (gangrene) in people with critical limb ischaemia Ⓖ.

INCIDENCE/ PREVALENCE Peripheral arterial disease is more common in people aged over 50 years than in younger people, and is more common in men than women. The prevalence of peripheral arterial disease of the legs (assessed by non-invasive tests) is about 3% in people under the age of 60 years, but rises to over 20% in people over 75 years.[1] The overall annual incidence of intermittent claudication is 1.5–2.6/1000 men and 1.2–3.6/1000 women.[2]

AETIOLOGY/ RISK FACTORS Factors associated with the development of peripheral arterial disease include age, gender, cigarette smoking, diabetes mellitus, hypertension, hyperlipidaemia, obesity, and physical inactivity. The strongest associations are with smoking (RR 2.0–4.0) and diabetes (RR 2.0–3.0).[3] Acute limb ischaemia Ⓖ may result from thrombosis arising within a peripheral artery or from embolic occlusion.

PROGNOSIS The symptoms of intermittent claudication can resolve spontaneously, remain stable over many years, or progress rapidly to critical limb ischaemia Ⓖ. About 15% of people with intermittent claudication eventually develop critical leg ischaemia, which endangers the viability of the limb. The annual incidence of critical limb ischaemia in Denmark and Italy in 1990 was 0.25–0.45/1000 people.[4,5] Coronary heart disease is the major cause of death in people with peripheral arterial disease of the legs. Over 5 years, about 20% of people with intermittent claudication have a non-fatal cardiovascular event (myocardial infarction or stroke).[6] The mortality of people with peripheral arterial disease is two to three times higher than that of age and sex matched controls. Overall mortality after the diagnosis of peripheral arterial disease is about 30% after 5 years and 70% after 15 years.[6]

AIMS OF INTERVENTION To reduce symptoms (intermittent claudication), local complications (arterial leg ulcers, critical leg ischaemia), and general complications (myocardial infarction and stroke).

OUTCOMES **Primary outcome:** Initial claudication distanceⒼ. **Secondary outcomes:** Absolute claudication distanceⒼ, generic/disease specific quality of life, clinical end points (intervention rates, post-intervention morbidity/mortality), physiological measures (ankle brachial pressure index), and all cause cardiovascular morbidity/mortality).

METHODS *Clinical Evidence* search and appraisal December 2003.

QUESTION **What are the effects of treatments for people with chronic peripheral arterial disease?**

OPTION **ANTIPLATELET AGENTS**

Systematic reviews have found strong evidence that antiplatelet agents reduce major cardiovascular events over an average of about 2 years compared with control treatment. Systematic reviews have found that antiplatelet agents reduce the risk of arterial occlusion and revascularisation procedures compared with placebo or no treatment. The balance of benefits and harms is in favour of treatment for most people with symptomatic peripheral arterial disease, because as a group they are at much greater risk of cardiovascular events.

Benefits: **Peripheral arterial disease complications:** We found two systematic reviews.[7,8] The first systematic review (search date 1997, 42 RCTs; 9214 people with intermittent claudicationⒼ, bypass surgery of the leg, or peripheral artery angioplasty) found that antiplatelet treatment significantly reduced the risk of arterial occlusion over 19 months compared with no additional treatment (arterial occlusion: RRR 30%; $P < 0.00001$).[8] The second systematic review (search date 1998, 54 RCTs of antithrombotic drugs) found that aspirin significantly reduced arterial occlusion or revascularisation procedures at 3 months compared with placebo (1 RCT, 2810 people: OR at 3 months 0.46, 95% CI 0.27 to 0.77).[7] It found that ticlopidine (2 RCTs, 1302 people) significantly reduced arterial occlusion or revascularisation procedures compared with placebo at up to 7 years (OR 0.62, 95% CI 0.41 to 0.93).[7] **Cardiovascular events:** We found two systematic reviews.[8,9] The first review (search date 1997, 42 RCTs, 9506 people with peripheral arterial disease) found that antiplatelet treatment significantly reduced the combined outcome of vascular death, myocardial infarction, or stroke over an average of 2 years compared with control (280/4844 [6.0%] with antiplatelet treatment *v* 347/4662 [7.0%] with control; RR 0.78, 95% CI 0.67 to 0.90; NNT 61, 95% CI 38 to 153).[8] The second systematic review (search date 1999, 39 RCTs) found that antiplatelet treatment significantly reduced the combined end point of myocardial infarction, stroke, or vascular death compared with control (6.5% with antiplatelet treatment *v* 8.1% with control; OR 0.78, 95% CI 0.63 to 0.96).[9]

Harms: One earlier systematic review (later updated;[8] original search date 1990, 35 RCTs, 8098 people with peripheral arterial disease) found no significant difference between antiplatelet and control treatment in the risk of non-fatal major bleeds (14/2545 [0.55%] *v* 9/2243 [0.40%]; RR 1.37, 95% CI 0.60 to 3.16).[10] The second review (search date 1999) found no significant difference between antiplatelet treatment and placebo in major bleeding (39 RCTs; 8449 people; 47/4349 [1%] with antiplatelet treatment *v* 33/4100 [< 1%] with placebo; OR 1.40, 95% CI 0.90 to 2.20).[9] The review also found no significant difference between aspirin and other antiplatelet agents in major bleeding (68/3467 [2%] with aspirin *v* 59/3561 [2%] with other antiplatelet agents; RR 1.18, 95% CI 0.84 to 1.67). The number of events was too low to exclude a clinically important increase in major bleeding.[9,10] Across a wide range of people, antiplatelet agents have been found to significantly increase the risk of major haemorrhage. **Intracranial haemorrhage:** These are uncommon, but they are often fatal or cause substantial disability in survivors. We found one relevant systematic review (search date 1997)[11] in which people were randomised to aspirin or control treatment for at least 1 month. It found that aspirin produced a small increased risk of intracranial haemorrhage in about 1/1000 (0.1%) people treated for 3 years.[11] Our meta-analysis of the primary prevention RCTs found a somewhat smaller absolute overall excess of about 0.1/1000 (0.01%) people treated with aspirin a year. **Extracranial haemorrhage:** Major extracranial bleeds occur mainly in the gastrointestinal tract and may require hospital admission or blood transfusion, but do not generally result in permanent disability and are rarely fatal. We found one relevant systematic review of aspirin versus control with a scheduled treatment duration of at least 1 year. It found the relative excess risk of gastrointestinal bleeding with aspirin to be about 70% (OR 1.7, 95% CI 1.5 to 1.9).[12] A recent overview of 15 observational studies, including over 10 000 cases of upper gastrointestinal bleeding or perforation requiring admission to hospital, found the relative risk with aspirin to be 2.5 (95% CI 2.4 to 2.7). If only those studies that had a prospective (and so methodologically more rigorous) design were considered, the relative risk fell to 1.9 (95% CI 1.7 to 2.1), similar to that found in the RCTs.[13] Meta-analysis of primary prevention RCTs found a similar relative excess risk of major extracranial (mainly gastrointestinal) haemorrhage and an absolute excess of about 0.7 major extracranial haemorrhages per 1000 people treated with aspirin a year.

Comment: We found no evidence about the effects of combined clopidogrel and aspirin compared with a single antiplatelet agent in people with peripheral arterial disease. Peripheral arterial disease increases the risk of cardiovascular events, so for most people the risk of bleeding is outweighed by the benefits of regular antiplatelet use.

OPTION EXERCISE

Systematic reviews and subsequent RCTs in people with chronic stable claudication have found that regular exercise at least three times weekly for between 3 and 6 months improves total walking distance and maximal exercise time after 3–12 months compared with no exercise. One RCT found that a "stop smoking and keep walking" intervention increased the maximal walking distance compared with usual care at 12 months. One RCT found that vitamin E plus regular exercise increased walking duration compared with placebo at 6 months.

Benefits: **Walking exercise versus no exercise:** We found two systematic reviews comparing exercise versus no exercise in people with chronic stable intermittent claudication**G** (search dates 1996,[14] and not reported;[15] see comment below) and three subsequent RCTs.[16–18] The first review found that exercise programmes (at least 30 minutes of walking as far as claudication permits, at least 3 times/week, for 3–6 months in people also being treated with surgery, aspirin, or dipyridamole) significantly increased both the initial claudication distance**G** and the absolute claudication distance**G** compared with no exercise (initial claudication distance, 4 RCTs; 94 people; mean increase between exercise and no exercise: 139 m, 95% CI 31 m to 247 m; absolute claudication distance, 5 RCTs; 115 people; mean increase between exercise and no exercise 179 m, 95% CI 60 m to 298 m) after 3–12 months.[14] Control treatments were placebo tablets (2 RCTs) or "instructed to continue with normal lifestyle". The second review (10 RCTs, including all those in the first review) found that exercise increased maximal exercise time compared with no exercise after 12 weeks to 15 months' follow up (3 RCTs; 53 people: WMD 6.5 minutes, 95% CI 4.4 minutes to 8.7 minutes).[15] The first subsequent RCT (52 people) compared a 24 week programme of initially supervised, regular polestriding (walking exercise using modified ski poles) with a no exercise programme.[16] All participants received standard medical treatment. At 24 weeks, it found that regular exercise significantly increased exercise tolerance compared with no exercise on a controlled work treadmill test (tolerance to exercise, walking at 1.8 miles/hour with a 12% gradient: mean increase in exercise duration about 28 minutes with exercise programme *v* 11 minutes without exercise programme; $P < 0.0001$).[16] The second subsequent RCT (64 people, excluding people with rest pain or exertional angina) compared treadmill exercise three times weekly versus no exercise.[17] People in the exercise group were encouraged to exercise for up to 30 minutes with mild to moderate claudication pain. The RCT found that exercise significantly increased time to onset of claudication compared with no exercise after 12 weeks (3.3 minutes at baseline to 6.2 minutes with exercise *v* 2.9 minutes at baseline to 3.2 minutes with no exercise; $P = 0.01$). The third RCT (52 people with intermittent claudication) compared 4 treatments: polestriding exercise (45–60 minutes, 3 times/week for 24 weeks) plus vitamin E; polestriding exercise plus placebo; vitamin E alone; and placebo alone.[18] It found that exercise improved walking duration on a constant work-rate treadmill test compared with placebo alone at 6 months (walking duration: 804 seconds at baseline to 2020 seconds at 6 months with exercise *v* 612 seconds to 623 seconds with placebo; P value not reported). **Exercise as part of multicomponent intervention versus usual care or placebo:** We found two RCTs.[18,19] The first RCT (52 people with intermittent claudication) compared 4 treatments: polestriding exercise (45–60 minutes, 3 times weekly for 24 weeks) plus vitamin E; polestriding exercise plus placebo; vitamin E alone; and placebo alone.[18] It found that exercise plus vitamin E improved walking duration on a constant work-rate treadmill test compared with placebo alone at 6 months (walking duration 486 seconds at baseline to 1886 seconds at 6 months with exercise plus vitamin E *v* 612 seconds to 623 seconds with placebo; P value not reported). The second RCT (882 men with early peripheral vascular disease identified by population screening) compared a "stop smoking and keep walking" intervention package versus usual care (see comment below).[19] It found that the intervention significantly increased maximal walking distance compared with usual care at 12 months (23% with intervention *v* 15% with control; $P = 0.008$). It found no significant difference between intervention and usual care in intermittent claudication grade (Edinburgh Claudication Questionnaire: $P = 0.26$). **Different types of exercise:** All the RCTs included in the systematic reviews involved walking exercise. We found one RCT (67 people with moderate to severe intermittent claudication), which compared arm with leg exercise of similar intensity.[20] A third group of 15 people was non-randomly allocated to no exercise. The RCT found no significant difference between arm and leg exercises in improvement in initial claudication distance or absolute claudication distance, although both groups improved after 6 weeks (improvement in initial claudication distance: 122% with arm exercise *v* 93% with leg exercise; improvement in absolute claudication distance: 147% with arm exercise *v* 150% with leg exercise).

Harms: The reviews and subsequent RCTs did not report on harms of the exercise programmes.[14,16–20]

Comment: The RCTs in the systematic reviews had low withdrawal rates, but it is unclear whether those assessing the outcomes were blind to the group allocation. Concealment of the allocation to participants was not possible.[14,15] Most (5/6) exercise programmes in the second review occurred under supervision.[15] In the second RCT examining exercise as a part of a multicomponent intervention, participants in the intervention group received an educational package, a brochure about community physiotherapy services, and information on the benefits of smoking cessation. The general practitioners of these participants received a letter plus educational material, (including information about effects of smoking cessation, nicotine replacement products, and about peripheral arterial disease), and a recommendation to refer the person to community physiotherapy. The community physiotherapist received details about likely referrals. Physiotherapists provided a community based mobility programme for senior citizens, consisting of supervised or home based exercise sessions and advice to walk at least 30 minutes daily.[19] We found one further systematic review (search date 1993, 21 observational studies or RCTs of exercise, 564 people with peripheral arterial disease).[19] It calculated effects based on the differences in claudication distance before and after exercise treatment, but it made no allowance for any spontaneous improvement that might have occurred in the participants. It reported large increases with exercise in the initial claudication distance (126–351 m) and in the absolute claudication distance (325–723 m), but these estimates were based on observational data. An ongoing Australian RCT is examining the effect of exercise treatment in 1400 men.[15] The benefit from arm exercise remains unconfirmed, but suggests that improved walking may be caused by generally improved cardiovascular function rather than local changes in the peripheral circulation.

OPTION SMOKING CESSATION

RCTs of advice to stop smoking would be considered unethical. The consensus view is that smoking cessation improves symptoms in people with intermittent claudication. One systematic review of observational studies found inconclusive results from stopping smoking, both in terms of increasing absolute claudication distance and reducing the risk of symptom progression, compared with people who continue to smoke.

Benefits: RCTs of advice to stop smoking are considered unethical. The consensus view is that smoking cessation improves symptoms in people with intermittent claudication**G**. We found one systematic review (search date 1996, 4 observational studies, 866 people) of advice to quit cigarette smoking versus no advice.[14] One large observational study in the systematic review found no significant increase in absolute claudication distance**G** after cessation of smoking.[14] Two other studies found conflicting results about the risk of deteriorating from moderate to severe claudication in people who successfully quit smoking compared with current smokers. The fourth study provided no numerical results. Overall, the review found no good evidence to confirm or refute the consensus view that advice to stop smoking improves symptoms in people with intermittent claudication.

Harms: We found no RCTs.

Comment: None.

OPTION CILOSTAZOL

Six RCTs found that cilostazol improved claudication distance at 12–24 weeks compared with placebo. However, adverse effects of cilostazol were common in the RCTs, and included headache, diarrhoea, and palpitations. One RCT found limited evidence that cilostazol increased initial and absolute claudication distance compared with pentoxifylline.

Benefits: We found no systematic review. **Versus placebo:** We found one non-systematic meta-analysis (search date not reported, 6 RCTs; 1751 people with claudication for 6 months or more, treated for between 12 and 24 weeks, 90% were current or previous smokers, 27% had diabetes mellitus, 60% had hypertension)[21] and one additional RCT (see comment below).[22] The meta-analysis (5 published RCTs plus data from 1 RCT held on file by a pharmaceutical company) found that cilostazol 100 mg twice daily significantly increased mean maximal treadmill walking distance and pain free treadmill walking distance compared with placebo (maximal distance: 250 m at baseline to 350 m with cilostazol *v* 252 m at baseline to 302 m with placebo; $P < 0.001$; pain free distance: 127 m at baseline to 210 m with cilostazol *v* 132 m at baseline to 185 m with placebo; $P < 0.001$).[21] One of the RCTs included in the meta-analysis also evaluated a lower dose of cilostazol (100 mg/day).[23] It found no significant difference between this dose of cilostazol and placebo for mean maximum walking distance (167 m with cilostazol 100 mg/day *v* 141 m with placebo; $P = 0.18$). The additional RCT (81 people with stable intermittent claudication**G** for 6 months or more) found that cilostazol 100 mg twice daily significantly increased initial claudication distance**G** and absolute claudication distance**G** at 12 weeks compared with placebo (intention to treat analysis; initial distance: 112.5 m with cilostazol *v* 84.6 m with placebo; $P = 0.007$; absolute distance: 231.7 m with cilostazol *v* 152.1 m with placebo; $P = 0.002$).[22] **Versus pentoxifylline:** See benefits of pentoxifylline, p 146.[24]

Harms: Harms were not reported in the meta-analysis.[21] Two RCTs included in the meta-analysis found that cilostazol significantly increased the risk of withdrawal from the trial because of adverse effects or concerns about safety compared with placebo (1 RCT: 39/227 [17%] with cilostazol 200 mg *v* 24/239 [10%] with placebo; RR 1.71, 95% CI 1.06 to 2.75; NNH 14, 95% CI 8 to 111; 1 RCT: 22.6% with cilostazol 200 mg *v* 12.1% with cilostazol 100 mg *v* 10.1% with placebo, CI not reported).[23,24] The second of these RCTs found that cilostazol 200 mg increased withdrawal due to headache and cardiovascular events compared with placebo (headache: 4.5% with cilostazol 200 mg *v* 0% with placebo; cardiovascular event: 12/133 with cilostazol *v* 5/129 with placebo, CI not reported). The additional RCT found that cilostazol 100 mg increased gastrointestinal complaints compared with placebo (44% with cilostazol *v* 15% with placebo; CI not reported).[22] Cilostazol is a phosphodiesterase inhibitor; RCTs have found that other phosphodiesterase inhibitors (milrinone, vesnarinone) are associated with increased mortality in people with heart failure. However, results aggregated from other studies have not found an excess of cardiovascular events with cilostazol.[25]

Comment: The meta-analysis comparing cilostazol with placebo was not based on studies identified systematically, and hence the selection of studies may be biased.[21] However, the meta-analysis included all the studies identified by our own systematic search. Analysis was on an intention to treat basis. Although the overall results of cilostazol compared with placebo indicate a significant effect of cilostazol on increasing walking distance, the RCTs have some weakness in their methods, which may limit the applicability of the results.[22,24,26,27] Firstly, none of the RCTs evaluated cilostazol beyond 24 weeks. In addition, some of the RCTs had high withdrawal rates after randomisation (up to 29%).[26] In most of the RCTs withdrawals were more common with cilostazol than with placebo.[22–24,26,27] To allow for these problems, the authors performed intention to treat analyses using "last available observation carried forward". However, the analyses did not include people with no observations to carry forward, and the effect of the difference in withdrawals between the groups was not explored adequately. If people with worsening claudication were more likely to withdraw, then the observed differences might have been artefactual. We found one further trial, written in Chinese, which compared cilostazol versus dipyridamole in 32 people with peripheral vascular disease and type 2 diabetes.[28] This study is awaiting translation and appraisal for inclusion in *Clinical Evidence*. Although cilostazol appears promising, the balance of its benefits and harms remains unclear.

OPTION PENTOXIFYLLINE

One systematic review and one subsequent RCT found insufficient evidence to compare pentoxifylline versus placebo. One RCT found limited evidence that pentoxifylline was less effective at improving initial and absolute claudication distance compared with cilostazol.

Benefits: We found one systematic review (search date 1999)[29] and one subsequent RCT.[24] The review found two RCTs (192 people) that met its reliability criteria for inclusion, but did not pool results. Neither RCT in the review found any significant difference between pentoxifylline and placebo for change in initial claudication distance**G** or absolute claudication distance**G** (follow up time not reported; improvement in mean initial claudication distance for pentoxifylline *v* placebo +15 m, 95% CI –5 m to +35 m *v* –30 m, 95% CI –138 m to +78 m; improvement in mean absolute claudication distance +21 m, 95% CI –10 to +52 m *v* +69 m, 95% CI –44 m to +182 m).[29] The subsequent RCT (438 people; see comment below) compared three treatments: pentoxifylline, cilostazol, and placebo.[24] It similarly found no significant difference between pentoxifylline and placebo in the proportion of people who had no change or deterioration in the claudication distance (72/212 [34%] with pentoxifylline *v* 68/226 [30%] with placebo; RR 1.13, 95% CI 0.86 to 1.48).[24] **Versus cilostazol:** The subsequent RCT (see comment below) found that pentoxifylline significantly increased the proportion of people who had no change or deterioration in the claudication distance compared with cilostazol (72/212 [34%] with pentoxifylline *v* 47/205 [23%] with cilostazol; RR 1.48, 95% CI 1.08 to 2.03; ARR 11%, 95% CI 2.4% to 20.0%; NNT 9, 95% CI 5 to 42). It found that pentoxifylline was less effective at increasing the initial claudication distance (202 m with pentoxifylline *v* 218 m with cilostazol; mean difference –16 m; P = 0.0001), and the absolute claudication distance (308 m with pentoxifylline *v* 350 m with cilostazol; mean difference –42 m; P = 0.0005) compared with cilostazol after 24 weeks.[24]

Harms: The subsequent RCT found that pentoxifylline significantly increased the risk of withdrawal from the RCT because of adverse effects or concerns about safety compared with placebo (44/232 [19%] with pentoxifylline *v* 24/239 [10%] with placebo; RR 1.89, 95% CI 1.19 to 3.00; NNH 12, 95% CI 7 to 39).[24] Adverse effects of pentoxifylline included sore throat (14% with pentoxifylline *v* 7% with placebo), dyspepsia, nausea, diarrhoea (8% with pentoxifylline *v* 5% with placebo; P = 0.31), and vomiting.[24] No life threatening adverse effects of pentoxifylline have been reported, although to date RCTs have been too small to assess this reliably.

Comment: The subsequent RCT had a high withdrawal rate after randomisation, which could be a source of bias (60/232 [26%] with pentoxifylline *v* 61/237 [26%] with cilostazol).[24]

OPTION PERCUTANEOUS TRANSLUMINAL ANGIOPLASTY

Two small RCTs in people with mild to moderate intermittent claudication found limited evidence that percutaneous angioplasty improved walking distance after 6 months compared with no angioplasty but found no significant difference after 2 or 6 years. Two small RCTs identified by a systematic review and four additional RCTs in people with femoro-popliteal or aorto-iliac artery stenoses found no significant difference between angioplasty alone and angioplasty plus stent placement in patency rates, occlusion rates, or clinical improvement. The RCTs may lack power to rule out an important clinical effect. One systematic review found that in people with chronic progressive peripheral arterial disease percutaneous transluminal angioplasty was less effective in improving patency compared with surgery after 12–24 months but found no significant difference after 4 years. The review found no difference in mortality after 12–24 months.

Benefits: **Percutaneous transluminal angioplasty (PTA) versus no PTA:** We found one systematic review (search date not reported, 2 RCTs, 78 men and 20 women with mild to moderate intermittent claudication**G**) comparing PTA of the aorto-iliac or femoro-popliteal arteries with no angioplasty.[30] The first RCT identified by the review found that PTA significantly increased the median claudication distance after 6 months compared with no PTA, but found no significant difference in median claudication distance or quality of life after 2 years (median claudication distance at 6 months: 667 m *v* 172 m; $P < 0.05$).[31] The second RCT found that PTA significantly increased the absolute claudication distance**G** at 6 months compared with an exercise programme (130 m *v* 50 m; WMD 80 m; $P < 0.05$), but found no significant difference in absolute claudication distance after 6 years (180 m *v* 130 m; WMD 50 m; $P > 0.05$).[32,33] **PTA versus PTA plus stents:** We found one systematic review (search date 2002, 2 RCTs, 104 people with aorto-iliac or femoro-popliteal lesions on angiography)[34] and four additional RCTs comparing PTA versus PTA plus stent.[35–38] Of these four additional RCTs, two compared routine PTA and stenting versus PTA and selective stenting.[35,38] The remaining two RCTs compared PTA and stenting with PTA alone.[36,37] The RCTs in the systematic review used different techniques and different definitions of restenosis, and data were not pooled.[34] The first RCT in the review (51 people who had received an intravenous bolus of heparin and oral aspirin) found no significant difference in patency assessed by colour flow duplex ultrasound or in occlusion rate (patency: 62% with PTA plus stent *v* 74% with PTA alone; $P = 0.22$; occlusion rate: 5/24 [21%] with PTA plus stent *v* 2/27 [7%] with PTA alone; $P = 0.16$).[39] The second RCT in the review (53 people who had received an intravenous bolus of heparin and oral aspirin) found no significant difference in patency after 34 months' follow up (62% with PTA plus stent placement *v* 68.4% with PTA).[40] People in the PTA plus stent group also received preoperative intravenous heparin bolus 500 units plus 1 g aspirin. The first additional RCT (279 people with intermittent claudication and iliac artery stenosis) comparing routine versus selective stenting found no significant difference in reintervention rates (7% with routine stent *v* 4% with selective stent, 95% CI −2% to +9%).[35] The second additional RCT (227 people with severe claudication or limb threatening stenosis of the superficial femoral artery) comparing routine versus selective stenting found no significant difference in death or in restenosis after 1 year (death: 8% with PTA *v* 4% with PTA plus stent; $P = 0.4$; > 50% restenosis: 32.3% with PTA *v* 34.7% with PTA plus stent; $P = 0.85$).[38] The third additional RCT (32 people) found no significant difference between PTA plus stent and PTA alone in "clinical improvement" after 1 year (60% with PTA plus stent v 71% with PTA; P = 0.17).[37] The fourth additional RCT (141 people, 154 limbs) found no significant difference between PTA plus stent placement and PTA alone in patency, as determined by angiography after 1 year (63% of limbs with PTA plus stent placement v 63% with PTA).[36] **PTA versus surgery:** See benefits of bypass surgery, p 148.

Harms: The systematic review did not report on harms.[34] One of the additional RCTs found that routine stenting significantly increased the risk of local vascular events compared with selective stenting after 1 year (P = 0.017).[38] Prospective cohort studies have found that PTA complications include puncture site major bleeding (3.4%), pseudoaneurysms (0.5%), limb loss (0.2%), renal failure secondary to intravenous contrast (0.2%), cardiac complications such as myocardial infarction (0.2%), and death (0.2%).[41,42]

Comment: This limited evidence suggests transient benefit from angioplasty compared with no angioplasty. The longer term effects of angioplasty or stent placement on symptoms, bypass surgery, and amputation remain unclear, and the available RCTs are too small to rule out clinically important effects of stent placement. The long term patency of femoropopliteal angioplasties is poor, and there is no evidence that the addition of stents confers any additional benefit.[36,37,40] The small number of RCTs and their small sample sizes and methodological weaknesses suggests that further clinical trials are needed to establish clinical effects reliably.

OPTION BYPASS SURGERY

One systematic review found that surgery in people with chronic progressive peripheral arterial disease improved primary patency after 12–24 months compared with percutaneous transluminal angioplasty, but found no significant difference after 4 years. The review found no significant difference in mortality after 12–24 months. One systematic review in people with acute limb ischaemia found that surgery reduced the amputation rate and pain compared with thrombolysis, but it found no significant difference in mortality after 1 year. Although the consensus view is that bypass surgery is the most effective treatment for people with debilitating symptomatic peripheral arterial disease, we found inadequate evidence from RCTs reporting long term clinical outcomes to confirm this view.

Benefits: **Surgery versus exercise:** We found no RCTs. **Surgery versus percutaneous transluminal angioplasty (PTA):** We found one systematic review (search date 2001, 2 RCTs, 365 people with chronic progressive peripheral arterial disease), which found no significant difference between surgery and PTA in mortality after 12–24 months (OR 1.08, 95% CI 0.61 to 1.89).[43] The review found that surgery significantly improved patency after 12–24 months compared with PTA (OR 0.62, 95% CI 0.39 to 0.99), but found no significant difference in primary patency after 4 years (P = 0.14). **Surgery versus thrombolysis:** We found one systematic review (search date 2001, 1 RCT in people with acute limb ischaemia**G**), which compared surgery with thrombolysis using tissue plasminogen activator or urokinase.[43] The review found no significant difference in mortality after 1 year (OR 1.59, 95% CI 0.70 to 3.59). The review found that surgery significantly reduced the amputation rate and significantly reduced the proportion of people reporting ongoing ischaemic pain after 1 year compared with thrombolysis (amputation rate: OR 0.19, 95% CI 0.06 to 0.59; ongoing ischaemic pain: OR 0.30, 95% CI 0.17 to 0.50). **Surgery versus PTA plus stent placement:** We found no RCTs comparing surgery with PTA plus stent placement that reported long term outcomes.

Harms: Surgery increased early post-procedural complications compared with PTA. Among people having aorto-iliac surgery, perioperative mortality (within 30 days of the procedure) was 3.3%, and complications having a major health impact occurred in 8.3%.[44] Among people having infrainguinal bypass surgery, perioperative mortality was about 2% and serious complications occurred in 8%.[45] Among people having PTA with or without stent placement, perioperative mortality was about 1% and serious complications occurred in about 5%.[46]

Comment: The RCTs are small, have different follow up periods, and assessed different outcomes. Indirect comparisons from observational studies of proxy outcomes (primary patency rates) suggest that for aorto-iliac stenosis or occlusion, greater patency rates 5 years after intervention are achieved with surgery (6250 [89%] people) compared with PTA (1300 [34–85%] people) or compared with combined PTA and stent placement (816 [54–74%] people).[37,41,42] Too few people with infrainguinal lesions were included in the RCTs to provide good evidence about surgical management. Indirect comparisons of proxy outcomes in people with infrainguinal lesions suggest worse results after PTA (after 5 years, patency 38%, range 34–42%) compared with surgery (patency 80%).[47] Although the consensus view is that bypass surgery is the most effective treatment for people with debilitating symptomatic peripheral arterial disease, we found inadequate evidence from RCTs reporting long term clinical outcomes to confirm this view.

GLOSSARY

Absolute claudication distance Also known as the total walking distance; the maximum distance a person can walk before stopping.

Acute limb ischaemia An ischaemic process that threatens the viability of the limb, and is associated with pain, neurological deficit, inadequate skin capillary circulation, and/or inaudible arterial flow signals by Doppler examination. This acute process often leads to hospitalisation.

Critical limb ischaemia results in a breakdown of the skin (ulceration or gangrene) or pain in the foot at rest. Critical limb ischaemia corresponds to the Fontaine classification III and IV (see below).

Fontaine's classification I: asymptomatic; II: intermittent claudication (see below); II-a: pain free, claudication walking more than 200 m; II-b: pain free, claudication walking less than 200 m; III: rest/nocturnal pain; IV: necrosis/gangrene.

Initial claudication distance The distance a person can walk before the onset of claudication symptoms.

Intermittent claudication Pain, stiffness, or weakness in the leg that develops on walking, intensifies with continued walking until further walking is impossible, and is relieved by rest.

REFERENCES

1. Fowkes FGR, Housely E, Cawood EH, et al. Edinburgh Artery Study: prevalence of asymptomatic and symptomatic peripheral arterial disease in the general population. *Int J Epidemiol* 1991;20:384–392.
2. Kannel WB, McGee DL. Update on some epidemiological features of intermittent claudication. *J Am Geriatr Soc* 1985;33:13–18.
3. Murabito JM, D'Agostino RB, Silberschatz H, et al. Intermittent claudication: a risk profile from the Framingham Heart Study. *Circulation* 1997;96:44–49.
4. Catalano M. Epidemiology of critical limb ischemia: north Italian data. *Eur J Med* 1993;2:11–14.
5. Ebskov L, Schroeder T, Holstein P. Epidemiology of leg amputation: the influence of vascular surgery. *Br J Surg* 1994:81:1600–1603.
6. Leng GC, Lee AJ, Fowkes FG, et al. Incidence, natural history and cardiovascular events in symptomatic and asymptomatic peripheral arterial disease in the general population. *Int J Epidemiol* 1996;25:1172–1181.
7. Girolami B, Bernardi E, Prins MH, et al. Antithrombotic drugs in the primary medical management of intermittent claudication: a

meta-analysis. *Thromb Haemost* 1999;81:715–722. Search date 1998; primary sources Medline and hand searches.

8. Antithrombotic Trialists' Collaboration. Collaborative meta-analysis of randomised trials of antiplatelet therapy for prevention of death, myocardial infarction, and stroke in high risk patients. *BMJ* 2002; 324:71–86. Search date 1997; primary sources Medline, Embase, Derwent, Scisearch, Biosis, the Cochrane Stroke and Peripheral Vascular Disease Group Registers, hand searches of journals, abstracts, and proceedings of meetings, reference lists of trials and review articles, and personal contact with colleagues, including representatives of pharmaceutical companies.
9. Robless P, Mikhailidis D, Stansby G. Systematic review of antiplatelet therapy for the prevention of myocardial infarction, stroke, or vascular death in patients with peripheral vascular disease. *Br J Surg* 2001;88:787–800. Search date 1999; primary sources Medline, Embase, Antiplatelet Trialists Collaboration register of trials, Cochrane Controlled Trials Register, proceedings from vascular surgical society meetings (Vascular Surgical Society of Great Britain and Ireland, European Vascular Surgical Society, North American Society of Vascular Surgery), contact with pharmaceutical companies that market antiplatelet agents for details of any trials (Bristol Myers Squibb, Sanofi Winthrop).
10. Antiplatelet Trialists' Collaborative overview of randomized trials of antiplatelet therapy. I: prevention of death, myocardial infarction, and stroke by prolonged antiplatelet therapy in various categories of patients. BMJ 1994;308:81–106. Search date 1990; primary sources Medline, Current Contents, hand searches of reference lists of trials and review articles, journal abstracts and meeting proceedings, trial register of the International Committee on Thrombosis and Haemostasis, and personal contacts with colleagues and antiplatelet manufacturers.
11. He J, Whelton PK, Vu B, et al. Aspirin and risk of hemorrhagic stroke: a meta-analysis of randomized controlled trials. *JAMA* 1998;280:1930–1935. Search date 1997; primary sources Medline, the authors' reference files, and reference lists from original communications and review articles.
12. Derry S, Loke YK. Risk of gastrointestinal haemorrhage with long term use of aspirin: meta-analysis. *BMJ* 2000;321:1183–1187. Search date not reported; primary sources Medline, Embase, and reference lists from previous review papers and retrieved trials.
13. García Rodríguez LA, Hernández-Díaz S, De Abajo FJ. Association between aspirin and upper gastrointestinal complications: systematic review of epidemiologic studies. *Br J Clin Pharmacol* 2001;52:563–571.
14. Girolami B, Bernardi E, Prins M, et al. Treatment of intermittent claudication with physical training, smoking cessation, pentoxifylline, or nafronyl: a meta-analysis. *Arch Intern Med* 1999;159:337–345. Search date 1996; primary sources Medline and hand searches of reference lists.
15. Leng GC, Fowler B, Ernst E. Exercise for intermittent claudication. In: The Cochrane Library, Issue 3, 2000. Oxford: Update Software. Search date not reported; primary sources Cochrane Peripheral Vascular Diseases Group trials register, Embase, reference lists of relevant articles, and personal contact with principal investigators of trials.
16. Langbein WE, Collins EG, Orebaugh C, et al. Increasing exercise tolerance of persons limited by claudication pain using polestriding. *J Vasc Surg* 2002;35:887–893.
17. Tsai JC, Chan P, Wong CH, et al. The effects of exercise training on walking function and perception of health status in elderly patients with peripheral arterial occlusive disease. *J Intern Med* 2002;252:448–455.
18. Collins EG, Langbein WE, Orebaugh C et al. Polestriding exercise and vitamin E management of peripheral vascular disease. *Med Sci Sports Exerc* 2003;35:384–393.
19. Fowler B, Jamrozik K, Norman P, et al. Improving maximum walking distance in early peripheral arterial disease: randomised controlled trial. *Aust J Physiother* 2002;48:269–275.
20. Walker RD, Nawaz S, Wilkinson CH, et al. Influence of upper- and lower-limb exercise training on cardiovascular function and walking distances in patients with intermittent claudication. *J Vasc Surg* 2000;31:662–669.
21. Regensteiner JG, Ware JE, McCarthy WJ, et al. Effect of cilostazol on treadmill walking, community-based walking ability, and health-related quality of life in patients with intermittent claudication due to peripheral arterial disease: meta-analysis of six randomized controlled trials. *J Am Geriatr Soc* 2002;50:1939–1946.
22. Dawson D, Cutler B, Meeisner M, et al. Cilostazol has beneficial effects in treatment of intermittent claudication. *Circulation* 1998;98:678–686.
23. Strandness DE, Dalman RL, Panian S, et al. Effect of cilostazol in patients with intermittent claudication: a randomized, double-blind, placebo controlled study. *Vasc Endovasc Surg* 2002;36:83–91.
24. Dawson DL, Cutler BS, Hiatt WR, et al. A comparison of cilostazol and pentoxifylline for treating intermittent claudication. *Am J Med* 2000;109:523–530.
25. Hiatt WR. Medical treatment of peripheral arterial disease and claudication. *N Engl J Med* 2001;344:1608–1621.
26. Money SR, Herd A, Isaacsohn JL, et al. Effect of cilostazol on walking distances in patients with intermittent claudication caused by peripheral vascular disease. *J Vasc Surg* 1998;27:267–275.
27. Beebe HG, Dawson D, Cutler B, et al. A new pharmacological treatment for intermittent claudication. *Arch Intern Med* 1999;159:2041–2050.
28. Yuan G-H, Gao Y, Feng Q, et al. Clinical evaluation of cilostazol in treatment of peripheral vascular disease with type 2 diabetes. *Chin J Clin Pharmacol* 1999;15:425–430.
29. De Backer TL, Vander Stichele RH, Warie HH, et al. Oral vasoactive medication in intermittent claudication: utile or futile? *Eur J Clin Pharmacol* 2000;56:199–206. Search date 1999; primary sources Medline, International Pharmaceutical Abstracts, The Cochrane Library, direct contact with marketing companies and key authors, snowballing and Science Citation Index search.
30. Fowkes FG, Gillespie IN. Angioplasty (versus non surgical management) for intermittent claudication. In: The Cochrane Library, Issue 3, 2002. Oxford: Update Software. Search date not reported; primary sources Cochrane Peripheral Vascular Diseases Group Trials Register, Embase, reference lists of relevant articles and conference proceedings, and personal contact with principal investigators of trials.
31. Whyman MR, Fowkes FGR, Kerracher EMG, et al. Randomized controlled trial of percutaneous transluminal angioplasty for intermittent claudication. *Eur J Vasc Endovasc Surg* 1996;12:167–172.
32. Creasy TS, McMillan PJ, Fletcher EWL, et al. Is percutaneous transluminal angioplasty better than exercise for claudication? Preliminary results of a prospective randomized trial. *Eur J Vasc Surg* 1990;4:135–140.
33. Perkins JMT, Collin J, Creasy TS, et al. Exercise training versus angioplasty for stable claudication. Long and medium term results of a prospective, randomized trial. *Eur J Vasc Endovasc Surg* 1996;11:409–413.
34. Bachoo P, Thorpe P. Endovascular stents for intermittent claudication. The Cochrane Library Issue 2, 2003. Oxford: Update Software. Search date 2002; primary sources Cochrane Peripheral Vascular Diseases Group Trials Register, Medline, Embase, hand searches of the *J Vasc Interv Radiol*, proceedings from vascular surgery and radiological

society meetings, bibliographies, and contact with authors of published trials and manufacturers of endovascular stents.

35. Teteroo E, van der Graef Y, Bosch J, et al. Randomized comparison of primary stent placement versus primary angioplasty followed by selective stent placement in patients with iliac artery occlusive disease. *Lancet* 1998;351:1153–1159.
36. Cejna M, Thurnher S, Illiasch H, et al. PTA versus Palmaz stent placement in femeropopliteal artery obstructions: a multicenter prospective randomized study. *J Vasc Interv Radiol* 2001;12:23–31.
37. Zdanowski Z, Albrechtsson U, Lundin A, et al. Percutaneous transluminal angioplasty with or without stenting for femoropopliteal occlusions? A randomized controlled study. *Int Angiol* 1999;18:251–255.
38. Becquemin JP, Favre JP, Marzelle J, et al. Systematic versus selective stent placement after superficial femoral artery balloon angioplasty: a multicenter prospective randomised study. *J Vasc Surg* 2003;37:487–494.
39. Vroegindeweij D, Vos L, Tielbeek A, et al. Balloon angioplasty combined with primary stenting versus balloon angioplasty alone in femoropopliteal obstructions: a comparative randomized study. *Cardiovasc Intervent Radiol* 1997;20:420–425.
40. Grimm J, Muller-Hulsbeck S, Jahnke T, et al. Randomized study to compare PTA alone versus PTA with Palmaz stent placement for femoropopliteal lesions. *J Vasc Interv Radiol* 2000;12:935–942.
41. Becker GJ, Katzen BT, Dake MD. Noncoronary angioplasty. *Radiology* 1989;170:921–940.
42. Matsi PJ, Manninen HI. Complications of lower-limb percutaneous transluminal angioplasty: a prospective analysis of 410 procedures on 295 consecutive patients. *Cardiovasc Intervent Radiol* 1998;21:361–366.
43. Leng GC, Davis M, Baker D. Bypass surgery for chronic lower limb ischemia. The Cochrane Library Issue 2, 2002. Oxford: Update Software. Search date 2001; primary sources Cochrane Peripheral Vascular Diseases Group Trials Register, Medline, Embase, reference lists of various articles, and contact with trial investigators.
44. De Vries SO, Hunink MG. Results of aortic bifurcation grafts for aortoiliac occlusive disease: a meta-analysis. *J Vasc Surg* 1997;26:558–569. Search date 1996; primary sources Medline and hand searches of review articles, original studies, and a vascular surgery textbook.
45. Johnston KW, Rae M, Hogg-Johnston SA, et al. Five-year results of a prospective study of percutaneous transluminal angioplasty. *Ann Surg* 1987;206:403–413.
46. Bosch J, Hunink M. Meta-analysis of the results of percutaneous transluminal angioplasty and stent placement for aortoiliac occlusive disease. *Radiology* 1997;204:87–96. Search date not reported; primary sources Medline and hand searches of reference lists.
47. Johnson KW. Femoral and popliteal arteries: reanalysis of results of balloon angioplasty. *Radiology* 1992;183:767–771.

Paul Bachoo
Consultant Vascular Surgeon
Aberdeen Royal Infirmary
Aberdeen
UK

Competing interests: None declared.

Stroke management

Search date January 2004

Elizabeth Warburton

QUESTIONS

INTERVENTIONS

To be covered in future updates
Early supported discharge from hospital and other issues pertaining to stroke service organisation
Other treatments for acute ischaemic stroke (corticosteroids, fibrinogen depleting agents, glycerol, haemodilution techniques)
Prevention of deep venous thrombosis/pulmonary embolism in people with stroke

See glossary G

Key Messages

Specialised care in stroke

- **Specialised care (specialist stroke rehabilitation)** One systematic review found that specialist stroke rehabilitation reduced death or dependency after a median follow up of 1 year compared with conventional (less specialised) care. Prospective observational data suggest that these findings may be reproducible in routine clinical settings. A second systematic review found no significant difference between care based on in-hospital care pathways and standard care in death or dependency rates. However, these results were based on one small RCT, which may have lacked power to detect clinically important effects. One small subsequent pilot study found no significant difference between intensive monitoring and usual stroke unit care in rates of poor outcome at 3 months but found that intensive monitoring reduced mortality.

Medical treatment in stroke

- **Aspirin** One systematic review in people with ischaemic stroke confirmed by computerised tomography scan found that aspirin taken within 48 hours of stroke onset reduced death or dependency at 6 months and increased the proportion of people making a complete recovery compared with placebo.

- **Immediate systemic anticoagulation** One systematic review comparing systemic anticoagulants (unfractionated heparin, low molecular weight heparin, heparinoids, oral anticoagulants, or specific thrombin inhibitors) with usual care without systemic anticoagulants found no significant difference in death or dependence after 3–6 months. One systematic review found no significant difference between anticoagulants (unfractionated and low molecular weight heparin) and aspirin in death or dependency at 3–6 months for all people with stroke or for the subset of people who also had atrial fibrillation. Systematic reviews provided evidence that systemic anticoagulation reduced the risk of symptomatic deep venous thrombosis in people with ischaemic stroke, but increased the risk of intracranial haemorrhage or extracranial haemorrhage.
- **Thrombolysis (increases overall mortality and fatal haemorrhages but reduces dependency in survivors; beneficial effects on dependency do not extend to streptokinase)** One systematic review in people with confirmed ischaemic stroke found that thrombolysis reduced the risk of the composite outcome of death or dependency after 1–6 months compared with placebo. However, it increased the risk of death from intracranial haemorrhage measured in the first 7–10 days and risk of death after 1–6 months. The excess in deaths was offset by fewer people being alive but dependent 6 months after stroke onset, and the net effect was a reduction in people who were dead or dependent. Systematic reviews that undertook meta-analyses for specific thrombolytic agents found that benefits and harms of recombinant tissue plasminogen activator were similar to the overall results. However, streptokinase increased mortality compared with placebo, and this harm was not offset by reduced dependency in survivors. Results of the reviews may not extrapolate to people with the mildest or most severe strokes.
- **Neuroprotective agents (calcium channel antagonists, γ-aminobutyric acid agonists, lubeluzole, glycine antagonists, tirilazad, N-methyl-D-aspartate antagonists)** RCTs found no evidence that calcium channel antagonists, lubeluzole, γ-aminobutyric acid agonists, tirilazad, glycine antagonists, or N-methyl-D-aspartate antagonists significantly improved clinical outcomes compared with placebo. One systematic review found that lubeluzole increased the risk of having Q-T prolongation to more than 450 milliseconds on electrocardiography compared with placebo.
- **Acute reduction in blood pressure** One systematic review in people with acute stroke found insufficient evidence about the effects of lowering blood pressure compared with placebo on clinical outcomes. However, other studies found conflicting results. Two RCTs have suggested that people treated with antihypertensive agents may have a worse clinical outcome and increased mortality.

Surgery: intracerebral haematoma

- **Evacuation** We found that the balance between benefits and harms has not been clearly established for the evacuation of supratentorial haematomas. We found no evidence from RCTs on the role of evacuation or ventricular shunting in people with infratentorial haematoma whose consciousness level is declining.

DEFINITION	Stroke is characterised by rapidly developing clinical symptoms and signs of focal, and at times global, loss of cerebral function lasting more than 24 hours or leading to death, with no apparent cause other than that of vascular origin.[1] Ischaemic stroke is stroke caused by vascular insufficiency (such as cerebrovascular thromboembolism) rather than haemorrhage.
INCIDENCE/ PREVALENCE	Stroke is the third most common cause of death in most developed countries.[2] It is a worldwide problem; about 4.5 million people die from stroke each year. Stroke can occur at any age, but half of all strokes occur in people over 70 years old.[3]
AETIOLOGY/ RISK FACTORS	About 80% of all acute strokes are ischaemic, usually resulting from thrombotic or embolic occlusion of a cerebral artery.[4] The remainder are caused either by intracerebral or subarachnoid haemorrhage.
PROGNOSIS	About 10% of all people with acute ischaemic strokes will die within 30 days of stroke onset.[5] Of those who survive the acute event, about 50% will experience some level of disability after 6 months.[6]

AIMS OF INTERVENTION	To minimise impairment, disability, secondary complications, and adverse effects from treatment.
OUTCOMES	Risk of death or dependency (generally assessed as the proportion of people dead or requiring physical assistance for transfers, mobility, dressing, feeding, or toileting 3–6 months after stroke onset);[6] quality of life.
METHODS	*Clinical Evidence* search and appraisal January 2004.

QUESTION What are the effects of specialised care in people with stroke?

OPTION SPECIALISED CARE

One systematic review found that specialist stroke rehabilitation reduced death or dependency after a median follow up of 1 year compared with conventional (less specialised) care. Prospective observational data suggest that these findings may be reproducible in routine clinical settings. A second systematic review found no significant difference between care based on in-hospital care pathways and standard care in death or dependency rates. However, these results were based on one small RCT, which may have lacked power to detect clinically important effects. One small subsequent pilot study found no significant difference between intensive monitoring and usual stroke unit care in rates of poor outcome at 3 months but found that intensive monitoring reduced mortality.

Benefits: We found one systematic review comparing specialised stroke rehabilitation versus conventional care,[7] one systematic review comparing integrated care pathway**G** versus conventional multidisciplinary care in hospital,[8] and one subsequent RCT[9] comparing intensive monitoring versus conventional stroke unit care. In most RCTs in the first review (search date 2001, 23 RCTs, 4911 people with stroke), the specialised stroke rehabilitation unit consisted of a designated area or ward, although some trials used a mobile "stroke team". People in these trials were usually transferred to stroke unit care within the first or second week after stroke onset. It found that stroke rehabilitation units significantly reduced death or dependency after a median follow up of 1 year compared with alternative, less organised care (AR 60.5% without stroke unit *v* 55.8% with stroke unit; ARR 4.7%, 95% CI 1.6% to 7.8%; NNT 21, 95% CI 13 to 63; OR 0.78, 95% CI 0.68 to 0.89 (see figure 1, p 165)).[7] The duration of stay was calculated differently for many of the trials, so heterogeneity among results limits generalisability. However, overall, duration of stay in the stroke unit was about 6 days (95% CI 2 to 10 days) shorter than duration of stay in a non-stroke unit setting. Two RCTs included in the review extended follow up to 5 years post stroke. The review found that organised stroke unit care significantly reduced death or dependency at 5 years compared with alternative care (2 RCTs; 223/286 [78%] with organised stroke unit care *v* 214/249 [86%] with alternative care; RR 0.91, 95% CI 0.84 to 0.99).[7] One RCT (220 people) included in the review found that care in a combined acute and rehabilitation unit increased the proportion of people able to live at home 10 years after their stroke compared with care in general wards (ARI 11.0%, 95% CI 1.9% to 20.0%; NNT 9, 95% CI 5 to 52).[13] The second systematic review (search date 2001, 3 RCTs, 340 people) compared care based on in-hospital care pathways versus standard care.[8] It found no significant difference in the combined outcome of death or dependency or death alone at 6 months (death or dependency: 1 RCT, 76 people; OR 1.36, 95% CI 0.68 to 2.72; death alone: 1 RCT, 76 people; OR 1.77, 95% CI 0.61 to 5.14). However, the meta-analysis may have lacked power to detect clinically important differences in effect. The subsequent RCT (54 people with acute ischaemic stroke) was a small pilot study that compared care in a stroke care monitoring unit (intensive monitoring of temperature, oxygen saturation, blood pressure, and electrocardiogram) versus conventional stroke unit care.[9] It found no significant difference between treatments in rates of "poor outcome" at 3 months but found that monitoring significantly reduced mortality (poor outcome defined as modified Rankin score ≥ 4 or Barthel Index < 60, or need for institutionalised care: 7/27 [25.9%] with monitoring *v* 13/27 [48.1%] with conventional care; P = 0.16; mortality: 1/27 [3.7%] with monitoring *v* 7/27 [25.9%] with conventional care; OR 0.11, 95% CI 0.02 to 0.96). The RCT may not have been large enough to detect clinically important differences in function.

Harms: No detrimental effects attributable to stroke units were reported.[7–9]

Comment: Although the proportional reduction in death or dependency seems larger with thrombolysis (see thrombolysis option, p 155), stroke unit care is applicable to most people with stroke, whereas thrombolysis is applicable only to a small proportion. The systematic review did not provide evidence about which aspects of the multidisciplinary approach led to improved outcome,[7] although one limited retrospective analysis of one of the RCTs found that several factors, including early mobilisation, increased use of oxygen, intravenous saline solutions, and antipyretics, might have been responsible.[14] Most RCTs excluded the most mild and severe strokes. Since publication of the systematic review,[7] prospective observational data have been collected in one large series of over 14 000 people in 80 Swedish hospitals.[15] In this series, people admitted to stroke units had reduced dependence at 3 months (RRR 6%, 95% CI 1% to 11%). Although biases are inherent in such observational data, the findings suggest that the results of the meta-analysis may be reproducible in routine clinical settings. One review examined the characteristics of 11 controlled trials identified by the first systematic review,[7] which found benefit from stroke units.[16] It found that most effective units described similar management in terms of: medical, nursing, and treatment assessment; early mobilisation, treatment of hypoxia, hyperglycaemia, and suspected infection; and coordinated goal directed rehabilitation policies.[16] The authors of the review suggested that these elements might form the benchmark for general stroke unit care and future studies.

QUESTION What are the effects of medical treatment in acute ischaemic stroke?

OPTION THROMBOLYSIS

One systematic review in people with confirmed ischaemic stroke found that thrombolysis reduced the risk of the composite outcome of death or dependency after 1–6 months compared with placebo. However, it increased the risk of death from intracranial haemorrhage measured in the first 7–10 days and risk of death after 1–6 months. The excess in deaths was offset by fewer people being alive but dependent 6 months after stroke onset, and the net effect was a reduction in people who were dead or dependent. Systematic reviews that undertook meta-analyses for specific thrombolytic agents found that benefits and harms of recombinant tissue plasminogen activator were similar to the overall results. However, streptokinase increased mortality compared with placebo, and this harm was not offset by reduced dependency in survivors. Results of the reviews may not extrapolate to people with the mildest or most severe strokes.

Benefits: **Any thrombolytic:** We found one systematic review (search date 1999, 17 RCTs, 5216 highly selected people[10]) comparing intravenous or intra-arterial thrombolysis versus placebo given soon after the onset of stroke. In the systematic review, all trials used computerised tomography or magnetic resonance imaging before randomisation to exclude intracranial haemorrhage or other non-stroke disorders. Results for three different thrombolytic agents (streptokinase, urokinase, and recombinant tissue plasminogen activator) were included. Two RCTs used the intra-arterial route and the rest used the intravenous route. Thrombolysis significantly reduced the composite risk of death or dependency compared with no thrombolysis at the end of the studies (1–6 months: ARR 4.2%, 95% CI 1.2% to 7.2%; NNT 24, 95% CI 14 to 83) (see figure 1, p 165) (see figure 2, p 166).[10] **Recombinant tissue plasminogen activator:** The systematic review meta-analyzed trials assessing intravenous recombinant tissue plasminogen activator and found that recombinant tissue plasminogen activator significantly reduced death or dependency compared with no thrombolysis at the end of the studies (ARR 5.7%, 95% CI 2.0% to 9.4%; RR 0.90; 95% CI 0.84 to 0.96; NNT 18, 95% CI 11 to 50). **Streptokinase:** The systematic review[10] (described above) did not meta-analyze data from trials assessing streptokinase. However, we found a second review that included the same streptokinase RCTs that were included in the first review (4 RCTs, search date not reported, 1292 people with acute ischaemic stroke), which found no significant difference between streptokinase and placebo in the proportion of people who were dead or dependent at 3 months (RR 0.99, 95% CI 0.92 to 1.06).[17]

Harms: **Any thrombolytic:** In the first systematic review, thrombolysis increased fatal intracranial haemorrhage measured in the first 7–10 days, and increased the risk of death by the end of follow up (fatal intracranial haemorrhage: ARI 4.4%, 95% CI 3.4% to 5.4%; RRI 396%, 95% CI 220% to 668%; NNH 23, 95% CI 19 to 29; death at 1–6 months: ARI 3.3%, 95% CI 1.2% to 5.4%; RRI 23%, 95% CI 10% to 38%; NNH 30, 95% CI 19 to 83).[10] This excess of deaths was offset by fewer people being alive but dependent 6 months after stroke onset. The net effect was a reduction in the proportion of people who were dead or dependent. **Recombinant tissue plasminogen activator:** Meta-analysis also found that recombinant tissue plasminogen activator significantly increased fatal intracranial haemorrhage at 7–10 days (ARI 2.9%, 95% CI 1.7% to 4.1%; RRI 259%, 95% CI 102% to 536%; NNH 34, 95% CI 24 to 59).[10] **Streptokinase:** The second systematic review found that streptokinase significantly increased mortality compared with placebo after 3 months (RR 1.46, 95% CI 1.24 to 1.73) and that the combination of aspirin plus streptokinase significantly increased mortality compared with placebo at 3 months (P = 0.005).[17]

Comment: In the first systematic review, there was no significant heterogeneity of treatment effect overall, but heterogeneity of results was noted for the outcomes of death, and death or dependency at final follow up among the eight trials of intravenous recombinant tissue plasminogen activator.[10] Explanations may include the combined use of antithrombotic agents (aspirin or heparin within the first 24 hours of thrombolysis), stroke severity, the presence of early ischaemic changes on computerised tomography scan, and the time from stroke onset to randomisation. Most trials reported outcomes at 3 months; only one trial reported 1 year outcome data.[18] We found little evidence about which people are most and least likely to benefit from thrombolysis. A subgroup analysis suggested that thrombolysis may be more beneficial if given within 3 hours of symptom onset, but the duration of the "therapeutic time window" could not be determined reliably. A recent preliminary pooling of three RCTs (1734 people) suggested that recombinant tissue plasminogen activator given between 3 and 6 hours may reduce death or dependency in some people compared with placebo.[19] However, there is currently no consensus about giving thrombolysis after 3 hours.

Newer magnetic resonance imaging techniques, such as diffusion/perfusion weighted imaging, may be helpful in patient selection, but studies using these techniques have so far been small.[20] Several trials of different thrombolytic regimens are underway.[21] One meta-analysis published after the search date for this issue of *Clinical Evidence* was identified during editing.[22] It suggested that early intravenous recombinant tissue plasminogen activator improved clinical outcomes compared with placebo.

OPTION ASPIRIN

One systematic review in people with ischaemic stroke confirmed by computerised tomography scan found that aspirin taken within 48 hours of stroke onset reduced death or dependency at 6 months and increased the proportion of people making a complete recovery compared with placebo.

Benefits: **Early use of aspirin:** We found one systematic review (search date 2002, 3 RCTs, 40 850 people with definite or presumed ischaemic stroke), which compared aspirin started within 14 days of the stroke versus placebo.[23] Most (> 98%) of the data in the systematic review came from two large RCTs of aspirin 160–300 mg daily started within 48 hours of stroke onset.[11,12] Most people had an ischaemic stroke confirmed by computerised tomography scan before randomisation, but people who were conscious could be randomised before computerised tomography scan if the stroke was very likely to be ischaemic on clinical grounds. Treatment duration varied from 10–28 days. The review found that aspirin started within the first 48 hours of acute ischaemic stroke reduced death or dependency at 6 months' follow up and increased the proportion of people making a complete recovery (death or dependency: 3 RCTs, 40 850 people; RR 0.97, 95% CI 0.95 to 0.99 (see figure 1, p 165); complete recovery: 2 RCTs, 40 541 people; RR 1.04, 95% CI 1.01 to 1.07). We found a second meta-analysis[24] of the two large RCTs.[11,12] It found that aspirin significantly reduced further stroke or death compared with placebo (ARR 0.90%, 95% CI 0.75% to 1.85%; NNT 111, 95% CI 54 to 133).[24] The effect was similar across subgroups (older *v* younger; male *v* female; impaired consciousness or not; atrial fibrillation or not; blood pressure; stroke subtype; timing of computerised tomography scanning). **Long term treatment:** See aspirin under stroke prevention, p 167.

Harms: Aspirin caused an excess of about two intracranial and four extracranial haemorrhages per 1000 people treated, but these small risks were more than offset by the reductions in death and disability from other causes both in the short term[23] and in the long term.[25] Common adverse effects of aspirin (such as dyspepsia and constipation) were dose related.[26]

Comment: We found no clear evidence that any one dose of aspirin is more effective than any other in the treatment of acute ischaemic stroke. One recent meta-regression analysis of the dose–response effect of aspirin on stroke found a uniform effect of aspirin in a range of doses from 50–1500 mg daily.[27] People unable to swallow safely after a stroke may be given aspirin as a suppository.

OPTION IMMEDIATE SYSTEMIC ANTICOAGULATION

One systematic review comparing systemic anticoagulants (unfractionated heparin, low molecular weight heparin, heparinoids, oral anticoagulants, or specific thrombin inhibitors) with usual care without systemic anticoagulants found no significant difference in death or dependence after 3–6 months. One systematic review found no significant difference between anticoagulants

(unfractionated and low molecular weight heparin) and aspirin in death or dependency at 3–6 months for all people with stroke or for the subset of people who also had atrial fibrillation. Systematic reviews provided evidence that systemic anticoagulation reduced the risk of symptomatic deep venous thrombosis in people with ischaemic stroke, but increased the risk of intracranial haemorrhage or extracranial haemorrhage.

Benefits: **Death or dependency:** We found one systematic review (search date 1999, 21 RCTs, 23 427 people)[28] comparing anticoagulants with usual care, one systematic review (search date 2000, 4 RCTs, 16 558 people treated within 14 days of acute ischaemic stroke)[29] comparing anticoagulants with aspirin, and one subsequent RCT.[30] The first systematic review compared unfractionated heparin, low molecular weight heparin, heparinoids, oral anticoagulants, or specific thrombin inhibitors with usual care without systemic anticoagulants.[28] Over 80% of the data came from one trial, which randomised people with any severity of stroke to either subcutaneous heparin or placebo, usually after exclusion of haemorrhage by computerised tomography scan.[12] The systematic review found no significant difference in the proportion of people dead or dependent in the treatment and control groups at the end of follow up (3–6 months after the stroke: ARR +0.4%, 95% CI –0.9% to +1.7%; RRR 0%, 95% CI –2% to +3%).[28] There was no clear short or long term benefit of anticoagulants in any prespecified subgroups (stroke of presumed cardioembolic origin *v* others; different anticoagulants). The second systematic review found no significant difference in death or dependency at 3–6 months between anticoagulants (unfractionated and low molecular weight heparin) and aspirin (OR 1.07, 95% CI 0.99 to 1.15).[29] Results were similar in the subgroup of people with atrial fibrillation (OR 1.10, 95% CI 0.90 to 1.35). The review found no significant difference in death or dependency between unfractionated heparin plus aspirin and aspirin alone, either for all people or for the subgroup of people with atrial fibrillation (1 RCT, all people: OR 1.00, 95% CI 0.92 to 1.09; people with atrial fibrillation: OR 1.00, 95% CI 0.92 to 1.09). The subsequent RCT randomised 404 people to one of four different doses of certoparin (a low molecular weight heparin) within 12 hours of stroke onset.[30] It found no difference in neurological outcome between the four groups 3 months after treatment. **Deep venous thrombosis and pulmonary embolism:** We found four systematic reviews.[28,29,31,32] The first systematic review (search date 1999, 10 small heterogeneous RCTs, 22 000 people) assessed anticoagulants in 916 people at high risk of deep venous thrombosis after their stroke.[28] Anticoagulation reduced deep vein thrombosis and symptomatic pulmonary emboli compared with control (deep venous thrombosis: ARR 29%, 95% CI 24% to 35%; RRR 64%, 95% CI 54% to 71%; NNT 3, 95% CI 2 to 4; pulmonary embolism: ARR 0.3%, 95% CI 0.1% to 0.6%; RRR 38%, 95% CI 16% to 54%; NNT 333, 95% CI 167 to 1000). No RCT performed investigations in all people to rule out silent events. The frequency of reported pulmonary emboli was low and varied among RCTs, so there may have been under-ascertainment. Two other systematic reviews (search dates 1999[32] and 2001,[31] same 5 RCTs in each review, 705 people with acute ischaemic stroke) found that low molecular weight heparins or heparinoids significantly reduced deep venous thrombosis compared with unfractionated heparin (AR 13% with low molecular weight heparins or heparinoids *v* 22% with unfractionated heparin; ARR 9.0%, 95% CI 4.5% to 16.0%). The number of events was too small to compare the effects of low molecular weight heparins or heparinoids with unfractionated heparin on death, intracranial haemorrhage, or functional outcome in survivors. The fourth systematic review (search date 2000, 2 RCTs) found that anticoagulants (unfractionated and low molecular weight heparin) significantly reduced symptomatic deep vein thrombosis during the treatment period compared with aspirin (OR 0.19, 95% CI 0.07 to 0.58). It found no significant difference in symptomatic pulmonary embolism (OR 0.85, 95% CI 0.55 to 1.32).[29]

Harms: One systematic review found that anticoagulation slightly increased symptomatic intracranial haemorrhages within 14 days of starting treatment compared with control (ARI 0.93%, 95% CI 0.68% to 1.18%; RRI 163%, 95% CI 95% to 255%; NNH 108, 95% CI 85 to 147).[28] The large trial of subcutaneous heparin found that this effect was dose dependent (symptomatic intracranial haemorrhage by using medium dose compared with low dose heparin for 14 days: RRI 143%, 95% CI 82% to 204%; NNH 97, 95% CI 68 to 169).[12] The review also found a dose dependent increase in major extracranial haemorrhages after 14 days of treatment with anticoagulants (ARI 0.91%, 95% CI 0.67% to 1.15%; RRI 231%, 95% CI 136% to 365%; NNH 109, 95% CI 87 to 149).[28] One systematic review (search date 2000, 4 RCTs) found that anticoagulants (unfractionated and low molecular weight heparin) significantly increased symptomatic intracranial haemorrhage compared with aspirin (OR 2.27, 95% CI 1.49 to 3.46).[29] It found that the increase was greater with higher dose compared with lower dose anticoagulants (high dose: OR 3.24, 95% CI 2.09 to 5.04; low dose: OR 1.29, 95% CI 0.72 to 2.32). One RCT identified by this systematic review[29] found no difference between dalteparin and aspirin for people with acute stroke and atrial fibrillation in adverse events, including symptomatic or asymptomatic intracerebral haemorrhage, progression of symptoms, or early or late death.[33] As in the systematic review,[28] the RCT comparing different doses of certoparin found that intracranial haemorrhage occurred more often in those receiving a higher dose of anticoagulant.[30] However, the overall proportion of people experiencing haemorrhagic complications in the RCT may have been artificially lowered because the study protocol was changed during the trial period so as to exclude people with early ischaemic changes on computerised tomography scan.

Comment: Alternative treatments to prevent deep venous thrombosis and pulmonary embolism after acute ischaemic stroke include aspirin and compression stockings. The evidence relating to these will be reviewed in future *Clinical Evidence* updates.

OPTION BLOOD PRESSURE REDUCTION

One systematic review in people with acute stroke found insufficient evidence about the effects of lowering blood pressure compared with placebo on clinical outcomes. However, other studies found conflicting results. Two RCTs have suggested that people treated with antihypertensive agents may have a worse clinical outcome and increased mortality.

Benefits: **Any hypertensive:** We found one systematic review (search date 2000, 5 RCTs, 281 people with acute stroke) comparing blood pressure lowering treatment with placebo.[34] Several different antihypertensive agents were used. The trials collected insufficient clinical data to allow an analysis of the relation between changes in blood pressure and clinical outcome to be carried out.

Harms: Two placebo controlled RCTs have suggested that people treated with antihypertensive agents may have a worse clinical outcome and increased mortality.[35,36] The first RCT (295 people with acute ischaemic stroke) compared nimodipine (a calcium channel antagonist) versus placebo.[35] The RCT was stopped prematurely because of an excess in unfavourable neurological outcomes in the nimodipine treated group.

Exploratory analyses confirmed that this negative correlation was related to reductions in mean arterial blood pressure (CI not reported; P = 0.02) and diastolic blood pressure (P = 0.0005). The second RCT (302 people with acute ischaemic stroke) assessed β blockers (atenolol or propranolol).[36] There was a non-significant increase in death for people taking β blockers, and no difference in the proportion of people achieving a good outcome. Although treatment with calcium channel antagonists in these trials was intended for neuroprotection, blood pressure was lower in the treatment group in several trials.

Comment: Population based studies suggest a direct and continuous association between blood pressure and the risk of recurrent stroke.[37] However, acute blood pressure lowering in acute ischaemic stroke may lead to increased cerebral ischaemia. The systematic review[34] identified several ongoing RCTs. We identified one additional ongoing RCT not included in the review.[38] Calcium channel antagonists are both antihypertensive agents and neuroprotective agents. They are considered specifically in the neuroprotective agents option, p 160.

OPTION NEUROPROTECTIVE AGENTS

RCTs found no evidence that calcium channel antagonists, lubeluzole, γ-aminobutyric acid agonists, tirilazad, glycine antagonists, or N-methyl-D-aspartate antagonists significantly improved clinical outcomes compared with placebo. One systematic review found that lubeluzole increased the risk of having Q-T prolongation to more than 450 milliseconds on electrocardiography compared with placebo.

Benefits: **Calcium channel antagonists:** We found two systematic reviews comparing calcium channel antagonists with placebo.[39,40] The first review (search date 1999, 28 RCTs, 7521 people with acute ischaemic stroke) found that calcium channel antagonists did not significantly reduce the risk of poor outcome (including death) at the end of the follow up period compared with placebo (ARI of poor outcome +4.9%, 95% CI –2.5% to +7.3%; RRI +4%, 95% CI –2% to +9%).[39] The second review (search date 1999)[40] included one additional RCT (454 people)[41] that was stopped prematurely because of publication of the first review.[39] Inclusion of its data did not change the results of the first review. **γ-Aminobutyric acid agonists:** We found one systematic review (search date not reported, 3 RCTs, 1002 people with acute ischaemic stroke)[42] and two subsequent RCTs.[43,44] The systematic review found no significant difference between piracetam (a γ-aminobutyric acid agonist) and control in the proportion of people dead or dependent at the end of follow up (ARI +0.2%, 95% CI –6.0% to +6.4%; RRI 0%, 95% CI –11% to +9%).[42] Similar results were found in the two subsequent RCTs.[43,44] The first subsequent RCT (1360 people with acute stroke) found no significant difference between clomethiazole (a γ-aminobutyric acid agonist) and placebo in functional independence (ARR +1.5%, 95% CI –4.0% to +6.6%; RRR +3%, 95% CI –7% to +13%).[43] The second subsequent RCT (1198 people with major acute ischaemic stroke treated within 12 hours) found no significant difference between clomethiazole and placebo in neurological recovery at 3 months (Barthel index ≥ 60: 42/586 [7.1%] with clomethiazole *v* 46/583 [7.9%] with placebo; OR 0.81, 95% CI 0.62 to 1.05).[44] **Lubeluzole:** We found one systematic review (search date 2001, 5 RCTs, 3510 people) that compared lubeluzole (5, 10, or 20 mg daily for 5 days) with placebo.[45] It found no significant difference between any dose of lubeluzole and placebo in death or dependency at the end of follow up (after 4–12 weeks' follow up: AR 54.6% with lubeluzole *v* 53.4% with placebo; ARI +1.2%, 95% CI –2.5% to +6.2%). **Glycine antagonists (gavestinel):** We found one systematic review (search date 2001, 8 RCTs, 3751 people).[46] It found no significant difference in death or dependency or in mortality between gavestinel and placebo after 1–3 months (death or dependency: OR 1.04, 95% CI 0.91 to 1.18; death: OR 1.12, 95% CI 0.95 to 1.32). We found two RCTs.[47,48] One RCT (1804 conscious people with limb weakness assessed within 6 hours of stroke onset) found no significant difference between gavestinel and placebo in survival and outcome at 3 months, as measured using the Barthel index (ARR +1.0%, 95% CI –3.5% to +6.0%).[47] The second RCT (1367 people with predefined level of limb weakness and functional independence before stroke) also found no significant difference in survival and outcome at 3 months, measured using the Barthel index (ARI +1.9%, 95% CI –3.8% to +6.4%).[48] **N-methyl-D-aspartate antagonists:** We found one systematic review (search date 2001, 10 RCTs, 6317 people).[46] It found no significant difference in death or dependence (presented as a combined outcome) between N-methyl-D-aspartate antagonists**G** and placebo (OR 1.05, 95% CI 0.95 to 1.16). Two recent RCTs assessing the N-methyl-D-aspartate antagonist Selfotel found no significant difference in the proportion of people with a Barthel index over 60, but data were limited as the trials were terminated because of adverse outcomes after only 31% of the total planned patient enrolment.[49] Similarly, an RCT comparing the N-methyl-D-aspartate antagonist aptiganel with placebo was terminated early because of lack of efficacy and a potential imbalance in mortality.[50] The RCT found a larger proportion of people with favourable outcomes in the placebo group and a non-significant trend favouring placebo in mortality.[50] **Tirilazad:** We found one systematic review (search date 2001, 6 RCTs, 1757 people with acute ischaemic stroke) comparing tirilazad (a steroid derivative) with placebo.[51] Tirilazad increased death and disability at 3 months' follow up when measured using the expanded Barthel index (OR 1.23, CI 1.01 to 1.51).[51]

Harms: **Calcium channel antagonists:** In the systematic review of calcium channel antagonists, indirect and limited comparisons of intravenous versus oral administration found no significant difference in adverse events (ARI of adverse events, iv *v* oral: +2.3%, 95% CI –0.9% to +3.7%; RRI +17%, 95% CI –3% to +41%).[39] **γ-Aminobutyric acid agonists:** In the systematic review of piracetam, there was a non-significant increase in death with piracetam compared with placebo, which was no longer apparent after correction for imbalance in stroke severity.[42] The second subsequent RCT (1198 people) found that clomethiazole significantly increased somnolence and rhinitis compared with placebo (somnolence: 50.6% with clomethiazole *v* 12.7% with placebo; rhinitis: 6.3% with clomethiazole *v* 1.9% with placebo; P value not reported).[44] **Lubeluzole:** The systematic review of lubeluzole found that, at any dose, lubeluzole was associated with a significant increase in the risk of having a heart conduction disorder (Q-T prolongation to more than 450 mseconds on electrocardiography) at the end of follow up (AR 11.9% with lubeluzole *v* 9.7% with control; ARI 2.2%, 95% CI 0.1% to 4.2%; NNH 45, 95% CI 23 to 1000).[45] Lubeluzole did not significantly increase heart rhythm disorders (atrial fibrillation, ventricular tachycardia or fibrillation, torsade de pointes) at the end of the scheduled follow up (OR 1.28, 95% CI 0.97 to 1.69). **Glycine antagonists (gavestinel):** The systematic review did not report on harms.[46] **N-methyl-D-aspartate antagonists:** The trials of Selfotel were terminated after enrolling 567 people because of greater early mortality in the Selfotel groups. The systematic review did not report on harms.[49] **Tirilazad:** The systematic review of tirilazad found an increased risk of injection site phlebitis compared with placebo (ARI 12.2%, 95% CI 8.7% to 15.7%).[51]

Comment: The effects of the cell membrane precursor citicholine have been assessed in small trials, and a systematic review is in progress.[52] Systematic reviews are being developed for antioxidants and for excitatory amino acid modulators.[53] Several RCTs are ongoing, including one of intravenous magnesium sulphate[54] and another of diazepam (a γ-aminobutyric acid agonist).[55]

QUESTION **What are the effects of surgical treatment for intracerebral haematomas?**

OPTION **EVACUATION**

We found that the balance between benefits and harms has not been clearly established for the evacuation of supratentorial haematomas. We found no evidence from RCTs on the role of evacuation or ventricular shunting in people with infratentorial haematoma whose consciousness level is declining.

Benefits: **For supratentorial haematomas:** We found three systematic reviews.[56–58] The first review (search date 1998)[56] and second review (search date 1997)[57] both assessed the same four RCTs comparing surgery (craniotomy in 3 trials and endoscopy in 1 trial) with best medical treatment in 354 people with primary supratentorial intracerebral haemorrhage. The second review also assessed information from case series.[57] Overall, neither review found significant short or long term differences between surgical and medical treatment for death or disability (ARI +3.3%, 95% CI –5.9% to +12.5%; RRI +5%, 95% CI –7% to +19%). The third review (search date 1999)[58] included several analyses. The first analysis included results from seven RCTs (530 people), including two RCTs not included in either of the first two systematic reviews. The overall results are similar to those of the first two systematic reviews, with no significant difference in death or disability for surgically treated people (ARI +3.5%, 95% CI –4.4% to +11.4%). A further analysis of results from only recent, post-computerised tomography, well constructed, balanced trials (5 trials, 224 people in total) did not find a significant difference between the two groups (ARR +9.3%, 95% CI –2.6% to +21.2%). **For infratentorial haematomas:** We found no evidence from systematic reviews or RCTs on the role of surgical evacuation or ventricular shunting.[59]

Harms: The two earlier reviews undertook subgroup analyses separating results for craniotomy and endoscopy. They found that for the 254 people randomised to craniotomy rather than best medical treatment, there was increased death and disability (ARI 12.0%, 95% CI 1.8% to 22.0%; RRI 17%, 95% CI 2% to 34%; NNH 8, 95% CI 5 to 56).[56,57] For the 100 people randomised to endoscopy rather than best medical practice, there was no significant effect on death and disability (RRR 24%, 95% CI –2% to +44%). The third systematic review did not evaluate these adverse outcomes.[58]

Comment: Current practice is based on the consensus that people with infratentorial (cerebellar) haematomas whose consciousness level is declining probably benefit from evacuation of the haematoma. We identified one ongoing multicentre trial comparing a policy of "early surgical evacuation" of haematoma versus "initial conservative treatment" in people with spontaneous intracerebral haemorrhage.[60]

GLOSSARY

Integrated care pathway A model of care that includes definition of therapeutic goals and specification of a timed plan designed to promote multidisciplinary care, improve discharge planning, and reduce the duration of hospital stay.

N-methyl-D-aspartate antagonist Glutamate can bind to N-methyl-D-aspartate receptors on cell surfaces. One hypothesis proposed that glutamate released during a stroke can cause further harm to neurones by stimulating the N-methyl-D-aspartate receptors. N-methyl-D-aspartate antagonists block these receptors.

Substantive changes

Neuroprotective agents: Glycine antagonists One systematic review added.[46] Categorisation unchanged.
Neuroprotective agents: N-methyl-D-aspartate antagonist One systematic review added.[46] Categorisation unchanged.
Immediate systemic anticoagulation Evidence re-appraised and categorisation changed to trade-off between benefits and harms.

REFERENCES

1. Hatano S. Experience from a multicentre stroke register: a preliminary report. *Bull World Health Organ* 1976;54:541–553.
2. Bonita R. Epidemiology of stroke. *Lancet* 1992;339:342–344.
3. Bamford J, Sandercock P, Dennis M, et al. A prospective study of acute cerebrovascular disease in the community: the Oxfordshire community stroke project, 1981–1986. 1. Methodology, demography and incident cases of first ever stroke. *J Neurol Neurosurg Psychiatry* 1988;51:1373–1380.
4. Bamford J, Dennis M, Sandercock P, et al. A prospective study of acute cerebrovascular disease in the community: the Oxfordshire community stroke project, 1981–1986. 2. Incidence, case fatality rates and overall outcome at one year of cerebral infarction, primary intracerebral and subarachnoid haemorrhage. *J Neurol Neurosurg Psychiatry* 1990;53:16–22.
5. Bamford J, Dennis M, Sandercock P, et al. The frequency, causes and timing of death within 30 days of a first stroke: the Oxfordshire community stroke project. *J Neurol Neurosurg Psychiatry* 1990;53:824–829.
6. Wade DT. Functional abilities after stroke: measurement, natural history and prognosis. *J Neurol Neurosurg Psychiatry* 1987;50:177–182.
7. Stroke Unit Trialists' Collaboration. Organised inpatient (stroke unit) care for stroke. In: The Cochrane Library, Issue 4, 2003. Chichester, UK: John Wiley & Sons, Ltd. Search date 2001; primary sources Cochrane Stroke Group Specialised Trials Register and hand searches of reference lists of relevant articles and personal contact with colleagues.
8. Kwan J, Sandercock P. In hospital care pathways for stroke (Cochrane Review). In: The Cochrane Library, Issue 4, 2003. Chichester, UK: John Wiley & Sons, Ltd. Search date 2001; primary sources Cochrane Stroke Group Specialised Trials Register, Cochrane Controlled Trials Register, Medline, Embase Cinahl, Index to Scientific and Technical Proceedings, Healthstar, *J Manage Care* (later renamed the *J Integr Care*, and reference lists.
9. Sulter G, Elting JW, Langedijk M, et al. Admitting acute ischemic stroke patients to a stroke care monitoring unit versus a conventional stroke unit. *Stroke* 2003;34:101–104.
10. Wardlaw JM, del Zoppo G, Yamaguchi T. Thrombolysis for acute ischaemic stroke. In: The Cochrane Library, Issue 4, 2003. Chichester, UK: John Wiley & Sons, Ltd. Search date 1999; primary sources Cochrane Stroke Group Specialised Register of Controlled Trials, Embase, hand searches of relevant journals and references listed in relevant papers, and personal contact with pharmaceutical companies and principal investigators of trials.
11. CAST (Chinese Acute Stroke Trial) Collaborative Group. Randomised placebo-controlled trial of early aspirin use in 20 000 patients with acute ischaemic stroke. *Lancet* 1997;349:1641–1649.
12. International Stroke Trial Collaborative Group. The International Stroke Trial (IST): a randomised trial of aspirin, heparin, both or neither among 19 435 patients with acute ischaemic stroke. *Lancet* 1997;349:1569–1581.
13. Indredavik B, Bakke RPT, Slordahl SA, et al. Stroke unit treatment. 10-year follow-up. *Stroke* 1999;30:1524–1527.
14. Indredavik B, Bakke RPT, Slordahl SA, et al. Treatment in a combined acute and rehabilitation stroke unit. Which aspects are most important. *Stroke* 1999;30:917–923.
15. Stegmayr B, Asplund K, Hulter-Asberg K, et al. Stroke units in their natural habitat: can results of randomized trials be reproduced in routine clinical practice? For the risk-stroke collaboration. *Stroke* 1999;30:709–714.
16. Langhorne P, Pollock A in conjunction with the Stroke Unit Trialists' Collaboration. What are the components of effective stroke unit care? *Age Ageing* 2002;31:365–371. Search date not reported; primary source Cochrane Review.
17. Cornu C, Boutitie F, Candelise L, et al. Streptokinase in acute ischemic stroke: an individual patient data meta-analysis: the thrombolysis in acute stroke pooling project. *Stroke* 2000;31:1555–1560.
18. Kwiatkowski T, Libman R, Frankel M, et al. Effects of tissue plasminogen activator for acute ischemic stroke at one year. National Institute of Neurological Disorders and stroke recombinant tissue plasminogen activator stroke study group. *N Engl J Med* 1999;340:1781–1787.
19. Ringleb PA, Schellinger PD, Schranz C, et al. Thrombolytic therapy within 3 to 6 hours after onset of ischemic stroke. Useful or harmful? *Stroke* 2002;33:1437–1441.
20. Parsons MW, Barber PA, Chalk J, et al. Diffusion- and perfusion-weighted MRI response to thrombolysis in stroke. *Ann Neurol* 2002;51:28–37.
21. Internet Stroke Center. http://www.strokecenter.org/trials (last accessed 6 January 2005).
22. Hacke W, Donnan G, Fieschi C, et al. Association of outcome with early stroke treatment: pooled analysis of ATLANTIS, ECASS, and NINDS rt-PA stroke trials. *Lancet* 2004;363:768–774.
23. Gubitz G, Sandercock P, Counsell C. Antiplatelet therapy for acute ischaemic stroke. In: The Cochrane Library, Issue 4, 2003. Chichester, UK: John Wiley & Sons, Ltd. Search date 2002; primary sources Cochrane Stroke Group Specialised Register of Controlled Trials, the Register of the Antiplatelet Trialists' Collaboration, MedStrategy, and personal contact with pharmaceutical companies.
24. Chen Z, Sandercock P, Pan H, et al. Indications for early aspirin use in acute ischemic stroke: a combined analysis of 40 000 randomized patients from the Chinese Acute Stroke Trial and the International Stroke Trial. *Stroke* 2000;31:1240–1249.
25. Antithrombotic Trialists' Collaboration. Collaborative meta-analysis of randomised trials of antiplatelet therapy for prevention of death, myocardial infarction, and stroke in high risk patients. *BMJ* 2002;324:71–86. Search date 1997; primary sources Medline, Embase, Derwent, Scisearch,

Biosis, Cochrane Stroke Group Controlled Trials Register, Cochrane Peripheral Vascular Disease Group Controlled Trials Register, hand searches of journals, abstracts, and proceedings of meetings, reference lists from relevant articles, and personal contact with colleagues and pharmaceutical companies.

26. Slattery J, Warlow CP, Shorrock CJ, et al. Risks of gastrointestinal bleeding during secondary prevention of vascular events with aspirin — analysis of gastrointestinal bleeding during the UK-TIA trial. *Gut* 1995;37:509–511.
27. Johnson ES, Lanes SF, Wentworth CE, et al. A metaregression analysis of the dose–response effect of aspirin on stroke. *Arch Intern Med* 1999;159:1248–1253.
28. Gubitz G, Counsell C, Sandercock P, et al. Anticoagulants for acute ischaemic stroke. In: The Cochrane Library, Issue 4, 2003. Chichester, UK: John Wiley & Sons, Ltd. Search date 1999; primary sources Cochrane Stroke Group Specialised Register of Controlled Trials, trials register held by the Antithrombotic Therapy Trialists' Collaboration, MedStrategy, and personal contact with pharmaceutical companies.
29. Berge E, Sandercock P. Anticoagulants versus antiplatelet agents for acute ischaemic stroke (Cochrane Review). In: The Cochrane Library, Issue 4, 2003. Chichester, UK: John Wiley & Sons, Ltd. Search date: 2000; primary sources Cochrane Stroke Group Trials Register, the Cochrane Controlled Trials Register, the trials register held by the Antithrombotic Therapy Trialists' Collaboration, Medline, Embase.
30. Diener H, Ringelstein E, von Kummer R, et al. Treatment of acute ischemic stroke with the low-molecular-weight heparin certoparin: results of the TOPAS Trial. *Stroke* 2001;32:22–29.
31. Counsell C, Sandercock P. Low-molecular-weight heparins or heparinoids versus standard unfractionated heparin for acute ischaemic stroke. In: The Cochrane Library, Issue 4, 2003. Chichester, UK: John Wiley & Sons, Ltd. Search date 2001; primary sources Cochrane Stroke Group Specialised Trials Register, MedStrategy, and personal contact with pharmaceutical companies.
32. Bath P, Iddenden R, Bath F. Low-molecular-weight heparins and heparinoids in acute ischemic stroke: a meta-analysis of randomized controlled trials. *Stroke* 2000;31:1770–1778. Search date 1999; primary sources Cochrane Stroke Group Database of Trials in Acute Stroke, Cochrane Library, and hand searches of reference lists of identified publications.
33. Berge E, Abdelnoor M, Nakstad P, et al. Low-molecular-weight heparin versus aspirin in people with acute ischaemic stroke and atrial fibrillation: a double-blind randomised study. HAEST Study Group. Heparin in Acute Embolic Stroke Trial. *Lancet* 2000;355:1205–1210.
34. Blood pressure in Acute Stroke Collaboration (BASC). Interventions for deliberately altering blood pressure in acute stroke. In: The Cochrane Library, Issue 4, 2003. Chichester, UK: John Wiley & Sons, Ltd. Search date 2000; primary sources Cochrane Stroke Group Specialised Register of Controlled Trials, Cochrane Library (CDSR, CCTR), Medline, Embase, Bids, ISI-Science Citation Index, hand searches of reference lists of existing reviews and the ongoing trials section of the journal *Stroke*, and personal contact with research workers in the field and pharmaceutical companies.
35. Wahlgren NG, MacMahon DG, DeKeyser J, et al. Intravenous nimodipine west European stroke trial (INWEST) of nimodipine in the treatment of acute ischaemic stroke. *Cerebrovasc Dis* 1994;4:204–210.
36. Barer DH, Cruickshank JM, Ebrahim SB, et al. Low dose beta blockade in acute stroke (BEST trial): an evaluation. *BMJ* 1988;296:737–741.
37. Rodgers A, MacMahon S, Gamble G. Blood pressure and risk of stroke patients with cerebrovascular disease. *BMJ* 1996;313:147.
38. Schrader J, Rothemeyer M, Luders S, et al. Hypertension and stroke — rationale behind the ACCESS trial. *Basic Res Cardiol* 1998;93(suppl 2):69–78.
39. Horn J, Limburg M. Calcium antagonists for acute ischemic stroke. In: The Cochrane Library, Issue 4, 2003. Chichester, UK: John Wiley & Sons, Ltd. Search date 1999; primary sources Cochrane Stroke Group Specialised Register of Controlled Trials and personal contact with trialists.
40. Horn J, Limburg M. Calcium antagonists for ischemic stroke: a systematic review. *Stroke* 2001;32:570–576. Search date 1999; primary sources Cochrane Collaboration Stroke Group Specialized Register of Controlled Trials, and personal contact with principal investigators and company representatives.
41. Horn J, de Haan R, Vermeulen M, et al. Very Early Nimodipine Use in Stroke (VENUS). A randomized, double-blind, placebo-controlled trial. *Stroke* 2001;32:461–465.
42. Ricci S, Celani MG, Cantisani AT, et al. Piracetam for acute ischaemic stroke (Cochrane Review). In: The Cochrane Library, Issue 4, 2003. Chichester, UK: John Wiley & Sons, Ltd. Search date not reported; primary sources Cochrane Stroke Review Group trials register, Medline, Embase, BIDIS ISI, hand searches of relevant journals, and personal contact with the manufacturer.
43. Wahlgren NG, Ranasinha KW, Rosolacci T, et al. Clomethiazole acute stroke study (CLASS): results of a randomised, controlled trial of clomethiazole versus placebo in 1360 acute stroke patients. *Stroke* 1999;30:21–28.
44. Lyden P, Shuaib A, Ng K, et al. Clomethiazole Acute Stroke Study in Ischemic Stroke (CLASS-I) final results. *Stroke* 2002;33:122–129.
45. Gandolfo C, Sandercock P, Conti M. Lubeluzole for acute ischaemic stroke. In: The Cochrane Library, Issue 4, 2003. Chichester, UK: John Wiley & Sons, Ltd. Search date 2001; primary sources Cochrane Stroke Group Specialised Register of Controlled Trials, Cochrane Controlled Trials Register (CENTRAL/CCTR), Medline, Embase, Pascal BioMed, Current Contents, hand searches of all references in relevant papers, and personal contact with Janssen Research Foundation.
46. Muir KW, Lees KR. Excitatory amino acid antagonists for acute stroke (Cochrane Review). In: The Cochrane Library, Issue 2, 2004. Chichester, UK: John Wiley & Sons, Ltd.
47. Lees K, Asplund K, Carolei A, et al. Glycine antagonist (gavestinel) in neuroprotection (GAIN International) in people with acute stroke: a randomised controlled trial. *Lancet* 2000;355:1949–1954.
48. Sacco R, DeRosa J, Haley E Jr, et al, for the GAIN Americas Investigators. Glycine antagonist in neuroprotection for patients with acute stroke. GAIN Americas: a randomized controlled trial. *JAMA* 2001;285:1719–1728.
49. Davis S, Lees K, Albers G, et al, for the ASSIST Investigators. Selfotel in acute ischemic stroke. Possible neurotoxic effects of an NMDA antagonist. *Stroke* 2000;31:347–354.
50. Albers GW, Goldstein LB, Hall D, et al. Aptiganel hydrochloride in acute ischemic stroke. A randomised controlled trial. *JAMA* 2001;286:2673–2682.
51. The Tirilazad International Steering Committee. Tirilazad for acute ischaemic stroke. In: The Cochrane Library, Issue 4, 2003. Chichester, UK: John Wiley & Sons, Ltd. Search date 2001; primary sources Cochrane Stroke Group Specialised Trials Register, Cochrane Controlled Trials Register (CENTRAL/CCTR), the Cochrane Library, hand searches of a publication on the quality of acute stroke RCTs, and personal contact with Pharmacia & Upjohn.
52. Saver JL, Wilterdink J. Choline precursors for acute and subacute ischemic and hemorrhagic stroke

(Protocol for a Cochrane Review). In: The Cochrane Library, Issue 4, 2003. Chichester, UK: John Wiley & Sons, Ltd.

53. Cochrane Stroke Review Group. Department of Clinical Neurosciences, Western General Hospital, Crewe Road, Edinburgh, UK EH4 2XU. http://www.dcn.ed.ac.uk/csrg (last accessed 6 January 2005).
54. Muir KW, Lees KR. IMAGES. Intravenous magnesium efficacy in stroke trial [abstract]. *Cerebrovasc Dis* 1996;6:75–73.
55. Lodder J, van Raak L, Kessels F, et al. Early GABA-ergic activation study in stroke (EGASIS). *Cerebrovasc Dis* 2000;10(suppl 2):80.
56. Prasad K, Shrivastava A. Surgery for primary supratentorial intracerebral haemorrhage. In: The Cochrane Library, Issue 4, 2003. Chichester, UK: John Wiley & Sons, Ltd. Search date 1998; primary sources Cochrane Stroke Group Trials Register and hand searches of reference lists of articles identified, three relevant monographs, and issues of *Curr Opin Neurol Neurosurg* and *Neurosurg Clin N Am*.
57. Hankey G, Hon C. Surgery for primary intracerebral hemorrhage: is it safe and effective? A systematic review of case series and randomised trials. *Stroke* 1997;28:2126–2132. Search date 1997; primary sources Medline, and hand searches of reference lists of identified articles, published epidemiological studies, and reviews.
58. Fernandes HM, Gregson B, Siddique S, et al. Surgery in intracerebral hemorrhage: the uncertainty continues. *Stroke* 2000;31:2511–2516. Search date 1999; primary sources Ovid databases (unspecified), Medline, and hand searches of the reference lists of identified articles and relevant cited references.
59. Warlow CP, Dennis MS, van Gijn J, et al, eds. Treatment of primary intracerebral haemorrhage. In: *Stroke: a practical guide to management*. Oxford: Blackwell Science, 1996:430–437.
60. Mendelow A. International Surgical Trial in Intracerebral Haemorrhage (ISTICH). *Stroke* 2000;31:2539.

Elizabeth Warburton
Consultant in Stroke Medicine
Neuroscience's
Addenbrookes Hospital, Cambridge, UK

Competing interests: EAW has received funding for a stroke nurse from Servier and has also been reimbursed for attending a stroke conference.

We would like to acknowledge the previous contributors of this chapter, including Gord Gubitz and Peter Sandercock.

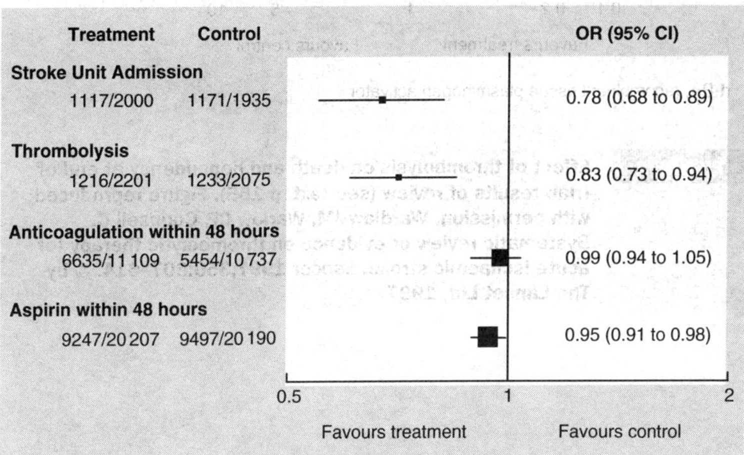

FIGURE 1 **Proportional effects on "death or dependency" at the end of scheduled follow up: results of systematic reviews.[7,10–12] Data refer only to benefits and not to harms (see text, p 157).**

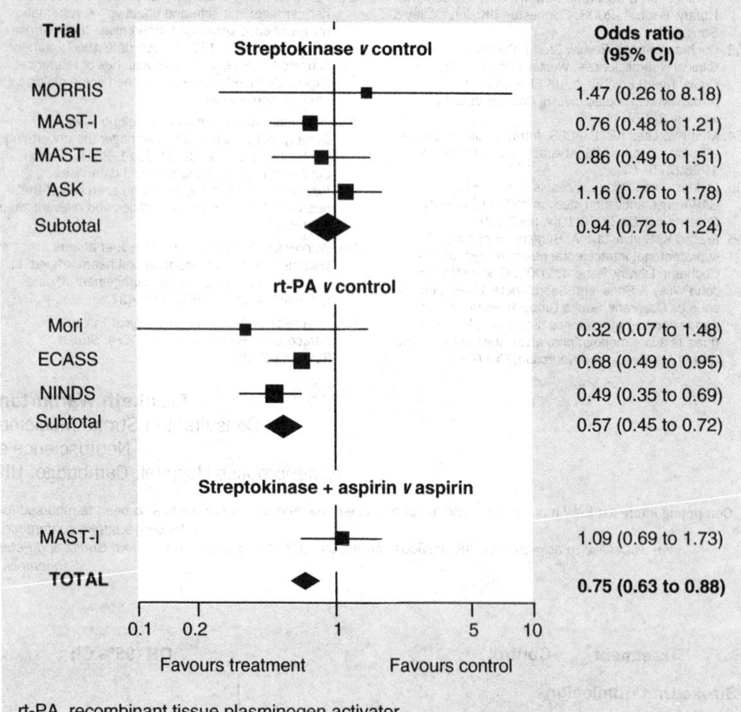

FIGURE 2 **Effect of thrombolysis on death and dependency at end of trial: results of review (see text, p 155). Figure reproduced with permission. Wardlaw JM, Warlow CP, Counsell C. Systematic review of evidence on thrombolytic therapy for acute ischaemic stroke. *Lancet* 1997;350:607–614. © by The Lancet Ltd, 1997.**

Stroke prevention

Search date September 2003

Gregory YH Lip, Peter Rothwell, and Cathie Sudlow

QUESTIONS

INTERVENTIONS

See glossary Ⓖ

Key Messages

In people with a prior stroke or transient ischaemic attack

- **Antiplatelet treatment** One systematic review found that prolonged antiplatelet treatment reduced the risk of serious vascular events including stroke in people with prior stroke or transient ischaemic attack compared with placebo or no antiplatelet treatment.
- **Blood pressure reduction** One systematic review and two subsequent large RCTs found that blood pressure lowering treatment reduced stroke and other major vascular events in people with a prior stroke or transient ischaemic attack, whether or not they were hypertensive. Two additional smaller RCTs in people with a prior stroke or transient ischaemic attack found no significant difference between atenolol and placebo in stroke, but these RCTs may have lacked power to detect clinically important differences.
- **Carotid endarterectomy in people with moderately severe (50–69%) symptomatic carotid artery stenosis** Evidence from a pooled analysis of individual patient data from three RCTs found that carotid endarterectomy reduced stroke and death compared with no endarterectomy in symptomatic people with 50–69% carotid stenosis.
- **Carotid endarterectomy in people with severe (> 70%) symptomatic carotid artery stenosis** Evidence from a pooled analysis of three RCTs found that carotid endarterectomy reduced stroke and death compared with no endarterectomy in symptomatic people with more than 70% carotid stenosis, although no benefit was found in people with near-occlusion. Benefit in symptomatic people with more than 70% stenosis was greater than in people with lower grade stenosis.
- **Cholesterol reduction** Systematic reviews of large RCTs found that statins reduced major vascular events, including stroke, compared with placebo in people with prior stroke or transient ischaemic attack. RCTs found no evidence that non-statin treatments reduced stroke compared with placebo or no treatment.
- **Carotid endarterectomy in people with asymptomatic but severe carotid artery stenosis** Two systematic reviews found that carotid endarterectomy reduced perioperative stroke, death, and subsequent ipsilateral stroke in people with asymptomatic but severe stenosis. However, because the risk of stroke without surgery in asymptomatic people is relatively low, the benefit from surgery is small.
- **Alternative antiplatelet regimens to aspirin (no evidence that any regimen more or less effective than aspirin alone)** Systematic reviews and subsequent RCTs found no good evidence that any antiplatelet regimen was superior to aspirin for long term secondary prevention of serious vascular events but found that clopidogrel was a safe and effective alternative to aspirin.
- **Carotid or vertebral percutaneous transluminal angioplasty** RCTs provided insufficient evidence about the effects of carotid or vertebral percutaneous transluminal angioplasty or stenting compared with medical treatment or carotid endarterectomy in people with a recent carotid or vertebral territory transient ischaemic attack or non-disabling ischaemic stroke who have severe stenosis of the ipsilateral carotid or vertebral artery.
- **Different blood pressure lowering regimens (no evidence that any regimen more or less effective than any other)** We found no RCTs comparing different blood pressure lowering regimens specifically among people with a prior stroke or transient ischaemic attack. Systematic reviews of RCTs in people with hypertension or vascular disease found little difference in stroke between regimens based on diuretics, angiotensin converting enzyme inhibitors, β blockers or calcium channel blockers. There was a direct relationship between the relative risk of stroke outcomes and the blood pressure reduction achieved.
- **Carotid endarterectomy in people with moderate (30–49%) symptomatic carotid artery stenosis** Evidence from a pooled analysis of individual patient data from three RCTs suggested that carotid endarterectomy was of no benefit in symptomatic people with 30–49% stenosis.

- **Carotid endarterectomy in people with symptomatic near-occlusion of the carotid artery** Three RCTs provided limited evidence that carotid endarterectomy increased the risk of stroke or death due to surgery in symptomatic people with near-occlusion of the ipsilateral carotid artery.
- **High dose versus low dose aspirin (no additional benefit but may increase harms)** One systematic review and one subsequent RCT found that low dose aspirin (75–150 mg/day) was as effective as higher doses for preventing serious vascular events. It found insufficient evidence that doses lower than 75 mg daily were as effective. Systematic reviews found no evidence of an association between aspirin dose and risk of intracranial, major extracranial, or gastrointestinal haemorrhage. RCTs found that high dose aspirin (500–1500 mg/day) increased the risk of upper gastrointestinal upset compared with medium dose aspirin (75–325 mg/day).
- **Anticoagulation in people in sinus rhythm** Systematic reviews found no significant difference between anticoagulation and placebo or antiplatelet treatment for preventing recurrent stroke after presumed ischaemic stroke in people in normal sinus rhythm. Anticoagulants increased the risk of fatal intracranial and extracranial haemorrhage compared with placebo. High intensity anticoagulation increased the risk of major bleeding compared with antiplatelet treatment.
- **Carotid endarterectomy in people with less than 30% symptomatic carotid artery stenosis** Evidence from a pooled analysis of individual patient data from three RCTs suggested that carotid endarterectomy increased the risk of stroke or death due to surgery in symptomatic people with less than 30% carotid stenosis.

In people with atrial fibrillation and a prior stroke or transient ischaemic attack

- **Oral anticoagulation** One systematic review found that adjusted dose warfarin reduced the risk of stroke compared with control in people with previous stroke or transient ischaemic attack. The best time to begin anticoagulation after an ischaemic stroke is unclear. One systematic review provided insufficient evidence to compare warfarin versus aspirin.
- **Aspirin** One systematic review of one RCT found no significant difference between aspirin and placebo in stroke or death in people with previous stroke or transient ischaemic attack. One systematic review provided insufficient evidence to compare aspirin versus warfarin.

In people with atrial fibrillation without a prior stroke or transient ischaemic attack

- **Aspirin in people with contraindications to anticoagulants** One systematic review found that aspirin reduced the risk of stroke compared with placebo, but another review found no significant difference. These findings support the use of aspirin in people with atrial fibrillation and contraindications to anticoagulants.
- **Oral anticoagulation** One systematic review found that warfarin reduced fatal and non-fatal ischaemic stroke compared with placebo, provided there was a low risk of bleeding and careful monitoring. The people in the review had a mean age of 69 years. One overview in people less than 65 years old found no significant difference in the annual stroke rate between warfarin and placebo.

DEFINITION Prevention in this context is the long term management of people with a prior stroke or transient ischaemic attack, and of people at high risk of stroke Ⓖ for other reasons such as atrial fibrillation. **Stroke:** See definition under stroke management, p 152. **Transient ischaemic attack:** This is similar to a mild ischaemic stroke except that symptoms last for less than 24 hours.[1]

INCIDENCE/ PREVALENCE See incidence/prevalence under stroke management, p 152.

AETIOLOGY/ RISK FACTORS See aetiology under stroke management, p 152. Risk factors for stroke include prior stroke or transient ischaemic attack, increasing age, hypertension, diabetes, cigarette smoking, and emboli associated with atrial fibrillation, artificial heart valves, or myocardial infarction. The relation with cholesterol is less clear. One overview of prospective studies among healthy middle aged people found no association between total cholesterol and overall stroke risk.[2] However, one review of prospective observational studies in eastern Asian people found that cholesterol was positively associated with ischaemic stroke but negatively associated with haemorrhagic stroke.[3]

PROGNOSIS People with a history of stroke or transient ischaemic attack are at high risk of all vascular events, such as myocardial infarction, but are at particular risk of subsequent stroke (about 10% in the first year and about 5% each year thereafter); see figure 1, p 193, and figure 1 in secondary prevention of ischaemic cardiac events, (Web only).[4,5] People with intermittent atrial fibrillation treated with aspirin should be considered at similar risk of stroke, compared with people with sustained atrial fibrillation treated with aspirin (rate of ischaemic stroke/year: 3.2% with intermittent *v* 3.3% with sustained).[6]

AIMS OF INTERVENTION To prevent death or disabling stroke, as well as other serious non-fatal outcomes, especially myocardial infarction, with minimal adverse effects from treatment.

OUTCOMES Stroke, myocardial infarction; mortality, and dependency.

METHODS *Clinical Evidence* search and appraisal September 2003. Options authored by Cathie Sudlow were searched September 2003 (including hand searches of vascular, neurology, and general medical journals). The six journals that contained the largest number of relevant papers were hand searched (search dates 1994–2000).

QUESTION What are the effects of preventive interventions in people with prior stroke or transient ischaemic attack?

OPTION BLOOD PRESSURE REDUCTION VERSUS NO BLOOD PRESSURE REDUCTION

Cathie Sudlow

One systematic review and two subsequent large RCTs found that blood pressure lowering treatment reduced stroke and other major vascular events in people with a prior stroke or transient ischaemic attack, whether or not they were hypertensive. Two additional smaller RCTs in people with a prior stroke or transient ischaemic attack found no significant difference between atenolol and placebo in stroke, but these RCTs may have lacked power to detect clinically important differences.

Benefits: We found one systematic review,[7] one non-systematic review[8] that identified two additional RCTs[9,10] and two subsequent RCTs[11,12] comparing antihypertensive treatment versus placebo, no treatment, or usual care in people with a prior stroke or transient ischaemic attack (TIA) or at high risk of stroke. The systematic review (search date not stated, 9 RCTs, 6753 people with a prior stroke or transient ischaemic attack) found that antihypertensive treatment significantly reduced stroke and major cardiovascular events compared with placebo, no treatment, or usual care over 2–7 years (stroke: RR 0.72, 95% CI 0.61 to 0.85; major cardiovascular events: RR 0.79, 95% CI 0.68 to 0.91).[7] Over 80% of people in the review were included in a single large RCT, the results of which have only been published in preliminary form.[13] The first additional RCT identified by the non-systematic review[8] (1473 people with non-disabling ischaemic stroke or TIA within previous 3 months) found no significant difference in combined fatal and non-fatal stroke between atenolol 50 mg daily and placebo after mean follow up of 32 months (52/732 [7.1%] with atenolol v 62/741 [8.4%] with placebo; HR 0.84, 95% CI 0.58 to 1.22).[10] The second additional RCT (720 people within three weeks of a stroke or TIA) found no significant difference in major stroke between atenolol 50 mg daily and placebo after mean follow up of 28 months (major stroke: 74/372 [19.9%] with atenolol v 69/348 [19.8%] with placebo; RR 0.79, 95% CI 0.54 to 1.16).[9] However, these two additional RCTs may have lacked power to detect clinically important differences. The first subsequent RCT (6105 people with a prior stroke or transient ischaemic attack) compared four years of the angiotensin converting enzyme inhibitor perindopril plus indapamide (added at the discretion of the treating physician) versus placebo.[11] It found that active treatment reduced blood pressure by 9/4 mm Hg and reduced stroke and major vascular events compared with placebo but did not significantly reduce mortality (stroke: RR 0.72, 95% CI 0.62 to 0.83; major vascular events: RR 0.74, 95% CI 0.66 to 0.84; mortality: RR 0.96, 95% CI 0.82 to 1.12). Relative risks were similar irrespective of baseline blood pressure (hypertensive or not) and the type of qualifying cerebrovascular event (ischaemic or haemorrhagic). Treatment with perindopril and indapamide produced significantly larger reductions in blood pressure, stroke and major vascular events than treatment with perindopril alone (average BP reduction: perindopril and indapamide 12/5 mm Hg, perindopril alone 5/3 mm Hg; stroke: perindopril and indapamide RR 0.57, 95% CI 0.46 to 0.70, perindopril alone RR 0.95, 95% CI 0.77 to 1.19; major vascular events: perindopril and indapamide RR 0.60, 95% CI 0.51 to 0.71, perindopril alone RR 0.96, 95% CI 0.80 to 1.15). The relative risks were consistent with those that would be predicted for the blood pressure reductions achieved.[11] The second subsequent RCT (9297 people at high risk of vascular disease, 1013 [11%] with a prior stroke or transient ischaemic attack) found that the angiotensin converting enzyme inhibitor ramipril reduced blood pressure by 3/2 mm Hg and significantly reduced stroke and major vascular events at 4.5 years compared with placebo (stroke: RR 0.68, 95% CI 0.56 to 0.84; major vascular events: RR 0.78, 95% CI 0.70 to 0.86).[12] Subsequent analysis found that relative risks were similar in people with and without a prior stroke or transient ischaemic attack and in those with and without hypertension at baseline (P = 0.21 between previous people with stroke and no previous stroke).[14]

Harms: The additional RCTs identified by the non-systematic review[8] found that atenolol increased the proportion of people reporting any adverse effect leading to discontinuation of study treatment compared with placebo (first RCT: 108/732 [15%] with atenolol *v* 56/741 [8%] with placebo; second RCT: 17% atenolol *v* 10% placebo; significance of either comparison not reported). The first subsequent RCT found a slight excess of premature cessation of all study tablets in the active treatment group (714/3051 [23%] active v 636/3054 [21%] placebo).[11]

Comment: In the second subsequent RCT, the timing of drug intake in relation to blood pressure measurement may have led to an underestimate of the effects of ramipril on blood pressure compared with other blood pressure lowering trials. For, unlike most other large trials of blood pressure lowering, treatment in this RCT was given in the evening, with blood pressure measurements taken during daytime study visits.[15] A substudy of 24 hour blood pressure recordings in 38 patients demonstrated that ramipril reduced BP more at night than during the day, and reduced the average 24 hour blood pressure by 10/4 mm Hg compared with placebo.[15] This would suggest that similar blood pressure reductions were achieved in the second and third RCTs, producing similar relative reductions in stroke. One systematic review of the effects of different blood pressure lowering drug regimens in people with hypertension, diabetes or vascular disease (including those with a prior stroke or transient ischaemic attack) found that the relative risks of stroke and other major vascular outcomes (apart from heart failure) were proportional to the blood pressure reduction achieved.[16] This suggests that, in general, the more the blood pressure is reduced, the greater the benefit, and that it is probably the size of the blood pressure reduction rather than the specific drug regimen used that determines the benefit. Observational studies in healthy middle aged and elderly people as well as in those with a history of a cerebrovascular event found no evidence of a threshold of systolic or diastolic blood pressure below which there was no reduction in stroke, at least down as far as about 115/75 mm Hg.[17–19] It seems appropriate to be particularly cautious lowering blood pressure in people with known severe stenosis of the carotid or vertebral arteries, because of concerns about the possibility of precipitating a recurrent stroke.[20]

OPTION DIFFERENT BLOOD PRESSURE LOWERING REGIMENS

Cathie Sudlow

We found no RCTs comparing different blood pressure lowering regimens specifically among people with a prior stroke or transient ischaemic attack. Systematic reviews of RCTs in people with hypertension or vascular disease found little difference in stroke between regimens based on diuretics, angiotensin converting enzyme inhibitors, β blockers or calcium channel blockers. There was a direct relationship between the relative risk of stroke outcomes and the blood pressure reduction achieved.

Benefits: We found no RCTs or reviews that looked solely at prevention in people who have had a prior stroke or transient ischaemic attack (TIA). We found three systematic reviews that compared the effects of different first-line blood pressure lowering regimens on stroke and other vascular outcomes in people with hypertension or vascular disease.[16,21,22] None of these reviews presented results separately for people with previous stroke or TIA. The first systematic review (search date 1997, 5 RCTs, 17 952 people with hypertension) evaluated first-line treatment and found that thiazide diuretics (low or high dose) reduced stroke and cardiovascular events after 1 to 10 years compared with β blockers but the reduction was not statistically significant (stroke: 107/8862 [1.2%] with diuretics v 130/8984 [1.4%] with β blockers, RR 0.84, 95% CI 0.65 to 1.08; total cardiovascular events: 431/8862 [4.9%] with diuretics v 495/8984 [10.2%] with β blockers; RR 0.88, 95% CI 0.78 to 1.00).[21] The second systematic review (search date 2002, 42 RCTs, 192 478 people with hypertension including people with diabetes, older adults, cerebrovascular disease, and renal disease, the proportion with previous stroke or TIA was not reported) compared low dose diuretics (starting dose generally 12.5–25 mg chlorthalidone or hydrochlorthiazide) with other first-line therapies (based on diuretics, angiotensin converting enzyme inhibitors, angiotensin receptor blockers, calcium antagonists, diuretics and α blockers and including placebo).[22] The mean duration of the included RCTs was 3 to 4 years. From a combination of direct and indirect comparisons, it found no evidence that first-line treatment with β blockers, angiotensin converting enzyme inhibitors, calcium channel blockers, angiotensin receptor blockers, or α blockers was significantly better than low dose diuretics for any outcome. The third systematic review (search date 2003, 29 RCTs, 162 341 people, the proportion with previous stroke or TIA was not reported) also assessed the effects on major cardiovascular outcomes of different blood pressure lowering regimens (based on angiotensin converting enzyme inhibitors, calcium antagonists, diuretics and β blockers) using only direct randomised comparisons.[16] The mean duration of follow up ranged from 2.0 to 8.4 years. Most people had pre-existing cardiovascular disease or more than one cardiovascular risk factor at baseline. In the analysis diuretics and β blockers were combined. It found that calcium antagonists reduced stroke compared with diuretics or β blockers but the decrease was of borderline significance (RR 0.93, 95% CI 0.86 to 1.00). It found that calcium antagonists reduced stroke compared with angiotensin converting enzyme inhibitors, but the decrease was of borderline significance (RR 0.89, 95% CI 0.80 to 0.99). It found that diuretics or β blockers reduced stroke compared with angiotensin converting enzyme inhibitors but the decrease was of borderline significance (RR 0.92, 95% CI 0.85 to 1.00). The relative risk of stroke was directly proportional to the difference between randomised groups in achieved blood pressure reduction.[16]

Harms: The first systematic review found that withdrawal due to adverse effects was significantly more common with β blockers than with thiazide diuretics (924/8984 [10.3%] with β blockers v 624/8862 [7.0%] with diuretics; RR 1.45, 95% CI 1.32 to 1.59).[21] See harms under blood pressure reduction, p 171.

Comment: None.

OPTION CHOLESTEROL REDUCTION

Cathie Sudlow

Systematic reviews of large RCTs found that statins reduced major vascular events, including stroke, compared with placebo in people with prior stroke or transient ischaemic attack. RCTs found no evidence that non-statin treatments reduced stroke compared with placebo or no treatment.

Benefits: Statins: We found three systematic reviews and one meta-analysis that assessed the effect of statins on stroke in various different populations.[23–26] None of these reviews presented results separately for people with previous stroke or transient ischaemic attack. The most recent systematic review (search date not stated) identified 30 RCTs assessing the effect on stroke of statins compared with placebo but it did not present pooled results from these RCTs.[25] Over 90% of the stroke outcomes were recorded in 8 large RCTs. These eight RCTs (70 000 people including middle aged men without coronary heart disease and older high risk people) were subsequently included in a meta-analysis.[26] The meta-analysis found that statins (simvastatin, pravastatin and atorvastatin) significantly reduced the combined outcome of fatal or non-fatal stroke compared with placebo (1195/35 614 [3.4%] with statin v 1468/35 598 [4.1%] with placebo; OR 0.81, 95% CI 0.75 to 0.87).[26] It found that reducing LDL cholesterol by 0.6 to 1.0 mmol/L reduced the relative risk of a fatal or non-fatal stroke by about one fifth. The largest RCT included in this meta-analysis compared simvastatin 40 mg daily versus placebo in over 20 000 people with a history of or at high- risk of vascular disease.[27] It included over 3000 people with a history of ischemic stroke or TIA, over 4000 with a pre-treatment cholesterol below 5.0 mmol/L, and almost 6000 aged over 70 years. It found that simvastatin reduced stroke, major vascular events (major coronary events, strokes, and coronary or non-coronary revascularisations), and deaths over 5 years compared with placebo (stroke: AR 4% with simvastatin v 6% with placebo; RR 0.75, 95% CI 0.66 to 0.85; major vascular events: AR 20% with simvastatin v 25% with placebo; RR 0.76, 95% CI 0.72 to 0.81; deaths: AR 13% with simvastatin v 15% with placebo; RR 0.87, 95% CI 0.81 to 0.94). The relative reduction in major vascular events was similar among those with different pre-treatment concentrations of cholesterol and triglycerides, among all age groups included, and regardless of prior history of coronary artery disease, ischaemic stroke or TIA, ischaemic heart disease, peripheral arterial disease or diabetes.[27] The results of systematic reviews that also included the smaller statin trials were similar.[23–25] The first of these reviews (search date 1995, 14 RCTs) found that reducing mean total cholesterol with a statin by 21% over an average of 4 years reduced the relative odds of stroke by 24%.[23] The second of these reviews (search date not stated, 16 RCTs, 39 065 people) found that statins reduced total stroke compared with placebo (372/22 014

[1.69%] with statins v 474/17 051 [2.78%] with control; OR 0.77, 95% CI 0.67 to 0.87).[24] Systematic reviews have also shown that the reduction in relative risks both of stroke and of coronary heart disease are proportional to the size of the reduction in LDL cholesterol and are smaller in the first two years of treatment than in subsequent years.[24,25] **Non-statin treatments:** We found no systematic reviews or RCTs that reported results separately for people with previous stroke or TIA. We found one overview,[28] one additional RCT[30] and two subsequent RCTs[29,31] that assessed the outcome of stroke. The overview (11 RCTs) compared reducing cholesterol with a non-statin treatment (fibrate, resin, or diet) versus placebo or no treatment.[28] It found no significant difference between a non-statin treatment and placebo in the risk of stroke (OR 0.99, 95% CI 0.82 to 1.21). The additional RCT (532 men who had a previous stroke or TIA) found no significant difference between clofibrate and placebo in death after 3.5 years (AR 13% with clofibrate *v* 19% with placebo; P value not reported).[30] The first subsequent RCT (2531 men with coronary heart disease) found no significant difference between gemfibrozil and placebo in the risk of stroke (AR 5% with gemfibrozil *v* 6% with placebo; RRR +25%, 95% CI –6% to +47%).[29] The second subsequent RCT (3090 patients with previous myocardial infarction or stable angina including 58 people with previous stroke or TIA) found no significant difference between bezafibrate (400 mg) and placebo in the risk of stroke after follow up for about 6 years (AR 4.6% with bezafibrate v 5.0% with placebo; P = 0.66).[31]

Harms: Statins: Although it has been suggested that statins may increase haemorrhagic stroke,[3,23] the largest statin RCT found no evidence that simvastatin increased haemorrhagic stroke.[27] A meta-analysis of cancer incidence in major statin trials found no excess risk of cancer with statins.[32] The large statin RCTs did not find any significant excess of serious adverse events with statins.[27,32–36] Non-statin treatments: The RCT comparing gemfibrozil with placebo found no significant excess of serious adverse events with treatment.[29] The RCT comparing bezafibrate with placebo found similar adverse effect rates for treatments.[31]

Comment: An RCT comparing atorvastatin versus placebo in 4700 people with minor stroke or TIA is in progress.[37] A planned overview of individual participant data from all RCTs of cholesterol reduction aims to summarise the effects of reducing cholesterol in different groups of people, including those with a prior stroke or TIA.[38]

OPTION ANTIPLATELET TREATMENT VERSUS NO ANTIPLATELET TREATMENT

Cathie Sudlow

One systematic review found that prolonged antiplatelet treatment reduced the risk of serious vascular events in people with prior stroke or transient ischaemic attack compared with placebo or no antiplatelet treatment.

Benefits: We found one systematic review (search date 1997, 195 RCTs, 135 640 people at high risk of vascular disease: previous stroke or transient ischaemic attack (TIA), acute stroke, ischaemic heart disease, heart failure, cardiac valve disease, atrial fibrillation, peripheral arterial disease, diabetes, and haemodialysis) comparing antiplatelet treatment (mostly aspirin) versus placebo or no antiplatelet treatment.[39] It found that in people with prior stroke or TIA (21 RCTs, 18 270 people) antiplatelet treatment reduced serious vascular events (stroke, myocardial infarction, or vascular death) compared with placebo or no antiplatelet treatment after 3 years (AR 18% with antiplatelet *v* 21% with placebo or no antiplatelet treatment; OR 0.78, 95% CI 0.73 to

0.85). Antiplatelet treatment also reduced the separate outcomes of stroke, myocardial infarction, vascular death, and death (see figure 1, p 193). For every 1000 people with a prior stroke or TIA treated for about 3 years, antiplatelet treatment prevented 25 non-fatal strokes, six non-fatal myocardial infarctions, and 15 deaths.[39]

Harms: The systematic review found that antiplatelet treatment in people with prior stroke or TIA increased major extracranial haemorrhage (haemorrhages requiring hospital admission or blood transfusion) and intracranial haemorrhage compared with no antiplatelet treatment (intracranial haemorrhage: AR 0.64% with antiplatelet *v* 0.56% with no antiplatelet; OR 1.2, CI not reported; major extracranial haemorrhage: AR 0.97% with antiplatelet *v* 0.47% with no antiplatelet; OR 2.0, CI not reported).[39] We found one systematic review (search date 1999, 24 RCTs) that assessed the effects of aspirin on gastrointestinal bleeding.[40] It found that aspirin increased gastrointestinal bleeding compared with placebo or no aspirin (OR 1.68, 95% CI 1.51 to 1.88). Another systematic review (search date 1997, 16 RCTs, 55 462 people) found that aspirin increased intracranial haemorrhage by about one event per 1000 people treated for 3 years.[41]

Comment: In people at high risk of vascular disease, including those with a prior ischaemic stroke or TIA, the large absolute reductions in serious vascular events produced by antiplatelet treatment far outweighed any absolute hazards.

OPTION HIGH DOSE VERSUS LOW DOSE ASPIRIN

Cathie Sudlow

One systematic review and one subsequent RCT found that low dose aspirin (75–150 mg/day) was as effective as higher doses for preventing serious vascular events. It found insufficient evidence that doses lower than 75 mg daily were as effective. Systematic reviews found no evidence of an association between aspirin dose and risk of intracranial, major extracranial, or gastrointestinal haemorrhage. RCTs found that high dose aspirin (500–1500 mg/day) increased the risk of upper gastrointestinal upset compared with medium dose aspirin (75–325 mg/day).

Benefits: We found one systematic review (search date 1997; 7225 people at high risk of vascular disease in RCTs comparing different doses of aspirin; about 60 000 people at high risk of vascular disease, excluding those with acute stroke, in RCTs comparing different doses of aspirin versus placebo or no aspirin) that compared the effects of higher versus lower dose aspirin on stroke.[39] and one subsequent RCT that compared the effects of higher versus lower dose aspirin.[42] The systematic review found no significant difference between aspirin 500–1500 mg daily and 75–325 mg daily in serious vascular events (stroke, myocardial infarction, or vascular death; OR 0.97, 95% CI 0.79 to 1.19). It also found that doses of 75 mg or more did not reduce serious vascular events compared with doses lower than 75 mg (OR 1.08, 95% CI 0.90 to 1.31). However, the comparison lacked power to exclude a clinically important difference. The systematic review also found that different aspirin doses reduced serious vascular events compared with placebo or no antiplatelet treatment by similar amounts for the higher daily doses but by a smaller amount for very low doses (higher doses, 500–1500 mg/day *v* placebo or no antiplatelet treatment: OR 0.81, 95% CI 0.75 to 0.87; 160–325 mg/day *v* placebo or no antiplatelet treatment: OR 0.74, 95% CI 0.69 to 0.80; 75–150 mg/day *v* placebo or no antiplatelet treatment: OR 0.68, 95% CI 0.59 to 0.79; lower doses, < 75 mg/day *v* placebo or no antiplatelet treatment: OR 0.87, 95% CI 0.74 to 1.03). See figure 2 in secondary prevention of ischaemic cardiac events, (Web only). People with acute stroke were excluded from these analyses. The results in people with prior stroke or transient ischaemic attack were not presented separately. The subsequent RCT (2849 people scheduled for carotid endarterectomy, most of whom had prior stroke or transient ischaemic attack) compared low dose aspirin (81 and 325 mg/day) versus high dose aspirin (650 and 1300 mg/day).[42] It found that high dose aspirin increased the combined outcome of stroke, myocardial infarction, and death after 3 months compared with low dose aspirin (AR 8.4% with high dose v 6.2% with low dose; RR 1.34, 95% CI 1.03 to 1.75).[42]

Harms: **Extracranial haemorrhage:** The systematic review found that the proportional increase in risk of major extracranial haemorrhage was similar with all daily aspirin doses. In direct comparisons, 75–325 mg aspirin did not increase major extracranial haemorrhage compared with doses lower than 75 mg (AR 2.5% with 75–325 mg/day *v* 1.8% with < 75 mg/day; P > 0.05).[39] We found one systematic review (search date 1999, 24 RCTs) of the effects of aspirin on gastrointestinal bleeding.[40] Indirect comparisons in a meta-regression analysis found no association between dose of aspirin and risk of gastrointestinal bleeds. RCTs directly comparing different daily doses of aspirin have found a trend toward more gastrointestinal haemorrhage and a significant increase in upper gastrointestinal symptoms with high (500–1500 mg) than with medium (75–325 mg) doses (upper gastrointestinal symptoms: OR 1.3, 95% CI 1.1 to 1.5), but no significant difference in these outcomes between 283 mg and 30 mg daily.[42–44] We found one systematic review of observational studies (search date 2001, 5 studies) of the effects of different doses of aspirin on the risk of upper gastrointestinal complications (bleeding, perforation, or upper gastrointestinal event leading to hospital admission or visit to specialist).[45] It found greater risks of upper gastrointestinal complications with doses of aspirin greater than 300 mg daily. **Intracranial haemorrhage:** We found one systematic review (search date 1997, 16 RCTs, 55 462 people) of the effects of aspirin on intracranial haemorrhage.[41] It found no clear variation in risk with the dose of aspirin used. Three RCTs directly compared different daily doses of aspirin and found no significant differences in the risk of intracranial haemorrhage, but they lacked power to detect clinically important differences.[42–44]

Comment: None.

OPTION ALTERNATIVE ANTIPLATELET REGIMENS TO ASPIRIN

Cathie Sudlow

Systematic reviews and subsequent RCTs and have found no good evidence that any antiplatelet regimen was superior to aspirin for long term secondary prevention of serious vascular events but found that clopidogrel was a safe and effective alternative to aspirin.

Benefits: **Thienopyridines (clopidogrel and ticlopidine) versus aspirin:** We found two systematic reviews (search dates 1997[39] and 1999[46]) and one subsequent RCT[47] that compared thienopyridines versus aspirin. The first systematic review (4 RCTs, 3791 people at high risk of vascular disease) found no significant difference between ticlopidine and aspirin in serious vascular events (stroke, myocardial infarction, or vascular death: AR 21% with ticlopidine *v* 23% with aspirin; OR 0.88, 95% CI is 0.75 to 1.03).[39] It also found that the risk of serious vascular events was similar with clopidogrel and aspirin (1 RCT, 19 185 people: AR 10% with clopidogrel *v* 11% with aspirin; OR 0.90, 95% CI 0.82 to 0.99). The second systematic review (4 RCTs) found that ticlopidine or clopidogrel marginally reduced vascular events after about 2 years compared with aspirin (OR 0.91, 95% CI 0.84 to 0.98; ARR 1.1%, 95% CI 0.2% to 1.9%).[46] The subsequent RCT (1809 African Americans with a recent non-cardioembolic ischaemic stroke) compared ticlopidine (500 mg/day) versus aspirin (650 mg/day) over two years and found no significant difference between these treatments in the primary outcome of recurrent stroke, myocardial infarction or vascular death (AR 14.7% with ticlopidine v 12.3% with aspirin, HR 1.22, 95% CI 0.94 to 1.57).[47] **Dipyridamole plus aspirin:** We found one systematic review (search date 1997, 25 relevant RCTs, 10 404 people) comparing dipyridamole plus aspirin versus aspirin alone.[39] It found no significant difference in serious vascular events (stroke, myocardial infarction, or vascular death) between dipyridamole plus aspirin and aspirin alone (AR 11.8% with combination treatment *v* 12.4% with aspirin alone; OR 0.94, 95% CI 0.83 to 1.06). Effects on stroke were not certain. Overall, the systematic review found that combination treatment reduced non-fatal strokes (183/5198 [3.5%] v 236/5206 [4.5%]; OR 0.76).[39] Most non-fatal stroke events (109 and 158 of the total) were recorded in one larger RCT (about 6000 people with a prior ischaemic stroke or TIA) comparing aspirin (50 mg daily) versus modified release dipyridamole (400 mg daily) versus both versus neither.[48] Combination treatment did not reduce stroke compared with aspirin alone in other trials.[39] These conflicting results may be because of the very low aspirin dose in the larger trial, the antihypertensive effect of dipyridamole, or chance. Triflusal versus aspirin: We found one systematic review and one subsequent RCT that compared triflusal versus aspirin.[39,49] The systematic review (3 RCTs, 2675 people at high risk of vascular events of whom 400 had a history of ischaemic stroke or TIA) found no significant difference between triflusal and aspirin in vascular events (AR 10% with triflusal v 10% with aspirin; OR 0.93, 95% CI 0.72 to 1.19).[39] The subsequent RCT (2113 people with a recent ischaemic stroke or TIA) found no significant difference between triflusal and aspirin in the primary outcome of ischaemic stroke, myocardial infarction or vascular death (AR 13.1% with triflusal v 12.4% with aspirin; HR 1.09, 95% CI 0.85 to 1.38).[49] However, the RCT lacked power to rule out a clinically important difference between treatments.

Harms: **Thienopyridines (clopidogrel and ticlopidine):** The second systematic review comparing thienopyridines versus aspirin found that the thienopyridines reduced gastrointestinal haemorrhage and upper gastrointestinal symptoms compared with aspirin (gastrointestinal haemorrhage: OR 0.71, 95% CI 0.59 to 0.86; indigestion, nausea, or vomiting: OR 0.84, 95% CI 0.78 to 0.90).[46] However, thienopyridines increased the incidence of skin rash and diarrhoea compared with aspirin (skin rash: clopidogrel *v* aspirin OR 1.3, 95% CI 1.2 to 1.5; ticlopidine *v* aspirin OR 2.2, 95% CI 1.7 to 2.9; diarrhoea: clopidogrel *v* aspirin OR 1.3, 95% CI 1.2 to 1.6; ticlopidine *v* aspirin OR 2.3, 95% CI 1.9 to 2.8). Ticlopidine (but not clopidogrel) increased neutropenia compared with aspirin (OR 2.7, 95% CI 1.5 to 4.8). Observational studies have found ticlopidine to be associated with thrombocytopenia and thrombotic thrombocytopenic purpura.[50,51] The subsequent RCT comparing aspirin and ticlopidine found that aspirin increased gastrointestinal tract haemorrhage compared with ticlopidine, but the increase was not statistically significant (0.9% with aspirin v 0.4% with ticlopidine, P = 0.39).[47] It found that ticlopidine increased diarrhoea, thrombocytopenia and neutropenia compared with aspirin, but the difference was not statistically significant (diarrhoea: 0.3% with ticlopidine v 0.2% with aspirin, P = 0.69; thrombocytopenia: 0.3% with ticlopidine v 0.2% with aspirin, P = 0.69; neutropenia: 3.4% with ticlopidine v 2.2% with aspirin, P = 0.12). **Dipyridamole plus aspirin:** One RCT found that combination treatment with dipyridamole plus aspirin was discontinued more frequently for adverse effects than was aspirin alone.[48] Triflusal versus aspirin: The subsequent RCT found a lower risk of haemorrhage with triflusal compared with aspirin (intracranial or major extracranial haemorrhage: 1.9% with triflusal v 4.0% with aspirin; HR 0.48, 95% CI 0.28 to 0.82; any haemorrhage: 16.7% with triflusal v 25.2% with aspirin; OR 0.76, 95% CI 0.67 to 0.86).[49]

Comment: Two large RCTs have assessed the effects of adding clopidogrel to aspirin for up to a year among a total of about 15 000 high risk ischemic heart disease patients (see benefits of antiplatelet treatments in angina [unstable], [Web only]).[52,53] Two further large RCTs are assessing the effects of clopidogrel plus aspirin versus aspirin alone among patients with acute myocardial infarction and among high vascular risk patients (including those with a prior ischemic stroke or transient ischaemic attack).[54,55] Another large RCT is comparing clopidogrel plus aspirin versus clopidogrel alone in 7600 high risk patients with a recent ischaemic stroke or TIA considered to be of atherothrombotic origin.[56] One ongoing RCT is comparing effects of oral anticoagulation, aspirin plus dipyridamole, and aspirin alone among 4500 people with a prior transient ischaemic attack or minor ischaemic stroke.[57]

OPTION ANTICOAGULATION IN PEOPLE IN SINUS RHYTHM

Cathie Sudlow

Systematic reviews found no significant difference between anticoagulation and placebo or antiplatelet treatment for preventing recurrent stroke after presumed ischaemic stroke in people in normal sinus rhythm. Anticoagulants increased the risk of fatal intracranial and extracranial haemorrhage compared with placebo. High intensity anticoagulation increased the risk of major bleeding compared with antiplatelet treatment.

Benefits: **Versus placebo:** We found one systematic review (search date 2002, 11 RCTs, 2487 people in sinus rhythm with previous non-embolic presumed ischaemic stroke or transient ischaemic attack, mean duration 1.9 years).[58] It found no significant difference between oral anticoagulants (warfarin, dicoumarol, or phenindione) and placebo or no treatment for death or dependency, serious vascular events (stroke, myocardial infarction or vascular death), or mortality (death or dependency: ARR +4%, 95% CI –6% to +14%; RR 0.95, 95% CI 0.82 to 1.09; serious vascular events: ARR +1%, 95% CI –7% to +8%; RR 0.98, 95% CI 0.82 to 1.18; death: ARR +1%, 95% CI –4% to +5%; RR 0.97, 95% CI 0.81 to 1.16). **Versus antiplatelet treatment:** We found one systematic review (search date 2001, 4 RCTs, 1870 people) comparing long term (> 6 months) treatment with oral anticoagulants (warfarin, phenprocoumarin, or acenocoumarol [nicoumalone]) versus antiplatelet treatment in people with a history of transient ischaemic attack or minor stroke of presumed arterial (non-cardiac) origin in the past 6 months.[59] It found no significant difference between high intensity (international normalised ratio [INR**G**] 3.0–4.5) or low intensity (INR 2.1–3.5) anticoagulation compared with antiplatelet treatment for preventing recurrent stroke (low intensity anticoagulation *v* antiplatelet treatment: ARR +0.2%, 95% CI –4.0% to +4.3%; RR 0.96, 95% CI 0.38 to 2.42; high intensity anticoagulation *v* antiplatelet treatment: ARR –0.1%, 95% CI –1.7% to +1.5%; RR 1.02, 95% CI 0.49 to 2.13).

Harms: **Versus placebo:** The systematic review found that anticoagulants significantly increased the risk of fatal intracranial haemorrhage and of major extracranial haemorrhage compared with control (fatal intracranial haemorrhage: ARI 2%, 95% CI 0% to 4%; RR 2.51, 95% CI 1.12 to 5.60; major extracranial haemorrhage: ARI 3%, 95% CI 3% to 5%; RR 3.45, 95% CI 1.82 to 6.54).[58] **Versus antiplatelet treatment:** The review comparing anticoagulants versus antiplatelet treatment found no significant difference in risk of major intracranial or extracranial bleeding between low intensity anticoagulation (INR 2.1–3.6) and antiplatelet treatment (RR 1.19, 95% CI 0.59 to 2.41).[59] However, high intensity anticoagulation (INR 3.0–4.5) significantly increased the risk of major intracranial or extracranial bleeding (RR 1.08, 95% CI 1.03 to 1.20).

Comment: **Versus placebo:** Most trials in the systematic review had major problems with their methods, including poor monitoring of anticoagulation.[58] Most were completed before introducing routine computerised tomography scanning, which means that people with primary haemorrhagic strokes could have been included. The systematic review could not therefore provide a reliable and precise overall estimate of the balance of risk and benefit regarding death or dependency. Versus antiplatelet treatment: Ongoing RCTs (including several thousand people with a non-cardioembolic ischaemic stroke or TIA) are comparing medium intensity oral anticoagulation (INR 2.0–3.0) versus aspirin.[60–62]

OPTION CAROTID ENDARTERECTOMY FOR PEOPLE WITH RECENT CAROTID TERRITORY ISCHAEMIA

Peter Rothwell

Evidence from a pooled analysis of individual patient data from three RCTs in people with symptomatic carotid artery stenosis suggested that carotid endarterectomy increased the risk of stroke or death due to surgery in people with less than 30% stenosis, was of no benefit in people with 30–49% stenosis, and was of increasing benefit in people with higher grade stenosis. The RCTs found that carotid endarterectomy is of greatest benefit in people with more than 70% stenosis, although it may be ineffective in people with near-occlusion. Two systematic reviews found that carotid endarterectomy reduced perioperative stroke, death, and subsequent ipsilateral stroke in people with asymptomatic but severe stenosis. However, because the absolute risk of stroke in asymptomatic people is relatively low, the benefit from surgery is small. One systematic review found no evidence that eversion carotid endarterectomy is more beneficial than conventional carotid endarterectomy.

Benefits: **People with symptomatic stenosis:** We found one pooled analysis[63] of individual patient data from the three large RCTs (4 publications) that examined the effects of endarectomy in people with symptomatic carotid stenosis.[64–67] The RCTs used different methods to measure the degree of carotid stenosis, studied different populations, and used different definitions of outcome events. However, the pooled analysis adjusted for these differences. The pooled analysis (3 RCTs, 6092 people, 35 000 person years of follow up) found that surgery increased the 5 year risk of any stroke or surgical death in people with less than 30% stenosis, had no significant effect in patients with 30–49% stenosis, was of some benefit in patients with 50–69% stenosis, and was highly beneficial in patients with 70% or more stenosis without near-occlusion (< 30% stenosis, 1746 people: RR 1.17, 95% CI 0.90 to 1.43; 30–49% stenosis, 1429 people: RR 0.90, 95% CI 0.75 to 1.04; 50–69% stenosis, 1549 people: RR 0.72, 95% CI 0.58 to 0.86; ≥ 70% stenosis without near-occlusion, 1095 people: RR 0.52, 95% CI 0.40 to 0.64).[63] However, there was no evidence of benefit in people with the most severe disease (near-occlusion of ipsilateral carotid artery, 262 people: RR compared with control 0.98, 95% CI 0.61 to 1.59). **People with asymptomatic stenosis:** We found two systematic reviews (search dates 1998) assessing carotid endarterectomy for asymptomatic carotid stenosis (no carotid territory transient ischaemic attack or minor stroke within the past few months).[68,69] One review included results from five RCTs (2440 people).[68] The other review included results from 2203 people from four of these five RCTs, after excluding the fifth RCT because of weak methods.[69] Both reviews found similar results. Carotid endarterectomy reduced the risk of perioperative stroke, death, or subsequent ipsilateral stroke compared with medical treatment only (for the review of 4 RCTs:[69] AR 4.9% over 3 years in the surgical group v 6.8% in the medical group; ARR 1.9%, 95% CI 0.1% to 3.9%; NNT 52, 95% CI 26 to 1000; for the review of 5 RCTs:[68] 4.7% over 3 years in the surgical group v 7.4% in the medical group; ARR 2.7%, 95% CI 0.8% to 4.6%; NNT 37, 95% CI 22 to 125). Although the risk of perioperative stroke or death from carotid surgery for people with asymptomatic stenosis appears to be lower than in people with symptomatic stenosis, the risk of stroke or death without surgery in asymptomatic people is low and so the absolute benefit from surgery is small, and for most people the balance of risk and benefit from surgery remains unclear.[68,69] **Eversion carotid endarterectomy versus conventional carotid endarterectomy:** We found one systematic review (search date 1999, 5 RCTs, 2645 people, 2590 carotid arteries) that compared eversion carotid endarterectomy versus conventional carotid endarterectomy**G** performed either with primary closure or patch angioplasty.[70] Overall, the review found no significant differences in the rate of perioperative stroke, stroke or death, local complication rate, and rate of neurological events (for stroke or death: AR 1.7% with eversion v 2.6% with conventional; ARR +0.9%, 95% CI –0.3% to +2.1%; for stroke: AR 1.4% with eversion v 1.7% with conventional, ARR +0.3%, 95% CI –0.7% to +1.3%).

Harms: **People with symptomatic stenosis:** The pooled analysis (3248 people randomised to surgery a median of 6 days after randomisation) reported 229 strokes or deaths within 30 days of surgery (7.1%, 95% CI 6.3 to 8.1).[63] Operative risk was not related to the degree of stenosis. The risk of death within 30 days of endarterectomy was 1.1% (36/3248; 95% CI 0.8% to 1.5%), and among 209 people who had an operative stroke 20 people (9.6%) died (95% CI 5.9% to 14.4%). One earlier systematic review (search date 1996, 36 studies) identified several risk factors for operative stroke and death from carotid endarterectomy, including female sex, occlusion of the contralateral internal carotid artery, stenosis of the ipsilateral external carotid artery, and systolic blood pressure greater than 180 mm Hg.[71] One systematic review (search date 2000, 103 studies including 6 RCTs, case series and routinely collected data) examining harms of carotid endarterectomy found that operative risk of stroke and death was highest in people with cerebral TIA or stroke and in people with re-stenosis, and lowest in people with ocular ischaemic events and asymptomatic stenosis (symptomatic stenosis v asymptomatic stenosis, 59 studies: OR 1.62, 95% CI 1.45 to 1.81; re-stenosis v primary surgery, 6 studies: OR 1.95, 95% CI 1.21 to 3.16; ocular events only v asymptomatic stenosis, 15 studies: OR 0.75, 95% CI 0.50 to 1.14).[72] It found that emergency surgery immediately after a TIA or stroke was associated with a major increase in operative risk compared with elective surgery performed a few days later (OR 4.9, 95% CI 3.4 to 7.1).[72] Endarterectomy is also associated with other postoperative complications, including wound infection (3%), wound haematoma (5%), and lower cranial nerve injury (5–7%).[32] **People with asymptomatic stenosis:** Given the low prevalence of severe carotid stenosis in the general population, there is concern that screening and surgical intervention in asymptomatic people may result in more strokes than it prevents.[73]

Comment: **People with symptomatic stenosis**: The RCTs included in the pooled analysis found different results.[64–67] However, this was due to differences in the methods of measurement of the degree of carotid stenosis on the pre-randomisation catheter angiograms (the method used in one

RCT[64] produced higher values than the method used in the other trials.[65,66,74]) and differences in the definitions of outcome events. Meta-analyses of the overall trial results have been reported but these took no account of the differences between the trials.[75,76] The subsequent pooled analysis of individual participant data corrected for these differences in methods, after which there were no clinically or statistically significant differences between the results of the three trials.[63] The degree of carotid stenosis was the single most important factor influencing effects of endarterectomy.[63] Subgroup analyses of the pooled data from the three RCTs[64–67] showed that benefits of carotid endarterectomy were greatest within 2 weeks of an ischaemic event (excluding emergency surgery and surgery in patients with major disabling stroke) and that benefits reduced if surgery was delayed (interaction; P = 0.009).[77] There was also evidence of reduced benefit in women (interaction; P = 0.003) and trend towards increasing benefit with age (P = 0.03). These observations were consistent across the individual trials. **People with asymptomatic stenosis:** A large RCT of endarterectomy versus medical treatment alone [78] has recently been completed and has presented preliminary results based on approximately 3000 randomised patients. The results and conclusions were broadly in keeping with those of the systematic reviews of the previous smaller RCTs.[68,69] "Prophylactic" endarterectomy for people undergoing coronary bypass surgery: It is common practice for endarterectomy for asymptomatic stenosis to be performed as a "prophylactic" procedure either prior to or during coronary artery bypass surgery because of the high risk of stroke in this group (stroke after coronary artery bypass graft overall: 1.71%; risk of stroke in people with asymptomatic stenosis: 3%).[79] We found no RCTs of endarterectomy for this indication. One systematic review (search date 2002, 97 RCTs) of outcomes following staged and synchronous carotid endarterectomy and coronary artery bypass reported overall operative risks of stroke and death of 10%.[80]

OPTION CAROTID AND VERTEBRAL PERCUTANEOUS TRANSLUMINAL ANGIOPLASTY

Peter Rothwell

RCTs provided insufficient evidence about effects of carotid or vertebral percutaneous transluminal angioplasty or stenting compared with medical treatment or carotid endarterectomy in people with a recent carotid or vertebral territory transient ischaemic attack or non-disabling ischaemic stroke who have severe stenosis of the ipsilateral carotid or vertebral artery.

Benefits: **Carotid percutaneous transluminal angioplasty versus endarterectomy:** We found one large RCT[81] and one small RCT that was stopped prematurely.[82] The larger RCT (504 people with a recent carotid territory transient ischaemic attack or non-disabling ischaemic stroke with stenosis of the ipsilateral carotid artery) compared "best medical treatment" plus carotid percutaneous transluminal angioplasty (PTA) versus "best medical treatment" plus carotid endarterectomy.[81] It found no significant difference between endovascular treatment and surgery for disabling stroke or death within 30 days of first treatment (AR for disabling stroke or death 6.4% with PTA *v* 5.9% with surgery; AR for stroke lasting more than 7 days or death 10.0% with PTA *v* 9.9% with surgery). The trial found no significant difference between treatments for ipsilateral stroke rate up to 3 years after randomisation (adjusted HR 1.04, 95% CI 0.63 to 1.70; P = 0.9). A small RCT of 23 people was stopped after 17 people had received allocated treatment because of a high procedural risk of stroke in the angioplasty group compared with the endarterectomy group (5/7 *v* 0/10, P = 0.03).[82] **Carotid angioplasty plus stenting versus endarterectomy:** We found three RCTs in symptomatic people.[83–85] The first RCT (219 people with carotid stenosis of 60–90%) found that carotid stenting significantly increased the combined outcome of ipsilateral stroke, procedure related death, or vasular death at 1 year compared with carotid endarterectomy (12.1% with stent *v* 3.6% with endarterectomy, $P = 0.022$).[83] The second RCT (104 people with > 70% carotid stenosis) found no significant difference between carotid angioplasty plus stenting and carotid endarterectomy for death or cerebral ischaemia (1 transient ischaemic attack with angioplasty *v* 1 death for endarterectomy; P not reported).[84] The third RCT was stopped prematurely due to slow enrolment (307 people, either asymptomatic with > 80% stenosis, or symptomatic with > 50% stenosis and considered to have a high operative risk with endarterectomy).[85] It found that endarterectomy significantly increased the risk of death, stroke or myocardial infarction at 30 days (9/156 [5.8%] with angioplasty plus stent v 19/151 [12.6%] with endarterectomy, $P < 0.05$).[85] **Vertebral artery angioplasty:** The RCT also compared vertebral angioplasty versus "best medical treatment" in 16 people, but did not provide enough data for reliable estimates of efficacy to be made.[81]

Harms: The RCT comparing carotid angioplasty versus endarterectomy found that cranial neuropathy was more common with endarterectomy (22 people [8.7%] undergoing endarterectomy *v* 0 people after angioplasty; $P < 0.0001$).[81] Major groin or neck haematoma occurred less often after angioplasty than after endarterectomy (3 people with angioplasty [1.2%] *v* 17 people with endarterectomy [6.7%]; $P < 0.0015$).[81] Harms data are not yet available from the other trials, which are still to be published in full.[17,83]

Comment: The RCTs comparing angioplasty versus endarterectomy had low power, and results lacked precision.[81] Several ongoing RCTs are comparing carotid endarterectomy versus primary stenting in people with recently symptomatic severe carotid stenosis. **Carotid percutaneous transluminal angioplasty:** The two RCTs comparing angioplasty (with or without stenting) and endarterectomy suggest that angioplasty with or without stenting is associated with a higher procedural risk than endarterectomy, and a higher rate of restenosis during follow up.[83,84] However, improvements in cerebral protection devices may reduce the procedural risks,[86] and several other RCTs comparing angioplasty plus stenting with cerebral protection versus endarterectomy are currently ongoing. The use of angioplasty is likely to increase in future, but trial results will help to decide whether increased use will be confined to people in whom endarterectomy is technically difficult.

QUESTION What are the effects of preventive anticoagulant and antiplatelet treatment in people with atrial fibrillation and prior stroke or transient ischaemic attack?

Gregory YH Lip

OPTION ANTICOAGULANT AND ANTIPLATELET TREATMENT

One systematic review found that adjusted dose warfarin reduced the risk of stroke compared with control in people with previous stroke or transient ischaemic attack. The best time to begin anticoagulation after an ischaemic stroke is unclear. One systematic review provided insufficient evidence to compare warfarin versus aspirin. One systematic review of one RCT found no significant diference between aspirin and placebo in stroke or death in people with previous stroke or transient ischaemic attack.

Benefits: **Adjusted dose warfarin versus placebo:** We found one systematic review (search date 1999[87], 1 RCT,[88] 439 people with previous stroke or TIA) that compared adjusted dose warfarin with a control in which people could self select to take aspirin. Target international normalised ratio (INR)**G** was 2.9. The RCT found that adjusted dose warfarin significantly reduced the risk of stroke compared with control (20/225 [8.9%] with warfarin v 50/214 [23.4%] with control; ARR 14.5%, 95% CI 7.7% to 21.3%; NNT 7, 95% CI 5 to 13). **Adjusted dose warfarin versus minidose warfarin: We found one** RCT (115 people with ischaemic stroke in the previous 1–6 months).[89] It found no significant difference between conventional (target INR 2.2–3.5) and low intensity (target INR 1.5–2.1) warfarin in ischaemic stroke rate after mean follow up of around 1 year (AR 1/55 [1.1%] with conventional intensity *v* 2/60 [1.7%] with low intensity warfarin).[89] The RCT was terminated prematurely because of significantly more bleeding complications with conventional intensity warfarin (see harms and comment, below). **Adjusted dose warfarin versus aspirin:** We found one systematic review (search date 1999)[87] which cited one RCT[88] comparing warfarin with aspirin. However, this comparison was not randomised, and therefore did not meet inclusion criteria for this chapter. **Adjusted dose warfarin versus other antiplatelet treatments:** We found one systematic review (search date 1999, 1 RCT,[90] 916 people within 15 days of stroke onset) comparing warfarin (target INR 2.0–3.5) versus indobufen.[87] It found no significant difference in the rate of recurrent stroke between treatments (5% for indobufen *v* 4% for warfarin; ARR +1.0%, 95% CI –1.7% to +3.7%).[87] Adjusted dose warfarin versus other anticoagulants: We found one RCT (3410 people with atrial fibrillation and at least one other risk factor for stroke, 24% with previous stroke or TIA), which compared open-label warfarin (INR 2.0–3.0) versus the oral thrombin inhibitor, ximelagatran (fixed dose, 36 mg twice daily).[91] It found no significant difference in stroke between warfarin and ximelagatran in a subgroup (822 people) with previous stroke or TIA after mean follow up of 17 months (5.1% per year with warfarin v 3.8% per year with ximelagatran, P = 0.313). **Aspirin versus placebo:** We found one systematic review (search date 1999, 1 RCT, 782 people with atrial fibrillation and prior stroke or TIA).[92] It found no significant difference between aspirin and placebo for stroke or death (stroke: OR 0.89, 95% CI 0.64 to 1.24; death: OR 0.95, 95% CI 0.69 to 1.31).

Harms: The major risk associated with anticoagulants and antiplatelet agents was haemorrhage. In the overview assessing elderly people with variable risk factors for stroke, the absolute risk of major bleeding was 1.0% for placebo, 1.0% for aspirin, and 1.3% for warfarin.[93] Another systematic review found the absolute risk of intracranial haemorrhage increased from 0.1% a year with control to 0.3% a year with warfarin, but the difference was not significant.[87] The absolute risks were three times higher in people who had bled previously. Both bleeding and haemorrhagic stroke were more common in people aged over 75 years. The risk of death after a major bleed was 13–33%, and risk of subsequent morbidity in those who survived a major bleed was 15%. The risk of bleeding was associated with an INR greater than 3, fluctuating INRs, and uncontrolled hypertension. In a systematic review (search date not stated, 2 RCTs) major extracranial bleeding was more frequent with anticoagulation treatment than with placebo (ARI 4.9%, 95% CI 1.6% to 8.2%; RR 6.2, 95% CI 1.4 to 27.1; NNH 20, 95% CI 12 to 63).[94] The studies were too small to define the rate of intracranial haemorrhage (none occurred). In a systematic review (search date not stated) comparing anticoagulants versus antiplatelet treatment, major extracranial bleeding was more frequent with anticoagulation (ARI 4.9%, 95% CI 1.6% to 8.2%; RR 6.4, 95% CI 1.5 to 28.1; NNH 20, 95% CI 12 to 63).[95] The studies were too small to define the rate of intracranial haemorrhage (in 1 RCT, none of the people on anticoagulant and 1 person on aspirin had an intracranial bleed). In the systematic review of oral anticoagulants versus placebo in low risk people, the number of intracranial haemorrhages was small, with a non-significant increase in the treatment group (5 in the treatment group and 2 in the control group).[96] Likewise, in the systematic review assessing antiplatelet treatment in low risk people with atrial fibrillation, too few haemorrhages occurred to characterise the effects of aspirin.[97] One more recent systematic review found no evidence that warfarin significantly increased the risk of major haemorrhage compared with placebo among people with no prior TIA or stroke (5 RCTs, 2415 people: ARI for major haemorrhage warfarin *v* placebo +0.8%, 95% CI –1.3% to +2.9%).[92] However, if people with prior stroke or TIA were included then warfarin significantly increased major haemorrhage (6 RCTs: ARI warfarin *v* placebo 1.3%, 95% CI 0.4% to 2.2%; NNH 77, 95% CI 45 to 250). The systematic review found no evidence of a difference in major haemorrhage between warfarin and aspirin; warfarin and any antiplatelet agent; warfarin and low dose warfarin plus aspirin; and low molecular weight heparin and placebo. However, the review may have lacked power to detect a clinically important difference.[92] One small RCT (157 people) found that full dose anticoagulation (target INR 2.0–2.6) plus aspirin significantly increased haemorrhagic complications compared with aspirin alone (13/76 [17%] with fluindione plus aspirin *v* 2/81[2.5%] with fluindione alone; P = 0.0021).[98] **Adjusted dose warfarin versus minidose warfarin:** One RCT (115 people) found that conventional intensity warfarin significantly increased major haemorrhagic complications compared with low intensity warfarin after about 1 year (6/55 [10.9%] with conventional v 0/60 [0%] with low intensity; P = 0.01).[89]

Comment: **Adjusted dose warfarin versus minidose warfarin:** The RCT comparing conventional versus low intensity warfarin found no significant difference between treatments.[89] This may be due to insufficient power; premature termination of the trial because of significantly more bleeding complications in the conventional intensity anticoagulation group; the low rate of ischaemic stroke observed in both groups in this population, possibly contributed to by different ethnicity from original anticoagulation trial cohorts; or the similar anticoagulation range reached in the two groups (1.9 with low intensity *v* 2.2 with conventional).[89] **Timing of anticoagulation:** The best time to start anticoagulation after an ischaemic stroke is unclear, but aspirin reduces the risk of recurrent stroke in such people with or without atrial fibrillation, suggesting that it is reasonable to use aspirin until it is considered safe to start oral anticoagulants.[99] See also comments in anticoagulant and antiplatelet treatment in people with atrial fibrillation in people without prior stroke or TIA.

QUESTION **What are the effects of preventive anticoagulant and antiplatelet treatment in people with atrial fibrillation and without prior stroke or transient ischaemic attack?**

Gregory YH Lip

OPTION **ANTICOAGULANT AND ANTIPLATELET TREATMENT**

One systematic review found that warfarin reduced fatal and non-fatal ischaemic stroke compared with placebo, provided there was a low risk of bleeding and careful monitoring. The people in the review had a mean age of 69 years. One overview in people less than 65 years old found no significant difference in the annual stroke rate between warfarin and placebo. One

systematic review found that aspirin reduced the risk of stroke compared with placebo, but another review found no significant difference. These findings support the use of aspirin in people with atrial fibrillation and contraindications to anticoagulants.

Benefits: **Adjusted dose warfarin versus placebo in people at high risk of stroke:** We found two systematic reviews examining the effect of warfarin in different groups of people with atrial fibrillation at high risk of stroke**G**.[87,92] The first systematic review (search date 1999, 6 RCTs, 2900 people at high risk, 80% without previous stroke or TIA, 45% had hypertension) compared adjusted dose warfarin versus placebo or control.[87] In one RCT (439 people) included in the review, people in the control group could self select aspirin. Target international normalised ratio (INR)**G** varied among RCTs (2.0–2.6 in primary prevention RCTs). The review found that adjusted dose warfarin significantly reduced the risk of stroke (ARR 4.0%, 95% CI 2.3% to 5.7%; NNT 25, 95% CI 18 to 43). For people without prior stroke or TIA (5 RCTs, 2462 people) the relative risk of stroke was reduced by 59% (ARR 2.7% per year, NNT for 1 year was 37, 95% CI not reported). The second systematic review (search date 1999, 14 RCTs) identified the same trials of warfarin compared with placebo and found similar results.[92] **Adjusted dose warfarin versus minidose warfarin in people at high risk of stroke:** We found one RCT that compared low, fixed dose warfarin plus aspirin versus standard adjusted dose warfarin;[100] three RCTs that compared adjusted dose warfarin versus low dose warfarin plus aspirin;[101–103] and one RCT that compared conventional intensity warfarin versus low intensity warfarin.[89] The first RCT (1044 people with atrial fibrillation at high risk of stroke) found that adjusted dose warfarin (target international normalised ratio [INR] 2.0–3.0) significantly reduced the combined rate of ischaemic stroke or systemic embolism, and reduced disabling or fatal stroke compared with low, fixed dose warfarin (target INR 1.2–1.5) plus aspirin (325 mg/day) (stroke or embolism: ARR 6.0%, 95% CI 3.4% to 8.6%; NNT 17, 95% CI 12 to 29; disabling or fatal stroke: ARR 3.9%, 95% CI 1.6% to 6.1%; NNT 26, 95% CI 16 to 63).[100] The three RCTs comparing adjusted dose warfarin versus low dose warfarin plus aspirin[101–103] were stopped prematurely when the results of the earlier trial[100] were published. Analyses of the optimal anticoagulation intensity for stroke prevention in atrial fibrillation found that stroke risk was substantially increased at INR levels below 2.[104,105] **Adjusted dose warfarin versus aspirin at high risk of stroke:** We found one systematic review comparing warfarin versus different antiplatelet regimens in people at high risk of stroke[87] and one subsequent individual patient meta-analysis.[106] The systematic review (search date 1999, 4 primary prevention RCTs, 7037 people of adjusted dose warfarin versus aspirin in high risk people (45% had hypertension).[87] Target INR varied among RCTs (2.0–4.5 in primary prevention RCTs). Adjusted dose warfarin reduced the overall risk of stroke compared with aspirin (ARR 2.9%, 95% CI 0.9% to 4.8%; NNT 34, 95% CI 21 to 111). The effect varied widely among the five RCTs, none of which were blinded. The recent individual patient meta-analysis (5 RCTs of primary and secondary prevention, 2633 people at high risk of ischaemic stroke, 76% without previous stroke or TIA) compared full dose oral anticoagulation (largely coumarin derivatives) versus aspirin (75–325 mg).[106] It found that anticoagulation significantly decreased strokes compared with aspirin in people at high risk of ischaemic stroke (ARR 3.3% per year). **Adjusted dose warfarin versus other antiplatelet treatment in people at high risk of stroke:** We found no systematic review or RCTs in people with AF and no previous stroke or TIA. Adjusted dose warfarin versus other anticoagulants in people at high risk of stroke: We found one RCT (3410 people with atrial fibrillation and one or more stroke risk factors, 76% without previous stroke or TIA) that compared open-label warfarin (INR 2.0–3.0) with the oral thrombin inhibitor, ximelagatran (fixed dose, 36 mg twice daily).[91] It found no significant difference between warfarin and ximelagatran for stroke or systemic embolism in a subgroup (2588 people) without previous stroke after mean follow up of 17 months (56/2240 person years [2.3% per year] with ximelagatran v 40/2446 person years [1.6% per year] with warfarin; ARR +0.7%, 95% CI –0.1% to +1.4%, RR 0.71, 95% CI 0.48 to 1.07). **Oral anticoagulant versus oral anticoagulant plus aspirin in people at high risk of stroke:** We found one RCT (157 people at high risk) that compared oral fluindione (active dose 5–25 mg) versus fluindione plus aspirin (100 mg).[98] It found no significant difference between fluindione alone and fluindione plus aspirin for a combined outcome of stroke, myocardial infarction, systemic arterial embolism, vascular death, or haemorrhagic complications after mean follow up of 8 months (2/81 [2.5%] with fluindione *v* 5/76 [6.6%] with fluindione plus aspirin; P = 0.21). The study was insufficiently powered to detect clinically important differences between treatments. **Minidose warfarin plus aspirin in people at moderate risk of stroke:** We found one RCT (668 people with persistent or permanent AF, low–medium risk defined as ≤ 4% risk of stroke) that compared warfarin 1.25 mg plus aspirin 75 mg daily versus no anticoagulation.[107] It found that warfarin plus aspirin reduced stroke and stroke or TIA compared with no anticoagulation after about 33 months, but the decrease was not significant (stroke: 32/334[9.6%] with warfarin plus aspirin v 41/334[12.3%] with no treatment, P = 0.28; stroke or TIA: 11.7% with warfarin plus aspirin v 16.5% with no anticoagulation, P = 0.09).[12] **Anticoagulants in people at low risk of stroke:** We found one systematic review[96] and one overview[93] comparing warfarin versus placebo in people with atrial fibrillation and a variety of stroke risks. Both reviews included the same five RCTs. The overview (2461 people) found that, for people younger than 65 years with atrial fibrillation (but no history of hypertension, stroke, TIA, or diabetes), the annual stroke rate was the same with warfarin or placebo (subgroup analysis among 17% of people on warfarin and 15% on placebo; stroke rate 1% per year in each group).[93] The systematic review (search date 1999, 2313 people with no prior stroke or TIA, mean age 69 years, 20% aged > 75 years; 45% had hypertension, 15% diabetes, and 15% a prior history of myocardial infarction) found that warfarin (INR 2.0–2.6) reduced fatal and non-fatal ischaemic stroke, reduced all ischaemic strokes or intracranial haemorrhage, and reduced the combined outcome of disabling or fatal ischaemic stroke or intracranial haemorrhage compared with placebo after mean follow up of 1.7 years (fatal and non-fatal ischaemic stroke: ARR 4.0%, 95% CI 2.4% to 5.6%; NNT 25, 95% CI 18 to 42; all ischaemic strokes or intracranial haemorrhage: ARR 4.5%, 95% CI 2.8% to 6.2%; NNT 22, 95% CI 16 to 36; combined outcome: ARR 1.8%, 95% CI 0.5% to 3.1%; NNT 56, 95% CI 32 to 200).[96] **Antiplatelet treatment in people at low risk of stroke:** We found two systematic reviews in people with atrial fibrillation at low risk of stroke.[87,97] The first review (search date 1999, 2 RCTs, 1680 people with either paroxysmal or sustained non-valvular atrial fibrillation confirmed by electrocardiogram but without previous stroke or TIA, 30% aged > 75 years) compared aspirin versus placebo.[97] It found that aspirin did not significantly reduce ischaemic stroke, all stroke, all disabling or fatal stroke, or the composite end point of stroke, myocardial infarction, or vascular death after mean follow up of 1.3 years (ischaemic stroke: OR 0.71, 95% CI 0.46 to 1.10; ARR +1.6%, 95% CI –0.5% to +3.7%; all stroke: OR 0.70, 95% CI 0.45 to 1.08; ARR +1.8%, 95% CI –0.5% to +3.9%; all disabling or fatal stroke: OR 0.88, 95% CI 0.48 to 1.58; ARR +0.4%, 95% CI –1.2% to +2.0%; composite end point: OR 0.76, 95% CI 0.54 to 1.05; ARR +2.3%, 95% CI

–0.4% to +5.0%). The second systematic review (search date 1999) included three RCTs of primary prevention.[87] The average rate of stroke among people taking placebo was 5.2% per year. Meta-analysis of the three RCTs found that antiplatelet treatment reduced the risk of stroke compared with placebo after mean follow up from 1.2–2.3 years (ARR 2.2%, 95% CI 0.3% to 4.1%; NNT 45, 95% CI 24 to 333).

Harms: **Adjusted dose warfarin versus minidose warfarin in people at high risk of stroke:** One RCT (115 people) found that conventional intensity warfarin significantly increased major haemorrhagic complications compared with low intensity warfarin after about 1 year (6/55 [10.9%] with conventional v 0/60 [0%] with low intensity; P = 0.01).[89] Adjusted dose warfarin versus other anticoagulants in people at high risk of stroke: One RCT (3410 people, 76% with no previous stroke or TIA) comparing open-label warfarin (INR 2.0–3.0) versus the oral thrombin inhibitor, ximelagatran (fixed dose, 36 mg twice daily) found that ximelagatran significantly reduced any haemorrhage (major plus minor) compared with warfarin but found no significant difference between treatments in rates of major haemorrhage (any haemorrhage: 29.8% per year with warfarin v 25.8% per year with ximelagatran, P = 0.007; major haemorrhage: 1.8% per year with warfarin v 1.3% per year with ximelagatran, P = 0.23).[91] It found that ximelagatran significantly increased the proportion of people with raised serum alanine aminotransferase (> 3 times normal) compared with warfarin (107/1704 [6%] with ximelagatran v 14/1703 [1%] with warfarin, P < 0.0001). Minidose warfarin plus aspirin versus no anticoagulant in people at low–moderate risk of stroke: One RCT (688 people) found that low dose warfarin plus aspirin significantly increased bleeding complications compared with no treatment after a mean follow up of 33 months (19/334 [5.7%] with warfarin plus aspirin v 4/334 [1.2%] with no treatment, P = 0.003).[107] There were no deaths from bleeding complications. See also harms of anticoagulant and antiplatelet treatment in people with atrial fibrillation in people with prior stroke or TIA, p 183.

Comment: The three risk strata used above have been identified based on evidence derived from one overview of five RCTs[93] and one subsequent RCT.[100] Most reviews have stratified effects of treatment in terms of these risk categories. However, one recent systematic review (search date 1999), which did not stratify for perceived risk, has suggested that RCTs may be too heterogeneous to determine effects of long term oral anticoagulation compared with placebo among people with non-rheumatic atrial fibrillation.[108] The review (search date 1999, 5 RCTs, 3298 people) has found results that conflict with those of previous reviews.[108] The review questions the methods and highlights the heterogeneity of RCTs of oral anticoagulation in people with non-rheumatic atrial fibrillation. People in the RCTs were highly selected (< 10%, range 3–40% of eligible people were randomised); many were excluded after assessments for the absence of contraindications and physicians' refusal to enter them into the study. Many of the studies were not double blinded, and in some studies there was poor agreement between raters for "soft" neurological end points. The frequent monitoring of warfarin treatment under trial conditions and motivation of people/investigators was probably more than that seen in usual clinical practice. The review has suggested that considerable uncertainty remains about benefits of long term anticoagulation in people with non-rheumatic atrial fibrillation. The review has different inclusion and exclusion criteria than previously published reviews, having excluded data from two RCTs and including a trial not included in previous reviews.[100] Unlike previous reviews, the recent systematic review did not stratify people for perceived stroke risk and identified no significant difference between anticoagulant and placebo with either a fixed effects model or a random effects model, which was employed to account for heterogeneity of underlying trials (fixed effects: OR 0.74, 95% CI 0.39 to 1.40 for stroke deaths; OR 0.86, 95% CI 0.16 to 1.17 for vascular deaths; random effects: OR 0.79, 95% CI 0.61 to 1.02 for combined fatal and non-fatal events).[108] The publication of this review has led to debate and uncertainty about clinical effectiveness of long term anticoagulation in people with non-rheumatic atrial fibrillation. Decisions to treat should be informed by considering trade offs between benefits and harms, and each person's treatment preferences.[109–114] We found net benefit of anticoagulation for people in atrial fibrillation who have had a TIA or stroke, or who are over 75 years of age and at a high risk of stroke. We found less clear cut evidence for those aged 65–75 years and at high risk, and for those with moderate risk (i.e. > 65 years and not in a high risk group or < 65 years with clinical risk factors) or for those at low risk (< 65 years with no other risk factors). The benefits of warfarin in the RCTs may not translate into effectiveness in clinical practice.[108,115,116] In the RCTs, most strokes in people randomised to warfarin occurred while they were not in fact taking warfarin, or were significantly underanticoagulated at the time of the event. A recent systematic review (search date not stated, 410 people) identified three trials comparing the outcomes of people treated with anticoagulants in the community versus the pooled results of the RCTs.[117] The authors confirmed that people who undergo anticoagulation for atrial fibrillation in actual clinical practice are generally older and have more comorbid conditions than people enrolled in RCTs. However, both groups had similar rates of stroke and major bleeding. This risk of minor bleeding was higher in the community group, and it was suggested that these people may require more intensive monitoring in routine practice.

GLOSSARY

Conventional carotid endarterectomy This is more commonly employed and involves a longitudinal arteriotomy of the carotid artery.

Eversion carotid endarterectomy This involves a transverse arteriotomy and reimplantation of the carotid artery.

International normalised ratio (INR) A value derived from a standardised laboratory test that measures the effect of an anticoagulant such as warfarin. The laboratory materials used in the test are calibrated against internationally accepted standard reference preparations, so that variability between laboratories and different reagents is minimised. Normal blood has an INR of 1. Therapeutic anticoagulation often aims to achieve an INR value of 2.0–3.5.

People at high risk of stroke People of any age with a previous transient ischaemic attack or stroke, or a history of rheumatic vascular disease, coronary artery disease, congestive heart failure, and impaired left ventricular function or echocardiography; and people aged 75 years and over with hypertension, diabetes, or both.

People at moderate risk of stroke People aged over 65 years who are not in the high risk group; and people aged under 65 years with clinical risk factors, including diabetes, hypertension, peripheral arterial disease, and ischaemic heart disease.

People at low risk of stroke All other people aged less than 65 years with no history of stroke, transient ischaemic attack, embolism, hypertension, diabetes, or other clinical risk factors.

REFERENCES

1. Hankey GJ, Warlow CP. *Transient ischaemic attacks of the brain and eye*. London: WB Saunders, 1994.
2. Prospective Studies Collaboration. Cholesterol, diastolic blood pressure, and stroke: 13 000 strokes in 450 000 people in 45 prospective cohorts. *Lancet* 1995;346:1647–1653.
3. Eastern Stroke and Coronary Heart Disease Collaborative Research Group. Blood pressure, cholesterol, and stroke in eastern Asia. *Lancet* 1998;352:1801–1807.
4. Warlow CP, Dennis MS, Van Gijn J, et al. Predicting recurrent stroke and other serious vascular events. In: *Stroke. A practical guide to management*. Oxford: Blackwell Science, 1996:545–552.
5. Antiplatelet Trialists' Collaboration. Collaborative overview of randomised trials of antiplatelet therapy — I: prevention of death, myocardial infarction, and stroke by prolonged antiplatelet therapy in various categories of patients. *BMJ* 1994;308:81–106. Search date 1990; primary sources Medline, Current Contents, hand searches

of journals, reference lists, and conference proceedings, and contact with authors of trials and manufacturers.
6. Hart RG, Pearce LA, Rothbart RM, et al. Stroke with intermittent atrial fibrillation: incidence and predictors during aspirin therapy. Stroke Prevention in Atrial fibrillation Investigators. *J Am Coll Cardiol* 2000;35:183–187.
7. The INDANA Project Collaborators. Effect of antihypertensive treatment in patients having already suffered from stroke. *Stroke* 1997;28:2557–2562. Search date not stated; primary sources electronic medical databases; survey of specialised and general medical journals and congress proceedings and consultanting experts.
8. PROGRESS Management Committee. Blood pressure lowering for the secondary prevention of stroke: rationale and design for PROGRESS. *J Hypertension* 1996; 14(suppl 2): S41–S46.
9. Eriksson S, Olofsson BO, Wester PO for the TEST study group: Atenolol in secondary prevention after stroke. *Cerebrovasc Dis* 1995,5:21–25.
10. Dutch TIA Trial Study Group: Trial of secondary prevention with atenolol after transient ischaemic attack or non-disabling ischaemic stroke. *Stroke* 1993,24:543–548.
11. PROGRESS Collaborative Group. Randomised trial of a perindopril-based blood-pressure-lowering regimen among 6105 individuals with previous stroke or transient ischaemic attack. *Lancet* 2001;358;1033–1041.
12. The Heart Outcomes Prevention Evaluation Study Investigators. Effects of an angiotensin–converting–enzyme inhibitor, ramipril, on cardiovascular events in high-risk patients. *New Engl J Med* 2000;342:145–153.
13. PATS Collaborating Group. Post-stroke antihypertensive treatment study: a preliminary result. *Chinese Med J* 1995;108:710–717.
14. Bosch J, Yusuf S, Pogue J, et al. Use of ramipril in preventing stroke: double blind randomised trial. *BMJ* 2002;324:1–5.
15. Svensson P, de Faire U, Sleight P, et al. Comparative effects of ramipril on ambulatory and office blood pressures. A HOPE substudy. *Hypertension* 2001;38:e28–e32.
16. Blood Pressure Lowering Treatment Trialists' Collaboration. Effects of different blood-pressure lowering regimens on major cardiovascular events: results of prospectively-designed overviews of randomised trials. *Lancet* 2003;362: 1527–1535. Search date 2003; primary sources not stated in review but used methods of Blood Pressure Lowering Treatment Trialists' Collaboration.
17. Prospective Studies Collaboration. Age–specific relevance of usual blood pressure to vascular mortality: a meta-analysis of individual data for one million adults in 61 prospective studies. *Lancet* 2002;360:1903–1913. Search date: not stated; primary sources Medline, Embase, abstracts of meetings, contact with investigators.
18. Rodgers A, MacMahon S, Gamble G, et al, for the United Kingdom Transient Ischaemic Attack Collaborative Group. Blood pressure and risk of stroke in patients with cerebrovascular disease. *BMJ* 1996;313:147.
19. Neal B, Clark T, MacMahon S, et al, on behalf of the Antithrombotic Trialists' Collaboration. Blood pressure and the risk of recurrent vascular disease. *Am J Hypertension* 1998;11:25A–26A.
20. Staessan JA, Wang J. Blood-pressure lowering for the secondary prevention of stroke. *Lancet* 2001;358:1026–1027.
21. Wright JM, Lee C-H, Chambers GK. Systematic review of antihypertensive therapies: does the evidence assist in choosing a first-line drug? *Can Med Assoc J* 1999;161:25–32. Search date 1997; primary sources Medline, Cochrane Library (Issue 2, 1998), and references from previous meta-analyses published between 1980 and 1997.
22. Psaty BM, Lumley T, Furberg CD, et al. Health outcomes associated with various antihypertensive therapies used as first-line agents. A network meta-analysis. *JAMA* 2003;289:2534–2544. Search date: 2002; primary sources Medline, previous meta-analyses and journal reviews.
23. Hebert PR, Gaziano JM, Chan KS, et al. Cholesterol lowering with statin drugs, risk of stroke, and total mortality: an overview of randomized trials. *JAMA* 1997;278:313–321. Search date 1995; primary sources electronic databases, reference lists, authors of trials and funding agencies. Cholesterol and Current Events (CARE) data added in 1996.
24. Di Maschio R, Marchioli R, Tognoni G. Cholesterol reduction and stroke occurrence: an overview of randomized clinical trials. *Cerebrovasc Dis* 2000;10:85–92. Search date: not stated; primary sources not stated.
25. Law MR, Wald NJ, Rudnicka AR. Quantifying effect of statins on low density lipoprotein cholesterol, ischaemic heart disease, and stroke: systematic review and meta-analysis. *BMJ* 20043;326:1423–1427. Search date: 2002; primary sources Medline, Cochrane and Web of Science databases.
26. Armitage J. Cholesterol lowering for the prevention of stroke. *Practical Neurology* 2003;3: 224–233.
27. Heart Protection Study Collaborative Group. MRC/BHF Heart Protection Study of cholesterol lowering with simvastatin in 20 536 high-risk individuals: a randomised placebo-controlled trial. *Lancet* 2002;360:7–22.
28. Hebert PR, Gaziano M, Hennekens CH. An overview of trials of cholesterol lowering and risk of stroke. *Arch Intern Med* 1995;155:50–55.
29. Rubins HB, Robins SJ, Collins D, et al. Gemfibrozil for the secondary prevention of coronary heart disease in men with low levels of high-density lipoprotein cholesterol. *N Engl J Med* 1999;341:410–418.
30. Anonymous. The treatment of cerebrovascular disease with clofibrate. Final report of the Veterans' Administration Cooperative Study of Atherosclerosis, neurology section. *Stroke* 1973;4:684–693.
31. The BIP Study Group. Secondary prevention by raising HDL–cholesterol and reducing triglycerides in patients with coronary artery disease. The Bezafibrate Infarction Prevention (BIP) Study. *Circulation* 2000;102:21–27.
32. Bond R, Narayan S, Rothwell PM, et al. Clinical and radiological risk factors for operative stroke and death in the European Carotid Surgery Trial. *Eur J Vasc Endovasc Surg* 2002;23:108–116.
33. The Long-term Intervention with Pravastatin in Ischaemic Disease (LIPID) study group. Prevention of cardiovascular events and death with pravastatin in patients with coronary heart disease and a broad range of initial cholesterol levels. *N Engl J Med* 1998;339:1349–1357.
34. Scandinavian Simvastatin Survival Study Group. Randomised trial of cholesterol lowering in 4444 patients with coronary heart disease: the Scandinavian Simvastatin Survival Study. *Lancet* 1994;344: 1383–1389.
35. The ALLHAT Officers and Coordinators for the ALLHAT Collaborative Research Group. Major outcomes in moderatly hypercholesterolemic, hypertensive patients randomized to pravastatin vs usual care. The antihypertensive and lipid-lowering treatment to prevent heart attack trial (ALLHAT-LLT). *JAMA* 2002;288:2998–3007.
36. Sever PS, Dahlf B, Poulter NR, et al. for the ASCOT investigators. Prevention of coronary and stroke events with atorvastatin in hypertensive patients who have average or lower-than-average cholesterol concentrations, in the Anglo-Scandinavian cardiac outcomes trial-loipid lowering arm (ASCOT-LLA): a multicentre randomised controlled trial. *Lancet* 2003;361:1149–1158.
37. http://www.strokecenter.org/trials/TrialDetail.asp?ref=67&browse=prevent (last accessed 3 December 2003).
38. Cholesterol Treatment Trialists' Collaboration. Protocol for a prospective collaborative overview of

all current and planned randomized trials of cholesterol treatment regimens. *Am J Cardiol* 1995;75:1130–1134.
39. Antithrombotic Trialists' Collaboration. Collaborative meta-analysis of randomised trials of antiplatelet therapy for prevention of death, myocardial infarction, and stroke in high risk patients. *BMJ* 2002;324:71–86. Corrections: *BMJ* 2002;324:141. Search date 1997; primary sources Medline, Embase, Derwent, SciSearch, Biosis, searching the trials registers of the Cochrane Stroke and Peripheral Vascular Disease Groups trials registers, and hand searches of selected journals, proceedings of meetings, reference lists of trials and review articles, and personal contact with colleagues and representatives of pharmaceutical companies.
40. Derry S, Loke YK. Risk of gastrointestinal haemorrhage with long term use of aspirin: meta-analysis. *BMJ* 2000;321:1183–1187. Search date 1999; primary sources Medline, Embase, and hand searches of reference lists from previous review papers and retrieved trials.
41. He J, Whelton PK, Vu B, et al. Aspirin and risk of hemorrhagic stroke. A meta-analysis of randomised controlled trials. *JAMA* 1998;280:1930–1935. Search date 1997; primary sources Medline and hand searches of reference lists of relevant articles.
42. Taylor DW, Barnett HJM, Haynes RB, et al, for the ASA and Carotid Endarterectomy (ACE) Trial Collaborators. Low-dose and high-dose acetylsalicylic acid for patients undergoing carotid endarterectomy: a randomised controlled trial. *Lancet* 1999;353:2179–2184.
43. The Dutch TIA Study Group. A comparison of two doses of aspirin (30 mg vs 283 mg a day) in patients after a transient ischaemic attack or minor ischaemic stroke. *N Engl J Med* 1991;325:1261–1266.
44. Farrell B, Godwin J, Richards S, et al. The United Kingdom transient ischaemic attack (UK-TIA) aspirin trial: final results. *J Neurol Neurosurg Psychiatry* 1991;54:1044–1054.
45. Garc a Rodr guez LA, Hernández-D az S, de Abajo FJ. Association between aspirin and upper gastrointestinal complications. Systematic review of epidemioligic studies. *Br J Clin Pharmacol* 2001;52;563–571. Search date 2001; primary sources Medline and hand searches of reference lists of reviews.
46. Hankey GJ, Sudlow CLM, Dunbabin DW. Thienopyridine derivatives (ticlopidine, clopidogrel) versus aspirin for preventing stroke and other serious vascular events in high vascular risk patients. In: The Cochrane Library, Issue 1, 2004. Chichester, UK: John Wiley & Sons, Ltd. Search date 1999; primary sources Cochrane Stroke Group Trials Register, Antithrombotic Trialists' Collaboration database, and personal contact with the Sanofi pharmaceutical company.
47. Gorelick PB, Richardson d, Kelly M, et al. Aspirin and ticlopidine for prevention of recurrent stroke in black patients. A randomized trial. *JAMA* 2003;289:2947–2957.
48. Diener HC, Cunha L, Forbes C, et al. European secondary prevention study 2: dipyridamole and acetylsalicylic acid in the secondary prevention of stroke. *J Neurol Sci* 1996;143:1–13.
49. Mat as–Guiu J, Ferro JM, Alvarez–Sab n J, et al. Comparison of triflusal and aspirin for prevention of vascular events in patients after cerebral infarction. The TACIP Study: a randomized, double–blind, multicenter trial. *Stroke* 2003;34:840–848.
50. Moloney BA. An analysis of the side effects of ticlopidine. In: Hass WK, Easton JD, eds. *Ticlopidine, platelets and vascular disease*. New York: Springer, 1993:117–139.
51. Bennett CL, Davidson CJ, Raisch DW, et al. Thrombotic thrombocytopenic purpura associated with ticlopidine in the setting of coronary artery stents and stroke prevention. *Arch Int Med* 1999;159:2524–2528.
52. The Clopidogrel in Unstable Angina to Prevent Recurrent Events (CURE) Trial Investigators. Effects of clopidogrel in addition to aspirin in patients with acute coronary syndromes without ST-segment elevation. *N Engl J Med* 2001;345:494–502.
53. Steinhubl SR, Berger PB, Mann JT, et al. for the CREDO Investigators. Early and sustained dual oral antiplatelet therapy following percutaneous coronary intervention. A randomized controlled trial. *JAMA* 2002; 288:2411–2420.
54. Second Chinese Cardiac Study (CCS-2) Collaborative Group. Rationale, design and organisation of the Second Chinese Cardiac Study (CCS-2): a randomised trial of clopidogrel plus aspirin, and of metoprolol, among patients with suspected acute myocardial infarction. *J Cardiovasc Risk* 2000;7:435–441.
55. http://www.clinicaltrials.gov/ct/show/NCT00050817?order=1
56. Major ongoing stroke trials: Management of ATherothrombosis with Clopidogrel in High-risk patients with recent transient ischemic attack or ischemic stroke (MATCH). *Stroke* 2002; 33:1733.
57. De Schryver ELLM, on behalf of the European/Australian Stroke Prevention in Reversible Ischaemia Trial (ESPRIT) Group. Design of ESPRIT: an international randomized trial for secondary prevention after non-disabling cerebral ischaemia of arterial origin. *Cerebrovasc Dis* 2000;10:147–150.
58. Sandercock P, Mielke O, Liu M, et al. Anticoagulants for preventing recurrence following presumed non-cardioembolic ischaemic stroke or transient ischaemic attack. In: The Cochrane Library, Issue 1, 2004. Chichester, UK: John Wiley & Sons, Ltd. Search date 2002; primary sources Cochrane Stroke Group Trials Register, and contact with companies marketing anticoagulant agents.
59. Algra A, De Schryver ELLM, van Gijn J, et al. Oral anticoagulants versus antiplatelet therapy for preventing further vascular events after transient ischaemic attack or minor stroke of presumed arterial origin (Cochrane Review). In: The Cochrane Library, Issue 1, 2004. Chichester, UK: John Wiley & Sons, Ltd. Search date 2001; primary sources Cochrane Stroke Group Trials Register and personal contact with authors of published trials.
60. Major ongoing stroke trials: Warfarin vs Aspirin for Symptomatic Intracranial Disease (WASID). *Stroke* 2002;33:1737.
61. Internet Stroke Center. http://www.strokecenter.org/trials/
62. De Schryvfer E, for the ESPRIT Study Group. ESPRIT: mild anticoagulation, acetylsalicylic acid plus dipyridamole or acetylsalicylic acid alone after cerebral ischaemia of arterial origin [abstract]. *Cerebrovasc Dis* 1998;8(suppl 4):83.
63. Rothwell PM, Gutnikov SA, Eliasziw M, et al, for the Carotid Endarterectomy Trialists' Collaboration. Analysis of pooled data from the randomised controlled trials of endarterectomy for symptomatic carotid stenosis. *Lancet* 2003;361:107–116.
64. European Carotid Surgery Trialists' Collaborative Group. Randomised trial of endarterectomy for recently symptomatic carotid stenosis: final results of the MRC European carotid surgery trial. *Lancet* 1998;351:1379–1387.
65. North American Symptomatic Carotid Endarterectomy Trial Collaborators. Beneficial effect of carotid endarterectomy in symptomatic patients with high-grade carotid stenosis. *N Engl J Med* 1991;325:445–453.
66. Barnett HJ, Taylor DW, Eliasziw M, et al. Benefit of carotid endarterectomy in patients with symptomatic moderate or severe stenosis. North American symptomatic carotid endarterectomy trial collaborators. *N Engl J Med* 1998;339:1415–1425.
67. Mayberg MR, Wilson E, Yatsu F, et al, for the Veterans Affairs Cooperative Studies Program 309 Trialist Group. Carotid endarterectomy and prevention of cerebral ischaemia in symptomatic carotid stenosis. *JAMA* 1991;266:3289–3294.
68. Benavente O, Moher D, Pham B. Carotid endarterectomy for asymptomatic carotid stenosis: a meta-analysis. *BMJ* 1998;317:1477–1480. Search date 1998; primary sources Medline, Cochrane

Controlled Trials Register, Ottawa Stroke Trials Register, Current Contents, and hand searches.

69. Chambers BR, You RX, Donnan GA. Carotid endarterectomy for asymptomatic carotid stenosis. In: The Cochrane Library, Issue 1, 2004. Chichester, UK: John Wiley & Sons, Ltd. Search date 1998; primary sources Cochrane Stroke Group Trials Register, Medline, Current Contents, hand searches of reference lists, and contact with researchers in the field.
70. Cao PG, De Rango P, Zannetti S, et al. Eversion versus conventional carotid endarterectomy for preventing stroke. In: The Cochrane Library, Issue 1, 2004. Chichester, UK: John Wiley & Sons, Ltd. Search date 1999; primary sources Medline, Cochrane Stroke Group Trials Register, hand searches of surgical journals and conference proceedings, and contact with experts.
71. Rothwell P, Slattery J, Warlow C. Clinical and angiographic predictors of stroke and death from carotid endarterectomy: systematic review. *BMJ* 1997;315:1571–1577. Search date 1996; primary sources Medline, Cochrane Collaboration Stroke database, and hand searches of reference lists.
72. Bond R, Rerkasem K, Rothwell PM. A systematic review of the risks of carotid endarterectomy in relation to the clinical indication and the timing of surgery. *Stroke* 2003;34:2290–3301. Search date: 2000; primary sources previous review, Medline, Embase, reference lists, and hand searching of six journals with the highest number of relevant articles.
73. Whitty C, Sudlow C, Warlow C. Investigating individual subjects and screening populations for asymptomatic carotid stenosis can be harmful. *J Neurol Neurosurg Psychiatry* 1998;64:619–623.
74. Rothwell PM, Gibson RJ, Slattery J, et al. Equivalence of measurements of carotid stenosis: a comparison of three methods on 1001 angiograms. *Stroke* 1994;25:2435–2439.
75. Cina C, Clase C, Haynes R. Carotid endarterectomy for symptomatic stenosis. In: The Cochrane Library, Issue 1, 2004. Chichester, UK: John Wiley & Sons, Ltd. Search date 1999; primary sources Cochrane Stroke Group Specialised Register of Trials, Medline, Embase, Healthstar, Serline, Cochrane Controlled Trials Register, DARE, and Best Evidence.
76. Goldstein LB, Hasselblad V, Matchar DB, et al. Comparison and meta-analysis of randomised trials of endarterectomy for symptomatic carotid artery stenosis. *Neurology* 1995;45:1965–1970.
77. Rothwell PM, Gutnikov SA, Mayberg MR, et al. A pooled analysis of individual patient data from trials of endarterectomy for symptomatic carotid stenosis: efficacy of surgery in important subgroups. *Stroke* 2001;32:328.
78. Halliday A, Thomas D, Manssfield A. The asymptomatic carotid surgery trial (ACST). Rationale and design. *Eur J Vascular Surg* 1994;8:703–710.
79. Naylor AR, Mehta Z, Rothwell PM, et al. Carotid artery disease and stroke during coronary artery bypass surgery: a critical review of the literature. *Eur J Vasc Endovasc Surg* 2002;23:283–294. Search date: 2000; primary sources Pubmed, manual searches of European Journal of Vascular and Endovascular Surgery, Journal of Vascular Surgery, Stroke, Annals of Thoracic Surgery, Journal of Thoracic and Cardiothoracic Surgery, reference lists.
80. Naylor AR, Cuffe RL, Rothwell PM, et al. A systematic review of outcomes following staged and synchronous carotid endarterectomy and coronary artery bypass. *Eur J Vasc Endovasc Surg* 2003;25: 380–389. Search date: 2002; primary sources Pubmed, manual searches of European Journal of Vascular and Endovascular Surgery, Journal of Vascular Surgery, Stroke, Annals of Thoracic Surgery, Journal of Thoracic and Cardiothoracic Surgery, reference lists.
81. CAVATAS Investigators. Endovascular versus surgical treatment in patents with carotid stenosis in the Carotid and Vertebral Artery Transluminal Angioplasty Study (CAVATAS): a randomised trial. *Lancet* 2001;357;1729–1737.
82. Naylor AR, Bolia A, Abbott RJ, et al. Randomized study of carotid angioplasty and stenting versus carotid endarterectomy: a stopped trial. *Journal of Vascular Surgery* 1998;28:326–334.
83. Alberts M.J, for the Publications Committee of the WALLSTENT. Results of a multicantre prospective randomised trial of carotid artery stenting vs. carotid endarterectomy. *Stroke* 2001;32:325.
84. Brooks WH, McClure RR, Jones MR, et al. Carotid angioplasty and stenting versus carotid endarterectomy: randomized trial in a community hospital. *J Am Coll Cardiol* 2001;38:1589–1595.
85. Yadav JS for the SAPPHIRE Investigators. Stenting with Angioplasty with Protection in Patients at High Risk for Endarterectomy: the SAPHIRE Study. *Circulation* 2002;106:2.
86. Reimers B, Corvaja N, Moshiri S, et al. Cerebral protection with filter devices during carotid artery stenting. *Circulation* 2001;104:12–15.
87. Hart R, Benavente O, McBride R, et al. Antithrombotic therapy to prevent stroke in patients with atrial fibrillation: a meta-analysis. *Ann Intern Med* 1999;131:492–501. Search date 1999; primary sources Medline, Cochrane Database, and Antithrombotic Trialists' Collaboration database.
88. Secondary prevention in non-rheumatic atrial fibrillation after transient ischaemic attack or minor stroke. EAFT(European Atrial Fibrillation Trial) Study Group. *Lancet* 1993;342:1255–1262.
89. Yamaguchi T. Optimal intensity of warfarin therapy for secondary prevention of stroke in patients with non-valvular atrial fibrillation: a multicenter, prospective randomised trial. Japanese Nonvalvular Atrial Fibrillation-Embolism Secondary Prevention Cooperative Study Group. *Stroke* 2000;31:817–821.
90. Morocutti C, Amabile G, Fattapposta F, et al, for the SIFA Investigators. Indobufen versus warfarin in the secondary prevention of major vascular events in non-rheumatic atrial fibrillation. *Stroke* 1997;28:1015–1021.
91. Executive Steering Committee on behalf of the SPORTIF III Investigators* Stroke prevention with the oral direct thrombin inhibitor ximelagatran compared with warfarin in patients with non-valvular atrial fibrillation (SPORTIF III): randomised controlled trial. *Lancet* 2003;362:1691–1698.
92. Segal JB, McNamara RL, Miller MR, et al. Anticoagulants or antiplatelet therapy for non-rheumatic atrial fibrillation and flutter. In: The Cochrane Library, Issue 1, 2004. Chichester, UK: John Wiley & Sons, Ltd. Search date 1999; primary sources Medline, Embase, Cochrane Heart Group Trials Register, hand searches of selected journals and conference proceedings, and contact with experts.
93. Atrial Fibrillation Investigators. Risk factors for stroke and efficacy of antithrombotic therapy in atrial fibrillation. *Arch Intern Med* 1994;154:1449–1457.
94. Koudstaal P. Anticoagulants for preventing stroke in patients with non-rheumatic atrial fibrillation and a history of stroke or transient ischemic attacks. In: The Cochrane Library, Issue 1, 2004. Chichester, UK: John Wiley & Sons, Ltd. Search date not stated; primary source Cochrane Stroke Group Trials Register and contact with trialists.
95. Koudstaal P. Anticoagulants versus antiplatelet therapy for preventing stroke in patients with non-rheumatic atrial fibrillation and a history of stroke or transient ischemic attacks. In: The Cochrane Library, Issue 1, 2004. Chichester, UK: John Wiley & Sons Ltd. Search date not stated; primary sources Cochrane Stroke Group Trials Register and contact with trialists.
96. Benavente O, Hart R, Koudstaal P, et al. Oral anticoagulants for preventing stroke in patients with non-valvular atrial fibrillation and no previous history of stroke or transient ischemic attacks. In: The Cochrane Library, Issue 1, 2004. Chichester, UK: John Wiley & Sons, Ltd. Search date 1999; primary sources Cochrane Stroke Group Specialised Register

of Trials, Medline, Antithrombotic Trialists' Collaboration database, and hand searches of reference lists of relevant articles.
97. Benavente O, Hart R, Koudstaal P, et al. Antiplatelet therapy for preventing stroke in patients with non-valvular atrial fibrillation and no previous history of stroke or transient ischemic attacks. In: The Cochrane Library, Issue 1, 2004. Chichester, UK: John Wiley & Sons, Ltd. Search date 1999; primary sources Medline, Cochrane Specialised Register of Trials, and hand searches of reference lists of relevant articles.
98. Lechat P, Lardoux H, Mallet A, et al. Anticoagulant (fluindione)–aspirin combination in patients with high risk atrial fibrillation. A randomised trial (Fluindione, fibrillation Auriculaire, Aspirin et Contraste Spontane; FFAACS). *Cerebrovasc Dis* 2001;12:245–252.
99. Chen ZM, Sandercock P, Pan HC, et al. Indications for early aspirin use in acute ischemic stroke: a combined analysis of 40 000 randomized patients from the Chinese acute stroke trial and the international stroke trial. On behalf of the CAST and IST collaborative groups. *Stroke* 2000;31:1240–1249.
100. Stroke Prevention in Atrial Fibrillation Investigators. Adjusted-dose warfarin versus low-intensity, fixed-dose warfarin plus aspirin for high-risk patients with atrial fibrillation: stroke prevention in atrial fibrillation III randomised clinical trial. *Lancet* 1996;348:633–638.
101. Pengo V, Zasso Z, Barbero F, et al. Effectiveness of fixed minidose warfarin in the prevention of thromboembolism and vascular death in nonrheumatic atrial fibrillation. *Am J Cardiol* 1998;82:433–437.
102. Gullov A, Koefoed B, Petersen P, et al. Fixed minidose warfarin and aspirin alone and in combination vs adjusted-dose warfarin for stroke prevention in atrial fibrillation. Second Copenhagen Atrial Fibrillation, Aspirin, and Anticoagulation Study. *Arch Intern Med* 1998;158:1513–1521.
103. Hellemons B, Langenberg M, Lodder J, et al. Primary prevention of arterial thrombo-embolism in non-rheumatic atrial fibrillation in primary care: randomised controlled trial comparing two intensities of coumarin with aspirin. *BMJ* 1999;319:958–964.
104. The European Atrial Fibrillation Trial Study Group. Optimal oral anticoagulant therapy in patients with non-rheumatic atrial fibrillation and recent cerebral ischemia. *N Engl J Med* 1995;333:5–10.
105. Hylek EM, Skates SJ, Sheehan MA, et al. An analysis of the lowest effective intensity of prophylactic anticoagulation for patients with non-rheumatic atrial fibrillation. *N Engl J Med* 1996;335:540–546.
106. Van Walraven C, Hart RG, Singer DE, et al. Oral anticoagulants vs aspirin in nonvalvular atrial fibrillation. An individual patient meta-analysis. *JAMA* 2002;288:2441–2448.
107. Edvardsson N, Juul-Moller S, Omblus R, et al. Effects of low-dose warfarin and aspirin versus no treatment on stroke in a medium-risk patient population with atrial fibrillation. *J Intern Med* 2003;254:95–101.
108. Taylor F, Cohen H, Ebrahim S. Systematic review of long term anticoagulation or antiplatelet treatment in patients with non-rheumatic atrial fibrillation. *BMJ* 2001;322:321–326. Search date 1999; primary sources Cochrane Central database, Embase, Medline, Cinahl, Sigle, hand searches of reference lists, and personal contact with experts.
109. Lip G. Thromboprophylaxis for atrial fibrillation. *Lancet* 1999;353:4–6.
110. Ezekowitz M, Levine J. Preventing stroke in patients with atrial fibrillation. *JAMA* 1999;281:1830–1835.
111. Hart R, Sherman D, Easton D, et al. Prevention of stroke in patients with non-valvular atrial fibrillation. *Neurology* 1998;51:674–681.
112. Feinberg W. Anticoagulation for prevention of stroke. *Neurology* 1998;51(suppl 3):20–22.
113. Albers G. Choice of antithrombotic therapy for stroke prevention in atrial fibrillation. Warfarin, aspirin, or both? *Arch Intern Med* 1998;158:1487–1491.
114. Nademanee K, Kosar E. Long-term antithrombotic treatment for atrial fibrillation. *Am J Cardiol* 1998;82:37N–42N.
115. Green CJ, Hadorn DC, Bassett K, et al. Anticoagulation in chronic non-valvular atrial fibrillation: a critical appraisal and meta-analysis. *Can J Cardiol* 1997;13:811–815.
116. Blakely J. Anticoagulation in chronic non-valvular atrial fibrillation: appraisal of two meta-analyses. *Can J Cardiol* 1998;14:945–948.
117. Evans A, Kalra L. Are the results of randomized controlled trials on anticoagulation in patients with atrial fibrillation generalizable to clinical practice? *Arch Intern Med* 2001;161:1443–1447. Search date not stated; primary sources Medline, Cochrane Library, and hand searches of reference lists of relevant retrieved articles.

Gregory YH Lip
Consultant Cardiologist and Professor of Cardiovascular Medicine, Director of Haemostasis Thrombosis and Vascular Biology Unit
City Hospital
Birmingham
UK

Peter Rothwell
Reader in Clinical Neurology
Department of Clinical Neurology
Oxford
UK

Cathie Sudlow
Wellcome Clinician Scientist and Senior Lecturer
Division of Clinical Neurosciences
University of Edinburgh
Edinburgh
UK

Competing interests: CS on one occasion received a fee from Sanofi-Synthelabo for giving a talk at a GP meeting. PR none declared. GYHL has received research funding and honoraria from various pharmaceutical companies in relation to atrial fibrillation and antithrombotic therapy, for meetings and educational symposia. In addition he is a member of advisory boards and one trial steering committee for Astra Zeneca.
The following previous contributors of this topic would also like to be acknowledged: Colin Baigent, Gord Gubitz, Peter Sandercock, and Bethan Freestone.

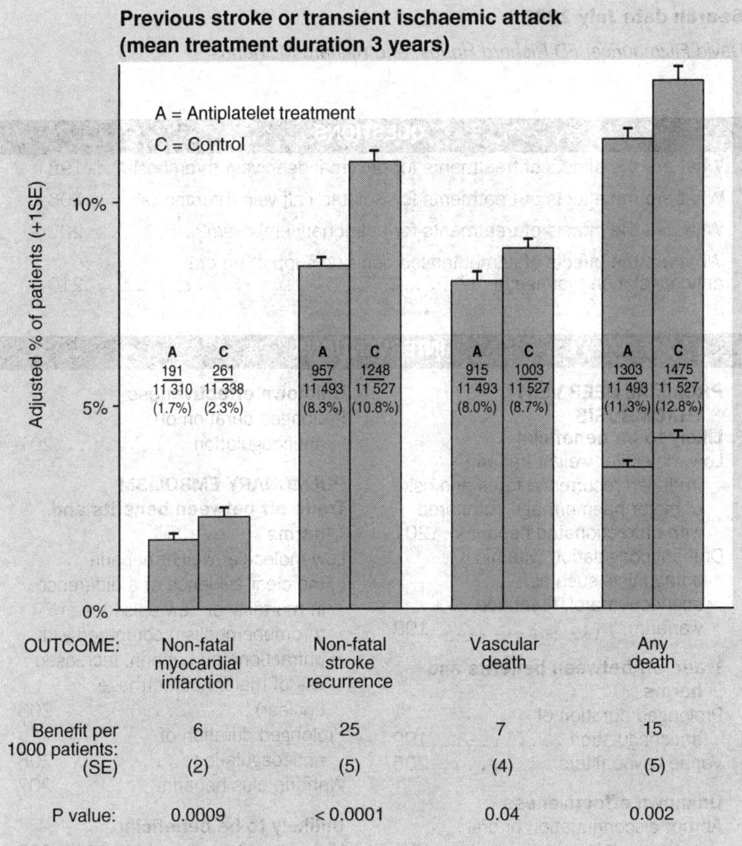

FIGURE 1 **Absolute effects of antiplatelet treatment on various outcomes in 21 trials in people with a prior (presumed ischaemic) stroke or transient ischaemic attack. The columns show the absolute risks over 3 years for each outcome. The error bars represent standard deviations. In the "any death" column, non-vascular deaths are represented by lower horizontal lines (see text, p 174). Adapted with permission.[4]**

Thromboembolism

Search date July 2003

David Fitzmaurice, FD Richard Hobbs, and Richard McManus

QUESTIONS

INTERVENTIONS

To be covered in future updates

Aspirin
Oral antithrombotic agents (such as glycoprotein IIb/IIIa antagonists)
Thromboembolism in pregnancy

See glossary Ⓖ

Key Messages

Proximal deep vein thrombosis

- **Low molecular weight heparin (reduced recurrence and reduced risk of major haemorrhage compared with unfractionated heparin)** Systematic reviews found that low molecular weight heparin reduced the incidence of recurrent thromboembolic disease in people with proximal deep vein thrombosis and decreased the risk of major haemorrhage over 3–6 months compared with unfractionated heparin. Two subsequent RCTs in people with proximal deep vein thrombosis receiving oral anticoagulation, some considered at high risk of pulmonary embolism, found no significant difference in pulmonary embolism or mortality at 12 days or recurrent venous thromboembolism over 2 years between adding low molecular weight heparin and adding unfractionated heparin. One of the RCTs also found no significant difference in rates of clinically important bleeding between low molecular weight heparin and unfractionated heparin. The reviews found no significant difference in thrombocytopenia between low molecular weight heparin and unfractionated heparin. One subsequent open label RCT found no significant difference in recurrent deep vein thrombosis at two years between low molecular weight heparin and unfractionated heparin.
- **Oral anticoagulants (vitamin K antagonists such as acenocoumarol, flutamide, warfarin)** We found no RCTs comparing vitamin K antagonists such as acenocoumarol, flutamide, and warfarin versus placebo. One RCT found that fewer people had recurrence of proximal deep vein thrombosis within 6 months with acenocoumarol (nicoumalone) plus intravenous unfractionated heparin as initial treatment than with acenocoumarol alone; as a result, the trial was stopped. One systematic review found no significant difference between oral anticoagulation and long term low molecular weight heparin in recurrent thromboembolism, major haemorrhage, or mortality.
- **Prolonged duration of anticoagulation** Two systematic reviews and one large subsequent RCT found fewer deep vein thrombosis recurrences with up to 48 months compared with up to 24 weeks' duration of anticoagulation with vitamin K antagonists. Another systematic review and two additional open label RCTs found no significant difference in the risk of deep vein thrombosis recurrences between longer and shorter duration of anticoagulation, but their results were limited by the use of indirect comparisons and by lack of power. One review found limited evidence that prolonged compared with shorter anticoagulation increased major haemorrhage, but another review and one large subsequent RCT found no significant difference in major haemorrhage. The absolute risk of recurrent venous thromboembolism decreases with time, but the relative risk reduction with treatment remains constant. Harms of treatment, including major haemorrhage, continue during prolonged treatment. Individuals have different risk profiles, and it is likely that the optimal duration of anticoagulation will vary.
- **Venae cavae filters** One RCT in people with proximal deep vein thrombosis considered at high risk of pulmonary embolism, all receiving oral anticoagulation, found that venae cavae filters reduced rates of pulmonary embolism at 12 days compared with no filters. However, the difference in rates of pulmonary embolism was not significant at 2 years, and venae cavae filters increased rates of recurrent deep vein thrombosis at 2 years.
- **Abrupt discontinuation of oral anticoagulation** One RCT in people who had received warfarin for 3–6 months provided insufficient evidence to compare abrupt withdrawal of warfarin versus an additional month of warfarin at a fixed low dose of 1.25 mg daily.
- **Compression stockings** We found no RCTs of standard compression stockings for treating people with proximal deep vein thrombosis. One RCT found that made to measure knee length graduated compression stockings reduced post-thrombotic syndrome over 5–8 years compared with no stockings.

- **High intensity oral anticoagulation** One RCT found that bleeding rates with warfarin treatment were increased by higher international normalised ratio target ranges (international normalised ratio 3.0–4.5), but recurrence rates were not significantly different compared with a lower range (international normalised ratio 2.0–3.0).
- **Home treatment with short term low molecular weight heparin** One systematic review of weak RCTs found no significant difference in recurrence of thromboembolism between heparin treatment at home and in hospital.
- **Low molecular weight heparin versus oral anticoagulation (long term)** One systematic review found no significant difference between long term low molecular weight heparin and oral anticoagulation in recurrent thromboembolism, major haemorrhage, or mortality.
- **Once daily versus twice daily low molecular weight heparin** Systematic reviews found no significant difference between once and twice daily low molecular weight heparin in recurrent thromboembolism or mortality at 10 days or 3 months. However, the reviews may have been underpowered to detect a clinically important difference because of low rates of recurrent thromboembolism and mortality in the trials.

Isolated calf vein thrombosis

- **Warfarin (reduced rate of proximal extension compared with no treatment in people who had received initial heparin and wore compression stockings)** One RCT, in people who had received initial intravenous unfractionated heparin (international normalised ratio 2.5–4.2) and wore compression stockings, found that warfarin reduced rates of proximal extension compared with no further treatment.
- **Prolonged duration of anticoagulation** One open label RCT found no significant difference in recurrent thromboembolism or rates of major haemorrhage between 6 and 12 weeks of warfarin. The absolute risk of recurrent venous thromboembolism decreases with time, but the relative risk reduction with treatment remains constant. Harms of treatment, including major haemorrhage, continue during prolonged treatment. Individuals have different risk profiles and it is likely that the optimal duration of anticoagulation will vary.

Pulmonary embolism

- **Low molecular weight heparin (no clear evidence of a difference in mortality or new episodes of thromboembolism compared with unfractionated heparin, increased risk of major haemorrhage unclear)** One RCT in people with symptomatic pulmonary embolism who did not receive thrombolysis or embolectomy found no significant difference between low molecular weight heparin and unfractionated heparin in mortality or new episodes of thromboembolism. Another RCT in people with proximal deep vein thrombosis without clinical signs or symptoms of pulmonary embolism, but with high probability lung scan findings, found that low molecular weight heparin reduced the proportion of people with new episodes of venous thromboembolism compared with intravenous heparin. The RCTs found no significant difference in major haemorrhage between low molecular weight heparin and unfractionated heparin, but may have been underpowered to detect a clinically important difference.
- **Prolonged duration of anticoagulation** We found no direct evidence in people with pulmonary embolism about the optimum duration of anticoagulation. Evidence for duration of treatment has been extrapolated from RCTs in people with proximal deep vein thrombosis and any venous thromboembolism, which found that longer courses of anticoagulation reduced recurrence compared with shorter courses but may increase the risk of major haemorrhage.
- **Warfarin plus heparin** One small RCT in people with pulmonary embolism found that warfarin plus heparin reduced mortality at 1 year compared with no anticoagulation.

- **High intensity anticoagulation** We found no direct evidence in people with pulmonary embolism about the optimum intensity of anticoagulation. Evidence for intensity of treatment has been extrapolated from RCTs in people with proximal deep vein thrombosis and any venous thromboembolism, which found that bleeding rates were increased by higher international normalised ratio target ranges (international normalised ratio 3.0–4.5), but recurrence rates were not significantly different compared with a lower range (international normalised ratio 2.0–3.0).
- **Thrombolysis** Systematic reviews and one subsequent RCT found no significant difference in mortality between thrombolysis plus heparin and heparin alone, and found that thrombolysis may increase the incidence of intracranial haemorrhage. RCTs identified by a systematic review found no significant difference in mortality or recurrent pulmonary embolism among different thrombolytics.

Computerised decision support

- **Computerised decision support in oral anticoagulation** We found no RCTs comparing computerised decision support versus usual management of oral anticoagulation that used clinically important outcomes (major haemorrhage or death). One systematic review and four subsequent RCTs found that, compared with usual care, the use of computerised decision support in oral anticoagulation increased the time spent in the target international normalised range. Another subsequent RCT found no significant difference between computerised decision support and standard manual support in the time spent in the target international normalised ratio range.

DEFINITION **Venous thromboembolism** is any thromboembolic event occurring within the venous system, including deep vein thrombosis and pulmonary embolism. **Deep vein thrombosis** is a radiologically confirmed partial or total thrombotic occlusion of the deep venous system of the legs sufficient to produce symptoms of pain or swelling. **Proximal deep vein thrombosis** affects the veins above the knee (popliteal, superficial femoral, common femoral, and iliac veins). **Isolated calf vein thrombosis** is confined to the deep veins of the calf and does not affect the veins above the knee. **Pulmonary embolism** is radiologically confirmed partial or total thromboembolic occlusion of pulmonary arteries, sufficient to cause symptoms of breathlessness, chest pain, or both. **Post-thrombotic syndrome** is oedema, ulceration, and impaired viability of the subcutaneous tissues of the leg occurring after deep vein thrombosis. **Recurrence** refers to symptomatic deterioration owing to a further (radiologically confirmed) thrombosis, after a previously confirmed thromboembolic event, where there had been an initial partial or total symptomatic improvement. **Extension** refers to a radiologically confirmed new, constant, symptomatic intraluminal filling defect extending from an existing thrombosis.

INCIDENCE/ PREVALENCE We found no reliable study of the incidence or prevalence of deep vein thrombosis or pulmonary embolism in the UK. A prospective Scandinavian study found an annual incidence of 1.6–1.8/1000 people in the general population.[1,2] One post mortem study estimated that 600 000 people develop pulmonary embolism each year in the USA, of whom 60 000 die as a result.[3]

AETIOLOGY/ RISK FACTORS Risk factors for deep vein thrombosis include immobility, surgery (particularly orthopaedic), malignancy, smoking, pregnancy, older age, and inherited or acquired prothrombotic clotting disorders.[4] The oral contraceptive pill is associated with increased risk of death due to venous thromboembolism (ARI with any combined oral contraception: 1–3/million women a year).[5] The principal cause of pulmonary embolism is a deep vein thrombosis.[4]

PROGNOSIS The annual recurrence rate of symptomatic calf vein thrombosis in people without recent surgery is over 25%.[6,7] Proximal extension develops in 40–50% of people with symptomatic calf vein thrombosis.[8] Proximal deep vein thrombosis may cause fatal or non-fatal pulmonary embolism, recurrent venous thrombosis, and the post-thrombotic syndrome. One case series (462 people) published in 1946 found 5.8% mortality from pulmonary emboli in people in a maternity hospital with untreated deep vein thrombosis.[9] One non-systematic review of observational studies found that, in people after recent surgery who have an asymptomatic deep calf vein thrombosis, the rate of fatal pulmonary embolism was 13–15%.[10] The incidence of other complications without treatment is not known. The risk of recurrent venous thrombosis and complications is increased by thrombotic risk factors.[11]

AIMS OF INTERVENTION To reduce acute symptoms of deep vein thrombosis and to prevent morbidity and mortality associated with thrombus extension, post-thrombotic syndrome, and pulmonary embolisation; to reduce recurrence; to minimise any adverse effects of treatment.

OUTCOMES Rates of symptomatic recurrence, post-thrombotic syndrome, symptomatic pulmonary embolism, and death. Proxy outcomes include radiological evidence of clot extension or pulmonary embolism. **For computerised decision support:** Time spent in the target international normalised range.

METHODS *Clinical Evidence* search and appraisal July 2003. Observational studies were used for estimating incidence, prevalence, and adverse event rates. RCTs were included only if participants were included and outcomes defined on the basis of objective tests, and if the trial provided dose ranges (with adjusted dosing schedules for oral anticoagulation and unfractionated heparin) and independent, blinded outcome assessment.

QUESTION What are the effects of treatments for proximal deep vein thrombosis?

OPTION ORAL ANTICOAGULATION (VITAMIN K ANTAGONISTS SUCH AS ACENOCOUMAROL, FLUTAMIDE, WARFARIN)

We found no RCTs comparing vitamin K antagonists such as acenocoumarol, flutamide, and warfarin versus placebo. One RCT found that fewer people had recurrence of proximal deep vein thrombosis within 6 months with acenocoumarol (nicoumalone) plus intravenous unfractionated heparin as initial treatment than with acenocoumarol alone; as a result, the trial was stopped. One systematic review found no significant difference between oral anticoagulation and long term low molecular weight heparin in recurrent thromboembolism, major haemorrhage, or mortality.

Benefits: **Versus placebo:** We found no systematic review or RCTs. **Acenocoumarol (nicoumalone) plus intravenous unfractionated heparin versus acenocoumarol alone:** We found no systematic review. One RCT (120 people with proximal deep vein thrombosis) found that fewer people had recurrence at interim analysis at 6 months with combined intravenous unfractionated heparin plus acenocoumarol than with acenocoumarol alone; as a result, the trial was stopped. The difference in recurrence did not quite reach significance (4/60 [7%] with combined treatment *v* 12/60 [20%] with warfarin alone; P = 0.058; see comment below).[12] **Versus low molecular weight heparin:** See benefits of low molecular weight heparin, p 202.

Harms: **Warfarin:** Two non-systematic reviews of RCTs and cohort studies found annual bleeding rates of 0–5% (fatal bleeding) and 2–8% (major bleeds) with warfarin (absolute numbers not reported).[13,14] Rates depended on how bleeding was defined and the intensity of anticoagulation. **Acenocoumarol plus intravenous unfractionated heparin versus acenocoumarol alone:** In the RCT comparing acenocoumarol plus heparin versus acenocoumarol alone, one person in the combined treatment group committed suicide at 6 months.[12] There were two cancer related deaths, confirmed by post mortem examination, in the group treated with warfarin alone: one in week 11 and the other in week 12. **Versus low molecular weight heparin:** See harms of low molecular weight heparin, p 203.

Comment: **Acenocoumarol plus intravenous unfractionated heparin versus acenocoumarol alone for initial treatment:** It is unclear why the RCT was stopped early when it found no significant difference in recurrence between groups. The lower recurrence rates with combined intravenous unfractionated heparin plus acenocoumarol compared with acenocoumarol alone suggest that it may have been considered unethical to continue the trial.

OPTION PROLONGED DURATION OF ANTICOAGULATION

Two systematic reviews and one large subsequent RCT found fewer deep vein thrombosis recurrences with up to 48 months compared with up to 24 weeks' duration of anticoagulation with vitamin K antagonists. Another systematic review and two additional open label RCTs found no significant difference in the risk of deep vein thrombosis recurrences between longer and shorter duration of anticoagulation, but their results were limited by the use of indirect comparisons and by lack of power. One review found limited evidence that prolonged compared with shorter anticoagulation increased major haemorrhage, but another review and one large subsequent RCT found no significant difference in major haemorrhage. The absolute risk of recurrent venous thromboembolism decreases with time, but the relative risk reduction with treatment remains constant. Harms of treatment, including major haemorrhage, continue during prolonged treatment. Individuals have different risk profiles and it is likely that the optimal duration of anticoagulation will vary.

Benefits: We found three systematic reviews,[15–17] one subsequent RCT,[18] and two additional open label RCTs.[19,20] The first review (search date 2000, 4 RCTs, 1500 people) included two RCTs of people with a first episode of venous thromboembolism, one RCT in people with a second episode of venous thromboembolism, and one RCT in people with acute proximal deep vein thrombosis.[15] All of the RCTs assessed warfarin. The periods of treatment compared were different in all four RCTs: 4 weeks versus 3 months, 6 weeks versus 6 months, 3 months versus 27 months, and 6 months versus 4 years. In all RCTs, warfarin doses were adjusted to achieve an international normalised ratio❻ of 2.0–3.0. The review found that prolonged 3–48 months treatment with warfarin significantly reduced thromboembolic complications compared with shorter warfarin treatment (AR 7/758 [0.9%] in the long arm *v* 91/742 [12.3%] in the short arm; RR 0.08, 95% CI 0.04 to 0.16; NNT 9, 95% CI 8 to 12). However, it found no significant reduction in mortality between prolonged and shorter treatment (AR 37/758 [4.9%] in the long arm *v* 50/742 [6.7%] in the short arm; RR 0.72, 95% CI 0.48 to 1.08).[15] The second systematic review (search date not stated, 7 RCTs, 2304 people) included three of the same RCTs as the first systematic review plus four RCTs that had been excluded from the first systematic review on methodological grounds (either because of problems with blinding of outcomes or lack of an objective test to confirm thromboembolism).[16] All of the RCTs assessed warfarin. This review also found that longer duration of warfarin reduced the risk of recurrent thromboembolism compared with shorter courses of warfarin treatment (74/1156 [6.4%] events per person with longer duration *v* 127/1148 [11.1%] with shorter duration; RR 0.60, 95% CI 0.45 to 0.79; NNT 22, 95% CI 15 to 43). The third systematic review (search date 2001) identified 16 RCTs, including all seven RCTs identified by the earlier reviews and two prospective cohort studies (3186 people with proximal deep vein thrombosis or pulmonary embolism).[17] It divided RCTs into short (4–6 weeks), medium (3 months) and long (4–6 months) duration of anticoagulation. The review did not directly compare longer versus shorter duration of anticoagulation; rather it calculated summary incidences for each time period. It found that, in all three groups, the incidence of recurrent venous thromboembolism reduced over time after the first episode. At 9–18 months from the first episode, the recurrence rate was equivalent in all three groups. In indirect comparisons, the review found no significant difference in the incidence of recurrent thromboembolism between long and short duration of anticoagulation (reported as non-significant, CI not reported), but it may have been underpowered to detect a clinically important difference. It found that, in the 3–6 months after a first episode, the incidence of recurrent venous thromboembolism was highest in the group of people treated for a long duration (3.96%, 95% CI 0.47% to 14.3%) compared with short (1.23%, 95% CI 0.79% to 1.83%) and medium (1.19%, 95% CI 0.91% to 1.53%) durations. The subsequent RCT (508 adults with idiopathic deep vein thromboembolism or pulmonary embolism who had received oral anticoagulation for a median 6.5 months, 40% of whom had experienced a previous thrombosis) compared continuing warfarin ≤10 mg daily to achieve an international normalised ratio target of 1.5–2.0 versus placebo. The trial aimed for a 4 year follow up, but it was terminated early (mean follow up 2.1 years) because warfarin significantly reduced recurrent venous thrombosis compared with placebo (14/255 [5%] with warfarin *v* 37/253 [15%]; HR 0.36, 95% CI 0.19 to 0.67).[18] This RCT may overstate the effect of long term low intensity warfarin. It is difficult to draw conclusions about the effects of long term warfarin in people with a first deep vein thrombosis from this trial because 40% of the people included in the trial had experienced a previous thrombosis.[18] The first open label RCT (736 people, including 539 with proximal deep vein thrombosis, pulmonary embolism, or both) comparing fluindione for 3 months versus 6 months found no significant difference in the risk of recurrent thromboembolism, although the confidence interval was wide (AR 21/270 [7.8%] with 3 months *v* 23/269 [8.6%] with 6 months; ARR +0.8%, 95% CI −3.9% to +5.4%; RR 0.93, 95% CI 0.53 to 1.65).[19] The second open label RCT (267 people with a first episode of symptomatic proximal deep vein thrombosis) compared warfarin or acenocoumarol treatment for 3 months versus 12 months.[20] It found no significant difference in recurrence of venous thromboembolism over a mean of 3 years between longer and shorter treatment (21/134 [15.7%] with 12 months *v* 21/133 [15.8%] with 3 months; RR 0.99, 95% CI 0.57 to 1.73). However, it found that mean time to recurrence was shorter with 3 months' than with 12 months' treatment (11.2 months with 3 months *v* 16 months with 12 months; no further data reported).[20]

Harms: **Haemorrhage:** The reviews included studies with different periods of treatment, and the populations studied had different types of venous thromboembolism (see benefits above). The first review found that prolonged anticoagulation significantly increased the risk of major haemorrhage**G** compared with shorter regimens (19/758 [2.5%] with prolonged anticoagulation *v* 4/742 [0.5%] with shorter anticoagulation; OR 3.75, 95% CI 1.63 to 8.62).[15] The second review found a greater risk of major haemorrhage with prolonged compared with shorter anticoagulation regimens, but the difference was not significant (10/917 [1.1%] with prolonged anticoagulation *v* 6/906 [0.7%] with shorter anticoagulation; RR 1.43, 95% CI 0.51 to 4.01).[16] The third review gave no information on risk of major haemorrhage.[17] The subsequent RCT found no significant difference in rates of major haemorrhage over a mean 2.1 years between continuity low intensity warfarin and placebo (5/255 [2%] with warfarin *v* 2/253 [0.8%] with placebo; P = 0.25).[18]

Comment: The absolute risk of recurrent venous thromboembolism decreases with time, whereas the relative risk reduction with treatment remains constant. Observed recurrence of venous thromboembolism is therefore dependent on length of follow up. Harms of treatment, including major haemorrhage, continue during prolonged treatment. Individuals have different risk profiles, and it is likely that the optimal duration of anticoagulation will vary.

OPTION HIGH INTENSITY ORAL ANTICOAGULATION

One RCT found that bleeding rates with warfarin treatment were increased by higher international normalised ratio target ranges (international normalised ratio 3.0–4.5), but recurrence rates were not significantly different compared with a lower range (international normalised ratio 2.0–3.0).

Benefits: We found one RCT (96 people with a first episode of idiopathic venous thromboembolism) comparing international normalised ratio**G** targets of 2.0–3.0 versus 3.0–4.5 over 12 weeks' treatment with warfarin after an initial course of intravenous heparin.[21] It found similar recurrence rates at 10 months for both international normalised ratio target ranges (1/47 [2.1%] with lower range *v* 1/49 [2.0%] with higher range; $P > 0.05$), but found significantly fewer haemorrhagic events with the lower target range (2/47 [4.3%] with lower range *v* 11/49 [22.4%] with higher range; ARR 18%, 95% CI 5% to 32%; RR 0.19, 95% CI 0.04 to 0.81; NNT 6, 95% CI 4 to 23).[21]

Harms: Two non-systematic reviews of RCTs and cohort studies found annual bleeding rates of 0–5% (fatal bleeding) and 2–8% (major bleeds) with warfarin (absolute numbers not reported).[13,14] Rates depended on how bleeding was defined and the intensity of anticoagulation.

Comment: None.

OPTION ABRUPT DISCONTINUATION OF ORAL ANTICOAGULATION

One RCT in people who had received warfarin for 3–6 months provided insufficient evidence to compare abrupt withdrawal of warfarin versus an additional month of warfarin at a fixed low dose of 1.25 mg daily.

Benefits: One RCT (41 people with proximal deep vein thrombosis who had received intravenous heparin for 3–5 days followed by warfarin for 3–6 months) compared abrupt withdrawal of warfarin versus an additional month of warfarin at a fixed low dose of 1.25 mg daily.[22] It found similar recurrence with abrupt compared with gradual discontinuation (3 people with abrupt withdrawal *v* 1 person with gradual withdrawal; CI not reported).[22]

Harms: The RCT gave no information on adverse effects.[22]

Comment: None.

OPTION LOW MOLECULAR WEIGHT HEPARIN VERSUS UNFRACTIONATED HEPARIN

Systematic reviews found that low molecular weight heparin reduced the incidence of recurrent thromboembolic disease in people with proximal deep vein thrombosis and decreased the risk of major haemorrhageG** over 3–6 months compared with unfractionated heparin. Two subsequent RCTs in people with proximal deep vein thrombosis receiving oral anticoagulation, some considered at high risk of pulmonary embolism, found no significant difference in pulmonary embolism or mortality at 12 days or recurrent venous thromboembolism over 2 years between adding low molecular weight heparin**

and adding unfractionated heparin. One of the RCTs also found no significant difference in rates of clinically important bleeding between low molecular weight heparin and unfractionated heparin. The reviews found no significant difference in thrombocytopenia between low molecular weight heparin and unfractionated heparin. One subsequent open label RCT found no significant difference in recurrent deep vein thrombosis at two years between low molecular weight heparin and unfractionated heparin.

Benefits: **Versus each other:** We found one systematic review[23] and two subsequent RCTs[24,25] in people with symptomatic proximal deep vein thrombosis, and one systematic review[26] in people with symptomatic venous thromboembolism, which included two RCTs in people with proximal deep vein thrombosis. The first review (search date 1994, 10 RCTs, 1424 people) found that, over 3–6 months, low molecular weight heparin (LMWH**G**) significantly reduced symptomatic thromboembolic complications compared with unfractionated heparin (5 RCTs: 17/540 [3%] with LMWH *v* 36/546 [7%] with unfractionated heparin; RR 0.47, 95% CI 0.27 to 0.82) and mortality (21/540 [4%] with LMWH *v* 39/546 [7%] with unfractionated heparin; RR 0.53, 95% CI 0.31 to 0.90).[23] The second review[26] (search date not stated, 16 open label and blinded RCTs, 6042 people with symptomatic venous thromboembolism) included two RCTs[27,28] in people with proximal deep vein thrombosis published after the search date of the first review. Results for people with proximal deep vein thrombosis alone were not analysed separately by the review.[26] The first RCT (961 people, open label) compared LMWH twice daily for 1 week versus LMWH once daily for 4 weeks versus intravenous unfractionated heparin.[27] It found that both LMWH regimens significantly increased thrombus regression at 21 days compared with unfractionated heparin (167/312 [53.5%] with once daily LMWH *v* 129/321 [40.2%] with unfractionated heparin; RR 1.29, 97.5% CI 1.08 to 1.53; 175/328 [53.4%] with twice daily LMWH *v* 129/321 [40.2%] with unfractionated heparin; RR 1.28, 97.5% CI 1.08 to 1.52). It found that twice daily LMWH significantly reduced recurrent thromboembolism at 90 days compared with unfractionated heparin (7/388 [1.8%] with twice daily LMWH *v* 24/375 [6.4%] with unfractionated heparin; RR 0.28, 97.5% CI 0.11 to 0.74), but found no significant difference between once daily LMWH and unfractionated heparin (13/374 [3.5%] with once daily LMWH *v* 24/375 [6.4%] with unfractionated heparin; RR 0.55, 97.5% CI 0.24 to 1.16). The second RCT (538 people, open label) compared fixed dose LMWH versus adjusted dose unfractionated heparin for 12 days.[28] It found no significant difference in thrombus regression at 7–15 days between LMWH and unfractionated heparin (RR 0.93, 95% CI 0.82 to 1.05). It also found that LMWH significantly reduced the composite end point of death, recurrent venous thromboembolism, or major bleeding at 6 months compared with unfractionated heparin (18/265 [7%] with LMWH *v* 35/273 [13%] with unfractionated heparin; RR 0.53, 95% CI 0.31 to 0.90).[28] The first subsequent RCT (294 people with proximal deep vein thrombosis, open label) compared three interventions: LMWH twice daily given mainly at home (outpatients), intravenous unfractionated heparin given in hospital, and subcutaneous heparin calcium given at home.[24] Heparin was given for 14 days and simultaneous anticoagulation with warfarin was given for at least 3 months. It found no significant difference in recurrent deep vein thrombosis (6/98 [6%] with unfractionated heparin *v* 6/97 [6%] with LMWH *v* 7/99 [7%] with subcutaneous heparin calcium).[24] The second subsequent open label, multicentre RCT involved 400 adults with venography confirmed proximal deep vein thrombosis considered at high risk of pulmonary embolism, 197 (49%) of whom had concurrent pulmonary embolism diagnosed within 48 hours of admission.[25] It compared four interventions in a two by two factorial design: low molecular weight heparin versus unfractionated heparin plus venae cavae filters**G** versus no filters for 8–12 days. Heparin was given for 8–12 days plus all participants received oral anticoagulation with warfarin or acenocoumarol for at least 3 months. There was no significant association between the type of heparin and use or not of filters (reported as non-significant, CI not reported); results for heparin and filters were analysed separately (see filters for comparison of filters versus no filters, p 205). The RCT performed a completer analysis maintaining initial treatment allocation in the analysis; data were not available for 28/400 (7%) of people. It found no significant difference in pulmonary embolism (2% with LMWH *v* 4% with unfractionated heparin; OR 0.38, 95% CI 0.10 to 1.38) or mortality at 12 days (2% with LMWH *v* 3% with unfractionated heparin; OR 0.69, 95% CI 0.20 to 2.46). It also found no significant difference in recurrent thromboembolism over 2 years (16.6% with LMWH *v* 15.8% with unfractionated heparin; OR 1.05, 95% CI 0.62 to 1.75).See systematic anticoagulation under stroke management, p 152.

Harms: **Haemorrhage:** We found two systematic reviews.[23,26] The first review found that unfractionated heparin was associated with significantly higher rates of clinically important bleeding compared with LMWH (21/759 [3%] with unfractionated heparin *v* 6/753 [0.8%] with LMWH; RR 3.47, 95% CI 1.41 to 8.55).[23] The second review (16 RCTs, 6055 people with proximal deep vein thrombosis or pulmonary embolism) also found that significantly fewer people taking LMWH had major haemorrhage**G** compared with people taking unfractionated heparin (OR 0.56, 95% CI 0.38 to 0.83; absolute results presented graphically). The first subsequent RCT found no episodes of major bleeding in people receiving LMWH or unfractionated heparin.[24] The second subsequent RCT found no significant difference between LMWH and unfractionated heparin in rates of major bleeding (7/195 [3.6%] with LMWH *v* 8/205 [3.9%] with unfractionated heparin; OR 0.90, 95% CI 0.33 to 2.49).[25] **Thrombocytopenia:** We found one systematic review[29] and one subsequent RCT.[30] The review (3306 people treated for at least 5 days) found no significant difference between LMWH and unfractionated heparin in the risk of thrombocytopenia (RR 0.85, 95% CI 0.45 to 1.62).[29] The subsequent RCT (1137 people with symptomatic venous thromboembolism, open label) assessed the risk of thrombocytopenia with three treatments: LMWH for 5–7 days; LMWH for 26–30 days; or unadjusted dose unfractionated heparin for 5–7 days.[30] It found that short term LMWH was associated with less thrombocytopenia compared with long term LMWH or unfractionated heparin (0/388 [0%] with short term LMWH *v* 2/374 [0.53%] with long term LMWH *v* 2/375 [0.53%] with unfractionated heparin). The RCT did not assess the significance of the difference between groups.

Comment: **Studies assessing harm:** These varied in their diagnostic criteria and definitions of adverse events, making interpretation difficult.

OPTION LOW MOLECULAR WEIGHT HEPARIN VERSUS ORAL ANTICOAGULATION (LONG TERM)

One systematic review found no significant difference between long term low molecular weight heparin and oral anticoagulation in recurrent thromboembolism, major haemorrhage, or mortality.

Benefits: We found one systematic review (search date 2001, 7 RCTs, 1137 people with proximal deep vein thrombosis treated initially with low molecular weight heparin [LMWH**G**] or unfractionated heparin for 5–10 days) comparing oral anticoagulation versus LMWH for 3 months.[31] It found no significant difference between LMWH and oral anticoagulation in mortality (21/568 [3.7%] with LMWH *v* 14/569 [2.5%] with oral anticoagulants; OR 1.51, 95% CI 0.77 to 2.97) or recurrent symptomatic thromboembolism over 3–6 months (27/568 [4.8%] with LMWH *v* 38/569 [6.7%] with oral anticoagulants; OR 0.70, 95% CI 0.42 to 1.16).[31]

Harms: The review found that LMWH significantly reduced major haemorrhageⒼ compared with long term oral anticoagulation (7 RCTs; 5/568 [0.9%] with LMWH *v* 14/569 [2.5%] with oral anticoagulation; OR 0.38, 95% CI 0.15 to 0.94). However, the review performed a separate analysis of RCTs that clearly concealed randomisation and were double blinded or where the assessor was blinded to outcome measures. When only these RCTs were included, it found no significant difference in major haemorrhage between long term LMWH and oral anticoagulation (3 RCTs; 4/236 [1.7%] with long term LMWH *v* 5/241 [2.1%] with anticoagulation; OR 0.80, 95% CI 0.21 to 3.00).[31]

Comment: **Studies assessing harm:** These varied in their diagnostic criteria and definitions of adverse events, making interpretation difficult.

OPTION ONCE DAILY VERSUS TWICE DAILY LOW MOLECULAR WEIGHT HEPARIN

Systematic reviews found no significant difference between once and twice daily low molecular weight heparin in recurrent thromboembolism or mortality at 10 days or 3 months. However, the reviews may have been underpowered to detect a clinically important difference because of low rates of recurrent thromboembolism and mortality in the trials.

Benefits: We found two systematic reviews (search date 1999[32], search date 2001[33], 5 RCTs, 1522 adults with symptomatic proximal deep vein thrombosis) comparing once versus twice daily low molecular weight heparin (LMWHⒼ) for 5–10 days.[32,33] Both systematic reviews included the same five RCTs and found similar results. However, the first review[32] included more RCTs in its meta-analyses so we report these results here. The reviews found no significant difference between once and twice daily LMWH in the proportion of people with symptomatic or asymptomatic venous thromboembolism at 10 days or 3 months (symptomatic venous thromboembolism at 10 days: 5 RCTs, 7/742 [0.9%] with once daily *v* 9/766 [1.2%] with twice daily; OR 0.82, 95% CI 0.26 to 2.49; at 3 months: 3 RCTs, 26/614 [4.2%] with once daily *v* 32/642 [5.1%] with twice daily; OR 0.85, 95% CI 0.48 to 1.49).[32] They also found no significant difference in mortality at 10 days or 3 months between once and twice daily LMWH, although mortality at 10 days was higher in people taking once daily LMWH (5 RCTs: 7/750 [0.9%] with once daily *v* 1/772 [0.1%] with twice daily; OR 6.73, 95% CI 0.85 to 305; at 3 months: 2 RCTs, 20/614 [3.3%] with once daily *v* 20/646 [3.1%] with twice daily; OR 1.05, 95% CI 0.53 to 2.09). The reviews may have been underpowered to detect a clinically important difference between once daily and twice daily LMWH because of low rates of recurrent thromboembolism and mortality in the trials.

Harms: The first review found no significant difference in rates of major bleeding between once and twice daily LMWH (10/750 [1.3%] with once daily *v* 9/772 [1.2%] with twice daily; OR 1.16, 95% CI 0.42 to 3.24).

Comment: Increased convenience but the potential for lower efficacy are elements to consider when deciding on once compared with twice daily regimens.

OPTION HOME TREATMENT WITH SHORT TERM LOW MOLECULAR WEIGHT HEPARIN

One systematic review of weak RCTs found no significant difference in recurrence of thromboembolism between heparin treatment at home and in hospital.

Benefits: We found one systematic review (search date 2000, 3 RCTs, 1104 people).[34] Two of the RCTs in the systematic review compared LMWH at home versus unfractionated heparin in hospital, and the other RCT compared LMWH both at home and in hospital. The RCTs had methodological problems, including high exclusion rates and partial hospital treatment in the home treatment arms. The systematic review found no significant difference between treatments in recurrence of thromboembolism or mortality.[34]

Harms: The systematic review found no significant difference between treatments in minor bleeding or major haemorrhage❻.[34]

Comment: None.

OPTION COMPRESSION STOCKINGS

We found no RCTs of standard compression stockings for treating people with proximal deep vein thrombosis. One RCT found that made to measure knee length graduated compression stockings significantly reduced post-thrombotic syndrome over 5–8 years compared with no stockings.

Benefits: We found no systematic review but found one RCT (194 people with a first episode of venogram proven proximal deep vein thrombosis who had received initial treatment with heparin followed by 3 months' treatment with oral anticoagulants) comparing made to measure knee length graduated compression stockings (see comment below) versus no stockings for 2 years.[35] Median follow up was 76 months (range 60–96 months). It found that, compared with no stockings, compression stockings significantly reduced mild to moderate post-thrombotic syndrome (19/94 [20%] with compression stockings *v* 46/94 [47%] with no stockings; $P < 0.001$) and severe post-thrombotic syndrome (11/100 [11%] with stockings *v* 23/100 [23%] with no stockings; $P < 0.001$).[35]

Harms: The RCT gave no information on harms.[35]

Comment: The compression stockings evaluated in the RCT were made to measure rather than the standard sized stockings generally used in clinical practice.[35]

OPTION VENAE CAVAE FILTERS

One RCT in people with proximal deep vein thrombosis considered at high risk of pulmonary embolism, all receiving oral anticoagulation, found that venae cavae filters reduced rates of pulmonary embolism at 12 days compared with no filters. However, the difference in rates of pulmonary embolism was not significant at 2 years, and venae cavae filters increased rates of recurrent deep vein thrombosis at 2 years.

Benefits: We found one open label multicentre RCT (400 adults from 44 centres in France with venography confirmed proximal deep vein thrombosis considered at high risk of pulmonary embolism; 197/400 [49%] had concurrent pulmonary embolism diagnosed within 48 hours of admission).[25] The RCT compared four interventions in a two by two factorial design: venae cavae filters❻ (four different types) versus no filters plus low molecular weight heparin (LMWH Ⓖ) versus unfractionated heparin for 8–12 days. Heparin was given for 8–12 days plus all participants received oral anticoagulation with warfarin or acenocoumarol for at least 3 months. There was no significant association between the type of heparin and use or not of filters (reported as non-significant, CI not reported); results for heparin and filters were analysed separately (see LMWH for comparison of LMWH v unfractionated heparin, p 202). The RCT found that venae cavae filters significantly reduced the incidence of pulmonary embolism at 12 days (2/200 [1%] with filter *v* 9/200 [5%] without filter; OR 0.22, 95% CI 0.05 to 0.90). However, it found no significant difference in pulmonary embolism at 2 years (6/200 [3%] with filters *v* 12/200[6%] with no filters; OR 0.50, 95% CI 0.19 to 1.33), and found that venae cavae filters significantly increased rates of recurrent thromboembolism over 2 years (37/200 [19%] with filters *v* 21/200 [11%] with no filters; OR 1.87, 95% CI 1.10 to 3.20). It also found no significant difference in mortality at 2 years (43/200 [22%] with filters *v* 40/200 [20%] with no filters; OR 1.10, 95% CI 0.72 to 1.70).

Harms: The RCT found no significant difference between venae cavae filters and no filters in major bleeding (17/200 [9%] with filters *v* 22/200 [11%] with no filters; OR 0.77, 95% CI 0.41 to 1.45).[25]

Comment: None.

QUESTION What are the effects of treatment for isolated calf vein thrombosis?

OPTION ANTICOAGULATION

We found no RCTs comparing heparin versus placebo, warfarin versus placebo, or heparin plus warfarin versus placebo. One RCT, in people who had received initial intravenous unfractionated heparin (international normalised ratio > 2.5–4.2) and wore compression stockings, found that warfarin reduced rates of proximal extension compared with no further treatment.

Benefits: **Versus placebo:** We found no RCTs comparing heparin versus placebo, warfarin versus placebo, or heparin plus warfarin versus placebo. **Warfarin plus heparin versus warfarin alone:** We found no systematic review. We found one RCT (51 people), which compared intravenous unfractionated heparin (international normalised ratio Ⓖ 2.5–4.2) for at least 5 days with or without 3 months of warfarin.[6] All participants also wore compression stockings. It found that heparin plus warfarin significantly reduced proximal extension of clot at 1 year compared with heparin alone (1/23 [4%] people with heparin plus warfarin *v* 9/28 [32%] people with heparin alone; ARR 28%, 95% CI 9% to 47%).

Harms: **Warfarin plus heparin versus warfarin alone:** The RCT found that two people taking warfarin plus heparin had clinically important bleeding.[6] No-one taking warfarin alone had clinically important bleeding. See harms of anticoagulation under treatments for proximal deep vein thrombosis, p 198.

Comment: Many reported cases of isolated calf vein thrombosis are asymptomatic but detected radiologically for research purposes. We found limited evidence about the clinical importance of asymptomatic calf vein thrombosis. Similarly, studies into the incidence of pulmonary embolism associated with isolated calf vein thrombosis detected asymptomatic embolism by ventilation–perfusion scanning, and the clinical relevance of these findings is unclear.

OPTION **PROLONGED DURATION OF ANTICOAGULATION**

One open label RCT found no significant difference in recurrent thromboembolism or rates of major haemorrhage between 6 and 12 weeks of warfarin. The absolute risk of recurrent venous thromboembolism decreases with time, but the relative risk reduction with treatment remains constant. Harms of treatment, including major haemorrhage, continue during prolonged treatment. Individuals have different risk profiles, and it is likely that the optimal duration of anticoagulation will vary.

Benefits: We found one open label RCT (736 people with proximal deep vein thrombosis, pulmonary embolism, or isolated calf vein thrombosis, 197 with isolated calf vein thrombosis) comparing 6 weeks versus 12 weeks of warfarin. A pre-planned analysis in people with isolated calf vein thrombosis found no significant difference in recurrence of venous thromboembolism (AR 2/105 [1.9%] with 6 weeks *v* 3/92 [3.3%] with 12 weeks; RR 0.58, 95% CI 0.10 to 3.36).[19]

Harms: The RCT found no significant difference in rates of haemorrhage between 6 weeks and 12 weeks of warfarin in people with isolated calf vein thrombosis (AR 13/105 [12.4%] with 6 weeks *v* 19/92 [20.6%] with 12 weeks; RR 0.59, 95% CI 0.31 to 1.26).[19]

Comment: Many reported cases of isolated calf vein thrombosis are asymptomatic but detected radiologically for research purposes. We found limited evidence about the clinical importance of asymptomatic calf vein thrombosis. Similarly, studies into the incidence of pulmonary embolism associated with isolated calf vein thrombosis detected asymptomatic embolism by ventilation–perfusion scanning, and the clinical relevance of these findings is unclear (see also comment about prolonged duration of anticoagulation under proximal deep vein thrombosis, p 201).

QUESTION **What are the effects of treatments for pulmonary embolism?**

OPTION **ANTICOAGULATION**

We found no RCTs comparing heparin versus placebo, warfarin versus placebo, or heparin plus warfarin versus heparin alone or versus warfarin alone. One small RCT found that heparin plus warfarin reduced mortality at 1 year compared with no anticoagulation.

Benefits: We found no RCTs comparing heparin versus placebo, warfarin versus placebo, or heparin plus warfarin versus heparin alone or versus warfarin alone. **Heparin plus warfarin versus no anticoagulation:** We found no systematic review. We found one RCT (published 1960; 35 people with pulmonary embolism) comparing heparin plus warfarin versus no anticoagulation.[36] It found that anticoagulation significantly reduced mortality at 1 year compared with no anticoagulation (0/16 [0%]; deaths with anticoagulation *v* 5/19 [26%] deaths with no anticoagulation: NNT 4, 95% CI 2 to 16).

Harms: **Heparin plus warfarin versus no anticoagulation:** The RCT gave no information on adverse effects.[36]

Comment: None.

OPTION **PROLONGED DURATION OF ANTICOAGULATION**

We found no direct evidence in people with pulmonary embolism about the optimum duration of anticoagulation. Evidence for duration of treatment has been extrapolated from RCTs in people with proximal deep vein thrombosis and any venous thromboembolism, which found that longer courses of anticoagulation reduced recurrence compared with shorter courses but may increase the risk of major haemorrhage.

Benefits: We found no direct evidence in people with pulmonary embolism (see comment below).

Harms: We found no direct evidence (see comment below).

Comment: We found no direct evidence in people with pulmonary embolism. Evidence for intensity and duration of treatment has been extrapolated from RCTs in people with proximal deep vein thrombosis and any venous thromboembolism. These trials found that longer courses of anticoagulation reduced recurrence compared with shorter courses (see benefits of anticoagulation under treatments for proximal deep vein thrombosis, p 198) but may increase the risk of major haemorrhage.

OPTION **HIGH INTENSITY ANTICOAGULATION**

We found no direct evidence in people with pulmonary embolism about the optimum intensity of anticoagulation. Evidence for intensity of treatment has been extrapolated from RCTs in people with proximal deep vein thrombosis and any venous thromboembolism, which found that bleeding rates were increased by higher international normalised ratio target ranges (international normalised ratio 3.0–4.5), but recurrence rates were not significantly different compared with a lower range (international normalised ratio 2.0–3.0).

Benefits: We found no direct evidence (see comment below).

Harms: We found no direct evidence (see comment below).

Comment: Evidence for intensity of treatment has been extrapolated from RCTs in people with proximal deep vein thrombosis and any venous thromboembolism. These trials found that recurrence rates were not significantly different with higher international normalised ratio**G** target ranges (international normalised ratio 3.0–4.5) compared with a lower range (international normalised ratio 2.0–3.0), but bleeding rates were increased by higher international normalised ratio target ranges.

OPTION **LOW MOLECULAR WEIGHT HEPARIN VERSUS UNFRACTIONATED HEPARIN**

One RCT, in people with symptomatic pulmonary embolism who did not receive thrombolysis or embolectomy, found no significant difference between low molecular weight heparin and unfractionated heparin in mortality or new episodes of thromboembolism. Another RCT in people with proximal deep vein thrombosis without clinical signs or symptoms of pulmonary embolism but with high probability lung scan findings found that low molecular weight heparin reduced the proportion of people with new episodes of venous thromboembolism compared with intravenous heparin. The RCTs found no significant difference in major haemorrhage between low molecular weight heparin and unfractionated heparin but may have been underpowered to detect a clinically important difference.

Benefits: We found no systematic review but found two RCTs.[37,38] The first RCT (612 people with symptomatic pulmonary embolism who did not receive thrombolysis or embolectomy) found no significant difference in mortality or recurrent thromboembolism between low molecular weight heparin (LMWH**G** — tinzaparin) and intravenous heparin (mortality: AR 12/304 [3.9%] with tinzaparin *v* 14/308 [4.5%] with heparin; P = 0.7; recurrent thromboembolism: AR 5/304 [1.6%] with tinzaparin *v* 6/308 [1.9%] with heparin; P = 0.8).[37] The second RCT (200 people with proximal deep vein thrombosis without clinical signs or symptoms of pulmonary embolism but with high probability lung scan findings) found that fixed dose LMWH given once daily significantly reduced the proportion of people with new episodes of venous thromboembolism compared with dose adjusted intravenous heparin (AR 0/97 [0%] with LMWH *v* 7/103 [6.8%] with iv heparin; P = 0.01).[38]

Harms: The first RCT comparing LMWH versus unfractionated heparin found no significant difference in the rate of major haemorrhage**G** (3/304 [1.0%] with LMWH *v* 5/308 [1.6%] with unfractionated heparin; P = 0.5).[39] The second RCT also found no significant difference in the risk of major haemorrhage (1/97 [1%] with LMWH *v* 2/103 [2%] with iv heparin; P = 0.6).[38] See harms of anticoagulation under treatments for proximal deep vein thrombosis, p 198. However, in both RCTs, the incidence of major haemorrhage was low and the number of people is likely to have been too small to detect a clinically important difference.[37,38]

Comment: None.

OPTION THROMBOLYSIS

Systematic reviews and one subsequent RCT found no significant difference in mortality between thrombolysis plus heparin and heparin alone, and found that thrombolysis may increase the incidence of intracranial haemorrhage. RCTs identified by a systematic review found no significant difference in mortality or recurrent pulmonary embolism among different thrombolytics.

Benefits: We found three systematic reviews,[39–41] one subsequent RCT,[42] and one large, non-randomised trial (see comment below).[43] **Plus heparin versus heparin alone:** All three reviews (search date 1998,[39] search date 2000,[40] and search date not reported[41]) identified the same nine RCTs (461 adults) comparing adding various thrombolytic agents to heparin versus heparin alone. The first review did not perform a meta-analysis and is not considered further.[39] The second systematic review found no significant difference in mortality or recurrence of pulmonary embolism between people treated with thrombolysis plus intravenous heparin compared with intravenous heparin alone (mortality: AR 11/241 [5%] with thrombolysis *v* 17/220 [8%] with heparin; RR 0.63, 95% CI 0.32 to 1.23; recurrent thromboembolism: AR 11/223 [5%] with thrombolysis *v* 19/205 [9%] with heparin; RR 0.59, 95% CI 0.30 to 1.18).[40] The third review also found no significant difference in a composite end point of death, recurrence of pulmonary embolism or major bleeding between thrombolysis plus heparin and heparin alone (56/241 [23%] *v* 57/220 [26%]; RR 0.9, 95% CI 0.57 to 1.32).[41] The subsequent RCT (256 people) comparing alteplase plus heparin versus placebo plus heparin for 2 days found no significant difference in in-hospital mortality over a mean 16.7 days (4/118 [3.4%] with alteplase plus heparin *v* 3/118 [2.2%] with heparin alone; P = 0.71).[42] However, it also found that people given heparin alone were significantly more likely to receive rescue thrombolysis than people given heparin plus alteplase (P = 0.004). This makes the results difficult to interpret.[42] **Versus each other:** One systematic review identified six RCTs (491 people) comparing different thrombolytic agents versus each other.[39] The review did not perform a meta-analysis. It found no significant difference in mortality or recurrent pulmonary embolism among different thrombolytics in the individual RCTs.

Harms: **Plus heparin versus heparin alone:** Two of the reviews[40,41] assessed haemorrhagic complications of thrombolysis, and we found one additional review (search date not reported).[44] The reviews defined "major haemorrhage"Ⓖ differently (see comment below). The first review found that thrombolysis plus heparin significantly increased the risk of major haemorrhage compared with heparin alone (33/241 [14%] with thrombolysis plus heparin *v* 14/220 [6%] with heparin alone, RR 1.76, 95% CI 1.04 to 2.98).[40] These results were robust to sensitivity analyses assessing methodological quality of study (high compared with low), and whether people were in shock or not in shock. The second review also found that thrombolysis plus heparin increased the risk of major haemorrhage compared with heparin alone (31/241 [12.9%] with thrombolysis plus heparin *v* 19/220 [8.6%] with heparin alone; RR 1.49, 95% CI 0.85 to 2.81).[41] The third review (16 RCTs, 1120 people) found a similar range of major bleeding event rates with thrombolysis compared with thrombolytics plus heparin or heparin alone (0–48% with thrombolytics *v* 0–45% with thrombolytics plus heparin *v* 0–27% with heparin alone; CI not reported).[44] It also found similar rates of major bleeding events with different thrombolytics (9–14%). It found that intravenous thrombolytics increased the proportion of people who had an intracranial haemorrhage compared with heparin (896 people; 1.2% with thrombolytics [half of which were fatal] *v* 0% with heparin alone).[44]

Comment: **Plus heparin versus heparin alone:** The three systematic reviews mentioned in the benefits section included only small RCTs and provide no evidence of benefit from thrombolysis with evidence of increased major haemorrhage. One additional, non-randomised trial (719 people), which excluded people with shock, found limited evidence that thrombolytics reduced overall mortality (8/169 [5%] with thrombolytics *v* 61/550 [11%] with heparin; RR 0.43, 95% CI 0.21 to 0.87) and recurrent pulmonary embolism over 30 days compared with heparin (13/169 [8%] with thrombolytics *v* 103/550 [19%] with heparin; RR 0.25, 95% CI 0.13 to 0.51).[43] However, these results should be interpreted with caution as people receiving heparin were older and more likely to have underlying cardiac or pulmonary disease than those receiving thrombolytics. **Definition of major haemorrhage:** The first review defined major haemorrhage as "intracranial or retroperitoneal haemorrhage or other bleeding requiring blood transfusion or surgery".[40] The second review defined major haemorrhage as "bleeding where it was fatal, intracranial, associated with a decrease in the haemoglobin level of at least 2 g/dl, or it required a transfusion of 2 or more units of red blood cells".[41]

QUESTION What are the effects of computerised decision support on oral anticoagulation management?

OPTION COMPUTERISED DECISION SUPPORT

We found no RCTs comparing computerised decision support versus usual management of oral anticoagulation that used clinically important outcomes (major haemorrhage or death). One systematic review and four subsequent RCTs found that, compared with usual care, the use of computerised decision

support in oral anticoagulation increased the time spent in the target international normalised range. Another subsequent RCT found no significant difference between computerised decision support and standard manual support in the time spent in the target international normalised ratio range.

Benefits: **Clinical outcomes:** We found no systematic review and no RCTs. **Laboratory outcomes:** We found one systematic review[45] and five subsequent RCTs.[46–50] The review (search date 1997, 9 RCTs, 1336 people) included eight RCTs using warfarin and one using heparin.[45] The computer systems advised the doses for initiation of anticoagulation (2 RCTs) and for maintenance of anticoagulation (6 RCTs). Follow up was short (15 days to 12 months). Indications for treatment included cardiac diseases and venous thrombosis. The outcome reported by seven RCTs (693 people) in the systematic review was the proportion of days within the target range of anticoagulation. The review found that computerised decision support**G** increased the time that the international normalised ratio**G** was in the target range compared with usual care (OR 1.29, 95% CI 1.12 to 1.49). Reanalysis, excluding one trial that introduced significant heterogeneity, found similar results (OR for remaining RCTs 1.25, 95% CI 1.08 to 1.45). The first subsequent RCT (285 people) compared a computerised decision support dosing system versus physician adjusted dosing in five hospitals.[46] People who were taking warfarin for at least 6 days were selected and followed for at least 3 months (results not analysed by intention to treat, results from 254 people [89%] analysed). People managed by computerised decision support spent significantly more time with their international normalised ratio in the target range than people managed conventionally (63% with computerised decision support *v* 53% with conventional management; $P < 0.05$).[46] The second subsequent RCT (244 people) compared a package of care that included computerised decision support versus traditional hospital outpatient management.[47] The intervention was based in primary care: a practice nurse clinic that included near patient international normalised ratio testing and computerised decision support. It found significantly more time spent in the target range after 12 months with packaged care versus traditional outpatient management (69% with packaged care *v* 57% with traditional care; $P < 0.001$), but found no significant difference in the proportion of tests in range (61% with packaged care *v* 51% with traditional care; reported as non-significant, no further data reported) or in the point prevalence of tests in range (71% with packaged care *v* 62% with traditional care; reported as non-significant, no further data reported).[47] The third subsequent RCT (101 people receiving oral anticoagulation after heart valve replacement) compared a computerised decision support system versus standard manual monitoring of international normalised ratio over 315 days.[48] It found no significant difference in the proportion of international normalised ratios in the target range or time spent in the target range (no further data and no mean follow up time reported). It found that people had significantly fewer dose changes with computerised than with standard manual monitoring (31% with computerised *v* 47% with manual; $P = 0.02$). The fourth subsequent RCT (335 people receiving initiation, 916 people receiving maintenance anticoagulation treatment for a variety of indications) compared a computerised decision support system for both dosing and appointment scheduling versus standard manual monitoring by "expert physicians".[49] It found that significantly more people managed by computerised decision support achieved a stable international normalised ratio in the first month and spent more time with their international normalised ratio in the target range over 3 months than people managed by standard monitoring (achieved stable range: 39% with computerised decision support *v* 27% with standard monitoring; $P < 0.01$, remained in range: 71% with computerised decision support *v* 68% with standard monitoring;

P < 0.001). The fifth subsequent RCT (122 people on warfarin after hip replacement) compared usual care versus computerised decision support.[50] Only initiation of warfarin was studied. It found that computerised decision support significantly reduced the mean time taken to reach therapeutic levels of anticoagulation compared with usual care (2.8 days with computerised decision support *v* 4.7 days with usual care; P = 0.002).[50]

Harms: One systematic review (search date 1997, 9 RCTs, 1336 people) found major haemorrhages**G** in 14/700 (2%) people with computerised decision support compared with 25/636 (4%) in the standard monitoring group.[45] Most of the events occurred in one study, making meta-analysis inappropriate. One RCT found no significant difference in overall mortality or serious adverse events with computerised decision support versus usual care.[46]

Comment: We found limited evidence (from small trials with short follow up of proxy outcomes) on the use of computerised decision support in oral anticoagulation management. Computerised decision support for oral anticoagulation seems to be at least as effective as human performance in terms of time spent in the target international normalised ratio range. It is not clear if this will translate to improved clinical outcomes. Larger and longer trials that measure clinical outcomes (particularly harms) are needed.

GLOSSARY

Computerised decision support system A computer program that provides advice on the significance and implications of clinical findings or laboratory results.

International normalised ratio (INR) A value derived from a standardised laboratory test that measures the effect of an anticoagulant. The laboratory materials used in the test are calibrated against internationally accepted standard reference preparations, so that variability between laboratories and different regions is minimised. Normal blood has an international normalised ratio of 1. Therapeutic anticoagulation often aims to achieve an international normalised ratio value of 2.0–3.5.

Low molecular weight heparin (LMWH) is made from heparin using chemical or enzymatic methods. The various formulations of LMWH differ in mean molecular weight, composition, and anticoagulant activity. As a group, LMWHs have distinct properties and it is not yet clear if one LMWH will behave exactly like another. Some LMWHs given subcutaneously do not require monitoring.

Major haemorrhage Exact definitions vary between studies but usually a major haemorrhage is one involving intracranial, retroperitoneal, joint, or muscle bleeding leading directly to death or requiring admission to hospital to stop the bleeding or provide a blood transfusion. All other haemorrhages are classified as minor.

Venae cavae filters Devices inserted in the inferior vena cava to prevent the migration of blood clots from the peripheral veins to the pulmonary circulation system.

REFERENCES

1. Nordstrom M, Linblad B, Bergqvist D, et al. A prospective study of the incidence of deep-vein thrombosis within a defined urban population. *Arch Intern Med* 1992;326:155–160.
2. Hansson PO, Werlin L, Tibblin G, et al. Deep vein thrombosis and pulmonary embolism in the general population. *Arch Intern Med* 1997;157:1665–1670.
3. Rubinstein I, Murray D, Hoffstein V. Fatal pulmonary emboli in hospitalised patients: an autopsy study. *Arch Intern Med* 1988;148:1425–1426.
4. Hirsh J, Hoak J. Management of deep vein thrombosis and pulmonary embolism. *Circulation* 1996;93:2212–2245.
5. Farley TMM, Meirik O, Chang CL, et al. Effects of different progestogens in low oestrogen oral contraceptives on venous thromboembolic disease. *Lancet* 1995;346:1582–1588.
6. Lagerstedt C, Olsson C, Fagher B, et al. Need for long term anticoagulant treatment in symptomatic calf vein thrombosis. *Lancet* 1985;334:515–518.
7. Lohr J, Kerr T, Lutter K, et al. Lower extremity calf thrombosis: to treat or not to treat? *J Vasc Surg* 1991;14:618–623.
8. Kakkar VV, Howe CT, Flanc C, et al. Natural history of postoperative deep vein thrombosis. *Lancet* 1969;ii:230–232.
9. Zilliacus H. On the specific treatment of thrombosis and pulmonary embolism with anticoagulants, with a particular reference to the post thrombotic sequelae. *Acta Med Scand* 1946;s171:1–221.
10. Giannoukas AD, Labropoulos N, Burke P, et al. Calf deep vein thrombosis: a review of the literature. *Eur J Vasc Endovasc Surg* 1995;10:398–404.
11. Lensing AWA, Prandoni P, Prins MH, et al. Deep-vein thrombosis. *Lancet* 1999;353:479–485.

12. Brandjes DPM, Heijboer H, Buller HR, et al. Acenocoumarol and heparin compared with acenocoumarol alone in the initial treatment of proximal-vein thrombosis. *N Engl J Med* 1992;327:1485–1489.
13. Landefeld CS, Beyth RJ. Anticoagulant related bleeding: clinical epidemiology, prediction, and prevention. *Am J Med* 1993;95:315–328.
14. Levine MN, Hirsh J, Landefeld CS, et al. Haemorrhagic complications of anticoagulant treatment. *Chest* 1992;102(suppl):352–363.
15. Hutten BA, Prins MH. Duration of treatment with vitamin K antagonists in symptomatic venous thromboembolism. In: The Cochrane Library, Issue 3, 2003. Oxford: Update Software. Search date 2000; primary sources Medline, Embase, hand searches of relevant journals, and personal contacts.
16. Pinede L, Duhaut P, Cucherat M, et al. Comparison of long versus short duration of anticoagulant therapy after a first episode of venous thromboembolism: a meta-analysis of randomized, controlled trials. *J Intern Med* 2000;247:553–562. Search date not stated; primary sources Medline, Embase, Cochrane Controlled Trials Register, and hand searches of reference lists.
17. van Dongen CJJ, Vink R, Hutten BA, et al. The incidence of recurrent venous thromboembolism after treatment with vitamin K antagonists in relation to time since first event. *Arch Intern Med* 2003;163:1285–1293. Search date 2001, primary sources Medline, Embase, hand searches of reference lists of pertinent articles, and personal contact with colleagues.
18. Ridker PM, Goldhaber SZ, Danielson E, et al. Long-term low-intensity warfarin therapy for the prevention of recurrent venous thromboembolism. *N Engl J Med* 2003;348:1425–1434.
19. Pinede L, Ninet J, Duhaut P, et al. Comparison of 3 and 6 months of oral anticoagulant therapy after a first episode of proximal deep vein thrombosis or pulmonary embolism and comparison of 6 and 12 weeks of therapy after isolated calf deep vein thrombosis. *Circulation* 2001;103:2453–2460.
20. Agnelli G, Prandoni P, Santamaria MG, et al. Three months versus one year of oral anticoagulant therapy for idiopathic deep venous thrombosis. Warfarin Optimal Duration Italian Trial Investigators. *N Engl J Med* 2001;345:165–169.
21. Hull R, Hirsh J, Jay RM, et al. Different intensities of oral anticoagulant therapy in the treatment of proximal vein thrombosis. *N Engl J Med* 1982;307:1676–1681.
22. Ascani A, Iorio A, Agnelli G. Withdrawal of warfarin after deep vein thrombosis: effects of a low fixed dose on rebound thrombin generation. *Blood Coagul Fibrinolysis* 1999;10:291–295.
23. Lensing AWA, Prins MH, Davidson BL, et al. Treatment of deep venous thrombosis with low-molecular weight heparins. *Arch Intern Med* 1995;155:601–607. Search date 1994; primary sources Medline, and manual and hand searches of references.
24. Belcaro G, Nicolaides AN, Cesarone MR, et al. Comparison of low-molecular-weight heparin, administered primarily at home, with unfractionated heparin, administered in hospital, and subcutaneous heparin, administered at home for deep-vein thrombosis. *Angiology* 1999;50:781–787.
25. Decousus H, Leizorovicz A, Parent F, et al. A clinical trial of vena caval filters in the prevention of pulmonary embolism in patients with proximal deep-vein thrombosis. Prevention du Risque d'Embolie Pulmonaire par Interruption Cave Study Group. *N Engl J Med* 1998;338:409–415.
26. Van der Heijden JF, Prins MH, Buller HR. For the initial treatment of venous thromboembolism: are all low-molecular-weight heparin compounds the same? *Thromb Res* 2000;10:V121–V130. Search date not stated; primary sources Medline, Embase, and Current Contents.
27. Breddin HK, Hach-Wunderle V, Nakov R, et al. Effects of a low-molecular-weight heparin on thrombus regression and recurrent thromboembolism in patients with deep-vein thrombosis. *N Engl J Med* 2001;344:626–631.
28. Harenberg J, Schmidt JA, Koppenhagen K, et al. Fixed-dose, body weight-independent subcutaneous LMW heparin versus adjusted dose unfractionated intravenous heparin in the initial treatment of proximal venous thrombosis. EASTERN Investigators. *Thromb Haemost* 2000;83:652–656.
29. Dolovich LR, Ginsberg JS, Douketis JD, et al. A meta-analysis comparing low-molecular-weight heparins with unfractionated heparin in the treatment of venous thromboembolism. *Arch Intern Med* 2000;160:181–188. Search date 1996; primary sources Medline, HEALTH, The Cochrane Library, and hand searches of references.
30. Lindhoff-Last E, Nakov R, Misselwitz F, et al. Incidence and clinical relevance of heparin-induced antibodies in patients with deep vein thrombosis treated with unfractionated or low-molecular-weight heparin. *Br J Haematol* 2002;118:1137–1142.
31. Van Der Heijden JF, Hutten BA, Buller HR, et al. Vitamin K antagonists or low-molecular-weight heparin for the long term treatment of symptomatic venous thromboembolism. In: The Cochrane Library, Issue 3, 2003. Oxford: Update Software. Search date 2001; primary sources Medline, Embase, Current Contents, hand searches of relevant journals, and personal contacts.
32. Couturaud F, Julian JA, Kearon C. Low molecular weight heparin administered once versus twice daily in patients with venous thromboembolism: a meta-analysis. *Thromb Haemost* 2001;86:980–984. Search date 1999; primary sources Medline, The Cochrane Library, hand searches of reference lists, and personal files of local experts.
33. van Dongen CJ, MacGillavry MR, Prins MH. Once versus twice daily LMWH for the initial treatment of venous thrombosis. In: The Cochrane Library, Issue 3, 2003. Oxford: Update Software. Search date 2001, primary sources Specialised Register of the Cochrane Peripheral Vascular Diseases Group to May 2001, the Cochrane Controlled Trials Register to Issue 1, 2002), hand searches of other relevant journals and cross-references, and personal contact with experts.
34. Schraibman IG, Milne AA, Royle EM. Home versus in-patient treatment for deep vein thrombosis. In: The Cochrane Library, Issue 3, 2003. Oxford: Update Software. Search date 2000; primary sources Medline, Embase, Cochrane Controlled Trials Register, and hand searches of relevant journals.
35. Brandjes DPM, Büller HR, Heijboer H, et al. Randomised trial of effect of compression stockings in patients with symptomatic proximal-vein thrombosis. *Lancet* 1997;349:759–762.
36. Barrit DW, Jordan SC. Anticoagulant drugs in the treatment of pulmonary embolism: a controlled trial. *Lancet* 1960;i:1309–1312.
37. Simonneau G, Sors H, Charbonnier B, et al. A comparison of low-molecular weight heparin with unfractionated heparin for acute pulmonary embolism. *N Engl J Med* 1997;337:663–669.
38. Hull RD, Raskob GE, Brant RF, et al. Low-molecular-weight heparin vs heparin in the treatment of patients with pulmonary embolism. American–Canadian Thrombosis Study Group. *Arch Intern Med* 2000;160:229–236.
39. Arcasoy SM, Kreit JW. Thrombolytic therapy for pulmonary embolism. A comprehensive review of current evidence. *Chest* 1999;115:1695–1707. Search date 1998; primary sources Medline and hand searches of reference lists of retrieved articles.
40. Thabut G, Thabut D, Myers RP, et al Thrombolytic therapy of pulmonary embolism: a meta-analysis. *J Am Coll Cardiol* 2002;40:1660–1667. Search date 2000, primary sources Medline, Embase, Current Contents, hand searches of reference lists of articles retrieved, and personal contact with experts in the field and manufacturers of thrombolytic agents.
41. Agnelli G, Becattini C, Kirschstein T. Thrombolysis vs heparin in the treatment of pulmonary embolism: A clinical outcome-based meta-analysis *Arch Intern*

Med 2002;162:2537–2541. Search date not reported, primary sources Medline and hand searches of reference lists of articles retrieved.
42. Konstantinides S, Geibel A, Heusel G, et al. Heparin plus alteplase compared with heparin alone in patients with submassive pulmonary embolism. *N Engl J Med* 2002;347:1143–1150.
43. Konstantinides S, Geibel A, Olschewski M, et al. Association between thrombolytic treatment and the prognosis of haemodynamically stable patients with major pulmonary embolism: results of a multicentre registry. *Circulation* 1997;96:882–888.
44. Levine MN, Goldhaber SZ, Gore JM, et al. Haemorrhagic complications of thrombolytic therapy in the treatment of myocardial infarction and venous thromboembolism. *Chest* 1995;108:291S–301S. Search date not stated; primary sources not stated.
45. Chatellier G, Colombet I, Degoulet P. An overview of the effect of computer-assisted management of anticoagulant therapy on the quality of anticoagulation. *Int J Med Inf* 1998;49:311–320. Search date 1997; primary source Medline.
46. Poller L, Shiach CR, MacCallum PK, et al. Multicentre randomised study of computerised anticoagulant dosage. European Concerted Action on Anticoagulation. *Lancet* 1998;352:1505–1509.
47. Fitzmaurice DA, Hobbs FDR, Murray ET, et al. Oral anticoagulation management in primary care with the use of computerized decision support and near-patient testing. Randomized Controlled Trial. *Arch Intern Med* 2000;160:2343–2348.
48. Ageno W, Turpie AG. A randomized comparison of a computer-based dosing program with a manual system to monitor oral anticoagulant therapy. *Thromb Res* 1998;91:237–240.
49. Manotti C, Moia M, Palareti G, et al. Effect of computer-aided management on the quality of treatment in anticoagulated patients: a prospective, randomized, multicenter trial of APROAT (Automated PRogram for Oral Anticoagulant Treatment). *Haematologica* 2001;86:1060–1070.
50. Motykie GD, Mokhtee D, Zebala LP, et al. The use of a Bayseian Forecasting Model in the management of warfarin therapy after total hip arthroplasty. *J Arthroplasty* 1999;14:988–993.

David Fitzmaurice
Senior Lecturer
Department of Primary Care and General Practice
The Medical School
University of Birmingham
Birmingham
UK

Richard F D Hobbs
Professor
Department of Primary Care and General Practice
The Medical School
University of Birmingham
Birmingham
UK

Richard McManus
Clinical Senior Lecturer
Department of Primary Care and General Practice
The Medical School
University of Birmingham
Birmingham
UK

Competing interests: DF has received reimbursement for attendance at scientific meetings from Leo Laboratories who make tinzaparin — a low molecular weight heparin. The Department of Primary Care and General Practice at the University of Birmingham, where the authors work, has a computerised decision support programme that is commercially available. FDRH is a member of the European Society of Cardiology (ESC) Working Party on Heart Failure, Treasurer of the British Society for Heart Failure, and Chair of the British Primary Care Cardiovascular Society (PCCS). He has received travel sponsorship and honoraria from several multinational biotechnology and pharmaceutical companies with cardiovascular products for plenary talks and attendance at major cardiology scientific congresses and conferences. RM none declared.

Varicose veins

Search date March 2004

Paul Tisi

QUESTIONS

INTERVENTIONS

See glossary G

Key Messages

- **Surgery (more effective than injection sclerotherapy)** We found no RCTs comparing surgery versus no treatment or compression stockings. RCTs have found that surgery reduced varicose vein recurrence and incidence of new varicose veins at 1–10 years compared with injection sclerotherapy.
- **Compression stockings** One crossover RCT found no significant difference in symptoms between compression stockings for 4 weeks and no treatment in people with varicose veins. However, the study may have lacked power to detect clinically important effects. One systematic review found that, in pregnant women with varicose veins, sodium tetradecyl sulphate sclerotherapy improved symptoms and cosmetic appearance of varicose veins compared with compression stockings after 6–24 months.
- **Injection sclerotherapy** One systematic review found no RCTs that compared injection sclerotherapy versus no treatment. One systematic review found that, in pregnant women with varicose veins, sodium tetradecyl sulphate sclerotherapy improved symptoms and the cosmetic appearance of varicose veins compared with compression stockings after 6–24 months. One RCT found no significant difference between polidocanol and sodium tetradecyl sulphate for improving the appearance of varicose veins at 16 weeks. One RCT reported a similar incidence of new varicose veins at 5 or 10 years with standard dose conventional sclerotherapy, high dose conventional sclerotherapy, and foam sclerotherapy. RCTs found that injection sclerotherapy was less effective at reducing varicose vein recurrence and incidence of new varicose veins at 1–10 years compared with surgery.

DEFINITION Although we found no consistent definition of varicose veins,[1] the term is commonly taken to mean veins that are distended and tortuous. Any vein may become varicose, but the term "varicose veins" conventionally applies to varices of the superficial leg veins. The condition is caused by poorly functioning valves within the lumen of the veins. Blood flows from the deep to the superficial venous systems through these incompetent valves, causing persistent superficial venous hypertension, which leads to varicosity of the superficial veins. Common sites of valvular incompetence include the saphenofemoral and saphenopopliteal junctions and perforating veins connecting the deep and superficial venous systems along the length of the leg. Sites of venous incompetence are determined by clinical examination, handheld Doppler, or duplex ultrasound. Symptoms of varicose veins include distress about cosmetic appearance, pain, itch, limb heaviness, and cramps. This review focuses on uncomplicated, symptomatic varicose veins. We have excluded treatments for chronic venous ulceration and other complications. We have also excluded studies that solely examine treatments for small, dilated veins in the skin of the leg, known as thread veins, spider veins, or superficial telangiectasia.

INCIDENCE/ PREVALENCE One large US cohort study found the biannual incidence of varicose veins to be 2.6% in women and 2.0% in men.[2] Incidence was constant over the age of 40 years. The prevalence of varicose veins in Western populations has been estimated in one study to be about 25–30% among women and 10–20% in men.[3] A recent Scottish cohort study has, however, found a higher prevalence of varices of the saphenous trunks and their main branches in men than in women (40% men and 32% women).[4]

AETIOLOGY/ RISK FACTORS One large case control study found that women with two or more pregnancies were at increased risk of varicose veins compared with women with fewer than two pregnancies (RR about 1.2–1.3 after adjustment for age, height, and weight).[2] It found that obesity was also a risk factor, although only among women (RR about 1.3). One narrative systematic review found insufficient evidence on the effects of other suggested risk factors, including genetic predisposition, prolonged sitting or standing, tight undergarments, low fibre diet, constipation, deep vein thrombosis, and smoking.[3]

PROGNOSIS We found no reliable data on prognosis, nor on the frequency of complications, which include chronic inflammation of affected veins (phlebitis), venous ulceration, and rupture of varices.

AIMS OF INTERVENTION To reduce symptoms, improve appearance, and prevent recurrence and complications, with minimal adverse effects.

OUTCOMES Symptoms, including pain, ache, itch, heaviness, cramps, and cosmetic distress or cosmetic appearance (self or physician rated); quality of life; recurrence rates; complications of treatment, including haematoma formation; pigmentation; ulceration; superficial thrombophlebitis; and deep venous and pulmonary thromboembolism. Retreatment rates were only considered if other outcomes were unavailable, and are described only in comments.

METHODS *Clinical Evidence* search and appraisal March 2004.

QUESTION What are the effects of treatments in adults with varicose veins?

OPTION COMPRESSION STOCKINGS

One crossover RCT found no significant difference in symptoms between compression stockings for 4 weeks and no treatment in people with varicose veins. However, the study may have lacked power to detect clinically important effects. One systematic review found that, in pregnant women with varicose veins, sodium tetradecyl sulphate sclerotherapy improved symptoms and cosmetic appearance of varicose veins compared with compression stockings after 6–24 months.

Benefits: **Versus no treatment:** We found one crossover RCT (72 people aged < 65 years with ≥2 of the following symptoms: pain, heaviness, itch, night cramps, swelling, or cosmetic distress).[5] People with a history of deep vein thrombosis were excluded. The study did not specify the sites of venous incompetence. It compared four treatments: a pharmacological agent (O-[beta-hydroxyethyl]-rutoside, 1 g/day orally), placebo alone, stockings plus placebo, and stockings plus the drug. Stockings were fitted to apply a pressure of 30–40 mm Hg to each ankle. Each treatment was given for 4 weeks before crossover to another treatment. The trial found no significant difference between stockings plus placebo and placebo alone for any symptom scores after each treatment (analysis not by intention to treat; 6 people excluded from analysis; symptom scores measured on 100 point visual analogue scale [high score = more severe]; pain: mean score 35 with stockings *v* 38 with placebo, P = 0.06; heaviness: 34 with stockings *v* 36 with placebo, P = 0.39; itch: 32 with stockings *v* 31 with placebo, P = 0.56; swelling: 28 with stockings *v* 35 with placebo, P = 0.13; night cramps: 22 with stockings *v* 25 with placebo, P = 0.24; cosmetic distress: 43 with stockings *v* 41 with placebo, P = 0.43). The RCT may have lacked power to detect clinically important effects. **Versus injection sclerotherapy:** See benefits of injection sclerotherapy, p 217. **Versus surgery:** See benefits of surgery, p 218.

Harms: The RCT did not report on harms of compression stockings.

Comment: **Versus no treatment:** The RCT did not report whether investigators were blinded to treatment allocation.[5] Reliability of results could be reduced because previous treatments might continue to have effects, even after crossover. The study did not report the duration of any washout period, which may have reduced such an effect between treatment periods.

OPTION INJECTION SCLEROTHERAPY

One systematic review found no RCTs that compared injection sclerotherapy versus no treatment. One systematic review found that, in pregnant women with varicose veins, sodium tetradecyl sulphate sclerotherapy improved symptoms and cosmetic appearance of varicose veins compared with compression stockings after 6–24 months. One RCT found no significant difference between polidocanol and sodium tetradecyl sulphate for improving the appearance of varicose veins at 16 weeks. One RCT reported a similar incidence of new varicose veins at 5 or 10 years with standard dose conventional sclerotherapy, high dose conventional sclerotherapy, and foam sclerotherapy. RCTs found that injection sclerotherapy was less effective at reducing varicose vein recurrence and incidence of new varicose veins at 1–10 years compared with surgery.

Benefits: **Versus no treatment:** One systematic review (search date 2002) found no RCTs.[1] **Versus compression stockings:** One systematic review (search date 2002) found one RCT (101 pregnant women with primary or recurrent varicose veins), which compared sclerotherapy using sodium tetradecyl sulphate versus compression stockings.[1] It found that sclerotherapy significantly improved symptoms and cosmetic appearance compared with compression stockings after 6–24 months (RR for improved symptoms and cosmetic appearance 1.61, 95% CI 1.19 to 2.18). **Versus surgery:** See benefits of surgery, p 218. **Different types of sclerosant:** One systematic review (search date 2002) found no RCTs reporting clinical outcomes in people with varicose veins.[1] We found one subsequent RCT.[6] This RCT (87 people with a total of 109 varicose veins; 55 veins 1–3 mm diameter; 54 veins 3–6 mm diameter) excluded people with saphenofemoral or saphenopopliteal incompetence.[6] Each vein, rather than each person, was randomly allocated to injection sclerotherapy with either polidocanol or sodium tetradecyl sulphate. The strength of solution depended on the size of vein being treated (veins 1–3 mm diameter: polidocanol 1% or sodium tetradecyl sulphate 0.5%; veins 3–6 mm diameter: polidocanol 3% or sodium tetradecyl sulphate 1.5%). The study found no significant difference between polidocanol and sodium tetradecyl sulphate in change in photographic appearance of either size group of veins 16 weeks after treatment (scale of 1–5 [1 = worse than pretreatment photograph; 5 = complete disappearance]; mean score for veins 1–3 mm diameter: 4.6 with sodium tetradecyl sulphate *v* 4.4 with polidocanol, P = 0.83; mean score for veins 3–6 mm diameter: 4.5 with sodium tetradecyl sulphate *v* 4.7 with polidocanol, P = 0.58). **Foam sclerotherapy versus conventional sclerotherapy:** We found one RCT in 887 people with uncomplicated varicose veins and long saphenous incompetence, with or without perforator incompetence.[7] It compared six treatment arms: standard dose conventional sclerotherapy (1–2 mL 2% or 3% sodium tetradecyl sulphate according to vein calibre, with 2–3 weeks' compression after sclerotherapy); high dose conventional sclerotherapy (3–6 mL 3% sodium tetradecyl sulphate, with 1–2 weeks' compression); foam sclerotherapy**G** (foaming agent plus 3% sodium tetradecyl sulphate); ligation**G**; stab avulsion**G**; and ligation plus sclerotherapy.[7] The RCT found that the incidence of new veins was similar with foam sclerotherapy, standard dose conventional sclerotherapy, and high dose conventional sclerotherapy at 5 and 10 years (AR for new veins at 5 years: 48% with standard dose sclerotherapy *v* 41% with high dose sclerotherapy *v* 44% with foam sclerotherapy; AR for new veins at 10 years: 56% with standard dose sclerotherapy *v* 49% with high dose sclerotherapy *v* 51% with foam sclerotherapy; significance not reported). We found one RCT (88 people with long saphenous incompetence), which compared sclerotherapy with 3% polidocanol foam versus 3% polidocanol liquid.[8] The RCT did not report on clinical outcomes other than harms (see harms below).

Harms: **Versus compression stockings:** The systematic review did not report on harms.[1] **Different types of sclerosant:** The RCT only reported local reactions.[6] It found that both treatments were associated with similar rates of ecchymosis (70% of veins treated with sodium tetradecyl sulphate *v* 58% with polidocanol), hyperpigmentation (64% with sodium tetradecyl sulphate *v* 53% with polidocanol), and thrombosis (46% with sodium tetradecyl sulphate *v* 42% with polidocanol; significance not reported for any comparison). Polidocanol reduced local urticaria and skin necrosis compared with sodium tetradecyl sulphate (skin necrosis 7% with sodium tetradecyl sulphate *v* 0% with polidocanol; urticaria 36% with sodium tetradecyl sulphate *v* 23% with polidocanol; significance not reported). **Foam sclerotherapy versus conventional sclerotherapy:** The first RCT did not discuss harms.[7] The second RCT found that skin inflammation was similarly common with polidocanol foam and polidocanol liquid (2/45 with foam *v* 3/43 with liquid; P value not reported).[8] **Versus surgery:** See harms of surgery, p 219.

Comment: **Versus surgery:** See comment under surgery, p 218. **Different types of sclerosant:** The subsequent RCT also included a further 42 patients with telangiectasia (veins < 1 mm diameter).[6] These were excluded from the results.

OPTION SURGERY VERSUS NON-SURGICAL TREATMENT

We found no RCTs comparing surgery versus no treatment or compression stockings. RCTs found that surgery reduced varicose vein recurrence and incidence of new varicose veins at 1–10 years compared with injection sclerotherapy.

Benefits: **Versus no treatment:** We found no RCTs. **Versus compression stockings:** We found no RCTs. **Versus injection sclerotherapy:** We found four RCTs comparing surgical versus non-surgical treatments for varicose veins.[7,9–11] The first RCT (164 people with symptomatic primary varicose veins, aged 21–65 years) compared surgery versus injection sclerotherapy (polidocanol 30 mg/mL; 0.5–0.75 mL injected into each varicosity, repeated after 1–2 weeks if required).[9] People were allocated to treatments without regard for site of venous incompetence (53 legs with saphenofemoral or saphenopopliteal incompetence alone; 97 legs with saphenofemoral or saphenopopliteal incompetence combined with perforator incompetence; 17 legs with perforator incompetence only). Among people allocated to surgery, the surgical technique depended on the site of venous incompetence (see comment below). It found that surgery increased the proportion of people who were free of varicose veins at 5 years compared with injection sclerotherapy (AR for freedom from varicose vein at 5 years: 55% with surgery *v* 3% with sclerotherapy; significance not reported; see comment below). The second RCT (249 people with varicose veins but no prior treatment, aged 15–64 years) compared surgery versus injection sclerotherapy.[10] The study did not specify the proportions of people with saphenofemoral, saphenopopliteal, or perforator incompetence. The extent and type of surgery depended on the site of venous incompetence (see comment below). The trial did not report on symptoms, quality of life, or recurrence (see comment below). The third RCT (82 people aged over 18 years) compared sclerotherapy (3% polidocanol; repeat treatments at 2 and/or 4 weeks as necessary) versus avulsion**G** under local anaesthetic.[11] People with saphenofemoral or deep venous incompetence were excluded. Sclerotherapy significantly increased recurrence at 1 and 2 years compared with avulsion (AR for recurrence at 1 year: 25% with sclerotherapy *v* 2.1% with avulsion; RR 12, 95% CI 1.62 to 88.7; AR for recurrence at 2 years: 37.5% with sclerotherapy *v* 2.1% with avulsion; RR 18, 95% CI 2.5 to 129.5). The fourth RCT, in 887 people with long saphenous incompetence, with or without perforator incompetence (see above), compared six treatments: standard dose conventional sclerotherapy (148 people); high dose conventional sclerotherapy (136 people); foam sclerotherapy**G** (150 people); ligation**G** (155 people); stab avulsion (144 people); and combined ligation and high dose conventional sclerotherapy (154 people).[7] Avulsion or ligation with or without sclerotherapy reduced the incidence of new varicose veins at 5 and 10 years compared with sclerotherapy alone, although it was not clear whether differences were significant (AR for new veins at 5 years: 48% with standard dose sclerotherapy *v* 41% with high dose sclerotherapy *v* 44% with foam sclerotherapy *v* 34% with ligation *v* 40% with stab avulsion *v* 37% with ligation plus sclerotherapy; AR for new veins at 10 years: 56% standard dose sclerotherapy *v* 49% high dose sclerotherapy *v* 51% foam sclerotherapy *v* 38% ligation *v* 41% stab avulsion *v* 37% ligation plus sclerotherapy; no significance tests reported).

Harms: **Versus injection sclerotherapy:** The first RCT reported postoperative wound infection in 6% and symptoms of sural or saphenous nerve injury in 10% of surgically treated patients (rates not reported in sclerotherapy group).[9] Five people (proportion not reported) in the sclerotherapy group had migratory thrombophlebitis and 28% developed haematoma (rates not reported in surgical group). Duration of sick leave was greater with surgery than with sclerotherapy (mean duration 20 days with surgery *v* 1 day with sclerotherapy; significance not reported). One person in the surgical arm had a symptomatic pulmonary embolism that resolved without complications. No thromboembolic events occurred in the sclerotherapy group. The second RCT reported that one person in the surgically treated group had severe bronchospasm under anaesthetic.[10] The 5 year follow up to this study reported that during surgery one person had a myocardial infarction and one person had a pulmonary embolus.[12] The third RCT found no significant difference in phlebitis between avulsion and sclerotherapy at 2 weeks (12% with avulsion *v* 27% with sclerotherapy; P = 0.07).[11] Sclerotherapy reduced telangiectasia (thread veins) at 2 years compared with avulsion (6.2% with avulsion *v* 0% with sclerotherapy; P = 0.039). The fourth RCT did not discuss harms.[7]

Comment: **Versus injection sclerotherapy:** The effects of surgery versus injection sclerotherapy or other treatments may vary according to the sites of venous incompetence. However, none of the identified RCTs reported relative effects with regard to sites of venous incompetence. In the surgical groups of the first two RCTs, varicose veins from saphenofemoral or saphenopopliteal incompetence were treated by ligation and stripping**G**, while incompetent perforator veins were treated by avulsion.[9,10] The first RCT did not report whether the investigators were blinded to treatment allocation.[9] It was not clear whether analysis was by intention to treat. The follow up rate at 5 years was about 77%. The second RCT found that surgery reduced retreatment rates compared with sclerotherapy at 3 years (14% with surgery *v* 22% with sclerotherapy; significance not reported).[10] The 5 year follow up of the same RCT also found that surgery reduced retreatment rates (24.2% with surgery *v* 40% with sclerotherapy; significance not reported; no blinding of assessors).[12]

GLOSSARY

Avulsion Used to treat multiple varicosities after saphenofemoral or saphenopopliteal ligation or in patients with perforator incompetence. Small incisions are made in the skin overlying each varicosity and the affected vein interrupted or excised.

Foam sclerotherapy A new technique in which a standard sclerosant is mixed with air to create a foam. This is then injected into the varicosities under ultrasound guidance.

Ligation Involves tying off a vein close to the site of incompetence to prevent blood flowing from the deep to the superficial system.

Sclerosant An injected solution which displaces blood from the vein, causing inflammation of the vein wall and occlusion. Commonly used sclerosants include sodium tetradecyl sulphate (sotradecol) and polidocanol (also called aetoxysclerol; aethoxysclerol; aethoxyskerol, or hydroxypolyaethoxydodecan).

Stripping A wire, plastic, or metal rod is passed through the lumen of the saphenous vein and is used to strip the entire vein out of the leg. This disconnects any superficial veins from the deep venous system.

REFERENCES

1. Tisi PV, Beverley CA. Injection sclerotherapy for varicose veins (Cochrane Review). In: The Cochrane Library, Issue 2, 2004. Chichester, UK: John Wiley & Sons, Ltd. Search date 2002; primary sources Embase, Medline, hand searches of references and relevant journals, and contact with manufacturers.
2. Brand FN, Dannenberg AL, Abbott RD, et al. The epidemiology of varicose veins: the Framingham study. *Am J Prev Med* 1988;4:96–101.
3. Kurz X, Kahn SR, Abenhaim L, et al. Chronic venous disorders of the leg: epidemiology, outcomes, diagnosis and management. Summary of an evidence-based report of the VEINES* task force. *Int Angiol* 1999;18:83–102.
4. Evans CJ, Fowkes FG, Ruckley CV, et al. Prevalence of varicose veins and chronic venous insufficiency in men and women in the general population. *J Epidemiol Community Health* 1999;53:149–153.
5. Anderson JH, Geraghty JG, Wilson YT, et al. Paroven and graduated compression hosiery for superficial venous insufficiency. *Phlebology* 1990;5:271–276.
6. Goldman MP. Treatment of varicose and telangiectatic leg veins: double blind prospective comparative trial between aethoxyskerol and sotradecol. *Dermatol Surg* 2002;28:52–55.
7. Belcaro G, Cesarone MR, Di Renzo A, et al. Foam-sclerotherapy, surgery, sclerotherapy, and combined treatment for varicose veins: a 10-year prospective, randomized, controlled trial (VEDICO Trial). *Angiology* 2003;54:307–315.
8. Hamel-Desnos C, Desnos P, Wollmann J-C, et al. Evaluation of the efficacy of polidocanol in the form of foam compared with liquid form in sclerotherapy of the greater saphenous vein: initial results. *Dermatol Surg* 2003;29:1170–1175.
9. Einarsson E, Eklof B, Neglen P. Sclerotherapy or surgery as treatment for varicose veins: a prospective randomized study. *Phlebology* 1993;8:22–26.
10. Chant ADB, Jones HO, Weddell JM. Varicose veins: a comparison of surgery and injection/compression sclerotherapy. *Lancet* 1972;2:1188–1191.
11. de Roos K, Nieman FHM, Martino Neumann HA. Ambulatory phlebectomy versus compression sclerotherapy: results of a randomized controlled trial. *Dermatol Surg* 2003;29:221–226.
12. Beresford SAA, Chant ADB, Jones HO, et al. Varicose veins: a comparison of surgery and injection/compression sclerotherapy. *Lancet* 1978;29:921–924.

Paul Tisi
Consultant Vascular Surgeon
Bedford Hospital, Bedford, UK

Competing interests: None declared.

Absence seizures in children

Search date September 2004

Ewa Posner

QUESTIONS

INTERVENTIONS

*We found no RCT evidence comparing valproate or ethosuximide versus placebo but there is consensus belief that valproate and ethosuximide are beneficial in typical absence seizures

See glossary G

Key Messages

Treatments

- **Ethosuximide*** We found one systematic review. It found no RCTs comparing ethosuximide versus placebo. There is, however, consensus that ethosuximide is beneficial, although it is associated with rare but serious adverse effects, including aplastic anaemia, skin reactions, and renal and hepatic impairment. The review found three small RCTs comparing ethosuximide versus valproate. It found no significant difference between ethosuximide and valproate in clinical response (as determined by either electroencephalogram or telemetry recordings, or observer reports of seizure frequency). The review found no RCTs comparing ethosuximide versus other anticonvulsants.
- **Lamotrigine** One RCT in children and adolescents who had previously benefited from lamotrigine found that lamotrigine increased the proportion of children who remained seizure free compared with placebo. However, lamotrigine was associated with serious skin reactions. We found no RCTs comparing lamotrigine versus other anticonvulsants.
- **Valproate*** We found one systematic review. It found no RCTs comparing valproate versus placebo. There is, however, consensus that valproate (sodium valproate or valproic acid) is beneficial, although it is associated with rare but serious adverse effects, including behavioural and cognitive abnormalities, liver necrosis, and pancreatitis. The review found three small RCTs comparing valproate versus ethosuximide. It found no significant difference between valproate and ethosuximide in clinical response (as determined by either electroencephalogram or telemetry recordings, or observer reports of seizure frequency). The review found no RCTs comparing valproate versus other anticonvulsants.
- **Gabapentin** One RCT found no significant difference between gabapentin and placebo in the frequency of typical absence seizures. However, the study may have lacked power to detect clinically important effects.

DEFINITION Absence seizures are sudden, frequent episodes of unconsciousness lasting a few seconds and are often accompanied by simple automatisms or clonic, atonic, or autonomic components. Typical absence seizures display a characteristic electroencephalogram showing regular symmetrical generalised spike and wave complexes with a frequency of 3 Hz and usually occur in children with normal development and intelligence. Typical absence seizures are often confused with complex partial seizures, especially in cases of prolonged seizure with automatisms. However, the abrupt ending of typical absence seizures, without a postictcal phase, is the most useful clinical feature in distinguishing the two types. Typical absence seizures should not be confused with atypical absence seizures, which differ markedly in electroencephalogram findings and ictal behaviour, and usually present with other seizure types in a child with a background of learning disability and severe epilepsy.[1] Typical absence seizures may be the sole seizure type experienced by a child. If this is the case and the child is of normal development and has no structural lesions, the child is said to have childhood absence epilepsy. Alternatively, typical absence seizures may coexist in children with other epileptic syndromes Ⓖ, such as juvenile myoclonic epilepsy or juvenile absence epilepsy, in which other seizure types are also present. This differentiation into typical versus atypical seizures is important, as the natural history and response to treatment varies in the two groups. Interventions for atypical absence seizures or for absence seizures secondary to structural lesions are not included in this chapter.

INCIDENCE/ PREVALENCE About 10% of seizures in children with epilepsy are typical absence seizures.[1] Annual incidence has been estimated at 0.7–4.6/100 000 people in the general population and 6–8/100 000 in children aged 0–15 years. Prevalence is 5–50/100 000 people in the general population.[2] Age of onset ranges from 3–13 years, with a peak at 6–7 years.

AETIOLOGY/ RISK FACTORS The cause of childhood absence epilepsy is presumed to be genetic. Seizures can be triggered by hyperventilation in susceptible children. Some anticonvulsants, such as phenytoin, carbamazepine, and vigabatrin are associated with an increased risk of absence seizures.

PROGNOSIS In childhood absence epilepsy, in which typical absence seizures are the only type of seizures suffered by the child, seizures generally cease spontaneously by 12 years of age or sooner. Less than 10% of children develop infrequent generalised tonic clonic seizures and it is very rare for them to continue having absence seizures.[3] In other epileptic syndromes Ⓖ (in which absence seizures may coexist with other types of seizure) prognosis is varied, depending on the syndrome. Absence seizures have a significant impact on quality of life. The episode of unconsciousness may occur at any time, and usually without warning. Affected children need to take precautions to prevent injury during absences and refrain from activities that would put them at risk if seizures occurred (e.g. climbing heights, swimming unsupervised, or cycling on busy roads). Often, school staff members are the first to notice the recurrent episodes of absence seizures, and treatment is generally initiated because of the adverse impact on learning.

AIMS OF INTERVENTION Cessation or decrease in the frequency of seizures, with minimum adverse effects of treatment.

OUTCOMES Seizure frequency measured as normalisation of the electroencephalogram; adverse effects of treatment with anticonvulsants. We found no studies assessing quality of life.

METHODS *Clinical Evidence* search and appraisal September 2004.

QUESTION **What are the effects of treatments for typical absence seizures in children?**

OPTION **VALPROATE**

We found one systematic review. It found no RCTs comparing valproate versus placebo. There is, however, consensus that valproate (sodium valproate or valproic acid) is beneficial, although it is associated with rare but serious adverse effects, including behavioural and cognitive abnormalities, liver necrosis, and pancreatitis. The review found three small RCTs comparing valproate versus ethosuximide. It found no significant difference between

valproate and ethosuximide in clinical response (as determined by either electroencephalogram or telemetry recordings, or observer reports of seizure frequency). The review found no RCTs comparing valproate versus other anticonvulsants.

Benefits: We found one systematic review (search date 2003).[4] **Versus placebo:** The review found no RCTs.[4] **Versus ethosuximide:** The review[4] found three small RCTs.[5–7] Results from the RCTs could not be pooled because each assessed different outcomes. The first RCT (28 treatment na ve children and adolescents aged 4–15 years with typical absence seizures) compared sodium valproate versus ethosuximide for up to 4 years.[5] Response was measured by 6 hour telemetry at two intervals 6 months apart, and parent and teacher reports of seizure frequency. The RCT found no significant difference in overall improvement between sodium valproate and ethosuximide (AR for > 50% decrease in the seizure frequency over 6 months: 12/14 [85.7%] with sodium valproate *v* 11/13 [84.6%] with ethosuximide; RR 1.01, 95% CI 0.74 to 1.39). The second RCT (45 children and adolescents aged 3–18 years with absence seizures, including children with other seizure types, children refractory to anticonvulsant treatment, and children who had not previously received any anticonvulsant treatment [treatment na ve children]) compared valproic acid versus ethosuximide followed by a crossover after 6 weeks.[6] Response to treatment was defined as no generalised spike wave discharges on 12 hour telemetered electroencephalogram. The RCT found no significant difference in response between valproic acid and ethosuximide at 6 weeks (na ve: 6/7 [86%] with valproic acid *v* 4/9 [44 %] with ethosuximide; RR 1.93, 95% CI 0.88 to 4.25; refractory: 3/15 [20%] with valproic acid *v* 4/14 [29%] with ethosuximide; RR 0.70, 95% CI 0.19 to 2.59). The third RCT (20 children aged 5–8 years) compared sodium valproate versus ethosuximide for up to 2 years in children with recent (< 6 months) onset of absence seizures.[7] Seizure frequency was assessed using electroencephalogram recordings and parent completed record cards. The RCT found no significant difference in complete remission of seizures between sodium valproate and ethosuximide (AR for remission of seizures [time to follow up not reported]: 7/10 [70%] with sodium valproate *v* 8/10 [80%] with ethosuximide; RR 0.88, 95% CI 0.53 to 1.46).[7] **Versus other anticonvulsants:** The review found no RCTs.[4]

Harms: Common adverse effects associated with valproate include dyspepsia, weight gain, tremor, transient hair loss, and haematological abnormalities. Rare adverse effects include behavioural and cognitive abnormalities, potentially fatal liver necrosis, and pancreatitis.[1] One RCT included in the review reported adverse events in children who had not previously received any anticonvulsant treatment.[6] The adverse events with valproate and ethosuximide included nausea, vomiting, poor appetite, drowsiness, dizziness, headache, and leukopenia. Transient thrombocytopenia occurred in two children with valproate. No child withdrew from the trial because of these events. Another RCT included in the review reported acute pancreatitis (1 child) and weight gain not responding to dietary restriction (1 child) with sodium valproate, and drowsiness (1 child receiving a high dose of ethosuximide).[5] The third RCT reported infrequent adverse events with both sodium valproate (transient nausea and vomiting, decreased number of platelets without thrombocytopenia) and ethosuximide (tiredness).[7]

Absence seizures in children

Comment: The RCTs comparing sodium valproate versus ethosuximide suggest a beneficial effect with sodium valproate and ethosuximide.[5–7] We found one study (crossover, 35 children: 19 with typical absence seizures, 14 with mixed seizures, 1 with astatic seizures, and 1 with generalised seizures) comparing sodium valproate versus ethosuximide or placebo for 4 weeks.[8] It found no significant difference in clinical effectiveness between sodium valproate and ethosuximide.[8]

OPTION ETHOSUXIMIDE

We found one systematic review. It found no RCTs comparing ethosuximide versus placebo. There is, however, consensus that ethosuximide is beneficial, although it is associated with rare but serious adverse effects, including aplastic anaemia, skin reactions, and renal and hepatic impairment. The review found three small RCTs comparing ethosuximide versus valproate. It found no significant difference between ethosuximide and valproate in clinical response (as determined by either electroencephalogram or telemetry recordings, or observer reports of seizure frequency). The review found no RCTs comparing ethosuximide versus other anticonvulsants.

Benefits: We found one systematic review (search date 2003).[4] **Versus placebo:** The review found no RCTs.[4] **Versus valproate:** See benefits of valproate, p 223. **Versus other anticonvulsants:** The review found no RCTs.[4]

Harms: Common adverse effects associated with ethosuximide include gastrointestinal disturbances, anorexia, weight loss, drowsiness, photophobia, headache, and behaviour and psychotic disturbances. Rare adverse effects include aplastic anaemia, serious skin reactions, and renal and hepatic impairment.[1] **Versus valproate:** See harms of valproate, p 223.

Comment: None.

OPTION LAMOTRIGINE

One RCT in children and adolescents who had previously benefited from lamotrigine found that lamotrigine increased the proportion of children who remained seizure free compared with placebo. However, lamotrigine was associated with serious skin reactions. We found no RCTs comparing lamotrigine versus other anticonvulsants.

Benefits: We found one systematic review (search date 2003).[4] **Versus placebo:** The review[4] found no RCTs in unselected children or adolescents with typical absence seizures, but it found one RCT in children and adolescents, in whom lamotrigine had previously been shown to be clinically effective.[9] The RCT (29 children and adolescents aged 3–15 years) with newly diagnosed typical absence seizures, in whom lamotrigine was clinically effective) compared lamotrigine versus placebo for four weeks.[9] Response was measured with 24 hour ambulatory electroencephalogram and a hyperventilation test**G** during the electroencephalogram. The RCT found that lamotrigine significantly increased the proportion of children who remained seizure free for 4 weeks compared with placebo (AR for remaining seizure free: 64% with lamotrigine *v* 21% with placebo; $P = 0.03$). **Versus other anticonvulsants:** The review found no RCTs.[4]

Harms: **Versus placebo:** The RCT reported abdominal pain, headache, nausea, anorexia, dizziness, and hyperkinesia with lamotrigine.[9] Skin rash was reported in 10/29 (35%) children, but only in one did the investigator consider it to be causally related to lamotrigine. The children from this

RCT were recruited into an open label continuation study (252 children; 43 [17%] with absence seizures), which looked at long term tolerability of lamotrigine.[10] A high proportion of these children (125/252 [50%]) discontinued, mostly because of inadequate response or for administrative reasons. The average duration of lamotrigine exposure was 96.7 weeks. The study found that the most common adverse events were dizziness (23/252 [9.1%]), somnolence (20/252 [7.9%]), nausea (16/252 [6.3%]), vomiting (13/252 [5.2%]), and headache (13/252 [5.2%]). We also found two open label add-on studies (study participants were receiving treatment for absence seizures at the time of enrolment and continue the treatment during the study) that reported on adverse events with lamotrigine.[11,12] The first add-on study (117 children aged 0–17 years with various drug resistant epilepsies) reported adverse events in 25/117 (21%) children during treatment with lamotrigine, including skin rash (mainly in children also receiving sodium valproate), ataxia, drowsiness, headache, and vomiting. Skin rash was reported as the main adverse event, occurring in 12 children (10 children were receiving valproic acid) 1–18 days after initiation of lamotrigine. No correlation was found with lamotrigine blood levels.[12] The second add-on study (285 children aged < 13 years with refractory epilepsies and ≥ 2 seizure types) found that rash was the most common adverse event leading to discontinuation of lamotrigine (total withdrawal rate 36/285 [12.6%]; withdrawal because of rash 21/285 [7.4%] from the study).[11]

Comment: The RCT randomised a group of children who responded to treatment with lamotrigine in an open label trial (potentially introducing selection bias).[9]

OPTION GABAPENTIN

One RCT found no significant difference between gabapentin and placebo in the frequency of typical absence seizures. However, the study may have lacked power to detect clinically important effects.

Benefits: We found no systematic review. **Versus placebo:** We found one RCT (33 children aged 4–16 years with absence seizures) comparing gabapentin (15–20 mg/kg daily) versus placebo.[13] The study consisted of a 2 week double blind treatment phase followed by a 6 week open label phase. Response was assessed as the change from baseline in seizure frequency (measured with quantified electroencephalogram) after 2 weeks. The RCT found no significant difference between gabapentin and placebo in frequency of typical absence seizures after 2 weeks. However, the trial may have lacked power to detect clinically important effects (see comment below). **Versus other anticonvulsants:** We found no RCTs.

Harms: The RCT found that somnolence and dizziness were the most frequent adverse events.[13] All reported adverse events were mild to moderate and no children withdrew from the study because of adverse events of treatment. This is consistent with the adverse effect profile of gabapentin reported by one other study.[14]

Comment: The RCT was of short duration and used relatively small doses of gabapentin.[13] The target dosage range was 15–20 mg/kg daily, although the current maintenance dose used in children with other types of epilepsy is 30 mg/kg daily.

Absence seizures in children

GLOSSARY

Epileptic syndrome The term used in the classification of childhood seizure disorders. It relates to a recognisable clinical and electroencephalogram pattern.

Hyperventilation test The test is performed by asking a child to breathe slowly and deeply for 3 minutes. In 90% of children with childhood absence epilepsy this will precipitate an absence attack.

REFERENCES

1. Panayiotopoulos CP. Treatment of typical absence seizures and related epileptic syndromes. *Paediatr Drugs* 2001;3:379–403.
2. Duncan JS, Panayiotopoulos CP. Typical absences and related epileptic syndromes. London: Churchill Communications Europe, 1995.
3. Panayiotopoulos CP. *A clinical guide to epileptic syndromes and their treatment*. Oxfordshire, UK: Bladon Medical Publishing, 2002:132.
4. Posner EB, Mohamed K, Marson AG. Ethosuximide, sodium valproate or lamotrigine for absence seizures in children and adolescents (Cochrane Review). In: The Cochrane Library, Issue 3, 2003. Oxford: Update Software. Search date 2003; primary sources Cochrane Epilepsy Group trials register, the Cochrane Central Register of Controlled Trials, Medline, Embase, and contact with various drug companies.
5. Callaghan N, O'Hare J, O'Driscoll D, et al. Comparative study of ethosuximide and sodium valproate in the treatment of typical absence seizures (petit mal). *Dev Med Child Neurol* 1982;24:830–836.
6. Sato S, White BG, Penry JK, et al. Valproic acid versus ethosuximide in the treatment of absence seizures. *Neurology* 1982;32:157–163.
7. Martinovic Z. Comparison of ethosuximide with sodium valproate as monotherapies of absence seizures. In: Parsonage M, et al. *Advances in epileptology: 14th Epilepsy International Symposium*. New York: Raven Press, 1983:301–305.
8. Suzuki M, Maruyama H, Ishibashi Y, et al. The clinical efficacy of sodium dipropylacetate and ethosuximide for infantile epilepsy by double-blind method: especially focusing on pure minor seizure. *Igakunoayum* 1972;82:470–488.
9. Frank LM, Enlow T, Holmes GL, et al. Lamictal (lamotrigine) monotherapy for typical absence seizures in children. *Epilepsia* 1999;40:973–979.
10. Duchowny M, Gilman J, Messenheimer J, et al. Long-term tolerability and efficacy of lamotrigine in pediatric patients with epilepsy. *J Child Neurol* 2002;17:278–285.
11. Besag FM, Wallace SJ, Dulac O, et al. Lamotrigine for the treatment of epilepsy in childhood. *J Pediatr* 1995;127:991–997.
12. Schlumberger E, Chavez F, Palacios L, et al. Lamotrigine in treatment of 120 children with epilepsy. *Epilepsia* 1994;35:359–367.
13. Trudeau V, Myers S, LaMoreaux L, et al. Gabapentin in naïve childhood absence epilepsy: results from two double-blind, placebo-controlled, multicenter studies. *J Child Neurol* 1996;11:470–475.
14. Anhut H, Ashman P, Feuerstein TJ, et al. Gabapentin (Neurontin) as add-on therapy in patients with partial seizures: a double-blind, placebo-controlled study. *Epilepsia* 1994;35:795–801.

Ewa Posner
Specialist Registrar in Paediatrics
Royal Victoria Infirmary
Newcastle upon Tyne
UK

Competing interests: None declared.

Acute otitis media in children

Search date February 2004

Paddy O'Neill and Tony Roberts

QUESTIONS

INTERVENTIONS

Key Messages

Treatments

- **Ibuprofen** One RCT in children aged 1–6 years receiving antibiotic treatment found that ibuprofen reduced earache as assessed by parental observation after 2 days compared with placebo.
- **Paracetamol** One RCT in children aged 1–6 years receiving antibiotic treatment found that paracetamol reduced earache as assessed by parental observation after 2 days compared with placebo.
- **Antibiotics (compared with placebo)** We found four systematic reviews comparing antibiotics versus placebo in acute otitis media. The reviews used different inclusion criteria and outcome measures. One review in children aged 4 months to 18 years found a reduction in symptoms with a range of antibiotics (cephalosporins, erythromycin, penicillins, trimethoprim–sulfamethoxazole [co-trimoxazole]) after 7–14 days of treatment compared with placebo. Another review in children younger than 2 years found no significant difference in clinical improvement after 7 days between antibiotics (penicillins, sulphonamides, amoxicillin/clavulanic acid [co-amoxiclav]) and placebo alone or placebo plus myringotomy. A third review in children aged 4 weeks to 18 years found that antibiotics (ampicillin, amoxicillin) reduced clinical failure rate within 2–7 days compared with placebo or observational treatment. The fourth review in children aged 6 months to 15 years found that, compared with placebo, the early use of antibiotics (erythromycin, penicillins) reduced the proportion of children still in pain 2–7 days after presentation, and reduced the risk of developing contralateral acute otitis media. This review also found that antibiotics increased the risk of vomiting, diarrhoea, or rashes.

- **Choice of antibiotic regimen** One systematic review in children aged 4 months to 18 years found no significant difference between a range of antibiotics in rate of treatment success at 7–14 days or of middle ear effusion at 30 days. Another systematic review in children aged 4 weeks to 18 years found no significant difference between antibiotics in clinical failure rates within 3–14 days. The second review also found that adverse effects, primarily gastrointestinal, were more common with cefixime than with amoxicillin or ampicillin, and were more common with amoxicillin/clavulanate (original formulation) than with azithromycin. Systematic reviews of placebo controlled RCTs have found that antibiotics increase the risk of vomiting, diarrhoea, and rashes.
- **Immediate compared with delayed antibiotic treatment** One RCT in children aged 6 months to 10 years found that immediate antibiotic treatment reduced the number of days of earache, ear discharge, and amount of daily paracetamol used after the first 24 hours of illness compared with delayed antibiotic treatment, but found no significant difference between groups in daily pain scores. It also found that immediate antibiotic treatment increased diarrhoea compared with delayed antibiotic treatment. Systematic reviews of placebo controlled RCTs have found that antibiotics increase the risk of vomiting, diarrhoea, and rashes.
- **Longer compared with short courses of antibiotics** One systematic review and two subsequent RCTs have found that 10 day courses of antibiotics reduce treatment failure, relapse, and reinfection at 8–19 days compared with 5 day courses, but found no significant difference between groups at 20–42 days. Systematic reviews of placebo controlled RCTs have found that antibiotics increase the risk of vomiting, diarrhoea, and rashes.
- **Myringotomy** One RCT in infants aged 3 months to 1 year found higher rates of persistent infection and lower rates of otoscopic recovery in children treated with myringotomy**G** plus placebo compared with children receiving antibiotic only. A second RCT in children aged 2–12 years found no significant difference between myringotomy only, amoxicillin only, and no treatment in reduction of pain at 24 hours or 7 days. A third RCT found higher rates of initial treatment failure (resolution of symptoms within 12 hours) with myringotomy plus placebo than with antibiotic only, for severe episodes of acute otitis media in children aged 2–12 years.

Preventing recurrence

- **Xylitol chewing gum or syrup** One RCT found that xylitol syrup or chewing gum reduced the proportion of children with at least one episode of acute otitis media compared with control. It found no significant difference between xylitol lozenges and control gum. It found that more children taking xylitol withdrew because of abdominal pain or other unspecified reasons compared with control.
- **Antibiotic prophylaxis (long term)** One systematic review in children and adults found that long term antibiotic prophylaxis reduced recurrence of acute otitis media compared with placebo. One subsequent RCT in children aged 3 months to 6 years found no significant difference between antibiotic prophylaxis and placebo in prevention of recurrence. A second subsequent RCT found that amoxicillin, but not sulfisoxazole reduced recurrence of acute otitis media within 6 months compared with placebo. The systematic review provided insufficient evidence on adverse effects of long term antibiotic prophylaxis, although one subsequent RCT reported that adverse effects included diarrhoea, vomiting, and thrombocytopenia. We found insufficient evidence on which antibiotic to use, for how long, and how many episodes of acute otitis media justify starting preventive treatment.
- **Tympanostomy (ventilation tubes)** One small RCT found that tympanostomy**G** tube insertion reduced the mean number of episodes of acute otitis media during the first 6 month period after treatment compared with myringotomy**G** alone or no surgery, but not during the subsequent 18 months. It also found a non-significant trend toward more recurrent infections and worse hearing after tube extrusion in those treated with tympanostomy. It found more tympanosclerosis in ears that received ventilating tubes compared with those that received myringotomy alone or no surgery.

DEFINITION Otitis media is an inflammation in the middle ear. Subcategories include acute otitis media (AOM), recurrent AOM, and chronic suppurative otitis media. AOM is the presence of middle ear effusion in conjunction with rapid onset of one or more signs or symptoms of inflammation of the middle ear. AOM presents with systemic and local signs, and has a rapid onset. The diagnosis is made on the basis of signs and symptoms, principally ear pain in the presence of a cloudy or bulging eardrum (and immobility of the eardrum if pneumatic otoscopy is performed). Erythema is a moderately useful sign for helping to establish the diagnosis. If the eardrum has a normal colour, then risk of AOM is low.[1] Uncomplicated AOM is limited to the middle ear cleft.[2] The persistence of an effusion beyond 3 months without signs of infection defines otitis media with effusion (also known as "glue ear"; see otitis media with effusion, p 624). Chronic suppurative otitis media is characterised by continuing inflammation in the middle ear causing discharge (otorrhoea) through a perforated tympanic membrane (see chronic suppurative otitis media, p 578).

INCIDENCE/ PREVALENCE AOM is common and has a high morbidity and low mortality in otherwise healthy children. In the UK, about 30% of children under 3 years of age visit their general practitioner with AOM each year, and 97% receive antimicrobial treatment.[3] By 3 months of age, 10% of children have had an episode of AOM. It is the most common reason for outpatient antimicrobial treatment in the USA.[4]

AETIOLOGY/ RISK FACTORS The most common bacterial causes for AOM in the USA and UK are *Streptococcus pneumoniae*, *Haemophilus influenzae*, and *Moraxella catarrhalis*.[3] Similar pathogens are found in Colombia.[5] The incidence of penicillin resistant *S pneumoniae* has risen, but rates differ between countries. The most important risk factors for AOM are young age and attendance at day care centres, such as nursery schools. Other risk factors include being white; male sex; a history of enlarged adenoids, tonsillitis, or asthma; multiple previous episodes; bottle feeding; a history of ear infections in parents or siblings; and use of a soother or pacifier. The evidence for an effect of environmental tobacco smoke is controversial.[3]

PROGNOSIS Without antibiotic treatment AOM symptoms improve in 24 hours in about 60% of children, and in about 80% of children the condition resolves in about 3 days. Suppurative complications occur in about 0.12% of children if antibiotics are withheld.[6] Serious complications are rare in otherwise healthy children but include hearing loss, mastoiditis Ⓖ, meningitis, and recurrent attacks.[3] The World Health Organization estimates that each year 51 000 children under the age of 5 years die from complications of otitis media in developing countries.[7]

AIMS OF INTERVENTION To reduce the severity and duration of pain and other symptoms; to prevent complications; to minimise adverse effects of treatment.

OUTCOMES Pain control (in infants this can be assessed by surrogate measures such as parental observation of distress/crying and analgesic use); incidence of complications such as deafness (usually divided into short and long term hearing loss), recurrent attacks of AOM, mastoiditis Ⓖ, and meningitis; resolution of otoscopic appearances; incidence of adverse effects of treatment.

METHODS *Clinical Evidence* search and appraisal February 2004.

QUESTION What are the effects of treatments?

OPTION ANALGESICS

One RCT in children aged 1–6 years receiving antibiotic treatment found that ibuprofen or paracetamol reduced earache as assessed by parental observation after 2 days compared with placebo.

Benefits: We found no systematic review but found one RCT (219 children aged 1–6 years with otoscopically diagnosed acute otitis media and receiving antibiotic treatment with cefaclor for 7 days), which compared the effect of treatment three times daily with ibuprofen or paracetamol versus placebo for 48 hours on earache (otalgia) and related outcomes.[8] It found that ibuprofen significantly reduced the incidence of earache after 2 days as assessed by parental observation compared with placebo (AR 5/71 [7%] with ibuprofen *v* 19/75 [25%] with placebo; RR 0.28, 95% CI 0.11 to 0.71; NNT 5, 95% CI 3 to 15), as did paracetamol (AR 7/73 [10%] with paracetamol *v* 19/75 [25%] with placebo;

RR 0.38, 95% CI 0.17 to 0.85; NNT 6, 95% CI 3 to 28). The RCT found no difference between paracetamol and ibuprofen in reducing earache, and no difference between ibuprofen, paracetamol, or placebo in other outcomes (appearance of the tympanic membrane; rectal temperature; and parental assessment of appetite, sleep, and playing activity).

Harms: The RCT found that 11 children experienced mild nausea, vomiting, and abdominal pain (5 [7%] taking ibuprofen *v* 3 [4%] taking paracetamol *v* 3 [4%] taking placebo). None were withdrawn from treatment.[8]

Comment: The evidence from this RCT is limited because the assessment of the child's pain relief was based on parental observation using a scale of 0 or 1.[8] The paracetamol versus placebo result has been recalculated by *Clinical Evidence* from data in the original publication, and corrects the stated conclusions of the RCT.

OPTION ANTIBIOTICS

We found four systematic reviews comparing antibiotics versus placebo in acute otitis media. The reviews used different inclusion criteria and outcome measures. One review in children aged 4 months to 18 years found a reduction in symptoms with a range of antibiotics (cephalosporins, erythromycin, penicillins, trimethoprim–sulfamethoxazole [co-trimoxazole]) after 7–14 days of treatment compared with placebo. Another review in children younger than 2 years found no significant difference in clinical improvement after 7 days between antibiotics (penicillins, sulphonamides, amoxicillin/clavulanic acid [co-amoxiclav]) and placebo alone or placebo plus myringotomyⒼ**. A third review in children aged 4 weeks to 18 years found that antibiotics (ampicillin, amoxicillin) reduced clinical failure rate within 2–7 days compared with placebo or observational treatment. The fourth review in children aged 6 months to 15 years found that, compared with placebo, the early use of antibiotics (erythromycin, penicillins) reduced the proportion of children still in pain 2–7 days after presentation, and reduced the risk of developing contralateral acute otitis media. This review also found that antibiotics increased the risk of vomiting, diarrhoea, or rashes.**

Benefits: **Versus placebo or no treatment:** We found four systematic reviews.[2,9–11] The first systematic review (search date 1992, 33 RCTs, 5400 children aged 4 months to 18 years) identified four RCTs (535 children) comparing antibiotics versus placebo in children receiving analgesics or other symptomatic relief.[9] Acute otitis media (AOM) was defined as bulging or opacification of the tympanic membrane with or without erythema, accompanied by at least one of the following signs: fever, otalgia, irritability, otorrhoea, lethargy, anorexia, vomiting, diarrhoea, and absent or poor mobility of the tympanic membrane. It found a significant increase in the rate of resolution of symptoms with a range of antibiotics (cephalosporins, erythromycin, penicillins, trimethoprim–sulfamethoxazole [co-trimoxazole]) after 7–14 days of treatment compared with placebo (ARI 13.7%, 95% CI 8.2% to 19.2%; NNT 7, 95% CI 5 to 12).[9] The second systematic review (search date 1997, 741 children aged < 2 years) identified four RCTs comparing antibiotics (penicillins, sulphonamide, amoxicillin/clavulanic acid [co-amoxiclav]) versus placebo alone or versus placebo plus myringotomy**Ⓖ**.[10] Three RCTs based diagnosis of AOM on otoscopic appearance of the tympanic membrane and clinical signs of acute infection, and one RCT based diagnosis on otoscopy findings alone. The systematic review found no significant difference between antibiotics and placebo in symptomatic improvement within 7 days (OR 1.31, 95% CI 0.83 to 2.08). The third systematic review (search date 1999, 5 RCTs, 1518 children aged 4 weeks to 18 years) compared the effects of antibiotics (ampicillin, amoxicillin) versus placebo or observation.[2] AOM was defined as the presence of middle ear effusion in conjunction with rapid onset of one or more signs or symptoms of inflammation of the middle ear, and was categorised as uncomplicated AOM when limited to the middle ear cleft. Clinical failure was defined as the presence of pain, fever, middle ear effusion, clinical signs of otitis media, or suppurative complications such as mastoiditis**G**. The review found that antibiotics (ampicillin, amoxicillin) significantly reduced clinical failure rate within 2–7 days compared with placebo or observational treatment (ARR 12.3%, 95% CI 2.8% to 21.8%; NNT 8, 95% CI 5 to 36). The fourth systematic review (search date 2000, 8 RCTs, 2287 children aged 6 months to 15 years) compared early use of antibiotics (erythromycin, penicillins, sulphonamides) versus placebo.[11] AOM was defined as acute earache with at least one abnormal eardrum, otoscopic middle ear effusion, and general signs and symptoms. Pain was assessed using parental report/score card/diary or clinician assessment at 4 days. The review found that antibiotics significantly reduced the proportion of children still in pain 2–7 days after presentation compared with placebo (182/1169 [15.6%] with antibiotics *v* 248/1118 [22.2%] with placebo; ARR 6.6%, 95% CI 3.4% to 9.8%; RR 0.30, 95% CI 0.19 to 0.40; NNT 15, 95% CI 11 to 30). In addition, it found that significantly fewer children experienced contralateral AOM with antibiotics (35/329 [10.6%] with antibiotics *v* 56/337 [16.6%] with placebo; ARR 5.9%, 95% CI 1.0% to 10.8%; RR 0.65, 95% CI 0.45 to 0.94). The review found no significant difference between groups in the rate of subsequent recurrence of AOM (187/864 [21.6%] with antibiotics *v* 175/804 [21.8%] with placebo; RR 0.99, 95% CI 0.83 to 1.19), abnormal tympanometry at 1 month (85/234 [36.3%] with antibiotics *v* 91/238 [38.2%] with placebo; RR 0.94, 95% CI 0.74 to 1.19), or abnormal tympanometry at 3 months (38/182 [20.9%] with antibiotics *v* 49/188 [26.1%] with placebo; RR 0.80, 95% CI 0.55 to 1.16). Four RCTs (717 children) reported pain outcomes (parental report of pain or symptom diary) 24 hours after presentation. All four RCTs found no significant difference in pain outcomes between antibiotics and placebo (RR 1.02, 95% CI 0.85 to 1.22). The review found only one reported case of mastoiditis in the included RCTs, which occurred in a penicillin treated group.[11]

Harms: Two systematic reviews gave no information on adverse events.[9,10] The third systematic review found that adverse effects, primarily gastrointestinal, were more common in children taking cefixime than in children taking amoxicillin or ampicillin (5 RCTs, total number of participants not reported; ARI 8.4%, 95% CI 3.8% to 13.1%; NNH 12, 95% CI 8 to 27) and were more common in children taking amoxicillin/clavulanate (original formulation) than in those taking azithromycin (3 RCTs, total number of participants not reported; ARI –18.0, 95% CI –28.0 to –8.0; NNH 6, 95% CI 4 to 13).[2] The fourth systematic review found that antibiotics significantly increased the risk of vomiting, diarrhoea, or rashes (AR 57/345 [17%] with antibiotics *v* 38/353 [11%] with placebo; RR 1.55, 95% CI 1.11 to 2.16; NNH 17, 95% CI 9 to 152).[11]

Comment: One systematic review[9] excluded two placebo controlled trials that were included in another review[11] because they included myringotomy**G** as part of the treatment. This may have biased the results in favour of antibiotic treatment and may explain the higher absolute risk reduction quoted in the first review.[9] Another systematic review commented on the difficulty in performing meta-analyses because of the varying criteria between studies for defining AOM and outcome measures.[2] The results of systematic reviews that compare antibiotics versus placebo may vary because of differences in entry criteria and outcome measures. One quasi-randomised trial from Sweden conducted in 1954 comparing the effects of antibiotics versus placebo found no cases of mastoiditis**G** in the penicillin treated group and 17% of cases in the control group.[12] Therefore, in populations in which the incidence of complicating mastoiditis is high, antibiotic treatment would be advised.

OPTION CHOICE OF ANTIBIOTIC REGIMEN

One systematic review in children aged 4 months to 18 years found no significant difference between a range of antibiotics in rate of treatment success at 7–14 days or of middle ear effusion at 30 days. Another systematic review in children aged 4 weeks to 18 years found no significant difference between antibiotics in clinical failure rates within 3–14 days. The second review also found that adverse effects, primarily gastrointestinal, were more common with cefixime than with amoxicillin or ampicillin, and were more common with amoxicillin/clavulanate (original formulation) than with azithromycin. Systematic reviews of placebo controlled RCTs have found that antibiotics increase the risk of vomiting, diarrhoea, and rashes.

Benefits: We found two systematic reviews.[2,9] One systematic review (search date 1992, 33 RCTs, 5400 children aged 4 months to 18 years) compared a range of antibiotics (cephalosporins, erythromycin, penicillins, trimethoprim–sulfamethoxazole [co-trimoxazole]).[9] Acute otitis media was defined as bulging or opacification of the tympanic membrane with or without erythema, accompanied by at least one sign (fever, otalgia, irritability, otorrhoea, lethargy, anorexia, vomiting, diarrhoea, poor or absent mobility of the tympanic membrane). Treatment success was defined as absence of all presenting signs and symptoms of acute otitis media at the evaluation point closest to 7–17 days after start of treatment. The systematic review found no significant differences between different antibiotics in rate of treatment success at 7–14 days or of middle ear effusion at 30 days. The second systematic review (search date 1999) found no significant difference between penicillin and ampicillin or amoxicillin in clinical failure rates within 7–14 days (3 RCTs, 491 children aged 4 weeks to 18 years; clinical failure rate difference +4.5%, 95% CI –1.8% to +10.7%).[2] The review also found no significant difference in clinical failure rates within 3–7 days between cefaclor and ampicillin or amoxicillin (4 RCTs, 56 children aged 4 weeks to 18 years; clinical failure rate difference –5.4%, 95% CI –15.2% to +4.4%). Clinical failure was defined as the presence of pain, fever, middle ear effusion, clinical signs of otitis media, or suppurative complications such as mastoiditis**G**.

Harms: See harms of antibiotics, p 231.

Comment: None.

OPTION IMMEDIATE COMPARED WITH DELAYED ANTIBIOTIC TREATMENT

One RCT in children aged 6 months to 10 years found that immediate antibiotic treatment reduced the number of days of earache, ear discharge, and amount of daily paracetamol used after the first 24 hours of illness compared with delayed antibiotic treatment, but found no significant difference between groups in daily pain scores. It also found that immediate antibiotic treatment increased diarrhoea compared with delayed antibiotic treatment. Systematic reviews of placebo controlled RCTs have found that antibiotics increase the risk of vomiting, diarrhoea, and rashes.

Benefits: We found one RCT (315 children aged 6 months to 10 years) comparing immediate versus delayed antibiotic (amoxicillin or erythromycin) use.[13] Acute otitis media was defined as acute otalgia and otoscopic evidence of acute inflammation of the ear drum, such as dullness or cloudiness with erythema, bulging, or perforation. Immediate antibiotic treatment was defined as a prescription given to parents at the initial consultation. Delayed antibiotic treatment was defined as follows: parents were asked to wait 72 hours after seeing the doctor before using the prescription, and to use the prescription only if the child still had substantial otalgia or fever, or was not starting to get better. Earache was assessed from daily diary of symptoms and perceived severity of pain scores (1 = no pain to 10 = extreme pain). The RCT found that, after the first 24 hours of illness, immediate antibiotic use significantly reduced the duration of earache (mean difference –1.10 days, 95% CI –0.54 days to –1.48 days), duration of ear discharge (mean difference –0.66 days, 95% CI –0.19 days to –1.13 days), number of disturbed nights (mean difference –0.72 days, 95% CI –0.30 days to –1.13 days), number of days crying (mean difference –0.69 days, 95% CI –0.31 days to –1.08 days), and the number of teaspoons of paracetamol used (mean difference –0.52 teaspoons daily, 95% CI –0.26 to –0.79 teaspoons daily) compared with delayed antibiotic use. The RCT found no significant difference between groups in mean daily pain score (mean difference –0.16, 95% CI –0.42 to +0.11), number of daily episodes of distress (mean difference –0.12, 95% CI –0.34 to +0.11), or days of absence from school (mean difference –0.18 days, 95% CI –0.76 days to +0.41 days).

Harms: The RCT found that immediate treatment significantly increased diarrhoea compared with delayed treatment (AR 25/135 [19%] with immediate *v* 14/150 [9%] with delayed; RR 1.9, 95% CI 1.08 to 3.66; NNH 11, 95% CI 5 to 125), but had no significant effect on rash (AR 6/133 [5%] with immediate *v* 8/149 [5%] with delayed; RR 0.84, 95% CI 0.30 to 2.36).[13] See harms of antibiotics, p 231.

Comment: None.

OPTION LONGER COMPARED WITH SHORT COURSES OF ANTIBIOTICS

One systematic review and two subsequent RCTs have found that 10 day courses of antibiotics reduce treatment failure, relapse, and reinfection at 8–19 days compared with 5 day courses, but found no significant difference between groups at 20–42 days. Systematic reviews of placebo controlled RCTs have found that antibiotics increase the risk of vomiting, diarrhoea, and rashes.

Benefits: We found one systematic review[14] and two subsequent RCTs.[15,16] The systematic review (search date 1998, 30 RCTs, 8215 children aged 4 weeks to 18 years with acute otitis media) found that treatment failure, relapse, or reinfection at an early evaluation (8–19 days) was significantly more likely with shorter courses of antibiotics (5 days) than with longer courses (8–10 days) (OR 1.52, 95% CI 1.17 to 1.98).[14] However, by 20–30 days there were no significant differences between treatment groups (OR 1.22, 95% CI 0.98 to 1.54). The first subsequent RCT (385 younger children with newly diagnosed acute otitis media, mean age 13.3 months, range 4.0–30.0 months) compared amoxicillin/clavulanate for 10 days (3 times a day) versus 5 days (3 times a day) followed by 5 days of placebo.[15] Clinical success or failure was assessed at 12–14 days and again at 28–42 days after starting treatment. Intention to treat analysis found that the 10 day regimen significantly increased clinical success on days 12–14 compared with the 5 day regimen (AR 158/186 [85%] for 10 days *v* 141/192 [73%] for 5 days; RR 1.16, 95% CI 1.04 to 1.28; NNT 8, 95% CI 5 to 30). However, by days 28–42 there was no significant difference in clinical success between the two groups (AR 108/185 [58%] for 10 days *v*

102/190 [54%] for 5 days; RR 1.09, 95% CI 0.91 to 1.30). The second subsequent RCT compared cefpodoxime/proxetil twice daily at 8 mg/kg daily for 10 days versus cefpodoxime/proxetil for 5 days followed by 5 days of placebo. It found that success rates were higher with the 10 day compared with the 5 day treatment group after 12–14 days (AR 199/222 [90%] for 10 days *v* 180/226 [80%] for 5 days; RR 1.13, 95% CI 1.04 to 1.22; NNT 10, 95% CI 6 to 30), but no significant difference was found after 28–42 days (AR 149/222 [67%] for 10 days *v* 141/226 [62%] for 5 days; RR 1.08, 95% CI 0.94 to 1.23).[16]

Harms: The systematic review and the two subsequent RCTs found no difference with short versus long courses of antibiotics in diarrhoea and/or vomiting and rash.[14–16] See harms of antibiotics, p 231.

Comment: None.

OPTION MYRINGOTOMY

One RCT in infants aged 3 months to 1 year found higher rates of persistent infection and lower rates of otoscopic recovery in children treated with myringotomy plus placebo compared with children receiving antibiotic only. A second RCT in children aged 2–12 years found no significant difference between myringotomy only, amoxicillin only, and no treatment in reduction of pain at 24 hours or 7 days. A third RCT found higher rates of initial treatment failure (resolution of symptoms within 12 hours) with myringotomy plus placebo than with antibiotic only, for severe episodes of acute otitis media in children aged 2–12 years.

Benefits: We found no systematic review but found three RCTs.[17–19] The first RCT (105 infants aged 3 months to 1 year with acute otitis media [AOM]) compared three treatments: antibiotic only (amoxicillin/clavulanic acid [co-amoxiclav]), myringotomy**G** plus placebo, and myringotomy plus antibiotic (co-amoxiclav).[17] AOM was defined as the presence of middle ear effusion and bulging (with or without redness of the tympanic membrane) associated with recent irritability or fever. The RCT found that those in the myringotomy plus placebo group had higher rates of persistent ear infection at 9–11 days compared with those receiving antibiotic alone (21/30 [70%] with myringotomy plus placebo *v* 2/30 [7%] with antibiotic alone; NNH 3, 95% CI 2 to 12) and lower rates of otoscopic recovery (7/32 [23%] with myringotomy plus placebo *v* 18/32 [60%] with antibiotic alone; NNH 3, 95% CI 2 to 5). The second RCT (171 children aged 2–12 years with AOM) compared no treatment, myringotomy only, amoxicillin (250 mg 3 times daily for 7 days) only, and amoxicillin plus myringotomy.[18] Diffuse redness, bulging of the eardrum, or both were taken as decisive. The RCT found no significant difference in pain between myringotomy only, amoxicillin only, and no treatment at 24 hours or after 7 days (pain at 24 hours: 26/36 [72%] with myringotomy *v* 34/47 [72%] with amoxicillin *v* 29/40 [72%] with no treatment; pain after 7 days: 31/35 [89%] with myringotomy *v* 43/46 [93%] with amoxicillin *v* 34/38 [90%] with no treatment).[18] The third RCT (536 infants and children aged between 7 months and 12 years with severe AOM or recurrent AOM) compared treatment with amoxycillin (40 mg/kg/day in 3 divided doses for 14 days) only, amoxicillin plus myringotomy, or myringotomy plus placebo.[19] AOM was diagnosed on the basis of fever, otalgia, or irritability with redness and/or bulging of the eardrum. An episode of AOM was classified as severe or non-severe according to the child's temperature and an otalgia score. The RCT found significantly higher rates of initial treatment failure (no resolution of symptoms within 12 hours) for severe episodes of AOM in children aged 2–12 years treated with myringotomy plus placebo compared with amoxicillin only (23.4% with placebo plus myringotomy *v* 4.1% with amoxicillin only).

Harms: The first RCT reported that, in those patients who had no diarrhoea at the start of the study, 7/60 [11.7%] receiving augmentin had three or more loose or watery bowel movements a day, as compared with 0/30 [0%] patients in the myringotomy**G** plus placebo group (P = 0.05).[17] The second RCT reported no difference in harms between the two groups.[18] The third RCT did not comment on adverse effects beyond treatment failures in the three arms of the study.[19]

Comment: Two RCTs provided results in the form of children or ears as the unit measured. Because randomisation was based on children, the figures reported here exclude those based on ears.[17,18]

QUESTION What are the effects of interventions to prevent recurrence?

OPTION ANTIBIOTIC PROPHYLAXIS (LONG TERM)

One systematic review in children and adults found that long term antibiotic prophylaxis reduced recurrence of acute otitis media compared with placebo. One subsequent RCT in children aged 3 months to 6 years found no significant difference between antibiotic prophylaxis and placebo in prevention of recurrence. A second subsequent RCT found that amoxicillin, but not sulfisoxazole reduced recurrence of acute otitis media within 6 months compared with placebo. The systematic review provided insufficient evidence on adverse effects of long term antibiotic prophylaxis, although one subsequent RCT reported that adverse effects included diarrhoea, vomiting, and thrombocytopenia. We found insufficient evidence on which antibiotic to use, for how long, and how many episodes of acute otitis media justify starting preventive treatment.

Benefits: **Versus placebo:** We found one systematic review[20] and two subsequent RCTs.[21,22] The systematic review (search date 1993) identified 33 RCTs comparing antibiotics versus placebo in prevention of recurrent acute otitis media (AOM) and otitis media with effusion.[20] Nine of the RCTs (945 people) examined recurrent AOM only. It was not clear from the review which of the studies referred only to children; four either included the word "children" in the title or appeared in paediatric journals. Most studies defined recurrent AOM as at least three episodes of AOM in 6 months. The most commonly used antibiotics were amoxicillin, trimethoprim–sulfamethoxazole (co-trimoxazole), and sulfamethoxazole given for 3 months to 2 years. All nine studies found a lower rate of recurrence with antibiotic treatment, although in seven of the studies the difference was not significant. Overall, the review found that antibiotics significantly reduced recurrence of AOM (AR of recurrence/person/month: 8% with antibiotics *v* 19% with placebo; ARR 11%, 95% CI 3% to 19%; NNT/month to prevent 1 acute episode 9, 95% CI 5 to 33). The first subsequent RCT (194 children aged 3 months to 6 years with 3 documented episodes of AOM within the preceding 6 months) compared amoxicillin (20 mg/kg/day) versus placebo.[21] The children were followed up monthly if they were asymptomatic or within 3–5 days if they had symptoms of upper respiratory tract infection for up to 90 days. The RCT found no significant difference between antibiotics and placebo in preventing recurrent AOM (RR of remaining AOM free, diagnosed by otoscopy and tympanometry 1.00, 95% CI 0.66 to 1.52 using completer analysis, 36 children lost to follow up). Calculations including those children lost to follow up yielded similar results whether the outcomes were assumed in favour of placebo or in favour of antibiotics. The second subsequent RCT (117 children with either a first episode of AOM before 6 months of age or two episodes before the first birthday) compared antibiotic treatment (amoxicillin 20 mg/kg/day or sulfisoxazole 50 mg/kg/day) versus placebo for 6 months.[22] The RCT found that amoxicillin significantly reduced recurrence compared with placebo at 6 months (freedom from AOM: 70% with amoxicillin *v* 32% with placebo; P < 0.01). Sulfisoxazole also reduced recurrence compared with placebo, but this difference was not significant (10% with sulfisoxazole *v* 29% with placebo; P value not reported). **Choice of antibiotic:** The systematic review found no significant difference in rate of recurrence between antibiotics.[20]

Harms: The second subsequent RCT reported adverse reactions, including vomiting, diarrhoea, rash, and thrombocytopaenia.[22] The number of infants affected within each treatment was not reported. Discontinuation rates for adverse reactions were similar among all treatment groups (2/40 [5.0%] with amoxycillin *v* 0/36 [0%] with sulfisoxazole *v* 2/41 [4.9%] with placebo; P value not reported). The study reported that no serious adverse reactions to amoxicillin, sulfisoxazole, or placebo occurred.

Comment: We found insufficient evidence on which antibiotic to use, for how long, and how many episodes of acute otitis media justify starting preventive treatment. In the second subsequent RCT, compliance with treatment varied between treatment groups.[22] The mean duration of treatment was 120.5 days for the amoxicillin group, 86.6 days for the sulfisoxazole group, and 98.6 days for the placebo group. The reported differences in outcome may be attributable to differences in duration of treatment.

OPTION XYLITOL CHEWING GUM OR SYRUP

One RCT found that xylitol syrup or chewing gum reduced the proportion of children with at least one episode of acute otitis media compared with control. It found no significant difference between xylitol lozenges and control gum. It found that more children taking xylitol withdrew because of abdominal pain or other unspecified reasons compared with control.

Benefits: We found no systematic review but found one RCT (857 children, 54% boys aged 6 months to 7 years) comparing xylitol (either as chewing gum, syrup, or lozenges) versus control (syrup or chewing gum) for 3 months.[23] The RCT randomised children into two groups according to their ability to chew gum. Children who could chew gum received xylitol gum (8.4 g/day, 179 children), xylitol lozenges (10 g/day, 176 children), or control gum (xylitol 0.5 g/day, 178 children). Children who could not chew gum received xylitol syrup (10 g/day, 159 children) or control syrup (0.5 g/day, 165 children). Each time the child showed any signs of acute respiratory infection, acute otitis media (AOM) was excluded using tympanometry and otoscopy. In the first group, xylitol gum significantly reduced the proportion of children with at least one episode of AOM compared with control gum (AR 29/179 [16%] with xylitol gum *v* 49/178 [28%] with control gum; RR 0.59, 95% CI 0.39 to 0.89; NNT 8, 95% CI 5 to 36), but it found no significant difference between xylitol lozenges and control gum (AR 39/176 [22%] with lozenges *v* 49/178 [28%] with control gum; RR 0.81, 95% CI 0.56 to 1.16). In the second group, xylitol syrup significantly reduced the proportion of children with at least one episode of AOM compared with control syrup (AR 46/159 [29%] with xylitol syrup *v* 68/165 [41%] with control syrup; RR 0.70, 95% CI 0.52 to 0.95; NNT 8, 95% CI 4 to 53).

Harms: The RCT found that significantly more children taking xylitol lozenges or syrup withdrew from the trial compared with control treatment (26/176 [15%] with xylitol lozenges *v* 8/178 [5%] with control gum; P < 0.001; 30/159 [19%] with xylitol syrup *v* 17/165 [10%] with control syrup; P < 0.03).[23] Most withdrawals were because of either an unwillingness to take the intervention, having left the area, or abdominal discomfort. We found no evidence on the long term effects of xylitol.

Comment: The children in this study received xylitol or the control intervention five times daily — a regimen that might be difficult to maintain in the long term.[23] The incidence of AOM in those who withdrew from the trial was not described; therefore, the reported effect of xylitol may be underestimated or overestimated.

OPTION TYMPANOSTOMY (VENTILATION TUBES)

One small RCT found that tympanostomy tube insertion reduced the mean number of episodes of acute otitis media during the first 6 month period after treatment compared with myringotomy alone or no surgery, but not during the subsequent 18 months. It also found a non-significant trend toward more recurrent infections and worse hearing after tube extrusion in those treated with tympanostomy. It found more tympanosclerosis in ears that received ventilating tubes compared with those that received myringotomy alone or no surgery.

Benefits: We found no systematic review but found one RCT.[24] The RCT (44 children aged 9 months to 7 years with bilateral recurrent acute otitis media (AOM) of equal severity in each ear despite over 3 months of antibiotic prophylaxis) compared tympanostomy**G** with ventilation tube insertion into a randomly selected ear, with the contralateral ear receiving either no surgery, or myringotomy**G** alone. Recurrent AOM was defined as the recurrent presence (more than 4 episodes) of otalgia with red and bulging tympanic membranes. The RCT found that tympanostomy tube insertion significantly reduced the mean number of episodes of AOM during the first 6 months after treatment compared with myringotomy alone or no surgery (actual mean difference: 0.6% with myringotomy alone *v* 1.8% with no surgery; difference in mean number of episodes –1.2, 95% CI –2.2 to –0.9). However, the RCT found that tympanostomy tube insertion did not significantly reduce the mean number of episodes of AOM during the subsequent 18 months (actual mean difference: 0.8% with myringotomy *v* 0.8% with no surgery; difference in mean number of episodes 0%, 95% CI –0.3 to +0.3).[24]

Harms: The RCT reported a non-significant trend (P = 0.30) toward more recurrent infections and worse hearing in ears that had received tympanostomy**G** tubes, which became apparent after tube extrusion.[24] Anatomical abnormalities (tympanosclerosis, atrophy, or retraction and chronic perforation, though not thought to be clinically significant) were more common in the ears receiving tympanostomy tubes. There was significantly more tympanosclerosis in ears that received tympanostomy tubes than in those that received myringotomy**G** alone (35/61 [57.4%] with tympanostomy tubes *v* 5/26 [19.2%] with myringotomy alone; P = 0.004) or no surgery (35/61 [57.4%] with tympanostomy tubes *v* 2/27 [7.4%] with no surgery; P ≤ 0.0001). At the 2 year evaluation the hearing was poorer in ears with anatomical abnormalities.

Comment: The RCT included some children with otitis media with effusion, although the results concerning benefits presented here refer only to those children in the study with recurrent AOM. It was not possible from the data available to differentiate the evidence on harms into children with recurrent AOM compared with otitis media with effusion. Medical treatment and antibiotic prophylaxis were allowed "whenever indicated". It was not possible from the data presented to tell whether the different groups differed in the amount of medical treatment and prophylactic antibiotics.

Acute otitis media in children

GLOSSARY

Mastoiditis The presence of infection in mastoid cavity.
Myringotomy The surgical creation of a perforation in tympanic membrane.
Tympanostomy The surgical creation of a perforation in tympanic membrane for the purpose of inserting a ventilation tube.

REFERENCES

1. Rothman R, Owens T, Simel DL. Does this child have acute otitis media? *JAMA* 2003;290:1633–1640.
2. Marcy M, Takata G, Shekelle P, et al. *Management of Acute Otitis Media. Evidence Report/Technology Assessment No. 15.* (Prepared by the Southern California Evidence Based Practice Centre under contract No. 290–97–0001.) AHRQ Publication No. 01-E010. Rockville, MD: Agency for Healthcare Research and Quality, May 2001. Search date 1999; primary sources Medline, Cochrane library, Health STAR, International Pharmaceutical Abstracts, CINAL, BIOSS, and EMBASE.
3. Froom J, Culpepper L, Jacobs M, et al. Antimicrobials for acute otitis media? A review from the International Primary Care Network. *BMJ* 1997;315:98–102.
4. Del Mar C, Glasziou P, Hayem M. Are antibiotics indicated as initial treatment for children with acute otitis media? A meta-analysis. *BMJ* 1997;314:1526–1529. Search date 1994; primary sources Medline and Current Contents.
5. Berman S. Otitis media in developing countries. *Pediatrics* 1995;96:126–131.
6. Rosenfeld RM. Natural history of untreated otitis media. *Laryngoscope* 2003;113:1645–1657.
7. World Health Organization. *World Development Report 1993: Investing in Health.* Oxford: Oxford University Press, 1993:215–222.
8. Bertin L, Pons G, d'Athis P, et al. A randomized double blind multicentre controlled trial of ibuprofen versus acetaminophen and placebo for symptoms of acute otitis media in children. *Fundam Clin Pharmacol* 1996;10:387–392.
9. Rosenfeld RM, Vertrees JE, Carr J, et al. Clinical efficacy of antimicrobial drugs for acute otitis media: meta-analysis of 5400 children from thirty-three randomised trials. *J Pediatr* 1994;124:355–367. Search date 1992; primary sources Medline and Current Contents.
10. Damoiseaux RA, van Balen FAM, Hoes AW, et al. Antibiotic treatment of acute otitis media in children under two years of age: evidence based? *Br J Gen Pract* 1998;48:1861–1864. Search date 1997; primary sources Medline, Embase, and hand searched references.
11. Glasziou PP, Del Mar CB, Sanders SL, et al. Antibiotics for acute otitis media in children. In: The Cochrane Library, Issue 1, 2004. Chichester, UK: John Wiley & Sons, Ltd. Search date 2000; primary sources Medline, Current Contents, reference lists, Cochrane Controlled Trials Register, and Index Medicus.
12. Rudberg, RD. Acute otitis media: comparative therapeutic results of sulphonamide and penicillin administered in various forms. *Acta Otolaryngol* 1954;113(suppl):1–79.
13. Little P, Gould C, Williamson I, et al. Pragmatic randomised controlled trial of two prescribing strategies for childhood acute otitis media. *BMJ* 2001;322:336–342.
14. Kozyrskyj AL, Hildes-Ripstein GE, Longstaffe SEA, et al. Short course antibiotics for acute otitis media. In: The Cochrane Library, Issue 1, 2004. Chichester, UK: John Wiley & Sons, Ltd. Search date 1998; primary sources Medline, Embase, Science Citation Index, Current Contents, hand searches of reference lists, and personal contacts.
15. Cohen R, Levy C, Boucherat M, et al. A multicenter randomized, double blind trial of 5 versus 10 days of antibiotic therapy for acute otitis media in young children. *J Pediatr* 1998;133:634–639.
16. Cohen R, Levy C, Boucherat M, et al. Five vs. ten days of antibiotic therapy for acute otitis media in young children. *Pediatr Infect Dis J* 2000;19:458–463.
17. Engelhard D, Cohen D, Strauss N, et al. Randomised study of myringotomy, amoxycillin/clavulanate, or both for acute otitis media in infants. *Lancet* 1989;2:141–143.
18. van Buchem FL, Dunk JH, van't Hof MA. Therapy of acute otitis media: myringotomy, antibiotics, or neither? A double blind study in children. *Lancet* 1981;318:883–887.
19. Kaleida PH, Casselbrant ML, Rockette HE, et al. Amoxicillin or myringotomy or both for acute otitis media: results of a randomised clinical trial. *Pediatrics* 1991;87:466–474.
20. Williams RL, Chalmers TC, Stange KC, et al. Use of antibiotics in preventing recurrent acute otitis media and in treating otitis media with effusion: a meta-analytic attempt to resolve the brouhaha. *JAMA* 1993;270:1344–1351. [Erratum in *JAMA* 1994;27:430]. Search date 1993; primary sources Medline and Current Contents.
21. Roark R, Berman S. Continuous twice daily or once daily amoxycillin prophylaxis compared with placebo for children with recurrent acute otitis media. *Pediatr Infect Dis J* 1997;16:376–378.
22. Teele DW, Klein JO, Word BM, et al. Antimicrobial prophylaxis for infants at risk for recurrent acute otitis media. *Vaccine* 2001;19(suppl 1):S140–S143.
23. Uhari M, Kontiokari T, Niemela MA. Novel use of xylitol sugar in preventing acute otitis media. *Pediatrics* 1998;102:879–884.
24. Le CT, Freeman DW, Fireman BH. Evaluation of ventilating tubes and myringotomy in the treatment of recurrent or persistent otitis media. *Pediatr Infect Dis J* 1991;10:2–11.

Paddy O'Neill
General Practitioner
Norton Medical Centre
Stockton on Tees
UK

Tony Roberts
Clinical Effectiveness Advisor and
Honorary Research Fellow
South Tees Hospitals Trust
North Tees Primary Care Trust
and The University of Durham
UK

Competing interests: None declared.

Asthma and other wheezing disorders in children

Search date June 2003

Duncan Keeley and Michael McKean

QUESTIONS

INTERVENTIONS

Asthma and other wheezing disorders in children

*In the absence of RCT evidence, categorisation based on observational evidence and strong consensus belief that oxygen is beneficial

See glossary G

Key Messages

Treating acute asthma in children

- **Oxygen** An RCT comparing oxygen treatment with no oxygen treatment in acute severe asthma would be considered unethical. One prospective cohort study and clinical experience support the need for oxygen in acute asthma.
- **High dose inhaled corticosteroids** We found one systematic review that identified four RCTs comparing high dose inhaled with oral corticosteroids in children. Three RCTs found no significant difference in hospital admission with nebulised budesonide or dexamethasone compared with oral prednisolone in children with mild to moderate asthma. One RCT in children with moderate to severe asthma found that, compared with inhaled fluticasone, oral prednisolone reduced hospital admission and improved lung function at 4 hours. A subsequent RCT in children aged 4–16 years found that, compared with oral prednisolone, nebulised fluticasone improved lung function over 7 days. Another RCT in children aged 5–16 years admitted to hospital with severe asthma found no significant difference with nebulised budesonide compared with oral prednisolone in lung function at 24 hours or 24 days after admission.
- **Inhaled ipratropium bromide added to β_2 agonists (in emergency room)** One systematic review has found that, compared with β_2 agonist alone, multiple doses of inhaled ipratropium bromide plus an inhaled β_2 agonist (fenoterol or salbutamol) reduced hospital admissions and improved lung function in children aged 18 months to 17 years with severe asthma exacerbations. In children with mild to moderate asthma exacerbations, a single dose of inhaled ipratropium bromide plus a β_2 agonist (fenoterol, salbutamol, or terbutaline) compared with a β_2 agonist alone improved lung function for up to 2 hours, but did not reduce hospital admissions.
- **Metered dose inhaler plus spacer devices for delivery of β_2 agonists (as effective as nebulisers)** One systematic review in children with acute but not life threatening asthma, who were old enough to use a spacer, has found no significant difference in hospital admission rates with a metered dose inhaler plus a spacer versus nebulisation for delivering β_2 agonists (fenoterol, salbutamol, or terbutaline) or β agonist (orciprenaline). Children using a metered dose inhaler with a spacer may have shorter stays in emergency departments, less hypoxia, and lower pulse rates compared with children receiving β_2 agonist by nebulisation.
- **Systemic corticosteroids** One systematic review has found that systemic corticosteroids increase the likelihood of early discharge and reduce the frequency of relapse within 1–3 months in children hospitalised with acute asthma.

- **Intravenous theophylline** One systematic review found that in children aged 1–19 years admitted to hospital with severe asthma, intravenous theophylline improved lung function and symptom scores 6–8 hours after treatment compared with placebo, but found no significant difference in number of bronchodilator treatments required or length of hospital stay. A subsequent RCT in children aged 1–17 years admitted to an intensive care unit with severe asthma found that, compared with controls, intravenous theophylline decreased the time to reach a clinical asthma score of 3 or less but found no significant difference in length of stay in the intensive care unit.
- **Inhaled ipratropium bromide added to salbutamol (after initial stabilisation)** One RCT in children admitted to hospital with initially stabilised severe asthma found no significant difference in clinical asthma scores during the first 36 hours with nebulised ipratropium bromide compared with placebo added to salbutamol (a β_2 agonist) and corticosteroid (hydrocortisone or prednisone).

Single agent prophylaxis in childhood asthma

- **Inhaled corticosteroids** One systematic review has found that, compared with placebo, prophylactic inhaled corticosteroids improve symptoms and lung function in children with asthma. Several RCTs have found that inhaled corticosteroids slightly reduce growth rate compared with placebo, although studies with long term follow up suggest attainment of normal adult height. Inhaled corticosteroids have been associated with rare reports of adrenal suppression. One RCT in children aged 6–16 years found no significant difference in improvement of asthma symptoms with inhaled beclometasone compared with theophylline, but found less use of bronchodilators and oral corticosteroids with inhaled beclometasone. Small RCTs have found inhaled corticosteroids to be more effective than sodium cromoglicate in improving symptoms and lung function. RCTs in children aged 5–16 years have found that, compared with inhaled long acting β_2 agonists (salmeterol) or inhaled nedocromil, inhaled corticosteroids (beclometasone, budesonide, or fluticasone) improve symptoms and lung function in children with asthma.
- **Inhaled nedocromil** Two RCTs in children aged 6–12 years found that, compared with placebo, inhaled nedocromil reduces asthma symptom scores, asthma severity, bronchodilator use, and improves lung function. One large RCT in children aged 5–12 years with mild to moderate asthma found no significant difference between nedocromil and budesonide or placebo in lung function, hospital admission rate, or the symptom score on diary cards, but found that budesonide was superior to nedocromil, and that nedocromil was superior to placebo in several measures of asthma symptoms and morbidity.
- **Oral montelukast** One RCT in children aged 6–14 years found that, compared with placebo, oral montelukast (a leukotriene receptor antagonist) increased from baseline the mean morning forced expiratory volume in 1 second and reduced the total daily β_2 agonist use, but found no significant difference in daytime asthma symptom score or in nocturnal awakenings with asthma. Another RCT in children aged 2–5 years found that, compared with placebo, oral montelukast improved average daytime symptom scores and reduced the need for rescue oral steroid courses, but found no significant difference in average overnight asthma symptom scores. We found no RCTs directly comparing oral montelukast with inhaled corticosteroids.
- **Inhaled salmeterol** Two RCTs in children aged 4–14 years found that, compared with placebo, inhaled salmeterol improved lung function but found conflicting evidence about reduced use of salbutamol. One RCT comparing inhaled salmeterol with beclometasone found that salmeterol was associated with a significant deterioration in bronchial reactivity.

- **Oral theophylline** One small RCT in children aged 6–15 years found that, compared with placebo, oral theophylline increased mean morning peak expiratory flow rate and reduced the mean number of acute night time attacks and doses of bronchodilator used. Another RCT in children aged 6–16 years found no significant difference in improvement of asthma symptoms with oral theophylline compared with inhaled beclometasone, but found greater use of bronchodilators and oral corticosteroids with theophylline over 1 year. Theophylline has serious adverse effects (cardiac arrhythmia, convulsions) if therapeutic blood concentrations are exceeded.
- **Inhaled sodium cromoglicate** One systematic review found insufficient evidence for prophylactic treatment with sodium cromoglicate in children aged less than 1 year to 18 years. Several small comparative RCTs found sodium cromoglicate to be less effective than inhaled corticosteroids in improving symptoms and lung function.

Additional prophylactic treatments in childhood asthma inadequately controlled by standard dose inhaled corticosteroids

- **Increased dose of inhaled beclometasone** One RCT in children aged 6–16 years taking inhaled beclometasone (a corticosteroid) comparing the addition of a second dose of beclometasone with placebo found no significant difference in lung function, symptom scores, exacerbation rates, or bronchial reactivity but found a reduction in growth velocity at 1 year.
- **Inhaled salmeterol** One RCT in children aged 6–16 years found that addition of salmeterol (a long acting β_2 agonist) increased peak expiratory flow rates in the first few months of treatment but found no increase after 1 year. A second short term RCT in children aged 4–16 years also found increased morning peak expiratory flow rates and more symptom free days at 3 months with addition of salmeterol.
- **Oral montelukast** One crossover RCT in children aged 6–14 years with persistent asthma who had been taking inhaled budesonide for at least 6 weeks found that, compared with addition of placebo, oral montelukast (a leukotriene receptor antagonist) reduced asthma exacerbations over 4 weeks. This difference was statistically significant but modest in clinical terms.
- **Oral theophylline** One small RCT found that addition of theophylline, compared with placebo, to previous treatment increased the proportion of symptom free days and reduced the use of additional orciprenaline (a β agonist) and additional corticosteroid (beclometasone or prednisolone) over 4 weeks. We found insufficient evidence to weigh these short term benefits and possible long term harms.

Treating acute wheeze in infants

- **Addition of ipratropium bromide to fenoterol** One RCT identified by a systematic review in infants aged 3–24 months found that addition of ipratropium bromide to fenoterol (a long acting β_2 agonist) compared with fenoterol alone reduced the proportion of infants receiving further treatment 45 minutes after initial treatment.
- **Inhaled salbutamol** One RCT in infants aged 3 months to 2 years found that, compared with placebo, nebulised salbutamol (a short acting β_2 agonist) improved respiratory rate but found no significant difference in hospital admission. Another RCT that included infants aged less than 18 months to 36 months found no significant difference in change from baseline in clinical symptom scores with nebulised salbutamol versus placebo.
- **Short acting β_2 agonists delivered by metered dose inhaler/spacer versus nebuliser** Two RCTs in children aged up to 5 years found no significant difference in hospital admissions with delivery of salbutamol through a metered dose inhaler plus spacer versus nebulised salbutamol. Another RCT in infants aged 1–24 months found no significant difference in improvement of symptoms with delivery of terbutaline through a metered dose inhaler plus spacer compared with nebulised terbutaline. Nebulised β_2 agonists may cause tachycardia, tremor, and hypokalaemia.

- **High dose inhaled corticosteroids** One systematic review found that high dose inhaled corticosteroids compared with placebo reduced the requirement for oral corticosteroids, but the difference was not statistically significant. The review also found a clear preference for the inhaled corticosteroids by the children's parents over placebo. The clinical importance of these results is unclear.
- **Inhaled ipratropium bromide** We found no RCTs comparing inhaled ipratropium bromide compared with placebo for treating acute wheeze.
- **Oral prednisolone** One small RCT found no significant difference in daily symptom scores with oral prednisolone (a corticosteroid) versus placebo.

Prophylaxis in wheezing infants

- **Oral salbutamol** One RCT identified by a systematic review in infants aged 3–14 months found that oral salbutamol (a short acting β_2 agonist) compared with placebo reduced treatment failures.
- **Higher dose inhaled budesonide** One RCT in infants aged 6–30 months found that higher prophylactic doses of inhaled budesonide (a corticosteroid) compared with placebo reduced symptoms and the proportion of children with acute wheezing episodes during a 12 week period but found no significant reduction in the proportion of wheezing episodes per infant. Another RCT in infants aged 11–36 months found that higher prophylactic doses of inhaled budesonide reduced the proportion of days requiring oral prednisolone, and symptoms of wheezing and sleep disturbance, but found no significant improvement for cough. Higher doses of inhaled corticosteroids have the potential for adverse effects.
- **Inhaled ipratropium bromide** One small RCT identified by a systematic review found no significant difference in relief of symptoms with nebulised ipratropium bromide compared with placebo. The study may have lacked power to exclude a clinically important difference between treatments.
- **Inhaled salbutamol** Two RCTs identified by a systematic review in infants aged up to 2 years found no significant improvement in symptoms with inhaled salbutamol (a short acting β_2 agonist) compared with placebo.
- **Lower dose inhaled budesonide** Three RCTs found no clear evidence of effectiveness with lower prophylactic doses of inhaled budesonide (a corticosteroid) in children aged 1 week to 6 years with recurrent wheeze.
- **Addition of inhaled beclometasone to salbutamol** One RCT found no significant improvement in symptoms with addition of inhaled beclometasone (a corticosteroid) compared with placebo to inhaled salbutamol (a short acting β_2 agonist).

DEFINITION Differentiation between asthma and non-asthmatic viral associated wheeze may be difficult; persisting symptoms and signs between acute attacks are suggestive of asthma, as are a personal or family history of atopic conditions such as eczema and hay fever. **Childhood asthma** is characterised by chronic or recurrent cough and wheeze. The diagnosis is confirmed by demonstrating reversible airway obstruction, preferably on several occasions over time, in children old enough to perform peak flow measurements or spirometry. Diagnosing asthma in children requires exclusion of other causes of recurrent respiratory symptoms. Acute asthma is a term used to describe a severe exacerbation of asthma symptoms accompanied by tachycardia and tachypnoea. The aim of prophylactic treatments in asthma is to minimise persistent symptoms and prevent acute exacerbations. **Wheezing in infants** is characterised by a high pitched purring or whistling sound produced mainly on the out breath and is commonly associated with an acute viral infection such as bronchiolitis (see bronchiolitis, p 280) or asthma. These are not easy to distinguish clinically.

INCIDENCE/ PREVALENCE **Childhood asthma:** Surveys have found an increase in the proportion of children diagnosed with asthma. The increase is higher than can be explained by an increased readiness to diagnose asthma. One questionnaire study from Aberdeen, Scotland, surveyed 2510 children aged 8–13 years in 1964 and 3403 children in 1989. Over the 25 years, the diagnosis of asthma rose from 4% to 10%.[1] The increase in the prevalence of childhood asthma from the 1960s to 1980s was accompanied by an increase in hospital admissions over the same period. In England and Wales this was a sixfold increase.[2] **Wheezing in infants** is common and seems to be increasing, although the magnitude of any increase is not clear.

One Scottish cross-sectional study (2510 children aged 8–13 years in 1964 and 3403 children in 1989) found that the prevalence of wheeze rose from 10% in 1964 to 20% in 1989, and episodes of shortness of breath rose from 5% to 10% over the same period.[1] Difficulties in defining clear groups (phenotypes) and the transient nature of the symptoms, which often resolve spontaneously, have confounded many studies.

AETIOLOGY/ RISK FACTORS **Childhood asthma:** Asthma is more common in children with a personal or family history of atopy, increased severity and frequency of wheezing episodes, and presence of variable airway obstruction or bronchial hyperresponsiveness. Precipitating factors for symptoms and acute episodes include infection, house dust mites, allergens from pet animals, exposure to tobacco smoke, and anxiety. **Wheezing in infants:** Most wheezing episodes in infancy are precipitated by viral respiratory infections.

PROGNOSIS **Childhood asthma:** A British longitudinal study of children born in 1970 found that 29% of 5 year olds wheezing in the past year were still wheezing at the age of 10 years.[3] Another study followed a group of children in Melbourne, Australia from the age of 7 years (in 1964) into adulthood. The study found that a large proportion (73%) of 14 year olds with infrequent symptoms had few or no symptoms by the age of 28 years, whereas two thirds of those 14 year olds with frequent wheezing still had recurrent attacks at the age of 28 years.[4] **Wheezing in infants:** One cohort study (826 infants followed from birth to 6 years) suggests that there may be at least three different prognostic categories for wheezing in infants: "persistent wheezers" (14% of total, with risk factors for atopic asthma such as elevated immunoglobulin E levels and a maternal history of asthma), who initially suffered wheeze during viral infections, and in whom the wheezing persisted into school age; "transient wheezers" (20% of total, with reduced lung function as infants but no early markers of atopy), who also suffered wheeze during viral infections but stopped wheezing after the first 3 years of life; and "late onset wheezers" (15% of total), who did not wheeze when aged under 3 years but had developed wheeze by school age.[5] Another retrospective cohort study found that 14% of children with one attack and 23% of children with four or more attacks in the first year of life had experienced at least one wheezing illness in the past year at the age of 10 years.[3] Administering inhaled treatments to young children can be difficult. Inconsistencies in results could reflect the effects of the differences in the drugs used, delivery devices used, dosages used, and the differences in the pattern of wheezing illnesses and treatment responses among young children.

AIMS OF INTERVENTION To reduce or abolish cough and wheeze; to attain best possible lung function; to reduce the risk of severe attacks; to minimise sleep disturbance and absence from school; to minimise adverse effects of treatment; and to allow normal growth.

OUTCOMES **Childhood asthma:** Wheeze, cough, nights disturbed by asthma, days lost from school or normal activities, diary card symptom scores, frequency of use of short acting β_2 agonists for symptom control, lung function tests (peak expiratory flow rates and forced expiratory volume in 1 second), airway hyperresponsiveness (measured using methacholine challenge tests), rates of health service use (emergency consultations, casualty attendances, hospital admissions). In acute episodes — blood oxygen saturation, admission rate from casualty, duration of admission, need for intensive care or intubation, mortality. **Wheezing in infants:** There are no suitable objective outcome parameters by which a response can be adequately measured, as clinical assessment of an infant's lung function is impractical. Symptoms and signs are usually subjective, vary between observers, and can be affected by short term changes. The main outcomes used in trials include: respiratory rate, work of breathing (suprasternal/sternal/intercostal/subcostal recession, grunting, nasal flare, and head bobbing), agitation, and oxygen saturations. Parental preference is considered to be a relevant outcome.

METHODS *Clinical Evidence* search and appraisal June 2003. We have excluded studies with heterogeneous groups of infants (those that included infants with bronchiolitis, episodic viral wheeze**G** and chronic, persistent wheeze).

QUESTION What are the effects of treatments for acute asthma in children?

Duncan Keeley

OPTION OXYGEN

An RCT comparing oxygen treatment with no oxygen treatment in acute severe asthma would be considered unethical. One prospective cohort study and clinical experience support the need for oxygen in acute asthma.

Benefits: We found no systematic review or RCTs (see comment below). One double blind, prospective cohort study (280 children) found that decreased oxygen saturation upon entry to an emergency department was correlated with increased treatment with intravenous aminophylline**G** and corticosteroids, and increased rates of hospital admission or subsequent readmission (arterial oxygen saturation ≤ 91% *v* arterial oxygen saturation ≥ 96%: OR 35, 95% CI 11 to 150; for arterial oxygen saturation 92–95% *v* ≥ 96%: OR 4.2, 95% CI 2.2 to 8.8).[6]

Harms: We found no evidence about harms.

Comment: An RCT of oxygen versus no oxygen treatment in acute severe asthma would be considered unethical. The cohort study does not address directly whether oxygen should be given therapeutically but it does suggest, along with clinical experience, that oxygen should continue to be given promptly to children with acute asthma.[6]

OPTION INHALED IPRATROPIUM BROMIDE ADDED TO β_2 AGONISTS

One systematic review has found that, compared with β_2 agonist alone, multiple doses of inhaled ipratropium bromide plus an inhaled β_2 agonist (fenoterol or salbutamol) reduced hospital admissions and improved lung function in children aged 18 months to 17 years with severe asthma exacerbations. In children with mild to moderate asthma exacerbations, a single dose of inhaled ipratropium bromide plus a β_2 agonist (fenoterol, salbutamol, or terbutaline) compared with a β_2 agonist alone improved lung function for up to 2 hours, but did not reduce hospital admissions. One subsequent RCT in children admitted to hospital with initially stabilised severe asthma found no significant difference in clinical asthma scores during the first 36 hours with nebulised ipratropium bromide compared with placebo added to salbutamol and corticosteroid (hydrocortisone or prednisone).

Benefits: We found one systematic review[7] and one subsequent RCT.[8] **Single dose:** The systematic review (search date 2000, 13 RCTs, children aged 18 months to 17 years with acute asthma)[7] found that in children with mild to moderate exacerbations, adding a single dose of inhaled ipratropium bromide to inhaled β_2 agonists (fenoterol, salbutamol**G**, or terbutaline) versus the β_2 agonist alone significantly improved forced expiratory volume in 1 second (FEV_1) at 1 hour (3 RCTs: standardised mean difference 0.57, 95% CI 0.21 to 0.93) and at 2 hours (3 RCTs: standardised mean difference 0.53, 95% CI 0.17 to 0.90), but found no significant reduction in hospital admission (3 RCTs: RR 0.93, 95% CI 0.65 to 1.32).[7] **Multiple doses:** The systematic review found that in children with mild, moderate, or severe exacerbations, adding multiple doses of inhaled ipratropium bromide to an inhaled β_2 agonist (fenoterol or salbutamol) improved FEV_1 (4 RCTs: WMD 9.7% of predicted FEV_1, 95% CI 5.7% to 13.7%, 1 hour after last ipratropium bromide inhalation) and reduced hospital admissions (6 RCTs: RR 0.75, 95% CI 0.62 to 0.89; NNT 13, 95% CI 8 to 32). Subgroup analysis found a significant reduction in children with only severe exacerbations (baseline FEV_1 < 50% of predicted or change of 7–9 in baseline clinical score after last combined inhalation; RR 0.71, 95% CI 0.58 to 0.89; NNT 7, 95% CI 5 to 20).[7] The subsequent RCT (80 children and adolescents aged 1–18 years admitted to hospital with moderate to severe asthma, FEV_1 25–85% predicted or clinical asthma score**G** of 3–9, initially stabilised in emergency department) compared addition of nebulised ipratropium bromide versus placebo (sodium chloride) to nebulised salbutamol and intravenous hydrocortisone or oral prednisone.[8] The RCT found no significant difference between groups during the first 36 hours in clinical asthma scores, oxygen saturation, or number of nebulisations needed.

Harms: The systematic review found no significant increase in risk of nausea (3 RCTs: RR 0.59, 95% CI 0.30 to 1.14), vomiting (3 RCTs: RR 1.03, 95% CI 0.37 to 2.87), or tremor (4 RCTs: RR 1.01, 95% CI 0.63 to 1.63) in children treated with multiple doses of ipratropium bromide.[7] The subsequent RCT found a significant increase in heart rate with ipratropium bromide compared with placebo (P = 0.01).[8]

Comment: None.

OPTION METERED DOSE INHALER PLUS SPACER DEVICES VERSUS NEBULISERS FOR DELIVERING β_2 AGONISTS

One systematic review, in children with acute but not life threatening asthma who were old enough to use a spacer, has found no significant difference in hospital admission rates with a metered dose inhaler plus a spacer compared with nebulisation for delivery of β_2 agonists (fenoterol, salbutamol, or terbutaline) or β agonist (orciprenaline). Children using a metered dose inhaler with a spacer may have shorter stays in emergency departments, less hypoxia, and lower pulse rates compared with children receiving β_2 agonist by nebulisation.

Benefits: We found one systematic review (search date 2001, 13 RCTs, 880 children with acute asthma but excluding life threatening asthma) comparing a spacer/holding chamber attached to a metered dose inhaler versus single or a multiple treatment with nebuliser for delivery of β_2 agonists (fenoterol, salbutamol**G**, or terbutaline) or β agonist (orciprenaline**G**).[9] The review found no significant difference between spacer and multiple treatments with nebulisers in hospital admission rates (OR 0.65, 95% CI 0.40 to 1.06). It found a significant increase in pulse rate with nebulisers (WMD 7.8% from baseline, 95% CI 5.3% to 10.2%). One RCT (152 children ≥ 2 years) included in the review found that the time spent in the emergency department was shorter in children using metered dose inhaler plus spacer (WMD –37 minutes, 95% CI –50 minutes to –24 minutes).[10] Two small RCTs included in the review comparing delivery of β_2 agonists (salbutamol or terbutaline) through a spacer versus single treatment with nebuliser found less deterioration in blood gases with the spacer.[9]

Harms: The systematic review found no significant deterioration in any of the outcome measures with delivery of β_2 agonists using metered dose inhaler plus a spacer versus nebulisation.[9]

Comment: These findings suggest that, in children old enough to use a spacer, metered dose inhaler with spacer could be substituted for nebulisation in the treatment of acute asthma in emergency departments and hospital wards.

OPTION SYSTEMIC CORTICOSTEROIDS

One systematic review has found that, compared with placebo, systemic corticosteroids increase the likelihood of discharge after 4 hours and reduce the frequency of relapse within 1–3 months in children hospitalised with acute asthma.

Benefits: **Versus placebo:** We found one systematic review (search date 2002) evaluating effects of systemic corticosteroids in children and adolescents with acute asthma.[11] The review found that oral corticosteroids significantly increased discharge from hospital at first review after 4 hours and reduced relapse within 3 months compared with placebo (2 RCTS, 210 children, mean age 5 years; discharge at first review after 4 hours: OR 7.00, 95% CI 2.98 to 16.45; NNT 3, 95% CI 2 to 8; relapse within 1–3 months: OR 0.19, 95% CI 0.07 to 0.55; NNT 3, 95% CI 2 to 7).[11] The review found no significant difference between oral or intravenous corticosteroids and placebo in mean length of hospital stay (3 RCTs, 132 children, mean age range 4–10 years; mean length of hospital stay: WMD –8.75 hours, 95% CI –19.23 hours to +1.74 hours), pulmonary function (2 RCTs, 64 children, mean age range 9–12 years; pulmonary function, % predicted peak expiratory flow rate: WMD +7.21, 95% CI –7.01 to +21.25). The corticosteroids used in the studies were oral or intravenous prednisolone, intravenous hydrocortisone, or intravenous methylprednisolone. **Oral corticosteroids versus high dose inhaled corticosteroids:** See benefits of high dose inhaled corticosteroids, p 247.

Harms: The studies included in the systematic review did not formally address the issue of harms.[11] We found few reports of adverse effects with short courses of systemic corticosteroids. **Varicella infection:** Several case reports have associated systemic corticosteroid treatment with severe varicella infection. One case control study (167 cases, 134 controls) in otherwise immunocompetent children with complicated and uncomplicated varicella infection did not find significant risk attributable to corticosteroid exposure (OR 1.6, 95% CI 0.2 to 17.0), but it was too small to exclude a clinically important risk.[12]

Comment: The studies included in the systematic review[11] probably excluded the most severely ill children; this was explicitly stated in one study. The authors of the review comment on the surprising paucity of evidence from RCTs for this accepted standard intervention. RCTs of systemic steroids versus placebo in severe acute asthma would now be considered unethical.

OPTION HIGH DOSE INHALED CORTICOSTEROIDS

We found one systematic review that identified four RCTs comparing high dose inhaled with oral corticosteroids in children. Three RCTs found no significant difference in hospital admissions with nebulised budesonide or dexamethasone compared with oral prednisolone in children with mild to moderate asthma. One RCT in children with moderate to severe asthma found that, compared with inhaled fluticasone, oral prednisolone reduced hospital admissions and improved lung function at 4 hours. A subsequent RCT in children aged 4–16 years found that, compared with oral prednisolone, nebulised fluticasone improved lung function over 7 days. Another RCT in children aged 5–16 years admitted to hospital with severe asthma found no significant difference with nebulised budesonide compared with oral prednisolone in lung function at 24 hours or 24 days after admission.

Benefits: **Versus oral corticosteroids:** We found one systematic review (search date 2000, 4 RCTs),[13] one subsequent RCT,[14] and one additional RCT.[15] The systematic review compared effects of initial treatment with high dose inhaled corticosteroids versus oral corticosteroids in hospital emergency departments on admission rates.[13] The results from the four RCTs were not pooled because of marked heterogeneity between studies. One RCT (100 children with moderate to severe asthma, aged 5–16 years, mean initial forced expiratory volume in 1 second, 45%) compared fluticasone (2 mg through metered dose inhaler with spacer) versus prednisone (2 mg/kg orally).[16] It found that prednisone reduced hospital admission (31% with fluticasone *v* 10% with prednisone; P = 0.01) and increased mean forced expiratory volume in 1 second at 4 hours (9% with fluticasone *v* 19% with prednisone; P ≤ 0.001).[16] The second RCT (111 children with mild to moderate asthma, aged 1–17 years) compared dexamethasone (1.5 mg/kg through nebuliser) versus prednisone (2 mg orally).[17] It found no significant difference between nebulised dexamethasone and oral prednisone in rates of hospital admission (12/56 [21%] with dexamethasone *v* 17/55 [31%] with prednisone; ARR +9.5%, 95% CI –8.0% to +21.0%; RR 0.69, 95% CI 0.36 to 1.27), but found fewer relapses with nebulised dexamethasone within 48 hours after discharge (0/44 [0%] *v* 6/38 [16%]; ARR –16.0%, 95% CI –27.0% to –4.5%); however, all children in the RCT received a 5 day course of prednisone (2 mg/kg/day) on discharge.[17] Two other RCTs (104 children with mild to moderate asthma) compared budesonide (800 μg through nebuliser at 1, 30, and 60 minutes; 1600 μg through turbohaler) versus prednisolone (2 mg/kg orally).[18,19] Overall, no significant differences were found between the groups in admission rates (OR for inhaled corticosteroids *v* oral corticosteroids 0.49, 95% CI 0.22 to 1.07).[18,19] The subsequent RCT (321 children aged 4–16 years, peak expiratory flow rate 40–75% predicted) compared nebulised fluticasone (1 mg twice daily for 7 days) versus oral prednisolone (2 mg/kg for 4 days then 1 mg/kg for 3 days). It found that nebulised fluticasone versus oral prednisolone significantly improved mean morning peak expiratory flow rate over 7 days (difference 9.5 L/minute, 95% CI 2.0 L/minute to 17.0 L/minute). No significant differences were found in symptom scores, withdrawals, or adverse events.[14] The additional RCT (46 children, aged 5–16 years, admitted to hospital with severe exacerbations of asthma) compared nebulised budesonide (2 mg/hour) with oral prednisolone (2 mg/kg) at admission and after 24 hours.[15] It found no significant difference between groups in flow expiratory volume in 1 second at 24 hours, or at 3 and 24 days after admission. All children in this trial were treated with budesonide (800 μg/day) after discharge from hospital.

Harms: The systematic review found no significant adverse effects with inhaled corticosteroids.[13] The subsequent RCT found no significant difference in the profile of adverse events between inhaled fluticasone and oral prednisolone, except a slightly higher frequency of oral candidiasis with fluticasone (8% with fluticasone *v* 3% with prednisolone).[14]

Comment: These RCTs suggest that high dose inhaled corticosteroids may be substituted for oral corticosteroids in the initial phase of treatment of moderately severe acute asthma. This may be useful for children who vomit oral corticosteroids or for children with frequent exacerbations where there is concern about the cumulative dose of oral steroids. One RCT was funded by the manufacturers of fluticasone.[14]

OPTION INTRAVENOUS THEOPHYLLINE

One systematic review found that in children aged 1–19 years admitted to hospital with severe asthma, intravenous theophylline improved lung function and symptom scores 6–8 hours after treatment compared with placebo, but found no significant difference in the number of bronchodilator treatments required or length of hospital stay. A subsequent RCT in children aged 1–17

years admitted to the intensive care unit with severe asthma found that, compared with controls, intravenous theophylline decreased the time to reach a clinical asthma score of 3 or less but found no significant difference in length of stay in the intensive care unit.

Benefits: We found one systematic review[20] and one subsequent RCT.[21] The systematic review (search date 2001, 7 RCTs, 380 children and adolescents aged 1–19 years admitted to hospital with severe asthma, flow expiratory volume in 1 second 35–45% predicted) compared the effects of intravenous theophylline versus placebo on lung function (measured as change from baseline in flow expiratory volume in 1 second).[20] The review found that at 6–8 hours, intravenous theophylline versus placebo significantly improved lung function (2 RCTs; WMD 8.4%, 95% CI 0.8% to 15.9%) and clinical symptom scores (WMD –0.71, 95% CI –0.82 to –0.60) but found no significant difference in the number of nebulised bronchodilator treatments required (2 RCTs; WMD +0.15; 95% CI –0.52 to +0.83) or length of hospital stay (3 RCTs; WMD +4.29; 95% CI –4.16 to +12.74). The subsequent RCT (47 children aged 1–17 years admitted to intensive care unit with severe asthma receiving salbutamol**G**, ipratropium, and methylprednisolone) compared intravenous theophylline versus controls on time to reach a clinical asthma score of 3 or less.[21] The RCT found that intravenous theophylline significantly decreased the time to reach a clinical asthma score of 3 or less compared with control (18.6 hours with theophylline *v* 31 hours with control; $P < 0.05$) but found no significant difference in length of stay in the intensive care unit.

Harms: The systematic review found that theophylline significantly increased the risk of vomiting (5 RCTs; RR 3.69, 95% CI 2.15 to 6.33) compared with placebo, but found no significant differences for headache, tremor, seizures, and arrhythmia. There were no deaths reported in the included studies.[20] The subsequent RCT found significantly higher incidence of emesis with theophylline and tremor with controls (both $P < 0.05$).[21] Theophylline can cause serious adverse effects (cardiac arrhythmia or convulsions) if therapeutic blood concentrations are exceeded.

Comment: None.

QUESTION What are the effects of single agent prophylaxis in childhood asthma?

Duncan Keeley

OPTION INHALED CORTICOSTEROIDS

One systematic review has found that, compared with placebo, prophylactic inhaled corticosteroids improve symptoms and lung function in children with asthma. Several RCTs have found that inhaled corticosteroids slightly reduce growth rate compared with placebo, although studies with long term follow up suggest attainment of normal adult height. Inhaled corticosteroids have been associated with rare reports of adrenal suppression. One RCT in children aged 6–16 years found no significant difference in improvement of asthma symptoms between inhaled beclometasone and theophylline, but found less use of bronchodilators and oral corticosteroids with inhaled beclometasone. Small RCTs have found inhaled corticosteroids to be more effective than sodium cromoglicate in improving symptoms and lung function. RCTs in children aged 5–16 years have found that inhaled corticosteroids (beclometasone, budesonide, or fluticasone) versus inhaled long acting β_2 agonist (salmeterol) or inhaled nedocromil improve symptoms and lung function in children with asthma.

Benefits: **Versus placebo:** We found one systematic review (search date 1996, 24 RCTs, 1087 children, 10/24 RCTs in preschool children, duration 4–88 weeks) comparing effects of regular inhaled corticosteroids (betamethasone, beclometasone, budesonide, flunisolide, or fluticasone) versus placebo on asthma symptoms (see comment below), concomitant drug use, and peak expiratory flow rate (PEFR).[22] It found that corticosteroids significantly improved symptom score (overall weighted relative improvement in symptom score 50%, 95% CI 49% to 51%), reduced β_2 agonist use (RR 0.37, 95% CI 0.36 to 0.38), reduced oral corticosteroid use (RR 0.68, 95% CI 0.66 to 0.70), and improved peak flow rate (weighted mean improvement in PEFR 11% predicted, 95% CI 9.5% to 12.5%). **Versus theophylline:** We found no systematic review. We found one RCT (195 children aged 6–16 years, followed for 12 months) comparing inhaled beclometasone (360 μg/day) versus oral theophylline.[23] It found no significant difference with inhaled beclometasone versus oral theophylline in the mean asthma symptom score (0 = no symptoms, 6 = incapacitating symptoms: mean score 0.5–0.8 for beclometasone *v* 0.6–0.9 for theophylline) with less use of bronchodilators and oral corticosteroids with inhaled beclometasone.[23] **Versus sodium cromoglicate:** We found no systematic review. We found four RCTs comparing inhaled corticosteroids (betamethasone, budesonide, fluticasone) versus inhaled sodium cromoglicate.[24–27] One RCT (20 children aged 6–14 years) found that betamethasone versus sodium cromoglicate significantly improved symptoms and lung function (mean PEFRs; $P < 0.001$).[24] The second RCT (crossover, 75 children aged 5–15 years) found that budesonide or fluticasone versus sodium cromoglicate significantly reduced bronchodilator use ($P < 0.05$) and lung function (forced expiratory volume in 1 second [FEV_1]; $P < 0.01$).[25] The third RCT (unblinded, 335 children aged 2–6 years) found that budesonide versus sodium cromoglicate significantly reduced the rate of asthma exacerbations over 52 weeks ($P \leq 0.001$). Asthma exacerbations were defined as use of systemic corticosteroids or additional maintenance treatment, emergency department or urgent care visit, or admission to hospital.[26] The fourth RCT (unblinded, multicentre, 225 children aged 4–12 years) found that fluticasone versus sodium cromoglicate significantly improved mean percentage PEFR (at 6–8 weeks; $P = 0.0001$) and symptoms (at 6–8 weeks; $P < 0.05$) but found no significant difference for relief medication use or FEV_1.[27] **Versus nedocromil:** We found no systematic review. We found one RCT (1041 children aged 5–12 years, with mild to moderate asthma, mean prestudy FEV_1 94% predicted, all using salbutamol Ⓖ for asthma symptoms) that compared inhaled budesonide (200 μg twice daily) and inhaled nedocromil (8 mg twice daily) versus placebo for 4–6 years.[28] It found no significant difference with budesonide compared with nedocromil or placebo in lung function, hospital admission rate, or the symptom score on diary cards but found that budesonide was superior to nedocromil, and that nedocromil was superior to placebo in several measures of asthma symptoms and morbidity (see table 1, p 265). The mean change in post-bronchodilator FEV_1 over the study period was not significantly different among the three groups. **Versus inhaled long acting β_2 agonists:** We found no systematic review but found two RCTs of beclometasone (200 μg twice daily) versus salmeterol (50 μg twice daily) for 1 year.[29,30] The first RCT (67 children aged 6–16 years) found that beclometasone was more effective than salmeterol in improving FEV_1 (mean change of FEV_1 −4.5% of predicted with salmeterol, 95% CI −9.0% to +0.1% *v* +10% with beclometasone, CI not reported; mean difference beclometasone *v* salmeterol 14.2%, 95% CI 8.3% to 20.0%), reducing the use of rescue salbutamol (0.44 uses/day with salmeterol *v* 0.07 uses/day with beclometasone; $P \leq 0.001$).[29] Both treatments improved symptom scores (before trial

3% of children asymptomatic with salmeterol *v* 6% with beclometasone; at 1 year 36% with salmeterol *v* 55% with beclometasone) and PEFR (improvement in morning PEFR 49 L/minute with salmeterol *v* 61 L/minute with beclometasone), but there was no significant difference between treatments at 1 year. There were two exacerbations in the beclometasone group compared with 17 in the salmeterol group.[29] The second RCT (241 children aged 6–14 years) compared beclometasone (81 children) versus salmeterol (80 children) versus placebo (80 children).[30] It found that beclometasone reduced airway hyperresponsiveness more than salmeterol (methacholine PC20 36 hours after study medication 12 months into the study: 2.1 mg/mL with beclometasone *v* 0.9 mg/mL with salmeterol; $P = 0.009$). Beclometasone versus placebo reduced rescue bronchodilator use (92% with beclometasone *v* 83% with placebo days and nights without need for salbutamol; $P \leq 0.001$) and treatment withdrawals because of exacerbations (5 with beclometasone *v* 15 with placebo; $P = 0.03$). Salmeterol versus placebo did not significantly reduce the use of a rescue bronchodilator (88% with salmeterol *v* 83% with placebo days and nights without need for salbutamol; $P = 0.09$) or treatment withdrawals because of exacerbations (15 with salmeterol *v* 15 with placebo; $P = 0.55$). Both salmeterol and beclometasone improved FEV_1 compared with placebo, but the difference between beclometasone and salmeterol was not significant (10% with beclometasone *v* 10% with salmeterol *v* 5% with placebo). **Versus oral montelukast:** We found no RCTs comparing inhaled corticosteroids versus oral montelukast in children. A systematic review of mainly adult studies comparing inhaled corticosteroids with leukotriene receptor antagonists found similar exacerbation rates, but greater improvement in lung function and symptoms with inhaled steroids.[31] See benefits section of leukotriene antagonists in adults with mild to moderate, persistent asthma option in asthma in adults topic, p 1891.

Harms: **Versus placebo:** One systematic review (search date 1996) found no significant difference with inhaled corticosteroids (betamethasone, budesonide, flunisolide, or fluticasone) versus placebo in adrenal function (12 RCTs) and found clinical cases of oral candidiasis (4 RCTs).[22] Case reports[32] and a national survey of paediatricians and endocrinologists[33] have indicated the possibility of adrenal suppression leading to adrenal crisis associated with hypoglycaemia in children on high dose inhaled corticosteroids. Most cases involved fluticasone, in daily doses of 500–2000 μg. Observational studies have found little or no biochemical evidence of change in bone metabolism with inhaled corticosteroids.[34,35] Two cross-sectional studies using a slit lamp to screen for lenticular changes in children taking long term inhaled corticosteroids (beclometasone, budesonide) found no posterior subcapsular cataracts.[36,37] The systematic review identified eight RCTs reporting growth velocity and found no significant difference with inhaled corticosteroids versus placebo.[22] One systematic review (search date 1993, 21 studies) reported height for age in 810 children with asthma treated with oral or inhaled corticosteroids. It found no evidence of growth impairment with inhaled beclometasone (12 studies, 331 children).[38] A second systematic review (search date 1999, 3 RCTs) identified one RCT (94 children, aged 7–9 years) comparing effect of inhaled beclometasone (400 μg/day) versus placebo on growth as a primary outcome measure in children with recurrent viral induced wheeze.[39] It found a significant decrease in growth with beclometasone versus placebo (mean growth at end of 7 month treatment period, 2.7 cm with beclometasone *v* 3.7 cm with placebo; 95% CI −1.4 cm to −0.6 cm; $P < 0.0001$) and found no significant catch up growth during a follow up 4 month washout period.[40] We found one large subsequent RCT that evaluated the effects of inhaled budesonide on growth in children with mild asthma.[41] The RCT found that children receiving budesonide grew less than children receiving placebo over 3 years (1 RCT, 3195 children aged 5–17 years; mean difference in growth per year: –0.43 cm, 95% CI –0.54 cm to –0.32 cm; P < 0.0001). The differences in growth rate were similar between children under 11 years treated with budesonide 200 µg per day (–0.45 cm per year, 95% CI –0.56 cm to –0.34 cm; P< 0.0001) and children over 11years being treated with budesonide 400 µg per day (–0.40 cm per year, 95% CI –0.66 cm to –0.14 cm; P = 0.003). In children less than 11 years being treated with 200 µg per day, the effect was more pronounced during the first year (–0.58 cm per year, 95% CI –0.76 cm to –0.40 cm; P < 0.0001) than during the third year (–0.33 cm per year, 95% CI –0.52 cm to –0.14 cm; P = 0.0005).[41] **Versus theophylline or sodium cromoglicate:** One RCT compared inhaled beclometasone (360 µg/day) versus oral theophylline for 1 year.[23] It found a significantly higher rate of growth (more notable in boys) in the theophylline group (mean rate of growth in prepubescent boys 4.3 cm/year with beclometasone *v* 6.2 cm/year with theophylline). This effect was not sufficient to be noticed by the children or by their parents, and no child was withdrawn from the study on this account.[23] One controlled, prospective study compared 216 children treated with budesonide (400–600 µg/day) with 62 children treated with theophylline or sodium cromoglicate over 3–5 years' follow up.[42] No significant changes in growth velocity were found at doses up to 400 µg/day (5.5 cm/year with budesonide *v* 5.6 cm/year with controls). The adult height of 142 of these budesonide treated children (mean treatment period 9.2 years, mean dosage 412 µg/day) was compared with 18 controls never treated with inhaled corticosteroids and 51 healthy siblings. There were no significant differences. Children in all groups attained their target adult height (mean difference between measured and target adult height: +0.3 cm, 95% CI –0.6 cm to +1.2 cm for budesonide treated children; –0.2 cm, 95% CI –2.4 cm to +2.1 cm for control children with asthma; +0.9 cm, 95% CI –0.4 cm to +2.2 cm for healthy siblings).[43] Two RCTs found no clinically relevant differences between inhaled corticosteroids (betamethasone, budesonide) and sodium cromoglicate.[24,26] One RCT found that budesonide versus fluticasone or sodium cromoglicate significantly reduced growth (decrease in height standard deviation score > 2 standard deviation compared with mean height standard deviation score change during preceding year; P < 0.05).[25] Another RCT found that a higher proportion of children taking sodium cromoglicate withdrew because of adverse events (breathlessness and wheeze, burning sensation in chest, sore throat, sickness) compared with fluticasone.[27] **Versus nedocromil:** A large RCT (1041 children with mild to moderate asthma) compared budesonide (400 µg/day) versus nedocromil versus placebo with 4–6 years' follow up.[28] The mean increase in height in the budesonide group was 1.1 cm less than in the placebo group (22.7 cm with budesonide *v* 23.8 cm with placebo; P = 0.005); the difference occurred mainly within the first year of treatment.[28] **Versus inhaled long acting β_2 agonists:** Two RCTs comparing beclometasone with salmeterol found slowing in linear growth with beclometasone (growth over year of treatment 5.4 cm[29] and 6.1 cm[30] in the salmeterol groups; 4.0 cm[29] and 4.7 cm[30] in the beclometasone groups; P = 0.004;[29] P = 0.007[30]). One RCT comparing inhaled beclometasone versus salmeterol found that symptom improvement in the salmeterol group was accompanied by significant deterioration in bronchial reactivity, indicating a failure to control underlying bronchial inflammation.[29]

Comment: Treatment with inhaled corticosteroids should be reviewed regularly and the dose gradually reduced to the lowest that is compatible with good symptom control.

OPTION INHALED SODIUM CROMOGLICATE

One systematic review found insufficient evidence for prophylactic treatment with inhaled sodium cromoglicate in children aged 1–18 years. Several small comparative RCTs found sodium cromoglicate to be less effective than inhaled corticosteroids in improving symptoms and lung function.

Benefits: **Versus placebo:** We found one systematic review (search date 1999, 24 RCTs, about 1000 children aged 0–18 years with moderate to severe asthma) comparing inhaled sodium cromoglicate versus placebo.[44] The RCTs differed in design, severity of asthma, number of children included, age of children, duration of intervention, and follow up period. The review found heterogeneity between RCTs but did not separately analyse RCTs in terms of asthma severity, age of children, or the outcome measured. The review found that sodium cromoglicate versus placebo significantly improved symptom scores for cough (point estimate not reported; 95% CI 0.11 to 0.26) and wheeze (point estimate not reported; 95% CI 0.13 to 0.27) but also found significant publication bias by the absence of small, negative trials (P = 0.01 for cough and wheeze). The review concluded that there is insufficient evidence for prophylactic treatment with sodium cromoglicate in children with asthma. **Versus inhaled corticosteroids:** See benefits of inhaled corticosteroids, p 250.

Harms: **Versus placebo:** Fifteen RCTs included in the systematic review reported adverse effects described as minor and of low incidence, including cough, bitter taste, wheezing, sneezing, throat irritation, and perioral eczema.[44] **Versus inhaled corticosteroids:** See harms of inhaled corticosteroids, p 251.

Comment: The conclusions of the systematic review[44] have been criticised in correspondence and the assertion made that analysis of trials using sodium cromoglicate by spinhaler in children over 5 years of age was consistent with a beneficial effect of sodium cromoglicate compared with placebo.[45]

OPTION INHALED NEDOCROMIL

Two RCTs in children aged 6–12 years found that, compared with placebo, inhaled nedocromil reduces asthma symptom scores, asthma severity, bronchodilator use, and improves lung function. One large RCT in children aged 5–12 years with mild to moderate asthma found no significant difference between nedocromil and budesonide or placebo in lung function, hospital admission rate, or the symptom score on diary cards, but found that budesonide was superior to nedocromil, and that nedocromil was superior to placebo in several measures of asthma symptoms and morbidity.

Benefits: We found no systematic review. **Versus placebo:** We found two RCTs.[46,47] The first RCT (209 children and adolescents aged 6–7 years allowed to continue using usual medication) compared inhaled nedocromil (4 mg 4 times daily) versus placebo for 12 weeks. Symptoms were recorded by the children in daily diary cards, including scoring day and night time asthma and cough severity, use of all medication, and morning and evening peak expiratory flow rates. The RCT found that inhaled nedocromil versus placebo significantly reduced total symptom scores, clinician assessed asthma severity, β_2 agonist use, and improved lung function (forced expiratory volume in 1 second).[46] The second RCT (parallel group study, 79 children aged 6–12 years recovering from acute asthma and allowed to use inhaled bronchodilators) compared inhaled nedocromil (2 mg 3 times daily) versus placebo for 12 weeks.[47] Symptoms were recorded by the children in daily diary cards, including day and night time asthma severity, morning and evening peak expiratory flow rates, and usage of bronchodilators. The RCT found that after 6 weeks, inhaled nedocromil versus placebo significantly improved (from baseline) the morning peak expiratory flow rate (difference, 20 L/minute; P = 0.036), evening peak expiratory flow rate (difference, 22 L/minute; P = 0.033), night time asthma score (difference on a 5 point scale, 0.48; P = 0.001), and daytime asthma score (difference on a 5 point scale, 0.38; P = 0.03). The RCT found no significant difference before 6 weeks of treatment. **Versus inhaled corticosteroids:** See benefits of inhaled corticosteroids, p 250.

Harms: **Versus placebo:** Sore throat and headache were reported marginally more often with nedocromil than placebo in the first RCT.[46] The second RCT found no significant difference between nedocromil and placebo in adverse event rates except for more frequent respiratory adverse events with placebo.[47] **Versus inhaled corticosteroids:** See harms of inhaled corticosteroids, p 251.

Comment: None.

OPTION INHALED LONG ACTING β_2 AGONISTS

Two RCTs in children aged 4–14 years found that, compared with placebo, inhaled salmeterol improved lung function but found conflicting evidence about reduced use of salbutamol. One RCT comparing inhaled salmeterol with beclometasone found that salmeterol was associated with a significant deterioration in bronchial reactivity.

Benefits: We found no systematic review. **Versus placebo:** We found two RCTs.[30,48] The first RCT (241 children aged 6–14 years with clinically stable asthma and < 1 month of prior glucocorticoid use) compared inhaled salmeterol (80 children) versus beclometasone (81 children) versus placebo (80 children) for 1 year.[30] The RCT found that salmeterol versus placebo significantly improved lung function (mean change in forced expiratory volume in 1 second as a percentage of predicted, 10% with salmeterol *v* 5% with placebo; P < 0.001) but found no significant difference in the use of rescue salbutamol**G** (P = 0.09) or withdrawals because of exacerbations (P = 0.55).[30] The second RCT (parallel group study, 207 children aged 4–11 years with asthma diagnosed according to American Thoracic Society guidelines, forced expiratory volume in 1 second [without medication] 50–80% predicted) compared inhaled salmeterol (50 µg twice daily) versus placebo for 12 weeks.[48] The RCT found that salmeterol significantly improved lung function compared with placebo (change in mean morning peak expiratory flow 25 L/minute with salmeterol *v* 13.2 L/minute with placebo; P < 0.001; change in mean evening peak expiratory flow 20 L/minute with salmeterol *v* 10.1 L/minute with placebo; P = 0.01) and reduced salbutamol use (–0.8 with salmeterol *v* –0.3 with placebo; P = 0.004). It found no significant difference in the number of nights without awakenings between salmeterol and placebo.[48] **Versus inhaled corticosteroids:** See benefits of inhaled corticosteroids, p 250.

Harms: **Versus placebo:** One RCT found no evidence of adverse effects from salmeterol over 1 year.[30] The second RCT found no significant difference between salmeterol and placebo for adverse effects.[48] **Versus inhaled corticosteroids:** See harms of inhaled corticosteroids, p 251. Long acting β_2 agonists occasionally cause tremor or tachycardia.

Comment: Monotherapy with long acting β_2 agonists is not advised because of the possibility of significant deterioration in bronchial reactivity indicating a failure to control underlying bronchial inflammation (see harms of inhaled corticosteroids, p 251).

OPTION ORAL THEOPHYLLINE

One small RCT in children aged 6–15 years found that, compared with placebo, oral theophylline increased mean morning peak expiratory flow rate and reduced the mean number of acute night time attacks and doses of bronchodilator used. Another RCT in children aged 6–16 years found no significant difference in improvement of asthma symptoms with oral theophylline compared with inhaled beclometasone, but found greater use of bronchodilators and oral corticosteroids with theophylline over 1 year. Theophylline has serious adverse effects (cardiac arrhythmia, convulsions) if therapeutic blood concentrations are exceeded.

Benefits: We found no systematic review. **Versus placebo:** We found one RCT (crossover study, 24 children aged 6–15 years experiencing at least 2 night awakenings/week) comparing once daily oral sustained release theophylline (mean theophylline level of 11.2 mg/L) versus placebo for 6 weeks.[49] The RCT found that theophylline versus placebo significantly increased mean morning peak expiratory flow (244 L/minute with theophylline *v* 207 L/minute with placebo; $P < 0.001$) and significantly reduced the mean number of acute night time attacks (3.2 with theophylline *v* 10.7 with placebo; $P < 0.001$) and the mean number of doses of bronchodilator used (6.5 with theophylline *v* 23.7 with placebo; $P < 0.001$). **Versus inhaled corticosteroids:** See benefits of inhaled corticosteroids, p 250.

Harms: **Versus placebo:** One RCT found significantly higher rates of gastric symptoms including dyspepsia, nausea, and vomiting with oral sustained release theophylline versus placebo (30% with theophylline *v* 6% with placebo; $P < 0.001$).[49] One systematic review (search date not stated, 12 studies, 340 children) of the behavioural and cognitive effects of theophylline found no evidence of significant adverse effects.[50] Theophylline has serious adverse effects (cardiac arrhythmia, convulsions) if therapeutic blood concentrations are exceeded.[51] **Versus inhaled corticosteroids:** See harms of inhaled corticosteroids, p 251.

Comment: None.

OPTION ORAL LEUKOTRIENE RECEPTOR ANTAGONISTS

One RCT in children aged 6–14 years found that, compared with placebo, oral montelukast increased from baseline the mean morning forced expiratory volume in 1 second and reduced the total daily β_2 agonist use, but found no significant difference in daytime asthma symptom score or in nocturnal awakenings with asthma. Another RCT in children aged 2–5 years found that, compared with placebo, oral montelukast improved average daytime symptom scores and reduced the need for rescue oral steroid courses, but found no significant difference in average overnight asthma symptom scores. We found no RCTs directly comparing oral montelukast with inhaled corticosteroids.

Benefits: We found no systematic review. **Versus placebo:** We found two RCTs.[52,53] The first RCT (parallel group study, 336 children aged 6–16 years with mean forced expiratory volume in 1 second 72% predicted, concomitant inhaled steroid treatment in 33% of placebo group and 39% of montelukast group) compared oral montelukast (5 mg/day) versus placebo for 8 weeks.[52] The RCT found that montelukast versus placebo significantly increased (from baseline) the mean morning flow expiratory volume in 1 second (8.2% with montelukast *v* 3.6% with placebo; $P < 0.001$) and significantly reduced the total daily β_2 agonist use (reduced by 13% with montelukast and increased by 9.5% with placebo; $P = 0.01$).[52] The RCT found no significant difference between montelukast versus placebo in daytime asthma symptom score or in nocturnal awakenings with asthma.[52] The second RCT (parallel group study, 689 children aged 2–5 years, concomitant inhaled steroid treatment in 29% of the placebo group, 27% of the montelukast group, 2 : 1 ratio montelukast : placebo group) compared oral montelukast (4 mg/day) versus placebo for 12 weeks.[53] The RCT found that montelukast versus placebo significantly improved average daytime symptom scores (improved by 0.37 with montelukast *v* 0.26 with placebo on a 6 point scale; $P = 0.003$) and reduced the need for rescue oral steroid courses (needed in 19% with montelukast *v* 28% with placebo; $P = 0.008$). The RCT found no significant difference between montelukast versus placebo in average overnight asthma symptom scores.[53] **Versus inhaled corticosteroids:** We found no RCTs comparing oral montelukast versus inhaled corticosteroids directly.

Harms: **Versus placebo:** Two RCTs found no significant difference in the incidence of adverse effects with montelukast versus placebo.[52,53]

Comment: None.

QUESTION What are the effects of additional prophylactic treatments in childhood asthma inadequately controlled by standard dose inhaled corticosteroids?

Duncan Keeley

OPTION INCREASED DOSE OF INHALED CORTICOSTEROID

One RCT in children aged 6–16 years taking inhaled beclometasone comparing the addition of a second dose of inhaled corticosteroid (beclometasone) with placebo found no significant difference in lung function, symptom scores, exacerbation rates, or bronchial reactivity but found a reduction in growth velocity at 1 year.

Benefits: We found no systematic review but found one RCT (177 children, age 6–16 years, 1 year of follow up, mean pre-bronchodilator flow expiratory volume in 1 second 86% predicted) comparing beclometasone (200 μg twice daily), salmeterol (50 μg twice daily), and placebo in children already taking beclometasone (200 μg twice daily).[54] No significant differences were found at 1 year in lung function (mean change in flow expiratory volume in 1 second 5.8% of predicted, 95% CI 2.9% to 8.7% with double dose beclometasone *v* 4.3%, 95% CI 2.1% to 6.5% with placebo), symptom scores, exacerbation rates, bronchial reactivity, or changes in airway responsiveness (1.30 units of methacholine, 95% CI 0.73 to 1.87 with salmeterol *v* 0.80, 95% CI 0.33 to 1.27 with placebo). No benefit of either adding salmeterol or a second dose of beclometasone was found in this group of children, whose compliance with pre-existing medication was good.

Harms: Growth was significantly slower in children receiving higher dose inhaled corticosteroids (3.6 cm, 95% CI 3.0 cm to 4.2 cm with double dose beclometasone *v* 5.1 cm, 95% CI 4.5 cm to 5.7 cm with salmeterol *v* 4.5 cm, 95% CI 3.8 cm to 5.2 cm with placebo).

Comment: Higher dose inhaled corticosteroids are frequently used, despite lack of evidence of benefit. In some children, higher prescribed doses may compensate for poor compliance or incorrect inhaler technique.

OPTION ADDITION OF REGULAR LONG ACTING β_2 AGONIST

One RCT in children aged 6–16 years found that addition of inhaled salmeterol (a long acting β_2 agonist) increased peak expiratory flow rates in the first few months of treatment but found no increase after 1 year. A second short term RCT in children aged 4–16 years also found increased morning peak expiratory flow rates and more symptom free days at 3 months with addition of salmeterol.

Benefits: We found no systematic review but found two RCTs.[54,55] One RCT (177 children) found that at 1 year the addition of inhaled salmeterol did not improve lung function, airway responsiveness, symptom scores, exacerbation rates, or bronchial reactivity.[54] Salmeterol versus placebo increased mean morning peak expiratory flow rates slightly after 3 months (difference: +12 L/minute). There were no significant differences in symptom scores at any time. The second RCT (210 children aged 4–16 years, 12 weeks' follow up, mean morning peak flow expiratory rate 79% predicted) compared salmeterol (50 µg twice daily) versus placebo in children inadequately controlled on inhaled corticosteroids (average dose 750 µg/day).[55] At 12 weeks, mean morning peak expiratory flow rate (relative to the predicted peak flow expiratory rate) was 4% higher in the salmeterol group. Mean evening peak expiratory flow rate was not significantly different. The median proportion of symptom free days improved more with salmeterol than with placebo (60% with salmeterol *v* 30% with placebo for the third month of treatment).

Harms: The RCTs found no significant adverse effects associated with salmeterol.[54,55]

Comment: The second RCT was organised and funded by the manufacturer of salmeterol. Studies of adults with poor control on low dose inhaled corticosteroids have found greater benefit with additional long acting β_2 agonists than with higher doses of inhaled steroid (see salmeterol v high dose inhaled corticosteroids in the chapter on asthma in adults, p 1891).

OPTION ADDITION OF ORAL THEOPHYLLINE

One small RCT found that addition of theophylline, compared with placebo, to previous treatment increased the proportion of symptom free days and reduced the use of additional β agonist (orciprenaline) and additional corticosteroid (beclometasone or prednisolone) over 4 weeks. We found insufficient evidence to weigh these short term benefits and possible long term harms.

Benefits: We found no systematic review but found one RCT (double blind crossover trial, 33 children, age 6–19 years, recruited from a hospital asthma clinic, 22 children using inhaled beclometasone [mean 533 µg/day], 11 using oral prednisolone [mean 30 mg alternate days]).[43] It found that the addition for 4 weeks of oral theophylline (serum concentration 10–20 µg/mL) versus placebo increased the mean number of symptom free days (63% with theophylline *v* 42% with placebo; $P \leq 0.01$). Inhaled β agonist (orciprenaline🅖) was needed twice as often with placebo (0.5 doses/day with theophylline *v* 1.0 with placebo; $P \leq 0.01$). Additional daily prednisolone was needed by fewer children while on theophylline than while on placebo (3/32 [9%] with theophylline *v* 10/32 [31%] with placebo; P = 0.02).

Harms: In the RCT, short term adverse effects included mild transient headache and nausea in six children after the crossover from placebo to the theophylline dose that they had previously tolerated.[56]

Comment: One child was excluded from the analysis because of poor compliance. The RCT was too brief to assess long term harms.

OPTION ADDITION OF ORAL LEUKOTRIENE RECEPTOR ANTAGONISTS

One crossover RCT in children aged 6–14 years with persistent asthma who had been taking inhaled budesonide for at least 6 weeks found that, compared with addition of placebo, oral montelukast (a leukotriene receptor antagonist) reduced asthma exacerbations over 4 weeks. This difference was statistically significant but modest in clinical terms.

Benefits: We found no systematic review but found one crossover RCT (279 children aged 6–14 years previously treated with inhaled corticosteroid for at least 6 weeks, with mean forced expiratory volume in 1 second 78% predicted after 1 month run-in with budesonide 200 μg) comparing adding oral montelukast versus placebo to inhaled budesonide over 4 weeks.[57] It found fewer asthma exacerbation days (decrease from baseline peak flow of > 20%, or increase from baseline of β_2 agonist use of > 70%) with montelukast versus placebo (12.2% with montelukast *v* 15.9% with placebo; P = < 0.001). No significant differences were found in quality of life measurements, global evaluations, or asthma attacks requiring unscheduled medical intervention or treatment with oral corticosteroid.

Harms: The RCT found no significant difference with montelukast versus placebo in asthma exacerbation, upper respiratory tract infection, headache, cough, pharyngitis, and fever.[57]

Comment: The RCT in children was brief (4 weeks treatment).[57] We found one large RCT of montelukast added to beclometasone in adults with inadequately controlled asthma that found benefit over a 16 week period.[58] Both RCTs were funded by the manufacturers of montelukast.

QUESTION What are the effects of treatments for acute wheezing in infants?

Michael McKean

OPTION SHORT ACTING β_2 AGONISTS

One RCT in infants aged 3 months to 2 years found that nebulised salbutamol improved respiratory rate and clinical symptom score compared with placebo but found no significant difference in hospital admission. Another RCT that included infants aged less than 18 months to 36 months found no significant difference in change from baseline in clinical symptom scores with nebulised salbutamol compared with placebo. Two RCTs in children aged up to 5 years found no significant difference in hospital admission with delivery of salbutamol through a metered dose inhaler plus spacer compared with nebulised salbutamol. Another RCT in infants aged 1–24 months found no significant difference in improvement of symptoms with delivery of terbutaline through a metered dose inhaler plus spacer compared with nebulised terbutaline. Nebulised β_2 agonists may cause tachycardia, tremor, and hypokalaemia.

Benefits: **Nebulised salbutamol versus placebo:** We found one systematic review (search date not stated)[59] that identified two RCTs in children with an acute exacerbation of wheeze in hospital emergency room settings.[60,61] One RCT (28 infants aged 3 months to 2 years) compared nebulised salbutamol**G** (0.3 mg/kg in 2 doses over 1 hour) versus placebo on respiratory rate and symptom score (assessment of heart rate, respiratory rate, wheeze, and accessory muscle score).[60] The RCT found that nebulised salbutamol versus placebo significantly improved respiratory rate (WMD –5.10 breaths/minute, 95% CI –9.45 breaths/minute to –0.75 breaths/minute) and total clinical symptom score for heart rate, respiratory rate, wheezing, and accessory muscle use (clinical symptom score on scale 0 [none] to 3 [severe], WMD –2.50, 95% CI –3.88 to –1.12) but found no significant difference in hospital admission (OR 1.95, 95% CI 0.27 to 13.98).[60] The second RCT (28 infants aged < 18 months and 13 infants aged 18–36 months with acute wheeze) found no significant difference in change from baseline in clinical symptom scores with nebulised salbutamol (2 doses of 0.15 mg/kg) versus placebo groups. Some improvement was observed in children aged more than 18 months, but this was not statistically significant.[61] **Delivery through metered dose inhaler versus nebuliser:** We found no systematic review. We found three RCTs comparing delivery of short acting β_2 agonists through metered dose inhaler versus nebuliser.[62–64] The first RCT (64 children aged 1–5 years with acute recurrent wheezing) found no significant difference in hospital admissions with delivery of salbutamol (50 μg/kg) through a metered dose inhaler plus spacer versus nebulised salbutamol (150 μg/kg).[62] The second RCT (42 infants, mean age < 2 years with acute wheezing) found no significant difference in hospital admissions with delivery of salbutamol (400 μg) through a metered dose inhaler plus spacer versus nebulised salbutamol (2.5 mg).[63] The third RCT (34 infants aged 1–24 months) found no significant difference in the rate of improvement from baseline of a clinical score (assessing respiratory rate, wheezing, retractions, degree of cyanosis, colour, and pulse oximetry data) with delivery of terbutaline (500 μg) through a metered dose inhaler plus spacer versus nebulised terbutaline (4 mg).[64]

Harms: **Nebulised salbutamol versus placebo:** The systematic review did not comment on any adverse effects of nebulised salbutamol in infants with acute wheezing.[59] Nebulised β_2 agonists may cause tachycardia, tremor, and hypokalaemia.[63] **Delivery through metered dose inhaler versus nebuliser:** Three RCTs found no clinically significant adverse events.[62–64]

Comment: None.

OPTION INHALED IPRATROPIUM BROMIDE

We found no RCTs comparing inhaled ipratropium bromide with placebo. One RCT identified by a systematic review in infants aged 3–24 months found that addition of ipratropium bromide to fenoterol compared with fenoterol alone reduced the proportion of infants receiving further treatment 45 minutes after initial treatment.

Benefits: **Versus placebo:** We found no systematic review and no RCTs. **Addition to long acting β_2 agonist:** We found one systematic review (search date not stated), which identified one RCT in infants aged under 2 years with wheeze.[65] The RCT (61 infants aged 3–24 months with acute wheeze) found that addition of ipratropium bromide (50 μg) to fenoterol (0.1 mg/kg) versus fenoterol (0.1 mg/kg) alone significantly reduced the proportion of infants receiving further treatment 45 minutes after initial treatment (OR 0.22, 95% CI 0.08 to 0.61).

Harms: The systematic review found no evidence of harm specific to the use of ipratropium bromide.[65]

Comment: The results of the review do not support the widespread, indiscriminate use of anticholinergic agents in the treatment of children under the age of 2 years with airways obstruction and wheeze. It is possible that infants did obtain symptomatic relief but that this was not always identified by the outcomes chosen.

OPTION ORAL CORTICOSTEROIDS

One small RCT found no significant difference in daily symptom scores with oral prednisolone compared with placebo.

Benefits: We found no systematic review. We found one RCT (38 acutely wheezing infants aged 3–17 months with wheezing episode lasting ≥ 48 hours, including 30 infants who had previously been admitted to hospital with wheeze)[66] comparing oral prednisolone (2 mg/kg/day) versus placebo given for 5 days during an acute wheezing episode. It found no significant difference in daily symptom scores (cough, wheeze, breathlessness) for the 56 acute wheezing episodes studied.[66]

Harms: The RCT found no adverse effects.[66]

Comment: None.

OPTION HIGH DOSE INHALED CORTICOSTEROIDS

One systematic review found that high dose inhaled corticosteroids compared with placebo reduced the requirement for oral corticosteroids but the difference was not statistically significant. The review also found a clear preference for the inhaled corticosteroids by the children's parents over placebo. The clinical importance of these results is unclear.

Benefits: We found one systematic review (search date not stated, 2 RCTs in infants with acute viral wheeze**G**).[67] The primary outcome for the review was wheeze episodes requiring oral corticosteroids. The review found that episodic high dose inhaled corticosteroids (budesonide, beclometasone) reduced the need for oral corticosteroids compared with placebo, but the difference was not statistically significant (2 crossover RCTs, 67 infants; RR 0.53, 95% CI 0.27 to 1.04). The review also found a clear preference for the inhaled corticosteroids by the children's parents over placebo (2 crossover RCTs, 67 infants; RR 0.64, 95% CI, 0.48 to 0.87).[67]

Harms: The systematic review did not report any adverse events. See harms of inhaled corticosteroids, p 251.[67]

Comment: Most of the RCTs included in the systematic review were carried out before the 1990s, when it was commonly thought that wheeze was synonymous with asthma and different patterns of wheeze in young children were seldom recognised. Although there is some evidence to support the use of high dose inhaled corticosteroids in acute episodes of viral wheeze, the practicalities of delivering treatment may limit applicability.

QUESTION What are the effects of prophylactic treatments for wheezing in infants?

Michael McKean

OPTION INHALED IPRATROPIUM BROMIDE

One small RCT identified by a systematic review found no significant difference in relief of symptoms with nebulised ipratropium bromide compared with placebo. The study may have lacked power to exclude a clinically important difference between treatments.

Benefits: We found one systematic review (search date not stated),[65] which found one RCT of high quality, although the power of the RCT was low.[68] The RCT (crossover, 23 infants aged 4–23 months) compared nebulised ipratropium bromide versus placebo or sodium cromoglicate. The RCT found no significant difference in relief of symptoms, as defined by diary cards, for ipratropium bromide versus placebo (OR 0.60, 95% CI 0.19 to 1.88).[68]

Harms: The RCT reported no significant adverse effects with ipratropium bromide.[68]

Comment: The study may have lacked power to exclude a clinically important difference between treatments. We found insufficient data to support the use of ipratropium bromide as a prophylactic agent for wheezing in infants.

OPTION SHORT ACTING β_2 AGONISTS

Two RCTs identified by a systematic review in infants aged up to 2 years found no significant improvement in symptoms with inhaled salbutamol compared with placebo. Another RCT identified by the same systematic review in infants aged 3–14 months found that oral salbutamol compared with placebo reduced treatment failures.

Benefits: We found one systematic review (search date not stated), which identified three RCTs in infants aged under 2 years with recurrent wheeze but no apparent history of acute viral bronchiolitis.[59] **Inhaled short acting β_2 agonists:** One RCT (crossover, 80 infants aged < 1 year with persistent or recurrent wheeze and a personal or family history of atopy) compared inhaled salbutamol**Ⓖ** (200 μg/day) versus placebo for 4 weeks. It found no significant difference between salbutamol versus placebo in symptoms (recorded in a diary) or lung function.[69] Another RCT (29 infants aged 2–18 months with a history of recurrent wheeze) compared inhaled salbutamol (600 μg) plus inhaled beclometasone (300 μg) versus inhaled salbutamol (600 μg) alone or placebo for 6 weeks.[70] It found no significant improvement in symptoms (cough, wheezing, sleep problems, expectorations) with salbutamol versus placebo.[70] **Oral short acting β_2 agonists:** One RCT (59 infants aged 3–14 months with at least 1 previous wheezy episode) compared oral salbutamol plus placebo, placebo plus prednisolone, and placebo plus placebo for 14 days.[71] It found that oral salbutamol versus placebo significantly reduced treatment failures (RR 2.51, 95% CI 1.09 to 5.79) and found no significant difference between salbutamol alone and the combination of salbutamol plus prednisolone.[71]

Harms: **Inhaled short acting β_2 agonists:** The RCTs did not report any adverse events.[69,70] **Oral short acting β_2 agonists:** The RCTs did not report any adverse events.[71]

Comment: None.

OPTION INHALED CORTICOSTEROIDS

Three RCTs found no clear evidence of effectiveness with lower prophylactic doses of inhaled corticosteroids (budesonide) in children aged 1 week to 6 years with recurrent wheeze. One RCT in infants aged 6–30 months found that higher prophylactic doses of inhaled corticosteroids (budesonide) compared with placebo reduced symptoms and the proportion of children with acute wheezing episodes during a 12 week period but found no significant reduction in the proportion of wheezing episodes per infant. Another RCT in infants aged 11–36 months found that higher prophylactic doses of inhaled corticosteroid

(budesonide) reduced the proportion of days requiring oral prednisolone and symptoms of wheezing and sleep disturbance, but found no significant improvement for cough. Higher doses of inhaled corticosteroids have the potential for adverse effects. One RCT found no significant improvement in symptoms with the addition of inhaled beclometasone compared with placebo to inhaled salbutamol.

Benefits: We found one systematic review (search date not stated)[67] and four additional RCTs.[72–75] **Lower dose versus placebo:** The systematic review identified one RCT.[76] The RCT (57 children aged 8 months to 6 years) found no significant difference after 4 months in acute episodes of wheeze with inhaled budesonide (400 µg/day by metered dose inhaler) versus placebo.[76] The RCT did not analyse infants separately. The first additional RCT (29 infants aged 4–17 months with recurrent wheeze) found that inhaled budesonide (150 µg through a metered dose inhaler) versus placebo significantly improved some symptoms (breathlessness, daytime wheeze, daytime cough) but not others (night time wheeze and cough), and found no significant difference in the need for bronchodilators.[74] The second additional RCT (60 infants aged 1–42 weeks ready for discharge after an episode of acute viral bronchiolitis requiring hospital admission) compared inhaled budesonide (200 µg/day through a metered dose inhaler) versus placebo for 12 months.[75] Symptoms of coughing and wheezing were recorded in a diary kept by parents. The RCT found no significant difference after 6 months in symptoms of coughing and wheezing with inhaled budesonide versus placebo.[75] **Higher dose versus placebo:** One additional RCT (40 infants aged 6–30 months with severe asthma) compared nebulised budesonide (1 mg twice daily) versus placebo for 12 weeks.[72] The RCT found that nebulised budesonide versus placebo significantly reduced the proportion of children with acute wheezing episodes (40% with budesonide *v* 83% with placebo; $P < 0.01$), incidence of daytime wheezing (2.2% with budesonide *v* 11.6% with placebo; $P < 0.05$), and incidence of night time wheezing (0.6% with budesonide *v* 6.5% with placebo; $P < 0.01$) but did not significantly reduce the number of acute wheezing episodes per child (0% with budesonide *v* 1% with placebo; $P = 0.13$). The second additional RCT (77 infants aged 11–36 months with moderate to severe recurrent wheezing) compared inhaled budesonide (400 µg twice daily) versus placebo for 12 weeks.[73] The RCT found that budesonide versus placebo significantly improved symptom scores from baseline for wheezing and sleep disturbance ($P < 0.05$ for both symptoms) but found no significant difference for cough or for restriction in physical activity because of coughing or wheezing. It also found that inhaled budesonide versus placebo significantly reduced the proportion of days requiring oral prednisolone.[73] **Addition of inhaled corticosteroid to short acting β_2 agonist:** We found one RCT (31 infants aged 13–18 months with recurrent wheeze) comparing the addition of inhaled beclometasone (200 µg twice daily) to inhaled salbutamol**G** (taken when needed) versus addition of inhaled placebo to inhaled salbutamol (as needed).[76] It found no significant difference between adding beclometasone versus placebo in clinical score, number of salbutamol doses, sleep disturbance, or number of symptom free days.[77]

Harms: The RCTs did not report any adverse events.[72–77] Higher doses of inhaled corticosteroids have the potential for adverse effects (see harms of inhaled corticosteroids, p 251).

Comment: None.

GLOSSARY

Aminophylline A stable combination of theophylline and ethylenediamine; the ethylenediamine is added to increase the solubility of theophylline in water.

Clinical asthma score is used to assess asthma severity. It involves five clinical variables (respiratory rate, wheezing, inspiratory–expiratory ratio, indrawing, dyspnoea), which are scored 0, 1, or 2. The scores for each variable are added together with a possible total score of 10.[78]

Orciprenaline is known as metaproterenol in USA; it is a non-selective β agonist.

Salbutamol is known as albuterol in USA; it is a short acting selective β_2 agonist.

Viral wheeze is defined as wheeze in association with nasal congestion and discharge but minimal or no intercurrent lower respiratory tract symptoms.

REFERENCES

1. Russell G, Ninan TK. Respiratory symptoms and atopy in Aberdeen school children: evidence from two surveys 25 years apart. *BMJ* 1992;304:873–875.
2. Kabesh M, Von Mutius E. Epidemiology and public health. In: Silverman M ed. *Childhood asthma and other wheezing disorders*. 2nd ed. London: Arnold, 2002.
3. Park ES, Golding J, Carswell F, et al. Pre-school wheezing and prognosis at 10. *Arch Dis Child* 1986;61:642–646.
4. Kelly WJW, Hudson I, Phelan PD, et al. Childhood asthma in adult life: a further study at 28 years of age. *BMJ* 1987;294:1059–1062.
5. Martinez FD, Wright AL, Taussig L, et al. Asthma and wheezing in the first six years of life. *N Engl J Med* 1995;333:133–138.
6. Geelhoed GC, Landau LI, Le Souef PN. Evaluation of SaO2 as a predictor of outcome in 280 children presenting with acute asthma. *Ann Emerg Med* 1994;23:1236–1241.
7. Plotnick LH, Ducharme FM. Combined inhaled anticholinergics and β_2 agonists in the initial management of acute paediatric asthma. In: The Cochrane Library, Issue 2, 2003. Chichester, UK: John Wiley & Sons, Ltd. Search date 2000; primary sources Medline, Embase, Cinahl, hand searches of bibliographies of references, and contact with pharmaceutical companies for details of unpublished trials and personal contacts.
8. Goggin N, Macarthur C, Parkin PC. Randomized trial of the addition of ipratropium bromide to albuterol and corticosteroid therapy in children hospitalized because of an acute asthma exacerbation. *Arch Pediatr Adolesc Med* 2001;155:1329–1334.
9. Cates CJ. Holding chambers versus nebulisers for β-agonist treatment of acute asthma. In: The Cochrane Library, Issue 2, 2003. Chichester, UK: John Wiley & Sons, Ltd. Search date 2001; primary sources Medline and Cochrane Airways Review Group Register.
10. Chou KJ, Cunningham SJ, Crain EF. Metered-dose inhalers with spacers vs nebulizers for pediatric asthma. *Arch Pediatr Adolesc Med* 1995;149:201–205.
11. Smith M, Iqbal S, Elliott TM, et al. Corticosteroids for hospitalised children with acute asthma (Cochrane Review). In: The Cochrane Library, Issue 2, 2003. Chichester, UK: John Wiley & Sons, Ltd. Date of most recent amendment: 15 December 2002. Date of most recent substantive amendment: 30 October 2002.
12. Patel H, Macarthur C, Johnson D. Recent corticosteroids use and the risk of complicated varicella in otherwise immunocompetent children. *Arch Pediatr Adolesc Med* 1996;150:409–414.
13. Edmonds ML, Camargo CA Jr, Pollack CV Jr, et al. Early use of inhaled corticosteroids in the emergency department treatment of acute asthma. In: The Cochrane Library, Issue 2, 2003. Chichester, UK: John Wiley & Sons, Ltd. Search date 2000; primary sources Cochrane Airways Group Register, and hand searches of bibliographies.
14. Manjra AI, Price J, Lenney W, et al. Efficacy of nebulised fluticasone propionate compared with oral prednisolone in children with an acute exacerbation of asthma. *Respir Med* 2000;94:1206–1214.
15. Matthews EE, Curtis PD, McLain B, et al. Nebulized budesonide versus oral steroid in severe exacerbations of childhood asthma. *Acta Paediatr* 1999;88:841–843.
16. Schuh S, Resiman J, Alshehri M, et al. A comparison of inhaled fluticasone and oral prednisone for children with severe acute asthma. *N Engl J Med* 2000;343:689–694.
17. Scarfone RJ, Loiselle JM, Wiley JF II, et al. Nebulized dexamethasone versus oral prednisone in the emergency treatment of asthmatic children. *Ann Emerg Med* 1995;26:480–486.
18. Volowitz B, Bentur L, Finkelstein Y, et al. Effectiveness and safety of inhaled corticosteroids in controlling acute asthma attacks in children who were treated in the emergency department: a controlled comparative study with oral prednisolone. *J Allergy Clin Immunol* 1998;102:1605–1609.
19. Devidayal S, Singhi S, Kumar L, et al. Efficacy of nebulized budesonide compared to oral prednisolone in acute bronchial asthma. *Acta Paediatr* 1999;88:835–840.
20. Mitra A, Bassler D, Ducharme FM. Intravenous aminophylline for acute severe asthma in children over 2 years using inhaled bronchodilators. In: The Cochrane Library, Issue 2, 2003. Chichester, UK: John Wiley & Sons, Ltd. Search date 2001; primary sources Cochrane Airways Group Register and reference lists of relevant articles.
21. Ream RS, Loftis LL, Albers GM, et al. Efficacy of IV theophylline in children with severe status asthmaticus. *Chest* 2001;119:1480–1488.
22. Calpin C, Macarthur C, Stephens D, et al. Effectiveness of prophylactic inhaled steroids in childhood asthma: a systematic review of the literature. *J Allergy Clin Immunol* 1997;100:452–457. Search date 1996; primary source Medline.
23. Tinkelman DG, Reed C, Nelson H, et al. Aerosol beclomethasone diproprionate compared with theophylline as primary treatment of chronic, mild to moderately severe asthma in children. *Pediatrics* 1993;92:64–77.
24. Ng SH, Dash CH, Savage SJ. Betamethasone valerate compared with sodium cromoglycate in asthmatic children. *Postgrad Med J* 1977;53:315–320.
25. Kannisto S, Voutilainen R, Remes K, et al. Efficacy and safety of inhaled steroid and cromone treatment in school-age children: a randomized pragmatic pilot study. *Pediatr Allergy Immunol* 2002;13:24–30.
26. Leflein JG, Szefler SJ, Murphy KR, et al. Nebulized budesonide inhalation suspension compared with cromolyn sodium nebulizer solution for asthma in young children: results of a randomized outcomes trial. *Pediatrics* 2002;109:866–872.
27. Price JF, Weller PH. Comparison of fluticasone propionate and sodium cromoglycate for the treatment of childhood asthma (an open parallel group study). *Respir Med* 1995;89:363–368.

28. The Childhood Asthma Management Program Research Group. Long-term effects of budesonide or nedocromil in children with asthma. *N Engl J Med* 2000;343:1054–1063.
29. Verberne A, Frost C, Roorda R, et al. One year treatment with salmeterol compared with beclomethasone in children with asthma. *Am J Respir Crit Care Med* 1997;156:688–695.
30. Simons FER and the Canadian Beclomethasone Diproprionate–Salmeterol Xinafoate Study Group. A comparison of beclomethasone, salmeterol and placebo in children with asthma. *N Engl J Med* 1997;337:1659–1665.
31. Ducharme FM, Hicks GC. Anti-leukotriene agents compared to inhaled corticosteroids in the management of recurrent and/or acute asthma. In: The Cochrane Library, Issue 2, 2003. Chichester, UK: John Wiley & Sons, Ltd. Search date 1999; primary sources Medline, Embase, Cinahl, hand searches of reference lists, and personal contact with colleagues and internal headquarters of leukotriene producers.
32. Drake AJ, Howells RJ, Shield JPH, et al. Symptomatic adrenal insufficiency presenting with hypoglycaemia in children with asthma receiving high dose inhaled fluticasone proprionate. *BMJ* 2002;324:1081–1083.
33. Todd GR, Acerini CL, Ross-Russell R, et al. Survey of adrenal crisis associated with inhaled corticosteroids in the United Kingdom. *Arch Dis Child* 2002;87:457–461.
34. Wolthers OD, Riis BJ, Pedersen S. Bone turnover in asthmatic children treated with oral prednisolone or inhaled budesonide. *Pediatr Pulmonol* 1993;16:341–346.
35. Reilly SM, Hambleton G, Adams JE, et al. Bone density in asthmatic children treated with inhaled corticosteroids. *Arch Dis Child* 2001;84:183–184.
36. Simons FE, Persaud MP, Gillespie CA, et al. Absence of posterior subcapsular cataracts in young patients treated with inhaled corticosteroids. *Lancet* 1993;342:776–778.
37. Abuektish F, Kirkpatrick JN, Russell G. Posterior subcapsular cataract and inhaled steroid therapy. *Thorax* 1995;50:674–676.
38. Allen DB, Mullen M, Mullen B. A meta-analysis of the effect of oral and inhaled steroids on growth. *J Allergy Clin Immunol* 1994;93:967–976. Search date 1993; primary sources literature searches of leading medical journals 1956–1993.
39. Sharek PJ, Bergman DA. Beclomethasone for asthma in children: effects on linear growth. In: The Cochrane Library, Issue 2, 2003. Chichester, UK: John Wiley & Sons, Ltd. Search date 1999; primary source Cochrane Airways Group Asthma Trials Register.
40. Doull IJ, Freezer NJ, Holgate ST. Growth of prepubertal children with mild asthma treated with inhaled beclometasone dipropionate. *Am J Resp Crit Care Med* 1995;151:1715–1719.
41. Pauwels RA, Pedersen S, Busse WW, et al. Early intervention with budesonide in mild persistent asthma: a randomised, double-blind trial. *Lancet* 2003;361:1071–1076.
42. Agertoft L, Pedersen S. Effects of long-term treatment with an inhaled corticosteroid on growth and pulmonary function in asthmatic children. *Respir Med* 1994;88:373–381.
43. Agertoft L, Pedersen S. Effect of long-term treatment with inhaled budesonide on adult height in children with asthma. *N Engl J Med* 2000;343:1064–1069.
44. Tasche M, Uijen J, Bernsen R, et al. Inhaled disodium cromoglycate (DSCG) as maintenance therapy in children with asthma: a systematic review. *Thorax* 2000;55:913–920. Search date 1999; primary sources Medline, Embase, Cochrane Controlled Trials Register, database of manufacturers of disodium cromoglicate, and hand searched references.
45. Edwards A, Holgate S, Howell J, et al. Sodium cromoglycate in childhood asthma [Letter]. *Thorax* 2001;56:331.
46. Armenio L, Baldini C, Bardare M, et al. Double blind placebo controlled study of nedocromil sodium in asthma. *Arch Dis Child* 1993;68:193–197.
47. Edwards AM, Lyons J, Weinberg E, et al. Early use of inhaled nedocromil sodium in children following an acute episode of asthma. *Thorax* 1999;54:308–315.
48. Weinstein S, Pearlman D, Bronsky E, et al. Efficacy of salmeterol xinafoate powder in children with chronic persistent asthma. *Ann Allergy Asthma Immunol* 1998;81:51–58.
49. Pedersen S. Treatment of nocturnal asthma in children with a single dose of sustained release theophylline taken after supper. *Clin Allergy* 1985;15:79–85.
50. Stein MA, Krasowski M, Leventhal BL, et al. Behavioural and cognitive effects of theophylline and caffeine. *Arch Pediatr Adolesc Med* 1996;50:284–288. Search date not stated; primary sources Medline, Psychlit, Dissertation Abstracts, and hand searched references.
51. Tsiu SJ, Self TH, Burns R. Theophylline toxicity: update. *Ann Allergy* 1990;64:241–257.
52. Knorr B, Matz J, Bernstein JA, et al. Montelukast for chronic asthma in 6–14 year old children. *JAMA* 1998;279:1181–1186.
53. Knorr B, Franchi LM, Bisgaard H, et al. Montelukast, a leukotriene receptor antagonist for the treatment of persistent asthma in children aged 2–5 years. *Pediatrics* 2001;108:E48.
54. Verberne A, Frost C, Duiverman E, et al. Addition of salmeterol versus doubling the dose of beclomethasone in children with asthma. *Am J Respir Crit Care Med* 1998;158:213–219.
55. Russell G, Williams DAJ, Weller P, et al. Salmeterol xinafoate in children on high dose inhaled steroids. *Ann Allergy Asthma Immunol* 1995;75:423–428.
56. Nassif EG, Weinberger M, Thompson R, et al. The value of maintenance theophylline in steroid dependent asthma. *N Engl J Med* 1981;304:71–75.
57. Simons FER, Villa JR, Lee BW, et al. Montelukast added to budesonide in children with persistent asthma: a randomized double blind crossover study. *J Pediatr* 2001;138:694–698.
58. Laviolette M, Malmstrom K, Lu S, et al. Montelukast added to inhaled beclomethasone in treatment of asthma. *Am J Respir Crit Care Med* 1999;160:1862–1868.
59. Chavasse R, Seddon P, Bara A, et al. Short acting beta agonists for recurrent wheeze in children under 2 years of age. In: The Cochrane Library, Issue 2, 2003. Chichester, UK: John Wiley & Sons, Ltd. Search date not stated; primary sources Medline and Pubmed.
60. Bentur L, Canny GJ, Shields MD, et al. Controlled trial of nebulised albuterol in children younger than 2 years of age with acute asthma. *Pediatrics* 1992;89:133–137.
61. Prahl P, Petersen NT, Hornsleth A. Beta$_2$-agonists for the treatment of wheezy bronchitis. *Ann Allergy* 1986;57:439–441.
62. Ploin D, Chapuis FR, Stamm D, et al. High-dose albuterol by metered dose inhaler plus a spacer device versus nebulization in preschool children with recurrent wheezing: a double-blind randomized equivalence trial. *Pediatrics* 2000;106:311–317.
63. Mandelberg A, Tsehori S, Houri S, et al. Is nebulized aerosol treatment necessary in the pediatric emergency department? *Chest* 2000;117:1309–1313.
64. Closa RM, Ceballos JM, Gomez-Papi A, et al. Efficacy of bronchodilators administered by nebulizers versus spacer devices in infants with acute wheezing. *Pediatr Pulmonol* 1998;26:344–348.
65. Everard ML, Bara A, Kurian M, et al. Anticholinergic drugs for wheeze in children under the age of two years. In: The Cochrane Library, Issue 2, 2003. Chichester, UK: John Wiley & Sons, Ltd. Search date not stated; primary sources Cochrane Airways Group Register and hand searches of respiratory care and paediatric journals.

66. Webb M, Henry R, Milner AD. Oral corticosteroids for wheezing attacks under 18 months. *Arch Dis Child* 1986;61:15–19.
67. McKean M, Ducharme F. Inhaled steroids for episodic viral wheeze of childhood. In: The Cochrane Library, Issue 2, 2003. Chichester, UK: John Wiley & Sons, Ltd. Search date not stated; primary sources Cochrane Airways Group Register and reference lists of articles.
68. Henry RL, Hiller EJ, Milner AD, et al. Nebulised ipratropium bromide and sodium cromoglycate in the first two years of life. *Arch Dis Child* 1984;59:54–57.
69. Chavasse RJ, Bastian-Lee Y, Richter H, et al. Inhaled salbutamol for wheezy infants: a randomised controlled trial. *Arch Dis Child* 2000;82:370–375.
70. Kraemer R, Graf Bigler U, Casaulter Aebischer C, et al. Clinical and physiological improvement after inhalation of low-dose beclomethasone dipropionate and salbutamol in wheezy infants. *Respiration* 1997;64:342–349.
71. Fox GF, Marsh MJ, Milner AD. Treatment of recurrent acute wheezing episodes in infancy with oral salbutamol and prednisolone. *Eur J Pediatr* 1996;155:512–516.
72. de Blic J, Delacourt C, Le Bourgeois M, et al. Efficacy of nebulized budesonide in treatment of severe infantile asthma: a double-blind study. *J Allergy Clin Immunol* 1996;98:14–20.
73. Bisgaard H, Munck SL, Nielsen JP, et al. Inhaled budesonide for treatment of recurrent wheezing in early childhood. *Lancet* 1990;336:649–651.
74. Noble V, Ruggins NR, Everard ML, et al. Inhaled budesonide for chronic wheezing under 18 months of age. *Arch Dis Child* 1992;67:285–288.
75. Fox GF, Everard ML, Marsh MJ, et al. Randomised controlled trial of budesonide for the prevention of post-bronchiolitis wheezing. *Arch Dis Child* 1999;80:343–347.
76. Wilson N, Sloper K, Silverman M. Effect of continuous treatment with topical corticosteroid on episodic viral wheeze in preschool children. *Arch Dis Child* 1995;72:317–320.
77. Barrueto L, Mallol J, Figueroa L. Beclomethasone dipropionate and salbutamol by metered dose inhaler in infants and small children with recurrent wheezing. *Pediatr Pulmonol* 2002;34:52–57.
78. Parkin PC, Macarthur C, Saunders NR, et al. Development of clinical asthma score for use in hospitalized children between 1 and 5 years of age. *J Clin Epidemiol* 1996;49:821–825.

Duncan Keeley
General Practitioner
Thame
UK

Michael McKean
Consultant in Respiratory Paediatrics
Newcastle-upon-Tyne
UK

Competing interests: DK has received occasional consultancy fees or assistance with organisation of, or travel to, meetings from companies including Allen and Hanburys, Astra, MSD, Zeneca, 3M, and Boots. MM none declared.

TABLE 1 **Comparison of inhaled budesonide, nedocromil, and placebo over 4–6 years on several measures of asthma symptoms and morbidity (see text, p 249).[28]**

Intervention	Budesonide (311 children)	Nedocromil (312 children)	Placebo (418 children)
Prednisone courses per 100 person years	70	102	122
Urgent care visits due to asthma per 100 person years	12	16	22
Hospital admissions due to asthma per 100 person years	2.5	4.3	4.4
Beclometasone or other asthma medications added	6.6%	17.1%	18.7%

Attention deficit hyperactivity disorder in children

Search date May 2004

Deborah Pritchard

QUESTIONS

INTERVENTIONS

See glossary G

Key Messages

Treatments

- **Atomoxetine** Four RCTs found that atomoxetine reduced symptoms of attention deficit hyperactivity disorder compared with placebo after up to 9 weeks of treatment. The RCTs found that atomoxetine decreased appetite and increased nausea, vomiting, asthenia, dyspepsia, infection, and pruritus compared with placebo.
- **Dexamfetamine sulphate** Two systematic reviews and one subsequent RCT found limited evidence that dexamfetamine improved some behavioural outcomes compared with placebo. One systematic review found insufficient evidence to compare the effects of dexamfetamine versus methylphenidate. One RCT found limited evidence that, in children already taking dexamfetamine or methylphenidate, adding clonidine reduced conduct symptoms of ADHD compared with added placebo after 6 weeks.
- **Methylphenidate** One systematic review and subsequent RCTs found that methylphenidate reduced core symptoms of attention deficit hyperactivity disorder in the short term compared with placebo, but disturbed sleep and appetite. The review found insufficient to compare the effects of methylphenidate versus dexamfetamine or tricyclic antidepressants. The review also found limited evidence that methylphenidate versus psychological/behavioural treatment improved symptoms in the medium term, but the clinical importance of these findings is unclear. One small RCT provided insufficient evidence to compare clonidine alone; methylphenidate alone, and the combination. A second RCT found limited evidence that, in children already taking dexamfetamine or methylphenidate, added clonidine reduced conduct symptoms of ADHD compared with added placebo after 6 weeks.
- **Methylphenidate plus psychological/behavioural treatment** One systematic review found inconsistent results for combination treatments (methylphenidate plus psychological/behavioural treatment) compared with placebo in children with attention deficit hyperactivity disorder. A second systematic review found that combination treatments improved attention deficit hyperactivity disorder symptoms compared with psychological/behavioural treatments alone. It also suggested that combined medication management plus intensive behavioural treatment was better than medication management alone.

- **Clonidine** Limited evidence from one systematic review suggested that clonidine reduced core attention deficit hyperactivity disorder symptoms compared with placebo, but the clinical importance of these findings is unclear. One small RCT provided insufficient evidence to compare clonidine alone; methylphenidate alone, and the combination. A second RCT found limited evidence that, in children already taking dexamfetamine or methylphenidate, added clonidine reduced conduct symptoms of ADHD compared with added placebo after 6 weeks.
- **Psychological/behavioural treatment** One systematic review of two small RCTs provided insufficient evidence to assess the effects of psychological/behavioural treatment compared with standard care. One large subsequent RCT found no significant difference between psychological/behavioural treatment and standard care in behaviour rating scales.

DEFINITION Attention deficit hyperactivity disorder (ADHD) is "a persistent pattern of inattention and hyperactivity and impulsivity that is more frequent and severe than is typically observed in people at a comparable level of development" (DSM-IV).[1] Inattention, hyperactivity, and impulsivity are commonly known as the core symptoms(G) of ADHD. Symptoms must be present for at least 6 months, observed before the age of 7 years, and "clinically important impairment in social, academic, or occupational functioning" must be evident in more than one setting. The symptoms must not be better explained by another disorder, such as an anxiety disorder(G), mood disorder, psychosis, or autistic disorder.[1] The World Health Organization's *International statistical classification of diseases and related health problems* (ICD-10)[2] uses the term "hyperkinetic disorder" for a more restricted diagnosis. It differs from the DSM-IV classification[3] as all three problems of attention, hyperactivity, and impulsiveness must be present, more stringent criteria for "pervasiveness" across situations must be met, and the presence of another disorder is an exclusion criterion. The evidence presented in this topic largely relates to children aged 5 years and above. There is a paucity of evidence of efficacy and safety of treatments in pre-school children.

INCIDENCE/ PREVALENCE Prevalence estimates of ADHD vary according to the diagnostic criteria used and the population sampled. DSM-IV prevalence estimates among school children range from 3–5%,[1] but other estimates vary from 1.7–16.0%.[4,5] No objective test exists to confirm the diagnosis of ADHD, which remains a clinical diagnosis. Other conditions frequently co-exist with ADHD. Oppositional defiant disorder(G) is present in 35% (95% CI 27% to 44%) of children with ADHD, conduct disorder(G) in 26% (95% CI 13% to 41%), anxiety disorder in 26% (95% CI 18% to 35%), and depressive disorder(G) in 18% (95% CI 11% to 27%).[6]

AETIOLOGY/ RISK FACTORS The underlying causes of ADHD are not known.[6] There is limited evidence that it has a genetic component.[7–9] Risk factors also include psychosocial factors.[10] There is increased risk in boys compared with girls, with ratios varying from 3 : 1[6] to 4 : 1.[3]

PROGNOSIS More than 70% of hyperactive children may continue to meet criteria for ADHD in adolescence, and up to 65% of adolescents may continue to meet criteria for ADHD in adulthood.[5] Changes in diagnostic criteria cause difficulty with interpretation of the few outcome studies. One cohort of boys followed up for an average of 16 years found a ninefold increase in antisocial personality disorder and a fourfold increase in substance misuse disorder.[7]

AIMS OF INTERVENTION To reduce inattention, hyperactivity, and impulsivity; and to improve psychosocial and educational functioning in affected children and adolescents, with minimal adverse effects of treatment.

OUTCOMES Measures of children's behaviour, such as Conners Teacher's Rating Scales(G); school performance, such as School Situations Questionnaire(G); self rated symptoms; adverse effects.

METHODS *Clinical Evidence* update search and appraisal May 2004.

QUESTION What are the effects of treatments for attention deficit hyperactivity disorder in children?

OPTION METHYLPHENIDATE

One systematic review and subsequent RCTs found that methylphenidate reduced core symptoms of attention deficit hyperactivity disorder in the short term compared with placebo, but disturbed sleep and appetite. The review found insufficient to compare the effects of methylphenidate versus dexamfetamine or tricyclic antidepressants. The review also found limited evidence that methylphenidate versus psychological/behavioural treatment improved symptoms in the medium term, but the clinical importance of these findings is unclear. One small RCT provided insufficient evidence to compare clonidine alone; methylphenidate alone, and the combination. A second RCT found limited evidence that, in children already taking dexamfetamine or methylphenidate, added clonidine reduced conduct symptoms of ADHD compared with added placebo after 6 weeks.

Benefits: We found one systematic review (search date 2000)[11] and four subsequent RCTs examining effects on symptoms.[12–15] Most studies were conducted in the USA, used a diagnosis of attention deficit disorder (DSM-III) or attention deficit hyperactivity disorder (ADHD; DSM-IIIR or DSM-IV), and included children aged 5–18 years, mostly recruited from psychiatric and other hospital outpatient clinics. We found one systematic review (search date not reported), which examined effects on later substance abuse.[16] It found no RCTs. **Versus placebo:** We found one systematic review that did not pool results from 13 rigorously selected short term RCTs (1177 children aged 5–18 years).[11] Three RCTs (99 children) found no significant difference in core symptoms❻ between methylphenidate and placebo. The other 10 RCTs found that compared with placebo, methylphenidate compared with placebo (dose range 0.56–0.72 mg/kg/day or 5–35 mg/day for trials reporting in those units) significantly improved the scores on Conners Teacher's Rating Scale❻ hyperactivity index ($P < 0.05$); (see table 1, p 277). The same systematic review found similar results in 17 other RCTs (643 children), which were less stringent in terms of homogeneity of participants, outcome measures, and methodological quality. The first subsequent RCT (parallel design, 276 children aged 6–12 years with ADHD but excluding children with Tourette's syndrome, ongoing seizure disorder, or psychotic disorder, and girls who had reached menarche) compared conventional (3 times/day dosing) and sustained release (once daily dosing) formulations of methylphenidate versus placebo.[12] The RCT found that methylphenidate significantly improved attention and behaviour at school compared with placebo (measured using mean teacher rated Abbreviated Inattention/Overactivity with Aggression (IOWA) Conners I/O rating scale [see table 1, p 277]) throughout the 4 week period of the study. It found no significant difference between conventional and sustained release formulations of methylphenidate. The second subsequent RCT (crossover design, 68 children aged 6–12 years) found similar benefit for slow release methylphenidate compared with placebo, and broad equivalence with conventional methylphenidate (see table 1, p 277).[13] Two other subsequent RCTs (crossover design, 1 RCT in 45 adolescents mean age 13.8 years and 1 RCT in 136 boys aged 7–12 years) also found that methylphenidate was significantly more effective at improving symptoms scores compared with placebo (both measured by the IOWA Connor's rating) (see table 1, p 277).[14,15] **Versus dexamfetamine [dexamphetamine]:** The systematic review[11] identified four poorly reported crossover RCTs (224 children, aged 5–18 years) comparing methylphenidate (dose range 0.6–4.5 mg/kg/day or 20 mg/day for trials reporting in those units) versus dexamfetamine (dose range 0.39–2.6 mg/kg/day or 10 mg/day for trials reporting in those units) but, because of heterogeneity, could not pool their results. Three RCTs (99 children, aged 5–12 years) found no significant difference between methylphenidate and dexamfetamine in the outcomes of interest (see table 1, p 277). The other RCT found improvement with methylphenidate compared with dexamfetamine for teacher reported, but not parent reported, outcomes. No firm conclusions can be drawn from these studies. **Versus clonidine or combined treatment:** See benefits of clonidine versus methylphenidate or combined treatment, p 271. **Versus tricyclic antidepressants:** The systematic review[11] identified, but could not pool, the results of two poorly reported crossover RCTs (105 children) comparing methylphenidate (dose 0.4 mg/kg/day or mean 20 mg/day for trials reporting in those units) versus imipramine (dose 1–2 mg/kg/day or mean 65 mg/day for trials reporting in those units). One RCT (75 children) found no significant difference in clinical outcomes after 1 year (see table 1, p 277). The other RCT (30 children) found that methylphenidate was less effective at improving some but not all outcomes in the short term compared with imipramine. No firm conclusions can be drawn from these studies. **Versus psychological/behavioural treatment:** We found one systematic review (search date 2000) that identified four RCTs comparing methylphenidate versus psychological/behavioural treatment❻.[11] Three of the RCTs (192 children aged 5–12 years) were poorly reported and compared a variety of psychological/behavioural treatments (individual cognitive training❻ over 12 weeks; parent and teacher training; behaviour treatment for 8 weeks) versus methylphenidate (5–60 mg/day). Overall, these three RCTs found limited evidence that, in the medium term (12–52 weeks), methylphenidate improved symptoms compared with psychological/behavioural treatment (see table 1, p 277). The fourth RCT (579 children aged 7–10 years) compared medication treatment (144 children, double blind titration of methylphenidate dose, switched to alternative medication after 28 days if response unsatisfactory, mean initial dose 30.5 mg/day) versus intensive behavioural management versus combined medication and intensive behavioural management versus standard community care.[17] A total of 74% of the children in the medication group were taking methylphenidate at the end of the study. Initial results were not reported as the number of children who improved, but only as P values. Methylphenidate improved some, but not all, of the symptoms of attention deficit disorder compared with psychological/behaviour treatment. Subsequent secondary analysis has developed these findings (see comment below).

Harms: The systematic review did not combine results on harms because of heterogeneity and incomplete data reporting.[11] It presented the number of RCTs that had found significant results. **Versus placebo:** The following symptoms were found by at least one RCT included in the systematic review to be significantly more common in children receiving methylphenidate: sleep disorders, anorexia or appetite disturbance, headache, motor tics, irritability, and abdominal pain (see table 2, p 279). Two of the subsequent RCTs[12,13] reported similar adverse effects. The fourth and fifth subsequent RCTs did not report on adverse effects.[14,15] We found no good evidence of effects of methylphenidate on growth rates in children. **Versus dexamfetamine:** Out of the four RCTs identified by the systematic review, two RCTs reported no significant difference with methylphenidate and dexamfetamine for anorexia or appetite disturbance and one RCT reported no significant difference in motor tics, abdominal pain, and irritability. **Versus clonidine or combined treatment:** See harms of clonidine versus methylphenidate or combined treatment, p 272. **Versus psychological/behavioural treatment:** The one large RCT comparing medication with intensive behavioural treatment❻ found that, of the children receiving either medication management or combined medication and intensive behavioural treatment, 50% reported mild adverse effects, 11% had moderate adverse effects, and 3% experienced severe adverse effects.[17] The study did not report adverse effects of non-drug intervention but did report that six out of 11 reported severe adverse effects (depression, worrying, or irritability, with some children reporting more than 1) could have been because of non-medication factors.

Comment: **Versus psychological/behavioural treatment:** The fourth RCT comparing medication versus intensive behavioural treatment is the largest and most rigorous currently available RCT of ADHD treatments.[17] Subsequent secondary analysis suggests that 56% of the children taking medication improved compared with 34% in the behavioural treatment group.[18] There is also a suggestion that children with comorbid behaviour problems (oppositional defiant disorder❻/conduct disorder❻) show a stronger response to medication than those without comorbid behaviour problems, and that children with ADHD and anxiety disorders❻ were likely to respond equally well to behavioural or medication treatments.[19] There are some concerns about the methods used in the RCT and caution should be exercised when using the results of secondary analysis as they are more susceptible to bias than the primary outcome analyses.[20] It should also be noted that the principal outcome measures were rating scales based on impressions of parents and teachers; they did not include the children's views or direct measures of their response to treatment. Long term effects on psychosocial adjustment, educational success, or behavioural improvement are unclear. We found no evidence about methylphenidate for preschool children.[21] **Conners Teacher's Rating Scale:** The abbreviated Conners Teacher's Rating Scale has been used widely in treatment studies and has been researched, validated, and standardised to measure treatment effects in ADHD.[22] However, the clinical importance of the effect of methylphenidate versus placebo on the abbreviated Conners Teacher's Rating Scale remains unclear.

OPTION DEXAMFETAMINE SULPHATE

Two systematic reviews and one subsequent RCT found limited evidence that dexamfetamine improved some behavioural outcomes compared with placebo. One systematic review found insufficient evidence to compare the effects of dexamfetamine versus methylphenidate. One RCT found limited evidence that, in children already taking dexamfetamine or methylphenidate, adding clonidine reduced conduct symptoms of ADHD compared with added placebo after 6 weeks.

Benefits: **Versus placebo:** We found two systematic reviews[5,21] and a subsequent RCT.[23] The first systematic review (search date 1997, 4 RCTs, 61 children aged 6–12 years, [dexamphetamine] 0.46–0.75 mg/kg/day) found that dexamfetamine significantly improved outcomes measured by the abbreviated Conners Teacher's Rating Scale❻ compared with placebo (WMD –4.8 points, 95% CI –6.4 points to –2.9 points).[21] The second later systematic review (search date 1997, 3 RCTs, 150 children aged 6–16 years, dexamfetamine 5–20 mg/day) only evaluated longer term studies (> 12 weeks).[5] It found some evidence of positive outcomes (including improved concentration and hyperactivity) with dexamfetamine compared with placebo. However, some methodological problems were identified with the RCTs in this review.[5] The subsequent RCT (crossover design, 35 children aged 6–12 years) found significant improvement with slow release formulation of dexamfetamine compared with placebo on two rating scales (including the hyperactivity index of the Conners Teacher's Rating Scale; $P < 0.001$).[23] **Versus methylphenidate:** See benefits of methylphenidate, p 268. **Versus clonidine or combined treatment:** See benefits of clonidine versus methylphenidate or combined treatment, p 271.

Harms: **Versus placebo:** Two RCTs identified by the first systematic review reported people withdrawing from the trial because of adverse events.[21] The second systematic review found that dexamfetamine significantly increased anorexia and appetite disturbance in three RCTs.[5] The subsequent RCT reported decreased appetite, weight loss, and sleep disturbance in children taking dexamfetamine.[23] **Versus methylphenidate:** See harms of methylphenidate versus clonidine or combined treatment, p 269. **Versus clonidine or combined treatment:** See harms of clonidine versus methylphenidate or combined treatment, p 272.

Comment: See comment of methylphenidate for the principal outcome measures, p 270.

OPTION CLONIDINE

Limited evidence from one systematic review suggested that clonidine reduced core attention deficit hyperactivity disorder symptoms compared with placebo, but the clinical importance of these findings is unclear. One small RCT provided insufficient evidence to compare clonidine alone; methylphenidate alone, and the combination. A second RCT found limited evidence that, in children already taking dexamfetamine or methylphenidate, added clonidine reduced conduct symptoms of ADHD compared with added placebo after 6 weeks.

Benefits: **Versus placebo:** We found one systematic review (search date 1999, 6 RCTs, 143 children, mean age 11 years, dose of clonidine 0.1–0.24 mg/day for 4–12 weeks).[24] One of the six RCTs included in the meta-analysis comparing clonidine versus placebo conducted by the review was a comparison of clonidine versus methylphenidate,[25] rather than versus placebo, and the rating scales of the clinical features of attention deficit hyperactivity disorder completed by parents, teachers, and clinicians were combined in the systematic review. The review found that clonidine was more effective than placebo at improving combined rating scores (effect size 0.58, 95% CI 0.27 to 0.89). The clinical importance of this result is unclear (see comment below), and the results should be treated with caution. **Versus methylphenidate or combined treatment:** We found no systematic review but found two RCTs.[25,26] The first, small RCT (3 groups of 8 boys aged 6–16 years with attention deficit hyperactivity disorder and either comorbid oppositional defiant disorder**G** or conduct disorder**G**) compared three interventions: clonidine (mean dose 0.17 mg/day), methylphenidate (mean dose 35 mg/day), and clonidine plus methylphenidate.[25] Most outcomes were not significantly different among the three groups. However, methylphenidate significantly improved the teacher reported score compared with clonidine (School Situations Questionnaire**G**; $P < 0.0003$). The clinical importance of this isolated result is unclear. The second RCT (67 children, aged 6–14 years with comorbid oppositional defiant disorder or conduct disorder who were already taking either dexamfetamine [dexamphetamine] or methylphenidate) compared additional clonidine versus additional placebo.[26] It defined improvement using an unconventionally stringent cut-off (38% reduction from baseline in parent reported symptoms for conduct and 43% reduction in parent reported symptoms for hyperactivity, using the

Hyperactive Index). At 6 weeks, it found that added clonidine significantly improved response rate for conduct compared with added placebo. It found no significant difference between treatments in response rate for hyperactivity (conduct response: 21/37 [57%] with added clonidine v 6/29 [21%] with added placebo; $P < 0.01$; hyperactive index response: 13/37 [35%] with added clonidine v 5/29 [17%] with added placebo; $P \leq 0.16$).[26]

Harms: **Versus placebo:** The systematic review[23] included information from 10 studies of harms. Not all were high quality RCTs, and their results are difficult to interpret. In children taking clonidine, nine of 10 studies found sedation in children; six studies found increased irritability. Electrocardiographs were recorded in two placebo controlled RCTs, which found no abnormalities. **Versus methylphenidate or combined treatment:** The first RCT (24 boys) found that two out of eight children on clonidine and four out of eight children on a combination of clonidine and methylphenidate developed bradycardia.[24] The second RCT (67 children already taking psychostimulants [dexamfetamine or methylphenidate]) found no significant difference between treatments for insomnia, daydreaming or staring, decreased appetite, sadness, euphoria, nightmares, stomach aches, headaches, nail-biting or tics (data not provided, P values not stated).[26] However, it found that, compared with placebo, adding clonidine significantly reduced lack of interest in others and lack of talking with others; irritability, proneness to crying and anxiety (rates not provided, $P<0.05$ for each outcome). It found that clonidine significantly increased drowsiness and dizziness compared with placebo during treatment (rates not provided, $P<0.05$), although these symptoms resolved within 6 weeks.

Comment: The systematic review[24] noted larger effect sizes in smaller and lower quality studies. Inclusion of the RCT of clonidine versus methylphenidate[25] in the systematic review creates difficulties in using that review to indicate the effects of clonidine versus placebo. The RCT[25] had a larger effect size than most other included studies, and it is likely to have inflated the final result of the meta-analysis. The results used by the systematic review for that RCT were not described in the original RCT report, and may have been a less reliable comparison of baseline and end of the study measures rather than a rigorous comparison of randomly allocated groups. Harms were reported as the number of studies that recorded a specific adverse effect or not rather than the number of children experiencing adverse effects.

OPTION ATOMOXETINE *New*

Four RCTs found that atomoxetine reduced symptoms of attention deficit hyperactivity disorder compared with placebo after up to 9 weeks of treatment. The RCTs found that atomoxetine decreased appetite and increased nausea, vomiting, asthenia, dyspepsia, infection, and pruritus compared with placebo.

Benefits: **Versus placebo:** We found no systematic review. We found four RCTs (reported in 3 papers), which found that atomoxetine significantly reduced symptoms measured by the Attention Deficit Hyperactivity Disorder Rating Scale (ADHD-RS**G**) at doses above 0.5 mg/kg twice daily (see table 3, p 279).[27–29] **Versus methylphenidate:** We found no systematic review or RCTs.

Harms: **Versus placebo:** The first RCT found that infection and pruritus increased with higher doses (infection: 1/83 [1.2%] with placebo v 0/44 [0%] with atomoxetine 0.5 mg/kg/day v 5/84 [6.0%] with atomoxetine 1.2 mg/kg/day v 6/83 [7.2%] with atomoxetine 1.8 mg/kg/day; pruritus:

0/83 [0%] with placebo *v* 0/44 [0%] with atomoxetine 0.5 mg/kg/day *v* 1/84 [1.2%] with atomoxetine 1.2 mg/kg/day *v* 5/83 [6.0%] with atomoxetine 1.8 mg/kg/day).[27] The second RCT found that atomoxetine significantly decreased appetite and significantly increased nausea, vomiting, asthenia, and dyspepsia compared with placebo (decreased appetite: 17/85 [20.0%] with atomoxetine *v* 5/85 [5.9%] with placebo; P = 0.02; vomiting: 13/85 [15.3%] with atomoxetine *v* 1/85 [1.2%] with placebo; P = 0.001; nausea: 10/85 [11.8%] with atomoxetine *v* 2/85 [2.4%] with placebo; P = 0.04; asthenia: 9/85 [10.6%] with atomoxetine *v* 1/85 [1.2%] with placebo; P = 0.02; dyspepsia: 8/85 [9.4%] with atomoxetine *v* 0/85 [0%] with placebo; P = 0.007).[28] The fourth and fifth RCTs were reported together.[29] They found that atomoxetine significantly decreased appetite compared with placebo (21.7% with atomoxetine *v* 7.3% with placebo; P < 0.05).[29] Further analyses of these two RCTs found no significant difference between treatments for cardiovascular adverse effects (palpitations, tachycardia, murmur, extrasystole, and bradycardia; P > 0.2 for all outcomes).[30] **Versus methylphenidate:** We found no RCTs.

Comment: We found two additional RCTs (reported together in a single paper) that compared atomoxetine versus placebo and focused on effects of discontinuation.[31] The paper reported results only for participants who completed the discontinuation phase of either study. The total number of participants randomised to treatments was not described, so we have not discussed results further. Atomoxetine is metabolised by the CYP 2D6 system of the liver. People with poor metabolism by this pathway may eliminate this drug more slowly and may be at greater risk of adverse effects.

OPTION PSYCHOLOGICAL/BEHAVIOURAL TREATMENT

One systematic review of two small RCTs provided insufficient evidence to assess the effects of psychological/behavioural treatment compared with standard care. One large subsequent RCT found no significant difference between psychological/behavioural treatment and standard care in behaviour rating scales.

Benefits: **Versus standard care:** We found one systematic review (search date 1997, 2 RCTs, 50 children aged 6–13 years)[21] and one subsequent RCT.[17] The systematic review found no significant difference between psychological/behavioural treatment**G** and standard care (medication, psychotherapy, or both as provided by the community health provider) in Conners Teacher's Rating Scales (SMD –0.40 points, 95% CI –1.28 points to +0.48 points) or parent ratings (1 RCT, 26 children, WMD –3.8 points, CI –9.6 points to +2.0 points). The RCTs identified by the systematic review were small and the clinical importance of these results is unclear. The subsequent RCT (290 children) found no significant difference between intensive behavioural treatments**G** for 14 months duration and standard community care (medication, psychotherapy, or both as provided by the community health provider).[17] In children with comorbid anxiety disorders**G**, the RCT found that intensive behavioural treatment resulted in better clinical outcomes. The results of this trial should be interpreted with caution, because of its weak problems. **Versus methylphenidate:** See benefits of methylphenidate, p 268.

Harms: **Versus standard care:** The systematic review and subsequent RCT did not make any comment about adverse effects.[17,21] **Versus methylphenidate:** See harms of methylphenidate, p 269.

Comment: **Versus standard care:** Children in the trials had different comorbid diagnoses, presentations, and clinical needs. Secondary analysis of one RCT[17] suggests possible small benefit with intensive behavioural treatment compared with standard community care (34% of children improved with intensive behavioural treatment v 25% with standard community care).[13] However, caution should be exercised in interpreting the results of secondary analysis as they are more susceptible to bias than the primary outcome analyses. **Versus methylphenidate:** See comments of methlynphenidate.[20]

OPTION METHYLPHENIDATE PLUS PSYCHOLOGICAL/BEHAVIOURAL TREATMENT

One systematic review found inconsistent results for combination treatments (methylphenidate plus psychological/behavioural treatment) compared with placebo in children with attention deficit hyperactivity disorder. A second systematic review found that combination treatments improved attention deficit hyperactivity disorder symptoms compared with psychological/ behavioural treatments alone. It also suggested that combined medication management plus intensive behavioural treatment was better than medication management alone.

Benefits: **Versus control/placebo:** We found one systematic review (search date 1997, 3 RCTs, 35 children aged 5–13 years).[21] It found that combination of methylphenidate with psychological/behavioural treatments**G** significantly improved parent ratings of attention deficit hyperactivity disorder compared with placebo or control (ADHD; Conners Parent's Rating Scale; WMD −7.3, 95% CI −12.3 to −2.4), but not teacher ratings of ADHD (Conners Teacher's Rating Scale**G**; WMD +3.8, 95% CI −2.0 to +9.6). The clinical importance of these findings is unclear.[21] **Versus psychological/behavioural treatments alone:** We found one systematic review (search date 2000, 11 RCTs, 428 children aged 5–18 years).[11] It found that methylphenidate plus behavioural treatments significantly improved ADHD behaviours, symptoms, and measures of academic achievement compared with behavioural treatments alone (see table 1, p 277). No significant difference was found in social skills or in measures of the relationship between parents and children.[11] The review separately assessed one RCT,[17] which found that combined drug plus intensive behavioural treatment significantly improved three out of five measures of ADHD core symptoms**G**, one out of three measures of aggression/oppositional behaviour, one out of three measures of anxiety depression, and one out of three measures of academic achievement compared with intensive behavioural treatment alone.[17]

Harms: The RCTs did not report any adverse effects. See harms of methylphenidate, p 269.

Comment: The RCT[17] is the largest and most methodologically rigorous study of ADHD treatments, with high standards for reporting and follow up of nearly all children (see comment under methylphenidate, p 270).[20] The results of a secondary analysis of this RCT[12] suggest that children with ADHD and comorbid anxiety respond equally well to medication management or intensive behavioural treatment (see comment about secondary analysis under methylphenidate, p 270);[19] but secondary analysis indicated that combined medication management plus intensive behavioural treatment was better than medication management alone.[19]

GLOSSARY

ADHD-RS (ADHD Rating Scale) an 18 point rating scale that is based on the 18 DSM-IV diagnostic criteria, which include a subjective assessment of inattention, hyperactivity, and impulsivity.

Anxiety disorder A range of conditions with features including apprehension, motor tension, and autonomic overactivity.

Behavioural treatment Treatment using insights from learning theory to achieve specific changes in behaviour. It is usually highly structured. It can be used with either children with attention deficit hyperactivity disorder or their parents/carers.

Cognitive training Brief structured treatment aimed at changing dysfunctional beliefs.

Conduct disorder Conduct disorders include a repetitive pattern of antisocial, aggressive, or defiant conduct that violate age appropriate social expectations.[2]

Conners Teacher's Rating Scales Widely used rating scales for assessment of symptoms of attention deficit hyperactivity disorder used extensively in both clinical work and epidemiological studies. There are 10 item parent and teacher questionnaires that can be used for children aged 3–17 years.

Core symptoms Inattention, hyperactivity, and impulsivity are commonly known as the core symptoms of attention deficit hyperactivity disorder.[5]

Depressive disorder Characterised by persistent low mood, loss of interest and enjoyment, and reduced energy.

Oppositional defiant disorder The presence of markedly defiant, disobedient, provocative behaviour, but without the severely dissocial or aggressive acts seen in conduct disorder.[2]

Psychological/behavioural treatments Includes any of the following methods: contingency management methods (e.g. behaviour modification); cognitive-behavioural therapy; individual psychotherapy; parent training or education; teacher training and education; parent and family counselling/therapy; social skills training; and electroencephalogram, biofeedback, or relaxation treatment.

School Situations Questionnaire A teacher completed questionnaire that measures the pervasiveness of child behaviour problems across 12 school situations.[32]

Substantive changes

Methylphenidate One systematic review added.[16] Conclusion unchanged.

Clonidine One RCT added.[26] Benefits and harms data enhanced. Conclusion unchanged.

REFERENCES

1. American Psychiatric Association. *Diagnostic and statistical manual of mental disorders (DSM-IV)*, 4th ed. Washington, DC: American Psychiatric Association, 1994.
2. World Health Organization. *International statistical classification of diseases and related health problems*, 10th rev ed. Geneva: World Health Organization, 1994.
3. Taylor E, Sergeant J, Doepfner M, et al. Clinical guidelines for hyperkinetic disorder. European Society for Child and Adolescent Psychiatry. *Eur Child Adolesc Psychiatry* 1998;7:184–200.
4. Goldman LS, Genel M, Bezman RJ, et al. Diagnosis and treatment of attention-deficit/hyperactivity disorder in children and adolescents. Council on Scientific Affairs, American Medical Association. *JAMA* 1998;279:1100–1107.
5. Jadad AR, Boyle M, Cunningham C, et al. *Treatment of attention-deficit/hyperactivity disorder*. Evidence report/technology assessment No 11. (Prepared by McMaster University under Contract No. 290–97-0017). Rockville MD: Agency for Health Care Policy and Research and Quality, 1999. Search date 1997; primary sources Medline, Cinahl, Healthstar, Psychinfo, Embase, The Cochrane Library, hand searches of reference lists, and contact with organisations funding research on attention deficit hyperactivity disorder and researchers. http://hstat.nlm.hih.gov/hq/Hquest/screen/DirectAccess/db/3143 (last accessed 24 February 2005).
6. Green M, Wong M, Atkins D, et al. *Diagnosis and treatment of attention-deficit/hyperactivity disorder in children and adolescents*. Council on Scientific Affairs, American Medical Association. Technical Review No. 3 (Prepared by Technical Resources International, Inc. under Contract No. 290–94-2024.). Rockville MD: Agency for Health Care Policy and Research, AHCPR Publication No. 99–0050, 1999.
7. Finkel MF. The diagnosis and treatment of the adult attention deficit hyperactivity disorders. *Neurologist* 1997;3:31–44.
8. Hertzig MEE, Farber EAE. *Annual progress in child psychiatry and child development, 1996*. New York: Brunner/Mazel Inc, 1997:602.
9. Kaminester DD. Attention deficit hyperactivity disorder and methylphenidate: when society misunderstands medicine. *McGill J Med* 1997;3:105–114.
10. Taylor E, Sandberg S, Thorley G, et al. *The epidemiology of childhood hyperactivity. Maudsley monographs*. London: Institute of Psychiatry, 1991:33.
11. Lord J, Paisley S. *The clinical effectiveness and cost-effectiveness of methylphenidate for hyperactivity in childhood*. London: National Institute for Clinical Excellence, Version 2, August 2000. Search date 2000; primary sources Jadad et al,[5] Medline, Cinahl, Healthstar, Psychinfo, and Embase.
12. Wolraich ML, Greenhill LL, Pelham W, et al. Randomized, controlled trial of OROS methylphenidate once a day in children with attention-deficit/hyperactivity disorder. *Pediatrics* 2001;108:883–892.

13. Pelham WE, Gnagy EM, Burrows-MacLean L, et al. Once-a-day Concerta methylphenidate versus three-times-daily methylphenidate in laboratory and natural settings. *Pediatrics* 2001;107:E105.
14. Evans SW, Pelham WE, Smith BH, et al. Dose-response effects of methylphenidate on ecologically valid measures of academic performance and classroom behavior in adolescents with ADHD. *Exp Clin Psychopharmacol* 2001;9:163–175.
15. Pelham WE, Hoza B, Pillow DR, et al. Effects of methylphenidate and expectancy on children with ADHD: behavior, academic performance, and attributions in a summer treatment program and regular classroom settings. *J Consult Clin Psychol* 2002;70:320–335.
16. Wilens TE, Faraone SV, Biederman J, et al. Does stimulant therapy of attention-deficit/hyperactivity disorder beget later substance abuse? A meta-analytic review of the literature. *Pediatrics* 2003;111:179–185. Search date not reported.
17. Jensen PS, Arnold LE, Richters JE, et al. A 14-month randomized clinical trial of treatment strategies for attention-deficit/hyperactivity disorder. The MTA Cooperative Group. Multimodal Treatment Study of Children with ADHD. *Arch Gen Psychiatry* 1999;56:1073–1086.
18. Swanson JM, Kraemer HC, Hinshaw SP, et al. Clinical relevance of the primary findings of the MTA: success rates based on severity of ADHD and ODD symptoms at the end of treatment. *J Am Acad Child Adolesc Psychiatry* 2001;40:168–179.
19. Jensen PS, Hinshaw SP, Kraemer HP, et al. ADHD comorbidity findings from MTA study: comparing comorbid subgroups. *J Am Acad Child Adolesc Psychiatry* 2001;40:147–158.
20. Boyle MH, Jadad AR. Lessons from large trials: the MTA study as a model for evaluating the treatment of childhood psychiatric disorder. *Can J Psychiatry* 1999;44:991–998.
21. Miller A, Lee SK, Raina P, et al. A review of therapies for attention-deficit/hyperactivity disorder. Canadian Coordinating Office for Health Technology Assessment, 1998. Search date 1997; primary sources Medline, Current Contents, hand searches of review articles, textbooks, British Columbia Methylphenidate Survey, and Intercontinental Medical Statistics for information on drug prescription and utilization in Canada.
22. Goyette CH, Conners CK, Ulrich RF. Normative data on revised Conners Parent and Teacher Rating scales. *J Abnorm Child Psychol* 1978;6:221–236.
23. James RS, Sharp WS, Bastain TM, et al. Double-blind, placebo-controlled study of single-dose amphetamine formulations in ADHD. *J Am Acad Child Adolesc Psychiatry* 2001;40:1268–1276.
24. Connor DF, Fletcher KE, Swanson JM. A meta-analysis of clonidine for symptoms of attention-deficit hyperactivity disorder. *J Am Acad Child Adolesc Psychiatry* 1999;38:1551–1559. Search date 1999; primary sources Medline; Psychinfo; Current Contents; Social and Behavioral Sciences; Current Contents Clinical Medicine; and hand searches of non-peer reviewed research reports, book chapters, chapter bibliographies, and individual report references.
25. Connor DF, Barkley RA, Davis HT. A pilot study of methylphenidate, clonidine, or the combination in ADHD comorbid with aggressive oppositional defiant or conduct disorder. *Clin Pediatr (Phila)* 2000;39:15–25.
26. Hazell PL, Stuart JE. A randomized controlled trial of clonidine added to psychostimulant medication for hyperactive and aggressive children. *J Am Acad Child Adolesc Psychiatry* 2003;42;886–894.
27. Michelson D, Faries D, Wernicke J, et al. Atomoxetine in the treatment of children and adolescents with attention-deficit/hyperactivity disorder: a randomized, placebo-controlled, dose-response study. *Pediatrics* 2001;108:E83. http://pediatrics.aappublications.org/cgi/reprint/108/5/e83 (last accessed 24 February 2005).
28. Michelson D, Allen AJ, Busner J, et al. Once-daily atomoxetine treatment for children and adolescents with attention deficit hyperactivity disorder: a randomized, placebo-controlled study. *Am J Psychiatry* 2002;159:1896–1901.
29. Spencer T, Heiligenstein JH, Biederman J, et al. Results from 2 proof-of-concept, placebo-controlled studies of atomoxetine in children with attention-deficit/hyperactivity disorder. *J Clin Psychiatry* 2002;63:1140–1147.
30. Wernicke JF, Faries D, Girod D, et al. Cardiovascular effects of atomoxetine in children, adolescents, and adults. *Drug Saf* 2003;26:729–740.
31. Wernicke JF, Adler L, Spencer T, et al. Changes in symptoms and adverse events after discontinuation of atomoxetine in children and adults with attention deficit/hyperactivity disorder: a prospective, placebo-controlled assessment. *J Clin Psychopharmacol* 2004;24:30–35.
32. Barkley RA. *Attention-deficit hyperactivity disorder: a handbook for diagnosis and treatment.* New York: Guilford Press, 1990.

Deborah Pritchard
Medicines and Healthcare Products Regulatory Agency (MHRA)
London
UK

Competing interests: None declared. The opinions expressed are those of the author and not those of the Medicines and Healthcare Products Regulatory Agency.

TABLE 1 **Methylphenidate studies (see text, p 268).[11–15]**

Ref	Intervention	Outcome		
11	MPH *v* placebo 13 RCTs	**Core symptoms score:**		
		Study author (year)	MPH (mean) *v* placebo (mean)	SMD (95% CI)
		Brown (1988)	17.33 *v* 24.50	–2.09 (–3.17 to –1.01)
		McBride (1988)	9.56 *v* 16.42	–1.06 (–1.42 to –0.69)
		Rapport (1989)	6.53 *v* 13.27	–1.26 (–1.72 to –0.81)
		Fischer (1991)	8.40 *v* 13.70	–0.76 (–0.98 to –0.53)
		Fitzpatrick (1992)	7.30 *v* 13.60	–0.85 (–1.51 to –0.18)
		DuPaul (1993)	7.16 *v* 15.84	–1.70 (–2.29 to –1.12)
		Klorman (1994)	6.50 *v* 14.00	–1.45 (–1.80 to –1.09)
		Buitelaar (1996)	18.00 *v* 22.00	–0.59 (–1.47 to +0.29)
		Lufi (1997)	30.85 *v* 32.60	–0.12 (–0.74 to +0.50)
		Hoeppner (1997)	8.20 *v* 13.54	–0.68 (–1.08 to –0.28)
		Manos (1999)	56.12 *v* 64.38	–0.60 (–1.03 to –0.16)
		Zeiner (1999)	8.83 *v* 14.69	–0.92 (–1.40 to –0.43)
		Pliszka (2000)	12.80 *v* 15.40	–0.32 (–0.96 to +0.32)
	MPH *v* dexamphetamine 3 RCTs	**Core symptoms score:**		
		Study author (year)	MPH (mean) *v* dexamphetamine (mean)	SMD (95% CI)
		Arnold (1978)	73.55 *v* 70.26	0.53 (0.01 to 1.06)
		Efron (1997)	56.14 *v* 58.76	–0.25 (–0.50 to 0)
		Pelham (1990)	2.30 *v* 1.70	+0.34 (–0.25 to +0.94)
	MPH *v* TCAs 1 study	**Core symptoms score:**		
		Study author (year)	MPH (mean) *v* TCAs (mean)	SMD (95% CI)
		Quinn (1975)	8.30 *v* 8.07	+0.05 (–0.41 to +0.50)
	MPH *v* psychological/behavioural treatments 2 RCTs	**Core symptoms score:**		
		Study author (year)	MPH (mean) *v* psychological/ behavioural treatments (mean)	SMD (95% CI)
		Brown (1985)	15.0 *v* 15.7	–0.22 (–1.10 to +0.66)
		Klein (1997)	1.2 *v* 2.10	–0.93 (–1.48 to –0.39)

TABLE 1 continued

Ref	Intervention	Outcome
	MPH plus psychological/behavioural treatments 2 RCTs	**Core symptoms score:** Study author (year) — MPH (mean) *v* MPH + psychological/behavioural treatments (mean) — SMD (95% CI) Brown (1985) — 15.10 *v* 15.00 — +0.02 (–0.85 to +0.90) Klein (1997) — 0.21 *v* 1.20 — –1.35 (–1.93 to –0.78)
12	IR-MPH 3 times/day *v* SR-MPH once daily *v* placebo	**Inattention/overactivity score (from baseline to end of study):** From 9.74 to 5.98 with SR-MPH *v* from 9.94 to 6.35 with IR-MPH *v* from 10.28 to 9.77 with placebo **Oppositional/defiant score (from baseline to end of study):** From 4.34 to 2.74 with SR-MPH *v* from 3.83 to 2.50 with IR-MPH *v* from 5.44 to 5.21 with placebo P < 0.001 for both interventions *v* placebo for all outcomes
13	IR-MPH 3 times/day *v* SR-MPH once daily *v* placebo	**Inattention/overactivity score (at end of study):** 5.00 with MPH 3 times/day *v* 4.69 with MPH once daily *v* 10.34 with placebo **Oppositional/defiant score (at end of study):** 1.99 with MPH 3 times/day *v* 1.81 with MPH once daily *v* 5.09 with placebo **Abbreviated Conners score (at end of study):** 7.94 with MPH 3 times/day *v* 7.82 with MPH once daily *v* 16.40 with placebo
14	MPH 10, 20, or 30 mg 3 times/day *v* placebo	**Inattention/overactivity score:** 2.7 with 10 mg *v* 1.7 with 20 mg *v* 1.2 with 30 mg *v* 4.4 with placebo **Oppositional/defiant score:** 1.3 with 10 mg *v* 0.9 with 20 mg *v* 0.6 with 30 mg *v* 2.5 with placeboP < 0.05 for all doses *v* placebo for all outcomes
15	MPH 0.3 mg/kg *v* placebo Q to A: Is this 3 times/day?	**Inattention/overactivity score:**0.5 with MPH *v* 1.9 with placeboP < 0.001 for MPH *v* placebo for both outcomes 1.8 with MPH *v* 3.5 with placebo **Oppositional/defiant score:**

IR, immediate release; MPH, methylphenidate; Ref, reference; SMD, standardised mean difference; SR, sustained release; TCA, tricyclic antidepressant.

TABLE 2 The number of RCTs reporting significant adverse effects with methylphenidate versus placebo (see text, p 269).[11] Published with permission ©NICE 2000.

Adverse effect	Number of trials
Anorexia or appetite disturbance	7/12 (58%)
Motor tics	1/2 (50%)
Irritability	2/9 (22%)
Sleep disorder	4/20 (20%)
Abdominal pain	2/10 (20%)
Headache	2/10 (20%)

TABLE 3 Placebo controlled RCTs of atomoxetine (see text, p 272).[27–29]

Ref	Population and Intervention	Mean difference (95% CI) in ADHD-RS score between treatment and placebo
27	0.5, 1.2, 1.8 mg/kg ATX twice daily *v* placebo Duration: 8 weeks 297 people aged 8–18 years	–4.1 (–9.0 to +0.8) with 0.5 mg/kg *v* –7.8 (–11.6 to –4.0) with 1.2 mg/kg *v* –7.7 (–11.6 to –3.8) with 1.8 mg/kg
28	ATX 1.0 mg/kg once daily *v* placebo	–7.8 (–11.2 to –4.4)
29	ATX 1.5 mg/kg twice daily *v* placebo	–10.1 (–14.5 to –5.7)
29	ATX 1.5 mg/kg twice daily *v* placebo	–8.5 (–13.0 to –4.0)

ADHD-RS, Attention Deficit Hyperactivity Disorder Rating Scale; ATX, atomoxetine.

Bronchiolitis in children

Search date October 2003

Juan Manuel Lozano

QUESTIONS

INTERVENTIONS

See glossary G

Key Messages

Prevention

- **Respiratory syncytial virus immunoglobulins or palivizumab (monoclonal antibody) in children at high risk** One systematic review has found that, in children born prematurely, in children with bronchopulmonary dysplasia, and in children with a combination of risk factors, prophylactic respiratory syncytial virus immunoglobulin or palivizumab (monoclonal antibody) reduces admission rates to hospital and intensive care units compared with placebo or no prophylaxis. Treatment duration varied between 4 and 6 months.
- **Nursing interventions (cohort segregation, handwashing, gowns, masks, gloves, and goggles) in children admitted to hospital** We found no RCTs about the effects of these interventions to prevent spread of bronchiolitis to other children.

Treatment

- **Bronchodilators (inhaled salbutamol, inhaled adrenaline [epinephrine])** Systematic reviews found that inhaled bronchodilators improved overall clinical scores in the short term (up to 24 hours after treatment) compared with placebo in children treated in hospital, emergency departments, and outpatient clinics. However, only one of two available systematic reviews pooled the clinical scores across trials, and although it found a statistically significant improvement in score in the short term, the clinical meaning of this finding is uncertain. They found no significant difference in admission rates between bronchodilators and placebo and no clinically important improvement in oxygen saturation. Subsequent RCTs found no evidence that nebulised adrenaline (epinephrine) improved short term outcomes during the first 4 days of illness in infants, the rate of hospital admission, the duration of hospital stay, or the time to resolution of illness compared with 0.9% sodium chloride. Four RCTs provided insufficient evidence of a difference between nebulised adrenaline and nebulised salbutamol in clinical severity, rate of hospital admission, or duration of admission.

- **Corticosteroids** RCTs provided limited and inconclusive evidence on the effects of corticosteroids compared with placebo.
- **Respiratory syncytial virus immunoglobulins, pooled immunoglobulins, or palivizumab (monoclonal antibody)** One systematic review has found that, in children born prematurely or children with bronchopulmonary dysplasia, prophylactic respiratory syncytial virus immunoglobulin or palivizumab (monoclonal antibody) given monthly reduces hospital admission and admission to intensive care compared with placebo or no prophylaxis. Treatment duration varied between 4 and 6 months.
- **Ribavirin** One systematic review found no significant difference between ribavirin and placebo in mortality, risk of respiratory deterioration, or duration of hospital stay in children admitted to hospital with respiratory syncytial virus bronchiolitis. It found limited evidence that ribavirin reduced the duration of mechanical ventilation. Two subsequent RCTs found no significant difference between ribavirin and placebo in duration of hospital stay or admission rate because of lower respiratory tract symptoms during the first year after the acute episode, or in the frequency of recurrent wheezing illness over 1 year of follow up.

DEFINITION Bronchiolitis is a virally induced acute bronchiolar inflammation that is associated with signs and symptoms of airway obstruction. Diagnosis is based on clinical findings. Clinical manifestations include fever, rhinitis (inflammation of the nasal mucosa), tachypnoea (rapid breathing), expiratory wheezing, cough, rales, use of accessory muscles, apnoea (absence of breathing), dyspnoea (difficulty in breathing), alar flaring (flaring of the nostrils), and retractions (indrawing of the intercostal soft tissues on inspiration). Disease severity Ⓖ of bronchiolitis may be classified clinically as mild, moderate, or severe.

INCIDENCE/ PREVALENCE Bronchiolitis is the most common lower respiratory tract infection in infants, occurring in a seasonal pattern with highest incidence in the winter in temperate climates,[1] and in the rainy season in warmer countries. Each year in the USA about 21% of infants have lower respiratory tract disease and 6–10/1000 infants are admitted to hospital for bronchiolitis (1–2% of children < 12 months of age).[2] The peak rate of admission occurs in infants aged 2–6 months.[3]

AETIOLOGY/ RISK FACTORS Respiratory syncytial virus is responsible for bronchiolitis in 70% of cases. This figure reaches 80–100% in the winter months. However, in early spring, parainfluenza virus type 3 is often responsible.[1]

PROGNOSIS **Morbidity and mortality:** Disease severity is related to the size of the infant, and to the proximity and frequency of contact with infective infants. Children at increased risk of morbidity and mortality are those with congenital heart disease, chronic lung disease, history of premature birth, hypoxia, and age less than 6 weeks.[4] Other factors associated with a prolonged or complicated hospital stay include a history of apnoea or respiratory arrest, pulmonary consolidation seen on a chest radiograph, and (in North America) people of Native American or Inuit race.[5] The risk of death within 2 weeks is high for children with congenital heart disease (3.4%) or chronic lung disease (3.5%) as compared with other groups combined (0.1%).[4] Rates of admission to intensive care units (range 31–36%) and need for mechanical ventilation (range 11–19%) are similar among all high risk groups.[4] The percentage of these children needing oxygen supplementation is also high (range 63–80%).[4] In contrast, rates of intensive care unit admission (15%) and ventilation (8%) in children who do not have high risk characteristics are markedly lower.[6] **Long term prognosis:** Information on long term prognosis varies among studies. One small prospective study of two matched cohorts (25 children with bronchiolitis; 25 children without) found no evidence that bronchiolitis requiring outpatient treatment is associated with an increased risk of asthma in the long term.[7] Possible confounding factors include variation in illness severity, smoke exposure, and being in overcrowded environments.[8] We found one prospective study in 50 randomly selected infants admitted with bronchiolitis, followed up by questionnaires for 5 years and a visit in the fifth year. It found a doubling of asthma incidence compared with the general population, although there was large (30%) loss to follow up and no matched control group.[9]

AIMS OF INTERVENTION To decrease morbidity and mortality, shorten hospital stay, and prevent transmission of infection, with minimal adverse effects.

OUTCOMES Death rate; rates of hospital admission; rate of intubation or admission to intensive care units; clinical score (clinical score is a subjective, unvalidated measure that is based on judgements made by the clinician); rates of clinical and serological infection. Oxygen saturation is a proxy outcome, and is reported here although the clinical significance and sensitivity of this outcome are unclear.

METHODS *Clinical Evidence* search and appraisal October 2003.

QUESTION What are the effects of prophylactic measures in high risk children?

OPTION RESPIRATORY SYNCYTIAL VIRUS IMMUNOGLOBULINS OR PALIVIZUMAB (MONOCLONAL ANTIBODY)

One systematic review has found that, in children born prematurely or children with bronchopulmonary dysplasia, prophylactic respiratory syncytial virus immunoglobulin or palivizumab (monoclonal antibody) given monthly reduces hospital admission and admission to intensive care compared with placebo or no prophylaxis. Treatment duration varied between 4 and 6 months.

Benefits: We found one systematic review (search date 1999, 4 RCTs, 2598 children) comparing monthly respiratory syncytial virus immunoglobulin (RSV Ig) or palivizumab (monoclonal antibody) with placebo or no prophylaxis.[10] Three of the RCTs used intravenous RSV Ig and one used intramuscular palivizumab. Treatment duration varied between 4 and 6 months. Two of the RCTs using RSV Ig were open label and both used no prophylaxis as the control intervention. The systematic review found that RSV Ig or palivizumab reduced admission to hospital compared with placebo (95/1535 [6%] with RSV Ig or palivizumab *v* 138/1063 [13%] with placebo; OR 0.48, 95% CI 0.37 to 0.64) and to the intensive care unit (27/1535 [2%] with RSV Ig or palivizumab *v* 43/1063 [4%] with placebo; OR 0.47, 95% CI 0.29 to 0.77). It found no significant difference in mechanical ventilation (16/1535 [1%] for RSV Ig or palivizumab *v* 14/1063 [1%] with placebo; OR 0.99, 95% CI 0.48 to 2.07). Follow up duration varied across RCTs in the systematic review from 150 days up to 17 months.[10]

Harms: See harms of immunoglobulins, p 288.

Comment: Premature infants included in the RCTs were children under 6 months old, with gestational age at birth of less than either 32 or 35 weeks. Children with bronchopulmonary dysplasia were under 2 years old and were still having treatment for this disorder. Planned subgroup analysis in the review found that prophylaxis significantly reduced hospital admission in children whose only risk factor was prematurity (OR 0.27, 95% CI 0.15 to 0.49) and in children with bronchopulmonary dysplasia alone (OR 0.54, 95% CI 0.37 to 0.80), but not in children with cardiac comorbidity alone (OR 0.64, 95% CI 0.37 to 1.10).[10] A cost-effectiveness analysis suggests that the clinical effect of palivizumab when used in all children who meet the licensed indication for it is small, and its benefits are likely to be more clinically relevant in children at the highest risk.[11]

QUESTION **What are the effects of measures to prevent transmission in hospital?**

OPTION **NURSING INTERVENTIONS (COHORT SEGREGATION, HANDWASHING, GOWNS, MASKS, GLOVES, AND GOGGLES)**

We found no RCTs about the effects of these interventions to prevent spread of bronchiolitis to other children.

Benefits: We found no systematic review and no RCTs of sufficient quality examining effects of cohort segregation(G), handwashing, gowns, masks, gloves, or goggles, used either singly or in combination, on nosocomial transmission of bronchiolitis in children (see comment below).

Harms: **Cohort segregation:** Potential risks associated with cohort segregation include misdiagnosing respiratory syncytial virus infection and putting non-infected people at risk by subsequent placement into the wrong cohort. **Handwashing:** Dermatitis is a potential adverse effect of repeated handwashing with some products, affecting care providers. **Other interventions:** No harms reported.

Comment: Handwashing is a well established technique for reducing cross-infection in other contexts, and so RCTs may not be ethically feasible. **Single nursing interventions:** We found four observational studies comparing nosocomial infection rates in separate series of children before and after introduction of cohort segregation, handwashing, gowns and masks, and goggles.[12–15] No study adjusted results for variations in baseline incidence. Three studies found a lower incidence of transmission after introduction of cohort segregation alone, handwashing alone, and eye–nose goggles alone.[12–14] The fourth study found no significant difference in transmission after introducing gowns and masks.[15] **Combinations of nursing interventions:** We found one RCT (58 medical personnel caring for children admitted with bronchiolitis), which found no significant difference in nosocomial infection rate in staff when they used gowns and masks in addition to handwashing (5/28 [18%] of those using gowns, masks, and handwashing *v* 4/30 [13%] in the control group; RR 1.3, 95% CI 0.4 to 3.6).[16] The RCT did not report transmission rates in the children. One non-randomised prospective trial (233 children at risk of severe nosocomial infection) compared transmission rates in wards using different nursing policies.[17] It found that a combination of cohort segregation, gowns, and gloves reduced nosocomial transmission rates compared with all other policies (cohort segregation alone, gown and gloves alone, no special precautions) taken together. However, the control interventions did not remain constant throughout the trial, the results were based on an interim analysis, and the definition of "at risk" children was not stated clearly.

QUESTION **What are the effects of treatments for children with bronchiolitis?**

OPTION **BRONCHODILATORS (INHALED SALBUTAMOL, INHALED ADRENALINE [EPINEPHRINE])**

Systematic reviews found that inhaled bronchodilators improved overall clinical scores in the short term (up to 24 hours after treatment) compared with placebo in children treated in hospital, emergency departments, and outpatient clinics. However, only one of two available systematic reviews pooled the clinical scores across trials, and although it found a statistically

significant improvement in score in the short term, the clinical meaning of this finding is uncertain. They found no significant difference in admission rates between bronchodilators and placebo and no clinically important improvement in oxygen saturation. Subsequent RCTs found no evidence that nebulised adrenaline (epinephrine) improved short term outcomes during the first 4 days of illness in infants, the rate of hospital admission, the duration of hospital stay, or the time to resolution of illness compared with 0.9% sodium chloride. Four RCTs provided insufficient evidence of a difference between nebulised adrenaline and nebulised salbutamol in clinical severity, rate of hospital admission, or duration of admission.

Benefits: **Versus placebo:** We found two systematic reviews[18,19] and five subsequent RCTs.[20–24] The first review (search date 1998, 8 RCTs, 485 children) evaluated children in outpatient clinics or the emergency department and after admission to hospital.[18] The second review (search date 1995, 5 RCTs, 251 children) considered children treated in outpatient clinics only.[19] Four RCTs were common to both reviews. The first review found that, in the short term, bronchodilators improved clinical scores in children with mild and moderately severe bronchiolitis (lack of improvement in clinical score, bronchodilator *v* placebo; RR 0.76, 95% CI 0.60 to 0.95).[18] The second review found that bronchodilators significantly improved oxygen saturation, but by a clinically unimportant amount (mean difference in oxygen saturation: 1.2%, 95% CI 0.8% to 1.6%),[19] while the first review found results for oxygen saturation that were too varied to allow pooling.[18] Both reviews found no significant difference in admission rates between bronchodilators and placebo in children treated in outpatient clinics or emergency departments (admission rates: RR 0.85, 95% CI 0.47 to 1.53;[18] 23/97 [24%] with bronchodilator *v* 21/90 [23%] with placebo; RR 1.0, 95% CI 0.6 to 1.7[19]). The first subsequent RCT (38 infants without previous wheezing episodes) compared a single dose (3 mg in 3 mL) of nebulised levo-adrenaline (epinephrine) with 0.9% sodium chloride placebo during the first 4 days of their respiratory illness.[20] It found no significant differences in respiratory and heart rates, oxygen saturation, and the RDAI**G** measured during the 60 minutes after treatment (results reported graphically). The second subsequent RCT (149 hospitalised infants without previous history of wheezing and with a clinical diagnosis of acute viral bronchiolitis) compared nebulisations of racemic adrenaline (0.03 mL/kg/dose of a 2.25% solution), salbutamol (0.03 mL/kg/dose of a 5 mg/mL solution), and placebo (0.03 mL/kg/dose of 0.9% sodium chloride) given every 1–6 hours, at the discretion of the attending medical team. There were no significant differences in the length of hospital stay (placebo *v* adrenaline: mean difference +3.5 hours, 95% CI –18.6 hours to +25.6 hours; placebo *v* salbutamol: mean difference +1.9 hours, 95% CI –18.3 hours to +22.1 hours) or in the mean time to normal oxygenation, adequate fluid intake, RDAI of 4 or less, or infrequent nebulisations.[21] The third subsequent RCT (75 infants with a clinical diagnosis of bronchiolitis presenting to 1 admitting unit) compared two doses of nebulised adrenaline (2 mL of a 1 : 1000 solution diluted to 5 mL with 0.9% sodium chloride) versus placebo (nebulised 0.9% sodium chloride). It found no significant difference in the frequency of admission to hospital (19/38 [50%] with adrenaline *v* 23/37 [62%] with placebo; RR 0.80, 95% CI 0.54 to 1.21).[22] The fourth subsequent RCT (129 infants with a clinical diagnosis of bronchiolitis, discharged directly home after an emergency department visit) compared oral salbutamol 0.1 mg/kg/dose versus oral placebo given three times daily for a maximum of 7 days or until complete resolution of bronchiolitis symptoms.[23] The RCT found no significant difference in the time to resolution of illness or in the frequency of admission to hospital (mean time to resolution of illness: 8.9 days with salbutamol *v* 8.4 days with placebo; $P = 0.5$; frequency of admission: 4/64 [6%] with salbutamol *v* 5/65 [8%] with placebo; RR 0.81, 95% CI 0.20 to 2.90).[23] The fifth subsequent RCT (194 infants admitted to hospital with a first episode of wheezing and a clinical diagnosis of bronchiolitis) compared three 4 mL doses of 1% nebulised adrenaline versus placebo (0.9% sodium chloride) given at 4 hour intervals after hospital admission.[24] It found no significant difference in the duration of hospital stay (adrenaline 58.8 hours, 95% CI 49.4 hours to 70.0 hours *v* placebo 69.5 hours, 95% CI 59.3 hours to 81.4 hours). **Compared with other treatments:** We found four RCTs comparing nebulised adrenaline versus salbutamol, which provided insufficient evidence to conclude a clinically significant difference between the two (see table 1, p 291).[21,25–27]

Harms: **Versus placebo:** The first review reported tachycardia, increased blood pressure, decreased oxygen saturation, flushing, hyperactivity, prolonged cough, and tremor after use of bronchodilators.[18] The review did not report the frequency of adverse effects. The second review gave no information on adverse effects.[19] Two subsequent RCTs reported that there were no adverse effects with treatment.[22,23] One subsequent RCT comparing racemic adrenaline, salbutamol, and placebo reported asymptomatic transient (< 1 hour) tachycardia, mild hypertension, and slight tremor which were equally frequent in all treatment groups (absolute numbers not reported).[21] One subsequent RCT also reported that nebulised adrenaline increased heart rate compared with placebo 60 minutes after the last treatment (mean heart rate: 151 beats/minute with adrenaline *v* 138 beats/minute with placebo; $P < 0.001$).[24] **Compared with other treatments:** One RCT reported a higher incidence of pallor in children treated with adrenaline than in those receiving salbutamol (at 30 minutes: 10/20 [50%] with adrenaline *v* 3/21 [14%] with salbutamol; RR 3.50, 95% CI 1.12 to 10.90; NNH 3, 95% CI 2 to 8).[26] The other RCTs gave no information on adverse effects.[20,25,27]

Comment: Only one of two available systematic reviews pooled the clinical scores across trials.[18] Although it found a statistically significant improvement in score in the short term, the clinical meaning of this finding is uncertain. One review found significant heterogeneity among RCTs in the effects of bronchodilators on oxygen saturation.[18] None of the RCTs considered respiratory failure as an outcome. Discrepancies in primary studies included differences in study populations such as inclusion of sedated children, short duration of follow up, and validity of clinical scores. Bronchodilators may improve the clinical appearance of a child through a general stimulatory effect rather than by improving respiratory function.[28]

OPTION CORTICOSTEROIDS

RCTs provided limited and inconclusive evidence on the effects of corticosteroids compared with placebo.

Benefits: **Short term effects:** We found one systematic review (search date 1999, 6 RCTs, 347 children in hospital),[29] six additional RCTs[30–35] and five subsequent RCTs[36–40] of corticosteroids compared with placebo in children with bronchiolitis. Three of the additional RCTs had been mentioned in the systematic review but were excluded because of data inconsistency,[33] treatment outside hospital,[34] or failure to report the outcome markers sought by the systematic review.[35] The systematic review found no significant difference in the mean duration of hospital stay (5 RCTs, 229 children: WMD −0.43 days, 95% CI −1.05 days to +0.18 days). Sensitivity analyses found similar results in the RCTs with clearly identified randomisation methods (4 RCTs, 253 children: WMD –0.35 days, 95% CI –0.84 days to +0.14 days), and after exclusion of RCTs that included children with previous wheezing (4 RCTs, 264 children: WMD –0.29 days, 95% CI –0.71 days to +0.13 days).[29] Results of the review comparing effects of corticosteroids versus placebo on clinical symptoms were difficult to interpret (see comment below). The RCTs in the systematic review reported different clinical scales at varying times after starting treatment. The scales usually included measurements of oxygen saturation, wheezing, accessory muscle use, and respiratory rate. Results reported 72 hours after starting treatment were too heterogeneous for analysis. Three RCTs (197 children) provided results 24 hours after starting treatment. The pooled standardised effect size from these three RCTs indicated that corticosteroids produced a significant improvement compared with placebo.[29] However, the clinical importance of such an improvement is not clear because different scales were combined across RCTs. All six additional RCTs and three of the five subsequent RCTs that compared clinical scores found no significant benefit from corticosteroids (see table 2, p 292).[30–37,40] **Long term effects:** We found three small RCTs with long term follow up (3 years,[41] 3–5 years,[42] and 2 years[43]), which used telephone questionnaires to examine the effect of corticosteroids during the acute episode on subsequent wheezing. Two of the three RCTs did not detect any benefit from corticosteroids.[41,42] The third was an open label RCT, in which 117 hospitalised infants (mean age 2.6 months, requiring hospital treatment because of respiratory syncytial virus bronchiolitis) were allocated to be in a control group (41 infants), and received inhaled budesonide for 7 days (40 infants) or inhaled budesonide for 2 months (36 infants).[43] However, this RCT had several problems that compromised its validity (see comment below).

Harms: The acute adverse effects of oral corticosteroids are well documented, and include hyperglycaemia and immunosuppression.[44] The RCTs did not give information on these.[30–40] See harms of corticosteroids in asthma and other wheezing disorders of childhood, p 239.

Comment: The evidence presented in the systematic review[29] is difficult to interpret because some of the RCTs did not exclude children with a history of wheezing who may have asthma, a condition likely to respond to corticosteroids. The clinical scales used in the RCTs included oxygen saturation, but the clinical relevance of changes in this parameter are unclear. Even if the results are accepted at face value, the clinical significance of an effect size is unclear. Furthermore, nine RCTs with more than double the number of children were not included in the meta-analysis. All of these RCTs, except one, did not find a benefit of corticosteroids, and the single RCT that did, only observed a transient improvement in clinical score at one time point. Another systematic review is underway (Lozano JM, personal communication, 2003). We found inadequate evidence to evaluate the effects of systemic compared with inhaled corticosteroids. The open label RCT comparing two different regimens of inhaled budesonide in hospitalised children had several problems that further compromised its validity.[43] Diagnosis of asthma was based only on a telephone survey; the children were not assessed to establish whether they had received additional interventions or exposures that could explain the results.

OPTION RIBAVIRIN

One systematic review found no significant difference between ribavirin and placebo in mortality, risk of respiratory deterioration, or duration of hospital stay in children admitted to hospital with respiratory syncytial virus bronchiolitis. It found limited evidence that ribavirin reduced the duration of

mechanical ventilation. Two subsequent RCTs found no significant difference between ribavirin and placebo in duration of hospital stay or admission rate because of lower respiratory tract symptoms during the first year after the acute episode, or in the frequency of recurrent wheezing illness over 1 year of follow up.

Benefits: We found one systematic review (search date 2000, 10 small RCTs)[47] and two subsequent RCTs.[48,49] The review found that, in children and infants hospitalised with respiratory syncytial virus bronchiolitis, ribavirin (tribavirin) did not significantly reduce mortality, respiratory deterioration, or duration of hospital stay compared with placebo (death: 5/86 [6%] with ribavirin *v* 7/72 [10%] with placebo; RR 0.61, 95% CI 0.21 to 1.75; respiratory deterioration: 4/56 [7%] with ribavirin *v* 11/60 [18%] with placebo; RR 0.42, 95% CI 0.15 to 1.17; duration of hospital stay WMD: –1.9 days with ribavirin *v* placebo, RR 95% CI –0.9 to +4.6 days). However, it found that ribavirin significantly reduced duration of ventilation compared with placebo (mean reduction in duration with ribavirin *v* placebo 1.2 days, 95% CI 0.2 days to 3.4 days).[47] The high mortality in both groups may have been because of severe disease at baseline. The first subsequent RCT (40 hospitalised infants who received ribavirin or placebo within 12 hours of admission) found no significant difference in outcomes measured during the acute episode, such as the duration of oxygen supplementation or duration of hospital stay (duration of oxygen supplementation: 2.72 days with ribavirin *v* 1.92 days with placebo; mean difference +0.80 days, 95% CI –0.73 days to +2.32 days; duration of hospital stay: 4.94 days with ribavirin *v* 3.36 days with placebo; mean difference +1.58 days, 95% CI –0.18 days to +3.35 days).[48] The RCT also followed the infants for 1 year after the initial episode. It found no significant difference in admission rates for recurrent lower respiratory illness or in use of bronchodilators (admission for recurrent lower respiratory tract infection: 2/16 [13%] with ribavirin *v* 3/19 [16%] with placebo; RR 0.79, 95% CI 0.15 to 4.17; use of bronchodilators: 5/16 [31%] with ribavirin *v* 8/19 [42%] with placebo; RR 0.74, 95% CI 0.30 to 1.82). However, the study may have lacked power to rule out a clinically important difference.[48] A second, open label RCT (45 previously healthy infants < 180 days old and hospitalised because of severe respiratory syncytial virus-confirmed bronchiolitis) compared nebulised ribavirin (60 mg/mL over three 2-hour periods for a total of 6 g/100 mL every 24 hours for 3 days) versus no ribavirin. It found no significant difference in the frequency of recurrent wheezing illness over 1 year of follow up (15/24 [63%] with ribavirin *v* 17/21 [81%] with placebo; RR 0.78, 95% CI 0.53 to 1.12).[49]

Harms: We found no results from prospective studies. The systematic review[47] and the two RCTs did not report harms.[48,49] We found case reports of headaches and contact lens dysfunction in carers.[50] Ribavirin has been reported to be associated with acute bronchospasm in treated children. The standard aerosol is sticky, and clogging of ventilatory equipment has been reported.[51]

Comment: We found one small prospective study comparing pulmonary function tests in 54 children previously randomised to inpatient treatment with ribavirin or placebo.[52] It found no evidence of long term differences in outcome, although the study was not sufficiently powered to rule out a clinically important difference.

OPTION RESPIRATORY SYNCYTIAL VIRUS IMMUNOGLOBULINS, POOLED IMMUNOGLOBULINS OR PALIVIZUMAB (MONOCLONAL ANTIBODY)

Small RCTs provided insufficient evidence to compare immunoglobulins or palivizumab versus albumin solution or versus 0.9% sodium chloride in children admitted to hospital with bronchiolitis.

Benefits: We found no systematic review, but found five RCTs (four using albumin solution as control, one using 0.9% sodium chloride, 335 children in total).[53–57] Two RCTs used pooled immunoglobulins, two RCTs used respiratory syncytial virus immunoglobulin (RSV Ig), and one RCT used palivizumab (synthetic monoclonal antibody). Neither of the RCTs using RSV Ig found evidence that RSV Ig shortened duration of hospital stay compared with albumin (in high risk children**G**; mean duration of hospital stay: 8.41 days with RSV Ig *v* 8.89 days with albumin; P = NS; in non-high risk children: mean stay 4.58 days with RSV Ig *v* 5.52 days with albumin; P = NS; CI values not reported).[53,54] The third RCT (35 children) found no evidence that palivizumab reduced duration of hospital stay, duration of ventilation, or duration of supplemental oxygen treatment (duration of hospital stay: mean 14.5 days, 95% CI 12.4 days to 16.6 days with palivizumab *v* 11.5 days, 95% CI 10.0 days to 13.0 days with placebo; P = 0.25; duration of ventilation: mean 8.8 days, 95% CI 6.5 days to 11.1 days with palivizumab *v* 6.2 days with placebo, 95% CI 4.7 days to 7.7 days; P = 0.45; duration of treatment with supplemental oxygen: mean 12.3 days, 95% CI 10.0 days to 14.6 days with palivizumab *v* 9.5 days, 95% CI 7.9 days to 11.1 days with placebo; P = 0.47).[55] Neither of the remaining RCTs found any evidence that pooled immunoglobulins improved outcome in children with bronchiolitis.[56,57]

Harms: The RCTs found that RSV Ig was associated with elevation in liver enzymes and anoxic spells (no frequencies provided).[53] One open label RCT (249 children) of prophylactic RSV Ig found that adverse effects occurred in about 3% of treated children.[10] The RCT and a subsequent analysis of the data found that effects included increased respiratory rate, mild fluid overload during the first infusion, urticarial reaction at the infusion site, mild decreases in oxygen saturation, and fever (no frequencies provided).[10,58]

Comment: Four RCTs used albumin as control. The effects of albumin in bronchiolitis are not known.

GLOSSARY

Cohort segregation Children infected with different viral strains are segregated from each other and treated separately, with the aim of preventing cross-infection.

Disease severity Mild: not requiring admission to hospital. Moderate: requiring admission to hospital but not intubation. Severe: requiring intubation or artificial ventilation.

High risk children Premature infants with or without bronchopulmonary dysplasia, or infants and children with congenital heart disease.

RDAI Respiratory Distress Assessment Instrument.

REFERENCES

1. Phelan P, Olinsky A, Robertson C. *Respiratory illness in children*. 4th ed. London: Blackwell Scientific Publications, 1994.
2. Gruber W. Bronchiolitis. In: Long S, Pickering L, Prober C, eds. *Principles and practice of pediatric infectious diseases*. 1st ed. New York: Churchill Livingstone, 1997:1821.
3. Glezen WP, Taber LH, Frank AL, et al. Risk of primary infection and reinfection with respiratory syncytial virus. *Am J Dis Child* 1986;140:543–546.
4. Navas L, Wang E, de Carvalho V, et al. Improved outcome of respiratory syncytial virus infections in a high-risk hospitalized population of Canadian children. *J Pediatr* 1992;121:348–354.
5. Wang EEL, Law BJ, Stephens D, et al. Pediatric Investigators Collaborative Network on Infections in

Canada (PICNIC) study of morbidity and risk factors with RSV disease. *J Pediatr* 1995;126:212–219.
6. Wang EEL, Law BJ, Boucher F, et al. Pediatric Investigators Collaborative Network on Infections in Canada (PICNIC) study of admission and management variation in patients hospitalized with respiratory syncytial viral lower respiratory infection. *J Pediatr* 1996;129:390–395.
7. McConnochie KM, Mark JD, McBride JT, et al. Normal pulmonary function measurements and airway reactivity in childhood after mild bronchiolitis. *J Pediatr* 1985;107:54–58.
8. McConnochie KM, Roghmann KJ. Parental smoking, presence of older siblings and family history of asthma increase risk of bronchiolitis. *Am J Dis Child* 1986;140:806–812.
9. Sly PD, Hibbert ME. Childhood asthma following hospitalization with acute viral bronchiolitis in infancy. *Pediatr Pulmonol* 1989;7:153–158.
10. Wang EEL, Tang NK. Immunoglobulin for preventing respiratory syncytial virus infection. In: The Cochrane Library, Issue 3, 2003. Oxford: Update Software. Search date 1999; primary sources Cochrane Acute Respiratory Infections Trials Register, Medline, and abstracts from the Pediatric Academy Meetings and the Intersciences Conference on Antimicrobial Agents and Chemotherapy from 1994–1997.
11. Simpson S, Burls A. *A systematic review of the effectiveness and cost-effectiveness of palivizumab (Synagis®) in the prevention of respiratory syncytial virus (RSV) infection in infants at high risk of infection*. Birmingham: West Midlands Health Technology Assessment Group, University of Birmingham, 2001.
12. Krasinski K, LaCouture R, Holzman R, et al. Screening for respiratory syncytial virus and assignment to a cohort at admission to reduce nosocomial transmission. *J Pediatr* 1990;116:894–898.
13. Isaacs D, Dickson H, O'Callaghan C, et al. Handwashing and cohorting in prevention of hospital acquired infections with respiratory syncytial virus. *Arch Dis Child* 1991;66:227–231.
14. Gala CL, Hall CB, Schnabel KC, et al. The use of eye-nose goggles to control nosocomial respiratory syncytial virus infection. *JAMA* 1986;256:2706–2708.
15. Hall CB, Douglas RG. Nosocomial respiratory syncytial virus infections: should gowns and masks be used? *Am J Dis Child* 1981;135:512–515.
16. Murphy D, Todd JK, Chao RK, et al. The use of gowns and masks to control respiratory illness in pediatric hospital personnel. *J Pediatr* 1981;99:746–750.
17. Madge P, Paton JY, McColl JH, et al. Prospective controlled study of four infection-control procedures to prevent nosocomial infection with respiratory syncytial virus. *Lancet* 1992;340:1079–1083.
18. Kellner JD, Ohlsson A, Gadomski AM, et al. Bronchodilators for bronchiolitis. In: The Cochrane Library, Issue 3, 2003. Oxford: Update Software. Search date 1998; primary sources Medline, Embase, Reference Update, reference lists of articles, and files of the authors.
19. Flores G, Horwitz RI. Efficacy of beta 2-agonists in bronchiolitis: a reappraisal and meta-analysis. *Pediatrics* 1997;100:233–239. Search date 1995; primary sources Medline and hand searches of references and selected journals.
20. Abul-Ainine A, Luyt D. Short term effects of adrenaline in bronchiolitis: a randomised controlled trial. *Arch Dis Child* 2002;86:276–279.
21. Patel H, Platt RW, Pekeles GS, et al. A randomized, controlled trial of the effectiveness of nebulized therapy with epinephrine compared with albuterol and saline in infants hospitalized for acute viral bronchiolitis. *J Pediatr* 2002;141:818–824.
22. Hariprakash S, Alexander J, Carroll W, et al. Randomized controlled trial of nebulized adrenaline in acute bronchiolitis. *Pediatr Allergy Immunol* 2003;14:134–139.
23. Patel H, Gouin S, Platt RW. Randomized, double-blind, placebo-controlled trial of oral albuterol in infants with mild-to-moderate acute viral bronchiolitis. *J Pediatr* 2003;142:509–514.
24. Wainwright C, Altamirano L, Cheney M, et al. A multicenter, randomized, double-blind, controlled trial of nebulized epinephrine in infants with acute bronchiolitis. *N Engl J Med* 2003;349:27–35.
25. Sanchez I, De Koster J, Powell RE, et al. Effect of racemic epinephrine and salbutamol on clinical score and pulmonary mechanics in infants with bronchiolitis. *J Pediatr* 1993;122:145–151.
26. Menon K, Sutcliffe T, Klassen TP. A randomized trial comparing the efficacy of epinephrine with salbutamol in the treatment of acute bronchiolitis. *J Pediatr* 1995;126:1004–1007.
27. Reijonen T, Korppi M, Pitkakangas S, et al. The clinical efficacy of nebulized racemic epinephrine and albuterol in acute bronchiolitis. *Arch Pediatr Adolesc Med* 1995;149:686–692.
28. Gadomski AM, Lichenstein R, Horton L, et al. Efficacy of albuterol in the management of bronchiolitis. *Pediatrics* 1994;93:907–912.
29. Garrison MM, Christakis DA, Harvey E, et al. Systemic corticosteroids in infant bronchiolitis: a meta-analysis. *Pediatrics* 2000;105:e44. Search date 1999; primary sources Medline, Embase, and Cochrane Clinical Trials Registry.
30. Richter H, Seddon P. Early nebulized budesonide in the treatment of bronchiolitis and the prevention of postbronchiolitic wheezing. *J Pediatr* 1998;132:849–853.
31. Bulow SM, Nir M, Levin E. Prednisolone treatment for respiratory syncytial virus infection: a randomized controlled trial of 147 infants. *Pediatrics* 1999;104:77.
32. Tal A, Bavilski C, Yohai D, et al. Dexamethasone and salbutamol in the treatment of acute wheezing in infants. *Pediatrics* 1983;71:13–18.
33. Connolly JH, Field CM, Glasgow JF, et al. A double blind trial of prednisolone in epidemic bronchiolitis due to respiratory syncytial virus. *Acta Paediatr Scand* 1969;58:116–120.
34. Berger I, Argaman Z, Schwartz SB. Efficacy of corticosteroids in acute bronchiolitis: short-term and long-term follow-up. *Pediatr Pulmonol* 1998;26:162–166.
35. Leer JA, Green JL, Heimlich EM, et al. Corticosteroid treatment in bronchiolitis. A controlled collaborative study in 297 infants and children. *Am J Dis Child* 1969;117:495–503.
36. Goebel J, Estrada B, Quinonez J, et al. Prednisolone plus albuterol versus albuterol alone in mild to moderate bronchiolitis. *Clin Pediatr* 2000;39:213–220.
37. Cade A, Brownlee KG, Conway SP, et al. Randomised placebo controlled trial of nebulised corticosteroids in acute respiratory syncytial viral bronchiolitis. *Arch Dis Child* 2000;82:126–130.
38. Schuh S, Coates AL, Binnie R, et al. Efficacy of oral dexamethasone in outpatients with acute bronchiolitis. *J Pediatr* 2002;140:27–32.
39. Buckingham SC, Jafri HS, Bush AJ, et al. A randomized, double-blind, placebo-controlled trial of dexamethasone in severe respiratory syncytial virus (RSV) infection: effects on RSV quantity and clinical outcome. *J Infect Dis* 2002;185:1222–1228.
40. van Woensel JBM, van Aalderen WMC, de Weerd W, et al. Dexamethasone for treatment of patients mechanically ventilated for lower respiratory tract infection caused by respiratory syncytial virus. *Thorax* 2003;58:383–387.
41. Reijonen TM, Kotaniemi-Syrjanen A, Korhonen K, et al. Predictors of asthma three years after hospital admission for wheezing in infancy. *Pediatrics* 2000;106:1406–1412.
42. Van Woensel JBM, Kimpen JLL, Sprikkelman AB, et al. Long-term effects of prednisolone in the acute phase of bronchiolitis caused by respiratory syncytial virus. *Pediatr Pulmonol* 2000;30:92–96.
43. Kajosaari M, Syvanen P, Forars M, et al. Inhaled corticosteroids during and after respiratory syncytial virus-bronchiolitis may decrease subsequent asthma. *Pediatr Allergy Immunol* 2000;11:198–202.

44. Schimmer BP, Parker KL. Adrenocorticotropic hormone; adrenocortical steroids and their synthetic analogs; inhibitors of the synthesis and actions of adrenocortical hormones. In: Hardman JG, Limbird LE, eds *Goodman & Gilman's the pharmacological basis of therapeutics*. 10th ed. New York: McGraw-Hill, 2001:1649–1677.
45. Friis B, Andersen P, Brenoe E, et al. Antibiotic treatment of pneumonia and bronchiolitis: a prospective randomised study. *Arch Dis Child* 1984;59:1038–1045.
46. Chambers HF. Antimicrobial agents. General considerations. In: Hardman JG, Limbird LE, eds *Goodman & Gilman's the pharmacological basis of therapeutics*. 10th ed. New York: McGraw-Hill, 2001:1143–1170.
47. Randolph AG, Wang EEL. Ribavirin for respiratory syncytial virus lower respiratory tract infection. In: The Cochrane Library, Issue 3, 2003. Oxford: Update Software. Search date 2000; primary sources Medline, hand searches of references, and contact of noted experts.
48. Everard ML, Swarbrick A, Rigby AS, et al. The effect of ribavirin to treat previously healthy infants admitted with acute bronchiolitis on acute and chronic respiratory morbidity. *Respir Med* 2001;95:275–280.
49. Edell D, Khoshoo V, Ross G, et al. Early ribavirin treatment of bronchiolitis: effect on long-term respiratory morbidity. *Chest* 2002;122:935–939.
50. Edelson PJ. Reactions to ribavirin. *Pediatr Infect Dis J* 1991;10:82.
51. Johnson EM. Developmental toxicity and safety evaluations of ribavirin. *Pediatr Infect Dis J* 199 7;9(suppl):85–87.
52. Long CE, Voter KZ, Barker WH, et al. Long term follow-up of children hospitalized with respiratory syncytial virus lower respiratory tract infection and randomly treated with ribavirin or placebo. *Pediatr Infect Dis J* 1997;16:1023–1028.
53. Rodriguez WJ, Gruber WC, Welliver RC, et al. Respiratory syncytial virus (RSV) immune globulin intravenous therapy for RSV lower respiratory tract infection in infants and young children at high risk for severe RSV infections. *Pediatrics* 1997;99:454–461.
54. Rodriguez WJ, Gruber WC, Groothuis JR, et al. Respiratory syncytial virus immune globulin treatment of RSV lower respiratory tract infection in previously healthy children. *Pediatrics* 1997;100:937–942.
55. Malley R, DeVincenzo J, Ramilo O, et al. Reduction of respiratory syncytial virus (RSV) in tracheal aspirates in intubated infants by use of humanized monoclonal antibody to RSV F protein. *J Infect Dis* 1998;178:1555–1561.
56. Hemming VG, Rodriguez W, Kim HW, et al. Intravenous immunoglobulin treatment of respiratory syncytial virus infections in infants and young children. *Antimicrob Agents Chemother* 1987;31:1882–1886.
57. Rimensberger PC, Burek-Kozlowska A, Morell A, et al. Aerosolized immunoglobulin treatment of respiratory syncytial virus infection in infants. *Pediatr Infect Dis J* 1996;15:209–216.
58. Groothuis JR, Levin MJ, Rodriguez W, et al. Use of intravenous gamma globulin to passively immunize high-risk children against respiratory syncytial virus: safety and pharmacokinetics. *Antimicrob Agents Chemother* 1991;35:1469–1473.

Juan Manuel Lozano
Titular Professor
Department of Paediatrics and Clinical Epidemiology Unit School of Medicine
Universidad Javeriana
Bogotá DC
Colombia

Competing interests: None declared. *We would like to acknowledge the previouscontributors of this chapter including Nancy Tang and Elaine Wang.*

TABLE 1 Studies of adrenaline (epinephrine) compared with salbutamol in bronchiolitis: results of RCTs (see text, p 284).

Ref	Allocation/blinding	Intervention	Number of children	Outcome	Results
21	Random/blinded	Nebulised racemic adrenaline or salbutamol	101 inpatients	Length of hospital stay; time to normal oxygenation, adequate fluid intake, RDAI < 4, or infrequent nebulisations	No differences
25	Random/blinded, crossover design	Nebulised racemic adrenaline or salbutamol	24 inpatients	Clinical score at 20–30 minutes	Improvement with adrenaline
26	Random/blinded	Nebulised adrenaline or salbutamol	42 emergency room patients	Pulse oximetry; RDAI scores at 30, 60, and 90 minutes; admission rate	Transient effect at 60 minutes; fewer admissions
27	Random/blinded, factorial design	Nebulised racemic adrenaline, salbutamol or saline placebo	100 emergency room patients	RDAI and RACS scores at 15 and 30 minutes	Unclear differences

RACS, Respiratory Assessment Change Score; RDAI, Respiratory Distress Assessment Instrument; Ref, reference.

TABLE 2 **Studies of corticosteroids compared with placebo in bronchiolitis: results of RCTs (see text, p 285).**

Ref	Allocation/blinding	Intervention	Number of children	Outcome	Results
30	Random/blinded	Nebulised budesonide	40	Clinical score and condition at 6 months	No benefit
31	Random/blinded	Prednisolone/ methylprednisolone	147	Hospital stay; supportive measures in hospital; condition at 1 month and 1 year after discharge	No benefit
32	Random/blinded, factorial design	Dexamethasone/placebo Salbutamol/placebo	32	Clinical score and hospital stay	No benefit
34	Random/blinded	Prednisolone	95	Duration of illness after hospitalisation	No benefit
35	Random/blinded	All had salbutamol; prednisone	38	Clinical score; oxygen saturation; condition at 7 days and 2 years later	No benefit
37	Random/blinded	Betamethasone	297	Nine respiratory tract signs; fever and complications after admission	No benefit
37	Random/blinded	All children received salbutamol (oral or inhaled) prednisolone	48	Bronchiolitis score at day 2	Transient effect only on day 2
33	Random/blinded	Budesonide	161	Hospital stay; time taken to be symptom free; readmission rates; GP consultation	No benefit
38	Random/blinded	Oral dexamethasone	70	Clinical score and admission rate	Improvement in clinical score and admission rate
39	Random/blinded	iv dexamethasone/placebo	41	Number ventilator, ICU, or hospital days	No benefit
40	Random/blinded	iv dexamethason	B2	Duration of mechanical ventilation	No benefit

GP, general practitioner; ICU, intensive care unit; Ref, reference.

Cardiorespiratory arrest in children

Search date February 2004

Kate Ackerman and David Creery

QUESTIONS

INTERVENTIONS

*Although we found no direct evidence to support their use, widespread consensus holds that, on the basis of indirect evidence and extrapolation from adult data, these interventions should be universally applied to children who have arrested. Placebo controlled trials would be considered unethical.

See glossary

Key Messages

- **Bag–mask ventilation** We found no RCTs. One non-randomised controlled trial found no significant difference in survival or neurological outcome between endotracheal intubation and bag–mask ventilation in children with non-submersion cardiorespiratory arrest requiring airway management in the community.
- **Bystander cardiopulmonary resuscitation** It is widely accepted that cardiopulmonary resuscitation and ventilation should be undertaken in children who have arrested. Placebo controlled trials would be considered unethical. One systematic review of observational studies has found that children whose arrest was witnessed and who received bystander cardiopulmonary resuscitation were more likely to survive to hospital discharge compared with no bystander cardiopulmonary resuscitation. We found no RCTs on the effects of training parents to perform cardiopulmonary resuscitation.
- **Intubation** We found no RCTs. One controlled trial found no significant difference in survival or neurological outcome between endotracheal intubation and bag–mask ventilation in children with non-submersion cardiorespiratory arrest.
- **Airway management and ventilation; direct current cardiac shock (for ventricular fibrillation or pulseless ventricular tachycardia); intravenous adrenaline (epinephrine) at standard dose** Although we found no direct evidence to support their use, widespread consensus based on indirect evidence and extrapolation from adult data holds that these interventions should be universally applied to children who have arrested. Placebo controlled trials would be considered unethical.
- **Intravenous adrenaline at high dose; intravenous sodium bicarbonate; intravenous calcium; training parents to perform cardiopulmonary resuscitation** We found no RCTs or prospective observational studies on the effects of these interventions in children who have arrested in the community.

Cardiorespiratory arrest in children

DEFINITION This chapter deals with non-submersion, out of hospital cardiorespiratory arrest in children, which is defined as a state of pulselessness and apnoea occurring outside of a medical facility and not caused by submersion in water.[1]

INCIDENCE/ PREVALENCE We found 12 observational studies (3 prospective, 9 retrospective) reporting the incidence of non-submersion out of hospital cardiorespiratory arrest in children (see table 1, p 300).[2–13] Two studies reported the incidence in both adults and children, and ten reported the incidence in children alone.[2–13] Incidence in the general population ranged from 2.2–5.7/100 000 people a year (mean 3.1, 95% CI 2.1 to 4.1). Incidence in children ranged from 6.9–18.0/100 000 children a year (mean 10.6, 95% CI 7.1 to 14.1).[8] One prospective study (300 children) found that about 50% of out of hospital cardiorespiratory arrests occurred in children under 12 months, and about two thirds occurred in children under 18 months.[11]

AETIOLOGY/ RISK FACTORS We found 26 observational studies reporting the causes of non-submersion pulseless arrests in a total of 1574 children. The commenest causes were undetermined (as in sudden infant death syndrome**G**) (39%), trauma (18%), chronic disease (7%), and pneumonia (4%) (see table 2, p 300).[1,3–12,14–28]

PROGNOSIS We found no observational studies that investigated non-submersion arrests alone. We found 27 studies (5 prospective, 22 retrospective; total of 1754 children) that reported out of hospital arrest.[1–12,14–28] The overall survival rate following out of hospital arrest was 5% (87 children). Nineteen of these studies (1140 children) found that of the 48 surviving children, 12 (25%) had no or mild neurological disability and 36 (75%) had moderate or severe neurological disability. We found one systematic review (search date 1997), which reported outcomes after cardiopulmonary resuscitation for both in hospital and out of hospital arrests in children of any cause, including submersion.[29] Studies were excluded if they did not report survival. The review found evidence from prospective and retrospective observational studies that out of hospital arrest of any cause in children has a poorer prognosis than arrest within hospital (132/1568 [8%] children survived to hospital discharge after out of hospital arrest *v* 129/544 [24%] children after in hospital arrests). About half of the survivors were involved in studies that reported neurological outcome. Of these, survival with "good neurological outcome" (i.e. normal or mild neurological deficit) was higher in children who arrested in hospital compared with those who arrested elsewhere (60/77 [78%] surviving children in hospital *v* 28/68 [41%] elsewhere).[29]

AIMS OF INTERVENTION To improve survival and minimise neurological sequelae.

OUTCOMES Out of hospital death rate; rate of death in hospital without return of spontaneous circulation; return of spontaneous circulation with subsequent death in hospital; and return of spontaneous circulation with successful hospital discharge with mild, moderate, severe, or no neurological sequelae; adverse effects of treatment.

METHODS *Clinical Evidence* search and appraisal February 2004, including a search for observational studies. In addition, the authors searched citation lists of retrieved articles and relevant review articles. Studies reporting out of hospital arrest in adults that listed "adolescent" as a MeSH heading were also reviewed. Both authors reviewed the retrieved studies independently and differences were resolved by discussion. Studies were excluded if data relating to submersion could not be differentiated from non-submersion data (except where we found no data relating exclusively to non-submersion arrest; in such cases we have included studies that did not differentiate these types of arrest and indicated their limitation in this regard). Some features of cardiorespiratory arrest in adults appear to be different from arrest in children, so studies were excluded if data for adults could not be differentiated from data for children.

QUESTION What are the effects of treatments for non-submersion out of hospital cardiorespiratory arrest?

OPTION AIRWAY MANAGEMENT AND VENTILATION

It is widely accepted, based on indirect evidence and extrapolation from adult data, that good airway management and rapid ventilation should be undertaken in a child who has arrested, and it would be considered unethical to test its role in a placebo controlled trial. We found no RCTs or prospective observational studies of airway management and ventilation.

Benefits: We found no systematic review, RCTs, or observational studies of sufficient quality.

Harms: We found no prospective evidence.

Comment: It is widely accepted, based on indirect evidence and extrapolation from adult data, that good airway management and rapid ventilation should be undertaken in a child who has arrested, and it would be considered unethical to test its role in a placebo controlled trial.

OPTION INTUBATION VERSUS BAG–MASK VENTILATION

We found no RCTs. One non-randomised controlled trial found no significant difference in survival or neurological outcome between endotracheal intubation and bag–mask ventilation in children with non-submersion cardiorespiratory arrest requiring airway management in the community.

Benefits: We found no systematic review or RCTs. We found one non-randomised controlled trial (830 children requiring airway management in the community, including 98 children who had arrested after submersion) comparing bag–mask ventilation versus endotracheal intubation (given by paramedic staff trained in these techniques).[30] Treatments were allocated on alternate days. Analysis was by intention to treat (see comment below). The trial found no significant difference in rates of survival or good neurological outcome (normal, mild deficit, or no change from baseline function) between the two treatment groups in children with non-submersion cardiorespiratory arrest (105/349 [30%] survived with bag–mask ventilation *v* 90/373 [24%] with intubation; good neurological outcome achieved in 80/349 [23%] of children with bag–mask ventilation *v* 70/373 [19%] with intubation).

Harms: The trial found that time spent at the scene of the arrest was longer when intubation was intended, and this was the only significant determinant of a longer total time from dispatch of paramedic team to arrival at hospital (mean time at scene: 9 minutes with bag–mask *v* 11 minutes with intubation; $P < 0.001$; mean total time: 20 minutes with bag–mask *v* 23 minutes with intubation; $P < 0.001$).[30] However, it found no significant difference between bag–mask ventilation and intubation in complications (complications in 727 children for whom data were available: gastric distension 31% with bag–mask *v* 7% with intubation; $P = 0.20$; vomiting 14% *v* 14%; $P = 0.82$; aspiration 14% *v* 15%; $P = 0.84$; oral or airway trauma 1% with bag–mask *v* 2% with intubation; $P = 0.24$). A total of 186 children across both treatment groups were thought by paramedical staff to be successfully intubated. Of these, oesophageal intubation occurred in three children (2%); the tube became dislodged in 27 children (14%; unrecognised in 12 children, recognised in 15); right main bronchus intubation occurred in 33 children (18%); and an incorrect size of tube was used in 44 children (24%). Death occurred in all but one of the children with oesophageal intubation or unrecognised dislodging of the tube.[30]

Comment: **Population characteristics:** The baseline characteristics of children did not differ significantly between groups in age, sex, ethnicity, or cause of arrest. The trial did not report the frequency of pulseless arrest**G** compared with that of respiratory arrest**G**. **Intention to treat:** Intubation and bag–mask ventilation were not mutually exclusive in the trial.[30] The trial protocol allowed bag–mask ventilation before intubation and after unsuccessful intubation. Of 420 children allocated to intubation, 115 received bag–mask ventilation before intubation, 128 received bag–mask ventilation after attempted intubation, four were lost to follow up, and the remainder received intubation that was believed to be successful. Of 410 children allocated to bag–mask ventilation, 10 children were intubated successfully (although in violation of study protocol), nine received bag–mask ventilation after attempted intubation, six were lost to follow up, and the remainder received bag–mask ventilation in accordance with study protocol.[30]

OPTION INTRAVENOUS ADRENALINE (EPINEPHRINE)

Intravenous adrenaline (epinephrine) at "standard dose" (0.01 mg/kg) is a widely accepted treatment for establishing return of spontaneous circulation and it would be considered unethical to test its role in a placebo controlled trial. We found no RCTs or prospective observational studies in children who have arrested in the community comparing adrenaline versus placebo or comparing standard or single doses versus high or multiple doses of adrenaline.

Benefits: We found no systematic review, RCTs, or prospective observational studies on the effects of intravenous adrenaline.

Harms: We found no prospective evidence.

Comment: Intravenous adrenaline (epinephrine) at "standard dose" (0.01 mg/kg) is a widely accepted treatment for establishing return of spontaneous circulation and it would be considered unethical to test its role in a placebo controlled trial. **High versus low dose:** Two small retrospective observational studies (128 people) found no evidence of a difference in survival to hospital discharge between low or single dose and high or multiple dose adrenaline, although the studies were too small to rule out an effect.[8,12]

OPTION INTRAVENOUS SODIUM BICARBONATE

We found no RCTs or observational studies of sufficient quality on the effects of intravenous bicarbonate in out of hospital cardiorespiratory arrest in children.

Benefits: We found no systematic review, RCTs, or observational studies of sufficient quality.

Harms: We found no prospective evidence.

Comment: Sodium bicarbonate is widely believed to be effective in arrest associated with hyperkalaemic ventricular tachycardia or fibrillation, but we found no prospective evidence supporting this.

OPTION INTRAVENOUS CALCIUM

We found no RCTs or observational studies of sufficient quality on the effects of intravenous calcium in out of hospital cardiorespiratory arrest in children.

Benefits: We found no systematic review, RCTs, or observational studies of sufficient quality.

Harms: We found no prospective evidence.

Comment: Calcium is widely believed to be effective in arrest associated with hyperkalaemic ventricular tachycardia or fibrillation, but we found no prospective evidence supporting this.

OPTION BYSTANDER CARDIOPULMONARY RESUSCITATION

It is widely accepted that cardiopulmonary resuscitation and ventilation should be undertaken in children who have arrested. Placebo controlled trials would be considered unethical. One systematic review of observational studies has found that children whose arrest was witnessed and who received bystander cardiopulmonary resuscitation were more likely to survive to hospital discharge compared with no bystander cardiopulmonary resuscitation. We found no RCTs on the effects of training parents to perform cardiopulmonary resuscitation.

Benefits: We found no RCTs. We found one systematic review (search date 1997, 1420 children who had arrested outside hospital) of prospective and retrospective observational studies.[29] This concluded that survival was improved in children who were witnessed to arrest and received cardiopulmonary resuscitation from a bystander. Of 150 witnessed arrests outside hospital, 28/150 (19%) survived to hospital discharge. Of those children who received bystander cardiopulmonary resuscitation, 20/76 (26%) survived to discharge compared with 8/74 (11%) in children whose arrest was witnessed but who did not receive cardiopulmonary resuscitation.[29] The review did not report survival rates in children whose arrests were not witnessed, but the overall survival rate for out of hospital cardiac arrest was 8%. **Training parents to perform cardiopulmonary resuscitation:** We found no systematic review, RCTs, or prospective observational studies examining the effects of training parents to perform cardiopulmonary resuscitation in children who have arrested outside hospital.

Harms: Potential harms include injury resulting from unnecessary chest compression after respiratory arrest with intact circulation.

Comment: Cardiopulmonary resuscitation was not randomly allocated and children resuscitated may be systematically different from those who did not receive resuscitation. The apparent survival rates for witnessed arrests and arrests with bystander initiated cardiopulmonary resuscitation may be artificially high because of inappropriate evaluation of true arrest. However, assuming confounding variables were evenly distributed between groups, then the best estimate of the benefit of cardiopulmonary resuscitation is a 15% absolute increase in the probability that children will be discharged alive from hospital. It is widely accepted that cardiopulmonary resuscitation and ventilation should be undertaken in children who have arrested. Placebo controlled trials would be considered unethical.

OPTION DIRECT CURRENT CARDIAC SHOCK

It is widely accepted that children who arrest outside hospital and are found to have ventricular fibrillation or pulseless ventricular tachycardia should receive direct current cardiac shock treatment. Placebo controlled trials would be considered unethical. We found no RCTs or prospective observational studies on the effects of direct current cardiac shock in children who have arrested in the community, regardless of the heart rhythm.

Benefits: We found no systematic review, RCTs, or observational studies of sufficient quality.

Harms: We found no prospective evidence.

Comment: It is widely accepted that children who arrest outside hospital and are found to have ventricular fibrillation or pulseless ventricular tachycardia should receive direct current cardiac shock treatment. Placebo controlled trials would be considered unethical. **In children with ventricular fibrillation:** One retrospective study (29 children with ventricular fibrillation who had arrested out of hospital from a variety of causes, including submersion) found that of 27 children who were defibrillated, 11 survived (5 with no sequelae, 6 with severe disability). The five children with good outcome all received defibrillation within 10 minutes of arrest (time to defibrillation not given for those who died). Data on the two children who were not defibrillated were not presented.[31] **In children with asystole:** One retrospective study in 90 children with asystole**G** (including those who had arrested after submersion) found that 49 (54%) had received direct current cardiac shock treatment. None of the children survived to hospital discharge, regardless of whether direct current cardiac shock was given.[32] We found one systematic review of observational studies that recorded electrocardiogram rhythm (search date 1997, 1420 children who had arrested outside hospital).[29] Bradyasystole**G** or pulseless electrical activity**G** were found in 73%, whereas ventricular fibrillation or pulseless ventricular tachycardia**G** were found in 10%.[29] The review found that survival after ventricular fibrillation or ventricular tachycardia arrest was higher than after asystolic arrest in children. Survival to discharge reported in the systematic review was 39/802 (5%) for children with initial rhythm asystole**G** and 30% (29/97) with initial rhythm ventricular fibrillation**G** or ventricular tachycardia.[29]

GLOSSARY

Asystole The absence of cardiac electrical activity.
Bradyasystole Bradycardia clinically indistinguishable from asystole.
Initial rhythm asystole The absence of cardiac electrical activity at initial determination.
Initial rhythm ventricular fibrillation Electrical rhythm is ventricular fibrillation at initial determination.
Pulseless arrest Absence of palpable pulse.
Pulseless electrical activity The presence of cardiac electrical activity in absence of a palpable pulse.
Pulseless ventricular tachycardia Electrical rhythm of ventricular tachycardia in absence of a palpable pulse.
Respiratory arrest Absence of respiratory activity.
Sudden infant death syndrome The sudden unexpected death of a child, usually between the ages of 1 month and 1 year, for which a thorough postmortem examination does not define an adequate cause of death. Near miss sudden infant death syndrome refers to survival of a child after an unexpected arrest of unknown cause.

REFERENCES

1. Schindler MB, Bohn D, Cox PN, et al. Outcome of out of hospital cardiac or respiratory arrest in children. *N Engl J Med* 1996;335:1473–1479.
2. Broides A, Sofer S, Press J. Outcome of out of hospital cardiopulmonary arrest in children admitted to the emergency room. *Isr Med Assoc J* 2000;2:672–674.
3. Eisenberg M, Bergner L, Hallstrom A. Epidemiology of cardiac arrest and resuscitation in children. *Ann Emerg Med* 1983;12:672–674.
4. Applebaum D, Slater PE. Should the Mobile Intensive Care Unit respond to pediatric emergencies? *Clin Pediatr (Phila)* 1986;25:620–623.
5. Tsai A, Kallsen G. Epidemiology of pediatric prehospital care. *Ann Emerg Med* 1987;16:284–292.
6. Thompson JE, Bonner B, Lower GM. Pediatric cardiopulmonary arrests in rural populations. *Pediatrics* 1990;86:302–306.
7. Safranek DJ, Eisenberg MS, Larsen MP. The epidemiology of cardiac arrest in young adults. *Ann Emerg Med* 1992;21:1102–1106.
8. Dieckmann RA, Vardis R. High-dose epinephrine in pediatric out of hospital cardiopulmonary arrest. *Pediatrics* 1995;95:901–913.

9. Kuisma M, Suominen P, Korpela R. Paediatric out of hospital cardiac arrests — epidemiology and outcome. *Resuscitation* 1995;30:141–150.
10. Ronco R, King W, Donley DK, et al. Outcome and cost at a children's hospital following resuscitation for out of hospital cardiopulmonary arrest. *Arch Pediatr Adolesc Med* 1995;149:210–214.
11. Sirbaugh PE, Pepe PE, Shook JE, et al. A prospective, population-based study of the demographics, epidemiology, management, and outcome of out of hospital pediatric cardiopulmonary arrest. *Ann Emerg Med* 1999;33:174–184.
12. Friesen RM, Duncan P, Tweed WA, et al. Appraisal of pediatric cardiopulmonary resuscitation. *Can Med Assoc J* 1982;126:1055–1058.
13. Hu SC. Out of hospital cardiac arrest in an Oriental metropolitan city. *Am J Emerg Med* 1994;12:491–494.
14. Barzilay Z, Somekh E, Sagy M, et al. Pediatric cardiopulmonary resuscitation outcome. *J Med* 1988;19:229–241.
15. Bhende MS, Thompson AE. Evaluation of an end-tidal CO_2 detector during pediatric cardiopulmonary resuscitation. *Pediatrics* 1995;95:395–399.
16. Brunette DD, Fischer R. Intravascular access in pediatric cardiac arrest. *Am J Emerg Med* 1988;6:577–579.
17. Clinton JE, McGill J, Irwin G, et al. Cardiac arrest under age 40: etiology and prognosis. *Ann Emerg Med* 1984;13:1011–1015.
18. Hazinski MF, Chahine AA, Holcomb GW, et al. Outcome of cardiovascular collapse in pediatric blunt trauma. *Ann Emerg Med* 1994;23:1229–1235.
19. Losek JD, Hennes H, Glaeser P, et al. Prehospital care of the pulseless, nonbreathing pediatric patient. *Am J Emerg Med* 1987;5:370–374.
20. Ludwig S, Kettrick RG, Parker M. Pediatric cardiopulmonary resuscitation. A review of 130 cases. *Clin Pediatr (Phila)* 1984;23:71–75.
21. Nichols DG, Kettrick RG, Swedlow DB, et al. Factors influencing outcome of cardiopulmonary resuscitation in children. *Pediatr Emerg Care* 1986;2:1–5.
22. O'Rourke PP. Outcome of children who are apneic and pulseless in the emergency room. *Crit Care Med* 1986;14:466–468.
23. Rosenberg NM. Pediatric cardiopulmonary arrest in the emergency department. *Am J Emerg Med* 1984;2:497–499.
24. Sheikh A, Brogan T. Outcome and cost of open- and closed-chest cardiopulmonary resuscitation in pediatric cardiac arrests. *Pediatrics* 1994;93:392–398.
25. Suominen P, Rasanen J, Kivioja A. Efficacy of cardiopulmonary resuscitation in pulseless paediatric trauma patients. *Resuscitation* 1998;36:9–13.
26. Suominen P, Korpela R, Kuisma M, et al. Paediatric cardiac arrest and resuscitation provided by physician-staffed emergency care units. *Acta Anaesthesiol Scand* 1997;41:260–265.
27. Torphy DE, Minter MG, Thompson BM. Cardiorespiratory arrest and resuscitation of children. *Am J Dis Child* 1984;138:1099–1102.
28. Walsh R. Outcome of pre-hospital CPR in the pediatric trauma patient [abstract]. *Crit Care Med* 1994;22:A162.
29. Young KD, Seidel JS. Pediatric cardiopulmonary resuscitation: a collective review. *Ann Emerg Med* 1999;33:195–205. Search date 1997; primary sources Medline and bibliographic search.
30. Gausche M, Lewis RJ, Stratton SJ, et al. Effect of out of hospital pediatric endotracheal intubation on survival and neurological outcome. *JAMA* 2000;283:783–790.
31. Mogayzel C, Quan L, Graves JR, et al. Out of hospital ventricular fibrillation in children and adolescents: causes and outcomes. *Ann Emerg Med* 1995;25:484–491.
32. Losek JD, Hennes H, Glaeser PW, et al. Prehospital countershock treatment of pediatric asystole. *Am J Emerg Med* 1989;7:571–575.

Kate Ackerman
The Children's Hospital
Boston
USA

David Creery
Children's Hospital of Eastern Ontario
Ottawa
Canada

Competing interests: None declared.

TABLE 1 **Incidence of non-submersion out of hospital cardiorespiratory arrest in children* (see text, p 294).**

Ref	Location	Year	Patient Population	Incidence/ 100 000 people in total population	Incidence/ 100 000 children
12	Manitoba, Canada	1982	Children (1mo - 16y)	2.9	ND
3	King County, USA	1983	Children (< 18y)	2.4	9.9
4	Jerusalem, Israel	1986	Children (≤ 14y)	2.5	6.9
5	Fresno, USA	1987	Children (< 19y)	5.7	ND
6	Midwestern USA	1990	Children (< 18y)	4.7	ND
7	King County, USA	1992	Adults and children	2.4	10.1
13	Taipei, Taiwan	1994	Adults and children	1.3	ND
8	San Francisco, USA	1995	Children (< 18y)	2.2	16.1
9	Helsinki, Finland	1995	Children (< 16y)	1.4	9.1
10	Birmingham, USA	1995	Children (≤ 13y)	ND	6.9
11	Houston, USA	1999	Children (≤ 17y)	4.9	18.0
2	Southern Israel	2000	Children (≤ 12y)	3.5	7.8

*Incidence represents arrests per 100 000 population per year. mo, months; ND, no data; y, years.

TABLE 2 **Causes of non-submersion out of hospital cardiorespiratory arrest in children* (see text, p 294).[1,3–12,14–28]**

Cause	Number of arrests (%)	Number of survivors (%)
Undetermined	691 (43.9)	1 (0.1)
Trauma	311 (19.8)	10 (3.2)
Chronic disease	126 (8.0)	9 (7.1)
Pneumonia	75 (4.8)	6 (8.0)
Non-accidental injury	23 (1.5)	2 (8.7)
Aspiration	20 (1.3)	0 (0)
Overdose	19 (1.2)	3 (15.8)
Other	309 (19.6)	28 (9.1)
Total	**1574 (100)**	**59 (3.7)**

*Figures represent the numbers of arrests/survivors in Children with each diagnosis.

Constipation in children

Search date August 2003

Gregory Rubin

QUESTIONS

INTERVENTIONS

CONSTIPATION

Trade off between benefits and harms

Unknown effectiveness

Covered elsewhere in *Clinical Evidence*

Constipation in adults, p 491

*Not widely licensed for use in children. Clinical use in adults was recently restricted because of heart rhythm abnormalities. See comments on cisapride under gastro-oesophageal reflux in children, p 354.

Key Messages

Constipation

- **Cisapride with or without magnesium oxide** Two RCTs in people aged 2–18 years found that cisapride improved stool frequency and symptoms of constipation after 8–12 weeks of treatment in an outpatient setting compared with placebo. One RCT in children aged 1–7 years with chronic constipation found that combined treatment with cisapride and magnesium oxide significantly improved stool frequency after 3–4 weeks of treatment in an outpatient setting compared with magnesium oxide alone. We found no evidence from primary care settings. Use of cisapride has been restricted in some countries because of adverse cardiac effects.
- **Biofeedback training** One systematic review found no significant difference between biofeedback plus conventional treatment and conventional treatment alone in children with persisting defecation disorders at 12 months.
- **Increased dietary fibre** We found no systematic review or RCTs on the effects of increasing dietary fibre.
- **Osmotic laxatives** We found no RCTs that compared osmotic laxatives versus placebo in children. Two small RCTs found no significant difference in stool frequency or consistency between lactulose and lactitol after 2–4 weeks in children aged 8 months to 16 years. One of the RCTs found that lactulose increased abdominal pain and flatulence compared with lactitol. A third RCT in non-breastfed constipated infants found no difference between different strengths of lactulose.
- **Stimulant laxatives** One systematic review found no reliable RCTs comparing stimulant laxatives versus placebo or other treatments.

Constipation in children

DEFINITION **Constipation** is characterised by infrequent bowel evacuations; hard, small faeces; or difficult or painful defecation. The frequency of bowel evacuation varies from person to person.[1] According to the Rome II diagnostic criteria for childhood defecation disorders, functional constipation can be defined as "either having hard or pellet-like stools for the majority of stools or firm stools two or less times per week in the absence of structural, endocrine or metabolic diseases".[2] Some studies reported in this chapter used other diagnostic criteria.[3] **Encopresis** is defined as involuntary bowel movements in inappropriate places at least once a month for 3 months or more, in children aged 4 years and older.[4]

INCIDENCE/ PREVALENCE Constipation with or without encopresis is common in children. It accounts for 3% of consultations to paediatric outpatient clinics and 25% of paediatric gastroenterology consultations in the USA.[5] Encopresis has been reported in 2% of children at school entry. The peak incidence is at 2–4 years of age.

AETIOLOGY/ RISK FACTORS No cause is discovered in 90–95% of children with constipation. Low fibre intake and a family history of constipation may be associated factors.[6] Psychosocial factors are often suspected, although most children with constipation are developmentally normal.[5] Chronic constipation can lead to progressive faecal retention, distension of the rectum, and loss of sensory and motor function. Organic causes for constipation are uncommon, but include Hirschsprung's disease (1/5000 births; male to female ratio of 4 : 1; constipation invariably present from birth), cystic fibrosis, anorectal physiological abnormalities, anal fissures, constipating drugs, dehydrating metabolic conditions, and other forms of malabsorption.[5] This chapter aims to cover children in whom no underlying cause is identified.

PROGNOSIS Childhood constipation can be difficult to treat and often requires prolonged support, explanation, and medical treatment. In one long term follow up study of children presenting under the age of 5 years, 50% recovered within 1 year and 65–70% recovered within 2 years; the remainder required laxatives for daily bowel movements or continued to soil for several years.[5] It is not known what proportion continue to have problems into adult life, although adults presenting with megarectum or megacolon often have a history of bowel problems from childhood.

AIMS OF INTERVENTION To remove faecal impaction and to restore a bowel habit in which stools are soft and passed without discomfort; to ensure self toileting and passing stools in appropriate places.

OUTCOMES Number of defecations per week; gut transit time as measured by timing the passage of radio-opaque pellets, which may be ingested within a gelatin capsule; use of laxatives; stool consistency; pain; difficulty in defecation; blood in stool; number of soilings per month.

METHODS *Clinical Evidence* search and appraisal August 2003 using the following keywords: constipation, encopresis, diet therapy, diagnosis, therapy, psychology, stimulant laxatives, dietary fibre, and lactulose. The search was limited to infants and children. Trials were selected for inclusion if they focused on the management of constipation or encopresis, or both; if they were relevant to primary health care; and if they included children without an organic cause for constipation.

QUESTION **What are the effects of treatments for constipation?**

OPTION **CISAPRIDE**

Two RCTs in people aged 2–18 years found that cisapride improved stool frequency and symptoms of constipation after 8–12 weeks of treatment in an outpatient setting compared with placebo. One RCT in children aged 1–7 years with chronic constipation found that combined treatment with cisapride and magnesium oxide significantly improved stool frequency after 3–4 weeks of treatment in an outpatient setting compared with magnesium oxide alone. We found no evidence from primary care settings. Use of cisapride has been restricted in some countries because of adverse cardiac effects.

Benefits: We found no systematic review but found three RCTs.[7–9] **Versus placebo:** One RCT (69 children and young adults aged 4–18 years, attending hospital with constipation, defined as pain, difficulty in defecation, or ≤ 3–4 bowel movements/week for at least 3 months in the absence of a history of bowel disease) found that cisapride 0.3 mg/kg daily (as a syrup) significantly increased stool frequency and decreased gut transit time after 8 weeks compared with placebo (mean stool frequency/week 6.75 with cisapride *v* 1.31 with placebo).[7] The second RCT (40 children aged 2–16 years with a history of chronic constipation referred to a paediatric hospital gastroenterology clinic) found significant benefit for cisapride compared with placebo at 12 weeks, measured by a composite of improved stool frequency, absence of faecal soiling, and no use of other laxatives (improvement in composite index 14/20 [70%] with cisapride *v* 7/20 [35%] with placebo; RR 2.00, 95% CI 1.03 to 3.88; NNT 3, 95% CI 1 to 24).[8] **Cisapride plus magnesium oxide versus magnesium oxide alone:** The third RCT (84 children aged 1–7 years, attending hospital with chronic constipation, defined as fewer than 2 spontaneous bowel movements/week for at least 1 month in the absence of any underlying medical condition or concomitant drug use) compared cisapride 0.2 mg/kg three times daily (as a syrup) plus magnesium oxide (125 mg 3 times daily for children weighing less than 20 kg and 250 mg 3 times daily for children weighing more than 20 kg) versus magnesium oxide alone.[9] Both groups showed a similar increase in stool frequency after 1 week of treatment (30/44 [68%] with cisapride plus magnesium oxide v 23/40 [58%] with magnesium oxide alone; P = 0.369). Although the number of children responding to magnesium oxide alone remained constant after 1–2 weeks of therapy, the number of those responding to the combined treatment was significantly greater after 4 weeks (40/44 [91%] with cisapride plus magnesium oxide *v* 27/40 [68%] with magnesium oxide alone; P = 0.013). No significant difference between the two treatment groups was found regarding stool consistency (softened in 29/44 [66%] children treated with cisapride plus magnesium oxide *v* 27/40 [68%] children treated with magnesium oxide; no change in 11 children of each treatment group; P = 0.876) or the incidence of blood in the stools (3 children in each treatment group; P = 1.0) after 4 weeks.

Harms: **Versus placebo:** The RCTs comparing the use of cisapride versus placebo did not report harms (see comment below).[7,8] **Cisapride plus magnesium oxide versus magnesium oxide alone:** Adverse events reported in the RCT comparing cisapride plus magnesium oxide versus magnesium oxide alone were minimal, limited to gastrointestinal upset, and showed no significant difference between the two treatment groups (adverse effects occurred in 2–4 children [5–9%] receiving combined treatment *v* 1–2 children [3–5%] in the group receiving monotherapy). None of the children in the study reported any arrhythmia-related symptoms.[9]

Comment: Use of cisapride has been restricted in some countries because of its association with heart rhythm abnormalities in adults. See comments on cisapride under gastro-oesophageal reflux in children, p 354.

OPTION INCREASED DIETARY FIBRE

We found no systematic review or RCTs on the effects of increasing dietary fibre.

Benefits: We found no systematic review or RCTs.

Harms: We found no RCTs.

Comment: None.

OPTION OSMOTIC LAXATIVES

We found no RCTs that compared osmotic laxatives versus placebo in children. Two small RCTs found no significant difference in stool frequency or consistency between lactulose and lactitol after 2–4 weeks in children aged 8 months to 16 years. One of the RCTs found that lactulose increased abdominal pain and flatulence compared with lactitol. A third RCT in non-breastfed constipated infants found no difference between different strengths of lactulose.

Benefits: **Versus placebo:** We found no systematic review and no placebo controlled RCTs of osmotic laxatives in children. **Versus each other:** We found two small RCTs[10,11] comparing the effects of lactitol versus lactulose on stool frequency and consistency and a third RCT[12] comparing the effects of two different dosages of lactulose in infants. The first RCT (51 children, aged 8 months to 16 years visiting a physician for chronic idiopathic constipation) found no significant difference in stool frequency or consistency between lactitol and lactulose at 4 weeks (stool frequency per week increased from 2.5 to 5.6 with lactitol *v* 2.0 to 4.8 for lactulose; significance not reported; stool consistency normal or soft in 15/23 [65%] children with lactitol *v* 16/19 [84%] with lactulose; reported as non-significant, no other data).[10] The second RCT (39 children, aged 11 months to 13 years) compared lactitol 150–350 mg/kg daily versus lactulose 150 mg/kg daily over 2 weeks.[11] It found no significant difference in stool frequency between lactulose and lactitol (stool frequency in both groups was 1–1.5/day). A third RCT (220 non-breastfed, constipated infants aged 0–6 months) compared 2% and 4% lactulose mixed with an artificial milk preparation.[12] At 14 days, over 90% of parents in both groups reported easy passage of normal or thin consistency stools. However, the RCT did not compare outcomes between treatment groups.

Harms: **Versus each other:** The first RCT found that significantly fewer children taking lactitol had abdominal pain or flatulence compared with lactulose (abdominal pain: 22% with lactitol *v* 58% with lactulose; $P < 0.005$; flatulence: 30% with lactitol *v* 63% with lactulose; $P < 0.01$).[10]

Comment: **Versus each other:** The benefits shown in the third RCT are comparisons of outcomes before and after treatment, and were not necessarily a result of the treatments.[12]

OPTION STIMULANT LAXATIVES

One systematic review found no reliable RCTs comparing stimulant laxatives versus placebo or other treatments.

Benefits: **Versus placebo or alternative treatment:** We found one systematic review (search date 2001), which found no RCTs of adequate methodological rigour comparing stimulant laxatives versus either placebo or alternative treatment in children (see comment below).[13] We found no subsequent placebo controlled RCTs of the effects of stimulant laxatives in children.

Harms: None identified.

Comment: **Versus placebo or alternative treatment:** The studies identified by the review were all comparative, used multiple interventions, and had small sample sizes.[13] One quasi-randomised study (using last hospital number digit to allocate patients) in 37 children (aged 3–12 years) with chronic constipation found that senna was significantly less effective in achieving daily bowel movements after 6 months than mineral oil concentrate (9/18 [50%] with senna *v* 16/19 [89%] with mineral oil;

$P < 0.05$) and less effective in reducing involuntary faecal soiling after 6 months (8/18 [44%] children continuing to soil with senna v 1/19 [5%] with mineral oil; RR 8.44, 95% CI 1.52 to 16.70).[14] No significant differences were found in the number of children with at least one recurrence of constipation symptoms during the treatment period (16/18 [89%] with senna v 12/19 [66%] with mineral oil; RR 0.71, 95% CI 0.48 to 1.04).

OPTION BIOFEEDBACK TRAINING

One systematic review found no significant difference between biofeedback plus conventional treatment and conventional treatment alone at 12 months.

Benefits: We found one systematic review (search date 2001, 8 RCTs).[3] The review found no significant difference in rates of persisting problems between conventional treatment plus biofeedback and conventional treatment alone at 12 months (OR 1.34, 95% CI 0.92 to 1.94). There was heterogeneity of borderline significance ($P = 0.087$). One included RCT (41 children) found a different trend from the other seven RCTs for reasons that were not apparent.[15] After exclusion of this RCT, results were no longer heterogeneous. Meta-analysis excluding this RCT found that biofeedback plus conventional treatment increased rates of persisting problems compared with conventional treatment alone (OR 1.59, 95% CI 1.07 to 2.35; heterogeneity $P = 0.53$).

Harms: None reported.

Comment: In the systematic review, sample sizes were generally small, and interventions and outcomes varied among trials.[3]

REFERENCES

1. Nelson R, Wagget J, Lennard-Jones JE, et al. Constipation and megacolon in children and adults. In: Misiewicz JJ, Pounder RE, Venables CW, eds. *Diseases of the gut and pancreas*. 2nd ed. Oxford: Blackwell Science, 1994;843–864.
2. Rasquin-Weber A, Hymen PE, Cucchiara S, et al. Childhood functional gastrointestinal disorders. *Gut* 1999;45(Suppl II):1160–1168.
3. Brazzelli M, Griffiths P. Behavioural and cognitive interventions with or without other treatments for defaecation disorders in children (Cochrane Review). In: The Cochrane Library, Issue 3, 2003. Chichester, UK: John Wiley & Sons, Ltd. Search date 2001; primary sources Cochrane Incontinence Group Trials Register, Cochrane Controlled Trials Register, hand searching of journals, and the Enuresis Resource and Information Centre Register.
4. American Psychiatric Association. *Diagnostic and statistical manual of mental disorders*. 4th ed. Washington, DC: American Psychiatric Association, 1994.
5. Loening-Baucke V. Chronic constipation in children. *Gastroenterology* 1993;105:1557–1563.
6. Roma E, Adamidis D, Nikolara R, et al. Diet and chronic constipation in children: the role of fiber. *J Pediatr Gastroenterol Nutr* 1999;28:169–174.
7. Halibi IM. Cisapride in the management of chronic pediatric constipation. *J Pediatr Gastroenterol Nutr* 1999;28:199–202.
8. Nurko MD, Garcia-Aranda JA, Worona LB, et al. Cisapride for the treatment of constipation in children: a double blind study. *J Pediatr* 2000;136:35–40.
9. Ni YH, Lin CC, Chang SH, et al. Use of cisapride with magnesium oxide in chronic pediatric constipation. *Acta Paediatr Taiwan* 2001;42:345–349.
10. Pitzalis G, Mariani P, Chiarini-Testa MR, et al. Lactitol in chronic idiopathic constipation of childhood. *Pediatr Med Chir* 1995;17:223–226.
11. Martino AM, Pesce F, Rosati U. The effects of lactitol in the treatment of intestinal stasis in childhood. *Minerva Pediatr* 1992;44:319–323.
12. Hejlp M, Kamper J, Ebbesen F, et al. Infantile constipation and allomin-lactulose. Treatment of infantile constipation in infants fed with breast milk substitutes: a controlled trial of 2% and 4% allomin-lactulose. *Ugeskr Laeger* 1990;152:1819–1822.
13. Price KJ, Elliott TM. What is the role of stimulant laxatives in the management of childhood constipation and soiling? In: The Cochrane Library, Issue 3, 2003. Chichester, UK: John Wiley & Sons, Ltd Search date 2001; primary sources Cochrane database of randomised controlled clinical trials, hand searching of paediatric journals, and contact with experts in the field.
14. Sondheimer JM, Gervaise EP. Lubricant versus laxative in the treatment of chronic functional constipation of children: a comparative study. *J Pediatr Gastroenterol Nutr* 1982;1:223–226.
15. Loening-Baucke V. Modulation of abnormal defecation dynamics by biofeedback treatment in chronically constipated children with encopresis. *J Pediatr* 1990;116:214–222.

Gregory Rubin
Professor of Primary Care
University of Sunderland, Sunderland, UK

Competing interests: None declared.

Croup

Search date November 2003

David Johnson

QUESTIONS

INTERVENTIONS

See glossary G

Key Messages

Mild croup

- **Dexamethasone (oral single dose)** One RCT found that, compared with placebo, a single oral dose of dexamethasone (0.15 mg/kg) reduced the proportion of children with mild croup seeking additional medical attention for ongoing croup symptoms within 7–10 days. We found no RCTs evaluating single versus multiple doses of dexamethasone, or other corticosteroids in children with mild croup.
- **Decongestants (oral)** We found no systematic review, RCTs, or prospective cohort studies on oral decongestants in children with mild croup.

- **Humidification** We found no systematic review, RCTs, or observational studies evaluating the effects of humidification in children with mild croup.
- **Antibiotics** We found no systematic review, RCTs, or prospective cohort studies evaluating any type of antibiotic in children with mild croup. However, there is widespread consensus that antibiotics do not shorten the clinical course of a disease that is predominantly viral in origin.

Moderate to severe croup

- **Adrenaline (epinephrine) (nebulised)** Three RCTs found that, compared with placebo, nebulised racemic adrenaline (epinephrine) 2.25% improved croup score within 30 minutes after starting treatment. One of these RCTs found that, by 2 hours, the treatment effect of adrenaline (epinephrine) had largely disappeared. None of the RCTs reported adverse effects suggesting myocardial insufficiency, nor any evidence suggesting that treatment increases cardiac demand (for example, following treatment, the heart rate did not rise). However, we found one well documented case report of a previously normal child with severe croup who sustained a small myocardial infarction after being treated with three adrenaline (epinephrine) nebulisations within 1 hour. One small RCT found no significant difference between nebulised racemic adrenaline (epinephrine) and heliox (helium–oxygen mixture) in overall mean change in croup scores over 4 hours in children already treated with humidified oxygen and intramuscular dexamethasone 0.6 mg/kg.
- **Budesonide, nebulised (compared with placebo)** One systematic review found that, compared with placebo, nebulised budesonide improved croup score at 6, 12, and 24 hours and reduced the need for adrenaline (epinephrine) treatment in children with moderate to severe croup. One RCT found that, compared with placebo, nebulised budesonide, 2 mg administered every 12 hours improved the time to a two point improvement in children's croup score.
- **Dexamethasone (compared with placebo)** One systematic review found that, compared with placebo, dexamethasone improved croup score at 6, 12, and 24 hours and reduced the need for adrenaline (epinephrine) treatment in children with moderate to severe croup. One subsequent RCT found that, compared with placebo, a single oral dose of dexamethasone 0.6 mg/kg reduced the proportion of children seeking additional medical attention for ongoing croup symptoms within 7 days.
- **Dexamethasone, oral (compared with nebulised budesonide)** One RCT found no significant difference between oral dexamethasone 0.6 mg/kg and nebulised budesonide 2 mg in the proportion of children treated with adrenaline (epinephrine) or admitted to hospital after 1 week. Another RCT found no significant difference between oral dexamethasone 0.6 mg/kg and nebulised budesonide 2 mg in the proportion of children treated with adrenaline (epinephrine) after 1 hour or admitted to hospital at 24 hours. This RCT also found that, compared with placebo, both oral dexamethasone and nebulised budesonide reduced hospital admission at 24 hours. Although oral dexamethasone and nebulised budesonide appear to be equivalent, it is preferable to use oral dexamethasone because nebulisation usually causes prolonged agitation and crying, which worsens the child's respiratory distress, and it takes on average 15 minutes to deliver nebulised budesonide compared with 1–2 minutes with oral dexamethasone.
- **Dexamethasone, intramuscular (compared with nebulised budesonide for croup scores)** One RCT found that, compared with nebulised budesonide, intramuscular dexamethasone 0.6 mg/kg improved croup scores at 5 hours but found no significant difference in hospital admission. In this RCT, those children randomised to receive budesonide did not receive a placebo intramuscular injection, but had an elastic bandage placed on their thigh to aid in masking. Therefore it is possible that masking may not have been maintained, potentially biasing the study's result.

- **Oxygen** We found no systematic review, RCTs, or any analytical observational studies evaluating the effects of oxygen in children with moderate to severe croup. An RCT of oxygen versus no oxygen in children with severe croup would be considered unethical. There is widespread consensus that oxygen is beneficial in children with severe respiratory distress. Given the lack of harm and the compelling logic for administering oxygen in children with severe respiratory distress, oxygen will continue to be administered to these children. One RCT found no significant difference in mean change from baseline in croup score with heliox (helium 70%, oxygen 30%) compared with oxygen 30% alone, but was too small to detect reliably a clinically important difference.
- **L-adrenaline (epinephrine) compared with racemic adrenaline (epinephrine)** One small RCT reported no significant difference in overall improvement in croup scores between L-adrenaline (epinephrine) (1 : 1000, 5 mL) and racemic adrenaline (epinephrine) (2.25%, 5 mL).
- **β_2 Agonists, short-acting (nebulised)** We found no systematic review, RCTs, or observational studies evaluating the effects of nebulised short acting β_2 agonists in children with moderate to severe croup. Although there is neither empirical evidence showing benefit nor a clear theoretical reason for using nebulised short acting β_2 agonists, in some communities, a significant proportion of children with croup are treated with nebulised short acting β_2 agonists.
- **Decongestants (oral)** We found no systematic review, RCTs, or prospective cohort studies evaluating the effects of any oral decongestant in children with moderate to severe croup.
- **Dexamethasone (different doses and routes of administration)** One RCT found no significant difference between single oral dexamethasone doses of 0.6 mg/kg and 0.3 mg/kg or between 0.3 mg/kg and 0.15 mg/kg for the need for adrenaline (epinephrine) after 1 hour, remaining in the short stay unit at 24 hours, or returning for care for croup symptoms following discharge. A systematic review (including studies using several different corticosteroids other than dexamethasone) found that the higher the dose administered, the greater the difference in the proportion of children reported to be improved between the corticosteroid and placebo groups. Two RCTs found no significant difference between intramuscular and oral dexamethasone 0.6 mg/kg for resolution of symptoms, unscheduled return for medical care, or after reassessment with further treatment with corticosteroid, adrenaline (epinephrine), and/or hospital admission. In both RCTs, children randomised to receive oral dexamethasone did not receive a placebo intramuscular injection, but had an elastic bandage placed on their thigh to aid in masking. Therefore, it is possible that masking may not have been maintained, potentially biasing the studies results.
- **Dexamethasone (oral) plus budesonide (nebulised)** One RCT found no significant difference in mean change from baseline in croup score within 4 hours between nebulised budesonide 2 mg added to oral dexamethasone 0.6 mg/kg and oral dexamethasone 0.6 mg/kg alone.
- **Heliox (helium–oxygen mixture)** One RCT found no significant difference in mean change from baseline in croup score with heliox (helium 70%, oxygen 30%) compared with oxygen 30% alone, both delivered by humidification for 20 minutes. However, this RCT, was too small to detect reliably a clinically important difference. Another RCT found no significant difference between nebulised racemic adrenaline (epinephrine) and heliox (helium–oxygen mixture) in overall mean change in croup scores over 4 hours in children already treated with humidified oxygen and intramuscular dexamethasone 0.6 mg/kg.
- **Humidification** One RCT found no significant difference between humidification and controls in mean change in croup scores at 2 hours in children who had already received a single oral dose of dexamethasone 0.6 mg/kg. In this RCT, humidification was delivered by a corrugated tube held to the child's face by a parent. Another RCT found no significant difference in improvement in croup scores at 12 hours between placing children with croup in a high humidity atmosphere (87–95%) in a humidified tent, and room air. One small case series of children with croup reported scalds from hot humidified air.

- **Nebulised adrenaline (epinephrine) alone compared with intermittent positive pressure breathing** One crossover RCT in 14 children aged 4 months to 5 years admitted to hospital with minimum inspiratory stridor at rest found no significant difference in overall improvement in croup scores between nebulised adrenaline (epinephrine) plus intermittent positive pressure breathing at 15–17 cm pressure and nebulised adrenaline (epinephrine) alone.
- **Antibiotics** We found no systematic reviews, RCTs, or prospective cohort studies that examined the benefit of any type of antibiotics in children with croup. However, there is strong consensus belief that antibiotics do not shorten the clinical course of a disease that is predominantly viral in origin. This statement does not apply if bacterial tracheitis is suspected.

Impending respiratory failure due to severe croup

- **Adrenaline (epinephrine) (nebulised)** We found no systematic review or RCTs evaluating the effects of adrenaline (epinephrine) in children with impending respiratory failure in severe croup. An RCT of adrenaline (epinephrine) versus no adrenaline (epinephrine) would be considered unethical. One cohort study in children with acute upper airway obstruction found that nebulised L adrenaline (epinephrine) improved mean croup score and reduced carbon dioxide levels. Another cohort study found that nebulised racemic adrenaline (epinephrine) reduced both stridor and paradoxical breathing.
- **Corticosteroids** One systematic review found that, compared with placebo, treatment with corticosteroids significantly reduced the rate of endotracheal intubation. One RCT in intubated children showed that, compared with placebo, treatment with prednisolone (1 mg/kg via nasogastric tube every 12 hours until 24 hours after extubation) significantly reduced the duration of intubation and the need for reintubation.
- **Oxygen** We found no systematic review, RCTs, or any analytical observational studies evaluating the effects of oxygen in children with impending respiratory failure in severe croup. An RCT of oxygen versus no oxygen in children with severe croup would be considered unethical. There is widespread consensus that oxygen is beneficial in children with severe respiratory distress.
- **Heliox (helium–oxygen mixture)** We found no systematic review, RCTs, or any analytical observational studies evaluating the effects of heliox (helium–oxygen mixture) in children with impending respiratory failure in severe croup.
- **Antibiotics** We found no systematic reviews, RCTs, or prospective cohort studies that examined the benefit of any type of antibiotics in children with croup. However, there is strong consensus belief that antibiotics do not shorten the clinical course of a disease that is predominantly viral in origin. This statement does not apply if bacterial tracheitis is suspected.
- **Sedatives** We found no systematic review or RCTs evaluating the effects of sedatives in children with impending respiratory failure in severe croup. One prospective cohort study showed that children with severe croup who were treated with sedatives had decreased croup scores but no decrease in transcutaneous carbon dioxide pressure. This suggests that sedatives decrease respiratory effort without improving ventilation.

DEFINITION Croup is characterised by the abrupt onset, most commonly at night, of a barking cough, inspiratory stridor, hoarseness, and respiratory distress due to upper airway obstruction. Croup symptoms are often preceded by symptoms of upper respiratory tract infection-like symptoms. The most important diagnoses to differentiate from croup include bacterial tracheitis, epiglottitis, and the inhalation of a foreign body. Some investigators distinguish subtypes of croup;[1–3] the subtypes most commonly distinguished are acute laryngotracheitis and spasmodic croup. Children with acute laryngotracheitis have an antecedent upper respiratory tract infection, are usually febrile, and are thought to have more persistent symptoms. Children with spasmodic croup do not have an antecedent upper respiratory tract infection, are afebrile, have recurrent croup, and are thought to have more transient symptoms. However, there is little empirical evidence justifying the view that spasmodic croup responds differently from acute laryngotracheitis. **Population:** For this review, we have included children up to the age of 12 years with croup; no attempt has been made to exclude spasmodic croup. We could not find definitions of clinical severity that are either widely accepted or rigorously derived. For this review, we have elected to use definitions derived by a committee consisting of a range of specialists and sub-specialists during the development of a clinical practise guideline from Alberta Medical Association (Canada).[4] The definitions of severity have been correlated with the Westley croup score**G**,[5] since it is the most widely used clinical score, and its validity and reliability have been well demonstrated.[6,7] **Mild croup:** Occasional barking cough, none to limited stridor at rest, and none to mild suprasternal and/or intercostal indrawing (retractions of the skin of the chest wall), corresponding to a Westley croup score of 0–2. **Moderate croup:** Frequent barking cough, easily audible stridor at rest, and suprasternal and sternal wall retraction at rest, but no or little distress or agitation, corresponding to a Westley croup score of 3–5. **Severe croup:** Frequent barking cough, prominent inspiratory and — occasionally — expiratory stridor, marked sternal wall retractions, decreased air entry on auscultation, and significant distress and agitation, corresponding to a Westley croup score of 6–11. **Impending respiratory failure:** Barking cough (often not prominent), audible stridor at rest (occasionally can be hard to hear), sternal wall retractions (may not be marked), usually lethargic or decreased level of consciousness, and often dusky complexion without supplemental oxygen, corresponding to a Westley croup score of > 11. When having severe respiratory distress, a young child's compliant chest wall "caves in" during inspiration, causing unsynchronised chest and abdominal wall expansion (paradoxical breathing**G**). Approximately 85% of children attending general emergency departments, by this classification scheme, have mild croup, and less than 1% have severe croup (unpublished prospective data obtained from 21 Alberta general emergency departments).

INCIDENCE/ PREVALENCE Croup has an average annual incidence of 3% and accounts for 5% of emergent admissions to hospital in children under 6 years of age in North America (unpublished population based data from Calgary Health Region, Alberta, Canada, 1996–2000).[8] One retrospective Belgian study found that 16% of 5–8 year old children had suffered from croup at least once during their life, and 5% had experienced recurrent croup (3 or more episodes).[9] We are not aware of epidemiological studies establishing the incidence of croup in other parts of the world.

AETIOLOGY/ RISK FACTORS Croup occurs most commonly in children between 6 months and 3 years of age, but can also occur in children as young as 3 months and as old as 12–15 years of age.[8] Croup is extremely rare in adults.[10] Croup occurs predominantly in late autumn, but can occur during any season, including summer.[8] Croup is caused by a variety of viral agents and, occasionally, by *Mycoplasma pneumoniae*.[8] Parainfluenza accounts for 75% of all cases, with the commonest type being parainfluenza type 1. The remaining proportion of cases are largely accounted for by respiratory syncytial virus, metapneumovirus, influenza A and B, adenovirus, and mycoplasma.[8,11–13] Viral invasion of the laryngeal mucosa leads to inflammation, hyperaemia, and oedema.[1] This leads to narrowing of the subglottic region. Children compensate for this narrowing by breathing more quickly and deeply. In children with more severe illness, as the narrowing progresses, their increased effort at breathing becomes counterproductive, airflow through the upper airway becomes turbulent (stridor), their compliant chest wall begins to cave in during inspiration, resulting in paradoxical breathing, and consequently the child becomes fatigued. With these events — if untreated — the child becomes hypoxic and hypercapnoeic, which eventually results in respiratory failure and arrest.[14,15]

PROGNOSIS Croup symptoms resolve in the majority of children within 48 hours.[16] However, a small percentage of children with croup have symptoms that persist for up to 1 week.[16] Hospitalisation rates vary significantly between communities but, on average, less than 5% of all children with croup are admitted to hospital.[17–20] Of those admitted to hospital, only 1–3% are intubated.[21–24] Mortality is low; in one 10-year study, less than 0.5% of intubated children died.[22] Uncommon complications of croup include pneumonia, pulmonary oedema, and bacterial tracheitis.[25–27]

AIMS OF INTERVENTION To minimise the duration and severity of disease episodes, with minimal adverse effects.

OUTCOMES Rate and duration of airway intubation; rate and duration of hospitalisation; rate of return to healthcare practitioner following an episode; adverse effects of treatment; change in clinical severity over time (as measured by a range of clinical scores); change in upper airway obstruction (as measured by a number of pathophysiological measurement tools).

METHODS Clinical Evidence search and appraisal November 2003. The only intervention for which a significant number of RCTs have been published is corticosteroids. Therefore, for all other interventions, we also searched for analytical observational studies and included RCTs, regardless of size.

QUESTION What are the effects of treatments in children with mild croup?

OPTION CORTICOSTEROIDS

One RCT found that, compared with placebo, a single oral dose of dexamethasone (0.15 mg/kg) reduced the proportion of children with mild croup seeking additional medical attention for ongoing croup symptoms within 7–10 days. We found no RCTs evaluating single versus multiple doses of dexamethasone or other corticosteroids in children with mild croup.

Benefits: We found no systematic review on corticosteroids only in children with mild croup. **Oral dexamethasone versus placebo:** We found one RCT in children with mild croup symptoms.[28] The RCT found that, compared with placebo, a single oral dose of dexamethasone 0.15 mg/kg significantly reduced the proportion of children seeking additional medical attention for ongoing croup symptoms within 7 to 10 days (1 RCT, 100 children aged 4–10 years presenting with mild croup without stridor and chest wall indrawing at rest; proportion seeking additional medical attention within 7–10 days: 0/50 [0%] with oral dexamethasone *v* 8/50 [16%] with placebo; ARR 16%, 95% CI 6% to 26%; NNT 6, 95% CI 4 to 17). In this RCT, mild croup was defined as symptoms not requiring hospital admission. In general, children presenting with stridor and chest wall retractions were excluded from this study.[28] **Single versus multiple doses:** We found no systematic review or RCTs. **Other corticosteroids:** We found no systematic review or RCTs.

Harms: We found insufficient evidence on adverse effects of corticosteroids in children with mild croup. The only RCT in children with mild croup that we identified did not report in adverse events.[28]

Comment: We found one RCT in which children were broadly described as having "mild" croup.[29] However, we did not include it in this review because it included children with stridor at rest and chest wall indrawing, who would qualify as having "moderate" croup according to the definitions used for this review.

OPTION HUMIDIFICATION

We found no systematic review, RCTs, or observational studies evaluating the effects of humidification in children with mild croup.

Benefits: We found no systematic review, RCTs, or observational studies evaluating the effects of humidification in children with mild croup.

Harms: We found no studies evaluating the potential adverse events associated with humidification treatment in children with mild croup.

Comment: Although humidification has been widely used as a treatment for croup since the 1800s,[30] surprisingly little evidence exists regarding whether or not it is effective.

OPTION ANTIBIOTICS

We found no systematic review, RCTs, or prospective cohort studies evaluating any type of antibiotic in children with mild croup. However, there is widespread consensus that antibiotics do not shorten the clinical course of a disease that is predominantly viral in origin.

Benefits: We found no systematic review, RCTs, or prospective cohort studies evaluating antibiotics in children with mild croup.

Harms: We found no studies evaluating potential adverse events associated with antibiotics in children with mild croup.

Comment: The routine use of antibiotics in children with croup is not recommended because the vast majority of cases of croup are of viral origin.[31–35] Surveys of practice patterns demonstrate that in some communities, 30–80% of children with croup are treated with antibiotics.[36–38]

OPTION ORAL DECONGESTANTS

We found no systematic review, RCTs, or prospective cohort studies on oral decongestants in children with mild croup.

Benefits: We found no systematic review, RCTs, or prospective cohort studies on oral decongestants in children with mild croup.

Harms: We found no studies evaluating potential adverse events associated with oral decongestants in children with mild croup.

Comment: Although there is little evidence of benefit from use of oral decongestants in children with croup, surveys of practice patterns demonstrate that in some communities a significant proportion of children with croup are treated with oral decongestants.[38]

QUESTION What are the effects of treatment in children with moderate to severe croup?

OPTION NEBULISED ADRENALINE (EPINEPHRINE)

Three RCTs found that, compared with placebo, nebulised racemic adrenaline (epinephrine) 2.25% improved croup score within 30 minutes after starting treatment. One of these RCTs found that, by 2 hours, the treatment effect of adrenaline (epinephrine) had largely disappeared. None of the RCTs reported adverse complications suggesting myocardial insufficiency, nor any evidence suggesting that treatment increases cardiac demand. However, we found one well documented case report of a previously normal child with severe croup who sustained a small myocardial infarction after being treated with three adrenaline (epinephrine) nebulisations within 1 hour. One small RCT found no significant difference between nebulised racemic adrenaline (epinephrine) and heliox (helium–oxygen mixture) in overall mean change in croup scores over 4 hours in children already treated with humidified oxygen and intramuscular dexamethasone 0.6 mg/kg. One small RCT reported no significant difference in overall improvement in croup scores between L-adrenaline (epinephrine) (1 : 1000, 5 mL) and racemic adrenaline (epinephrine) (2.25%, 5 mL). One crossover RCT in 14 children aged 4 months to 5 years admitted to hospital with minimum inspiratory stridor at rest found no significant difference in overall improvement in croup scores between nebulised adrenaline (epinephrine) plus intermittent positive pressure breathing at 15–17 cm pressure and nebulised adrenaline (epinephrine) alone.

Benefits: We found no systematic review but found five small RCTs.[5,39–43] **Versus placebo:** The first RCT found that, compared with placebo, nebulised racemic adrenaline (epinephrine) 2.25% (0.5 mL/kg via nebuliser) significantly improved croup score at 30 minutes after inhalation (1 RCT, 54 children aged 4 months to 11 years with combined Taussig croup score**G**/Westley croup score**G** 2–9 [possible range 0–15]; mean change from baseline croup score: –2.7 with adrenaline [epinephrine] *v* –1.1 with placebo; P = 0.003).[39] The second RCT found that, compared with placebo, nebulised racemic adrenaline (epinephrine) 2.25% (0.5 mL) administered by intermittent positive pressure breathing (IPPB) significantly improved croup scores at 10 minutes and 30 minutes after treatment but found no significant difference at 120 minutes (1 RCT, 20 children aged 4 months to 12 years admitted to an intensive care high humidity mist room with Westley croup score 3–6; change in mean baseline croup score: adrenaline [epinephrine], 3.9 pretreatment, 1.7 at 10 minutes [P < 0.01], 1.7 at 30 minutes [P < 0.01], 3.3 at 120 minutes [NS]; placebo, 4.1 pretreatment, 3.7 at 10 minutes, 3.1 at 30 minutes, 3.8 at 120 minutes, all NS).[5] The third RCT found that, compared with placebo, nebulised racemic adrenaline (epinephrine) 2.25% (dose weight adjusted) administered by IPPB significantly improved croup score at 20 minutes after initiation of treatment (1 RCT, 13 children aged 5 months to 11 years, admitted to hospital with croup [Taussig croup score, 5–12, possible range 0–14]; mean change from baseline croup score: estimated treatment difference 3.6, 95% CI 2.5 to 4.7; P < 0.001; mean, SD, group treatment differences, and P value calculated by the author from individual patient data supplied in the published paper[40] for this RCT). **Versus heliox (helium–oxygen mixture):** One small RCT found no significant difference between nebulised racemic adrenaline (epinephrine) and heliox in overall mean change in croup scores over 4 hours in children with moderate to severe croup already treated with humidified oxygen and intramuscular dexamethasone 0.6 mg/kg (1 RCT, 29 children aged 6 months to 3 years evaluated in a paediatric emergency department and intensive care unit with croup [modified Taussig croup score 5–9, possible range 0–14]; mean change in croup scores between 2 groups at 4 hours: P = 0.13; results presented graphically).[41] However, after 30 minutes the mean croup scores for children treated with heliox were consistently lower than the mean croup scores in the adrenaline (epinephrine) group. The difference in the mean scores continued to increase until 180 minutes (results presented graphically).[41] In this RCT the children were treated with either one or two normal saline nebulisations, followed by the delivery of 70% helium/30% oxygen for 3 hours or, one or two racemic adrenaline (epinephrine) nebulisations (2.25%, 0.5 mL), followed by the delivery of 100% oxygen for 3 hours, both delivered through a tight-fitting mask. The second nebulisation was ordered at the discretion of the attending physician, based on whether the child had continued respiratory distress. Only a respiratory therapist not otherwise involved in the study was aware of study assignment. Children were assessed using the modified croup score at 30, 60, 90, 120, 150, 180, and 240 minutes following initiation of therapy.[41] **L-Adrenaline versus racemic adrenaline (epinephrine):** One small RCT in 31 children aged 6 months to 6 years evaluated in an emergency department with croup (modified Downes and Raphaely croup score**G** ≥ 6, possible range 0–10) found no significant difference in overall improvement in croup scores between L-adrenaline (epinephrine) (1 : 1000, 5 mL) and racemic adrenaline (epinephrine) (2.25%, 5 mL).[43] However, this RCT did not report actual P values but reported mean croup scores (at baseline, 5, 15, 30, 60, 90, and 120 minutes), mean heart rate, and blood pressure. The mean scores for the L-adrenaline (epinephrine) group were slightly lower than for the racemic adrenaline (epinephrine) group.[43] **Nebulisation alone versus with intermittent positive pressure breathing:** We found one crossover RCT, in 14 children aged 4 months to 5 years admitted to hospital with croup (minimum inspiratory stridor at rest).[42] The RCT reported no significant difference in overall improvement in croup scores between delivery of adrenaline (epinephrine) 2.25% (0.25 mL) by nebulisation alone and delivery of adrenaline (epinephrine) by nebulisation plus IPPB (15–17 cm pressure).[42] However, this RCT did not report actual P values for differences in treatment effect but reported Westley croup scores (at baseline, 30, 60, 90, and 120 minutes).[42]

Harms: The RCTs reported no adverse effects and in particular observed no increase in heart rate or respiratory rate with adrenaline (epinephrine).[39–43] We found one case report of a previously normal 11 year old child with severe croup treated with three nebulised doses of racemic adrenaline (epinephrine) (2.25%, 0.5 mL) within 60 minutes. During administration of the third dose, the child developed ventricular tachycardia. Treatment was discontinued, and normal sinus rhythm returned. The child was later demonstrated to have normal cardiac anatomy, and clear evidence of a myocardial infarction based on persistently abnormal ECG, elevated CPK-MB levels, and an abnormal nuclear stress test.[44]

Comment: We found one small RCT in 20 children aged 5 months to 5 years, evaluated either in the emergency department or in hospital, with croup. Children were treated with either nebulised racemic adrenaline (epinephrine) (2.25%, 0.5 mL) with IPPB or nebulised placebo with IPPB.[45] Assessment occurred immediately before and 15 minutes after treatment. The RCT found that eight out of 10 treated with adrenaline (epinephrine) and five out of 10 treated with placebo had a reduction in clinical score of 2 or more, which was interpreted as "significant improvement", but details of quantitative data are not available.[45]

OPTION NEBULISED BUDESONIDE

One systematic review found that, compared with placebo, nebulised budesonide improved croup score at 6, 12, and 24 hours and reduced the need for adrenaline (epinephrine) treatment in children with moderate to severe croup. One RCT found that, compared with placebo, nebulised budesonide, 2 mg administered every 12 hours, improved the time to a two point improvement in children's croup score. Two RCTs found that, compared with nebulised budesonide 1 mg or 4 mg, intramuscular dexamethasone 0.6 mg/kg improved croup scores at 5 or 12 hours. One of these RCTs found no significant difference in hospital admission between nebulised budesonide 4 mg and intramuscular dexamethasone 0.6 mg/kg. One RCT found no significant difference in mean change from baseline in croup score within 4 hours between nebulised budesonide 2 mg added to oral dexamethasone 0.6 mg/kg and oral dexamethasone 0.6 mg/kg alone

Benefits: **Versus placebo:** We found two systematic reviews.[46,47] One systematic review (search date 1997) found that, compared with placebo, nebulised budesonide significantly improved croup score at 6, 12, and 24 hours (change from baseline croup score budesonide *v* placebo: at 6 hours, 5 RCTs, 327 children; WMD –1.34, 95% CI –1.71 to –0.96; at 12 hours, 2 RCTs, 71 children; WMD –1.33, 95% CI –1.96 to –0.70; at 24 hours, 1 RCT, 35 children; WMD –2.03, 95% CI –3.63 to –0.43).[46] It found that, compared with placebo, budesonide significantly reduced the need for adrenaline (epinephrine) treatment (ARR 9%, 95% CI 2% to 16%). The review also found that, compared with placebo, corticosteroids (budesonide [nebulised], dexamethasone [oral]) significantly reduced the length of time spent in the emergency department (5 RCTs,

596 children; time spent in the emergency department: WMD 11 hours, 95% CI −18 hours to + 4 hours; test for overall effect: P = 0.0005) and length of hospital stay (6 RCTs, 698 children; length of hospital stay: WMD 16 hours, 95% CI −31 hours to +1 hour; test for overall effect: P < 0.00001).[46] All estimates had significant heterogeneity between trials. Croup was defined as a syndrome consisting of hoarseness, barking cough, and stridor; an alternative diagnosis of acute stridor was excluded.[46] The second systematic review (search date 1999) included RCTs irrespective of diagnostic criteria used, symptom severity, or the study setting and pooled the results of RCTs on nebulised budesonide and dexamethasone, but did not separately assess the effect of budesonide alone.[47] The review identified one additional RCT on budesonide not included in the first systematic review. The RCT found that, compared with placebo, nebulised budesonide 2 mg administered every 12 hours significantly improved the time to a two point improvement in children's croup score (82 hospitalised children aged 6 months to 8 years, time to 2 point improvement in croup score: P = 0.01) Croup scores were assessed at baseline, then at 2, 6, 12, 24, 36, and 48 hours following treatment.[48] **Versus oral dexamethasone:** See benefits of oral dexamethasone, p 316. **Versus intramuscular dexamethasone:** See benefits of intramuscular dexamethasone, p 316. **Plus oral dexamethasone:** See benefits of oral dexamethasone, p 316.

Harms: The systematic reviews we identified did not report on adverse outcomes.[46,47]

Comment: None.

OPTION DEXAMETHASONE

One systematic review found that, compared with placebo, dexamethasone improved croup score at 6, 12, and 24 hours and reduced the need for adrenaline (epinephrine) treatment in children with moderate to severe croup. One subsequent RCT found that, compared with placebo, a single oral dose of dexamethasone 0.6 mg/kg reduced the proportion of children seeking additional medical attention for ongoing croup symptoms within 7 days. One RCT found no significant difference between single oral dexamethasone doses of 0.6 mg/kg and 0.3 mg/kg or between 0.3 mg/kg and 0.15 mg/kg for the need for adrenaline (epinephrine) after 1 hour, remaining in the short stay unit at 24 hours, or returning for care for croup symptoms following discharge. A systematic review (including studies using several different corticosteroids other than dexamethasone) found that the higher the dose administered, the greater the difference in the proportion of children reported to be improved between the corticosteroid and placebo groups. Two RCTs found no significant difference between intramuscular and oral dexamethasone 0.6 mg/kg for resolution of symptoms, unscheduled return for medical care, or after reassessment with further treatment with corticosteroid, adrenaline (epinephrine), and/or hospital admission. In both RCTs, children randomised to receive oral dexamethasone did not receive a placebo intramuscular injection, but had an elastic bandage placed on their thigh to aid in masking. One RCT found that, compared with nebulised budesonide, intramuscular dexamethasone 0.6 mg/kg improved croup scores at 5 hours but found no significant difference in hospital admission. In this RCT, those children randomised to receive budesonide did not receive a placebo intramuscular injection, but had an elastic bandage placed on their thigh to aid in masking. Therefore, it is possible that masking may not have been maintained, potentially biasing the study's result. One RCT found no significant difference between oral dexamethasone 0.6 mg/kg and nebulised budesonide 2 mg in the proportion of children treated with adrenaline (epinephrine) or admitted to hospital after 1 week. Another RCT found no significant difference between

oral dexamethasone 0.6 mg/kg and nebulised budesonide 2 mg in the proportion of children treated with adrenaline (epinephrine) after 1 hour or admitted to hospital at 24 hours. This RCT also found that, compared with placebo, both oral dexamethasone and nebulised budesonide reduced hospital admission at 24 hours. Although oral dexamethasone and nebulised budesonide appear to be equivalent, it is preferable to use oral dexamethasone because nebulisation usually causes prolonged agitation and crying, which worsens the child's respiratory distress, and it takes on average 15 minutes to deliver nebulised budesonide compared with 1–2 minutes with oral dexamethasone. One RCT found no significant difference in mean change from baseline in croup score within 4 hours between nebulised budesonide 2 mg added to oral dexamethasone 0.6 mg/kg and oral dexamethasone 0.6 mg/kg alone.

Benefits: We found three systematic reviews[46,47,49] and five subsequent RCTs.[29,50–53] **Versus placebo:** One systematic review (search date 1997) found that, compared with placebo, dexamethasone (im, oral) significantly improved croup score at 6, 12, and 24 hours (change from baseline croup score dexamethasone *v* placebo: at 6 hours, 7 RCTs, 365 children; WMD −1.07, 95% CI −1.20 to −0.93; at 12 hours, 5 RCTs, 146 children; WMD −0.91, 95% CI −1.09 to −0.73; at 24 hours, 4 RCTs, 73 children; WMD −1.21, 95% CI −1.58 to −0.83).[46] It found that, compared with placebo, dexamethasone significantly reduced the need for adrenaline (epinephrine) treatment (ARR 12%, 95% CI 4% to 20%). It also found that, compared with placebo, corticosteroids (budesonide [nebulised], dexamethasone [im, oral]) significantly reduced length of time spent in the emergency department (5 RCTs, 596 children; time spent in emergency department: WMD −11 hours, 95% CI −18 hours to + 4 hours; test for overall effect: P = 0.0005) and length of hospital stay (6 RCTs, 698 children; length of hospital stay: WMD −16 hours, 95% CI −31 hours to +1 hour; test for overall effect: P < 0.00001). All estimates had significant heterogeneity between trials. Croup was defined as a syndrome consisting of hoarseness, barking cough, and stridor; an alternative diagnosis of acute stridor was excluded.[46] The second systematic review (search date 1999) included RCTs irrespective of diagnostic criteria used, symptom severity, or the study setting and pooled the results of RCTs on nebulised budesonide and dexamethasone, but did not separately assess the effect of dexamethasone alone.[47] One subsequent RCT found that, compared with placebo, a single oral dose of dexamethasone (0.6 mg/kg, maximum dose 10 mg) significantly reduced the proportion of children seeking additional medical attention for ongoing croup symptoms within 7 days (1 RCT, 3 arm study, 264 children aged 6 months to 6 years presenting with barking cough, stridor, and/or hoarseness for fewer than 48 hours; seeking additional medical attention within 7 days: 7/87 [8%] with oral dexamethasone *v* 18/88 [20%] with placebo; ARR 12%, 95% CI 2% to 23%; NNT 8, 95% CI 4 to 45).[29] This RCT also included comparison with nebulised dexamethasone 160 μg. It found no significant difference between nebulised dexamethasone 160 μg and placebo in the proportion of children seeking additional medical help (19/91 [20%] *v* 18/88 [20%]; ARR 0%). However, the dose of nebulised dexamethasone of 160 μg is extremely small. In this RCT, a modified Westley croup score**G** (Westley croup score 0–5) was used to assess croup severity; the stridor section of the score was altered to include 1 point if the subject had stridor only with agitation or excitement.[29] **Oral dexamethasone dose:** We found one systematic review (search date 1987, 10 studies, 1 286 children).[49] The review included studies using different types of corticosteroids, and the authors converted all steroids to cortisone dose equivalents for a 12.5 kg child (doses used ranged from 4.2 mg to 267 mg cortisone or approximately 0.05 mg/kg to 0.66 mg/kg dexamethasone). The cortisone dose equivalent was plotted relative to the difference in the proportion of children improved between the steroid and placebo groups. The review found that the higher the dose of corticosteroid administered, the greater the difference in the proportion of children reported to be improved between the corticosteroid and placebo groups.[49] One RCT identified by another systematic review[46] found no significant difference between single oral dexamethasone doses of 0.6 mg/kg and 0.3 mg/kg for the outcomes of the need for adrenaline (epinephrine) after 1 hour, remaining in the short stay unit at 24 hours, or returning for care for croup symptoms following discharge (1 RCT, 120 children aged 6 months to 14 years with stridor and chest wall retractions at rest and croup score ≥3 [croup score range not available]; need for adrenaline [epinephrine] after 1 hour: 1/31 [3%] with 0.6 mg/kg dexamethasone *v* 0/29 [0%] 0.3 mg/kg dexamethasone; ARR 3%, 95% CI –9% to +16%; remaining in the short stay unit at 24 hours: 2/31 [6%] with 0.6 mg/kg dexamethasone *v* 2/29 [7%] *v* 0.3 mg/kg dexamethasone; ARR 0%, 95% CI –16% to +15%; returning for care for croup symptoms following discharge: 3/31 [10%] 0.6 mg/kg dexamethasone *v* 2/29 [7%] with 0.3 mg/kg dexamethasone; ARR 3%, 95% CI –14% to +19%).[54] It also found no significant difference between single oral dexamethasone doses of 0.3 mg/kg and 0.15 mg/kg for the same outcomes (need for adrenaline [epinephrine] after 1 hour: 0/31 [0%] with 0.3 mg/kg dexamethasone *v* 0/29 [0%] with 0.15 mg/kg dexamethasone; ARR 0%, 95% CI –12% to +11%; remaining in the short stay unit at 24 hours: 0/31 [0%] with 0.3 mg/kg dexamethasone *v* 1/29 [3%] with 0.15 mg/kg dexamethasone; ARR –3%, 95% CI –17% to +8%; returning for care for croup symptoms following discharge: 1/31 [3%] with 0.3 mg/kg dexamethasone *v* 1/29 [3%] with 0.15 mg/kg dexamethasone; ARR 0%, 95% CI –14% to +13%).[54] However, this RCT did not report either the individual or an overall test for differences. **Intramuscular versus oral dexamethasone:** One subsequent RCT found no significant difference between intramuscular and oral dexamethasone 0.6 mg/kg for resolution of symptoms, unscheduled return for medical care, or after reassessment with further treatment with corticosteroid, adrenaline (epinephrine), and/or admission to hospital within 72 hours (1 RCT, 277 children aged 3 months to 12 years evaluated in an emergency department with croup; symptoms not completely resolved: 64/139 [46%] with intramuscular dexamethasone *v* 72/138 [52%] with oral dexamethasone; ARI 6%, 95% CI –6% to +18%; unscheduled return for medical care: 45/139 [32%] with intramuscular dexamethasone *v* 35/138 [25%] with oral dexamethasone; ARR 7%, 95% CI –4% to +18%; returned for reassessment and treated with corticosteroid, adrenaline [epinephrine], and/or admitted to hospital: 11/139 [8%] with intramuscular dexamethasone *v* 12/138 [9%] with oral dexamethasone; ARI 1%, 95% CI –6% to +7%).[51] Another subsequent RCT found no significant difference between intramuscular dexamethasone and oral dexamathasone 0.6 mg/kg for initial hospital admission, unscheduled return visit to medical care within 24 hours, and further treatment with corticosteroid, adrenaline (epinephrine), and/or admission to hospital (1 RCT, 277 children aged 3 months to 12 years evaluated in an emergency department with croup; symptoms not completely resolved at 24 hours: 64/139 [46%] with intramuscular dexamethasone *v* 72/138 [52%] with oral dexamathasone; ARI 6%, 95% CI –6% to +18%; unscheduled return visit to medical care within 24 hours: 45/139 [32%] with intramuscular dexamethasone *v* 35/138 [25%] with oral dexamathasone; ARR 7%, 95% CI –4% to +18%; and further treatment with corticosteroid, adrenaline [epinephrine], and/or admission to hospital: 11/139 [8%] with intramuscular dexamethasone *v* 12/138 [9%] with oral dexamathasone; ARI 1%, 95% CI –6% to

+7%).[52] In both RCTs, children randomised to receive oral dexamethasone did not receive a placebo intramuscular injection, but had an elastic bandage placed on their thigh to aid in masking.[51,52] **Intramuscular dexamethasone versus nebulised budesonide:** One RCT identified by systematic review[46] found that, compared with nebulised budesonide 4 mg, intramuscular dexamethasone 0.6 mg/kg significantly improved croup score at 5 hours but found no significant difference in hospital admission (mean croup score at 5 hours: –2.9 with intramuscular dexamethasone *v* –2.0 with nebulised budesonide; estimated treatment difference –0.9, 95% CI –1.5 to –0.3; P = 0.003; hospital admission: 11/47 [23%] with intramuscular dexamethasone *v* 18/48 [38%] with nebulised budesonide; OR 0.5, 95% CI 0.2 to 1.2; P = 0.18). In this RCT, those children randomised to receive budesonide did not receive a placebo intramuscular injection, but had an elastic bandage placed on their thigh to aid in masking. Therefore, it is possible that masking may not have been maintained, potentially biasing the study's results.[55] This RCT evaluated the relationship between subtypes of croup (spasmodic croup, acute laryngotracheitis, or a mixed presentation) and treatment effect. The RCT found that the type of croup did not qualitatively alter the differences between treatment groups for either hospitalisation rates, the number of additional treatments, or the change in the Westley croup score (quantitative data not available).[55] We found one subsequent RCT published in Danish with an abstract in English.[50] It found that, compared with nebulised budesonide 1 mg, intramuscular dexamethasone 0.6 mg/kg significantly improved croup score at 6 hours and 12 hours (1 RCT, 59 children aged 3 months to 6 years hospitalised for croup, improvement in Westley croup score with intramuscular dexamethasone *v* nebulised budesonide: P = 0.001 at 6 hours; P = 0.0004 at 12 hours; means and CIs not provided). Information about how blinding was carried out was not available in the abstract.[50] **Oral dexamethasone versus nebulised budesonide:** We found two RCTs.[53,54] The results of one RCT are reported under oral dexamethasone plus nebulised budesonide below.[53] Another RCT[54] identified by systematic review[46] found no significant difference between oral dexamethasone 0.6 mg/kg and nebulised budesonide 2 mg in the proportion of children treated with adrenaline (epinephrine) after 1 hour or admitted to hospital at 24 hours (1 RCT, 3 arm study, 80 children aged 5 months to 13 years with croup score ≥ 3 [range not available], evaluated in an emergency department with croup [croup score range not provided]; treatment with adrenaline [epinephrine] after 1 hour: 0/23 with oral dexamathasone *v* 0/27 with nebulised budesonide; ARR 0%, 95% CI –12% to +14%; hospital admission at 24 hours: 2/23 [8.7%] with oral dexamathasone *v* 5/27 [18.5%] with nebulised budesonide; ARR 10%, 95% CI –9% to +28%).[56] The RCT also found that, compared with placebo, treatment with oral dexamethasone or nebulised budesonide significantly reduced hospital admission at 24 hours (hospital admission at 24 hours: 9% with oral dexamethasone *v* 19% with nebulised budesonide *v* 50% with placebo; P < 0.05).[56] **Oral dexamethasone plus nebulised budesonide:** One subsequent RCT found no significant difference between oral dexamethasone 0.6 mg/kg alone and oral dexamethasone 0.6 mg/kg plus nebulised budesonide 2 mg in mean change from baseline in croup score within 4 hours (1 RCT, 198 children aged 3 months to 5 years with Westley croup score 2–7; mean change from baseline in croup score: –2.4 with oral dexamethasone; –2.3 with nebulised budesonide; –2.4 with dexamathasone plus budesonide; estimated treatment differences [clinically important = 1]: oral dexamethasone *v* nebulised budesonide –0.12, 95% CI –0.53 to +0.29; oral dexamethasone *v* oral dexamethasone plus nebulised budesonide

0.02, 95% CI –0.39 to +0.43; nebulised budesonide *v* oral dexamethasone plus nebulised budesonide 0.14, 95% CI –0.27 to +0.55).[53] This RCT also found no significant difference between nebulised budesonide alone, oral dexamethasone alone, and nebulised budesonide plus oral dexamethasone in the proportion of children treated with adrenaline (epinephrine) (2/65 [3%] with budesonide *v* 2/69 [3%] with dexamethasone *v* 2/64 [3%] with budesonide + dexamethasone; P = 1.00) or admitted to hospital after 1 week (0/65 [0%] with budesonide *v* 1/68 [0%] with dexamethasone *v* 0/64 [0%] with budesonide plus dexamethasone; P = 1.00).

Harms: **Versus placebo:** Two systematic reviews did not report on adverse outcomes.[46,47] One subsequent RCT did not report on adverse outcomes.[29] **Oral dexamethasone dose:** One systematic review and one subsequent RCT did not report on adverse outcomes.[49,54] **Intramuscular versus oral dexamethasone:** Two subsequent RCTs did not report on adverse outcomes.[51,52] **Intramuscular dexamethasone versus nebulised budesonide:** One RCT[55] identified by systematic review[46] reported that no children in any of the treatment groups had adverse effects. One subsequent RCT did not report on adverse outcomes.[50] **Oral dexamethasone versus nebulised budesonide:** One RCT[56] identified by systematic review[46] did not report on adverse outcomes. **Oral dexamethasone plus nebulised budesonide:** One subsequent RCT reported that one child developed oral thrush following treatment with budesonide, one child developed hives, another child was reported to show violent behaviour following treatment with oral dexamethasone, and one child was reported to be more hyperactive than usual following treatment with both oral dexamethasone and nebulised budesonide.[53]

Comment: **Oral dexamethasone dose:** Regarding the issue of what dose of dexamethasone to use, the one published RCT which focused on this topic enrolled only a relatively small number of children, with relatively mild croup. Consequently, this study is probably underpowered to detect a clinically important difference, especially in children with more severe disease. **Oral dexamethasone versus nebulised budesonide:** Although from the results of two RCTs, oral dexamethasone and nebulised budesonide appear to be equivalent, there are several practical reasons for preferentially using oral dexamethasone. Important clinical considerations include the stress involved for the child (nebulisation usually causes prolonged agitation and crying, which worsens the child's respiratory distress) and the time required to deliver the drugs (on average oral administration takes 1–2 minutes, whereas nebulisation requires 15 minutes). In addition, the overall cost of nebulisation is higher because nebuliser apparatus and nursing time are required.

OPTION OXYGEN

We found no RCTs or observational studies evaluating the effects of oxygen in children with moderate to severe croup. An RCT of oxygen versus no oxygen in children with severe croup would be considered unethical. There is widespread consensus that oxygen is beneficial in children with severe respiratory distress. One RCT found no significant difference in mean change from baseline in croup score with heliox (helium 70%, oxygen 30%) compared with oxygen 30% alone, both delivered by humidification for 20 minutes. This RCT was too small to detect reliably a clinically important difference.

Benefits: **Versus no oxygen treatment:** We found no systematic review, RCTs, or any analytical observational studies evaluating the effects of oxygen in children with moderate to severe croup. An RCT of oxygen versus no oxygen in children with severe croup would be considered unethical. We found one prospective cohort study that demonstrated that children with croup can have hypoxia, even in the absence of severe upper airway obstruction, apparently due to intrapulmonary shunting.[57] This study did not attempt to find out if administration of oxygen decreases respiratory effort. **Versus heliox (helium–oxygen mixture):** See benefits of heliox (helium–oxygen mixture), p 320.

Harms: **Versus no oxygen treatment:** We found no observational studies evaluating adverse events associated with treatment with oxygen in children with moderate to severe croup. **Versus heliox (helium–oxygen mixture):** See harms of heliox (helium–oxygen mixture), p 320.

Comment: There is compelling logic for administering oxygen in children with severe respiratory distress, and no evidence of harm.

OPTION HELIOX (HELIUM–OXYGEN MIXTURE)

One RCT found no significant difference in mean change from baseline in croup score with heliox (helium 70%, oxygen 30%) compared with oxygen 30% alone, both delivered by humidification for 20 minutes. This RCT was too small to detect reliably a clinically important difference. Another RCT found no significant difference between nebulised racemic adrenaline (epinephrine) and heliox in overall mean change in croup scores over 4 hours in children already treated with humidified oxygen and intramuscular dexamethasone 0.6 mg/kg.

Benefits: **Versus oxygen alone:** We found one RCT.[58] It found no significant difference in mean change from baseline in croup score with heliox (helium 70%, oxygen 30%) compared with oxygen 30% alone, both delivered by humidification for 20 minutes (1 RCT, 15 children aged 6 months to 4 years evaluated in an emergency department with croup [modified Westley croup score**G** approximately 1–5, possible range 0–16]; mean change from baseline in croup score: –2.25 with heliox *v* –1.42 with oxygen alone; P = 0.32).[58] Children were assessed using the modified croup score at baseline and then 20 minutes following initiation of treatment. This RCT was too small to detect reliably a clinically important difference. **Versus nebulised adrenaline (epinephrine):** See benefits of nebulised adrenaline (epinephrine), p 313.

Harms: **Versus oxygen alone:** We found one RCT, which did not report any adverse events.[58] Potential adverse effects include hypoxia secondary to inadequate oxygen concentrations in the heliox mix, and hypothermia secondary to prolonged administration of heliox. **Versus nebulised adrenaline (epinephrine):** See harms of nebulised adrenaline (epinephrine), p 314.

Comment: None.

OPTION HUMIDIFICATION

One RCT found no significant difference between humidification and controls in mean change in croup scores at 2 hours in children who had already received a single oral dose of dexamethasone 0.6 mg/kg. In this RCT, humidification was delivered by a corrugated tube held to the child's face by a parent. Another RCT found no significant difference in improvement in croup scores at 12 hours between placing children with croup in a high humidity atmosphere (87–95%) in a humidified tent, and room air. One small case series of children with croup reported scalds from hot humidified air.

Benefits: We found no systematic review. **Humidified oxygen:** We found one RCT comparing humidified oxygen delivered through a "mist stick" versus controls (no humidified oxygen) in children with moderate croup who had received a single oral dose of dexamethasone 0.6 mg/kg.[59] It found no significant difference between the two groups in overall mean change in croup scores at 2 hours (1 RCT, 71 children aged 3 months to 6 years evaluated in an emergency department with croup [Westley croup score🅖 2–7]; mean change from baseline in croup score: humidified oxygen *v* controls, P = 0.39; actual mean score numbers not available).[59] The croup score was reassessed at 30, 60, 90, and 120 minutes after initiation of treatment (all non-significant). Humidified oxygen was delivered through a corrugated tube held to the child's face by a parent. The concentration of oxygen used was not stated and the actual percentage humidity delivered to each child was not measured. **Humidified air:** We found one RCT, which found no significant difference in improvement in croup scores at 12 hours between placing children with croup in a high humidity atmosphere (87–95%) in a humidified tent, and room air (1 RCT, 16 children 6 months to 5 years admitted to hospital with croup; mean Westley croup score at 12 hours: 3.00 with humidification *v* 3.75 with room air; P value not available, reported in RCT as not significant).[60] The Westley croup score was reassessed at 1, 2, 3, 4, 5, 6, and 12 hours after initiation of treatment (all NS).[60]

Harms: The two RCTs that we identified did not report on adverse events.[59,60] We found a small case series of children with croup who suffered scalds from hot humidified air.[61] We found no reports of bronchospasm or hyponatraemia associated with humidification, nor of complications resulting from exposure to contaminated humidifiers, although there have been reports of both bacterial and fungal contamination of humidifiers.[62]

Comment: We found one RCT, which was published only in abstract form,[63] and one small unblinded cohort study,[64] neither of which have been reviewed here. Although humidification has been a widely used and accepted treatment for croup since the 1800s, little evidence exists regarding whether or not it is effective.[30]

OPTION β_2 AGONISTS, SHORT ACTING (NEBULISED)

We found no systematic review, RCTs, or observational studies evaluating the effects of nebulised short acting β_2 agonists in children with moderate to severe croup. Although there is neither empirical evidence showing benefit nor a clear theoretical reason for using nebulised short acting β_2 agonists, in some communities a significant proportion of children with croup are treated with nebulised short acting β_2 agonists.

Benefits: We found no systematic review, RCTs, or prospective cohort studies evaluating the effects of nebulised short acting β_2 agonists in children with moderate to severe croup.

Harms: We found no case reports of adverse events in children associated with treatment with nebulised short acting β_2 agonists.

Comment: Although there is neither empirical evidence showing benefit nor a clear theoretical reason for using nebulised short acting β_2 agonists,[31–34] surveys of practice patterns demonstrate that — in some communities — a significant proportion of children with croup are treated with nebulised short acting β_2 agonists.[37,38,65]

OPTION ANTIBIOTICS

We found no RCTs, or prospective cohort studies on antibiotics in children with moderate to severe croup. However, there is strong consensus that antibiotics do not shorten the clinical course of a disease that is predominantly viral in origin. This does not apply if bacterial tracheitis is suspected.

Benefits: We found no systematic reviews, RCTs, or prospective cohort studies on antibiotics in children with moderate to severe croup.

Harms: We found two published case reports of children initially diagnosed with croup who were treated with both dexamethasone and antibiotics for several days. One child was later diagnosed as having herpetic tracheitis and the other as having candida laryngotracheitis.[66,67]

Comment: The routine use of antibiotics in children with croup is widely assumed to be of no benefit because the vast majority of cases of croup are of viral origin.[31–34] An exception to this rule occurs in children who have more severe distress with signs and symptoms consistent with bacterial tracheitis. Although bacterial tracheitis should be a consideration in only a small percentage of children, surveys of practice patterns demonstrate that in some communities 30–80% of children with croup are treated with antibiotics.[36–38]

OPTION ORAL DECONGESTANTS

We found no RCTs or prospective cohort studies evaluating the effects of any oral decongestants in children with moderate to severe croup.

Benefits: We found no systematic review, RCTs, or prospective cohort studies on oral decongestants in children with moderate to severe croup.

Harms: We found no studies evaluating the adverse effects of oral decongestants in children with moderate to severe croup.

Comment: Although there is little evidence of benefit from oral decongestants, surveys of practice patterns demonstrate that in some communities a significant proportion of children with croup are treated with oral decongestants.[38]

QUESTION What are the effects of treatments in children with impending respiratory failure due to severe croup?

OPTION NEBULISED ADRENALINE (EPINEPHRINE)

We found no RCTs on adrenaline (epinephrine) in children with impending respiratory failure due to severe croup. An RCT of adrenaline (epinephrine) versus no adrenaline (epinephrine) would be considered unethical. One cohort study in children with acute upper airway obstruction found that nebulised L-adrenaline (epinephrine) improved mean croup score and reduced carbon dioxide levels. Another cohort study found that nebulised racemic adrenaline (epinephrine) reduced stridor and paradoxical breathing.

Benefits: We found no systematic review or RCTs evaluating the effects of adrenaline (epinephrine) in children with impending respiratory failure due to severe croup. An RCT of adrenaline (epinephrine) versus no adrenaline (epinephrine) in children with impending respiratory failure would be considered unethical. We found two cohort studies in children treated with adrenaline (epinephrine) for acute upper airway obstruction.[68,69] The first cohort study assessed and monitored the severity of airway obstruction using the Westley croup score**G** and continuous transcutaneous carbon dioxide pressure monitoring.[69] It found that in children with acute upper airway obstruction, nebulised L-adrenaline (epinephrine) (1 : 1000, 0.2 mL/kg) significantly improved mean croup score and reduced carbon dioxide levels (1 cohort study, 17 children aged 8 months to 5 years admitted to a paediatric intensive care unit with croup; mean Westley croup score: 12.4 before treatment *v* 5.3

after L-adrenaline [epinephrine] treatment; $P \leq 0.001$; mean transcutaneous carbon dioxide pressure monitoring: 51.0 mm Hg before treatment *v* 42.8 mm Hg after L-adrenaline [epinephrine] treatment; $P \leq 0.001$).[69] The second cohort study assessed the severity of airway obstruction using a respiratory inductance plethysmograph to measure thoracoabdominal asynchrony (paradoxical breathing**G**), which was expressed as a phase angle ranging from 0–180°.[68] It found that in children with acute upper airway obstruction, nebulised racemic adrenaline (epinephrine) (0.03 mL/kg, concentration not provided) significantly reduced mean phase angles (1 cohort study, 17 children aged 1 month to 4 years admitted to a paediatric intensive care unit with croup; mean phase angles: 83.6° before treatment *v* 38.3° after adrenaline [epinephrine] treatment; $P = 0.001$). This cohort study also reported a high association between the phase angle and the degree of stridor.[68]

Harms: One cohort study found no significant increase in heart rate or respiratory rate in children treated with racemic adrenaline (epinephrine).[69] Six children eventually needed intubation.[69] The second cohort study found no significant increase in heart rate or respiratory rate in children treated with racemic adrenaline (epinephrine).[68] One child was intubated.[68]

Comment: In children with severe impending respiratory failure, nebulised adrenaline (epinephrine) causes rapid improvement which can forestall the need for intubation. Although the effect of adrenaline (epinephrine) is relatively transient, it provides a "window of opportunity" for corticosteroid therapy to take effect.

OPTION ANTIBIOTICS

We found no RCTs or prospective cohort studies on antibiotics in children with impending respiratory failure due to severe croup. However, there is strong consensus that antibiotics do not shorten the clinical course of a disease that is predominantly viral in origin. This does not apply if bacterial tracheitis is suspected.

Benefits: We found no systematic reviews, RCTs, or prospective cohort studies on antibiotics in children with impending respiratory failure due to severe croup.

Harms: We found no studies evaluating adverse effects of antibiotics in children with impending respiratory failure due to severe croup.

Comment: The routine use of antibiotics in children with croup is widely assumed to be of no benefit because the vast majority of cases of croup are of viral origin.[31–34] An exception to this rule occurs in those children who have more severe distress with signs and symptoms consistent with bacterial tracheitis. Although bacterial tracheitis should be a consideration in only a small percentage of children, surveys of practice patterns demonstrate that in some communities, 30–80% of children with croup are treated with antibiotics.[36–38]

OPTION CORTICOSTEROIDS

One systematic review found that, compared with placebo, treatment with corticosteroids significantly reduced the rate of endotracheal intubation. This review included studies using different types of corticosteroids and routes of administration; the authors converted all steroids to cortisone dose equivalents for a 12.5 kg child (doses used ranged from 4.2–267 mg

cortisone). One RCT in intubated children showed that, compared with placebo, treatment with prednisolone (1 mg/kg via nasogastric tube every 12 hours until 24 hours after extubation) significantly reduced the duration of intubation and the need for reintubation.

Benefits: **Versus placebo:** We found one systematic review (search date 1987) and one subsequent RCT.[49,70] The review found that, compared with placebo, treatment with corticosteroids significantly reduced the rate of endotracheal intubation (9 studies, 1126 children; rate of endotracheal intubation: 1/575 [0.2%] *v* 7/551 [1.3%]; ARR 1.1%, 95% CI 0.1% to 2.1%).[49] This review included studies using different types of corticosteroids and routes of administration (dexamethasone [im, sc, oral]; methylprednisolone [im]; prednisolone [oral]), and the authors converted all steroids to cortisone dose equivalents for a 12.5 kg child (doses used ranged from 4.2–267 mg or approximately 0.05 mg/kg to 0.66 mg/kg dexamethasone).[49] The subsequent RCT found that, compared with placebo, prednisolone (1 mg/kg via nasogastric tube every 12 hours until 24 hours after extubation) significantly reduced the duration of intubation and the need for reintubation (1 RCT, 70 children, median duration in hours: 98, 95% CI 85 to 113 *v* 138, 95% CI 118 to 160) and the need for reintubation (2/38 [5%] *v* 11/32 [34%]; ARR 34%, 95% CI 26% to 42%; NNT 3, 95% CI 2 to 4).[70]

Harms: **Versus placebo:** One systematic review found that none of the studies analysed reported on adverse effects.[49] The subsequent RCT did not report on adverse events, although two of the children enrolled and randomised to the placebo group were later diagnosed as having bacterial tracheitis and were excluded from analysis.[70]

Comment: None.

OPTION HELIOX (HELIUM–OXYGEN MIXTURE)

We found no systematic review, RCTs, or any analytical observational studies evaluating the effects of heliox (helium–oxygen mixture) in children with impending respiratory failure due to severe croup.

Benefits: We found no systematic review, RCTs, or any analytical observational studies evaluating the effects of heliox (helium–oxygen mixture) in children with impending respiratory failure due to severe croup.

Harms: We found no studies evaluating the adverse effects of heliox (helium–oxygen mixture) in children with impending respiratory failure due to severe croup.

Comment: The theoretical advantage of heliox is that oxygen combined with helium is less dense than either room air or 100% oxygen. Lower density allows laminar, rather than turbulent, gas flow in a narrow airway. Because laminar flow is more efficient, children with a narrow airway can be better ventilated, potentially preventing respiratory failure.

OPTION OXYGEN

We found no RCTs or observational studies evaluating the effects of oxygen in children with impending respiratory failure due to severe croup. An RCT of oxygen versus no oxygen in children with severe croup would be considered unethical. There is widespread consensus that oxygen is beneficial in children with severe respiratory distress.

Benefits: We found no systematic review, RCTs, or observational studies evaluating the effects of oxygen in children with impending respiratory failure due to severe croup. An RCT of oxygen versus no oxygen in children with severe croup would be considered unethical. There is widespread consensus that oxygen is beneficial in children with severe respiratory distress.

Harms: We found no studies evaluating the adverse effects of oxygen in children with impending respiratory failure due to severe croup. There are unlikely to be any significant complications resulting from administration of oxygen to children with severe respiratory distress.

Comment: Children with impending respiratory failure are typically hypoxic, and administration of oxygen helps to prevent hypoxic cell injury. There is compelling logic for administering oxygen in children with severe respiratory distress and no evidence of harm.

OPTION SEDATIVES

We found no systematic review or RCTs evaluating the effects of sedatives in children with impending respiratory failure in severe croup. One prospective cohort study found that children with severe croup treated with sedatives had decreased croup scores, but found no corresponding decrease in transcutaneous PCO_2. This suggests that sedatives decrease respiratory effort without improving ventilation.

Benefits: We found no systematic review or RCTs evaluating the effects of sedatives in children with impending respiratory failure in severe croup.

Harms: We found no systematic review or RCTs evaluating the effects of sedatives in children with impending respiratory failure in severe croup.

Comment: We found one prospective cohort study in children with impending respiratory failure who were continuously monitored using clinical scores and transcutaneous carbon dioxide measurements.[69] The cohort study showed that children treated with chloral hydrate 30–40 mg/kg over 4–6 hours had significantly improved croup scores, but found no corresponding decrease in transcutaneous carbon dioxide measurements (1 cohort study, 17 children aged 8 months to 5 years with croup [severe to impending respiratory failure, mean Westley croup score**G** 12]; mean change from baseline in croup scores: 11.2 before chloral hydrate *v* 6.5 after chloral hydrate; $P < 0.001$; mean transcutaneous carbon dioxide level: 46.5 mm Hg before chloral hydrate *v* 47.3 mm Hg after chloral hydrate; reported as no significant difference, P value not available). This cohort study also showed that nebulised adrenaline (epinephrine) 1 : 1000 (2 mL/10 kg) significantly improved both the croup scores and transcutaneous carbon dioxide (both $P < 0.001$).[69] We found no analytical studies evaluating the effects of other sedatives in children with impending respiratory failure in severe croup. Although sedative therapy is no longer accepted as standard therapy for children with croup,[31–34] and there is no empirical evidence demonstrating benefit, sedatives are still occasionally used in hospitalised children to treat children with more severe croup.[69,71]

GLOSSARY

Downes and Raphaely croup score[72] Total score ranging from 0–10 points. Five component items make up the score:

- Inspiratory breath sounds (0 = normal, 1 = harsh with rhonchi, 2 = delayed)
- Stridor (0 = normal, 1 = inspiratory, 2 = inspiratory and expiratory)
- Cough (0 = none, 1 = hoarse cry, 2 = bark)
- Retractions/nasal flaring (0 = normal, 1 = suprasternal/present, 2 = suprasternal and intercostal/present)

Cyanosis (0 = none, 1 = in room air, 2 = in FIO_2 0.4).

Paradoxical breathing (thoracoabdominal asynchrony) occurs in young children with severe respiratory distress. Typically, in well people the abdomen and chest expand and contract in a synchronised fashion with respiration. Children compensate for narrowing of their upper airway by increasing their work of breathing, which increases intrapleural pressure and the rate of airflow through the upper airway. With greater increases in pleural pressure, during inspiration, young children's compliant chest wall begins to collapse as the abdomen protrudes, owing to diaphragmatic contraction. This thoracoabdominal asynchrony is commonly referred to as paradoxical breathing.

Taussig croup score[41] Total score ranging from 0–14 points. Five component items make up the score:

Colour (0 = normal, 1 = dusky, 2 = cyanotic in air, 3 = cyanotic in 30–40% oxygen)
Air entry (0 = normal, 1 = mildly diminished, 2 = moderately diminished, 3 = substantially diminished)
Retractions (0 = none, 1 = mild, 2 = moderate, 3 = severe)
Level of consciousness (0 = normal, 1 = restlessness, 2 = lethargy [depression])
Stridor (0 = none, 1 = mild, 2 = moderate, 3 = severe [or no stridor in the presence of other signs of severe obstruction]).

Westley croup score[4] Total score ranging from 0–17 points. Five component items make up the score:

Stridor (0 = none, 1 = with agitation only, 2 = at rest)
Retractions (0 = none, 1 = mild, 2 = moderate, 3 = severe)
Air entry (0 = normal, 1 = decreased, 2 = markedly decreased)
Cyanosis (0 = none, 4 = cyanosis with agitation, 5 = cyanosis at rest)
Level of consciousness (0 = normal [including asleep], 5 = disorientated).

REFERENCES

1. Cherry JD. Croup (laryngitis, laryngotracheitis, spasmodic croup, and laryngotracheobronchitis). In: Feigin R. CJ ed. *Textbook of pediatric infectious diseases*. 3rd ed, Vol. 1. Philadelphia, PA: WB Saunders Company, Harcourt Brace Jovanovich, Inc, 1992: 209–220.
2. Cherry JD. The treatment of croup: continued controversy due to failure of recognition of historic, ecologic, and clinical perspectives. *J Pediatr* 1979;94:352–354.
3. Tunnessen W, Feinstein A. The steroid–croup controversy: an analytic review of methodologic problems. *J Pediatr* 1980;96:751–756.
4. "Croup" Working Committee. Guideline for the Diagnosis and Management of Croup. Alberta Medical Association Clinical Practise Guidelines (Canada). http://www.albertadoctors.org/bcm/ama/amawebsite.nsf/AllDocSearch/87256DB000705C3F87256E05005534E2/$File/CROUP.PDF?OpenElement
5. Westley CR, Ross EK, Brooks JG. Nebulized racemic epinephrine by IPPB for the treatment of croup. *Am J Dis Child* 1978;132:484–487.
6. Klassen TP, Feldman ME, Watters LK, et al. Nebulized budesonide for children with mild-to-moderate croup. *N Engl J Med* 1994;331:285–289.
7. Klassen TP, Rowe RC. The croup score as an evaluative instrument in clinical trials [abstract]. *Arch Pediatr Adolesc Med* 1995;149:60.
8. Denny F, Murphy TF, Clyde WA Jr, et al. Croup: an 11-year study in a pediatric practice. *Pediatrics* 1983;71:871 – 876.
9. Van Bever HP, Wieringa MH, Weyler JJ, et al. Croup and recurrent croup: their association with asthma and allergy. An epidemiological study on 5–8-year-old children. *Eur J Pediatr* 1999;158:253–257.
10. Tong MC, Chu MC, Leighton SE, et al. Adult croup. *Chest* 1996;109:1659–1662.
11. Chapman RS, Henderson FW, Clyde WA Jr, et al. The epidemiology of tracheobronchitis in pediatric practice. *Am J Epidemiol* 1981;114:786–797.
12. Glezen WP, Loda FA, Clyde WAJ, et al. Epidemiologic patterns of acute lower respiratory disease of children in a pediatric group practice. *J Pediatr* 1971;78:397–406.
13. Williams JV, Harris PA, Tollefson SJ, et al. Human metapneumovirus and lower respiratory tract disease in otherwise healthy infants and children. *N Engl J Med* 2004;350:443–450.
14. Davis GM. An examination of the physiological consequences of chest wall distortion in infants with croup. In: *Medical science*. Calgary: University of Calgary, 1985:90.
15. Davis GM, Cooper DM, Mitchell I. The measurement of thoraco-abdominal asynchrony in infants with severe laryngotracheobronchitis. *Chest* 1993;103:1842–1848.
16. Johnson DW, Williamson J. Croup: duration of symptoms and impact on family functioning. *Pediatr Res* 2001;49:83A.
17. Phelan PD, Landau LI, Olinksy A. Respiratory illness in children. Oxford: Blackwell Science, 1982: 32–33.
18. To T, Dick P, Young W. Hospitalization rates of children with croup in Ontario. *J Paediatr Child Health* 1996;1:103–108.
19. Johnson DW, Williamson J. Health care utilization by children with croup in Alberta. *Pediatr Res* 2003;53:185A.
20. Dawson KP, Mogridge N, Downward G. Severe acute laryngotracheitis in Christchurch 1980–90. *N Z Med J* 1991;104:374–375.
21. Sofer S, Dagan R, Tal A. The need for intubation in serious upper respiratory tract infection in pediatric patients (a retrospective study). *Infection* 1991;19:131–134.
22. McEniery J, Gillis J, Kilham H, et al. Review of intubation in severe laryngotracheobronchitis. *Pediatrics* 1991;87:847–853.
23. Sendi K, Crysdale WS, Yoo J. Tracheitis: outcome of 1,700 cases presenting to the emergency department during two years. *J Otolaryngol* 1992;21:20–24.
24. Tan AK, Manoukian JJ. Hospitalized croup (bacterial and viral); the role of rigid endoscopy. *J Otolaryngol* 1992;21:48–53.
25. Super DM, Cartelli NA, Brooks LJ, et al. A prospective randomized double-blind study to evaluate the effect of dexamethasone in acute laryngotracheitis. *J Pediatr* 1989;115:323–329.

26. Kanter RK, Watchko JF. Pulmonary edema associated with upper airway obstruction. *Am J Dis Child* 1984;138:356–358.
27. Edwards KM, Dundon MC, Altemeier WA. Bacterial tracheitis as a complication of viral croup. *Pediatr Infect Dis* 1983;2:390–391.
28. Geelhoed GC, Turner J, Macdonald WB. Efficacy of a small single dose of oral dexamethasone for outpatient croup: a double blind placebo controlled clinical trial. *BMJ* 1996;313:140–142.
29. Luria JW, Gonzalez-del-Rey JA, DiGiulio GA, et al. Effectiveness of oral or nebulized dexamethasone for children with mild croup. *Arch Pediatr Adolesc Med* 2001;155:1340–1345.
30. Marchessault V. Historical review of croup. *J Paediatr Child Health* 2001;6:721–723.
31. Kaditis AG, Wald ER. Viral croup: current diagnosis and treatment. *Pediatr Infect Dis J* 1998;17:827–834.
32. Klassen TP. Croup. A current perspective. *Pediatr Clin North Am* 1999;46:1167–1178.
33. Brown JC. The management of croup. *Br Med Bull* 2002;61:189–202.
34. Geelhoed GC. Croup. *Pediatr Pulmonol* 1997;23:370–374.
35. Parainfluenza viral infections. In: Pickering L, ed. *Red book: 2003 report of the Committee on Infectious Diseases*. Elk Grove Village, IL: American Academy of Pediatrics, 2003:454–455.
36. Stephan U, Wiesemann HG, Hanssler L, et al. Are corticosteroids necessary in treatment of croup? Therapiewoche 1984;34:1518–1522.
37. Gonzalez de Dios J, Ramos Lizana J, Lopez Lopez C. Laryngitis epidemic (893 cases of acute laryngotracheitis and spastic croup). II. Clinical, diagnostic and therapeutic aspects. *An Esp Pediatr* 1990;32:417–422. [In Spanish]
38. Johnson D, Williamson J, Craig W, et al. Management of croup: practise variation among 21 Alberta Hospitals. *Pediatr Res* 2004;55:113A.
39. Kristjansson S, Berg-Kelly K, Winso E. Inhalation of racemic epinephrine in the treatment of mild and moderately severe croup. Clinical symptom score and oxygen saturation measurements for evaluation of treatment effects. *Acta Paediatr* 1994;83:1156–1160.
40. Taussig LM, Castro O, Beaudry PH, et al. Treatment of laryngotracheobronchitis (croup). Use of intermittent positive-pressure breathing and racemic epinephrine. *Am J Dis Child* 1975;129:790–793.
41. Weber JE, Chudnofsky CR, Younger JG, et al. A randomized comparison of helium–oxygen mixture (Heliox) and racemic epinephrine for the treatment of moderate to severe croup. *Pediatrics* 2001;107:e96.
42. Fogel JM, Berg IJ, Gerber MA, et al. Racemic epinephrine in the treatment of croup: nebulization alone versus nebulization with intermittent positive pressure breathing. *J Pediatr* 1982;101:1028–1031.
43. Waisman Y, Klein BL, Boenning DA, et al. Prospective randomized double-blind study comparing L-epinephrine and racemic epinephrine aerosols in the treatment of laryngotracheitis (croup). *Pediatrics* 1992;89:302–306.
44. Butte MJ, Nguyen BX, Hutchison TJ, et al. Pediatric myocardial infarction after racemic epinephrine administration. *Pediatrics* 1999;104:e9.
45. Gardner HG, Powell KR, Roden VJ, et al. The evaluation of racemic epinephrine in the treatment of infectious croup. *Pediatrics* 1973;52:52–55.
46. Ausejo M, Saenz A, Pham B, et al. Glucocorticoids for croup. In: The Cochrane Library. Issue 4, 2003. Chichester, UK: John Wiley & Sons, Ltd. Search date 1997. Primary sources The Cochrane Controlled Trials Register, MEDLINE and EMBASE. This review has also been published in *BMJ* 1999; 319:595–600.
47. Griffin S, Ellis S, Fitzgerald-Barron A, et al. Nebulised steroid in the treatment of croup: a systematic review of randomised controlled trials. *Br J Gen Pract* 2000;50:135–141. Search date 1999; primary sources Cochrane Controlled Trials Register, Medline, Embase, and Cinahl.
48. Roberts GW, Master VV, Staugas RE, et al. repeated dose inhaled budesonide in the treatment of croup versus placebo. *J Paediatr Child Health* 1999;35:170–171.
49. Kairys SW, Olmstead EM, O'Connor GT. Steroid treatment of laryngotracheitis: a meta-analysis of the evidence from randomized trials. *Pediatrics* 1989;83:683–693. Search date 1987; primary source Medline.
50. Pedersen LV, Dahl M, Falk-Petersen HE, et al. Inhaled budesonide versus intramuscular dexamethasone in the treatment of pseudo-croup. *Ugeskr Laeger* 1998;160:2253–2256. [In Danish]
51. Rittichier KK, Ledwith CA. Outpatient treatment of moderate croup with dexamethasone: intramuscular versus oral dosing. *Pediatrics* 2000;106:1344–1348.
52. Donaldson D, Poleski D, Knipple E, et al. Intramuscular versus oral dexamethasone for the treatment of moderate-to-severe croup: a randomized, double-blind trial. *Acad Emerg Med* 2003;10:16–21.
53. Klassen TP, Craig WR, Moher D, et al. Nebulized budesonide and oral dexamethasone for treatment of croup: a randomized controlled trial. *JAMA* 1998;279:1629–1632.
54. Geelhoed GC, Macdonald WB. Oral dexamethasone in the treatment of croup: 0.15 mg/kg versus 0.3 mg/kg versus 0.6 mg/kg. *Pediatr Pulmonol* 1995;20:362–368.
55. Johnson DW, Jacobson S, Edney PC, et al. A comparison of nebulized budesonide, intramuscular dexamethasone, and placebo in moderately severe croup. *N Engl J Med* 1998;339:498–503.
56. Geelhoed GC, Macdonald WB. Oral and inhaled steroids in croup: a randomized, placebo-controlled trial. *Pediatr Pulmonol* 1995;20:355–361.
57. Newth CJ, Levison H, Bryan AC. The respiratory status of children with croup. *J Pediatr* 1972;81:1068–1073.
58. Terregino CA, Nairn SJ, Chansky ME, et al. The effect of Heliox on croup: a pilot study. *Acad Emerg Med* 1998;5:1130–1133.
59. Neto GM, Kentab O, Klassen TP, et al. A randomized controlled trial of mist in the acute treatment of moderate croup. *Acad Emerg Med* 2002; 9:873–879.
60. Bourchier D, Dawson KP, Fergusson DM. Humidification in viral croup: a controlled trial. *Aust Paediatr J* 1984;20:289–291.
61. Greally P, Cheng K, Tanner MS, et al. Children with croup presenting with scalds. *BMJ* 1990;301:113.
62. Solomon WR. Fungus aerosols arising from cold-mist vaporizers. *J Allergy Clin Immunol* 1974;54:222–228.
63. Jamshidi PB, Kemp JS, Peter JR, et al. The effect of humidified air in mild to moderate croup: evaluation using croup scores and respiratory inductance plethysmograph. *Pediatr Res* 2001;49:79A.
64. Lenney W, Milner AD. Treatment of acute viral croup. *Arch Dis Child* 1978;53:704–706.
65. Hampers LC, Faries SG. Practice variation in the emergency management of croup. *Pediatrics* 2002;109:505–508.
66. Mancao MY, Sindel LJ, Richardson PH, et al. Herpetic croup: two case reports and a review of the literature. *Acta Paediatr* 1996;85:118–120.
67. Burton DM, Seid AB, Kearns DB, et al. Candida laryngotracheitis: a complication of combined steroid and antibiotic usage in croup. *Int J Pediatr Otorhinolaryngol* 1992;23:171–175.
68. Sivan Y, Deakers TW, Newth CJ. Thoracoabdominal asynchrony in acute upper airway obstruction in small children. *Am Rev Respir Dis* 1990;142:540–544.
69. Fanconi S, Burger R, Maurer H, et al. Transcutaneous carbon dioxide pressure for monitoring patients with severe croup. *J Pediatr* 1990;117:701–705.

70. Tibballs J, Shann FA, Landau LI. Placebo-controlled trial of prednisolone in children intubated for croup. *Lancet* 1992;340:745–748.
71. Kuusela A-L, Vesikari T. A randomized double-blind, placebo-controlled trial of dexamethasone and racemic epinephrine in the treatment of croup. *Acta Paediat Scand* 1988;77:99–104.
72. Downes JJ, Raphaely RC. Pediatric intensive care. *Anesthesiology* 1975;43:238–250.

David Johnson
Associate Professor
Department of Pediatrics, University of Calgary, Calgary, Canada

Competing interests: David Johnson has authored seven of the abstracts, randomized trials, or meta-analysis referenced in this review.

Depression in children and adolescents

Search date January 2004

Philip Hazell

QUESTIONS

INTERVENTIONS

See glossary

Key Messages

- In the light of emerging evidence and consensus on harms data on some of the pharmacological treatments included in this review since the time of writing, and the current FDA sponsored meta-analysis of safety data, this chapter will be undergoing review in its next updated version. These data relate to increased risks of suicide and self harm with some pharmacological agents. In the interim, practitioners should be guided by the recommendations and warnings issued by their national drug regulatory authorities with respect to the prescribing of antidepressants to juveniles.

Treatments

- **Cognitive behavioural therapy (in children and adolescents with mild to moderate depression)** One systematic review in children and adolescents with mild to moderate depression found that cognitive behavioural therapy improved symptoms compared with non-specific support.
- **Interpersonal therapy (in adolescents with mild to moderate depression)** Two RCTs found that interpersonal therapy increased recovery rate after 12 weeks in adolescents with mild to moderate depression compared with clinical monitoring or waiting list control.
- **Selective serotonin reuptake inhibitors** Three RCTs provided limited evidence that fluoxetine improved symptoms of depression compared with placebo. One RCT found that, in adolescents with major depression, paroxetine improved response rate after 8 weeks compared with placebo. Another RCT in people with major depression (aged 12–20 years) found no significant difference in effects on improvement rates between paroxetine and clomipramine, although it may have lacked power to detect clinically important effects. Pooled analysis of two RCTs found

that, in children and adolescents with major depression, sertraline improved depressive symptoms compared with placebo, but this improvement was clinically small. We found no RCTs on other selective serotonin reuptake inhibitors. RCTs found that adverse effects such as dizziness, sleepiness, headache, tremor, and gastrointestinal symptoms are common with selective serotonin reuptake inhibitors, although adverse effect profiles vary among different drugs in the class. Selective serotonin reuptake inhibitors are frequently associated with dizziness, light-headedness, drowsiness, poor concentration, nausea, headache, and fatigue if treatment is reduced or stopped. On the basis of unpublished data, regulatory authorities in both the UK and the USA have recommended that paroxetine should not be prescribed for people under 18 years of age.

- **Cognitive behavioural therapy (in adolescents with major depression or dysthymia with depressed parents)** One RCT in depressed adolescents with major depression or dysthymia with depressed parents found no significant difference in recovery from depression between cognitive behavioural therapy plus usual care and usual care alone over 2 years.
- **Electroconvulsive therapy** We found no RCTs on electroconvulsive therapy in children and adolescents with depression.
- **Family therapy** We found insufficient evidence in children and adolescents about the effects of family therapy.
- **Intravenous clomipramine (in adolescents)** One small RCT found that, in non-suicidal adolescents, intravenous clomipramine improved depression scores at 6 days compared with placebo. However, the trial was too small and brief for us to draw reliable conclusions.
- **Lithium** One small RCT in children with depression and a family history of bipolar affective disorder found no significant difference between lithium and placebo in global assessment or depression scores after 6 weeks. However, the study may have lacked power to detect clinically important effects.
- **Monoamine oxidase inhibitors** One small RCT provided insufficient evidence to compare the reversible monoamine oxidase inhibitor, moclobemide, versus placebo in children aged 9–15 years with major depression, some of whom had a comorbid disorder. We found no RCTs on non-reversible monoamine oxidase inhibitors in children or adolescents.
- **Specific psychological treatments other than cognitive behavioural therapy** We found insufficient evidence in children and adolescents about the effects of specific psychological treatments other than cognitive behavioural therapy.
- **St John's Wort (*Hypericum perforatum*)** We found no RCTs on St John's Wort (*Hypericum perforatum*) in children or adolescents with depression.
- **Venlafaxine** One small RCT in children and adolescents with major depression receiving psychotherapy found no significant difference between venlafaxine and placebo in improvement of depressive symptoms after 6 weeks. However, the study may have lacked power to detect clinically important effects.
- **Tricyclic antidepressants (in adolescents)** One systematic review in adolescents and children found no significant difference in depression scores between oral tricyclic antidepressants (amitriptyline, desipramine, imipramine, nortriptyline) and placebo after 4–10 weeks. However, subgroup analyses found that oral tricyclic antidepressants improved symptoms compared with placebo in adolescents but not children. There was no significant difference in rates of remission. The review also found that oral tricyclic antidepressants were associated with adverse effects. One RCT found no significant difference in improvement rates between oral clomipramine and paroxetine after 8 weeks.
- **Tricyclic antidepressants (in children)** Subgroup analyses in one systematic review found no significant difference between oral tricyclic antidepressants (amitriptyline, desipramine, imipramine, nortriptyline) and placebo in children with depression. The review also found that oral tricyclic antidepressants were associated with adverse effects.

DEFINITION Compared with adult depression (see depressive disorders, p 1238), depression in children (6–12 years) and adolescents (13–18 years) may have a more insidious onset, may be characterised more by irritability than sadness, and occurs more often in association with other conditions such as anxiety, conduct disorder, hyperkinesis, and learning problems.[1] The term "major depression" is used to distinguish discrete episodes of depression from mild, chronic (1 year or longer) low mood, or irritability, which is known as "dysthymia".[1] The severity of depression may be defined by the level of impairment and the presence or absence of psychomotor changes and somatic symptoms (see depressive disorders, p 1238). In some studies, severity of depression is defined according to cut-off scores on depression rating scales. A manic episode is defined by abnormally and persistently elevated, expansive, or irritable mood. Additional symptoms may include grandiosity, decreased need for sleep, pressured speech, flight of ideas, distractibility, psychomotor agitation, and impaired judgement.[2]

INCIDENCE/ PREVALENCE Estimates of prevalence of depression among children and adolescents in the community range from 2–6%.[3,4] Prevalence tends to increase with age, with a sharp rise at around the onset of puberty. Pre-adolescent boys and girls are affected equally by the condition, but in adolescents, depression is more common among girls than boys.[5]

AETIOLOGY/ RISK FACTORS The aetiology is uncertain, but may include genetic vulnerability,[6] childhood events, and current psychosocial adversity.[1]

PROGNOSIS In children and adolescents, the recurrence rate after a first depressive episode is 40%.[7] Young people experiencing a moderate to severe depressive episode may be more likely than adults to have a manic episode within the following few years.[1,8] Trials of treatments for child and adolescent depression have found high rates of response to placebo (as much as two thirds of people in some inpatient studies) suggesting that episodes of depression may be self limiting in many cases.[9] A third of young people who experience a depressive episode will make a suicide attempt at some stage, and 3–4% will die from suicide.[1]

AIMS OF INTERVENTION To improve mood, social and occupational functioning, and quality of life; to reduce morbidity and mortality; to prevent recurrence of depressive disorder; with minimal adverse effects.

OUTCOMES In children and adolescents, there are developmentally specific pseudo-continuous outcome measuresⒼ such as the Children's Depression Rating Scale and the Children's Depression Inventory, although some studies of adolescents use scales developed for use in adults such as the Hamilton Rating Scale for Depression. Pseudo-continuous outcome measures reported by parents, such as the Children's Depression Inventory for Parents, are also used. Categorical outcomes are sometimes expressed as people no longer meeting specified criteria for depression on a structured psychiatric interview such as the Kiddie-SADS, which combines data from children and their parents. Global improvement in symptoms as judged by an investigator is sometimes reported using the Clinical Global Impressions Scale or the Clinical Global Assessment Scale (see table 1, p 341).

METHODS *Clinical Evidence* search and appraisal January 2004.

QUESTION What are the effects of treatments?

OPTION TRICYCLIC ANTIDEPRESSANTS

One systematic review in adolescents and children found no significant difference in depression scores between oral tricyclic antidepressants (amitriptyline, desipramine, imipramine, nortriptyline) and placebo after 4–10 weeks. However, subgroup analyses found that oral tricyclic antidepressants improved symptoms compared with placebo in adolescents, but not in children. There was no significant difference in rates of remission. The review also found that oral tricyclic antidepressants were associated with adverse effects. One RCT found no significant difference in improvement rates

between oral clomipramine and paroxetine after 8 weeks. One small RCT found that, in non-suicidal adolescents, intravenous clomipramine improved depression scores at 6 days compared with placebo. However, the trial was too small and brief for us to draw reliable conclusions.

Benefits: **Oral tricyclic antidepressants versus placebo:** We found one systematic review (search date 2000, 13 RCTs, 506 children and adolescents aged 6–18 years, severity of depression not reported).[9] It found no significant difference in overall improvement between oral tricyclic antidepressants (amitriptyline, desipramine, imipramine, and nortriptyline) and placebo after 4–10 weeks (OR 0.84, 95% CI 0.56 to 1.25). Subgroup analyses found that tricyclic antidepressants significantly reduced symptoms compared with placebo in adolescents (7 RCTs; 351 people; effect size SMD –0.47, 95% CI –0.92 to –0.02). However, there was no significant difference in children (3 RCTs; 65 people; effect size SMD +0.15, 95% CI –0.64 to +0.34). **Oral tricyclic antidepressants versus selective serotonin reuptake inhibitors:** See benefits of selective serotonin reuptake inhibitors (paroxetine versus the predominantly serotonergic tricyclic antidepressant clomipramine), p 333. **Pulsed intravenous clomipramine:** We found one RCT (16 non-suicidal adolescent outpatients, aged 14–18 years, with major depression [21-item Hamilton Rating Scale for Depression score ≥ 18]), which compared pulsed intravenous clomipramine**G** 200 mg versus placebo.[10] It found that intravenous clomipramine significantly reduced Hamilton Rating Scale for Depression scores compared with placebo at 6 days (mean reduction in score: 15.0 with clomipramine *v* 9.0 with placebo; $P < 0.05$). However, it found no significant difference in remission rate (remission defined as ≥ 50% decrease in Hamilton Rating Scale for Depression scores; AR 7/8 [88%] with iv clomipramine *v* 3/8 [38%] with placebo; $P = 0.06$).[10] The study may have lacked power to detect a clinically important effect.

Harms: **Oral tricyclic antidepressants:** The systematic review found that tricyclic antidepressants were more commonly associated with vertigo (OR 8.47, 95% CI 1.40 to 51.00), orthostatic hypotension (OR 4.77, 95% CI 1.11 to 20.50), tremor (OR 6.29, 95% CI 1.78 to 22.17), and dry mouth (OR 5.19, 95% CI 1.15 to 23.50) than placebo.[9] The review found no significant differences between tricyclic antidepressants and placebo in tiredness (OR 1.52, 95% CI 0.63 to 3.67), sleep problems (OR 1.87, 95% CI 0.84 to 4.14), headache (OR 1.15, 95% CI 0.68 to 1.95), palpitations (OR 1.20, 95% CI 0.17 to 8.68), perspiration (OR 2.01, 95% CI 0.39 to 10.44), constipation (OR 1.94, 95% CI 0.72 to 5.24), or problems with micturition (OR 0.30, 95% CI 0.01 to 7.89). **Pulsed intravenous clomipramineG:** The RCT did not report any adverse effects.[10]

Comment: We found single case reports and case series of toxicity and mortality from tricyclic antidepressants in overdose and therapeutic doses.[11] The death rate has been estimated at 0.4/100 000 prescriptions.[12] While very rare, any such risk has been considered unacceptable when there are safer alternatives. Further research is needed to determine long term effects of intravenous clomipramine. In the light of emerging evidence and consensus on harms data on some of the pharmacological treatments included in this review since the time of writing, and the current FDA sponsored meta-analysis of safety data, this chapter will be undergoing review in its next updated version. These data relate to increased risks of suicide and self harm with some pharmacological agents. In the interim, practitioners should be guided by the recommendations and warnings issued by their national drug regulatory authorities with respect to the prescribing of antidepressants to juveniles.

OPTION MONOAMINE OXIDASE INHIBITORS

One small RCT provided insufficient evidence to compare the reversible monoamine oxidase inhibitor, moclobemide, versus placebo in children aged 9–15 years with major depression, some of whom had a comorbid disorder. We found no RCTs on non-reversible monoamine oxidase inhibitors in children or adolescents.

Benefits: We found no systematic review. **Reversible monoamine oxidase inhibitors:** We found one small RCT (20 Turkish children aged 9–15 years with major depression, including 13 children with a comorbid disorder) comparing moclobemide versus placebo for 5 weeks.[13] The RCT found that moclobemide significantly improved clinician rated scale scores (Clinical Global Impressions Scale — investigator assessment of severity of depression, adverse effects, and global recovery) compared with placebo after 5 weeks but not on parent rated (Children's Depression Inventory for Parents) and self reported measures (Children's Depression Inventory).[13] The small sample size limits the conclusions that may be drawn from this RCT.[13] **Non-reversible monoamine oxidase inhibitors:** We found no RCTs.

Harms: The RCT found no significant difference in adverse events assessed using Clinical Global Impression of adverse effects scale and self assessed adverse effects forms between moclobemide and placebo.[13] We found no information on the safety of moclobemide usage in children younger than 9 years.

Comment: In the light of emerging evidence and consensus on harms data on some of the pharmacological treatments included in this review since the time of writing, and the current FDA sponsored meta-analysis of safety data, this chapter will be undergoing review in its next updated version. These data relate to increased risks of suicide and self harm with some pharmacological agents. In the interim, practitioners should be guided by the recommendations and warnings issued by their national drug regulatory authorities with respect to the prescribing of antidepressants to juveniles.

OPTION SELECTIVE SEROTONIN REUPTAKE INHIBITORS

Three RCTs provided limited evidence that fluoxetine improved symptoms of depression compared with placebo. One RCT found that, in adolescents with major depression, paroxetine improved response rate after 8 weeks compared with placebo. Another RCT in people with major depression (aged 12–20 years) found no significant difference in effects on improvement rates between paroxetine and clomipramine, although it may have lacked power to detect clinically important effects. Pooled analysis of two RCTs found that, in children and adolescents with major depression, sertraline improved depressive symptoms compared with placebo, but this improvement was clinically small. We found no RCTs on other selective serotonin reuptake inhibitors. RCTs found that adverse effects such as dizziness, sleepiness, headache, tremor, and gastrointestinal symptoms are common with selective serotonin reuptake inhibitors, although adverse effect profiles vary among different drugs in the class. Selective serotonin reuptake inhibitors are frequently associated with dizziness, light-headedness, drowsiness, poor concentration, nausea, headache, and fatigue if treatment is reduced or stopped. On the basis of unpublished data, regulatory authorities in both the UK and the USA have recommended that paroxetine should not be prescribed for people under 18 years of age.

Benefits: **Fluoxetine:** We found one systematic review (search date 1998,[14] 2 RCTs[15,16]) and one subsequent RCT.[17] The systematic review did not pool results.[14] The first RCT identified by the review (40 adolescents aged 13–18 years, of whom 30 completed the trial, severity of depression not reported) found no significant difference in the mean number of depression symptoms or psychosocial functioning (Clinical Global Impressions Scale) between fluoxetine 20–60 mg and placebo after 8 weeks (RR of failure to improve: 1.00, 95% CI 0.36 to 2.75).[15] The second RCT identified by the review (96 children and adolescents aged 7–17 years with major depression) found that fluoxetine 20 mg significantly improved depression symptoms according to the self reported Children's Depression Rating Scale compared with placebo after 8 weeks (proportion with improved Clinical Global Impressions Scale: 27/48 [56%] with fluoxetine *v* 16/48 [33%] with placebo; RR of failure to improve: 0.66, 95% CI 0.45 to 0.96; proportion with improved self reported Children's Depression Rating Scale: 34% with fluoxetine *v* 18% with placebo; P < 0.01).[16] The subsequent RCT (219 children and adolescents aged 8–17 years with major depression) found no significant difference between fluoxetine and placebo in response defined a priori on the Children's Depression Rating Scale at 8 weeks (response defined as ≥ 30% improvement in score: 71/109 [65%] with fluoxetine *v* 54/101 [54%] with placebo; P = 0.093).[17] The RCT found that fluoxetine significantly improved scores on the Children's Depression Rating Scale or Clinical Global Impressions Severity Scale compared with placebo at 8 weeks (difference in mean improvement with fluoxetine *v* placebo; Children's Depression Rating Scale: 7.1, 95% CI 3.3 to 10.9; Clinical Global Impressions Severity Scale: 0.6, 95% CI 0.3 to 1.0). **Paroxetine:** We found two RCTs. The first RCT (180 adolescents aged 12–18 years, of whom 133 completed the trial, severity of depression score of at least 12 on the Hamilton Rating Scale for Depression and < 60 on the Children's Global Assessment Scale) compared effects of paroxetine 20–40 mg, imipramine (gradual upward titration to 200–300 mg), and placebo for 8 weeks with respect to end point response (Hamilton Rating Scale for Depression score ≤ 8 or a 50% reduction from baseline score) and change from baseline score (Hamilton Rating Scale for Depression).[18] The RCT did not include a direct statistical comparison of paroxetine versus imipramine. The RCT found that paroxetine significantly improved response rate compared with placebo (AR for failure to respond: 37% with paroxetine *v* 54% with placebo; ARI 17%, CI not reported; RR 0.68, 95% CI 0.49 to 0.95; P = 0.02). The second RCT (121 people aged 12–20 years with major depression) compared paroxetine versus clomipramine.[19] The RCT found no significant difference in rates of improvement after 8 weeks of treatment (achieving a score of 2 ["much" improved] or 1 ["very much" improved] on the Clinical Global Impressions Scale: 35/59 [59%] with paroxetine *v* 32/55 [58%] with clomipramine; P = 0.71). However, the trial may have lacked power to detect clinically important differences. **Sertraline:** We found two RCTs (376 children and adolescents aged 6–17 years; Children's Depression Rating Scale [Revised] score ≥ 45; Clinical Global Impression of Illness Scale score ≥ 4), which compared sertraline (25 mg/day titrated up to 200 mg/day) versus placebo for 10 weeks.[20] Pooled analysis of the RCTs found that sertraline significantly reduced depressive symptoms and improved response rate compared with placebo after 10 weeks (mean reduction in Children's Depression Rating Scale [Revised] score: 30.24 with sertraline *v* 25.83 with placebo; P = 0.001; response rate defined as ≥ 40% reduction in Children's Depression Rating Scale [Revised] score: 128/185 [69%] with sertraline *v* 106/179 [59%] with placebo; CI not reported, P = 0.05; NNT 10, CI not reported). **Other selective serotonin reuptake inhibitors:** We found no RCTs.

Harms: **Selective serotonin reuptake inhibitors in general:** A discontinuation syndrome after abrupt stopping or reduction in the dose of selective serotonin reuptake inhibitors has been described in a series of six cases.[21] The most frequent symptoms included dizziness, lightheadedness, drowsiness, poor concentration, nausea, headache, and fatigue.[21] **Fluoxetine:** One of the RCTs included in the systematic review found more weight loss with fluoxetine than with placebo (data not reported).[15] The other included RCT did not report on adverse effects.[16] The subsequent RCT found that headache was reported significantly more often with fluoxetine than with placebo (P = 0.017).[17] **Paroxetine:** The first RCT reported more serious adverse events with paroxetine compared with placebo (12% with paroxetine *v* 2% with placebo).[18] The most common adverse events were somnolence (17% with paroxetine *v* 3% with placebo) and tremor (11% with paroxetine *v* 2% with placebo) but no statistical analyses were reported. The second RCT found significantly fewer adverse effects with paroxetine than with clomipramine (31/63 [49%] with paroxetine *v* 40/58 [69%] with clomipramine; P = 0.027).[19] The most common adverse events were dizziness (6.3% with paroxetine *v* 34.5% with clomipramine; P value not reported), headache (17.5% with paroxetine *v* 24.1% with clomipramine; P value not reported), and nausea (11.1% with paroxetine *v* 24.1% with clomipramine; P value not reported). On the basis of unpublished data, regulatory authorities in both the UK and USA have recommended that paroxetine should not be prescribed for people under 18 years of age.[22] **Sertraline:** The RCTs reported that the following adverse effects affected at least 5% of people and were at least twice as frequent with sertraline than placebo: insomnia (20% with sertraline *v* 8% with placebo), diarrhoea (11% with sertraline *v* 4% with placebo), anorexia (10% with sertraline *v* 2% with placebo), vomiting (9% with sertraline *v* 4% with placebo), agitation (8% with sertraline *v* 2% with placebo), urinary incontinence (7% with sertraline *v* 0% with placebo), and purpura (6% with sertraline *v* 1% with placebo). No statistical analyses were reported for these outcomes.[20]

Comment: In the light of emerging evidence and consensus on harms data on some of the pharmacological treatments included in this review since the time of writing, and the current FDA sponsored meta-analysis of safety data, this chapter will be undergoing review in its next updated version. These data relate to increased risks of suicide and self harm with some pharmacological agents. In the interim, practitioners should be guided by the recommendations and warnings issued by their national drug regulatory authorities with respect to the prescribing of antidepressants to juveniles.

OPTION VENLAFAXINE

One small RCT in children and adolescents with major depression receiving psychotherapy found no significant difference between venlafaxine and placebo in improvement of depressive symptoms after 6 weeks. However, the study may have lacked power to detect clinically important effects.

Benefits: We found one systematic review (search date 1998,[14] 1 RCT[23]). The RCT (33 children and adolescents aged 8–17 years with major depression receiving psychotherapy) compared venlafaxine (37.5–75.0 mg/day in divided doses) versus placebo for 6 weeks.[23] It found no significant difference in improvement of depressive symptoms with venlafaxine compared with placebo (Children's Depression Inventory: P = 0.37; Hamilton Rating Scale for Depression: P = 0.50; Children's Depression Rating Scale: P = 0.48).

Harms: The RCT reported nausea in a subgroup of participants aged ≥13 years.[23]

Comment: The RCT may have lacked power to rule out a clinically important difference. In the light of emerging evidence and consensus on harms data on some of the pharmacological treatments included in this review since the time of writing, and the current FDA sponsored meta-analysis of safety data, this chapter will be undergoing review in its next updated version. These data relate to increased risks of suicide and self harm with some pharmacological agents. In the interim, practitioners should be guided by the recommendations and warnings issued by their national drug regulatory authorities with respect to the prescribing of antidepressants to juveniles.

OPTION LITHIUM

One small RCT in children with depression and a family history of bipolar affective disorder found no significant difference between lithium and placebo in global assessment or depression scores after 6 weeks. However, the study may have lacked power to detect clinically important effects.

Benefits: We found no systematic review. We found one RCT (30 children aged 6–12 years, with non-bipolar depression and family history of bipolar affective disorder), which compared lithium with placebo for 6 weeks.[24] The RCT found no significant difference between lithium and placebo (global assessment: P = 0.07; 9 depression items of the Kiddie-SADS interview: P = 0.91).

Harms: Of the 17 children randomised to lithium treatment, four were withdrawn because of adverse effects (3 had confusion, 1 had nausea and vomiting).[24]

Comment: The RCT may have lacked power to rule out a clinically important difference. It is not routine practice to give lithium alone to depressed children. Lithium is sometimes used to augment antidepressants and to prevent mania from developing with antidepressant use, but we found no RCTs of lithium for this indication.

OPTION ST JOHN'S WORT (*HYPERICUM PERFORATUM*)

We found no RCTs on St John's Wort (*Hypericum perforatum*) in children or adolescents with depression.

Benefits: We found no systematic review and no RCTs.

Harms: We found no RCTs.

Comment: None.

OPTION ELECTROCONVULSIVE THERAPY

We found no RCTs on electroconvulsive therapy in children and adolescents with depression.

Benefits: We found no systematic review and no RCTs.

Harms: We found no specific evidence on harms in children and adolescents. Known adverse effects in adults include memory impairment. See electroconvulsive therapy under depressive disorders, p 1238.

Comment: None.

OPTION SPECIFIC PSYCHOLOGICAL TREATMENTS

One systematic review in children and adolescents with mild to moderate depression found that cognitive behavioural therapy improves symptoms compared with non-specific support. One subsequent RCT in adolescents with major depression or dysthymia with depressed parents, found no significant

difference in recovery from depression between cognitive behavioural therapy plus usual care and usual care alone over 2 years. Two RCTs found that interpersonal therapy increased recovery rate after 12 weeks in adolescents with mild to moderate depression compared with clinical monitoring or waiting list control. We found insufficient evidence that family therapy or group treatments other than cognitive behavioural therapy are effective for depression in children and adolescents.

Benefits: **Cognitive behavioural therapy:** We found one systematic review (search date 1997, 6 RCTs, 376 children and adolescents with mild to moderate depression) of cognitive behavioural therapy**G** versus other treatments ranging from waiting list control to supportive psychotherapy,[25] and one subsequent RCT.[26] The systematic review found that cognitive behavioural therapy significantly increased the rate of resolution of symptoms of depression compared with other treatments (OR 3.2, 95% CI 1.9 to 5.2; NNT 4, 95% CI 3 to 5).[25] The subsequent RCT (88 adolescents aged 13–18 years with major depression or dysthymia who had depressed parents) compared cognitive behavioural therapy (16 sessions) plus usual care versus usual care alone.[26] The RCT found no significant difference in recovery rate between cognitive behavioural therapy plus usual care and usual care alone at 2 years (≥8 weeks with few or no depressive symptoms: 13/41 [31.7%] with cognitive behavioural therapy plus usual care *v* 14/47 [29.8%] with usual care alone; RR and P value not reported). A factor that could have contributed to the absence of a treatment effect was the higher level of impairment in the participants compared with other RCTs. **Interpersonal therapy:** We found two small RCTs, which compared 12 weekly sessions of interpersonal therapy**G** versus clinical monitoring or waiting list control in adolescents with depression.[27,28] The first RCT (48 adolescents aged 12–18 years with major depressive disorder) found that interpersonal therapy significantly increased recovery rate compared with clinical monitoring (Hamilton Rating Scale for Depression < 6 or Beck Depressive Inventory score < 9: 18/24 [75%] with interpersonal therapy *v* 11/24 [46%] with clinical monitoring alone; RR 1.64, 95% CI 1.00 to 2.68; ARR 29%, 95% CI 3% to 56%).[27] The second RCT (46 adolescents with major depression) found no significant difference in the proportion of adolescents not manifesting severe depression between interpersonal therapy and being on a waiting list (defined by a cut-off score on the Children's Depression Inventory: 17/19 [89%] with interpersonal therapy *v* 12/18 [67%] with waiting list; RR 1.33, 95% CI 0.94 to 1.93; ARR +22%, 95% CI –3% to +49%).[28] However, if the Children's Depression Inventory score was considered as a continuous measure, then the mean Children's Depression Inventory score was significantly lower after interpersonal therapy than with waiting list ($P < 0.01$). **Attachment based family therapy:** We found one RCT (32 adolescents aged 13–17 years with major depression), which compared 6 weeks of attachment based family therapy**G** versus 6 weeks of waiting list control.[29] It found no significant difference in remission rates between attachment based family therapy and waiting list control at 6 weeks (people no longer meeting criteria for major depression on the Kiddie-SADS interview: 13/16 [81%] with attachment based family therapy *v* 7/15 [47%] on the waiting list; RR 1.74, 95% CI 0.97 to 3.14). However, the study may have lacked the power to detect a clinically important difference between groups. **Systemic behavioural family therapy:** We found one RCT (78 adolescents with major depressive disorder), which compared systemic behavioural family therapy**G** versus non-specific supportive therapy.[30] The RCT found no significant difference in remission rates (combination of no longer meeting DSM-III-R criteria for major depression as determined by the Kiddie-SADS interview and Beck Depression Inventory score < 9: 29% with systemic behavioural family therapy *v* 34% with non-specific supportive therapy). **Group administered cognitive behavioural therapy:** We found one RCT (123 adolescents aged 14–18 years with major depression or dysthymia), which compared group administered cognitive behavioural therapy versus waiting list control.[31] It found that cognitive behavioural therapy significantly increased the remission rate (as determined by Longitudinal Interval Follow-up Evaluation Interview for DSM-III-R diagnoses: 46/69 [67%] with group cognitive behavioural therapy *v* 13/27 [48%] with waiting list control; $P < 0.05$). **Group therapeutic support versus group social skills training:** We found one RCT (66 adolescents aged 13–17 years, of whom 47 completed the protocol; 58 with major depression in the past year, 8 with dysthymia in the past year), which compared group therapeutic support versus group social skills training.[32] In 26 adolescents whose Kiddie-SADS scores were in the clinical range in the week before treatment, the RCT found no significant difference in remission rates (score of < 4 on Kiddie-SADS dysphoria and anhedonia symptoms: 8/16 [50%] with group therapeutic support *v* 4/10 [40%] with group social skills training; RR and P value not reported).

Harms: The RCTs did not report any adverse events.[26–28,30–35] We found no report of harms specifically for children and adolescents.

Comment: In the first RCT of interpersonal therapy**G**, sessions were augmented by telephone contact.[27] No long term trials of pure treatment have been reported. However, we found one prospective study, in which 107 adolescents with depression had been randomised to cognitive behavioural therapy**G**, systemic behavioural family therapy**G**, or non-directive supportive therapy**G**.[36] After the initial trial phase of 16 weeks, they were allowed booster treatments and also had access to open treatment in any modality for the 2 years of follow up. They were assessed at 3 monthly intervals for the first 12 months and then again at 24 months. The study found no significant difference between groups in depressive symptoms (of 104 adolescents for whom there were sufficient follow up data, 38% experienced sustained recovery, 21% experienced persistent depression, and 41% had a relapsing course).[36]

GLOSSARY

Attachment based family therapy A brief structured psychotherapy directed to adolescents and their parents or caregivers. It aims to repair attachment while promoting the autonomy of the adolescent. The treatment has five specific tasks; the focus of the family is shifted from "fixing" the individual to improving family relationships; an alliance is established with the individual; parental empathy for the individual is enhanced by exploring the parents' own stressors and history of attachment failure; the individual is encouraged to express previously unexpressed anger about core conflicts; and the individual is encouraged to make successful connections outside the home (e.g. at school, with peers, and at work).

Cognitive behavioural therapy A brief structured treatment (20 sessions over 12–16 weeks) aimed at changing the dysfunctional beliefs and negative automatic thoughts that characterise depressive disorders.[37] Cognitive behavioural therapy requires a high level of training for the therapist, and has been adapted for children and adolescents suffering from depression. A course of treatment is characterised by 8–12 weekly sessions, in which the therapist and the child collaborate to solve current difficulties. The treatment is structured and often directed by a manual. Treatment generally includes cognitive elements, such as the challenging of negative thoughts, and behavioural elements, such as structuring time to engage in pleasurable activity.

Interpersonal therapy A standardised form of brief psychotherapy (usually 12–16 weekly sessions) intended primarily for outpatients with unipolar non-psychotic depressive disorders. It focuses on improving the individual's interpersonal functioning and identifying the problems associated with the onset of the depressive episode.[38] In children and adolescents, interpersonal therapy has been adapted for adolescents to address common adolescent developmental issues, for example separation from parents, exploration of authority in relationship to parents, development of dyadic interpersonal relationships, initial experience with the death of a relative or friend, and peer pressure.

Non-directive supportive therapy Helping people to express feelings, and clarify thoughts and difficulties; therapists suggest alternative understandings and do not give direct advice but try to encourage people to solve their own problems.

Pseudo-continuous outcome measure The strict definition of a continuous outcome is one measured on a scale that is continuously variable, good examples being height or systolic blood pressure. In addition, there is an assumption that an increase in 1 unit in one region is equivalent to an increase of 1 unit in another region of the scale. In the case of psychometric scales made up of a series of questions the latter assumption is not always valid, in which case the scale may be referred to as a pseudo-continuous measure. Caution needs to be applied in interpreting the magnitude of change reported on such measures.

Pulsed intravenous clomipramine An intravenous loading procedure for clomipramine.

Systemic behavioural family therapy A combination of two treatment approaches that have been used effectively for dysfunctional families. In the first phase of treatment, the therapist clarifies the concerns that brought the family into treatment, and provides a series of reframing statements designed to optimise engagement in therapy and identification of dysfunctional behaviour patterns (systemic therapy). In the second phase, the family members focus on communication and problem solving skills and the alteration of family interactional patterns (family behavioural therapy).

REFERENCES

1. Birmaher B, Ryan ND, Williamson DE, et al. Childhood and adolescent depression: a review of the past 10 years, Part I. *J Am Acad Child Adolesc Psychiatry* 1996;35:1427–1439.
2. American Psychiatric Association. *Diagnostic and statistical manual of mental disorders, 4th ed.* Washington DC: American Psychiatric Association, 1994;328.
3. Costello EJ, Angold A, Burns BJ, et al. The Great Smoky Mountains Study of Youth. Goals, design, methods, and the prevalence of DSM-III-R disorders. *Arch Gen Psychiatry* 1996;53:1129–1136.
4. Costello EJ. Developments in child psychiatric epidemiology. *J Am Acad Child Adolesc Psychiatry* 1989;28:836–841.
5. Lewinsohn PM, Rohde P, Seely JR. Major depressive disorder in older adolescents: prevalence, risk factors, and clinical implications. *Clin Psychol Rev* 1998;18:765–794.
6. Rice F, Harold G, Thapar A. The genetic aetiology of childhood depression: a review. *J Child Psychol Psychiatry* 2002;43:65–79.
7. Birmaher B, Williamson DE, Dahl RE, et al. Clinical presentation and course of depression in youth: does onset in childhood differ from onset in adolescence? *J Am Acad Child Adolesc Psychiatry* 2004;43:63–70.
8. Geller B, Fox LW, Fletcher M. Effect of tricyclic antidepressants on switching to mania and on the onset of bipolarity in depressed 6-12-year-olds. *J Am Acad Child Adolesc Psychiatry* 1993;32:43–50.
9. Hazell P, O'Connell D, Heathcote D, et al. Tricyclic drugs for depression in children and adolescents. In: The Cochrane Library, Issue 4, 2003. Chichester, UK: John Wiley & Sons, Ltd. Search date 2000; primary sources Medline, Embase, Excerpta Medica, Cochrane Depression, Anxiety and Neurosis Review Group Trials Register, hand searching of relevant studies and the Journal of American Academy of Child and Adolescent Psychiatry, and personal contact with authors of relevant studies in progress.
10. Sallee FR, Vrindavanam NS, Deas-Nesmith D, et al. Pulse intravenous clomipramine for depressed adolescents: double-blind, controlled trial. *Am J Psychiatry* 1997;154:668–673.
11. Anon. Sudden death in children treated with a tricyclic antidepressant. *Med Lett Drugs Ther* 1990;32:53.
12. Werry JS, Biederman J, Thisted R, et al. Resolved: cardiac arrhythmias make desipramine an unacceptable choice in children. *J Am Acad Child Adolesc Psychiatry* 1995;34:1239–1245.
13. Avci A, Diler RS, Kibar M, et al. Comparison of moclobemide and placebo in young adolescents with major depressive disorder. *Ann Med Sci* 1999;8:31–40.
14. Williams JW, Mulrow CD, Chiquette E, et al. A systematic review of newer pharmacotherapies for depression in adults: evidence report summary. *Ann Intern Med* 2000;132:743–756. Search date 1998; primary sources Medline, Embase, Psychlit, Lilacs, Psyindex, Sigle, Cinahl, Biological Abstracts, Cochrane Controlled Trials, hand searches, and personal contacts.
15. Simeon JG, Dinicola VF, Ferguson HB, et al. Adolescent depression: a placebo-controlled fluoxetine treatment study and follow-up. *Prog Neuropsychopharmacol Biol Psychiatry* 1990;14:791–795.
16. Emslie GJ, Rush AJ, Weinberg WA, et al. A double-blind, randomized, placebo-controlled trial of fluoxetine in children and adolescents with depression. *Arch Gen Psychiatry* 1997;54:1031–1037.
17. Emslie GJ, Heiligenstein JH, Wagner KD, et al. Fluoxetine for acute treatment of depression in children and adolescents: a placebo-controlled, randomized clinical trial. *J Am Acad Child Adolesc Psychiatry* 2002;41:1205–1215.
18. Keller MB, Ryan ND, Strober M, et al. Efficacy of paroxetine in the treatment of adolescent major depression: a randomized, controlled trial. *J Am Acad Child Adolesc Psychiatry* 2001;40:762–772.
19. Braconnier A, Le Coent R, Cohen D. Paroxetine versus clomipramine in adolescents with severe major depression: a double-blind, randomized, multicenter trial. *J Am Acad Child Adolesc Psychiatry* 2003;42:22–29.
20. Wagner KD, Ambrosini P, Rynn M, et al. Efficacy of sertraline in the treatment of children and adolescents with major depressive disorder: two randomized controlled trials. *JAMA* 2003;290:1033–1041.

21. Diler RS, Avci A. Selective serotonin reuptake inhibitor discontinuation syndrome in children: six case reports. *Curr Ther Res Clin Exp* 2002;63:188–197.
22. Riddle MA. Paroxetine and the FDA. *J Am Acad Child Adolesc Psychiatry* 2004;43:128–130.
23. Mandoki MW, Tapia MR, Tapia MA, et al. Venlafaxine in the treatment of children and adolescents with major depression. *Psychopharmacol Bull* 1997;33:149–154.
24. Geller B, Cooper TB, Zimerman B, et al. Lithium for prepubertal depressed children with family history predictors of future bipolarity: a double-blind, placebo-controlled study. *J Affect Disord* 1998;51:165–175.
25. Harrington R, Whittaker J, Shoebridge P, et al. Systematic review of efficacy of cognitive behavioural therapies in childhood and adolescent depressive disorder. *BMJ* 1998;316:1559–1563. Search date 1997; primary sources Medline, Psychlit, Cochrane, and hand searches of reference lists, book chapters, conference proceedings, and relevant journals in the field.
26. Clarke GN, Hornbrook M, Lynch F, et al. Group cognitive-behavioral treatment for depressed adolescent offspring of depressed patients in a health maintenance organization. *J Am Acad Child Adolesc Psychiatry* 2002;41:305–313.
27. Mufson L, Weissman MM, Moreau D, et al. Efficacy of interpersonal psychotherapy for depressed adolescents. *Arch Gen Psychiatry* 1999;56:573–579.
28. Rossello J, Bernal G. The efficacy of cognitive-behavioral and interpersonal treatments for depression in Puerto Rican adolescents. *J Consult Clin Psychol* 1999;67:734–745.
29. Diamond GS, Reis BF, Diamond GM, et al. Attachment-based family therapy for depressed adolescents: a treatment development study. *J Am Acad Child Adolesc Psychiatry* 2002;41:1190–1196.
30. Brent DA, Holder D, Kolko D, et al. A clinical psychotherapy trial for adolescent depression comparing cognitive, family, and supportive therapy. *Arch Gen Psychiatry* 1997;54:877–885.
31. Clarke GN, Rohde P, Lewinsohn PM, et al. Cognitive-behavioral treatment of adolescent depression: efficacy of acute group treatment and booster sessions. *J Am Acad Child Adolesc Psychiatry* 1999;38:272–279.
32. Fine S, Forth A, Gilbert M, et al. Group therapy for adolescent depressive disorder: a comparison of social skills and therapeutic support. *J Am Acad Child Adolesc Psychiatry* 1991;30:79–85.
33. Lewinsohn PM, Clarke GN. Psychosocial treatments for adolescent depression. *Clin Psychol Rev* 1999;19:329–342.
34. Reinecke MA, Ryan NE, DuBois DL. Cognitive-behavioral therapy of depression and depressive symptoms during adolescence: a review and meta-analysis. *J Am Acad Child Adolesc Psychiatry* 1998;37:26–34.
35. Mendez Carrillo FX, Moreno PJ, Sanchez-Meca J, et al. Effectiveness of psychological treatment for child and adolescent depression: a qualitative review of two decades of research. *Psicol Conductual* 2000;8:487–510.
36. Birmaher B, Brent DA, Kolko D, et al. Clinical outcome after short-term psychotherapy for adolescents with major depressive disorder. *Arch Gen Psychiatry* 2000;57:29–36.
37. Haaga DAF, Beck AT. Cognitive therapy. In: Paykel ES, ed. *Handbook of affective disorders*. Edinburgh: Churchill Livingstone, 1992;511–523.
38. Klerman GL, Weissman H. Interpersonal psychotherapy. In: Paykel ES, ed. *Handbook of affective disorders*. Edinburgh: Churchill Livingstone, 1992;501–510.

Philip Hazell
Conjoint Professor of Child and Adolescent Psychiatry/Director Child and Youth Mental Health Service
University of Newcastle
Newcastle
Australia

Competing interests: The author has been paid a fee by Pfizer, the manufacturer of sertraline, for speaking to general practitioners about the evidence for the treatment of depression in young people. The author's service has been in receipt of funding from Eli Lilly to participate in a relapse prevention trial of atomoxetine for attention deficit hyperactivity disorder.

TABLE 1 Summary of outcome measures commonly used in trials of treatments for depression in children and adolescents (see text, p 331).

Outcome measure	Description	Scoring system
Children's Depression Rating Scale (Revised)	Semistructured interview with child, supplemented with information from parents or significant others. Assesses 17 symptoms including those that serve as DSM criteria for depressive disorders. Based on how child has felt over previous 2 weeks. Can be used as a screening instrument for depression, a confirmatory diagnostic tool, and a measure of treatment response in children. Good inter-rater (0.74–0.96) and test–retest (0.80–0.96) reliability, sound internal consistency (0.70), and insensitive to age of child.	Items scored on a scale of 1 (least difficulties) to 5 or 7 (greatest difficulties). The summary score (range 17–113) is then transformed into a t score. Scores < 55 are unlikely to be associated with depressive disorder, scores 55–64 indicate possible risk, and scores > 65 are likely to be associated with depressive disorder.
Children's Depression Inventory	Self report questionnaire (administrator may read aloud while child completes) consisting of 27 items. For each item the child chooses 1 of 3 statements describing how they have felt over the previous 2 weeks. Covers most DSM criteria for depressive disorder. Can be used as a screening instrument for depression, a confirmatory diagnostic tool, and a measure of treatment response in children. Variable test–retest reliability (0.38–0.87) but sound internal consistency (0.59–0.88).	Items scored on a scale of 0 (least difficulties) to 2 (greatest difficulties). An aggregate score (range 0–54) of ≥ 11 is associated with depressive disorder (sensitivity 0.67, specificity 0.60). Items load onto 5 factors including dysphoric mood, acting out, loss of personal and social interest, self depreciation, and vegetative symptoms.
Hamilton Rating Scale for Depression (Revised)	Designed to assess adult depressive symptomatology but has been widely used with adolescent populations. Clinician rating based on interview with person and a self report problem inventory. Can be used as a screening instrument for depression, a confirmatory diagnostic tool, and a measure of treatment response. Excellent inter-rater reliability (> 0.90), and moderate to good internal consistency (0.45–0.90).	Items are scored on a 3–5 point scale of 0 (absent) to 2 or 4 (clearly present/severe). An aggregate score (range 0–64) of 11 is indicative of a diagnosis of depression.
Children's Depression Inventory for Parents	Modified version of the Children's Depression Inventory. Completed by parents, it describes the child over the previous 2 weeks. May be used as a confirmatory diagnostic tool and is sensitive to treatment response. Moderate test–retest reliability (0.54–0.75), and sound internal consistency (0.82–0.85). Parents generally moderate to good total score correlation (0.54–0.64), but parent–child correlation is variable (0.03–0.74).	Items scored on a scale of 0 (least difficulties) to 2 (greatest difficulties). An aggregate score (range 0–54) of ≥ 12 is associated with depressive disorder but does not discriminate well between depression and other psychiatric conditions (sensitivity 0.87, specificity 0.24).

TABLE 1 continued

Outcome measure	Description	Scoring system
Kiddie Schedule for Affective Disorders and Schizophrenia (Kiddie-SADS)	Semistructured diagnostic interview for children and adolescents, completed with child and parents. Covers most childhood disorders. Current and lifetime assessment versions are available. Used in research trials as a standard method of diagnostic assessment. Good inter-rater reliability (0.86–0.89). Moderate to good test–retest reliability of individual items (0.41–0.81), and for categorical depression diagnosis (0.54). Moderate internal consistency of depression items (0.60–0.84).	Items are scored on a 2 or 3 point scale (not present, subthreshold/threshold). Some versions include a 0–6 scale to assess severity (not at all/normal to extreme).
Clinical Global Impressions Scale	Clinician ratings to assess overall severity of symptoms with reference to baseline functioning. Inter-rater reliability is high when clinicians are trained, and test–retest reliability is moderate to good.	Consists of three global measures: Severity of illness (scale 1–7; normal to extremely ill); Global improvement (scale 1–7; very much improved to very much worse); and the Efficacy index (scale 1–4; compares improvement in symptoms with adverse effects, from none to outweighs therapeutic effect). Higher scores indicate more severe symptomatology and impairment, or little change from pretreatment baseline.
Depression Checklist scores	Includes 10 major symptoms of depression, as used by DSM-III, and as appropriate for children. Each symptom category is anchored by characteristic behaviours of that symptom. The symptom category is assessed as positive if any of the presentations are evident. Has been used as a confirmatory diagnostic tool and a measure of treatment response. No information available regarding reliability or consistency.	Total scores (range 0–10) reflect the number of depressive symptoms. Follows a DSM approach to diagnosis, such that if a child has sufficient symptoms that reach threshold for a period of 1 month and represent a change from their usual behaviour then they can be diagnosed with depression.
Longitudinal Interval Follow-up Evaluation Interview for DSM-III-R	Clinician rated semistructured interview with patient that assesses the longitudinal course of mental illness. Excellent inter-rater reliability for psychiatric symptom ratings and global assessment scores (0.90).	Sections are rated on various scales that range upwards from 1 and have variable end points. Low scores indicate no symptomatology/high functioning and high scores indicate severe symptomatology/diagnostic

Gastroenteritis in children

Search date August 2004

Jacqueline Dalby-Payne and Elizabeth Elliott

QUESTIONS

INTERVENTIONS

Key Messages

Treatments

- **Oral rehydration solutions (as effective as iv fluids)** One systematic review and two additional RCTs in children with mild to moderate dehydration in developed countries found no significant difference between oral rehydration solutions and intravenous fluids in duration of diarrhoea, time spent in hospital, or weight gain at discharge. One small RCT in children with mild to moderate dehydration managed in the emergency department found that oral rehydration reduced length of stay in the department. However, it did not significantly reduce rate of hospital admission compared with intravenous fluids. One RCT in children with severe dehydration in a developing country found that oral rehydration solutions reduced the duration of diarrhoea and increased weight gain at discharge, and were associated with fewer adverse effects compared with intravenous fluids.
- **Lactose-free feeds (reduces duration of diarrhoea)** One systematic review and three of five subsequent RCTs found limited evidence that lactose-free feeds reduced the duration of diarrhoea in children with mild to severe dehydration compared with feeds containing lactose. The remaining two subsequent RCTs found no significant difference between lactose-free and lactose containing feeds in diarrhoea duration.
- **Loperamide (reduces duration of diarrhoea, but adverse effects unclear)** Two RCTs found that, in children with mild to moderate dehydration, loperamide reduces the duration of diarrhoea compared with placebo. Another RCT found no significant difference between loperamide and placebo in the duration of diarrhoea. We found insufficient evidence to assess the risk of adverse effects.
- **Nasogastric rehydration (as effective as iv fluids)** Two RCTs conducted in the USA compared nasogastric with intravenous rehydration fluids and found different results. One small RCT, in children with moderate dehydration, found limited evidence that nasogastric rehydration fluids reduced the duration of diarrhoea and length of hospital stay compared with intravenous fluids. The second, larger RCT found no significant difference in stool output between nasogastric and intravenous fluids. However, it found a greater percentage weight gain with intravenous fluids. It found that more attempts at reinsertion were required for intravenous catheters compared with nasogastric catheters.

- **Clear fluids (other than oral rehydration solutions)** We found no systematic review or RCTs comparing "clear fluids" (water, carbonated drinks, and translucent fruit juices) versus oral rehydration solutions for treatment of acute gastroenteritis.

DEFINITION Acute gastroenteritis is caused by infection of the gastrointestinal tract, commonly caused by a virus. It is characterised by rapid onset of diarrhoea with or without vomiting, nausea, fever, and abdominal pain.[1] In children, the symptoms and signs can be non-specific.[2] Diarrhoea is defined as the frequent passage of unformed liquid stools.[3] Regardless of the cause, the mainstay of management of acute gastroenteritis is provision of adequate fluids to prevent and treat dehydration. In this chapter we examine the benefits and harms of different treatments irrespective of cause.

INCIDENCE/ PREVALENCE Worldwide, about 3–5 billion cases of acute gastroenteritis occur in children under 5 years of age each year.[4] In the UK, acute gastroenteritis accounts for 204/1000 general practitioner consultations in children under 5 years of age.[5] Gastroenteritis leads to hospital admission in 7/1000 children under 5 years of age a year in the UK[5] and 13/1000 in the USA.[6] In Australia, gastroenteritis accounts for 6% of all hospital admissions in children under 15 years of age.[7]

AETIOLOGY/ RISK FACTORS In developed countries, acute gastroenteritis is predominantly caused by viruses (87%), of which rotavirus is most common;[8–11] bacteria cause most of the remaining cases, predominantly *Campylobacter*, *Salmonella*, *Shigella*, and *Escherichia coli*. In developing countries, bacterial pathogens are more frequent, although rotavirus is also a major cause of gastroenteritis.

PROGNOSIS Acute gastroenteritis is usually self limiting but if untreated can result in morbidity and mortality secondary to water and electrolyte losses. Acute diarrhoea causes 4 million deaths a year in children under 5 years of age in Asia (excluding China), Africa, and Latin America, and over 80% of deaths occur in children under 2 years of age.[12] Although death is uncommon in developed countries, dehydration secondary to gastroenteritis is a significant cause of morbidity and need for hospital admission.[6,7,13]

AIMS OF INTERVENTION To reduce the duration of diarrhoea and quantity of stool output, and duration of hospital stay; to prevent and treat dehydration; to promote weight gain after rehydration; to prevent persistent diarrhoea associated with lactose intolerance**G**.

OUTCOMES Total stool volume; duration of diarrhoea (time until permanent cessation); failure rate of oral rehydration treatment (as defined by individual RCTs); weight gain after rehydration; length of hospital stay; mortality.

METHODS *Clinical Evidence* search and appraisal August 2004.

QUESTION **What are the effects of treatments for acute gastroenteritis?**

OPTION **CLEAR FLUIDS (OTHER THAN ORAL REHYDRATION SOLUTIONS)**

We found no systematic review or RCTs comparing "clear fluids" (water, carbonated drinks, and translucent fruit juices) versus oral rehydration solutions for treatment of acute gastroenteritis.

Benefits: We found no systematic review or RCTs of "clear fluids" compared with oral rehydration solutions (see comment below).

Harms: We found no RCTs.

Comment: In this chapter, oral rehydration solutions are defined as glucose plus electrolyte or food (e.g. rice) based electrolyte solutions. Fruit juices and carbonated drinks are low in sodium and potassium, and usually have a high sugar content, which can exacerbate diarrhoea.

OPTION ORAL REHYDRATION SOLUTIONS

One systematic review and two additional RCTs in children with mild to moderate dehydration in developed countries found no significant difference between oral rehydration solutions and intravenous fluids in duration of diarrhoea, time spent in hospital, or weight gain at discharge. One small RCT in children with mild to moderate dehydration managed in the emergency department found that oral rehydration reduced length of stay in the department. However, it did not significantly reduce rate of hospital admission compared with intravenous fluids. One RCT in children with severe dehydration in a developing country found that oral rehydration solutions reduced the duration of diarrhoea and increased weight gain at discharge, and were associated with fewer adverse effects compared with intravenous fluids.

Benefits: **Mild to moderate dehydration:** We found one systematic review[14] (search date 1993, 4 RCTs,[15–18] 223 children in developed countries with acute gastroenteritis, most with mild to moderate dehydration and in hospital), two additional RCTs,[19,20] and one subsequent RCT[21] comparing oral rehydration solutions versus intravenous fluids (see table 1, p 350). The review and the additional RCTs found no significant difference between oral and intravenous fluids in the duration of diarrhoea, time spent in hospital, or weight gain at discharge. If children responded poorly to oral fluids, they were given intravenous fluids, which was used as a measure of failure of oral fluids. However, the failure rate of intravenous treatment was not recorded. The subsequent RCT (34 children managed in the emergency department) did not report on duration of diarrhoea, length of hospital stay, or weight gain.[21] However, it found that oral rehydration significantly reduced length of stay in the emergency department compared with intravenous fluids, but found no significant difference for rate of admission to hospital (mean length of stay in emergency department: 225 minutes with oral rehydration *v* 358 minutes with iv rehydration; $P < 0.01$; rate of admission to hospital: 11% with oral rehydration *v* 25% with iv rehydration; $P = 0.2$). **Severe dehydration:** We found no systematic review. We found one RCT (470 children in Iran with acute gastroenteritis with severe dehydration) comparing oral rehydration solutions versus intravenous fluids (see table 1, p 350).[22] It found that oral treatment significantly reduced the duration of diarrhoea and increased weight gain at discharge compared with intravenous rehydration (mean duration: 4.8 days with oral rehydration *v* 5.5 days with iv rehydration; difference 0.7 days; $P < 0.01$; percentage increase in admission weight: 9% with oral rehydration *v* 7% with iv rehydration; $P < 0.001$). Failure of oral treatment (defined as the need to move to iv treatment) occurred in 1/236 children (0.4%, CI not reported). It found no significant difference in mortality between oral and intravenous fluids (2/236 [1%] with oral rehydration *v* 5/234 [2%] with iv rehydration; RR 0.40, 95% CI 0.08 to 2.02). Causes of death were not reported.

Harms: **Mild to moderate dehydration:** The systematic review reported no adverse effects.[14] One additional RCT (100 children in Afghanistan) reported fever and rigors in 9/50 (18%) children receiving intravenous fluids compared with none receiving oral fluids.[19] **Severe dehydration:** The RCT in children in Iran found that significantly more children receiving intravenous treatment vomited during the first 6 hours of rehydration (47/236 [20%] with oral rehydration *v* 70/234 [30%] with iv rehydration; RR 0.64, 95% CI 0.46 to 0.89).[22] There was no significant difference in the risk of peri-orbital oedema or abdominal distension (peri-orbital oedema: RR 0.99, 95% CI 0.25 to 3.92; abdominal distension: RR 8.90, 95% CI 0.48 to 164.00). Phlebitis at the injection site requiring antibiotics occurred in 5/234 (2%) children. Subgroup analysis of 58 children with hypernatraemia in this RCT found that fewer children taking oral fluids developed seizures during rehydration compared with intravenous fluids, although the difference did not quite reach significance (2/34 [6%] with oral rehydration v 6/24 [25%] with iv rehydration; RR 0.23, 95% CI 0.05 to 1.07).[22]

Comment: The quality of the RCTs was difficult to assess because of poor reporting. One RCT reported the method of allocation concealment[21] and two reported the method of randomisation.[19,21] Blinding of outcomes was impossible owing to the nature of the intervention. All RCTs used intention to treat analysis. The RCT in children managed in the emergency department was small and may have lacked power to detect clinically important effects.[21]

OPTION NASOGASTRIC REHYDRATION

Two RCTs conducted in the USA compared nasogastric with intravenous rehydration fluids and found different results. One small RCT, in children with moderate dehydration, found limited evidence that nasogastric rehydration fluids reduced the duration of diarrhoea and length of hospital stay compared with intravenous fluids. The second, larger RCT found no significant difference in stool output between nasogastric and intravenous fluids. However, it found a greater percentage weight gain with intravenous fluids. It found that more attempts at reinsertion were required for intravenous catheters compared with nasogastric catheters.

Benefits: **Versus intravenous fluids:** We found no systematic review. We found two RCTs conducted in the USA in children with gastroenteritis.[23,24] The first small RCT (24 children with moderate dehydration, aged 2–24 months) found that nasogastric rehydration significantly reduced the duration of diarrhoea and length of hospital stay compared with intravenous fluids (duration of diarrhoea after admission: 23.3 hours with nasogastric fluids v 43.9 hours with iv fluids; $P < 0.05$; hospital stay: 1.8 days with nasogastric fluids v 2.8 days with iv fluids; $P < 0.05$).[23] One of the 12 children in the nasogastric rehydration group was not able to be adequately hydrated and required intravenous fluids. The second RCT (96 children with moderate dehydration, aged 3–36 months) found that intravenous fluids significantly increased the percentage body weight gain compared with nasogastric rehydration. However, it found no significant difference in absolute weight gain (percentage increase in body weight: 2.21% with nasogastric fluids v 3.58% with iv fluids; $P = 0.007$; absolute weight gain: 220 g with nasogastric fluids v 350 g with iv; P value not reported).[24] It found no significant difference in stool output (no data reported). Nasogastric rehydration failed in 1/48 (2%) children.

Harms: The first RCT found that nasogastric rehydration reduced complications compared with intravenous fluids.[23] It found that the most common complication with intravenous fluids group was infiltration at the catheter site (children required a mean 1.9 iv catheters). The second RCT found that 2/46 (4.3%) children in the nasogastric rehydration group required a second attempt at tube placement whereas 13/44 (61.4%) children in the intravenous fluids group required additional attempts at intravenous catheterisation.[24] Other complications of treatment were not reported.

Comment: The quality of the RCTs was difficult to assess because of poor reporting.[23,24] The method of allocation concealment or blinding of outcome assessment was not reported in either RCT. Intention to treat analysis was not performed in one RCT.[24] Nasogastric rehydration was safe and effective with a low failure rate. Despite the small sample size, statistically and clinically significant benefits from nasogastric rehydration were shown in one RCT.[23] In the larger RCT, outcomes (duration of diarrhoea and stay in hospital) for which nasogastric rehydration was found beneficial in the smaller RCT were not reported.[24] The beneficial effect of intravenous fluids on weight gain is difficult to interpret and suggests that rehydration may be quicker with intravenous than nasogastric fluids.

OPTION LOPERAMIDE

Two RCTs found that, in children with mild to moderate dehydration, loperamide reduces the duration of diarrhoea compared with placebo. Another RCT found no significant difference between loperamide and placebo in the duration of diarrhoea. We found insufficient evidence to assess the risk of adverse effects.

Benefits: We found no systematic review. We found five RCTs in children with acute diarrhoea (701 children, most with mild to moderate dehydration) (see table 2, p 352).[25–30] Of the three RCTs that assessed the duration of diarrhoea, two[25,27] found that loperamide significantly reduced duration of diarrhoea compared with placebo (largest RCT, 315 children; risk of having diarrhoea at 24 hours, 36/100 [36%] with loperamide *v* 112/203 [55%] with placebo; RR 0.83, 95% CI 0.73 to 0.94).[25] Another RCT found no significant difference.[26] The results of other outcomes are included in table 2, p 352.

Harms: Four RCTs reported no adverse effects from loperamide.[25–27,29] One RCT found significantly more mild abdominal distension, excessive sleep, and lethargy in children taking loperamide compared with placebo (3/16 [19%] with loperamide 0.8 mg/kg *v* 1/18 [6%] with loperamide 0.4 mg/kg *v* 0/18 [0%] with placebo; RR loperamide *v* placebo 4.90, 95% CI 0.28 to 86.00). Adverse effects caused one child to withdraw from the trial.[28] We found one evidence based guideline that identified case studies reporting lethargy, intestinal ileus, respiratory depression, and coma, especially in infants.[2]

Comment: We found insufficient evidence to estimate accurately the risk of adverse effects of loperamide in children.

OPTION LACTOSE-FREE FEEDS

One systematic review and three of five subsequent RCTs found limited evidence that lactose-free feeds reduced the duration of diarrhoea in children with mild to severe dehydration compared with feeds containing lactose. The remaining two subsequent RCTs found no significant difference between lactose-free and lactose containing feeds in diarrhoea duration.

Benefits: We found one systematic review (search date not reported, 13 RCTs, 873 children with mild to severe dehydration)[30] and five subsequent RCTs[31–35] comparing feeds containing lactose versus lactose-free feed (see table 3, p 353). The review was limited by flaws in its methods (see comment below). It found that feeds containing lactose significantly increased "treatment failure" compared with lactose-free feeds (89/399 [22%] with lactose *v* 56/474 [12%] with lactose-free; RR 2.1, 95% CI 1.6 to 2.7). The definition of treatment failure varied among trials and included increasing severity or persistence of diarrhoea or recurrence of dehydration. It found that lactose-free feeds significantly reduced the mean duration of diarrhoea compared with feeds containing lactose (9 RCTs; 826 children with mild or no dehydration receiving oral rehydration treatment; 92 hours with lactose *v* 88 hours with lactose-free; SMD

0.2; P = 0.001). When the three RCTs that included children given additional solid food were excluded, it found that lactose-free feeds significantly reduced the duration of diarrhoea compared with feeds containing lactose (6 RCTs, 604 children, 95 hours with lactose v 82 hours with lactose-free; SMD 0.3; P < 0.001). Children receiving lactose-free feeds had significantly reduced stool frequency compared with feeds containing lactose (4 RCTs, 387 children, 4.0 stool movements/day with lactose v 3.5 stool movements/day with lactose-free; SMD 0.3; P < 0.004). Total stool volume was greater in children who received feeds containing lactose (4 RCTs, 209 children; SMD 0.4; P = 0.002). Differences in weight gain during treatment could not be assessed because of the use of solid food in two studies and considerable heterogeneity among studies. Of the five subsequent RCTs,[31–35] three found that lactose-free feeds significantly reduced the duration of diarrhoea compared with feeds containing lactose (see table 3, p 353).[31,34,35] The other two found no significant difference.[32,33] The results of other outcomes are summarised in table 3, p 353.

Harms: The one RCT assessing adverse effects reported none in the treatment or control groups.[33]

Comment: Although the systematic review stated criteria for inclusion and exclusion of RCTs, only published studies were included and the method of determining RCT quality was not reported.[28] There was considerable heterogeneity among studies, which limits the validity of the meta-analyses. Lactose-free feeds were superior to feeds containing lactose for the duration of diarrhoea. Differences for other outcomes, although statistically significant, were not clinically important.

GLOSSARY

Lactose intolerance Malabsorption of lactose can occur for a short period after acute gastroenteritis because of mucosal damage and temporary lactase deficiency.

Substantive changes

Lactose-free feeds One RCT added;[35] benefits data enhanced and categorisation unchanged.

REFERENCES

1. Armon K, Elliott EJ. Acute gastroenteritis. In: Moyer VA, Elliott EJ, Davis RL, eds. *Evidence based pediatrics and child health, 2nd edition*. London: BMJ Books, 2004;377–392.
2. American Academy of Pediatrics (APP). Practice parameter: the management of acute gastroenteritis in young children. American Academy of Pediatrics, Provisional Committee on Quality Improvement, Subcommittee on Acute Gastroenteritis. *Pediatrics* 1996;97:424–435.
3. Critchley M. *Butterworths medical dictionary, second edition*. London: Butterworths, 1986.
4. OPCS. *Mid-1993 population estimates for England and Wales*. London: HMSO, 1994.
5. OPCS. *Morbidity statistics from general practice. Fourth national study, 1991–1992*. London: HMSO, 1993.
6. Glass RI, Lew JF, Gangarosa RE, et al. Estimates of morbidity and mortality rates for diarrheal diseases in American children. *J Pediatr* 1991;118:S27–S33.
7. Elliott EJ, Backhouse JA, Leach JW. Pre-admission management of acute gastroenteritis. *J Paediatr Child Health* 1996;32:18–21.
8. Conway SP, Phillips RR, Panday S. Admission to hospital with gastroenteritis. *Arch Dis Child* 1990;65:579–584.
9. Finkelstein JA, Schwartz JS, Torrey S, et al. Common clinical features as predictors of bacterial diarrhea in infants. *Am J Emerg Med* 1989;7:469–473.
10. DeWitt TG, Humphrey KF, McCarthy P. Clinical predictors of acute bacterial diarrhea in young children. *Pediatrics* 1985;76:551–556.
11. Ferson MJ. Hospitalisations for rotavirus gastroenteritis among children under five years of age in New South Wales. *Med J Aust* 1996;164:273–276.
12. Anonymous. *A manual for the treatment of diarrhoea. Programme for the control of diarrhoeal diseases*. Geneva: WHO, 1990.
13. Conway SP, Phillips RR, Panday S. Admission to hospital with gastroenteritis. *Arch Dis Child* 1990;65:579–584.
14. Gavin N, Merrick N, Davidson B. Efficacy of glucose-based oral rehydration therapy. *Pediatrics* 1996;98:45–51. Search date 1993; primary sources Medline and experts and organisations involved in diarrhoea treatment contacted.
15. Santosham M, Daum RS, Dillman L, et al. Oral rehydration therapy of infantile diarrhea: a controlled study of well-nourished children hospitalized in the United States and Panama. *N Engl J Med* 1982;306:1070–1076.
16. Listernick R, Zieserl E, Davis AT. Outpatient oral rehydration in the United States. *Am J Dis Child* 1986;140:211–215.
17. Tamer AM, Friedman LB, Maxwell SR, et al. Oral rehydration of infants in a large urban US medical center. *J Pediatr* 1985;107:14–19.

18. Issenman RM, Leung AK. Oral and intravenous rehydration of children. *Can Fam Physician* 1993;39:2129–2136.
19. Singh M, Mahmoodi A, Arya LS, et al. Controlled trial of oral versus intravenous rehydration in the management of acute gastroenteritis. *Indian J Med Res* 1982;75:691–693.
20. Martin de Pumarejo M, Lugo CE, Alvarez-Ruiz JR, et al. Oral rehydration: experience in the management of patients with acute gastroenteritis in the emergency room at the Dr. Antonio Ortiz pediatric hospital. *Bol Assoc Med PR* 1990;82:227–233.
21. Atherly-John YC, Cunningham SJ, Crain EF. A randomized trial of oral vs intravenous rehydration in a pediatric emergency department. *Arch Pediatr Adolesc Med* 2002;156:1240–1243.
22. Sharifi J, Ghavami F, Nowrouzi Z, et al. Oral versus intravenous rehydration therapy in severe gastroenteritis. *Arch Dis Child* 1985;60:856–860.
23. Gremse DA. Effectiveness of nasogastric rehydration in hospitalized children with acute diarrhoea. *J Paediatr Gastroenterol Nutr* 1995;21;145–148.
24. Nager AL, Wang VJ. Comparison of nasogastric and intravenous methods of rehydration in pediatric patients with acute dehydration. *Pediatrics* 2002;109:566–572.
25. Diarrhoeal Diseases Study Group (UK). Loperamide in acute diarrhoea in childhood: results of a double blind, placebo controlled multicentre clinical trial. *BMJ Clin Res Ed* 1984;289:1263–1267.
26. Owens JR, Broadhead R, Hendrickse RG, et al. Loperamide in the treatment of acute gastroenteritis in early childhood. Report of a two centre, double-blind, controlled clinical trial. *Ann Trop Paediatr* 1981;1:135–141.
27. Kassem AS, Madkour AA, Massoud BZ, et al. Loperamide in acute childhood diarrhoea: a double blind controlled trial. *J Diarrhoeal Dis Res* 1983;1:10–16.
28. Karrar ZA, Abdulla MA, Moody JB, et al. Loperamide in acute diarrhoea in childhood: results of a double blind, placebo controlled clinical trial. *Ann Trop Paediatr* 1987;7:122–127.
29. Bowie MD, Hill ID, Mann MD. Loperamide for treatment of acute diarrhoea in infants and young children. A double-blind placebo-controlled trial. *S Afr Med J* 1995;85:885–887.
30. Brown KH, Peerson JM, Fontaine O. Use of nonhuman milks in the dietary management of young children with acute diarrhea: a meta-analysis of clinical trials. *Pediatrics* 1994;93:17–27. Search date not reported; primary sources Medline, hand searches of reference lists, and contact with researchers.
31. Allen UD, McLeod K, Wang EE. Cow's milk versus soy-based formula in mild and moderate diarrhea: a randomized, controlled trial. *Acta Paediatr* 1994;83:183–187.
32. Clemente YF, Tapia CC, Comino AL, et al. Lactose-free formula versus adapted formula in acute infantile diarrhea. *An Esp Pediatr* 1993;39:309–312.
33. Lozano JM, Cespedes JA. Lactose vs. lactose free regimen in children with acute diarrhoea: a randomized controlled trial. *Arch Latinoam Nutr* 1994;44:6–11.
34. Fayad IM, Hashem M, Husseine A, et al. Comparison of soy-based formulas with lactose and with sucrose in the treatment of acute diarrhoea in infants. *Arch Pediatr Adolesc Med* 1999;153:675–680.
35. Wall CR, Webster J, Quirk P, et al. The nutritional management of acute diarrhea in young infants: effect of carbohydrate ingested. *J Pediatr Gastroenterol Nutr* 1994;19:170–174.

Jacqueline Dalby-Payne
Consultant Paediatrician
The Children's Hospital at Westmead
Sydney
Australia

Elizabeth Elliott
Associate Professor
Discipline of Paediatrics and Child Health
University of Sydney
Consultant Paediatrician
The Children's Hospital at Westmead
Sydney
Australia

Competing interests: None declared.

TABLE 1 **Oral versus intravenous fluids in mild to moderate[15–21] and severe dehydration[22] (see text, p 345).**

Intervention (saline concentration in %, unless otherwise stated)	Participants (age)	Duration of diarrhoea (days)	Stay in hospital (days)	Weight gain	Stool output (mL/kg body weight)	Failure of oral treatment (defined as the need to revert to iv treatment)*
Oral versus iv fluids in mild to moderate dehydration						
ORS (90, 50) *v* iv[15]	52 children from USA and 94 children in Panama with acute diarrhoea (3–24 months)	NS	NR	NS	USA: ORS (90) *v* iv (NS); ORS (50) *v* iv (193 *v* 112; $P < 0.02$) Panama: ORS (90) *v* iv (90 *v* 168; $P < 0.001$); ORS (50) *v* iv (NS)	1/98 (1%)
ORS (60) *v* iv[16]	29 children with acute diarrhoea (3–24 months)	NR	NR	NS	NR	2/15 (13%)
ORS (75, 50) *v* iv[17]	100 children with acute diarrhoea (3–33 months)	NR	NS	NS	NR	3/50 (6%)
ORS (45, 74) *v* iv[18]	42 children with acute diarrhoea (6–31 months)	NR	NR	NS	NR	4/22 (18%)
ORS (3.5 g/L) *v* iv[19]	100 children with acute diarrhoea (mean age 11 years)	NS	NR	NS	NR	NR
ORS (75) *v* iv[20]	31 children with acute diarrhoea (mean age 4–5 years)	NS	NR	NS	NR	NR

TABLE 1 continued

Intervention (saline concentration in %, unless otherwise stated)	Participants (age)	Duration of diarrhoea (days)	Stay in hospital (days)	Weight gain	Stool output (mL/kg body weight)	Failure of oral treatment (defined as the need to revert to iv treatment)*
ORS (NR) v iv[21]	34 children with acute diarrhoea (3 months to 17 years)	NR	NR	NR	NR	3/18 (17%)
Oral versus iv fluids in severe dehydration						
ORS (80, 40) *v* iv[22]	470 children with acute diarrhoea (1–18 months)	ORS < iv (4.8 *v* 5.5; P < 0.01)	NR	ORS > iv (8.9% *v* 7.3%; P < 0.001)	NR	1/236 (0.4%)

*Although this outcome measures treatment failure of oral treatment it is not a comparative outcome as the number of children responding poorly to intravenous treatment was not recorded. iv, intravenous; NR, not reported; NS, non-significant; ORS, oral rehydration solution

TABLE 2 **Loperamide in mild to moderate dehydration: results of placebo controlled RCTs (see text, p 347).[25–29]**

Intervention (loperamide dose mg/kg/day)	Participants (age)	Duration of diarrhoea	Stay in hospital	Weight gain	Stool output
Loperamide (0.4, 0.8) *v* placebo[25]	315 children with acute diarrhoea and mild to moderate dehydration (3 months to 3 years)	L < placebo; risk of having diarrhoea at 24 hours; RR 0.83, 95% CI 0.73 to 0.94.	NS	L > placebo; children with increased weight at 3 days: loperamide 0.8 mg *v* 0.4 mg *v* placebo: 58% *v* 51% *v* 36%	NR
Loperamide (0.2) *v* placebo[26]	50 children with acute diarrhoea (1–4 years)	NS	NS	NS	NR
Loperamide (0.2) *v* placebo[27]	100 children with acute diarrhoea and mild to moderate dehydration (< 2 years)	L < placebo; 59.1 hours *v* 81.1 hours; $P < 0.05$	NR	NS	NS
Loperamide (0.4, 0.8) *v* placebo[28]	53 children with acute diarrhoea (3 months to 3 years)	NR	NR	L > placebo; children with increased weight at 3 days: loperamide 0.8 mg *v* 0.4 mg *v* placebo: 88% *v* 50% *v* 39%; RR 0.53, 95% CI 0.29 to 0.97	NR
Loperamide (0.8) *v* placebo[29]	185 children with acute gastroenteritis and mild to moderate dehydration (3–18 months).	NR	NS	NR	NR

L, loperamide; NR, not reported; NS, non-significant.

TABLE 3 **Feeds containing lactose versus lactose-free feeds in children with mild to severe dehydration: results of subsequent RCTs (see text, p 347).[31–34]**

Intervention	Participants (age)	Duration of diarrhoea	Weight gain	Total stool output (mL/kg body weight)	Treatment failure
Cow's milk *v* soy-based formula[31]	76 children with acute diarrhoea and mild to moderate dehydration (2–12 months)	L > LF; 6.6 days *v* 4.5 days; $P < 0.01$	NS	NR	NS
Lactose *v* lactose-free formula[32]	60 children with acute diarrhoea (< 1 year)	NS	NS	NR	NR
Lactose *v* lactose-free formula[33]	52 children with acute diarrhoea and mild to moderate dehydration (1–24 months)	NS	NS	NR	NS
Soy-based formula with lactose *v* soy-based formula with sucrose[34]	200 boys with acute diarrhoea (3–18 months)	L > LF; 39 hours *v* 23 hours; $P < 0.001$	NS	L > LF; mean 164 (95% CI 131 to 208) *v* 69 (95% CI 55 to 87); $P < 0.001$	NS
Lactose-free *v* low lactose *v* lactose formula[35]	91 children with acute gastroenteritis (< 24 months)	L > LF; 38 hours *v* 25 hours; $P < 0.03$	L < LF; 7.48 kg *v* 7.84 kg; $P < 0.05$	NR	NR

NR, not recorded; NS, non-significant; L, lactose-containing; LF, lactose-free.

Gastro-oesophageal reflux in children

Search date September 2003

Yadlapalli Kumar and Rajini Sarvananthan

QUESTIONS

INTERVENTIONS

*Not widely licensed for use in children. Clinical use in adults has been restricted because of heart rhythm abnormalities.

See glossary G

Key Messages

- **Feed thickeners in infants** One systematic review of feed thickeners found no RCTs in newborn infants. One RCT in infants aged 14–120 days found that a pre-thickened infant formula reduces regurgitation, choking and gagging, and coughing within a week without causing constipation. One small RCT in infants aged 1–16 weeks found no significant difference between carob flour and placebo thickening after 1 week, although the study may have lacked power to detect a clinically important difference.
- **Sodium alginate** Two RCTs in infants and in children under 2 years found that sodium alginate reduced the frequency of regurgitation at 8–14 days compared with placebo. A third small RCT of children under 17 years of age comparing sodium alginate with metoclopramide and with placebo found no significant difference between treatments.
- **Domperidone** One small RCT provided insufficient evidence about the effects of domperidone in children with gastro-oesophageal reflux.
- **H_2 antagonists** Two small RCTs provided insufficient evidence about the effects of H_2 antagonists in children with gastro-oesophagael reflux. Neither RCT reported clinically meaningful results.
- **Metoclopramide** We found insufficient evidence from three small RCTs about the clinical effects of metoclopramide compared with placebo or other treatments.
- **Proton pump inhibitors** We found no RCTs of proton pump inhibitors for gastro-oesophageal reflux in children.
- **Surgery** We found no RCTs of surgery for gastro-oesophageal reflux in children.
- **Positioning (left lateral or prone)** Three crossover RCTs in children aged under 6 months found limited evidence that prone or left lateral positioning improved oesophageal pH variables compared with supine positioning. Both prone and left lateral positions may be associated with a higher risk of sudden infant death syndrome compared with supine positioning.
- **Cisapride** One systematic review found no significant difference between cisapride and placebo in the proportion of children with improved symptoms at the end of treatment. Cisapride has been withdrawn or restricted in several countries because of an association with heart rhythm abnormalities.

Clin Evid 2005;13:354–361.

DEFINITION Gastro-oesophageal reflux disease is the passive transfer of gastric contents into the oesophagus due to transient or chronic relaxation of the lower oesophageal sphincter.[1] A survey of 69 children (median age 16 months) with gastro-oesophageal reflux disease attending a tertiary referral centre found that presenting symptoms were recurrent vomiting (72%), epigastric and abdominal pain (36%), feeding difficulties (29%), failure to thrive (28%), and irritability (19%).[2] However, results may not be generalisable to younger children or children presenting in primary care, who make up the majority of cases. Over 90% of children with gastro-oesophageal reflux disease have vomiting before 6 weeks of age.[1]

INCIDENCE/ PREVALENCE Gastro-oesophageal regurgitation is considered a problem if it is frequent, persistent, and is associated with other symptoms such as increased crying, discomfort with regurgitation, and frequent back arching.[1,3] A cross-sectional survey of parents of 948 infants attending 19 primary care paediatric practices found that regurgitation of at least one episode a day was reported in 51% of infants aged 0–3 months. "Problematic" regurgitation occurred in significantly fewer infants (14% *v* 51%; $P < 0.001$).[3] Peak regurgitation reported as "problematic" was reported in 23% of infants aged 6 months.[3]

AETIOLOGY/ RISK FACTORS Risk factors for gastro-oesophageal reflux disease include immaturity of the lower oesophageal sphincter, chronic relaxation of the sphincter, increased abdominal pressure, gastric distension, hiatus hernia, and oesophageal dysmotility.[1] Premature infants and children with severe neurodevelopmental problems or congenital oesophageal anomalies are particularly at risk.[1]

PROGNOSIS Regurgitation is considered benign, and most cases resolve spontaneously by 12–18 months of age.[4] In a cross-sectional survey of 948 parents, the peak age for reporting four or more episodes of regurgitation was at 5 months of age (23%), which decreased to 7% at 7 months ($P < 0.001$). One cohort study found that infants with frequent spilling Ⓖ in the first 2 years of life (90 days or more in the first 2 years) were more likely to have symptoms of gastro-oesophageal reflux at 9 years of age than those with no spilling (RR 2.3, 95% CI 1.3 to 4.0).[5] The prevalence of "problematic" regurgitation also reduced from 23% in infants aged 6 months to 3.25% in infants aged 10–12 months.[3] Rare complications of gastro-oesophageal reflux disease include oesophagitis with haematemesis and anaemia, respiratory problems (such as cough, apnoea, and recurrent wheeze), and failure to thrive.[1] A small comparative study (40 children) suggested that, when compared with healthy children, infants with gastro-oesophageal reflux disease had slower development of feeding skills and had problems affecting behaviour, swallowing, food intake, and mother–child interaction.[6]

AIMS OF INTERVENTION To relieve symptoms, maintain normal growth, prevent complications such as oesophagitis, and minimise adverse effects of treatment.

OUTCOMES Clinical condition (in terms of improvement in symptoms of vomiting and regurgitation); growth; parental distress; and incidence of complications (e.g. oesophagitis). Reflux Index, a measure of the percentage of time with a low oesophageal pH (frequently < pH 4), is a surrogate outcome that is often used in RCTs. Clinical interpretation of the resulting data is problematic. We have only reported Reflux Index findings where clinical outcomes are unavailable.

METHODS *Clinical Evidence* search and appraisal September 2003. The authors also searched Cinahl for studies on incidence and prevalence. Studies did not often discuss whether breastfeeding was also undertaken or withdrawn in treatment groups. Presence or absence of concomitant breastfeeding may have confounded study results.

QUESTION **What are the effects of treatments for symptomatic gastro-oesophageal reflux?**

OPTION **DIFFERENT SLEEP POSITIONS IN INFANTS**

Three crossover RCTs in children aged under 6 months found limited evidence that prone or left lateral positioning improved oesophageal pH variables compared with supine positioning. Both prone and left lateral positions may be associated with a higher risk of sudden infant death syndrome compared with supine positioning.

Benefits: We found no systematic review or RCTs on the effect of posture on clinical symptoms, but found three small crossover RCTs on the effect of posture on oesophageal pH variables such as Reflux Index.[7–9] The first RCT (crossover, 24 infants, age < 5 months) assessed four sleep positions (supine, prone, left lateral, right lateral) over 48 hours; for the first 24 hours, the infant was held horizontally, and for the remaining 24 hours the infant's head was elevated.[7] It found that the prone and left lateral positions significantly reduced the Reflux Index over 48 hours compared with the supine and right lateral positions ($P < 0.001$); it found no significant difference in the Reflux Index with horizontal positioning compared with head elevation. The second RCT (crossover, 15 infants, age < 6 months) alternated placing infants for 2 hours in a prone position (head elevated in a harness) and placing infants for 2 hours in a supine position (in an infant seat where the head and trunk were elevated to 60°) after a feed of apple juice.[8] It found that prone positioning significantly reduced the Reflux Index over 72 normal hours compared with supine positioning ($P < 0.001$). The third RCT (crossover, 18 infants, < 37 weeks gestation but > 7 days old) compared prone versus left lateral versus right lateral positions over 24 hours. It found that prone and left lateral positions significantly reduced Reflux Index compared with right lateral position ($P < 0.001$), the number of reflux episodes ($P < 0.001$), and duration of longest reflux episode ($P < 0.001$).[9]

Harms: The RCTs gave no information on adverse effects (see comment below).[7–9]

Comment: All three RCTs measured the surrogate outcome of Reflux Index, and it is difficult to interpret the clinical importance of the observed changes.[7–9] The results of these RCTs should be interpreted with caution because oesophageal pH variable may change over time, and the results were not assessed before crossover. Both prone and left lateral positioning have been associated with an increased risk of sudden infant death syndrome (see sudden infant death syndrome for prone positioning, p 434). One large, prospective cohort study found that the left lateral sleeping position compared with the supine position increased the risk of sudden infant death syndrome (at 2 months, adjusted OR 6.6, 95% CI 1.7 to 25.2).[10]

OPTION FEED THICKENERS IN INFANTS

One systematic review of feed thickeners found no RCTs in newborn infants. One RCT in infants aged 14–120 days found that a pre-thickened infant formula reduces regurgitation, choking and gagging, and coughing within a week without causing constipation. One small RCT in infants aged 1–16 weeks found no significant difference between carob flour and placebo thickening after 1 week, although the study may have lacked power to detect a clinically important difference.

Benefits: We found one systematic review (search date 2001), full-term infants < 28 days of age and preterm infants up to 44 weeks postmenstrual corrected age)[11] and two RCTs in older infants.[12,13] The review identified no RCTs that reported results separately for neonates. **Versus placebo:** The first RCT (20 infants aged 1–16 weeks with regurgitation > 5 times daily, receiving formula feeds, parental reassurance and prone positioning) compared carob flour thickened feeds with placebo thickening (Saint John's bread, which is free of fibre and polysaccharides).[12] It found no significant difference in regurgitation rates between carob flour and placebo thickening after 1 week of treatment (mean regurgitation score 2.2 with carob flour *v* 3.3 with placebo; $P = 0.14$). The second RCT (104 infants aged 14–120 days, with regurgitation ≥ 5 times a day) compared pre-thickened milk formula (Enfamil AR®) versus standard milk formula.[13] It found that thickened feed significantly reduced regurgitation after feeding and the volume regurgitated compared with placebo at 1 and 5 weeks (% decrease in feeds that were followed by regurgitation, 1 week: –34% with thickened feed *v* –22% with standard feed, P = 0.045; week 5: –38% with thickened feed *v* –24% with standard feed, P = 0.036; decrease in regurgitation volume, 1 week: –4.5% with thickened feed *v* –3.4% with standard feed, P = 0.035; week 5: –4.6% with thickened feed *v* –3.4% with standard feed, P = 0.050). It found that thickened feed significantly reduced the percentage of feeds with choke-gag reflux**G** at 1 and 5 weeks (1 week decrease from baseline: 27% with thickened feed *v* 15% with control, P = 0.004; 5 week decrease from baseline significant in favour of thickened feed: P = 0.049, no other data provided).

Harms: The second RCT (104 infants) found no significant difference in discontinuation rates between thickened feed and control (discontinuation: 13% with thickened feed *v* 20% with standard formula, P not reported).[13] It is not clear in the paper what the babies who discontinued from standard formula moved on to. One RCT (24 children, age 0–6 months with gastro-oesophageal reflux disease), assessing the effects of feed thickeners on cough, found that feeds thickened with dry rice cereal significantly increased coughing after feeding compared with isocaloric unthickened feeds (mean cough salvos/hour 3.1 with thickened feeds *v* 2.0 with unthickened feeds; P = 0.034).[14]

Comment: The clinical significance of changes in regurgitation scores in the first RCT is unclear.[12] One small crossover RCT (24 infants, age 5–11 months) found that carob flour significantly reduced a symptom score and the frequency of vomiting recorded by parents compared with traditional formula thickened with rice after 2 weeks (symptom score: mean relative reduction 70% with carob flour *v* 49% with traditional formula plus rice, P < 0.01; frequency of vomiting as recorded by parents, P < 0.05).[15] The results of this crossover RCT should be treated with caution because symptoms may change over time and the results were not assessed before crossover.[15]

OPTION SODIUM ALGINATE

Two RCTs in infants and in children under 2 years found that sodium alginate reduced the frequency of regurgitation at 8–14 days compared with placebo. A third small RCT of children under 17 years of age comparing sodium alginate with metoclopramide and with placebo found no significant difference between treatments.

Benefits: We found no systematic review but we found three RCTs.[16–18] The first RCT (90 infants aged 0–12 months attending 25 general practices) found that aluminium-free alginate reduced the number of episodes of vomiting after 14 days and increased the number of symptom free days compared with placebo (median number of episodes in previous 24 hours: 3.0 with alginate *v* 5.0 with placebo, P = 0.009; at least 10% symptom free days: 31% with alginate *v* 11% with placebo, P = 0.027).[16] The second RCT (20 children, mean age 28 months) found that sodium alginate reduced the total number of reflux episodes per 24 hours, as detected with pH monitoring, compared with baseline (episodes: alginate 131.6 at baseline to 65.0 after treatment; placebo 87 at baseline to 91 post-treatment; between treatment comparisons were not reported).[17] The third RCT (30 children aged 4 months to 17 years) found no significant difference in the frequency of regurgitation episodes over 24 hours with sodium alginate, metoclopramide, or placebo given before a meal (episode defined as pH < 4) or in Reflux Index over 24 hours (reported as non-significant; no further data reported).[18]

Harms: One RCT found no significant difference in adverse effects between aluminium-free alginate and placebo.[16] One other RCT found no adverse effects.[17]

Comment: The high sodium content of sodium alginate may be inappropriate in preterm babies.[19]

OPTION CISAPRIDE

One systematic review found no significant difference between cisapride and placebo in the proportion of children with improved symptoms or in prevalence of oesophagitis at the end of treatment. Cisapride has been withdrawn or restricted in several countries because of an association with life-threatening heart rhythm abnormalities.

Benefits: We found one systematic review (search date 2002, 10 RCTs, 415 children aged up to 5 years).[20] It found no significant difference between cisparide and placebo at 2–8 weeks in vomiting score or endoscopically confirmed oesophagitis (5 RCTs, 156 children: standardised WMD in vomiting score –0.18; 95% CI –0.51 to +0.15; oesophagitis, 2 RCTs, 37 children: RR 0.80, 95% CI 0.40 to 1.61).[20]

Harms: The systematic review found no significant difference between cisapride and placebo in adverse events (6 RCTs: RR 1.16; 95% CI 0.95 to 1.41).[20] Adverse effects included fever, insomnia, nervousness, irritability, diarrhoea, vomiting, eructations, cough, upper respiratory tract infection, and asthma. One of the included RCTs (68 children aged 6 months to 4 years) assessed mean corrected QTc on electrocardiograph and found no significant difference between cisapride and placebo.[21] See comment below.

Comment: The authors of the systematic review stated that, in view of the small number of children analysed, there was still uncertainty about the beneficial effect of cisapride. They estimated that a minimum sample size of 120 children per treatment arm would be required to detect a 30% reduction in vomiting with cisapride. Limitations in the identified RCTs included incomplete reporting of study design, lack of clear description of methods used to randomise children, and adverse effects not reported as clearly or completely as the benefits. Cisapride has been withdrawn or its use restricted in several countries because of an increased frequency of heart rhythm abnormalities that are associated with sudden death.[22] One case control study (201 children, age 1–12 months) found that cisapride significantly prolonged the QTc interval on electrocardiogram in a subgroup of infants younger than 3 months, but in older infants the difference was not significant.[23] A second case control study (252 infants) found similar results.[24] A third case control study (120 children) found prolonged QT interval in some normal children with or without cisapride.[25] Gastrointestinal adverse effects (borborygmi, cramps, and diarrhoea) occurred in 2% of infants.[23] Rash, pruritus, urticaria, bronchospasm, extrapyramidal effects, headache, dose-related increases in urinary frequency, hyperprolactinaemia, and reversible liver function abnormalities were extremely rare. Most macrolide antibiotics and cimetidine elevate plasma cisapride levels and may increase the clinical risk.[23]

OPTION DOMPERIDONE

One small RCT provided insufficient evidence about the effects of domperidone in children with gastro-oesophageal reflux.

Benefits: We found no systematic review. One small RCT (17 children, age 5 months to 11 years) found no significant difference in symptoms (vomiting, spitting, irritability, heartburn, coughing, choking), as assessed by daily parent record or Reflux Index, after 4 weeks of treatment between domperidone and placebo.[26] The RCT might have been too small to exclude a clinically important difference.

Harms: The RCT found that four children taking domperidone had mild self limiting diarrhoea compared with two children taking placebo.[26]

Comment: None.

OPTION H_2 ANTAGONISTS

Two small RCTs provided insufficient evidence about the effects of H_2 antagonists on children with gastro-oesophageal reflux.

Benefits: We found no systematic review but found two small RCTs.[27,28] The first RCT (double blind, 37 children aged 1 month to 14 years with gastro-oesophageal reflux disease complicated by oesophagitis, 32 analysed) found that cimetidine 30–40 mg/kg daily significantly increased the proportion of children who improved compared with placebo at 12 weeks (67.4% improved in clinical score from baseline with cimetidine v 29.6% with placebo; $P < 0.01$).[27] The clinical score was developed for the study and the clinical importance of this result is unclear. The second small RCT (27 children, aged 3–14 years with gastro-oesophageal reflux disease) compared different doses of cimetidine but reported only physiological outcomes (gastric pH, gastric acid suppression).[28] We found no RCTs of ranitidine in children.

Harms: The RCTs found no adverse effects.[27,28]

Comment: Both RCTs were small and provide insufficient evidence about clinical effects. Cimetidine has been reported to cause bradycardia in a small subgroup of people and may increase cisapride plasma levels.[23] Uncontrolled studies of ranitidine have reported bronchospasm, acute dystonic reactions, sinus node dysfunction, bradycardia, and vasovagal reactions.[23]

OPTION METOCLOPRAMIDE

We found insufficient evidence from three small RCTs about the clinical effects of metoclopramide compared with placebo or other treatments.

Benefits: We found no systematic review but found three RCTs.[18,29,30] The first RCT (crossover; 30 infants aged 1–9 months receiving formula feed) found that metoclopramide 1 mg/kg four times daily significantly reduced the Reflux Index over 2 weeks compared with placebo ($P < 0.001$), but it found no significant difference in average daily symptoms (see comment below).[29] A second RCT (44 infants aged under 1 year) found no significant difference in the Reflux Index at 14 days between metoclopramide 0.2 mg three times daily and placebo before a meal.[30] A third RCT (30 infants aged 4 months to 17 years) compared three treatments: metoclopramide sodium alginate, and placebo (see benefits of sodium alginate, p 357).[18]

Harms: The RCTs gave no information on adverse effects.[18,29,30]

Comment: The results of the crossover RCT should be treated with caution as it did not assess the effects of metoclopramide versus placebo before crossover.[29] In the second RCT 5/44 (11%) of infants withdrew from the study, three because of lack of efficacy and two for unknown reasons; the results given are not intention to treat.[30] One observational study (42 infants), which assessed the effect of metoclopramide 0.2 mg or 0.3 mg on pH parameters, found that metoclopramide was associated with dystonia in one infant and increased irritability in three infants.[31]

OPTION PROTON PUMP INHIBITORS

We found no RCTs of proton pump inhibitors for gastro-oesophageal reflux in children.

Benefits: We found no systematic review or RCTs on proton pump inhibitors. One small case series did not report clinical outcomes.[32]

Harms: We found no systematic review or RCTs.

Comment: Proton pump inhibitors have been reported to cause hepatitis, and omeprazole chronically elevates serum gastrin.[32]

OPTION SURGERY

We found no RCTs of surgery for gastro-oesophageal reflux in children.

Benefits: We found no systematic review or RCT.

Harms: A retrospective review (106 children) of modified Nissen's fundoplication found a failure rate of 8% and, when neurologically impaired children were included, a long term mortality of 8%.[33] If only neurologically normal children were considered, then the mortality was 2% in the immediate postoperative period and 3% on long term follow up (3 deaths in 62 children; all deaths were in children with congenital abnormalities).

Comment: We found a case series of 22 children who had undergone anterior gastric fundoplication.[34] Twenty children (91%) remained asymptomatic at 2 years. Complications of surgical treatment include dumping, retching, intestinal obstruction, "gas bloat", and recurrence of gastro-oesophageal reflux disease.[19]

GLOSSARY

Spilling When liquid or substance in small particles falls or spills out of the mouth.

Choke-gag reflux Regurgitation of food into the pharynx and upper oesophagus that causes choking and gagging as the person tries to protect the airway in an automatic reflex action.

REFERENCES

1. Herbst JJ. *Textbook of Gastroenterology and Nutrition in Infancy*. 2nd ed. New York: Raven Press, 1989:803–813.
2. Lee WS, Beattie RM, Meadows N, et al. Gastro-oesophageal reflux: Clinical profiles and outcome. *J Paediatr Child Health* 1999;35:568–571.
3. Nelson SP, Chen EH, Syniar GM, et al. Prevalence of symptoms of gastroesophageal reflux during infancy. *Arch Pediatr Adolesc Med* 1997;151:569–572.
4. Vandenplas Y, Belli D, Benhamou P, et al. A critical appraisal of current management practices for infant regurgitation — recommendations of a working party. *Eur J Pediatr* 1997;156:343–357.
5. Martin JA, Pratt N, Kennedy D, et al. Natural history and familial relationships of infant spilling to 9 years of age. *Paediatrics* 2002;109:1061–1067.
6. Mathisen B, Worrall L, Masel J, et al. Feeding problems in infants with gastro-oesophageal reflux disease: a controlled study. *J Paediatr Child Health* 1999;35:163–169.
7. Tobin JM, McCloud P, Cameron DJS. Posture and gastro-oesophageal reflux: a case for left lateral positioning. *Arch Dis Child* 1997;76:254–258.
8. Orenstein SR, Whitington PF. Positioning for prevention of infant gastroesophageal reflux. *J Pediatr* 1983;103:534–537.
9. Ewer AK, James ME, Tobin JM. Prone and left lateral positioning reduce gastro-oesophageal reflux in preterm infants. *Arch Dis Child Fetal Neonatal Ed* 1999;81:F201–205.

10. Dwyer T, Ponsonby AB, Newman NM, et al. Prospective cohort study of prone sleeping position and sudden infant death syndrome. *Lancet* 1991;337:1244–1247.
11. Huang RC, Forbes DA, Davies MW. Feed thickener for newborn infants with gastro-oesophageal reflux. In: The Cochrane Library, Issue 3, 2003. Oxford: Update software. Search date 2001; primary sources Medline, Cochrane Controlled Trials Register, Cochrane Library, Cinahl, conference and symposia proceedings published in *Paediatric Research* 1990–1994, and conference proceedings for the European Society for Paediatric Gastroenterology and Nutrition and the North American Society for Paediatric Gastroenterology and Nutrition.
12. Vandenplas Y, Hachimi-Idrissi S, Casteels A, et al. A clinical trial with an "anti-regurgitation" formula. *Eur J Pediatr* 1994;153:419–423.
13. Vanderhoof JA, Moran JR, Harris CL, Merkel KL, Orenstein SR. Efficacy of a pe-thickened infant formula: a multicenter, double-blind, randomized, placebo-controlled parallel group trial in 104 infants with symptomatic gastroesophageal reflux. *Clin Pediatr* 2003;42:483–495.
14. Orenstein SR, Shalaby TM, Putnam PE. Thickening feedings as a cause of increased coughing when used as therapy for gastroesophageal reflux in infants. *J Pediatr* 1992;121:913–915.
15. Borrelli O, Salvia G, Campanozzi A, et al. Use of a new thickened formula for treatment of symptomatic gastroesophageal reflux in infants. *Ital J Gastroenterol Hepatol* 1997;29:237–242.
16. Miller S. Comparison of the efficacy and safety of a new aluminium-free paediatric alginate preparation and placebo in infants with recurrent gastro-oesophageal reflux. *Curr Med Res Opin* 1999;15:160–168.
17. Buts JP, Barudi C, Otte JB. Double-blind controlled study on the efficacy of sodium alginate (Gaviscon) in reducing gastroesophageal reflux assessed by 24 hour continuous pH monitoring in infants and children. *Eur J Pediatr* 1987;146:156–158.
18. Forbes D, Hodgson M, Hill, R. The effects of gaviscon and metoclopramide in gastroesophageal reflux in children. *J Pediatr Gastroenterol Nutr* 1986;5:556–559.
19. Davies AEM, Sandhu BK. Diagnosis and treatment of gastro-oesophageal reflux. *Arch Dis Child* 1995;73:82–86.
20. Dalby-Payne JR, Morris AM, Craig JC. Meta-analysis of randomized controlled trials on the benefits and risks of using cisapride for the treatment of gastroesophageal reflux in children. *J Gastroenterol Hepatol* 2003;18:196–202. Search date 2002. Primary sources Medline, Embase, Cochrane Controlled Trials Register, bibliographies of identified trials and correspondence with manufacturer.
21. Levy J, Hayes C, Kern J et al. Does cisapride influence cardiac rhythm? Results of a United States multicenter, double-blind, placebo-controlled paediatric study. *J Pediatr Gastroenterol Nutr* 2001;32: 458–63.
22. WHO Pharmaceuticals Newsletter, No.3, 2000. http://www.who.int/medicines/library/pnewslet/pn32000.html (last accessed 17 February 2004).
23. Vandenplas Y, Belli DC, Benatar A, et al. The role of cisapride in the treatment of pediatric gastroesophageal reflux. *J Pediatr Gastroenterol Nutr* 1999;28:518–528.
24. Benatar A, Feenstra A, Decraene T, et al. Effects of cisapride on corrected QT interval, heart rate, and rhythm in infants undergoing polysomnography. *Pediatrics* 2000;106:E85.
25. Ramirez-Mayans J, Garrido-Garcia LM, Huerta-Tecanhuey A, et al. Cisapride and QTc interval in children. *Pediatrics* 2000;106:1028–1030.
26. Bines JE, Quinlan JE, Treves S, et al. Efficacy of domperidone in infants and children with gastroesophageal reflux. *J Pediatr Gastroenterol Nutr* 1992;14:400–405.
27. Cucchiara S, Gobio-Casali L, Balli F, et al. Cimetidine treatment of reflux esophagitis in children: An Italian multicentre study. *J Pediatr Gastroenterol Nutr* 1989;8:150–156.
28. Lambert J, Mobassaleh M, Grand RJ. Efficacy of cimetidine for gastric acid suppression in pediatric patients. *J Pediatr* 1992;120:474–478.
29. Tolia V, Calhoun J, Kuhns L, et al. Randomized, double-blind trial of metoclopramide and placebo for gastroesophageal reflux. *J Pediatr* 1989;115:141–145.
30. Bellisant E, Duhamel JF, Guillot M, et al. The triangular test to assess the efficacy of metoclopramide in gastroesophageal reflux. *Clin Pharm Ther* 1997;61:377–384.
31. Hyams JS, Leichtner AM, Zamett LO, et al. Effect of metoclopramide on prolonged intraoesophageal pH testing in infants with gastroesophageal reflux. *J Pediatr Gastroenterol Nutr* 1986;5:716–720.
32. Gunasekaran TS, Hassall EG. Efficacy and safety of omeprazole for severe gastroesophageal reflux in children. *J Pediatr* 1993;123:148–154.
33. Spillane AJ, Currie B, Shi E. Fundoplication in children: Experience with 106 cases. *Aust NZ J Surg* 1996;66:753–756.
34. Bliss D, Hirschl R, Oldham K, et al. Efficacy of anterior gastric fundoplication in the treatment of gastroesophageal reflux in infants and children. *J Paediatr Surg* 1994;29:1071–1075.

Yadlapalli Kumar
Consultant Paediatrician
Royal Cornwall Hospital
Treliske
Truro
Cornwall
UK

Rajini Sarvananthan
Lecturer in Paediatrics
Faculty of Medicine
Universiti Kebangsaan Malaysia
Kuala Lumpar
Malaysia

Competing interests: None declared.

Infantile colic

Search date September 2004

Teresa Kilgour and Sally Wade

QUESTIONS

INTERVENTIONS

Key Messages

Treatments

- **Whey hydrolysate milk** One small RCT found limited evidence that replacing cows' milk formula with whey hydrolysate formula reduced crying recorded in a parental diary.
- **Dicycloverine (dicyclomine)** Two systematic reviews of RCTs of variable quality found limited evidence that dicycloverine reduced crying in infants with colic compared with placebo. RCTs found that dicycloverine increased drowsiness, constipation, and loose stools compared with placebo, but the difference did not reach significance. Case reports of harms in infants have included breathing difficulties, seizures, syncope, asphyxia, muscular hypotonia, and coma.
- **Advice to reduce stimulation** One RCT found limited evidence that advice to reduce stimulation (by not patting, lifting, or jiggling the baby, or by reducing auditory stimulation) reduced crying after 7 days in infants under 12 weeks compared with an empathetic interview giving no advice. However, we were unable to draw reliable conclusions from this small study.
- **Car ride simulation** One RCT found no significant difference between car ride simulation plus reassurance; counselling mothers about specific management techniques (responding to crying with gentle soothing motion, avoiding over stimulation, using a pacifier, and prophylactic carrying) plus reassurance; and reassurance alone, in terms of maternal anxiety or hours of infant crying over 2 weeks.
- **Casein hydrolysate milk** Two RCTs found insufficient evidence about the effects of replacing cows' milk formula with casein hydrolysate hypoallergenic formula. Another small RCT found that substituting soya or cows' milk with casein hydroysate formula was less effective at reducing the duration and extent of crying with focused counselling.
- **Cranial osteopathy** We found no RCTs on the effects of cranial osteopathy in infants with colic.

- **Focused counselling** One RCT found no significant difference between counselling mothers about specific management techniques (responding to crying with gentle soothing motion, avoiding over stimulation, using a pacifier, and prophylactic carrying) plus reassurance; car ride simulation plus reassurance; and reassurance alone, in terms of maternal anxiety or hours of infant crying over 2 weeks. Another small RCT found that counselling decreased the duration and extent of crying compared with substitution of soya or cows' milk with casein hydrolysate formula.
- **Herbal tea** One small RCT found that herbal tea (containing extracts of camomile, vervain, licorice, fennel, and balm mint in a sucrose solution) improved symptoms of colic rated by parents at 7 days compared with sucrose solution alone. However, we were unable to draw reliable conclusions from this small study.
- **Infant massage** One RCT found no significant difference between massage and a crib vibrator for colic related crying or parental rating of symptoms of infantile colic, but it may have lacked power to detect a clinically important difference.
- **Low lactose milk** Four small crossover RCTs provided insufficient evidence on the effects of low lactose milk in infants with colic.
- **Soya based infant feeds** One small RCT found that soya based infant feeds reduced the duration of crying in infants with colic compared with standard cows' milk formula. However, we were unable to draw reliable conclusions from this small study.
- **Spinal manipulation** Two RCTs found insufficient evidence about the effects of spinal manipulation.
- **Sucrose solution** One small crossover RCT found limited evidence that sucrose solution improved symptoms of colic as rated by parents after 12 days compared with placebo. However, we were unable to draw reliable conclusions from this small study.
- **Advice to increase carrying** One RCT found no significant difference in daily crying time between advice to carry the infant, even when not crying, for at least an additional 3 hours a day and general advice (to carry, check baby's nappy, feed, offer pacifier, place baby near mother, or use background stimulation such as music).
- **Simethicone (activated dimeticone)** One RCT found no significant difference between simethicone and placebo in colic rated by carers. Another RCT found no significant difference between simethicone and placebo in improvement as rated by parental interview, 24 hour diary, or behavioural observation. Another poor quality RCT found that simethicone reduced the number of crying attacks on days 4–7 of treatment compared with placebo. One RCT found insufficient evidence to compare simethicone with spinal manipulation.

DEFINITION Infantile colic is defined as excessive crying in an otherwise healthy baby. The crying typically starts in the first few weeks of life and ends by 4–5 months. Excessive crying is defined as crying that lasts at least 3 hours a day, for 3 days a week, for at least 3 weeks.[1] Due to the natural course of infantile colic, it can be difficult to interpret trials which do not include a placebo or have no treatment group for comparison.

INCIDENCE/ PREVALENCE Infantile colic causes one out of six families (17%) to consult a health professional. One systematic review of 15 community based studies found a wide variation in prevalence, which depended on study design and method of recording.[2] Two prospective studies identified by the review yielded prevalence rates of 5% and 19%.[2] One RCT (89 breast and formula fed infants) found that, at 2 weeks of age, the prevalence of crying more than 3 hours a day was 43% among formula fed infants and 16% among breast fed infants. The prevalence at 6 weeks was 12% (formula fed) and 31% (breast fed).[3]

AETIOLOGY/ RISK FACTORS The cause is unclear and, despite its name, infantile colic may not have an abdominal cause. It may reflect part of the normal distribution of infantile crying. Other possible explanations are painful intestinal contractions, lactose intolerance, gas, or parental misinterpretation of normal crying.[1]

PROGNOSIS Infantile colic improves with time. One study found that 29% of infants aged 1–3 months cried for more than 3 hours a day, but by 4–6 months of age the prevalence had fallen to 7–11%.[4]

AIMS OF INTERVENTION	To reduce infant crying and distress, and the anxiety of the family, with minimal adverse effects of treatment.
OUTCOMES	Presence and duration of colic, as determined by frequency and duration of crying, measured on dichotomous, ordinal, or continuous scales; parents' perceptions of severity, recorded in a diary.
METHODS	*Clinical Evidence* search and appraisal September 2004. The contributors also searched Cinahl up to 1999 for publications using reduction in crying or colic as the main outcome. Trials were excluded for the following reasons: infants studied had normal crying patterns, infants were older than 6 months, interventions lasted less than 3 days, trials had no control groups, or had low scores on the Jadad scale❻.[5]

QUESTION **What are the effects of treatments for infantile colic?**

OPTION **DICYCLOVERINE (DICYCLOMINE)**

Two systematic reviews of RCTs of variable quality found limited evidence that dicycloverine reduced crying in infants with colic compared with placebo. RCTs found that dicycloverine increased drowsiness, constipation, and loose stools compared with placebo, but the difference did not reach significance. Case reports of harms in infants have included breathing difficulties, seizures, syncope, asphyxia, muscular hypotonia, and coma.

Benefits: We found two systematic reviews.[1,6] The first systematic review (search date 1996)[1] identified five RCTs (134 infants) comparing the effect of dicycloverine❻ versus placebo on crying or the presence of colic. It found that dicycloverine (most frequently 5 mg 4 times daily) significantly reduced crying over about 1 week's treatment compared with placebo (5 RCTs; effect size 0.46, 95% CI 0.33 to 0.60).[1] The clinical importance of this result is unclear (see comment below). The second systematic review (search date 1999)[6] identified three RCTs included in the first systematic review,[1] but did not pool results. One RCT[7] identified by the review found that dicycloverine significantly reduced colic compared with placebo (cherry syrup) (elimination of colic: 63% with dicycloverine *v* 25% with placebo; RR 0.50, 95% CI 0.28 to 0.88).[6] The other two RCTs identified by the review used definitions of colic that included symptoms but not duration and frequency, and reported results in terms of clinical scores.[6] The review reported that both RCTs found significantly better mean clinical scores with dicycloverine compared with placebo (P values not reported).

Harms: Two of five RCTs[8,9] in the systematic reviews[1,6] assessed harms of dicycloverine❻ compared with placebo. The first RCT (crossover design, 30 infants) found more drowsiness with dicycloverine compared with placebo (4/30 [13%] with dicycloverine *v* 1/30 [3%] with placebo; ARI +10%, 95% CI –4% to +24%).[8] The second RCT (crossover design, 25 infants) found more loose stools or constipation in infants taking dicycloverine compared with placebo (3/25 [12%] with dicycloverine *v* 1/25 [4%] with placebo; ARI +8%, 95% CI –7% to +23%).[9] Case reports of harms in infants have included breathing difficulties, seizures, syncope, asphyxia, muscular hypotonia, and coma.[10]

Comment: The first review is limited because it pooled different outcome measures from RCTs and included crossover studies that only report outcomes after crossover.[1] The crossover design is unlikely to provide valid evidence because infantile colic has a naturally variable course, and the effects of dicycloverine❻ may continue even after a washout period.[11] Only one RCT identified by the reviews stated measures to make the control syrup taste the same as the drug syrup.[8]

OPTION SIMETHICONE (ACTIVATED DIMETICONE [DIMETHICONE])

One RCT found no significant difference between simethicone and placebo in colic rated by carers. Another RCT found no significant difference between simethicone and placebo in improvement as rated by parental interview, 24 hour diary, or behavioural observation. Another poor quality RCT found that simethicone reduced the number of crying attacks on days 4–7 of treatment compared with placebo. One RCT found insufficient evidence to compare simethicone with spinal manipulation.

Benefits: **Versus placebo:** We found two systematic reviews (search dates 1996,[1] 1999,[6] same 3 RCTs in each review, 136 infants) comparing the effect of simethicone🅖 versus placebo on the duration of crying or the presence of colic. The first RCT identified by the reviews (double blind, crossover, 83 infants aged 2–8 weeks) compared 0.3 mL of simethicone versus placebo before feeds.[12] It found no significant difference in colic when rated by carers (28% improved with simethicone *v* 37% with placebo *v* 20% with both; effect size for simethicone versus placebo –0.10, 95% CI –0.27 to +0.08).[1,12] The second RCT identified by the reviews (double blind, crossover trial, 27 infants aged 2–8 weeks) found no significant difference between simethicone and placebo in improvement as rated by parental interview, 24 hour diary, or behavioural observation (effect size +0.06, 95% CI –0.17 to +0.28) (see comment below).[1,13] The third, poor quality, RCT identified by the reviews (26 infants aged 1–12 weeks) reported no details on how cases of colic were defined.[14] It found that simethicone significantly reduced the number of crying attacks on days 4–7 of treatment compared with placebo (effect size 0.54, 95% CI 0.21 to 0.87).[1,14] **Versus spinal manipulation:** See benefits of spinal manipulation, p 370.

Harms: **Versus placebo:** None of the RCTs reported adverse effects with either simethicone🅖 or placebo.[12–14] **Versus spinal manipulation:** See benefits of spinal manipulation.

Comment: The crossover design of two of the RCTs limits their validity, as they did not report results before crossover and infantile colic has a naturally variable course; therefore the effects of simethicone🅖 may continue even after a washout period.[12,13]

OPTION SOYA BASED INFANT FEEDS (COMPARED WITH COWS' MILK)

One small RCT found that soya based infant feeds reduced the duration of crying in infants with colic compared with standard cows' milk formula. However, we were unable to draw reliable conclusions from this small study.

Benefits: We found two systematic reviews (search dates 1996[1] and 1999,[6] 2 RCTs). One RCT (19 infants) included in the review found that soya based infant feeds🅖 significantly reduced the duration of crying compared with standard cows' milk formula (4.3–12.7 hours with soya based infant feeds *v* 17.3–20.1 hours with cows' milk; mean difference –10.3 hours, 95% CI –16.2 hours to –4.3 hours) (see comment below).[15] The second RCT in the review provided insufficient evidence, as it considered infants admitted to hospital for colic and used weak methods (Jadad scale 1🅖).[16]

Harms: No harms were reported in the RCTs.[15,16]

Comment: In the first RCT, mothers were not told which milk the babies received, but differences between the milks may have been detected from smell and texture.[15] We were unable to draw reliable conclusions from the second small RCT.

OPTION CASEIN HYDROLYSATE MILK (COMPARED WITH COWS' MILK)

Two RCTs found insufficient evidence about the effects of replacing cows' milk formula with casein hydrolysate hypoallergenic formula. Another small RCT found that substituting soya or cows' milk with casein hydroysate formula was less effective at reducing the duration and extent of crying with focused counselling.

Benefits: **Versus cows' milk:** We found two systematic reviews (search dates 1996[1] and 1999[6]), which identified the same two RCTs.[17,18] The first RCT (double blind, crossover, 17 infants) included in the reviews studied the effect of each of three changes of infant diet over 4 days.[17] Bottle fed infants received casein hydrolysate milk**G** and cows' milk alternately. By the third change, it found no notable difference in the incidence of colic between groups. A total of 8/17 (47%) infants left the study before completion. The second RCT (122 infants) included in the reviews compared bottle fed infants (38 infants) given casein hydrolysate milk (active diet) versus cows' milk formula, and breast fed infants (77 infants) with mothers on a hypoallergenic diet**G** (active diet) versus controls on an unmodified diet.[18] A total of 54 infants received the active diet, but the RCT did not specify which of these were bottle fed and which were breast fed. The RCT pooled the results of breast and bottle fed babies and found that the active diet reduced infant distress as measured by parents on a validated chart compared with control diet (distress reduction: 39% [95% CI 25% to 50%] with active diet *v* 16% [95% CI 0% to 30%] with control diet; P = 0.012). The number of bottle fed infants was too small to establish or exclude important effects in infants bottle fed casein hydrolysate milk versus cows' milk. **Casein hydrolysate milk versus counselling:** See benefits of focused counselling, p 368.

Harms: No harms were reported in the RCTs.[17,18]

Comment: None.

OPTION WHEY HYDROLYSATE FORMULA (COMPARED WITH COWS' MILK FORMULA)

One small RCT found limited evidence that replacing cows' milk formula with whey hydrolysate formula reduced crying recorded in a parental diary.

Benefits: We found two systematic reviews (search dates 1996[1] and 1999[6]) and one subsequent RCT.[19] The systematic reviews found no RCTs of adequate quality. The subsequent, double blind RCT (43 infants) found that whey hydrolysate formula**G** reduced the time that babies cried each day compared with standard cows' milk formula, measured by a validated parental diary (crying reduced by 63 minutes/day, 95% CI 1 minute/day to 127 minutes/day; P = 0.05).[19] Parents may not have been blind to the intervention. When asked, six indicated that they were aware of allocation, but two of these falsely identified the formula. When these infants' results were removed from the analysis, the crying time with whey hydrolysate formula was still significantly reduced compared with standard cows' milk formula (crying reduced by 58 minutes/day; P = 0.03).[19]

Harms: No harms were identified in the subsequent RCT.[19]

Comment: None.

OPTION LOW LACTOSE (LACTASE TREATED) MILK

Four small crossover RCTs provided insufficient evidence on the effects of low lactose milk in infants with colic.

Benefits: We found two systematic reviews (search dates 1996[1] and 1999,[6] 2 RCTs) and two additional RCTs.[20,21] The first RCT included in the reviews (double blind, crossover, 10 weaned infants) compared four interventions: bottle feeding using pooled breast milk; low lactose (lactase treated) breast milk; cows' milk; and low lactose (lactase treated) cows' milk.[22] It found no evidence that low lactose milk reduced the timing, severity, or duration of colic recorded by parents lactase treated milks, ($P > 0.05$; compared with all measures).[22] The second RCT (12 breast fed infants) included in the reviews compared low lactose versus placebo drops given within 5 minutes of feeding.[6] It found no significant difference in time spent feeding, sleeping, or crying. The first additional RCT (crossover, 13 infants) compared low lactose milk versus placebo treated milk.[20] It found a significant reduction in crying time with low lactose milk (1.1 hours/day, 95% CI 0.2 hours/day to 2.1 hours/day); however, caution should be applied in interpreting the results because of the small number of infants in the trial and the crossover design (see comments below). The second additional RCT (crossover, 53 infants) found that low lactose formula/breast milk reduced crying time after crossover at 25 days compared with untreated formula/breast milk, but the difference was not significant (median 11.0 hours with lactase *v* 14.1 hours with no lactase; median difference in crying time 23%; $P = 0.09$).[21]

Harms: No harms were reported in the RCTs.[1,6,20,21]

Comment: It is difficult to draw firm conclusions from these RCTs.[1,6,20,21] The babies were not selected on the basis of confirmed lactose intolerance. The crossover design of three of the RCTs limits their validity and clinical utility because infantile colic has a naturally variable course.[20–22]

OPTION SUCROSE SOLUTION

One small crossover RCT found limited evidence that sucrose solution improved symptoms of colic as rated by parents after 12 days compared with placebo. However, we were unable to draw reliable conclusions from this small study.

Benefits: We found one systematic review (search date 1999,[6] 1 RCT[23]). The small crossover RCT (19 infants) included in the review compared 2 mL of 12% sucrose solution versus placebo given to babies when they continued to cry despite comforting.[23] Parents, blind to the intervention, scored the effect of the treatment on a scale of 1–5. Treatments were crossed over after 3–4 days and again after 6–8 days. The RCT found that sucrose significantly increased parent rated improvement after 12 days compared with placebo (12/19 [63%] with sucrose *v* 1/19 [5%] with placebo; ARI 58%, 95% CI 10% to 89%; NNT 2, 95% CI 1 to 10; RR 12, 95% CI 3 to 19; see comment below).[23]

Harms: No harms were reported in the RCT.[23]

Comment: We were unable to draw reliable conclusions from this study because of the small sample size and crossover study design.

OPTION HERBAL TEA

One small RCT found that herbal tea (containing extracts of camomile, vervain, licorice, fennel, and balm mint in a sucrose solution) improved symptoms of colic rated by parents at 7 days compared with sucrose solution alone. However, we were unable to draw reliable conclusions from this small study.

Benefits: We found two systematic reviews (search dates 1996[1] and 1999,[6] 1 RCT[24]). The RCT (68 infants) included in the reviews compared herbal tea (containing extracts of camomile, vervain, licorice, fennel, and balm mint in a sucrose solution) versus sucrose solution alone given by parents up to three times daily in response to episodes of colic (see comment below).[24] Allocation was known only to the pharmacist, and the taste and smell of the tea and placebo were similar. Parents rated the response using a symptom diary. The RCT found that, at 7 days, herbal tea eliminated colic significantly more frequently than sucrose solution (number of colic free infants: 19/33 [58%] with herbal tea *v* 9/35 [26%] with sucrose; ARI 32%, 95% CI 7% to 53%; RR 2.2, 95% CI 1.3 to 3.1; NNT 3, 95% CI 2 to 14).

Harms: No harms were reported in the RCT.[24]

Comment: The RCT did not state the exact proportion of the herbs used in the preparation.[24] We were unable to draw reliable conclusions from this study due to small sample size.

OPTION FOCUSED COUNSELLING

One RCT found no significant difference between counselling mothers about specific management techniques (responding to crying with gentle soothing motion, avoiding over stimulation, using a pacifier, and prophylactic carrying) plus reassurance; car ride simulation plus reassurance; and reassurance alone, in terms of maternal anxiety or hours of infant crying over 2 weeks. Another small RCT found that counselling decreased the duration and extent of crying compared with substitution of soya or cows' milk with casein hydrolysate formula.

Benefits: **Counselling plus reassurance versus car ride simulation plus reassurance versus reassurance alone:** We found two systematic reviews (search dates 1996[1] and 1999,[6] 1 RCT). The RCT (38 infants) assessed maternal anxiety and the hours of crying each day by questionnaire.[25] The RCT compared three interventions: counselling mothers about specific management techniques (responding to crying with gentle soothing motion, avoiding over stimulation, using a pacifier, and prophylactic carrying) plus reassurance**G** and support; car ride simulation device plus reassurance and support; and reassurance and support alone. It found no significant difference among groups in maternal anxiety or hours of infant crying over 2 weeks (mean hours of crying: results presented graphically, P value not provided; mean maternal anxiety score: results presented graphically, P value not provided).[25]
Counselling versus elimination of cows' milk protein: We found two systematic reviews (search dates 1996[1] and 1999,[6], 1 RCT). The RCT (20 infants) found that counselling parents to respond to their baby's cries by feeding, holding, offering a pacifier, stimulating, or putting the baby down to sleep, decreased the duration and extent of crying significantly more than substitution of soya or cows' milk with casein hydrolysate**G** formula (mean decrease in crying, recorded by parent diary, 2.1 hours/day with counselling *v* 1.2 hours/day with dietary change; P = 0.05).[26]

Harms: No harms were reported in the RCTs.[25,26]

Comment: None.

OPTION CAR RIDE SIMULATION

One RCT found no significant difference between car ride simulation plus reassurance; counselling mothers about specific management techniques (responding to crying with gentle soothing motion, avoiding over stimulation, using a pacifier, and prophylactic carrying) plus reassurance; and reassurance alone, in terms of maternal anxiety or hours of infant crying over 2 weeks.

Benefits: **Car ride simulation plus reassurance versus counselling plus reassurance versus reassurance alone:** See benefits of focused counselling, p 368.

Harms: **Car ride simulation plus reassurance versus counselling plus reassurance versus reassurance alone:** See harms of focused counselling, p 366. No harms were reported in the RCT.[25]

Comment: None.

OPTION ADVICE TO INCREASE CARRYING

One RCT found no significant difference in daily crying time between advice to carry the infant, even when not crying, for at least an additional 3 hours a day and general advice (to carry, check baby's nappy, feed, offer pacifier, place baby near mother, or use background stimulation such as music).

Benefits: **Advice to increase carrying versus general advice:** We found two systematic reviews (search dates 1996[1] and 1999,[6] 1 RCT). The RCT (66 infants) included in the reviews compared advising mothers of babies with colic to carry their infant, even when not crying, for at least an additional 3 hours a day versus general advice (to carry, check baby's nappy, feed, offer pacifier, place baby near mother, or use background stimulation such as music).[27] Women in the "advice to carry" group carried their babies for 4.5 hours daily compared with 2.6 hours daily in the general advice group. The RCT found no significant difference in daily crying time (mean difference 3 minutes less, 95% CI 37 minutes less to 32 minutes more).[27]

Harms: No harms were reported in the RCT.[27]

Comment: None.

OPTION ADVICE TO REDUCE STIMULATION

One RCT found limited evidence that advice to reduce stimulation (by not patting, lifting, or jiggling the baby, or by reducing auditory stimulation) reduced crying after 7 days in infants under 12 weeks compared with an empathetic interview giving no advice. However, we were unable to draw reliable conclusions from this small study.

Benefits: **Advice to reduce stimulation versus no advice:** We found two systematic reviews (search dates 1996[1] and 1999,[6] 1 RCT). The RCT (42 infants, median age 10 weeks) included in the reviews compared advising mothers to reduce stimulation (by not patting, lifting, or jiggling the baby, or reducing auditory stimulation) versus empathetic interview giving no advice.[28] For infants under 12 weeks, advice to reduce stimulation significantly improved a change rating scale for more infants compared with no advice (after 7 days: 14/15 [93%] improved with advice *v* 6/12 [50%] with control; ARI 43%, 95% CI 8% to 49%; RR 1.9,

95% CI 1.2 to 2.0; NNT 2, 95% CI 2 to 13).[28] Improvement in the change rating scale was defined as a score of +2 or better on a scale from –5 to +5 that indicated a perceived change in crying since the start of the trial. It is unclear whether this scale has been validated (see comment below).

Harms: No harms were reported in the RCT.[28]

Comment: Mothers given advice to reduce stimulation were also given permission to leave their infants if they felt that they could no longer tolerate the crying. It is unclear whether the improved change score represents a true change in the hours that the baby cried, or altered maternal perception.

OPTION CRANIAL OSTEOPATHY

We found no RCTs on the effects of cranial osteopathy in infants with colic.

Benefits: We found no systematic review and no RCTs on the effects of cranial osteopathy**G** in infants with colic.

Harms: We found no RCTs.

Comment: None.

OPTION INFANT MASSAGE

One RCT found no significant difference between massage and a crib vibrator for colic related crying or parental rating of symptoms of infantile colic, but it may have lacked power to detect a clinically important difference.

Benefits: **Versus usual care:** We found no systematic reviews or RCTs. **Versus other care:** We found no systematic reviews. We found one RCT (58 infants, 47% with colic; see comment below) comparing massage versus a crib vibrator over a 4 week period.[29] Infant massage (performed 3 times daily) included gentle stroking of the skin over different parts of the head, body, and limbs, using olive oil and while maintaining eye contact. The crib vibrator was used for 25 minute periods at least three times daily (see comment below). Colic symptom ratings were obtained from parental diaries of crying. The RCT found no significant difference between massage and a crib vibrator for colic related crying or parental rating of symptoms (AR for less colicky crying: 64% with massage *v* 52% with crib vibrator; P = 0.24).[29]

Harms: No harms were reported in the RCT.[29]

Comment: Only 47% of infants in the RCT had colic, so the results may not apply specifically to infants with colic.[29] The RCT stated that "use of a crib vibrator was chosen for control intervention or placebo treatment because it had been ineffective in a previous study".[29] It is unclear whether reduced crying in this RCT reflects the natural course of infantile colic or the specific effect of interventions.[29] The RCT may have lacked power to detect clinically important effects.

OPTION SPINAL MANIPULATION

Two RCTs found insufficient evidence about the effects of spinal manipulation.

Benefits: **Versus simethicone (activated dimeticone [dimethicone]):** We found no systematic review. We found one RCT (41 infants), which compared 2 weeks of spinal manipulation**G** versus 2 weeks of daily treatment with simethicone**G**; parents recorded length of crying in a colic diary.[30] The RCT found that spinal manipulation significantly reduced crying compared with simethicone (mean reduction in crying for days 4–7: 2.4 hours with spinal manipulation *v* 1.0 hours with simethicone; P = 0.04).[30] Parents were not blinded to treatment allocation. **Versus holding:** We found no systematic review. We found one RCT (86 infants), which compared spinal palpation by a chiropractor versus holding of the infant by a nurse (in each case 3 times over 8 days).[31] The parents, who were blind to the intervention, rated symptom severity on a five point scale and recorded crying in a diary. The RCT found no significant difference between spinal palpation and holding for crying reduction (by day 8, mean reduction 3.1 hours for both groups; P = 0.98).

Harms: No harms were reported in the RCTs.[30,31]

Comment: It is unclear whether reduced crying reflected the effects of interventions or spontaneous improvement.

GLOSSARY

Casein hydrolysate milk Contains casein protein; it is used in the same way as soya based infant feeds.
Cranial osteopathy Involves gentle manipulation of the tissues of the head by an osteopath.
Dicycloverine (dicyclomine) This has direct antispasmodic action on the gastrointestinal tract and anticholinergic effects, which are similar to atropine.
Hypoallergenic diet In bottle fed infants, a hypoallergenic diet uses a casein hydrolysate formula. In breast fed infants, a hypoallergenic diet involves a maternal diet free of artificial colourings, preservatives, and additives, and low in common allergens (e.g. milk, egg, wheat, and nuts).
Jadad scale This measures factors that have an impact on trial quality. Poor description of the factors, rated by low figures, is associated with greater estimates of effect. The scale includes three items: was the study described as randomised? (0–2); was the study described as double blind? (0–2); was there a description of withdrawals and dropouts? (0–1).[5]
Reassurance Informing the parent that infantile colic is a self limiting condition resolving by 3–4 months of age, and is not caused by disease or any fault in parental care.
Simethicone (activated dimeticone [dimethicone]) This has defoaming properties, which can aid dispersion of gas in the gastrointestinal tract.
Soya based infant feeds Contain proteins from soya beans; the feeds are used as lactose free vegetable milks for those with lactose or cows' milk protein intolerance.
Spinal manipulation Chiropractic manual treatment of the infant's vertebral column.
Whey hydrolysate milk Contains whey protein; it is used in the same way as soya based infant feeds

REFERENCES

1. Lucassen PLBJ, Assendelft WJJ, Gubbels JW, et al. Effectiveness of treatments for infantile colic: a systematic review. *BMJ* 1998;316:1563–1569. Search date 1996: primary sources Cochrane Controlled Trials Register, Embase, Medline, and hand searches of reference lists.
2. Lucassen PLBJ, Assendelft WJJ, Van Eijk JTHM, et al. Systematic review of the occurrence of infantile colic in the community. *Arch Dis Child* 2001;84:398–403. Search date 1998; primary sources Embase and Medline.
3. Lucas A, St James-Roberts I. Crying, fussing and colic behaviour in breast and bottle-fed infants. *Early Hum Dev* 1998;53:9–19.
4. St James-Roberts I, Halil A. Infant crying patterns in the first year: normal community and clinical findings. *J Child Psychol Psychiatry* 1991;32:951–968.
5. Jadad AR, Moore RA, Carroll D, et al. Assessing the quality of reports of randomized clinical trials: is blinding necessary? *Control Clin Trials* 1996;17:1–12.
6. Garrison MM, Christakis DA. A systematic review of treatments for infant colic. *Pediatrics* 2000;106:184–190. Search date 1999; primary sources Medline, Cochrane Clinical Trials Registry, hand searches of reference lists, and authors.
7. Weissbluth M, Christoffel KK, Davis AT. Treatment of infantile colic with dicyclomine hydrochloride. *J Pediatr* 1984:104:951–955.
8. Hwang CP, Danielsson B. Dicyclomine hydrochloride in infantile colic. *BMJ* 1985;291:1014.
9. Gruinseit F. Evaluation of the efficacy of dicyclomine hydrochloride ("Merbentyl") syrup in the treatment of infantile colic. *Curr Med Res Opin* 1977;5:258–261.
10. Williams J, Watkin Jones R. Dicyclomine: worrying symptoms associated with its use in some small babies. *BMJ* 1984;288:901.
11. Fleiss JL. The crossover study. In: Fleiss JL, ed. *The design and analysis of clinical experiments.* New York: Wiley and Sons, 1986.

12. Metcalf TJ, Irons TG, Sher LD, et al. Simethicone in the treatment of infantile colic: a randomized, placebo-controlled, multicenter trial. *Pediatrics* 1994;94:29–34.
13. Danielsson B, Hwang CP. Treatment of infantile colic with surface active substance (simethicone). *Acta Paediatr Scand* 1985;74:446–450.
14. Sethi KS, Sethi JK. Simethicone in the management of infant colic. *Practitioner* 1988;232:508.
15. Campbell JPM. Dietary treatment of infantile colic: a double-blind study. *J R Coll Gen Pract* 1989;39:11–14.
16. Lothe L, Lindbert T, Jakobsson I. Cow's milk formula as a cause of infantile colic: a double-blind study. *Pediatrics* 1982;70:7–10.
17. Forsythe BWC. Colic and the effect of changing formulas: a double blind, multiple-crossover study. *J Pediatr* 1989;115:521–526.
18. Hill DJ, Hudson IL, Sheffield LJ, et al. A low allergen diet is a significant intervention in infantile colic: results of a community based study. *J Allergy Clin Immunol* 1995;96:886–892.
19. Lucassen PLBJ, Assendelft WJJ, Gubbels LW, et al. Infantile colic: crying time reduction with a whey hydrolysate; a double blind, randomized placebo-controlled trial. *Pediatrics* 2000;106:1349–1354.
20. Kearney PJ, Malone AJ, Hayes T, et al. A trial of lactase in the management of infant colic. *J Hum Nutr Diet* 1998;11:281–285.
21. Kanabar D, Randhawa M, Clayton P. Improvement of symptoms of infant colic following reduction of lactose load with lactase. *J Hum Nutr Diet* 2001,14;359–363.
22. Stahlberg MR, Savilahti E. Infantile colic and feeding. *Arch Dis Child* 1986;61:1232–1233.
23. Markestad T. Use of sucrose as a treatment for infant colic. *Arch Dis Child* 1997;77:356–357.
24. Weizman Z, Alkrinawi S, Goldfarb D, et al. Herbal teas for infantile colic. *J Pediatr* 1993;123:670–671.
25. Parkin PC, Schwartz CJ, Manuel BA. Randomised controlled trial of three interventions in the management of persistent crying of infancy. *Pediatrics* 1993;92;197–201.
26. Taubman B. Parental counselling compared with elimination of cow's milk or soy milk protein for the treatment of infant colic syndrome: a randomized trial. *Pediatrics* 1988;81:756–761.
27. Barr RG, McMullen SJ, Spiess H, et al. Carrying as a colic "therapy": a randomized controlled trial. *Pediatrics* 1991;87:623–630.
28. McKenzie S. Troublesome crying in infants: effect of advice to reduce stimulation. *Arch Dis Child* 1991;66:1416–1420.
29. Huhtala V, Lehtonen L, Heinonen R, et al. Infant massage compared with crib vibrator in the treatment of colicky infants. *Pediatrics* 2000;105:e84.
30. Wiberg JMM, Nordsteen J, Nilsson N. The short term effect of spinal manipulation in the treatment of infant colic: a randomized controlled clinical trial with a blinded observer. *J Manipulative Physiol Ther* 1999;22:517–522.
31. Olafsdottir E, Forshei S, Fluge G, et al. Randomised controlled trial of infant colic treated with chiropractic spinal manipulation. *Arch Dis Child* 2001;84:138–141.

Teresa Kilgour
Staff Grade Community Paediatrician
City Hospitals Sunderland
Sunderland
UK

Sally Wade
Staff Grade Community Paediatrician
Archer Street Clinic
Darlington
UK

Competing interests: None declared.

Measles: prevention

Search date July 2004

Nitu Sengupta, Helen Bedford, David Elliman, and Robert Booy

QUESTIONS

INTERVENTIONS

See glossary

Key Messages

Measles vaccination

- **Monovalent measles vaccine or combined MMR vaccine (reduced incidence of measles and child mortality compared with placebo or no vaccine)** We found no RCTs comparing the clinical effects of combined measles, mumps, and rubella (MMR) versus no vaccine or placebo. One large RCT, one quasi randomised trial, one large retrospective cohort study, and several observational studies found that monovalent vaccine reduced the incidence of measles. Mass population cohort studies and other observational studies also consistently found important reductions in child mortality after measles vaccination. Observational studies found that measles vaccination programmes were followed by a reduction in the incidence of subacute sclerosing panencephalitis. Several features of measles infection occur or are suspected to occur after the vaccine, but we found no studies comparing rates of occurrence between people with naturally acquired measles and those who have been vaccinated. Severe complications are rare with measles immunisation. One non-systematic review found that, compared with placebo, measles vaccination increased the incidence of fever and febrile seizures, although febrile seizures are rare and do not progress into afebrile seizures. Observational studies found that aseptic meningitis, a rare complication, increased after mass vaccination with the L-Z and Urabe strains of MMR, but no increased incidence has been reported with Jeryl Lynn, Hoshino, or Rubini strains. Observational studies found that both measles vaccination and naturally acquired measles increased the incidence of idiopathic thrombocytopenic purpura. Observational studies found no association between the incidence of asthma in healthy children and MMR vaccination. They also found no significant change in the incidence of Guillain–Barré syndrome, autism, diabetes, or inflammatory bowel disease as a result of measles vaccination. Anaphylaxis has been reported after vaccination with MMR, but this is extremely rare.
- **Comparative effects of combined MMR and monovalent measles vaccine** We found no RCTs comparing the clinical effects of MMR versus monovalent vaccines in children. Seroconversion rates are similar with both vaccines.

Measles: prevention

DEFINITION Measles is an infectious disease caused by a ribonucleic acid paramyxovirus. The illness is characterised by an incubation period of 6–19 days (median 13 days);[1] a prodromal period of 2–4 days with upper respiratory tract symptoms; conjunctivitis, Koplik's spots on mucosal membranes, and high fever; followed by a widespread maculopapular rash that persists, with fever, for 5–6 days.

INCIDENCE/ PREVALENCE Incidence varies according to vaccination coverage. Worldwide, there are an estimated 30 million cases of measles each year,[2] but the incidence is only 0–10/100 000 people in countries with widespread vaccination programmes such as the USA, UK, Mexico, India, China, Brazil, and Australia.[3] In the USA, before licensing of effective vaccines, more than 90% of people were infected by the age of 15 years. After licensing in 1963, incidence fell by about 98%.[4] The mean annual incidence in Finland was 366/100 000 in 1970,[5] but declined to about zero by the late 1990s.[6] Similarly, the annual incidence declined to almost zero in Chile, the English speaking Caribbean, and Cuba during the 1990s when vaccination programmes were introduced.[7,8]

AETIOLOGY/ RISK FACTORS Measles is highly contagious and spreads through airborne droplets. As with most other infectious diseases, risk factors include overcrowding and low herd immunity**G**. Newborn babies have a lower risk of measles than do older infants, owing to protective maternalantibodies, although in recent US outbreaks maternal antibody protection was lower than expected.[4] Antibody levels are lower in babies born to immunised mothers compared with offspring of naturally infected mothers.[9,10]

PROGNOSIS The World Health Organization estimated that measles caused 777 000 deaths and 27.5 million disability adjusted life years in 2000.[11] **Disease in healthy people:** In developed countries, most prognostic data come from the prevaccination era and from subsequent outbreaks in non-vaccinated populations. The overall rate of complications in the UK was 6.7% before the introduction of measles vaccination. Encephalitis affected 1.2/1000 diseased people, and respiratory complications in 38/1000 diseased people.[12] Other complications before the introduction of the vaccine included seizures, with or without fever, affecting 5/1000 people with measles.[13] Idiopathic thrombocytopenic purpura has been reported, but the frequency is not known. Subacute sclerosing panencephalitis (SSPE) is an inevitably fatal, progressive degenerative disorder of the central nervous system with a mean onset 7–10 years after measles infection. It is more common when measles occurs under the age of 1 year (18/100 000 in children < 1 year of age *v* 4/100 000 overall), as identified by a passive reporting system set up in England and Wales to monitor the incidence of SSPE.[14] Between 1989–1991 in the USA, measles resurgence among young children (< 5 years) who had not been immunised led to 55 622 cases, with more than 11 000 hospital admissions and 166 deaths.[15–17] Measles complications include diarrhoea (9%), pneumonia (6%), and acute encephalitis (about 0.14%).[17] Measles during pregnancy results in higher risk of premature labour[18] but no proven increase in congenital anomalies.[19] **Disease in malnourished or immunocompromised people:** In malnourished people, particularly those with vitamin A deficiency, measles case fatality can be as high as 25%. Immunocompromised people have a higher morbidity and mortality. Children younger than 5 years, and adults older than 20 years, have a higher risk of severe complications and death.[15,20] In the period 1974–1984, four UK centres reported that 15/51 (29%) deaths in children in their first remission from leukaemia resulted from measles.[21] Another report reviewing cases from the same four UK centres between 1973 and 1986 found that five out of 17 cases of measles in children with malignancies proved fatal.[22] At least 5 out of 36 (14%) measles associated deaths in 1991 in the USA were in HIV infected persons.[15] Worldwide, measles is a major cause of blindness, and causes 5% of deaths in young children (< 5 years).[23]

AIMS OF INTERVENTION To prevent measles, with minimal adverse effects.

OUTCOMES Rates of clinically apparent measles and measles related complications, including death. If no clinical outcomes were available then we reported rates of seroconversion**G** because it is highly correlated with vaccine efficacy**G**. Rates of adverse effects of vaccination: acute fever, febrile seizures, inflammatory bowel disease, developmental regression**G**, autism, aseptic meningitis, idiopathic thrombocytopenic purpura, arthritis and arthralgia, anaphylaxis, asthma, subacute sclerosing panencephalitis, and Guillain–Barré syndrome.

METHODS *Clinical Evidence* search and appraisal July 2004. The authors also searched World Health Organization, US Communicable Disease Control, Eurosurveillance website, UK Health Protection Agency websites, and hand searched national and international policy documents. For additional information on vaccine strains and branding, . Where possible, original articles were sought and critiqued in preference to non-systematic reviews. Comprehensive or systematic reviews were included. We included studies involving vaccine strains that are currently widely used. For additional information on vaccine strains and branding, . In the benefits section comparing different vaccines and schemes, we included RCTs and stronger observational studies, because after the high clinical efficacy against measles shown in early RCTs, further RCTs have been considered unethical (see benefits of measles vaccination, p 375). We included a selection of recent population outbreak studies to demonstrate the ongoing effect of measles on mortality; the studies included represent only a small proportion of reports available. In the harms sections, we included RCTs and robust observational studies (see harms, p 377).

QUESTION What are the effects of measles vaccination?

OPTION MONOVALENT MEASLES VACCINE OR COMBINED MMR VACCINE VERSUS PLACEBO OR NO VACCINE

We found no RCTs comparing the clinical effects of combined measles, mumps, and rubella (MMR) versus no vaccine or placebo. One large RCT, one quasi randomised trial, one large retrospective cohort study, and several observational studies found that monovalent vaccine reduced the incidence of measles. Mass population cohort studies and other observational studies also consistently found important reductions in child mortality after measles vaccination. Observational studies found that measles vaccination programmes were followed by a reduction in the incidence of subacute sclerosing panencephalitis. Several features of measles infection occur or are suspected to occur after the vaccine, but we found no studies comparing rates of occurrence between people with naturally acquired measles and those who have been vaccinated. Severe complications are rare with measles immunisation. One non-systematic review found that, compared with placebo, measles vaccination increased the incidence of fever and febrile seizures, although febrile seizures are rare and do not progress into afebrile seizures. Observational studies found that aseptic meningitis, a rare complication, increased after mass vaccination with the L-Z and Urabe strains of MMR, but no increased incidence has been reported with Jeryl Lynn, Hoshino, or Rubini strains. Observational studies found that both measles vaccination and naturally acquired measles increased the incidence of idiopathic thrombocytopenic purpura. Observational studies found no association between the incidence of asthma in healthy children and MMR vaccination. They also found no significant change in the incidence of Guillain–Barré syndrome, autism, diabetes, or inflammatory bowel disease as a result of measles vaccination. Anaphylaxis has been reported after vaccination with MMR, but this is extremely rare.

Benefits: **Measles:** We found no systematic reviews. We found no RCTs comparing the clinical effects of MMR**G** versus no vaccine or placebo. We found one RCT from the USA[24] and one quasi randomised controlled trial from the UK of monovalent measles vaccine versus placebo or no vaccines.[25] We also found one large retrospective cohort study[26] and several other large observational studies[5,27,28] assessing measles infection rates in vaccinated compared with unvaccinated children. All found that measles vaccination reduced measles infection rates. The RCT carried out in the USA assessed measles infection rates in children receiving two doses of killed vaccine followed by one dose of either live (combined schedule) or killed vaccine given at monthly intervals (strain not specified).[24] Infection rates were then compared with those in two groups of children receiving three doses of placebo at the same intervals. It was found that, over 14 months, protection was offered best by the "combined" schedule, with 96% efficacy (95% CI 94.7% to 97.2%). The quasi randomised trial conducted in the UK followed 36 211 children aged 10 months to 2 years for 9 months.[25] Children were allocated according to birth date to live vaccine alone (9538 children); killed vaccine (E-E-B strain) followed by live vaccine (SWZ strain; 10 434 children); or no vaccination (16 239 children). The trial found an 85% efficacy over 6 months' follow up in children who had been vaccinated with either live vaccine alone or killed vaccine followed by live vaccine compared with unvaccinated controls (20 cases per 1000 children vaccinated *v* 134 cases per 1000 unvaccinated children). Follow up of a subset of these children (live vaccine group [7889 children]; killed/live vaccine [8171 children], and unvaccinated [5593 children]) found an increase in protective effect 2 years and 9 months after vaccination (94% live vaccine *v* 88% killed/live vaccine) after exposure to two major epidemics.[25] After 15 years' follow up (at 12–27 years after recruitment) of 9106 children, there was a higher incidence of measles in the unvaccinated group.[29] The difference between vaccinated and unvaccinated children remained after controlling for subsequent vaccination in initial placebo groups, but it did not remain after controlling for growing herd immunity**G** after mass vaccination (AR 0.3/1000 person years with vaccine *v* 1/1000 person years with no vaccine; $P < 0.001$). The overall protective efficacy was high (92%, 95% CI 86 to 95%) between 1976 and 1990.[29] The large retrospective cohort study of the entire US population from 1985–1992 compared measles infection rates in children who were vaccinated versus rates in children whose parents had declined vaccination (17 390 cases from a vaccinated population of 51 264 140 to 52 377 192 from 1985–1992 *v* 2827 measles cases from an unvaccinated population of 234 040 to 245 887 from 1985–1992).[26] The cohort study did not state what proportion of vaccinated children received monovalent or MMR vaccine, although MMR was already widely used in the USA by 1985. The study found that, although overall measles incidence was low because of herd immunity, vaccination significantly reduced measles infection compared with no vaccination (RR of measles in unvaccinated *v* vaccinated 4–170, depending on age group and year of survey). We also found many population based studies from different countries with different health care systems and different socioeconomic and demographic distributions.[5,28,30–32] These studies consistently found that measles vaccination is associated with a steep decline in measles. In most resource rich countries, 95% of the population must be vaccinated to eliminate measles. In countries with greater population density, coverage may need to reach 99% to eliminate measles.[33] One time series from the World Health Organization found a global decline in reported measles incidence (which underestimates true incidence) from about 4 500 000 a year in 1980 to about 1 000 000 a year in 2000.[27] The decline was associated with the rise in reported measles vaccination coverage from about 10% in 1980 to about 80% in 2000. One population based time series of measles incidence from Finland found that, in a population of about 5 million people, after the introduction of a live monovalent vaccination programme (1975–1981) the number of new measles cases each year fell from an average of 2074 cases in 1977–1981 to 44 cases in 1985.[5] New cases declined to almost zero by the mid 1990s. Shortly after introducing the MMR programme in Finland in 1982, rubella and mumps incidence also fell to almost zero. One cross sectional study in a Brazilian city, which was repeated before and after a measles vaccination campaign in 1987 (8163 people, strain not stated), found that reported measles incidence fell from 222/

100 000 in 1987 to 2.7/100 000 in 1988.[28] However, measles outbreaks in countries with high vaccine coverage**G** can still occur. During 1999–2000 in The Netherlands, a measles outbreak took place in a school in which only 7% of the children were vaccinated.[34] Eventually, 94% of unvaccinated people from closed communities were affected, amounting to 3292 cases. Although The Netherlands had one of the lowest rates of measles disease with high vaccine coverage (96%), the epidemic was attributed to the presence of small unvaccinated pockets. **Mortality:** We found one systematic review (search date not reported, 10 cohort studies, 2 case control studies),[35] one subsequent cohort study,[36] and three population based outbreak studies (two published reports[37,38] and a personal communication) evaluating the effects of monovalent measles vaccination on mortality. The systematic review found that live monovalent measles vaccination in seven developing countries reduced all cause mortality in vaccinated children by 30–80% compared with unvaccinated children, depending on follow up period and country.[35] The subsequent cohort study compared a group of children in Bangladesh vaccinated with live Schwarz strain monovalent measles vaccine versus age matched unvaccinated children (8135 matched pairs).[36] It found a significant reduction in mortality with vaccination (16 270 children aged 9–60 months at vaccination; RR for death at 43 months 0.54, 95% CI 0.45 to 0.65). In Campania, Italy, where MMR vaccine coverage was less than 70%, a measles outbreak of 1571 cases was reported in 2002.[37] The outbreak led to 594 hospitalisations and four deaths. From December 1999 to June 2000, an outbreak of measles in Dublin, Ireland, lead to 1115 notifications and 111 measles related paediatric admissions.[38] Only a third of the children who were over the age of 15 months (the age recommended for MMR vaccination) were vaccinated, and all three deaths reported occurred in unvaccinated children. In contrast, a 2001–2002 measles outbreak in Coburg, Germany, where vaccine uptake was around 77%, resulted in 1191 cases and 43 hospitalisations, but no deaths (A Siedler, personal communication, 2004). **Subacute sclerosing panencephalitis:** Wherever it has been monitored, subacute sclerosing panencephalitis (SSPE) has exhibited a major fall in prevalence after the introduction of measles containing vaccines.[39–42] A case control study found that a history of measles vaccination was less likely among people with SSPE than among healthy controls (OR 0.25, 95% CI 0.05 to 0.54).[43] We found no other studies for MMR vaccine, but SSPE is uncommon where any measles containing vaccine is in widespread use. No measles virus recovered from brain biopsies of 19 people who suffered SSPE were linked to a vaccine like strain.[44]

Harms: **Acute fever and febrile seizures:** We found one non-systematic review,[45] one RCT,[46] one cohort study,[47] and one observational study of a population based surveillance programme reporting fever due to vaccination in otherwise healthy children.[48] The review (search date 1998) reported that up to 5% of non-immune people develop moderate to high fever (≥ 38.6 °C) within 7–21 days of vaccination.[45] The RCT (crossover design) assessed the acute adverse effects of MMR**G** compared with placebo in 1162 twins (460 children aged 1 year, of whom 1.3% had previously been vaccinated; 702 aged ≥ 2 years, 95% of whom had previously been vaccinated or experienced measles).[46] One member of each twin pair was randomly selected and allocated to MMR vaccination followed 3 weeks later by placebo. The other twin was allocated to the opposite combination. The RCT found that, among children aged 14–18 months, MMR significantly increased the incidence of moderate fever (range 38.6°C to 39.5°C) within 21 days (25% with MMR *v* 6% with placebo; OR 3.28, 95% CI 2.23 to 4.82) and high fever (> 39.5°C; 7% with MMR *v* 3% with placebo; OR 2.83, 95% CI 1.47 to 5.45). Among children older than 6 years there was no significant difference in incidence rates of fever (5 per 1000 in children receiving vaccine or placebo; P > 0.10). One retrospective cohort study in 679 942 children from four health maintenance organisations**G** in the USA found that children who had received MMR (strains not listed) were significantly more likely to experience febrile seizures 8–14 days after receiving MMR compared with children of the same age who had not been vaccinated (ARI 25–34 additional seizures per 100 000 immunised children; RR 2.83, 95% CI 1.44 to 5.55; ARI estimated by comparison with background seizure risk in all children aged 12–24 months: 0.025%; NNH 4000; CI not reported).[47] The study found no significant difference in febrile seizures during the first week (RR 1.73, 95% CI 0.72 to 4.15) or 15–30 days after vaccination (RR 0.97, 95% CI 0.49 to 1.95). The study followed up 562 children with febrile convulsions (22 within 7–21 days of MMR, 18 within 0–7 days of diphtheria, tetanus, and pertussis [DTP**G**], 1 after both vaccines and 521 whose seizures occurred outside these periods following vaccination). It found that, in comparing MMR or DTP versus no vaccine, there was no significant difference in the risk of developing subsequent seizures (RR 0.65, 95% CI 0.32 to 1.35). No child with a febrile seizure after vaccination went on to develop afebrile seizures. Similarly, among 273 children with febrile convulsions in one of the four participating organisations, the study found no evidence that MMR vaccination before seizure significantly increased the risk of learning disability or developmental delay compared with no vaccination before seizure (RR after adjusting for age at first febrile seizure 0.56, 95% CI 0.07 to 4.20). It found no significant increase in afebrile seizures after MMR vaccination ((within15–30 days of MMR: RR 0.48, 95% CI 0.05 to 4.64). We found a population based passive surveillance of harms of MMR in all 1.8 million people vaccinated over a 14 year period in Finland.[48] Surveillance relied on health care personnel's awareness of the programme and their reporting of adverse events felt to be associated with MMR. Advertisements of the programme appeared in seminars, the media, and the medical press. Acute reactions were more likely to have been reported than long term effects. Fever was associated with MMR in 277 children (AR 15 per 100 000 vaccinees or 9.2 per 100 000 doses). Febrile seizures were reported in 52 children (AR 17 per million doses), of which 28 could have been caused by MMR (9 per million doses) according to predefined clinical and serological criteria. These are gross underestimates compared with the US retrospective study,[47] and suggest an inadequacy of the Finnish study for detecting relatively minor events.[48] We found one self controlled case series**G**, which examined the incidence of febrile convulsions after MMR vaccination.[49] It found an increased risk of hospital admission 6–11 days after receiving MMR vaccine at between 12 and 24 months of age (AR 50 per 100 000; ARI 33 additional seizures per 100 000 doses), but not in the period 15–35 days after the Jeryl Lynn containing vaccine. In the same period after vaccination with the Urabe containing vaccine, it found an absolute risk of febrile seizures or aseptic meningitis of 91 per 100 000 vaccinees with an attributable risk of 38 per 100 000 vaccinees compared with no vaccination. **Aseptic meningitis:** Observational studies using differing methods have reported a wide range of risk estimations for aseptic meningitis after MMR vaccination (AR 7 to 250 per million vaccines), even in the same country.[50] Using self controlled case series in the UK, the risk of aseptic meningitis was assessed for MMR vaccines containing either Urabe or Jeryl Lynn mumps vaccine virus strains.[49] The case series found that the vaccine increased the risk of aseptic meningitis 15–35 days after receiving Urabe containing vaccines (AR 67 per million, ARI 63 per million vaccinated children). No cases of aseptic meningitis were reported with the Jeryl Lynn containing

MMR vaccine. This latter finding was confirmed using similar methodology in a US study.[51] An observational study in part of Brazil, based on hospital admissions before and after a mass immunisation campaign using Urabe containing MMR, found that MMR significantly increased the risk of aseptic meningitis 3–5 weeks after vaccination (RR 30.4, 95% CI 11.5 to 80.8; attributable risk 71 per million doses; 32 cases in 452 344 doses).[52] A case cross over study**G** of hospitalised children found no significant risk of developing aseptic meningitis with the Jeryl Lynn or the Rubini strains of the vaccine (RR 0.6, 95% CI 0.18 to 1.97), but found an increased risk after vaccination with the Urabe or Hoshino strains, particularly in the third week after vaccination (RR 15.6, 95% CI 5.9 to 41.2).[53] However, the assignment of vaccine strains was based on assuming a pattern of provider usage rather than individual records, and there was no evidence that this assumption was tested. Reported cases of aseptic meningitis increased during a mass MMR immunisation campaign using the Leningrad-Zagreb (L-Z) mumps strain in Brazil in 1997, compared with the previous 2 years (28.7 cases per 10 000 person weeks *v* 4.5 cases per 10 000 person weeks).[54] The absolute risk of aseptic meningitis 15–35 days after vaccination was 29 per 100 000 doses. Other causes of aseptic meningitis were not ruled out and therefore the attributable risk could not be calculated, but the temporal pattern of increase in cases suggests that most were due to the vaccine. The risk of aseptic meningitis following L-Z containing MMR seems to be higher than that following both Urabe and Jeryl Lynn containing vaccines. Similar findings were reported after a mass immunisation campaign with L-Z vaccine in two states in Brazil in 1998.[55] The incidence of aseptic meningitis increased compared with the previous 2 years. The estimated attributable risk of aseptic meningitis after vaccination ranged from 52 per million to 160 per million vaccinations, depending on the criteria used. **Idiopathic thrombocytopenic purpura:** Naturally acquired measles and measles vaccination have been associated with idiopathic thrombocytopenic purpura (ITP). We found two self controlled case series, the second including the cases from the first.[49,56] In these studies, vaccination records were linked with computerised hospital admission records, and the incidence of ITP during a risk period (0–42 days after MMR vaccine) was compared with the incidence outside this risk period. ITP significantly increased after MMR vaccination (AR 45 per million people, ARI 31 per million people; RR 3.27, 95% CI 1.49 to 7.16). The study included 14 children who had had a first episode of ITP before MMR immunisation. Although three of these children had further episodes of ITP, none were within 6 weeks of immunisation.[49,56] A case control study carried out in the UK found that MMR was associated with an increased incidence of ITP within 6 weeks of administration (ARI 40 per million vaccinees, 95% CI 11 per million to 47 per million).[57] **Arthritis and arthralgia:** One crossover RCT in twin children found that vaccination with MMR, given either at 14–18 months of age or 6 years of age, significantly increased the risk of developing arthralgia compared with placebo (14–18 months: OR 3.66, CI 1.74 to 7.70; $P < 0.001$).[46] The duration of arthralgia was not described, but it is implied that it was mild. **Anaphylaxis:** Anaphylaxis after MMR has been reported, albeit infrequently.[58] We found no accurate figures. During the 1994 measles rubella vaccine campaign in the UK, 5.8 million children (5–16 years of age) were vaccinated. Passive surveillance using "yellow cards"**G** identified 123 reports of children with signs or symptoms of allergic reactions in varying degrees of severity, but with no deaths or anaphylaxis within 24 hours of vaccination.[59] The absolute risk is therefore 15 per million doses. If confined to anaphylactic reactions, the rate was 1 per 100 000 doses.[60] **Asthma and eczema:** We found three cohort studies[61–63] and one case control study.[64] The studies, all of which had weak methods, found no evidence of an association between MMR and asthma or eczema. The first cohort study in four health maintenance organisations in the USA compared the MMR immunisation status of children with diagnosed and treated asthma.[61] Inclusion criteria were children with asthma after the age of 1 year. Children also had to be enrolled with the health maintenance organisation at birth and remain so until at least the age of 18 months. The median age of last follow up for the whole group of children was 28 months. The median age of first episode of asthma was 11 months. It found no significant difference in the risk of developing asthma after MMR vaccination (RR 0.97, 95% CI 0.91 to 1.04). It found no significant change in these figures when only those children with asthma requiring emergency room attendance or hospital admission were included. Although the duration of follow up was relatively short the authors argue that this was probably long enough to pick up most cases.[61] The second cohort study, carried out in the USA, assessed children who had been enrolled in an earlier case control study of infant wheezing and compared the incidence of asthma in children who had been vaccinated with MMR vaccine versus those who had not.[62] 1778 children aged 3–7 years were included of which 881 had wheezed in infancy and 897 had not. The study found no significant difference in the proportion of children who had asthma between vaccinated and unvaccinated children (33/383 [8%] of vaccinated *v* 125/1395 [9%] of unvaccinated; adjusted OR 1.19, 95% CI 0.78 to 1.82). Secondary analysis also found no significant difference in the incidence of asthma in children with a history of infant wheezing (adjusted OR 1.20, 95% CI 0.55 to 2.63) or with no history of infantile wheezing (adjusted OR 1.05, 95% CI 0.65 to 1.70; absolute numbers not reported). The third cohort study, using a General Practice Research Database in the UK, (29238 children) assessed the incidence of asthma/wheeze and eczema following MMR vaccination.[63] Only children without asthma, wheeze, or eczema prior to immunisation were enrolled. The study found a significant increase in the risk of asthma and eczema after MMR vaccination (asthma 1753/16470 children vaccinated over 69602 person years; adjusted OR 2.20, 95% CI 1.50 to 3.21; eczema: 1884/14353 children over 59520 person years). The difference between the groups in asthma incidence was only evident in children who consulted their doctor less frequently. This raises the possibility that some of the children within this very small group may have had undiagnosed asthma. Furthermore, only 1.6% of children in the study were unvaccinated, which makes the results difficult to interpret. The case control study carried out in New Zealand in children aged 7–9 years, and diagnosed with asthma, found no significant association between MMR vaccine and diagnosed asthma (OR 1.43, 95% CI 0.85 to 2.41).[64] The authors of this report concluded that there may be some under diagnosis of children with asthma. **Diabetes mellitus:** We found one population based study of children born in Denmark between 1990 and 2000, which used hospital records (initially inpatient only and then all hospital attendances) to calculate the number of children who developed type 1 diabetes mellitus and compared the incidence of diabetes between vaccinated and unvaccinated children.[65] The authors stated that using hospital records would account for over 90% of children with diabetes in Denmark. They found that 681 children out of 739,694 enrolled (4 720 517 person years) had type 1 diabetes. The study found no significant difference in the incidence of diabetes between children who had received MMR and those who had not (RR 1.14, 95% CI 0.90 to 1.45). **Guillain–Barré syndrome:** Guillain–Barré syndrome has been reported after vaccination with measles containing vaccines.[45] In the 1994–1995 Measles-Rubella campaign in UK, three cases of Guillain–Barré syndrome were reported, but this is well within the expected background rate.[59] A retrospective study of Finnish hospital discharges in people who developed Guillain–Barré syndrome looked at vaccination records over a 4 year period and found no cases of Guillain–Barré syndrome within 6 weeks of immunisation.[48] The shortest interval was 10 weeks and was in a person who also suffered an infectious illness during this interval. **Developmental regression or autistic spectrum disorders:** We found one non-systematic review of observational studies,[66] one case control study (624 cases of autistic spectrum disorders Ⓖ),[67] one large retrospective cohort study (738 cases of autistic spectrum disorders),[68] and two additional population surveillance studies (498 cases of autistic spectrum disorders analysed in two studies[69,70] and an estimated total population of 1.8 million vaccinated people in the other study[48]). None of the studies found an association between MMR vaccine and autistic spectrum disorders. The non-systematic review (search date not reported) found no causal relationship between MMR and autism.[66] The review included two large cross sectional time series,[71,72] which reported that the incidence of autism increased independently of MMR coverage. They found no association between MMR vaccination and autism. The first cross sectional time series was carried out among kindergarten children in California in 1999.[71] It looked at children born between 1980–1994 and immunised with MMR by 17 months or 24 months, and compared these figures with autism cases referred to the state developmental services department over the same time (absolute figures not reported). It found that MMR coverage at 24 months rose slightly (from 72% in 1980 to 82% in 1994; 14% proportional rise). Referral rates for new autism cases increased disproportionately in the same period (from 44/100 000 births in 1980 to 208/100 000 live births in 1994; a 373% proportional rise). The authors of the report found it difficult to attribute the large increase in referral rates to the small rise in immunisation rates. However, referral rates to the department may not reflect accurately the incidence of autistic syndromes. The second cross sectional time series was carried out in the UK.[72] It found that, during the period 1988–1993, the risk of autism among boys increased, whereas MMR coverage remained almost constant at about 97% (AR of first diagnosis of autism aged 2–5 years: 8 per 100 000, 95% CI 4 to 14 per 100 000 for children born in 1988 *v* 29 per 100 000, 95% CI 20 to 43 per 100 000 for children born in 1993; 305 cases of autism over just greater than 3 million person years at risk).[72] The case control study (624 children with autism aged 3–10 years and 1824 age, sex, and school/region matched controls) also found no significant association between measles vaccination and autism.[67] The study assessed vaccination at certain ages and compared rates of autism in vaccinated children with those in healthy unvaccinated controls. When age of MMR vaccination was divided into "on time" vaccination (before 18 months of age) compared with not vaccinated, MMR vaccination before 24 months of age compared with not vaccinated, and vaccination before 36 months of age compared with not vaccinated, only the latter analysis was significant (93% of children with autism were vaccinated at 36 months compared with 91% of control children; OR 1.49, 95% CI 1.04 to 2.14). In practice, most children receive MMR vaccine by the age of 2–3 years. The apparent increase in the risk of autism in the analysis at 36 months is thought to be an artefact resulting from the requirement for MMR vaccination of autistic children before entering special education programmes at the age of 36 months. Non-autistic children who are not vaccinated before the age of 2–3 years will generally not be vaccinated until they enrol in school at around age 5 years. The large retrospective cohort study (537 303 children born in Denmark between January 1991 and December 1998; 2 129 864 person years exposure) found no association between MMR vaccination and autistic spectrum disorders (82% of population vaccinated; RR of autistic disorder in vaccinated *v* non-vaccinated children 0.92, 95% CI 0.68 to 1.24; RR of other autistic spectrum disorder in vaccinated *v* non-vaccinated children 0.83, 95% CI 0.65 to 1.07).[68] It also found no association between autistic spectrum disorder and age at time of vaccination (P = 0.23), time since vaccination (P = 0.42), or calendar date of vaccination (P = 0.06). Results remained unchanged when children with autistic disorders due to fragile X syndrome, tuberous sclerosis, congenital rubella, or Angelman's syndrome were included. However, it is possible that the young age of some children at the close of the study may have biased the results against an association. It is not possible to ascertain from the published data whether this potential bias was allowed for. The first population surveillance study used records at child development centres and special schools to identify 498 children diagnosed with autism before the age of 5 years born in eight health districts in the UK between 1979 and 1998.[69] It was found that the incidence of autism increased over this period. However, there was no change in the rate of increase after the start of the MMR vaccination programme. Using the same methods and birth cohort, but including fewer districts (473 children diagnosed with autism before the age of 5 years), the proportion of children with autism who had developmental regression**G** or bowel symptoms was assessed.[70] The study found no significant change in these proportions during this time period (P value for trend = 0.50 and 0.47, respectively). The second long term population surveillance study from Finland was based on passive reporting and found no cases of vaccination related developmental regression among 1.8 million people vaccinated with MMR.[48] However, events that did not result in hospital admission or were not temporally closely associated with the vaccination may not have been reported in this study. This would particularly apply to conditions such as autism, and so it is not possible to draw any conclusions from this study about a possible link between MMR and autism spectrum disorders in either the long or the short term. **Inflammatory bowel disease:** We found one non-systematic review,[45] one cohort study,[73] one population surveillance study,[48] one case control study,[74] and one case series.[75] None of the studies found an association between MMR and inflammatory bowel disease. The non-systematic review (search date 1998, 6 large observational studies from different developed countries) found no evidence of an association between inflammatory bowel disease and measles vaccine (meta-analysis not performed).[45] The retrospective cohort study compared rates of ulcerative colitis, Crohn's disease, and inflammatory bowel disease (assessed by postal questionnaire) in 7616 people who had received live monovalent measles vaccination with rates in people who had not received measles vaccination by the age of 5 years (mean age at vaccination 17.6 months, standard deviation 7.4 months).[73] Participants were those available from an original population based cohort of all 16 000 children born in the first week of 1970 in the UK. The study found no significant difference in the risk of developing ulcerative colitis, Crohn's disease, or inflammatory bowel disease among people (aged 26 years at the time of the study) who had received monovalent measles vaccine and those who had not, whether or not the result was adjusted for sex, socioeconomic status, or crowding (AR for Crohn's disease 0.25% with vaccine *v* 0.31% without; adjusted OR 0.7, 95% CI 0.3 to 1.6; AR for ulcerative colitis 0.16% with vaccine *v* 0.27% without; adjusted OR 0.6, 95% CI 0.2 to 1.6; AR for inflammatory bowel disease 0.41% with vaccine *v* 0.58% without; adjusted OR 0.6, 95% CI 0.3 to 1.2). The long term population based passive surveillance study from Finland found no cases of inflammatory bowel disease associated with vaccination in 1.8 million people vaccinated with MMR followed up for 14 years but, as discussed earlier, there are major limitations to the methodology of this study.[48] The case control study included 142 people in the USA with definite or probable inflammatory bowel disease from members of four health maintenance organisations (67 people with ulcerative colitis and 75 people with Crohn's disease).[74] Cases (people with inflammatory bowel disease) were identified by computerised search of electronic records and manual abstraction of medical records from 1958–1989 for three organisations and from 1979–1989 for the remaining one. The date of data collection is not clear and so the potential age range was not reported; people who were not members of the health maintenance organisation between 6 months of age and disease onset were excluded. The study found that people with inflammatory bowel disease were not more likely to have received MMR than people without inflammatory bowel disease taken from the same health maintenance organisation and matched for sex and year of birth (OR for Crohn's disease 0.40, 95% CI 0.08 to 2.00; OR for ulcerative colitis 0.80, 95% CI 0.18 to 3.56; OR for all inflammatory bowel disease 0.59, 95% CI 0.21 to 1.69). The study similarly found no association between other measles containing vaccines, Crohn's disease, ulcerative colitis, or all inflammatory bowel disease. The analysis in the paper compared MMR or other measles containing vaccines versus no measles containing vaccine. The other measles containing vaccines are almost certain to be single measles vaccine, but this was not made explicit in the paper and so it is deemed inappropriate to comment further. The case series raised the question of a possible relation between MMR and developmental regression in 12 children with bowel symptoms.[75] The series was retrospective (parents surveyed up to 8 years after vaccination), small, lacked a control group, and was selective in its sample. The authors stated that it does not prove a link or causal association between MMR vaccination and their postulated syndrome of autism and enterocolitis.

Comment: **Benefits:** RCTs comparing the clinical effects of MMR**G** versus no vaccine or placebo are deemed unethical because of the existing evidence of efficacy of measles vaccine and the harms associated with naturally acquired measles. **Harms:** Results of studies assessing fever in children vaccinated against measles should be interpreted in light of the very high prevalence of acute fever in children with measles infection.[46,76,77] A large proportion of the literature on adverse events after immunisation is based on passive reporting, albeit enhanced.[48] This has major limitations. Events may be under reported and yet events that are reported may not be linked to the intervention. For example, a case series postulated a possible causal association between MMR and a syndrome of autism and enterocolitis, despite no evidence being found to prove this association.[75] Such studies can flag up issues for further investigation but cannot be used as definitive evidence either of size of risk or even causal association, as they are only hypothesis generating. We found two observational studies that compared the incidence of autism following monovalent measles vaccine versus that following MMR vaccine.[78,79] Both studies had methodological flaws that meant we were unable to draw conclusions about the effects of monovalent versus MMR vaccine on the risk of autism. The case-control study included small numbers (21 cases and 42 controls) and there was a low response rate from parents of people in the control group (58%), which may have led to bias.[78] The other observational study recruited members of a parents' organisation and conducted a time-trend analysis in people with autism aged from 6–40 years. The analysis was made at a single point in time. It is likely that the characteristics of the older members of the group would be different from those of the younger ones, which makes a time trend analysis difficult to interpret. The inclusion of a self selected group of people also makes the results subject to bias.

OPTION MMR VERSUS MONOVALENT MEASLES VACCINE

We found no RCTs comparing the clinical effects of MMR versus monovalent vaccines in children. Seroconversion rates are similar with both vaccines.

Benefits: We found no RCTs comparing clinical effects of MMR**G** versus monovalent vaccine. We found two RCTs comparing rates of measles seroconversion**G** after live MMR (Schwarz measles plus Urabe Am 9 mumps plus RA 27/3 rubella) versus Schwarz strain monovalent measles vaccine. The first RCT (420 children with no clinical history of measles or mumps, mean age about 15 months) found similar seroconversion rates in both groups after 6 weeks (92.6% with MMR *v* 96.8% with monovalent measles).[77] The second RCT (319 children, mean age 13 months) also found similar seroconversion rates in both groups at 6 weeks (93% with MMR *v* 92% with Schwarz strain monovalent measles vaccine).[80]

Harms: The first RCT found no significant difference in fever incidence rates (fever after MMR 38.3%; after measles vaccine 37.8%; $P > 0.05$). The RCT is likely to have been underpowered to detect other clinically important adverse effects.

Comment: MMR**G** vaccine also protects against mumps and rubella, which cause serious complications in non-immune people. Mumps causes orchitis, pancreatitis, meningoencephalitis, sensorineural deafness, infertility, and rarely death. Rubella acquired during the first trimester can cause fetal death or severe fetal damage with deafness, blindness, heart defects, liver, spleen, and brain damage. The use of MMR rather than monovalent measles, mumps, and rubella vaccines provides earlier protection against all three diseases. Use of single vaccines also requires more injections over a longer period of time, which may lower uptake rates thereby increasing prevalence of these diseases. **Measles risk after seroconversion:** One systematic review of cohort studies (search date 1995) examined risk of measles infection at least 21 days after vaccine induced seroconversion**G** (monovalent or polyvalent vaccine).[81] It identified 10 studies that met inclusion criteria. In the subset of six cohort studies examining live vaccine, in which vaccination status was cross checked against medical records, risk of clinical measles infection in children who had seroconverted after vaccination was zero (0 infections from 2061 people exposed; CI not reported).

GLOSSARY

Autistic spectrum disorders are defined by early onset (< 36 months) difficulties in social reciprocity and communication as well as restrictive, repetitive behaviour. The disorders include autistic disorder, childhood disintegrative disorder, Rett's syndrome, and Asperger's disorder.

Case cross over study is in effect the same as a self controlled case series, in which each person serves as his or her own control.

Combined measles, mumps, and rubella (MMR) vaccine Vaccine with components that aim to raise immunity to measles, mumps, and rubella infections. Contains live attenuated measles virus.

Developmental regression is defined as loss of acquired developmental skills.

DTP Diphtheria, tetanus, and pertussis combined vaccine.

Health maintenance organisation (HMO) These are medical centres in the USA that have primary, secondary, and tertiary medical care facilities and are generally funded by private health care insurance. The relevance of HMOs is their participation in the Vaccine Safety Datalink (VSD) project set up by the Centres for Disease Control and Prevention (CDC) in 1991. This project links medical event information, vaccine history, and selected demographic information from the computerised databases of four staff HMOs: Group Health Co-operative of Puget Sound in Seattle, Kaiser Permanate Northwest in

Portland, Kaiser Permanante Medical Care Program of North California in Oakland, and Southern California Kaiser Permanante in Los Angeles.

Herd immunity Background level of immunity in the community. A high level of herd immunity reduces risk of infection even in non-immune individuals, because there is no pool of at risk individuals who may transmit the infectious agent.

Self controlled case series A case series in which people act as their own controls by comparing event rates within a defined time period of exposure with earlier and/or later periods.[49]

Seroconversion Development in the blood of specific antimeasles antibody. Seroconversion is often used as a proxy for clinical efficacy.

Vaccine coverage Prevalence of vaccination in the community.

Vaccine efficacy An estimate of the proportional reduction in cases associated with the use of a vaccine. Efficacy % = (1 – [attack rate in vaccinated/attack rate in unvaccinated] x 100).

Yellow cards A passive reporting system, in which a health professional becomes aware of a significant adverse event after a medication has been administered and reports this to the UK Committee on Safety of Medicines using a yellow card.

Substantive changes

Measles vaccination: benefits Three population based studies reporting that measles vaccination is associated with a steep decline in measles added.[30–32] Evidence strengthened; categorisation unchanged.

Measles vaccination: benefits Three population based studies assessing the effects of measles outbreaks in vaccinated compared with unvaccinated cohorts added (two published[37,38] and one reported in personal correspondence). Evidence strengthened; categorisation unchanged.

Measles vaccination: harms Observational studies assessing the association between MMR and asthma or eczema,[62,63] type 1 diabetes,[65] and autism[67] added. Harms data enhanced; categorisation unchanged.

REFERENCES

1. Richardson M, Elliman D, MaGuire H, et al. Evidence base of incubation periods, periods of infectiousness and exclusion policies for the control of communicable diseases in schools and preschools. *Pediatr Infect Dis J* 2001;20:380–391.
2. Immunisation plus reducing measles mortality. http://www.unicef.org/programme/health/document/meastrat.pdf (last accessed 5 February 2004).
3. Immunisation plus reducing measles mortality. http://www.who.int/vaccines-surveillance/graphics/htmls/meainc.htm (last accessed 5 February 2004).
4. Center for Disease Control. *Epidemiology and prevention of vaccine-preventable diseases.* Atlanta: CDC, 2000.
5. Peltola H, Heinonen P, Valle M, et al. The elimination of indigenous measles, mumps and rubella from Finland by a 12-year, two-dose vaccination program. *N Engl J Med* 1994;331:1397–1402.
6. Peltola H, Davidkin I, Valle M, et al. No measles in Finland. *Lancet* 1997;350:1364–1365.
7. de Quadros CA, Olive J, Hersh BS, et al. Measles elimination in the Americas: evolving strategies. *JAMA* 1996;275:224–229.
8. Pan American Health Organization. Surveillance in the Americas. *Wkly Bull* 1995;1.
9. Pabst HF, Spady DW, Marusyk RG, et al. Reduced measles immunity in infants in a well-vaccinated population. *Pediatr Infect Dis J* 1992;11:525–529.
10. Brugha R, Ramsay M, Forsey T, et al. A study of maternally derived measles antibody in infants born to naturally infected and vaccinated women. *Epidemiol Infect* 1996;117:519–524.
11. WHO. *World Health Report, 2001:statistical annex.* Geneva: WHO, 2001.
12. Miller DL. Frequency of complications of measles, 1963. Report on a National Inquiry by the Public Health Laboratory Service in Collaboration with the Society of Medical Officers of Health. *BMJ* 1964;2:75–78.
13. Miller CL. Severity of notified measles. *BMJ* 1978;1:1253–1255.
14. Farrington CP. Subacute sclerosing panencephalitis in England and Wales: transient effects and risk estimates. *Stat Med* 1991;10:1733–1744.
15. Atkinson WL, Hadler SC, Redd SB, et al. Measles surveillance: United States, 1991. *MMWR Morb Mortal Wkly Rep* 1992;41:1–12.
16. MMWR Current Trends Measles: United States, 1989 and first 20 weeks of 1990. *MMWR Morb Mortal Wkly Rep* 1990;39:353–363.
17. MMWR Current Trends Measles: United States, 1990. *MMWR Morb Mortal Wkly Rep* 1991;40:369–372.
18. Siegel M, Fuerst HT. Low birth weight and maternal virus diseases. *JAMA* 1966;197:680–684.
19. Siegel M. Congenital malformations following chickenpox, measles, mumps and hepatitis. Results of a cohort study. *JAMA* 1973;226:1521–1524.
20. van den Hoof S, Conyn-van Spaendonck MA, van Steenbergen JE. Measles epidemic in the Netherlands, 1999–2000. *J Infect Dis* 2002;186:1483–1486.
21. Gray MM, Hann IM, Glass S, et al. Mortality and morbidity caused by measles in children with malignant disease attending four major treatment centres: a retrospective review. *BMJ* 1987;295:19–22.
22. Kernahan J, McQuillin J, Craft AW. Measles in children who have malignant disease. *BMJ* 1987;295:15–18.
23. WHO Child Health http://www.who.int/child-adolescent-health/OVERVIEW/Child_Health/child_epidemiology.htm (last accessed 28 January 2004).
24. Guinee VF, Henderson DA, Casey HL, et al. Cooperative measles vaccine field trial. I. Clinical efficacy. *Pediatrics* 1966;37:649–665.
25. Anonymous. Vaccination against measles: clinical trial of live measles vaccine given alone and live

vaccine preceded by killed vaccine. Second report to the medical research council by the measles vaccines committee. *BMJ* 1968;2:449–452.
26. Salmon DA, Haber M, Gangarosa E, et al. Health consequences of religious and philosophical exemptions from immunization laws: individual and societal risk of measles. *JAMA* 1999;282:47–53.
27. WHO. Measles global annual reported incidence and MCV coverage. http://www.who.int/vaccines-surveillance/graphics/htmls/IncMeas.htm (last accessed 28 January 2004).
28. Pannuti CS, Moraes JC, Souza VA, et al. Measles antibody prevalence after mass immunization in Sao Paulo, Brazil. *Bull World Health Organ* 1991;69:557–560.
29. Ramsay ME, Moffatt D, O'Connor M. Measles vaccine: a 27-year follow up. *Epidemiol Infect* 1994;112:409–412.
30. de Quadros CA, Izurieta H, Carrasco P, Brana M, Tambini G. Progress toward measles eradication in the region of the Americas. *J Infect Dis* 2003;187(suppl 1):S102–S110.
31. Ramsay ME, Jin L, White J, Litton P, Cohen B, Brown D. The elimination of indigenous measles transmission in England and Wales. *J Infect Dis* 2003;187(suppl 1):S198–S207.
32. McFarland JW, Mansoor OD, Yang B. Accelerated measles control in the western Pacific region. *J Infect Dis* 2003;187(suppl 1):S246–S251.
33. Anderson RM, May RM. Static aspects of eradication and control. In: *Infectious diseases of humans dynamics and control*. Oxford: Oxford Science Publications 88, 1992.
34. van den Hof S, Meffre CM, Conyn-van Spaendonck MA, et al. Measles outbreak in a community with very low vaccine coverage, the Netherlands. *Emerg Infect Dis* 2001;7(suppl 3):593–597.
35. Aaby P, Samb B, Simondon F, et al. Non-specific beneficial effect of measles immunisation: analysis of mortality studies from developing countries. *BMJ* 1995;311:481–485. Search date not reported; primary source Medline.
36. Koenig MA, Khan B, Wojtynak B. Impact of measles vaccination on childhood mortality in rural Bangladesh. *Bull World Health Organ* 1990;68:441–447.
37. CDC. Measles epidemic attributed to inadequate vaccination coverage: Campania, Italy, 2002. *MMWR Morb Mortal Wkly Rep* 2003;52:1044–1047.
38. McBrien J, Murphy J, Gill D, Cronin M, O'Donovan C, Cafferkey MT. Measles outbreak in Dublin, 2000. *Pediatr Infect Dis J* 2003;22:580–584.
39. Sussman J, Compston DAS. Subacute sclerosing panencephalitis in Wales. *Q J Med* 1994;87:23–34.
40. Beersma MFC, Galama JMD, Van Druten HAM, et al. Subacute sclerosing panencephalitis in the Netherlands: 1976–1990. *Int J Epidemiol* 1992;21:583–589.
41. Anlar B, Köse G, G<umlat>rer Y, et al. Changing epidemiological features of subacute sclerosing panencephalitis. *Infection* 2001;29:192–195.
42. Bojinova VS, Dimova PS, Belopitova LD, et al. Clinical and epidemiological characteristics of subacute sclerosing panencephalitis in Bulgaria during the past 25 years (1978–2002). *Eur J Paediatr Neurol* 2004;8:89–94.
43. Halsey NA, Modlin JF, Jabbour JT, et al. Risk factors in subacute sclerosing panencephalitis: a case-control study. *Am J Epidemiol* 1980;111:415–424.
44. Lynn R, Nicoll A, Rahi J, et al, eds. Royal College of Paediatrics and Child Health British Paediatric Surveillance Unit 14th Annual Report 1999–2000. http://bpsu.inopsu.com/bpsuar2000final.pdf.
45. Duclos P, Ward BJ. Measles vaccines: a review of adverse events. *Drug Saf* 1998;6:435–454. Search date 1998; primary sources Stratton RS, Howe CJ, Johnston Jr RB. Adverse events associated with childhood vaccines: evidence bearing on causality. Washington DC: National Academy Press 1994 for papers published before 1994; for articles published after 1994 primary sources WHO Collaborating Centre for International Drug Monitoring Database, discussion groups, advisory committee documents, and other unspecified databases.
46. Virtanen M, Peltola H, Paunio M, et al. Day-to-day reactogenicity and the healthy vaccinee effect of measles–mumps–rubella vaccination. *Pediatrics* 2000;106:e62.
47. Barlow WE, Davis RL, Glasser JW. The risk of seizures after receipt of whole cell pertussis or measles mumps and rubella vaccine. *N Engl J Med* 2001;345:656–661.
48. Patja A, Davidkin I, Kurki T, et al. Serious adverse events after measles–mumps–rubella vaccination during a fourteen year prospective follow up. *Pediatr Infect Dis J* 2000;19:1127–1134.
49. Farrington P, Pugh S, Colville A, et al. A new method for active surveillance of adverse events from diphtheria/tetanus/pertussis and measles/mumps/rubella vaccines. *Lancet* 1995;345:567–569.
50. Miller E, Goldacre M, Pugh S, et al. Risk of aseptic meningitis after measles, mumps, and rubella vaccine in UK children. *Lancet* 1993;341:979.
51. Black S, Shinefield H, Ray P, et al. Risk of hospitalization because of aseptic meningitis after measles-mumps-rubella vaccination in one- to two-year-old children: an analysis of the Vaccine Safety Datalink (VSD) Project. *Pediatr Infect Dis J* 1997;16:500–503.
52. Dourado I, Cunha S, Teixeira MG, et al. Outbreak of aseptic meningitis associated with mass vaccination with a urabe-containing measles-mumps-rubella vaccine: implications for immunization programs. *Am J Epidemiol* 2000;151:524–530.
53. Ki M, Park T, Yi S G, et al. Risk analysis of aseptic meningitis after measles-mumps-rubella vaccination in Korean children by using a case-crossover design. *Am J Epidemiol* 2003;157:158–165.
54. de Silveira CM, Kmetzsch CI, Mohrdieck R, et al. The risk of aseptic meningitis associated with the Leningrad-Zagreb mumps vaccine strain following mass vaccination with measles-mumps-rubella, Rio Grande do Sul, Brazil 1997. *Int J Epidemiol* 2002;31:978–982.
55. Da Cunha SS, Rodrigues LC, Barreto ML, et al. Outbreak of aseptic meningitis and mumps after mass vaccination with MMR vaccine using the Leningrad-Zagreb mumps strain. *Vaccine* 2002:20:1106–1112.
56. Miller E, Waight P, Farrington CP, et al. Idiopathic thrombocytopenic purpura and MMR vaccine. *Arch Dis Child* 2001;84:227–229.
57. Black C, Kaye JA, Jick, H. MMR vaccine and idiopathic thrombocytopaenic purpura. *Br J Clin Pharmacol* 2003;55:107–111.
58. Stratton KR, Howe CJ, Johnston RB, eds. *Adverse events associated with childhood vaccines. Evidence bearing on causality*. Washington DC: National Academy Press, 1994.
59. Committee on Safety of Medicines and Medicines Control Agency. Adverse reactions to measles rubella vaccine. *Curr Prob Pharmacovigil* 1995;25:9–10.
60. Salisbury DM, Campbell H, Edwards B. *Measles Rubella Immunisation Campaign in England "One Year On"*. London: Department of Health, November 1995.
61. DeStefano D, Gu P, Kramarz BI, et al. Childhood vaccinations and risk of asthma. *Pediatr Infect Dis J* 2002;21:498–504.
62. Maher JE, Mullooly JP, Drew L, DeStefano F. Infant vaccinations and childhood asthma among full-term infants. *Pharmacoepidemiol Drug Saf* 2004;13:1–9.
63. McKeever TM, Lewis SA, Smith C, Hubbard R. Vaccination and allergic disease: a birth cohort study. *Am J Public Health* 2004;94:985–989.
64. Wickens K, Crane J, Kemp T, et al. A case-control study of risk factors for asthma in New Zealand children. *Aust N Z J Public Health* 2001;25:44–49.
65. Hviid A, Stellfeld M, Wohlfahrt J, Melbye M. Childhood vaccination and type 1 diabetes. *N Engl J Med* 2004;350:1398–1404.

66. Institute of Medicine. *Immunization safety review: measles–mumps–rubella vaccine and autism.* Washington DC: National Academy Press, 2001. http://books.nap.edu/books/0309074479/html/index.html (last accessed 28 January 2004).
67. DeStefano F, Bhasin TK, Thompson WW, Yeargin-Allsopp M, Boyle C. Age at first measles-mumps-rubella vaccination in children with autism and school-matched control subjects: a population-based study metropolitan Atlanta. *Pediatrics* 2004;113:259–266.
68. Madsen KM, Hviid A, Vestergaard M, et al. A population-based study of measles, mumps, and rubella vaccination and autism. *N Engl J Med* 2002;347:1477–1482.
69. Taylor B, Miller E, Farrington CP, et al. Autism and measles, mumps, and rubella vaccine: no epidemiological evidence for a causal association. *Lancet* 1999;353:2026–2029.
70. Taylor B, Miller E, Lingam R, et al. Measles, mumps, and rubella vaccination and bowel problems or developmental regression in children with autism: a population study. *BMJ* 2002;324:393–396.
71. Dales L, Hammer SJ, Smith N. Time trends in autism and in MMR immunization coverage in California. *JAMA* 2001;285:1183–1185.
72. Kaye JA, del Mar Melero-Montes M, Jick H. Mumps, measles, and rubella vaccine and the incidence of autism recorded by general practitioners: a time trend analysis. *BMJ* 2001;322:460–463.
73. Morris DL, Montgomery SM, Thompson NP. Measles vaccination and inflammatory bowel disease: a National British Cohort study. *Am J Gastroenterol* 2000;95:3507–3512.
74. Davis RL, Kramarz P, Bohlke K, et al. Measles–mumps–rubella and other measles containing vaccines do not increase risk for inflammatory bowel disease: a case control study from the Vaccine Safety Datalink project. *Arch Pediatr Adolesc Med* 2001;155:354–359.
75. Wakefield AJ, Murch SH, Anthony A, et al. Ileal–lymphoid–nodular hyperplasia, non-specific colitis, and pervasive developmental disorder in children. *Lancet* 1998;351:637–641.
76. Ceyhan M, Kanra G, Erdem G, et al. Immunogenicity and efficacy of one dose measles–mumps–rubella (MMR) vaccine at twelve months of age as compared to monovalent measles vaccination at nine months followed by MMR revaccination at fifteen months of age. *Vaccine* 2001;19:4473–4478.
77. Edees S, Pullan CR, Hull D. A randomised single blind trial of a combined mumps measles rubella vaccine to evaluate serological response and reactions in the UK population. *Public Health* 1991;105:91–97.
78. Takahashi H, Suzumura S, Shirakizawa F, et al. An epidemiological study on Japanese autism concerning routine childhood immunization history. *Jpn J Infect Dis* 2003;56:114–117.
79. Chen W, Landau S, Sham P, Fombonne E. No evidence for links between autism, MMR and measles virus. *Psychol Med* 2004;34:543–553.
80. Robertson CM, Bennet VJ, Jefferson N, et al. Serological evaluation of a measles, mumps, and rubella vaccine. *Arch Dis Child* 1988;63:612–616.
81. Anders J, Jacobson R, Poland G, et al. Secondary failure rates of measles vaccines: a meta-analysis of published studies. *Pediatr Infect Dis J* 1996;15:62–66. Search date 1995; primary sources Medline (English language only), hand searches of references cited in initialsearch and references cited within first generation references.

Helen Bedford
Dr
Centre for Paediatric Epidemiology
Institute of Child Health
London
UK

Nitu Sengupta
Dr
Queen Mary School of Medicine and
Dentistry, Barts and The London
London
UK

David Elliman
Dr
Islington PCT and
Great Ormond Street Hospital
London
UK

Robert Booy
Professor
Queen Mary School of Medicine and
Dentistry, Barts and The London
London
UK

Competing interests: HB, RB & DE have in the past received money from vaccine manufacturers to attend symposia and conduct research. RB also acts as a consultant to a number of vaccine manufacturers. NS: none declared.

Migraine headache in children

Search date August 2004

Nick Barnes, Guy Millman, and Elizabeth James

QUESTIONS

INTERVENTIONS

See glossary G

Key Messages

Treatments for acute attacks

- **$5HT_1$ antagonists (e.g. Triptans)** Two RCTs provided insufficient evidence that nasal sumatriptan reduced symptoms of migraine, but found that sumatriptan increased taste disturbance compared with placebo. One RCT found no significant difference in pain relief between oral rizatriptan and placebo.
- **Antiemetics** We found no RCTs of antiemetics in children with migraine headache.
- **Codeine phosphate** We found no RCTs.
- **Non-steroidal anti-inflammatory drugs** We found no reliable RCTs assessing the effects of non-steroidal anti-inflammatory drugs in children and adolescents with migraine headache.
- **Paracetamol** We found no RCTs of sufficient quality addressing the effects of paracetamol (acetaminophen) in children or adolescents with migraine headache.

Prophylaxis

- **Stress management** One small RCT provided limited evidence that a stress management programme improved headache severity and frequency compared with no stress management at 1 month.
- **Dietary manipulation** We found no RCTs of sufficient quality in children and adolescents with migraine headache.
- **Pizotifen** We found no RCTs of sufficient quality.
- **Progressive muscle relaxation** We found no RCTs of sufficient quality examining effects of progressive muscle relaxation in children with migraine headache.
- **Thermal biofeedback** We found no RCTs of sufficient quality examining effects of thermal biofeedback in children with migraine headache.
- **β blockers** One RCT found that propranolol increased perception of benefit compared with placebo. However, one RCT found no significant difference in migraine episodes and another RCT found that propranolol increased headache duration compared with placebo.

DEFINITION Migraine is defined by the International Headache Society (IHS) as a recurrent headache that occurs with or without aura**G** and lasts 2–48 hours.[1] It is usually unilateral in nature, pulsating in quality, of moderate or severe intensity, and is aggravated by routine physical activity. Nausea, vomiting, photophobia, and phonophobia are common accompanying symptoms. This topic focuses on children younger than 18 years. Diagnostic criteria for children are broader than criteria for adults, allowing for a broader range of duration and a broader localisation of the pain (see table 1, p 395).[2] Diagnosis is difficult in young children, because the condition is defined by subjective symptoms. Studies that do not explicitly use criteria that are congruent with IHS diagnostic criteria (or revised IHS criteria in children < 15 years of age) have been excluded from this topic.

INCIDENCE/ PREVALENCE Migraine occurs in 3–10% of children,[3–7] and currently affects 50/1000 school age children in the UK and an estimated 7.8 million children in the European Union.[8] Studies in developed countries suggest that migraine is the most common diagnosis among children presenting with headache to a medical practitioner. It is rarely diagnosed in children under 2 years of age because of the symptom based definition, but increases steadily with age thereafter.[1,9,10] It affects boys and girls similarly before puberty, but after puberty girls are more likely to suffer from migraine.[4,6,10] See incidence/prevalence of migraine headache, p 1622.

AETIOLOGY/ RISK FACTORS The cause of migraine headaches is unknown. We found few reliable data identifying risk factors or measuring their effects in children. Suggested risk factors include stress, foods, menses, and exercise in genetically predisposed children and adolescents.[10,11]

PROGNOSIS We found no reliable data about prognosis of childhood migraine headache diagnosed by IHS criteria. It has been suggested that more than half the children will have spontaneous remission after puberty.[10] It is believed that migraine that develops during adolescence tends to continue in adult life, although attacks tend to be less frequent and severe in later life.[12] We found one longitudinal study from Sweden (73 children with "pronounced" migraine and mean age onset 6 years) with over 40 years follow up, which predated the IHS criteria for migraine headache.[13] It found that migraine headaches had ceased before the age of 25 years in 23% of people. However, by the age of 50 years, more than 50% of people continued to have migraine headaches. We found no prospective data examining long term risks in children with migraine.

AIMS OF INTERVENTION To provide relief from symptoms; to prevent recurrent attacks in the long term, and to minimise the disruption of childhood activities, with minimal adverse effects.

OUTCOMES Pain scores (usually on visual analogue scales); migraine recurrence; functional indicators (such as time off school, behavioural scores, sleep scores, and sleep satisfaction); any adverse effects of treatment. Migraine index is a validated scale for measuring severity in adult migraine. Its validity in children is unclear.

METHODS *Clinical Evidence* search and appraisal August 2004.

QUESTION **What are the effects of treatments for acute attacks of migraine headache in children?**

OPTION **PARACETAMOL**

We found no RCTs of sufficient quality addressing the effects of paracetamol (acetaminophen) in children or adolescents with migraine headache.

Benefits: We found no systematic review or RCTs of sufficient quality (see comment below).

Harms: We found no RCTs. See paracetamol poisoning for symptoms and treatment of paracetamol overdose, p 1756.

Comment: We found one three way crossover RCT (106 children) comparing paracetamol, ibuprofen, and placebo. The RCT had high withdrawal rates (17%) and did not report results before crossover.[14] This may have introduced bias because of continued treatment effects after crossover, and because of unequal withdrawals among groups.

OPTION NON-STEROIDAL ANTI-INFLAMMATORY DRUGS

We found no reliable RCTs assessing the effects of non-steroidal anti-inflammatory drugs in children and adolescents with migraine headache.

Benefits: We found no systematic review or reliable RCTs.

Harms: We found no RCTs.

Comment: We found one three arm crossover RCT (106 children) comparing paracetamol, ibuprofen, and placebo. It was excluded because it had methodological flaws that compromised the validity of its results, including failure to report results before crossover.[14]

OPTION CODEINE PHOSPHATE

We found no RCTs.

Benefits: We found no systematic review or RCTs addressing the effects of codeine phosphate in children or adolescents with migraine headache.

Harms: We found no RCTs. Known adverse effects of codeine include nausea, vomiting, constipation, drowsiness, potential for respiratory depression in overdose, difficulty for micturition, and dry mouth.

Comment: None.

OPTION $5HT_1$ ANTAGONISTS (E.G. TRIPTANS)

Two RCTs provided insufficient evidence that nasal sumatriptan reduced symptoms of migraine, but found that sumatriptan increased taste disturbance compared with placebo. One RCT found no significant difference in pain relief between oral rizatriptan and placebo.

Benefits: **Sumatriptan versus placebo:** We found two RCTs.[15,16] The first RCT (653 children aged 12–17 years) compared three different doses of nasal sumatriptan (5, 10, or 20 mg) with placebo.[15] It found that nasal sumatriptan increased complete resolution of headache compared with placebo at 2 hours, although the result was significant only for the lowest dose (74/118 [63%] with 20 mg; 85/133 [64%] with 10 mg; 84/128 [66%] with 5 mg; 69/131 [53%] with placebo; $P < 0.05$ for 5 mg *v* placebo, but not for other doses *v* placebo).[15] The second RCT (129 children aged 8–17 years) had a crossover design. It compared nasal sumatriptan (10 mg for body weight 20–39 kg; 20 mg for body weight > 39 kg) with placebo.[16] Results before crossover (94 children included in pre-crossover analysis) found that nasal sumatriptan significantly increased relief of headache (measured as a 2 point fall from baseline on a 5 point scale where 5 = severe and 1 = no pain) compared with placebo at 2 hours (headache relief: 34/46 [74%] with sumatriptan *v* 16/48 [33%] with placebo; $P < 0.001$).[16] **Rizatriptan versus placebo:** We found one RCT (360 children aged 12–17 years), which compared oral rizatriptan versus placebo.[17] It found no significant difference between rizatriptan and placebo for partial or complete pain relief at 2 hours (pain free: 48/149 [32%] with rizatriptan *v* 40/142 [28%] with placebo; $P = 0.47$; partial pain relief: 98/149 [66%] with rizatriptan *v* 80/142 [56%] with placebo; $P = 0.08$).[17] It found that rizatriptan significantly reduced nausea and somnolence compared with placebo (nausea at 1 hour: AR 26% with rizatriptan *v* 37% with placebo; $P = 0.044$; nausea at 1.5 hours: AR 22% with rizatriptan *v* 35% with placebo; $P = 0.016$; nausea at 4 hours: AR 16% with rizatriptan *v* 27% with placebo; $P = 0.036$; somnolence: AR 5.6% with rizatriptan *v* 1.8% with placebo; $P < 0.05$).

Harms: **Sumatriptan versus placebo:** The first RCT found that taste disturbance was more common with sumatriptan compared with placebo (19% with 5 mg *v* 30% with 10 mg *v* 26% with 20 mg *v* 2% with placebo).[15] The second RCT also reported that taste disturbance was more common with sumatriptan compared with placebo (results after crossover: 29% with sumatriptan *v* 3% with placebo; $P < 0.001$).[16] However, neither study found any significant differences for other adverse effects. **Rizatriptan versus placebo:** The RCT reported that one child taking rizatriptan developed transient jaundice and hyperglycaemia, which resolved within 1 week.[17]

Comment: **Sumatriptan versus placebo:** We found one RCT (only the abstract published).[18] It could not, therefore, be assessed adequately. A second double blind, placebo controlled, crossover RCT did not report results before crossover and had a high withdrawal rate (26%), and it has, therefore, been excluded.[19] We found one small crossover RCT (14 children aged 6.4–9.8 years).[20] However, it did not present results before crossover, and so has been excluded. **Rizatriptan versus placebo:** In the RCT comparing rizatriptan with placebo 360 children were originally enrolled. Of these, 64 children did not receive placebo or rizatriptan, the reasons for which were not reported. Seven children subsequently withdrew, although reasons for stopping treatment were not reported.

OPTION ANTIEMETICS

We found no RCTs of antiemetics in children with migraine headache.

Benefits: We found no systematic review or RCTs.

Harms: We found no RCTs.

Comment: None.

QUESTION What are the effects of prophylaxis for migraine in children?

OPTION β BLOCKERS

One RCT found that propranolol increased perception of benefit compared with placebo. However, one RCT found no significant difference in migraine episodes and another RCT found that propranolol increased headache duration compared with placebo.

Benefits: We found no systematic review. **Versus placebo:** We found three small RCTs that compared propranolol versus placebo.[21–23] The first RCT (double blind, crossover, 32 children aged 7–16 years) found that propranolol (60–120 mg/day divided in 3 doses) significantly increased perception of benefit compared with placebo during a 3 month period (report of "some benefit" before crossover: 13/13 [100%] with propranolol *v* 4/15 [27%] with placebo; $P < 0.001$).[21] However, reliability may be limited because 13% of people were lost to follow up. The second RCT (double blind, crossover, 53 children aged 9–15 years) compared propranolol 40–120 mg daily with placebo.[22] It found that propranolol significantly increased headache duration compared with placebo (results before crossover; mean duration of headache: 436 minutes with propranolol *v* 287 minutes with placebo; $P < 0.01$). The third RCT (double blind, crossover, 33 children aged 6–12 years) found no significant difference in the number of episodes of migraine between propranolol 3 mg/kg daily and placebo at 3 months (results before crossover; mean number of headaches: 14.9 with propranolol v 13.3 with placebo; P = 0.47).[23] In five people in whom migraine was thought to be provoked by food, diet was restricted to avoid those foods (no details about type of foods reported). This may have confounded apparent treatment effects.

Harms: The first RCT reported insomnia in 2/13 (18%) children taking propranolol, but did not report on adverse effects in the placebo group.[21] The second RCT found no significant difference in adverse effects between placebo and propranolol (12 children affected in each group).[22] Adverse effects in both groups included abdominal pain, increased appetite, worsening of headaches, and fatigue. However, the trial was too small to yield reliable information about harms. The third trial did not report on adverse effects.[23] All RCTs probably lacked power to detect clinically important differences.

Comment: None.

OPTION PIZOTIFEN

We found no RCTs of sufficient quality.

Benefits: We found no systematic review or RCTs of sufficient quality.

Harms: We found no systematic review or RCTs that met International Headache Society (IHS) criteria for migraine (see comment below).

Comment: We found one RCT (47 children aged 7–14 years) comparing pizotifen with placebo.[24] It pre-dated the IHS diagnostic criteria for migraine and people in this study would not all fulfil the current IHS definition. The study has, therefore, been excluded. We found one further RCT comparing pizotifen with placebo.[25] It has only been published in abstract form and so we could not reliably review its methods.

OPTION DIETARY MANIPULATION

We found no RCTs of sufficient quality in children and adolescents with migraine headache.

Benefits: We found no systematic review and no RCTs of sufficient quality (see comment below).

Harms: We found no RCTs.

Comment: We found one small RCT (39 children allocated to treatment), which attempted to investigate effects of excluding dietary vasoactive amines**G** on morbidity related to migraine.[26] However, the study predated the International Headache Society criteria for migraine and a large proportion (33%) of eligible children were excluded before randomisation. The study has, therefore, been excluded.

OPTION THERMAL BIOFEEDBACK

We found no RCTs of sufficient quality examining effects of thermal biofeedback in children with migraine headache.

Benefits: We found no systematic review and no RCTs of sufficient quality (see comment below).

Harms: We found no RCTs.

Comment: We found two RCTs with more than 10 people in each treatment arm.[27,28] However, the first had high loss to follow up (46%),[27] and the second was published only as a conference abstract.[28]

OPTION **PROGRESSIVE MUSCLE RELAXATION**

We found no RCTs of sufficient quality examining effects of progressive muscle relaxation in children with migraine headache.

Benefits: We found no systematic review and no RCTs of sufficient quality (see comment below).

Harms: We found no RCTs.

Comment: We found one RCT (99 people aged 9–17 years), which compared progressive muscle relaxation**G** with psychological counselling.[29] However, high loss to follow up (30%) precluded reliable conclusions.

OPTION **STRESS MANAGEMENT**

One small RCT provided limited evidence that a stress management programme improved headache severity and frequency compared with no stress management at 1 month.

Benefits: We found no systematic review. We found one RCT (87 people, aged 11–18 years).[30] It found that a self administered stress management**G** programme reduced headache severity and frequency compared with both a stress management programme delivered by the clinic, and with no stress management at 1 month (16/24 [67%] improved with self administered treatment *v* 10/23 [44%] with treatment delivered by the clinic *v* 6/25 [24%] with no stress management; $P < 0.01$ for differences among all three groups).[30]

Harms: The RCT did not report on harms.[30]

Comment: None.

GLOSSARY

Aura A premonitory sensation or warning experienced before the start of a migraine headache.

Dietary manipulation A change in diet aimed specifically at reducing or removing from the diet a foodstuff that is thought to provoke migraine headache.

Dietary vasoactive amines Dietary amines (protein subunits) that may have an effect on cerebral vascular tone.

Progressive muscle relaxation Volitional muscle relaxation aimed at altering the perception of symptoms such as headache.

Stress management Coping or relaxation strategies that aim to alter the perception of symptoms.

Thermal biofeedback A treatment in which an individual attempts to alter their skin temperature by responding to feedback about their skin temperature.

Substantive changes

$5HT_1$ antagonists One crossover RCT added;[16] benefits data enhanced but categorisation unchanged.

REFERENCES

1. Headache Classification Committee of the International Headache Society. Classification and diagnostic criteria for headache disorders, cranial neuralgias and facial pain. *Cephalalgia* 1988;8(suppl 7):1–96.
2. Winner P, Martinez W, Mate L, et al. Classification of pediatric migraine: proposed revisions to the IHS criteria. *Headache* 1995;35:407–410.
3. Hockaday JM, Barlow CF. Headache in children. In: Olesen J, Tfelt-Hansen P, Welch KMA, eds. *The headaches*. New York: Raven Press, 1993:795–808.
4. Bille B. Migraine in schoolchildren. *Acta Paediatr* 1962;51(suppl 136):1–151.
5. Goldstein M, Chen TC. The epidemiology of disabling headache. *Adv Neurol* 1982;33:377–390.
6. Abu-Arefeh I, Russell G. Prevalence of headache and migraine in schoolchildren. *BMJ* 1994;309:765–769.
7. Ueberall M. Sumatriptan in paediatric and adolescent migraine. *Cephalalgia* 2001;21(suppl 1):21–24.
8. Evers S. Drug treatment of migraine in children. A comparative review. *Paediatr Drugs* 1999;1:7–18.
9. Migraine. In: Behrman RE, Kliegman RM, Jenson HB, eds. *Nelson textbook of pediatrics*. 16th ed. Philadelphia: Saunders, 2000:1832–1834.
10. Amery WK, Vandenbergh V. What can precipitating factors teach us about the pathogenesis of migraine? *Headache* 1987;27:146–150.
11. Blau JN, Thavapalan M. Preventing migraine: a study of precipitating factors. *Headache* 1988;28:481–483.
12. Pearce JMS. Migraine. In: Weatherall DJ, Ledingham JGG, Warrell DA, eds. *Oxford textbook of medicine*. Oxford: Oxford University Press 1996:4024–4026.
13. Bille B. A 40-year follow-up of school children with migraine. *Cephalalgia* 1997;17:488–491.
14. Hamalainen ML, Hoppu K, Valkeila E, et al. Ibuprofen or acetaminophen for the acute treatment of migraine in children. *Neurology* 1997;48:103–107.
15. Winner P, Rothner AD, Saper J, et al. A randomized, double-blind, placebo-controlled study of sumatriptan nasal spray in the treatment of acute migraine in adolescents. *Pediatrics* 2000;106:989–997.
16. Ahonen K, Hamalainen ML, Rantala H, et al. Nasal sumatriptan is effective in treatment of migraine attacks in children. A randomized trial. *Neurology* 2004;62:883–887.
17. Winner P, Lewis D, Visser WH, et al. Rizatriptan 5 mg for the acute treatment of migraine in adolescents: a randomised, double-blind, placebo-controlled study. *Headache* 2002;42:49–55.
18. Korsgard AG. The tolerability, safety and efficacy of oral sumatriptan 50 mg and 100 mg for the acute treatment of migraine in adolescents. *Cephalalgia* 1995;15(suppl 16):99.
19. Hamalainen ML, Hoppu K, Santavuori P. Sumatriptan for migraine attacks in children: a randomized placebo-controlled study. Do children with migraine respond to oral sumatriptan differently from adults? *Neurology* 1997;48:1100–1103.
20. Ueberall MA, Wenzel D. Intranasal sumatriptan for the acute treatment of migraine in children. *Neurology* 1999;52:1507–1510.
21. Ludviggson J. Propranolol used in the prophylaxis of migraine in children. *Acta Neurol Scand* 1974;50:109–115.
22. Forsythe WI, Gillies D, Sills MA. Propranolol ("Inderal") in the treatment of childhood migraine. *Dev Med Child Neurol* 1984;26:737–741.
23. Olness K, Macdonald JT, Uden DL. Comparison of self-hypnosis and propranolol in the treatment of juvenile classic migraine. *Pediatrics* 1987;79:593–597.
24. Gillies D, Sills M, Forsythe I. Pizotifen (Sanomigran) in childhood migraine. A double-blind controlled trial. *Eur Neurol* 1986;25:32–35.
25. Salmon MA. Pizotifen (BC.105. Sanomigran) in the prophylaxis of childhood migraine. *Cephalalgia* 1985;5(suppl 3):178. [Abstract]
26. Salfield SAW, Wardley BL, Houlsby WT, et al. Controlled study of exclusion of dietary vasoactive amines in migraine. *Arch Dis Child* 1987;62:458–460.
27. Labbe EL, Williamson DA. Treatment of childhood migraine using autogenic feedback training. *J Consult Clin Psychol* 1984;52:968–976.
28. Andrasik F, Attanasio V, Blanchard EB, et al. Behavioural treatment of pediatric migraine headache. In: Andrasik F (Chair), Recent developments in the assessment and treatment of headache. Symposium conducted at the annual meeting of the Association for Advancement of Behaviour Therapy, Philadelphia, PA, 1984.
29. McGrath PJ, Humphreys P, Goodman JT, et al. Relaxation prophylaxis for childhood migraine: a randomised placebo-controlled trial. *Dev Med Child Neurol* 1988;30:626–631.
30. McGrath PJ, Humphreys P, Keene D, et al. The efficacy of a self-administered treatment for adolescent migraine. *Pain* 1992;49:321–324.

Nick Barnes
Specialist Registrar Paediatrics
John Radcliffe Hospital
Oxford
UK

Guy Millman
Specialist Registrar
Paediatric Neurology
Manchester Children's Hospital
Manchester
UK

Elizabeth James
General Practitioner
Didcot Health Centre
Didcot
UK

Competing interests: None declared.

TABLE 1 International Headache Society criteria for migraine.[1] (Text in parenthesis indicates suggested revisions for children < 15 years of age.[2])

At least 5 episodes **without aura** fulfilling **all** of criteria **1–3:**		OR	At least 2 episodes **with aura** fulfilling at least **three** of criteria **1–4:**	
1.	Headache lasting 2–48 hours (30 minutes–48 hours)		1.	One or more fully reversible aura symptoms including focal cortical, brain stem dysfunction, or both
2.	Headache meeting at least two of the following criteria: a) Unilateral or bilateral (either frontal or temporal) distribution of pain b) Throbbing c) Moderate to severe intensity d) Aggravated by routine physical activity		2.	At least one aura symptom that develops gradually over more than 4 minutes, or 2 or more symptoms that occur in succession
3.	At least one of the following symptoms while headache is present: a) Nausea, vomiting, or both b) Photophobia, phonophobia, or both		3.	No aura symptoms lasting more than 60 minutes
			4.	Headache follows aura within 60 minutes

Neonatal jaundice

Search date November 2003

Anthony Kwaku Akobeng

QUESTIONS

INTERVENTIONS

To be covered in future updates
Antenatal anti-D immunoglobulin
Continuous versus intermittent phototherapy
Immunoglobulin infusion for isoimmune haemolytic jaundice
Intrauterine blood transfusion
Lamp colour in phototherapy
Phenobarbitone
Position change versus static position in phototherapy
Routine intravenous fluids during phototherapy

*Although we found no RCTs, there is a general consensus that exchange transfusion is effective in reducing serum bilirubin levels

Key Messages

- **Exchange transfusion** We found no RCTs on the effects of exchange transfusion versus no treatment or versus phototherapy. There is general consensus that exchange transfusion is effective in reducing serum bilirubin levels and in preventing neuro-developmental sequelae. In most of the RCTs comparing other interventions, exchange transfusion was used successfully to reduce serum bilirubin levels when those interventions failed to control the rise of serum bilirubin.
- **Phototherapy** Two RCTs found that both conventional phototherapy and fibreoptic phototherapy reduced neonatal jaundice more effectively than no treatment. One systematic review (which included quasi-randomised as well as randomised controlled trials) and one subsequent RCT found that conventional phototherapy was more effective than fibreoptic phototherapy, although subgroup analysis in the systematic review found no significant difference between groups in preterm infants. No trials included in the review evaluated the impact of either phototherapy method on parent–infant bonding. One RCT found a greater effect with double conventional compared with single conventional phototherapy, whilst another RCT found no significant difference between double fibreoptic and single conventional phototherapy. One systematic review (which included quasi-randomised as well as randomised controlled trials) found no significant difference between fibreoptic plus conventional and conventional phototherapy alone in additional phototherapy, exchange transfusion, or percentage change in bilirubin after 24 hours, although it noted a trend favouring the fibreoptic plus conventional group. Most trials did not report kernicterus as an outcome. We found insufficient evidence on the adverse effects of phototherapy.
- **Albumin infusion** We found no RCTs on the effects of albumin infusion versus no treatment or versus other treatment.
- **Home versus hospital phototherapy** We found no RCTs on the effects of home phototherapy versus no treatment or versus hospital phototherapy.

Clin Evid 2005;13:396–401.

DEFINITION Neonatal jaundice refers to the yellow colouration of the skin and sclera of newborn babies that results from hyperbilirubinaemia.

INCIDENCE/ PREVALENCE Jaundice is the most common condition requiring medical attention in newborn babies. About 50% of term and 80% of preterm babies develop jaundice in the first week of life.[1] Jaundice is also a common cause of readmission to hospital after early discharge of newborn babies.[2] Jaundice usually appears 2–4 days after birth and disappears 1–2 weeks later, usually without the need for treatment.

AETIOLOGY/ RISK FACTORS In most infants with jaundice, there is no underlying disease and the jaundice is termed physiological. Physiological jaundice occurs when there is accumulation of unconjugated bilirubin in the skin and mucous membranes. It typically presents on the second or third day of life and results from the increased production of bilirubin (due to increased circulating red cell mass and a shortened red cell lifespan) and the decreased excretion of bilirubin (due to low concentrations of the hepatocyte binding protein, low activity of glucuronyl transferase, and increased enterohepatic circulation) that normally occur in newborn babies. In some infants, unconjugated hyperbilirubinaemia may be associated with breast feeding (breast milk jaundice), and this typically occurs after the third day of life. Although the exact cause of breast milk jaundice is not clear, it is generally believed to be due to an unidentified factor in breast milk. Non-physiological causes include blood group incompatibility (Rhesus or ABO problems), other causes of haemolysis, sepsis, bruising, and metabolic disorders. Gilbert's and Crigler-Najjar syndromes are rare causes of neonatal jaundice.

PROGNOSIS In the newborn baby, unconjugated bilirubin can penetrate the blood–brain barrier and is potentially neurotoxic. Unconjugated hyperbilirubinaemia can, therefore, result in neuro-developmental sequelae including the development of kernicterus. Kernicterus is brain damage arising from the deposition of bilirubin in brain tissue. However, the exact level of bilirubin that is neurotoxic is unclear, and kernicterus at autopsy has been reported in infants in the absence of markedly elevated levels of bilirubin.[3] Recent reports suggest a resurgence of kernicterus in countries in which this complication had virtually disappeared.[4] This has been attributed mainly to early discharge of newborns from hospital.

AIMS OF INTERVENTION To prevent the development of bilirubin-associated neuro-developmental sequelae; to reduce serum bilirubin levels; with minimal adverse effects.

OUTCOMES Mortality; hearing loss; incidence of kernicterus and other neuro-developmental sequelae; adverse events due to treatment (including effects on parent–infant bonding); duration of treatment; failure of treatment (defined as the need to use other forms of treatment); length of hospital stay; need for transfusion; changes in serum bilirubin levels.

METHODS *Clinical Evidence* search and appraisal November 2003. This chapter focuses on interventions for treating unconjugated hyperbilirubinaemia. The prevention of this condition, and the specific treatment of its underlying causes, is not covered. Conjugated hyperbilirubinaemia, a condition that may indicate an underlying liver or biliary tract disorder, is beyond the scope of this chapter.

QUESTION What are the effects of treatments for unconjugated hyperbilirubinaemia in term and preterm infants?

OPTION PHOTOTHERAPY

Two RCTs found that both conventional phototherapy and fibreoptic phototherapy reduced neonatal jaundice more effectively than no treatment. One systematic review (which included quasi-randomised as well as randomised controlled trials) and one subsequent RCT found that conventional phototherapy was more effective than fibreoptic phototherapy, although subgroup analysis in the systematic review found no significant difference between groups in preterm infants. No trials included in the review evaluated the impact of either phototherapy method on parent–infant bonding. One RCT found a greater effect with double conventional compared with single conventional phototherapy, whilst another RCT found no significant difference between double fibreoptic and single conventional phototherapy. One systematic review (which included quasi-randomised as well as randomised

controlled trials) found no significant difference between fibreoptic plus conventional and conventional phototherapy alone in additional phototherapy, exchange transfusion, or percentage change in bilirubin after 24 hours, although it noted a trend favouring the fibreoptic plus conventional group. Most trials did not report kernicterus as an outcome. We found insufficient evidence on the adverse effects of phototherapy.

Benefits:

Conventional phototherapy versus no treatment: We found no systematic review but found one RCT.[5] The RCT compared conventional phototherapy using daylight fluorescent lamps versus no treatment in three birth weight groups: less than 2000 g; 2000–2499 g; and 2500 g and over. Exchange transfusion was given at predetermined serum bilirubin levels in each group. The RCT examined prevention of hyperbilirubinaemia in the lowest birth weight group, and treatment of established hyperbilirubinaemia in the remaining two groups. Only the results of treatment of established hyperbilirubinaemia are reported here. The RCT found that in the 2000–2499 g birth weight group (141 infants, serum bilirubin ≥ 10 mg/dL, average 12.4 mg/dL) phototherapy significantly reduced the proportion of infants with higher maximal serum bilirubin levels compared with no treatment (serum bilirubin ≥ 15 mg/dL: 18.6% with phototherapy *v* 42.3% with no treatment; P = 0.002). Overall, it found that phototherapy significantly decreased the proportion of infants with exchange transfusion compared with no treatment (4.3% with phototherapy *v* 25.4% with no treatment; P < 0.001). On subgroup analysis, it found that in non-haemolytic jaundice, phototherapy significantly decreased exchange transfusion compared with no treatment, but it found no significant difference between groups in haemolytic jaundice (non-haemolytic: 1.9% with phototherapy *v* 27.5% with no treatment, P = 0.0002; haemolytic: 16.7% with phototherapy *v* 22.2% with no treatment, reported as not significant). The RCT found that in the 2500 g or over birth weight group (276 infants, serum bilirubin ≥ 13 mg/dL, average 15.6–15.7 mg/dL) phototherapy significantly reduced mean serum bilirubin levels until 24 hours after the cessation of therapy compared with no treatment (results presented graphically; P value not reported). Overall, it found no significant difference between phototherapy and no treatment in the proportion of infants with exchange transfusion (10% with phototherapy *v* 16.9% with no treatment; reported as not significant). On subgroup analysis, it found that in non-haemolytic jaundice, phototherapy significantly decreased exchange transfusion compared with no treatment, but it found no significant difference between groups in haemolytic jaundice (non-haemolytic: 2.9% with phototherapy *v* 17.3% with no treatment, P = 0.05; haemolytic: 17.1% with phototherapy *v* 16.7% with no treatment, reported as not significant).[5] A subsequent report of the RCT noted that there were two deaths before hospital discharge (2000–2499 g group: 1 with phototherapy *v* 1 with no treatment; ≥ 2500 g group: none).[6] A further follow up report of the RCT found no significant difference in either of the two birth weight groups between treatment groups in cerebral palsy or other motor abnormalities (clumsiness, hypotonia, abnormal movement) after 1 and 6 years.[7]

Fibreoptic phototherapy versus no treatment: We found one systematic review (search date 2000; term and preterm infants; randomised and quasi-randomised trials; see comment below).[8] The review found one RCT (46 term infants, haemolysis excluded) that compared fibreoptic phototherapy (Wallaby system) versus no treatment. Conventional phototherapy was commenced if the serum bilirubin reached predetermined levels. The review found that, compared with no treatment, fibreoptic phototherapy significantly increased the percentage change in serum bilirubin per hour (WMD –0.44%, 95% CI –0.21% to –0.67%) and the percentage change after 24 hours of treatment (WMD –10.7%, 95% CI –3.26% to –18.14%).[8] It found that infants in the fibreoptic phototherapy group were less likely to require conventional phototherapy, but this did not reach significance (0/23 [0%] with fibreoptic phototherapy v 3/23 [13%] with no treatment: RR 0.14, 95% CI 0.01 to 2.62). **Conventional versus fibreoptic phototherapy:** We found one systematic review (search date 2000; term and preterm infants; randomised and quasi-randomised trials; see comment below)[8] and one subsequent RCT.[9] The review found that conventional phototherapy significantly increased the percentage change of serum bilirubin after 24 and 48 hours of treatment compared with fibreoptic phototherapy (24 hours: 5 trials, 203 infants; WMD 3.59%, 95% CI 1.27% to 5.92%; 48 hours: 4 trials, 183 infants; WMD 10.79%, 95% CI 8.33% to 13.26%).[8] It also found that fibreoptic phototherapy significantly increased the use of additional phototherapy compared with conventional phototherapy (8 trials; 52/366 [14%] with fibreoptic v 35/390 [9%] with conventional; RR 1.68, 95% CI 1.18 to 2.38). It found no significant difference between fibreoptic and conventional phototherapy in the use of exchange transfusion (3 trials; 4/97 [4%] with fibreoptic v 3/117 [3%] with conventional; RR 1.62, 95% CI 0.38 to 6.93). In a subgroup analysis of preterm babies only, it found no significant difference between fibreoptic phototherapy and conventional phototherapy in the duration of phototherapy (3 trials, 232 infants; WMD +2 hours, 95% CI –3.5 hours to +7.52 hours), use of additional phototherapy (5 trials; 3/148 [2%] with fibreoptic v 3/156 [2%] with conventional; RR 1.07, 95% CI 0.27 to 4.27), percentage change in serum bilirubin after 24 hours of treatment (1 trial, 20 infants; WMD +1.7%, 95% CI –2.65% to +6.05%), and repeat phototherapy for rebound jaundice (3 trials; 10/122 [8%] with fibreoptic v 5/121 [4%] with conventional; RR 2.00, 95% CI 0.71 to 5.63).[8] The subsequent RCT (109 term infants, birth weight ≥2500 g, haemolysis excluded) found that conventional daylight phototherapy significantly increased the rate of decline of serum bilirubin and significantly decreased treatment duration compared with fibreoptic phototherapy (bilirubin decline rate: 0.15 ± 0.06 mg/dL/hour with conventional v 0.1 ± 0.05 mg/dL/hour with fibreoptic, $P < 0.05$; duration of phototherapy: 49.4 ± 14.4 hours with conventional v 61 ± 13.1 hours with fibreoptic; $P < 0.05$).[9] **Double versus single phototherapy:** We found one systematic review (search date 2000; term and preterm infants; randomised and quasi-randomised trials; see comment below)[8] and one additional RCT.[10] The systematic review found one RCT (86 term infants, haemolysis excluded) comparing double fibreoptic phototherapy (infants wrapped in 2 BiliBlankets) versus single conventional phototherapy.[8] It found no significant difference between groups in duration of treatment (WMD +2.24 hours, 95% CI –10.68 hours to +15.16 hours), percentage change in serum bilirubin per hour (WMD –0.04%, 95% CI –0.17% to +0.09%), percentage change in serum bilirubin per day (WMD +2.82%, 95% CI –1.84% to +7.48%), and the use of repeat phototherapy for rebound jaundice (RR 1.05, 95% CI 0.07 to 16.22).[8] The review also compared double phototherapy using a combination of fibreoptic plus conventional phototherapy versus conventional phototherapy alone. It found no significant difference between fibreoptic plus conventional phototherapy and single conventional phototherapy in exchange transfusion (1 trial; 0/19 [0%] with fibreoptic plus conventional v 2/23 [8%] with conventional; RR 0.24, 95% CI 0.01 to 4.72), additional phototherapy (1 trial; 0/90 [0%] with fibreoptic plus conventional v 4/90 [4%] with conventional; RR 0.11, 95% CI 0.01 to 2.02), and percentage change in serum bilirubin after 24 or 48 hours (1 trial, 26 infants; 24 hours: WMD –3.2%, 95% CI –17.2% to +10.8%; 48 hours: WMD –9.2%, 95% CI –25.02% to +6.62%), although it noted a trend favouring the fibreoptic plus conventional group. It found no significant difference between fibreoptic plus conventional phototherapy and single conventional phototherapy in repeat phototherapy for rebound jaundice (6 trials; 36/232 [16%] with fibreoptic plus conventional *v* 30/240 [13%] with conventional; RR 1.29, 95% CI 0.85 to 1.95).[8] The additional RCT (51 term infants, birth weight ≥ 2500 g, haemolysis included) compared double conventional phototherapy using daylight fluorescent lamps versus single conventional phototherapy.[10] It found that double conventional phototherapy reduced serum bilirubin significantly faster during the first 24 hours compared with single conventional phototherapy (0.22 ± 0.12 mg/dL/hour with double *v* 0.14 ± 0.10 mg/dL/hour with single; P = 0.02). It found a trend for double conventional phototherapy to reduce bilirubin faster on the second day but this did not reach significance (P = 0.06). It found that double conventional phototherapy significantly reduced duration of treatment compared with single conventional phototherapy (34.9 ± 12.6 hours *v* 43.7 ± 17.5 hours; P = 0.039). It did not report on kernicterus or other long term outcomes.

Harms: Most RCTs did not report on adverse events. **Conventional versus fibreoptic phototherapy:** In the systematic review, one small trial found that transepidermal water loss (sweating) was significantly higher in infants treated with fibreoptic devices compared with conventional phototherapy, and one small trial found no significant difference between fibreoptic and conventional phototherapy in mothers developing migraine during their infant's treatment with phototherapy.[8] However, the clinical significance of this is uncertain. One RCT reported transient erythema (1/50 [2%] with conventional *v* 1/50 [2%] with fibreoptic) and mild watery stools not leading to dehydration (3/50 [6%] with conventional *v* 3/50 [6%] with fibreoptic).[9] **Double versus single phototherapy:** One RCT found no significant difference between double conventional and single conventional phototherapy in weight reduction, frequency of stooling, or fever.[10]

Comment: As well as including RCTs, the systematic review also included quasi-randomised controlled trials, all of which used alternate or sequential allocation.[8] This may limit the validity of its conclusions. Two different fibreoptic devices were used by trials included in the review: BiliBlanket and Wallaby. The irradiance of the Wallaby phototherapy system and BiliBlanket are different, and the irradiance setting of the BiliBlanket was not the same in different trials.[8] Conventional phototherapy varied between trials, with trials using either halogen or fluorescent lamps, emitting white light, blue light, or a mixture of the two.[8] Inclusion criteria in the trials varied, with some excluding infants with haemolysis and others including them. No trials including infants with haemolysis reported separate data for this group, and the review was unable to do a planned subgroup analysis on this group.[8] Phototherapy was instituted at different serum bilirubin levels in different trials. Outcomes of trials included in the review were reported mainly in terms of changes in serum bilirubin levels; the incidence of kernicterus was not reported in any of the trials.[8] No trials were identified to support or refute the view that fibreoptic devices interfere less with infant care or impact less on parent–child bonding.[8]

OPTION HOME PHOTOTHERAPY

We found no RCTs on the effects of home phototherapy versus no treatment or versus hospital phototherapy.

Benefits: **Versus no treatment:** We found no systematic review or RCTs. **Versus hospital phototherapy:** We found no systematic review or RCTs.

Harms: We found no RCTs.

Comment: None.

OPTION ALBUMIN INFUSION

We found no RCTs on the effects of albumin infusion versus no treatment or versus other treatment.

Benefits: **Versus no treatment:** We found no systematic review or RCTs. **Versus other treatment:** We found no systematic review or RCTs.

Harms: We found no RCTs.

Comment: None.

OPTION EXCHANGE TRANSFUSION

We found no RCTs on the effects of exchange transfusion versus no treatment or versus phototherapy. There is general consensus that exchange transfusion is effective in reducing serum bilirubin levels and in preventing neuro-developmental sequelae. In most of the RCTs comparing other interventions, exchange transfusion was used successfully to reduce serum bilirubin levels when those interventions failed to control the rise of serum bilirubin.

Benefits: **Versus no treatment:** We found no systematic review or RCTs (see comment below). **Versus phototherapy:** We found no systematic review or RCTs.

Harms: We found no RCTs.

Comment: There is general consensus that exchange transfusion is effective in reducing serum bilirubin levels and preventing neuro-developmental sequelae. In most of the RCTs comparing other interventions, exchange transfusion was used successfully to reduce serum bilirubin levels when those interventions failed to control the rise of serum bilirubin.

REFERENCES

1. Kumar RK. Neonatal jaundice. An update for family physicians. *Aust Fam Physician* 1999;28:679–682.
2. Gale R, Seidman DS, Stevenson DK. Hyperbilirubinemia and early discharge. *J Perinatol* 2001;21:40–43.
3. Turkel SB, Guttenberg ME, Moynes DR, et al. Lack of identifiable risk factors for kernicterus. *Pediatrics* 1980;66:502–506.
4. Hansen TWR. Kernicterus in term and near-term infants — the specter walks again. *Acta Paediatr* 2000;89:1155–1157.
5. Brown AK, Kim MH, Wu PYK, et al. Efficacy of phototherapy in prevention and management of neonatal hyperbilirubinemia. *Pediatrics* 1985;75:393–400.
6. Lipsitz PJ, Gartner LM, Bryla DA. Neonatal and infant mortality in relation to phototherapy. *Pediatrics* 1985;75:422–426.
7. Scheidt PC, Bryla DA, Nelson KB et al. Phototherapy for neonatal hyperbilirubinemia: six-year follow-up of the National Institute of Child Health and Human Development clinical trial. *Pediatrics* 1990;85:455–463.
8. Mills JF, Tudehope D. Fibreoptic phototherapy for neonatal jaundice (Cochrane Review). In: The Cochrane Library. Issue 2, 2003. Oxford: Update Software. Search date 2000; primary sources Cochrane Controlled Trials Register, Medline, Embase, reference lists, conference proceedings, and personal communications with authors.
9. Sarici SU, Alpay F, Dundaroz MR, et al. Fibreoptic phototherapy versus conventional daylight phototherapy for hyperbilirubinemia of term newborns. *Turk J Pediatr* 2001; 43: 280–285.
10. Nuntnarumit P, Naka C. Comparison of the effectiveness between the adapted-double phototherapy versus conventional-single phototherapy. *J Med Assoc Thai* 2002;85:S1159–S1166.

Anthony Akobeng
Consultant Paediatrician
Central Manchester and Manchester
Children's University Hospitals
Manchester
UK

Competing interests: None declared.

Nocturnal enuresis in children

Search date February 2003

Natalie Lyth and Sara Bosson

QUESTIONS

INTERVENTIONS

Key Messages

- **Enuresis alarm plus dry-bed training (as effective as enuresis alarm alone)** One systematic review has found limited evidence that a higher proportion of children achieve 14 consecutive dry nights with alarm plus dry bed training than with no treatment. A second systematic review found no significant difference between alarm plus dry bed training and alarm alone for achieving 14 consecutive dry nights.
- **Desmopressin (in short term)** One systematic review has found that desmopressin reduces bedwetting by at least one night per week and increases the chance of attaining initial success (14 consecutive dry nights) compared with placebo. The review found insufficient evidence comparing either intranasal versus oral administration of desmopressin or desmopressin versus tricyclic drugs. There was some evidence that higher doses of desmopressin were more likely to reduce the number of wet nights during treatment compared with lower doses. The review found no difference between desmopressin and enuresis alarms in the number of children achieving initial success, although one RCT found that, after 3 months of treatment, enuresis alarms were better than desmopressin at reducing the number of wet nights per week. We found insufficient evidence about effects of desmopressin in the long term.
- **Dry bed training (in short term)** One systematic review has found that a greater proportion of children achieved 14 consecutive dry nights with dry bed training than with no treatment.
- **Enuresis alarm (in short and long term)** One systematic review has found that enuresis alarms increase initial success rates compared with no treatment and that 31–61% of children using alarms were still dry at 3 months. The review found that children using an alarm were nine times less likely to relapse than were children taking desmopressin. We found limited evidence from one small RCT that dry bed training reduced bedwetting compared with an enuresis alarm after initial treatment and after 6 months. One systematic review found no significant difference between

alarm plus dry bed training and alarm alone for achieving 14 consecutive dry nights. Two RCTs found that adding intranasal desmopressin to treatment with an alarm reduced bedwetting in the short term (3–4 weeks) compared with treatment with alarm alone. However, one RCT found no significant difference between treatment with intranasal desmopressin plus alarm and treatment with placebo plus alarm on long term follow up at 6 months.

- **Laser acupuncture (as effective as desmopressin in one RCT)** One RCT found no difference between laser acupuncture and intranasal desmopressin in the number of wet nights in children aged over 5 years.
- **Standard home alarm clock (in short term)** One RCT found that a higher proportion of children achieved 14 consecutive dry nights with standard home alarm clock than with waking after 3 hours' sleep.
- **Dry bed training (in long term)** One systematic review has found no significant long term difference in the proportion of dry nights between dry bed training and no treatment. However, one small RCT showed some long-term advantages of dry bed training.
- **Standard home alarm clock (in long term)** One RCT found no significant difference in the proportion of dry nights achieved at 3 months between standard home alarm clock and waking after 3 hours' sleep.
- **Ultrasound** We found no RCTs. One small controlled trial in children aged 6–14 years found that ultrasound increased the proportion of dry nights for up to 12 months compared with control.
- **Adding desmopressin to an alarm (in long term)** One systematic review found that desmopressin plus alarm was better at reducing the number of wet nights per week during treatment compared with alarm alone or alarm plus placebo, although there was no significant difference between alarm plus desmopressin and alarm alone in the rate of initial success.
- **Tricyclic drugs (imipramine, desipramine)** One systematic review has found that tricyclic drugs (imipramine, desipramine) increase the chance of attaining 14 consecutive dry nights compared with placebo, although tricyclic drugs increased adverse effects such as anorexia, anxiety reaction, constipation, depression, diarrhoea, dizziness, drowsiness, dry mouth, headache, irritability, lethargy, sleep disturbance, upset stomach, and vomiting compared with placebo. We found no good studies comparing tricyctic drugs versus desmopressin. The review found no significant difference between imipramine and an enuresis alarm during the treatment period, but it found limited evidence that an alarm reduced bedwetting after the treatment had stopped compared with imipramine.

DEFINITION Nocturnal enuresis is the involuntary discharge of urine at night in the absence of congenital or acquired defects of the central nervous system or urinary tract in a child aged 5 years or older.[1] Disorders that have bedwetting as a symptom (termed "nocturnal incontinence") can be excluded by a thorough history, examination, and urinalysis. "Monosymptomatic" nocturnal enuresis is characterised by night time symptoms only and accounts for 85% of cases. Nocturnal enuresis is defined as primary if the child has not been dry for a period of more than 6 months, and secondary if such a period of dryness preceded the onset of wetting.

INCIDENCE/ PREVALENCE Between 15% and 20% of 5 year olds, 7% of 7 year olds, 5% of 10 year olds, 2–3% of 12–14 year olds, and 1–2% of people aged 15 years and over wet the bed twice per week on average.[2]

AETIOLOGY/ RISK FACTORS Nocturnal enuresis is associated with several factors, including small functional bladder capacity, nocturnal polyuria, and arousal dysfunction. Linkage studies have identified associated genetic loci on chromosomes 8q, 12q, 13q, and 22q11.[3–6]

PROGNOSIS Nocturnal enuresis has widely differing outcomes, from spontaneous resolution to complete resistance to all current treatments. About 1% of adults remain enuretic. Without treatment, about 15% of children with enuresis become dry each year.[7] We found no RCTs on the best age at which to start treatment in children with nocturnal enuresis. Anecdotal experience suggests that reassurance is sufficient below the age of 7 years. Behavioural treatments, such as alarms, require motivation and commitment from the child and a parent. Anecdotal experience suggests that children under the age of 7 years may not exhibit the commitment needed.

AIMS OF INTERVENTION To stay dry on particular occasions (e.g. when visiting friends); to reduce the number of wet nights; to reduce the impact of the enuresis on the child's lifestyle; to initiate successful continence; to avoid relapse, with minimal adverse effects.

OUTCOMES Rate of initial success (defined as 14 consecutive dry nights); average number of wet nights per week; number of relapses after initial success; average number of wet nights after treatment has ceased.

METHODS *Clinical Evidence* search and appraisal February 2003.

QUESTION What are the effects of interventions for relief of symptoms?

OPTION DESMOPRESSIN

One systematic review has found that desmopressin reduces bedwetting by at least one night per week and increases the chance of attaining initial success (14 consecutive dry nights) compared with placebo. The review found insufficient evidence comparing either intranasal versus oral administration of desmopressin or desmopressin versus tricyclic drugs. There was some evidence that higher doses of desmopressin were more likely to reduce the number of wet nights during treatment compared with lower doses. The review found no difference between desmopressin and enuresis alarms in the number of children achieving initial success, although one RCT found that, after 3 months of treatment, enuresis alarms were better than desmopressin at reducing the number of wet nights per week. One systematic review found that desmopressin plus alarm was better at reducing the number of wet nights per week during treatment compared with alarm alone or alarm plus placebo, although there was no significant difference in the rate of initial success.

Benefits: We found one systematic review (search date 2002, 41 RCTs, 2760 children).[8] **Versus placebo:** The systematic review identified 28 RCTs that compared desmopressin versus placebo.[8] It found that desmopressin (10–60 μg) significantly reduced the number of wet nights per week during treatment compared with placebo (desmopressin 20 μg; pooled WMD –1.34, 95% CI –1.57 to –1.11). Ten of the RCTs assessed the rate of initial success (14 consecutive dry nights) and found that desmopressin significantly increased the chance of initial success compared with placebo (RR for success with desmopressin [20 μg] *v* placebo 1.2, 95% CI 1.1 to 1.3) (see table 1, p 410). **Intranasal versus oral desmopressin:** The review found one RCT that compared intranasal desmopressin versus oral desmopressin.[8] The review found insufficient evidence comparing intranasal versus oral administration of desmopressin. **Versus tricyclic drugs:** The review found two RCTs that compared desmopressin versus tricyclic drugs.[8] It found insufficient evidence comparing desmopressin versus either amitriptyline or imipramine. **Versus enuresis alarm:** The review found three RCTs that compared desmopressin versus enuresis alarms.[8] It found no significant difference between desmopressin and alarm in the number of children achieving initial success (RR 1.34, 95% CI 0.94 to 1.91). However, one RCT (50 children) found that desmopressin significantly reduced the number of wet nights per week during the first week of treatment (RR –1.70, 95% CI –2.96 to –0.44) compared with alarm, although after 3 months of treatment enuresis alarms were significantly better than desmopressin at reducing the number of wet nights per week (RR 1.40, 95% CI 0.14 to 2.66). **Plus enuresis alarm:** The review found two RCTs that compared alarm plus desmopressin versus alarm alone.[8] It found that alarm plus desmopressin was significantly better at reducing the number of wet nights per week during treatment compared with alarm alone (RR –1.35, 95% CI –2.32 to –0.38). However, the review also found no significant difference between alarm plus desmopressin and alarm alone in the rate of initial success (RR 0.88, 95% CI 0.52 to 1.50). The review found two RCTs (149 children) that compared alarm plus desmopressin versus alarm plus placebo.[8] It found that alarm plus desmopressin was significantly better at reducing the number of wet nights per week during treatment compared with alarm plus placebo (RR –1.00, 95% CI –1.56 to –0.44). However, the review also found no significant difference between alarm plus desmopressin and alarm plus placebo in the rate of initial success (RR 1.12, 95% CI 0.83 to 1.51). **Versus laser acupuncture:** See benefits of laser acupuncture, p 408. **Lower versus higher doses of desmopressin:** The review found eight RCTs that compared different doses of desmopressin.[8] It found some evidence that higher doses were more likely to reduce the number of wet nights during treatment compared with lower doses (wet nights with desmopressin 20 μg *v* desmopressin 60 μg; WMD –0.72, 95% CI –0.3 to –0.14). However, there was no difference between doses in the rate of initial success.

Harms: The systematic review reported nasal discomfort, headache, nosebleeds, bad taste, rash, sight disturbance, and anorexia.[8] Rarely, water intoxication has been reported.[14]

Comment: The systematic review included only studies of interventions used to remedy either primary or secondary nocturnal enuresis (incontinence was excluded by medical examination or explicitly mentioned in the inclusion/exclusion criteria of included RCTs), and included a systematic measurement of baseline wetting (with one exception) and outcomes. Many of the included RCTs were of poor quality.[8]

OPTION TRICYCLIC DRUGS (IMIPRAMINE, DESIPRAMINE)

One systematic review has found that tricyclic drugs (imipramine, desipramine) increase the chance of attaining 14 consecutive dry nights compared with placebo, although tricyclic drugs increased adverse effects such as anorexia, anxiety reaction, constipation, depression, diarrhoea, dizziness, drowsiness, dry mouth, headache, irritability, lethargy, sleep disturbance, upset stomach, and vomiting compared with placebo. We found no good studies comparing tricyclic drugs versus desmopressin. The review found no significant difference between imipramine and an enuresis alarm during the treatment period, but found limited evidence that an alarm reduced bedwetting compared with imipramine after the treatment had stopped.

Benefits: We found one systematic review (search date 1997, 22 RCTs, 1100 children).[9] Many of the trials were of poor quality. **Versus placebo:** The review identified 10 RCTs comparing the effect of imipramine versus placebo on mean number of wet nights per week.[9] It found that imipramine significantly reduced bedwetting by one night per week compared with placebo (WMD –0.84 nights, 95% CI –1.21 nights to –0.47 nights) The review also found that imipramine (4 RCTs) and desipramine (1 RCT) significantly increased the chance of attaining 14 consecutive dry nights compared with placebo (imipramine: RR 5.0, 95% CI 2.4 to 10.4; desipramine: RR 3.60, 95% CI 1.07 to 11.81) (see table 1, p 410). **Versus enuresis alarm:** The review (3 small RCTs, 103 children) found no significant difference in mean number of wet nights per week between imipramine and an enuresis alarm during the treatment period.[9] However, after treatment was stopped, two of the three RCTs found that the enuresis alarm reduced bedwetting compared with imipramine (WMD in number of dry nights per week: 1.03 nights, 95% CI 0.19 nights to 1.87 nights).[9] **Versus desmopressin:** We found no good studies comparing tricyclic drugs versus desmopressin.

Harms: The systematic review reported that tricyclic drugs increased adverse effects compared with placebo.[9] Effects included anorexia, anxiety reaction, burning sensation, constipation, depression, diarrhoea, dizziness, drowsiness, dry mouth, headache, irritability, lethargy, sleep disturbance, upset stomach, and vomiting. The review also found that tricyclic drugs increased adverse effects compared with desmopressin (AR for adverse effects: 83/480 [17.3%] with tricyclic drugs *v* 41/579 [7.1%] with desmopressin). Tricyclic drugs have been reported as fatal in overdose.

Comment: None.

OPTION ENURESIS ALARM

One systematic review has found that enuresis alarms increase initial success rates compared with no treatment, and that 31–61% of children using alarms were still dry at 3 months. We found limited evidence from one small RCT that dry bed training reduced bedwetting compared with an enuresis alarm after initial treatment and after 6 months. One systematic review found no significant difference between alarm plus dry bed training and alarm alone for achieving 14 consecutive dry nights. One systematic review found that desmopressin plus alarm was better at reducing the number of wet nights per week during treatment compared with alarm alone or alarm plus placebo, although there was no significant difference in the rate of initial success.

Benefits: **Versus no treatment:** We found one systematic review (search date 1997, 4 RCTs).[10] It found that significantly more children achieved 14 consecutive dry nights with enuresis alarm than with no treatment and that 31–61% were still dry at 3 months (see table 1, p 410). **Versus dry bed training:** See benefits of dry bed training, p 407. **Plus dry bed training:** See benefits of alarm plus dry bed training, p 407. **Versus desmopressin:** See benefits of desmopressin, p 404. **Plus desmopressin versus alarm plus placebo:** See benefits of desmopressin, p 404.

Harms: One systematic review found that adverse effects of alarms were limited to minor inconvenience because of alarm malfunction or disturbance.[12] One systematic review reported that adverse affects included fright, false alarms, and waking of other people in the house.[10] However, it was unable to estimate the frequency of these events.

Comment: None.

OPTION STANDARD HOME ALARM CLOCK

One RCT found that a standard home alarm clock, set to wake the child immediately before their usual time of enuresis, reduced bedwetting compared with a strategy of routinely waking the child after 3 hours' sleep, but it found no significant difference in the proportion of dry nights at 3 months.

Benefits: We found no systematic review but found one RCT.[11] It found that significantly more children achieved 14 consecutive dry nights with a standard home alarm clock to wake the child immediately before their usual time of enuresis compared with a strategy of routinely waking the child after 3 hours' sleep, but it found no significant difference in the proportion of dry nights at 3 months (see table 1, p 410).

Harms: No adverse effects were reported in the RCT.[11]

Comment: None.

OPTION DRY BED TRAINING

Two RCTs found that dry bed training reduced bedwetting in the short term compared with no treatment, although we found insufficient reliable evidence about long term effects. We found limited evidence from one small RCT that dry bed training reduced bedwetting compared with an enuresis alarm after initial treatment and after 6 months.

Benefits: We found one systematic review (search date 1996, 1 RCT, 45 children)[12] and one subsequent small RCT (36 people).[13] **Versus no treatment:** The review found that significantly more children achieved 14 consecutive dry nights with dry bed training**G** than with no treatment, although it found no long term advantage (see table 1, p 410). The subsequent small RCT compared three groups: dry bed training, alarm, and no treatment.[13] It found that, within the 16 week treatment period, dry bed training decreased bedwetting compared with no treatment (see table 1, p 410). However, it was not clear whether this difference was significant. **Versus enuresis alarm:** The subsequent small RCT described above found that dry bed training decreased bedwetting compared with alarm both during treatment and 6 months after treatment (see table 1, p 410).[13] However, it was not clear whether this difference was significant. **Plus enuresis alarm:** See benefits of enuresis alarm plus dry bed training, p 407.

Harms: Neither the review[12] nor the subsequent RCT[13] reported on harms.

Comment: The small RCT was conducted in children from families with low socioeconomic status, and reported lower success rates compared with other trials.[13] This may reduce the generalisability of results.

OPTION ENURESIS ALARM PLUS DRY BED TRAINING

One systematic review has found limited evidence that a higher proportion of children achieve 14 consecutive dry nights with alarm plus dry bed training than with no treatment. A second systematic review found no significant difference between alarm plus dry bed training and alarm alone for achieving 14 consecutive dry nights.

Benefits: **Versus no treatment:** We found one systematic review (search date 1996, 1 RCT, 45 children).[12] It found that significantly more children achieved 14 consecutive dry nights with dry bed training plus an alarm than with no treatment (1 RCT; RR 10, 95% CI 2.69 to 37.24) (see table 1, p 410). **Versus alarm alone:** We found one systematic review (search date 1997, 5 RCTs, 220 children).[10] It found no significant difference between alarm plus dry bed training and alarm alone for achieving 14 consecutive dry nights (RR for not achieving 14 consecutive dry nights 1.03, 95% CI 0.65 to 1.65).

Harms: See harms of dry bed training, p 407. See harms of enuresis alarm, p 406.

Comment: None.

OPTION ULTRASOUND

We found no RCTs of ultrasound in children with primary nocturnal enuresis. We found one small controlled trial in children aged 6–14 years, which found that ultrasound reduced the number of wet nights compared with control in both the short and long term.

Benefits: We found no systematic review of RCTs of ultrasound in children with primary nocturnal enuresis.

Harms: We found no RCTs.

Comment: We found one controlled trial (35 children with primary nocturnal enuresis, aged 6–14 years) comparing ultrasound (27 children) versus control (8 children treated without the apparatus being switched on).[15] Ultrasound treatment was applied daily to lumbosacral skin for 10 sessions. The trial found that ultrasound versus control reduced the number of wet nights per week at 1 week, 3 months, 6 months, and 12 months after treatment ($P < 0.05$ at all times). The study did not find any adverse effects.[15]

OPTION LASER ACUPUNCTURE

One RCT found no significant difference between laser acupuncture and intranasal desmopressin in reduction of wet nights in children aged over 5 years.

Benefits: We found no systematic review. **Versus no treatment:** We found no RCTs. **Versus desmopressin:** We found one RCT (40 children aged > 5 years with primary nocturnal enuresis) comparing laser acupuncture versus intranasal desmopressin (20–40 μg for 3 months).[16] Laser acupuncture was applied to seven predefined acupuncture areas for 30 seconds per session for 10–15 sessions. Complete response was defined as a reduction in the number of wet nights of at least 90%. At 6 months the RCT found no significant difference between laser acupuncture and intranasal desmopressin in reduction in wet nights (complete responders: 65% with laser acupuncture *v* 75% with desmopressin).

Harms: The RCT did not find any adverse effects with either laser acupuncture or intranasal desmopressin.[16]

Comment: Laser acupuncture treatment may not be widely available.

GLOSSARY

Dry bed training A multicomponent behavioural programme for treatment of nocturnal enuresis in children. Elements of the programme are directed at increasing bladder capacity, strengthening the sphincter, and encouraging rapid movement from bed to toilet.

REFERENCES

1. Forsythe WI, Butler R. 50 years of enuretic alarms; a review of the literature. *Arch Dis Child* 1991;64:879–885.
2. Blackwell C. *A guide to enuresis: a guide to treatment of enuresis for professionals*. Bristol: Eric, 1989.
3. Eiberg H. Total genome scan analysis in a single extended family for primary nocturnal enuresis: evidence for a new locus (ENUR 3) for primary nocturnal enuresis on chromosome 22q11. *Eur Urol* 1998;33:34–36.
4. Eiberg H. Nocturnal enuresis is linked to a specific gene. *Scand J Urol Nephrol* 1995;173(suppl):15–17.
5. Arnell H, Hjalmas M, Jagervall G, et al. The genetics of primary nocturnal enuresis: inheritance and suggestion of a second major gene on chromosome 12q. *J Med Genet* 1997;34:360–365.
6. Eiberg H, Berendt I, Mohr J. Assignment of dominant inherited nocturnal enuresis (ENUR 1) to chromosome 13q. *Nat Genet* 1995;10:354–356.
7. Forsythe WI, Redmond A. Enuresis and spontaneous cure rate of 1129 enuretics. *Arch Dis Child* 1974;49:259–263.
8. Glazener CMA, Evans JHC. Desmopressin for nocturnal enuresis in children. In: The Cochrane Library, Issue 3, 2002. Oxford: Update Software. Search date March 2002; primary sources Medline, Embase, Amed, Assia, Bids, Cinahl, Psychlit, Sigle, and DHSS data.
9. Glazener CMA, Evans JHC. Tricyclic and related drugs for nocturnal enuresis in children. In: The Cochrane Library, Issue 1, 2003. Oxford: Update Software. Search date 1997; primary sources Medline, Embase, Amed, Assia, Bids, Cinahl, Psychlit, Sigle, and DHSS data.
10. Glazener CMA, Evans JHC. Alarm interventions for nocturnal enuresis in children (Cochrane Review). In: The Cochrane Library, Issue 1, 2003. Oxford: Update Software. Search date 1997; primary sources Medline, Embase, Amed, Assia, Bids, Cinahl, Psychlit, Sigle, and DHSS data.
11. El-Anany FG, Maghraby HA, Shaker SED, et al. Primary nocturnal enuresis: a new approach to conditioning treatment. *Urology* 1999;53:405–409.
12. Lister-Sharp D, O'Meara S, Bradley M, et al. University of York. NHS Centre for Reviews and Dissemination. August 1997. *A systematic review of the effectiveness of interventions for managing childhood nocturnal enuresis*. CRD Report 11. Search date 1996; primary sources Cochrane Library, Medline, Embase, and Psychlit.

13. Nawaz S, Griffiths P, Tappin D. Parent-administered modified dry-bed training for childhood nocturnal enuresis: evidence for superiority over urine-alarm conditioning when delivery factors are controlled. *Behav Intervent* 2002;17:247–260.
14. Robson WL, Leung AK. Side effects and complications of treatment with desmopressin for enuresis. *J Natl Med Assoc* 1994;86:775–778.
15. Kosar A, Akkus S, Savas S, et al. Effect of ultrasound in the treatment of primary nocturnal enuresis. *Scand J Urol Nephrol* 2000;34:361–365.
16. Radmayr C, Schlager A, Studen M, et al. Prospective randomised trial using laser acupuncture versus desmopressin in the treatment of nocturnal enuresis. *Eur Urol* 2001;40:201–205.

Natalie Lyth
Associate Specialist Child Health
Hambleton and Richmondshire Primary Care Trust
Thirsk
UK

Sara Bosson
Staff Grade Community Paediatrician
Weston Area Health Trust
Weston-Super-Mare
UK

Competing interests: SB, none declared. NL has been reimbursed for attending a symposium by Ferring Pharmaceuticals, the manufacturer of Desmotabs (desmopressin).

TABLE 1 **Treatments for enuresis: advantages and disadvantages (see text, p 406).**

	Short term relief of symptoms (14 consecutive dry nights)	Long term relief of symptoms	Evidence	Advantages	Disadvantages
Desmopressin (intranasal)[8]	RR *v* placebo 1.2, 95% CI 1.1 to 1.3	No better than placebo after completion of treatment	Meta-analysis of 10 RCTs	Effective within days, few adverse effects with appropriate pretreatment advice	Case reports of water intoxication
Tricyclic drugs (imipramine)[9]	RR *v* placebo 5.0, 95% CI 2.4 to 10.4	No better than placebo (RR 1.1)	Meta-analysis of 4 RCTs	Effective within days	Risk of lethal overdose, frequent significant adverse effects
Enuresis alarm[10]	RR *v* no treatment 3.7, 95% CI 2.6 to 5.3	31–61% still dry at 3 months. Nine times less likely relapse than with desmopressin	Meta-analysis of 4 RCTs	Safe	Takes longer to become dry, needs good cooperation from child and family
Standard home alarm clock[11]	77.1% *v* 61.8% with waking after 3 hours' sleep (RR 1.3; $P = 0.03$)	No better at 3 months than waking after 3 hours' sleep (66% dry *v* 56%; $P = 0.19$)	1 RCT, 125 people	Safe, does not require bed wetting to initiate alarm	None reported
Dry bed training[12]	RR *v* no treatment 2.5, 95% CI 0.55 to 11.4	No better than no treatment (RR 0.4, 95% CI 0.14 to 1.13)	1 good quality RCT, 45 people	Safe	Requires high degree of motivation
Dry bed training[13]	66% *v* 25% for alarm and *v* 8% for no treatment ($P < 0.001$)	58% v 17% for alarm remained completely dry 6 months after completion of dry bed training	1 small RCT, 36 children		
Dry bed training plus alarm[12]	RR *v* no treatment 10, 95% CI 2.69 to 37.24	No better than alarm alone (RR 1.0, 95% CI 0.7 to 1.5)	1 RCT, 45 people	Safe	Requires an even greater input from the family than either treatment alone

Nosebleeds in children

Search date February 2004

Gerald McGarry

QUESTIONS

INTERVENTIONS

Key Messages

- **Antiseptic cream versus no treatment** One RCT found that chlorhexidine/neomycin cream reduced nosebleeds compared with no treatment at 8 weeks.
- **Antiseptic cream versus cautery** One small RCT found no significant difference in nosebleeds between chlorhexidine/neomycin cream and silver nitrate cautery at 8 weeks. However, the study may have lacked power to detect clinically important differences between treatments. Some children found the smell and taste of the antiseptic cream unpleasant. All children found cautery painful despite the use of local anaesthesia.
- **Cautery plus antiseptic cream** One small RCT found insufficient evidence about the effects of silver nitrate cautery plus chlorhexidine/neomycin cream compared with chlorhexidine/neomycin cream alone.
- **Cautery versus no treatment** We found no RCTs about the effects of this intervention.

Nosebleeds in children

DEFINITION Recurrent idiopathic epistaxis is recurrent, self limiting, nasal bleeding for which no specific cause is identified. There is no consensus on the frequency or severity of recurrences.

INCIDENCE/ PREVALENCE A cross-sectional study of 1218 children (aged 11–14 years) found that 9% had frequent episodes of epistaxis.[1] It is likely that only the most severe episodes are considered for treatment.

AETIOLOGY/ RISK FACTORS In children, most epistaxis occurs from the anterior part of the septum in the region of Little's area.[2] Initiating factors include local inflammation, mucosal drying, and local trauma (including nose picking).[2] Epistaxis caused by other specific local (e.g. tumours) or systemic factors (e.g. clotting disorders) is not considered here.

PROGNOSIS Recurrent epistaxis is less common in people over 14 years old, and many children "grow out" of this problem.

AIMS OF INTERVENTION To reduce the number and severity of epistaxis episodes; to minimise adverse effects of treatment.

OUTCOMES Number and severity of epistaxis episodes.

METHODS *Clinical Evidence* search and appraisal February 2004.

QUESTION **What are the effects of treatments for recurrent idiopathic epistaxis in children?**

OPTION **ANTISEPTIC CREAMS**

One RCT found that chlorhexidine/neomycin cream reduced nosebleeds compared with no treatment at 8 weeks. One small RCT found no significant difference in nosebleeds between chlorhexidine/neomycin cream and silver nitrate cautery at 8 weeks, although the study may have lacked power to detect a clinically important effect. Some children found the smell and taste of antiseptic cream unpleasant. All children found cautery painful, despite the use of local anaesthesia. One small RCT found insufficient evidence about the effects of silver nitrate cautery plus chlorhexidine/neomycin cream versus chlorhexidine/neomycin cream alone.

Benefits: We found no systematic review. **Versus no treatment:** We found one RCT (103 children aged 3–13 years with recurrent epistaxis for a mean of 20 months, unblinded design) that compared antiseptic cream (chlorhexidine hydrochloride 0.1%, neomycin sulphate 3250 U/g) applied to both nostrils twice daily for 4 weeks versus no treatment.[3] It found that antiseptic cream significantly increased the proportion of children who had complete resolution of bleeding compared with no treatment at 8 weeks (no bleeding in past 4 weeks: 26/47 [55%] with antiseptic cream *v* 12/41 [29%] with no treatment; RR 0.53, 95% CI 0.31 to 0.91; NNT 4, 95% CI 3 to 9). **Versus cautery:** We found one small RCT (48 children aged 3–14 years with at least 1 episode of epistaxis during the previous 4 weeks and a "history of repeated epistaxis"), which compared antiseptic cream (chlorhexidine hydrochloride 0.1%, neomycin sulphate 3250 U/g) applied to both nostrils twice daily for 4 weeks versus silver nitrate cautery.[4] Cautery was undertaken in secondary care using silver nitrate applied on a stick to prominent vessels or bleeding points. The RCT found no significant difference in the proportion of children with complete resolution of bleeding at 8 weeks (no bleeding during the past 4 weeks: 12/24 [50%] with antiseptic cream *v* 13/24 [54%] with cautery; RR 0.92, 95% CI 0.54 to 1.59). It also found similar rates of partial success with antiseptic cream compared with cautery at 8 weeks (proportion of children with 50% reduction in number of bleeds during the past 4 weeks: 4/24 [16.6%] with antiseptic cream v 3/24 [12.5%] with cautery) and failure at 8 weeks (proportion of children with less than 50% reduction in number of bleeds in past 4 weeks: 7/24 [29%] with antiseptic cream v 6/24 [25%] with cautery). **Plus cautery:** See benefits of silver nitrate cautery, p 413.

Harms: **Versus no treatment:** The RCT comparing antiseptic cream with no treatment gave no information about adverse effects.[3] Some commercial antiseptic creams contain arachis (peanut) oil, and the RCT excluded all children with peanut allergies.[3] **Versus cautery:** The RCT comparing antiseptic cream with cautery found no adverse reactions with antiseptic cream, but some children found the smell and taste unpleasant (no further data reported).[4] Chlorhexidine/neomycin cream may cause occasional skin reactions. All children undergoing cautery experienced pain, even with 5% cocaine as a local anaesthetic.[4]

Comment: See comment under silver nitrate cautery, p 413.

OPTION SILVER NITRATE CAUTERY

We found no RCTs comparing silver nitrate cautery with no treatment. One small RCT found no significant difference in nosebleeds between silver nitrate cautery and antiseptic cream at 8 weeks, although the study may have lacked power to detect a clinically important effect. Some children found the smell and taste of antiseptic cream unpleasant. All children found cautery painful, despite the use of local anaesthesia. One small RCT found insufficient evidence about the effects of silver nitrate cautery plus chlorhexidine/neomycin cream versus chlorhexidine/neomycin cream alone.

Benefits: We found no systematic review. **Versus no treatment:** We found no RCTs. **Versus antiseptic cream:** See benefits of antiseptic creams, p 412. **Plus antiseptic cream:** One RCT (40 adults, 24 children) compared once only silver nitrate cautery plus chlorhexidine hydrochloride 0.1%/neomycin sulphate 3250 U/g cream twice daily for 2 weeks versus antiseptic cream alone.[5] The RCT did not provide discrete results in children and included too few children to draw conclusions.

Harms: **Versus no treatment:** We found no RCTs. **Versus antiseptic cream:** See harms of antiseptic creams, p 413. **Plus antiseptic cream:** The RCT did not report harms.[5] Recognised complications of cautery include pain and septal perforation, although the incidence of septal perforation following unilateral cautery in children is not known.

Comment: Both RCTs involving silver nitrate cautery were undertaken in the context of secondary care.[4,5] Silver nitrate cautery is also used in primary care. It is unknown whether complication rates differ. Simultaneous bilateral cautery in children is not recommended because of an expected increased risk of perforation.

REFERENCES

1. Rodeghiero F, Castaman G, Dini E. Epidemiological investigation of the prevalence of von Willebrand's disease. *Blood* 1987;69:454–459.
2. Watkinson JC. Epistaxis. In: Kerr AG, Mackay IS, Bull TR, eds. *Scott-Brown's Otolaryngology, Volume 4 Rhinology*. Oxford: Butterworth-Heinemann, 1997;18:1–19.
3. Kubba H, MacAndie C, Botma M, et al. A prospective, single blind, randomized controlled trial of antiseptic cream for recurrent epistaxis in childhood. *Clin Otolaryngol* 2001;26:465–468.
4. Ruddy J, Proops DW, Pearman K, et al. Management of epistaxis in children. *Int J Paediatr Otorhinolaryngol* 1991;21:139–142.
5. Murthy P, Nilssen ELK, Rao S, et al. A randomised clinical trial of antiseptic nasal carrier cream and silver nitrate cautery in the treatment of recurrent anterior epistaxis. *Clin Otolaryngol* 1999;228–231.

Gerald McGarry
Consultant Otorhinolaryngologist Honorary Clinical Senior Lecturer
Glasgow Royal Infirmary, Glasgow, UK

Competing interests: None declared. *We would like to acknowledge the previous contributors of this chapter, including Martin Burton and Robert Walton.*

Perinatal asphyxia

Search date June 2004

William McGuire

QUESTIONS

INTERVENTIONS

See glossary

Key Messages

Treatments

- **Antioxidants** One systematic review found insufficient evidence from two small RCTs about the effects of antioxidants in infants with perinatal asphyxia.
- **Calcium channel blockers** We found no RCTs on the effects of calcium channel blockers in infants with asphyxia.
- **Corticosteroids** We found no RCTs on the effects of corticosteroids in infants with perinatal asphyxia.
- **Fluid restriction** We found no RCTs on the effects of fluid restriction in infants with perinatal asphyxia.
- **Hyperventilation** We found no RCTs on the effects of hyperventilation in infants with perinatal asphyxia.
- **Magnesium sulphate** We found no RCTs on the effects of magnesium sulphate in infants with asphyxia.
- **Mannitol** One small RCT provided insufficient evidence on the effects of mannitol in infants with asphyxia.
- **Opiate antagonists** One small RCT identified by a systematic review did not report on the effects of opiate antagonists, mortality or neurodevelopmental outcomes in infants with perinatal asphyxia.
- **Prophylactic anticonvulsants** One systematic review of three small, methodologically flawed RCTs found no significant difference in mortality or neurodevelopmental outcomes between barbiturates and no drug treatment in term infants with perinatal asphyxia.

DEFINITION The clinical diagnosis of perinatal asphyxia is based on several criteria, the two main ones being: evidence of cardiorespiratory and neurological depression, defined as an Apgar score**G** of less than 7 at 5 minutes after birth; and evidence of acute hypoxic compromise with acidaemia, defined as an arterial blood pH of less than 7 or base excess greater than 12 mmol/L.[1] In many settings, especially in resource poor countries, it may be impossible to assess fetal or neonatal acidaemia. Signs of "hypoxic-ischaemic" encephalopathy (neonatal encephalopathy) or other organ dysfunction can also be part of the clinical picture. In the immediate postpartum period when resuscitation is being undertaken, it may not be possible to determine whether the neurological and cardiorespiratory depression is secondary to hypoxia-ischaemia, or to another condition such as feto-maternal infection or metabolic disease. However, these features often take time to develop and are therefore not useful in deciding the immediate management of infants with suspected perinatal asphyxia. In addition, neonatal encephalopathy may have a variety of causes which may be unrelated to an hypoxia-ischaemic event.[2–4]

INCIDENCE/ PREVALENCE Estimates of the incidence of perinatal asphyxia vary depending on the definitions used. In resource rich countries the incidence of severe perinatal asphyxia (causing death or severe neurological impairment) is about 1/1000 live births.[5,6] In resource poor countries, perinatal asphyxia is probably much more common. Data from hospital based studies in such settings suggest an incidence of 5–10/1000 live births.[7–9] This probably represents an underestimate of the true community incidence of perinatal asphyxia in resource poor countries.

AETIOLOGY/ RISK FACTORS Perinatal asphyxia may occur *in utero*, during labour and delivery, or in the immediate postnatal period. There are numerous causes, including placental abruption, cord compression, transplacental anaesthetic or narcotic administration, intrauterine pneumonia, severe meconium aspiration, congenital cardiac or pulmonary anomalies, and birth trauma. Postnatal asphyxia can be caused by an obstructed airway, maternal opiates which can cause respiratory depression, or congenital sepsis.

PROGNOSIS Worldwide, perinatal asphyxia is a major cause of death and of acquired brain damage in newborn infants.[9] The prognosis depends on the severity of the asphyxia. Only a minority of infants with severe encephalopathy after perinatal asphyxia survive without handicap.[5] However, there are limited population based data on long term outcomes after perinatal asphyxia, such as cerebral palsy, developmental delay, visual and hearing impairment, and learning and behavioural problems. After an asphyxial event, there may be an opportunity to intervene to minimise brain damage. The first phase of brain damage, early cell death, results from primary exhaustion of the cellular energy stores. Early cell death can occur within minutes. Immediate resuscitation to restore oxygen supply and blood circulation aims to limit the extent of this damage. A secondary phase of neuronal injury may occur several hours after the initial insult. The mechanisms believed to be important in this process include oxygen free radical production, intracellular calcium entry, and apoptosis. Treatments during the post-resuscitation phase aim to block these processes thereby limiting secondary cell damage and minimising the extent of any brain damage.

AIMS OF INTERVENTION To minimise brain and other organ damage with minimal adverse effects.

OUTCOMES **Primary outcomes:** Death before hospital discharge; incidence of severe neurodevelopmental disability**G** assessed at greater than 12 months of age using a validated tool. **Secondary outcomes:** Severity of hypoxic-ischaemic encephalopathy**G** assessed using a validated tool.[10]

METHODS *Clinical Evidence* search and appraisal June 2004. We searched primary sources to July 2004, and the Cochrane Library Issue 3, 2004.

QUESTION **What are the effects of interventions in term or near term newborns with perinatal asphyxia?**

OPTION **ANTIOXIDANTS**

One systematic review found insufficient evidence from two small RCTs about the effects of antioxidants in infants with perinatal asphyxia.

Benefits: **Allopurinol versus no drug treatment:** We found one systematic review (search date not reported, 1 RCT).[11] The RCT (22 neonates [> 36 weeks' gestation] with asphyxia) compared allopurinol 40 mg/kg versus no drug treatment. It found no significant difference in mortality between groups (AR for death: 2/11 [18.2%] with allopurinol *v* 6/11 [54.5%] with no drug treatment; RR, NNT, or P values not reported).[12] It is likely that the RCT was too small to detect a clinically relevant effect (see comment below). The review also included data on long term neurodevelopmental outcomes that were reported in a conference abstract. There was no significant difference between treatments in the composite outcome of rates of death or developmental delay (method of assessment not reported, AR for death or developmental delay: 4/11 [36.4%] with allopurinol *v* 7/11 [63.6%] with no drug treatment; P = 0.39). ***Miltiorrhizae* versus citicoline (cytidine diphosphate choline):** We found one systematic review (search date not reported, 1 RCT).[11] The RCT (63 neonates with perinatal asphyxia) compared *miltiorrhizae* (a Chinese herb with antioxidative properties) versus citicoline (also an antioxidant).[13] It found a significant reduction in the risk of death or neurological abnormality (assessed using the Chinese neonatal behavioural neurological assessment scores, further details not reported) with *miltiorrhizae* compared with citicoline (AR for death or neurological abnormality: 6/35 [17.1%] with *miltiorrhizae* *v* 13/28 [46.4%] with citicoline; RR 0.37, 95% CI 0.16 to 0.81).

Harms: **Allopurinol versus no drug treatment:** The RCT reported no adverse effects.[12] ***Miltiorrhizae* versus citicoline:** The RCT did not report on harms.[13]

Comment: Free radicals are recognised as an important cause of brain damage in infants who have suffered an asphyxial injury.[14] In theory, antioxidants might therefore prevent free radical neuronal damage after perinatal asphyxia. The small RCT comparing allopurinol with no drug treatment found that infants treated with allopurinol had improved cerebral perfusion and electrical brain activity.[12] This intervention may be worth further assessment. The results of the RCT comparing *miltiorrhizae* with citicoline suggest that *miltiorrhizae* improves outcomes (or that citicoline worsens outcomes).[13] The systematic review cautioned that for both RCTs there was insufficient information on allocation concealment, method of randomisation, and blinding of assessors to determine trial quality and validity of the findings.

OPTION CALCIUM CHANNEL BLOCKERS

We found no RCTs on the effects of calcium channel blockers in infants with asphyxia.

Benefits: We found no systematic review or RCTs.

Harms: We found no RCTs.

Comment: The use of calcium channel blockers has been associated with clinically important hypotension in severely asphyxiated newborn infants.[15] In one small case series four term(G) infants (> 36 weeks' gestation) with asphyxia received a continuous infusion of nicardipine. The heart rate increased in all four infants and mean arterial blood pressure fell in three. Two infants had a sudden and marked fall in blood pressure, together with severe impairment of skin blood flow and a concurrent fall in cerebral blood flow.[15]

OPTION CORTICOSTEROIDS

We found no RCTs on the effects of corticosteroids in infants with perinatal asphyxia.

Benefits: We found no systematic review or RCTs.

Harms: We found no RCTs.

Comment: Although corticosteroids may reduce cerebral oedema, data from studies in older children or adults with cerebral hypoxia, and from animal studies, have not shown that steroids improve neurological outcomes.[16,17] In a small case series of newborn infants with birth asphyxia treated with dexamethasone, there was no evidence of an effect on cerebral perfusion pressure.[18]

OPTION FLUID RESTRICTION

We found no RCTs on the effects of fluid restriction in infants with perinatal asphyxia.

Benefits: We found no systematic review or RCTs.

Harms: We found no RCTs.

Comment: Current recommendations to restrict fluid input are based mainly on data from the treatment of adults and older children, or from animal models of cerebral hypoxia.[19] The rationale is that fluid restriction may limit cerebral oedema, which may be important in the pathogenesis of brain damage after perinatal asphyxia. However, there is concern that excessive fluid restriction may cause dehydration and hypotension, resulting in decreased cerebral perfusion and further brain damage.

OPTION HYPERVENTILATION

We found no RCTs on the effects of hyperventilation in infants with perinatal asphyxia.

Benefits: We found no systematic review or RCTs.

Harms: We found no RCTs.

Comment: Hyperventilation induced hypocapnoea causes cerebral vasoconstriction.[20] Although this might be associated with a compensatory increase in oxygen extraction in the brain, vasoconstriction may potentially worsen regional cerebral ischaemia.

OPTION MAGNESIUM SULPHATE

We found no RCTs on the effects of magnesium sulphate in infants with asphyxia.

Benefits: We found no systematic review or RCTs (see comment below).

Harms: We found no RCTs.

Comment: We found one RCT (33 infants with severe birth asphyxia) that compared magnesium sulphate infusion 250 mg/kg daily plus dopamine 5 μg/kg/minute infusion versus no drug treatment for 3 days.[21] It found no significant difference in mortality between the groups (AR 2/17 [12%] with magnesium sulphate plus dopamine *v* 1/16 [6%] with no drug treatment; $P > 0.99$; RR and NNT not reported). There were no data on long term neurodevelopmental outcomes. The RCT found that magnesium sulphate plus dopamine significantly improved a composite outcome (defined as survival with normal cranial computed tomography and electroencephalography results and establishment of oral feeding by 14 days of age) compared with no drug treatment (AR for positive response: 12/17 [70.6%] with magnesium sulphate plus dopamine *v* 5/16 [31.3%] with no drug treatment; P = 0.04). There were no significant differences in blood pressure or heart rate between treatments.[21]

OPTION MANNITOL

One small RCT provided insufficient evidence on the effects of mannitol in infants with asphyxia.

Benefits: **Versus no drug treatment:** We found one small RCT (25 term**G** [> 36 weeks' gestation] neonates with asphyxia), which compared mannitol (a single dose of 1 g/kg) versus no drug treatment.[22] There was no significant difference in mortality between the groups (AR 4/12 [33.3%] with mannitol *v* 4/13 [30.7%] with no drug treatment; RR, NNT, and P values not reported). There were no data on long term neurodevelopmental outcomes.

Harms: The RCT did not report on harms.[22]

Comment: None.

OPTION OPIATE ANTAGONISTS

One small RCT identified by a systematic review did not report on the effects of opiate antagonists, mortality or neurodevelopmental outcomes in infants with perinatal asphyxia.

Benefits: We found one systematic review (search date 2003).[23] The review identified one RCT, which did not report on mortality or neurodevelopmental outcomes (see comment below).

Harms: The RCT identified in the systematic review did not report on harms.[23]

Comment: The RCT identified by the review[23] (193 infants with 1 minute Apgar scores**G** ≤ 6) compared intramuscular naloxone (about 0.4 mg/kg) versus placebo (saline solution injection).[24] The RCT did not report on mortality or neurodevelopmental outcomes. It found no significant difference in respiratory rate and heart rate at 24 hours after birth. However, it did find that naloxone improved active muscle tone of upper and lower limbs compared with placebo (significance not reported).

OPTION PROPHYLACTIC ANTICONVULSANTS

One systematic review of three small, methodologically flawed RCTs found no significant difference in mortality or neurodevelopmental outcomes between barbiturates and no drug treatment in term infants with perinatal asphyxia.

Benefits: **Versus no drug treatment:** We found one systematic review (search date 2001, 3 RCTs, 110 term**G** infants, > 36 weeks' gestation), which compared barbiturate (thiopental or phenobarbitone) versus no drug treatment.[25] It found no significant difference in mortality, or in rates of severe neurodevelopmental disability**G** in the 77 survivors (3 RCTs: AR for death: 12/58 [20.6%] with barbiturate *v* 10/52 [19.2%] with no drug treatment; RR 1.06, 95% CI 0.50 to 2.27; AR for severe neurodevelopmental disability: 9/40 [22.5%] with barbiturate *v* 14/37 [37.8%] with no drug treatment; RR 0.61, 95% CI 0.30 to 1.22).

Harms: The RCTs did not report on harms.[25]

Comment: The three RCTs were small and had methodological weaknesses including lack of allocation concealment, lack of blinding, and lack of placebo control.

GLOSSARY

Apgar score Quantitative score usually measured at 1, 5, and 10 minutes after birth. The infant's heart rate, respiratory effort, muscle tone, response to stimulation (usually pharyngeal suctioning), and colour are assessed. For each of these five components, assessors award a maximum of 2 points for normal, 1 point for poor, and 0 points for bad. An Apgar score of less than 7 indicates moderate neuro/cardiorespiratory depression and a score of less than 3 indicates severe depression. The Apgar score is less reliable in premature infants, in whom it directly correlates with gestation.
Developmental quotient Assessed by means of a validated tool, usually Bayley Scales of Infant Development: Psychomotor Developmental Index and Mental Developmental Index
Hypoxic-ischaemic encephalopathy (neonatal encephalopathy) is an abnormal neuro-behavioural state in newborn infants. It is described clinically by stages (see definition, p 415).[10] **Stage 1 (mild)** hyper-alertness, hyper-reflexia, dilated pupils, tachycardia, and absence of seizures. **Stage 2 (moderate)** lethargy, hyper-reflexia, contraction of the pupils, bradycardia, seizures, hypotonia with weak suck, and Moro. **Stage 3 (severe)** stupor, flaccidity, seizures, small pupils which react poorly to light, decreased stretch reflexes, hypothermia, and absent Moro.
Near term Greater than 34 completed weeks' gestation and less than 37 weeks' gestation.
Severe neurodevelopmental disability Is defined as any one or combination of the following: non-ambulant cerebral palsy, developmental delay (developmental quotient (see above) < 70), auditory and visual impairment.
Term Greater than 36 completed weeks' gestation.

Substantive changes

Opiate antagonists One systematic review added, which provided no new evidence.[23] Categorisation unchanged.

REFERENCES

1. MacLennan A. A template for defining a causal relation between acute intrapartum events and cerebral palsy: international consensus statement. *BMJ* 1999;319:1054–1059.
2. Badawi N, Kurinczuk JJ, Keogh JM, et al. Antepartum risk factors for newborn encephalopathy: the Western Australian case-control study. *BMJ* 1998;317:1549–1553.
3. Badawi N, Kurinczuk JJ, Keogh JM, et al. Intrapartum risk factors for newborn encephalopathy: the Western Australian case-control study. *BMJ* 1998;317:1554–1558.
4. Ellis M, Manandar N, Manandar DS, et al. Risk factors for neonatal encephalopathy in Kathmandu, Nepal, a developing country: unmatched case-control study. *BMJ* 2000;320:1229–1236.
5. Levene ML, Kornberg J, Williams TH. The incidence and severity of post-asphyxial encephalopathy in full-term infants. *Early Hum Dev* 1985;11:21–26.
6. Thornberg E, Thiringer K, Odeback A, et al. Birth asphyxia: incidence, clinical course and outcome in a Swedish population. *Acta Paediatr* 1995;84:927–932.
7. Airede AI. Birth asphyxia and hypoxic-ischaemic encephalopathy: incidence and severity. *Ann Trop Paediatr* 1991;11:331–335.
8. Oswyn G, Vince JD, Friesen H. Perinatal asphyxia at Port Moresby General Hospital: a study of incidence, risk factors and outcome. *P N G Med J* 2000;43:110–120.
9. Jones G, Steketee RW, Black RE, et al. How many child deaths can we prevent this year? *Lancet* 2003;362:65–71.
10. Sarnat HB, Sarnat MS. Neonatal encephalopathy following fetal distress. A clinical and electroencephalographic study. *Arch Neurol* 1976;33:696–705.
11. Whitelaw A. Systematic review of therapy after hypoxic-ischaemic brain injury in the perinatal period. *Semin Neonatol* 2000;5:33–40. Search date not reported.
12. Van Bel F, Shadid M, Moison RM, et al. Effect of allopurinol on postasphyxial free radical formation, cerebral hemodynamics, and electrical brain activity. *Pediatrics* 1998;101:185–193.
13. Wang XL, Yu SL, Yu T, et al. Treatment of neonatal hypoxic ischaemic encephalopathy (HIE) with compound *Salvia miltiorrhizae* and citicoline: a comparative study in China. *Singapore Paediatr J* 1997;39:120–123.
14. Inder TE, Volpe JJ. Mechanisms of perinatal brain injury. *Semin Neonatol* 2000;5:3–16.
15. Levene MI, Gibson NA, Fenton AC, et al. The use of a calcium-channel blocker, nicardipine, for severely asphyxiated newborn infants. *Dev Med Child Neurol* 1990;32:567–574.
16. Alderson P, Roberts I. Corticosteroids for acute traumatic brain injury. In: The Cochrane Library. Issue 3, 2004. Chichester, UK: John Wiley & Sons, Ltd. Search date 2002. Primary sources Cochrane Injuries Group Specialised Register, CCTR, Medline and Embase.
17. Altman DI, Young RS, Yagel SK. Effects of dexamethasone in hypoxic-ischemic brain injury in the neonatal rat. *Biol Neonate* 1984;46:149–156.
18. Levene MI, Evans DH. Medical management of raised intracranial pressure after severe birth asphyxia. *Arch Dis Child* 1985;60:12–16.

19. Donn SM, Goldstein GW, Schork MA. Neonatal hypoxic-ischemic encephalopathy: current management practices. *J Perinatol* 1988;8:49–52.
20. Rosenberg AA. Response of the cerebral circulation to hypocarbia in postasphyxia newborn lambs. *Paediatr Res* 1992;32:537–541.
21. Ichiba H, Tamai H, Negishi H, et al. Randomized controlled trial of magnesium sulfate infusion for severe birth asphyxia. *Pediatr Int* 2002;44:505–509.
22. Adhikari M, Moodley M, Desai PK. Mannitol in neonatal cerebral oedema. *Brain Dev* 1990;12:349–351.
23. McGuire W, Fowlie PW, Evans DJ. Naloxone for preventing morbidity and mortality in newborn infants of greater than 34 weeks' gestation with suspected perinatal asphyxia. (Cochrane review). In: The Cochrane Library, Issue 3, 2004. Chichester, UK: John Wiley & Sons, Ltd. Search date 2003. Primary sources the Cochrane Central Register of Controlled Trials, Medline, Embase, conference proceedings, and previous reviews.
24. Chernick V, Manfreda J, De Booy V, et al. Clinical trial of naloxone in birth asphyxia. *J Pediatr* 1988;113:519–525.
25. Evans DJ, Levene MI. Anticonvulsants for preventing mortality and morbidity in full term newborns with perinatal asphyxia (Cochrane Review). In: The Cochrane Library, Issue 3, 2004. Oxford: Update Software. Search date 2001. Primary Sources Medline, Embase, CCTR and handsearch of conference abstracts.

William McGuire
Dr
Tayside Institute of Child Health
Ninewells Hospital and Medical School
Dundee
UK

Competing interests: None declared.

Reducing pain during blood sampling in infants

Search date May 2003

Deborah Pritchard

QUESTIONS

INTERVENTIONS

To be covered in future updates

Interventions in children over 1 year old

See glossary Ⓖ

Key Messages

Reducing pain related distress during heel puncture

- **Holding (skin to skin) versus swaddling in term infants** RCTs found that holding reduced crying during heel puncture compared with swaddling in term infants.
- **Oral glucose** RCTs found that oral glucose reduced pain responses (particularly the duration of crying) in preterm and term infants compared with water or no treatment.
- **Oral sucrose** Systematic reviews and additional RCTs found good evidence in preterm infants and limited evidence in term infants that oral sucrose reduced pain responses (particularly the duration of crying) compared with water or no treatment. One RCT found that sucrose did not appear to increase the benefit of holding. Three RCTs in term infants found that sucrose plus pacifier was more effective than pacifier alone, although one RCT in preterm infants found no significant difference in pain score between a pacifier dipped in sucrose and pacifier alone. One RCT found insufficient evidence about the effects of oral sucrose compared with lidocaine–prilocaine emulsion in term infants undergoing heel puncture.
- **Other sweeteners** RCTs have found that other sweeteners (hydrogenated glucose or an artificial sweetener, 10 parts cyclamate and 1 part saccharin) reduce pain scores and the percentage of time spent crying in term infants compared with water.

Reducing pain during blood sampling in infants

- **Pacifiers** RCTs in term and preterm infants have found that pacifiers given before heel puncture reduce pain responses compared with no treatment.
- **Positioning (tucking arms and legs) in preterm infants** One RCT found limited evidence that pain responses were reduced by tucking the arms and legs into a mid-line flexed position during heel puncture.
- **Rocking** We found limited evidence that rocking reduces pain related stress compared with placebo.
- **Multiple doses of sweet solution** One small RCT found no significant difference in pain of heel puncture between multiple and single doses of sucrose.
- **Swaddling** One small RCT found no significant difference in pain responses from swaddling compared with no swaddling.
- **Breast milk or breast feeding** RCTs found no evidence that breast milk or breast feeding during heel puncture reduced pain responses or crying in neonates compared with water.
- **Prone position** One RCT found no significant difference in pain score between prone position and either side or supine position during heel puncture.
- **Topical anaesthetics** Systematic reviews and additional RCTs found no evidence of reduced pain responses, particularly crying, following heel puncture with topical anaesthetic (lidocaine, lidocaine–prilocaine emulsion, or tetracaine [amethocaine]) compared with placebo.
- **Warming** Two RCTs in term infants found no benefit of warming before heel puncture.

Reducing pain related distress during venepuncture

- **Breast feeding** One RCT found that breast feeding during venepuncture reduced pain responses compared with oral water or being held. The RCT found no significant difference in pain response between breast feeding and oral glucose.
- **Oral glucose** RCTs have found that oral glucose reduces pain responses (particularly the duration of crying) in term and preterm infants compared with water or no treatment. One RCT found no significant difference in pain scores between sucrose and glucose.
- **Oral sucrose** RCTs have found that oral sucrose reduces pain responses (particularly the duration of crying) in term and preterm infants compared with water or no treatment. One RCT found no significant difference in pain between sucrose and glucose.
- **Pacifiers** One RCT found that pacifiers reduced pain responses compared with water or no treatment in term infants undergoing venepuncture.
- **Topical anaesthetics** Four RCTs found limited evidence that lidocaine–prilocaine emulsion reduced pain responses to venepuncture compared with placebo. Two RCTs found that tetracaine (amethocaine) gel reduced pain and crying during venepuncture compared with placebo.
- **Other sweeteners** We found no RCTs of other sweeteners for venepuncture.

DEFINITION Methods of sampling blood in infants include heel puncture, venepuncture, and arterial puncture. Heel puncture involves lancing of the lateral aspect of the infant's heel, squeezing the heel, and collecting the pooled capillary blood. Venepuncture involves aspirating blood through a needle from a peripheral vein. Arterial blood sampling is not discussed in this review. RCTs in this review were performed in a hospital care setting and the evidence relates to preterm and ill infants who have multiple blood tests, rather than infants undergoing heel puncture tests for routine screening. The results therefore cannot be applied to routine screening heel puncture tests in healthy infants.

INCIDENCE/ PREVALENCE Almost every infant in the developed world undergoes heel puncture to screen for metabolic disorders (e.g. phenylketonuria). Many infants have repeated heel punctures or venepunctures to monitor blood glucose or haemoglobin. Preterm or ill neonates may undergo 1–21 heel punctures or venepunctures per day.[1–3] These punctures are likely to be painful. Heel punctures comprise 61–87% and venepunctures comprise 8–13% of the invasive procedures performed on ill infants. Analgesics are rarely given specifically for blood sampling procedures, but 5–19% of infants receive analgesia for other indications.[2,3] In one study, comfort measures were provided during 63% of venepunctures and 75% of heel punctures.[3]

AETIOLOGY/ RISK FACTORS Blood sampling in infants can be difficult to perform, particularly in preterm or ill infants. Young infants may have increased sensitivity and more prolonged responses to pain than older age groups.[4] Factors that may affect the infant's pain responses include postconceptional age, previous pain experience, and procedural technique.

PROGNOSIS Pain caused by blood sampling is associated with acute behavioural and physiological deterioration.[4] Experience of pain during heel puncture seems to heighten pain responses during subsequent blood sampling.[5] Other adverse effects of blood sampling include bleeding, bruising, haematoma, and infection.

AIMS OF INTERVENTION To obtain an adequate blood sample with minimal pain for the infant and minimal adverse effects of treatments.

OUTCOMES We found no easily administered, widely accepted assessment of pain in infants. Where available, we have analysed the proportion of infants crying, or the duration of crying. Other pain related responses measured in the studies included facial expressions (the number of specific expressions, or the duration of those expressions), heart rate, and transcutaneous oxygen saturation levels. Studies used composite scales composed of behavioural and cardiorespiratory signs of pain related distress, or both, only some of which have been validated, such as the Premature Infant Pain Profile Ⓖ scale. We have not pooled differences in pain related responses or for different pain scales. The assessment of pain is difficult in pre-verbal children. Pain assessment methods varied in the RCTs, and a validated scale was not always used. Some measurements (e.g. facial expression) are difficult to score objectively. In many RCTs, blinding was not possible (e.g. where pacifiers were used).

METHODS *Clinical Evidence* search and appraisal May 2003, and additional hand searches by contributors.

QUESTION What are the effects of interventions to reduce pain related distress during heel puncture?

OPTION ORAL SWEET SOLUTIONS

RCTs have found that oral sucrose, glucose, or other sweeteners reduce pain responses in preterm and term infants (particularly the duration of crying when given 2 minutes before blood sampling) compared with water or no treatment. Evidence for sucrose in term infants was more limited; less than half of the RCTs found an effect. One small RCT found no significant difference between multiple and single doses of sucrose in pain scores for heel puncture. We found no clear evidence that any one sugar is superior to the others. There was weak evidence that solutions of 24% or more were more effective. Three RCTs in term infants found that sucrose plus pacifier was more effective than pacifier alone, but one RCT found no effect in preterm infants.

Benefits: **Sucrose:** We found one systematic review (search date 2001,[6] 4 RCTs[7–10]) and three additional RCTs[11–13] comparing oral sucrose (0.05–2.00 mL of 7.5–70%) versus water or no treatment in preterm newborns. All seven RCTs found that sucrose (24–70%) significantly reduced pain responses and pain scores compared with water. Three of these seven RCTs also found that the time spent crying during the procedure and the total duration of crying was significantly reduced with sucrose (25% and 50%).[7,9,13] One RCT found no significant difference between 15% sucrose and water.[13] We found one systematic review (search date 2001,[6] 7 RCTs[9,10,14–18]) and 12 additional RCTs[11–13,19–28] comparing oral sucrose (0.05–2.00 mL of 7.5–70%) versus water or no treatment in term newborns. Eight of the 19 RCTs found that sucrose (12–70%) significantly reduced pain scores compared with water.[10,12,15,17,23–26] Eight of the 19 RCTs found that sucrose decreased the percentage of time spent crying compared with water.[14,15,17,19–21,24,28] Nine of the 19 RCTs found that sucrose significantly reduced crying time (mean or median differences 16–90 seconds).[9,16,18,22–27] Two of the 19 RCTs found a significant difference only for infants given 25–50% sucrose and not for those given lower concentrations.[13,16] One RCT used a low concentration of sucrose (2 mL of 7.5%), and found no significant difference in duration of crying.[29] **Sucrose plus pacifier:** We found three RCTs comparing a pacifier**G** dipped in 12–24% sucrose or table sugar crystals versus pacifier dipped in water.[27,28,30] One RCT was in preterm infants.[30] It found no significant difference in pain responses (mean Premature Infant Pain Profile [PIPP] score**G**) between pacifier dipped in 12–24% sucrose or table sugar crystals and pacifier dipped in water.[30] Two RCTs were in term infants.[27,28] Both RCTs found that pacifier dipped in 12–24% sucrose or table sugar crystals reduced crying time compared with pacifier dipped in water.[27,28] **Sucrose plus holding:** We found one RCT (94 term infants) comparing sucrose, sucrose plus holding, holding with water, and water alone.[15] It found that pain scores and duration of crying decreased in the holding group compared with no holding and in the sucrose groups compared with no sucrose, but the differences were of borderline significance. There was no evidence of an interaction between sucrose and holding ($P = 0.37$). We found no RCTs in preterm infants. **Glucose:** We found four systematic reviews (search dates 1995,[31] 2001,[6] 1998,[32] 2000;[33] 2 RCTs [14,34]), three additional RCTs, and one subsequent RCT.[26,35–37] One of the additional RCTs (crossover, 17 infants) was in preterm infants.[35] It found that 10% glucose significantly reduced mean pain scores compared with no treatment. Two RCTs identified by the systematic reviews, two additional RCTs, and one subsequent RCT were in term infants.[14,26,34,35,37] All five RCTs compared glucose (1–2 mL of 10–33% solution) with water or no treatment before heel puncture.[14,26,34,35] Two RCTs found fewer infants cried with 30% glucose compared with water or no treatment.[34,35] One RCT found that 30% glucose significantly reduced crying time (75% decrease) compared with no treatment, but it found no significant difference in crying time (50% decrease) between 10% glucose and no treatment (50% decrease).[34] One RCT found no significant difference in mean crying time between 12% glucose and water.[14] One RCT found a significant reduction in pain scores with 33% glucose compared with no treatment.[37] One RCT found no significant difference in mean crying time or pain scores between 12.5% glucose and water (pain: mean PIPP score reduced by 2.5; $P < 0.001$).[26] **Glucose plus pacifier:** We found three RCTs comparing a pacifier dipped in 10–33% glucose versus no treatment, water, glucose alone, or pacifier alone.[26,36,37] One crossover RCT was in preterm infants.[36] It found that glucose plus pacifier significantly reduced the mean pain score compared with no treatment (glucose plus pacifier *v* no treatment: reduction in mean PIPP score 3.6 for glucose plus pacifier; $P = 0.001$).[36] Two RCTs were in term infants.[26,37] The RCTs found that glucose (12.5% and 33%, respectively) dipped pacifiers significantly reduced crying time and pain score compared with glucose alone, water, or no treatment.[26,37] **Other sweeteners:** We found three systematic reviews (search dates 1995,[31] 2001,[6] 1998;[32] 1 RCT[17]) and one additional RCT in term infants.[38] The RCT in the review found that hydrogenated glucose**G** significantly decreased pain scores, duration of first cry, and percentage of time spent crying compared with water, but found no significant difference compared with sucrose.[17] The additional RCT (120 term infants) comparing an artificial sweetener (10 parts cyclamate and 1 part saccharin) with water found small but significant differences in percentage of time crying and pain scores.[38] We found no RCTs in preterm infants.

Concentration of glucose or sucrose: We found two systematic reviews (search dates 2001[6] and 1998;[32] 1 RCT[34]) and six additional RCTs of the effects of glucose or sucrose concentration in heel puncture.[14,16,17,22,34,39] We found no RCTs solely in preterm infants. We found one RCT of 60 term and preterm infants.[34] It found no significant difference between 10% and 30% glucose in the duration of crying or in the proportion of babies who cried at all (no crying: 40% with 10% glucose *v* 53% with 30% glucose; P > 0.05). Three RCTs were in term infants.[14,16,17] One RCT (75 neonates) found that increasing concentrations of sucrose (2 mL of 12.5%, 25%, and 50%) produced significantly greater reductions in duration of crying.[16] The other two RCTs (56 infants) found no difference in duration of crying with different sucrose concentrations (2 mL of 25–50% or 12–25% sucrose).[14,17] **Multiple doses of sweeteners:** We found one RCT (32 preterm neonates, mean gestation 31 weeks), which compared a single dose (0.5 mL) of 24% sucrose 2 minutes before heel puncture versus three doses given 2 minutes before the procedure, immediately before the procedure, and during the procedure.[11] Pain scores measured at five points during the procedure were significantly different only at the latest time. We found no RCTs in term infants. **Sucrose versus glucose:** We found two RCTs (226 term infants undergoing heel puncture) comparing glucose versus sucrose.[22,26] One RCT found that 30% sucrose reduced crying time by a mean of 30 seconds compared with 30% glucose (P = 0.006).[22] The second RCT found no significant difference between 12.5% sucrose and 12.5% glucose.[26] We found no RCTs in preterm infants. **Sucrose versus breast milk:** We found one small RCT (20 term infants).[28] It found that sucrose plus pacifier significantly reduced the percentage of time crying compared with colostrum plus pacifier. We found no RCTs in preterm infants.

Harms: No adverse effects from oral sucrose or glucose administered to full term or preterm infants were reported in any of the RCTs. Transient choking and oxygen desaturation have been associated with the administration of oral sweeteners (directly into the mouth and when administered on a pacifier).[40] The safety of repeated oral administration of sucrose or glucose has not been adequately investigated. There is no evidence that repeated dosing with sweeteners leads to conditioning. Theoretical adverse effects include hyperglycaemia and necrotising enterocolitis.

Comment: There is concern that parents, impressed with the calming effect of sweeteners, may continue to use it at home. This could be harmful in high concentrations or repeated doses. Some studies were crossover RCTs, which may produce biased estimates of the effect of sucrose if neonates become habituated to pain or if the washout period between interventions is too short.[7,9,12] Only some RCTs reported adequate concealment of allocation.[7,8,11,15,23,35,39] In one study, it was uncertain whether infants were randomly allocated.[20] Most had blinded measurement of at least some of the pain responses, particularly crying, on the basis of independent audio or video tape recordings. One RCT had no blinded outcome assessment.[9] We found inadequate evidence about the benefits or harms of repeated administration of sucrose or glucose for repeated blood sampling.

OPTION BREAST MILK OR BREAST FEEDING

RCTs found no evidence that breast milk or breast feeding reduced pain responses or crying in neonates undergoing heel puncture compared with water. One RCT found no evidence that breast milk plus pacifier was more effective than pacifier alone. One RCT found that breast feeding reduced pain responses compared with swaddling in the cot.

Benefits: **Breast milk:** We found one systematic review (search date 1998,[32] 2 RCTs,[18,34] 126 preterm and term neonates undergoing heel puncture) and two subsequent RCTs (177 term infants)[25,38] comparing breast milk or colostrums (1–2 mL) versus water. None found a significant effect of breast milk on duration of crying[18,25,34,38] or proportion of infants not crying.[34] **Breast milk plus pacifier:** One RCT (20 term infants) found no significant difference between infants given a pacifier**Ⓖ** dipped in breast milk versus a pacifier dipped in water.[28] **Breast feeding:** One RCT compared term infants who were held and breast fed with infants given water or breast milk in their cot (62 term infants).[25] No significant effect was found for breast feeding compared with water or breast milk on the duration of crying. Another RCT (30 term infants) compared breast feeding with being swaddled in the cot.[41] Breast feeding decreased the duration of grimacing (mean 17.2 seconds in breastfed *v* 83.3 seconds in swaddled babies) and the duration of crying (mean 8.8 seconds breastfed *v* 72.7 seconds).

Harms: None reported.

Comment: Concealment of allocation was not clearly stated in any RCT. Assessment of pain responses was blind in two RCTs[25,38] and not clearly stated in two other RCTs.[18,34]

OPTION TOPICAL ANAESTHETICS

Systematic reviews and additional RCTs found no evidence of reduced pain responses, particularly crying, following heel puncture with topical anaesthetic (lidocaine, lidocaine–prilocaine emulsion, or tetracaine [amethocaine]) compared with placebo.

Benefits: **Lidocaine or lidocaine–prilocaine emulsion:** We found three systematic reviews (search dates 1996,[42] 1998,[32] and 1998;[43] 5 RCTs[44–48]) and one additional RCT,[1] comparing lidocaine or lidocaine–prilocaine emulsion versus placebo in neonates undergoing heel puncture. Treatments were usually given 30–60 minutes before heel puncture, with the exception of one RCT that randomised infants to eight application times (10–120 minutes before heel puncture).[47] The six RCTs used different assessments of pain responses. Three RCTs included 186 preterm neonates,[1,44,45] and three RCTs included 192 infants who were mainly term neonates.[46–48] None of the RCTs found a significant difference in pain scores between lidocaine or lidocaine–prilocaine emulsion and placebo. One RCT found no significant difference between lidocaine–prilocaine emulsion and placebo in the proportion of infants who cried during the procedure (54/56 [96%] *v* 52/54 [96%]).[47] **Tetracaine (amethocaine) versus placebo:** One RCT (60 infants, median gestation 36 weeks, undergoing heel puncture using an automated device) found no significant difference between tetracaine and placebo in pain score or the proportion of infants who cried (20/30 [67%] with tetracaine *v* 13/29 [45%]; ARI +22%, 95% CI –4% to +47%).[49] **Topical anaesthetic versus sucrose:** We found no studies of topical anaesthetic versus sweet solutions for heel puncture. **Topical anaesthetic versus pacifiers:** We found no RCTs.

Harms: We found six RCTs (250 infants), which reported absence of adverse reactions to lidocaine–prilocaine emulsion or to placebo, or no difference in minor, transient local reactions.[1,46–48,50,51] One cohort study (500 neonates) found unusual cutaneous effects associated with lidocaine–prilocaine emulsion in four neonates under 32 weeks' gestation.[52] Methaemoglobinaemia can occur with the prilocaine constituent of lidocaine–prilocaine emulsion. Levels of methaemoglobin over 25–30% can cause clinical symptoms of hypoxia.[53] We found one systematic review (search date 1996, 12 RCTs or cohort studies, > 355 neonates)[42] and two subsequent RCTs (167 neonates)[1,53] of lidocaine–prilocaine emulsion for heel puncture, venepuncture, circumcision, or lumbar puncture. All but one of these studies found mean methaemoglobin levels less than 1.5% in neonates given lidocaine–prilocaine emulsion. The other RCT (47 preterm and term infants given lidocaine–prilocaine emulsion) found that the highest mean methaemoglobin levels (2.3%, range 0.6–6.2%) occurred after 15 days of repeated doses of lidocaine–prilocaine emulsion.[52] A systematic review found two case reports of neonates who were treated with oxygen at methaemoglobin levels of 12% and 16%.[42] No local skin reactions were seen after application of tetracaine or placebo in the 140 neonates studied.

Comment: Some of the studies reported adequate concealment of allocation.[51,54–56] Three RCTs used videotaped recordings of pain responses to blind assessors to the intervention.[50,51,54,55] In the other RCTs, although placebo ointment was used, pain responses were assessed by observers at the time of the procedure, rather than by scoring of video film. Deduction of treatment allocation may have been possible in the studies including lidocaine–prilocaine emulsion because of the smell and skin blanching caused by lidocaine–prilocaine emulsion. One study excluded 25% of children who had high behaviour scores before puncture, and presented results only for selected subgroups.[50] The findings of this study may be difficult to generalise.

OPTION PACIFIERS

Eight RCTs have found reduced pain responses in term and preterm infants given pacifiers compared with no treatment before heel puncture. Three RCTs found weak evidence that pacifiers dipped in sucrose reduced pain responses compared with pacifiers alone.

Benefits: **Pacifier alone:** We found one systematic review (search date 2001,[6] 1 RCT[30]) and seven additional RCTs comparing pacifiers Ⓖ versus no treatment (445 infants, of whom 271 were preterm).[24,30,36,57–60] Four of the RCTs were crossover trials.[30,36,57,58] Pacifiers were given 2–5 minutes before heel puncture. RCTs found that pacifiers significantly reduced pain responses[36,45,59] or the percentage of time spent in a distressed, fussy, or awake state compared with no pacifiers.[58,59] In the three RCTs in term infants, those given a pacifier cried for significantly less time,[24,57,60] spent less time in fussy or awake states,[60] or had reduced pain score.[57] However, reductions were not significant for all measures of pain; in one study grimacing was not significantly reduced by the pacifier[24] and, in another, the pain score was similar during the procedure but fell more quickly in babies given pacifiers.[57] **Pacifier plus multimodal sensory stimulation:** We found two RCTs.[36,37] They found that a pacifier plus multimodal sensory stimulation (pacifer plus glucose, massage, visual, and auditory stimulation) during heel puncture significantly reduced the pain score when compared with no treatment,[36] or pacifier alone, or glucose plus pacifier.[37] One RCT (crossover, 17 preterm infants) found a mean Premature Infant Pain Profile score Ⓖ reduction when compared with no pacifier (7.15; $P < 0.001$) and when compared with glucose plus pacifer, pacifier alone, or glucose alone (mean Premature Infant Pain Profile score reduction 2.6–4.55; $P < 0.01$ for each of the 3 comparisons).[36] Another RCT found that multimodal sensory stimulation was even more effective than glucose plus pacifier in reducing pain scores in term infants.[37] **Pacifiers plus sucrose:** See benefits of oral sweet solutions, p 423.

Harms: No adverse effects were reported in any of the studies. The use of pacifiers has been associated with transient choking and oxygen desaturation.

Comment: None of the studies explicitly defined the method of allocation to pacifier or no treatment. Three RCTs blinded assessors to the intervention by analysing audio tapes of crying during the procedure.[36,58,60] Measurement of pain responses on the basis of facial expressions were not blinded to the pacifiers or music intervention.

OPTION PHYSICAL CONTACT (HOLDING, ROCKING, POSITIONING, SWADDLING, WARMING, AND PRIOR HANDLING)

We found insufficient evidence from one small RCT about the effects of swaddling. Two RCTs have found that holding reduces crying during heel puncture compared with swaddling. One RCT found that sucrose did not appear to modify the effect of holding. We found limited evidence that rocking reduces pain related stress compared with placebo. One RCT found limited evidence that pain responses were reduced by tucking the arms and legs into a mid-line flexed position during heel puncture, or by avoiding stressful handling before heel puncture. One RCT found no significant difference in pain score between prone position and either side or supine position during heel puncture. Two RCTs found no effect of warming before heel puncture.

Benefits: **Swaddling versus no swaddling:** We found no systematic review but found one small crossover RCT (15 neonates).[61] It found no significant difference in facial expressions of pain or arousal state between swaddling immediately after heel puncture and no swaddling.[61] **Holding versus swaddling:** We found no systematic review but found two RCTs (124 term infants undergoing heel puncture).[15,62] One RCT (30 infants) compared holding the baby with skin to skin contact versus being swaddled in a crib.[62] It found that holding significantly reduced crying and grimacing compared with swaddling (proportion crying during procedure 8% *v* 45%; ARR 37%, CI not reported; NNT 3, 95% CI 2 to 13). **Rocking:** We found no systematic review but found two RCTs comparing rocking versus no intervention.[8,60] One RCT (44 preterm infants, 25–34 weeks' gestation) compared 0.05 mL water given before heel puncture versus simulated rocking using a respirator attached to an air mattress.[8] The study found no significant differences in facial expressions of pain. The other RCT (40 term neonates) compared no intervention with being held vertically and rocked by the examiner.[60] The study found that rocking reduced the duration of crying ($P = 0.05$) during the procedure and the risk of persistent crying (2/20 [10%] with rocking *v* 9/20 [45%] with no intervention; ARR 35%, CI 10% to 60%; NNT 3, 95% CI 2 to 10). **Positioning:** We found no systematic review but found four RCTs comparing positioning, swaddling, or stressful handling versus no intervention.[30,61,63,64] One crossover RCT (122 preterm infants, 25–34 weeks' gestation, undergoing heel puncture) compared prone position versus side or supine position.[30] The study found no significant difference in the mean pain score. Another RCT (crossover, 30 preterm neonates, 25–35 weeks' gestation) compared facilitative tucking during and after heel puncture (defined as the gentle containment of arms and legs in a flexed, mid-line position) versus no intervention.[63] The RCT found a significant reduction in the total crying time and time to quietening (mean cry duration 2.2 *v* 0.3 minutes; $P < 0.001$). The fourth RCT (48 mainly preterm infants, mean gestation < 35 weeks) compared handling (as if being prepared for a lumbar puncture) with avoidance of handling for 10 minutes prior to heel puncture.[64] The study found that prior handling increased facial expressions of pain, the proportion of time crying, and crying at all during the 2 minutes after heel puncture (21/21 [100%] handled babies cried *v* 21/27 [78%]

non-handled babies; ARR +22%; CI –24% to +68%). **Warming:** We found one systematic review (search date 1998,[32] 1 RCT[65]) and one subsequent RCT.[66] The RCT identified by the review compared 57 term infants undergoing heel puncture on 80 occasions with an automated lancet with (41 infants) or without (40 infants) prior warming of the heel. The heel was warmed for 10 minutes with a gel pack at 40 °C. It found no significant difference in the proportion of infants who grimaced and cried between warming and not warming (14/41 [34%] *v* 10/40 [25%]; RR 1.4, 95% CI 0.7 to 2.7). Sampling time was slightly longer in the warmed heels (median time 44 seconds, interquartile range 25–62 seconds *v* 40 seconds, interquartile range 28–72 seconds), but the number of repeat punctures was slightly lower (5/41 [12%] *v* 8/40 [20%]; RR 0.6, 0.2 to 1.7). The subsequent RCT (100 preterm infants) found no significant difference in the crying time or number of repeated punctures after heel warming compared with no warming.[66]

Harms: No adverse events were reported for any of these interventions.

Comment: **Holding:** Assessment of crying was based on analysis of audio or videotape recordings and was blind to the sucrose intervention but not to holding.[15,62] Assessments based on facial expressions were not blind to the intervention. **Rocking:** The method of allocation to rocking or standard care was adequate in one study[8] and unclear in the other.[59] Both studies used blinded assessment of pain responses based on video[8] and audio tape[60] recordings. **Position, swaddling, and prior handling:** None of the studies explicitly reported the method of allocation to the interventions, and only the study comparing handling versus no handling assessed pain responses blind to the intervention.[64] **Warming:** The method of allocation was not reported and assessment of outcomes was not blind to the intervention.

QUESTION What are the effects of interventions to reduce pain related distress during venepuncture?

OPTION ORAL SWEET SOLUTIONS

RCTs have found that oral sucrose or glucose reduce pain responses (particularly the duration of crying) compared with water, topical anaesthetic or no treatment in term and preterm infants undergoing venepuncture. One RCT found that 25% glucose was more effective than 10% glucose. We found no RCTs of other sweetners.

Benefits: **Sucrose:** We found two systematic reviews (search dates 1995,[31] 2001;[6] 2 RCTs[39,67]) and one additional RCT.[68] One RCT (28 infants) in the review was in preterm infants.[67] It found that 24% sucrose reduced crying time compared with water but found no significant difference between 12% sucrose and water (20 infants: mean duration of crying 19 seconds with 24% sucrose *v* 73 seconds with water). One RCT identified by the review and the additional RCT were in term infants.[39,68] Both RCTs (201 infants) found that 24–30% sucrose significantly reduced the duration of crying and pain scores compared with water or no treatment. **Glucose:** We found four RCTs comparing 2 mL of 10–30% glucose versus water in infants undergoing venepuncture.[35,39,69,70] One RCT (60 infants) was in preterm infants.[69] It found that 25% glucose significantly reduced the duration of crying compared with water but found no significant difference between 10% glucose and water (mean duration of crying: 40.5 seconds [SD 38.98] with 25% glucose *v* 68.9 seconds [SD 44.15] with 10% glucose *v* 85.5 seconds [SD 44.1] with water). Three RCTs were in term infants.[35,39,70] The first RCT (60 infants) found that glucose significantly reduced pain scores compared with water but found no difference in the proportion of infants crying (46% with glucose *v* 39% with water).[35] The second RCT (75 infants) found significantly reduced median pain scores with glucose compared with water or no treatment (median pain score difference 2 [glucose 5, water 7], 95% CI 1 to 4; P = 0.005).[39] The third RCT (201 infants) compared 30% glucose plus placebo on the skin versus lidocaine–prilocaine topical anaesthetic cream plus oral water.[70] It found that glucose significantly improved Premature Infant Pain Profile (PIPP) scoreⒼ and duration of pain compared with topical anaesthetic cream (PIPP scores: 4.6 with glucose *v* 5.7 with anaesthetic cream, P = 0.0314; median duration of crying: 1 second with glucose *v* 18 seconds with topical anaesthetic, P < 0.001). It also found that glucose significantly reduced the proportion of infants thought to have pain (defined as PIPP > 6: 19.3% with glucose *v* 41.7% with anaesthetic cream, P = 0.0007). **Other sweeteners:** We found no RCTs of other sweeteners for venepuncture. **Concentration of glucose or sucrose:** One RCT found that 25% glucose significantly reduced the duration of crying compared with 10% glucose (40.5 seconds *v* 68.9 seconds).[69] **Sucrose versus glucose:** One RCT (150 term infants) found no significant difference between 30% sucrose and 30% glucose in pain scores.[39]

Harms: No adverse effects from oral sucrose or glucose administered to full term or preterm infants were reported in any of the RCTs. Transient choking and oxygen desaturation have been associated with the administration of oral sweeteners (directly into the mouth and when administered on a pacifier).[40] The safety of repeated oral administration of sucrose or glucose has not been adequately investigated. Theoretical adverse effects include hyperglycaemia and necrotising enterocolitis.

Comment: See comment under oral sweet solutions with heel puncture, p 425.

OPTION TOPICAL ANAESTHETICS

Four RCTs found limited evidence that lidocaine–prilocaine emulsion reduced pain responses to venepuncture compared with placebo. Two RCTs found that tetracaine (amethocaine) gel reduced pain and crying during venepuncture compared with placebo.

Benefits: **Lidocaine–prilocaine emulsion:** We found two systematic reviews (search dates 1996[42] and 1998;[32] 2 RCTs[54,71]) and two additional RCTs[50,51], which compared lidocaine–prilocaine emulsion versus placebo in infants undergoing venepuncture. One RCT (120 term infants) found that lidocaine–prilocaine emulsion significantly reduced the duration of crying and pain score at 15 seconds after venepuncture compared with placebo, but found no significant difference in pain score 60 seconds after venepuncture (median duration of crying: 12 seconds *v* 31 seconds; P < 0.05; pain score: Neonatal Facial Coding System scoreⒼ 287 *v* 374; P = 0.02).[54] The second RCT (60 children) found that 19/28 in the lidocaine–prilocaine emulsion group and 14/28 in the placebo group did not cry at all during the procedure.[71] The study did not measure duration of crying or pain score. The third RCT (41 infants and toddlers) found that lidocaine–prilocaine emulsion significantly reduced behavioural pain score compared with placebo (P < 0.01).[50] The fourth RCT (19 preterm infants) found no significant difference in pain or total duration of crying between lidocaine–prilocaine emulsion and placebo (pain assessed using Neonatal Facial Coding System score, mean difference 0, 95% CI −2.00 to +1.75; median difference in duration of crying: −22 seconds, 95% CI −96 seconds to +24 seconds).[51] **Tetracaine (amethocaine) versus placebo:** Two RCTs (80 preterm and term neonates undergoing venepuncture) found that tetracaine significantly reduced pain scores and the proportion who cried compared with placebo (4/19 [21%] with tetracaine *v* 15/20 [75%] with placebo; ARR 54%, 95% CI 2% to 80%; NNT 2, 95% CI 1 to 4).[55,56] **Topical anaesthetic versus sucrose:** We found one RCT (55 venepunctures in 51 term neonates), which compared lidocaine–prilocaine emulsion versus 24% sucrose versus lidocaine–prilocaine emulsion plus sucrose versus water.[68] Crying was taped and assessed blind to treatment. Lidocaine–prilocaine emulsion alone was reported to be less effective than sucrose alone or lidocaine–prilocaine emulsion plus sucrose, but analyses were not presented. **Topical anaesthetic versus oral glucose:** See oral sweet solutions, p 429. **Topical anaesthetic versus pacifiers:** We found no RCTs.

Harms: See harms under topical anaesthetics with heel puncture, p 426.

Comment: Some of the studies reported adequate concealment of allocation.[46,47,49] One RCT used videotaped recordings of pain responses to blind assessors to the intervention.[49]

OPTION PACIFIERS

One RCT found that pacifiers reduced pain responses compared with water or no treatment in term infants undergoing venepuncture.

Benefits: We found one RCT (100 term infants undergoing venepuncture) comparing a pacifier**G** or a pacifier plus sucrose versus no treatment or 2 mL water orally in infants.[67] The study found a significant reduction in the pain score during the procedure (median difference in 10 point pain score 5 for pacifiers alone *v* water and 6 for pacifiers plus sucrose *v* water; $P < 0.0001$).

Harms: The RCT reported no adverse effects.[67] The use of pacifiers has been associated with transient choking and oxygen desaturation.

Comment: The RCT did not explicitly define the method of allocation to pacifier or no treatment.[67]

OPTION BREAST FEEDING

One RCT found that breast feeding during venepuncture reduced pain responses compared with oral water or being held. The RCT found no significant difference in pain response between breast feeding and oral glucose

Benefits: We found no systematic reviews but we found one RCT.[72] The RCT (180 term infants) compared four treatments while the infant was held in its mother's arms during venepuncture: breast feeding, no intervention, sterile water, and 30% glucose plus pacifier. It found that breast feeding significantly reduced pain response compared with holding alone or sterile water (median premature infant pain profile score**G**: 4.5 with breast feeding *v* 13 with holding *v* 12 with sterile water; $P < 0.0001$ for breast feeding *v* holding; $P < 0.0001$ for breast feeding *v* sterile water). It found no significant difference in pain response between breast feeding and glucose (median premature infant pain profile score 4.5 with breast feeding *v* 4 with glucose, $P = 0.28$).

Harms: The RCT found no adverse effects.[72]

Comment: Blinding was impossible in the RCT because of the nature of the interventions.[72]

Reducing pain during blood sampling in infants

GLOSSARY

Hydrogenated glucose syrup An aqueous solution of hydrogenated part hydrolysed starch composed of a mixture of mainly maltitol with sorbitol and hydrogenated oligosaccharides and polysaccharides. Preparations containing a minimum 98% maltitol are known as maltitol syrup.

Neonatal Facial Coding System (NFCS) score Facial coding system used to evaluate pain responses in full term and preterm infants. Presence or absence of six facial actions (e.g. eyes squeezed shut, deepening of the naso-labial furrow) is recorded.

Pacifier A device with a teat that a baby sucks on for comfort. Some pacifiers can deliver a liquid to the baby. Also known as a "dummy", "soother", or "plug" in some countries.

Premature Infant Pain Profile (PIPP) score A seven item composite scale that scores behavioural and cardiorespiratory pain responses coded 0 to 3 (maximum score 21).

REFERENCES

1. Stevens B, Johnston C, Taddio A, et al. Management of pain from heel lance with lidocaine–prilocaine (EMLA) cream: is it safe and efficacious in preterm infants? *J Dev Behav Pediatr* 1999;20:216–221.
2. Johnston CC, Collinge JM, Henderson SJ, et al. A cross-sectional survey of pain and pharmacological analgesia in Canadian neonatal intensive care units. *Clin J Pain* 1997;13:308–312.
3. Porter FL, Anand KJS. Epidemiology of pain in neonates. *Res Clin Forum* 1998;20:9–18.
4. Anand K, Stevens BJ, McGrath PJ. *Pain in neonates.* Amsterdam: Elsevier Science BV, 2000.
5. Taddio A, Gurguis MG, Koren G. Lidocaine-prilocaine cream versus tetracaine gel for procedural pain in children. *Ann Pharmacother* 2002;36:687–692.
6. Stevens B, Yamada J, Ohlsson A. Sucrose for analgesia in newborn infants undergoing painful procedures. In: The Cochrane Library, Issue 3, 2002. Oxford: Update Software. Search date 2001; primary sources Medline, Embase, Reference Update, Cochrane Library, and hand searches of personal files, bibliographies, recent neonatal and pain journals, and conference proceedings.
7. Bucher HU, Moser T, von Siebenthal K, et al. Sucrose reduces pain reaction to heel lancing in preterm infants: a placebo-controlled, randomized and masked study. *Pediatr Res* 1995;38:332–335.
8. Johnston CC, Stremler RL, Stevens BJ, et al. Effectiveness of oral sucrose and simulated rocking on pain response in preterm neonates. *Pain* 1997;72:193–199.
9. Ramenghi LA, Wood CM, Griffith GC, et al. Reduction of pain response in premature infants using intraoral sucrose. *Arch Dis Child Fetal Neonatal Ed* 1996;74:F126–F128.
10. Gibbins SA. Efficacy and safety of sucrose for procedural pain relief in preterm and term neonates. *Dissert Abstract Int* 2001;62–04B:1804.
11. Johnston CC, Stremler R, Horton L, et al. Effect of repeated doses of sucrose during heel stick procedure in preterm neonates. *Biol Neonate* 1999;75:160–166.
12. Mellah D, Gourrier E, Merbouche S, et al. Analgesia with saccharose during heel capillary prick. A randomized study in 37 newborns of over 33 weeks of amenorrhea. *Arch Pediatr* 1999;6:610–616 [in French].
13. Storm H, Fremming A. Food intake and oral sucrose in preterms prior to heel prick. *Acta Paediatr* 2002;91:555–560.
14. Abad Massanet F, Diaz Gomez NM, Domenech Martinez E, et al. Analgesic effect of oral sweet solution in newborns. *An Esp Pediatr* 1995;43:351–354.
15. Gormally S, Barr RG, Wertheim L, et al. Contact and nutrient caregiving effects on newborn infant pain responses. *Dev Med Child Neurol* 2001;43:28–38.
16. Haouari N, Wood C, Griffiths G, et al. The analgesic effect of sucrose in full term infants: a randomised controlled trial. *BMJ* 1995;310:1498–1500.
17. Ramenghi LA, Griffith GC, Wood CM, et al. Effect of non-sucrose sweet tasting solution on neonatal heel prick responses. *Arch Dis Child Fetal Neonatal Ed* 1996;74:F129–F131.
18. Ors R, Ozek E, Baysoy G, et al. Comparison of sucrose and human milk on pain response in newborns. *Eur J Pediatr* 1999;158:63–66.
19. Blass EM, Hoffmeyer LB. Sucrose as an analgesic for newborn infants. *Pediatrics* 1991;87:215–218.
20. Blass EM. Pain-reducing properties of sucrose in human newborns. *Chem Senses* 1995;20:29–35.
21. Blass EM. Milk-induced hypoalgesia in human newborns. *Pediatrics* 1997:99:825–829.
22. Isik U, Ozek E, Bilgen H, et al. Comparison of oral glucose and sucrose solutions on pain response in neonates. *J Pain* 2000;1:275–278.
23. Overgaard C, Knudsen A. Pain-relieving effect of sucrose in newborns during heel prick. *Biol Neonate* 1999;75:279–284.
24. Blass EM, Watt LB. Suckling- and sucrose-induced analgesia in human newborns. *Pain* 1999;83:611–623.
25. Bilgen H, Ozek E, Cebeci D, et al. Comparison of sucrose, expressed breast milk, and breast-feeding on the neonatal response to heel prick. *J Pain* 2001;2:301–305.
26. Akman I, Zek E, Bilgen H, et al. Sweet solutions and pacifiers for pain relief in newborn infants. *J Pain* 2002;3:199–202
27. Greenberg CS. A sugar-coated pacifier reduces procedural pain in newborns. *Pediatr Nurs* 2002;28:271–277.
28. Blass EM, Miller LW. Effects of colostrum in newborn humans: dissociation between analgesic and cardiac effects. *J Dev Behav Pediatr* 2001;22:385–390.
29. Rushforth JA, Levene MI. Effect of sucrose on crying in response to heel stab. *Arch Dis Child* 1993;69:388–389.
30. Stevens B, Johnston C, Franck L, et al. The efficacy of developmentally sensitive interventions and sucrose for relieving procedural pain in very low birth weight neonates. *Nurs Res* 1999;48:35–43.
31. Stevens B, Taddio A, Ohlsson A, et al. The efficacy of sucrose for relieving procedural pain in neonates: a systematic review and meta-analysis. *Acta Paediatr* 1997;86:837–842. Search date 1995; primary sources Medline, Embase, Reference Update, and hand searches of personal files, bibliographies, most recent neonatal and pain journals, and conference proceedings.
32. Ohlsson A, Taddio A, Jadad AR, et al. Evidence-based decision making, systematic reviews and the Cochrane collaboration: implications for neonatal analgesia. In: Anand K, Stevens B, McGrath PJ, eds. *Pain in Neonates*. Amsterdam: Elsevier Science BV, 2000:251–268. Search date 1998; primary sources Medline, Cochrane Library, hand searches of personal files, and reference lists.
33. Bauer K, Versmold H. Oral sugar solutions in pain therapy of neonates and premature infants. *Z Geburtshilfe Neonatol* 2001;205:80–85. Search date 2000; primary source PubMed.

34. Skogsdal Y, Eriksson M, Schollin J. Analgesia in newborns given oral glucose. *Acta Paediatr* 1997;86:217–220.
35. Eriksson M, Gradin M, Schollin J. Oral glucose and venepuncture reduce blood sampling pain in newborns. *Early Hum Dev* 1999;55:211–218.
36. Bellieni CV, Buonocore G, Nenci A, et al. Sensorial saturation: an effective analgesic tool for heel-prick in preterm infants: a prospective randomized trial. *Biol Neonate* 2001;80:15–18.
37. Bellieni CV, Bagnoli F, Perrone S, et al. Effect of multisensory stimulation on analgesia in term neonates: a randomized controlled trial. *Pediatr Res* 2002;51:460–463.
38. Bucher HU, Baumgartner R, Bucher N, et al. Artificial sweetener reduces nociceptive reaction in term newborn infants. *Early Hum Dev* 2000:59:51–60.
39. Carbajal R, Chauvet X, Couderc S, et al. Randomised trial of analgesic effects of sucrose, glucose, and pacifiers in term neonates. *BMJ* 1999;319:1393–1397.
40. Horitz N. Does oral glucose reduce the pain of neonatal procedure? *Arch Dis Child* 2002;80–81.
41. Gray L, Miller LW, Philipp BL, et al. Breastfeeding is analgesic in healthy newborns. *Pediatrics* 2002;109:590–593.
42. Taddio A, Ohlsson A, Einarson TR, et al. A systematic review of lidocaine–prilocaine cream (EMLA) in the treatment of acute pain in neonates. *Pediatrics* 1998;101:E1. Search date 1996; primary sources Medline, Embase, Reference Update, and hand searches of personal files and meeting proceedings.
43. Essink-Tjebbes CM, Hekster YA, Liem KD, et al. Topical use of local anesthetics in neonates. *Pharm World Sci* 1999;21:173–176. Search date 1998; primary source Medline.
44. Ramaioli F, Amice De D, Guzinska K, et al. EMLA cream and the premature infant [abstract]. *Int Monitor Reg Anaesthesia* 1993;59.
45. Stevens B, Johnston C, Taddio A, et al. *The safety and efficacy of EMLA for heel lance in premature neonates.* International Association for the Study of Pain, 8th World Congress on Pain, Vancouver, Canada 1996;239:181–182.
46. Rushforth JA, Griffiths G, Thorpe H, et al. Can topical lignocaine reduce behavioural response to heel prick? *Arch Dis Child Fetal Neonatal Ed* 1995;72:F49–F51.
47. Larsson BA, Jylli L, Lagercrantz H, et al. Does a local anaesthetic cream (EMLA) alleviate pain from heel-lancing in neonates? *Acta Anaesthesiol Scand* 1995;39:1028–1031.
48. Wester U. Analgesic effect of lidocaine ointment on intact skin in neonates. *Acta Paediatr* 1993;82:791.
49. Jain A, Rutter N, Ratnayaka M. Topical amethocaine gel for pain relief of heel prick blood sampling: a randomised double blind controlled trial. *Arch Dis Child Fetal Neonatal Ed* 2001;84:F56–F59.
50. Robieux I, Kumar R, Radhakrishnan S, et al. Assessing pain and analgesia with a lidocaine–prilocaine emulsion in infants and toddlers during venipuncture. *J Pediatr* 1991;118:971–973.
51. Acharya AB, Bustani PC, Phillips JD, et al. Randomised controlled trial of eutectic mixture of local anaesthetics cream for venepuncture in healthy preterm infants. *Arch Dis Child Fetal Neonatal Ed* 1998;78:F138–F142.
52. Gourrier E, Karoubi P, el Hanache A, et al. Use of EMLA cream in a department of neonatology. *Pain* 1996;68:431–434.
53. Brisman M, Ljung BM, Otterbom I, et al. Methaemoglobin formation after the use of EMLA cream in term neonates. *Acta Paediatr* 1998;87:1191–1194.
54. Larsson BA, Tannfeldt G, Lagercrantz H, et al. Alleviation of the pain of venepuncture in neonates. *Acta Paediatr* 1998;87:774–779.
55. Jain A, Rutter N. Does topical amethocaine gel reduce the pain of venepuncture in newborn infants? A randomised double blind controlled trial. *Arch Dis Child Fetal Neonatal Ed* 2000;83:F207–F210.
56. Moore J. No more tears: a randomized controlled double-blind trial of Amethocaine gel vs. placebo in the management of procedural pain in neonates. *J Adv Nurs* 2001;34:475–482.
57. Bo LK, Callaghan P. Soothing pain-elicited distress in Chinese neonates. *Pediatrics* 2000:105:E49.
58. Corbo MG, Mansi G, Stagni A, et al. Nonnutritive sucking during heelstick procedures decreases behavioral distress in the newborn infant. *Biol Neonate* 2000;77:162–167.
59. Field T, Goldson E. Pacifying effects of nonnutritive sucking on term and preterm neonates during heelstick procedures. *Pediatrics* 1984;74:1012–1015.
60. Campos RG. Rocking and pacifiers: two comforting interventions for heelstick pain. *Res Nurs Health* 1994;17:321–331.
61. Fearon I, Kisilevsky BS, Hains SMJ, et al. Swaddling after heel lance: age-specific effects on behavioural recovery in preterm infants. *J Dev Behav Pediatr* 1997;18:222–232.
62. Gray L, Watt L, Blass EM. Skin-to-skin contact is analgesic in healthy newborns. *Pediatrics* 2000;105(1):e14.
63. Corff KE, Seideman R, Venkataraman PS, et al. Facilitated tucking: a nonpharmacologic comfort measure for pain in preterm neonates. *J Obstet Gynecol Neonatal Nurs* 1995;24:143–147.
64. Porter FL, Wolf CM, Miller JP. The effect of handling and immobilization on the response to acute pain in newborn infants. *Pediatrics* 1998;102:1383–1389.
65. Barker DP, Willetts B, Cappendijk VC, et al. Capillary blood sampling: should the heel be warmed? *Arch Dis Child Fetal Neonatal Ed* 1996;74:F139–F140.
66. Janes M, Pinelli J, Landry S, et al. Comparison of capillary blood sampling using an automated incision device with and without warming the heel. *J Perinatol* 2002;22:154–158.
67. Abad F, Diaz NM, Domenech E, et al. Oral sweet solution reduces pain-related behaviour in preterm infants. *Acta Paediatr* 1996;85:854–858.
68. Abad F, Diaz-Gomez NM, Domenech E, et al. Oral sucrose compares favourably with lidocaine–prilocaine cream for pain relief during venepuncture in neonates. *Acta Paediatr* 2001;90:160–165.
69. Deshmukh LS, Udani RH. Analgesic effect of oral glucose in preterm infants during venipuncture: a double blind, randomized, controlled trial. *J Trop Pediatr* 2002;48:138–141.
70. Gradin M, Eriksson M, Holmqvist G, et al. Pain reduction at venepuncture in newborns: oral glucose compared with local anesthetic cream. *Pediatrics* 2002;110:1053–1057.
71. Lindh V, Wiklund U, Hakansson S. Assessment of the effect of EMLA during venipuncture in the newborn by analysis of heart rate variability. *Pain* 2000;86:247–254.
72. Carbajal R, Veerapen S, Couderc S, et al. Analgesic effect of breast feeding in term neonates: randomised controlled trial. *BMJ* 2003;326:13.

Deborah Pritchard
Medical Assessor (Paediatrics)
Medicines and Healthcare Products
Regulatory Agency
London
UK

Competing interests: None declared.

Sudden infant death syndrome

Search date July 2004

David Creery and Angelo Mikrogianakis

QUESTIONS

INTERVENTIONS

*Observational evidence only; RCTs unlikely to be conducted.

See glossary G

Key Messages

Reducing the risk

- **Advice to avoid prone sleeping** One non-systematic review and 12 observational studies found that eight campaigns encouraging non-prone positioning and seven campaigns involving, among other recommendations, advice to encourage non-prone sleeping positions were followed by a reduced incidence of sudden infant death syndrome.
- **Advice to avoid tobacco smoke exposure*** One non-systematic review and four observational studies found limited evidence that campaigns to reduce several risk factors for sudden infant death, which included tobacco smoke exposure, were followed by a reduced incidence of sudden infant death syndrome. One observational study found that smoking was associated with an increased risk of sudden infant death.
- **Advice to avoid bed sharing*** One observational study found that a campaign to reduce several risk factors for sudden infant death, which included advice to avoid bed sharing, was followed by a reduced incidence of sudden infant death syndrome. However, it is not clear whether effects were specifically due to the advice to avoid bed sharing.
- **Advice to avoid over heating or over wrapping*** One non-systematic review and one observational study found limited evidence that campaigns to reduce several risk factors for sudden infant death, which included over wrapping and over heating, were followed by a reduced incidence of sudden infant death syndrome. However, it is not clear whether effects were specifically due to the advice to avoid over wrapping or over heating.
- **Advice to avoid soft sleeping surfaces*** We found no evidence on the effects of advice to avoid soft sleeping surfaces in the prevention of sudden infant death syndrome.
- **Advice to breastfeed*** One non-systematic review and three observational studies found that campaigns to reduce several risk factors for sudden infant death, which included advice to breastfeed, were followed by a reduced incidence of sudden infant death syndrome. However, it is not clear whether effects were specifically due to the advice to breastfeed.
- **Advice to promote soother use*** One systematic review found insufficient evidence on soother use in the prevention of sudden infant death syndrome.

*Observational evidence only; RCTs unlikely to be conducted.

DEFINITION Sudden infant death syndrome (SIDS) is the sudden death of an infant aged under 1 year that remains unexplained after review of the clinical history, examination of the scene of death, and postmortem.

INCIDENCE/ PREVALENCE The incidence of SIDS has varied over time and among nations (incidence per 1000 live births of SIDS in 1996: The Netherlands 0.3, Japan 0.4, Canada 0.5, England and Wales 0.7, USA 0.8, and Australia 0.9).[1]

AETIOLOGY/ RISK FACTORS By definition, the cause of SIDS is not known. Observational studies have found an association between SIDS and several risk factors, including prone sleeping**G** position,[2,3] prenatal or postnatal exposure to tobacco smoke,[4] soft sleeping surfaces,[5,6] hyperthermia/over wrapping**G** (see tables A, B, and C on web extra),[7,8] bed sharing (particularly with mothers who smoke),[9,10] lack of breast-feeding,[11,12] and lack of soother**G** use.[7,13] The incidence of SIDS is increased in the siblings of that infant.[14,15]

PROGNOSIS Prognosis is not applicable.

AIMS OF INTERVENTION To reduce the incidence of SIDS, with minimal adverse effects of interventions.

OUTCOMES Incidence of SIDS; rates of exposure to known risk factors for SIDS; adverse effects of interventions, measured directly or by quality of life questionnaires.

METHODS *Clinical Evidence* search and appraisal July 2004.

QUESTION **What are the effects of interventions to reduce the risk of sudden infant death syndrome?**

OPTION **ADVICE TO AVOID PRONE SLEEPING**

One non-systematic review and 12 observational studies found that eight campaigns encouraging non-prone positioning and seven campaigns involving, among other recommendations, advice to encourage non-prone sleeping positions were followed by a reduced incidence of sudden infant death syndrome.

Benefits: We found no systematic review and no RCTs comparing advice to avoid prone sleeping**G** positions versus no such advice (see comment below). **National advice campaigns:** We found one non-systematic review of national campaigns (3 observational studies, 1 of which has also been reported separately[16]),[12] and 12 additional observational studies conducted after national advice campaigns (see comment below).[9,17–28] The review and additional observational studies describe eight campaigns that delivered advice to avoid prone positioning alone (see table 1, p 441),[17–19,21,22,24–26] and seven campaigns that provided advice to avoid a combination of different risk factors, including prone positioning (see table 2, p 442).[9,12,16,20,23,27,28] The review and additional observational studies all found that the incidence of sudden infant death syndrome (SIDS) was reduced after the campaigns (see table 1, p 441) (see table 2, p 442). One of the additional observational studies found that the incidence of prone positioning (a risk factor for SIDS) decreased significantly after the campaign (from 54% before the campaign to 5% after the campaign; $P < 0.001$).[27]

Harms: No increased frequency of adverse effects of non-prone positioning were reported in one non-systematic review and 13 observational studies of advice to avoid prone sleeping**G**.[12,16–28] Two studies found no increase in the risk of inhaling vomitus associated with non-prone positioning.[26,29] Three observational studies documented a temporal relationship between advice to avoid prone sleeping and an increase in the incidence of occipital plagiocephaly without synostosis**G**,[30–32] whereas one of the observational studies found that the incidence of other forms of plagiocephaly with synostosis remained constant.[30]

Comment: The review of SIDS risk factor reduction campaigns in Norway, Denmark, and Sweden reported that the campaign in Norway provided advice to avoid prone sleeping**G** plus advice to avoid tobacco smoke exposure.[12] However, the original paper describing the Norwegian campaign reported that this campaign only provided advice to avoid prone sleeping.[16] One of the additional observational studies reported that the incidence of SIDS was declining before the campaign started, and hence the reduction attributable to advice provided by the campaign is not clear.[9,20] A second additional observational study did not report on how advice was provided or exactly which SIDS risk factors were targeted, and it did not describe details of the advice given to avoid exposure to cigarette smoke (i.e. prenatally, postnatally, or both; maternal smoking alone or smoking by other household members as well).[23] A third additional observational study did not specify whether the advice to stop smoking was given to mothers or other family members and what advice was given regarding avoidance of over heating.[27] Systematic reviews of observational studies have found an association between prone sleeping position and an increased risk of SIDS, leading to the initiation of non-prone sleep campaigns in several countries.[2,3] RCTs investigating the effects of advice to avoid prone positioning may be considered unethical, given the existing observational evidence; they would also be difficult to conduct, given the extremely large units of randomisation required and the high level of pre-existing public awareness regarding the risks associated with prone positioning in sleep.

OPTION ADVICE TO AVOID TOBACCO SMOKE EXPOSURE

One non-systematic review and four observational studies found limited evidence that campaigns to reduce several risk factors for sudden infant death, which included tobacco smoke exposure, were followed by a reduced incidence of sudden infant death syndrome. One observational study found that smoking was associated with an increased risk of sudden infant death.

Benefits: We found no systematic review and no RCTs comparing advice to avoid tobacco smoke exposure versus no such advice (see comment below). **National advice campaigns:** We found one non-systematic review of national campaigns (3 observational studies, 1 of which has also been reported separately[16]),[12] and four additional observational studies after national advice campaigns (see table 2, p 442).[9,20,23,27,28] The review and additional observational studies found that the campaigns were all followed by a reduced incidence of sudden infant death syndrome (SIDS) during the data collection periods (see table 2, p 442). However, the campaigns included other advice in addition to avoiding tobacco smoke exposure, and in some countries the incidence of SIDS had started to fall before the campaign started (see comment under advice to avoid prone sleeping, p 436). The first additional observational study found that the population attributable risk**G** of SIDS associated with maternal smoking alone was 44% (prevalence 19%; OR 5.17, 95% CI 3.13 to 8.55), and for maternal smoking plus bed sharing it was 33% (prevalence 5%; OR 11.1, 95% CI 5.85 to 21.1).[9,20] The third additional observational study found that the percentage of mothers not smoking during pregnancy increased significantly after the campaign (from 77% before the campaign to 82% after the campaign; $P < 0.01$).[27] The fourth additional observational study found that maternal smoking in Kanagawa province in Japan decreased from 9.4% before the campaign to 0% after the campaign.[28]

Harms: None of the studies we found reported evidence on harms of a reduction in infant tobacco smoke exposure.

Comment: RCTs investigating the effects of advice to reduce infant tobacco smoke exposure would be difficult to conduct, given the extremely large units of randomisation required and the high level of pre-existing public awareness regarding the risks associated with tobacco smoke exposure.

OPTION ADVICE TO AVOID SOFT SLEEPING SURFACES

We found no evidence on the effects of advice to avoid soft sleeping surfaces in the prevention of sudden infant death syndrome.

Benefits: We found no systematic review, RCTs, or observational studies of sufficient quality (see comment below).

Harms: None of the studies we found reported evidence on harms of advice to avoid soft sleeping surfaces.

Comment: RCTs investigating the effects of advice to avoid soft sleeping surfaces would be difficult to conduct, given the extremely large units of randomisation required.

OPTION ADVICE TO AVOID OVER HEATING OR OVER WRAPPING

One non-systematic review and one observational study found limited evidence that campaigns to reduce several risk factors for sudden infant death, which included over wrapping and over heating, were followed by a reduced incidence of sudden infant death syndrome. However, it is not clear whether effects were specifically due to the advice to avoid over wrapping or over heating.

Benefits: We found no systematic review and no RCTs comparing advice to avoid over heating or over wrapping**G** versus no such advice (see comment below). **National advice campaigns:** We found one non-systematic review of national campaigns (3 observational studies, 1 of which has also been reported separately[16]),[12] and one additional observational study after a national advice campaign (see table 2, p 442).[27] Two of the national advice campaigns reported in the review and the additional observational study provided advice to avoid over heating or over wrapping plus advice to avoid other risk factors for sudden infant death syndrome (see comment under advice to avoid prone sleeping, p 436).[12,27] The third campaign reported by the review did not provide advice on over heating or over wrapping.[16] The review and additional observational study found that the campaigns were all followed by a reduction in the incidence of sudden infant death syndrome during the data collection periods (see table 2, p 442).[12,27]

Harms: None of the studies we found reported evidence on harms of advice to avoid over heating or over wrapping**G**.

Comment: RCTs investigating the effects of advice to avoid over heating or over wrapping**G** would be difficult to conduct, given the extremely large units of randomisation required.

OPTION ADVICE TO AVOID BED SHARING

One observational study found that a campaign to reduce several risk factors for sudden infant death, which included advice to avoid bed sharing, was followed by a reduced incidence of sudden infant death syndrome. However, it is not clear whether effects were specifically due to the advice to avoid bed sharing.

Benefits: We found no systematic review and no RCTs comparing advice to avoid bed sharing versus no advice (see comment below). **National advice campaigns:** We found one observational study, which reported the results of a national campaign that provided advice to avoid bed sharing, to avoid prone sleeping**G**, to avoid exposing infants to tobacco smoke from any source either during pregnancy or for the first year of life, and to breastfeed if possible (see comment below) (see table 2, p 442).[9,20] The observational study found that the incidence of sudden infant death syndrome (SIDS) reduced after the campaign (see table 2, p 442), and that the population attributable risk**G** for SIDS associated with maternal smoking plus bed sharing was 33% (prevalence 5%; OR 11.1, 95% CI 5.85 to 21.10).[20]

Harms: None of the studies we found reported evidence on harms associated with advice to avoid bed sharing.

Comment: The observational study reported that advice to avoid bed sharing was introduced after the main campaign had started.[9,20] The study also reported that the incidence of SIDS was declining before the campaign started, and hence the reduction attributable to advice provided by the campaign is not clear.[20] RCTs investigating the effects of advice to avoid bed sharing would be difficult to conduct, given the extremely large units of randomisation required.

OPTION ADVICE TO BREASTFEED

One non-systematic review and three observational studies found that campaigns to reduce several risk factors for sudden infant death, which included advice to breastfeed, were followed by a reduced incidence of sudden infant death syndrome. However, it is not clear whether effects were specifically due to the advice to breastfeed.

Benefits: We found no systematic review and no RCTs comparing advice to encourage breastfeeding versus no such advice in order to reduce the incidence of sudden infant death syndrome (SIDS; see comment below). **National advice campaigns:** We found one non-systematic review of national campaigns (3 observational studies, 1 of which has also been reported separately[16]),[12] and three additional observational studies after national advice campaigns (see table 2, p 442).[9,20,27,28] The review and additional observational studies found that the campaigns were all followed by a reduced incidence of SIDS during the data collection periods (see table 2, p 442). However, the campaigns included advice other than advice to encourage breastfeeding, and in some countries the incidence of SIDS had started to fall before the campaign started (see comment under advice to avoid prone sleeping, p 436). The second additional observational study found that the incidence of not breastfeeding reduced significantly after the campaign (from 21% before the campaign to 7% after the campaign; $P < 0.001$).[27] The third additional observational study found that rates of breastfeeding only in Kanagawa province in Japan increased from 53.1% to 67.3% after the campaign.[28]

Harms: None of the studies we found reported evidence on harms associated with advice to encourage breastfeeding.

Comment: RCTs investigating the effects of promotion of breastfeeding would be unethical, given the evidence of benefits associated with breastfeeding.

OPTION ADVICE TO PROMOTE SOOTHER USE

One systematic review found insufficient evidence on soother use in the prevention of sudden infant death syndrome.

Benefits: We found no systematic review and no RCTs comparing advice to encourage use of a soother**G** versus no such advice to reduce the incidence of sudden infant death syndrome (see comment below). **National advice campaigns:** We found no observational studies after national advice campaigns. **Other observational studies:** We found one systematic review (search date 2000) that identified four case control studies.[33] All four studies included in the review found an association between increased soother use and reduced risk of sudden infant death syndrome, but none of the studies concluded that the association was causal.

Harms: The studies we found provided no evidence on harms of soother**G** use.

Comment: RCTs investigating the effects of advice to promote soother**G** use would be difficult to conduct, given the extremely large units of randomisation required.

GLOSSARY

Occipital plagiocephaly with or without synostosis Flattening of the occipital bone, with or without a malformation of the corresponding cranial suture line.

Over wrapping Wrapping/bundling of infants in excessive amounts of clothing or bedding, resulting in sweating, raised core temperature, or both.

Population attributable risk A measure of the disease rate in exposed people, compared with that in unexposed people, multiplied by the prevalence of exposure to the risk factor in the population.

Prone sleeping Sleeping on one's front.

Soother (dummy, pacifier) An object placed in the infant's mouth for the sole purpose of providing comfort.

REFERENCES

1. Canadian Bureau of Reproductive and Child Health/Laboratory Centre for Disease Control/Canadian Perinatal Surveillance System (CPSS); Fact sheet: http://www.hc-sc.gc.ca/hpb/lcdc/brch/factshts/sids_e.html (last accessed 30 June 2004).
2. Beal SM, Finch CF. An overview of retrospective case-control studies investigating the relationship between prone sleeping position and SIDS. *J Paediatr Child Health* 1991;27:334–339.
3. American Academy of Pediatrics AAP Task Force on Infant Positioning and SIDS. Positioning and SIDS. *Pediatrics* 1992;89:1120–1126.
4. Anderson HR, Cook DG. Passive smoking and sudden infant death syndrome: review of the epidemiological evidence. *Thorax* 1997;52:1003–1009.
5. Mitchell EA, Thompson JM, Ford RP, et al. Sheepskin bedding and the sudden infant death syndrome. New Zealand Cot Death Study Group. *J Pediatr* 1998;133:701–704.
6. Ponsonby AL, Dwyer T, Gibbons LE, et al. Factors potentiating the risk of sudden infant death syndrome associated with the prone position. *N Engl J Med* 1993;329:377–382.
7. Fleming PJ, Blair PS, Bacon C, et al. Environment of infants during sleep and risk of the sudden infant death syndrome: results of the 1993–5 case-control study for confidential enquiry into stillbirths and deaths on infancy. Confidential Enquiry into Stillbirths and Deaths Regional Coordinators and Researchers. *BMJ* 1996;313:191–195.
8. Ponsonby AL, Dwyer T, Gibbons LE, et al. Thermal environment and sudden infant death syndrome: case-control study. *BMJ* 1992;304:277–282.
9. Mitchell EA, Tuohy PG, Brunt JM, et al. Risk factors for sudden infant death syndrome following the prevention campaign in New Zealand: a prospective study. *Pediatrics* 1997;100:835–840.
10. Scragg R, Mitchell EA, Taylor BJ, et al. Bed sharing, smoking, and alcohol in the sudden infant death syndrome. New Zealand Cot Death Study Group. *BMJ* 1993;307:1312–1318.
11. Mitchell EA, Taylor BJ, Ford RP, et al. Four modifiable and other major risk factors for cot death: the New Zealand study. *J Paediatr Child Health* 1992;28(suppl 1):S3–S8.
12. Wennergren G, Alm B, Oyen N, et al. The decline in the incidence of SIDS in Scandinavia and its relation to risk-intervention campaigns. Nordic Epidemiological SIDS Study. *Acta Paediatr* 1997;86:963–968.
13. L'Hoir MP, Engelberts AC, van Well GT, et al. Risk and preventive factors for cot death in The Netherlands, a low-incidence country. *Eur J Pediatr* 1998;157:681–688.
14. Oyen N, Skjaerven R, Irgens LM. Population-based recurrence risk of sudden infant death syndrome compared with other infant and fetal deaths. *Am J Epidemiol* 1996;144:300–305.
15. Guntheroth WG, Lohmann R, Spiers PS. Risk of sudden infant death syndrome in subsequent siblings. *J Pediatr* 1990;116:520–524.
16. Haaland K, Thoresen M. Crib death, sleeping position and temperature. *Tidsskr Nor Laegeforen* 1992;112:1466–1470. [In Norwegian]
17. Schellscheidt J, Ott A, Jorch G. Epidemiological features of sudden infant death after a German intervention campaign in 1992. *Eur J Pediatr* 1997;156:655–660.
18. Skadberg BT, Morild I, Markestad T. Abandoning prone sleeping: effect on the risk of sudden infant death syndrome. *J Pediatr* 1998;132:340–343.
19. Wigfield RE, Fleming PJ, Berry PJ, et al. Can the fall in Avon's sudden infant death rate be explained by changes in sleeping position? *BMJ* 1992;304:282–283.
20. Mitchell EA, Aley P, Eastwood J. The national cot death prevention program in New Zealand. *Aust J Public Health* 1992;16:158–161.
21. Markestad T, Skadberg B, Hordvik E, et al. Sleeping position and sudden infant death syndrome (SIDS): effect of an intervention programme to avoid prone sleeping. *Acta Paediatr* 1995;84:375–378.

22. Vege A, Rognum TO, Opdal SH. SIDS — changes in the epidemiological pattern in Eastern Norway 1984–1996. *Forensic Sci Int* 1998;93:155–166.
23. Adams EJ, Chavez GF, Steen D, et al. Changes in the epidemiologic profile of sudden infant death syndrome as rates decline among California infants: 1990–1995. *Pediatrics* 1998;102:1445–1451.
24. Mitchell EA, Ford RP, Taylor BJ, et al. Further evidence supporting a causal relationship between prone sleeping position and SIDS. *J Paediatr Child Health* 1992;28(suppl 1):S9–S12.
25. Dwyer T, Ponsonby AL, Blizzard L, et al. The contribution of changes in the prevalence of prone sleeping position to the decline in sudden infant death syndrome in Tasmania. *JAMA* 1995;273:783–789.
26. Spiers PS, Guntheroth WG. Recommendations to avoid the prone sleeping position and recent statistics for sudden infant death syndrome in the United States. *Arch Pediatr Adolesc Med* 1994;148:141–146.
27. Kiechl-Kohlendorfer U, Peglow UP, Kiechl S, et al. Epidemiology of sudden infant death syndrome (SIDS) in the Tyrol before and after an intervention campaign. *Wien Klin Wochenschr* 2001;113:27–32.
28. Sawaguchi T, Nishida H, Fukui F, et al. Study on social responses (encouraging public awareness) to sudden infant death syndrome: evaluation of SIDS prevention campaigns. *Forensic Sci Int* 2002;130(suppl):S78–S80.
29. Malloy M. Trends in postneonatal aspiration deaths and reclassification of sudden infant death syndrome: impact of the "Back to Sleep" program. *Pediatrics* 2002;109:661–665.
30. Kane AA, Mitchell LE, Craven KP, et al. Observations on a recent increase in plagiocephaly without synostosis. *Pediatrics* 1996;97:877–885.
31. Gonzalez de Dios J, Moya M, Jimenez L, et al. Increase in the incidence of occipital plagiocephaly. *Rev Neurol* 1998;27:782–784. [In Spanish]
32. Christensen L, <coslash>stergaard JR, Nørholt SE. Positional plagiocephaly. *Ugeskr Laeger* 2002;165:46–50. [In Danish]
33. Zotter H, Kerbl R, Kurz R, Muller W. Pacifier use and sudden infant death syndrome: should health professionals recommend pacifier use based on present knowledge? *Wien Klin Wochenschr* 2002;114:791–794. Search date 2000; primary sources Medline and Pubmed.

David Creery
Head, Paediatric Intensive Care

Angelo Mikrogianakis
Children's Hospital of Eastern Ontario
Ottawa
Canada

Competing interests: None declared.

TABLE 1 **Observational studies after national campaigns providing advice to avoid prone sleeping positions (see text, p 435).**

Country/reference	Dissemination	SIDS incidence/1000 live births (95% CI)		Number of infants	Risk of prone sleeping after campaign (95% CI)
		From	To		
Germany (West)[17]	Not specified	1.56	0.92	59 cases, 156 controls	OR 11.7 (5.3 to 26.2)
Germany, North Rhine–Westphalia[17]		2.17	1.33		
Norway[18]	Health professional education Media campaign	3.5 (2.64 to 4.36)	0.3 (0.05 to 0.54)	6 cases, 493 controls	OR 42.0 (5 to 390)
UK, Avon[19]	Maternal education Health professional education	3.5	1.7	32 cases, 70 controls, 152 population based controls	NA
Norway/Hordaland[21]	Health professional education Media campaign	3.5	1.6	30 cases, 123 controls	OR 11.3 (3.6 to 36.5)
Norway[22]	Health professional education Media campaign	2	0.6	200 cases	NA
New Zealand[24]	Maternal education Health professional education Media campaign	4	3.1	485 cases, 1800 controls	NA
Australia[25]	Maternal education Health professional education	3.8 (3.5 to 4.2)	1.5 (0.9 to 2.2)	449 cases	NA
USA[26]	Media campaign	2.36	2.02	233 cases	NA

NA, not available; SIDS, sudden infant death syndrome.

TABLE 2 **Observational studies after national campaigns providing advice to avoid several sudden infant death syndrome risk factors including prone sleeping positions (see text, p 435).**

Country/ year of start	Data collection	Advice to avoid or encourage	Dissemination	SIDS incidence/ 1000 live births (95% CI)		Number of infants	Risk (95% CI)
				From	To		
Norway 1989[12,16]	1992–95	Avoid prone sleeping	Newspapers National media broadcasts Midwives Other healthcare professionals Presentation at a SIDS prevention conference	2.3	0.6	244 cases 869 controls	Adjusted OR prone sleeping 5.4 (2.8 to 10.5)
Denmark 1991[12]	1992–95	Avoid prone sleeping, tobacco smoke, over wrapping	Not described	1.6	0.2	244 cases 869 controls	Adjusted OR prone sleeping 5.4 (2.8 to 10.5)
Sweden 1992[12]	1992–95	Avoid prone sleeping, tobacco smoke, over wrapping Encourage breast feeding	Not described	1.0	0.4		

TABLE 2 continued

Country/ year of start	Data collection	Advice to avoid or encourage	Dissemination	SIDS incidence/ 1000 live births (95% CI)		Number of infants	Risk (95% CI)
				From	To		
New Zealand 1990[9,20]	1991–93	Avoid prone sleeping, tobacco smoke (any source; during pregnancy/first year of life) bed sharing Encourage breast feeding	Parents antenatal classes Postnatal wards Healthcare professionals Conferences Journals Public newspapers TV programmes	4.1	2.1	127 cases 922 controls	Not reported
California 1990–1995[23]		Avoid prone sleeping, cigarette smoking	Public	2.69 (black infants) 1.04 (other infants)	2.15 (black infants) 0.61 (other infants)	3508 cases	Not reported
Austria 1994–1995[27]		Avoid prone sleeping, smoking, over heating Encourage breast feeding	Parents antenatal classes, maternity wards, routine health checks Public newspapers Radio/TV	1984–1994: 1.83	1995: 0.4 1996–1998 unchanged	160 cases	Not reported
Japan 1996[28]	1995 and 1998		Medical professional education Encourage Maternal education	0.44	0.33	Not reported	Not reported

SIDS, sudden infant death syndrome.

Urinary tract infection in children

Search date January 2004

James Larcombe

QUESTIONS

INTERVENTIONS

ACUTE URINARY TRACT INFECTION

Likely to be beneficial

Antibiotics (more effective than placebo)* . . . 447

Oral antibiotics (as effective as initial intravenous antibiotics in children without severe vesicoureteric reflux or renal scarring) . . . 449

Unknown effectiveness

Immediate empirical antibiotic treatment (unclear benefit compared with delayed treatment based on microscopy and culture) . . . 447

Unlikely to be beneficial

Longer (7–14 days) courses of initial intravenous antibiotics (no more effective than shorter [3–4 days] courses of intravenous antibiotics in children with acute pyelonephritis). . . . 450

Longer (7–14 days) courses of oral antibiotics (no more effective than shorter [2–4 days] courses for non-recurrent lower urinary tract infections in the absence of renal tract abnormality) . . . 448

Likely to be ineffective or harmful

Prolonged delay in treatment (> 4 days) . . . 447

Single dose of oral antibiotics (less effective than longer course [7–10 days]) . . . 448

PREVENTION OF RECURRENCE

Likely to be beneficial

Immunotherapy . . . 452

Prophylactic antibiotics . . . 451

Unknown effectiveness

Surgical correction of moderate to severe vesicoureteric reflux (grades III–IV) with bilateral nephropathy . . . 453

Unlikely to be beneficial

Surgical correction of minor functional anomalies . . . 453

Surgical correction of moderate to severe vesicoureteric reflux with adequate glomerular filtration rate (similar benefits to medical management) . . . 453

*Based on consensus. Placebo controlled RCTs would be considered unethical.

See glossary G

Key Messages

Acute urinary tract infection

- **Antibiotics (more effective than placebo)*** There is consensus that antibiotics are likely to be beneficial compared with placebo. Placebo controlled trials of antibiotics for symptomatic acute urinary tract infection in children are considered unethical.
- **Oral antibiotics (as effective as initial intravenous antibiotics in children without severe vesicoureteric reflux or renal scarring)** One RCT identified by a systematic review found no significant difference between oral cephalosporins alone and a regimen of 3 days of intravenous cephalosporins plus continued oral cephalosporins in duration of fever, reinfection rate, renal scarring, or extent of

scarring in children aged 2 years or younger with a first confirmed urinary tract infection. The RCT found weak evidence that in children with grades III–IV reflux, initial intravenous treatment plus oral treatment may reduce renal scarring compared with oral treatment alone at 6 months.

- **Immediate empirical antibiotic treatment (unclear benefit compared with delayed treatment based on microscopy and culture)** We found no RCTs comparing early empirical treatment with delayed treatment based on the results of microscopy or culture in acute urinary tract infection in children. Retrospective analysis of one RCT found no significant difference in risk of renal scarring between cephalosporin treatment within 24 hours compared with 24 hours after the onset of fever in children under 2 years of age with urinary tract infections.
- **Longer (7–14 days) courses of initial intravenous antibiotics (no more effective than shorter [3–4 days] courses of intravenous antibiotics in children with acute pyelonephritis)** One systematic review found no significant difference between long (7–14 days) and short (3–4 days) courses of initial intravenous antibiotics in persistence of bacteriuria after treatment, recurrent urinary tract infection at 6–12 months, or renal scarring at 3–6 months in children with acute pyelonephritis.
- **Longer (7–14 days) courses of oral antibiotics (no more effective than shorter [2–4 days] courses for non-recurrent lower urinary tract infections in the absence of renal tract abnormality)** One systematic review found no significant difference between longer courses (7–14 days) and shorter courses (2–4 days) of the same oral antibiotic in cure rate at 7 days after treatment in children with no history of renal tract abnormality and judged not to have acute pyelonephritis❻. Another systematic review found no significant difference between 7–14 day courses and 3 day courses of any antibiotic in cure rate. However, longer courses may be associated with more adverse effects.
- **Prolonged delay in treatment (> 4 days)** We found no RCTs. Five retrospective studies found that medium to long term delays (4 days to 7 years) in treatment may be associated with an increased risk of renal scarring.
- **Single dose of oral antibiotics (less effective than longer course [7–10 days])** One systematic review found that single dose oral amoxicillin decreased cure rate at 3–30 days compared with a longer (10 days) course of oral amoxicillin. Another systematic review found that single day or single dose regimens increased treatment failure compared with 7–14 day courses of any antibiotic.

Prevention of recurrence

- **Immunotherapy** One RCT in children with recurrent urinary tract infection found that adding pidotimod (an immunotherapeutic agent) to antibiotic treatment reduced recurrence compared with adding placebo.
- **Prophylactic antibiotics** One systematic review found limited evidence that prophylactic antibiotics (co-trimoxazole, nitrofurantoin, given for 10 weeks to 12 months) reduced urinary tract infection recurrence in children compared with placebo or no treatment. One RCT found that nitrofurantoin reduced recurrence of urinary tract infection over 6 months compared with trimethoprim. However, more children discontinued treatment with nitrofurantoin because of adverse effects. We found no RCTs evaluating the optimum duration of prophylactic antibiotics.
- **Surgical correction of moderate to severe vesicoureteric reflux (grades III–IV) with bilateral nephropathy** One small RCT found a non-significantly greater decline in glomerular filtration rate over 10 years with medical treatment compared with surgery in children with moderate to severe bilateral vesicoureteric reflux and bilateral nephropathy.
- **Surgical correction of minor functional anomalies** We found no RCTs. One observational study suggested that children with minor anomalies do not develop renal scarring and therefore may not benefit from surgery.

- **Surgical correction of moderate to severe vesicoureteric reflux with adequate glomerular filtration rate (similar benefits to medical management)** One systematic review found no significant difference between surgical and medical management (prophylactic antibiotic treatment) in urinary tract infections or their complications from after 1–5 years in children with moderate to severe vesicoureteric reflux, although surgery abolished reflux. One subsequent RCT, reporting 10 years' follow-up, found that new renal scars rarely occurred with either management strategy after 5 years.

DEFINITION Urinary tract infection (UTI) is defined by the presence of a pure growth of more than 10^5 colony forming units of bacteria per millilitre of urine. Lower counts of bacteria may be clinically important, especially in boys and in specimens obtained by urinary catheter. Any growth of typical urinary pathogens is considered clinically important if obtained by suprapubic aspiration. In practice, three age ranges are usually considered on the basis of differential risk and different approaches to management: children under 1 year; young children (1–4, 5, or 7 years, depending on the information source); and older children (up to 12–16 years). Recurrent UTI is defined as a further infection by a new organism. Relapsing UTI is defined as a further infection with the same organism.

INCIDENCE/ PREVALENCE Boys are more susceptible before the age of 3 months; thereafter the incidence is substantially higher in girls. Estimates of the true incidence of UTI depend on rates of diagnosis and investigation. At least 8% of girls and 2% of boys will have a UTI in childhood.[1]

AETIOLOGY/ RISK FACTORS The normal urinary tract is sterile. Contamination by bowel flora may result in urinary infection if a virulent organism is involved or if the child is immunosuppressed. In neonates, infection may originate from other sources. *Escherichia coli* accounts for about 75% of all pathogens. *Proteus* is more common in boys (about 30% of infections). Obstructive anomalies are found in 0–4% and vesicoureteric reflux in 8–40% of children being investigated for their first UTI.[2] One meta-analysis of 12 cohort studies (537 children admitted to hospital for UTI, 1062 kidneys) found that 36% of all kidneys had some scarring on DMSA scintigraphyⒼ and that 59% of children with vesicoureteric reflux on micturating cystourethography had at least one scarred kidney (pooled positive likelihood ratio 1.96, 95% CI 1.51 to 2.54; pooled negative likelihood ratio 0.71, 95% CI 0.58 to 0.85). There was evidence of heterogeneity in likelihood ratios among studies. The authors concluded that vesicoureteric reflux is a weak predictor of renal damage in children admitted to hospital.[3] Thus, although vesicoureteric reflux is a major risk factor for adverse outcome, other factors, some of which have not yet been identified, are also important. Vesicoureteric reflux itself runs in families: in one review article, the incidence of reflux in siblings ranged from 26% (a cohort of asymptomatic siblings) to 86% (siblings with a history of urinary tract infection) compared with a rate of less than 1% in the normal population.[4] Although some gene variants appear to be more common in children who suffer renal damage, no clear link has yet been established between specific genes and an adverse outcome.[5] Local or systemic immune problems are also likely to be factors in the development of urinary tract infection.

PROGNOSIS After first infection, about 50% of girls have a further infection in the first year and 75% within 2 years.[6] We found no figures for boys, but a review suggests that recurrences are common under 1 year of age, but rare subsequently.[7] Renal scarring occurs in 5–15% of children within 1–2 years of their first UTI, although 32–70% of these scars are noted at the time of initial assessment.[2] The incidence of renal scarring rises with each episode of infection in childhood.[8] Retrospective analysis of an RCT comparing oral versus intravenous antibiotics found that new renal scarring after a first UTI was more common in children with vesicoureteric reflux than in children without reflux (logistic regression model; AR of scarring: 16/107 [15%] with reflux *v* 10/165 [6%] without reflux; RR 2.47, 95% CI 1.17 to 5.24).[9] A study (287 children with severe vesicoureteric reflux treated either medically or surgically for any UTI) evaluated the risk of renal scarring with serial DMSA scintigraphyⒼ over 5 years. It found that younger children (aged < 2 years) were at greater risk of renal scarring than older children regardless of treatment for the infection (AR for deterioration in DMSA scan over 5 years: 21/86 [24%] for younger children *v* 27/201 [13%] for older children; RR 1.82, 95% CI 1.09 to 3.03).[10] One prospective study found that children of all ages who presented with symptoms of pyelonephritisⒼ were likely to have renal abnormalities (abnormal initial scans in 34/65 [52%] children).[11] Another prospective study found that the highest rates of renal scarring after pyelonephritis Ⓖ occurred between 1–5 years of age.[12] A further prospective study by the same team found that children aged over 1 year had more abnormalities on DMSA scans at 3 months after an episode of pyelonephritis (54/129 [42%] older children *v* 22/91 [24%] younger children; RR 1.73, 95% CI 1.14 to 2.63).[13] They noted conflicting results in previous literature on this subject.[14] They also found that girls were more likely than boys to develop scarring on DMSA scan at 3 months after an episode of pyelonephritis (67/171 [39%] girls *v* 9/49 [18%] boys; RR 2.13, 95% CI 1.15 to 3.96).[13] Renal scarring is associated with future complications: poor renal growth, recurrent adult pyelonephritis, impaired glomerular function, early hypertension, and end stage renal failure.[14–17] A combination of recurrent UTI, severe vesicoureteric reflux, and the presence of renal scarring at first presentation is associated with the worst prognosis. One prospective observational study assessed the persistence of scarring on DMSA scans in children with a first UTI.[18] Grading of scars was as follows: mild (< 25% of kidney affected), moderate (25–50% of kidney), and severe (> 50% of kidney). The study found that vesicoureteric reflux was associated with more persistent scarring at 6 months (in children with severe scarring on initial scan: 7/8 [88%] with reflux had a persisting lesion *v* 1/7 [14%] without reflux; RR 6.13, 95% CI 0.98 to 38.00; in children with mild to moderate scarring on initial scan: 3/8 [38%] with reflux had a persisting lesion *v* 5/31 [16%] without reflux; RR 2.70, 95% CI 0.81 to 9.10).[18] The study also found that vesicoureteric reflux was associated with a higher risk of pyelonephritis on the initial scan (RR for pyelonephritis with reflux *v* without reflux 1.62, 95% CI 1.14 to 2.31).

AIMS OF INTERVENTION To relieve acute symptoms; to eliminate infection; and to prevent recurrence, renal damage, and long term complications.

OUTCOMES **Short term:** clinical symptoms and signs (dysuria, frequency, and fever); urine culture; incidence of new renal scars. **Long term:** incidence of recurrent infection; prevalence of renal scarring; renal size and growth; renal function; prevalence of hypertension and renal failure.

METHODS *Clinical Evidence* search and appraisal January 2004.

QUESTION What are the effects of treatment of acute urinary tract infection in children?

OPTION ANTIBIOTICS VERSUS PLACEBO

There is consensus that antibiotics are likely to be beneficial compared with placebo. Placebo controlled trials of antibiotics for symptomatic acute urinary tract infection in children are considered unethical.

Benefits: We found no systematic reviews or RCTs.

Harms: We found no RCTs.

Comment: Placebo controlled trials would be considered unethical because there is a strong consensus that antibiotics are likely to be beneficial. The improved response seen with longer compared with very short courses of antibiotics is indirect evidence that antibiotics are likely to be more effective than no treatment.

OPTION IMMEDIATE EMPIRICAL VERSUS DELAYED ANTIBIOTIC TREATMENT

We found no RCTs comparing early empirical treatment with delayed treatment based on the results of microscopy or culture in acute urinary tract infection in children. Retrospective analysis of one RCT found no significant difference in risk of renal scarring between cephalosporin treatment within 24 hours compared with 24 hours after the onset of fever in children under 2 years of age with urinary tract infections. Five retrospective studies found that medium to long term delays (4 days to 7 years) in treatment may be associated with an increased risk of renal scarring.

Benefits: We found no RCTs comparing immediate empirical treatment with treatment that is delayed while awaiting the results of microscopy or culture. We found one RCT that compared oral cefixime for 14 days (double dose on day 1) versus intravenous cefotaxime for 3 days plus oral cefixime for the succeeding 11 days for urinary tract infection in children under 2 years.[9] Retrospective analysis of its results found no evidence that children treated 24 hours after the onset of fever with either regime were at greater risk of renal scarring than children presenting within 24 hours (9/99 [9%] of children presenting before 24 hours *v* 19/159 [12%] of children presenting later; RR 1.3, 95% CI 0.6 to 2.7; P = 0.29).

Harms: The RCT did not report on any adverse effects.[9]

Comment: Five retrospective observational studies found increased rates of scarring in children in whom diagnosis was delayed between 4 days (in acute urinary tract infection) to 7 years (when a child presented with chronic non-specific symptoms).[2]

OPTION LONGER VERSUS SHORT COURSES OF ORAL ANTIBIOTICS

One systematic review found no significant difference between longer courses (7–14 days) and shorter courses (2–4 days) of the same oral antibiotic in cure rate at 7 days after treatment in children with no history of renal tract abnormality and judged not to have acute pyelonephritis. Another systematic review found no significant difference between 7–14 day courses and 3 day courses of any antibiotic in cure rate. However, longer courses may be associated with more adverse effects. One systematic review found that single dose oral amoxicillin decreased cure rate at 3–30 days compared with a longer (10 days) course of oral amoxicillin. Another systematic review found that single day or single dose regimens increased treatment failure compared with 7–14 day courses of any antibiotic.

Benefits: We found two systematic reviews that included trials comparing longer versus short course of the same antibiotic (search dates 1999[19] and 2002[20]). Both reviews included the following antibiotics: amoxicillin, nitrofurantoin, trimethoprim/sulfadiazine, nalidixic acid, pivmecillinam, nitrofurantoin, amoxicillin/clavulanic acid, and cefuroxime. We found a third systematic review (search date 2001, 17 RCTs) that compared longer with shorter courses of any antibiotic.[21] **Versus single dose and short course:** The first review (17 RCTs, children and adolescents aged < 18 years with uncomplicated cystitis) included single dose drug regimens.[19] It found that longer (≥ 5 days) courses of antibiotic increased microbiological cure rate between 3–30 days after start of treatment compared with short (≤ 4 days) course (difference in cure rates 7.9%, 95% CI 2.1% to 13.8%).[19] However, studies were statistically heterogeneous and meta-analysis may not have been appropriate. The review found that longer (10 days) amoxicillin course increased microbiological cure rate between 3–30 days after enrolment compared with single dose amoxicillin (4 RCTs: difference in cure rate for longer *v* short course 13%, 95% CI 4% to 24%; NNT with longer course for cure 8, 95% CI 5 to 25; no statistical heterogeneity among studies in meta-analysis). However, it found no significant difference between longer (7–10 days) and shorter course or single dose (≤ 3 days) co-trimoxazole for microbiological cure (6 RCTs: difference in cure rate for longer *v* short course +6.2%, 95% CI −3.7% to +16.2%). The second systematic review excluded single dose regimens.[20] The third systematic review similarly found that 7–14 day courses of any antibiotic reduced treatment failure compared with single day or single dose regimens (RR 2.73, 95% CI 1.38 to 5.40).[21] Compared with any short course, including single day or single dose regimens, it found that longer courses reduced treatment failure (RR 1.94, 95% CI 1.19 to 3.15).[21] **Versus short course, but not single dose or single day regimens:** The second review (search date 2002, 10 RCTs, 652 children and adolescents aged 3 months to 18 years with urinary tract infections [UTI] and asymptomatic infection) excluded antibiotic courses of less than 2 days' duration.[20] All studies in the review excluded children with known renal tract abnormalities or acute pyelonephritis**G** and all included children with a history of recurrent UTI. The review found no significant difference between longer (7–14 days) and short (2–4 days) antibiotic courses for microbiological cure within 7 days of treatment (8 RCTs: RR of positive urine culture ≤ 7 days after treatment for longer *v* short courses 1.06, 95% CI 0.64 to 1.76).[20] It also found no significant difference between longer and shorter courses in UTI recurrence 1–15 months after treatment (10 RCTs: RR 0.95, 95% CI 0.70 to 1.29). The review found no significant difference between longer (7–14 days) and short (2–4 days) courses of sulphonamides, such as co-trimoxazole, for persistence of UTI after treatment or recurrence of UTI 10 days to 15 months after treatment (6 RCTs, 233 children: RR of UTI at end of treatment 0.80, 95% CI 0.45 to 1.41; RR of recurrent UTI 0.96, 95% CI 0.64 to 1.44).[20] The third review found no significant difference between 7–14 day courses and 3 day courses of any antibiotic for treatment failure (RR 1.36, 95% CI 0.68 to 2.72).[21]

Harms: The first systematic review reported that dose related adverse effects, such as neutropenia with β-lactam antibiotics, seemed to increase in frequency with the length of administration.[19] The second systematic review found no significant difference between short and longer courses for antibiotic resistant UTI (persistent resistant bacteriuria at the end of treatment, 1 RCT: RR 0.57, 95% CI 0.32 to 1.01; resistant recurrent UTI, 3 RCTs: RR 0.39, 95% CI 0.12 to 1.29).[20]

Comment: The studies included in the reviews differed in the lengths of treatment and antibiotics used; the definitions of cure, relapse, and reinfection; and the diagnostic criteria for pyelonephritis**G** or complicated UTI. Comparisons were made both for the whole group and for subgroups. In the first review, treatment groups were compared with fixed or random effects models, based on statistical analysis of the heterogeneity of the groups.[19] The second review included an unspecified number of children with asymptomatic bacteriuria.[20] The clinical importance of treating this group remains unclear. Several factors may reduce the generalisability of results to all children with lower UTI. First, the review excluded children with acute pyelonephritis only, which may not have excluded all cases of upper UTI. Second, all the RCTs in the second review included children with recurrent UTI, who have higher rates of treatment failure than children with no history of UTI.[20] Finally, many studies included in the reviews were in children attending outpatient departments and emergency rooms. Response to treatment may be different in this group compared with unselected populations.[21]

OPTION ORAL VERSUS INITIAL INTRAVENOUS ANTIBIOTICS

One RCT identified by a systematic review found no significant difference between oral cephalosporins alone and a regimen of 3 days of intravenous cephalosporins plus continued oral cephalosporins in duration of fever, reinfection rate, renal scarring, or extent of scarring in children aged 2 years or younger with a first confirmed urinary tract infection. The RCT found weak evidence that in children with grades III–IV reflux, initial intravenous treatment plus oral treatment may reduce renal scarring compared with oral treatment alone at 6 months.

Benefits: We found one systematic review (search date 2002),[22] which identified one RCT (309 children, aged ≤ 2 years, fever > 38.2 °C, with a first urinary tract infection confirmed from catheter specimen) that was sufficiently powered to produce meaningful results.[9] The RCT compared oral cefixime for 14 days (double dose on day 1) with initial intravenous cefotaxime for 3 days plus 11 days of oral cefixime.[9] It found no significant difference between treatments in mean duration of fever, reinfection rate, incidence of renal scarring, and mean extent of scarring (fever duration: 24.7 hours with oral treatment *v* 23.9 hours with initial iv treatment, WMD +0.80 hours, 95% CI –4.41 hours to +6.01 hours; symptomatic reinfection rate within 6 months: 7/140 [5%] with oral treatment *v* 11/147 [7%] with initial iv treatment, RR 0.67, 95% CI 0.27 to 1.67; renal scarring: 15/132 [11%] with oral treatment *v* 11/140 [8%] with initial iv treatment, RR 1.45, 95% CI 0.63 to 3.03; mean proportion of renal parenchyma with damage at 6 months: 7.9% with oral treatment *v* 8.6% with initial iv treatment, WMD –0.70%, 95% CI –1.74% to +0.34%).[22] Post hoc subgroup analysis found no significant difference in renal scarring at 6 months between oral and initial intravenous antibiotics in children with or without vesicoureteric reflux (with reflux: RR 1.88, 95% CI 0.83 to 4.24; without reflux: RR 0.80, 95% CI 0.23 to 2.73).[9] However, in children with more severe reflux (grades III–IV❻), subgroup analysis found that initial intravenous treatment reduced the risk of renal scarring at 6 months compared with oral antibiotics (new renal scarring on DMSA❻ scan within 6 months: 8/24 [33%] with oral treatment *v* 1/22 [5%] with initial iv treatment; ARI 29%, 95% CI 8% to 49%; NNH 3, 95% CI 2 to 13).[9]

Harms: The RCT[9] identified by the systematic review[22] did not report on adverse effects.

Comment: The adequately powered RCT identified by the review[22] excluded 3/309 [1%] children because investigators considered that the severity of symptoms in these children warranted intravenous treatment.[9]

OPTION LONGER VERSUS SHORT COURSES OF INITIAL INTRAVENOUS ANTIBIOTICS IN CHILDREN WITH PYELONEPHRITIS

One systematic review found no significant difference between long (7–14 days) and short (3–4 days) courses of initial intravenous antibiotics in persistence of bacteriuria after treatment, recurrent urinary tract infection at 6–12 months, or renal scarring at 3–6 months in children with acute pyelonephritis.

Benefits: We found one systematic review (search date 2002, 4 RCTs, 480 children with acute pyelonephritis❻) comparing long (7–14 days) with short (3–4 days) regimens involving initial intravenous antibiotics (ceftriaxone with or without netilmicin, or temocillin, given for 3–4 days and followed by either oral antibiotics or further iv antibiotics).[22] The review found no significant difference between long and short courses in persistent bacteriuria after treatment (3 RCTs, 251 people: RR 3.09, 95% CI 0.13 to 74.55). The review also found no significant difference between long and short courses in recurrent urinary tract infection within 6–12 months, or persisting renal parenchymal defects at 3–6 months (recurrent urinary tract infection, 4 RCTs, 480 children: RR 1.15, 95% CI 0.52 to 2.51; persisting renal parenchymal defects, 3 RCTs, 315 children: 0.99, 95% CI 0.72 to 1.37). Subgroup analyses found no significant difference in persisting renal parenchymal defects on DMSA scintigraphy❻) between long and short courses for children with or without vesicoureteric reflux or in children under 1 year of age or over

1 year of age (with reflux, 2 RCTs, 81 children: RR 0.99, 95% CI 0.56 to 1.74; without reflux, 2 RCTs, 175 children: RR 1.19, 95% CI 0.81 to 1.76; age < 1 year, 1 RCT,[13] 91 children: RR 1.46, 95% CI 0.71 to 3.01; age ≥1 year, 1 RCT,[13] 129 children: 0.89, 95% CI 0.55 to 3.05).[22]

Harms: The review reported solely on rate of gastrointestinal adverse effects.[22] It found no significant difference in gastrointestinal adverse effects between long and short courses (2 RCTs: RR 1.29, 95% CI 0.55 to 3.05).

Comment: None.

QUESTION What are the effects of interventions to prevent recurrence?

OPTION PROPHYLACTIC ANTIBIOTICS

One systematic review found limited evidence that prophylactic antibiotics (co-trimoxazole, nitrofurantoin, given for 10 weeks to 12 months) reduced urinary tract infection recurrence in children compared with placebo or no treatment. One RCT found that nitrofurantoin reduced recurrence of urinary tract infection over 6 months compared with trimethoprim. However, more children discontinued treatment with nitrofurantoin because of adverse effects. We found no RCTs evaluating the optimum duration of prophylactic antibiotics.

Benefits: **Versus no prophylaxis:** We found one systematic review (search date 2002).[23] The systematic review (3 RCTs, 151 children aged < 18 years at risk of urinary tract infection [UTI] but without a renal tract abnormality or major neurological, urological, or muscular disease) compared the effects of antibiotics (nitrofurantoin, co-trimoxazole) with placebo or no treatment on risk of recurrent UTI.[23] There was variation between the RCTs in the duration of antibiotic prophylaxis (10 weeks to 12 months) and method of concealment (see comment below). The review found that antibiotics reduced the risk of recurrent UTI compared with placebo or no treatment (RR 0.36, 95% CI 0.16 to 0.77).[23] **Comparison of antibiotics:** We found one systematic review (search date 2002, 1 RCT) comparing nitrofurantoin with trimethoprim.[23] It found that nitrofurantoin reduced recurrence of UTI over 6 months compared with trimethoprim (RR 0.48, 95% CI 0.25 to 0.92; NNT 5, 95% CI 3 to 33). **Duration of prophylaxis:** We found no RCTs evaluating the optimum length of prophylaxis even in children with vesicoureteric reflux (although 2 studies of prolonged acute treatment were identified).[24]

Harms: **Versus no prophylaxis:** No adverse effects were reported in the RCTs included in the systematic review.[23] **Comparison of antibiotics:** One RCT found that more children discontinued treatment with nitrofurantoin compared with trimethoprim because of adverse effects, including nausea, vomiting, or stomach ache (RR 3.17, 95% CI 1.36 to 7.37; NNH 5, 95% CI 3 to 13).[23] One study found that although gastrointestinal flora were affected by treatment, *E coli* (cultured from rectal swabs from 70% of children) remained sensitive to the prophylactic antibiotic co-trimoxazole).[25] However, another study found that children who had recently received co-trimoxazole for 4 weeks or more were more likely to have resistant *E coli* isolates than those who had received no antibiotics (OR 23.4, 95% CI 12.0 to 47.6).[26]

Comment: The systematic review was thorough but the RCTs it identified had weak methods.[23] None of the RCTs included in the systematic review used intention to treat analyses. Only one had adequate concealment and only one specified the outcome measures. It may not be possible clinically to identify children who are at high risk of recurrent UTIs and long term damage.[27] Routine prophylaxis until the results of investigations are known may, therefore, be warranted, but we found no good evidence about the benefits or harms of antibiotic prophylaxis.

OPTION IMMUNOTHERAPY

One RCT in children with recurrent urinary tract infection found that adding pidotimod (an immunotherapeutic agent) to antibiotic treatment reduced recurrence compared with adding placebo.

Benefits: We found two RCTs.[28,29] We found one RCT (double blind, 60 children aged 2–8 years with recurrent urinary tract infection [UTI]) comparing pidotimod versus placebo when added to standard antibiotic treatment.[28] The study included a further 60 day phase, using half dose pidotimod compared with half dose placebo. The RCT found that adding pidotimod reduced relapse rates compared with adding placebo at 60 days (4/30 [13%] with added pidotimod *v* 13/30 [43%] with added placebo; $P < 0.05$).[28] We found one open pilot RCT (40 girls with recurrent UTI), which compared nitrofurantoin versus an antigenic extract of *E coli*.[29] It found no significant difference in the incidence of UTIs (clinical and microbiological confirmation) between the two treatments during 6 months of active treatment or during the subsequent 6 months' follow up (AR during active treatment: 3/17 [17.6%] with nitrofurantoin *v* 4/21 [19.0%] with antigenic extract; $P = 0.91$; AR during follow up: 4/17 [23.5%] with nitrofurantoin *v* 3/21 [14.3%] with antigenic extract; $P = 0.78$; analysis by non-conservative intention to treat).

Harms: In the RCT of pidotimod, the only adverse effects recorded were thought to be attributable to concomitant antibiotic treatment.[28] The open pilot study found no significant difference in withdrawal rates between the antigenic extract of *E coli* (1/22 [5%] children) and nitrofurantoin (1/18 [6%] children).[29]

Comment: **Intravenous immunoglobulin:** We found one systematic review (search date 1997, 15 RCTs), which compared intravenous immunoglobulin**G** prophylaxis with placebo or no treatment.[30] It found that intravenous immunoglobulin prophylaxis reduced serious infections, including UTIs, in preterm and low birth weight neonates (RR for all serious infections 0.80, 95% CI 0.68 to 0.94; NNT 24, 95% CI 15 to 83).[30] The dose varied from 120 mg/kg to 1 g/kg. The number of treatments varied from one to seven. The specific effect on UTIs was not reported. We found no evidence for or against the suggestion that preparations with specific antibodies against common pathogens are more beneficial.[31] The greatest benefits were noted in units with higher nosocomial infection**G** rates. It remains unclear whether intravenous immunoglobulin is only justified where infection control policies have failed to reduce the infection rate.[30] Preterm and low birth weight neonates might have greater immune deficiency than other neonates and might be expected to gain more from treatment with immunoglobulin. **Other immunotherapeutic agents:** We found one non-randomised, age matched study in 10 otherwise healthy girls (aged 5–11 years) with recurrent UTI who were given intramuscular injections of inactivated uropathogenic bacteria. It found that the girls who had received the inactivated uropathogenic bacteria had reduced frequency of subsequent UTI compared with 10 other age matched girls with UTI who had not received the inactivated bacteria preparation.[32] This study is limited by its non-randomised design and small sample size. We found another study (40 children aged 3–12 years with recurrent UTI caused by *E coli* and no anatomical or functional impairments of the urinary tract) comparing prophylactic antibiotics (amoxicillin with clavulanic acid or cephalosporins) versus prophylactic antibiotics plus an immunomodulator with *E coli* antigens for 3 months followed up for 3 months after the end of treatment.[33] The method of randomisation was not reported. The study found that urinary secretory immunoglobulin A levels, initially low in both groups, were raised 3 months after the end of treatment with antibiotics plus immunomodulator but not with antibiotics alone. It also found that antibiotics plus immunomodulator reduced recurrences over 6 months compared with antibiotics alone (recurrences: 2/25 [8%] with antibiotics plus immunomodulator *v* 8/13 [61%] with antibiotics alone).[33]

OPTION SURGICAL CORRECTION FOR MINOR FUNCTIONAL ANOMALIES

We found no RCTs. One observational study suggested that children with minor anomalies do not develop renal scarring and therefore may not benefit from surgery.

Benefits: We found no systematic review or RCTs.

Harms: Potential harms include the usual risks of surgery.

Comment: One small prospective observational study (271 children) suggested that children with minor anomalies do not develop renal scarring and therefore may not benefit from surgery.[34] Renal scars were present in more children with moderate degrees of vesicoureteric reflux than in children with minor anomalies (8/20 [40%] with moderate degrees of vesicoureteric reflux *v* 0/6 [0%] with minor anomalies). In the presence of major anomalies, the prevention of urinary tract infections is not the prime motive of surgical intervention.

OPTION SURGICAL CORRECTION FOR MODERATE TO SEVERE VESICOURETERIC REFLUX

One systematic review found no significant difference between surgical and medical management (prophylactic antibiotic treatment) in urinary tract infections or their complications from after 1–5 years in children with moderate to severe vesicoureteric reflux, although surgery abolished reflux. One subsequent RCT, reporting 10 years' follow-up, found that new renal scars rarely occurred with either management strategy after 5 years. One small RCT found a non-significantly greater decline in glomerular filtration rate over 10 years with medical treatment compared with surgery in children with moderate to severe bilateral vesicoureteric reflux and bilateral nephropathy.

Benefits: **Versus medical management, short to medium term outcome (≤ 5 years):** We found one systematic review (search date 2003, 8 RCTs, 947 children with moderate to severe [grades III–V**G**] vesicoureteric reflux), which compared surgical correction plus subsequent antibiotic cover (for 1–24 months; most commonly 6 months) versus medical management (continuous prophylactic antibiotics: co-trimoxazole, trimethoprim, or nitrofurantoin).[35] It found no significant differences in subsequent urinary tract infection (UTI) at 2 years or 4–5 years (UTI at 2 years, 4 RCTs, 341 children: 33/164 [20%] with surgery *v* 36/177 [20%] with medical treatment, RR 1.07, 95% CI 0.55 to 2.09; UTI at 4–5 years, 3 RCTs, 479 children: 90/244 [37%] with surgery *v* 86/235 [35%] with medical treatment, RR 0.99, 95% CI 0.79 to 1.26). However, it found that surgery significantly reduced clinically diagnosed febrile UTI by 5 years (2 RCTs, 429 children: RR 0.43, 95% CI 0.27 to 0.70).[35] It found that surgery abolished reflux in a greater proportion of children than 4–5 years of medical management (93–99% after surgical correction *v* 16–49% spontaneous resolution during 4–5 years of medical management). It found no significant difference between surgery and medical treatment in new and progressive renal scarring at 5 years assessed using DMSA**G** scans (3 RCTs, 468 children: RR 1.05, 95% CI 0.85 to 1.29). **Longer term outcome (10 years):** We found two RCTs that assessed longer term outcome.[36,37] The first RCT (223 children aged < 11 years at entry, with grades III–V**G** vesicoureteric reflux, glomerular filtration rate ≥ 70 mL/minute/1.73 m^2) compared surgery with medical management (as above) over 10 years.[36] It found only one case of new scarring between 5 and 10 years in either group, and found no significant difference in the development of new scars at 10 years (5–10 years: 1/149 [0.67%] with surgery *v* 1/153 [0.65%] with medical treatment; 10 years: 22/110 [20%] with surgery *v* 20/113 [18%] medical treatment; RR 1.10, 95% CI 0.64 to 1.93). The second RCT (25 boys and 27 girls aged 1–12 years with bilateral vesicoureteric reflux [grades III–V] and bilateral nephropathy) found a steady decline in glomerular filtration rate over 10 years in children on medical treatment compared with surgery but the difference was not significant (see table 1, p 457).[37] The RCT was too small to detect a clinically important effect.

Harms: The systematic review (search date 2003) found that adverse effects were not well reported in the identified RCTs.[35] Risks with surgery may include those of any operative procedure under general anaesthetic, as well as specific postoperative complications. Two RCTs (3 papers) reported rates of postoperative obstruction to the urinary tract.[38–40] The European arm of a multinational RCT found postoperative urinary tract obstruction in 10/151 children (6.6%), with an increased risk of severe scarring after obstruction (RR 23.83, 95% CI 5.05 to 112.42).[39] The study did not report on the clinical consequences of these radiological findings. The US arm of the same multinational RCT found that 7/9 (78%) children who had postoperative obstruction developed evidence of renal scarring on DMSA scintigraphy**G**.[38] The second RCT found that none (0/70) of the children who had surgery developed postoperative pelvi-calyceal obstruction.[40] Risks of medical management may include adverse effects of antibiotic treatment and antibiotic resistance.

Comment: Surgery is usually considered only in children with more severe vesicoureteric reflux (grades III–V**G**), who are less likely to experience spontaneous resolution.[7,41] It has been suggested that the best results are obtained by centres handling the greatest number of children.[42] **Other clinical outcomes after surgery:** The review could not perform a meta-analysis on other outcome measures (renal growth, end stage renal failure, development of hypertension, and glomerular filtration rates) because of the differences between studies in reporting data.[35] Individual trials reporting on these measures found no differences, though the numbers of adverse outcomes were small. **Effects of surgery in children with vesicoureteric reflux and nephropathy:** One of the RCTs in the systematic review[35] compared corrective surgery with medical management (as above) over 4 years in children with more severe disease at the point of entry into the study (25 boys and 27 girls aged 1–12 years with bilateral vesicoureteric reflux [grades III–V] and bilateral nephropathy, glomerular filtration rate ≥ 20 mL/minute/1.73m^2 [more commonly children with rates of 20–70 mL/minute/1.73m^2 are excluded]).[37] It found no significant difference in development of new scars between surgical and medical treatment (AR 8/50 [16%] kidneys with corrective surgery *v* 7/54 [13%] kidneys with medical treatment; RR 1.20, 95% CI 0.47 to 3.40).[37] The RCT found that, over a period of 4 years, 20/54 (37%) kidneys of children in the medical group had spontaneous resolution to no or minimal vesicoureteric reflux (grades 0 or I) and that corrective surgery was possible without complications in 47/50 (94%) kidneys in the surgical group (ARI 57%, 95% CI 47% to 69%).[37] We found one prospective cohort study (226 children aged 5 days to 12 years who presented with UTI and vesicoureteric reflux [grades III–IV]) with follow up of 10–41 years.[14] It found that surgery increased resolution of reflux compared with medical treatment (AR of resolution from age 8–14 years on micturating cystourethrography: 29/33 [88%] with surgery *v* 134/193 [69%] with medical treatment; ARI 19%, 95% CI 6% to 31%). The study did not compare clinical outcomes.

Endoscopic surgical management (sub-ureteric implantation of inert or hypo-allergenic substances) versus medical management: The systematic review[35] identified one RCT[43] that compared endoscopic techniques (sub-ureteric implantation of a co-polymer) with versus medical management (continuous antibiotic prophylaxis). The RCT (60 children aged ≥1) found that surgery increased risk of UTI compared with antibiotics over 1 year, but the difference was not significant (RR 7.15, 95% CI 0.42 to 121.05).[43] At 1 year, 27/39 (69%) children managed by endoscopic sub-ureteric implantation of a co-polymer and 8/21 (38%) children managed medically showed resolution of vesicoureteric reflux, defined as the presence of no or Grade I reflux.[43] Children with failed endoscopic treatment had formal open surgery.[43] We found several studies comparing radiological outcomes between different endoscopic procedures, but no other studies that compared endoscopic surgery with medical management, or that assessed clinical outcomes.

GLOSSARY

DMSA scintigraphy A scan following intravenous injection of a radioisotope solution, which is excreted by the kidneys. The scan yields information about the structure and function of the urinary tract.

Intravenous immunoglobulins Immunoglobulin preparations derived from donated human plasma containing antibodies prevalent in the general population.

Nosocomial infection Definitions vary but typically an infection arising at least 48–72 hours after admission to hospital. The infection may have been acquired from other people, hospital staff, the hospital environment, or from pre-existing subclinical infection.

Pyelonephritis Inflammation of the kidney and its pelvis caused by bacterial infection.

Severity of vesicoureteric reflux: Grade I Reflux into ureters only. **Grade II** Reflux into ureters, pelvis, and calyces. **Grade III** Mild to moderate dilatation or tortuosity of ureters and mild to moderate dilatation of pelvis, but little or no forniceal blunting. **Grade IV** As grade III, but with complete obliteration of forniceal angles, yet maintenance of papillary impressions in calyces. **Grade V** Gross dilatation of ureters, pelvis, and calyces, and papillary impressions in calyces obliterated.

Substantive changes

Oral versus initial intravenous antibiotics One systematic review added;[22] categorisation unchanged.

Longer versus short courses of initial intravenous antibiotics in children with pyelonephritis One systematic review added;[22] categorisation unchanged but benefits data enhanced.

Surgical correction for vesicoureteric reflux One systematic review added;[35] categorisation unchanged but benefits data enhanced.

REFERENCES

1. Hellstrom A, Hanson E, Hansson S, et al. Association between urinary symptoms at 7 years old and previous urinary tract infections. *Arch Dis Child* 1991;66:232–234.
2. Dick PT, Feldman W. Routine diagnostic imaging for childhood urinary tract infections: a systematic overview. *J Pediatr* 1996;128:15–22. Search date 1994; primary sources Medline, Current Contents, and hand searches of article bibliographies.
3. Gordon I, Barkovics M, Pindoria S, et al. Primary vesicoureteric reflux as a predictor of renal damage in children hospitalized with urinary tract infection: a systematic review and meta-analysis. *J Am Soc*

Nephrol 2003;14:739–744. Search date 2002; primary sources Medline, Embase, and hand searches using authors' names.
4. Chertin B, Puri P. Familial vesicoureteral reflux. *J Urol* 2003;169:1804–1808.
5. Wennerstrom M, Hansson S, Jodal U, et al. Primary and acquired renal scarring in boys and girls with urinary tract infection. *J Pediatr* 2000;136:30–34.
6. Smellie JM, Katz G, Gruneberg RN. Controlled trial of prophylactic treatment in childhood urinary tract infection. *Lancet* 1978;ii:175–178.
7. Jodal U, Hansson S, Hjalmas K. Medical or surgical management for children with vesico-ureteric reflux? *Acta Paediatr Suppl* 1999;431:53–61.
8. Jodal U. The natural history of bacteriuria in childhood. *Infect Dis Clin North Am* 1987;1:713–729.
9. Hoberman A, Wald ER, Hickey RW, et al. Oral versus initial intravenous therapy for urinary tract infections in young febrile children. *Pediatrics* 1999;104:79–86.
10. Piepsz A, Tamminen-Mobius T, Reiners C, et al. Five-year study of medical and surgical treatment in children with severe vesico-ureteric reflux dimercaptosuccinic acid findings. International Reflux Study Group in Europe. *Eur J Pediatr* 1998;157:753–758.
11. Rosenberg AR, Rossleigh MA, Brydon MP, et al. Evaluation of acute urinary tract infection in children by dimercaptosuccinic acid scintigraphy: a prospective study. *J Urol* 1992;148:1746–1749.
12. Benador D, Benador N, Slozman D, et al. Are younger patients at higher risk of renal sequelae after pyelonephritis? *Lancet* 1997;349:17–19.
13. Benador D, Neuhaus TJ, Papazyan J-P, et al. Randomised controlled trial of three day versus 10 day intravenous antibiotics in acute pyelonephritis: effect on renal scarring. *Arch Dis Child* 2001;84;241–246.
14. Smellie JM, Prescod NP, Shaw PJ, et al. Childhood reflux and urinary infection: a follow-up of 10–41 years in 226 adults. *Pediatr Nephrol* 1998;12:727–736.
15. Berg UB. Long-term follow-up of renal morphology and function in children with recurrent pyelonephritis. *J Urol* 1992;148:1715–1720.
16. Martinell J, Claeson I, Lidin-Janson G, et al. Urinary infection, reflux and renal scarring in females continuously followed for 13–38 years. *Pediatr Nephrol* 1995;9:131–136.
17. Jacobson S, Eklof O, Erikkson CG, et al. Development of hypertension and uraemia after pyelonephritis in childhood: 27 year follow up. *BMJ* 1989;299:703–706.
18. Biggi A, Dardanelli L, Cussino P, et al. Prognostic value of the acute DMSA scan in children with first urinary tract infection. *Pediatr Nephrol* 2001;16:800–804.
19. Tran D, Muchant DG, Aronoff SC. Short-course versus conventional length antimicrobial therapy for uncomplicated lower urinary tract infections in children: a meta-analysis of 1279 patients. *J Pediatr* 2001;139;93–99. Search date 1999; primary sources Medline, and reference lists of identified studies.
20. Michael M, Hodson EM, Craig JC, et al. Short versus standard duration oral antibiotic therapy for acute urinary tract infection in children (Cochrane review). In: The Cochrane Library, Issue 4, 2003. Oxford: Update Software. Search date 2002; primary sources Medline, Embase, Cochrane Library, hand searches of reference lists of identified RCTs, and contact with investigators in the field.
21. Keren R, Chan E. A meta-analysis of randomized, controlled trials comparing short- and long-course antibiotic therapy for urinary tract infections in children. *Pediatrics* 2002;109:e70. Search date 2001; primary sources Medline, Cochrane Controlled Trials Register, hand searches of references, and contact with experts. Limited to English language published articles.
22. Bloomfield P, Hodson EM, Craig JC. Antibiotics for acute pyelonephritis in children. (Cochrane Review). In: The Cochrane Library, Issue 1, 2004. Chichester, UK: John Wiley & Sons, Ltd. Search date 2002; primary sources Cochrane Register of Controlled Trials, Medline, Embase, reference lists, and abstracts from conference proceedings.
23. Williams GJ, Lee A, Craig JC. Long-term antibiotics for preventing recurrent urinary tract infection in children. In: The Cochrane Library, Issue 4, 2003. Oxford: Update Software. Search date 2002; primary sources Medline, Embase, Cochrane Controlled Trials Register, reference lists in reviews, and contact with experts.
24. Garin EH, Campos A, Homsy Y. Primary vesico-ureteral reflux: a review of current concepts. *Pediatr Nephrol* 1998;12:249–256.
25. Smellie JM, Gruneberg RN, Leakey A, et al. Long term low dose co-trimoxazole in prophylaxis of childhood urinary tract infection: clinical aspects/bacteriological aspects. *BMJ* 1976;2:203–208.
26. Allen UD, MacDonald N, Fuite L, et al. Risk factors for resistance to "first-line" antimicrobials among urinary tract isolates of *Escherichia coli* in children. *CMAJ* 1999;160:1436–1440.
27. Greenfield SP, Ng M, Gran J. Experience with vesicoureteric reflux in children: clinical characteristics. *J Urol* 1997;158:574–577.
28. Clemente E, Solli R, Mei V, et al. Therapeutic efficacy and safety of pidotimod in the treatment of urinary tract infections in children. *Arzneimittelforschung* 1994;44:1490–1494.
29. Lettgen B. Prevention of urinary tract infections in female children. *Curr Ther Res* 1996;57:464–475.
30. Ohlsson A, Lacy JB. Intravenous immunoglobulin for preventing infection in pre-term and/or low-birth-weight infants. In: The Cochrane Library, Issue 4, 2001. Oxford: Update Software. Search date 1997; primary sources Medline, Embase, Cochrane Library, Reference Update, Science Citation Index, and hand searches of reference lists of identified RCTs and personal files.
31. Weisman LE, Cruess DF, Fischer GW. Opsonic activity of commercially available standard intravenous immunoglobulin preparations. *Pediatr Infect Dis J* 1994;13:1122–1125. [Erratum in: *Pediatr Infect Dis J* 1995;14:349.]
32. Nayir A, Emre S, Sirin A, et al. The effects of vaccination with inactivated uropathogenic bacteria in recurrent urinary tract infections of children. *Vaccine* 1995;13:987–990.
33. Czerwionka-Szarflarska M, Pawlowska M. Uro-vaxom in the treatment of recurrent urinary tract infections in children. *Pediatr Pol* 1996;71:599–604. [In Polish]
34. Pylkannen J, Vilska J, Koskimies O. The value of childhood urinary tract infection in predicting renal injury. *Acta Paediatr Scand* 1981;70:879–883.
35. Wheeler D, Vimalachandra D, Hodson EM, et al. Antibiotics and surgery for vesicoureteric reflux: a meta-analysis of randomised controlled trials. *Arch Dis Child* 2003;88:688–694. Search date 2003; primary sources Medline, Embase, Cochrane Trials Register, reference lists, and contact with researchers in the field.
36. Olbing H, Smellie JM, Jodal U, et al. New renal scars in children with severe VUR: a 10-year study of randomized treatment. *Pediatr Nephrol* 2003;18:1128–1131.
37. Smellie JM, Barratt TM, Chantler C, et al. Medical versus surgical treatment in children with severe bilateral vesicoureteric reflux and bilateral nephropathy: a randomized controlled trial. *Lancet* 2001;357:1329–1333.
38. Weiss R, Duckett J, Spitzer A. Results of a randomized clinical trial of medical versus surgical management of infants and children with grades III and IV primary vesico-ureteral reflux (United States): the international reflux study in children. *J Urol* 1992;148:1667–1673.
39. Jodal U, Koskimies O, Hanson E, et al. Infection pattern in children with vesicoureteral reflux

randomly allocated to operation or long-term antibacterial prophylaxis. *J Urol* 1992;148:1650–1652.
40. Birmingham Reflux Study Group. A prospective trial of operative versus non-operative treatment of severe vesicoureteric reflux in children: five years' observation. *BMJ* 1987;295:237–241.
41. Sciagra R, Materassi M, Rossi V, et al. Alternative approaches to the prognostic stratification of mild to moderate primary vesicoureteral reflux in children. *J Urol* 1996;155:2052–2056.
42. Smellie JM. Commentary: management of children with severe vesicoureteral reflux. *J Urol* 1992;148:1676–1678.
43. Capozza N, Caione P. Dextranomer/hyaluronic acid copolymer implantation for vesico-ureteric reflux: a randomized comparison with antibiotic prophylaxis. *J Pediatr* 2002;140:230–234.

James Larcombe
General Practitioner, Sedgefield and
Regional Research Fellow
NHSE Northern and Yorkshire
Sedgefield
UK

Competing interests: None declared.

TABLE 1 **Average glomerular filtration rates in children with bilateral vesicoureteric reflux and bilateral nephropathy at the commencement of the study, at 4 years, and at 10 years after randomisation to medical or surgical management (see text, p 453).[37]**

Mean GFR (mL/minute)	At entry	At 4 years	At 10 years
Medical management	72.4	70.2	68.3
Surgical management	71.7	73.7	74.1
Difference in change in GFR from entry (95% CI)	–	+7.1% (–6.4% to +20.6%)	+8.9% (–10.3% to +28.2%)

GFR, glomerular filtration rate.

Anal fissure (chronic)

Search date January 2004

Marion Jonas and John Scholefield

QUESTIONS

INTERVENTIONS

To be covered in future updates
Nifedipine for chronic anal fissure
Treatments for acute anal fissure

*Based on limited evidence and consensus opinion
See glossary G

Key Messages

- **Internal anal sphincterotomy** One systematic review found that internal anal sphincterotomy improved fissure healing compared with topical glyceryl trinitrate after 6 weeks to 2 years. One systematic review found that internal anal sphincterotomy reduced fissure persistence compared with botulinum A toxin-haemagglutinin complex at 12 months. One systematic review found no significant difference between internal anal sphincterotomy and anal stretch in persistence of fissures, and found that both procedures healed 70–95% of fissures. However, it found that anal stretch increased rates of flatus incontinence compared with internal anal sphincterotomy. One systematic review found no significant difference between open and closed internal anal sphincterotomy in persistence of fissures. One small RCT found no significant difference between internal anal sphincterotomy and anal advancement flap in patient satisfaction or fissure healing.
- **Anal advancement flap (as effective as internal anal sphincterotomy based on 1 small RCT)** One small RCT found no significant difference between lateral internal anal sphincterotomy and anal advancement flap in patient satisfaction or fissure healing.
- **Topical glyceryl trinitrate** One systematic review and one subsequent RCT found limited evidence from heterogeneous RCTs that topical glyceryl trinitrate reduced persistence of fissures compared with placebo. Results were difficult to interpret because of differing durations and doses of treatments. Consensus opinion regards glyceryl trinitrate as an effective first line treatment for chronic anal fissure. One systematic review found that internal anal sphincterotomy improved fissure healing compared with topical glyceryl trinitrate after 6 weeks to 2 years. One systematic review found no significant difference in fissure persistence between topical glyceryl trinitrate ointment and botulinum A toxin-hc injection after 2 months. Two RCTs found no significant difference between glyceryl trinitrate ointment and a glyceryl

trinitrate patch in fissure healing after 8–12 weeks. Two RCTs found no significant difference between topical glyceryl trinitrate and topical diltiazem in fissure healing at 8 weeks.

- **Anal stretch (as effective as internal anal sphincterotomy but higher rates of flatus incontinence)** One systematic review found no significant difference between internal anal sphincterotomy and anal stretch in persistence of fissures. It found that both procedures healed 70–95% of fissures. Anal stretch increased rates of flatus incontinence compared with internal anal sphincterotomy.
- **Botulinum A toxin-haemagglutinin complex** One systematic review found no significant difference in fissure persistence between botulinum A toxin-haemagglutinin and placebo or topical glyceryl nitrate at 2 months. One systematic review and one additional RCT found no significant difference between high and low dose botulinum A toxin-haemagglutinin complex after 2–3 months. One systematic review found that botulinum A toxin-haemagglutinin complex significantly increased fissure persistence compared with anal sphincterotomy at 12 months.
- **Botulinum A toxin-haemagglutinin complex plus nitrates** We found no RCTs comparing botulinum A toxin-haemagglutinin complex plus nitrates versus placebo. One small RCT found that botulinum A toxin-haemagglutinin complex plus topical isosorbide dinitrate three times daily increased fissure healing at 6 weeks compared with botulinum A toxin-haemagglutinin complex alone. It found no significant difference at 8 or 12 weeks.
- **Diltiazem** We found no placebo controlled RCTs. Two RCTs found no significant difference between topical diltiazem and topical glyceryl trinitrate in fissure healing at 8 weeks. One small RCT identified by a systematic review found no significant difference in fissure persistence after 8 weeks between oral diltiazem and topical diltiazem but that adverse events were more common with oral diltiazem.
- **Indoramin** One RCT found no significant difference between oral indoramin and placebo in fissure healing after 6 weeks, but it may have been too small to detect a clinically important difference.

DEFINITION Anal fissure is a split or tear in the lining of the distal anal canal. It is a painful condition often associated with fresh blood loss from the anus and perianal itching. **Acute anal fissures** have sharply demarcated, fresh mucosal edges, often with granulation tissue at the base. The majority of acute fissures will heal spontaneously, or with increased oral fluid and dietary fibre intake as well as laxatives where there is a history of constipation. Fissures persisting for longer than 6 weeks are generally defined as chronic. **Chronic anal fissures** have margins that are indurated, with less granulation tissue; the muscle fibres of the internal anal sphincter may be seen at the base. These require intervention in order to heal.

INCIDENCE/ PREVALENCE Anal fissures are common in all age groups, but we found no reliable evidence about incidence.

AETIOLOGY/ RISK FACTORS Low intake of dietary fibre may be a risk factor for the development of acute anal fissure.[1] People with anal fissure often have raised resting anal canal pressures with anal spasm.[2,3] Men and women are equally affected by anal fissure, and up to 11% of women develop anal fissure after childbirth.[4]

PROGNOSIS Placebo controlled studies found that 70–90% of untreated "chronic" fissures did not heal during the study.[5,6]

AIMS OF INTERVENTION To relieve symptoms (pain, bleeding, and irritation); to heal the fissure; to minimise adverse effects of treatment.

OUTCOMES Proportion of people with fissure healing (intact anal mucosal lining); symptom score for intensity of symptoms of pain, bleeding, and irritation (typically a linear visual analogue scale that consists of an unmarked 100 mm horizontal line, the left end of which represents absence of symptoms and the right end represents the worst symptoms imaginable; a vertical mark is made across this line by the person with the fissure); proportion of people reporting adverse effects of treatment.

METHODS *Clinical Evidence* search and appraisal January 2004.

QUESTION **What are the effects of treatments for chronic anal fissure?**

OPTION **TOPICAL GLYCERYL TRINITRATE**

One systematic review and one subsequent RCT found limited evidence from heterogeneous RCTs that topical glyceryl trinitrate reduced persistence of fissures compared with placebo. Results were difficult to interpret because of differing durations and doses of treatments. Consensus opinion regards glyceryl trinitrate as an effective first line treatment for chronic anal fissure. One systematic review found that internal anal sphincterotomy improved fissure healing compared with topical glyceryl trinitrate after 6 weeks to 2 years. One systematic review found no significant difference in fissure persistence between topical glyceryl trinitrate ointment and botulinum A toxin-hc injection after 2 months. Two RCTs found no significant difference between glyceryl trinitrate ointment and a glyceryl trinitrate patch in fissure healing after 8–12 weeks. Two RCTs found no significant difference between topical glyceryl trinitrate and topical diltiazem in fissure healing at 8 weeks.

Benefits: **Versus placebo:** We found one systematic review (search date 2003, 7 RCTs, 694 people)[7] and one subsequent RCT.[8] The systematic review found that topical glyceryl trinitrate (GTN**G**) significantly reduced persistence of fissure compared with placebo, although results were statistically heterogeneous (OR 0.64, 95% CI 0.44 to 0.92).[7] The subsequent RCT (200 people) found no significant difference in healing or pain between GTN (0.1%, 0.2%, or 0.4% twice daily) and placebo after 8 weeks of treatment (AR for healing: 62/133 [46.6%] with all GTN treatments *v* 18/48 [37.5%] with placebo, P = 0.3; pain scores not reported: 0.1% GTN *v* placebo, P = 0.40; 0.2% GTN *v* placebo, P = 0.34; 0.4% GTN *v* placebo, P = 0.64).[8] **Versus internal anal sphincterotomy:** We found one systematic review (search date 2003, 4 RCTs, 249 people).[7] It found that GTN significantly increased persistence of anal fissure compared with internal anal sphincterotomy (OR 8.97, 95% CI 4.75 to 16.94). **Versus botulinum A toxin-haemagglutinin complex:** See benefits of botulinum A toxin-haemagglutinin complex, p 462. **GTN ointment versus GTN patch: We found one systematic review** (search date 2003, 1 RCT, 42 people)[7] and one subsequent RCT.[9] The review found no significant difference between GTN ointment and GTN patch in persistence of chronic anal fissure at 8 weeks (OR 1.00, 95% CI 0.29 to 3.39). The subsequent RCT (89 people) found no significant difference between GTN ointment (0.2%, 3 times daily) and a GTN patch in fissure healing after 12 weeks of treatment (82 people included in analysis; AR for healing: 27/34 [79%] with GTN ointment *v* 39/48 [81%] with GTN patch, P = 1.0; RR and CI not reported).[9] **Versus topical diltiazem:** We found one systematic review (search date 2003, 1 RCT, 72 people; 60 included in analysis)[7] and one subsequent RCT.[10] The review found no significant difference in fissure persistence between GTN (0.2% ointment applied twice daily for 6–8 weeks) and topical diltiazem (2% cream applied twice daily for 6–8 weeks) at 8 weeks (OR 0.66, 95% CI 0.22 to 2.01). The subsequent RCT (43 people) found no significant difference in fissure healing between GTN (0.5% ointment applied twice daily) and topical diltiazem (2% ointment applied twice daily) after 8 weeks (AR for healing 18/21 [86%] with GTN ointment *v* 19/22 [90%] with diltiazem, P > 0.95; RR and CI not reported).[10]

Harms: **Versus placebo:** The systematic review found that topical GTN significantly increased the risk of headaches compared with placebo (11 RCTs, including 1 RCT in people with acute anal fissure and 3 RCTs in children; 767 people; OR 4.09, 95% CI 2.54 to 6.60).[7] The subsequent RCT also found that GTN increased the risk of headache compared with placebo (51/133 [38.3%] with GTN *v* 6/48 [12.5%] with placebo; P value not reported).[8] **Versus internal anal sphincterotomy:** The systematic review found that GTN significantly increased the risk of headache compared with sphincterotomy (4 RCTs, 227 people; OR 36.65, 95% CI 9.72 to 138.21).[7] The review also found that GTN significantly reduced the risk of flatus incontinence compared with sphincterotomy (4 RCTs, 161 people; OR 0.23, 95% CI 0.02 to 2.07). **Versus botulinum A toxin-haemagglutinin complex:** See harms of botulinum A toxin-haemagglutinin complex, p 463. **GTN ointment versus GTN patch:** The systematic review found no significant difference between GTN ointment and GTN patch in the risk of headaches (1 RCT, 42 people; OR 1.54, 95% CI 0.42 to 5.61).[7] **Versus diltiazem:** The systematic review found that GTN significantly increased all adverse events and significantly increased headache compared with diltiazem (1 RCT, 60 people; all adverse events: OR 3.63, 95% CI 1.23 to 10.73; headache: OR 4.07, 95% CI 1.37 to 12.14).[7]

Comment: Results of the RCTs are difficult to interpret because of differences between trials in entry criteria, in the doses and durations of GTN treatments used, and in the advice and application of topical GTN. The review included studies in which participants had a history of pain for at least 4 weeks, or pain of shorter duration but similar episodes in the past.[7] It excluded RCTs in people with atypical fissures. We found insufficient evidence about the optimal duration and dose of topical GTN treatment. Entry criteria may have varied among the trial centres in multicentre RCTs. The authors, therefore, believe that some of the single centre RCTs, which have tightly controlled entry criteria and dosage regimens, probably reflect the effectiveness of GTN more accurately than the multicentre RCTs. Consensus opinion regards GTN as being an effective first line treatment for chronic anal fissures.

OPTION DILTIAZEM

We found no placebo controlled RCTs. Two RCTs found no significant difference between topical diltiazem and topical glyceryl trinitrate in fissure healing at 8 weeks. One small RCT identified by a systematic review found no significant difference in fissure persistence after 8 weeks between oral diltiazem and topical diltiazem but that adverse events were more common with oral diltiazem.

Benefits: **Versus placebo:** We found one systematic review (search date, 2003), which found no RCTs.[7] **Topical diltiazem versus topical glyceryl trinitrate:** See benefits of topical glyceryl trinitrate, p 460. **Oral versus topical diltiazem:** We found one systematic review (search date 2003, 1 RCT, 50 people), which found no significant difference between oral diltiazem 60 mg twice daily and 2% topical diltiazem gel in fissure persistence after 8 weeks of treatment (OR 3.20, 95% CI 1.00 to 10.20).[7]

Harms: **Oral versus topical diltiazem:** The RCT included in the review found that oral diltiazem significantly increased adverse events, which included nausea, vomiting, headache, rash, and altered smell, compared with topical diltiazem (AR 8/24 [33%] with oral diltiazem *v* 0/26 with topical diltiazem; OR calculated by review 32.48, 95% CI 1.77 to 597.56).[7,11]

Comment: We found insufficient evidence about the optimal duration of diltiazem treatment. The role of diltiazem in treating fissures previously failing to heal with glyceryl trinitrate is unclear.

OPTION INDORAMIN

One RCT found no significant difference between oral indoramin and placebo in fissure healing after 6 weeks, but it may have been too small to detect a clinically important difference.

Benefits: **Versus placebo:** We found no systematic review. We found one small RCT (23 people with chronic anal fissures).[12] It found no significant difference between oral indoramin 20 mg twice daily and placebo for fissure healing at 6 weeks (AR for healing: 1/14 [7%] with indoramin *v* 2/9 [22%] with placebo; RR 0.30, 95% CI 0.03 to 3.05; see comment below). The RCT did not provide comparative data between treatments for pain scores.

Harms: The RCT reported that indoramin caused adverse effects in 7/14 (50%) people.[12]

Comment: The RCT was small and may have lacked adequate power to detect a clinically important difference.[12] It found that the single fissure that healed with indoramin recurred after 3 months.

OPTION BOTULINUM A TOXIN-HAEMAGGLUTININ COMPLEX (BOTULINUM A TOXIN-HC)

One systematic review found no significant difference in fissure persistence between botulinum A toxin-haemagglutinin and placebo or topical glyceryl nitrate at 2 months. One systematic review and one additional RCT found no significant difference between high and low dose botulinum A toxin-haemagglutinin complex after 2–3 months. One systematic review found that botulinum A toxin-haemagglutinin complex significantly increased fissure persistence compared with anal sphincterotomy at 12 months.

Benefits: **Versus placebo:** We found one systematic review (search date 2003, 2 RCTs, 74 people).[7] The review found no significant difference in fissure persistence between botulinum A toxin-haemagglutinin complex (botulinum A toxin-hc; 20 U Botox preparation) injection and placebo injection into the anal sphincter after 2 months (OR 0.75, 95% CI 0.32 to 1.77).[7] However, the results were statistically heterogeneous. **Versus topical glyceryl trinitrate (GTN):** We found one systematic review (search date 2003, 2 RCTs, 107 people).[7] The review found no significant difference in fissure persistence between botulinum A toxin-hc injection (5 U or 20 U Botox preparation) and topical GTN ointment (6 weeks treatment with 0.3% or 0.2%) after 2 months (OR 0.48, 95% CI 0.21 to 1.10).[7] However, results were statistically heterogeneous, perhaps because the doses of treatment differed between the two trials. **Versus internal anal sphincterotomy:** We found one systematic review (search date 2003, 1 RCT, 111 people).[7] It found that botulinum A toxin-hc (0.3 U/kg) significantly increased fissure persistence compared with anal sphincterotomy at 12 months (OR 5.57, 95% CI 1.52 to 20.42).[7] **Different doses of botulinum A toxin-hc:** We found one systematic review (search date 2003, 1 RCT, 150 people)[7] and one additional RCT.[13] The review found no significant difference in fissure persistence between higher dose botulinum A toxin-hc (30 U Botox preparation; retreatment with 50 U after 1 month) and lower dose botulinum A toxin-hc (20 U Botox preparation; retreatment with 30 U after 1 month) after 2 months (OR 2.87, 95% CI 0.73 to 11.25).[7] Similarly, the additional RCT (50 people) found no significant difference in fissure healing between higher dose botulinum A toxin-hc (40 U) and lower dose botulinum A toxin-hc (20 U) after 3 months (AR for healing: 20/25 [80%] with higher dose *v* 19/25 [76%] with lower dose; RR 1.10, 95% CI 0.78 to 1.41).[13] It was not clear why this study was excluded from the review. **Plus nitrates:** See benefits of botulinum A toxin-hc plus nitrates, p 463.

Harms: **Versus placebo:** The systematic review found no significant difference in adverse effects between botulinum A toxin-hc and placebo (1 RCT, 44 people; OR 1.00, 95% CI 0.24 to 4.10).[7] **Versus topical GTN:** The systematic review found that botulinum A toxin-hc was significantly less likely to cause headache compared with GTN (2 RCTs, 107 people; OR 0.11, 95% CI 0.01 to 0.93).[7] **Versus internal anal sphincterotomy:** The systematic review found that botulinum A toxin-hc was significantly less likely to cause minor incontinence compared with anal sphincterotomy (1 RCT, 111 people; OR 0.05, 95% CI 0.00 to 0.85).[7] The RCT also found that internal anal sphincterotomy significantly delayed return to daily activities compared with botulinum A toxin-hc (14.8 days with sphincterotomy *v* 1.0 day with botulinum A toxin-hc; P < 0.0001).[15] **Different doses botulinum A toxin-hc:** The RCT identified by the systematic review found that mild flatus incontinence was more common with higher than with lower dose botulinum A toxin-hc at 2 weeks after injection (5/75 [7%] with higher dose *v* 0/75 [0%] with lower dose; RR and CI values not reported).[14] The additional RCT found flatus incontinence in 6% of people for less than 2 weeks, and faecal incontinence in 4% of people for 1 week.[13] Early pilot studies reported complications associated with the use of botulinum A toxin-hc, including pain, bleeding, sepsis associated with injection, and faecal incontinence, in up to 7% of people.[16,17]

Comment: Recurrent fissure may occur after treatment is discontinued.

OPTION BOTULINUM A TOXIN-HAEMAGGLUTININ COMPLEX (BOTULINUM A TOXIN-HC) PLUS NITRATES

We found no RCTs comparing botulinum A toxin-haemagglutinin complex plus nitrates versus placebo. One small RCT found that botulinum A toxin-haemagglutinin complex plus topical isosorbide dinitrate three times daily increased fissure healing at 6 weeks compared with botulinum A toxin-haemagglutinin complex alone. It found no significant difference at 8 or 12 weeks.

Benefits: **Versus placebo:** We found no RCTs. **Versus botulinum A toxin-haemagglutinin complex (botulinum A toxin-hc) alone:** We found one RCT (30 people with anal fissures that had not healed with topical isosorbide dinitrate alone), which found that botulinum A toxin-hc Ⓖ injection (20 U) followed by topical isosorbide dinitrate (2.5 mg 3 times daily) significantly increased fissure healing compared with botulinum A toxin-hc injection alone at 6 weeks (healing: 10/15 [67%] with botulinum A toxin-hc plus isosorbide dinitrate *v* 3/15 [20%] with botulinum A toxin-hc alone; ARI 47%, 95% CI 11% to 82%; RR 3.30, 95% CI 1.14 to 9.75; NNT 3, 95% CI 2 to 5).[18] It found no significant difference at 8 and 12 weeks after treatment (healing at 8 weeks: 11/15 [73%] with botulinum A toxin-hc plus isosorbide dinitrate *v* 9/15 [60%] with botulinum A toxin-hc alone; P value reported as non-significant; healing at 12 weeks: 11/15 [73%] with botulinum A toxin-hc plus isosorbide dinitrate *v* 10/15 [66%] with botulinum A toxin-hc alone; P value reported as non-significant).

Harms: The RCT did not report on harms.[18] See harms of botulinum A toxin-haemagglutinin complex, p 463.

Comment: The RCT was small and may have lacked power to detect statistically significant differences at 8 and 12 weeks.[18]

OPTION INTERNAL ANAL SPHINCTEROTOMY

One systematic review found that internal anal sphincterotomy improved fissure healing compared with topical glyceryl trinitrate after 6 weeks to 2 years. One systematic review found that internal anal sphincterotomy reduced fissure persistence compared with botulinum A toxin-haemagglutinin complex at 12 months. One systematic review found no significant difference between internal anal sphincterotomy and anal stretch in persistence of fissures, and found that both procedures healed 70–95% of fissures. However, it found that anal stretch increased rates of flatus incontinence compared with internal anal sphincterotomy. One systematic review found no significant difference between open and closed internal anal sphincterotomy in persistence of fissures. One small RCT found no significant difference between internal anal sphincterotomy and anal advancement flap in patient satisfaction or fissure healing.

Benefits: **Versus topical glyceryl trinitrate:** See benefits of topical glyceryl trinitrate, p 460. **Versus botulinum A toxin-haemagglutinin complex:** See benefits of botulinum A toxin-haemagglutinin complex, p 462. **Versus anal stretch:** We found one systematic review (search date not reported; data pooled for end points of persistence of fissure and postoperative incontinence of flatus; 6 RCTs, 386 people), which compared internal anal sphincterotomy versus anal stretch**G**.[19] It found that both internal anal sphincterotomy and anal stretch healed 70–95% of fissures. The review found no significant difference between anal stretch and internal anal sphincterotomy in persistence of fissures (6 RCTs; RR 1.16, 95% CI 0.65 to 2.08; see comment below). **Open versus closed internal anal sphincterotomy:** The systematic review found no significant difference between open and closed internal anal sphincterotomy in persistence of fissures (2 RCTs; RR 1.61, 95% CI 0.28 to 9.28; see comment below).[19] **Versus anal advancement flap:** We found no systematic review. We found one RCT (40 people), which found no significant difference between internal anal sphincterotomy and anal advancement flap**G** in patient satisfaction or fissure healing at 3 months (people reporting themselves "dissatisfied" 3/20 [15%] with sphincterotomy v 3/20 [15%] with anal advancement, people "satisfied" or reporting the result as "excellent" 17/20 [85%] with sphincterotomy v 17/20 [85%] with anal advancement; P value not reported; fissures healed: 20/20 [100%] with sphincterotomy *v* 17/20 [85%] with anal advancement flap; P = 0.12).[20]

Harms: **Versus topical glyceryl trinitrate:** See harms of topical glyceryl trinitrate, p 460. **Versus botulinum A toxin-hc:** See harms of botulinum A toxin-haemagglutinin complex, p 463. **Versus anal stretch:** The systematic review found that anal stretch significantly increased rates of flatus incontinence compared with internal anal sphincterotomy (4 RCTs; RR 6.63, 95% CI 2.06 to 21.3; see comment below).[19] **Open versus closed internal anal sphincterotomy:** The review found no significant difference between open and closed lateral internal anal sphincterotomy in the risk of postoperative flatus incontinence (2 RCTs; RR 0.79, 95% CI 0.29 to 2.13; see comment below).[19] **Versus anal advancement flap:** In the RCT (40 people), no person experienced incontinence after either anal sphincterotomy or after anal advancement flap.[20]

Comment: Only two outcomes were considered by the systematic review: persistence of the fissure and flatus incontinence.[19] Other outcomes (e.g. complications related to wound healing) may be relevant. The review reported that, in contrast to the evidence from randomised studies, four retrospective observational studies found that anal stretch significantly increased fissure persistence compared with internal anal sphincterotomy (RR 1.89, 95% CI 1.28 to 2.81).[19] More evidence is needed to establish effects on fissure healing of anal advancement flap compared with anal sphincterotomy.

GLOSSARY

Anal advancement flap Edges of the fissure are excised and healthy anal mucosa is mobilised to cover the defect.

Anal stretch Traditionally index and middle fingers of each hand inserted into the anal canal and pulled in opposite directions, the stretch held for 1 minute.

Botulinum A toxin-haemagglutinin complex (botulinum A toxin-hc) A formulation of botulinum A toxin and haemagglutinin for injection. Different preparations are used at different doses for the same indication and the strength (in units) of one preparation may not be equivalent to that of another preparation labelled as containing the same number of units.

Internal anal sphincterotomy Incision in the internal anal sphincter either posteriorly or laterally, but more commonly laterally, and usually "tailored" to the length of the fissure.

Topical glyceryl trinitrate (GTN) Usually applied as 0.2–0.3% ointment.

REFERENCES

1. Jensen SL. Diet and other risk factors for fissure-in-ano. Prospective case control study. *Dis Colon Rectum* 1988;31:770–773.
2. Gibbons CP, Read NW. Anal hypertonia in fissures: cause or effect? *Br J Surg* 1986;73:443–445.
3. Lund JN, Scholefield JH. Internal sphincter spasm in anal fissure. *Br J Surg* 1997;84:1723–1724.
4. Martin JD. Postpartum anal fissure. *Lancet* 1953;i:271–273.
5. Lund JN, Scholefield JH. A randomised, prospective, double-blind, placebo-controlled trial of glyceryl trinitrate ointment in the treatment of anal fissure. *Lancet* 1997;349:11–14.
6. Carapeti EA, Kamm MA, McDonald PJ, et al. Randomised controlled trial shows that glyceryl trinitrate heals anal fissures, higher doses are not more effective, and there is a high recurrence rate. *Gut* 1999;44:727–730.
7. Nelson R. Non surgical therapy for anal fissure (Cochrane Review). In: The Cochrane Library, Issue 2, 2004. Chichester, UK: John Wiley & Sons, Ltd. Search date 2003; primary sources PubMed, the Cochrane Library, the CCCG specialised trials register, search of reference lists, proceedings of relevant meetings, and discussions with authors published in the field.
8. Scholefield JH, Bock JU, Marla B, et al. A dose finding study with 0.1%, 0.2%, and 0.4% glyceryl trinitrate ointment in patients with chronic anal fissures. *Gut* 2003;52:264–269.
9. Colak T, Ipek T, Urkaya N, et al. A randomised study comparing systematic transdermal treatment and local application of glyceryl trinitrate ointment in the management of chronic anal fissure. *Eur J Surg* 2002;588:188–122.
10. Bielecki K, Kolodziejczak M. A prospective randomised trial of diltiazem and glyceryltrinitrate ointment in the treatment of chronic anal fissure. *Colorectal Dis* 2003;5:256–257.
11. Jonas M, Neal KR, Abercrombie JF, et al. A randomized trial of oral vs. topical diltiazem for chronic anal fissures. *Dis Colon Rectum* 2001;44:1074–1078.
12. Pitt J, Dawson PM, Hallan RI, et al. A double-blind randomized placebo-controlled trial of oral indoramin to treat chronic anal fissure. *Colorectal Dis* 2001;3:165–168.
13. Jost W, Schrank B. Chronic anal fissures treated with botulinum toxin injections: a dose-finding study with Dysport. *Colorectal Dis* 1999;1:26–29.
14. Brisindi G, Maria G, Sganga G, et al. Effectiveness of higher doses of botulinum toxin to induce healing in patients with chronic anal fissures. *Surgery* 2002;131:179–184.
15. Mentes BB, Irkorucu O, Akin M, et al. Comparison of botulinum toxin injection and lateral internal sphincterotomy for the treatment of chronic anal fissure. *Dis Colon Rectum* 2003;46:232–237.
16. Jost WH. One hundred cases of anal fissure treated with botulin toxin: early and long-term results. *Dis Colon Rectum* 1997;40:1029–1032.
17. Jost WH, Schanne S, Mlitz H, et al. Perianal thrombosis following injection therapy into the external anal sphincter using botulinum toxin. *Dis Colon Rectum* 1995;38:781.
18. Lysy J, Israelit-Yatzkan Y, Sestiery-Ittah M, et al. Topical nitrates potentiate the effect of botulinum toxin in the treatment of patients with refractory anal fissure. *Gut* 2001;48:221–224.
19. Nelson R. Operative procedures for fissure in ano. In: The Cochrane Library, Issue 3, 2004. Oxford: Update Software. Search date 2001; primary sources Cochrane Library, Medline, the Internet, and hand searches of cited reference lists from included reports.
20. Leong AF, Seow-Choen F. Lateral sphincterotomy compared with anal advancement flap for chronic anal fissure. *Dis Colon Rectum* 1995;38:69–71.

Marion Jonas
Specialist Registrar, General Surgery

John Scholefield
Professor of Surgery
University of Nottingham, Nottingham, UK

Competing interests: MJ none declared. JS has received commercial funding for research and for attending symposia.

Appendicitis

Search date October 2003

John Simpson and William Speake

QUESTIONS

INTERVENTIONS

Key Messages

Treatments

- **Adjuvant antibiotics** One systematic review and one subsequent RCT in children and adults with simple or complicated appendicitis undergoing appendicectomy have found that prophylactic antibiotics reduce wound infections and intra-abdominal abscesses compared with no antibiotics. Subgroup analysis from the systematic review has found that antibiotics reduce the number of wound infections in children with complicated appendicitis compared with no antibiotics. However, subgroup analysis from the systematic review found no significant difference in the number of wound infections between antibiotics and no antibiotics in children with simple appendicitis. One subsequent RCT in children with simple appendicitis found no significant difference with antibiotic prophylaxis compared with no antibiotic prophylaxis in wound infections, but the RCT may have been too small to exclude a clinically important difference.
- **Laparoscopic surgery versus open surgery (in children)** One systematic review has found that, in children, laparoscopic surgery reduced the number of wound infections and the length of hospital stay compared with open surgery, but found no significant difference in postoperative pain, time to mobilisation, or proportion of intra-abdominal abscesses.
- **Antibiotics versus surgery** One small RCT in adults with suspected appendicitis found that conservative treatment with antibiotics reduced pain and morphine consumption for the first 10 days compared with appendicectomy. However, the RCT found that 35% of people treated with antibiotics were readmitted within 1 year with acute appendicitis and subsequently underwent appendicectomy.
- **Laparoscopic surgery versus open surgery (in adults)** One systematic review and one subsequent RCT have found that laparoscopic surgery in adults reduces wound infections, postoperative pain, duration of hospital stay, and time taken to return to work compared with open surgery. However, the systematic review found that laparoscopic surgery increased postoperative intra-abdominal abscesses compared with open surgery.

- **Open surgery versus no treatment** We found no RCTs comparing open surgery versus no surgery.
- **Stump inversion at open appendicectomy** One RCT found no significant difference between stump inversion and simple ligation in wound infection, length of hospital stay, or intra-abdominal abscesses. Another RCT found that stump inversion increased wound infections compared with simple ligation, but found no significant difference between groups for intra-abdominal abscesses or length of hospital stay.

DEFINITION	Acute appendicitis is acute inflammation of the vermiform appendix.
INCIDENCE/ PREVALENCE	The incidence of acute appendicitis is falling, although the reason for this is unclear. The reported lifetime risk of appendicitis in the USA is 8.7% in men and 6.7% in women,[1] and there are about 60 000 cases reported annually in England and Wales. Appendicitis is the most common surgical emergency requiring operation.
AETIOLOGY/ RISK FACTORS	The cause of appendicitis is uncertain, although various theories exist. Most relate to luminal obstruction, which prevents escape of secretions and inevitably leads to a rise in intraluminal pressure within the appendix. This can lead to subsequent mucosal ischaemia, and the stasis provides an ideal environment for bacterial overgrowth. Potential causes of the obstruction are faecoliths, often because of constipation, lymphoid hyperplasia, or caecal carcinoma.[2]
PROGNOSIS	The prognosis of untreated appendicitis is unknown, although spontaneous resolution has been reported in at least 1/13 (8%) episodes.[3] The recurrence of appendicitis after conservative management,[3,4] and recurrent abdominal symptoms in certain people,[5] suggests that chronic appendicitis and recurrent acute or subacute appendicitis may also exist.[6] The standard treatment for acute appendicitis is appendicectomy. RCTs comparing treatment with no treatment would be regarded as unethical. The mortality from acute appendicitis is less than 0.3%, rising to 1.7% after perforation.[7] The most common complication of appendicectomy is wound infection, occurring in 5–33% of cases.[8] Intra-abdominal abscess formation occurs less frequently, in 2% of appendicectomies.[9] A perforated appendix in childhood does not appear to have subsequent negative consequences on female fertility.[10]
AIMS OF INTERVENTION	To reduce pain; prevent postoperative infection; shorten hospital stay; and hasten return to normal activity.
OUTCOMES	Wound infection rates; intra-abdominal infection rates; postoperative pain; return of bowel function; return to normal activity; mortality.
METHODS	*Clinical Evidence* search and appraisal October 2003.

QUESTION What are the effects of medical treatment for acute appendicitis?

OPTION ANTIBIOTICS

We found no RCTs comparing antibiotics versus placebo or no treatment. One small RCT in adults with suspected appendicitis found that conservative treatment with antibiotics reduced pain and morphine consumption for the first 10 days compared with appendicectomy. However, the RCT found that 35% of people treated with antibiotics were readmitted within 1 year with acute appendicitis and subsequently had an appendicectomy.

Benefits: **Versus no treatment:** We found no systematic review and no RCTs comparing antibiotics versus placebo or no treatment. **Versus surgery:** We found one RCT (40 adults with suspected appendicitis), which compared antibiotic treatment (iv cefotaxime 2 g twice daily plus tinidazole 800 mg/day for 2 days followed by oral ofloxacin 200 mg twice daily plus tinidazole 500 mg twice daily for 8 days) versus open appendicectomy.[4] It found that antibiotics significantly reduced pain in the period from 12 hours to 10 days after initiation of treatment compared with appendicectomy ($P < 0.01$; other data presented graphically) and significantly reduced morphine consumption ($P < 0.001$).

Harms: **Versus no treatment:** We found no systematic review and no RCTs. **Versus surgery:** The RCT (40 adults with suspected appendicitis) found that all people treated conservatively with antibiotics were discharged from hospital within 48 hours, except one who had surgery for generalised peritonitis after a perforation of the appendix 12 hours after randomisation to receive antibiotic treatment.[4] The RCT found that 7/20 (35%) people who received conservative management were readmitted with acute appendicitis and had an appendicectomy within 1 year (mean 7 months, range 3–12 months). The RCT found that there was one wound infection in the surgically treated group, and that no deaths occurred with either treatment.

Comment: Inclusion criteria for the RCT included typical symptoms and signs of acute appendicitis, such as positive findings on ultrasound, and raised neutrophil/C reactive protein levels on blood assays.

QUESTION What are the effects of surgical treatment for acute appendicitis?

OPTION OPEN SURGERY

We found no systematic review or RCTs of open surgery compared with no treatment. One RCT in adults with suspected appendicitis found that conservative treatment with antibiotics reduced pain and morphine consumption compared with appendicectomy for the first 10 days after starting treatment. However, it found that 35% of people treated with antibiotics were readmitted within 1 year with acute appendicitis and subsequently underwent appendicectomy.

Benefits: **Versus no treatment:** We found no systematic review or RCTs of open surgery versus no treatment. **Versus antibiotics:** See benefits of antibiotics, p 467.

Harms: **Versus no treatment:** We found no RCTs. **Versus antibiotics:** See harms of antibiotics, p 468.

Comment: Surgery is now a well established treatment. An RCT that compares open surgery versus no treatment is unlikely to be conducted due to ethical concerns.

OPTION LAPAROSCOPIC SURGERY VERSUS OPEN SURGERY

One systematic review and one subsequent RCT have found that laparoscopic surgery in adults reduces wound infections, postoperative pain, duration of hospital stay, and time taken to return to work compared with open surgery. However, the systematic review found that laparoscopic surgery increased postoperative intra-abdominal abscesses compared with open surgery. The review found that, in children, laparoscopic surgery reduced the number of wound infections and the length of hospital stay compared with open surgery, but found no significant difference in postoperative pain, time to mobilisation, or proportion of intra-abdominal abscesses.

Benefits: We found one systematic review (search date 2002)[11] and one subsequent RCT[12] comparing laparoscopic surgery versus open surgery. **In adults:** The systematic review found that laparoscopic surgery significantly reduced the number of wound infections compared with open surgery, but significantly increased the number of postoperative intra-abdominal abscesses (wound infections: 34 RCTs, 4324 adults; 86/2213 [4%] with laparoscopic surgery *v* 161/2111 [8%] with open surgery; OR 0.47, 95% CI 0.36 to 0.62; abscesses: 34 RCTs, 4373 adults; 41/2239 [2%] with laparoscopic surgery *v* 13/2134 [< 1%] with open surgery; OR 2.77, 95% CI 1.61 to 4.77).[11] The review also found that laparoscopic surgery significantly reduced pain on the first postoperative day, and reduced the length of hospital stay and time taken to return to work (reduction in pain measured using a 100 mm visual analogue scale: 8 mm, 95% CI 3 mm to 13 mm; reduction in length of hospital stay: 0.7 days, 95% CI 0.4 days to 1.0 days; reduction in time to return to work: 3 days, 95% CI 1 day to 5 days). The subsequent RCT (200 adults with suspected appendicitis) found that laparoscopic surgery significantly reduced pain on the second and seventh postoperative days compared with open surgery (pain assessed on a visual analogue scale [1 = no pain; 10 = unbearable pain]; mean pain score on day 2: 2.79 with laparoscopic surgery *v* 4.77 with open surgery, P < 0.001; mean pain score on day 7: 1.26 with laparoscopic surgery *v* 1.95 with open surgery, P < 0.001).[12] The RCT found that laparoscopic surgery significantly reduced the time to return to full activity compared with open surgery (15.85 days *v* 19.65 days, P < 0.01), although it found no significant difference in incidence of postoperative complications or in length of hospital stay between laparoscopic and open surgery (postoperative complications: 9/96 [9.4%] with laparoscopic surgery *v* 7/104 [6.7%] with open surgery, P > 0.05; length of hospital stay: 4.7 days with laparoscopic surgery *v* 5.0 days with open surgery; difference stated as not significant). **In children:** The systematic review (5 RCTs, 436 children aged 1–16 years) found that laparoscopic surgery significantly reduced the number of wound infections and the length of hospital stay compared with open surgery (wound infections: 5 RCTs, 436 children; OR 0.22, 95% CI 0.08 to 0.61; difference in hospital stay: 1 RCT, difference of –0.7 days, 95% CI –1.1 days to –0.3 days).[11] The review found no significant difference between laparoscopic surgery and open surgery for intra-abdominal abscesses, in postoperative pain, and in the time to mobilisation (intra-abdominal abscesses: 5 RCTs, 436 children: 1/220 [0.45%] with laparoscopic appendicectomy *v* 1/216 [0.46%] with conventional appendicectomy; OR 1.00, 95% CI 0.06 to 16.50; postoperative pain: 2 RCTs, 124 children; difference in visual analogue scale –0.068 cm, 95% CI –0.797 cm to +0.660 cm; time to mobilisation: 1 RCT, 58 children; difference of –0.25 days, 95% CI –0.65 days to +0.15 days).

Harms: The review did not report any further data on harms.[11]

Comment: The systematic review included people with a clinical diagnosis of acute appendicitis and provided no information on preoperative imaging or the use of perioperative antibiotics.[11] Analyses were performed on an intention to treat basis. Studies reporting a negative appendicectomy[G] rate of more than 50% were excluded. The number of trials looking specifically at paediatric practice is small and, as in the adult studies, not all outcomes were assessed in all trials. Most trials were unblinded and, in addition, heterogeneity was present in most analyses, although not for wound infections or intra-abdominal abscesses. The definition and reporting of additional operative or postoperative complications was inconsistent. One RCT included in the review subsequently presented results from a subset of 25 children aged 4–15 years with complicated appendicitis.[13] It found no significant difference between laparoscopic and open surgery in the length of hospital stay or time to return to normal activities. It found two major complications (one pelvic abscess and one entero-cutaneous fistula) in 13 people receiving laparoscopic surgery compared with no major complications in 12 people receiving open surgery. In the subsequent RCT, participants were required to stay in hospital for a minimum of 3 days.[12]

OPTION STUMP INVERSION AT OPEN APPENDICECTOMY

One RCT found no significant difference between stump inversion and simple ligation in wound infection, length of hospital stay, or intra-abdominal abscesses. Another RCT found that stump inversion increased wound infections compared with simple ligation, but found no significant difference between groups for intra-abdominal abscesses or length of hospital stay.

Benefits: We found no systematic review but found two RCTs.[14,15] The first RCT (735 people aged 14–91 years with complicated or simple appendicitis Ⓖ) compared double invagination (purse string with Z stitch, 374 people) versus simple ligation of the stump (361 people).[14] The RCT found no significance difference in wound infection, length of hospital stay, or intra-abdominal abscesses between double invagination and simple ligation (wound infection: 33/374 [8.8%] with double invagination v 30/361 [8.3%] with simple ligation; length of hospital stay: 4.6 days with double invagination v 4.9 days with simple ligation; intra-abdominal abscesses: 6/374 [1.6%] with double invagination v 2/361 [< 1%] with simple ligation). The second RCT (134 people aged 4–90 years) compared simple ligation versus double invagination.[15] The RCT found a significantly higher incidence of wound infection with double invagination compared with simple ligation but found no significant difference for intra-abdominal abscesses or length of hospital stay (wound infection: 4/55 [7.3%] with double invagination v 0/79 [0%] with simple ligation, $P = 0.017$; abscesses: 1 in each group; length of hospital stay: median 5 days for both groups).

Harms: In the two RCTs, postoperative adhesive ileus was seen more frequently in the double invagination groups (6/374 [1.6%] with double invagination v 1/361 [< 1%] with simple ligation, $P < 0.05$;[14] 1/55 [1.8%] with double invagination v 0/79 [0%] with simple ligation[15]). No other specific complications were documented.[14,15]

Comment: Increased complications after invagination are believed to be due to longer operative time. Both trials comment on potential caecal distortion after invagination of the appendix stump, which has mimicked caecal cancer on subsequent contrast imaging — a further potential hazard of stump invagination.[14,15]

QUESTION What are the effects of adjuvant treatments for acute appendicitis?

OPTION ADJUVANT ANTIBIOTICS

One systematic review and one subsequent RCT in children and adults with simple or complicated appendicitis undergoing appendicectomy have found that prophylactic antibiotics reduce wound infections and intra-abdominal abscesses compared with no antibiotics. Subgroup analysis from the systematic review has found that antibiotics reduce the number of wound infections in children with complicated appendicitis compared with no antibiotics. However, subgroup analysis from the systematic review found no significant difference in the number of wound infections between antibiotics and no antibiotics in children with simple appendicitis. One subsequent RCT in children with simple appendicitis found no significant difference with antibiotic prophylaxis compared with no antibiotic prophylaxis in wound infections, but the RCT may have been too small to exclude a clinically important difference.

Benefits: **Versus placebo or no treatment:** We found one systematic review (search date 2000, 44 RCTs or CCTs, 9298 adults and children having an appendicectomy with either simple appendicitis or complicated appendicitis❻)[9] and one subsequent RCT, which compared antibiotic prophylaxis versus placebo or no prophylaxis.[16] The review found that perioperative systemic antibiotic prophylaxis significantly reduced wound infections and intra-abdominal abscesses compared with no antibiotic prophylaxis (wound infections, 20 RCTs/CCTs: 287/4326 [7%] with antibiotics *v* 632/4317 [15%] with no antibiotics; OR 0.32, 95% CI 0.24 to 0.42; see comment below; intra-abdominal abscesses, 8 RCTs/CCTs: 16/2211 [< 1%] with antibiotics *v* 39/2257 [2%] with no antibiotics; OR 0.35, 95% CI 0.13 to 0.91).[9] Subgroup analysis found that, in people with simple appendicitis, antibiotic prophylaxis significantly reduced wound infections and intra-abdominal abscesses compared with no antibiotics (wound infections, 26 RCTs/CCTs: 113/2610 [4%] with antibiotics *v* 286/2707 [11%] with no antibiotics; OR 0.37, 95% CI 0.30 to 0.46; intra-abdominal abscesses, 8 RCTs/CCTs: 9/1433 [< 1%] with antibiotics *v* 22/1535 [1%] with no antibiotics; OR 0.46, 95% CI 0.23 to 0.94). A subgroup analysis in people with complicated appendicitis found that antibiotic prophylaxis significantly reduced wound infections but found no significant difference in intra-abdominal abscesses (wound infections, 24 RCTs/CCTs: 121/645 [19%] with antibiotics *v* 175/507 [35%] with no antibiotics; OR 0.28, 95% CI 0.21 to 0.38; intra-abdominal abscesses, 3 RCTs/CCTs: 3/262 [1%] with antibiotics *v* 4/205 [2%] with no antibiotics; OR 0.54, 95% CI 0.12 to 2.43). The review also found no significant difference in wound infections between topical antibiotics and placebo (52/339 [15%] with topical antibiotics *v* 61/340 [18%] with placebo; OR 0.77, 95% CI 0.49 to 1.23). **In children:** The systematic review (7 RCTs, 987 children aged 0–15 years with either simple or complicated appendicitis) found no significant difference between perioperative systemic antibiotic prophylaxis and no antibiotic prophylaxis in wound infections or intra-abdominal abscesses (wound infections: 23/548 [4%] with antibiotics *v* 34/542 [6%] with no antibiotics; OR 0.64, 95% CI 0.37 to 1.10; intra-abdominal abscesses: 1/142 [< 1%] with antibiotics *v* 5/141 [4%] with no antibiotics; OR 0.25, 95% CI 0.05 to 1.26; see comment below).[9] Subgroup analysis in children with simple appendicitis found no significant difference between treatments in wound infections, although in children with complicated appendicitis, antibiotic prophylaxis significantly reduced wound infections (simple appendicitis, 3 RCTs/CCTs: 7/347 [2%] with antibiotics *v* 8/357 [2%] with no antibiotics; OR 0.92, 95% CI 0.33 to 2.57; complicated appendicitis, 3 RCTs/CCTs: 5/134 [4%] with antibiotics *v* 15/119 [13%] with no antibiotics; OR 0.31, 95% CI 0.12 to 0.77). The subsequent RCT (108 children with simple appendicitis) compared three treatments: no antibiotic, one antibiotic dose (1 g ceftriaxone), and 5 days of regular antibiotics (1 g/day ceftriaxone).[16] The RCT reported that only one wound infection occurred, and this was in a child who received no antibiotics (other numerical data not provided).

Harms: Several harms have been considered in the benefits section. The review and RCT did not report any further data on harms.[9,16]

Comment: The systematic review did not distinguish between antibiotic regimens or between different antibiotic drugs.[9] These issues are being addressed in a systematic review to be published in the future. There were limited numbers of children in the systematic review and RCT; therefore, the results may lack statistical power.[9,16] The review found insufficient data to provide subgroup analysis for numbers of intra-abdominal abscesses in children with either simple or complicated appendicitis.[9] The benefit of antibiotics for simple appendicitis in children is unclear. The review did not report on preoperative imaging studies.[9]

GLOSSARY

Complicated appendicitis Perforated or gangrenous appendicitis or the presence of a periappendicular abscess.

Simple appendicitis Clinically normal or inflamed appendix, in the absence of gangrene, perforation, or abscess around the appendix.

Negative appendicectomy Term used for an operation performed for suspected appendicitis, in which the appendix is found to be normal on histological evaluation.

REFERENCES

1. Addiss DG, Shaffer N, Fowler BS, et al. The epidemiology of appendicitis and appendectomy in the United States. *Am J Epidemiol* 1990;132:910–925.
2. Larner AJ. The aetiology of appendicitis. *Br J Hosp Med* 1988;39:540–542.
3. Cobben LP, de van Otterloo AM, Puylaert JB. Spontaneously resolving acute appendicitis: frequency and natural history in 60 patients. *Radiology* 2000;215:349–352.
4. Eriksson S, Granstrom L. Randomized controlled trial of appendicectomy versus antibiotic therapy for acute appendicitis. *Br J Surg* 1995;82:166–169.
5. Barber MD, McLaren J, Rainey JB. Recurrent appendicitis. *Br J Surg* 1997;84:110–112.
6. Mattei P, Sola JE, Yeo CJ. Chronic and recurrent appendicitis are uncommon entities often misdiagnosed. *J Am Coll Surg* 1994;178:385–389.
7. Velanovich V, Satava R. Balancing the normal appendectomy rate with the perforated appendicitis rate: implications for quality assurance. *Am Surg* 1992;58:264–269.
8. Krukowski ZH, Irwin ST, Denholm S, et al. Preventing wound infection after appendicectomy: a review. *Br J Surg* 1988;75:1023–1033.
9. Andersen BR, Kallehave FL, Andersen HK. Antibiotics versus placebo for prevention of postoperative infection after appendectomy. In: The Cochrane Library, Issue 4, 2003. Chichester, UK: John Wiley & Sons, Ltd. Search date 2000; primary sources Cochrane Controlled Trials Register, Medline, Embase, Cochrane Colorectal Cancer Group Specialised Register, and hand searches of reference lists of identified trials.
10. Andersson R, Lambe M, Bergstrom R. Fertility patterns after appendicectomy: historical cohort study. *BMJ* 1999;318:963–967.
11. Sauerland SR, Lefering R, Neugebauer EAM. Laparoscopic versus open surgery for suspected appendicitis. In: The Cochrane Library, Issue 4, 2003. Chichester, UK: John Wiley & Sons, Ltd. Search date 2002; primary sources The Cochrane Library, Medline, Embase, Scisearch, and Biosis.
12. Milewczyk M, Michalik M, Ciesielski M.A prospective, randomized, unicenter study comparing laparoscopic and open treatments of acute appendicitis. *Surg Endosc* 2003;17:1023–1028.
13. Lintula H, Kokki H, Vanamo K, et al. Laparoscopy in children with complicated appendicitis. *J Pediatr Surg* 2002;37:1317–1320.
14. Engstrom L, Fenyo G. Appendicectomy: assessment of stump invagination versus simple ligation: a prospective, randomized trial. *Br J Surg* 1985;72:971–972.
15. Jacobs PP, Koeyers GF, Bruyninckx CM. Simple ligation superior to inversion of the appendiceal stump; a prospective randomized study. *Ned Tijdschr Geneeskd* 1992;136:1020–1023. [in Dutch]
16. Gorecki WJ, Grochowski JA. Are antibiotics necessary in nonperforated appendicitis in children? A double blind randomised controlled trial. *Med Sci Monit* 2001;7:289–292.

John Simpson
Lecturer in Surgery
University of Nottingham
Nottingham
UK

William Speake
Specialist Registrar
Division of Gastrointestinal Surgery
University Hospital Nottingham
Nottingham
UK

Competing interests: None declared.

Cholecystitis (acute)

Search date December 2003

Julie Margenthaler, Douglas Schuerer, and Robb Whinney

QUESTIONS

INTERVENTIONS

See glossary

Key Messages

- **Early cholecystectomy** Four RCTs found that operation before the scheduled date because of recurrent or worsening symptoms was necessary in 13–19% of people receiving delayed cholecystectomy (open or laparoscopic cholecystectomy after 6–8 weeks). The RCTs found no significant difference between early (within 72 hours) and delayed cholecystectomy (open or laparoscopic) in intraoperative or postoperative complications, but found that early cholecystectomy reduced hospital stay. Two RCTs found that early laparoscopic cholecystectomy increased duration of operation compared with delayed laparoscopic cholecystectomy but reduced use of analgesics. The RCTs found no significant difference between early and delayed laparoscopic cholecystectomy in the rate of conversion to open cholecystectomy.
- **Laparoscopic cholecystectomy** One RCT found that observation alone had a failure rate after 8 years of 30%, but found no difference in the rate of gallstone related complications (recurrent cholecystitis, pancreatitis, intractable pain) or emergency admissions for pain compared with cholecystectomy (open or laparoscopic). Three RCTs found that laparoscopic cholecystectomy reduced hospital stay, and found limited evidence that it reduced duration of surgery and intraoperative/postoperative complications compared with open cholecystectomy. One RCT found no difference between conventional laparoscopic cholecystectomy and minilaparoscopic cholecystectomy in use of analgesics, hospital stay, and rates of conversion to open cholecystectomy. Duration of surgery was marginally shorter with conventional laparoscopic cholecystectomy.
- **Minilaparoscopic cholecystectomy** One RCT found no difference between minilaparoscopic and conventional laparoscopic cholecystectomy in use of analgesics, hospital stay, and rates of conversion to open cholecystectomy. Duration of surgery was marginally longer with minilaparoscopic cholecystectomy.

- **Open cholecystectomy** One RCT found that observation alone had a failure rate after 8 years of 30%, but found no difference in the rate of gallstone related complications (recurrent cholecystitis, pancreatitis, intractable pain) or emergency admissions for pain compared with cholecystectomy (open or laparoscopic). Three RCTs found that open cholecystectomy increased hospital stay and found limited evidence that it increased duration of surgery and intraoperative/postoperative complications compared with laparoscopic cholecystectomy.
- **Observation alone** One RCT found that observation alone had a failure rate after 8 years of 30%, but found no difference in the rate of gallstone related complications (recurrent cholecystitis, pancreatitis, intractable pain) or emergency admissions for pain compared with cholecystectomy (open or laparoscopic).

DEFINITION **Acute cholecystitis** results from obstruction of the cystic duct usually by a gallstone followed by distension and subsequent chemical or bacterial inflammation of the gallbladder. People with acute cholecystitis usually have unremitting right upper quadrant pain, anorexia, nausea, vomiting, and fever. About 95% of people with acute cholecystitis have gallstones (calculous cholecystitis) and 5% lack gallstones (acalculous cholecystitis).[1] Severe acute cholecystitis may lead to necrosis of the gallbladder wall known as gangrenous cholecystitis. This review does not include people with acute cholangitis, which is a severe complication of gallstone disease and generally a result of bacterial infection.

INCIDENCE/ PREVALENCE The incidence of acute cholecystitis among people with gallstones is unknown. Twenty per cent of people admitted to hospital for biliary tract disease have acute cholecystitis.[1] The number of cholecystectomies carried out for acute cholecystitis has increased from the mid 1980s to the early 1990s, especially in elderly people.[2] Acute calculous cholecystitis is three times more common in women than men up to the age of 50 years, and about 1.5 times more common in women than men thereafter.[1]

AETIOLOGY/ RISK FACTORS Acute calculous cholecystitis seems to be caused by obstruction of the cystic duct by a gallstone or local mucosal erosion and inflammation caused by a stone, but cystic duct ligation alone does not produce acute cholecystitis in animal studies. The role of bacteria in the pathogenesis of acute cholecystitis is not clear; positive cultures of bile or gallbladder wall are found in 50–75% of cases.[3,4] The cause of acute acalculous cholecystitis is uncertain and may be multifactorial, including increased susceptibility to bacterial colonisation of static gallbladder bile.[1]

PROGNOSIS Complications of acute cholecystitis include perforation of the gallbladder, pericholecystic abscess, and fistula caused by gallbladder wall ischaemia and infection. In the USA, the overall mortality from untreated complications is about 20%.[5]

AIMS OF INTERVENTION To reduce mortality and morbidity relating to acute cholecystitis, with minimal adverse effects of treatment.

OUTCOMES Mortality at 30 days, persistent pain, intolerance to food, recurrent attacks of cholecystitis, quality of life, and adverse effects of treatment. Some outcomes relate to surgery: duration of surgery, need for nasogastric tube, need for/duration of analgesics, need for antibiotics, rate of surgical complications (bile duct injuries, pancreatitis, other), and duration of hospital stay. Postoperative fall in haemoglobin and conversion of a planned laparoscopic cholecystectomy Ⓖ to an open cholecystectomy Ⓖ are surrogate outcomes.

METHODS *Clinical Evidence* search and appraisal December 2003. None of the RCTs stated whether participants had calculous or acalculous cholecystitis. The RCTs excluded people unable to undergo surgery because of comorbid conditions (recent myocardial infarction, severe chronic obstructive pulmonary disease or respiratory insufficiency, end stage metastatic disease, and multi system organ failure) and contraindications for cholecystectomy (use of antiplatelet therapy that could not safely be discontinued during the perioperative period).

QUESTION **What are the effects of treatments for acute cholecystitis?**

OPTION **LAPAROSCOPIC CHOLECYSTECTOMY**

One RCT found that observation alone had a failure rate after 8 years of 30%, but found no difference in the rate of gallstone related complications (recurrent cholecystitis, pancreatitis, intractable pain) or emergency admissions for pain compared with cholecystectomy (open or laparoscopic). Three RCTs found that laparoscopic cholecystectomy reduced hospital stay and found limited evidence that it reduced duration of surgery and intraoperative and postoperative complications compared with open cholecystectomy. One RCT found no difference between conventional laparoscopic cholecystectomy and minilaparoscopic cholecystectomy in use of analgesics, hospital stay, and rates of conversion to open cholecystectomy. Duration of surgery was marginally shorter with conventional laparoscopic cholecystectomy.

Benefits: **Versus no treatment:** We found no systematic review or RCTs comparing laparoscopic cholecystectomy**G** versus no treatment. We found one RCT (64 people with acute cholecystitis) comparing (laparoscopic or open) cholecystectomy versus observation alone.[6] In the cholecystectomy group, 27/31 (87%) people had the operation at a median of 3.6 months after randomisation. After 8 years, 10/33 (30%) people, who were originally randomised to observation, had undergone cholecystectomy (failure rate). In the cholecystectomy group, 4/31 (13%) refused operation on the grounds of freedom from symptoms ($P < 0.0001$). **Versus open cholecystectomy:G**. We found no systematic review, but found three RCTs.[7–9] All three RCTs found that laparoscopic cholecystectomy improved intraoperative and postoperative outcomes compared with open cholecystectomy. The first RCT (271 people with acute cholecystitis) compared laparoscopic (146 people) versus open (97 people) cholecystectomy.[7] The rate of conversion from laparoscopic to open cholecystectomy was 27%. The people randomised to receive open cholecystectomy were on average 10 years older than people receiving laparoscopic cholecystectomy ($P < 0.001$), and had a significantly higher incidence of comorbid conditions ($P = 0.002$) and gangrenous cholecystitis ($P = 0.03$). The RCT found that, compared with open cholecystectomy, laparoscopic cholecystectomy significantly reduced duration of surgery (mean 60 minutes with laparoscopic *v* 90 minutes with open cholecystectomy; $P < 0.00001$), use of nasogastric tube (51% with laparoscopic *v* 94% with open cholecystectomy; $P < 0.0001$), mean use of analgesia (75 mg pethidine with laparoscopic *v* 175 mg with open cholecystectomy; $P < 0.0001$; 1 g oral metamizole with laparoscopic *v* 3 g with open cholecystectomy; $P < 0.0001$), and hospital stay (3 days with laparoscopic *v* 7 days with open cholecystectomy; $P < 0.0001$). The second RCT (63 people with acute cholecystitis) compared laparoscopic versus open cholecystectomy.[8] The rate of conversion from laparoscopic to open cholecystectomy was 16%. The RCT found that laparoscopic cholecystectomy significantly reduced hospital stay compared with open cholecystectomy (4 days with laparoscopic *v* 14 days with open cholecystectomy; $P = 0.0063$). It found no significant difference in duration of surgery between laparoscopic and open cholecystectomy (mean 108 minutes with laparoscopic *v* 99 minutes with open cholecystectomy; $P = 0.49$). The third RCT (230 people with acute cholecystitis) reported a conversion rate from laparoscopic to open cholecystectomy of 5/109 (4.4%). It found no significant difference in duration of surgery between laparoscopic and open cholecystectomy, although laparoscopic cholecystectomy tended to be slightly shorter

(95 ± 43.7 minutes with laparoscopic cholecystectomy v 102.3 ± 46.3 minutes with open cholecystectomy; P value reported as non-significant).[9] Similarly, the RCT found no significant difference in mean fall in haemoglobin postoperatively between laparoscopic and open cholecystectomy, although the mean fall was smaller in the laparoscopic cholecystectomy group (mean fall in haemoglobin: 1.9 g/L in the open cholecystectomy group v 1.1 g/L in the laparoscopic cholecystectomy group; P = 0.6). Postoperative hospital stay was shorter in the laparoscopic cholecystectomy group (8.5 ± 3.9 days in the open cholecystectomy group v 5.8 ± 4.2 days in the laparoscopy group; P value not reported). **Versus minilaparoscopic cholecystectomy:** See benefits of minilaparoscopic cholecystectomy, p 477.

Harms: **Versus no treatment:** The RCT comparing cholecystectomy versus observation found no significant difference in the overall rate of gallstone related events (complications or emergency admissions for pain; 6/31 [19%] with cholecystectomy v 12/33 [36%] with observation; P = 0.16).[6] Similarly, the RCT found no significant difference in the rates of major or minor operative complications in people receiving cholecystectomy comparing people randomised to cholecystectomy versus people randomised to observation (major complication rate: 3/27 [11%] in the group randomised to cholecystectomy v 1/10 [10%] in the group randomised to observation; minor complication rate: 7/27 [26%] in the group randomised to cholecystectomy v 1/10 [10%] in the group randomised to observation; P = 0.66 for difference in overall postoperative complications between the two groups). Major complications included bile duct injuries or haemorrhage, whereas minor complications included wound infection, subphrenic collections, or miscellaneous infections (urinary and respiratory). The RCT found no gallstone related deaths in either group. **Versus open cholecystectomy:** The first RCT found no significant difference between laparoscopic cholecystectomy**G** and open cholecystectomy in the proportion of people with postoperative complications (24/146 [16%] with laparoscopic v 25/97 [26%] with open; reported as non-significant, CI not reported).[7] Complications were classified as surgical infections (wound infection, subphrenic, or subhepatic abscess), non-infectious surgical (bile duct injury or haemorrhage), remote infections (urinary or respiratory), and miscellaneous (atelectasis or deep vein thrombosis). The second RCT found that laparoscopic cholecystectomy significantly reduced postoperative complications compared with open cholecystectomy (major complications: 0% with laparoscopic v 23% with open cholecystectomy; minor complications: 3% with laparoscopic v 19% with open cholecystectomy; P = 0.0048 for overall complication rate comparing laparoscopic v open cholecystectomy).[8] Major complications included myocardial infarction, pneumonia and sepsis, femoral artery embolism, serious wound infection, late incisional hernia requiring surgical repair, adhesive intestinal obstruction within 1 month of cholecystectomy, and retained common bile duct stone. Minor complications included diarrhoea, urinary infection, and confusion. The RCT found no deaths or bile duct injuries in either treatment group. The third RCT found higher complication rates with open cholecystectomy compared with laparoscopic cholecystectomy (overall complication rate: 26/116 [22.4%] with open cholecystectomy v 14/109 [12.8%] with laparoscopic cholecystectomy; intraoperative complication rate: 12/116 [10.3%] with open cholecystectomy v 8/109 [7.3%] with laparoscopic cholecystectomy; postoperative complication rate: 14/116 [12%] with open cholecystectomy v 6/109 [5.5%] with laparoscopic cholecystectomy, P values not reported).[9] Intraoperative complications included haemorrhage, bile duct injury, and passing of stones; postoperative complications were defined as haemorrhage, pneumonia, thrombosis, bile duct stones, bile leakage, or wound infections. **Versus minilaparoscopic cholecystectomy:** See harms of minilaparoscopic cholecystectomy, p 478.

Comment: None of the RCTs differentiated between calculous and acalculous cholecystitis. **Versus open cholecystectomy:** The first RCT found that laparoscopic surgery was associated with fewer complications if undertaken by more experienced surgeons.[7] Open cholecystectomy is primarily required in people who have a fistula from the gallbladder into the bile duct or intestine and in some people who have perforation and abscess in the right upper quadrant. Conversion from laparoscopic to open cholecystectomy is needed if the laparoscopic procedure cannot be completed without risking injury to surrounding structures or when bleeding cannot be stopped. We found one systematic review in people with symptomatic gallstones, which did not differentiate between people with and without acute cholecystitis.[10] The review (search date 1995) indirectly compared outcomes in people who had laparoscopic cholecystectomy (98 case series or RCTs, 78 747 people with symptomatic gallstones) versus outcomes in people who had open cholecystectomy (28 case series or RCTs, 12 973 people treated with open cholecystectomy). It found that laparoscopic cholecystectomy was associated with lower mortality (86–91/100 000 with laparoscopic *v* 660–740/100 000 with open cholecystectomy; CI not reported) but a higher rate of bile duct injury (36–47/10 000 with laparoscopic *v* 19–29/10 000 with open cholecystectomy; CI not reported).

OPTION OPEN CHOLECYSTECTOMY

One RCT found that observation alone had a failure rate after 8 years of 30%, but found no difference in the rate of gallstone related complications (recurrent cholecystitis, pancreatitis, intractable pain) or emergency admissions for pain compared with cholecystectomy (open or laparoscopic). Three RCTs found that open cholecystectomy increased hospital stay and found limited evidence that it increased duration of surgery and intraoperative and postoperative complications compared with laparoscopic cholecystectomy.

Benefits: **Versus no treatment:** We found no systematic review or RCTs only comparing open cholecystectomy versus no treatment (see benefits of laparoscopic cholecystectomy, p 475). **Versus laparoscopic cholecystectomy:** See benefits of laparoscopic cholecystectomy, p 475.

Harms: **Versus no treatment:** See harms of laparoscopic cholecystectomy, p 476. **Versus laparoscopic cholecystectomy:** See harms of laparoscopic cholecystectomy, p 476.

Comment: **Versus laparoscopic cholecystectomy:** See comments under laparoscopic cholecystectomy, p 477.

OPTION MINILAPAROSCOPIC CHOLECYSTECTOMY

One RCT found no difference between minilaparoscopic and conventional laparoscopic cholecystectomy in use of analgesics, hospital stay, and rates of conversion to open cholecystectomy. Duration of surgery was marginally longer with minilaparoscopic cholecystectomy.

Benefits: **Versus no treatment:** We found no systematic review and no RCTs comparing minilaparoscopic cholecystectomy Ⓖ versus no treatment. **Versus conventional laparoscopic cholecystectomy:** We found one

RCT (69 people with acute cholecystitis) comparing minilaparoscopic cholecystectomy (2–3 mm diameter instruments) versus conventional laparoscopic cholecystectomy (5 mm diameter instruments).[11] It found no significant difference between minilaparoscopic and conventional laparoscopic cholecystectomy in the rate of conversion to open cholecystectomy**G** (7.9% with minilaparoscopic *v* 6.5% with conventional laparoscopic cholecystectomy; P = 0.597). It found that a similar proportion of people needed postoperative antiemetics plus analgesics (30/35 [86%] with minilaparoscopic *v* 22/29 [76%] with conventional laparoscopic; P value not reported), and found no significant difference between minilaparoscopic and conventional laparoscopic cholecystectomy in duration of hospital stay (mean 4.3 days with minilaparoscopic *v* 4.2 days with conventional laparoscopic cholecystectomy; P value reported as non-significant, CI not reported). Similarly, the RCT found no significant difference in duration of surgery between minilaparoscopic cholecystectomy and conventional laparoscopic cholecystectomy, but the operation tended to be marginally longer with minilaparoscopic cholecystectomy (mean 113.8 minutes with minilaparoscopic *v* 98.2 minutes with conventional laparoscopic; P = 0.056).

Harms: The RCT found no major complications (common bile duct injury, bile leakage, intra-abdominal bleeding, abscess formation) associated with minilaparoscopic or conventional laparoscopic cholecystectomy (see comment below).[11] It found similar rates of minor complications (wound infection, short term postoperative ileus, bleeding from the subumbilical port site) between the two treatment groups (4/35 [11%] with minilaparoscopic cholecystectomy *v* 2/29 [7%] with conventional laparoscopic cholecystectomy; P value not reported).

Comment: The RCT may have been underpowered to detect clinically important adverse effects.[11] To date, there is no formal training in minilaparoscopy outside of traditional laparoscopic training. Most published studies using minilaparoscopy come from either non-US centres or large academic centres in the USA, which allows no estimate of the extent of its use outside this setting.

OPTION EARLY VERSUS DELAYED CHOLECYSTECTOMY

Four RCTs found that operation before the scheduled date because of recurrent or worsening symptoms was necessary in 13–19% of people receiving delayed cholecystectomy (open or laparoscopic cholecystectomy after 6–8 weeks). The RCTs found no significant difference between early (within 72 hours) and delayed cholecystectomy (open or laparoscopic) in rates of intraoperative or postoperative complications, but found that early cholecystectomy reduced hospital stay. Two RCTs found that early laparoscopic cholecystectomy increased duration of operation compared with delayed laparoscopic cholecystectomy but reduced use of analgesics. The RCTs found no significant difference between early and delayed laparoscopic cholecystectomy in the rate of conversion to open cholecystectomy.

Benefits: We found no systematic review. **Early versus delayed open cholecystectomy:** We found two RCTs comparing early versus delayed open cholecystectomy**G**.[12,13] The first RCT (165 people with acute cholecystitis) compared early (mean time to operation 1.6 days) versus delayed (mean time to operation 2.6 months) open cholecystectomy.[12] Operation before the scheduled date because of peritonitis, jaundice, cholangitis, or empyema was necessary in 10/82 (13%) people assigned to delayed open cholecystectomy. The RCT found no significant difference in duration of symptoms between people randomised to receive early versus delayed open cholecystectomy (mean 2.2 days with early surgery *v* 2.3 days with delayed surgery; P value reported as non-significant). Similarly, the RCT found no significant difference in duration of surgery (mean 93 minutes with early surgery *v* 85 minutes with delayed surgery; P > 0.10). However, it found that early open cholecystectomy significantly reduced hospital stay compared with delayed open cholecystectomy (10.7 days with early surgery *v* 18.2 with delayed surgery, mean difference 7.5 days; P < 0.001). The second RCT (192 people) compared early open cholecystectomy (mean time to operation 2.5 days) versus delayed open cholecystectomy (mean time to operation not reported).[13] Operation before the scheduled date because of worsening or recurrent symptoms was necessary in 15/91 (14%) people assigned to delayed open cholecystectomy. The RCT found that early open cholecystectomy significantly reduced hospital stay (9.1 days with early surgery *v* 15.5 days with delayed surgery; P < 0.05). **Early versus delayed laparoscopic cholecystectomy:** We found two RCTs comparing early versus delayed laparoscopic cholecystectomy**G**.[14,15] The first RCT (104 people) compared early (within 24 hours of admission) versus delayed (after 6–8 weeks) laparoscopic cholecystectomy.[14] In people assigned to delayed laparoscopic cholecystectomy, operation before the scheduled date because of worsening or recurrent symptoms was necessary in 8/51 (16%) people, and 5/51 (10%) people did not have surgery after successful conservative treatment. The RCT found no significant difference in the rate of conversion to open cholecystectomy between early and delayed laparoscopic cholecystectomy (21% with early surgery *v* 24% with delayed surgery; P = 0.74), or use of postoperative analgesics (2 doses pethidine with early surgery *v* 1 dose pethidine with delayed surgery; P = 0.14). However, the RCT found that early laparoscopic cholecystectomy significantly increased duration of operation compared with delayed laparoscopic cholecystectomy (122.8 minutes with early surgry *v* 106.6 minutes with delayed surgery, P < 0.04). The second RCT (99 people) compared early laparoscopic cholecystectomy (median time to operation 63 hours) versus delayed laparoscopic cholecystectomy (median time to operation 67 days).[15] Operation before the scheduled date was necessary in 8/41 (19.5%) people assigned to delayed laparoscopic cholecystectomy, five because of peritonitis and three because of persistent fever. The RCT found no significant difference in the rate of conversion to open cholecystectomy between early and delayed laparoscopic cholecystectomy, although more people receiving delayed laparoscopic cholecystectomy converted to open cholecystectomy (5/45 [11%] with early surgery *v* 9/41 [23%] with delayed surgery; P = 0.174). The RCT found that early laparoscopic cholecystectomy significantly increased duration of operation compared with delayed surgery (mean 135 minutes with early surgery *v* 105 minutes with delayed surgery; P = 0.022). However, it found that early laparoscopic cholecystectomy significantly reduced use of analgesics (mean 1 dose with early surgery *v* 2 doses with delayed surgery; P < 0.004) and total hospital stay (6 days with early surgery *v* 11 days with delayed surgery; P < 0.001) compared with delayed laparoscopic cholecystectomy.

Harms: **Early versus delayed open cholecystectomy:** In the first RCT, 11/82 (15%) people undergoing delayed cholecystectomy had recurrent symptoms during the waiting period (5 with acute cholecystitis, 2 with acute pancreatitis, 4 with biliary colic).[12] The RCT found similar rates of intraoperative complications between early and delayed open cholecystectomy, and found no significant difference between early and delayed open cholecystectomy in the proportion of people with postoperative complications (14% with early surgery *v* 17% with delayed surgery; P value reported as non-significant). There were no deaths in people receiving early open cholecystectomy and one death in people receiving delayed surgery. The second RCT found no significant difference between early and delayed open cholecystectomy in rates of intraoperative and postoperative complications (15% in all groups; P value reported as not significant). There were no deaths in people receiving early open cholecystectomy and one death in people receiving delayed. The complications in both RCTs included pneumonia, wound infection, wound dehiscence, incisional hernia, intra-abdominal abscess, mesenteric thrombosis, pancreatitis, myocardial infarction, and transient psychosis. **Early versus delayed laparoscopic cholecystectomy:** The first RCT found no significant difference in postoperative complications between early and delayed laparoscopic cholecystectomy (5/53 [9%] with early surgery *v* 3/38 [8%] with delayed surgery; P = 0.80).[14] Postoperative complications included subphrenic collection, bile leak from the cystic duct stump, superficial wound infection, and postoperative respiratory failure requiring mechanical ventilation for 3 days. The second RCT found no significant difference in the proportion of people with postoperative complications between early and delayed laparoscopic cholecystectomy (6/45 [13%] with early surgery *v* 12/41 [29%] with delayed surgery; P = 0.07). Postoperative complications included wound infection, bile leak, intra-abdominal fluid collection, chest infection, urinary tract infection, bile duct injury, intra-abdominal bleeding, retained ductal stone, ileus, and atrial fibrillation.

Comment: People with acute cholecystitis who have multiple comorbid conditions and relative contraindications for cholecystectomy may be treated with antibiotics, a low fat diet, and, in some instances, a cholecystostomy tube. Because of high rates of recurrent cholecystitis, most patients undergo a delayed cholecystectomy when their comorbid conditions are better controlled. Only one of the RCTs gave information on the number of people who did not undergo surgery because of successful conservative treatment.[14] **Early versus delayed open cholecystectomy:** Surgeons in the RCTs had a variety of experience. In the first RCT, open cholecystectomies were carried out by staff surgeons and senior residents only, with 85% of the operations carried out by one of the authors of the RCT.[12] In the second RCT, open cholecystectomies were carried out by a large number of surgeons of "varied experience".[13] **Early versus delayed laparoscopic cholecystectomy:** All laparoscopic cholecystectomies were carried out by "experienced surgeons" who had carried out ≥50 previous laparoscopic cholecystectomies in one RCT[14] and ≥300 in the other.[15]

GLOSSARY

Laparoscopic cholecystectomy involves removal of the gallbladder using a projection camera and 5–10 mm trocar ports. Conversion from laparascopic to open cholecystectomy is needed if the laparoscopic procedure cannot be completed without risking injury to surrounding structures or when bleeding cannot be stopped. Open cholecystectomy is required in people who have a fistula from the gallbladder into the bile duct or intestine, and in some people who have perforation and abscess in the right upper quadrant.

Minilaparoscopic cholecystectomy involves removal of the gallbladder using a projection camera and 2–3 mm trocar ports.

Open cholecystectomy involves removal of the gallbladder via laparotomy. Open cholecystectomy is required in people who have a fistula from the gallbladder into the bile duct or intestine, and in some people who have perforation and abscess in the right upper quadrant.

REFERENCES

1. Indar AA, Beckingham IJ. Acute cholecystitis. *BMJ 2002;*325:639–643.
2. Diettrick NA, Cacioppo JC, Davis RP. The vanishing elective cholecystectomy. *Arch Surg* 1988;810:123–126.
3. Fukunaga FH. Gallbladder bacteriology, histology and gallstones: study of unselected cholecystectomy specimens in Honolulu. *Arch Surg* 1973;169:106–110.
4. Lou MA, Mandal AK, Alexander JL, et al. Bacteriology of the human biliary tract and the duodenum. *Arch Surg* 1997;965:112–116.
5. Isch JH, Finnernan JC, Nahrwold DL. Perforation of the gallbladder. *Am J Gastroenterol* 1971;55:451–458.
6. Vetrhus M, Soreide O, Nesvik I, Sondenaa K. Acute cholecystitis: delayed surgery or observation. A randomized clinical trial. *Scand J Gastroenterol* 2003;38:985–990.
7. Eldar S, Sabo E, Nash E, et al. Laparoscopic versus open cholecystectomy in acute cholecystitis. *Surg Laparosc Endosc* 1997;7:407–414.
8. Kiviluoto T, Siren J, Luukkonen P, et al. Randomised trial of laparoscopic versus open cholecystectomy for acute and gangrenous cholecystitis. *Lancet* 1998;351:321–325.
9. Schiedeck THK, Schulte T, Gunarsson R, Bruch HP. Laparoscopic cholecystectomy in acute cholecystitis. *Minim Invasive Chirurg* 1997;6:48–51.
10. Shea JA, Healey MJ, Berlin JA, et al. Mortality and complications associated with laparoscopic cholecystectomy: a meta-analysis. *Ann Surg* 1996;224:609–620. Search date 1995; primary sources Medline and hand searches of bibliographies.
11. Hsieh CH. Early minilaparoscopic cholecystectomy in patients with acute cholecystitis. *Am J Surg* 2003;185:344–348.
12. Jarvinen HJ, Hastbacka J. Early cholecystectomy for acute cholecystitis. *Ann Surg* 1980;191:501–505.
13. Norrby S, Herlin P, Holmin T, et al. Early or delayed cholecystectomy in acute cholecystitis? A clinical trial. *Br J Surg* 1983;70:163–165.
14. Lai BS, Kwong KH, Leung KL, et al. Randomized trial of early versus delayed laparoscopic cholecystectomy for acute cholecystitis. *Br J Surg* 1998;85:764–767.
15. Lo CM, Liu CL, Fan ST, et al. Prospective randomized study of early versus delayed laparoscopic cholecystectomy for acute cholecystitis. *Ann Surg* 1998;227:461–467.

Julie Margenthaler
Resident in Surgery
Barnes Jewish Hospital
St. Louis, MO
USA

Douglas Schuerer
Assistant Professor of Surgery
Washington University School of Medicine
St Louis, MO
USA

Robb Whinney
Assistant Professor of Surgery
Washington University School of Medicine
St Louis, MO
USA

Competing interests: None declared.

Colonic diverticular disease

Search date February 2004

John Simpson and Robin Spiller

QUESTIONS

INTERVENTIONS

See glossary G

Key Messages

Treatment for uncomplicated diverticular disease

- **Rifaximin (plus dietary fibre supplementation *v* dietary fibre supplementation alone)** Two RCTs in people with uncomplicated diverticular disease found that rifaximin plus dietary fibre supplementation improved symptoms compared with dietary fibre supplementation alone after 12 months of treatment.
- **Bran and ispaghula husk** One small RCT in people with uncomplicated diverticular disease found no significant difference between bran or ispaghula husk and placebo in symptom relief after 16 weeks.
- **Elective surgery** We found no RCTs of elective open or laparoscopic colonic resection in people with uncomplicated diverticular disease.
- **Lactulose** One small RCT in people with uncomplicated diverticular disease found no significant difference between lactulose and a high fibre diet in self rated improvement after 12 weeks.
- **Methylcellulose** One small RCT in people with uncomplicated diverticular disease found no significant difference between methylcellulose and placebo in mean symptom scores after 3 months.

Treatment to prevent complications

- **Increased fibre intake** We found no RCTs examining complication rates after advice to consume a high fibre diet or of dietary fibre supplementation.
- **Mesalazine (after an attack of acute diverticulitis)** One methodologically flawed RCT provided insufficient evidence about effects of mesalazine compared with no treatment in people previously treated for an episode of acute diverticulitis.

Clin Evid 2005;13:482–490.

Treatment for acute diverticulitis

- **Medical treatment** We found no RCTs comparing medical treatment versus placebo in people with acute diverticulitis. One small RCT found no significant difference between intravenous cefoxitin and intravenous gentamicin plus intravenous clindamycin in rates of clinical cure. Observational studies in people with acute diverticulitis have found low mortality with medical treatment, but found that recurrence rates may be high.
- **Surgery (for diverticulitis complicated by generalised peritonitis)** We found no RCTs comparing surgery versus no surgery or versus medical treatment. One RCT found no significant difference in mortality between acute resection and transverse colostomy of the sigmoid colon. A second RCT found no significant difference in mortality between primary and secondary sigmoid colonic resection, but found that primary resection reduced rates of postoperative peritonitis and emergency reoperation. We found no RCTs comparing open versus laparoscopic surgery.

DEFINITION Colonic diverticula are mucosal out pouchings through the large bowel wall. They are often accompanied by structural changes (elastosis of the taenia coli, muscular thickening, and mucosal folding). They are usually multiple and occur most frequently in the sigmoid colon. If diverticula are associated with symptoms, then this is termed diverticular disease**G**. If asymptomatic, then the condition is known as diverticulosis**G**.

INCIDENCE/ PREVALENCE In the UK the incidence of diverticulosis increases with age; about 5% of people are affected in their fifth decade of life and about 50% by their ninth decade.[1] Diverticulosis is common in developed countries, although there is a lower prevalence of diverticulosis in Western vegetarians consuming a diet high in roughage.[2] Diverticulosis is almost unknown in rural Africa and Asia.[3]

AETIOLOGY/ RISK FACTORS There is an association between low fibre diets and diverticulosis of the colon.[3] Prospective observational studies have found that both physical activity and a high fibre diet are associated with a lower risk of developing diverticular disease.[4,5] Case control studies have found an association between perforated diverticular disease and non-steroidal anti-inflammatory drugs, corticosteroids, and opiate analgesics, whereas calcium antagonists have a protective effect.[6–9] People in Japan, Singapore, and Thailand develop diverticula that affect mainly the right side of the colon.[10]

PROGNOSIS Symptoms will develop in 10–25% of people with diverticula at some point in their lives.[1] It is unclear why some people develop symptoms and some do not. Even after successful medical treatment of acute diverticulitis**G** almost two thirds of people suffer recurrent pain in the lower abdomen.[11] Recurrent diverticulitis is observed in 7–42% of people with diverticular disease, and after recovery from the initial attack the calculated yearly risk of suffering a further episode is 3%.[12] About half of recurrences occur within 1 year of the initial episode and 90% occur within 5 years.[13] Complications of diverticular disease (perforation, obstruction, haemorrhage, and fistula formation) are each seen in about 5% of people with colonic diverticula when followed up for 10–30 years.[14] In the UK the incidence of perforation is 4 cases per 100,000 people per year, leading to approximately 2000 cases annually.[15] Intra-abdominal abscess formation is also a recognised complication.

AIMS OF INTERVENTION To reduce mortality, symptoms, and complications, with minimal adverse effects.

OUTCOMES Subjective gastrointestinal symptoms assessed by the use of questionnaires. Admission and readmission rates as a result of diverticular disease and its complications. Incidence of diverticulitis, haemorrhage, perforation, abscess, fistula formation, and mortality. Stool weight and transit time are surrogate outcomes.

METHODS *Clinical Evidence* search and appraisal February 2004.

QUESTION **What are the effects of treatments for uncomplicated diverticular disease?**

OPTION **BRAN AND ISPAGHULA HUSK**

One small RCT in people with uncomplicated diverticular disease found no significant difference between bran or ispaghula husk and placebo in symptom relief after 16 weeks.

Benefits: **Versus placebo:** We found no systematic review, but found one crossover RCT comparing fibre supplements versus placebo.[16] The crossover RCT (76 people with uncomplicated diverticular disease, no other gastrointestinal disorders, and no prior abdominal operations) compared three treatments: bran crispbread (6.99 g/day fibre), ispaghula husk drink (a bulk forming laxative; 9.04 g/day fibre), and placebo (2.34 g/day fibre). It found no significant differences among treatments for pain score (score range: 0 = least severe, 100 = most severe), lower bowel symptom score (combination of the pain score and sensation of incomplete emptying, straining, stool consistency, flatus, and aperients taken; score range: 0 = least severe, 110 = most severe), or general symptom score (including nausea, vomiting, dyspepsia, belching, and abdominal distension; score range: 0 = least severe, 55 = most severe; see comment below) after 16 weeks (pain scores after treatment: 15.2 with bran *v* 19.5 with ispaghula husk *v* 17.5 with placebo; P value not reported; lower bowel symptom scores after treatment: 39.7 with bran *v* 41.3 with ispaghula husk *v* 45.0 with placebo; P value not reported; general symptom scores after treatment: 6.7 with bran *v* 8.1 with ispagula husk *v* 7.6 with placebo; P value not reported). The RCT found that both active treatments significantly reduced straining at stool, increased wet stool weight and stool frequency, and significantly softened the stools after 16 weeks compared with placebo (straining: bran *v* placebo, $P < 0.01$; ispaghula husk *v* placebo, $P < 0.001$; wet stool weight: both active treatments *v* placebo, $P < 0.001$; stool frequency: both active treatments *v* placebo, $P < 0.001$; stool softening: both active treatments *v* placebo, $P < 0.001$; CI not reported for any comparison).[16]

Harms: No significant adverse effects were reported in the RCT.[16]

Comment: In the RCT, 18/76 (24%) people withdrew from the trial and analysis of data was not by intention to treat.[16] The RCT did not specify the exact number of people receiving each treatment, precluding calculations of relative risk and confidence interval. People in the RCT had been investigated to exclude coexisting abdominal pathology but the extent of the investigations was not stated.[16]

OPTION **METHYLCELLULOSE**

One small RCT in people with uncomplicated diverticular disease found no significant difference between methylcellulose and placebo in symptom scores at 3 months.

Benefits: **Versus placebo:** We found no systematic review but found one RCT (30 people with symptomatic diverticular disease and no other gastrointestinal disease) that compared methylcellulose (500 mg twice daily) versus placebo.[17] It found no significant difference between treatments on mean symptom score at 3 months (see comment below; mean symptom score 13.0 with methylcellulose *v* 16.7 with placebo; difference in means –3.7, 95% CI –8.9 to +1.5).

Harms: None reported.

Comment: The score used to assess symptoms and signs was not described clearly, but included barium enema results.[17] The range of the score was 0–50, where 0 meant least severe symptoms and 50 meant most severe. The RCT was small and of short duration, and both the methylcellulose and placebo treatments were associated with an improvement in symptom scores. Diverticular disease was confirmed by barium enema but the extent of other investigations to exclude comorbidity was not stated.

OPTION LACTULOSE

One small RCT in people with uncomplicated diverticular disease found no significant difference between lactulose and a high fibre diet in self rated improvement after 12 weeks.

Benefits: We found no systematic review. **Versus placebo:** We found no RCTs. **Versus high fibre diet:** We found one RCT (43 people with diverticular disease and no other abdominal pathology) comparing lactulose (15 mL twice daily) versus a high fibre diet (30–40 g/day fibre).[18] It found no significant difference in the proportion of people who reported their symptoms to be much improved after 12 weeks (see comment below; 7/20 [35%] with lactulose *v* 9/21 [43%] with high fibre diet; RR 0.80, 95% CI 0.34 to 1.77).

Harms: The RCT found a non-significant increase in the risk of new symptoms with high fibre diet compared with lactulose (12/21 [57%] with high fibre diet *v* 9/20 [45%] with lactulose; RR 1.30, 95% CI 0.70 to 2.34).[18] The symptoms were described as minor but no further details were provided. The RCT found that 2/20 (10%) people taking lactulose withdrew from the trial because of symptoms: one with abdominal pain and one with nausea.

Comment: Although "much improved" was used as an outcome by the RCT, this term was not defined clearly.[18] People were investigated to exclude coexisting abdominal pathology but the extent of the investigations was not stated.

OPTION ANTIBIOTICS (RIFAXIMIN)

Two RCTs in people with uncomplicated diverticular disease found that rifaximin plus dietary fibre supplementation improved symptoms compared with dietary fibre supplementation alone after 12 months of treatment.

Benefits: We found no systematic review but found two RCTs.[19,20] The first RCT (168 people with uncomplicated diverticular disease**G**) compared dietary fibre supplementation (glucomannan 2 g/day) plus oral rifaximin**G** (400 mg twice daily) versus dietary fibre supplementation (glucomannan 2 g/day) plus placebo.[19] Both treatments were given for 7 days each month for 1 year (see comment below). The RCT found that dietary fibre supplementation plus rifaximin significantly increased the proportion of people with no symptoms or only mild symptoms after 12 months of treatment (69% with rifaximin *v* 39% with placebo; P = 0.001; results presented graphically; absolute numbers not provided). The RCT found no significant difference between treatments in the severity of diarrhoea, tenesmus, or upper abdominal pain (absolute data and significance testing not reported). The second open RCT (968 people with diverticular disease) compared dietary fibre supplementation (glucomannan 4 g/day) plus rifaximin (400 mg twice daily for 7 days every month) versus dietary fibre supplementation alone (glucomannan 4 g/day).[20] The RCT found that dietary fibre supplementation plus rifaximin improved global symptom score significantly more than dietary fibre supplementation alone at 12 months (global symptom score assessed on six clinical variables: upper abdominal pain/discomfort, lower abdominal pain/discomfort, bloating, tenesmus, diarrhoea, and abdominal tenderness; each variable rated from 0 [no symptoms] to 3 [severe] and summed for a total maximum score of 18; score changed from 6.5 at baseline to 1.0 with dietary fibre supplementation plus rifaximin v 6.3 at baseline to 2.0 with dietary fibre supplementation alone; P = 0.003).

Harms: The first RCT did not report on harms.[19] In the second open RCT, 10 people (1.68%) taking rifamixin plus glucomannan and 5 (1.34%) taking glucomannan alone experienced adverse effects (nausea, headache, and weakness).[20]

Comment: One RCT reported that 17/168 (10%) people did not complete the trial, although analysis was not by intention to treat.[19] For each treatment group, 2/84 (2%) people were withdrawn because of acute diverticulitis❻.

OPTION **ELECTIVE SURGERY**

We found no RCTs of elective open or laparoscopic colonic resection in people with uncomplicated diverticular disease.

Benefits: We found no systematic review or RCTs.

Harms: We found no data on harms of elective surgery in people with diverticular disease❻.

Comment: None.

QUESTION **What are the effects of treatments to prevent complications of diverticular disease?**

OPTION **ADVICE TO INCREASE FIBRE INTAKE**

We found no RCTs examining complication rates after advice to consume a high fibre diet or dietary fibre supplementation.

Benefits: We found no systematic review or RCTs.

Harms: We found no RCTs.

Comment: Fibre is often used with the aim of preventing complications in people with diverticular disease❻ because observational studies have found that the disease is less frequent in populations with high fibre intake (see incidence/prevalence, p 483).

OPTION **MESALAZINE**

One methodologically flawed RCT provided insufficient evidence about effects of mesalazine compared with no treatment in people previously treated for an episode of acute diverticulitis.

Benefits: **Versus no treatment:** We found no systematic review, but found one RCT (166 people previously treated for an episode of mild/moderate diverticulitis) compared 8 weeks of treatment with oral mesalazine (400 mg twice daily) versus no treatment.[21] People in both groups had received intramuscular sulbactam–ampicillin (1.5 g twice daily) and oral rifaximinⒼ (400 mg twice daily) for 7 days before randomisation. The RCT found that mesalazine reduced symptomatic recurrence at 4 years compared with no treatment (12/81 [15%] with mesalazine *v* 39/85 [46%] with no treatment; RR 0.32, 95% CI 0.18 to 0.57; NNT 4, 95% CI 3 to 6).[21] See comment below.

Harms: The RCT found that abdominal pain was more common with mesalazine than no treatment (13/81 [16%] with mesalazine *v* 4/85 [5%] with no treatment; RR 3.40, 95% CI 1.16 to 10.00; NNH 8, 95% CI 4 to 70).[21]

Comment: The RCT provided insufficient information on several factors.[21] The recurrence of inflammation was diagnosed according to unspecified clinical and laboratory criteria. Methods for determining symptom scores, including the assessment and diagnosis of pain, were not reported. Forty-five people did not complete the study, but there was no difference in withdrawal rate between groups (3 people died, 9 people had a severe complication of diverticular disease, and 33 were withdrawn because of "poor" adherence to treatment [poor adherence was not defined]).[21] One non-randomised controlled trial (218 people with at least 2 episodes of acute diverticulitisⒼ in the previous year, 193 analysed) compared treatment with rifaximin (400 mg twice daily for 7 days followed by 400 mg twice daily for 7 days/month) plus mesalazine (800 mg three times daily for 7 days followed by 800 mg twice daily for 7 days/month) versus rifaximin alone (400 mg twice daily for 7 days followed by 400 mg twice daily for 7 days/month).[22] It found that rifaximin plus mesalazine significantly increased the proportion of people who were symptom free at 12 months compared with rifaximin alone (89/104 [86%] with rifaximin plus mesalazine *v* 44/89 [49%] with rifaximin alone; $P < 0.0005$).

QUESTION **What are the effects of treatments for acute diverticulitis?**

OPTION **MEDICAL TREATMENT**

We found no RCTs comparing medical treatment versus placebo in people with acute diverticulitis. One small RCT found no significant difference between intravenous cefoxitin and intravenous gentamicin plus intravenous clindamycin in rates of clinical cure. Observational studies in people with acute diverticulitis have found low mortality with medical treatment, but found that recurrence rates may be high.

Benefits: We found no systematic review. **Versus placebo:** We found no RCTs. **Versus other medical treatments:** We found one RCT (51 people with a clinical diagnosis of acute diverticulitisⒼ who did not need immediate surgery) that compared intravenous cefoxitin (1–2 g every 6 hours) versus intravenous gentamicin (1.7 mg/kg loading dose followed by 1.0–1.4 mg/kg every 8 hours) plus intravenous clindamycin (total dose of 2400–2700 mg/day in 3 or 4 equal doses).[23] It found no significant difference in clinical cure rate (see comment below; 27/30 [90%] with cefoxitin *v* 18/21 [86%] with gentamicin plus clindamycin; RR 1.10, 95% CI 0.85 to 1.30).

Harms: In the RCT, toxicity (possibly antibiotic related) occurred with both treatments, although the proportion of people affected was not significantly different between treatments (2/30 [7%] with cefoxitin *v* 3/21 [14%] with gentamicin plus clindamycin; RR 0.47, 95% CI 0.09 to 2.56).[23]

Comment: Clinical cure was defined as complete resolution of symptoms and signs associated with diverticulitis plus discharge from hospital without recurrence for at least 6 weeks or complete resolution of symptoms and signs plus having had an elective surgical procedure with primary anastomosis in the absence of colostomy without septic complications.[23] We found many observational studies of medical treatment for acute diverticulitis, with variable follow up periods (1–12 years), which consistently report low mortality (0–5%).[12,24–26] These observational trials also reported that 7–42% of people treated medically suffer recurrent episodes of acute diverticulitis.

OPTION SURGERY

We found no RCTs comparing surgery versus no surgery or versus medical treatment. One RCT found no significant difference in mortality between acute resection and transverse colostomy of the sigmoid colon. A second RCT found no significant difference in mortality between primary and secondary sigmoid colonic resection, but found that primary resection reduced rates of postoperative peritonitis and emergency reoperation. We found no RCTs comparing open versus laparoscopic surgery.

Benefits: We found no systematic review. **Surgery versus placebo or medical treatment:** We found no RCTs. **Comparison of types of open surgery:** We found two RCTs.[27,28] Both were small and may have lacked power to detect clinically important effects. The first RCT (62 people with diffuse peritonitis complicating perforated acute diverticulitis**G** of the left colon; median age 72 years) compared acute sigmoid colonic resection**G** versus no acute resection (acute transverse colostomy, suture, and omental covering of a visible perforation).[27] The RCT found no significant difference between acute sigmoid colonic resection and no acute resection in mortality within 30 days (mortality: 8/31 [26%] with acute resection *v* 6/31 [19%] with no acute resection; RR 1.30, 95% CI 0.52 to 3.39). However, subgroup analysis of people with purulent peritonitis (46 people) found that acute sigmoid colonic resection significantly increased postoperative mortality compared with no acute resection (6/25 [24%] with acute resection *v* 0/21 [0%] with no acute resection; ARI 24.0%, 95% CI 4.5% to 44.0%). Subgroup analysis of people with faecal peritonitis (16 people) found no significant difference between acute sigmoid colonic resection and no acute resection in postoperative mortality (2/6 [33%] with acute resection *v* 6/10 [60%] with no acute resection; RR 0.60, 95% CI 0.16 to 1.92; see comment below). This subgroup analysis probably lacked power to detect a clinically important difference. The second RCT (105 people with generalised peritonitis complicating sigmoid diverticulitis; mean age 66 years) compared primary versus secondary sigmoid colonic resection.[28] Primary resection involved surgical removal of the affected sigmoid colon plus either formation of an end colostomy, or formation of a primary colorectal anastomosis with or without a proximal defunctioning colostomy**G**. Secondary resection involved initial closing of any visible bowel perforations plus the formation of a defunctioning colostomy. A second (definitive) procedure was then undertaken at a later date to perform a sigmoid colon resection plus a colorectal anastomosis with or without a defunctioning colostomy. The RCT found that primary sigmoid colonic resection significantly reduced rates of postoperative peritonitis after the initial procedure and significantly reduced rates of emergency reoperation compared with secondary sigmoid colonic resection (postoperative peritonitis: 1/55 [2%] with primary resection *v* 10/44 [23%] with secondary resection; RR 0.09, 95% CI 0.01 to 0.70; NNT 5, 95% CI 3 to 12; emergency reoperation:

2/55 [4%] with primary resection *v* 9/48 [19%] with secondary resection; RR 0.19, 95% CI 0.04 to 0.90; NNT 7, 95% CI 4 to 35). The RCT found no significant difference between treatments in mortality (13/55 [24%] with primary resection *v* 9/48 [19%] with secondary resection; RR 1.30, 95% CI 0.60 to 2.70; see comment below). **Open surgery versus laparoscopic surgery:** We found no RCTs.

Harms: The first RCT found no significant difference between acute resection and no acute resection in rates of cardiopulmonary complications, thromboembolism, mental confusion, or other complications including wound dehiscence, wound infection but no dehiscence, intraperitoneal abscess formation, ileus, colo-cutaneous fistula, and revision of colostomy (cardiopulmonary complications: 13/31 [42%] with acute resection *v* 14/31 [45%] with no acute resection; RR 0.90, 95% CI 0.53 to 1.63; thromboembolism: 3/31 [9.7%] with acute resection *v* 5/31 [16%] with no acute resection; RR 0.60, 95% CI 0.16 to 2.30; mental confusion: 4/31 [13%] with acute resection *v* 4/31 [13%] with no acute resection; RR 1.00, 95% CI 0.27 to 3.65).[27] The second RCT found no significant difference between treatments in rates of wound complications, extra-abdominal septic complications, or extra-abdominal non-septic complications (wound complications: 20/55 [36%] with primary resection *v* 23/48 [48%] with secondary resection; RR 0.80, 95% CI 0.48 to 1.20; extra-abdominal septic complications: 11/55 [20%] with primary resection *v* 12/48 [25%] with secondary resection; RR 0.80, 95% CI 0.39 to 1.65; extra-abdominal non-septic complications: 26/55 [47%] with primary resection *v* 21/48 [44%] with secondary resection; RR 1.08, 95% CI 0.71 to 1.65).[28]

Comment: The first RCT was conducted in a single centre and took 14 years to recruit 62 people.[27] The second RCT was conducted in 17 centres and took 7 years to recruit 105 people.[28] Both studies were small and may have lacked power to detect a significant difference between treatments. The high complication rates reported are not surprising in predominantly elderly people after a perforation of the large bowel. The wide spectrum of presentation and operative treatment options for acute complicated diverticulitis makes RCTs difficult to perform.

GLOSSARY

Acute diverticulitis This condition occurs when a diverticulum becomes acutely inflamed. There may be general symptoms and signs of infection (including fever and rapid heart rate) with or without local symptoms and signs (pain and localised tenderness, usually in the lower left abdomen, sometimes with a mass that can be felt on abdominal or rectal examination).

Acute sigmoid colonic resection Immediate resection of the sigmoid colon, involving end colostomy of the proximal bowel and creating a mucus fistula with the distal bowel or oversewing the rectal stump.

Defunctioning colostomy Stoma created to divert faecal flow, such that faeces no longer flows through the anus.

Diverticular disease This term is used to describe diverticula associated with any symptoms.[29] Symptoms commonly include abdominal pain and alteration in bowel habit. Diverticular disease may be complicated by abscess formation, fistulae, perforation, obstruction, or haemorrhage.

Diverticulosis The presence of diverticula that are asymptomatic. Most people with sigmoid colonic diverticula have no symptoms.

Rifaximin A rifamycin antibacterial drug with antimicrobial actions similar to those of rifampicin. It is marketed predominantly in Italy.

REFERENCES

1. Parks TG. Natural history of diverticular disease of the colon. *Clin Gastroenterol* 1975;4:53–69.
2. Gear JS, Ware A, Fursdon P, et al. Symptomless diverticular disease and intake of dietary fibre. *Lancet* 1979;1:511–514.
3. Painter NS, Burkitt DP. Diverticular disease of the colon, a 20th Century problem. *Clin Gastroenterol* 1975;4:3–21.
4. Aldoori WH, Giovannucci EL, Rimm EB, et al. Prospective study of physical activity and the risk of symptomatic diverticular disease in men. *Gut* 1995;36:276–282.
5. Aldoori WH, Giovannucci EL, Rimm EB, et al. A prospective study of diet and the risk of symptomatic diverticular disease in men. *Am J Clin Nutr* 1994;60:757–764.
6. Campbell K, Steele RJ. Non-steroidal anti-inflammatory drugs and complicated diverticular disease: a case-control study. *Br J Surg* 1991;78:190–191.
7. Morris CR, Harvey IM, Stebbings WS, et al. Anti-inflammatory drugs, analgesics and the risk of perforated colonic diverticular disease. *Br J Surg* 2003;90:1267–1272.
8. Morris CR, Harvey IM, Stebbings WS, et al. Do calcium channel blockers and antimuscarinics protect against perforated colonic diverticular disease? A case control study. *Gut* 2003;52:1734–1737.
9. Morris CR, Harvey IM, Stebbings WS, et al. Epidemiology of perforated colonic diverticular disease. *Postgrad Med J* 2002;78:654–658.
10. Sugihara K, Muto T, Morioka Y, et al. Diverticular disease of the colon in Japan. A review of 615 cases. *Dis Colon Rectum* 1984;27:531–537.
11. Munson KD, Hensien MA, Jacob LN, et al. Diverticulitis. A comprehensive follow-up. *Dis Colon Rectum* 1996;39:318–322.
12. Haglund U, Hellberg R, Johnsen C, et al. Complicated diverticular disease of the sigmoid colon. An analysis of short and long term outcome in 392 patients. *Ann Chir Gynaecol* 1979;68:41–46.
13. Parks TG, Connell AM. The outcome in 455 patients admitted for treatment of diverticular disease of the colon. *Br J Surg* 1970;57:775–778.
14. Boles RS, Jordon SM. The clinical significance of diverticulosis. *Gastroenterology* 1958;35:579–581.
15. Hart AR, Kennedy HJ, Stebbings WS, et al. How frequently do large bowel diverticula perforate? An incidence and cross-sectional study. *Eur J Gastroenterol Hepatol* 2000;12:661–665.
16. Ornstein MH, Littlewood ER, Baird IM, et al. Are fibre supplements really necessary in diverticular disease of the colon? A controlled clinical trial. *BMJ* 1981;282:1353–1356.
17. Hodgson WJ. The placebo effect. Is it important in diverticular disease? *Am J Gastroenterol* 1977;67:157–162.
18. Smits BJ, Whitehead AM, Prescott P. Lactulose in the treatment of symptomatic diverticular disease: a comparative study with high-fibre diet. *Br J Clin Pract* 1990;44:314–318.
19. Papi C, Ciaco A, Koch M, et al. Efficacy of rifaximin in the treatment of symptomatic diverticular disease of the colon. A multicentre double-blind placebo-controlled trial. *Aliment Pharmacol Ther* 1995;9:33–39.
20. Latella G, Pimpo MT, Sottili S, et al. Rifaximin improves symptoms of acquired uncomplicated diverticular disease of the colon. *Int J Colorectal Dis* 2003;18:55–62.
21. Trespi E, Colla C, Panizza P, et al. Therapeutic and prophylactic role of mesalazine (5-ASA) in symptomatic diverticular disease of the colon. 4-year follow-up results. *Minerva Gastroenterol Dietol* 1999;45:245–252.
22. Tursi A, Brandimarte G, Daffina R. Long-term treatment with mesalazine and rifaximin versus rifaximin alone for patients with recurrent attacks of acute diverticulitis of colon. *Dig Liver Dis* 2002;34:510–515.
23. Kellum JM, Sugerman HJ, Coppa GF, et al. Randomized, prospective comparison of cefoxitin and gentamicin–clindamycin in the treatment of acute colonic diverticulitis. *Clin Ther* 1992;14:376–384.
24. Larson DM, Masters SS, Spiro HM. Medical and surgical therapy in diverticular disease: a comparative study. *Gastroenterology* 1976;71:734–737.
25. Sarin S, Boulos PB. Long-term outcome of patients presenting with acute complications of diverticular disease. *Ann R Coll Surg Engl* 1994;76:117–120.
26. Farthmann EH, Ruckauer KD, Haring RU. Evidence-based surgery: diverticulitis — a surgical disease? *Langenbecks Arch Surg* 2000;385:143–151.
27. Kronborg O. Treatment of perforated sigmoid diverticulitis: a prospective randomised trial. *Br J Surg* 1993;80:505–507.
28. Zeitoun G, Laurent A, Rouffet F, et al. Multicentre, randomized clinical trial of primary versus secondary sigmoid resection in generalized peritonitis complicating sigmoid diverticulitis. *Br J Surg* 2000;87:1366–1374.
29. Kohler L, Sauerland S, Neugebauer E. Diagnosis and treatment of diverticular disease: results of a consensus development conference. The Scientific Committee of the European Association for Endoscopic Surgery. *Surg Endosc* 1999;13:430–436.

John Simpson
Lecturer in Surgery
Department of General Surgery
University Hospital Nottingham
Nottingham
UK

Robin Spiller
Professor of Gastroenterology
Division of Gastroenterology
University Hospital Nottingham
Nottingham
UK

Competing interests: None declared.

Constipation in adults

Search date December 2003

Frank Frizelle and Murray Barclay

QUESTIONS

INTERVENTIONS

See glossary G

Covered elsewhere in *Clinical Evidence*

Constipation in children, p 301

Key Messages

Lifestyle advice in adults with idiopathic chronic constipation

- **Lifestyle advice** We found no RCTs of lifestyle advice in adults with idiopathic chronic constipation.

Bulking agents in adults with idiopathic chronic constipation

- **Ispaghula husk (psyllium)** One RCT identified by a systematic review found that ispaghula husk increased the frequency of bowel movements and improved overall symptoms compared with placebo after 2 weeks. We found limited evidence from two RCTs that ispaghula husk improved symptoms compared with lactulose at 4 weeks. One RCT provided insufficient evidence to compare ispaghula husk versus macrogol 3350. One RCT found no clinically important difference between ispaghula husk and docusate in frequency of bowel movements, stool consistency, straining, or pain after 2 weeks.
- **Bran** We found no RCTs of sufficient quality comparing bran versus placebo in adults with idiopathic chronic constipation.

Stool softeners in adults with idiopathic chronic constipation

- **Paraffin; seed oils/arachis oil** We found no RCTs in adults with idiopathic chronic constipation.

Osmotic laxatives in adults with idiopathic chronic constipation

- **Macrogols** Three RCTs identified by a systematic review and one small additional RCT found that macrogols (polyethylene glycols) improved symptoms after 2–20 weeks compared with placebo. One RCT found insufficient evidence to compare macrogol 3350 versus ispaghula husk. One systematic review and one subsequent RCT found that macrogols improved global satisfaction and severity of constipation at 4 weeks compared with lactulose.
- **Lactulose** We found limited evidence from two RCTs that lactulose improved symptoms compared with placebo. We found limited evidence from two RCTs that lactulose was less effective in improving symptoms at 4 weeks than ispaghula husk. Three RCTs identified by systematic reviews compared lactulose versus lactitol and found different results. Two RCTs found no significant difference in effectiveness at 2–4 weeks and one RCT found that lactulose was less effective than lactitol in increasing bowel movement frequency at 2 weeks. One RCT identified by a systematic review and one subsequent RCT found that lactulose was less effective than macrogols in improving global satisfaction and severity of constipation at 4 weeks.
- **Lactitol** One small crossover RCT identified by a systematic review found that lactitol increased the frequency of bowel movements compared with placebo after 4 weeks. Three RCTs identified by systematic reviews compared lactitol versus lactulose and found different results. Two RCTs found no significant difference in frequency of bowel movements at 2–4 weeks and one RCT found that lactitol increased frequency of bowel movements at 2 weeks compared with lactulose.
- **Magnesium salts; phosphate enemas; sodium citrate enemas** We found no RCTs in adults with idiopathic chronic constipation.

Stimulant laxatives in adults with idiopathic chronic constipation

- **Dantron** We found no RCTs of dantron in adults with idiopathic chronic constipation. Animal studies have suggested that dantron may be carcinogenic. Its use is, therefore, recommended only in people who are terminally ill.
- **Docusate** One systematic review identified no RCTs of sufficient quality comparing docusate versus placebo. One RCT identified by a systematic review found no clinically important difference between docusate and ispaghula husk in frequency of bowel movements, stool consistency, straining, or pain after 2 weeks.
- **Bisacodyl; glycerol/glycerin suppositories; picosulphate (picosulfate); senna** We found no RCTs in adults with idiopathic chronic constipation.

DEFINITION Bowel habits and perception of bowel habit vary widely within and among populations, making constipation difficult to define strictly. The Rome II criteria Ⓖ is a standardised tool that diagnoses chronic constipation on the basis of two or more of the following symptoms for at least 12 weeks in the preceding year: straining at defaecation on at least a quarter of occasions; stools that are lumpy/hard on at least a quarter of occasions; sensation of incomplete evacuation on at least a quarter of occasions; and three or fewer bowel movements a week.[1] In practice, however, diagnostic criteria are less rigid and are in part dependent on perception of normal bowel habit. Typically, chronic constipation might be diagnosed when a person has bowel actions twice a week or less, for two consecutive weeks, especially in the presence of features such as straining at stool, abdominal discomfort, and sensation of incomplete evacuation. In this chapter, we have included all RCTs that stated that all participants had chronic constipation, whether or not this diagnosis was made according to strict Rome II criteria. Where the definitions of constipation in the RCTs differ markedly from those presented here, we have made this difference explicit. In this chapter, we deal with chronic constipation that is not caused by a specific underlying disease (sometimes known as idiopathic constipation) in adults aged over 18 years. We have excluded studies in pregnant women and in people with constipation associated with underlying specific organic diseases such as autonomic neuropathy, spinal cord injury, bowel obstruction, and paralytic ileus.

INCIDENCE/ PREVALENCE Twelve million general practitioner prescriptions were written for laxatives in England in 2001.[2] Prevalence data are limited by small samples and problems with definition. One UK survey of 731 women found that 8.2% had constipation meeting Rome II criteria, and 8.5% defined themselves as being constipated.[3] A larger survey (1892 adults) found that 39% of men and 52% of women reported straining at stool on more than a quarter of occasions.[4] Prevalence rises in the elderly. Several surveys from around the world suggest that in a community setting, prevalence among the elderly is about 20%.[4–7]

AETIOLOGY/ RISK FACTORS One systematic review found that factors associated with increased risk of constipation included low fibre diet, low fluid intake, reduced mobility, and consumption of drugs such as opioids and anticholinergic antidepressants.[8]

PROGNOSIS Untreated constipation may lead to faecal impaction, particularly in elderly and confused people.[9] Constipation has been suggested as a risk factor for haemorrhoids and colorectal cancer, but evidence of causality is lacking.[9]

AIMS OF INTERVENTION To relieve symptoms of constipation, to restore normal bowel habit, and to improve quality of life, with minimal adverse effects.

OUTCOMES Symptoms (frequency of bowel movements, straining at defaecation, hard/lumpy stools, sensation of incomplete evacuation/tenesmus); use of laxatives; cure of constipation (based on Rome II criteria or self or practitioner's report).

METHODS Clinical Evidence search and appraisal December 2003.

QUESTION What are the effects of lifestyle advice in adults with idiopathic chronic constipation?

OPTION LIFESTYLE ADVICE OR CHANGE OF LIFESTYLE

We found no RCTs of lifestyle advice in adults with idiopathic chronic constipation.

Benefits: We found no systematic review or RCTs.

Harms: We found no RCTs.

Comment: None.

QUESTION What are the effects of bulking agents in adults with idiopathic chronic constipation?

OPTION BRAN

We found no RCTs of sufficient quality comparing bran versus placebo in adults with idiopathic chronic constipation.

Benefits: **Versus placebo:** We found one systematic review (search date 1995), which identified no RCTs of sufficient quality.[10] We found no subsequent RCTs.

Harms: The systematic review gave no information on adverse effects.[10]

Comment: None.

OPTION ISPAGHULA HUSK (PSYLLIUM)

One RCT identified by a systematic review found that ispaghula husk increased the frequency of bowel movements and improved overall symptoms compared with placebo after 2 weeks. We found limited evidence from two RCTs that ispaghula husk improved symptoms compared with lactulose at 4 weeks. One RCT provided insufficient evidence to compare ispaghula husk versus macrogol 3350. One RCT found no clinically important difference between ispaghula husk and docusate in frequency of bowel movements, stool consistency, straining, or pain after 2 weeks.

Benefits: We found two systematic reviews (search dates 1995[10] and 2001[8]). **Versus placebo:** The second review[8] found one RCT (201 people, mean 2.3 bowel movements/week, mean age 49 years, 183 completed the trial). The RCT found that 3.6 g ispaghula husk three times daily significantly increased the frequency of bowel movements after 2 weeks compared with placebo (median bowel movements/week: 7.0 with ispaghula *v* 4.5 with placebo, $P < 0.05$; abdominal pain/discomfort better, assessed using 3 point Likert scale with options better, the same, or worse: 21/35 [60%] with ispaghula *v* 12/26 [46%] with placebo, $P = 0.035$).[11] It also assessed symptoms of straining and constipation as "better", "the same", or "worse" than baseline. It found that, compared with placebo, ispaghula husk significantly increased the proportion of people whose symptoms were "better" (straining "better": 59/70 [84%] with ispaghula *v* 36/63 [57%] with placebo, $P = 0.003$; self assessment that constipation was "better": 90/101 [89%] with ispaghula *v* 46/95 [48%] with placebo; $P < 0.001$). **Versus lactulose:** The first systematic review[10] identified one RCT.[12] The RCT (112 outpatients, mean age 50 years) found that 3.5 g ispaghula twice daily significantly increased the frequency of bowel movements after 4 weeks compared with 15 mL lactulose twice daily (7.8/week with ispaghula *v* 6.6/week with lactulose; $P < 0.05$).[12] It found that a similar proportion of people had straining at stool (no straining: 21/45 [47%] with ispaghula *v* 15/48 [31%] with lactulose; P value not reported) and clinical improvement (defined by practitioner's report of overall clinical impression of symptom severity; much improved on Clinical Global Improvement score: 29/45 [64%] with ispaghula *v* 33/48 [69%] with lactulose; P value not reported). The second review[8] identified one RCT (see comment below).[13] The RCT (394 people presenting to their general practitioner with constipation; 90% had constipation > 7 days) compared 3.5 g ispaghula husk twice daily (224 people) versus other laxatives chosen at the discretion of the general practitioner (170 people, of whom 91 received lactulose).[13] Constipation was defined on the basis of self report of perceived reduction in bowel frequency or difficulty in passing stool over the previous week. Subgroup analysis found that the proportion of movements with hard stools was lower with ispaghula husk than with lactulose at 4 weeks (18% with ispaghula *v* 27% with lactulose; P value not reported). **Versus macrogols:** The second systematic review[8] identified one RCT published only as an abstract (120 people in hospital, mean age 50 years). It found that 13.7 g macrogol 3350 plus electrolytes twice daily significantly increased "overall effectiveness" compared with 3.5 g ispaghula twice daily at 2 weeks (92% with macrogol 3350 *v* 73% with ispaghula; $P = 0.005$). "Overall effectiveness" was not defined in the review and no further details were available.[8] **Versus docusate:** The second review[8] identified one RCT (170 people aged 20–70 years, 90% female, mean age 37 years). It found that 5.1 g ispaghula husk twice daily significantly increased the frequency of bowel movements in the second week compared with 100 mg docusate sodium twice daily but found no significant difference between straining at stool or pain with bowel motions (frequency: 3.5/week with ispaghula husk *v* 2.9/week with docusate, P = 0.02; straining: P = 0.29; pain: P = 0.15).[14] The difference in frequency of bowel movements was small, and is likely to be of little clinical importance.

Harms: **Versus placebo:** The review gave no information on adverse effects.[10] **Versus lactulose:** One RCT identified by the earlier review[10] found that fewer people had soiling at the time of the first bowel motion with ispaghula husk than with lactulose (soiling: 2.1% with ispaghula *v* 8.3% with lactulose; P value not reported).[13] It found that fewer people had abdominal pain over 4 weeks with ispaghula than with lactulose (weeks 1–2: 32% with ispaghula *v* 41% with lactulose; weeks 3–4: 15% with ispaghula *v* 22% with lactulose; P value not reported). **Versus macrogols:** The review gave no information on adverse effects.[8] **Versus docusate:** The review and included RCT gave no information on adverse effects.[8,14]

Comment: Reported adverse effects of ispaghula include flatulence, abdominal distension, and a feeling of bloating. However, we were unable to estimate reliably the frequency of these effects. It is not clear why the second review[8] did not include the RCT[12] that was identified by the first review.[10]

QUESTION What are the effects of stool softeners in adults with idiopathic chronic constipation?

OPTION PARAFFIN

We found no RCTs of paraffin in adults with idiopathic chronic constipation.

Benefits: We found no systematic review or RCTs.

Harms: We found no RCTs.

Comment: Paraffin reduces absorption of fat soluble vitamins (vitamins A, D, E, and K). However, we found no reliable evidence to measure the risk of vitamin deficiency with paraffin in people with chronic constipation.

OPTION SEED OILS/ARACHIS OIL

We found no RCTs of seed oils or arachis oil in adults with idiopathic chronic constipation.

Benefits: We found no systematic review or RCTs.

Harms: We found no RCTs.

Comment: Arachis oil is derived from peanuts, and is therefore contraindicated in people with peanut allergy.

QUESTION What are the effects of osmotic laxatives in adults with idiopathic chronic constipation?

OPTION LACTITOL

One small crossover RCT identified by a systematic review found that lactitol increased the frequency of bowel movements compared with placebo after 4 weeks. Three RCTs identified by systematic reviews compared lactitol versus

lactulose and found different results. Two RCTs found no significant difference in frequency of bowel movements at 2–4 weeks and one RCT found that lactitol increased frequency of bowel movements at 2 weeks compared with lactulose.

Benefits: **Versus placebo:** We found one systematic review (search date 1996,[9] 1 crossover RCT,[15] 43 people recruited in nursing homes passing ≤ 3 bowel movements/week, mean age 84 years). The RCT found that 20 g lactitol four times daily significantly increased the number of bowel movements compared with placebo in the third and fourth week of treatment before crossover (absolute numbers presented graphically; $P < 0.001$).[15] **Versus lactulose:** We found two systematic reviews (search date 1996,[9] search date 2001[8]), which between them identified three RCTs (see comment below). The first RCT (60 people in nursing homes, mean age 79 years) found that 15 g lactitol daily significantly increased the number of bowel movements at 2 weeks compared with 15 mL lactulose daily (5.5/week with lactitol *v* 4.9/week with lactulose; $P = 0.0001$).[9] The second RCT (61 people, mean age 54 years, 57 people analysed) found no significant difference between lactitol (20 g/day for 3 days then 10 g/day) and lactulose (30 mL syrup [20.1 g]/day for 3 days then 20 mL syrup [13.4 g]/day) in frequency of bowel movements over 4 weeks (6.7/week with lactitol *v* 7.4/week with lactulose; P value reported as non-significant).[16] The third RCT (60 people taking laxatives, mean age 60 years) found no significant difference between lactitol (mean dose 20 g/day) and lactulose 20 mL syrup daily in frequency of bowel movement at 2 weeks (6.09/week with lactitol *v* 5.53/week with lactulose; $P > 0.05$).[17]

Harms: **Versus placebo:** The review gave no information on adverse effects.[9] **Versus lactulose:** The second RCT found that lactitol significantly reduced the proportion of people with adverse effects compared with lactulose (10/32 [31%] with lactitol *v* 16/26 [62%] with lactulose; $P = 0.02$).[16] The third RCT found no significant difference between lactitol and lactulose in adverse events or other symptoms (bloating, flatulence, nausea, cramping, or diarrhoea).[8]

Comment: **Versus lactulose:** Further details may be available in *Clinical Evidence* when we have translated the third RCT into English.[17]

OPTION LACTULOSE

We found limited evidence from two RCTs that lactulose improved symptoms compared with placebo. We found limited evidence from two RCTs that lactulose was less effective in improving symptoms at 4 weeks than ispaghula husk. Three RCTs identified by systematic reviews compared lactulose versus lactitol and found different results. Two RCTs found no significant difference in effectiveness at 2–4 weeks and one RCT found that lactulose was less effective than lactitol in increasing bowel movement frequency at 2 weeks. One RCT identified by a systematic review and one subsequent RCT found that lactulose was less effective than macrogols in improving global satisfaction and severity of constipation at 4 weeks.

Benefits: We found three systematic reviews that included trials of lactulose (search dates 1995,[10] 1996,[9] and 2001[8]). **Versus placebo:** Between them the reviews identified four RCTs. The first RCT (24 recruited outpatients, mean age 28 years) found that high dose lactulose (60 mL four times/day) significantly increased the frequency of bowel movements compared with placebo after 1 week (4.5/week with lactulose *v* 2.8/week with placebo; $P < 0.05$).[10] The second RCT (47 people in a nursing home, mean age 85 years, 42 analysed) found that lactulose (30 mL four times/day) significantly reduced five symptoms (cramping, griping, flatulence, tenesmus, and bloating) compared with placebo at 12 weeks (P = 0.04).[9] It found no significant difference in the number of bowel movements (4.9/week with lactulose *v* 3.6/week with placebo; P = 0.10). The third RCT (103 people, mean age > 60 years) did not report on our outcomes of interest.[9] For a description of the fourth RCT, see comment below. **Versus ispaghula husk:** See benefits of ispaghula husk, p 494. **Versus lactitol:** See benefits of lactitol, p 496. **Versus macrogols:** The most recent review[8] identified one RCT[18] and we found one subsequent RCT.[19] The RCT identified by the review (115 people passing < 3 stools/week, straining at stool, or both) found that lactulose 20 g daily was significantly less effective than macrogol 3350 26 g daily in increasing the number of weekly bowel movements (0.9 with lactulose *v* 1.3 with macrogol 3350; P = 0.005), easing stool evacuation (scored as 0 for easy to 4 for very difficult: absolute mean score: 1.0 with lactulose *v* 0.5 with macrogol 3350; P < 0.001), and improving global satisfaction at 1 month (satisfaction scored as 0 for terrible–10 for excellent: 5.2 with lactulose *v* 7.4 with macrogol 3500; P < 0.001).[18] The subsequent RCT (85 elderly people) found that macrogol (10 g PEG 4000 daily) significantly increased the proportion of people with complete remission of constipation compared with lactulose (15 ml daily) at two and four weeks (2 weeks: 63.6% with PEG 4000 *v* 39.0% with lactulose, P < 0.01; 4 weeks: 69% with PEG 4000 *v* 42.1% with lactulose, P < 0.01).[19]

Harms: **Versus placebo:** The reviews gave no information on adverse effects.[9,10] **Versus ispaghula husk:** See harms of ispaghula husk, p 495. **Versus lactitol:** See harms of lactitol, p 496. **Versus macrogols:** The RCT identified by the review found one adverse event (depression) leading to withdrawal with lactulose compared with two adverse events (acute diarrhoea) with macrogol 3350.[18] It found that macrogol 3350 increased the frequency of liquid stools compared with lactulose over 4 weeks (mean number of loose stools over 4 weeks: 2.4 with macrogol 3350 *v* 0.6 with lactulose; P = 0.001). The subsequent RCT found no significant difference in adverse effects between macrogol and lactulose (11.7% with PEG 4000 *v* 16.1% with lactulose; P > 0.05).[19]

Comment: **Versus placebo:** The most recent review[8] also identified one crossover RCT,[20] but it was not clear whether results were reported before the crossover. The RCT (55 people) compared lactulose versus placebo in a crossover design with 4 week treatment periods and a 2 week washout. It found that 30 mL lactulose significantly improved complete or partial treatment success compared with placebo (23/29 [79%] with lactulose *v* 17/26 [65%] with placebo; P < 0.01). More detailed results may be available when this RCT is translated.[20]

OPTION MACROGOLS (POLYETHYLENE GLYCOLS)

Three RCTs identified by a systematic review and one small additional RCT found that macrogols (polyethylene glycols) improved symptoms after 2–20 weeks compared with placebo. One RCT found insufficient evidence to compare macrogol 3350 versus ispaghula husk. One systematic review and one subsequent RCT found that macrogols improved global satisfaction and severity of constipation at 4 weeks compared with lactulose.

Benefits: **Versus placebo:** We found one systematic review (search date 2001,[8] 3 RCTs[21–23]) and one additional RCT.[24] The first RCT identified by the review (70 adults aged 18–73 years meeting Rome diagnostic criteria for chronic constipation(G) who had previously received a 4 week course of macrogol 4000 14.6 g twice daily) found that continued macrogol 4000 (14.6 g twice daily) significantly increased the proportion of people who were "asymptomatic" at 20 weeks compared with placebo (70% with macrogol 4000 *v* 20% with placebo; P < 0.001).[21] "Asymptomatic" was defined as three bowel movements or more a week, no use of laxatives, no straining at defaecation, feeling of complete evacuation, and no hard/pellet-like stools. Analysis did not seem to be by intention to treat; significantly more people taking macrogol 4000 completed the trial (70% with macrogol 4000 *v* 30% with placebo; P < 0.01).[21] The second RCT identified by the review (151 chronically constipated people with ≤ 2 bowel movements during the 7 day run in period, mean age 47 years, 144 analysed) found that 17 g of macrogols significantly increased the frequency of bowel movements and increased the number of satisfactory bowel movements (defined by self report) compared with dextrose placebo after 14 days (number of bowel movements in week 2: 4.5 with macrogols *v* 2.7 with placebo, P < 0.001; satisfactory bowel movements: 68% with macrogols *v* 46% with placebo, P < 0.001).[22] The third RCT identified by the review (55 people with < 2 bowel movements a week for > 12 months, mean age 42 years, 48 people analysed) compared twice daily macrogols versus placebo.[23] It found that macrogols significantly increased the number of bowel movements per week, and decreased straining at defaecation compared with placebo at 8 weeks (bowel movements/week: 4.8 with macrogols *v* 2.8 with placebo, P < 0.002; marked straining: 8% with macrogols *v* 41% with placebo; P < 0.03).[23] The additional small cross-over RCT (34 people randomised, aged 20–60 years, 31 people analysed) found that macrogol 3350 (69.6 g/L; 500 mL/day) increased the frequency of bowel motions at 1 week compared with placebo, but the statistical significance was not reported for the pre-crossover period (13.56/week with macrogols *v* 5.53/week with placebo).[24] **Versus ispaghula husk:** See benefits of ispaghula husk, p 494. **Versus lactulose:** See benefits of lactulose, p 496.

Harms: **Versus placebo:** The first RCT identified by the review found no significant difference between macrogol 4000 and placebo in adverse events (number of events: nausea: 22/33 with macrogol *v* 17/37 with placebo; vomiting: 1 event in each group; anal pain: 5/33 with macrogol *v* 0/37 with placebo; presence of fresh blood in stool [indicating damage to anorectal mucosa]: 7/33 with macrogol *v* 2/37 with placebo; epigastric pain/discomfort: 13/33 with macrogol *v* 16/37 with placebo).[21] The second RCT identified by the review found no significant difference between macrogols and placebo in adverse events.[22] The third RCT in the review found no significant difference in abdominal symptoms at 8 weeks between macrogols and placebo (abdominal pain: 24% with macrogols *v* 35% with placebo; abdominal bloating: 48% with macrogols *v* 70% with placebo; flatulence: 20% with macrogols *v* 39% with placebo; borborygmi: 32% with macrogols *v* 13% with placebo; P values not reported).[23] The subsequent RCT did not report adverse effects by treatment group.[24] **Versus ispaghula husk:** See harms of ispaghula husk, p 495. **Versus lactulose:** See harms of lactulose, p 496.

Comment: One RCT (266 ambulatory people in general practice, mean age 51 years, 85% female) compared four different macrogol regimens over 4 weeks: macrogol 3350 (5.9 g/day); macrogol 3350 (11.8 g/day); macrogol 4000 (10 g/day), and macrogol 4000 (20 g/day).[25] It found no significant difference among treatments in bowel frequency, but found that standard dose polyethylene glycol 3350 (5.9 g) significantly increased the proportion of people with stools of normal consistency compared with maximum dose macrogol 3350 and maximum dose macrogol 4000 (P < 0.001).[25]

OPTION MAGNESIUM SALTS

We found no RCTs of magnesium salts in adults with idiopathic chronic constipation.

Benefits: We found no systematic review and no RCTs.

Harms: We found no RCTs.

Comment: None.

OPTION PHOSPHATE ENEMAS (RECTAL PHOSPHATES)

We found no RCTs of phosphate enemas in adults with idiopathic chronic constipation.

Benefits: We found no systematic review and no RCTs.

Harms: We found no RCTs.

Comment: None.

OPTION SODIUM CITRATE ENEMAS (RECTAL SODIUM CITRATE)

We found no RCTs of sodium citrate enemas in adults with idiopathic chronic constipation.

Benefits: We found no systematic review and no RCTs.

Harms: We found no RCTs.

Comment: None.

QUESTION What are the effects of stimulant laxatives in adults with idiopathic chronic constipation?

OPTION BISACODYL

We found no RCTs of bisacodyl in adults with idiopathic chronic constipation.

Benefits: We found no systematic review and no RCTs.

Harms: We found no RCTs.

Comment: None.

OPTION DANTRON

We found no RCTs of dantron in adults with idiopathic chronic constipation. Animal studies have suggested that dantron may be carcinogenic. Its use is, therefore, recommended only in people who are terminally ill.

Benefits: We found no systematic review and no RCTs (see comment below).

Harms: We found no RCTs.

Comment: Animal studies have suggested that dantron may be carcinogenic. Its use is, therefore, recommended only in people who are terminally ill.

OPTION **DOCUSATE**

One systematic review identified no RCTs of sufficient quality comparing docusate versus placebo. One RCT identified by a systematic review found no clinically important difference between docusate and ispaghula husk in frequency of bowel movements, stool consistency, straining, or pain after 2 weeks.

Benefits: **Versus placebo:** We found one systematic review (search date 1995) that identified no RCTs of sufficient quality.[10] **Versus ispaghula husk:** See benefits of ispaghula husk, p 494.

Harms: **Versus placebo:** The review gave no information on adverse effects.[10] **Versus ispaghula husk:** See harms of ispaghula husk, p 495.

Comment: None.

OPTION **GLYCEROL/GLYCERIN SUPPOSITORIES**

We found no RCTs of glycerol/glycerin suppositories in adults with idiopathic chronic constipation.

Benefits: We found no systematic review and no RCTs.

Harms: We found no RCTs.

Comment: None.

OPTION **SENNA**

We found no RCTs of the effects of senna in adults with idiopathic chronic constipation.

Benefits: We found no systematic review and no RCTs.

Harms: We found no RCTs.

Comment: None.

OPTION **PICOSULPHATE (PICOSULFATE)**

We found no RCTs of picosulphate in adults with idiopathic chronic constipation.

Benefits: We found no systematic review and no RCTs (see comment below).

Harms: We found no RCTs.

Comment: Picosulphate is a powerful stimulant laxative. Use is usually restricted to people with severe constipation or to clear the bowel of stool before surgery or radiological or endoscopic investigation.

GLOSSARY

Rome II criteria (updated 1999) Rome criteria for constipation require two or more of the following symptoms to be present for at least 12 weeks out of the preceding 12 months: straining at defaecation on at least a quarter of occasions; stools are lumpy/hard on at least a quarter of occasions; sensation of incomplete evacuation on at least a quarter of occasions; and three or fewer bowel movements a week.[1]

REFERENCES

1. Thompson WG, Longstreth GF, Drossman DA, et al. Functional bowel disorders and functional abdominal pain. *Gut* 1999;45;43–47.
2. Prescription cost analysis. Department of Health. 2001. http://www.doh.gov.uk/stats/pca2001.xls (last accessed 28 November 2003).

3. Probert CS, Emmett PM, Heaton KW. Some determinants of whole-gut transit time: a population-based study. *QJM* 1995;88:311–315.
4. Heaton KW. Cleave and the fibre story. *J R Nav Med Serv* 1980;66:5–10.
5. Donald IP, Smith RG, Cruikshank JG, et al. A study of constipation in the elderly living at home. *Gerontology* 1985;31:112–118.
6. Campbell AJ, Busby WJ, Horwath CC. Factors associated with constipation in a community based sample of people aged 70 years and over. *J Epidemiol Community Health* 1993;47:23–26.
7. Talley NJ, Fleming KC, Evans JM, et al. Constipation in an elderly community: a study of prevalence and potential risk factors. *Am J Gastroenterol* 1996;91:19–25.
8. NHS Centre for Reviews and Dissemination Effectiveness of laxatives in adults. *Effective Health Care* 2001;7. Search date 2001; primary sources Medline, Embase, Psychinfo, Cochrane Library, Cinahl, International Pharmaceutical Abstracts, Amed, and contact with manufacturers and relevant experts.
9. Petticrew M, Watt I, Sheldon T. Systematic review of the effectiveness of laxatives in the elderly. *Health Technol Assess* 1997;1:1–52. Search date 1996; primary sources recent systematic review by Tramonte et al 1997,[10] Medline, Biological Abstracts, Microdex, bibliographies, text books, contact with manufacturers of laxatives, Embase, Psychlit, Cochrane Library, Cinahl, International Pharmaceutical Abstracts, and Amed.
10. Tramonte SM, Brand MB, Mulrow CD, et al. The treatment of chronic constipation in adults: a systematic review. *J Gen Intern Med* 1997;12:15–24. Search date 1995; primary sources Medline, Biological Abstracts, Micromedex (a drug information service), hand searches of bibliographies of identified articles and textbooks, and personal contact with laxative manufacturers in North America and authors.
11. Fenn GC, Wilkinson PD, Lee CE, et al. A general practice study of the efficacy of Regulan in functional constipation. *Br J Clin Pract* 1986;40:192–197.
12. Rouse M, Chapman N, Mahapatra M, et al. An open, randomised, parallel group study of lactulose versus ispaghula in the treatment of chronic constipation in adults. *Br J Clin Pract* 1991;45:28–30.
13. Dettmar PW, Sykes J. A multi-centre, general practice comparison of ispaghula husk with lactulose and other laxatives in the treatment of simple constipation. *Curr Med Res Opin* 1998;14:227–233.
14. McRorie JW, Daggy BP, Morel JG, et al. Psyllium is superior to decusate sodium for treatment of chronic constipation. Aliment Pharmacol Ther 1998;12:491–497.
15. Vanderdonckt J, Coulon J, Denys W, et al. Study of the laxative effect of lactitol (Importal) in an elderly institutionalized but not bedridden, population suffering from constipation. *J Clin Exp Gerontol* 1990;21:171–189.
16. Hammer B, Ravelli GP. Chronische funktionelle Obstipation. [Chronic functional constipation Lactitol maintenance dose, a multicentre comparative study with lactulose] *Ther Schweiz* 1992;8:328–335. [In German]
17. Heitland W, Mauersberger H. Untersuchung der laxativen Wirkung von Lactitol gneegen Lactulose in einer offenen, randomisererten Vergleichssudie. [Study of the laxative effect of Lactitol as opposed to lactulose in an open, randomized comparative study.] *Schweiz Rundsch Med Prax* 1988;77:493–495. [In German]
18. Attar A, Lemann M, Ferguson A, et al. Comparison of a low dose polyethylene glycol electrolyte solution with lactulose for treatment of chronic constipation. *Gut* 1999;44:226–230.
19. Zhang CQ, Zhang GW, Zhang KL, et al. Clinical evaluation of polyethylene glycol 4000 in treatment of functional constipation in elderly patients. World Chin J Digesto; 2003;11:1399–1401.
20. Castillo R, Nardi G, Simhan D. La lactulosa en el tratamiento de la constipacion cronica idiopatica. *Pren Med Argent* 1995;82:173–176.
21. Corazziari E, Badiali D, Bazzocchi G, et al. Long term efficacy, safety, and tolerability of low daily doses of isosmotic polyethylene glycol electrolyte balanced solution (PMF-100) in the treatment of functional chronic constipation. *Gut* 2000;46:522–526.
22. DiPalma JA, DeRidder PH, Orlando RC, et al. A randomized, placebo-controlled, multicenter study of the safety and efficacy of a new polyethylene glycol laxative. *Am J Gastroenterol* 2000;95:446–450.
23. Corazziari E, Badiali D, Habib FI, et al. Small volume isosmotic polyethylene glycol electrolyte balanced solution (PMF-100) in treatment of chronic nonorganic constipation. *Dig Dis Sci* 1996;41:1636–1642.
24. Baldonedo YC, Lugo E, Uzcategui AA, et al. Evaluation and use of polyethylene glycol in patients with constipation. Journal of the Venezuelan Society of Gastroenterology 1991;45:294–297.
25. Chaussade S, Minic M. Comparison of efficacy and safety of two doses of two different polyethylene glycol–based laxatives in the treatment of constipation. Aliment Pharmacol Ther 2003;7:165–172.

Frank Frizelle
Professor of Colorectal Surgery
Christchurch Hospital and School of Medicine
Christchurch
New Zealand

Murray Barclay
Gastroenterologist and Clinical Pharmacologist
Christchurch Hospital and School of Medicine
Christchurch
New Zealand

Competing interests: None declared. *We would like to acknowledge the previous contributors of this chapter, including Bazian Ltd.*

Gastro-oesophageal reflux disease

Search date July 2003

Paul Moayyedi, Brendan Delaney, and David Forman

QUESTIONS

INTERVENTIONS

Key Messages

Initial treatment

- **H_2 receptor antagonists** One systematic review has found that H_2 receptor antagonists reduce the risk of persisting oesophagitis compared with placebo, but are not as effective as proton pump inhibitors.
- **Proton pump inhibitors** One systematic review, one additional RCT, and one subsequent RCT found that proton pump inhibitors increase healing compared with placebo or H_2 receptor antagonists. One systematic review found that esomeprazole 40 mg daily increased healing at 4 weeks compared with omeprazole 20 mg daily. RCTs have found no significant differences in clinical benefit among other proton pump inhibitors.
- **Antacids/alginates** Two RCTs provided limited evidence that antacids reduced symptom scores at 4–8 weeks compared with placebo, but neither found a significant difference in endoscopic healing. We found limited evidence on the effects of antacids compared with H_2 receptor antagonists. The first RCT found no significant difference between antacids compared with cimetidine in endoscopic healing at 8 weeks. The second RCT found that antacids were less effective for heartburn symptoms compared with ranitidine at 12 weeks.
- **Lifestyle advice** Small RCTs provided insufficient evidence on the effects of raising the head of the bed or weight loss for the treatment of reflux oesophagitis. We found no RCTs on the effects of reducing coffee intake, stopping smoking, reducing alcohol intake, or reducing fatty food intake.

- **Motility stimulants** One RCT found that cisapride increased endoscopic healing compared with placebo at 12 weeks. The use of cisapride has been restricted in some countries because of concerns about heart rhythm abnormalities. We found no RCTs of domperidone or metoclopramide.

Maintenance treatment

- **Proton pump inhibitors** RCTs have found that proton pump inhibitors reduce relapse in people with healed reflux oesophagitis compared with placebo or H_2 receptor antagonist at 6–18 months. One systematic review has found that standard dose lansoprazole (30 mg/day) was as effective as omeprazole (20 mg/day) for maintaining healing at 12 months. However, the systematic review and one subsequent RCT provided evidence that lower dose lansoprazole (15 mg/day) was less effective than higher dose lansoprazole (30 mg/day), omeprazole, or esomeprazole for maintaining healing for up to 12 months.
- **Laparoscopic surgery** One systematic review found no fully published RCTs comparing laparoscopic surgery versus medical treatment for maintenance of remission. Two RCTs found no significant difference between open and laparoscopic fundoplication for remission at 3 months to 2 years. One RCT found that laparoscopic treatment was associated with surgical complications, although the rate was lower than with open surgery.
- **Open surgery** RCTs have found that open Nissen fundoplication compared with medical treatment improved the endoscopic grade of oesophagitis in people with chronic gastro-oesophageal reflux disease and oesophagitis at between 3 and 38 months. However, longer term follow up from one of these RCTs found no significant difference in endoscopic appearance between surgery and medical treatment at 10 years. Two RCTs found no significant difference between open and laparoscopic fundoplication for remission at 3 months to 2 years. One RCT found that mortality was higher with open surgery than with medical treatment. One RCT found that complication rates were higher with open than with laparoscopic surgery.
- **Antacids/alginates** We found no RCTs on the effects of antacids/alginates on the long term management of reflux oesophagitis.
- **H_2 receptor antagonists** One RCT found no significant difference between ranitidine and placebo for relapse of oesophagitis at 6 months in people with previously healed reflux oesophagitis. RCTs have found that H_2 receptor antagonists are less effective than proton pump inhibitors for maintaining remission up to 12 months.
- **Lifestyle advice** We found no RCTs on the effects of lifestyle advice on the long term management of reflux oesophagitis.
- **Motility stimulants** Three RCTs have found that cisapride compared with placebo improved maintenance of healing at 6–12 months. Two further RCTs found no evidence of a difference, but they might have lacked power to detect a clinically significant effect. The use of cisapride has been restricted in some countries because of concerns about effects on heart rhythms. We found no RCTs comparing other prokinetic drugs with placebo or each other in people with gastro-oesophageal reflux disease and oesophagitis.

DEFINITION Gastro-oesophageal reflux disease (GORD) is defined as reflux of gastroduodenal contents into the oesophagus, causing symptoms that are sufficient to interfere with quality of life.[1] People with GORD often have symptoms of heartburn and acid regurgitation.[2] GORD can be classified according to the results of upper gastrointestinal endoscopy. Currently the most validated method is the Los Angeles classification, where an endoscopy showing mucosal breaks in the distal oesophagus indicate the presence of oesophagitis, which is graded in severity from grade A (mucosal breaks of < 5 mm in the oesophagus) to grade D (circumferential breaks in the oesophageal mucosa).[1,3] Alternatively, severity may be graded according to the Savary–Miller classification (grade I: linear, non-confluent erosions, to grade IV: severe ulceration or stricture).

INCIDENCE/ PREVALENCE Surveys from Europe and the USA suggest that 20–25% of the population have symptoms of GORD, and 7% have heartburn daily.[4,5] In primary care settings, about 25–40% of people with GORD have oesophagitis on endoscopy, but most have endoscopy negative reflux disease.[3]

AETIOLOGY/ RISK FACTORS We found no evidence of clear predictive factors for GORD. Obesity is reported to be a risk factor for GORD but epidemiological data are conflicting.[6,7] Smoking and alcohol are also thought to predispose to GORD, but observational data are limited.[7,8] It has been suggested that some foods, such as coffee, mints, dietary fat, onions, citrus fruits, or tomatoes, may predispose to GORD.[9] However, we found insufficient data on the role of these factors. We found limited evidence that drugs that relax the lower oesophageal sphincter, such as calcium channel blockers, may promote GORD.[10] Twin studies suggest that there may be a genetic predisposition to GORD.[8]

PROGNOSIS GORD is a chronic condition, with about 80% of people relapsing once medication is discontinued.[11] Many people therefore require long term medical treatment or surgery. Endoscopy negative reflux disease remains stable, with a minority of people developing oesophagitis over time.[12] However, people with severe oesophagitis may develop complications such as oesophageal stricture or Barrett's oesophagus.[1]

AIMS OF INTERVENTION To relieve reflux symptoms, increase healing rates, and reduce the complications of GORD, such as stricture formation; to improve quality of life; to minimise adverse effects of treatment.

OUTCOMES Frequency and severity of symptoms; quality of life. Healing rates (assessed endoscopically in people with oesophagitis), which have been shown to be closely associated with clinical outcomes.[13,14] pH measurement of reflux is an intermediate outcome that is often used in RCTs, but it is difficult to interpret clinically. We excluded RCTs based solely on this outcome.

METHODS *Clinical Evidence* search and appraisal July 2003.

QUESTION What are the effects of interventions in the initial treatment of gastro-oesophageal reflux disease associated with oesophagitis?

OPTION LIFESTYLE ADVICE

Small RCTs provided insufficient evidence on the effects of raising the head of the bed or weight loss for the treatment of reflux oesophagitis. We found no RCTs on the effects of reducing coffee intake, stopping smoking, reducing alcohol intake, or reducing fatty food intake.

Benefits: We found no systematic review. **Raising the head of the bed:** One RCT (71 people aged 22–77 years with endoscopically diagnosed gastro-oesophageal reflux [grade C]) compared raising the head of the bed (to produce a 10° slope) versus not raising the head of the bed in people additionally randomised to ranitidine (150 mg twice daily) versus placebo for 6 weeks.[15] It found that, in people taking placebo, raising the head of the bed increased participant reported improvement compared with not raising the head of the bed at 6 weeks (grading of improvement not specified; 10/17 [59%] with bed raised *v* 4/14 [29%] without; significance of individual comparisons not reported). The benefit of raising the head of the bed was increased in people taking ranitidine (13/15 [87%] with ranitidine + raised head of bed *v* 10/17 [59%] with placebo + raised head of bed; significance not stated). Endoscopic appearances were not significantly different among any of the four groups. **Weight loss:** One RCT (20 people with gastro-oesophageal reflux confirmed by 24 hour pH measurement, mean body mass index 31.4 kg/m^2) compared a low calorie diet (430 kcal/day for the first 6 weeks) plus advice and support for 6 months versus standard instructions about reflux disease and general advice to lose weight.[16] It found no significant difference between groups in symptoms or the number of episodes of reflux (analysis not by intention to treat; 19 people in analysis; no further data reported), but the study may have lacked power to detect a clinically significant difference. **Reducing coffee intake; stopping smoking; reducing alcohol intake; reducing fatty food intake:** We found no RCTs on these lifestyle measures.

Harms: We found no RCTs.

Comment: None.

OPTION ANTACIDS/ALGINATES

Two RCTs provided limited evidence that antacids reduced symptom scores at 4–8 weeks compared with placebo, but neither found a significant difference in endoscopic healing. We found limited evidence on the effects of antacids compared with H_2 receptor antagonists. The first RCT found no significant difference between antacids compared with cimetidine in endoscopic healing at 8 weeks. The second RCT found that antacids were less effective for heartburn symptoms compared with ranitidine at 12 weeks.

Benefits: We found no systematic review. **Versus placebo:** We found two RCTs.[17,18] The first RCT (91 people with gastro-oesophageal reflux disease and endoscopically confirmed oesophagitis grade A–C) compared antacids (1 tablet aluminium hydroxide/magnesium carbonate 1 hour after meals and at bedtime) versus cimetidine (400 mg twice daily) versus placebo for 8 weeks.[17] It found that antacids significantly reduced the number of days with reflux symptoms compared with placebo and reduced the median symptom score (days with reflux: 5 days *v* 13 days, $P < 0.05$; symptom score: measured on a 100 mm visual analogue scale [100 mm = worst score]: 8 with antacids *v* 33 with placebo). However, it found no significant difference in endoscopic healing at 8 weeks (8/27 [30%] with antacids *v* 6/29 [21%] with placebo). The second, smaller RCT (32 people with gastro-oesophageal reflux disease and oesophagitis confirmed by pH monitoring and an acid perfusion test) compared antacids (15 mL doses of aluminium and magnesium hydroxide 7 times daily) versus placebo for 4 weeks.[18] The results of this RCT may be biased in favour of antacids because 11 people who had no heartburn symptoms after taking placebo for 1 week were eliminated from the analysis. It found no significant difference between antacids and placebo in the frequency or severity of reflux or in endoscopic healing at 4 weeks, although it may have lacked power to exclude a clinically significant effect. **Versus H_2 receptor antagonists:** We found two RCTs.[17,18] The first RCT (91 people, described above) found no significant difference between antacids and cimetidine in endoscopic healing at 8 weeks (8/27 [30%] people taking antacids *v* 11/29 [38%] people taking cimetidine).[17] The second RCT (155 people with oesophagitis up to grade D) found that calcium carbonate (750 mg as needed) was significantly less effective than ranitidine for reducing the frequency and severity of heartburn after 1 week (150 mg twice daily) (results presented graphically; $P < 0.05$).[19] Subgroup analysis in people with erosive oesophagitis of grade A or greater (73 people) found that calcium carbonate significantly reduced the proportion of people with endoscopic healing at 12 weeks compared with ranitidine (10/35 [29%] with calcium carbonate *v* 21/38 [55%] with ranitidine; RR 0.52, 95% CI 0.28 to 0.94).

Harms: One of the RCTs (91 people) found that six people in the antacid group reported transient constipation after 4 weeks of treatment.[17] One RCT (32 people) found that antacids caused increased gastrointestinal adverse effects, including diarrhoea, nausea, vomiting, occult blood in the stool, gas, constipation, and duodenal ulcer, compared with controls

(12% with antacids v 3% with ranitidine; P = 0.056).[18] One person taking antacids developed a duodenal ulcer. The RCT also found that a smaller proportion of people had headache, dizziness, insomnia, malaise, fatigue, weakness, chills, and nervousness with antacids versus placebo (1% with antacids v 4% with ranitidine), but the difference was not significant (P = 0.37).

Comment: None.

OPTION MOTILITY STIMULANTS

One RCT found that cisapride increased endoscopic healing compared with placebo at 12 weeks. The use of cisapride has been restricted in some countries because of concerns about heart rhythm abnormalities. We found no RCTs of domperidone or metoclopramide.

Benefits: We found no systematic review but found one RCT (177 people with uncomplicated gastro-oesophageal reflux disease and oesophagitis) comparing cisapride (10 or 20 mg 4 times daily) versus placebo for 12 weeks.[20] It found that cisapride 20 mg significantly increased endoscopic healing of oesophagitis compared with placebo at 12 weeks (analysis not by intention to treat; 20 people excluded from analysis: 26/51 [51%] healed with cisapride 20 mg v 21/51 [41%] with 10 mg v 20/55 [36%] with placebo; $P < 0.05$; no further data reported.) We found no RCTs comparing metoclopramide or domperidone with placebo or other prokinetic drugs.

Harms: In some countries, use of cisapride has been restricted because of concerns about heart rhythm abnormalities that are associated with sudden death.[21] The RCT found no significant difference between cisapride and placebo in any adverse effects.[20] Common adverse events included diarrhoea (16.4% cisapride 20 mg v 12.5% cisapride 10 mg v 8.3% placebo), headache (11.5% v 16.1% v 26.7%), and constipation (6.6% v 10.7% v 6.7%).

Comment: None.

OPTION H_2 RECEPTOR ANTAGONISTS

One systematic review has found that H_2 receptor antagonists reduce the risk of persisting oesophagitis compared with placebo, but are not as effective as proton pump inhibitors.

Benefits: **Versus placebo:** We found one systematic review (search date not reported; 10 RCTs, 2171 people) comparing H_2 receptor antagonists versus placebo in people with oesophagitis.[22] It found that H_2 receptor antagonists significantly decreased the risk of persistent oesophagitis compared with placebo (time to outcome not stated: RR of oesophagitis persisting with H_2 receptor antagonists v placebo 0.79, 95% CI 0.72 to 0.87; NNT 6, 95% CI 5 to 10). **Versus proton pump inhibitors:** See benefits of proton pump inhibitors for initial treatment of gastro-oesophageal reflux disease, p 507.

Harms: The systematic review did not report on harms.[22]

Comment: A systematic review evaluating drug treatment in the short term management of oesophagitis is currently being conducted.[23]

OPTION PROTON PUMP INHIBITORS

One systematic review, one additional RCT, and one subsequent RCT found that proton pump inhibitors increase healing compared with placebo or H_2 receptor antagonists. One systematic review found that esomeprazole 40 mg daily increased healing at 4 weeks compared with omeprazole 20 mg daily. RCTs have found no significant differences in clinical benefit among other proton pump inhibitors.

Benefits: **Versus placebo:** We found one systematic review (search date not reported; 4 RCTs, 380 people with gastro-oesophageal reflux disease and oesophagitis) comparing proton pump inhibitors versus placebo.[22] It found that proton pump inhibitors were more effective than placebo for preventing persistence of oesophagitis (RR for persistence 0.31, 95% CI 0.13 to 0.75; time to outcome not specified; NNT 2, 95% CI 1 to 5). **Versus H_2 receptor antagonists:** The same systematic review (search date not reported, 16 RCTs, 2321 people), one additional RCT, and one subsequent RCT compared proton pump inhibitors with H_2 receptor antagonists.[22,24,25] The systematic review found that proton pump inhibitors significantly decreased persistent oesophagitis compared with H_2 receptor antagonists (RR 0.5, 95% CI 0.43 to 0.58; NNT 4, 95% CI 3 to 4; time to outcome not stated).[22] Both the additional and the subsequent RCT found similar results.[24,25] The additional RCT (177 people with Savary–Miller stages 2–4 oesophagitis) found that lansoprazole (15 mg/day and 30 mg/day) significantly increased endoscopically confirmed healing compared with ranitidine (150 mg daily) at 28 days (33/60 [55%] with lansoprazole 15 mg *v* 44/55 [80%] with lansoprazole 30 mg *v* 20/50 [40%] with ranitidine, $P < 0.01$ for lansoprazole 15 mg *v* ranitidine; $P < 0.001$ for lansoprazole 30 mg *v* ranitidine).[24] The subsequent RCT (221 people with equivalent to > Savary–Miller stage 2 oesophagitis) found that pantoprazole (20 mg and 40 mg daily) significantly increased endoscopically confirmed healing compared with nizatidine (150 mg daily) at 4 and 8 weeks (4 weeks: 48/75 [64%] with pantoprazole 40 mg *v* 43/70 [61%] with pantoprazole 20 mg *v* 16/72 [22%] with ranitidine; $P < 0.001$ for both doses of pantoprazole *v* nizatidine; 8 weeks: 58/70 [83%] with pantoprazole 40 mg *v* 57/72 [79%] with pantoprazole 20 mg *v* 29/70 [41%] with nizatidine; $P < 0.001$ for both doses of pantoprazole *v* nizatidine).[25] **Versus each other:** We found two systematic reviews (search dates 2000)[26,27] and three subsequent RCTs[28–30] comparing different proton pump inhibitors in people with reflux oesophagitis. The reviews found similar results, although results in the second review were reported more clearly and covered additional comparisons.[27] The second review found that esomeprazole (40 mg/day) significantly increased healing at 4 weeks compared with omeprazole (20 mg once daily) (3 RCTs; healing rate 1814/2446 [74%] with esomeprazole *v* 1583/2431 [65%] with omeprazole; RR 1.14, 95% CI 1.10 to 1.18; NNT 13, 95% CI 9 to 17). The review found no significant difference between lansoprazole (30 mg) and omeprazole (20 mg) at 4 weeks (5 RCTs; healing rate 704/972 [72%] with lansoprazole v 692/979 [71%] with omeprazole; RR 1.02, 95% CI 0.97 to 1.08). The review found no significant difference between pantoprazole (40 mg) and omeprazole (20 mg) or between rabeprazole (20 mg) and omeprazole (20 mg) at 4 weeks (pantoprazole *v* omeprazole, 3 RCTs, healing rate: 388/574 [68%] with pantoprazole *v* 325/474 [69%] with omeprazole; RR 0.99, 95% CI 0.91 to 1.07; rabeprazole *v* omeprazole, healing rate: 81/100 [81%] with rabeprazole *v* 83/102 [81%] with omeprazole; RR 1.00, 95% CI 0.87 to 1.14).[27] The first subsequent RCT (328 people with grade I oesophagitis) comparing pantoprazole (20 mg once daily) versus omeprazole (20 mg once daily) found no significant difference between treatments in healing rate at 8 weeks or symptom relief at 4 weeks (symptom relief: 77% with pantoprazole *v* 84% with omeprazole; no further data reported; healing rates: 90% with pantoprazole *v* 95% with omeprazole; OR 0.62, 95% CI 0.34 to 1.13).[28] The second subsequent RCT (461 people with symptomatic grade I–IV oesophagitis) compared three interventions: omeprazole (20 mg/day modified release tablets); lansoprazole (30 mg/day); and pantoprazole (40 mg/day).[29] It found no significant difference between omeprazole and lansoprazole or pantoprazole in complete resolution of heartburn symptoms at 8 weeks (89% heartburn free with pantoprazole *v* 87% with omeprazole *v* 81% with lansoprazole; ARR for omeprazole *v* pantoprazole +2%, 90% CI –4.6% to +7.6%; ARI for omeprazole *v* lansoprazole +6%, 90% CI –0.8% to +12.8%). The third subsequent RCT (251 people with symptomatic grade II–III oesophagitis) found no significant difference between rabeprazole (20 mg/day) and omeprazole (40 mg/day) in complete relief of heartburn, regurgitation, or epigastric pain after 3 days (analysis not by intention to treat; relief of heartburn 99/118 [84%] with rabeprazole *v* 96/116 [83%] with omeprazole; ARI +1.1%, 95% CI –8.4% to +10.7%; no regurgitation 101/112 [90%] with rabeprazole *v* 102/115 [89%] with omeprazole; ARI +1.5%, 95% CI –6.5% to +9.5%; no epigastric pain 89/112 [80%] with rabeprazole *v* 99/115 [86%] with omeprazole; ARR +6.6%, 95% CI –3.2% to +16.4%).[30]

Harms: The systematic review gave no information on harms.[22] **Versus H_2 receptor antagonists:** The additional RCT found no significant difference in adverse effects between lansoprazole and ranitidine (AR for any adverse effect: 21% with lansoprazole 15 mg *v* 12% with lansoprazole 30 mg *v* 20% with ranitidine, P not reported).[24] The subsequent RCT found no significant difference in adverse effects between pantoprazole and nizatidine (AR for any adverse effect: 49% with pantoprazole 20 mg *v* 54% with pantoprazole 40 mg *v* 59% with nizatidine).[25] The most common adverse effects were headache and diarrhoea (headache: 10/80 [13%] with pantoprazole 20 mg *v* 15/81 [19%] with pantoprazole 40 mg *v* 19/82 [23%] with nizatidine; diarrhoea: 8/80 [10%] with pantoprazole 20 mg *v* 6/81 [7%] with pantoprazole 40 mg *v* 9/82 [11%] with nizatidine).[25] **Versus each other:** The subsequent RCT found similar rates of adverse events with pantoprazole and omeprazole (any adverse event: 57% with pantoprazole *v* 50% with omeprazole; severe adverse events: 10% *v* 13%; nausea 8% *v* 7%; diarrhoea 5% *v* 6%; headache 6% *v* 3%).[28]

Comment: A systematic review evaluating drug treatment in the short term management of oesophagitis is currently being conducted.[23]

QUESTION What are the effects of interventions in the maintenance treatment of gastro-oesophageal reflux disease associated with oesophagitis?

OPTION LIFESTYLE ADVICE

We found no RCTs on the effects of lifestyle advice on the long term management of reflux oesophagitis.

Benefits: We found no systematic review or RCTs.

Harms: We found no RCTs.

Comment: None.

OPTION ANTACIDS/ALGINATES

We found no RCTs on the effects of antacids/alginates on the long term management of reflux oesophagitis.

Benefits: We found no systematic review or RCTs.

Harms: See benefits of antacids/alginates for the initial treatment of gastro-oesophageal reflux disease, p 505.

Comment: None.

OPTION MOTILITY STIMULANTS

Three RCTs have found that cisapride compared with placebo improved maintenance of healing at 6–12 months. Two further RCTs found no evidence of a difference, but they might have lacked power to detect a clinically significant effect. The use of cisapride has been restricted in some countries because of concerns about heart rhythm abnormalities. We found no RCTs comparing other prokinetic drugs with placebo or each other in people with gastro-oesophageal reflux disease and oesophagitis.

Benefits: We found no systematic review. We found five RCTs (1398 people) comparing cisapride (up to 40 mg/day) versus placebo for 6–12 months.[31–35] Two RCTs found no significant difference between treatments in the maintenance of endoscopic healing,[33,35] and three RCTs found that cisapride significantly increased maintenance of healing (see table 1, p 515).[31,32,34] We found no RCTs comparing other prokinetic drugs with placebo for maintanence treatment in people with gastro-oesophageal reflux disease and healed oesophagitis.

Harms: See motility stimulants for initial treatment of gastro-oesophageal reflux disease, p 506.

Comment: None.

OPTION H_2 RECEPTOR ANTAGONISTS

One RCT found no significant difference between ranitidine and placebo for relapse of oesophagitis at 6 months in people with previously healed reflux oesophagitis. RCTs have found that H_2 antagonists are less effective than proton pump inhibitors for maintaining remission at up to 12 months.

Benefits: **Versus placebo:** We found no systematic review. We found one RCT (69 people with endoscopically healed oesophagitis) comparing ranitidine (150 mg at bedtime) versus placebo for 6 months.[36] It found no significant difference between ranitidine and placebo in relapse rates at 6 months (8 people excluded from analysis: 14/33 [42%] with ranitidine *v* 10/28 [36%] with placebo; CI and P value not reported). **Versus proton pump inhibitors:** See benefits of proton pump inhibitors for maintenance treatment in gastro-oesophageal reflux disease, p 510.

Harms: The RCT found that four people, all taking placebo, reported adverse effects (rashes, transient headache, transient parasthaesia).[36] RCTs have shown similar rates of adverse events between H_2 receptor antagonists and placebo.[37]

Comment: None.

OPTION PROTON PUMP INHIBITORS

RCTs have found that proton pump inhibitors reduce relapse in people with healed reflux oesophagitis compared with placebo or H_2 receptor antagonist at 6–18 months. One systematic review has found that standard dose lansoprazole (30 mg/day) was as effective as omeprazole (20 mg/day) for maintaining healing at 12 months. However, the systematic review and one subsequent RCT provided evidence that lower dose lansoprazole (15 mg/day) was less effective than higher dose lansoprazole (30 mg/day), omeprazole, or esomeprazole for maintaining healing for up to 12 months.

Benefits: **Versus placebo:** We found one systematic review (search date 2000, 7 RCTs, 1320 people with healed oesophagitis),[26] four subsequent RCTs,[38–41] and one additional RCT.[42] The systematic review did not pool results.[26] All seven RCTs included in the review found that proton pump inhibitors (rabeprazole 10 or 20 mg/day; omeprazole 10 or 20 mg/day; lansoprazole 15 or 30 mg/day) reduced relapse rate at 6 months compared with placebo (results reported graphically; RR about 0.1 to about 0.8). The subsequent and additional RCTs found similar results (see table 2, p 516). **Versus H_2 receptor antagonists:** We found one systematic review that compared proton pump inhibitors versus ranitidine (search date 2000, 5 RCTs, 638 people with healed oesophagitis)[26] and one additional RCT.[43] The systematic review did not pool results.[26] All five RCTs included in the review found that proton pump inhibitors (omeprazole 10 or 20 mg/day; lansoprazole 15 or 30 mg/day) reduced relapse rate compared with ranitidine at 6 months (results reported graphically: RR about 0.1 to about 0.6). The additional RCT (264 people with healed oesophagitis and no symptoms of gastro-oesophageal reflux) found that omeprazole (10 mg/day) increased remission rate compared with ranitidine (150 mg twice daily) at 12 months (AR 68% with omeprazole *v* 39% with ranitidine; RR 1.43, 95% CI 1.26 to 1.57).[43] **Versus each other:** We found one systematic review (search date 2001, 12 RCTs),[44] one additional RCT,[45] and two subsequent RCTs.[46,47] The review found that lansoprazole (15 mg/day) was less effective for maintaining healing than esomeprazole (20 mg/day), higher dose lansoprazole (30 mg/day), or omeprazole (20 mg/day) (esomeprazole 20 mg *v* lansoprazole 15 mg: 1 RCT, 1224 people; RR for maintaining healing at 6 months 1.09, 95% CI 1.02 to 1.17; lansoprazole 30 mg *v* lansoprazole 15 mg: 7 RCTs, 1505 people; RR at 12 months 1.12, 95% CI 1.05 to 1.18; omeprazole 20 mg *v* lansoprazole 15 mg: 1 RCT, 597 people; RR at 12 months 1.19, 95% CI 1.10 to 1.30).[44] However, the review found no significant difference between higher dose lansoprazole (30 mg/day) and omeprazole (20 mg/day) for maintenance of healing at 12 months (2 RCTs, 859 people; RR 1.01, 95% CI 0.96 to 1.06). The additional RCT (243 people with healed oesophagitis) found no significant difference between rabeprazole (10 or 20 mg/day) and omeprazole (20 mg/day) for relapse rates at 12 months (12 months: AR 5% with 10 mg rabeprazole, 4% with 20 mg rabeprazole, 5% with 20 mg omeprazole).[45] The first subsequent RCT (137 people with healed grade I–III oesophagitis) found no significant difference between daily low dose lansoprazole (15 mg) and alternate day full dose lansoprazole (30 mg) for oesophagitis recurrence at 6 months (AR 12.1% with daily low dose lansoprazole *v* 19.0% with alternate day full dose lansoprazole; OR 1.31; 95% CI 0.57 to 3.02).[46] The second subsequent RCT (1236 people with healed Los Angeles classification grade A–D oesophagitis) found that esomeprazole (20 mg/day) significantly increased remission rates compared with lansoprazole (15 mg daily) over 6 months (83% with esomeprazole *v* 74% with lansoprazole, $P < 0.0001$).[47]

Harms: See benefits of proton pump inhibitors for initial treatment in gastro-oesophageal reflux disease, p 507. **Versus each other:** One subsequent RCT found that rates of withdrawal due to adverse events were similar with esomeprazole and lansoprazole (4.7% with esomeprazole *v* 5.2% with lansoprazole, P not reported).[47] It found that the most common adverse event was diarrhoea (5.7% with esomeprazole *v* 6.8% with lansoprazole, P not reported).

Comment: Limited evidence from cohort studies and small RCTs has suggested that long term proton pump inhibitor treatment may be associated with atrophic gastritis in people with *Helicobacter pylori*.[48–50] Gastric atrophy is a risk factor for gastric cancer.[51] However, we found no reliable evidence of long term clinical effects of proton pump inhibitors on gastric cancer rates in people with gastro-oesophageal reflux disease and oesophagitis. One crossover RCT (233 people with upper gastrointestinal disorders; 214 with gastro-oesophageal reflux disease, whose symptoms were controlled with proton pump inhibitors) compared 4 weeks' treatment with omeprazole versus rabeprazole. Post-crossover analysis found that a similar proportion of people preferred each of the treatments over the other (data and P value for overall comparison not reported).[52]

OPTION OPEN SURGERY

RCTs have found that open Nissen fundoplication improves the endoscopic grade of oesophagitis compared with medical treatment in people with chronic gastro-oesophageal reflux disease and oesophagitis at between 3 and 38 months. However, longer term follow up from one RCT found no significant difference in endoscopic appearance between surgery and medical treatment at 10 years. Two RCTs found no significant difference between open and laparoscopic fundoplication for remission at 3 months to 2 years. One RCT found that complication rtes with higher with open than with laparoscopic surgery. The benefit of antireflux surgery in controlling symptoms must be balanced against the small risk of operative mortality (< 1%) associated with this procedure.

Benefits: **Versus medical treatment:** We found one systematic review (search date 1999, 4 RCTs, 518 people with chronic gastro-oesophageal reflux disease [GORD] and oesophagitis).[53] Three included RCTs compared open antireflux surgery versus antacids and H_2 receptor antagonists in people with severe or complicated GORD. All reported that surgery significantly reduced reflux and improved the endoscopic grade of oesophagitis compared with medical treatment (see table 3, p 517). Ten years' follow up of one of the RCTs included in the review (239/247 people originally enrolled) found no significant difference in endoscopic appearance between open surgery and medical treatment (mean endoscopic grade 1.80 with surgery *v* 1.89 with medical treatment; P = 0.76).[54] The fourth RCT in the review (298 people randomised, 255 analysed) compared open antireflux surgery versus omeprazole (20 mg/day) over 5 years.[55] It defined treatment failure as one or more of: moderate or severe heartburn or acid regurgitation; oesophagitis > grade 2; moderate or severe dysphagia; and required or preferred alternative treatment (omeprazole or surgery). It found that surgery significantly reduced treatment failure compared with omeprazole at 5 years (20/103 [19%] with surgery *v* 49/114 [43%] with omeprazole, P < 0.001). **Open surgery versus laparoscopic surgery:** We found two RCTs.[56,57] The first RCT (148 people with persistent GORD and oesophagitis following medical treatment) found no significant difference between open and laparoscopic Nissen fundoplication in symptomatic remission at 3 months (35 people excluded from end point analysis: 98% remission with open surgery *v* 97% with laparoscopic surgery; reported as non-significant; no further data reported).[56] The second RCT (42 people with GORD) also found no clear difference in symptoms or endoscopically defined remission at 2 years with open compared with laparoscopic Nissen fundoplication (analysis not by intention to treat; endoscopic remission: all people receiving laparoscopic surgery were in remission *v* all but 2 people with open surgery, number of people in analysis not reported; symptoms [4 people excluded from analysis]: 79% free of heartburn with laparoscopic surgery *v* 58% with open surgery; 95% free of regurgitation in both groups; significance not assessed).[57]

Harms: **Versus medical treatment:** One RCT included in the review reported significantly higher mortality with surgery compared with medical treatment, mainly because of cardiovascular disease during long term follow up (RR 1.57, 95% CI 1.01 to 2.46).[54] The systematic review reported that one included RCT found that open Nissen fundoplication significantly increased early satiety, inability to belch, and inability to vomit compared with medical treatment.[53] **Versus laparoscopic surgery:** The first RCT found that overall complication rate (including splenectomy, pneumothorax, subphrenic abscess, wound infection, cicatricial hernia) was higher with open compared with laparoscopic Nissen fundoplication (6/57 [11%] people with laparoscopy *v* 10/46 [22%] with open Nissen fundoplication).[56] The second RCT did not report on operative complications.[57]

Comment: The benefit of antireflux surgery in controlling symptoms must be balanced against the very small operative mortality (< 1%) associated with this procedure.[58]

OPTION LAPAROSCOPIC SURGERY

One systematic review identified no fully published RCTs comparing laparoscopic surgery versus medical treatment for maintenance of remission. Two RCTs found no significant difference in remission between open and laparoscopic fundoplication at 3 months to 2 years. One RCT found that laparoscopic treatment was associated with surgical complications, although the rate was lower than with open surgery.

Benefits: **Laparoscopic surgery versus medical treatment:** We found one systematic review (search date 1999).[53] It identified no fully published RCTs that examined effects on symptoms or endoscopically defined healing (see comment below). **Laparoscopic surgery versus open surgery:** See benefits of open surgery, p 511.

Harms: **Versus medical treatment:** We found insufficient evidence to compare harms of laparoscopic surgery versus medical treatment. **Versus open surgery:** See harms of open surgery, p 512.

Comment: The review identified one RCT (90 people with severe gastro-oesophageal reflux disease for at least 6 months) that was published as an abstract only.[53] It found similar results for laparoscopic surgery compared with proton pump inhibitors for quality of life at 3 months (scale not reported).

REFERENCES

1. Dent J, Brun J, Fendrick AM, et al. An evidence-based appraisal of reflux disease management: the Genval Workshop Report. *Gut* 1999;44(suppl 2):S1–S16.
2. Klauser AG, Schindlbeck NE, Muller-Lissner SA. Symptoms in gastro-oesophageal reflux disease. *Lancet* 1990;335:205–208.
3. Armstrong D, Bennett JR, Blum AL, et al. The endoscopic assessment of esophagitis: a progress report on observer agreement. *Gastroenterology* 1996;111:85–92.
4. Kay L, Jorgensen T. Epidemiology of upper dyspepsia in a random population. *Scand J Gastroenterol* 1994;29:1–6.

5. Isolauri J, Laippala P. Prevalence of symptoms suggestive of gastro-oesophageal reflux disease in an adult population. *Ann Med* 1995;27:67–70.
6. Lagergren J, Bergstrom R, Nyren O. No relation between body mass and gastro-oesophageal reflux symptoms in a Swedish population based study. *Gut* 2000;47:26–29.
7. Locke GR III, Talley NJ, Fett SL, et al. Risk factors associated with symptoms of gastroesophageal reflux. *Am J Med* 1999;106:642–649.
8. Romero Y, Cameron AJ, Locke GR III, et al. Familial aggregation of gastroesophageal reflux in patients with Barrett's esophagus and esophageal adenocarcinoma. *Gastroenterology* 1997;113:1449–1456.
9. Terry P, Lagergren J, Wolk A, et al. Reflux-inducing dietary factors and risk of adenocarcinoma of the esophagus and gastric cardia. *Nutr Cancer* 2000;38:186–191.
10. Lagergren J, Bergstrom R, Adami HO, et al. Association between medications that relax the lower esophageal sphincter and risk for esophageal adenocarcinoma. *Ann Intern Med* 2000;133:165–175.
11. Dent J, Yeomans ND, Mackinnon M, et al. Omeprazole v ranitidine for the prevention of relapse of reflux oesophagitis. A controlled double blind trial of their efficacy and safety. *Gut* 1994;35:590–598.
12. Trimble KC, Douglas S, Pryde A, et al. Clinical characteristics and natural history of symptomatic but not excess gastro-esophageal reflux. *Dig Dis Sci* 1995;40:1098–1104.
13. Hatlebakk JG, Berstad A. Prognostic factors for relapse of reflux oesophagitis and symptoms during 12 months of therapy with lansoprazole. *Aliment Pharmacol Ther* 1997;11:1093–1099.
14. Vakil NB, Shaker R, Johnson DA, et al. The new proton pump inhibitor esomeprazole is effective as a maintenance therapy in GERD patients with healed erosive oesophagitis: a 6-month, randomized, double-blind, placebo-controlled study of efficacy and safety. *Aliment Pharmacol Ther* 2001;15:927–935.
15. Harvey RF, Hadley N, Gill TR, et al. Effects of sleeping with the bed-head raised and of ranitidine in patients with severe peptic oesophagitis. *Lancet* 1987;2:1200–1203.
16. Kjellin A, Ramel S, Rossner S, et al. Gastroesophageal reflux in obese patients is not reduced by weight reduction. *Scand J Gastroenterol* 1996;31:1047–1051.
17. Farup PG, Weberg R, Berstad A, et al. Low-dose antacids versus 400 mg cimetidine twice daily for reflux oesophagitis. *Scand J Gastroenterol* 1990;25:315–320.
18. Graham DY, Patterson DJ. Double-blind comparison of liquid antacid and placebo in the treatment of symptomatic reflux esophagitis. *Dig Dis Sci* 1983;28:559–563.
19. Earnest D, Robinson M, Rodriguez-Stanley S, et al. Managing heartburn at the "base" of the GERD "iceberg": effervescent ranitidine 150 mg bd provides faster and better heartburn relief than antacids. *Aliment Pharmacol Ther* 2000;14:911–918.
20. Richter JE, Long JF. Cisapride for gastrooesophageal reflux disease: a placebo-controlled, double-blind study. *Am J Gastroenterol* 1995;90:423–430.
21. Piquette RK. Torsade de pointes induced by cisapride/clarithromycin interaction. *Ann Pharmacother* 1999;33:22–26.
22. Delaney B, Moayyedi P. *Dyspepsia. Health Care Needs Assessment*, 4th ed. Stevens A, Raftery J (eds). NHS Executive, 2002 (in press) http://hcna.radcliffe-oxford.com/dyspepsia.htm (last accessed 17 February 2003). Search date not reported; primary sources are a recent systematic review funded by the NHS R&D HTA programme, three recently published Cochrane reviews, and abstracts of recently completed trials.
23. Preston C, Donnellan C, Moayyedi P. Medical treatments for the short term management of reflux oesophagitis (protocol for a Cochrane Review). In: The Cochrane Library, Issue 2, 2002. Oxford: Update Software.
24. Petite JP, Aucomte A, Barbare JC, et al. Lansoprazole versus ranitidine in the treatment of reflux oesophagitis. A multi-centre study. *Med Chir Dig* 1991–20,No. 8.
25. Kovacs TOG, Wilcox CM, Devault K, et al. Comparison of the efficacy of pantoprazole vs. nizatidine in the treatment of erosive oesophagitis: a randomized, active-controlled, double-blind study. *Aliment Pharmacol Ther* 2002;16:2043–2052.
26. Caro JJ, Salas M, Ward A. Healing and relapse rates in gastro-oesophageal reflux disease treated with the newer proton-pump inhibitors lansoprazole, rabeprazole and pantoprazole compared with omeprazole, ranitidine and placebo: evidence from randomized controlled trials. *Clin Ther* 2001;23:998–1017. Search date 2000; primary sources Medline and hand searches of reference lists
27. Edwards SJ, Lind T, Lundell L. Systematic review of proton pump inhibitors for the acute treatment of reflux oesophagitis. *Aliment Pharmacol Ther* 2001;15:1729–1736. Search date 2000; primary sources Medline, Embase, Biosis, and AstraZeneca internal database.
28. Bardhan KD, van Rensburg C. Comparable clinical efficacy and tolerability of 20 mg pantoprazole and 20 mg omeprazole in patients with grade I reflux oesophagitis. *Aliment Pharmacol Ther* 2001;15:1585–1591.
29. Mulder C, Westerveld B, Smit J, et al. A double blind, randomized comparison of omeprazole Multiple Unit Pellet System (MUPS) 20 mg, lansoprazole 30 mg and pantoprazole 40 mg in symptomatic reflux oesophagitis followed by 3 months of omeprazole MUPS maintenance treatment: a Dutch multicentre trial. *Eur J Gastroenterol Hepatol* 2002;14:649–656.
30. Holtmann G, Bytzer P, Metz M, et al. A randomized, double blind, comparative study of standard dose rabeprazole and high dose omeprazole in gastro-oesophageal reflux disease. *Aliment Pharmacol Ther* 2002:16;479–485.
31. Toussaint J, Gossuin A, Deruyttere M, et al. Healing and prevention of relapse of reflux oesophagitis by cisapride. *Gut* 1991;32:1280–1285.
32. Blum AL, Adami B, Bouzo MH, et al. Effect of cisapride on relapse of esophagitis. A multinational, placebo-controlled trail in patients healed with an antisecretory drug. *Dig Dis Sci* 1993;38:551–560.
33. McDougall NI, Watson RGP, Collins JSA, et al. Maintenance therapy with cisapride after healing of erosive oesophagitis: a double blind placebo controlled trial. *Aliment Pharmacol Ther* 1997;11:487–495.
34. Hatlebakk JG, Johnsson F, Vilien M, et al. The effect of cisapride in maintaining symptomatic remission in patients with gastro-oesophageal reflux disease. *Scand J Gastroenterol* 1997;32:1100–1106.
35. Tytgat GNJ, Hansen OJA, Carling L, et al. Effect of cisapride on relapse of reflux oesophagitis, healed with an antisecretory drug. *Scand J Gastroenterol* 1992;27:175–183.
36. Koelz HR, Birchler R, Bretholz A, et al. Healing and relapse of reflux esophagitis during treatment with ranitidine. *Gastroenterology* 1986;91:1198–1205.
37. Freston JW. Cimetidine. I. Developments, pharmacology, and efficacy. *Ann Intern Med* 1982;97:573–580.
38. Birbara C, Breiter J, Perdomo C, et al. Rabeprazole for the prevention of recurrent erosive or ulcerative gastro-oesophageal reflux disease. *Eur J Gastroenterol Hepatol* 2000;12:889–897.
39. Caos A, Moskovitz M, Dayal Y, et al. Rabeprazole for the prevention of pathological and symptomatic relapse of erosive or ulcerative gastroesophageal reflux disease. *Am J Gastroenterol* 2000;95:3081–3088.
40. Johnson DA, Benjamin SB, Vakil NB, et al. Esomeprazole once daily for 6 months is effective therapy for maintaining healed erosive esophagitis

and for controlling gastroesophageal reflux symptoms: a randomised, double-blind, placebo-controlled study of efficacy and safety. *Am J Gastroenterol* 2001;96:27–34.
41. Vakil NB, Shaker R, Johnson DA, et al. The new proton pump inhibitor esomeprazole is effective as a maintenance therapy in GERD patients with healed erosive esophagitis: a 6-month randomized, double-blind, placebo-controlled study of efficacy and safety. *Aliment Pharmacol Ther* 2001;15:927–935.
42. Bardhan KD, Cherian P, Vaishnavi A, et al. Erosive oesophagitis: outcome of repeated long term maintenance treatment with low dose omeprazole 10 mg or placebo. *Gut* 1998;43:458–464.
43. Festen HPM, Schenk E, Tan G, et al. Omeprazole versus high-dose ranitidine in mild gastro-oesophageal reflux disease: short- and long-term treatment. *Am J Gastroenterol* 1999;94:931–936.
44. Edwards S, Lind T, Lundell L. Systematic review of proton pump inhibitors for the maintenance of healed reflux oesophagitis. *J Drug Assess* 2002;5:165–178. Search date 2001; primary sources Embase, Medline, and Astra Zeneca's internal database.
45. Thjodleifsson B, Beker JA, Dekkers C, et al. Rabeprazole versus omeprazole in preventing relapse of erosive or ulcerative gastroesophageal reflux disease. *Dig Dis Sci* 2000;45:845–853.
46. Baldi F, Morselli-Labate A, Cappiello R, et al. Daily low-dose versus alternate day full-dose lansoprazole in the maintenance treatment of reflux oesophagitis. *Am J Gastroenterol* 2002;97:1358–1364.
47. Lauritsen K, Deviere J, Bigard MA, et al. Esomeprazole 20 mg and lansoprazole 15 mg in maintaining healed reflux oesophagitis: Metropole study results. *Aliment Pharmacol Ther* 2003;17:333–341.
48. Kuipers EJ, Lundell L, Klinkenberg-Knol EC, et al. Atrophic gastritis and *Helicobacter pylori* infection in patients with reflux esophagitis treated with omeprazole or fundoplication. *N Engl J Med* 1996;334:1018–1022.
49. Eissele R, Brunner G, Simon B, et al. Gastric mucosa during treatment with lansoprazole: *Helicobacter pylori* is a risk factor for argyrophil cell hyperplasia. *Gastroenterology* 1997;112:707–717.
50. Lundell L, Miettinen P, Myrvold HE, et al. Lack of effect of acid suppression therapy on gastric atrophy. *Gastroenterology* 1999;117:319–326.
51. Uemura N, Okamoto S, Yamamoto S, et al. *Helicobacter pylori* infection and the development of gastric cancer. *N Engl J Med* 2001;345:784–789.
52. Johnson M, Guiford S, Libretto S, et al. Patients have preferences: a multicentre, double-blind, crossover study comparing rabeprazole and omeprazole. *Curr Med Res Opin* 2002;18:303–310.
53. Allgood PC, Bachmann M. Medical or surgical treatment for chronic gastro-oesophageal reflux? A systematic review of published evidence of effectiveness. *Eur J Surg* 2000;166:713–721. Search date 1999; primary sources Medline, Embase, Science Citation Index, hand searches of eight key journals and reference lists, and authors and experts contacted.
54. Lundell L, Miettinen P, Myrvold HE, et al. Long-term management of gastro-oesophageal reflux disease with omeprazole or open antireflux surgery: results of a prospective randomised clinical trial. *Eur J Gastroenterol Hepatol* 2000;12:879–887.
55. Lundell L, Miettinen P, Myrvold HE, et al. Continued (5-year) follow-up of a randomized clinical study comparing antireflux surgery and omeprazole in gastroesophageal reflux disease. *J Am Coll Surg* 2001;192:172–181.
56. Spechler SJ, Lee E, Ahnen D, et al. Long-term outcome of medical and surgical therapies for gastroesophageal reflux disease. *JAMA* 2001;285:2331–2338.
57. Bias JE, Bartelsman JFWM, Bonjer HJ, et al. Laparoscopic or conventional Nissen fundoplication for gastro-oesophageal reflux disease: randomized clinical trial. *Lancet* 2000;355:170–174.
58. Trastek VF, Deschamps C, Allen MS, et al. Uncut Collis–Nissen fundoplication: learning curve and long-term results. *Ann Thorac Surg* 1998;66:1739–1744.
59. Heikkinen T-J, Haukipuro K, Bringman S, et al. Comparison of laparoscopic and open Nissen fundoplication 2 years after operation. *Surg Endosc* 2000;14:1019–1023.

Paul Moayyedi
Professor
Department of Medicine
Gastroenterology
McMaster University, Ontario, Canada

Brendan Delaney
Professor
Department of Primary Care and General Practice University of Birmingham Medical School, Birmingham, UK

David Forman
Professor
Upper Gastrointestinal and Pancreatic Diseases Cochrane Group University Cochrane Group University of Leeds, Leeds, UK

Competing interests: PM has received lecture and consultancy fees from Astra Zeneca and Wyeth Laboratories. DF has received lecture fees and consultancy fees from Astra Zeneca and lecture fees from Wyeth and Takeda. BD has received fees for speaking at conferences and educational meetings from Astra Zeneca and Axcan.

TABLE 1 **Summary of RCTs comparing cisapride versus placebo for maintenance treatment in people with reflux oesophagitis (see text, p 509).**

Ref	Intervention	Number of people	Duration (months)	Remission with cisapride	Remission with placebo	RR for remaining in remission with cisapride *v* placebo (95 % CI)
30	Cisapride 10 mg twice daily	80 people with healed oesophagitis after cisapride 40 mg/day given for at least 8 wks	6	28/37 (76%)	25/43 (58%)	1.30 (0.95 to 1.79)
31	Cisapride 10 mg twice daily*	443 people with complete endoscopic resolution of active reflux oesophagitis after treatment with an acid antisecretory agent	12	98/149 (66%)	70/143 (49%)	1.35 (1.10 to 1.64)
32	Cisapride 20 mg/day	42 people with healed oesophagitis after omeprazole 20 mg twice daily for 8–14 wks	6	0/21 (0%)	4/21 (19%)	0.81 (0.66 to 1.00)
33	Cisapride 20 mg twice daily†	535 people without reflux or with mild reflux oesophagitis after 4–8 weeks treatment with either H^2 receptor antagonists or proton pump inhibitors	6	74/176 (42%)	65/184 (35%)	1.19 (0.92 to 1.54)
34	Cisapride 20 mg twice daily	298 people with oesophagitis	6	Absolute numbers not reported (55 %)	Absolute numbers not reported (79 %)	CI and P value not reported

*This trial also evaluated cisapride 20 mg at night with similar results to those with cisapride 10 mg twice daily.
†This trial also evaluated cisapride 20 mg daily with similar results to those with cisapride 20 mg twice daily.
Ref, reference. References 30 and 31 used oesophagitis recurrence as the main end point; references 32–34 used reflux symptom recurrence as the main end-point; data from reference 34 was estimated from life tables presented in the results section and is not actual data given in the papers.

TABLE 2 **Further RCTs comparing proton pump inhibitors with placebo for maintenance treatment in people with reflux oesophagitis (see text, p 510).**

Ref	Drug evaluated	Duration (months)	Remission in PPI arm	Remission in placebo arm	RR of remission with PPI v placebo (95% CI)
37	Rabeprazole 20 mg/day	12	80/93 (86%)	29/99 (29%)	2.94 (2.13 to 4.00)
38	Rabeprazole 20 mg/day	12	62/69 (90%)	20/70 (29%)	3.13 (2.17 to 4.55)
39	Esomeprazole 40 mg/day	6	77/82 (94%)	22/77 (29%)	3.33 (2.33 to 4.76)
40	Esomeprazole 40 mg/day	6	81/92 (88%)	27/94 (29%)	3.00 (2.22 to 4.17)
41	Omeprazole 10 mg/day*	18	66/130 (51%)	14/133 (11%)	5.00 (2.86 to 8.33)
37	Rabeprazole 10 mg/day*	12	72/93 (77%)	29/99 (29%)	2.63 (1.92 to 3.70)
38	Rabeprazole 10 mg/day*	12	51/70 (73%)	20/70 (29%)	2.56 (1.72 to 3.85)
39	Esomeprazole 20 mg/day*	6	76/82 (93%)	22/77 (29%)	3.23 (2.27 to 4.55)
40	Esomeprazole 20 mg/day*	6	77/98 (78%)	27/94 (29%)	2.70 (1.96 to 3.85)

*Maintenance dose.
PPI, proton pump inhibitor; Ref, reference.

TABLE 3 **Summary of RCTs comparing open antireflux surgery versus medical treatment for maintenance of remission in people with gastro-oesophageal reflux disease and oesophagitis (see text, p 511).**

Ref	Patient population	Intervention	Follow up (months)	Outcome assessed	Result
53	Adults with complicated GORD	88 antacids + ranitidine 77 continuous antacids + ranitidine 82 open Nissen fundoplication	12	Reduction in grade of oesophagitis at 12 months	Surgery significantly more effective than medical treatment (P 0.003; no further data reported)
53	Adults with severe GORD	16 antacids 10 Belsey–Mark IV repair 5 anterior fundoplication + Hills posterior gastropexy	38	Absence of reflux at 1 year using the acid perfusion test	11/15 (73%) with surgery *v* 3/16 (19%) with antacids (OR 11.9, 95% CI 2.1 to 65.2)
53	Adults with GORD and asthma	30 placebo 30 cimetidine 30 posterior gastropexy	3	pH testing for absence of reflux	Not intention to treat: 25/26 (96%) with surgery *v* 3/27 (11%) with control (OR 200, 95% CI 19.4 to 2059)
54	Adults with healed reflux oesophagitis	155 omeprazole 20 mg/day 155 open antireflux surgery	36	Endoscopic remission	Not intention to treat; 103/119 (87%) with surgery *v* 111/113 (83%) with omeprazole (OR not stated)

GORD, gastro-oesophageal reflux disease; Ref, reference.

Helicobacter pylori infection

Search date October 2004

Brendan Delaney, Paul Moayyedi, and David Forman

QUESTIONS

INTERVENTIONS

PREVENTION OF GASTRIC CANCER
Unknown effectiveness
H pylori eradication for prevention of gastric cancer (adenocarcinoma) 527

TREATING NON-ULCER DYSPEPSIA
Beneficial
H pylori eradication for non-ulcer dyspepsia 528

TREATING DYSPEPSIA
Beneficial
H pylori eradication in people with uninvestigated dyspepsia (more effective than placebo and as effective as endoscopy based management)* 528

DIFFERENT ERADICATION TREATMENTS
Likely to be beneficial
Quadruple regimen (as effective as triple regimen). 531
Three day quadruple regimen (as effective as 1 week triple regimen but with fewer adverse effects).531
Triple regimen (more effective than dual regimen). 529
Two week triple regimen (more effective than 1 week triple regimen) 532

Unknown effectiveness
Different triple regimens (relative effects on clinical outcomes unclear) 530

*Endoscopy should not be delayed in people at risk of malignancy
See glossary G

Key Messages

Treating duodenal ulcer

- ***H pylori* eradication for healing and preventing recurrence of duodenal ulcer** One systematic review found that *H pylori* eradication treatment increased duodenal ulcer healing compared with no treatment, and that *H pylori* eradication treatment plus 1 month of antisecretory drug treatment increased duodenal ulcer healing compared with antisecretory drugs alone for 1 month. It also found that eradication treatment reduced recurrence compared with no treatment, although there was no significant difference in recurrence between eradication treatment plus antisecretory drug treatment for 1 month compared with ongoing antisecretory maintenance treatment alone in people with healed duodenal ulcers. One systematic review found that *H pylori* eradication treatment reduced the risk of bleeding compared with ulcer healing treatment alone, or compared with ulcer treatment plus subsequent antisecretory maintenance treatment in people with duodenal or gastric ulcer.

Treating gastric ulcer

- ***H pylori* eradication for preventing recurrence of gastric ulcer** One systematic review found no significant difference in healing between *H pylori* eradication treatment plus antisecretory drugs and antisecretory drugs alone. It found that *H pylori* eradication treatment reduced recurrence compared with no treatment. One systematic review found that *H pylori* eradication treatment reduced the risk of bleeding compared with ulcer healing treatment alone, or compared with ulcer treatment plus subsequent antisecretory maintenance treatment in people with duodenal or gastric ulcer.

Treating NSAID ulcers

- ***H pylori* eradication for healing of NSAID related peptic ulcers** One RCT found no significant difference between *H pylori* eradication and antisecretory treatment alone in healing of peptic ulcer in people who were taking NSAIDs and had bleeding peptic ulcers.

Preventing NSAID ulcers with previous ulcers or dyspepsia

- ***H pylori* eradication for prevention of NSAID related peptic ulcers in people with previous ulcers or dyspepsia** One RCT found that, in people with *H pylori* infection and taking non-steroidal anti-inflammatory drugs who had previous ulcers or dyspepsia, *H pylori* eradication treatment reduced the risk of developing new peptic ulcers compared with omeprazole at 6 months. Another RCT found that, in people with *H pylori* infection and with a previous bleeding ulcer, *H pylori* eradication was less effective than maintenance treatment with omeprazole in preventing a recurrent bleeding peptic ulcer in people taking naproxen, but there was no significant difference between treatments in people taking low dose aspirin.

Preventing NSAID ulcers without previous

- ***H pylori* eradication for the prevention of non-steroidal anti-inflammatory drug (NSAID) related peptic ulcers in people without previous ulcers (more effective than placebo and as effective as antisecretory treatment)** One RCT found that *H pylori* eradication treatment reduced the risk of non-steroidal anti-inflammatory drug (NSAID) related peptic ulcers compared with no treatment in people without previous ulcers. Another RCT found that *H pylori* eradication reduced the risk of NSAID related peptic ulcers compared with placebo, but was not significantly different from antisecretory treatment alone.

Preventing GORD

- ***H pylori* eradication in *H pylori* positive people with gastro-oesophageal reflux disease** Two RCTs in *H pylori* positive people with gastro-oesophageal reflux disease found no significant difference between *H pylori* eradication treatment and placebo in symptoms over 2 years.

Treating MALT

- ***H pylori* eradication for gastric B cell lymphoma** We found no RCTs of *H pylori* eradication treatment in people with B cell gastric lymphoma. Observational studies provided limited evidence that 60–93% of people with localised, low grade B cell lymphoma experience tumour regression in response to *H pylori* eradication treatment, possibly avoiding, or delaying, the need for radical surgery, radiotherapy, or chemotherapy.

Prevention of gastric cancer

- ***H pylori* eradication for prevention of gastric cancer (adenocarcinoma)** One RCT in people positive for *H pylori* found no significant difference in the risk of gastric cancer between eradication treatment and placebo at 7.5 years. In people with gastric atrophy or intestinal metaplasia, one RCT found that *H pylori* eradication increased the regression of high risk lesions compared with no eradication. However, the RCT did not assess the effects of eradication treatment on development of gastric cancer. We found consistent evidence from observational studies of an association between *H pylori* infection and increased risk of distal gastric adenocarcinoma.

Treating non-ulcer dyspepsia

- ***H pylori* eradication for non-ulcer dyspepsia** One systematic review in people with non-ulcer dyspepsia found that *H pylori* eradication reduced dyspeptic symptoms at 3–12 months compared with placebo.

Treating dyspepsia

- ***H pylori* eradication in people with uninvestigated dyspepsia (more effective than placebo and as effective as endoscopy based management)** One RCT in people with *H pylori* found that *H pylori* eradication increased relief from dyspeptic symptoms at 1 year compared with placebo. One systematic review and one subsequent RCT in people at low risk of gastrointestinal malignancy found no significant difference in dyspepsia between *H pylori* testing plus eradication compared with management based on initial endoscopy after 1 year. However, delaying endoscopy is not safe in people at increased risk of gastrointestinal malignancy.

Different eradication treatments

- **Quadruple regimen (as effective as triple regimen)** Two RCTs found that quadruple treatments were as effective as triple treatments for eradication of *H pylori* in people with or without a history of duodenal ulcer.
- **Three day quadruple regimen (as effective as 1 week triple regimen but with fewer adverse effects)** One RCT comparing a 3 day quadruple regimen versus a 1 week triple regimen found no significant difference in *H pylori* eradication at 6 weeks. However, it found that people taking the 3 day quadruple regimen experienced fewer days of adverse effects.
- **Triple regimen (more effective than dual regimen)** We found no systematic review or RCTs of the effects of triple regimens compared with dual regimens on dyspeptic symptom scores, proportion of individuals with symptoms, quality of life, or mortality. One systematic review found that triple regimens eradicated *H pylori* from more people than dual regimens.
- **Two week triple regimen (more effective than 1 week triple regimen)** One systematic review found that 14 days of treatment with proton pump inhibitor based triple regimens increased *H pylori* eradication rates compared with 7 days of treatment with the same regimen.
- **Different triple regimens (relative effects on clinical outcomes unclear)** We found no systematic review or RCTs of the effects of different triple regimens on dyspeptic symptom scores, proportion of individuals with symptoms, quality of life, or mortality. One systematic review found that increasing the clarithromycin dose in a triple regimen containing amoxicillin increased *H pylori* eradication. However, increasing the clarithromycin dose in a triple regimen containing metronidazole had no significant additional effect on *H pylori* eradication. Another systematic review found that a triple regimen of metronidazole plus clarithromycin plus ranitidine bismuth increased eradication at 5–7 days compared with a triple regimen containing amoxicillin plus clarithromycin plus ranitidine bismuth.

DEFINITION *Helicobacter pylori* is a Gram negative flagellated spiral bacterium found in the stomach. Infection with *H pylori* is predominantly acquired in childhood. *H pylori* infection is not associated with a specific type of dyspeptic symptom. The organism is associated with lifelong chronic gastritis and may cause other gastroduodenal disorders.[1] *H pylori* can be identified indirectly by serology or by the C13 urea breath test. The urea breath test is more accurate than serology, with a sensitivity and specificity greater than 95%, and indicates active infection, whereas serology may lack specificity and cannot be used reliably as a test of active infection. Thus, the urea breath test is the test of choice where prevalence, and hence predictive value of serology may be low, or where a "test of cure" is required. In some areas stool antigen tests, which have a similar performance to the urea breath test are now available. This chapter focuses on *H pylori* positive people throughout.

INCIDENCE/ PREVALENCE In the developed world, *H pylori* prevalence rates vary with year of birth and social class. Prevalence in many developed countries tends to be much higher (50–80%) in individuals born before 1950 compared with prevalence (< 20%) in individuals born more recently.[2] In many developing countries, the infection has a high prevalence (80–95%) irrespective of the period of birth.[3] Adult prevalence is believed to represent the persistence of a historically higher rate of infection acquired in childhood, rather than increasing acquisition of infection during life.

AETIOLOGY/ RISK FACTORS Overcrowded conditions associated with childhood poverty lead to increased transmission and higher prevalence rates. Adult reinfection rates are low — less than 1% a year.[3]

PROGNOSIS *H pylori* infection is believed to be causally related to the development of duodenal and gastric ulceration, B cell gastric lymphoma Ⓖ, and distal gastric cancer. About 15% of people infected with *H pylori* will develop a peptic ulcer, and 1% of people will develop gastric cancer during their lifetime.[4] One systematic review of observational studies (search date 2000, 16 studies, 1625 people)[5] found that the frequency of peptic ulcer disease in people taking non-steroidal anti-inflammatory drugs (NSAIDs) was greater in those who were *H pylori* positive than in those who were *H pylori* negative (peptic ulcer: 341/817 [41.7%] in *H pylori* positive NSAID users *v* 209/808 [25.9%] in *H pylori* negative NSAID users, OR 2.12, 95% CI 1.68 to 2.67).

AIMS OF INTERVENTION Eradication of *H pylori*; improvement in dyspeptic symptoms; improvement in ulcer healing; reduction in ulcer recurrence and complications; reduced mortality from peptic ulcer complications of gastric cancer; improved quality of life.

OUTCOMES Eradication rates of *H pylori*; dyspeptic symptom scores and proportion of people with symptoms; rates of ulcer healing, recurrence, and complications; quality of life; mortality; adverse effects of treatment.

METHODS *Clinical Evidence* search and appraisal October 2004.

QUESTION What are the effects of *H pylori* eradication treatment in people with a proven duodenal ulcer?

OPTION ERADICATION TREATMENT IN PEOPLE WITH A PROVEN DUODENAL ULCER

One systematic review found that *H pylori* eradication treatment increased duodenal ulcer healing compared with no treatment, and that *H pylori* eradication treatment plus 1 month of antisecretory drug treatment increased duodenal ulcer healing compared with antisecretory drugs alone for 1 month. It also found that eradication treatment reduced recurrence compared with no treatment, although there was no significant difference in recurrence between eradication treatment plus antisecretory drug treatment for 1 month compared with ongoing antisecretory maintenance treatment alone in people with healed duodenal ulcers. One systematic review found that *H pylori* eradication treatment reduced the risk of bleeding compared with ulcer healing treatment alone, or compared with ulcer treatment plus subsequent antisecretory maintenance treatment in people with duodenal or gastric ulcer.

Benefits: **Endoscopic healing:** We found one systematic review (search date 2002).[6] It found that eradication treatment plus antisecretory drugs**G** for 1 month significantly improved healing compared with antisecretory drugs alone for 1 month (34 RCTs, 3910 people; AR for healing: 83% with eradication treatment plus antisecretory drugs for 1 month *v* 81% with antisecretory drugs alone for 1 month; RR for ulcer persistence 0.66, 95% CI 0.58 to 0.76; NNT for persistence 14, 95% CI 11 to 20). It found that eradication treatment alone also significantly improved healing compared with no treatment (2 RCTs, 207 people; AR for healing: 76% with eradication treatment *v* 42% with no treatment: RR for persistence 0.37, 95% CI 0.25 to 0.53; NNT 3, 95% CI 2 to 4). **Prevention of recurrence:** We found one systematic review (search date 2002).[6] It found no significant difference in recurrence after ulcer healing between eradication treatment plus antisecretory drugs for 1 month and ongoing maintenance antisecretory drugs alone (4 RCTs, 319 people; AR: 12% with eradication treatment plus antisecretory drugs for 1 month *v* 16% with ongoing maintenance antisecretory drugs alone; RR for eradication treatment plus antisecretory drugs *v* antisecretory drugs alone 0.73, 95% CI 0.42 to 1.25). It found that eradication treatment alone significantly reduced recurrence compared with no treatment (26 RCTs, 2434 people; AR: 14% with eradication treatment *v* 64% with no treatment; RR 0.19, 95% CI 0.15 to 0.26). However, results were heterogeneous, because of differing eradication regimens and lengths of follow up. Subgroup analysis found that proton pump inhibitor**G** containing eradication regimens significantly reduced recurrence compared with no treatment (5 RCTs, 531 people; AR: 8% with eradication treatment *v* 65% with no treatment; RR 0.14, 95% CI 0.09 to 0.20). **Prevention of bleeding:** We found one systematic review (search date 2000, 7 RCTs), which compared *H pylori* eradication versus ulcer treatment alone or versus ulcer treatment plus subsequent antisecretory maintenance treatment in people with duodenal ulcer or gastric ulcer.[7] The review found that *H pylori* eradication significantly reduced the risk of bleeding compared with ulcer treatment with antisecretory drugs alone (4 RCTs, 262 people; 6/133 [5%] with eradication *v* 28/129 [22%] with ulcer treatment alone; RR 0.20, 95% CI 0.11 to 0.53; NNT 6, 95% CI 4 to 11), and *H pylori* eradication also significantly reduced the risk of bleeding compared with ulcer treatment plus antisecretory treatment (3 RCTs, 470 people; 4/257 [1.6%] with eradication *v* 12/213 [5.6%] with ulcer treatment plus antisecretory treatment; RR 0.30, 95% CI 0.09 to 0.77; NNT 25, 95% CI 13 to 167). **Prevention of perforation or obstruction:** We found no systematic review and no RCTs.

Harms: One systematic review (search date 2002, 39 RCTs, 5066 people with duodenal ulcer or gastric ulcers) found that eradication treatment significantly increased adverse events compared with antisecretory drugs**Ⓖ** or no treatment (AR: 22% with eradication treatment *v* 8% with antisecretory drugs or no treatment; RR 2.28, 95% CI 1.72 to 3.02).[6] It did not perform separate meta-analyses for people with duodenal ulcer and gastric ulcer. One systematic review (search date 1995) found that minor adverse effects are common with bismuth**Ⓖ** (40% of people), metronidazole (39%), clarithromycin (22%), and tinidazole (7%).[8] Discontinuation of treatment because of severe adverse effects is rare (bismuth 4%, metronidazole 2%, clarithromycin 1%, and tinidazole < 1%).

Comment: We excluded analyses that grouped people by *H pylori* status at the end of the trial. Observational evidence from RCTs suggests that duodenal ulcer recurrence rates 1 year after treatment are lower in people with successful *H pylori* eradication treatment (in the review of US RCTs, recurrence rates were: 20%, 95% CI 14% to 26%, in people cured of *H pylori* *v* 56%, 95% CI 50% to 61%, for people remaining infected).[9] The recurrence rate in non-US trials was lower than the recurrence rate found in the US trials (6% for people cured of *H pylori*). The difference in recurrence rates between US and non-US studies may be explained partially by the marked loss to follow up in the US trials (9–41%). However, countries with low prevalence of *H pylori* infection also have a low prevalence of duodenal ulcers, but a greater proportion of those ulcers arise from causes other than *H pylori*; therefore, eradication may be less effective where *H pylori* prevalence is low. Poor adherence to *H pylori* eradication treatment and the use of less effective regimens may lead to increased antibiotic resistance in *H pylori*, but we found no direct evidence to support this. The harms of *H pylori* eradication treatment are mainly the minor short term effects of the antibiotics, particularly nausea from metronidazole or clarithromycin, and diarrhoea. Bismuth**Ⓖ** may turn the stools black.

QUESTION **What are the effects of *H pylori* eradication treatment for people with a proven gastric ulcer?**

OPTION **ERADICATION TREATMENT IN PEOPLE WITH A PROVEN GASTRIC ULCER**

One systematic review found no significant difference in healing between *H pylori* eradication treatment plus antisecretory drugs and antisecretory drugs alone. It found that *H pylori* eradication treatment reduced recurrence compared with no treatment. One systematic review found that *H pylori*

eradication treatment reduced the risk of bleeding compared with ulcer healing treatment alone, or compared with ulcer treatment plus subsequent antisecretory maintenance treatment in people with duodenal or gastric ulcer.

Benefits: **Endoscopic healing:** We found one systematic review (search date 2002).[6] It found no significant difference in healing between eradication treatment plus antisecretory drugs**G** and antisecretory drugs alone (13 RCTs, 1469 people; AR: 78% with eradication treatment plus antisecretory drugs *v* 87% with antisecretory drugs alone; RR for ulcer persistence 1.32, 95% CI 0.92 to 1.90). The review found no RCTs comparing eradication treatment versus no treatment in people with gastric ulcers. **Prevention of recurrence:** We found one systematic review (search date 2002).[6] It found that eradication treatment significantly reduced recurrence compared with no treatment (9 RCTs, 774 people; AR: 12% with eradication treatment *v* 40% with no treatment; RR 0.31, 95% CI 0.19 to 0.48; NNT 3, 95% CI 3 to 5). The review found no RCTs comparing eradication treatment versus maintenance antisecretory treatment. **Prevention of bleeding:** See benefits under effects of eradication treatment for H pylori in people with a proven duodenal ulcer, p 522. **Prevention of other complications:** We found no systematic review or RCTs.

Harms: See harms under effects of eradication treatment for H pylori in people with a proven duodenal ulcer, p 523.

Comment: None.

QUESTION What are the effects of *H pylori* eradication treatment in people with non-steroidal anti-inflammatory drug (NSAID) related peptic ulcers?

OPTION ERADICATION TREATMENT IN PEOPLE WITH NSAID RELATED PEPTIC ULCERS

One RCT found no significant difference between *H pylori* eradication and antisecretory treatment alone in healing of peptic ulcer in people who were taking NSAIDs and had bleeding peptic ulcers.

Benefits: We found one RCT comparing *H pylori* eradication treatment versus proton pump inhibitor**G** alone in people with non-steroidal anti-inflammatory drug related peptic ulcer.[10] The RCT (195 people with *H pylori*, using non-steroidal anti-inflammatory drugs and with bleeding peptic ulcers) found no significant difference in healing rate between *H pylori* eradication treatment (bismuth**G** subcitrate plus tetracycline plus metronidazole plus omeprazole) and omeprazole alone at 8 weeks (AR for healing: 77/93 [83%] with eradication treatment *v* 88/102 [86%] with omeprazole alone; P = 0.50; analysis by intention to treat).[10]

Harms: The RCT did not report on harms.[10]

Comment: None.

QUESTION What are the effects of *H pylori* eradication treatment for preventing non-steroidal anti-inflammatory drug (NSAID) related peptic ulcers in people with previous ulcers or dyspepsia

OPTION ERADICATION TREATMENT FOR PREVENTING NON-STEROIDAL ANTI-INFLAMMATORY DRUG RELATED PEPTIC ULCERS IN PEOPLE WITH PREVIOUS ULCERS OR DYSPEPSIA

One RCT found that, in people with *H pylori* infection and taking non-steroidal anti-inflammatory drugs who had previous ulcers or dyspepsia, *H pylori* eradication treatment reduced the risk of developing new peptic ulcers

compared with omeprazole at 6 months. Another RCT found that, in people with *H pylori* infection and with a previous bleeding ulcer, *H pylori* eradication was less effective than maintenance treatment with omeprazole in preventing a recurrent bleeding peptic ulcer in people taking naproxen, but there was no significant difference between treatments in people taking low dose aspirin.

Benefits: We found two RCTs.[11,12] The first RCT (102 people with *H pylori* and taking non-steroidal anti-inflammatory drug [NSAIDs], with a history of dyspepsia or peptic ulceration, but without active ulcers) compared a quadruple eradication regimen**G** versus omeprazole alone. It found that eradication treatment significantly reduced the cumulative 6 month risk of peptic ulcer compared with omeprazole alone (cumulative 6 month risk of ulcer: 12.1% with eradication treatment *v* 34.4% with omeprazole alone; P = 0.009).[11] It also found that eradication treatment reduced the cumulative 6 month risk of bleeding peptic ulcer compared with omeprazole alone (cumulative 6 month risk of bleeding ulcer: 4.2% with eradication treatment *v* 27.1% with omeprazole alone; P = 0.003). The second RCT (250 people taking low dose aspirin and 150 people taking naproxen, with a bleeding peptic ulcer that healed with omeprazole treatment, and *H pylori*) compared a 1 week triple eradication regimen**G** (bismuth**G** subcitrate plus tetracycline plus metronidazole) versus maintenance treatment with omeprazole for 6 months.[12] It found that in people taking naproxen, *H pylori* eradication treatment was associated with a significantly higher cumulative 6 month risk of developing a bleeding ulcer than omeprazole. It found no significant difference between groups in people taking aspirin (recurrent bleeding ulcer in people taking naproxen: 18.8% with eradication treatment *v* 4.4% with omeprazole; ARR 14.4%, 95% CI 4.4% to 24.4%; recurrent bleeding ulcer in people taking aspirin: 1.9% with eradication treatment *v* 0.9% with omeprazole; absolute difference +1.0%, 95% CI –1.9% to +3.9%; see comment below).

Harms: The RCTs did not report on harms.

Comment: Given the much lower risk of bleeding with low dose aspirin compared with naproxen, the RCT[12] may have been underpowered with respect to aspirin, although a large absolute affect can be excluded.

QUESTION **What are the effects of *H pylori* eradication treatment for preventing non-steroidal anti-inflammatory drug (NSAID) related peptic ulcers in people without previous ulcers?**

OPTION **ERADICATION TREATMENT FOR PREVENTING NON-STEROIDAL ANTI-INFLAMMATORY DRUG RELATED PEPTIC ULCERS IN PEOPLE WITHOUT PREVIOUS ULCERS**

One RCT found that *H pylori* eradication treatment reduced the risk of non-steroidal anti-inflammatory drug (NSAID) related peptic ulcers compared with no treatment in people without previous ulcers. Another RCT found that *H pylori* eradication reduced the risk of NSAID related peptic ulcers compared with placebo, but was not significantly different from antisecretory treatment alone.

Benefits: We found two RCTs.[13,14] The first RCT (100 *H pylori* positive people requiring non-steroidal anti-inflammatory drug [NSAID] treatment, and without any history of peptic ulceration or gastric surgery) compared a 1 week triple eradication regimen**G** versus no treatment, before 8 weeks of NSAID treatment.[13] It found that *H pylori* eradication treatment significantly reduced the risk of peptic ulceration at 8 weeks compared with no eradication treatment (AR for ulcer: 3/45 [7%] with eradication treatment *v* 12/47 [26%] without eradication treatment; P = 0.01). The second RCT (832 people with *H pylori* and no history of ulcer, requiring treatment with an NSAID) compared four treatments: 1 week of *H pylori* triple eradication treatment❻; 1 week of *H pylori* triple eradication treatment plus 4 weeks of omeprazole; omeprazole alone for 5 weeks; and placebo for 5 weeks.[14] All active treatments were significantly more effective at preventing peptic ulcers at 5 weeks than placebo, but there was no significant difference among active treatments (AR for ulcer: 2/161 [1.2%] with eradication treatment alone *v* 2/173 [1.2%] with eradication treatment plus maintenance omeprazole *v* 0/155 [0%] with omeprazole alone *v* 10/171 [5.8%] with placebo; P < 0.05 for each active treatment *v* placebo; analysis not by intention to treat).

Harms: The RCTs did not report on harms.

Comment: None.

QUESTION **What are the effects of *H pylori* eradication treatment in people with proved gastro-oesophageal reflux disease?**

OPTION **ERADICATION TREATMENT IN PEOPLE WITH GASTRO-OESOPHAGEAL REFLUX DISEASE**

Two RCTs in *H pylori* positive people with gastro-oesophageal reflux disease found no significant difference between *H pylori* eradication treatment and placebo in symptoms over 2 years.

Benefits: We found no systematic review but found two RCTs.[15,16] The first RCT (190 *H pylori* positive people with gastro-oesophageal reflux disease [GORD] but no duodenal ulcer) compared *H pylori* eradication treatment versus placebo. It found no significant difference in symptomatic relapse between groups over 1 year (83% in both groups; difference 0%, 95% CI –11% to +11%).[15] The second RCT (1558 *H pylori* positive people) compared *H pylori* eradication versus placebo in pre-specified subgroups with and without symptoms of GORD at baseline.[16] At 2 years, it found no significant difference in heartburn or reflux between eradication treatment and placebo in people with symptoms of GORD at baseline (heartburn: OR 0.90, 95% CI 0.71 to 1.14; reflux: OR 0.89, 95% CI 0.62 to 1.29).

Harms: The RCTs provided insufficient evidence about the harms of *H pylori* eradication treatment in people with GORD.[15,16] Case control studies have found an increased risk of reflux symptoms after *H pylori* eradication.[17] However, discontinuation of antisecretory treatment❻ after *H pylori* eradication might have unmasked symptoms of coexisting GORD.

Comment: None.

QUESTION **What are the effects of *H pylori* eradication treatment in people with B cell lymphoma of the stomach?**

OPTION **ERADICATION TREATMENT IN PEOPLE WITH B CELL LYMPHOMA OF THE STOMACH**

We found no RCTs of *H pylori* eradication treatment in people with B cell gastric lymphoma. Observational studies provided limited evidence that 60–93% of people with localised, low grade B cell lymphoma experience tumour regression in response to *H pylori* eradication treatment, possibly avoiding, or delaying, the need for radical surgery, radiotherapy, or chemotherapy.

Benefits: We found no systematic review and no RCTs.

Harms: We found no RCTs.

Comment: Treatment options for primary gastric lymphoma include surgery, radiotherapy, chemotherapy, and *H pylori* eradication. We found no direct comparative studies. We found six prospective cohort studies of *H pylori* eradication in people with localised, low grade lymphomas.[18] Tumour regression occurred in 60–93% of people, but responses were sometimes delayed and some people relapsed within 1 year of treatment. A further uncontrolled study (28/34 [82%] people with B cell gastric lymphoma**G** who were found to be *H pylori* positive and were given eradication treatment) found that 14/28 people (50%, 95% CI 31% to 69%) achieved complete remission at 18 months' follow up.[19]

QUESTION **What are the effects of *H pylori* eradication treatment on the risk of developing gastric cancer?**

OPTION **ERADICATION TREATMENT FOR PREVENTION OF GASTRIC CANCER**

One RCT in people positive for *H pylori* found no significant difference in the risk of gastric cancer between eradication treatment and placebo at 7.5 years. In people with gastric atrophy or intestinal metaplasia, one RCT found that *H pylori* eradication increased the regression of high risk lesions compared with no eradication. However, the RCT did not assess the effects of eradication treatment on development of gastric cancer. We found consistent evidence from observational studies of an association between *H pylori* infection and increased risk of distal gastric adenocarcinoma.

Benefits: **In people positive for *H pylori*:** We found no systematic review. We found one RCT (1630 healthy people positive for *H pylori*, without macroscopic lesions on endoscopy).[20] It found no significance difference in the risk of gastric cancer between eradication treatment and placebo at 7.5 years (7/817 [0.86%] with eradication treatment *v* 11/813 [1.35%] with placebo; HR 0.63, 95% CI 0.24 to 1.62). **In people at high risk of gastric cancer:** We found no systematic review or RCTs of the effects of *H pylori* eradication on the development of gastric cancer in people at high risk. One RCT (852 people with gastric atrophy or intestinal metaplasia found at screening endoscopy) compared four treatments: *H pylori* eradication treatment, β carotene, ascorbic acid, and placebo.[21] It found that *H pylori* eradication treatment significantly increased lesion regression compared with no eradication treatment (calculated by multivariate modelling) for both atrophy (RR 4.8, 95% CI 1.6 to 14.2) and intestinal metaplasia (RR 3.1, 95% CI 1.0 to 9.3; no absolute numbers reported).

Harms: Neither RCT reported on harms.[20,21] We found no RCTs in people at risk of gastric cancer.

Comment: In the first RCT, post-hoc analysis suggested that gastric cancer may only develop in people with pre-cancerous lesions at baseline. We found one systematic review of nested case control studies (search date 1999, 12 studies, 1228 cases, 3406 controls).[22] In the absence of trial data, this is the best evidence of an association between *H pylori* infection and gastric cancer. The review found that, overall, there was a significant association between *H pylori* infection and the subsequent development of gastric cancer (OR 2.36, 95% CI 1.98 to 2.81). The review found no significant association between *H pylori* and cardia cancer (OR 0.99, 95% CI 0.72 to 1.35), but did find a significant association for non-cardia cancer (OR 2.97, 95% CI 2.34 to 3.77). The review also found a strong interaction with age and time from sample collection. *H pylori* does not colonise areas of cancer, intestinal metaplasia, or atrophy, and antibodies may be lost with increasing age. Prospective studies with a short time period between the collection of the serum sample and the development of the cancer, or retrospective studies, may underestimate the association. The review found a significant association between *H pylori* and non-cardia (distal) cancer where the time from sampling to cancer was more than 10 years (OR 5.93, 95% CI 3.41 to 10.3).[22]

QUESTION **What are the effects of *H pylori* eradication treatment in people with proved non-ulcer dyspepsia?**

OPTION **ERADICATION TREATMENT IN PEOPLE WITH PROVED NON-ULCER DYSPEPSIA**

One systematic review in people with non-ulcer dyspepsia found that *H pylori* eradication reduced dyspeptic symptoms at 3–12 months compared with placebo.

Benefits: We found one systematic review (search date 2002, 12 RCTs, 2903 people with *H pylori* and non-ulcer dyspepsia), which found that *H pylori* eradication significantly improved dyspeptic symptoms at 3–12 months compared with placebo (AR for symptoms: 1004/1593 [63%] with eradication treatment *v* 927/1310 [70%] with placebo; RR 0.91, 95% CI 0.86 to 0.95; NNT 15, 95% CI 10 to 31).[23] Three RCTs (839 people) in the systematic review found no significant difference between *H pylori* eradication treatment and placebo in quality of life at 12 months (WMD –0.25, 95% CI –3.49 to +2.99).[23]

Harms: See harms of eradication treatment for H pylori in people with a proved duodenal ulcer, p 523. We found two RCTs that assessed whether *H pylori* eradication treatment increases the prevalence of oesophagitis in people with non-ulcer dyspepsia.[24,25] They found no significant difference between *H pylori* eradication treatment and placebo in endoscopically assessed oesophagitis (5.7% with eradication treatment *v* 2.9% with placebo; ARI +2.8%, 95% CI –0.5% to +6.0%; RR 2.1, 95% CI 0.9 to 4.6). No trial evaluated individual dyspeptic symptoms, so the effect on reflux symptoms cannot be estimated separately from epigastric pain.

Comment: None.

QUESTION **What are the effects of *H pylori* eradication treatment in people with uninvestigated dyspepsia?**

OPTION **ERADICATION TREATMENT IN PEOPLE WITH UNINVESTIGATED DYSPEPSIA**

One RCT in people with *H pylori* found that *H pylori* eradication increased relief from dyspeptic symptoms at 1 year compared with placebo. One systematic review and one subsequent RCT in people at low risk of gastrointestinal malignancy found no significant difference in dyspepsia between *H pylori* testing plus eradication compared with management based on initial endoscopy after 1 year. However, delaying endoscopy is not safe in people at increased risk of gastrointestinal malignancy.

Benefits: ***H pylori* eradication versus placebo:** We found one RCT (294 people with dyspeptic symptoms and confirmed *H pylori* infection), which found that *H pylori* eradication treatment significantly increased the proportion of people who were free of dyspeptic symptoms at 1 year compared with placebo (41/145 [28%] with eradication treatment v 22/149 [15%] with placebo; difference 13%, 95% CI 4% to 24%; P = 0.008).[26] **Initial *H pylori* testing plus eradication treatment versus management based on initial endoscopy:** We found one systematic review[27] and one subsequent RCT.[28] The systematic review (search date 2002, 4 RCTs, 1412 people with dyspepsia not considered to be at high risk of gastrointestinal malignancy; see comment below) found no significant difference between *H pylori* testing plus eradication treatment and endoscopy based management in the proportion of people with dyspepsia at 1 year (173/707 [24%] with *H pylori* testing and eradication treatment v 179/705 [25%] with endoscopy based management; RR 0.94, 95% CI 0.71 to 1.25).[27] The subsequent RCT (270 people consulting their general practitioner with dyspepsia and without "alarm symptoms"; see comment below) found no significant difference in symptom improvement between *H pylori* "test and treat" management and people receiving endoscopy based management at 1 year (dyspeptic symptoms evaluated on a 5 point Likert scale; scores depicted graphically; P = 0.51 for mean overall score comparison).[28] It found no significant difference between the groups in improvement of quality of life at 1 year (evaluated using the RAND-36 questionnaire; scores depicted graphically; P > 0.05 for median score comparison in all 9 components).

Harms: The systematic review gave no information on adverse effects.[27] Two of the RCTs in the review found that a small proportion of people given *H pylori* eradication treatment discontinued treatment because of short term adverse effects, which were not specified (14/104 [13%] people in the first RCT[29] and 4/80 [5%] in the second RCT[30]). The subsequent RCT did not reported on harms.[28]

Comment: The results of the systematic review[27] and subsequent RCT[28] were in people at low risk of gastrointestinal malignancy and are not applicable to all people with dyspepsia. People with "alarm" symptoms (dysphagia, weight loss, jaundice, epigastric mass, or anaemia), or over the age of 55 years, with either continuous epigastric pain or first onset of symptoms in the previous year, may have a significant risk of upper gastrointestinal malignancy and may benefit from prompt endoscopy. Two of the RCTs in the review were conducted in a hospital setting and the third, conducted in primary care, is not yet published in full.[31] One of the RCTs in the review, conducted in a hospital setting, stipulated that all eligible people with dyspepsia who were consulting with a general medical practitioner should be included, but the other entered only routine referrals. The results of the review might not apply directly to primary care, where people with less severe dyspepsia might be treated and *H pylori* eradication rates might be lower, and the reassuring or anxiety provoking effect of specialist consultation might not be replicated.[27]

QUESTION Do eradication treatments differ in their effects?

OPTION TRIPLE REGIMENS

We found no systematic review or RCTs of the effects of triple regimens compared with dual regimens on dyspeptic symptom scores, proportion of individuals with symptoms, quality of life, or mortality. One systematic review found that triple regimens eradicated *H pylori* from more people than dual regimens.

Benefits: **Duodenal ulcer complication rates:** We found no systematic review or RCTs. **Eradication rates:** We found one systematic review (search date 1995; 19 RCTs of omeprazole plus amoxicillin [amoxycillin] versus omeprazole plus amoxicillin plus bismuth**G**; 17 RCTs of dual regimens**G** containing a proton pump inhibitor**G** versus triple regimens**G**).[8] No formal meta-analysis was performed, but dual regimens eradicated *H pylori* from fewer people compared with triple regimens (2 antibiotics plus either a proton pump inhibitor or bismuth) (results presented graphically).

Harms: See harms under effects of eradication treatment for H pylori in people with a proved duodenal ulcer, p 522.

Comment: Many RCTs of *H pylori* eradication treatment have methodological problems, such as lack of a gold standard for defining cure, and many are published only as an abstract. A systematic review comparing eradication treatments for *H pylori* eradication is in progress.[31] Factors that might influence the choice of eradication treatment for an individual also include ease of adherence, potential harms, allergy or sensitivity, drug resistance, and cost.

OPTION DIFFERENT TRIPLE REGIMENS

We found no systematic review or RCTs of the effects of different triple regimens on dyspeptic symptom scores, proportion of individuals with symptoms, quality of life, or mortality. One systematic review found that increasing the clarithromycin dose in a triple regimen containing amoxicillin increased *H pylori* eradication. However, increasing the clarithromycin dose in a triple regimen containing metronidazole had no significant additional effect on *H pylori* eradication. Another systematic review found that a triple regimen of metronidazole plus clarithromycin plus ranitidine bismuth increased eradication at 5–7 days compared with a triple regimen containing amoxicillin plus clarithromycin plus ranitidine bismuth.

Benefits: **Clinical outcomes and duodenal ulcer complication rates:** We found no systematic review and no direct comparison of the effect of different triple regimens**G** on clinical outcomes or complication rates. **Eradication rates:** We found two systematic reviews comparing different triple regimens.[32,33] The first systematic review (search date 1998, 4 RCTs) found that a higher clarithromycin dose 500 mg twice daily in combination with a proton pump inhibitor**G** and amoxicillin (amoxycillin) significantly increased *H pylori* eradication compared with using a lower clarithromycin dose 250 mg twice daily in the combination (90% with clarithromycin 500 mg *v* 80% with clarithromycin 250 mg; RR 0.89, 95% CI 0.81 to 0.97; NNT 11, 95% CI 6 to 38).[32] The review found no significant difference between clarithromycin 500 mg twice daily and clarithromycin 250 mg twice daily, in combination with a proton pump inhibitor and metronidazole, in eradication rates (89% with clarithromycin 500 mg *v* 87% with clarithromycin 250 mg; RR 0.98, 95% CI 0.93 to 1.04). The second systematic review (search date 2000, 8 RCTs, 1139 people) found that ranitidine bismuth**G** 400 mg daily plus clarithromycin 250 mg plus metronidazole 400 mg twice daily significantly increased eradication at 5–7 days compared with ranitidine 400 mg daily plus clarithromycin 500 mg twice daily plus amoxicillin 1000 mg twice daily (499/565 [88%] with ranitidine bismuth plus clarithromycin plus metronidazole *v* 467/574 [81%] with ranitidine plus clarithromycin plus amoxicillin; RR 1.09, 95% CI 1.03 to 1.14).[33] **Antibiotic resistance:** We found one systematic review (search date 1995, 19 RCTs, 1006 people with metronidazole sensitive *H pylori*, 452 with metronidazole resistant *H pylori*)[8] and one subsequent RCT,[34] in which data were analyzed to examine effects of resistance on eradication rate.

The review found that nitroimidazole based regimens achieved *H pylori* eradication in significantly fewer people with strains showing nitroimidazole resistance in the laboratory than in people with sensitive strains (99%, 95% CI 97% to 100% eradication in people with sensitive strains *v* 69%, 95% CI 60% to 77% in people with resistant strains).[8] The subsequent RCT (33 people with a proven duodenal ulcer and *H pylori* infection, and primary metronidazole resistance, and 81 without resistance) found that metronidazole resistance significantly decreased the *H pylori* eradication rate with an omeprazole plus metronidazole plus clarithromycin regimen (77/81 [95.1%] without resistance *v* 25/33 [75.8%] with metronidazole resistance; RR 0.79, 95% CI 0.62 to 0.93).[34]

Harms: See harms under effects of eradication treatment for H pylori in people with a proved duodenal ulcer, p 523.

Comment: The systematic review assessing nitroimidazole resistance concluded that clinically important reduction of eradication rates is unlikely if the proportion of resistant strains is below 15–25%.[8] Systematic reviews of *H pylori* eradication treatments are difficult to interpret (see triple regimens, p 529).

OPTION QUADRUPLE REGIMENS

Two RCTs in people with *H pylori* infection found that quadruple treatments were as effective as triple treatments for eradication of *H pylori* in people with or without a history of duodenal ulcer. One subsequent RCT comparing a 3 day quadruple regimen versus a 1 week triple regimen found no significant difference in *H pylori* eradication at 6 weeks. However, it found that people taking the 3 day quadruple regimen experienced fewer days of adverse effects.

Benefits: We found no systematic review and three RCTs.[35–37] The first RCT (405 people with *H pylori* infection and dyspepsia but no duodenal ulcer or oesophagitis on endoscopy) compared three treatments: triple treatment for 7 days (pantoprazole 40 mg plus amoxicillin 1000 mg plus clarithromycin 500 mg all twice daily for 7 days); quadruple treatment for 7 days (pantoprazole 40 mg twice daily plus bismuth**G** subcitrate 108 mg 4 times daily plus tetracycline 500 mg 4 times daily plus metronidazole 200 mg 3 times daily and 400 mg at night); and a different triple treatment for 14 days (bismuth subcitrate 108 mg 4 times daily plus tetracycline 500 mg 4 times daily plus metronidazole 200 mg 3 times daily and 400 mg at night).[35] It found no significant difference between the triple and quadruple 7 day regimens in eradication rates at 8 weeks (intention to treat analysis; eradication: 110/134 [82.1%] with 7 day quadruple treatment *v* 104/134 [77.6%] with 7 day triple treatment; ARI 4.5%, 95% CI –5.1% to +14.1%; P = 0.4). The 7 day quadruple regimen significantly improved eradication rate compared with the 14 day triple regimen at 8 weeks (110/134 [82.1%] with 7 day quadruple treatment *v* 95/137 [69.3%] with 14 day triple treatment; ARI 12.8%, 95% CI 2.7% to 22.8%; P = 0.01). The second RCT (299 people with *H pylori* infection and a current or previous duodenal ulcer) compared a 10 day course of quadruple treatment (bismuth biskalcitrate 420 mg plus metronidazole 375 mg plus tetracycline 375 mg taken 4 times daily plus 20 mg omeprazole twice daily) versus a 10 day course of triple treatment (omeprazole 20 mg plus amoxicillin 1000 mg plus clarithromycin 500 mg all twice daily).[36] It found no significant difference between treatments in eradication rate 2 months after treatment (121/138 [87.7%] with quadruple treatment *v* 114/137 [83.2%] with triple treatment; ARI +4.5%, 95% CI –3.9% to +12.8%;

P = 0.29). One RCT (118 people with active duodenal ulcer at endoscopy) compared a 3 day quadruple regimen (lansoprazole plus clarithromycin plus metronidazole plus bismuth subcitrate) versus a 7 day triple regimen (lansoprazole plus clarithromycin plus metronidazole).[37] It found no significant difference in *H pylori* eradication at 6 weeks (50/58 [86.2%] with 3 day quadruple treatment *v* 52/60 [86.7%] with 7 day triple treatment; RR 0.99, 95% CI 0.79 to 1.09).

Harms: The first RCT found that the proportion of people stopping treatment because of adverse effects was similar with 7 day quadruple treatment**Ⓖ** (3%) and 7 day triple treatment**Ⓖ** (2%), but higher with 14 day triple treatment (9%; no statistical comparison reported).[35] The second RCT did not discuss harms.[36] The RCT comparing a 3 day quadruple regimen versus a 1 week triple regimen found that people taking the 3 day regimen experienced significantly fewer days of bitter taste, bowel disturbance, malaise, and dark stools (mean: 2.54 days with 3 day quadruple treatment *v* 4.58 days with 7 day triple treatment; $P < 0.001$).[37] See harms under effects of eradication treatment for H pylori in people with proved duodenal ulcer, p 523.

Comment: The rationale for quadruple regimens**Ⓖ** is that they can be used as second line treatment, giving different antibiotics than those commonly given with current triple treatments**Ⓖ**, thus reducing the likelihood of resistance.

OPTION DURATION OF *H PYLORI* ERADICATION TREATMENT

One systematic review found that 14 days of treatment with proton pump inhibitor based triple regimens increased *H pylori* eradication rates compared with 7 days of treatment with the same regimen.

Benefits: **Duodenal ulcer complication rates:** We found no systematic review and no RCTs. **Eradication rates:** We found one systematic review[38] and one subsequent RCT.[37] The review (search date 1999, 7 RCTs, 906 people) compared 14 days' treatment with proton pump inhibitor**Ⓖ** based triple regimens**Ⓖ** versus 7 days' treatment with proton pump inhibitor based triple regimens.[38] It found that 14 days' treatment significantly increased *H pylori* eradication rates compared with 7 days' treatment (339/470 [72.1%] with 7 days' treatment *v* 353/436 [81.0%] with 14 days' treatment; RR 0.89, 95% CI 0.83 to 0.96; NNT 11, 95% CI 7 to 33).

Harms: See harms under effects of eradication treatment for H pylori in people with a proved duodenal ulcer, p 523. The systematic review found insufficient data to report harms.[38]

Comment: The systematic review only considered regimens containing clarithromycin plus either metronidazole or amoxicillin.[38] The risk of failure of a 7 day regimen as opposed to a 14 day regimen in any particular individual will relate to the local prevalence of antibiotic resistance, as 14 day regimens may overcome resistance to one of the antibiotics used. As longer regimens have a longer duration of minor adverse effects, the balance between local failure rate and adverse effects must be decided on the basis of locally validated data.

GLOSSARY

Antisecretory treatment A treatment that reduces the production of acid by the stomach. These may either be H_2 receptor antagonists or proton pump inhibitors.

Bismuth A compound containing bismuth, such as bismuth subsalicylate or ranitidine bismuth citrate.

Dual regimens *H pylori* eradication regimen consisting of two components: an antisecretory agent and an antibiotic.

MALT "Mucosa associated lymphoid tissue" is constitutionally found in the intestine but not in the stomach. MALT lymphoma is also known as B cell gastric lymphoma.
Proton pump inhibitor A drug that directly inhibits the mechanism within the stomach that secretes acid, such as esomeprazole, lansoprazole, omeprazole, or rabeprazole.
Quadruple regimens *H pylori* eradication regimen consisting of a proton pump inhibitor plus bismuth plus metronidazole plus tetracycline.
Triple regimens *H pylori* eradication regimen consisting of three components. The original "triple regimen" was bismuth subsalicylate plus metronidazole plus either amoxicillin (amoxycillin) or tetracycline. Now the term usually applies to a proton pump inhibitor plus two antibiotics.

Substantive changes

Eradication treatment in people with a proven duodenal ulcer One systematic review added;[6] categorisation unchanged.
Eradication treatment in people with a proved gastric ulcer One systematic review added;[6] categorisation unchanged.
Eradication treatment in people with gastro-oesophageal reflux disease One RCT added;[16] categorisation unchanged.
Eradication treatment for prevention of gastric cancer One RCT added;[20] categorisation unchanged.

REFERENCES

1. Nguyen TN, Barkun AN, Fallone CA. Host determinants of *Helicobacter pylori* infection and its clinical outcome. *Helicobacter* 1999;4:185–197.
2. Harvey RF, Spence RW, Lane JA, et al. Relationship between the birth cohort pattern of *Helicobacter pylori* infection and the epidemiology of duodenal ulcer. *Q J Med* 2002;95:519–525.
3. Axon AT. *Helicobacter pylori* infection. *J Antimicrob Chemother* 1993;32(suppl A):61–68.
4. Graham DY. Can therapy ever be denied for *Helicobacter pylori* infection? *Gastroenterology* 1997;113:S113–S117.
5. Huang J-Q, Sridhar S, Hunt RH. Role of *Helicobacter pylori* infection and non-steroidal anti-inflammatory drugs in peptic ulcer disease: a meta-analysis. *Lancet* 2002;359:14–22. (Search date 2000, data sources, Medline, Cochrane database, hand searching).
6. Ford AC, Delaney BC, Forman D, et al. Eradication therapy in *Helicobacter pylori* positive peptic ulcer disease: systematic review and economic analysis. *Am J Gastroenterol* 2004;99:1833–1855. Search date 2002.
7. Sharma VK, Sahai AV, Corder FA, et al. *Helicobacter pylori* eradication is superior to ulcer healing with or without maintenance therapy to prevent further ulcer haemorrhage. *Aliment Pharmacol Ther* 2001;15:1939–1947. Search date 2000; primary sources Medline and conference abstracts.
8. Penston JG, McColl KEL. Eradication of *Helicobacter pylori*: an objective assessment of current therapies. *Br J Clin Pharmacol* 1997;43:223–243. Search date 1995; primary sources Medline and conference abstracts.
9. Laine L, Hopkins RJ, Girardi LS. Has the impact of *Helicobacter pylori* therapy on ulcer recurrence in the United States been overstated? A meta-analysis of rigorously designed trials. *Am J Gastroenterol* 1998;93:1409–1415. Search date 1996; primary sources Medline, conference abstracts, and pharmaceutical companies (US trials only).
10. Chan FKL, Sung JJY, Suen R, et al. Does eradication of *Helicobacter pylori* impair healing of nonsteroidal anti-inflammatory drug associated bleeding peptic ulcers? A prospective randomized study. *Aliment Pharmacol Ther* 1998;12:1201–1205.
11. Chan FKL, To KF, Wu JCY, et al. Eradication of *Helicobacter pylori* and risk of peptic ulcers in patients starting long term treatment with non-steroidal anti-inflammatory drugs: a randomized trial. *Lancet* 2002;359:9–13.
12. Chan FKL, Chung SCS, Suen BY, et al. Preventing recurrent upper gastrointestinal bleeding in patients with *Helicobacter pylori* infection who are taking low-dose aspirin or naproxen. *N Engl J Med* 2001;344:967–973.
13. Chan FKL, Sung JJY, Chung SCS, et al. Randomised trial of eradication of *Helicobacter pylori* before non-steroidal anti-inflammatory drug therapy to prevent peptic ulcers. *Lancet* 1997;350:975–979.
14. Labenz J, Blum AL, Bolten WW, et al. Primary prevention of diclofenac associated ulcers and dyspepsia by omeprazole or triple therapy in *Helicobacter pylori* positive patients: a randomised, double blind, placebo controlled, clinical trial. *Gut* 2002;51:329–335.
15. Moayyedi P, Bardhan C, Young L, et al. *Helicobacter pylori* eradication does not exacerbate reflux symptoms in gastroesophageal reflux disease. *Gastroenterology* 2001;121:1120–1126.
16. Harvey RF, Lane JA, Murray LJ, et al. Randomised controlled trial of the effects of *Helicobacter pylori* infection and its eradication on heartburn and gastro-oesophageal reflux: Bristol helicobacter project. *BMJ* 2004;328:1417.
17. Labenz J, Blum AL, Bayerdorffer E, et al. Curing *Helicobacter pylori* infection in patients with duodenal ulcer may provoke reflux esophagitis. *Gastroenterology* 1997;112:1442–1447.
18. Roher HD, Vereet PR, Wormer O, et al. *Helicobacter pylori* in the upper gastrointestinal tract: medical or surgical treatment of gastric lymphoma? *Langenbecks Arch Surg* 2000;385:97–105. Search date not reported; primary sources Medline and hand searches.
19. Steinbach G, Ford R, Glober G, et al. Antibiotic treatment of gastric lymphoma of mucosa-associated lymphoid tissue. An uncontrolled trial. *Ann Intern Med* 1999;131:88–95.
20. Wong B, Lam SK, Wong WM, et al. *Helicobacter pylori* eradication to prevent gastric cancer in a high-risk region of China: a randomized controlled trial. *JAMA* 2004;291:187–194
21. Correa P, Fontham ETH, Bravo JC, et al. Chemoprevention of gastric dysplasia: randomized trial of antioxidant supplements and anti-*Helicobacter pylori* therapy. *J Natl Cancer Inst* 2000;92:1881–1888.
22. *Helicobacter* and Cancer Collaborative Group. Gastric cancer and *Helicobacter pylori*: a combined analysis of 12 case control studies nested within prospective cohorts. *Gut* 2001;49:347–353. Search date 1999; primary sources Medline and contact with investigators.
23. Soo S, Moayyedi P, Deeks J, et al. Eradication of *Helicobacter pylori* for non-ulcer dyspepsia. In: The

Cochrane Library, Issue 3, 2003. Oxford: Update Software. Search date 2002; Cochrane Controlled Trials Register primary sources Medline, Embase, Cinahl, SIGLE, hand searches of reference lists, and personal contact with experts in the field and pharmaceutical companies.
24. Blum AL, Talley NJ, O'Morain C, et al. Lack of effect of treating *Helicobacter pylori* infection in patients with nonulcer dyspepsia. *N Engl J Med* 1998;339:1875–1881.
25. Koelz HR, Arnold R, Stolte M, et al. Treatment of *Helicobacter pylori* (HP) does not improve symptoms of functional dyspepsia. *Gastroenterology* 1998;114:A182.
26. Chiba N, Veldhuyzen van Zanten SJO, Sinclair P, et al. Treating *Helicobacter pylori* infection in primary care patients with uninvestigated dyspepsia: the Canadian adult dyspepsia empiric treatment *Helicobacter pylori* positive (CADET-Hp) randomised controlled trial. *BMJ* 2002;324:1012.
27. Delaney BC, Moayyedi P, Forman D. Initial management strategies for dyspepsia (Cochrane Review). In: The Cochrane Library, Issue 3, 2003. Oxford: Update Software. Search date 2002; primary sources Medline, Embase, Science Citation Index, conference abstracts, and survey of experts.
28. Arents NLA, Thijs JC, van Zwet AA, et al. Approach to treatment of dyspepsia in primary care. A randomised trial comparing 'test and treat' with prompt endoscopy. *Arch Intern Med* 2003;163:1606–1612.
29. Lassen AT, Pedersen FM, Bytzer P, et al. *Helicobacter pylori* "test and eradicate" or prompt endoscopy for management of dyspeptic patients. A randomised controlled trial with one year follow-up. *Lancet* 2000;356:455–460.
30. Heaney A, Collins JSA, Watson RGP, et al. A prospective randomised trial of a "test and treat" policy versus endoscopy based management in young *Helicobacter pylori* positive patients with ulcer-like dyspepsia, referred to a hospital clinic. *Gut* 1999;45:186–190.
31. Forman D, Bazzoli F, Bennett C, et al. Therapies for the eradication of *Helicobacter pylori*. Protocol for a Cochrane Review. In: The Cochrane Library, Issue 3, 2003. Oxford: Update Software.
32. Huang JQ, Hunt RH. The importance of clarithromycin dose in the management of *Helicobacter pylori* infection: a meta-analysis of triple therapies with a proton pump inhibitor, clarithromycin and amoxycillin or metronidazole. *Aliment Pharmacol Ther* 1999;13:719–729. Search date 1998; primary sources Medline and conference abstracts.
33. Janssen M, Van Oijen A, Verbeek A, et al. A systematic comparison of triple therapies for treatment of *Helicobacter pylori* infection with proton pump inhibitor/ranitidine bismuth citrate plus clarithromycin and either amoxicillin or a nitroimidazole. *Aliment Pharmacol Ther* 2001;15:613–624. Search date 2000; primary sources Medline and hand searches of reference lists and meetings abstracts.
34. Lind T, Peal MFU. The Mach 2 study: role of omeprazole in eradication of *Helicobacter pylori* with 1-week triple therapies. *Gastroenterology* 1999;116:248–253.
35. Katelaris PH, Forbes GM, Talley NJ, et al. A randomized comparison of quadruple and triple therapies for *Helicobacter pylori* eradication: the QUADRATE study. *Gastroenterology* 2002;123:1763–1769.
36. Laine L, Hunt R, El Zimaity H, et al. Bismuth-based quadruple therapy using a single capsule of bismuth biskalcitrate, metronidazole, and tetracycline given with omeprazole versus omeprazole, amoxicillin, and clarithromycin for eradication of *Helicobacter pylori* in duodenal ulcer patients: a prospective, randomized, multicenter, North American trial. *Am J Gastroenterol* 2003;98:562–567.
37. Wong B, Wang W, Wong W, et al. Three-day lansoprazole quadruple therapy for *Helicobacter pylori*-positive duodenal ulcers: a randomised controlled study. Aliment Pharmacol Ther 2001;15:843–849.
38. Calvet X, Garcia N, Lopez T, et al. A meta-analysis of short versus long therapy with a proton pump inhibitor, clarithromycin and either metronidazole or amoxycillin for treating *Helicobacter pylori* infection. *Aliment Pharmacol Ther* 2000;14:603–609. Search date 1999; primary sources Medline and conference proceedings.

Brendan Delaney
Department of Primary Care
and General Practice
University of Birmingham
Birmingham
UK

Paul Moayyedi
McMaster University
Hamilton
Canada

David Forman
Cochrane Upper Gastrointestinal
and Pancreatic Disease
Collaborative Review Group
University of Leeds
Leeds
UK

Competing interests: BD has received fees for speaking at conferences and educational meetings from Astra Zeneca, Eisai, and Axcan. DF has received consulting fees from Astra Zeneca, Wyeth, and TAP-TAKEDA. PM has accepted fees for speaking from Astra Zeneca, Wyeth, Mareda, and Abbott Laboratories.

Inguinal hernia

Search date September 2004

Sanjay Purkayastha, Thanos Athanasiou, Paris Tekkis, Ara Darzi

QUESTIONS

INTERVENTIONS

To be covered in future updates
Conservative interventions (e.g. trusses, belts)
Laparoscopic TEP versus TAPP repair

*Based on clinical experience and consensus

See glossary

Key Messages

Unilateral inguinal hernia

- **Open mesh repair (reduced recurrence compared with open suture repair, with no increase in surgical complications)** We found no systematic review, RCTs, or cohort studies of sufficient quality comparing open mesh repair versus expectant management. One systematic review found that open mesh repair reduced inguinal hernia recurrence and slightly reduced the length of hospital stay compared with open suture repair. The review and one subsequent RCT found no significant difference in surgical complications between open mesh and open suture repair. One systematic review and three subsequent RCTs found that open mesh repair increased the overall recovery time compared with totally extraperitoneal (TEP) laparoscopic repair and found limited evidence that open mesh repair slightly increased hospital stay and postoperative pain. They found no significant difference between open mesh repair and TEP laparoscopic repair in either recurrence or most postoperative complications, although the systematic review and one RCT found limited evidence that open mesh repair increased postoperative haematoma compared with TEP laparoscopic repair. One systematic review found that open mesh repair increased postoperative pain at 3 months and time to return to usual activities compared with transabdominal preperitoneal (TAPP) laparoscopic repair. It found insufficient evidence to compare the effects of open mesh repair versus TAPP laparoscopic repair on recurrence rates. One subsequent RCT found that open mesh repair increased postoperative pain and length of hospital stay compared with TAPP laparoscopic repair. Adverse effects of open mesh repair and TAPP laparoscopic repair were similar, although the review found that open mesh repair decreased the risk of seroma and increased postoperative numbness and superficial infection compared with TAPP laparoscopic repair.
- **Totally extraperitoneal (TEP) laparoscopic repair (reduced pain and time to return to usual activities compared with open repair)** We found no systematic review, RCTs, or cohort studies of sufficient quality comparing totally extraperitoneal (TEP) laparoscopic repair versus expectant management. One systematic review and three subsequent RCTs found that TEP laparoscopic repair decreased the overall recovery time compared with open mesh repair and found limited evidence that TEP laparoscopic repair slightly reduced hospital stay and postoperative pain compared with open mesh repair. They found no significant difference between open mesh repair and TEP laparoscopic repair in either recurrence or most postoperative complications, although the systematic review and one RCT found limited evidence that TEP laparoscopic repair reduced postoperative haematoma compared with open mesh repair. One systematic review found that TEP laparoscopic repair reduced pain after 3 months and reduced length of hospital stay slightly compared with open suture repair, but found no significant difference in risk of recurrence or time to return to normal activities. One subsequent RCT found no significant difference between TEP laparoscopic repair and open suture repair in recurrence, length of hospital stay, or groin pain. Adverse effects were similar for TEP laparoscopic and open suture repair, although the review found that TEP laparoscopic repair increased the risk of seroma but decreased the risk of infection compared with open suture repair.
- **Transabdominal preperitoneal (TAPP) laparoscopic repair (reduced pain and time to return to usual activities compared with open mesh repair)** We found no systematic review, RCTs, or cohort studies of sufficient quality comparing transabdominal preperitoneal (TAPP) laparoscopic repair versus expectant management. One systematic review found that TAPP laparoscopic repair reduced postoperative pain at 3 months, and time to return to usual activities compared with open mesh repair. It found insufficient evidence to compare effects of TAPP laparoscopic repair versus open mesh repair on recurrence rates. One subsequent RCT found that TAPP laparoscopic repair reduced postoperative pain and length of hospital stay compared with open mesh repair. Adverse effects of open mesh repair and TAPP laparoscopic repair were similar, although TAPP laparoscopic repair increased the risk of seroma and decreased postoperative numbness and superficial infection compared with open mesh repair. One systematic review and subsequent RCTs

found that TAPP laparoscopic repair decreased postoperative pain and time to return to usual activities compared with open suture repair. The systematic review found limited evidence that TAPP laparoscopic repair reduced recurrence compared with open suture repair, although two subsequent RCTs found no significant difference. Adverse effects of TAPP laparoscopic repair and open suture repair were similar.

- **Open suture repair (conventional, well established surgical technique but less effective for improving clinically important outcomes than open mesh repair, TEP laparoscopic repair or TAPP laparoscopic repair)*** Clinical experience and consensus opinion suggest that surgery is effective for primary unilateral inguinal hernia. Open suture repair is a well established surgical technique. However, we found no systematic review, RCTs, or cohort studies of sufficient quality comparing open suture repair versus expectant management. One systematic review found that open suture repair was less effective at reducing inguinal hernia recurrence than open mesh repair and that it increased length of hospital stay. The review and one subsequent RCT found no significant difference in surgical complications between open suture repair and open mesh repair. One systematic review found that open suture repair increased pain after 3 months and increased length of hospital stay slightly compared with totally extraperitoneal (TEP) laparoscopic repair, but found no significant difference in risk of recurrence or time to return to normal activities, whereas one subsequent RCT found no significant difference between TEP laparoscopic repair and open suture repair in recurrence, length of hospital stay, or groin pain. Adverse effects were similar for TEP laparoscopic repair and open suture repair, although the review found that open suture repair decreased the risk of seroma but increased the risk of infection compared with TEP laparoscopic repair. One systematic review and subsequent RCTs found that open suture repair increased postoperative pain, and time to return to usual activities compared with transabdominal preperitoneal (TAPP) laparoscopic repair. The systematic review found limited evidence that open suture repair was less effective at reducing recurrence compared with TAPP laparoscopic repair, although two subsequent RCTs found no significant difference. Adverse effects of open suture repair and TAPP laparoscopic repair were similar.
- **Expectant management** We found no systematic review, RCTs, or cohort studies of sufficient quality of expectant management in people with unilateral inguinal hernia.

Bilateral inguinal hernia

- **Open mesh repair (may reduce length of hospital stay compared with open suture repair)** We found no systematic review, RCTs, or cohort studies of sufficient quality comparing open mesh repair versus expectant management in people with bilateral inguinal hernia. One systematic review found limited evidence that open mesh repair reduced length of hospital stay compared with open suture repair but found insufficient evidence to compare other clinical effects. One systematic review found limited evidence that open mesh repair increased the time taken to return to normal activities and postoperative superficial infection compared with transabdominal preperitoneal laparoscopic repair. It found insufficient evidence to compare other clinical effects and insufficient evidence to compare clinical effects of open mesh repair versus totally extraperitoneal laparoscopic repair.
- **Open suture repair (conventional, well established surgical technique but may be less effective in improving clinically important outcomes than open mesh repair or TAPP laparoscopic repair)*** Clinical experience and consensus opinion suggest that surgical intervention is an effective treatment for bilateral inguinal hernia. Open suture repair is a well established surgical technique. However, we found no systematic review, RCTs, or cohort studies of sufficient quality comparing open suture repair versus expectant management in people with bilateral inguinal hernia. One systematic review found limited evidence that open suture repair increased length of hospital stay compared with open mesh repair but found

insufficient evidence to compare other clinical effects. One systematic review found limited evidence that open suture repair increased the time taken to return to normal activities compared with transabdominal preperitoneal laparoscopic repair. It found insufficient evidence to compare other clinical effects, and found insufficient evidence to compare clinical effects of open suture repairs versus totally extraperitoneal laparoscopic repair.

- **Transabdominal preperitoneal (TAPP) laparoscopic repair (may reduce time to return to normal activities compared with open repair)** We found no systematic review, RCTs, or cohort studies of sufficient quality comparing transabdominal preperitoneal (TAPP) laparoscopic repair versus expectant management in people with bilateral inguinal hernia. One systematic review found limited evidence that TAPP laparoscopic repair reduced the time taken to return to normal activities compared with open suture repair or open mesh repair, and that TAPP laparoscopic repair reduced postoperative superficial infection compared with open mesh repair. It found insufficient evidence to compare other clinical effects.
- **Expectant management** We found no systematic review, RCTs, or cohort studies of sufficient quality of expectant management in people with bilateral inguinal hernia.
- **Totally extraperitoneal (TEP) laparoscopic repair** We found no systematic review, RCTs, or cohort studies of sufficient quality comparing totally extraperitoneal laparoscopic (TEP) repair versus expectant management in people with bilateral inguinal hernia. One systematic review found insufficient evidence to compare clinical effects of TEP laparoscopic repair versus open suture and open mesh repairs.

Recurrent inguinal hernia

- **Open mesh repair (slightly reduced length of hospital stay compared with open suture repair; other effects uncertain)** We found no systematic review, RCTs, or cohort studies of sufficient quality comparing open mesh repair versus expectant management. One systematic review found limited evidence that open mesh repair slightly reduced length of hospital stay compared with open suture repair in people with recurrent inguinal hernia. However, the review found insufficient evidence to compare effects on pain, time to return to usual activities, further recurrence, or other complications of surgery. One systematic review found limited evidence that open mesh repair increased the time taken to return to normal activities compared with transabdominal preperitoneal and totally extraperitoneal laparoscopic repair techniques, but it found insufficient evidence to compare other clinical effects.
- **Open suture repair (conventional, well established surgical technique but may be less effective in improving clinically important outcomes than open mesh repair or TAPP laparoscopic repair)*** Clinical experience and consensus opinion suggest that surgery is an effective treatment for recurrent inguinal hernia. Open suture repair is a well established surgical technique. However, we found no systematic review, RCTs, or cohort studies of sufficient quality comparing open suture repair versus expectant management. One systematic review found limited evidence that open suture repair slightly increased length of hospital stay compared with open mesh repair in people with recurrent inguinal hernia but found insufficient evidence to compare effects on pain, time to return to usual activities, further recurrence, or other complications of surgery. One systematic review found limited evidence that open suture repair increased the time taken to return to normal activities compared with transabdominal preperitoneal laparoscopic repair. It found insufficient evidence to compare other clinical effects and insufficient data to compare benefits of open suture repair versus totally extraperitoneal laparoscopic repair.
- **Totally extraperitoneal (TEP) laparoscopic repair (may reduce time to return to normal activities compared with open mesh repair; other effects uncertain)** We found no systematic review, RCTs, or cohort studies of sufficient quality comparing totally extraperitoneal (TEP) laparoscopic repair versus expectant management in people with recurrent inguinal hernia. One systematic review found limited evidence that TEP laparoscopic repair reduced the time taken to return to normal activities compared with open mesh repair. However, it found insufficient evidence to compare other clinical effects and insufficient data to compare the effects of TEP laparoscopic repair versus open suture repair.

- **Transabdominal preperitoneal (TAPP) laparoscopic repair (may reduce time to return to normal activities compared with open repair; other effects uncertain)** We found no systematic review, RCTs, or cohort studies of sufficient quality comparing transabdominal preperitoneal laparoscopic repair versus expectant management. One systematic review found limited evidence that transabdominal preperitoneal laparoscopic repair reduced the time taken to return to normal activities compared with open suture repair and open mesh repair in people with recurrent inguinal hernia but found insufficient evidence to compare other clinical effects.
- **Expectant management** We found no systematic review, RCTs, or cohort studies of sufficient quality of expectant management in people with recurrent inguinal hernia.

DEFINITION Inguinal hernia is an out-pouching of peritoneum, with or without its contents, which occurs through the muscles of the anterior abdominal wall at the level of the inguinal canal, in the groin. It almost always occurs in men, because of the inherent weakness of the abdominal wall where the spermatic cord passes through the inguinal canal. A portion of bowel may become caught in the peritoneal pouch, and present as a lump in the groin. The hernia may extend into the scrotum, and can cause discomfort or ache. Primary hernias relate to the first presentation of a hernia and are distinct from recurrent hernias. A hernia is described as reducible if it occurs intermittently (e.g. on straining or standing) and can be pushed back into the abdominal cavity and is irreducible if it remains permanently outside the abdominal cavity. Inguinal hernia is usually a long standing condition and diagnosis is made clinically, on the basis of these typical symptoms and signs. The condition may occur in one groin (unilateral hernia) or both groins simultaneously (bilateral hernia), and may recur after treatment (recurrent hernia). Occasionally, hernia may present acutely because of complications (see prognosis below). In this chapter we deal only with non-acute, uncomplicated inguinal hernias in adults. Clinical experience and consensus opinion suggest that surgical intervention is an effective treatment for inguinal hernia. However, surgery is associated with complications (see outcomes below), therefore, much of this chapter examines the relative effectiveness and safety of different surgical techniques. Inguinal hernias are frequently classified as direct or indirect, depending on whether the hernia sac bulges directly through the posterior wall of the inguinal canal (direct hernia), or rather passes through the internal inguinal ring alongside the spermatic cord, and follows the course of the inguinal canal (indirect hernia). However, none of the studies that we identified distinguished between these two types of inguinal hernia. Identified studies gave little detail about the severity of hernia among included participants. In general, studies explicitly excluded people with irreducible or complicated hernia, large hernia (extending into the scrotum), or serious co-morbidity, and those at high surgical risk (e.g. because of coagulation disorders).

INCIDENCE/PREVALENCE We found one nationally mandated guideline, which reported that 105 000 people (about 0.2% of people) develop an inguinal hernia each year in England and Wales.[1] Inguinal hernia is usually repaired surgically in resource rich countries. Surgical audit data therefore provide reasonable estimates of incidence, and support estimates of this order of magnitude. National statistical survey data from England reported that about 70 000 inguinal hernia repairs were undertaken in public health care settings in England in 2002–2003.[2] Similarly, in the USA estimates based on cross-sectional data suggest that about 700 000 inguinal hernia repairs were undertaken in 1993.[3] A national survey of general practices covering about 1% of the population of England and Wales in 1991–1992 found that about 95% of people presenting to primary care settings with inguinal hernia were male.[4] It found that the incidence rose from about 11/10 000 person-years in men aged 16–24 years to about 200/10 000 person-years in men aged 75 years or above.

AETIOLOGY/RISK FACTORS Age and male sex are risk factors (see incidence/prevalence above). Chronic cough and manual labour involving heavy lifting are conventionally regarded as risk factors because they lead to high intra-abdominal pressure. Obesity has also been suggested to be a risk factor. However, we found no reliable data to quantify these risks.

PROGNOSIS We found few reliable data on untreated prognosis. Strangulation, intestinal obstruction, and infarction are the most important acute complications of untreated hernia and are potentially life threatening. National statistics from England found that 5% of primary inguinal hernia repairs were undertaken as emergencies (presumably because of acute complications) in 1998–1999.[2] Older age, longer duration of hernia, and longer duration of irreducibility are thought to be risk factors for acute complication,[5] although we found no reliable data to quantify these effects.

AIMS OF INTERVENTION To prevent recurrence; to alleviate symptoms; to allow return to normal activities; to improve quality of life; to prevent acute hernia complications, while minimising adverse effects of treatment.

OUTCOMES **Benefits:** Hernia recurrence; hernia complications; quality of life; length of hospital stay; time to return to normal activities; pain. **Harms:** Adverse effects of surgery: seroma; haematoma; numbness; infection; vascular injury; visceral injury; wound hernia or dehiscence; surgical mortality; and other complications of intervention.

METHODS *Clinical Evidence* search and appraisal September 2004. For the option on expectant management(G), we also searched for cohort studies.

QUESTION What are the effects of elective treatment for primary unilateral inguinal hernia?

OPTION EXPECTANT MANAGEMENT

We found no systematic review, RCTs, or cohort studies of sufficient quality of expectant management in people with unilateral inguinal hernia.

Benefits: **Versus open suture repair, open mesh repair, or laparoscopic repair:** We found no systematic review, RCTs, or cohort studies of sufficient quality.

Harms: **Versus open suture repair, open mesh repair, or laparoscopic repair:** We found no systematic review, RCTs, or cohort studies of sufficient quality.

Comment: Expectant management(G) might be considered a reasonable strategy in people who have only mild symptoms, and in whom the risk of hernia complications is low (see prognosis, p 539) or operative risk is high. However, we found no reliable evidence about the benefits and risks of expectant management compared with surgery.

OPTION OPEN MESH REPAIR

We found no systematic review, RCTs, or cohort studies of sufficient quality comparing open mesh repair versus expectant management. One systematic review found that open mesh repair reduced inguinal hernia recurrence and slightly reduced the length of hospital stay compared with open suture repair. The review and one subsequent RCT found no significant difference in surgical complications between open mesh and open suture repair. One systematic review and three subsequent RCTs found that open mesh repair increased the overall recovery time compared with totally extraperitoneal (TEP) laparoscopic repair and found limited evidence that open mesh repair slightly increased hospital stay and postoperative pain. They found no significant difference between open mesh repair and TEP laparoscopic repair in either recurrence or most postoperative complications, although the systematic review and one RCT found limited evidence that open mesh repair increased postoperative haematoma compared with TEP laparoscopic repair. One systematic review found that open mesh repair increased postoperative pain at 3 months and time to return to usual activities compared with transabdominal preperitoneal (TAPP) laparoscopic repair. It found insufficient evidence to compare the effects of open mesh repair versus TAPP laparoscopic repair on recurrence rates. One subsequent RCT found that open mesh repair increased postoperative pain and length of hospital stay compared with TAPP laparoscopic repair. Adverse effects of open mesh repair and TAPP

laparoscopic repair were similar, although the review found that open mesh repair decreased the risk of seroma and increased postoperative numbness and superficial infection compared with TAPP laparoscopic repair.

Benefits: **Versus expectant management:** We found no systematic review, RCTs, or cohort studies of sufficient quality. **Versus open suture repair:** We found one systematic review (search date 2000)[6] and one subsequent RCT.[7] The review found that open mesh repair significantly reduced hernia recurrence and duration of hospital stay compared with open suture repair**G** (hernia recurrence: 18 RCTs, predominantly people with unilateral hernia [see comment below], 4532 people; OR 0.37, 95% CI 0.26 to 0.51; duration of hospital stay: 17 RCTs, 3733 people; weighted mean reduction in length of stay: 0.28 days, 95% CI 0.22 days to 0.35 days).[6] However, the difference in hospital stay was small and may be of limited importance to people having surgery. The review found limited evidence that open mesh repair**G** significantly reduced the risk of continuing postoperative pain after 3 months and reduced time to return to usual activities compared with open suture repair (continuing pain after 3 months: 9 RCTs, 2393 people; OR 0.68, 95% CI 0.47 to 0.98; time to return to normal activities: 8 RCTs, 1279 people; HR 0.81, 95% CI 0.73 to 0.91), although trial results were heterogeneous, suggesting that these effects may be dependent on factors other than surgical method alone (see comment below). The subsequent RCT (100 men, 5 of whom had bilateral inguinal hernia [see comment below]) found no significant difference between open mesh repair and open suture repair in time to return to normal activity (5.1 weeks in both groups; difference 0 weeks, 95% CI –1.6 weeks to +1.6 weeks).[7] The RCT reported that two hernias had recurred in each group after up to 4 years' follow up. **Versus TAPP laparoscopic repair:** See benefits of TAPP laparoscopic repair, p 545. **Versus TEP laparoscopic repair:** See benefits of TEP laparoscopic repair, p 543.

Harms: **Versus expectant management:** We found no systematic review, RCTs, or cohort studies of sufficient quality. **Versus open suture repair:** The systematic review found no significant difference between open mesh repair**G** and open suture repair**G** in haematoma, seroma, superficial infection, life threatening surgical complications, deep or mesh infection, persisting numbness after 3 months, or mortality, although serious events and death were rare in both groups (haematoma: 13 RCTs, 3072 people; OR 0.93, 95% CI 0.68 to 1.26; seroma: 11 RCTs, 3045 people; OR 1.52, 95% CI 0.92 to 2.52; superficial infection: 16 RCTs, 3516 people: OR 1.24, 95% CI 0.84 to 1.84; life threatening complication/deep infection: 14 RCTs, 3508 people; OR 1.00, 95% CI 0.20 to 4.95; persisting numbness: 3 RCTs, 602 people; OR 0.70, 95% CI 0.29 to 1.72; death: 6 RCTs, 1564 people; OR 1.35, 95% CI 0.65 to 2.80).[6] The subsequent RCT (100 men) similarly found no significant difference between open mesh repair and open suture repair in haematoma, infection, and seroma, although it may have lacked power to detect clinically important differences between groups.[7] **Versus TAPP laparoscopic repair:** See harms of TAPP laparoscopic repair, p 546. **Versus TEP laparoscopic repair:** See harms of TEP laparoscopic repair, p 544.

Comment: The systematic review found that results for persisting pain after 3 months and time to return to usual activities were heterogeneous and highly sensitive to one RCT in each case.[6] The reasons for heterogeneity among studies may include use of different variants of the suturing and mesh repair, different participant characteristics, differing experience of operating surgeons, or differing methods of outcome measurement among studies. When the analyses were adjusted for heterogeneity, the results were no longer significant (persisting pain: random effects model; OR 0.86, 95% CI 0.43 to 1.73; time to return to work: sensitivity analysis excluding 1 RCT; HR 0.89, 95% CI 0.80 to 1.00). The systematic review included people with unilateral, bilateral, or recurrent femoral or inguinal hernia. However, the numbers of people with bilateral or recurrent hernias were small, and the number with femoral hernia was negligible. Overall results are therefore applicable to people with unilateral inguinal hernia. Separate meta-analyses were performed in people with recurrent or bilateral hernia, and are presented below (see questions on primary bilateral inguinal hernia, p 547 and recurrent inguinal hernia, p 551). The subsequent RCT also included a small proportion of men with bilateral inguinal hernia and did not present results separately in men with unilateral hernia.[7] However, this is unlikely to affect applicability of results. The study was small compared with the systematic review, and probably lacked power to detect differences in recurrence rate between groups.

OPTION OPEN SUTURE REPAIR

Clinical experience and consensus opinion suggest that surgery is effective for primary unilateral inguinal hernia. Open suture repair is a well established surgical technique. However, we found no systematic review, RCTs, or cohort studies of sufficient quality comparing open suture repair versus expectant management. One systematic review found that open suture repair was less effective at reducing inguinal hernia recurrence than open mesh repair and that it increased length of hospital stay. The review and one subsequent RCT found no significant difference in surgical complications between open suture repair and open mesh repair. One systematic review found that open suture repair increased pain after 3 months and increased length of hospital stay slightly compared with totally extraperitoneal (TEP) laparoscopic repair, but found no significant difference in risk of recurrence or time to return to normal activities, whereas one subsequent RCT found no significant difference between TEP laparoscopic repair and open suture repair in recurrence, length of hospital stay, or groin pain. Adverse effects were similar for TEP laparoscopic repair and open suture repair, although the review found that open suture repair decreased the risk of seroma but increased the risk of infection compared with TEP laparoscopic repair. One systematic review and subsequent RCTs found that open suture repair increased postoperative pain, and time to return to usual activities compared with transabdominal preperitoneal (TAPP) laparoscopic repair. The systematic review found limited evidence that open suture repair was less effective at reducing recurrence compared with TAPP laparoscopic repair, although two subsequent RCTs found no significant difference. Adverse effects of open suture repair and TAPP laparoscopic repair were similar.

Benefits: **Versus expectant management:** We found no systematic review, RCTs, or cohort studies of sufficient quality. **Versus open mesh repair:** See benefits of open mesh repair, p 541. **Versus TAPP laparoscopic repair:** See benefits of TAPP laparoscopic repair, p 545. **Versus TEP laparoscopic repair:** See benefits of TEP laparoscopic repair, p 543.

Harms: **Versus expectant management:** We found no systematic review, RCTs, or cohort studies of sufficient quality. **Versus open mesh repair:** See harms of open mesh repair, p 541. **Versus** TAPP laparoscopic repair repairⓖ: See harms of TAPP laparoscopic repair, p 546. **Versus TEP laparoscopic repair:** See harms of TEP laparoscopic repair, p 544.

Comment: Open suture repairⓖ is a well established method of management for people with inguinal hernias.

OPTION **TOTALLY EXTRAPERITONEAL (TEP) LAPAROSCOPIC REPAIR**

We found no systematic review, RCTs, or cohort studies of sufficient quality comparing totally extraperitoneal (TEP) laparoscopic repair versus expectant management. One systematic review and three subsequent RCTs found that TEP laparoscopic repair decreased the overall recovery time compared with open mesh repair and found limited evidence that TEP laparoscopic repair slightly reduced hospital stay and postoperative pain compared with open mesh repair. They found no significant difference between open mesh repair and TEP laparoscopic repair in either recurrence or most postoperative complications, although the systematic review and one RCT found limited evidence that TEP laparoscopic repair reduced postoperative haematoma compared with open mesh repair. One systematic review found that TEP laparoscopic repair reduced pain after 3 months and reduced length of hospital stay slightly compared with open suture repair, but found no significant difference in risk of recurrence or time to return to normal activities. One subsequent RCT found no significant difference between TEP laparoscopic repair and open suture repair in recurrence, length of hospital stay, or groin pain. Adverse effects were similar for TEP laparoscopic and open suture repair, although the review found that TEP laparoscopic repair increased the risk of seroma but decreased the risk of infection compared with open suture repair.

Benefits: **Versus expectant management:** We found no systematic review, RCTs, or cohort studies of sufficient quality. **Versus open suture repair:** We found one systematic review (search date 2002)[8] and one subsequent RCT.[9] The review found that totally extraperitoneal (TEP) laparoscopic repair**Ⓖ** significantly reduced persisting pain after 3 months compared with open suture repair**Ⓖ** (persisting pain: 2 RCTs, 515 people; OR 0.22, 95% CI 0.14 to 0.35).[8] However, it found no significant difference between TEP laparoscopic repair and open suture repair in risk of recurrence or time to return to normal activities (recurrence: 5 RCTs, 1519 people; OR 0.67, 95% CI 0.38 to 1.18; time to return to usual activities: 1 RCT, 94 people; HR 0.78, 95% CI 0.52 to 1.17). The review found that TEP laparoscopic repair significantly reduced length of hospital stay compared with open suture repair, although the difference was small (4 RCTs, 1338 people; weighted mean reduction in length of stay: 0.34 days, 95% CI 0.22 days to 0.45 days). The subsequent RCT (261 people) found no significant difference in length of hospital stay, recurrence, or groin pain between TEP laparoscopic repair and open suture repair after 2 years (244 people in analysis; median hospital stay: 1 day with laparoscopic repair *v* 1 day with open suture repair; P value not reported; recurrence: 5/119 [4%] with TEP laparoscopic repair *v* 0/125 [0%] with open suture repair; $P > 0.05$; groin pain: 14/119 [12%] with TEP laparoscopic repair *v* 8/125 [6%] with open suture repair; $P > 0.05$).[9] **Versus open mesh repair:** We found one systematic review (search date 2002)[8] and three subsequent RCTs.[10–12] The review found that TEP laparoscopic repair significantly reduced persisting pain after 3 months and time to return to usual activities compared with open mesh repair**Ⓖ** (persisting pain: 3 RCTs, 350 people; OR 0.13, 95% CI 0.05 to 0.34; time to return to usual activities: 4 RCTs, 409 people; HR 0.26, 95% CI 0.21 to 0.33).[8] However, it found no significant difference between TEP laparoscopic repair and open mesh repair in risk of recurrence (6 RCTs, 678 people; OR 0.97, 95% CI 0.34 to 2.77). The review found that TEP laparoscopic repair significantly reduced length of hospital stay compared with open mesh repair, although the difference was small (5 RCTs, 622 people; weighted mean reduction in length of stay: 0.34 days, 95% CI 0.23 days to 0.45 days). The first subsequent RCT (299 people with unilateral hernia, of whom 297 had inguinal hernia and about 85% had primary hernia) compared TEP laparoscopic repair versus two different open mesh repair techniques.[10] It found that TEP laparoscopic repair significantly reduced the time to full recovery (assessed by participant's perception) compared with open mesh repair techniques (14 days with TEP laparoscopic repair *v* about 24–28 days with open mesh repair; P < 0.0001). It found no significant difference between TEP laparoscopic repair and open mesh repair in recurrence rate (about 2% with TEP laparoscopic repair *v* about 1% with open mesh repair; P value not reported). The second subsequent RCT (185 people with inguinal hernia, of whom 130 had primary unilateral hernia, 10 had bilateral hernia, and 28 had recurrent hernia; 19 people excluded from analyses) found no significant difference in postoperative pain or recurrence at 1 year (2/76 [2.6%] with TEP laparoscopic repair *v* 0/85 [0%] with open mesh repair; P = 0.23).[12] However, it found that TEP laparoscopic repair significantly reduced time to return to work compared with open mesh repair (mean: 8 days with TEP laparoscopic repair *v* 11 days with open mesh repair; P = 0.003). The third subsequent RCT (134 people with inguinal hernia, of whom 95 had primary unilateral hernia and the remainder had bilateral or recurrent hernia) found that TEP laparoscopic repair significantly reduced pain on the first postoperative day, hospital stay, and time to return to normal activities (mean pain score on visual analogue scale from 0–10: 2.73 with TEP laparoscopic repair *v* 4.61 with open mesh repair; mean hospital stay: 1.80 days with TEP laparoscopic repair *v* 2.73 days with open mesh repair; mean time to return to normal activities: 10.8 days with TEP laparoscopic repair *v* 15.2 days with open mesh repair; P = 0.001 for all comparisons).[11] However, treatment effects may have been confounded by baseline differences between groups. A greater proportion of people receiving TEP laparoscopic repair had bilateral or recurrent hernias than in the open mesh repair group.

Harms: **Versus expectant management:** We found no systematic review, RCTs, or cohort studies of sufficient quality. **Versus open suture repair:** The systematic review found no significant difference between TEP laparoscopic repair**G** and open suture repair**G** in haematoma or vascular injury (haematoma: 3 RCTs, 1337 people; OR 1.27, 95% CI 0.70 to 2.33; vascular injury: 3 RCTs, 1279 people; OR 0.55, 95% CI 0.06 to 5.30).[8] However, it found that TEP laparoscopic repair significantly increased seroma and reduced superficial infection compared with open suture repair (seroma: 3 RCTs, 1279 people; OR 7.65, 95% CI 2.33 to 25.09; superficial infection: 3 RCTs, 1279 people; OR 0.14, 95% CI 0.03 to 0.61). No cases of deep infection (2 RCTs, 1098 people) or visceral injury (2 RCTs, 1098 people) were reported with either TEP laparoscopic repair or open suture repair. The review reported that the risk of persisting numbness after 3 months was not estimable. The subsequent RCT found no significant difference in complications between TEP laparoscopic repair and open suture repair (7 cases with TEP laparoscopic repair *v* 4 with open suture repair; P value not reported).[9] Six people in the TEP group had severe pain and one person had epididymitis, whereas two people in the open suture group had severe pain, one person had gastroenteritis, and one person had a fever of unknown cause. **Versus open mesh repair:** The systematic review found that TEP laparoscopic repair significantly reduced haematoma compared with open mesh repair**G** (4 RCTs, 526 people; OR 0.26, 95% CI 0.14 to 0.48).[8] It found no significant difference between TEP laparoscopic and open mesh repair in seroma, superficial infection, or persisting numbness after 3 months (seroma: 4 RCTs, 526 people; OR 1.12, 95% CI 0.24 to 5.09; superficial infection: 5 RCTs, 526 people; OR 2.03, 95% CI 0.21 to 19.85; numbness after 3 months: 3 RCTs, 302 people; OR 0.21, 95% CI 0.04 to 1.21). No case of deep infection (3 RCTs, 311 people), vascular injury (3 RCTs,

323 people), or visceral injury (2 RCTs, 298 people) was reported with either TEP laparoscopic repair or open mesh repair. The first subsequent RCT found no significant difference between TEP laparoscopic repair and two types of open mesh repair in overall early complications (including haematoma, seroma, infection, and numbness; P = 0.34 for differences between the three groups).[10] The second subsequent RCT found no significant difference in overall perioperative complications (including visceral or vascular injury).[12] Common postoperative complications were pain, haematoma, and numbness. Haematoma and numbness were significantly more common with open mesh repair than with TEP laparoscopic repair (haematoma: 7/74 [10%] with TEP laparoscopic repair *v* 16/68 [24%] with open mesh repair; P = 0.03; numbness: 8/71 [11%] with TEP laparoscopic repair *v* 38/47 [81%] with open mesh repair; P < 0.00001). Testicular pain was significantly more common with TEP laparoscopic repair than with open mesh repair (19/62 [31%] with TEP laparoscopic repair *v* 6/79 [8%] with open mesh repair; P = 0.003). The third subsequent RCT found that haematoma or seroma and groin pain were the most common surgical complications, and occurred with similar frequency between groups (haematoma/ seroma: 5 events with TEP laparoscopic repair *v* 3 events with open mesh repair; groin pain: 4 events with TEP laparoscopic repair *v* 2 events with open mesh repair).[11] However, event rates were too small to detect clinically important differences between groups.

Comment: The systematic review excluded people with non-inguinal hernias, but it did include a small proportion of people with recurrent or bilateral hernias).[8] Overall results are therefore applicable to people with unilateral inguinal hernia. Separate meta-analyses were performed for recurrent and bilateral hernia, and are presented below (see questions on primary bilateral inguinal hernia, p 547 and recurrent inguinal hernia, p 551). Similarly, the subsequent RCTs included a minority of people with recurrent or bilateral inguinal hernia, or femoral hernia. We have reported on overall results of these studies, because results are likely to be generalisable to people with primary unilateral inguinal hernia.

OPTION TRANSABDOMINAL PREPERITONEAL (TAPP) LAPAROSCOPIC REPAIR

We found no systematic review, RCTs, or cohort studies of sufficient quality comparing transabdominal preperitoneal (TAPP) laparoscopic repair versus expectant management. One systematic review found that TAPP laparoscopic repair reduced postoperative pain at 3 months, and time to return to usual activities compared with open mesh repair. It found insufficient evidence to compare effects of TAPP laparoscopic repair versus open mesh repair on recurrence rates. One subsequent RCT found that TAPP laparoscopic repair reduced postoperative pain and length of hospital stay compared with open mesh repair. Adverse effects of open mesh repair and TAPP laparoscopic repair were similar, although TAPP laparoscopic repair increased the risk of seroma and decreased postoperative numbness and superficial infection compared with open mesh repair. One systematic review and subsequent RCTs found that TAPP laparoscopic repair decreased postoperative pain and time to return to usual activities compared with open suture repair. The systematic review found limited evidence that TAPP laparoscopic repair reduced recurrence compared with open suture repair, although two subsequent RCTs found no significant difference. Adverse effects of TAPP laparoscopic repair and open suture repair were similar.

Benefits: **Versus expectant management:** We found no systematic review, RCTs, or cohort studies of sufficient quality. **Versus open suture repair:** We found one systematic review (search date 2002)[8] and two subsequent RCTs.[13,14] The systematic review found that transabdominal preperitoneal (TAPP) laparoscopic repair**G** significantly reduced recurrence, length of hospital stay, time to return to usual activities, and persisting pain after 3 months compared with open suture repair**G**, although the effect on length of hospital stay was slight (recurrence: 16 RCTs, 2259 people; OR 0.45, 95% CI 0.28 to 0.72; length of hospital stay: 13 RCTs, 1586 people; weighted mean reduction 0.10 days, 95% CI 0.02 days to 0.17 days; time to return to usual activities: 7 RCTs, 728 people; HR 0.50, 95% CI 0.43 to 0.58; persisting pain after 3 months: 8 RCTs, 1233 people; OR 0.35, 95% CI 0.24 to 0.50).[8] The first subsequent RCT (176 people, 152 of whom had unilateral inguinal hernia and 24 of whom had bilateral inguinal hernia) found no significant difference between TAPP laparoscopic repair and open suture repair in recurrence rate, although the RCT may have lacked power to detect a clinically important difference (recurrence: 2/86 [2.3%] with TAPP laparoscopic repair *v* 1/90 [1.1%] with open suture repair; P value not reported).[13] The second RCT (multicentre trial, 1042 people with primary unilateral inguinal hernia) found that TAPP laparoscopic repair significantly reduced postoperative pain in the first week (determined by self reporting using a visual analogue scale; $P < 0.001$).[14] It also found limited evidence that TAPP laparoscopic repair reduced the amount of sick leave required by participants (loss to follow up for sick leave 18%; median duration: 10 days with TAPP laparoscopic repair *v* 14 days with open suture repair; $P < 0.001$). It found no significant difference in recurrence at 3 months (1.2% with TAPP laparoscopic repair *v* 0.6% with open suture repair; $P = 0.339$). **Versus open mesh repair:** We found one systematic review (search date 2000)[8] and one subsequent RCT.[15] The review found no significant difference between TAPP laparoscopic repair and open mesh repair**G** in hernia recurrence (12 RCTs, 1830 people; OR 1.01, 95% CI 0.58 to 1.85). However, results were heterogeneous, suggesting that the possibility of a beneficial or adverse effect on recurrence cannot be reliably excluded (see comment below). It found that TAPP laparoscopic repair significantly reduced time to return to usual activities and persisting pain after 3 months compared with open mesh repair (time to return to usual activities: 7 RCTs, 876 people; HR 0.63, 95% CI 0.55 to 0.72; persisting pain after 3 months: 7 RCTs, 1348 people; OR 0.59, 95% CI 0.43 to 0.83). TAPP laparoscopic repair significantly increased length of hospital stay compared with open mesh repair, although the effect was slight (length of hospital stay: 12 RCTs, 1657 people; weighted mean increase 0.15 days, 95% CI 0.09 days to 0.21 days). The subsequent RCT (50 people) found that TAPP laparoscopic repair reduced the length of hospital stay and postoperative pain compared with open mesh repair (length of hospital stay: 1.52 days with TAPP *v* 2.24 days with open mesh; $P < 0.05$; postoperative pain at 24 hours [on a 100 point scale: 0 = least pain, 100 = most severe pain]: 20.92 with TAPP *v* 37.24 with open mesh; $P < 0.05$).[15] There were no recurrences in either group after a mean follow up of 13.5 months.

Harms: **Versus expectant management:** We found no systematic review, RCTs, or cohort studies of sufficient quality. **Versus open suture repair:** The systematic review found no significant difference in haematoma, superficial infection, or deep infection between TAPP laparoscopic**G** and open suture repair**G** (haematoma: 15 RCTs, 2061 people; OR 1.18, 95% CI 0.81 to 1.73; superficial infection: 12 RCTs, 1992 people; OR 0.47, 95% CI 0.21 to 1.04; deep infection: 7 RCTs, 1248 people; OR 0.98, 95% CI 0.06 to 15.7).[8] It found that TAPP laparoscopic repair significantly increased risk of seroma compared with open suture repair (10 RCTs, 1424 people; OR 1.93, 95% CI 1.25 to 2.99) but significantly reduced risk of numbness (persisting numbness after 3 months: 5 RCTs, 871 people; OR 0.20, 95% CI 0.09 to 0.43). The first subsequent RCT (176 people) found no significant difference between TAPP laparoscopic and open suture repair in seroma, haematoma, or wound infection, although it may have lacked power to detect clinically important differences (seroma or haematoma: 4% with TAPP laparoscopic repair *v* 3% with open suture repair; infection: 1% with TAPP laparoscopic repair *v* 2% with open suture repair).[13] The second subsequent RCT similarly found no significant difference between TAPP laparoscopic and open suture repair in overall complication rate at 1 week (14.7% with TAPP laparoscopic repair *v* 18.3% with open suture repair; $P = 0.113$). TAPP laparoscopic repair was associated with significantly fewer cases of haematoma or seroma than open suture repair (combined rate: 9.1% with TAPP laparoscopic repair *v* 14.7% with open suture repair; $P < 0.01$). **Versus open mesh repair:** The systematic review found no significant difference in haematoma or deep infection between TAPP laparoscopic and open mesh repair Ⓖ (haematoma: 10 RCTs, 1485 people; OR 0.77, 95% CI 0.56 to 1.04; deep infection: 10 RCTs, 1537 people; OR 0.16, 95% CI 0.00 to 8.03).[8] It found that TAPP laparoscopic repair significantly increased the risk of seroma compared with open mesh repair (10 RCTs, 1499 people; OR 2.47, 95% CI 1.44 to 4.24). However, TAPP laparoscopic repair significantly reduced the risk of superficial infection and numbness compared with open mesh repair (superficial infection: 10 RCTs, 1583 people; OR 0.36, 95% CI 0.23 to 0.59; numbness: 7 RCTs, 1288 people; OR 0.18, 95% CI 0.10 to 0.33). The subsequent RCT reported that two people in the TAPP laparoscopic group had pain, swelling, and purulent discharge 12 and 15 months after the operation.[15] One person in the open mesh group had scrotal haematoma and one person had superficial wound infection.

Comment: The systematic review excluded people with non-inguinal hernias, but it did include a small proportion of people with recurrent or bilateral hernias.[8] Overall results are likely to be applicable to people with unilateral inguinal hernia. Separate meta-analyses were performed in people with recurrent or bilateral hernia, and are presented below (see questions on primary bilateral inguinal hernia, p 547 and recurrent inguinal hernia, p 551). Similarly, the subsequent RCTs included a minority of people with recurrent or bilateral inguinal hernia, or femoral hernia. We have reported on overall results of these RCTs, because results are likely to be generalisable to people with primary unilateral inguinal hernia. **Versus open mesh repair:** The systematic review reported a lack of consistency in results for recurrence among included RCTs.[8] Reasons for heterogeneity may include use of different variants of the surgical techniques, different participant characteristics, differing experience of operating surgeons, or differing methods of outcome measurement among studies.

QUESTION **What are the effects of elective treatment for primary bilateral inguinal hernia?**

OPTION **EXPECTANT MANAGEMENT**

We found no systematic review, RCTs, or cohort studies of sufficient quality of expectant management in people with bilateral inguinal hernia.

Benefits: **Versus open suture repair, open mesh repair, or laparoscopic repair:** We found no systematic review, RCTs, or cohort studies of sufficient quality.

Harms: **Versus open suture repair, open mesh repair, or laparoscopic repair:** We found no systematic review, RCTs, or cohort studies of sufficient quality.

Comment: Expectant management might be considered a reasonable strategy in people who have only mild symptoms, and in whom the risk of hernia complications is low (see prognosis, p 539) or operative risk is high. However, we found no reliable evidence about the benefits and risks of expectant management compared with surgery.

OPTION OPEN MESH REPAIR

We found no systematic review, RCTs, or cohort studies of sufficient quality comparing open mesh repair versus expectant management in people with bilateral inguinal hernia. One systematic review found limited evidence that open mesh repair reduced length of hospital stay compared with open suture repair but found insufficient evidence to compare other clinical effects. One systematic review found limited evidence that open mesh repair increased the time taken to return to normal activities and postoperative superficial infection compared with transabdominal preperitoneal laparoscopic repair. It found insufficient evidence to compare other clinical effects and insufficient evidence to compare clinical effects of open mesh repair versus totally extraperitoneal laparoscopic repair.

Benefits: **Versus expectant management:** We found no systematic review, RCTs, or cohort studies of sufficient quality. **Versus open suture repair:** We found one systematic review (search date 2000).[6] It found limited evidence from a small meta-analysis of two RCTs (46 people with bilateral inguinal hernia) that open mesh repair significantly reduced length of hospital stay compared with open suture repair (WMD in length of stay: 1.52 days, 95% CI 0.70 days to 2.33 days). However, it found no significant difference between techniques in time to return to normal activities, persisting pain after 3 months, or recurrence (time to return to normal activities: 1 RCT, 10 people; HR 1.47, 95% CI 0.43 to 5.09; persisting pain: 1 RCT, 10 people; OR 12.18, 95% CI 0.22 to 665.00; recurrence: 2 RCTs, 46 people; OR 0.70, 95% CI 0.05 to 9.60). **Versus totally extraperitoneal (TEP) laparoscopic repair:** See benefits of TEP laparoscopic repair, p 549. **Versus transabdominal preperitoneal (TAPP) laparoscopic repair:** See benefits of TAPP laparoscopic repair, p 550.

Harms: **Versus expectant management:** We found no systematic review, RCTs, or cohort studies of sufficient quality. **Versus open suture repair:** The review found no significant difference between open mesh repair and open suture repair in risk of haematoma or seroma (haematoma: 2 RCTs, 46 people; OR 0.47, 95% CI 0.08 to 2.83; seroma: 2 RCTs, 46 people; OR 7.30, 95% CI 0.36 to 146.00).[6] **Versus TEP laparoscopic repair:** See harms of TEP laparoscopic repair, p 549. **Versus TAPP laparoscopic repair:** See harms of TAPP laparoscopic repair, p 550.

Comment: The meta-analyses comparing open mesh repair versus open suture repair for people with bilateral hernia were based on very few data. Therefore, the incidence of several clinically important outcomes could not be estimated. Similarly, many of the results lacked power to detect clinically important differences in outcomes. Confidence intervals were wide and the lack of significance for these results should not be taken to imply a lack of clinically important difference between surgical techniques.

OPTION OPEN SUTURE REPAIR

Clinical experience and consensus opinion suggest that surgical intervention is an effective treatment for bilateral inguinal hernia. Open suture repair is a well established surgical technique. However, we found no systematic review,

RCTs, or cohort studies of sufficient quality comparing open suture repair versus expectant management in people with bilateral inguinal hernia. One systematic review found limited evidence that open suture repair increased length of hospital stay compared with open mesh repair but found insufficient evidence to compare other clinical effects. One systematic review found limited evidence that open suture repair increased the time taken to return to normal activities compared with transabdominal preperitoneal laparoscopic repair. It found insufficient evidence to compare other clinical effects, and found insufficient evidence to compare clinical effects of open suture repairs versus totally extraperitoneal laparoscopic repair.

Benefits: **Versus expectant management:** We found no systematic review, RCTs, or cohort studies of sufficient quality. **Versus open mesh repair:** See benefits of open mesh repair, p 548. **Versus totally extraperitoneal (TEP) laparoscopic repair:** See benefits of TEP laparoscopic repair, p 549. **Versus transabdominal preperitoneal (TAPP) laparoscopic repair:** See benefits of TAPP laparoscopic repair, p 550.

Harms: **Versus expectant management:** We found no systematic review, RCTs, or cohort studies of sufficient quality. **Versus open mesh repair:** See harms of open mesh repair, p 548. **Versus TEP laparoscopic repair:** See harms of TEP laparoscopic repair, p 549. **Versus TAPP laparoscopic repair:** See harms of TAPP laparoscopic repair, p 550.

Comment: Clinical experience and consensus opinion suggest that surgical intervention is an effective treatment for bilateral inguinal hernia. Open suture repair is a well established surgical technique.

OPTION TOTALLY EXTRAPERITONEAL (TEP) LAPAROSCOPIC REPAIR

We found no systematic review, RCTs, or cohort studies of sufficient quality comparing totally extraperitoneal laparoscopic (TEP) repair versus expectant management in people with bilateral inguinal hernia. One systematic review found insufficient evidence to compare clinical effects of TEP laparoscopic repair versus open suture and open mesh repairs.

Benefits: **Versus expectant management:** We found no systematic review, RCTs, or cohort studies of sufficient quality. **Versus open mesh repair:** We found one systematic review (search date 2002).[8] It found no significant difference between totally extraperitoneal (TEP) laparoscopic repair**G** and open mesh repair**G** in either return to usual activities or persisting pain after 3 months (time to return to usual activities: 2 RCTs, 34 people; OR 0.68, 95% CI 0.32 to 1.45; persisting pain: 1 RCT, 19 people; OR 3.28, 95% CI 0.02 to 708.00). The review found insufficient evidence to compare effects of TEP laparoscopic repair versus open mesh repair on recurrence. **Versus open suture repair:** We found one systematic review.[8] It found insufficient evidence to compare effects of TEP laparoscopic repair versus open suture repair**G** on time to return to usual activities, recurrence, or persisting pain after 3 months.

Harms: **Versus expectant management:** We found no systematic review, RCTs, or cohort studies of sufficient quality. **Versus open mesh repair:** The review found no significant difference between TEP laparoscopic repair**G** and open mesh repair**G** for haematoma or persisting numbness after 3 months (haematoma: 1 RCT, 19 people; OR 3.28, 95% CI 0.02 to 708.00; persisting numbness: 1 RCT, 19 people; OR 3.28, 95% CI 0.02 to 708.00).[8] **Versus open suture repair:** The review found insufficient data to compare harms of TEP laparoscopic repair versus open suture repair**G**.[8]

Comment: The meta-analyses comparing laparoscopic versus open surgery for people with bilateral hernia were based on very few data. Therefore, the incidence of several clinically important outcomes could not be estimated. Similarly, many of the results lacked power to detect clinically important differences in outcomes. Confidence intervals were wide and the lack of significance for these results should not be taken to imply a lack of clinically important difference between surgical techniques.

OPTION TRANSABDOMINAL PREPERITONEAL (TAPP) LAPAROSCOPIC REPAIR

We found no systematic review, RCTs, or cohort studies of sufficient quality comparing transabdominal preperitoneal (TAPP) laparoscopic repair versus expectant management in people with bilateral inguinal hernia. One systematic review found limited evidence that TAPP laparoscopic repair reduced the time taken to return to normal activities compared with open suture repair or open mesh repair, and that TAPP laparoscopic repair reduced postoperative superficial infection compared with open mesh repair. It found insufficient evidence to compare other clinical effects.

Benefits: **Versus expectant management:** We found no systematic review, RCTs, or cohort studies of sufficient quality. **Versus open mesh repair:** We found one systematic review (search date 2002).[8] It found limited evidence from a meta-analysis of small RCTs that TAPP laparoscopic repair**G** significantly reduced time to return to normal activities compared with open mesh repair**G** (5 RCTs, 79 people; OR 0.44, 95% CI 0.27 to 0.73). However, it found no significant difference between TAPP laparoscopic and open mesh repair in length of hospital stay or persisting pain after 3 months (length of hospital stay: 5 RCTs, 100 people; WMD –0.20 days, 95% CI –0.40 days to 0.00 days; persisting pain: 2 RCTs, 74 people; OR 0.80, 95% CI 0.29 to 2.22). The review did not report on recurrence rates. **Versus open suture repair:** We found one systematic review.[8] It found limited evidence from a small meta-analysis that TAPP laparoscopic repair significantly reduced time to return to normal activities compared with open suture repair**G** (3 RCTs, 59 people with bilateral inguinal hernia; OR 0.52, 95% CI 0.31 to 0.88). However, it found no significant difference between TAPP laparoscopic repair and open suture repair in length of hospital stay or persisting pain at 3 months (length of hospital stay: 4 RCTs, 97 people; WMD –0.05 days, 95% CI –0.17 days to +0.07 days; persisting pain: 2 RCTs, 63 people; OR 0.38, 95% CI 0.10 to 1.43). The review did not report on recurrence rates.

Harms: **Versus expectant management:** We found no systematic review, RCTs, or cohort studies of sufficient quality. **Versus open mesh repair:** The review found no significant difference in haematoma, seroma, or persisting numbness between TAPP laparoscopic repair**G** and open mesh repair**G** in people with bilateral inguinal hernia (haematoma: 4 RCTs, 90 people; OR 0.84, 95% CI 0.27 to 2.64; seroma: 4 RCTs, 90 people; OR 2.86, 95% CI 0.79 to 10.35; numbness: 3 RCTs, 84 people; OR 0.18, 95% CI 0.04 to 0.81).[8] However, TAPP laparoscopic repair significantly reduced superficial infection compared with open mesh repair (4 RCTs, 90 people; OR 0.22, 95% CI 0.07 to 0.69). **Versus open suture repair:** The review found no significant difference in haematoma, seroma, superficial infection, or visceral injury between TAPP laparoscopic repair and open suture repair**G** in people with bilateral inguinal hernia (haematoma: 4 RCTs, 97 people; OR 1.26, 95% CI 0.37 to 4.29; seroma: 3 RCTs, 82 people; OR 0.85, 95% CI 0.24 to 3.04; superficial infection: 4 RCTs, 97 people: OR 0.97, 95% CI 0.08 to 11.59; visceral injury: 3 RCTs, 82 people; OR 5.16, 95% CI 0.09 to 286.00).[8]

Comment: The meta-analyses comparing laparoscopic versus open surgery for people with bilateral hernia were based on few data. Therefore, the incidence of several clinically important outcomes could not be estimated. Similarly, many of the results lacked power to detect clinically important differences in outcomes. Confidence intervals were wide and the lack of significance for these results should not be taken to imply a lack of clinically important difference between techniques.

QUESTION What are the effects of elective treatment for recurrent inguinal hernia?

OPTION EXPECTANT MANAGEMENT

We found no systematic review, RCTs, or cohort studies of sufficient quality of expectant management in people with recurrent inguinal hernia.

Benefits: **Versus open suture, open mesh, or laparoscopic repair:** We found no systematic review, RCTs, or cohort studies of sufficient quality.

Harms: **Versus open suture, open mesh, or laparoscopic repair:** We found no systematic review, RCTs, or cohort studies of sufficient quality.

Comment: Expectant management**G** might be considered a reasonable strategy in people who have only mild symptoms, and in whom the risk of hernia complications is low (see prognosis, p 539) or operative risk is high. However, we found no reliable evidence about the benefits and risks of expectant management compared with surgery.

OPTION OPEN MESH REPAIR

We found no systematic review, RCTs, or cohort studies of sufficient quality comparing open mesh repair versus expectant management. One systematic review found limited evidence that open mesh repair slightly reduced length of hospital stay compared with open suture repair in people with recurrent inguinal hernia. However, the review found insufficient evidence to compare effects on pain, time to return to usual activities, further recurrence, or other complications of surgery. One systematic review found limited evidence that open mesh repair increased the time taken to return to normal activities compared with transabdominal preperitoneal and totally extraperitoneal laparoscopic repair techniques, but it found insufficient evidence to compare other clinical effects.

Benefits: **Versus expectant management:** We found no systematic review, RCTs, or cohort studies of sufficient quality. **Versus open suture repair:** We found one systematic review (search date 2000).[6] It found that open mesh repair**G** significantly reduced length of hospital stay, although the effect was small (2 RCTs, 59 people with recurrent inguinal hernia; weighted mean reduction in length of hospital stay: 0.41 days, 95% CI 0.07 days to 0.75 days). It found no significant difference between open mesh repair and open suture repair**G** in risk of further recurrence, persisting pain after 3 months, or time to return to usual activities (recurrence: 2 RCTs, 59 people; OR 1.79, 95% CI 0.39 to 8.23; persisting pain: 2 RCTs, 49 people; OR 1.05, 95% CI 0.19 to 5.82; return to usual activities: 2 RCTs, 33 people; HR 0.88, 95% CI 0.44 to 1.74). However, these analyses were unlikely to have adequate power to detect clinically important effects. **Versus totally extraperitoneal (TEP) laparoscopic repair:** See benefits of TEP laparoscopic repair, p 553. **Versus transabdominal preperitoneal (TAPP) laparoscopic repair:** See benefits of TAPP laparoscopic repair, p 553.

Harms: **Versus expectant management:** We found no systematic review, RCTs, or cohort studies of sufficient quality. **Versus open suture repair:** The review found no significant differences between open mesh repairⓖ and open suture repairⓖ in haematoma, superficial infection, life threatening visceral or vascular injury, deep infection, numbness, or mortality (haematoma: OR 0.98, 95% CI 0 to 16.53; superficial infection: OR 5.29, 95% CI 0.10 to 289.31; life threatening complication/deep infection: OR 1.47, 95% CI 0.08 to 25.46; numbness persisting > 3 months: OR 1.73, 95% CI 0.29 to 10.16; mortality: OR 0.07, 95% CI 0 to 1.28).[6] However, confidence intervals were wide, reflecting the low power of these analyses. Clinically important differences between treatments may not have been detected. **Versus TEP laparoscopic repair:** See harms of TEP laparoscopic repair, p 553. **Versus TAPP laparoscopic repair:** See harms of TAPP laparoscopic repair, p 554.

Comment: None.

OPTION OPEN SUTURE REPAIR

Clinical experience and consensus opinion suggest that surgery is an effective treatment for recurrent inguinal hernia. Open suture repair is a well established surgical technique. However, we found no systematic review, RCTs, or cohort studies of sufficient quality comparing open suture repair versus expectant management. One systematic review found limited evidence that open suture repair slightly increased length of hospital stay compared with open mesh repair in people with recurrent inguinal hernia but found insufficient evidence to compare effects on pain, time to return to usual activities, further recurrence, or other complications of surgery. One systematic review found limited evidence that open suture repair increased the time taken to return to normal activities compared with transabdominal preperitoneal laparoscopic repair. It found insufficient evidence to compare other clinical effects and insufficient data to compare benefits of open suture repair versus totally extraperitoneal laparoscopic repair.

Benefits: **Versus expectant management:** We found no systematic review, RCTs, or cohort studies of sufficient quality. **Versus open mesh repair:** See benefits of open mesh repair, p 551. **Versus totally extraperitoneal (TEP) laparoscopic repair:** See benefits of TEP laparoscopic repair, p 553. **Versus transabdominal preperitoneal (TAPP) repair:** See benefits of TAPP laparoscopic repair, p 553.

Harms: **Versus expectant management:** We found no systematic review, RCTs, or cohort studies of sufficient quality. **Versus open mesh repair:** See harms of open mesh repair, p 552. **Versus TEP laparoscopic repair:** See harms of TEP laparoscopic repair, p 553. **Versus TAPP laparoscopic repair:** See harms of TAPP laparoscopic repair, p 554.

Comment: Open suture repairⓖ is a well established method of management for people with inguinal hernias.

OPTION TOTALLY EXTRAPERITONEAL (TEP) LAPAROSCOPIC REPAIR

We found no systematic review, RCTs, or cohort studies of sufficient quality comparing totally extraperitoneal (TEP) laparoscopic repair versus expectant management in people with recurrent inguinal hernia. One systematic review found limited evidence that TEP laparoscopic repair reduced the time taken to return to normal activities compared with open mesh repair. However, it found insufficient evidence to compare other clinical effects and insufficient data to compare the effects of TEP laparoscopic repair versus open suture repair.

Benefits: **Versus expectant management:** We found no systematic review, RCTs, or cohort studies of sufficient quality. **Versus open mesh repair:** We found one systematic review (search date 2002).[8] It found limited evidence from one small RCT that TEP laparoscopic repair**G** significantly reduced time to return to usual activities compared with open mesh repair**G** (1 RCT, 40 people; OR 0.14, 95% CI 0.05 to 0.36). However, it found no significant difference between TEP laparoscopic repair and open mesh repair for persisting pain after 3 months or for recurrence (persisting pain: 1 RCT, 36 people; OR 0.19, 95% CI 0.01 to 3.32; recurrence: 1 RCT, 36 people; OR 0.23, 95% CI 0.01 to 4.48). **Versus open suture repair:** We found one systematic review.[8] It found insufficient data to compare benefits of TEP laparoscopic repair versus open suture repair**G**.

Harms: **Versus expectant management:** We found no systematic review, RCTs, or cohort studies of sufficient quality. **Versus open mesh repair:** The systematic review found limited evidence from one small RCT that TEP laparoscopic repair**G** significantly reduced haematoma compared with open mesh repair**G** (36 people; OR 0.15, 95% CI 0.03 to 0.87).[8] **Versus open suture repair:** The systematic review found no RCTs reporting on haematoma or seroma.[8]

Comment: The meta-analyses comparing laparoscopic versus open surgery for people with recurrent hernia were based on very few data. Therefore, the incidence of several clinically important outcomes, particularly complications, could not be estimated. Similarly, many of the results lacked power to detect clinically important differences in outcomes. Confidence intervals were wide and the lack of significance for these results should not be taken to imply a lack of clinically important difference between surgical techniques.

OPTION TRANSABDOMINAL PREPERITONEAL (TAPP) LAPAROSCOPIC REPAIR

We found no systematic review, RCTs, or cohort studies of sufficient quality comparing transabdominal preperitoneal laparoscopic repair versus expectant management. One systematic review found limited evidence that transabdominal preperitoneal laparoscopic repair reduced the time taken to return to normal activities compared with open suture repair and open mesh repair in people with recurrent inguinal hernia but found insufficient evidence to compare other clinical effects.

Benefits: **Versus expectant management:** We found no systematic review, RCTs, or cohort studies of sufficient quality. **Versus open mesh repair:** We found one systematic review (search date 2002).[8] It found that transabdominal preperitoneal (TAPP) laparoscopic repair**G** significantly reduced time to return to usual activities compared with open mesh repair**G** (5 RCTs, 114 people; OR 0.55, 95% CI 0.37 to 0.80). However, it found no significant difference between TAPP laparoscopic and open mesh repair in length of hospital stay, persisting pain after 3 months, or further recurrence (length of hospital stay: 5 RCTs, 190 people; WMD +0.02 days; 95% CI –0.13 days to +0.17 days; persisting pain after 3 months: 3 RCTs, 153 people; OR 1.22, 95% CI 0.49 to 3.03; recurrence: 5 RCTs, 190 people; OR 1.20, 95% CI 0.43 to 3.32). **Versus open suture repair:** We found one systematic review (search date 2002).[8] It found that TAPP laparoscopic repair reduced time to return to usual activities compared with open suture repair**G**, although the difference was not significant (3 RCTs, 57 people with recurrent inguinal hernia; HR 0.70, 95% CI 0.41 to 1.20). It found no significant difference between TAPP laparoscopic repair and open suture repair in length of hospital stay, persisting pain after 3 months, or further recurrence (length of hospital stay: 4 RCTs, 92 people; weighted mean difference +0.08 days, 95% CI –0.25 days to +0.41 days; persisting pain after 3 months: 2 RCTs, 53 people; OR 0.18, 95% CI 0 to 9.42; recurrence: 4 RCTs, 93 people; OR 0.31, 95% CI 0.04 to 2.26).

Harms: **Versus expectant management:** We found no systematic review, RCTs, or cohort studies of sufficient quality. **Versus open mesh repair:** The review found that TAPP laparoscopic repair**G** significantly reduced persisting numbness after 3 months compared with open mesh repair**G** (4 RCTs, 162 people; OR 0.18, 95% CI 0.05 to 0.69).[8] However, it found no significant difference in haematoma, seroma, superficial infection, or visceral injury (haematoma: 4 RCTs, 182 people; OR 1.04, 95% CI 0.43 to 2.54; seroma: 4 RCTs, 176 people; OR 2.06, 95% CI 0.83 to 5.11; superficial infection: 4 RCTs, 182 people; OR 0.45, 95% CI 0.14 to 1.44; visceral injury: 3 RCTs, 103 people; OR 5.47, 95% CI 0.10 to 294.00). No cases of deep infection or vascular injury occurred in either group (deep infection: 2 RCTs, 182 people; vascular injury: 3 RCTs, 103 people). **Versus open suture repair:** The systematic review found no significant difference in haematoma, seroma, superficial infection, deep infection, or persisting numbness after 3 months (haematoma: 4 RCTs, 93 people; OR 1.70, 95% CI 0.42 to 6.84; seroma: 4 RCTs, 93 people; OR 2.14, 95% CI 0.21 to 22.16; superficial infection: 4 RCTs, 93 people; OR 0.18, 95% CI 0 to 9.42; deep infection: 2 RCTs, 68 people; OR 0.15, 95% CI 0 to 7.71; numbness: 2 RCTs, 53 people; OR 0.16, 95% CI 0.02 to 1.70).[8] No cases of vascular or visceral injury occurred in either group (4 RCTs, 93 people).

Comment: The meta-analyses comparing laparoscopic versus open surgery for people with recurrent hernia were based on few data.[8] Therefore, the incidence of several clinically important outcomes, particularly complications, could not be estimated. Similarly, many of the results lacked power to detect clinically important differences in outcomes. Confidence intervals were wide and the lack of significance for these results should not be taken to imply a lack of clinically important differences between surgical techniques.

GLOSSARY

Expectant management A policy of no active intervention.

Open mesh repair An open operation, in which a synthetic mesh is inserted across the posterior wall of the inguinal canal. Variants include the Lichtenstein and Stoppa procedures. The technique may be performed under local or regional anaesthetic.

Open suture repair An open operation to repair (using sutures) the weakness in the muscles and fascia through which the hernia sac has protruded. There are many variants of the technique (e.g. Bassini, McVay Maloney, and Shouldice procedures). The technique is commonly performed under local or regional anaesthetic.

Totally extraperitoneal (TEP) laparoscopic repair Does not involve entering the peritoneum with the laparoscope. The technique is usually performed under general anaesthetic.

Transabdominal preperitoneal (TAPP) laparoscopic repair Involves entering the peritoneum with the laparoscope, although the repair itself (done with a mesh) is undertaken anterior to the peritoneum. The technique is usually performed under general anaesthetic.

Substantive changes

Totally extraperitoneal laparoscopic repair in unilateral inguinal hernia One new RCT found no significant difference in outcomes between totally extraperitoneal laparoscopic repair and open suture repair;[9] categorisation unchanged.

Transabdominal preperitoneal laparoscopic repair in unilateral inguinal hernia One new RCT found that transabdominal preperitoneal laparoscopic repair reduced hospital stay and postoperative pain compared with open mesh repair;[15] categorisation unchanged.

REFERENCES

1. NICE. Guidance on the use of laparoscopic surgery for inguinal hernia. January 2001. http://www.nice.org.uk/pdf/Laphernias_Full_guidance.pdf (last accessed 30 July 2004).
2. Department of Health. Hospital Episode Statistics, England: Financial year 2002–03. > (last accessed 30 July 2004) http:www.dh.gov.uk/assetRoot/04/06/73/91/04067391.pdf.
3. Rutkow IM, Robbins AW. Demographic, classificatory, and socioeconomic aspects of hernia repair in the United States. *Surg Clin North Am* 1993;73:413–426.
4. Royal College of General Practitioners. *Morbidity statistics from general practice. Fourth national study.* London: HMSO, 1995.
5. Rai S, Chandra SS, Smile SR. A study of the risk of strangulation and obstruction in groin hernias. *Aust N Z J Surg* 1998;68:650–654.
6. Scott NW, McCormack K, Graham P, Go PMNYH, Ross SJ, Grant AM on behalf of the EU Hernia Trialists Collaboration. Open Mesh versus Non-Mesh for Groin Hernia repair (Cochrane Review). In: *The Cochrane Library*, Issue 3, 2004. Chichester, UK: John Wiley & Sons, Ltd. Search date 2000; primary sources Medline, the Cochrane Central Controlled Trials Registry, relevant websites, search of reference lists, communication with authors of trials and specialists.
7. Koukourou A, Lyon W, Rice J, et al. Prospective randomized trial of polypropylene mesh compared with nylon darn in inguinal hernia repair. *Br J Surg* 2001;88:931–934.
8. McCormack K, Scott NW, Go PMNYH, Ross S, Grant AM on behalf of the EU Hernia Trialists Collaboration. Laparoscopic techniques versus open techniques for inguinal hernia repair (Cochrane Review). In: *The Cochrane Library*, Issue 3, 2004. Chichester, UK: John Wiley & Sons, Ltd. Search date 2002; primary sources Medline, Embase, the Cochrane Central Controlled Trials Registry, search of reference lists, communication with authors of trials and specialists, website check.
9. Wennstrom I, Berggren P, Akerud L, et al. Equal results with laparoscopic and Shouldice repairs of primary inguinal hernia in men. Report from a prospective randomised study. *Scand J Surg* 2004;93:34–36.
10. Bringman S, Ramel S, Heikkinen TJ, et al. Tension-free inguinal hernia repair: TEP versus mesh-plug versus Lichtenstein. A prospective randomized controlled trial. *Ann Surg* 2003;237:142–147.
11. Colak T, Akca T, Kanik A, et al. Randomized clinical trial comparing laparoscopic totally extraperitoneal approach with open mesh repair in inguinal hernia. *Surg Laparosc Endosc Percutan Tech* 2003;13:191–195.
12. Andersson B, Hallen M, Leveau P, et al. Laparoscopic extraperitoneal inguinal hernia repair versus open mesh repair: a prospective randomized controlled trial. *Surgery* 2003; 133:464–472.
13. Lorenz D, Stark E, Oestreich K, et al. Laparoscopic hernioplasty versus conventional hernioplasty (Shouldice): results of a prospective randomized trial. *World J Surg* 2000;24:739–746.
14. Berndsen F, Arvidsson D, Enander LK, et al. Postoperative convalescence after inguinal hernia surgery: prospective randomized multicenter study of laparoscopic versus Shouldice inguinal hernia repair in 1042 patients. *Hernia* 2002;6:56–61.
15. Anadol ZA, Ersoy E, Taneri F, et al. Outcome and cost comparison of laparoscopic transabdominal preperitoneal hernia repair versus Open Lichtenstein technique. *J Laparoendosc Adv Surg Tech A* 2004;14:159–163.

Sanjay Purkayastha
Clinical Research Fellow
Department of Surgical Oncology and Technology
Imperial College, London, UK

Paris Tekkis
Senior Lecturer
Department of Surgical Oncology and Technology
Imperial College, London, UK

Thanos Athanasiou
Locum Consultant
St Mary's Hospital NHS Trust
Department of Cardiothoracic Surgery, London, UK

Ara Darzi
Professor of Surgery and Head of Department
Department of Surgical Oncology and Technology
Imperial College, London, UK

Competing interests: None declared.

We would like to acknowledge the previous contributors of this chapter, including Bazian Ltd.

Irritable bowel syndrome

Search date June 2004

Gregory Rubin, Niek de Wit and Roger H Jones

QUESTIONS

INTERVENTIONS

Key Messages

Treatments

- **Antidepressants (amitriptyline, clomipramine, desipramine, doxepin, mianserin, trimipramine)** One systematic review found limited evidence from low to moderate quality RCTs that antidepressants (amitriptyline, clomipramine, desipramine, doxepin, mianserin, trimipramine) reduced symptoms of irritable bowel syndrome compared with placebo in the short term. It was not clear whether the effects on irritable bowel syndrome were independent of the effects on psychological symptoms.
- **Smooth muscle relaxants (cimetropium bromide, hyoscine butyl bromide, mebeverine hydrochloride, otilonium bromide, pinaverium bromide, trimebutine)** One systematic review found limited evidence that smooth muscle relaxants (cimetropium bromide, hyoscine butyl bromide, mebeverine hydrochloride, otilonium bromide, pinaverium bromide, trimebutine) improved symptoms compared with placebo. One subsequent RCT found no significant difference between alverine and placebo in improvement in abdominal pain, although the study may have lacked power to detect a clinically important effect. One RCT identified by a systematic review found that mebeverine was less effective for symptoms than alosetron in women with diarrhoea predominant irritable bowel syndrome, although there are concerns that alosetron may be associated with ischaemic colitis.
- **$5HT_4$ receptor agonists (tegaserod)** One systematic review found that in women with constipation predominant irritable bowel syndrome, tegaserod improved symptoms compared with placebo. It found insufficient evidence about the effects of tegaserod in men. One subsequent RCT found that in adults with irritable bowel syndrome and without diarrhoea, tegaserod improved symptoms compared with placebo. The systematic review and the RCT found that tegaserod increased diarrhoea compared with placebo.

- **Alosetron** One systematic review found that alosetron (a $5HT_3$ receptor antagonist) improved symptoms in women with diarrhoea predominant irritable bowel syndrome compared with placebo or mebeverine. However, alosetron is associated with adverse effects, particularly constipation, and has been restricted in some countries because of concerns that it may be associated with ischaemic colitis. The systematic review provided insufficient evidence about the effects of alosetron in men.
- **$5HT_3$ receptor antagonists other than alosetron** We found no RCTs examining $5HT_3$ receptor antagonists other than alosetron.
- **Fibre supplementation** One systematic review found limited evidence that fibre supplementation improved symptoms of irritable bowel syndrome and irritable bowel syndrome related constipation.

DEFINITION Irritable bowel syndrome (IBS) is a chronic non-inflammatory condition characterised by abdominal pain, altered bowel habit (diarrhoea or constipation), and abdominal bloating, but with no identifiable structural or biochemical disorder. Symptom based criteria, such as the Manning criteria (see table 1, p 563),[1] the Rome I criteria (see table 2, p 563),[2] and the Rome II criteria (see table 3, p 563),[3] aid diagnosis but their main use is in defining populations in clinical trials. The Rome criteria also subcategorise IBS according to predominant symptoms (diarrhoea, constipation, or alternating between diarrhoea and constipation). In practice, the division between constipation predominant and diarrhoea predominant IBS may not be clear-cut in all people. Restriction of trial entry to a subcategory of IBS limits the generalisability of study results.

INCIDENCE/ PREVALENCE Estimates of incidence and prevalence vary depending on the diagnostic criteria used to define IBS. One cross-sectional postal survey (4476 people aged 20–69 years) in Teeside, UK, defined IBS as recurrent abdominal pain on more than six occasions during the previous year plus two or more of the Manning criteria (see table 1, p 563).[4] It estimated prevalence in the UK to be 16.7% (95% CI 15.4% to 18.0%) overall, with a prevalence of 22.8% (95% CI 20.8% to 24.8%) among women and 10.5% (95% CI 8.9% to 12.1%) among men.[4] A cross-sectional postal survey (4500 people aged > 17 years) in Australia found prevalences of IBS of 13.6% (95% CI 12.3% to 14.8%) using the Manning criteria (see table 1, p 563), 6.9% (95% CI 6.0% to 7.8%) using the Rome I criteria (see table 2, p 563), and 4.4% (95% CI 3.5% to 5.1%) using the Rome II criteria (see table 3, p 563).[5]

AETIOLOGY/ RISK FACTORS The pathophysiology of IBS is not certain. Studies on the aetiology of IBS have been descriptive or retrospective, and are of limited reliability. Suggested aetiological factors include: abnormal gastrointestinal motor function,[6–8] enhanced visceral perception,[9–11] psychosocial factors such as a history of childhood abuse,[12] genetic predisposition,[13–15] and a history of enteric mucosal inflammation.[16,17] We found no reliable prospective data to measure these associations.

PROGNOSIS A retrospective study reviewed the medical records of people with IBS (112 people aged 20–64 years when diagnosed with IBS at the Mayo Clinic, USA, in 1961–1963). IBS was defined as the presence of abdominal pain associated with either disturbed defecation or abdominal distension and the absence of organic bowel disease.[18] Over a 32 year period, death rates were similar among people with IBS compared with age and gender matched controls. One postal survey (4432 adults aged 20–69 years) found that people with IBS are significantly more likely to have had a cholecystectomy than controls (OR 1.9, 95% CI 1.2 to 3.2).[4] A paper reporting on the same survey population (2238 women aged 20–69 years) found that women with IBS were significantly more likely to have had a hysterectomy than controls (OR 1.6, 95% CI 1.1 to 2.2).[19] We found no reliable estimates of the duration of IBS if left untreated.

AIMS OF INTERVENTION To improve symptoms and reduce disability, with minimal adverse effects.

OUTCOMES Severity of IBS symptoms (in particular abdominal pain, constipation, diarrhoea, bloating, and urgency of defecation) using validated self report instruments, including: Adequate Relief;[20] the Irritable Bowel Severity Scoring System;[21] the Gastrointestinal Symptom Rating Scale;[22,23] the Functional Bowel Disorder Severity Index;[24] the IBS Symptom Questionnaire;[24] Quality of Life and Global Impact of IBS; the Irritable Bowel Syndrome Quality of Life Measurement;[25,26] the Irritable

Bowel Syndrome Quality of Life Questionnaire;[27] the Digestive Health Status Instrument;[28] the Functional Digestive Disorder Quality of Life Questionnaire;[29] the Irritable Bowel Syndrome Health Related Quality of Life questionnaire.[30] Adverse effects of treatment.

METHODS *Clinical Evidence* search and appraisal June 2004.

QUESTION What are the effects of treatments in people with irritable bowel syndrome?

OPTION ANTIDEPRESSANT MEDICATION

One systematic review found limited evidence from low to moderate quality RCTs that antidepressants (amitriptyline, clomipramine, desipramine, doxepin, mianserin, trimipramine) reduced symptoms of irritable bowel syndrome compared with placebo in the short term. It was not clear whether the effects on irritable bowel syndrome were independent of the effects on psychological symptoms.

Benefits: We found one systematic review (search date 1998; 8 RCTs solely in people with irritable bowel syndrome; 575 people).[31] It found that antidepressants (amitriptyline, clomipramine, desipramine, doxepin, mianserin, trimipramine) significantly improved symptoms compared with placebo after 6 weeks (262 people in 7 RCTs with dichotomous outcomes defined as "improvement in abdominal pain" or "response to treatment": OR 4.2, 95% CI 2.3 to 7.9; ARR 32%, 95% CI 15% to 48%; NNT 3, 95% CI 2 to 7; 575 people in 8 RCTs with continuous outcome measures for abdominal pain: SMD 0.9, 95% CI 0.6 to 1.2). We found no subsequent RCTs.

Harms: The systematic review did not analyse combined data on adverse effects, but did report on one RCT (25 people), in which mianserin significantly increased fatigue compared with placebo (80% with mianserin *v* 14% with placebo; P value not reported).[31] Of the other studies in the review, six RCTs did not assess adverse effects and one RCT did not describe adequately how adverse effects were recorded.[31]

Comment: The review reported that the studies were short term and of low to moderate quality. In addition, the studies did not adjust for the effects of antidepressants on underlying depression, which could account for some of the benefits of antidepressants in people with irritable bowel syndrome.

OPTION SMOOTH MUSCLE RELAXANTS

One systematic review found limited evidence that smooth muscle relaxants (cimetropium bromide, hyoscine butyl bromide, mebeverine hydrochloride, otilonium bromide, pinaverium bromide, trimebutine) improved symptoms compared with placebo. One subsequent RCT found no significant difference between alverine and placebo in improvement in abdominal pain, although the study may have lacked power to detect a clinically important effect. One RCT identified by a systematic review found that mebeverine was less effective for symptoms than alosetron in women with diarrhoea predominant irritable bowel syndrome, although there are concerns that alosetron may be associated with ischaemic colitis.

Benefits: **Versus placebo:** We found one systematic review (search date 1999, 23 RCTs in which at least 51% of people had irritable bowel syndrome; 1888 people)[32] and one subsequent RCT.[33] The review found that smooth muscle relaxants (cimetropium bromide, hyoscine butyl bromide, mebeverine hydrochloride, otilonium bromide, pinaverium bromide, trimebutine) significantly increased global improvement, reduced pain, and improved abdominal distension compared with placebo (global improvement: 21 RCTs, 1852 people; OR 2.13, 95% CI 1.77 to 2.58; improvement in pain: 11 RCTs, 1135 people; OR 1.65, 95% CI 1.30 to 2.10; improvement in abdominal distension: 6 RCTs, 885 people; OR 1.46, 95% CI 1.10 to 1.94).[32] However, the review found no significant difference between smooth muscle relaxants and placebo for constipation (4 RCTs, 230 people; OR 0.89, 95% CI 0.60 to 1.31). The subsequent RCT (107 people with Rome II irritable bowel syndrome (see table 3, p 563)) compared 12 weeks of treatment with alverine citrate 120 mg three times daily versus placebo.[33] The main efficacy outcomes were abdominal pain scores recorded at each clinical visit (at recruitment, after a 2 week run in period, and after 4, 6, 10, and 12 weeks of treatment) and on self reported diary cards completed during the run in period, between visits at weeks 4 and 6, and between visits at weeks 10 and 12. The RCT found no significant difference in symptoms between alverine citrate and placebo over 12 weeks of treatment (AR for symptom improvement: 66% with alverine citrate *v* 58% with placebo; $P = 0.5$; no further data reported; percentage reduction in mean daily diary scores for abdominal pain from diary card 1 to diary card 3: 43.7% with alverine citrate *v* 33.3% with placebo; $P > 0.5$), but it may have lacked power to exclude a clinically important effect. **Versus $5HT_3$ receptor antagonists:** See benefits of 5HT3 antagonists, p 560.

Harms: The systematic review found no significant difference in adverse events between smooth muscle relaxants and placebo (18 RCTs, 1384 people; mean percentage of people with adverse events: 14% with smooth muscle relaxants *v* 10% with placebo; $P = 0.08$).[32] The subsequent RCT reported no serious adverse effects with alverine.[33]

Comment: Heterogeneity in inclusion criteria among identified trials in the review may limit the reliability of the meta-analysis.[32] Some of the included trials did not use standard diagnostic criteria and many used poorly validated outcome measures. The review excluded studies on dicyclomine and peppermint oil, citing a high risk of adverse effects. It also excluded trials of propantheline, so the results might not apply to all smooth muscle relaxants.

OPTION $5HT_4$ RECEPTOR AGONISTS

One systematic review found that in women with constipation predominant irritable bowel syndrome, tegaserod improved symptoms compared with placebo. It found insufficient evidence about the effects of tegaserod in men. One subsequent RCT found that in adults with irritable bowel syndrome and without diarrhoea, tegaserod improved symptoms compared with placebo. The systematic review and the RCT found that tegaserod increased diarrhoea compared with placebo.

Benefits: We found one systematic review (search date 2002; 8 RCTs [4 RCTs published as abstracts only]; 5320 people [mainly women]; see comment below)[34] and one subsequent RCT which compared tegaserod with placebo.[35] In the systematic review, seven RCTs (5234 people) were in people with constipation predominant irritable bowel syndrome (IBS) and one RCT (86 people) was in people with diarrhoea predominant IBS. The review found that tegaserod (4 or 12 mg/day) significantly increased the proportion of people who improved (see comment below) compared with placebo after 12 weeks (tegaserod 12 mg; 4 RCTs in people with constipation predominant IBS: 685/1603 [42.7%] with tegaserod *v* 573/1591 [36.0%] with placebo; RR 1.19, 95% CI 1.09 to

1.29; NNT 14, 95% CI 10 to 33; tegaserod 4 mg; 3 RCTs in people with constipation predominant IBS: 327/846 [38.7%] with tegaserod *v* 281/839 [33.5%] with placebo; RR 1.15, 95% CI 1.02 to 1.31; NNT 20, 95% CI 10 to 100). The subsequent RCT (647 people with Rome II IBS) compared tegaserod 6 mg twice daily with placebo.[35] The RCT excluded people whose primary bowel symptom was diarrhoea. The primary outcome was satisfactory relief from symptoms, recorded at weekly intervals during a 2 week run in and 12 week treatment period, using a telephone interactive voice response system. It found that tegaserod significantly increased the proportion of people reporting improvement in the previous week (34% with tegaserod *v* 23% with placebo; OR 1.8, 95% CI 1.3 to 2.4).

Harms: The systematic review found that tegaserod significantly increased the proportion of people with diarrhoea compared with placebo (3 RCTs; AR for diarrhoea: 103/1320 [7.8%] with tegaserod 12 mg *v* 37/1301 [2.8%] with placebo; RR 2.75, 95% CI 1.90 to 3.97; NNH 20).[34] The systematic review reported no serious drug related adverse events and no reported cases of ischaemic colitis. The subsequent RCT also found that tegaserod increased the proportion of people with diarrhoea compared with placebo but the statistical significance was not reported (9.2% with tegaserod 6 mg twice daily *v* 1.3% with placebo).[35]

Comment: The RCTs were mainly in women (about 90% of participants) and results may not, therefore, generalise to men with IBS. The trials identified by the review were not of adequate duration to determine whether the benefits of tegaserod remain in the long term. In the four RCTs included in the meta-analysis, participants were asked to rate their global assessment of relief (i.e. overall quality of life and IBS symptoms) as "completely relieved", "considerably relieved", "somewhat relieved", "unchanged", or "worse" each week. Participants reporting that they were "completely" or "considerably" relieved in at least 50% of the last four assessments or "somewhat relieved" in 100% of the last four assessments were considered to have improved. We found a second systematic review (search date not reported), which combined six studies in a narrative synthesis with no meta-analysis.[36] Five of these studies had used an outcome measure of interest, all five were included in the first systematic review.

OPTION 5HT$_3$ RECEPTOR ANTAGONISTS

One systematic review found that alosetron improved symptoms in women with diarrhoea predominant irritable bowel syndrome compared with placebo or mebeverine. However, alosetron is associated with adverse effects, particularly constipation, and has been restricted in some countries because of concerns that it may be associated with ischaemic colitis. The systematic review provided insufficient evidence about the effects of alosetron in men. We found no RCTs examining other 5HT$_3$ receptor antagonists.

Benefits: **Alosetron versus placebo:** We found one systematic review (search date 2002; 5 RCTs; 2675 people; mainly women; see comment below).[37] Most people (75%) had diarrhoea predominant irritable bowel syndrome. It found that alosetron (≥ 2 mg/day) significantly improved symptoms compared with placebo after 12 weeks' treatment (OR for improvement [see comment below] 1.85, 95% CI 1.57 to 2.18). The review reported that the benefits of alosetron disappeared when treatment was stopped (follow up scores not reported in the review). **Alosetron versus mebeverine:** We found one systematic review (1

RCT; 623 people; mainly women; see comment below).[37] It found that alosetron (≥ 2 mg/day) significantly improved symptoms compared with mebeverine after 12 weeks' treatment (OR 1.69, 95% CI 1.42 to 2.32). **Other $5HT_3$ receptor antagonists:** We found no RCTs of sufficient quality.

Harms: Alosetron has been restricted in some countries because of concerns that it may be associated with ischaemic colitis. In the systematic review, two cases of ischaemic colitis were reported in people taking alosetron, with an estimated prevalence of 0.1%.[37] **Alosetron versus placebo:** The systematic review found that adverse events and constipation were significantly more common with alosetron than with placebo (5 RCTs, 2675 people; OR for adverse effects 1.58, 95% CI 1.34 to 1.85; OR for constipation 6.11, 95% CI 4.82 to 7.82).[37] **Alosetron versus mebeverine:** The systematic review found that constipation was significantly more common with alosetron than with mebeverine, but there was no significant difference in overall adverse events between treatments (1 RCT, 623 women; OR for constipation 10.59, 95% CI 9.15 to 12.25; OR for adverse effects 1.22, 95% CI 0.87 to 1.69).

Comment: The studies included in the review evaluated either global improvement of symptoms, or abdominal discomfort or pain. In the meta-analysis, participants were considered improved if they reported positive outcome (e.g. adequate relief) on at least 50% of occasions during each study.[37] The efficacy of alosetron in men is unclear, because 94.5% of participants in the RCTs included in the review were women.

OPTION FIBRE SUPPLEMENTATION

One systematic review found limited evidence that fibre supplementation improved symptoms of irritable bowel syndrome and irritable bowel syndrome related constipation.

Benefits: We found one systematic review (search date 2002, 17 RCTs, 1363 people with irritable bowel syndrome) of fibre supplementation.[38] It found that soluble fibre (psyllium, ispaghula, and polycarbophil) significantly improved global symptoms and constipation compared with placebo (improvement in global symptoms, 8 RCTs: RR 1.55, 95% CI 1.35 to 1.78; improvement in constipation, 2 RCTs: RR 1.60, 95% CI 1.06 to 2.42; both results statistically heterogeneous). It found that insoluble fibre (corn fibre and wheat bran) improved constipation compared with placebo (6 RCTs: RR 1.54, 95% CI 1.10 to 2.14). It found no significant difference between insoluble fibre and placebo for global symptoms (improvement in global symptoms compared with each other, 4 RCTs: RR 0.89, 95% CI 0.72 to 1.11).

Harms: The systematic review found that soluble fibre significantly increased abdominal pain compared with placebo (improvement in pain, 3 RCTs: RR 0.67, 95% CI 0.47 to 0.95, result significantly heterogeneous).[38] It found no significant difference between insoluble fibre and placebo for abdominal pain (6 RCTs: RR 0.87, 95% CI 0.69 to 1.08).

Comment: The authors of the systematic review[38] commented on the heterogeneity of the studies, the variability in outcome measures employed, small sample sizes, and the variable quality of the studies. None of the studies included in the review were set in primary care.

Substantive changes

$5HT_4$ receptor agonists One RCT added.[35] Categorisation unchanged.
Fibre supplementation One systematic review added.[38] Categorisation unchanged.

REFERENCES

1. Manning AP, Thompson WG, Heaton KW, et al. Towards positive diagnosis of the irritable bowel. *BMJ* 1978;2:653–654.
2. Thompson WG, Dotevall G, Drossman DA. Irritable bowel syndrome: guidelines for diagnosis. *Gastroenterol Int* 1989;2:92–95.
3. Drossman DA, Thompson WG, Talley NJ, et al. Identification of sub-groups of functional gastrointestinal disorders. *Gastroenterol Int* 1990;3:159–172.
4. Kennedy TM, Jones RH. Epidemiology of cholecystectomy and irritable bowel syndrome in a UK population. *Br J Surg* 2000;87:1658–1663. [Erratum in *Br J Surg* 2001;88:1021]
5. Boyce PM, Koloski NA, Talley NJ. Irritable bowel syndrome according to varying diagnostic criteria: are the new Rome II criteria unnecessarily restrictive for research and practice? *Am J Gastroenterol* 2000;95:3176–3183. [Erratum in *Am J Gastroenterol* 2001;96:1319]
6. Prior A, Maxton DG, Whorwell PJ. Anorectal manometry in irritable bowel syndrome: differences between diarrhoea and constipation predominant subjects. *Gut* 1990;31:458–462.
7. Gorard DA, Libby GW, Farthing MJ. Ambulatory small intestinal motility in "diarrhoea" predominant irritable bowel syndrome. *Gut* 1994;35:203–210.
8. Kellow JE, Philips SF. Altered small bowel motility in irritable bowel syndrome is correlated with symptoms. *Gastroenterology* 1987;92:1885–1893.
9. Mayer EA, Gebhart GF. Basic and clinical aspects of visceral hyperalgesia. *Gastroenterology* 1994;107:271–293.
10. Mertz H, Morgan V, Tanner G, et al. Regional cerebral activation in irritable bowel syndrome and control subjects with painful and nonpainful rectal distention. *Gastroenterology* 2000;118:842–848.
11. Mertz H, Naliboff B, Munakata J, et al. Altered rectal perception is a biological marker of patients with irritable bowel syndrome. *Gastroenterology* 1995;109:40–52. [Erratum in *Gastroenterology* 1997;113:1054]
12. Delvaux M, Denis P, Allemand H. Sexual abuse is more frequently reported by IBS patients than by patients with organic digestive diseases or controls. Results from a multicentre inquiry. *Eur J Gastroenterol Hepatol* 1997;9:345–352.
13. Locke GR 3rd, Zinsmeister AR, Talley NJ, et al. Familial associations in adults with functional gastrointestinal disorders. *Mayo Clin Proc* 2000;75:907–912.
14. Levy RL, Jones KR, Whitehead WE, et al. Irritable bowel syndrome in twins: heredity and social learning both contribute to etiology. *Gastroenterology* 2001;121:799–804.
15. Morris-Yates A, Talley NJ, Boyce PM, et al. Evidence of a genetic contribution to functional bowel disorder. *Am J Gastroenterol* 1998;93:1311–1317.
16. Collins SM. Is the irritable gut an inflamed gut? *Scand J Gastroenterol Suppl* 1992;27:102–105.
17. Gwee KA, Leong YL, Graham C, et al. The role of psychological and biological factors in postinfective gut dysfunction. *Gut* 1999;44:400–406.
18. Owens DM, Nelson DK, Talley NJ. The irritable bowel syndrome: long-term prognosis and the physician–patient interaction. *Ann Intern Med* 1995;122:107–112.
19. Kennedy TM, Jones RH. The epidemiology of hysterectomy and irritable bowel syndrome in a UK population. *Int J Clin Pract* 2000;54:647–650.
20. Mangel AW, Hahn B, Heath AT, et al. Adequate relief as an endpoint in clinical trials in irritable bowel syndrome. *J Int Med Res* 1998;26:76–81.
21. Francis CY, Morris J, Whorwell PJ. The irritable bowel severity scoring system: a simple method of monitoring irritable bowel syndrome and its progress. *Aliment Pharmacol Ther* 1997;11:395–402.
22. Revicki DA, Wood M, Wiklund I, et al. Reliability and validity of the Gastrointestinal Symptom Rating Scale in patients with gastroesophageal reflux disease. *Qual Life Res* 1998;7:75–83.
23. Svedlund J, Sjodin I, Dotevall G. GSRS — a clinical rating system for gastrointestinal symptoms in patients with irritable bowel syndrome and peptic ulcer disease. *Dig Dis Sci* 1988;33:129–134.
24. Drossman DA, Li Z, Toner BB, et al. Functional bowel disorders. A multicenter comparison of health status and development of illness severity index. *Dig Dis Sci* 1995;40:986–995.
25. Patrick DL, Drossman DA, Frederick IO, et al. Quality of life in persons with irritable bowel syndrome: development and validation of a new measure. *Dig Dis Sci* 1998;43:400–411.
26. Drossman DA, Patrick DL, Whitehead WE, et al. Further validation of the IBS-QOL: a disease-specific quality-of-life questionnaire. *Am J Gastroenterol* 2000;95:999–1007.
27. Hahn BA, Kirchdoerfer LJ, Fullerton S, et al. Evaluation of a new quality of life questionnaire for patients with irritable bowel syndrome. *Aliment Pharmacol Ther* 1997;11:547–552.
28. Shaw M, Talley NJ, Adlis S, et al. Development of a digestive health status instrument: tests of scaling assumptions, structure and reliability in a primary care population. *Aliment Pharmacol Ther* 1998;12:1067–1078.
29. Chassany O, Marquis P, Scherrer B, et al. Validation of a specific quality of life questionnaire for functional digestive disorders. *Gut* 1999;44:527–533.
30. Wong E, Guyatt GH, Cook DJ, et al. Development of a questionnaire to measure quality of life in patients with irritable bowel syndrome. *Eur J Surg Suppl* 1998;583:50–56.
31. Jackson JL, O'Malley PG, Tomkins G, et al. Treatment of functional gastrointestinal disorders with antidepressant medications: a meta-analysis. *Am J Med* 2000;108:65–72. Search date 1998; primary sources Medline, Psychlit, Embase, Cochrane Controlled Trials Register, Cochrane Database of Systematic Reviews, Federal Research in Progress, and hand searches of references of reviewed articles.
32. Poynard T, Regimbeau C, Benhamou Y. Meta-analysis of smooth muscle relaxants in the treatment of irritable bowel syndrome. *Aliment Pharmacol Ther* 2001;15:355–361. Search date 1999; primary sources Medline, Current Contents and hand searches of general reviews, an overview of relevant meta-analyses and reference lists of published RCTs, and personal contact with pharmaceutical companies.
33. Mitchell SA, Mee AS, Smith GD, et al. Alverine citrate fails to relieve the symptoms of irritable bowel syndrome: results of a double-blind, randomized, placebo-controlled trial. *Aliment Pharmacol Ther* 2002;16:1187–1195.
34. Evans BW, Clark WK, Moore DJ, et al. Tegaserod for the treatment of irritable bowel syndrome (Cochrane Review). In: The Cochrane Library, Issue 2, 2004. Chichester, UK: John Wiley & Sons, Ltd. Search date 2002.
35. Nyhlin H, Bang C, Elsborg L, et al. A double-blind placebo-controlled randomized study to evaluate the efficacy, safety and tolerability of tegaserod in patients with irritable bowel syndrome. *Scand J Gastroenterol* 2004;39:119–126. Search date 2002; primary sources Medline.
36. Jones BW, Moore DJ, Robinson SM, et al. A systematic review of tegaserod for the treatment of irritable bowel syndrome. *J Clin Pharm Ther* 2002;27:343–352. Search date not reported.
37. Cremonini F, Delgado-Aros S, Camilleri M. Efficacy of alosetron in irritable bowel syndrome: a meta-analysis of randomized controlled trials. *Neurogastroenterol Motil* 2003;15:79–86. Search date 2002; primary sources Medline, Embase and hand searches of the cross-references included in the studies retrieved.
38. Bijkerk CJ, Muris JW, Knottnerus JA, et al. Systematic review: the roles of different types of fibre in the treatment of irritable bowel syndrome. *Aliment Pharmacol Ther* 2004;19:245–251.

Irritable bowel syndrome

Niek de Wit
Associate professor
Julius center for health sciences and primary care
University medical center Utrecht
Universiteitsweg
Utrecht
The Netherlands

Gregory Rubin
Professor of Primary Care
Centre for Primary and Community Care,
University of Sunderland
Sunderland
UK

Roger Jones
Wolfson Professor of General Practice
Department of General Practice
Guy's, King's, and St Thomas's Medical School
King's College
London
UK

Competing interests: The authors have advised several pharmaceutical companies on the development of therapies for irritable bowel syndrome. GR has been reimbursed by Novartis for attending conferences and has received research funding from them. GR has shares in GlaxoSmithKline. NdW is co-author of one systematic review (ref 38) that is referenced in this paper.

TABLE 1 Manning criteria.

Recurrent abdominal pain and two or more of the following:
- Relief of pain with defecation
- More frequent stools at the onset of pain
- Looser stools at the onset of pain
- Visible abdominal distension
- Passage of mucus per rectum
- A sensation of incomplete evacuation

TABLE 2 Rome I criteria.

Abdominal pain or discomfort that is one or more of the following:
- Relieved with defecation
- Associated with a change in frequency of stool
- Associated with a change in consistency of stool
Plus two or more of the following for at least 25% of occasions or days:
- Altered stool frequency
- Altered stool form
- Passage of mucus
- Bloating or a feeling of abdominal distension

TABLE 3 Rome II criteria.

At least 12 weeks (which need not be consecutive) in the preceding 12 months of abdominal discomfort or pain that has 2 of 3 features:
- Relieved by defecation
- Onset associated with a change in frequency of stool
- Onset associated with a change in form (appearance) of stool
The following cumulatively support the diagnosis of IBS:
- Abnormal stool frequency (> 3 daily or < 3 weekly)
- Abnormal stool form (lumpy/hard or loose/watery)
- Abnormal stool passage (straining, urgency, feeling of incomplete evacuation)
- Passage of mucus
- Bloating or feeling of abdominal distension

Pancreatic cancer

Search date May 2003

Bazian Ltd

QUESTIONS

INTERVENTIONS

To be covered in future updates

Adjuvant chemoimmunotherapy for resectable disease

Adjuvant chemoradiotherapy for resectable disease

Adjuvant local chemotherapy for resectable disease

Treatments for advanced disease

*RCTs comparing surgery versus no surgery may be considered unethical in people with pancreatic cancer that is considered suitable for complete tumour resection

See glossary

Key Messages

Surgical treatments in people with resectable pancreatic cancer

- **Pancreaticoduodenectomy (Whipple's procedure)** We found no RCTs comparing pancreaticoduodenectomy (Whipple's procedure) with non-surgical treatment in people with resectable pancreatic cancer, although such studies may be considered unethical. Observational data provide limited evidence that surgery may reduce mortality compared with non-surgical treatment, although results may be confounded by differences in disease stage. Small RCTs found no significant difference in quality of life or survival at 5 years between pancreaticoduodenectomy and pylorus preserving pancreaticoduodenectomy.
- **Pylorus preserving pancreaticoduodenectomy (compared with Whipple's procedure)** Small RCTs found no significant difference between pylorus preserving surgery and classical pancreaticoduodenectomy (Whipple's procedure) for overall quality of life at 1 year or survival at 5 years in people with resectable tumours. However, the studies may have lacked power to exclude clinically important differences for these outcomes.

Adjuvant treatments in people with completely resected pancreatic cancer

- **Systemic fluorouracil based chemotherapy** One RCT has found that adjuvant fluorouracil based chemotherapy improves median survival by about 1 year compared with no adjuvant chemotherapy in people with resected pancreatic cancer. However, this RCT and a second RCT found no significant difference in 5 year survival. The second RCT found that adjuvant fluorouracil based chemotherapy increased ≥ Grade 2 leukopenia, anorexia, and nausea or emesis compared with no chemotherapy. A third RCT did not compare chemotherapy alone with no chemotherapy directly.
- **Systemic gemcitabine based chemotherapy** One systematic review found insufficient evidence about effects of adjuvant gemcitabine compared with no adjuvant chemotherapy in people with resected pancreatic cancer.

DEFINITION	In this chapter, the term "pancreatic cancer" refers to primary adenocarcinoma of the pancreas. Other pancreatic malignancies, such as carcinoid tumour, are not considered. Symptoms of pancreatic cancer include pain, jaundice, nausea, weight loss, loss of appetite, and symptoms of gastrointestinal obstruction and diabetes. Pancreatic cancer is staged from I to IV according to disease spread. Stage I disease is limited to the pancreas, duodenum, bile duct, or peri-pancreatic tissues, with no distant metastases or regional lymph node involvement. Stages II–IV describe disease that has spread more extensively or become metastatic. A pancreatic tumour is considered resectable if there is a possibility that surgery could remove all cancerous tissue completely. Early stage tumours in the tail or body of the pancreas are more likely to be resectable than the more common, later stage cancers in the head of the pancreas. Other factors that influence resectability include proximity of the tumour to major blood vessels and perceived peri-operative risk.
INCIDENCE/ PREVALENCE	Pancreatic cancer is the eighth most common cancer in the UK with an annual incidence in England and Wales of about 12/100 000.[1] It is the fourth most common cause of cancer death in higher income countries, responsible for about 30 000 deaths each year in the USA.[2] Prevalence is similar in men and women, with 5–10% presenting with resectable disease.[3]
AETIOLOGY/ RISK FACTORS	Pancreatic cancer is more likely in people who smoke and have high alcohol intake. Dietary factors, such as lack of fruit and vegetables, are also reported risk factors.[4] One meta-analysis of observational studies found that people with diabetes mellitus of more than 5 years' duration are more likely to develop pancreatic cancer compared with the general population.[5] However, estimates of the magnitude of increased risk vary. Additional risk factors include pancreatitis and, in some cases, a family history.[1]
PROGNOSIS	Prognosis is poor. One year survival is about 12%, with 5 year survival ranging from less than 1% in those with advanced cancer at presentation to 5% in those with early stage cancer at presentation.[1,6]
AIMS OF INTERVENTION	In early stage (resectable) pancreatic cancer: to improve survival and quality of life. In advanced pancreatic cancer: treatment aims to improve symptoms and quality of life.
OUTCOMES	One and 5 year survival; quality of life; symptoms; and adverse effects of treatment.
METHODS	*Clinical Evidence* search and appraisal May 2003.

QUESTION **What are the effects of surgical treatments in people with pancreatic cancer that is considered suitable for complete tumour resection?**

OPTION **PANCREATICODUODENECTOMY (WHIPPLE'S PROCEDURE)**

We found no RCTs comparing pancreaticoduodenectomy (Whipple's procedure Ⓖ) versus non-surgical treatment in people with resectable pancreatic cancer, although such studies may be considered unethical. Observational data provide limited evidence that surgery may reduce mortality compared with

non-surgical treatment, although results may have been confounded by differences in disease stage. Small RCTs found no significant difference in quality of life or survival at 5 years between pancreaticoduodenectomy and pylorus preserving pancreaticoduodenectomy.

Benefits: **Versus non-surgical treatment:** We found no RCTs in people with resectable (early stage) pancreatic cancer (see comment below). **Versus pylorus preserving pancreaticoduodenectomy:** See benefits of pylorus preserving pancreaticoduodenectomy, p 566.

Harms: We found no RCTs.

Comment: RCTs comparing surgery versus non-surgical treatment would be considered unethical in people with tumours that are considered suitable for resection. One large cohort study (100 313 people with pancreatic cancer) found that people having pancreatectomy lived longer than people not treated surgically (5 year survival, 23% with surgery *v* 5% without surgery).[7] However, results may have been confounded by differences in disease stage between those having surgery and those treated without surgery.

OPTION PYLORUS PRESERVING PANCREATICODUODENECTOMY

Small RCTs found no significant difference between pylorus preserving pancreaticoduodenectomy and standard pancreaticoduodenectomy (Whipple's procedure) for overall quality of life at 1 year, survival at 5 years, or adverse events in people with resectable tumours. However, the studies may have lacked power to exclude clinically important differences for these outcomes.

Benefits: **Versus standard pancreaticoduodenectomy (Whipple's procedure):** We found one systematic review (search date 2000, 2 RCTs, 108 people with pancreatic cancer)[9] and two additional RCTs.[10,11] The systematic review compared standard pancreaticoduodenectomy (Whipple's procedure**G**) versus pylorus preserving pancreaticoduodenectomy.[9] The first small RCT identified by the review (38 people with resectable head of pancreas or peri-ampullary cancer) did not report on cancer recurrence, quality of life, or survival.[8] The second RCT identified by the review (77 people with head of pancreas or peri-ampullary cancer) found no significant difference between techniques after a median follow up of 1.1 years (61 people included in analysis; median survival: 24 months with pylorus preserving surgery *v* 16 months with Whipple's procedure; $P = 0.29$).[12] The first additional RCT (48 people with resectable head of pancreas or peri-ampullary cancer) found no significant difference between pylorus preserving surgery and Whipple's procedure for global quality of life scores at 2–60 weeks (quality of life measured by 100 point EORTC-QLQ-30 score; results presented graphically, score in both groups about 50 preoperatively and 35 at 60 weeks; $P > 0.05$).[10] The second additional RCT (40 people with head of pancreas or peri-ampullary cancer) found no significant difference between procedures for 5 year survival (20% with pylorus preserving surgery *v* 13% with Whipple's procedure). However, the study may have lacked power to exclude a clinically important difference.[11]

Harms: The first RCT identified by the review found no significant difference in peri-operative blood loss between pylorus preserving surgery and Whipple's procedure (mean blood loss 451 mL with pylorus preserving surgery *v* 687 mL with Whipple's procedure; $P > 0.2$; CI for difference not reported).[8] It also found no significant differences between treatments for peri-operative death (1 person with pylorus preserving surgery v 0 with Whipple's procedure), biliary leak (0 in both groups); pancreatitis (1 in both groups), wound infection (1 in both groups), cardiovascular events (0 with pylorus preserving surgery v 1 with Whipple's procedure), or upper gastrointestinal bleeding (0 with pylorus preserving surgery v 1 with Whipple's procedure). However, the RCT may have lacked power to exclude clinically important differences for these outcomes. Delayed gastric emptying was more common with pylorus preserving surgery (6 people with pylorus preserving surgery v 1 with Whipple's procedure).[8] The second RCT identified by the review found no significant differences between the techniques for delayed gastric emptying (32% with pylorus preserving surgery v 45% with Whipple's procedure), fistula (2% with pylorus preserving surgery v 3% with Whipple's procedure), wound infection (7% with pylorus preserving surgery v 8% with Whipple's procedure), or peri-operative mortality (2.7% with pylorus preserving surgery v 5% with Whipple's procedure).[12] The first additional RCT also found that complication rates were similar in both groups (wound infection: 3 people with pylorus preserving surgery v 4 people with Whipple's procedure; pneumonia: 2 people with pylorus preserving surgery v 3 people with Whipple's procedure; peritonitis 1 person in both groups; and sepsis 0 people with pylorus preserving surgery v 2 people with Whipple's procedure).[10] The second additional RCT reported similar complications and frequencies to the other trials. Differences between procedures were not significant for any of these complications except gastric atony (6 people with pylorus preserving surgery v 1 person with Whipple's procedure; $P < 0.05$).[11]

Comment: The RCTs may have lacked power to detect clinically important differences between procedures.

QUESTION **What are the effects of adjuvant treatments in people with completely resected pancreatic cancer?**

OPTION **ADJUVANT SYSTEMIC GEMCITABINE BASED CHEMOTHERAPY**

One systematic review found insufficient evidence about the effects of adjuvant gemcitabine compared with no adjuvant chemotherapy in people with resected pancreatic cancer.

Benefits: **Versus no adjuvant chemotherapy:** We found one systematic review examining the effects of gemcitabine based chemotherapy in people with resected pancreatic cancer (search date 2000).[1] It identified no RCTs comparing adjuvant gemcitabine versus no adjuvant chemotherapy or placebo (see comment below).

Harms: The systematic review identified two studies that assessed harms of gemcitabine from both controlled and uncontrolled clinical trials.[1] Both studies included people with non-pancreatic tumours. The studies found that gemcitabine was associated with the following grade 3–4 toxicities: anaemia (about 7%), leukopenia (about 9%), neutropenia (about 25%), and thrombocytopenia (5–7%).

Comment: This option excludes adjuvant gemcitabine combined with radiotherapy or immunotherapy, which will be covered in future updates.

OPTION **ADJUVANT SYSTEMIC FLUOROURACIL BASED CHEMOTHERAPY**

One small multicentre RCT has found that adjuvant fluorouracil based chemotherapy improved median survival from about 1 year to about 2 years compared with no adjuvant chemotherapy in people with resected pancreatic

cancer. However, this RCT and a second RCT found no significant difference in 5 year survival between adjuvant chemotherapy with fluorouracil based chemotherapy and no chemotherapy. The RCTs found that chemotherapy was commonly associated with adverse events such as leukopenia, nausea and vomiting, alopecia, and anorexia.

Benefits: **Versus no adjuvant chemotherapy:** We found three RCTs assessing effects of fluorouracil based chemotherapy after successful surgical resection❻.[13–15] The first RCT (multicentre trial in 61 people: 47 with resected pancreatic cancer and 14 with carcinoma of the papilla of Vater) compared chemotherapy (6 cycles of fluorouracil 500 mg/m^2, doxorubicin 40 mg/m^2, and mitomycin C 6 mg/m^2 once every 3 weeks) versus no adjuvant chemotherapy. It found that chemotherapy significantly improved median survival compared with no adjuvant treatment (intention to treat analysis: median survival 23 months with chemotherapy *v* 11 months without chemotherapy; P = 0.04). However, there was no difference for 5 year survival (4% with chemotherapy *v* 8% without chemotherapy; P = 0.10; CI not reported). The study may have lacked power to detect clinically important differences in 5 year survival.[13] The second RCT (508 people with pancreaticobiliary cancer including 92 people with pancreatic cancer, 72 people with bile duct cancer, and 41 people with ampulla of Vater cancer who had had successful surgical resection) compared adjuvant chemotherapy (mitomycin C plus 5-fluorouracil) versus no chemotherapy.[14] Chemotherapy consisted of two 5 day courses of intravenous chemotherapy with mitomycin C 6 mg/m^2 and 5-fluorouracil 310 mg/m^2, followed by oral 5-fluorouracil 100 mg/m^2 daily from 5 weeks postoperatively until disease recurrence. People with pancreatic cancer had had different surgical techniques. Subgroup analysis in people with pancreatic cancer found no significant difference in 5 year survival between adjuvant chemotherapy and no adjuvant chemotherapy (median survival: 17.8% with chemotherapy *v* 26.6% with no chemotherapy, P = 0.45). The third RCT (541 people with resected pancreatic cancer) compared four adjuvant strategies: chemotherapy (425 mg/m^2 fluorouracil plus folinic acid 20 mg/m^2), chemoradiotherapy, chemoradiotherapy plus the chemotherapy regimen, and observation only. It did not report results for adjuvant chemotherapy alone compared with no adjuvant chemotherapy (see comment below).[15]

Harms: The first RCT reported that one person died of chemotherapy associated sepsis.[13] Other adverse effects of chemotherapy included non-fatal sepsis (4 people), alopecia (11 people), leukopenia less than 2.5 x 10^9/L white cells (occurred 5 times overall), cardiotoxicity (2 people), and nephrotoxicity (2 people). After 3 months, four people experienced nausea and vomiting with chemotherapy compared with none in the control group. The second RCT (508 people with resected pancreaticobiliary cancer) found that chemotherapy significantly increased leukopenia, anorexia, and nausea or vomiting compared with no chemotherapy (grade ≥ 2 leukopenia: 12.9% with chemotherapy *v* 3% with no chemotherapy; grade ≥ 2 anorexia: 22.4% with chemotherapy *v* 13.9% with no chemotherapy; grade ≥ 2 nausea/vomiting: 12.9% with chemotherapy *v* 6.9% with no chemotherapy, P < 0.05 for each comparison).

Comment: This option excludes adjuvant fluorouracil combined with radiotherapy or immunotherapy, which will be covered in future updates. The first RCT included only people under 75 years old with high performance status (Karnofsky score > 60).[13] Six of 30 people allocated to chemotherapy received no chemotherapy and 17 did not complete all six cycles of treatment. The third RCT found that chemoradiotherapy significantly improved survival compared with no chemoradiotherapy (median survival: 19.7 months with chemoradiotherapy *v* 14.0 months with no chemoradiotherapy; HR 0.66, 95% CI 0.52 to 0.83).[15] It was not possible from this analysis to establish whether effects were due to chemotherapy or concomitant radiotherapy.

GLOSSARY

Successful surgical resection Surgery is defined as successful if, after resection, no residual disease is observed macroscopically or histologically in the tumour resection margins.

Whipple's procedure Radical pancreaticoduodenectomy involving removal of the pancreas, duodenum, and gastric pylorus.

REFERENCES

1. Ward S, Morris E, Bansback N, et al. A rapid and systematic review of the clinical effectiveness and cost-effectiveness of gemcitabine for the treatment of pancreatic cancer. *Health Technol* Assess 2001;5:1–70. Search date 2000; primary sources Medline, Embase, Science Citation Index, Cochrane Library, NHS CRD, NHS EED, NHS HTA, Pubmed, OHE HEED, National and International Research Registers, and contact with HTA agencies.
2. Jemal PA, Murray T, Samuels A. Cancer statistics, 2003. *CA Cancer J Clin* 2003;53:5–26.
3. Maisey N, Chau I, Cunningham D, et al. Multicenter randomized Phase III trial comparing protracted venous infusion (PVI) fluorouracil (5-FU) with PVI 5-FU plus mitomycin in inoperable pancreatic cancer. *J Clin Oncol* 2002;20:3130–3136.
4. Working Group on Diet and Cancer. Nutritional aspects of the development of cancer. (Committee on Medical Aspects of Food and Nutrition Policy; no. 48.) London: Department of Health, 1998.
5. Everhart, J, Wright, D. Diabetes mellitus as a risk factor for pancreatic cancer. A meta-analysis. *JAMA* 1995;273:1605–1609.
6. Bramhall SR, Allum WH, Jones AG, et al. Treatment and survival in 13,560 patients with pancreatic cancer: an epidemiological study in the West Midlands. *Br J Surg* 1995;82:111–115.
7. Sener SF, Fremgen A, Menck HR, et al. Pancreatic cancer: a report of treatment and survival trends for 100,313 patients diagnosed from 1985–1995, using the National Cancer Database. *J Am Coll Surg* 1999;189:1–7.
8. Lin PW, Lin YJ. Prospective randomized comparison between pylorus-preserving and standard pancreaticoduodenectomy. *Br J Surg* 1999;86:603–607.
9. Schafer M, Stengel P, Demartines N, et al. Pancreatic excisions for chronic pancreatitis and cancer: their rationale for "factual" surgery. Evidence-based medicine. *Journal de Chirurgie* 2001;138:325–335. Search date 2000; primary sources Medline and hand searches of reference lists [In French].
10. Wenger F, Jacobi C, Haubold K, et al. Gastrointestinal quality of life after duodenopancreatectomy in pancreatic carcinoma. Preliminary results of a prospective randomized study: pancreatoduodenectomy or pylorus-preserving pancreatoduodenectomy. [German] *Chirurg* 1999;70:1454–1459.
11. Paquet K-J. Comparison of Whipple's pancreaticoduodenectomy with the pylorus-preserving pancreaticoduodenectomy — a prospectively controlled, randomized long-term trial. *Chirurg Gastroenterol* 1998;14:54–58.
12. Seiler C, Wagner M, Sadowski C, et al. Randomized prospective trial of pylorus-preserving vs. Classic duodenopancreatectomy (Whipple procedure): initial clinical results. *J Gastrointest Surg* 2000;4:443–452.
13. Bakkevold KE, Arnesjo B, Dahl O, et al. Adjuvant combination chemotherapy (AMF) following radical resection of carcinoma of the pancreas and papilla of Vater — results of a controlled, prospective, randomised multicentre study. *Eur J Cancer* 1993;29A:698–703.
14. Takada T, Amano H, Yasuda H, et al. Is postoperative adjuvant chemotherapy useful for gallbladder carcinoma? A Phase III multicenter prospective randomized controlled trial in patients with resected pancreaticobiliary carcinoma. *Cancer* 2002;95:1685–1695.
15. Neoptolemos JP, Dunn JA, Stocken DD, et al. Adjuvant chemoradiotherapy and chemotherapy in resectable pancreatic cancer: a randomised controlled trial. *Lancet* 2001;358:1576–1585.

Bazian Ltd
London
UK

Competing interests: None declared.

Stomach cancer

Search date September 2003

Charles Bailey

QUESTIONS

INTERVENTIONS

RADICAL V CONSERVATIVE SURGERY

Likely to be beneficial

Complete tumour resection* 571
Subtotal gastrectomy for resectable distal tumours (as effective as total gastrectomy) 572

Unknown effectiveness

Radical versus conservative lymphadenectomy 574

Likely to be ineffective or harmful

Removal of adjacent organs 573

ADJUVANT CHEMOTHERAPY

Likely to be beneficial

Adjuvant chemotherapy 574

To be covered in future updates

Addition of bacterial and fungal extracts to adjuvant chemotherapy
Adjuvant radiotherapy
Endoscopic mucosal resection for early gastric cancer
Regional chemotherapy

*Observational evidence only; RCTs unlikely to be conducted.

See glossary

Key Messages

Radical v conservative surgery

- **Complete tumour resection** RCTs of complete tumour resection are unlikely to be conducted. Observational studies and multivariate analysis of RCTs have found a strong association between survival and complete resection of the primary tumour.
- **Subtotal gastrectomy for resectable distal tumours (as effective as total gastrectomy)** Two RCTs in people with primary tumours in the distal stomach found no significant difference in 5 year survival or postoperative mortality between total and subtotal gastrectomy.
- **Radical versus conservative lymphadenectomy** Two large RCTs found no significant difference in 5 year survival rates between radical and conservative lymphadenectomy. However, confounding factors may have affected reliability of results, and we found conflicting data from subgroup analyses of prospective cohort studies.
- **Removal of adjacent organs** One RCT found no significant difference between radical gastrectomy plus splenectomy and radical gastrectomy alone in 5 year survival rates or postoperative mortality. The RCT found that radical gastrectomy plus splenectomy significantly increased the number of postoperative infections compared with radical gastrectomy alone. Retrospective analyses of observational studies and RCTs in people with stomach cancer found that removal of additional organs (spleen and distal pancreas) increased morbidity and mortality compared with no organ removal.

Adjuvant chemotherapy

- **Adjuvant chemotherapy** One large systematic review and two subsequent RCTs found that adjuvant chemotherapy increased survival compared with surgery alone. Two subsequent RCTs found no significant difference between adjuvant chemotherapy and surgery alone in 5 year survival.

DEFINITION Stomach cancer is usually an adenocarcinoma arising in the stomach and includes tumours arising at or just below the gastro-oesophageal junction (type II and III junctional tumours). Tumours are staged according to degree of invasion and spread (see table 1, p 577). Only non-metastatic stomach cancers are considered in this chapter.

INCIDENCE/ PREVALENCE The incidence of stomach cancer varies among countries and by gender (incidence per 100 000 population a year in Japanese men is about 80, Japanese women 30, British men 18, British women 10, white American men 11, white American women 7).[1] Incidence has declined dramatically in North America, Australia, and New Zealand since 1930, but the decline in Europe has been slower.[2] In the USA, stomach cancer remains relatively common among particular ethnic groups, especially Japanese–Americans and some Hispanic groups. The incidence of cancer of the proximal stomach and gastro-oesophageal junction is rising rapidly in many European populations and in North America.[3,4] The reasons for this are poorly understood.

AETIOLOGY/ RISK FACTORS Distal stomach cancer is strongly associated with lifelong infection with *Helicobacter pylori* and poor dietary intake of antioxidant vitamins (A, C, and E).[5,6] In Western Europe and North America, distal stomach cancer is associated with relative socioeconomic deprivation. Proximal stomach cancer is strongly associated with smoking (OR about 4),[7] and is probably associated with gastro-oesophageal reflux, obesity, high fat intake, and medium to high socioeconomic status.

PROGNOSIS Invasive stomach cancer (stages T2–T4) is fatal without surgery. Mean survival without treatment is less than 6 months from diagnosis.[8,9] Intramucosal or submucosal cancer (stage T1) may progress slowly to invasive cancer over several years.[10] In the USA, over 50% of people recently diagnosed with stomach cancer have regional lymph node metastasis or involvement of adjacent organs. The prognosis after macroscopically and microscopically complete resection (R0) is related strongly to disease stage Ⓖ, particularly penetration of the serosa (stage T3) and lymph node involvement. Five year survival rates range from over 90% in intramucosal cancer to about 20% in people with stage T3N2 disease (see table 1, p 577). In Japan, the 5 year survival rate for people with advanced disease is reported to be about 50%, but the explanation for the difference remains unclear. Comparisons between Japanese and Western practice are confounded by factors such as age, fitness, and disease stage, as well as by tumour location, because many Western series include gastro-oesophageal junction adenocarcinoma, which is associated with a much lower survival rate after surgery.

AIMS OF INTERVENTION To prevent progression; extend survival; and relieve symptoms, with minimal adverse effects.

OUTCOMES Survival; quality of life; adverse effects of treatment.

METHODS *Clinical Evidence* search and appraisal September 2003. Hand searches of conference proceedings and consultations with experts were used to identify relevant studies. In many instances, we have separated trials and results from different geographical areas because of differences in baseline risk and demographics, and possible differences in response to treatments. However, the meaning of terms to describe such populations, such as "Western" and "Asian", were not clearly defined in many identified studies.

QUESTION **What are the effects of radical versus conservative surgical resection?**

OPTION **COMPLETE VERSUS INCOMPLETE TUMOUR RESECTION**

RCTs of complete tumour resection are unlikely to be conducted. Observational studies and multivariate analysis of RCTs have found a strong association between survival and complete resection of the primary tumour.

Benefits: We found no systematic review or RCTs directly comparing complete versus incomplete tumour resection or positive versus clear microscopic resection margins (see comment below). Multivariate risk factor analysis of RCTs and retrospective cohort studies found that failure to achieve microscopically clear resection margins was associated with a poor outcome independently of other indicators of tumour spread and behaviour.[11–13]

Harms: We found no systematic review or RCTs.

Comment: Current consensus is that improving long term survival is best achieved by complete resection of the primary tumour with microscopic confirmation of clear resection margins ("curative" gastrectomy). We found two observational studies comparing surgery versus no surgery.[8,9] They found that people who did not undergo resection (generally those with the most advanced disease and highest co-morbidity) had a near zero 5 year survival, and mean survival without treatment from time of diagnosis was found to be less than 6 months. In view of this evidence it is unlikely that an RCT of surgery versus no surgery or complete versus incomplete tumour removal would be carried out.

OPTION TOTAL VERSUS SUBTOTAL GASTRECTOMY FOR RESECTABLE DISTAL TUMOURS

Two RCTs in people with primary tumours in the distal stomach found no significant difference in 5 year survival or postoperative mortality between total and subtotal gastrectomy.

Benefits: **Five year survival:** We found no systematic review, but found two RCTs (787 people, 4 publications) comparing total versus subtotal Ⓖ gastrectomy.[14–17] Neither RCT used blinded allocation. The first RCT (648 people aged < 76 years with a resectable tumour and a macroscopic proximal margin of more than 6 cm) compared total versus subtotal gastrectomy.[14,15] All people involved in the RCT had a regional lymphadenectomy (D2). The RCT found no significant difference between total and subtotal gastrectomy in the incidence of microscopic resection margin involvement or in 5 year survival (microscopic resection margin involvement: 15/315 [4.8%] with subtotal gastrectomy *v* 6/303 [2.0%] with total gastrectomy; ARI +2.8%, 95% CI –0.1% to +9.6%; Kaplan–Meier 5 year survival estimates 65% for subtotal *v* 62% for total gastrectomy; HR 0.89, 95% CI 0.68 to 1.17). Multivariate analysis found that after adjustment for covariates, the type of stomach surgery had no significant effect on 5 year survival (HR 1.01, 95% CI 0.76 to 1.33). The second RCT (169 people with potentially curable distal stomach cancer) compared total versus subtotal gastrectomy and found no significant difference in 5 year survival (48% in each group; CI not reported).[16,17] **Quality of life:** We found no RCTs that examined quality of life with total versus subtotal gastrectomy in people with resectable distal tumours.

Harms: **Postoperative morbidity:** Morbidity included intra-abdominal sepsis, chest infections, wound sepsis, and fistulae. The first RCT found no significant difference between subtotal and total gastrectomy in postoperative morbidity or length of hospital stay (postoperative morbidity: 29/320 [9%] with subtotal gastrectomy *v* 40/304 [13%] with total gastrectomy; RR 0.67, 95% CI 0.44 to 1.08; hospital stay: 13.8 days for subtotal *v* 15.4 days for total gastrectomy).[14,15] The second RCT also found no significant difference in postoperative morbidity (32/93 [34%] for subtotal gastrectomy *v* 25/76 [32%] for total gastrectomy; RR 1.05, 95% CI 0.68 to 1.60).[16,17] **Postoperative mortality:** The first RCT found no significant difference in postoperative mortality (4/320 [1%]

with subtotal gastrectomy *v* 7/304 [2%] with total gastrectomy; RR 0.54, 95% CI 0.16 to 1.84). The second RCT also found no significant difference in postoperative mortality (3/93 [3.2%] with subtotal gastrectomy *v* 1/76 [1.3%] with total gastrectomy; RR 2.45, 95% CI 0.26 to 23.01). Nearly all non-randomised studies that we identified reported higher mortality with total gastrectomy than with subtotal gastrectomy, but total gastrectomy tended to be performed in people with more extensive disease.

Comment: Infiltration of the proximal resection margin by microscopic tumour deposits is perceived as a problem in people with poorly differentiated "diffuse" cancer of the distal stomach undergoing distal subtotal gastrectomy. Some surgeons have therefore recommended total gastrectomy "de principe"Ⓖ for these tumours. The two RCTs found similar survival after total and subtotal gastrectomy in people with primary tumours in the distal stomach.[14–17] Both RCTs recruited otherwise fit people, which may explain the low postoperative mortality.

OPTION REMOVAL OF ADJACENT ORGANS

One RCT found no significant difference between radical gastrectomy plus splenectomy and radical gastrectomy alone in 5 year survival rates or postoperative mortality. The RCT found that radical gastrectomy plus splenectomy significantly increased the number of postoperative infections compared with radical gastrectomy alone. Retrospective analyses of observational studies and RCTs in people with stomach cancer found that removal of additional organs (spleen and distal pancreas) increased morbidity and mortality compared with no organ removal.

Benefits: We found no systematic review. We found one RCT (187 people, aged 25–80 years), which compared radical (D2) gastrectomy plus splenectomy versus radical gastrectomy alone.[18] It found no significant difference in 5 year survival rates (42% with gastrectomy plus splenectomy *v* 36% with gastrectomy alone; $P > 0.5$; absolute numbers not provided).

Harms: The RCT (187 people) found that gastrectomy plus splenectomy significantly increased the number of postoperative infections compared with radical gastrectomy alone (fever > 38 °C, $P < 0.04$; pulmonary infections, $P < 0.008$; subphrenic abscesses, $P < 0.05$), but found no significant difference in postoperative mortality (4/90 [4%] with gastrectomy plus splenectomy *v* 3/97 [3%] with gastrectomy alone; RR 1.40, 95% CI 0.33 to 6.24).[18] Retrospective analyses of RCTs and cohort studies in which removal of the spleen and distal pancreas had been performed routinely during radical total gastrectomy (D2)Ⓖ (see table 2, p 577), and at the surgeon's discretion during non-radical total gastrectomy (D1), found that removal of the spleen or distal pancreas was associated with increased perioperative mortality (OR about 2) and no evidence of improved long term survival.[19,20]

Comment: Some advocates of radical surgery have suggested routine removal of the spleen and distal pancreas to ensure complete regional lymph node dissection during total gastrectomy. Current consensus is that removal of adjacent organs is justified only when necessary to ensure complete tumour removal, or when required because of trauma during surgery. An RCT has started in Japan to evaluate the role of splenectomy in total gastrectomy for proximal gastric cancer.[21]

OPTION **RADICAL VERSUS CONSERVATIVE LYMPHADENECTOMY**

Two large RCTs found no significant difference in 5 year survival rates between radical and conservative lymphadenectomy. However, confounding factors may have affected the reliability of results, and we found conflicting data from subgroup analyses of prospective cohort studies.

Benefits: We found no systematic review but found two RCTs comparing radical lymphadenectomy (D2)Ⓖ versus conservative lymphadenectomy (D1)Ⓖ.[22,23] The first RCT (711 people) found no significant difference in 5 year survival rates (45% with conservative lymphadenectomy *v* 47% with radical lymphadenectomy; ARR +2.0%, 95% CI –5.6% to +9.6%).[22] The second RCT (400 people) also found no significant difference in 5 year survival rates (35% with conservative lymphadenectomy *v* 33% with radical lymphadenectomy; HR 1.10, 95% CI 0.87 to 1.39, see comment below).[23]

Harms: The two large RCTs comparing radical versus conservative lymphadenectomy found increased perioperative mortality with the more extensive operation.[22,23] In the first RCT (711 people) the difference in mortality almost achieved significance (10% with D2 resection *v* 6% with D1 resection; P = 0.06). The second RCT (400 people) found significantly higher mortality with D2 than with D1 resection (13% with D2 *v* 6% with D1; P < 0.04). In both of these large RCTs the excess mortality may have been due to associated pancreatic and splenic removal, rather than the radical lymphadenectomy.[22,23]

Comment: The RCTs were conducted by surgeons with limited prior experience and training in D2 resection, and results may have been affected by both learning curve effects[24] and failure to apply the assigned treatment (contamination and non-compliance).[25] Subgroup analysis from the second RCT found a possible advantage for D2 resection in people with stage II and IIIA disease (corresponding to T1N2M0, T2N1M0, T3N0M0, T2N2M0, T3N1M0, and T4N0M0), particularly in those people who did not have additional organ removal.[23] One large prospective cohort study (1654 people with gastric cancer) found no benefit from D2 resection (defined within this study as > 25 lymph nodes removed; 300 people) compared with D1 resection (≤ 25 nodes removed; 1096 people) in the entire cohort of people with gastric cancer after 10 years' follow up. Subgroup analysis found that there may be a beneficial effect of D2 compared with D1 resection in the subgroup of people with stage II tumours (230 people; RR of long term survival 1.8, 95% CI 1.3 to 2.7).[26] Cohort studies comparing radical versus conservative lymphadenectomy are affected by numerous biases, particularly selection bias, where surgeons reserve D2 surgery for younger or fitter people, or where recent D2 operations are compared with historical D1 controls; differing definitions of "limited" and "extended"; and stage migration biasⒼ. These biases make the interpretation of observational data difficult.

QUESTION **What are the effects of adjuvant chemotherapy?**

OPTION **ADJUVANT CHEMOTHERAPY**

One large systematic review and two subsequent RCTs found that adjuvant chemotherapy increased survival compared with surgery alone. Two subsequent RCTs found no significant difference between adjuvant chemotherapy and surgery alone in 5 year survival.

Benefits: **Versus surgery alone:** We found one systematic review (search date 1999)[27] and four subsequent RCTs,[28–31] which compared adjuvant chemotherapy**G** versus surgery alone. The review (search date 2000, 20 RCTs, 3658 people; see comment below) found that adjuvant chemotherapy compared with surgery alone significantly reduced the risk of death (HR 0.82, 95% CI 0.75 to 0.89). The first subsequent RCT (137 people with gastric adenocarcinoma and positive lymph nodes) compared adjuvant chemotherapy versus surgery alone and found that adjuvant chemotherapy significantly increased median survival time (31 months [range 7 to > 60 months] with adjuvant chemotherapy *v* 18 months [range 2 to > 60 months] with surgery alone; $P < 0.01$; HR for death 1.96, 95% CI 1.32 to 2.92).[28] The second subsequent RCT (274 people with gastric adenocarcinoma T3, T4 or N1, N2) found no significant difference between adjuvant chemotherapy and surgery alone in 5 year survival (overall survival: 52% with adjuvant chemotherapy *v* 48% with surgery alone; HR 0.93, 95% CI 0.65 to 1.34).[29] The third subsequent RCT (139 people) compared three groups: surgery plus hyperthermic intraperitoneal chemotherapy; surgery plus normothermic intraperitoneal chemotherapy; and surgery alone.[30] It found that surgery plus hyperthermic chemotherapy (mitomycin C plus cisplatin at 42 °C) significantly increased overall 5 year survival rates versus surgery alone ($P = 0.01$; result presented graphically), and that surgery plus hyperthermic chemotherapy also significantly increased overall 5 year survival rates compared with surgery plus normothermic chemotherapy (mitomycin C plus cisplatin at 37 °C) ($P = 0.05$; result presented graphically). Subgroup analysis found that these results were consistent for people with advanced disease (T3 or node positive), but in people with less advanced disease (T2 or node negative) subgroup analysis found no significant difference in overall 5 year survival rates. The fourth subsequent RCT (252 people with serosa negative gastric cancer) found no significant difference in 5 year survival between adjuvant chemotherapy and surgery alone (91.2% with adjuvant chemotherapy *v* 86.1% with surgery alone, $P = 0.13$).[31]

Harms: The review did not report on harms.[27] Two RCTs included in the review reported toxicity (mainly nausea and vomiting) in 53% of people.[32,33] Serious toxicity was usually because of cardiac or cumulative haematological problems; treatment related mortality was 1–2%. Two subsequent RCTs reported no significant difference in postoperative complications with adjuvant chemotherapy.[30,31]

Comment: Two RCTs[34,35] included in the systematic review[27] may have been duplicate versions of the same RCT. Many more recent adjuvant chemotherapy regimens have not been evaluated fully in RCTs. One further meta-analysis has been identified, which is awaiting translation.[36] Preoperative superselective intra-arterial chemotherapy may not be available outside of specialist centres.

GLOSSARY

Adjuvant chemotherapy Treatment with cytotoxic drugs given in addition to surgery in an attempt to achieve cure.

Disease stage Surgical and microscopic assessment of the primary tumour. Microscopic spread to distant sites can be detected only by radical surgery, creating a potential bias.

Conservative lymphadenectomy (D1) Removal of perigastric lymph nodes — lymph nodes that lie adjacent to the stomach.

Radical lymphadenectomy (D2) Removal of regional lymph nodes — lymph nodes that lie along the blood vessels that supply the stomach.

Stage migration bias Apparent increase in stage specific survival without influencing overall survival caused by recategorisation of the stage after removal of diseased lymph nodes.

Subtotal distal gastrectomy Removal of lower part (usually two thirds or four fifths) of the stomach.
Total gastrectomy Removal of the whole stomach.
Total gastrectomy "de principe" Total gastrectomy where it is not technically necessary to remove a distal tumour; this technique is used to minimise the risk of resection line involvement or later second cancer of the gastric stump.

REFERENCES

1. Whelan SL, Parkin DM, Masuyer E, eds. *Trends in cancer incidence and mortality* (IARC scientific publication no. 102). Lyon: IARC Scientific Publications, 1993.
2. Cancer Research Campaign. *Factsheet 18*. London: Cancer Research Campaign, 1993.
3. Powell J, McConkey CC. Increasing incidence of adenocarcinoma of the gastric cardia and adjacent sites. *Br J Cancer* 1990;62:440–443.
4. Devesa SS, Blot WJ, Fraumeni JF Jr. Changing patterns in the incidence of esophageal and gastric carcinoma in the United States. *Cancer* 1998;83:2049–2053.
5. EUROGAST study group. An international association between *Helicobacter pylori* infection and gastric cancer. *Lancet* 1993;341:1359–1362.
6. Buiatti E, Palli D, Decarli A, et al. A case-control study of gastric cancer and diet in Italy. II Association with nutrients. *Int J Cancer* 1990;45:896–901.
7. Rios-Castellanos E, Sitas F, Shepherd NA, et al. Changing pattern of gastric cancer in Oxfordshire. *Gut* 1992;33:1312–1317.
8. Boddie AW Jr, McMurtrey MJ, Giacco GG, et al. Palliative total gastrectomy and esophagogastrectomy: an evaluation. *Cancer* 1983;51:1195–2000.
9. McCulloch P. Should general surgeons treat gastric carcinoma? An audit of practice and results. *Br J Surg* 1994;81:417–420.
10. Kohli Y, Kawai K, Fujita S. Analytical studies of the growth of human gastric cancer. *J Clin Gastroenterol* 1981;3:129–133.
11. Maruyama K, Okabayashi K, Kinoshita T. Progress in gastric cancer surgery in Japan and its limits of radicality. *World J Surg* 1987;11:418–425.
12. Jakl RJ, Miholic J, Koller R, et al. Prognostic factors in adenocarcinoma of the cardia. *Am J Surg* 1995;169:316–319.
13. Allum WH, Hallissey MT, Kelly KA. Adjuvant chemotherapy in operable gastric cancer: 5 year follow-up of the first British Stomach Cancer Group trial. *Lancet* 1989;1:571–574.
14. Bozzetti F, Marubini E, Bonfanti G, et al. Total versus subtotal gastrectomy: surgical morbidity and mortality rates in a multicenter Italian randomized trial. *Ann Surg* 1997;226:613–620.
15. Bozzetti F, Marubini E, Bonfanti G, et al. Subtotal versus total gastrectomy for gastric cancer: five-year survival rates in a multicenter randomized Italian trial. *Ann Surg* 1999;230:170–178.
16. Gouzi JL, Huguier M, Fagniez PL, et al. Gastrectomie totale contre gastrectomie partielle pour adeno-cancer de l'antre. Une etude francaise prospective controlee. *Ann Chir* 1989;43:356–360.
17. Gouzi JL, Huguier M, Fagniez PL, et al. Total versus subtotal gastrectomy for adenocarcinoma of the gastric antrum. A French prospective controlled study. *Ann Surg* 1989;209:162–166.
18. Csendes A, Burdiles P, Rojas J, et al. A prospective randomised study comparing D2 total gastrectomy versus D2 total gastrectomy plus splenectomy in 187 patients with gastric carcinoma. *Surgery* 2002;131:401–407.
19. Bonenkamp JJ, Songun I, Hermans J, et al. Randomised comparison of morbidity after D1 and D2 dissection for gastric cancer in 996 Dutch patients. *Lancet* 1995;345:745–748.
20. Cuschieri A, Fayers P, Fielding J, et al. Postoperative morbidity and mortality after D1 and D2 resections for gastric cancer: preliminary results of the MRC randomised controlled surgical trial. *Lancet* 1996;347:995–999.
21. Sano T, Yamanoto S, Sasako M. Randomized controlled trial to evaluate splenectomy in total gastrectomy for proximal gastric cancer. *Jpn J Clin Oncol* 2002;32:363–364.
22. Bonenkamp JJ, Hermans J, Sasako M, et al. Extended lymph-node dissection for gastric cancer. Dutch Gastric Cancer Group. *N Engl J Med* 1999;340:908–914.
23. Cuschieri A, Weedon S, Fielding J, et al. Patient survival after D1 and D2 resections for gastric cancer: long-term results of the MRC randomised surgical trial. *Br J Cancer* 1999;79:1522–1530.
24. Parikh D, Chagla L, Johnson M, et al. D2 gastrectomy: lessons from a prospective audit of the learning curve. *Br J Surg* 1996;83:1595–1599.
25. Bunt AMG, Hermans J, Boon MC, et al. Evaluation of the extent of lymphadenectomy in a randomised trial of Western versus Japanese style surgery in gastric cancer. *J Clin Oncol* 1994;12:417–422.
26. Siewert JR, Bottcher K, Stein HJ, et al. Relevant prognostic factors in gastric cancer: ten-year results of the German Gastric Cancer Study. *Ann Surg* 1998;228:449–461.
27. Mari E, Floriani I, Tinazzi A, et al. Efficacy of adjuvant chemotherapy after curative resection for gastric cancer: a meta-analysis of published randomised trials. A study of the GISCAD (Gruppo Italiano per lo Studio dei Carcinomi dell'Apparato Digerente). *Ann Oncol* 2000;11:837–843. Search date 2000; primary sources Medline, Embase, Cancerlit, and hand searched references.
28. Neri B, Cini G, Andreoli F, et al. Randomized trial of adjuvant chemotherapy versus control after curative resection for gastric cancer: 5-year follow-up. *Br J Cancer* 2001;84:878–880.
29. Bajetta E, Buzzoni R, Mariani L, et al. Adjuvant chemotherapy in gastric cancer: 5-year results of a randomised study by the Italian Trials in Medical Oncology (ITMO) Group. *Ann Oncol* 2002;13:299–307.
30. Yonemura Y, De Aretxabala X, Fujimura T, et al. Intraoperative chemohyperthermic peritoneal perfusion as an adjuvant to gastric cancer: final results of a randomized controlled study. *Hepato-gastroenterology* 2001;48:1776–1782.
31. Nashimoto A, Nakajima T, Furukawa H, et al. Randomized trial of adjuvant chemotherapy with mitomycin, Fluorouracil, and Cytosine arabinoside followed by oral Fluorouracil in serosa-negative gastric cancer: Japan Clinical Oncology Group 9206–1. *J Clin Oncol* 2003;21:2282–2287.
32. Coombes RC, Schein PS, Chilvers CE, et al. A randomised trial comparing adjuvant 5-fluoro-uracil, doxorubicin and mitomycin C with no treatment in operable gastric cancer. International Collaborative Cancer Group. *J Clin Oncol* 1990;8:1362–1369.
33. Hallissey MT, Dunn JA, Ward LC, et al. The second British Stomach Cancer Group trial of adjuvant radiotherapy or chemotherapy in advanced gastric cancer: 5 year follow-up. *Lancet* 1994;343:1309–1312.
34. Alcobendas F, Milla A, Estape J, et al. Mitomycin C as an adjuvant in resected gastric cancer. *Ann Surg* 1983;198:13–17.
35. Grau JJ, Estape J, Alcobendas F. Positive results of adjuvant mitomycin C in resected gastric cancer: a randomised trial on 134 patients. *Eur J Cancer* 1993;29A:340–342.
36. Panzini I, Gianni L, Fattori P, et al. Adjuvant chemotherapy in gastric cancer: a meta-analysis of randomized trials and a comparison with previous meta-analyses. *Tumori* 2002;88:21–27.

Stomach cancer

Charles Bailey
Clinical Research Fellow
Department of Surgery, Oncology, and Technology Imperial College
London
UK

Competing interests: None declared.
The previous contributor of this topic would also like to be acknowledged: Peter McCulloch.

TABLE 1 Staging of stomach cancer (see text, p 571).

Stage	Description
T1	Involvement of mucosa ± submucosa
T2	Involvement of muscularis propria
T3	Involvement of serosa but no spread to adjacent organs
T4	Involvement of adjacent organs
N0	No lymph node involvement
N1	Local (perigastric) nodes involved
N2	Regional nodes involved
N3	More distant intra-abdominal nodes involved
M0	No metastases
M1	Metastases

TABLE 2 Different types of surgical resection for stomach cancer (see text, p 573).

Resection	Description
R0	Removal of all detectable tumour, with a margin of healthy tissue confirmed microscopically: synonymous with "curative" resection.
R1	Incomplete removal, with histological evidence of cancer at the resection margin.
R2	Incomplete removal, with macroscopically obvious remnants of the main tumour: synonymous with "palliative" resection.
D1	Removal of all or part of the stomach, together with local (perigastric) nodes.
D2	Removal of all or part of the stomach, together with local and regional nodes, which lie along the branches of the coeliac axis.
D3/D4	More radical lymph node resection, including removal of para-aortic nodes and nodes within the small bowel mesentery.

Chronic suppurative otitis media

Search date November 2003

Jose Acuin

QUESTIONS

INTERVENTIONS

Key Messages

Adults

- **Topical antibiotics** We found no RCTs with long term follow up. Two RCTs found limited evidence that topical quinolone antibiotics improved otoscopic appearances compared with placebo in adults with chronic suppurative otitis media. Six RCTs found no clear evidence of clinically important differences among topical antibiotics in adults. One systematic review found that topical antibiotics were more effective than systemic antibiotics for reducing otoscopic features of chronic suppurative otitis media. One RCT found no significant difference between topical ceftizoxime plus systemic ceftizoxime and systemic ceftizoxime alone. One RCT found no significant difference between preoperative topical antibiotics and no preoperative treatment in people undergoing tympanoplasty. Short term topical antibiotics have been associated with few adverse events in RCTs. Uncontrolled case studies have reported vestibular ototoxicity after topical non-quinolone antibiotics.
- **Ear cleansing (aural toilet)** We found no RCTs comparing ear cleansing versus no treatment in adults.
- **Systemic antibiotics** We found insufficient evidence about the effects of systemic antibiotics compared with placebo, no treatment, each other, or topical antiseptics. One systematic review found that systemic antibiotics were less effective than topical antibiotics in reducing otoscopic features of chronic suppurative otitis media. Two RCTs found no significant difference between systemic plus topical antibiotics and topical antibiotics alone, although a third RCT found that topical quinolone was more effective than oral plus topical non-quinolones. We found no evidence about long term treatment.

- **Topical antibiotics plus topical steroids** One systematic review found insufficient evidence from three RCTs about effects on symptoms of topical antibiotics plus topical steroids compared with placebo or topical steroids alone.
- **Topical antiseptics** We found no systematic reviews and no RCTs comparing topical antiseptics versus placebo or no treatment. One RCT in adults found no significant difference between topical antiseptics plus ear cleansing under microscopic control and either topical or oral antibiotics. One RCT found no significant difference in resolution of ear discharge between topical povidone–iodine and topical quinolone. The RCTs were too small to establish or exclude a clinically important effect from topical antiseptics in adults.
- **Topical steroids** We found no RCTs comparing topical steroids versus placebo or no treatment.
- **Tympanoplasty with or without mastoidectomy** We found no RCTs comparing tympanoplasty with or without mastoidectomy versus no surgery for chronic suppurative otitis media without cholesteatoma.

Children

- **Ear cleansing** One systematic review found insufficient evidence from two RCTs to compare a simple form of ear cleansing versus no ear cleansing in children with chronic suppurative otitis media.
- **Systemic antibiotics** RCTs found insufficient evidence about the effects of systemic antibiotics in children with chronic suppurative otitis media.
- **Topical antibiotics** We found no systematic reviews and no RCTs comparing topical antibiotics versus placebo in children. One RCT with a high drop-out rate found that topical ciprofloxacin increased the proportion of children with no discharge at 10–21 days compared with a combination of framycetin, gramicidin, and dexamethasone eardrops.
- **Topical antibiotics plus topical steroids** Small RCTs found insufficient evidence to compare topical antibiotics plus topical steroids versus cleansing only or topical antiseptics. One RCT with a high drop-out rate found that topical ciprofloxacin increased the proportion of children with no discharge at 10–21 days compared with a combination of framycetin, gramicidin, and dexamethasone eardrops.
- **Topical antiseptics** Two RCTs found no significant difference in otorrhoea between topical antiseptics and control after 2 weeks. One RCT found no significant difference in otorrhoea between topical antiseptics and topical antibiotic plus steroid. However, the RCTs were too small to exclude a clinically important effect.
- **Topical steroids** We found no RCTs comparing topical steroids versus placebo or no treatment in children.
- **Tympanoplasty with or without mastoidectomy** We found no RCTs comparing tympanoplasty with or without mastoidectomy versus no surgery for chronic suppurative otitis media without cholesteatoma.

DEFINITION Chronic suppurative otitis media is persistent inflammation of the middle ear or mastoid cavity. Synonyms include "chronic otitis media (without effusion)", chronic mastoiditis, and chronic tympanomastoiditis. Chronic suppurative otitis media is characterised by recurrent or persistent ear discharge (otorrhoea) over 2–6 weeks through a perforation of the tympanic membrane. Typical findings also include thickened granular middle ear mucosa, mucosal polyps, and cholesteatoma🅖 within the middle ear. Chronic suppurative otitis media is differentiated from chronic otitis media with effusion, in which there is an intact tympanic membrane with fluid in the middle ear but no active infection. Chronic suppurative otitis media does not include chronic perforations of the eardrum that are dry, or only occasionally discharge, and have no signs of active infection.

INCIDENCE/ PREVALENCE The worldwide prevalence of chronic suppurative otitis media is 65–330 million people. Between 39–200 million (60%) suffer from clinically significant hearing impairment. Otitis media was estimated to have caused 28 000 deaths and loss of over 2 million Disability Adjusted Life Years🅖 in 2000,[1] 94% of which were in developing countries. Most of these deaths were probably due to chronic suppurative otitis media because acute otitis media is a self limiting infection. Estimates of prevalence are shown in table A on web extra.[2–32]

AETIOLOGY/ RISK FACTORS Chronic suppurative otitis media is assumed to be a complication of acute otitis media, but the risk factors for chronic suppurative otitis media are not clear. Frequent upper respiratory tract infections and poor socioeconomic conditions (overcrowded housing,[33] hygiene, and nutrition) may be related to the development of chronic suppurative otitis media.[34,35] Improvement in housing, hygiene, and nutrition in Maori children was associated with a halving of the prevalence of chronic suppurative otitis media between 1978 and 1987.[36] Also see acute otitis media, p 227.

PROGNOSIS Most children with chronic suppurative otitis media have mild to moderate hearing impairment (about 26–60 dB increase in hearing thresholds) based on surveys among children in Africa, Brazil,[37] India,[38] and Sierra Leone,[39] and among the general population in Thailand.[40] In many developing countries, chronic suppurative otitis media represents the most frequent cause of moderate hearing loss (40–60 dB).[41] Persistent hearing loss during the first 2 years of life may increase learning disabilities and poor scholastic performance.[42] Spread of infection may lead to life threatening complications such as intracranial infections and acute mastoiditis.[43] The frequency of serious complications fell from 20% in 1938 to 2.5% in 1948 and is currently estimated to be about 0.24% in Thailand and 1.8% in Africa. This is believed to be associated with increased use of antibiotic treatment, tympanoplasty, and mastoidectomy**G**.[44–46] Cholesteatoma is another serious complication that has been found in a variable proportion of people with chronic suppurative otitis media (range 0–60%).[47–50] In the West, the incidence of cholesteatoma is low (in 1993 in Finland the age standardised incidence of cholesteatoma was eight new cases per 100 000 population/year).[51]

AIMS OF INTERVENTION To improve symptoms of otorrhoea; heal perforations; improve hearing; and reduce complications, with minimum adverse effects of treatment.

OUTCOMES **Dichotomous variables:** Proportion of people with otorrhoea measured subjectively or by otoscopy; with tympanic perforation; hearing loss; intra- and extracranial complications; death; or adverse effects. The correlation between subjective cessation of otorrhoea and otoscopic findings was poor in one RCT.[52] Many RCTs used compound outcomes (e.g. otoscopic finding of otorrhoea or otoscopic finding of inflammation in the middle ear). **Continuous variables:** Duration of otorrhoea free periods; severity of hearing loss. "Otoscopic activity" refers to appearances on otoscopy such as active discharge from the middle ear and inflammation of the middle ear mucosa.

METHODS *Clinical Evidence* search and appraisal November 2003, including a search for observational studies on surgery. We found one systematic review (search date 1996, 24 RCTs, 1660 people) of treatments for chronic suppurative otitis media.[53] It did not analyse results for children and adults separately. We have excluded all studies that included both adults (aged ≥ 16) and children (aged ≤ 10),[54–57] or which failed to specify the age of participants.[58,59] The RCTs varied in their definitions of chronic suppurative otitis media and measurements of severity. All RCTs were brief (7 days to 3 weeks). Most had inadequate methods for us to draw reliable conclusions (see main text for descriptions). Participants with cholesteatoma were excluded from most, but not all, trials. All trials excluded people with impending serious complications.

QUESTION **What are the effects of treatments for chronic suppurative otitis media in adults?**

OPTION **EAR CLEANSING (AURAL TOILET)**

We found no RCTs comparing ear cleansing versus no treatment in adults.

Benefits: We found one systematic review (search date 1996), which found no RCTs in adults comparing ear cleansing**G** versus no treatment.[53]

Harms: We found no RCTs.

Comment: Techniques of ear cleansing vary considerably. In Western countries, microsuction of the external and middle ear under microscopic control by a trained operator is the standard method of ear cleansing. Microscopic examination of the ear with ear cleansing is an important aspect of diagnosis of persistent otorrhoea. RCTs comparing ear cleansing versus no treatment would probably be considered unethical.

OPTION TOPICAL ANTIBIOTICS

We found no RCTs with long term follow up. Two RCTs found limited evidence that topical quinolone antibiotics improved otoscopic appearances compared with placebo in adults with chronic suppurative otitis media. Six RCTs found no clear evidence of clinically important differences among topical antibiotics in adults. One systematic review found that topical antibiotics were more effective than systemic antibiotics for reducing otoscopic features of chronic suppurative otitis media. One RCT found no significant difference between topical ceftizoxime plus systemic ceftizoxime and systemic ceftizoxime alone. One RCT found no significant difference between preoperative topical antibiotics and no preoperative treatment in people undergoing tympanoplasty. Short term topical antibiotics have been associated with few adverse events in RCTs. Uncontrolled case studies have reported vestibular ototoxicity after topical non-quinolone antibiotics.

Benefits: **Versus placebo:** We found no systematic review but found two small RCTs in adults.[60,61] Both RCTs found that quinolone topical antibiotics improved otorrhoea compared with placebo, but both RCTs had weak methods. The first RCT (50 adults with chronic suppurative otitis media but no cholesteatoma **G** in a hospital clinic in Thailand) found that, after 7 days, topical ciprofloxacin in 0.9% sodium chloride (5 drops 0.25 g/L 3 times/day for 7 days) significantly reduced persistent signs on otoscopic examination compared with topical 0.9% sodium chloride (3/19 [16%] had persistent signs with ciprofloxacin *v* 14/16 [88%] with 0.9% sodium chloride solution; RR 0.18, 95% CI 0.06 to 0.52; NNT 2, 95% CI 2 to 3).[60] The RCT lasted only 7 days, had 30% loss to follow up (15/50), and did not clearly describe the methods of randomisation and allocation concealment. The second RCT (51 adults with chronic suppurative otitis media without cholesteatoma in a hospital clinic in Israel; 60 ears) compared 3 weeks' treatment with topical ciprofloxacin versus topical tobramycin versus a dilute antiseptic solution (1% aluminium acetate), which was used as a placebo.[61] It found that ciprofloxacin significantly reduced the proportion of people with unimproved otorrhoea compared with diluted aluminium acetate (4/19 [21%] with ciprofloxacin *v* 10/17 [59%] with diluted aluminium acetate; OR 0.21, 95% CI 0.06 to 0.80; NNT 3, 95% CI 2 to 18). The RCT found that tobramycin did not significantly reduce otorrhoea compared with control (5/18 [28%] with tobramycin *v* 10/17 [59%] with control; OR 0.29, 95% CI 0.08 to 1.09). This RCT randomised people to treatments, but presented results in terms of number of ears. The 1% aluminium acetate may not have been an inert control (see topical antiseptics, p 583). **Versus each other:** We found one systematic review (search date 1996,[53] 4 RCTs, 406 adults) and two subsequent RCTs (see table 1, p 593).[61,66] Three RCTs found no clear difference between the otoscopic response with a topical quinolone (ciprofloxacin) and that with topical non-quinolones (gentamicin, tobramycin, and polymyxin–neomycin–hydrocortisone). The three RCTs comparing different topical non-quinolone antibiotics found no significant difference in the proportion of people who still had a wet ear on otoscopy at the end of treatment (see table 1, p 593).[67–69] **Versus systemic antibiotics:** See benefits of systemic antibiotics, p 584. **Versus topical antiseptics:** See benefits of topical antiseptics, p 583. **Added to systemic antibiotics:** We found one RCT (248 adults), which compared topical ceftizoxime (2 g/day) versus 0.9% sodium chloride solution among people who were given intramuscular ceftizoxime for 7 days.[70] It found no significant difference at the end of treatment between the two groups in terms of improvement of symptoms and otoscopic findings (improvement 96% with topical ceftizoxime *v* 93% with 0.9% sodium chloride; RR and CI not reported). **Added to non-antibiotic treatments:** We found one RCT (101 adults about to undergo tympanoplasty**G**), which compared preoperative topical ofloxacin instilled for 10 minutes, preoperative topical ofloxacin instilled for 3 minutes, or no preoperative topical treatment.[71] It found no significant difference among groups for closure of tympanic perforations (28/33 with 10 minutes ofloxacin; 27/33 with 3 minutes ofloxacin; 31/35 with no treatment). However, the study may have lacked power to detect clinically important differences.

Harms: **Topical antibiotics versus placebo:** One systematic review found that adverse drug reaction rates in RCTs were low and did not vary appreciably among antibiotics.[53] The adverse events included *Candida* infections, dizziness, itching, stinging, and earache. One subsequent small RCT found no reported adverse events with topical ciprofloxacin used for 7 days in 19 ears.[60] Another subsequent RCT (322 people) found no significant difference in adverse event rate with topical ciprofloxacin versus topical polymyxin-B plus neomycin plus hydrocortisone (24/165 [15%] with ciprofloxacin *v* 12/153 [8%] with topical polymyxin-B plus neomycin plus hydrocortisone; RR 1.86, 95% CI 0.96 to 3.60).[66] Vertigo was reported by two people with topical ciprofloxacin and by none using topical polymyxin-B plus neomycin plus hydrocortisone. **Ototoxic effects of topical antibiotics:** We found one systematic review[53] and two subsequent RCTs[55,60] in adults and children, which examined hearing before and after topical antibiotics. The systematic review (search date 1996, 11 RCTs)[53] found negligible or no change in hearing after topical antibiotics. Three RCTs in adults and children[54,55,60] found no case of worsened hearing in those who were given topical ciprofloxacin or topical aminoglycoside. One RCT found deterioration of the audiogram in only one person with topical polymyxin-B plus neomycin plus hydrocortisone after 6–12 days (0/157 with topical ciprofloxacin *v* 1/138 with topical polymyxin-B plus neomycin plus hydrocortisone; OR 0.12, 95% CI 0.002 to 5.99).[66] The clinical importance of this difference is unclear.

Comment: There is consensus that topical antibiotics must be combined with thorough ear cleansing to be effective. We found no evidence about long term effects on complications. The comparative RCTs were small and their quality variable. We found no clear evidence from RCTs of ototoxicity from any topical antibiotic. Evidence about ototoxicity is based only on the assessment of audiograms after short term exposure to the antibiotics, and uncontrolled case studies have reported ototoxicity associated with some topical non-quinolone antibiotics for 7–120 days.[68,69,72] Most of the people in the observational studies had vestibular rather than cochlear symptoms, suggesting that the evidence from audiograms and hearing tests may not exclude ototoxicity. Most topical non-quinolone antibiotics have license restrictions against prolonged use, or use in people with perforation of the ear drum.

OPTION TOPICAL ANTIBIOTICS PLUS TOPICAL STEROIDS

One systematic review found insufficient evidence from three RCTs about effects on symptoms of topical antibiotics plus topical steroids compared with placebo or topical steroids alone.

Benefits: **Versus placebo:** We found one systematic review (search date 1996,[53] 2 RCTs,[52,73] 196 people, no pooling of results) of combined topical antibiotics plus steroid for 4–6 weeks compared with placebo.

Both RCTs found that topical antibiotics plus steroid significantly reduced persistent otorrhoea compared with control. The first RCT (123 adults with chronic suppurative otitis media, no cholesteatoma, and no open mastoid cavity) found that significantly fewer people had otoscopically active otitis media after treatment with gentamicin plus hydrocortisone than with placebo (appearance of active otitis: 33/64 [52%] people with treatment *v* 44/59 [75%] with placebo; OR 0.38, 95% CI 0.18 to 0.78).[52] Similar results were found in 42 other people who had an open mastoid cavity. The second RCT (31 adults) also found that gentamicin plus hydrocortisone reduced active otitis media on otoscopy compared with placebo at the end of 4 weeks of treatment (6/17 [35%] with treatment *v* 11/14 [79%] with placebo; OR 0.18, 95% CI 0.05 to 0.75).[73] **Versus topical steroid:** The systematic review[53] identified one RCT (64 adults),[67] which found that topical gentamicin plus hydrocortisone reduced the proportion of people with persistent activity on otoscopy compared with betametasone after 3 weeks of treatment (6/30 [20%] with gentamicin–hydrocortisone *v* 17/24 [71%] with betametasone; RR 0.28, 95% CI 0.13 to 0.60; NNT 2, 95% CI 2 to 4).

Harms: See harms of topical antibiotics, p 582.

Comment: See comment under topical antibiotics, p 582.

OPTION TOPICAL ANTISEPTICS (ALUMINIUM ACETATE, BORAX, BORIC ACID, HYDROGEN PEROXIDE, IODINE POWDER)

We found no systematic reviews and no RCTs comparing topical antiseptics versus placebo or no treatment. One RCT in adults found no significant difference between topical antiseptics plus ear cleansing under microscopic control and either topical or oral antibiotics. One RCT found no significant difference in resolution of ear discharge between topical povidone–iodine and topical quinolone. The RCTs were too small to establish or exclude a clinically important effect from topical antiseptics in adults.

Benefits: **Versus placebo:** We found no systematic review and no RCT. **Versus topical antibiotics:** We found one systematic review (search date 1996,[53] 1 RCT,[74] 51 adults) and one subsequent RCT.[75] The RCT identified by the review compared three treatments: topical antiseptics, topical antibiotics, and oral antibiotics.[74] It found no significant difference between topical antiseptics (boric acid and iodine powder plus ear cleansing **G** under microscopic vision) and topical antibiotics (gentamicin or chloramphenicol) in persistent activity on otoscopy (13/20 [65%] with topical antiseptics *v* 15/18 [83%] with topical antibiotics; OR 0.40, 95% CI 0.10 to 1.66).[74] The subsequent RCT (40 people over 10 years of age in India) compared 10 days treatment with 5% topical povidone–iodine (3 drops three times daily) versus 0.3% topical ciprofloxacin.[75] It found similar proportions of people with resolution of discharge after 4 weeks (14/19 [74%] with povidone *v* 18/21 [86%] with ciprofloxacin; P value not reported). **Versus systemic antibiotics:** See benefits of systemic antibiotics, p 584.

Harms: Adverse effects included dizziness and local pain. The systematic review found negligible or no changes in hearing acuity after topical treatment.[53] In the subsequent RCT comparing topical povidone–iodine versus topical ciprofloxacin, none of the participants developed allergic reactions or deterioration of audiometric thresholds.[75]

Comment: The available evidence from RCTs in adults is insufficient to establish or exclude a clinically important effect from topical antiseptics.

OPTION TOPICAL STEROIDS

We found no RCTs in adults comparing topical steroids versus placebo or no treatment.

Benefits: We found no systematic review or RCTs.

Harms: We found no systematic review or RCTs.

Comment: Topical steroids have been used in combination with topical antibiotics (see topical antibiotics, p 581).

OPTION SYSTEMIC ANTIBIOTICS

We found insufficient evidence about the effects of systemic antibiotics compared with placebo, no treatment, each other, or topical antiseptics. One systematic review found that systemic antibiotics were less effective than topical antibiotics in reducing otoscopic features of chronic suppurative otitis media. Two RCTs found no significant difference between systemic plus topical antibiotics and topical antibiotics alone, although a third RCT found that topical quinolone was more effective than oral plus topical non-quinolones. We found no evidence about long term treatment.

Benefits: **Versus placebo in people receiving no other treatment:** We found one systematic review (search date 1996), which found no RCTs investigating the effects of systemic antibiotics in adults receiving no other treatment.[53] **Versus topical antibiotics:** We found one systematic review (search date 1996,[53] 5 RCTs, 271 adults) (see table 2, p 594).[74,76–79] All RCTs found a better response with topical antibiotics than with systemic antibiotics. The topical antibiotics used were ofloxacin, ciprofloxacin, gentamicin, and chloramphenicol. The systemic antibiotics were oral cefalexin, cloxacillin, amoxicillin, ofloxacin, ciprofloxacin, co-amoxiclav, and intramuscular gentamicin. The systematic review found that, overall, topical antibiotics were more effective than systemic antibiotics at reducing otoscopic features of chronic suppurative otitis media by the end of the trials (34/153 [22%] with topical antibiotics v 77/138 [56%] with systemic antibiotics; OR 0.23, 95% CI 0.14 to 0.37). **Versus topical antiseptics:** We found one systematic review (search date 1996, 2 RCTs, 152 people).[53] The first RCT (51 adults) compared three treatments: oral antibiotics (cefalexin, flucloxacillin, cloxacillin, or amoxicillin according to bacterial sensitivity), topical antiseptics (boric acid and iodine powder plus ear cleansing**G** under microscopic vision), and topical antibiotics (gentamicin or chloramphenicol).[74] It found no significant difference between oral antibiotics and topical antiseptics in the rate of persistent activity on otoscopy (8/13 [62%] with oral antibiotics v 13/20 [65%] with topical antiseptics v 15/18 [83%] with topical antibiotics; for oral antibiotic v topical antiseptic: OR 0.87, 95% CI 0.21 to 3.61). The second RCT (119 people with an age range from 11–79 years) found no significant difference between topical hydrogen peroxide or boric acid for 10–20 days versus various systemic antibiotics (choice based on sensitivity results, administered orally or intravenously) for otoscopically persistent discharge or inflamed mucosa at the end of treatment (33/71 [46%] with systemic antibiotic v 29/48 [60%] with topical antiseptic: OR 0.58, 95% CI 0.28 to 1.19). The confidence interval was too large to exclude a clinically important difference. **Systemic antibiotics versus other systemic antibiotics:** We found one systematic review (search date 1996,[53] 1 RCT, 75 adults) and two subsequent RCTs.[80,81] The RCT in the systematic review found no clear evidence of differences between oral ciprofloxacin (500 mg twice daily) and amoxicillin–clavulanate (500 mg 3 times daily) given for 5–10 days in persistent otoscopic activity at 3–4 weeks (16/40 [40%] with ciprofloxacin *v* 22/35 [63%] with amoxicillin–clavulanate; OR 0.41, 95% CI 0.16 to 1.00). The first subsequent RCT (190 adults) found no significant difference between oral cefotiam hexetil and amoxicillin–clavulanate given for 10 days in persistent otoscopic abnormality after the end of treatment (37/94 [39%] with cefotiam *v* 33/94 [35%] with amoxicillin–clavulanate; OR 1.20, 95% CI 0.67 to 2.16; see comment below).[80] The second subsequent RCT (30 adults, 22 analysed) compared oral levofloxacin (500 mg once daily) versus oral co-amoxiclav (675 mg three times daily) for 10 days.[81] It found no significant difference between treatments in the proportion of people with no discharge at 15 days (9/10 [90%] *v* 6/12 [50%]; P value not reported). The RCT may have been too small to detect a clinically important difference. **Added to other non-antibiotic treatments:** We found one systematic review (search date 1996,[53] 1 RCT,[82] 26 adults) comparing systemic antibiotics versus placebo in people receiving other forms of treatment. The RCT (26 adults having mastoidectomy/tympanoplasty Ⓖ) found that intravenous ceftazidime (2 g 12 hours preoperatively and 1–2 g 8 hourly for 5 days postoperatively) reduced the proportion of people with otorrhoea on otoscopy or with positive *Pseudomonas aeruginosa* cultures at 2 months compared with no antibiotic (1/14 [7%] with iv ceftazidime *v* 7/12 [58%] with no antibiotic; OR 0.10, 95% CI 0.02 to 0.51).[82] Although randomisation was thorough, groups are likely to have been unbalanced for baseline severity, with more people in the antibiotic arm having only tympanoplasty. **Added to topical antibiotics:** We found one systematic review (search date 1996,[53] 2 RCTs,[76,82] 100 adults). The first included RCT found no significant difference in otorrhoea at 2 weeks with topical ciprofloxacin with and without oral ciprofloxacin given for 5–10 days (5/20 [25%] with oral ciprofloxacin *v* 3/20 [15%] with no oral ciprofloxacin; OR 1.84, 95% CI 0.40 to 8.49).[76] The second RCT found no significant difference in otorrhoea at the end of treatment with topical gentamicin–hydrocortisone (for 4 weeks) with and without oral metronidazole given for 2 weeks (6/14 [43%] with metronidazole *v* 6/16 [38%] without metronidazole; OR 1.24, 95% CI 0.29 to 5.23).[83] **Oral plus topical non-quinolone antibiotics versus topical quinolone antibiotics alone:** We found one RCT (80 adults, 89 ears),[84] which found that topical ofloxacin (0.3%) reduced the proportion of ears exhibiting persistent signs (ear pain, discharge, or inflammation on otoscopic examination) after 2 weeks compared with oral amoxicillin (amoxycillin) plus topical chloramphenicol (33% of ears with ofloxacin *v* 63% of ears with oral amoxicillin plus topical chloramphenicol; number of ears examined not reported; $P < 0.001$). The RCT randomised people but analysed the number of ears with persistent otorrhoea.

Harms: The systematic review found that adverse effects of systemic antibiotics include *Candida* infections, headache, nausea, and allergic reactions.[53] One RCT (80 adults) reported ototoxicity (defined as an elevation in bone conduction thresholds, speech reception thresholds of ≥ 5 dB, or both) with amoxicillin–chloramphenicol but not with ciprofloxacin (absolute numbers not reported).[84] The RCT comparing oral levofloxacin versus oral co-amoxiclav found no adverse effects.[81]

Comment: We found one further, recent RCT comparing quinolone with non-quinolone antibiotics, which is being translated for consideration in future *Clinical Evidence* updates.[85]

OPTION — TYMPANOPLASTY WITH OR WITHOUT MASTOIDECTOMY

We found no RCTs comparing tympanoplasty with or without mastoidectomy versus no surgery for chronic suppurative otitis media without cholesteatoma.

Benefits: We found no systematic review and no RCTs.

Harms: We found no RCTs.

Comment: We found many retrospective cohort studies. One of these (41 people with bilateral chronic suppurative otitis media operated on at one unit in Italy) compared hearing in ears that had previous tympanoplasty versus hearing in contralateral ears treated without surgery.[86] The hearing in both operated and non-operated ears progressively deteriorated, but the rate of decline was significantly slower in operated ears. Tympanoplasty**G** can be combined with mastoidectomy**G** when the possibility of restoring some functional hearing without jeopardising surgical clearance of the disease exists. Observational studies have found that the success of surgery depends on several factors: age, technical skill of the surgeon,[87] availability of remnant eardrum and ossicles,[88] and type of mastoidectomy performed. The success rate for sealing a tympanic perforation with a graft can be 90–95%. Hearing deficit may be corrected in about 50–70% of operated ears.[89–91]

QUESTION **What are the effects of treatments for chronic suppurative otitis media in children?**

OPTION **EAR CLEANSING**

One systematic review found insufficient evidence from two RCTs to compare a simple form of ear cleansing versus no ear cleansing in children with chronic suppurative otitis media.

Benefits: **Versus no treatment:** We found one systematic review (search 1996,[53] 2 RCTs,[92,93] 658 children), which found no significant difference in persistent otorrhoea or persistent ear drum perforation between a simple form of ear cleansing**G** and no ear cleansing over 3–16 weeks (persisting otorrhoea, 2 RCTs; 125/170 [74%] with ear cleansing *v* 91/114 [80%] with no treatment; OR 0.63, 95% CI 0.36 to 1.12; persisting tympanic perforations, 1 RCT;[92] 125/144 [87%] *v* 63/73 [87%]; OR 1.04, 95% CI 0.46 to 2.38).

Harms: The review did not provide any evidence about the adverse effects of ear cleansing.

Comment: Techniques of ear cleansing vary considerably. In some countries, microsuction of the external and middle ear under microscopic control by a trained operator is a standard method of ear cleansing. In other countries, cleansing of the external auditory canal may be performed by parents, carers, or peers by dry mopping with cotton wool on orange sticks around four times daily. Both RCTs were performed in areas with a high prevalence of chronic suppurative otitis media (Solomon Islands[92] and Kenya[93]). The first RCT followed all the randomised children for 6 weeks but presented results as number of ears with persistent otorrhoea.[92] The second RCT randomised 145 schools but analysed the numbers of children with persistent otorrhoea.[93] It followed children for 16 weeks, but analysed results only for the 72% of the children who completed the RCT. Neither study described allocation concealment methods. In one RCT,[23] the randomisation process was described, but outcome assessors were not blinded to treatment allocation. The results of the meta-analysis in the systematic review[53] need to be approached with care because it combined results from the first RCT for the numbers of ears with persistent signs at 6 weeks with results from the second RCT for the number of children with persistent signs after 16 weeks. There was significant heterogeneity between the two RCTs in the effect of ear cleansing on otorrhoea (P = 0.02). Overall, we found no good evidence of benefit from simple ear cleansing, but the evidence is not strong enough to exclude a clinically important benefit.

OPTION TOPICAL ANTIBIOTICS

We found no systematic reviews and no RCTs comparing topical antibiotics versus placebo in children. One RCT with a high drop-out rate found that topical ciprofloxacin increased the proportion of children with no discharge at 10–21 days compared with a combination of framycetin, gramicidin, and dexamethasone eardrops.

Benefits: **Versus placebo:** We found no systematic reviews and no RCTs comparing topical antibiotics versus placebo in children. **Versus each other:** We found one systematic review (search date 1996[53]), which identified no RCTs exclusively in children with chronic suppurative otitis media. **Versus oral antibiotics:** We found one systematic review (search date 2000[94]), which identified no RCTs in children. **Versus topical antibiotics plus topical steroids:** We found one RCT (147 children aged 1–14 years with at least 2 weeks of otorrhoea and eardrum perforation, 36 dropped out, see comment below), which compared 0.3% topical ciprofloxacin versus a combination of framycetin (0.5%) plus gramicidin plus dexamethasone eardrops (5 drops twice daily for 9 days).[95] All ears were gently syringed with povidone–iodine (0.5%) prior to instillation of topical antibiotics. The RCT found that ciprofloxacin significantly increased cure rates compared with the combination treatment after 10–21 days (cured defined as absence of discharge: 42/55 [76.4%] with ciprofloxacin *v* 29/56 [51.8%] with combination; P = 0.009). It found no significant difference between treatments in size of perforation (P = 0.59) or hearing impairment (P = 0.62). However, results may have been confounded by different antibiotics being administered in either treatment arm.

Harms: The RCT comparing ciprofloxacin versus combination treatment reported that 21 children (18.9%) reported minor adverse reactions including bitter taste, ear pain, and transient dizziness (bitter taste: 8 children with ciprofloxacin *v* 6 with combination; ear pain: 3 with ciprofloxacin *v* 2 with combination; transient dizziness: 2 with ciprofloxacin *v* 1 with combination; P value not reported).[95]

Comment: We found no RCTs evaluating ototoxicity from any topical antibiotic. Evidence about ototoxicity is based only on the assessment of audiograms after short term exposure to the antibiotics, and uncontrolled case studies have reported ototoxicity associated with use of some topical non-quinolone antibiotics for 7–120 days.[96–98] Most of the people in the observational studies had vestibular rather than cochlear symptoms, suggesting that the evidence from audiograms and hearing tests may not exclude ototoxicity. Most topical non-quinolone antibiotics have license restrictions against prolonged use, or use in people with perforation of the eardrum. The RCT comparing topical ciprofloxacin with combination ear drops had a high drop-out rate (almost 25%).[94]

OPTION TOPICAL ANTIBIOTICS PLUS TOPICAL STEROIDS

Small RCTs found insufficient evidence to compare topical antibiotics plus topical steroids versus cleansing only or topical antiseptics. One RCT with a high drop-out rate found that topical ciprofloxacin increased the proportion of children with no discharge at 10–21 days compared with a combination of framycetin, gramicidin, and dexamethasone eardrops.

Benefits: **Versus placebo:** We found one systematic review (search date 1996,[53] 1 RCT,[92] 50 children, 67 ears) comparing combined topical antibiotics plus steroid (topical dexamethasone 0.05%, framycetin sulphate 0.5%, gramicidin 0.005%) versus ear cleansing**G** only. The RCT found no significant difference between topical antibiotics plus steroid and ear cleansing only in the proportion of ears with unchanged otorrhoea on otoscopy after 6 weeks (17/41 [42%] with topical antibiotic plus steroid plus ear cleansing *v* 13/26 [50%] with ear cleansing alone; OR 0.71, 95% CI 0.27 to 1.90). **Versus topical antiseptics:** We found one systematic review (search date 1996,[53] 1 RCT,[92] 55 children, 73 ears), which found no significant difference between topical antiseptic (boric acid 2% in 20% alcohol, 3 drops to each ear, 4 times daily after ear cleansing) and topical antibiotic plus steroid (dexamethasone 0.05%, framycetin sulphate 0.5%, gramicidin 0.005%) in the proportion of ears with persistent otorrhoea (12/32 [38%] with topical antiseptic *v* 17/41 [41%] with topical antibiotic plus steroid; OR 0.85, 95% CI 0.33 to 2.17). **Versus topical steroid or topical antibiotics alone:** See benefits of topical antibiotics in children, p 587.

Harms: **Versus placebo or topical antiseptics:** The RCTs did not provide any evidence about harms.[53] **Versus topical steroid or topical antibiotics alone:** See harms of topical antibiotics in children, p 587.

Comment: One RCT[23] found no difference in effectiveness between topical antibiotics with steroids and ear cleansing alone. However, this study was small, did not report methods for allocation concealment and blinding, and randomised children but analysed ears. We found no RCTs or systematic reviews about long term effects on complications. See comment under topical antibiotics, p 587.

OPTION **TOPICAL ANTISEPTICS (ALUMINIUM ACETATE, BORAX, BORIC ACID, HYDROGEN PEROXIDE, IODINE POWDER)**

Two RCTs found no significant difference in otorrhoea between topical antiseptics and control. One RCT found no significant difference in otorrhoea between topical antiseptics and topical antibiotic plus steroid. However, the RCTs were too small to exclude a clinically important effect.

Benefits: **Versus placebo:** We found no systematic review but found two RCTs.[92,99] The first RCT (60 children with otorrhoea in a hospital clinic in South Africa, 67 ears) compared aluminium acetate solutions of varying concentrations (13.00% *v* 3.25% *v* 1.30%).[99] The most dilute solution was considered to be inactive. Results were obtained for 56 (84%) ears. The RCT found no significant difference in dry ears after 2 weeks (21/26 [81% of ears] with 13% aluminium acetate *v* 15/20 [75%] with a 3.25% aluminium acetate *v* 5/10 [50%] with 1.3% aluminium acetate; P = 0.18). The second RCT (43 children, 58 ears) found no significant difference between topical antiseptic (boric acid 2% in 20% alcohol, 3 drops to each ear, 4 times daily after ear cleansing **G**) and ear cleansing alone in the proportion of children with unchanged otoscopic appearance after 6 weeks (12/32 [38%] with topical antiseptic *v* 13/26 [50%] with ear cleansing alone; OR 0.61, 95% CI 0.22 to 1.71).[92] **Versus topical antibiotic plus steroid:** See benefits of topical antibiotics plus topical steroids, p 587. **Versus systemic antibiotics:** See benefits of systemic antibiotics in children, p 589.

Harms: Adverse effects included dizziness and local pain. The systematic review found negligible or no changes in hearing acuity after topical treatment.[53]

Comment: We found small studies, which found no difference in the short term effects of topical antiseptics compared with systemic antibiotics (see systemic antibiotics, p 589). The available evidence is insufficient to establish or exclude a clinically important effect from topical antiseptics.

OPTION TOPICAL STEROIDS

We found no RCTs comparing topical steroids versus placebo or no treatment in children.

Benefits: We found no systematic review or RCTs.

Harms: We found no RCTs.

Comment: None.

OPTION SYSTEMIC ANTIBIOTICS

RCTs found insufficient evidence about the effects of systemic antibiotics in children with chronic suppurative otitis media.

Benefits: **Versus placebo in children receiving no other treatment:** We found one systematic review (search date 1996),[53] which found no RCTs investigating the effects of systemic antibiotics in children receiving no other treatment. **Versus topical antibiotics:** We found one systematic review (search date 1996, no RCTs) and no subsequent RCTs.[53] **Versus topical antiseptics:** One systematic review (search date 1996) found no RCTs.[53] **Versus each other:** We found one systematic review (search date 1996,[53] 1 RCT, 36 children) and one subsequent RCT.[100] The systematic review found no significant difference in otoscopic evidence of otorrhoea between intravenous mezlocillin and intravenous ceftazidime at the end of treatment (otoscopic evidence of otorrhoea: 0/17 [0%] with mezlocillin *v* 0/19 [0%] with ceftazidime).[53] The subsequent RCT (30 children) found no significant difference in success rates (complete disappearance of discharge) and days to disappearance between ceftazidime and aztreonam (disappearance of discharge: 84.6% with ceftazidime *v* 67.0% with aztreonam; P value reported as not significant; days to disappearance of discharge: 7.9 days with ceftazidime *v* 8.4 days with aztreonam).[100] **Added to non-antibiotic treatments:** We found one systematic review (search date 1996,[53] 1 RCT,[101] 33 children). The RCT (33 children having ear cleansing by suctioning and debridement for 1–2 weeks) found that intravenous antibiotic (mezlocillin or ceftazidime for 3–21 days) significantly reduced persistent otorrhoea detected at otoscopy after 6 months compared with no antibiotic (0/21 [0%] with iv antibiotic *v* 11/12 [92%]; OR 0.02, 95% CI 0.004 to 0.08). **Added to topical antibiotics:** We found one systematic review (search date 1996,[53] 1 RCT[92]). The RCT (62 children, 81 ears, all treated with ear cleansing plus drops containing dexamethasone 0.05%, framycetin sulphate 0.5%, gramicidin 0.005%) found no significant difference between oral clindamycin (15 mg/kg daily) and no clindamycin on the proportion of ears with unchanged otoscopic otorrhoea after 6 weeks (23/40 [58%] with clindamycin *v* 17/41 [41%] without clindamycin; OR 1.88, 95% CI 0.79 to 4.48).[92]

Harms: The systematic review found that (in all age groups) adverse effects of systemic antibiotics included *Candida* infections, headache, nausea, and allergic reactions.[53]

Comment: We found no clear evidence from RCTs that systemic antibiotics differ in their effectiveness. The studies in children found similar results to those in adults.

OPTION TYMPANOPLASTY WITH OR WITHOUT MASTOIDECTOMY

We found no RCTs in children comparing tympanoplasty with or without mastoidectomy versus no surgery for chronic suppurative otitis media without cholesteatoma.

Benefits: We found no systematic review and no RCTs.

Harms: We found no RCTs.

Comment: We found no evidence from RCTs, but found numerous retrospective observational studies. Tympanoplasty is often combined with mastoidectomy whenever the possibility of restoring some functional hearing without jeopardising surgical clearance of the disease exists. Observational studies have found that the success of surgery depends on several factors (age, technical skill of the surgeon,[102] presence of middle ear discharge,[103] type of mastoidectomy performed, and technique of middle ear construction[87]). Success rate for sealing a tympanic perforation with a graft can be 90–95%. Hearing deficit may be corrected in about 50–70% of operated ears.[89–91]

GLOSSARY

Cholesteatoma An accumulation of epithelial debris in the middle ear cavity that can arise congenitally or can be acquired. The tissue is probably derived from skin. It grows slowly but can erode and destroy adjacent structures (ossicles, the mastoid, the inner ear, or the bone leading to the intracranial cavity) potentially leading to persistent pain and otorrhoea, hearing loss, dizziness, facial nerve paralysis, and intracranial infection.
Disability Adjusted Life Year (DALY) A measure of the impact of a condition, designed to include the loss attributable to premature death and the loss caused by a disability of known duration and severity. One DALY is equivalent to the loss of 1 year of healthy life.
Ear cleansing Also known as aural toilet, this consists of mechanical removal of ear discharge and other debris from the ear canal and middle ear by mopping with cotton pledgets, wicking with gauze, flushing with sterile solution, or suctioning. This can be done with an otomicroscope or under direct vision with adequate illumination of the middle ear.
Mastoidectomy A general term used to describe various surgical procedures that are usually used to remove abnormal parts of the mastoid bone and surrounding structures, or to allow access to the middle ear.
Tympanoplasty A general term used to describe various surgical repairs of the eardrum or ossicles of the middle ear to improve hearing in people with conductive deafness.

REFERENCES

1. World Health Report, 2000. http://www.who.int/whr/2001/archives/2000/en/pdf/Annex4-en.pdf (last accessed 21 July 2003).
2. Bastos I, Reimer A, Ingvarsson L, et al. Chronic otitis media and hearing loss among school children in a refugee camp in Angola. *J Audiol Med* 1995;4:1–11.
3. Bastos I, Reimer A, Lundgren K. Chronic otitis media and hearing loss in otitis in urban schoolchildren in Angola — a prevalence study. *J Audiol Med* 1993;2:129–140.
4. Manni JJ. Lema PN. Otitis media in Dar es Salaam, Tanzania. *J Laryngol Otol* 1987;101:222–228.
5. Bastos I, Mallya J, Ingvarsson L, et al. Middle ear disease and hearing impairment in northern Tanzania. A prevalence study of schoolchildren in the Moshi and Monduli districts. *Int J Pediatr Otorhinolaryngol* 1995;32:1–12.
6. McPherson B, Holborow CA. A study of deafness in West Africa: the Gambian Hearing Health Project. *Int J Pediatr Otorhinolaryngol* 1985;10:115–135.
7. Pisacane A, Ruas I. Bacteriology of otitis media in Mozambique. *Lancet* 1982;1:1305.
8. Halama AR, Voogt GR, Musgrave GM. Prevalence of otitis media in children in a black rural community in Venda (South Africa). *Int J Pediatr Otorhinolaryngol* 1986;11:73–77.
9. Hatcher J, Smith A, Mackenzie I, et al. A prevalence study of ear problems in school children in Kiambu district, Kenya, May 1992. *Int J Pediatr Otorhinolaryngol* 1995;33:197–205.
10. Okeowo PA. Observations on the incidence of secretory otitis media in children. *J Trop Pediatr* 1985;31:295–298.
11. Bal I, Hatcher J. Results of Kenyan Prevalence Survey. *Her Net News* 1992;4:1–2. In Berman S. Otitis media in developing countries. *Pediatrics* 1996;1:126–130.
12. Cohen D, Tamir D. The prevalence of middle ear pathologies in Jerusalem school children. *Am J Otol* 1989;19:456–459.
13. Podoshin L, Fradis M, Ben-David Y, et al. Cholesteatoma: an epidemiologic study among members of kibbutzim in northern Israel. *Ann Otol Rhinol Laryngol* 1986;95:365–368.
14. Bafaqeeh SA, Zakzouk S, Muhaimed HA, et al. Relevant demographic factors and hearing impairment in Saudi children: epidemiological study. *J Laryngol Otol* 1994;108:294–298.
15. Noh KT, Kim CS. The changing pattern of otitis media in Korea. *Int J Pediatr Otorhinolaryngol* 1985;9:77–87.

16. Kim CS, Jung HW, Yoo KY. Prevalence and risk factors of chronic otitis media in Korea: results of a nation-wide survey. *Acta Otolaryngol* 1993;113:369–375.
17. Jacob A, Rupa V, Job A, et al. Hearing impairment and otitis media in a rural primary school in South India. *Int J Pediatr Otorhinolaryngol* 1997;39:133–138.
18. Elango S, Purohit GN, Hashim M, et al. Hearing loss and ear disorders in Malaysian school children. *Int J Pediatr Otorhinolaryngol* 1991;22:75–80.
19. Lee L, Cao W, Xu F. Disability among the elderly in China: analysis of the national sampling survey of disability in 1987. *Chin Med J* 1997;110:236–237.
20. Dang Hoang S, Nhan Trung S, Le T, et al. Prevalence of chronic otitis media in a randomly selected population sampled in two communities in Southern Vietnam. Proceedings of Copenhagen Otitis Media Conference, June 1–5, 1997;Abstr 13.
21. Garrett J, Stewart J. Hearing loss and otitis media in Guam: impact of professional services. *Asia Pac J Public Health* 1989;3:213–218.
22. Dever G, Stool S, Manning S, et al. Otitis oceania: middle ear disease in the Pacific basin. *Ann Otol Rhinol Laryngol* 1990;99(suppl 149):25–27.
23. Elango S, Purohit GN, Hashim M, et al. Hearing loss and ear disorders in Malaysian school children. *Int J Pediatr Otorhinolaryngol* 1991;22:75–80.
24. Eason R, Harding F, Nicholson R, et al. Chronic suppurative otitis media in the Solomon Islands: a prospective microbiological, audiometric and therapeutic survey. *N Z Med J* 1986;99:812–815.
25. Dever G, Stool S, Manning S, et al. Otitis oceania: middle ear disease in the Pacific basin. *Ann Otol Rhinol Laryngol* 1990;99(suppl 149):25–27.
26. Bastos I, Reimer A, Andreasson L. Middle ear disease and hearing loss among urban children and orphans in Bauru, Brazil. A prevalence study. *J Audiol Med* 1994.
27. Browning GG, Gatehouse S. *The prevalence of middle ear disease in the adult British population. Clin Otolaryngol* 1992;17:317–321.
28. Alho OP, Jokinen K, Laitakari K, et al. Chronic suppurative otitis media and cholesteatoma. Vanishing diseases among Western populations? *Clin Otolaryngol* 1997;22:358–361.
29. Pedersen CB, Zachau-Christiansen B. Chronic otitis media and sequelae in the population of Greenland. *Scand J Soc Med* 1988;16:15–19.
30. Nelson SM, Berry RI. Ear disease and hearing loss among Navajo children — a mass survey. *Laryngoscope* 1994;94:316–323.
31. Canterbury D. Changes in hearing status of Alaskan natives. *Ann Otol Rhinol Laryngol* 1990;99(suppl):22–23.
32. Sunderman J, Dyer H. Chronic ear disease in Australian aborigines. *Med J Aust* 1984;140:708–711.
33. Homoe P. Otitis media in Greenland. Studies on historical, epidemiological, microbiological, and immunological aspects. *Int J Circumpolar Health* 2001;60(suppl 2):1–54.
34. Tos M. Sequelae of secretory otitis media and the relationship to chronic suppurative otitis media. *Ann Otol Rhino Laryngol* 1990;99:18–19.
35. Daly KA, Hunter LL, Levine SC, et al. Relationships between otitis media sequelae and age. *Laryngoscope* 1998;108:1306–1310.
36. New Zealand Health Technology Assessment Clearing House. Screening programmes for the detection of otitis media with effusion and conductive hearing loss in pre-school and new entrant school children: a critical appraisal of the literature (NZHTA REPORT 3). Christchurch, New Zealand, June 1998. http://nzhta.chmeds.ac.nz/screen.htm (last accessed 21 July 2003). Search date 1998; primary sources English language articles in Medline, Cinahl, HealthSTAR, Current Contents (combined files), Cochrane Library Database of Abstracts of Reviews of Effectiveness, NHS Economic Evaluation Database, New Zealand Bibliographic Network, New Zealand Ministry of Health publications, United States National Institute of Health publications, Catalogues of New Zealand medical libraries, and publications and current projects by the International Network of Agencies for Health Technology Assessment (INAHTA).
37. Bastos I. Otitis media and hearing loss among children in developing countries. Malmo: University of Malmo, 1994.
38. Jacob A, Rupa V, Job A, et al. Hearing impairment and otitis media in a rural primary school in south India. *Int J Pediatr Otorhinolaryngol* 1997;39:133–138.
39. Seely DR, Gloyd SS, Wright AD, et al. Hearing loss prevalence and risk factors among Sierra Leonean Children. *Arch Otolaryngol Head Neck Surg* 1995;121:853–858.
40. Antarasena S, Antarasena N, Lekagul S, et al. The epidemiology of deafness in Thailand. *Otolaryngol Head Neck Surg* 1988;3:9–13.
41. Muya EW, Owino O. *Special education in Africa: research abstracts*. Nairobi: UNESCO;1986.
42. Teele DW, Klein JO, Chase C, et al. Otitis media in infancy and intellectual ability, school achievement, speech, and language at age 7 years. Greater Boston Otitis Media Study Group. *J Infect Dis* 1990;162:685–694.
43. Osma U, Cureoglu S, Hosoglu S. The complications of chronic otitis media: report of 93 cases. *J Laryngol Otol* 2000;114:97–100.
44. Kenna M. Incidence and prevalence of complications of otitis media. *Ann Otol Rhinol Laryngol* 1990;99(suppl 149):38–39.
45. Berman S. Otitis media in developing countries. *Pediatrics* 1995;96:126–131.
46. Sorensen H. Antibiotics in suppurative otitis media. *Otolaryngol Clin North Am* 1977;10:45–50.
47. Mahoney JL. Mass management of otitis media in Zaire. *Laryngoscope* 1980;90:1200–1208.
48. Noh KT, Kim CS. The changing pattern of otitis media in Korea. *Int J Pediatr Otorhinolaryngol* 1985;9:77–87.
49. Nelson SM, Berry RI. Ear disease and hearing loss among Navajo children — a mass survey. *Laryngoscope* 1994;94:316–323.
50. Muhaimeid H, Zakzouk S, Bafaqeeh SA. Epidemiology of chronic suppurative otitis media in Saudi children. *Int J Pediatr Otorhinolaryngol* 1993;26:101–108.
51. Alho OP, Jokinen K, Laitakari K, et al. Chronic suppurative otitis media and cholesteatoma. Vanishing diseases among Western populations? *Clin Otolaryngol Allied Sci* 1997;22:358–361.
52. Browning GG, Gatehouse S, Calder IT. Medical management of active chronic otitis media: a controlled study. *J Laryngol Otol* 1988;102:491–495.
53. Acuin J, Smith A, Mackenzie I. Interventions for chronic suppurative otitis media. In: The Cochrane Library. Issue 4, 2001. Oxford: Update Software. Search date 1996; primary sources Medline, Hearing network database, handsearches, and experts.
54. Ozagar A, Koc A, Ciprut A, et al. Effects of topical otic preparations on hearing in chronic otitis media. *Otolaryngol Head Neck Surg* 1997;117:405–408.
55. De Miguel Martinez I, Vasallo M Jr, Ramos MA. Antimicrobial therapy in chronic suppurative otitis media. *Acta Otorrinolaringol Esp* 1999;50:15–19.
56. Rotimi V, Olabiyi D, Banjo T, et al. Randomised comparative efficacy of clindamycin, metronidazole, and lincomycin, plus gentamicin in chronic suppurative otitis media. *West Afr J Med* 1990;9:89–97.
57. Tutkun A, Ozagar A, Koc A, et al. Treatment of chronic ear disease — Topical ciprofloxacin vs topical gentamicin. *Arch Otolaryngol Head Neck Surg* 1995;121:1414–1416.
58. Tong MC, Woo JK, van Hasselt CA. A double-blind comparative study of ofloxacin otic drops versus neomycin-polymyxin B-hydrocortisone otic drops in the medical treatment of chronic suppurative otitis media. *J Laryngol Otol* 1996;110:309–314.

59. Clayton M, Osborne J, Rutherford D, et al. A double-blind, randomized, prospective trial of a topical antiseptic versus a topical antibiotic in the treatment of otorrhea. *Clin Otolaryngol* 1990;15:7–10.
60. Kasemsuwan L, Clongsuesuek P. A double blind, prospective trial of topical ciprofloxacin versus normal saline solution in the treatment of otorrhoea. *Clin Otolaryngol* 1997;22:44–46.
61. Fradis M, Brodsky A, Ben David J, et al. Chronic otitis media treated topically with ciprofloxacin or tobramycin. *Arch Otolaryngol Head Neck Surg* 1997;123:1057–1060.
62. Gyde MC, Randall RF. Comparative double-blind study of trimethoprim-sulfacetamide-polymyxin B and of gentamicine in the treatment of otorrhoea. *Ann Otolaryngol Chir Cervicofac* 1978;95:43–55.
63. Gyde M. A double-blind comparative study of trimethoprim-polymyxin B versus trimethoprim-sulfacetamide-polymyxin B otic solutions in the treatment of otorrhea. *J Laryngol Otol* 1981;95:251–259.
64. Gyde MC, Norris D, Kavalec EC. The weeping ear: clinical re-evaluation of treatment. *J Int Med Res* 1982;10:333–340.
65. Llorente J, Sabater F, Maristany M, et al. Multicenter comparative study of the effectiveness and tolerance of topical ciprofloxacine (0.3%) versus topical gentamicine (0.3%) in the treatment of chronic suppurative otitis media without cholesteatoma. *An Otorrinolaringol Ibero Am* 1995;5:521–533.
66. Miro N, Perello E, Casamitjana F, et al. Controlled multicenter study on chronic suppurative otitis media treated with topical applications of ciprofloxacin 0.2% solution in single-dose containers or combination of polymyxin B, neomycin, and hydrocortisone suspension. *Otolaryngol Head Neck Surg* 2000;23:617–623.
67. Crowther JA, Simpson D. Medical treatment of chronic otitis media: steroid or antibiotic with steroid ear-drops? *Clin Otolaryngol* 1991;6:142–144.
68. Marias J, Rutka JA. Ototoxicity and topical eardrops. *Clin Otolaryngol* 1998;23:360–367.
69. Leliever WC. Topical gentamicin-induced positional vertigo. *Otolaryngol Head Neck Surg* 1985;93:553–555.
70. Mira E, Benazzo M. Uso topico delle cefalosporine nel trattamento delle otiti medie purulente: valutazione della ceftizoxima (eposerin®). *Riv Ital Otorinolaringol Audiol Foniat* 1992;12:219–225.
71. Tong MC, Yue V, Ku PK, et al. Preoperative topical ofloxacin solution for tympanoplasty: a randomized, controlled study. *Otol Neurotol* 2002;23:18–20.
72. Longridge NS. Topical gentamicin vestibular toxicity. *J Otolaryngol* 1994;23:444–446.
73. Picozzi G, Browning G, Calder I. Controlled trial of gentamicin and hydrocortisone ear drops in the treatment of active chronic otitis media. *Clin Otolaryngol* 1983;8:367–368.
74. Browning G, Picozzi G, Calder I, et al. Controlled trial of medical treatment of active chronic otitis media. *BMJ* 1983;287:1024.
75. Jaya C, Job A, Mathai E et al. Evaluation of topical povidone–iodine in chronic suppurative otitis media. *Arch Otolaryngol Head Neck Surg* 2003;129:1098–1100
76. Esposito S, D'Errico G, Montanaro C. Topical and oral treatment of chronic otitis media with ciprofloxacin. *Arch Otolaryngol Head Neck Surg* 1990;116:557–559.
77. Esposito S, D'Errico G, Mantanaro C. Topical ciprofloxacin vs. intramuscular gentamicin for chronic otitis media. *Arch Otolaryngol Head Neck Surg* 1992;118:842–844.
78. Povedano Rodriguez V, Seco Pinero M, Jurado Ramos A, et al. Eficacia del ciprofloxacino topico en el tratamiento de la otorrea cronica. *Acta Otorrinolaryngologica Espantildeola* 1995;46:15–18.
79. Yuen P, Lau S, Chau P, et al. Ofloxacin eardrop treatment for active chronic suppurative otitis media: prospective randomized study. *Am J Otol* 1994;15:670–673.
80. Cannoni M, Bonfils P, Sednaoui P, et al. Cefotiam hexetil versus amoxicillin/clavulanic acid for the treatment of chronic otitis media in adults. *Med Mal Infect* 1997;27:915–921.
81. Gonzalez A, Galindo T. Estudio abierto del tratamiento de otitis media cronica con levofloxacino vs amoxicillina /clavulanato. *Invest Med Int* 2001;28:33–36.
82. Lildholdt T, Felding J, Juul A, et al. Efficacy of perioperative ceftazidime in the surgical treatment of chronic otitis media due to *Pseudomonas aeruginosa*. *Arch Otorhinolaryngol* 1986;243:167–169.
83. Picozzi G, Browning G, Calder I. Controlled trial of gentamicin and hydrocortisone ear drops with and without systemic metronidazole in the treatment of active chronic otitis media. *Clin Otolaryngol* 1984;9:305.
84. Supiyaphun P, Kerekhanjanarong V, Koranasophonepun J, et al. Comparison of ofloxacin otic solution with oral amoxycillin plus chloramphenicol ear drop in treatment of chronic suppurative otitis media with acute exacerbation. *J Med Assoc Thai* 2000;83:61–68.
85. Baba S, Ito H, Kinoshita H, et al. Comparative study of cefmetazole and cefazolin in the treatment of suppurative otitis media. *Jpn J Antibiot* 1982;35:1523–1552.
86. Colletti V, Fiorino FG, Indelicato T. Surgery vs natural course of chronic otitis media. Long term hearing evaluation. *Acta Otolaryngol* 1991;111:762–768.
87. Soldati D, Mudry A. Cholesteatoma in children: techniques and results. *Int J Pediatr Otorhinolaryngol* 2000;52:269–276.
88. Chang CC, Chen MK. Canal-wall-down tympanoplasty with mastoidectomy for advanced cholesteatoma. *J Otolaryngol* 2000;29:270–273.
89. Vartiainen E, Kansanen M. Tympanomastoidectomy for chronic otitis media without choleasteatoma. *Otolaryngol Head Neck Surg* 1992;106:230–234.
90. Mishiro Y, Sakagami M, Takahashi Y, et al. Tympanoplasty with and without mastoidectomy for non-cholesteatomatous chronic otitis media. *Eur Arch Otorhinolaryngol* 2001;258:13–15.
91. Berenholz LP, Rizer FM, Burkey JM, et al. Ossiculoplasty in canal wall down mastoidectomy. *Otolaryngol Head Neck Surg* 2000;123:30–33.
92. Eason R, Harding E, Nicholson R, et al. Chronic suppurative otitis media in the Solomon Islands: a prospective, microbiological, audiometric and therapeutic survey. *N Z Med J* 1986;99:812–815.
93. Smith A, Hatcher J, Mackenzie I, et al. Randomised controlled trial of treatment of chronic suppurative otitis media in Kenyan schoolchildren. *Lancet* 1996;348:1128–1133.
94. Abes G, Espallardo N, Tong M et al. A systematic review of the effectiveness of ofloxacin otic solution for the treatment of suppurative otitis media. *ORL J Otorhinolaryngol Relat Spec* 2003; 65:106–116. Search date 2000; primary sources Medline, Cochrane Library, Centerwatch Clinical Trial Listing Service, Trial Banks, Research and Researcher Registry: Queen's University, hand searches of collaborators' local libraries and references lists of retrieved articles.
95. Couzos S, Lea T, Mueller R et al. Effectiveness of ototopical antibiotics for chronic suppurative otitis media in Aboriginal children: a community-based, multicentre, double-blind randomised controlled trial. *Med J Aust* 2003;179:185–190.
96. Marias J, Rutka JA. Ototoxicity and topical eardrops. *Clin Otolaryngol* 1998;23:360–367.
97. Leliever WC. Topical gentamicin-induced positional vertigo. *Otolaryngol Head Neck Surg* 1985;93:553–555.
98. Longridge NS. Topical gentamicin vestibular toxicity. *J Otolaryngol* 1994;23:444–446.
99. Thorp MA, Gardiner IB, Prescott CA. Burow's solution in the treatment of active mucosal chronic suppurative otitis media: determining an effective dilution. *J Laryngol Otol* 2000;114:432–436.

100. Somekh E, Cordova Z. Ceftazidime versus aztreonam in the treatment of pseudomonal chronic suppurative otitis media in children. *Scand J Infect Dis* 2000;32:197–199.

101. Fliss D, Dagan R, Houri Z, et al. Medical management of chronic suppurative otitis media without cholesteatoma in children. *J Pediatr* 1990;116:991–996.

102. Darrouzet V, Duclos JY, Portmann D, et al. Preference for the closed technique in the management of cholesteatoma of the middle ear in children: a retrospective study of 215 consecutive patients treated over 10 years. *Am J Otol* 2000;21:474–481.

103. Tos M, Stangerup SE, Orntoft S. Reasons for reperforation after tympanoplasty in children. *Acta Otolaryngol Suppl* 2000;543:143–146.

Jose Acuin
Associate Professor
De La Salle University Health Sciences Campus, Dasmarinas Cavite, Philippines

Competing interests: None declared.

TABLE 1 **RCTs of topical antibiotics versus each other (see text, p 581).**

Ref	Population with CSOM (people/ears, age setting)	Comparison	Absolute results*	OR
Different topical non–quinolone antibiotics *v* each other				
62	Adults, 57 ears, France, Variable duration	Topical 0.3% gentamicin *v* topical trimethoprim–sulfacetamide–polymyxin B	4/30 (13%) 5/27(19%)	1.47 (0.36 to 6.03)
63	27 ears, France, 7–14 days	Topical trimethoprim–sulfacetamide–polymyxin B *v* topical trimethoprim–polymyxin B	4/13 (31%) 8/14 (57%)	0.36 (0.08 to 1.59)
64	14 adults, France, 30–40 years, 2 weeks	Topical 0.3% gentamicin *v* topical colistin–neomycin–hydrocortisone	1/8 (13%) 1/6 (17%)	0.73 (0.04 to 13.45)
Topical quinolone *v* topical non–quinolone antibiotics				
65	308 adults, Spain, 30 days	Topical 0.3% ciprofloxacin *v* topical 0.3% gentamicin	8/159 (5%) 9/149 (6%)	0.82 (0.31 to 2.19)
66	322 adults, 14–71 years, Spain, 6–12 days	Topical ciprofloxacin *v* topical polymyxin B–neomycin–hydrocortisone	22/168 (13%) 37/154 (24%)	0.48 (0.28 to 0.85) ITT 0.67 (0.30 to 1.51) on protocol
61	40 adults, Clinics in Israel, 3 weeks	Topical ciprofloxacin *v* topical tobramycin	10/19 (53%) 8/18 (44%)	1.38 (0.39 to 4.91)

*Outcomes for all RCTs are the proportion of people with wet ear on otoscopic examination and with negative culture, usually measured at the end of treatment. COSM, chronic suppurative otitis media; ITT, intention to treat analysis; OR, odds ratio; Ref, reference.

TABLE 2 RCTs of topical antibiotics versus systemic antibiotics (see text, p 584).

Ref	Population with chronic suppurative otitis media	Comparison	Persistent otorrhoea	
			Absolute results	OR
74	Adults Scottish hospital clinic	Topical gentamicin or chloramphenicol *v* various systemic antibiotics	11/18 (61%) *v* 8/13 (62%)	0.98 (0.23 to 4.15)
75	60 adults 5–10 days	Topical ciprofloxacin *v* oral ciprofloxacin	3/20 (15%) *v* 12/20 (60%)	0.15 (0.04 to 0.54)
76	60 adults 5–10 days	Topical ciprofloxacin *v* im gentamicin	5/30 (17%) *v* 17/30 (57%)	0.15 (0.05 to 0.49)
77	60 adults 10 days	Topical ciprofloxacin *v* oral ciprofloxacin	5/30 (17%) *v* 15/30 50%)	0.23 (0.08 to 0.56)
78	60 adults 7 days	Topical ciprofloxacin *v* oral amoxicillin/clavulanate	7/30 (57%) *v* 20/30 (67%)	0.18 (0.07 to 0.49)

im, intramuscular; Ref, reference.

Ear wax

Search date December 2003

George Browning

QUESTIONS

INTERVENTIONS

*Although many practitioners consider these to be standard treatments, we found no RCTs of these interventions.

See glossary G

Key Messages

- **Ear syringing** There is consensus that ear syringing is effective, but we found no RCTs comparing ear syringing alone versus no treatment or versus other treatment. RCTs provided insufficient evidence to assess syringing after the use of wax softeners. Reported complications of ear syringing include otitis externa, perforation of the ear drum, damage to the skin of the external canal, tinnitus, pain, and vertigo.
- **Manual removal (other than ear syringing)** We found no RCTs about mechanical methods of removing ear wax other than syringing, although many practitioners consider these to be standard treatments.
- **Wax softeners** Two RCTs provided inconclusive evidence about the effects of wax softeners compared with no treatment, saline, or placebo (sterile water). The first RCT in elderly people with impacted wax found that a proprietary wax softening agent containing arachis oil/chlorobutanol/*p*-dichlorobenzene reduced the proportion of ears requiring syringing compared with no treatment, but found no significant difference between the proprietary wax softening agent and saline/sterile water. It also found no significant difference between sodium bicarbonate and either no treatment or saline/sterile water in the proportion of ears requiring syringing. Another RCT in children found no significant difference in the proportion of ears requiring syringing between either docusate sodium or triethanolamine and saline. RCTs found no consistent evidence that any one type of wax softener was superior to the others. RCTs also provided insufficient evidence to assess wax softeners prior to syringing.

DEFINITION	Ear wax is normal and becomes a problem only if it produces deafness, pain, or other aural symptoms. Ear wax may also need to be removed if it prevents inspection of the ear drum. The term "impacted wax"Ⓖ is used in different ways, and can merely imply the coexistence of wax obscuring the ear drum with symptoms in that ear.[1]
INCIDENCE/ PREVALENCE	We found four surveys of the prevalence of impacted wax.[2-5] The studies were carried out in a variety of populations and used a variety of definitions of impacted wax; prevalence ranged from 7–35%. It is unclear how these figures relate to prevalence in the general population.
AETIOLOGY/ RISK FACTORS	Factors that prevent the normal extrusion of wax from the ear canal (e.g. wearing a hearing aid, using cotton buds to clean ears) increase the chance of ear wax accumulating.
PROGNOSIS	Most ear wax emerges from the external canal spontaneously; one RCT that included a no treatment group found that 32% of ears with impacted wax showed spontaneous resolution after 5 days.[1] Without impaction or adherence to the drum, there is likely to be minimal, if any, hearing loss.
AIMS OF INTERVENTION	To relieve symptoms or to allow examination by completely removing impacted wax or obstructing waxⒼ; and to soften impacted wax to ease mechanical removal.
OUTCOMES	Proportion of people (or ears) with relief of hearing loss or discomfort; subjective assessment of amount of wax remaining. **After use of wax softeners for ear wax removal:** proportion of people requiring mechanical removal to improve symptoms; perceived ease of mechanical removal (measured, for example, by the volume of water used to accomplish successful syringing).
METHODS	*Clinical Evidence* search and appraisal December 2003.

QUESTION What are the effects of methods to remove symptomatic ear wax?

OPTION WAX SOFTENERS

Two RCTs provided inconclusive evidence about the effects of wax softeners compared with no treatment, saline, or placebo (sterile water). The first RCT in elderly people with impacted wax found that a proprietary wax softening agent containing arachis oil/chlorobutanol/*p*-dichlorobenzene reduced the proportion of ears requiring syringing compared with no treatment, but found no significant difference between the proprietary wax softening agent and saline/sterile water. It also found no significant difference between sodium bicarbonate and either no treatment or saline/sterile water in the proportion of ears requiring syringing. Another RCT in children found no significant difference in the proportion of ears requiring syringing between either docusate sodium or triethanolamine and saline. RCTs found no consistent evidence that any one type of wax softener was superior to the others. RCTs also provided insufficient evidence to assess wax softeners prior to syringing.

Benefits: We found one systematic review (search date 2003, 8 RCTs, 537 people) comparing wax softeners versus placebo, no treatment, or each other.[6] The review selected RCTs in which the primary outcome was the proportion of ears with sufficient clearance of the external auditory canal to make further mechanical clearance (syringing) unnecessary. The review did not perform a meta-analysis because of heterogeneity among the trials identified in treatments used, duration, methods, and outcome assessments.[6] **Versus placebo or no treatment:** The review[6] identified two RCTs.[1,7] The first RCT identified by the review included 113 people recruited from a hospital for the elderly with impacted waxⒼ in one or both ears.[1] Ears were randomly allocated to treatment by the nursing staff with a proprietary softening agent (arachis oil/chlorobutanol/*p*-dichlorobenzene), sodium bicarbonate plus glycerol plus sterile water, placebo (sterile water alone), or no treatment. People already using ear drops and people with other pathology of the ear canal or ear drum were excluded. The RCT found that the proprietary softening agent significantly reduced the proportion of ears that required syringing compared with no treatment (31/40 [78%] with wax softener *v* 36/38 [95%] with no treatment; $P < 0.05$), but found no significant difference between the proprietary softening agent and sterile water (31/40 [78%] with wax softener *v* 30/38 [79%] with sterile water; P value reported as non-significant, CI not reported; see comment below).[1] The RCT also found no significant difference in the proportion of ears that required syringing between sodium bicarbonate plus glycerol plus water and either no treatment, or water (P values reported as non-significant, CI not reported).[1] The second RCT (48 children) identified by the review compared either docusate sodium or triethanolamine versus saline. It found no significant difference in the proportion of ears that required syringing between either of the wax softeners and saline (docusate sodium *v* saline; RR 1.07, 95% CI 0.17 to 6.64; triethanolamine *v* saline; RR 3.29, 95% CI 0.80 to 13.57).[6] **Versus each other:** The review[6] identified two RCTs[1,8] and two quasi-randomised trials[9,10] comparing different wax softeners. We also found one additional RCT[11] and one quasi-randomised trial.[12] The trials were conducted in a variety of settings. All but one RCT[1] had design deficiencies that could lead to bias. The trials varied in size from 36 people (72 ears) to 160 people (286 ears). The most common outcomes were a subjective assessment of the amount of wax remaining, the need for further mechanical clearance (syringing), or the perceived ease of syringing. The RCTs found no consistent evidence that any one type of wax softener was clinically superior to any other (see table 1, p 600). **Prior to syringing:** The review[6] identified one RCT[13] and we found four additional RCTs[14–17] and one quasi-randomised trial[18] comparing various wax softeners given prior to ear syringing versus each other or versus no treatment (see table 2, p 604). The trials varied in size from 50 people (50 ears) to 130 people (224 ears). All had design deficiencies that could lead to bias. Two of the RCTs found differences in wax clearance among wax softeners, and another two RCTs found no overall difference (see table 2, p 604). The fifth RCT compared oily drops plus syringing versus oily drops alone and assessed improvement in hearing.[17] The RCT did not relate improvements in hearing to amount of wax removed. It found that oily drops plus syringing significantly increased the proportion of people with improved hearing compared with oily drops alone.[17] However, oily drops may impair baseline hearing level, which may have biased the results in favour of the intervention. This makes the RCT difficult to interpret. The quasi-randomised trial found no significant difference between water instilled for 15 minutes and oil instilled nightly for 3 days, but the statistical tests performed may have been inadequate.[18]

Harms: **Versus placebo or no treatment:** The first RCT found no cases of irritation in people using a wax softener.[1] The second RCT gave no information on adverse effects of the wax softeners compared with saline; it found that 10/48 [21%] of children experienced pain during irrigation.[7] **Versus each other:** Three RCTs gave no information on adverse effects (see table 1, p 600). Two RCTs found single cases of irritation, pain, itching, buzzing, or dislike of smell in people using wax softeners. One RCT found that the frequency of adverse effects, including pain, irritation, giddiness, and dislike of smell, was similar in people using arachis oil/chlorobutanol/*p*-dichlorobenzene compared with a proprietary agent (Otocerol® — the composition of which was not reported).[8] **Prior to syringing:** Three RCTs found no cases of irritation in people using a wax softener (see table 1, p 600). The other two RCTs gave no information on adverse effects.

Comment: When assessing the proportion of ears that did not require syringing in the first RCT[1], the review[6] included both people whose ears were "moderately clear" and "completely clear" in its calculation. However, in the RCT, only ears that were completely clear were not syringed; we have therefore reported figures from the original RCT[1] above. We found no good evidence about the optimal duration of treatment. Most trials did not use rigorous methods of randomisation, and did not control for degree of ear canal occlusion at randomisation. Many trials were sponsored by companies that manufactured only one of the products being tested, but the possibility of publication bias (failure to publish unfavourable results) has not been assessed. The inclusion criteria for the RCTs were not always clear: many stated that the participants had impacted wax without defining this.

OPTION MECHANICAL METHODS

We found no RCTs about mechanical methods of removing ear wax, although many practitioners consider these to be standard treatments. There is consensus that ear syringing is effective, but we found no RCTs comparing ear syringing alone versus no treatment or versus other treatment. RCTs provided insufficient evidence to assess syringing after the use of wax softeners. Reported complications of ear syringing include otitis externa, perforation of the ear drum, damage to the skin of the external canal, tinnitus, pain, and vertigo.

Benefits: We found no systematic review and no RCTs comparing mechanical methods alone versus no treatment or alternative treatment. **After use of wax softeners:** See benefits of wax softeners, p 596.

Harms: One survey found that 38% of 274 general practitioners reported complications in people receiving syringing, including otitis externa, perforation of the ear drum, damage to the skin of the external canal, tinnitus, pain, and vertigo.[19] We found no study of the incidence of these complications, or the effect of training and experience. People may experience dizziness during syringing or when wax is removed by suction. **After use of wax softeners:** See harms of wax softeners, p 597.

Comment: There is consensus that syringing is effective and that training can reduce complications, but we found no reliable evidence. Mechanical techniques other than syringing include manual removal under direct vision, with or without a microscope, using suction, probes, or forceps. These methods require specific training and access to appropriate equipment.

GLOSSARY

Impacted wax Wax that has been compressed in the ear canal, completely obstructing the lumen. In practice, many RCTs define impaction as the presence of symptoms associated with wax obscuring the ear drum.

Obstructing wax Wax that obscures direct vision of the ear drum.

REFERENCES

1. Keane EM, Wilson H, McGrane D, et al. Use of solvents to disperse ear wax. *Br J Clin Pract* 1995;49:7–12.
2. Kalantan KA, Abdulghani H, Al-Taweel AA, et al. Use of cotton tipped swab and cerumen impaction. *Ind J Otol* 1999;5:27–31.
3. Minja BM, Machemba A. Prevalence of otitis media, hearing impairment and cerumen impaction among school children in rural and urban Dar es Salaam, Tanzania. *Int J Pediatr Otorhinolaryngol* 1996;37:29–34.
4. Swart SM, Lemmer R, Parbhoo JN, et al. A survey of ear and hearing disorders amongst a representative sample of Grade 1 school children in Swaziland. *Int J Pediatr Otorhinolaryngol* 1995;32:23–34.
5. Lewis-Cullinan C, Janken JK. Effect of cerumen removal on the hearing ability of geriatric patients. *J Adv Nurs* 1990;15:594–600.
6. Burton MJ, Dorée CJ. Ear drops for the removal of ear wax (Cochrane Review). In: The Cochrane Library, Issue 4, 2003. Chichester, UK: John Wiley & Sons, Ltd. Search date 2003, primary sources Cochrane ENT Group Register, Cochrane Central Register of Controlled Trials, Medline, Embase, and hand searches of reference lists of all trials retrieved.
7. Meehan P, Isenhour JL, Reeves R, Wrenn K. Ceruminolysis in the pediatric patient: a prospective, double-blinded, randomized controlled trial. *Acad Emerg Med* 2002;9:521–522.

8. Jaffe G, Grimshaw J. A multicentric clinical trial comparing Otocerol with Cerumol as cerumenolytics. *J Int Med Res* 1978;6:241–244.
9. Lyndon S, Roy P, Grillage MG, et al. A comparison of the efficacy of two ear drop preparations ("Aurax" and "Earex") in the softening and removal of impacted ear wax. *Curr Med Res Opin* 1992;13:21–25.
10. Fahmy S, Whitefield M. Multicentre clinical trial of Exterol as a cerumenolytic. *Br J Clin Pract* 1982;36:197–204.
11. Carr MM, Smith RL. Ceruminolytic efficacy in adults versus children. *J Otolaryngol* 2001;30:154–156.
12. Dummer DS, Sutherland IA, Murray JA. A single-blind, randomized study to compare the efficacy of two ear drop preparations ("Andax" and "Cerumol") in the softening of ear wax. *Curr Med Res Opin* 1992;13:26–30.
13. Singer AJ, Sauris E, Viccellio AW. Ceruminolytic effects of docusate sodium: a randomized controlled trial. *Ann Emerg Med* 2000;36:228–232.
14. Amjad AH, Scheer AA. Clinical evaluation of cerumenolytic agents. *Eye Ear Nose Throat Mon* 1975;54:76–77.
15. Chaput de Saintonge DM, Johnstone CI. A clinical comparison of triethanolamine polypeptide oleate-condensate ear drops with olive oil for the removal of impacted wax. *Br J Clin Pract* 1973;27:454–455.
16. Fraser JG. The efficacy of wax solvents: *in vitro* studies and a clinical trial. *J Laryngol Otol* 1970;84:1055–1064.
17. Memel D, Langley C, Watkins C, et al. Effectiveness of ear syringing in general practice: a randomised controlled trial and patients' experiences. *Br J Gen Pract* 2002;52:906–911.
18. Eekhof JA, de Bock GH, Le Cessie S, et al. A quasi-randomised controlled trial of water as a quick softening agent of persistent earwax in general practice. *Br J Gen Pract* 2001;51:635–637.
19. Sharp JF, Wilson JA, Ross L, et al. Ear wax removal: a survey of current practice. *BMJ* 1990;301:1251–1252.

George Browning
Professor of Otorhinolaryngology
MRC Institute of Hearing Research, Glasgow, UK

Competing interests: None declared. *The following previous contributors of this topic would also like to be acknowledged: Martin Burton, Elizabeth Mogg.*

TABLE 1 Effects of wax softeners: results of comparative RCTs (see text, p 596).[1,8–12]

Ref	Wax softener	Administration	Selection characteristic; setting	Number of people (ears)	Randomisation; blinding	Outcome	Results	Adverse effects
1	(a) Arachis oil Chlorobutanol *p*-dichlorobenzene (Cerumol®) (b) Sodium bicarbonate (in glycerol) (c) Sterile water (d) No treatment	4 drops twice a day for 5 days	Impacted ear(s); hospital	113 recruited; 97 completed (155)	Randomisation (technique not described) Double blind (active treatments)	Residual wax; 3 tiered clinical rating scale	No significant difference between (a) and (b) in proportion of ears completely clear at 5 days (22% with (a) *v* 21% with (b); reported as NS, CI not reported)	No cases of irritation
8	(a) Ethyleneoxide-polyoxypropylene glycol Choline salicylate (b) Arachis oil Chlorobutanol *p*-dichlorobenzene (Cerumol®)		Impacted or hardened wax; general practice	50 (100)	Not stated; single blind	Residual wax, colour, and consistency; objective hearing; global impression of efficiency	No significant difference in any outcome between (a) and (b) (reported as NS, CI not reported), for example (b) In treatments reduces residual was in approx 50% of ears.	Two irritation with (a); one itch, one buzzing with (b)

TABLE 1 continued

Ref	Wax softener	Administration	Selection characteristic; setting	Number of people (ears)	Randomisation; blinding	Outcome	Results	Adverse effects
9	(a) Ethyleneoxide-polyoxypropylene glycol, Choline salicylate (Audax) (b) Arachis oil Almond oil Rectified camphor oil (Earex)	Drops to fill ear twice a day for 4 days	Symptoms requiring wax softener; general practice	36 (72)	Not stated; not blind	Degree of impaction No significant difference between (a) and (b) in proportion with no or mild impaction (27/38 with (a) *v* 17/34 with (b); reported as NS, CI not reported. Need for syringing; ease of syringing; global impression of efficiency	(a) better than (b); easy removal: 37/38 *v* 19/30 $P < 0.005$	One irritation with one disliked smell of (b)
10	(a) 5% urea hydrogen peroxide in glycerol (b) Glycerol	5–10 drops twice a day for 1 week	Ear wax problems; ENT department	40 (80)	Alternation; double blind	Need for syringing; ease of syringing	(a) significantly better than (b); proportion of ears not requiring syringing: 35/40 *v* 20/40; P	Not assessed

TABLE 1 continued

Ref	Wax softener	Administration	Selection characteristic; setting	Number of people (ears)	Randomisation; blinding	Outcome	Results	Adverse effects
10	(a) 5% urea hydrogen peroxide in glycerol (b) Arachis oil, Chlorobutanol, *p*-dichlorobenzene (Cerumol®)	5–10 drops twice a day for 1 week	Ear wax problems; ENT department	50 (100)	Alternation; double blind	Need for syringing; ease of syringing	(a) better than (b); proportion ears not requiring syringing 20/50 *v* 5/50; $P < 0.001$	Not assessed
10	(a) 5% urea hydrogen peroxide in glycerol (b) Arachis oil, Chlorobutanol, *p*-dichlorobenzene, (Cerumol®)	5–10 drops twice a day for a week	Ear wax problems; general practice	160 (286)	Alternation; double blind	Need for syringing; ease of syringing	(a) significantly better than (b); proportion ears not requiring syringing or where syrininging easy: 146/157 *v* 93/129; $p < 0.001$	Not assessed
11	(a) Otocerol® (b) Arachis oil, Chlorobutanol, *p*-dichlorobenzene (Cerumol®)	Three consecutive nights	For whom a wax softener would normally be prescribed; general practice	106 (not stated)	Random allocation; double blind	3 tiered clinical rating scale	No significant difference; 38/53 *v* 33/53 (reported as NS, CI npt reported)	Pain; irritation; giddiness; smell (with (a)reg; 7/53 with (b) 10/53)

TABLE 1 continued

Ref	Wax softener	Administration	Selection characteristic; setting	Number of people (ears)	Randomisation; blinding	Outcome	Results	Adverse effects
12	(a) 10% aqueous sodium bicarbonate (b) 2.5% aqueous acetic acid	Daily applications for 14 days	Incidentally noted wax Paediatric and adult ENT departments	60 (138)	Randomisation strategy not stated; blind selection of bottles by the person. Observers blind	Otoscopic score of degree of wax	No significant difference in change in impaction (reported as NS, CI not reported) scores	Pain in 2/34 people with (b).

ENT, ear, nose and throat; Ref, reference; NS, non–significant.

TABLE 2 Effects of wax softeners prior to syringing: results of comparative RCTs (see text, p 596).[13–18]

Ref	Wax softener	Administration	Selection characteristic; setting	Number of people (ears)	Randomisation; blind	Outcome	Results	Adverse effects
13	(a) Triethylamine polypeptide (b) Docusate sodium (Waxol®)	One dose 15 minutes before syringing	Partial or totally accluding wax	50 (50)	Random order; not blind	Visualisation of tympanic membrane	(b) significantly better than (a) (22/27 [82%] *v* 8/23 [35%])	None reported in either group
14	(a) Triethanolamine polypeptide oleate condensate (b) Carbamide peroxide	One dose 30 minutes before syringing	Hard or impacted wax; setting unclear	80 (not stated)	Random allocation; double blind	Amount of wax removed by syringing assessed on 4 tiered clinical rating scale proportion with excellent or good results	(a) better than (b); success: 33/40 ears *v* 7/40 but (b) normally used as multiple installations CI not reported	None reported
15	(a) Triethanolamine polypeptide oleate condensate (b) Olive oil	One dose 20 minutes before syringing	Impacted wax suitable for syringing; hospital outpatient department	67 (not stated)	Random order; double blind	Amount of wax removed by syringing assessed on a 3 tiered clinical rating scale	No significant difference overall (20/32 *v* 21/35 reported as NS, CI not reported); (a) needed significantly less water	Non assessed

TABLE 2 continued

Ref	Wax softener	Administration	Selection characteristic; setting	Number of people (ears)	Randomisation; blind	Outcome	Results	Adverse effects
16	(a) Arachis oil Chlorobutanol *p*-dichlorobenzene (Cerumol®) (b) Docusate sodium (Waxsol®) (c) Olive oil *v* (d) Sodium bicarbonate (inglycerol)	Ear canal filled for 15 minutes, once daily every 3 days	Bilateral hard and occluding wax; geriatric hospital	124 (248)	Each participant was allocated (d) in one randomly chosen ear and treatment with (a), (b), or (c) in the other ear. Double blind.	Number of ears in which forceful syringing failed	(a) significantly better than (d), 1/24 *v* 5/24; $P < 0.05$. No significant difference between (b) and (d) 3/24 *v* 5/24; P reported as NS, CI not reported. No significant difference between (c) and (d); 2/24 *v* 4/24; P reported as NS, CI not reported. No significant difference among (a), (b), or (c); P reported as NS, CI not reported.	Not assessed
17	(a) Oily drops plus syringing (b) Oily drops alone	Not described	One or both ear drums completely obscured by wax; general practice	44 participants had one ear syringed, 70 had both open label.	Improved in hearing by ≥10db	(a) significantly better than (b), 18/53 [34%] *v* 1/61 [2%]; $P < 0.001$	However, results may be biased in favour of (a) as olive oil may in fact impair baseline hearing.	Not assessed
18	(a) Water, cotton ear plug (b) Oil, cotton ear plug	(a) 15 minutes (b) nightly for 3 days	Persistent wax after five syringing attemps; general practice	130 (224)	Quasi-randomised (year of birth); not blind	Number of attempts needed to clear	No significant difference; however, statistical tests performed may have been inadequate	Not assessed

Ref, reference.

Menière's disease

Search date February 2004

Adrian James and Marc Thorp

QUESTIONS

INTERVENTIONS

See glossary G

Key Messages

Treatments for acute attacks

- **Anticholinergics; benzodiazepines; betahistine** We found no RCTs on the effects of these interventions in treating acute attacks of Menière's disease.

Interventions to prevent acute attacks and delay disease progression

- **Betahistine (for vertigo or tinnitus)** Seven RCTs provided insufficient evidence to compare betahistine versus placebo in terms of their effects on frequency and severity of attacks of vertigo, tinnitus, and aural fullness. Two small RCTs in people with definite or possible Menière's disease found no significant difference in tinnitus between betahistine and trimetazidine. One of these RCTs found that trimetazidine reduced the intensity of vertigo compared with betahistine, but the other RCT found no significant difference in vertigo intensity between trimetazidine and betahistine.
- **Diuretics** One small crossover RCT provided insufficient evidence about the effects of triamterene plus hydrochlorothiazide on hearing, vertigo, or tinnitus. We found no evidence on their effects on disease progression.
- **Trimetazidine** We found no RCTs comparing trimetazidine versus placebo in Menière's disease. Two small RCTs in people with definite or possible Menière's disease found no significant difference in tinnitus between betahistine and trimetazidine. One of these RCTs found that trimetazidine reduced the intensity of vertigo compared with betahistine, but the other RCT found no significant difference in vertigo intensity between trimetazidine and betahistine. We found no evidence on the effects of trimetazidine on disease progression.

- **Betahistine (for hearing loss)** Four RCTs in people with possible Menière's disease found no significant difference between betahistine and placebo in change in hearing assessed by pure tone audiograms. Two small RCTs in people with definite or possible Menière's disease found no significant difference in hearing between betahistine and trimetazidine.
- **Lithium** Two small crossover RCTs in people with possible Menière's disease provided insufficient evidence to compare lithium versus placebo in terms of their effects on vertigo, tinnitus, aural fullness, or hearing, although they found that lithium was associated with tremor, thirst, and polyuria in some people.
- **Aminoglycosides; dietary modification; psychological support; vestibular rehabilitation** We found no RCTs on the effects of these interventions in preventing attacks of Menière's disease or delaying disease progression.

DEFINITION Menière's disease is characterised by recurrent episodes of spontaneous rotational vertigo, sensorineural hearing loss, tinnitus, and a feeling of fullness or pressure in the ear. It may be unilateral or bilateral. Acute episodes can occur in clusters of about 6–11 a year, although remission may last several months.[1] The diagnosis is made clinically.[2] It is important to distinguish Menière's disease from other types of vertigo that might occur independently with hearing loss and tinnitus, and respond differently to treatment (e.g. benign positional vertigo, acute labyrinthitis). Strict diagnostic criteria help to identify the condition. In this chapter we applied the classification of the American Academy of Otolaryngology — Head and Neck Surgery to assess the diagnostic rigour used in RCTs (see table 1, p 613).[3–5]

INCIDENCE/ PREVALENCE Menière's disease is most common between 40–60 years of age, although younger people may be affected.[6,7] In Europe, the incidence is about 50–200/ 100 000 a year. A survey of general practitioner records of 27 365 people in the UK found an incidence of 43 affected people in a 1 year period (157/100 000).[8] Diagnostic criteria were not defined in this survey. A survey of over 8 million people in Sweden found an incidence of 46/100 000 a year with diagnosis strictly based on the triad of vertigo, hearing loss, and tinnitus.[9] From smaller studies, the incidence appears lower in Uganda[10] and higher in Japan (350/100 000, based on a national survey of hospital attendances during a single week).[7]

AETIOLOGY/ RISK FACTORS Menière's disease is associated with endolymphatic hydrops (raised endolymph pressure in the membranous labyrinth of the inner ear),[11] but a causal relationship remains unproven.[12] Specific disorders associated with hydrops (such as temporal bone fracture, syphilis, hypothyroidism, Cogan's syndrome, and Mondini dysplasiaⒼ) can produce symptoms similar to those of Menière's disease.

PROGNOSIS Menière's disease is progressive but fluctuates unpredictably. It is difficult to distinguish natural resolution from the effects of treatment. Significant improvement in vertigo is usually seen in the placebo arm of RCTs.[13,14] Acute attacks of vertigo often increase in frequency during the first few years after presentation and then decrease in frequency in association with sustained deterioration in hearing.[6] In most people, vertiginous episodes eventually cease completely.[15] In one 20 year cohort study in 34 people, 28 (82%) people had at least moderate hearing loss (mean pure tone hearing loss > 50 dB)[1] and 16 (47%) developed bilateral disease. Symptoms other than hearing loss improve in 60–80% of people irrespective of treatment.[16]

AIMS OF INTERVENTION To prevent attacks of Menière's disease; to reduce the severity of vertigo in acute attacks; to relieve chronic symptoms of hearing loss and tinnitus; to improve quality of life, with minimum adverse effects of treatment.

OUTCOMES Frequency and severity of acute attacks of vertigo; hearing acuity; severity of tinnitus; sensation of aural fullness; functional impairment and quality of life; adverse effects of treatment.

METHODS *Clinical Evidence* search and appraisal February 2004. We excluded studies with loss to follow up of over 20%. We excluded RCTs that did not use American Academy of Otolaryngology — Head and Neck Surgery diagnostic criteria.[3–5]

QUESTION **What are the effects of treatments for acute attacks?**

OPTION **ANTICHOLINERGICS**

We found no RCTs about the effects of anticholinergics for acute attacks of Menière's disease.

Benefits: We found no systematic review and no RCTs. We found one non-randomised trial (see comment below).[17]

Harms: The non-randomised trial gave no information on adverse effects.[17]

Comment: The non-randomised trial (37 people with definite Menière's disease) compared an anticholinergic (glycopyrrolate 2 mg twice daily as required) versus placebo for 4 weeks.[17] It found that glycopyrrolate significantly reduced the severity of vertigo and its impact on quality of life compared with placebo (Dizziness Handicap Inventory, a validated symptom score,[18] change from baseline to end of trial: 76 to 37 points with glycopyrrolate *v* 73 to 75 points with placebo; $P < 0.001$). The lack of randomisation means that this result should be interpreted with caution.

OPTION **BENZODIAZEPINES**

We found no RCTs about the effects of benzodiazepines for acute attacks of Menière's disease.

Benefits: We found no systematic review or RCTs.

Harms: We found no RCTs.

Comment: None.

OPTION **BETAHISTINE**

We found no RCTs about the effects of betahistine for acute attacks of Menière's disease.

Benefits: We found no systematic review or RCTs.

Harms: We found no RCTs.

Comment: One observational study conducted in 1940 found that intravenous histamine was associated with a reduced severity of acute attacks of Menière's disease.[19]

QUESTION **What are the effects of interventions to prevent acute attacks and delay disease progression?**

OPTION **DIURETICS**

One small crossover RCT provided insufficient evidence about the effects of triamterene plus hydrochlorothiazide on hearing, vertigo, or tinnitus. We found no evidence on their effects on disease progression.

Benefits: We found no systematic review but found one crossover RCT (33 people with possible Menière's disease) comparing a diuretic (triamterene 50 mg plus hydrochlorothiazide 25 mg) versus placebo.[20] It found no significant audiological change in hearing over 17 weeks (P > 0.2). However, the trial may have lacked power to detect a clinically important difference. The trial provided insufficient data to assess effects on vertigo and tinnitus (see comment below).

Harms: The RCT gave no information on adverse effects.[20]

Comment: In the RCT the frequency of vertigo attacks was reduced and tinnitus was unchanged, but valid statistical analyses cannot be performed because the study presented only the mean values for categorical data.[20]

OPTION TRIMETAZIDINE

We found no RCTs comparing trimetazidine versus placebo to prevent attacks of Menière's disease. Two small RCTs in people with definite or possible Menière's disease found no significant difference between trimetazidine and betahistine in hearing or tinnitus. One of these RCTs found that trimetazidine reduced the intensity of vertigo compared with betahistine, but the other RCT found no significant difference in vertigo intensity between trimetazidine and betahistine. We found no evidence on the effects of trimetazidine on disease progression.

Benefits: We found no systematic review. **Versus placebo:** We found no RCTs. **Versus betahistine:** We found two RCTs.[21,22] The first RCT (20 people with definite or probable Menière's disease) compared trimetazidine (20 mg three times daily) versus betahistine (8 mg three times daily) over 3 months.[21] It found no significant difference in hearing, tinnitus, aural fullness, or quality of life (RR for improved quality of life 1.0, 95% CI 0.34 to 2.93). Trimetazidine significantly increased the proportion of people reporting that the duration of vertigo was "substantially better or cured" or reporting that the intensity of vertigo was "substantially better or cured" compared with betahistine (vertigo improved: RR 1.8, 95% CI 1.0 to 3.2; vertigo intensity: RR 1.7, 95% CI 1.0 to 2.8). Trimetazidine also significantly improved the global impression of vertigo scale compared with betahistine, but it is not clear whether this scale has been validated (RR for improvement 2.5, 95% CI 1.17 to 5.3).[21] The second RCT (45 people with possible Menière's disease) compared trimetazidine (20 mg three times daily) versus betahistine (12 mg three times daily) over 2 months and found no significant difference in hearing or tinnitus.[22] A beneficial effect of trimetazidine on vertigo intensity was reported, but this was not confirmed by analysis of the available data (P = 0.23; 2 sided Fisher's exact test).[22]

Harms: No significant adverse effects were reported in the RCTs.[21,22]

Comment: None.

OPTION BETAHISTINE

Seven RCTs in people with probable or possible Menière's disease provided insufficient evidence to compare betahistine versus placebo in terms of their effects on frequency and severity of attacks of vertigo, tinnitus, and aural fullness. Four of the RCTs found no significant difference between betahistine and placebo in change in hearing assessed by pure tone audiograms. Two small RCTs in people with definite or possible Menière's disease found no significant difference between trimetazidine and betahistine in hearing or

tinnitus. One of these RCTs found that trimetazidine reduced the intensity of vertigo compared with betahistine, but the other RCT found no significant difference in vertigo intensity between trimetazidine and betahistine.

Benefits: **Versus placebo:** We found one systematic review[23] (search date 1999, 6 RCTs,[13,24–28] 162 people) and one subsequent RCT[29] that compared betahistine versus placebo in people with Menière's disease. The review did not include a meta-analysis because of heterogeneity among trials (see comment below).[23] The first RCT identified by the review (30 people with possible Menière's disease) found that betahistine (8 mg three times daily) significantly reduced the severity of vertigo after 6 weeks compared with placebo (P = 0.0001), tinnitus (P = 0.001), and aural fullness (P = 0.02).[24] The second RCT identified by the review (35 people with possible Menière's disease, crossover design, see comment below) found no significant difference between betahistine (24 mg three times daily in a slow release formulation) and placebo in tinnitus (P = 0.68) or aural fullness (P = 0.63) after 16 weeks.[13] Vertigo was not adequately assessed. The third RCT identified by the review (16/36 people had a possible diagnosis of Menière's disease) found no significant difference between betahistine (18 mg twice daily) and placebo after 2 weeks on the proportion of people reporting improved vertigo or tinnitus (vertigo: RR 1.17, 95% CI 0.86 to 1.58; tinnitus: RR 2.4, 95% CI 0.11 to 51.32).[25] The fourth RCT identified by the review (10 people with possible Menière's disease) found no significant difference between betahistine (8 mg three times daily) and placebo in the proportion of people with improved vertigo, tinnitus, or aural fullness over 6–12 months (improved vertigo: RR 5.0, 95% CI 0.3 to 84).[26] None of the RCTs found any change in hearing as assessed by pure tone audiograms.[13,24–26] The remaining two RCTs identified by the review reported insufficient detail to confirm reliably that the participants had Menière's disease.[27,28] The subsequent RCT (81 people with possible or probable Menière's disease) found that betahistine (8 mg twice daily) significantly reduced the frequency of attacks of vertigo and increased the proportion of people reporting a reduction in severity of vertigo over 3 months compared with placebo (results presented graphically; decrease in vertigo attacks: about 65% with betahistine *v* about 20% with placebo, P < 0.05; reduced intensity score read from graph: about 67% with betahistine *v* about 30% with placebo, P < 0.03).[29] However, the results should be interpreted with caution because it was not clear whether other outcomes were assessed but not reported. The RCT did not report the number of people with each outcome, severity of symptoms, or effects on hearing.[29] **Versus trimetazidine:** See benefits of trimetazidine, p 609.

Harms: **Versus placebo:** None of the RCTs identified by the review reported any significant adverse effects.[23] The subsequent RCT (81 people) found that betahistine increased headache compared with placebo (5/41 [12.2%] with betahistine *v* 0/40 [0%] with placebo; P value and CI not reported).[29] It found no significant difference between treatments for overall adverse effects (28% with betahistine *v* 22% with placebo; P value and CI not reported). **Versus trimetazidine:** No significant adverse effects were reported in the RCTs.[21,22]

Comment: The systematic review reported that "we found no trials with a low risk of methodological bias which used the highest level of diagnostic criteria and outcome measures".[23] It stated that the lack of diagnostic certainty made it inappropriate to combine results.[23] Bias from selective reporting of outcome measures cannot be excluded in the subsequent RCT comparing betahistine versus placebo.[29] **Crossover studies:** These are difficult to interpret if used to evaluate the effects of treatments on conditions that fluctuate in intensity or if interventions have prolonged effects.[30] Menière's disease is not a stable condition and it is unknown whether any effects of betahistine are prolonged.

OPTION LITHIUM

Two small crossover RCTs in people with possible Menière's disease provided insufficient evidence to compare lithium versus placebo in terms of their effects on vertigo, tinnitus, aural fullness, or hearing, although they found that lithium was associated with tremor, thirst, and polyuria in some people.

Benefits: We found no systematic review but found two crossover RCTs (50 people with possible Menière's disease) of lithium versus placebo.[31,32] They reported no difference in vertigo, tinnitus, aural fullness, or hearing, but no analysable results were presented.

Harms: In the RCTs, serum lithium concentration was checked every 2 weeks to reduce the risk of adverse effects.[31,32] Two people withdrew from one RCT because of adverse effects from lithium (tremor, thirst, polyuria).[31]

Comment: The crossover RCT design may be inappropriate because Menière's disease is not stable and it is not clear whether the lithium is free of other effects.[31,32] Dosage was adjusted to maintain serum lithium concentration between 0.7–1.1 mmol/L.

OPTION DIETARY MODIFICATION

We found no RCTs about the effects of dietary modification in preventing attacks of Menière's disease on delaying disease progression.

Benefits: We found no systematic review or RCTs.

Harms: We found no RCTs.

Comment: It has been suggested that a low salt diet reduces endolymphatic pressure in endolymphatic hydrops,[33] but we found no evidence from RCTs to support or refute this.

OPTION AMINOGLYCOSIDES

We found no RCTs about the effects of aminoglycosides in preventing attacks of Menière's disease on delaying disease progression.

Benefits: We found no systematic review or RCTs.

Harms: Aminoglycosides have been reported to be associated with a risk of severe disruption of balance (including oscillopsia Ⓖ) and sensorineural hearing loss.[34]

Comment: Aminoglycosides have been used in severe bilateral Menière's disease,[35–37] but we found no evidence from RCTs to support or to refute this.

OPTION PSYCHOLOGICAL SUPPORT

We found no RCTs about the effects of psychological support, such as reassurance, in preventing attacks of Menière's disease on delaying disease progression.

Benefits: We found no systematic review or RCTs.

Harms: We found no RCTs.

Comment: Symptomatic improvement is seen with all treatments for Menière's disease, including placebo[16,31] or being put on a waiting list for surgery.[38] Such improvements may be attributed to the psychological support of receiving treatment, but have not been distinguished from improvements attributable to the natural history of Menière's disease.

OPTION VESTIBULAR REHABILITATION

We found no RCTs about the effects of vestibular rehabilitation in prevening attacks of Menière's disease on delaying disease progression.

Benefits: We found no systematic review or RCTs.

Harms: We found no RCTs.

Comment: None.

GLOSSARY

Cogan's syndrome Episodic vertigo of the Menière's type, hearing loss, and interstitial keratitis, without syphilis.[5]

Mondini dysplasia A congenital deformity of the cochlea in which only the basal turns are present.

Oscillopsia A disabling disturbance of the vestibulo-ocular reflex, manifest as oscillating vision typically with head movement.

Vestibular rehabilitation Involves a series of exercises intended to improve the sense of balance through controlled movements of the head and body.[39] It is usually recommended for stable vestibular disorders.[40]

REFERENCES

1. Friberg U, Stahle J, Svedberg A. The natural course of Menière's disease. *Acta Otolaryngol Suppl* 1984;406:72–77.
2. Kitahara M. Concepts and diagnostic criteria of Menière's disease. In: Kitahara M, ed. *Menière's disease*. Tokyo: Springer-Verlag, 1990:3–12.
3. Alford BR. Menière's disease: criteria for diagnosis and evaluation of therapy for reporting. Report of subcommittee on equilibrium and its measurement. *Trans Am Acad Ophthalmol Otolaryngol* 1972;76:1462–1464.
4. Pearson BW, Brackmann DE. Committee on Hearing and Equilibrium guidelines for reporting treatment results in Menière's disease. *Otolaryngol Head Neck Surg* 1985;93:578–581.
5. Committee on Hearing and Equilibrium. Guidelines for the diagnosis and evaluation of therapy in Menière's disease. *Otolaryngol Head Neck Surg* 1995;113:181–185.
6. Moffat DA, Ballagh RH. Menière's disease. In: Kerr AG, Booth JB, eds. *Scott-Brown's otolaryngology*. 6th ed. Oxford: Butterworth-Heinemann, 1997.
7. Watanabe I. Incidence of Menière's disease, including some other epidemiological data. In: Oosterveld WJ, ed. *Menière's disease: a comprehensive appraisal*. Chichester: Wiley, 1983:9–23.
8. Cawthorne T, Hewlett AB. Menière's disease. *Proc Royal Soc Med* 1954;47:663–670.
9. Stahle J, Stahle C, Arenberg IK. Incidence of Menière's disease. *Arch Otolaryngol* 1978;104:99–102.
10. Nsamba C. A comparative study of the aetiology of vertigo in the African. *J Laryngol Otol* 1972;86:917–925.
11. Hallpike C, Cairns H. Observations on the pathology of Menière's syndrome. *J Laryngol Otol* 1938;53:625–655.
12. Ruckenstein MJ, Harrison RV. Cochlear pathology in Menière's disease. In: Harris JP, ed. *Menière's disease*. The Hague: Kugler Publications, 1999:195–202.
13. Schmidt JT, Huizing EH. The clinical drug trial in Menière's disease with emphasis on the effect of betahistine SR. *Acta Otolaryngol* 1992;497(suppl):1–189.
14. Moser M, Ranacher G, Wilmot TJ, et al. A double-blind clinical trial of hydroxyethylrutosides in Menière's disease. *J Laryngol Otol* 1984;98:265–272.
15. Silverstein H, Smouha E, Jones R. Natural history versus surgery for Menière's disease. *Otolaryngol Head Neck Surg* 1989;100:6–16.
16. Torok N. Old and new in Menière's disease. *Laryngoscope* 1977;87:1870–1877.
17. Storper IS, Spitzer JB, Scanlan M. Use of glycopyrrolate in the treatment of Menière's disease. *Laryngoscope* 1998;108:1442–1445.
18. Jacobson GP, Newman CW. The development of the Dizziness Handicap Inventory. *Arch Otolaryngol Head Neck Surg* 1990;116:424–427.
19. Sheldon CH, Horton BT. Treatment of Menière's disease with histamine administered intravenously. *Proceedings of the Staff Meetings of the Mayo Clinic* 1940;15:17–21.
20. van Deelen GW, Huizing EH. Use of a diuretic (Dyazide) in the treatment of Menière's disease. A double-blind cross-over placebo-controlled study. *ORL J Otorhinolaryngol Relat Spec* 1986;48:287–292.
21. Kluyskens P, Lambert P, D'Hooge D. Trimetazidine versus betahistine in vestibular vertigo. A double blind study. *Ann Otolaryngol Chir Cervicofac* 1990;107(suppl 1):11–19. [In French]
22. Martini A, De Domenico F. Trimetazidine versus betahistine in Menière's disease. A double blind method. *Ann Otolaryngol Chir Cervicofac* 1990;107(suppl 1):20–27. [In French]
23. James AL, Burton MJ. Betahistine for Menière's disease or syndrome. In: The Cochrane Library, Issue 3, 2002. Oxford: Wiley. Search date 1999; primary sources Cochrane Controlled Trials Register, Medline, Embase, Index Medicus, and hand searches of reference lists.

24. Salami A, Dellepiane M, Tinelle E, et al. Studio a doppia cecita' tra cloridrato di betaistina e placebo nel trattamento delle sindromi Menieriformi. *Valsalva* 1984;60:302–312. [In Italian]
25. Okamato K, Hazeyama F, Taira T, et al. Therapeutic results of betahistine in Menière's disease with statistical analysis. *Iryo* 1968;22:650–666. [In Japanese]
26. Ricci V, Sittoni V, Nicora M. Valutazione terapeutica e tollerabilita del chloridrato di betaistina (Microser) in confronto a placebo nella malattia di Menière. *Riv Ital Ornitolog Audiolog Foniat* 1987;7:347–350.
27. Burkin A. Betahistine treatment of Menière's syndrome. *Clin Med* 1967;74:41–48.
28. Elia JC. Double-blind evaluation of a new treatment for Menière's syndrome. *JAMA* 1966;196:187–189.
29. Mira E, Guidetti G, Ghilardi L, et al. Betahistine dihydrochloride in the treatment of peripheral vestibular vertigo. *Eur Arch Otorhinolaryngol* 2003;260:73–77.
30. Fleiss JL. The crossover study. In: *The design and analysis of clinical experiments.* Chichester: Wiley, 1984.
31. Thomsen J, Bech P, Prytz S, et al. Menière's disease: lithium treatment (demonstration of placebo effect in a double blind cross-over trial). *Clin Otolaryngol* 1979;4:119–123.
32. Thomsen J, Bech P, Geisler A, et al. Lithium treatment of Menière's disease: results of a double-blind cross-over trial. *Acta Otolaryngol* 1976;82:294–296.
33. Furstenburg AC, Richardson G, Lathrop FD. Menière's disease. Addenda to medical therapy. *Arch Otolaryngol* 1941;34:1083–1092.
34. Balyan FR, Taibah A, De Donato G, et al. Titration streptomycin therapy in Menière's disease: long-term results. *Otolaryngol Head Neck Surg* 1998;118:261–266.
35. Wilson WR, Schuknecht HF. Update on the use of streptomycin therapy for Menière's disease. *Am J Otol* 1980;2:108–111.
36. Graham MD. Bilateral Menière's disease. Treatment with intramuscular titration streptomycin sulfate. *Otolaryngol Clin North Am* 1997;30:1097–1100.
37. Shea JJ, Ge X, Orchik DJ. Long-term results of low dose intramuscular streptomycin for Menière's disease. *Am J Otol* 1994;15:540–544.
38. Kerr AG, Toner JG. A new approach to surgery for Menière's disease: talking about surgery. *Clin Otolaryngol* 1998;23:263–264.
39. Dix MR. The rationale and technique of head exercises in the treatment of vertigo. *Acta Otorhinolaryngol Belg* 1979;33:370–384.
40. Clendaniel RA, Tucci DL. Vestibular rehabilitation strategies in Menière's disease. *Otolaryngol Clin North Am* 1997;30:1145–1158.

Adrian James
Department of Otolaryngology,
Southmead Hospital
Bristol
UK

Marc Thorp
Department of Otolaryngology
Corner Brook Newfoundland
Canada

Competing interests: None declared.

TABLE 1 American Academy of Otolaryngology — Head and Neck Surgery definition of the certainty of diagnosis of Menière's disease (see text, p 607).[3–5]

Certain	Definite Menière's disease plus postmortem confirmation
Definite	Two or more episodes of vertigo* plus audiometrically confirmed sensorineural hearing loss; tinnitus or aural fullness plus other causes excluded
Probable	One episode of vertigo* plus audiometrically confirmed sensorineural hearing loss plus tinnitus or aural fullness; other causes excluded
Possible	Episodes of vertigo* with no hearing loss, or sensorineural hearing loss with dysequilibrium; other causes excluded

*Defined as spontaneous, rotational vertigo lasting more than 20 minutes.

Middle ear pain and trauma during air travel

Search date March 2004

Simon Janvrin

QUESTIONS

INTERVENTIONS

Key Messages

- **Oral decongestants in adults** One RCT in adult passengers with a history of ear pain during air travel found limited evidence that oral pseudoephedrine decreased symtoms of barotrauma during air travel compared with placebo. One other RCT in adult passengers with a history of ear pain during air travel found limited evidence that oral pseudoephedrine decreased ear pain and hearing loss compared with placebo.
- **Oral decongestants in children** One small RCT in children up to the age of 6 years found no significant difference between oral pseudoephedrine and placebo in ear pain at take off or landing.
- **Topical nasal decongestants** One small RCT in adults with a history of ear pain during air travel found no significant difference between oxymetazoline nasal spray and placebo in symptoms of barotrauma.

DEFINITION	The effects of air travel on the middle ear can include ear drum pain, vertigo, hearing loss, and ear drum perforation.
INCIDENCE/ PREVALENCE	The prevalence of symptoms depends on the altitude, type of aircraft, and characteristics of the passengers. One point prevalence study found that 20% of adult and 40% of child passengers had negative pressure in the middle ear after flight, and that 10% of adults and 22% of children had auroscopic evidence of damage to the ear drum.[1] We found no data on the incidence of perforation, which seems to be extremely rare in commercial passengers.
AETIOLOGY/ RISK FACTORS	During aircraft descent, the pressure in the middle ear drops relative to that in the ear canal. A narrow, inflamed, or poorly functioning Eustachian tube impedes the necessary influx of air. As the pressure difference between the middle and outer ear increases, the ear drum is pulled inward.
PROGNOSIS	In most people symptoms resolve spontaneously. Experience in military aviation shows that most ear drum perforations will heal spontaneously.[2]
AIMS OF INTERVENTION	To prevent ear pain and trauma during air travel.
OUTCOMES	Incidence and severity of pain and hearing loss; incidence of perforation of ear drum; barotrauma Ⓖ.
METHODS	*Clinical Evidence* search and appraisal March 2004.

QUESTION What are the effects of preventive interventions?

OPTION ORAL DECONGESTANTS

One RCT in adult passengers with a history of ear pain during air travel found limited evidence that oral pseudoephedrine decreased symptoms of barotrauma during air travel compared with placebo. One other RCT in adult passengers with a history of ear pain during air travel found limited evidence that oral pseudoephedrine decreased ear pain and hearing loss compared with placebo. One small RCT in children up to the age of 6 years found no significant difference between oral pseudoephedrine and placebo in ear pain at take off or landing.

Benefits: We found no systematic review. We found three RCTs comparing oral pseudoephedrine versus placebo.[3–5] Two RCTs in adult passengers, with a history of ear pain during air travel, compared oral pseudoephedrine (120 mg given at least 30 minutes before flight) versus placebo.[3,4] Those with acute or chronic ear problems were excluded. Both RCTs assessed outcomes by a post-flight questionnaire returned by mail. The first RCT (150 adults) compared three treatments: oral pseudoephedrine; oxymetazoline nasal spray; or placebo.[3] The RCT found that pseudoephedrine significantly decreased the proportion of people with symptoms of barotrauma Ⓖ compared with placebo (ear pain, blockage, hearing loss, dizziness/vertigo, tinnitus: 14/41 [34%] with pseudoephedrine *v* 29/41 [71%] with placebo; RR 0.48, 95% CI 0.29 to 0.67).[3] The second RCT (190 adults) found that pseudoephedrine significantly reduced ear pain (25/96 [26%] with pseudoephedrine *v* 43/94 [46%] with placebo; P = 0.007) and hearing loss compared with placebo (20/96 [21%] with pseudoephedrine *v* 38/94 [40%] with placebo; P = 0.006).[4] The third RCT (50 children up to the age of 6 years) compared oral pseudoephedrine versus placebo.[5] It found no significant difference in ear pain between children taking pseudoephedrine or placebo at either take off or landing.

Harms: Adverse effects reported by the first RCT included drowsiness (4/41 [10%] with pseudoephedrine *v* 2/41 [5%] with placebo), dry mouth (4/41 [10%] *v* 1/41 [2%]), nasal irritation (1/41 [2%] *v* 0/41 [0%]), stomach upset (1/41 [2%] *v* 0/41 [0%]), and headache (0/41 [0%] *v* 1/41 [2%]).[3] The second RCT reported drowsiness (7/96 [7.3%] with pseudoephedrine v 2/94 [2.2%] with placebo) and nausea and dry mouth (4.2% v 4.3%).[4] The third RCT found more children taking pseudoephedrine were drowsy on take off compared with placebo (30/50 [60%] with pseudoephedrine v 11/41 [27%] with placebo; P = 0.003).[5]

Comment: None.

OPTION TOPICAL NASAL DECONGESTANTS

One small RCT in adults with a history of ear pain during air travel found no significant difference with oxymetazoline nasal spray versus placebo in symptoms of barotrauma.

Benefits: We found no systematic review. We found one RCT in adults with a history of ear pain during air travel, which compared oxymetazoline nasal spray, oral pseudoephedrine, or placebo during air travel.[3] Outcomes were assessed by a post-flight questionnaire returned by mail. The RCT (150 people) found no significant difference in symptoms of barotrauma(G) between oxymetazoline versus placebo (ear pain, blockage, hearing loss, dizziness/vertigo, tinnitus: 64% of people with oxymetazoline v 71% of people with placebo; P = 0.695).[3]

Harms: Adverse effects included nasal irritation (6/42 [14%] with oxymetazoline v 0/41 [0%] with placebo), drowsiness (1/42 [2%] v 2/41 [5%]), dry mouth (1/42 [2%] v 1/41 [2%]), stomach upset (1/42 [2%] v 0/41 [0%]), and headache (1/42 [2%] v 1/41 [2%]).[3]

Comment: The RCT may have been too small to rule out an effect of topical decongestants.

GLOSSARY

Barotrauma Symptoms caused by changes of atmospheric pressure are called barotrauma. In the ear these include ear drum pain, vertigo, hearing loss, tinnitus and ear drum perforation.

REFERENCES

1. Stangerup S-E, Tjernstrom O, Klokke M, et al. Point prevalence of barotitis in children and adults after flight, and the effect of autoinflation. *Aviat Space Environ Med* 1998;69:45–49.
2. O'Reilly BJ. Otorhinolaryngology. In: Ernsting J, Nicholson AN, Rainford DJ, eds. *Aviation Medicine*. 3rd edition. Oxford: Butterworth-Heinemann, 1999:319–336.
3. Jones JS, Sheffield W, White LJ, et al. A double-blind comparison between oral pseudoephedrine and topical oxymetazoline in the prevention of barotrauma during air travel. *Am J Emerg Med* 1998;16:262–264.
4. Csortan E, Jones J, Haan M, et al. Efficacy of pseudoephedrine for the prevention of barotrauma during air travel. *Ann Emerg Med* 1994;23:1324–1327.
5. Buchanan BJ, Hoagland J, Fischer PR. Pseudoephedrine and air travel-associated ear pain in children. *Arch Pediatr Adolesc Med* 1999;153:466–468.

Simon Janvrin
Civil Aviation Authority, West Sussex, UK

Competing interests: None declared.

Otitis externa

Search date March 2004

Daniel Hajioff

QUESTIONS

INTERVENTIONS

See glossary G

Key Messages

Treatment of otitis externa

- **Topical aluminium acetate drops (as effective as topical anti-infective agents)** We found no RCTs that compared topical aluminium acetate versus placebo. One RCT in people with acute diffuse otitis externa found no significant difference between aluminium acetate drops and topical polymyxin–neomycin–hydrocortisone drops in time to clinical cure or clinical cure rate at 4 weeks.
- **Topical anti-infective agents (antibiotics or antifungals with or without steroids)** One RCT found that methylprednisolone–neomycin drops improved symptoms and signs compared with placebo at 28 days. Two RCTs found no significant difference in cure rate between topical quinolones and other topical anti-infective agents. One RCT found that triamcinolone–neomycin drops improved resolution rates compared with hydrocortisone–neomycin–polymyxin B drops. Two RCTs found limited evidence that neomycin–dexamethasone–acetic acid spray improved clinical cure compared with topical anti-infective drops that did not contain acetic acid. We found no RCTs on the effects of topical anti-infective agents versus oral antibiotics. One RCT found limited evidence of no significant difference between topical anti-infective ointment plus oral co-trimoxazole and topical anti-infective ointment alone in symptom severity, symptom duration, and cure rate. One RCT in people with acute diffuse otitis externa found no significant difference between topical polymyxin-neomycin-hydrocortisone drops and aluminium acetate drops in time to clinical cure or cure rate at 4 weeks.
- **Topical steroids** One RCT in people with mild or moderate acute or chronic otitis externa found that topical budesonide improved symptoms and signs compared with placebo. We found no RCTs of topical steroids compared with topical anti-infective agents. One RCT found no significant difference in symptom scores between low potency steroid (topical hydrocortisone) and high potency steroid (topical hydrocortisone butyrate) after 1 week.

- **Oral antibiotics** We found no RCTs of oral antibiotics compared with placebo or topical anti-infective agents. One RCT found limited evidence of no significant difference between oral co-trimoxazole plus topical anti-infective ointment and topical anti-infective ointment alone in symptom severity, symptom duration, and cure rate.
- **Specialist aural toilet** We found no RCTs that compared specialist aural toilet versus no aural toilet. One RCT found no significant difference between an ear wick plus anti-infective drops versus ribbon gauze impregnated with anti-infective ointment in resolution rates after 4 weeks.
- **Topical acetic acid (insufficient evidence to demonstrate effectiveness versus placebo)** We found no RCTs comparing topical acetic acid versus placebo. One RCT in adults with acute diffuse otitis externa found that topical steroids plus antibiotics and topical acetic acid plus steroids reduced the duration of symptoms, increased overall cure rates, and reduced recurrence compared with acetic acid alone.
- **Oral antibiotics plus topical anti-infective agents (no better than topical anti-infective agents alone)** One RCT found limited evidence of no significant difference between oral co-trimoxazole plus topical anti-infective ointment and topical anti-infective ointment alone in symptom severity, symptom duration, and cure rate.

DEFINITION Otitis externa is inflammation, often with infection, of the external ear canal. This inflammation is usually generalised throughout the ear canal, so it is often referred to as "diffuse otitis externa". The present topic excludes localised inflammations such as furuncles. Otitis externa has acute (< 6 weeks), chronic (> 3 months), and necrotising (malignant) forms. Acute otitis externa may present as a single episode, or recur. It causes severe pain with aural discharge and associated hearing loss.[1] If the ear canal is visible, it appears red and inflamed. Chronic otitis externa may result in canal stenosis with associated hearing loss, for which it may be difficult to fit hearing aids. Necrotising otitis externa is defined by destruction of the temporal bone, usually in people with diabetes or in people who are immunocompromised, and can be life threatening.[2] In this chapter, we look at empirical treatment of acute and chronic otitis externa only.

INCIDENCE/ PREVALENCE Otitis externa is common in all parts of the world. The incidence is not known precisely, but 10% of people are thought to have been affected at some time.[3] The condition affects children but is more common in adults. It accounts for a large proportion of the workload of otolaryngology departments, but milder cases are often managed in primary care.[3]

AETIOLOGY/ RISK FACTORS Otitis externa may be associated with local or generalised eczema of the ear canal. It is more common in swimmers, in humid environments, in people with an absence of ear wax or narrow external ear canals, in hearing aid users, and after mechanical trauma.[4]

PROGNOSIS We found few reliable data. Many cases of otitis externa resolve spontaneously over several weeks or months. Acute episodes have a tendency to recur, although the risk of recurrence is unknown. Experience suggests that chronic inflammation affects a small proportion of people after a single episode of acute otitis externa, and may rarely lead to canal stenosis.[1]

AIMS OF INTERVENTION To improve or abolish symptoms; to prevent recurrence and complications, with minimal adverse effects.

OUTCOMES Severity and duration of signs and symptoms (pain, discharge, hearing loss, redness); rates of resolution or cure (defined as complete resolution of signs and symptoms); prevention of recurrence; ability to use hearing aids; quality of life; adverse effects of treatment.

METHODS *Clinical Evidence* search and appraisal March 2004. We excluded RCTs with a follow up of less than 80%. We also excluded RCTs with a follow up of less than 1 month, so that we could assess rates of sustained resolution and recurrence.

QUESTION **What are the effects of empirical treatment?**

OPTION **ORAL ANTIBIOTICS**

We found no RCTs of oral antibiotics compared with placebo or topical anti-infective agents. One RCT found limited evidence of no significant difference between oral co-trimoxazole plus topical anti-infective ointment and topical anti-infective ointment alone in symptom severity, symptom duration, and cure rate.

Benefits: We found no systematic review. **Versus placebo:** We found no RCTs. **Versus topical anti-infective agents:** We found no RCTs. **Plus topical anti-infective agents:** One double blind RCT (105 people with any severity of acute diffuse otitis externa on otoscopy) compared 5 days of oral co-trimoxazole versus placebo in a primary care setting.[5] Both groups also received repeated applications of ointment containing triamcinolone, neomycin, and gramicidin, and had suction of the external canal if discharge was present. The RCT found no significant difference between groups in symptom severity scores, duration of symptoms, or cure rate (improvement in mean symptom severity score on scale ranging from 1 [no symptoms] to 5 [severe symptoms]: 0.72 with added oral co-trimoxazole *v* 0.69 with added placebo; $P > 0.4$; mean duration of symptoms: 3.1 days with added oral co-trimoxazole *v* 3.1 days with placebo; $P > 0.5$; cure rates: 18/47 [38%] with added oral co-trimoxazole *v* 21/53 [40%] with placebo; $P > 0.8$).[5]

Harms: The RCT did not report on harms.[5]

Comment: None.

OPTION **TOPICAL ANTI-INFECTIVE AGENTS (ANTIBIOTICS OR ANTIFUNGALS WITH OR WITHOUT STEROIDS)**

One RCT found that methylprednisolone–neomycin drops improved symptoms and signs compared with placebo at 28 days. Two RCTs found no significant difference in cure rate between topical quinolones and other topical anti-infective agents. One RCT found that triamcinolone–neomycin drops improved resolution rates compared with hydrocortisone–neomycin–polymyxin B drops. Two RCTs found limited evidence that neomycin–dexamethasone–acetic acid spray improved clinical cure compared with topical anti-infective drops that did not contain acetic acid. We found no RCTs on the effects of topical anti-infective agents versus oral antibiotics. One RCT found limited evidence of no significant difference between topical anti-infective ointment plus oral co-trimoxazole and topical anti-infective ointment alone in symptom severity, symptom duration, and cure rate. One RCT in people with acute diffuse otitis externa found no significant difference between topical polymyxin-neomycin-hydrocortisone drops and aluminium acetate drops in time to clinical cure or cure rate at 4 weeks.

Benefits: We found no systematic review. **Versus placebo:** One double blind RCT (40 people in secondary care with mild, moderate, or severe, acute or chronic diffuse otitis externa) compared methylprednisolone–neomycin drops versus placebo drops for 10 days.[6] All people in the RCT had "cleansing" of their external ear canals (details not reported). The RCT found that methylprednisolone–neomycin drops significantly improved symptoms compared with placebo at 28 days ("good" response: 11/20 [55%] with methylprednisolone–neomycin drops *v* 2/20 [10%] with placebo; $P < 0.001$) **Versus oral antibiotics:** We found no RCTs. **Plus oral antibiotics:** See benefits of oral antibiotics, p 619. **Versus each other:** We found four RCTs.[7–10] Three RCTs compared preparations containing a quinolone versus other agents.[7–9] The first, a double blind RCT (842 people with mild to severe acute diffuse otitis externa on otoscopy), compared ciprofloxacin drops with or without hydrocortisone versus polymyxin–neomycin–hydrocortisone drops in a primary care setting for 1 week.[7] People in both groups received suction or mopping of discharge if present. The RCT found no significant difference between ciprofloxacin alone, ciprofloxacin–hydrocortisone, and polymyxin–neomycin–hydrocortisone at 14–28 days' follow up (improvement or resolution: 222/239 [93%] with ciprofloxacin *v* 212/236 [90%] with ciprofloxacin–hydrocortisone *v* 198/228 [87%] with polymyxin–neomycin–hydrocortisone; P values not reported).[7] The second RCT (single blind, 601 people with any severity of acute diffuse otitis externa on otoscopy) compared ofloxacin drops versus neomycin–hydrocortisone–polymyxin B drops in a primary care setting for 10 days.[8] At 1 month, it found no significant difference between groups for clinical or microbiological cure (clinical cure: 215/242 [89%] with ofloxacin *v* 206/232 [89%] with neomycin–hydrocortisone–polymyxin B drops, P = 0.86; microbiological cure: 85/93 [91%] with ofloxacin *v* 97/103 [94%] with neomycin–hydrocortisone–polymyxin B drops, P = 0.77; no further data reported). A third RCT is being translated and will be included in future updates of *Clinical Evidence*.[9] The fourth RCT (double blind, 55 people with moderate to severe acute or chronic diffuse otitis externa on otoscopy, in a secondary care setting) compared drops containing hydrocortisone–neomycin sulphate and polymyxin B versus drops containing triamcinolone–neomycin undecenoate for 1 month or until resolution of all symptoms and signs.[10] All people received microsuction of their ears if discharge was present. The RCT found that triamcinolone–neomycin drops significantly improved resolution rates compared with hydrocortisone–neomycin–polymyxin B drops at 1 month (resolution: 27/34 [79%] with triamcinolone–neomycin *v* 10/21 [47%] with hydrocortisone–neomycin–polymyxin B; P < 0.01).[10] **Antibiotic–steroid–acetic acid spray versus antibiotic–steroid drops:** We found two RCTs.[11,12] One single blind RCT (60 people with any severity of acute or chronic diffuse otitis externa on otoscopy) compared neomycin–dexamethasone–acetic acid spray versus framycetin–gramicidin–dexamethasone drops in a primary care setting for 10 days.[11] At 1 month, the neomycin–dexamethasone–acetic acid spray significantly improved symptoms and signs compared with the framycetin–gramicidin–dexamethasone drops (symptom free: 26/32 [81.3%] with neomycin–dexamethasone–acetic acid spray *v* 6/26 [23.1%] with framycetin–gramicidin–dexamethasone drops, P < 0.0001; free of clinical signs: 17/32 [53.1%] with neomycin–dexamethasone–acetic acid spray *v* 10/28 [37.0%] with framycetin–gramicidin–dexamethasone drops, P < 0.05). A second, unblinded RCT (187 people with any severity of acute or chronic diffuse otitis externa on otoscopy) compared neomycin–dexamethasone–acetic acid spray versus neomycin–hydrocortisone–polymyxin B drops in a primary care setting for 10 days.[12] It found no significant difference between groups in the proportion of people with improved global symptom scores at 10 days and at 1 month (at 10 days: 86/91 [94.5%] improved with neomycin–dexamethasone–acetic acid spray *v* 79/85 [92.9%] with neomycin–hydrocortisone–polymyxin B drops, P > 0.5; at 1 month: 54/86 [62.8%] improved with neomycin–dexamethasone–acetic acid spray *v* 48/81 [59.3%] with neomycin–hydrocortisone–polymyxin B drops, P > 0.5).[12] However, compared with neomycin–hydrocortisone–polymyxin B drops, neomycin–dexamethasone–acetic acid spray significantly increased the proportion of people considered to have "good" improvement in signs at 10 days (48/91 [52.7%] with neomycin–dexamethasone–acetic acid spray *v*

31/85 [36.5%] with neomycin–hydrocortisone–polymyxin B drops, P < 0.05). **Versus topical steroids:** We found no RCTs. **Versus topical aluminium acetate:** See benefits of topical aluminium acetate, p 622.

Harms: Versus each other: One RCT found no significant difference between ofloxacin drops and neomycin–hydrocortisone–polymyxin B drops in rates of local pruritus, dizziness, or vertigo (local pruritus: 25/158 [15.8%] with ofloxacin *v* 18/156 [11.5%] with neomycin–hydrocortisone–polymyxin B, P = 0.33; dizziness or vertigo: 4/158 [2.5%] with ofloxacin *v* 2/156 [1.3%] with neomycin–hydrocortisone–polymyxin B, P value not reported).[8] Antibiotic-steroid-acetic acid spray versus antibiotic-steroid drops: One RCT reported that 6/32 (18.8%) people using neomycin–dexamethasone–acetic acid spray and 3/26 (11.5%) people using framycetin–gramicidin–dexamethasone drops reported local stinging or burning in the first few days of treatment (significance not reported), which did not affect adherence.[11] The other RCTs did not report on harms.[7,9,10,12]

Comment: None.

OPTION TOPICAL STEROIDS

One RCT in people with mild or moderate acute or chronic otitis externa found that topical budesonide improved symptoms and signs compared with placebo. We found no RCTs of topical steroids compared with topical anti-infective agents. One RCT found no significant difference in symptom scores between low potency steroid (topical hydrocortisone) and high potency steroid (topical hydrocortisone butyrate) after 1 week.

Benefits: We found no systematic review. **Versus placebo:** We found one double blind RCT (60 people with mild or moderate acute or chronic diffuse otitis externa on otoscopy).[13] People with complete occlusion of the external ear canal were excluded. The RCT compared budesonide drops versus placebo drops in a secondary care setting for 7 days.[13] Ear discharge was treated by suction in both groups. The RCT found that budesonide drops significantly improved symptoms and signs compared with placebo after 10 days (change from baseline in a global clinical score ranging from 0 [no symptoms/signs] to 3 [severe symptoms/signs]: −2.29 with budesonide *v* +0.23 with placebo; P = 0.001). **Versus topical anti-infective agents:** We found no RCTs. **Low versus high potency steroids:** One double blind RCT (55 people with any severity of acute or chronic diffuse otitis externa on otoscopy) compared low potency steroid drops (1% hydrocortisone) versus high potency steroid drops (hydrocortisone-17-α-butyrate) in a secondary care setting.[14] It found no significant difference between treatments in symptom scores after 1 week of treatment (score ranging from 0 [no symptoms] to 3 [severe symptoms]: 0.84 with low potency steroid drops *v* 0.80 with high potency steroid drops; P > 0.2).[14]

Harms: **Versus placebo:** The RCT found no significant difference in the frequency of local or systemic adverse events between groups (30% with budesonide *v* 27% with placebo).[13] **Low versus high potency steroids:** The RCT did not report on harms.[14]

Comment: None.

OPTION TOPICAL ALUMINIUM ACETATE DROPS

We found no RCTs that compared topical aluminium acetate versus placebo. One RCT in people with acute diffuse otitis externa found no significant difference between aluminium acetate drops and topical polymyxin–neomycin–hydrocortisone drops in time to clinical cure or clinical cure rate at 4 weeks.

Benefits: We found no systematic review. **Versus placebo:** We found no RCTs. **Versus topical anti-infective agents:** One RCT (126 people with any severity of acute diffuse otitis externa on otoscopy) compared aluminium acetate drops versus polymyxin–neomycin–hydrocortisone drops in a primary care setting for 14 days.[15] People in both groups had discharge removed if present (no further details of technique provided). The RCT found no significant difference between groups in clinical cure rate at 4 weeks or mean time to clinical resolution (clinical cure rate: 59/65 [91%] with aluminium acetate *v* 49/61 [80%] with polymyxin–neomycin–hydrocortisone, $P > 0.2$; mean time to clinical resolution: 9.4 days with aluminium acetate *v* 11.1 days with polymyxin–neomycin–hydrocortisone; $P > 0.2$).

Harms: The RCT did not report on harms.[15]

Comment: None.

OPTION TOPICAL ACETIC ACID

We found no RCTs comparing topical acetic acid versus placebo. One RCT in adults with acute diffuse otitis externa found that topical steroids plus antibiotics and topical acetic acid plus steroids reduced the duration of symptoms, increased overall cure rates, and reduced recurrence compared with acetic acid alone.

Benefits: Versus placebo: We found no systematic review and no RCTs. Versus topical steroids plus antibiotics: We found one RCT (213 adults in primary care with any severity of diffuse acute otitis externa on otoscopy), which compared three treatments: acetic acid drops, triamcinolone–acetic acid drops, and dexamethasone–neomycin–polymixin drops.[16] All groups received aural toilet**G** (suction or expandable sponge wick) as required. It found that acetic acid alone significantly increased time to recovery, reduced cure rate at 21 days, and significantly increased the risk of recurrence between 21 and 48 days compared with topical steroids plus antibiotics (median time to recovery: 8.0 days with acetic acid v 6.0 days with steroid–antibiotic drops, P value not stated; cure: 40/65 [62%] with acetic acid v 63/73 [86%] with steroid plus antibiotic; OR for steroid plus antibiotic v acetic acid 3.9, 95% CI 1.7 to 9.1; recurrence: 21/47 [45%] with acetic acid v 14/68 [21%] with steroid plus antibiotic; OR for steroid plus antibiotic v acetic acid 0.4, 95% CI 0.2 to 1.0). Versus topical acetic acid plus steroids: We found one RCT (213 adults in primary care with any severity of diffuse acute otitis externa on otoscopy), which is described above.[16] It found that acetic acid alone significantly increased time to recovery, reduced cure rate at 21 days, and significantly increased recurrence rate compared with topical acetic acid plus steroids (median time to recovery: 8.0 days with acetic acid v 7.0 days with acetic acid plus steroids; cure: 40/65 [62%] with acetic acid v 54/61 [89%] with acetic acid plus steroid; OR for acetic acid plus steroid v acetic acid 4.8, 95% CI 1.9 to 12.3; recurrence: 21/47 [45%] with acetic acid v 15/57 [26%] with acetic acid plus steroid; OR for acetic acid plus steroid v acetic acid 0.3, 95%CI 0.1 to 0.7).

Harms: In the RCT, 74% of participants reported at least one adverse effect.[16] Adverse effects included local burning, pain, and irritation, although the study reported no significant difference among the treatment groups (no data presented).

Comment: None.

OPTION SPECIALIST AURAL TOILET

We found no RCTs that compared specialist aural toilet versus no aural toilet. One RCT found no significant difference between an ear wick plus anti-infective drops versus ribbon gauze impregnated with anti-infective ointment in resolution rates after 4 weeks.

Benefits: We found no systematic review. **Versus no aural toilet⊖:** We found no RCTs. **Comparison of different types of aural toilet:** One RCT in a secondary care setting (94 people with moderate to severe acute diffuse otitis externa on otoscopy) compared an ear wick plus anti-infective drops (framycetin–gramicidin–dexamethasone or flumetasone) removed after 3 days versus ribbon gauze impregnated with anti-infective ointment (framycetin–gramicidin or triamcinolone–gramicidin–neomycin–nystatin) removed after 3 days.[17] It found no significant difference between groups in resolution rates at 4 weeks (resolution defined as absence of symptoms and signs: 30/47 [64%] with ear wick v 33/47 [70%] with ribbon gauze; P = 0.58).

Harms: No adverse effects were reported.[17]

Comment: The results of studies may not be generalisable to settings where professionals have not been trained to provide specialist aural toilet.

GLOSSARY

Aural toilet Aural toilet is usually performed in a secondary (specialist) setting and includes dry mopping of the ear canal or suction. These can be performed using a head light or microscope, which allows cleaning of the more medial areas of the ear canal.

Topical acetic acid New option added. Categorised as Unknown effectiveness.

REFERENCES

1. Agius AM, Pickles JM, Burch KL. A prospective study of otitis externa. *Clin Otolaryngol* 1992;17:150–154.
2. Doroghazi RM, Nadol JB, Hyslop NE, et al. Invasive external otitis. Report of 21 cases and review of the literature. *Am J Med* 1981;71:603–618.
3. Raza SA, Denholm SW, Wong JC. An audit of the management of otitis externa in an ENT casualty clinic. *J Laryngol Otol* 1995;109:130–133.
4. Hirsh BE. Infections of the external ear. *Am J Otolaryngol* 1992;17:207.
5. Yelland MJ. The efficacy of oral cotrimoxazole in the treatment of otitis externa in general practice. *Med J Aust* 1993;158:697–699.
6. Cannon SJ, Grunwaldt E. Treatment of otitis externa with a tropical steroid–antibiotic combination. *Eye Ear Nose Throat Mon* 1967;46:1296–1302.
7. Pistorius B, Westberry K, Drehobl M, et al. Prospective, randomized, comparative trial of ciprofloxacin otic drops, with or without hydrocortisone, vs. polymyxin B–neomycin–hydrocortisone otic suspension in the treatment of acute diffuse otitis externa. *Infect Dis Clin Pract* 1999;8:387–395.
8. Jones RN, Milazzo J, Seidlin M. Ofloxacin otic solution for treatment of otitis externa in children and adults. *Arch Otolaryngol Head Neck Surg* 1997;123:1193–1200.
9. Sabater F, Maristany M, Mensa J, et al. Prospective double-blind randomized study of the efficacy and tolerance of topical ciprofloxacin vs topical gentamicin in the treatment of simple chronic otitis media and diffuse external otitis [in Spanish]. *Acta Otorrinolaringol Esp* 1996;47:217–220.
10. Worgan D. Treatment of otitis externa. Report of a clinical trial. *Practitioner* 1969;202:817–820.
11. Smith RB, Moodie J. A general practice study to compare the efficacy and tolerability of a spray ("Otomize") versus a standard drop formulation ("Sofradex") in the treatment of patients with otitis externa. *Curr Med Res Opin* 1990;12:12–18.
12. Smith RB, Moodie J. Comparative efficacy and tolerability of two antibacterial/anti-inflammatory formulations ("Otomize" spray and ("Otosporin" drops) in the treatment of otitis externa in general practice. *Curr Med Res Opin* 1990;11:661–667.
13. Jacobsson S, Karlsson G, Rigner P, et al. Clinical efficacy of budesonide in the treatment of eczematous external otitis. *Eur Arch Otorhinolaryngol* 1991;248:246–249.
14. Buch-Rasmussen A. Hydrocortisone alcoholic solution in eczematous external otitis. *J Int Med Res* 1979;7:449–451.
15. Lambert IJ. A comparison of the treatment of otitis externa with Otosporin and aluminium acetate: a report from a services practice in Cyprus. *J R Coll Gen Pract* 1981;31:291–294.
16. van Balen FAM, Smit, WM, Zuithoff NPA, et al. Clinical efficacy of three common treatments in acute otitis externa in primary care: randomized control trial. *BMJ* 2003;327:1201–1203.
17. Pond F, McCarty D, O'Leary S. Randomized trial on the treatment of oedematous acute otitis externa using ear wicks or ribbon gauze: clinical outcome and cost. *J Laryngol Otol* 2002;116:415–419.

Daniel Hajioff
Specialist Registrar
Department of Otolaryngology, Charing Cross Hospital, London, UK

Competing interests: None declared.

Otitis media with effusion

Search date March 2004

Ian Williamson

Key Messages

Prevention

- **Modifying risk factors to prevent otitis media with effusion** We found no RCTs on the effects of interventions aimed at modifying risk factors, such as passive smoking and bottle feeding, in preventing otitis media with effusion.

Treatment

- **Autoinflation (with purpose-manufactured nasal balloon)** One systematic review found that autoinflation with a purpose-manufactured nasal balloon improved effusion compared with no treatment. Some children may find autoinflation difficult. We found no evidence on other methods of autoinflation.
- **Ventilation tubes plus adenoidectomy/adenotonsillectomy** We found one systematic review, which found that ventilation tubes and adenoidectomy alone or in combination were equally effective and reduced mean hearing impairment by less than 12 decibels. The clinical significance of this hearing improvement was variable. One RCT from the review, which subsequently reported outcomes after 5 years, found that the use of ventilation tubes plus adenoidectomy/adenotonsillectomy was more effective than adenoidectomy/adenotonsillectomy or ventilation tubes alone; all of these surgical interventions were more effective than no treatment in reducing duration of otitis media with effusion. Two subsequent RCTs found different effects on language development with ventilation tubes compared with watchful waiting. A third subsequent RCT found that early insertion of ventilation tubes reduced behavioural problems at 9 months compared with watchful waiting.

- **Corticosteroids (intranasal)** One small RCT found no significant difference between intranasal corticosteroids alone compared with placebo for resolution of effusion. A second small RCT found limited evidence that intranasal corticosteroids plus antibiotics improved symptoms compared with antibiotics alone.
- **Antibiotics (oral)** One systematic review found limited evidence that antibiotics improved short term outcomes compared with placebo or no treatment. However, a second systematic review of higher quality and incorporating six RCTs from the first review found no significant difference between antibiotics and placebo. A third systematic review found limited evidence from four RCTs that antibiotics plus oral corticosteroids improved resolution rates compared with antibiotics alone. Another small RCT in the same review found limited evidence that antibiotics plus intranasal corticosteroids improved symptoms compared with antibiotics alone. Adverse effects with antibiotics (mainly nausea, vomiting, and diarrhoea) were reported in 2–32% of children.
- **Mucolytics** One systematic review found no significant difference between 1–3 month courses of carbocisteine or carbocisteine lysine and placebo or no treatment, in resolution of effusion. Three small RCTs of bromhexine versus placebo found inconclusive results.
- **Antihistamines plus oral decongestants** One systematic review found no significant difference between antihistamines plus oral decongestants compared with placebo in clearance of effusion after 4 weeks.
- **Corticosteroids (oral)** One systematic review found no significant difference between oral corticosteroids and placebo in clearance of effusion after 2 weeks. It found limited evidence that oral corticosteroids plus antibiotics improved resolution rates compared with antibiotics alone.
- **Adenoidectomy alone; adenotonsillectomy alone; autoinflation (with other devices); tonsillectomy; ventilation tubes alone** We found insufficient evidence on the effects of these interventions.

DEFINITION Otitis media with effusion (OME), or "glue ear", is serous or mucoid but not mucopurulent fluid in the middle ear. Children usually present with hearing loss and speech problems. In contrast to those with acute otitis media (see chapter, p 227), children with OME do not suffer from acute ear pain, fever, or malaise. Hearing loss is usually mild and often identified when parents express concern regarding their child's behaviour, performance at school, or language development.

INCIDENCE/ PREVALENCE OME is commonly seen in paediatric practice and accounts for 25–35% of all cases of otitis media.[1] One study in the UK found that, at any time, 5% of children aged 5 years had persistent (at least 3 months) bilateral hearing loss associated with OME.[2] The prevalence declines considerably beyond 6 years of age.[3] About 50–80% of children aged 4 years have been affected by OME some time in the past.[3,4] One study estimated that, between the ages of 2 months and 2 years, 91.1% of young children will have one episode of middle ear effusion, and 52.2% will have bilateral involvement.[5] OME is the most common reason for referral for surgery in children in the UK. The number of consultations for otitis media increased by 150% between 1975 and 1990. Middle ear effusions also occur infrequently in adults after upper respiratory tract infection or after air travel. They may persist for weeks or months after an episode of acute otitis media.[6] OME is estimated to account for 25–35% of all cases of otitis media.

AETIOLOGY/ RISK FACTORS Contributory factors include upper respiratory tract infection and narrow upper respiratory airways.[6,7] Case control studies have identified risk factors, including age 6 years or younger at first onset, day care centre attendance, large number of siblings, low socioeconomic group, frequent upper respiratory tract infection, bottle feeding, and household smoking.[3,6] These factors may be associated with about twice the risk of developing OME.[7]

PROGNOSIS Data from one prospective study of children aged 2–4 years showed that 50% of OME cases resolved within three months and 95% within a year.[8] In 5% of preschool children, OME (identified by tympanometric screening) persists for at least 1 year.[8,9] One cohort study of 3 year olds found that 65% of OME cases cleared within three months.[9] Most children aged 6 years or older will not have further problems.[2] The disease is ultimately self limiting in most cases.[2,5,10]

However, one large cohort study (534 children) found that middle ear disease increased reported hearing difficulty at 5 years of age (OR 1.44, 95% CI 1.18 to 1.76) and was associated with delayed language development in children up to 10 years of age.[11] Hearing loss is the most common complication of OME. Most children with OME have fluctuating or persistent hearing deficits with mild to moderate degrees of hearing loss, averaging 27 decibels. The type of hearing loss is usually conductive, but may be sensorineural, or both. The sensorineural type is usually permanent.[12] Tympanic membrane perforation, tympanosclerosis, otorrhoea, and cholesteatoma occur more frequently among children with OME than those without OME. These conditions are especially common among children with OME who have had a myringotomy with ventilation tube placement.[13]

AIMS OF INTERVENTION To improve hearing and wellbeing; to avoid poor behavioural, speech, and educational development; to prevent recurrent earache and otitis media, with minimal adverse effects.

OUTCOMES Resolution of effusion (both speed and completeness) assessed by otoscopy, tympanometry, or global clinical assessment; hearing impairment, assessed by audiometry or tympanometry (although the positive predictive value of these tests has been reported as low as 49%);[14] developmental and behavioural tests; language and speech development; adverse effects of treatment. Patient centred outcomes in children with OME (e.g. disability or quality of life) need further development and evaluation.

METHODS *Clinical Evidence* search and appraisal March 2004.

QUESTION What are the effects of preventive interventions?

OPTION MODIFYING RISK FACTORS

We found no RCTs on the effects of risk factor interventions aimed at modifying risk factors, such as passive smoking and bottle feeding, in preventing otitis media with effusion.

Benefits: We found no systematic review or RCTs of interventions aimed at modifying risk factors for otitis media with effusion (see comment below).

Harms: We found no RCTs.

Comment: There is good epidemiological evidence that the risk of otitis media with effusion is increased by passive smoking,[3] bottle feeding,[5] low socioeconomic group, and exposure to a large number of other children.[14] Feasible preventive interventions may include strategies to reduce household smoking and encourage breast feeding.

QUESTION What are the effects of pharmacological, mechanical, and surgical treatments?

OPTION ANTIBIOTICS (ORAL)

One systematic review found limited evidence that antibiotics improved short term outcomes compared with placebo or no treatment. However, a second systematic review of higher quality and incorporating six RCTs from the first review found no significant difference between antibiotics and placebo. A third systematic review found limited evidence from four RCTs that antibiotics plus oral corticosteroids improved resolution rates compared with antibiotics alone. Another small RCT in the same review found limited evidence that antibiotics plus intranasal corticosteroids improved symptoms compared with antibiotics alone. Adverse effects with antibiotics (mainly nausea, vomiting, and diarrhoea) were reported in 2–32% of children.

Benefits: **Versus placebo:** We found two systematic reviews.[14,15] The first systematic review (search date 1992, 10 RCTs, 1041 children with otitis media with effusion, age range not reported) reported RCTs which were heterogeneous in study design. Eight RCTs compared antimicrobial drugs (amoxicillin with or without clavulanic acid, cefaclor, erythromycin, sulfisoxazole, sulfamethoxazole, or trimethoprim) versus placebo or no treatment. One RCT compared antimicrobial drugs (erythromycin plus sulfisoxazole, cefaclor, and amoxicillin) versus each other and placebo and one RCT compared an antibiotic (trimethoprim–sulfamethoxazole [co-trimoxazole]) versus antihistamine plus decongestant plus antitussic.[14] Treatment duration varied from 2–5 weeks. Follow up was from 10–60 days. At up to 1 month, antimicrobial treatment significantly increased resolution of effusion (assessed by pneumatic otoscopy, tympanometry, and audiometry) compared with placebo or no treatment (pooled ARR for non-resolution with antibiotics *v* placebo or no treatment: 14%, 95% CI 4% to 24%). The second systematic review (search date 1997, 8 RCTs [including 6 of the RCTs from the first review], 1292 children with otitis media with effusion, age range not reported) compared antibiotics versus placebo and found no significant difference in cure rate over 2–5 weeks (cure rate: 179/813 [22%] with antibiotics *v* 85/479 [18%] with placebo; ARI of cure: +4.3%, 95% CI –0.1% to +8.6%).[15] **Antibiotics plus corticosteroids:** See benefits of corticosteroids, p 627.

Harms: The systematic reviews did not report rates of adverse events in children on placebo or no treatment.[14,15] Adverse events were frequent with antibiotics. For amoxicillin, diarrhoea was reported in 20–30% and rashes in 3–5% of children. For amoxicillin–clavulanic acid (co-amoxiclav), diarrhoea was reported in 9%, nausea and vomiting in 4%, and skin rashes and urticaria in 3% of children.[14,16] For antibiotics overall, nausea and vomiting, diarrhoea, or both were reported in 2–32% of children, and cutaneous reactions were reported in fewer than 5%.[16] Adherence to long courses of antibiotics was poor. Prescribing antibiotics for minor illness encouraged further consultations[17] and antibiotic resistance.[18]

Comment: The second systematic review[15] contained a methodological criticism of the first review[14] and pointed out that pooling data from studies with and without placebo controls introduced a significant bias towards antibiotic efficacy.

OPTION CORTICOSTEROIDS

One systematic review found no significant difference between oral corticosteroids and placebo in clearance of effusion after 2 weeks. It found limited evidence that oral corticosteroids plus antibiotics improved resolution rates compared with antibiotics alone. One small RCT found no significant difference between intranasal corticosteroids alone compared with placebo for resolution of effusion. A second small RCT found limited evidence that intranasal corticosteroids plus antibiotics improved symptoms compared with antibiotics alone.

Benefits: We found one systematic review (search date 2002, 10 RCTs, 718 children in secondary care and selected [air force base] settings).[19] **Oral corticosteroids versus placebo:** The systematic review identified three RCTs (108 children) comparing oral corticosteroids (either prednisone or dexamethasone) versus placebo. Presence of effusion was assessed clinically by pneumatic otoscopy, tympanometry, and audiometry after 7–14 days of treatment. The review found no significant difference in mean improvement at 2 weeks after treatment (AR of clearance compared with placebo +21%, 95% CI –3% to +44%).

Longer term effects were not sufficiently recorded for inclusion. **Oral corticosteroids plus antibiotic:** The systematic review identified four RCTs (274 children) comparing antibiotic (cefixime, amoxycillin, or sulfisoxazole) plus oral corticosteroids (betamethasone or prednisone) versus antibiotic alone.[19] Time to measurement of results varied from 1 week to 6 months. The review found a significant difference in clearance rates with combined treatment compared with antibiotic alone (ARR for non-clearance *v* antibiotic alone at 2 weeks 32%, 95% CI 20% to 50%, P < 0.01). Longer term effects were not sufficiently recorded for inclusion. **Intranasal corticosteroids versus placebo:** The systematic review identified one RCT (45 children), which found no significant difference between intranasal dexamethasone and placebo in persistence of effusion at 3 weeks (OR 2.12, 95% CI 0.65 to 6.90).[20] **Intranasal corticosteroids plus antibiotics:** The systematic review identified one RCT (59 children aged 3–11 years), which found that intranasal corticosteroids plus antibiotics significantly reduced effusions at 4 weeks (P < 0.05), 8 weeks (P < 0.05), and 12 weeks (P < 0.01) compared with antibiotics plus placebo.[21]

Harms: The six RCTs in the review reporting on adverse events found no severe or lasting adverse effects of corticosteroids.[19] The other RCTs mentioned mild possible adverse effects of corticosteroids, such as vomiting, diarrhoea, dermatitis, transient nasal stinging, and epistaxis.

Comment: The trials in the review were small and showed significant heterogeneity.[19] Use of secondary care populations weakens the applicability of results to primary care.

OPTION ANTIHISTAMINES PLUS ORAL DECONGESTANTS

One systematic review found no significant difference between antihistamines plus oral decongestants compared with placebo in clearance of effusion in children with otitis media with effusion after 4 weeks.

Benefits: We found one systematic review (search date 1992, 4 large RCTs, 1202 infants and older children, age range not reported).[14] The review found no significant difference between 4 weeks of treatment with antihistamine plus oral decongestants compared with placebo in effusion clearance rate, as assessed by history, otoscopy, and tympanometry (mean difference –0.009, 95% CI –0.036 to +0.054).

Harms: Adverse effects of antihistamines include hyperactivity, insomnia, drowsiness, behavioural change, blood pressure variability, and seizures.[14] One RCT in healthy volunteers found that decongestant nose drops given for 3 weeks or more led to iatrogenic rhinitis.[22]

Comment: The RCTs in the review included clinically heterogeneous groups (e.g. infants and older children) and selected individuals from ambulatory care or waiting lists.[14] However, the review suggested that the evidence could be generalised to a child of any age.

OPTION MUCOLYTICS

One systematic review found no significant difference between 1–3 month courses of carbocisteine or carbocisteine lysine and placebo or no treatment in resolution of effusion. Three small RCTs of bromhexine versus placebo found inconclusive results.

Benefits: We found one systematic review (search date 1993, 6 RCTs, 428 children aged 3–11 years and 2 adults) comparing 15–90 days' treatment with carbocisteine, carbocisteine lysine, or both, compared with placebo or no treatment.[23] The review found that mucolytics were associated more frequently with complete resolution but the difference with the control group was not significant (178 children; 80/81 [99%] with treatment *v* 54/98 [55%] with placebo; OR 2.25, 95% CI 0.97 to 5.22). Three small RCTs (155 children and 195 ears) comparing another mucolytic (bromhexine) with placebo found inconclusive results.[24–26]

Harms: The review gave no information on adverse effects.[23]

Comment: The RCTs in the review were heterogeneous in their clinical outcomes and treatment duration.[23] However, the RCTs combined in the meta-analysis were homogeneous regarding dosage and outcome.

OPTION AUTOINFLATION

One systematic review found that autoinflation with a purpose-manufactured nasal balloon improved effusion compared with no treatment. Some children may find autoinflation difficult. We found no evidence on other methods of autoinflation.

Benefits: We found one systematic review (search date not reported, 6 RCTs, 435 children, age range not reported) comparing autoinflation versus no treatment (see comment below).[27] Three RCTs (386 children) found that children using purpose-manufactured nasal balloons were more likely than controls to improve within 1 week to 3 months using tympanometric and audiometric criteria (OR 3.53, 95% CI 2.03 to 6.14).[27] We found no systematic review and no RCTs on other methods of autoinflation (such as inflating a carnival blower through the nostril or forcible exhalation through the nostrils, with closed mouth, into an anaesthetic mask with a flow meter attachment).

Harms: The review found no reports of serious adverse effects.[27]

Comment: The quality of the review's evidence is limited by several weaknesses. Most trials seemed not to use intention to treat analysis, and beneficial effects were noted only when adherence was 70% or greater.[27] Outcome assessments were not blinded, and follow up was short. The RCTs also varied in their outcome measures: being effusion free, improved tympanogram, or improvement in hearing. The eustachian tubes can be inflated by several methods, including blowing up a balloon through a plastic tube inserted into the nostril. In one RCT, 12% of children aged 3–10 years were unable to use the balloon.[28] The studies to date have had methodological problems (different devices, selection criteria, duration of treatment, outcome measures, etc.), so the data is suggestive rather than conclusive. Autoinflation may be used as a short-term measure — its long-term efficacy is unknown. Empirical use of autoinflation is reasonable, especially in older children, because it is associated with minimal adverse effects. Studies have been done using the Otovent autoinflation device. There is insufficient evidence for other autoinflation devices.

OPTION SURGERY

We found one systematic review, which found that ventilation tubes and adenoidectomy alone or in combination were equally effective and reduced mean hearing impairment by less than 12 decibels. The clinical significance of this hearing improvement was variable. One RCT from the review, which subsequently reported outcomes after 5 years, found that ventilation tubes plus adenoidectomy/adenotonsillectomy was more effective than adenoidectomy/adenotonsillectomy or ventilation tubes alone, and all of these surgical interventions were more effective than no treatment in reducing

duration of otitis media with effusion. Two subsequent RCTs found different effects on language development with ventilation tubes compared with watchful waiting. A third subsequent RCT found that early insertion of ventilation tubes reduced behavioural problems at 9 months compared with watchful waiting. We found no good evidence on the effects of tonsillectomy alone or any evidence of additional benefit of adenotonsillectomy over adenoidectomy alone.

Benefits: **Ventilation tubes (e.g. grommets; also known as tympanostomy tubes) versus adenoidectomy:** We found one systematic review (search date 1992, 19 RCTs)[10] and one subsequent report after 5 years of an RCT included in the review,[29] and three subsequent RCTs.[13,30,31] The review concluded that ventilation tubes and adenoidectomy alone or in combination were equally effective and reduced mean hearing impairment by less than 12 decibels. The clinical significance of this hearing improvement was variable.[10] Nine RCTs reported the data per child (1508 children) and 10 reported data per ear (1452 children). None were placebo controlled, although some RCTs used children who had received ventilation tubes in one ear only and in these cases the operated and non-operated ears were compared against each other (see comment below). Outcomes were mean change in audiometry, tympanometry, and clinical and otoscopic evidence of otitis media with effusion (OME). One of the RCTs within the review subsequently reported outcomes after 5 years.[29] The RCT (228 children aged 2–9 years) compared adenotonsillectomy or adenoidectomy (analysed together) versus neither procedure. All children had a ventilation tube inserted into one randomly chosen ear. Outcomes were mean audiometric change, and tympanometric and otoscopic clearance assessed over 6 months to 10 years after treatment and reported per ear. The three subsequent RCTs assessed treatment with ventilation tubes alone by comparing the use of ventilation tubes with watchful waiting,[30] early versus delayed insertion of ventilation tubes,[31] and early insertion of bilateral ventilation tubes versus watchful waiting.[13] **Ventilation tubes alone:** The 5 year follow up of an RCT within the review found that median duration of glue ear was reduced from 7.8 years without treatment to 4.9 years with ventilation tubes.[29] The first and second subsequent RCTs studied children under the age of 3 years and the main outcomes reported were speech and language development rather than hearing or persistence of effusion.[30,31] The first subsequent RCT (187 children aged 16–24 months) found that treatment with ventilation tubes improved verbal comprehension and expressive language compared with watchful waiting (significance not reported).[30] The second subsequent RCT (429 children aged ≤ 3 years with persistent effusion and mild to moderate hearing loss) compared early versus delayed insertion of ventilation tubes.[31] It found no significant effect on language development measured on a range of scales. The third subsequent RCT (182 children, mean age 2.9 years) found that early insertion of bilateral ventilation tubes significantly reduced behavioural problems at 9 months compared with watchful waiting using the Richman behaviour check list**G** (percentage ≥ 10 on Richman score: 25/84 [30%] of children with bilateral ventilation tubes *v* 31/66 [47%] of children with watchful waiting; RR 0.63, 95% CI 0.30 to 0.96).[13] **Adenoidectomy alone:** The review reported a mean of less than 12 decibels short term improvement in hearing after adenoidectomy (CI not reported).[10] The 5 year follow up of the included RCT found that median duration of OME was reduced from 7.8 years without treatment to 4 years with adenoidectomy alone.[29] **Ventilation tubes plus adenoidectomy:** The review found that adenoidectomy gave little additional benefit over ventilation tubes alone in terms of mean short term hearing gain, which varied from 1.1–2.6 decibels.[10] The 5 year follow up of an RCT within the review found improved tympanometric and otoscopic clearance when combining adenoidectomy/adenotonsillectomy with ventilation tubes versus ventilation tubes alone or no treatment. Median duration of OME assessed tympanometrically was reduced from 7.8 years without treatment to 2.8 years with adenoidectomy/adenotonsillectomy plus ventilation tubes.[29] **Tonsillectomy:** The review found no good quality RCTs for tonsillectomy alone in OME.[10] **Adenotonsillectomy:** One RCT in the review found that adding tonsillectomy gave no benefit over adenoidectomy alone in the treatment of children with OME.[10]

Harms: We found one systematic review (search date 1999), which found that transient otorrhoea was a common complication of ventilation tube insertion (7 studies, 1522 children: incidence 16%, 95% CI 14% to 18%) and even more so later (23 studies, 5491 people: incidence 26%, 95% CI 25% to 27%).[32] Recurrent ear discharge was also common (7 studies, 1144 children: incidence 7.4%, 95% CI 6.0% to 9.0%) and often became chronic (3 studies, 451 children: incidence 3.8%, 95% CI 2.0% to 6.0%). **Ventilation tubes alone:** A systematic review of observational and experimental studies (search date 1998) of the complications after ventilation tube insertion found a reported prevalence of tympanosclerosis in 39–65% of treated ears as opposed to 0–10% of untreated ears.[33] Partial atrophy was noted in 16–73% of treated ears and in 5–31% of those untreated. Atelectasis ranged from 10–37% of treated ears as opposed to 1–20% of those untreated, and attic retraction was noted in 10–52% of treated ears and 29–40% of those untreated. The average hearing loss associated with these abnormalities was less than 5 decibels. The rate of otorrhoea after swimming in children with ventilation tubes is low, particularly in non-divers, and protection to the ear confers no proven benefit.[34] **Adenotonsillectomy:** Deaths have been reported in 1/16 700 to 1/25 000 children for adenotonsillectomy (no figures reported for adenoidectomy alone) and postoperative haemorrhage occurred in 0.5%.[35]

Comment: Myringotomy is usually performed together with ventilation tube insertion but is not effective on its own.[10] The validity of using operated and non-operated ventilation tube insertion as intervention and control as described in the systematic review is uncertain and the more recent studies have randomised children rather than ears.[10] The second subsequent RCT reported that the groups were not equivalent at baseline, with an initially higher level of educational development in children in the watchful waiting group.[30] The third subsequent RCT had low withdrawal rates (17/90 [18%] with watchful waiting *v* 9/92 [9%] with early surgery) but no intention to treat analysis.[13] About half of children who have ventilation tubes inserted will have reinsertion within 5 years.[36] Resolution after surgery takes longer in younger children and in those whose parents smoke, irrespective of treatment.[13]

GLOSSARY

Richman behaviour check list A 12 item derivation of the Behaviour Screening questionnaire.

REFERENCES

1. Eden A, Fireman P, Stool SE. Otitis media with effusion: sorting out the options. *Patient Care* 2000;29:32–56.
2. Williamson IG, Dunleavey J, Bain J, et al. The natural history of otitis media with effusion: a three year study of the incidence and prevalence of abnormal tympanograms in four SW Hampshire infant and first schools. *J Laryngol Otol* 1994;108:930–934.
3. Casselbrant ML, Brostoff LM, Cantekin EI, et al. Otitis media with effusion in preschool children. *Laryngoscope* 1985;95:428–436.
4. Zielhuis GA, Rach GH, Van den Broek P. The occurrence of otitis media with effusion in Dutch pre-school children. *Clin Otolaryngol* 1990;15:147–153.
5. Paradise JL, Rockette HE, Colborn DK, et al. Otitis media in 2253 Pittsburgh area infants: prevalence and risk factors during the first two years of life. *Pediatrics* 1997;99:318–333.

6. Teele D, Klein J, Rosner B. Epidemiology of otitis media during the first seven years of life in children in greater Boston: a prospective, cohort study. *J Infect Dis* 1989;160:83–94.
7. Haggard M, Hughes E. Objectives, values and methods of screening children's hearing — a review of the literature. London: HMSO, 1991.
8. Zeilhuis GA, Rach GH, Broek PV. Screening for otitis media with effusion in pre-school children. *Lancet* 1989;1:311–314.
9. Fiellau-Nikolajsen M. Tympanometry in three year old children: prevalence and spontaneous course of MEE. *Ann Otol Rhinol Laryngol* 1980;89(Suppl 68):233–237.
10. University of York. Centre for Reviews and Dissemination. 1992. The treatment of persistent glue ear in children. Effective Health Care 1(4). Search date 1992; primary sources Bids, Medline, and Embase.
11. Bennett KE, Haggard MP. Behaviour and cognitive outcomes in middle ear disease. *Arch Dis Child* 1999;80:28–35.
12. Lim DJ. Recent advances in otitis media. *Ann Otol Rhinol Laryngol Suppl* 2002;199:1–124.
13. Wilks J, Maw R, Peters TJ, et al. Randomised controlled trial of early surgery versus watchful waiting for glue ear: the effect on behavioural problems in pre-school children. *Clin Otol* 2000;25:209–214.
14. Stool SE, Berg SO, Berman S, et al. Otitis media with effusion in young children: clinical practice guideline number 12. AHCPR Publication 94–0622. Rockville, Maryland: Agency for Health Care Policy and Research, Public Health Service, United States Department of Health and Human Services, July 1994. Search date 1992; primary sources online database of National Library of Medicine and 10 specialised bibliographic databases.
15. Cantekin EI, McGuire TW. Antibiotics are not effective for otitis media with effusion: reanalysis of meta-analysis. *Otorhinolaryngol Nova* 1998;8:214–222. Search date 1997; primary sources RCTs in refereed journals and proceedings published between 1980 and 1997 in English language publications.
16. Computerised clinical information system. Denver, Colorado: Micromedex, June 1993.
17. Little P, Gould C, Williamson I, et al. Reattendance and complications in a randomised trial of prescribing strategies for sore throat: the medicalising effect of prescribing antibiotics. *BMJ* 1997;315:350–352.
18. Wise R, Hart T, Cars O, et al. Antimicrobial resistance is a major threat to public health [Editorial]. *BMJ* 1998;317:609–610.
19. Butler CC, van der Voort JH. Oral or topical nasal steroids for hearing loss associated with otitis media with effusion in children. In: The Cochrane Library, Issue 4, 2002. Oxford: Update Software. Search date 2002; primary sources Cochrane Controlled Trials Register, Embase, and Medline.
20. Shapiro GG, Bierman CW, Furukawa CT, et al. Treatment of persistent eustachian tube dysfunction with aerosolized nasal dexamethasone phosphate versus placebo. *Ann Allergy* 1982;49:81–85.
21. Tracy TM, Demain JG, Hoffman KM, et al. Intranasal beclomethasone as an adjunct to treatment of chronic middle ear effusion. *Ann Allergy Asthma Immunol* 1998;80:198–206.
22. Graf P. Rhinitis medicamentosa: aspects of pathophysiology and treatment. *Eur J Allergy Clin Immunol* 1997;52(Suppl 40):28–34.
23. Pignataro O, Pignataro LD, Gallus G, et al. Otitis media with effusion and S-carboxymethylcysteine and/or its lysine salt: a critical overview. *Int J Pediatr Otorhinolaryngol* 1996;35:231–241. Search date 1993; primary sources Medline, Embase, and Biosis.
24. Van der Merwe J, Wagenfeld DJ. The negative effects of mucolytics in otitis media with effusion. *S Afr Med J* 1987;72:625–626.
25. Stewart IA, Guy AM, Allison RS, et al. Bromhexine in the treatment of otitis media with effusion. *Clin Otolaryngol* 1985;10:145–149.
26. Roydhouse N. Bromhexine for otitis media with effusion. *N Z Med J* 1981;94:373–375.
27. Reidpath DD, Glasziou PP, Del Mar C. Systematic review of autoinflation for treatment of glue ear in children. *BMJ* 1999;318:1177–1178. Search date not reported; primary sources Medline, Cochrane Library, and pharmaceutical company database.
28. Blanshard JD, Maw AR, Bawden R. Conservative treatment of otitis media with effusion by autoinflation of the middle ear. *Clin Otolaryngol* 1993;18:188–192.
29. Maw R, Bawden R. Spontaneous resolution of severe chronic glue ear in children and the effect of adenoidectomy, tonsillectomy, and insertion of ventilation tubes. *BMJ* 1993;306:756–760.
30. Rovers MM, Stratman H, Ingels K, et al. The effect of ventilation tubes on language development in infants with otitis media with effusion: a randomised trial. *Pediatrics* 2000;106:e42.
31. Paradise J, Feldman HM, Campbell TF, et al. Effect of early or delayed insertion of tympanostomy tubes for persistent otitis media on developmental outcomes at the age of three years. *N Engl J Med* 2001;344:1179–1187.
32. Kay DJ, Nelson M, Rosenfeld RM. Meta-analysis of tympanostomy tube sequelae. *Otolaryngol Head Neck Surg* 2001;124:374–380. Search date 1999; primary sources Medline and hand searches.
33. Schilder AG. Assessment of complications of the conditions and of the treatment of otitis media with effusion. *Int J Pediatr Otolaryngol* 1999;49:S247–S251. Search date 1998; primary sources not reported.
34. Carbonell R, Ruiz-Garcia V. Ventilation tubes after surgery with otitis media with effusion or acute otitis media and swimming. Systematic review and meta-analysis. *Int J Pediatr Otorhinolaryngol* 2002;66:281–289.
35. Yardley MP. Tonsillectomy, adenoidectomy and adenotonsillectomy; are they safe day case procedures? *J Laryngol Otol* 1992;106:299–300.
36. Maw AR. Development of tympanosclerosis in children with otitis media with effusion and ventilation tubes. *J Laryngol Otol* 1991;105:614–617.

Ian Williamson
Senior Lecturer in Primary Medical Care
The University of Southampton
Southampton
UK

Competing interests: None declared.

Seasonal allergic rhinitis

Search date September 2003

Aziz Sheikh, Sukhmeet Singh Panesar, and Sangeeta Dhami

QUESTIONS

INTERVENTIONS

See glossary Ⓖ

Key Messages

Quality of life

- **Oral fexofenadine** Of all the oral antihistamines, only fexofenadine has been shown in RCTs to improve quality of life as well as rhinitis symptoms compared with placebo.
- **Oral leukotriene receptor antagonists** One systematic review provided good evidence that montelukast improved quality of life compared with placebo.
- **Oral leukotriene receptor antagonists plus oral antihistamines** One systematic review has found that montelukast plus loratadine improves quality of life compared with placebo. However, it found no evidence that combined treatment was any more effective than loratadine or montelukast alone.
- **Intranasal antihistamines; intranasal ipratropium bromide; oral decongestants; oral decongestants plus oral antihistamines; other oral antihistamines** We found no RCTs evaluating the effects of these interventions on quality of life.

Rhinitis symptoms

- **Oral antihistamines** Numerous RCTs have found that oral antihistamines (acrivastine, azatadine, brompheniramine, cetirizine, ebastine, loratadine, desloratadine, or mizolastine) improve rhinitis symptoms compared with placebo. Drowsiness, sedation, and somnolence were the most commonly reported adverse effects.
- **Oral pseudoephedrine plus oral antihistamines** RCTs have found that pseudoephedrine plus oral antihistamines (fexofenadine, acrivastine, cetirizine, terfenadine, triprolidine, loratadine, or azatadine) improve overall symptoms of seasonal allergic rhinitis compared with pseudoephedrine or oral antihistamine or placebo alone. The most common adverse effects reported with combination treatment were headache and insomnia.
- **Intranasal levocabastine** RCTs found that intranasal levocabastine improved symptoms of seasonal allergic rhinitis compared with placebo.
- **Oral leukotriene receptor antagonists** One systematic review provided good evidence that montelukast improved nasal symptoms compared with placebo. One RCT provided inconclusive evidence about effects of pranlukast compared with placebo.
- **Oral leukotriene receptor antagonists plus oral antihistamines** One systematic review has found that montelukast plus loratadine improves nasal symptoms compared with placebo. However, it found no evidence that combined treatment was any more effective than loratadine or montelukast alone.
- **Oral astemizole** RCTs have found that astemizole improves rhinitis symptoms compared with placebo but astemizole has been associated with prolongation of the QTc interval, and may induce ventricular arrhythmias.
- **Oral terfenadine** RCTs have found conflicting results about the effectiveness of terfenadine compared with placebo on rhinitis symptoms. Terfenadine is associated with risk of fatal cardiac toxicity if used in conjunction with macrolide antibiotics, oral antifungal agents, or grapefruit juice.
- **Intranasal azelastine** RCTs have found conflicting results about effectiveness of intranasal azelastine compared with placebo on symptoms of seasonal allergic rhinitis. Two small RCTs found no significant difference in nasal symptoms between intranasal antihistamines (azelastine, levocabastine) and oral antihistamines (cetirizine, terfenadine).
- **Intranasal ipratropium bromide** We found no systematic review or published RCTs.

DEFINITION Seasonal allergic rhinitis is a symptom complex that may affect several organ systems. Symptoms will typically consist of seasonal sneezing, nasal itching, nasal blockage, and watery nasal discharge.[1] Eye symptoms (red eyes, itchy eyes, and tearing) are common. Other symptoms may include peak seasonal coughing, wheezing, and shortness of breath, oral allergy syndrome (manifesting as an itchy swollen oropharynx on eating stoned fruits), and systemic symptoms such as tiredness, fever, a pressure sensation in the head, and itchiness. Confirming the presence of pollen hypersensitivity using objective allergy tests such as skin prick tests, detection of serum specific IgE, and nasal provocation challenge testing may improve diagnostic accuracy.

INCIDENCE/ PREVALENCE Seasonal allergic rhinitis is found throughout the world. Epidemiological evidence suggests that there is considerable geographical variation in its prevalence. Prevalence is highest in socioeconomically developed countries, where the condition may affect as much as 25% of the population.[2–4] Prevalence and severity are increasing. It is thought that improved living standards and reduced risk of childhood infections may lead to immune deviation of T helper cells in early life, which may increase susceptibility to seasonal allergic rhinitis (the so called "hygiene hypothesis").[5,6] Although people of all ages may be affected, the peak age of onset is adolescence.[7]

AETIOLOGY/ RISK FACTORS The symptoms of seasonal allergic rhinitis are caused by an IgE mediated type 1 hypersensitivity reaction to grass, tree, or weed pollen. Allergy to other seasonal aeroallergens such as fungal spores may also provoke symptoms. Typically, symptoms become worse during the relevant pollen season and in the open, when pollen exposure is increased. Risk factors include a personal or family history of atopy or other allergic disorders, male sex, birth order (increased risk being seen in first born), and small family size.[8,9]

PROGNOSIS Seasonal allergic rhinitis may impair quality of life, interfering with work, sleep, and recreational activities.[10] Other allergic problems such as asthma and eczema frequently coexist, adding to the impact of rhinitis.[11]

AIMS OF INTERVENTION Treatments for seasonal allergic rhinitis aim to minimise or eliminate symptoms, optimise quality of life, and reduce the risk of developing coexistent disease.

OUTCOMES We extracted data on the following outcomes: quality of life, days off school/work, rhinitis symptom scores (as described in studies), medication usage and medication usage scores (as defined in studies), and adverse effects. Although most of these outcome measures have face validity, few have been formally validated. Few studies used validated quality of life measures.

METHODS *Clinical Evidence* search and appraisal September 2003.

QUESTION What are the effects of treatments for symptoms of seasonal allergic rhinitis?

OPTION ORAL ANTIHISTAMINES

Only fexofenadine has been shown in RCTs to improve quality of life as well as rhinitis symptoms, although astemizole has been associated with prolongation of the QTc interval, and may induce ventricular arrhythmias. RCTs have found conflicting results about the effectiveness of terfenadine compared with placebo on rhinitis symptoms. Terfenadine is associated with the risk of fatal cardiac toxicity if used with macrolide antibiotics, oral antifungal agents, or grapefruit juice. Numerous RCTs have found that other oral antihistamines (acrivastine, azatadine, brompheniramine, cetirizine, desloratidine, ebastine, loratadine, and mizolastine) improve rhinitis symptoms compared with placebo. Drowsiness, sedation, and somnolence were the most commonly reported adverse effects of oral antihistamines.

Benefits: We found no systematic review. We found numerous RCTs comparing oral antihistamines versus placebo or other antihistamines, but only three RCTs evaluated quality of life as an outcome measure.[12–14] Most of the RCTs used symptom scores to evaluate the effectiveness of oral antihistamines on rhinitis symptoms (see tables A, B, and C on web extra). **Acrivastine:** Three RCTs found that acrivastine 16–32 mg daily significantly reduced rhinitis symptoms compared with placebo.[15–17] **Astemizole:** Eight RCTs found that astemizole (10 mg once daily or 10 or 25 mg once weekly) reduced overall symptoms compared with placebo.[18–25] One RCT did not specify either the dose of treatment or the frequency of its administration.[25] **Azatadine:** One small RCT (crossover, 38 people aged > 12 years with both asthma and rhinitis) found no significant difference in rhinitis symptoms between adding azatadine (1 mg twice daily) or placebo to the existing treatment regimen (not specified).[26] **Brompheniramine:** Two large RCTs comparing brompheniramine 8–24 mg daily versus terfenadine 60–120 mg daily or placebo found that brompheniramine significantly improved rhinitis symptoms compared with placebo.[27,28] **Cetirizine:** Eight RCTs found that cetirizine 10 mg daily significantly improved rhinitis symptoms compared with placebo.[29–36] One additional RCT (470 people) found that levocetirizine (2.5, 5, and 10 mg once daily for 2 weeks) significantly reduced sneezing, rhinorrhoea, nasal pruritus, and ocular pruritus compared with placebo over the 2 weeks (difference in mean total 4 symptom score compared with placebo: 0.91 with 2.5 mg; 1.11 with 5 mg; 1.61 with 10 mg; $P < 0.001$).[37] **Ebastine:** We found three RCTs comparing ebastine 10–40 mg daily versus placebo[38–40] and one

RCT comparing ebastine 10 or 20 mg daily versus loratadine 10 mg daily versus placebo.[39] All four RCTs found that ebastine significantly improved rhinitis symptoms compared with placebo.[38–41] **Fexofenadine:** We found nine RCTs.[12–14,41–46] Three of these RCTs reported on quality of life. The first RCT (multicentre, 845 people aged 12–65 years with history of seasonal allergic rhinitis and positive skin test to an unspecified allergen) compared fexofenadine 120 or 180 mg daily versus placebo over 2 weeks.[12] Outcomes were assessed using Rhinoconjunctivitis Quality of Life Questionnaire**G** score; work, classroom, and daily activity impairment (Work Productivity and Activity Impairment instrument**G**) and general health (SF-36 Health Survey**G**). The RCT found that fexofenadine significantly improved quality of life ($P \leq 0.006$) and reduced work and daily activity impairment ($P \leq 0.004$) compared with placebo. The RCT found no significant difference in classroom impairment between fexofenadine and placebo. The second RCT (multicentre, 1948 people aged 11–68 years with 2 year history of seasonal allergic rhinitis and positive skin test to grass and tree allergens) also found that fexofenadine 120 mg daily significantly improved quality of life ($P \leq 0.05$) and reduced work impairment ($P \leq 0.05$) compared with placebo.[13] The third RCT (multicentre, 688 people aged 12–75 years with a 2 year history of seasonal allergic rhinitis and a positive skin test for grass, tree pollen, or both) compared fexofenadine 120 mg daily with loratadine 10 mg daily or placebo over 2 weeks.[14] The RCT found that fexofenadine significantly improved quality of life ($P < 0.005$) and 24 hour reflective symptom scores ($P < 0.0001$) compared with placebo.[14] The remaining six RCTs did not report on quality of life. All the RCTs found that fexofenadine 80–240 mg daily significantly improved rhinitis symptoms compared with placebo.[41–46] **Loratadine:** Ten RCTs comparing loratadine versus placebo or other antihistamines (clemastine, mequitazine, terfenadine) found that loratadine reduced rhinitis symptom scores more than placebo.[47–56] One further RCT (337 people aged ≥ 12 years or with 2 year history of seasonal allergic rhinitis) found that, over 2 weeks, desloratadine 5 mg daily reduced total rhinitis symptom score more than placebo ($P < 0.01$).[57] **Desloratadine:** We found one systematic review (search date 2002, 4 RCTs of people with seasonal allergic rhinitis)[58] and one additional RCT comparing desloratadine versus placebo or other antihistamines.[59] The systematic review found that desloratadine significantly reduced the total symptom score, total nasal symptoms, total non-nasal symptoms, and self assessed congestion scores compared with placebo ($P \leq 0.05$ for all comparisons).[58] One additional RCT (337 people aged ≥ 12 years or with 2 year history of seasonal allergic rhinitis) found that over 2 weeks desloratadine 5 mg daily was significantly faster at reducing total rhinitis symptom score compared with placebo ($P < 0.01$).[54] **Mizolastine:** Two RCTs found that mizolastine 10 or 15 mg daily significantly reduced physician rated overall symptom scores compared with placebo ($P < 0.005$). They found no significant difference between mizolastine 5 mg daily and placebo.[59,60] **Terfenadine:** We found 15 RCTs comparing terfenadine versus placebo or other antihistamines.[30,33,38,50–52,60–68] Eight of the RCTs found that terfenadine significantly reduced overall subject rated symptom scores compared with placebo.[50–52,60–64] The seven other RCTs found no significant difference in subject rated overall rhinitis symptom scores between terfenadine and placebo.[30,33,38,65–68] **Other antihistamines:** We found no RCTs. **Oral versus intranasal antihistamines:** See benefits of intranasal antihistamines, p 637.

Harms: Most of the RCTs reported drowsiness, sedation, or somnolence as a common adverse effect (see tables A, B, and C on web extra). **Astemizole:** Astemizole has been associated with prolongation of the

QTc interval, and thus has the potential to induce ventricular arrhythmias.[69] **Fexofenadine:** Two RCTs did not report specifically on any adverse effects.[12,13] One RCT found no significant difference in adverse effects between fexofenadine and placebo or loratadine.[14] **Desloratadine:** One RCT found no significant difference in adverse effects between desloratadine and placebo.[54] **Terfenadine:** Terfenadine is associated with risk of fatal cardiac toxicity if used in conjunction with macrolide antibiotics, oral antifungal agents, or grapefruit juice.[70] **Other antihistamines:** We found one cohort study (postmarketing surveillance of fexofenadine, acrivastine, cetirizine, and loratadine involving 43 363 people; the main outcome measure was sedation or drowsiness).[71] It found significantly higher incidence of sedation for acrivastine (OR 2.79, 95% CI 1.69 to 4.58; $P < 0.0001$) and cetirizine (OR 3.53, 95% CI 2.07 to 5.42; $P < 0.0001$) compared with loratadine. However, it found no difference between fexofenadine and loratadine (OR 0.63, 95% CI 0.36 to 1.11; $P = 0.1$). No increase in risk of accident or injury was found with any of the four antihistamines.[71]

Comment: None.

OPTION INTRANASAL ANTIHISTAMINES

We found no systematic review or RCTs evaluating the effects of intranasal antihistamines on quality of life. One meta-analysis of 11 RCTs (10 unpublished) has found that intranasal levocabastine improves symptoms of seasonal allergic rhinitis compared with placebo. Four RCTs found conflicting results on effectiveness of intranasal azelastine compared with placebo on symptoms of seasonal allergic rhinitis. Two small RCTs found no significant difference in nasal symptoms between intranasal antihistamines (azelastine, levocabastine) and oral antihistamines (cetirizine, terfenadine).

Benefits: We found no systematic review or RCTs evaluating the effect of intranasal antihistamines on quality of life. **Levocabastine versus placebo:** We found one meta-analysis (11 RCTs, only 1 published study, total of 693 people, no significant heterogeneity found across individual studies) comparing the global effectiveness of intranasal levocabastine with placebo.[72] Global effectiveness was defined as response or no response of rhinitis symptoms to treatment, assessed by study investigators. The meta-analysis found that the global effectiveness of levocabastine was significantly better than placebo (pooled OR 2.30, 95% CI 1.70 to 3.11; $P < 0.001$). One of two additional levocabastine RCTs not included in the meta-analysis found that levocabastine significantly reduced subject rated rhinitis symptoms compared with placebo over a 4 week period ($P < 0.05$).[73] The second levocabastine trial was small (16 people).[74] It found no significant difference in symptoms between the active and placebo treated groups. **Azelastine versus placebo:** We found four RCTs comparing effects of azelastine with placebo on rhinitis symptoms.[75–78] The first RCT (160 people aged 18–65 years with a history of seasonal allergic rhinitis of at least 3 years) compared intranasal azelastine 1.12 mg daily with intranasal beclomethasone 0.4 mg daily or placebo for 2 weeks.[75] Six symptoms (sneezing, nasal itching, rhinorrhoea, nasal stuffiness, eye itching, and watery eyes) were scored daily by the participants. The RCT found that azelastine significantly reduced subject rated rhinitis symptom scores compared with placebo ($P < 0.05$; summary data not reported). The second RCT (multicentre, 262 people aged > 12 years with a history of seasonal allergic rhinitis for at least 2 years and positive skin test for unspecified seasonal allergens) compared intranasal azelastine 0.52–1.04 mg daily with oral chlorpheniramine 24 mg daily versus placebo for 4 weeks.[76] Efficacy was measured as changes from baseline in total and major symptom complex severity scores. Symptoms included runny nose or sniffles; itchy nose; watery eyes; itchy eyes, ears, throat or palate; cough; postnasal drip; stuffiness; nose blows; and sneezes. The RCT found no significant difference between azelastine and placebo in total subject rated symptom scores 4 weeks after randomisation. The third RCT (30 people aged 18–53 years with 2 year history of seasonal allergic rhinitis and positive skin test to grass or Parietaria) found no significant difference between intranasal azelastine 0.28–0.56 mg daily and placebo in symptoms scores (summary data and P value not reported).[77] The fourth RCT (99 people, aged 19–61 years with a history of seasonal allergic rhinitis of at least 1 year) found that azelastine decreased symptoms compared with placebo at 7 days, although statistical significance depended on how "response" was defined (decrease in total ocular and nasal scores by ≥ 50%, with fewer than 3 cetirizine rescue tablets in the first 7 days: 43% with azelastine *v* 30% with placebo; P = 0.18; decrease of total ocular and nasal scores by ≥ 50% at day 7, with no cetirizine rescue tablets: 49% with azelastine *v* 28% with placebo; P = 0.04).[78] **Intranasal versus oral antihistamines:** We found two small double blind RCTs comparing intranasal antihistamines versus oral antihistamines.[79,80] Both RCTs found no significant difference in nasal symptoms between intranasal antihistamines (azelastine, levocabastine) and oral antihistamines (cetirizine, terfenadine).

Harms: No serious adverse effects were reported in these trials. Frequency of adverse effects was similar in treatment and placebo arms. The most common adverse effects were sinusitis and headache.

Comment: **Intranasal versus oral antihistamines:** The two RCTs comparing intranasal versus oral antihistamines may have been underpowered to detect any significant difference between these two classes of treatment.[79,80]

OPTION ORAL DECONGESTANTS

We found no systematic review or RCTs evaluating the effect of oral decongestants on quality of life. RCTs have found that pseudoephedrine plus oral antihistamines (fexofenadine, acrivastine, cetirizine, terfenadine, triprolidine, loratadine, desloratadine, or azatadine) improve overall symptoms of seasonal allergic rhinitis compared with pseudoephedrine, oral antihistamine, or placebo. The most common adverse effects reported with combination treatment were headache and insomnia.

Benefits: We found no systematic review or RCTs evaluating the effect of oral decongestants on quality of life. We found no RCTs only comparing oral decongestants with placebo. We found 10 RCTs comparing the effects of oral decongestants plus oral antihistamines with either decongestant alone, antihistamine alone, or placebo on rhinitis symptoms.[77–86] **Pseudoephedrine plus fexofenadine:** The first RCT (651 people aged 12–65 years with positive skin prick to ragweed extract and clinical response to antihistamines) compared sustained release pseudoephedrine (120 mg twice daily) plus fexofenadine (60 mg twice daily) with pseudoephedrine (120 mg twice daily) or fexofenadine (60 mg twice daily) for 2 weeks.[77] The RCT found that pseudoephedrine plus fexofenadine reduced symptom scores for sneezing (P < 0.0001); itchy nose and palate, throat, or both (P = 0.002); and itchy, watery, red eyes (P = 0.0006) compared with pseudoephedrine alone. Pseudoephedrine plus fexofenadine reduced nasal congestion scores compared with fexofenadine alone (P = 0.0005).[77] **Pseudoephedrine plus acrivastine:** The second RCT (multicentre, double blind, 702 people aged ≥ 12 years with a history of seasonal allergic rhinitis symptoms during the ragweed pollen season of at least 2 years and a positive skin test for ragweed antigen) compared pseudoephedrine 60 mg daily plus acrivastine 8 mg daily versus pseudoephedrine 60 mg daily or acrivastine 8 mg daily or placebo for 2 weeks.[78] The RCT found that pseudoephedrine plus acrivastine reduced the mean nasal congestion scores ($P < 0.001$) compared with acrivastine and improved the mean diary symptom scores from baseline when compared with acrivastine alone, pseudoephedrine alone, or placebo ($P < 0.01$). **Pseudoephedrine plus cetirizine:** The third RCT (687 people aged 12–65 years with history of pollen associated allergic rhinitis and positive skin test to unspecified seasonal allergens) compared sustained release pseudoephedrine (120 mg twice daily) plus cetirizine (5 mg twice daily) versus pseudoephedrine alone or cetirizine alone.[79] The main outcome measure was based on five symptoms (blocked nose, sneezing, runny nose, itchy nose, and itchy eyes) assessed by participants over the 2 week treatment period. The RCT found that pseudoephedrine plus cetirizine improved symptoms of sneezing, runny nose, itchy nose, and itchy eyes ($P < 0.001$ for all outcomes). However, it had no effect on blocked nose compared with pseudoephedrine or cetirizine alone. **Pseudoephedrine plus terfenadine:** The fourth RCT (41 people, pollen sensitivity status not reported) found that sustained release pseudoephedrine (120 mg twice daily) plus terfenadine (60 mg twice daily) improved overall symptoms ($P < 0.05$) when assessed by both the physician and the participant compared with terfenadine alone (60 mg twice daily).[80] **Pseudoephedrine plus triprolidine:** The fifth RCT (crossover, 40 people aged 22–47 years with clinical history of seasonal allergic rhinitis and positive skin test to mixed grasses, flowers, moulds, trees, house dust extract, and house dust mite) compared pseudoephedrine (60 mg 3 times daily) plus triprolidine (2.5 mg 3 times daily) with pseudoephedrine alone, triprolidine alone, or placebo for 10 weeks. Efficacy was measured with participant assessed symptom score. The RCT found that pseudoephedrine plus triprolidine gave the lowest sneezing, runny nose, and eye irritation score but pseudoephedrine alone gave the lowest blocked nose score.[81] **Pseudoephedrine plus loratadine or desloratadine:** The sixth RCT (multicentre, 847 people aged 12–60 years with history of moderate or severe seasonal allergic rhinitis and positive skin test to ragweed and other prevalent seasonal allergens) compared pseudoephedrine 240 mg daily plus loratadine 10 mg daily versus pseudoephedrine alone, loratadine alone, or placebo for 2 weeks. The RCT found that pseudoephedrine plus loratadine or loratadine alone reduced total symptom scores ($P \leq 0.01$) compared with pseudoephedrine or placebo.[82] The seventh RCT (multicentre, 435 people aged 12–60 years with history of moderate to severe symptoms of seasonal allergic rhinitis and positive skin test to unspecified allergens) compared modified release pseudoephedrine (120 mg twice daily) plus loratadine (5 mg twice daily) versus pseudoephedrine alone, loratadine alone, or placebo. The RCT found that pseudoephedrine plus loratadine improved mean total symptom scores compared with pseudoephedrine alone or placebo ($P < 0.05$).[83] The eighth RCT (1018 people) compared three treatments; desloratadine 5 mg plus pseudoephedrine 240 mg once daily, desloratadine alone, and pseudoephedrine alone.[84] It found that desloratadine plus pseudoephedrine significantly decreased mean morning and evening self assessed nasal congestion scores ($P < 0.01$) and morning nasal congestion scores ($P < 0.01$) at 15 days compared with desloratadine alone or pseudoephedrine alone. It found no significant difference between single treatments in mean nasal congestion scores.[84] **Pseudoephedrine plus azatadine:** The ninth RCT (65 people aged 14–72 years with severe seasonal allergic rhinitis assessed with by symptom scoring method) compared pseudoephedrine 60 mg twice daily plus azatadine 1 mg twice daily with pseudoephedrine alone or placebo for 2 weeks. The RCT found that pseudoephedrine plus azatadine improved signs and symptoms of seasonal allergic rhinitis compared with placebo (74% people with pseudoephedrine plus azatadine *v* 29% people with placebo).[85] The 10th RCT (80 people randomised, 65 analysed) compared azatadine maleate 1 mg plus pseudoephedrine sulphate 60 mg twice daily versus placebo.[86] It found that pseudoephedrine plus azatadine increased the proportion of people with "excellent" self and physician rated improvement (> 75% improvement from baseline) compared with placebo at 2 weeks, but the statistical significance was not reported (self rated excellent improvement: 77% with azatadine plus pseudoephedrine *v* 23% with placebo; physician rated excellent improvement: 74% with azatadine plus pseudoephedrine *v* 19% with placebo). **Other decongestants:** We found no RCTs.

Harms: **Pseudoephdrine plus fexofenadine:** The first RCT found no significant difference in the incidence of adverse effects between pseudoephedrine plus fexofenadine and pseudoephedrine alone.[77] It found that pseudoephedrine plus fexofenadine significantly increased adverse effects compared with fexofenadine alone ($P < 0.001$). Headache and insomnia were the most commonly reported adverse effects. **Pseudoephedrine plus acrivastine:** The second RCT found that pseudoephedrine plus acrivastine increased adverse effects (dry mouth, somnolence, nervousness, insomnia) compared with placebo.[78] **Pseudoephedrine plus cetirizine:** The third RCT found no significant difference in the incidence of adverse effects between pseudoephedrine plus cetirizine compared with pseudoephedrine alone or cetirizine alone.[79] **Pseudoephedrine plus terfenadine:** The fourth RCT did not compare the incidence of adverse effects between pseudoephedrine plus terfenadine and terfenadine alone.[80] Terfenadine has been associated with serious adverse events (see harms of oral antihistamines, p 636). **Pseudoephedrine plus triprolidine:** The fifth RCT reported drowsiness with pseudoephedrine plus triprolidine and triprolidine alone.[81] Dry mouth was reported with pseudoephedrine plus triprolidine and pseudoephedrine alone. **Pseudoephedrine plus loratadine:** The sixth RCT found higher incidence of adverse effects (headache, dry mouth) with pseudoephedrine plus loratadine and pseudoephedrine alone compared with placebo ($P \leq 0.05$).[82] The seventh RCT found no significant difference in adverse effects between pseudoephedrine plus loratadine and pseudoephedrine alone.[83] It found a significantly higher incidence of adverse effects (insomnia, dry mouth) with the pseudoephedrine plus loratadine compared with either loratadine alone or placebo ($P = 0.01$).[83] **Pseudoephedrine plus desloratidine:** The eighth RCT found a higher rate of insomnia with pseudoephedrine alone than desloratadine alone or desloratadine plus pseudoephedrine (7.9% with pseudoephedrine alone *v* 0.6% with loratadine alone *v* 4.8% with pseudoephedrine plus loratadine, P value not reported).[84] However, rates of discontinuing treatment because of adverse events were similar with pseudoephedrine plus desloratadine and pseudoephedrine alone. **Pseudoephedrine plus azatadine:** The ninth RCT did not compare the incidence of adverse effects between pseudoephedrine plus azatadine and placebo.[85] The 10th RCT reported that three people had adverse effects (1 person with nervousness and 1 person with raised blood pressure with azatadine plus pseudoephedrine, and 1 person with palpitations and nervousness with placebo).[86]

Comment: None.

OPTION **INTRANASAL IPRATROPIUM BROMIDE**

We found no systematic review or fully published RCTs.

Benefits: We found no systematic review or fully published RCTs comparing intranasal ipratropium bromide with placebo for seasonal allergic rhinitis (see comment below).

Harms: We found no systematic review or RCTs.

Comment: We found one RCT reported as an abstract only.[87] The RCT (429 people) compared intranasal ipratropium bromide (84 mg/nostril given 4 times daily) with placebo for 3 weeks during the ragweed season. It found that ipratropium bromide significantly reduced the severity (P = 0.002) and duration (P = 0.008) of rhinorrhoea during the 3 weeks of treatment compared with placebo. This benefit was maintained during periods of high pollen count. The RCT found no significant difference between ipratropium bromide and placebo for symptoms of nasal congestion, sneezing, or postnasal drip.

OPTION ORAL LEUKOTRIENE RECEPTOR ANTAGONISTS

One systematic review provides good evidence that an oral leukotriene receptor antagonist, montelukast, improves nasal symptoms and quality of life compared with placebo. Three RCTs identified by a systematic review have found that montelukast plus loratadine improves nasal symptoms and quality of life compared with placebo, although they found no evidence that combined treatment was any more effective than loratadine or montelukast alone. One RCT found inconclusive evidence about effects of pranlukast compared with placebo on symptoms.

Benefits: **Montelukast alone:** We found one systematic review (search date 2003, 5 RCTs) that did not pool results.[88] The first RCT in the review (1302 people aged 15–81 years) compared three treatments: montelukast 10 mg daily, loratadine 10 mg daily, and placebo.[55] It found that montelukast significantly improved daytime nasal symptoms and quality of life compared with placebo (symptoms rated from 0 [none] to 3 [bothersome most of the time/very bothersome some of the time]; mean difference compared with placebo: –0.13, 95% CI –0.21 to –0.06; quality of life assessed by improvement in Rhinoconjunctivitis Quality of Life Questionnaire score Ⓖ: –0.89 with montelukast *v* –0.65 with placebo; P = 0.003). The RCT did not directly compare montelukast versus loratadine. The second RCT in the review (907 people aged 15–82 years with seasonal allergic rhinitis for ≥ 2 years and positive skin test), carried out in the autumn, compared montelukast 10 mg daily, loratadine 10 mg daily, montelukast plus loratadine, and placebo.[56] Montelukast significantly improved daytime nasal symptom scores and quality of life compared with placebo (mean difference from baseline versus placebo: –0.23, 95% CI –0.35 to –0.11; P < 0.001; difference in Rhinoconjunctivitis Quality of Life Questionnaire score: –1.09, 95% CI –1.26 to –0.92; P < 0.02). The third RCT in the review (1214 nonsmoking people) compared the same three treatments (montelukast 10 mg, loratadine 10 mg, and placebo) and used the same outcome measures.[89] It found that montelukast significantly improved daytime nasal symptoms, night time symptoms, and rhinoconjunctivitis quality of life over 2 weeks (mean difference, daytime nasal symptoms: –0.09, 95% CI –0.16 to –0.03; night time symptoms [difficulty getting to sleep, night time wakenings, and nasal congestion on wakening] all scored from 0 to 3: –0.08, 95% CI –0.13 to –0.02; Rhinoconjunctivitis Quality of Life Questionnaire score:–0.24, 95% CI –0.38 to –0.11) The fourth RCT in the review (460 people aged 15–75 years) compared four treatments: montelukast 10 mg daily, montelukast 20 mg daily; montelukast 10 mg daily plus loratadine 10 mg daily; loratadine 10 mg daily; and placebo.[90] It found no significant difference in daytime nasal symptoms score between montelukast alone and placebo at 2 weeks (difference in daytime symptom score using the same outcome measures: –0.11 with 10 mg; –0.04 with 20 mg, P value not reported in review). The fifth RCT in the review (62 people) compared four treatments: montelukast 10 mg daily; montelukast 10 mg daily plus loratadine 10 mg daily; fluticasone nasal spray; and placebo.[91] It found that montelukast alone significantly reduced daytime nasal symptoms compared with placebo at 6–8 weeks (improvement in symptoms [absolute score on 0 to 4 scale]: 1.1; P = 0.03). **Montelukast plus oral antihistamines:** We found one systematic review (search date 2003; 3 RCTs).[88] The identified RCTs compared montelukast 10 mg daily plus loratadine 10 mg daily versus montelukast 10 or 20 mg daily, loratadine 10 mg daily, or placebo. The review did not pool results. The first RCT in the review (460 people aged 15–75 years) found that montelukast plus loratadine significantly improved daytime nasal symptoms and quality of life at 2 weeks compared with placebo (daytime nasal symptoms: P < 0.05; improvement in Rhinoconjunctivitis Quality of Life Score: 0.36; P < 0.05). The second RCT in the review (907 people aged 15–82 years with seasonal allergic rhinitis for ≥ 2 years and positive skin test) was carried out in the autumn.[56] It found that montelukast plus loratadine significantly improved nasal symptom scores at 2 weeks compared with placebo but not compared with montelukast alone or loratadine alone (*v* placebo, combination: –0.32, 95% CI –0.42 to –0.21; P < 0.001; montelukast alone: –1.09, 95% CI –1.26 to –0.92; *v* loratadine alone: –0.26, 95% CI –0.37 to –0.16). It found that montelukast plus loratadine significantly improved quality of life compared with placebo. However, it found no significant difference in quality of life between montelukast plus loratadine and either montelukast alone or loratadine alone (improvement in Rhinoconjunctivitis Quality of Life Questionnaire score, montelukast plus loratadine *v* placebo: 1.16, 95% CI 1.03 to 1.29; P < 0.001). The third RCT in the review (62 people) compared four treatments: montelukast 10 mg daily plus loratadine 10 mg daily; montelukast 10 mg daily; fluticasone nasal spray; and placebo.[91] It found that montelukast plus loratadine significantly reduced daytime nasal symptoms compared with placebo at 6–8 weeks (P < 0.001). **Other oral leukotriene receptor antagonists:** We found one systematic review (search date not reported),[92] which identified one RCT.[93] The RCT (484 people) compared four treatments: pranlukast 300 or 600 mg daily; loratadine 10 mg daily and placebo.[93] It found that pranlukast 300 mg significantly reduced symptoms at 4 weeks compared with placebo. However, it found no significant difference between pranlukast 600 mg and placebo at 4 weeks (pranlukast 300 mg *v* placebo; P value not reported; pranlukast 600 mg *v* placebo; results and P value not reported).

Harms: Neither of the two systematic reviews assessed harms.[88,92] RCTs found no significant difference in adverse effects among montelukast plus loratadine, montelukast alone, loratadine alone, and placebo.[55,56,90] One RCT found no significant difference in adverse effects between montelukast plus loratadine, montelukast alone, loratadine alone, and placebo.[94]

Comment: **Other oral leukotriene receptor antagonists:** It is unclear why the RCT found that the lower dose of pranlukast significantly reduced symptoms compared with placebo, while the larger dose did not. These results should be interpreted with caution.[93]

GLOSSARY

Rhinoconjunctivitis Quality of Life Questionnaire is widely used in clinical trials to evaluate problems associated with rhinoconjunctivitis such as nose and eye symptoms by adults. It has 28 questions in seven domains (activity limitations, sleep problems, non-nasal/eye symptoms, practical problems, nose symptoms, eye symptoms, and emotional function) and is in both self administered and interviewer administered formats. People are asked to recall their experiences during the previous week and to give their responses on a seven point scale.[95]

SF-36 Health Survey includes one multi-item scale that assesses eight health concepts: limitations in physical activities because of health problems; limitations in social activities because of physical or emotional problems; limitations in usual role activities because of physical health problems; bodily pain; general mental health (psychological distress and wellbeing); limitations in usual role activities because of emotional problems; vitality (energy and fatigue); and general health perceptions. The survey was constructed for self administration by people aged 14 years or older, and for administration by a trained interviewer in person or by telephone.[96]

Work Productivity and Activity Impairment instrument is a questionnaire designed to measure work and activity impairment in adults during the previous 7 days. It is constructed for self administration or for use by interviewer in person or by telephone. The number of items varies between six and nine, depending on the version used.

REFERENCES

1. Lund VJ, Aaronsen D, Bousquet J, et al. International consensus report on the diagnosis and management of rhinitis. *Allergy* 1994;49:1–34.
2. The International Study of Asthma and Allergies in Childhood Steering Committee. Worldwide variation in prevalence of symptoms of asthma, allergic rhinoconjunctivitis, and atopic eczema: ISAAC. *Lancet* 1998;351:1225–1232.
3. Shamssain MH, Shamsian N. Prevalence and severity of asthma, rhinitis, and atopic eczema: the North East study. *Arch Dis Child* 1999;81:313–317.
4. Sibbald B, Rink E. Epidemiology of seasonal and perennial rhinitis; clinical presentation and medical history. *Thorax* 1991;46:895–901.
5. Fleming DM, Crombie DL. Prevalence of asthma and hay fever in England and Wales. *BMJ* 1987;294:279–283.
6. Durham SR. Summer hay fever. In: Durham SR, ed. *ABC of allergies*. London: BMJ Books, 1998:16–18.
7. Scadding GK, Church MK. Rhinitis. In: Holgate ST, Church MK, Lichtenstein LM, eds. *Allergy* 2nd ed. London: Mosby, 2001:55–76.
8. Parikh A, Scadding GK. Seasonal allergic rhinitis. *BMJ* 1997;314:1392.
9. Ross AM, Fleming DM. Incidence of allergic rhinitis in general practice, 1981–92. *BMJ* 1994;308:897–900.
10. Blaiss MS. Quality of life in allergic rhinitis. *Ann Allergy Asthma Immunol* 1999;83:449–454.
11. Sheikh A. Asthma and coexistent disease. *Asthma Gen Pract* 1998;6:17–18.
12. Meltzer EO, Casale TB, Nathan RA, et al. Once-daily fexofenadine HCl improves quality of life and reduces work and activity impairment in patients with seasonal allergic rhinitis. *Ann Allergy Asthma Immunol* 1999;83;311–317.
13. Tanner LA, Reilly M, Meltzer EO, et al. Effect of fexofenadine HCl on quality of life and work, classroom, and daily activity impairment in patients with seasonal allergic rhinitis. *Am J Manag Care* 1999;5:S235–S247.
14. Van Cauwenberge P, Juniper EF. Comparison of the efficacy, safety and quality of life provided by fexofenadine hydrochloride 120 mg, loratadine 10 mg and placebo administered once daily for the treatment of seasonal allergic rhinitis. *Clin Exp Allergy* 2000;30:891–899.
15. Leonhardt L, Gale NM, Gibbs TG. Placebo-controlled randomised evaluation of acrivastine in seasonal allergic rhinitis. *Acta Therap* 1988;14:241–248.
16. Bruno G, D'Amato G, Del Giacco GS, et al. Prolonged treatment with acrivastine for seasonal allergic rhinitis. *J Int Med Res* 1989;17:40B–46B.
17. Williams BO, Hull H, McSorley P, et al. Efficacy of acrivastine plus pseudoephedrine for symptomatic relief of seasonal allergic rhinitis due to mountain cedar. *Ann Allergy* 1996;76:432–438.
18. Franke W, Messinger D. Double-blind multicenter controlled clinical study comparing the efficacy of picumast dihydrochloride versus astemizole and placebo in patients with seasonal allergic rhinitis. *Drug Res* 1989;39:1360–1363.
19. Howarth PH, Emanuel MB, Holgate ST. Astemizole, a potent histamine H_1 -receptor antagonist: effect in allergic rhinoconjunctivitis, on antigen and histamine induced skin weal responses and relationship to serum levels. *Br J Clin Pharmacol* 1984;18:1–8.
20. Knight A. Astemizole — a new, non-sedating antihistamine for hayfever. *J Otolaryngol* 1985;14:85–88.
21. Oei HD. Double-blind comparison of loratadine (SCH 29851), astemizole, and placebo in hay fever with special regard to onset of action. *Ann Allergy* 1988;61:436–439.
22. Malmberg H, Holopainen E, Grahne B, et al. Astemizole in the treatment of hay fever. *Allergy* 1983;38:227–231.
23. Howarth PH, Holgate ST. Comparative trial of two non-sedative H_1 antihistamines, terfenadine and astemizole, for hay fever. *Thorax* 1984;39:668–672.
24. Callier J, Engelen RF, Ianniello I, et al. Astemizole (R 43 512) in the treatment of hay fever. an international double-blind study comparing a weekly treatment (10 mg and 25 mg) with a placebo. *Curr Ther Res* 1981;29:24–35.
25. Sooknundun M, Kacker SK, Sundaram KR. Treatment of allergic rhinitis with a new long-acting H_1 receptor antagonist: astemizole. *Ann Allergy* 1987;58:78–81.
26. Yan K, Harvey P, Pincus R. Trial of azatadine maleate (Zadine) in allergic asthma and rhinitis. *Clin Trials J* 1986;3:304–308.
27. Thoden WR, Druce HM, Furey SA, et al. Brompheniramine maleate: a double-blind, placebo-controlled comparison with terfenadine for symptoms of allergic rhinitis. *Am J Rhin* 1998;12:293–299.
28. Klein GL, Littlejohn T, Lockhart EA, et al. Brompheniramine, terfenadine, and placebo in allergic rhinitis. *Ann Allergy Asthma Immunol* 1996;77:365–370.
29. Ciprandi G, Passalacqua G, Mincarini M, et al. Continuous versus on demand treatment with cetirizine for allergic rhinitis. *Ann Allergy Asthma Immunol* 1997;79:507–511.
30. Ciprandi G, Tosca M, Ricca V, et al. Cetirizine treatment of rhinitis in children with pollen allergy: evidence of its antiallergic activity. *Clin Exp Allergy* 1997;27:1160–1166.
31. Grant JA, Nicodemus CF, Findlay SR, et al. Cetirizine in patients with seasonal rhinitis and concomitant asthma: prospective, randomized, placebo-controlled trial. *J Allergy Clin Immunol* 1995;95:923–932.
32. Lockey RF, Widlitz MD, Mitchell DQ, et al. Comparative study of cetirizine and terfenadine versus placebo in the symptomatic management of seasonal allergic rhinitis. *Ann Allergy Asthma Immunol* 1996;76:448–454.

33. Sabbah A, Daele J, Wade AG, et al. Comparison of the efficacy, safety and onset of action of mizolastine, cetirizine and placebo in the management of seasonal allergic rhinoconjunctivitis. *Ann Allergy Asthma Immunol* 1999;83:319–325.
34. Tarchalska-Krynska B, Zawisa E. Clinical assessment of cetirizine. *Polski Tygodnik Lekarski* 1990;45:123–126.
35. Murray JJ, Nathan RA, Bronsky EA, et al. Comprehensive evaluation of cetirizine in the management of seasonal allergic rhinitis: impact on symptoms, quality of life, productivity, and activity impairment. *Allergy Asthma Proc* 2002;6:391–398.
36. Noonan MJ, Raphael GD, Nayak A, et al. The health-related quality of life effects of once-daily cetirizine HCl in patients with seasonal allergic rhinitis: a randomized double-blind, placebo-controlled trial. *Clin Exp Allergy* 2003;33:351–358.
37. Leynadier F, Mees K, Arendt C, Pinelli ME. Efficacy and safety of levocetirizine in seasonal allergic rhinitis. *Acta Otorhinolayrngol Belg* 2001;55:305–312.
38. Ankier SI, Warrington SJ. A double-blind placebo-controlled study of the efficacy and tolerability of ebastine against hayfever in general practice patients. *J Int Med* 1989;226:453–458.
39. Storms WW. Clinical studies of the efficacy and tolerability of ebastine 10 or 20 mg once daily in the treatment of seasonal allergic rhinitis in the US. Adis International Limited. *Drugs* 1996;52:20–25
40. Frank H Jr, Gillen M, Rohatagi SS, et al. A double-blind, placebo-controlled study of the efficacy and safety of ebastine 20 mg once daily given with and without food in the treatment of seasonal allergic rhinitis. *J Clin Pharmacol* 2002;42:1097–1104.
41. Ratner PH, Lim JC, Georges GC. Comparison of once-daily ebastine 20mg, ebastine 10mg, loratadine 10mg, and placebo in the treatment of seasonal allergic rhinitis. *J Allergy Clin Immunol* 2000;105:1101–1107.
42. Howarth PH, Stern MA, Roi L, et al. Double-blind, placebo-controlled study comparing the efficacy and safety of fexofenadine hydrochloride (120 and 180 mg once daily) and cetirizine in seasonal allergic rhinitis. *J Allergy Clin Immunol* 1999;104:927–933.
43. Bronsky EA, Falliers CJ, Kaiser HB, et al. Effectiveness and safety of fexofenadine, a new nonsedating H_1 -receptor antagonist, in the treatment of fall allergies. *Allergy Asthma Proc* 1998;19:135–141.
44. Casale TB, Andrade C, Qu R. Safety and efficacy of once-daily fexofenadine HCl in the treatment of autumn seasonal allergic rhinitis. *Allergy Asthma Proc* 1999;20:193–198.
45. Bernstein DI, Schoenwetter WF, Nathan RA, et al. Efficacy and safety of fexofenadine hydrochloride for treatment of seasonal allergic rhinitis. *Ann Allergy Asthma Immunol* 1997;79:443–448.
46. Wilson AM, Haggart E, Sims EJ, et al. Effects of fexofenadine and desloratadine on subjective and objective measures of nasal congestion in seasonal allergic rhinitis. *Clin Exp Allergy* 2002;32:1504–1509.
47. Gutkowski A, Bedard P, Del Carpio J, et al. Comparison of the efficacy and safety of loratadine, terfenadine, and placebo in the treatment of seasonal allergic rhinitis. *J Allergy Clin Immunol* 1988;81:902–907.
48. Del Carpio J, Kabbash L, Turenne Y, et al. Efficacy and safety of loratadine (10 mg once daily), terfenadine (60 mg twice daily), and placebo in the treatment of seasonal allergic rhinitis. *J Allergy Clin Immunol* 1989;84:741–746.
49. Bruttmann G, Pedrali P. Loratadine (SCH_2 9851) 40 mg once daily versus terfenadine 60 mg twice daily in the treatment of seasonal allergic rhinitis. *J Int Med Res* 1987;15:63–70.
50. Irander K, Odkvist LM, Ohlander B. Treatment of hay fever with loratadine — a new non-sedating antihistamine. *Allergy* 1990;45:86–91.
51. Skassa-Brociek W, Bousquet J, Montes F, et al. Double-blind placebo-controlled study of loratadine, mequitazine, and placebo in the symptomatic treatment of seasonal allergic rhinitis. *J Allergy Clin Immunol* 1988;81:725–730.
52. Dockhorn RJ, Bergner A, Connell JT. Safety and efficacy of loratadine (Sch-29851): a new non-sedating antihistamine in seasonal allergic rhinitis. *Ann Allergy* 1987;58:407–411.
53. Horak F, Bruttmann G, Pedrali P, et al. A multicentric study of loratadine, terfenadine and placebo in patients with seasonal allergic rhinitis. *Arzneimittel-Forsch* 1988;38:124–128.
54. Berger WE, Schenkel EJ, Mansfield LE, and the Desloratadine Study group. Safety and efficacy of desloratadine 5mg in asthma patients with seasonal allergic rhinitis and nasal congestion. *Ann Allergy Asthma Immunol* 2002;89:485–491
55. Philip G, Malmstrom K, Hampel FC Jr, et al., for the Montelukast Spring Rhinitis Group. Montelukast for treating seasonal allergic rhinitis: a randomized, double-blind, placebo-controlled trial performed in the spring. *Clin Exp Allergy* 2002;32:1020–1028.
56. Nayak A, Philip G, Lu S, et al., and the Montelukast Fall Rhinitis Investigator Group. Efficacy and tolerability of montelukast alone or in combination with loratadine in seasonal allergic rhinitis: a multicenter, randomized, double-blind, placebo-controlled trial performed in the fall. *Ann Allergy Asthma Immunol* 2002;88:592–600.
57. Meltzer EO, Prenner BM, Nayak A, Desloratadine Study Group. Efficacy and tolerability of once-daily 5mg desloratadine, an H-1 receptor antagonist with seasonal allergic rhinitis: assessment during the spring and fall seasons. *Clin Drug Invest* 2001;21:25–32.
58. Limon L, Kockler DR. Desloratadine: a nonsedating antihistamine. *Ann Pharmacother* 2003;37:237–246. Search date 2002; primary sources Medline, reference lists, and Schering Corporation.
59. Stern M, Blondin-Ertzbischoff P, Murrieta-Aguttes M, et al. Rapid and sustained efficacy of mizolastine 10 mg once daily in seasonal allergic rhinitis. *J Int Med Res* 1998;26:292–303.
60. Leynadier F, Bousquet J, Murrieta M, et al. Efficacy and safety of mizolastine in seasonal allergic rhinitis. The Rhinase Study Group. *Ann Allergy* 1996;76:163–168.
61. Boerner D, Metz K, Eberhardt R, et al. A placebo-controlled comparison of the efficacy and tolerability of picumast dihydrochloride and terfenadine in patients with seasonal allergic rhinitis. *Arzneimittel-Forsch* 1989;39:1356–1359.
62. Kagan G, Dabrowicki E, Huddlestone L. A double-blind trial of terfenadine and placebo in hay fever using a substitution technique for non-responders. *J Int Med Res* 1980;8:404–407.
63. Brandon ML, Weiner M. Clinical studies of terfenadine in seasonal allergic rhinitis. *Arzneimittel-Forsch* 1982;32:1204–1205.
64. Brooks CD, Karl KJ, Francom SF. Profile of ragweed hay fever symptom control with terfenadine started before or after symptoms are established. *Clin Exp Allergy* 1990;20:21–26.
65. Simpson RJ. Budesonide and terfenadine, separately and in combination, in the treatment of hay fever. *Ann Allergy* 1994;73:497–502.
66. Van Bavel J, Findlay SR, Hampel FC, et al. Intranasal fluticasone propionate is more effective than terfenadine tablets for seasonal allergic rhinitis. *Arch Int Med* 1994;154:2699–2704.
67. Bronsky EA, Dockhorn RJ, Meltzer EO, et al. Fluticasone propionate aqueous nasal spray compared with terfenadine tablets in the treatment of seasonal allergic rhinitis. *J Allergy Clin Immunol* 1996;97:915–921.
68. Darnell R, Pecoud A, Richards DH. A double-blind comparison of fluticasone propionate aqueous nasal spray, terfenadine tablets and placebo in the treatment of patients with seasonal allergic rhinitis to grass pollen. *Clin Exp Allergy* 1994;24:1144–1150.

69. Committee on Safety of Medicines. Astemizole (Hismanal): only available on prescription. Important new contraindications and interactions. http://www.mca.gov.uk / (last accessed 9 June 2003).
70. Committee on Safety of Medicines. Terfenadine: Information for Doctors and Pharmacists, http://www.mca.gov.uk/aboutagency/regframework/csm/csmhome.htm (last accessed 9 June 2003).
71. Mann RD, Pearce GL, Dunn N, et al. Sedation with "non-sedating" antihistamines: four prescription-event monitoring studies in general practice. *BMJ* 2000;320:1184–1187.
72. Schuermans V, Lewi PJ, Gypen LM, et al. Meta-analysis of the global evaluation of levocabastine nasal spray versus placebo. *Drug Inf J* 1993;27:575–584.
73. Hampel FC, Martin BG, Dolen J, et al. Efficacy and safety of levocabastine nasal spray for seasonal allergic rhinitis *Am J Rhinology* 1999;13:55–62.
74. Di Lorenzo G, Gervasi F, Drago A, et al. Comparison of the effects of fluticasone propionate, aqueous nasal spray and levocabastine on inflammatory cells in nasal lavage and clinical activity during the pollen season in seasonal rhinitics. *Clin Exp Allergy* 1999;29:1367–1377.
75. Newson-Smith G, Powell M, Baehre M, et al. A placebo controlled study comparing the efficacy of intranasal azelastine and beclomethasone in the treatment of seasonal allergic rhinitis. *Eur Arch Otorhinolaryngol* 1997;254:236–241.
76. LaForce C, Dockhorn RJ, Prenner BM, et al. Safety and efficacy of azelastine nasal spray (Astelin NS) for seasonal allergic rhinitis: a 4-week comparative multicenter trial. *Ann Allergy Asthma Immunol* 1996;76:181–188.
77. Ciprandi G, Ricca V, Passalacqua G, et al. Seasonal rhinitis and azelastine: long- or short-term treatment? *J Allergy Clin Immunol* 1997;99:301–307.
78. Duarte C, Baéhre M, Gharakhanian S, Leynadier F, and the French Azelastine Group. Treatment of severe seasonal rhinoconjunctivitis by a combination of azelastine nasal spray and eye drops: a double-blind, double-placebo study. *J Invest Allergol Clin Immunol* 2001;11:34–40.
79. Mosges R, Klimek L, Spaeth J, et al. Topical versus systemical treatment with antihistamines in seasonal allergic rhinitis. *Allergologi* 1995;18:145–150. [In German]
80. Bahmer F, Ruprecht KW. Safety and efficacy of topical levocabastine compared with oral terfenadine. *Ann Allergy* 1994;72:429–434.
81. Sussman GL, Mason J, Compton D, et al. The efficacy and safety of fexofenadine HCl and pseudoephedrine alone and in combination in seasonal allergic rhinitis. *J Allergy Clin Immunol* 1999;104:100–106.
82. Dockhorn RJ, Williams BO, Sanders RL. Efficacy of acrivastine with pseudoephedrine in treatment of allergic rhinitis due to ragweed. *Ann Allergy Asthma Immunol* 1996;76:204–208.
83. Grosclaude M, Mees K, Pinelli ME, et al. Cetirizine and pseudoephedrine retard, given alone or in combination with seasonal allergic rhinitis. *Rhinology* 1997;35:67–73.
84. Schenkel E, Corren J , Murray JJ. Efficacy of once-daily desloratadine/pseudoephedrine for relief of nasal congestion. *Allergy Asthma Proc* 2002;23:325–330.
85. Panda NK, Mann SBS. Comparative efficacy and safety of terfenadine with pseudoephedrine and terfenadine alone in allergic rhinitis. *Otolaryngol Head Neck Surg* 1998;118:253–255.
86. Tarasido JC. Azatadine maleate/pseudoephedrine sulfate repetabs versus placebo in the treatment of severe seasonal allergic rhinitis. *J Int Med Res* 1980;8:391–394.
87. Busse W, Biondi R, Casale T, et al. Randomised double-blind, parallel placebo-controlled multi-centre trial of ipratropium bromide nasal spray 0.06% in patients with seasonal allergic rhinitis. *Ann Allergy Asthma Immunol* 1999;82:109. [Abstract]
88. Gonyeau MJ, Partisano AM. A clinical review of montelukast in the treatment of seasonal allergic rhinitis. *Formulary* 2003;38:368–378. Search date: 1990–2003; primary sources Medline, Embase, and PreMedline.
89. van Adelsberg J, Philip G, LaForce CF, et al. Randomized controlled trial evaluating the clinical benefit of montelukast for treating spring seasonal allergic rhinitis. *Ann Allergy Asthma Immunol* 2003;90:214–222.
90. Meltzer EO, Malmstrom K, Lu S, et al. Concomitant montelukast and loratadine as treatment for seasonal allergic rhinitis — a randomised placebo-controlled clinical trial. *J Allergy Clin Immunol* 2000;105:917–922.
91. Pullerits T, Praks L, Ristioja V, et al Comparison of a nasal glucocorticoid, antileukotriene and a combination of antileukotriene and antihistamine the treatment of seasonal allergic rhinitis. *J Allergy Clin Immunol* 2002;109:949–955.
92. Nathan RA. Pharmacotherapy for allergic rhinitis: a critical review of leukotriene receptor antagonists compared with other treatments. *Ann Allergy Asthma Immunol* 2003;90:182–190. Search date not stated, primary sources Medline and hand searches of relevant conference proceedings.
93. Grossman J, Ratner PH, Nathan R, et al. Pranlukast, an oral leukotriene receptor antagonist, relieves symptoms in patients with seasonal allergic rhinitis. *J Allergy Clin Immunol* 1997;99:S443.
94. Bronsky E, Boggs P, Findlay S, et al. Comparative efficacy and safety of a once-daily loratadine–pseudoephedrine combination versus its components alone and placebo in the management of seasonal allergic rhinitis. *J Allergy Clin Immunol* 1995;96:139–147.
95. Measurement of health related quality of life: adult rhinoconjunctivitis. http://www.qoltech.co.uk/Rhinocon.htm (last accessed 9 June 2003).
96. Ware JJ, Sherbourne CD. The MOS 36-item short-form health survey (SF-36). I. Conceptual framework and item selection. *Med Care* 1992;30;473–483.

Aziz Sheikh
Professor of Primary Care Research & Development Division of Community Health Sciences: GP Section
University of Edinburgh, Edinburgh, UK

Sukhmeet Singh Panesar
Medical Student
Imperial College London, London, UK

Sangeeta Dhami
General Practitioner
Edinburgh, UK

Competing interests: None declared.

Sinusitis (acute)

Search date August 2004

Kim Ah-See

QUESTIONS

INTERVENTIONS

See glossary G

Key Messages

Clinically diagnosed

- **Antibiotics** Three RCTs found no good evidence that amoxicillin, with or without clavulanate, reduced or cured symptoms compared with placebo in people with clinically diagnosed acute sinusitis, who had not had radiological or bacteriological confirmation of disease. Two RCTs found that amoxicillin, with or without clavulanate, increased diarrhoea compared with placebo. We found no RCTs examining effects of other antibiotics (co-trimoxazole, cephalosporins, azithromycin, and erythromycin) compared with placebo or each other.
- **Antihistamines** We found no RCTs examining clinical effects of antihistamines in people with clinically diagnosed acute sinusitis.
- **Decongestants** We found no RCTs examining clinical effects of topical or systemic decongestants in people with clinically diagnosed acute sinusitis.
- **Topical steroids** We found no RCTs examining clinical effects of topical steroids in people with clinically diagnosed acute sinusitis.

Radiologically or bacteriologically confirmed

- **Cephalosporins and macrolides (fewer adverse effects than amoxicillin or amoxicillin–clavulanate)** We found no RCTs comparing cephalosporins or macrolides with placebo. One systematic review and two subsequent RCTs in people with radiologically or bacteriologically confirmed acute sinusitis found no significant difference in clinical resolution between amoxicillin or amoxicillin–clavulanate and cephalosporins or macrolides. However, cephalosporins and macrolides caused fewer adverse effects than amoxicillin and amoxicillin–clavulanate. One RCT found no significant difference in clinical improvement or clinical cure between cefaclor (a cephalosporin) and azithromycin (a macrolide).
- **Amoxicillin and amoxicillin–clavulanate (more adverse effects than cephalosporins or macrolides)** One systematic review identified two RCTs in people with radiologically or bacteriologically confirmed acute maxillary sinusitis, which found that amoxicillin improved early clinical cure rate compared with placebo, but was associated with more frequent adverse effects, mainly gastrointestinal. One systematic review and two subsequent RCTs in people with radiologically or bacteriologically confirmed acute sinusitis found no significant difference in clinical resolution between amoxicillin or amoxicillin–clavulanate and cephalosporins or macrolides. However, amoxicillin and amoxicillin–clavulanate caused more adverse effects.
- **Antihistamines** We found no RCTs examining the effects of antihistamines in people with radiologically or bacteriologically confirmed acute sinusitis.
- **Decongestants** We found no RCTs examining the effects of decongestants in people with radiologically or bacteriologically confirmed acute sinusitis.
- **Different dosages of antibiotics** One RCT in people with radiologically or bacteriologically confirmed acute sinusitis found no significant difference in clinical resolution rates or adverse events between two and three daily doses of cefaclor. We found no RCTs of other antibiotics comparing different dosage regimens.
- **Topical steroids** We found no RCTs examining the effects of topical steroids in people with radiologically or bacteriologically confirmed acute sinusitis.
- **Long course antibiotic regimens (no more effective than short course regimens, and more adverse effects)** RCTs in people with confirmed acute sinusitis found no significant difference in clinical resolution rates between 6–10 day courses and 3–5 day courses of azithromycin, telithromycin, co-trimoxazole or cefuroxime (a cephalosporin) up to 3 weeks after treatment. RCTs found similar rates of adverse effects and diarrhoea between longer and shorter courses of azithromycin and telithromycin. One RCT found that adverse effects, which were mainly gastrointestinal, were more frequent with a longer course of cefuroxime than with a shorter course of cefuroxime.

DEFINITION Acute sinusitis is defined pathologically, by transient inflammation of the mucosal lining of the paranasal sinuses lasting less than 4 weeks. Clinically, it is characterised by nasal congestion, rhinorrhoea Ⓖ, facial pain, hyposmia Ⓖ, sneezing, and, if more severe, additional malaise and fever. The diagnosis is usually made clinically (on the basis of history and examination, but without radiological or bacteriological investigation). Clinically diagnosed acute sinusitis is less likely to be caused by bacterial infection than is acute sinusitis confirmed by radiological or bacteriological investigation.[1] In this chapter, we have excluded studies in children, in people with symptoms for more than 4 weeks (chronic sinusitis), and in people with symptoms after facial trauma. We have made it clear in each section whether we are dealing with clinically diagnosed acute sinusitis or acute sinusitis that has been confirmed by bacteriological or radiological investigation, because the effects of treatment may be different in these groups.

INCIDENCE/ PREVALENCE Each year in Europe, 1–5% of adults are diagnosed with acute sinusitis by their general practitioner.[2] Extrapolated to the British population, this is estimated to cause 6 million restricted working days a year.[3,4] Most people with acute sinusitis are assessed and treated in a primary care setting. The prevalence varies according to whether diagnosis is made on clinical grounds or on the basis of radiological or bacteriological investigation.

AETIOLOGY/ RISK FACTORS One systematic review (search date 1998) reported that about 50% of people with a clinical diagnosis of acute sinusitis have bacterial sinus infection.[1] The usual pathogens in acute bacterial sinusitis are *Streptococcus pneumoniae* and *Haemophilus influenzae*, with occasional infection with *Moraxella catarrhalis*. Preceding viral upper respiratory tract infection is often the trigger for acute bacterial sinusitis,[5] with about 0.5% of common colds becoming complicated by the development of acute sinusitis.[6]

PROGNOSIS One meta-analysis of RCTs found that up to two thirds of people with acute sinusitis had spontaneous resolution of symptoms without active treatment.[7] One non-systematic review reported that people with acute sinusitis are at risk of chronic sinusitis and irreversible damage to the normal mucociliary mucosal surface.[8] One further non-systematic review reported rare life-threatening complications such as orbital cellulitis**Ⓖ** and meningitis after acute sinusitis.[9] However, we found no reliable data to measure these risks.

AIMS OF INTERVENTION To relieve symptoms as quickly as possible, with minimal adverse effects.

OUTCOMES Symptom scores; time to self reported symptom resolution; time to clinical resolution (defined by examiner). In the identified studies, clinical improvement and clinical cure were often used as outcome measures. "Clinical improvement" was defined as improvement in clinical state as rated by the assessor or by the participant. "Clinical cure" was defined as resolution of symptoms as rated by assessor or participant.

METHODS *Clinical Evidence* search and appraisal August 2004.

QUESTION What are the effects of treatments in people with clinically diagnosed acute sinusitis?

OPTION ANTIBIOTICS

Three RCTs found no good evidence that amoxicillin, with or without clavulanate, reduced or cured symptoms compared with placebo in people with clinically diagnosed acute sinusitis, who had not had radiological or bacteriological confirmation of disease. Two RCTs found that amoxicillin, with or without clavulanate, increased diarrhoea compared with placebo. We found no RCTs examining effects of other antibiotics (co-trimoxazole, cephalosporins, azithromycin, and erythromycin) compared with placebo or each other.

Benefits: **Amoxicillin versus placebo:** We found two RCTs in people with an exclusively clinical diagnosis of acute sinusitis, without reliance on radiological or bacteriological investigations.[10,11] The first RCT (416 people in a primary care setting) compared amoxicillin (500 mg 3 times daily) versus placebo for 10 days. It found no significant difference between amoxicillin and placebo in treatment success at the end of treatment (treatment success defined by absent or mild symptoms: 35% with amoxicillin *v* 29% with placebo; RR 1.14, 95% CI 0.92 to 1.42). The second RCT (150 people with clinically diagnosed acute maxillary sinusitis in a primary care setting) compared three antibiotics (amoxicillin, doxycycline, and penicillin) versus placebo.[11] It found that amoxicillin increased recovery rates compared with placebo at 2 weeks but the statistical significance was not reported (recovery assessed by telephone: 18/23 [78%] with amoxicillin *v* 39/59 [66%] with placebo). **Amoxicillin–clavulanate versus placebo:** We found one RCT (252 adults recruited from general practices and outpatient clinics).[12] It found no significant difference between 6 days of amoxicillin–clavulanate and placebo for time to return to normal activities (HR adjusted for specified variables 0.99, 95% CI 0.68 to 1.45). **Co-trimoxazole, cephalosporins, azithromycin, or erythromycin versus placebo:** We found no RCTs. **Versus each other:** We found no RCTs.

Harms: **Amoxicillin versus placebo:** The first RCT found that diarrhoea was significantly more common with amoxicillin compared with placebo (29% with amoxicillin *v* 19% with placebo; RR 1.28, CI 1.05 to 1.57).[10] The second RCT did not report adverse effects separately for amoxicillin compared with placebo.[11] **Amoxicillin–clavulanate versus placebo:** The subsequent RCT found that amoxicillin–clavulanate significantly increased diarrhoea at 7 days and non-significantly increased diarrhoea at 14 days compared with placebo (7 days: OR 3.89, 95% CI 2.09 to 7.25; 14 days: OR 1.71, 95% CI 0.91 to 3.23).[12] **Co-trimoxazole, cephalosporins, azithromycin, or erythromycin versus placebo:** We found no RCTs. **Versus each other:** We found no RCTs.

Comment: The RCTs may have lacked adequate follow up to detect clinically important differences between amoxicillin and placebo.

OPTION DECONGESTANTS, TOPICAL STEROIDS, AND ANTIHISTAMINES

We found no RCTs examining clinical effects of topical or systemic decongestants, topical steroids, or antihistamines in people with clinically diagnosed acute sinusitis.

Benefits: **Decongestants; topical steroids; antihistamines:** We found no RCTs.

Harms: We found no RCTs.

Comment: None.

QUESTION What are the effects of antibiotics in people with radiologically or bacteriologically confirmed acute sinusitis?

OPTION AMOXICILLIN AND AMOXICILLIN–CLAVULANATE

One systematic review identified two RCTs in people with radiologically or bacteriologically confirmed acute maxillary sinusitis, which found that amoxicillin improved early clinical cure rate compared with placebo, but was associated with more frequent adverse effects, mainly gastrointestinal. One systematic review and two subsequent RCTs in people with radiologically or bacteriologically confirmed acute sinusitis found no significant difference in clinical resolution between amoxicillin or amoxicillin–clavulanate and cephalosporins or macrolides. However, amoxicillin and amoxicillin–clavulanate caused more adverse effects.

Benefits: **Amoxicillin versus placebo:** We found two systematic reviews (search date 1998, number of relevant RCTs not reported, 761 adults with acute uncomplicated sinusitis;[1] and search date 1998, 2 RCTs, 344 adults with acute sinusitis[13]). The first review did not report separately on effects of amoxicillin compared with placebo.[1] The second review found that 7–10 days of amoxicillin significantly increased complete symptom resolution compared with placebo (2 RCTs; OR 2.24, 95% CI 1.40 to 3.56).[13] **Amoxicillin–clavulanate versus placebo:** The first review with the most recent search date did not report separately on the effects of amoxicillin–clavulanate compared with placebo.[1] The second review found no RCTs.[13] **Versus cephalosporin and macrolides:** See benefits of cephalosporins and macrolides, p 650.

Harms: **Amoxicillin versus placebo:** Both RCTs included in the earlier review[13] found that antibiotics significantly increased adverse effects (mainly gastrointestinal) compared with placebo (first RCT,[14] diarrhoea: 47% with amoxicillin *v* 11% with placebo; P = 0.001; second RCT,[15] all adverse effects: 28% with amoxicillin *v* 9% with placebo; P <0.001).

Comment: One of the RCTs that compared amoxicillin with placebo was a three arm trial, which also examined effects of penicillin. We have not reported results in the penicillin group.

OPTION CEPHALOSPORINS AND MACROLIDES

We found no RCTs comparing cephalosporins or macrolides with placebo. One systematic review and two subsequent RCTs in people with radiologically or bacteriologically confirmed acute sinusitis found no significant difference in clinical resolution between amoxicillin or amoxicillin–clavulanate and cephalosporins or macrolides. However, cephalosporins and macrolides caused fewer adverse effects than amoxicillin and amoxicillin–clavulanate. One RCT found no significant difference in clinical improvement or clinical cure between cefaclor (a cephalosporin) and azithromycin (a macrolide).

Benefits: **Versus placebo:** We found two systematic reviews (search dates 1998[1] and 1998[13]). The first review did not report separately on the effects of cephalosporins and macrolides compared with placebo.[1] The second review found no RCTs comparing these antibiotics with placebo.[13] We found no subsequent RCTS. **Versus amoxicillin:** The second systematic review found 10 RCTs (1590 adults), which compared penicillin antibiotics (including amoxicillin) versus cephalosporins, macrolides (clarithromycin, spiramycin, azithromycin, roxithromycin, pristamycin, and erythromycin), or minocycline in people with radiologically or bacteriologically confirmed acute maxillary sinusitis.[13] It found no significant difference in clinical resolution rate between newer non-penicillins and the penicillin antibiotics (OR 0.85, 95% CI 0.70 to 1.08). **Versus amoxicillin–clavulanate:** The second review (10 RCTs, 3957 adults)[13] and two subsequent RCTs[16,17] compared amoxicillin–clavulanate versus macrolides or cephalosporins. The second systematic review found no significant difference in clinical resolution rate between amoxicillin–clavulanate and the other antibiotics (OR 0.90, 95% CI 0.76 to 1.08). The first subsequent RCT (941 adults) found no significant difference in cure rates between amoxicillin–clavulanate (500–125 mg 3 times daily for 10 days) and azithromycin (500 mg daily for 3 or 6 days) at 28 days (cure rate 71.5% with amoxicillin–clavulanate *v* 71.5% with 3 days of azithromycin *v* 74.1% for 6 days of azithromycin; 97.5% CI for difference: –8.4% to + 8.3% for 3 days and –5.6% to +10.9% for 6 days of azithromycin).[16] The second subsequent RCT (607 adults with acute maxillary sinusitis at baseline, 423 people analysed on a per protocol basis, see comment below) found no significant difference in cure rate between amoxicillin–clavulanate and telithromycin (800 mg for 5 or 10 days) at 17–24 days follow up (cure rate 74.5% with amoxicillin–clavulanate *v* 75.3% with 5 days of telithromycin *v* 72.9% with 10 days of telithromycin; 95% CI for difference: –9.9% to +11.7% with 5 days and –1.6%, 95% CI –12.7% to +9.5% with 10 days of telithromycin).[17] **Macrolides versus cephalosporins:** The second systematic review[13] identified one RCT (496 people).[18] It found no significant difference between azithromycin (500 mg once daily for 3 days) and cefaclor (250 mg 3 times daily for 10 days) in clinical improvement or resolution of symptoms after 11–15 days (clinical improvement or clinical resolution: 228/245 [93%] with azithromycin *v* 233/241 [97%] with cefaclor; P value not reported).

Harms: **Versus placebo:** We found no RCTs. **Versus amoxicillin:** The systematic review found that the risk of stopping treatment because of adverse effects was lower with cephalosporins and macrolides (clarithromycin, spiramycin, azithromycin, roxithromycin, pristamycin, and erythromycin) than with penicillins (OR 0.54, 95% CI 0.29 to 1.00).[13] **Versus amoxicillin–clavulanate:** The systematic review found that the risk of stopping treatment because of adverse effects was lower with cephalosporins and macrolides than with amoxicillin–clavulanate (OR 0.37, 95% CI 0.26 to 0.52).[13] The first subsequent RCT found that amoxicillin–clavulanate significantly increased adverse effects compared with azithromycin (51% with amoxicillin–clavulanate *v* 31% with 3 days of azithromycin *v* 38% with 6 days of azithromycin; P value not reported).[16] The most common adverse effect was diarrhoea, which was more frequent with amoxicillin–clavulanate (32% with amoxicillin–clavulanate *v* 17% with 3 days of azithromycin *v* 21% with 6 days of azithromycin; P value not reported). The second subsequent RCT found similar rates of adverse effects between amoxicillin–clavulanate and 5 or 10 days of telithromycin (42% with amoxicillin–clavulanate *v* 47% with 5 days of telithromycin *v* 43% with 10 days of telithromycin; P value not reported).[17] It found no significant difference between treatments for diarrhoea (5% with amoxicillin–clavulanate *v* 1.6% with 5 days of telithromycin *v* 3.1% with 10 days of telithromycin; P value not reported). **Macrolides versus cephalosporins:** One RCT comparing azithromycin versus cefaclor found no significant difference in adverse effects between treatments (11% with azithromycin *v* 10% with cefaclor; P = 0.82).[18] The most common adverse effects gastrointestinal symptoms (9.4% with azithromycin *v* 5.7% with cefaclor).

Comment: **Versus amoxicillin–clavulanate:** In the second subsequent RCT people were excluded from analysis owing to major protocol violations (insufficient duration of treatment, incorrect diagnosis, or missing data).[17] Exclusion rates were similar among treatment groups (65/202 [32%] with amoxicillin–clavulanate *v* 55/201 [27%] with 5 days of telithromycin *v* 64/204 [31%] with 10 days of telithromycin).

OPTION LONG COURSE ANTIBIOTIC REGIMENS

RCTs in people with confirmed acute sinusitis found no significant difference in clinical resolution rates between 6–10 day courses and 3–5 day courses of azithromycin, telithromycin, co-trimoxazole or cefuroxime (a cephalosporin) up to 3 weeks after treatment. RCTs found similar rates of adverse effects and diarrhoea between longer and shorter courses of azithromycin and telithromycin. One RCT found that adverse effects, which were mainly gastrointestinal, were more frequent with a longer course of cefuroxime than with a shorter course of cefuroxime.

Benefits: **Macrolides:** We found two RCTs that compared longer versus shorter courses of azithromycin or telithromycin.[16,17] Neither RCT was designed to compare longer versus shorter courses of the same antibiotic. The first RCT (936 adults) compared 3 and 6 days of azithromycin with amoxicillin–clavulanate.[16] It found similar cure rates between the shorter compared with longer courses of azithromycin (71.5% with 3 days *v* 74.1% with 6 days; P value not reported). The second RCT (607 adults with acute maxillary sinusitis at baseline, 423 people analysed on a per protocol basis) compared 5 and 10 days of telithromycin with amoxicillin–clavulanate.[17] It found similar cure rates between the shorter compared with longer courses of telithromycin (75.3% with 5 days *v* 72.9% with 10 days; P value not reported). **Co-trimoxazole:** One RCT (80 people with confirmed sinusitis) found no significant difference in clinical resolution or improvement between a 10 day and a 3 day course of co-trimoxazole at 14 days' follow up (AR for resolution or improvement about 76% in each group; CI not reported; P = 0.45).[19] **Cephalosporins:** One RCT (401 people with confirmed sinusitis) found no significant difference in clinical resolution rates between a 10 day and a 5 day course of cefuroxime 11–18 days after treatment (73% with 10 day course *v* 74% with 5 day course; ARR with shorter course +1.0%, 90% CI −7.5% to +8.5%).[2]

Harms: **Azithromycin:** The RCT comparing 3 and 6 days of azithromycin found similar rates of overall adverse effects and diarrhoea between the shorter and longer courses (all adverse effects: 31.1% with 3 days *v* 37.6% with 6 days; diarrhoea: 17.0% with 3 days *v* 21.2% with 6 days, P values not reported).[16] **Telithromycin:** The RCT comparing 5 and 10 days of telithromycin found similar rates of overall adverse effects and diarrhoea between the shorter and longer courses (all adverse effects: 42.2% with 5 days *v* 46.9% with 10 days; diarrhoea: 19.3% with 5 days *v* 20.5% with 10 days; P values not reported).[17] **Co-trimoxazole:** The RCT found no significant difference in adverse events between a 3 day and a 10 day course of co-trimoxazole (CI not reported; P = 0.2).[19] **Cephalosporins:** The RCT found that a larger proportion of people on the 10 day course of cefuroxime reported minor adverse effects, mainly gastrointestinal, compared with the 5 day course of cefuroxime (11.8% with 10 day course *v* 5.8% with 5 day course; significance not reported).[2]

Comment: None.

OPTION DIFFERENT DOSAGES OF ANTIBIOTICS

One RCT in people with radiologically or bacteriologically confirmed acute sinusitis found no significant difference in clinical resolution rates or adverse events between two and three daily doses of cefaclor. We found no RCTs of other antibiotics comparing different dosage regimens.

Benefits: **Amoxicillin, amoxicillin–clavulanate, azithromycin, erythromycin, and co-trimoxazole:** We found no RCTs comparing different daily dosing regimens of the same antibiotic. **Cephalosporins:** One RCT (298 people with confirmed acute sinusitis) compared different daily dose regimens of the same cephalosporin.[20] It found no significant difference in clinical resolution rates between cefaclor 500 mg three times daily and cefaclor 750 mg twice daily at 14 days follow up (clinical resolution rate: 95.7% with 500 mg 3 times daily *v* 97.3% with 750 mg twice daily; CI not reported; P = 0.333).

Harms: The RCT found no significant difference in adverse event rates between cefaclor 500 mg three times daily and cefaclor 750 mg twice daily (adverse event rate: 24.7% with 750 mg twice daily *v* 32% with 500 mg 3 times daily; CI not reported, P = 0.162).[20]

Comment: None.

OPTION DECONGESTANTS, TOPICAL STEROIDS, AND ANTIHISTAMINES

We found no RCTs examining the effects of decongestants, topical steroids, or antihistamines in people with radiologically or bacteriologically confirmed acute sinusitis.

Benefits: **Decongestants; topical steroids; antihistamines:** We found no RCTs.

Harms: We found no RCTs.

Comment: None.

GLOSSARY

Hyposmia Reduced, not absent, sense of smell.

Orbital cellulitis Inflammation of the soft tissues in and around the eye socket.

Rhinorrhoea Discharge from the nasal cavity.

Substantive changes

Amoxycillin and amoxicillin–clavulanate (clinically confirmed acute sinusitis) One RCT added.[12] Categorisation unchanged.

Cephalosporins and macrolides (radiologically or bacteriologically confirmed acute sinusitis) Two RCTs added.[16,17] Categorisation unchanged.

Long versus short course antibiotics Two RCTs added.[16,17] Categorisation unchanged. Benefits and harms data enhanced.

REFERENCES

1. Benninger MS, Sedory Holzer SE, Lau J. Diagnosis and treatment of uncomplicated acute bacterial rhinosinusitis: summary of the Agency for Health Care Policy and Research evidence-based report. *Otolaryngol Head Neck Surg* 2000;122:1–7. Search date 1998; primary sources Medline and bibliographies or retrieved articles.
2. Dubreuil C, Gehanno P, Goldstein F, et al. Treatment of acute maxillary sinusitis in adult outpatients: comparison of a five versus ten day-course of cefuroxime axetil. *Med Malad Infect* 2001;31:70–78.
3. Kennedy DW. International conference on sinus terminology, staging, therapy. *Ann Otol Rhinol Laryngol* 1995;104:10.
4. Jones NS. Rhinosinusitis. In: *Statements of clinical effectiveness in otorhinolaryngology*. London British Association of Otorhinolaryngologists, Head and Neck Surgeons, 1998:21–31.
5. Henry DC, Moller DJ, Adelglass J, et al. Comparison of sparfloxacin and clarithromycin in the treatment of acute bacterial maxillary sinusitis. Sparfloxacin Multicenter AMS Study Group. *Clin Ther* 1999;21:340–352.
6. Low DE, Desrosiers M, McSherry J, et al. A practical guide for the diagnosis and treatment of acute sinusitis. *CMAJ* 1997;156(suppl 6):S1–S14.
7. de Ferranti SD, Ioannidis JP, Lau J, et al. Are amoxycillin and folate inhibitors as effective as other antibiotics for acute sinusitis? A meta-analysis. *BMJ* 1998;317:632–637.
8. Goodman GM, Slavin RG. Medical management in adults of chronic sinus disease. *Immunol Allergy Clin North Am* 1994;14:69–87.
9. Ramsey PG, Weymuller EA. Complications of bacterial infection of the ears, paranasal sinuses, and oropharynx in adults. *Emerg Med Clin North Am* 1985;3:143–160.
10. De Sutter AI, De Meyere MJ, Christiaens TC, et al. Does amoxicillin improve outcomes in patients with purulent rhinorrhea? A pragmatic randomized double-blind controlled trial in family practice. *J Fam Pract* 2002;51:317–323.
11. Varonen H, Kunnamo I, Savolainen S, et al. Treatment of acute rhinosinusitis diagnosed by clinical criteria or ultrasound in primary care: a placebo-controlled randomised trial. *Scand J Prim Health Care* 2003;21:121–126.
12. Bucher HC, Tschudi P, Young J, et al. Effect of amoxicillin–clavulanate in clinically diagnosed acute rhinosinusitis: a placebo-controlled, double-blind, randomized trial in general practice. *Arch Intern Med* 2003;163:1793–1798.
13. Williams JW, Aguilar C, Makela M, et al. Antibiotics for acute maxillary sinusitis (Cochrane Review). In: The Cochrane Library, Issue 3, 2004. Oxford: Update Software. Search date 2001; primary sources Medline, Embase, search of bibliographies of included studies, and discussion with pharmaceutical companies.
14. Lindbaek M, Hjortdahl P, Johnsen ULH. Randomised, double blind, placebo controlled trial of penicillin V and amoxycillin in treatment of acute sinus infections in adults. *BMJ* 1996;313:325–329.
15. Van Buchem FL, Knottnerus JA, Schrijnemaekers VJJ, et al. Primary-care-based randomised placebo-controlled trial of antibiotic treatment in acute maxillary sinusitis. *Lancet* 1997;349:683–687.
16. Henry DC, Riffer E, Sokol WN, et al. Randomized double-blind study comparing 3- and 6-day regimens of azithromycin with a 10-day amoxicillin–clavulanate regimen for treatment of acute bacterial sinusitis. *Antimicrob Agents Chemother* 2003;47:2770–2774.
17. Luterman M, Tellier G, Lasko B, et al. Efficacy and tolerability of telithromycin for 5 or 10 days vs amoxicillin/clavulanic acid for 10 days in acute maxillary sinusitis. *Ear Nose Throat J* 2003;82:576–590.
18. O'Doherty B. An open comparative study of azithromycin versus cefaclor in the treatment of patients with upper respiratory tract infections. *J Antimicrob Chemother* 1996;37(suppl C):71–81.
19. Williams JW Jr, Holleman DR Jr, Samsa GP, et al. Randomized controlled trial of 3 vs 10 days of trimethoprim/sulfamethoxazole for acute maxillary sinusitis. *JAMA* 1995;273:1015–1021.
20. Turik M, Watkins M, Johns D Jr. Double-masked, randomized, parallel-group comparison of cefaclor AF and cefaclor in the treatment of acute bacterial sinusitis. *Curr Ther Res Clin Exp* 1997;58:227–239.

Kim Ah-See
Consultant Otolaryngologist-Head and Neck Surgeon
Aberdeen Royal Infirmary
Aberdeen
UK

Competing interests: None declared.

Tinnitus

Search date February 2004
Angus Waddell

QUESTIONS

INTERVENTIONS

Key Messages

- **Tricyclic antidepressants** One systematic review of one RCT in people with depression and chronic tinnitus found that tricyclic antidepressants (nortriptyline) improved tinnitus related disability and symptoms of depression at 6 weeks, but found no significant difference in self reported tinnitus severity compared with placebo. One small RCT in people with tinnitus but without depression found that a greater proportion of people rated themselves as improved with tricyclic antidepressants (amitriptyline) compared with placebo at 6 weeks. Tricyclic antidepressants are associated with adverse effects such as dry mouth, blurred vision, and constipation.
- **Benzodiazepines (alprazolam)** One systematic review found limited evidence from one RCT that alprazolam, a benzodiazepine, improved self reported tinnitus severity after 12 weeks. Benzodiazepines can have adverse effects that may outweigh potential benefits.
- **Psychotherapy** One systematic review found insufficient evidence about the effects of cognitive behavioural treatment, relaxation therapy, education, or biofeedback compared with other or no treatment in people with chronic tinnitus.
- **Carbamazepine** One systematic review of one RCT found no significant difference between carbamazepine and placebo in tinnitus severity at 30 days. Treatment with carbamazepine was associated with an increased risk of dizziness, nausea, and headaches.
- **Acupuncture; baclofen; cinnarizine; electromagnetic stimulation; ginkgo biloba; hyperbaric oxygen; hypnosis; lamotrigine; low power laser; nicotinamide; tinnitus masking devices; zinc** We found insufficient evidence about the effects of these interventions.

DEFINITION Tinnitus is defined as the perception of sound, which does not arise from the external environment, from within the body (e.g. vascular sounds), or from auditory hallucinations related to mental illness. This review is concerned with tinnitus, where tinnitus is the only, or the predominant, symptom in an affected person.

INCIDENCE/ PREVALENCE Up to 18% of the general population in industrialised countries are mildly affected by chronic tinnitus, and 0.5% report tinnitus having a severe effect on their ability to lead a normal life.[1]

AETIOLOGY/ RISK FACTORS Tinnitus may occur as an isolated idiopathic symptom or in association with any type of hearing loss. Tinnitus may be a particular feature of presbycusis, noise induced hearing loss, Menière's disease Ⓖ (see Menière's disease, p 606), or the presence of an acoustic neuroma. In people with toxicity from aspirin or quinine, tinnitus can occur while hearing thresholds remain normal. Tinnitus is also associated with depression, although it may be unclear whether the tinnitus is a manifestation of the depressive illness or a factor contributing to its development.[2]

PROGNOSIS Tinnitus may have an insidious onset, with a long delay before clinical presentation. It may persist for many years or decades, particularly when associated with a sensorineural hearing loss. In Menière's disease, both the presence and intensity of tinnitus can fluctuate. Tinnitus may cause disruption of sleep patterns, an inability to concentrate, and depression.[3]

AIMS OF INTERVENTION To reduce the loudness and intrusiveness of the tinnitus and to reduce its impact on daily life, with minimum adverse effects from treatment.

OUTCOMES The number of people with resolution of tinnitus; tinnitus loudness (assessed by a visual analogue scale, symptom scores, or by audiometric matching); impact of tinnitus measured by estimates of interference with activities of daily life or with emotional state.

METHODS *Clinical Evidence* search and appraisal February 2004.

QUESTION **What are the effects of treatments for chronic tinnitus?**

OPTION **TRICYCLIC ANTIDEPRESSANTS**

One systematic review of one RCT in people with depression and chronic tinnitus found that tricyclic antidepressants (nortriptyline) improved tinnitus related disability and symptoms of depression at 6 weeks, but found no significant difference in self reported tinnitus severity improvement compared with placebo. One small RCT in people with tinnitus but without depression found that a greater proportion of people rated themselves as improved with tricyclic antidepressants (amitriptyline) compared with placebo at 6 weeks. Tricyclic antidepressants are associated with adverse effects such as dry mouth, blurred vision, and constipation.

Benefits: We found one systematic review (search date 1998, 1 RCT, 92 people with tinnitus and depression or depressive symptoms but no bipolar disorder or other mental health diagnosis)[4] and one subsequent RCT.[5] The RCT identified by the review found that nortriptyline (titrated to maintain therapeutic blood levels for depression) significantly improved measures of depression and tinnitus related disability score.[4] However, the RCT found no significant difference in the proportion of people reporting overall improvement in tinnitus severity after 6 weeks (AR for improvement: 43% with nortriptyline *v* 30% with placebo; P = 0.2; raw data not reported).[6] The subsequent RCT (37 people with no history of depression) found that a greater proportion of people rated themselves as "improved" with amitriptyline (50 mg/night for 1 week followed by 100 mg/night for 5 weeks) than with placebo after 6 weeks (19/20 [95%] "improved" on amitriptyline *v* 2/17 [12%] with placebo; OR 8.1, 95% CI 5.6 to 10.6). There was no significant difference between treatment groups in the frequency of occurrence of tinnitus (figures not reported).[5]

Harms: The systematic review did not report on harms.[4] The subsequent RCT found mild sedation and dryness of the mouth lasting for 1–2 weeks but reported no major adverse effects.[5] Other studies have established that common adverse effects of tricyclic antidepressants include dry mouth, blurred vision, and constipation (see harms of tricyclic antidepressants under depressive disorders, p 1238).

Comment: The subsequent RCT may have lacked power to detect clinically important effects on the frequency of occurrence of tinnitus.[5]

OPTION BENZODIAZEPINES

One systematic review found limited evidence from one RCT that alprazolam, a benzodiazepine, improved self reported tinnitus severity after 12 weeks. Benzodiazepines can have side effects that may outweigh potential benefits.

Benefits: We found one systematic review (search date 1995, 1 RCT, 40 people).[7] It found that alprazolam (initially 0.5 mg/night) significantly improved reported tinnitus severity compared with placebo after 12 weeks (reported improvement: 13/17 [76%] with alprazolam *v* 1/19 [5%] with placebo; RR 14.5, 95% CI 2.1 to 53.0), but interpretation of these results is difficult (see comment below).[8]

Harms: The RCT reported that two (10%) people receiving alprazolam withdrew from the trial because of excessive tiredness.[8] Long term use of benzodiazepines can lead to dependence (see harms of benzodiazepines under generalised anxiety disorder, p 1277).

Comment: The RCT used dose adjustment of alprazolam but no dose adjustment of placebo, potentially biasing the results because of a difference in the attention given to people in the two groups.[8] Another systematic review (search date 1998) found three other studies that used weaker methods; none of the studies provided evidence that benzodiazepines improved symptoms of tinnitus compared with placebo.[4]

OPTION CARBAMAZEPINE

One systematic review of one RCT found no significant difference between carbamazepine and placebo in tinnitus severity at 30 days. Carbamazepine was associated with an increased risk of dizziness, nausea, and headaches.

Benefits: We found one systematic review (search date 1995, 1 RCT, 48 people).[7] The RCT identified by the review found no significant difference between carbamazepine (150 mg 3 times daily for 30 days) and placebo in self reported improvement in tinnitus severity after 30 days' treatment (2/24 [8%] improved with carbamazepine *v* 3/24 [13%] with placebo; RR 0.67, 95% CI 0.12 to 3.60).[9]

Harms: The RCT found that carbamazepine significantly increased the number of people reporting adverse effects compared with placebo (including dizziness, nausea, and headaches; 25/34 [63%] with carbamazepine *v* 1/24 [4%] with placebo; RR 17.6, 95% CI 2.6 to 121.0).[9]

Comment: A more recent systematic review (search date 1998) found four additional RCTs comparing carbamazepine versus placebo.[4] All were appraised in the earlier review,[7] but were excluded from the initial review on methodological grounds.

OPTION LAMOTRIGINE

One small crossover RCT found no significant difference in tinnitus loudness or annoyance between lamotrigine and placebo. However, the RCT may have lacked power to detect a clinically important effect.

Benefits: We found one crossover RCT comparing lamotrigine versus placebo (33 people, see comment).[10] The RCT found no significant difference between lamotrigine (25 mg/day for 2 weeks, 50 mg/day for 2 weeks, and then 100 mg/day for 4 weeks) and placebo in tinnitus loudness or annoyance measured on a five point scale (11/31 [35%] people improved with lamotrigine *v* 6/31 [19%] people with placebo; RR 1.80, 95% CI 0.78 to 4.34; see comment).

Harms: One person withdrew from the lamotrigine group due to nausea, vomiting, and headache, and one person withdrew from the placebo group due to dizziness and rash.[10]

Comment: Post-crossover results are difficult to interpret due to the possibility of a persistence of treatment effect after crossover. The RCT may have lacked power to detect a clinically important effect.[10]

OPTION NICOTINAMIDE

One systematic review of one RCT found no significant difference between nicotinamide and placebo in tinnitus severity at 30 days. However, the RCT may have lacked power to detect a clinically important effect.

Benefits: We found one systematic review (search date 1998, 1 RCT, 48 people).[4] The RCT included in the review found no significant difference between nicotinamide (70 mg 3 times daily for 30 days) and placebo in subjective improvement after 30 days' treatment (2/24 [8%] with nicotinamide *v* 3/24 [13%] with placebo; RR 0.7, 95% CI 0.1 to 3.6).[11]

Harms: The systematic review found no significant difference between nicotinamide and placebo in the proportion of people reporting headache (4/24 [16%] with nicotinamide *v* 1/24 [4%] with placebo; RR 4.0, 95% CI 0.5 to 33.2) or dizziness (2/24 [8%] *v* 0/24 [0%]; ARI +0.08, 95% CI –0.06 to +0.20).[4]

Comment: The RCT may have lacked power to detect a clinically important effect.[11]

OPTION CINNARIZINE

One systematic review of one RCT found no significant difference between cinnarizine and placebo in tinnitus severity. However, the RCT may have lacked power to detect a clinically important effect.

Benefits: We found one systematic review (search date 1998, 1 RCT, 30 people).[4] It found no significant difference between cinnarizine (25 mg 3 times daily for 10 weeks) and placebo in subjective improvement (1/10 [10%] improved with cinnarizine *v* 1/20 [5%] with placebo; RR 2.00, 95% CI 0.14 to 29.00; see comment below).[12]

Harms: The RCT did not report harms.[12]

Comment: The RCT did not specify the follow up period and may have lacked power to detect a clinically important effect.[12]

OPTION ZINC

One systematic review of one RCT found no significant difference between zinc and placebo in tinnitus severity at 8 weeks. However, the RCT may have lacked power to detect a clinically important effect.

Benefits: We found one systematic review (search date 1998, 1 RCT, 50 people).[4] It found no significant difference between zinc (100 mg 3 times daily for 8 weeks) and placebo in reported tinnitus severity after 8 weeks' treatment (2/23 [9%] people improved with zinc v 2/25 [8%] people with placebo; RR 1.10, 95% CI 0.16 to 7.00; see comment below).[13]

Harms: The systematic review did not report harms.[13]

Comment: The RCT may have lacked power to detect a clinically important effect.[13]

OPTION BACLOFEN

One systematic review of one RCT found no significant difference between baclofen and placebo in tinnitus severity. However, the trial may have lacked power to detect a clinically important effect.

Benefits: We found one systematic review (search date 1998, 1 RCT, 63 people).[4] It found no significant difference between baclofen (10 mg twice daily increasing to 30 mg twice daily for 3 weeks) and placebo in subjective improvement (3/31 [10%] improved with baclofen v 1/32 [3%] with placebo; RR 3.10, 95% CI 0.34 to 28.00; see comment below).[14]

Harms: The RCT included in the review did not report harms.[14]

Comment: The RCT did not specify the follow up period and may have lacked power to detect a clinically important effect.[14]

OPTION ACUPUNCTURE

One systematic review found insufficient evidence about the effects of acupuncture.

Benefits: We found one systematic review (search date 1998, 6 studies, 185 people).[15] The review included one quasi-randomised RCT,[16] two open RCTs,[12,17] two crossover RCTs,[18,19] and one blinded RCT.[20] All studies were small and brief. The blinded RCT (54 people) found no significant difference between acupuncture (25 sessions over 2 months) and sham acupuncture (superficial penetration at random non-acupuncture points) in tinnitus loudness on a pooled visual analogue score (4% improvement with acupuncture v 1% deterioration with placebo, P value not reported).[20] The first crossover RCT identified by the review (14 people) found that acupuncture significantly increased the number of people who reported a reduction in tinnitus loudness after one session of treatment compared with sham acupuncture (5/14 [36%] with acupuncture v 0/14 [0%] with sham acupuncture; $P = 0.05$).[18] The second crossover RCT (20 people) found no significant difference between acupuncture and placebo on a pooled visual analogue score of subjective tinnitus severity after 3 weeks ($P = 0.22$).[19]

Harms: The review did not report on adverse effects.[15]

Comment: None.

OPTION PSYCHOTHERAPY

One systematic review found insufficient evidence about the effects of cognitive behavioural treatment, relaxation therapy, education, or biofeedback, compared with other or no treatment in people with chronic tinnitus.

Benefits: We found one systematic review (search date 1998, 8 RCTs, 269 people) of different psychotherapeutic approaches (cognitive behavioural treatment, relaxation therapy, education/information, biofeedback).[21] The review had important methodological problems that compromise its validity (see comments below). It found significant reductions in subjective loudness and tinnitus annoyance for a combination of different psychotherapeutic approaches at 3 months or more post-treatment compared with pre-treatment scores (SMD for subjective loudness 0.68, 95% CI 0.62 to 0.74; SMD for tinnitus annoyance 0.83, 95% CI 0.82 to 0.84).

Harms: The review did not report harms.[21]

Comment: Despite many studies on psychotherapeutic measures to treat tinnitus, the evidence for benefit remains limited. Many of the RCTs suffer from weak methods, high withdrawal rates, and pooled or surrogate outcome measures. The systematic review pooled study results across arms of trials, losing the benefits of randomisation and increasing the risk of bias. Pre-treatment to post-treatment effect sizes do not allow comparison of psychotherapy with no treatment or any other treatment.[21] The review did not report which interventions were used as control in the RCTs.

OPTION ELECTROMAGNETIC STIMULATION/EAR CANAL MAGNETS

Three small RCTs found insufficient evidence to compare electromagnetic stimulation versus placebo. One RCT found no significant difference between simple ear canal magnets and placebo on tinnitus symptoms after 4 weeks.

Benefits: **Electromagnetic stimulation:** We found no systematic review, but found three small RCTs (136 people) comparing electromagnetic stimulation with placebo.[22–24] The first RCT (58 people) found that electromagnetic stimulation significantly increased the number of people who had improved tinnitus compared with placebo (14/31 [45%] with electromagnetic stimulation *v* 2/23 [9%] with placebo; RR 5.2, 95% CI 1.3 to 20.6; see comment below).[23] The second RCT (48 people) found no significant difference between electromagnetic stimulation and placebo in tinnitus sensation levels after 1 week (6/24 [25%] with electromagnetic stimulation *v* 6/24 [25%] with placebo; RR 1.00, 95% CI 0.39 to 2.59).[22] The third RCT (20 people; see comment below) used a crossover design and did not report results before the crossover.[24] **Magnets:** We found no systematic review but found one RCT (49 people).[25] The RCT found no significant difference between a simple ear canal magnet (neodymium, iron, and boron) and placebo (same material but unmagnetised) in tinnitus symptoms after 4 weeks' treatment (AR for symptom improvement: 7/26 [27%] with magnet *v* 4/23 [17%] with placebo; RR 1.50, 95% CI 0.53 to 4.50).

Harms: **Electromagnetic stimulation:** The RCTs reported no adverse effects associated with electromagnetic stimulation.[22–24] **Magnets:** The RCT did not report on harms.[25]

Comment: **Electromagnetic stimulation:** The first RCT, which did not specify the length of follow up, reported that 4/58 (7%) people withdrew from the trial and that the analysis was not by intention to treat.[23] The crossover RCT found no significant difference with electrical suppression compared with a placebo device in reducing tinnitus severity (2/20 [10%] active device *v* 4/20 [20%] with placebo device; P = NS).[24]

OPTION HYPNOSIS

One RCT found no significant difference between hypnosis and counselling for symptom severity at 3 months.

Benefits: We found one systematic review (search date 1995)[7] and one additional RCT.[26] The review found no RCTs that met its inclusion criteria. The additional RCT (92 people who were pre-selected to be suggestible to hypnosis) found no significant difference between three sessions teaching self hypnosis and control (a single counselling session) in symptom severity scores after 3 months (24/44 [55%] improved with hypnosis *v* 23/42 [55%] with counselling; RR 1.00, 95% CI 0.68 to 1.46). The RCT also found no significant difference in the number of people reporting worsened tinnitus (11/44 [25%] with hypnosis *v* 14/42 [32%] with counselling; RR 0.8, 95% CI 0.4 to 1.5).

Harms: No adverse effects were reported.[7,26]

Comment: None.

OPTION LOW POWER LASER

One RCT found no significant difference between low power laser and placebo for symptom severity at 1 month.

Benefits: We found no systematic review but found one RCT.[27] The RCT (49 people) found no significant difference between laser (50 mW directed towards the mastoid bone) and placebo in the number of people reporting improved tinnitus symptoms after 1 month (2/25 [8%] with laser *v* 7/24 [29%] with placebo; RR 0.27, 95% CI 0.06 to 1.20).[27]

Harms: No adverse effects were reported.[27]

Comment: None.

OPTION TINNITUS MASKING DEVICES

One small RCT identified by a systematic review found no significant difference between a masking device and placebo in tinnitus symptoms at 12 weeks.

Benefits: We found one systematic review (search date 1998, 2 RCTs).[4] The first RCT (21 people) found no significant difference in intensity of tinnitus symptoms between a masking device**G** and placebo at 12 weeks (7/21 [33%] improved with the masking device; 5/21 [24%] improved with the placebo; RR 1.40, 95% CI 0.55 to 3.55).[28] The second RCT was of insufficient quality to include in this review (see comment below).[29]

Harms: The RCT found that 2/21 (10%) people reported worsened tinnitus with a masking device.[28]

Comment: The excluded RCT had a high withdrawal rate (67%) and was unblinded.[29]

OPTION GINKGO BILOBA

We found no good quality RCTs of ginkgo biloba for tinnitus.

Benefits: We found no good quality RCTs (see comment).

Harms: We found no good quality RCTs.

Comment: We found one systematic review (search date 1998) which found four RCTs comparing gingko biloba versus placebo.[30] However, we excluded these RCTs on the basis of poor methodology (pseudo-randomisation, unblinded assessors, selection of participants by previous positive response to gingko biloba), or high withdrawal rate.[31] One subsequent RCT (1121 people) was also excluded due to high withdrawal rate (36%).[32]

OPTION HYPERBARIC OXYGEN

We found no systematic review or RCTs on the effects of hyperbaric oxygen for people with tinnitus.

Benefits: We found no systematic review or RCTs.

Harms: We found no RCTs.

Comment: None.

GLOSSARY

Masking device A small device similar to a behind-the-ear hearing aid, which produces a broad frequency noise. It is thought to hide the noise of the tinnitus.
Menière's disease A condition characterised by episodic vertigo, tinnitus, and sensorineural hearing loss.
Presbycusis Age related hearing loss.

REFERENCES

1. Coles RR. Epidemiology of tinnitus (1). *J Laryngol Otol* 1984;9(suppl):7–15.
2. Sullivan MD, Katon W, Dobie R, et al. Disabling tinnitus: association with affective disorder. *Gen Hosp Psychiatry* 1988;10:285–291.
3. Zoger S, Svedlund J, Holgers KM. Psychiatric disorders in tinnitus patients without severe hearing impairment: 24 month follow-up of patients at an audiological clinic. *Audiology* 2001;40:133–140.
4. Dobie RA. A review of randomized clinical trials in tinnitus. *Laryngoscope* 1999;109:1202–1211. Search date 1998; primary sources Medline and hand searches.
5. Bayar N, Boke B, Turan E, et al. Efficacy of amitriptyline in the treatment of subjective tinnitus. *J Otolaryngol* 2001;30:300–303.
6. Dobie RA, Sakai CS, Sullivan MD, et al. Antidepressant treatment of tinnitus patients: report of a randomized clinical trial and clinical prediction of benefit. *Am J Otol* 1993;14:18–23.
7. Schilter B, Jäger B, Heerman R, et al. Pharmacological and psychological treatment options in chronic subjective tinnitus: a meta-analysis of effective treatments. *HNO* 2000;48:589–597. [In German] Search date 1995; primary sources Medline, Psyindex, Psychlit, and hand searches including German, English, and French language papers.
8. Johnson RM, Brummett R, Schleuning A. Use of alprazolam for relief of tinnitus. A double-blind study. *Arch Otolaryngol Head Neck Surg* 1993;119:842–845.
9. Hulshof JH, Vermeij P. The value of carbamazepine in the treatment of tinnitus. *ORL J Otorhinolaryngol Relat Spec* 1985;47:262–266.
10. Simpson JJ, Gilbert AM, Weiner GM, et al. The assessment of lamotrigine, an antiepileptic drug, in the treatment of tinnitus. *Am J Otol* 1999;20:627–631.
11. Hulshof JH, Vermeij P. The effect of nicotinamide on tinnitus: a double-blind controlled study. *Clin Otolaryngol* 1987;12:211–214.
12. Podoshin L, Ben-David Y, Fradis M, et al. Idiopathic subjective tinnitus treated by biofeedback, acupuncture and drug therapy. *Ear Nose Throat J* 1991;70:284–289.
13. Paaske PB, Pedersen CB, Kjems G, et al. Zinc in the management of tinnitus. Placebo-controlled trial. *Ann Otol Rhinol Laryngol* 1991;100:647–649.
14. Westerberg BD, Roberson JB Jr, Stach BA. A double-blind placebo-controlled trial of baclofen in the treatment of tinnitus. *Am J Otol* 1996;17:896–903.
15. Park J, White AR, Ernst E. Efficacy of acupuncture as a treatment for tinnitus: a systematic review. *Arch Otolaryngol Head Neck Surg* 2000;126:489–492. Search date 1998; primary sources Medline, Cochrane Controlled Trials Register, Embase, and Ciscom.
16. Axelsson A, Andersson S, Gu LD. Acupuncture in the management of tinnitus: a placebo-controlled study. *Audiology* 1994;33:351–360.
17. Furugard S, Hedin PJ, Eggertz A, et al. Acupuncture worth trying in severe tinnitus. *Lakartidningen* 1998;95:1922–1928.
18. Marks NJ, Emery P, Onisiphorou C. A controlled trial of acupuncture in tinnitus. *J Laryngol Otol* 1984;98:1103–1109.
19. Hansen PE, Hansen JH, Bentzen O. Acupuncture therapy of chronic unilateral tinnitus. A double-blind cross-over study. *Ugeskr Laeger* 1981;143:2888–2890.
20. Vilholm OJ, Moller K, Jorgensen K. Effect of traditional Chinese acupuncture on severe tinnitus: a double-blind, placebo-controlled, clinical investigation with open therapeutic control. *Br J Audiol* 1998;32:197–204.
21. Andersson G, Lyttkens L. A meta-analytic review of psychological treatments for tinnitus. *Br J Audiol* 1999;33:201–210. Search date 1998; primary sources Medline and psychological abstracts.
22. Fiedler SC, Pilkington H, Willatt DJ. Electromagnetic stimulation as a treatment of tinnitus: a further study[abstract]. *Clin Otolaryngol* 1998;23:270.
23. Roland NJ, Hughes JB, Daley MB, et al. Electromagnetic stimulation as a treatment of tinnitus: a pilot study. *Clin Otolaryngol* 1993;18:278–281.
24. Dobie RA, Hoberg KE, Rees TS. Electrical tinnitus suppression: a double-blind crossover study. *Otolaryngol Head Neck Surg* 1986;95:319–333.
25. Coles R, Bradley P, Donaldson I, et al. A trial of tinnitus therapy with ear-canal magnets. *Clin Otolaryngol* 1991;16:371–372.
26. Mason JD, Rogerson DR, Butler JD. Client centred hypnotherapy in the management of tinnitus — is it better than counselling? *J Laryngol Otol* 1996;110:117–120.
27. Mirz F, Zachariae R, Andersen SE, et al. The low-power laser in the treatment of tinnitus. *Clin Otolaryngol* 1999;24:346–354.
28. Erlandsson S, Ringdahl A, Hutchins T, et al. Treatment of tinnitus: a controlled comparison of masking and placebo. *Br J Audiol* 1987;21:37–44.
29. Stephens SDG, Corcoran AL. A controlled study of tinnitus masking. *Br J Audiol* 1985;19:159–167.
30. Ernst E, Stevinson C. Ginkgo biloba for tinnitus: a review. *Clin Otolaryngol* 1999;24:164–167. Search date 1998; primary sources Medline, Embase, The Cochrane Library, contact with manufacturers, and hand search of reference lists.

31. Morgenstern C, Biermann E.Long-term treatment of tinnitus with the special gingko extract, Egb 761. *Fortschr Med* 1997;115:57–58.[in German]

32. Drew S, Davies E. Effectiveness of ginkgo biloba in treating tinnitus: double blind, placebo controlled trial. *BMJ* 2001;322:73–75.

Angus Waddell
Consultant Otolaryngologist
Great Western Hospital
Swindon
UK

Competing interests: None declared.
We would like to acknowledge the previous contributors of this chapter, including Richard Canter.

Tonsillitis

Search date December 2003

William McKerrow

QUESTIONS

INTERVENTIONS

Key Messages

- **Tonsillectomy compared with antibiotics in children** Two systematic reviews that included the same two RCTs in children found insufficient evidence to compare surgical versus medical treatment. One subsequent RCT in less severely affected children found that surgery reduced the frequency of throat infection compared with medical treatment over 3 years. It suggested that the modest benefit may be outweighed by the morbidity associated with the surgery in populations with a low incidence of tonsillitis.
- **Tonsillectomy compared with antibiotics in adults** We found no RCTs evaluating tonsillectomy in adults.

Tonsillitis

DEFINITION Tonsillitis is an infection of the parenchyma of the palatine tonsils. The definition of severe recurrent tonsillitis is arbitrary, but recent criteria have defined tonsillitis as five or more episodes of true tonsillitis a year, symptoms for at least a year, and episodes that are disabling and prevent normal functioning.[1] The definition does not include tonsillitis due to infectious mononucleosis, which usually occurs as a single episode. However, acute tonsillitis in this situation may be followed by recurrent tonsillitis in some people. Tonsillitis may occur in isolation or as part of a generalised pharyngitis. The clinical distinction between tonsillitis and pharyngitis is unclear in the literature, and the condition is often referred to simply as "acute sore throat". A sore throat lasting for 24–48 hours as part of the prodrome of minor upper respiratory tract infection is excluded from this definition. Diagnosis of acute tonsillitis is primarily clinical, with the main interest being in whether the illness is viral or bacterial, this being of relevance if antibiotics are being considered. Studies have attempted to distinguish viral from bacterial sore throat on clinical grounds, but the results are conflicting, suggesting a lack of reliable diagnostic criteria. Investigations to assist with this distinction include throat swabs and serological tests, including the rapid antigen test and the antistreptolysin O titre. Rapid antigen testing is convenient and popular in North America but has doubtful sensitivity (61–95%), at least when measured against throat swab results, although specificity is higher (88–100%).[1]

INCIDENCE/ PREVALENCE Recurrent sore throat has an incidence in general practice in the UK of 100 per 1000 population a year.[2] Acute tonsillitis is more common in childhood.

AETIOLOGY/ RISK FACTORS Common bacterial pathogens include β haemolytic and other streptococci. Bacteria are cultured only from a minority of people with tonsillitis. The role of viruses is uncertain. In tonsillitis associated with infectious mononucleosis, the most common infective agent is the Epstein–Barr virus (present in 50% of children and 90% of adults with the condition). Cytomegalovirus infection may also result in the clinical picture of infectious mononucleosis, and the differential diagnosis also includes toxoplasmosis, HIV, hepatitis A, and rubella.[3]

PROGNOSIS We found no good data on the natural history of tonsillitis or recurrent sore throat in children or adults. People in RCTs randomised to medical treatment (courses of antibiotics as required) have shown a tendency towards improvement over time.[4,5] Recurrent severe tonsillitis results in considerable morbidity, including time lost from school or work. The most common complication of acute tonsillitis is peritonsillar abscess, but we found no good evidence on its incidence. Rheumatic fever and acute glomerulonephritis are recognised complications of acute tonsillitis associated with group A β haemolytic streptococci. These diseases are rare in developed countries, but do occasionally occur. They are still a common problem in certain populations, notably Australian Aboriginals, and may be effectively prevented in closed communities by the use of penicillin. A systematic review found no evidence that aggressive antibiotic treatment of acute sore throat in the developed world was useful in the prevention of these diseases.[6]

AIMS OF INTERVENTION To abolish tonsillitis; to reduce the frequency and severity of recurrent throat infections; to improve general wellbeing, behaviour, and educational achievement, with minimal adverse effects.

OUTCOMES Number and severity of episodes of tonsillitis or sore throat; requirement for antibiotics and analgesics; time off work or school; behaviour, school performance, general wellbeing; morbidity and mortality of surgery; and adverse effects of drugs.

METHODS *Clinical Evidence* search and appraisal December 2003.

QUESTION **What are the effects of tonsillectomy in children and adults with severe tonsillitis?**

OPTION **TONSILLECTOMY VERSUS ANTIBIOTICS**

Two systematic reviews that included the same two RCTs in children found insufficient evidence to compare surgical versus medical treatment. One subsequent RCT in less severely affected children found that surgery reduced the frequency of throat infection compared with medical treatment over 3

years. It suggested that the modest benefit may be outweighed by the morbidity associated with the surgery in populations with a low incidence of tonsillitis. We found no RCTs evaluating tonsillectomy versus antibiotics in adults.

Benefits: We found two systematic reviews (search dates 1997[7] and 1998[8]) and one subsequent RCT.[9] **Children:** Both reviews identified the same two RCTs as being the only ones that met quality inclusion criteria (see comment below).[4,5] The smaller RCT involved 91 children who fulfilled criteria for "severe tonsillitis" (7 episodes in the preceding year, 5 episodes/year in the preceding 2 years, or 3 episodes/year in the preceding 3 years).[4] It compared three treatments: tonsillectomy alone (27 children); adenotonsillectomy (16 children); or intermittent courses of antibiotics as needed (48 children). Sixteen children were withdrawn from the non-surgical group by their parents and underwent surgery, and children who developed infections after surgery received antibiotics as necessary for each episode of infection. Secondary outcome measures, such as time off school, were also considered. The RCT found that children with tonsillectomy experienced significantly fewer throat infections than those with antibiotics, amounting to an average of three fewer throat infections in the first 2 years, but by the third year the difference was no longer significant, (year 1: 1.24 episodes per person *v* 3.09 episodes per person, $P = 0.001$; year 2: 1.61 *v* 2.66, $P = 0.001$; year 3: 1.77 *v* 2.20, $P > 0.05$). The larger RCT (246 "less severely affected" children than in the smaller RCT [4]) is published only in abstract form.[5] Some children in this study also underwent adenoidectomy. The limited data available provide no evidence of a difference between surgical and medical treatment. The first systematic review concluded that the risk of adverse effects was such that the use of tonsillectomy was not supportable from the available evidence.[7] The second review concluded that it was not possible to determine the effectiveness of tonsillectomy from these RCTs because of the significant baseline differences between the people assigned to surgical and non-surgical treatment and the impossibility of eliminating any effect from the adenoidectomy additionally carried out on some of the included children.[8] One subsequent RCT (328 children with a history of milder recurrent episodes of throat infection than in the smaller RCT [4]) stratified children according to history and age.[9] Children with no apparent indication for adenoidectomy (recurrent or persistent otitis media or obstructing adenoids) were randomised to tonsillectomy, adenotonsillectomy, or medical treatment (3 way trial, 177 children). Children with any apparent indication for adenoidectomy were randomised to adenotonsillectomy or medical treatment (2 way trial, 151 children). In both populations, outcomes were significantly better with surgery compared with medical treatment (children without indication for adenoidectomy [3 way trial]: mean number of moderate or severe episodes/year during 3 years' follow up: 0.09 with tonsillectomy [$P = 0.002$] *v* 0.08 with adenotonsillectomy [$P = 0.003$] *v* 0.33 with medical treatment; in children with indication for adenotonsillectomy [2 way trial]: 0.07 with adenotonsillectomy *v* 0.28 with medical treatment [$P < 0.001$]; see comment below).[9] **Adults:** The reviews found no RCTs that evaluated tonsillectomy in adults with recurrent tonsillitis or sore throats.

Harms: **Tonsillectomy:** The risks of tonsillectomy include those associated with general anaesthesia and those specific to the procedure (bleeding, pain, otalgia, and, rarely, nasopharyngeal stenosis). The subsequent RCT found that 16/203 children who had surgery (8%) suffered complications.[9] One suffered anaesthetic induction trismus and possible incipient malignant hyperthermia; three children had intraoperative haemorrhage with one of them needing reintervention under anaesthesia; and one child required a posterior nasopharyngeal pack and admission to intensive care. Seven children (3.4%) developed postoperative haemorrhage and five of these were readmitted to hospital, one requiring transfusion. The mean duration of postoperative sore throat was 6.3 days (range 0–21 days).[9] The overall complication rate in the smaller RCT (91 children)[4] was 14% (all were "readily managed or self limiting") compared with 2–8% in one Scottish tonsillectomy audit.[10] Haemorrhage, either primary (in the immediate postoperative period) or secondary, occurred in 4% of children studied in the larger RCT[5] and fewer than 1% of children in the Scottish tonsillectomy audit.[10] **Antibiotics:** In the smaller RCT (91 children), erythematous rashes occurred in 4% of children in the non-surgical group while taking penicillin.[4] Other adverse effects of antibiotics include allergic reactions and the promotion of resistant bacteria. One RCT found that, for people with milder episodes of sore throat, the prescribing of antibiotics compared with no initial prescription significantly increased the proportion of people who returned to see their physician in the short term because of sore throat (716 people with sore throat and an abnormal physical sign; return rate 38% with initial antibiotics *v* 27% without; adjusted HR for return 1.39, 95% CI 1.03 to 1.89).[11] The subsequent RCT found that rates of erythematous rash were similar in children from the surgical and control groups (4/190 [2%] in surgery groups *v* 3/138 [2%] in control groups).[9] We found no evidence of adverse effects on the immune system following tonsillectomy.

Comment: In the subsequent RCT, 79% of the children allocated to tonsillectomy and 78.8% of those assigned to adenotonsillectomy had surgery within 90 days of the randomisation.[9] In the control groups, 12/60 (20%) children in the three way RCT and 19/78 (24%) with an indication for adenoidectomy eventually underwent surgery. Although a significant reduction was found in the mean number of episodes of throat illnesses with surgical interventions, rates of illness in the control groups were low.[9] The authors of the RCT concluded that the benefits of surgery may be outweighed by the risks of surgery in populations with a low incidence of illness, such as the population of children included in the RCT.[9] **Background:** Tonsillectomy is one of the most frequently performed surgical procedures in the UK, particularly in children, and accounts for about 20% of all operations performed by otolaryngologists.[10] Adenoidectomy is now performed with tonsillectomy only when there is a specific indication to remove the adenoids as well as the tonsils. **Quality of the evidence:** In the smaller RCT[4] included in the reviews, there were significant baseline differences between groups before treatment, and the authors pooled the results of tonsillectomy and adenotonsillectomy making it impossible to assess the effectiveness of tonsillectomy alone. The systematic reviews came to broadly the same conclusions, but the weighting of the evidence was different. The earlier review did not quantify the evidence for the adverse effects mentioned, although it concluded that because of adverse effects tonsillectomy was not supported.[7] The principal author of the original RCT[4] defends its conclusions in the Comments and Criticisms section in the current issue of the Cochrane Review.[8] He argues that the baseline differences between cases in the control and treatment groups which were not accounted for in the randomisation are irrelevant to the outcome. Furthermore, he contends that the effect of adenoidectomy in some members of the treatment group could not have accounted for the difference in outcome in that group. The subsequent RCT in less severely affected children[9] was designed and run at the same time as the other RCTs discussed,[4,5] but the authors did study tonsillectomy separately from adenoidectomy, and the conclusions are more robust. **Gaps in the evidence:** We found no RCT that found improved general wellbeing, development, or behaviour, despite suggestions that these are influenced by tonsillectomy.[10] We found no RCTs addressing long term effects of tonsillectomy. **New**

techniques: Various newer techniques for tonsillectomy have been described and are in use, including ultrasonic dissection, cold ablation, laser tonsillectomy, and diathermy tonsillectomy. These are currently being assessed, and possible benefits and harms have not yet been fully evaluated. Adjuvant treatment may reduce adverse effects, and various modalities are being studied.[12]

REFERENCES

1. Management of sore throat and indications for tonsillectomy. National Clinical Guideline No 34. Scottish Intercollegiate Guidelines Network, Edinburgh.
2. Shvartzman P. Careful prescribing is beneficial. *BMJ* 1994;309:1101–1102.
3. Papesch M, Watkins R. Epstein Barr virus infectious mononucleosis. *Clin Otolaryngol* 2001;26:3–8.
4. Paradise JL, Bluestone CD, Bachman RZ, et al. Efficacy of tonsillectomy for recurrent throat infection in severely affected children. *N Engl J Med* 1984;310:674–683.
5. Paradise JL, Bluestone CD, Rogers KD, et al. Comparative efficacy of tonsillectomy for recurrent throat infection in more versus less severely affected children [abstract]. *Pediatr Res* 1992;31:126A.
6. Del Mar CB, Glasziou PP, Spinks AB. Antibiotics for sore throat (Cochrane Review). In: The Cochrane Library, Issue 4, 2003. Chichester, UK: John Wiley & Sons, Ltd. Search date 1999; primary sources Medline, The Cochrane Library, the Cochrane collection of hand searched trials and reference lists.
7. Marshall T. A review of tonsillectomy for recurrent throat infection. *Br J Gen Pract* 1998;48:1331–1335. Search date 1997; primary sources Cochrane Library and Medline.
8. Burton MJ, Towler B, Glasziou P. Tonsillectomy versus non-surgical treatment for chronic/recurrent acute tonsillitis. In: The Cochrane Library, Issue 4, 2003. Chichester, UK: John Wiley & Sons, Ltd. Search date 1998; primary sources Medline, Embase, Cochrane Controlled Trials Register, and hand searched references.
9. Paradise JL, Bluestone CD, Colborne DK, et al. Tonsillectomy and adenotonsillectomy for recurrent throat infection in moderately affected children. *Pediatrics* 2002;110:7–15.
10. Blair RL, McKerrow WS, Carter NW, et al. The Scottish tonsillectomy audit. *J Laryngol Otol* 1996;110(suppl 20):1–25.
11. Little P, Gould C, Williamson I, et al. Reattendance and complications in a randomised trial of prescribing strategies for sore throat: the medicalising effect of prescribing antibiotics. *BMJ* 1997;315:350–352.
12. Steward DL, Chung SJ. The role of adjuvant therapies and techniques in tonsillectomy. *Curr Opin Otolaryngol Head Neck Surg* 2000;8:186–192.

William McKerrow
Consultant Otolaryngologist
Raigmore Hospital
Inverness
UK

Competing interests: None declared.
We would like to acknowledge the previous contributor for this chapter, Martin Burton.

Diabetic nephropathy

Search date December 2003

Michael Shlipak

QUESTIONS

INTERVENTIONS

To be covered in future updates

Calcium channel blockers

Statins

See glossary

Key Messages

Type 1 diabetes and early nephropathy

- **Angiotensin converting enzyme inhibitors (progression to late nephropathy)** One systematic review found that, compared with placebo or controls, angiotensin converting enzyme inhibitors (captopril, lisinopril, enalapril, perindopril, and ramipril) reduced progression to macroalbuminuria and increased regression to normoalbuminuria in normotensive people with type 1 diabetes and microalbuminuria. We found no systematic review or RCTs comparing effects of angiotensin converting enzyme inhibitors versus placebo in people with type 1 diabetes and early nephropathy for the outcomes mortality (all cause), incidence of end stage renal disease, or incidence of cardiovascular events (stroke, heart failure, myocardial infarction).
- **Glycaemic control (progression to late nephropathy)** One systematic review found that, compared with conventional control, intensive glycaemic control reduced progression of nephropathy in people with type 1 diabetes and either normal albumin excretion or microalbuminuria. The review found no significant difference between intensive glycaemic control and conventional control in the incidence of severe hypoglycaemia, but found higher incidence of diabetic ketoacidosis in people treated with continuous subcutaneous insulin infusion compared with conventional multiple injection treatment. We found no systematic review or RCT evaluating effects of glycaemic control in people with type 1 diabetes and early nephropathy for the outcomes of mortality, or incidence of cardiovascular events (stroke, heart failure, myocardial infarction).
- **Angiotensin II receptor antagonists** We found no systematic review or RCTs comparing effects of angiotensin II receptor antagonists versus placebo in people with type 1 diabetes and early nephropathy for outcomes of interest. Long term placebo controlled RCTs would not be ethical because of the established benefits of angiotensin converting enzyme inhibitors and similarity between these two drug classes. We found no RCTs comparing angiotensin II receptor antagonists versus angiotensin converting enzyme inhibitors in people with type 1 diabetes and early nephropathy.
- **Lipid lowering** We found no systematic review or RCTs on lipid lowering in people with type 1 diabetes and early nephropathy for the outcomes of progression to late nephropathy, mortality (all cause), incidence of end stage renal disease, or incidence of cardiovascular events (stroke, heart failure, myocardial infarction).
- **Protein restriction** We found no systematic review or RCTs comparing effects of low protein diet versus usual diet in people with type 1 diabetes and early nephropathy for the outcomes of progression to late nephropathy, mortality (all cause), incidence of end stage renal disease, or incidence of cardiovascular events (stroke, heart failure, myocardial infarction).
- **Tight control of blood pressure** We found no systematic review or RCTs comparing tight control of blood pressure versus conventional control in people with type 1 diabetes and early nephropathy for the outcomes of progression to late nephropathy, mortality (all cause), incidence of end stage renal disease, or incidence of cardiovascular events (stroke, heart failure, myocardial infarction).

Type 1 diabetes and late nephropathy

- **Captopril** One RCT in people with type 1 diabetes and late nephropathy found that, compared with placebo, captopril (an angiotensin converting enzyme inhibitor) reduced the combined outcome of renal transplant, end stage renal disease, or death over 3 years. We found no systematic review or RCTs comparing effects of captopril versus placebo in people with type 1 diabetes and late nephropathy for the outcome of incidence of cardiovascular events (stroke, heart failure, myocardial infarction) or on effects of other angiotensin converting enzyme inhibitors for the outcomes of interest.

- **Angiotensin II receptor antagonists** We found no systematic review or RCTs comparing effects of angiotensin II receptor antagonists versus placebo in people with type 1 diabetes and late nephropathy for outcomes of mortality (all cause), incidence of end stage renal disease, or incidence of cardiovascular events (stroke, heart failure, myocardial infarction). Long term placebo controlled RCTs would not be ethical because of the established benefits of angiotensin converting enzyme inhibitors and similarity between these two drug classes. We found no RCTs comparing angiotensin II receptor antagonists with angiotensin converting enzyme inhibitors in people with type 1 diabetes and late nephropathy.
- **Glycaemic control** We found no systematic review or RCTs comparing intensive glycaemic control with conventional glycaemic control in people with type 1 diabetes and late nephropathy for the outcomes of mortality (all cause), incidence of end stage renal disease, or incidence of cardiovascular events (stroke, heart failure, myocardial infarction).
- **Lipid lowering** We found no systematic review or RCT evaluating effects of lipid lowering in people with type 1 diabetes and late nephropathy for the outcomes of mortality, incidence of end stage renal disease, or incidence of cardiovascular events (stroke, heart failure, myocardial infarction).
- **Protein restriction** One small RCT found that, compared with usual protein intake, a low protein diet significantly reduced the cumulative incidence of end stage renal disease or death over 4 years in people with type 1 diabetes and late nephropathy. This RCT was small, and neither participants nor study investigators could be blinded to the randomisation owing to the nature of the intervention. We found no systematic review or RCTs comparing effects of low protein diet versus usual diet in people with type 1 diabetes and late nephropathy for the outcome of incidence of cardiovascular events (stroke, heart failure, myocardial infarction).
- **Tight control of blood pressure** We found no systematic review or RCT evaluating effects of tight blood pressure control versus conventional control in people with type 1 diabetes and late nephropathy for the outcomes of mortality, incidence of end stage renal disease, or incidence of cardiovascular events (stroke, heart failure, myocardial infarction).

Type 2 diabetes and early nephropathy

- **Angiotensin converting enzyme inhibitors** One RCT found that, compared with placebo, enalapril significantly reduced progression to late nephropathy. One RCT comparing ramipril versus placebo with subgroup analysis in people with diabetes and early nephropathy found that ramipril reduced the combined outcome of myocardial infarction, stroke, or cardiovascular death. One systematic review in people with diabetes and nephropathy, which did not stratify the results by the type of diabetes, found that, compared with placebo, angiotensin converting enzyme inhibitors significantly reduced progression to late nephropathy in people with diabetes and microalbuminuria over 3 years. We found no systematic review or RCTs comparing angiotensin converting enzyme inhibitors versus placebo in people with type 2 diabetes and early nephropathy for the outcomes of mortality (all cause), incidence of end stage renal disease, or incidence of cardiovascular events (stroke, heart failure, myocardial infarction).
- **Irbesartan (progression to late nephropathy)** One RCT in people with type 2 diabetes, hypertension, and microalbuminuria found that, compared with placebo, an angiotensin II receptor antagonist irbesartan 300 mg reduced progression from early to late nephropathy over 2 years, but found no significant decrease with irbesartan 150 mg. We found no systematic review or RCTs comparing angiotensin II receptor antagonists versus placebo in people with type 2 diabetes and early nephropathy for the outcomes of mortality (all cause), incidence of end stage renal disease, or incidence of cardiovascular events (stroke, heart failure, myocardial infarction).

- **Tight control of blood pressure (progression to late nephropathy)** One RCT found that, in people with type 2 diabetes, early nephropathy, and baseline blood pressure within the normal range, a lower diastolic blood pressure target (10 mm Hg below baseline) significantly reduced progression from microalbuminuria to overt albuminuria over 5 years compared with a moderate diastolic blood pressure target (80–89 mm Hg). We found no systematic review or RCTs on tight blood pressure control in people with type 2 diabetes and early nephropathy for the outcomes of progression to late nephropathy, mortality (all cause), incidence of end stage renal disease, or incidence of cardiovascular events (stroke, heart failure, myocardial infarction).
- **Glycaemic control** We found no systematic review or RCTs evaluating effects of glycaemic control in people with type 2 diabetes and early nephropathy for the outcomes of progression to late nephropathy, mortality, incidence of end stage renal disease, or incidence of cardiovascular events (stroke, heart failure, myocardial infarction).
- **Lipid lowering** We found no systematic review or RCTs on lipid lowering in people with type 2 diabetes and early nephropathy for the outcomes of progression to late nephropathy, mortality (all cause), incidence of end stage renal disease, or incidence of cardiovascular events (stroke, heart failure, myocardial infarction).
- **Protein restriction** We found no systematic review or RCTs on protein restriction in people with type 2 diabetes and early nephropathy for the outcomes of progression to late nephropathy, mortality (all cause), incidence of end stage renal disease, or incidence of cardiovascular events (stroke, heart failure, myocardial infarction).

Type 2 diabetes and late nephropathy

- **Losartan (progression to end stage renal disease)** We found two RCTs comparing angiotensin II receptor antagonists versus placebo for the outcomes of progression to end stage renal disease, cardiovascular events, and all cause mortality. One RCT in people with type 2 diabetes and late nephropathy found that, compared with placebo, losartan reduced progression to end stage renal disease over 3.4 years but found no significant difference in fatal or non-fatal cardiovascular events or death from any cause. Another RCT in people with type 2 diabetes and late nephropathy found no significant difference between irbesartan and placebo in progression to end stage renal disease or death from any cause over 2.6 years. It also found that irbesartan significantly reduced the incidence of congestive heart failure compared with placebo, but no significant difference for a composite cardiovascular outcome, cardiovascular death, myocardial infarction, cerebrovascular accident, or cardiac revascularisation. In both RCTs, angiotensin II receptor antagonist was discontinued if hyperkalemia occurred.
- **Angiotensin converting inhibitors** We found no systematic review or RCTs comparing angiotensin converting enzyme inhibitors versus placebo in people with type 2 diabetes and late nephropathy for the outcomes of mortality (all cause), incidence of end stage renal disease, or incidence of cardiovascular events (stroke, heart failure, myocardial infarction).
- **Glycaemic control** We found no systematic review or RCTs on glycaemic control in people with type 2 diabetes and late nephropathy for the outcomes of mortality (all cause), incidence of end stage renal disease, or incidence of cardiovascular events (stroke, heart failure, myocardial infarction).
- **Lipid lowering** We found no systematic review or RCTs on lipid lowering in people with type 2 diabetes and late nephropathy for the outcomes of mortality (all cause), incidence of end stage renal disease, or incidence of cardiovascular events (stroke, heart failure, myocardial infarction).
- **Protein restriction** We found no systematic review or RCTs on protein restriction in people with type 2 diabetes and late nephropathy for the outcomes of mortality (all cause), incidence of end stage renal disease, or incidence of cardiovascular events (stroke, heart failure, myocardial infarction).

- **Tight control of blood pressure** We found no systematic review or RCTs on tight blood pressure control in people with type 2 diabetes and late nephropathy for the outcomes of mortality (all cause), incidence of end stage renal disease, or incidence of cardiovascular events (stroke, heart failure, myocardial infarction).

DEFINITION Diabetic nephropathy is a clinical syndrome characterised by albuminuria on at least two occasions that are separated by 3–6 months, in people with diabetes. Diabetic nephropathy is usually accompanied by hypertension, progressive rise in proteinuria, and decline in renal function. In type 1 diabetes, five stages have been proposed**G**. Of these stages, stages 1 and 2 are equivalent to pre-clinical nephropathy and are detected only by imaging or biopsy. Stage 3 is synonymous with early nephropathy, the clinical term used in this chapter. Stage 4 nephropathy is also known clinically as late nephropathy, and this term will be used for the remainder of this chapter. Stage 5 represents the progression to end stage renal disease. **Population:** For the purpose of this review, we have included people with diabetes and both early nephropathy, synonymous with microalbuminuria, usually defined by albuminuria level of 30–300 mg/day (or albumin/creatinine ratio of 30–300 mg/g [3.4–34 mg/mmol]), and late nephropathy, synonymous with macroalbuminuria, characterised by albuminuria > 300 mg/day (or albumin/creatinine ratio > 300 mg/g [34 mg/mmol]). The treatment of people with diabetes and end stage renal disease is not covered in this chapter.

INCIDENCE/ PREVALENCE In 1997, the worldwide prevalence of diabetes was 124 million and is expected to increase to 221 million in 2010.[1] In the UK, 1.4 million people had been diagnosed with diabetes in 1998, and estimates suggest 1 million more have diabetes, but have not yet been diagnosed.[2] After 20 years of diabetes, the cumulative risk of proteinuria is 27% in type 2 and 28% in type 1.[3] In both type 1 and type 2 diabetes, the overall prevalence of microalbuminuria and macroalbuminuria is about 30–35%.[4] In addition, the incidence of diabetic nephropathy is increasing, in part due to the growing epidemic of type 2 diabetes and increased life expectancies; for example, in the USA, the incidence has increased by 150% in the past decade.[5]

AETIOLOGY/ RISK FACTORS Duration of diabetes, older age, male gender, smoking status, and poor glycaemic control have all been found to be risk factors in the development of nephropathy.[6,7] In addition, certain ethnic groups seem to be at greater risk for developing diabetic nephropathy. Microalbuminuria is less pathognomonic among type 2 diabetics, because hypertension, which commonly complicates type 2 diabetes, can also cause microalbuminuria. Hypertension can also cause renal insufficiency, so the time to development of renal insufficiency can be shorter in type 2 diabetes than in type 1. For people who have an atypical course, renal biopsy may be advisable. In addition, there are some differences in the progression of type 1 and type 2 diabetic nephropathy. In type 2 diabetics, albuminuria is more often present at diagnosis. Hypertension is also more common in type 2 diabetic nephropathy. Finally, microalbuminuria is less predictive of late nephropathy in type 2 diabetics compared with type 1.[8]

PROGNOSIS People with microalbuminuria are at increased risk for progression to macroalbuminuria and end stage renal disease. The course of renal function is similar between type 1 and type 2 diabetes. The natural history of diabetic nephropathy is better defined in type 1 than type 2 diabetes. In type 2 diabetes, the course can be more difficult to predict, primarily because the date of onset of diabetes is less commonly known and comorbid conditions can contribute to renal disease. Without specific interventions, about 80% of people with type 1 diabetes and 20–40% of people with type 2 diabetes with microalbuminuria will progress to macroalbuminuria.[9] Diabetic nephropathy is associated with poor outcomes. Diabetic nephropathy is the most common cause of end stage renal disease in the UK, accounting for 20% of all cases[10] whereas, in the USA, diabetes accounts for 48% of all new cases of end stage renal disease.[11] People with type 1 diabetes and proteinuria have been found to have a 40-fold greater risk of mortality than people without proteinuria.[12] The prognostic significance of proteinuria is less extreme in type 2 diabetes, although people with proteinuria do have a four-fold risk of death compared with people without proteinuria.[13] In addition, increased cardiovascular risk has been associated with albuminuria in people with diabetes.[14] African Americans, Native Americans, and Mexican Americans have a much higher risk of developing end stage renal disease in the setting of diabetes compared with white people.[9,15] In the USA, African American people with diabetes progress to end stage renal disease at a significantly more rapid rate than white poeple with diabetes.[16] In England, the rates for initiating treatment for end stage renal disease are 4.2 and 3.7 times higher for African Caribbeans and Indo Asians compared with white people.[17] The Pima tribe of Native Americans, located in southwestern USA, have much higher rates of diabetic nephropathy compared with white people, and also progress to end stage renal disease at a faster rate.[18]

AIMS OF INTERVENTION To prevent death and complications of chronic renal failure and the need for chronic dialysis or transplantation (end stage renal disease), with minimal adverse events.

OUTCOMES **Early nephropathy:** Progression to late nephropathy (proteinuria determined by albumin excretion rate > 300 mg/g [34 mg/mmol]); mortality (all cause); incidence of end stage renal disease; or incidence of cardiovascular events (stroke, heart failure, myocardial infarction). **Late nephropathy:** Mortality (all cause); incidence of end stage renal disease; or incidence of cardiovascular events (stroke, heart failure, myocardial infarction). **Excluded outcomes:** Change or doubling of serum creatinine as a surrogate marker.

METHODS *Clinical Evidence* search and appraisal December 2003. The inclusion criteria for studies for this review are quantitative systematic reviews or RCTs with at least 10 outcomes in the placebo group. We excluded RCTs that only reported a mean change in proteinuria as an outcome.

QUESTION What are the effects of treatments in people with type 1 diabetes and early nephropathy?

OPTION ANGIOTENSIN CONVERTING ENZYME INHIBITORS

One systematic review found that, compared with placebo or controls, angiotensin converting enzyme inhibitors (captopril, lisinopril, enalapril, perindopril, and ramipril) reduced progression to macroalbuminuria and increased regression to normoalbuminuria in normotensive people with type 1 diabetes and microalbuminuria. We found no systematic review or RCTs comparing effects of angiotensin converting enzyme inhibitors versus placebo in people with type 1 diabetes and early nephropathy for the outcomes mortality (all cause), incidence of end stage renal disease, or incidence of cardiovascular events (stroke, heart failure, myocardial infarction).

Benefits: We found one systematic review (search date not reported), which found that, compared with placebo or controls, angiotensin converting enzyme (ACE) inhibitors significantly reduced progression to macroalbuminuria and increased regression to normoalbuminuria in normotensive people with type 1 diabetes and microalbuminuria (individual patient data meta-analysis from 12 trials; 698 people; progression to macroalbuminuria: OR 0.38, 95% CI 0.25 to 0.57; $P < 0.001$; regression to normoalbuminuria: OR 3.07, 95% CI 2.15 to 4.44).[19] The included ACE inhibitors were captopril, lisinopril, enalapril, perindopril, and ramipril. We found no systematic review or RCTs comparing effects of ACE inhibitors versus placebo in people with type 1 diabetes and early nephropathy for the outcomes of mortality (all cause), incidence of end stage renal disease, or incidence of cardiovascular events (stroke, heart failure, myocardial infarction).

Harms: The systematic review did not report on evidence about harms of ACE inhibitors in people with type 1 diabetes and microalbuminuria.[19]

Comment: None.

OPTION ANGIOTENSIN II RECEPTOR ANTAGONISTS

We found no systematic review or RCTs comparing effects of angiotensin II receptor antagonists versus placebo in people with type 1 diabetes and early nephropathy for outcomes of interest. Long term placebo controlled RCTs would not be ethical because of the established benefits of angiotensin

converting enzyme inhibitors and similarity between these two drug classes. We found no RCTs comparing angiotensin II receptor antagonists versus angiotensin converting enzyme inhibitors in people with type 1 diabetes and early nephropathy.

Benefits: We found no systematic review or RCTs comparing effects of angiotensin II receptor antagonists with placebo in people with type 1 diabetes and early nephropathy for the outcomes of progression to late nephropathy: mortality (all cause), incidence of end stage renal disease, or incidence of cardiovascular events (stroke, heart failure, myocardial infarction). Long term placebo controlled RCTs would not be ethical in people with type 1 diabetes and nephropathy because of the established benefits of angiotensin converting enzyme (ACE) inhibitors and similarity between these two drug classes. **Versus ACE inhibitors:** We found no RCTs comparing angiotensin II receptor antagonists versus ACE inhibitors in people with type 1 diabetes and early nephropathy.

Harms: We found no RCTs.

Comment: None.

OPTION PROTEIN RESTRICTION

We found no systematic review or RCTs comparing effects of low protein diet versus usual diet in people with type 1 diabetes and early nephropathy for the outcomes of progression to late nephropathy, mortality (all cause), incidence of end stage renal disease, or incidence of cardiovascular events (stroke, heart failure, myocardial infarction).

Benefits: We found no systematic review or RCTs comparing effects of low protein diet with usual diet in people with type 1 diabetes and early nephropathy for the outcomes of interest.

Harms: We found no RCTs.

Comment: None.

OPTION GLYCAEMIC CONTROL

One systematic review found that, compared with conventional control, intensive glycaemic control reduced progression of nephropathy in people with type 1 diabetes and early nephropathy. The review found no significant difference between intensive glycaemic control and conventional control in the incidence of severe hypoglycaemia, but found higher incidence of diabetic ketoacidosis in people treated with continuous subcutaneous insulin infusion compared with conventional multiple injection treatment. We found no systematic review or RCTs comparing intensive glycaemic control versus conventional glycaemic control in people with type 1 diabetes and early nephropathy for the outcomes of mortality (all cause), incidence of end stage renal disease, or incidence of cardiovascular events (stroke, heart failure, myocardial infarction).

Benefits: One systematic review (search date 1991, 16 RCTs) found that, compared with conventional control, intensive glycaemic control significantly reduced progression of nephropathy in people with type 1 diabetes and either normal albumin excretion or microalbumuria (7 RCTs, 266 people; nephropathy progression: OR 0.34, 95% CI 0.20 to 0.58; $P < 0.001$).[20] We found no systematic review or RCTs comparing intensive glycaemic control versus conventional glycaemic control in people with type 1 diabetes and early nephropathy for the outcomes of mortality (all cause), incidence of end stage renal disease, or incidence of cardiovascular events (stroke, heart failure, myocardial infarction).

Harms: The review found no significant difference between intensive glycaemic control and conventional control in the incidence of severe hypoglycaemia (6 trials; severe hypoglycaemia increased by 9.1 episodes/100 person years, 95% CI –1.4 to 19.6).[3] The review also found a significantly higher incidence of diabetic ketoacidosis in people treated with continuous subcutaneous insulin infusion compared with conventional multiple injection treatment (3 trials, 99 people; ketoacidosis increased by 12.6 episodes/100 person years, 95% CI 8.7 to 16.5).[20]

Comment: None.

OPTION TIGHT CONTROL OF BLOOD PRESSURE

We found no systematic review or RCTs comparing tight control of blood pressure versus conventional control in people with type 1 diabetes and early nephropathy for the outcomes of progression to late nephropathy, mortality (all cause), incidence of end stage renal disease, or incidence of cardiovascular events (stroke, heart failure, myocardial infarction).

Benefits: We found no systematic review or RCTs comparing tight control of blood pressure versus conventional control in people with type 1 diabetes and early nephropathy for the outcomes of interest.

Harms: We found no RCTs.

Comment: None.

OPTION LIPID LOWERING

We found no systematic review or RCTs on lipid lowering in people with type 1 diabetes and early nephropathy for the outcomes of progression to late nephropathy, mortality (all cause), incidence of end stage renal disease, or incidence of cardiovascular events (stroke, heart failure, myocardial infarction).

Benefits: We found no systematic review or RCTs on lipid lowering in people with type 1 diabetes and early nephropathy for the outcomes of interest.

Harms: We found no RCTs.

Comment: None.

QUESTION What are the effects of treatments in people with type 1 diabetes and late nephropathy?

OPTION ANGIOTENSIN CONVERTING ENZYME INHIBITORS

One RCT in people with type 1 diabetes and late nephropathy found that, compared with placebo, captopril (an angiotensin converting enzyme inhibitor) reduced the combined outcome of renal transplant, end stage renal disease, or death over 3 years. We found no systematic review or RCTs comparing effects of captopril versus placebo in people with type 1 diabetes and late nephropathy for the outcome of incidence of cardiovascular events (stroke, heart failure, myocardial infarction) or on effects of other angiotensin converting enzyme inhibitors for the outcomes of interest.

Benefits: We found one RCT,[21] which found that captopril significantly reduced the combined outcome of renal transplant, end stage renal disease, or death over 3 years compared with placebo (1 RCT, 409 people; combined outcome of renal transplant, end stage renal disease, or death: 23/207 [11%] with captopril *v* 42/202 [21%] with placebo;

RR 0.5, 95% CI 0.18 to 0.70).[21] Diabetic nephropathy was defined as a urinary protein excretion rate > 500 mg/day and serum creatinine ≤ 2.5 mg/dL (221 μmol/L).[21] We found no systematic review or RCTs comparing effects of captopril with placebo for the outcome of incidence of cardiovascular events (stroke, heart failure, myocardial infarction) or on effects of other angiotensin converting enzyme inhibitors.

Harms: One RCT found that, in people with type 1 diabetes and early nephropathy, hyperkalemia occurred in three (1.5%) participants taking angiotensin converting enzyme inhibitors, and none of the participants taking placebo.[21]

Comment: None.

OPTION ANGIOTENSIN II RECEPTOR ANTAGONISTS

We found no systematic review or RCTs comparing effects of angiotensin II receptor antagonists versus placebo in people with type 1 diabetes and late nephropathy for outcomes of mortality (all cause), incidence of end stage renal disease, or incidence of cardiovascular events (stroke, heart failure, myocardial infarction). Long term placebo controlled RCTs would not be ethical because of the established benefits of angiotensin converting enzyme inhibitors and similarity between these two drug classes. We found no RCTs comparing angiotensin II receptor antagonists versus angiotensin converting enzyme inhibitors in people with type 1 diabetes and late nephropathy.

Benefits: We found no systematic review or RCTs comparing effects of angiotensin II receptor antagonists versus placebo in people with type 1 diabetes and late nephropathy for the outcomes of interest. Long term placebo controlled RCTs would not be ethical in people with type 1 diabetes and nephropathy because of the established benefits of angiotensin converting enzyme inhibitors and similarity between these two drug classes. **Versus angiotensin converting enzyme inhibitors:** We found no RCTs comparing angiotensin II receptor antagonists versus angiotensin converting enzyme inhibitors in people with type 1 diabetes and late nephropathy.

Harms: We found no RCTs.

Comment: None.

OPTION PROTEIN RESTRICTION

One small RCT found that, compared with usual protein intake, a low protein diet significantly reduced the cumulative incidence of end stage renal disease or death over 4 years in people with type 1 diabetes and late nephropathy. This RCT was small, and neither participants nor study investigators could be blinded to the randomisation owing to nature of the intervention. We found no systematic review or RCTs comparing effects of low protein diet versus usual diet in people with type 1 diabetes and late nephropathy for the outcome of incidence of cardiovascular events (stroke, heart failure, myocardial infarction).

Benefits: We found one small RCT, which found that, compared with usual protein intake, a low protein diet significantly reduced the cumulative incidence of end stage renal disease or death over 4 years in people with type 1 diabetes and late nephropathy (1 RCT, 82 people aged 18–60 years; cumulative incidence of end stage renal disease or death: 4/41 [10%] with low protein diet *v* 11/41 [27%] with usual protein intake; RR 0.23, 95% CI 0.07 to 0.72).[22] The causes of death were heart failure or myocardial infarction.[22] This RCT was small, and neither participants nor study investigators could be blinded to the randomisation owing to the nature of the intervention. We found no systematic review or RCTs comparing effects of low protein diet with usual diet in people with type 1 diabetes and late nephropathy for the outcome of incidence of cardiovascular events (stroke, heart failure, myocardial infarction).

Harms: The RCT did not report on evidence about harms of protein restriction in people with type 1 diabetes and late nephropathy.[22]

Comment: We found one systematic review (search date 1994, 5 randomised, controlled or time-controlled crossover studies), which included four trials (78 patients) with late, and one trial (30 patients) with early nephropathy.[23] The review found that, compared with usual protein diet, a low protein diet significantly slowed the increase in urinary albumin level or the decline in glomerular filtration rate or creatinine clearance in people with type 1 diabetes and late nephropathy (5 trials, 108 people; RR 0.56, 95% CI 0.40 to 0.77). The diets ranged from 0.5–0.85 g of protein/kg body weight per day in the intervention groups, and follow up ranged from 9–33 months. The review did not discuss the clinical relevance of these findings.

OPTION GLYCAEMIC CONTROL

We found no systematic review or RCTs comparing intensive glycaemic control with conventional glycaemic control in people with type 1 diabetes and late nephropathy for the outcomes of mortality (all cause), incidence of end stage renal disease, or incidence of cardiovascular events (stroke, heart failure, myocardial infarction).

Benefits: We found no systematic review or RCTs comparing intensive glycaemic control versus conventional glycaemic control in people with type 1 diabetes and late nephropathy for the outcomes of interest.

Harms: We found no RCTs.

Comment: None.

OPTION TIGHT CONTROL OF BLOOD PRESSURE

We found no systematic review or RCTs comparing tight control of blood pressure versus conventional control in people with type 1 diabetes and late nephropathy for the outcomes of mortality (all cause), incidence of end stage renal disease, or incidence of cardiovascular events (stroke, heart failure, myocardial infarction).

Benefits: We found no systematic review or RCTs comparing tight control of blood pressure with conventional control in people with type 1 diabetes and early or late nephropathy for the outcomes of interest.

Harms: We found no RCTs.

Comment: None.

OPTION LIPID LOWERING

We found no systematic review or RCTs on lipid lowering in people with type 1 diabetes and late nephropathy for the outcomes of mortality (all cause), incidence of end stage renal disease, or incidence of cardiovascular events (stroke, heart failure, myocardial infarction).

Benefits: We found no systematic review or RCTs on lipid lowering in people with type 1 diabetes and late nephropathy for the outcomes of interest.

Harms: We found no RCTs.

Comment: None.

QUESTION What are the effects of treatments in people with type 2 diabetes and early nephropathy?

OPTION ANGIOTENSIN CONVERTING ENZYME INHIBITORS

One RCT found that, compared with placebo, enalapril significantly reduced progression to late nephropathy. One RCT comparing ramipril versus placebo with subgroup analysis in people with diabetes and early nephropathy found that ramipril reduced the combined outcome of myocardial infarction, stroke, or cardiovascular death. One systematic review in people with diabetes and nephropathy, which did not stratify the results by the type of diabetes, found that, compared with placebo, angiotensin converting enzyme inhibitors significantly reduced progression to late nephropathy in people with diabetes and microalbuminuria over 3 years. We found no systematic review or RCTs comparing angiotensin converting enzyme inhibitors versus placebo in people with type 2 diabetes and early nephropathy for the outcomes of mortality (all cause), incidence of end stage renal disease, or incidence of cardiovascular events (stroke, heart failure, myocardial infarction).

Benefits: We found one systematic review (search date 1999)[24] and two subsequent RCTs.[25,26] The systematic review evaluated the effects of angiotensin converting enzyme inhibitors in people with diabetes and nephropathy, but did not stratify the results by the type of diabetes.[24] It found that, compared with placebo, angiotensin converting enzyme inhibitors significantly reduced progression to late nephropathy in people with diabetes and microalbuminuria over 3 years (9 RCTs, 642 people, mean age 36 years; progression to macroalbuminuria: RR 0.35, 95% CI 0.24 to 0.53). The first subsequent RCT compared ramipril versus placebo and included a subgroup analysis in 1140 people with diabetes and early nephropathy.[25] Within the subgroup, the RCT found that ramipril was associated with a significant reduction in the combined outcome of myocardial infarction, stroke, or cardiovascular death (specific odds ratios were not reported). The outcome of total mortality was not reported separately for people with diabetes and early nephropathy. However, the RCT found that ramipril reduced the risk of mortality in the diabetic subgroup (196/1808 [10.8%] with ramipril *v* 248/1769 [14.0%] with placebo; $P = 0.004$). The second subsequent RCT found that, compared with placebo, enalapril significantly reduced the risk of progression to late nephropathy over 5 years (6/49 [12.2%] with enalapril *v* 19/45 [42.2%] with placebo; $P < 0.005$; ARR 30%, 95% CI 15% to 45%; $P < 0.001$).[26]

Harms: The systematic review and one subsequent RCT did not report on harms.[24,26] One subsequent found a greater incidence of cough on ramipril 133/1808 (7%) compared with placebo 37/1769 (2%); P value not reported.[25]

Comment: None.

OPTION ANGIOTENSIN II RECEPTOR ANTAGONISTS

One RCT in people with type 2 diabetes, hypertension, and microalbuminuria found that, compared with placebo, an angiotensin II receptor antagonist irbesartan 300 mg reduced progression from early to late nephropathy over 2 years but found no significant decrease with irbesartan 150 mg. We found no systematic review or RCTs comparing angiotensin II receptor antagonists with

placebo in people with type 2 diabetes and early nephropathy for the outcomes of mortality (all cause), incidence of end stage renal disease, or incidence of cardiovascular events (stroke, heart failure, myocardial infarction).

Benefits: We found one RCT, which found that, compared with placebo, irbesartan 300 mg significantly reduced progression to late nephropathy over 2 years in people with type 2 diabetes, hypertension and microalbuminuria, but found no significant decrease with irbesartan 150 mg (1 RCT, 590 people; progression from early to late nephropathy: 10/194 [5.2%] with irbesartan 300 mg *v* 30/201 [14.9%] with placebo; HR 0.30, 95% CI 0.14 to 0.61; $P < 0.001$; 19/195 [9.7%] with irbesartan 150 mg *v* 30/201 [14.9%]; HR 0.61, 95% CI 0.34 to 1.08; $P = 0.08$). Early nephropathy (microalbuminuria) was defined as an albumin excretion rate of 20–200 μg/minute and late nephropathy as albumin excretion rate > 200 μg/minute.[27] We found no systematic review or RCTs comparing angiotensin II receptor antagonists versus placebo in people with type 2 diabetes and early nephropathy for the outcomes of mortality (all cause), incidence of end stage renal disease, or incidence of cardiovascular events (stroke, heart failure, myocardial infarction).

Harms: The RCT found no significant difference in the proportion of people permanently discontinuing medication (1 RCT, 590 people; 14.9% with combined doses of irbesartan *v* 18.9% with placebo; $P = 0.21$).[27]

Comment: None.

OPTION PROTEIN RESTRICTION

We found no systematic review or RCTs on protein restriction in people with type 2 diabetes and early nephropathy for the outcomes of progression to late nephropathy, mortality (all cause), incidence of end stage renal disease, or incidence of cardiovascular events (stroke, heart failure, myocardial infarction).

Benefits: We found no systematic review or RCTs on protein restriction in people with type 2 diabetes and early nephropathy for the outcomes of interest.

Harms: We found no RCTs.

Comment: None.

OPTION GLYCAEMIC CONTROL

We found no systematic review or RCTs on glycaemic control in people with type 2 diabetes and early nephropathy for the outcomes of progression to late nephropathy, mortality (all cause), incidence of end stage renal disease, or incidence of cardiovascular events (stroke, heart failure, myocardial infarction).

Benefits: We found no systematic review or RCTs on glycaemic control in people with type 2 diabetes and early nephropathy for the outcomes of interest.

Harms: We found no RCTs.

Comment: None.

OPTION TIGHT CONTROL OF BLOOD PRESSURE

One RCT found that, in people with type 2 diabetes, early nephropathy, and baseline blood pressure within the normal range, a lower diastolic blood pressure target (10 mm Hg below baseline) significantly reduced progression from microalbuminuria to overt albuminuria over 5 years compared with a

moderate diastolic blood pressure target (80–89 mm Hg). We found no systematic review or RCTs on tight blood pressure control in people with type 2 diabetes and early nephropathy for the outcomes of progression to late nephropathy, mortality (all cause), incidence of end stage renal disease, or incidence of cardiovascular events (stroke, heart failure, myocardial infarction).

Benefits: We found no systematic review but found one RCT.[28] It found that, in people with type 2 diabetes, early nephropathy, and baseline blood pressure within the normal range, a lower diastolic blood pressure target significantly reduced progression from microalbuminuria to overt albuminuria over 5 years compared with a moderate diastolic blood pressure target (480 people aged 40–74 years; $P = 0.02$; results presented graphically).[28] The lower diastolic blood pressure target was 10 mm Hg below baseline diastolic blood pressure and moderate diastolic blood pressure target was 80–89 mm Hg. We found no systematic review or RCTs on tight blood pressure control in people with type 2 diabetes and early nephropathy for the outcomes of progression to late nephropathy, mortality (all cause), incidence of end stage renal disease, or incidence of cardiovascular events (stroke, heart failure, myocardial infarction).

Harms: The RCT did not evaluate adverse effects of lower target diastolic blood pressure compared with moderate target diastolic blood pressure in people with type 2 diabetes and baseline blood pressure within the normal range.[28]

Comment: None.

OPTION LIPID LOWERING

We found no systematic review or RCTs on lipid lowering in people with type 2 diabetes and early nephropathy for the outcomes of progression to late nephropathy, mortality (all cause), incidence of end stage renal disease, or incidence of cardiovascular events (stroke, heart failure, myocardial infarction).

Benefits: We found no systematic review or RCTs on lipid lowering in people with type 2 diabetes and early nephropathy for the outcomes of interest.

Harms: We found no RCTs.

Comment: None.

QUESTION What are the effects of treatments in people with type 2 diabetes and late nephropathy?

OPTION ANGIOTENSIN CONVERTING ENZYME INHIBITORS

We found no systematic review or RCTs comparing angiotensin converting enzyme inhibitors versus placebo in people with type 2 diabetes and late nephropathy for the outcomes of mortality (all cause), incidence of end stage renal disease, or incidence of cardiovascular events (stroke, heart failure, myocardial infarction).

Benefits: We found no systematic review or RCTs comparing angiotensin converting enzyme inhibitors with placebo in people with type 2 diabetes and late nephropathy for the outcomes of interest.

Harms: We found no RCTs.

Comment: None.

OPTION ANGIOTENSIN II RECEPTOR ANTAGONISTS

We found two RCTs comparing angiotensin II receptor antagonists versus placebo for the outcomes of progression to end stage renal disease, cardiovascular events, and all cause mortality. One RCT in people with type 2 diabetes and late nephropathy found that, compared with placebo, losartan reduced progression to end stage renal disease over 3.4 years, but found no significant difference in fatal or non-fatal cardiovascular events or death from any cause. Another RCT in people with type 2 diabetes and late nephropathy found no significant difference between irbesartan and placebo in progression to end stage renal disease, or death from any cause over 2.6 years. It also found that irbesartan significantly reduced the incidence of congestive heart failure compared with placebo, but no significant difference for a composite cardiovascular outcome, cardiovascular death, myocardial infarction, cerebrovascular accident, or cardiac revascularisation. In both RCTs, angiotensin II receptor antagonist was discontinued if hyperkalemia occurred.

Benefits: We found no systematic review but found two RCTs comparing angiotensin II receptor antagonists versus placebo for the outcomes of progression to end stage renal disease, cardiovascular events, and all cause mortality.[29,30] The first RCT found that, compared with placebo, losartan significantly reduced progression to end stage renal disease over 3.4 years, but found no significant difference in fatal or non-fatal cardiovascular events or death from any cause (1 RCT, 1513 people with type 2 diabetes and urine albumin/creatinine ratio ≥ 300 mg/g [34 mg/mmol] and serum creatinine levels between 1.3–3.0; progression to end stage renal disease: 147/751 [19.6%] with losartan *v* 194/762 [25.5%] with placebo; RR 0.72, 95% CI 0.58 to 0.89; ARR 2.3 cases/100 person years; fatal or non-fatal cardiovascular events: 247/751 [32.9%] with losartan *v* 268/762 [35.2%] with placebo; RR 0.94, 95% CI 0.81 to 1.08; death from any cause: 158/751 [21%] with losartan *v* 155/762 [20.3%] with placebo; RR 1.03, 95% CI 0.85 to 1.26).[29] Late nephropathy was defined as urine albumin/creatinine ratio of 300 mg/g (34 mg/mol) or higher and serum creatinine levels between 1.3 and 3.0 mg/dL. Both losartan and placebo were taken in addition to conventional antihypertensive treatment (calcium channel blockers, diuretics, alpha blockers, beta blockers).[29] The second RCT found no significant difference between irbesartan and placebo in progression to end stage renal disease, or death from any cause over 2.6 years in people with type 2 diabetes and late nephropathy (1715 people with type 2 diabetes, hypertension, and proteinuria > 900 mg [median 2.9 g/day] and serum creatinine 1.0–3.0 mg/dL; progression to end stage renal disease: 82/579 [14.2%] with irbesartan *v* 101/569 [17.8%] with placebo; RR 0.77, 95% CI 0.57 to 1.03; P = 0.07; death from any cause: RR 0.92, 95% CI 0.69 to 1.23).[30] A second publication of this RCT[30] reported that irbesartan significantly reduced the incidence of congestive heart failure compared with placebo (80/579 [14%] with irbesartan *v* 113/569 [20%] with placebo; RR 0.72, 95% CI 0.52 to 1.00; P = 0.048), but found no significant difference for a composite cardiovascular outcome (259/579 [45%] with irbesartan *v* 284/569 [50%] with placebo; RR 0.90, 95% CI 0.74 to 1.10; P > 0.2), cardiovascular death (52/579 [9%] with irbesartan *v* 46/569 [8%] with placebo; RR 1.08, 95% CI 0.72 to 1.60; P > 0.2), myocardial infarction (48/579 [8%] with irbesartan *v* 51/569 [9%] with placebo; RR 0.90, 95% CI 0.60 to 1.33; P > 0.2), cerebrovascular accident (30/579 [5%] with irbesartan *v* 28/569 [5%] with placebo; RR 1.01, 95% CI 0.61 to 1.67; P > 0.2), or cardiac revascularisation (31/579 [5%] with irbesartan *v* 39/569 [7%] with placebo; RR 0.80, 95% CI 0.49 to 1.30; P > 0.2).[31]

Diabetic nephropathy

Harms: One RCT found that a lower proportion of people discontinued medication with losartan compared with placebo (1 RCT, 1513 people; 46.5% with losartan *v* 53.5% with placebo; absolute numbers and statistical significance data not provided).[29] In this RCT, medication was discontinued if hyperkalemia occurred (1.1 % with losartan *v* 0.5% with placebo; absolute numbers and statistical significance data not provided). In the second RCT, medication was stopped because of hyperkalaemia (1 RCT, 1715 people; hyperkalaemia 11/579 [1.9%] with irbesartan *v* 2/569 [0.4%] with placebo; P = 0.01).[30]

Comment: In both RCTs (RENAAL and IDNT), the primary outcome was a composite end point of the doubling of serum creatinine, end stage renal disease, or death.[29,30] In each RCT, the angiotensin II receptor antagonist (losartan or irbesartan) significantly reduced the incidence of the primary outcome compared with placebo. In this review, we have focused only on the clinical outcomes of end stage renal disease, cardiovascular events, and death.

OPTION PROTEIN RESTRICTION

We found no systematic review or RCTs on protein restriction in people with type 2 diabetes and late nephropathy for the outcomes of mortality (all cause), incidence of end stage renal disease, or incidence of cardiovascular events (stroke, heart failure, myocardial infarction).

Benefits: We found no systematic review or RCTs on protein restriction in people with type 2 diabetes and late nephropathy for the outcomes of interest.

Harms: We found no RCTs.

Comment: None.

OPTION GLYCAEMIC CONTROL

We found no systematic review or RCTs on glycaemic control in people with type 2 diabetes and late nephropathy for the outcomes of mortality (all cause), incidence of end stage renal disease, or incidence of cardiovascular events (stroke, heart failure, myocardial infarction).

Benefits: We found no systematic review or RCTs on glycaemic control in people with type 2 diabetes and late nephropathy for the outcomes of interest.

Harms: We found no RCTs.

Comment: None.

OPTION TIGHT CONTROL OF BLOOD PRESSURE

We found no systematic review or RCTs on tight blood pressure control in people with type 2 diabetes and late nephropathy for the outcomes of mortality (all cause), incidence of end stage renal disease, or incidence of cardiovascular events (stroke, heart failure, myocardial infarction).

Benefits: We found no systematic review or RCTs on tight blood pressure control in people with type 2 diabetes and late nephropathy for the outcomes of interest.

Harms: We found no RCTs.

Comment: None.

OPTION LIPID LOWERING

We found no systematic review or RCTs on lipid lowering in people with type 2 diabetes and late nephropathy for the outcomes of mortality (all cause), incidence of end stage renal disease, or incidence of cardiovascular events (stroke, heart failure, myocardial infarction).

Benefits: We found no systematic review or RCTs on lipid lowering in people with type 2 diabetes and late nephropathy for the outcomes of interest.

Harms: We found no RCTs.

Comment: None.

GLOSSARY

Stages of progression of nephropathy in type 1 diabetes:

Stage 1 is characterised by renal hypertrophy and hyperfiltration, and is present at the time of diagnosis of type 1 diabetes.[32]

Stage 2 is typically asymptomatic, lasting for an average of 10 years. The earliest notable changes are renal hypertrophy seen on renal ultrasound and an increase in the glomerular filtration rate due to hyperfiltration. At this stage, the kidneys demonstrate typical histologic abnormalities, including diffuse thickening of the glomerular and tubular basement membranes. Glomerular and tubuloepithelial cell hypertrophy are also evident. About one third of patients who develop these changes will develop microalbuminuria.

Stage 3 develops an average of 10 years after the onset of diabetes. Patients develop microalbuminuria (defined as a urine albumin excretion greater than 30 mg/day but less than 300 mg/day. The development of microalbuminuria is the earliest clinically detectable evidence of diabetic nephropathy. At this stage, serum creatinine level is typically normal. About 80% of people who develop microalbuminuria will progress to overt proteinuria. This proportion may be decreasing in the current era as a result of aggressive early treatment with ACE inhibitors and angiotensin receptor blockers. Microalbuminuria is well correlated with renal biopsy findings, particularly nodular glomerulosclerosis. The diagnosis of microalbuminuria is traditionally made with a 24 hour urine collection to measure urine albumin using radioimmunoassay or enzyme linked immunosorbent assays. An alternate and easier method to detect microalbuminuria is measurement of the albumin to creatinine ratio in a spot urine specimen. A ratio between 0.03 and 0.3 (mg albumin/mg creatinine) or 30–300 mg/g (mg albumin/g creatinine) [3.4–34 mg/mmol] is well correlated with 24 hour collections, and is now the preferred screening test for diabetic nephropathy.[33]

Stage 4 or late nephropathy occurs 15–20 years after the onset of diabetes. Urine albumin increases beyond microalbuminuria to macroalbuminuria (> 300 mg/day or > 200 μg/minute). It is at this stage that glomerular filtration rate declines and urine protein excretion increases to > 500 mg/day. The glomerular filtration rate declines on average 0.5–1.0 mL/minute/month. Blood pressure also rises, probably reflecting renal parenchymal disease in sodium retention. Histologically, renal fibrosis becomes more evident. Mesangial expansion develops resulting in diffuse and nodular glomerulosclerosis. The degree of mesangial expansion correlates well with increases in urine albumin excretion and loss of renal function.

Stage 5 or the development of end stage renal disease, occurs a median of 7 years from the development of persistent proteinuria.

REFERENCES

1. Amos AF, McCarty DJ, Zimmet P. The rising global burden of diabetes and its complications: estimates and projections to the year 2010. *Diabet Med* 1997;14(suppl 5):S1–S85.
2. Diabetes UK. Who gets diabetes and what causes it? http://www.diabetes.org.uk/diabetes/get.htm (last accessed 16 August 2004).
3. Hasslacher C, Ritz E, Wahl P, et al. Similar risks of nephropathy in patients with type I or type II diabetes mellitus. *Nephrol Dial Transplant* 1989;4:859–863.
4. Parving HH, Osterby R, Ritz E. Diabetic nephropathy. In: Brenner BM, ed. *The kidney*. Philadelphia: WB Saunders, 2000:1731–1773.
5. Remuzzi G, Schieppati A, Ruggenenti P. Clinical practice. Nephropathy in patients with type 2 diabetes. *N Engl J Med* 2002;346:1145–1151.
6. Marcantoni C, Ortalda V, Lupo A, et al. Progression of renal failure in diabetic nephropathy. *Nephrol Dial Transplant* 1998;13(suppl 8):16–19.

7. Ballard DJ, Humphrey LL, Melton LJ, 3rd, et al. Epidemiology of persistent proteinuria in type II diabetes mellitus. Population-based study in Rochester, Minnesota. *Diabetes* 1988;37:405–412.
8. Powers A. Diabetes mellitus. In: Braunwald E, Fauci AS, Kasper DL, et al eds. *Harrison's principles of internal medicine*. New York: McGraw-Hill, 2001.
9. Molitch ME, DeFronzo RA, Franz MJ, et al. Nephropathy in diabetes. *Diabetes Care* 2004;27(suppl 1):S79–S83.
10. Ansell D, Feest T. *UK renal registry report*. Bristol: UK Renal Registry, 2001.
11. USRDS. *2000 annual data report*. Bethesda, MD: National Institutes of Health, National Institute of Diabetes and Digestive and Kidney Diseases, 2000.
12. Borch-Johnsen K, Andersen PK, Deckert T. The effect of proteinuria on relative mortality in type 1 (insulin-dependent) diabetes mellitus. *Diabetologia* 1985;28:590–596.
13. Morrish NJ, Stevens LK, Head J, et al. A prospective study of mortality among middle-aged diabetic patients (the London Cohort of the WHO Multinational Study of Vascular Disease in Diabetics) I: Causes and death rates. *Diabetologia* 1990;33:538–541.
14. Mogensen CE. Microalbuminuria, blood pressure and diabetic renal disease: origin and development of ideas. *Diabetologia* 1999;42:263–285.
15. Mokdad AH, Ford ES, Bowman BA, et al. Diabetes trends in the US: 1990–1998. *Diabetes Care* 2000;23:1278–1283.
16. Hsu CY, Lin F, Vittinghoff E, Shlipak MG. Racial differences in the progression from chronic renal insufficiency to end-stage renal disease in the United States. *J Am Soc Nephrol* 2003;14:2902–2907.
17. Roderick PJ, Raleigh VS, Hallam L, Mallick NP. The need and demand for renal replacement therapy in ethnic minorities in England. *J Epidemiol Community Health* 1996;50:334–339.
18. Lemley KV. A basis for accelerated progression of diabetic nephropathy in Pima Indians. *Kidney Int Suppl* 2003:S38–S42.
19. ACE Inhibitors in Diabetic Nephropathy Trialist Group. Should all patients with type 1 diabetes mellitus and microalbuminuria receive angiotensin-converting enzyme inhibitors? A meta-analysis of individual patient data [comment]. *Ann Intern Med* 2001;134:370–379. Search date not reported; primary source Medline.
20. Wang PH, Lau J, Chalmers TC. Meta-analysis of effects of intensive blood-glucose control on late complications of type I diabetes. *Lancet* 1993;341:1306–1309. Search date 1991; primary sources not reported.
21. Lewis EJ, Hunsicker LG, Bain RP, Rohde RD. The effect of angiotensin-converting-enzyme inhibition on diabetic nephropathy. The Collaborative Study Group. *N Engl J Med* 1993;329:1456–1462.
22. Hansen HP, Tauber-Lassen E, Jensen BR, et al. Effect of dietary protein restriction on prognosis in patients with diabetic nephropathy. *Kidney Int* 2002;62:220–228.
23. Pedrini MT, Levey AS, Lau J, et al. The effect of dietary protein restriction on the progression of diabetic and nondiabetic renal diseases: a meta-analysis. *Ann Intern Med* 1996;124:627–632. Search date 1994; primary source Medline.
24. Kshirsagar AV, Joy MS, Hogan SL, et al. Effect of ACE inhibitors in diabetic and nondiabetic chronic renal disease: a systematic overview of randomized placebo-controlled trials. *Am J Kidney Dis* 2000;35:695–707. Search date 1999; primary source Medline.
25. Heart Outcomes Prevention Evaluation Study Investigators. Effects of ramipril on cardiovascular and microvascular outcomes in people with diabetes mellitus: results of the HOPE study and MICRO-HOPE substudy. *Lancet* 2000;355:253–259.
26. Ravid M, Savin H, Jutrin I, et al. Long-term effects of ACE inhibition on development of nephropathy in diabetes mellitus type II. *Kidney Int Suppl* 1994;45:S161en164.
27. Parving HH, Lehnert H, Brochner-Mortensen J, et al. The effect of irbesartan on the development of diabetic nephropathy in patients with type 2 diabetes. *N Engl J Med* 2001;345:870–878.
28. Schrier RW, Estacio RO, Esler A, et al. Effects of aggressive blood pressure control in normotensive type 2 diabetic patients on albuminuria, retinopathy and strokes. *Kidney Int* 2002;61:1086–1097.
29. Brenner BM, Cooper ME, de Zeeuw D, et al. Effects of losartan on renal and cardiovascular outcomes in patients with type 2 diabetes and nephropathy. *N Engl J Med* 2001;345:861–869.
30. Lewis EJ, Hunsicker LG, Clarke WR, et al. Renoprotective effect of the angiotensin-receptor antagonist irbesartan in patients with nephropathy due to type 2 diabetes. *N Engl J Med* 2001;345:851–860.
31. Berl T, Hunsicker LG, Lewis JB, et al. Cardiovascular outcomes in the Irbesartan Diabetic Nephropathy Trial of patients with type 2 diabetes and overt nephropathy. *Ann Intern Med* 2003;138:542–549.
32. Fioretto P, Steffes MW, Brown DM, Mauer SM. An overview of renal pathology in insulin-dependent diabetes mellitus in relationship to altered glomerular hemodynamics. *Am J Kidney Dis* 1992;20:549–558.
33. Eknoyan G, Hostetter T, Bakris GL, et al. Proteinuria and other markers of chronic kidney disease: a position statement of the national kidney foundation (NKF) and the National Institute of Diabetes and Digestive and Kidney Diseases (NIDDK). *Am J Kidney Dis* 2003;42:617–622.

Michael Shlipak
Associate Professor of Medicine
Epidemiology & Biostatistics, San Francisco
VA Medical Center
San Francisco
USA

Competing interests: None declared.

Foot ulcers and amputations in diabetes

Search date September 2003

Dereck Hunt and Hertzel Gerstein

QUESTIONS

INTERVENTIONS

Key Messages

Preventive interventions

- **Screening and referral to foot care clinics** One RCT found that a diabetes screening and protection programme (involving referral to a foot clinic if high risk features were present) reduced the risk of major amputation compared with usual care after 2 years.
- **Education** One systematic review found insufficient evidence about the effects of patient education for preventing foot ulcers, serious foot lesions, or amputation.
- **Therapeutic footwear** In people with diabetes and previous diabetic foot ulcer, one RCT found no significant difference in rates of foot ulceration between therapeutic footwear and usual footwear.

Treatments

- **Pressure off-loading with non-removable cast** RCTs found that pressure off-loading with total contact casting or non-removable fibreglass casts improved healing of non-infected diabetic foot ulcers compared with traditional dressing changes, removable cast walkers or half shoes, or specialised cloth shoes.
- **Human skin equivalent** One RCT found that human skin equivalent increased ulcer healing rates compared with saline moistened gauze in people with chronic neuropathic non-infected foot ulcers.

Foot ulcers and amputations in diabetes

- **Systemic hyperbaric oxygen (for infected ulcers)** One RCT identified by a systematic review found that systemic hyperbaric oxygen plus usual care reduced amputation rates at 10 weeks compared with usual care alone in people with severely infected diabetic foot ulcers, but one small RCT found no significant difference between treatments in major amputation rates. The second RCT but may have been too small to detect a clinically important difference.
- **Topical growth factors** One systematic review found that topical growth factors increased healing rates compared with placebo in people with non-infected diabetic foot ulcers.
- **Cultured human dermis** One systematic review found insufficient evidence of the effects of cultured human dermis on ulcer healing in people with non-infected diabetic foot ulcers.
- **Pressure off-loading with felted foam or pressure relief half shoe** One RCT found no significant difference in time to ulcer healing between a pressure off-loading felted foam dressing and a pressure relief half shoe.
- **Systemic hyperbaric oxygen (for non-infected non-ischaemic ulcers)** One small RCT found no significant difference between hyperbaric oxygen plus usual care and usual care alone in ulcer healing at 4 weeks in people with non-infected, neuropathic, non-ischaemic ulcers.

DEFINITION	Diabetic foot ulceration is full thickness penetration of the dermis of the foot in a person with diabetes. Ulcer severity is often classified using the Wagner system. Grade 1 ulcers are superficial ulcers involving the full skin thickness but no underlying tissues. Grade 2 ulcers are deeper, penetrating down to ligaments and muscle, but not involving bone or abscess formation. Grade 3 ulcers are deep ulcers with cellulitis or abscess formation, often complicated with osteomyelitis. Ulcers with localised gangrene are classified as Grade 4 and those with extensive gangrene involving the entire foot are classified as Grade 5.
INCIDENCE/ PREVALENCE	Studies conducted in Australia, Finland, the UK, and the USA have reported the annual incidence of foot ulcers among people with diabetes as 2.5–10.7%, and the annual incidence of amputation as 0.25–1.8%.[1–10]
AETIOLOGY/ RISK FACTORS	Long term risk factors for foot ulcers and amputation include duration of diabetes, poor glycaemic control, microvascular complications (retinopathy, nephropathy, and neuropathy) and peripheral vascular disease. The strongest predictors of foot complications are altered foot sensation, foot deformities, and previous foot ulcer or amputation.[1–10]
PROGNOSIS	People with diabetes are at risk of foot ulcers, infections, and vascular insufficiency. Amputation is indicated if these are severe or do not improve with conservative treatment. As well as affecting quality of life, these complications account for a large proportion of the healthcare costs of diabetes. For people with healed diabetic foot ulcers, the 5 year cumulative rate of ulcer recurrence is 66% and of amputation is 12%.[11]
AIMS OF INTERVENTION	To prevent diabetic foot complications, including ulcers and amputations; and to improve ulcer healing and prevent amputations where ulcers already exist, with minimum adverse effects.
OUTCOMES	Rates of development or recurrence of foot ulcers or major foot lesions; rate of amputation (surgical removal of all or part of the lower extremity; major amputation🅖 or minor amputation🅖; time ulcers take to heal, or the proportion healed in a given period; rates of hospital admission; rates of foot infection; adverse effects of treatment.
METHODS	*Clinical Evidence* search and appraisal September 2003.

QUESTION What are the effects of preventive interventions?

OPTION SCREENING AND REFERRAL TO FOOT CARE CLINIC

One RCT found that a diabetes screening and protection programme (involving referral to a foot clinic if high risk features were present) reduced the risk of major amputation compared with usual care after 2 years.

Benefits: We found one systematic review (search date 1998, 1 RCT, 2002 people attending a general diabetes clinic).[12] The RCT compared a diabetes screening and protection programme with usual care over 2 years.[13] People in the diabetes screening and protection programme were screened for deficits in pedal pulses, light touch, and vibration sensation. People with persistent abnormal findings were referred to the diabetic foot clinic if they had a history of foot ulcer, were found to have a low ankle–brachial index (< 0.75), or were noted to have foot deformities. The clinic provided podiatry and protective shoes as well as education regarding foot care. Usual care consisted of the normal follow up for people in the clinic, who could be referred to the foot care clinic by a healthcare professional. The RCT found that the diabetes screening and protection programme reduced major amputation**G** compared with usual care (AR 0.1% with the diabetes programme *v* 1.2% with usual care; ARR 1.1%, 95% CI 0.4% to 1.9%; NNT 91, 95% CI 53 to 250).

Harms: The RCT did not report adverse effects.[13]

Comment: None.

OPTION **THERAPEUTIC FOOTWEAR**

In people with diabetes and previous diabetic foot ulcer, one RCT found no significant difference in rates of foot ulceration between therapeutic footwear and usual footwear.

Benefits: We found one systematic review (search date 1998), which identified no RCTs (see comment below).[12] We found one subsequent RCT (400 people with diabetes mellitus and previous foot ulcer but without severe deformity, mean age 62 years) comparing three treatments over 2 years: extra-depth and extra-width therapeutic shoes fitted with customised cork inserts, therapeutic shoes fitted with polyurethane inserts, and usual footwear.[14] The RCT found no significant difference in foot ulceration rates between therapeutic footwear and usual footwear (AR for foot ulceration 15% with cork insert *v* 14% with polyurethane insert *v* 17% with usual footwear; RR cork insert *v* usual footwear 0.88, 95% CI 0.51 to 1.52; RR polyurethane insert *v* usual footwear 0.85, 95% CI 0.48 to 1.48).

Harms: The RCT did not report adverse effects.[14]

Comment: The systematic review[12] identified one non-randomised controlled trial.[15] The trial alternately allocated 69 people with a previous diabetic foot ulcer to either an intervention group (in which people received therapeutic shoes) or to a control group (in which people continued to wear their ordinary shoes).[15] Therapeutic shoes were manufactured according to the Towey guidelines (deep enough to fit customised insoles and toe deformities, and made with soft thermoformable leather along with semirocker soles). All participants received information on foot care and footwear. After 1 year, the trial found that wearing therapeutic shoes reduced ulcer recurrence compared with ordinary shoes (27% with therapeutic shoes *v* 58% with ordinary shoes; ARR 31%, 95% CI 7% to 55%; NNT 4, 95% CI 2 to 14). The trial did not report any adverse effects associated with therapeutic shoes. Alternate allocation increases the possibility of confounding.

OPTION **EDUCATION**

One systematic review found insufficient evidence of the effects of education programmes for prevention of diabetic foot ulcers.

Benefits: We found one systematic review (search date 2001, three RCTs, one quasi randomised trial).[16] The first RCT in the review (352 people with diabetes attending 4 primary care teams, randomised by primary care team) compared structured care (a patient education session about foot care plus patient follow up reminders plus prompts to healthcare providers to examine feet and provide education) with usual care (not described).[17] It found that structured care reduced "serious foot lesions" (based on the Seattle Wound Classification Scale**G**)[18] compared with usual care after 12 months (OR 0.41, 95% CI 0.16 to 1.00). The second RCT in the review (266 people with diabetes attending primary care) compared foot care education (nine sessions on foot care and skin hygiene, diabetes, risk factors, diet, and weight management) with usual care.[19] It found no significant difference in ulcer and amputation rates (combined) after 1.5 years (10/127 [8%] with foot care education *v* 16/139 [12%] with usual care; OR 0.66, 95% CI 0.30 to 1.49). The third RCT in the review (530 people with diabetes without any obvious need for foot care) compared education from a podiatrist (45 minute session covering footwear, hygiene, toenail cutting, emollient cream, avoiding risk, foot gymnastics, and preventive podiatric care) plus podiatric visits of 30–60 minutes' duration for 1 year with written foot care instructions.[20,21] It found no significant difference in amputation and ulcer rates between foot education plus podiatric visits and written foot care instructions after 7 years (amputation rate: 1/267 with education plus podiatric visits *v* 0/263 with written foot care instructions; P value undefined; ulcer rate: 0.6% with education plus podiatric visits *v* 0.6% with written instructions; P = 1.0) The quasi randomised trial in the review (227 people with diabetes, allocated according to social security number) compared a single 1 hour educational class about foot care with routine diabetes education.[22] It found that the educational session reduced ulcer recurrences and major amputation after 2 years (ulcer recurrence: 4.5% for foot care education *v* 14.7% for routine education; RR 0.31, 95% CI 0.15 to 0.65; NNT 10, 95% CI 6 to 26; major amputation: 2.8% for foot care education *v* 10.2% for routine education; RR 0.28, 95% CI 0.11 to 0.70; NNT 14, 95% CI 8 to 50).

Harms: The systematic review did not report harms.[16]

Comment: The studies included in the systematic review were of poor methodological quality.[16] The flaws included the following: only one trial had blinded outcome assessment; one trial made no comment on loss to follow up; some studies offered no comment on concealment of randomisation; the trials did not use an intention to treat approach; and the eligibility criteria with respect to risk of ulceration were described adequately in only one trial.

QUESTION What are the effects of treatments?

OPTION PRESSURE OFF-LOADING

RCTs found that pressure off-loading with total contact casting or non-removable fibreglass casts improved healing of non-infected diabetic foot ulcers compared with traditional dressing changes, removable cast walkers or half shoes, or specialised cloth shoes. One RCT found no significant difference in time to ulcer healing between a pressure off-loading felted foam dressing and a pressure relief half shoe.

Benefits: We found one systematic review (search date 1998, one relevant RCT, 40 people with diabetes and plantar foot ulcers but no signs of infection or gangrene)[23] and three subsequent RCTs.[24–26] **Versus traditional**

dressing changes: The RCT in the review compared total contact casting**G** versus traditional dressing changes.[27] Casts were applied by an experienced physical therapist, changed after 5–7 days, and then every 2–3 weeks until healing occurred. Control participants were provided with accommodative footwear and crutches or a walker, and were instructed to complete wet to dry dressing changes 2–3 times daily. The RCT found that total contact casting significantly increased ulcer healing and reduced infection compared with traditional dressing changes (ulcer healing: 91% with total contact casting *v* 32% with traditional dressing; ARR 59%, 95% CI 31% to 87%; NNT 2, 95% CI 1 to 3; infection: 0/21 with total contact casting *v* 5/19 with traditional dressing; $P < 0.05$).[27] **Versus removable casts/shoes:** The first subsequent RCT (63 people with diabetes mellitus and non-infected neuropathic plantar foot ulcers) compared three treatments: total contact casting, removable cast walker, and a half shoe.[24] All participants had weekly visits for wound care and debridements. The RCT found that total contact casting increased ulcer healing compared with removable cast walkers or half shoes after 12 weeks (89% with total contact casting *v* 61% with removable cast walker or half-shoe; ARR 28%, 95% CI 5% to 51%; NNT 4, 95% CI 2 to 19). The second subsequent RCT (50 people with diabetes mellitus and non-infected neuropathic plantar foot ulcers) compared non-removable fibreglass casts with specialised cloth shoes with rigid soles and off-loading insoles over 30 days.[25] All participants had dressing changes every 2 days. It found that non-removable fibreglass casts improved ulcer healing compared with specialised cloth shoes (50% of ulcers healed with fibreglass casts *v* 21% with specialised cloth shoes; ARR 29%, 95% CI 1.4% to 57%; NNT 4, 95% CI 2 to 72). **Pressure off loading felted foam dressings versus a pressure relief half shoe:** The third subsequent RCT (61 people with diabetes mellitus and a neuropathic plantar forefoot ulcer) compared pressure off-loading felted foam dressings with a pressure relief half shoe over at least 10 weeks.[26] The RCT found no significant difference in time to ulcer healing (79.6 days with felted foam *v* 83.2 days with a half shoe, $P = 0.61$).

Harms: The RCT identified in the systematic review found that 3/21 (14%) people treated with total contact casting developed fungal infections requiring topical treatment. This did not prevent continued casting.[27] The other RCTs reported no adverse effects.[24–26]

Comment: Soft tissue infections and osteomyelitis are contraindications to total contact casting.

OPTION CULTURED HUMAN DERMIS

One systematic review found insufficient evidence about the effects of cultured human dermis on ulcer healing in people with non-infected diabetic foot ulcers.

Benefits: We found one systematic review (search date 1998, 2 RCTs, 331 people) comparing topical application of cultured human dermis substitute**G** (weekly for 8 weeks) plus usual care versus usual care alone in people attending hospital outpatient clinics with diabetic foot ulcers with no signs of infection or severe vascular compromise.[23] All participants received wound debridement and were encouraged to avoid weight bearing on the affected limb. The review found no significant difference in ulcer healing at 12 weeks between cultured human dermis compared with usual care (+21% increase in ulcer healing with cultured human dermis compared with usual care at 12 weeks, 95% CI −13% to +36%).

Harms: One RCT identified by the systematic review found no significant difference between cultured human dermis and usual care in the rates of ulcer infections, and no effect on haematology or serum chemistry values or glycaemic control.[23] The other RCT found no significant differences in wound infection rates.

Comment: Cultured human dermis may not be widely available.

OPTION HUMAN SKIN EQUIVALENT

One RCT found that human skin equivalent increased ulcer healing rates compared with saline moistened gauze in people with chronic neuropathic non-infected foot ulceration.

Benefits: We found no systematic review. We found one RCT (208 people aged 18–80 years with diabetes mellitus and chronic neuropathic non-infected foot ulceration) comparing human skin equivalent**G** (Graftskin applied weekly for a maximum of 5 weeks) with saline moistened gauze (applied weekly).[28] It found that human skin equivalent improved ulcer healing compared with saline moistened gauze after 12 weeks (56% with human skin equivalent *v* 38% with saline moistened gauze; ARI 18%, 95% CI 5% to 33%; RR 1.5, 95% CI 1.1 to 2.0; NNT 6, 95% CI 3 to 20).

Harms: The RCT found no significant serious adverse effects.[28] Wound infections and cellulitis were equally frequent in both groups. Osteomyelitis and amputations were less frequent in people receiving human skin equivalent (osteomyelitis: 2.7% with human skin equivalent *v* 10.4% with saline moistened gauze; amputations: 6.3% with human skin equivalent *v* 15.6% with saline moistened gauze).

Comment: Human skin equivalent may not be widely available.

OPTION TOPICAL GROWTH FACTORS

One systematic review found that topical growth factors increased healing rates compared with placebo in people with non-infected diabetic foot ulcers.

Benefits: We found one systematic review (search date 1998, 6 RCTs) comparing four different topical growth factors**G** versus placebo in people attending hospital outpatient clinics with diabetic foot ulcers who were free of signs of infection or severe vascular compromise. All participants received wound debridement and were encouraged to avoid weight bearing on the affected limb. The systematic review did not pool the results from the RCTs.[23] Two of the identified RCTs include fewer than 10 people per treatment arm, and are excluded from this summary. The first RCT (65 people) found that treatment with a topical growth factor (arginine–glycine–aspartic acid matrix) twice weekly for up to 10 weeks increased healing rates compared with placebo (AR for non-healing: 65% with matrix *v* 92% with placebo; ARR 27%, 95% CI 6% to 48%; NNT 4, 95% CI 2 to 15; P = 0.02).[29] The second RCT (118 people) found that treatment with platelet derived growth factor (30 μg/g once daily for up to 20 weeks) increased healing rates compared with placebo (AR for non-healing: 52% with platelet derived growth factor *v* 75% with placebo; ARR 23%, 95% CI 5% to 41%; NNT 5, 95% CI 3 to 14; P = 0.01).[30] The third RCT (382 people) found that platelet derived growth factor (100 μg/g once daily for up to 20 weeks) increased healing rates compared with placebo (AR for non-healing: 50% with platelet derived growth factor *v* 65% with placebo; ARR 15%, 95% CI 2% to 28%; NNT 7, 95% CI 4 to 42; P = 0.007).[31] The fourth RCT (81 people) found that CT-102 increased healing compared with placebo (non-healing: 20% with CT-102 *v* 71% with placebo; ARR 51%, 95% CI 19% to 84%; NNT 2, 95% CI 1 to 5; P = 0.01).[32]

Harms: The systematic review reported no growth factor related adverse effects.[23]

Comment: These therapeutic agents are not widely available and may be expensive. There has been little long term follow up of people treated with these growth factors.

OPTION SYSTEMIC HYPERBARIC OXYGEN

One RCT identified by a systematic review found that systemic hyperbaric oxygen⊕ plus usual care reduced amputation rates at 10 weeks compared with usual care alone in people with severely infected diabetic foot ulcers. One small RCT found no significant difference in major amputation rates⊕ between systemic hyperbaric oxygen plus usual care compared with usual care alone, although it may have been too small to detect a clinically important difference. One small RCT in people with non-infected neuropathic foot ulcers found no significant difference between hyperbaric oxygen plus usual care and usual care alone in ulcer healing at 4 weeks.

Benefits: **Infected foot ulcers** We found one systematic review (search date 1998, 1 RCT)[23] and one additional RCT.[33] The RCT in the systematic review (70 people with severe infected diabetic foot ulcers with full thickness gangrene or abscess, or a large infected ulcer that had not healed after 30 days) compared systemic hyperbaric oxygen⊕ (daily 90 minute sessions at 2.2–2.5 atmospheres) plus usual care (aggressive debridement, broad spectrum iv antibiotics, revascularisation if indicated, and optimised glycaemic control) versus usual care alone.[34] After 10 weeks, systemic hyperbaric oxygen plus usual care significantly reduced rates of major amputation compared with usual care alone (8.6% with systemic hyperbaric oxygen *v* 33% with usual care alone; RR 0.26, 95% CI 0.16 to 0.92; ARR 24%, 95% CI 4% to 45%; NNT 5, 95% CI 2 to 23). The additional RCT (30 people with chronic infected foot ulcers) compared usual care alone (including debridement, iv antibiotics, and optimised glycaemic control) versus usual care plus four treatments with systemic hyperbaric oxygen (8 x 45 minutes sessions at 3 atmospheres pressure) over 2 weeks.[33] It found no significant difference in the risk of major amputation, although it may have lacked power to detect a clinically important effect (13.3% with systemic hyperbaric oxygen *v* 46.7% with usual care alone; ARR +33%, 95% CI –1.6% to +68%). **Non-infected non-ischaemic ulcers** One small RCT (28 people with neuropathic foot ulcers) compared systemic hyperbaric oxygen therapy (90 minute sessions at 2.5 atmospheres twice daily for 2 weeks) plus usual care versus usual care alone.[35] It found no significant difference in the proportion of completely healed ulcers or in reduction in ulcer size at 4 weeks (completely healed: 2/14 [14%] with hyperbaric treatment *v* 0/13 [0%] with control, P not reported; reduction of ulcer surface area: 62% with hyperbaric treatment *v* 22% with control, P not reported).

Harms: In the RCT identified by the systematic review, two people developed symptoms of barotraumatic otitis, but this did not interrupt treatment.[34]

Comment: The smaller RCTs comparing hyperbaric oxygen with usual care may have been too small to rule out a clinically important effect.[33,35]

GLOSSARY

Cultured human dermis consists of neonatal fibroblasts cultured *in vitro* onto a bioabsorbable mesh to produce a living, metabolically active tissue containing normal dermal matrix proteins and cytokines.

Human skin equivalent consists of two allogenic layers containing human skin cells. One layer is formed by dermal cells (human fibroblasts) and the second layer is formed by epidermal cells. Human skin equivalent produces cytokines and growth factors involved in the skin healing process.

Major amputations are above or below knee amputations.

Minor amputations involve partial removal of a foot, including toe or forefoot resections.

Pressure off-loading refers to the use of different techniques designed to minimise the amount of force applied to the ulcer site.

Seattle wound classification system is used to standardise the description of diabetic foot ulcers. It has 10 categories, from superficial wound (category 1) to deep wound involving infection and tissue necrosis (category 10).[18]

Systemic hyperbaric oxygen refers to exposing a patient to a high oxygen, high pressure environment designed to improve oxygen delivery to the ulcer site.

Topical growth factors are synthetically produced factors specifically designed to promote cellular proliferation or matrix production at an ulcer site.

Total contact casting is the application of a layer of plaster over the foot and lower leg, designed to distribute pressure evenly over the entire plantar aspect of the foot to reduce exposure of plantar ulcers to pressure, even when the person is walking.

REFERENCES

1. Rith-Najarian SJ, Stolusky T, Gohdes DM. Identifying diabetic patients at high risk for lower-extremity amputation in a primary health care setting. *Diabetes Care* 1992;15:1386–1389.
2. Veves A, Murray HJ, Young MJ, et al. The risk of foot ulceration in diabetic patients with high foot pressure: a prospective study. *Diabetologia* 1992;35:660–663.
3. Young MJ, Breddy JL, Veves A, et al. The prediction of diabetic neuropathic foot ulceration using vibration perception thresholds: a prospective study. *Diabetes Care* 1994;17:557–560.
4. Humphrey ARG, Dowse GK, Thoma K, et al. Diabetes and nontraumatic lower extremity amputations. Incidence, risk factors, and prevention: a 12 year follow-up study in Nauru. *Diabetes Care* 1996;19:710–714.
5. Lee JS, Lu M, Lee VS, et al. Lower-extremity amputation: incidence, risk factors, and mortality in the Oklahoma Indian Diabetes Study. *Diabetes* 1993;42:876–882.
6. Lehto S, Ronnemaa T, Pyorala K, et al. Risk factors predicting lower extremity amputations in patients with NIDDM. *Diabetes Care* 1996;19:607–612.
7. Moss SE, Klein R, Klein B. Long-term incidence of lower-extremity amputations in a diabetic population. *Arch Fam Med* 1996;5:391–398.
8. Nelson RG, Gohdes DM, Everhart JE, et al. Lower-extremity amputations in NIDDM: 12 year follow-up study in Pima Indians. *Diabetes Care* 1988;11:8–16.
9. Boyko ED, Ahroni JH, Stensel V, et al. A prospective study of risk factors for diabetic foot ulcer. The Seattle diabetic foot study. *Diabetes Care* 1999;22:1036–1042.
10. Abbott CA, Carrington AL, Ashe H, et al. The North-West Diabetes Foot Care Study: incidence of, and risk factors for, new diabetic foot ulceration in a community-based patient cohort. *Diabet Med* 2002;19:377–384.
11. Apelqvist J, Larsson J, Agardh CD. Long-term prognosis for diabetic patients with foot ulcers. *J Intern Med* 1993;233:485–491.
12. Mason J, O'Keeffe C, McIntosh A, et al. A systematic review of foot ulcer in patients with type 2 diabetes mellitus. I: prevention. *Diabet Med* 1999;16:801–812. Search date 1998; primary sources Cochrane Controlled Trials Register, Medline, Embase, Cinahl, Healthstar, Psychlit, Science Citation, Social Science Citation, Index to Scientific and Technical Conference Proceedings (ISI), HMIC database, and Sigle.
13. McCabe CJ, Stevenson RC, Dolan AM. Evaluation of a diabetic foot screening and protection programme. *Diabet Med* 1998;15:80–84.
14. Reiber GE, Smith DG, Wallace C, et al. Effect of therapeutic footwear on foot reulceration in patients with diabetes: a randomized controlled trial. *JAMA* 2002;287:2552–2558.
15. Uccioli L, Faglia E, Monticone G, et al. Manufactured shoes in the prevention of diabetic foot ulcers. *Diabetes Care* 1995;18:1376–1378.
16. Valk GD, Kriegsman DMW, Assendelft WJJ. Patient education for preventing diabetic foot ulceration. A systematic review. *Endocrinol Metab Clin North Am* 2002;31:633–658. Search date 2001; primary sources Cochrane Controlled Trials Register, the Wounds Group Speciliased Trials Register, and the reference list of all relevant studies.
17. Litzelman DK, Slemenda CW, Langefeld CD, et al. Reduction of lower extremity clinical abnormalities in patients with non-insulin-dependent diabetes mellitus. *Ann Intern Med* 1993;119:36–41.
18. Pecoraro RE, Reiber GE. Classification of wounds in diabetic amputees. *Wounds* 1990;2:65–73.
19. Bloomgarden ZT, Karmally W, Metzger MJ, et al. Randomized controlled trial of diabetic patient education: improved knowledge without improved metabolic status. *Diabetes Care* 1987;10:263–272.
20. Hamalainen H, Ronnemaa T, Toikka T, et al. Long-term effects of one year of intensified podiatric activities on foot-care knowledge and self-care habits in patients with diabetes. *Diabetes Educ* 1998;24:734–740.
21. Ronnemaa T, Hamalainen H, Toikka T, et al. Evaluation of the impact of podiatrist care in the primary prevention of foot problems in diabetic subjects. *Diabetes Care* 1997;20:1833–1837.
22. Malone JM, Snyder M, Anderson G, et al. Prevention of amputation by diabetic education. *Am J Surg* 1989;158:520–524.
23. Mason J, O'Keeffe C, Hutchinson A, et al. A systematic review of foot ulcer in patients with type 2 diabetes mellitus. II: treatment. *Diabet Med* 1999;16:889–909. Search date 1998; primary sources Cochrane Controlled Trials Register, Medline, Embase, Cinahl, Healthstar, Psychlit, Science Citation, Social Science Citation, Index to Scientific and Technical Conference Proceedings (ISI), HMIC database, and Sigle.
24. Armstrong DG, Nguyen HC, Lavery LA, et al. Off-loading the diabetic foot wound: a randomized clinical trial. *Diabetes Care* 2001;24:1019–1022.
25. Caravaggi C, Faglia E, De Giglio R, et al. Effectiveness and safety of a nonremovable fiberglass off-bearing cast versus a therapeutic shoe in the treatment of neuropathic foot ulcers: a randomized study. *Diabetes Care* 2000;23:1746–1751.

26. Zimny S, Meyer MF, Schatz H, et al. Applied felted foam for plantar pressure relief is an efficient therapy in neuropathic diabetic foot ulcers. *Exp Clin Endocrinol Diabetes* 2002;110:325–328.
27. Mueller MJ, Diamond JE, Sinacore DR, et al. Total contact casting in treatment of diabetic plantar ulcers. *Diabetes Care* 1989;12:384–388.
28. Veves A, Falanga V, Armstrong DG, et al. Graftskin, a human skin equivalent, is effective in the management of noninfected neuropathic diabetic foot ulcers: a prospective randomized multicenter clinical trial. *Diabetes Care* 2001;24:290–295.
29. Steed DL, Ricotta JJ, Prendergast JJ, et al. Promotion and acceleration of diabetic ulcer healing by arginine-glycine-aspartic acid (RGD) peptide matrix. *Diabetes Care* 1995;18:39–46.
30. Steed DL, and the Diabetic Ulcer Study Group. Clinical evaluation of recombinant human platelet-derived growth factor for the treatment of lower extremity diabetic ulcers. *J Vasc Surg* 1995;21:71–81.
31. Wieman TJ, Smiell JM, Su Y. Efficacy and safety of a topical gel formulation of recombinant human platelet-derived growth factor-BB (Becaplermin) in patients with chronic neuropathic diabetic ulcers. *Diabetes Care* 1998;21:822–827.
32. Holloway G, Steed D, DeMarco M, et al. A randomized controlled dose response trial of activated platelet supernatant, topical CT-102 in chronic, non-healing diabetic wounds. *Wounds* 1993;5:198–206.
33. Doctor N, Pandya S, Supe A. Hyperbaric oxygen therapy in diabetic foot. *J Postgrad Med* 1992;38:112–114.
34. Faglia E, Favales F, Aldeghi A, et al. Adjunctive systemic hyperbaric oxygen therapy in treatment of severe prevalently ischemic diabetic foot ulcer. *Diabetes Care* 1996;19:1338–1343.
35. Kessler L, Bilbault P, Ortega F, et al. Hyperbaric oxygenation accelerates the healing rate of nonischemic chronic diabetic foot ulcers: a prospective randomized study. *Diabetes Care* 2003;26:2378–2382.

Dereck Hunt
Assistant Professor of Medicine

Hertzel Gerstein
Professor of Medicine
McMaster University
Hamilton, Ontario
Canada

Competing interests: None declared.

Glycaemic control in type 1 diabetes

Search date September 2003

Amaryllis Campbell

QUESTIONS

INTERVENTIONS

Key Messages

Interventions in adolescents

- **Educational interventions (compared with controls)** We found no systematic review or RCTs evaluating a specific type of education or using HbA1c as the only method for measuring glycated haemoglobin. One systematic review found that, compared with controls, different educational and psychosocial interventions in adolescents with type 1 diabetes produced a small improvement in quality of life and glycated haemoglobin (measured using a variety of methods). However, most of the RCTs in the review were small studies, most of the interventions lacked any theoretical basis, and many of the outcome measures were not validated or standardised. We found no systematic review or RCTs evaluating the effects of education in adolescents with type 1 diabetes on the incidence of hypoglycaemia, diabetic ketoacidosis, neuropsychological impairment, weight gain, or fluid retention.
- **Different frequencies of insulin administration** We found no systematic review or RCTs specifically evaluating the effects of frequency of insulin administration in adolescents with type 1 diabetes for the outcomes of rate of rise of glycated haemoglobin (measured as HbA1c), quality of life, incidence of and mortality from hypoglycaemia or diabetic ketoacidosis, weight gain, fluid retention, neuropsychological impairment, or all cause mortality.

- **Different frequencies of self blood glucose monitoring** We found no systematic review or RCTs specifically evaluating the effects of frequency of self blood glucose monitoring in adolescents with type 1 diabetes for the outcomes of rate of rise of glycated haemoglobin (measured as HbA1c), quality of life, incidence of and mortality from hypoglycaemia or diabetic ketoacidosis, weight gain, fluid retention, neuropsychological impairment, or all cause mortality.
- **Intensive treatment programmes (compared with conventional treatment programmes)** We found no systematic review or RCTs specifically in adolescents comparing intensive treatment programmes with conventional treatment programmes for the outcomes of rate of rise of glycated haemoglobin (measured as HbA1c), quality of life, incidence of and mortality from hypoglycaemia or diabetic ketoacidosis, weight gain, fluid retention, neuropsychological impairment, or all cause mortality.

Interventions in adults

- **Continuous subcutaneous insulin infusion (compared with multiple daily subcutaneous insulin injections)** One crossover RCT found that, compared with multiple daily subcutaneous injections of a quick acting insulin analogue insulin aspart, delivery of insulin aspart by continuous subcutaneous infusion improved glycated haemoglobin levels (measured as HbA1c) and quality of life scores at 16 weeks in people with type 1 diabetes and longstanding poor glycaemic control. This RCT found more episodes of mild hypoglycaemia per patient week with continuous subcutaneous infusion but found no significant difference in incidence of severe hypoglycaemia at 16 weeks. Another RCT found no significant difference at 9 months between continuous subcutaneous infusion of insulin lispro and multiple daily injections of insulin lispro in glycated haemoglobin (measured as HbA1c), quality of life scores, or hypoglycaemia in people with type 1 diabetes previously receiving two or more insulin injections a day. The potential disadvantages of continuous subcutaneous insulin infusion include the risk of diabetic ketoacidosis owing to disconnection or malfunction of the pump and infection.
- **Intensive treatment programmes (compared with conventional treatment programmes)** One RCT identified by a systematic review and two RCTs found that, compared with conventional treatment programmes, intensive treatment programmes reduced glycated haemoglobin levels at follow up varying from 1 to 10 years. The two RCTs reported different findings on quality of life measures and hypoglycaemia. One RCT found no significant difference between intensive and conventional treatment programmes in diabetes related quality of life but found an increase in incidence of severe hypoglycaemia with intensive treatment programmes. The other RCT found that, compared with conventional treatment, intensive treatment improved diabetes dependent quality of life but found no significant difference in the perceived frequency of hypoglycaemia. One systematic review found that compared with conventional treatment, intensive treatment increased hypoglycaemia, diabetic ketoacidosis (when the treatment programme involved the use of insulin pumps), and mortality associated with acute complications of intensive treatment but found no significant difference in all cause mortality.
- **Different frequencies of self blood glucose monitoring** We found no systematic review or RCTs specifically evaluating the effects of frequency of self blood glucose monitoring in adults with type 1 diabetes for the outcomes of rate of rise of glycated haemoglobin (measured as HbA1c), quality of life, incidence of and mortality from hypoglycaemia or diabetic ketoacidosis, weight gain, fluid retention, neuropsychological impairment, or all cause mortality.
- **Educational interventions (compared with controls)** One RCT identified by a systematic review found no significant difference in glycated haemoglobin (measured as HbA1c) levels at 18 months between education in self monitoring of blood glucose, self management education, or usual care but was incompletely reported and may have lacked power to detect clinically important differences. We found no systematic review or RCTs specifically comparing the effects of group versus individual educational interventions or secondary care versus primary care educational interventions in adults with type 1 diabetes for the outcomes of interest. Given the nature of type 1 diabetes and the central importance of self management of the

condition, all individuals with type 1 diabetes will have received some education at diagnosis; most studies of the effects of education will therefore be examining the impact of subsequent educational interventions. It may be difficult to separate out the effects of individual components of what typically will be a complex package of care, including elements of education, self management training, psychological support, and optimisation of insulin regimes.

DEFINITION The term diabetes mellitus encompasses a group of disorders characterised by chronic hyperglycaemia with disturbances of carbohydrate, fat, and protein metabolism resulting from defects of insulin secretion, insulin action, or both. The World Health Organization definition now recognises diabetes as a progressive disorder of glucose metabolism in which individuals may move between normoglycaemia, impaired glucose tolerance, or impaired fasting glycaemia and frank hyperglycaemia. Type 1 diabetes occurs when the pancreas produces too little insulin or no insulin at all, because of destruction of the pancreatic islet β cells, usually attributable to an autoimmune process. Markers of autoimmune destruction (autoantibodies to islet cells, autoantibodies to insulin, or autoantibodies to both islet cells and insulin, and to glutamic acid decarboxylase) can be found in 85–90% of individuals with type 1 diabetes when fasting diabetic hyperglycaemia is first detected.[1] The definition of type 1 diabetes also includes individuals with β cell destruction who are prone to ketoacidosis but for which no specific cause can be found. However it excludes those forms of β cell destruction for which a specific cause can be found (e.g. cystic fibrosis, pancreatitis, cancer of the pancreas).[2] Type 2 diabetes results from defects in both insulin secretion and insulin action. The risk of type 2 diabetes increases with age and lack of physical activity, and occurs more frequently in individuals with obesity, hypertension, and dyslipidaemia (the metabolic syndrome). It occurs more frequently in women with previous gestational diabetes. There is also evidence of a familial predisposition. Type 2 diabetes is not covered in this chapter. **Diagnosis:** In the presence of symptoms (such as thirst, passing increased volumes of urine, blurring of vision, and weight loss) diabetes may be diagnosed on the basis of a single random elevated plasma glucose ($\geq$ 11.1 mmol/L). In the absence of symptoms the diagnosis should be based on at least one additional blood glucose result in the diabetic range, either from a random sample, or fasting (plasma blood glucose $\geq$ 7.0 mmol/L) or from the oral glucose tolerance test (plasma blood glucose $\geq$ 11.1 mmol/L 2 hours after a 75 g glucose load).[2] **Population:** For the purpose of this chapter, we have included adolescents and adults with type 1 diabetes, but excluded pregnant women and people who are acutely unwell for example after surgery or myocardial infarction.

INCIDENCE/ PREVALENCE It is estimated that slightly more than 218 000 people develop type 1 diabetes worldwide annually, of whom about 40% are children. The incidence varies considerably between populations, with 60 000 new cases occurring annually in Europe, 45 000 new cases in the South East Asian region, 36 000 new cases in North America, and the lowest number of new cases, 6,900 annually, in the African region.[3] There seems to be a worldwide increase in the incidence of type 1 diabetes in both high and low incidence populations.[4] The prevalence of type 1 diabetes is currently estimated as 5.3 million people worldwide, and also varies between populations, reflecting both the variation in incidence rates and differing population structures and mortality.[3]

AETIOLOGY/ RISK FACTORS Two main aetiological forms of type 1 diabetes are recognised. Autoimmune diabetes mellitus results from autoimmune mediated destruction of the β cells of the pancreas. The rate of destruction varies, but all individuals with this form of diabetes eventually become dependent on insulin for survival. Peak incidence of autoimmune diabetes is during childhood and adolescence but it may occur at any age. There is a genetic predisposition and people with this type of diabetes may have other autoimmune disorders.[5] Certain viruses have been associated with β cell destruction, including rubella, Coxsackie B, and cytomegalovirus. Other environmental factors are probably also contributory, but these are poorly defined and understood. Idiopathic diabetes (in which the cause is unidentified) is more common in individuals of African and Asian origin.[2]

PROGNOSIS Untreated, most people with type 1 diabetes, particularly those with autoimmune diabetes mellitus, will experience increasing blood glucose levels, progressing to ketoacidosis or non-ketotic hyperosmolar states resulting in coma and death. The course of idiopathic diabetes may be more varied with some people experiencing permanent lack of insulin and a tendency to ketoacidosis, although in others the requirement for insulin treatment may fluctuate.[2] However most people with type 1 diabetes require insulin for survival, and are described as insulin dependent. The long term effects of diabetes include retinopathy, nephropathy, and neuropathy. Individuals with diabetes mellitus are also at increased risk of cardiovascular, cerebrovascular, and peripheral vascular disease. Good glycaemic control can reduce the risk of developing diabetic complications.[6]

AIMS OF INTERVENTION To control blood glucose levels; to maximise quality of life; to prevent diabetic emergencies, such as ketoacidosis. To maintain HbA1c levels within the target range in order to slow disease progression and to reduce risk of micro- and macrovascular complications. To minimise adverse effects of treatment.

OUTCOMES **Primary outcomes:** Change in glycated haemoglobin (measured as HbA1c); quality of life; incidence of and mortality from hypoglycaemia; incidence of and mortality from diabetic ketoacidosis; weight gain; fluid retention; neuropsychological impairment. **Secondary outcomes:** all cause mortality; change in glycated haemoglobin (not measured as HbA1c). **Excluded outcomes:** Long term outcomes such as development of retinopathy, nephropathy, neuropathy, and cardiovascular disease.

METHODS *Clinical Evidence* search and appraisal September 2003. Studies for inclusion were identified by an initial search for systematic reviews and meta-analyses. Where a good quality systematic review was available a further search was conducted for RCTs from the date of the review only. Where a meta-analysis had not been performed the individual RCTs identified by the review were re-appraised and their results reported individually. Some identified RCTs were excluded owing to short follow up time (< 12 weeks for studies with HbA1c as primary outcome, < 12 months for studies of educational or behavioural modification), incomplete follow up (< 80%), or unclear reporting of methodology (especially for studies of educational interventions). Measuring glycated haemoglobin HbA1c is now the standard method for monitoring glycaemic control. Therefore, studies using measures of glycaemic control other than HbA1c have only been included where studies using HbA1c as a measure for glycated haemoglobin are unlikely to be conducted. Crossover trials were included only if results were reported at the end of the initial treatment period before crossover. Reference lists were searched for further systematic reviews or RCTs not identified by the initial search. Educational interventions are defined as interventions, single, or multiple, that provide information, self management programmes, or both. Interventions primarily focused on the organisational aspects of delivery of care have been excluded. Educational interventions for adults and adolescents have been considered separately, as adolescents are generally acknowledged to have different educational needs from adults and poorer glycaemic control. Studies testing the effects of multiple intervention programmes without an education component have been excluded.

QUESTION **What are the effects of interventions in adolescents with type 1 diabetes?** New

OPTION **INTENSIVE TREATMENT PROGRAMMES IN ADOLESCENTS** New

We found no systematic review or RCTs specifically in adolescents comparing intensive treatment programmes with conventional treatment programmes for the outcomes of rate of rise of glycated haemoglobin (measured as HbA1c), quality of life, incidence of and mortality from hypoglycaemia or diabetic ketoacidosis, weight gain, fluid retention, neuropsychological impairment, or all cause mortality.

Benefits: We found no systematic review or RCTs specifically evaluating the effects of multiple intervention programmes with an education component in adolescents with type 1 diabetes for the outcomes of interest.

Harms: We found no systematic review RCTs in adolescents for the clinical outcomes of interest.

Comment: Glycaemic control typically worsens in adolescence, owing to a combination of physical and psychological change and development (see comments on educational interventions, p 698). Although in theory the complex changes that occur in adolescence might best be addressed through multiple intervention programmes which combine an educational element with behavioural training, psychosocial support, and intensification of treatment, it may in practice be difficult to engage some adolescents in such programmes.

OPTION EDUCATION IN ADOLESCENTS New

We found no systematic review or RCTs evaluating a specific type of education or using HbA1c as the only method for measuring glycated haemoglobin. One systematic review found that, compared with controls, different educational and psychosocial interventions in adolescents with type 1 diabetes produced a small improvement in quality of life and glycated haemoglobin (measured using a variety of methods). However, most of the RCTs in the review were small studies, most of the interventions lacked any theoretical basis, and many of the outcome measures were not validated or standardised. We found no systematic review or RCTs evaluating the effects of education in adolescents with type 1 diabetes on the incidence of hypoglycaemia, diabetic ketoacidosis, neuropsychological impairment, weight gain, or fluid retention.

Benefits: **Educational interventions versus controls:** We found no systematic review or RCTs evaluating a specific type of education or method of delivery. We found one systematic review (search date 1999), which evaluated the effects of different educational and psychosocial interventions in adolescents with type 1 diabetes and included studies using different measurements for glycated haemoglobin levels and quality of life.[7] The authors of this review conducted meta-analyses using effect sizes. The review found that, compared with controls, educational interventions produced a small improvement in quality of life (8 RCTs, data on total number of people and age range not availabl; mean effect size 0.37, 95% CI 0.19 to 0.55). The authors state that in the behavioural sciences, effect sizes of about 0.2 would be considered small, 0.5 to be medium, and those greater than 0.8 to be large. The review also found that, compared with controls, educational interventions reduced glycated haemoglobin (12 RCTs, 573 adolescents mean age range 9.0–14.5 years; mean effect size +0.33, 95% CI –0.04 to +0.70 equivalent to a reduction in HbA1c of 0.6%; P value not reported).[7] Most of the RCTs identified by this systematic review were small studies, lacking sufficient power to detect small to medium effect sizes. They were characterised by a wide variety of interventions and a lack of standardised or validated outcome measures. Most of them were conducted in the USA, and their findings may not be generalisable to other populations or settings. We found no systematic review or RCTs in adolescents with type 1 diabetes for other clinical outcomes of interest.

Harms: **Educational interventions versus controls:** One systematic review did not report any data on adverse events or outcomes.[7]

Comment: Adolescents are generally acknowledged to have different educational needs to adults. Adolescence has also been shown to be associated with a worsening of glycaemic control and the onset and progression of complications of diabetes. Although some of this deterioration may be because of the physiological changes of puberty some is undoubtedly because of changes in self care behaviour.[7] Educational interventions seem to have the potential to improve outcomes in adolescence but there is little evidence on which to base recommendations about specific educational approaches in terms of their content or setting.

OPTION DIFFERENT FREQUENCIES OF SELF BLOOD GLUCOSE MONITORING IN ADOLESCENTS New

We found no systematic review or RCTs specifically evaluating the effects of frequency of self blood glucose monitoring in adolescents with type 1 diabetes for the outcomes of rate of rise of glycated haemoglobin (measured as HbA1c), quality of life, incidence of and mortality from hypoglycaemia or diabetic ketoacidosis, weight gain, fluid retention, neuropsychological impairment, or all cause mortality.

Benefits: We found no systematic review or RCTs specifically evaluating the effects of frequency of self blood glucose monitoring in adolescents with type 1 diabetes for clinical outcomes of interest.

Harms: We found no systematic review RCTs in adolescents for the clinical outcomes of interest.

Comment: Maintaining blood glucose levels as close to the normal range as possible has been shown to delay or reduce the onset of long term complications of diabetes in adults, and frequent blood glucose monitoring, in conjunction with other elements of an intensive treatment programme, has been shown to improve glycaemic control.[6] However it is well recognised that adolescence is a time when metabolic control typically worsens as young people start to take responsibility for managing their own diabetes. Frequent blood glucose monitoring may not be a priority for young people developing a more independent and less structured lifestyle and wanting to fit in with their peer group. Currently there is little good evidence on which to base advice to adolescents about the optimum frequency of self blood glucose monitoring.

OPTION DIFFERENT FREQUENCIES OF INSULIN ADMINISTRATION IN ADOLESCENTS New

We found no systematic review or RCTs specifically evaluating the effects of frequency of insulin administration in adolescents with type 1 diabetes for the outcomes of rate of rise of glycated haemoglobin (measured as HbA1c), quality of life, incidence of and mortality from hypoglycaemia or diabetic ketoacidosis, weight gain, fluid retention, neuropsychological impairment, or all cause mortality.

Benefits: We found no systematic review or RCTs specifically evaluating the effects of frequency of insulin administration in adolescents with type 1 diabetes for the outcomes of interest.

Harms: We found no systematic review RCTs in adolescents for the clinical outcomes of interest.

Comment: Adolescence is a period of rapid physical and psychological change when insulin regimes are likely to need reviewing and adapting in order to maintain good glycaemic control. However we were unable to find good quality data on the risks and benefits of different frequency insulin regimes in adolescents.

QUESTION What are the effects of interventions in adults with type 1 diabetes? New

OPTION INTENSIVE TREATMENT PROGRAMMES IN ADULTS New

One RCT identified by a systematic review and two RCTs found that, compared with conventional treatment programmes, intensive treatment programmes reduced glycated haemoglobin levels at follow up varying from 1 to 10 years.

The two RCTs reported different findings on quality of life measures and hypoglycaemia. One RCT found no significant difference between intensive and conventional treatment programmes in diabetes related quality of life but found an increase in incidence of severe hypoglycaemia with intensive treatment programmes. The other RCT found that, compared with conventional treatment, intensive treatment improved diabetes dependent quality of life but found no significant difference in the perceived frequency of hypoglycaemia. One systematic review found that compared with conventional treatment, intensive treatment increased hypoglycaemia, diabetic ketoacidosis (when the treatment programme involved the use of insulin pumps), and mortality associated with acute complications of intensive treatment but found no significant difference in all cause mortality.

Benefits: **Intensive treatment programmes versus conventional treatment programmes:** We found one systematic review (search date 2002),[8] one additional RCT,[6,9] and one subsequent RCT.[10] The systematic review identified one RCT comparing intensive treatment programmes versus controls (see below).[11] The RCT found that, compared with controls, intensive treatment programmes significantly reduced HbA1c levels at 1.5, 3.0, 5.0, 7.5, and 10.0 years (102 people, mean age 31 ± 7.4 years, attending an outpatient clinic; mean reduction in HbA1c *v* controls: 1.5% at 1.5 years, figures extrapolated from graph, no SEM given; 1.6 ± 0.1% at 3.0 years; 1.5 ± 0.1% at 5.0 years; 1.4 ± 0.7% at 7.5 years; 1.1 ± 0.6% at 10.0 years; $P < 0.01$ for all outcomes).[11] People in the intensive treatment programme were recommended multiple insulin injections and frequent blood glucose monitoring with goals for home blood glucose levels set individually, and an overall target HbA1c of 7%. Telephone contact was made every 2 weeks or more frequently initially if needed, with review in the clinic every 2 months. People in the control group were advised to monitor their blood glucose and adjust their insulin to achieve lower blood glucose levels; the goal of treatment was to reduce blood glucose without giving rise to serious hypoglycaemia. The additional RCT, which did not use HbA1c as a measure for glycated haemoglobin, found that, compared with conventional treatment regimens, intensive treatment significantly reduced glycated haemoglobin (1 RCT, 1441 people mean age 27 ± 7 years: median of all quarterly HbA1 values for year 9 of the study: 7.0% with intensive treatment regimens *v* 9.2% with conventional treatment; $P < 0.001$).[6] The RCT found no significant difference in quality of life between intensive and conventional treatment programmes as assessed by the Diabetes Quality of Life Measure (DQOL), the Symptom Checklist-90R, the Medical Outcome Study 36 Item Short Form Survey (SF-36), and intercurrent psychosocial events.[9] Intensive treatment programme consisted of multiple daily injections of insulin or continuous subcutaneous insulin infusion, with the dosage adjusted according to the results of blood glucose self monitoring performed at least four times daily, dietary intake, and anticipated exercise, in order to meet pre-set blood glucose targets. Conventional treatment consisted of one or two subcutaneous insulin injections daily, daily self monitoring of urine or blood glucose, and education about diet and exercise. People in the intensive treatment group were seen at their study centre every month and contacted more frequently by telephone to review and adjust their treatment; people in the conventional treatment group were seen and examined every 3 months. The subsequent RCT compared immediate insulin dose adjustment training to enable dietary freedom (Dose Adjustment for Normal Eating [DAFNE] training) with a waiting list control group attending insulin dose adjustment training 6 months later.[10] DAFNE training consisted of a 5 day training course providing people with the skills to match insulin dose to desired carbohydrate intake on a meal by meal basis. The RCT found that, compared with delayed training in insulin dose adjustment to enable dietary freedom, immediate insulin dose adjustment training significantly improved HbA1c levels and led to a small improvement in diabetes dependent quality of life at 6 months and the improvement was maintained at 1 year (1 RCT, 169 adults with type 1 diabetes and moderate or poor glycaemic control defined as HbA1c 7.5–12%, mean age 40 years; improvement in HbA1c at 6 months: mean difference between groups 1.0%, 95% CI 0.5% to 1.4%; $P < 0.0001$; improvement in HbA1c at 12 months: mean difference between groups 0.5%, 95% CI 0.2% to 0.9%; $P = 0.001$; mean difference between groups in Diabetes Quality Of Life scale at 6 months: 0.4, 95% CI –0.1 to +0.9; $P < 0.01$; at 12 months: quantitative values not reported; on the Diabetes Quality of Life scale possible scores range from –9 = maximum negative impact of diabetes to +9 = maximum positive impact of diabetes).[10]

Harms: **Intensive treatment programmes versus usual care:** One systematic review (search date 2002)[8] did not report any quantified data on harms of intensive treatment programmes. One RCT identified by the review found that, compared with controls, a higher proportion of people receiving intensive treatment experienced at least one hypoglycaemic episode at 3 and 5 year follow up (1 RCT, 102 people, mean age 31 ± 7.4 years, attending an outpatient clinic; proportion of people experiencing at least 1 hypoglycaemic episode at 3 years: 57% with intensive treatment *v* 23% with controls; $P < 0.01$; at 5 years: 77% with intensive treatment *v* 56% with controls; $P < 0.05$; at 10 years: 86% with intensive treatment *v* 73% with controls; P values and absolute numbers not reported).[11] This RCT also reported on the proportion of people experiencing diabetic ketoacidosis (at 7.5 years: 1 episode of diabetic ketoacidosis with intensive treatment *v* 2 episodes with controls; at 10 years: 1 episode of diabetic ketoacidosis with education *v* 4 episodes with controls; P values not reported). No data on mortality were reported.[11] One additional RCT found an increased incidence of severe hypoglycaemia with intensive treatment compared with control treatment (1 RCT, 1441 people, mean age 27 ± 7 years; 62 hypoglycaemic episodes in which assistance was required per 100 patient years with intensive treatment *v* 19 hypoglycaemic episodes per 100 patient years with control treatment; $P < 0.001$).[6] The RCT found no significant difference between intensive and control treatment in the event rate for diabetic ketoacidosis (2.0 episodes per 100 patient years with intensive treatment *v* 1.8 episodes per 100 patient years with conventional treatment; $P > 0.7$), measures of neuropsychological impairment or all cause mortality (7 deaths with intensive treatment *v* 4 deaths with control treatment; P value not reported).[6] Over a 9 year study period, the RCT found an excess weight gain of 4.75 kg with intensive treatment compared with control treatment, with about half the excess weight gain occurring in the first year (3.3 kg weight gain with intensive treatment *v* 1.2 kg weight gain with control treatment; $P < 0.0001$).[12] The subsequent RCT comparing immediate insulin dose adjustment training to enable dietary freedom (Dose Adjustment for Normal Eating [DAFNE] training) with a waiting list control group attending insulin dose adjustment training 6 months later found no significant difference in the perceived frequency of hypoglycaemia between the two groups (1 RCT, 169 adults with type 1 diabetes and moderate or poor glycaemic control defined as HbA1c 7.5–12.0%, mean age 40 years; mean difference in perceived hypoglycaemia score –0.23, 95% CI –0.68 to +0.21; $P = 0.31$, on a scale of 0–6 where higher scores indicate a higher perceived frequency of hypoglycaemia).[10] This RCT did not report on other outcomes of interest. We also found a second systematic review (search date 1995, 14 RCTs, which included the additional RCT above, 1028 adults with type 1 diabetes randomised to intensive treatment and 1039 to conventional treatment) that conducted meta-analyses for adverse outcomes of intensive treatment in people with type 1 diabetes.[13] The systematic review found that, compared with conventional treatment, intensive treatment significantly increased the risk of hypoglycaemia (14 RCTs, 2067 people, combined odds ratio for hypoglycaemia 2.99, 95% CI 2.45 to 3.64; P < 0.0001)[13] and of diabetic ketoacidosis (14 RCTs, 2067 people, combined OR 1.74, 95% CI 1.27 to 2.38, P = 0.0003).[13] The review found a higher risk of diabetic ketoacidosis with intensive treatment involving insulin pumps compared with conventional treatment (8 RCTs, 311 people, OR 7.20, 95% CI 2.95 to 17.58; P < 0.0001), no significant difference between intensive treatment involving multiple insulin injection compared with conventional treatment (1 RCT, 102 people, plus 3 RCTs, 148 people, where no episodes of diabetic ketoacidosis occurred, OR 1.13, 95% CI 0.15 to 8.35; P = 0.09), and no significant difference between intensive treatment where a choice was offered between insulin pumps and multiple insulin injections compared with conventional treatment (3 RCTs, 1511 people, OR 1.28, 95% CI 0.90 to 1.83; P = 0.17).[13] The systematic review found no significant difference in all cause mortality between conventional treatment and intensive treatment (14 RCTs, 2067 people, OR 1.40, 95% CI 0.65 to 3.02; P = 0.39) but found a significant increase in mortality that was potentially associated with acute complications of intensive treatment (7 deaths with intensive treatment *v* 0 deaths with conventional treatment, 5 deaths attributed to diabetic ketoacidosis and 2 sudden deaths in young people, OR not defined; P = 0.007).[13] We found no systematic review or RCTs reporting on the effects of intensive treatment programmes on fluid retention.

Comment: The additional RCT (Diabetes Control and Complications Trial) provided convincing evidence of the benefits of intensive insulin treatment in improving glycaemic control, although the intervention group also received intensive education, monitoring, and follow up so that improvements in glycaemic control may not be attributable solely to the effects of intensified insulin treatment.[6] The results, which represent a large investment of time and resources in a secondary care setting, may not be reproducible outside the study setting, or in primary care. Most intensive interventions to improve glycaemic control are likely to involve modification of treatment as well as an educational programme and training in self management. The outcome of studies testing intensive treatment programmes suggest that they may be more effective than interventions which are more narrowly focused on intensification of treatment or education alone. However, better glycaemic control is associated with higher rates of hypoglycaemia, which may not be acceptable to some people with type 1 diabetes, although the Diabetes Control and Complications Trial did not find any difference in quality of life for intensively treated people compared with those receiving conventional treatment.

OPTION EDUCATION IN ADULTS New

One RCT identified by a systematic review found no significant difference in glycated haemoglobin (measured as HbA1c) levels at 18 months between education in self monitoring of blood glucose, self management education, or usual care but was incompletely reported and may have lacked power to detect clinically important differences. We found no systematic review or RCTs specifically comparing the effects of group versus individual educational interventions or secondary care versus primary care educational interventions in adults with type 1 diabetes for the outcomes of interest. Given the nature of type 1 diabetes and the central importance of self management of the condition, all individuals with type 1 diabetes will have received some education at diagnosis; most studies of the effects of education will therefore be examining the impact of subsequent educational interventions. It may be

difficult to separate out the effects of individual components of what typically will be a complex package of care, including elements of education, self management training, psychological support, and optimisation of insulin regimes.

Benefits: **Educational interventions versus controls:** We found one systematic review (search date 2002)[8] that identified one RCT specifically assessing the effects of education alone.[14] The RCT identified by the review found no significant difference in HbA1c levels at 18 months between education in self monitoring of blood glucose, self management education, or usual care (1 RCT, 37 adults aged > 17 years, attending an outpatient clinic; mean reduction in HbA1c: 2.1% with education plus self blood glucose monitoring *v* 2.0% with self monitoring of blood glucose alone *v* 2% with education alone *v* 0.8% with usual care). The RCT was incompletely reported and may have been underpowered to detect clinically important differences.[14] We found no systematic review or RCTs comparing the effects of group education versus controls, group education versus individual education, or secondary care versus primary care based education in adults with type 1 diabetes for the outcomes of interest.

Harms: **Educational interventions versus controls:** One RCT identified by a systematic review did not report any data on the incidence of hypoglycaemia, diabetic ketoacidosis, or all cause mortality for education in self monitoring of blood glucose, self management education, or usual care.[14]

Comment: Given the nature of type 1 diabetes and the central importance of self management of the condition, all individuals with type 1 diabetes will have received some education at diagnosis; most studies of the effects of education will therefore be examining the impact of subsequent educational interventions. We found few studies examining the effects of an education programme only, perhaps because of the difficulty of separating out one element of what typically will be a complex package of care, including elements of education, self management training, psychological support, and optimisation of insulin regimes. The effects of intensive multiple intervention programmes are considered separately. Education in groups might seem to offer advantages in terms of cost, time, and mutual support for group members but we were unable to find any good quality evidence either for or against group education.

OPTION DIFFERENT FREQUENCIES OF SELF BLOOD GLUCOSE MONITORING IN ADULTS New

We found no systematic review or RCTs specifically evaluating the effects of frequency of self blood glucose monitoring in adults with type 1 diabetes for the outcomes of rate of rise of glycated haemoglobin (measured as HbA1c), quality of life, incidence of and mortality from hypoglycaemia or diabetic ketoacidosis, weight gain, fluid retention, neuropsychological impairment, or all cause mortality.

Benefits: We found no systematic review or RCTs specifically evaluating the effects of frequency of self blood glucose monitoring in adults with type 1 diabetes. For the outcomes of rate of rise of glycated haemoglobin (measured as HbA1c), quality of life, incidence of and mortality from hypoglycaemia or diabetic ketoacidosis, weight gain, fluid retention, neuropsychological impairment, or all cause mortality.

Harms: We found no systematic review or RCTs specifically evaluating the effects of frequency of blood glucose monitoring in adults with type 1 diabetes for the outcomes of interest.

Comment: One RCT (the Diabetes Control and Complications Trial; see benefits of intensive treatment programmes, p 700) has established the effectiveness of frequent blood glucose monitoring (4 tests/day) as part of an intensive package of care that included intensive insulin treatment, the self adjustment of treatment in line with pre-set blood glucose targets, and monthly clinic visits with telephone review between visits. It did not aim to assess the effectiveness of intensive blood glucose monitoring in isolation. Although regular self monitoring of blood glucose is recommended to people with type 1 diabetes there are no reliable data on which to base advice about optimum frequency of self blood glucose testing.

OPTION CONTINUOUS SUBCUTANEOUS INSULIN INFUSION New

One crossover RCT found that, compared with multiple daily subcutaneous injections of a quick acting insulin analogue insulin aspart, delivery of insulin aspart by continuous subcutaneous infusion improved glycated haemoglobin levels (measured as HbA1c) and quality of life scores at 16 weeks in people with type 1 diabetes and longstanding poor glycaemic control. This RCT found more episodes of mild hypoglycaemia per patient week with continuous subcutaneous infusion but found no significant difference in incidence of severe hypoglycaemia at 16 weeks. Another RCT found no significant difference at 9 months between continuous subcutaneous infusion of insulin lispro and multiple daily injections of insulin lispro in glycated haemoglobin (measured as HbA1c), quality of life scores, or hypoglycaemia in people with type 1 diabetes previously receiving two or more insulin injections a day. The potential disadvantages of continuous subcutaneous insulin infusion include the risk of diabetic ketoacidosis owing to disconnection or malfunction of the pump and infection.

Benefits: **Continuous subcutaneous insulin infusion versus multiple daily subcutaneous insulin injections:** We found two RCTs.[15,16] One crossover RCT found that, compared with multiple daily subcutaneous injections of a quick acting insulin analogue insulin aspart, delivery of insulin aspart by continuous subcutaneous infusion significantly improved glycated haemoglobin levels (measured as HbA1c) and quality of life scores at 16 weeks in people with type 1 diabetes and longstanding poor glycaemic control (1 crossover RCT, 79 people aged 18–70 years with HbA1c > 8.5% in the preceding 6 months; mean difference in HbA1c between continuous subcutaneous infusion and multiple daily subcutaneous injections at first crossover, –0.84%, 95% CI –1.3% to –0.36%; P = 0.002; quality of life scores using SF-36 for general health: +5.9 with continuous subcutaneous infusion *v* –1.2 with multiple daily subcutaneous injections; P = 0.048; quality of life scores using SF-36 for mental health: +5.2 with continuous subcutaneous infusion *v* –0.6 with multiple daily subcutaneous injections; P = 0.05).[15] The second RCT found no significant difference between continuous subcutaneous infusion of insulin lispro and multiple daily injections of insulin lispro in glycated haemoglobin (measured as HbA1c) or quality of life scores at 9 months in people with type 1 diabetes previously receiving two or more insulin injections a day (1 RCT, 27 people aged 18–60 years with diabetes for at least 2 years; overall baseline adjusted treatment effect for HbA1c between continuous subcutaneous infusion and multiple daily injection +0.08%, 95% CI –0.23 to +0.39; P > 0.10; mean difference between continuous subcutaneous insulin infusion and multiple daily insulin injections for quality of life scores using the Diabetes Quality of Life Scale: Satisfaction subscale +7.2, 95% CI –3.4 to +17.9; P > 0.10; Impact subscale +1.6, 95% CI –4.6 to +7.7; P > 0.10; Diabetic worry subscale +5.4, 95% CI –6.7 to + 17.6; P > 0.10; Social worry subscale –4.3, 95% CI

−18.8 to +10.1; P > 0.10; Global health subscale +0.9, 95% CI −12.7 to +14.4; P > 0.10; overall difference using MANOVA not significant, P > 0.10).[16] We found no systematic review or RCTs evaluating the effects of continuous subcutaneous insulin infusion for other clinical outcomes of interest.

Harms: **Continuous subcutaneous insulin infusion versus multiple daily subcutaneous insulin injections:** One RCT found no significant difference in the incidence of severe hypoglycaemia, defined as hypoglycaemia requiring help from another person, at 16 weeks in people treated with a quick acting insulin analogue, insulin aspart, by continuous subcutaneous insulin infusion compared with delivery of insulin aspart by multiple daily subcutaneous injection (1 crossover RCT, 79 people aged 18–70 years; number of severe hypoglycaemic episodes 3/39 [8%] with continuous subcutaneous infusion *v* 6/40 [15%] with multiple daily subcutaneous injections; P = 0.48). However, the RCT also found that a higher proportion of people experienced mild hypoglycaemia, defined as a self blood glucose monitoring value of 3.9 mmol/L or less, in the continuous subcutaneous infusion group compared with multiple daily subcutaneous injections group (difference between treatments in episodes of mild hypoglycaemia per patient week: 0.99, 95% CI 0.11 to 1.87; P = 0.028).[15] One episode of ketoacidosis occurred in both groups and change in weight was similar in both groups (change in weight: 0.60 ± 2.94 kg with continuous subcutaneous infusion group *v* 0.88 ± 2.74 kg with multiple daily subcutaneous injections; P = 0.68).[15] The second RCT found no significant difference in the rate of reported hypoglycaemia over 9 months in people treated with insulin lispro by continuous subcutaneous infusion compared with multiple daily injections of insulin lispro (1 RCT, 27 people aged 18–60 years; mean number of hypoglycaemic events: 8.0 with continuous subcutaneous infusion *v* 7.4 with multiple daily injections; P > 0.10).[16]

Comment: The Diabetes Control and Complications Trial (see benefits of intensive treatment programmes, p 700) demonstrated the benefits of intensive insulin treatment in improving glycaemic control and reducing the incidence of long term complications of diabetes. However, there are potential short term disadvantages to intensive insulin treatment in terms of the need for multiple injections, an increased risk of hypoglycaemia, and, in the case of continuous subcutaneous insulin infusion, the potential hazards, and inconvenience associated with the pump itself (diabetic ketoacidosis owing to disconnection or malfunction of the pump, infection, siting of the device, etc). The available evidence suggests that intensive treatment does not significantly impair quality of life in the short to medium term, but data about longer term and less common outcomes, especially with regard to continuous subcutaneous insulin infusion are lacking.

REFERENCES

1. Verge CF, Gianini R, Kawasaki E, et al. Predicting type I diabetes in first-degree relatives using a combination of insulin, GAD, and ICA512bdc/IA-2 autoantibodies. *Diabetes* 1996;45:926–933.
2. World Health Organization. *Definition, diagnosis and classification of diabetes mellitus and its complications: report of a WHO consultation*. 1999. Geneva.
3. International Diabetes Federation. *Diabetes atlas*. 2000.
4. Onkamo P, Vaananen S, Karvonen M, et al. Worldwide increase in incidence of Type I diabetes – the analysis of the data on published incidence trends. *Diabetologia* 1999;42:1395–1403.
5. Betterle C, Zanette F, Pedini B, et al. Clinical and subclinical organ-specific autoimmune manifestations in type 1 (insulin-dependent) diabetic patients and their first-degree relatives. *Diabetologia* 1984;26:431–436.
6. The Diabetes Control and Complications Trial Research Group. The effect of intensive treatment of diabetes on the development and progression of long-term complications in insulin-dependent diabetes mellitus. *New Engl J Med* 1993;329:977–986.
7. Hampson SE, Skinner TC, Hart J, et al. Effects of educational and psychosocial interventions for adolescents with diabetes mellitus: a systematic review. *Health Technol Assess* 2001;5:No10.
8. Loveman E, Cave C, Green C, et al. The clinical and cost-effectiveness of patient education models for diabetes: a systematic review and economic evaluation. *Health Technol Assess* 2003;7:No22.

9. The Diabetes Control and Complications Trial Research Group. Influence of intensive diabetes treatment on quality-of-life outcomes in the Diabetes Control and Complications Trial. *Diabetes Care* 1996;19:195–203.
10. DAFNE Study Group. Training in flexible, intensive insulin management to enable dietary freedom in people with type 1 diabetes: dose adjustment for normal eating (DAFNE) randomised controlled trial. *BMJ* 2002;325:746–749.
11. Reichard P, Britz A, Cars I, et al. The Stockholm Diabetes Intervention Study (SDIS): 18 months' results. *Acta Med Scand* 1988;224:115–122.
12. The Diabetes Control and Complications Trial Research Group. Influence of intensive diabetes treatment on body weight and composition of adults with type 1 diabetes in the Diabetes Control and Complications Trial. *Diabetes Care* 2001;24:1711–1721.
13. Egger M, Davey Smith G, Stettler C, et al. Risks of adverse effects of intensified treatment in insulin-dependent diabetes mellitus: a meta-analysis. *Diabet Med* 1997;14:919–928.
14. Terent A, Hagfall O, Cederholm U. The effect of education and self-monitoring of blood glucose on glycosylated hemoglobin in type I diabetes. A controlled 18-month trial in a representative population. *Acta Med Scand* 1985;217:47–53.
15. DeVries JH, Snoek FJ, Kostense PJ, et al. A randomized trial of continuous subcutaneous insulin infusion and intensive injection therapy in type 1 diabetes for patients with long-standing poor glycemic control. *Diabetes Care* 2002;25:2074–2080.
16. Tsui E, Barnie A, Ross S, et al. Intensive insulin therapy with insulin lispro: a randomized trial of continuous subcutaneous insulin infusion versus multiple daily insulin injection. *Diabetes Care* 2001;24:1722–1727.

Amaryllis Campbell
General Practitioner
Arun Adur and Worthing PCT
UK

Competing interests: None declared.

Obesity

Search date April 2004

David E Arterburn, David E DeLaet, and David R Flum

QUESTIONS

INTERVENTIONS

DRUG TREATMENTS IN OBESE ADULTS

Trade off between benefits and harms

Diethylpropion 714
Fluoxetine 715
Mazindol 714
Orlistat 715
Phentermine 713
Sibutramine alone 711

Unknown effectiveness

Sibutramine plus orlistat (insufficient evidence to compare with sibutramine alone) 711

SURGERY IN MORBIDLY OBESE ADULTS

Likely to be beneficial

Gastric bypass (increased weight loss compared with gastroplasty or gastric banding) 719
Laparoscopic bariatric surgery (reduced wound infections and risk of incisional hernias compared with open bariatric surgery, no significant difference in weight loss) 721

Trade off between benefits and harms

Bariatric surgery (more effective for clinically important weight loss in morbidly obese adults than non-surgical treatment but operative complication rates common) 717

Unknown effectiveness

Biliopancreatic diversion (no studies comparing biliopancreatic diversion versus other bariatric techniques) 721
Gastric banding (less effective in reducing weight than gastric bypass; insufficient evidence to assess benefits and harms compared with gastroplasty) . . 718
Gastroplasty (less effective in reducing weight than gastric bypass; insufficient evidence to assess benefits and harms compared with gastric banding) 721

To be covered in future updates

Ephedra

Covered elsewhere in *Clinical Evidence*

Lifestyle interventions to achieve weight loss in the general population: see changing behaviour, p 89

See glossary G

Key Messages

Drug treatments in obese adults

- **Diethylpropion** One systematic review found that, in people having lifestyle interventions, diethylpropion promoted modest weight loss compared with placebo in obese adults. The review provided insufficient evidence to compare diethylpropion versus other agents. We found two case reports describing pulmonary hypertension and psychosis with diethylpropion. We found insufficient evidence on weight regain and long term safety. A European Commission review concluded that a link between diethylpropion and heart and lung problems could not be excluded.
- **Fluoxetine** One systematic review found that, in people having lifestyle interventions, fluoxetine promoted modest weight loss compared with placebo in obese adults. We found insufficient evidence on weight regain and long term safety of fluoxetine in obesity. One systematic review of antidepressant treatment found an association between selective serotonin reuptake inhibitors such as fluoxetine and uncommon but serious adverse events, including bradycardia, bleeding, granulocytopenia, seizures, hyponatraemia, hepatotoxicity, serotonin syndrome, and extrapyramidal effects.
- **Mazindol** One systematic review found that, in people having lifestyle interventions, mazindol promoted modest weight loss compared with placebo in obese adults. The review provided insufficient evidence to compare mazindol versus other agents. We found one case report of pulmonary hypertension diagnosed 1 year after stopping treatment with mazindol. We found one case series of mazindol in people with stable cardiac disease that reported cardiac events such as atrial fibrillation and syncope. We found insufficient evidence on weight regain and long term safety.
- **Orlistat** Systematic reviews and subsequent RCTs found that, in people on a low calorie diet, orlistat modestly increased weight loss at 6–12 months compared with placebo in obese adults, in both those who did and who did not have diabetes, hyperlipidaemia, and hypertension. One RCT in obese people with hypercholesterolaemia found that orlistat plus fluvastatin increased weight loss compared with orlistat or fluvastatin alone. Another RCT found that orlistat was less effective than sibutramine in achieving weight loss. Adverse effects such as oily spotting from the rectum, flatulence, and faecal urgency occurred in a high proportion of people taking orlistat. We found insufficient evidence on weight regain and long term safety.
- **Phentermine** One systematic review found that, in people having lifestyle interventions, phentermine promoted modest weight loss compared with placebo in obese adults. RCTs identified by the review provided insufficient evidence to compare phentermine versus other agents. We found insufficient evidence on weight regain and long term safety with phentermine. A European Commission review concluded that a link between phentermine and heart and lung problems could not be excluded.
- **Sibutramine alone** Systematic reviews and subsequent RCTs found that, in people having dietary interventions with or without exercise, sibutramine promoted modest weight loss at 8 weeks, 6 months, and 1 year compared with placebo in obese adults, in both those who did and who did not have diabetes, hypertension, hyperlipidaemia, or binge eating disorder. RCTs in obese adults who had lost weight by taking sibutramine found limited evidence that sibutramine was more effective than placebo for weight maintenance. Other RCTs found that weight regain occurred when sibutramine was discontinued. One RCT found that sibutramine achieved greater weight loss than orlistat or metformin. RCTs provided insufficient evidence to compare sibutramine versus other agents. Sibutramine was temporarily suspended from the market in Italy for use in obesity because of concerns about severe adverse reactions, including arrhythmias, hypertension, and two deaths resulting from cardiac arrest. Two RCTs found no significant difference in the incidence of valvular heart disease between sibutramine and placebo, although these trials may have lacked power to detect a clinically important difference.
- **Sibutramine plus orlistat (insufficient evidence to compare with sibutramine alone)** One RCT provided insufficient evidence to compare sibutramine plus orlistat versus sibutramine alone.

Surgery in morbidly obese adults

- **Gastric bypass (increased weight loss compared with gastroplasty or gastric banding)** RCTs provided moderate evidence that gastric bypass promoted greater weight loss than either gastroplasty or gastric banding. Five RCTs identified by a systematic review found that gastric bypass increased weight loss compared with horizontal gastroplasty. Two RCTs identified by the review found that gastric bypass increased weight loss at 1–3 years compared with vertical banded gastroplasty but another two RCTs found no significant difference between the procedures. One small RCT identified by the review found limited evidence of greater weight loss with gastric bypass than with gastric banding or vertical banded gastroplasty. Another small RCT identified by the review found that gastric bypass increased the proportion of people with 50% weight loss at 18 months compared with vertical banded gastroplasty or gastrogastrostomy. Perioperative mortalities were similar for these procedures. Postoperative complications were common and varied by type of procedure performed.
- **Laparoscopic bariatric surgery (reduced wound infections and risk of incisional hernias compared with open bariatric surgery, no significant difference in weight loss)** Five RCTs found no significant difference in weight loss between open and laparoscopic bariatric procedures. The RCTs found consistent evidence that laparoscopic surgery reduced the incidence of wound and incisional hernia complications compared with open surgery. They found more limited evidence that laparoscopic procedures decreased length of hospital stay compared with open procedures; but data are insufficient to draw conclusions about other complication rates.
- **Bariatric surgery (more effective for clinically important weight loss in morbidly obese adults than non-surgical treatment but operative complication rates common)** One RCT and one cohort study in morbidly obese adults identified by three systematic reviews found that bariatric surgery (horizontal gastroplasty, vertical banded gastroplasty, gastric bypass, or gastric banding) was more effective than non-surgical treatment in increasing weight loss in people with morbid obesity. The cohort study found that, on average, bariatric surgery for obesity resulted in weight losses of 25–44 kg after 1–2 years (compared with matched participants who did not have surgery) and sustained weight loss of 20 kg up to 8 years later. The risk of death from bariatric surgery is estimated to be 0–1.5%. Operative and postoperative complications are common and vary with the type of bariatric procedure performed. The reviews identified no RCTs and we found no observational studies of sufficient quality comparing biliopancreatic diversion versus non-surgical treatment.
- **Biliopancreatic diversion (no studies comparing biliopancreatic diversion versus other bariatric techniques)** Three systematic reviews identified no RCTs and we found no observational studies of sufficient quality comparing biliopancreatic diversion versus other bariatric procedures.
- **Gastric banding (less effective in reducing weight than gastric bypass; insufficient evidence to assess benefits and harms compared with gastroplasty)** One small RCT identified by a systematic review found limited evidence that gastric banding was less effective than gastric bypass in reducing weight. Two RCTs found inconclusive results regarding weight loss with gastric banding compared with vertical banded gastroplasty. There were no postoperative deaths in either RCT. Postoperative complications were common and varied by type of procedure performed. There is insufficient evidence to recommend one procedure over the other.
- **Gastroplasty (less effective in reducing weight than gastric bypass; insufficient evidence to assess benefits and harms compared with gastric banding)** Two RCTs found inconclusive results regarding weight loss with vertical banded gastroplasty compared with gastric banding. Five RCTs identified by a systematic review found that horizontal gastroplasty was less effective than gastric bypass for

increasing weight loss. Four RCTs identified by the review found that vertical banded gastroplasty was less effective than gastric bypass in increasing weight loss at 1–3 years but another two RCTs found no significant difference between the procedures. Perioperative mortalities were similar for these procedures. Postoperative complications were common and varied by type of procedure performed. There is insufficient evidence to recommend one procedure over another.

DEFINITION Obesity is a chronic condition characterised by an excess of body fat. It is most often defined by the body mass index**G** (BMI), a mathematical formula that is highly correlated with body fat. BMI is weight in kilograms divided by height in metres squared (kg/m^2). Worldwide, adults with BMIs between 25–30 kg/m^2 are categorised as overweight, and those with BMIs above 30 kg/m^2 are categorised as obese.[1,2] Nearly 5 million US adults used prescription weight loss medication between 1996 and 1998. A quarter of users were not overweight. Inappropriate use of prescription medication is more common among women, white people, and Hispanic people.[3] The National Institutes of Health in the USA has issued guidelines for obesity treatment, which indicate that all obese adults (BMI > 30 kg/m^2) and all adults with a BMI of 27 kg/m^2 or more and concomitant risk factors or diseases are candidates for drug treatment.[1] Morbidly obese adults (BMI > 40 kg/m^2) and all adults with a BMI of 35 kg/m^2 or more and concomitant risk factors are candidates for bariatric surgery.

INCIDENCE/ PREVALENCE Obesity has increased steadily in many countries since 1900. In the UK in 2001, it was estimated that 21% of men and 24% of women were obese.[4] In the past decade alone, the prevalence of obesity in the USA has increased from 22.9% between 1988 and 1994, to 30.5% between 1999 and 2000.[5]

AETIOLOGY/ RISK FACTORS Obesity is the result of long term mismatches in energy balance where daily energy intake exceeds daily energy expenditure.[6] Energy balance is modulated by a myriad of factors, including metabolic rate, appetite, diet, and physical activity.[7] Although these factors are influenced by genetic traits, the increase in obesity prevalence in the past few decades cannot be explained by changes in the human gene pool, and is more often attributed to environmental changes that promote excessive food intake and discourage physical activity.[7,8] Less commonly, obesity may also be induced by drugs (e.g. high dose glucocorticoids), or be secondary to a variety of neuroendocrine disorders such as Cushing's syndrome and polycystic ovary syndrome.[9]

PROGNOSIS Obesity is a risk factor for several chronic diseases, including hypertension, dyslipidaemia, diabetes, cardiovascular disease, sleep apnoea, osteoarthritis, and some cancers.[1] The relationship between increasing body weight and mortality is curvilinear, where mortality is highest among adults with very low body weight (BMI**G** < 18.5 kg/m^2) and among adults with the highest body weight (BMI > 35 kg/m^2).[2] Results from five prospective cohort studies and 1991 national statistics suggest that the number of annual deaths attributable to obesity among US adults is about 280 000.[10] Obese adults also have more annual admissions to hospitals, more outpatient visits, higher prescription drug costs, and worse health related quality of life than normal weight adults.[11,12]

AIMS OF INTERVENTION To achieve realistic gradual weight loss, and prevent the morbidity and mortality associated with obesity, without undue adverse effects.

OUTCOMES Reduction in mortality; adverse effects of treatment. We found no studies that assessed the primary outcome of reduction in mortality associated with obesity. Proxy measures assessed in studies included mean weight loss (kg), proportion of people losing 5% or more of baseline body weight, and proportion of people maintaining weight loss.

METHODS *Clinical Evidence* search and appraisal April 2004. We did not perform a search for observational studies of bariatric surgery. However, we have included all observational studies of bariatric surgery identified by systematic reviews. We have excluded RCTs with greater than 30% loss to follow up unless they performed an intention to treat analysis. However, such RCTs may be included in the meta-analyses of systematic reviews. Two systematic reviews[13,14] and two cohort studies[15,16] of bariatric surgery were published after the search date of our review. They are mentioned in the comments and will be reported in full in the next issue of *Clinical Evidence*.

QUESTION What are the effects of drug treatments in adults with obesity?

OPTION SIBUTRAMINE

Systematic reviews and subsequent RCTs found that, in people having dietary interventions with or without exercise, sibutramine promoted modest weight loss at 8 weeks, 6 months, and 1 year compared with placebo in obese adults, in both those who did and who did not have diabetes, hypertension, hyperlipidaemia, or binge eating disorder. RCTs in obese adults who had lost weight by taking sibutramine found limited evidence that sibutramine was more effective than placebo for weight maintenance. Other RCTs found that weight regain occurred when sibutramine was discontinued. One RCT found that sibutramine achieved greater weight loss than orlistat or metformin. RCTs provided insufficient evidence to compare sibutramine versus other agents or sibutramine plus orlistat versus sibutramine alone. Sibutramine was temporarily suspended from the market in Italy for use in obesity because of concerns about severe adverse reactions, including arrhythmias, hypertension, and two deaths resulting from cardiac arrest. Two RCTs found no significant difference in the incidence of valvular heart disease between sibutramine and placebo, although these trials may have lacked power to detect a clinically important difference.

Benefits: **Sibutramine versus placebo:** We found one systematic review (search date 2002, 29 RCTs in people with body mass index**G** 25–40 kg/m^2, some with diabetes, hypertension, hyperlipidaemia, or binge eating disorder)[17] and one subsequent RCT.[18] The review meta-analyzed data for groups of RCTs with similar study duration, method of analysis, and duration of follow up.[17] All of the meta-analyses found that sibutramine significantly increased weight loss compared with placebo. The review found that sibutramine 10–15 mg daily significantly increased weight loss at 8–12 weeks compared with placebo (7 RCTs, 546 people; WMD –2.78 kg, 95% CI –3.29 kg to –2.26 kg). Trials of 16–24 weeks' duration, all comparing sibutramine 10–15 mg daily versus placebo, were meta-analyzed in three subgroups because of significant heterogeneity among the trials in methods of analysis. The weighted mean difference in weight loss between sibutramine and placebo ranged from –3.43 kg, 95% CI –4.50 to –2.36 to –6.03 kg, 95% CI –7.36 to –4.70 kg; people who completed the trial had the greatest weight loss. The review also found that sibutramine 10–15 mg daily significantly increased weight loss at 45–54 weeks compared with placebo (5 RCTs, 2188 people; WMD –4.45 kg, 95% CI –5.29 to –3.62 kg). The review found similar rates of weight loss in trials that specifically recruited obese adults with type 2 diabetes mellitus, hypertension, or hyperlipidaemia and trials in obese adults who did not have co-morbidities.[17] The subsequent RCT (60 obese adults with binge eating disorder) compared sibutramine 15 mg daily versus placebo for 12 weeks.[18] It found that sibutramine significantly increased weight loss at 12 weeks compared with placebo (7.4 kg weight loss with sibutramine *v* 1.4 kg weight gain with placebo; $P < 0.001$). One RCT identified by the review assessed sibutramine for weight maintenance.[17] Participants with greater than 5% weight loss at the completion of 6 months' treatment with sibutramine 10 mg daily were randomised to continue to receive sibutramine 10–20 mg daily or placebo for 18 months (467 people). The RCT was limited by only 56% follow up at 2 years. It found that sibutramine maintained significantly more weight loss at 2 years compared with placebo (WMD –4.0 kg, 95% CI –5.6 kg to –2.4). Two RCTs identified by the review assessed weight regain after discontinuation of treatment in people who had successful weight loss after 6 months' treatment with sibutramine. People regained 43% of lost body weight at

6 months (40 people) and 55% of lost body weight at 18 months (115 people).[17] **Sibutramine versus orlistat or metformin:** We found no systematic review but found one RCT (150 obese women) comparing three treatments: sibutramine 20 mg daily; orlistat (120 mg 3 times daily); and metformin (850 mg twice daily) for 6 months.[19] All people were also instructed to follow a reduced calorie diet of 25 kcal/kg of ideal body weight. The RCT found that sibutramine achieved greater weight loss than either orlistat or metformin (–13.0 kg with sibutramine *v* –8.0 kg with orlistat *v* –9.0 kg with metformin; sibutramine *v* orlistat and sibutramine *v* metformin $P < 0.0001$). **Sibutramine versus other agents:** We found one systematic review (search date 1999), which identified no RCTs comparing sibutramine versus diethylpropion, fluoxetine, mazindol, orlistat, or phentermine.[20] **Sibutramine plus orlistat:** We found no systematic review but found one RCT (34 women who had completed 1 year of sibutramine plus lifestyle modification), which compared sibutramine 10–15 mg daily plus orlistat (120 mg 3 times daily) versus sibutramine plus placebo for weight maintenance.[21] Only 76% of the women completed the study. Mean body weight did not change significantly in either group over a 16 week period (+0.1 kg with sibutramine plus orlistat *v* +0.5 kg with sibutramine plus placebo).

Harms: **Sibutramine versus placebo:** We found one systematic review[17] and two additional RCTs[22,23] that assessed adverse effects of sibutramine. The review found that sibutramine increased blood pressure (mean increase: systolic blood pressure: –0.2 mm Hg at 8–12 weeks, range from –1.6 to +5.6 mm Hg at 16–24 weeks in several RCTs, and range from +4.6 mm Hg at 44–54 weeks; diastolic blood pressure: range from +1.6 mm Hg at 8–12 weeks, –0.8 to +1.7 mmHg at 16–24 weeks, and +2.8 mm Hg at 44–54 weeks in several RCTs).[17] It also found that sibutramine significantly increased heart rate compared with placebo (increase in heart rate: 1.3 beats/minute at 8–12 weeks, 0.75–5.9 beats/minute at 16–24 weeks, and 5.9 beats/minute at 44–54 weeks).[17] Sibutramine was also associated with increased levels in total and low density lipoprotein cholesterol levels at 16–24 weeks compared with placebo (increase in total cholesterol: –1.9 to +1.8 mg/dL; increase in low density lipoprotein cholesterol 0.6 to 2.6 mg/dL); but no increase at 44–54 weeks.[17] Common adverse effects were headache, nausea, constipation, insomnia, and dry mouth, occurring in 20.4% of people taking sibutramine compared with 3.4% of people on placebo ($P < 0.01$).[17] We found two RCTs that assessed the effects of sibutramine on heart valve function.[22,23] Both of these RCTs may have been too small to detect clinically important adverse effects. The first RCT (210 obese people) compared sibutramine versus placebo for 12 months.[22] It found no significant difference in the incidence of valvular disease between sibutramine and placebo (3/133 [2.3%] with sibutramine 15–20 mg/day *v* 2/77 [2.6%] with placebo; OR 0.87, 90% CI 0.19 to 3.97). The trial did not report on efficacy. The second RCT (184 obese people) compared sibutramine 10 or 20 mg daily versus placebo.[23] It reported no change in valvular appearance on echocardiogram in any group (no statistical comparisons between or within groups reported).[23] We found no evidence about adverse effects after more than 1 year of treatment. Sibutramine was temporarily suspended from the market in Italy in March 2002 in response to 50 reported adverse reactions, including seven severe adverse reactions (tachycardia, hypertension, and arrhythmia) and two deaths resulting from cardiac arrest. The Central European Committee for Proprietary Medicinal Products (CPMP) completed a review of sibutramine in June 2002, and concluded that the risk benefit profile of sibutramine remains in favour of benefit; it therefore lifted the suspension in August 2002.[24] To date, searches of the websites of other regulatory authorities, including the Medicines Control Agency, UK; the Food and Drug Administration, USA;

Health, Canada; and the Therapeutics Goods Administration, Australia, found that no other countries have taken any regulatory actions against the drug. **Sibutramine versus orlistat or metformin:** The RCT reported dry mouth, insomnia, constipation, and hypertension with sibutramine, and abdominal discomfort with orlistat and metformin.[19] **Sibutramine versus other agents:** The systematic review gave no information on adverse effects.[20] **Sibutramine plus orlistat:** The RCT found that people who received sibutramine plus orlistat experienced more soft stools, bowel movements, oily evacuation, and more faecal urge than sibutramine alone (soft stools: 50.0% with sibutramine plus orlistat *v* 9.1% with sibutramine alone; increased frequency of bowel movements: 50.0% with sibutramine plus orlistat *v* 9.1% with sibutramine alone; oily evacuation: 42.9% with sibutramine plus orlistat *v* 0% with sibutramine alone; more faecal urgency: 42.9% with sibutramine plus orlistat *v* 9.1% with sibutramine alone).[21]

Comment: Most of the people treated with sibutramine received additional dietary interventions, and many also have received an exercise intervention. The review suggested that weight loss with sibutramine is associated with both positive and negative changes in cardiovascular and metabolic risk factors.[17] Sibutramine has been associated with increases in systolic and diastolic blood pressure, heart rate, and total as well as low density lipoprotein cholesterol; it has conversely been associated with modest decreases in triglyceride levels, fasting serum glucose levels, glycosylated haemoglobin levels, and modest increases in high density lipoprotein cholesterol levels.[17]

OPTION PHENTERMINE

One systematic review found that, in people having lifestyle interventions, phentermine promoted modest weight loss compared with placebo in obese adults. RCTs identified by the review provided insufficient evidence to compare phentermine versus other agents. We found insufficient evidence on weight regain and long term safety with phentermine. A European Commission review concluded that a link between phentermine and heart and lung problems could not be excluded.

Benefits: **Phentermine versus placebo:** We found one systematic review (search date 1999, 6 RCTs, 368 people) comparing phentermine 15–30 mg daily versus placebo in obese adults, with mean follow up of 13.2 weeks (range 2–24 weeks).[20] The review found that phentermine produced significantly more weight loss than placebo (effect size: < 0.6 [information presented graphically]; mean difference in weight loss between phentermine and placebo in the six RCTs ranged from 0.6–6.0 kg). **Phentermine versus diethylpropion:** The review also found that phentermine significantly increased weight loss compared with diethylpropion (1 RCT, 99 people: mean weight loss 8.3 kg with phentermine *v* 6.3 kg with diethylpropion; effect size: 0.57, CI not reported).[20] **Phentermine versus mazindol:** See benefits of mazindol, p 714. **Phentermine versus other drugs:** The review found no RCTs comparing phentermine versus diethylpropion, fluoxetine, orlistat, or sibutramine.[20]

Harms: The systematic review gave no information on adverse effects.[20] Phentermine given alone has not been associated with valvular heart disease.[25] A European Commission review reported that, although no new safety problems were identified with phentermine, a link between phentermine and heart and lung problems could not be totally excluded.[26]

Comment: Most of the people treated with phentermine received additional lifestyle interventions.[20] High withdrawal rates have been reported for phentermine.

OPTION MAZINDOL

One systematic review found that, in people having lifestyle interventions, mazindol promoted modest weight loss compared with placebo in obese adults. The review provided insufficient evidence to compare mazindol versus other agents. We found one case report of pulmonary hypertension diagnosed 1 year after stopping treatment with mazindol. We found one case series of mazindol in people with stable cardiac disease that reported cardiac events such as atrial fibrillation and syncope. We found insufficient evidence on weight regain and long term safety.

Benefits: **Mazindol versus placebo:** We found one systematic review (search date 1999, 22 RCTs, 906 people) comparing mazindol 1–3 mg daily versus placebo in obese adults with mean follow up of 11 weeks (range 2–20 weeks).[20] The review found that mazindol significantly increased weight loss compared with placebo (effect size: < 0.5; absolute data presented graphically; mean difference in weight loss between mazindol and placebo in the 22 RCTs ranged from 0.1–7.3 kg). **Mazindol versus other drugs:** The review also compared mazindol versus other agents.[20] Three RCTs identified by the review found no significant difference in weight loss between mazindol and diethylpropion (mean 6.7 kg with mazindol *v* 5.1 with diethylpropion; effect size: +0.31, 95% CI –0.07 to +0.69). One RCT identified by the review found that mazindol significantly increased weight loss compared with phentermine (mean 6.7 kg *v* 5.5 kg; effect size: 0.12, CI not reported). The review found no RCTs comparing mazindol versus diethylpropion, fluoxetine, orlistat, or sibutramine.

Harms: The systematic review gave no information on adverse effects.[20] We found a single case report of pulmonary hypertension diagnosed 12 months after stopping mazindol that had been taken for 10 weeks.[27] One case series of mazindol in people with stable cardiac disease reported several cardiac events (3 episodes of atrial fibrillation and 2 of syncope in 15 people receiving mazindol for 12 weeks).[28] The frequency of serious adverse events with this agent remains unclear.

Comment: Most of the people treated with mazindol received additional lifestyle interventions.[20]

OPTION DIETHYLPROPION

One systematic review found that, in people having lifestyle interventions, diethylpropion promoted modest weight loss compared with placebo in obese adults. The review provided insufficient evidence to compare diethylpropion versus other agents. We found two case reports describing pulmonary hypertension and psychosis with diethylpropion. We found insufficient evidence on weight regain and long term safety. A European Commission review concluded that a link between diethylpropion and heart and lung problems could not be excluded.

Benefits: **Diethylpropion versus placebo:** We found one systematic review (search date 1999, 9 RCTs, 353 people) comparing diethylpropion 75 mg daily versus placebo in obese adults with mean follow up of 17.6 weeks (range 6–52 weeks).[20] The review found that diethylpropion significantly increased weight loss compared with placebo (effect size: < 0.55 [information presented graphically]; mean difference in weight loss between diethylpropion and placebo in the 9 RCTs ranged from 1.6–11.5 kg). **Diethylpropion versus mazindol:** See benefits of mazindol, p 714. **Diethylpropion versus phentermine:** See benefits of phentermine, p 713. **Diethylpropion versus other drugs:** The review identified no RCTs comparing diethylpropion versus fluoxetine, orlistat, or sibutramine.[20]

Harms: The systematic review gave no information on adverse effects.[20] Case reports have described pulmonary hypertension and psychosis in users of diethylpropion.[29,30] The frequency of serious adverse events with diethylpropion remains unclear. A European Commission review of the risks and benefits of diethylpropion concluded that randomised trials do not adequately show efficacy for weight loss.[26] Although no new safety problems were identified with diethylpropion, the Commission commented that a link between diethylpropion and heart and lung problems could not be totally excluded.

Comment: Most of the people treated with diethylpropion received additional lifestyle interventions.[20]

OPTION FLUOXETINE

One systematic review found that, in people having lifestyle interventions, fluoxetine promoted modest weight loss compared with placebo in obese adults. We found insufficient evidence on weight regain and long term safety of fluoxetine in obesity. One systematic review of antidepressant treatment found an association between selective serotonin reuptake inhibitors such as fluoxetine and uncommon but serious adverse events, including bradycardia, bleeding, granulocytopenia, seizures, hyponatraemia, hepatotoxicity, serotonin syndrome, and extrapyramidal effects.

Benefits: **Fluoxetine versus placebo:** We found one systematic review (search date 1999, 11 RCTs, 1219 people) comparing fluoxetine 32.5–60.0 mg daily versus placebo in obese adults with mean follow up of 27.5 weeks (range 6–60 weeks).[20] The review found that fluoxetine produced significant weight loss compared with placebo (effect size: < 0.45 [information presented graphically]; mean difference in weight loss between fluoxetine and placebo in the 11 RCTs ranged from 0.2–7.4 kg). **Fluoxetine versus other drugs:** The review identified no RCTs comparing fluoxetine versus diethylpropion, mazindol, orlistat, phentermine, or sibutramine.[20]

Harms: The systematic review gave no information on adverse effects.[20] One older systematic review (search date 1998) of antidepressant treatment (for other indications) found that selective serotonin reuptake inhibitors were associated with a 10–15% incidence of anxiety, diarrhoea, dry mouth, headache, and nausea.[31] The review also found an association between selective serotonin reuptake inhibitors and uncommon but serious adverse events, including bradycardia, bleeding, granulocytopenia, seizures, hyponatraemia, hepatotoxicity, serotonin syndromeⒼ, and extrapyramidal effectsⒼ.

Comment: Most of the people treated with fluoxetine received additional lifestyle interventions.[20]

OPTION ORLISTAT

Systematic reviews and subsequent RCTs found that, in people on a low calorie diet, orlistat modestly increased weight loss at 6–12 months compared with placebo in obese adults, in both those who did and who did not have diabetes, hyperlipidaemia, and hypertension. One RCT in obese people with hypercholesterolaemia found that orlistat plus fluvastatin increased weight loss compared with orlistat or fluvastatin alone. Another RCT found that orlistat was less effective than sibutramine in achieving weight loss. Adverse effects such as oily spotting from the rectum, flatulence, and faecal urgency occurred in a high proportion of people taking orlistat. We found insufficient evidence on weight regain and long term safety.

Benefits: **Orlistat versus placebo:** We found one systematic review (search date 2002),[32] and one subsequent RCT[33] comparing orlistat versus placebo. The review (19 RCTs) meta-analyzed results from RCTs with similar study design, dose of orlistat, and duration of follow up.[32] All of the meta-analyses found that orlistat at all doses significantly increased modest weight loss at 6 months to 1 year compared with placebo. For example, orlistat 60 or 120 mg 3 times daily significantly increased weight loss at 1 year compared with placebo (2 RCTs, 910 people: WMD –2.44 kg, 95% CI –3.40 kg to –1.47 kg with 60 mg; 3 RCTs, 1789 people: WMD –3.19 kg (95% CI –3.98 kg to –2.40 kg with 120 mg). However, the meta-analyses found no significant difference in weight loss at 3 months between orlistat and placebo. For example, one meta-analysis found no significant difference between orlistat 50–60 mg 3 times daily and placebo in weight loss at 3 months (2 RCTs, 133 people: WMD –1.24 kg, 95% CI –2.65 kg to +0.16 kg). Similar beneficial results were found comparing the efficacy of orlistat at greater and lesser durations of treatment. The review performed separate meta-analyses comparing orlistat versus placebo in people with defined obesity related comorbidities such as type 2 diabetes mellitus, hyperlipidaemia, or multiple cardiovascular risk factors (impaired glucose tolerance/diabetes, dyslipidaemia, or hypertension) and found similar results. The subsequent RCT (343 obese people with non-insulin dependent diabetes) found that orlistat (120 mg 3 times daily) significantly increased weight loss compared with placebo at 6 months (mean weight loss: 4.24 kg with orlistat *v* 2.58 with placebo; $P = 0.0003$).[33] The review identified one RCT comparing orlistat versus placebo for weight maintenance.[32] After 6 months of diet alone, people received orlistat (30, 60, or 120 mg 3 times daily) or placebo for 1 year. The RCT found that orlistat 120 mg significantly reduced weight regain at 1 year compared with placebo. However, it found no significant difference in weight regain between orlistat at other doses and placebo (percentage of weight regained: 32.4% with orlistat 120 mg *v* 47.2% with orlistat 60 mg *v* 53.3% with orlistat 30 mg *v* 56.0% with placebo; $P < 0.001$ for orlistat 120 mg *v* placebo, P reported as non-significant for other doses, CI not reported).[32] **Orlistat plus fluvastatin:** We found no systematic review but found one RCT (99 obese people with hypercholesterolaemia) that compared four treatments over 1 year: orlistat (120 mg 3 times daily); fluvastatin (80 mg 4 times daily); orlistat (120 mg 3 times daily) plus fluvastatin (80 mg 4 times daily); and placebo.[34] It found that orlistat plus fluvastatin significantly increased weight loss compared orlistat alone, fluvastatin alone, or placebo (mean weight loss: 11.4 kg with orlistat plus fluvastatin *v* 8.6 kg with orlistat *v* 8.0 kg with fluvastatin *v* 7.6 kg with placebo; $P < 0.05$). **Orlistat plus sibutramine:** See benefits of sibutramine, p 711. **Versus other drugs:** We found one systematic review (search date 1999), which identified no RCTs comparing orlistat versus diethylpropion, fluoxetine, mazindol, phentermine or sibutramine.[20] We found one subsequent RCT comparing orlistat versus sibutramine (see benefits of sibutramine, p 711).[21]

Harms: **Versus placebo:** Gastrointestinal adverse events such as loose stools, increased defaecation, abdominal pain, nausea and vomiting, oily spotting from the rectum, flatulence, and faecal urgency were more common with orlistat than placebo (48–95% with orlistat 120 mg 3 times daily *v* 18–68% with placebo).[32] The first subsequent RCT (343 people with type 2 diabetes mellitus) found that orlistat significantly increased gastrointestinal adverse effects and increased withdrawals because of adverse effects compared with placebo (gastrointestinal effects: 65% with orlistat *v* 37% with placebo; withdrawals: 4.7% with orlistat *v* 2.9% with placebo; P values not reported).[33] **Orlistat plus sibutramine:** See harms of sibutramine, p 712. **Versus sibutramine:** See harms of sibutramine, p 712.

Comment: People treated with orlistat also undertook a low calorie diet.[32] Because of the high rates of gastrointestinal adverse effects associated with orlistat, authors have queried whether blinded evaluation is possible.[21] At the end of a double blinded 16 week trial, 22/26 [85%] people correctly identified their treatment group.

QUESTION **What are the effects of bariatric surgery in adults with morbid obesity?**

OPTION **BARIATRIC SURGERY VERSUS NON-SURGICAL TREATMENT**

One RCT and one cohort study in morbidly obese adults identified by three systematic reviews found that bariatric surgery (horizontal gastroplasty, vertical banded gastroplasty, gastric bypass, or gastric banding) was more effective than non-surgical treatment in increasing weight loss in people with morbid obesity. The cohort study found that, on average, bariatric surgery for obesity resulted in weight losses of 25–44 kg after 1–2 years (compared with matched participants who did not have surgery) and sustained weight loss of 20 kg up to 8 years later. The risk of death from bariatric surgery is estimated to be 0–1.5%. Operative and postoperative complications are common and vary with the type of bariatric procedure performed. The reviews identified no RCTs and we found no observational studies of sufficient quality comparing biliopancreatic diversion versus non-surgical treatment.

Benefits: We found three systematic reviews of bariatric surgery (search dates 2001,[35] 2003[36,37]), all of which identified the same single RCT and multicentre cohort study with matched controls comparing bariatric surgery (horizontal gastroplasty**G**, vertical banded gastroplasty**G**, gastric bypass**G**, or gastric banding**G**) versus non-surgical treatment. The RCT and cohort study both suggested that bariatric surgery was more effective than non-surgical treatment for weight loss in adults with morbid obesity. The RCT (57 adults ≥ 60% overweight) identified by the reviews compared horizontal gastroplasty versus a very low calorie diet (500 kcal, 34 g protein daily) for 24 months. It found that horizontal gastroplasty significantly reduced body weight at 24 months compared with a very low calorie diet (32 kg with gastroplasty *v* 9 kg with very low calorie diet; $P < 0.05$). However, it found no significant difference in the proportion of people who had a net weight loss of 10 kg at 5 years (30% with horizontal gastroplasty *v* 17% with a very low calorie diet; P value reported as non-significant, CI not reported). The multicentre cohort study (2188 people) identified by the reviews[35–37] compared bariatric surgery versus usual care.[38] Eligible participants self selected either a bariatric surgery group or a non-surgical (usual care) group. Each person who selected surgical treatment was matched on 18 clinical variables with a person from the non-surgical group. Each surgeon determined the surgical procedure offered: vertical banded gastroplasty (> 70%), gastric bypass (6%), or gastric banding (23%). Usual care was according to local practice and usually did not include pharmacotherapy. The cohort study found that people who had surgery lost significantly more weight than people receiving usual care at 1 year (mean weight loss: 44.0 kg with gastric bypass [68 people] *v* 30.7 kg with vertical banded gastroplasty [834 people] *v* 25.8 kg with gastric banding [255 people] *v* 1.6 kg with usual care [1031 people]; $P < 0.0001$ for all surgical groups *v* usual care). The differences in weight loss between groups remained significant at 8 years (mean percentage of body weight lost: 16.3% with surgery [232 people] *v* 0.9% weight gained with usual care [251 people]; mean difference in weight 20.7 kg; $P < 0.01$).

Harms: The RCT reported no deaths related to surgery and no-one required re-operation.[35–37] As of 31 January 2001 the cohort study reported five postoperative deaths in 2010 people (0.25%); three deaths owing to leakage, one owing to technical mistake during laparoscopic surgery, and one owing to postoperative myocardial infarction.[38] It reported that 2.2% of people required re-operation. One systematic review evaluated 38 surgical case series of bariatric surgery, which included people with both substantial comorbid conditions and mild health problems, and found that perioperative mortalities were low and similar across bariatric procedures: 0–1.5% among people who received gastric bypass**G**, gastroplasty**G**, or gastric banding**G**.[37] Perioperative complications were common, including: subphrenic abscess (7%), atelectasis or pneumonia (4%), wound infection (4%), and pulmonary symptoms (6.2%).

Comment: The cohort study will not be able to report on total mortality until 2004–2006.[38] Horizontal gastroplasty**G** is less often performed worldwide, because of evidence of greater weight loss and comparable complication rates with gastric bypass**G**. Two systematic reviews were published after the search date of our review.[13,14] These reviews did not identify any additional RCTs comparing bariatric surgery versus non-surgical techniques. Two cohort studies were published after our search date, which compared bariatric surgery versus non-surgical treatment in morbidly obese adults.[15,16] The first study (1035 people having surgery and 5746 having non-surgical treatment) found significantly lower mortality over a mean of 5.3 years in people having surgery compared with people having non-surgical treatment (0.68% with surgery *v* 6.17% with non-surgical treatment; RR 0.11; 95% CI 0.04 to 0.27).[15] The second cohort study (3328 people having surgery and 62 781 having non-surgical interventions) also found significantly lower mortality at 15 years' follow up in people having surgery compared with non-surgical treatment (12% with surgery *v* 16% with non-surgical treatment; adjusted HR 0.67; 95% CI 0.54 to 0.85).[16] This study also found 2% mortality at 30 days in people having surgery.[16]

OPTION GASTRIC BANDING VERSUS OTHER BARIATRIC SURGICAL TECHNIQUES

One small RCT identified by a systematic review found limited evidence that gastric banding was less effective than gastric bypass in reducing weight. Two RCTs found inconclusive results regarding weight loss with gastric banding compared with vertical banded gastroplasty. There were no postoperative deaths in either RCT. Postoperative complications were common and varied by type of procedure performed. There is insufficient evidence to recommend one procedure over the other.

Benefits: **Gastric banding versus gastric bypass:** See benefits of gastric bypass, p 719. **Gastric banding versus vertical banded gastroplasty:** We found one systematic review (search date 2001, 1 RCT)[35] and one subsequent RCT.[39] The RCT (59 adults with body mass index**G** [BMI] ≥ 40 or BMI ≥ 37 with associated comorbidity) identified by the review found that people having gastric banding**G** had smaller weight loss at 1 year compared with people having vertical banded gastroplasty**G** (results not reported), but at 5 years people having gastric banding had lost more weight (43 kg with gastric banding *v* 35 kg with vertical banded gastroplasty; CI not reported).[35] The subsequent RCT (200 adults with BMI 40–50) found that significantly fewer people having gastric banding had an excellent or good result (defined as residual excess weight of < 50%) at 2 years compared with people having vertical banded gastroplasty (35% with gastric banding *v* 74% with vertical banded gastroplasty; P < 0.001) Success rates were lower with gastric banding at 3 years, but the difference did not quite reach significance (25% with gastric banding *v* 63% with vertical banded gastroplasty; P = 0.056).[39]

Harms: **Gastric banding versus gastric bypass:** See harms of gastric bypass, p 720. **Gastric banding versus vertical banded gastroplasty:** The first RCT reported one death from each group during the follow up period but neither death was attributed to the surgery. Re-operations occurred in 33% of people having vertical banded gastroplasty**G** and 10% of people having gastric banding**G**. Gastroesophageal reflux was more common in people having vertical banded gastroplasty compared with people having gastric banding (14.8% with gastroplasty *v* 11.5% with gastric banding).[35] No deaths were reported in the second RCT.[39] It found that gastric banding significantly increased the proportion of people who required re-operation compared with vertical banded gastroplasty (25% with gastric banding *v* 0% with vertical banded gastroplasty; $P < 0.05$). It also found that gastric banding significantly increased late complications, such as pouch dilatation, pouch-to-fundus fistula, symptomatic reflux disease, and gastric bezoar compared with vertical banded gastroplasty (33% with gastric banding *v* 14% with gastroplasty; $P < 0.001$).[39]

Comment: None.

OPTION GASTRIC BYPASS VERSUS OTHER BARIATRIC SURGICAL TECHNIQUES

RCTs provided moderate evidence that gastric bypass promoted greater weight loss than either gastroplasty or gastric banding. Five RCTs identified by a systematic review found that gastric bypass increased weight loss compared with horizontal gastroplasty. Two RCTs identified by the review found that gastric bypass increased weight loss at 1–3 years compared with vertical banded gastroplasty but another two RCTs found no significant difference between the procedures. One small RCT identified by the review found limited evidence of greater weight loss with gastric bypass than with gastric banding or vertical banded gastroplasty. Another small RCT identified by the review found that gastric bypass increased the proportion of people with 50% weight loss at 18 months compared with vertical banded gastroplasty or gastrogastrostomy. Perioperative mortalities were similar for these procedures. Postoperative complications were common and varied by type of procedure performed.

Benefits: We found one systematic review (search date 2001, 9 RCTs, 962 people) comparing gastric bypass**G** versus vertical banded or horizontal gastroplasty**G**.[35] **Gastric bypass versus horizontal gastroplasty:** The review identified five RCTs (384 morbidly obese people) that compared gastric bypass versus horizontal gastroplasty.[35] All of the RCTs found that gastric bypass significantly increased weight loss compared with horizontal gastroplasty. Trials reported an average of 35–42% weight loss with gastric bypass compared with 16–29% with horizontal gastroplasty at 12 months ($P < 0.05$ in all RCTs). **Gastric bypass versus vertical banded gastroplasty, gastric banding, or gastrogastrostomy:** The review identified four RCTs that compared gastric bypass versus vertical banded gastroplasty and two RCTs that compared three interventions.[35] The first RCT (42 adults with body mass index**G** ≥ 40) found that gastric bypass significantly increased weight loss compared with vertical banded gastroplasty at 12 months (percentage weight loss: 78% with gastric bypass *v* 52% with vertical banded gastroplasty: $P < 0.05$). The second RCT (40 adults > 44 kg overweight) also found that gastric bypass significantly increased weight loss compared with vertical banded gastroplasty at 12 months, 2 years, and 3 years (12 months: 68% with gastric bypass *v* 43% with vertical banded gastroplasty; $P < 0.001$; 2 years: 66% with gastric bypass *v* 39% with vertical banded gastroplasty; $P < 0.001$; 3 years: 62% with gastric bypass *v* 37% with vertical banded gastroplasty; $P < 0.001$). The other two RCTs (109 adults, 32 with body mass index ≥ 40) found no significant difference in weight loss between the two procedures at 36 months, 3 years, and 5–6 years. The fifth RCT (77 adults) compared three interventions: gastric bypass, gastric banding**G**, or vertical banded gastroplasty. It found greater mean excess weight loss at 18 months with gastric bypass than with vertical banded gastroplasty or gastric banding (77% with gastric bypass *v* 65% with gastric banding *v* 60% with vertical banded gastroplasty; CI not reported). The sixth RCT (310 people) also compared three procedures: gastric bypass (99 adults), vertical banded gastroplasty (106 adults), or gastrogastrostomy (105 adults). It found that gastric bypass significantly increased the proportion of people who had a successful outcome (defined as 50% weight loss: 67% with gastric bypass *v* 48% with vertical banded gastroplasty *v* 17% with gastrogastrostomy; $P < 0.001$).[35]

Harms: **Gastric bypass versus vertical banded gastroplasty:** Three RCTs comparing gastric bypass**G** versus vertical banded gastroplasty**G** identified by the review reported no deaths.[35] One RCT comparing gastric bypass versus vertical banded gastroplasty reported no deaths in the vertical banded gastroplasty group but two deaths (10%) in the gastric bypass group, occurring after 3 days and 12 months owing to presumed arrhythmia. **Gastric bypass versus horizontal gastroplasty:** Four RCTs comparing gastric bypass versus horizontal gastroplasty identified by the review reported no operative mortality.[35] The fifth RCT reported two deaths: one 6 days after gastroplasty owing to anastomotic leak and cerebrovascular accident and one death within 30 days after gastric bypass owing to pulmonary embolism. The type of postoperative complications differed for these procedures. People having gastric bypass had symptomatic ulcer disease (25%), intractable vomiting and stomal stenosis (25%), marginal ulcers of jejunal side of gastrojejunostomy (5%), cholelithiasis (13%), and peptic gastroesophagitis (33%). People having vertical banded gastroplasty had superficial stomal erosions (5%), cholelithiasis (24%), and peptic gastroesophagitis (18%). One RCT found that significantly more people having gastric bypass had dumping syndrome (28% with gastric bypass *v* 0% with horizontal gastroplasty; $P < 0.05$) or heartburn (59% with gastric bypass *v* 32% with horizontal gastroplasty; $P < 0.05$). Other early and late complications varied little between procedures; however, one RCT reported that 32% of people having gastric bypass and 42% having gastroplasty had some form of postoperative complication.[35] **Gastric bypass versus gastric banding or vertical banded gastroplasty:** The RCT comparing gastric bypass, vertical banded gastroplasty, and gastric banding**G** reported one death (group not specified).[35] One person who had vertical banded gastroplasty required re-operation (4%) for staple disruption, while 44% of people having gastric banding required re-operation for inadequate weight loss, nutritional disorder, or increased vomiting. **Gastric bypass versus vertical banded gastroplasty or gastrogastrostomy:** The RCT comparing gastric bypass, vertical banded gastroplasty, and gastrogastrostomy identified by the review reported two postoperative deaths (groups not specified), one from complications of a subsequent cholecystectomy, and one from carcinoma of the colon.[35] Early and late complication rates were similar among procedures.

Comment: Two systematic reviews were published after our search date, both of which concluded that gastric bypass**G** results in greater weight loss than vertical banded gastroplasty**G**.[13,14]

OPTION GASTROPLASTY VERSUS OTHER BARIATRIC SURGICAL TECHNIQUES

Two RCTs found inconclusive results regarding weight loss with vertical banded gastroplasty compared with gastric banding. Five RCTs identified by a systematic review found that horizontal gastroplasty was less effective than gastric bypass for increasing weight loss. Four RCTs identified by the review found that vertical banded gastroplasty was less effective than gastric bypass in increasing weight loss at 1–3 years but another two RCTs found no significant difference between the procedures. Perioperative mortalities were similar for these procedures. Postoperative complications were common and varied by type of procedure performed. There is insufficient evidence to recommend one procedure over another.

Benefits: **Gastroplasty versus gastric banding:** See benefits of gastric banding, p 718. **Gastroplasty versus gastric bypass:** See benefits of gastric bypass, p 719.

Harms: **Gastroplasty versus gastric banding:** See harms of gastric banding, p 719. **Gastroplasty versus gastric bypass:** See harms of gastric bypass, p 720.

Comment: Two systematic reviews were published after our search date, and these reviews both concluded that vertical banded gastroplasty**Ⓖ** results in less weight loss than gastric bypass**Ⓖ**.[13,14]

OPTION BILIOPANCREATIC DIVERSION VERSUS OTHER BARIATRIC SURGICAL TECHNIQUES

Three systematic reviews identified no RCTs and we found no observational studies of sufficient quality comparing biliopancreatic diversion versus other bariatric procedures.

Benefits: We found three systematic reviews (search dates 2001,[35] 2003[36,37]), which identified no RCTs comparing biliopancreatic diversion**Ⓖ** versus other bariatric surgery techniques.

Harms: We found no RCTs.

Comment: None.

OPTION OPEN VERSUS LAPAROSCOPIC BARIATRIC SURGERY

Five RCTs found no significant difference in weight loss between open and laparoscopic bariatric procedures. The RCTs found consistent evidence that laparoscopic surgery reduced the incidence of wound and incisional hernia complications compared with open surgery. They found more limited evidence that laparoscopic procedures decreased length of hospital stay compared with open procedures; but data are insufficient to draw conclusions about other complication rates.

Benefits: We found one systematic review (search date 2001, 3 RCTs, 256 people with morbid obesity)[35] and two subsequent RCTs[40,41] comparing open versus laparoscopic techniques. **Open versus laparoscopic gastric banding:** The review identified one RCT (50 adults with body mass index**Ⓖ** ≥ 40) that found no significant difference in weight loss between open and laparoscopic gastric banding**Ⓖ** at 12 months (34.4 kg with open *v* 35.0 kg with laparoscopic; P reported as non-significant).[35] **Open versus laparoscopic gastric bypass:** The review identified two RCTs and we found one subsequent RCT that found no significant difference in weight loss at 1 and 2 years between open and laparoscopic gastric bypass**Ⓖ**.[35,40] The first RCT (155 people) identified by the review found no significant difference in weight loss at 1 year (62% with open *v* 68% with laparoscopic; P = 0.07). The second RCT (51 people) identified by the review also found no significant difference in body mass index (BMI) at 1 year (reduction in BMI: 13 kg/m^2 with open *v* 14 kg/m^2 with laparoscopic; reported as non-significant, CI not reported in review). The subsequent RCT (104 people with morbid obesity) found no significant difference in weight loss at a mean 23 months between open and laparoscopic techniques (reported as non-significant, results presented graphically).[40] **Open versus laparoscopic vertical banded gastroplasty:** The review identified no RCTs.[35] One subsequent RCT (30 adults with body mass index 40–50) found similar weight loss between open and laparoscopic vertical banded gastroplasty**G** at 12 months (mean: 55% with open *v* 47% with laparoscopic; CI not reported).[41]

Harms: **Open versus laparoscopic gastric banding:** One of the RCTs reported no deaths.[35] The review found no significant difference in surgical complications between the two procedures (reported as non-significant, CI not reported in the review), although people having open gastric banding**G** had more incisional hernia complications (12% with open *v* 0% with laparoscopic). Re-admissions and overall length of hospital stay were significantly higher in people having open compared with laparoscopic procedures (re-admissions: 60% with open *v* 24% with laparoscopic; hospital stay: 11.8 days with open *v* 7.8 days with laparoscopic; P < 0.05 for both outcomes). **Open versus laparoscopic gastric bypass:** The RCTs reported four postoperative deaths: one owing to malignant hyperthermia, one owing to possible pulmonary thromboembolism (laparoscopic), one owing to intestinal obstruction (laparoscopic), and one owing to evisceration.[35,40] The review found no significant difference between open and laparoscopic bypass in the proportion of people who had major surgical complications (9.2% of people with open *v* 7.6% of people with laparoscopic; P = 0.78).[35] In all three RCTs identified by the review, minor complications (including vomiting, colicky pain, and wound infection) were not significantly different between groups.[35] The subsequent RCT found that open gastric bypass**G** was associated with a significantly higher rate of late complications (including eventrations, abscess, intestinal obstruction, and pancreatitis) compared with laparoscopic bypass (24% with open *v* 11% with laparoscopic; P < 0.05).[40] Operating time was longer for the laparoscopic procedure in two RCTs and longer for the open procedure in one RCT. Hospital stay was significantly shorter for the laparoscopic procedure in all three RCTs (4–8 days with open *v* 3–5 days with laparoscopic; P < 0.05). **Open versus laparoscopic vertical banded gastroplasty:** The RCT reported no deaths.[41] Operating time was significantly longer for the laparoscopic procedure (2.10 hours with open *v* 1.45 hours with laparoscopic; P = 0.002), but average hospital stay was not significantly different (4 days for both techniques). Two people, one in each group, developed a fistula at the gastric partition that required re-operation. Two people having open gastroplasty**G** developed abdominal wall hernias at 12 months.

Comment: One systematic review was published after our search date, which also concluded that laparoscopic procedures result in fewer wound complications or incisional hernias than open procedures.[14]

GLOSSARY

Biliopancreatic diversion There are two different types of biliopancreatic diversion. Standard biliopancreatic diversion surgically removes the lower third of the stomach and then forms a connection with the remaining stomach pouch with a portion a small intestine beyond where the stomach was originally attached. Biliopancreatic diversion with duodenal switch divides the stomach vertically and removes the left half, leaving the connection between the stomach and the duodenum of the small intestine intact. A length of intestine is also removed and the duodenum is reconnected further down the small intestine. The aim is to increase weight loss by reducing calories and decreasing nutrient absorption.

Body mass index (BMI) Expressed as weight in kilograms divided by height in metres squared (kg/m^2). In the USA and UK, individuals with body mass indexes of 25–30 kg/m^2 are considered overweight; those with body mass indexes above 30 kg/m^2 are considered obese.

Extrapyramidal effects Include acute dystonia, a Parkinsonism-like syndrome, and akathisia.

Gastric banding involves placing an adjustable band around the upper portion of the stomach. The band is connected to a reservoir, which the surgeon can tighten or loosen, by the infusion of varying amounts of a saline solution. The newly created upper pouch will only allow the person to consume small amounts of food at a time.

Gastric bypass The roux-en-Y gastric bypass procedure involves dividing the stomach and creating a small pouch, which is then closed using several rows of staples. The remaining portion of the stomach is not removed but is "bypassed" and plays a diminished role in the digestive process. A Y-shaped portion of the small intestine is then attached to the pouch. The volume the new stomach pouch is capable of holding is about 25 g. The aim is to increase weight loss by reducing calories, altering gastrointestinal appetite hormones, and decreasing nutrient absorption.

Gastroplasty Vertical banded gastroplasty involves stapling the front of the stomach to the back of the stomach along a vertical plane, partitioning the stomach into two, unequal parts which connect through a small (about 0.5 cm) opening. This allows the partially digested food to move from the small stomach pouch into the rest of the stomach and then the intestines. The newly created upper pouch will only allow the person to consume small amounts of food at a time.

Serotonin syndrome Clinical features include agitation, ataxia, diaphoresis, diarrhoea, fever, hyper-reflexia, myoclonus, shivering, and changes in mental status. The occurrence and severity of syndrome does not seem to be dose related.

REFERENCES

1. National Institutes of Health. *Clinical guidelines on the identification, evaluation, and treatment of overweight and obesity in adults: the Evidence Report*. Bethesda, Maryland: US Department of Health and Human Services, 1998.
2. World Health Organization. *Obesity: preventing and managing the global epidemic*. Report of a WHO consultation. WHO Technical Series: World Health Organization, 2000; No. 894. Geneva.
3. Khan LK, Serdula MK, Bowman BA, et al. Use of prescription weight loss pills among U.S. adults in 1996–1998. *Ann Intern Med* 2001;134:282–286.
4. Obesity statistics. British Heart Foundation Statistics Website. Source: Health Survey for England 2001. Available at: http://www.dphpc.ox.ac.uk/bhfhprg/ (last accessed 15 November 2004).
5. Flegal KM, Carroll MD, Ogden CL, et al. Prevalence and trends in obesity among US adults, 1999–2000. *JAMA* 2002;288:1723–1727.
6. Schwartz MW, Woods SC, Porte D, et al. Central nervous system control of food intake. *Nature* 2000;404:661–671.
7. Weinsier RL, Hunter GR, Heini AF, et al. The etiology of obesity: relative contribution of metabolic factors, diet, and physical activity. *Am J Med* 1998;105:145–150.
8. French SA, Story M, Jeffery RW. Environmental influences on eating and physical activity. *Annu Rev Public Health* 2001;22:309–335.
9. Bray GA. Obesity: etiology. In: UpToDate, issue 8/1, 2000. Wellesley, MA: UpToDate Inc.
10. Allison DB, Fontaine KR, Manson JE, et al. Annual deaths attributable to obesity in the United States. *JAMA* 1999;282:1530–1538.
11. Quesenberry CP, Caan B, Jacobson A. Obesity, health services use, and health care costs among members of a health maintenance organization. *Arch Intern Med* 1998;158:466–472.
12. Kushner RF, Foster GD. Obesity and quality of life. *Nutrition* 2000;16:947–952.
13. Shekelle PG, Morton SC, Maglione M, et al. Pharmacological and surgical treatment of obesity. Summary, Evidence Report/Technology Assessment No. 103. (Prepared by the Southern California-RAND Evidence-based Practice Center, under Contract No 290-02-0003.) AHRQ Publication No 04-E028-1. Rockville, MD: Agency for Healthcare Research and Quality. July 2004. Search date 2003; primary sources Medline, Cochrane Controlled Clinical Trials Register Database, reference lists of relevant reviews.
14. Buchwald H, Avidor Y, Braunwald E, et al. Bariatric surgery: a systematic review and meta-analysis. *JAMA* 2004;292:1727–1737. Search date 2003; primary sources Medline, Current Contents, the Cochrane Library databases, and manual reference checks of all articles on bariatric surgery published in the English language between 1990–2003.
15. Christou NV, Sampalis JS, Liberman M, et al. Surgery decreases long-term mortality, morbidity, and health care use in morbidly obese patients. *Ann Surg* 2004;240:416–424.
16. Flum DR, Dellinger EP. Impact of gastric bypass operation on survival: a population-based analysis. *J Am Coll Surg* 2004;199:543–551.
17. Arterburn DE, Crane PK, Veenstra DL. The efficacy and safety of sibutramine for weight loss: a systematic review. *Arch Intern Med* 2004;164:994–1003. Search date 2002; primary sources Medline, Embase, the Cochrane Library, Agricola, Biosis previews, Cinahl, Current Contents, International Pharmaceutical Abstracts, the Science Citation Index, the Social Science Citation Index, hand searches of reference lists of all previous reviews of sibutramine, contact with key authors in the field to identify unpublished and ongoing trials,

and with pharmaceutical industry representatives from Abbott Laboratories, North Chicago, Ill, for additional unpublished data.
18. Appolinario JC, Bacaltchuk J, Sichieri R, et al. A randomized, double-blind, placebo-controlled study of sibutramine in the treatment of binge-eating disorder. *Arch Gen Psychiatry* 2003;60:1109–1116.
19. Gokcel A, Gumurdulu Y, Karakose H, et al. Evaluation of the safety and efficacy of sibutramine, orlistat and metformin in the treatment of obesity. *Diabetes Obes Metab* 2002;4:49–55.
20. Haddock CK, Poston WSC, Dill PL, et al. Pharmacotherapy for obesity: a quantitative analysis of four decades of published randomized clinical trials. *Int J Obes* 2002;26:262–273. Search date 1999; primary sources Medline, Psychinfo, hand searches, and personal contact with individual authors.
21. Wadden TA, Berkowitz RI, Womble LG, et al. Effects of sibutramine plus orlistat in obese women following 1 year of treatment by sibutramine alone: a placebo-controlled trial. *Obes Res* 2000;8:431–437.
22. Zannad F, Gille B, Grentzinger A, et al. Effects of sibutramine on ventricular dimensions and heart valves in obese patients during weight reduction. *Am Heart J* 2002;144:508–515.
23. Bach DS, Rissanen AM, Mendel CM, et al. Absence of cardiac valve dysfunction in obese patients treated with sibutramine. *Obes Res* 1999;7:363–369.
24. Health Sciences Authority. Centre for Pharmaceutical Administration. Drug Alerts. Updates Report on Sibutramine. Information page. http://www.hsa.gov.sg/html/business/0000000000000001560.html#1 (last accessed 15 November 2004).
25. Gaasch WH, Aurigemma GP. Valvular heart disease induced by anorectic drugs. In: UpToDate, issue 8/3, 2003. Wellesley, MA: UpToDate Inc.
26. Medicines Control Agency. Committee on Safety in Medicines. Important safety message: European withdrawal of anorectic agents/appetite suppressants: new legal developments, no new safety issues: licences for phentermine and amfepramone being withdrawn May 2001. Information page. http://www.mca.gov.uk/ourwork/monitorsafequalmed/safetymessages/anorectic.htm (last accessed 15 November 2004).
27. Hagiwara M, Tsuchida A, Hyakkoku M, et al. Delayed onset of pulmonary hypertension associated with an appetite suppressant, mazindol: a case report. *Jpn Circ* 2000;64:218–221.
28. Bradley MH, Blum NJ, Scheib RJ. Mazindol in obesity with known cardiac disease: a clinical evaluation. *J Int Med Res* 1974;2:347–349.
29. Thomas SH, Butt AY, Corris PA, et al. Appetite suppressants and primary pulmonary hypertension in the United Kingdom. *Br Heart J* 1995;74:660–663.
30. Little JD, Romans SE. Psychosis following readministration of diethylpropion: a possible role for kindling? *Int Clin Psychopharmacol* 1993;8:67–70.
31. Mulrow CD, Williams JW Jr, Trivedi M, et al. Treatment of depression: newer pharmacotherapies. *Psychopharmacol Bull* 1998;34:409–795. Search date 1998; primary sources the Cochrane Collaboration Depression, Anxiety and Neurosis (CCDAN) Review Group register of trials, and bibliographies of trial and review articles.
32. O'Meara S, Riemsma R, Shirran L, et al. A systematic review of the clinical effectiveness of orlistat used for the management of obesity. *Obes Rev* 2004;5:51–68. Search date 2002; primary sources Amed, Biosis, British Nursing Index, the Cochrane Library, Cinahl, Dare, DH-Data, Econlit, Embase, Helmis, HTA database, Index to Scientific and Technical Proceedings, King's Fund Database, Medline, the National Research Register, NHS Economic Evaluation Database, Office of Health Economics Health Economic Evaluations Database, Science Citation Index, Social Science Citation Index, hand searches of bibliographies of retrieved studies, Internet searches, and contact with experts in the field.
33. Halpern A, Mancini MC, Suplicy H, et al. Latin-American trial of orlistat for weight loss and improvement in glycaemic profile in obese diabetic patients. Diabetes Obes Metab 2003;5:180–188.
34. Derosa G, Mugellini A, Ciccarelli L, et al. Randomized, double-blind, placebo-controlled comparison of the action of orlistat, fluvastatin, or both on anthropometric measurements, blood pressure, and lipid profile in obese patients with hypercholesterolemia prescribed a standardized diet. *Clin Ther* 2003;25:1107–1122.
35. Colquitt J, Clegg A, Sidhu M, et al. Surgery for morbid obesity (Cochrane Review). The Cochrane Library, Issue 1, 2004. Chichester, UK: John Wiley & Sons, Ltd. Search date 2001; primary sources Cochrane Controlled Trials Register, Medline, Pubmed, Embase, Psychinfo, Cinahl, Science and Social Sciences Citation Index, British Nursing Index, Web of Science Proceedings, Biosis, Amed, National Research Register, hand searches of reference lists of relevant articles and journals, and contact with experts in the field.
36. Lefevre F, Aronson N. Special report: the relationship between weight loss and changes in morbidity following bariatric surgery for morbid obesity. *TEC Bulletin* 2003; 18(9). Search date 2003; primary sources Medline, manual reviews of bibliographies of selected references, pertinent Cochrane Reviews and review of Current Contents.
37. McTigue KM, Harris R, Hemphill B, et al. Screening and interventions for obesity in adults: summary of the evidence for the U.S. Preventive Services Task Force. *Ann Intern Med* 2003;139:933–949. Search date 2003; primary sources Medline and the Cochrane Library January 1994 to February 2003.
38. Sjostrom L. *Surgical treatment of obesity: an overview and results from the SOS study*. In: Bray G, Bouchard C, eds. The handbook of obesity: clinical applications, 2nd ed. New York, NY: Marcel Dekker, Inc, 2004;372–376.
39. Morino M, Toppino M, Bonnet G, et al. Laparoscopic adjustable silicone gastric banding versus vertical banded gastroplasty in morbidly obese patients: a prospective randomized controlled clinical trial. *Ann Surg* 2003;238:835–841; discussion 841–842.
40. Lujan JA, Frutos MD, Hernandez Q, et al. Laparoscopic versus open gastric bypass in the treatment of morbid obesity: a randomized prospective study. *Ann Surg* 2004;239:433–437.
41. Davila-Cervantes A, Borunda D, Dominguez-Cherit G, et al. Open versus laparoscopic vertical banded gastroplasty: a randomized controlled double blind trial. *Obes Surg* 2002;12:812–818.

David Arterburn
Assistant Professor of Medicine
University of Cincinnati
Institute for Health Policy
and Health Services Research
and the Cincinnati Department of Veterans
Affairs
Cincinnati
USA

Obesity

David DeLaet
Adjunct Assistant Professor
of Medicine
University of Cincinnati
Department of Internal Medicine
Cincinnati
USA

David Flum
Assistant Professor
University of Washington
Department of Surgery
Seattle
USA

Competing interests: None declared. The views expressed in this article are those of the authors and do not necessarily represent the views of the US Department of Veterans Affairs.

We would like to acknowledge the previous contributors of this chapter, including Polly Hitchcock-Noel and Cynthia Mulrow.

Prevention of cardiovascular events in diabetes

Search date October 2003

Ronald Sigal, Janine Malcolm, and Hilary Meggison

QUESTIONS

INTERVENTIONS

Trade off between benefits and harms

Unknown effectiveness

*No RCT but observational evidence suggests some benefit.

See glossary G

Key Messages

Smoking cessation

- **Smoking cessation** We found no RCTs on promotion of smoking cessation specifically in people with diabetes. Observational evidence and extrapolation from evidence in people without diabetes suggest that promotion of smoking cessation is likely to reduce cardiovascular events.

Blood pressure

- **Antihypertensive treatment (compared with no antihypertensive treatment)** One systematic review and RCTs have found that blood pressure lowering with antihypertensive agents in people with diabetes and hypertension reduces cardiovascular morbidity and mortality compared with no antihypertensive treatment.
- **Lower target blood pressures** Large RCTs including people with diabetes and hypertension have found that control of blood pressure to a target diastolic blood pressure of no more than 80 mm Hg reduces the risk of major cardiovascular events. One RCT in normotensive people with diabetes found that intensive blood pressure lowering reduced cerebral vascular events but found no significant difference in cardiovascular death, myocardial infarction, congestive heart failure, or all cause mortality.
- **Different antihypertensive drugs** Systematic reviews and RCTs have found that angiotensin converting enzyme inhibitors, diuretics, β blockers, and calcium channel blockers all reduce cardiovascular morbidity and mortality in people with diabetes and hypertension. However, there are differences in the types of adverse effects reported with different antihypertensive drugs. RCTs have found that people taking atenolol gained more weight than those taking captopril, an increase in risk of congestive heart failure with lisinopril or amlodipine compared with chlorthalidone, a higher frequency of headache with diltiazem compared with diuretics or β blockers, and a higher rate of withdrawal from treatment because of adverse effects with atenolol compared with losartan.

Dyslipidaemia

- **Statins** One systematic review and RCTs have found that statins reduce cardiovascular morbidity and mortality compared with placebo.
- **Aggressive versus moderate lipid lowering with statins** One RCT found that, compared with usual care, treatment with atorvastatin to achieve a target low density lipoprotein concentration below 2.6 mmol/L (< 100 mg/dL) reduces cardiovascular morbidity and mortality. Another RCT found no significant difference between a lower target low density lipoprotein (1.55–2.20 mmol/L) using lovastatin, along with cholestyramine if necessary, and a moderate target low density lipoprotein (3.36–3.62 mmol/L) in 4 year event rate for myocardial infarction and death.
- **Fibrates** One RCT found that gemfibrozil reduced cardiovascular events over 5 years compared with placebo whereas another smaller RCT found no significant difference. One RCT found that bezafibrate reduced cardiovascular events compared with placebo.
- **Low versus standard statin dose in older people** One RCT found no significant difference in cardiovascular events between low dose pravastatin (5 mg/day) and standard dose pravastatin (10–20 mg/day) over 4 years.

Prevention of cardiovascular events in diabetes

Antiplatelet drugs

- **Adding glycoprotein IIb/IIIa inhibitors to heparin in acute coronary syndromes** We found no RCTs comparing glycoprotein IIb/IIIa inhibitors versus no antiplatelet treatment. One RCT in people presenting with unstable angina or acute myocardial infarction without ST segment elevation found that addition of tirofiban (a glycoprotein IIb/IIIa inhibitor) to heparin reduced the composite outcome of death, myocardial infarction, or refractory ischaemia at 180 days compared with heparin alone. This RCT found no significant difference between tirofiban plus heparin and heparin alone in risk of bleeding in people already taking aspirin.
- **Clopidogrel** We found no RCTs comparing only clopidogrel versus placebo. One RCT in people with diabetes and with recent ischaemic stroke, myocardial infarction, or established peripheral arterial disease found no significant difference between clopidogrel and aspirin at 28 days in cardiovascular events. This RCT also found a lower proportion of people hospitalised for a bleeding event with clopidogrel than with aspirin.
- **Prophylactic aspirin** One systematic review found that, compared with controls, antiplatelet treatment mainly with aspirin did not significantly reduce the combined risk of non-fatal myocardial infarction, non-fatal stroke, death from a vascular cause, or death from an unknown cause in people with diabetes and cardiovascular disease diagnosis. The review found that antiplatelet treatment was associated with an increase in the risk of major extracranial haemorrhage and haemorrhagic stroke, but the results for people with diabetes were not reported separately.
- **Adding clopidogrel to aspirin in acute coronary syndromes** One RCT in people presenting with unstable angina or non-Q-wave myocardial infarction and also taking aspirin found no significant reduction in cardiovascular events after 12 months with addition of clopidogrel compared with placebo. This RCT also found a higher proportion of major bleeds with addition of clopidogrel than with placebo.

Blood glucose control

- **Intensive versus conventional glycaemic control** One systematic review found that, compared with conventional glycaemic control, intensive glycaemic control for more than 2 years reduced the occurrence of first major cardiovascular event in people with type 1 diabetes. Two RCTs found no significant difference in cardiovascular morbidity and mortality with intensive compared with conventional glycaemic control in people with type 2 diabetes. These RCTs also found an increase in weight gain and hypoglycaemic episodes with intensive compared with conventional treatment.
- **Metformin versus diet alone in overweight or obese people with type 2 diabetes** One RCT in overweight or obese people with type 2 diabetes found that intensive treatment with metformin compared with conventional treatment with diet alone reduced myocardial infarction but not stroke over 5 years. This RCT found no significant increase in major hypoglycaemic episodes in the metformin group compared with the diet only group.

Multiple risk factor treatment

- **Intensive multiple risk factor treatment** One RCT found that, compared with conventional treatment according to clinical guidelines, intensive treatment of multiple risk factors with strict treatment goals in people with type 2 diabetes and microalbuminuria reduced cardiovascular disease over 8 years. Multiple risk factor treatment included simultaneously targeting diet, exercise, glycaemic control, blood pressure, treatment of microalbuminuria, and antiplatelet treatment. We found no systematic review or RCTs comparing treatment of multiple risk factors with treatment of a single risk factor for cardiovascular outcomes.

Revascularisation

- **Coronary artery bypass graft (CABG) compared with percutaneous transluminal coronary angioplasty (PTCA)** One systematic review found that, in people with diabetes, CABG reduced all cause mortality at 4 years after initial revascularisation compared with PTCA, but found no significant difference at 6.5 years. One large RCT in people with diabetes and multivessel coronary artery disease has found that CABG reduces mortality or myocardial infarction within 8 years compared with PTCA. Another smaller RCT found a non-significant reduction in mortality with CABG compared with PTCA at 4 years.
- **Stent plus glycoprotein IIb/IIIa inhibitors in people undergoing PTCA** RCTs in people with diabetes undergoing PTCA have found that the combination of stent and a glycoprotein IIb/IIIa inhibitor reduces cardiovascular morbidity and mortality compared with stent plus placebo.
- **CABG compared with PTCA plus stent** One RCT in people with diabetes and multivessel coronary artery disease found no significant difference, at time of discharge, between CABG and PTCA plus stent in cardiovascular morbidity or mortality but found an increase in risk of stroke. However, the same RCT found that, compared with PTCA plus stent, CABG reduced cardiovascular risk at 1 year.
- **PTCA compared with thrombolysis** We found no systematic review or RCTs comparing PTCA versus thrombolysis for prevention of cardiovascular events in people with diabetes. One RCT, in people with diabetes presenting with an acute myocardial infarction, found no significant difference between PTCA and thrombolysis with alteplase in single outcome of death or composite outcome of death, reinfarction, or disabling stroke at 30 days.

DEFINITION **Diabetes mellitus:** See definition under glycaemic control in type 1 diabetes, p 696. **Cardiovascular disease (CVD):** Atherosclerotic disease of the heart and/or the coronary, cerebral, or peripheral vessels leading to clinical events such as acute myocardial infarction**G**, congestive heart failure, sudden cardiac death, stroke, gangrene, and/or need for revascularisation procedures. **Population:** In previous versions of *Clinical Evidence* we attempted to differentiate between primary and secondary prevention in this topic. However, in middle aged and older people with type 2 diabetes this distinction may not be clinically important. We are not aware of any intervention that has been shown to be effective in secondary prevention but ineffective in primary prevention, or vice versa, in people with diabetes. In most cases a large proportion of people with diabetes entered into CVD prevention trials are middle aged and older with additional CVD risk factors, and a large portion of these actually have undiagnosed CVD.

INCIDENCE/ PREVALENCE Diabetes mellitus is a major risk factor for CVD. In the USA, a survey of deaths in 1986 suggested that 60–75% of people with diabetes die from cardiovascular causes.[1] The annual incidence of CVD is increased in people with diabetes (men: RR 2–3; women: RR 3–4, adjusted for age and other cardiovascular risk factors).[2] About 45% of middle aged and older white people with diabetes have evidence of coronary artery disease compared with about 25% of people without diabetes in the same populations. In a Finnish population based cohort study (1059 people with diabetes and 1373 people without diabetes, aged 45–64 years), the 7 year risk of acute myocardial infarction was as high in adults with diabetes without previous cardiac disease (20.2/100 person years) as it was in people without diabetes with previous cardiac disease (18.8/100 person years).[3]

AETIOLOGY/ RISK FACTORS Diabetes mellitus increases the risk of CVD. Cardiovascular risk factors in people with diabetes include conventional risk factors (age, prior CVD, cigarette smoking, hypertension, dyslipidaemia, sedentary lifestyle, family history of premature CVD) and more diabetes specific risk factors (elevated urinary protein excretion, poor glycaemic control). Conventional risk factors for CVD contribute to an increase in the relative risk of CVD in people with diabetes to about the same extent as in those without diabetes. One prospective cohort study (164 women and 235 men with diabetes [mean age 65 years] and 437 women and 1099 men without diabetes [mean age 61 years] followed for mortality for a mean of 3.7 years after acute myocardial infarction) found that significantly more people with diabetes died compared with people without diabetes (116/399 [29%] with diabetes *v* 204/1536 [13%] without diabetes; RR 2.2, 95% CI 1.8 to 2.7).[4] It also found that the mortality risk after myocardial infarction associated with diabetes was higher for women than for men (adjusted HR 2.7, 95% CI 1.8 to 4.2 for women *v* 1.3,

95% CI 1.0 to 1.8 for men). Physical inactivity is a significant risk factor for cardiovascular events in both men and women. Another cohort study (5125 women with diabetes) found that participation in little (< 1 hour/week) or no physical activity compared with physical activity for at least 7 hours a week was associated with doubling of the risk of a cardiovascular event.[5] A third cohort study (1263 men with diabetes, mean follow up 12 years) found that low baseline cardiorespiratory fitness increased overall mortality compared with moderate or high fitness (RR 2.9, 95% CI 2.1 to 3.6), and overall mortality was higher in those reporting no recreational exercise in the previous 3 months than in those reporting any recreational physical activity in the same period (RR 1.8, 95% CI 1.3 to 2.5).[6] The absolute risk of CVD is almost the same in women as in men with diabetes. Diabetes specific cardiovascular risk factors include the duration of diabetes during adulthood (the years of exposure to diabetes before age 20 years add little to the risk of CVD); raised blood glucose concentrations (reflected in fasting blood glucose or HbA1c**G**); and any degree of microalbuminuria (albuminuria 30–299 mg/24 hours).[7] People with diabetes and microalbuminuria have a higher risk of coronary morbidity and mortality than do people with normal levels of urinary albumin and a similar duration of diabetes (RR 2–3).[8,9] Clinical proteinuria increases the risk of mortality from cardiac events in people with type 2 diabetes (RR 2.61, 95% CI 1.99 to 3.43)[10] and type 1 diabetes (RR 9)[7,11,12] compared with people with the same type of diabetes who have normal albumin excretion. An epidemiological analysis of people with diabetes enrolled in the Heart Outcomes Prevention Evaluation cohort study (3498 people with diabetes and at least 1 other cardiovascular risk factor, age > 55 years, of whom 1140 [32%] had microalbuminuria at baseline; 5 years' follow up) found higher risk for major cardiovascular events in those with microalbuminuria (albumin : creatinine ratio [ACR] ≥ 2.0 mg/mmol) than in those without microalbuminuria (adjusted RR 1.97, 95% CI 1.68 to 2.31), and for all cause mortality (RR 2.15, 95% CI 1.78 to 2.60).[13] It also found an association between ACR and the risk of major cardiovascular events (ACR 0.22–0.57 mg/mmol: RR 0.85, 95% CI 0.63 to 1.14; ACR 0.58–1.62 mg/mmol: RR 1.11, 95% CI 0.86 to 1.43; ACR 1.62–1.99 mg/mmol: RR 1.89, 95% CI 1.52 to 2.36).

PROGNOSIS Diabetes mellitus increases the risk of mortality or serious morbidity after a coronary event (RR 1.5–3.0).[2,3,14,15] This excess risk is partly accounted for by increased prevalence of other cardiovascular risk factors in people with diabetes. A systematic review (search date 1998, 15 prospective cohort studies) found that, in people with diabetes admitted to hospital for acute myocardial infarction, "stress hyperglycaemia" was associated with significantly higher mortality in hospital compared with lower blood glucose levels (RR 1.7, 95% CI 1.2 to 2.4).[16] One large prospective cohort study (91 285 men aged 40–84 years) found higher all cause and coronary heart disease (CHD) mortality at 5 years' follow up in men with diabetes than in men without coronary artery disease or diabetes (age adjusted RR 3.3, 95% CI 2.6 to 4.1 in men with diabetes and without coronary artery disease *v* RR 2.3, 95% CI 2.0 to 2.6 in healthy people; RR 5.6, 95% CI 4.9 to 6.3 in men with coronary artery disease but without diabetes *v* RR 2.2, 95% CI 2.0 to 2.4 in healthy people; RR 12.0, 95% CI 9.9 to 14.6 in men with both risk factors *v* RR 4.7, 95% CI 4.0 to 5.4 in healthy people).[17] Multivariate analysis did not materially alter these associations. Diabetes mellitus alone is associated with a twofold increase in risk for all cause death, with a threefold increase in risk of death from CHD, and, in people with pre-existing CHD, with a 12-fold increase in risk of death from CHD compared with people with neither risk factor.[17]

AIMS OF INTERVENTION To reduce mortality and morbidity from cardiovascular disease with minimum adverse effects.

OUTCOMES Incidence of fatal or non-fatal acute myocardial infarction; congestive heart failure; sudden cardiac death; coronary revascularisation; stroke; gangrene; angiographic evidence of coronary, cerebral, vascular, or peripheral arterial stenosis; all cause mortality.

METHODS *Clinical Evidence* search and appraisal October 2003. We searched for systematic reviews and RCTs with at least 10 confirmed clinical cardiovascular events among people with diabetes. Studies reporting only intermediate end points (e.g. regression of plaque on angiography, lipid changes) were not included. Most of the evidence comes from subgroup analyses of large RCTs that included people with diabetes. As with all subgroup analyses, and studies with small numbers, these results must be interpreted as suggestive rather than definitive.

QUESTION What are the effects of promoting smoking cessation in people with diabetes?

OPTION PROMOTING SMOKING CESSATION

We found no RCTs on promotion of smoking cessation specifically in people with diabetes. Observational evidence and extrapolation from people without diabetes suggest that promotion of smoking cessation is likely to reduce cardiovascular events.

Benefits: We found no systematic review or RCTs on promotion of smoking cessation specifically in people with diabetes.

Harms: We found no RCTs.

Comment: Observational studies have found that cigarette smoking is associated with increased cardiovascular death in people with diabetes. Smoking cessation in people without diabetes has been found to be associated with reduced risk. People with diabetes are likely to benefit from smoking cessation at least as much as people who do not have diabetes but have other risk factors for cardiovascular events (see smoking cessation under secondary prevention of ischaemic cardiac events, [Web only]).

QUESTION What are the effects of controlling blood pressure in people with diabetes?

OPTION ANTIHYPERTENSIVE TREATMENT VERSUS NO ANTIHYPERTENSIVE TREATMENT

One systematic review and RCTs have found that, in people with diabetes and hypertension, blood pressure lowering with antihypertensive agents reduces cardiovascular morbidity and mortality compared with no antihypertensive treatment.

Benefits: We found two systematic reviews,[18,19] and one meta-analysis of major RCTs.[20] The second systematic review (search date 2002) did not attempt to pool the results of RCTs identified.[19] We found four RCTs,[21–24] that were subsequent to the first systematic review.[18] The first systematic review (search date 2000) found that, compared with controls, blood pressure lowering with antihypertensive agents significantly reduced mortality but found no significant effect on myocardial infarction (6 RCTs, 7572 people with diabetes with or without diagnosis of cardiovascular disease [CVD], aged > 50 years; mortality: 10 deaths/1000 person years in treatment arms *v* 19 deaths/1000 person years in control arms; RR 0.51, 95% CI 0.38 to 0.69; myocardial infarction: 14/1000 person years in treatment arms *v* 16/1000 person years in control arms; rate ratio 0.76, 96% CI 0.51 to 1.01).[18] A meta-analysis of large RCTs of angiotensin converting enzyme (ACE) inhibitors and β blockers found that, compared with placebo, both ACE inhibitors and β blockers reduced risk of all cause mortality (6 RCTs of ACE inhibitors *v* placebo, 2398 people with diabetes and left ventricular dysfunction; all cause mortality: RR 0.84, 95% CI 0.070 to 1.0; 3 RCTs of β blockers *v* placebo, 1883 people with diabetes, all cause mortality: RR 0.77, 95% CI 0.61 to 0.96).[20] The first subsequent RCT found that, compared with placebo, antihypertensive treatment with nitrendipine or enalapril with or without hydrochlorothiazide significantly reduced all cardiovascular events over a median of 2 years but found no significant difference for all cause mortality (1 RCT, 495 people with diabetes without a diagnosis of CVD, aged ≥ 60 years with blood pressure 165–220/< 95 mm Hg; all CVD events over median 2 years: 13/252 [5.2%] with antihypertensive treatment *v* 31/240 [12.9%] with placebo; ARR 8%, 95% CI 3% to 10%; RR 0.4, 95% CI 0.21 to 0.75; NNT 13, 95% CI 10 to 31; all cause mortality: 16/252 [6.3%] with antihypertensive treatment *v* 26/240 [10.8%] with placebo; ARR +4.5%, 95% CI –0.7% to +7.4%; RR 0.59, 95% CI 0.32 to 1.06).[21] The second subsequent RCT found no significant difference between antihypertensive treatment with irbesartan or amlodipine and placebo in cardiovascular composite outcomes over 2.6 years (1 RCT, 1715 people with type 2 diabetes, hypertension and nephropathy, aged 30–70 years; 172/579 [30%] with irbesartan *v* 161/569 [28%] with placebo; HR 0.90, 95% CI 0.74 to 1.10; 161/567 [28%] with amlodipine *v* 161/569 [28%] with placebo; HR 1.00, 95% CI 0.83 to 1.21; 172/579 [30%] with irbesartan *v* 161/567 [28%] with amlodipine; HR 0.90, 95% CI 0.74 to 1.10).[25] The third subsequent RCT found no significant difference between antihypertensive treatment with irbesartan and placebo in non-fatal cardiovascular events over 2 years (1 RCT, 590 people with type 2 diabetes, microalbuminuria, and hypertension, mean age 58 years; 8/194 [4.1%] with irbesartan *v* 17/201 [8.5%] with placebo; RR 0.49, 95% CI 0.22 to 1.10).[23] The fourth subsequent RCT found that, compared with placebo, antihypertensive treatment with ramipril significantly reduced major cardiovascular events and death from any cause over 4.5 years (1 RCT, 3 arm study, 9541 people aged ≥ 55 years with diabetes and additional CVD risk factors such as diagnosed coronary vascular disease, current smoker, hypercholesterolaemia, hypertension, or microalbuminuria; major cardiovascular event such as coronary vascular disease death, acute myocardial infarction**G**, or stroke: 277/1808 [15.3%] with ramipril *v* 351/1769 [19.8%] with placebo; RR 0.75, 95% CI 0.64 to 0.88; ARR 4.5%; NNT 22, 95% CI 14 to 43; death from any cause: 196/1808 [10.8%] with ramipril *v* 248/1769 [14.0%] with placebo; RR 0.76, 95% CI 0.67 to 0.92; ARR 3.2%; NNT 32, 95% CI 19 to 98).[24] The relative effect of ramipril was present in all subgroups regardless of hypertensive status, microalbuminuria, type of diabetes, and nature of diabetes treatment (diet, oral agents, or insulin). The RCT also compared vitamin versus placebo and found no significant effect on morbidity or mortality.[24,26,27]

Harms: The systematic review[18] and first subsequent RCT[21] gave no information on adverse effects. An earlier report of the second subsequent RCT[25] had stated that the RCT found a significantly higher incidence of hyperkalaemia resulting in discontinuation of treatment with irbesartan than with amlodipine or placebo (11/579 [1.9%] with irbesartan *v* 3/567 [0.5%] with amlodipine *v* 2/569 [0.4%] with placebo; P = 0.01 for both comparisons).[22] The third subsequent RCT stated that significantly more people had "serious adverse events" with irbesartan than with placebo but it did not state what they were (15.4% with irbesartan *v* 22.8% with placebo).[23] The fourth subsequent RCT found that cough was 5% more frequent with the ACE inhibitor (ramipril) than with placebo.[24]

Comment: None.

OPTION DIFFERENT ANTIHYPERTENSIVE DRUGS

Systematic reviews and RCTs have found that angiotensin converting enzyme inhibitors, diuretics, β blockers, and calcium channel blockers all reduce cardiovascular morbidity and mortality in people with diabetes and hypertension. However, there are differences in the types of adverse effects reported for different antihypertensive drugs. RCTs have found that people taking atenolol gained more weight than those taking captopril, an increase in

risk of congestive heart failure with lisinopril compared with chlorthalidone, a higher frequency of headache with diltiazem than with diuretics or β blockers, and a higher rate of withdrawal from treatment because of adverse effects with atenolol than with losartan.

Benefits: We found two systematic reviews,[19,28] and two subsequent RCTs.[29,30] The first systematic review (search date 2002) did not attempt to pool the results of RCTs identified.[19] We have reported the results of the second systematic review (search date 2000),[28] the relevant RCTs identified by the first systematic review[19] and the two subsequent RCTs.[29,30] **Angiotensin converting enzyme (ACE) inhibitors versus calcium channel blockers:** One systematic review[28] identified two RCTs comparing ACE inhibitors (fosinopril, enalapril) versus calcium channel blockers (amlodipine, nisoldipine) in people with diabetes without a diagnosis of cardiovascular disease (CVD).[31,32] The review found that ACE inhibitors significantly reduced combined cardiovascular events compared with calcium channel blockers but it found no significant reduction in acute myocardial infarction**G**, stroke, or death in people with diabetes without a diagnosis of CVD (2 RCTs; combined cardiovascular events — cardiovascular death, acute myocardial infarction, congestive heart failure, stroke, pulmonary infarction, angina: 34/424 [8%] with ACE inhibitors *v* 70/426 [16%] with calcium channel blockers; ARR 8%, 95% CI 4% to 13%; RR 0.49, 95% CI 0.33 to 0.72; NNT 13, 95% CI 7 to 25; death: 17/424 [4.0%] with ACE inhibitors *v* 22/426 [5.2%] with calcium channel blockers; ARR 1%; RR 0.78, 95% CI 0.42 to 1.44; acute myocardial infarction: 15/424 [4%] with ACE inhibitors *v* 38/426 [9%] with calcium channel blockers; ARR 5%, 95% CI 2% to 9%; RR 0.40, 95% CI 0.22 to 0.71; NNT 19, 95% CI 12 to 46; stroke: 11/424 [2.6%] with ACE inhibitors *v* 21/426 [4.9%] with calcium channel blockers; ARR 2.3%; RR 0.53, 95% CI 0.26 to 1.08).[31,32] The subsequent RCT compared ACE inhibitors (enalapril, lisinopril), calcium channel blockers (felodipine, isradipine), β blockers (atenolol, metoprolol, pindolol), and diuretics (hydrochlorothiazide plus amiloride).[33] It found that, compared with calcium channel blockers, ACE inhibitors significantly reduced fatal and non-fatal myocardial infarctions (1 RCT, 719 people with diabetes without a diagnosis of CVD, mean age 76 years, mean blood pressure 190/99 mm Hg; 17/235 [7%] with ACE inhibitors *v* 32/231 [14%] with calcium channel blockers; RR 0.51, 95% CI 0.28 to 0.92). However, it found no significant difference between groups in the incidence of major cardiovascular events over 4 years (major cardiovascular events per 1000 person years: 64.2 with ACE inhibitors *v* 67.7 with calcium channel blockers *v* 75.0 with β blockers or diuretics). **ACE inhibitors versus β blockers:** One RCT[34] identified in a systematic review[28] found no significant difference between captopril and atenolol in number of cardiovascular events over 8.4 years (1 RCT, 758 people with diabetes without a diagnosis of CVD; cardiovascular events: 102/400 [25.5%] with captopril *v* 75/358 [20.9%] with atenolol; ARI +5%, 95% CI –1% to +11%; RR 1.22, 95% CI 0.94 to 1.58). **ACE inhibitors versus β blockers or diuretics:** One RCT[35] identified by the systematic review[28] found that, compared with diuretics or β blockers, captopril significantly reduced acute myocardial infarction, stroke, or death (1 RCT, 572 people with or without a diagnosis of CVD; acute myocardial infarction, stroke, or death: 46/263 [17.5%] with diuretics/β blockers *v* 35/309 [11.3%] with captopril; RR 0.65, 95% CI 0.43 to 0.97). **ACE inhibitors or calcium channel blockers versus diuretics:** One RCT found no significant difference between lisinopril or amlodipine and chlorthalidone in 6 year fatal cardiac heart disease, non-fatal myocardial infarction, fatal and non-fatal stroke, or all cause mortality (1 RCT, 12 063 people with diabetes and established hypertension, aged ≥ 55 years; primary outcome of non-fatal myocardial infarction plus coronary heart disease death: chlorthalidone *v* lisinopril: RR 1.00, 95% CI 0.87 to 1.14; amlodipine *v* chlorthalidone: RR 1.04, 95% CI 0.94 to 1.14; absolute numbers for the diabetic subgroup not reported, results presented graphically).[36] **Angiotensin II receptor antagonists versus β blockers:** One RCT found that, compared with atenolol, losartan significantly reduced composite cardiovascular outcomes over 4 years (1 RCT, 1195 people with diabetes with or without a diagnosis of CVD, aged 55–80 years; composite cardiovascular outcomes — mortality, stroke, and myocardial infarction: 103/586 [17.6%] with losartan *v* 139/609 [22.8%] with atenolol; RR 0.77, 95% CI 0.61 to 0.97; NNT 19, 95% CI 11 to 142).[37] **Calcium channel blockers versus diuretics or β blockers:** One RCT identified by the systematic review[19] found no significant difference between diltiazem and conventional antihypertensive treatment with diuretic, β blocker, or a combination of the two in fatal or non-fatal stroke, myocardial infarction, and other cardiovascular death (1 RCT, 727 people with diabetes and diastolic pressure ≥ 100 mm Hg on 2 occasions, aged 50–74 years; fatal or non-fatal stroke, myocardial infarction, and other cardiovascular death: 44/351 [12.5%] with diltiazem *v* 44/376 [11.7%] with conventional treatment; RR 1.07, 95% CI 0.72 to 1.59.[38] One subsequent RCT found no significant difference between modified release verapamil and a diuretic or β blocker in the composite outcomes of myocardial infarction, stroke, or cardiovascular death over 3 years (3239 people with diabetes and hypertension with or without CVD diagnosis, aged ≥ 55 years, myocardial infarction, stroke, or cardiovascular death: 101/1616 [6.3%] with verapamil *v* 116/1623 [7.1%] with diuretic or β blocker; RR 0.86, 95% CI 0.66 to 1.12).[29] A second subsequent RCT found no significant difference between nifedipine and co-amilozide (amiloride plus hydrochlorothiazide) in composite outcome of cardiovascular death, myocardial infarction, heart failure, or stroke over a mean of 4 years (1302 people with diabetes and hypertension with or without CVD diagnosis, aged 55–80 years; cardiovascular death, myocardial infarction, heart failure, or stroke: 54/651 [8.3%] with nifedipine *v* 55/655 [8.4%] with co-amilozide, RR 0.99, 95% CI 0.69 to 1.4).[30]

Harms: **ACE inhibitors versus calcium channel blockers:** One systematic review[28] and a subsequent RCT[33] gave no information on adverse effects. **ACE inhibitors versus β blockers:** One RCT identified in the systematic review found that people taking atenolol gained more weight than did those taking captopril (3.4 kg with atenolol *v* 1.6 kg with captopril; P = 0.02).[34] Over the first 4 years of the trial people allocated to atenolol had higher mean HbA1c**G** (7.5% with atenolol *v* 7.0% with captopril; P = 0.004). However, no significant difference was found between groups over the subsequent 4 years. No significant difference was found between atenolol and captopril in rates of hypoglycaemia, lipid concentrations, tolerability, blood pressure lowering, or prevention of disease events. **ACE inhibitors versus β blockers or diuretics:** One RCT gave no information on adverse effects.[35] **ACE inhibitors or calcium channel blockers versus diuretics:** One RCT found an increased risk of congestive heart failure with lisinopril than with chlorthalidone (RR 1.22, 95% CI 1.05 to 1.42) and with amlodipine than with chlorthalidone (RR 1.42, 95% CI 1.23 to 1.64).[36] A previous report for this RCT described an increased risk of combined coronary vascular disease events with doxazosin than with chlorthalidone when these agents were used to treat hypertension (coronary heart disease, death, non-fatal myocardial infarction, stroke, angina, coronary revascularisation, congestive heart failure, and peripheral arterial disease: RR 1.24, 95% CI 1.12 to 1.38).[39] The doxazosin arm of the RCT was terminated because of this increase in risk.[39] **Angiotensin II receptor antagonists versus β blockers:** One RCT found that discontinuation of treatment because of adverse effects was less common with losartan than with atenolol (2/586 [0.3%] with losartan v 9/609 [1.5%] with atenolol; RR 0.23, 95% CI 0.05 to 1.06; P = 0.065).[37] Adverse events that occurred with significantly greater frequency with losartan than with atenolol were bradycardia (1% with atenolol v 9% with losartan; P < 0.0001), cold extremities (4% with atenolol v 6% with losartan; P < 0.0001), albuminuria (5% with atenolol v 6% with losartan; P = 0.0002), hyperglycaemia (5% with atenolol v 7% with losartan; P = 0.007), asthenia/fatigue (15% with atenolol v 17% with losartan; P = 0.001), back pain (10% with atenolol v 12% with losartan; P = 0.004), dyspnoea (10% with atenolol v 14% with losartan; P < 0.0001), and lower extremity oedema (12% with atenolol v 14% with losartan; P = 0.002).[37] **Calcium channel blockers versus diuretics or β blockers:** One RCT identified by the systematic review[19] found significantly greater frequency of headache with diltiazem than with diuretics or β blockers (8.5% with diltiazem v 5.7% with diuretics or β blockers; P < 0.001).[38] One subsequent RCT found a higher frequency of withdrawal from the study because of constipation with calcium channel blockers than with β blockers or diuretics (216/8179 [2.6%] with calcium channel blockers v 28/8297 [0.3%] with β blockers or diuretics).[29] The second subsequent RCT did not comment on adverse effects of treatment.[30]

Comment: The evidence suggests that thiazide-like diuretics, β blockers, ACE inhibitors, and calcium channel blockers all significantly reduce cardiovascular events in people with diabetes. The results of one large RCT cast doubt on the conclusions of earlier, smaller studies suggesting that ACE inhibitors are superior to calcium channel blockers.[36] The RCT indicates that chlorthalidone is at least as effective as an ACE inhibitor as initial treatment for hypertension in terms of prevention of major cardiovascular events.[36] It is unclear whether ACE inhibitors and β blockers are equivalent. In most RCTs, combination treatment with more than one agent was required to achieve target blood pressures. One large RCT found that the ACE inhibitor ramipril, which reduces urinary protein excretion, also reduced cardiovascular morbidity and mortality in older diabetic people with other cardiac risk factors.[24] The relative cardioprotective effect of the ACE inhibitor was present to the same extent in people with or without hypertension, and with or without microalbuminuria.

OPTION TARGET BLOOD PRESSURE

Large RCTs including people with diabetes and hypertension have found that tighter control of blood pressure to a target diastolic blood pressure of no more than 80 mm Hg or less reduces the risk of major cardiovascular events. One RCT in normotensive people with diabetes found that intensive blood pressure lowering reduced cerebral vascular accidents but found no significant difference in cardiovascular death, myocardial infarction, congestive heart failure, or all cause mortality.

Benefits: We found no systematic review but found three RCTs.[34,40–42] The first RCT found that, compared with moderate target blood pressure (≤ 180/105 mm Hg), tight target blood pressure (≤ 150/85 mm Hg) significantly reduced fatal or non-fatal acute myocardial infarction**G** and stroke but found no significant difference for peripheral vascular events over 8.4 years (1 RCT, 1148 people with hypertension managed with atenolol or captopril; fatal or non-fatal acute myocardial infarction: 107/758 [14%] with tight blood pressure target v 83/390 [21%] with moderate blood pressure target; RR 0.66, 95% CI 0.51 to 0.86, NNT 14, 95% CI 9 to 35; stroke: 38/758 [5.0%] with tight blood pressure target v 34/390 [8.7%] with moderate blood pressure target; RR 0.58, 95% CI 0.37 to 0.90; NNT 27, 95% CI 18 to 116; peripheral vascular events: 8/758 [1.1%] with tight blood pressure target v 8/390 [2.1%] with moderate blood pressure target; RR 0.52, 95% CI 0.20 to 1.36).[34,40] The second RCT found that the risk of major cardiovascular events was reduced by 50% over 3.8 years with a target diastolic blood pressure of 80 mm Hg or less compared with a target blood pressure of 90 mm Hg or less (1 multicentre RCT, 3 arm study, 1501 people with hypertension managed with felodipine, ACE inhibitors, β blockers, or diuretics; major cardiovascular events: 22/499 [4.4%] with target blood pressure ≤80 mm Hg v 45/501 [9.0%] with target blood pressure ≤90 mm Hg; RR 0.5, 95% CI 0.3 to 0.8; NNT 22, 95% CI 16 to 57).[41] The third RCT found a significantly lower incidence of cerebral vascular accidents with a target diastolic blood pressure of 10 mm Hg below baseline using nisoldipine or enalapril compared with unchanged baseline diastolic blood pressure of 80–89 mm Hg with placebo over 5.3 years (1 RCT, 480 people with type 2 diabetes and baseline blood pressure < 140/90 mm Hg being managed with nisoldipine or enalapril; cerebral vascular accidents: 4/237 [1.7%] with target diastolic blood pressure of 10 mm Hg below baseline v 13/243 [5.4%] with unchanged baseline diastolic blood pressure of 80–89 mm Hg; OR 3.29, CI 1.06 to 10.25; NNT 27, 95% CI 14 to 255).[42] The RCT found no significant difference in cardiovascular death, myocardial infarction, congestive heart failure, or all cause mortality. The RCT also found that, in a subgroup of people with type 2 diabetes and peripheral arterial disease at baseline (ankle : brachial index < 0.90), intensive blood pressure lowering to a mean of 128/75 mm Hg compared with no blood pressure reduction significantly reduced major cardiovascular events (1 RCT, 53 people, CVD death, non-fatal myocardial infarction, non-fatal stroke, heart failure requiring hospital admission, or pulmonary infarction: 3/22 [13.6%] with intensive blood pressure lowering v 12/31 [38.7%] with no blood pressure reduction; ARR 0.25%, 95% CI 0.03 to 0.47, NNT 4, 95% CI 2 to 37).[43]

Harms: We found no good evidence of a threshold below which it is harmful to lower blood pressure. One RCT found that a significantly greater proportion of people gained weight with atenolol than with captopril (mean weight gain over 9 years: 3.4 kg with atenolol v 1.6 kg with captopril; P = 0.02) but it found no significant difference in hypoglycaemia or weight gain with tight blood pressure control (≤150/85 mm Hg) compared with moderate blood pressure control (≤180/105 mm Hg).[34,40] The second RCT comparing tight versus moderate blood pressure control did not provide information on adverse effects.[41] The third RCT in normotensive people gave no information on adverse effects.[42]

Comment: Aggressive lowering of blood pressure in people with diabetes and hypertension reduces cardiovascular morbidity and mortality. In most trials, combination treatment with more than one agent was required to achieve target blood pressures.

QUESTION **What are the effects of treating dyslipidaemia in people with diabetes?**

OPTION **FIBRATES**

One RCT found that gemfibrozil reduced cardiovascular events over 5 years compared with placebo. Another smaller RCT found no significant difference. One RCT found that bezafibrate reduced cardiovascular events compared with placebo.

Benefits: We found two systematic reviews (search date 2000[18] and search date not reported[44]). Neither of these systematic reviews included pooling or summary estimates across the fibrate trials. We have reported results of individual RCTs identified by at least one of the systematic reviews. One RCT found that gemfibrozil did not significantly reduce myocardial infarction or cardiac death over 5 years compared with placebo (1 RCT, 135 men aged 40–55 years with diabetes without a diagnosis of cardiovascular disease [CVD]: 2/59 [3.4%] events with gemfibrozil *v* 8/76 [10.5%] with placebo; ARR +7.1%, 95% CI −2.1% to +16.8%; RR 0.32, 95% CI 0.07 to 1.46).[45] A second RCT found that, compared with placebo, gemfibrozil 1200 mg daily significantly reduced coronary heart disease, death, stroke, or non-fatal acute myocardial infarction Ⓖ over 5 years (1 RCT, 769 people aged < 74 years with diabetes and CVD diagnosis: 105/388 [27%] events with gemfibrozil *v* 141/381 [37%] events with placebo; HR 0.68, 95% CI 0.53 to 0.88).[46] A third RCT found that bezafibrate significantly reduced myocardial infarction or new ischaemic changes on electrocardiogram over 3 years compared with placebo (1 RCT, 164 people aged 35–65 years with type 2 diabetes without a diagnosis of CVD; 5/64 [7.8%] events with bezafibrate *v* 16/64 [25%] events with placebo; ARR 17.2%, 95% CI 4.6% to 30.1%; RR 0.31, 95% CI 0.12 to 0.80; NNT 6, 95% CI 5 to 20).[47] A fourth RCT found no significant difference in the proportion of people who either had myocardial infarction or died after 39 months of treatment between fenofibrate 200 mg daily and placebo (1 RCT, 418 people with diabetes and with or without CVD diagnosis, mean age 57 years; 15/207 [7.2%] events with fenofibrate *v* 21/211 [9.9%] events with placebo; ARR +2.7%, 95% CI −2.8% to +8.3%; RR 0.73, 95% CI 0.39 to 1.37).[48] This RCT was underpowered for myocardial infarction and death, but there were trends toward reduced risk of myocardial infarction with fenofibrate (9 with fenofibrate *v* 12 with placebo) and death (6 with fenofibrate *v* 9 with placebo). A benefit for fenofibrate in reducing myocardial infarction and death is suggested and certainly cannot be excluded.

Harms: The systematic reviews[18,44] did not comment on adverse effects. One RCT reported no significant difference between fenofibrate and placebo in gallbladder symptoms (0.5% with fenofibrate *v* 1.4% with placebo), liver toxicity (1.5% with fenofibrate *v* 0% with placebo), muscle pain (0% with fenofibrate *v* 0.5% with placebo), joint pain (3.4% with fenofibrate *v* 2.5% with placebo), or cancer (2.4% with fenofibrate *v* 3.3% with placebo).[48]

Comment: None.

OPTION STATINS

One systematic review and RCTs have found that statins reduce cardiovascular morbidity and mortality compared with placebo. One RCT found that treatment with atorvastatin to achieve a target low density lipoprotein below 2.6 mmol/L reduces cardiovascular morbidity and mortality compared with usual care. Another RCT found no significant difference between use of lovastatin, plus cholestyramine if necessary, to achieve lower target low density lipoprotein of 1.55–2.20 mmol/L and a moderate target low density lipoprotein of 3.36–3.62 mmol/L in 4 year event rate for myocardial infarction and death. One RCT found no significant difference in cardiovascular events in older people with low dose pravastatin 5 mg daily and standard dose pravastatin 10–20 mg daily over 4 years.

Benefits: We found one systematic review,[18] five subsequent RCTs,[49–53] and one additional RCT.[54] We also found a systematic review that did not conduct a meta-analysis for RCTs evaluating statins, but provided a commentary on the quality of data on people with diabetes included in such trials (see comment below).[44] **Versus placebo:** The systematic review (search date 2000) found that pravastatin or simvastatin significantly reduced cardiovascular events over 6 years compared with placebo (3 RCTs,[55–57] 1570 people: 34 events per 1000 person years with statins *v* 44 events with placebo per 1000 person years; RR 0.77, 95% CI 0.62 to 0.96; person years needed to treat 120, 95% CI 61 to 4856).[18] One RCT identified in the systematic review found no significant difference between lovastatin and placebo in myocardial infarction, unstable angina, or sudden cardiac death over 5 years (4/84 [4.8%] events with lovastatin *v* 6/71 [8.5%] events with placebo; ARR +3.7%, 95% CI –5.6% to +11.9%; RR 0.56, 95% CI 0.16 to 1.91).[58] The first subsequent RCT found that, compared with placebo, simvastatin significantly reduced all cause mortality, non-fatal myocardial infarction, coronary heart disease (CHD), death, total stroke, or any revascularisation over 5 years in people with diabetes aged 40–80 years regardless of whether or not they had previous vascular disease (1 RCT, among the 1981 people in the trial with diabetes and previous CHD: 325/972 [33.4%] events with simvastatin *v* 381/1009 [37.8%] events with placebo; ARR 4.3%; NNT 23, 95% CI 12 to 897; among 1070 people with diabetes and previous non-coronary vascular disease but without previous CHD: major cardiovascular disease [CVD] events: 141/551 [25.6%] with simvastatin *v* 171/519 [32.9%] with placebo; ARR 7.5%; NNT 14, 95% CI 8 to 49; among 2912 people with diabetes but no previous CHD or other vascular disease: major CVD events: 135/1455 [9.3%] with simvastatin *v* 196/1457 [17.2%] with placebo; ARR 4.2, NNT 24, 95% CI 16 to 53).[49] By the end of the study 38% of those allocated to placebo were taking a statin not used in the study.[49] The second subsequent RCT found that fluvastatin significantly reduced cardiac death, non-fatal myocardial infarction, and reintervention over 4 years compared with placebo (1 RCT, 202 people aged 18–80 years with diabetes and a diagnosis of CVD: 26/120 [21%] events with fluvastatin *v* 31/82 [37.8%] events with placebo; ARR 0.161, 95% CI 0.033 to 0.290; NNT 7, 95% CI 4 to 30).[50] The third subsequent RCT found no significant difference in cardiac death or non-fatal myocardial infarction between pravastatin 40 mg daily and placebo over 4.8 years (1 RCT, 3638 people aged ≥55 years with type 2 diabetes and additional CHD risk factors; CHD death plus non-fatal myocardial infarction: RR 0.89, 95% CI 0.71 to 1.10; absolute numbers not reported, results presented graphically).[51] Baseline low density lipoprotein (LDL) cholesterol was required to be in the range 3.1–4.9 mmol/L for people with no known CHD and 2.6–3.3 mmol/L for those with previously diagnosed CHD. Usual care could include lipid lowering agents at the primary care physician's discretion.[51] The fourth subsequent RCT found no significant difference in cardiovascular death or myocardial infarction between atorvastatin 10 mg daily and placebo over 3 years (1 RCT, 2532 people aged 40–79 years with diabetes, hypertension, total cholesterol ≤6.5 mmol/L and at least 2 other cardiovascular risk factor but without coronary artery disease diagnosis; cardiovascular death, or myocardial infarction: RR 0.84, 95% CI 0.55 to 1.28).[52] **Aggressive versus moderate lipid lowering:** One RCT[59] identified by a systematic review[18] found no significant difference between aggressive lipid lowering and moderate lipid lowering in 4 year event rate for myocardial infarction and death (1 RCT, 116 people aged 21–74 years with type 2 diabetes and a diagnosis of CVD; 4 year event rate for death: 6.5 with aggressive lipid lowering *v* 9.6 with moderate lipid lowering; RR 0.67, 99% CI 0.12 to 3.75; 4 year event rate for myocardial infarction: 4.8 with aggressive lipid lowering *v* 11.6 with moderate lipid lowering; RR 0.40, 99% CI 0.07 to 2.47). The RCT used lovastatin and cholestyramine as necessary to achieve the targets for aggressive lipid lowering (LDL cholesterol 1.55–2.20 mmol/L [60–85 mg/dL]) and moderate lipid lowering (LDL cholesterol

3.36–3.62 mmol/L [130–140 mg/dL]). This RCT had limited power because of the small number of people enrolled who had diabetes.[59] A subsequent RCT found that, compared with usual care, treatment with atorvastatin to achieve a target LDL of below 2.6 mmol/L (< 100 mg/dL) significantly reduced the risk of all cause mortality, non-fatal myocardial infarction, unstable angina, congestive heart failure, revascularisation, and stroke over 3 years (1 RCT, 313 people with a diagnosis of CVD, mean age 58 years: RRR 0.42; P = 0.0001; results presented graphically). The atorvastatin dose was titrated from 10 mg daily to a maximum of 80 mg daily to achieve a target LDL cholesterol of below 2.6 mmol/L. Usual care consisted of treatment by the family practitioner, which could include diet, exercise, weight loss and/or drug treatment including lipid lowering agents; 14% of people in the usual care group received any lipid lowering agents.[53] **Low versus standard statin dose in older people:** One subsequent RCT found no significant difference in cardiovascular events between low dose pravastatin 5 mg daily and standard dose pravastatin 10–20 mg daily over 4 years (1 RCT, 199 people aged > 60 years with diabetes: 17/104 [16.3%] events with low dose pravastatin *v* 15/95 [15.8%] events with standard dose pravastatin; ARR +0.006%, 95% CI –0.097 to +0.108).[54]

Harms: **Versus placebo:** One systematic review (search date 2000) did not report on adverse effects.[18] The first subsequent RCT evaluated the effects of simvastatin compared with placebo on adverse outcomes other than cardiovascular events in people with diabetes.[49] The RCT found no significant difference between simvastatin and placebo for withdrawal from treatment because of elevated liver enzymes (48 [0.5%] with simvastatin *v* 35 [0.3%] with placebo), muscle symptoms (49 [0.5%] with simvastatin *v* 50 [0.5%] with placebo), or hospital admission due to chronic obstructive pulmonary disease/asthma (132 [1.3%] with simvastatin *v* 150 [1.5%] with placebo). The second subsequent RCT conducted a safety analysis for fluvastatin compared with placebo in 1640 people. It found no significant difference between fluvastatin and placebo in the proportion of people withdrawing from treatment (174/822 [21%] with fluvastatin *v* 196/818 [24%] with placebo; RR 0.88, 95% CI 0.74 to 1.06).[50] The third subsequent RCT specifically stated that no data on adverse effects were collected.[51] The fourth subsequent RCT found no significant difference in serious adverse events or liver enzyme changes between those allocated atorvastatin and those allocated placebo.[52] **Aggressive versus moderate lipid lowering:** One RCT did not report any adverse events.[59] The subsequent RCT found no significant difference between atorvastatin and usual care in the proportion of people withdrawn from the study because of elevated liver enzymes.[53] **Low versus standard statin dose in older people:** One RCT comparing low versus standard pravastatin dose found no significant difference in adverse events between groups.[54]

Comment: We found one RCT that is of major importance.[49] The RCT is interesting because it was not necessary to have an abnormal lipid profile or prior vascular disease to be enrolled and it provides the first clear evidence that statin treatment is effective for primary prevention of CVD.[49] The relative risk reductions for major cardiovascular events were similar with or without previous CHD, and with lower and higher initial LDL cholesterol. The results of this RCT suggest that treatment with a statin is likely to be beneficial in most diabetic people who are at significant risk of CHD, regardless of initial LDL level and regardless of whether they have previous CVD. Furthermore, this and other studies provided stronger evidence for the value of treatment with statins per se, rather than for targeting any specific LDL cholesterol level. Besides this RCT,[49] most published RCTs with sufficient power to detect effects on cardiovascular events have enrolled comparatively few people with diabetes or have excluded them altogether. The available evidence is, therefore, based almost entirely on subgroup analyses of larger trials in which there was generally little information regarding the type and duration of diabetes, severity of complications, and metabolic control.[44] The statin versus placebo trial published after both systematic reviews was terminated early due to high efficacy of atorvastatin in the overall study population (HR for cardiovascular death plus non-fatal myocardial infarction 0.64, 95% CI 0.050 to 0.083).[52] Although the difference was not significant in the diabetic subgroup, the confidence intervals for diabetic and non-diabetic subgroups overlapped one another. Several large ongoing trials are evaluating the effects of fibrates in people with diabetes.

QUESTION What are the effects of antiplatelet drugs in people with diabetes?

OPTION PROPHYLACTIC ASPIRIN

One systematic review found that, compared with controls, antiplatelet treatment mainly with aspirin did not significantly reduce the combined risk of non-fatal myocardial infarction, non-fatal stroke, death from a vascular cause, or death from an unknown cause in people with diabetes and cardiovascular disease diagnosis. The review found that antiplatelet treatment was associated with an increase in the risk of major extracranial haemorrhage and haemorrhagic stroke, but the results for people with diabetes were not reported separately.

Benefits: We found one systematic review (search date 1997),[60] and one additional RCT.[61] The review found that, compared with controls, antiplatelet treatment mainly with aspirin did not significantly reduce the combined risk of non-fatal myocardial infarction, non-fatal stroke, death from a vascular cause, or death from an unknown cause (9 RCTs, 4961 people with diabetes and cardiovascular disease [CVD] diagnosis; 403/2568 [15.7%] with antiplatelet treatment *v* 426/2558 [16.7%] with control; RR 0.94, 95% CI 0.83 to 1.07). This non-significant 6% relative risk reduction was in contrast to the finding of highly significant 25% relative risk reduction for the same outcomes in the full meta-analysis (people with or without diabetes combined).[60] The largest RCT included in the systematic review found that aspirin 650 mg daily significantly reduced fatal or non-fatal myocardial infarction but not stroke over 5 years compared with placebo (1 RCT, 3711 people aged 18–70 years with diabetes; fatal or non-fatal myocardial infarction: 241/1856 [13%] with aspirin *v* 283/1855 [15%] with placebo; RR 0.851, 95% CI 0.726 to 0.998; NNT 44, 95% CI 22 to 3490; fatal or non-fatal stroke: 92/1856 [5%] with aspirin *v* 78/1855 [4%] with placebo; RR 1.179, 95% CI 0.878 to 1.583 [calculated by *Clinical Evidence*]).[62] The additional RCT found that aspirin significantly reduced the risk of acute myocardial infarction**G** over 5 years compared with placebo (1 RCT, 533 male physicians with diabetes but no diagnosis of CVD: 11/275 [4.0%] with aspirin *v* 26/258 [10.1%] with placebo; RR 0.39, 95% CI 0.20 to 0.79; NNT 16, 95% CI 12 to 47).[61] **Versus clopidogrel:** See benefits of clopidogrel, p 741. **Aspirin plus clopidogrel:** See benefits of clopidogrel, p 741.

Harms: In the systematic review, doses of aspirin ranged from 75–1500 mg daily. Most RCTs used aspirin 75–325 mg daily.[60] Doses higher than 325 mg daily increased the risk of haemorrhagic adverse effects without improving preventive efficacy. No difference in efficacy or adverse effects was found in the dose range 75–325 mg daily. The systematic review found that antiplatelet treatment was associated with a 50% relative increase in the risk of major extracranial haemorrhage and a 22% relative increase in risk of haemorrhagic stroke. These results were for the overall meta-analysis; results were not reported separately for the people with diabetes.[60] The largest RCT in people with diabetes within the systematic review (3711 people with diabetes, duration 5 years) found no significant increase in the risks of vitreous, retinal, gastrointestinal, or cerebral haemorrhage with aspirin 650 mg daily compared with placebo.[62] The additional RCT found no significant difference in adverse events between aspirin and placebo.[61]

Comment: We found insufficient evidence to define precisely which people with diabetes should be treated with aspirin. The risk of CVD is low before 30 years of age; most white adults with diabetes aged over 30 years are at increased risk of CVD. Widely accepted contraindications to aspirin treatment include aspirin allergy, bleeding tendency, anticoagulant treatment, recent gastrointestinal bleeding, and clinically active liver disease.[63]

OPTION CLOPIDOGREL

We found no RCTs comparing only clopidogrel versus placebo. One RCT in people with diabetes and with recent ischaemic stroke, myocardial infarction, or established peripheral arterial disease found no significant difference between clopidogrel and aspirin at 28 days in cardiovascular events. This RCT also found a lower proportion of people hospitalised for a bleeding event with clopidogrel than with aspirin. One RCT in people presenting with unstable angina or non-Q-wave myocardial infarction and also taking aspirin found no significant reduction in cardiovascular events after 12 months with addition of clopidogrel compared with placebo. This RCT also found a higher proportion of major bleeds with clopidogrel than with placebo.

Benefits: **Versus placebo:** We found no RCTs comparing only clopidogrel versus placebo. **Versus aspirin:** One RCT in people in people with diabetes and with recent ischaemic stroke, myocardial infarction, or established peripheral arterial disease found no significant difference between clopidogrel and aspirin at 28 days in cardiovascular events (1 RCT, 3866 people, mean age 64 years; angina, vascular death, myocardial infarction, all cause stroke, and readmission to hospital for ischaemic events: 299/1914 [15.6%] with clopidogrel *v* 345/1952 [17.7%] with aspirin; ARR +2.1%, 95% CI –0.3% to +4.4%; RR 0.88, 95% CI 0.77 to 1.02).[64] **Adding clopidogrel to aspirin:** One RCT in people presenting with unstable angina or non-Q-wave myocardial infarction and also taking aspirin found no significant reduction in cardiovascular events after 12 months with addition of clopidogrel compared with placebo (1 RCT, 2840 people with diabetes, mean age 64 years; cardiovascular death, non-fatal myocardial infarction, or stroke at 12 months: 200/1405 [14.2%] with clopidogrel *v* 240/1435 [16.7%] with placebo; RR 0.85, 95% CI 0.71 to 1.01).[65] People were randomised within 24 hours of an acute event and were given either given clopidogrel 300 mg bolus then 75 mg daily plus aspirin 75–325 mg daily or placebo plus aspirin.[65]

Harms: **Versus placebo:** One RCT found that a significantly lower proportion of people were hospitalised for a bleeding event with clopidogrel than with aspirin at 28 days (1 RCT, 3866 people, mean age 64 years; hospital admission for a bleeding event: 34/1914 [1.8%] with clopidogrel *v* 55/1952 [2.8%] with aspirin; RRR 37.0%, 95% CI 3.8% to 58.7%; P = 0.031).[64] **Adding clopidogrel to aspirin:** One RCT in people presenting with unstable angina or non-Q-wave myocardial infarction and also taking aspirin found a significantly higher proportion of major bleeds with clopidogrel than with placebo (3.7% with clopidogrel *v* 2.7% with placebo; RR 1.38, 95% CI 1.13 to 1.67; P = 0.001).[65]

Comment: None.

OPTION GLYCOPROTEIN IIB/IIIA INHIBITORS

We found no RCTs comparing glycoprotein IIb/IIIa inhibitors versus no antiplatelet treatment. One RCT in people presenting with unstable angina or acute myocardial infarction without ST segment elevation found that the addition of tirofiban (a glycoprotein IIb/IIIa inhibitor) to heparin reduced the composite outcome of death, myocardial infarction, or refractory ischaemia at 180 days compared with heparin alone. This RCT found no significant difference between tirofiban plus heparin and heparin alone in risk of bleeding in people already taking aspirin.

Benefits: We found no RCTs comparing glycoprotein IIb/IIIa inhibitors versus no antiplatelet treatment. **Adding glycoprotein IIb/IIIa inhibitors to heparin:** One RCT, in people with diabetes presenting with unstable angina or acute myocardial infarction**G** without ST segment elevation, found that addition of tirofiban (a glycoprotein IIb/IIIa inhibitor) to heparin compared with heparin alone significantly reduced the composite outcome of death, myocardial infarction, or refractory ischaemia at 180 days (1 RCT, 362 people already taking aspirin, mean age 65 years: 19/169 [11.2%] with tirofiban plus heparin *v* 37/193 [19.2%] with heparin alone; ARR 8.0%, 95% CI 0.7% to 15.3%; RR 0.586, 95% CI 0.351 to 0.980; P = 0.03; NNT 13, 95% CI 7 to 146).[66] **Adjunct to percutaneous coronary revascularisation:** See benefits of intracoronary stenting plus glycoprotein IIb/IIIa inhibitors, p 746.

Harms: **Adding glycoprotein IIb/IIIa inhibitors to heparin:** One RCT found no significant difference between tirofiban plus heparin and heparin alone in risk of bleeding in people already taking aspirin (9.5% with tirofiban plus heparin *v* 8.3% with heparin alone; RR 1.16, 95% CI 0.56 to 2.39).[66]

Comment: None.

QUESTION What are the effects of blood glucose control in prevention of cardiovascular disease in people with diabetes?

OPTION BLOOD GLUCOSE CONTROL

One systematic review found that, compared with conventional glycaemic control, intensive glycaemic control for more than 2 years reduced the occurrence of first major cardiovascular event in people with type 1 diabetes. Two RCTs found no significant difference in cardiovascular morbidity and mortality with intensive compared with conventional glycaemic control in people with type 2 diabetes. These RCTs also found an increase in weight gain and hypoglycaemic episodes with intensive compared with conventional treatment. One RCT in overweight or obese people with type 2 diabetes found that intensive treatment with metformin compared with conventional treatment with diet alone reduced myocardial infarction but not stroke over 5 years. This RCT found no significant increase in major hypoglycaemic episodes in the metformin group compared with the diet only group.

Benefits: We found one systematic review (search date 1996),[67] and three subsequent RCTs.[68–70] **Intensive versus conventional glycaemic control in type 1 diabetes:** The systematic review found that, compared with conventional glycaemic control, intensive glycaemic control for more than 2 years significantly reduced the occurrence of first major cardiovascular event in people with type 1 diabetes (6 RCTs, 1731 people aged 30–42 years with type 1 diabetes; first major cardiovascular event: 27/961 [2.8%] events with intensive control v 55/970 [5.7%] events with conventional glycaemic control; OR 0.55, 95% CI 0.35 to 0.88).[67] Major macrovascular events were defined as fatal or non-fatal myocardial infarction, sudden cardiac death, revascularisation procedure, angina with confirmed coronary artery disease, stroke, lower limb amputation, peripheral arterial events, and peripheral vascular disease. Conventional glycaemic control consisted of one or two daily injections of insulin without self adjustment of insulin dosage according to blood or urine glucose monitoring results. Intensive glycaemic control consisted of three or more injections of insulin with the dosage adjusted according to self monitoring of blood glucose levels.[67] **Intensive versus conventional glycaemic control in type 2 diabetes:** One RCT in people with type 2 diabetes found no significant difference between intensive and conventional glycaemic control in myocardial infarction or stroke over 5 years (1 RCT, 1138 people with type 2 diabetes but without a diagnosis of cardiovascular disease [CVD], mean age 54 years; myocardial infarction: 387/2729 [14.2%] with intensive control v 186/1138 [16.3%] with conventional control; RR 0.84, 95% CI 0.71 to 1.00; P = 0.052; stroke: 148/2729 [5.4%] with intensive control v 55/1138 [4.8%] with conventional control; RR 1.11, 95% CI 0.81 to 1.51).[69] Another RCT in people with type 2 diabetes found no significant difference between intensive insulin treatment with a stepped plan designed to achieve near normal blood sugar levels and standard once daily insulin injection in the rate of new cardiovascular events over 27 months (1 RCT, 153 men with type 2 diabetes, mean age 60 years, many of whom had previous cardiovascular events; new cardiovascular events: 24/75 [32%] with intensive treatment v 16/80 [20%] with standard treatment; RR 1.60, 95% CI 0.92 to 2.50).[70] **Metformin versus diet alone in overweight or obese people with type 2 diabetes:** One RCT in overweight or obese people with type 2 diabetes found that intensive treatment with metformin compared with conventional treatment with diet alone significantly reduced myocardial infarction but not stroke over 5 years (1 RCT, 753 people without a diagnosis of CVD, mean age 53 years; myocardial infarction: 39/342 [11%] with metformin v 73/411 [18%] with diet alone; RR 0.61, 95% CI 0.41 to 0.89; stroke: 12/342 [3.5%] with metformin v 23/411 [5.6%] with diet alone; RR 0.59, 95% CI 0.29 to 1.18).[68]

Harms: **Intensive versus conventional glycaemic control in type 1 diabetes:** The systematic review did not comment on harms.[67] The largest RCT included in the review found that weight gain and waist to hip ratio were significantly increased in the intensive treatment group compared with conventional treatment (weight gain: P ≤ 0.001; waist to hip ratio: P = 0.02).[71] **Intensive versus conventional glycaemic control in type 2 diabetes:** One RCT found that intensive treatment significantly increased weight gain and hypoglycaemic episodes compared with conventional treatment (P < 0.0001).[69] A second RCT found significantly higher mild and moderate hypoglycaemic events with intensive treatment compared with conventional treatment (16.5 events a patient a year with intensive treatment v 1.5 events a patient a year with conventional treatment; P < 0.001). However, it was noted that some hypoglycaemic episodes may not have been detected in the conventional treatment group because of less frequent measurement of blood glucose levels.[70] **Metformin versus diet alone in overweight or obese people with type 2 diabetes:** One RCT found no significant increase in major hypoglycaemic episodes in the metformin group compared with the diet only group (0.6% with metformin v 0.7% with diet only).[68]

Comment: The role of intensive glucose lowering in primary prevention of cardiovascular events remains unclear. However, such treatment clearly reduces the risk of microvascular disease and does not increase the risk of CVD. The potential of the largest RCT in people with type 2 diabetes to show an effect of tighter glycaemic control was limited by the small difference achieved in median HbA1c**G** between intensive and conventional treatment and the relatively low risk of CVD.[68,69] In contrast, in another primary prevention trial, a larger 1.9% difference in median HbA1c was achieved between groups, but the young age of the participants and consequent low incidence of cardiovascular events limited the power of the study to detect an effect of treatment on incidence of CVD.[71,72] The RCT of insulin in type 2 diabetes included men with a high baseline risk of cardiovascular events and achieved a 2.1% absolute difference in HbA1c.[70] The RCT was small and the observed difference between groups could have arisen by chance.

QUESTION **What are the effects of treating multiple risk factors in prevention of cardiovascular disease in people with diabetes?**

OPTION **INTENSIVE MULTIPLE RISK FACTOR TREATMENT**

We found no systematic review or RCTs comparing treatment of multiple risk factors with treatment of a single risk factor for cardiovascular outcomes. One RCT found that, compared with conventional treatment according to clinical guidelines, intensive treatment of multiple risk factors with strict treatment goals in people with type 2 diabetes and microalbuminuria reduces cardiovascular disease over 8 years. Multiple risk factor treatment included simultaneously targeting diet, exercise, glycaemic control, blood pressure, treatment of microalbuminuria, and antiplatelet treatment.

Benefits: We found no systematic review or RCTs comparing treatment of multiple risk factors with treatment of a single risk factor for cardiovascular outcomes. **Intensive versus conventional treatment:** We found one RCT comparing intensive treatment of multiple risk factors versus conventional treatment of multiple risk factors.[73] The RCT found that, compared with conventional treatment, intensive treatment of multiple risk factors in people with type 2 diabetes and microalbuminuria significantly reduced cardiovascular disease (CVD) over 8 years (1 RCT, 160 people including 39 with CVD diagnosis, mean age 55 years; combined outcome of death from CVD, non-fatal myocardial infarction, non-fatal stroke, revascularisation, or amputation: HR 0.47, 95% CI 0.24 to 0.73; ARR 20.0%, 95% CI 5.7% to 34.0%, NNT 5, 95% CI 3 to 18). The intensive treatment group received a stepwise treatment plan with strict treatment goals and included behaviour modification (diet, exercise, smoking cessation) and drug treatment for aggressive management of blood glucose, blood pressure, dyslipidaemia, microalbuminuria, and aspirin treatment for people with ischaemic CVD. The conventional treatment group received treatment for multiple risk factors according to clinical guidelines from their general practitioner.

Harms: **Intensive versus conventional treatment:** The RCT did not specifically evaluate adverse events.[73] It found no significant difference in the incidence of minor episodes of hypoglycaemia between intensive and conventional treatment of multiple risk factors (42/80 [53%] with intensive treatment *v* 39/80 [49%] with conventional treatment; P = 0.5). Severe hypoglycaemia requiring assistance from another person occurred at some point in 5/80 (6.3%) people in the intensive treatment group and in 12/80 (15%) people in the conventional treatment group. One person in the intensive treatment group was hospitalised for a bleeding ulcer.[73]

Comment: **Intensive versus conventional treatment:** All people in the RCT had microalbuminuria at baseline so their cardiovascular risk would have been higher than in people with diabetes without microalbuminuria. However, the conventional treatment group received high quality care, based on guidelines, and the risk reductions from the intensive treatment might have been greater if the comparison had been with "usual care" in the community.[73]

QUESTION **What are the effects of revascularisation procedures in people with diabetes?**

OPTION CORONARY ARTERY BYPASS VERSUS PERCUTANEOUS TRANSLUMINAL ANGIOPLASTY

One systematic review found that, in people with diabetes, coronary artery bypass graft (CABG) reduced all cause mortality at 4 years after initial revascularisation compared with percutaneous transluminal coronary angioplasty (PTCA) but found no significant difference at 6.5 years. One large RCT in people with diabetes and multivessel coronary artery disease has found that CABG reduces mortality or myocardial infarction within 8 years compared with PTCA. Another smaller RCT found a non-significant reduction in mortality with CABG compared with PTCA at 4 years. One RCT in people with diabetes and multivessel coronary artery disease found no significant difference, at time of discharge, between CABG and PTCA plus stent in cardiovascular morbidity or mortality but found an increase in risk of stroke. However, the same RCT found that, compared with PTCA plus stent, CABG reduced cardiovascular risk at 1 year.

Benefits: **Without stenting:** One systematic review (search date 2001) found that, in people with diabetes, coronary artery bypass graft (CABG) significantly reduced all cause mortality at 4.0 years after initial revascularisation compared with percutaneous transluminal coronary angioplasty (PTCA) but it found no significant difference at 6.5 years (3 RCTs: 537 people with diabetes; all cause mortality at 4.0 years: ARR 8.6%, 95% CI 2.2% to 15.0%; P < 0.01; all cause mortality at 6.5 years; ARR 3.9%, 95% CI –17.0% to 25.0%; P = 0.71).[74] The systematic review identified four RCTs. Two RCTS reported results at 4.0 and 6.5 years, one only at 4.0 years and one only at 6.5 years.[74] Two RCTs identified by the systematic review compared CABG versus PTCA, without stenting or a glycoprotein IIb/IIIa inhibitor.[75,76] The first RCT found that CABG significantly reduced the proportion of people who died or suffered Q wave myocardial infarction over a mean of 7.7 years compared with PTCA (1 RCT, 353 people with diabetes and 2 or 3 vessel coronary disease, mean age 62 years: 60/173 [34.7%] with CABG *v* 85/170 [50%] with PTCA; ARR 15%, 95% CI 5% to 26%; RR 0.69, 95% CI 0.54 to 0.89; NNT 7, 95% CI 4 to 20).[75] This survival benefit was confined to those receiving at least one internal mammary graft. The second RCT found no significant difference in mortality 4 years after CABG or PTCA (1 RCT, 125 people, mean age 61 years; mortality: 8/63 [12.5%] with CABG *v* 14/62 [22.6%] with PTCA; RR 0.56, 95% CI 0.25 to 1.25; ARR +9.9%, 95% CI –3.4% to +23.1%).[76] **With stenting:** One RCT found no significant difference in people with diabetes treated with CABG or PTCA in short term risks (up to discharge) of composite end point of death, myocardial infarction, repeat CABG, and repeat PTCA (1 RCT, 208 people with diabetes and 2 or 3 vessel coronary disease; composite outcome of death, myocardial infarction, repeat CABG, and repeat PTCA: 9/96 [9.4%] with CABG *v* 11/112 [9.8%] with PTCA; RR 1.05, 95% CI 0.45 to 2.42).[77]

Harms: **Without stenting:** The systematic review did not report on harms.[74] One RCT found higher inhospital mortality among people with diabetes (1.2% after CABG *v* 0.6% after PTCA) and myocardial infarction during the initial admission to hospital (5.8% after CABG *v* 1.8% after PTCA), but these differences were not found to be significant.[75] The second RCT did not report on harms.[76] **With stenting:** One RCT found a significant increase in risk of stroke with CABG compared with PTCA (4 with CABG *v* 0 with PTCA plus stent; P = 0.04). However, at 1 year the same RCT also found a significantly higher incidence of the composite end point with PTCA plus stenting (1 RCT, 208 people with diabetes and 2 or 3 vessel coronary disease; composite outcome of death, myocardial infarction, repeat CABG, and repeat PTCA: 41/112 [36%] with PTCA plus stent *v* 15/96 [15.6%] with CABG; RR 2.34, 95% CI 1.38 to 3.96; NNH 5, 95% CI 4 to 11).[77]

Comment: None.

OPTION PERCUTANEOUS TRANSLUMINAL CORONARY ANGIOPLASTY COMPARED WITH THROMBOLYSIS

We found no systematic review or RCTs comparing percutaneous transluminal coronary angioplasty versus thrombolysis for prevention of cardiovascular events in people with diabetes. One RCT, in people with diabetes presenting with an acute myocardial infarction, found no significant difference between percutaneous transluminal coronary angioplasty and thrombolysis with alteplase in single outcome of death or composite outcome of death, reinfarction, or disabling stroke at 30 days.

Benefits: We found no systematic review or RCTs comparing percutaneous transluminal coronary angioplasty (PTCA) versus thrombolysis for prevention of cardiovascular events in people with diabetes. **In people presenting with acute myocardial infarction:** One RCT found no significant difference between PTCA and thrombolysis with alteplase in single outcome of death or composite outcome of death, reinfarction, or disabling stroke at 30 days (1 RCT, 177 people with diabetes, mean age 65 years, presenting with acute myocardial infarction**G** within 12 hours of chest pain onset; single outcome of death: 8/99 [8.1%] after PTCA *v* 5/78 [6.4%] after alteplase; RR 1.26, 95% CI 0.43 to 3.71; composite outcome of death, reinfarction, or disabling stroke: 11/99 [11%] after PTCA *v* 13/78 [17%] after alteplase; RR 0.67, 95% CI 0.32 to 1.41).[78] The RCT found no significant difference in 30 day mortality among people with diabetes (8/99 [8.1%] after PTCA *v* 5/78 [6.4%] after alteplase).

Harms: **In people presenting with acute myocardial infarction:** One RCT did not report on adverse effects of PTCA and thrombolysis with alteplase.[68]

Comment: None.

OPTION INTRACORONARY STENTING PLUS GLYCOPROTEIN IIB/IIIA INHIBITORS

RCTs in people with diabetes undergoing percutaneous transluminal coronary angioplasty have found that the combination of stent and a glycoprotein IIb/IIIa inhibitor reduces cardiovascular morbidity and mortality compared with stent plus placebo.

Benefits: We found one non-systematic review of individual patient data[79] and two subsequent RCTS.[80,81] **Versus placebo:** The non-systematic review[79] pooled data from three placebo controlled trials of percutaneous coronary intervention: EPILOG,[82] EPISTENT,[83–85] and EPIC.[86] The non-systematic review found that, compared with placebo, abciximab (a glycoprotein IIb/IIIa inhibitor) significantly reduced overall mortality at 1 year (1462 people with diabetes, mean age 60.9 years; mortality: 22/888 [2.5%] with abciximab *v* 26/574 [4.5%] with placebo; 0.547, 95% CI 0.313 to 0.956; P = 0.03).[79] The first subsequent RCT found that, compared with placebo, eptifibatide (a glycoprotein IIb/IIIa inhibitor) significantly reduced the composite outcome of death or myocardial infarction but found no significant difference for single outcome of death at 1 year (1 RCT, 466 people with diabetes undergoing non-urgent coronary stent implantation, mean age 62 years; composite outcome of death or myocardial infarction: 18/232 [7.8%] with eptifibatide *v* 31/234 [13.4%] with placebo; HR 0.57, 95% CI 0.32 to 1.02; P = 0.001; single outcome of mortality: 3/232 [1.3%] with eptifibatide *v* 8/234 [3.5%] with placebo; HR 0.37, 95% CI 0.10 to 1.41; P = 0.28).[81] **Comparison of glycoprotein IIb/IIIa inhibitors:** The second subsequent RCT found no significant difference between tirofiban and abciximab in composite outcomes of death or myocardial infarction at 30 days and 6 months, or overall mortality at 1 year (1 RCT, 1117 people with diabetes having percutaneous coronary interventions, mean age 62 years; composite outcomes of death or myocardial infarction: at 30 days: 33/560 [5.9%] with tirofiban *v* 29/557 [5.2%] with abciximab; HR 1.14, 95% CI 0.69 to 1.87; P = 0.6; at 6 months: 46/560 [8.2%] with tirofiban *v* 42/557 [7.5%] with abciximab; HR 1.09, 95% CI 0.72 to 1.65; P = 0.7; overall mortality at 1 year: 2.9% with tirofiban *v* 2.1% with abciximab; P = 0.4, absolute numbers not reported).[80]

Harms: **Versus placebo:** One non-systematic review of individual patient data found that there was slightly greater bleeding in people given abciximab than in those given placebo (major bleeding: 4.3% with abciximab *v* 3.0% with placebo; minor bleeding: 6.9% with abciximab *v* 6.3% with placebo; intracranial haemorrhage: 0% with abciximab *v* 0.17% with placebo). None of these differences were significant.[79] The subsequent RCT report on any adverse events associated with eptifibatide.[70] **Comparison of glycoprotein IIb/IIIa inhibitors:** One RCT found no significant difference between abciximab and tirofiban in major bleeding events (P = 0.725).[81]

Comment: For people with diabetes undergoing percutaneous procedures, the combination of stent and glycoprotein IIb/IIIa inhibitor reduces restenosis rates and serious morbidity. It is unclear whether these adjunctive treatments would reduce morbidity, mortality, and restenosis associated with percutaneous revascularisation procedures to the levels seen with coronary artery bypass grafting. The study comparing abciximab versus tirofiban and the study comparing eptifibatide versus placebo were both insufficiently powered to detect reductions in major cardiovascular events in the subgroups of people with diabetes.

GLOSSARY

Acute myocardial infarction is infarction that occurs when circulation to a region of the heart is obstructed and necrosis is occurring; clinical symptoms include severe pain, pallor, perspiration, nausea, dyspnoea, and dizziness. Myocardial infarction is gross necrosis of the myocardium as a result of interruption of blood supply usually caused by atherosclerosis of the coronary arteries; myocardial infarction without pain or other symptoms (silent infarction) is common in people with diabetes.

HbA1c The haemoglobin A1c test is the most common laboratory test of glycated haemoglobin (haemoglobin that has glucose irreversibly bound to it). HbA1c provides an indication of the "average" blood glucose over the preceding 3 months. The HbA1c is a weighted average over time of the blood glucose level; many different glucose profiles can produce the same level of HbA1c.

REFERENCES

1. Geiss LS, Herman WH, Smith PJ. Mortality in non-insulin-dependent diabetes. In: Harris MI, ed. *Diabetes in America*. 2nd ed. Bethesda, MD: National Institutes of Health, 1995:233–255.
2. Wingard DL, Barrett-Connor E. Heart disease and diabetes. In: Harris MI, ed. *Diabetes in America*. 2nd ed. Bethesda, MD: National Institutes of Health, 1995:429–448.
3. Haffner SM, Lehto S, Ronnemaa T, et al. Mortality from coronary heart disease in subjects with type 2 diabetes and in nondiabetic subjects with and without prior myocardial infarction. *N Engl J Med* 1998;339:229–234.
4. Mukamai KJ, Nesto RW, Cohen MC, et al. Impact of diabetes on long-term survival after acute myocardial infarction. *Diabetes Care* 2001;24:1422–1427.
5. Hu FB, Stampfer MJ, Solomon C, et al. Physical activity and risk for cardiovascular events in diabetic women. *Ann Intern Med* 2001;134:96–105.
6. Wei M, Gibbons LW, Kampert JB, et al. Low cardiorespiratory fitness and physical inactivity as predictors of mortality in men with type 2 diabetes. *Ann Intern Med* 2000;132:605–611.
7. Krolewski AS, Warram JH, Freire MB. Epidemiology of late diabetic complications. A basis for the development and evaluation of preventive programs. *Endocrinol Metab Clin North Am* 1996;25:217–242.
8. Messent JW, Elliott TG, Hill RD, et al. Prognostic significance of microalbuminuria in insulin-dependent diabetes mellitus: a twenty-three year follow-up study. *Kidney Int* 1992;41:836–839.
9. Dinneen SF, Gerstein HC. The association of microalbuminuria and mortality in non-insulin-dependent diabetes mellitus: a systematic overview of the literature. *Arch Intern Med* 1997;157:1413–1418. Search date 1995; primary sources Medline, SciSearch, and hand searching of bibliographies.
10. Valmadrid CT, Klein R, Moss SE, et al. The risk of cardiovascular disease mortality associated with microalbuminuria and gross proteinuria in persons with older-onset diabetes mellitus. *Arch Intern Med* 2000;160:1093–1100.
11. Borch Johnsen K, Andersen PK, Deckert T. The effect of proteinuria on relative mortality in type 1 (insulin-dependent) diabetes mellitus. *Diabetologia* 1985;28:590–596.
12. Warram JH, Laffel LM, Ganda OP, et al. Coronary artery disease is the major determinant of excess mortality in patients with insulin-dependent diabetes mellitus and persistent proteinuria. *J Am Soc Nephrol* 1992;3(suppl 4):104–110.
13. Gerstein Hertzel C, Johannes FE, Qilong Yi, et al. Albuminuria and risk of cardiovascular events, death and heart failure in diabetic and nondiabetic individuals. *JAMA* 2001;286:421–426.
14. Behar S, Boyko V, Reicher-Reiss H, et al. Ten-year survival after acute myocardial infarction: comparison of patients with and without diabetes. SPRINT Study Group. Secondary Prevention Reinfarction Israeli Nifedipine Trial. *Am Heart J* 1997;133:290–296.
15. Mak KH, Moliterno DJ, Granger CB, et al. Influence of diabetes mellitus on clinical outcome in the thrombolytic era of acute myocardial infarction: GUSTO-I Investigators: global utilization of streptokinase and tissue plasminogen activator for occluded coronary arteries. *J Am Coll Cardiol* 1997;30:171–179.
16. Capes SE, Hunt D, Malmberg K, et al. Stress hyperglycaemia and increased risk of death after myocardial infarction in patients with and without diabetes: a systematic overview. *Lancet* 2000;355:773–778. Search date 1998; primary sources Medline, Science Citation Index, hand searches of bibliographies of relevant articles, and contact with experts in the field.
17. Lotufo PA, Gazziano M, Chae CU, et al. Diabetes and all-cause coronary heart disease mortality among US male physicians. *Arch Intern Med* 2001;161:242–247.
18. Huang ES, Meigs JB, Singer DE. The effect of interventions to prevent cardiovascular disease in patients with type 2 diabetes mellitus. *Am J Med* 2001;111:633–642. Search date 2000; primary sources Medline and reference lists.
19. Vijan S, Hayward RA. Treatment of hypertension in type 2 diabetes mellitus: blood pressure goals, choice of agents, and setting priorities in diabetes care. *Ann Intern Med* 2003;138:593–602. Search date 2002; primary sources Cochrane Library, Medline, references from meta-analyses, review articles, and expert recommendation.
20. Shekelle PG, Rich MW, Morton SC, et al. Efficacy of angiotensin-converting enzyme inhibitors and beta-blockers in the management of left ventricular systolic dysfunction according to race, gender, and diabetic status: a meta-analysis of major clinical trials. *J Am Coll Cardiol* 2003;41:1529–1538.
21. Tuomilehto J, Rastenyte D, Birkenhäger WH, et al. Effects of calcium-channel blockade in older patients with diabetes and systolic hypertension. *N Engl J Med* 1999;340:677–684.
22. Lewis EJ, Hunsicker LG, Clark WR, et al. Renoprotective effect of the angiotensin receptor antagonist irbesartan in patients with nephropathy due to type 2 diabetes. *N Engl J Med* 2001:345:851–860.
23. Parving HH, Lehnert H, Brochner-Mortensen J, et al. The effect of irbesartan on the development of diabetic nephropathy in patients with type 2 diabetes. *N Engl J Med* 2001;345:870–878.
24. Heart Outcomes Prevention Evaluation (HOPE) Study Investigators. Effects of ramipril on cardiovascular and microvascular outcomes in people with diabetes mellitus: results of the HOPE study and the MICRO-HOPE substudy. *Lancet* 2000;355:253–259.
25. Berl T, Hunsicker LG, Lewis JB, et al. Cardiovascular outcomes in the Irbesartan Diabetic Nephropathy Trial of patients with type 2 diabetes and overt nephropathy. *Ann Intern Med* 2003;138:542–549.
26. Bosch J, Yusuf S, Pogue J, et al. Use of ramipril in preventing stroke: double blind randomized trial. *BMJ* 2002;324:699–702.
27. Lonn E, Roccaforte R, Yi Q, et al. Effect of long-term therapy with ramipril in high-risk women. *J Am Coll Cardiol* 2002;40:693–702.
28. Pahor M, Psaty BM, Alderman MH, et al. Therapeutic benefits of ACE inhibitors and other antihypertensive drugs in patients with type 2 diabetes. *Diabetes Care* 2000;23:888–892. Search date 2000; primary source Medline.
29. Black HR, Elliott WJ, Grandits G, et al. Principal results of the Controlled Onset Verapamil Investigation of Cardiovascular End Points (CONVINCE) trial. *JAMA* 2003;289:2073–2082.
30. Mancia G, Brown M, Castaigne A, et al. Outcomes with nifedipine GITS or Co-amilozide in hypertensive diabetics and nondiabetics in Intervention as a Goal in Hypertension (INSIGHT). *Hypertension* 2003;41:431–436.
31. Tatti P, Pahor M, Byington RP, et al. Outcome results of the Fosinopril versus Amlodipine Cardiovascular Events randomised Trial (FACET) in patients with hypertension and NIDDM. *Diabetes Care* 1998;21:597–603.
32. Estacio RO, Jeffers BW, Hiatt WR, et al. The effect of nisoldipine as compared with enalapril on cardiovascular events in patients with non-insulin-dependent diabetes and hypertension. *N Engl J Med* 1998;338:645–652.
33. Lindholm LH, Hansson L, Ekbom T, et al. Comparison of antihypertensive treatment in preventing cardiovascular events in elderly diabetic patients:

results from the Swedish trial in old patients with hypertension – 2. *J Hypertens* 2000;18:1671–1675.
34. UK Prospective Diabetes Study Group. Efficacy of atenolol and captopril in reducing risk of macrovascular and microvascular complications in type 2 diabetes: UKPDS 39. *BMJ* 1998;317:713–720.
35. Niskanen L, Hedner T, Hansson L, et al. Reduced cardiovascular morbidity and mortality in hypertensive diabetic patients on first-line therapy with an ACE inhibitor compared with diuretic/beta-blocker-based treatment regiment, a subanalysis of the Captopril Prevention Project. *Diabetes Care* 2001;24:2091–2096.
36. ALLHAT Officers and Coordinators for the ALLHAT Collaborative Research Group. Major outcomes in high-risk hypertensive patients randomized to angiotensin-converting enzyme inhibitor or calcium channel blocker vs diuretic: The Antihypertensive and Lipid-Lowering Treatment to Prevent Heart Attack Trial (ALLHAT). *JAMA* 2002;288:2981–2997.
37. Lindholm LH, Ibsen H, Dahlof B, et al. Cardiovascular morbidity and mortality in patients with diabetes in the Losartan Intervention For Endpoint reduction in hypertension study (LIFE): a randomized trial against atenolol. *Lancet* 2002;359:1004–1010.
38. Hansson L, Hedner T, Lund-Johansen P, et al. Randomized trial of effects of calcium antagonists compared with diuretics and beta-blockers on cardiovascular morbidity and mortality in hypertension: the Nordic Diltiazem (NORDIL) study. *Lancet* 2000;356:359–365.
39. ALLHAT Collaborative Research Group. Major cardiovascular events in hypertensive patients randomised to doxazosin vs chlorthalidone: the antihypertensive and lipid-lowering treatment to prevent heart attack trial (ALLHAT). *JAMA* 2000;283:1967–1975.
40. UK Prospective Diabetes Study Group. Tight blood pressure control and risk of macrovascular and microvascular complications in type 2 diabetes: UKPDS 38. *BMJ* 1998;317:703–713.
41. Hansson L, Zanchetti A, Carruthers SG, et al. Effects of intensive blood-pressure lowering and low-dose aspirin in patients with hypertension: principal results of the Hypertension Optimal Treatment (HOT) randomised trial. *Lancet* 1998;351:1755–1762.
42. Schrier RW, Estacio RO, Esler A, et al. Effects of aggressive blood pressure control in normotensive type 2 diabetic patients on albuminuria, retinopathy and strokes. *Kidney Int* 2002;6:1086–1097.
43. Mehler PS, Coll JR, Estacio R, et al. Intensive blood pressure control reduces the risk of cardiovascular events in patients with peripheral arterial disease and type 2 diabetes. *Circulation* 2003;107:753–756.
44. Gami AS, Montori VM, Erwin PJ, et al. Systematic review of lipid lowering for primary prevention of coronary heart disease in diabetes. *BMJ* 2003;326:528–529. Search date not reported; primary source Medline.
45. Koskinen P, Manttari M, Manninen V, et al. Coronary heart disease incidence in NIDDM patients in the Helsinki Heart Study. *Diabetes Care* 1992;15:820–825.
46. Rubins HB, Robins SJ, Collins D, et al. Diabetes, plasma insulin, and cardiovascular disease: subgroup analysis from the Department of Veterans Affairs high-density lipoprotein intervention trial (VA-HIT). *Arch Intern Med* 2002;162:2597–2604.
47. Elkeles RS, Diamond JR, Poulter C, et al. Cardiovascular outcomes in type 2 diabetes. A double-blind placebo-controlled study of bezafibrate: the St Mary's, Ealing, Northwick Park Diabetes Cardiovascular Disease Prevention (SENDCAP) Study. *Diabetes Care* 1998;21:641–648.
48. Diabetes Atherosclerosis Interventions Study Investigators. Effect of fenofibrate on progression of coronary-artery disease in type 2 diabetes: The Diabetes Atherosclerosis Interventions Study, a randomized study. *Lancet* 2001;357:905–910.
49. Collins R, Armitage J, Parish S, et al. MRC/BHF Heart Protection Study of cholesterol-lowering with simvastatin in 5963 people with diabetes: a randomised placebo-controlled trial. *Lancet* 2003;361:2005–2016.
50. Serruys P, Feyter P, Macaya C, et al. Fluvastatin for the prevention of cardiac events following successful first percutaneous coronary intervention. *JAMA* 2002;287:3215–3222.
51. The ALLHAT officers and coordinators for the ALLHAT Collaborative research group. Major outcomes in moderately hypercholesterolemic, hypertensive patients randomized to pravastatin versus usual care. *JAMA* 2002;288:2998–3007.
52. Sever PS, Dahlof B, Poulter NR, et al. Prevention of coronary and stroke events with atorvastatin in hypertensive patients who have average or lower-than-average cholesterol concentrations, in the Anglo-Scandinavian Cardiac Outcomes Trial – Lipid Lowering Arm (ASCOT-LLA): a multicentre randomised controlled trial. *Lancet* 2003;361:1149–1158.
53. Athyros V, Papageorgiou A, Mercouris B, et al. Treatment with atorvastatin to the National Cholesterol Educational Program goal versus "usual" care in secondary coronary heart disease prevention. The GREek Atorvastatin and Coronary-heart-disease Evaluation (GREACE) study. *Curr Med Res Opin* 2002;18:220–228.
54. Ito H, Yasuyoshi O, Yasuo O, et al. A comparison of low versus standard dose pravastatin therapy for the prevention of cardiovascular events in the elderly: the Pravastatin anti-atherosclerosis trial in the elderly (PATE). *J Atheroscler Thromb* 2001;8:33–44.
55. Pyorala K, Pedersen TR, Kjekshus J, et al. Cholesterol lowering with simvastatin improves prognosis of diabetic patients with coronary heart disease. A subgroup analysis of the Scandinavian Simvastatin Survival Study (4S). *Diabetes Care* 1997;20:614–620.
56. The Long-term Intervention with Pravastatin in Ischemic Disease (LIPID) Study Program. Prevention of cardiovascular events and death with pravastatin in patients with coronary heart disease and a broad range of initial cholesterol levels. *N Engl J Med* 1998;339:1349–1357.
57. Sacks FM, Pfeffer MA, Moye LA, et al. The effect of pravastatin on coronary events after myocardial infarction in patients with average cholesterol levels. Cholesterol and Recurrent Events Trial investigators. *N Engl J Med* 1996;335:1001–1009.
58. Downs JR, Clearfield M, Weis S, et al. Primary prevention of acute coronary events with lovastatin in men and women with average cholesterol levels: results of AFCAPS/TexCAPS. Air Force/Texas Coronary Atherosclerosis Prevention Study. *JAMA* 1998;279:1615–1622.
59. Hoogwerf BJ, Waness A, Cressman W, et al. Effects of aggressive cholesterol lowering and low-dose anticoagulation on clinical and angiographic outcomes in patients with diabetes. The Post Coronary Artery Bypass Graft Trial. *Diabetes* 1999;48:1289–1294.
60. Antithrombotic Trialists' Collaboration. Collaborative meta-analysis of randomised trials of antiplatelet therapy for prevention of death, myocardial infarction, and stroke in high risk patients. *BMJ* 2002;324:71–86. [Erratum in: *BMJ* 2002;324:141]. Search date 1997; primary sources Medline, Embase, Derwent, Scisearch, and Biosis.
61. Steering Committee of the Physicians' Health Study Research Group. Final report on the aspirin component of the ongoing Physicians' Health Study. *N Engl J Med* 1989;321:129–135.
62. ETDRS Investigators. Aspirin effects on mortality and morbidity in patients with diabetes mellitus. *JAMA* 1992;268:1292–1300.
63. American Diabetes Association. Aspirin therapy in diabetes. *Diabetes Care* 1997;20:1772–1773.
64. Bhatt DL, Marso SP, Hirsch AT, et al. Amplified benefit of clopidogrel versus aspirin in patients with diabetes mellitus. *Am J Cardiol* 2002;90:625–628.

65. The Clopidogrel in Unstable Angina to Prevent Recurrent Events Trial Investigators. Effects of clopidogrel in addition to aspirin in patients with acute coronary syndromes without ST-segment elevation. *N Engl J Med* 2001;345:494–502.
66. Theroux P, Alexander J, Pharand C, et al. Glycoprotein IIb/IIIa receptor blockade improves outcomes in diabetic patients presenting with unstable angina/Non-ST-elevation myocardial infarction results from the platelet receptor inhibitor in ischemic syndrome management in patients limited by unstable signs and symptoms. *Circulation* 2000;102:2466–2472.
67. Lawson ML, Gerstein HC, Tsui E, et al. Effect of intensive therapy on early macrovascular disease in young individuals with type 1 diabetes. A systematic review and meta-analysis. *Diabetes Care* 1999;22:B35–B39. Search date 1996; primary sources Medline, Citation Index, personal files, and bibliographies of all retrieved articles.
68. UK Prospective Diabetes Study Group. Effect of intensive blood-glucose control with metformin on complications in overweight patients with type 2 diabetes (UKPDS 34). *Lancet* 1998;352:854–865.
69. UK Prospective Diabetes Study Group. Intensive blood-glucose control with sulphonylureas or insulin compared with conventional treatment and risk of complications in patients with type 2 diabetes (UKPDS 33). *Lancet* 1998;352:837–853.
70. Abraira C, Colwell J, Nuttall F, et al. Cardiovascular events and correlates in the Veterans Affairs Diabetes Feasibility Trial: Veterans Affairs Cooperative Study on glycemic control and complications in type II diabetes. *Arch Intern Med* 1997;157:181–188.
71. DCCT Research Group. Effect of intensive diabetes management on macrovascular events and risk factors in the Diabetes Control and Complications Trial. *Am J Cardiol* 1995;75:894–903.
72. DCCT Research Group. The effect of intensive treatment of diabetes on the development and progression of long-term complications in insulin-dependent diabetes mellitus. *N Engl J Med* 1993;329:977–986.
73. Gaede P, Vedel P, Larsen N, et al. Multifactorial intervention and cardiovascular disease in patients with type 2 diabetes. *N Engl J Med* 2003;348:383–393.
74. Hoffman SN, TenBrook JA, Wolf MP, et al. A meta-analysis of randomized controlled trials comparing coronary artery bypass graft with percutaneous transluminal coronary angioplasty: one- to eight-year outcomes. *J Am Coll Cardiol* 2003;41:1293–1304. Search date 2001; primary source Medline.
75. The BARI Investigators. Seven-year outcome in the Bypass Angioplasty Revascularization Investigation (BARI) by treatment and diabetic status. *J Am Coll Cardiol* 2000;35:1122–1129.
76. Kurbaan AS, Bowker TJ, Ilsley CD, et al. Difference in the mortality of the CABRI diabetic and nondiabetic populations and its relation to coronary artery disease and the revascularization mode. *Am J Cardiol* 2001;87:947–950.
77. Abizaid A, Costa MA, Centemero M, et al. Clinical and economic impact of diabetes mellitus on percutaneous and surgical treatment of multivessel coronary disease patients: insights form the arterial revascularization therapy study (ARTS) trial. *Circulation* 2001;104:533–538.
78. Hasdai D, Granger CB, Srivatsa S, et al. Diabetes mellitus and outcome after primary coronary angioplasty for acute myocardial infarction: lessons from the GUSTO-IIb angioplasty study. *J Am Coll Cardiol* 2000;35:1502–1512.
79. Bhatt DL, Marso SP, Lincoff AM, et al. Abciximab reduces mortality in diabetics following percutaneous coronary intervention. *J Am Coll Cardiol* 2000;35:922–928.
80. Roffi M, Moliterno D, Meier B, et al. Impact of different platelet glycoprotein IIb/IIIa receptor inhibitors among diabetic patients undergoing percutaneous coronary intervention. *Circulation* 2002;105:2730–2736.
81. Labinaz M, Madan M, O'Shea JO, et al. Comparison of one-year outcomes following coronary artery stenting in diabetic versus nondiabetic patients (from the Enhanced Suppression of the Platelet IIb/IIIa Receptor With Integrilin Therapy [ESPRIT] Trial). *Am J Cardiol* 2002;90;585–590.
82. Kleiman NS, Lincoff AM, Kereiakes DJ, et al. Diabetes mellitus, glycoprotein IIb/IIIa blockade, and heparin: evidence for a complex interaction in a multicenter trial. EPILOG Investigators. *Circulation* 1998;97:1912–1920.
83. Marso SP, Lincoff AM, Ellis SG, et al. Optimizing the percutaneous interventional outcomes for patients with diabetes mellitus: results of the EPISTENT (Evaluation of platelet IIb/IIIa inhibitor for stenting trial) diabetic substudy. *Circulation* 1999;100:2477–2484.
84. The EPISTENT Investigators. Randomised placebo-controlled and balloon-angioplasty-controlled trial to assess safety of coronary stenting with use of platelet glycoprotein-IIb/IIIa blockade. Evaluation of platelet IIb/IIIa inhibitor for stenting. *Lancet* 1998;352:87–92.
85. Topol EJ, Mark DB, Lincoff AM, et al. Outcomes at 1 year and economic implications of platelet glycoprotein IIb/IIIa blockade in patients undergoing coronary stenting: results from a multicentre randomised trial. EPISTENT Investigators. Evaluation of Platelet IIb/IIIa Inhibitor for Stenting. *Lancet* 1999;354:2019–2024. [Erratum in *Lancet* 2000;355:1104].
86. The EPIC Investigation. Use of a monoclonal antibody directed against the platelet glycoprotein IIb/IIIa receptor in high-risk coronary angioplasty. *N Engl J Med* 1994;330:956–961.

Ronald Sigal
Associate Professor of Medicine and Human Kinetics

Janine Malcolm
Clinical Scholar, Division of Endocrinology and Metabolism
University of Ottawa, Ontario, Canada

Hilary Meggison
Fellow, Critical Care
Ottawa Hospital, Ottawa, Canada

Competing interests: RS has received research support from Aventis, GlaxoSmithKline, Bristol-Myers-Squibb, Merck-Frosst and Boehringer-Ingelheim. He has received speaker's fees from Aventis, GlaxoSmithKline, Servier, Novo-Nordisk and Eli Lilly. He has been reimbursed by Merck-Frosst for organising a symposium. JM and HM have had travel expenses reimbursed by GlaxoSmithKline for attending a symposium.
We would like to acknowledge the previous contributors of this chapter, including Marie-France Levac.

Primary hypothyroidism

Search date December 2003

Birte Nygaard

QUESTIONS

INTERVENTIONS

CLINICAL (OVERT) HYPOTHYROIDISM

Beneficial

Levothyroxine (L-thyroxine)* 753

Unknown effectiveness

Levothyroxine (L-thyroxine) plus liothyronine (compared with L-thyroxine alone). 753

SUBCLINICAL HYPOTHYROIDISM

Unknown effectiveness

Levothyroxine (L-thyroxine) 754

*No RCT evidence, but there is clinical consensus that levothyroxine is beneficial in clinical (overt) hypothyroidism. A placebo controlled trial would be considered unethical.

See glossary Ⓖ

Key Messages

Clinical (overt) hypothyroidism

- **Levothyroxine (L-thyroxine)** We found no RCTs comparing levothyroxine versus placebo, although there is consensus that treatment is beneficial. Treating clinical (overt) hypothyroidism with thyroid hormone (levothyroxine) can induce hyperthyroidism and reduce bone mass in postmenopausal women and increase risk of atrial fibrillation.
- **Levothyroxine (L-thyroxine) plus liothyronine (compared with L-thyroxine alone)** Three small RCTs provided insufficient evidence of outcome improvement between a combination of levothyroxine plus liothyronine and levothyroxine alone. Treating clinical (overt) hypothyroidism with thyroid hormone (levothyroxine) can induce hyperthyroidism and reduce bone mass in postmenopausal women and increase the risk of atrial fibrillation.

Subclinical hypothyroidism

- **Levothyroxine (L-thyroxine)** One RCT in women with biochemically defined subclinical hypothyroidism found no significant difference between levothyroxine and placebo in overall symptom improvement at 1 year. The RCT may, however, have lacked power to exclude a clinically important difference between treatments. Another RCT found no significant difference in health related quality of life scores between levothyroxine and placebo. One RCT found inconclusive results about the effect of levothyroxine versus placebo on cognitive function in people with subclinical hypothyroidism. One RCT found that levothyroxine improved left ventricular function at 6 months compared with placebo. Treating subclinical hypothyroidism with thyroid hormone can induce hyperthyroidism and reduce bone mass in postmenopausal women and increase the risk of atrial fibrillation.

Primary hypothyroidism

DEFINITION

Hypothyroidism is characterised by low levels of blood thyroid hormone. **Clinical (overt) hypothyroidism** is diagnosed on the basis of characteristic clinical features consisting of mental slowing, depression, dementia, weight gain, constipation, dry skin, hair loss, cold intolerance, hoarse voice, irregular menstruation, infertility, muscle stiffness and pain, bradycardia, hypercholesterolaemia, combined with a raised blood level of thyroid stimulating hormone (TSH) (serum TSH levels > 12 mU/L), and a low serum thyroxine (T_4Ⓖ) level (serum T_4 < 60 nmol/L). **Subclinical hypothyroidism** is diagnosed when serum TSH is raised (serum TSH levels > 4 mU/L) but serum thyroxine is normal and there are no symptoms or signs, or only minor symptoms or signs, of thyroid dysfunction. **Primary hypothyroidism** is seen after destruction of the thyroid gland because of autoimmunity (the most common cause), or medical intervention such as surgery, radioiodine, and radiation. **Secondary hypothyroidism** is seen after pituitary or hypothalamic damage, and results in insufficient production of TSH. Secondary hypothyroidism is not covered in this review. **Euthyroid sick syndrome** is diagnosed when tri-iodothyronine (T_3Ⓖ) levels are low, serum thyroxine is low, and TSH levels are normal or low. Euthyroid sick syndrome is not covered in this review.

INCIDENCE/ PREVALENCE

Hypothyroidism is more common in women than in men (in the UK, female : male ratio of 6 : 1). One study (2779 people in the UK with a median age of 58 years) found the incidence of clinical (overt) hypothyroidism was 40/10 000 women per year and 6/10 000 men per year. The prevalence was 9.3% in women and 1.3% in men.[1] In areas with high iodine intake, the incidence of hypothyroidism can be higher than in areas with normal or low iodine intake. In Denmark, where there is moderate iodine insufficiency, the overall incidence of hypothyroidism is 1.4/10 000 per year increasing to 8/10 000 per year in people older than 70 years.[2] The incidence of subclinical hypothyroidism increases with age. Up to 10% of women over the age of 60 years have subclinical hypothyroidism (evaluated from data from the Netherlands and USA).[3,4]

AETIOLOGY/ RISK FACTORS

Primary thyroid gland failure can occur as a result of chronic autoimmune thyroiditis, radioactive iodine treatment, or thyroidectomy. Other causes include drug adverse effects (e.g. amiodarone and lithium), transient hypothyroidism due to silent thyroiditis, subacute thyroiditis, or postpartum thyroiditis.

PROGNOSIS

In people with subclinical hypothyroidism, the risk of developing overt hypothyroidism is described in the UK Whickham Survey (25 years' follow up; for women: OR 8, 95% CI 3 to 20; for men: OR 44, 95% CI 19 to 104; if both a raised TSH and positive antithyroid antibodies were present; for women: OR 38, 95% CI 22 to 65; for men: OR 173, 95% CI 81 to 370). For women, the survey found an annual risk of 4.3% per year (if both raised serum TSH and antithyroid antibodies were present), 2.6% per year (if raised serum TSH was present alone); the minimum number of people with raised TSH and antithyroid antibodies who would need treating to prevent this progression to clinical (overt) hypothyroidism in one person over 5 years is 5–8.[1] **Cardiovascular disease:** A large cross-sectional study (25 862 people with serum TSH between 5.1–10 mU/L) found significantly higher mean total cholesterol concentrations in hypothyroid people compared with euthyroid people (5.8 *v* 5.6 mmol/L).[3] Another study (124 elderly women with subclinical hypothyroidism, 931 euthyroid women) found a significantly increased risk of myocardial infarction in women with subclinical hypothyroidism (OR 2.3, 95% CI 1.3 to 4.0) and of aortic atherosclerosis (OR 1.7, 95% CI 1.1 to 2.6).[4] **Mental health:** Subclinical hypothyroidism is associated with depression.[5] People with subclinical hypothyroidism may have depression that is refractory to both antidepressant drugs and thyroid hormone alone. Memory impairment, hysteria, anxiety, somatic complaints, and depressive features without depression have been described in people with subclinical hypothyroidism.[6]

AIMS OF INTERVENTION

To eliminate the symptoms of hypothyroidism and maximise quality of life.

OUTCOMES

Quality of life and neuropsychological impairments (evaluated by congestive function tests, memory tests, reaction time, self rating mood scales, and depression scores); cardiovascular disease (episodes of atrial fibrillation and ischaemic events); cardiac function (evaluated by echocardiography); changes in body composition (measured by osteodensitometry or bioimpedance measurements); prevention of progression from subclinical to overt hypothyroidism; adverse effects of treatments (bone mass, fracture rate, development of hyperthyroidism).

METHODS

Clinical Evidence search and appraisal December 2003, with an additional manual search of reference lists.

QUESTION **What are the effects of treatments for clinical (overt) hypothyroidism?**

OPTION **LEVOTHYROXINE (L-THYROXINE) FOR CLINICAL (OVERT) HYPOTHYROIDISM**

We found no RCTs comparing levothyroxine versus placebo, although there is consensus that treatment is beneficial. Treating clinical (overt) hypothyroidism with thyroid hormone (levothyroxine) can induce hyperthyroidism and reduce bone mass in postmenopausal women and increase the risk of atrial fibrillation.

Benefits: We found no RCTs comparing levothyroxine versus placebo in people with clinical hypothyroidism, although there is consensus that treatment is beneficial (see comment below).

Harms: We found no RCTs comparing levothyroxine versus placebo in people with clinical hypothyroidism. Over-treatment with levothyroxine may cause hyperthyroidism. **Fracture rate:** One longitudinal observational study (1180 people on levothyroxine followed for an average of 8.6 years) found no significant increase in fracture rate between levothyroxine and control.[7] **Bone mass:** We found one systematic review (search date not stated, 13 RCTs) in a total of 441 premenopausal women and 317 postmenopausal women.[8] All women had received prolonged levothyroxine treatment with reduced serum TSH concentration but normal T_4 and T_3Ⓖ values. In premenopausal women (average age 40 years, treated with levothyroxine 164 µg/day for 8.5 years leading to suppressed serum TSH) the review found no significant difference between levothyroxine and control in bone mass after 8.5 years (2.7% less bone mass with levothyroxine *v* control; P value reported as non significant). In postmenopausal women (average age 61.2 years, treated with levothyroxine 171 µg/day for 9.9 years leading to suppressed serum TSH), it found that levothyroxine significantly reduced bone mass compared with control after 9.9 years (bone mass 9.0% lower with levothyroxine than control, 95% CI 2.4% to 15.7%). **Atrial fibrillation:** We found no analytical study directly evaluating the effects of levothyroxine for the outcome of atrial fibrillation. We found one cohort study evaluating the incidence of atrial fibrillation in people aged over 60 years with low serum TSH concentrations (≤ 0.1 mU/L). The cohort study found that low serum TSH concentrations were associated with an increased risk of atrial fibrillation (diagnosed by electrocardiogram) at 10 years (61 people with low TSH [36 taking a thyroid hormone], 1576 people with normal TSH [46 taking a thyroid hormone]; incidence of atrial fibrillation: 28 per 1000 person years with low TSH values v 11 per 1000 person years with normal TSH values; 13/61 [21.3%] with low TSH values v 133/1576 [8.4%] with normal TSH values; RR 2.53, 95% CI 1.52 to 4.20; RR calculated by *Clinical Evidence*).[9]

Comment: A placebo controlled trial would be considered unethical.

OPTION **LEVOTHYROXINE (L-THYROXINE) PLUS LIOTHYRONINE FOR CLINICAL (OVERT) HYPOTHYROIDISM**

Three small RCTs provided insufficient evidence of outcome improvement between a combination of levothyroxine plus liothyronine and levothyroxine alone. Treating clinical (overt) hypothyroidism with thyroid hormone (levothyroxine) can induce hyperthyroidism and reduce bone mass in postmenopausal women and increase the risk of atrial fibrillation.

Benefits: We found three RCTs of people with clinical hypothyroidism who had been treated for at least 6 months with levothyroxine, comparing a reduced dose of levothyroxine plus liothyronine versus levothyroxine alone.[10–12] The first RCT (110 people with clinical hypothyroidism; crossover design) found that the combined treatment had significantly higher total General Health Questionnaire 28 scores (GHQ28: 0 = best score, 86 = poorest score) compared with levothyroxine alone at 10 weeks (mean GHQ score: 21.2 with levothyroxine plus liothyronine v 18.3 with levothyroxine alone; P = 0.033).[10] No significant differences were seen in cognitive function evaluated by several cognitive tests. No titration of the levothyroxine or liothyronine dose were made and this resulted in a significant difference in serum thyroid stimulating hormone (TSH) between the combined treatment and thyroxine alone (serum TSH: 3.1 mU/l with levothyroxine plus liothyronine v 1.5 mU/l with levothyroxine alone; P < 0.001). The second RCT (40 people with clinical hypothyroidism and depression) found no significant difference in SCL–90 scores (a measure of depression: 0 = best score, 90 = poorest score) or CES–D scores (a measure of depression: 0 = best score, 60 = poorest score) between levothyroxine plus liothyronine and levothyroxine alone at 15 weeks (mean CES-D scores: 24.8 at baseline to 14.4 with levothyroxine plus liothyronine v 17.5 at baseline to 12.8 with levothyroxine alone; P value for mean changes in scores = 0.284; mean SCL-90 scores: 44.9 at baseline to 27.5 with levothyroxine plus liothyronine v 34.4 at baseline to 19.1 with levothyroxine alone; P value for mean changes in scores = 0.656).[11] The third RCT (46 people with clinical hypothyroidism) found no significant difference in improvement of a hypothyroid specific HRQL questionnaire (a general health questionnaire; 27 = best outcome and 145 = worst outcome) between levothyroxine plus liothyronine and levothyroxine alone at 16 weeks (mean HRQL scores: 66 at baseline to 50 with levothyroxine plus liothyronine v 77 at baseline to 58 with levothyroxine alone; P value for mean changes in scores = 0.54).[12] In one of the 13 neurophysiological tests (grooved peg board Ⓖ) a significant difference was seen favouring the control group (2% increase in score on the combined therapies, compared with 2% fall in score on levothyroxine; P = 0.03).

Harms: See harms of levothyroxine for clinical hypothyroidism, p 753.

Comment: None.

QUESTION What are the effects of treatments for subclinical hypothyroidism?

OPTION LEVOTHYROXINE (L-THYROXINE) FOR SUBCLINICAL HYPOTHYROIDISM

One RCT in women with biochemically defined subclinical hypothyroidism found no significant difference between levothyroxine and placebo in overall symptom improvement at 1 year. The RCT may, however, have lacked power to exclude a clinically important difference between treatments. Another RCT found no significant difference in health related quality of life scores between levothyroxine and placebo. One RCT found inconclusive results about the effect of levothyroxine versus placebo on cognitive function in people with subclinical hypothyroidism. One RCT found that levothyroxine improved left ventricular function at 6 months compared with placebo. Treating subclinical hypothyroidism with thyroid hormone can induce hyperthyroidism and reduce bone mass in postmenopausal women and increase the risk of atrial fibrillation.

Benefits: **General symptoms:** We found two RCTs.[13,14] The first RCT compared levothyroxine (50 μg/day) versus placebo in 33 women with increased thyroid stimulating hormone (TSH), normal serum thyroxine and normal free T_4 and T_3**G**, and on average, two of the following symptoms: muscle cramps, dry skin, cold intolerance, fatigue, or constipation.[13] Physical examination revealed no signs of hypothyroidism, apart from dry or coarse skin, which was present in about 50% of women in each group. The RCT examined the effects of treatment on general symptoms (evaluated by a questionnaire in participants stating if they were feeling better, unchanged, or worse) for 1 year. It found no significant difference in overall symptom improvement between levothyroxine and placebo (8/17 [47%] people with levothyroxine *v* 3/16 [19%] people with placebo; P = 0.14, recalculated by *Clinical Evidence*).[13] The second RCT (40 women with increased TSH and normal T_4) compared levothyroxine versus placebo for 6 months. The RCT found no significant difference between levothyroxine and placebo in health related quality of life scores at 6 months (Hospital Anxiety and Depression Scale, 0 = best score and 42 = poorest score: 12 at baseline to 9 with levothyroxine v 12 at baseline to 9 with placebo; and the 30-item General Health Questionnaire, 0 = best score and 30 = poorest score: 5 at baseline to 2 with levothyroxine v 5 at baseline to 0 with placebo; P = 0.9).[14] **Cognitive function:** We found one RCT (37 people, aged > 55 years, TSH > 6.0 mU/L, normal T_4, T_3, and thyroxine binding globulin) comparing levothyroxine (25 μg/day for 4 weeks then 50 μg/day) versus placebo for 10 months. It found no significant difference between levothyroxine and placebo in any outcome except in one psychometric memory score based on a battery of cognitive function tests evaluating memory (the composition memory score**G**: P = 0.01).[15] No firm conclusions could be drawn from these findings. **Cardiac function:** We found one RCT (20 people with increased TSH, and normal T_4 and T_3 for least 1 year) which compared the effects of levothyroxine (50 μg/day) versus placebo on cardiac function for 1 year.[16] Cardiac function was evaluated by conventional two-dimensional Doppler echocardiography and ultrasonic videodensitometry. The RCT found that levothyroxine significantly improved left ventricular function compared with placebo at 6 months (increased isovolumic relaxation time, P < 0.03; peak A, P < 0.01; pre-ejection/ejection time ratio, P < 0.03; cyclic variation index, P < 0.05).[16]

Harms: **General symptoms:** The first RCT did not report on adverse effects.[13] The second RCT found a significant worsening in anxiety scores with levothyroxine versus placebo (P = 0.03).[14] **Cognitive function:** In the RCT, 2/18 (11%) people taking levothyroxine withdrew because of complications (1 had increased angina and 1 had new onset atrial fibrillation).[15] **Cardiac function:** The RCT did not report on adverse effects.[16]

Comment: None.

GLOSSARY

T_3 is used as an abbreviation for endogenous tri-iodothyronine in medical and biochemical reports.

T_4 is used as an abbreviation for endogenous thyroxine in medical and biochemical reports.

Grooved peg board is a board consisting of 25 holes, where each peg fits into only one hole; the test measures the time to put all the pegs in the right holes.

Composition memory score is the average score for the Logical Memory and Word Learning tests.

REFERENCES

1. Vanderpump MP, Tunbridge WM, French JM, et al. The incidence of thyroid disorder in the community: a twenty-year follow-up of the Whickham survey. *Clin Endocriniol (Oxf)* 1995;43:55–68.
2. Laurberg P, Bülow Pedersen I, Pedersen KM, et al. Low incidence rate of overt hypothyroidism compared with hyperthyroidism in an area with moderately low iodine intake. *Thyroid* 1999;9:33–38.
3. Canaris GJ, Manowitz NR, Mayor G, et al. The Colorado thyroid disease prevalence study. *Arch Intern Med* 2000;160:526–533.
4. Hak AE, Pols HA, Visser TJ, et al. Subclinical hypothyroidism is an independent risk factor for atherosclerosis and myocardial infarction in elderly women: the Rotterdam Study. *Ann Intern Med* 2000;132:270–278.
5. Haggerty JJ, Stern RA, Mason GA, et al. Subclinical hypothyroidism: a modifiable risk factor for depression? *Am J Psychiatry* 1993;150:508–510.
6. Monzani F, Del Guerra P, Caraccio N, et al. Subclinical hypothyroidism: neurobehavioral features and beneficial effect of L-thyroxine treatment. *Clin Invest* 1993;71:367–371.
7. Leese GP, Jung RT, Guthrie C, et al. Morbidity in patients on L-thyroxine: a comparison of those with a normal TSH to those with a suppressed TSH. *Clin Endocrinol* 1992;37:500–503.
8. Faber J, Galløe AM. Changes in bone mass during prolonged subclinical hyperthyroidism due to L-thyroxine treatment: a meta-analysis. *Eur J Endocrinol* 1994;130:350–356. Search date not stated; primary sources Medline and hand searches of references from literature and abstracts published at international endocrinological meetings 1985–1992.
9. Sawin CT, Geller A, Wolf PA, et al. Low serum thyrotropin concentrations as a risk factor for atrial fibrillation in older persons. *N Engl J Med* 1994;331:1249–1252.
10. Walsh JP, Shiels L, Lim EEM, et al. Combined thyroxine/liothyronine treatment does not improve well-being, quality of life or cognitive function compared to thyroxine alone: a randomized controlled trial in patients with primary hypothyroidism. *J Clin Endocrinol Metab* 2003;88:4543–4550.
11. Sawka AM, Gerstein HC, Marriott MJ, et al. Does a combination regime of thyroxine (T4) and 3,5,3_-triiodothyronine improve depression symptoms better than T4 alone in patients with hypothyroidism? Results of a double-blind, randomized controlled trial. *J Clin Endocrinol Metab* 2003;88:4551–4555.
12. Clyde PW, Harari AE, Getka EJ, et al. Combined levothyroxine plus liothyronine compared with levothyroxine alone in primary hypothyroidism, A randomized controlled trial. *JAMA* 2003;290:2952–2960.
13. Cooper DS, Halpern R, Wood LC, et al. L-thyroxine therapy in subclinical hypothyroidism. *Ann Intern Med* 1984;101:18–24.
14. Kong WM, Sheikh MH, Lumb PJ, et al. A 6-month randomized trial of thyroxine treatment in woman with mild subclinical hypothyroidism. *Am J Med* 2002;112:348–354.
15. Jaeschke R, Guyatt G, Gerstein H, et al. Does treatment with L-thyroxine influence health status in middle-aged and older adults with subclinical hypothyroidism? *J Gen Intern Med* 1996;11:744–749.
16. Monzani F, Bello VD, Caraccio N, et al. Effect of levothyroxine on cardiac function and structure in subclinical hypothyroidism: a double blind placebo-controlled study. *J Clin Endocrinol Metab* 2001;86:1110–1115.

Birte Nygaard
University of Copenhagen
Copenhagen
Denmark

Competing interests: None declared.
The following previous contributor of this topic would also like to be acknowledged: Lars Kristensen.

Acute anterior uveitis

Search date February 2004

André Curi, Kimble Matos, and Carlos Pavesio

QUESTIONS

INTERVENTIONS

Unknown effectiveness

Non-steroidal anti-inflammatory drug eye drops 760

Steroid eye drops 758

To be covered in future updates

Mydriatics

Oral steroids

Slow taper of drug treatment

Subconjunctival steroid injection

Treatment of chronic iridocyclitis

See glossary G

Key Messages

- **Non-steroidal anti-inflammatory drug eye drops** One RCT found no significant difference between non-steroidal anti-inflammatory drug and placebo eye drops in clinical cure rate after 21 days. Three RCTs found no significant difference between non-steroidal anti-inflammatory drugs and steroid eye drops in clinical cure rate after 14 or 21 days.
- **Steroid eye drops** Steroid eye drops have been standard treatment for anterior uveitis since the early 1950s. However, we found insufficient evidence from RCTs about their effects in people with acute anterior uveitis. One small RCT found no significant difference with steroid (betamethasone phosphate/clobetasone butyrate) eye drops compared with placebo eye drops in symptom severity after 14 or 21 days. Two RCTs found no significant difference between prednisolone and rimexolone in the anterior chamber cell count (a marker of disease severity). One RCT found that prednisolone increased the proportion of people with fewer than five anterior chamber cells per examination field compared with loteprednol after 28 days. The results of a second RCT comparing prednisolone with loteprednol were difficult to interpret. RCTs found that rimexolone and loteprednol were less likely than prednisolone to be associated with increased intraocular pressure, although differences were not statistically significant. Three RCTs found no significant difference between steroid and non-steroidal anti-inflammatory drug eye drops in clinical cure rate after 14 or 21 days.

Acute anterior uveitis

DEFINITION	Anterior uveitis is inflammation of the uveal tract, and includes iritis and iridocyclitis**G**. It can be classified according to its clinical course into acute or chronic anterior uveitis, or according to its clinical appearance into granulomatous or non-granulomatous anterior uveitis. **Acute anterior uveitis** is characterised by an extremely painful red eye, often associated with photophobia and occasionally with decreased visual acuity. **Chronic anterior uveitis** is defined as inflammation lasting over 6 weeks. It is usually asymptomatic, but many people have mild symptoms during exacerbations.
INCIDENCE/ PREVALENCE	Acute anterior uveitis is rare with an annual incidence of 12/100 000 population.[1] It is particularly common in Finland (annual incidence 22.6/100 000 population, prevalence 68.7/100 000 population), probably owing to genetic factors such as the high frequency of HLA-B27 in the Finnish population.[2] It is equally common in men and women, and more than 90% of cases occur in people older than 20 years of age.[2,3]
AETIOLOGY/ RISK FACTORS	No cause is identified in 60–80% of people with acute anterior uveitis. Systemic disorders that may be associated with acute anterior uveitis include ankylosing spondylitis, Reiter's syndrome, juvenile chronic arthritis, Kawasaki syndrome, infectious uveitis, Behçet's syndrome, inflammatory bowel disease, interstitial nephritis, sarcoidosis, multiple sclerosis, Wegener's granulomatosis, Vogt-Koyanagi-Harada syndrome, and masquerade syndromes**G**. Acute anterior uveitis also occurs in association with HLA-B27 expression not linked to any systemic disease, or it may be the manifestation of an isolated eye disorder such as Fuchs' iridocyclitis, Posner-Schlossman syndrome, or Schwartz syndrome. Acute anterior uveitis may occur after surgery or as an adverse drug or hypersensitivity reaction.[2,3]
PROGNOSIS	Acute anterior uveitis is often self limiting, but we found no evidence about how often it resolves spontaneously, in which people, or over what length of time. Complications include posterior synechiae**G**, cataract, glaucoma, and chronic uveitis. In a study of 154 people (232 eyes) with acute anterior uveitis (119 people HLA-B27 positive), visual acuity was better than 20/60 in 209/232 eyes (90%), and 20/60 or worse in 23/232 eyes (10%), including worse than 20/200 (classified as legally blind) in 11/232 eyes (5%).[4]
AIMS OF INTERVENTION	To reduce inflammation; to relieve pain; and to prevent complications and loss of visual acuity, with minimal adverse effects.
OUTCOMES	Degree of inflammation using scores that register a range of different variables as markets of disease severity: number of anterior chamber cells per examination field; flare in the anterior chamber; keratic precipitates; ciliary flush; and severity of symptoms (photophobia and pain).
METHODS	*Clinical Evidence* search and appraisal February 2004.

QUESTION What are the effects of anti-inflammatory eye drops?

OPTION STEROID EYE DROPS

Steroid eye drops have been standard treatment for anterior uveitis since the early 1950s. However, we found insufficient evidence from RCTs about their effects in people with acute anterior uveitis. One small RCT found no significant difference with steroid (betamethasone phosphate/clobetasone butyrate) eye drops compared with placebo eye drops in symptom severity after 14 or 21 days. Two RCTs found no significant difference between prednisolone and rimexolone in the anterior chamber cell count (a marker of disease severity). One RCT found that prednisolone increased the proportion of people with fewer than five anterior chamber cells per examination field compared with loteprednol after 28 days. The results of a second RCT comparing prednisolone with loteprednol were difficult to interpret. RCTs found that rimexolone and loteprednol were less likely than prednisolone to be associated with increased intraocular pressure, although differences were not statistically significant. RCTs found no significant difference between steroid and non-steroidal anti-inflammatory drug eye drops in clinical cure rate after 14 or 21 days.

Benefits: We found no systematic review. **Versus placebo:** We found one RCT (60 people) that compared three treatments: betamethasone phosphate 1% (2 drops every 2 hours), clobetasone butyrate 0.1% (2 drops every 2 hours), and placebo.[5] The RCT found no significant difference with steroid (betamethasone phosphate/clobetasone butyrate) compared with placebo eye drops in symptom severity after 14 or 21 days (results presented graphically; see comment below). **Versus each other:** We found two papers reporting four RCTs.[6,7] Two RCTs compared prednisolone 1% versus rimexolone 1% eye drops.[6] The larger RCT (183 people) found no significant difference in the number of anterior chamber cells per examination field after 28 days (see comment below; 0.4 cells per examination field with rimexolone *v* 0.2 cells per examination field with prednisolone, difference 0.2 cells per examination field, CI not reported; P = 0.16). The smaller RCT (83 people) also found no significant difference in the number of anterior chamber cells per examination field after 28 days (see comment below; 0.3 cells per examination field with rimexolone *v* 0.2 cells per examination field with prednisolone, difference 0.1 cells per examination field; CI not reported; P = 0.40).[6] Two RCTs compared prednisolone 1% versus loteprednol 0.5% eye drops.[7] The larger RCT (175 people) found that prednisolone significantly increased the proportion of people with fewer than five anterior chamber cells per examination field after 28 days compared with loteprednol (5 people lost to follow up; 77/89 [87%] with prednisolone *v* 58/81 [72%] with loteprednol; RR 1.20, 95% CI 1.03 to 1.42; NNT 7, 95% CI 4 to 35). The smaller RCT (70 people) found more people had fewer than five anterior chamber cells per examination field with prednisolone compared with loteprednol but the difference was not significant (see comment below).[7] **Versus non-steroidal anti-inflammatory drug eye drops:** See topical non-steroidal anti-inflammatory drug eye drops, p 760.

Harms: Widely known adverse effects of topical steroid eye drops include local irritation, hyperaemia, oedema, and blurred vision. Rarely, topical eye drops have been associated with glaucoma, cataract, and herpes simplex keratitis. In the RCTs, adverse events were generally mild, resolved without treatment, and did not result in permanent damage.[5–7] In the smaller RCT comparing loteprednol versus prednisolone eye drops, 4/70 (6%) people were withdrawn because of adverse effects: cystoid macular oedema and ocular symptoms in the loteprednol group, and interstitial keratitis and increased age related macular degeneration in the prednisolone group.[7] **Raised intraocular pressure:** The largest RCT's found clinically significant increases in intraocular pressure (defined as > 10 mm Hg from baseline) more frequently with prednisolone versus rimexolone and with prednisolone versus loteprednol, although the differences were not statistically significant (11/94 [12%] people with prednisolone *v* 6/89 [7%] people with rimexolone; RR 1.7, 95% CI 0.7 to 4.5;[6] 6/91 [7%] people with prednisolone *v* 1/84 [1%] people with loteprednol; RR 5.5, 95% CI 0.7 to 45.0[7]).

Comment: Topical steroids have been standard treatment for anterior uveitis since the early 1950s, especially for people with acute or severe uveitis. **Versus placebo:** In the RCT comparing steroid eye drops versus placebo, 12/60 (20%) people did not complete the trial and analysis of data was not by intention to treat.[5] Of these, 4/12 (33%) people were withdrawn from the placebo group because of the severity of their anterior uveitis. The trial was too small to rule out any clinically important effect of topical steroids. **Versus each other:** In the RCTs comparing prednisolone versus rimexolone, people were excluded from analysis for a variety of reasons (23/183 [13%] in the larger RCT and 8/93 [9%] in the smaller RCT).[6] The smaller RCT of prednisolone versus loteprednol enrolled people in the USA and UK; however, it only reported results for the subgroup of people recruited from the USA.[7] This makes the results difficult to interpret.

OPTION NON-STEROIDAL ANTI-INFLAMMATORY DRUG EYE DROPS

One RCT found no significant difference between non-steroidal anti-inflammatory drug and placebo eye drops in clinical cure rate after 21 days. Three RCTs found no significant difference between non-steroidal anti-inflammatory drug and steroid eye drops in clinical cure rate after 14 or 21 days.

Benefits: We found no systematic review. **Versus placebo:** We found one RCT (100 people) that compared three types of eye drops: non-steroidal anti-inflammatory drug (NSAID) (tolmetin 5%), steroid (prednisolone 0.5%), and placebo (sterile saline 0.9%).[8] People were asked to instil two drops every 2 hours during the waking period plus atropine 1% eye drops once daily. The RCT found no significant difference between NSAIDs and placebo eye drops in clinical cure rate after 21 days (15/32 [47%] with tolmetin *v* 16/32 [50%] with placebo; RR 0.9, 95% CI 0.6 to 1.6). **Versus steroids:** We found three RCTs.[8,9,10] The first RCT (described above)[8] formed no significant difference between NSAID and steroid eye drops in clinical cure rate after 21 days (see comment below; 15/32 [47%] with tolmetin *v* 22/32 [69%] with prednisolone; RR 0.7, 95% CI 0.4 to 1.1) The second RCT (71 people) compared three treatments: prednisolone disodium phosphate 0.5%, betamethasone disodium phosphate 0.1%, and tolmetin sodium dihydrate 5%.[9] People were asked to instil one drop every 2 hours during waking hours, and all received atropine 1% eye drops once daily. The RCT found no significant difference between the NSAID (tolmetin sodium dihydrate) and steroid (prednisolone disodium phosphate/betamethasone disodium phosphate) eye drops in clinical cure rate after 21 days (see comment below; 12/21 [57%] people with tolmetin sodium dihydrate *v* 31/39 [79%] with prednisolone disodium phosphate/betamethasone disodium phosphate; RR 1.4, 95% CI 0.9 to 2.1).[9] The third RCT (49 people) compared NSAID eyedrops (indometacin [indomethacin] 0.1%) steroid (dexamethasone 1%) eye drops given six times daily.[10] Most people (equal numbers in each group) also received atropine eye drops three times daily. The RCT found a lower proportion of people clinically cured after 14 days with indometacin but the difference was of borderline significance (see comment below; 12/25 [48%] people with indometacin *v* 18/24 [75%] people with dexamethasone; RR 0.6, 95% CI 0.4 to 1.0).

Harms: In the second RCT 6/20 people (30%) receiving NSAID eye drops reported a transient stinging sensation in their eyes.[9] In the third RCT, more people receiving indometacin reported eye irritation, although the difference was not significant (7/25 [28%] with indometacin *v* 3/24 [13%] with dexamethasone; RR 2.2, 95% CI 0.7 to 7.8).[10]

Comment: Two RCTs used "clinical cure" as an outcome measure, although neither defined this term.[8,9] The third RCT defined "clinical cure" as absence of clinical signs or symptoms suggestive of inflammation.[10] The RCT comparing NSAID with placebo eye drops reported that 6/71 people (8%) did not complete the trial,[8] and the second reported that 11/71 (15%) people did not complete the trial.[9] Neither of these RCTs analysed data by intention to treat.

GLOSSARY

Iridocyclitis Inflammation of both iris and ciliary body. Cells are present in the anterior chamber and in the vitreous.

Iritis Inflammation of the iris. Cells are seen in the anterior chamber but not in the vitreous.

Masquerade syndromes Comprise a group of disorders that occur with intraocular inflammation and are often misdiagnosed as a chronic idiopathic uveitis.

Posterior synechiae Adhesions between the iris and the lens capsule.

REFERENCES

1. Darrel RW, Wagner HP, Kurland CT. Epidemiology of uveitis: incidence and prevalence in a small urban community. *Arch Ophthalmol* 1962;68:501–514.
2. Paivonsalo-Hietanen T, Tuominen J, Vaahtoranta-Lehtonen H, et al. Incidence and prevalence of different uveitis entities in Finland. *Acta Ophthalmol Scand* 1997;75:76–81.
3. Rosenbaum JT. Uveitis. An internist's view. *Arch Intern Med* 1989;149:1173–1176.
4. Linssen A, Meenken C. Outcomes of HLA-B27-positive and HLA-B27-negative acute anterior uveitis. *Am J Ophthalmol* 1995;120:351–361.
5. Dunne JA, Travers JP. Topical steroids in anterior uveitis. *Trans Ophthalmol Soc UK* 1979;99:481–484.
6. Foster CS, Alter G, DeBarge RL, et al. Efficacy and safety of rimexolone 1% ophthalmic suspension vs prednisolone acetate in the treatment of uveitis. *Am J Ophthalmol* 1996;122:171–182.
7. The Loteprednol Etabonate US Uveitis Study Group. Controlled evaluation of loteprednol etabonate and prednisolone acetate in the treatment of acute anterior uveitis. *Am J Ophthalmol* 1999;127:537–544.
8. Young BJ, Cunninghan WF, Akingbehin T. Double-masked controlled clinical trial of 5% tolmetin versus 0.5% prednisolone versus 0.9% saline in acute endogenous nongranulomatous anterior uveitis. *Br J Ophthalmol* 1982;66:389–391.
9. Dunne JA, Jacobs N, Morrison A, et al. Efficacy in anterior uveitis of two known steroids and topical tolmetin. *Br J Ophthalmol* 1985;69:120–125.
10. Sand BB, Krogh E. Topical indometacin, a prostaglandin inhibitor, in acute anterior uveitis. A controlled clinical trial of non-steroid versus steroid anti-inflammatory treatment. *Acta Ophthalmol* 1991;69:145–148.

André Curi
Clinical Research Fellow
Moorfields Eye Hospital
London
UK

Kimble Matos
Research Fellow
Moorfields Eye Hospital
London
UK

Carlos Pavesio
Consultant Ophthalmic Surgeon
Moorfields Eye Hospital
London
UK

Competing interests: None declared.

Age related macular degeneration

Search date July 2004

Jennifer Arnold

QUESTIONS

INTERVENTIONS

To be covered in future updates
Corticosteroids
Antiangiogenesis agents

See glossary G

Key Messages

Prevention of progression

- **Antioxidant vitamin and zinc supplementation** One systematic review found modest evidence from one large RCT that, in people with early to late age related macular degeneration, antioxidant vitamins plus zinc supplements reduced the risk of progression and vision loss over 6 years compared with placebo.
- **Laser to drusen** Two RCTs provided insufficient evidence to assess whether laser to drusen decreased incidence of late age related macular degeneration, choroidal neovascularisation, or geographic atrophy. The first RCT found that threshold laser treatment improved visual acuity after 2 years compared with no treatment, but not compared with subthreshold treatment. The second, larger RCT found no significant difference between laser and no treatment in visual acuity after 1 year. However, subgroup analysis found improved visual acuity where laser treatment had reduced the number of drusen by 50% or more. The RCT also found that, in people with unilateral (but not bilateral) drusen, laser increased the short term incidence of choroidal neovascularisation compared with no treatment.

Treatment

- **Photodynamic treatment with verteporfin** Two systematic reviews in people with age related macular degeneration found that photodynamic treatment with verteporfin reduced the risk of moderate or severe loss of visual acuity and of legal blindness after 1–2 years in people with vision better than 20/100 or 20/200 compared with placebo. Photodynamic treatment with verteporfin was associated with an initial loss of vision and photosensitive reactions in a small proportion of people.

- **Thermal laser photocoagulation** Four large RCTs found that, in people with well demarcated exudative age related macular degeneration, thermal laser photocoagulation reduced severe visual loss after 2–5 years compared with no treatment, but was associated with an immediate and permanent reduction in visual acuity. Choroidal neovascularisation recurred within 3 years in about half of those treated. One small RCT provided insufficient evidence to compare thermal laser photocoagulation versus submacular surgery.
- **External beam radiation** Two large, high quality RCTs and one smaller RCT found no significant difference between low dose external beam radiation and observation alone in moderate visual loss. However, one large RCT and one smaller RCT found that low dose external beam radiation reduced the degree of visual loss compared with placebo. Another smaller RCT found no significant difference in visual loss between high dose external beam radiation and observation. We found insufficient evidence on long term safety, although RCTs found no evidence of toxicity to the optic nerve or retina after 12–24 months.
- **Submacular surgery** Two small RCTs provided insufficient evidence about the effects of submacular surgery.
- **Subcutaneous interferon alfa-2a** One large RCT found that, compared with placebo, subcutaneous interferon alfa-2a (an antiangiogenesis drug) increased visual loss after 1 year, although the difference was not significant. The RCT also found evidence of serious ocular and systemic adverse effects.

DEFINITION Age related macular degeneration (AMD) has two clinical stages: **early AMD** marked by drusen**G** and pigmentary change, and usually associated with normal vision; and **late or sight threatening AMD** associated with a decrease in central vision. Late stage AMD has two forms: **atrophic (or dry) AMD,** characterised by geographic atrophy**G**; and **exudative (or wet) AMD**, characterised by choroidal neovascularisation**G**, which eventually causes a disciform scar.

INCIDENCE/ PREVALENCE AMD is a common cause of blindness registration in industrialised countries. Atrophic AMD is more common than the more sight threatening exudative AMD, affecting about 85% of people with AMD.[1] Late (sight threatening) AMD is found in about 2% of all people aged over 50 years, and incidence rises with age (0.7–1.4% of people aged 65–75 years; 11–19% of people aged > 85 years).[2–4]

AETIOLOGY/ RISK FACTORS Proposed hypotheses for the cause of AMD involve vascular factors and oxidative damage coupled with genetic predisposition.[5] Age is the strongest risk factor. Ocular risk factors for the development of exudative AMD include the presence of soft drusen**G**, macular pigmentary change, choroidal neovascularisation in the other eye, and previous cataract surgery.[6] Systemic risk factors include hypertension, smoking, and a family history of AMD.[5,7,8] Hypertension, diet (especially intake of antioxidant micronutrients), and oestrogen are suspected as causal agents, but the effects of these factors remain unproved.[5]

PROGNOSIS AMD impairs central vision, which is required for reading, driving, face recognition, and all fine visual tasks. **Atrophic AMD** progresses slowly over many years, and time to legal blindness**G** is highly variable (usually about 5–10 years).[9,10] **Exudative AMD** is more often threatening to vision; 90% of people with severe visual loss**G** owing to AMD have the exudative type. This condition usually manifests with a sudden worsening and distortion of central vision. One study estimated (based on data derived primarily from cohort studies) that the risk of developing exudative AMD in people with bilateral soft drusen**G** was 1–5% at 1 year and 13–18% at 3 years.[11] The observed 5 year rate in a population survey was 7%.[12] Most eyes (estimates vary from 60–90%) with exudative AMD progress to legal blindness and develop a central defect (scotoma) in the visual field.[13–16] Peripheral vision is preserved, allowing the person to be mobile and independent. The ability to read with visual aids depends on the size and density of the central scotoma and the degree to which the person retains sensitivity to contrast. Once exudative AMD has developed in one eye, the other eye is at high risk (cumulative estimated incidence: 10% at 1 year, 28% at 3 years, and 42% at 5 years).[17]

AIMS OF INTERVENTION To minimise loss of visual acuity and central vision; to preserve the ability to read with or without visual aids; to optimise quality of life; to minimise adverse effects of treatment.

OUTCOMES Visual acuity; rates of legal blindness(G); contrast sensitivity; quality of life; visual fields; rate of progression to late AMD; rate of adverse effects of treatment. Visual acuity is measured using special eye charts (logMAR charts, usually the Early Treatment of Diabetic Retinopathy Study [ETDRS] chart), although many studies do not specify which chart was used. In this review, it may be assumed that the logMAR chart has been used unless otherwise stated. Stable vision is usually defined as loss of two lines or less on the ETDRS chart. Moderate visual loss(G) is defined as a loss of greater than three lines and severe visual loss(G) is defined as a loss of greater than six lines. Loss of vision to legal blindness (< 20/200) is also used as an outcome.

METHODS *Clinical Evidence* search and appraisal July 2004.

QUESTION **What are the effects of interventions to prevent progression of age related macular degeneration?**

OPTION **ANTIOXIDANT VITAMIN AND MINERAL SUPPLEMENTS**

One systematic review found modest evidence from one large RCT that, in people with early to late age related macular degeneration, antioxidant vitamins plus zinc supplements reduced the risk of progression and vision loss over 6 years compared with placebo.

Benefits: We found one systematic review (search date 2001, 7 RCTs, 4119 people).[18] Six of the trials reported were small with inconsistent results and these studies are not considered further. The remaining, large RCT identified by the review (3640 people aged 55–80 years) included people with at least moderate drusen(G) in both eyes or choroidal neovascularisation(G) or geographic atrophy(G) in one eye.[19] It compared four treatments: placebo, zinc (total daily dose, zinc 80 mg plus copper 2 mg), antioxidants (total daily dose, vitamin C 500 mg plus vitamin E 400 IU plus beta-carotene 15 mg), and zinc plus antioxidants. The RCT defined progression to advanced age related macular degeneration (AMD) as the development of choroidal neovascularisation or geographic atrophy. It found that, compared with placebo, zinc plus antioxidants significantly reduced the proportion of people progressing to advanced AMD (OR 0.72, 99% CI 0.52 to 0.98) or moderate vision loss(G) (OR 0.73, 99% CI 0.54 to 0.99) over a 6 year period.[19] Fifteen of 1063 (1.4%) people with early AMD (moderate bilateral drusen) developed advanced AMD (5 year incidence 1.5%) and the effect of supplementation compared with placebo was found to be higher when these people were excluded (antioxidants plus zinc: OR 0.66, 99% CI 0.47 to 0.91; zinc alone: OR 0.71, 99% CI 0.52 to 0.99; antioxidants alone: OR 0.76, 99% CI 0.55 to 1.05).[19]

Harms: In the large RCT, 71% of people were taking 75% or more of their tablets at 5 years.[19] There was little evidence of harm in the large RCT, although it found a significant increase in yellow skin discolouration in people taking antioxidants (151/1823 [8.3%] with antioxidants *v* 108/1798 [6.0%] with placebo; OR 1.4, 95% CI 1.1 to 1.8; $P < 0.01$). It also found a significant increase in admission to hospital for genitourinary complications (urinary tract infection, prostatic hyperplasia, and stress incontinence in women) in people taking zinc (134/1783 [7.5%] with zinc *v* 90/1838 [4.9%] with placebo; OR 1.6, 95% CI 1.2 to 2.1; $P < 0.01$). Harmful effects of long term supplementation with the dosages used in the RCT cannot be ruled out.[19] High dose zinc supplements may result in gastrointestinal intolerance. Studies in people with other conditions suggest that in people with high risk of lung cancer (smokers and people working with asbestos) beta-carotene further increases the risk of lung cancer.[20,21]

Comment: The high dosages given in this study cannot be achieved by dietary intake alone. The study was conducted in relatively well nourished Americans (57% of people were taking zinc or antioxidant vitamins before enrolment, and 67% took additional multivitamin supplements to recommended daily allowance levels during the study). Trials in populations with different nutritional statuses are required. We found no evidence on the effects of supplements in people with no AMD or early signs of the disease (early drusen❻ only) or established late AMD (choroidal neovascularisation❻ or geographic atrophy❻) in both eyes. An allied systematic review (search date 2002) found no evidence that supplements prevent AMD in people with no signs of the disease.[22] Results are awaited from four large ongoing studies in the USA and Australia that address this question.

OPTION LASER TO DRUSEN

Two RCTs provided insufficient evidence to assess whether laser to drusen decreased incidence of late age related macular degeneration, choroidal neovascularisation, or geographic atrophy. The first RCT found that threshold laser treatment improved visual acuity after 2 years compared with no treatment, but not compared with subthreshold treatment. The second, larger RCT found no significant difference between laser and no treatment in visual acuity after 1 year. However, subgroup analysis found improved visual acuity where laser treatment had reduced the number of drusen by 50% or more. The RCT also found that, in people with unilateral (but not bilateral) drusen, laser increased the short term incidence of choroidal neovascularisation compared with no treatment.

Benefits: **Versus no treatment:** We found no systematic review. We found two RCTs (4 publications).[23–26] The first RCT (229 eyes, 75 people with unilateral drusen❻ and 77 people with bilateral drusen❻; see comment below) compared three treatments: diode laser❻ at a threshold level (visible burns; 63 eyes), diode laser at a subthreshold level (invisible burns; 57 eyes), and no laser treatment (109 eyes).[23] It found that laser treatment at either level (threshold or subthreshold) significantly increased visual acuity compared with no laser treatment after 2 years (improvement of ≥ 2 lines: 12/105 [11%] with laser treatment *v* 0/91 [0%] with no treatment; NNT 9, 95% CI 6 to 25). The RCT found no significant difference between threshold and subthreshold treatment in visual acuity after 2 years (improvement of ≥ 2 lines: 8/56 [14%] with threshold treatment *v* 4/49 [8%] with subthreshold treatment; RR 1.80, 95% CI 0.56 to 5.50). The second RCT (120 eyes with unilateral drusen, 312 eyes with bilateral drusen, 276 people; see comment below) compared argon-green laser❻ versus no laser treatment.[24–26] It found no significant difference between laser treatment and no laser treatment in visual acuity after 1 year (AR for improvement of ≥ 1 line: 60/167 [36%] with laser treatment *v* 48/183 [26%] with no laser treatment; RR 1.40, 95% CI 1.00 to 1.88; AR for reduction of ≥ 1 line: 44/167 [26%] with laser treatment *v* 65/183 [36%] with no laser treatment; RR 0.70, 95% CI 0.54 to 1.02). Three smaller RCTs, which did not meet *Clinical Evidence* inclusion criteria, found results which were consistent with the larger RCTs cited above.[27–29]

Harms: Macular laser treatment may induce choroidal neovascularisation (CNV❻) and retinal atrophy. The first RCT found no significant difference between threshold and subthreshold laser treatment in the proportion of eyes with CNV after 24 months (7/56 [12%] with threshold laser treatment *v* 4/49 [8%] with subthreshold laser treatment; RR 1.50, 95% CI 0.45 to 4.68).[23] In the second RCT, early analysis found that in the subgroup of people with unilateral drusen❻, argon-green laser❻ significantly increased the incidence of CNV compared with no laser treatment (estimated 12 month incidence: 10/59 [17%] with laser treatment *v* 2/61 [3%] with no laser treatment; $P < 0.05$; CI not reported; see comment below).[25] Both RCTs found that laser induced retinal atrophy was uncommon, with 2/120 (2%) treated eyes affected in one study,[25] and 1/105 (1%) treated eyes affected in the other.[23]

Comment: Both the RCTs sought to minimise CNV**G** by using low intensity and subthreshold laser burns and by positioning laser burns at a distance (generally > 500 μm) from the fovea centre. The first RCT reported that 196/229 (86%) eyes completed 24 months' follow up, although it is not clear whether analysis of data was by intention to treat.[23] The second RCT ceased enrolment and treatment prematurely because of a higher incidence of CNV within the first 12 months in people receiving laser treatment with unilateral (but not with bilateral) drusen**G**.[24–26] The second RCT reported that 351/432 (81%) eyes completed 12 months' follow up, although analysis of data was not by intention to treat and people with CNV were excluded.[24,25] It found limited evidence from a subgroup analysis that improved visual acuity was more likely with a greater reduction in drusen after 1 year (AR for improvement of ≥ 1 line: 36/77 [48%] in eyes with ≥ 50% reduction in drusen *v* 24/90 [27%] in eyes with < 50% reduction; RR 1.80, 95% CI 1.16 to 2.66). There is now considerable interest in preventive strategies for people with high risk drusen. One model estimates that a preventive measure of 10% efficacy in people with bilateral drusen would more than halve the risk of developing legal blindness**G** relative to current treatment.[30] Other RCTs of laser to drusen are either ongoing[31] or planned.[23,24]

QUESTION **What are the effects of treatments for exudative age related macular degeneration?**

OPTION **PHOTODYNAMIC TREATMENT WITH VERTEPORFIN**

Two systematic reviews in people with age related macular degeneration found that photodynamic treatment with verteporfin reduced the risk of moderate or severe loss of visual acuity and of legal blindness after 1–2 years in people with vision better than 20/100 or 20/200 compared with placebo. Photodynamic treatment with verteporfin was associated with an initial loss of vision and photosensitive reactions in a small proportion of people.

Benefits: We found two systematic reviews (search date 2002,[32] and not reported[33]). Both reviews identified the same two RCTs (948 people with new and recurrent subfoveal choroidal neovascularisation [CNV**G**] owing to age related macular degeneration), which compared photodynamic treatment**G** with verteporfin**G** (6 mg/m^2 body surface area) versus placebo (photodynamic treatment with 5% dextrose solution).[34,35] Treatments were repeated as necessary every 3 months. The first systematic review performed a meta-analysis and found that photodynamic treatment with verteporfin significantly reduced the risk of moderate**G** and severe visual loss**G** compared with placebo at 24 months (moderate visual loss**G**: OR 0.77, 95% CI 0.69 to 0.87; severe visual loss: OR 0.62, 95% CI 0.50 to 0.76).[32] The second systematic review did not perform a meta-analysis because of baseline differences between the two trials (see comment below).[33] However, it re-examined data for the outcome of legal blindness**G** (< 20/200). It found that, in both RCTs, photodynamic treatment reduced the risk of legal blindness compared with placebo at 24 months (first RCT:[34] 165/402 [41%] with photodynamic treatment with verteporfin *v* 114/207 [55%] with placebo; ARR 14%, 95% CI 6% to 22%; second RCT:[35] 26/225 [26%] with photodynamic treatment with verteporfin *v* 50/114 [44%] with placebo; ARR 18%, 95% CI 7% to 28%).

Harms: Verteporfin**G** is a photosensitive dye and care must be taken to avoid leakage into surrounding tissues during infusion and exposure to bright light soon after treatment. Advice in the study was to avoid light for 48 hours, but some photosensitive reactions were observed in treated people after 3–5 days.[32] The treatment was well tolerated but was more likely than the control intervention to cause a transient decrease in vision, injection site reactions, photosensitivity, and infusion related low back pain. Severe vision decrease**G** (> 20 letters or 4 lines) was recorded in 3/402 (< 1%) people in the first RCT[34] and in 10/225 (4%) people in the second RCT[35] within 7 days of treatment, although some visual recovery occurred in most cases. The risk seems to be higher in people with occult and no classic**G** CNV**G**.

Comment: There were important differences in the populations recruited into the RCTs. The first RCT included people with some classic**G** CNV and vision of about 20/40 to 20/200.[34] The second RCT included people with better vision or with no evidence of classic CNV and vision better than 20/100.[35] The first systematic review performed subgroup analyses based on baseline CNV lesion classification.[32] It found greater benefit in people with only classic lesions (RR of moderate vision loss**G** at 24 months for photodynamic treatment**G** *v* placebo: 0.88, 95% CI 0.74 to 1.04 if occult CNV was present; 0.42, 95% CI 0.30 to 0.60 if occult CNV was absent). However, it found that the amount of classic CNV in the lesion had no significant effect on the benefit from treatment (RR of moderate vision loss at 24 months for photodynamic treatment: 0.77, 95% CI 0.64 to 0.92 if no classic CNV was present; 0.93, 95% CI 0.77 to 1.14 if classic CNV consisted of 1–49% of the lesion; 0.60, 95% CI 0.48 to 0.75 if classic CNV consisted of ≥ 50% of the lesion; P = 0.066). Exploratory analysis of data from both trials suggests that baseline lesion size might be an important predictor of effect.[36] Most people treated with photodynamic treatment with verteporfin**G** will continue to lose visual acuity. Although benefit was shown for people with vision better than 20/100 or 20/200, it is not known what the impact of treatment is on those with poorer vision.

OPTION THERMAL LASER PHOTOCOAGULATION

Four large RCTs found that, in people with well demarcated exudative age related macular degeneration, thermal laser photocoagulation reduced severe visual loss after 2–5 years compared with no treatment, but was associated with an immediate and permanent reduction in visual acuity. Choroidal neovascularisation recurred within 3 years in about half of those treated. One small RCT provided insufficient evidence to compare thermal laser photocoagulation versus submacular surgery.

Benefits: **Versus no treatment:** We found no systematic review. We found four large open label multicentre RCTs in selected populations with exudative age related macular degeneration comparing laser photocoagulation**G** versus no treatment (see table 1, p 775).[13–16,37–39] We also found four smaller RCTs that included a wider range of people.[40–43] All four large RCTs found that laser treatment significantly reduced the risk of severe visual loss**G** compared with no treatment after 3 years' follow up. Participants differed in terms of the position of the choroidal neovascularisation (CNV**G**) on the retina, whether far from, near to, or under the centre of fixation (extrafoveal,[13,15] juxtafoveal,[16,37] or subfoveal[14,38,39]). The RCT of extrafoveal CNV found that laser photocoagulation significantly reduced severe visual loss compared with no treatment (see table 1, p 775).[13,15] Results were similar in eyes with juxtafoveal CNV (see table 1, p 775) (see comment below).[16,37] The two RCTs in people with subfoveal CNV also found that laser photocoagulation reduced severe visual loss compared with no treatment, although it was associated with an immediate and permanent loss of visual acuity in some people in the treated groups.[14] The RCTs found that choiroidal neovascularisation recurred in 39-54% of people within 3 years and that 76% of people with classic CNV had recurrence at 5 years. Of the four smaller RCTs, one RCT (127 eyes) found that fovea sparing laser photocoagulation significantly reduced the risk of deteriorating visual acuity compared with no treatment (AR for loss of < 3 lines after 12 months: 28/68 [41%] with laser treatment *v* 12/59 [20%] with no treatment; RR 2.00, 95% CI 1.13 to 3.61; NNT 5, 95% CI 3 to 16).[40] The other three RCTs found no significant difference between scatter (non-confluent) laser photocoagulation and no treatment in occult CNV, but may have lacked power to detect clinically important effects.[41–43]

Versus submacular surgery: See benefits of submacular surgery, p 770.

Harms: Laser destroys new vessels and surrounding retina, and the resultant scar causes a corresponding defect in the central visual field. If the laser is applied to subfoveal lesions, or if the laser burn spreads to the fovea, visual acuity will be impaired. Two of the RCTs described immediate loss of visual acuity with laser treatment (an average loss of 3 lines).[14,39] We found no evidence of other adverse effects.

Comment: The RCT examining effects of laser in eyes with juxtafoveal CNVⒼ found evidence from subgroup analysis that benefit may be limited to eyes with CNV that is of the pure classicⒼ type (no occult element) on fluorescein angiography (237/496 [48%] of randomised eyes; OR 2.2, 95% CI 1.4 to 3.4).[16,37] We found two RCTs comparing different laser wavelengths for photocoagulation of CNV.[44,45] Neither found a significant difference between krypton-red and argon-green laserⒼ in visual acuity after a maximum of 5 years. The benefits of laser photocoagulationⒼ depend on accurate, complete treatment requiring high quality angiography and trained, experienced practitioners.[13–16,37–39] The risk of immediate loss of visual acuity with laser photocoagulation may limit its acceptability.

OPTION EXTERNAL BEAM RADIATION

Two large, high quality RCTs and one smaller RCT found no significant difference between low dose external beam radiation and observation alone in moderate visual loss. However, one large RCT and one smaller RCT found that low dose external beam radiation reduced the degree of visual loss compared with placebo. Another smaller RCT found no significant difference in visual loss between high dose external beam radiation and observation. We found insufficient evidence on long term safety, although RCTs found no evidence of toxicity to the optic nerve or retina after 12–24 months.

Benefits: **Low dose external beam radiation:** We found no systematic review. We found three large[46–48] and two smaller RCTs.[49,50] The first large RCT (205 people with new subfoveal choroidal neovascularisation [CNVⒼ]) found no significant difference between external beam radiation to the macula (8 fractions of 2 Gy) and placebo in the risk of moderate visual lossⒼ 1 year after treatment (51% with external beam radiation *v* 53% with placebo; P = 0.88; see comment below).[46] The second large RCT (203 people) found no significant difference between external beam radiation (6 fractions of 2 Gy) and observation in the risk of moderate or severe visual lossⒼ 1 or 2 years after treatment (moderate visual loss: 53/93 [57%] with external beam radiation *v* 52/91 [57%] with observation at 12 months; P = 0.91; 61/87 [70%] with external beam radiation *v* 71/87 [82%] with observation at 24 months; P = 0.08; severe visual loss: 26/93 [28%] with external beam radiation *v* 37/91

[41%] with observation at 12 months; P = 0.06; 31/87 [36%] with external beam radiation *v* 44/87 [51%] with observation at 24 months; P = 0.29).[47] The third large RCT (161 people) found that external beam radiation (4 fractions of 2 or 4 Gy) significantly reduced the mean number of lines of vision lost compared with placebo (1 Gy) 18 months after treatment (mean number of lines of vision lost: 1.73 with total of 8 Gy radiation *v* 3.23 with placebo; P = 0.011; 1.93 with total of 16 Gy *v* 3.23 with placebo; P = 0.05).[48] The two smaller RCTs also found different results.[49,50] The first of these (83 people) found no significant difference between external beam radiation (7 fractions of 2 Gy) and placebo (sham radiation) in visual acuity after 12 months (mean number of lines lost: 4.14 with external beam radiation *v* 3.39 with placebo; P = 0.35) or in angiographic outcomes (lesion size/progression of CNV, see comment below).[49] The second small RCT found that low dose external beam radiation significantly reduced mean visual loss after 2 years compared with observation (1 RCT, 101 people; P < 0.0001; CI and absolute numbers not reported).[50] **High dose external beam radiation:** We found no systematic review. We found one RCT.[51] The RCT (74 people with new subfoveal CNV) compared external beam radiation (4 fractions of 6 Gy) delivered to the macula versus observation.[51] It found no significant difference between treatments in the risk of moderate or severe visual loss after 12 months (32.0% with external beam radiation *v* 52.2% with observation; ARR +20%, 95% CI –4% to +44%; absolute numbers not reported).

Harms: **Low dose external beam radiation:** The five RCTs[46–50] found that there were no radiation related adverse events up to 24 months' follow up, although one study[47] noted decreased tear film production and stability in the treated group. **High dose external beam radiation:** The RCT reported that no harms were observed.[51]

Comment: In the first RCT, no treatment benefit was detected for subgroups of people classified as having some classic**G** CNV**G** (83 people, 41 treated, 42 control) or occult only lesions (122 people, 60 treated, 62 control) on the basis of fluorescein angiography (occult lesions: 47% with radiotherapy treatment *v* 49% with placebo; P = 0.80; classic/mixed lesions: 58% with radiotherapy treatment *v* 58% with placebo; P = 0.47).[46] In the first RCT, we could not replicate the percentages presented in the paper from the raw data provided for cataract and dry eye symptom results.[47] Results for the third RCT are only expressed as change in the mean vision, and percentages with moderate**G** or severe vision loss**G** are not given.[48] We also found one small exploratory RCT[52] of high dose external beam radiation that was under powered but found similar results to the larger RCT cited above.[51] Radiotherapy is potentially toxic to the retina, optic nerve, lens, and lacrimal system, with toxic effects sometimes manifesting up to 2 years after treatment.[53] The biological effects of external beam radiation, both benefits and harms, depend on the dose in each fraction, the number of fractions delivered, and the time between each fraction. Total doses of up to 25 Gy, delivered in daily fractions of 2 Gy or less, are generally claimed not to cause damage to the retina or optic nerve. Uncontrolled pilot studies suggest that the main risks using the present dosing and delivery techniques are cataract formation (2/41 [5%] people in one series)[54] and transient dry eye symptoms (10/75 [13%] in a second case series).[55] One case series using total doses of 16–20 Gy in fraction sizes of 4–5 Gy found radiation toxicity of the optic nerve, retina, or choroid in 20/231 (9%) eyes after 12–24 months.[56] Another case series of proton beam radiation found radiation retinopathy in 11/27 (41%) eyes exposed to higher doses after 12 months.[57] A two centre case series of people treated with external beam radiation (5–10 fractions of 2 Gy/

fraction) reported an abnormal choroidal vascular growth pattern associated with macular bleeding and exudation, and marked loss of visual acuity.[58] This change was detected in 12/95 (12%) people in the first centre and 7/98 (7%) people in the second centre after 12 months. Experience from pilot studies and case series suggests that, although higher radiation doses may be more effective in inducing regression of CNV, they carry an increased risk of sight threatening toxicity. RCTs with less than 2 years' follow up may miss important adverse effects.

OPTION SUBMACULAR SURGERY

Two small RCTs provided insufficient evidence about the effects of submacular surgery.

Benefits: **Versus no treatment:** We found no systematic review or RCTs. **Versus laser photocoagulation:** We found no systematic review. We found one small exploratory RCT that found no significant difference between submacular surgery**G** and laser photocoagulation**G** in the proportion of eyes with improved visual acuity after 2 years (70 people with recurrent subfoveal choroidal neovascularisation**G** after previous laser photocoagulation treatment) defined as visual acuity better than or no more than 1 line worse than baseline as measured on a modified Bailey-Lovie chart (14/28 [50%] with surgery *v* 20/31 [65%] with laser treatment; RR 0.80, 95% CI 0.49 to 1.22).[59] However, the study may have lacked power to detect a clinically important effect. **Versus other surgical techniques:** We found no systematic review. We found one RCT (80 eyes with exudative age related macular degeneration [AMD]) comparing submacular surgery plus subretinal injection of tissue plasminogen activator versus submacular surgery plus subretinal injection of a control solution (balanced salt solution).[60] It found no significant difference between techniques in the proportion of eyes with any visual improvement (5/40 [12%] with surgery plus tissue plasminogen activator *v* 6/40 [15%] with surgery plus control; RR 0.80, 95% CI 0.28 to 2.51) or with fluorescein angiographic evidence of active choroidal neovascularisation after 1 year (7/40 [18%] with surgery plus tissue plasminogen activator *v* 8/40 [20%] with surgery plus control; RR 0.90, 95% CI 0.35 to 2.18). However, confidence intervals were wide and the study may have lacked power to detect clinically important effects.

Harms: Submacular surgery**G** may threaten vision itself or necessitate further surgical intervention. However, we found no information on the frequency of adverse events. The largest case series of people with AMD and non-AMD treated with submacular surgery reported cataract formation (in < 40%), retinal detachment (5–8%), recurrent new vessel formation (18–35% within 12 months), and macular complications (no rates reported).[61]

Comment: Most evidence for submacular surgery**G** currently comes from small uncontrolled case series (< 50 people with AMD) with short follow up times, often including people with other types of macular degeneration. These series found that few people with AMD had improved vision with surgery.[53,61] Comparing results is difficult because of evolving surgical techniques, changes in outcome measures, and variations in follow up. Several large open label RCTs are currently recruiting and will compare standardised surgical technique versus no treatment in new and haemorrhagic choroidal neovascularisation**G** in people with AMD (Bressler S, personal communication, 1999). Other surgical techniques are being developed in volunteers, including macular translocation and retinal pigment epithelial transplantation, but these have yet to be evaluated formally.

OPTION SUBCUTANEOUS INTERFERON ALFA-2A

One large RCT found that, compared with placebo, subcutaneous interferon alfa-2a (an antiangiogenesis drug) increased visual loss after 1 year, although the difference was not significant. The RCT also found evidence of serious ocular and systemic adverse effects.

Benefits: We found no systematic review. We found one RCT (481 people with age related macular degeneration and subfoveal choroidal neovascularisationⒼ) comparing three doses of subcutaneous interferon alfa-2a (1.5, 3, and 6 million IU 3 times/week for 1 year) versus placebo.[62] It found that interferon alfa-2a at all doses was associated with a non-significant reduction in visual acuity after 52 weeks compared with placebo (see comment below; AR for reduction of ≥ 3 lines: 142/286 [50%] with interferon alfa-2a *v* 40/105 [38%] with placebo; RR 1.20, 95% CI 0.90 to 1.62).[62]

Harms: Adverse effects of interferon alfa-2a were common and potentially severe in this RCT[62] and in other poorer quality RCTs, which did not meet *Clinical Evidence* inclusion criteria. Effects included fatigue and influenza-like symptoms, gastrointestinal symptoms (including nausea, diarrhoea, and loss of appetite), and central and peripheral nervous system effects (including headaches and dizziness). Although at least one adverse event was reported in 90/105 (86%) people taking placebo, the proportion of people on active treatment who suffered adverse effects increased with dose, as did the severity of adverse effects. The RCT reported that 20/286 (7%) people receiving interferon alfa-2a developed interferon associated retinopathy (retinal haemorrhages or cotton wool spots).[62]

Comment: In the RCT, 90/481 (18%) of people did not complete the trial and analysis of data was not by intention to treat.[62] There is widespread interest in safe, effective antiangiogenesis drugs for prophylaxis in exudative age related macular degeneration. Several drugs are currently under clinical study. RCTs are currently investigating the use of intraocular or periocular steroids and antivascular endothelial growth factor.

GLOSSARY

Choroidal neovascularisation (CNV) New vessels in the choroid, classified by fluorescein angiography: in terms of its position in relation to the fovea — extrafoveal, juxtafoveal, or subfoveal; in terms of its appearance — classic (well defined) or occult (poorly defined); and in terms of its borders — well demarcated or poorly demarcated.

Drusen Small, yellow, bright objects, often near the macula, seen by ophthalmoscopy. They are located under the basement membrane of the retinal pigment epithelium. They are present in many older people with normal vision, but a greater proportion of large drusen indicate higher risk of subsequent loss of acuity from age related macular degeneration.

Geographic atrophy A feature of atrophic age related macular degeneration, characterised by atrophy of the retina and inner choroidal layers at the macular leaving only the deep choroidal vessels visible.

Laser (diode, krypton, argon-green) Lasers used in ophthalmology that produce focused light of different specific wavelengths.

Laser photocoagulation Treatment using a thermal (hot) laser to photocoagulate the retina. When used to ablate or treat a choroidal neovascularisation (CNV), the treatment is generally confluent over the CNV. Fovea-sparing laser photocoagulation is confluent laser applied in an annulus around fixation. Scatter or non-confluent laser photocoagulation is applied in a grid.

Legal blindness Visual acuity less than 20/200. A reading of 20/200 (or 6/60 in metric) on the Snellen chart means that a person can see at 20 feet (or 6 m) what a normally sighted person can see at 200 feet (or 60 m).

Age related macular degeneration

Moderate vision loss Loss of three or more lines of distance vision measured on a special eye chart, corresponding to a doubling of the visual angle.
Photodynamic treatment A two step procedure of intravenous infusion of a photosensitive dye followed by application of a non-thermal laser that activates the dye. The treatment aims to cause selective closure of the choroidal new vessels.
Predominantly classic choroidal neovascularisation Choroidal neovascularisation in which more than 50% of lesion area consists of classic choroidal neovascularisation on fluorescein angiography.
Severe vision loss Loss of six or more lines of distance vision measured on a special eye chart, corresponding to a quadrupling of the visual angle.
Submacular surgery Removal of haemorrhage, choroidal neovascularisation, or both after vitrectomy.
Verteporfin A photosensitive dye used in photodynamic treatment.

Substantive changes

External beam radiation Recategorisation to Unknown effectiveness based on review of the existing evidence.

REFERENCES

1. Bressler SB, Bressler NM, Fine SL. Age-related macular degeneration. *Surv Ophthalmol* 1988;32:375–413.
2. Klein R, Klein BEK, Linton KLP. Prevalence of age-related maculopathy: the Beaver Dam Eye Study. *Ophthalmology* 1992;99:933–943.
3. Vingerling JR, Dielemans I, Hofman A, et al. The prevalence of age-related maculopathy in the Rotterdam study. *Ophthalmology* 1995;102:205–210.
4. Mitchell P, Smith W, Attebo K, et al. Prevalence of age-related maculopathy in Australia. The Blue Mountains Eye Study. *Ophthalmology* 1995;102:1450–1460.
5. Evans JR. Risk factors for age-related macular degeneration. *Prog Retin Eye Res* 2001;20:227–253.
6. Wang, JJ, Klein R, Smith W, et al. Cataract surgery and the 5-year incidence of late-stage age-related maculopathy: pooled findings from the Beaver Dam and Blue Mountains eye studies. *Ophthalmology* 2003;110:1960–1067.
7. Pieramici DJ, Bressler SB. Age-related macular degeneration and risk factors for the development of choroidal neovascularization in the fellow eye. *Curr Opin Ophthalmol* 1998;9:38–46.
8. Smith W, Assink J, Klein R, et al. Risk factors for age-related macular degeneration: pooled findings from three continents. *Ophthalmology* 2001;108:697–704.
9. Maguire P, Vine AK. Geographic atrophy of the retinal pigment epithelium. *Am J Ophthalmol* 1986;102:621–625.
10. Sarks JP, Sarks SH, Killingsworth M. Evolution of geographic atrophy of the retinal pigment epithelium. *Eye* 1988;2:552–577.
11. Holz FG, Wolfensberger TJ, Piguet B, et al. Bilateral macular drusen in age-related macular degeneration: prognosis and risk factors. *Ophthalmology* 1994;101:1522–1528.
12. Klein R, Klein BEK, Jensen SC, et al. The five-year incidence and progression of age-related maculopathy. The Beaver Dam Eye study. *Ophthalmology* 1997;104:7–21.
13. Macular Photocoagulation Study Group. Argon laser photocoagulation for neovascular maculopathy: five-year results from randomized clinical trials. *Arch Ophthalmol* 1991;109:1109–1114.
14. Macular Photocoagulation Study Group. Laser photocoagulation of subfoveal neovascular lesions of age-related macular degeneration: updated findings from two clinical trials. *Arch Ophthalmol* 1993;111:1200–1209.
15. Macular Photocoagulation Study Group. Argon laser photocoagulation for neovascular maculopathy. Three-year results from randomized clinical trials. *Arch Ophthalmol* 1986;104:694–701.
16. Macular Photocoagulation Study Group. Laser photocoagulation for juxtafoveal choroidal neovascularisation. Five-year results from randomized clinical trials. *Arch Ophthalmol* 1994;112:500–509.
17. Macular Photocoagulation Study Group. Risk factors for choroidal neovascularisation secondary to age-related macular degeneration. Arch Ophthalmol 1997;115:741–747.
18. Evans JR. Antioxidant vitamin and mineral supplements for age-related macular degeneration (Cochrane Review). In: The Cochrane Library, Issue 2, 2004. Chichester, UK: John Wiley & Sons, Ltd. Search date 2001; primary sources Medline, Embase, Cochrane Controlled Trials Register, Science Citation Index, hand searches of reference lists of relevant trials, and personal communication with investigators of included studies.
19. Age-related Eye Disease Study Research Group. A randomised placebo-controlled clinical trial of high-dose supplementation with vitamins C and E, beta carotene, and zinc for age-related macular degeneration and vision loss: AREDS report no 8. *Arch Ophthalmol* 2001;119:1417–1436.
20. The Alpha-tocopherol, Beta Carotene Cancer Prevention Study Group. The effect of vitamin E and beta carotene on the incidence of lung cancer and other cancers in male smokers. *N Engl J Med* 1994;330:1029–1035.
21. Omenn GS, Goodman GE, Thornquist MD, et al. Effects of a combination of beta carotene and vitamin A on lung cancer and cardiovascular disease. *N Engl J Med* 1996;334:1150–1155.
22. Evans JR, Henshaw K. Antioxidant vitamin and mineral supplementation for preventing age-related macular degeneration (Cochrane Review). In: The Cochrane Library, Issue 2, 2004. Chichester, UK: John Wiley & Sons, Ltd. Search date 2002; primary sources Medline, Embase, Cochrane Controlled Trials Register, Science Citation Index, hand searches of reference lists of relevant trials, and personal communication with investigators and experts in the field.
23. Olk, RJ, Friberg TR, Stickney KL, et al. Therapeutic benefits of infrared (810 nm) diode laser macular grid photocoagulation in prophylactic treatment of nonexudative age-related macular degeneration: two-year results of a randomized pilot study. *Ophthalmology* 1999;106:2082–2090.
24. Ho CA, Maguire MG, Yoken J, et al. The Choroidal Neovascularization Prevention Trial Research Group. Laser-induced drusen reduction improves visual function at 1 year. *Ophthalmology* 1999;106:1367–1373.
25. The Choroidal Neovascularization Prevention Trial Research Group. Laser treatment in eyes with large

drusen. Short-term effects seen in a pilot randomized clinical trial. *Ophthalmology* 1998;105:11–23.

26. The Choroidal Neovascularization Prevention Trial Research Group. Laser treatment in fellow eyes with large drusen: updated findings from a pilot randomized clinical trial. *Ophthalmology* 2003;110:971–978.
27. Little HL, Showman JM, Brown BW. A pilot randomized controlled study on the effect of laser photocoagulation of confluent soft macular drusen. *Ophthalmology* 1997;104:623–631.
28. Frennesson C, Nilsson SEG. Prophylactic laser treatment in early age-related maculopathy reduced the incidence of exudative complications. *Br J Ophthalmol* 1998;82:1169–1174.
29. Figueroa MS, Regueras A, Bertrand J, et al. Laser photocoagulation for macular soft drusen. Updated results. *Retina* 1997;17:378–384.
30. Lanchoney DM, Maguire MG, Fine SL. A model of the incidence and consequences of choroidal neovascularisation secondary to age-related macular degeneration. Comparative effects of current treatment and potential prophylaxis on visual outcomes in high-risk patients. *Arch Ophthalmol* 1998;116:1045–1052.
31. Owens SL, Guymer RH, Gross-Jendroska M, et al. Fluorescein angiographic abnormalities after prophylactic macular photocoagulation for high-risk age-related maculopathy. *Am J Ophthalmol* 1999;127:681–687.
32. Wormald R, Evans J, Smeeth L, et al. Photodynamic therapy for neovascular age-related macular degeneration (Cochrane Review). In: The Cochrane Library, Issue 3, 2003. Chichester, UK: John Wiley & Sons, Ltd. Search date 2002; primary sources Cochrane Central Register of Controlled Trials, Medline, Embase, Science Citation Index, personal Communication with authors, and hand searches of reference lists of relevant studies for further trials.
33. Husereau DR, Shukla VB, Skidmore B, et al. Photodynamic therapy with verteporfin for the treatment of neovascular age-related macular degeneration: a clinical assessment. Ottawa: Canadian Coordinating Office for Health Technology Assessment; 2002. Technology report no 31. Search date not reported; primary sources Medline, Embase, Healthstar, Pascal, Scisearch, Toxline, The Cochrane Library, Pubmed, personal contact with experts in the field and with drug manufacturers, Grey Literature Searches, Current Contents Search, ADIS LMS Drug Alerts, Pharmaceutical News Index, bibliographic searches, and hand searches.
34. Bressler NM, Treatment of Age-Related Macular Degeneration with Photodynamic Therapy (TAP) Study Group. Photodynamic therapy of subfoveal choroidal neovascularisation in age-related macular degeneration with verteporfin: two-year results of 2 randomized clinical trials: TAP report 2. *Arch Ophthalmol* 2001;119:198–207.
35. Verteporfin In Photodynamic Therapy Study Group. Verteporfin therapy of subfoveal choroidal neovascularization in age-related macular degeneration: two-year results of a randomized clinical trial including lesions with occult with no classic choroidal neovascularization: verteporfin in photodynamic therapy report 2. *Am J Ophthalmol* 2001;131:541–560.
36. Blinder KJ, Bradley S, Bressler NM, et al. Effect of lesion size, visual acuity, and lesion composition on visual acuity change with and without verteporfin therapy for choroidal neovascularisation secondary to age-related macular degeneration: TAP and VIP report no. 1. *Am J Ophthalmol* 2003;136:407–418.
37. Macular Photocoagulation Study Group. Occult choroidal neovascularization. Influence on visual outcome in patients with age-related macular degeneration. *Arch Ophthalmol* 1996;114:400–412.
38. Macular Photocoagulation Study Group. Persistent and recurrent neovascularization after laser photocoagulation for subfoveal choroidal neovascularization of age-related macular degeneration. *Arch Ophthalmol* 1994;112:489–499.
39. Macular Photocoagulation Study Group. Visual outcome after laser photocoagulation for subfoveal choroidal neovascularization secondary to age-related macular degeneration. The influence of initial lesion size and initial visual acuity. *Arch Ophthalmol* 1994;112:480–488.
40. Coscas G, Soubrane G, Ramahefasolo C, et al. Perifoveal laser treatment for subfoveal choroidal new vessels in age-related macular degeneration. Results of a randomized clinical trial. *Arch Ophthalmol* 1991;109:1258–1265.
41. Bressler NM, Maguire MG, Murphy PL, et al. Macular scatter ("grid") laser treatment of poorly demarcated subfoveal choroidal neovascularisation in age-related macular degeneration. Results of a randomised pilot trial. *Arch Ophthalmol* 1996;114:1456–1464.
42. Arnold J, Algan M, Soubrane G, et al. Indirect scatter laser photocoagulation to subfoveal choroidal neovascularization in age-related macular degeneration. *Graefes Arch Clin Exp Ophthalmol* 1997;235:208–216.
43. Barondes MJ, Pagliarini S, Chisholm IH, et al. Controlled trial of laser photocoagulation of pigment epithelial detachments in the elderly: 4 year review. *Br J Ophthalmol* 1992;76:5–7.
44. Macular Photocoagulation Study Group. Evaluation of argon green vs krypton red laser for photocoagulation of subfoveal choroidal neovascularisation in the Macular Photocoagulation Study. *Arch Ophthalmol* 1994;112:1176–1184.
45. Willan AR, Cruess AF, Ballantyne M. Argon green vs krypton red laser photocoagulation for extrafoveal choroidal neovascularization secondary to age-related macular degeneration: 3-year results of a multicentre randomized trial. *Can J Ophthalmol* 1996;31:11–17.
46. The Radiation Therapy for Age-related Macular Degeneration (RAD) Study Group. A prospective randomized double-masked trial on radiation therapy for neovascular age-related macular degeneration (RAD) study. *Ophthalmology* 1999;106:2239–2247.
47. Hart PM, Chakravarthy U, Mackenzie G, et al. Visual outcomes in the subfoveal radiotherapy study: a randomized controlled trial of teletherapy for age-related macular degeneration. *Arch Ophthalmol* 2002;120:1029–1038.
48. Valmaggia C, Reis G, Ballinari P. Radiotherapy for subfoveal choroidal neovascularization in age-related macular degeneration: a randomized clinical trial. *Am J Ophthalmol* 2002;133:521–529.
49. Marcus DM, Sheils W, Johnson MH, et al. External beam irradiation of subfoveal choroidal neovascularization complicating age-related macular degeneration: one-year results of a prospective, double-masked, randomized clinical trial. *Arch Ophthalmol* 2001;119:171–180.
50. Kobayashi H, Kobayashi K. Age-related macular degeneration: long-term results of radiotherapy for subfoveal neovascular membranes. *Am J Ophthalmol* 2000;130:617–635.
51. Bergink GJ, Hoyng CB, Van der Maazen RW, et al. A randomized controlled clinical trial on the efficacy of radiation therapy in the control of subfoveal choroidal neovascularization in age-related macular degeneration: radiation versus observation. *Graefes Arch Clin Exp Ophthalmol* 1998;236:321–325.
52. Char DH, Irvine AI, Posner MD, et al. Randomized trial of radiation for age-related macular degeneration. *Am J Ophthalmol* 1999;127:574–578.
53. Ciulla TA, Danis RP, Harris A. Age-related macular degeneration: a review of experimental treatments. *Surv Ophthalmol* 1998;43:134–146.
54. Hart PM, Chakravarthy U, MacKenzie G, et al. Teletherapy for subfoveal choroidal neovascularisation of age-related macular degeneration: results of follow up in a non-randomised study. *Br J Ophthalmol* 1996;80:1046–1050.

55. Finger PT, Berson A, Sherr D, et al. Radiation therapy for subretinal neovascularization. *Ophthalmology* 1996;103:878–889.
56. Mauget-Faysse M, Chiquet C, Milea D, et al. Long term results of radiotherapy for subfoveal choroidal neovascularisation in age-related macular degeneration. *Br J Ophthalmol* 1999;83:923–928.
57. Flaxel CJ, Fridrichsen EJ, Osborn Smith J, et al. Proton beam irradiation of subfoveal choroidal neovascularisation in age-related macular degeneration. *Eye* 2000;14:155–164.
58. Spaide RF, Leys A, Herrmann-Delemazure B, et al. Radiation-associated choroidal neovasculopathy. *Ophthalmology* 1999;106:2254–2260.
59. Submacular Surgery Trials Pilot Study Investigators. Submacular surgery trials randomized pilot trial of laser photocoagulation versus surgery for recurrent choroidal neovascularization secondary to age-related macular degeneration: I. Ophthalmic outcomes. Submacular surgery trials pilot study report number 1. *Am J Ophthalmol* 2000;130:387–407.
60. Lewis H, Van der Brug MS. Tissue plasminogen activator-assisted surgical excision of subfoveal choroidal neovascularization in age-related macular degeneration: a randomized, double-masked trial. *Ophthalmology* 1997;104:1847–1851.
61. Thomas MA, Dickinson JD, Melberg NS, et al. Visual results after surgical removal of subfoveal choroidal neovascular membranes. *Ophthalmology* 1994;101:1384–1396.
62. Pharmacological Therapy for Macular Degeneration Study Group. Interferon alfa-2a is ineffective for patients with choroidal neovascularization secondary to age-related macular degeneration: results of a prospective randomized placebo-controlled clinical trial. *Arch Ophthalmol* 1997;115:865–872.

Jennifer Arnold
Consultant Ophthalmologist
Marsden Eye Specialists
Parramatta
New South Wales
Australia

Competing interests: JA was a clinical investigator in the study of photodynamic treatment using verteporfin, funded by Novartis/QLT, and has been supported by Novartis for attendance at conferences and symposia.

TABLE 1 Laser photocoagulation of choroidal neovascularisation (CNV) versus observation in exudative age related macular degeneration: results of Macular Photocoagulation Study Group RCTs (see text, p 767).

Site of CNV (type of laser)	Number of eyes	Severe visual loss (6 or more lines)	Vision level; treated *v* control	Rate of recurrence in treated eyes
Extrafoveal CNV (argon-blue-green)[13,15]	236	RR 1.5 at 6 months to 5 years; $P = 0.001$	≥ 20/40 at 3 years; 33% *v* 22%	54% at 5 years
Juxtafoveal CNV (krypton-red)[16,37]	496	RR 1.2 at 6 months to 5 years; $P = 0.04$	≥ 20/40 at 3 years; 13% *v* 7%	76% at 5 years (classic CNV only)
New subfoveal CNV (argon-green or krypton)[14,38,39]	373	20% treated *v* 37% control at 2 years; $P < 0.01$	> 20/200 at 4 years; 12% *v* 11%	44% at 3 years
Recurrent subfoveal CNV (argon-green or krypton)[14,38,39]	206	9% treated *v* 28% control at 2 years; $P = 0.03$	> 20/200 at 3 years; 25% *v* 12%	39% at 3 years

CNV, choroidal neovascularisation.

Bacterial conjunctivitis

Search date February 2004

Justine Smith

QUESTIONS

INTERVENTIONS

See glossary Ⓖ

Key Messages

- **Antibiotic treatment in culture positive bacterial conjunctivitis** One systematic review and two subsequent RCTs found that antibiotics (polymyxin–bacitracin, ciprofloxacin, ofloxacin, levofloxacin, or moxifloxacin) increase rates of clinical and microbiological cure compared with placebo. Four RCTs found no significant difference between different antibiotics in clinical or microbiological cure. One RCT found that fusidic acid increased clinical cure rate compared with chloramphenicol. One RCT found that topical netilmicin increased clinical cure rate compared with topical gentamicin. One RCT found that topical levofloxacin increased microbiological cure rate, but not clinical cure rate, compared with topical ofloxacin.
- **Empirical antibiotic treatment of suspected bacterial conjunctivitis** One systematic review found limited evidence from one RCT that topical norfloxacin increased rates of clinical and microbiological improvement or cure after 5 days compared with placebo. RCTs comparing different topical antibiotics versus each other found no significant difference in rates of clinical or microbiological cure. One RCT found no significant difference between topical polymyxin–bacitracin ointment and oral cefixime for clinical or microbiological improvement or cure.

Clin Evid 2005;13:776–781.

DEFINITION	Conjunctivitis is any inflammation of the conjunctiva, generally characterised by irritation, itching, foreign body sensation, and watering or discharge. Bacterial conjunctivitis may often be distinguished from other types of conjunctivitis by the presence of a yellow–white mucopurulent discharge. There is also usually a papillary reaction (small bumps with fibrovascular cores on the palpebral conjunctiva, appearing grossly as a fine velvety surface). Bacterial conjunctivitis is usually bilateral. Treatment is often based on clinical suspicion that the conjunctivitis is bacterial, without waiting for results of microbiological investigations. In this topic, we have therefore distinguished effects of empirical treatment from effects of treatment in people with culture positive bacterial conjunctivitis. This review covers only non-gonococcal bacterial conjunctivitis.
INCIDENCE/ PREVALENCE	We found no good evidence on the incidence or prevalence of bacterial conjunctivitis.
AETIOLOGY/ RISK FACTORS	Conjunctivitis may be infectious (caused by bacteria or viruses) or allergic. In adults, bacterial conjunctivitis is less common than viral conjunctivitis, although estimates vary widely (viral conjunctivitis has been reported to account for 8–75% of acute conjunctivitis).[1-3] *Staphylococcus* species are the most common pathogens for bacterial conjunctivitis in adults, followed by *Streptococcus pneumoniae* and *Haemophilus influenzae*.[4,5] In children, bacterial conjunctivitis is more common than viral, and is mainly caused by *Haemophilus influenzae*, *Streptococcus pneumoniae*, and *Moraxella catarrhalis*.[6,7]
PROGNOSIS	Most bacterial conjunctivitis is self limiting. One systematic review (search date 2001) found clinical cure or significant improvement with placebo within 2–5 days in 64% of people (99% CI 54% to 73%).[8] Some organisms cause corneal or systemic complications, or both. Otitis media may develop in 25% of children with *H influenzae* conjunctivitis,[9] and systemic meningitis may complicate primary meningococcal conjunctivitis in 18% of people.[10]
AIMS OF INTERVENTION	To achieve rapid cure of infection, and to prevent complications, with minimum adverse effects of treatment.
OUTCOMES	Time to cure or improvement. **Clinical signs/symptoms:** hyperaemia, discharge, papillae, follicles, chemosis, itching, pain, and photophobia. Most studies used a numbered scale to grade signs and symptoms. Some studies also included evaluation by investigators and participants regarding success of treatment. **Culture results:** These are proxy outcomes usually expressed as the number of colonies, sometimes with reference to a threshold level. Results were often classified into categories such as eradication, reduction, persistence, and proliferation.
METHODS	*Clinical Evidence* search and appraisal February 2004.

QUESTION **What are the effects of antibiotics in adults and children with bacterial conjunctivitis?**

OPTION **EMPIRICAL TREATMENT WITH ANTIBIOTICS IN PEOPLE WITH SUSPECTED BACTERIAL CONJUNCTIVITIS**

One systematic review found limited evidence from one RCT that topical norfloxacin increased rates of clinical and microbiological improvement or cure after 5 days compared with placebo. RCTs comparing different topical antibiotics versus each other found no significant difference in rates of clinical or microbiological cure. One RCT found no significant difference between topical polymyxin–bacitracin ointment and oral cefixime for clinical or microbiological improvement or cure.

Benefits: **Versus placebo:** We found one systematic review (search date 2001, 1 RCT, 284 adults; 50% of participants were culture positive) comparing topical norfloxacin versus placebo (see table A on web extra).[8] It found that norfloxacin significantly increased rates of clinical and microbiological improvement or cure after 5 days compared with placebo (88%, 95% CI 81% to 93% with norfloxacin *v* 72%, 95% CI 63% to 79% with placebo; $P < 0.01$; see comment below). **Versus each other:** We found no systematic review but found 22 RCTs conducted in adults and children (see table A on web extra).[11–29] These RCTs found no significant difference between different topical antibiotics in rates of clinical or microbiological cure. **Versus oral antibiotics:** We found one RCT (80 children).[30] It found no significant difference between polymyxin–bacitracin ointment plus oral placebo and topical placebo plus oral cefixime in clinical improvement or bacteriological failure rates (failure rate: 15/40 [37.5%] with cefixime *v* 7/40 [17.5%] with polymyxin–bacitracin; $P = 0.07$).

Harms: **Versus placebo:** One RCT identified by the review reported minor adverse events in 4.2% of people for norfloxacin compared with 7.1% for placebo (P value not reported).[5] One non-systematic review reported four cases of aplastic anaemia with topical chloramphenicol and three cases of Stevens–Johnson syndrome with topical sulphonamides.[31] However, the review did not report the number of people using these drugs, making it difficult to exclude other possible causes of aplastic anaemia. **Versus each other:** See table A on web extra.[11–29]

Comment: The placebo controlled RCT identified by the review did not assess the effect of topical antibiotics on antibiotic resistance.[5] Most other trials included children as well as adults, and the ratio of children to adults was usually not specified. The comparisons of lomefloxacin versus chloramphenicol and fusidic acid, the comparison of norfloxacin versus fusidic acid, and the comparison of tobramycin versus fusidic acid, were single blind. One RCT found that a significantly greater proportion of participants rated topical tobramycin as more inconvenient than the viscous preparation of fusidic acid, because of a difference in the frequency of administration.[27] The RCT also found that adherence among children was significantly higher with fusidic acid.

OPTION ANTIBIOTICS IN PEOPLE WITH CULTURE POSITIVE BACTERIAL CONJUNCTIVITIS

One systematic review and two subsequent RCTs found that topical antibiotics (polymyxin–bacitracin, ciprofloxacin, ofloxacin, levofloxacin, or moxifloxacin) increase rates of both clinical and microbiological cure compared with placebo. Four RCTs found no significant difference between different antibiotics in clinical or microbiological cure. One RCT found that fusidic acid increased clinical cure rate compared with chloramphenicol. One RCT found that topical netilmicin increased clinical cure rate compared with topical gentamicin. One RCT found that topical levofloxacin increased microbiological cure rate, but not clinical cure rate, compared with topical ofloxacin.

Benefits: **Versus placebo:** We found one systematic review (search date 2000, 3 RCTs) in people with culture positive bacterial conjunctivitis, which compared antibiotics (polymyxin–bacitracin, ciprofloxacin, and ofloxacin) versus placebo (see table A on web extra),[8] and two subsequent RCTs.[32,33] The first RCT identified by the review (84 children with culture proven *H influenzae* or *S pneumoniae* bacterial conjunctivitis) found that topical polymyxin–bacitracin significantly increased clinical cure after 3–5 days compared with placebo, but found no significant difference after 8–10 days (3–5 days: 62% with antibiotic *v* 28% with placebo; $P < 0.02$; 8–10 days: 91% with antibiotic *v* 72% with placebo; $P > 0.05$).[34] The RCT found that topical polymyxin–bacitracin significantly increased microbiological cure rates after both 3–5 days and 8–10 days compared with placebo. The second RCT (177 people, age not specified) found that topical ciprofloxacin significantly increased microbiological cure rates after 3 days compared with placebo (132/140 [94%] with antibiotic *v* 22/37 [59%] with placebo; RR 1.59, 95% CI 1.21 to 2.08).[35] The third RCT identified by the review, which compared antibiotics versus placebo, is published only in abstract form.[36] The first subsequent RCT (249 people aged 2–91 years, of whom 117 were culture positive) compared topical levofloxacin versus placebo.[32] It found that levofloxacin significantly increased microbiological and clinical cure after 5 days of treatment (microbiological cure: 90% with levofloxacin *v* 53% with placebo; CI not reported; $P < 0.001$; clinical cure: 77% with antibiotic *v* 60% with placebo; CI not reported; $P = 0.026$). The second subsequent RCT (73 people aged 1–89 years, 51 of whom were culture positive) found that a 3 day treatment of topical moxifloxacin significantly increased microbiological and clinical cure compared with placebo about 1 week after starting treatment (microbiological cure: 78% with antibiotic *v* 39% with placebo, CI not reported; $P = 0.005$; clinical cure: 93% with antibiotic *v* 63% with placebo; CI not reported; $P = 0.009$).[33] The study did not state whether or not analysis was restricted only to people with culture positive bacterial conjunctivitis. **Versus each other:** We found no systematic review but found seven RCTs (see table A on web extra).[35,37–42] The first RCT (139 children) found that fusidic acid significantly increased clinical cure rate compared with chloramphenicol (85% with fusidic acid *v* 48% with chloramphenicol; $P < 0.0001$).[37] The second RCT (251 people) found no significant difference in reduction or eradication of bacteria between ciprofloxacin and tobramycin after 7 days (94.5% with ciprofloxacin *v* 91.9% with tobramycin; $P > 0.5$).[35] The third RCT (141 children) found no significant difference in clinical cure between ciprofloxacin and tobramycin (87% with ciprofloxacin *v* 90% with tobramycin; $P > 0.05$) or in microbiological cure rate (90% with ciprofloxacin *v* 84% with tobramycin; $P = 0.29$) after 7 days.[38] The fourth RCT (156 children) compared three treatments: trimethoprim–polymyxin, gentamicin, and sulfacetamide (sulphacetamide).[39] It found no significant difference in clinical cure rate between any of the treatments (84% with trimethoprim–polymyxin *v* 88% with gentamicin *v* 89% with sulfacetamide; $P > 0.1$) or in microbiological cure rate (83% with trimethoprim–polymyxin *v* 68% with gentamicin *v* 72% with sulfacetamide; $P > 0.1$) after 2–7 days. The fifth RCT (40 people) found no significant difference in symptom resolution between lomefloxacin and ofloxacin after 7 days (88% with lomefloxacin *v* 75% ofloxacin; $P < 0.08$).[40] The sixth RCT (121 people) found that topical netilmicin (0.3%) administered as one or two drops to affected eyes four times daily significantly increased clinical cure rate after both 5 and 10 days compared with 0.3% topical gentamicin ($P = 0.01$ after 5 days; $P = 0.001$ after 10 days; other results presented graphically).[41] The seventh RCT (423 adults and children entered, 208 included in per protocol analysis) found that topical levofloxacin 0.5% for 5 days significantly increased microbiological cure rate but found no significant difference in clinical cure rate at 6–10 days compared with topical ofloxacin 0.3% (microbiological cure: 89% with levofloxacin *v* 80% with ofloxacin; $P = 0.034$; clinical cure: 76% with levofloxacin *v* 76% with ofloxacin; $P > 0.05$).[42]

Harms: **Versus placebo:** See table A on web extra. **Versus each other:** The following minor adverse effects of topical antibiotics compared with each other were reported in RCTs that included people with suspected bacterial conjunctivitis: punctuate epithelial erosions (35% for tobramycin *v* 20% for ciprofloxacin); bad taste (20% for norfloxacin *v* 6% for fusidic acid); stinging (50% for norfloxacin *v* 37% for fusidic acid); and burning (33% with gentamicin *v* 20% with lomefloxacin; 1.45% with levofloxacin *v* 0.97% with ofloxacin).[13,17,18,42] (see table A on web extra).

Comment: None of the RCTs addressed the effect on antibiotic resistance of using topical antibiotics in bacterial conjunctivitis, which would be of interest given the self limiting nature of the disease. The age of the study participants was not always specified and no RCTs reported any patient orientated outcomes or assessed rates of reinfection. In most of the RCTs, people were randomised and began treatment before their culture results were available, and people with negative baseline culture results were excluded from the efficacy analyses.

REFERENCES

1. Wishart PK, James C, Wishart MS, et al. Prevalence of acute conjunctivitis caused by chlamydia, adenovirus, and herpes simplex virus in an ophthalmic casualty department. *Br J Ophthalmol* 1984;68:653–655.
2. Fitch CP, Rapoza PA, Owens S, et al. Epidemiology and diagnosis of acute conjunctivitis at an inner-city hospital. *Ophthalmology* 1989;96:1215–1220.
3. Woodland RM, Darougar S, Thaker U, et al. Causes of conjunctivitis and keratoconjunctivitis in Karachi, Pakistan. *Trans R Soc Trop Med Hygiene* 1992;86:317–320.
4. Seal DV, Barrett SP, McGill JI. Aetiology and treatment of acute bacterial infection of the external eye. *Br J Ophthalmol* 1982;66:357–360.
5. Miller IM, Wittreich J, Vogel R, et al, for the Norfloxacin-Placebo Ocular Study Group. The safety and efficacy of topical norfloxacin compared with placebo in the treatment of acute bacterial conjunctivitis. *Eur J Ophthalmol* 1992;2:58–66.
6. Gigliotti F, Williams WT, Hayden FG, et al. Etiology of acute conjunctivitis in children. *J Pediatr* 1981;98:531–536.
7. Weiss A, Brinser JH, Nazar-Stewart V. Acute conjunctivitis in childhood. *J Pediatr* 1993;122:10–14.
8. Sheikh A, Hurwitz B, Cave J. Antibiotics versus placebo for acute bacterial conjunctivitis. In: The Cochrane Library, Issue 2, 2003. Oxford: Update Software. Search date 2001; primary sources Cochrane Controlled Trials Register, Medline, bibliographies of identified trials, Science Citation Index, and personal contacts with investigators and pharmaceutical companies.
9. Bodor FF. Conjunctivitis-otitis media syndrome: more than meets the eye. *Contemp Pediatr* 1989;6:55–60.
10. Barquet N, Gasser I, Domingo P, et al. Primary meningococcal conjunctivitis: report of 21 patients and review. *Rev Infect Dis* 1990;12:838–847.
11. Kettenmeyer A, Jauch A, Boscher M, et al. A double-blind double-dummy multicenter equivalence study comparing topical lomefloxacin 0.3% twice daily with norfloxacin 0.3% four times daily in the treatment of acute bacterial conjunctivitis. *J Clin Res* 1998;1:75–86.
12. Agius-Fernandez A, Patterson A, Fsadni M, et al. Topical lomefloxacin versus topical chloramphenicol in the treatment of acute bacterial conjunctivitis. *Clin Drug Invest* 1998;15:263–269.
13. Montero J, Casado A, Perea E, et al. A double-blind double-dummy comparison of topical lomefloxacin 0.3% twice daily with topical gentamicin 0.3% four times daily in the treatment of acute bacterial conjunctivitis. *J Clin Res* 1998;1:29–39.
14. Adenis JP, Arrata M, Gastaud P, et al. Etude randomisee multicentrique acide fusidique gel ophtalmique et rifamycine collyre dans les conjonctivites aigues. *J Fr Ophtalmol* 1989;12:317–322.
15. Huerva V, Ascaso FJ, Latre B, et al. Tolerancia y eficacia de la tobramicina topica vs cloranfenicol en el tratamiento de las conjuntivitis bacterianas. *Ciencia Pharmaceutica* 1991;1:221–224.
16. Gallenga PE, Lobefalo L, Colangelo L, et al. Topical lomefloxacin 0.3% twice daily versus tobramycin 0.3% in acute bacterial conjunctivitis: a multicenter double-blind phase III study. *Ophthalmologica* 1999;213:250–257.
17. Alves MR, Kara JN. Evaluation of the clinical and microbiological efficacy of 0.3% ciprofloxacin drops and 0.3% tobramycin drops in the treatment of acute bacterial conjunctivitis. *Rev Bras Oftalmol* 1993;52:371–377.
18. Wall AR, Sinclair N, Adenis JP. Comparison of Fucithalmic (fusidic acid viscous eye drops 1%) and Noroxin (norfloxacin ophthalmic solution 0.3%) in the treatment of acute bacterial conjunctivitis. *J Clin Res* 1998;1:316–325.
19. Behrens-Baumann W, Quentin CD, Gibson JR, et al. Trimethoprim-polymyxin B sulphate ophthalmic ointment in the treatment of bacterial conjunctivitis: a double-blind study versus chloramphenicol ophthalmic ointment. *Curr Med Res Opin* 1988;11:227–231.
20. Van-Rensburg SF, Gibson JR, Harvey SG, Burke CA. Trimethoprim-polymyxin ophthalmic solution versus chloramphenicol ophthalmic solution in the treatment of bacterial conjunctivitis. *Pharmatherapeutica* 1982;3:274–277.
21. Gibson JR. Trimethoprim-polymyxin B ophthalmic solution in the treatment of presumptive bacterial conjunctivitis — a multicentre trial of its efficacy versus neomycin-polymyxin B-gramicidin and chloramphenicol ophthalmic solutions. *J Antimicrob Chemother* 1983;11:217–221.
22. Genee E, Schlechtweg C, Bauerreiss P, et al. Trimethoprim-polymyxin eye drops versus neomycin-polymyxin-gramicidin eye drops in the treatment of presumptive bacterial conjunctivitis — a double-blind study. *Ophthalmologica* 1982;184:92–96.
23. Malminiemi K, Kari O, Latvala M-L, et al. Topical lomefloxacin twice daily compared with fusidic acid in acute bacterial conjunctivitis. *Acta Ophthalmol Scand* 1996;74:280–284.
24. Carr WD. Comparison of Fucithalmic (fusidic acid viscous eye drops 1%) and Chloromycetin Redidrops (chloramphenicol eye drops 0.5%) in the treatment of acute bacterial conjunctivitis. *J Clin Res* 1998;1:403–411.
25. Horven I. Acute conjunctivitis. A comparison of fusidic acid viscous eye drops and chloramphenicol. *Acta Ophthalmol* 1993;71:165–168.
26. Hvidberg J. Fusidic acid in acute conjunctivitis. Single-blind, randomized comparison of fusidic acid and chloramphenicol viscous eye drops. *Acta Ophthalmol* 1987;65:43–47.
27. Jackson WB, Low DE, Dattani D, et al. Treatment of acute bacterial conjunctivitis: 1% fusidic acid viscous drops vs. 0.3% tobramycin drops. *Can J Ophthalmol* 2002;37:228–237.
28. Sinclair, Leigh DA. A comparison of fusidic acid viscous eye drops and chloramphenicol eye ointment in acute conjunctivitis. *Curr Ther Res* 1988;44;468–474.
29. The Trimethoprim-Polymyxin B Sulphate Ophthalmic Ointment Study Group. Trimethoprim-polymyxin B sulphate ophthalmic ointment versus chloramphenicol ophthalmic ointment in the treatment of bacterial conjunctivitis – a review of four clinical studies. *J Antimicrob Chemother* 1989; 23: 261–266.
30. Wald ER, Greenberg D, Hoberman A. Short term oral cefixime therapy for treatment of bacterial conjunctivitis. *Pediatr Infect Dis J* 2001;20:1039–1042.
31. Stern GA, Killingsworth DW. Complications of topical antimicrobial agents. *Int Ophthalmol Clin* 1989;29:137–142.
32. Hwang DG, Schanzlin DJ, Rotberg MH et al. A phase III, placebo controlled clinical trial of 0.5%

levofloxacin ophthalmic solution for the treatment of bacterial conjunctivitis. *Br J Ophthalmol* 2003;87:1004–1009.
33. Gross RD, Lichtenstein SJ, Schlech BA. Early clinical and microbiological responses in the treatment of bacterial conjunctivitis with moxifloxacin ophthalmic solution 0.5% (vigamox) using BID dosing. *Todays Ther Trends* 2003;21:227–237.
34. Gigliotti G, Hendley JO, Morgan J, et al. Efficacy of topical antibiotic therapy in acute conjunctivits in children. *J Pediatr* 1984; 104:623–626.
35. Leibowitz HM. Antibacterial effectiveness of ciprofloxacin 0.3% ophthalmic solution in the treatment of bacterial conjunctivitis. *Am J Ophthalmol* 1991;112:29S–33S.
36. Ofloxacin Study Group III. A placebo-controlled clinical study of the fluoroquinolone ofloxacin in patients with external infection. *Invest Ophthalmol Vis Sci* 1990;31:572.
37. Van Bijsterveld OP, El Batawi Y, Sobhi FS, et al. Fusidic acid in infections of the external eye. *Infection* 1987;15:16–19.
38. Gross RD, Hoffman RO, Lindsay RN. A comparison of ciprofloxacin and tobramycin in bacterial conjunctivitis is children. *Clin Pediatr* 1997;36:435–444.
39. Lohr JA, Austin RD, Grossman M, et al. Comparison of three topical antimicrobials for acute bacterial conjunctivitis. *Pediatr Infect Dis J* 1988;7:626–629.
40. Tabbara KF, El-Sheik HF, Monowarul Islam SM, et al. Treatment of acute bacterial conjunctivitis with topical lomefloxacin 0.3% compared to topical ofloxacin 0.3%. *Eur J Ophthalmol* 1999; 9:269–275.
41. Papa V, Aragona P, Scuderi AC, et al. Treatment of acute bacterial conjunctivitis with topical netilmicin. *Cornea* 2002;21:43–47.
42. Schwab IR, Friedlaender M, McCulley J, et al, and the Levofloxacin Bacterial Conjunctivitis Active Control Study Group. A phase III clinical trial of 0.5% levofloxacin ophthalmic solution versus 0.3% ofloxacin ophthalmic solution for the treatment of bacterial conjunctivitis. *Ophthalmology* 2003;110:457–465.

Justine Smith
Assistant Professor of Ophthalmology
Casey Eye Institute Oregon Health & Science University
Portland
USA

Competing interests: None declared.

Cataract

Search date November 2003

David Allen

QUESTIONS

INTERVENTIONS

See glossary G

Key Messages

- **Manual extracapsular extraction (better than intracapsular extraction)** One RCT found that manual extracapsular extraction plus intraocular lens implant improved visual acuity and quality of life compared with intracapsular extraction plus aphakic glasses. The RCT also found a higher rate of complications with intracapsular extraction plus aphakic glasses than with a manual extracapsular extraction plus intraocular lens implant. The RCT and a systematic review of observational studies found that a higher proportion of people had complications with manual extracapsular extraction than with phaco extracapsular extraction.
- **Phaco extracapsular extraction (better than manual extracapsular extraction)** We found no systematic review or RCTs comparing phaco extracapsular extraction versus no extraction. One RCT identified by a systematic review found improved vision up to 1 year after phaco extracapsular extraction plus foldable posterior chamber intraocular lens implant compared with manual extracapsular extraction plus rigid posterior chamber intraocular lens implant. The RCT and a systematic review of observational studies found that a higher proportion of people had complications with manual extracapsular extraction than with phaco extracapsular extraction.

DEFINITION	**Cataracts** are cloudy or opaque areas in the lens of the eye (which should usually be completely clear). This results in changes that can impair vision. **Age related (or senile) cataract** is defined as cataract occurring in people over 16 years of age in the absence of known mechanical, chemical, or radiation trauma. This chapter covers treatment for age related cataract. It does not cover cataract in people with diabetes mellitus or recurrent uveitis; these conditions can affect the surgical outcome.
INCIDENCE/ PREVALENCE	Cataract accounts for over 40% of blindness worldwide — causing blindness in about 38 million people.[2] In a rural setting in the USA in the 1970s, the prevalence of visually significant cataract ranged from approximately 5% at the age of 65 years to around 50% in people older than 75 years.[3] The incidence of non-age related cataract within this population is so small that this can be taken as the effective incidence of age related cataract.
AETIOLOGY/ RISK FACTORS	Diet, smoking,[4] and exposure to ultraviolet light[5] are thought to be risk factors in the development of age related cataract. In addition, some people may have a genetic predisposition to development of age related cataract.[6]
PROGNOSIS	Age related cataract progresses with age, but at an unpredictable rate. Cataract surgery is indicated when the chances of significant visual improvement outweigh the risks of a poor surgical outcome. It is not dependent on reaching a specific visual acuity standard. Cataract surgery may also be indicated where the presence of cataract makes it hard to treat or monitor concurrent retinal disease, such as diabetic retinopathy.
AIMS OF INTERVENTION	To restore vision and to improve quality of life with minimal adverse effects of treatment.
OUTCOMES	Uncorrected visual acuity; corrected visual acuity; speed and stability of visual rehabilitation; quality of life (including frequency and severity of accidents); adverse effects of treatment such as endophthalmitis, vitreous loss, cystoid macular oedema and induced astigmatism**G**, retinal detachment.
METHODS	*Clinical Evidence* search and appraisal November 2003.

QUESTION **What are the effects of surgery for age related cataract without other ocular co-morbidity?**

OPTION **MANUAL EXTRACAPSULAR CATARACT EXTRACTION**

One RCT found that manual extracapsular extraction plus intraocular lens implant improved visual acuity and quality of life compared with intracapsular extraction plus aphakic glasses. The RCT also found a higher rate of complications with intracapsular extraction plus aphakic glasses than with manual extracapsular extraction plus intraocular lens implant. The RCT and a systematic review of observational studies found that a higher proportion of people had complications with manual extracapsular extraction than with phaco extracapsular extraction.

Benefits: **Versus no extraction:** We found no systematic review or RCTs comparing manual extracapsular extraction**G** versus no extraction. There is consensus that the clinical and quality of life benefits of modern cataract removal are such that an RCT that includes non-intervention would be unethical. **Versus intracapsular extraction:** We found one RCT comparing manual extracapsular extraction plus intraocular lens implant versus intracapsular extraction plus aphakic glasses, with follow up lasting 1 year.[7–10] The RCT found that manual extracapsular extraction plus intraocular lens implant significantly improved visual acuity and quality of life compared with intracapsular extraction plus aphakic glasses (1 RCT, 3400 people aged range 40–75 years: best corrected vision 20/40 or better at 1 year: 1420/1474 [96.3%] with manual extracapsular extraction *v* 1271/1401 [90.7%] with intracapsular extraction; $P < 0.00001$; visual function and quality of life as assessed using a specifically designed and validated questionnaire showed an effect size difference 12 months after surgery of 0.61 in favour of manual extracapsular extraction in general visual function; 99% CI 0.33 to 0.89; $P < 0.00001$). In the study an effect size of 0.5 was considered "medium" and one of 0.8 was considered "large". **Versus phaco extracapsular extraction🅖:** See benefits of phaco extracapsular extraction, p 784.

Harms: **Versus intracapsular extraction:** The RCT followed patients for 1 year and then reviewed random samples of the participants at 3 and 4 years.[7–10] It found a significantly higher rate of complications with intracapsular extraction plus aphakic glasses than with manual extracapsular extraction plus intraocular lens implant (clinical cystoid macular oedema🅖 at 6 months after surgery: 70/1558 [4%] *v* 26/1559 [2%]; RR 2.7, 95% CI 1.7 to 4.3; cumulative complications over the first year after surgery: 203/1401 [14%] *v* 113/1474 [8%]; RR 2.7, 95% CI 1.7 to 4.3; 4 year incidence of grade II or III [grading: I minor peripheral opacity only; II present in central zone with mild obscuration of fundus detail; III as II but with marked obscuration of fundus detail] posterior capsule opacification🅖 in a sample of the manual extracapsular extraction patients: 43/327 [13.1%]; 95% CI 9.7% to 17.3%). **Versus phaco extracapsular extraction:** See harms of phaco extracapsular extraction, p 785.

Comment: The RCT is particularly relevant to the developing world.[7–10] The setting was a high volume service with experienced surgeons, and therefore the findings should be generalised with caution. The use of different forms of optical correction in the two treatment arms (intraocular lens implant and aphakic glasses) will have accounted for some of the difference in visual acuity and outcomes. The posterior capsule opacification rate was less than might be expected given the techniques and intraocular lenses in use in the study.

OPTION PHACO EXTRACAPSULAR EXTRACTION (PHACOEMULSIFICATION)

We found no systematic review or RCTs comparing phaco extracapsular extraction versus no extraction. One RCT identified by a systematic review found improved vision up to 1 year after phaco extracapsular extraction plus foldable posterior chamber intraocular lens implant compared with manual extracapsular extraction plus rigid posterior chamber intraocular lens implant. The RCT and a systematic review of observational studies found that a higher proportion of people had complications with manual extracapsular extraction than with phaco extracapsular extraction.

Benefits: **Versus no extraction:** We found no systematic review or RCTs comparing phaco extracapsular extraction🅖 versus no extraction. There is consensus that the clinical and quality of life benefits of modern cataract removal are such that an RCT that includes non-intervention would be unethical. **Versus manual extracapsular extraction:** We found one systematic review (search date 2001),[11] which identified one RCT that met the inclusion criteria.[12] The RCT (476 people aged over 40 years, mean age 72.3 years in the manual extracapsular extraction🅖 group *v* 71.1 years in the phaco extracapsular extraction group) found that phaco extracapsular extraction plus foldable posterior chamber intraocular lens implant significantly improved vision up to 1 year after surgery compared with manual extracapsular extraction plus rigid posterior chamber intraocular lens implant (proportion achieving good combined vision and refraction results at 6 weeks: 164/237 [69%] with phaco *v* 128/225 [57%] with manual; OR 1.22, 95% CI 1.06 to 1.40; proportion achieving 20/30 vision unaided: at 3 weeks 80/244 [33%] with phaco *v* 26/229 [11%] with manual; OR 2.89, 95% CI 1.93 to

4.33; at 1 year 87/224 [39%] with phaco v 42/215 [20%] with manual; OR 1.99, 95% CI 1.45 to 2.73). Primary outcome measure was visual acuity (20/30 or better and refraction within 1 dioptre of planned); secondary outcome measure was unaided visual acuity.[11]

Harms: **Versus no extraction:** We found no systematic review or RCTs. **Versus manual extracapsular extraction:** The RCT identified by the systematic review[11] found that a significantly greater proportion of people had complications with manual extracapsular extraction❻ than with phaco extracapsular extraction❻ (complications during surgery: 48/233 [21%] with manual v 17/246 [7%] with phaco, $P < 0.0001$; posterior capsule opacification❻ at 1 year: 68/232 [29%] with manual v 48/245 [20%] with phaco, OR 1.7, 95% CI 1.1 to 2.7; laser capsulotomy rates: absolute numbers not given, OR 2.1, 95% CI 1.0 to 4.5; suture removal within 3 months of surgery: 85/232 [37%] with manual extracapsular extraction v 8/245 [3%] with phaco extracapsular extraction, $P < 0.0001$).[12] As primary outcomes, the RCT evaluated capsule rupture and vitreous loss❻ during surgery, and astigmatism and posterior capsule opacification during 1 year of follow up. As secondary outcomes it evaluated perioperative difficulties and other complications.[12] We also found another systematic review (search date not stated; earliest and latest papers cited dated 1979 and 1991; 90 observational studies) assessing complications following manual extracapsular cataract extraction with posterior chamber intraocular lens implantation, phaco extracapsular cataract extraction with posterior chamber intraocular lens implantation, or intracapsular cataract extraction with flexible anterior chamber intraocular lens implantation.[13] Major complications found by the systematic review were endophthalmitis❻ (16 studies, 30 656 eyes: 0.13%, 95% CI 0.09% to 0.17%), retinal detachment (42 studies, 33 603 eyes: 0.7%, 95% CI 0.6% to 0.8%), and bullous keratopathy (27 studies, 15 971 eyes: 0.3%, 95% CI 0.2% to 0.4%). Less serious complications showing statistically significant differences ($P < 0.05$) — all in favour of phaco extracapsular extraction — were as follows: angiographic cystoid macular oedema❻ (phaco 2.62% [2 studies, 873 eyes] v manual 8.91% [2 studies, 393 eyes]); iris trauma (phaco 0.7% [2 studies, 2033 eyes] v manual 4.0% [6 studies, 1314 eyes]); and vitreous loss (phaco 0.24% [4 studies, 2732 eyes] v manual 1.08% [22 studies, 7284 eyes]).

Comment: Phaco extracapsular extraction has largely superseded manual extracapsular cataract extraction in the developed world, based on clinical experience. The one RCT is therefore important as a randomised study of the two techniques.[12] The study was specifically designed to employ surgeons who were experienced in both techniques. The target level of postoperative vision was more demanding than in the earlier observational studies reported in the other systematic review.[13]

GLOSSARY

Cystoid macular oedema is not true oedema but a condition in which fluid accumulates in cyst-like spaces in the outer plexiform layer of the retina. It is usually self limiting but can result in permanent reduction in visual acuity. It is thought to be associated with breakdown of the blood–retina barrier and is more common after complicated surgery.

Endophthalmitis is literally inflammation of some or all parts of the eye. It is normally, if not qualified as in this chapter, taken to be caused by postoperative infection.

Induced astigmatism is the change in refractive power of the cornea along different meridians as a result of the change in shape caused by surgical incisions.

Intracapsular extraction is removal of the entire lens and capsule.

Manual extracapsular extraction is removal of the anterior capsule and lens contents (nucleus and cortex) *en bloc* without using ultrasound or other methods of breaking up the nucleus before removal. The posterior capsule is left behind. This technique is commonly referred to as "extracapsular extraction".

Phaco extracapsular extraction (phacoemulsification) is use of ultrasound to break up the lens nucleus for less invasive extraction through a smaller incision. The posterior capsule is left behind as in manual extracapsular extraction. This technique is commonly referred to as "phacoemulsification".

Posterior capsule opacification is opacification of the posterior capsule (which is left behind at the end of an extracapsular or phaco cataract extraction). When it occurs it is usually progressive and can result in reduced visual function. Grading: I minor peripheral opacity only; II present in central zone with mild obscuration of fundus detail; III as II but with marked obscuration of fundus detail.

Vitreous loss is loss of the vitreous gel that normally fills the posterior segment (behind the lens) of the eye. Its loss during intracapsular cataract surgery, or in the presence of rupture of the posterior capsule in extracapsular surgery can give rise to potentially sight threatening complications.

REFERENCES

1. The Royal College of Ophthalmologists Cataract Surgery Guidelines. February 2001. www.rcophth.ac.uk/publications/guidelines (last accessed 22 March 2004).
2. Thylefors B, Negrel AD, Pararajasegaram R, et al. Global data on blindness. *Bull World Health Organ* 1995;73:115–121.
3. Leibowitz HM, Krueger DE, Maunder LR, et al. The Framingham Eye Study monograph: an ophthalmological and epidemiological study of cataract, glaucoma, diabetic retinopathy, macular degeneration, and visual acuity in a general population of 2631 adults, 1973–1975. *Surv Ophthalmol* 1980;24(suppl):335–610.
4. Flaye DE, Sullivan KN, Cullinan TR, et al. Cataracts and cigarette smoking: the City Eye Study. *Eye* 1989;3:379–384.
5. Taylor HR, West SK, Rosenthal FS, et al. Effect of ultraviolet radiation on cataract formation. *N Engl J Med* 1988;319:1429–1433.
6. Heiba IM, Elston RC, Klein BEK, et al. Evidence for a major gene for cortical cataract. *Invest Ophthalmol Vis Sci* 1995;36:227–235.
7. Natchiar GN, Thulasiraj RD, Negrel AD, et al. The Madurai intraocular lens study. I: a randomized clinical trial comparing complications and vision outcomes of intracapsular cataract extraction and extracapsular cataract extraction with posterior chamber intraocular lens. *Am J Ophthalmol* 1998;125:1–13.
8. Prajna V, Chandrakanth KS, Kim R, et al. The Madurai intraocular lens study. II: clinical outcomes. *Am J Ophthalmol* 1998;125:14–25.
9. Fletcher A, Vijaykumar V, Thulasiraj RD, et al. The Madurai intraocular lens study. III: visual functioning and quality of life outcomes. *Am J Ophthalmol* 1998;125:26–35.
10. Prajna V, Ellwein LB, Selvaraj S, et al. The Madurai intraocular lens study. IV: posterior capsule opacification. *Am J Ophthalmol* 2000;130:304–309.
11. Snellingen T, Evans JR, Ravilla T, et al. Surgical interventions for age related cataract. In: The Cochrane Library, Issue 1, 2003. Oxford: Update Software. Search date 2001; primary sources Cochrane Controlled Trials Register, Medline, Embase, and hand searches of reference lists of identified trials and personal contact with investigators and experts in the field.
12. Minassian DC, Rosen P, Dart JKG, et al. Extracapsular cataract extraction compared with small incision surgery by phacoemulsification: a randomized trial. *Br J Ophthalmol* 2001;85:822–829
13. Powe NR, Schein OD, Gieser SC, et al. Synthesis of the literature on visual acuity and complications following cataract extraction with intraocular lens implantation. *Arch Ophthalmol* 1994;112:239–252. Search date not stated; primary sources Medline and hand searches of the bibliographies of identified articles and personal contact with experts in the field.

David Allen
Consultant Eye Surgeon
Sunderland Eye Infirmary
Sunderland
UK

Competing interests: The author has had travel and accommodation expenses reimbursed by several companies manufacturing intraocular lenses and phacoemulsification machines.

Diabetic retinopathy

Search date January 2004

Simon Harding

QUESTIONS

INTERVENTIONS

DIABETIC RETINOPATHY

Beneficial

Control of diabetes (see glycaemic control in type 1 diabetes, p 694)

Control of hypertension (see primary prevention, [Web only])

Macular photocoagulation in people with clinically significant macular oedema 790

Peripheral retinal laser photocoagulation in people with preproliferative *(moderate/severe non-proliferative)* retinopathy and maculopathy 789

Peripheral retinal laser photocoagulation in people with proliferative retinopathy. 789

Likely to be beneficial

Grid photocoagulation to zones of retinal thickening in people with diabetic maculopathy 790

Unknown effectiveness

Macular photocoagulation in people with maculopathy but without clinically significant macular oedema 790

Peripheral retinal laser photocoagulation in people with background or preproliferative (*non-proliferative*) retinopathy without maculopathy 789

VITREOUS HAEMORRHAGE

Likely to be beneficial

Vitrectomy in people with severe vitreous haemorrhage and proliferative retinopathy (if performed early) 792

Unknown effectiveness

Vitrectomy in people with maculopathy. 792

To be covered in future updates

Corticosteroids in people with maculopathy

Drug treatment in diabetic retinopathy

Covered elsewhere in *Clinical Evidence*

Prevention of diabetic retinopathy (see glycaemic control in type 1 diabetes, p 694)

In this chapter terms used in the UK are written in normal text, and visual acuities are presented in units of metres; where terms used in the USA are different they are written in italics and visual acuities are presented in units of feet (see table 1, p 794).

See glossary G

Key Messages

Diabetic retinopathy

- **Control of diabetes** See glycaemic control in type 1 diabetes, p 694.
- **Control of hypertension** See primary prevention, [Web only].
- **Macular photocoagulation to macular microaneurysus in people with clinically significant macular oedema** One large RCT found that laser photocoagulation to the macula reduced visual loss at 3 years in eyes with macular oedema plus mild to moderate diabetic retinopathy compared with no treatment. There was some evidence of greater benefit in eyes with better vision. Subgroup analysis found that focal laser treatment reduced visual loss in eyes with clinically significant macular oedema, particularly in people in whom the centre of the macula was involved or imminently threatened.

- **Peripheral retinal laser photocoagulation in people with preproliferative (moderate/severe non-proliferative*) retinopathy and maculopathy** RCTs in eyes with preproliferative retinopathy and maculopathy found that peripheral retinal photocoagulation reduced the risk of severe visual loss at 5 years compared with no treatment.
- **Peripheral retinal laser photocoagulation in people with proliferative retinopathy** RCTs have found that peripheral retinal photocoagulation reduced the risk of severe visual loss at 2–3 years compared with no treatment. One RCT in eyes with high risk proliferative diabetic retinopathy found that low intensity argon laser reduced vitreous haemorrhage and macular oedema compared with standard intensity argon laser. It found no significant difference between treatments for visual acuity, although it may have lacked power to detect clinically important effects.
- **Grid photocoagulation to zones of retinal thickening in people with diabetic maculopathy** One RCT found that grid photocoagulation improved visual acuity in treated eyes at 12 months and at 24 months compared with no treatment. Photocoagulation reduced the risk of moderate visual loss by 50–70% compared with no treatment.
- **Macular photocoagulation in people with maculopathy but without clinically significant macular oedema** We found no RCTs of macular photocoagulation in this population.
- **Peripheral retinal laser photocoagulation in people with background or preproliferative (non-proliferative*) retinopathy without maculopathy** We found no RCTs in people with background or preproliferative retinopathy without maculopathy.

Vitreous haemorrhage

- **Vitrectomy in people with severe vitreous haemorrhage and proliferative retinopathy (if performed early)** One RCT found that early vitrectomy reduced visual loss at 1, 2, and 3 years in eyes with severe vitreous haemorrhage and proliferative retinopathy compared with deferred (for 1 year) vitrectomy.
- **Vitrectomy in people with maculopathy** We found no RCTs.

*Terms in italics indicate US definitions

DEFINITION	Diabetic retinopathy is characterised by varying degrees of microaneurysms, haemorrhages, exudates *(hard exudates)*, venous changes, new vessel formation, and retinal thickening. It can involve the peripheral retina, the macula, or both. The range of severity of retinopathy includes background *(mild non-proliferative)*, preproliferative *(moderate/severe non-proliferative)*, proliferative and advanced retinopathy**G**. Involvement of the macula can be focal, diffuse, ischaemic**G**, or mixed.
INCIDENCE/ PREVALENCE	Diabetic eye disease is the most common cause of blindness in the UK, responsible for 12% of registrable blindness in people aged 16–64 years.[1]
AETIOLOGY/ RISK FACTORS	Risk factors include age, duration and control of diabetes, raised blood pressure, and raised serum lipids.[2]
PROGNOSIS	Natural history studies from the 1960s found that at least half of people with proliferative diabetic retinopathy progressed to Snellen visual acuity**G** of less than 6/60 (*20/200*) within 3–5 years.[3–5] After 4 years' follow up, the rate of progression to less than 6/60 *(20/200)* visual acuity in the better eye was 1.5% in people with type 1 diabetes, 2.7% in people with non-insulin requiring type 2 diabetes, and 3.2% in people with insulin requiring type 2 diabetes.[6]
AIMS OF INTERVENTION	To prevent visual disability, partial sight and blindness; to improve quality of life, with minimum adverse effects.
OUTCOMES	Visual acuity (measured using a Snellen chart, unless otherwise stated**G**). Incidence of visual disability (visual acuity 6/24 [*20/80*] or worse in the better eye), partial sight registration (visual acuity 6/60 [*20/200*] or worse in the better eye), and registrable blindness (visual acuity 3/60 [*10/200*] or worse in the better eye). Much of the published data used eyes as the unit of analysis rather than people. Significant loss of vision is often defined as loss of two or more Snellen lines of

acuity (vision measured on standard Snellen chart) roughly equivalent to doubling of the visual angle (visual angle is the angle subtended at the eye of the smallest letter visible by that eye) — a measure used extensively in research.

METHODS *Clinical Evidence* search and appraisal January 2004. Additional papers were identified from manual searches. Figures for numbers needed to treat and numbers needed to harm refer to the number of eyes rather than patients.

QUESTION **What are the effects of treatments for diabetic retinopathy?**

OPTION **PERIPHERAL RETINAL LASER PHOTOCOAGULATION**

RCTs found that peripheral retinal photocoagulation reduced the risk of severe visual loss in eyes with preproliferative (*moderate/severe non-proliferative*) retinopathy and maculopathy, proliferative retinopathy, and proliferative retinopathy with high risk characteristics compared with no treatment. We found no RCTs in people with preproliferative (*moderate/severe non-proliferative*) retinopathy without maculopathy. We found no evidence that one type of laser is better than another. One RCT in eyes with high risk proliferative diabetic retinopathy found that low intensity argon laser reduced vitreous haemorrhage and macular oedema compared with standard intensity argon laser, although the study may have lacked power to detect clinically important effects on visual acuity.

Benefits: **Versus no treatment:** We found no systematic review, but found six RCTs (7 publications) (see table 2, p 795),[7–13] which recruited people with different grades of diabetic retinopathy, and compared different regimens of peripheral retinal photocoagulation versus no treatment or versus deferred treatment. Two RCTs recruited only people with proliferative diabetic retinopathy**Ⓖ**; both found that peripheral photocoagulation significantly reduced the risk of blindness after 2 or 3 years compared with no treatment (see table 2, p 795).[7,8] Two large RCTs recruited people with either preproliferative (*moderate/severe non-proliferative*) or proliferative retinopathy**Ⓖ**).[9,10,13] Both found that early photocoagulation decreased the risk of severe visual loss at 5 years compared with no early photocoagulation, but in one of the RCTs the rate of severe visual loss was low and the effect was not significant (see table 2, p 795). A subgroup analysis[14] of one of these RCTs[10,13] found that the benefit was significant in people with type 2 diabetes and with severe preproliferative (*severe non-proliferative*) or early proliferative retinopathy without high risk characteristics**Ⓖ** (data presented graphically). The other two RCTs recruited only people with preproliferative (*moderate/severe non-proliferative*) diabetic retinopathy, but most of the people in these RCTs had diabetic maculopathy.[11,12] Both RCTs found that peripheral photocoagulation significantly reduced the risk of visual deterioration at 5 years compared with no treatment. We found no RCTs of photocoagulation in people with preproliferative (*moderate/severe non-proliferative*) retinopathy who have not yet developed maculopathy (see table 2, p 795). **Different types of laser:** We found no systematic review. A large multicentre RCT found no difference in effectiveness between krypton red and argon laser in the treatment of proliferative diabetic retinopathy with new vessels on the disc.[15] A smaller RCT (42 eyes with proliferative diabetic retinopathy) compared argon with double frequency YAG lasers and found no difference in rates of regression of new vessels after mean follow up of 29 months.[16] **Low versus standard intensity laser:** We found one RCT (50 people; 65 eyes with high risk proliferative diabetic retinopathy), which compared low intensity argon laser (minimum energy to produce barely visible blanching of the epithelium, median 235 mW; mean follow up of 22.4

months) versus standard intensity argon laser (median 450 mW; mean follow up of 21.6 months).[17] It found no significant difference between treatments in visual acuity (mean visual acuity on logMAR chart**G** 0.18 in eyes treated with low intensity laser *v* 0.27 in eyes treated with standard intensity laser, P = 0.231).

Harms: Adverse effects were reported as more common in the photocoagulation arm and include loss of visual field and visual acuity,[16,18,19] increased glare,[20] reduced contrast[20,21] and colour sensitivity,[22] temporary choroidal effusion, anterior uveitis, worsening macular oedema, and pain during treatment. Most studies were too small to provide accurate estimates of the frequency of these adverse effects, and they probably overestimate the risks because they used old treatment protocols. In one RCT, using an argon treatment protocol that has since been modified in current practice, constriction of visual field to within 45° of fixation occurred in 5% of eyes (NNH 20), constriction within 30° in 0%, and loss of vision by two or more Snellen lines in 3% (NNH 33; data presented graphically, no CIs reported).[9] **Fractionation:** One RCT found that adverse effects (including exudative retinal detachment, choroidal detachment, and angle closure) were reduced if photocoagulation was administered in multiple sessions spaced over time rather than in a single session.[23] **Different types of laser:** We found no clear evidence of different rates of complications with different lasers. Argon blue/green causes temporarily reduced colour sensation in treating surgeons. Dye laser[24] and orange laser (600 nm)[25] may be more painful than argon for peripheral retinal photocoagulation.[23] **Low versus standard intensity laser:** The RCT comparing low versus high intensity laser found that low intensity laser significantly reduced clinically significant macular oedema and vitreous haemorrhage**G** compared with standard intensity laser, but found no significant difference for choroidal detachment or neurotrophic keratopathy (clinically significant macular oedema: 1 eye treated with low intensity laser *v* 7 with standard intensity, P = 0.023; vitreous haemorrhage: no eyes *v* 6 eyes, P = 0.009; choroidal detachment: no eyes *v* 3 eyes, P = 0.103; neurotrophic keratopathy: no eyes *v* 2 eyes, P = 0.224).[17]

Comment: Limited prospective observational data suggest that peripheral retinal photocoagulation should be repeated until there is evidence of regression.[25] We found no evidence that theoretical advantages with certain lasers are reflected in significant improvements in clinical outcomes. Studies of visual field loss do not consider field loss before laser photocoagulation; one study found significant field loss in people with diabetes before laser compared with people without diabetes ($P < 0.01$).[26] We found one meta-analysis[27] comparing photocoagulation versus no treatment for diabetic retinopathy; its results are difficult to interpret because it was not based on a published systematic review, it did not include the largest RCT,[10] and it included one RCT of macular photocoagulation.[28]

OPTION MACULAR LASER PHOTOCOAGULATION FOR MACULOPATHY

RCTs found that laser photocoagulation to the macula reduces visual loss at 2–3 years in eyes with macular oedema plus mild to moderate preproliferative *(moderate/severe non-proliferative)* diabetic retinopathy compared with no treatment. There was some evidence of greater benefit in eyes with better vision. Subgroup analysis in one large RCT found that focal laser treatment reduced visual loss in eyes with clinically significant macular oedema compared with no treatment, particularly in people in whom the centre of the macula was involved or imminently threatened. Effects of photocoagulation in other categories of maculopathy remain unclear. We found no evidence that one type of laser is better than another in diabetic maculopathy.

Benefits: **Versus no treatment:** We found no systematic review. We found three RCTs comparing macular argon laser photocoagulation with no treatment in eyes with maculopathy, two used focal treatment to microaneurysms,[28–30] and one used a grid to zones of thickened retina.[31] **Focal treatment to microaneurysms:** The first RCT (39 people with symmetrical macular oedema and preproliferative [*moderate/severe non-proliferative*] diabetic retinopathy**G**), found no significant difference in the incidence of visual deterioration between photocoagulation and no treatment after 2 years, but the study may have lacked power to detect a clinically important difference (visual deterioration of completing eyes: 7/30 [23%] eyes with laser *v* 13/30 [43%] eyes with no treatment; RR 0.54, 95% CI 0.25 to 1.16).[28] The second and much larger RCT (2244 people with macular oedema plus mild to moderate preproliferative retinopathy) compared focal laser treatment**G** using an argon laser versus no treatment.[30] It found that laser photocoagulation significantly reduced the risk of moderate visual loss compared with no treatment after 3 years (RR 0.50, 95% CI 0.47 to 0.53; NNT 8 eyes, 95% CI 7 eyes to 12 eyes). Subgroup analysis found that focal laser treatment was significantly more effective in eyes with clinically significant macular oedema**G**, particularly in people in whom the centre of the macula was involved or imminently threatened.[13,32] The benefit was less in eyes with less extensive macular oedema. However, this may have been because both groups had low rates of visual loss from baseline. **Grid laser to zones of retinal thickening:** The third RCT (160 eyes with diffuse maculopathy with or without clinically significant macular oedema) found that grid laser photocoagulation**G** significantly reduced loss of visual acuity compared with no treatment at 12 months (RR 0.84; NNT 4 eyes, 95% CI 3 eyes to 9 eyes) and at 24 months (RR 0.78, 95% CI 0.60 to 0.96; NNT 3 eyes, 95% CI 2 eyes to 7 eyes).[31] Photocoagulation reduced the risk of moderate visual loss (defined as a doubling of the visual angle, equivalent to loss of about two Snellen lines) by 50–70%.[30,31] **Different types of laser:** We found no systematic review. Several small RCTs have found no difference between argon, diode, krypton red, and dye lasers in people with diabetic maculopathy.

Harms: Uncontrolled studies reported that loss of contrast sensitivity and visual acuity occurred after direct application of the laser to the centre of the fovea. We found no accurate estimates of the frequency of adverse effects. **Focal treatment to microaneurysms:** The largest RCT found no significant difference in the frequency of immediate visual loss in treated compared with untreated people.[30] One prospective observational study reported a 40% reduction in macular function measured using the pattern electroretinogram in people undergoing focal argon paramacular treatment.[33] Other complications include laser damage to the centre of the fovea and induction of choroidal neovascularisation, but we found no reliable data on frequency. **Grid laser to zones of retinal thickening:** In the relevant RCT, paracentral grid-like scotomas or haze were visible to most people treated with grid photocoagulation, but the data were insufficient to estimate the frequency of this effect.[31]

Comment: The benefits of laser photocoagulation are less notable in people with maculopathy than in those with proliferative retinopathy. RCTs are needed to compare efficacy and harm of focal and grid laser protocols**G**. We found no evidence that theoretical advantages of certain types of laser result in significant improvements in clinical outcomes. The RCT examining grid laser to zones of retinal thickening had some loss to follow up.[31] The 12 month analysis was conducted on 149 people and the 24 month analysis on 79 people.

QUESTION What are the effects of treatments for vitreous haemorrhage?

OPTION VITRECTOMY

One RCT with 4 years' follow up found that vitrectomy reduced visual loss if performed early in people with vitreous haemorrhage, especially in those with severe proliferative retinopathy. Its role in people with both vitreous haemorrhage and diabetic maculopathy remains unclear.

Benefits: We found no systematic review. **In retinopathy:** We found one RCT comparing early vitrectomy versus deferral of vitrectomy for 1 year in 616 eyes with proliferative retinopathy and recent severe vitreous haemorrhage**G** (reducing visual acuity to ≤2/60 [*5/200*]).[34] At 1, 2, and 3 years after treatment, eyes in the early treatment group were significantly more likely to have visual acuity of at least 6/12 (*20/40*) than those in the deferred treatment group (at 2 years: RR with vitrectomy *v* deferred vitrectomy for visual acuity 6/12 or better 0.84; ARR 10%; NNT 10, 95% CI 6 to 29; see comment below). **In maculopathy:** We found no RCTs.

Harms: A retrospective study of 260 eyes treated with vitrectomy reported neovascular glaucoma in 6%, retinal detachment in 8%, and cataract in 27%.[35] Glaucoma was more likely in people with associated preoperative retinal detachment. In one RCT, the use of preoperative intravitreal tissue plasminogen activator failed to reduce the rate of complications in 56 patients undergoing vitrectomy for the complications of proliferative diabetic retinopathy.[36]

Comment: Four year follow up data were available for 370/616 eyes in the RCT.[34] Subgroup analyses found a greater benefit in people with type 1 diabetes than in those with type 2 diabetes, and found greater benefit in people with more severe levels of proliferative retinopathy (visual acuity at least 10/20: 59% with early treatment and 35% with deferred treatment in people with type 1 diabetes *v* 14% with early treatment and 11% with deferred treatment in people with type 2 diabetes; 44% with early treatment and 40% with deferred treatment in eyes with least severe new vessels *v* 35% with early treatment and 10% with deferred treatment in eyes with very severe new vessels).[37]

GLOSSARY

Advanced retinopathy Retinopathy characterised by tractional retinal detachment (see below), vitreous haemorrhage obscuring fundus details, or both.

Background retinopathy *(mild non-proliferative)* Characterised by microaneurysms, small haemorrhages, and exudates *(hard exudates)*.

Clinically significant macular oedema Characterised by one or more of the following: retinal thickening at or within 500 µm of the centre of the fovea; exudates *(hard exudates)* at or within 500 µm of the centre of the fovea when accompanied by retinal thickening; one or more disc area(s) of thickening extending to within one disc diameter of the centre of the fovea. This is a clinical feature of maculopathy common to many eyes with maculopathy and indicates a significant threat to vision.

Diffuse exudative maculopathy Characterised by thickened oedematous retina at the fovea, often with cystic changes.

Focal exudative maculopathy Characterised by exudates *(hard exudates)* within one disc diameter of the centre of the fovea or circinate rings of exudates *(hard exudates)* within the macula.

Focal laser treatment Laser applied directly to microaneurysms.

Grid laser treatment Laser applied in a grid pattern to zones of retinal thickening, zones of capillary non-perfusion, or both.

High risk characteristics (1) New vessels at the disc extending over at least a third of the disc area; and/or (2) new vessels at the disc extending over less than a third of the disc area or new vessels elsewhere extending over at least half of the disc area, both in the presence of vitreous or pre-retinal haemorrhage.

Ischaemic maculopathy Characterised by zones of capillary non-perfusion visible only on fluorescein angiography but often inferred from presence of deep blot haemorrhages within the fovea.

logMAR chart A tool for measuring visual acuity, similar to but more precise than a Snellen chart. The chart is typically read at 4 m and scored from the total number of letters read. A score of 1.0 is equivalent to Snellen acuity 6/60 and indicates that all 5 letters on the top line, but no others, were read. A score of 0.1 is equivalent to Snellen acuity 6/6.

Preproliferative retinopathy Mild, moderate, or severe *(moderate or severe non-proliferative)* depending on number/location of lesions; characterised by cotton wool spots, deep round haemorrhages, venous beading, loops and reduplication, and intraretinal microvascular anomalies.

Proliferative retinopathy Characterised by new vessels at the disc or elsewhere.

Snellen visual acuity The Snellen chart usually includes letters, numbers, or pictures printed in lines of decreasing size, which are read or identified from a fixed distance; distance visual acuity is usually measured from a distance of 6 m *(20 feet)*. The Snellen visual acuity is written as a fraction: 6/18 means that from 6 m away the best line that can be read is a line that could normally be read from a distance of 18 m away.

Tractional retinal detachment Fibrous scar tissue between the vitreous humour and retina pulls the retina away from the underlying retinal pigment epithelium. This type of retinal detachment is most common in the proliferative diabetic retinopathy.

Vitrectomy The vitreous is the normally clear gelatinous material that fills most of the inside of the eye. The vitreous can be affected by bleeding, inflammatory cells, debris, or scar tissue. Vitrectomy involves removal of the abnormal vitreous material.

Vitreous haemorrhage Bleeding into the vitreous of the eye from blood vessels arising from the retina.

REFERENCES

1. Evans J, Rooney C, Ashwood F, et al. Blindness and partial sight in England and Wales: April 1990–March 1991. *Health Trends* 1996;28:5–12.
2. Ebeling P, Koivisto VA. Occurrence and interrelationships of complications in insulin-dependent diabetes in Finland. *Acta Diabetol* 1997;34:33–38.
3. Beetham WP. Visual prognosis of proliferating diabetic retinopathy. *Br J Ophthalmol* 1963;47:611–619.
4. Caird FI, Burditt AF, Draper GJ. Diabetic retinopathy: a further study of prognosis for vision. *Diabetes* 1968;17:121–123.
5. Deckert T, Simonsen SE, Poulsen JE. Prognosis of proliferative retinopathy in juvenile diabetes. *Diabetes* 1967;10:728–733.
6. Klein R, Klein BEK, Moss SE. The Wisconsin epidemiologic study of diabetic retinopathy: an update. *Aust NZ J Ophthalmol* 1990;18:19–22.
7. British Multicentre Study Group. Proliferative diabetic retinopathy: treatment with xenon arc photocoagulation. *BMJ* 1977;i:739–741.
8. Hercules BL, Gayed II, Lucas SB, et al. Peripheral retinal ablation in the treatment of proliferative diabetic retinopathy: a three-year interim report of a randomised, controlled study using the argon laser. *Br J Ophthalmol* 1977;61:555–563.
9. Diabetic Retinopathy Study Research Group. DRS group 8: photocoagulation treatment of proliferative diabetic retinopathy. *Ophthalmology* 1981;88:583–600.
10. Flynn HW Jr, Chew EY, Simons BD, et al. Pars plana vitrectomy in the Early Treatment Diabetic Retinopathy Study. ETDRS report number 17. *Ophthalmology* 1992;99:1351–1357.
11. British Multicentre Study Group. Photocoagulation for diabetic maculopathy: a randomized controlled clinical trial using the xenon arc. *Diabetes 1983*;32:1010–1016.
12. Patz A, Schatz H, Berkow JW, et al. Macular edema — an overlooked complication of diabetic retinopathy. *Trans Am Acad Ophthalmol Otol* 1973;77:34–42.
13. Early Treatment Diabetic Retinopathy Study Research Group. Early photocoagulation for diabetic retinopathy: ETDRS report 9. *Ophthalmology* 1991;98:766–785.
14. Ferris F. Early photocoagulation in patients with either type I or type II diabetes. *Trans Am Ophthalmol Soc* 1996;94:505–537.
15. Bandello F, Brancato R, Lattanzio R, et al. Double-frequency Nd:YAG laser vs argon-green laser in the treatment of proliferative diabetic retinopathy: randomized study with long-term follow-up. *Lasers Surg Med* 1996;19:173–176.
16. Blankenship GW. A clinical comparison of central and peripheral argon laser panretinal photocoagulation for proliferative diabetic retinopathy. *Ophthalmology* 1988;95:170–177.
17. Bandello F, Brancato R, Menchini U, et al. Light panretinal photocoagulation (LPRP) versus classic panretinal photocoagulation (CPRP) in proliferative diabetic retinopathy. *Semin Ophthalmol* 2001;16:12–18.
18. Pearson AR, Tanner V, Keightey SJ, et al. What effect does laser photocoagulation have on driving visual fields in diabetics? *Eye* 1998;12:64–68.
19. Theodossiadis GP. Central visual field changes after panretinal photocoagulation in proliferative diabetic retinopathy. *Ophthalmologica* 1990;201:71–78.
20. Mackie SW, Walsh G. Contrast and glare sensitivity in diabetic patients with and without pan-retinal photocoagulation. *Ophthalmic Physiol Opt* 1998;18:173–181.
21. Khosla PK, Rao V, Tewari HK, et al. Contrast sensitivity in diabetic retinopathy after panretinal photocoagulation. *Ophthalmic Surg* 1994;25:516–520.

22. Birch J, Hamilton AM. Xenon arc and argon laser photocoagulation in the treatment of diabetic disc neovascularization. Part 2: effect on colour vision. *Trans Ophthalmol Soc UK* 1981;101:93–99.
23. Doft BH. Single versus multiple treatment sessions of argon laser panretinal photocoagulation for proliferative diabetic retinopathy. *Ophthalmology* 1982;89:772–779.
24. Seiberth V, Schatanek S, Alexandridis E. Panretinal photocoagulation in diabetic retinopathy: argon versus dye laser coagulation. *Graefes Arch Clin Exp Ophthalmol* 1993;231:318–322.
25. Cordeiro MF, Stanford MR, Phillips PM, et al. Relationship of diabetic microvascular complications to outcome in panretinal photocoagulation treatment of proliferative diabetic retinopathy. *Eye* 1997;11:531–536.
26. Buckley S. Field loss after pan retinal photocoagulation with diode and argon lasers. *Doc Ophthalmol* 1992;82:317–322.
27. Duffy SW, Rohan TE, Altman DG. A method for combining matched and unmatched binary data: application to randomized, controlled trials of photocoagulation in the treatment of diabetic retinopathy. *Am J Epidemiol* 1989;130:371–378.
28. Blankenship GW. Diabetic macular edema and argon laser photocoagulation: a prospective randomized study. *Ophthalmology* 1979;86:69–75.
29. The Krypton Argon Regression Neovascularization Study Research Group. Randomized comparison of krypton versus argon scatter photocoagulation for diabetic disc neovascularization: the krypton argon regression neovascularization study report number 1. *Ophthalmology* 1993;100:1655–1664.
30. Early Treatment Diabetic Retinopathy Study Research Group. Photocoagulation for diabetic macular edema. *Arch Ophthalmol* 1985;103:1796–1806.
31. Olk RJ. Modified grid argon (blue–green) laser photocoagulation for diffuse diabetic macular edema. *Ophthalmology* 1986;93:938–950.
32. Anonymous. Focal photocoagulation treatment of diabetic macular edema: relationship of treatment effect to fluorescein angiographic and other retinal characteristics at baseline: ETDRS report 19. *Arch Ophthalmol* 1995;113:1144–1155.
33. Ciavarella P, Moretti G, Falsini B, et al. The pattern electroretinogram (PERG) after laser treatment of the peripheral or central retina. *Curr Eye Res* 1997;16:111–115.
34. Diabetic Retinopathy Vitrectomy Study Group. Early vitrectomy for severe vitreous hemorrhage in diabetic retinopathy. Four-year results of a randomized trial: diabetic retinopathy vitrectomy study report 5. *Arch Ophthalmol* 1990;108:958–964.
35. Sima P, Zoran T. Long-term results of vitreous surgery for proliferative diabetic retinopathy. *Doc Ophthalmol* 1994;87:223–232.
36. Le Mer Y, Korobelnik, JF, Morel C, et al. TPA-assisted vitrectomy for proliferative diabetic retinopathy: results of a double-masked, multicenter trial. *Retina* 1999;19:378–382.
37. The Diabetic Retinopathy Vitrectomy Study Research Group. Early vitrectomy for severe proliferative diabetic retinopathy in eyes with useful vision. Results of a randomized trial. Diabetic Retinopathy Vitrectomy Study Report 3. *Ophthalmology* 1988;95:1307–1320.

Simon Harding
Consultant Ophthalmologist
St Paul's Eye Unit, Royal Liverpool
University Hospital
Liverpool
UK

Competing interests: None declared.

TABLE 1 Equivalent UK and US terminology, where different.

UK terminology	US terminology
Background retinopathy	*Mild non-proliferative retinopathy*
Preproliferative retinopathy	*Moderate non-proliferative retinopathy*
Severe preproliferative retinopathy	*Severe non-proliferative retinopathy*
Exudate	*Hard exudate*
Snellen visual acuity measured in metres (e.g. 6/24)	*Snellen visual acuity measured in feet (e.g. 20/80)*

TABLE 2 **RCTs of peripheral photocoagulation versus no treatment in people with diabetic retinopathy (see text, p 789).**

Ref	Number of people (eyes)	Degree of retinopathy*: Preproliferative (*non-proliferative*)	Proliferative	Diabetic maculopathy	Comparison	Outcome (at time)	Result* (analyses by number of eyes) (95% CI)
7	100 (200)	No	All (bilateral)		Peripheral xenon arc *v* no treatment	Blindness by last assessment (mean around 2 years)	5/100 *v* 17/100 RR 0.29 (0.11 to 0.77) NNT 9 (5 to 31)
8	94 (188)	No	All (bilateral)		Peripheral argon laser *v* no treatment	Blindness (3 years)	7/94 (7%) *v* 36/94 (38%) RR 0.19 (0.09 to 0.41) NNT 3 (3 to 6)
9	1742 (3484)	Yes if bilateral	Yes	Yes	Peripheral + focal photocoagulation *v* no treatment	Severe visual loss (5 years)	90/650 (14%) *v* 171/519 (33%) RR 0.42 (0.34 to 0.53) NNT 6 (5 to 7)
13	3711 (7422)	Yes	Yes	Yes	Various early photocoagulation regimens *v* deferred photocoagulation	Severe visual loss (5 years)	2.6% *v* 3.7%† HR 0.77 (0.56 to 1.06)
10	As above	As above	As above	As above	As above	Vitrectomy rate‡ (5 years)	2.3% *v* 4.0%†

TABLE 2 continued

Ref	Number of people (eyes)	Degree of retinopathy*: Preproliferative (*non-proliferative*)	Degree of retinopathy*: Proliferative	Degree of retinopathy*: Diabetic maculopathy	Comparison	Outcome (at time)	Result* (analyses by number of eyes) (95% CI)
11	99 (198)	Yes	No	All	Peripheral xenon arc *v* no treatment	Visual deterioration (5 years)	19/60 (32%) *v* 39/60 (55%) RR 0.49 (0.32 to 0.74) NNT 3 (2 to 7)
12	63 (126)	Yes if bilateral	No	Yes	Peripheral laser *v* no treatment	Visual deterioration (26 months)	4/63 (6%) *v* 40/63 (63%) RR 0.10 (0.04 to 0.26) NNT 2 (2 to 3)

In these columns, a blank means that the RCT did not explicitly state whether included people had that characteristic. 'All': only people with that characteristic were included; 'Yes': some people with that characteristic were included; 'No': all people with that characteristic were explicitly excluded.
*Where necessary, relative risks were calculated by *Clinical Evidence* using absolute risks reported in each RCT.
†RCT reported percentages and did not provide absolute numbers. Hazard ratio taken from the published report based on Cox proportional hazards model.
‡The indication for vitrectomy changed halfway through the RCT. Initially vitrectomy was performed only after onset of severe visual loss. Later, it was performed 1–6 months after severe vitreous haemorrhage.

Glaucoma

Search date July 2004

Rajiv Shah and Richard Wormald

QUESTIONS

INTERVENTIONS

To be covered in future updates

Early detection of glaucoma (opportunistic case finding, population screening)

*No placebo controlled RCTs but strong consensus that treatments are effective

See glossary G

Key Messages

Primary open angle glaucoma

- **Laser trabeculoplasty plus medical treatment (compared with no initial treatment or medical treatment alone)** One RCT in people with newly diagnosed primary open angle or pseudoexfoliation glaucoma found that initial treatment with laser trabeculoplasty plus topical medical treatment to lower intraocular pressure reduced progression of glaucoma compared with no initial treatment at 6 years. One RCT found that, compared with medical treatment alone, combined treatment with initial laser trabeculoplasty followed by medical treatment reduced intraocular pressure and deterioration in optic disc appearance, and improved visual fields after a mean of 7 years.
- **Topical medical treatment (some RCTs included people with primary open angle glaucoma or ocular hypertension alone)** One systematic review and one subsequent RCT in people with primary open angle glaucoma or ocular hypertension alone provided limited evidence that medical treatments reduced intraocular pressure compared with placebo or close observation at between 3 months and 5 years' follow up. However, they found no significant difference between medical treatment and placebo in visual field loss at 1–3 years' follow up. However, one large subsequent RCT found that in people with ocular hypertension, but no evidence of

glaucomatous damage, topical medical treatment reduced the risk of developing primary open angle glaucoma after 5 years compared with close observation. One RCT found that, compared with medical treatment alone, initial laser trabeculoplasty followed by medical treatment reduced intraocular pressure and deterioration in optic disc appearance, and improved visual fields after a mean of 7 years. Two RCTs found that surgical trabeculectomy reduced both visual field loss and intraocular pressures compared with medical treatment, but found no significant difference between treatments in visual acuity after about 5 years. One RCT in people with primary open angle glaucoma, pigmentary glaucoma, or pseudoexfoliative glaucoma found no significant difference between initial medical treatment and initial surgical trabeculectomy in visual field loss at 5 years. It found that loss of visual acuity was greater with initial surgical trabeculectomy, but the significance of this finding was not reported.

- **Surgical trabeculectomy** Two RCTs found that surgical trabeculectomy reduced visual field loss and intraocular pressure compared with medical treatment, but found no significant difference between treatments in visual acuity after about 5 years. One RCT in people with primary open angle glaucoma, pigmentary glaucoma, or pseudoexfoliation glaucoma found no significant difference between initial medication and initial surgical trabeculectomy in visual field loss at 5 years. It found that loss of visual acuity was greater with surgical trabeculectomy, but the significance of this difference was not reported. Two RCTs found that surgical trabeculectomy reduced intraocular pressure compared with laser trabeculoplasty, but found mixed effects for changes in visual acuity and visual field loss after 5–7 years. Surgical trabeculectomy has been reported to be associated with a reduction in central vision.
- **Laser trabeculoplasty (compared with surgical trabeculectomy)** Two RCTs found that surgical trabeculectomy reduced intraocular pressure compared with laser trabeculoplasty, but found mixed effects for changes in visual acuity after 5–7 years.

Lowering intraocular pressure

- **Medical treatment** One RCT found that both surgical and medical treatment, either singly or combined, reduced progression of visual field loss after 8 years compared with no treatment.
- **Surgical treatment** One RCT found that both surgical and medical treatment, either singly or combined, reduced progression of visual field loss after 8 years compared with no treatment, but found that surgery increased cataract formation after 8 years.

Acute angle closure glaucoma

- **Medical treatment*** We found no placebo controlled RCTs, but consensus suggests that medical treatments are effective for acute angle closure glaucoma. One small RCT found no significant difference in intraocular pressure after 2 hours with low dose pilocarpine versus an intensive pilocarpine regimen versus pilocarpine ocular inserts. We found no RCTs of other medical treatments.
- **Surgical treatment*** We found no placebo controlled RCTs, but consensus suggests that surgical treatments are effective for acute angle closure glaucoma. One small RCT found no significant difference between surgical iridectomy and laser iridotomy in visual acuity or intraocular pressure after 3 years.

*No placebo controlled RCTs but strong consensus that treatments are effective

DEFINITION Glaucoma is a group of diseases characterised by progressive optic neuropathy. It is usually bilateral but asymmetric and may occur at any intraocular pressure. All forms of glaucoma show optic nerve damage (cupping and/or pallor) associated with peripheral visual field loss. **Primary open angle glaucoma** occurs in people with an open anterior chamber drainage angle**G** and no secondary identifiable cause. Knowledge of the natural history of these conditions is incomplete, but it is thought that the problem starts with an intraocular pressure that is too high for the optic nerve. However, in a significant proportion of people with glaucoma (about 40%) intraocular pressure is within the statistically defined normal range. The term ocular hypertension generally applies to eyes with an intraocular pressure greater than the statistical upper limit of normal (about 21 mm Hg). However, only a relatively small proportion of eyes with raised intraocular pressure have an optic nerve that is vulnerable to its effects (about 10%). However, because intraocular pressure is the main and only modifiable risk factor for the disease, studies on the effectiveness of reducing intraocular pressure often include people who have both ocular hypertension and primary open angle glaucoma. Previously, trialists were anxious about withholding active treatment in overt primary open angle glaucoma, and so many placebo or no treatment trials selected people just with ocular hypertension. Trials comparing treatments often include both people with primary open angle glaucoma and people with ocular hypertension, but in these the outcome is usually intraocular pressure alone. **Normal tension glaucoma** occurs in people with intraocular pressures that are consistently below the statistical upper limit of normal (21 mm Hg; 2 standard deviations above the population mean). **Acute angle closure glaucoma** is glaucoma resulting from a rapid and severe rise in intraocular pressure caused by physical obstruction of the anterior chamber drainage angle.

INCIDENCE/ PREVALENCE Glaucoma occurs in 1–2% of white people aged over 40 years, rising to 5% at 70 years. Primary open angle glaucoma accounts for two thirds of those affected, and normal tension glaucoma for about a quarter.[1,2] In black people glaucoma is more prevalent, presents at a younger age with higher intraocular pressures, is more difficult to control, and is the main irreversible cause of blindness in black populations of African origin.[1,3] Glaucoma related blindness is responsible for 8% of new blind registrations in the UK.[4]

AETIOLOGY/ RISK FACTORS The major risk factor for developing primary open angle glaucoma is raised intraocular pressure. Lesser risk factors include family history and ethnic origin. The relationship between systemic blood pressure and intraocular pressure may be an important determinant of blood flow to the optic nerve head and, as a consequence, may represent a risk factor for glaucoma.[5] Systemic hypotension, vasospasm (including Raynaud's disease and migraine), and a history of major blood loss have been reported as risk factors for normal tension glaucoma in hospital based studies.[6] Risk factors for acute angle closure glaucoma include family history, female sex, being long sighted, and cataract. A recent systematic review did not find any evidence supporting the theory that routine pupillary dilatation with short acting mydriatics was a risk factor for acute angle closure glaucoma.[7]

PROGNOSIS Advanced visual field loss is found in about 20% of people with primary open angle glaucoma at diagnosis,[8] and is an important prognostic factor for glaucoma related blindness.[9] Blindness due to glaucoma results from gross loss of visual field or loss of central vision. Once early field defects have appeared, and where the intraocular pressure is greater than 30 mm Hg, untreated people may lose the remainder of the visual field in 3 years or less.[10] As the disease progresses, people with glaucoma have difficulty moving from a bright room to a darker room, and judging steps and kerbs. Progression of visual field loss is often slower in normal tension glaucoma. Acute angle glaucoma leads to rapid loss of vision, initially from corneal oedema and subsequently from ischaemic optic neuropathy.

AIMS OF INTERVENTION To prevent progression of visual field loss and to minimise adverse effects of treatment.

OUTCOMES Visual acuity; visual fields; onset of glaucoma. Optic disc cupping and intraocular pressure are surrogate outcomes.

METHODS *Clinical Evidence* search and appraisal July 2004.

QUESTION **What are the effects of treatments for established primary open angle glaucoma?**

OPTION **LASER TRABECULOPLASTY**

One RCT in people with newly diagnosed primary open angle or pseudoexfoliation glaucoma found that initial treatment with laser trabeculoplasty plus topical medical treatment to lower intraocular pressure reduced progression of glaucoma compared with no initial treatment at 6 years. One RCT found that, compared with medical treatment alone, combined

treatment with initial laser trabeculoplasty followed by medical treatment reduced intraocular pressure and deterioration in optic disc appearance, and improved visual fields after a mean of 7 years. Two RCTs found that surgical trabeculectomy reduced intraocular pressure compared with laser trabeculoplasty, but found mixed effects for changes in visual acuity after 5–7 years.

Benefits: **Versus no treatment:** We found one RCT (255 people, age 50–80 years, newly detected primary open angle glaucoma or pseudoexfoliation glaucoma, previously untreated), which compared laser trabeculoplasty**G** plus topical betaxolol hydrochloride versus no initial treatment.[11] The progression of glaucoma was defined by objective visual field changes and/or optic disc changes in one or both eyes of the person. Disc changes were assessed by two masked graders using flicker chronoscopy. Visual field changes were determined by using pattern deviation glaucoma change probability maps. On average, treatment reduced intraocular pressure by 25% from baseline, whereas intraocular pressure was unchanged from baseline in the control group. The RCT found that laser trabeculoplasty plus topical betaxolol hydrochloride significantly reduced the proportion of people with progression of glaucoma after 6 years compared with control (definite visual field and optic disc progression: 58/129 [45%] with treatment *v* 78/126 [62%] with control; P = 0.007). It found that the average time to progression was longer with laser trabeculoplasty plus topical betaxolol hydrochloride than with control (median time to progression: 66 months with treatment *v* 48 months with control; P value not reported).[11] **Versus medical treatment:** We found one RCT (203 people), which compared medical treatment alone versus combined treatment (initial laser trabeculoplasty followed by medical treatment).[12] It found that combined treatment significantly reduced intraocular pressure, improved visual fields, and reduced deterioration in optic disc appearance compared with medical treatment alone after a mean of 7 years (intraocular pressure: 1.2 mm Hg greater reduction with combined treatment, P = 0.001; visual fields: 0.6 dB greater improvement with combined treatment, P < 0.001; deterioration in optic disc appearance: P = 0.005).[12] **Versus surgical trabeculectomy:** See benefits of surgical trabeculectomy, p 802.

Harms: Adverse effects of laser trabeculoplasty**G** are mild and include a transient rise in intraocular pressure (> 5 mm Hg in 91/271 [34%] people) and formation of peripheral anterior synechiae**G** (in 93/271 [34%] people).[12] In the RCT comparing treatment with laser trabeculoplasty plus topical betaxolol hydrochloride versus no initial treatment, there was a significantly more rapid development of lens opacities in the treatment group (results presented graphically; P = 0.002).[11]

Comment: The first RCT was a multicentre trial with multiple observers, although it is not clear whether these observers were masked to the intervention.[12]

OPTION TOPICAL MEDICAL TREATMENT

One systematic review and one subsequent RCT in people with primary open angle glaucoma or ocular hypertension alone provided limited evidence that medical treatments reduced intraocular pressure compared with placebo or close observation at between 3 months and 5 years' follow up. However, they found no significant difference between medical treatment and placebo in visual field loss at 1–3 years' follow up. However, one large subsequent RCT found that in people with ocular hypertension, but no evidence of glaucomatous damage, topical medical treatment reduced the risk of developing primary open angle glaucoma after 5 years compared with close observation. One RCT found that, compared with medical treatment alone,

initial laser trabeculoplasty followed by medical treatment reduced intraocular pressure and deterioration in optic disc appearance, and improved visual fields after a mean of 7 years. Two RCTs found that surgical trabeculectomy reduced both visual field loss and intraocular pressures compared with medical treatment, but found no significant difference between treatments in visual acuity after about 5 years. One RCT in people with primary open angle glaucoma, pigmentary glaucoma, or pseudoexfoliative glaucoma found no significant difference between initial medical treatment and initial surgical trabeculectomy in visual field loss at 5 years. It found that loss of visual acuity was greater with initial surgical trabeculectomy, but the significance of this finding was not reported.

Benefits: **Versus placebo or no treatment:** We found one systematic review (search date 1991, 16 RCTs; see comment below)[13] and two subsequent RCTs.[14,15] The systematic review included RCTs of people with primary open angle glaucoma, primary open angle glaucoma or ocular hypertension, and ocular hypertension alone.[13] It found that medical treatment significantly reduced mean intraocular pressure after a minimum follow up of 3 months or longer compared with placebo (6 RCTs, 452 people; mean reduction in intraocular pressure 4.9 mm Hg, 95% CI 2.5 mm Hg to 7.3 mm Hg). The review found no significant difference between medical treatment and placebo in visual field loss after follow up of 1 year or longer (3 RCTs, 306 people; pooled OR for any worsening of visual field loss 0.75, 95% CI 0.42 to 1.35). The first subsequent large RCT (1636 people, age 40–80 years, mean intraocular pressure 24–32 mm Hg in one eye and 21–32 mm Hg in the other eye, and no evidence of glaucomatous damage) compared topical treatment (any commercially available topical ocular hypotensive medication) versus close observation.[14] The development of primary open angle glaucoma was defined as a reproducible visual field abnormality or optic disc deterioration in one or both eyes. Disc and visual field changes were determined by masked certified readers and then by a masked end point committee. The average reduction in intraocular pressure was 22.5 ± 9.9% with topical treatment compared with 4 ± 11.6% with control (significance not reported). The RCT found that topical treatment significantly reduced the incidence of primary open angle glaucoma over 5 years compared with control (4.4% with treatment *v* 9.5% with control; HR 0.40, 95% CI 0.27 to 0.59; see comment below). The second subsequent RCT (356 people with intraocular pressure between 22 mm Hg and 35 mm Hg and no evidence of visual field damage) compared betaxolol versus placebo.[15] Conversion to glaucoma was based on visual field change only. The RCT found that betaxolol significantly reduced intraocular pressure compared with placebo, but found no significant difference in the incidence of glaucoma between groups after 3 years (intraocular pressure 21.6 mm Hg with betaxolol *v* 23.7 mm Hg with placebo, $P < 0.0001$; AR for developing glaucoma 5/135 [3.7%] with betaxolol *v* 6/132 [4.5%] with placebo, $P = 0.8$). There was a relatively high withdrawal rate (101/356 [28%]) from the study, which prevented analysis after 5 years. **Versus laser trabeculoplasty:** See benefits of laser trabeculoplasty, p 800. **Versus surgical trabeculoplasty:** See benefits of surgical trabeculoplasty, p 802.

Harms: Systemic adverse effects of topical treatments are uncommon but may be serious, including exacerbation of chronic obstructive airways disease after use of non-selective topical β blockers. Non-selective topical β blockers can also cause systemic hypotension and reduction in resting heart rate.[16] The first subsequent RCT in people with ocular hypertension found that a significantly higher percentage of people in the treatment group reported ocular symptoms (57% with treatment *v* 47% with control; $P < 0.001$) or symptoms affecting the skin, hair, or nails

(23% with treatment v 18% with control; P < 0.001).[14] The most common symptoms affecting the eyes were dryness, tearing, and itching. The second subsequent RCT reported similar rates of withdrawal because of intolerance to treatment in both groups (8/182 [4.4%] with betaxolol v 7/174 [4.0%] with placebo; significance not reported).[15]

Comment: The systematic review did not report separately the inclusion/exclusion criteria or the topical medical treatments or regimens used in the placebo controlled RCTs included.[13] It reported that in general, over all included studies (102 RCTs), treatment schedules and selection and eligibility criteria varied widely. The first subsequent RCT in people with ocular hypertension noted that the results did not imply that all people with borderline or elevated intraocular pressure should receive medication; rather, decisions should be based on individual circumstances and individual risk factors for developing primary open angle glaucoma.[14] The European Glaucoma Prevention Study is due to present its findings soon.

OPTION SURGICAL TRABECULECTOMY

Two RCTs found that surgical trabeculectomy reduced visual field loss and intraocular pressure compared with medical treatment, but found no significant difference between treatments in visual acuity after about 5 years. One RCT in people with primary open angle glaucoma, pigmentary glaucoma, or pseudoexfoliation glaucoma found no significant difference between initial medication and initial surgical trabeculectomy in visual field loss at 5 years. It found that loss of visual acuity was greater with surgical trabeculectomy, but the significance of this difference was not reported. Two RCTs found that surgical trabeculectomy reduced intraocular pressure compared with laser trabeculoplasty, but found mixed effects for changes in visual acuity and visual field loss after 5–7 years. Surgical trabeculectomy has been reported to be associated with a reduction in central vision.

Benefits: We found no systematic review. **Versus medical treatment:** We found three RCTs.[17–19] The first RCT (116 people) compared surgical trabeculectomy**G** (followed by medical treatment when indicated) versus medical treatment (followed by trabeculectomy when medical treatment did not work).[18] It found no significant difference between treatments in visual acuity (P = 0.44; other results presented graphically; CI not reported), but found that trabeculectomy significantly reduced visual field loss compared with medical treatment (P = 0.03; other results presented graphically; CI not reported) after a mean of 4.6 years. The second RCT (186 people) compared three treatments: medical treatment (pilocarpine ± timolol ± a sympathomimetic), laser trabeculoplasty**G**, and surgical trabeculectomy.[17] It found that surgical trabeculectomy significantly reduced intraocular pressures compared with medical treatment or laser trabeculoplasty (P = 0.0001; other results presented graphically; CI not reported), but found no significant difference between treatments in visual acuity after 5 years (results presented graphically; P reported as not significant). The third RCT was a large multicentre trial (607 people newly diagnosed with primary open angle glaucoma, pigmentary glaucoma, or pseudoexfoliation glaucoma), which compared medical treatment versus surgical trabeculectomy (with or without 5 fluorouracil) as initial treatments (see comment below).[19] It found no significant difference between groups in visual field loss after 5 years (measured using visual field scores, score range 0 = normal to 20 = end stage glaucoma; visual field scores adjusted for cataract extraction: 0.28 units worse with initial surgical treatment; P = 0.07). Progression of visual field loss was similar with both treatments after 5 years (AR for worsening of visual field score by 3 units: 11% with medical treatment v 14% with surgical treatment; significance not reported). Loss of visual acuity was greater in the surgical group at

5 years, but the significance of this difference was not reported (AR for 15 letter or greater loss of visual acuity at 5 years: 3.9% with medical treatment *v* 7.2% with surgical treatment; significance not reported). Both treatments reduced intraocular pressure, but the reduction was significantly greater in the surgical group (results presented graphically; P reported as significant). **Versus laser trabeculoplasty:** We found two RCTs.[17,20] The first RCT (789 eyes with advanced glaucoma; 451 black people, 325 white people) compared surgical trabeculectomy versus laser trabeculoplasty as initial treatments.[20] Initial surgical trabeculectomy was followed by laser trabeculoplasty and repeat surgical trabeculectomy as required; initial laser trabeculoplasty was followed by surgical trabeculectomy as required. Race–treatment interactions were found to be significant for the primary outcome measures, and therefore results were analysed by race. Subgroup analysis found that in black people initial laser trabeculoplasty significantly improved vision compared with surgical trabeculectomy (both visual acuity and visual field; $P < 0.01$; other results presented graphically; CI not reported), although in white people the RCT found no significant difference between treatments in vision after 7 years (results presented graphically). The RCT also found that in both black people and white people surgical trabeculectomy reduced intraocular pressure compared with laser trabeculoplasty (significance not reported; results presented graphically). The second RCT compared three treatments: medical treatment, laser trabeculoplasty, and surgical trabeculectomy and is described above.[17]

Harms: Surgical trabeculectomy**Ⓖ** is associated with a reduction in central vision. In one observational study, 83% of people lost two lines of Snellen visual acuity.[21] One RCT in people with normal tension glaucoma has found that treatment, including trabeculectomy, compared with no treatment, significantly increased cataract formation after 8 years (see harms of lowering intraocular pressure in normal tension glaucoma, p 804).[22,23]

Comment: **Versus medical treatment:** In the third RCT, participants who did not achieve their target intraocular pressure went on to receive laser trabeculoplasty.[19] The RCT reported that about 8% of participants in both groups failed to achieve their intraocular pressure target. **Versus initial laser trabeculoplasty:** Ten year follow up of the first RCT[20] has been published, but it is not reported here because of a high loss to follow up.[24]

QUESTION What are the effects of lowering intraocular pressure in people with normal tension glaucoma?

OPTION MEDICAL AND SURGICAL TREATMENTS

One RCT found that both surgical and medical treatment, either singly or combined, reduced progression of visual field loss after 8 years compared with no treatment, but found that surgery increased cataract formation after 8 years.

Benefits: We found no systematic review. We found one RCT (140 eyes in 140 people), which compared treatment to reduce intraocular pressure by 30% (with drugs or trabeculectomy**Ⓖ**, or both; 61 eyes) versus no treatment (79 eyes).[22] Progression of visual field loss was defined by deepening of an existing scotoma**Ⓖ**, a new or expanded field defect coming close to central vision, or a fresh scotoma in a previously normal part of the visual field. Optic disc changes were photographed and independently assessed by two ophthalmologists. The RCT found that treatment significantly reduced progression of visual field loss after 8 years compared with no treatment (7/61 [12%] eyes with treatment *v* 28/79 [35%] eyes with no treatment; RR 0.32, 95% CI 0.15 to 0.70; NNT 5, 95% CI 3 to 9).[22]

Harms: The RCT found that treatment (drugs ± trabeculectomy**G**) significantly increased cataract formation after 8 years compared with no treatment (23/61 [38%] with treatment *v* 11/79 [14%] with no treatment; RR 2.7, 95% CI 1.4 to 5.1; NNH 4, 95% CI 2 to 10).[22] Subgroup analysis found that the excess risk of cataract formation was confined to those people treated surgically (P = 0.0001). See harms of surgical trabeculectomy, p 803.

Comment: A companion paper[23] to the RCT[22] suggests that the favourable effect of intraocular pressure lowering treatment versus no treatment is evident only when the cataract inducing effect of trabeculectomy**G** is removed. Not all cases of normal pressure glaucoma progress when untreated (40% have not progressed at 5 years).[23]

QUESTION **What are the effects of treatment for acute angle closure glaucoma?**

OPTION **MEDICAL TREATMENT**

We found no placebo controlled RCTs, but consensus suggests that medical treatments are effective for acute angle closure glaucoma. One small RCT found no significant difference in intraocular pressure after 2 hours with low dose pilocarpine versus an intensive pilocarpine regimen versus pilocarpine ocular inserts. We found no RCTs of other medical treatments.

Benefits: **Pilocarpine versus placebo:** We found one systematic review (search date 2002), which identified no placebo controlled RCTs (see comment below).[25] **Low dose versus high dose pilocarpine drops versus pilocarpine ocular inserts:** We found one systematic review (search date 2002).[25] It identified one RCT (77 eyes) that compared three groups: initial treatment with low dose pilocarpine (2% pilocarpine drops applied to the eye twice in 1 hour); intensive pilocarpine (4% pilocarpine drops applied to the eye every 5 minutes for 1 hour or longer); and pilocarpine ocular inserts (releasing 40 μg pilocarpine/hour).[26] All of the people in the RCT also received treatment with acetazolamide (500 mg iv). The RCT reported no significant difference between groups in intraocular pressures after 2 hours (further data and P value not reported). **Other medical treatments:** We found no RCTs.

Harms: **Low dose versus high dose pilocarpine drops versus pilocarpine ocular inserts:** The RCT identified by the review reported that ocular inserts were associated with local discomfort (statistical data not reported).[26]

Comment: RCTs of pilocarpine versus placebo would be considered unethical. There is consensus that medical treatment with pressure lowering drugs (especially those that can be given parenterally, such as iv acetazolamide) are effective in acute angle closure glaucoma. We found no evidence from RCTs to support or challenge this view.

OPTION **SURGICAL TREATMENT**

We found no placebo controlled RCTs, but consensus suggests that surgical treatments are effective for acute angle closure glaucoma. One small RCT found no significant difference between surgical iridectomy and laser iridotomy in visual acuity or intraocular pressure after 3 years.

Benefits: **Surgical or laser procedure versus placebo:** We found one systematic review (search date 2002), which identified no placebo controlled RCTs (see comment below).[25] **Surgical peripheral iridectomy versus Nd:YAG laser iridotomy:** We found one systematic review (search date

2002, 1 RCT that met *Clinical Evidence* inclusion criteria).[25] The RCT identified by the review (48 people with uniocular acute angle closure glaucoma) compared peripheral iridectomy versus Nd:YAG laser iridotomy**G**.[6] It found no significant difference in visual acuity (0.30 logMAR units with peripheral iridectomy *v* 0.57 logMAR units with laser iridotomy; statistical data not reported) and no significant difference in intraocular pressure (intraocular pressure < 21 mm Hg: 15/21 [70%] with peripheral iridectomy *v* 19/27 [72%] with laser iridotomy; RR 1.02, 95% CI 0.71 to 1.46) after 3 years.

Harms: The systematic review did not report on harms.[25] Surgical iridectomy**G** involves an open operation on the eye, with risk of serious complications, including intraocular infection or haemorrhage. We found no published evidence quantifying these risks. Nd:YAG laser iridotomy**G** is associated with haemorrhage from the iris, pressure spikes, and corneal oedema.[27] Nd:YAG and argon laser iridotomy can produce focal, non-progressive lens opacity.[28] In one non-randomised controlled trial, iris haemorrhage was more common with the Nd:YAG laser but pupil distortion, iritis, and late blockage were more common with the argon laser.[29]

Comment: We found no placebo controlled RCTs of surgical treatment of acute angle closure glaucoma, but consensus suggests that surgical treatments are effective. Management of acute angle closure glaucoma is aimed at restoring flow of aqueous humour to the anterior chamber angle and adjacent trabecular meshwork. One non-randomised controlled trial found that the mean number of laser burns required to penetrate the iris was six with the Nd:YAG laser and 73 with the argon laser.[29]

GLOSSARY

Drainage angle Area in the anterior chamber of the eye where the iris meets the sclera, and where fluid from the aqueous humour drains via the trabecular meshwork.

Laser iridotomy Involves making a hole in the base of the iris (without opening the eye) using either an argon or Nd:YAG laser.

Laser trabeculoplasty Laser trabeculoplasty is performed with a laser, using a contact lens with an internal mirror, which allows focal burning of the pigmented trabecular meshwork.

Scotoma Visual field defect consisting of an area of partial or complete loss of vision, surrounded by an area of normal vision.

Surgical iridectomy Opening the eye at the corneal limbus and removing a triangle of tissue from the base of the iris.

Synechiae Adhesions between the iris and surrounding structures, which can form following inflammation. Synechiae may form between the iris and the lens or between the iris and the inner surface of the cornea.

Trabeculectomy A microsurgical procedure in which a partial thickness trapdoor in the sclera is elevated at its junction with the cornea under the conjunctiva. Under the trapdoor, a small hole is fashioned from the sclera to the anterior chamber. This allows drainage of aqueous into the subconjunctival space. An iridectomy is performed at the site of the hole in the sclera.

Substantive changes

Topical medical treatment for primary open angle glaucoma One RCT added;[15] categorisation unchanged.

Surgical trabeculectomy for primary open angle glaucoma One RCT added;[19] categorisation unchanged.

Medical treatments for acute angle closure glaucoma One systematic review added;[25] categorisation unchanged.

Surgical iridectomy and laser iridotomy for acute angle closure glaucoma One systematic review added;[25] categorisation unchanged.

REFERENCES

1. Sommer A, Tielsch JM, Katz J, et al. Relationship between intraocular pressure and primary open angle glaucoma among white and black Americans. *Arch Ophthalmol* 1991;109:1090–1095.
2. Coffey M, Reidy A, Wormald R, et al. The prevalence of glaucoma in the west of Ireland. *Br J Ophthalmol* 1993;77:17–21.
3. Leske MC, Connell AM, Wu SY, et al. Incidence of open-angle glaucoma: the Barbados Eye Studies. The Barbados Eye Studies Group. *Arch Ophthalmol* 2001;119:89–95.
4. Government Statistical Service. *Causes of blindness and partial sight amongst adults*. London: HMSO, 1988.
5. Tielsch JM, Katz J, Quigley HA, et al. Diabetes, intraocular pressure, and primary open-angle glaucoma in the Baltimore Eye Survey. *Ophthalmology* 1995;102:48–53.
6. Fleck BW, Wright E, Fairley EA. A randomised prospective comparison of operative peripheral iridectomy and Nd:YAG laser iridotomy treatment of acute angle closure glaucoma: 3 year visual acuity and intraocular pressure control outcome. *Br J Ophthalmol* 1997;81:884–888.
7. Pandit RJ, Taylor R. Mydriasis and glaucoma: exploding the myth. A systematic review. *Diabet Med* 2000;17:693–699.
8. Sheldrick JH, Ng C, Austin DJ, et al. An analysis of referral routes and diagnostic accuracy in cases of suspected glaucoma. *Ophthalmic Epidemiol* 1994;1:31–38.
9. Fraser S, Bunce C, Wormald R, et al. Deprivation and late presentation of glaucoma: case-control study. *BMJ* 2001;322:639–643.
10. Jay JL, Murdoch JR. The rates of visual field loss in untreated primary open angle glaucoma. *Br J Ophthalmol* 1993;77:176–178.
11. Heijl A, Leske MC, Bengtsson B, et al. Reduction of intraocular pressure and glaucoma progression: results from the Early Manifest Glaucoma Trial. *Arch Ophthalmol* 2002;120:1268–1279.
12. Glaucoma Laser Trial Group. The glaucoma laser trial (GLT) and glaucoma laser trial follow-up study: results. *Am J Ophthalmol* 1995;120:718–731.
13. Rossetti L, Marchetti I, Orzalesi N, et al. Randomised clinical trials on medical treatment of glaucoma: are they appropriate to guide clinical practice? *Arch Ophthalmol* 1993;111:96–103. Search date 1991; primary source Medline.
14. Kass MA, Heuer DK, Higginbotham EJ, et al. The Ocular Hypertension Treatment Study: a randomized trial determines that topical ocular hypotensive medication delays or prevents the onset of primary open-angle glaucoma. *Arch Ophthalmol* 2002;120:701–713.
15. Kamal D, Garway-Heath D, Ruben S, et al. Results of the betaxolol versus placebo treatment trial in ocular hypertension. *Graefes Arch Clin Exp Ophthalmol* 2003;241:196–203.
16. Diamond JP. Systemic adverse effects of topical ophthalmic agents: implications for older patients. *Drugs Aging* 1997;11:352–360.
17. Migdal C, Gregory W, Hitchins R, et al. Long-term functional outcome after early surgery compared with laser and medicine in open angle glaucoma. *Ophthalmology* 1994;101:1651–1657.
18. Jay JL, Allan D. The benefit of early trabeculectomy versus conventional management in primary open angle glaucoma relative to severity of disease. *Eye* 1989;3:528–535.
19. Feiner L, Piltz-Seymour JR; Collaborative Initial Glaucoma Treatment Study. Collaborative Initial Glaucoma Treatment Study: a summary of results to date. *Curr Opin Ophthalmol* 2003;14:106–111.
20. The AGIS investigators. The Advanced Glaucoma Intervention Study (AGIS): 4. Comparison of treatment outcomes within race. Seven year results. *Ophthalmology* 1998;105:1146–1164.
21. Costa UP, Smith M, Spaeth GL, et al. Loss of vision after trabeculectomy. *Ophthalmology* 1993;100:599–612.
22. Collaborative Normal-tension Glaucoma Study Group. Comparison of glaucomatous progression between untreated patients with normal-tension glaucoma and patients with therapeutically reduced intraocular pressure. *Am J Ophthalmol* 1998;126:487–497.
23. Collaborative Normal-tension Glaucoma Study Group. The effectiveness of intraocular pressure reduction in the treatment of normal-tension glaucoma. *Am J Ophthalmol* 1998;126:498–505.
24. Ederer F, Gaasterland DA, Dally LG, et al. The Advanced Glaucoma Intervention Study (AGIS): 13. Comparison of treatment outcomes within race: 10-year results. *Ophthalmology* 2004;111:651–664.
25. Saw SM, Gazzard G, Friedman DS. Interventions for angle-closure glaucoma: an evidence-based update. *Ophthalmology* 2003;110:1869–1878; quiz 1878–1879, 1930. Search date 2002; primary sources MEDLINE, PubMed, EMBASE, Cochrane Collaborations, hand search of reference lists of important articles.
26. Edwards RS. A comparative study of Ocusert Pilo 40, intensive pilocarpine and low-dose pilocarpine in the initial treatment of primary acute angle-closure glaucoma. *Curr Med Res Opin* 1997;13:501–509.
27. Fleck BW, Dhillon B, Khanna V, et al. A randomised, prospective comparison of Nd:YAG laser iridotomy and operative peripheral iridectomy in fellow eyes. *Eye* 1991;5:315–321.
28. Pollack IP, Robin AL, Dragon DM, et al. Use of neodymium:YAG laser to create iridotomies in monkeys and humans. *Trans Am Ophthalmol Soc* 1984;82:307–328.
29. Moster MR, Schwartz LW, Spaeth GL, et al. Laser iridectomy. A controlled study comparing argon and neodymium:YAG. *Ophthalmology* 1986;93:20–24.

Rajiv Shah
Ophthalmic Surgeon
Department of Ophthalmology
St Vincent's Hospital, Sydney, Australia

Richard Wormald
Consultant Ophthalmic Surgeon
Moorfields Eye Hospital, London, UK

Competing interests: RS none declared. RW has received honoraria for speaking and attending meetings from various pharmaceutical companies producing treatments for glaucoma including Alcon, Allergan, and Pfizer.

We would like to acknowledge the previous contributors of this chapter including: Jeremy Diamond, Colm O'Brien.

Ocular herpes simplex

Search date August 2003

Nigel H Barker

QUESTIONS

INTERVENTIONS

See glossary G

Key Messages

Treating epithelial keratitis

- **Interferons** One systematic review found that topical interferons (alpha or beta) increase healing after 7 and 14 days compared with placebo. The review found no significant difference between a topical interferon and a topical antiviral agent in healing after 7 days, but found that a topical interferon increased healing after 14 days. The review also found that topical interferon plus a topical antiviral agent increased healing compared with a topical antiviral agent alone after 14 days. "Healing" was not clearly defined.
- **Topical antiviral agents** One systematic review has found that topical antivirals (idoxuridine or vidarabine) increase healing after 14 days compared with placebo, and that trifluridine or aciclovir increase healing compared with idoxuridine after 7 and 14 days. The review has also found that antiviral treatment plus debridement increases healing after 7 days compared with either treatment alone. It found no significant difference in healing at 14 days between antiviral treatment plus debridement and antiviral treatment alone. It also found no significant difference between topical antiviral agents and topical interferon in healing after 7 days, but found that topical interferon increased healing after 14 days. The review also found that adding topical interferon to a topical antiviral agent increased healing compared with the antiviral agent alone. "Healing" was not clearly defined.
- **Debridement** One systematic review has found no significant difference between debridement and no treatment. The review has also found that debridement plus antiviral treatment improves healing at 7 days compared with either treatment alone. This difference remained significant at 14 days for combined treatment compared with debridement alone.

Treating stromal keratitis

- **Topical corticosteroids** One RCT in people receiving topical antiviral treatment found that topical corticosteroids reduced progression and shortened the duration of stromal keratitis compared with placebo.
- **Oral aciclovir** One RCT in people receiving topical corticosteroids plus topical antiviral treatment found no significant difference between oral aciclovir and placebo in rates of treatment failure at 16 weeks.

Preventing recurrence of epithelial or stromal keratitis

- **Long term (1 year) oral aciclovir** One large RCT in people with at least one previous episode of epithelial or stromal keratitis found that long term oral aciclovir reduced recurrence after 1 year compared with placebo.
- **Short term (3 weeks) oral aciclovir** One RCT in people with epithelial keratitis receiving a topical antiviral agent (trifluridine) found no significant difference between short term prophylaxis with oral aciclovir and placebo in the rate of stromal keratitis or iritis at 1 year.

Preventing ocular herpes simplex in people with corneal grafts

- **Oral aciclovir** One small RCT found limited evidence that prophylactic use of oral aciclovir reduced recurrence and improved graft survival compared with placebo.

DEFINITION Ocular herpes simplex is usually caused by herpes simplex virus type 1 (HSV-1) but also occasionally by the type 2 virus (HSV-2). Ocular manifestations of HSV are varied and include blepharitis (inflammation of the eyelids), canalicular obstruction, conjunctivitis, epithelial keratitis, stromal keratitis(G), iritis, and retinitis. HSV infections are classified as neonatal, primary (HSV in a person with no previous viral exposure), and recurrent (previous viral exposure with humoral and cellular immunity present).

INCIDENCE/ PREVALENCE Infections with HSV are usually acquired in early life. A US study found antibodies against HSV-1 in about 50% of people with high socioeconomic status and 80% of people with low socioeconomic status by the age of 30 years.[1] However, only about 20–25% of people with HSV antibodies had any history of clinical manifestations of ocular or cutaneous herpetic disease.[2] Ocular HSV is the most common cause of corneal blindness in high income countries and is the most common cause of unilateral corneal blindness in the world.[3] A 33 year study of the population of Rochester, Minnesota, found the annual incidence of new cases of ocular herpes simplex was 8.4/100 000 (95% CI 6.9 to 9.9) and the annual incidence of all episodes (new and recurrent) was 20.7/100 000 (95% CI 18.3 to 23.1).[4] The prevalence of ocular herpes was 149 cases/100 000 population (95% CI 115 to 183). Twelve per cent of people had bilateral disease.[4]

AETIOLOGY/ RISK FACTORS Epithelial keratitis results from productive, lytic viral infection of the corneal epithelial cells. Stromal keratitis and iritis are thought to result from a combination of viral infection and compromised immune mechanisms. Observational evidence (346 people with ocular HSV in the placebo arm of an RCT) found that the risk of developing stromal keratitis was 4% in people with no previous history of stromal keratitis (RR 1.0) compared with 32% (RR 10, 95% CI 4.32 to 23.38) with previous stromal keratitis, but that a history of epithelial keratitis was not a risk factor for recurrent epithelial keratitis.[5] Age, sex, ethnicity, and previous experience of non-ocular HSV disease were not associated with an increased risk of recurrence.[5]

PROGNOSIS HSV epithelial keratitis tends to resolve spontaneously within 1–2 weeks. In a trial of 271 people treated with topical trifluorothymidine and randomly assigned to receive either oral aciclovir or placebo, the epithelial lesion had resolved completely or was at least less than 1 mm after 1 week of treatment with placebo in 89% of people and after 2 weeks in 99% of people.[6] Stromal keratitis or iritis occurs in about 25% of people following epithelial keratitis.[7] The effects of HSV stromal keratitis include scarring, tissue destruction, neovascularisation, glaucoma, and persistent epithelial defects. Rate of recurrence of ocular herpes for people with one episode is 10% at 1 year, 23% at 2 years, and 50% at 10 years.[8] The risk of recurrent ocular HSV infection (epithelial or stromal) has also been found to increase with the number of previous episodes reported (2 or 3 previous episodes: RR 1.41, 95% CI 0.82 to 2.42; 4 or more previous episodes: RR 2.09, 95% CI 1.24 to 3.50).[5] Of corneal grafts performed in Australia over a 10 year period, 5% were in people with visual disability or with actual or impending corneal perforation following stromal ocular herpes simplex. The recurrence of HSV in a corneal graft has a major effect on graft survival. The Australian Corneal Graft Registry has found that, in corneal grafts performed for HSV keratitis, there was at least one HSV recurrence in 58% of corneal grafts that failed over a follow up period of 9 years.[9]

AIMS OF INTERVENTION To reduce the morbidity of HSV keratitis and iritis; to reduce the risk of recurrent disease; and to improve corneal graft survival after penetrating keratoplasty**G**.

OUTCOMES Healing time; severity and duration of symptoms; severity of complications; rates of recurrence; corneal graft survival.

METHODS *Clinical Evidence* search and appraisal August 2003.

QUESTION What are the effects of treatments in people with epithelial keratitis?

OPTION TOPICAL ANTIVIRAL AGENTS

One systematic review has found that topical antivirals (idoxuridine or vidarabine) increase healing after 14 days compared with placebo, and that trifluridine or aciclovir increase healing compared with idoxuridine after 7 and 14 days. The review has also found that antiviral treatment plus debridement increases healing after 7 days compared with either treatment alone. It found no significant difference in healing at 14 days between antiviral treatment plus debridement and antiviral treatment alone. It also found no significant difference between topical antiviral agents and topical interferon in healing after 7 days, but found that topical interferon increased healing after 14 days. The review also found that adding topical interferon to a topical antiviral agent increased healing compared with the antiviral agent alone. "Healing" was not clearly defined.

Benefits: We found one systematic review (search date 2000, 96 RCTs, 4991 people; see comment below).[10] **Versus placebo:** The review found that idoxuridine significantly increased healing after 7 days compared with placebo (10 RCTs; OR 4.05, 95% CI 2.60 to 6.30; see comment below) and after 14 days (2 RCTs; OR 4.17, 95% CI 1.33 to 13.00).[10] The review also compared vidarabine versus placebo and found no significant difference in healing after 7 days (numerical data not reported), but found that vidarabine significantly increased healing after 14 days (1 RCT; OR 5.40, 95% CI 1.42 to 20.5). **Versus each other:** The review found that compared with idoxuridine, trifluridine significantly increased healing after 7 days (3 RCTs; OR 4.74, 95% CI 2.52 to 8.91) and after 14 days (4 RCTs; OR 6.83, 95% CI 3.02 to 15.5).[10] The review also found that aciclovir significantly increased healing after 7 days compared with idoxuridine (8 RCTs; OR 5.33, 95% CI 3.33 to 8.53) and after 14 days (11 RCTs; OR 3.71, 95% CI 2.27 to 6.08), but found no significant difference between vidarabine and idoxuridine in healing after 7 days (3 RCTs; OR 1.24, 95% CI 0.72 to 2.00) or after 14 days (3 RCTs; OR 1.24, 95% CI 0.65 to 2.37). **Antiviral treatment plus physical debridement:** See benefits of debridement, p 810. **Antiviral treatment versus topical interferons:** See benefits of interferons, p 810. **Antiviral treatment plus topical interferons:** See benefits of interferons, p 810.

Harms: The review did not report harms.[10]

Comment: The outcome measure "healing" was not clearly defined.[10] The review reported that the number of people involved in the comparison of vidarabine versus placebo was small, although it did not provide any absolute numbers.

OPTION **DEBRIDEMENT**

One systematic review has found no significant difference between debridement and no treatment. The review has also found that debridement plus antiviral treatment improves healing at 7 days compared with either treatment alone. This difference remained significant at 14 days for combined treatment compared with debridement alone.

Benefits: We found one systematic review (search date 2000, 96 RCTs, 4991 people).[10] **Debridement alone:** The review compared different types of physicochemical debridement versus no treatment and found no significant difference in healing after 7 days (2 RCTs; OR 1.62, 95% CI 0.72 to 3.61) or after 14 days (1 RCT; OR 2.12, 95% CI 0.38 to 12.0).[10] **Debridement plus antiviral treatment:** The review found that physicochemical debridement plus an antiviral agent significantly increased healing after 7 days compared with physicochemical debridement alone (7 RCTs; OR 2.08, 95% CI 1.17 to 3.71) and after 14 days (2 RCTs; OR 10.81, 95% CI 1.81 to 64.5).[10] The review also found that physicochemical debridement plus an antiviral agent significantly increased healing compared with antiviral treatment alone after 7 days (7 RCTs; OR 2.01, 95% CI 1.21 to 3.34), but found no significant difference in healing after 14 days (significance testing not reported). One RCT identified by the review compared debridement plus aciclovir versus debridement plus idoxuridine and found no significant difference in healing after 7 or 14 days (CI not reported).

Harms: None reported.

Comment: The review found that all methods of debriding the corneal epithelium produced similar rates of re-epithelialisation.[10] The variety of treatments used in the review limits the applicability of the summary results. The review included "healed" as an outcome measure without clearly defining this term.

OPTION **INTERFERONS**

One systematic review has found that topical interferons (alpha or beta) increase healing after both 7 and 14 days compared with placebo. The review found no significant difference between topical interferon and a topical antiviral agent in healing after 7 days, but found that topical interferon increased healing after 14 days. The review also found that topical interferon plus a topical antiviral agent increased healing compared with a topical antiviral agent alone after 14 days. "Healing" was not clearly defined.

Benefits: We found one systematic review (search date 2000, 96 RCTs, 4991 people).[10] **Versus placebo:** The review found that topical interferons (alpha or beta) significantly increased healing after 7 days (3 RCTs; OR 2.09, 95% CI 1.15 to 3.81; see comment below) and after 14 days compared with placebo (2 RCTs; OR 3.43, 95% CI 1.30 to 9.02).[10] **Different concentrations:** One RCT identified by the review found no significant difference between low concentration interferon (< 1 MU/mL) and higher concentrations of interferon in healing after 7 days (1 RCT; OR 0.21, 95% CI 0.02 to 2.42).[10] The RCT may have been too small to exclude a clinically important difference. **Versus topical antivirals:** The review found no significant difference in healing after 7 days between topical interferon and topical antiviral agents (2 RCTs; OR 1.18, 95% CI 0.29 to 4.75), but found that topical interferon significantly increased healing compared with a topical antiviral agent after 14 days (3 RCTs; OR 3.48, 95% CI 1.06 to 11.4).[10] **Topical interferons plus antiviral agents:** The review found that topical interferon plus a topical antiviral agent significantly increased healing compared with a topical antiviral agent alone (usually trifluridine) after 7 days (8 RCTs; OR 13.3, 95% CI 7.41 to 23.9) but found no significant difference in healing after 14 days (5 RCTs; OR 2.62, 95% CI 0.91 to 7.57).[10]

Harms: The review did not report on harms.[10]

Comment: The outcome measure "healing" was not clearly defined.[10]

QUESTION What are the effects of treatments in people with stromal keratitis?

OPTION TOPICAL CORTICOSTEROIDS

One RCT in people receiving topical antiviral treatment found that topical corticosteroids reduced progression and shortened the duration of stromal keratitis compared with placebo.

Benefits: We found one RCT (106 people; see comment below) comparing topical prednisolone sodium phosphate (in decreasing concentrations over 10 weeks) versus placebo.[11] All participants received topical trifluridine. It found that prednisolone significantly reduced the persistence or progression of stromal inflammation and shortened the duration of stromal keratitis**G** compared with placebo (median 26 days with corticosteroid *v* median 72 days with placebo; difference 46 days, 95% CI 14 to 58 days).

Harms: In the RCT, nine people in the steroid group reported adverse effects.[11] Four people developed dendritic epithelial keratitis**G** and were removed from the trial. Four people developed toxic responses to trifluridine after week 5. These people were not withdrawn but the trifluridine was stopped. One person developed an epithelial defect and was withdrawn. Adverse events were reported in six people receiving placebo. All six were withdrawn from the study (1 person developed dendritic keratitis, 3 people developed an epithelial defect, and 2 people developed allergic conjunctivitis attributed to trifluorothymidine within the first 9 days of the trial).

Comment: The trial did not specify whether or not intention to treat analysis was performed.[11]

OPTION ORAL ACICLOVIR

One RCT in people receiving topical corticosteroids plus topical antiviral treatment found no significant difference between oral aciclovir and placebo in rates of treatment failure at 16 weeks.

Benefits: We found one RCT (104 people with herpes simplex virus stromal keratitis**G** receiving concomitant topical corticosteroids and a topical antiviral agent [trifluridine]) of oral aciclovir.[12] The primary outcome was time to treatment failure, defined as worsening or no improvement of stromal keratitis or an adverse event. The RCT found no significant difference between aciclovir in median time to treatment failure compared with placebo (84 days with aciclovir *v* 62 days with placebo; P = 0.46; CI not reported), or in reported rates of treatment failure by week 16 (38/51 [75%] with aciclovir *v* 39/53 [74%] with placebo; RR 1.01, 95% CI 0.78 to 1.24).[12]

Harms: The RCT found that two people in the placebo group developed adverse effects attributed to trifluridine (epithelial keratopathy in 1 person and an allergic reaction in the other).[12] Other adverse effects reported included pneumonia with possible pulmonary embolus (1 person), congestive heart failure (1 person), diarrhoea (1 person), oedema of the lower extremities (1 person), and anaemia (1 person). Adverse reactions reported in the aciclovir group included toxicity to trifluorothymidine (1 person) and headache (1 person).

Comment: None.

QUESTION What are the effects of interventions to prevent recurrence of ocular herpes simplex?

OPTION ORAL ACICLOVIR

One large RCT in people with at least one previous episode of epithelial or stromal keratitis found that long term oral aciclovir reduced recurrence after 1 year compared with placebo. One RCT in people with epithelial keratitis receiving a topical antiviral agent (trifluridine) found no significant difference between short term prophylaxis with oral aciclovir and placebo in the rate of stromal keratitis or iritis at 1 year.

Benefits: We found no systematic review. We found two RCTs.[6,13] **Long term (1 year) oral aciclovir:** The first RCT (703 immunocompetent people aged ≥12 years who had epithelial or stromal ocular herpes simplex virus in one or both eyes within the preceding 12 months) compared oral aciclovir (400 mg twice daily for 1 year) versus placebo.[13] It found that aciclovir treatment significantly reduced the risk of any type of recurrence after 1 year (19% with aciclovir *v* 32% with placebo; RR 0.55, 95% CI 0.41 to 0.75). Prespecified subgroup analysis (337 people with at least 1 previous episode of stromal keratitis) found that aciclovir significantly reduced the risk of stromal keratitis**Ⓖ** compared with placebo, but only in people who had at least one prior episode (14% with aciclovir *v* 28% with placebo; RR 0.48, 95% CI 0.29 to 0.80). The RCT found no rebound in the rate of ocular herpes simplex virus in the 6 months after stopping treatment. **Short term (3 weeks) oral aciclovir:** The second RCT (287 people with epithelial keratitis**Ⓖ** all treated with topical trifluridine) compared a 3 week course of oral aciclovir versus placebo.[6] It found no significant difference in the rate of stromal keratitis or iritis (11% with aciclovir *v* 10% with placebo; RR 1.04, 95% CI 0.52 to 2.10), and no significant difference in the cumulative risk of developing stromal keratitis or iritis at 1 year of follow up (12% with aciclovir *v* 11% with placebo; P = 0.92; CI not reported).

Harms: The RCT of long term treatment found that adverse effects (mostly gastrointestinal problems) were uncommon and occurred with similar frequency in both groups.[13] Thirty two people (15 aciclovir *v* 17 placebo) discontinued treatment because of adverse effects. The most common adverse effect reported was gastrointestinal upset (7 aciclovir *v* 9 placebo).

Comment: None.

QUESTION What are the effects of interventions to prevent recurrence of ocular herpes simplex in people with corneal grafts?

OPTION ORAL ACICLOVIR

One small RCT found limited evidence that prophylactic use of oral aciclovir reduced recurrence and improved graft survival compared with placebo.

Benefits: We found no systematic review. We found one small non-blinded RCT (22 people, 23 eyes, who had received keratoplasty**G**), which compared oral aciclovir (800 or 1000 mg, 4 or 5 times orally daily, tapered during the first 12 months, for a maximum of 15 months) versus placebo.[14] Oral aciclovir was started before surgery or on the first day after surgery. The RCT found that oral aciclovir significantly reduced the number of recurrences of ocular herpes simplex compared with placebo after a mean follow up of 17 months in people receiving aciclovir and 21 months in those receiving placebo (0% with aciclovir *v* 44% with placebo; $P < 0.01$), and also that aciclovir significantly reduced the number of eyes with graft failure compared with usual care (14% with aciclovir treated eyes *v* 56% with placebo; $P < 0.05$; CI not provided).

Harms: None reported.

Comment: None.

GLOSSARY

Epithelial keratitis Inflammation of the cells that form the surface layer of the cornea.
Keratoplasty A procedure in which diseased corneal tissue is removed and replaced by donor corneal material.
Stromal keratitis Inflammation of the middle layer of the cornea. The stroma forms 90% of the corneal substance. It lies between the epithelium and Bowman's membrane anteriorly and Desçemet's membrane and the endothelium posteriorly.

REFERENCES

1. Nahmias AJ, Lee FK, Beckman-Nahmias S. Sero-epidemiological and sociological patterns of herpes simplex virus infection in the world. *Scand J Infect Dis Suppl* 1990;69:19–36.
2. Kaufman HE, Rayfield MA, Gebhardt BM. Herpes simplex viral infections. In: Kaufman HE, Baron BA, McDonald MB, eds. *The Cornea*. 2nd ed. Woburn, MA: Butterworth-Heinemann, 1997.
3. Dawson CR, Togni B. Herpes simplex eye infections: clinical manifestations, pathogenesis, and management. *Surv Ophthalmol* 1976;21:121–135.
4. Liesegang TJ, Melton LJ III, Daly PJ, et al. Epidemiology of ocular herpes simplex. Incidence in Rochester, Minnesota, 1950 through 1982. *Arch Ophthalmol* 1989;107:1155–1159.
5. Herpetic Eye Disease Study Group. Predictors of recurrent herpes simplex virus keratitis. *Cornea* 2001;20:123–128.
6. The Herpetic Eye Disease Study Group. A controlled trial of oral acyclovir for the prevention of stromal keratitis or iritis in patients with herpes simplex virus epithelial keratitis. The Epithelial Keratitis Trial. *Arch Ophthalmol* 1997;115:703–712.
7. Wilhelmus KR, Coster DJ, Donovan HC, et al. Prognosis indicators of herpetic keratitis. Analysis of a five-year observation period after corneal ulceration. *Arch Ophthalmol* 1981;99:1578–1582.
8. Liesegang TJ. Epidemiology of ocular herpes simplex. Natural history in Rochester, Minnesota, 1950 through 1982. *Arch Ophthalmol* 1989;107:1160–1165.
9. Williams KA, Muehlberg SM, Lewis RF, et al. *The Australian Corneal Graft Registry:1996 Report*. Adelaide: Mercury Press, 1997.
10. Wilhelmus KR. Interventions for herpes simplex virus epithelial keratitis. In: The Cochrane Library, Issue 3, 2001. Oxford: Update Software. Search date 2000; primary sources Medline, Central, Embase, Index medicus, Excerpta Medica Ophthalmology, Cochrane Eyes and Vision Group specialised register, The Cochrane Controlled Trials Register, hand searching of reference lists of primary reports, review articles, and corneal textbooks, and conference proceedings pertaining to ocular virology.
11. Wilhelmus KR, Gee L, Hauck WW, et al. Herpetic Eye Disease Study. A controlled trial of topical corticosteroids for herpes simplex stromal keratitis. *Ophthalmology* 1994;101:1883–1895.
12. Barron BA, Gee L, Hauck WW, et al. Herpetic Eye Disease Study. A controlled trial of oral acyclovir for herpes simplex stromal keratitis. *Ophthalmology* 1994;101:1871–1882.
13. Herpetic Eye Disease Study Group. Acyclovir for the prevention of recurrent herpes simplex virus eye disease. *N Engl J Med* 1998;339:300–306.
14. Barney NP, Foster CS. A prospective randomized trial of oral acyclovir after penetrating keratoplasty for herpes simplex keratitis. *Cornea* 1994;13:232–236.

Nigel H Barker
Consultant Ophthalmologist
Warrens Eye Centre
Manor Lodge, St Michael
Barbados

Competing interests: None declared.

HIV infection

Search date July 2003

Martin Talbot

QUESTIONS

INTERVENTIONS

Covered elsewhere in *Clinical Evidence*

Preventing mother to child transmission (see HIV: mother to child transmission, p 823).

Prophylaxis against specific opportunistic infections (see HIV: prevention of opportunistic infections, p 834).

*Based on observational studies and indirectly from RCTs in other settings

Key Messages

Prevention

- **Early diagnosis and treatment of sexually transmitted diseases** One RCT has found that early diagnosis and treatment of sexually transmitted diseases reduces the risk of acquiring HIV infection over 2 years.
- **Postexposure prophylaxis in healthcare workers** One case control study found limited evidence suggesting that postexposure prophylaxis with zidovudine may reduce the risk of HIV infection over 6 months. Evidence from other settings suggests that combining several antiretroviral drugs is likely to be more effective than zidovudine alone.
- **Presumptive mass treatment of sexually transmitted diseases** One RCT found no significant difference in the incidence of HIV over 20 months between presumptive mass treatment for sexually transmitted diseases and no treatment.

Treatment

- **Three antiretroviral drug regimens (compared with two antiretroviral drug regimens)** One systematic review has found that, compared with two antiretroviral drug regimens, three drug regimens reduce disease progression or death. Some of the reviewed trials included a non-nucleoside reverse transcriptase inhibitor as a third drug, and some a protease inhibitor.
- **Two antiretroviral drug regimens (compared with single antiretroviral drug regimens)** Large RCTs, with follow up of 1–3 years, have found that two drug regimens (zidovudine plus another nucleoside analogue or protease inhibitor drug) reduce the risk of new AIDS defining illnesses and death compared with zidovudine alone. Adverse events were common in all treatment groups.

- **Early versus delayed antiretroviral treatment with multidrug regimens** One systematic review compared early versus delayed antiretroviral treatment, but the RCTs were all started when zidovudine was the only drug available. Overall, the systematic review found no significant difference in the risk of AIDS free survival or overall survival with extended follow up. We found no RCTs exploring this question with two or three drug regimens.
- **Four antiretroviral drug regimens (compared with three antiretroviral drug regimens)** We found no systematic review or RCTs comparing four antiretroviral drug regimens with three antiretroviral drug regimens for clinical outcomes.

DEFINITION HIV infection refers to infection with the human immunodeficiency virus type 1 or type 2. Clinically, this is characterised by a variable period (average around 8–10 years) of asymptomatic infection, followed by repeated episodes of illness of varying and increasing severity as immune function deteriorates. The type of illness varies greatly by country, availability of specific treatments for HIV, and prophylaxis for opportunistic infections.

INCIDENCE/ PREVALENCE Worldwide estimates suggest that, by June 2001, about 51 million people had been infected with HIV, about 16 million people had died as a result, and about 16 000 new HIV infections were occurring each day.[1] About 90% of HIV infections occur in the developing world.[1] Occupationally acquired HIV infection in healthcare workers has been documented in 95 definite and 191 possible cases, although this is likely to be an underestimate.[2]

AETIOLOGY/ RISK FACTORS The major risk factor for transmission of HIV is unprotected heterosexual or homosexual intercourse. Other risk factors include needlestick injury, sharing drug injecting equipment, and blood transfusion. An HIV infected woman may also transmit the virus to her baby. This has been reported in 15–30% of pregnant women with HIV infection. Not everyone who is exposed to HIV will become infected, although risk increases if exposure is repeated, at high dose, or through blood. There is at least a two to five times greater risk of HIV infection among people with sexually transmitted diseases.[3]

PROGNOSIS Without treatment, about half of people infected with HIV will become ill and die from AIDS over about 10 years. A meta-analysis of 13 cohort studies from Europe and the USA looked at 12 574 treatment naïve people starting highly active antiretroviral therapy with a combination of at least three drugs.[4] During 24 310 person years of follow up, 1094 people developed AIDS or died. Baseline CD4 cell count and baseline HIV-1 viral load were associated with the probability of progression to AIDS or death. Other independent predictors of poorer outcome were advanced age, infection through injection drug use, and a previous diagnosis of AIDS. The CD4 cell count at initiation was the dominant prognostic factor in people starting highly active antiretroviral therapy. Genetic factors have been shown to affect response to antiretroviral treatment, but were not considered in the meta-analysis.[4]

AIMS OF INTERVENTION To reduce transmission of HIV; to prevent or delay the onset of AIDS, as manifested by opportunistic infections and cancers; to increase survival; to minimise loss of quality of life caused by inconvenience and adverse effects of current regimens.

OUTCOMES Incidence of HIV infection, new AIDS diseases, and adverse events; mortality; quality of life.

METHODS *Clinical Evidence* search and appraisal July 2003. In addition, we contacted experts in the field, and reviewed abstract books and CDs for conferences held since 1995. Trials were included if they were designed to detect differences in clinical end points. Where trials using clinical end points were unavailable, we included trials using surrogate markers known to denote higher risk of disease progression. Many trials of new treatments are of short duration, which may reflect the fact that many new drugs have only short term effects. We have included evidence on single and two drug antiretroviral regimens, because it may be useful in countries where three drug treatment is not widely available.

QUESTION What are the effects of preventative interventions?

OPTION EARLY DETECTION AND TREATMENT OF SEXUALLY TRANSMITTED DISEASES

One RCT has found that early diagnosis and treatment of sexually transmitted diseases reduces the risk of acquiring HIV infection over 2 years

Benefits: We found no systematic review. One RCT randomised 12 communities in Tanzania (about 12 000 people) to intervention or no intervention.[5] Intervention consisted of diagnosis and treatment of sexually transmitted diseases (STDs) at a local health centre (within 90 minutes' walking distance), provision of free condoms during the current STD episode, and health education by healthcare workers trained in STD case management. The RCT found that intervention significantly reduced the risk of acquiring HIV over 2 years (RR 0.58, 95% CI 0.42 to 0.79).

Harms: Syndromic case management (treating people for the most likely causes of their symptoms and signs) may result in wrong or unnecessary treatment. The RCT gave no information on this.[5]

Comment: There is a clear biological mechanism for the synergistic effect of STDs on HIV transmission, and for STD control as an HIV control strategy. The inflammation associated with STDs increases HIV shedding in genital secretions, and treating STDs reduces this inflammation.[6] Syndromic management of STDs is more commonly used in resource limited settings. In other settings, a microbiological diagnosis is usually made, allowing specific treatment. The trial, randomised by the community and analysed by the individual, uses regression analysis in an attempt to overcome the associated cluster bias, but it is unclear whether this is successful.

OPTION PRESUMPTIVE SEXUALLY TRANSMITTED DISEASE TREATMENT

One RCT found no significant difference in the incidence of HIV over 20 months between presumptive mass treatment for sexually transmitted diseases and no treatment.

Benefits: We found no systematic review. One RCT randomised 10 communities in Uganda (about 12 000 people) to intervention or no intervention.[7] Intervention consisted of treating all adults with several drugs for sexually transmitted diseases (STDs) every 10 months. Although the prevalence of some STDs fell in intervention communities, there was no significant difference in the incidence of HIV between intervention and control communities over 20 months of follow up (incidence of HIV in both groups about 1.5/100 person years; RR intervention *v* control 0.97, 95% CI 0.81 to 1.16).

Harms: Mass treatment means that many uninfected people will be unnecessarily treated for STDs, exposing them to risks of adverse drug reactions and possibly of drug resistance. The RCT gave no information on this.[7]

Comment: The negative finding of the RCT has several possible explanations other than ineffectiveness of the intervention: a high incidence of symptomatic STDs between rounds of mass treatment; a low population risk for treatable STDs; and intense exposure to HIV.[7] The trial, randomised by the community and analysed by the individual, used regression analysis in an attempt to overcome the associated cluster bias, but it is unclear whether this was successful. As many as 80% of STDs are unrecognised or asymptomatic.[8] The variable efficacy of these two interventions may reflect the epidemiological properties of mature versus emerging epidemics. Health seeking behaviour clearly will have an impact. Many sexually transmitted infections are unrecognised or asymptomatic and the analysis of these trials, using regression analysis in an attempt to overcome cluster bias, may have an effect on the reported outcomes.[9]

OPTION POSTEXPOSURE PROPHYLAXIS IN HEALTHCARE WORKERS

One case control study found limited evidence suggesting that postexposure prophylaxis with zidovudine may reduce the risk of HIV infection over 6 months. Evidence from other settings suggests that combining several antiretroviral drugs is likely to be more effective than zidovudine alone.

Benefits: We found no systematic review or RCTs. **Zidovudine alone:** One case control study from the USA and France evaluated outcomes in 31 health workers who acquired HIV infection after occupational exposure, and outcomes in 679 controls who did not acquire HIV infection despite occupational exposure.[10] This study included people followed up for at least 6 months after exposure. HIV infection was less likely in people who received postexposure prophylaxis compared with those who did not (reduction in OR by 81%, 95% CI 43% to 94%). It found that the risk of seroconversion increased with severity of exposure; for example, a penetrating injury with a hollow, bloody needle carried the greatest risk. **Zidovudine plus other antiretroviral drugs:** We found no studies of postexposure prophylaxis using combinations of antiretroviral drugs.

Harms: Short term toxicity (including fatigue, nausea, and vomiting) and gastrointestinal discomfort have been reported by 50–75% of people taking zidovudine and caused 30% to discontinue postexposure prophylaxis.[11] Treatment studies suggest that the frequency of adverse effects is higher in people taking a combination of antiretroviral drugs (reported in 50–90%), which may reduce adherence to postexposure prophylaxis (24–36% discontinued). The risk of drug interactions is also increased. Severe adverse effects, including hepatitis and pancytopenia, have been reported in people taking combination postexposure prophylaxis, but the incidence is not known.

Comment: Case control studies are considered sufficient because experimental studies are hard to justify ethically, and are logistically difficult because of the low rate of seroconversion in exposed people. A summary of 25 studies (22 seroconversions in 6955 exposed people) found that the risk of HIV transmission after percutaneous exposure was 0.32% (95% CI 0.18% to 0.45%) and that the risk after mucocutaneous exposure was 0.03% (95% CI 0.006% to 0.19%).[2] Indirect evidence for postexposure prophylaxis comes from animal studies[10] and from a placebo controlled RCT of zidovudine in pregnant women,[12] which found a reduced frequency of mother to child HIV transmission, presumed to be caused in part by postexposure prophylaxis. RCTs have found that combinations of two, three, or more antiretroviral drugs are more effective than single drug regimens in suppressing viral replication. There is also an unquantified risk that zidovudine alone may not prevent transmission of zidovudine resistant strains of HIV. This constitutes the rationale for combining antiretroviral drugs for postexposure prophylaxis.

QUESTION What are the effects of different antiretroviral drug treatment regimens?

OPTION TWO ANTIRETROVIRAL DRUGS REGIMENS VERSUS ONE DRUG REGIMENS

Large RCTs, with follow up of 1–3 years, have found that two drugs regimens (zidovudine plus another nucleoside analogue or protease inhibitor drug) reduce the risk of new AIDS defining illnesses and death compared with ziduvudine alone. Adverse events were common in all treatment groups.

Benefits: We found one systematic review,[13] two additional RCTs,[14,15] and one subsequent RCT[16] comparing two drugs versus one drug regimens. The systematic review (search date not reported, 6 RCTs, 7700 people) compared zidovudine plus didanosine or zidovudine plus zalcitabine versus zidovudine alone.[13] Participants entered the trials with various stages of infection and were followed for an average of 29 months, during which time 2904 people developed progressive disease and 1850 died. The combined drug regimens significantly delayed disease progression compared with single drug regimens (RR for disease progression with addition of didanosine 0.74, 95% CI 0.67 to 0.82; RR with addition of zalcitabine 0.86, 95% CI 0.78 to 0.94) and death (RR with addition of didanosine 0.72, 95% CI 0.64 to 0.82; RR with addition of zalcitabine 0.87, 95% CI 0.77 to 0.98). After 3 years, the estimated percentages of people who were alive and without a new AIDS event were 53% for zidovudine plus didanosine versus 49% for zidovudine plus zalcitabine versus 44% for zidovudine alone; the percentages alive were 68% versus 63% versus 59%. The first additional RCT (940 people) comparing zalcitabine plus saquinavir (a protease inhibitor) versus either drug as monotherapy found that combination treatment significantly reduced clinical disease (RR 0.51, 95% CI 0.36 to 0.72) or death (RR 0.32, 95% CI 0.16 to 0.64) at 1 year.[14] The second additional RCT (1895 people with CD4 positive T cell counts 25–250/mm^3) found that adding lamivudine (a nucleoside analogue) to regimens containing zidovudine (zidovudine alone in 62%, zidovudine plus didanosine or zalcitabine in the rest) significantly reduced the risk of AIDS or death over about 1 year (HR 0.42, 95% CI 0.32 to 0.57).[15] The subsequent RCT (996 people who had never received antiretroviral treatment) compared zidovudine plus indinavir (a protease inhibitor) versus either zidovudine or indinavir alone.[16] It found that combination treatment significantly reduced the rate of progression to AIDS compared with zidovudine alone after a median follow up of 1 year (combination *v* zidovudine: RR 0.30, 95% CI 0.18 to 0.50). It found no significant difference between combination treatment and indinavir alone (RR 0.77, 95% CI 0.72 to 2.32).

Harms: Adverse effects such as anaemia and neutropenia were common in all groups in all of the RCTs cited above. Up to a third of participants experienced a serious adverse event, with the highest rates in people with lower CD4 counts. Adverse events led to cessation of blind treatment in about a third of participants. The addition of didanosine to zidovudine increased the risks of nausea (RR 1.8, 95% CI 1.1 to 2.9), abdominal pain (RR 1.6, 95% CI 1.0 to 2.7), and pancreatitis (RR 4.6, 95% CI 1.0 to 22.0) compared with zidovudine alone. Addition of zalcitabine increased the risk of neuropathy (RR 2.2, 95% CI 1.4 to 3.6).[13] Addition of lamivudine did not significantly increase the rate of adverse events.[15] The subsequent RCT found that frequent adverse effects in all three treatment groups were abdominal pain, fever, asthenia/fatigue, and malaise.[16] Both indinavir alone and indinavir plus zidovudine versus zidovudine significantly increased the risk of kidney stone formation (40/332 [12%] with indinavir or indinavir plus zidovudine *v* 13/332 [4%] with zidovudine; RR 3.08, 95% CI 1.72 to 5.29; NNH 12, 95% CI 6 to 36). Overall, 2.9% of people permanently discontinued some or all of their study treatment because of adverse effects before an AIDS related clinical event.[17]

Comment: Two drug regimens often allow substantial residual viral replication in an environment where drug resistant variants have selective advantage. Resistance to these drugs tends to develop over several months to years.[17] The relevance of this is not fully understood but prior use of, and measurable resistance to, nucleoside analogue reverse transcriptase inhibitors tends to be associated with poorer virological response to new regimens that include drugs of this class.[18–20]

OPTION THREE ANTIRETROVIRAL DRUGS REGIMENS VERSUS TWO DRUGS REGIMENS

One systematic review has found that, compared with two antiretroviral drugs regimens, three drugs regimens reduce disease progression or death. Some of the reviewed trials included a non-nucleoside reverse transcriptase inhibitor as a third drug, and some a protease inhibitor.

Benefits: We found one systematic review (search date 2001, 54 RCTs, 4558 people) comparing different drug regimens.[21] The review identified 12 RCTs comparing three versus two drugs regimens. Some of the reviewed trials included a non-nucleoside reverse-transcriptase inhibitor as a third drug, and some a protease inhibitor. The review found that triple therapy significantly improved clinical outcomes compared with double therapy after less than 2 years of follow up (9 RCTs, disease progression or death: OR 0.6, 95% CI 0.5 to 0.8). The largest RCT identified by the review (3485 people with CD4 counts of 50–350/mm^3 who had low exposure to zidovudine) compared zidovudine plus zalcitabine plus saquinavir versus zidovudine plus zalcitabine or zidovudine plus saquinavir.[22] It found that triple therapy significantly reduced the risk of AIDS or death (RR of AIDS or death 0.50; CI not reported; P = 0.0001). Health related quality of life did not change significantly over 48 weeks for individuals in the triple therapy group for mental health (P = 0.146) but did for physical health (P = 0.008).[22]

Harms: In the included RCT, about 25% of people in each group had nausea, 10% diarrhoea, 10% vomiting, 10% headache, 4% abdominal pain, and 3% peripheral neuropathy.[23] There was no significant difference between people taking three versus two drugs in other adverse effects (fever, asthenia, anorexia, rash, pruritus, myalgia, insomnia, anaemia, buccal mucosa ulceration, and dyspepsia). Although metabolic toxicity and lipodystrophy are well recognised as side effects in adults,[24] in children the prevalence of clinical lipodystrophy is not yet reliably established. One trial in children comparing three drugs versus two drugs regimens, with the addition of nelfinavir, reported that the incidence of minor adverse events (vomiting, diarrhoea, cutaneous reaction, fever, and anaemia) was similar with nelfinavir and placebo groups per 100 child years (84.8 with nelfinavir, 84.4 with placebo; P = 0.26).[25] However, all diarrhoea events occurred in the nelfinavir group (P = 0.01).

Comment: Few of the trials used clinical end points. Longer term follow up of people taking protease inhibitors has found abnormal fat distribution, hyperglycaemia, and raised triglyceride and cholesterol concentrations. The clinical significance of these changes is uncertain. Many drugs interact with protease inhibitors because of inhibition of cytochrome P450. There is an urgent need for large RCTs in children. The relevance of lipodystrophy and other metabolic changes in growing children is uncertain. Treatment of children should, wherever possible, be undertaken by experts in paediatric HIV infection.

OPTION FOUR ANTIRETROVIRAL DRUGS VERSUS THREE DRUGS REGIMENS

We found no systematic review or RCTs comparing four antiretroviral drugs regimens with three antiretroviral drugs regimens for clinical outcomes.

Benefits: We found no systematic review or RCTs comparing four antiretroviral drugs regimens with three antiretroviral drugs regimens for clinical outcomes.

Harms: We found no systematic review or RCTs comparing four antiretroviral drugs regimens with three antiretroviral drugs regimens for clinical outcomes.

Comment: Clearly, adherence to therapy, which is such an important strategy in minimising the development of viral resistance, becomes more difficult with more complex regimens. Side effects and drug interactions with four antiretroviral drug regimens are as yet poorly documented phenomena. The RCTs comparing three versus two antiretroviral drugs regimens, or four versus two antiretroviral drugs regimens, point to superior antiviral effects of an increasing number of antiretroviral agents. Many of the studies involving four antiretroviral drugs, in fact, refer to the addition of a low dose of ritonavir to three antiretroviral drugs in order to boost the effect of other antiretroviral drugs. The question of four versus three antiretroviral drug regimens for clinical end points remains unresolved.

OPTION EARLY VERSUS DELAYED ANTIRETROVIRAL TREATMENT

One systematic review compared early versus delayed antiretroviral treatment, but the RCTs were all started when zidovudine was the only drug available. Overall, the systematic review found no significant difference in the risk of AIDS free survival or overall survival with extended follow up. We found no RCTs exploring this question with two or three drug regimens.

Benefits: We found one systematic review (search date not reported, 5 RCTs, 7722 people with asymptomatic HIV mainly with CD4 counts > 200/mm^3) comparing zidovudine given immediately versus zidovudine deferred until the early signs of AIDS.[26] It found that immediate treatment significantly increased AIDS free survival compared with deferred treatment at 1 year (78/4431 [1.76%] with immediate zidovudine *v* 131/3291 [3.98%] with deferred zidovudine; OR 0.52, 95% CI 0.39 to 0.68), but the difference was not significant at the end of the RCTs (median follow up of 50 months; 1026/4431 [23.2%] with immediate zidovudine *v* 882/3291 [26.8%] with deferred zidovudine; OR 0.96, 95% CI 0.87 to 1.05). Overall survival was similar in the two groups at 1 year (24/4431 [5.4%] with immediate zidovudine *v* 18/3291 [5.5%] with deferred zidovudine; OR 1.22, 95% CI 0.67 to 2.25) and at the end of the RCTs (734/4431 [16.6%] with immediate zidovudine *v* 617/3291 [18.7%] with deferred zidovudine; OR 1.04, 95% CI 0.93 to 1.16).

Harms: A meta-analysis presented pooled toxicity data in terms of events per 100 patient years.[27] In asymptomatic people, early treatment conferred a small but significant increase in the risk of anaemia (RR of haemoglobin < 8.0 g/dL; early *v* deferred treatment 2.1, 95% CI 1.1 to 4.1;

AR 0.4 events per 100 person years). There was also a small increase in risk of neutropenia with early treatment (AR 1.1 events per 100 person years; CI not reported; P = 0.07). In symptomatic people, the excess incidence of severe anaemia probably reflected the high doses of zidovudine (1200–1500 mg/day; RR of severe anaemia, high *v* low dose 3.6, 95% CI 1.3 to 10). The authors advised that the toxicity results should be interpreted cautiously, because the results varied considerably.

Comment: No new trials on this question are ongoing. With three drug regimens, rates of AIDS and death are currently low and treatment is known to be beneficial up to and over a 2 year period (see benefits of three drugs regimens, p 819). Many people feel sufficiently certain about when to start treatment — based on evidence about HIV pathogenesis, resistance, immune regeneration with treatment, and long term adverse effects — and so would not consider randomisation to immediate versus deferred treatment. Decisions on when to initiate multidrug treatment are currently based on our understanding of how HIV induces immune damage, the capacity for immune regeneration while on treatment, the toxicity and inconvenience of treatment, and the risk of resistance, rather than on results of RCTs.

REFERENCES

1. United Nations AIDS website. http://www.unaids.org (last accessed 19 February 2004).
2. Public Health Laboratory Services. *Occupational transmission of HIV. Summary of published reports.* London: PHLS, December 1997.
3. Centers for Disease Control and Prevention. HIV prevention through early detection and treatment of other sexually transmitted diseases – United States. *MMWR Morb Mortal Wkly Rep* 1998;47:RR12.
4. Egger M, May M, Chene G, et al. Prognosis of HIV-1-infected patients starting highly active antiretrviral therapy: a collaborative analysis of prospective studies. *Lancet* 2002;360:119–128.
5. Grosskurth H, Mosha F, Todd J, et al. Impact of improved treatment of sexually transmitted diseases on HIV infection in rural Tanzania: randomised controlled trial. *Lancet* 1995;346:530–536.
6. Cohen MS, Hoffman IF, Royce RA, et al. Reduction of concentration of HIV-1 in semen after treatment of urethritis: implications for prevention of sexual transmission of HIV-1. *Lancet* 1997;349:1868–1873.
7. Wawer MJ, Sewankambo NK, Serwadda D, et al. Control of sexually transmitted diseases for AIDS prevention in Uganda: a randomised community trial. *Lancet* 1999;353:525–535.
8. Wilkinson D, Abdool Karim SS, Harrison A, et al. Unrecognised sexually transmitted infections in rural South African women: a hidden epidemic. *Bull World Health Organ* 1999;77:22–28.
9. Wilkinson, D, Rutherford, G. Population-based interventions for reducing sexually-transmitted infections, including HIV infection (Cochrane Review). In *The Cochrane Library.* Issue 4, 2003. Chichester, UK: John Wiley & Sons, Ltd. Search date 2000; primary sources Cochrane Controlled Trials Register, Medline, Embase, conference abstracts, reference lists, contact with authors and experts in the field.
10. Centers for Disease Control and Prevention. Public health service guidelines for the management of health-care worker exposures to HIV and recommendations for post exposure prophylaxis. *MMWR Morb Mortal Wkly Rep* 1998;47:RR7.
11. Cardo DM, Culver DH, Ciesielski CA, et al. Case-control study of HIV seroconversion in health care workers after percutaneous exposure. *N Engl J Med* 1997;337:1485–1490.
12. Connor EM, Sperling RS, Gelber R, et al. Reduction of maternal–infant transmission of human immunodeficiency virus type 1 with zidovudine treatment: paediatric AIDS clinical trials group protocol 076 study group. *N Engl J Med* 1994;331:1173–1180.
13. HIV Trialists' Collaborative Group. Zidovudine, didanosine, and zalcitabine in the treatment of HIV infection: meta-analyses of the randomised evidence. *Lancet* 1999;353:2014–2015. Search date not reported; primary sources Medline, hand searches of conference proceedings, and personal contact with investigators and pharmaceutical companies.
14. Haubrich R, Lalezari J, Follansbee SE, et al. Improved survival and reduced clinical progression in HIV-infected patients with advanced disease treated with saquinavir plus zalcitabine. *Antivir Ther* 1998;3:33–42.
15. CAESAR Co-ordinating Committee. Randomized trial of addition of lamivudine or lamivudine plus loviride to zidovudine-containing regimens for patients with HIV-1 infection: the CAESAR trial. *Lancet* 1997;349:1413–1421.
16. Lewi DS, Suleiman JM, Uip DE, et al. Randomized, double-blind trial comparing indinavir alone, zidovudine alone and indinavir plus zidovudine in antiretroviral therapy-naïve HIV-infected individuals with CD4 cells counts between 50 and 250/mm^3. *Rev Inst Med Trop Sao Paulo* 2000;42:27–36.
17. Brun-Vezinet F, Boucher C, Loveday C, et al. HIV-1 viral load, phenotype, and resistance in a subset of drug-naïve participants from the Delta trial. *Lancet* 1997;350:983–990.
18. D'Aquila RT, Johnson VA, Welles SL, et al. Zidovudine resistance and HIV-1 disease progression during antiretroviral therapy. *Ann Intern Med* 1995;122:401–408.
19. Ledergerber B, Egger M, Opravil M, et al. Clinical progression and virological failure on highly active antiretroviral therapy in HIV-1 patients: a prospective cohort study. *Lancet* 1999;353:863–868.
20. Staszewski S, Miller V, Sabin CA, et al. Virological response to protease inhibitor therapy in an HIV clinic cohort. *AIDS* 1999;13:367–373.
21. Jordan R, Gold L, Cummins C, et al. Systematic review and meta-analysis of evidence for increasing numbers of drugs in antiretroviral therapy. *BMJ* 2002;324:757–760. Search date 2001; primary sources Medline, the Cochrane Library, Embase, CINAHL, PsychLIT, Healthstar, appropriate internet sites such as AIDSTRIALS, citation lists, and contact with pharmaceutical companies.
22. Revicki DA, Moyle G, Stellbrink HJ, et al. Quality of life outcomes of combination zalcitabine–zidovudine,

saquinavir–zidovudine, and saquinavir–zalcitabine–zidovudine therapy for HIV-infected adults with CD4 cell counts between 50 and 350/mm^3. *AIDS* 1999;13:851–858

23. Stellbrink H-J, Hawkins D, Clumeck N, et al. Randomized, multicentre phase III study of saquinavir plus zidovudine plus zalcitabine in previously untreated or minimally pretreated HIV-infected patients. *Clin Drug Invest* 2000;20:295–307.
24. Mascolini M. Metabolic toxicities and side-effects. Managing the metabolic side-effects of anti-retroviral therapy. *HIV Treat Bull* 2002;3:21–32.
25. Anonymous. PENTA comparison of dual nucleoside-analogue reverse transcriptase inhibitor regimens with and without nelfinavir in children with HIV-1 who have not previously been treated: the PENTA 5 randomised trial. *Lancet* 2002;359:733–740.
26. Darbyshire J, Foulkes M, Peto R, et al. Immediate versus deferred zidovudine (AZT) in asymptomatic or mildly symptomatic HIV infected adults. In: The Cochrane Library, Issue 4, 2003. Chichester, UK: John Wiley & Sons, Ltd. Search date not reported; primary sources Medline, hand searches of conference abstracts, and contact with investigators and pharmaceutical companies.
27. Ioannidis JP, Cappelleri JC, Lau J, et al. Early or deferred zidovudine therapy in HIV-infected patients without an AIDS-defining illness: a meta-analysis. *Ann Intern Med* 1995;122:856–866. Search date 1994; primary sources Medline, AIDSLine, AIDSTrials, AIDSDrugs, CHEMID, hand searches of current contents, and international conferences on AIDS.

Martin Talbot
Consultant Physician in Genito-urinary Medicine/HIV and Director of Undergraduate Medical Education
Sheffield Teaching Hospitals
Sheffield
UK

Competing interests: None declared.

We would like to acknowledge the previous contributors of this chapter, including Margaret Johnson, Andrew Philips, David Wilkinson, and Bazian Ltd.

HIV: mother to child transmission

Search date January 2004

Jimmy Volmink and Unati Mahlati

QUESTIONS

INTERVENTIONS

Key Messages

Reducing transmission of HIV

- **Antiretroviral drugs** One systematic review found that zidovudine reduced the incidence of HIV in infants compared with placebo. One RCT identified by the review found that longer courses of zidovudine given to mother and infant reduced the incidence of HIV in infants compared with shorter courses of zidovudine. One RCT found that nevirapine given to the mother and to her newborn reduced the risk of HIV transmission compared with zidovudine. One RCT found no additional advantage in giving nevirapine to the mother and baby when transmission rates were already reduced by mothers receiving standard antiretroviral treatment. One RCT found that zidovudine plus lamivudine given in the antenatal, intrapartum, and postpartum periods, or during the intrapartum and postpartum periods, reduced the risk of transmission of HIV at 6 weeks compared with placebo. One RCT found no significant difference in newborn HIV infection rates between nevirapine monotherapy and zidovudine plus lamivudine given to the mother during labour and to the mother and baby after delivery. However, one RCT found that nevirapine plus zidovudine given twice daily to babies for 7 days after birth reduced HIV transmission at 6 to 8 weeks compared with a single dose of nevirapine given to babies immediately after birth.
- **Avoiding breast feeding (provided there is access to clean water and health education)** One RCT in women with HIV who had access to clean water and health education found that, compared with breast feeding, formula feeding reduced the incidence of HIV in infants at 24 months without increasing mortality.
- **Elective caesarean section** One RCT provided limited evidence that elective caesarean section reduced the incidence of HIV in infants at 18 months compared with vaginal delivery.
- **Immunotherapy** One RCT found no significant difference in HIV transmission to infants from mothers taking zidovudine and either HIV hyperimmune globulin or immunoglobulin without HIV antibody. However, the study may have been too small to detect a clinically important difference.
- **Vaginal microbicides** One systematic review, which identified no RCTs, provided insufficient evidence to assess the effects of vaginal microbicides on the transmission of HIV to infants.

- **Vitamin supplements** Three RCTs found that vitamin A supplements given to HIV positive pregnant women had no significant effect on the risk of HIV infection in their infants compared with either placebo or no vitamin A. One RCT found that multivitamins given to mothers during pregnancy and lactation had no significant effect on HIV infection in their infants compared with placebo.

DEFINITION Mother to child transmission of HIV infection is defined as transmission of HIV infection from an infected mother to her child during gestation, labour, or through breast feeding in infancy. HIV-1Ⓖ infection may be transmitted from mother to child,[1] although HIV-2Ⓖ is rarely transmitted in this way.[2] Infected children usually have no symptoms or signs of HIV at birth, but develop them over subsequent months or years.[3]

INCIDENCE/ PREVALENCE A review of 13 cohort studies found that the risk of mother to child transmission of HIV without antiviral treatment is on average about 15–20% in Europe, 15–30% in the USA, and 25–35% in Africa.[4] The risk of transmission is estimated to be 15–30% during pregnancy, with an additional risk of about 10–20% postpartum through breast feeding.[5] UNAIDS estimates that 2.5 million children under the age of 5 years are living with HIV/AIDS. Of these, over 80% are in sub-Saharan Africa.[6] In 2003 alone, an estimated 700 000 children under 15 years of age (75% in sub-Saharan Africa) were newly infected with HIV.[6]

AETIOLOGY/ RISK FACTORS Transmission of HIV to children is more likely if the mother has a high viral load.[1,7,8] Women with detectable viraemia (by p24 antigen or culture) have double the risk of transmitting HIV-1Ⓖ to their infants than those who do not.[1] Prospective studies have also found that breast feeding is a risk factor for mother to child transmission of HIV.[9,10] Other risk factors include sexually transmitted diseases, chorioamnionitis, prolonged rupture of membranes, vaginal mode of delivery, low CD4 count, advanced maternal HIV disease, obstetric events increasing bleeding (episiotomy, perineal laceration, and intrapartum haemorrhage), young maternal age, and history of stillbirth.[6,11–15]

PROGNOSIS About 25% of infants infected with HIV progress rapidly to AIDS or death in the first year. Some survive beyond 12 years of age.[3] One European study found a mortality of 15% in the first year of life and a mortality of 28% by the age of 5 years.[16] A recent study reported that, in children under 5 years of age in sub-Saharan Africa, HIV accounted for 2% of deaths in 1990 and almost 8% in 1999.[17] Five countries (Botswana, Namibia, Swaziland, Zambia, and Zimbabwe) had rates of HIV attributable mortality in excess of 30/1000 in children under the age of 5 years.

AIMS OF INTERVENTION To reduce mother to child transmission of HIV and improve infant survival, with minimal adverse effects.

OUTCOMES HIV infection status of the child; infant morbidity and mortality; maternal morbidity and mortality; adverse effects of treatment for mother and infant.

METHODS *Clinical Evidence* search and appraisal January 2004.

QUESTION What are the effects of measures to reduce mother to child transmission of HIV?

OPTION ANTIRETROVIRAL DRUGS

One systematic review found that zidovudine reduced the incidence of HIV in infants compared with placebo. One RCT identified by the review found that longer courses of zidovudine given to mother and infant reduced the incidence of HIV in infants compared with shorter courses of zidovudine. One RCT found that nevirapine given to the mother and to her newborn reduced the risk of HIV transmission compared with zidovudine. One RCT found no additional advantage in giving nevirapine to the mother and baby when transmission rates were already reduced by mothers receiving standard antiretroviral treatment. One RCT found that zidovudine plus lamivudine given in the antenatal, intrapartum, and postpartum periods, or during the intrapartum and postpartum periods, reduced the risk of transmission of HIV at 6 weeks compared with placebo. One RCT found no significant difference in newborn HIV infection rates between nevirapine monotherapy and zidovudine plus

lamivudine given to the mother during labour and to the mother and baby after delivery. However, one RCT found that nevirapine plus zidovudine given twice daily to babies for 7 days after birth reduced HIV transmission at 6 to 8 weeks compared with a single dose of nevirapine given to babies immediately after birth.

Benefits: **Zidovudine versus placebo:** We found one systematic review (search date 2001, 4 RCTs, 1585 women) that compared zidovudine given to the mother before, during, or after labour versus placebo.[18] In one of the included RCTs, infants of mothers receiving zidovudine were also given zidovudine for 6 weeks after birth.[19] The review found that zidovudine significantly reduced the incidence of HIV in infants compared with placebo (4 RCTs AR 85/687 [12.3%] with zidovudine *v* 165/692 [24%] with placebo; RR 0.52, 95% CI 0.41 to 0.65). The results remained significant when the RCT of zidovudine that used the most intensive regimen[19] was excluded from the analysis (combined results of sensitivity analysis: AR 70/495 [14%] with less intensive regimens *v* 119/507 [23%] with placebo; RR 0.60, 95% CI 0.46 to 0.79).[20–22] The review found that zidovudine significantly reduced HIV transmission to infants among both breast feeding and non-breast feeding mothers (breast feeding mothers: RR 0.62, 95% CI 0.46 to 0.85; non-breast feeding: RR 0.50, 95% CI 0.30 to 0.85; results calculated after exclusion of the RCT with the most intensive regimen).[18] The RCTs included in the review are also individually described (see table 1, p 833). **Alternative zidovudine regimens:** We found one systematic review (search date 2001).[18] It identified one RCT (1437 women), which compared four different zidovudine regimens. Zidovudine was given to mothers from a specific time in gestation until delivery and to the infant until a specific age: "short–short" course (mother from 35 weeks, infant for up to 3 days); "long–long" (mother from 28 weeks, infant for up to 6 weeks); "short–long" (mother from 35 weeks, infant for up to 6 weeks); and "long–short" (mother from 28 weeks, infant for up to 3 days).[23] The RCT found that a "long–long" course significantly reduced HIV in infants compared with a "short–short" course (AR 9/220 [4%] with "long–long" course *v* 24/229 [10%] with "short–short" course; RR 0.39, 95% CI 0.19 to 0.82). As the "short–short" regimen seemed not to reduce transmission of HIV, it was discontinued at the first interim analysis. The trial found no significant difference between a "long–long" and "short–long" course (26/401 [7%] with "long–long" *v* 29/338 [9%] with "short–long" course; RR 0.76, 95% CI 0.45 to 1.25) or between a "long–long" and "long–short" course (26/401 [7%] with "long–long" *v* 16/340 [5%] with "long–short" course; RR 1.37, 95% CI 0.75 to 2.50). **Zidovudine versus nevirapine:** The systematic review[18] identified one unblinded RCT (626 women from a predominantly breast feeding population in Uganda), which compared zidovudine versus nevirapine.[24] It found that nevirapine (given to mothers as a single oral dose at the onset of labour and to infants as a single dose within 72 hours of birth) significantly reduced HIV in infants compared with zidovudine (given orally to women during labour and to their newborns for 7 days after birth) at 14–16 weeks (AR 37/246 [15%] with nevirapine *v* 65/250 [26%] with zidovudine; RR 0.58, 95% CI 0.40 to 0.83). Follow up of this RCT found that nevirapine significantly reduced HIV-1Ⓖ infection and HIV-1 infection or death compared with zidovudine at age 18 months (HIV-1 infection: 15.7% with nevirapine *v* 25.8% with zidovudine; HR 0.59, 95% 0.41 to 0.84; ARR 10.1%, 95% CI 3.5% to 16.6%; HIV-1 infection or death: 20.7% with nevirapine *v* 30.7% with zidovudine; RR 37%, 95% CI 13% to 54%).[25] **Nevirapine added to standard antiretroviral treatment:** One RCT compared nevirapine (given to mothers as a single oral dose at the onset of labour and to infants as a single dose within 72 hours of birth) versus placebo among 1506 non-breast feeding women in the USA, Europe, Brazil, and the Bahamas, who were already receiving standard antiretroviral treatment.[26] It found no significant difference between nevirapine and placebo in HIV risk in infants after 6 months (AR 9/631 [1.4%] with nevirapine *v* 10/617 [1.6%] with placebo; ARR–0.2, 95% CI –1.5 to +1.2; RR 0.88, 95% CI 0.36 to 2.15). The trial was stopped early because it was considered unlikely that a clinically important effect could be detected given the low overall HIV transmission rate. Only 1270 (84.3%) women eventually received the study treatment. **Combination antiretroviral regimens versus placebo:** One RCT (1797 predominantly breast feeding women in South Africa, Uganda, and Tanzania) compared zidovudine plus lamivudine versus placebo.[27] This combination of antiretroviral drugs significantly reduced the risk of HIV transmission at 6 weeks compared with placebo when given in the antenatal (from 36 weeks), intrapartum, and postpartum (to mother and baby for 1 week) periods (regimen A) (AR 16/281 [5.7%] with zidovudine plus lamivudine *v* 40/261 [15.3%] with placebo; RR 0.37, 95% CI 0.21 to 0.65; NNT 11, 95% CI 7 to 24) and during the intrapartum and postpartum periods (regimen B) (AR 24/270 [8.9%] with zidovudine plus lamivudine *v* 40/261 [15.3%] with placebo; RR 0.58, 95% CI 0.36 to 0.94; NNT 16, 95% CI 9 to 126). The RCT found that zidovudine plus lamivudine given during the intrapartum period alone (regimen C) did not significantly affect the risk of transmission at 6 weeks (AR 40/282 [14.2%] with zidovudine plus lamivudine *v* 40/261 [15.3%] with placebo; RR 0.93, 95% CI 0.62 to 1.40). However, survival analysis found no significant difference in the incidence of HIV infection in infants at 18 months (14.9%, 95% CI 9.4% to 22.8% with regimen A; 18.1%, 95% CI 12.1% to 26.2% with regimen B; 20.0%, 95% CI 12.9% to 30.1% with regimen C; and 22.2%, 95% CI 15.9% to 30.2% with placebo; P values not reported). It also found no significant difference in infant mortality at 18 months (10.1% with regimen A, 14.2% with regimen B, 12.8% with regimen C, and 13.4% with placebo; P = 0.40). **Single drug versus combination antiretroviral regimens:** Two RCTs compared nevirapine monotherapy versus combination antiretroviral regimens.[28,29]. The first RCT (1317 women in South Africa) compared nevirapine (given to the mother during labour and to the mother and baby within 48 hours of delivery) versus zidovudine plus lamivudine (given to the mother during labour and to the mother and baby for 1 week after birth).[28] It found no significant difference between nevirapine and zidovudine plus lamivudine in HIV infection rate at 8 weeks (excluding intrauterine infection: AR 5.7% with nevirapine *v* 3.6% with zidovudine plus lamivudine; P = 0.11; overall infection rate: 12.3% with nevirapine *v* 9.3% with zidovudine plus lamivudine; P = 0.11). The second RCT (1119 babies born to HIV positive Malawian women) assessed postexposure prophylaxis by comparing a single dose of nevirapine given to babies immediately after birth versus nevirapine plus zidovudine twice daily for 7 days after birth.[29] It found that nevirapine plus zidovudine significantly reduced HIV transmission rate at 6–8 weeks compared with nevirapine alone for babies regardless of their HIV status at birth (overall HIV transmission rate at 6–8 weeks: 15.3% with nevirapine plus zidovudine *v* 20.9% with nevirapine; P = 0.03; HIV transmission rate at 6–8 weeks for babies not infected at birth: 7.7% with nevirapine plus zidovudine *v* 12.1% with nevirapine; OR 0.60, 95% CI 0.37 to 0.97).

Harms: **Zidovudine versus placebo:** The review found that intensive zidovudine significantly increased the risk of neonatal haematological toxicity compared with placebo (RR 1.86, 95% CI 1.18 to 2.94; specific effects undefined). No significant difference was found between less intensive regimens and placebo (RR 0.77, 95% CI 0.44 to 1.35).[18] Infants who received the most intensive regimen and were followed for 18 months had mild reversible anaemia that resolved by 12 weeks of age.[30] The same trial in uninfected infants followed for a median of 4.2 years found no significant difference between zidovudine and placebo in growth patterns, immunological parameters, or the occurrence of childhood cancers.[31] **Alternative zidovudine regimens:** The RCT found that the rate of serious adverse events in mothers and infants was similar for all regimens. The rates of severe anaemia in infants were "long–long" 1%, "long–short" 0%, "short–long" 0.3%, and "short–short" 1.3%.[23] **Zidovudine versus nevirapine:** The RCT of zidovudine versus nevirapine found no significant difference in serious adverse effects or death at either 8 weeks or 18 months (serious adverse effects defined as fatal or life threatening, permanently disabling, requiring inpatient admission, a congenital anomaly, cancer or overdose, or otherwise judged to be serious by the onsite clinician; serious adverse effects in the first 8 weeks: mothers 3.6% with zidovudine *v* 4.9% with nevirapine, P = 0.443; infants 11.3% with zidovudine *v* 9.1% with nevirapine, P = 0.348; deaths in the first 8 weeks: mothers 1.0% with zidovudine *v* 0.0% with nevirapine; P = 0.081; infants 3.2% with zidovudine *v* 1.3% with nevirapine; P = 0.091; serious adverse effects up to 18 months: infants 31.4% with zidovudine *v* 34.1% with nevirapine; P = 0.476; deaths up to 18 months: infants 13.6% with zidovudine *v* 10.6% with nevirapine; P = 0.253).[24,25] **Combination antiretroviral regimens:** One RCT found similar rates of adverse effects between zidovudine plus lamivudine and placebo. For grade 3 and 4 laboratory events before week 6 (in relation to haemoglobin, leucocytes, lymphocytes, thrombocytes, creatinine, or transaminase levels) the rates in mothers were: regimen A 9%, regimen B 6%, regimen C 7%, and placebo 8%; the corresponding rates in babies were 5% in each of the groups. Congenital abnormalities for the four groups were: regimen A 7%, regimen B 8%, regimen C 6%, and placebo 7%. The rates for neurological events (up to 18 months) in infants were regimen A 2%, regimen B 4%, regimen C 4%, and placebo 3%.[27] **Single drug versus combination antiretroviral regimens:** Both RCTs found similar rates of adverse effects between nevirapine monotherapy and combination antiretroviral regimens.[28,29] The first RCT found that adverse effects in mothers included deaths (0.8% with nevirapine *v* 0.6% with zidovudine plus lamivudine), obstetric procedures (24% with nevirapine *v* 26% with zidovudine plus lamivudine), rash (0.6% with nevirapine *v* 0.8% with zidovudine plus lamivudine), and caesarean section (28% with nevirapine *v* 31% with zidovudine plus lamivudine). No hepatic or haematological adverse effects were reported for either group. Adverse effects in infants included deaths (3% in each), respiratory disorders (16% with nevirapine *v* 17% with zidovudine plus lamivudine), infections (8% with nevirapine *v* 9% with zidovudine plus lamivudine), hepatic adverse effects (3% in each), and rash (2% with nevirapine *v* 3% with zidovudine plus lamivudine). The second RCT found that adverse event rates were similar with the two postexposure prophylaxis regimens (deaths: 8.5% with nevirapine plus zidovudine *v* 11.8% with nevirapine; P = 0.08; grade 3–4 events: 7.8% with nevirapine plus zidovudine *v* 5.6% with nevirapine; P = 0.16).[30]

Comment: In the first RCT comparing nevirapine versus zidovudine plus lamivudine, all women received counselling on infant feeding practices and 42% in each group chose to breast feed.[28] In the second RCT comparing nevirapine versus nevirapine plus zidovudine, deaths were mainly attributable to HIV infection (e.g. pneumonia, septicaemia, meningitis, and gastroenteritis), while less than 1% of the grade 3–4 adverse events were judged to be related to the study drugs.[29]

OPTION AVOIDING BREAST FEEDING

One RCT in women with HIV who had access to clean water and health education found that, compared with breast feeding, formula feeding reduced the incidence of HIV in infants at 24 months without increasing mortality.

Benefits: We found no systematic review. We found one RCT (425 HIV-1 seropositive women with access to clean water and health education in Kenya), which found that formula feeding significantly reduced the proportion of infants with HIV at 24 months compared with breast feeding (AR 31/205 [15%] with formula feeding *v* 61/197 [31%] with breast feeding; RR 0.49, 95% CI 0.33 to 0.72; NNT 7, 95% CI 5 to 13).[5] Although infants were breast fed throughout the RCT, the greatest exposure to breast milk occurred during the first 6 months of life. The RCT found no significant difference in mortality between breast feeding and formula feeding at 24 months (AR: 39/204 [19%] with formula feeding *v* 45/197 [23%] with breast feeding; RR 0.84, 95% CI 0.57 to 1.23).[5]

Harms: The RCT did not report on adverse effects (see comment below).[5]

Comment: The RCT did not report on adherence to the intervention. In countries with high infant mortality, avoiding breast feeding may increase infant morbidity and mortality further through its effect on nutrition, immunity, maternal fertility, and birth spacing. Access to clean water and education when using formula feeds may explain the similar mortality in breast fed and formula fed infants. We are aware of ongoing trials investigating the effects of modifying breast feeding practices. In addition to avoiding breast feeding, these trials are evaluating the effects of exclusive breast feeding for a limited duration with abrupt weaning and inactivation of HIV in breast milk.

OPTION ELECTIVE CAESAREAN SECTION

One RCT provided limited evidence that elective caesarean section reduced the incidence of HIV in infants at 18 months compared with vaginal delivery.

Benefits: We found one systematic review (search date not stated, 1 RCT, 436 women), which compared elective caesarean section at 38 weeks versus vaginal delivery.[32] It found that caesarean section significantly reduced HIV transmission to infants at 18 months compared with vaginal delivery (AR 3/170 [3%] with caesarean section *v* 21/200 [11%] with vaginal delivery; RR 0.16, 95% CI 0.05 to 0.55; NNT 11, 95% CI 10 to 21).[32]

Harms: No serious adverse effects were reported in either group. Postpartum fever was significantly more common in women having caesarean section compared with vaginal delivery (15/225 [7%] with caesarean section *v* 2/183 [1%] with vaginal delivery; RR 6.1, 95% CI 1.5 to 22.0; NNH 18, 95% CI 16 to 50). Postpartum bleeding, intravascular coagulation, and severe anaemia were rare in both groups.[32]

Comment: About 15% of women withdrew from the RCT or were lost to follow up. None of the women breast fed, although this was not stated as a specific exclusion criterion. More women who gave birth by caesarean section versus vaginal delivery had received zidovudine during pregnancy (70% with caesarean section *v* 58% with vaginal delivery); this means that the observed difference between groups may not have been exclusively due to the different delivery methods.[32]

OPTION IMMUNOTHERAPY

One RCT found no significant difference in HIV transmission to infants from mothers taking zidovudine and either HIV hyperimmune globulin or immunoglobulin without HIV antibody. However, the study may have been too small to detect a clinically important difference.

Benefits: We found one systematic review (search date not stated, 1 RCT, 501 women), which compared HIV hyperimmune globulin versus immunoglobulin without HIV antibody given to women during pregnancy, the intrapartum period, and to their infants at birth.[32] Women in both groups received a standard course of zidovudine and no infants were breast fed. The RCT found no significant difference in transmission of HIV up to 6 months of age between HIV hyperimmune globulin and immunoglobulin without HIV antibody regimens (4.1% with HIV hyperimmune globulin *v* 6.0% with immunoglobulin without HIV antibody; CI not reported; P = 0.36).[32]

Harms: The trial reported no significant adverse effects.[32]

Comment: The low overall transmission rate (5%) in this study was much lower than the anticipated rate of greater than 15% used to calculate the appropriate sample size. The trial was unable to exclude a clinically important effect of HIV hyperimmune globulin on the number of children with HIV.[32]

OPTION VAGINAL MICROBICIDES

One systematic review, which identified no RCTs, provided insufficient evidence to assess the effects of vaginal microbicides on the transmission of HIV to infants.

Benefits: We found one systematic review (search date 2002).[33] It identified no RCTs, but found one quasi-randomised trial (see comment below).[34]

Harms: The review identified no RCTs (see comment below).[33]

Comment: The systematic review identified one quasi-randomised trial (898 women), which assessed the effectiveness of vaginal irrigation with chlorhexidine during labour for reducing the risk of transmission. HIV positive women at a hospital in Kenya were allocated to vaginal irrigation or no irrigation during alternate weeks (i.e. all women received cleansing in 1 week, then all women received no cleansing the following week, and so on).[34] The trial found no evidence of a lower rate of HIV transmission after vaginal cleansing versus no cleansing (AR 63/307 [20.5%] with vaginal cleansing *v* 64/295 [21.7%] without vaginal cleansing; RR 0.95, 95% CI 0.69 to 1.29). The trial reported no adverse effects in mothers or infants. In the trial, concealment of allocation was inadequate, and the analysis did not take into account the effect of clustering. Caution is therefore warranted in interpreting the study findings.[34]

OPTION VITAMIN SUPPLEMENTS

Three RCTs found that vitamin A supplements given to HIV positive pregnant women had no significant effect on the risk of HIV infection in their infants compared with either placebo or no vitamin A. One RCT found that multivitamins given to mothers during pregnancy and lactation had no significant effect on HIV infection in their infants compared with placebo.

Benefits: **Vitamin A:** We found one systematic review[35] (search date 2002, 2 RCTs,[36,37] 1813 women) and one subsequent RCT[38] comparing vitamin A supplements (with or without multivitamins) versus placebo given to mothers during the antenatal and intrapartum period. The review found no significant difference between vitamin A and placebo in HIV transmission to infants (AR 123/558 [22.0%] with vitamin A *v* 109/527 [20.7%] with placebo; RR 1.07, 95% CI 0.85 to 1.34).[35] The subsequent RCT (697 pregnant women with HIV in Malawi) compared vitamin A versus no vitamin A given from 18 to 28 weeks' gestation until delivery.[38] It found no significant difference between vitamin A and no vitamin A in perinatal HIV transmission at 6 weeks and 24 months (at 6 weeks: AR 26.6% with vitamin A *v* 27.8% with no vitamin A; P = 0.76; at 24 months: 27.7% with vitamin A *v* 32.8% with no vitamin A; P = 0.21). **Multivitamins:** We found one RCT.[36] It found no significant difference between multivitamins (given to mothers during pregnancy and lactation) and placebo in HIV transmission to infants at 6 weeks (AR 16% with multivitamins *v* 16% with placebo; RR 1.04, 95% CI 0.65 to 1.66).[36]

Harms: **Vitamin A:** The systematic review[35] found no evidence of an effect of vitamin A versus placebo on the incidence of stillbirth (RR 1.06, 95% CI 0.65 to 1.75); preterm birth either less than 34 weeks (RR 0.87, 95% CI 0.59 to 1.29) or less than 37 weeks (RR 0.90, 95% CI 0.74 to 1.10); or low birth weight (< 2500 g; RR 0.88, 95% CI 0.67 to 1.15). A follow up report[39] of one RCT[36] included in the review[35] found no significant difference between vitamin A and placebo on infant death by 24 months (AR 25.9% with vitamin A *v* 24.2% with placebo; RR 1.08, 95% CI 0.84 to 1.39). **Multivitamins:** Long term follow up[39] of one RCT[36] included in the review[35] found no significant difference between multivitamins and placebo in infant death at 24 months (AR 24.1% with multivitamins *v* 26.1% with placebo; RR 0.91, 95% CI 0.71 to 1.17).

Comment: The RCTs were performed because observational studies have found an association in pregnant women between transmission of HIV and low serum levels of vitamin A.[40] We found one subgroup analysis[38] of one RCT[36] that had been included in the systematic review.[35] The RCT originally compared four treatments taken throughout pregnancy and lactation in 1083 pregnant women with HIV-1Ⓖ in Tanzania: vitamin A alone, multivitamins excluding vitamin A, multivitamins plus vitamin A, or placebo.[36] Subgroup analysis among infants who were HIV negative at 6 weeks of age found that vitamin A taken during pregnancy and lactation increased the risk of HIV transmission through breast feeding when compared with placebo (AR 34.2% with vitamin A *v* 25.4% with placebo; RR 1.38, 95% CI 1.09 to 1.76).[39] However, there was no significant difference between multivitamins and placebo in HIV transmission from breast feeding (AR 30.7% with multivitamins *v* 29.0% with placebo; RR 1.04, 95% CI 0.82 to 1.32). One RCT found that giving vitamin A to pregnant women reduced both the number of low birth weight infants and also the number of infants with anaemia at 6 weeks postpartum.[39]

GLOSSARY

Human immunodeficiency virus type 1 (HIV-1) is the most common cause of HIV disease throughout the world.

Human immunodeficiency virus type 2 (HIV-2) is predominantly found in West Africa and is more closely related to the simian immunodeficiency virus than to HIV-1.

REFERENCES

1. John GC, Kreiss J. Mother-to-child transmission of human immunodeficiency virus type 1. *Epidemiol Rev* 1996;18:149–157.
2. Adjorlolo-Johnson G, De Cock KM, Ekpini E, et al. Prospective comparison of mother-to-child transmission of HIV-1 and HIV-2 in Abidjan, Ivory Coast. *JAMA* 1994;272:462–466.
3. Peckham C, Gibb D. Mother-to-child transmission of the human immunodeficiency virus. *N Engl J Med* 1995;333:298–302.
4. Working Group on MTCT of HIV. Rates of mother-to-child transmission of HIV-1 in Africa, America and Europe: results of 13 perinatal studies. *J Acquir Immune Defic Syndr* 1995;8:506–510.

5. Nduati R, John G, Mbori-Ngacha D, et al. Effect of breastfeeding and formula feeding on transmission of HIV-1: a randomized clinical trial. *JAMA* 2000;283:1167–1174.
6. UNAIDS/WHO. Report of the global HIV/AIDS epidemic. December 2003 estimates.
7. Mofenson LM. Epidemiology and determinants of vertical HIV transmission. *Semin Pediatr Infect Dis* 1994;5:252–256.
8. Khouri YF, McIntosh K, Cavacini L, et al. Vertical transmission of HIV-1: correlation with maternal viral load and plasma levels of CD4 binding site anti-gp 120 antibodies. *J Clin Invest* 1995;95:732–737.
9. Dunn DT, Newell ML, Ades AE, et al. Risk of human immunodeficiency virus type-1 transmission through breastfeeding. *Lancet* 1992;240:585–588.
10. Miotti PG, Taha ET, Newton I, et al. HIV transmission through breastfeeding: a study in Malawi. *JAMA* 1999;282:744–749.
11. Nair P, Alger L, Hines S, et al. Maternal and neonatal characteristics associated with HIV infection in infants of seropositive women. *J Acquir Immune Defic Syndr* 1993;6:298–302.
12. Minkoff H, Burns DN, Landesman S, et al. The relationship of the duration of ruptured membranes to vertical transmission of human immunodeficiency virus. *Am J Obstet Gynecol* 1995;173:585–589.
13. European Collaborative Study. Risk factors for mother-to-child transmission of HIV-1. *Lancet* 1992;339:1007–1012.
14. Mofenson LM. A critical review of studies evaluating the relationship of mode of delivery to perinatal transmission of human immunodeficiency virus. *Pediatr Infect Dis J* 1995;14:169–176.
15. Jamieson D, Sibailly TS, Sadek R, et al. HIV-1 viral load and other risk factors for mother- to-child transmission in a breastfeeding population in Cote d'Ivoire. *J Acquir Immune Defic Syndr*2003;34:430–436.
16. European Collaborative Study. Natural history of vertically acquired human immunodeficiency virus-1 infection. *Pediatrics* 1994;94:815–819.
17. Walker N, Schwartlander B, Bryce J. Meeting international goals in child survival and HIV/AIDS. *Lancet* 2002;360:284–289.
18. Brocklehurst P, Volmink J. Antiretrovirals for reducing the risk of mother-to-child transmission of HIV infection (Cochrane Review). In: The Cochrane Library, Issue 4, 2003. Chichester, UK: John Wiley & Sons, Ltd. Search date 2001; primary sources Cochrane Pregnancy and Childbirth Group Trials Register, Cochrane Controlled Trials Register, and conference abstracts.
19. Connor EM, Sperling RS, Gelber RD, et al. Reduction of maternal–infant transmission of human immunodeficiency type 1 with zidovudine treatment. *N Engl J Med* 1994;311:1173–1180.
20. Shaffer N, Chuachoowong R, Mock PA, et al. Short-course zidovudine for perinatal HIV-1 transmission in Bangkok, Thailand: a randomised controlled trial. *Lancet* 1999;353:773–780.
21. Wiktor SZ, Ekpini E, Karon JM, et al. Short-course oral zidovudine for prevention of mother-to-child transmission of HIV-1 in Abidjan, Cote d'Ivoire: a randomised trial. *Lancet* 1999;353:781–785.
22. Dabis F, Msellati P, Meda N, et al. Six-month efficacy, tolerance, and acceptability of a short regimen of oral zidovudine to reduce vertical transmission of HIV in breastfed children in Cote d'Ivoire and Burkina Faso: a double-blind placebo-controlled multicentre trial. *Lancet* 1999;353:786–792.
23. Lallemant M, Jourdain G, Le Couer S, et al. A trial of shortened zidovudine regimens to prevent mother-to-child transmission of human immunodeficiency virus type 1. *N Engl J Med* 2000;343:982–991.
24. Guay LA, Musoke P, Fleming T, et al. Intrapartum and neonatal single-dose nevirapine compared with zidovudine for prevention of mother-to-child transmission of HIV-1 in Kampala, Uganda: HIVNET 012 randomised trial. *Lancet* 1999;354:795–802.
25. Brooks Jackson J, Musoke P, Fleming T, et al. Intrapartum and neonatal single-dose nevirapine compared with zidovudine for prevention of mother-to-child transmission of HIV-1 in Kampala, Uganda:18 month follow-up of the HIVNET 012 randomised trial. *Lancet* 2003;362:859–868.
26. Dorenbaum A, Cunningham CK, Gelber RD, et al. Two-dose intrapartum/newborn nevirapine and standard antiretroviral therapy to reduce perinatal HIV transmission. A randomized trial. *JAMA* 2002;288:189–198.
27. Petra Study Team. Efficacy of three short-course regimens of zidovudine and lamivudine in preventing early and late transmission of HIV-1 from mother to child in Tanzania, South Africa, and Uganda (Petra study): a randomised, double-blind, placebo-controlled trial. *Lancet* 2002;359:1178–1186.
28. Moodley D, Moodley J, Coovadia H, et al. A multicenter randomized controlled trial of nevirapine versus a combination of zidovudine and lamivudine to reduce intrapartum and early postpartum mother-to-child transmission of human immunodeficiency virus type 1. *J Infect Dis* 2003;187:725–735.
29. Taha ET, Kumwenda N, Gibbons A, et al. Short post-exposure prophylaxis in newborn babies to reduce mother- to-child transmission of HIV-1: NVAZ randomized clinical trial. *Lancet* 2003;362:1171–1177.
30. Sperling RS, Shapiro DE, McSherry GD, et al. Safety of the maternal–infant zidovudine regimen utilized in the Pediatric AIDS Clinical Trial Group 076 Study. *AIDS* 1998;12:1805–1813.
31. Culnane M, Fowler MG, Lee S, et al. Lack of long term effects of *in utero* exposure to zidovudine among uninfected children born to HIV-infected women. *JAMA* 1999;281:151–157.
32. Brocklehurst P. Interventions for decreasing the risk of mother-to-child transmission of HIV infection. In: The Cochrane Library, Issue 4, 2003. Chichester, UK: John Wiley & Sons, Ltd. Search date not stated; primary sources Cochrane Pregnancy and Childbirth Group Trials Register and Cochrane Controlled Trials Register.
33. Shey Wiysonge CU, Brocklehurst P, Sterne JAC. Vaginal disinfection during labour for reducing the risk of mother-to-child transmission of HIV infection (Cochrane Review). In: The Cochrane Library, Issue 4, 2003. Chichester, UK: John Wiley & Sons, Ltd. Search date 2002; primary sources Cochrane Controlled Trials Register, Cochrane Pregnancy and Childbirth Group Trials Register, Pubmed, Embase, Aidsline, Lilacs, Aidstrials, Aidsdrugs, reference lists, conference abstracts, and contact with experts and pharmaceutical companies.
34. Gaillard P, Mwanyumba F, Verhofstede C, et al. Vaginal lavage with chlorhexidine during labour to reduce mother-to-child HIV transmission: clinical trial in Mombassa, Kenya. *AIDS* 2001;15:389–396.
35. Shey Wiysonge CU, Brocklehurst P, Sterne JAC. Vitamin A supplementation for reducing the risk of mother-to-child transmission of HIV infection (Cochrane Review). In: The Cochrane Library, Issue 4, 2003. Chichester, UK: John Wiley & Sons, Ltd. Search date 2002: primary sources Cochrane Controlled Trials Register, Cochrane Pregnancy and Childbirth Group Trials Register, Pubmed, Embase, Aidsline, Lilacs, Aidstrials, Aidsdrugs, Reference lists, Conference abstracts, contact with experts and pharmaceutical companies.
36. Fawzi WW, Msamanga G, Hunter D, et al. Randomized trial of vitamin supplements in relation to vertical transmission of HIV-1 in Tanzania. *J Acquir Immune Defic Syndr* 2000;23:246–254.
37. Coutsoudis A, Pillay K, Spooner E, et al. Randomized trial testing the effect of vitamin A supplementation on pregnancy outcomes and early, mother-to-child HIV-1 transmission in Durban, South Africa. *AIDS* 1999;13:1517–1524.
38. Fawzi WW, Msamanga GI, Hunter D, et al. Randomized trial of vitamin supplements in relation to transmission of HIV-1 through breastfeeding and early child mortality. *AIDS* 2002;16:1935–1944.

39. Kumwenda N, Miotti PG, Taha TE, et al. Antenatal vitamin A supplementation increases birth weight and decreases anemia among infants born to human immunodeficiency virus-infected women in Malawi. *Clin Infect Dis* 2002;35:618–624.

40. Fawzi WW, Hunter DJ. Vitamins in HIV disease progression and vertical transmission. *Epidemiology* 1998;9:457–466.

Jimmy Volmink
Professor and Chair of Primary Health Care
Faculty of Health Sciences
University of Cape Town
Cape Town
South Africa

Competing interests: None declared.

TABLE 1 **Placebo controlled trials of zidovudine to reduce mother to child transmission of HIV** **(see text, p 825).**

Ref	Participants	Maternal treatment	Infant treatment	Transmission rate	RR (95% CI)
Infants not breast fed					
18	477 women with confirmed HIV (60 centres in the USA and France)	*Antepartum* Orally 100 mg 5 times daily starting at 14–34 weeks' gestation *Intrapartum* 2 mg/kg iv over 1 hour then 1 mg/kg/hour until delivery	Orally 2 mg/kg every 6 hours for 6 weeks (given only to babies of mothers treated with ZDV)	At 18 months: placebo 26%, ZDV 8%	0.32 (0.18 to 0.59)
19	397 women with confirmed HIV-1 (2 centres in Bangkok and Thailand)	*Antepartum* Orally 300 mg twice daily from 36 weeks' gestation *Intrapartum* Orally 300 mg every 3 hours until delivery	Nil	At 6 months: placebo 19%, ZDV 9%	0.52 (0.30 to 0.85)
Infants breast fed					
20	280 women with confirmed HIV-1 (1 hospital in the Ivory Coast)	*Antepartum* Orally 300 mg twice daily from 36 weeks' gestation *Intrapartum* Orally 300 mg every 3 hours until delivery	Nil	At 3 months: placebo 25%, ZDV 16%	0.63 (0.38 to 1.05)
21	431 women with confirmed HIV-1 (Ivory Coast and Burkina Faso)	*Antepartum* Orally 250 or 300 mg twice daily from 36–38 weeks' gestation *Intrapartum* Orally single dose of 500 or 600 mg at onset of labour *Postpartum* Orally 250 or 300 mg twice daily for 7 days	Nil	At 6 months: placebo 28%, ZDV 18%	0.62 (0.40 to 0.95)

iv, intravenously; Ref, reference; ZDV, zidovudine.

HIV: prevention of opportunistic infections

Search date December 2003

John Ioannidis and David Wilkinson

QUESTIONS

INTERVENTIONS

Key Messages

- The absolute benefits of prophylactic regimens for opportunistic infections are probably smaller in people with HIV who are also talking highly active antiretroviral treatment (HAART). The rate of PCP, toxoplasmosis, and other opportunistic infections has been reduced by HAART.

PCP and toxoplasmosis prophylaxis

- **Atovaquone** We found no RCTs comparing atovaquone versus placebo. RCTs in people who are either intolerant of or fail to respond to trimethoprim–sulfamethoxazole found that atovaquone is as effective as dapsone or aerosolised pentamidine in preventing *P carinii* pneumonia (PCP). It would be unethical to perform a trial of atovaquone compared with placebo.
- **Azithromycin (alone or plus rifabutin, compared with rifabutin alone, for PCP prevention)** One RCT found that azithromycin, either alone or in combination with rifabutin, reduced the risk of *P carinii* pneumonia (PCP) compared with rifabutin alone in people receiving standard PCP prophylaxis.
- **Trimethoprim–sulfamethoxazole for PCP** Systematic reviews found that trimethoprim–sulfamethoxazole reduces the incidence of PCP compared with placebo or pentamidine. Two systematic reviews found that trimethoprim–sulfamethoxazole reduced incidence of PCP compared with dapsone (with or without pyrimethamine), although only one of these reviews found that the reduction was significant. One systematic review and one subsequent RCT found no significant difference between high and low dose trimethoprim–sulfamethoxazole for PCP prophylaxis, although adverse effects were more common with the higher dose.
- **Trimethoprim–sulfamethoxazole for toxoplasmosis** One RCT found no significant difference between trimethoprim–sulfamethoxazole and placebo for preventing toxoplasmosis. One systematic review has found no significant difference between trimethoprim–sulfamethoxazole and dapsone (with or without pyrimethamine) for preventing toxoplasmosis.

Tuberculosis prophylaxis

- **Antituberculosis prophylaxis versus placebo (in people with positive tuberculin test)** One systematic review found that in people who are HIV and tuberculin skin test positive, antituberculosis prophylaxis drugs reduced the frequency of tuberculosis compared with placebo over 2–3 years. The review found no evidence of benefit in people who are HIV positive but tuberculin skin test negative. One RCT found that the benefit of prophylaxis diminished with time after treatment was stopped.

- **Isoniazid for 6–12 months (*v* combination treatment for 2–3 months — longer treatment regimen, but similar benefits and fewer harms)** RCTs found no evidence of a difference in effectiveness between regimens using combinations of tuberculosis drugs for 2–3 months and those using isoniazid alone for 6–12 months. One RCT found that multidrug regimens increased the number of people with adverse reactions resulting in cessation of treatment.

Primary MAC prophylaxis

- **Azithromycin** One RCT found that azithromycin reduced the incidence of *M avium* complex (MAC) compared with placebo. One RCT found that both azithromycin and azithromycin plus rifabutin reduced the incidence of MAC compared with rifabutin alone.
- **Clarithromycin** One RCT found that clarithromycin reduced the incidence of *M avium* complex (MAC) compared with placebo. One RCT found that both clarithromycin and clarithromycin plus rifabutin reduced the incidence of MAC compared with rifabutin alone.
- **Rifabutin plus macrolides** One RCT found that rifabutin plus clarithromycin reduced the incidence of *M avium* complex (MAC) compared with rifabutin alone. One RCT found that azithromycin plus rifabutin reduced the incidence of MAC compared with azithromycin alone or rifabutin alone. One systematic review and two subsequent RCTs found that toxicity, including uveitis, was more common with combination therapy than with clarithromycin or rifabutin alone.

Secondary MAC prophylaxis

- **Clarithromycin, rifabutin, and ethambutol (more effective than clarithromycin plus clofazimine)** One RCT found that clarithromycin, rifabutin and ethambutol reduced MAC relapse compared with clarithromycin plus clofazimine.
- **Ethambutol added to clarithromycin plus clofazimine** One RCT found that adding ethambutol to clarithromycin and clofazimine reduced MAC relapse compared with clarithromycin plus clofazimine.
- **Rifabutin added to clarithromycin plus ethambutol** One RCT found no significant difference in survival by adding rifabutin to clarithromycin plus ethambutol in people with previous MAC.
- **Clofazimine added to clarithromycin and ethambutol (higher mortality than clofazimine plus ethambutol)** One RCT found that adding clarithromycin to clofazimine and ethambutol was associated with higher mortality compared with clofazimine plus ethambutol.

CMV, HSV, and VZV prophylaxis

- **Aciclovir (for HSV and VZV)** One systematic review found that aciclovir reduced HSV and VZV infection, and reduced overall mortality in people at different clinical stages of HIV infection compared with placebo. It found no reduction in CMV.
- **Oral ganciclovir (in people with severe CD4 delpetion)** One RCT found that oral ganciclovir reduced the incidence of cytomegalovirus (CMV) in people with severe CD4 depletion compared with placebo. It found that 26% of people who took ganciclovir developed severe neutropenia. A second RCT found no significant difference in prevention of CMV between ganciclovir and placebo.
- **Famciclovir (for recurrent HSV)** One small RCT found that famciclovir reduced the rate of viral shedding compared with placebo, but provided insufficient evidence on the effect of famciclovir on herpes simplex virus (HSV) recurrence.
- **Valaciclovir (less effective than aciclovir for CMV)** One RCT found that valaciclovir versus aciclovir reduced the incidence of CMV, but may be associated with increased mortality.

Primary fungal prophylaxis

- **Fluconazole or itraconazole** RCTs in people with advanced HIV disease found that both fluconazole and itraconazole reduced the incidence of invasive fungal infections compared with placebo. One RCT found that fluconazole reduced the incidence of invasive fungal disease and mucocutaneous candidiasis compared with clotrimazole. One RCT found no difference between high and low dose fluconazole. Azoles have been associated with congenital problems and potentially serious interactions with other drugs.

Secondary fungal prophylaxis

- **Itraconazole (for *Penicillium marneffei*)** Two RCTs found that itraconazole reduced the incidence of relapse of P marneffei infection and candidiasis compared with placebo.
- **Intraconazole (*v* fluconazole for maintenance treatment of cryptococcal meningitis)** One RCT found that itraconazole increased the risk of relapse of cryptococcal meningitis compared with fluconazole.

Discontinuing prophylaxis in people on HAART

- **Discontinuing prophylaxis for MAC in people with CD4 > 100/mm^3** Two RCTs in people with CD4 > 100/mm^3 taking HAART found that discontinuation of prophylaxis for MAC disease did not increase the incidence of MAC disease.
- **Discontinuing prophylaxis for PCP and toxoplasmosis in people with CD4 > 200/mm^3** One systematic review of two unblinded RCTs in people with CD4 > 200/mm^3 taking HAART found that discontinuation of prophylaxis did not increase the incidence of PCP. Two unblinded RCTs found that discontinuation of prophylaxis did not increase the incidence of toxoplasmosis.
- **Discontinuing prophylaxis for CMV in people with CD4 > 100/mm^3** We found insufficient evidence on the effects of discontinuation of maintenance treatment for CMV retinitis or other end organ disease in people with CD4 > 100/mm^3 taking HAART.

DEFINITION Opportunistic infections are intercurrent infections that occur in people infected with HIV. Prophylaxis aims to avoid either the first occurrence of these infections (primary prophylaxis) or their recurrence (secondary prophylaxis, maintenance treatment). This review includes *Pneumocystis carinii* pneumonia (PCP), *Toxoplasma gondii* encephalitis, *Mycobacterium tuberculosis*, *Mycobacterium avium* complex (MAC) disease, cytomegalovirus (CMV) disease (most often retinitis), infections from other herpesviruses (herpes simplex virus [HSV] and varicella zoster virus [VZV]), and invasive fungal disease (*Cryptococcus neoformans*, *Histoplasma capsulatum*, and *Penicillium marneffei*Ⓖ).

INCIDENCE/ PREVALENCE The incidence of opportunistic infections is high in people with immune impairment. Data available before the introduction of highly active antiretroviral treatment (HAART) suggest that, with a CD4 < 250/mm^3, the 2 year probability of developing an opportunistic infection is 40% for PCP, 22% for CMV, 18% for MAC, 6% for toxoplasmosis, and 5% for cryptococcal meningitis.[1] The introduction of HAART has reduced the rate of opportunistic infections. One cohort study found that the introduction of HAART decreased the incidence of PCP by 94%, CMV by 82%, and MAC by 64%, as presenting AIDS events. HAART decreased the incidence of events subsequent to the diagnosis of AIDS by 84% for PCP, 82% for CMV, and 97% for MAC.[2]

AETIOLOGY/ RISK FACTORS Opportunistic infections are caused by a wide array of pathogens and result from immune defects induced by HIV. The risk of developing opportunistic infections increases dramatically with progressive impairment of the immune system. Each opportunistic infection has a different threshold of immune impairment, beyond which the risk increases substantially.[1] Opportunistic pathogens may infect the immunocompromised host *de novo*, but usually they are simply reactivations of latent pathogens in such hosts.

PROGNOSIS Prognosis depends on the type of opportunistic infection. Even with treatment they may cause serious morbidity and mortality. Most deaths owing to HIV infection are caused by opportunistic infections.

AIMS OF INTERVENTION	To prevent the occurrence and relapse of opportunistic infections; to discontinue unnecessary prophylaxis; to minimise adverse effects of prophylaxis and loss of quality of life.
OUTCOMES	First occurrence and relapse of opportunistic infections and adverse effects of treatments. We have not considered neoplastic diseases associated with specific opportunistic infections.
METHODS	*Clinical Evidence* search and appraisal December 2003. We also reviewed abstract books/CDs for the following conferences held between 1995 and early 2001: European Clinical AIDS, HIV Drug Treatment, Interscience Conferences on Antimicrobial Agents and Chemotherapy, National Conferences on Human Retroviruses and Opportunistic Infections, and World AIDS Conference. We placed emphasis on systematic reviews and RCTs published after 1993.

QUESTION **What are the effects of prophylaxis for *P carinii* pneumonia (PCP) and toxoplasmosis?**

OPTION **TRIMETHOPRIM–SULFAMETHOXAZOLE**

Systematic reviews found that trimethoprim–sulfamethoxazole is more effective than pentamidine or placebo at reducing the incidence of PCP. One RCT found no significant difference between trimethoprim–sulfamethoxazole and placebo for preventing PCP or toxoplasmosis. Two systematic reviews found that trimethoprim–sulfamethoxazole reduced the incidence of PCP compared with dapsone (with or without pyrimethamine), although only one of these reviews found that the reduction was significant. One systematic review found no difference between trimethoprim–sulfamethoxazole and dapsone (with or without pyrimethamine) for incidence of toxoplasmosis. One systematic review and one subsequent RCT found no significant difference between high and low dose trimethoprim–sulfamethoxazole for PCP prophylaxis, although adverse effects were more common with the higher dose.

Benefits: We found two systematic reviews (search dates 1995[3] and not stated[4]) and two subsequent RCTs.[6,7] **Trimethoprim–sulfamethoxazole or pentamidie versus placebo:** The first systematic review analysed the effects of trimethoprim–sulfamethoxazole (co-trimoxazole) or pentamidine versus placebo. It found that prophylaxis with trimethoprim–sulfamethoxazole or pentamidine reduced the incidence of PCP compared with placebo (6 RCTs, [1 of trimethoprim–sulfamethoxazole, 5 of pentamidine] 823 people with advanced disease, *P carinii* events; RR 0.32, 95% CI 0.23 to 0.46).[3] The single RCT from the review that compared trimethoprim–sulfamethoxazole versus placebo (60 HIV positive people with a new diagnosis of Karposi's sarcoma) found that trimethoprim–sulfamethoxazole reduced the incidence of PCP over 24 months compared with placebo (0/30 [0%] with trimethoprim–sulfamethoxazole *v* 16/30 [53%] with placebo; significance not reported).[5] One subsequent RCT (545 people in sub-Saharan Africa with symptomatic disease; second or third clinical stage disease in the WHO staging system**G**; regardless of CD4 cell count) compared trimethoprim–sulfamethoxazole with placebo and found no significant difference in incidence of PCP or toxoplasmosis (no cases of PCP reported).[6] **Trimethoprim–sulfamethoxazole versus pentamidine:** The first systematic review found that trimethoprim–sulfamethoxazole significantly reduced the incidence of PCP compared with aerosolised pentamidine (14 RCTs, 2248 people, *P carinii* events; RR 0.58, 95% CI 0.45 to 0.75; absolute data not reported).[3] The second systematic review found no significant difference between trimethoprim–sulfamethoxazole and aerosolised pentamidine for preventing toxoplasmosis (13 RCTs, 2226 people; RR 0.78, 95% CI 0.55

to 1.11).[4] **Trimethoprim–sulfamethoxazole versus dapsone (with or without pyrimethamine):** The first systematic review found no significant difference between trimethoprim–sulfamethoxazole compared with dapsone (with or without pyrimethamine), although the incidence of PCP was lower in the trimethoprim–sulfamethoxazole group (8 RCTs; RR 0.61, 95% CI 0.34 to 1.10).[3] The second systematic review found that trimethoprim–sulfamethoxazole was significantly more effective in preventing PCP than dapsone/pyrimethamine (8 RCTs; RR 0.49, 95% CI 0.26 to 0.92).[4] It found no significant difference between trimethoprim–sulfamethoxazole and dapsone/pyrimethamine in preventing toxoplasmosis (13 RCTs; RR 1.17, 95% CI 0.68 to 2.04). **High versus low dose trimethoprim–sulfamethoxazole:** The first systematic review found no significant difference in the rate of PCP infection between lower dose (160/800 mg 3 times/week or 80/400 mg/day) and higher dose (160/800 mg/day) trimethoprim–sulfamethoxazole (failure rate per 100 person years was 1.8, 95% CI 1.0 to 3.3 with lower dose *v* 0.5, 95% CI 0 to 2.9 with higher dose; significance not reported).[3] One subsequent RCT (2625 people) also found no significant difference in the rate of PCP infection in people who received trimethoprim–sulfamethoxazole 160/800 mg daily compared with three times weekly (3.5 *v* 4.1 per 100 person years; RR 0.82, 95% CI 0.61 to 1.09; P = 0.16), or in the rate of toxoplasmosis (1.8 *v* 1.8 per 100 person years; RR 1.02, 95% CI 0.39 to 2.63).[7]

Harms: **Trimethoprim–sulfamethoxazole versus placebo:** One RCT in sub-Saharan Africa found that people on trimethoprim–sulfamethoxazole were less likely to suffer a serious event (death or hospital admission, irrespective of the cause) than those on placebo, regardless of their initial CD4 cell count (HR 0.57, 95% CI 0.43 to 0.75; P < 0.001).[6] Moderate neutropenia occurred more frequently with trimethoprim–sulfamethoxazole (neutropenia AR 62/271 [23%] with trimethoprim–sulfamethoxazole *v* 26/244 [10%] with placebo; RR 2.1, 95% 1.4 to 3.3; NNH 8, 95% CI 5 to 14). Two RCTs (largest 377 people) found that gradual initiation of trimethoprim–sulfamethoxazole may improve tolerance of the regimen compared with abrupt initiation.[8,9] Two RCTs (238 people, 50 people) found no significant benefit from acetylcysteine in preventing trimethoprim–sulfamethoxazole hypersensitivity reactions in HIV infected people.[10,11] **High versus low dose trimethoprim–sulfamethoxazole:** One systematic review found that severe adverse effects (predominantly rash, fever, and haematological effects leading to discontinuation within 1 year) occurred in more people taking higher doses of trimethoprim–sulfamethoxazole than in those taking lower doses (25% *v* 15%).[3] The RCT comparing high dose with low dose trimethoprim–sulfamethoxazole found that discontinuation because of adverse effects was significantly more common in people taking high doses of trimethoprim–sulfamethoxazole (RR 2.14; P < 0.001).[7] **Dapsone:** One systematic review found that adverse effects were more frequent with high doses than low doses of dapsone (29% *v* 12%).[3] Another systematic review (search date 1996, 16 trials, 4267 people) evaluating dapsone toxicity found no significant difference in mortality between dapsone and other prophylaxis (OR for mortality for dapsone *v* other prophylaxis 1.11, 95% CI 0.96 to 1.29).[12] **Pentamidine:** Bronchospasm occurred in 3% of people taking aerosolised pentamidine 300 mg monthly.[3]

Comment: **Concomitant coverage for toxoplasmosis:** Standard trimethoprim–sulfamethoxazole prophylaxis or dapsone should offer adequate coverage for toxoplasmosis. Pentamidine has no intrinsic activity against *T gondii*. Toxoplasmosis risk is probably clinically meaningful only with CD4 < 100/mm^3 and positive toxoplasma serology.[1]

Role of highly active antiretroviral treatment (HAART): We found more than 50 RCTs on the prophylaxis of PCP and/or toxoplasmosis, but their results should be interpreted with caution because they were conducted mostly before the advent and widespread use of HAART. Although this is unlikely to affect the comparative results, HAART has resulted in a large decrease in the rate of PCP, toxoplasmosis, and other opportunistic infections; therefore, the absolute benefits of these prophylactic regimens are probably smaller when used with HAART. **Prophylaxis in Africa:** Beneficial effects of trimethoprim–sulfamethoxazole in Africa may be largely because of prophylaxis for bacterial infections rather than PCP. The largest trial conducted in Africa found that trimethoprim–sulfamethoxazole significantly reduced mortality and hospital admissions.[6] However, a smaller trial (100 people) found no significant effect on mortality or hospital admission, although it may have lacked power to detect a significant difference (HR for death or hospital admission 1.10, 95% CI 0.57 to 2.13).[13]

OPTION ATOVAQUONE

We found no RCTs comparing atovaquone versus placebo. RCTs in people who are either intolerant of or fail to respond to trimethoprim–sulfamethoxazole found that atovaquone is as effective as dapsone or aerosolised pentamidine in preventing *P carinii* pneumonia (PCP). It would be unethical to perform a trial of atovaquone compared with placebo.

Benefits: We found no systematic review. **Versus placebo:** We found no RCTs. **Versus dapsone:** One RCT (1057 people intolerant of trimethoprim–sulfamethoxazole, of whom 298 had a history of PCP) found no significant difference between atovaquone 1500 mg daily compared with dapsone 100 mg daily (15.7 cases of PCP per 100 person years with atovaquone *v* 18.4 with dapsone; P = 0.20).[14] **Versus pentamidine:** One RCT (549 people intolerant of trimethoprim–sulfamethoxazole) compared high dose versus low dose atovaquone (1500 mg/day *v* 750 mg/day) versus monthly aerosolised pentamidine (300 mg). It found no significant difference between the groups in the incidence of PCP (26% *v* 22% *v* 17%) or mortality (20% *v* 13% *v* 18%) after a median follow up of 11.3 months.[15]

Harms: **Versus dapsone:** The RCT comparing atovaquone with dapsone found that the overall risk of stopping treatment because of adverse effects was similar in the two arms (RR 0.94, 95% CI 0.74 to 1.19).[14] Atovaquone was stopped more frequently than dapsone in people who were receiving dapsone at baseline (RR 3.78, 95% CI 2.37 to 6.01), and less frequently in people not receiving dapsone at baseline (RR 0.42, 95% CI 0.30 to 0.58).

Comment: See role of highly active antiretroviral treatment in comment under trimethoprim–sulfamethoxazole, p 839. In clinical practice, atovaquone is usually used in people who are either intolerant of or fail to respond to trimethoprim–sulfamethoxazole.

OPTION AZITHROMYCIN

One RCT found that azithromycin, either alone or in combination with rifabutin, reduced the risk of *P carinii* pneumonia (PCP) compared with rifabutin alone in people receiving standard PCP prophylaxis.

Benefits: We found no systematic review. **Versus placebo:** We found no RCTs. **Versus rifabutin:** We found one RCT (693 HIV-1 positive people) that compared azithromycin, rifabutin, and both drugs in combination in people who were already receiving standard PCP prophylaxis.[16] It found that there were significantly fewer cases of PCP in people taking either azithromycin or azithromycin plus rifabutin compared with rifabutin alone (RR azithromycin *v* rifabutin 0.54, 95% CI 0.32 to 0.94; RR azithromycin plus rifabutin *v* rifabutin 0.55, 95% CI 0.32 to 0.94).

Harms: Gastrointestinal adverse effects are common with azithromycin, but they are usually mild and do not lead to stopping treatment. The addition of rifabutin significantly increased the risk of stopping treatment (RR 1.67; P = 0.03).[17]

Comment: See role of highly active antiretroviral treatment in comment under trimethoprim–sulfamethoxazole, p 839. The low incidence of PCP infection in people taking highly active antiretroviral treatment means that the absolute benefit of prophylaxis is smaller.

QUESTION What are the effects of antituberculosis prophylaxis in people with HIV infection?

OPTION ANTITUBERCULOSIS PROPHYLACTIC REGIMENS VERSUS PLACEBO

One systematic review found that in people who are HIV and tuberculin skin test positive, antituberculosis prophylaxis drugs reduced the frequency of tuberculosis compared with placebo over 2–3 years. The review found no evidence of benefit in people who are HIV positive but tuberculin skin test negative. One RCT found that the benefit of prophylaxis diminished with time after treatment was stopped.

Benefits: We found one systematic review (search date 2000).[18] The systematic review identified seven RCTs in 4652 HIV positive adults from Haiti, Kenya, USA, Zambia, and Uganda.[18] All compared isoniazid (6–12 months) or combination treatment (rifampicin plus pyrazinamide, isoniazid plus rifampicin, or isoniazid plus rifampicin plus pyrazinamide) (2–3 months) with placebo. Mean follow up was 2–3 years, and the main outcomes, stratified by tuberculin skin test positivity, were tuberculosis (either microbiological or clinical) and death. Among tuberculin skin test positive adults, antituberculosis prophylaxis significantly reduced the incidence of tuberculosis (RR compared with placebo 0.24, 95% CI 0.14 to 0.40) and was associated with a non-significant reduction in the risk of death (RR compared with placebo 0.77, 95% CI 0.58 to 1.03). Among tuberculin skin test negative adults there was no significant difference in risk of tuberculosis (RR compared with placebo 0.87, 95% CI 0.56 to 1.36) or death (RR compared with placebo 1.07, 95% CI 0.88 to 1.30). One of the RCTs included in the systematic review (1053 Zambian adults; 161 tuberculin skin test positive, 517 negative, the rest unknown) comparing isoniazid versus rifampicin plus pyrazinamide versus placebo for up to 6 months has published results at 3 years' follow up.[19] Many people taking placebo were offered isoniazid after randomisation. Intention to treat analysis found that isoniazid or rifampicin plus pyrazinamide significantly reduced the risk of tuberculosis at 2.5 years compared with placebo (cumulative AR not provided; RR 0.55, 95% CI 0.32 to 0.93), although the benefit diminished over this time. We found one subsequent RCT published as a letter (see comment below).[20]

Harms: Data on adverse drug reactions were not always stratified by tuberculin skin test positivity. In the first review there was a significant increase in adverse drug reactions requiring cessation of treatment with isoniazid compared with placebo (RR 1.75, 95% CI 1.23 to 2.47).[18]

Comment: Without prophylaxis, people who are HIV and tuberculin skin test positive have a 50% or more lifetime risk of developing tuberculosis compared with a 10% lifetime risk in people who are HIV positive but tuberculin skin test negative.[21] Clinical features of tuberculosis may be atypical in people with HIV infection and diagnosis may be more difficult, disease progression more rapid, and outcome worse. The subsequent RCT published as a letter (237 HIV positive Haitian adults with negative tuberculin skin test) found no significant difference between isoniazid (300 mg) versus no treatment in mortality, or the incidence of AIDS or tuberculosis at 1 year.[20]

OPTION DIFFERENT ANTITUBERCULOSIS PROPHYLACTIC REGIMENS VERSUS EACH OTHER

RCTs found no evidence of a difference in effectiveness between regimens using combinations of tuberculosis drugs for 2–3 months and those using isoniazid alone for 6–12 months. One RCT found that multidrug regimens increased the number of people with adverse reactions resulting in cessation of treatment.

Benefits: We found no systematic review. We found six RCTs.[19,22–26] Three RCTs (750, 1583, and 393 people) compared isoniazid versus rifampicin/pyrazinamide in people who were HIV and tuberculin skin test positive.[22–24] All found no significant difference in rates of tuberculosis. The fourth RCT (1564 HIV and tuberculin skin test positive people from Uganda) compared three treatments (isoniazid alone, isoniazid plus rifampicin, and isoniazid, rifampicin and pyrazinamide) versus placebo.[25] It reported comparisons between each regimen versus placebo, but did not directly compare different regimens against each other (see comment below). The fifth RCT (133 adults, mixed tuberculin skin test positive and negative) comparing isoniazid for 12 months versus isoniazid plus rifampicin for 3 months found no significant difference in the incidence of tuberculosis (AR 4.2% with isoniazid *v* 2.1% with isoniazid plus rifampicin; RR 0.51, 95% CI 0.09 to 2.8).[26] The sixth RCT (1053 Zambian adults; 161 tuberculin skin test positive, 517 negative, the rest unknown) compared isoniazid for 6 months versus rifampicin plus pyrazinamide for 3 months versus placebo.[19] Many people in the placebo group were offered isoniazid after randomisation. Intention to treat analysis found no significant difference between isoniazid versus rifampicin plus pyrazinamide in the rate of tuberculosis at any time during a mean follow up of 3 years.

Harms: One RCT found that the proportion of people discontinuing treatment increased with the number of drugs given: isoniazid 1%, isoniazid plus rifampicin 2%, and all three drugs 6%.[23]

Comment: The fourth RCT compared each of three drug regimens versus placebo, but not versus each other.[25] It found that the risk of tuberculosis was significantly reduced with isoniazid alone (RR compared with placebo 0.33, 95% CI 0.14 to 0.77), and with isoniazid and rifampicin combined (RR compared with placebo 0.40, 95% CI 0.18 to 0.86). However, it found only a non-significant trend toward reduction with isoniazid, rifampicin, and pyrazinamide combined (RR compared with placebo 0.51, 95% CI 0.24 to 1.08). There is concern about emergence of rifampicin resistance if this drug is used in antituberculosis prophylaxis, although we found no reports of this. There is a theoretical risk that widespread, unsupervised use of isoniazid alone could promote resistance to this drug, although we found no evidence that this has happened.

QUESTION **What are the effects of prophylaxis for disseminated *M avium* complex (MAC) disease for people without previous MAC disease?**

OPTION **AZITHROMYCIN**

One RCT found that azithromycin reduced the incidence of *M avium* complex (MAC) compared with placebo. One RCT found that both azithromycin and azithromycin plus rifabutin reduced the incidence of MAC compared with rifabutin alone.

Benefits: We found no systematic review. **Versus placebo:** One RCT (174 people with AIDS and CD4 < 100/mm^3) found that azithromycin reduced the incidence of MAC compared with placebo (11% with azithromycin *v* 25% with placebo; P = 0.004).[27] **Versus rifabutin:** See benefits of rifabutin plus macrolides, p 844. **Versus rifabutin plus azithromycin:** See benefits of rifabutin plus macrolides, p 844.

Harms: Gastrointestinal adverse effects were more likely with azithromycin than with placebo (71/90 [79%] with azithromycin *v* 25/91 [28%] with placebo; NNH 2, CI not reported), but they were rarely severe enough to cause discontinuation of treatment (8% *v* 2% in the two arms; P = 0.14).[27] See also harms under rifabutin plus macrolides, p 844.

Comment: Prospective cohort studies found that the risk of disseminated MAC disease increased substantially with a lower CD4 count and was clinically important only for CD4 < 50/mm^3.[1] **Role of highly active antiretroviral treatment (HAART):** Most of the RCTs of MAC prophylaxis were conducted before the widespread use of HAART. HAART reduces the absolute risk of MAC infection. The absolute risk reduction of prophylactic regimens may be smaller when used in people treated with HAART.

OPTION **CLARITHROMYCIN**

One RCT found that clarithromycin reduced the incidence of *M avium* complex (MAC) compared with placebo. One RCT found that both clarithromycin and clarithromycin plus rifabutin reduced the incidence of MAC compared with rifabutin alone.

Benefits: **Versus placebo:** We found one systematic review (search date 1997) of prophylaxis and treatment of MAC.[28] It identified one RCT (682 people with advanced AIDS) that found that clarithromycin significantly reduced the incidence of MAC compared with placebo (6% with clarithromycin *v* 16% with placebo; HR 0.31, 95% CI 0.18 to 0.53). It found no significant difference in the death rate (32% *v* 41%; HR 0.75; P = 0.026).[29] **Versus rifabutin:** See benefits of rifabutin plus macrolides, p 844. **Versus rifabutin plus clarithromycin:** See benefits of rifabutin plus macrolides, p 844.

Harms: Adverse effects led to discontinuation of treatment in slightly more people taking clarithromycin than placebo (8% with clarithromycin *v* 6% with placebo; P = 0.45). More people taking clarithromycin suffered altered taste (11% *v* 2%) or rectal disorders (8% *v* 3%).[27] See also harms under rifabutin plus macrolides, p 844.

Comment: Prospective cohort studies found that the risk of disseminated MAC disease increased substantially with a lower CD4 count and was clinically important only for CD4 < 50/mm^3.[1] See role of highly active antiretroviral treatment in comment under azithromycin, p 841.

OPTION RIFABUTIN PLUS MACROLIDES

One RCT found that rifabutin plus clarithromycin reduced the incidence of *M avium* complex (MAC) compared with rifabutin alone. One RCT found that azithromycin plus rifabutin reduced the incidence of MAC compared with azithromycin alone or rifabutin alone. One systematic review and two subsequent RCTs found that toxicity, including uveitis, was more common with combination therapy than with clarithromycin or rifabutin alone.

Benefits: **Clarithromycin plus rifabutin:** We found no systematic review. One RCT (1178 people with AIDS) compared rifabutin versus clarithromycin versus clarithromycin plus rifabutin.[30] It found that the risk of MAC was significantly reduced in the clarithromycin alone group (RR 0.56 for clarithromycin *v* rifabutin; P = 0.005) and the combination group when compared with rifabutin alone (RR 0.43 for combination *v* rifabutin; P = 0.0003). There was no significant difference in the risk of MAC between the combination and clarithromycin arms (RR 0.79 combination *v* clarithromycin, P = 0.36). **Azithromycin plus rifabutin:** One RCT (693 HIV positive people) found that the combination of azithromycin plus rifabutin versus azithromycin alone or rifabutin alone reduced the incidence of MAC at 1 year (15.3% with rifabutin *v* 7.6% with azithromycin *v* 2.8% with combination; HR 0.53 azithromycin *v* rifabutin, P = 0.008; HR 0.28 combination *v* rifabutin, P < 0.001; HR 0.53 combination *v* azithromycin, P = 0.03).[17]

Harms: In one RCT, dose limiting toxicity was more likely with azithromycin plus rifabutin than with azithromycin alone (HR 1.67; P = 0.03).[17] In another RCT, adverse events occurred in 31% of people receiving the combination of clarithromycin and rifabutin compared with 16% on clarithromycin alone and 18% on rifabutin alone (P < 0.001).[30] Uveitis occurred in 42 people: 33 were on clarithromycin plus rifabutin, seven were on rifabutin alone, and two were on clarithromycin alone. **Uveitis:** We found one systematic review (search date 1994, 54 people with rifabutin associated uveitis).[31] It found that uveitis was dose dependent. It occurred from 2 weeks to more than 7 months after initiation of rifabutin treatment, and was more likely in people taking rifabutin and clarithromycin. In most people, uveitis resolved 1–2 months after discontinuation of rifabutin.

Comment: Prospective cohort studies found that the risk of disseminated MAC disease increased substantially with a lower CD4 count and was clinically important only for CD4 < 50/mm^3.[1] Clarithromycin may inhibit rifabutin metabolism; rifabutin may decrease levels of delavirdine and saquinavir. See role of highly active antiretroviral treatment in comment under azithromycin, p 841.

QUESTION What are the effects of prophylaxis for disseminated *M avium* complex (MAC) disease for people with previous MAC disease?

OPTION COMBINATION TREATMENT

One RCT found that adding ethambutol to clarithromycin and clofazimine reduced *M avium* complex (MAC) relapse compared with clarithromycin plus clofazimine. One RCT found that adding clofazimine to clarithromycin and ethambutol was associated with higher mortality. One RCT found that clarithromycin, rifabutin and ethambutol reduced MAC relapse compared with clarithromycin plus clofazimine. One RCT found no significant difference in survival by adding rifabutin to clarithromycin plus ethambutol.

Benefits: We found no systematic review but found four RCTs.[32–35] **Clarithromycin, clofazimine, and ethambutol versus clarithromycin and clofazimine:** The first RCT (95 people) found that the combination of clarithromycin 1000 mg daily, clofazimine, and ethambutol was associated with significantly fewer relapses of MAC than the combination of clarithromycin plus clofazimine without ethambutol (68% relapsed in 3 drug regimen *v* 12% in 2 drug regimen at 36 weeks; P = 0.004).[32] **Clarithromycin, clofazimine, and ethambutol versus clarithromycin and ethambutol:** The second RCT (106 people) found that the addition of clofazimine to clarithromycin and ethambutol did not improve clinical response and was associated with higher mortality (see harms below).[33] **Clarithromycin, rifabutin, and ethambutol versus clarithromycin and clofazimine:** The third RCT (144 people) found that the combination of clarithromycin, rifabutin, and ethambutol reduced the relapse rate of MAC compared with clarithromycin plus clofazimine.[34] **Clarithromycin and ethambutol versus rifabutin, clarithromycin, and ethambutol:** The fourth RCT (198 people) found no significant difference in survival between people taking clarithromycin plus ethambutol and people taking clarithromycin plus ethambutol plus rifabutin.[35]

Harms: The second RCT, which added clofazimine to clarithromycin plus rifabutin, found higher mortality in the clofazimine arm (62% with clofazimine *v* 38% without clofazimine; P = 0.012).[33] High doses of clarithromycin (1000 mg twice daily)[36,37] and clofazimine[33] increased mortality. One RCT (85 people) comparing clarithromycin 500 mg twice daily versus 1000 mg twice daily found that, after a median follow up of 4.5 months, more people died with the higher dose (17/40 [43%] with 1000 mg twice daily *v* 10/45 [22%] with 500 mg twice daily; ARI 20%, 95% CI 0.2% to 33%; NNH 5, 95% CI 3 to 470).[36] A similar difference was seen in another RCT (154 people).[37] Combinations of drugs may lead to increased toxicity. Optic neuropathy may occur with ethambutol, but has not been reported in RCTs in people with HIV, where the dose and symptoms were carefully monitored.[35,36]

Comment: The observed increased mortality associated with clofazimine and high doses of clarithromycin has led to avoidance of these drugs.

QUESTION **What are the effects of prophylaxis for cytomegalovirus (CMV), herpes simplex virus (HSV), and varicella zoster virus (VZV)?**

OPTION **GANCICLOVIR**

One RCT found that oral ganciclovir reduced the incidence of cytomegalovirus (CMV) in people with severe CD4 depletion compared with placebo. It found that 26% of people who took ganciclovir developed severe neutropenia. A second RCT found no significant difference in prevention of CMV between ganciclovir and placebo.

Benefits: We found no systematic review. **Versus placebo:** We found two RCTs.[38,39] The first RCT (725 people with a median CD4 count of 22/mm^3) found that oral ganciclovir halved the incidence of CMV compared with placebo (event rate 16% with ganciclovir *v* 30% with placebo; P = 0.001).[38] The second RCT (994 HIV-1 infected people with CD4 < 100/mm^3 and CMV seropositivity) found no significant difference in the rate of CMV in people taking oral ganciclovir compared with placebo (event rates 13.1 *v* 14.6 per 100 person years; HR 0.92, 95% CI 0.65 to 1.27).[39] Both RCTs found no significant difference in overall mortality.

Harms: In the first RCT, severe neutropenia that required granulocyte colony stimulating factor was more common with ganciclovir compared with placebo (24% v 9%).[38]

Comment: Differences in the results of RCTs may have arisen by chance or owing to protocol variability; for example, no baseline ophthalmologic examinations were performed in the second trial.[39] The low incidence of CMV disease in people taking highly active antiretroviral treatment, and the high rates of adverse events, means that the clinical value of oral ganciclovir in people who have not had active CMV disease is unclear.

OPTION ACICLOVIR

One systematic review found that aciclovir did not reduce the incidence of cytomegalovirus (CMV) disease, but reduced herpes simplex virus (HSV) and varicella zoster virus (VZV) infection and overall mortality in people at different clinical stages of HIV infection compared with placebo. One RCT found that valaciclovir reduced the incidence of CMV disease more than aciclovir, but non-significantly increased mortality.

Benefits: **Versus placebo:** We found one systematic review of individual patient data (search date not stated, 8 RCTs) in people with HIV infection (ranging from asymptomatic infection to full-blown AIDS).[40] It found no significant difference in protection against CMV disease between aciclovir compared with no treatment or placebo. However, aciclovir significantly reduced overall mortality (RR 0.81; $P = 0.04$) and HSV and VZV infections ($P < 0.001$ for both).[40] **Aciclovir versus valaciclovir:** One RCT (1227 CMV seropositive people with CD4 < 100/mm^3) compared valaciclovir, high dose aciclovir, and low dose aciclovir. It found increased mortality in the valaciclovir group, which did not reach statistical significance ($P = 0.06$).[41] The CMV rate was lower in the valaciclovir group than the aciclovir groups (12% v 18%; $P = 0.03$).

Harms: One RCT found that toxicity and early medication discontinuations were significantly more frequent in the valaciclovir arm (1 year discontinuation rate: 51% for valaciclovir v 46% for high dose aciclovir v 41% for low dose aciclovir).[39]

Comment: The survival benefit with aciclovir is unclear. The absolute risk reduction may be higher in people who have frequent HSV or VZV infections.

OPTION FAMCICLOVIR

One small RCT found that famciclovir reduced the rate of viral shedding compared with placebo, but provided insufficient evidence on the effect of famciclovir on herpes simplex virus (HSV) recurrence.

Benefits: We found no systematic review. One small crossover placebo controlled RCT (48 people) found that famciclovir suppressed HSV in people with frequent recurrences (HSV was isolated in 9/1071 [0.8%] famciclovir days v 122/1114 [10.9%] placebo days; $P < 0.001$).[42] Breakthrough reactivations on famciclovir were short lived and often asymptomatic.

Harms: Famciclovir was well tolerated, and the incidence of adverse effects was similar in both groups.

Comment: The conclusions of this study are difficult to interpret. The randomisation process allocated participants to groups, but the intention to treat analysis involved the number of days with symptoms rather than the number of participants who improved. There was no assessment of statistical significance of clinical outcomes. The trial's analysis is impeded by a high withdrawal rate

QUESTION What are the effects of prophylaxis for invasive fungal disease in people without previous fungal disease?

OPTION AZOLES

RCTs in people with advanced HIV disease found that both fluconazole and itraconazole reduced the incidence of invasive fungal infections compared with placebo. One RCT found that fluconazole reduced the incidence of invasive fungal disease and mucocutaneous candidiasis compared with clotrimazole. One RCT found no difference between high and low dose fluconazole. Azoles have been associated with congenital problems and potentially serious interactions with other drugs.

Benefits: We found no systematic review. **Fluconazole versus placebo:** One RCT (323 women with CD4 ≤ 300/mm^3) found that fluconazole significantly reduced the incidence of candidiasis compared with placebo (44% with fluconazole *v* 58% with placebo suffered at least 1 episode of candidiasis; RR 0.56, 95% CI 0.41 to 0.77).[43] **Itraconazole versus placebo:** We found three RCTs.[44–46] The first RCT (295 people with advanced HIV disease) found that itraconazole reduced the incidence of invasive fungal infections (P = 0.0007).[44] It found no significant effect on recurrent or refractory candidiasis. The second RCT (129 people with CD4 cell count < 200/mm^3) also found that itraconazole reduced invasive fungal infections compared with placebo after a median of about 40 weeks (AR 1.6% with itraconazole *v* 16.7% with placebo; RR 0.1; P = 0.003; CI not reported).[45] In the third RCT (344 people with CD4 cell count < 300/mm^3), itraconazole did not significantly reduce invasive fungal infections compared with placebo (AR 5.9% with itraconazole *v* 7.0% with placebo; P = 0.42).[46] However, the study may have lacked power to detect clinically important differences. **High dose versus low dose fluconazole:** One RCT (636 people) compared fluconazole 200 mg daily with 400 mg once weekly and found no difference in the rate of invasive fungal infections over a follow up of 74 weeks (8% *v* 6%; ARR +2.2%, 95% CI –1.7% to +6.%).[47] However, the incidence of candidiasis was twice as common in people taking the weekly dose. **Fluconazole versus clotrimazole troches:** One RCT found that fluconazole reduced the incidence of invasive fungal disease and mucocutaneous candidal infections compared with clotrimazole (4% *v* 11%; HR 3.3, 95% CI 1.5 to 7.6).[48]

Harms: Congenital anomalies have occurred in a few children born to mothers receiving fluconazole. Itraconazole is embryotoxic and teratogenic in animals. Trials have therefore excluded pregnant women. Azoles may interact with antiretroviral regimens.[49] Azole drugs inhibit the metabolism of some drugs such as terfenadine. Theoretically they may increase the risk of sudden death because of ventricular tachycardia.

Comment: Azoles effectively reduce invasive fungal disease. Any absolute benefit is probably even lower in people treated with highly active antiretroviral treatment. Lack of evidence of any survival benefit, potential for complex drug interactions with current antiretroviral regimens, and potential for developing resistant fungal isolates means that there is doubt about routine antifungal prophylaxis in HIV infected people without previous invasive fungal disease.

QUESTION **What are the effects of prophylaxis for invasive fungal disease in people with previous fungal disease?**

OPTION **AZOLES**

Two RCTs found that itraconazole reduced the incidence of relapse of *P marneffei* infection and candidiasis compared with placebo. One RCT found that itraconazole increased the relapse of cryptococcal meningitis compared with fluconazole. We found no RCTs on intraconazole for histoplasmosis.

Benefits: We found no systematic review. **Itraconazole versus placebo:** One RCT (71 people with AIDS in Asia) found that itraconazole significantly reduced the relapse of *P marneffei* infection**G** compared with placebo (0/36 [0%] with itraconazole *v* 20/35 [57%] with placebo relapsed within 1 year; P < 0.001).[50] A second RCT (44 people with HIV infection and candidiasis, treated with itraconazole 200 mg for 4 weeks before randomisation) compared prophylaxis with itraconazole versus placebo for 24 weeks. It found that itraconazole reduced relapse rates (5/24 [21%] with itraconazole v 14/20 [70%] with placebo; ARR 49%, 95% CI 19% to 64%; NNT 2, 95% CI 2 to 5) and increased the time interval before relapse occurred (median time to relapse: itraconazole 8.0 weeks v placebo 10.4 weeks; P = 0.001).[51] **Itraconazole versus fluconazole:** One RCT (108 people with HIV infection) found that fluconazole reduced relapses of successfully treated cryptococcal meningitis compared with itraconazole (13/57 [23%] with itraconazole v 2/51 [4%] with fluconazole; ARR 19%, 95% CI 6.2% to 31.7%; RR 0.17, 95% CI 0.04 to 0.71; NNT 5, 95% CI 3 to 16).[52] The trial was stopped early because of the higher rate of relapse with itraconazole.

Harms: In one RCT, discontinuation of itraconazole occurred in two people because of skin rashes, one because of severe anaemia, and one because of gastrointestinal effects compared with none taking fluconazole.[52]

Comment: Recurrent infection is common in people with previous *C neoformans*, *H capsulatum*, and *P marneffei* infections. Lifelong maintenance may be needed in the presence of immune impairment.

QUESTION **What are the effects of discontinuing prophylaxis against opportunistic pathogens in people on highly active antiretroviral treatment (HAART)?**

OPTION **DISCONTINUING PROPHYLAXIS FOR *P CARINII* PNEUMONIA (PCP) AND TOXOPLASMOSIS**

One systematic review of two unblinded RCTs in people with CD4 > 200/mm^3 taking HAART found that discontinuation of prophylaxis did not increase the incidence of PCP. Two unblinded RCTs found that discontinuation of prophylaxis did not increase the incidence of toxoplasmosis.

Benefits: **PCP:** We found one systematic review (search date 2001, 2 RCTs, 3584 people, 2 non-randomised controlled trials, and 10 studies with other designs) about the effects of discontinuing prophylaxis.[53] The review found a low incidence of PCP in people discontinuing both primary and secondary prophylaxis after a mean of 1.5 years (7/3035 [0.23%] with discontinuing primary prophylaxis and 1/549 [0.18%] discontinuing secondary prophylaxis; mean annual incidence over 1.5 years 0.23%, 95% CI 0.10% to 0.46%; no statistical heterogeneity among studies). Neither of the two RCTs identified in the review found any cases of PCP after discontinuation (first RCT: 587 people with satisfactory response to HAART, CD4 > 200/mm^3, and viral load < 5000 copies/mm^3 for > 3 months, AR for PCP or toxoplasma encephalitis at median 20 months 0%, whether or not prophylaxis continued;[54] second RCT: 708 people taking HAART, CD4 > 200/mm^3 for 3 months, AR for PCP at 6 months 0%).[55] **Toxoplasmosis:** We found two RCTs.[55,56] The first, which was included in the systematic review, found no cases of toxoplasma encephalitis at 6 months in people discontinuing prophylaxis (see PCP above).[55] The second RCT (302 people with a satisfactory response to HAART) compared discontinuation versus continuation of toxoplasma prophylaxis.[56] After a median of 10 months it found no episodes of toxoplasma encephalitis in either group.

Harms: The systematic review found no direct harms from discontinuing prophylaxis.[53]

Comment: The risk of PCP may increase after discontinuing prophylaxis in people who do not respond to antiretroviral treatment. We found no direct evidence of the effects of different HAART regimens on the risk of PCP or toxoplasmosis. Antiretroviral regimens with different mechanisms of action may have different clinical effects on opportunistic infections and HIV disease progression, despite inducing satisfactory suppression of HIV-1 replication and adequate CD4 responses. Also, CD4 cell count is an incomplete marker of immune reconstitution. It is possible that people with the same CD4 count may have different immune deficits regarding control of PCP and other opportunistic pathogens. An extensive amount of research is being conducted on other parameters of immune reconstitution, but the clinical implications are uncertain at present. One decision analysis based on the systematic review suggested that, in the long term, discontinuation of PCP prophylaxis in people who respond to HAART should result in fewer PCP episodes and fewer prophylaxis related adverse effects.[53]

OPTION DISCONTINUING PROPHYLAXIS FOR *M AVIUM* COMPLEX (MAC)

Two RCTs in people with CD4 > 100/mm^3 taking HAART found that discontinuation of prophylaxis for MAC disease did not increase the incidence of MAC disease.

Benefits: We found no systematic review but we found two RCTs. The first RCT (520 people without previous MAC disease, with CD4 > 100/mm^3 in response to HAART) compared azithromycin with placebo.[57] There were no episodes of confirmed MAC disease in either group over a median follow up of 12 months. The second RCT (643 people with CD4 > 100/mm^3 in response to HAART) compared azithromycin 1200 mg once weekly versus placebo. Over a median follow up of 16 months there was no significant difference in the incidence of MAC between the groups (2/321 [0.62%] with placebo *v* 0/322 [0%] with azithromycin; difference +0.5 events per 100 person years, 95% CI –0.2 to +1.2 events per 100 person years).[58]

Harms: In both RCTs, adverse effects leading to discontinuation of treatment were more common with azithromycin than with placebo (7% *v* 1%, P = 0.002; 8% *v* 2%, P < 0.001).[57,58]

Comment: It is not clear whether different antiretroviral regimens have different clinical effects on opportunistic infections and on the need for specific prophylaxis.

OPTION DISCONTINUING PROPHYLAXIS FOR CYTOMEGALOVIRUS (CMV)

We found insufficient evidence on the effects of discontinuation of maintenance treatment for CMV retinitis or other end organ disease in people with CD4 > 100/mm³ taking HAART.

Benefits: We found no systematic review or RCTs.

Harms: We found no evidence from systematic reviews or RCTs.

Comment: We found several small case series (see table 1, p 853).[59–68] Of the two studies with the longest follow-up, one found no relapses in 41 people after a mean of 20.4 months from discontinuing maintenance treatment[59] and the other found only 1 relapse among 36 people after a median follow up of 21 months from discontinuing treatment.[68] The relapse occurred in a person with immunological failure (CD4 62/mm³). However, another study with mean follow up of 14.5 months found five (29%) relapses among 17 participants who withdrew from maintenance; all of them occurred after the CD4 cell count had dropped again to below 50/mm³ (8 days/10 months after this event).[62] In one case series, 12/14 (86%) participants had evidence of immune reconstitution retinitis even before starting withdrawal of prophylaxis.[61] Worsening uveitis was associated with a substantial vision loss (> 3 lines) in three participants. It is difficult to conduct a RCT with adequate power to exclude modest differences in relapse rates. The observational evidence suggests that withdrawal of CMV maintenance treatment may be considered in selected people in whom CMV disease is in remission, CD4 > 100mm³, and HIV replication remains suppressed. We found no clear evidence on whether CMV viral load should be considered in the decision to withdraw from maintenance. One small case series found that relapses were associated with a drop in the CD4 cell count.[62] However, we found no randomised or other reliable evidence about when to restart CMV maintenance treatment.

GLOSSARY

***Penicillium marneffei* infection** A common opportunistic infection in South East Asia.

The WHO staging system for HIV infection and disease consists of a "clinical axis" that is represented by a sequential list of clinical conditions believed to have prognostic significance, which subdivides the course of HIV infection into four clinical stages; and a "laboratory axis" that subdivides each clinical stage into three strata according to CD4 cell count or total lymphocyte count.

REFERENCES

1. Gallant JE, Moore RD, Chaisson RE. Prophylaxis for opportunistic infections in patients with HIV infection. *Ann Intern Med* 1994;120:932–944.
2. Detels R, Tarwater P, Phair JP, et al. Effectiveness of potent antiretroviral therapies on the incidence of opportunistic infections before and after AIDS diagnosis. *AIDS* 2001;15:347–355.
3. Ioannidis JPA, Cappelleri JC, Skolnik PR, et al. A meta-analysis of the relative efficacy and toxicity of *Pneumocystis carinii* prophylactic regimens. *Arch Intern Med* 1996;156;177–188. Search date 1995; primary sources Medline and conference abstracts.
4. Bucher HC, Griffith L, Guyatt GH, et al. Meta-analysis of prophylactic treatments against *Pneumocystis carinii* pneumonia and toxoplasma encephalitis in HIV-infected patients. *J Acquir Immune Defic Syndr Hum Retrovirol* 1997;15:104–114. Search date not stated; primary sources Medline, Aidsline, Aidstrials, Aidsdrugs, screening the Proceedings of the International and European Conferences on AIDS, bibliographies of identified trials, and by contacting experts.
5. Fischl MA, Dickinson GM, La Voie L. Safety and efficacy of sulfamethoxazole and trimethoprim chemoprophylaxis for *Pneumocystis carinii* pneumonia in AIDS. *JAMA* 1988;259:1185–1189.
6. Anglaret X, Chene G, Attia A, et al. Early chemoprophylaxis with trimethroprim-sulphamethoxazole for HIV-1-infected adults in Abidjan, Cote d'Ivoire: a randomized trial. *Lancet* 1999;353:1463–1468.
7. El-Sadr W, Luskin-Hawk R, Yurik TM, et al. A randomized trial of daily and thrice weekly trimethoprim-sulfamethoxazole for the prevention of *Pneumocystis carinii* pneumonia in HIV-infected individuals. *Clin Infect Dis* 1999;29:775–783.
8. Leoung GS, Stanford JF, Giordano MF, et al. Trimethoprim-sulfamethoxazole (TMP-SMZ) dose escalation versus direct rechallenge for *Pneumocystis carinii* pneumonia prophylaxis in human immunodeficiency virus-infected patients with previous adverse reaction to TMP-SMZ. *J Infect Dis* 2001;184:992–997.
9. Para MF, Finkelstein D, Becker S, et al. Reduced toxicity with gradual initiation of

trimethoprim-sulfamethoxazole for *Pneumocystis carinii* pneumonia. *J Acquir Immune Defic Syndr* 2000;24:337–343.

10. Walmsley SL, Khorasheh S, Singer J, et al. A randomized trial of N-acetylcysteine for prevention of trimethoprim-sulfamethoxazole hypersensitivity reactions in *Pneumocystis carinii* pneumonia prophylaxis (CTN057). Canadian HIV Trials Network 057 Study Group. *J Acquir Immune Defic Syndr Hum Retrovirol* 1998;19:498–505.
11. Akerlund B, Tynell E, Bratt G, et al. N-acetylcysteine treatment and the risk of toxic reactions to trimethoprim-sulphamethoxazole in primary *Pneumocystis carinii* prophylaxis in HIV-infected patients. *J Infect* 1997;35:143–147.
12. Saillour-Glenisson F, Chene G, Salmi LR, et al. Effect of dapsone on survival in HIV-infected patients: a meta-analysis. *Rev Epidemiol Sante Publique* 2000;48:17–30. Search date 1996; primary sources Medline, Aidstrials, Aidsdrugs, registries of clinical trials, abstracts from international AIDS conferences and infectious diseases meetings, and consultation with active experts.
13. Maynart M, Lievre L, Sow PS, et al. Primary prevention with cotrimoxazole for HIV-1-infected adults: results of the pilot study in Dakar, Senegal. *J Acquir Immune Defic Syndr* 2001;26:130–136.
14. El Sadr WM, Murphy RL, Yurik TM, et al. Atovaquone compared with dapsone for the prevention of *Pneumocystis carinii* pneumonia in patients with HIV infection who cannot tolerate trimethoprim, sulfonamides, or both. Community Programs for Clinical Research on AIDS and the AIDS Clinical Trials Group. *N Engl J Med* 1998;339:1889–1895.
15. Chan C, Montaner J, Lefebre EA, et al. Atovaquone suspension compared with aerosolized pentamidine for prevention of *Pneumocystis carinii* in human immunodeficiency virus-infected subjects intolerant of trimethoprim or sulfonamides. *J Infect Dis* 1999;180:369–376.
16. Dunne MW, Bozzette S, McCutchan JA, et al. Efficacy of azithromycin in prevention of *Pneumocystis carinii* pneumonia: a randomized trial. California Collaborative Treatment Group. *Lancet* 1999;354:891–895.
17. Havlir DV, Dube MP, Sattler FR, et al. Prophylaxis against disseminated *Mycobacterium avium* complex with weekly azithromycin, daily rifabutin, or both. California Collaborative Treatment Group. *N Engl J Med* 1996;335:392–398.
18. Wilkinson D. Drugs for preventing tuberculosis in HIV infected persons. In: The Cochrane Library, Issue 4, 2001. Oxford: Update Software. Search date 2000; primary sources Cochrane Infectious Diseases Group Trials Register, Cochrane Controlled Trials Register Issue 3, Embase, and hand searched references.
19. Quigley MA, Mwinga A, Hosp M, et al. Long-term effect of preventive therapy for tuberculosis in a cohort of HIV infected Zambian adults. *AIDS* 2001;15:215–222.
20. Fitzgerald DW, Severe P, Joseph P, et al. No effect of isoniazid prophylaxis for purified protein derivative negative HIV-infected adults living in a country with endemic tuberculosis: results of a randomised trial. *J Acquir Immune Defic Syndr* 2001;28:305–307.
21. Selwyn PA, Hartel D, Lewis VA, et al. A prospective study of the risk of tuberculosis among intravenous drug users with human immunodeficiency virus infection. *N Engl J Med* 1989;320:545–550.
22. Halsey NA, Coberly JS, Desmormeaux J, et al. Randomised trial of isoniazid versus rifampicin and pyrazinamide for prevention of tuberculosis in HIV-1 infection. *Lancet* 1998;351:786–792.
23. Mwinga A, Hosp M, Godfrey-Faussett P, et al. Twice weekly tuberculosis preventive therapy in HIV infection in Zambia. *AIDS* 1998;12:2447–2457.
24. Gordin F, Chaisson RE, Matts JP, et al. Rifampin and pyrazinamide vs isoniazid for prevention of tuberculosis in HIV-infected persons: an international randomized trial. *JAMA* 2000;283:1445–1450.
25. Whalen CC, Johson JL, Okwera A, et al. A trial of three regimens to prevent tuberculosis in Ugandan adults with the human immunodeficiency virus. *N Engl Med* 1997;337:801–808.
26. Alfaro EM, Cuadra F, Solera J, et al. Assessment of two chemoprophylaxis regimens for tuberculosis in HIV-infected patients. *Med Clin* 2000;115:161–165.
27. Oldfield EC, Fessel WJ, Dunne MW, et al. Once weekly azithromycin therapy for prevention of *Mycobacterium avium* complex infection in patients with AIDS: a randomized, double-blind, placebo-controlled multicenter trial. *Clin Infect Dis* 1998;26:611–619.
28. Faris MA, Raasch RH, Hopfer RL, et al. Treatment and prophylaxis of disseminated *Mycobacterium avium* complex in HIV-infected individuals. *Ann Pharmacother* 1998;32:564–573. Search date 1997; primary sources Medline and Aidsline.
29. Pierce M, Crampton S, Henry D, et al. A randomized trial of clarithromycin as prophylaxis against disseminated *Mycobacterium avium* complex infection in patients with advanced immunodeficiency syndrome. *N Engl J Med* 1996;335:384–391.
30. Benson CA, Williams PL, Cohn DL, et al. Clarithromycin or rifabutin alone or in combination for primary prophylaxis of *Mycobacterium avium* complex disease in patients with AIDS: a randomized, double-blind, placebo-controlled trial. *J Infect Dis* 2000;181:1289–1297.
31. Tseng AL, Walmsley SL. Rifabutin-associated uveitis. *Ann Pharmacother* 1995;29:1149–1155. Search date 1994; primary sources Medline and hand searches of reference lists and conference abstracts.
32. Dube MP, Sattler FR, Torriani FJ, et al. A randomized evaluation of ethambutol for prevention of relapse and drug resistance during treatment of *Mycobacterium avium* complex bacteremia with clarithromycin-based combination therapy. *J Infect Dis* 1997;176:1225–1232.
33. Chaisson RE, Keiser P, Pierce M, et al. Clarithromycin and ethambutol with or without clofazimine for the treatment of bacteremic *Mycobacterium avium* complex disease in patients with HIV infection. *AIDS* 1997;11:311–317.
34. May T, Brel F, Beuscart C, et al. Comparison of combination therapy regimens for the treatment of human immunodeficiency virus-infected patients with disseminated bacteremia due to *Mycobacterium avium*. ANRS Trial 033 Curavium Group. Agence Nationale de Reserche sur le Sida. *Clin Infect Dis* 1997;25:621–629.
35. Gordin F, Sullam P, Shafran S, et al. A placebo-controlled trial of rifabutin added to a regimen of clarithromycin and ethambutol in the treatment of *M. avium* complex bacteremia. *Clin Infect Dis* 1999;28:1080–1085.
36. Cohn DL, Fisher EJ, Peng GT, et al. A prospective randomized trial of four three-drug regimens in the treatment of disseminated *Mycobacterium avium* complex disease in AIDS patients: excess mortality associated with high-dose clarithromycin. Terry Beirn Programs for Clinical Research on AIDS. *Clin Infect Dis* 1999;29:125–133.
37. Chaisson RE, Benson CA, Dube MP, et al. Clarithromycin therapy for bacteremic *Mycobacterium avium* complex disease: a randomized, double-blind, dose-ranging study in patients with AIDS. *Ann Intern Med* 1994;121:905–911.
38. Spector SA, McKinley GF, Lalezari JP, et al. Oral ganciclovir for the prevention of cytomegalovirus disease in persons with AIDS. Roche Cooperative Oral Ganciclovir Study Group. *N Engl J Med* 1996;334:1491–1497.
39. Brosgart CL, Louis TA, Hillman DW, et al. A randomized, placebo-controlled trial of the safety and efficacy of oral ganciclovir for prophylaxis of cytomegalovirus disease in HIV-infected individuals. Terry Beirn Community Programs for Clinical Research on AIDS. *AIDS* 1998;12:269–277.

40. Ioannidis JPA, Collier AC, Cooper DA, et al. Clinical efficacy of high-dose acyclovir in patients with human immunodeficiency virus infection: a meta-analysis of randomized individual patient data. *J Infect Dis* 1998;178:349–359. Search date not stated; primary sources Medline, abstract searching from major meetings, trial directories, and communication with experts, investigators of the identified trials, and industry researchers.
41. Feinberg JE, Hurwitz S, Cooper D, et al. A randomized, double-blind trial of valaciclovir prophylaxis for cytomegalovirus disease in patients with advanced human immunodeficiency virus infection. AIDS Clinical Trials Group Protocol 204/Glaxo Wellcome 123–014 International CMV Prophylaxis Study Group. *J Infect Dis* 1998;177:48–56.
42. Schacker T, Hu HL, Koelle DM, et al. Famciclovir for the suppression of symptomatic and asymptomatic herpes simplex virus reactivation in HIV-infected persons: a double-blind, placebo-controlled trial. *Ann Intern Med* 1998;128:21–28.
43. Schuman P, Capps L, Peng G, et al. Weekly fluconazole for the prevention of mucosal candidiasis in women with HIV infection: a randomized, double-blind, placebo-controlled trial. *Ann Intern Med* 1997;126:689–696.
44. McKinsey DS, Wheat LJ, Cloud GA, et al. Itraconazole prophylaxis for fungal infections in patients with advanced human immunodeficiency virus infection: randomized, placebo-controlled, double-blind study. National Institute of Allergy and Infectious diseases Mycoses Study Group. *Clin Infect Dis* 1999;28:1049–1056.
45. Chariyalertsak S, Supperatpinyo K, Sirisanthana T, et al. A controlled trial of itraconazole as primary prophylaxis for systemic fungal infections in patients with advanced human immunodeficiency virus infection in Thailand. *Clin Infect Dis* 2002;34:277–284.
46. Smith DE, Bell J, Johnson M, et al. A randomized, double-blind, placebo-controlled study of itraconazole capsules for the prevention of deep fungal infections in immunodeficient patients with HIV infection. *HIV Med* 2001;2:78–83.
47. Havlir DV, Dube MP, McCutchan JA, et al. Prophylaxis with weekly versus daily fluconazole for fungal infections in patients with AIDS. *Clin Infect Dis* 1998;27:253–256.
48. Powderly WG, Finkelstein DM, Feinberg J, et al. A randomized trial comparing fluconazole with clotrimazole troches for the prevention of fungal infections in patients with advanced human immunodeficiency virus infection. *N Engl J Med* 1995;332:700–705.
49. Tseng AL, Foisy MM. Management of drug interactions in patients with HIV. *Ann Pharmacother* 1997;31:1040–1058.
50. Supparatpinyo K, Perriens J, Nelson KE, et al. A controlled trial of itraconazole to prevent relapse of Penicillium marneffei infection in patients with the human immunodeficiency virus. *N Engl J Med* 1998;339:1739–1743.
51. Smith D, Midgley J, Gazzard B. A randomized, double-blind study of itraconazole versus placebo in the treatment and prevention of oral or oesophageal candidosis in patients with HIV infection. *Int J Clin Pract* 1999;53:349–352.
52. Saag MS, Cloud GA, Graybill JR, et al. A comparison of itraconazole versus fluconazole as maintenance therapy for AIDS associated cryptococcal meningitis. *Clin Infect Dis* 1999;28:291–296.
53. Trikalinos TA, Ioannidis JPA. Discontinuation of *Pneumocystis carinii* prophylaxis in patients infected with human immunodeficiency virus: a meta-analysis and decision analysis. *Clin Infect dis* 2001;33:1901–1909. Search date 2001; primary sources Medline, Aidsline, Embase, and abstracts from major meetings.
54. Lopez Bernaldo de Quiros JC, Miro JM, Pena JM, et al. A randomized trial of the discontinuation of primary and secondary prophylaxis against *Pneumocystis carinii* pneumonia after highly active antiretroviral therapy in patients with HIV infection. *N Engl J Med* 2001;344:159–167.
55. Mussini C, Pezzotti P, Govoni A, et al. Discontinuation of primary prophylaxis for *Pneumocystis carinii* pneumonia and toxoplasmic encephalitis in human immunodeficiency virus type I-infected patients: the changes in opportunistic prophylaxis study. *J Infect Dis* 2000;181:1635–1642.
56. Miro JM, Lopez JC, Podzamczer D, et al, and the GESIDA 04/98B study group. Discontinuation of toxoplasmic encephalitis prophylaxis is safe in HIV-1 and *T. gondii* co-infected patients after immunological recovery with HAART. Preliminary results of the GESIDA 04/98B study. In: Abstracts of the 7th Conference on Retroviruses and Opportunistic Infections, Alexandria, Virginia: Foundation for Retrovirology and Human Health. Abstract no. 230.
57. El-Sadr WM, Burman WJ, Grant LB, et al. Discontinuation of prophylaxis for *Mycobacterium avium* complex disease in HIV-infected patients who have a response to antiretroviral therapy. *N Engl J Med* 2000;342:1085–1092.
58. Currier JS, Williams PL, Koletar SL, et al. Discontinuation of Mycobacterium avium complex prophylaxis in patients with antiretroviral therapy-induced increases in CD4+ cell count. A randomized, double-blind, placebo-controlled trial. *Ann Intern Med* 2000;133:493–503.
59. Curi AL, Muralha A, Muralha L, et al. Suspension of anticytomegalovirus maintenance therapy following immune recovery due to highly active antiretroviral therapy. *Br J Ophthalmol* 2001;85:471–473.
60. Jouan M, Saves M, Tubiana R, et al. Discontinuation of maintenance therapy for cytomegalovirus in HIV-infected patients receiving highly active antiretroviral therapy. RESTIMOP study team. *AIDS* 2001;15:23–31.
61. Whitcup SM, Fortin E, Lindblad AS, et al. Discontinuation of anticytomegalovirus therapy in patients with HIV infection and cytomegalovirus retinitis. *JAMA* 1999;282:1633–1637.
62. Torriani FJ, Freeman WR, MacDonald JC, et al. CMV retinitis recurs after stopping treatment in virological and immunological failure of potent antiretroviral therapy. *AIDS* 2000;14:173–180.
63. Postelmans L, Gerald M, Sommereijns B, et al. Discontinuation of maintenance therapy for CMV retinitis in AIDS patients on highly active antiretroviral therapy. *Ocul Immunol Inflamm* 1999;7:199–203.
64. Jabs DA, Bolton SG, Dunn JP, et al. Discontinuing anticytomegalovirus therapy in patients with immune reconstitution after combination therapy. *Am J Opthalmol* 1998;126:817–822.
65. Vrabec TR, Baldassano VF, Whitcup SM. Discontinuation of maintenance therapy in patients with quiescent cytomegalovirus retinitis and elevated CD4+ counts. *Ophthalmology* 1998;105:1259–1264.
66. MacDonald JC, Torriani FJ, Morse LS, et al. Lack of reactivation of cytomegalovirus (CMV) retinitis after stopping CMV maintenance therapy in AIDS patients with sustained elevations in CD4 T cells in response to highly active antiretroviral therapy. *J Infect Dis* 1998;177:1182–1187.
67. Tural C, Romeu J, Sirera G, et al. Long-lasting remission of cytomegalovirus retinitis without maintenance therapy in human immunodeficiency virus-infected patients. *J Infect Dis* 1998;177:1080–1083.
68. Berenguer J, Gonzalez J, Pulido F, et al. Discontinuation of secondary prophylaxis in patients with cytomegalovirus retinitis who have responded to highly active antiretroviral therapy. *Clin Infect Dis* 2002;34:394–397.

HIV: prevention of opportunistic infections

John Ioannidis
Chairman
Department of Hygiene and Epidemiology
University of Ioannina School of Medicine, Ioannina, Greece

David Wilkinson
Pro Vice Chancellor and Vice President
Division of Health Sciences
University of South Australia, Adelaide, Australia

Competing interests: None declared.

We would like to acknowledge the previous contributors of this chapter, including Margaret Johnson and Andrew Phillips.

TABLE 1 **Observational studies of discontinuation of cytomegalovirus maintenance treatment in people with previous cytomegalovirus disease (see text, p 850).**

Ref	Criteria for discontinuation	Participants	Follow up (months)	Relapses
62*	CD4 >70	17	14.5 (mean)	5
63	CD4 ≥ 75	8	8 (median)	0
61	CD4 >150	14	16.4 (mean)	0
64	CD4 297 (median)	15	8 (median)	0
65	CD4 >100	8	11.4 (mean)	0
66*	CD4 183 (median)	11	5 (median)	0
67	CD4 >150 VL < 200/mL –ve CMV by PCR	7	9 (median)	0
59	CD4 > 143	41	20.4 (mean)	0
60	CD4 > 75 VL < 30 000/mL	48	11 (mean)	2
68	CD4 > 100 VL < 500 or CD4 >150 VL < 10 0000 copies/mL	36	21 (median)	1

Studies with more than five people are included. CD4 count is measured in cells/mm^3. *McDonald et al[66] is an early report of the same study followed by the Torriani et al[62] report. All relapses in the latter report occurred in people who had already experienced a decrease of CD4 to < 50 cells/mm^3. CMV, cytomegalovirus; PCR, polymerase chain reaction; Ref, reference; VL, viral load (HIV-1 RNA in plasma).

Pneumocystis pneumonia in people with HIV

Search date November 2004

Richard Bellamy

QUESTIONS

INTERVENTIONS

Covered elsewhere in *Clinical Evidence*

Prophylaxis for *Pneumocystis* pneumonia and other AIDS-related opportunistic infections (see HIV: prevention of opportunistic infections, p 834).

Key Messages

First line treatments

- **Atovaquone** We found no RCTs comparing atovaquone versus placebo or no treatment as the first line treatment for *Pneumocystis* pneumonia in people infected with HIV. One RCT found that atovaquone was less effective than trimethoprim–sulfamethoxazole. One RCT found that atovaquone was equally effective as intravenous pentamidine. Adverse effects requiring termination of treatment occurred less frequently with atovaquone than with trimethoprim–sulfamethoxazole or intravenous pentamidine.
- **Clindamycin–primaquine** We found no RCTs comparing clindamycin–primaquine versus placebo or no treatment as the first line treatment for *Pneumocystis* pneumonia in people infected with HIV. RCTs found clindamycin–primaquine was as effective as trimethoprim sulfamethoxazole and trimethoprim–dapsone and no significant difference in rates of serious adverse effects.
- **Pentamidine (aerosolised)** We found no RCTs comparing aerosolised pentamidine versus placebo or no treatment as first line treatment for *Pneumocystis* pneumonia in people infected with HIV. Two RCTs found no significant difference in mortality between aerosolised pentamidine and trimethoprim–sulfamethoxazole, but they found lower rates of serious adverse effects with aerosolised pentamidine. One RCT found no significant difference in mortality or treatment failure between aerosolised and intravenous pentamidine.

- **Pentamidine (intravenous)** We found no RCTs comparing intravenous pentamidine versus placebo or no treatment as first line treatment for *Pneumocystis* pneumonia in people infected with HIV. Two RCTs found no significant difference in mortality, treatment failure, or adverse effects between intravenous pentamidine and trimethoprim–sulfamethoxazole. However, a third RCT found that intravenous pentamidine increased mortality compared with trimethoprim–sulfamethoxazole. One RCT found no significant difference between intravenous pentamidine and atovaquone, but atovaquone caused fewer adverse effects requiring termination of treatment. One RCT found no significant difference in mortality or treatment failure between intravenous and aerosolised pentamidine.
- **Trimethoprim–dapsone** We found no RCTs comparing trimethoprim–dapsone versus placebo or no treatment as first line treatment for *Pneumocystis* pneumonia in people infected with HIV. RCTs have found that trimethoprim–dapsone was as effective as trimethoprim–sulfamethoxazole, with similar rates of adverse effects. One RCT found that trimethoprim–dapsone was as effective as clindamycin–primaquine.
- **Trimethoprim–sulfamethoxazole (co-trimoxazole)** We found no RCTs comparing trimethoprim–sulfamethoxazole versus placebo or no treatment as first line treatment for *Pneumocystis* pneumonia in people infected with HIV. One RCT found that trimethoprim–sulfamethoxazole was more effective than atovaquone. Two RCTs found no significant difference in mortality, treatment failure, or adverse effects between intravenous pentamidine and trimethoprim–sulfamethoxazole. However, a third RCT found that trimethoprim-sulfamethoxazole reduced mortality compared with intravenous pentamidine. RCTs have found that trimethoprim–sulfamethoxazole was as effective as clindamycin–primaquine and trimethoprim–dapsone, and aerosolised pentamidine. RCTs have found that adverse events requiring termination of treatment were more frequent with trimethoprim–sulfamethoxazole than atovaquone or aerosolised pentamidine.

Adjuvant corticosteroids in HIV

- **Adjuvant corticosteroids for moderate to severe *Pneumocystis* pneumonia** One systematic review found that adjuvant corticosteroids reduced mortality when used early in the treatment of moderate to severe *Pneumocystis* pneumonia (see definition, p 855).
- **Adjuvant corticosteroids for mild *Pneumocystis* pneumonia** We found insufficient evidence on the effects of adjuvant corticosteroids in the early treatment of mild *Pneumocystis* pneumonia in people infected with HIV (see definition, p 855).

Treatment if first line treatment fails

- **Treatment after failure of first line treatment** We found no systematic review and no RCTs comparing the effectiveness or adverse effects of different treatments after failure of first line treatment for *Pneumocystis* pneumonia in people infected with HIV. One systematic review of controlled studies, case series, and case reports suggested that clindamycin–primaquine may be more effective than alternative treatments in this situation.

DEFINITION *Pneumocystis* pneumonia (PCP) is caused by the opportunistic fungus *Pneumocystis jiroveci*. The infection occurs in people with impaired immune function. Most cases occur in people infected with HIV, in whom PCP is an AIDS defining illness. The pneumonia is generally classified as **mild** if P_aO_2 is greater than 70 mm Hg on room air, if the alveolar–arterial oxygen gradient is less than 35 mm Hg, or both. It is generally classified as **moderate/severe** if the P_aO_2 is less than 70 mm Hg, if the alveolar–arterial oxygen gradient is greater than 35 mm Hg, or both. This chapter focuses on the treatment of PCP in adults infected with HIV. Prevention of PCP is covered under HIV: prevention of opportunistic infections, p 834.

INCIDENCE/ PREVALENCE PCP is the most common AIDS defining illness in developed nations.[1] It is probably also common throughout the developing world, although the prevalence is harder to assess here because of difficulties in making the diagnosis. Before the widespread use of prophylaxis it was estimated that up to 80% of people with AIDS

Pneumocystis pneumonia in people with HIV

would eventually develop PCP.[2] Widespread use of prophylaxis against PCP and of highly active antiretroviral treatment has dramatically reduced the incidence of this infection (see HIV: prevention of opportunistic infections, p 834).

AETIOLOGY/ RISK FACTORS Risk factors for PCP include HIV infection, primary immune deficiencies, prematurity, cancer, use of immune suppressants after organ transplantation, and prolonged use of high dose corticosteroids. HIV infection is now responsible for the vast majority of cases of PCP. Among adults with HIV infection, those with a CD4 count below 200 cells per mm^3 are at highest risk, and the median CD4 count at diagnosis of PCP is about 50 cells per mm^3.[3]

PROGNOSIS It is generally believed that without treatment PCP would almost certainly be fatal in a person with AIDS. For ethical reasons, no studies have examined short term prognosis without treatment. People with AIDS and PCP frequently have other serious opportunistic infections, which can adversely affect their prognosis.

AIMS OF INTERVENTION To reduce mortality owing to PCP and minimise adverse effects of treatment.

OUTCOMES Mortality, treatment failure (requiring change of treatment), and adverse effects.

METHODS *Clinical Evidence* search and appraisal November 2004. We placed emphasis on systematic reviews of RCTs and large RCTs. We considered smaller RCTs and systematic reviews of non-controlled studies if large, placebo controlled RCTs were not available. Studies of the treatment of PCP can be hard to analyse because many participants swapped treatment arms if they did not respond to, or experienced toxicity with, their initial treatment allocation. Many studies allowed clinicians to use their own discretion when deciding if a change in treatment was warranted, without having rigorous, predefined criteria for the change. Some people may have changed treatments before they had adequate opportunity to respond to the initial treatment allocation. Mortality and treatment failure rates were usually compared on an intention to treat basis but many authors analysed adverse events using an on-treatment analysis. To ensure comparability between studies, all statistics comparing dichotomous outcomes were recalculated using $2 \times 2\ \chi^2$ tests with Yates' correction factor, except for comparisons where the sample size was less than 40, when Fisher's exact test was used. The studies reviewed in this chapter included only HIV infected people, except where otherwise specified. Most studies were carried out in the developed world, with an over-representation of white men. Although some studies included teenagers, there were few data from this group, and most studies excluded pregnant women and children; it was therefore hard to draw conclusions about the effects of treatment in these groups. Trimethoprim–sulfamethoxazole (TMP–SMX; co-trimoxazole) is generally regarded as the standard treatment for PCP, and most studies used this as their comparator.

QUESTION What are the effects of first line antipneumocystis treatments for *Pneumocystis* pneumonia in people infected with HIV?

OPTION TRIMETHOPRIM–SULFAMETHOXAZOLE (CO-TRIMOXAZOLE)

We found no RCTs comparing trimethoprim–sulfamethoxazole versus placebo or no treatment as first line treatment for *Pneumocystis* pneumonia in people infected with HIV. One RCT found that trimethoprim–sulfamethoxazole was more effective than atovaquone. Two RCTs found no significant difference in mortality, treatment failure, or adverse effects between intravenous pentamidine and trimethoprim–sulfamethoxazole. However, a third RCT found that trimethoprim-sulfamethoxazole reduced mortality compared with intravenous pentamidine. RCTs have found that trimethoprim–sulfamethoxazole was as effective as clindamycin–primaquine and trimethoprim–dapsone, and aerosolised pentamidine. RCTs have found that adverse events requiring termination of treatment were more frequent with trimethoprim–sulfamethoxazole than atovaquone or aerosolised pentamidine.

Benefits: We found no systematic review. **Versus placebo:** We found no RCTs. **Versus aerosolised pentamidine:** See benefits of aerosolised pentamidine, p 857. **Versus intravenous pentamidine:** See benefits of intravenous pentamidine, p 858. **Versus atovaquone:** See benefits of atovaquone, p 859. **Versus clindamycin–primaquine:** See benefits of clindamycin–primaquine, p 860. **Versus trimethoprim–dapsone:** See benefits of trimethoprim–dapsone, p 861.

Harms: We found no systematic review. The adverse effects requiring termination of treatment that most frequently occurred in people receiving trimethoprim–sulfamethoxazole were skin rashes, severe nausea and vomiting, raised liver enzymes, fever, and leucopaenia.[4–8] In some studies, nausea and vomiting were reported to occur in as many as 40% of people, causing termination of treatment in 5–10%.[4,5,7] Skin rashes occurred in as many as 30–45% of people, causing termination of treatment in 10–15%.[4,5,7,8] **Versus placebo:** We found no RCTs. **Versus aerosolised pentamidine:** See harms of aerosolised pentamidine, p 858. **Versus intravenous pentamidine:** See harms of intravenous pentamidine, p 859. **Versus atovaquone:** See harms of atovaquone, p 860. **Versus clindamycin–primaquine:** See harms of clindamycin–primaquine, p 861. **Versus trimethoprim–dapsone:** See harms of trimethoprim–dapsone, p 862.

Comment: None.

OPTION PENTAMIDINE (AEROSOLISED)

We found no RCTs comparing aerosolised pentamidine versus placebo or no treatment as first line treatment for *Pneumocystis* pneumonia in people infected with HIV. Two RCTs found no significant difference in mortality between aerosolised pentamidine and trimethoprim–sulfamethoxazole, but they found lower rates of serious adverse effects with aerosolised pentamidine. One RCT found no significant difference in mortality or treatment failure between aerosolised and intravenous pentamidine.

Benefits: We found no systematic review. **Versus placebo:** We found no RCTs. **Versus intravenous pentamidine:** We found one RCT (45 people with suspected *Pneumocystis* pneumonia [PCP], 38 people with confirmed PCP) comparing 600 mg daily of aerosolised pentamidine with 3 mg per kg daily of intravenous pentamidine (duration of treatment not reported). There was no significant difference in mortality between treatments (2/17 [11.8%] with aerosolised pentamidine *v* 0/21 [0%] with iv pentamidine; RR could not be calculated; $P = 0.19$, Fisher's exact test), nor was there a significant difference in rates of treatment failure (2/17 [11.8%] with aerosolised pentamidine *v* 4/21 [19.0%] with iv pentamidine; RR 0.62, 95% CI 0.13 to 2.98; $P = 0.67$, Fisher's exact test).[9] The wide confidence interval suggests that the trial had insufficient power to detect a clinically important difference between treatments. There was a significantly higher rate of early recrudescence in people treated with aerosolised pentamidine compared with intravenous pentamidine (7/20 [35%] with aerosolised pentamidine *v* 0/18 [0%] with iv pentamidine; $P = 0.009$, Fisher's exact test).[9] **Versus trimethoprim–sulfamethoxazole (TMP–SMX):** We found two RCTs.[4,5] The first RCT (46 people with confirmed PCP categorised as mild [P_aO_2 > 70 mm Hg on room air], of whom 45 [75%] were evaluated) compared 21 days (intended duration) of aerosolised pentamidine 600 mg daily versus trimethoprim 20 mg per kg daily plus sulfamethoxazole 100 mg per kg daily given intravenously in four doses. It found no significant difference in rates of treatment failure at the end of treatment (5/22 [22.7%] with pentamidine *v* 8/23 [34.8%] with TMP–SMX;

RR 0.65, 95% CI 0.25 to 1.69; P = 0.57).[4] The second RCT (367 adults with presumed PCP categorised as mild to moderate [alveolar–arterial oxygen gradient < 55 mm Hg on room air], diagnosis of PCP confirmed in 287 [80%]) compared a minimum of 10 days of aerosolised pentamidine 600 mg daily versus trimethoprim 15 mg per kg daily plus sulfamethoxazole 75 mg per kg daily given intravenously for at least 5 days followed by oral treatment. It found no significant difference in mortality at 35 days (12/182 [6.6%] with pentamidine *v* 17/185 [9.2%] with TMP–SMX; RR 0.72, 95% CI 0.35 to 1.46; P = 0.47). Rates of treatment failure were significantly higher with aerosolised pentamidine at the end of treatment (94/182 [51.6%] with pentamidine *v* 22/185 [11.9%] with TMP–SMX; RR 4.34, 95% CI 2.86 to 6.59; P < 0.001).[5]

Harms: We found no systematic review. **Versus placebo:** We found insufficient evidence. **Versus intravenous pentamidine:** The RCT found no significant difference in the rates of major adverse effects requiring termination of treatment (0/17 [0%] with aerosolised pentamidine *v* 3/21 [14.3%] with iv pentamidine; RR could not be calculated as no events occurred with aerosolised pentamidine; P = 0.24, Fisher's exact test). There were significantly fewer total adverse effects in those receiving aerosolised pentamidine (2/17 [11.8%] with aerosolised pentamidine *v* 11/21 [52.4%] with iv pentamidine; RR 0.22, 95% CI 0.06 to 0.88; P = 0.02, Fisher's exact test).[9] **Versus TMP–SMX:** In both RCTs, serious adverse effects occurred significantly less frequently with aerosolised pentamidine than with TMP–SMX (first RCT: 0/22 [0%] with pentamidine *v* 7/24 [29.2%] with TMP–SMX; RR could not be calculated as no events occurred with pentamidine; P = 0.02;[4] second RCT: 17/179 [9.5%] with pentamidine *v* 73/187 [39.0%] with TMP–SMX; RR 0.24, 95% CI 0.15 to 0.40; P < 0.001).[5]

Comment: Adverse effects in people receiving aerosolised pentamidine rarely require termination of treatment because systemic absorption of the drug is minimal.[4] **Versus TMP–SMX:** Both RCTs excluded people with severely impaired respiratory function. These people may be expected to have done less well with aerosolised pentamidine because of reduced drug delivery.[4,5]

OPTION PENTAMIDINE (INTRAVENOUS)

We found no RCTs comparing intravenous pentamidine versus placebo or no treatment as first line treatment for *Pneumocystis* pneumonia in people infected with HIV. Two RCTs found no significant difference in mortality, treatment failure, or adverse effects between intravenous pentamidine and trimethoprim–sulfamethoxazole. However, a third RCT found that intravenous pentamidine increased mortality compared with trimethoprim–sulfamethoxazole. One RCT found no significant difference between intravenous pentamidine and atovaquone, but atovaquone caused fewer adverse effects requiring termination of treatment. One RCT found no significant difference in mortality or treatment failure between intravenous and aerosolised pentamidine.

Benefits: We found no systematic review. **Versus placebo:** We found no RCTs. **Versus aerosolised pentamidine:** See benefits of aerosolised pentamidine, p 857. **Versus trimethoprim–sulfamethoxazole (TMP–SMX):** We found three RCTs (41,[6] 70,[7] and 163[8] people with confirmed *Pneumocystis* pneumonia [PCP]). The first RCT compared intravenous pentamidine 4 mg per kg daily for 21 days versus trimethoprim 20 mg per kg daily plus sulfamethoxazole 100 mg per kg daily given intravenously in four doses. It found no significant difference in mortality during treatment (1/20 [5.0%] with pentamidine *v* 5/20 [25.0%] with

TMP–SMX; RR 0.20, 95% CI 0.03 to 1.56; P = 0.18).[6] However, the wide confidence interval suggests that the trial had insufficient power to detect important differences in mortality. The second RCT compared intravenous pentamidine 4 mg per kg daily for 17–21 days versus trimethoprim 15–20 mg per kg daily plus sulfamethoxazole 75–100 mg per kg daily given intravenously until clinical improvement occurred, followed by oral treatment. It found significantly higher mortality and need for respiratory support with intravenous pentamidine at the end of treatment (13/33 [39.4%] with pentamidine *v* 5/36 [13.9%] with TMP–SMX; RR 2.84, 95% CI 1.13 to 7.10; P = 0.03).[7] The third RCT compared intravenous pentamidine 4 mg per kg daily for 21 days versus intravenous trimethoprim 20 mg per kg daily plus intravenous sulfamethoxazole 100 mg per kg daily. It found no significant difference in mortality at the end of treatment (18/68 [26.5%] with iv pentamidine *v* 30/92 [32.6%] with TMP–SMX; RR 0.81, 95% CI 0.50 to 1.33; P = 0.51) or in rates of treatment failure requiring change of treatment (27/68 [39.7%] with pentamidine *v* 39/92 [42.4%] with TMP–SMX; RR 0.94, 95% CI 0.64 to 1.37; P = 0.86).[8] **Versus atovaquone:** See benefits of atovaquone, p 859.

Harms: We found no systematic review. The adverse effects requiring termination of treatment that most frequently occurred in people receiving intravenous pentamidine were raised liver enzymes, raised serum creatinine, hyponatraemia, hypoglycaemia, leucopaenia, and rash.[6–8] **Versus placebo:** We found insufficient evidence. **Versus aerosolised pentamidine:** See harms of aerosolised pentamidine, p 858. **Versus TMP–SMX:** The first and third RCTs found no significant difference in rates of major adverse reactions (14/32 [43.8%] with pentamidine *v* 13/32 [40.6%] with TMP–SMX; RR 1.08, 95% CI 0.61 to 1.91; P = 1.00;[6] 17/68 [25%] with pentamidine *v* 31/92 [33.7%] with TMP–SMX; RR 0.74, 95% CI 0.45 to 1.23; P = 0.31).[8] In the second RCT, only one adverse event (in a person receiving pentamidine) required termination of treatment.[7] **Versus atovaquone:** See harms of atovaquone, p 860.

Comment: None.

OPTION ATOVAQUONE

We found no RCTs comparing atovaquone versus placebo or no treatment as the first line treatment for *Pneumocystis* pneumonia in people infected with HIV. One RCT found that atovaquone was less effective than trimethoprim–sulfamethoxazole. One RCT found that atovaquone was equally effective as intravenous pentamidine. Adverse effects requiring termination of treatment occurred less frequently with atovaquone than with trimethoprim–sulfamethoxazole or intravenous pentamidine.

Benefits: We found no systematic review. **Versus placebo:** We found no RCTs. **Versus trimethoprim–sulfamethoxazole (TMP–SMX):** We found one RCT (408 people with suspected *Pneumocystis* pneumonia [PCP], diagnosis histologically confirmed in 322 people) comparing oral atovaquone 750 mg three times daily for 21 days versus oral trimethoprim 320 mg three times daily plus oral sulfamethoxazole 1600 mg three times daily.[10] Among the people in whom PCP was confirmed, those receiving atovaquone had significantly higher rates of treatment failure at the end of treatment (28/138 [20.3%] with atovaquone *v* 10/146 [6.8%] with TMP–SMX; RR 2.96, 95% CI 1.50 to 5.87; P = 0.002) and mortality within 4 weeks of treatment completion (11/160 [6.9%] with atovaquone *v* 1/162 [0.6%] with TMP–SMX; RR 11.14, 95% CI 1.45 to 85.27; P = 0.008). **Versus intravenous**

pentamidine: We found one non-blinded RCT (144 people with suspected PCP, diagnosis confirmed in 109) comparing oral atovaquone 750 mg three times daily for 21 days versus intravenous pentamidine 3–4 mg per kg daily. Among those with confirmed PCP, there was no significant difference in rates of treatment failure at the end of treatment (16/56 [28.6%] with atovaquone *v* 9/53 [17.0%] with pentamidine; RR 1.68, 95% CI 0.81 to 3.47; P = 0.23).[11] The wide confidence interval suggests that the trial had insufficient power to detect a clinically important difference between treatments.

Harms: We found no systematic review. The adverse effects requiring termination of treatment that most frequently occurred in people receiving atovaquone were rash and raised liver enzymes.[10–12] **Versus placebo:** We found no RCTs. **Versus TMP–SMX:** In one RCT (reported in two papers) adverse effects requiring a change in treatment were significantly less frequent with atovaquone (19/203 [9.4%] with atovaquone *v* 50/205 [24.4%] with TMP–SMX; RR 0.38, 95% CI 0.23 to 0.63; P < 0.0001).[10,12] **Versus intravenous pentamidine:** In one RCT adverse events requiring termination of treatment were significantly less frequent with atovaquone (5/73 [6.8%] with atovaquone *v* 29/71 [40.8%] with pentamidine; RR 0.17, 95% CI 0.07 to 0.41; P < 0.0001).[11]

Comment: None.

OPTION CLINDAMYCIN–PRIMAQUINE

We found no RCTs comparing clindamycin–primaquine versus placebo or no treatment as the first line treatment for *Pneumocystis* pneumonia in people infected with HIV. RCTs found clindamycin–primaquine was as effective as trimethoprim–sulfamethoxazole and trimethoprim–dapsone and no significant difference in rates of serious adverse effects.

Benefits: We found no systematic review. **Versus placebo:** We found no RCTs. **Versus trimethoprim–sulfamethoxazole (TMP–SMX):** We found three RCTs (65,[13] 181,[14] and 87[15] people with confirmed *Pneumocystis* pneumonia [PCP]). The first RCT compared a 21 day course of clindamycin (600 mg given iv 4 times daily for 10 days followed by 450 mg given orally 4 times daily for 11 days) plus oral primaquine 15 mg daily versus trimethoprim 240 mg four times daily plus sulfamethoxazole 1200 mg four times daily given intravenously for the first 10 days then orally. Among the people in whom PCP was confirmed, there was no significant difference in rates of treatment failure at the end of treatment (3/27 [11.1%] with clindamycin–primaquine *v* 2/22 [9.1%] with TMP–SMX; RR 1.22, 95% CI 0.22 to 6.68; P = 0.81).[13] The wide confidence interval suggests that the trial had insufficient power to detect a clinically important difference between treatments. The second RCT compared a 21 day course of three treatments: oral clindamycin 600 mg three times daily plus oral primaquine 30 mg daily, oral trimethoprim 320 mg three times daily plus oral sulfamethoxazole 1600 mg three times daily, and oral trimethoprim 320 mg three times daily plus oral dapsone 100 mg daily. At 2 months, there was no significant difference between clindamycin–primaquine and TMP–SMX in mortality (2/58 [3.4%] with clindamycin–primaquine *v* 4/64 [6.3%] with TMP–SMX; RR 0.55, 95% CI 0.10 to 2.90; P = 0.77) or rates of therapeutic failure on or before day 21 (4/58 [6.9%] with clindamycin–primaquine *v* 6/64 [9.4%] with TMP–SMX; RR 0.74, 95% CI 0.22 to 2.48; P = 0.87).[14] The results of the third treatment arm are discussed under trimethoprim–dapsone (see benefits of trimethoprim–dapsone option, p 861). The third RCT compared 21 days (intended duration) of intravenous or oral clindamycin 450 mg four times daily plus oral primaquine 15 mg daily versus oral trimethoprim 320 mg three times daily plus intravenous or oral sulfamethoxazole 1600 mg four times daily. There was no significant difference in mortality at the end of treatment (1/45 [2.2%] with clindamycin–primaquine *v* 2/42 [4.8%] with TMP–SMX; RR 0.47, 95% CI 0.04 to 4.96; P = 0.95) or in rates of therapeutic failure at the end of treatment (11/45 [24.4%] with clindamycin–primaquine *v* 9/42 [21.4%] with TMP–SMX; RR 1.14, 95% CI 0.53 to 2.47; P = 0.94).[15] The wide confidence interval suggests that the trial had insufficient power to detect clinically important differences in mortality between treatments.

Harms: We found no systematic review. The adverse effects requiring termination of treatment that most frequently occurred in people receiving clindamycin–primaquine were rash, raised liver enzymes, leucopaenia, anaemia, and methaemoglobinaemia.[13–15] **Versus placebo:** We found insufficient evidence. **Versus TMP–SMX:** In the first two RCTs there was no significant difference in rates of adverse effects that required a change in treatment (6/27 [22.2%] with clindamycin–primaquine *v* 4/22 [18.2%] with TMP–SMX; RR 1.22, 95% CI 0.39 to 3.80; P = 0.99;[13] 19/58 [32.8%] with clindamycin–primaquine *v* 23/64 [35.9%] with TMP–SMX; RR 0.91, 95% CI 0.56 to 1.49; P = 0.86[14]). The third RCT reported lower rates of serious adverse events with clindamycin–primaquine, but this was not significant if the 2 x 2 χ^2 test with Yates' correction factor was performed (13/45 [28.9%] with clindamycin–primaquine *v* 21/42 [50.0%] with TMP–SMX; RR 0.58, 95% CI 0.33 to 1.00; P = 0.07).[15]

Comment: None.

OPTION TRIMETHOPRIM–DAPSONE

We found no RCTs comparing trimethoprim–dapsone versus placebo or no treatment as first line treatment for *Pneumocystis* pneumonia in people infected with HIV. RCTs have found that trimethoprim–dapsone was as effective as trimethoprim–sulfamethoxazole, with similar rates of adverse effects. One RCT found that trimethoprim–dapsone was as effective as clindamycin–primaquine.

Benefits: We found no systematic review. **Versus placebo:** We found no RCTs. **Versus trimethoprim–sulfamethoxazole (TMP–SMX):** We found two RCTs (60[16] and 181[14] people with confirmed *Pneumocystis* pneumonia [PCP]). The first study compared a 21 day course of oral trimethoprim 20 mg per kg daily plus oral dapsone 100 mg daily versus oral trimethoprim 20 mg per kg daily plus oral sulfamethoxazole 100 mg per kg daily. There was no significant difference in rates of treatment failure at the end of treatment (2/30 [6.7%] with trimethoprim (TMP)–dapsone *v* 3/30 [10.0%] with TMP–SMX; RR 0.67, 95% CI 0.12 to 3.71; P = 1.00).[16] The second RCT compared a 21 day course of three treatments: oral clindamycin 600 mg three times daily plus oral primaquine 30 mg daily, oral trimethoprim 320 mg three times daily plus oral sulfamethoxazole 1600 mg three times daily, and oral trimethoprim 320 mg three times daily plus oral dapsone 100 mg daily. At 2 months, there was no significant difference between TMP–dapsone and TMP–SMX in mortality (2/59 [3.4%] with TMP–dapsone *v* 4/64 [6.3%] with TMP–SMX; RR 0.54, 95% CI 0.10 to 2.85; P = 0.75) or in rates of therapeutic failure on or before day 21 (7/59 [11.9%] with TMP–dapsone *v* 6/64 [9.4%] with TMP–SMX; RR 1.27, 95% CI 0.45 to 3.55; P = 0.88).[14] The results of the third treatment arm are discussed below. **Versus clindamycin–primaquine:** The second RCT found no significant difference between TMP–dapsone and clindamycin–primaquine in mortality at 2 months (2/59 [3.4%] with TMP–dapsone v 2/58 [3.4%] with clindamycin–primaquine; RR 0.98, 95% CI 0.14 to 6.75; P = 0.62) or in rates of therapeutic failure on or before day 21 (7/59 [11.9%] with TMP–dapsone v 4/58 [6.9%] with clindamycin–primaquine; RR 1.72, 95% CI 0.53 to 5.56; P = 0.55).[14] The wide confidence interval suggests that the trial had insufficient power to detect a clinically important difference in mortality between treatments.

Harms: We found no systematic review. The adverse effects requiring termination of treatment that most frequently occurred in people receiving TMP–dapsone were rash, vomiting, and raised liver enzymes.[14,16] **Versus placebo:** We found insufficient evidence. **Versus TMP–SMX:** The first RCT reported lower rates of major adverse events with TMP–dapsone, although this did not reach statistical significance when the 2 x 2 χ^2 test with Yates' correction factor was used (9/30 [30.0%] with TMP–dapsone v 17/30 [56.7%] with TMP–SMX; RR 0.53, 95% CI 0.28 to 0.99; P = 0.07).[16] The second RCT found no significant difference in rates of adverse effects requiring a change in dose or treatment between TMP–dapsone and TMP–SMX (19/59 [32.2%] with TMP–dapsone v 23/64 [35.9%] with TMP–SMX; RR 0.90, 95% CI 0.55 to 1.47; P = 0.81).[14] **Versus clindamycin–primaquine:** The second RCT found no significant difference in the rate of adverse effects requiring a change in dose or treatment between TMP–dapsone and clindamycin–primaquine (19/59 [32.2%] with TMP–dapsone v 19/58 [32.8%] with clindamycin–primaquine; RR 0.98, 95% CI 0.58 to 1.66; P = 0.89).[14]

Comment: None.

QUESTION What are the effects of adjuvant corticosteroids in people receiving first line antipneumocystis treatments for *Pneumocystis* pneumonia in people infected with HIV?

OPTION ADJUVANT CORTICOSTEROIDS

One systematic review found that adjuvant corticosteroids reduced mortality when used early in the treatment of moderate to severe *Pneumocystis* pneumonia (see definition, p 855). We found insufficient evidence on the effects of adjuvant corticosteroids in the early treatment of mild *Pneumocystis* pneumonia.

Benefits: We found one systematic review[17] and two subsequent RCTs.[23,24] The review (search date 1991, 4 RCTs, 326 people with confirmed *Pneumocystis* pneumonia [PCP]) found that corticosteroids decreased mortality and respiratory failure in people with moderate to severe PCP (initial P_aO_2 < 70 mm Hg on room air or an alveolar–arterial gradient > 35 mm Hg), when initiated within 72 hours of starting specific antibiotic treatment.[17] No meta-analysis was performed. The largest RCT included in the review was not blinded. This trial (333 people with suspected PCP, 251 with confirmed or probable PCP were eligible for analysis) compared prednisone 40 mg twice daily for 5 days, followed by 40 mg daily for 5 days then 20 mg daily for the duration of antipneumocystis treatment (or equivalent dose of methylprednisolone) versus no adjuvant corticosteroid. After 31 days, those receiving corticosteroids had significantly lower mortality (13/123 [10.6%] with corticosteroids v 28/128 [21.9%] with no corticosteroids; RR 0.48, 95% CI 0.26 to 0.89; P = 0.02) and lower rates of respiratory failure (17/123 [13.8%] with corticosteroids v 38/128 [29.7%] with no corticosteroids; RR 0.47, 95% CI 0.28 to 0.78; P = 0.004). In people with mild PCP there was no significant difference in mortality (0/28 [0%] with corticosteroids *v* 1/34 [3.0%] with no corticosteroids; RR could not be calculated as no events occurred with corticosteroids; P = 0.92) or respiratory failure (1/28 [3.6%] with corticosteroids *v* 3/34 [8.8%] with no corticosteroids; RR 0.40, 95% CI 0.04 to 3.68; P = 0.75).[18] The three remaining RCTs included in the review were small (23, 37, and 41 people with probable or confirmed PCP).[19–22] The first subsequent RCT (non-blinded, 59 people with PCP and either a $P_aO_2 < 67.5$ mm Hg or $P_aCO_2 < 30$ mm Hg on room air) compared 10 days of intravenous methylprednisolone 0.5 mg per kg four times daily versus no adjuvant corticosteroid. The authors reported fewer deaths with methylprednisolone at the end of treatment, but this was not significant when the 2 x 2 χ^2 test with Yates' correction factor was used (3/30 [10.0%] with methylprednisolone *v* 9/29 [31.0%] with no corticosteroids; RR 0.32, 95% CI 0.10 to 1.07; P = 0.09).[23] Fewer people required mechanical ventilation with methylprednisolone (3/30 [10.0%] with methylprednisolone *v* 12/29 [41.4%] with no corticosteroid; RR 0.24, 95% CI 0.08 to 0.77; P = 0.01). The second subsequent RCT (78 people with HIV related PCP and either a $P_aO_2 < 70$ mm Hg breathing room air or an alveolar–arterial oxygen gradient > 40 mm Hg on oxygen) compared 21 days of intravenous methylprednisolone 40 mg twice daily versus placebo. There was no significant difference in mortality at the end of treatment (4/40 [10.0%] with methylprednisolone *v* 6/38 [15.8%] with placebo; RR 0.63, 95% CI 0.19 to 2.07; P = 0.67) or the need for mechanical ventilation at the end of treatment (3/40 [7.5%] with methylprednisolone *v* 5/38 [13.2%] with placebo; RR 0.57, 95% CI 0.15 to 2.22; P = 0.65).[24]

Harms: The systematic review found a small increase in the rate of infection in people treated with corticosteroids.[17] In the largest of the studies included in this review, the frequency of new herpetic lesions was higher in the corticosteroid group (32/123 [26.0%] with corticosteroid *v* 19/128 [14.8%] with no corticosteroid; RR 1.75, 95% CI 1.05 to 2.92; P = 0.04) and there was a non-significant increase in the occurrence of oral candida infections (65/123 [52.8%] with corticosteroid *v* 53/128 [41.4%] with no corticosteroid; RR 1.28, 95% CI 0.98 to 1.66; P = 0.09).[18] There was no significant difference in rates of serious opportunistic infections (cytomegalovirus disease, *Mycobacterium avium* bacteraemia, cryptococcosis, oesophageal candidosis, and Kaposi's sarcoma) (28/123 [22.8%] with corticosteroid *v* 27/128 [21.1%] with no corticosteroid; RR 1.08, 95% CI 0.68 to 1.72; P = 0.87).[18] The smaller RCTs included in the review found no significant increase in the risk of infection with corticosteroids, although one RCT reported a high overall rate of adverse events (3 opportunistic infections, 2 bacteraemias, 1 urinary tract infection, 1 upper gastrointestinal haemorrhage, and 2 acute psychoses among 19 people treated with methylprednisolone).[22] The first subsequent RCT found no significant difference in the number of people with a complicating condition (5/30 [16.7%] with methylprednisolone *v* 4/29 [13.8%] with no corticosteroid; RR 1.21, 95% CI 0.36 to 4.06; P = 0.96).[23] The second subsequent RCT found more superinfections with corticosteroids but this was not significant (33 with methylprednisolone *v* 24 with placebo; P = 0.51).[24]

Comment: In one of the RCTs that showed no benefit from the use of adjuvant corticosteroids, the methylprednisolone was started later than the antipneumocystis drugs (more than 3 days for most people).[22] This may explain the negative results of the study. We found no other RCTs on the use of corticosteroids after antipneumocystis drugs had failed and respiratory deterioration had already occurred.

QUESTION **What are the effects of treatments for *Pneumocystis* pneumonia in people infected with HIV who have not responded to first line antipneumocystis treatment?**

OPTION **TREATMENTS IN PEOPLE WHO HAVE NOT RESPONDED TO FIRST LINE ANTIPNEUMOCYSTIS TREATMENT**

We found no systematic review and no RCTs comparing the effectiveness or adverse effects of different treatments after failure of first line treatment for *Pneumocystis* pneumonia in people infected with HIV. One systematic review of controlled studies, case series, and case reports suggested that clindamycin–primaquine may be more effective than alternative treatments in this situation.

Benefits: We found no systematic review and no RCTs comparing different treatments for *Pneumocystis* pneumonia (PCP) in people infected with HIV who had experienced treatment failure with first line treatment.

Harms: We found no systematic review and no RCTs.

Comment: We found one systematic review (search date 1999, 27 controlled clinical trials, case series, or case reports) of treatment in people with PCP after failure of first line treatment. This included a meta-analysis (497 people with confirmed PCP, although 41 of these people did not have AIDS) comparing pentamidine, trimethoprim–sulfamethoxazole, clindamycin–primaquine, trimetrexate, eflornithine, and atovaquone. More people responded to clindamycin–primaquine than to the other treatments (42–44/48 [87.5–91.7%] with clindamycin–primaquine *v* 64/164 [39.0%] with pentamidine *v* 27/51 [52.9%] with trimethoprim–sulfamethoxazole *v* 47/159 [29.6%] with trimetrexate *v* 40/70 [57.1%] with eflornithine *v* 4/5 [80.0%] with atovaquone).[25] As these results were obtained from different cohort studies, it is difficult to make direct comparisons between the treatments, and the results should be interpreted with caution.

REFERENCES

1. Selik Rm, Starcher ET, Curran JW. Opportunistic diseases reported in AIDS patients: frequencies, associations and trends. *AIDS* 1987;1:175–182.
2. Glatt AE, Chirgwin K, Landesman SH. Treatment of infections associated with human immunodeficiency virus. *N Engl J Med* 1988;318:1439–1448.
3. Phair J, Munoz A, Detels R, et al. The risk of *Pneumocystis carinii* pneumonia in the acquired immunodeficiency syndrome. *N Engl J Med* 1990;322:161–165.
4. Arasteh KN, Vohringer HF, Heise WS, et al. Pentamidine aerosol vs cotrimoxazole in the treatment of slight to moderate *Pneumocystis carinii* pneumonia. *Drug Invest* 1994;8:321–330.
5. Montgomery AB, Feigal DW Jr, Sattler F, et al. Pentamidine aerosol versus trimethoprim–sulfamethoxazole for *Pneumocystis carinii* in acquired immune deficiency syndrome. *Am J Respir Crit Care Med* 1995;151:1068–1074.
6. Wharton JM, Coleman DL, Wofsy CB, et al. Trimethoprim–sulfamethoxazole or pentamidine for *Pneumocystis carinii* pneumonia in the acquired immunodeficiency syndrome. A prospective randomized trial. *Ann Intern Med* 1986;105:37–44.
7. Sattler FR, Cowan R, Nielsen DM, et al. Trimethoprim–sulfamethxazole compared with pentamidine for treatment of *Pneumocystis carinii* pneumonia in the acquired immunodeficiency syndrome. A prospective, noncrossover study. *Ann Intern Med* 1988;109:280–287.
8. Klein NC, Duncanson FP, Lenox TH, et al. Trimethoprim–sulfamethoxazole versus pentamidine for *Pneumocystis carinii* pneumonia in AIDS patients: results of a large prospective randomized treatment trial. *AIDS* 1992;6:301–305.
9. Conte JE Jr, Chernoff D, Feigal DW Jr, et al. Intravenous or inhaled pentamidine for treating *Pneumocystis carinii* pneumonia in AIDS. A randomized trial. *Ann Intern Med* 1990;113:203–209.
10. Hughes W, Leoung G, Kramer F, et al. Comparison of atovaquone (566C80) with trimethoprim–sulfamethxazole to treat *Pneumocystis carinii* pneumonia in patients with AIDS. *N Engl J Med* 1993;328:1521–1527.
11. Dohn MN, Weinberg WG, Torres RA, et al. Oral atovaquone compared with intravenous pentamidine for *Pneumocystis carinii* pneumonia in patients with AIDS. *Ann Intern Med* 1994;121:174–180.
12. Hughes WT, LaFon SW, Scott JD, et al. Adverse events associated with trimethoprim–sulfamethoxazole and atovaquone during the treatment of AIDS-related *Pneumocystis carinii* pneumonia. *J Infect Dis* 1995;171:1295–1301.
13. Toma E, Fournier S, Dumont M, et al. Clindamycin/primaquine versus trimethoprim–sulfamethoxazole as primary therapy for *Pneumocystis carinii* pneumonia in AIDS: a randomized, double-blind pilot trial. *Clin Infect Dis* 1993;17:178–184.
14. Safrin S, Finkelstein DM, Feinberg J, et al. Comparison of three regimens for treatment of mild to moderate *Pneumocystis carinii* pneumonia in patients with AIDS. A double-blind, randomized trial

of oral trimethoprim–sulfamethoxazole, dapsone-trimethoprim, and clindamycin–primaquine. ACTG 108 Study Group. *Ann Intern Med* 1996;124:792–802.
15. Toma E, Thorne A, Singer J, et al. Clindamycin with primaquine vs. trimethoprim–sulfamethoxazole therapy for mild and moderately severe *Pneumocystis carinii* pneumonia in patients with AIDS: a multicenter, double-blind, randomized trial (CTN 004). *Clin Infect Dis* 1998;27:524–530.
16. Medina I, Mills J, Leoung G, et al. Oral therapy for *Pneumocystis carinii* pneumonia in the acquired immunodeficiency syndrome. A controlled trial of trimethoprim–sulfamethoxazole versus trimethoprim–dapsone. *N Engl J Med* 1990;323:776–782.
17. Sistek CJ, Wordell CJ, Hauptman SP. Adjuvant corticosteroid therapy for *Pneumocystis carinii* pneumonia in AIDS patients. *Ann Pharmacother* 1992;26:1127–1133.
18. Bozzette SA, Sattler FR, Chiu J, et al. A controlled trial of early adjunctive treatment with corticosteroids for *Pneumocystis carinii* pneumonia in the acquired immunodeficiency syndrome. California Collaborative Treatment Group. *N Engl J Med* 1990;323:1451–1457.
19. Gagnon S, Boota AM, Fischl MA, et al. Corticosteroids as adjunctive therapy for severe *Pneumocystis carinii* pneumonia in the acquired immunodeficiency syndrome. A double-blind, placebo-controlled trial. *N Engl J Med* 1990;323:1444–1450.
20. Montaner JSG, Lawson LM, Levitt N, et al. Corticosteroids prevent early deterioration in patients with moderately severe *Pneumocystis carinii* pneumonia and the acquired immunodeficiency syndrome (AIDS). *Ann Intern Med* 1990;113:14–20.
21. Montaner JSG, Guillemi S, Quieffin J, et al. Oral corticosteroids in patients with mild *Pneumocystis carinii* pneumonia and the acquired immune deficiency syndrome (AIDS). *Tuber Lung Dis* 1993;74:173–179.
22. Clement M, Edison R, Turner J, et al. Corticosteroids as adjunctive therapy in severe *Pneumocystis carinii* pneumonia; a prospective, placebo-controlled trial. *Am Rev Respir Dis* 1989;139:A250.
23. Nielsen TL, Eeftinck Schattenkerk JK, Jensen BN, et al. Adjunctive corticosteroid therapy for *Pneumocystis carinii* pneumonia in AIDS: a randomized European multicenter open label study. *J Acquir Immune Defic Syndr Hum Retrovirol* 1992;5:726–731.
24. Walmsley S, Levinton C, Brunton J. A multicenter randomized double-blind placebo-controlled trial of adjunctive corticosteroids in the treatment of *Pneumocystis carinii* pneumonia complicating the acquired immune deficiency syndrome. *J Acquir Immune Defic Syndr Hum Retrovirol* 1995;8:348–357.
25. Smego RA Jr, Nagar S, Maloba B, et al. A meta-analysis of salvage therapy for *Pneumocystis carinii* pneumonia. *Arch Intern Med* 2001;161:1529–1533. Search date 1999; primary sources Medline plus hand searches of Index Medicus, Current Contents, bibliographies of articles, and major infectious disease textbooks.

Richard Bellamy
ObaapaVitA Trial Director
Kintampo Health Research Centre
Kintampo
Ghana

Competing interests: None declared.

TABLE 1 Summary of randomised controlled trials of interventions to treat *Pneumocystis* pneumonia in people infected with HIV.

Ref	Participants randomised	Treatments compared	Numbers analyzed in each arm	Mortality RR* (95% CI)	Respiratory and/or treatment failure RR* (95% CI)
4	46 people with confirmed PCP and $P_aO_2 > 70$ mm Hg on room air	Aerosolised pentamidine *v* TMP–SMX	22 *v* 23		0.65 (0.25–1.69)
5	367 people with confirmed or presumed PCP and alveolar–arterial oxygen gradient < 55 mm Hg	Aerosolised pentamidine *v* TMP–SMX	182 *v* 185	0.72 (0.35–1.46)	4.34 (2.86–6.59)
6	41 people with a proven first episode of PCP	Intravenous pentamidine *v* TMP–SMX	20 *v* 20	0.20 (0.03–1.56)	
7	70 people with confirmed or presumed PCP	Intravenous pentamidine *v* TMP–SMX	33 *v* 36		2.84 (1.13–7.10)
8	187 people with suspected PCP; only the 163 people in whom the diagnosis was confirmed were evaluated further	Intravenous pentamidine *v* TMP–SMX	68 *v* 92	0.81 (0.50–1.33)	0.94 (0.64–1.37)
9	45 patients with suspected PCP; only the 38 people in whom the diagnosis was confirmed and who gave consent were evaluated for treatment effectiveness	Aerosolised pentamidine *v* intravenous pentamidine	23 *v* 22		0.62 (0.13–2.98)
10,12	408 people with suspected PCP and alveolar–arterial oxygen gradient ≤ 45 mm Hg. Only the 322 people in whom the diagnosis was confirmed were evaluated further	Atovaquone *v* TMP–SMX	160 *v* 162	11.14 (1.45–85.27)	2.96 (1.50–5.87)

TABLE 1 continued

Ref	Participants randomised	Treatments compared	Numbers analyzed in each arm	Mortality RR* (95% CI)	Respiratory and/or treatment failure RR* (95% CI)
11	144 people with suspected PCP; only the 109 people in whom the diagnosis was confirmed were evaluated for treatment effectiveness	Atovaquone *v* intravenous pentamidine	56 *v* 53		1.68 (0.81–3.47)
13	65 people with a suspected first episode of PCP; only the 49 people in whom the diagnosis was confirmed were evaluated further	Clindamycin–primaquine *v* TMP–SMX	27 *v* 22		1.22 (0.22–6.68)
14	256 people with suspected PCP; only the 181 people in whom the diagnosis was confirmed were evaluated further	Clindamycin–primaquine *v* TMP–dapsone *v* TMP–SMX	58 *v* 59 *v* 64	C-P: 0.55 (0.10–2.90) TMP–dapsone: 0.54 (0.10–2.85)	C-P: 0.74 (0.22–2.48) TMP–dapsone: 1.27 (0.45–3.55)
15	116 people with suspected PCP; only the 87 people in whom the diagnosis was confirmed were evaluated further	Clindamycin–primaquine *v* TMP–SMX	45 *v* 42	0.47 (0.04–4.96)	1.14 (0.53–2.47)
16	60 people with a first episode of confirmed PCP and $P_aO_2 > 60$ mm Hg on room air	TMP–dapsone *v* TMP–SMX	30 *v* 30		0.67 (0.12–3.71)
18	333 people with suspected PCP; only the 251 with confirmed or probable PCP were evaluated further	Prednisone *v* no corticosteroid	123 *v* 128	0.48 (0.26–0.89)	0.47 (0.28–0.78)
19	24 people with suspected PCP; only the 23 people in whom the diagnosis was confirmed were evaluated further	Intravenous methylprednisolone *v* placebo	12 *v* 11	0.31 (0.11–0.85)	0.31 (0.11–0.85)

TABLE 1 continued

Ref	Participants randomised	Treatments compared	Numbers analyzed in each arm	Mortality RR* (95% CI)	Respiratory and/or treatment failure RR* (95% CI)
20,21	37 people with a first episode of confirmed PCP and arterial oxygen saturation ≥85% on room air	Prednisone *v* placebo	18 *v* 19		0.13 (0.02–0.95)
22	41 people with confirmed PCP and $P_aO_2 \leq 50$ mm Hg on room air	Intravenous methylprednisolone *v* placebo	19 *v* 22	1.16 (0.58–2.31)	
23	59 people with a first episode of confirmed PCP and either P_aO_2 < 67.5 mm Hg or P_aCO_2 < 30 mm Hg on room air	Intravenous methylprednisolone *v* no corticosteroid	30 *v* 29	0.32 (0.10–1.07)	0.24 (0.08–0.77)
24	120 people with suspected PCP and P_aO_2 < 70 mm Hg or alveolar–arterial oxygen gradient > 40 mm Hg. Only the 78 people in whom the diagnosis was confirmed were evaluated further	Intravenous methylprednisolone *v* placebo	40 *v* 38	0.63 (0.19–2.07)	0.57 (0.15–2.22)

*RR refers to the first treatment in comparison with the second. For reference 14 the RR refers to each treatment in comparison with TMP–SMX. For further details on the design, patient eligibility criteria, dose and duration of the treatments administered, length of follow up, and the definition of respiratory/treatment failure used in each study, please see the main text. Numbers analyzed are smaller than those enrolled in some cases because the study authors did not perform an intent to treat
SMX, sulfamethoxazole; TMP, trimethoprim; Ref, reference.

Amoebic dysentery

Search date January 2004

Leonila Dans and Elizabeth Martinez

QUESTIONS

INTERVENTIONS

*No placebo controlled RCTs. Categorisation based on consensus and evidence of similar effectiveness among these drugs

See glossary G

Key Messages

- **Metronidazole** We found no RCTs comparing metronidazole versus placebo. We found six RCTs comparing metronidazole versus tinidazole. Four RCTs found that tinidazole improved parasite clearance at 30 days compared with metronidazole. One RCT found no significant difference between metronidazole and tinidazole in parasite clearance at 30 days, while one RCT found similar parasite clearance with both treatments at 6 days. Five of the RCTs reported adverse effects; two of these RCTs found more adverse events with metronidazole than with tinidazole, whereas three RCTs found no significant difference in the rates of adverse effects between the two drugs.
- **Ornidazole** One RCT found that ornidazole improved parasite clearance compared with placebo. Nausea and vomiting were more common with ornidazole than with placebo, but the difference was not significant. Two RCTs found no significant difference between ornidazole and tinidazole or secnidazole for clearing parasites in children with amoebic dysentery.
- **Secnidazole** We found no RCTs comparing secnidazole versus placebo. One RCT found no significant difference between secnidazole and ornidazole in clearing parasites in children with amoebic dysentery.
- **Tinidazole** We found no RCTs comparing tinidazole versus placebo. We found six RCTs comparing metronidazole versus tinidazole. Four RCTs found that tinidazole improved parasite clearance at 30 days compared with metronidazole. One RCT found no significant difference between metronidazole and tinidazole in parasite clearance at 30 days, while one RCT found similar parasite clearance with both treatments at 6 days. Five of the RCTs reported adverse effects; two of these RCTs found more adverse effects with metronidazole than with tinidazole, whereas three RCTs found no significant difference in the rates of adverse effects between the two drugs. One RCT found no significant difference between tinidazole and ornidazole for clearing parasites in children with amoebic dysentery.

- **Emetine, paromomycin** We found no RCTs evaluating these interventions for the treatment of amoebic dysentery in endemic areas.

DEFINITION Amoebic dysentery is caused by a protozoan parasite *Entamoeba histolytica*. Invasive intestinal parasitic infection can result in symptoms of fulminant dysentery, with fever, chills, and bloody or mucous diarrhoea, abdominal discomfort, or diarrhoea containing blood or mucus alternating with periods of constipation or remission. This chapter focuses on amoebic dysentery only, and includes populations with both suspected and documented disease in endemic areas (areas in which levels of infection do not exhibit wide fluctuations through time).[1] Extraintestinal amoebiasis (e.g. amoebic liver abscess) and asymptomatic amoebiasis are not covered. The term "amoebic dysentery" encompasses people described as having symptomatic intestinal amoebiasis, amoebic colitis, amoebic diarrhoea, or invasive intestinal amoebiasis.

INCIDENCE/ PREVALENCE We found no accurate global prevalence data of *E histolytica* infection and amoebic dysentery. Estimates on the prevalence of *Entamoeba* infection range from 1–40% of the population in Central and South America, Africa, and Asia, and from 0.2–10.8% in endemic areas of developed countries such as the USA.[2–5] However, these estimates are difficult to interpret, mainly because infection can remain asymptomatic or go unreported,[6] and because many older reports do not distinguish *E histolytica* from a non-pathogenic, morphologically identical species *Entamoeba dispar*. Development and availability of more sophisticated methods (such as the ELISA based test) to differentiate the two species might give a more accurate estimate of its global prevalence.[7] Infection with *E histolytica* is a common cause of acute diarrhoea. One survey in Egypt found that 38% of people with acute diarrhoea in an outpatient clinic had amoebic dysentery.[8]

AETIOLOGY/ RISK FACTORS Ingestion of cysts from food or water contaminated with faeces is the main route of *E histolytica* transmission. Low standards of hygiene and sanitation, particularly those related to crowding, tropical climate, contamination of food and water with faeces, and inadequate disposal of faeces all account for the high rates of infection seen in developing countries.[9,10] It has been suggested that some animals, such as dogs, pigs, and monkeys, may act as reservoir hosts to the protozoa, but this has not been proven. In developed countries, risk factors include communal living, oral and anal sex, compromised immune system, and migration or travel from endemic areas.[9,11,12]

PROGNOSIS Amoebic dysentery may progress to amoeboma Ⓖ, fulminant colitis, toxic megacolon, colonic ulcers, and may lead to perforation.[13] Amoeboma may be mistaken for colonic carcinoma or pyogenic abscess. Amoebic dysentery may also result in chronic carriage and the chronic passing of amoebic cysts. Fulminant amoebic dysentery is reported to have 55–88% mortality.[14,15] It is estimated that over 500 million people are infected with *E histolytica* worldwide.[10] Between 40 000 to 100 000 will die each year, placing it second to malaria in mortality caused by protozoan parasites.[16]

AIMS OF INTERVENTION To reduce the infectious period, length of illness, risks of dehydration, risks of transmission to others, and rates of severe illness; to prevent complications and death.

OUTCOMES Mortality; quality of life; severity of diarrhoea (duration, time to formed stools, number of loose stools per day, stool volume); rate of complications (i.e. amoeboma, extension to pleural cavity, chronic cyst carriage); length of hospital stay; rate of hospital admission; relief of symptoms (i.e. cramps, nausea, vomiting); therapeutic cure (defined as absence of parasites in stools, disappearance of symptoms, and healing of ulcers); failure of treatment (defined as either persistence of symptoms or persistence of parasites, or both); and adverse effects of treatment.

METHODS *Clinical Evidence* search and appraisal January 2004.

QUESTION What are the effects of drug treatments for amoebic dysentery in endemic areas?

OPTION METRONIDAZOLE

We found no RCTs comparing metronidazole versus placebo. We found six RCTs comparing metronidazole versus tinidazole. Four RCTs found that tinidazole improved parasite clearance at 30 days compared with metronidazole. One RCT found no significant difference between metronidazole and tinidazole in parasite clearance at 30 days, while one RCT found similar parasite clearance with both treatments at 6 days. Five of the RCTs reported adverse effects; two of these RCTs found more adverse events with metronidazole than with tinidazole, whereas three RCTs found no significant difference in the rates of adverse effects between the two drugs.

Benefits: We found no systematic reviews. **Versus placebo:** We found no RCTs. **Versus tinidazole:** We found six RCTs.[17–22] Four RCTs[17–20] found that tinidazole significantly reduced failure rate (as defined by persistence of symptoms or parasites after 30 days) compared with metronidazole; one RCT[22] found no significant difference in 30 day failure rate between tinidazole and metronidazole, whereas one RCT[21] found similar failure rates for the two drugs at 6 days (see table 1, p 875). **Versus secnidazole, ornidazole, emetine, or paromomycin:** We found no RCTs.

Harms: **Versus tinidazole:** Two RCTs[19,22] reported significantly fewer adverse events (nausea, vomiting, abdominal pain, bitter taste, diarrhoea, generalised weakness, furry tongue, dark urine, loss of appetite, blurring of vision, headache, sleep disturbance, vertigo, skin rash, dysuria) with tinidazole than with metronidazole, whereas three RCTs[17,18,20] found no significant difference in adverse effects between treatments (see table 1, p 875). One RCT did not report adverse events.[21]

Comment: It is not clear whether two of the RCTs[19,20] involved the same group of people or different groups sampled from the same population. The quality of many of the RCTs, particularly those published before 1990, was difficult to assess because details of methods were often not described.

OPTION SECNIDAZOLE

We found no RCTs comparing secnidazole versus placebo. One RCT found no significant difference between secnidazole and ornidazole in clearing parasites in children with amoebic dysentery.

Benefits: We found no systematic reviews. **Versus placebo:** We found no RCTs. **Versus ornidazole:** We found one RCT (102 children with amoebic dysentery).[23] It found no significant difference between secnidazole 30 mg/kg daily for 3 days and ornidazole 15 mg/kg daily for 10 days in failure to clear parasites by 10 days after treatment (10/42 [23.8%] with ornidazole *v* 19/60 [31.7%] with secnidazole; RR 0.75, 95% CI 0.39 to 1.45). **Versus metronidazole, tinidazole, emetine, or paromomycin:** We found no RCTs.

Harms: **Versus ornidazole:** No adverse effects were observed with either secnidazole or ornidazole.[23]

Comment: None.

OPTION ORNIDAZOLE

One RCT found that ornidazole improved parasite clearance compared with placebo. Nausea and vomiting were more common with ornidazole than with placebo, but the difference was not significant. Two RCTs found no significant difference between ornidazole and tinidazole or secnidazole for clearing parasites in children with amoebic dysentery.

Benefits: We found no systematic reviews. **Versus placebo:** We found one RCT (55 people aged 5–92 years with amoebic dysentery).[24] It found that ornidazole 500 mg three times daily significantly reduced failure rate compared with placebo (AR for failure to clear parasites after 8–10 days: 7/35 [20.0%] with ornidazole *v* 20/20 [100%] with placebo; RR 0.43, 95% CI 0.29 to 0.63). **Versus tinidazole:** We found one RCT (40 children aged 1–13 years with amoebic dysentery).[25] It found no significant difference in treatment failure rate between ornidazole 50 mg/kg daily for 3 days and tinidazole 50 mg/kg daily for 3 days after 4 weeks (AR for failure to eradicate parasites: 0/18 [0%] with ornidazole *v* 1/17 [5.9%] with tinidazole; RR 3.17, 95% CI 0.14 to 72.80). **Versus secnidazole:** See benefits of secnidazole, p 871. **Versus metronidazole, ornidazole, emetine, or paromomycin:** We found no RCTs.

Harms: **Versus placebo:** Nausea and vomiting were more common with ornidazole than with placebo, although the difference was not significant (AR for adverse events: 3/35 [8.6%] with ornidazole *v* 0/20 [0%] with placebo; RR 4.08, 95% CI 0.22 to 75.25).[24] **Versus tinidazole:** The RCT reported mild vomiting in one person with ornidazole.[25] **Versus secnidazole:** See harms of secnidazole, p 871.

Comment: In the RCT comparing ornidazole versus tinidazole, most of the children had a concomitant helminthiasis**G** (presence of ascaris, trichuris, or ancylostoma: 17/20 [85%] in the tinidazole group *v* 18/20 [90%] in the ornidazole group).[25] Clinical outcomes in this RCT might have been masked by symptoms of concomitant helminthiasis.

OPTION TINIDAZOLE

We found no RCTs comparing tinidazole versus placebo. We found six RCTs comparing metronidazole versus tinidazole. Four RCTs found that tinidazole improved parasite clearance at 30 days compared with metronidazole. One RCT found no significant difference between metronidazole and tinidazole in parasite clearance at 30 days, while one RCT found similar parasite clearance with both treatments at 6 days. Five of the RCTs reported adverse effects; two of these RCTs found more adverse effects with metronidazole than with tinidazole, whereas three RCTs found no significant difference in the rates of adverse effects between the two drugs. One RCT found no significant difference between tinidazole and ornidazole for clearing parasites in children with amoebic dysentery.

Benefits: We found no systematic reviews. **Versus placebo:** We found no RCTs. **Versus metronidazole:** See benefits of metronidazole, p 871. **Versus ornidazole:** See benefits of ornidazole, p 872. **Versus secnidazole, emetine, or paromomycin:** We found no RCTs.

Harms: **Versus metronidazole:** See harms of metronidazole, p 871. **Versus ornidazole:** See harms of ornidazole, p 872.

Comment: None.

OPTION EMETINE

We found no RCTs evaluating emetine for the treatment of amoebic dysentery.

Benefits: We found no systematic reviews or RCTs comparing emetine versus placebo, metronidazole, tinidazole, secnidazole, ornidazole, or paromomycin.

Harms: We found no RCTs.

Comment: None.

OPTION PAROMOMYCIN

We found no RCTs evaluating paromomycin for the treatment of amoebic dysentery.

Benefits: We found no systematic reviews or RCTs comparing paromomycin versus placebo, metronidazole, tinidazole, secnidazole, ornidazole, or emetine.

Harms: We found no RCTs.

Comment: None.

GLOSSARY

Amoeboma A granulomatous lesion of the caecum or ascending colon caused by localised chronic *E histolytica* infection.
Helminthiasis Presence in the body of parasitic worms, including nematode worms such as *Ascaris*, *Trichuris*, and *Ancylostoma*.

REFERENCES

1. Anonymous. *Dictionary of epidemiology centre for the epidemiology of infectious disease*. Oxford: University of Oxford, UK, 1994/1995.
2. Rivera WI, Tachinaba H, Kanbara H. Field study on the distribution of *Entamoeba dispar* in the northern Philippines as detected by PCR. *Am J Trop Med Hyg* 1998; 59:916–21.
3. Haque R, Faruque AS, Hahn P, et al. Entamoeba and Entamoeba dispar infection in children in Bangladesh. *J Infect Dis* 1997;175:734–746.
4. Braga LL, Mendonca Y, Piva CA, et al. Seropositivity for and intestinal colonization with *Entamoeba histolytica* and *Entamoeba dispar* in individuals in Northern Brazil. *J Clin Microbiol* 1998;36:3044–3045.
5. Chacin-Bonilla L, Bonillla E, Parra AM, et al. Prevalence of *Entamoeba histolytica* and other intestinal parasites in a community in Venezuela. *Ann Trop Med Parasitol* 1992;86:373–380.
6. Anonymous. Amoebiasis. *Wkly Epidemiol Rec* 1997;72: 97–99.
7. Huston CD, Petri WA. Amoebiasis: clinical implications of the recognition of entamoeba dispar. *Curr Infect Dis Rep* 1999;1:441–447.
8. Abd-Alla MD, Ravdin JI. Diagnosis of amoebic colitis by antigen capture ELISA in patients presenting with acute diarrhoea in Cairo, Egypt. *Trop Med Int Health* 2002;7:365–370.
9. Davis, AN, Haque R, Petri WA. Update on protozoan parasites in the intestine. *Curr Opin Gastroenterol* 2002,18:10–14.
10. Lucas R, Upcroft JA. Clinical significance of the redefinition of the agent of amoebiasis. *Rev Latinoam Microbiol* 2001;43:183–187.
11. Petri WA, Singh U. Diagnosis and management of amebiasis. *Clin Infect Dis* 1999;29:1117–1125.
12. Stanley SL. Amoebiasis. *Lancet* 2003;361:1025–1034.
13. Haque R, Huston CD, Hughes M, et al. Amebiasis. *N Engl J Med* 2003; 348:1565–1573.
14. Singh B, Moodley J, Ramdial PK. Fulminant amoebic colitis: a favorable outcome. *Int Surg* 2001;8677–8681.
15. Vargas M, Pena A. Toxic amoebic colitis and amoebic colon perforation in children: an improved prognosis. *J Pediatr Surg* 1976;11:223–225.
16. Espinosa-Cantellano M, Martinez Palomo. Recent developments in amoebiasis research. *Curr Opin Infect Dis* 2000;13:45–456.
17. Singh G, Kumar S. Short course of single daily dosage treatment with tinidazole and metronidazole in intestinal amoebiasis: a comparative study. *Curr Med Res Opin* 1977;5:157–160.
18. Swami B, Lavakusulu D, Sitha Devi C. Tinidazole and metronidazole in the treatment of intestinal amoebiasis. *Curr Med Res Opin* 1977;5:152–156.
19. Misra NP, Gupta RC. A comparison of a short course of single daily dosage therapy of tinidazole with metronidazole in intestinal amoebiasis. *J Int Med Res* 1977;5:434–437.
20. Misra NP. A comparative study of tinidazole with metronidazole as a single daily dose of three days in symptomatic intestinal amoebiasis. *Drugs* 1978;5(suppl):19–22.
21. Chunge CN, Estambale BBA, Pamba HO, et al. Comparison of four nitriioimidazole compounds for treatment of symptomatic amoebiasis in Kenya. *East Afr Med J* 1989;66:724–726.
22. Misra NP, Laiq SM. Comparative trial of tinidazole and metronidazole in intestinal amoebiasis. *Curr Ther Res Dec* 1974;16:1255–1263.
23. Toppare MF, Kitapci F, Senses DA, et al. Ornidazole and secnidazole in the treatment of symptomatic intestinal amoebiasis in childhood. *Trop Doc* 1994:183–184.

24. Apt W, Perez C, Miranda C, Gabor M, Doren G. Tratiamento de la amebiasis intestinal y giardiasis con ornidazol [in Spanish]. *Rev Med Chile* 1983;111:1130–1133.

25. Panggabean A, Sutjipto A, Aldy D, et al. Tinidazole versus ornidazole in amebic dysentery in children (a double blind trial). *Paediatr Indones* 1980;20:229–235.

Leonila Dans
Associate Professor
Manila
Philippines

Elizabeth Martinez
Associate Professor
Manila
Philippines

Competing interests: None declared.

TABLE 1 **Failure rates and adverse events for trials of tinadazole versus metronidazole in people with amoebic dysentery (see text, p 871).**

Reference	Population	Failure rates* Tinadazole v metronidazole	Adverse events Tinadazole v metronidazole
17	60 people aged 16–55 years	2/27 [7.4%] v 12/29 [41.3%] RR 0.18, 95% CI 0.04 to 0.73	14/27 [51.9%] v 22/29 [75.9%] RR 0.68, 95% CI 0.45 to 1.04
18	60 people† mean age 30.5 years, range not stated	1/29 [3.4%] v 12/27 [44.4%] RR 0.08, 95% CI 0.01 to 0.56	15/29 [51.7%] v 10/27 [37.0%] RR 1.40, 95% CI 0.76 to 2.56
19	60 hospitalised people aged 16–60 years‡	3/30 [10.0%] v 14/30 [46.7%] RR 0.21, 95% CI 0.07 to 0.67	8/30 [26.7%] v 16/30 [53.3%] RR 0.50, 95% CI 0.25 to 0.99
20	60 hospitalised people aged 16–60 years‡	3/29 [10.3%] v 14/30 [46.7%] RR 0.22, 95% CI 0.07 to 0.69	8/29 [27.6%] v 16/30 [53.3%] RR 0.52, 95% CI 0.26 to 1.02
21	225 people aged 12–65 years§	78/123 [63.4%] v 60/102 [58.8%] Significance not reported	Not reported
22	60 people aged 16–50 years	7/30 [23.3%] v 8/30 [26.7%] RR 0.88, 95% CI 0.36 to 2.11	2/30 [6.7%] v 9/30 [30%] RR 0.22, 95% CI 0.05 to 0.94

*Failure rates defined as persistence of symptoms or parasites after 30 days in five trials [17–20,22] and as persistence of parasites after 6 days in one trial.[21] †*Entamoeba histolytica* present in stools. ‡It is not clear whether these RCTs involved the same group of people, or different groups sampled from the same population.[19,20] §Participants in one RCT[21] were randomised into four treatment groups: branded metronidazole, branded tinidazole, generic metronidazole, and generic tinidazole. The results presented here for this RCT are pooled for the branded and generic preparations of each drug.

Chickenpox

Search date March 2004

George Swingler

QUESTIONS

INTERVENTIONS

See glossary G

Key Messages

Prevention in healthy adults and children

- **Live attenuated vaccine in healthy children** Two RCTs identified by a systematic review found that live attenuated varicella vaccine reduced clinical chickenpox in healthy children compared with placebo, with no significant increase in adverse effects.
- **Zoster immune globulin versus human serum globulin in healthy children** One small RCT in children exposed to a sibling with chickenpox found that zoster immune globulin reduced the proportion of exposed children with clinical chickenpox at 20 days compared with human immune serum globulin.

- **Live attenuated vaccine in healthy adults** We found no RCTs in healthy adults on the effects of live attenuated varicella vaccine.

Prevention in immunocompromised adults and children

- **High dose aciclovir (> 3200 mg/day) in people with HIV infection** One systematic review in people with HIV infection found that high dose aciclovir (at least 3200 mg/day) reduced the risk of clinical chickenpox and reduced all cause mortality over 22 months' treatment compared with placebo.
- **Aciclovir in people with immunocompromise other than HIV** We found no RCTs on the effects of aciclovir in people with immunocompromise other than HIV.
- **Live attenuated vaccine in immunocompromised people** We found no RCTs in immunocompromised adults or children on the effects of live attenuated varicella vaccine.
- **Zoster immune globulin in immunocompromised adults** We found no RCTs on the effects of zoster immune globulin in immunocompromised adults.
- **Zoster immune globulin versus varicella zoster immune globulin in immunocompromised children** One RCT in immunocompromised children exposed to a sibling with chickenpox found no significant difference in clinical chickenpox with zoster immune globulin compared with varicella zoster immune globulin at 12 weeks.

Treatment in healthy adults and children

- **Oral aciclovir in healthy people (given < 24 hours of onset of rash)** Two systematic reviews found that oral aciclovir reduced the symptoms of chickenpox in healthy adults and children compared with placebo.
- **Oral aciclovir in healthy people (given > 24 hours after onset of rash)** One systematic review and one additional RCT found that oral aciclovir given beyond 24 hours after onset of rash did not reduce the symptoms of chickenpox compared with placebo.

Treatment in immunocompromised adults and children

- **Intravenous aciclovir for treatment of chickenpox in children with malignancy** Two RCTs compared intravenous aciclovir versus placebo in children with cancer. One large RCT found that aciclovir reduced clinical deterioration. The other smaller RCT found no significant difference in clinical deterioration.
- **Aciclovir in immunocompromised adults** We found no RCTs on the effects of aciclovir in immunocompromised adults.

DEFINITION Chickenpox is caused by primary infection with varicella zoster virus. In healthy people, it is usually a mild self limiting illness, characterised by low grade fever, malaise, and a generalised, itchy, vesicular rash.

INCIDENCE/ PREVALENCE Chickenpox is extremely contagious. Over 90% of unvaccinated people become infected, but infection occurs at different ages in different parts of the world: over 80% of people have been infected by the age of 10 years in the USA, the UK, and Japan, and by the age of 30 years in India, South East Asia, and the West Indies.[1,2]

AETIOLOGY/ RISK FACTORS Chickenpox is caused by exposure to varicella zoster virus.

PROGNOSIS **Infants and children:** In healthy children the illness is usually mild and self limiting. In the USA, death rates in infants and children (aged 1–14 years) with chickenpox are about 7/100 000 in infants and 1.4/100 000 in children.[3] In Australia, mortality with chickenpox is about 0.5–0.6/100 000 in children aged between 1 and 11 years, and about 1.2/100 000 in infants.[4] Bacterial skin sepsis is the most common complication in children under 5 years of age, and acute cerebellar ataxia is the most common complication in older children; both cause hospital admission in 2–3/10 000 children.[5] **Adults:** Mortality in adults is higher, at about 31/100 000.[3] Varicella pneumonia is the most common complication, causing 20–30 hospital admissions/10 000 adults.[5] Activation of latent varicella zoster virus infection can cause herpes zoster, also known as shingles (see postherpetic neuralgia, p 1026). **Cancer chemotherapy:** One case series (77 children with both cancer and chickenpox) found that more children receiving chemotherapy compared with those in remission developed progressive chickenpox with multiple organ involvement (19/60 [32%] with children receiving chemotherapy *v* 0/17 [0%] with children in remission) and more children died (4/60 [7%] with children receiving chemotherapy *v* 0/17 [0%] with children in remission).[6] **HIV infection:** One retrospective case series (45 children with AIDS) found that one in four children with AIDS who acquired chickenpox in hospital developed pneumonia and 5% died.[7] In a retrospective cohort study (73 children with HIV and chickenpox; 83% with symptomatic HIV), infection beyond 2 months occurred in 10 children (14%) and recurrent varicella zoster virus infections occurred in 38 children (55%). There was a strong association between an increasing number of recurrences and low CD4 cell counts.[8] Half of recurrent infections involved generalised rashes and the other half had zoster. **Newborns:** We found no cohort studies of untreated children with perinatal exposure to chickenpox. One cohort study (281 neonates receiving varicella zoster immune globulin Ⓖ because their mothers had developed a chickenpox rash during the month before or after delivery) found that 134 (48%) developed a chickenpox rash and 19 (14%) developed severe chickenpox.[9] Severe chickenpox occurred in neonates of mothers whose rash had started during the 7 days before delivery.

AIMS OF INTERVENTION To prevent clinical chickenpox (characterised by a rash); to reduce the duration of illness and complications of chickenpox.

OUTCOMES Development of clinical chickenpox; duration of illness (time to no new lesions, disappearance of fever); complications of chickenpox; mortality.

METHODS *Clinical Evidence* search and appraisal March 2004.

QUESTION **What are the effects of interventions to prevent chickenpox in healthy adults and children?**

OPTION LIVE ATTENUATED VARICELLA VACCINE

Two RCTs identified by a systematic review found that live attenuated varicella vaccine reduced clinical chickenpox in healthy children compared with placebo, with no significant increase in adverse effects. We found no RCTs in healthy adults.

Benefits: We found one systematic review (search date 2000, 2 RCTs).[10] **In healthy children:** The first RCT (914 healthy children aged 1–14 years) found that live attenuated varicella vaccine significantly reduced clinical chickenpox at 9 months (0/468 [0%] with vaccine *v* 38/446 [8.5%] with placebo; ARR 8.5%, 95% CI 6.1% to 11.5%; protection level 100%)[11] and at 2 years (1/163 [1%] with vaccine *v* 21/161 [13%] with placebo; OR 0.05, 95% CI 0.01 to 0.35).[12] The second RCT (327 healthy children aged 10–30 months) also found that live attenuated varicella vaccine significantly reduced clinical chickenpox after a mean of 29 months (AR 5/166 [3%] with vaccine *v* 41/161 [25%] with placebo; RR 0.12, 95% CI 0.05 to 0.29).[13] **In healthy adults:** The review found no RCTs assessing clinical outcomes in healthy adults.

Harms: The systematic review found that the only reported adverse effect with varicella vaccine was a non-significant increase in varicella-like papules or vesicles (AR 5.4% with vaccine *v* 3.7% with placebo; RR 1.45, 95% CI 0.53 to 4.0).[10] No children had fever or constitutional symptoms. One postmarketing analysis of a database of 89 753 vaccinated adults and children found no associations with any rare serious adverse events.[14] Another analysis found that the rate of serious adverse events was 2.9/100 000 doses.[15]

Comment: A new systematic review of vaccines for preventing varicella in children and adults is under way.[16] Aciclovir, varicella zoster immune globulin and zoster immune globulin are of questionable clinical importance for prevention in healthy people. Data from both healthy and immunocompromised people are presented elsewhere (see benefits of aciclovir in prevention, p 879 and benefits of zoster immune globulin in prevention, p 880).

QUESTION What are the effects of interventions to prevent chickenpox in immunocompromised adults and children?

OPTION LIVE ATTENUATED VARICELLA VACCINE

We found no RCTs in immunocompromised adults or children.

Benefits: We found no RCTs assessing clinical outcomes in people receiving cancer chemotherapy or in people with HIV.

Harms: We found no RCTs.

Comment: A new systematic review of vaccines for preventing varicella in children and adults is under way.[16]

OPTION ACICLOVIR (HIGH DOSE)

One systematic review in people with HIV infection found that high dose aciclovir (≥ 3200 mg/day) reduced the risk of clinical chickenpox and reduced all cause mortality over 22 months' treatment compared with placebo. We found no RCTs in people with other forms of immunocompromise.

Benefits: **In people with HIV:** We found one systematic review (search date not reported, 8 RCTs, 1792 people with different stages of HIV, median CD4 count 34–607/mm^3) comparing high dose aciclovir versus placebo.[17] Three of the RCTs were unpublished, including two pharmaceutical company trials. The review found that aciclovir (≥ 3200 mg/day for up to 22 months) significantly reduced clinical chickenpox (AR 14/895 [2%] with aciclovir *v* 54/897 [6%] with placebo; OR 0.29, 95% CI 0.13 to 0.63; NNT 23, 95% CI 17 to 39). All cause mortality was also reduced (HR 0.78, 95% CI 0.65 to 0.93; OR 0.75, 95% CI 0.57 to 1.00). The treatment effect did not vary significantly with CD4 count. We found no RCTs of lower doses of aciclovir in people with HIV. **In other immunocompromised people:** We found no RCTs of aciclovir in adults or children with other forms of immunocompromise.

Harms: The systematic review did not assess adverse effects (see harms under aciclovir for treatment, p 881).

Comment: None.

OPTION ZOSTER IMMUNE GLOBULIN

We found no RCTs on the effects of zoster immune globulin in immunocompromised adults, although one small RCT in healthy children found that zoster immune globulin reduced the proportion of children with clinical chickenpox compared with immune serum globulin. One RCT in immunocompromised children exposed to a sibling with chickenpox found no significant difference in clinical chickenpox with zoster immune globulin compared with varicella zoster immune globulin at 12 weeks.

Benefits: We found no systematic review. **Versus placebo:** We found no RCTs. **Versus immune serum globulin (ISG) in immunocompromised children:** We found no RCTs. **Versus varicella zoster immune globulin (VZIG) in immunocompromised children:** We found one RCT (164 immunocompromised children, mostly with leukaemia, exposed to a sibling with chickenpox) comparing zoster immune globulin (ZIG)Ⓖ (1.25 mL/10 kg) versus VZIGⒼ (1.25 mL/10 kg).[18] It found no significant difference in the proportion of children with clinical chickenpox at 12 weeks (AR 31/88 [37%] with ZIG *v* 36/81 [44%] with VZIG; RR 0.84, 95% CI 0.58 to 1.22).

Harms: None of the RCTs assessed adverse effects.

Comment: **Versus ISG in healthy children:** We found one small RCT (12 healthy susceptible children exposed to a sibling with recent onset of chickenpox) comparing ZIG (2 mL/10 kg) versus ISG (2 mL/10 kg).[19] It found that ZIG significantly reduced the proportion of children with clinical chickenpox at 20 days (AR 0/6 [0%] with ISG *v* 6/6 [100%] with ZIG; OR 0, 95% CI 0 to 0.28). In the absence of evidence in immunocompromised people, data on effects in healthy people may be of some use, but the applicability of the findings to immunocompromised people is questionable. The imprecise estimates might not exclude clinically important differences.

QUESTION What are the effects of treatments for chickenpox in healthy adults and children?

OPTION ACICLOVIR

Two systematic reviews found that oral acyclovir reduced the symptoms of chickenpox in healthy people compared with placebo. One systematic review and one additional RCT found that oral aciclovir given beyond 24 hours after onset of rash did not reduce the symptoms of chickenpox compared with placebo.

Benefits: **In healthy children:** We found one systematic review in children and adolescents (search date 2002, 3 RCTs, 979 children)[20] and one additional RCT in both children and adults.[21] The systematic review compared aciclovir versus placebo given within 24 hours of onset of rash in otherwise healthy children aged 0–18 years.[20] It did not perform a meta-analysis because of differences in age among participants. Two of the three RCTs included in the review found that aciclovir (20 mg/kg or 800 mg 4 times daily) significantly reduced the time to no new lesions compared with placebo (WMD 1.2 days, 95% CI 1.0 day to 1.5 days in the first RCT; WMD 1.1 days, 95% CI 0.5 days to 1.8 days in the second RCT). The remaining RCT found no significant difference in the time to no new lesions with aciclovir 10–20 mg/kg compared with placebo (WMD 0 days, 95% CI –0.5 days to +0.5 days). The number of days to no fever was significantly reduced by aciclovir in all three RCTs (first trial: WMD 1.1 days, 95% CI 0.9 days to 1.3 days; second trial: WMD 1.0 days, 95% CI 0.5 days to 1.5 days; third trial: WMD 1.3 days, 95% CI 0.6 days to 2.0 days).[20] We found one additional RCT that included children, adolescents, and adults (77 people).[21] It found that aciclovir started on the second day of the rash significantly reduced the time to no new lesions in children compared with starting on the third day (median 4 days when started on second day *v* 5 days when started on third day; P < 0.04) but found no significant difference in adolescents and adults. Earlier treatment significantly reduced the time to lowering of fever in adolescents (median 2–3 days when started on second day *v* 3–4 days when started on third day; P < 0.02) but not in children and adults. **In healthy adults:** We found one systematic review (search date 1997, 3 RCTs).[22] It did not perform a meta-analysis. The first RCT identified by the review (76 adults) compared early and late administration of aciclovir (800 mg 5 times daily) versus placebo. It found that aciclovir given within 24 hours of the rash significantly reduced the maximum number of lesions and the time to full crusting of lesions compared with placebo. It found no difference in time to full crusting of lesions if aciclovir was given 24–72 hours after the rash. The two remaining RCTs (total of 168 healthy adults) compared aciclovir given more than 24 hours after the onset of the rash versus placebo. Neither found a significant difference in the time to no new lesions, and did not provide numerical information on the time to lowering of fever. We found one additional RCT that included children, adolescents, and adults (see in healthy children above).[21]

Harms: The systematic review in children found no significant differences between treatment and control groups, or unfavourable trends in children taking aciclovir.[20]

Comment: The effect on the measured outcomes was small and of questionable clinical importance in healthy people who make an uneventful recovery without treatment.

QUESTION What are the effects of treatments for chickenpox in immunocompromised adults and children?

OPTION ACICLOVIR

Two RCTs compared intravenous aciclovir versus placebo in children with cancer. One large RCT found that aciclovir reduced clinical deterioration. The other smaller RCT found no significant difference in clinical deterioration. We found no RCTs on the effects of aciclovir in immunocompromised adults.

Benefits: **In immunocompromised children:** We found two placebo controlled RCTs of intravenous aciclovir in children with cancer receiving chemotherapy.[23,24] The largest RCT (50 children aged 1–14 years with chickenpox, 60% of whom had a rash for > 24 hours) found that significantly fewer children receiving aciclovir (500 mg/m^2 of body surface area) deteriorated clinically and were transferred to open label aciclovir compared with placebo, (1/25 [4%] with aciclovir *v* 12/25 [48%] with placebo; RR 0.08, 95% CI 0.01 to 0.59; NNT 3, 95% CI 2 to 4).[23] Analysis of the remaining children not moved to open label aciclovir found that aciclovir significantly reduced the time to full crusting of lesions (mean 5.7 days with aciclovir *v* 7.1 days with placebo; $P < 0.013$). It found no significant difference in lowering of fever. The second RCT (20 children, mean age 6.4 years) comparing aciclovir (500 mg/m^2 of body surface area) versus placebo found no significant difference in the proportion of children who deteriorated clinically and were moved to open label aciclovir (AR 1/8 [12.5%] with aciclovir *v* 5/12 [42%] with placebo; RR 0.30, 95% CI 0.04 to 2.1).[24] However, the RCT was too small to exclude a clinically important difference. **In immunocompromised adults:** We found no RCTs.

Harms: In the first RCT, two of 25 children on aciclovir developed transient elevated blood urea nitrogen levels, compared with two children with other transient minor adverse effects on placebo.[23] In the second RCT, no adverse events were observed in the eight children receiving aciclovir, except one child with a self limiting maculo-papular rash lasting 1 day.[24]

Comment: In the first RCT in immunocompromised children the exclusion from the subsequent analysis of children taking placebo who deteriorated clinically means that the effect of placebo may have been overestimated.[23]

GLOSSARY

Immune serum globulin (ISG) Immunoglobulin prepared from pooled human plasma.
Varicella zoster immune globulin (VZIG) Prepared from units of donor plasma selected for high titres of antibodies to varicella zoster virus.
Zoster immune globulin (ZIG) Prepared from the plasma of donors convalescing from herpes zoster (sustainable supplies are difficult to obtain).

REFERENCES

1. Lee BW. Review of varicella zoster seroepidemiology in India and Southeast Asia. *Trop Med Int Health* 1998;3:886–890.
2. Garnett GP, Cox MJ, Bundy DA, et al. The age of infection with varicella-zoster virus in St Lucia, West Indies. *Epidemiol Infect* 1993;110:361–372.
3. Preblud SR. Varicella: complications and costs. *Pediatrics* 1986;78:728–735.
4. Scuffman PA, Lowin AV, Burgess MA. The cost effectiveness of varicella vaccine programs for Australia. *Vaccine* 1999;18:407–415.
5. Guess HA, Broughton DD, Melton LJ, et al. Population-based studies of varicella complications. *Pediatrics* 1986;78:723–727.
6. Feldman S, Hughes WT, Daniel CB. Varicella in children with cancer: seventy-seven cases. *Pediatrics* 1975;56:388–397.
7. Leibovitz E, Cooper D, Giurgiutiu D, et al. Varicella-zoster virus infection in Romanian children infected with the human immunodeficiency virus. *Pediatrics* 1993;92:838–842.
8. von Seidlein L, Gillette SG, Bryson Y, et al. Frequent recurrence and persistence of varicella-zoster virus infections in children infected with human immunodeficiency virus type 1. *J Pediatr* 1996;128:52–57.
9. Miller E, Cradock-Watson JE, Ridehalgh MK. Outcome in newborn babies given anti-varicella-zoster immunoglobulin after perinatal maternal infection with varicella-zoster virus. *Lancet* 1989;2:371–373.
10. Skull SA, Wang EE. Varicella vaccination: a critical review of the evidence. *Arch Dis Child* 2001;85:83–90. Search date 2000; primary sources Medline, Embase, The Cochrane Library, reference lists, the internet for position papers from health oganisations, and vaccine product information.
11. Weibel RE, Neff BJ, Kuter BJ, et al. Live attenuated varicella virus vaccine. Efficacy trial in healthy children. *New Engl J Med* 1984;310:1409–1415.
12. Kuter BJ, Weibel RE, Guess HA, et al. Oka/Merck varicella vaccine in healthy children: final report of a 2-year efficacy study and 7-year follow-up studies. *Vaccine* 1991;9:643–647.
13. Varis T, Vesikari T. Efficacy of high-titer live attenuated varicella vaccine in healthy young children. *J Infect Dis* 1996;174:S330–S334.
14. Black S, Shinefield H, Ray P, et al. Postmarketing evaluation of the safety and effectiveness of varicella vaccine. *Pediatr Infect Dis J* 1999;18:1041–1046.
15. Wise RP, Salive ME, Braun MM, et al. Postlicensure safety surveillance for varicella vaccine. *JAMA* 2000;284:1271–1279.
16. Coole L, Law B, McIntyre P. Vaccines for preventing varicella in children and adults (Protocol for a Cochrane Review). In: The Cochrane Library, Issue 1, 2004. Chichester, UK: John Wiley & Sons, Ltd.
17. Ioannidis JP, Collier AC, Cooper DA, et al. Clinical efficacy of high-dose aciclovir in patients with human immunodeficiency virus infection: a meta-analysis of randomized individual patient data. *J Infect Dis* 1998;178:349–359. Search date not reported; primary sources Medline, hand searches of abstracts from meetings, trial directories, and communication with experts.
18. Zaia JA, Levin MJ, Preblud SR, et al. Evaluation of varicella-zoster immune globulin: protection of immunosuppressed children after household exposure to varicella. *J Infect Dis* 1983;147:737–743.
19. Brunell PA, Ross A, Miller LH, et al. Prevention of varicella by zoster immune globulin. *N Engl J Med* 1969;280:1191–1194.
20. Klassen TP, Belseck EM, Wiebe N, et al. Acyclovir for treating varicella in otherwise healthy children and adolescents (Cochrane Review). In: The Cochrane Library, Issue 4, 2002. Oxford: Update Software. Search date 2002; primary sources Cochrane Controlled Trials Register, Medline, Embase, PubMed, hand searches of reference lists, and contact with authors and pharmaceutical companies.
21. Balfour HH Jr, Edelman CK, Anderson RS, et al. Controlled trial of acyclovir for chickenpox evaluating time of initiation and duration of therapy and viral resistance. *Pediatr Infect Dis J* 2001;20:919–926.
22. Alfandari S. Second question: antiviral treatment of varicella in adult or immunocompromised patients. *Med Malad Infect* 1998;28:722–729. Search date 1997; primary sources Medline, Embase, and hand searches of reference lists and selected journals.
23. Nyerges G, Meszner Z, Gyarmati E, et al. Aciclovir prevents dissemination of varicella in immunocompromised children. *J Infect Dis* 1988;157:309–313.
24. Prober CG, Kirk LE, Keeney RE. Aciclovir therapy of chickenpox in immunosuppressed children: a collaborative study. *J Pediatr* 1982;101:622–625.

George Swingler
School of Child and Adolescent Health Red Cross Children's Hospital and the University of Cape Town, Cape Town, South Africa

Competing interests: None declared.

We would like to acknowledge the previous contributors of this chapter, including Jimmy Volmink.

Congenital toxoplasmosis

Search date March 2004

Piero Olliaro

QUESTIONS

INTERVENTIONS

Unknown effectiveness

See glossary Ⓖ

Key Messages

- **Antiparasitic drugs** Two systematic reviews of studies in women who seroconverted during pregnancy found insufficient evidence on the effects of current antiparasitic treatment compared with no treatment on mother or baby.

Congenital toxoplasmosis

DEFINITION Toxoplasmosis is caused by the parasite *Toxoplasma gondii*. Infection is asymptomatic or unremarkable in immunocompetent individuals, but leads to a lifelong antibody response. During pregnancy, toxoplasmosis can be transmitted across the placenta and may cause intrauterine death, neonatal growth retardation, mental retardation, ocular defects, and blindness in later life. Congenital toxoplasmosis (confirmed infection of the fetus or newborn) presents at birth: either as subclinical disease, which may evolve with neurological or ophthalmological disease later in life; or as a disease of varying severity, ranging from mild ocular damage to severe mental retardation.

INCIDENCE/ PREVALENCE Reported rates of toxoplasma seroprevalence vary among and within countries, as well as over time. The risk of primary infection is highest in young people, including young women during pregnancy. We found no cohort studies describing annual seroconversion rates in women of childbearing age nor incidence of primary infection. One systematic review (search date 1996) identified 15 studies that reported rates of seroconversion in non-immune pregnant women ranging from 2.4–16/1000 in Europe and from 2–6/1000 in the USA.[1] France began screening for congenital toxoplasmosis in 1978, and during the period 1980–1995 the seroconversion rate during pregnancy in non-immune women was 4–5/1000.[2]

AETIOLOGY/ RISK FACTORS Toxoplasma infection is usually acquired by ingesting either sporocysts (from unwashed fruit or vegetables contaminated by cat faeces) or tissue cysts (from raw or undercooked meat). The risk of contracting toxoplasma infection varies with eating habits, contact with cats and other pets, and occupational exposure.

PROGNOSIS One systematic review of studies conducted from 1983–1996 found no population based prospective studies of the natural history of toxoplasma infection during pregnancy.[1] One systematic review (search date 1997; 9 controlled, nonrandomised studies) found that untreated toxoplasmosis acquired during pregnancy was associated with infection rates in children of between 10–100%.[3] We found two European studies that correlated gestation at time of maternal seroconversion with risk of transmission and severity of disease at birth.[4,5] Risk of transmission increased with gestational age at maternal seroconversion, reaching 70–90% when seroconversion occurred after 30 weeks' gestation. In contrast, the risk of the infant developing clinical disease was highest when maternal seroconversion occurred early in pregnancy. The highest risk of developing early signs of disease (including chorioretinitis and hydrocephaly) was about 10%, recorded when seroconversion occurred between 24 and 30 weeks' gestation.[5] Infants with congenital toxoplasmosis and generalised neurological abnormalities at birth develop mental retardation, growth retardation, blindness or visual defects, seizures, and spasticity. Children with subclinical infection at birth may have cognitive, motor, and visual deficits, which may go undiagnosed for many years. One case control study (845 school children in Brazil) found mental retardation and retinochoroiditis to be significantly associated with positive toxoplasma serology (population attributable risk 6–9%).[6]

AIMS OF INTERVENTION To prevent transmission from mother to child, congenital infection, visual impairment, and neurological impairment in neonates and in later life, with minimum adverse effects.

OUTCOMES Incidence of spontaneous abortion, fetal infection, and overt neonatal disease (neurological and visual impairment); serological positivity in the newborn; adverse effects of treatment.

METHODS *Clinical Evidence* search and appraisal March 2004.

QUESTION What are the effects on mother and baby of treating toxoplasmosis during pregnancy?

OPTION ANTIPARASITIC DRUGS

Two systematic reviews of studies in women who seroconverted during pregnancy found insufficient evidence on the effects of current antiparasitic treatment compared with no treatment on mother or baby.

Benefits: We found two systematic reviews (search dates 1997)[3,7] and one study of case series.[8] The first review identified no RCTs.[3] It identified nine small cohort studies comparing treatments (spiramycin alone, pyrimethamine–sulphonamides, or a combination of the two treatments) versus no treatment.[3] Five of the studies identified by the review found that treating mothers significantly reduced fetal infection rates compared with no treatment ($P < 0.01$), the other four found no significant reduction in fetal infection. The second review had stricter inclusion criteria and identified no RCTs or observational studies of sufficient quality.[7] The study of case series of women treated with spiramycin or spiramycin plus pyrimethamine–sulphonamide found no evidence of a difference in outcomes (fetal infection, overt neonatal disease).[8] Comparing data from these studies was difficult because of different follow up periods.

Harms: Spiramycin and pyrimethamine–sulphonamides are reportedly well tolerated and non-teratogenic.[9] Sulpha drugs are known to carry a risk of kernicterus(G) in the newborn and should be avoided if possible in the third trimester; there is also a risk of bone marrow suppression, which can be reduced through concomitant use of folic acid.[9]

Comment: We found that the quality of evidence was poor. Studies included in the second systematic review were small and did not account for differences in gestation. Only two studies provided information about the control group and congenital infection was common in the treatment groups.[3] One decision analysis on screening and treatment for intrauterine toxoplasma infection has suggested that treatment may save the pregnancy without preventing infection in the neonate.[10] This may lead to an increase in congenital disease. Drug regimens of co-trimoxazole (trimethoprim plus sulfamethoxazole [sulphamethoxazole]), atovaquone, or fluoroquinolones, which are either used or being tested for secondary prophylaxis of toxoplasmosis in immunocompromised people (particularly those with HIV infection), have not been studied in pregnancy because their reproductive toxicity has not been properly documented. Finally, optimal duration of follow up is not established, although the longer the children are observed the higher the incidence of sequelae.

GLOSSARY

Kernicterus Cerebral toxicity caused by high levels of bilirubin in the neonate is known as kernicterus. Clinical effects include vomiting, lethargy, fever, and fits.

REFERENCES

1. Eskild A, Oxman A, Magnus P, et al. Screening for toxoplasmosis in pregnancy: what is the evidence of reducing a health problem? *J Med Screen* 1996;3:188–194. Search date 1996; primary sources Medline, Cochrane Pregnancy and Childbirth Database, and hand searched references.
2. Carme B, Tirard-Fleury V. Toxoplasmosis among pregnant women in France: seroprevalence, seroconversion and knowledge levels: trends 1965–1995. *Med Malad Infect* 1996;26:431–436.
3. Wallon M, Liou C, Garner P, et al. Congenital toxoplasmosis: systematic review of evidence of efficacy of treatment in pregnancy. *BMJ* 1999;318:1511–1514. Search date 1997; primary sources Medline, Embase, Pascal, Biological Abstracts, and personal communications.
4. Foulon W, Villena I, Stray-Pedersen B, et al. Treatment of toxoplasmosis during pregnancy: a multicenter study of impact on fetal transmission and children's sequelae at age 1 year. *Am J Obstet Gynecol* 1999;180:410–415.
5. Dunn D, Wallon M, Peyron F, et al. Mother-to-child transmission of toxoplasmosis: risk estimates for clinical counselling. *Lancet* 1999;353:1829–1833.
6. Caiaffa WT, Chiari CA, Figueiredo AR, et al. Toxoplasmosis and mental retardation: report of a case-control study. *Mem Inst Oswaldo Cruz* 1993;88:253–261.
7. Peyron F, Wallon M, Liou C, et al. Treatments for toxoplasmosis in pregnancy. In: The Cochrane Library, Issue 2, 2000. Oxford: Update Software. Search date 1997; primary sources Medline, Embase, Pascal, Biological Abstracts, and the Cochrane Controlled Trials Register.
8. Vergani P, Ghidini A, Ceruti P, et al. Congenital toxoplasmosis: efficacy of maternal treatment with spiramycin alone. *Am J Reprod Immunol* 1998;39:335–340.
9. Garland SM, O'Reilly MA. The risks and benefits of antimicrobial therapy in pregnancy. *Drug Saf* 1995;13:188–205.
10. Bader TJ, Macones GA, Asch DA. Prenatal screening for toxoplasmosis. *Obstet Gynecol* 1997;90:457–464.

Congenital toxoplasmosis

Piero Olliaro
Scientist/Manager
UNDP/World Bank/WHO Special Programme for Research and Training in Tropical Diseases CDS/TDR/World Health Organization
Geneva
Switzerland

Competing interests: None declared.

Dengue fever

Search date November 2004

Marissa M Alejandria

QUESTIONS

INTERVENTIONS

TREATMENTS

*Although we found no direct evidence to support their use, widespread consensus holds that intravenous fluid replacement with crystalloids should be used universally in children with dengue haemorrhagic fever or dengue shock syndrome because these conditions lead to an acute increase in vascular permeability that leads to plasma leakage, resulting in increased haematocrit and decreased blood pressure. Placebo controlled trials would be considered unethical.

See glossary G

Key Messages

Treatments

- **Intravenous fluids*** We found no RCTs comparing intravenous fluids versus placebo or no treatment. It is widely accepted that immediate fluid replacement should be undertaken in a child who has dengue haemorrhagic fever or dengue shock syndrome; it would be considered unethical to test its role in a placebo controlled trial.
- **Colloids (compared with crystalloids)** Two RCTs found no significant difference in mortality, recurrence of shock, or requirement for further infusions between crystalloids and colloids for acute resuscitation in Vietnamese children with dengue shock syndrome, but they are likely to have been underpowered to detect a clinically important difference.
- **Adding carbazochrome sodium sulfonate (AC-17) to standard intravenous fluids** One RCT in Thai children with dengue haemorrhagic fever/dengue shock syndrome found no significant difference in the development of shock, pleural effusion, and duration of hospitalization between adding carbazochrome sodium sulfonate and adding placebo to standard intravenous fluids. Another RCT with weak methods in Indonesian children with grade II dengue haemorrhagic fever found limited evidence that adding carbazochrome sodium sulfonate to standard intravenous fluids decreased the occurrence of pleural effusion compared with standard intravenous fluids alone.

- **Adding corticosteroids to standard intravenous fluids** Two RCTs in Thai and Indonesian children with dengue shock syndrome found no significant difference in mortality between adding corticosteroids to standard fluid replacement and adding placebo to standard fluid replacement. One open label RCT with weak methods in Burmese children with dengue shock syndrome found limited evidence that adding hydrocortisone to intravenous fluids reduced mortality compared with intravenous fluids alone.
- **Adding intravenous immunoglobulin to standard intravenous fluids** We found no published RCTs on the effects of intravenous immunoglobulin in people with dengue haemorrhagic fever or dengue shock syndrome. One unpublished RCT in Filipino children with dengue shock syndrome found that adding intravenous immunoglobulin to standard intravenous fluids reduced mortality compared with adding placebo to standard intravenous fluids.

*Although we found no direct evidence to support their use, widespread consensus holds that intravenous fluid replacement with crystalloids should be used universally in children with dengue haemorrhagic fever or dengue shock syndrome because these conditions lead to an acute increase in vascular permeability that leads to plasma leakage, resulting in increased haematocrit and decreased blood pressure. Placebo controlled trials would be considered unethical.

DEFINITION Dengue infection is a mosquito borne arboviral infection. The spectrum of dengue virus infection ranges from asymptomatic or undifferentiated febrile illness to dengue fever and dengue haemorrhagic fever or dengue shock syndrome. An important criterion to consider in the diagnosis of dengue infection is history of travel or residence in a dengue endemic area within 2 weeks of the onset of fever. **Dengue fever** is an acute febrile illness whose clinical presentation varies with age. Infants and young children may have an undifferentiated febrile disease with a maculopapular rash. Children aged 15 years or older and adults may have either a mild febrile illness or the classic incapacitating disease also called "breakbone fever" presenting with high fever of sudden onset and non-specific signs and symptoms of severe headache; pain behind the eyes; muscle, bone, or joint pains; nausea; vomiting; and rash. **Dengue haemorrhagic fever** is characterised by four criteria: acute onset of high fever; haemorrhagic manifestations evidenced by positive tourniquet testⒼ, skin haemorrhages, mucosal and gastrointestinal tract bleeding; thrombocytopenia; and evidence of plasma leakage manifested by a rise or drop in haematocrit, fluid in the lungs or abdomen, or hypoproteinaemia. Dengue haemorrhagic fever is classified into four grades of severity (see table 1, p 895).[1] Presence of thrombocytopenia and haemoconcentration differentiates dengue haemorrhagic fever grades I and II from dengue fever. Grades III and IV dengue haemorrhagic fever are considered **dengue shock syndrome.**[1] Plasma leakage is the major pathophysiological feature observed in dengue haemorrhagic fever.

INCIDENCE/ PREVALENCE Dengue fever and dengue haemorrhagic fever are public health problems worldwide, particularly in low-lying areas where *Aedes aegypti*, a domestic mosquito, is present. Cities near to the equator but high in the Andes are free of dengue because *Aedes* mosquitoes do not survive at high altitudes. Worldwide, an estimated 50–100 million cases of dengue fever and hundreds of thousands of dengue haemorrhagic fever occur yearly.[2] Endemic regions are the Americas, South East Asia, western Pacific, Africa, and the eastern Mediterranean. Major global demographic changes and their consequences (particularly increases in the density and geographic distribution of the vector with declining vector control; unreliable water supply systems; increasing non-biodegradable container and poor solid waste disposal; increased geographic range of virus transmission owing to increased air travel; and increased population density in urban areas) are responsible for the resurgence of dengue in the past century.[3,4] The World Health Organization estimates that global temperature rises of 1.0–3.5 °C can increase transmission by shortening the extrinsic incubation period of viruses within the mosquito, adding 20 000–30 000 more fatal cases annually.[5]

AETIOLOGY/ RISK FACTORS Dengue virus serotypes 1–4 (DEN 1, 2, 3, 4) belonging to the flavivirus genus are the aetiologic agents. These serotypes are closely related but antigenically distinct. *Ae aegypti*, the principal vector, transmits the virus to man. Dengue haemorrhagic fever and dengue shock syndrome typically occur in children under the age of 15 years, although dengue fever primarily occurs in adults and older children. Important risk factors influencing who will develop dengue haemorrhagic fever or severe disease during epidemics include the virus strain and serotype, immune status of the host, and age and genetic predisposition. There is evidence that sequential infection or pre-existing antidengue antibodies increases the risk of dengue haemorrhagic fever through antibody dependent enhancement.[3,4,6–8]

PROGNOSIS Dengue fever is an incapacitating disease but prognosis is favourable in previously healthy adults, although dengue haemorrhagic fever and dengue shock syndrome are major causes of hospital admission and mortality in children. Dengue fever is generally self limiting, with less than 1% case fatality. The acute phase of the illness lasts for 2–7 days but the convalescent phase may be prolonged for weeks associated with fatigue and depression, especially in adults. Prognosis in dengue haemorrhagic fever and dengue shock syndrome depends on prevention or early recognition and treatment of shock. Case fatality ranges from 2.5% to 5.0%. Once shock sets in, fatality may be as high as 12–44%.[9] In centres with appropriate intensive supportive treatment, fatality can be less than 1%. There is no specific antiviral treatment. The standard treatment is to give intravenous fluids to expand plasma volume. People usually recover after prompt and adequate fluid and electrolyte supportive treatment. The optimal fluid regimen, however, remains the subject of debate. This is particularly important in dengue, where one of the management difficulties is to correct hypovolaemia rapidly without precipitating fluid overload.

AIMS OF INTERVENTION To prevent mortality and improve symptoms, with minimal adverse effects.

OUTCOMES Mortality; recurrence of shock; symptom relief; renal failure; length of hospital stay; time to recovery; time off work; need for blood transfusion; fluid requirements; adverse effects (bleeding, fluid overload, hypersensitivity reactions, and secondary infections). Secondary outcomes include development of shock and development of pleural effusion.

METHODS *Clinical Evidence* search and appraisal November 2004. The author also retrieved additional material through hand searches and personal contact with experts in the field.

QUESTION What are the effects of supportive treatments for dengue haemorrhagic fever or dengue shock syndrome in children?

OPTION INTRAVENOUS FLUIDS

We found no RCTs comparing intravenous fluids versus placebo or no treatment. It is widely accepted that immediate fluid replacement should be undertaken in a child who has dengue haemorrhagic fever or dengue shock syndrome; it would be considered unethical to test its role in a placebo controlled trial. Two RCTs found no significant difference in mortality, recurrence of shock, or requirement for further infusions between crystalloids and colloids for acute resuscitation in Vietnamese children with dengue shock syndrome, but it is likely that they were underpowered to detect a clinically important difference.

Benefits: **Versus placebo or no treatment:** We found no RCTs (see comment below). **Crystalloids versus colloids:** We found no systematic review but found two RCTs (see comment below).[10,11] The first RCT (50 Vietnamese children aged 5–15 years with dengue shock syndrome) compared four intravenous fluid regimens for acute resuscitation: two crystalloid regimens (sodium chloride or Ringer's lactate solution, 25 children) and two colloid regimens (dextran 70 or gelafundin, 25 children).[10] Crystalloids or colloids were infused at a rate of 20 mL/kg for the first hour followed by 10 mL/kg for the second hour. All children then received further intravenous infusions on an open basis at the discretion of the attending physician according to World Health Organization guidelines. All children recovered with fluid resuscitation alone (no deaths in any group). The RCT found no significant difference among groups in recurrence of shock (median 1 episode in each group; $P = 0.46$) or requirement for further infusions of crystalloids ($P = 0.16$)

or colloids (P = 0.70) between the 2 hour infusion and full recovery from shock. Recovery from shock was defined as a pulse pressure of 20 mm Hg or greater. The RCT also found no significant difference among groups in median duration in shock (mean 1.5 hours with sodium chloride *v* 5.0 hours with Ringer's *v* 2.8 hours with dextran 70 *v* 7.0 hours with gelafundin; P = 0.36).[10] The second RCT (222 Vietnamese children, aged 1–15 years with dengue shock syndrome) also compared four intravenous fluid regimens for acute resuscitation: two crystalloid regimens (sodium chloride or Ringer's lactate solution, 111 children) and two colloid regimens (dextran 70 or gelafundin, 111 children).[11] The fluids were infused at a rate of 20 mL/kg for the first hour. All children then received further infusions of Ringer's lactate solution according to World Health Organization guidelines. However, children who failed to improve or who deteriorated were given additional colloid (dextran 70) infusions at the discretion of the attending physician. All children recovered with fluid resuscitation (no deaths in any group). The RCT found no significant difference between crystalloids and colloids in the proportion of children who had recurrence of shock (24/90 [27%] with colloids *v* 20/81 [25%] with crystalloids; RR 1.02, 95% CI 0.56 to 1.85). It also found no significant difference among groups in the total volume of fluid infused until full recovery from shock (P = 0.95) or in the proportion of children who required further infusions after the first hour (17/56 [30%] with sodium chloride *v* 20/55 [36%] with Ringer's *v* 17/55 [31%] with dextran 70 *v* 15/56 [27%] with gelafundin; P = 0.75).[11]

Harms: The first RCT found no adverse effects attributable to colloids or crystalloids, but it may have been underpowered to detect clinically important adverse effects.[10] In the second RCT, six children developed fever and chills after completing colloid treatment.[11] Two children receiving colloids had recurrence of shock, which responded to treatment with crystalloids. One child in the gelafundin group had severe epistaxis requiring transfusion and another child in the dextran group developed a large haematoma at a site of minor trauma. Thirty five children equally distributed among the four groups required diuretic treatment for 1 or 2 days after recovery from shock.[11]

Comment: It would be considered unethical to test the role of intravenous fluids in children with dengue haemorrhagic fever or dengue shock syndrome in a placebo controlled trial. Widespread consensus holds that intravenous fluid replacement with crystalloids should be universally used in children with dengue haemorrhagic fever or dengue shock syndrome because these conditions lead to an acute increase in vascular permeability that leads to plasma leakage, resulting in increased haematocrit and decreased blood pressure. The RCTs comparing crystalloids versus colloids are likely to have been underpowered to detect a clinically important difference in outcomes.[10,11] The RCTs measured outcomes at 1 or 2 hours after fluid infusion so a clinically important effect within the first hour of fluid resuscitation may have been overlooked. Regardless of whether colloid or crystalloid is more effective, if equal volumes are infused, there is no difference between them with regard to fluid overload.[12]

OPTION ADDING CORTICOSTEROIDS TO STANDARD INTRAVENOUS FLUIDS

Two RCTs in Thai and Indonesian children with dengue shock syndrome found no significant difference in mortality between adding corticosteroids to standard fluid replacement and adding placebo to standard fluid replacement.

One open label RCT with weak methods in Burmese children with dengue shock syndrome found limited evidence that adding hydrocortisone to intravenous fluids reduced mortality compared with intravenous fluids alone.

Benefits: We found no systematic review. We found three RCTs.[13–15] The first RCT (63 Thai children aged < 15 years with dengue shock syndrome receiving standard intravenous fluids) compared adding methylprednisolone sodium succinate (given as single bolus of 30 mg/kg) versus adding 5% dextrose in normal saline solution as placebo.[13] All children received crystalloids (either Ringer's lactate or 0.5% glucose in sodium chloride) given at a rate of 10–20 mL/kg adjusted to clinical and hydration status. Whole blood was given if there was a drop in haematocrit, and platelet concentrate was given if bleeding was uncontrolled. Haematocrit was monitored every 2–4 hours depending on the severity of shock and bleeding. The RCT found no significant difference in mortality between adding methylprednisolone and adding placebo to intravenous fluids (4/32 [12.5%] with methylprednisolone *v* 4/31 [12.9%] with placebo; RR 0.97, 95% CI 0.27 to 3.54). It also found no significant difference in duration of hospital stay (mean 7.3 days with methylprednisolone *v* 6.2 days with placebo; $P > 0.2$) or in the proportion of children who needed blood transfusion (11/32 [34%] with methylprednisolone *v* 8/31 [26%] with placebo; RR 1.51, 95% CI 0.51 to 4.46).[13] The second RCT (97 Indonesian children aged 1–10 years with dengue shock syndrome confirmed by serologic, virologic, or both examinations receiving standard intravenous fluids) compared adding hydrocortisone hemisuccinate (given iv as single dose of 50 mg/kg) versus adding sodium chloride as placebo.[14] It also found no significant difference in mortality between adding hydrocortisone and adding placebo (8/47 [17%] with hydrocortisone *v* 9/50 [18%] with placebo; RR 0.95, 95% CI 0.40 to 2.25) and no significant difference in mean fluid requirements between hydrocortisone and placebo (mean 2.3 L with hydrocortisone *v* 2.4 L with placebo; $P > 0.05$).[14] The third RCT (98 Burmese children, aged 1–8 years with serologically proved dengue shock syndrome, open label) compared adding hydrocortisone hemisuccinate to intravenous fluid regimens including crystalloids (normal saline, modified Ringer's lactate solution), plasma, and blood products versus intravenous fluid regimens alone (see comment below).[15] Hydrocortisone hemisuccinate was given intravenously in a single dose of 25 mg/kg on day 1, 15 mg/kg on day 2, and 10 mg/kg on day 3. It was unclear how many children received crystalloids and blood products alone or in combination.[15] The RCT found that adding hydrocortisone significantly reduced mortality compared with intravenous fluids alone (9/48 [19%] with hydrocortisone *v* 22/50 [44%] with intravenous fluids alone; RR 0.43, 95% CI 0.22 to 0.83; see comment below).[15]

Harms: In the first RCT, the frequency of episodes of infection (pneumonia, bacteraemia) and pulmonary haemorrhage were similar with methylprednisolone compared with placebo.[13] Three children taking methylprednisolone had convulsions. All survivors were followed up 2 weeks after treatment and sequelae rates, including haematomas, stiff joints, otitis media, abscesses, and gingivitis, were similar between the two groups.[13] The other two RCTs gave no information on adverse effects.[14,15]

Comment: The third RCT is an open trial with unclear randomisation scheme and allocation concealment, which could have overestimated the effect of adding hydrocortisone.[15] Baseline characteristics of the two groups were not comparable, with a greater proportion of children aged under 2 years and longer duration of shock in the children who did not receive steroids, which could have contributed to the higher mortality in these children. There is also a slight discrepancy between what is reported in the text of the article (see benefits above) and what is reported in the table about the number of children taking intravenous fluids alone who died; the figure reported in the table is 19/50, which gives a slightly different result (9/48 [19%] with hydrocortisone *v* 19/50 [38%] with intravenous fluids alone; RR 0.49, 95% CI 0.25 to 0.98). The other RCTs[13,14] did not find the mortality reduction found in the earlier RCT.[15] Differences in quality of methods in the RCTs and improvements in supportive care in the 1990s may account for the inconsistent results. A systematic review of corticosteroids in adults and children with dengue shock syndrome is in progress.[16] We found one unpublished systematic review (search date 1992,[17] 3 RCTs [described above],[13–15] 2 clinical trials,[18,19] 334 children with dengue haemorrhagic fever or dengue shock syndrome) that compared steroids versus placebo (personal communication, Thongpenyai Y, 2003).[17] The unpublished review found that trials were heterogeneous, but meta-analysis of the two RCTs (160 children with dengue shock syndrome) with adequate blinding and comparable groups at baseline found no significant difference in mortality between adding steroids to intravenous fluids and adding placebo (12/79 [15%] with steroids *v* 13/81 [16%] with placebo; OR 0.94, 95% CI 0.37 to 2.41).[17] Meta-analysis of all five studies also found no significant difference in mortality between adding steroids to standard intravenous fluids and intravenous fluids alone (AR 27/152 [18%] with steroids *v* 36/160 [22%] with placebo; pooled OR 0.65, 95% CI 0.35 to 1.19).[17]

OPTION ADDING INTRAVENOUS IMMUNOGLOBULIN TO STANDARD INTRAVENOUS FLUIDS

We found no published RCTs on the effects of intravenous immunoglobulin in people with dengue haemorrhagic fever or dengue shock syndrome. One unpublished RCT in Filipino children with dengue shock syndrome found that adding intravenous immunoglobulin to standard intravenous fluids reduced mortality compared with adding placebo to standard intravenous fluids.

Benefits: We found no systematic review or published RCTs (see comment below).

Harms: We found no published RCTs.

Comment: One unpublished, double blind RCT, conducted in a tertiary university teaching hospital in the Philippines (216 Filipino children, age 6 months to 14 years, 205 with serologically confirmed dengue shock syndrome) compared intravenous immunoglobulin (0.4 g/kg once daily for 3 days) versus placebo (personal communication, Frias MV, 2003).[20] All children received standard intravenous crystalloids as prescribed by World Health Organization guidelines. The RCT found that immunoglobulin significantly reduced mortality compared with placebo (18/108 [17%] with intravenous immunoglobulin *v* 31/108 [29%] with placebo; RR 0.58, 95% CI 0.35 to 0.97; NNT 8, 95% CI 4 to 102).[20] It found a similar duration of hospital stay between intravenous immunoglobulin and placebo. More children had a rash with intravenous immunoglobulin than with placebo but the difference was not significant (RR 1.6, 95% CI 0.95 to 2.68).[20]

OPTION ADDING CARBAZOCHROME SODIUM SULFONATE (AC-17) TO STANDARD INTRAVENOUS FLUIDS

One RCT in Thai children with dengue haemorrhagic fever/dengue shock syndrome found no significant difference in the development of shock, pleural effusion, and duration of hospitalization between adding carbazochrome sodium sulfonate and adding placebo to standard intravenous fluids. Another

RCT with weak methods in Indonesian children with grade II dengue haemorrhagic fever found limited evidence that adding carbazochrome sodium sulfonate to standard intravenous fluids decreased the occurrence of pleural effusion compared with standard intravenous fluids alone.

Benefits: We found no systematic review but found two RCTs.[21,22] The first RCT (95 Thai children aged 1.8–14.8 years with dengue haemorrhagic fever/dengue shock syndrome confirmed by serologic examinations and/or viral cultures, admitted before the onset of shock, receiving standard intravenous fluids) compared adding carbazochrome sodium sulfonate (AC-17) versus adding B vitamins as placebo.[21] Carbazochrome sodium sulfonate was given as an initial bolus injection followed by a continuous drip infusion for 3 days. The RCT found no significant difference in the development of shock during the course of treatment between adding carbazochrome sodium sulfonate to intravenous fluids and adding placebo to intravenous fluids (4/45 [8.9%] with carbazochrome sodium sulfonate *v* 3/50 [6%] with placebo; P = 0.44). It also found no significant difference between groups in the mean duration of hospital stay (mean: 4 days with carbazochrome sodium sulfonate *v* 4 days with placebo; reported as not significant, P value not reported) and in the overall development of pleural effusion (15/45 [33%] with carbazochrome sodium sulfonate *v* 15/50 [30%] with placebo; P = 0.89).[21] The RCT found no significant difference between groups in pleural effusion occurring on day 1, day 2, or day 3 after admission (day 1: 20% with carbazochrome sodium sulfonate *v* 14% with placebo; day 2: 31% *v* 28%; day 3: 20% *v* 14%; reported as not significant, P values not reported).[21] The second RCT (77 Indonesian children aged 6 months to 12 years with serologically confirmed grade II dengue haemorrhagic fever, receiving standard intravenous fluids; see comment below) compared adding carbazochrome sodium sulfonate versus adding 0.9% sodium chloride as placebo.[22] The RCT found no significant difference between groups in the development of pleural effusion on the first day after admission (13/37 [35%] with carbazochrome sodium sulfonate *v* 21/39 [54%] with placebo; P < 0.20) but it found that adding carbazochrome sodium sulfonate significantly decreased the development of pleural effusion compared with intravenous fluids alone on the second day after admission (8/38 [21%] with carbazochrome sodium sulfonate *v* 19/36 [53%] with placebo; P < 0.005) and on the third day after admission (5/37 [14%] with carbazochrome sodium sulfonate *v* 16/38 [42%] with placebo; P < 0.01).[22] The analysis was not by intention to treat.

Harms: In the first RCT the occurrence of bleeding during treatment was similar between the carbazochrome sodium sulfonate and placebo group (2/45 [2%] children with carbazochrome sodium sulfonate *v* 3/50 [6%] children with placebo).[21] All bleeding manifestations were mild; four children had epistaxis that needed local packing and one child had blood stained vomitus. None of the children needed a blood transfusion. The second RCT did not report on adverse effects.[22]

Comment: Neither RCT reported mortality as a primary outcome.[21,22] Only intermediate outcomes, such as the development of shock and pleural effusion as a marker of plasma leakage, were reported. The second RCT may have had methodologic flaws, which could have overestimated the treatment effect.[22] It did not report the randomization scheme and allocation concealment, how the identity of the experimental drug and the placebo were masked from the health care providers, or the baseline comparability of the two groups in terms of age and duration of illness prior to treatment.[22]

Dengue fever

GLOSSARY

Tourniquet test A test that is performed by inflating the blood pressure cuff to a point midway between systolic and diastolic pressures for 5 minutes. It involves then deflating the cuff, waiting for the skin to return to its normal colour, and then counting the number of petechiae visible in a 2.5 cm square in the ventral surface of the forearm. Twenty or more petechiae in square patch (6.25 cm^2) constitutes a positive tourniquet test.

REFERENCES

1. World Health Organization. Dengue hemorrhagic fever: diagnosis, treatment, prevention and control. Geneva: WHO 1997.
2. Pinheiro FP, Corber SJ. Global situation of dengue and dengue haemorrhagic fever, and its emergence in the Americas. *World Health Stat Q* 1997;50:161–168.
3. Gubler DJ. Dengue and dengue hemorrhagic fever. *Clin Microbiol Rev* 1998;11:480–494.
4. Guzman MG, Kouri G. Dengue: an update. *Lancet Infect Dis* 2002;2:33–42.
5. Githeko AK, Lindsay SW, Confalonieri UE, et al. Climate change and vector-borne diseases: a regional analysis. *Bull World Health Organ* 2000;78:1136–1147.
6. Cardosa MJ. Dengue haemorrhagic fever: questions of pathogenesis. *Curr Opin Infect Dis* 2000;13:471–475.
7. Morens DM. Antibody-dependent enhancement of infection and the pathogenesis of viral disease. *Clin Infect Dis* 1994;19:500–512.
8. Vaughn DW, Green S, Kalayanarooj S, et al. Dengue viremia titer, antibody response pattern, and virus serotype correlate with disease severity. *J Infect Dis* 2000;181:2–9.
9. Rigau-Perez JG, Clark GG, Gubler DJ, et al. Dengue and dengue hemorrhagic fever. *Lancet* 1998;352:971–977.
10. Dung NM, Day NPJ, Tam DTH, et al. Fluid replacement in dengue shock syndrome: a randomized, double-blind comparison of four intravenous-fluid regimens. *Clin Infect Dis* 1999;29:787–794.
11. Ngo NT, Cao XT, Kneen R, et al. Acute management of dengue shock syndrome: a randomized double-blind comparison of 4 intravenous fluid regimens in the first hour. *Clin Infect Dis* 2001;32:204–213.
12. Halstead SB, O'Rourke EJ. Editorial response: resuscitation of patients with dengue hemorrhagic fever/dengue shock syndrome. *Clin Infect Dis* 1999;29:795–796.
13. Tassniyom S, Vasanawathana S, Chirawatkul A, et al. Failure of high-dose methylprednisolone in established dengue shock syndrome: a placebo-controlled, double-blind study. *Pediatrics* 1993;92:111–115.
14. Sumarmo, Talogo W, Asrin A, et al. Failure of hydrocortisone to affect outcome in dengue shock syndrome. *Pediatrics* 1982;69:45–49.
15. Min M, Tin U, Aye M, et al. Hydrocortisone in the management of dengue shock syndrome. *Southeast Asian J Trop Med Public Health* 1975;6:573–579.
16. Panpanich R, Sornchai P, Kanjanaratanakorn K. Corticosteroids for treating dengue shock syndrome (protocol for a Cochrane Review). In: The Cochrane Library, Issue 4, 2004. Chichester, UK: John Wiley & Sons, Ltd.
17. Tongpenyai Y. Steroids in dengue hemorrhagic fever [dissertation]. Hamilton, ON, Canada: McMaster University 1992.
18. Pongpanich B, Bhanchet P, Phanichyakarn P, et al. Studies on dengue hemorrhagic fever. Clinical study: an evaluation of steroids as a treatment. *J Med Assoc Thai* 1973;56:6–14.
19. Sumarmo MSW, Martoatmodjo K. Clinical observations on dengue shock syndrome (An evaluation of steroid treatment). *Paediatr Indones* 1975;15:151–160.
20. Frias MV. The use of intravenous immunoglobulin in dengue shock syndrome: a randomized double-blind placebo-controlled trial [dissertation]. Manila, The Philippines: University of the Philippines College of Medicine 1999.
21. Tassniyom S, Vasanawathana S, Dhiensiri T, et al. Failure of carbazochrome sodium sulfonate (AC-17) to prevent dengue vascular permeability or shock: a randomized, controlled trial. *J Pediatr* 1997;131:525–528.
22. Funahara Y, Sumarmo, Shirahata A, et al. Protection against marked plasma leakage in dengue haemorrhagic fever by infusion of carbazochrome sodium sulfonate (AC-17). *Southeast Asian J Trop Med Public Health* 1987;18:356–361.

Marissa Alejandria
Associate Professor
Section of Infectious Diseases
Departments of Medicine
and Clinical Epidemiology
College of Medicine
University of the Philippines
Manila
The Philippines

Competing interests: None declared.

TABLE 1 World Health Organization grading of severity of dengue haemorrhagic fever.[1]

Grade	Description
Grade I	Fever accompanied by non-specific constitutional symptoms; the only haemorrhagic manifestation is a positive tourniquet test, easy bruising, or both
Grade II	Spontaneous bleeding in addition to the manifestations of Grade I, usually in the form of skin and other haemorrhages
Grade III	Circulatory failure manifested by a rapid, weak pulse and narrowing of pulse pressure or hypotension, with the presence of cold, clammy skin, and restlessness
Grade IV	Profound shock with undetectable blood pressure or pulse

Reproduced with permission of World Health Organization. Dengue haemorrhagic fever: diagnosis, treatment, prevention and control. Geneva: WHO 1997.

Diarrhoea in adults (acute)

Search date January 2004

Guy de Bruyn

QUESTIONS

INTERVENTIONS

See glossary

Clin Evid 2005;13:896–916.

Key Messages

Diarrhoea in developed countries

- **Antimotility agents** RCTs found that loperamide hydrochloride and loperamide oxide reduced the duration of diarrhoea and improved symptoms of acute diarrhoeal illness compared with placebo. One RCT found that diphenoxylate–atropine reduced rate of bowel actions compared with placebo but found no significant difference in median time to last stool. One RCT found more constipation-like periods in people taking loperamide hydrochloride and loperamide oxide 2 mg than in people taking placebo. However, it found no significant difference in constipation-like periods between loperamide oxide 1 mg and placebo.
- **Antibiotics (empirical use for mild–moderate diarrhoea)** RCTs found that antibiotics reduced the duration of diarrhoea and improved symptoms of acute diarrhoeal illness compared with placebo, and were more effective in eradicating pathogens from stool. One RCT found various self-limiting adverse effects in of people taking antibiotics, but these only led to discontinuation of treatment in people with rash. Bacterial resistance to *Campylobacter* developed in five people taking antibiotics.
- **Oral rehydration solutions** We found no systematic review or RCTs evaluating the effects of oral rehydration solutions for acute diarrhoea in adults living in developed countries.

Travellers' diarrhoea

- **Antimotility agents** Two RCTs found that loperamide hydrocholoride reduced the duration of diarrhoea compared with placebo. One of these RCTs also found that loperamide alone and trimethoprim–sulfamethoxazole alone were associated with similar durations of diarrhoea but that combination therapy with loperamide plus trimethoprim–sulfamethoxazole reduced the duration of diarrhoea compared with loperamide alone. Two RCTs found no significant difference in improvement of symptoms of acute diarrhoea between loperamide plus ciprofloxacin and ciprofloxacin.
- **Antibiotics (empirical use for mild–moderate diarrhoea** One systematic review, one subsequent RCT, and one additional RCT found that antibiotics reduced the duration of diarrhoea compared with placebo. The systematic review performed a meta-analysis of five RCTs and reported more adverse effects in people taking antibiotics compared with placebo, but none were judged to be serious.
- **Oral rehydration solutions** We found no systematic review or RCTs evaluating the effects of oral rehydration solutions on acute mild–moderate diarrhoea in adults from the developed world travelling to developing countries. One RCT found no significant difference in duration or diarrhoea or symptom control between loperamide plus oral rehydration solution and oral rehydration solution alone.

Mild–moderate diarrhoea in developing countries

- **Antimotility agents** RCTs found that lidamidine and loperamide improved symptoms of acute diarrhoea compared with placebo.
- **Antibiotics (empirical use)** Two RCTs with flawed methods found no significant difference in symptoms of acute mild–moderate diarrhoea between antibiotics and placebo in adults living in developing countries.
- **Citrate oral rehydration solution (compared with bicarbonate oral rehydration solution)** One RCT found no significant difference in stool output at 48 hours between citrate oral rehydration solution and bicarbonate oral rehydration solution.

Severe diarrhoea in developing countries

- **Amino acid oral rehydration solution** RCTs found modest clinical benefit with amino acid oral rehydration solution compared with standard oral rehydration solution in both in people with cholera and non-cholera diarrhoea.
- **Rice based oral rehydration solution** One systematic review found that rice based oral rehydration solution (ORS) reduced stool volume compared with standard ORS both in people with cholera and non-cholera diarrhoea. One additional RCT found that rice ORS reduced stool output compared with standard ORS.

- **Antibiotics (empirical use)** We found no systematic review or RCTs evaluating the effects of empirical use of antibiotics in treating severe diarrhoea in adults living in developing countries.
- **Antimotility agents** We found no systematic review or RCTs evaluating the effects of antimotility agents in treating severe diarrhoea in adults living in developing countries.
- **Bicarbonate oral rehydration solution** RCTs found no significant difference in total stool output or duration of diarrhoea between bicarbonate oral rehydration solution and standard or chloride oral rehydration solution.
- **Intravenous rehydration (compared with nasogastric tube rehydration or oral rehydration solution)** One small RCT found no significant difference in the duration of diarrhoea or total stool volume between enteral rehydration through a nasogastric tube and intravenous rehydration. We found no systematic review or RCTs comparing oral rehydration solution alone versus intravenous rehydration.
- **Reduced osmolarity oral rehydration solution** Three RCTs found modest and inconsistent effects of reduced osmolarity oral rehydration solution (ORS) on stool volume and duration of diarrhoea compared with standard ORS. Reduced osmolarity ORS was associated with an increased risk of non-symptomatic hyponatremia.

DEFINITION Diarrhoea is watery or liquid stools, usually with an increase in stool weight above 200 g daily and an increase in daily stool frequency. This chapter covers empirical treatment Ⓖ of suspected infectious diarrhoea in adults.

INCIDENCE/ PREVALENCE An estimated 4000 million cases of diarrhoea occurred worldwide in 1996, resulting in 2.5 million deaths.[1] In the USA, the estimated incidence for infectious intestinal disease is 0.44 episodes per person per year (1 episode per person every 2.3 years), resulting in about one consultation with a doctor per person every 28 years.[2] A recent community study in the UK reported an incidence of 19 cases per 100 person years, of which 3.3 cases per 100 person years resulted in consultation with a general practitioner.[3] Both estimates derive from population based studies including both adults and children. The epidemiology of travellers' diarrhoea Ⓖ is not well understood. Incidence is higher in travellers visiting developing countries, but it varies widely by location and season of travel.[4]

AETIOLOGY/ RISK FACTORS The cause of diarrhoea depends on geographical location, standards of food hygiene, sanitation, water supply, and season. Commonly identified causes of sporadic diarrhoea in adults in developed countries include *Campylobacter*, *Salmonella*, *Shigella*, *Escherichia coli*, *Yersinia*, protozoa, and viruses. No pathogens are identified in more than half of people with diarrhoea. In returning travellers, about 50% of episodes are caused by bacteria such as enterotoxigenic *E coli*, *Salmonella*, *Shigella*, *Campylobacter*, *Vibrio*, enteroadherent *E coli*, *Yersinia*, and *Aeromonas*.[5]

PROGNOSIS In developing countries, diarrhoea is reported to cause more deaths in children under 5 years of age than any other condition.[1] Few studies have examined which factors predict poor outcome in adults. In developed countries, death from infectious diarrhoea is rare, although serious complications, including severe dehydration and renal failure, can occur and may necessitate admission to hospital. Elderly people and those in long term care have an increased risk of death.[6]

AIMS OF INTERVENTION To reduce the infectious period, length of illness, risk of dehydration, risk of transmission to others, and rates of severe illness; and to prevent complications and death, with minimum adverse effects.

OUTCOMES Illness duration (time from start of treatment to last loose stool; time to first formed stool; duration of diarrhoea; duration of fever, duration of excretion of organisms); symptom control (number of loose stools a day; stool volume; relief of cramps, nausea and vomiting; incidence of vomiting; incidence of severe illness); microbiological efficacy (eradication of pathogens); presence of bacterial resistance; and rate of hospital admission.

METHODS *Clinical Evidence* search and appraisal January 2004.

QUESTION What are the effects of treatments for acute diarrhoea in adults living in developed countries? New

OPTION ANTIBIOTICS (EMPIRICAL USE)

RCTs found that antibiotics reduced the duration of diarrhoea and improved symptoms of acute diarrhoeal illness compared with placebo, and were more effective in eradicating pathogens from stool. One RCT found various self-limiting adverse effects in of people taking antibiotics, but these only led to discontinuation of treatment in people with rash. Bacterial resistance to *Campylobacter* developed in five people taking antibiotics.

Benefits: We found no systematic review but found 5 RCTs comparing empirical treatment with one or more antibiotics (ciprofloxacin, trimethoprim–sulfamethoxazole, nifuroxazide, ofloxacin, and pefloxacin) versus placebo or symptomatic treatment.[7–11] **Duration of diarrhoea or fever:** The first RCT (102 adults in France with acute diarrhoea**G** defined as > 3 watery stools per day) found that nifuroxazide (400 mg twice daily for 5 days) significantly reduced mean duration of diarrhoea compared with placebo (2.09 days with nifuroxazide *v* 3.26 days with placebo, P < 0.004).[7] The second RCT (202 adults in the US with acute diarrhoea defined as > 3 unformed stools in the previous 24 hours or > 2 unformed stools in the 8 hours before presentation) compared three interventions: ciprofloxacin (500 mg twice daily for 5 days), trimethoprim–sulfamethoxazole (160 to 800mg twice daily for 5 days), and placebo.[8] It found that ciprofloxacin significantly shortened the duration of diarrhoea compared with placebo (2.4 days with ciprofloxacin *v* 3.4 days with placebo, P < 0.0005). However, it found no significant difference between trimethoprim–sulfamethoxazole and placebo in the proportion of people who were cured or improved (P < 0.05), except on day 3. The third RCT (117 adults in Spain with acute gastroenteritis, defined as > 2 unformed stools in the previous 24 hours or > 2 in the previous 8 hours with fever, abdominal pain, urgency, or other gastrointestinal complaints) compared single dose ofloxacin 400 mg versus placebo.[9] It found no significant difference between ofloxacin and placebo in the average duration of diarrhoea (2.51 days with ofloxacin *v* 3.41 days with placebo, P = 0.117) but found that ofloxacin significantly reduced duration of fever compared with placebo (0.63 days with ofloxacin *v* 1.05 days with placebo, P = 0.02). The fourth RCT (173 adults in the UK with severe acute gastroenteritis, defined as > 4 fluid stools per 24 hours with at least one of the following symptoms: abdominal pain, fever, vomiting, myalgia, or headache) compared ciprofloxacin (500 mg twice daily for 5 days) versus placebo.[10] It found that ciprofloxacin significantly reduced duration of diarrhoea (2.2 days with ciprofloxacin *v* 4.6 days with placebo, P < 0.0001) and other gastrointestinal symptoms after treatment compared with placebo (1.9 days with ciprofloxacin *v* 4.3 days with placebo, P < 0.0001). The fifth RCT (82 adults in Croatia with acute bacterial gastroenterocolitis, defined as > 3 loose stools in 24 hours, fever > 38 °C, and at least one of the following symptoms: abdominal pain, nausea, or vomiting) compared 5 and 7 day regimens of pefloxacin 400 mg once daily versus symptomatic treatment (described as standard supportive regimen).[11] It found that both pefloxacin regimens reduced the mean duration of fever days compared with symptomatic treatment (3.3 days with 5 day pefloxacin *v* 5.0 days with symptomatic treatment, P < 0.001; 3.0 days with 7 day pefloxacin *v* 5.0 days with symptomatic treatment, P < 0.001). The RCT found no significant difference in the mean duration of fever days between the two pefloxacin regimens (P = 0.261). **Symptom control:** The first RCT found that the number of bowel movements per day was significantly smaller with nifuroxazide on day 1 compared with placebo (3.09 with nifuroxazide *v* 4.40 with placebo, P < 0.015) and day 2 (1.89 with nifuroxazide *v* 2.79 with placebo, P < 0.008) but the difference did not reach significance on day 3 of treatment (1.46 with nifuroxazide *v* 1.98 with placebo, P value reported as not significant, CI not reported).[7] The second (three-armed) RCT found that the proportion of people cured or improved was significantly increased by days 1, 3, 4, and 5 with ciprofloxacin compared with placebo (P < 0.05).[8] Although differences between trimethoprim–sulfamethoxazole and placebo were seen, only the difference on day 3 was significant (proportion of people cured or improved on day 3: 76% with trimethoprim–sulfamethoxazole *v* 58% with placebo, P < 0.05). The third RCT found no significant difference in the proportion of people with unchanged symptoms for more than 48 hours between ofloxacin and placebo (3/44 [7%] with ofloxacin *v* 6/46 [13%] with placebo, P = 0.485).[9] The fourth RCT found that ciprofloxacin significantly reduced the proportion of people with unresolved symptoms compared with placebo (3/81 [4%] with ciprofloxacin *v* 17/81 [21%] with placebo, P < 0.001).[10] The fifth RCT found that both pefloxacin regimens significantly reduced the average number of loose stools a day compared with symptomatic treatment (day 3: 3.0 with 5 day pefloxacin *v* 4.2 with symptomatic treatment, 3.0 with 7 day pefloxacin *v* 4.2 with symptomatic treatment; day 5: 1.5 with 5 day pefloxacin *v* 4.0 with symptomatic treatment, 1.6 with 7 day pefloxacin *v* 4.0 with symptomatic treatment; day 7: 1.2 with 5 day pefloxacin *v* 2.1 with symptomatic treatment, 1.4 with 7 day pefloxacin *v* 2.1 with symptomatic treatment; P < 0.001).[11] It found no significant difference in the average number of loose stools a day between the two pefloxacin regimens (P > 0.23). **Microbiological efficacy:** In the second RCT, 61 pathogens (mainly *Campylobacter*, *Shigella*, and *Salmonella*) were isolated from 57/202 (28%) participants.[8] The RCT found that ciprofloxacin was significantly more effective in eradication of pathogens than placebo (number of negative stool samples: 14/17 [82%] with ciprofloxacin *v* 4/19 [21%] with placebo, P < 0.001), or trimethoprim–sulfamethoxazole (number of negative stool samples: 14/17 [82%] with ciprofloxacin *v* 12/25 [48%] with trimethoprim–sulfamethoxazole, P < 0.001). In the third RCT, pathogens (mainly *Salmonella enteritidis*) were isolated from 72/117 (62%) participants.[9] The RCT found that ofloxacin was significantly more effective in eradication of pathogens after 2 days of treatment compared with placebo (number of people with negative stool samples after 2 days: 36/53 [68%] with ofloxacin *v* 23/56 [41%] with placebo, P = 0.0018). However, it found no significance difference in eradication of pathogens on day 15 with ofloxacin compared with placebo (number of people with negative stool samples on day 15: 33/43 [77%] with ofloxacin *v* 32/45 [71%] with placebo, P = 0.63). In the fourth RCT, pathogens (mainly *Campylobacter* and *Salmonella* species) were isolated from 141/162 (87%) of participants.[10] The RCT found that more people had negative stool samples on day 5 with ciprofloxacin than placebo (59/69 [86%] people with ciprofloxacin *v* 23/67 [34%] with placebo, P value not reported). It found no significant difference in eradication of pathogens six weeks after treatment between the two groups (8/67 [12%] with ciprofloxacin *v* 8/65 [12%] with placebo, P value not reported). In the fifth RCT, pathogens (mainly *S enteritidis* and *Salmonella typhimurium*) were isolated from all 82 (100%) participants.[11] The RCT found that both pefloxacin regimens were significantly more effective in eradication of pathogens from day 5 onwards compared with symptomatic treatment (number of people with negative stool samples on day 5: 18/20 [90%] with 5 day pefloxacin *v* 21/35 [60%] with symptomatic treatment, P = 0.049; 23/27 [93%] with 7 day pefloxacin *v* 21/35 [60%] with symptomatic treatment,

P = 0.017; day 7: 19/20 [95%] with 5 day pefloxacin *v* 22/35 [63%] with symptomatic treatment; 23/27 [93%] with 7 day pefloxacin *v* 22/35 [63%] with symptomatic treatment, P values reported as significant, CI not reported). Both pefloxacin regimens achieved eradication of pathogens in all 47 (100%) people one week after therapy compared with 29/35 (87%) people with symptomatic treatment (P value not reported). All participants had negative stool samples 4 weeks after treatment.

Harms: The first RCT found no adverse effects.[7] The second RCT reported 20 adverse effects with ciprofloxacin (4 people with headache, 4 with myalgia, 3 with sleep disturbances, 3 with nausea, 2 with rash, 1 each with vaginitis, dysphagia, dizziness, and a bitter taste); 23 with trimethoprim–sulfamethoxazole (8 people with headache, 4 with rash, 3 with dizziness, 3 with nausea, 2 with sleep disturbances, 1 each with dysuria, bloating, and a sour taste); 12 with placebo (5 people with headache, 2 with nausea, 2 with dizziness, 1 each with myalgias, dysuria, and rash). Complaints were self-limiting; however therapy was discontinued in people with rash.[8] Bacterial resistance to ciprofloxacin developed in 2/10 (20%) people and to trimethoprim–sulfamethoxazole in 3/14 (21%) people with *Campylobacter* isolates. The third RCT found no difference in adverse effects between treatment groups (1 person with headache in the ofloxacin group and 1 person with rash in the placebo group; no treatment required, P value not reported).[9] The fourth RCT found two adverse effects with ciprofloxacin that could be attributed to the treatment (1 each with unpleasant taste and vaginal thrush); the number of adverse effects in the placebo was not reported. No bacterial resistance developed during treatment.[10] The fifth RCT found no adverse effects requiring discontinuation of therapy with pefloxacin.[11]

Comment: The pathogenic organisms isolated from patients in each study varied and may partly explain variations in effect. Reported outcomes varied between trials, which precludes direct comparisons or summaries of treatment effect.

OPTION ANTIMOTILITY AGENTS

RCTs found that loperamide hydrochloride and loperamide oxide reduced the duration of diarrhoea and improved symptoms of acute diarrhoeal illness compared with placebo. One RCT found that diphenoxylate–atropine reduced rate of bowel actions compared with placebo but found no significant difference in median time to last stool. One RCT found more constipation-like periods in people taking loperamide hydrochloride and loperamide oxide 2 mg than in people taking placebo. However, it found no significant difference in constipation-like periods between loperamide oxide 1 mg and placebo.

Benefits: We found no systematic review but found six RCTs.[12–17] **Difenoxin:** We found no RCTs. **Diphenoxylate:** We found one RCT (152 adults with acute diarrhoea**G** for < 24 hours) comparing diphenoxylate–atropine versus placebo. It found that diphenoxylate significantly reduced the rate of bowel actions in the 24 hours after treatment (P = 0.05).[12] The RCT found no significant difference in median time to last loose stool (25 hours with diphemoxylate *v* 30 hours with placebo; P = 0.29). **Lidamidine:** We found no RCTs. **Loperamide hydrochloride:** We found two RCTs (409[14] and 261[15] adults with acute diarrhoea, defined as > 2 watery or loose stools in the previous 24 hours) with four study arms each, comparing loperamide hydrochloride versus placebo and versus two doses of loperamide oxide (1 mg and 2 mg). Both RCTs found that loperamide hydrochloride significantly reduced duration of diarrhoea compared with placebo (first RCT:[14] median time to complete relief of diarrhoea: 27 hours with loperamide hydrochloride *v* 45 hours 15 minutes with placebo, P = 0.006; second RCT:[15] median time to complete relief of diarrhoea: 17 hours 30 minutes with loperamide hydrochloride *v* 37 hours with placebo, P = 0.007). They found no significant difference among the groups on active treatment (first RCT: median time to complete relief of diarrhoea: 27 hours with loperamide hydrochloride *v* 23 hours 30 minutes with loperamide oxide 1 mg *v* 25 hours 30 minutes with loperamide oxide 2 mg, P > 0.7; second RCT: median time to complete relief of diarrhoea: 17 hours 30 minutes with loperamide hydrochloride *v* 18 hours with loperamide oxide 1 mg *v* 18 hours 30 minutes with loperamide oxide 2 mg, P > 0.8). **Loperamide oxide:** We found five RCTs comparing loperamide oxide versus placebo, or loperamide hydrochloride, or comparing different doses of loperamide oxide.[13–17] The first RCT (230 adults with > 2 watery or loose stools in the previous 24 hours) had three study arms and compared two doses of loperamide oxide (1 mg and 2 mg) with placebo.[13] It found that both doses significantly reduced duration of diarrhoea compared with placebo (median time to complete relief of diarrhoea: 27 hours 55 minutes with loperamide oxide 1 mg *v* 40 hours 35 minutes with placebo, P = 0.022; 25 hours with loperamide oxide 2 mg *v* 40 hours 35 minutes with placebo, P = 0.011). The second and third RCTs had four study arms each and compared two doses of loperamide oxide (1 mg and 2 mg) with placebo and loperamide hydrochloride.[14,15] Both RCTs found that both doses of loperamide oxide significantly reduced duration of diarrhoea compared with placebo (first RCT: median time to complete relief of diarrhoea: 23 hours 30 minutes with loperamide oxide 1 mg *v* 45 hours 15 minutes with placebo, P = 0.009; 25 hours 30 minutes with loperamide oxide 2 mg *v* 45 hours 15 minutes with placebo, P = 0.007; second RCT: median time to complete relief of diarrhoea: 18 hours with loperamide oxide 1 mg *v* 37 hours with placebo, P = 0.003; 18 hours 30 minutes with loperamide oxide 2 mg *v* 37 hours with placebo, P = 0.012) and found no significant difference between the groups on active treatment (see loperamide hydrochloride above). The fourth RCT (242 adults with acute diarrhoea, defined as > 3 loose or watery stools in the previous 24 hours) compared two doses of loperamide oxide (0.5 mg and 1 mg) with placebo.[16] It found that both doses of loperamide oxide significantly reduced duration of diarrhoea compared with placebo (median time to complete relief of diarrhoea: 25 hours 40 minutes with loperamide oxide 0.5 mg *v* 34 hours 15 minutes with placebo, P = 0.041; 26 hours 30 minutes with loperamide oxide 1 mg *v* 34 hours 15 minutes with placebo, P = 0.044). Investigators' ratings of overall efficacy of loperamide oxide 1 mg, using a 5 point scale, were significantly better than placebo (P = 0.008) but the difference did not reach significance between loperamide oxide 0.5 mg and placebo (P = 0.096). Similarly, patients' overall evaluations of the efficacy of treatment, using a 100 point visual analogue scale, were significantly better with loperamide oxide 1 mg compared with placebo (P = 0.003) but the difference did not reach significance between loperamide oxide 0.5 mg and placebo (P value reported as not significant, CI not reported). The fifth RCT (258 adults with acute diarrhoea, defined as ≥ 4 watery or loose stools within the previous 24 hours, and with diarrhoea for no more than 72 hours) compared four interventions: loperamide oxide 1 mg, 2 mg, 4 mg, or placebo. All were given an initial dose of two tablets and told to take another tablet on experiencing symptoms. All groups treated with loperamide had a quicker median time to relief of diarrhoea than groups treated with placebo, but there was no significant difference between three drug related groups (median time to first relief 28 hours 40 minutes placebo; 10 hours loperamide 1 mg; 12 hours 45 minutes loperamide 2 mg; 7 hours 30 minutes loperamide 4 mg).[17]

Harms: **Difenoxin:** We found no RCTs. **Diphenoxylate:** The RCT comparing diphenoxylate–atropine versus placebo did not report adverse events.[12] **Lidamidine:** We found no RCTs. **Loperamide hydrochloride:** The first RCT found significantly more constipation-like periods in people taking loperamide hydrochloride compared with placebo (25% v 7%, $P \leq 0.002$).[14] The second RCT (261 adults) compared loperamide oxide 1 mg with loperamide oxide 2 mg, with loperamide 2 mg, and with placebo.[15] Adverse events were mainly gastrointestinal (4 people on loperamide oxide 1 mg, 4 people on loperamide oxide 2 mg, 8 people on placebo, and 6 people on loperamide 2 mg; gastrointestinal adverse effects not specified). The significance of the difference between groups in adverse events was not reported. **Loperamide oxide:** The first RCT found that few adverse events were reported and all were mild or moderate (3/70 [4.3%] people on 1 mg loperamide oxide, 1/72 [1.4%] people on 2 mg loperamide oxide, 3/71 [4.2%] people on placebo).[13] The second RCT found significantly more constipation-like periods in people taking loperamide oxide 2 mg compared with placebo (24% v 7%, $P \leq 0.002$), but found no significant difference in people taking loperamide oxide 1 mg compared with placebo (16% v 7%, reported as not significant).[14] The third RCT (261 adults) compared loperamide oxide 1 mg with loperamide oxide 2 mg, with loperamide 2 mg, and with placebo.[15] Adverse events were mainly gastrointestinal (4 people on loperamide oxide 1 mg, 4 people on loperamide oxide 2 mg, 8 people on placebo, and 6 people on loperamide 2 mg; gastrointestinal adverse effects not specified). The significance of the difference between groups in adverse events was not reported. The fourth RCT (242 adults) found that more people on placebo than loperamide oxide reported adverse events but significance was not reported (16/80 [20%] people on placebo, 3/79 [4%] people on loperamide oxide 0.5 mg, 7/83 [8%] people on loperamide oxide 1 mg).[16] Abdominal cramps were the most frequently reported adverse effect in people taking placebo. In one person on placebo the cramps were noted as severe. The fifth RCT found that adverse events of any kind reported after non-leading questions were 13/66 (19.7%) for placebo, 7/64 (10.9%) for loperamide oxide 1 mg, 13/63 (20.6%) for loperamide oxide 2 mg, 14/65 (21.5%) for loperamide oxide 4 mg (significance of difference between groups not reported).[17] Significance of results was not reported. The number of people having a constipation-like period for ≥ 48 hours were: 11% with placebo, 10% with loperamide oxide 1 mg, 25% with loperamide oxide 2 mg, and 25% with loperamide oxide 4 mg). There was no significant difference between loperamide oxide and placebo.

Comment: None.

OPTION ORAL REHYDRATION SOLUTIONS

We found no systematic review or RCTs evaluating the effects of oral rehydration solutions for acute diarrhoea in adults living in developed countries.

Benefits: We found no systematic review and no RCTs.

Harms: We found no systematic review and no RCTs.

Comment: None.

QUESTION **What are the effects of treatments for acute mild–moderate diarrhoea in adults from the developed world travelling to developing countries?** New

OPTION **ANTIBIOTICS (EMPIRICAL USE)**

One systematic review, one subsequent RCT, and one additional RCT found that antibiotics reduced the duration of diarrhoea compared with placebo. The systematic review performed a meta-analysis of five RCTs and reported more adverse effects in people taking antibiotics compared with placebo, but none were judged to be serious.

Benefits: We found one systematic review[18] (search date 1999, 19 RCTs, 3157 people) and one subsequent RCT[19] comparing a variety of antibiotics versus placebo, versus a different dose of the same antibiotic, or versus another antibiotic in adults travelling from developed countries to developing countries. **Multiple destination studies (Central America, South America, Africa):** We found one systematic review,[18] which identified two RCTs,[20,21] and we found one subsequent RCT.[19] The first RCT identified by the review (142 US male military personnel in South America and West Africa with acute diarrhoea**G**) compared oral norfloxacin (400 mg twice daily for 5 days) versus oral trimethoprim–sulfamethoxazole (160/800 mg twice daily for 5 days).[20] It found no significant difference in duration of diarrhoea between norfloxacin and trimethoprim–sulfamethoxazole (mean number of days of diarrhoea after beginning treatment: 1.6 *v* 1.8, P = 0.37). Bacterial enteropathogens in stool samples were identified in 36/73 (49.3%) of the norfloxacin group and 27/69 (39.1%) of the trimethoprim–sulfamethoxazole group. In vitro resistance was found to trimethoprim–sulfamethoxazole in 20/74 (27%) of isolates tested but not to norfloxacin.[20] The second RCT identified by the review (447 Swedish travellers to Africa, Asia, or Latin America with acute diarrhoea) compared oral norfloxacin (400 mg twice daily for 3 days) versus placebo.[21] It found that norfloxacin significantly increased cure rates for diarrhoea after 3 days (≤1 loose stool/24 hours without additional symptoms) compared with placebo (34/48 [73.9%] *v* 18/48 [37.5%], P < 0.0001). The subsequent RCT (380 adult tourists in Guatemala, Mexico, and Kenya with acute diarrhoea defined as ≥3 unformed stools in 24 hours plus one additional sign of enteric infection) compared rifamixin (600 mg/day for 3 days) versus rifamixin (1200 mg/day for 3 days) versus placebo.[19] At 5 days' follow up median time since last unformed stool was significantly lower with rifamixin 600 mg/day and rifamixin 1200 mg/day compared with placebo (32.5 *v* 32.9 *v* 60.0 hours, P = 0.0001 for either rifamixin group *v* placebo). **Central America (Mexico, Belize):** One systematic review[18] identified 12 RCTs.[22–34] The first RCT (17 travellers from Houston, Texas to Mexico with ≥4 loose stools or ≥2 loose stools plus any of: ≥38.0 °C oral temperature, vomiting, or abdominal cramps during the previous 24 hour period) compared ciprofloxacin 250 mg twice daily for 3 days versus placebo.[22] It found that ciprofloxacin cured (≤1 loose stool/24 hours without additional symptoms) significantly more people after 48 hours compared with placebo (6/7 [86%] *v* 2/8 [25%], P = 0.04); produced significantly fewer loose stools per day (0.4 *v* 2.6, P = 0.03); significantly less mean time to cure from start of treatment (26 hours *v* 60 hours, P = 0.03). The second RCT (83 British troops having one or more loose stools in Belize) compared ciprofloxacin 500 mg (single dose) versus placebo.[23] It found that ciprofloxacin significantly improved diarrhoea compared with placebo (mean time to last liquid stool: 20.9 hours *v* 50.4 hours, P < 0.0001; mean time to last unformed stool: 24.8 hours *v* 53.5 hours, P < 0.0001). The other 10 RCTs were all carried out in the same centre in Guadalajara, Mexico, and are described in table 1, p 914.[24–34] **North and West Africa (Morocco, Egypt, the Gambia):** One systematic review[18] identified two RCTs.[34,35] The first RCT (106 Finnish tourists in Morocco with travellers' diarrhoea**G**, defined as ≥ 4 unformed stools in 24 hours or 3 unformed stools in 8 hours, plus ≥ 1 of: abdominal pain or spasms, nausea, vomiting, or fever) compared norfloxacin (400 mg twice daily for 3 days) versus placebo. It found that norflaxacin significantly reduced the mean duration of days with diarrhoea compared with placebo (1.2 days *v* 3.3 days, P < 0.01).[34] The second RCT (195 tourists in the Gambia with acute diarrhoea, defined as ≥ 1 watery or soft stool plus abdominal cramps, vomiting, or nausea) compared three interventions: fleroxacin (400 mg for 1 day), fleroxacin (400 mg/day for 2 days), and placebo.[35] It found that both 1 day and 2 day fleroxacin were significantly more effective than placebo in producing normal stool consistency at 48 hours' follow up (36/54 [67%] *v* 34/48 [71%] *v* 18/49 [37%], P < 0.01 between fleroxacin groups *v* placebo; no significant difference between fleroxacin groups, P value not reported). The proportion of people with total relief of diarrhoea was significantly larger in people taking fleroxacin at either dose compared with placebo, but there was no significant difference between different doses of fleroxacin (36 hours: 50% *v* 50% *v* 14%; 48 hours: 67% *v* 71% *v* 37% [absolute numbers not reported], P < 0.05 between fleroxacin groups *v* placebo; no significant difference between different doses of fleroxacin, P value not reported). Fleroxacin at either dose significantly increased the proportion of people cured of all symptoms compared with placebo, but there was no significant difference between different doses of fleroxacin (48 hours: 28/54 [52%] *v* 24/48 [50%] *v* 14/49 [29%]; P < 0.05 between fleroxacin groups *v* placebo; no significant difference between fleroxacin at different doses, P value not reported; 72 hours: > 80% *v* > 80% *v* 47% [numbers not reported], P < 0.01 between fleroxacin groups *v* placebo; no significant difference between fleroxacin groups, P value not reported). **Asia (India, Thailand):** One systematic review[18] identified two RCTs.[36,37] The first RCT (47 Danish tourists with diarrhoea in India) compared pivmecillinam (400 mg 3 times daily for 3 days) versus placebo. It found that pivmecillinam significantly reduced the duration of watery stools compared with placebo (< 24 hours' duration: 20/24 [83%] with pivmecillinam *v* 10/23 [43%] with placebo; 24–48 hours' duration: 6/24 [25%] *v* 8/23 [35%]; > 48 hours' duration: 0/24 [0%] *v* 6/23 [26%]; P < 0.05).[36] The second RCT (79 US military personnel in Thailand with acute diarrhoea, defined as ≥ 3 liquid bowel movements in 24 hours or 2 liquid movements plus fever, cramps, nausea, or vomiting) compared azithromycin 500 mg versus ciprofloxacin 500 mg. It found that mean duration of illness was similar in both groups (36.9 hours with azithromycin *v* 38.2 hours with ciprofloxacin, reported as similar, P value not reported.[37]

Harms: The systematic review[18] conducted a meta-analysis of five RCTs.[24,25,31,32,35] There were significantly more adverse effects in people taking antibiotics compared with placebo (OR 2.37, 95% CI 1.50 to 3.75). However, the adverse effects were not serious and resolved on withdrawal from the drug. **Multiple destination studies (Latin America, South America, Africa):** The first RCT stated that no adverse effects were reported.[20] The second RCT reported two adverse events with norfloxacin (constipation, heartburn: 2/19 [10.5%]) and seven adverse events in the placebo group (vertigo, headache, myalgia, constipation, and paraesthesia: 7/21 [33.3%]).[21] None of the people had norfloxacin resistant *E coli* before or after treatment; however, *E coli* resistant to other antibiotics was more frequent after treatment, particularly in the placebo group. The subsequent RCT found no significant difference in non-serious adverse effects (gastrointestinal related, headache) between groups (74/125 [59.2%] rifaximin 600 mg *v* 88/126 [69.8%] rifamixin 1200 mg *v* 90/129 [69.8%] placebo).[19] Fatigue was reported significantly more with rifaximin 1200 mg (P = 0.023, absolute data not reported). **Central America (Mexico, Belize):** The first RCT found that no adverse events were reported.[22] The second RCT found that no adverse events were reported.[23] See table 1, p 914 for adverse effects of treatment found at the centre in Guadalajara, Mexico.[24–33] **North and West Africa (Morocco, Egypt, the Gambia):** The first RCT (106 people) reported more mild adverse events with placebo compared with norfloxacin (18 cases with placebo *v* 7 cases with norfloxcacin; significance not reported).[34] The second RCT (safety analysis on 190 people out of 195), found that adverse events judged to be remotely, possibly, or probably related to the treatment were significantly more likely with fleroxacin-1 or fleroxacin-2 compared with placebo (25/64 [39%] with placebo, 36/61 [59%] with fleroxacin-1 [P < 0.05], and 42/65 [65%] with fleroxacin-2 [P < 0.05]).[35] The most common adverse event was fatigue. No adverse event was considered to be serious. **Asia (India, Thailand):** The RCTs did not report on adverse effects.[36,37]

Comment: One RCT (598 people ≥ 12 years old with acute diarrhoea lasting ≤ 5 days; only 70% of people had travellers' diarrhoea, the rest had non-travellers' diarrhoea) compared norfloxacin (400 mg twice daily) versus placebo. It found that norfloxacin significantly cured diarrhoea after 5 days (≤ 1 loose stool/24 hours without additional symptoms) compared with placebo (161/257 [63%] *v* 130/254 [51%], P = 0.003).[38] Differences in effectiveness of antibiotics between regions are likely to be due to local levels of antimicrobial resistance. As the prevalence of resistance steadily changes, it would be misleading to ascribe differences in efficacy to location.

OPTION ANTIMOTILITY AGENTS

Two RCTs found that loperamide hydrocholoride reduced the duration of diarrhoea compared with placebo. One of these RCTs also found that loperamide alone and trimethoprim–sulfamethoxazole alone were associated with similar durations of diarrhoea but that combination therapy with loperamide plus trimethoprim–sulfamethoxazole reduced the duration of diarrhoea compared with loperamide alone. Two RCTs found no significant difference in improvement of symptoms of acute diarrhoea between loperamide plus ciprofloxacin and ciprofloxacin.

Benefits: We found no systematic review but we found four RCTs.[29,39–41] **Loperamide hydrochloride versus placebo:** The first RCT (227 US school students attending summer school in Mexico, with ≥ 3 unformed stools in 24 hours, diarrhoea of ≤ 14 days' duration, and at least one of abdominal cramps, nausea, or vomiting) compared four interventions: loperamide hydrochloride 4 mg as loading dose and 2 mg on each loose bowel movement, single dose trimethoprim–sulfamethoxazole 300/1600 mg, trimethoprim–sulfamethoxazole 160/800 mg twice daily for 3 days, , combination trimethoprim–sulfamethoxazole 160 mg/800 mg twice daily for 3 days plus loperamide, and placebo. It found that mean duration of diarrhoea was significantly shorter with loperamide compared with placebo (33 hours *v* 58 hours, P ≤ 0.05).[29] Results from other arms of the RCT are presented under appropriate subheadings below. The second RCT (50 North American and Western European adult expatriates in Bangladesh, > 3 unformed stools during previous 24 hours, and ill for less than 72 hours) compared loperamide 2 mg after each loose stool with placebo.[39] It found that people treated with loperamide had significantly fewer stools on day 1 and 2 (figures presented graphically). **Loperamide hydrochloride alone versus**

trimethoprim–sulfamethoxazole: The four armed RCT (see above) found that mean duration of diarrhoea was similar in both groups (33 hours with loperamide and 36 hours with trimethoprim–sulfamethoxazole; significance not reported).[29] **Loperamide hydrochloride alone versus loperamide hydrochloride plus trimethoprim–sulfamethoxazole (combination treatment):** The four armed RCT found that combination treatment significantly reduced mean duration of diarrhoea compared with loperamide alone (33 hours *v* 16 hours, $P < 0.05$).[29] **Loperamide plus ciprofloxacin versus ciprofloxacin alone:** The first RCT (104 US military personnel with diarrhoea in Egypt) compared ciprofloxacin (500 mg twice daily for 3 days) plus loperamide (4 mg initial dose, then 2 mg for every loose stool, up to 16 mg/day) versus ciprofloxacin (500 mg twice daily for 3 days) plus placebo (taken for every loose stool, up to 8 caplets/day).[40] At 24 hours' follow up there was no significant difference in improvement (a 50% reduction in the daily number of stools compared with the previous 24 hours) or recovery (disappearance of all symptoms) between ciprofloxacin plus loperamide compared with ciprofloxacin plus placebo (41/50 [82%] *v* 36/54 [67%]; OR 2.3, 95% CI 0.8 to 6.3; $P = 0.08$). At 48 hours' follow up there was no significant difference in improvement or recovery (45/50 [92%] *v* 48/54 [89%]; OR not reported; $P > 0.2$). There was no significant difference in mean number of liquid stools after 24 and 48 hours' treatment between ciprofloxacin plus loperamide compared with ciprofloxacin plus placebo (24 hours: 1.9 *v* 2.6, $P = 0.19$; 48 hours: 3.1 *v* 4.0, $P = 0.19$).[40] The second RCT (142 military personnel with diarrhoea in Thailand) compared ciprofloxacin 750 mg plus loperamide (4 mg initial dose, followed by 2 mg after each loose stool, up to 16 mg/day) versus ciprofloxacin (500 mg twice daily for 3 days) plus loperamide (4 mg initial dose, followed by 2 mg after each loose stool, up to 16 mg/day) versus ciprofloxacin 750 mg plus placebo.[41] It found that there was no significant difference in the proportion of people fully recovered at 24, 48, and 72 hours between treatment groups (24 hours: 36% with single dose ciprofloxacin plus loperamide *v* 38% with 3 day ciprofloxacin plus loperamide *v* 36% with single dose ciprofloxacin plus placebo; 48 hours: 70% *v* 64% *v* 64%; 72 hours: 83% *v* 82% *v* 96%; P values not reported). It also found no significant difference between the three treatment groups in mean time until the last unformed stool (34 *v* 44 *v* 36 hours; P values not reported) and mean time until all symptoms were relieved (40 *v* 45 *v* 38 hours; P values not reported).[41]

Harms: The second RCT reported that 3 people treated with loperamide suffered from dizziness and 4 people suffered from constipation on loperamide compared with 3 taking placebo (significance not reported).[39]

Comment: None.

OPTION ORAL REHYDRATION SOLUTIONS

We found no systematic review or RCTs evaluating the effects of oral rehydration solutions on acute mild–moderate diarrhoea in adults from the developed world travelling to developing countries. One RCT found no significant difference in duration or diarrhoea or symptom control between loperamide plus oral rehydration solution and oral rehydration solution alone.

Benefits: We found no systematic review or RCTs.

Harms: We found no systematic review or RCTs.

Comment: One RCT (80 US students in Mexico) compared oral rehydration solution (500 mL initially, followed by 250 mL after each unformed stool, up to 1000 mL/day) plus loperamide (4 mg initially, followed by 2 mg after each unformed stool, up to 8 mg/day) versus loperamide alone for 48 hours.[42] It found no significant difference between groups in duration of diarrhoea or symptom control.

QUESTION What are the effects of treatments for acute mild–moderate diarrhoea in adults living in developing countries? New

OPTION ANTIBIOTICS (EMPIRICAL USE)

Two RCTs with flawed methods found no significant difference in symptoms of acute mild–moderate diarrhoea between antibiotics and placebo in adults living in developing countries.

Benefits: We found no systematic review but found an article reporting two Mexican RCTs which compared two different antibiotics versus placebo and versus trimethoprim–sulfamethoxazole.[43] The first RCT (307 adults with ≥ 3 unformed stools in 24 hours, of less than 72 hours duration and, if pre-treatment, stools contained ≥ 10 fecal leucocytes) compared trimethoprim–sulfamethoxazole 160/800 mg twice daily versus clioquinol 250 mg three times daily versus placebo. Analysis was not intention to treat (20 people were excluded from the analysis). It found no significant difference in mean number of unformed stools passed during the three day study (4.2 with trimethoprim–sulfamethoxazole *v* 4.2 with clioquniol *v* 5.3 with placebo; P value not reported). The second RCT (150 men with ≥ 4 unformed stools in the previous 24 hours, or 3 unformed stools in the previous 8 hours and one or more of fever, abdominal pain, faecal urgency, nausea, or vomiting of no more than 60 hours duration) compared three interventions: enoxacin, trimethoprim–sulfamethoxazole, and placebo. Analysis was not intention to treat (13 people were excluded from the analysis). Results were separated out into subgroups based on presence of pathogens before statistical analysis. It found no significant difference in the proportion of people who were well by 72 hours with enoxacin and with trimethoprim–sulfamethoxazole than with placebo (enoxacin 23/47 [49%] *v* trimethoprim–sulfamethoxazole 21/43 [49%] *v* placebo 16/49 [33%]; $P > 0.05$).[43]

Harms: The first RCT did not report on adverse events.[43] The second RCT reported four people suffered from adverse events leading to removal from the trial (one with light headedness, vertigo and photophobia, and one with moderate depression in the enoxacin group, and one person in the trimethoprim–sulfamethoxazole group with skin rash and one with moderate nervousness and abdominal pain).

Comment: None.

OPTION ANTIMOTILITY AGENTS

RCTs found that lidamidine and loperamide improved symptoms of acute diarrhoea compared with placebo.

Benefits: We found no systematic review but found two Mexican RCTs comparing antimotility agents versus placebo, versus each other, or comparing different doses of the same antimotility drug.[44,45] The first RCT (30 adults with acute diarrhoea**G**) found that lidamidine reduced the mean stool weight after 29 hours (435 g with lidamidine 4 mg *v* 364 g with lidamidine 2 mg *v* 576 g with placebo).[44] The second RCT (105 adults with acute diarrhoea) compared lidamidine versus loperamide versus placebo.[45] It found that there were fewer loose stools after 72 hours with lidamidine than with placebo (8.5 stools *v* 3.9 stools; P value not reported).

Harms: Constipation occurred in one person taking lidamidine compared with no-one taking placebo (1/35 [3%] with lidamidine *v* 0/35 [0%] with placebo).[45]

Comment: None.

OPTION ORAL REHYDRATION SOLUTIONS

One RCT found no significant difference in stool output at 48 hours between citrate oral rehydration solution and bicarbonate oral rehydration solution.

Benefits: We found no systematic review. We found one RCT comparing citrate oral rehydration solution (ORS) versus bicarbonate ORS.[46] The RCT (57 adults in Bangladesh with acute uncomplicated diarrhoea) found no significant difference between treatments in stool output over 48 hours (data reported as non-significant). Three people were excluded from the citrate group and four people from the bicarbonate ORS group mainly due to them being unable to be rehydrated orally because of persistent vomiting.

Harms: The RCT did not report on adverse events.[46]

Comment: None.

QUESTION What are the effects of treatments for acute severe diarrhoea in adults living in developing countries? New

OPTION ANTIBIOTICS (EMPIRICAL USE)

We found no systematic review or RCTs evaluating the effects of empirical use of antibiotics in treating severe diarrhoea in adults living in developing countries.

Benefits: We found no systematic review or RCTs.

Harms: We found no systematic review or RCTs.

Comment: See comment under oral rehydration solutions, p 909.

OPTION ANTIMOTILITY AGENTS

We found no systematic review or RCTs evaluating the effects of antimotility agents in treating severe diarrhoea in adults living in developing countries.

Benefits: We found no systematic review or RCTs.

Harms: We found no systematic review or RCTs.

Comment: None.

OPTION ORAL REHYDRATION SOLUTIONS

RCTs found modest clinical benefit with amino acid ROS compared with standard ORS in both cholera and non-cholera diarrhoea. RCTs found no significant difference in total stool output or duration of diarrhoea between bicarbonate oral rehydration solution and standard or chloride oral

rehydration solution. RCTs found modest and inconsistent effects of reduced-osmolarity ORS on stool volume and duration of diarrhoea compared with standard ORS. Reduced osmolarity ORS was associated with an increased risk of non-symptomatic hyponatremia. One systematic review found that rice-based ORS reduced stool volume compared with standard ORS in cholera and non-cholera diarrhoea. One small RCT found no significant difference in the duration of diarrhoea or total stool volume between enteral rehydration through a nasogastric tube and intravenous rehydration We found no systematic review or RCTs comparing oral rehydration solution alone versus intravenous rehydration.

Benefits: We found one systematic review (search date 1998, 4 RCTs, 694 adults)[47] and nine additional RCTs (see table A on web extra).[48–56] **Oral rehydration solutions (ORS) versus no rehydration:** We found no systematic review or RCTs. RCTs of oral rehydration versus no rehydration would be considered unethical. **Amino acid ORS:** We found no systematic review. We found two RCTs (97 men admitted to hospital with acute and severe dehydration from diarrhoea who received intravenous rehydration,[49] 108 men with diarrhoea < 48 hours' duration and severe dehydration[50]) comparing amino acid ORS versus standard ORS❻. In the RCT with intravenous rehydration, amino acid ORS was associated with a non-significant reduction in the total duration of diarrhoea and significantly reduced the total volume of stool compared with standard ORS.[49] The other RCT found that amino acid ORS improved weight gain, but not stool volume, compared with standard ORS in patients with cholera. For patients with non-cholera diarrhoea, amino acid ORS was associated with a reduction in stool volume, but not in weight gain.[50] **Bicarbonate ORS:** We found no systematic review. We found one small RCT (60 people with cholera and severe dehydration) comparing bicarbonate ORS versus an otherwise identical ORS, in which the bicarbonate was replaced with chloride.[51] The RCT found no significant difference in total stool output or duration of diarrhoea. We found two RCTs comparing bicarbonate versus standard ORS.[52,53] The first RCT (180 males with diarrhoea < 48 hours' duration) found no significant difference between treatments in the duration or volume of diarrhoea.[52] The second RCT (130 people with cholera) did not assess the significance of the difference between groups, although duration and volume of diarrhoea were greater with bicarbonate ORS than chloride ORS.[53] **Reduced osmolarity ORS:** We found no systematic review. We found three RCTs, which found a small and inconsistent effect on total volume of stool and duration of diarrhoea with reduced osmolarity ORS versus standard ORS.[54–56] **Rice based ORS:** We found one systematic review (search date 1998, 4 RCTs) in people with cholera and non-cholera diarrhoea.[47] The review found that, in adults with cholera, rice based ORS significantly reduced the 24 hour stool volume compared with standard ORS (4 RCTs, WMD −51 mL/kg, 95% CI −66 mL/kg to −36 mL/kg). One additional RCT found that both rice based ORS and low sodium rice based ORS significantly reduced stool output compared with standard ORS (4 L for rice based ORS *v* 5 L for standard ORS, $P < 0.02$; 3 L for low sodium rice based ORS *v* 5 L for standard ORS, $P < 0.05$).[56] **Oral rehydration versus intravenous rehydration:** We found no systematic review or RCTs comparing oral rehydration solution (ORS) alone versus intravenous rehydration. We found one small RCT (20 adults with cholera and severe dehydration) comparing enteral rehydration through a nasogastric tube versus intravenous rehydration.[48] Both groups received initial intravenous fluids for up to 90 minutes. The RCT found no significant difference in the total duration of diarrhoea (44 hours with iv fluids *v* 37 hours with nasogastric fluids; difference +7 hours, 95% CI −6 hours to +20 hours), total volume of stool passed (8.2 L *v* 11 L; difference −2.9 L), or duration of *Vibrio* excretion (1.1 days *v* 1.4 days; difference 0.3 days, 95% CI 0 days to 1 day).

Harms: **Amino acid ORS:** One RCT reported no episodes of hypernatraemiaⓖ or hyponatraemiaⓖ in people taking amino acid ORS or standard ORSⓖ.[50] **Bicarbonate ORS:** One RCT (130 people with cholera) reported that significantly more people taking standard ORS thought it tasted "bad" than those taking bicarbonate ORS (29% taking standard ORS *v* 13% taking bicarbonate ORS; CI not reported).[20] **Reduced osmolarity ORS:** Reduced osmolarity ORS significantly increased non-symptomatic hyponatraemia (OR 2.1, 95% CI 1.1 to 4.1) compared with standard ORS.[54] In RCTs evaluating symptomatic hyponatraemia, no cases were reported.[54,55]

Comment: All people with cholera received antibiotic treatment in addition to fluid treatment. Oral tetracycline or doxycycline were widely used, and were initiated at varying intervals after the start of oral rehydration. Response to ORS in people with cholera may not be comparable with response in people with less severe forms of diarrhoea.

GLOSSARY

Acute diarrhoea An episode of diarrhoea lasting 14 days or less.

Empirical treatment Therapy guided by professional experience, or given prior to or without reference to the results of microbiologic investigations.

Hypernatraemia An elevation in the concentration of sodium in serum above the normal range.

Hyponatraemia A reduction in the concentration of sodium in serum below the normal range.

Severe diarrhoea A diarrhoeal illness associated with profuse or dehydrating stool losses, blood, fever, or illness in infants, the elderly, or the immunocompromised.

Standard oral rehydration solution (ORS) An oral rehydration solution that includes citrate 10 mmol/L and glucose 111 mmol/L, and has an osmolarity of 311 mmol/L.

Travellers' diarrhoea Diarrhoea occurring during or shortly after travel in people who have crossed a national boundary.

Substantive changes

This chapter has been restructured to examine the effectiveness of treatments for acute diarrhoea in adults by severity and region.

Diarrhoea in developed countries: antibiotics (empirical use) One RCT added;[11] categorisation unchanged.

Diarrhoea in developed countries: antimotility agents Categorisation changed to Likely to be beneficial after re-evaluating the evidence.

Travellers' diarrhoea: antibiotics (empirical use) One subsequent RCT added;[19] categorisation unchanged.

Travellers' diarrhoea: antimotility agents Three RCTs added;[29,40,41] categorisation changed to Likely to be beneficial.

Mild–moderate diarrhoea in developing countries: antimotility agents Categorisation changed to Likely to be beneficial after re-evaluating the evidence.

REFERENCES

1. *The World Health Report 1997*. Geneva: World Health Organization, 1997:14–22.
2. Garthwright WE, Archer DL, Kvenberg JE. Estimates of incidence and costs of intestinal infectious diseases in the United States. *Public Health Rep* 1988;103:107–115.
3. Wheeler JG, Sethi D, Cowden JM, et al. Study of infectious intestinal disease in England: rates in the community, presenting to general practice, and reported to national surveillance. *BMJ* 1999;318:1046–1050.
4. Cartwright RY, Chahed M. Foodborne diseases in travellers. *World Health Stat Q* 1997;50:102–110.
5. Jiang ZD, Lowe B, Vernekar MP, et al. Prevalence of enteric pathogens among international travelers with diarrhea acquired in Kenya (Mobasa), India (Goa), or Jamaica (Montego Bay). *J Infect Dis* 2002;185:497–502.
6. Lew JF, Glass RI, Gangarosa RE, et al. Diarrheal deaths in the United States 1979 through 1987. *JAMA* 1991;265:3280–3284.

7. Bouree P, Chaput JC, Krainik F, et al. Double-blind controlled study of the efficacy of nifuroxazide versus placebo in the treatment of acute diarrhea in adults. *Gastroenterol Clin Biol* 1989;13:469–472. [in French]
8. Goodman LJ, Trenholme GM, Kaplan RL, et al. Empiric antimicrobial therapy of domestically acquired acute diarrhea in urban adults. *Arch Intern Med* 1990;150:541–546.
9. Noguerado A, Garcia-Polo I, Isasia T, et al. Early single dose therapy with ofloxacin for empirical treatment of acute gastroenteritis: a randomised, placebo-controlled double-blind clinical trial. *J Antimicrob Chemother* 1995;36:665–672.
10. Dryden MS, Gabb RJ, Wright SK. Empirical treatment of severe acute community-acquired gastroenteritis with ciprofloxacin. *Clin Infect Dis* 1996;22:1019–1025.
11. Troselj-Vukic B, Poljak I, Milotic R, et al. Efficacy of pefloxacin in the treatment of patients with acute infectious diarrhoea. *Clin Drug Invest* 2003;23:591–596.
12. Lustman F, Walters EG, Shroff NE, et al. Diphenoxylate hydrochloride (Lomotil) in the treatment of acute diarrhoea. *Br J Clin Pract* 1987;41:648–651.
13. Dettmer A. Loperamide oxide in the treatment of acute diarrhea in adults. *Clin Ther* 1994;16:972–980.
14. Hughes IW. First line treatment in acute non-dysenteric diarrhoea: clinical comparison of loperamide oxide, loperamide and placebo. *Br J Clin Pract* 1995;49:181–185.
15. Van den Eynden B, Spaepen W. New approaches to the treatment of patients with acute, nonspecific diarrhea: a comparison of the effects of loperamide and loperamide oxide. *Curr Ther Res* 1995;56:1132–1141.
16. Dreverman JWM, Van der Poel AJM. Loperamide oxide in acute diarrhoea: a double-blind, placebo-controlled trial. *Aliment Pharmacol Ther* 1995;9:441–446.
17. Cardon E, Van Elsen J, Frascio M, et al. Gut-selective opiates: the effect of loperamide oxide in acute diarrhoea in adults. The Diarrhoea Trialists Group. *Eur J Clin Res* 1995;7:135–144.
18. De Bruyn G, Hahn S, Borwick A. Antibiotic treatment for travellers' diarrhoea. In: The Cochrane Library, Issue 3, 2002. Oxford: Update Software. Search date 2000; primary sources The Cochrane Collaboration Trials Register (Issue 3, 1998), Medline, Embase, and hand searching and contact with experts.
19. Steffen R, Sack DA, Riopel L, et al. Therapy of travelers' diarrhea with rifaximin on various continents. *Am J Gastroenterol* 2003;98:1073–1078.
20. Thornton SA, Wignall SF, Kilpatrick ME, et al. Norfloxacin compared to trimethoprim/sulfamethoxazole for the treatment of travelers' diarrhea among U.S. military personnel deployed to South America and West Africa. *Mil Med* 1992;157:55–58.
21. Wiström J, Jertborn M, Hedström Sä, et al. Short-term self-treatment of travellers' diarrhoea with norfloxacin: a placebo-controlled study. *J Antimicrob Chemother* 1989;23:905–913.
22. Wiström J, Gentry LO, Palmgren AC, et al. Ecological effects of short-term ciprofloxacin treatment of travellers' diarrhoea. *J Antimicrob Chemother* 1992;30:693–706.
23. Salam I, Katelaris P, Leigh-Smith S, et al. Randomised trial of single-dose ciprofloxacin for travellers' diarrhoea. *Lancet* 1994;344:1537–1539.
24. DuPont HL, Reves RR, Galindo E, et al. Treatment of travelers' diarrhea with trimethoprim/sulfamethoxazole and with trimethoprim alone. *N Engl J Med* 1982;307:841–844.
25. Ericsson CD, DuPont HL, Sullivan P, et al. Bicozamycin, a poorly absorbable antibiotic, effectively treats travelers' diarrhea. *Ann Intern Med* 1983;98:20–25.
26. DuPont HL, Ericsson CD, Galindo E, et al. Furazolidone versus ampicillin in the treatment of traveler's diarrhea. *Antimicrob Agents Chemother* 1984;26:160–163.
27. Ericsson CD, Johnson PC, DuPont HL, et al. Role of a novel antidiarreal agent, BW942C, alone or in combination with trimethoprim-sulfamethoxazole in the treatment of traveler's diarrea. *Antimicrob Agents Chemother* 1986;29:1040–1046.
28. Ericsson CD, Johnson PC, DuPont HL, et al. Ciprofloxacin or trimethoprim-sulfamethoxazole as initial therapy for travelers' diarrea. *Ann Intern Med* 1987;106:216–220.
29. Ericsson CD, DuPont HL, Mathewson JJ. Treatment of traveler's diarrhea with sulfamethoxazole and trimethoprim and loperamide. *JAMA* 1990;263:257–261.
30. Ericsson CD, Nicholls-Vasquez I, DuPont HL, et al. Optimal dosing of trimethoprim-sulfamethoxazole when used with loperamide to treat travelers' diarrhea. *Antimicrob Agents Chemother* 1992;36:2821–2824.
31. DuPont HL, Ericsson CD, Mathewson JJ, et al. Oral aztreonam, a poorly absorbed yet effective therapy for bacterial diarrhea in US travelers to Mexico. *JAMA* 1992;267:1932–1935.
32. DuPont HL, Ericsson CD, Mathewson JJ, et al. Five versus three days of ofloxacin therapy for traveler's diarrhea: a placebo-controlled study. *Antimicrob Agents Chemother* 1992;36:87–91.
33. Ericsson CD, DuPont HL, Mathewson JJ. Single dose ofloxacin plus loperamide compared with single dose or three days of ofloxacin in the treatment of travelers' diarrhea. *J Travel Med* 1997;4:3–7.
34. Mattila L, Peltola H, Siitonen A, et al. Short-term treatment of traveler's diarrhea with norfloxacin: a double-blind, placebo-controlled study during two seasons. *Clin Infect Dis* 1993;17:779–782.
35. Steffen R, Jori R, DuPont HL, et al. Efficacy and toxicity of fleroxacin in the treatment of travelers' diarrhea. *Am J Med* 1993;94:182S–186S.
36. Christensen OE, Tuxen KK, Menday P. Treatment of travellers' diarrhoea with pivmecillinam [letter]. *J Antimicrob Chemother* 1988;22:570–571.
37. Kuschner RA, Trofa AF, Thomas RJ, et al. Use of azithromycin for the treatment of Campylobacter enteritis in travellers to Thailand, an area where ciprofloxacin resistance is prevalent. *Clin Infect Dis* 1995;21:536–541.
38. Wistrom J, Jertborn M, Ekwall E, et al. Empiric treatment of acute diarrheal disease with norfloxacin: a randomized, placebo-controlled study. Swedish Study Group. *Ann Intern Med* 1992;117:202–208.
39. Van Loon FPL, Bennish ML, Speelman P, et al Double blind trial of loperamide for treating acute watery diarrhoea in expatriates in Bangladesh. *Gut* 1989;30:492–495.
40. Taylor DN, Sanchez JL, Candler W, et al. Treatment of travelers' diarrhea: ciprofloxacin plus loperamide compared with ciprofloxacin alone. *Ann Intern Med* 1991;114:731–734.
41. Petruccelli BP, Murphy GS, Sanchez JL, et al. Treatment of traveler's diarrhea with ciprofloxacin and loperamide. *J Infect Dis* 1992;165:557–560.
42. Caeiro JP, DuPont HL, Albrecht H, et al. Oral rehydration therapy plus loperamide versus loperamide alone in the treatment of traveler's diarrhoea. *Clin Infect Dis* 1999;28:1286–1289.
43. De la Cabada FJ, DuPont HL, Gyr K, et al. Antimicrobial therapy of bacterial diarrhea in adult residents of Mexico — lack of an effect. *Digestion* 1992;53:134–141.
44. Heredia Diaz JG, Alcantara I, Solis A. Evaluation of the safety and effectiveness of WHR-1142A in the treatment of non-specific acute diarrhea. *Rev Gastroenterol Mex* 1979;44:167–73. [in Spanish]
45. Heredia Diaz JG, Kajeyama Escobar ML. Double-blind evaluation of the effectiveness of lidamidine hydrochloride (WHR-1142A) vs. loperamide vs. placebo in the treatment of acute diarrhea. *Salud Publica Mex* 1981;23:483–491. [in Spanish]

46. Ahmed SM, Islam MR, Butler T. Effective treatment of diarrhoeal dehydration with an oral rehydration solution containing citrate. *Scand J Infect Dis* 1986;18:65–70.
47. Fontaine O, Gore SM, Pierce NF. Rice-based oral rehydration solution for treating diarrhoea. In: The Cochrane Library, Issue 3, 2002. Oxford: Update Software. Search date 1998; primary sources Medline, Embase, Lilacs, Cochrane Controlled Trials Register, and Cochrane Infectious Diseases Group.
48. Pierce NF, Sack RB, Mitra RC, et al. Replacement of water and electrolyte losses in cholera by an oral glucose-electrolyte solution. *Ann Intern Med* 1969;70:1173–1181.
49. Patra FC, Sack DA, Islam A, et al. Oral rehydration formula containing alanine and glucose for treatment of diarrhoea: a controlled trial. *BMJ* 1989;298:1353–1356.
50. Khin-Maung-U, Myo-Khin, Nyunt-Nyunt-Wai, et al. Comparison of glucose/electrolyte and maltodextrin/glycine/glycyl-glycine/electrolyte oral rehydration solutions in cholera and watery diarrhoea in adults. *Ann Trop Med Parasitol* 1991;85:645–650.
51. Sarker SA, Mahalanabis D. The presence of bicarbonate in oral rehydration solution does not influence fluid absorption in cholera. *Scand J Gastroenterol* 1995;30:242–245.
52. Mazumder RN, Nath SK, Ashraf H, et al. Oral rehydration solution containing trisodium citrate for treating severe diarrhoea: controlled clinical trial. *BMJ* 1991;302:88–89.
53. Hoffman SL, Moechtar MA, Simanjuntak CH, et al. Rehydration and maintenance therapy of cholera patients in Jakarta: citrate-based versus bicarbonate-based oral rehydration salt solution. *J Infect Dis* 1985;152:1159–1165.
54. Alam NH, Majumder RN, Fuchs GJ. Efficacy and safety of oral rehydration solution with reduced osmolarity in adults with cholera: a randomised double-blind clinical trial. *Lancet* 1999;354:296–299.
55. Faruque ASG, Mahalanabis D, Hamadani JD, et al. Reduced osmolarity oral rehydration salt in cholera. *Scand J Infect Dis* 1996;28:87–90.
56. Bhattacharya MK, Bhattacharya SK, Dutta D, et al. Efficacy of oral hyposmolar glucose-based and rice-based oral rehydration salt solutions in the treatment of cholera in adults. *Scand J Gastroenterol* 1998;33:159–163.

Guy de Bruyn
Project Director
Perinatal HIV Research Unit, University of the Witwatersrand, Chris Hani Baragwanath Hospital
Johannesburg
South Africa

Competing interests: None declared.

TABLE 1 Effects of antibiotics for travellers' diarrhoea in Guadalajara, Mexico (see text).

Ref	Antibiotics	Participants	Duration of illness after therapy start	Adverse effects
Oflocacin				
32	Ofloxacin 300 mg twice a day for 5 days *v* 3 days *v* placebo	232 adults (66 *v* 81 *v* 79) (acute diarrhoea ≥ 4 unformed stools in 24 h or ≥ 3 unformed stools in 8 h, plus fever or other gastrointestinal complaint)	Mean: 39 h (P = NS compared with placebo) *v* 28 h (P < 0.05 compared with placebo) *v* 56 h	3/68 (4%) in 5 day group *v* 4/84 (5%) in 3 day group (insomnia, dizziness, dysgeusia [2 each], sleep disorder, nausea, vaginitis [1 each]. Two ofloxacin patients discontinued (nausea and vaginitis, and headache and rash)
33	Ofloxacin 400 mg single dose *v* ofloxacin 200 mg twice a day for 3 days *v* ofloxacin 400 mg single dose plus loperamide (4 mg then 2 mg after each loose stool)	166 adults (56 *v* 56 *v* 54) (≥ 3 unformed stools in 24 h plus one additional symptom of enteric disease)	Median: 14 h *v* 28 h *v* 0 h (P < 0.001)	No participants had a clinically important adverse reaction
Aztreonam				
31	Aztreonam 100 mg 3 times a day for 5 days *v* placebo	191 adults (98 *v* 93) (acute diarrhoea ≥ 4 unformed stools in 24 h or 3 in 8 h, plus ≥ 1 additional symptom [abdominal pain or cramps, nausea, vomiting, or fever])	Median: 33 h *v* 68 h (P = 0.0001)	18/98 (18%) *v* 12/93 (13%) experienced adverse effects (mild gastrointestinal complaints: 4 *v* 2; respiratory symptoms: 9 *v* 8) (NS; P value not reported)

TABLE 1 continued

Ref	Antibiotics	Participants	Duration of illness after therapy start	Adverse effects
Trimethoprim–sulfamethoxazole				
29	TMP-SMX (320/1600 mg) single dose *v* TMP-SMX (160/800 mg) twice a day for 3 days *v* loperamide HCl (4 mg initially, 2mg after each loose stool, ≤ 16 mg/day) *v* TMP-SMX (160/800 mg) twice a day for 3 days plus loperamide hydrochloride (4 mg initially, 2 mg after each loose stool, ≤ 16 mg/day) *v* placebo	227 adults (44 *v* 45 *v* 46 *v* 47 *v* 45) (≥ 3 unformed stools in 24 h plus one additional symptom of enteric disease)	Mean: 28 h *v* 36 h *v* 33 h *v* 16 h *v* 58 h ($P \leq 0.005$ compared with active treatments)	One person taking TMP-SMX for 3 days had a self-limiting rash
27	BW942C (20 mg initially then 10mg 5 times/day) *v* TMP-SMX (160/800mg twice a day) *v* BW942C (20 mg initially then 10 mg 5 times/day) plus TMP-SMX (160/800mg twice a day) *v* placebo; for 72 hours	134 adults (31 *v* 31 *v* 31 *v* 33) (acute diarrhoea ≥ 4 unformed stools in 24 h or 3 in 8 h, plus one additional symptom of enteric disease)	24 h (TMP-SMX) *v* 59 h (placebo), $P = 0.001$	9/32 (28.1%) BW942C *v* 2/31 TMP-SMX (6.5%) *v* 3/33 (9.1%) BW942C+TMP-SMX *v* 1/33 (3.0%) placebo (dizziness, light-headedness, restlessness, sleeplessness, difficulty concentrating, confusion or euphoria within the first 24 h)
28	Ciprofloxacin 500 mg v TMP-SMX (160/800 mg) *v* placebo twice a day for 5 days	181 adults (60 *v* 59 *v* 62) (acute diarrhoea ≥ 4 unformed stools in 24 h or 3 in 8 h plus ≥ 1 symptom of enteric disease)	Average: 29 h *v* 20 h *v* 81 h ($P \leq 0.001$ compared to active treatment)	2 ciprofloxacin (pruritis of the hands and eyes/swelling of hand and lips; vaginal infection) v 1 TMP-SMX (halos around lights)

TABLE 1 continued

Ref	Antibiotics	Participants	Duration of illness after therapy start	Adverse effects
30	TMP-SMX (160/800 mg bd for 3 days) plus loperamide (4 mg then 2 mg after each loose stool, ≤ 16 mg/day, for 3 days) *v* TMP-SMX (320/1600 mg single dose) plus loperamide (4mg then 2 mg after each loose stool, ≤ 16 mg/day, for 3 days) *v* TMP-SMX (320/1600 mg loading dose then 160/800mg bd for 5 doses) plus loperamide (4mg then 2mg after each loose stool, ≤16mg/day, for 3 days)	190 adults (62 *v* 64 *v* 64) (≥ 6 unformed stools in 24 h)	Time until 50% well: 11 h *v* 4 h *v* 0 h (P < 0.09 favouring group C); time until 75% well: 34 h *v* 33 h *v* 12 h (P < 0.09 favouring third group)	No participants reported a serious adverse effect
24	TMP-SMX (160/800 mg bd for 5 days) *v* TMP (200 mg bd for 5 days) *v* placebo	110 adults (37 *v* 38 *v* 35) (diarrhoea ≥ 4 unformed stools in 24 h or ≥ 3 in 8 h, plus ≥ 1 additional symptom of enteric disease)	29.2 h *v* 30.7 h *v* 92.8 h (P < 0.0001)	One (3%) of TMP group had minimal self limiting rash
Bicozamycin				
25	Bicozamycin (500mg 4 times/day for 3 days) *v* placebo	140 adults (72 *v* 68) (acute diarrhoea ≥ 4 unformed stools in 24 h plus one additional symptom of enteric disease)	28.2 h *v* 63.7 h (P = 0.00009)	Minor rash in 4/78 *v* 1/68. 1/72 had an eruption (erythematous macular patches)
Furazolidone *v* ampicillin				
26	Furazolidone (100 mg four times a day for 5 days) *v* ampicillin (500 mg four times a day for 5 days)	94 adults (47 *v* 47) (≥ 4 unformed stools in 24 h or 3 unformed stools in 8 h)	Mean: 57 h *v* 72 h (NS; P value not reported)	9/17 (52.9%) *v* 2/20 (10%) who had consumed alcohol had facial flusing. 12/47 (25.5%) taking furazaolidone had dark yellow urine.

h, hour; NS, not significant; Ref, reference; TMP, trimethoprim, TMP-SMX, trimethoprim–sulfamethoxazole.

Hepatitis B (prevention)

Search date October 2003

Kamran Siddiqi

QUESTIONS

INTERVENTIONS

Key Messages

In countries with high endemicity

- **Selective immunisation of high risk individuals (evidence only for children born to HBsAg positive mothers)** One non-systematic review of mainly observational studies with both plasma derived and recombinant vaccine, and three RCTs of plasma derived hepatitis B immunisation all found that immunisation prevented chronic carrier state compared with placebo or no treatment in children born to HBsAg positive mothers. One RCT found minor adverse events with immunisation; the other RCTs did not report on adverse events. We found no good evidence in other high risk groups. One cluster RCT found that selective immunisation in high risk individuals was less effective than universal immunisation of infants in preventing chronic carrier state and acute hepatitis events.
- **Universal immunisation of infants (limited evidence that it may be better than selective immunisation of high risk individuals)** One non-systematic review and four additional and subsequent RCTs provided evidence that universal (both recombinant and plasma derived) hepatitis B immunisation in infants in countries with high endemicity, compared with placebo, reduces acute hepatitis and development of a chronic carrier state for at least 15 years. Observational studies and one RCT found only minor adverse reactions after recombinant hepatitis B immunisation. One cluster RCT found universal immunisation with first plasma and then recombinant vaccine reduced the development of chronic carrier state and acute hepatitis events compared with immunisation of high risk groups.

Hepatitis B (prevention)

In countries with low endemicity

- **Selective immunisation of high risk individuals** One systematic review found that, in countries with low endemicity, plasma derived hepatitis B immunisation prevented acute hepatitis B and development of chronic carrier state in healthcare workers at high risk of exposure to bodily fluids. Three RCTs found that plasma derived hepatitis B immunisation prevented acute hepatitis B in homosexual men. One small RCT found no significant difference in hepatitis B events in heterosexual partners of infected people. Three RCTs of plasma derived immunisation in people on regular haemodialysis found potentially conflicting results. Two RCTs from France and Belgium found good protective efficacy against chronic carrier state. However, one large US based RCT found no good evidence of benefit. The systematic review of plasma derived vaccination found no significant difference between immunisation and placebo in the rate and severity of adverse events. One observational study showed a high prevalence of hepatitis B carrier state and low immunisation uptake in young homosexuals despite a national strategy to immunise high risk groups. Surveillance data from a national programme in Japan found that immunisation of neonates (with recombinant hepatitis B vaccine plus hepatitis B immunoglobulin [HBIG]) born to HBsAg positive mothers provided 95% protection against the development of a chronic carrier state. We found insufficient evidence to compare the effectiveness of selective immunisation in high risk individuals with other strategies.
- **Universal immunisation of infants** One historical cohort study found a reduction in the prevalence of hepatitis B chronic carrier state after universal immunisation. We found insufficient evidence to compare its effectiveness with other strategies. Two cohort studies and surveillance data did not report any links between hepatitis B immunisation and serious adverse events.
- **Comparative effectiveness of different strategies** We found no systematic reviews, RCTs, or observational studies comparing the effectiveness of different immunisation strategies in countries with low endemicity.
- **Universal immunisation of adolescents** We found insufficient evidence to assess the effects of universal adolescent immunisation, or to compare its effectiveness with other strategies. One observational study suggests minor adverse effects after hepatitis B immunisation in this group.

DEFINITION Hepatitis B is a viral infectious disease with an incubation period of 40–160 days. Acute hepatitis B infection is characterised by anorexia, vague abdominal discomfort, nausea and vomiting, jaundice, and occasional fever. Illness is associated with deranged liver function tests (especially raised alanine transaminases) and presence of serological markers of acute hepatitis B infection (e.g. hepatitis B surface antigen [HBsAg**G**], antiHBc IgM).[1]

INCIDENCE/ PREVALENCE The incidence of acute hepatitis B and prevalence of its chronic carrier state**G** varies widely across the globe. In areas with HBsAg prevalence ≥ 8%, e.g. South East Asia and Africa), more than half of the population becomes infected at some point in their lives.[2] In countries with low endemicity**G** (HBsAg prevalence < 2%, e.g. North America, western Europe, Australia), most of the population do not become infected.[2] Nearly a third of the world population has been infected by hepatitis B at some point, and at least 350 million people (5–6% of world population) are currently chronic carriers of hepatitis B infection.[3]

AETIOLOGY/ RISK FACTORS In countries with high endemicity, most infections occur during childhood from an infected mother to her baby (vertical transmission) or from one family member to another (horizontal transmission).[4] Horizontal transmission is thought to be an important route of hepatitis B infection during early childhood, and probably occurs mainly through unnoticed contact with blood from infected family members.[5] In countries with high endemicity, the proportion of chronic HBsAg carriage attributable to vertical transmission has been estimated at 5–50%.[6–8] The proportion of chronic HBsAg carriage attributable to horizontal transmission is not known, although one survey in China found that 27.2% of families had one or more HBsAg positive members.[8] In developed countries, most hepatitis B infection occurs later, from sexual activity, injection drug use, or occupational exposure. Less frequent causes of infection include household contact, regular haemodialysis, transmission from a healthcare professional, and receipt of organs or blood products.[9] The vaccination policy of a country is a large determinant of the risk of developing hepatitis B. Since the development of plasma derived hepatitis B vaccine in the early 1980s, subsequently replaced by recombinant vaccineⒼ, many countries have adopted a policy of universal immunisation of all infants. On the basis of disease burden, the World Health Organization recommended that hepatitis B vaccine be incorporated into routine infant and childhood immunisation programmes in countries with high endemicity by 1995 and in all countries by 1997.[10] However, in many countries with low endemicity, universal immunisation policy remains controversial and has still not been adopted.[11] Some of these countries have adopted a policy of selective immunisation of high risk individuals. Others have adopted a universal adolescent immunisation policy.

PROGNOSIS Hepatitis B infection resolves after the acute infection in 90–95% of cases. In the remainder (5–10%), it may result in several serious sequelae. Massive hepatic necrosis occurs in 1% of people with acute viral hepatitis, leading to a serious and often fatal condition called acute fulminant hepatitis. Between 2% and 10% of those infected as adults become chronic carriers, indicated by HBsAg persistence for more than 6 months. Chronic carriage is more frequent in those infected as children, and reaches up to 90% in those infected during the perinatal period.[1] Between 20% and 25% of chronic carriers develop a progressive chronic liver disease. In about one quarter to one third of cases, this progresses to cirrhosis and hepatocellular carcinoma.[12] These complications usually arise in older adults and are major causes of mortality in populations with high hepatitis B endemicity.[4] Observational studies suggest that in these countries almost 80% of chronic liver disease and cirrhosis is attributed to hepatitis B, and these complications lead to at least 1 million deaths every year worldwide.

AIMS OF INTERVENTION To reduce the risk of acquiring hepatitis B infection in susceptible people, while minimising adverse effects of interventions.

OUTCOMES Incidence of acute hepatitis B; prevalence of chronic carrier state; chronic liver disease; cirrhosis and hepatocellular carcinoma secondary to hepatitis B; mortality secondary to hepatitis B infection and its chronic sequelae; adverse events.

METHODS *Clinical Evidence* search and appraisal October 2003, including a search for observational studies. Where there were no good RCT data for a given comparison or outcome, we included the best available observational data. Both plasma derived and recombinant vaccines were included.

QUESTION What are the effects of immunisation in countries with high endemicity?

OPTION UNIVERSAL IMMUNISATION OF INFANTS

One non-systematic review and four additional and subsequent RCTs found that universal immunisation of infants (using either recombinant or plasma derived vaccines) reduces acute hepatitis and development of a chronic carrier state compared with placebo. The longest RCT found that universal immunisation protected at 15 years. Two historical cohort studies found reduced secondary mortality from hepatocellular carcinoma in children born after the introduction of a universal plasma derived hepatitis immunisation programme. One additional historical cohort study found a lower rate of related chronic liver disease, cirrhosis, and hepatocellular cancer after the introduction of a universal plasma derived immunisation programme. Three non-systematic reviews and one RCT found only minor adverse reactions after recombinant hepatitis B immunisation. One cluster RCT found universal immunisation with first plasma and then recombinant vaccine reduced the development of chronic carrier state and acute hepatitis events compared with immunisation of high risk groups.

Benefits: **Versus placebo or no immunisation:** We found one non-systematic review (search date 1989, 2 RCTs, 203 infants, aged less than 1 year),[13] three subsequent RCTs,[14–17] one additional RCT,[18] and three additional historical cohort studies,[19–21] comparing hepatitis B vaccine versus placebo or no vaccine. The review found that recombinant hepatitis B vaccine protected against development of the chronic carrier state**G** at both 9 months after immunisation (protective efficacy**G** 87%; 15/148 [10.1%] HBsAg**G** positive in the intervention group) and 15 months (protective efficacy 96%; 2/55 [3.6%] HBsAg positive in the intervention group).[13] Confidence limits and numbers of people in control group not reported. The first subsequent RCT, conducted in the Gambia (1864 infants), compared four doses of hepatitis B vaccine (recombinant or plasma derived) given along with the World Health Organization's recommended Expanded Program Immunisation**G** versus Expanded Program Immunisation only.[14,15] It found that hepatitis B vaccine plus Expanded Program Immunisation significantly protected against development of the chronic carrier state at 4 years after immunisation (protective efficacy 94%, 95% CI 84% to 98%; 4/720 [0.6%] HBsAg positive with intervention *v* 103/816 [13%] with placebo). It found the results were still significant after 9 years (protective efficacy 90%, 95% CI 79% to 95%; 4/677 [0.5%] HBsAg positive with intervention *v* 99/823 [12%] with placebo). The second subsequent RCT, conducted in China (649 children aged 3–36 months, with no serological markers for previous infection), compared three doses of plasma derived hepatitis B vaccine versus placebo.[16] It found that hepatitis B vaccine significantly protected children against development of the chronic carrier state at 5, 12, and 15 years after immunisation (5 year protective efficacy 100.0%, 0/152 [0%] HBsAg positive with immunisation *v* 24/190 [12.6%] with placebo, $P < 0.001$; 12 year protective efficacy 82.2%, 3/171 [1.8%] HBsAg positive with immunisation *v* 18/179 [10.1%] with placebo, $P < 0.01$; 15 year protective efficacy 88.0%, 1/52 [1.9%] HBsAg positive with immunisation *v* 9/154 [16.7%] with placebo, $P < 0.01$; CI not reported). The third subsequent RCT, also in China (513 children aged 3–36 months, with no serological markers for previous infection), compared three doses of plasma derived hepatitis B vaccine versus placebo.[17] It found that hepatitis B vaccine significantly protected children against development of the chronic carrier state at 12 years after immunisation (protective efficacy 92%; 1/167 [0.6%] HBsAg positive with immunisation *v* 14/183 [7.6%] with placebo; $P < 0.0001$, CI not reported). One additional RCT from Burundi (480 infants) compared the protective efficacy of a plasma derived hepatitis vaccine**G** versus placebo 1 year after immunisation.[18] It found that the vaccine significantly protected children from both acute hepatitis B events**G** (efficacy 100%; event rates 0/59 [0%] with immunisation *v* 5/59 [8.5%] with placebo; $P = 0.046$) and development of chronic carrier state (efficacy 100%; carrier rates 0/59 [0%] with hepatitis B vaccine *v* 4/59 [6.8%] with placebo; statistics not reported). One additional historical cohort study in Taiwan estimated the incidence of hepatocellular carcinoma in three historical cohorts (children born during 1981–1986 [17 million], children born during 1987–1990 [14 million], and children born during 1991–1994 [14 million]) 5–13 years after immunisation with a plasma vaccine.[19] The average annual incidence of hepatocellular carcinoma was significantly reduced in children born after the introduction of universal immunisation in 1984 (0.70 per 100 000 [95% CI 0.65 per 100 000 to 0.78 per 100 000] in the 1981–1986 cohort, 0.57 per 100 000 [95% CI 0.48 per 100 000 to 0.62 per 100 000] in the 1987–1990 cohort, and 0.36 per 100 000 [95% CI 0.23 per 100 000 to 0.48 per 100 000] in the 1991–1994 cohort; $P < 0.01$ for comparison between before and after the 1990 cohorts). Mortality secondary to hepatocellular carcinoma was also reduced in the 1991–1994 cohort compared with the two other cohorts combined (incidence of hepatocellular deaths before July 1990 0.72 per 1000 000 and after July 1990 0.33 per 1000 000; RR 0.51; $P < 0.001$; see comment below). The second additional historical cohort study (children aged 1–9 years) in Taiwan also found a lower hepatocellular carcinoma standardised mortality ratio after the vaccination programme with a plasma derived vaccine (1.25 [95% CI 0.70 to 2.25] in 1983 *v* 0.34 [95% CI 0.14 to 0.89] in 1993, comparative statistical results not reported).[20] This contrasted with no change in the adult standardised mortality ratio secondary to hepatocellular carcinoma during this period. The third additional historical cohort study (children, adolescents, and young people) assessed the impact of universal immunisation (initially with plasma and then with recombinant vaccine**G**) on related chronic liver disease, cirrhosis, and hepatocellular carcinoma in a town in southern Italy.[21] It found a decline in the prevalence of chronic carrier state 15 years after starting the immunisation programme (prevalence of HBsAg 8.3% during 1978–1983 *v* 1.0% in 1997, P < 0.001). It also reported a reduction in the prevalence of related chronic liver disease, cirrhosis, and hepatocellular carcinoma, but no numerical data were provided. **Versus selective immunisation in high risk individuals:** We found one cluster RCT in Italy (2 towns with a population of about 60 000 each), which compared a universal immunisation strategy**G** (all infants and adolescents) versus immunisation of high risk groups only (people living with chronic carriers, homosexual men, intravenous drug abusers, infants born to infected mothers, healthcare workers, commercial sex workers, people receiving transfusion and other blood products, people exposed to needle stick injuries, and people with chronic eczema and psoriasis).[22] It used plasma derived vaccine until 1987 and then recombinant vaccine. It found universal immunisation was associated with a bigger reduction in the incidence of hepatitis B (with universal immunisation, mean annual incidence of hepatitis B 63/100 000 during 1963–1990 and 3/100 000 during 1991–1993; with high risk group immunisation, mean annual incidence of hepatitis B 55/100 000 during 1963–1990 and 15/100 000 in 1991–1993). It also found universal immunisation was associated with lower prevalence of HBsAg positivity (13.4% in 1978 to 3.0% in 1993 with universal immunisation *v* 13.6% in 1978 to 7.4% with selective immunisation; statistical significance not reported).

Harms: **Versus placebo or no treatment:** The non-systematic review found that 10% of children (13 trials, 2096 enrolled) and 4% of neonates (11 trials, 1187 enrolled) had adverse reactions after hepatitis B recombinant immunisation. Sore arm (8.5%) in children and mild fever (2.5%) in neonates were the two most commonly reported symptoms.[13] It found no serious adverse reactions. We found two other non-systematic reviews that assessed connective tissue disorders**G** and recombinant vaccine.[23,24] The first review found two uncontrolled population based studies.[23] The first study (166 757 children in New Zealand) of plasma derived vaccine found that arthritis or arthralgia occurred in less than 1 episode in 10 000 vaccines. The second study of plasma derived vaccine (43 618 people in Alaska) found that arthritis or arthralgia lasting more than 3 days occurred in less than 1 episode in 3000 vaccines. It found weak evidence (case reports and case series) of a link between hepatitis B vaccine and serious connective tissue disorders. The second non-systematic review (search date 2000, number of studies not reported) found no evidence (from case series and case reports) of a causal link between systematic lupus erythrematosis and recombinant vaccine.[24] One RCT in Egypt (590 infants) compared the addition of three doses of hepatitis B vaccine (recombinant) plus routine immunisation starting at birth (group A) versus immunisation at 2 months (group B) versus routine immunisation only (group C).[25] It found infants who started hepatitis B immunisation at 2 months had a significantly higher proportion of minor adverse reaction compared with children immunised at birth or with routine immunisation alone (group A 5/178 [2.8%] had local reaction and 10/178 [5.6%] had fever *v* group

B 12/167 [7.2%] had local reaction and 12/167 [7.2%] had fever *v* group C 3/191 [1.6%] had local reaction and 4/191 [2.1%] had fever; P < 0.05 for group B *v* A and C) after the first dose. It found no serious adverse reactions in any group. One RCT found that infants immunised from birth onwards suffered less frequent adverse reactions than infants who received their first dose at the age of 2 months.[25] The RCT used strict inclusion criteria excluding underweight children and those with other disorders. The trial claimed to have lost only 10% of participants at follow up, with none because of adverse effects, but did not say how this was assessed. None of the reviews, RCTs, or cohort studies in the benefits section reported on harms.[14–21] **Versus selective immunisation of high risk individuals:** The RCT did not report any adverse effects with either intervention.[22]

Comment: **Versus placebo or no treatment:** All RCTs mentioned in the benefits section had above high loss to follow up.[13–21] This proportion was particularly high in one 15 year long study (83%) in China.[16] However, sensitivity analysis in the RCT conducted in the Gambia found immunisation reduced incidence of chronic carrier state after 9 years even after taking the 31% loss to follow up into account.[15] The study in Italy had possible misclassification bias as final diagnosis of hepatitis events were made only clinically by general practitioners and not validated.[21] **Versus selective immunisation of high risk individuals:** The cluster RCT in the two towns in southern Italy was possibly exposed to cross contamination and the effects of migration.[22] Despite these possible limitations, the difference between the declines in the incidences of hepatitis was overwhelmingly supportive toward universal immunisation strategy.

OPTION SELECTIVE IMMUNISATION OF HIGH RISK INDIVIDUALS

One non-systematic review of mainly observational studies with both plasma derived and recombinant vaccine, and three RCTs of plasma derived hepatitis B immunisation all found that immunisation prevented chronic carrier state compared with placebo or no treatment in children born to HBsAg positive mothers. One RCT found minor adverse events with immunisation; the other RCTs did not report on adverse events. We found no good evidence in other high risk groups. One cluster RCT found that selective immunisation in high risk individuals was less effective than universal immunisation of infants in preventing chronic carrier state and acute hepatitis events.

Benefits: **Versus placebo or no treatment:** We found one non-systematic review[26] and two additional RCTs.[27–29] The review (24 studies in infants; mainly individual, clinical, and epidemiological surveillance studies) assessed the protective efficacy**G** of both plasma derived and recombination vaccine in neonates born to mothers infected with hepatitis B.[26] The review did not do a meta-analysis owing to differences in study design. However, it found consistently high protective efficacy for both types of vaccines compared with placebo or historical controls in several studies. The first additional RCT, conducted in Taiwan, compared plasma derived vaccine with or without hepatitis B immunoglobulin (HBIG) versus no immunisation (group A vaccine alone, group B vaccine plus one dose of HBIG, group C vaccine plus two doses of HBIG, and group D no vaccine).[27] Infants receiving immunisation were more protected against HBsAg**G** compared with non-immunised children at 6 months (HBsAg positives in group A 9/38 [23.7%], efficacy 73.7%; P < 0.05; group B 4/36 [11.1%], efficacy 87.7%; reported as non-significant, but P value not reported; group C 2/38 [5.3%], efficacy 94.1%; P < 0.05, and group D 26/29 [90%]). It also found that adding HBIG significantly increased protection compared with vaccine only.[27] The second additional RCT, in China (208 children born to HBsAg positive mothers), compared two different brands of plasma derived vaccine with or without HBIG versus placebo in preventing the development of chronic carrier state**G** (group A placebo, group B vaccine produced by an international company, group C vaccine produced locally, and group D local vaccine plus HBIG).[28,29] It found that children receiving international vaccine brand were significantly less likely to develop the chronic carrier state than children who received placebo or the local brand after 6 months (prevalence of HBsAg: group A 24/55 [47%], group B 3/55 [5.4%], group C 12/56 [21%], and group D 2/27 [7%]; protective efficacy 87% [$P < 0.001$] in group B, 51% [$P < 0.03$] in group C, and 83% [$P < 0.003$] in group D), and at 5 years (prevalence of HBsAg: group A 19/31 [66%], group B 2/19 [11%]; protective efficacy 72%, group C 4/20 [22%] protective efficacy 38%; and group D 2/11 [12%]; P values not reported). It found similar protective efficacy in group B (international brand) and D (addition of HBIG to the local vaccine) in preventing hepatitis B carrier state (CI or P values not reported). **Versus universal immunisation of infants:** See benefits of universal immunisation of infants, p 919.[28,29]

Harms: **Versus placebo or no treatment:** In China, one RCT reported minor adverse reactions (5%, mainly irritability and rash) after immunisation of infants born to HBsAg positive mothers.[30] No further comparison with the control group was made. The other RCTs did not report on adverse events.[27–30] **Versus universal immunisation of infants:** See harms of universal immunisation of infants, p 921.

Comment: **Versus placebo or no treatment:** Two RCTs were conducted in China. Only 55% of women eligible for the trial agreed to take part in one RCT, which might make the results not representative of the population.[30] The other RCT, which lasted for 10 years, lost 56% of participants during follow up at 9 years.[28,29] Although groups were similar at baseline, this leads to attrition bias. One RCT in China (220 children born to HBsAg positive mothers) compared plasma derived vaccine against recombinant vaccine**G** (group A plasma derived vaccine only, group B plasma derived vaccine plus HBIG, group C recombinant vaccine 20 μg, and group D recombinant vaccine 10 μg) in preventing the development of chronic carrier state.[30] It found that recombinant vaccine in either dose with or without HBIG provided more protection (group A protective efficacy 51%, prevalence of HBsAg 12/49 [24.5%]; group B protective efficacy 82.6%, prevalence of HBsAg 4/46 [8.7%]; group C protective efficacy 92%, prevalence of HBsAg 2/50 [4%]; and group D protective efficacy 87%, prevalence of HBsAg 3/49 [6.1%]; no P values reported) against plasma derived vaccine after 12 months. **Versus universal immunisation of infants:** See comment of universal immunisation of infants, p 922.

QUESTION **What are the effects of immunisation in countries with low endemicity?**

OPTION **SELECTIVE IMMUNISATION OF HIGH RISK INDIVIDUALS**

One systematic review found that, in countries with low endemicity, plasma derived hepatitis B immunisation prevented acute hepatitis B and development of chronic carrier state in healthcare workers at high risk of exposure to bodily fluids. Three RCTs found that plasma derived hepatitis B immunisation prevented acute hepatitis B in homosexual men. One small RCT found no significant difference in hepatitis B events in heterosexual partners of infected people. Three RCTs of plasma derived immunisation in people on regular haemodialysis found potentially conflicting results. Two RCTs from France and Belgium found good protective efficacy against chronic carrier state. However, one large US based RCT found no good evidence of benefit.

Hepatitis B (prevention)

The systematic review of plasma derived vaccination found no significant difference between immunisation and placebo in the rate and severity of adverse events. One observational study showed a high prevalence of hepatitis B carrier state and low immunisation uptake in young homosexuals despite a national strategy to immunise high risk groups. Surveillance data from a national programme in Japan found that immunisation of neonates (with recombinant hepatitis B vaccine plus hepatitis B immunoglobulin) born to HBsAg positive mothers provided 95% protection against the development of a chronic carrier state. We found insufficient evidence to compare the effectiveness of selective immunisation in high risk individuals with other strategies in countries with low endemicity.

Benefits: **Versus placebo or no immunisation:** We found one systematic review (search date not reported, 4 RCTs, 2701 people) of plasma derived vaccines in healthcare workers.[31] It found that vaccination significantly reduced hepatitis B compared with placebo (OR 0.33, 95% CI 0.21 to 0.53; NNT estimated between 7–145 depending on the baseline incidence of hepatitis B). Mean length of follow up was 14.5 months. We found three RCTs in homosexual men.[32–34] The first RCT (800 homosexual men in the Netherlands) compared immunisation with plasma derived vaccine versus placebo for 21.5 months.[32] It found that immunisation significantly reduced the incidence of acute hepatitis infections compared with placebo (17/397 [4.3%] with immunisation *v* 56/403 [13.9%] with placebo; RR 0.31, 95% CI 0.18 to 0.52; NNT 11, 95% CI 8 to 18) among homosexual men. The second RCT (1083 homosexual men in the USA) compared hepatitis immunisation with plasma derived vaccine versus placebo.[33] It found that vaccine significantly protected against acute hepatitis B (acute hepatitis B: 13/448 [2.7%] with immunisation *v* 77/431 [21%] with placebo; $P < 0.0001$) and chronic carrier state**G** at the end of 2 years (protective efficacy**G** 87%; $P < 0.0001$; HBsAg**G** positive 12/448 [2.7%] with immunisation *v* 90/448 [23.5%] with placebo; OR 71.6; CI and P value not reported). The third RCT (1402 homosexual men in the USA) compared hepatitis B immunisation with plasma derived vaccine versus placebo.[34] It found that immunisation significantly reduced the risk of hepatitis B events compared with placebo 2 years after immunisation (hepatitis events: 58/482 [9%] with immunisation *v* 110/443 [21%] with placebo; $P < 0.001$). We found one RCT (160 partners of infected people) that assessed the post-exposure prophylactic efficacy of hepatitis B immunisation versus placebo among regular heterosexual partners of infected people.[35] It found no significant difference in the incidence of acute hepatitis events at 9 months (12/75 [16%] with immunisation and 13/71 [18.3%] with placebo; $P > 0.5$). We found three RCTs comparing hepatitis B immunisation versus placebo in people on haemodialysis.[36–38] The first RCT (138 people in France) found that immunisation with plasma derived vaccine significantly reduced events 12 months after immunisation (15/72 [21%] with immunisation *v* 29/66 [45%] with placebo; $P < 0.02$).[36] The second RCT (401 people in Belgium) of plasma derived vaccine found a large and significant reduction in the hepatitis B attack rates with immunisation in the 435 days assessment (7/197 [4%] with immunisation *v* 30/191 [18%] with placebo; protective efficacy 78%; $P = 0.00016$).[37] However, one large RCT (1311 people in the USA) of plasma derived vaccine did not find any significant difference in the incidence of acute hepatitis B events**G** between immunisation and placebo 2 years after immunisation (42/660 [6.4%] with immunisation *v* 35/651 [5.4%] with placebo; $P > 0.05$).[38] In Japan, where hepatitis B prevalence is about 1.4% and occurs mainly because of vertical transmission from infected mother to their neonates, a national immunisation programme (recombinant hepatitis B immunisation plus hepatitis B immunoglobulin) for neonates born to HBsAg positive mothers was introduced in 1986. Most expectant mothers (95.1%) were tested and this strategy protected most of the neonates born to infected mothers between 1986 and 1994 from developing a chronic carrier state (980/1030 [95.1%] of neonates born to infected mothers did not develop carrier state).[39] **Versus universal immunisation:** We found no systematic review, RCTs, or observational studies.

Harms: The systematic review of plasma derived hepatitis B immunisation in healthcare workers did not find any significant difference in incidence of adverse events (OR 1.13, 95% CI 0.95 to 1.35), severity of systemic adverse events (OR 1.60, 95% CI 0.64 to 4.04), or severity of local adverse events (OR 1.09, 95% CI 0.90 to 1.33) between vaccination and placebo.[31] The first RCT in homosexual men of plasma derived vaccine found no significant difference between the two groups (incidence of adverse events: 24.3% in the intervention group *v* 21.4% in the control group; difference not statistically significant; P value not reported).[33] The other two RCTs of plasma derived vaccine found a higher incidence of mild adverse reactions with immunisation compared with placebo.[32,34] One RCT found increased incidence of sore arm and dizziness after immunisation (sore arm: 8.9% with immunisation *v* 5.9% with placebo; dizziness: 2.6% with immunisation *v* 0.6% with placebo; $P < 0.001$) and the other RCT found a significant increase in sore arm (sore arm after first dose: 64% with immunisation *v* 45% with placebo; $P < 0.001$). One RCT in people receiving haemodialysis found a significantly higher incidence of adverse reactions with plasma derived vaccine immunisation compared with placebo (42% with immunisation *v* 22% with placebo; $P < 0.005$).[37] The other two RCTs in people receiving haemodialysis found no significant difference (3% with immunisation *v* 9% with placebo in the French RCT[36] and 13% with immunisation *v* 14% with placebo in the US RCT[38]). None of these RCTs found any serious adverse reactions. A retrospective study of post-marketing surveillance data in adults in the USA found that, compared with other vaccines, recombinant hepatitis B vaccine significantly increased risk of neuropathy (0.39 per million with recombinant hepatitis B vaccine *v* 0.12 per million with other vaccines; RR 3.3, 95% CI 1.4 to 8.0; $P < 0.01$), arthritis (0.88 per million with recombinant hepatitis B vaccine *v* 0.06 per million with other vaccines; RR 15, 95% CI 7 to 36; $P < 0.001$), multiple sclerosis (0.39 per million with recombinant hepatitis B vaccine *v* 0.01 per million with other vaccines; RR 19, 95% CI 7 to 442; $P < 0.001$), and other chronic adverse reactions.[40] However, such reactions are rare, and results should be interpreted with caution because of the retrospective nature of the study.

Comment: Both RCTs from the USA in homosexual men had high loss to follow up (19%[33] and 25%[34]) during 2 years, raising the possibility of bias. The RCT from the Netherlands lost 4.0–4.8% of participants during follow up.[32] All three RCTs had comparable groups in both intervention and control arms. However, one cross sectional study from the USA suggests poor uptake and high prevalence of chronic carrier state in this group despite a national high risk immunisation programme**G**.[41] This may be an underestimate of the actual problem, as only 62% were approached out of all eligible men, and only 62% of these agreed to take part in the study. One RCT found no advantage in providing post-exposure immunisation to the regular partners of people infected with hepatitis B identified during their hospital admission for recent jaundice.[35] The RCT was able to recruit only 75% of the eligible partners, which might make the results unrepresentative. One cohort study found that hepatitis B vaccine provides protection against the development of chronic carrier state in residents of mentally handicap institutions up to 11 years. However, nearly 51% of participants did not complete follow up in this study. The US based RCT in people on haemodialysis lost 35% of participants during follow up as opposed to 15% in the French RCT, and less than 1% in the Belgian RCT. The US trial also had a low event rate in both placebo and intervention arms compared with the other two trials. This may be the reason for not detecting any significant difference between the two groups.

OPTION UNIVERSAL IMMUNISATION OF INFANTS

One historical cohort study found a reduction in the prevalence of hepatitis B chronic carrier state after universal immunisation in countries with low endemicity. We found insufficient evidence to compare its effectiveness with other strategies. Two cohort studies and surveillance data did not report any links between hepatitis B immunisation and serious adverse reactions.

Benefits: **Versus placebo or no immunisation:** We found no RCTs assessing the efficacy of universal immunisation in countries with low endemicityⒼ of hepatitis B. One historical cohort study in Alaska (7 villages, 533 children aged ≤ 10 years) found a marked decline in the prevalence of chronic carrier stateⒼ after the adoption of universal immunisation strategy (prevalence of HBsAgⒼ 3.1% during 1982–1987 and 0% during 1993–1994, statistical significance not reported).[42] **Versus other immunisation strategies:** We found no systematic review, RCTs, or observational studies.

Harms: One retrospective cohort study in the USA (6515 children age < 6 years) of recombinant vaccineⒼ compared the incidence of adverse reactions in vaccinated versus unvaccinated children.[43] It found that children who received hepatitis B immunisation had higher rates of arthritis, acute ear infection, and pharyngitis compared with unvaccinated children (arthritis OR 5.91, 95% CI 1.05 to 33.14; acute ear infection OR 1.60, 95% CI 1.00 to 2.58; and pharyngitis OR 1.41, 95% CI 0.95 to 2.09). The results were adjusted for demographic differences, but absolute risk and exact number of events were not given. A second cohort study (conducted in the USA, 5655 children) of recombinant vaccine found no significant difference in the adverse events reported to health services in the first 21 days after birth between vaccinated and unvaccinated children (27/3302 [0.8%] with vaccinated *v* 26/2353 [1.1%] with unvaccinated, P = 0.28).[44] Fever, allergic reactions, seizures, or other neurological events were among the most common events in both groups. Post-marketing surveillance data of recombinant vaccine in USA during 1991–1995 found no unexpected adverse events in children given recombinant hepatitis B vaccine with or without other routine immunisation (no statistical analysis done).[45] It reported 18 neonatal deaths during 1991–1998 after hepatitis B immunisations,[46] but no causal link was established between these deaths and immunisation. Surveillance data from Italy (1991–2000) of recombinant vaccine reported 19 serious post-immunisation adverse events, none of which was linked to multiple sclerosis or any other serious neurological disease.[47] Surveillance data from the USA did not suggest any link between hepatitis B immunisation and neurological or other serious adverse reactions.[45,46]

Comment: The Alaskan study was only able to recruit 49% of children approached, which might make results unrepresentative.[42] Two studies (one cohort[44] and one case control[43]), both with a large sample size, found conflicting results. However, none reported any serious adverse reactions. Both studies did not validate their data from other sources. The case control study had a potential for non-response bias, as the people who participated may not be representative of the general population. The cohort study analyzed adverse events reported only to hospitals and may, therefore, have underestimated the frequency of events.

OPTION UNIVERSAL IMMUNISATION OF ADOLESCENTS

We found insufficient evidence to assess the effects of universal adolescent immunisation, or to compare its effectiveness with other strategies. One observational study suggests minor adverse effects after hepatitis B immunisation in this group.

Benefits: We found no systematic review or RCTs.

Harms: One study from the routine post-marketing vaccine surveillance system in Canada (41 494 students aged 11 years) found 69 adverse events.[48] The major categories were injection site reactions (23%), fainting (20%), and rashes (17%). There were four cases of arthritis and one instance of anaphylaxis. The study had no control group, which makes establishing causality difficult.

Comment: We found a cross sectional survey of hepatitis B infection markers in a random sample of 1215 pregnant women aged 15–44 years in British Columbia, Canada. From this cohort, researchers assessed the prevalence of HBsAg**G** among 15–19 year old girls, 7 years after the start of an adolescent vaccination programme (begun in 1992).[49] It reported no cases of HBsAg positivity in that age group. However, the prevalence of HBsAg among women aged 15–44 was 1.4% in the full cohort, which consisted mainly of people who had not been vaccinated under the programme.[49] The survey does not provide causal evidence on the efficacy of the adolescent immunisation strategy, but does suggest that the strategy may be protective against developing chronic carrier state.[49] We found no strong evidence on the effects of the adolescent immunisation strategy adopted in many parts of the USA and Canada. Evaluation of adolescent immunisation schemes in Canada did not include the primary outcome measures adopted in this review.[50] Surveillance data from the USA and Canada have reported few serious adverse reactions. The results are based on self reported events and had no control group.[48]

GLOSSARY

Acute hepatitis B events Any acute illness with raised liver enzymes (alanine aminotransferase [ALT] levels) and serological signs of acute hepatitis (HBsAg, antiHBc IgM).[51]

Chronic carrier state A person is considered a chronic carrier if the HBsAg has been persistently positive for more than 6 months.[51]

Connective tissue disorders These are multisystemic conditions secondary to an inflammatory response in the body against its own tissues resulting in damage and long term disability.[51]

Countries with high hepatitis B endemicity HBsAg prevalence 8% or higher.[41]

Countries with low hepatitis B endemicity HBsAg prevalence less than 2%.[52]

Expanded Program Immunisation Was launched by the World Health Organization in 1974, to provide systematic immunisation to all infants on a global scale.

HBsAg Hepatitis B surface antigen is a serological marker on the surface of hepatitis B virus. It indicates acute or chronic hepatitis B infection.[52]

Hepatitis vaccine Both types of vaccines (plasma derived vaccine rarely used now and yeast derived recombinant vaccine most commonly used).[52]

High risk immunisation strategy In this strategy hepatitis B vaccine is recommended in individuals and groups who are at high risk of hepatitis B because of their lifestyle, occupation, and other factors. These include close contact of a case or a carrier, babies born to infected mothers, parenteral drug misusers, individuals who change sexual partners frequently, homosexual or bisexual men, people with haemophilia, people on haemodialysis, healthcare workers, and residents of institutions for individuals with severe learning disabilities.[52]

Protective efficacy $[(R_1 - R_2)/R_1] \times 100$ where R_1 is the incidence of event in control population and R_2 is the incidence of event in the immunised population.[30] This is the same as the relative risk reduction.

Recombinant vaccine It contains HBsAg absorbed on aluminium hydroxide adjuvant and is prepared from yeast cells using recombinant DNA technology.[1]

Universal immunisation strategy In this strategy, routine hepatitis B immunisation is carried out for either all infants or adolescents through a national programme.[52]

REFERENCES

1. Department of Health. *Immunisation against infectious disease*. London: HMSO, 1996.
2. Kane M. Global programme for control of hepatitis B infection. *Vaccine* 1995;13(suppl 1):47–49.
3. Margolis HS. Hepatitis B virus infection. *Bull World Health Organ* 1998;76(suppl 2):152–153.
4. Kao JH, Chen DS. Global control of hepatitis B virus infection. *Lancet Infect Dis* 2002;2:395–403.
5. Kammerlander R, Zimmermann H. Transmission of hepatitis B. *Soz Praventivmed* 1998;43:S31–33,S105–107. [In French/German]
6. van Hattum J, Boland GJ, Jansen KG, Kleinpenning AS, van Bommel T, van Loon AM et al. Transmission profile of hepatitis B virus infection in the Batam region, Indonesia. Evidence for a predominantly horizontal transmission profile. *Adv Exp Med Biol* 2003;531:177–183.
7. Yao GB. Importance of perinatal versus horizontal transmission of hepatitis B virus infection in China. *Gut* 1996;38:S39–S42.
8. Yao JL. Perinatal transmission of hepatitis B virus infection and vaccination in China. *Gut* 1996; 38:S37–S38.
9. Lee WM. Hepatitis B virus infection (comment). *N Engl J Med* 1997;337:1733–1745.
10. World Health Organization. Hepatitis B vaccine. *Wkly Epidemiol Rec* 1991;11.
11. Edmunds WJ. Universal or selective immunisation against hepatitis B virus in the United Kingdom? A review of recent cost-effectiveness studies. *Commun Dis Public Health* 1998;1:221–228.
12. Maddrey WC. Hepatitis B: an important public health issue. *J Med Virol* 2000;61:362–366.
13. Andre FE. Summary of safety and efficacy data on a yeast-derived hepatitis B vaccine. *Am J Med* 1989;87:14S–20S.
14. Fortuin M, Chotard J, Jack AD, et al. Efficacy of hepatitis B vaccine in the Gambian expanded programme on immunisation. *Lancet* 1993;341:1129–1131.
15. Viviani S, Jack A, Hall AJ, et al. Hepatitis B vaccination in infancy in The Gambia: protection against carriage at 9 years of age. *Vaccine* 1999;17:2946–2950.
16. Liao SS, Li RC, Li H, et al. Long-term efficacy of plasma-derived hepatitis B vaccine: a 15-year follow-up study among Chinese children. *Vaccine* 1999;17:2661–2666.
17. Liao SS, Li RC, Li H, et al. Long-term efficacy of plasma-derived hepatitis B vaccine among Chinese children: a 12-year follow-up study. *World J Gastroenterol* 1999;5:165–166.
18. Perrin J, Coursaget P, Ntareme F, et al. Hepatitis B immunization of newborns according to a two dose protocol. *Vaccine* 1986;4:241–244.
19. Chang MH, Chen CJ, Lai MS, et al. Universal hepatitis B vaccination in Taiwan and the incidence of hepatocellular carcinoma in children. Taiwan Childhood Hepatoma Study Group. *N Engl J Med* 1997;336:1855–1859.
20. Lee CL, Ko YC. Hepatitis B vaccination and hepatocellular carcinoma in Taiwan. *Pediatrics* 1997;99:351–353.
21. Da Villa G, Piccinino F, Scolastico C, et al. Long-term epidemiological survey of hepatitis B virus infection in a hyperendemic area (Afragola, southern Italy): results of a pilot vaccination project. *Res Virol* 1998;149:263–270.
22. Da Villa G, Picciottoc L, Elia S, et al. Hepatitis B vaccination: universal vaccination of newborn babies and children at 12 years of age versus high risk groups. A comparison in the field. *Vaccine* 1995;13:1240–1243.
23. Arkachaisri T. Serum sickness and hepatitis B vaccine including review of the literature. *J Med Assoc Thail* 2002;85(suppl 2):607–612.
24. Hanslik T, Vaillant JN, Audrain L, et al. Systemic lupus erythematosus and risk of hepatitis B vaccination: from level of evidence to prescription. *Rev Med Interne* 2000;21:785–790. [In French]
25. Bassily S, Kotkat A, Gray G, et al. Comparative study of the immunogenicity and safety of two dosing schedules of hepatitis B vaccine in neonates. *Am J Trop Med Hygiene* 1995;53:419–422.
26. Andre FE, Zuckerman AJ. Review: protective efficacy of hepatitis B vaccines in neonates. *Med Virol* 1994;44:144–151.
27. Lo KJ, Tsai YT, Lee SD. Combined passive and active immunization for interruption of perinatal transmission of hepatitis B virus in Taiwan. *Hepatogastroenterology* 1985;32:65–68.
28. Xu ZY, Liu CB, Francis DP, et al. Prevention of perinatal acquisition of hepatitis B virus carriage using vaccine: preliminary report of a randomized, double-blind placebo-controlled and comparative trial. *Pediatrics* 1985;76:713–718.
29. Xu ZY, Duan SC, Margolis HS, Purcell RH, et al. Long-term efficacy of active postexposure immunization of infants for prevention of hepatitis B virus infection. United States-People's Republic of China Study Group on Hepatitis B. *J Infect Dis* 1995;171:54–60.
30. Halliday ML, Kang LY, Rankin JG, et al. An efficacy trial of a mammalian cell-derived recombinant DNA hepatitis B vaccine in infants born to mothers positive for HBsAg, in Shanghai, China. *Int J Epidemiol* 1992;21:564–573.
31. Jefferson T, Demicheli V, Deeks J, et al. Vaccines for preventing hepatitis B in health-care workers. In: The Cochrane Library, Issue 1, 2003. Oxford: Update Software. Search date not reported; primary sources Medline; Embase; The Cochrane Library; hand searches of *Vaccine* and reference lists; and contact with authors, researchers, and manufacturers.
32. Coutinho RA, Lelie N, Albrecht VL. Efficacy of a heat inactivated hepatitis B vaccine in male homosexuals: outcome of a placebo controlled double blind trial. *BMJ* 1983;286:1305–1308.
33. Szmuness W, Stevens CE, Zang EA, et al. A controlled clinical trial of the efficacy of the hepatitis B vaccine (Heptavax B): a final report. *Hepatology* 1981;1:377–385.
34. Francis DP, Hadler SC, Thompson SE, et al. The prevention of hepatitis B with vaccine. Report of the centers for disease control multi-center efficacy trial among homosexual men. *Ann Intern Med* 1982;97:362–366.
35. Roumeliotou-Karayannis A, Papaevangolou C, Tassopoulos N, et al. Post-exposure active immunoprophylaxis of spouses of acute viral hepatitis B patients. *Vaccine* 1985;3:31–34.
36. Crosnier J, Jungers P, Courouce AM. Randomised placebo-controlled trial of hepatitis B surface antigen vaccine in French haemodialysis units: II, haemodialysis patients. *Lancet* 1981;1:797–800.
37. Desmyter J, Colaert J, De Groote G, et al. Efficacy of heat-inactivated hepatitis B vaccine in haemodialysis patients and staff. Double-blind placebo-controlled trial. *Lancet* 1983;2:1323–1328.

38. Stevens CE, Alter HJ, Taylor PE, et al. Hepatitis B vaccine in patients receiving hemodialysis. Immunogenicity and efficacy. *N Engl J Med* 1984;311:496–501.
39. Noto H, Terao T, Ryou S, et al. Combined passive and active immunoprophylaxis for preventing perinatal transmission of the hepatitis B virus carrier state in Shizuoka, Japan during 1980–1994. *J Gastroenterol Hepatol* 2003;18:943–949.
40. Geier DA, Geier MR. Chronic adverse reactions associated with hepatitis B vaccination. *Ann Pharmacother* 2002;36:1970–1971.
41. MacKellar DA, Valleroy LA, Secura GM, et al. Two decades after vaccine license: hepatitis B immunization and infection among young men who have sex with men. *Am J Public Health* 2001;91:965–971.
42. Harpaz R, McMahon BJ, Margolis HS, et al. Elimination of new chronic hepatitis B virus infections: results of the Alaska immunization program. *J Infect Dis* 2000;181:413–418.
43. Fisher MA, Eklund SA, James SA, et al. Adverse events associated with hepatitis B vaccine in U.S. children less than six years of age, 1993 and 1994. *Ann Epidemiol* 2001;11:13–21.
44. Lewis E, Shinefield HR, Woodruff BA, et al. Safety of neonatal hepatitis B vaccine administration. *Pediatr Infect Dis J* 2001;20:1049–1054.
45. Niu MT, Davis DM, Ellenberg S. Recombinant hepatitis B vaccination of neonates and infants: emerging safety data from the Vaccine Adverse Event Reporting System. *Pediatr Infect Dis J* 1996;15:771–776.
46. Niu MT, Salive ME, Ellenberg SS. Neonatal deaths after hepatitis B vaccine: the vaccine adverse event reporting system, 1991–1998. *Arch Pediatr Adolesc Med* 1999;153:1279–1282.
47. Zanetti AR. Update on hepatitis B vaccination in Italy 10 years after its implementation. *Vaccine* 2001;19:2380–1283.
48. Dobson S, Scheifele D, Bell A. Assessment of a universal, school-based hepatitis B vaccination program [comment]. *JAMA* 1995;274:1209–1213.
49. Dawar M, Patrick DM, Bigham M, et al. Impact of universal preadolescent vaccination against hepatitis B on antenatal seroprevalence of hepatitis B markers in British Columbia women. *CMAJ* 2003;168:703–704.
50. Bell A. Universal hepatitis B immunization: the British Columbia experience. *Vaccine* 1995;13:S77–S81.
51. Andreoli TE, Carpenter CCJ, Griggs RC, et al (eds). *Cecil essentials of medicine*. Philadelphia: WB Saunders company, 1993.
52. Chin JE (ed). *Control of communicable diseases*. Washington: American Public Health Association, 2000.

Kamran Siddiqi
Dr
Nuffield Institute for Health
Leeds
UK

Competing interests: None declared.

Influenza

Search date July 2003

Lucy Hansen

QUESTIONS

INTERVENTIONS

Key Messages

- Conclusions from studies in people with laboratory confirmed influenza may not be extrapolated to people with clinically suspected influenza, who have not had laboratory confirmation of infection with influenza A or B. RCTs provided insufficient evidence to assess the effects of antiviral agents on reducing serious complications of influenza.
- **All antivirals for preventing serious influenza complications** We found insufficient evidence about the effects of antiviral agents on reducing serious complications of influenza
- **Oral amantadine for early treatment of influenza A in adults (duration of symptoms reduced)** One systematic review and three RCTs have found that oral amantadine reduces the duration of influenza A symptoms by about 1 day compared with placebo.
- **Orally inhaled zanamivir for early treatment of influenza A or B in adults (duration of symptoms reduced)** Two systematic reviews have found that orally inhaled zanamivir reduces the duration of influenza symptoms by about 1 day compared with placebo but a subsequent RCT found no significant difference between treatments. Complication rates and adverse effects were similar in people taking zanamivir and placebo.
- **Oral oseltamivir for early treatment of influenza A and B in adults (duration of symptoms reduced)** Two systematic reviews found that oseltamivir reduces the duration of symptoms by up to 1 day but one subsequent RCT found no significant difference between oseltamivir and placebo. Two RCTs found that oseltamivir increased nausea and vomiting compared with placebo.
- **Oral rimantadine for early treatment of influenza A in adults (duration of symptoms reduced)** One systematic review has found that oral rimantadine reduces the duration of influenza A symptoms by about 1 day compared with placebo. We found insufficient evidence about adverse effects in this setting.

DEFINITION Influenza is caused by infection with influenza viruses. Uncomplicated influenza is characterised by the abrupt onset of fever, chills, non-productive cough, myalgias, headache, nasal congestion, sore throat, and fatigue.[1] Influenza is usually diagnosed clinically. Not all people infected with influenza viruses become symptomatic, and not everybody with the above symptoms will have influenza. Between 40% and 85% of infections result in clinical illness depending on age and pre-existing immunity to the virus.[2]

INCIDENCE/ PREVALENCE In temperate areas, influenza activity typically peaks between late December and early March in the northern hemisphere and May and September in the southern hemisphere. In tropical areas, there is no temporal peak in influenza activity through the year.[3] The annual incidence of influenza varies yearly, and depends partly on the underlying level of population immunity to circulating influenza viruses.[1] One localised study in the USA found that serological conversion with or without symptoms occurred in 10–20% a year, with the highest infection rates in people aged under 20 years.[4] Attack rates are higher in institutions and in areas of overcrowding.[5]

AETIOLOGY/ RISK FACTORS Influenza viruses are transmitted primarily from person to person through respiratory droplets disseminated during sneezing, coughing, and talking.[1,6]

PROGNOSIS The incubation period of influenza is 1–4 days and infected adults are usually contagious from the day before symptom onset until 5 days after symptom onset. The signs and symptoms of uncomplicated influenza usually resolve within a week, although cough and fatigue may persist.[1] Complications include otitis media, bacterial sinusitis, secondary bacterial pneumonia, and, less commonly, viral pneumonia, respiratory failure, and exacerbations of underlying disease.[1,3] In the UK, 1.3% patients with influenza-like illness are hospitalised each year (95% CI 0.6% to 2.6%).[7] It is estimated that 300–400 deaths each year are attributable to influenza, rising to in excess of 29 000 during an epidemic.[7] The risk of hospitalisation is highest in people 65 years or older, in very young children, and in those with chronic medical conditions.[1,8,9] Over 90% of influenza related deaths during recent seasonal epidemics in the USA have been in people 65 years or older.[1] During influenza pandemics, morbidity and mortality may be high in younger age groups.[1] Severe illness is more common with influenza A infections than with influenza B infections.[1]

AIMS OF INTERVENTION To reduce the duration and severity of influenza signs and symptoms, and the risk of complications, and to minimise adverse effects of treatment.

OUTCOMES Severity and duration of symptoms; frequency and severity of complications of influenza; adverse effects of treatment.

METHODS *Clinical Evidence* search and appraisal July 2003. The authors searched Medline (1966–2001; major MeSH topics: amantadine and influenza, rimantadine and influenza; keywords: zanamivir, 4-guanidino-Neu5Ac2en, GG167, oseltamivir, GS4104, and Ro64-0796). Meeting abstracts were used to identify unpublished studies of zanamivir and oseltamivir. We included only systematic reviews and double blind RCTs of treatment versus placebo for naturally occurring influenza. We excluded RCTs and reviews of chemoprophylaxis of influenza, experimentally induced influenza, and reviews that combined RCTs of more than one agent. We only assessed people with laboratory confirmed influenza. For amantadine and rimantadine, we included only RCTs of influenza A. For zanamivir and oseltamivir, we included studies of influenza A or B. For zanamivir, we included only RCTs of orally inhaled drug and excluded intranasal drops plus oral inhalation unless oral inhalation results were reported separately. For amantadine, rimantadine, and oseltamivir we included only RCTs of oral administration. We excluded RCTs primarily on children younger than 12 years, those that used an antipyretic rather than a placebo as control, RCTs in which the delay from symptom onset to starting treatment was unclear, and RCTs without quantitative measures of clinical effectiveness.

QUESTION What are the effects of antiviral medications for early treatment of laboratory confirmed influenza in adults?

OPTION ORAL AMANTADINE

One systematic review and three RCTs have found that, in people with influenza A, oral amantadine reduces the duration of symptoms by about 1 day compared with placebo.

Benefits: We found one systematic review (search date 2002, 7 RCTs, 531 otherwise healthy people)[10] and three additional RCTs[11–13] of oral amantadine (usually started within 48 hours of symptom onset) versus placebo in people with influenza A (see table A on web extra). The review found that amantadine significantly reduced the duration of fever compared with placebo (temperature > 37.0 °C reduced by 1 day, 95% CI 0.7 days to 1.3 days). We found no RCTs of the effect of amantadine in preventing serious complications of influenza, such as pneumonia or exacerbation of chronic diseases. We found no RCTs of amantadine for treatment of influenza A in pregnant women, those with chronic disease, or in immunised people.

Harms: The review found no significant difference in the frequency of adverse effects between amantadine and placebo groups. However, the included RCTs contained little information about the relative adverse effects of amantadine compared with placebo when used for treatment of influenza A (see table A on web extra).[14–16] More evidence is available about the harms of amantadine when used for prophylaxis of influenza A (see comment below).

Comment: In vitro, amantadine has specific antiviral activity against influenza A but not influenza B viruses.[17] The RCTs used different outcome measures, and so summarising the results is difficult. Only one RCT examined amantadine in elderly people.[13] All RCTs considered only people with laboratory confirmed influenza A, and so the analyses were not by intention to treat. The proportion of influenza A isolates from the general population exhibiting resistance to amantadine has remained low.[18,19] Amantadine resistant influenza A viruses have not been found to be more virulent than non-resistant viruses.[3] The limited evidence from elderly and high risk groups makes it difficult to generalise results to these populations. A systematic review found that use of amantadine for prophylaxis of influenza A is associated with an increased incidence of gastrointestinal and central nervous system adverse effects compared with placebo.[10]

OPTION ORAL RIMANTADINE

One systematic review has found that oral rimantadine reduces the duration of symptoms by about 1 day compared with placebo in people with influenza A. We found insufficient evidence about adverse effects in this setting.

Benefits: We found one systematic review (search date 2002, 3 RCTs, 104 otherwise healthy adults)[10] and one small additional RCT[20] of rimantadine (usually started within 48 hours of symptom onset) compared with placebo in people with influenza A (see table A on web extra). The review found that rimantadine significantly reduced the duration of fever compared with placebo (temperature > 37.0 °C reduced by 1.3 days, 95% CI 0.8 days to 1.8 days). We found no RCTs of rimantadine for treatment of influenza A in people over 65 years of age, in pregnant women, in those with chronic disease, or in immunised people. We found no RCTs of the effect of rimantadine in preventing serious complications of influenza, such as pneumonia or exacerbation of chronic diseases.

Harms: The review found insufficient evidence about the adverse effects of rimantadine compared with placebo in people with influenza A.[10] One non-systematic review (340 adults treated for influenza) comparing rimantadine with placebo found that more people taking rimantadine had central nervous system symptoms, most commonly insomnia (10.8% *v* 8.6%; P value not reported); and gastrointestinal symptoms, most commonly abdominal pain and nausea (6.0% *v* 2.3%; P value not reported).[21] Additional evidence is available about adverse effects of rimantadine when used for prophylaxis of influenza A (see comment below).

Comment: In vitro studies have found that rimantadine has specific antiviral activity against influenza A but not influenza B viruses.[17] The RCTs used different outcome measures and so summarising results is difficult. Additional studies of rimantadine have been performed in Russia, but information in English is limited.[22] Viruses that are resistant to rimantadine show cross-resistance to amantadine, and *vice versa*.[18] Influenza A viruses resistant to rimantadine have not been found to be more virulent than non-resistant viruses.[3] The proportion of influenza A isolates from the general population exhibiting resistance to rimantadine (or amantadine) has remained low.[18,19] The limited evidence from elderly and high risk groups makes it difficult to generalise results to these populations. A systematic review found that use of rimantadine for prophylaxis of influenza A is associated with an increased incidence of gastrointestinal adverse effects compared with placebo.[10]

OPTION ORALLY INHALED ZANAMIVIR

Two systematic reviews have found that orally inhaled zanamivir reduces the duration of influenza symptoms by about 1 day compared with placebo in people with influenza A or B. One subsequent RCT found a similar but smaller effect, which was not statistically significant. Adverse effects were similar in people taking zanamivir and placebo.

Benefits: We found two systematic reviews (search date 2001,[7] >10 RCTs; and 2000,[23] 8 RCTs) and one subsequent RCT that compared inhaled zanamivir (usually started within 48 hours of symptom onset) versus placebo (see table B on web extra).[24] The reviews both analysed data on an intention to treat basis. The two systematic reviews largely included the same RCTs but some RCTs were unique to each review.[7,23] **Symptoms in overall populations:** One systematic review found that zanamivir reduced the median time to alleviation of symptoms by 1 day compared with placebo (about 5 days with zanamivir *v* about 6 days with placebo; difference –1 day, 95% CI –1.7 days to –0.4 days).[23] **Symptoms in healthy populations:** One systematic review found that zanamivir reduced the median time to alleviation of symptoms by 1 day compared with placebo (absolute mean duration not reported; difference: –0.8 days, 95% CI –1.31 days to –0.26 days).[7] The subsequent RCT (1023 military conscripts) found that zanamivir reduced the duration of symptoms compared with placebo but the difference was not statistically significant (median time to symptom alleviation: 2.0 days with zanamivir *v* 2.33 days with placebo; difference 0.33 days, 95% CI –0.17 days to +1.0 days, P = 0.08).[24] **Symptoms in high risk populations:** Both systematic reviews found that zanamivir reduced the median time to alleviation of symptoms compared with placebo in high risk people (difference in symptom duration in high risk defined as co-existing medical condition plus aged 65 years and older: 0.93 days, 95% CI –1.9 to +0.05 days;[7] reduction from about 8–7 days, difference with high risk defined as co-existing medical condition: 1.16 days, 95% CI 0.13 days to 2.19 days[23]). **Complications:** One systematic review found no significant difference between zanamivir and placebo in overall rates of complications or the need for antibiotics for complications (any complication: 35% with zanamivir *v* 38% with placebo, P = 0.61; need for antibiotics: 18% with zanamivir *v* 23% with placebo, P = 0.20).[23] It found no significant difference between zanamivir and placebo in complications requiring antibiotics in high risk people (70/391 [18%] with zanamivir *v* 97/412 [24%] with placebo; difference –8%, 95% CI –21% to +5% using random effects model because significant heterogeneity was present).[23]

Harms: Adverse effects were similar in people taking zanamivir compared with placebo (the inhaled lactose vehicle alone — see table B on web extra).[23] Observational evidence found that zanamivir may be associated with bronchospasm and worsening of underlying respiratory disease.[25]

Comment: Zanamivir is administered as an orally inhaled powder. In vitro studies have found that zanamivir has antiviral activity against both influenza A and B viruses.[26] RCTs have predominantly included people with influenza A (≥ 85%). Because of the short period for which zanamivir has been available, and the lack of optimal assays to detect resistant strains, we found insufficient evidence to comment on the development of viral resistance to zanamivir.[3,27–31] We found one RCT (525 people with obstructive airways disease and influenza) published in abstract form only.[32] It found that zanamivir significantly reduced time to symptom resolution compared with placebo (median reduction with zanamivir *v* placebo 1.5 days; P = 0.009). We found some observational evidence that zanamivir may be associated with bronchospasm and worsening of underlying respiratory disease.[25] However, one RCT published in abstract form found a small but significant increase in morning and evening peak expiratory flow rate with zanamivir compared with placebo (morning peak expiratory flow rate 12.9 L/minute higher with zanamivir *v* placebo, P = 0.011; evening peak expiratory flow rate 13.1 L/minute higher, P = 0.007).[32] It found a non-significant reduction between zanamivir and placebo in complications needing antibiotics or a change in respiratory medication (ARR 58% with zanamivir *v* placebo, P = 0.064).

OPTION ORAL OSELTAMIVIR

One systematic review found that oseltamivir reduces the duration of symptoms by up to 1 day but one subsequent RCT found a smaller difference between oseltamivir and placebo. Two RCTs found that oseltamivir increased nausea and vomiting compared with placebo.

Benefits: We found one systematic review (search date 2001, 8 RCTs);[7] and one subsequent RCT.[33] in people with laboratory confirmed influenza. Analysis in the review and the RCT was on an intention to treat basis. **Symptoms in healthy populations:** The systematic review (3 RCTs in 937 otherwise healthy people) found that oseltamivir significantly reduced the median time to alleviation of symptoms compared with placebo (absolute median duration not stated; difference: –20.69 hours, 95% CI –33.97 hours to –7.41 hours).[7] The subsequent RCT (478 healthy people with febrile illness during the influenza season) found a small difference between oseltamivir and placebo in the median duration of illness (83.5 hours with oseltamivir *v* 87.7 hours with placebo, P not reported).[33] Survival analysis found that oseltamivir significantly increased the proportion of people with alleviation of symptoms compared with placebo (P = 0.0355). **Symptoms in high risk people:** The systematic review (5 RCTs, 1134 people) found no significant difference between oseltamivir and placebo in the time to symptom alleviation (difference: –8.33 hours, 95% CI –33.69 hours to +17.03 hours, P value not reported).[7] **Complications:** One RCT (number of people not reported) identified by the systematic review (search date 2001) found no significant difference in the need for antibiotics for complications between oseltamivir and placebo (odds reduction 43%, no further details available in review, data from drug manufacturer).[7]

Harms: Nausea and vomiting were significantly more common in people receiving oseltamivir compared with placebo.[34,35] The subsequent RCT found no significant difference between oseltamivir and placebo in adverse events possibly or probably related to the study drug (21/134 [16%] with oseltamivir *v* 19/139[14%] with placebo, P = 0.56).[33]

Comment: Due to the short period for which oseltamivir has been available, and the lack of optimal assays to detect resistant strains, we found insufficient evidence about viral resistance to oseltamivir.[3,28,30,31]

REFERENCES

1. Cox NJ, Fukuda K. Influenza. *Infect Dis Clin North Am* 1998;12:27–38.
2. Fox JP, Cooney MK, Hall CE, et al. Influenza virus infections in Seattle families, 1975–1979. II. Pattern of infection in invaded households and relation of age and prior antibody to occurrence of infection and related illness. *Am J Epidemiol* 1982;116:228–242.
3. Bridges CB, Fukuda K, Uyeki TM, et al. Prevention and control of influenza: recommendations of the Advisory Committee on Immunization Practices (ACIP). *MMWR Recomm Rep* 2002;51(RR-3):1–31.
4. Sullivan KM, Monto AS, Longini IM. Estimates of the US health impact of influenza. *Am J Public Health* 1993;83:1712–1716.
5. Kilbourne ED. *Influenza*. New York: Plenum Medical Book Co, 1987:269–270.
6. Tablan OC, Anderson LJ, Arden NH, et al. Hospital Infection Control Practices Advisory Committee. Guideline for prevention of nosocomial pneumonia. *Infect Control Hosp Epidemiol* 1994;15:587–604.
7. Cooper NJ, Sutton AJ, Abrams KR, et al. Effectiveness of neuraminidase inhibitors in treatment and prevention of influenza A and B: systematic review and meta-analyses of randomised controlled trials. *BMJ* 2003;326:1235–1239. Search date 2001; primary sources Medline, Embase, Integrated Science Citation Index, PubMed, references, previous systematic reviews and meta-analysis, manufacturer's trial databases, and contact with drug companies
8. Neuzil KM, Mellen BG, Wright PF, et al. The effect of influenza on hospitalizations, outpatient visits, and courses of antibiotics in children. *N Engl J Med* 2000;342:225–231.
9. Izurieta HS, Thompson WW, Kramarz P, et al. Influenza and the rates of hospitalization for respiratory disease among infants and young children. *N Engl J Med* 2000;342:232–239.
10. Jefferson TO, Demicheli V, Deeks JJ, et al. Amantadine and rimantadine for preventing and treating influenza A in adults. In: The Cochrane Library, Issue 2, 2003. Oxford: Update Software. Search date 1997; primary sources Medline, Cochrane Controlled Trials Register, Embase, reviews of references of identified trials, and letters to manufacturers and authors.
11. Baker LM, Shock MP, Iezzoni DG. The therapeutic efficacy of Symmetrel (amantadine hydrochloride) in naturally occurring influenza A2 respiratory illness. *J Am Osteopath Assoc* 1969;68:1244–1250.
12. Galbraith AW, Schild AW, Schild GC, et al. The therapeutic effect of amantadine in influenza occurring during the winter of 1971–1972 assessed by double-blind study. *J R Coll Gen Pract* 1973;23:34–37.
13. Walters HE, Paulshock M. Therapeutic efficacy of amantadine HCl. *Mo Med* 1970;67:176–179.
14. Kitamoto O. Therapeutic effectiveness of amantadine hydrochloride in influenza A2: double-blind studies. *Jpn J Tuberc Chest Dis* 1968;15:17–26.
15. Kitamoto O. Therapeutic effectiveness of amantadine hydrochloride in naturally occurring Hong Kong influenza: double-blinded studies. *Jpn J Tuberc Chest Dis* 1971;17:1–7.
16. Van Voris LP, Betts RF, Hayden FG, et al. Successful treatment of naturally occurring influenza A/USSR/77 H_1 N1. *JAMA* 1981;245:1128–1131.
17. Tominack RL, Hayden FG. Rimantadine hydrochloride and amantadine hydrochloride use in influenza A virus infections. *Infect Dis Clin North Am* 1987;1:459–478.
18. Belshe RB, Burk B, Newman F, et al. Resistance of influenza A viruses to amantadine and rimantadine: results of one decade of surveillance. *J Infect Dis* 1989;159:430–435.
19. Ziegler T, Hemphill ML, Ziegler M-L, et al. Low incidence of rimantadine resistance in field isolates of influenza A viruses. *J Infect Dis* 1999;180:935–939.
20. Rabinovich S, Baldini JT, Bannister R. Treatment of influenza: the therapeutic efficacy of rimantadine HCl in a naturally occurring influenza A2 outbreak. *Am J Med Sci* 1969;257:328–335.
21. Soo W. Adverse effects of rimantadine: summary from clinical trials. *J Respir Dis* 1989;10(suppl.):S26–S31.
22. Zlydnikov DM, Kubar OI, Kovaleva TP, et al. Study of rimantadine in the USSR: a review of the literature. *Rev Infect Dis* 1981;3:408–421.
23. Burls A, Clark W, Stewart T, et al. Zanamivir for the treatment of influenza in adults: a systematic review and economic evaluation. *Health Technol Assess* 2002;6:1–87. Search date 2000; primary sources Cochrane Library, Medline, Embase, Science Citation Index, Glaxo Wellcome Clinical Trials Register, follow up of internet links, hand searches of Scrip, Federal

Drug Association submissions for new drug applications, conference abstracts, reference lists, and Glaxo Wellcome submission to NICE.
24. Puhakka T, Lehti H, Vainionpaa R, et al. Zanamivir: a significant reduction in viral load during treatment in military conscripts with influenza. *Scand J Infect Dis* 2003;35:52–58.
25. Henney JE. Revised labeling for zanamivir. *JAMA* 2000;284:1234.
26. Woods JM, Bethell RC, Coates JAV, et al. 4-guanidino-2,4-dideoxy-2,3-dehydro-N-acetylneuraminic acid is a highly effective inhibitor of both the sialidase (neuraminidase) and growth of a wide range of influenza A and B viruses *in vitro*. *Antimicrob Agents Chemother* 1993;37:1473–1479.
27. Read RC. Letter to the Editor. *Lancet* 1999;353:668–669.
28. Tisdale M. Monitoring of viral susceptibility: new challenges with the development of influenza NA inhibitors. *Rev Med Virol* 2000;10:45–55.
29. Gubareva LV, Kaiser L, Brenner MK, et al. Evidence for zanamivir resistance in an immunocompromised child infected with influenza B virus. *J Infect Dis* 1998;178:1257–1262.
30. Gubareva LV, Webster RG, Hayden FG. Detection of influenza virus resistance to neuraminidase inhibitors by an enzyme inhibition assay. *Antiviral Res* 2002;53:47–61.
31. Zambon M, Hayden FG. Position statement: global neuraminidase inhibitor susceptibility network. *Antiviral Res* 2001;49:147–156.
32. Berger W, Stein WJ, Sharp SJ, et al. Effect of inhaled zanamivir on pulmonary function and illness duration in asthma and/or chronic obstructive pulmonary disease (COPD) patients with influenza. *Ann Allergy Asthma Immunol* 2001;86:85.
33. Li L, Cai B, Wang M, et al. A double-blind, randomized, placebo-controlled multicenter study of oseltamivir phosphate for treatment of influenza infection in China. *Chin Med J* 2003;116:44–48.
34. Treanor JJ, Hayden FG, Vrooman PS, et al. Efficacy and safety of the oral neuraminidase inhibitor oseltamivir in treating acute influenza: a randomized controlled trial. *JAMA* 2000;283:1016–1024.
35. Nicholson KG, Aoki FY, Osterhaus ADME, et al. Efficacy and safety of oseltamivir in treatment of acute influenza: a randomized controlled trial. *Lancet* 2000;355:1845–1850.

Lucy Hansen
Locum Consultant Physician with Specialist interest in Immunology
Hairmyres Hospital
East Kilbride
UK

Competing interests: None declared.

We would like to acknowledge the previous contributors of this chapter, including Timothy Uyeki.

Leprosy

Search date November 2003

Diana Lockwood

QUESTIONS

INTERVENTIONS

*Observational evidence only; RCTs unlikely to be conducted

See glossary G

Key Messages

Prevention

- **Vaccination (Bacillus Calmette Guerin [BCG] vaccine; BCG plus killed *Mycobacterium leprae*; ICRC vaccine; *Mycobacterium w* vaccine)** One RCT evaluated four different vaccines and found that the largest effect was with ICRC vaccine and BCG plus killed *M leprae*, followed by BCG alone. The effectiveness of *Mycobacterium w* was only marginal. However, only for the vaccine BCG alone were the findings corroborated by large controlled clinical trials in different geographical areas with long term follow up. Only one RCT reported on harms of vaccination; it found these to be minimal.

Treatment

- **Multidrug treatment for multibacillary leprosy** We found no reliable comparisons of multidrug treatment with rifampicin plus clofazimine plus dapsone versus dapsone alone, or versus dapsone plus rifampicin, in people with multibacillary leprosy. Observational studies found that multidrug treatment improved skin lesions and was associated with a low relapse rate. The evidence on the incidence of adverse effects is poor. Multidrug treatment was not compared with dapsone alone because rising dapsone resistance rates would make such a study unethical.
- **Multidrug treatment for paucibacillary leprosy** We found no reliable comparisons of multidrug treatment with dapsone plus rifampicin versus dapsone alone in people with paucibacillary leprosy, and RCTs would probably be unethical because of rising rates of dapsone resistance. Observational studies found that multidrug treatment improved skin lesions and was associated with a low relapse rate. We found poor evidence on the incidence of adverse effects.

- **Multiple dose compared with single dose treatment for single skin lesion leprosy** One RCT found that multiple dose treatment with rifampicin monthly plus dapsone daily for 6 months achieved higher cure rates at 18 months than single dose treatment with rifampicin plus minocycline plus ofloxacin. Some improvement occurred in 99% of people in both groups. Adverse effects were similar with both regimens.

DEFINITION Leprosy is a chronic granulomatous disease caused by *Mycobacterium leprae*, primarily affecting the peripheral nerves and skin. The clinical picture depends on the individual's immune response to *M leprae*. At the tuberculoid end of the Ridley–Jopling scale, individuals have good cell mediated immunity and few skin lesions. At the lepromatous end of the scale, individuals have low reactivity for *M leprae*, causing uncontrolled bacterial spread and skin and mucosal infiltration. Peripheral nerve damage occurs across the spectrum. Nerve damage may occur before, during, or after treatment. Some people have no nerve damage, others develop anaesthesia of the hands and feet, which puts them at risk of developing neuropathic injury. Weakness and paralysis of the small muscles of the hands, feet, and eyes puts patients at risk of developing deformity and contractures. Loss of the fingers and toes is due to repeated injury in a weak, anaesthetic limb. These visible deformities cause stigmatisation. Classification is based on clinical appearance and bacterial index of lesions**G**. The World Health Organization field leprosy classification is based on the number of skin lesions: single lesion leprosy (1 lesion), paucibacillary leprosy (2–5 skin lesions), and multibacillary leprosy (> 5 skin lesions).[1]

INCIDENCE/ PREVALENCE Worldwide, about 720 000 new cases of leprosy are reported each year,[2] and about 2 million people have leprosy related disabilities. Six major endemic countries (India, Brazil, Myanmar, Madagascar, Nepal, and Mozambique) account for 88% of all new cases. Cohort studies show a peak of disease presentation between 10–20 years of age.[3] After puberty, there are twice as many cases in males as in females.

AETIOLOGY/ RISK FACTORS *M leprae* is discharged from the nasal mucosa of people with untreated lepromatous leprosy, and spreads, via the recipient's nasal mucosa, to infect their skin and nerves. It is a hardy organism and has been shown to survive outside human hosts in India for many months.[4] Risk factors for infection include household contact with a person with leprosy. We found no good evidence of an association with HIV infection, nutrition, or socioeconomic status.[5]

PROGNOSIS Complications of leprosy include nerve damage, immunological reactions, and bacillary infiltration. Without treatment, tuberculoid infection eventually resolves spontaneously. Most people with borderline tuberculoid and borderline lepromatous leprosy gradually develop lepromatous infection. Many people have peripheral nerve damage at the time of diagnosis, ranging from 15% in Bangladesh[6] to 55% in Ethiopia.[7] Immunological reactions can occur with or without antibiotic treatment. Further nerve damage occurs through immune mediated reactions (type 1 reactions) and neuritis**G**. Erythema nodosum leprosum**G** (type 2 reaction) is an immune complex mediated reaction causing fever, malaise, and neuritis, which occurs in 20% of people with lepromatous leprosy and 5% with borderline lepromatous leprosy.[8] Secondary impairments (wounds, contractures, and digit resorption) occur in 33–56% of people with established nerve damage.[9] We found no recent information on mortality.

AIMS OF INTERVENTION **Prevention:** To prevent infection. **Treatment:** To treat infection and improve skin lesions; to prevent relapse and complications (nerve damage and erythema nodosum leprosum). Prevention of complications such as ulcers and deformity may improve the quality of life for the individual and help reduce the severe stigmatisation that still accompanies leprosy.

OUTCOMES **Prevention:** Incidence of leprosy. **Treatment:** Clinical improvement, relapse rate, quality of life, adverse effects of treatment, and mortality.

METHODS *Clinical Evidence* search and appraisal November 2003, including a search for observational studies. The author identified additional references from hand searches of reference lists. RCTs of preventative interventions need a long follow up period, as the incubation period can be 2–15 years, depending on disease type. We excluded trials with less than 2 years' follow up.

QUESTION **What are the effects of interventions to prevent leprosy?**

OPTION **VACCINATION**

One RCT evaluated four different vaccines and found that the largest effect was with ICRC vaccine and bacillus Calmette Guerin (BCG) plus killed *M leprae*, followed by BCG alone. The effectiveness of *Mycobacterium w* was only marginal. However, only for BCG alone were the findings corroborated by large controlled clinical trials conducted in different geographical locations with long term follow up. Only one RCT reported on harms of vaccination; it found these to be minimal.

Benefits: We found no systematic review. **Different vaccines versus placebo:** We found one RCT, carried out in a leprosy endemic area with clinical leprosy as the outcome measure (see table A on web extra).[10] The RCT (double blind, 171 400 healthy people in India aged 1–65 years, follow up for 6–7 years) compared four vaccines (ICRC vaccine❻: 22 541 people; *Mycobacterium w* vaccine: 33 720 people; BCG: 38 213 people; and BCG plus killed *M leprae:* 38 229 people) versus normal saline (38 697 people). It included a statistical adjustment for the multiple comparisons against saline. All four vaccines significantly reduced the incidence of leprosy compared with saline. The most effective vaccines were ICRC vaccine (RRR 65.5%, 95% CI 48.0% to 77.0%) and BCG plus killed *M leprae* (RRR 64.0%, 95% CI 50.4% to 73.9%). BCG alone was also effective (RRR 34.1%, 95% CI 13.5% to 49.8%), whereas the significance of the effect of *Mycobacterium w* was marginal (RRR 25.7%, 95% CI 1.9% to 43.8%). **BCG versus no treatment or placebo:** In addition to the RCT mentioned above,[10] we found three controlled clinical trials conducted in different geographical locations comparing BCG alone versus placebo, carried out in leprosy endemic areas, with clinical leprosy as the outcome measure (see table A on web extra).[11–13] The controlled trials (in a total of over 39 000 children in Uganda, Myanmar, and Papua New Guinea) were quasi- or non-randomised, but had longer follow up than the RCT (13–16 years). They found that BCG significantly reduced the incidence of leprosy in all three countries (see table A on web extra). The degree of protection against leprosy varied between countries, with higher protection in Uganda than Myanmar. One of the trials also looked at mortality and found a significant reduction (442/2707 [16.3%] deaths from all causes with BCG *v* 489/2649 [18.5%] with saline; RR 0.89, 95% CI 0.79 to 0.99; NNT 47, 95% CI 24 to 997).[12] **BCG plus killed *M leprae* versus placebo:** In addition to the RCT mentioned above,[10] we found one further RCT carried out in leprosy endemic areas, with clinical leprosy as the outcome measure (see table A on web extra).[14] The RCT stratified people according to the presence of a BCG scar. Those with a scar or a possible scar (54 865 people) received either BCG, BCG plus killed *M leprae*, or placebo. This RCT (double blind, 121 020 healthy people in Malawi without history of previous leprosy or tuberculosis, severe malnutrition, or other severe illness, aged ≥ 3 months, follow up for 5–9 years) found that combined results for BCG and BCG plus killed *M leprae* indicated significantly reduced incidence of leprosy compared with placebo (combined analysis for BCG or BCG plus killed *M leprae* versus placebo; RR 0.51, 95% CI 0.26 to 0.99).[14] Those without a scar (66 155 people) received BCG or BCG plus killed *M leprae*. **ICRC vaccine versus placebo:** We found one RCT (see different vaccines *v* placebo, above).[10] ***Mycobacterium w* versus placebo:** We found one RCT (see different vaccines *v* placebo, above).[10] **Dose of vaccine:** The controlled trial performed in Myanmar compared two different concentrations of BCG vaccine versus no treatment.[13] The vaccine with the higher concentration of bacilli significantly reduced the incidence of leprosy over 14 years (3.8/1000 person years**G** with BCG *v* 5.4/1000 person years for controls; RRR 30%, 95% CI 19–40%). The vaccine with the lower concentration of bacilli had no significant protective effect (5.0/1000 person years with BCG *v* 5.6/1000 person years; RRR +11%, 95% CI –3% to +23%). The RCT performed in Malawi found no significant differences between a higher and a standard dose of killed *M leprae*.[14]

Harms: The RCT conducted in India found that "fluctuant adenitis" was minimal with all four vaccines used, and no other adverse effects were observed (numbers not reported).[10] The other trials did not report on harms.[11–14]

Comment: In the trial in Malawi, 7/82 people (9%) tested positive for HIV.[14] Eleven different batches of BCG were used. The number of people lost to follow up was high (26%), and the sample size may have been insufficient to rule out clinically important effects, given that there were multiple comparisons against placebo.[14]

QUESTION What are the effects of treatments for leprosy?

OPTION MULTIDRUG TREATMENT FOR PAUCIBACILLARY LEPROSY

We found no reliable comparison between multidrug treatment with dapsone plus rifampicin versus dapsone alone in people with paucibacillary leprosy, and RCTs would probably be unethical because of rising rates of dapsone resistance. Observational studies found that multidrug treatment improved skin lesions and was associated with a low relapse rate. We found poor evidence on the incidence of adverse effects.

Benefits: We found no systematic review or RCT (see comment below). We found seven observational studies assessing the effects of multidrug treatment (dapsone 100 mg/day plus rifampicin 600 mg monthly for 6 months), with follow up ranging from 6 months to 10 years (see table 1, p 944 and table 2, p 945).[15–22] The studies used different methods of assessment, making it difficult to compare results. **Skin lesions:** Three cohort studies reported rates of resolution of skin lesions (see comment below) (see table 1, p 944).[15–17,19] One study (499 people) found that resolution of lesions occurred in 38% of people after 1 year;[16] another (50 people) found that resolution occurred in 8% of people after 6 months.[15] The number of people with lesions that were clinically active after treatment ranged from 2–44%.[15–17] **Nerve impairment:** Two studies reported rates of new or worsening nerve impairment (see table 1, p 944).[17,19] One (499 people) found that new disabilities occurred in 2.5% of people, and worsening of existing disabilities occurred in 3.3% after 4 years.[19] The other study (130 people) found that the visible disabilities (World Health Organization grade II**G**) increased from 4% at enrolment to 7% after 8–10 years' follow up.[17] **Relapse:** Six studies reported relapse rates over a 3–8 year follow up period (see table 2, p 945).[17–22] The risk of relapse ranged from 0% over a mean of 4.1 years in Ethiopia[18] and 0.33% over 5 years (0.66/1000 person years) in China[22] to 2.5% over 4 years (6.5/1000 person years) in Malawi.[19] (It is clinically difficult to differentiate relapse from reaction in paucibacillary leprosy**G**.)

Harms: None of the studies formally monitored adverse effects. In one study, hepatitis due to rifampicin occurred in 1/130 people (0.8%), but the method of diagnosis was not reported.[17] In another study, 1/503 people (0.2%) suffered an "allergic reaction" to rifampicin and dapsone (details not reported).[16]

Comment: Because studies had shown that 30% of *M leprae* isolates were resistant to dapsone,[23] the World Health Organization introduced the combination of dapsone plus rifampicin urgently in 1982, without formal RCTs comparing it against dapsone.

OPTION MULTIDRUG TREATMENT FOR MULTIBACILLARY LEPROSY

We found no reliable comparisons between multidrug treatment with rifampicin plus clofazimine plus dapsone versus dapsone alone, or versus dapsone plus rifampicin, in people with multibacillary leprosy. Observational studies found that multidrug treatment improved skin lesions and was associated with a low relapse rate. The evidence on the incidence of adverse effects is poor. Multidrug treatment was not compared with dapsone alone because rising dapsone resistance rates would make such a study unethical.

Benefits: We found no systematic review or RCTs. We found six observational studies assessing the effects of multidrug treatment (monthly supervised rifampicin 600 mg and clofazimine 300 mg, plus daily unsupervised dapsone 100 mg and clofazimine 500 mg) for 24 months.[17,18,20,22,24,25] **Skin lesions:** One study in Thailand (53 people) found that 29% of lesions were still active at 3 years (see table 3, p 945).[17] **Nerve impairment:** The study in Thailand found that the proportion of people with visible deformity (World Health Organization grade II**G**) increased from 8% at enrolment to 13% at 8–10 years' follow up.[17] **Relapse:** Six observational studies reported relapse rates (see table 4, p 946),[17,18,20,22,24,25] which varied from 0/1000 person years**G** in Ethiopia to 20.4/1000 person years in India. In the study conducted in India, the overall relapse rate was 20/260 (7.7%) over about 8 years (20.4/1000 person years), and 18/20 (90%) relapses were in people with a bacterial index**G** greater than 4 at the start of treatment.[24]

Harms: Most studies did not report on adverse effects. Skin pigmentation may occur with clofazimine, which may be especially problematic in people with fair skin.

Comment: Only one study[24] stratified its results according to bacterial index. The World Health Organization study group on chemotherapy recommended that treatment be given for 24 months.[26] In 1998, the 7th Expert Committee gave the option of reducing the length of treatment from 24 months to 12 months.[1] We found no controlled trial to support this recommendation. We found one RCT (93 people with untreated lepromatous leprosy), which compared dapsone 50 mg daily plus daily rifampicin 450 mg versus dapsone 50 mg daily plus monthly rifampicin 1200 mg for the first 6 months of treatment.[27] It found no significant difference in clinical improvement between daily versus monthly rifampicin (40/47 [85%] with daily rifampicin *v* 43/46 [91%]; RR 0.91, 95% CI 0.62 to 1.03). Adverse effects were more common with daily than with monthly rifampicin, causing discontinuation in 8.5% of people with daily rifampicin compared with 0% with monthly rifampicin.[27] Multidrug treatment was not compared with dapsone alone because rising dapsone resistance rates would make such a study unethical.

OPTION MULTIPLE DOSE VERSUS SINGLE DOSE TREATMENT FOR SINGLE SKIN LESIONS

One RCT found that multiple dose treatment with rifampicin monthly plus dapsone daily for 6 months achieved higher cure rates at 18 months than single dose treatment with rifampicin plus minocycline plus ofloxacin. Some improvement occurred in 99% of people in both groups. Adverse effects were similar with both regimens.

Benefits: We found no systematic review. We found one RCT (1483 people with single skin lesions typical of paucibacillary leprosy**G**; see comment below) comparing single dose treatment with rifampicin 600 mg plus ofloxacin 400 mg plus minocycline 100 mg versus multiple dose treatment with dapsone 100 mg daily plus rifampicin 600 mg monthly for 6 months.[28] Outcomes measured at 18 months were based on a scoring system involving five measurements: disappearance of the lesion, reduction in hypopigmentation, reduction in the degree of infiltration, reduction in the size of the lesion, and improvement in sensation in the lesion. Treatment failure was defined as no change or an increase in the clinical score, and marked improvement was defined as a difference of 13 between the baseline and 18 month scores. The RCT found that multiple dose treatment significantly increased the proportion of people with marked improvement compared with single dose treatment (392/684 [57.3%] with multiple dose *v* 361/697 [51.8%] with single dose; P = 0.04) and with complete cure (374/684 [54.7%] *v* 327/697 [46.9%]; RR 1.17, 95% CI 1.05 to 1.28; NNT 13, 95% CI 8 to 40). There were 12 treatment failures (6 in each group), and 99.1% of people in both groups had some improvement by the end of the study.[28]

Harms: Allergic reactions (which were not specified) occurred in seven people (6 taking multiple dose *v* 1 taking single dose treatment), and gastrointestinal effects occurred in five people (2 taking multiple dose *v* 3 taking single dose treatment). There was no significant difference in the number of type 1 reactions**G** (7/697 [1.0%] with single dose treatment *v* 3/684 [0.4%] with multiple dose; ARI +0.6%, 95% CI –0.2% to +3.4%).

Comment: The RCT did not specify its diagnostic criteria and did not confirm the clinical diagnosis. The follow up of only 18 months for people in the single dose group is short for detection of relapse. Some infections in this group would have resolved spontaneously, and the absence of a placebo control group means that the treatment effect cannot be estimated.[28] Single dose treatment has previously been assessed in people with paucibacillary leprosy. One RCT (622 people in Zaïre) compared two single dose regimens: rifampicin 40 mg/kg plus clofazimine 1200 mg versus rifampicin 40 mg/kg plus clofazimine 100 mg plus dapsone 100 mg plus ethionamide 500 mg. It found that the overall relapse rate was 20.4/1000 person years**G**, which was substantially higher than the relapse rate found for 6 months' treatment with dapsone plus rifampicin (see dapsone plus rifampicin, p 941), or rifampicin plus dapsone plus clofazimine (see rifampicin plus dapsone plus clofazimine, p 941). However, single dose treatment has operational advantages in the field, particularly when people live in remote areas and are unable to attend a clinic for several months.[29]

GLOSSARY

Bacteriological index A measure of the density of *M leprae* in the skin. Slit skin smears are made at several sites, and the smears are stained and examined microscopically. The number of bacteria per high power field is scored on a logarithmic scale (0–6), and the index calculated by dividing the total score by the numbers of sites sampled.

Heaf grade 0 = 0–4 mm induration; 1 = 5–9; 2 = 10–14; 3 = 15–19; 4 = ≥ 20. A grade 3 or 4 test generally indicates infection with *M tuberculosis*, although the cut off point varies between countries.

ICRC vaccine A vaccine developed at the Indian Cancer Research Centre.

Multibacillary leprosy More than five skin lesions (WHO 1998, WHO expert committee on leprosy seventh report 874).

Neuritis Inflammation of a nerve, presenting with any of the following: spontaneous nerve pain, paraesthesia, tenderness, or sensory, motor or autonomic impairment.

Paucibacillary leprosy Between two and five skin lesions.
Person years at risk The number of new cases of disease in a specified time period divided by the number of person years at risk during that period (average number at risk of relapse multiplied by the length of observation)
Single lesion leprosy One skin lesion.
Type 1 (reversal) reaction A delayed type hypersensitivity reaction occurring at sites of *M leprae* antigen. It presents with acutely inflamed skin lesions and acute neuritis (nerve tenderness with loss of function).
Type 2 reaction or erythema nodosum leprosum An immunological complication of multibacillary leprosy presenting with short lived and recurrent crops of tender erythematous subcutaneous nodules that may ulcerate. There may be signs of systemic involvement with fever, and inflammation in lymph nodes, nerves, eyes, joints, testes, fingers, toes, or other organs.
World Health Organization disability grading A simple grading system for use in the field, mainly for collection of general data regarding disabilities.[1] Grade 0 = no anaesthesia, no visible deformity or damage; grade 1 = anaesthesia present, but no visible deformity or damage; grade 2 = visible deformity or damage present.

REFERENCES

1. WHO Expert Committee on Leprosy. *World Health Organ Tech Rep Ser* 1988;768:1–51.
2. World Health Organization. Leprosy global situation. *Wkly Epidemiol Rec* 2002;77:1–8.
3. Fine PE. Leprosy: the epidemiology of a slow bacterium. *Epidemiol Rev* 1982;4:161–188.
4. Desikan KV, Sreevatsa. Extended studies on the viability of *Mycobacterium leprae* outside the human body. *Lepr Rev* 1995;66:287–295.
5. Lienhardt C, Kamate B, Jamet P, et al. Effect of HIV infection on leprosy: a three-year survey in Bamako, Mali. *Int J Lepr Other Mycobact Dis* 1996;64:383–391.
6. Croft RP, Richardus JH, Nicholls PG, et al. Nerve function impairment in leprosy: design, methodology, and intake status of a prospective cohort study of 2664 new leprosy cases in Bangladesh (The Bangladesh Acute Nerve Damage Study). *Lepr Rev* 1999;70:140–159.
7. Saunderson P, Gelore S, Desta K, et al. The pattern of leprosy-related neuropathy in the AMFES patients in Ethiopia: definitions, incidence, risk factors and outcome. *Lepr Rev* 2000;71:285–308.
8. Pfaltzgraff R, Ramu G. Clinical leprosy. In: Hastings R ed. *Leprosy*. Edinburgh: Churchill Livingstone, 1994:237–287.
9. van Brakel WH. Peripheral neuropathy in leprosy and its consequences. *Lepr Rev* 2000;71:S146–S153.
10. Gupte MD, Vallishayee RS, Anantharaman DS, et al. Comparative leprosy vaccine trial in south India. *Indian J Lepr* 1998;70:369–388.
11. Brown JA, Stone MM, Sutherland I. BCG vaccination of children against leprosy in Uganda: results at end of second follow-up. *BMJ* 1968;1:24–27.
12. Bagshawe A, Scott GC, Russell DA, et al. BCG vaccination in leprosy: final results of the trial in Karimui, Papua New Guinea, 1963–79. *Bull World Health Organ* 1989;67:389–399.
13. Lwin K, Sundaresan T, Gyi MM, et al. BCG vaccination of children against leprosy: fourteen-year findings of the trial in Burma. *Bull World Health Organ* 1985;63:1069–1078.
14. Karonga Prevention Trial Group. Randomised controlled trial of single BCG, repeated BCG, or combined BCG and killed *Mycobacterium leprae* vaccine for prevention of leprosy and tuberculosis in Malawi. *Lancet* 1996;348:17–24.
15. Kar PK, Arora PN, Ramasastry CV, et al. A clinicopathological study of multidrug therapy in borderline tuberculoid leprosy. *J Indian Med Assoc* 1994;92:336–337.
16. Boerrigter G, Ponnighaus JM, Fine PE. Preliminary appraisal of a WHO-recommended multiple drug regimen in paucibacillary leprosy patients in Malawi. *Int J Lepr Other Mycobact Dis* 1988;56:408–417.
17. Dasananjali K, Schreuder PA, Pirayavaraporn C. A study on the effectiveness and safety of the WHO/MDT regimen in the northeast of Thailand; a prospective study, 1984–1996. *Int J Lepr Other Mycobact Dis* 1997;65:28–36.
18. Gebre S, Saunderson P, Byass P. Relapses after fixed duration multiple drug therapy: the AMFES cohort. *Lepr Rev* 2000;71:325–331.
19. Boerrigter G, Ponnighaus JM, Fine PE, et al. Four-year follow-up results of a WHO-recommended multiple-drug regimen in paucibacillary leprosy patients in Malawi. *Int J Lepr Other Mycobact Dis* 1991;59:255–261.
20. Schreuder PA. The occurrence of reactions and impairments in leprosy: experience in the leprosy control program of three provinces in northeastern Thailand, 1987–1995 [correction of 1978–1995]. I. Overview of the study. *Int J Lepr Other Mycobact Dis* 1998;66:149–158.
21. Chopra NK, Agarawal JS, Pandya PG. A study of relapse in paucibacillary leprosy in a multidrug therapy project, Baroda District, India. *Lepr Rev* 1990;61:157–162.
22. Li HY, Hu LF, Hauang WB, et al. Risk of relapse in leprosy after fixed duration multi-drug therapy. *Int J Lepr Other Mycobact Dis* 1997;65:238–245.
23. Ji B. Drug resistance in leprosy – a review. *Lepr Rev* 1985;56:265–278.
24. Girdhar BK, Girdhar A, Kumar A. Relapses in multibacillary leprosy patients: effect of length of therapy. *Lepr Rev* 2000;71:144–153.
25. Shaw IN, Natrajan MM, Rao GS, et al. Long-term follow up of multibacillary leprosy patients with high BI treated with WHO/MDT regimen for a fixed duration of two years. *Int J Lepr Other Mycobact Dis* 2000;68:405–409.
26. Chemotherapy of leprosy. Report of a WHO study group. WHO Technical Report Series, No 847, 1994
27. Yawalkar SJ, McDougall AC, Languillon J, et al. Once-monthly rifampicin plus daily dapsone in initial treatment of lepromatous leprosy. *Lancet* 1982;1:1199–1202.
28. Single-lesion Multicentre Trial Group. Efficacy of single-dose multidrug therapy for the treatment of single-lesion paucibacillary leprosy. *Indian J Leprosy* 1997;69:121en129.
29. Pattyn SR. A randomized clinical trial of two single-dose treatments for paucibacillary leprosy. *Lepr Rev* 1994;65:45–57.

Diana Lockwood
Consultant Leprologist
London School of Hygiene & Tropical Medicine and The Hospital for Tropical Diseases
London
UK

Competing interests: None declared.

TABLE 1 **Dapsone plus rifampicin in paucibacillary leprosy: clinical outcomes (see text, p 939).**

Ref	Location	Cohort size	Follow up (years)	Clinical outcome: Skin lesions	Clinical outcome: Nerve impairment
16,19	Malawi	499	1[16] 4[19]	**At 1 year[16]** *Not evident:* 180/473 (38.0%)[16] *Visible but not active:* 282/473 (59.6%)[16] *Visible and active:* 11/473 (2.3%)[16]	**At 4 years[19]** *New disabilities:* 12/484 (2.5%)[16] *Worsening of existing disabilities:* 16/484 (3.3%)[16]
15	India	50	0.5	*Inactive:* 4/50 (8%) *Marked improvement:* 16/50 (32%) *Regression (active):* 22/50 (44%) *Increased activity:* 8/50 (16%)	No data
17	Thailand	130	8–10	*Clinically active after treatment:* 27/123 (22%)	*Grade 2 disability:* At enrolment, 4% At follow up, 7% (absolute numbers not provided)

Ref, reference.

TABLE 2 Dapsone plus rifampicin in paucibacillary leprosy: relapse rates (see text, p 939).

Ref	Location	Cohort size	Treatment	Follow up (years)	Relapse rate
20	Thailand	420	MDT	About 5	8/393 (2.0%) 4.1/1000 PYAR (estimated as timescale not definite)
19	Malawi	499	MDT	4	12/484 (2.5%) 6.5/1000 PYAR
21	India	11 095	MDT (723 people received a second course)	3	21/10 995 (0.19%) PYAR not calculable as relapse rate for people receiving two courses was not presented separately
22	China	878 (who had not previously received chemotherapy)	MDT	5	0.66/1000 PYAR
17	Thailand	124	MDT	Mean 8.2	2/112 [1.8%] 2.0/1000 PYAR
18	Ethiopia	246	MDT	Mean 4.1	0

MDT, multidrug treatment; PYAR, person-years at risk; Ref, reference.

TABLE 3 Dapsone/rifampicin/clofazimine in multibacillary leprosy: clinical outcomes (see text, p 941).

				Clinical outcome	
Ref	Location	Cohort size	Follow up (years)	Skin lesions	Nerve impairment
17	Thailand	53	Range 10–12	Clinically active at about 3 years: 14/49 (29%)	Grade 2 disability: Start of treatment: 8% End of treatment: 13%

Ref, Reference.

TABLE 4 Dapsone/rifampicin/clofazimine in multibacillary leprosy: relapse rates (see text, p 941).

Ref	Location	Cohort size	Follow up (years)	Relapse rate
20	Thailand	220	3	2/198 (1.0%) 3.3/1000 PYAR
22	China	2318	10	0/1000 PYAR
17	Thailand	53 (12 with BI ≥ 5 at enrolment	8 (range 2–10)	0/1000 PYAR
18	Ethiopia	256 (57 people with BI > 4 at enrolment)	4.3 (range 0–8.6) 38% followed up for ≥ 5 years	0/1000 PYAR
24	India	260	Range 1–8	20/260 (7.6%) 20.4/1000 PYAR 18/20 (90%) with BI > 4 at enrolment
25	India	65	Range 1–8	1/46 (2.1%) 0.023/1000 PYAR

BI, bacterial index, PYAR, person years at risk; Ref, reference.

Lyme disease

Search date September 2003

Edward Hayes and Paul Mead

QUESTIONS

INTERVENTIONS

PREVENTION OF LYME DISEASE
Beneficial
Prophylactic antibiotics after *Ixodes scapularis* tick bites in Lyme disease endemic areas in North America 949

TREATMENT OF LYME DISEASE ARTHRITIS
Likely to be beneficial
Cefotaxime (more effective than penicillin)* 950
Ceftriaxone (more effective than penicillin)* 950
Doxycycline (as effective as amoxicillin plus probenecid). . .950
Penicillin (more effective than placebo). 950

TREATMENT OF LATE NEUROLOGICAL LYME DISEASE
Likely to be beneficial
Cefotaxime (more effective than penicillin)* 952

Unknown effectiveness
Ceftriaxone (in people with late neurological Lyme disease) . . .952
Ceftriaxone (in people with late neurological Lyme disease who had previously been treated) 952

Likely to be ineffective or harmful
Ceftriaxone plus doxycycline (in people with late neurological Lyme disease who had been previously treated) 952

*Based on subgroup analysis of RCTs

See glossary**G**

Key Messages

Prophylactic treatment of tick bite

- **Prophylactic antibiotics after *Ixodes scapularis* tick bites in Lyme disease endemic areas in North America** One systematic review in people with recognised *I scapularis* tick bites in the preceding 72 hours found that antibiotics reduced the risk of developing clinical Lyme disease compared with placebo, but the difference was not significant. One subsequent large RCT in people who had removed an attached *I scapularis* tick in the preceding 72 hours found that doxycycline reduced the proportion of people with erythema migrans at the site of the tick bite compared with placebo.

Treatment of Lyme arthritis

- **Cefotaxime (more effective than penicillin)** One RCT found weak evidence from a small subgroup analysis of people with Lyme arthritis that cefotaxime increased the proportion of people with full recovery compared with penicillin.
- **Ceftriaxone (more effective than penicillin)** One RCT found weak evidence from a small subgroup analysis of people with Lyme arthritis that ceftriaxone improved symptoms compared with penicillin.

- **Doxycycline (as effective as amoxicillin plus probenecid)** One RCT in people with Lyme arthritis found no significant difference between doxycycline and amoxicillin plus probenecid in resolution of Lyme arthritis.
- **Penicillin (more effective than placebo)** One RCT in people with Lyme arthritis has found that penicillin increases resolution of Lyme arthritis compared with placebo.

Treatment of late neurological Lyme disease

- **Cefotaxime (more effective than penicillin)** One RCT found weak evidence from a small subgroup analysis of people with late Lyme disease that cefotaxime improved symptoms of neuropathy compared with penicillin.
- **Ceftriaxone (in people with late neurological Lyme disease)** One RCT found insufficient evidence from a small subgroup analysis in people with late neurological Lyme disease about effects of ceftriaxone and cefotaxime.
- **Ceftriaxone (in people late neurological Lyme disease who had previously been treated)** One RCT in people with previously treated Lyme disease found no significant difference between ceftriaxone and placebo in cognitive functioning at 6 months. It found that ceftriaxone improved fatigue but blinding in this RCT was incomplete.
- **Ceftriaxone plus doxycycline (in people with late neurological Lyme disease who had been previously treated)** One RCT comparing ceftriaxone plus doxycycline with placebo in people with previously treated Lyme disease and persistent neurological symptoms found no significant difference in health related quality of life at interim analysis at 180 days.

DEFINITION Lyme disease is an inflammatory illness resulting from infection with spirochetes of the *Borrelia burgdorferi* genospecies transmitted to humans by ticks. Some infected people have no symptoms. The characteristic manifestation of early Lyme disease is erythema migrans: a circular rash at the site of the infectious tick attachment that expands over a period of days to weeks in 80–90% of people with Lyme disease. Early disseminated infection may cause secondary erythema migrans, disease of the nervous system (facial palsy or other cranial neuropathies, meningitis, and radiculoneuritis), musculoskeletal disease (arthralgia), and, rarely, cardiac disease (myocarditis or transient atrioventricular block). Untreated or inadequately treated Lyme disease can cause late disseminated manifestations weeks to months after infection. These late manifestations include arthritis, polyneuropathy, and encephalopathy. Diagnosis of Lyme disease is based primarily on clinical findings and a high likelihood of exposure to infected ticks. Serological testing is helpful in people with endemic exposure who have clinical findings consistent with later stage disseminated Lyme disease.

INCIDENCE/ PREVALENCE Lyme disease occurs in temperate regions of North America, Europe, and Asia. It is the most commonly reported vector borne disease in the USA, with over 23 000 cases reported a year.[1] Most cases occur in the north-eastern and north-central states, with a reported annual incidence in endemic states as high as 133/100 000 people.[1] In highly endemic communities, the incidence of Lyme disease may exceed 1000/100 000 people a year.[1] In some countries of Europe, the incidence of Lyme disease has been estimated to be over 100/100 000 people a year.[2] Foci of Lyme disease have been described in northern forested regions of Russia, in China, and in Japan.[3] Transmission cycles of *B burgdorferi* have not been described in tropical areas or in the southern hemisphere.[3]

AETIOLOGY/ RISK FACTORS Lyme disease is caused by infection with any of the *B burgdorferi* sensu lato genospecies. Virtually all cases of Lyme disease in North America are the result of infection with *B burgdorferi*. In Europe, Lyme disease may be caused by *B burgdorferi*, *B garinii*, or *B afzelii*. The infectious spirochetes are transmitted to humans through the bite of certain *Ixodes* ticks.[3] Humans who have frequent or prolonged exposure to the habitats of infected *Ixodes* ticks are at highest risk of acquiring Lyme disease. Individual risk depends on the likelihood of being bitten by infected tick vectors, which varies with the density of vector ticks in the environment, the prevalence of infection in ticks, and the extent of a person's contact with infected ticks. The risk of Lyme disease is often concentrated in focal areas. In the USA, risk is highest in certain counties within north-eastern and north-central states during the months of April to July.[2] People become infected when they engage in activities in wooded or bushy areas that are favourable habitats for ticks, and deer and rodent hosts. A vaccine based on recombinant outer surface protein Osp-A was licensed for use in the USA but later removed from the market.

PROGNOSIS Lyme disease is rarely fatal. Untreated Lyme arthritis resolves at a rate of 10–20% a year; over 90% of facial palsies due to Lyme disease resolve spontaneously, and most cases of Lyme carditis resolve without sequelae.[4] However, untreated Lyme disease can result in arthritis (50% of untreated people), meningitis or neuropathies (15% of untreated people), carditis (5–10% of untreated people with erythema migrans), and, rarely, encephalopathy.

AIMS OF INTERVENTION To prevent Lyme disease; to ameliorate or eliminate the symptoms of established Lyme disease; to reduce sequelae, with minimal adverse effects.

OUTCOMES **For prophylaxis:** incidence of Lyme disease, adverse events. **For treatment:** incidence, prevalence, or severity of symptoms and signs of short term manifestations; long term sequelae of infection; quality of life.

METHODS *Clinical Evidence* search and appraisal September 2003. Additional searches of authors' files.

QUESTION What are the effects of measures to prevent Lyme disease?

OPTION PROPHYLACTIC TREATMENT OF TICK BITE

One systematic review in people with recognised *I scapularis* tick bites in the preceding 72 hours found that antibiotics reduced the risk of developing clinical Lyme disease compared with placebo, but the difference was not significant. One subsequent large RCT in people who had removed an attached *I scapularis* tick in the preceding 72 hours found that doxycycline reduced the proportion of people with erythema migrans at the site of the tick bite compared with placebo.

Benefits: We found one systematic review[5] and one subsequent RCT[6] comparing prophylactic antibiotics versus placebo for the treatment of tick bite (see table 1, p 955). The review (search date 1995,[5] 3 RCTs,[7–9] 639 adults and children with recognised *I scapularis* tick bites in the preceding 72 hours; see comment below) found that prophylactic treatment with antibiotics (penicillin, amoxicillin [amoxycillin], and tetracycline) reduced the risk of developing clinical Lyme disease (erythema migrans) compared with placebo, but the difference was not significant (0/308 [0%] with antibiotics *v* 4/292 [1.4%] with placebo; ARR 1.4%, 95% CI 0% to 3%; OR 0, 95% CI 0 to 1.5; P = 0.12).[5] The subsequent large RCT (482 people ≥ 12 years old who had removed an attached *I scapularis* tick in the preceding 72 hours; see comment below) compared doxycycline (200 mg as a single dose) versus placebo with 6 weeks' follow up.[6] It found that doxycycline significantly reduced the proportion of people with erythema migrans at the site of the tick bite and the proportion of people with any evidence of Lyme disease compared with placebo (erythema migrans: 1/235 [0.4%] with doxycycline *v* 8/247 [3.2%] with placebo; ARR 2.8%, 95% CI 0.4% to 5.2%; NNT 36, 95% CI 20 to 250; any evidence of Lyme disease defined as erythema migrans at the site of the tick bite, or at other sites, or a viral-like illness with laboratory evidence of Lyme disease: 3/235 [1.3%] with doxycycline *v* 11/247 [4.5%] with placebo; ARR 3.2%, 95% CI 0.2% to 6.2%; NNT 31, 95% CI 16 to 500). None of the 431 people who had serum samples tested at study entry and 3 and 6 weeks later had asymptomatic seroconversion for antibody to *B burgdorferi*. Erythema migrans at the site of the tick bite only occurred if the removed tick was in the nymph stage, was partially engorged, and was estimated to be attached for more than 72 hours. A subgroup analysis found that in people who removed partially engorged nymphal ticks, doxycycline significantly reduced erythema migrans at the site of the tick bite compared with placebo (AR 1/78 [1.3%] with doxycycline *v* 8/81 [9.9%] with placebo; ARR 8.6%, 95% CI 1.4% to 15.8%; NNT 12, 95% CI 7 to 71).[6]

Harms: Two RCTs in the review found that penicillin and amoxycillin increased rash compared with placebo but the incidence was low (1 RCT: AR 1/27 [4%] with penicillin *v* 0/29 [0%] with placebo; 1 RCT: AR 2/205 [1%] with amoxicillin *v* 0/182 [0%] with placebo) (see table 1, p 955). The third RCT in the review found no adverse effects among persons who had been treated with antibiotics.[5] The subsequent RCT (309 people who recorded data on adverse events) found that doxycycline significantly increased nausea and vomiting compared with placebo. However, it found no significant difference between treatments for abdominal discomfort, diarrhoea, and dizziness (nausea and vomiting: 33/156 [21.0%] with doxycycline *v* 6/153 [3.9%] with placebo; ARI 17.2%, 95% CI 9.8% to 24.6%; NNH 6, 95% CI 4 to 10; abdominal discomfort: 11/156 [7.1%] with doxycycline *v* 6/153 [3.9%] with placebo; P = 0.34; diarrhoea: 6/156 [3.8%] with doxycycline *v* 6/153 [3.9%] with placebo; P = 0.79; dizziness: 4/156 [2.6%] with doxycycline *v* 1/153 [0.7%] with placebo; P = 0.37).[6]

Comment: The three RCTs included in the systematic review[5] and the subsequent RCT[6] were all conducted in Lyme disease endemic areas in North America. There is a possibility that people treated with antibiotics for tick bite may not develop erythema migrans but could progress to late stages of Lyme disease. However, none of the people who were treated with antibiotics in the RCTs had asymptomatic infection with *B burgdorferi*, or developed late manifestations of Lyme disease during follow up (ranging from 6 weeks to 3 years). The most recent and largest RCT found that for a baseline risk of 1% for contracting Lyme disease in the control group, the number needed to treat for a single dose of doxycycline 200 mg to prevent Lyme disease was 31.[6] The same RCT found that the number needed to harm for nausea or vomiting from this treatment was six; therefore, about five people would develop nausea or vomiting for every person in whom Lyme disease was prevented. People in the RCT with adult ticks, non-engorged ticks, or both did not develop Lyme disease, although Lyme disease can occur after the bite of an engorged adult tick. If treatment was limited to people with engorged nymphal ticks (NNT 12), then two people would develop nausea and less than one person would develop vomiting for every person in whom Lyme disease was prevented.

QUESTION What are the effects of antibiotic treatment for Lyme disease arthritis?

OPTION TREATMENT OF LYME DISEASE ARTHRITIS

One RCT in people with Lyme arthritis has found that penicillin increases resolution of Lyme arthritis compared with placebo. Another RCT in people with Lyme arthritis found no significant difference between doxycycline and amoxicillin plus probenecid in resolution of Lyme arthritis. One RCT found weak evidence from a small subgroup analysis of people with Lyme arthritis that ceftriaxone improved symptoms compared with penicillin. One RCT found weak evidence from a small subgroup analysis of people with Lyme arthritis that cefotaxime increased the proportion of people with full recovery compared with penicillin. Some people have developed symptoms of neuroborreliosis and inflammatory tissue reactions (Jarisch-Herxheimer reaction) after oral antibiotic treatment of Lyme arthritis.

Benefits: We found no systematic review. **People with Lyme arthritis:** We found two RCTs in people with Lyme disease arthritis.[10,11] The first RCT (40 people with Lyme disease arthritis) compared intramuscular benzathine penicillin versus saline placebo.[10] It found that penicillin significantly increased the proportion of people having complete resolution of the arthritis compared with placebo (AR 7/20 [35%] with penicillin *v* 0/20 [0%] with placebo; $P < 0.02$).[10] The second RCT (48 people with Lyme arthritis) compared oral doxycycline (100 mg twice daily for 30 days) versus oral amoxicillin (500 mg) plus probenecid (4 times daily for 30 days).[11] After 3 months, an intention to treat analysis found no significant difference between treatments in rates of arthritis (AR 18/25 [72%] with doxycycline *v* 16/23 [70%] with amoxicillin plus probenecid; RR 1.04, 95% CI 0.72 to 1.49). In the doxycycline group, one person had recurrence of arthritis and another developed polyneuropathy after treatment. In the amoxicillin plus probenecid group, one person had recurrent arthritis, two developed polyneuropathy, and two developed encephalopathy. **Subgroup analyses of people with Lyme arthritis:** We found three other RCTs in people with a variety of forms of late Lyme disease (including Lyme arthritis).[12–14] The first RCT (23 people with late Lyme disease, 70% with arthritis) compared ceftriaxone (2 g iv every 12 hours for 14 days) versus penicillin (4 MU iv every 4 hours for 10 days).[12] It found that ceftriaxone increased clinical improvement at 3 months but the difference was not significant (AR of improvement 12/13 [92%] with ceftriaxone *v* 5/10 [50%] with penicillin; RR 1.85, 95% CI 0.97 to 3.50). It found that, in a subgroup of people with arthritis, ceftriaxone increased the proportion of people with improved arthritis (AR 9/9 [100%] with ceftriaxone *v* 2/7 [29%] with penicillin; NNT 2, 95% CI 1 to 4). The second RCT (135 people with late Lyme disease, 73 with arthritis) compared cefotaxime (6 g/day for 8–10 days) versus penicillin G (20 MU/day for 8–19 days).[13] It found that cefotaxime significantly increased rates of full recovery 2 years after treatment compared with penicillin (AR 44/69 [64%] with cefotaxime *v* 25/66 [38%] with penicillin; RR 1.68, 95% CI 1.18 to 2.41; NNT 3, 95% CI 2 to 11). In the subgroup of people with arthritis, ceftriaxone significantly increased rates of full recovery compared with penicillin (17/39 [44%] with cefotaxime *v* 4/34 [12%] with penicillin; RR 3.7, 95% CI 1.4 to 9.9; NNT 4, 95% CI 2 to 10). The third RCT (62 people with disseminated Lyme disease, 13 people with Lyme arthritis) did not report separate results for the subgroup with arthritis. It compared intravenous ceftriaxone followed by oral amoxicillin plus probenecid versus oral cefixime plus probenecid.[14]

Harms: Some people have developed symptoms of neuroborreliosis**G** after oral antibiotic treatment of arthritis.[11] Jarisch-Herxheimer reactions**G** have been described in people treated for late Lyme disease. One RCT reported symptoms suggestive of a mild Jarisch-Herxheimer reaction in 12/44 (27%) of people treated with ceftriaxone and 1/10 (10%) of people with penicillin,[12] and one RCT reported "Herxheimer-like" reactions in 20.0% of people treated with penicillin and 40.5% of people treated with cefotaxime.[13] One RCT reported in an unspecified number of people with possible "Herxheimer-like" reactions, including fever, transient rash, and worsening of symptoms or cardiac arrhythmia, among people treated with cefixime and probenecid, and with ceftriaxone followed by amoxicillin.[14] It found no significant difference in the risk of developing a prolonged form of such reactions with ceftriaxone plus amoxicillin compared with cefixime plus probenecid (18/30 [60%] with ceftriaxone plus amoxicillin treatment *v* 12/30 [40%] with cefixime plus probenecid; RR 1.50, 95% CI 0.88 to 2.54).[14] Other harms include those expected from the antibiotics. In RCTs including people with Lyme arthritis, the following adverse effects were reported: diarrhoea and skin rash with ceftriaxone;[12] shock and colitis with penicillin; anaphylaxis and colitis with cefotaxime;[13] rash and gastrointestinal effects with amoxicillin and probenecid;[11] diarrhoea and rash with cefixime; and nausea, diarrhoea, and rash with ceftriaxone followed by amoxicillin.[14]

Comment: Results of the RCTs that presented results for subgroups of people with Lyme arthritis should be interpreted with caution as people with arthritis were not randomly assigned to treatment groups. The RCTs were small, and the type, dose, and regimen of antibiotics used varied between trials. The enrolment criteria also varied between trials. Only one RCT had a placebo control.[10] The proportion of people who respond in comparative RCTs is difficult to interpret because, without a placebo comparison, it is unclear how many people would have improved without treatment.

QUESTION **What are the effects of antibiotic treatment for late neurological Lyme disease?**

OPTION **TREATMENT OF LATE NEUROLOGICAL LYME DISEASE**

One RCT found weak evidence from a small subgroup analysis of people with late Lyme disease that cefotaxime improved symptoms of neuropathy compared with penicillin. A small subgroup analysis of one RCT in people with late neurological Lyme disease found no significant difference between ceftriaxone and cefotaxime in the proportion of people who were asymptomatic. However, the analysis may have lacked power to detect a clinically important effect. One RCT comparing ceftriaxone plus doxycycline versus placebo in people with previously treated Lyme disease and persistent late neurological symptoms found no significant difference in health related quality of life or cognitive function at interim analysis at 180 days. One RCT in people with previously treated Lyme disease found no significant difference between ceftriaxone and placebo in cognitive functioning at 6 months. It found that ceftriaxone improved fatigue, but blinding in this RCT was incomplete.

Benefits: **People with late neurological Lyme disease:** We found two RCTs comparing antibiotics with placebo in people previously treated for Lyme disease.[15,16] The first RCT (129 people, 78 people seropositive for *B burgdorferi*, 51 people who were seronegative) compared antibiotics (iv ceftriaxone 2 g/day for 30 days followed by oral doxycycline 100 mg twice daily for 60 days) versus placebo.[15] All participants had persistent symptoms including arthralgia, myalgia, neurocognitive changes, altered sensation, malaise, headache, and sleep disturbance. At 180 days, a planned interim analysis found no significant difference between antibiotics and placebo in improvement in mood, pain, cognitive functioning, or neuropsychological tests.[17] The analysis found that the chance of finding a significant difference in health related quality of life (measured by the SF-36 scale) after completion of the full study was less than 5%. The study was, therefore, terminated.[15] The second RCT (55 people seropositive for *B burgdorferi*) compared intravenous ceftriaxone (2 g/day for 28 days) versus placebo.[16] All participants had persistent fatigue 6 months after previous treatment with at least 3 weeks of antibiotics. It found that ceftriaxone significantly improved fatigue at 6 months compared with placebo. However, it found no significant difference in cognitive function (fatigue improved, defined as a decrease ≥0.7 units on modified Fatigue Severity Scale: 18/28 [64.0%] with ceftriaxone *v* 5/27 [18.5%] with placebo; RR 3.50; 95% CI 1.50 to 8.03; improved cognitive function defined as ≥25% improvement in Alpha–arithmetic Test score: 2/26 [8%] with ceftriaxone *v* 2/22

[9%] with placebo; P = 0.99). However, there was evidence of inadequate blinding, which may have influenced participants' perceptions of fatigue (71% of people receiving ceftriaxone correctly guessed their treatment). **Subgroup analyses in people with late neurological Lyme disease:** We found two RCTs that included people with late neurological Lyme disease and presented results separately for this group.[13,18] The first RCT (135 people with late Lyme disease, 93 with neuropathy) compared cefotaxime (6 g/day for 8–10 days) versus penicillin G (20 MU/day for 8–19 days).[13] Two years after treatment, cefotaxime significantly increased complete recovery compared with penicillin (44/69 [64%] with cefotaxime *v* 25/66 [38%] with penicillin; RR 1.68, 95% CI 1.18 to 2.41). Similar results were reported for the subgroup with neuropathy (35/49 [71%] with cefotaxime *v* 20/44 [46%] with penicillin; RR 1.57, 95% CI 1.09 to 2.27). The second RCT (33 people with Lyme neuroborreliosis of varying duration) compared ceftriaxone (2 g iv/day for 10 days) versus cefotaxime (2 g iv every 8 hours for 10 days).[18] Some of the people treated with ceftriaxone were asymptomatic before treatment, and so were excluded from analysis (3/17 [18%]). Of the remaining people, most (17/30 [57%]) had disease duration of over 30 days at study entry, and some (8/30 [27%]) had a duration over 60 days. The RCT found no significant difference between ceftriaxone and cefotaxime in the proportion of people who were asymptomatic after 8 months (8/14 [57%] with ceftriaxone *v* 9/16 [56%] with cefotaxime; RR 1.02, 95% CI 0.54 to 1.90).

Harms: See harms under treatments for Lyme disease arthritis, p 951. **People with late neurological Lyme disease:** The first RCT in people with previously treated Lyme disease found no significant difference in the overall rate of adverse events between antibiotic and placebo.[17] The second RCT in people with previously treated Lyme disease also found no significant difference between ceftriaxone and placebo in overall minor adverse event rates. However, it found that ceftriaxone increased diarrhoea compared with placebo (diarrhoea: 43% with ceftriaxone *v* 25% with placebo; P value not reported).[16] One person receiving ceftriaxone was admitted to hospital for anaphylaxis. **Subgroup analyses in people with late neurological Lyme disease:** In the other clinical trials of people with late neurological Lyme disease reported above, the following adverse effects were reported: shock and colitis with penicillin, and anaphylaxis and colitis with cefotaxime;[12] rash with cefotaxime, and fever, diarrhoea, and elevated liver enzymes with ceftriaxone.[18] One case control study found an association between biliary disease and ceftriaxone treatment of suspected late Lyme disease.[19]

Comment: The RCTs of previously untreated people either recruited people with late Lyme disease, some of whom had neurological manifestations, or people with Lyme neuroborreliosis, some of whom had late disease. Results presented for these subsets of study participants may be subject to undetected biases, because people with late neurological disease were not randomly assigned to treatment groups. None of these RCTs had a placebo treated control group. The antibiotics used in RCTs, as well as doses and schedules, varied between trials. The enrolment criteria also varied between trials.

GLOSSARY

Jarisch-Herxheimer reaction An inflammatory reaction in tissues induced by antibiotic treatment of spirochetal diseases, and believed to be caused by an immunological reaction to the release of spirochetal antigens.

Neuroborreliosis Central or peripheral neuropathy resulting from infection with *Borrelia* sp spirochetes.

REFERENCES

1. Centers for Disease Control and Prevention (CDC). Lyme disease — United States, 2001–2002. *MMWR Morb Mortal Wkly Rep* 2004;53:365–369.
2. O'Connel S, Granstorm M, Gray JS, et al. Epidemiology of European Lyme borreliosis. *Zentralbl Bakteriol* 1998;287:229–240.
3. Dennis DT. Epidemiology, ecology, and prevention of Lyme disease. In: Rahn DW, Evans J, eds. *Lyme disease*. Philadelphia: American College of Physicians, 1998:7–34.
4. Rahn DW, Evans J, eds. *Lyme disease*. Philadelphia: American College of Physicians, 1998.
5. Warshafsky S, Nowakowski J, Nadelman RB, et al. Efficacy of antibiotic prophylaxis for prevention of Lyme disease. *J Gen Intern Med* 1996;11:329–333. Search date 1995; primary sources Medline and hand searches of reference lists for English language papers.
6. Nadelman RB, Nowakowski J, Fish D, et al. Prophylaxis with single-dose doxycycline for the prevention of Lyme disease after an *Ixodes scapularis* tick bite. *N Engl J Med* 2001;345:79–84.
7. Costello CM, Steere AC, Pinkerton RE, et al. A prospective study of tick bites in an endemic area for Lyme disease. *J Infect Dis* 1989;159:136–139.
8. Shapiro ED, Gerber MA, Holabird NB, et al. A controlled trial of antimicrobial prophylaxis for Lyme disease after deer-tick bites. *N Engl J Med* 1992;327:1769–1773.
9. Agre F, Schwartz R. The value of early treatment of deer tick bites for the prevention of Lyme disease. *Am J Dis Children* 1993;147:945–947.
10. Steere AC, Green J, Schoen RT, et al. Successful parenteral penicillin therapy of established Lyme arthritis. *N Engl J Med* 1985;312:869–874.
11. Steere AC, Levin RE, Molloy PJ, et al. Treatment of Lyme arthritis. *Arthritis Rheum* 1994;37:878–888.
12. Dattwyler RJ, Halperin JJ, Volkman DJ, et al. Treatment of late Lyme borreliosis — randomized comparison of ceftriaxone and penicillin. *Lancet* 1998;1:1191–1194.
13. Hassler D, Zoller M, Haude H-D, et al. Cefotaxime versus penicillin in the late stage of Lyme disease — prospective, randomized therapeutic study. *Infection* 1990;18:16–20.
14. Oksi J, Nikoskelainen J, Vijanen MK. Comparison of oral cefixime and intravenous ceftriaxone followed by oral amoxicillin in disseminated Lyme borreliosis. *Eur J Clin Microbiol Infect Dis* 1998;17:715–719.
15. Klempner MS, Hu LT, Evans J, et al. Two controlled trials of antibiotic treatment in patients with persistent symptoms and a history of Lyme disease. *N Engl J Med* 2001;345:85–92.
16. Krupp LB, Hyman LG, Grimson R, et al. Study and Treatment Of Post Lyme disease (STOP-LD): a randomized double masked clinical trial. *Neurology* 2003;60:1923–1930.
17. Kaplan RF, Trevino RP, Johnson GM, et al. Cognitive function in post-treatment Lyme disease: do additional antibiotics help? *Neurology* 2003;60:1916–1922.
18. Pfister H-W, Preac-Mursic V, Wilske B, et al. Randomized comparison of ceftriaxone and cefotaxime in Lyme neuroborreliosis. *J Infect Dis* 1991;163:311–318.
19. Ettestad PJ, Campbell GL, Welbel SF, et al. Biliary complications in the treatment of unsubstantiated Lyme disease. *J Infect Dis* 1995;171:356–361.

Edward Hayes
Medical Epidemiologist

Paul Mead
Medical Epidemiologist

US Centers for Disease Control and Prevention
Fort Collins, Colorado
USA

Competing interests: None declared.

TABLE 1 Prophylactic treatment of tick bite with antibiotics; results of placebo controlled RCTs (see text, p 949).[6–9]

Ref	Population (all noticed tick bites < 72 hours prior to study enrolment)	Intervention	Number of people with any evidence of Lyme disease (antibiotic v placebo)	Adverse effects (antibiotic v placebo)
6	482 people aged ≥ 12 years	Doxycycline (200 mg single dose) versus placebo	3/235 (1%) v 11/247 (4%); ARR 3.2%, 95% CI 0.2% to 6.2%	Nausea: 24/156 (15.4%) v 4/153 (2.6%); ARI 12.8%, 95% CI 6.4% to 19.2%; NNH 8, 95% CI 6 to 16 Vomiting: 9/156 (5.8%) v 2/153 (1.3%); ARI 4.5%, 95% CI 0.3% to 8.6%; NNH 23, 95% CI 12 to 303)
7	68 people aged ≥ 5 years	Penicillin (250 mg qds for 10 days) versus placebo	0/32 (0%) v 1/36 (3%); ARR 2.8%, 95% CI –3.0% to +8.5%	Rash: 1/27 (4%) v 0/29 (0%)
8	372 people of any age	Amoxicillin (250 mg tds for 10 days) versus placebo	0/205 (0%) v 2/182 (1%); ARR 1.1%, 95% CI –0.3% to +2.5%	Rash possibly due to amoxicillin: 2/205 (1%) v 0/182 (0%)
9	184 people aged 3–19 years	Penicillin (250 mg qds for 10 days in people < 9 years) or tetracycline (250 mg qds for 10 days in people > 9 years) versus placebo	0/89 (0%) v 4/90 (4%); ARR 4.4%, 95% CI 0.1% to 8.8%	Hives reported in 1 person who received placebo

qds, four times daily; ref, reference; tds, three times daily.

Malaria: prevention in travellers

Search date March 2004

Ashley M Croft

QUESTIONS

INTERVENTIONS

Covered elsewhere in *Clinical Evidence*
Malaria (severe, life threatening), p 977

Key Messages

Non-drug prevention adults

- **Insecticide treated nets** We found no RCTs in travellers. One systematic review in adult and child residents of malaria endemic settings found that insecticide treated nets reduced the number of mild episodes of malaria and reduced child mortality.
- **Insecticide treated clothing in adults** Two RCTs in soldiers and refugee householders found that permethrin treated fabric (clothing or sheets) reduced the incidence of malaria.
- **Aerosol insecticides in adults** We found no RCTs on the effects of aerosol insecticides in preventing malaria in travellers. One large questionnaire survey in travellers found insufficient evidence on the effects of aerosol insecticides in preventing malaria. Two community RCTs in residents of malaria endemic areas found that indoor spraying of aerosol insecticides reduced clinical malaria.
- **Air conditioning and electric fans in adults** We found no RCTs on the effects of air conditioning or electric fans in preventing malaria in travellers. One large questionnaire survey found that air conditioning reduced the incidence of malaria. One small observational study found that electric ceiling fans reduced total catches of culicine mosquitos in indoor spaces but did not significantly reduce total catches of anopheline mosquitoes.
- **Full length clothing in adults** We found no RCTs on the effects of full length clothing in preventing malaria in travellers. One large questionnaire survey in travellers found that wearing trousers and long sleeved shirts reduced the incidence of malaria.
- **Mosquito coils and vaporising mats in adults** We found no RCTs on the effects of coils and vaporising mats in preventing malaria in travellers. One case-control study of coils in travellers found no evidence of a protective effect against malaria. One RCT of coils and one observational study of pyrethroid vaporising mats found that these devices reduced numbers of culicine mosquitoes in indoor spaces.
- **Smoke** We found no RCTs on the effects of smoke in preventing malaria. One controlled clinical trial found that smoke repelled mosquitoes during the evening.
- **Topical (skin applied) insect repellents in adults** We found no RCTs on the effects of topical (skin applied) insect repellents in preventing malaria in travellers. One small crossover RCT found that diethyltoluamide (DEET) preparations protected against mosquito bites. DEET has been reported to cause systemic and skin adverse reactions, particularly with prolonged use.
- **Acoustic buzzers in adults; biological control measures** We found no RCTs on the effects of these interventions.

Drug prophylaxis in adults

- **Atovaquone plus proguanil in adults** One RCT in migrants with limited immunity found that atovaquone plus proguanil reduced the proportion of people with malaria compared with placebo. One RCT found no significant difference between atovaquone plus proguanil and chloroquine plus proguanil in preventing malaria. One RCT of atovaquone plus proguanil versus mefloquine found no cases of clinical malaria throughout the trial, but found a higher rate of neuropsychiatric harm with mefloquine than with atovaquone plus proguanil. RCTs comparing adverse effects of atovaquone plus proguanil versus chloroquine plus proguanil found different results. One RCT found that atovaquone plus proguanil reduced adverse effects compared with mefloquine and chloroquine plus proguanil and had similar adverse effect rates compared with doxycycline. Another RCT found no significant difference in adverse events between atovaquone plus proguanil and chloroquine plus proguanil.
- **Doxycycline in adults** One RCT in soldiers and one RCT in migrants with limited immunity found that doxycycline reduced the risk of malaria compared with placebo. One of the RCTs found that doxycycline was associated with nausea and vomiting, diarrhoea, cough, headache, and unspecified dermatological symptoms over 13 weeks. We found no evidence on long term safety. One RCT found that doxycycline had fewer adverse effects than mefloquine or chloroquine plus proguanil and had similar adverse effect rates compared with atovaquone plus proguanil.

Malaria: prevention in travellers

- **Chloroquine plus proguanil in adults** One RCT found no significant difference between chloroquine plus proguanil and chloroquine plus sulfadoxine plus pyrimethamine in the incidence of *P falciparum* malaria. One RCT found no significant difference between chloroquine plus proguanil and proguanil alone in the incidence of *P falciparum* malaria. One RCT found no significant difference between chloroquine plus proguanil and atovaquone plus proguanil in preventing malaria. RCTs comparing adverse effects of chloroquine plus proguanil versus atovaquone plus proguanil found different results. One RCT found that chloroquine plus proguanil increased adverse effects compared with three other common antimalarial drug regimens (doxycycline, mefloquine, and atovaquone plus proguanil). Another RCT found no significant difference in adverse events between chloroquine plus proguanil and atovaquone plus proguanil.
- **Mefloquine in adults** One systematic review of one RCT in soldiers found that mefloquine reduced cases of malaria compared with placebo, and found that mefloquine had a protective efficacy of 100%. One RCT of mefloquine versus atovaquone plus proguanil found no cases of clinical malaria throughout the trial, but found a higher rate of neuropsychiatric harm with mefloquine compared with atovaquone plus proguanil. One RCT found that mefloquine had more adverse effects than doxycycline or atovaquone plus proguanil and had similar adverse event rates compared with chloroquine plus proguanil.
- **Chloroquine in adults** We found no RCTs on the effects of chloroquine in travellers. One RCT in Austrian workers residing in Nigeria found no significant difference between chloroquine and sulfadoxine plus pyrimethamine in the incidence of malaria after 6–22 months. *P falciparum* resistance to chloroquine is now established in most malaria endemic regions of the world.
- **Pyrimethamine plus dapsone in adults** We found no RCTs in travellers. One RCT in Thai soldiers found insufficient evidence to compare pyrimethamine plus dapsone versus proguanil plus dapsone. We found limited observational evidence that pyrimethamine plus dapsone may cause agranulocytosis.
- **Amodiaquine in adults** We found no RCTs on the effects of amodiaquine in preventing malaria in travellers. We found limited observational evidence that amodiaquine may cause neutropenia, liver damage, and hepatitis.
- **Sulfadoxine plus pyrimethamine in adults** We found no RCTs of sulfadoxine plus pyrimethamine alone. One RCT found no significant difference between chloroquine plus proguanil and chloroquine plus sulfadoxine plus pyrimethamine in the incidence of *P falciparum* malaria. One retrospective observational study suggested that sulfadoxine plus pyrimethamine was associated with severe cutaneous reactions.

Antimalaria vaccines

- **Vaccines** We found no RCTs in travellers. One systematic review of antimalaria vaccines in residents of malaria endemic areas found that the SPf66 vaccine reduced first attacks of malaria compared with placebo.

Prevention in child travellers

- **Mefloquine in children** We found no RCTs of the effects of mefloquine in preventing malaria in child travellers.
- **Topical (skin applied) insect repellents containing DEET in children** We found no RCTs on the effects of DEET in preventing malaria in child travellers. Case reports in young children found serious adverse effects with DEET.

Prevention in pregnant travellers

- **Insecticide treated nets in pregnant travellers** We found no RCTs on the effects of insecticide treated nets in preventing malaria in pregnant travellers. One RCT of pregnant residents of a malaria endemic area found insufficient evidence on the effects of permethrin treated nets in preventing malaria.
- **Antimalaria drugs in pregnant travellers; insecticide treated clothing in pregnant travellers; topical (skin applied) insect repellents in pregnant travellers** We found no RCTs on the effects of these interventions.

Prevention in airline pilots

- **Antimalaria drugs in airline pilots** We found no RCTs on the effects of antimalaria drugs in airline pilots.

DEFINITION Malaria is an acute parasitic disease of the tropics and subtropics, caused by the invasion and destruction of red blood cells by one or more of four species of the genus *Plasmodium*: *P falciparum*, *P vivax*, *P ovale*, and *P malariae*.[1] The clinical presentation of malaria varies according to the infecting species, and to the genetics, immune status, and age of the infected person.[2] The most severe form of human malaria is caused by *P falciparum*, in which variable clinical features include spiking fevers, chills, headache, muscular aching and weakness, vomiting, cough, diarrhoea, and abdominal pain; other symptoms related to organ failure may supervene, such as: acute renal failure, generalised convulsions, and circulatory collapse, followed by coma and death.[3,4] *P falciparum* accounts for over 50% of malaria infections in most East Asian countries, over 90% in sub-Saharan Africa, and almost 100% in Hispaniola.[5] Travellers are defined here as visitors from a malaria-free area to a malaria-endemic area, and who stay in the endemic area for less than 1 year.

INCIDENCE/ PREVALENCE Malaria is the most dangerous parasitic disease of humans, infecting around 5% of the world's population, and causing about one million deaths each year.[6] The disease is strongly resurgent, due to the effects of war, climate change, large-scale population movements, increased breeding opportunities for vector mosquitoes, rapidly spreading drug and insecticide resistance, and neglect of public health infrastructure.[1,7] Malaria is currently endemic in over 100 countries, which are visited by over 125 million international travellers each year.[4] Cases of malaria acquired by international travellers from industrialised countries probably number 25 000 annually; of these, about 10 000 are reported, and 150 are fatal.[8]

AETIOLOGY/ RISK FACTORS Humans acquire malaria from sporozoites transmitted by the bite of infected female anopheline mosquitoes.[9] When foraging, blood-thirsty female mosquitoes fly upwind searching for the scent trail of an attractive host.[10] Female anophelines are attracted to their human hosts over a range of between 7–20 metres, and through a variety of stimuli including exhaled carbon dioxide, lactic acid, other host odours, warmth, and moisture.[11] Larger people tend to be bitten by mosquitoes more than smaller individuals, and adults more often than infants and children.[11,12] Women get significantly more mosquito bites in trials than men.[13] Of about 3200 mosquito species so far described, some 430 belong to the genus *Anopheles*, and of these, around 70 anopheline species are known to transmit malaria, with about 40 species considered important vectors.[14] Malaria transmission does not usually occur at temperatures below 16 °C or above 35 °C, nor at altitudes greater than 3000 metres above sea level at the equator (lower elevations in cooler climates), because sporozoite development in the mosquito cannot take place.[15] The optimum conditions for transmission are a humidity of over 60% and an ambient temperature between 25–30 °C.[16] Most of the important vectors of malaria breed in small temporary collections of fresh surface water exposed to sunlight and with little predation, and in sites such as residual pools in drying river beds.[17] Although rainfall provides breeding sites for mosquitoes, excessive rainfall may wash away mosquito larvae and pupae.[18] Conversely, prolonged droughts may be associated with increased malaria transmission if they reduce the size and flow rates of large rivers sufficiently to produce suitable *Anopheles* breeding sites.[19] Anopheline mosquitoes vary in their preferred feeding and resting locations, although the majority bite in the evening and at night.[20] The *Anopheles* mosquito will feed by day only if unusually hungry.[21] *Anopheles* adults usually fly not more than 2–3 kilometres from their breeding sites, although a flight range of up to 7 kilometres has been observed.[22] Exceptionally, strong winds may carry *Anopheles* up to 30 kilometres or more.[11] In travellers, malaria risk is related to destination, activity, and duration of travel. A retrospective cohort study (5898 confirmed cases) in Italian travellers between 1989–1997 found the malaria incidence was 1.5/1000 from travel to Africa, 0.11/1000 from travel to Asia, and 0.04/1000 from Central–South America.[23] A survey of 2131 German travellers to sub-Saharan Africa found that solo travellers were at almost a 9-fold greater risk of infection than those on package tours.[24] A case control study (46 cases, 557 controls) reported that a visit to the tropics of more than 21 days doubles the malaria risk compared with visits lasting 21 days or less.[25]

PROGNOSIS Malaria can develop after just one anopheline mosquito bite.[26] Human malaria has a usual incubation period of between 10–14 days (*P falciparum*, *P vivax*, and *P ovale*) to around 28 days (*P malariae*).[27] Certain strains of *P vivax* and *P ovale* can have a much longer incubation period, of between 6–18 months.[19] Some 90% of malaria attacks in travellers occur at home.[28] People with any fever pattern should be considered to have malaria until proven otherwise, when they have been to endemic areas.[4,6,21,26,29] Once malaria infection occurs, older travellers are at higher risk of poor clinical outcomes and death. In US travellers between 1966–1987, the case fatality rate was 0.4% for people aged 0–19, 2.2% between ages 20–39, 5.8% between ages 40–69, and 30.3% for those aged 70–79.[30] Complications and death from malaria are mainly because of inappropriate therapy, or due to delay in the initiation of treatment.[31] If malaria is diagnosed and treated promptly, around 88% of previously healthy travellers will recover completely.[32]

AIMS OF INTERVENTION To reduce the risk of infection; to prevent illness and death, with minimal adverse effects of treatment.

OUTCOMES Rates of clinical malaria and death, and adverse effects of treatment. Proxy measures include numbers of mosquito bites and rates of mosquito catches in indoor areas. We found limited evidence linking numbers of mosquito bites and risk of malaria.[33]

METHODS *Clinical Evidence* search and appraisal March 2004. Additional hand searches by the author of his own files. All RCTs were appraised, irrespective of size. Evidence from case-control studies, and from one large questionnaire survey in European tourists, have been included in some sections where randomised studies did not exist, or where they did not address specific questions. In some sections, evidence of harms has been extracted from case series.

QUESTION What are the effects of non-drug preventative interventions in adult travellers?

OPTION AEROSOL INSECTICIDES IN ADULTS

We found no RCTs on the effects of aerosol insecticides in preventing malaria in travellers. One large questionnaire survey in travellers found insufficient evidence on the effects of aerosol insecticides in preventing malaria. Two community RCTs in residents of malaria endemic areas found that indoor spraying of aerosol insecticides reduced clinical malaria.

Benefits: We found no systematic review or RCTs in travellers (see comment below). Two community RCTs found that indoor residual spraying of synthetic pyrethroids reduced clinical malaria in lifelong residents of malaria endemic areas.[34,35]

Harms: We found no evidence of harms.

Comment: One large questionnaire survey (89 617 European tourists returning from East Africa) found that commercially available personal aerosol insecticides did not significantly reduce the incidence of malaria ($P = 0.55$).[36] Historically, indoor residual spraying has not been recommended for short stay travellers, but we found no evidence to support this.

OPTION BIOLOGICAL CONTROL MEASURES

We found no RCTs on the effects of biological control measures in preventing malaria in travellers.

Benefits: We found no systematic review or RCTs of biological control measures**G** in preventing malaria in travellers (see comment below).

Harms: We found no evidence of harms.

Comment: One systematic review (search date 1997) identified two cohort studies based on mosquito counts.[37] It found no evidence that growing the citrosa plant and encouraging natural predation of insects by erecting bird or bat houses reduced bites to humans from infected anopheline mosquitoes. The only known way to reduce mosquito populations naturally is to eliminate sources of standing water, such as blocked gutters, tree stump holes, and discarded tyres, cans, and bottles.[37]

OPTION AIR CONDITIONING AND ELECTRIC FANS

We found no RCTs on the effects of air conditioning or electric fans in preventing malaria in travellers. One large questionnaire survey in travellers found that air conditioning reduced the incidence of malaria. One small observational study found that electric ceiling fans reduced total catches of culicine mosquitoes but did not significantly reduce total catches of anopheline mosquitoes in indoor spaces.

Benefits: We found no systematic review or RCTs (see comment below).

Harms: We found no evidence of harms.

Comment: One questionnaire survey of 89 617 European tourists returning from East Africa measured malaria incidence with a two stage self completed questionnaire administered during the return flight, and again 12 weeks later. It found that sleeping in an air conditioned room significantly reduced the incidence of malaria ($P = 0.04$).[36] One cohort study (6 experimental huts in villages in Pakistan) of various antimosquito interventions found that an electric ceiling fan run at high speed significantly reduced total catches of blood fed culicine mosquitoes ($P < 0.05$), but did not significantly reduce total catches of blood fed anopheline mosquitoes.[38] These studies support the finding that mosquitoes are reluctant to fly in windy conditions,[39] but suggest that anopheline mosquitoes are more tolerant of air turbulence than culicine mosquitoes.

OPTION ACOUSTIC BUZZERS

We found no RCTs on the effects of acoustic buzzers to prevent malaria in adults.

Benefits: We found no systematic review and no RCTs with clinical malaria as an outcome.

Harms: We found no RCTs.

Comment: We found one non-randomised controlled trial (18 houses in Gabon) of a commercially available ultrasound emitting device. The trial lasted 6 weeks and used total mosquito catches as an outcome.[40] Most mosquitoes were culicine. It found no significant difference in mosquito catches between the ultrasound emitting device and a sham device ($P = 0.48$).[40]

OPTION MOSQUITO COILS AND VAPORISING MATS

We found no RCTs on the effects of coils and vaporising mats in preventing malaria in travellers. One case-control study of coils in travellers found no evidence of a protective effect against malaria. One RCT of coils and one observational study of pyrethroid vaporising mats found that these devices reduced numbers of culicine mosquitoes in indoor spaces.

Benefits: We found no systematic review and no RCTs that used clinical malaria as an outcome. We found one case-control study (603 British travellers to the Gambia between September and December, 48% of whom burnt mosquito coils), which found no significant difference in coil use among people with or without malaria (OR 0.65, 95% CI 0.32 to 1.34).[25]

Harms: We found no evidence of harms.

Comment: One RCT (18 houses in Malaysia) compared various mosquito coil formulations versus no treatment.[41] It found that treated coils reduced populations of mosquitoes by 75% but 85% of the mosquitoes collected were culicine.[41] One observational study of pyrethroid vaporising mats in six experimental huts in a Pakistan village setting found that the mats reduced total catches of blood fed mosquitoes by 56%.[38]

OPTION SMOKE

We found no RCTs on the effects of smoke in preventing malaria in travellers. One controlled clinical trial found that smoke repelled mosquitoes during the evening.

Benefits: We found no systematic review and no RCTs of smoke in preventing malaria. We found one controlled clinical trial (see comment below).[42]

Harms: There may be an irritant and toxic effect of smoke on the eyes and respiratory system, but this effect was not quantified in the controlled clinical trial.[42]

Comment: One controlled clinical trial, in which five small fires were tended on five successive evenings in a village in Papua New Guinea, found a smoke specific and species specific effect from different types of smoke.[42] Catches of one anopheline species were reduced by 84% by burning betelnut (95% CI 62% to 94%), 69% by burning ginger (95% CI 25% to 87%), and 66% by burning coconut husks (95% CI 17% to 86%).

OPTION INSECTICIDE TREATED NETS

We found no RCTs in travellers. One systematic review in adult and child residents of malaria endemic settings found that insecticide treated nets reduced the number of mild episodes of malaria and reduced child mortality.

Benefits: We found no systematic review and no RCTs in travellers. We found one systematic review (search date not reported), which identified 18 RCTs in malaria endemic settings (stable transmission area > 1 infective bite per person per year; non-traveller children and adults).[43] It found that nets sprayed or impregnated with a pyrethroid insecticide such as permethrin reduced the number of mild episodes of malaria compared with no nets or untreated nets over four to 29 months (insecticide treated nets *v* no nets: 2 RCTs; RRR 48%, 95% CI 41% to 54%; insecticide treated nets *v* untreated nets: 3 RCTs; RRR 39%, 95% CI 27% to 48%; see comment below) and child mortality (impregnated nets *v* no nets: 3 RCTs; RR 0.83, CI not reported; impregnated nets *v* untreated nets: 1 RCT; RR 0.77, CI not reported).[43] The review reported a summary risk difference of 5.6 deaths averted per 1000 children protected per year (4 RCTs; CI not reported).[43]

Harms: We found no evidence of harms.

Comment: In 7 RCTs included in the review, randomisation and allocation were done by individual (or household), whereas in 11 RCTs it was done by group (household, zones within 1 village, hamlets, villages, or blocks of villages).[43] Reported confidence intervals for protective efficacy are not corrected for cluster randomisation.[43] Permethrin remains active for about 4 months.[44] Although the analysis of insecticide treated nets was undertaken in non-traveller children and adults, the results may be generalisable to other groups such as travellers.

OPTION **INSECTICIDE TREATED CLOTHING**

Two RCTs in soldiers and refugee householders found that permethrin treated fabric (clothing or sheets) reduced the incidence of malaria.

Benefits: We found no systematic review but found two RCTs.[45,46] The first RCT (172 male Colombian soldiers patrolling a malaria endemic area for a mean of 4.2 weeks) found that permethrin impregnated uniforms significantly reduced the incidence of malaria compared with non-impregnated uniforms (3/86 [3%] *v* 12/86 [13%]; RR 0.25, 95% CI 0.07 to 0.85).[45] The second RCT (102 refugee households in northwestern Pakistan) found that permethrin treated wraps and top sheets significantly reduced the risk of falciparum malaria compared with placebo over 4 months (RR 0.56, 95% CI 0.41 to 0.78).[46]

Harms: The first RCT also included an analysis of permethrin impregnated uniforms versus non-impregnated uniforms in 286 soldiers patrolling a leishmaniasis endemic area for a mean 6.6 weeks.[45] It found that 2/229 (0.9%) participants wearing permethrin impregnated uniforms experienced irritation and itching. No comparative information was given for soldiers wearing non-impregnated uniforms.

Comment: In the first RCT, the entire uniform (hat, shirt, undershirt, trousers, socks) was treated with a single application of permethrin. All participants were instructed to wear the uniform continuously, day and night, with the sleeves rolled down. Each participant washed his own uniform two to three times during the study, using soap and water, but uniforms were not reimpregnated with permethrin. Topical (skin applied) insect repellents were not used. Trials in soldiers may not be generalisable to other travellers.

OPTION **FULL LENGTH CLOTHING**

We found no RCTs on the effects of full length clothing in preventing malaria in travellers. One large questionnaire survey in travellers found that wearing trousers and long sleeved shirts reduced the incidence of malaria.

Benefits: We found no systematic review or RCTs (see comment below). **Other lifestyle changes:** We found no studies (see comment below).

Harms: None.

Comment: We found one large questionnaire survey (89 617 European tourists returning from East Africa), which found that wearing long sleeved shirts and trousers significantly reduced the incidence of malaria ($P = 0.02$).[36] **Other lifestyle changes:** These include not travelling to malaria endemic regions during the rainy season (when most malaria transmission occurs) and not going outdoors in the evening or at night. Travellers who take day trips from a malaria free city to a malaria endemic region may be at minimal risk if they return to the city before dusk.[47] Some authors suggest wearing light rather than dark clothing, as insects prefer landing on dark surfaces.[47,48]

OPTION **TOPICAL (SKIN APPLIED) INSECT REPELLENTS**

We found no RCTs on the effects of topical (skin applied) insect repellents in preventing malaria in travellers. One small crossover RCT found that diethyltoluamide (DEET) preparations protected against mosquito bites. DEET has been reported to cause systemic and skin adverse reactions, particularly with prolonged use.

Benefits: We found no systematic review and no RCTs (see comment below).

Harms: We found a case series of systemic toxic reactions (confusion, irritability, insomnia) in US national park employees after repeated and prolonged use of DEET.[49] We found 14 case reports of contact urticaria and irritant contact dermatitis (mostly in soldiers) as a result of DEET.[36] The risk of absorption is especially high if DEET is left in the antecubital fossa overnight.[50] DEET also degrades certain plastics, such as spectacle frames.[51]

Comment: One small crossover RCT (4 people), involving successive random exposure to female culicine mosquitoes, compared six different controlled release preparations of DEET.[52] It found that all gave at least 95% protection against mosquito bites.[52] DEET is a broad spectrum repellent effective against mosquitoes, biting flies, chiggers, fleas, and ticks, and has been used for over 40 years.[37] Although most authorities would recommend the use of topical (skin applied) repellents in malaria endemic areas, the only evidence comes from small RCTs with non-clinical outcomes. Larger RCTs are needed to compare DEET versus other topical (skin applied) repellents and placebo in preventing malaria.

QUESTION What are the effects of drug prophylaxis in adult travellers?

OPTION CHLOROQUINE

We found no RCTs on the effects of chloroquine in travellers. One RCT in Austrian workers residing in Nigeria found no significant difference between chloroquine and sulfadoxine plus pyrimethamine in the incidence of malaria after 6–22 months. *P falciparum* resistance to chloroquine is now established in most malaria endemic regions of the world.

Benefits: We found no systematic review or RCTs in travellers. One RCT (173 Austrian industrial workers residing in Nigeria) found no significant difference between chloroquine and sulfadoxine plus pyrimethamine in the incidence of malaria after 6–22 months.[53]

Harms: The RCT found that chloroquine was associated with insomnia in 3/87 (3%) people.[54] Two people withdrew from the study because of adverse effects: one with skin rash and the other with visual disturbance. Retrospective questionnaire surveys have suggested that severe adverse effects are rare at prophylactic dosages.[54]

Comment: Alcohol consumption, other medication, and comorbidities can modify the effects of antimalaria drugs.[55,56] *P falciparum* resistance to chloroquine is now established in almost all malaria endemic regions of the world, although there are countries (principally in Central America and the Near East) where there has been no reported resistance.

OPTION CHLOROQUINE PLUS PROGUANIL

One RCT found no significant difference between chloroquine plus proguanil and chloroquine plus sulfadoxine plus pyrimethamine in the incidence of *P falciparum* malaria. One RCT found no significant difference between chloroquine plus proguanil and proguanil alone in the incidence of *P falciparum* malaria. One RCT found no significant difference between chloroquine plus proguanil and atovaquone plus proguanil in preventing malaria. RCTs comparing adverse effects of chloroquine plus proguanil versus atovaquone plus proguanil found different results. One RCT found that chloroquine plus proguanil increased adverse effects compared with three

other common antimalarial drug regimens (doxycycline, mefloquine, and atovaquone plus proguanil). Another RCT found no significant difference in adverse events between chloroquine plus proguanil and atovaquone plus proguanil.

Benefits: **Versus chloroquine plus sulfadoxine plus pyrimethamine:** We found one open label RCT (767 Scandinavian travellers to East Africa; 70% of trips were > 4 weeks; duration of follow up not reported) comparing chloroquine plus proguanil versus chloroquine plus sulfadoxine plus pyrimethamine.[57] It found no significant difference between treatments in rates of *P falciparum* malaria (4/384 [1%] *v* 3/383 [0.7%] travellers; RR 1.3, 95% CI 0.3 to 5.9).[57] **Versus proguanil alone:** We found one RCT (1625 Dutch travellers to Africa; 60% spent < 6 weeks in tropical areas).[58] It found no significant difference between chloroquine 300 mg weekly plus proguanil 200 mg daily and proguanil alone in incidence of *P falciparum* malaria four weeks after returning to the Netherlands (risk per 100 person months: chloroquine plus proguanil 2.8, 95% CI 0.9 to 10.1 *v* proguanil alone 6.0, 95% CI 2.6 to 14.0).[58] **Versus atovaquone plus proguanil:** See benefits of atovaquone plus proguanil in adults, p 968.

Harms: In the RCT conducted in Scandinavian travellers, adverse effects associated with chloroquine plus proguanil were nausea (3%), diarrhoea (2%), and dizziness (1%).[57] One cohort study (470 British soldiers in Belize) found that the risk of mouth ulcers almost doubled with chloroquine plus proguanil compared with proguanil alone (P = 0.025).[59] One RCT (623 non-immune travellers to sub-Saharan Africa) compared four chemoprophylaxis regimens started 17 days before travel and continued for 4 weeks after return: doxycycline; mefloquine; chloroquine plus proguanil; and atovaquone plus proguanil.[60] It found that chloroquine plus proguanil increased severe (required medical advice) adverse effects compared with the other three treatments, although the differences were not significant among treatments (19/153 [12%] with chloroquine plus proguanil *v* 16/153 [11%] with mefloquine *v* 9/153 [6%] with doxycycline *v* 11/164 [7%] with atovaquone plus proguanil; P = 0.14 for comparison of all 4 treatments). It found that chloroquine plus proguanil increased mild (trivial) to moderate (interferes with daily activity) adverse effects compared with the other three treatments (45% with chloroquine plus proguanil *v* 42% with mefloquine *v* 33% with doxycycline *v* 32% with atovaquone plus proguanil; P = 0.048 for comparison of all 4 treatments). See comment below.

Comment: The incidence of confirmed *P falciparum* malaria in both trials[57,58] was so low that a clinically important effect cannot be excluded. The RCT that compared adverse effects of four different drug regimens was not powered to assess malaria prevention.[60] It found no cases of malaria with any treatment. The RCT tested the difference between all four treatments but did not directly compare any two interventions versus each other.

OPTION DOXYCYCLINE

One RCT in soldiers and one RCT in migrants with limited immunity found that doxycycline reduced the risk of malaria compared with placebo. One of the RCTs found that doxycycline was associated with nausea and vomiting, diarrhoea, cough, headache, and unspecified dermatological symptoms over 13 weeks. We found no evidence on long term safety. One RCT found that doxycycline had fewer adverse effects than mefloquine or chloroquine plus proguanil and had similar adverse effect rates compared with atovaquone plus proguanil.

Benefits: We found no systematic review but found two RCTs.[61,62] The first RCT (136 Indonesian soldiers) compared doxycycline versus mefloquine versus placebo in a malaria endemic setting (see comment below).[61] It found that, in an area of drug resistance, doxycycline significantly reduced the risk of malaria compared with placebo after a 13 to 15 week prophylaxis period (AR 1/67 [2%] with doxycycline *v* 53/69 [77%] with placebo; RR 0.02, 95% CI 0.003 to 0.14; NNT 2, 95% CI 2 to 2). The second RCT (300 Indonesian migrants with limited immunity) comparing azithromycin versus doxycycline versus placebo found that doxycycline significantly reduced the incidence of malaria compared with placebo over 20 weeks (2/75 [3%] cases of *P falciparum* malaria with doxycycline *v* 29/77 [38%] with placebo; RR 0.07, 95% CI 0.02 to 0.29; NNT 3, 95% CI 2 to 4; 1/75 [2%] cases of *P vivax* malaria with doxycycline *v* 27/77 [35%] with placebo; RR 0.04, 95% CI 0.01 to 0.28).[62]

Harms: The first RCT found that doxycycline was associated with gastrointestinal symptoms (including nausea and vomiting, abdominal pain, and diarrhoea) in 16/67 (24%) soldiers, unspecified dermatological problems in 22/67 (33%), cough in 21/67 (31%), and headache in 11/67 (16%) over 13 weeks.[61] One questionnaire survey (383 returned Australian travellers taking doxycycline) found that 40% reported nausea or vomiting, 12% reported diarrhoea, and 9% of female travellers reported vaginitis.[63] Evidence from case reports suggests that, in sunny conditions, up to 50% of travellers using doxycycline may experience photoallergic skin rash.[64] One RCT (623 non-immune travellers to sub-Saharan Africa) compared four treatments.[60] It found that doxycycline reduced adverse effects compared with mefloquine and chloroquine plus proguanil, and had similar adverse effect rates compared with atovaquone plus proguanil (severe adverse effects: 12% with chloroquine plus proguanil *v* 11% with mefloquine *v* 7% with atovaquone plus proguanil *v* 6% with doxycycline; P = 0.14; mild to moderate adverse effects: 45% with chloroquine plus proguanil *v* 42% with mefloquine *v* 33% with doxycycline *v* 32% with atovaquone plus proguanil; P = 0.048 for comparison of all 4 treatments). See comment below.

Comment: Most drug trials in travellers have been in soldiers, and the results may not be generalisable to tourists or business travellers.[65,66] Both RCTs were three arm parallel studies. Only the doxycycline versus placebo comparisons are reported here.[61,62] The RCT that compared adverse effects of four different drug regimens was not powered to assess malaria prevention.[60] It found no cases of malaria with any treatment. The RCT tested the difference between all four treatments but did not directly compare any two interventions versus each other.

OPTION MEFLOQUINE

One systematic review of one RCT in soldiers found that mefloquine reduced cases of malaria compared with placebo, and found that mefloquine had a protective efficacy of 100%. One RCT of mefloquine versus atovaquone plus proguanil found no cases of clinical malaria throughout the trial, but found a higher rate of neuropsychiatric harm with mefloquine compared with atovaquone plus proguanil. One RCT found that mefloquine had more adverse effects than doxycycline or atovaquone plus proguanil and had similar adverse event rates compared with chloroquine plus proguanil.

Benefits: We found one systematic review[66] and one subsequent RCT.[67] **Versus placebo:** We found one systematic review (search date 2000), which identified one RCT (203 Indonesian soldiers) comparing mefloquine versus doxycycline versus placebo in a malaria endemic setting that assessed malaria incidence (see comment below).[66] It found that, compared with placebo, mefloquine had a protective efficacy of 100% after up to 15 weeks of treatment (95% CI 93% to 100%; malaria cases: 0 in 202 person-months of exposure with mefloquine *v* 53 in 109 person-months of exposure with placebo). **Versus atovaquone plus proguanil:** The subsequent RCT (976 people) compared mefloquine plus placebo versus atovaquone plus proguanil. It found no clinical cases of malaria among people included in the trial.[67]

Harms: The systematic review identified 10 RCTs (275 people) of mefloquine for 2–15 weeks of treatment.[66] It found no significant difference between mefloquine and alternative antimalaria prophylaxis (chloroquine or doxycycline) in withdrawal (29/863 [3%] with mefloquine *v* 20/798 [2%] with alternative prophylaxis; RR 1.32, 95% CI 0.75 to 2.31).[66] Commonly reported adverse effects associated with mefloquine were headache (16%), insomnia (15%), and fatigue (8%).[66] The review found over 500 case reports of mefloquine adverse effects, including four reports of death. These reports suggest that mefloquine is a potentially harmful drug for tourists and business travellers and requires more careful evaluation through an RCT in these groups.[66] The subsequent RCT (976 non-immune tourists and business travellers) found no significant difference in the risk of adverse events between mefloquine plus placebo and atovaquone plus proguanil (313/493 [63.5%] with atovaquone plus proguanil *v* 324/483 [67.1%] with mefloquine; ARR +2.6%, 95% CI –3.4% to +8.5%).[67] However, when adverse effects specifically attributable to the study drug were analysed, there were significantly more adverse effects caused by mefloquine than by atovaquone plus proguanil (204/483 [42%] with mefloquine *v* 149/493 [30%] with atovaquone plus proguanil; RR 1.40, 95% CI 1.18 to 1.66; NNH 9, 95% CI 6 to 17; see comment below). Specifically, mefloquine increased the incidence of "strange or vivid dreams" compared with atovaquone plus proguanil (66/483 [14%] *v* 33/493 [7%]), insomnia (65/483 [13%] *v* 15/493 [3%]), dizziness or vertigo (43/483 [9%] *v* 11/493 [2%]), anxiety (18/483 [4%] *v* 3/493 [1%]), depression (17/483 [4%] *v* 3/493 [1%]), visual difficulties (16/483 [3%] *v* 8/493 [2%]), and headache (19/493 [4%] *v* 32/483 [7%]).[67] Retrospective questionnaire surveys in tourists and business travellers found that sleep disturbance and psychosis were common.[68] One review of 74 dermatological case reports found that up to 30% of mefloquine users developed a maculopapular rash and 4–10% had pruritus.[69] Ten cohort studies in tourists found that more women than men experienced adverse effects (including dizziness, sleep disturbance, headache, diarrhoea, and nausea) with mefloquine.[63,68,70–77] One retrospective questionnaire survey of 93 668 European travellers to East Africa found that elderly travellers experienced fewer adverse reactions (not specified) with mefloquine than younger travellers ($P < 0.05$).[78] A review of 516 published case reports suggested that many of mefloquine's adverse effects could be explained as a posthepatic syndrome due to mefloquine use combined with concurrent insults to the liver (such as from alcohol, dehydration, an oral contraceptive pill, recreational drugs, and other liver damaging drugs), and that in some users mefloquine may also cause a symptomatic thyroid disturbance.[79] One RCT (623 non-immune travellers to sub-Saharan Africa) compared four treatments.[60] It found that mefloquine and chloroquine plus proguanil had similar adverse event rates and that both these treatments had higher severe adverse effects compared with doxycycline or atovaquone plus proguanil (severe adverse effects: 12% with chloroquine plus proguanil *v* 11% with mefloquine *v* 7% with atovaquone plus proguanil *v* 6% with doxycycline; $P = 0.14$; mild to moderate adverse effects: 45% with chloroquine plus proguanil *v* 42% with mefloquine *v* 33% with doxycycline *v* 32% with atovaquone plus proguanil; $P = 0.048$ for comparison of all 4 treatments). See comment below.

Comment: Trials in soldiers may not be generalisable to other travellers. The RCT in Indonesian soldiers was a three arm parallel RCT. It compared mefloquine (68 people) versus doxycycline (67 people) versus placebo (69 people). Only the comparison of mefloquine versus placebo is included here.[66] The subsequent RCT of mefloquine versus atovaquone plus proguanil suggested a higher rate of adverse effects with mefloquine than in previous studies, but this RCT only reported adverse events that occurred after starting active treatment, which was 3 weeks earlier in the mefloquine group than in the atovaquone plus proguanil group.

OPTION ATOVAQUONE PLUS PROGUANIL

One RCT in migrants with limited immunity found that atovaquone plus proguanil reduced the proportion of people with malaria compared with placebo. One RCT found no significant difference between atovaquone plus proguanil and chloroquine plus proguanil in preventing malaria in travellers. One RCT of mefloquine versus atovaquone plus proguanil found no cases of clinical malaria throughout the trial, but found a higher rate of neuropsychiatric harm with mefloquine than with atovaquone plus proguanil. RCTs comparing adverse effects of atovaquone plus proguanil versus chloroquine plus proguanil found different results. One RCT found that atovaquone plus proguanil reduced adverse effects compared with mefloquine and chloroquine plus proguanil and had similar adverse effect rates compared with doxycycline. Another RCT found no significant difference in adverse events between atovaquone plus proguanil and chloroquine plus proguanil.

Benefits: We found no systematic review, but found three RCTs.[67,80,81] **Versus placebo:** One RCT (299 Indonesian migrants with limited immunity) found that atovaquone plus proguanil significantly decreased the proportion of people with malaria compared with placebo at 24 weeks (AR 3/150 [2%] with atovaquone plus proguanil *v* 37/149 [25%] with placebo; P < 0.001).[80] **Versus chloroquine plus proguanil:** One multicentre RCT (1083 travellers) comparing atovaquone plus proguanil versus chloroquine plus proguanil found no significant difference in the incidence of malaria after 9 weeks (1/511 [0.2%] cases of *P ovale* malaria with atovaquone plus proguanil *v* 3/511 [0.6%] cases of *P falciparum* malaria with chloroquine plus proguanil; ARR 0.4%; RR 0.33, 95% CI 0.03 to 3.16).[81] **Versus mefloquine:** See benefits of mefloquine in adults, p 966.

Harms: **Versus placebo:** The RCT found that stomatitis (P < 0.001) and back pain (P = 0.009) occurred significantly more frequently in the atovaquone plus proguanil group, whereas abdominal pain (P = 0.02) and malaise (P = 0.01) occurred significantly more frequently with placebo (absolute numbers not given).[80] Most adverse events were described as mild or moderate. Four subjects had severe events that were possibly drug related (3 people with abdominal pain and 1 with skin rash).[80] **Versus chloroquine plus proguanil:** The multicentre RCT in travellers found no significant difference between atovaquone plus proguanil and chloroquine plus proguanil in one or more adverse events (311/511 [61%] with atovaquone plus proguanil *v* 329/511 [64%] with chloroquine plus proguanil; RR 0.95, 95% CI 0.85 to 1.04).[81] Common adverse effects were mainly gastrointestinal (atovaquone plus proguanil *v* chloroquine plus proguanil: diarrhoea 5% *v* 7%, mouth ulcers 4% *v* 5%, abdominal pain 3% *v* 6%, nausea 2% *v* 7%), neuropsychiatric (atovaquone plus proguanil *v* chloroquine plus proguanil: strange/vivid dreams 4% *v* 3%, dizziness 3% *v* 4%, insomnia 2% *v* 2%), and visual difficulties (2% *v* 2%).[81] One RCT (623 non-immune travellers to sub-Saharan Africa) compared four treatments.[60] It found that atovaquone plus proguanil reduced adverse effects compared with chloroquine plus proguanil but did not report the statistical significance of the difference (7% with atovaquone plus proguanil v 12% with chloroquine plus proguanil). **Versus mefloquine:** See harms of mefloquine in adults, p 967.

Comment: None.

OPTION AMODIAQUINE

We found no RCTs on the effects of amodiaquine in preventing malaria in travellers. We found limited observational evidence that amodiaquine may cause neutropenia, liver damage, and hepatitis.

Benefits: We found no systematic review and no RCTs in travellers.

Harms: One retrospective cohort study in 10 000 British travellers taking prophylactic amodiaquine for 6–13 weeks reported severe neutropenia in about 1/2000 users.[82] We found 28 case reports describing liver damage or hepatitis in travellers who had taken amodiaquine for about 2 months to treat or prevent malaria.[83–88]

Comment: Amodiaquine use is now restricted to treatment of malaria because of adverse effects.

OPTION PYRIMETHAMINE PLUS DAPSONE

We found no systematic review and no RCTs in travellers. One RCT in Thai soldiers found insufficient evidence to compare pyrimethamine plus dapsone versus proguanil plus dapsone. We found limited observational evidence that pyrimethamine plus dapsone may cause agranulocytosis.

Benefits: We found no systematic review and no RCTs in travellers. One RCT in Thai soldiers comparing pyrimethamine plus dapsone versus proguanil plus dapsone found no significant difference in *P falciparum* infection rates over 40 days (10.3% with proguanil plus dapsone *v* 11.3% with pyrimethamine plus dapsone; results presented graphically, P value not reported) but found a significantly lower *P vivax* infection rate with proguanil plus dapsone compared with pyrimethamine plus dapsone (1.6% *v* 12.4%; results presented graphically, $P < 0.001$).[89]

Harms: The RCT in Thai soldiers found that fewer than 2% reported any drug related symptoms from pyrimethamine plus dapsone.[89] One retrospective cohort study in 15 000 Swedish travellers taking pyrimethamine plus dapsone reported agranulocytosis in about 1/2000 users.[90]

Comment: None.

OPTION SULFADOXINE PLUS PYRIMETHAMINE

We found no RCTs of sulfadoxine plus pyrimethamine alone. One RCT found no significant difference between chloroquine plus proguanil and chloroquine plus sulfadoxine plus pyrimethamine in the incidence of *P falciparum* malaria. One retrospective observational study suggested that sulfadoxine plus pyrimethamine was associated with severe cutaneous reactions.

Benefits: We found no systematic review and no RCTs of sulfadoxine plus pyrimethamine alone. We found one RCT of sulfadoxine plus pyrimethamine plus chloroquine versus chloroquine plus proguanil (see benefits of chloroquine plus proguanil in adults, p 965).

Harms: One retrospective observational study in 182 300 US travellers taking prophylactic sulfadoxine plus pyrimethamine reported severe cutaneous reactions (erythema multiforme, Stevens–Johnson syndrome, toxic epidermal necrolysis) in 1/5000–8000 users, with a mortality of about 1/11 000–25 000 users.[90]

Comment: None.

QUESTION What are the effects of antimalaria vaccines in travellers?

OPTION VACCINES

We found no RCTs of the effects of antimalaria vaccines in travellers. One systematic review of antimalaria vaccines in residents of malaria endemic areas found that the SPf66 vaccine reduced first attacks of malaria compared with placebo.

Benefits: We found no systematic review or RCTs of antimalaria vaccines in travellers. One systematic review (search date 1999, 13 RCTs) of antimalaria vaccines in residents of malaria endemic areas found that the SPf66 vaccine significantly reduced the incidence of first attacks of *P falciparum* malaria compared with placebo after up to 2 years (1039/3718 [28%] with SPf66 *v* 1108/3681 [30%] with placebo; RR 0.90, 95% CI 0.84 to 0.96).[91]

Harms: The systematic review found that, in all but one of the RCTs of the SPf66 vaccine, fewer than 10% of recipients reported a systemic reaction (fever, headache, gastric symptoms, muscle pain, dizziness), and fewer than 35% reported a local reaction (inflammation, nodules, pain, erythema, pruritus, induration, injection site warmth).[91] The remaining RCT found a larger proportion of local cutaneous reactions, although these resolved within 24 hours with symptomatic treatment. It also reported higher systemic reaction rates after vaccination (11–16%), although rates after placebo were also higher (10–13%). Surveillance was also more intense than in the other RCTs.

Comment: None.

QUESTION What are the effects of preventative interventions in child travellers?

OPTION TOPICAL (SKIN APPLIED) INSECT REPELLENTS CONTAINING DEET IN CHILDREN

We found no RCTs on the effects of diethyltoluamide (DEET) in preventing malaria in child travellers. Case reports in young children found serious adverse effects with DEET.

Benefits: We found no systematic review or RCTs.

Harms: We found 13 case reports of encephalopathic toxicity in children aged under 8 years after excessive use (not clearly defined) of topical (skin applied) insect repellents containing DEET.[92,93]

Comment: Infants and young children have thinner skin and greater surface area to mass ratio.[94] Some authors advise that ethylhexanediol should be issued as a topical (skin applied) insect repellent in preference to DEET in children aged 1–8 years;[95] however, we found insufficient evidence.

OPTION MEFLOQUINE

We found no RCTs of the effects of mefloquine in preventing malaria in child travellers.

Benefits: We found no systematic review or RCTs.

Harms: Two RCTs in children and adults with symptomatic *P falciparum* malaria found that mefloquine was associated with less vomiting, nausea, anorexia, diarrhoea, and dizziness in children than in adults.[96,97] One RCT found that the incidence of early vomiting (< 1 hour) in children under 5 years of age was higher than in older children and adults (17% with children under 5 *v* 4% with older children and adults). However, in those children under 5 years of age who did not vomit their initial medication, late vomiting (> 1 hour) was less than in older children and adults (12% with children under 5 *v* 22% with older children and adults).[98]

Comment: None.

QUESTION What are the effects of antimalaria interventions in pregnant travellers?

OPTION INSECTICIDE TREATED NETS IN PREGNANT TRAVELLERS

We found no RCTs on the effects of insecticide treated nets in preventing malaria in pregnant travellers. One RCT of pregnant residents of a malaria endemic area found insufficient evidence on the effects of permethrin treated nets in preventing malaria.

Benefits: We found no systematic review or RCTs in pregnant travellers. We found one RCT (341 pregnant women living in Thailand, 3 sites in a malaria endemic area), which compared permethrin treated nets versus non-treated nets versus usual practice.[99] Two sites found no significant difference in the incidence of malaria with treated nets, whereas the third site found that treated nets significantly reduced the incidence of malaria.

Harms: We found no evidence relating to pregnant travellers. The RCT of permethrin treated nets in Thailand found no evidence of toxic effects to mother or fetus.[99]

Comment: One non-randomised controlled trial (3 pregnant women and 3 non-pregnant women) reported that pregnant women are twice as likely to be bitten by anopheline mosquitoes compared with non-pregnant women (mean bites per night: 6.3 for pregnant women *v* 3.1 for non-pregnant women; $P = 0.0002$).[100] Pregnant women are relatively immunosuppressed and are at greater risk of severe malaria than non-pregnant women.[101] Contracting malaria significantly increases the likelihood of losing the fetus.[102]

OPTION INSECTICIDE TREATED CLOTHING

We found no RCTs in pregnant travellers of the effects of impregnated clothing.

Benefits: We found no systematic review or RCTs.

Harms: We found little evidence relating to pregnant travellers. **Permethrin:** One RCT (341 pregnant women living in Thailand) of permethrin treated nets found no evidence of toxic effects to mother or fetus.[99] **Diethyltoluamide (DEET):** See harms of topical (skin applied) insect repellents in pregnant travellers, p 972.

Comment: See comment under insecticide treated nets in pregnant travellers, p 971.

OPTION TOPICAL (SKIN APPLIED) INSECT REPELLENTS

We found no RCTs in pregnant travellers. It is unclear which topical (skin applied) insect repellents are safe in pregnancy.

Benefits: We found no systematic review or RCTs.

Harms: We found little evidence in pregnant travellers. **Diethyltoluamide (DEET):** We found one case report indicating an adverse fetal outcome (mental retardation, impaired sensorimotor coordination, craniofacial dysmorphology) in a child whose mother had applied DEET daily throughout her pregnancy.[103] One RCT in pregnant women (897 refugees in a Thai forest area of low malaria endemicity) comparing DEET (median dose 214.2 g per pregnancy) versus a cosmetic cream found no differences in weekly reporting of headache, dizziness, or nausea and vomiting over 2–6 months.[104] It also found no adverse effects on infant survival, growth, or development at either birth or 1 year (survival 95.2% with DEET *v* 94.0% without DEET; $P = 0.57$; mean weight at 1 year 7983 g with DEET *v* 7984 g without DEET). Some animal studies have found that DEET crosses the placental barrier.[105] Animal studies of reproductive effects of DEET are inconclusive.[102,106]

Comment: See comment under insecticide treated nets in pregnant travellers, p 971. The RCT in refugees reported that DEET significantly increased the number of women reporting skin warmth (359/449 [80%] with DEET *v* 258/448 [58%] with cosmetic cream; RR 1.39, 95% CI 1.27 to 1.52), although the clinical significance of this is unclear.[104] Some authors advise that only plant derived skin applied insect repellents are safe in pregnancy because of a potential risk of mutagenicity from DEET.[95] However, we found no evidence on the effects of other repellents.

OPTION ANTIMALARIA DRUGS

We found no RCTs on the effects of antimalaria drugs in pregnant travellers. We found insufficient evidence on the safety of chloroquine, doxycycline, and mefloquine in pregnancy.

Benefits: We found one systematic review (search date 2000), which identified no RCTs in pregnant travellers.[107] It identified 15 RCTs of antimalaria drugs in pregnancy, all in residents of malaria endemic settings. It found that antimalaria prophylaxis significantly reduced the number of women infected at least once compared with no prophylaxis (5/167 [3%] *v* 37/170 [22%]; RR 0.14, 95% CI 0.06 to 0.34) and significantly reduced the number of episodes of fever (22/119 [18%] with prophylaxis *v* 45/108 [42%] with no prophylaxis; RR 0.42, 95% CI 0.27 to 0.66). It found no significant difference between antimalaria prophylaxis and no prophylaxis in the number of perinatal deaths (66/1494 [4%] *v* 64/1426 [4%]; RR 1.02, 95% CI 0.73 to 1.43) or preterm births (17/182 [9%] with prophylaxis *v* 22/175 [12%] with no prophylaxis; RR 0.75, 95% CI 0.42 to 1.35), but found that antimalaria prophylaxis resulted in significantly higher birth weight in the infant compared with no prophylaxis (OR 0.53, 95% CI 0.32 to 0.81).[107]

Harms: **Chloroquine:** One RCT (1464 pregnant long term residents of Burkina Faso) gave no information on adverse effects.[108] **Doxycycline:** Case reports have found that doxycycline taken in pregnancy or while breast feeding may damage fetal or infant bones or teeth.[54] **Mefloquine:** One RCT (339 long term Thai residents) found that mefloquine significantly increased the number of women reporting dizziness compared with placebo (28% with mefloquine *v* 14% with placebo; $P < 0.005$), but found no other significant adverse effects on the mother, the pregnancy, or on infant survival or development over 2 years' follow up.[109]

Comment: See comment under insecticide treated nets in pregnant travellers, p 971. Mefloquine is secreted in small quantities in breast milk, but it is believed that levels are too low to harm infants.[54]

QUESTION **What are the effects of antimalaria interventions in airline pilots?**

OPTION **ANTIMALARIA DRUGS IN AIRLINE PILOTS**

We found no RCTs on the effects of antimalaria drugs in airline pilots.

Benefits: We found no systematic review or RCTs (see comment below).

Harms: **Doxycycline:** One retrospective questionnaire survey (28 Israeli pilots) found that 39% experienced adverse effects from up to two months of doxycycline treatment (abdominal pain 7/28, fatigue 5/28; see comment below).[110] **Mefloquine:** One placebo controlled RCT of adverse effects (23 trainee commercial pilots) found no evidence that mefloquine significantly affected flying performance after 3 weeks of treatment (mean total number of errors recorded by the instrument coordination analyser 12.6 with mefloquine *v* 11.7 with placebo).[111] One retrospective questionnaire survey (15 Israeli non-aviator aircrew) found that 13% experienced adverse effects from mefloquine after up to 2 months of treatment (dizziness, nausea, and abdominal pain in 2/15, abdominal discomfort in 1/15; see comment below).[110]

Comment: Airline pilots are specified as a different group because as an occupational group they are subject to health and safety legislation that is highly prescriptive about certain drugs. One retrospective questionnaire survey (28 Israeli pilots taking doxycycline and 15 non-aviator crew taking mefloquine) found no cases of malaria at 4 weeks.[110]

GLOSSARY

Biological control measures Antimosquito interventions based on modifying the local flora or fauna.

REFERENCES

1. Weller PF. Protozoan infections. In: Dale DC, ed. *Infectious diseases.* New York: WebMD, 2003:651–675.
2. Pasvol V. Malaria. In: Cohen J, Powderly WG, eds. *Infectious diseases.* 2nd ed. London: Mosby, 2004:1579–1591.
3. Jong EC, McMullen R. *The travel and tropical medicine manual.* Philadelphia:Saunders, 2003.
4. World Health Organization. *International travel and health.* Geneva:WHO, 2003:30–148.
5. Funk-Baumann M. Geographic distribution of malaria at traveler destinations. In: Schlagenhauf P, ed. *Traveler's malaria.* Hamilton, Ontario: BC Decker, 2001:56–93.
6. White NJ. Malaria. In: Cook GC, Zumla AI, eds. *Manson's tropical diseases.* 21st ed. London: Saunders, 2003:1205–1295.
7. Martens P, Hall L. Malaria on the move: human population movement and malaria transmission. *Emerg Infect Dis* 2000;6:103–109.
8. Wellems TE, Miller LH. Two worlds of malaria. *N Engl J Med* 2003;349:1496–1498.
9. Krogstad DJ. Plasmodium species (malaria). In: Mandell GL, Bennett JE, Dolin R, eds. *Mandell, Douglas, and Bennett's principles and practice of infectious diseases.* 5th ed. New York: Churchill Livingstone,2000:2817–2831.
10. White GB. Medical acarology and entomology. In: Cook GC, Zumla AI, eds. *Manson's tropical diseases.* 21st ed. London: Saunders,2003:1717–1805.
11. Service MW, Townson H. The Anopheles vector. In: Warrell DA, Gilles HM, eds. *Essential malariology.* 4th ed. London: Arnold, 2002:59–84.
12. Goodyer LI. *Travel medicine for health professionals.* London: Pharmaceutical Press, 2004.

13. Golenda CF, Solberg VB, Burge R, et al. Gender-related efficacy difference to an extended duration formulation of topical N,N–diethyl–m–toluamide (DEET). *Am J Trop Med Hyg* 1999;60:654–657.
14. Renshaw M, Silver JB. Malaria, human. In: Service MW, ed. *Encyclopedia of arthropod-transmitted infections of man and domesticated animals*. New York: CABI Publishing, 2001:314–327.
15. Burkot TR,Graves PM. Malaria, babesiosis, theileriosis and related diseases. In: Eldridge BF, Edman JD, eds. *Medical entomology*. Dordrecht: Kluwer Academic Publishers, 2004:187–230.
16. Snow RS, Gilles HM. The epidemiology of malaria. In: Warrell DA, Gilles HM, eds. *Essential malariology*. 4th ed. London: Arnold,2002:85–106.
17. Peters W, Pasvol G. *Tropical medicine and parasitology*. 5th ed. London: 2002.
18. Gillies MT. Anopheline mosquitos: vector behaviour and bionomics. In: Wernsdorfer WH, McGregor I, eds. *Malaria: principles and practice of malariology*. Edinburgh: Churchill Livingstone,1988:453–485.
19. Taylor TE, Strickland GT. Malaria. In: Strickland GT, ed. *Hunter's tropical medicine and emerging infectious diseases*. 8th ed. Philadelphia: WB Saunders,2000:614–663.
20. Bradley DJ, Warrell DA. Malaria. In: Warrell DA, Cox TM, Firth JD, Benz EJ, eds. *Oxford textbook of medicine*. 4th ed. Oxford: Oxford University Press,2003:721–748.
21. Kassianos GC. *Immunization: childhood and travel health*. 4th ed. Oxford: Blackwell Science,2001.
22. Charlwood JD, Alecrim WA. Capture-recapture studies with the South American malaria vector Anopheles darlingi, Root. *Ann Trop Med Parasitol* 1989;83:569–576.
23. Romi R, Sabatinelli G, Majori G. Malaria epidemiological situation in Italy and evaluation of malaria incidence in Italian travelers. *J Travel Med* 2001;8:6–11.
24. Jelinek T, Loscher T, Nothdurft HD. High prevalence of antibodies against circumsporozoite antigen of *Plasmodium falciparum* without development of symptomatic malaria in travellers returning from sub-Saharan Africa. *J Infect Dis* 1996;174:1376–1379.
25. Moore DAJ, Grant AD, Armstrong M, et al. Risk factors for malaria in UK travellers. *Trans R Soc Trop Med Hygiene* 2004;98:55–63.
26. Winstanley P. Malaria: treatment. *J R Coll Physicians Lond* 1998;32:203–207.
27. Stürchler D. Global epidemiology of malaria. In: Schlagenhauf P, ed. *Traveler's malaria*. Hamilton, Ontario: BC Decker,2001:14–55.
28. Kain KC, Keystone JS. Malaria in travelers. Epidemiology, disease and prevention. *Infect Dis Clin North Am* 1998;12:267–284.
29. Hellgren U. Approach to the patient with malaria. In: Keystone JS, Kozarsky PE, Freedman DO, Nothdurft HD, Connor BA, eds. *Travel medicine*. London: Mosby,2004:169–274.
30. Greenberg AE, Lobel HO. Mortality from *Plasmodium falciparum* malaria in travelers from the United States, 1959 to 1987. *Ann Intern Med* 1990;113:326–327.
31. Grobusch MP. Self-diagnosis and self-treatment of malaria by the traveler. In: Keystone JS. Kozarsky PE, Freedman DO, Nothdurft HD, Connor BA, eds. *Travel medicine*. London: Mosby, 2004:157–167.
32. Miller SA, Bergman BP, Croft AM. Epidemiology of malaria in the British Army from 1982–1996. *J R Army Med Corps* 1999;145:20–22.
33. Beier JC, Oster CN, Onyango FK, et al. *Plasmodium falciparum* incidence relative to entomological inoculation rates at a site proposed for testing malaria vaccines in western Kenya. *Am J Trop Med Hyg* 1994;50:529–536.
34. Misra SP, Webber R, Lines J, et al. Spray versus treated nets using deltamethrin — a community randomized trial in India. *Trans R Soc Trop Med Hyg* 1999;93:456–457.
35. Rowland M, Mahmood P, Iqbal J, et al. Indoor residual spraying with alphacypermethrin controls malaria in Pakistan: a community-randomized trial. *Trop Med Int Health* 2000;5:472–481.
36. Schoepke A, Steffen R, Gratz N. Effectiveness of personal protection measures against mosquito bites for malaria prophylaxis in travellers. *J Travel Med* 1998;5:188–192.
37. Fradin MS. Mosquitoes and mosquito repellents: a clinician's guide. *Ann Intern Med* 1998;128:931–940. Search date 1997; primary sources Medline, the Internet, the Extension Toxicology Network database, hand searches of reference lists, and contact with distributors of natural insect repellents.
38. Hewitt SE, Farhan M, Urhaman H, et al. Self-protection from malaria vectors in Pakistan: an evaluation of popular existing methods and appropriate new techniques in Afghan refugee communities. *Ann Trop Med Parasitol* 1996;90:337–344.
39. Service MW. *Mosquito ecology: field sampling methods*. 2nd ed. London: Chapman and Hall, 1993.
40. Sylla el-HK, Lell B, Krsmsner PG. A blinded, controlled trial of an ultrasound device as mosquito repellent. *Wein Klin Wochenschr* 2000;112:448–450.
41. Yap HH, Tan HT, Yahaya AM, et al. Field efficacy of mosquito coil formulations containing d-allethrin and d-transallethrin against indoor mosquitoes especially *Culex quinquefasciatus*. *Southeast Asian J Trop Med Public Health* 1990;21:558–563.
42. Vernède R, van Meer MMM, Aplers MP. Smoke as a form of personal protection against mosquitoes, a field study in Papua New Guinea. *Southeast Asian J Trop Med Public Health* 1994;25:771–775.
43. Lengeler C. Insecticide treated bednets and curtains for preventing malaria. In: The Cochrane Library, Issue 1, 2004. Chichester, UK: John Wiley & Sons, Ltd. Search date not stated; primary sources Cochrane Infectious Diseases Group Trial Register, Medline, Embase, and hand searches of reference lists, relevant journals, and personal contact with funding agencies and manufacturers.
44. Winstanley P. Malaria: treatment. *J R Coll Physicians Lond* 1998;32:203–207.
45. Soto J, Medina F, Dember N, et al. Efficacy of permethrin-impregnated uniforms in the prevention of malaria and leishmaniasis in Colombian soldiers. *Clin Infect Dis* 1995;21:599–602.
46. Rowland M, Durrani N, Hewitt S, et al. Permethrin-treated *chaddars* and top-sheets: appropriate technology for protection against malaria in Afghanistan and other complex emergencies. *Trans R Soc Trop Med Hyg* 1999;93:465–472.
47. Juckett G. Malaria prevention in travelers. *Am Fam Physician* 1999;59:2523–2530.
48. Bradley DJ, Warhurst DC. Guidelines for the prevention of malaria in travellers from the United Kingdom. *Commun Dis Rep CDR Rev* 1997;7:R137–R152.
49. McConnell R, Fidler AT, Chrislip D. Everglades National Park health hazard evaluation report. Cincinatti, Ohio: US Department of Health and Human Services, Public Health Service, 1986. NIOSH Health Hazard Evaluation Report No. HETA-83–085-1757.
50. Lamberg SI, Mulrennan JA. Bullous reaction to diethyl toluamide (DEET) resembling a blistering insect eruption. *Arch Dermatol* 1969;100:582–586.
51. Curtis CF, Townson H. Malaria: existing methods of vector control and molecular entomology. *Br Med Bull* 1998;54:311–325.
52. Gupta RK, Rutledge LC. Laboratory evaluation of controlled-release repellent formulations on human volunteers under three climatic regimens. *J Am Mosq Control Assoc* 1989;5:52–55.
53. Stemberger H, Leimer R, Widermann G. Tolerability of long-term prophylaxis with Fansidar: a randomized double-blind study in Nigeria. *Acta Trop* 1984;41:391–399.

54. Petersen E. Malariaprofylakse. *Ugeskr Læger* 1997;159:2723–2730.
55. Gherardin T. Mefloquine as malaria prophylaxis. *Aust Fam Physician* 1999;28:310.
56. Schlagenhauf P. Mefloquine for malaria chemoprophylaxis 1992–1998: a review. *J Travel Med* 1999;6:122–133.
57. Fogh S, Schapira A, Bygbjerg IC, et al. Malaria chemoprophylaxis in travellers to east Africa: a comparative prospective study of chloroquine plus proguanil with chloroquine plus sulfadoxine-pyrimethamine. *BMJ* 1988;296:820–822.
58. Wetsteyn JCFM, de Geus A. Comparison of three regimens for malaria prophylaxis in travellers to east, central, and southern Africa. *BMJ* 1993;307:1041–1043.
59. Drysdale SF, Phillips-Howard PA, Behrens RH. Proguanil, chloroquine, and mouth ulcers. *Lancet* 1990;335:164.
60. Schlagenhauf P, Tschopp A, Johnson R, et al. Tolerability of malaria chemoprophylaxis in non-immune travellers to sub-Saharan Africa: multicentre, randomised, double blind, four arm study. *BMJ* 2003;327:1078–1081.
61. Ohrt C, Richie TL, Widjaja H, et al. Mefloquine compared with doxycycline for the prophylaxis of malaria in Indonesian soldiers. A randomized, double-blind, placebo-controlled trial. *Ann Intern Med* 1997;126:963–972.
62. Taylor WR, Richie TL, Fryauff DJ, et al. Malaria prophylaxis using azithromycin: a double-blind, placebo-controlled trial in Irian Jaya, Indonesia. *Clin Infect Dis* 1999;28:74–81.
63. Phillips MA, Kass RB. User acceptability patterns for mefloquine and doxycycline malaria chemoprophylaxis. *J Travel Med* 1996;3:40–45.
64. Leutscher PDC. Malariaprofylakse. *Ugeskr Læger* 1997;159:4866–4867.
65. Anonymous. Mefloquine and malaria prophylaxis [letter]. *Drug Ther Bull* 1998;36:20–22.
66. Croft AMJ, Garner P. Mefloquine for preventing malaria in non-immune adult travellers. In: The Cochrane Library, Issue 1, 2004. Chichester, UK: John Wiley & Sons, Ltd. Search date 2000; primary sources Cochrane Infectious Diseases Group Trial Register, Medline, Embase, Lilacs, Science Citation Index, hand searches of reference lists of articles, and personal contact with researchers in the subject of malaria chemoprophylaxis and drug companies.
67. Overbosch D, Schilthuis H, Bienzle U, et al. Atovaquone-proguanil versus mefloquine for malaria prophylaxis in nonimmune travelers: results from a randomized double-blind study. *Clin Infect Dis* 2001;33:1015–1021.
68. Barrett PJ, Emmins PD, Clarke PD, et al. Comparison of adverse events associated with use of mefloquine and combinations of chloroquine and proguanil as antimalarial prophylaxis: postal and telephone survey of travellers. *BMJ* 1996;313:525–528.
69. Smith HR, Croft AM, Black MM. Dermatological adverse effects with the antimalarial drug mefloquine: a review of 74 published case reports. *Clin Exp Dermatol* 1999;24:249–254.
70. Weinke T, Trautmann M, Held T, et al. Neuropsychiatric side effects after the use of mefloquine. *Am J Trop Med Hyg* 1991;45:86–91.
71. Bem L, Kerr L, Stuerchler D. Mefloquine prophylaxis: an overview of spontaneous reports of severe psychiatric reactions and convulsions. *J Trop Med Hyg* 1992;95:167–169.
72. Huzly D, Schönfeld C, Beurle W, et al. Malaria chemoprophylaxis in German tourists: a prospective study on compliance and adverse reactions. *J Travel Med* 1996;3:148–155.
73. Schlagenhauf P, Steffen R, Lobel H, et al. Mefloquine tolerability during chemoprophylaxis: focus on adverse event assessments, stereochemistry and compliance. *Trop Med Int Health* 1996;1:485–494.
74. Handschin JC, Wall M, Steffen R, et al. Tolerability and effectiveness of malaria chemoprophylaxis with mefloquine or chloroquine with or without co-medication. *J Travel Med* 1997;4:121–127.
75. Van Riemsdijk MM, van der Klauw MM, van Heest JAC, et al. Neuro-psychiatric effects of antimalarials. *Eur J Clin Pharmacol* 1997;52:1–6.
76. Micheo C, Arias C, Rovira A. Adverse effects and compliance with mefloquine or chloroquine + proguanil malaria chemoprophylaxis. *Proceedings of the Second European Conference on Travel Medicine*, Venice, Italy, 2000:29–31.
77. van Riemsdijk MM, Ditters JM, Sturkenboom MCJM, et al. Neuropsychiatric events during prophylactic use of mefloquine before travelling. *Eur J Clin Pharmacol* 2002;58:441–445.
78. Mittelholzer ML, Wall M, Steffen R, et al. Malaria prophylaxis in different age groups. *J Travel Med* 1996;4:219–223.
79. Croft AM, Herxheimer A. Adverse effects of the antimalaria drug, mefloquine: due to primary liver damage with secondary thyroid involvement? *BMC Public Health* 2002;2:6.
80. Ling J, Baird JK, Fryauff DJ, et al. Randomized, placebo-controlled trial of atovaquone/proguanil for the prevention of *Plasmodium falciparum* or *Plasmodium vivax* malaria among migrants to Papua, Indonesia. *Clin Infect Dis* 2002;35:825–833.
81. Hogh B, Clarke PD, Camus D, et al. Atovaquone-proguanil versus chloroquine-proguanil for malaria prophylaxis in non-immune travellers: a randomised, double-blind study. *Lancet* 2000;356:1888–1894.
82. Hatton CSR, Peto TEA, Bunch C, et al. Frequency of severe neutropenia associated with amodiaquine prophylaxis against malaria. *Lancet* 1986;1:411–414.
83. Neftel K, Woodtly W, Schmid M, et al. Amodiaquine induced agranulocytosis and liver damage. *BMJ* 1986;292:721–723.
84. Larrey D, Castot A, Pessayre D, et al. Amodiaquine-induced hepatitis. A report of seven cases. *Ann Intern Med* 1986;104:801–803.
85. Woodtli W, Vonmoos P, Siegrist P, et al. Amodiaquin-induzierte hepatitis mit leukopenie. *Schweiz Med Wochenschr* 1986;116:966–968.
86. Bernuau J, Larrey D, Campillo B, et al. Amodiaquine-induced fulminant hepatitis. *J Hepatol* 1988;6:109–112.
87. Charmot G, Goujon C. Hépatites mineures pouvant être duesà l'amodiaquine. *Bull Soc Pathol Exot* 1987;80:266–270.
88. Raymond JM, Dumas F, Baldit C, et al. Fatal acute hepatitis due to amodiaquine. *J Clin Gastroenterol* 1989;11:602–603.
89. Shanks GD, Edstein MD, Suriyamongkol V, et al. Malaria chemoprohylaxis using proguanil/dapsone combinations on the Thai-Cambodian border. *Am J Trop Med Hyg* 1992;46:643–648.
90. Miller KD, Lobel HO, Satriale RF, et al. Severe cutaneous reactions among American travelers using pyrimethamine-sulfadoxine for malaria prophylaxis. *Am J Trop Med Hyg* 1986;35:451–458.
91. Graves P, Gelband H. Vaccines for preventing malaria. In: The Cochrane Library, Issue 1, 2004. Chichester, UK: John Wiley & Sons, Ltd. Search date 1999; primary sources Cochrane Infectious Diseases Group Trials Register, Cochrane Controlled Trial Register, Medline, Embase, hand searches of reference lists, and personal contact with organisations and researchers in the field.
92. Osimitz TG, Murphy JV. Neurological effects associated with use of the insect repellent *N,N*-diethyl-*m*-toluamide (DEET). *J Toxicol Clin Toxicol* 1997;35:435–441.
93. De Garbino JP, Laborde A. Toxicity of an insect repellent: *N,N*-diethyl-*m*-toluamide. *Vet Hum Toxicol* 1983;25:422–423.
94. Are insect repellents safe [editorial]? *Lancet* 1988;ii:610–611.
95. Bouchaud O, Longuet C, Coulaud JP. Prophylaxie du paludisme. *Rev Prat* 1998;48:279–286.
96. Smithuis FM, van Woensel JBM, Nordlander E, et al. Comparison of two mefloquine regimens for treatment of *Plasmodium falciparum* malaria on the northeastern Thai-Cambodian border. *Antimicrob Agents Chemother* 1993;37:1977–1981.

97. Ter Kuile FO, Dolan G, Nosten F, et al. Halofantrine versus mefloquine in treatment of multidrug-resistant falciparum malaria. *Lancet* 1993;341:1044–1049.
98. Luxemburger C, Price RN, Nosten F, et al. Mefloquine in infants and young children. *Ann Trop Paediatr* 1996;16:281–286.
99. Dolan G, ter Kuile FO, Jacoutot V, et al. Bed nets for the prevention of malaria and anaemia in pregnancy. *Trans R Soc Trop Med Hyg* 1993;87:620–626.
100. Lindsay S, Ansell J, Selman C, et al. Effects of pregnancy on exposure to malaria mosquitoes. *Lancet* 2000;355:1972.
101. Suh KN, Keystone JS. Malaria prophylaxis in pregnancy and children. *Infect Dis Clin Pract* 1996;5:541–546.
102. Osimitz TG, Grothaus RH. The present safety assessment of DEET. *J Am Mosq Control Assoc* 1995;11:274–278.
103. Schaefer C, Peters PW. Intrauterine diethyltoluamide exposure and fetal outcome. *Reprod Toxicol* 1992;6:175–176.
104. McGready R, Hamilton KA, Simpson JA, et al. Safety of the insect repellent *N,N*-diethyl-*m*-toluamide (DEET) in pregnancy. *Am J Trop Med Hyg* 2001;65:285–289.
105. Blomquist L, Thorsell W. Distribution and fate of the insect repellent 14C-*N,N*-diethyl-*m*-toluamide in the animal body. II. Distribution and excretion after cutaneous application. *Acta Pharmacol Toxicol (Copenh)* 1977;41:235–243.
106. Samuel BU, Barry M. The pregnant traveler. *Infect Dis Clin North Am* 1998;12:325–354.
107. Garner P, Gülmezoglu AM. Prevention versus treatment for malaria in pregnant women. In: The Cochrane Library, Issue 1, 2004. Chichester, UK: John Wiley & Sons, Ltd. Search date 2000; primary sources Cochrane Infectious Diseases Group Trial Register, Cochrane Controlled Trials Register, Medline, Embase, hand searches of reference lists, and personal contact with researchers.
108. Cot M, Roisin A, Barro D, et al. Effect of chloroquine chemoprophylaxis during pregnancy on birth weight: results of a randomized trial. *Am J Trop Med Hyg* 1992;46:21–27.
109. Nosten F, ter Kuile F, Maelankiri L, et al. Mefloquine prophylaxis prevents malaria during pregnancy: a double-blind, placebo-controlled study. *J Infect Dis* 1994;169:595–603.
110. Shamiss A, Atar E, Zohar L, et al. Mefloquine versus doxycycline for malaria prophylaxis in intermittent exposure of Israeli Air Force aircrew in Rwanda. *Aviat Space Environ Med* 1996;67:872–873.
111. Schlagenhauf P, Lobel H, Steffen R, et al. Tolerance of mefloquine by Swissair trainee pilots. *Am J Trop Med Hyg* 1997;56:235–240.

Ashley M Croft
Director of Public Health
NATO Headquarters Rheindahlen, Mönchengladbach, Germany

Competing interests: None declared.

Malaria: severe, life threatening

Search date February 2004

Aika Omari and Paul Garner

QUESTIONS

INTERVENTIONS

See glossary G

*Based on consensus. RCTs would be considered unethical.

Key Messages

Antimalarial treatment for complicated falciparum malaria

- **Artemether (as effective as quinine)** Two systematic reviews and four subsequent RCTs found no significant difference in death rates between artemether and quinine in people with severe malaria. One of the reviews found no significant difference in the speed of coma recovery, fever clearance time, or neurological sequelae between artemether and quinine. The second review found no significant difference in neurological sequelae at recovery between artemether and quinine.
- **High initial dose quinine** (reduced parasite and fever clearance times, but no difference in mortality) One systematic review of three small RCTs in adults and children, and one subsequent RCT in children found no significant difference in mortality between quinine regimens with high initial quinine dose and those with no loading dose. The systematic review found that high initial dose quinine reduced parasite and fever clearance times compared with no loading dose. The subsequent RCT found no significant difference between high initial dose and no loading dose for recovery of consciousness or parasite clearance time. One small RCT included in the review found that high initial dose quinine increased transient partial hearing loss compared with no loading dose. Another small RCT in the review found no significant difference between treatments in neurological sequelae.
- **Quinine** We found no RCTs comparing quinine versus either placebo or no treatment, but international consensus recommends quinine for the treatment of severe falciparum malaria.

Malaria: severe, life threatening

- **Intramuscular versus intravenous quinine** One RCT in children found no significant difference between intramuscular and intravenous quinine in recovery times or death. However, the study may have lacked power to detect clinically important differences between treatments.
- **Intravenous artesunate versus quinine** One RCT found no significant difference in mortality between intravenous artesunate and quinine, but it may have been underpowered to detect a clinically important difference.
- **Rectal artemisinin and its derivatives** One systematic review of small RCTs found no significant difference in mortality between rectal artemisinin and quinine in people with severe malaria. One RCT found no significant difference in mortality between rectal dihydroartemisinin and quinine. We found no systematic review and no RCTs comparing rectal artesunate versus quinine.

Adjunctive treatment for complicated falciparum malaria

- **Desferrioxamine mesylate** One systematic review found limited evidence that the risk of persistent seizures in children with cerebral malaria was reduced with desferrioxamine mesylate compared with placebo.
- **Exchange blood transfusion** One systematic review found no suitable RCTs. A systematic review of case control studies found no significant difference in mortality between exchange transfusion plus antimalarial drugs and antimalarial drugs alone.
- **Initial blood transfusion** One systematic review found no significant difference in mortality between initial and expectant blood transfusion among clinically stable children (no respiratory distress or cardiac failure) with malarial anaemia, but found that adverse events were more common with initial blood transfusion. The review found no significant difference between transfusion and no transfusion for the combined outcome of death or severe adverse events. Transmission of hepatitis B or HIV was not reported. We found no RCTs examining the effects of transfusion in adults with malaria.
- **Dexamethasone** One systematic review found no significant difference in mortality between dexamethasone and placebo, but gastrointestinal bleeding and seizures were more common with dexamethasone.

DEFINITION Malaria is caused by protozoan infection of red blood cells with *Plasmodium falciparum* and comprises a variety of syndromes. This review deals with clinically complicated malaria (i.e. malaria that presents with life threatening conditions, including coma, severe anaemia, renal failure, respiratory distress syndrome, hypoglycaemia, shock, spontaneous haemorrhage, and convulsions). The diagnosis of cerebral malaria should be considered where there is encephalopathy in the presence of malaria parasites. A strict definition of cerebral malaria requires the presence of unrousable coma, and no other cause of encephalopathy (e.g. hypoglycaemia, sedative drugs), in the presence of *P falciparum* infection.[1] This review does not currently cover the treatment of malaria in pregnancy.

INCIDENCE/ PREVALENCE Malaria is a major health problem in the tropics, with 300–500 million clinical cases occurring annually, and an estimated 1.1–2.7 million deaths each year as a result of severe malaria.[2] Over 90% of deaths occur in children under 5 years of age, mainly from cerebral malaria and anaemia.[2] In areas where the rate of malaria transmission is stable (endemic), those most at risk of acquiring severe malaria are children under 5 years old, because adults and older children have partial immunity, which offers some protection. In areas where the rate of malaria transmission is unstable (non-endemic), severe malaria affects both adults and children. Non-immune travellers and migrants are also at risk of developing severe malaria.

AETIOLOGY/ RISK FACTORS Malaria is transmitted by the bite of infected female anopheline mosquitoes. Certain genes are associated with resistance to severe malaria. The human leukocyte antigens HLA-Bw53 and HLA-DRB1*1302 protect against severe malaria. However, associations of HLA antigens with severe malaria are limited to specific populations.[3,4] Haemoglobin S[3] and haemoglobin C[5] are also protective against severe malaria. Genes such as the tumour necrosis factor gene have also been associated with increased susceptibility to severe malaria (see aetiology under malaria: prevention in travellers, p 956).[6]

PROGNOSIS In children under 5 years of age with cerebral malaria, the estimated case fatality of treated malaria is 19%, although reported hospital case fatality may be as high as 40%.[1,7] Neurological sequelae persisting for more than 6 months occur in more than 2% of survivors, and include ataxia, hemiplegia, speech disorders, behavioural disorders, epilepsy, and blindness. Severe malarial anaemia has a case fatality rate higher than 13%.[7] In adults, the mortality of cerebral malaria is 20%; this rises to 50% in pregnancy, and neurological sequelae occur in about 3% of survivors.[8]

AIMS OF INTERVENTION To prevent death and cure the infection; to prevent long term disability; to minimise neurological sequelae resulting from cerebral malaria, with minimal adverse effects of treatment.

OUTCOMES Death; parasite clearance at day 7 or 14; parasite clearance time; fever clearance time; time to walking and drinking; coma recovery time; neurological sequelae at follow up; adverse events.

METHODS *Clinical Evidence* search and appraisal February 2004, including a search for observational studies. We applied the World Health Organization criteria for severe malaria when deciding which RCTs to include.[1]

QUESTION What are the effects of antimalarial treatments for complicated falciparum malaria in non-pregnant people?

OPTION QUININE VERSUS PLACEBO OR NO TREATMENT

We found no RCTs comparing quinine versus either placebo or no treatment, but international consensus recommends quinine for the treatment of severe falciparum malaria.

Benefits: Placebo controlled RCTs would be inappropriate in severe malaria (see comment below).

Harms: We found two observational studies on hypoglycaemia associated with quinine. One study in people with severe malaria treated with quinine in Thailand found a correlation between plasma quinine and insulin levels during hypoglycaemic episodes ($P = 0.007$).[9] One prospective cohort study in Zaire (9 children and 19 adults) treated severe malaria with intravenous quinine (average dose 8.5 mg base/kg over 1 hour every 8 hours).[10] Nine people developed significant hypoglycaemia (glucose < 2.8 mmol/L), which was associated with high plasma insulin levels. It is not clear from these studies whether hypoglycaemia was caused by malaria or by quinine administration.

Comment: The use of quinine to treat severe malaria was established before modern trial methods were developed. In a case series in Singapore (1944–1945), 15 adults with acute severe malaria were treated with continuous intravenous quinine.[11] Thirteen recovered and two comatose people died. In a non-comparative study conducted in Zaire (1987), intravenous quinine (10 mg/kg 8 hourly for 3 days) was given to 34 children (aged 7 months to 13 years) with severe or moderate falciparum malaria.[12] One child who was comatose on admission died. The mean parasite clearance time**G** was 59.6 hours. The mean fever clearance time**G** was 44.1 hours. Thirty three children were clinically well and had negative blood slides on day 7. Reviews[13,14] and consensus statements[1,15,16] recommend quinine for treatment of severe falciparum malaria, particularly in chloroquine resistant areas.

OPTION INTRAMUSCULAR VERSUS INTRAVENOUS QUININE

One RCT in children found no significant difference between intramuscular and intravenous quinine in recovery times or death. However, the study may have lacked power to detect clinically important differences between treatments.

Benefits: We found no systematic review. We found one RCT (59 Kenyan children < 12 years old in 1989–1990), which compared intramuscular versus intravenous quinine (20 mg salt/kg loading immediately followed by 10 mg salt/kg 12 hourly) versus standard dose intravenous quinine in severe falciparum malaria.[17] The RCT found no significant difference in mortality, mean parasite clearance timeⒼ or recovery time to drinking or walking, but may have lacked power to detect a clinically important difference (mortality: 3/20 [15%] deaths with im quinine *v* 1/18 [5.6%] with iv quinine; RR 2.7, 95% CI 0.3 to 23.7; mean parasite clearance time: 57 hours with im quinine *v* 58 hours with iv quinine; WMD –1.0 hours, 95% CI –12.2 hours to +10.2 hours; mean recovery times to drinking: 47 hours with im quinine *v* 32 hours with iv quinine; WMD +15 hours, 95% CI –5.6 hours to +35.6 hours; mean recovery times to walking: 98 hours with im quinine *v* 96 hours with iv quinine; WMD +2.0 hours, 95% CI –24.5 hours to +28.5 hours).

Harms: Neurological sequelae were reported in two children in the intramuscular group, and one child in the intravenous group had transient neurological sequelae that were not specified (2/20 [10%] with im quinine *v* 1/18 [5.6%] with iv quinine; RR 1.8, 95% CI 0.2 to 18.2).[17]

Comment: Quinine concentration profiles were similar with both routes of administration, and peak concentrations were achieved soon after intramuscular injection. The sample size might have been insufficient to rule out important clinical differences.[17]

OPTION HIGH INITIAL DOSE QUININE VERSUS NO LOADING DOSE

One systematic review of three small RCTs in adults and children, and one subsequent RCT in children found no significant difference in mortality between quinine regimens with high initial quinine dose and those with no loading dose. The systematic review found that high initial dose quinine reduced parasite and fever clearance times compared with no loading dose. The subsequent RCT found no significant difference between high initial dose and no loading dose for recovery of consciousness or parasite clearance time. One small RCT included in the review found that high initial dose quinine increased transient partial hearing loss compared with no loading dose. Another small RCT in the review found no significant difference between treatments in neurological sequelae.

Benefits: We found one systematic review (search date 2002, 3 RCTs, 92 people)[18] and one subsequent RCT.[19] The systematic review found no significant difference in mortality between high initial dose of quinine (20 mg salt/kg or 16 mg base/kg given im or iv) and no loading dose, followed in both groups by standard dose quinine (2 RCTs; 2/35 [5.7%] died with high initial dose *v* 5/37 [13.5%] with no loading dose; RR 0.43, 95% CI 0.09 to 2.15).[18] One of the included RCTs (39 children) found no significant difference between high initial dose and no loading dose in mean time to recover consciousness (14 hours with high initial dose *v* 13 hours with no loading dose; WMD +1.0 hours, 95% CI –8.8 hours to +10.8 hours).[17] Parasite clearance timeⒼ and fever clearance timeⒼ were shorter for the high initial dose quinine group than for the group with no loading dose (parasite clearance time: 2 RCTs, 67 people; WMD –7.4 hours, 95% CI –13.2 hours to –1.6 hours; fever clearance time: 2 RCTs, 68 people; WMD –11.1 hours, 95% CI –20.0 hours to –2.2 hours). The subsequent RCT (72 children aged 8 months to 15 years in Togo [1999–2000]) found no significant difference between high initial dose intravenous quinine regimen (20 mg quinine salt/kg over 4 hours, then 10 mg quinine salt/kg 12 hourly) and no loading dose (15 mg salt/kg 12 hourly) in mortality (2/35 [6%] with high initial dose *v* 2/37 [5%] with no loading dose; RR 1.06,

95% CI 0.16 to 7.1).[19] It found no significant difference between high initial dose and no loading dose for recovery of consciousness or parasite clearance time (recovery of consciousness: 35.5 hours with high initial dose v 28.6 hours with no loading dose; WMD +6.9 hours, 95% CI –0.6 hours to +14.4 hours; time to 100% parasite clearance: 48 hours with high initial dose v 60 hours with no loading dose; P value not reported).

Harms: The systematic review found no significant difference between high initial dose of quinine and no loading dose in rate of hypoglycaemia (2 RCTs; 4/35 [11%] hypoglycaemia with high initial dose v 3/37 [8%] with no loading dose; RR 1.39, 95% CI 0.32 to 6.00).[18] One RCT (33 people) included in the review found that high initial dose quinine significantly increased transient partial hearing loss compared with no loading dose (10/17 [59%] v 3/16 [19%]; RR 3.14, 95% CI 1.05 to 9.38).[20] One RCT (39 children) included in the review found no significant difference between high initial dose of quinine and no loading dose in neurological sequelae (1/18 [6%] high initial dose v 2/21 [10%] no loading dose; RR 0.58, 95% CI 0.06 to 5.91).[17]

Comment: The RCTs may have been too small to detect a clinically important difference.[17,19,20]

OPTION ARTEMETHER VERSUS QUININE

Two systematic reviews and four subsequent RCTs found no significant difference in death rates between artemether and quinine in people with severe malaria. One of the reviews found no significant difference in the speed of coma recovery, fever clearance time, or neurological sequelae between artemether and quinine. The second review found no significant difference in neurological sequelae at recovery between artemether and quinine.

Benefits: We found two systematic reviews[21,22] and four subsequent RCTs.[23–26] The first review (search date not reported, 7 RCTs, 1919 adults and children) analysed individual participant data.[21] It found no significant difference in mortality between intramuscular artemether and either intravenous or intramuscular quinine (im quinine in 1 RCT only) in severe falciparum malaria (mortality 136/961 [14%] with artemether v 164/958 [17%] with quinine; OR 0.80, 95% CI 0.62 to 1.02). Parasite clearance was faster with artemether than with quinine (HR 0.62, 95% CI 0.56 to 0.69). The review found no significant difference in the speed of coma recovery, fever clearance time**G**, or neurological sequelae between artemether and quinine (coma recovery time with quinine: HR 1.09, 95% CI 0.97 to 1.22; fever clearance time with quinine: HR 1.01, 95% CI 0.90 to 1.15; neurological sequelae: 81/807 [10%] with artemether v 91/765 [12%] with quinine; OR 0.82, 95% CI 0.59 to 1.15). It found that rates for the combined outcome of death or neurological sequelae were significantly lower for artemether than for quinine (OR 0.77, 95% CI 0.62 to 0.96; P = 0.02).[21] The second review (search date 1999, 11 RCTs, 2142 people) found a small significant reduction in mortality for intramuscular artemether compared with intravenous quinine (OR 0.72, 95% CI 0.57 to 0.91).[22] However, more rigorous analysis excluding three poorer quality RCTs found no significant difference in mortality (OR 0.79, 95% CI 0.59 to 1.05). The review found no significant difference in neurological sequelae at recovery between artemether and quinine (OR 0.8, 95% CI 0.52 to 1.25). The first subsequent RCT (105 people aged 15–40 years with cerebral malaria in Bangladesh) compared intramuscular artemether (160 mg initially, then 80 mg/kg once daily) versus intravenous quinine (loading dose 20 mg/kg, then 10 mg/kg 8 hourly).[23] It found no significant difference in death rates or neurological sequelae between artemether and quinine (death: 9/51 [18%] with artemether v 10/54 [19%] with quinine; OR 0.94, 95% CI 0.35 to 2.55; neurological sequelae: 3/51 [6%] with artemether v 1/54 [2%] with quinine; RR 3.18, 95% CI 0.34 to 29.56). Mean fever clearance time and coma recovery time were significantly longer for artemether than for quinine (fever clearance time: 58 hours with artemether v 47 hours with quinine; WMD 11.0 hours, 95% CI 1.6 hours to 20.4 hours; coma recovery time: 74 hours with artemether v 53 hours with quinine; WMD 20.8 hours, 95% CI 3.6 hours to 38.0 hours). There was no significant difference in mean parasite clearance time**G** between artemether and quinine (52 hours with artemether v 61 hours with quinine; WMD –8.6 hours, 95% CI –22.5 hours to +5.3 hours). The second subsequent RCT (41 children with severe malaria in Sudan, 40 analysed) compared intramuscular artemether (3.2 mg/kg loading dose, then 1.6 mg/kg daily) versus intravenous quinine (loading dose 20 mg/kg, then 10 mg/kg 8 hourly).[24] It found that artemether significantly increased fever clearance time but found no significant difference between artemether and quinine in time to parasite clearance (mean fever clearance time: 30.5 hours with artemether v 18 hours with quinine; P = 0.02; mean parasite clearance time: 16 hours with artemether v 22.4 hours with quinine; P > 0.05). It found that one child died with quinine compared with no deaths with artemether (0/20 [0%] with artemether v 1/21 [5%] with quinine; P value not reported). The third subsequent RCT (77 comatosed children aged 3 months to 15 years with cerebral malaria) compared intramuscular artemether (1.6 mg/kg 12 hourly) versus intravenous quinine (10 mg/kg 8 hourly).[25] It found no significant difference in death rates between artemether and quinine (3/38 [8%] with artemether v 2/39 [5%]; P value not reported). There was no significant difference in mean fever clearance time, coma recovery time, and parasite clearance time (fever clearance time: 31 hours with artemether v 36 hours with quinine; coma recovery time: 21 hours with artemether v 26 hours with quinine; parasite clearance time: 36 hours with artemether v 41 hours with quinine; P value not reported for any comparison). The fourth subsequent RCT (46 children age up to 14 years with severe malaria in India) compared intramuscular artemether (1.6 mg/kg 12 hourly) versus intravenous quinine (20 mg/kg 8 hourly).[26] It found no significant difference in mortality (5/23 [10.7%] with artemether v 6/23 [13.0%] with quinine; OR 0.79, 95% CI 0.2 to 3.06). It found that artemether significantly improved parasite clearance time and coma recovery time compared with quinine, but found no significant difference in fever clearance time (parasite clearance time: 40.9 hours with artemether v 51.9 hours with quinine, WMD –11.0 hours, 95% CI –14.47 hours to –7.53 hours; coma recovery time: 34.8 hours with artemether v 40.8 hours with quinine; WMD –6.0 hours, 95% CI –10.41 hours to –1.59 hours; fever clearance time: 44.5 hours with artemether v 45.9 hours with quinine; WMD –1.4 hours, 95% CI –5.71 hours to +2.91 hours).

Harms: The second review stated that not all studies reported on harms.[22] Among those that did, the size of proportion affected was small and similar between groups. The harms reported included nausea, vomiting, diarrhoea, abdominal pain, pruritus, urticaria, rash and injection site pain, and abscess. The second subsequent RCT found that one child treated with quinine developed hypoglycaemia (0/20 [0%] with artemether v 1/21 [5%] with quinine; P value not reported).[24] It reported no neurological problems in either treatment group after 28 days of follow up. The third subsequent RCT found no significant difference in transient neurological sequelae between artemether and quinine (2/38 [5%] with artemether v 1/39 [3%] with quinine; P value not reported).[25] The fourth subsequent RCT reported no important adverse effects with either artemether or quinine, and provided no details.[26]

Comment: The third subsequent RCT did not use loading doses of either artemether or quinine at the beginning of treatment.[25] Treatment allocation in the fourth subsequent RCT was quasi-randomised by date of admission.[26] We found a fifth subsequent RCT (52 people).[27] However, it was not clear whether participants had severe malaria, and outcomes were poorly reported.

OPTION RECTAL ARTEMISININ DERIVATIVES (ARTEMISININ, ARTESUNATE, OR DIHYDROARTEMISININ) VERSUS QUININE

One systematic review of small RCTs found no significant difference in mortality between rectal artemisinin and quinine in people with severe malaria. One RCT found no significant difference in mortality between rectal dihydroartemisinin and quinine in people with severe malaria. We found no systematic review and no RCTs comparing rectal artesunate versus quinine.

Benefits: **Rectal artemisinin versus quinine:** We found one systematic review (search date 1999, 3 RCTs) comparing rectal artemisinin versus quinine in severe malaria.[22] Two RCTs were conducted in Vietnam and one in Ethiopia (1996–1997). Meta-analysis found lower mortality with artemisinin and quicker coma recovery time, but the difference was not significant (mortality, 3 RCTs: 9/87 [10%] with artemisinin v 16/98 [16%] with quinine; RR 0.73, 95% CI 0.35 to 1.50; coma recovery, 2 RCTs, 59 people: WMD −9.0 hours, 95% CI −19.7 hours to +1.7 hours). Fever clearance time🅖 was not significantly different (no figures provided). **Rectal dihydroartemisin versus quinine:** We found one RCT (67 people aged 2–60 years with severe malaria in Kenya in 1998), which compared rectal dihydroartemisin (160 mg initially, then 80 mg for 2 days for people above 16 years; variable dosage depending on age in people less than 16 years) versus intravenous quinine (20 mg/kg initially, then 10 mg/kg 8 hourly).[28] It found no deaths with either treatment. It found that dihydroartemisinin significantly improved parasite clearance time compared with quinine, but found no significant difference in fever clearance time (parasite clearance: 38 hours with dihydroartemisinin v 49 hours with quinine; WMD −11 hours, 95% CI −14 hours to −7 hours; fever clearance time: 28 hours with dihydroartemisinin v 22 hours with quinine; WMD 6 hours, 95% CI 3 to 9 hours). **Rectal artesunate versus quinine:** We found no systematic review and no RCTs comparing rectal artesunate versus quinine.

Harms: **Rectal artemisinin versus quinine:** One RCT found that artemisinin significantly reduced the risk of hypoglycaemia compared with quinine (3/30 [10%] with artemisinin v 19/30 [63%] with quinine; RR 0.16, 95% CI 0.05 to 0.48).[29] **Rectal dihydroartemisin versus quinine:** One RCT found that dihydroartemisin significantly reduced tinnitus compared with quinine (1/30 [3%] with dihydroartemisinin v 10/37 [27%] with quinine; OR 0.09, 95% CI 0.01 to 0.78).[28]

Comment: The World Health Organization is currently conducting a trial of prompt administration of rectal artesunate for severe malaria by paramedical staff before referral to hospital (Gomes M, personal communication, 2004).

OPTION **INTRAVENOUS ARTESUNATE VERSUS QUININE**

One small RCT found no significant difference in mortality between intravenous artesunate and quinine, but it may have been underpowered to detect a clinically important difference.

Benefits: We found no systematic reviews. We found one RCT (113 adults with severe malaria in Thailand) comparing intravenous artesunate (2.4 mg/kg initially, 1.2 mg/kg 12 hours later, then 1.2 mg/kg daily) versus intravenous quinine (20 mg/kg initially, then 10 mg/kg 8 hourly).[30] It found no significant difference between treatments in mortality after 300 hours (7/59 [12%] artesunate *v* 12/54 [22%] quinine; RR 0.53, 95% CI 0.23 to 1.26). It found that artesunate significantly improved parasite clearance time, but found no significant difference in fever clearance time**G** or coma recovery time (parasite clearance time: 63 hours with artesunate *v* 76 hours with quinine; P = 0.019; fever clearance time: 41 hours with artesunate *v* 65 hours with quinine; P = 0.2; coma recovery time: 17 hours with artesunate *v* 18 hours with quinine; P = 0.6).

Harms: The RCT found that artesunate significantly reduced hypoglycaemia compared with quinine (6/59 [10%] with artesunate *v* 15/54 [28%] with quinine; RR 0.37, 95% CI 0.15 to 0.88).[30] It found that one person treated with artesunate developed an urticarial rash.

Comment: None.

QUESTION **What are the effects of adjunctive treatment for complicated falciparum malaria in non-pregnant people?**

OPTION **DESFERRIOXAMINE MESYLATE**

One systematic review found limited evidence that the risk of persistent seizures in children with cerebral malaria was reduced with desferrioxamine mesylate compared with placebo.

Benefits: **Versus placebo:** We found one systematic review (search date 2003, 2 RCTs, 435 children > 6 years of age with cerebral malaria treated with quinine) of desferrioxamine mesylate (100 mg/kg daily iv for 72 hours) versus placebo.[31] Both RCTs were conducted in Zambia (1990–1991). The review found no difference in overall mortality, but the meta-analysis may have been underpowered to detect a clinically important difference (39/217 [18%] with desferrioxamine *v* 28/218 [13%] with placebo; RR 1.40, 95% CI 0.89 to 2.18). The review found that desferrioxamine mesylate significantly reduced the risk of persistent seizures (93/168 [55.4%] with desferrioxamine *v* 115/166 [69.3%] with placebo; RR 0.80, 95% CI 0.67 to 0.95).

Harms: One RCT included in the review found no significant difference between desferrioxamine mesylate and placebo for phlebitis or recurrent hypoglycaemia (phlebitis: 26/172 [15%] with desferrioxamine *v* 20/172 [12%] with placebo; RR 1.30, 95% CI 0.76 to 2.24; recurrent hypoglycaemia: 43/172 [25%] with desferrioxamine *v* 29/172 [17%] with placebo; RR 1.48, 95% CI 0.97 to 2.26).[32]

Comment: The trials were probably underpowered to detect a clinically important difference in adverse events.

OPTION DEXAMETHASONE

One systematic review found no significant difference in mortality between dexamethasone and placebo, but gastrointestinal bleeding and seizures were more common with dexamethasone.

Benefits: **Versus placebo:** We found one systematic review (search date 1999, 2 RCTs, 143 people with severe/cerebral malaria treated with quinine), which compared dexamethasone versus placebo over 48 hours.[33] One RCT was conducted in Indonesia and the other in Thailand. The review found no significant difference in mortality (14/71 [20%] with dexamethasone *v* 16/72 [25%] with placebo; RR 0.89, 95% CI 0.47 to 1.68). One RCT found a longer mean time between start of treatment and coma resolution with dexamethasone (76 hours with dexamethasone *v* 57 hours with placebo; $P < 0.02$),[34] but the other RCT found no significant difference (83.4 hours with dexamethasone *v* 80.0 hours with placebo; WMD +3.4 hours, 95% CI −31.3 hours to +38.1 hours).[35]

Harms: The review found that dexamethasone significantly increased gastrointestinal bleeding and seizures compared with placebo (gastrointestinal bleeding: 7/71 [10%] with dexamethasone *v* 0/72 [0%] with placebo; RR 8.17, 95% CI 1.05 to 63.6; seizures: 1/71 [15.5%] with dexamethasone *v* 3/72 [4%] with placebo; RR 3.32, 95% CI 1.05 to 10.47).[33]

Comment: No effect of steroids on mortality was shown, but the trials were small. The effect of steroids on disability was not reported.

OPTION INITIAL BLOOD TRANSFUSION FOR TREATING MALARIAL ANAEMIA

One systematic review found no significant difference in mortality between initial and expectant blood transfusion among clinically stable children (no respiratory distress or cardiac failure) with malarial anaemia, but found that adverse events were more common with initial blood transfusion. The review found no significant difference between transfusion and no transfusion for the combined outcome of death or severe adverse events. Transmission of hepatitis B or HIV was not reported. We found no RCTs examining the effects of transfusion in adults with malaria.

Benefits: We found one systematic review (search date 1999, 2 RCTs, 230 children with malarial anaemia; packed cell volume range 12–17%).[36] The first RCT (116 children) compared initial blood transfusion versus conservative treatment in children from Tanzania, and the second RCT (114 children) compared blood transfusion versus iron supplements in children from the Gambia. Both trials excluded children who were clinically unstable with respiratory distress or signs of cardiac failure. Meta-analysis found fewer deaths in the transfused children, but the difference was not significant (1/118 [1%] with transfusion *v* 3/112 [3%] with control; RR 0.41, 95% CI 0.06 to 2.70). We found no RCTs examining the effects of transfusion in adults with malaria.

Harms: Coma and convulsions occurred more often after transfusion (8/118 [6.8%] with transfusion *v* 0/112 [0%] without transfusion; RR 8.6, 95% CI 1.1 to 66.0).[36] Seven of the eight adverse events occurred in one RCT. Meta-analysis combining deaths and severe adverse events found no significant difference between people who received transfusions and people who did not (8/118 [7%] with transfusion *v* 3/112 [3%] without transfusion; RR 2.5, 95% CI 0.7 to 9.3). Transmission of hepatitis B or HIV was not reported.

Comment: Studies were small, and loss to follow up was greater than 10%, both of which are potential sources of bias. In the first RCT, one child in the transfusion group and one child in the conservative treatment group required an additional transfusion after clinical assessment. In the second RCT, 10 children allocated to receive iron supplements later required transfusion when packed cell volume fell below 12% or they showed signs of respiratory distress.

OPTION EXCHANGE BLOOD TRANSFUSION

One systematic review found no suitable RCTs. A systematic review of case control studies found no significant difference in mortality between exchange transfusion plus antimalarial drugs and antimalarial drugs alone.

Benefits: We found one systematic review (search date 2001).[37] It found no suitable RCTs in people with malaria. We found no additional RCTs that met our inclusion criteria (see comment below).

Harms: We found no RCTs.

Comment: We found one systematic review of case control studies[37] and one small RCT.[38] The review (search date 2001, 8 studies, 279 people) found no significant difference in mortality between exchange transfusion plus antimalarial drugs and antimalarial drugs only (8 studies; OR for death 1.2, 95% CI 0.7 to 2.1).[37] Admission criteria for exchange transfusion varied in the included studies, but generally parasitaemia was greater than 10%, and most people had failed to improve after 24 hours of antimalarial treatment. The methods and volumes used for exchange transfusion also varied. Those who received exchange blood transfusions had higher mean levels of parasitaemia before treatment began (26% with exchange transfusion *v* 11% with no exchange transfusion; $P < 0.05$) and fulfilled more World Health Organization criteria for the diagnosis of severe malaria (mean 3.6 with exchange transfusion *v* 2.8 with no exchange transfusion; $P = 0.03$). The RCT compared exchange transfusion plus antimalarial drugs versus antimalarial drugs, but it included only eight people.[38]

GLOSSARY

Fever clearance time The time between commencing treatment and the temperature returning back to normal.

Parasite clearance time (PCT) The time between commencing treatment and the first negative blood test. PCT 50 is the time taken for parasites to be reduced to 50% of the first test value and PCT 90 is the time taken for parasites to be reduced to 10% of the first test value.

REFERENCES

1. World Health Organization. Severe falciparum malaria. World Health Organization, Communicable Diseases Cluster. *Trans R Soc Trop Med Hyg* 2000;94:S1–S90.
2. World Health Organization. WHO Expert Committee on Malaria: Twentieth report. 1998 Geneva Switzerland. *World Health Organ Tech Rep Ser* 2000;892:i–v:1–74.
3. Hill AVS. Malaria resistance genes: a natural selection. *Trans R Soc Trop Med Hyg* 1992;86:225–226.
4. Hill AVS. Genetic susceptibility to malaria and other infectious diseases: from the MHC to the whole genome. *Parasitology* 1996;112:S75–S84.
5. Modiano D, Luoni G, Sirima BS, et al. Haemoglobin C protects against clinical *Plasmodium falciparum* malaria. *Nature* 2001;414:305–308.
6. McGuire W, Hill AV, Allsopp CE, et al. Variation in the TNF-alpha promoter region associated with susceptibility to cerebral malaria. *Nature* 1994;371:508–510.
7. Murphy SC, Breman JG. Gaps in the childhood malaria burden in Africa: cerebral malaria, neurological sequelae, anemia, respiratory distress, hypoglycemia, and complications of pregnancy. *Am J Trop Med Hyg* 2001;64:S57–S67.
8. White NJ. Malaria. In: Cook GC, ed. *Manson's tropical diseases*. 20th ed. London: WB Saunders 1996:1087–1164.
9. White N, Warrell D, Chanthavanich P, et al. Severe hypoglycemia and hyperinsulinemia in falciparum malaria. *N Engl J Med* 1983;309:61–66.
10. Okitolonda W, Delacollette C, Malengreau M, et al. High incidence of hypoglycaemia in African patients treated with intravenous quinine for severe malaria. *BMJ* 1987;295:716–718.
11. Strahan JH. Quinine by continuous intravenous drip in the treatment of acute falciparum malaria. *Trans R Soc Trop Med Hyg* 1948;41:669–76.
12. Greenberg AE, Nguyen-Dinh P, Davachi F, et al. Intravenous quinine therapy of hospitalized children

with *Plasmodium falciparum* malaria in Kinshasa, Zaire. *Am J Trop Med Hyg* 1988;40:360–364.
13. Hall AP. The treatment of severe falciparum malaria. *Trans R Soc Trop Med Hyg* 1977;71:367–378.
14. Warrell DA. Treatment of severe malaria. *J R Soc Med* 1989;82(suppl 17):44–50.
15. World Health Organization. The use of antimalarial drugs. Report of a WHO Informal consultation, 13–17 November 2000 (WHO/CDS/RBM/2001.33). Geneva: World Health Organization, 2001.
16. Looareesuwan S, Olliaro P, White NJ, et al. Consensus recommendation on the treatment of malaria in Southeast Asia. *Southeast Asian J Trop Med Public Health* 1998;29:355–360.
17. Pasvol G, Newton CRJC, Winstanley PA, et al. Quinine treatment of severe falciparum malaria in African children: a randomized comparison of three regimens. *Am J Trop Med Hyg* 1991;45:702–713.
18. Lesi A, Meremikwu M. High first dose quinine for treating severe malaria. In: The Cochrane Library, Issue 2, 2003. Oxford: Update Software. Search date 2002; primary sources Cochrane Infectious Diseases Group specialised trials register, Cochrane Controlled Trials Register, Medline, Embase, Lilacs, conference proceedings, researchers working in the field, and hand searches of references.
19. Assimadi JK, Gbadoé AD, Agbodjan-Djossou O, et al. Intravenous quinine treatment of cerebral malaria in African children: comparison of a loading dose regimen to a regimen without loading dose [French]. *Arch Pediatr* 2002;9:587–594.
20. Tombe M, Bhatt KM, Obel AOK. Quinine loading dose in severe falciparum malaria at Kenyatta National Hospital, Kenya. *East Afr Med J* 1992;69:670–674.
21. Artemether Quinine Meta-analysis Study Group. A meta-analysis using individual patient data of trials comparing artemether with quinine in the treatment of severe falciparum malaria. *Trans R Soc Trop Med Hyg* 2001;95:637–650. Search date not reported; primary sources Medline, Cochrane, and discussions with an international panel of malaria clinical investigators.
22. McIntosh HM, Olliaro P. Artemisinin derivatives for treating severe malaria. In: The Cochrane Library, Issue 2, 2003. Oxford: Update Software. Search date 1999; primary sources Cochrane Infectious Diseases Group Trials Register, Medline, Bids, Science Citation Index, Embase, African Index Medicus, Lilacs, hand searches of reference lists and conference abstracts, and contact with organisations and researchers in the field and pharmaceutical companies.
23. Faiz A, Rahman E, Hossain A, et al. A randomized controlled trial comparing artemether and quinine in the treatment of cerebral malaria in Bangladesh. *Ind J Malariol* 2001;38:9–18.
24. Adam I, Idris HM, Mohamed-Ali AA, et al. Comparison of intramuscular artemether and intravenous quinine in the treatment of Sudanese children with severe falciparum malaria. *East Afr Med J* 2002;79:621–625.
25. Satti GM, Elhassan SH, Ibrahim SA. The efficacy of artemether versus quinine in the treatment of cerebral malaria. *J Egypt Soc Parasitol* 2002;32:611–623.
26. Huda SN, Shahab T, Ali SM, et al. A comparative clinical trial of artemether and quinine in children with severe malaria. *Indian Pediatr* 2003;40:939–945.
27. Singh NB, Bhagyabati Devi S, Singh TB, et al. Artemether vs quinine therapy in *Plasmodium falciparum* malaria in Manipur — a preliminary report. *J Communic Dis* 2001;33:83–87.
28. Esamai F, Ayuo P, Owino–Ongor W, et al. Rectal dihydroartemisinin versus intravenous quinine in the treatment of severe malaria: a randomised clinical trial. *East Afr Med J* 2000;77:273–278.
29. Birku Y, Makonnen E, Bjorkman A. Comparison of rectal artemisinin with intravenous quinine in the treatment of severe malaria in Ethiopia. *East Afr Med J* 1999;76:154–159.
30. Newton PN, Angus BJ, Chierakul W, et al. Randomized comparison of artesunate and quinine in the treatment of severe falciparum malaria. *Clin Infect Dis* 2003;37:7–16.
31. Smith HJ, Meremikwu M. Iron chelating agents for treating malaria. In: The Cochrane Library, Issue 2, 2003. Oxford: Update Software. Search date 2003; primary sources Trials Register of the Cochrane Infectious Diseases Group, Cochrane Controlled Trials Register, Medline, Embase, and hand searches of reference lists.
32. Thuma PE, Mabeza GF, Biemba G, et al. Effect of iron chelation therapy on mortality in children with cerebral malaria. *Trans R Soc Trop Med Hyg* 1998;92:214–218.
33. Prasad K, Garner P. Steroids for treating cerebral malaria. In: The Cochrane Library, Issue 2, 2003. Oxford: Update Software. Search date 1999; primary sources Trials Register of the Cochrane Infectious Diseases Group and Cochrane Controlled Trials Register.
34. Warrell DA, Looareesuwan S, Warrell MJ, et al. Dexamethasone proves deleterious in cerebral malaria. A double-blind trial in 100 comatose patients. *N Engl J Med* 1982;306:313–319.
35. Hoffman SL, Rustama D, Punjabi NH, et al. High-dose dexamethasone in quinine-treated patients with cerebral malaria: a double-blind, placebo-controlled trial. *J Infect Dis* 1988;158:325–331.
36. Meremikwu M, Smith HJ. Blood transfusion for treating malarial anaemia. In: The Cochrane Library, Issue 2, 2003. Oxford: Update Software. Search date 1999; primary sources Trials Register of the Cochrane Infectious Diseases Group, Embase, African Index Medicus, Lilacs, hand searches of reference lists, and contact with experts.
37. Riddle MS, Jackson JL, Sanders JW, et al. Exchange transfusion and an adjunct therapy in severe *Plasmodium falciparum* malaria: a meta-analysis. *Clin Infect Dis* 2002:34:1192–1198. Search date 2001; primary sources Medline, Embase, Fedrip, and the Cochrane Database of Clinical Trials.
38. Saddler M, Barry M, Ternouth I, et al. Treatment of severe malaria by exchange transfusion [letter]. *N Engl J Med* 1990;322:58.

Aika Omari
Dr (Specialist Registrar in Paediatrics)
Glan Clwyd Hospital
Rhyl, Denbighshire
UK

Paul Garner
Professor of Medicine
Liverpool School of Tropical Medicine
Liverpool
UK

Competing interests: None declared.

Malaria: uncomplicated, caused by *Plasmodium falciparum*

Search date September 2004

David Taylor-Robinson, Katharine Jones, and Paul Garner

QUESTIONS

INTERVENTIONS

Covered elsewhere in *Clinical Evidence*
Malaria: prevention in travellers, p 956
Malaria: severe, life threatening, p 977
See glossary G

Key Messages

Empirical treatment

- **Empirical treatment versus treatment of microscopy or rapid diagnostic test confirmed uncomplicated malaria** We found no RCTs comparing empirical treatment versus treatment of malaria confirmed by microscopy or rapid diagnostic tests.

Non-artemisinins v non-artemisinins

- **Chlorproguanil–dapsone (possibly more effective than sulfadoxine–pyrimethamine but with more serious adverse effects)** We found no RCTs reporting results for day 28 outcomes with chlorproguanil–dapsone compared with sulfadoxine–pyrimethamine. One RCT identified by a systematic review found lower rates of treatment failure at day 14 with chlorproguanil–dapsone compared with sulfadoxine–pyrimethamine. The review found no significant difference in rates of overall and serious adverse events between treatments. One RCT identified by the review found that a higher proportion of people taking chlorproguanil-dapsone had red blood cell disorders compared with sulfadoxine-pyrimethamine. The other RCT found a higher rate of adverse events leading to discontinuation of treatment with chlorproguanil–dapsone compared with sulfadoxine–pyrimethamine. We found no RCTs comparing a 3 day regimen of chlorproguanil–dapsone (with 2.0 mg chlorproguanil) versus amodiaquine.
- **Sulfadoxine–pyrimethamine plus amodiaquine (no proven benefit compared with sulfadoxine–pyrimethamine or amodiaquine alone)** One systematic review found no significant difference in rates of day 28 cure or adverse events between sulfadoxine–pyrimethamine plus amodiaquine and sulfadoxine–pyrimethamine alone although one RCT identified by the review found a shorter mean fever clearance time with the combination treatment compared with sulfadoxine–pyrimethamine alone. One additional RCT found higher rates of day 28 cure and mild to moderate adverse events with the combination treatment compared with sulfadoxine–pyrimethamine alone. One systematic review found no significant difference in cure rate at day 28, mean parasite clearance time, and fever clearance time between sulfadoxine–pyrimethamine plus amodiaquine and amodiaquine alone. Three subsequent RCTs found inconsistent results for cure rates and no significant difference in fever clearance times or rate of adverse events between combination treatment and amodiaquine alone. One RCT found that combination treatment reduced mean parasite clearance time compared with amodiaquine alone.
- **Sulfadoxine–pyrimethamine plus chloroquine (no proven benefit compared with sulfadoxine–pyrimethamine alone)** We found no RCTs reporting results for day 28 outcomes with sulfadoxine–pyrimethamine plus chloroquine compared with sulfadoxine–pyrimethamine alone. Two small RCTs provided insufficient evidence to determine whether there was any difference in rates of treatment failure at days 21 (first RCT) and 14 (second RCT) between treatments and gave no information on adverse events.

Artemisinins *v* non-artemisinins

- **Artesunate (3 days) plus amodiaquine (more effective than amodiaquine alone)** One systematic review found lower rates of parasitological failure at day 28 and gametocytaemia at day 7 with a 3 day regimen of artesunate plus amodiaquine compared with amodiaquine alone. It found no significant difference in serious adverse events between treatments. Amodiaquine is not used in South East Asia due to multidrug resistance.

- **Artesunate (3 days) plus sulfadoxine–pyrimethamine (more effective than sulfadoxine–pyrimethamine alone but limited evidence of effectiveness when compared with amodiaquine plus sulfadoxine–pyrimethamine)** One systematic review found that artesunate plus sulfadoxine–pyrimethamine reduced parasitological failure rate at day 28 and gametocytaemia rate at day 7 compared with sulfadoxine–pyrimethamine alone. It found no significant difference in adverse events between treatments. One additional RCT found no significant difference in treatment failure rate at day 28, mean fever clearance time, and adverse events between treatments. However, it found that combination treatment reduced gametocytaemia in people with an absence of gametocytes at study onset compared with sulfadoxine–pyrimethamine alone. One RCT found that artesunate (3 days) plus sulfadoxine–pyrimethamine significantly increased polymerase chain reaction unadjusted parasitological failure rate at day 28 compared with amodiaquine plus sulfadoxine–pyrimethamine. It found no significant difference in polymerase chain reaction adjusted results between treatments. Sulfadoxine-pyrimethamine and amodiaquine are not used in South East Asia due to multidrug resistance.
- **Artesunate (3 days) plus mefloquine (more effective than mefloquine alone)** Two systematic reviews found that artesunate plus mefloquine reduced treatment failure at day 28 compared with mefloquine alone. Two additional RCTs found that combination treatment reduced the proportion of people with gametocytaemia at day 21 compared with mefloquine alone. The first review reported major adverse effects in both groups, including acute psychosis, anxiety, palpitations, and sleep disturbance. The second review found no significant difference in the rates of serious adverse events between treatments. The additional RCTs found no serious adverse events. In South East Asia artesunate plus mefloquinine is used due to multidrug resistance. In regions where other antimalarial drugs have clinical effects, choosing artesunate plus mefloquine requires a trade off between the higher cure associated with mefloquine and its adverse effects.
- **Artemether–lumefantrine (6 doses)** We found no RCTs comparing a 6 dose regimen of artemether–lumefantrine versus chloroquine, amodiaquine, sulfadoxine–pyrimethamine, or mefloquine.
- **Artesunate (3 days) plus chlorproguanil–dapsone** We found no RCTs comparing a 3 day regimen of artesunate plus chlorproguanil–dapsone versus chlorproguanil–dapsone alone. Chloraproguanil-dapsone should not be used in South East Asia due to multidrug resistance.

Artemisinins: most effective regimen

- **Artemether–lumefantrine (6 doses) (more effective than a 4 dose regimen, but no significant difference compared with 3 day artesunate plus either mefloquine or amodiaquine)** One RCT found that six doses of artemether–lumefantrine given over 3 days increased treatment cure at 28 days compared with a 4 dose regimen. It found no serious adverse events and no adverse cardiovascular effects. One systematic review found no significant difference in parasitaemia at day 28 between six doses of artemether–lumefantrine and artesunate plus mefloquine. One RCT identified by the review found no significant difference in median parasite or fever clearance times between treatments. The review found no significant difference in mild to moderate or serious adverse events between treatments. One RCT found no significant difference in adequate clinical and parasitological response at day 14 between six doses of artemether–lumefantrine and artesunate plus amodiaquine. However, it found that six doses of artemether–lumefantrine reduced vomiting at days 1 and 2 compared with artesunate plus amodiaquine.

DEFINITION Malaria is a parasite transmitted by Anopheles mosquitoes. There are four types of human malaria, *falciparum*, *vivax*, *ovale*, and *malariae*, with *falciparum* being the most important cause of illness and death, and also known to develop resistance to antimalarial drugs.[2] This chapter covers treatments only for *falciparum* malaria and a population of adults and children living in endemic malarial areas, who, by definition, are exposed (seasonally or all year round) to malaria. It does not cover treatment of malaria in non-immune travellers, pregnant women, and people infected with HIV. Repeated falciparum malaria infections result in a temporary and incomplete immunity. Therefore, adults living in areas where malaria is common are often found to be "semi-immune", presenting with asymptomatic or chronic forms of malaria, with clinical episodes that are attenuated by their immunity. "**Severe malaria**" is defined as a form of symptomatic malaria with signs of vital organ disturbance (WHO 2000).[2] Any person with symptomatic malaria who does not develop any such signs is defined as having "**uncomplicated malaria**". This chapter assesses the effectiveness of antimalarial drugs only in people with uncomplicated malaria. Table 3, p 1008 provides an overview of the number of RCTs for each treatment and comparison included in this chapter.

INCIDENCE/ PREVALENCE Malaria is a major health problem in the tropics, with 300–500 million new clinical cases annually, most of them cases of uncomplicated malaria. An estimated 1.1–2.7 million deaths occur annually as a result of severe *falciparum* malaria.[2]

AETIOLOGY/ RISK FACTORS The malaria parasite is transmitted by infected Anopheles mosquitoes. Risk factors for developing the disease include exposure to infected mosquitoes (living in an endemic area; housing that allows mosquitoes to enter, and absence of mosquito nets; and living in an area where Anopheles mosquitoes can thrive). Risk factors in relation to severity of the illness relate to host immunity, determined mainly by exposure to the parasite, and therefore varying with level of transmission in the area and the age of the host. Malaria is uncommon in the first 6 months of life (fetal haemoglobin is protective); it is, however, common in children over 6 months of age. In areas of intense transmission, infection is attenuated by host immunity in older age groups, but with less intense transmission morbidity and mortality can be high in adults as well.

PROGNOSIS Uncomplicated malaria may progress to severe malaria, become chronic, or resolve with effective treatment or the development of improved immunity. The outcome is, therefore, dependent on host immunity and prompt access to effective treatment. In the absence of effective treatment, people with no or low immunity are at increased risk of developing severe malaria (see Malaria: severe, life threatening, p 977) resulting in high morbidity and mortality.

AIMS OF INTERVENTION To alleviate symptoms; to prevent progression to severe disease; to cure the infection; with minimal adverse effects.

OUTCOMES Clinical failureⒼ rate (defined as proportion of people with symptoms of malaria plus parasitaemia at or before day 28); clinical failure rate at time frames other than day 28 (where no 28 day evidence available); total failureⒼ rate (defined as clinical failure rate plus proportion of people with asymptomatic parasitaemia at day 28); parasitological failureⒼ rate (defined as proportion of people with parasitaemia at day 28), parasitological failure rate at time frames other than day 28 (where no 28 day evidence available), parasitological conversion rate, parasitological success rate, fever clearance time, gametocytaemiaⒼ rate, gametocyte clearance timeⒼ, rate of progression to severe disease, adverse effects requiring admission to hospital or discontinuation of treatment. Day 14 failure does not sufficiently predict treatment failureⒼ by day 28 in trials of drugs with a terminal elimination half life of more than a few days.[3] Some of the differences in rates of treatment failure at day 14 may result from differences in elimination kinetics between the drugs, whereas day 28 outcomes are less influenced by these effects. Therefore, we have identified day 28 treatment failure as the main outcome to assess drug effectiveness for this review. We reported results for outcomes of time frames shorter than 28 days only where no 28 day results were available.

METHODS *Clinical Evidence* search and appraisal September 2004. We searched the Cochrane Infectious Diseases Group's trials register, Cochrane Central Register of Controlled Trials (Central) published in The Cochrane Library (Issue 3, 2004), Medline from 1966, Embase from 1980, Lilacs from 1982, and used our systematic review and RCT search filters for MeSH headings for 'malaria' and key words including antimalarial drugs such as amodiaquine, artemether–lumefantrine (formerly benflumetol), artesunate, artesunate–mefloquine, chloroquine, chlorproguanil–dapsone, mefloquine, mefloquine–sulfadoxine–pyrimethamine, proguanil, and sulfadoxine–pyrimethamine. We conducted the search and identified the questions in collaboration with the World Health Organization Malaria Technical Guidelines Development Group who are currently developing evidence based guidelines for uncomplicated malaria treatment that draw explicitly on this chapter. Table 4, p 1009 outlines a possible pragmatic (but not evidence-based) decision making framework for applying the evidence. Policy changes for uncomplicated malaria in Africa now focus on how to replace current regimens, especially amodiaquine and sulfadoxine–pyrimethamine, which are now failing due to emerging drug resistance. This issue, however, is no longer relevant in South East Asia where high levels of multidrug resistance have been known to exist for some time and standard monotherapies are no longer in use. Therefore, South East Asia has been excluded from the question assessing these treatments (What are the effects of non-artemisinin treatments, compared with amodiaquine or sulfadoxine-pyrimethamine, in people living in endemic areas [excluding South East Asia]?, p 992).

QUESTION **What are the effects of empirical treatment of clinical malaria compared with treatment targeted to those with parasitaemia?** New

OPTION **EMPIRICAL TREATMENT** New

We found no RCTs comparing empirical treatment versus treatment of malaria confirmed by microscopy or rapid diagnostic tests.

Benefits: **Versus treatment of malaria confirmed by microscopy or rapid diagnostic tests:** We found no systematic review or RCTs comparing empirical treatment versus treatment of microscopy**G** or rapid diagnostic tests**G** confirmed malaria.

Harms: We found no RCTs.

Comment: Empirical treatment with antimalarial drugs in all people with fever used to be common in stable endemic areas. Current regimens are more expensive and so this policy is being questioned. However, testing everyone will also increase costs and burden health workers. In addition, there is a risk that treating only people with positive laboratory test results for malaria may delay treatment and people may default before test results can be obtained.

QUESTION **What are the effects of non-artemisinin treatments, compared with amodiaquine or sulfadoxine-pyrimethamine, in people living in endemic areas (excluding South East Asia)?** New

OPTION **SULFADOXINE–PYRIMETHAMINE PLUS CHLOROQUINE** New

We found no RCTs reporting results for day 28 outcomes with sulfadoxine–pyrimethamine plus chloroquine compared with sulfadoxine–pyrimethamine alone. Two small RCTs provided insufficient evidence to determine whether there was any difference in rates of treatment failure at days 21 (first RCT) and 14 (second RCT) between treatments and gave no information on adverse events.

Benefits: **Versus sulfadoxine–pyrimethamine:** We found one systematic review (search date 2001, no RCTs meeting our inclusion criteria, see comment below).[4] We found no additional RCTs meeting our inclusion criteria that reported on 28 day outcomes but found two RCTs with shorter follow up periods.[5,6] The first RCT (160 children and adults, Colombia) found a lower treatment failure**G** rate at day 21 with sulfadoxine-pyrimethanine plus chloroquine compared with sulfadoxine–pyrimethamine alone (11/64 [17%] with sulfadoxine-pyrimethanine plus chloroquine *v* 19/79 [26%] with sulfadoxine–pyrimethamine alone; no statistical data reported).[5] Similarly, the second RCT (71 children, Uganda) found a lower treatment failure rate at day 14 with sulfadoxine-pyrimethamine plus chloroquine compared with sulfadoxine–pyrimethamine alone (4/32 [13%] with combination treatment v 5/30 [17%] with sulfadoxine–pyrimethamine alone; no statistical data reported).[6]

Harms: **Versus sulfadoxine–pyrimethamine:** Neither RCT gave information on adverse events.[5,6]

Comment: The systematic review[4] identified two RCTs comparing sulfadoxine–pyrimethamine plus chloroquine versus sulfadoxine–pyrimethamine alone.[7,8] However, neither trial met our inclusion criteria. The first RCT (85 children aged < 12 years, Papua New Guinea) compared combination treatment using an atypical single dose chloroquine 10 mg/kg daily versus sulfadoxine–pyrimethamine alone.[7] The second RCT (405 children aged 1–10 years, The Gambia) had a high rate of loss to follow up (26% and 30%/treatment group).[8]

OPTION SULFADOXINE–PYRIMETHAMINE PLUS AMODIAQUINE New

One systematic review found no significant difference in rates of day 28 cure or adverse events between sulfadoxine–pyrimethamine plus amodiaquine and sulfadoxine–pyrimethamine alone although one RCT identified by the review found a shorter mean fever clearance time with the combination treatment compared with sulfadoxine–pyrimethamine alone. One additional RCT found higher rates of day 28 cure and mild to moderate adverse events with the combination treatment compared with sulfadoxine–pyrimethamine alone. One systematic review found no significant difference in cure rate at day 28, mean parasite clearance time, and fever clearance time between sulfadoxine–pyrimethamine plus amodiaquine and amodiaquine alone. Three subsequent RCTs found inconsistent results for cure rates and no significant difference in fever clearance times or rate of adverse events between combination treatment and amodiaquine alone. One RCT found that combination treatment reduced mean parasite clearance time compared with amodiaquine alone.

Benefits: **Versus sulfadoxine–pyrimethamine:** We found one systematic review (search date 2001,[4] 4 RCTs, 3 in Africa[9–11] and 1 in China,[12] 484 people) and one additional RCT (see table 1, p 1005).[13] Three RCTs identified by the systematic review found slightly higher cure rates at day 28 with sulfadoxine–pyrimethamine plus amodiaquine compared with sulfadoxine–pyrimethamine alone, although the overall difference did not reach significance.[4] Similarly, two RCTs (1 each in Uganda and China, overall 116 people) identified by the review found no significant difference in mean parasite clearance times between the two treatment groups.[9,12] However, the Chinese RCT (69 people) identified by the review found a significantly shorter mean fever clearance time with combination treatment compared with sulfadoxine–pyrimethamine alone.[12] The additional RCT (191 children aged under 10 years, Cameroon) found a significantly higher adequate clinical response with a negative smear at day 28 with sulfadoxine-pyrimethanine plus chloroquine compared with sulfadoxine–pyrimethamine alone.[13] Similarly, mean fever clearance time was significantly lower with combination treatment compared with sulfadoxine–pyrimethamine alone. **Versus amodiaquine:** We found one systematic review (search date 2001, 3 RCTs in China, Mozambique, and Uganda)[4] and three subsequent RCTs (see table 2, p 1006).[13–15] Two RCTs (150 people in China[12] and Mozambique[9]) identified by the review found higher parasitological cure rates at day 28 with sulfadoxine-pyrimethanine plus amodiaquine compared with amodiaquine alone. Due to the apparent heterogeneity between individual study results, the combined relative risk as assessed by several methods did not reach significance (see comment below).[9,12] The RCTs found a slightly shorter mean parasite clearance time with combination treatment compared with amodiaquine alone, although the difference did not reach significance. Similarly, the Chinese RCT (97 people) identified by the review found a shorter mean fever clearance time with combination treatment compared with amodiaquine alone, although the difference did not reach significance.[12] The first subsequent RCT (159 children aged 0.5–10.0 years, Nigeria) found no significant difference in cure rates at day 28 or mean fever clearance times between the two treatment groups.[14] However, mean parasite clearance time was significantly shorter with combination treatment compared with amodiaquine alone. The second subsequent RCT (127 children aged under 10 years, Cameroon) found a significantly higher adequate clinical response with negative smear at day 28 with combination treatment compared with amodiaquine alone.[13] However, the RCT found no significant difference in mean fever clearance time. The third subsequent RCT (235 children aged 6–59 months, Uganda) found a lower parasitological failure**G** rate at day 28 with combination treatment compared with amodiaquine alone although the results did not reach significance.[15]

Harms: **Versus sulfadoxine–pyrimethamine:** The Chinese RCT identified by the systematic review found no significant difference in the rate of adverse events between the two treatment groups (41.7% with sulfadoxine-pyrimethanine plus chloroquine *v* 42.9% with sulfadoxine–pyrimethamine alone; P value and absolute numbers not reported).[12] Sinus bradycardia and vomiting were the most frequent adverse events overall and were also more frequent with combination treatment compared with sulfadoxine–pyrimethamine alone (no statistical data reported). However, abdominal pain, headache, and dizziness were more common with sulfadoxine–pyrimethamine alone (no statistical data reported). The Ugandan RCT reported no serious adverse effects in either treatment group, whereas the RCT conducted in Mozambique gave no information on adverse events.[9,10] One RCT (400 people) measured haemoglobin and white blood cell count throughout the follow up period and found no significant difference between treatments.[10] The additional RCT found a significantly higher rate of fatigue, the most common adverse effect overall, with combination treatment compared with sulfadoxine–pyrimethamine (59/62 [95%] with combination treatment *v* 47/62 [76%] with sulfadoxine–pyrimethamine alone; $P < 0.05$).[13] Similarly, the RCT found higher rates of headache and vomiting with combination treatment compared with sulfadoxine–pyrimethamine alone (headache: 4/62 [6%] with combination treatment *v* 0/62 [0%] with sulfadoxine–pyrimethamine alone; $P < 0.05$; vomiting: 14/62 [23%] with combination treatment *v* 5/62 [8%] with sulfadoxine–pyrimethamine alone; $P < 0.05$). The RCT found an increased rate of pruritus with combination treatment compared with sulfadoxine–pyrimethamine alone, although the difference did not reach significance (9/62 [15%] with combination treatment *v* 3/62 [5%] with sulfadoxine–pyrimethamine alone; P value not reported). One person having sulfadoxine–pyrimethamine monotreatment presented with purulent vesicles in the thoracic region. **Versus amodiaquine:** The Chinese RCT reported a slightly higher rate of adverse events with combination treatment compared with amodiaquine alone (41.7% with combination treatment *v* 36% with amodiaquine alone; P value not reported).[12] Sinus bradycardia and vomiting were the most frequent adverse events overall and also more frequent with combination treatment compared with amodiaquine alone (no statistical data reported).

The Ugandan RCT reported no serious adverse effects in either treatment group, whereas the RCT conducted in Mozambique gave no information on adverse events.[9,10] The first subsequent RCT found three children with sleep disturbance secondary to pruritus but found no significant difference between treatments (2/75 with combination treatment *v* 1/82 with amodiaquine alone; P value not reported).[14] All other adverse reactions were reported as mild. The second subsequent RCT found no significant difference in fatigue between treatments (59/62 [95%] with combination treatment *v* 54/61 [89%] with amodiaquine alone; P value not reported) and cutaneous reactions (dermatitis in the hip area in 1 person and diffuse urticaria at day 5 in 1 person) in two people with amodiaquine alone (0/62 [0%] with combination treatment *v* 2/61[3%] with amodiaquine alone; P value not reported).[13] However, the third subsequent RCT reported both treatments to be well tolerated and found no serious adverse effects.[15]

Comment: **Versus amodiaquine:** The systematic review found significant heterogeneity between effect sizes for parasitological cure rates at day 28 between the two RCTs.[9,12] The reviewers found no significant difference between treatments when using a random effects model, or worst and best case scenarios assuming people lost to follow up were either all treatment failures🅖 or successes.[4]

OPTION CHLORPROGUANIL–DAPSONE (3 DOSE REGIMEN WITH 2.0 MG CHLORPROGUANIL) New

We found no RCTs reporting results for day 28 outcomes with chlorproguanil–dapsone compared with sulfadoxine–pyrimethamine. One RCT identified by a systematic review found lower rates of treatment failure at day 14 with chlorproguanil–dapsone compared with sulfadoxine–pyrimethamine. The review found no significant difference in rates of overall and serious adverse events between treatments. One RCT identified by the review found that a higher proportion of people taking chlorproguanil-dapsone had red blood cell disorders compared with sulfadoxine-pyrimethamine. The other RCT found a higher rate of adverse events leading to discontinuation of treatment with chlorproguanil–dapsone compared with sulfadoxine–pyrimethamine. We found no RCTs comparing a 3 day regimen of chlorproguanil–dapsone (with 2.0 mg chlorproguanil) versus amodiaquine.

Benefits: **Versus sulfadoxine–pyrimethamine:** We found one systematic review[16] (search date 2004, 2 multicentre RCTs in Africa[17,18], 2760 children) which identified only RCTs with a follow up period of 7 and 14 days. The first RCT (1850 children aged 1–10 years in Gabon, Kenya, Malawi, Nigeria, and Tanzania) identified by the review found a significantly lower rate of treatment failure🅖 at day 14 with chlorproguanil–dapsone compared with sulfadoxine–pyrimethamine (63/1366 [4.6%] with chlorproguanil–dapsone *v* 37/343 [10.8%] with sulfadoxine–pyrimethamine; RR 0.36, 95% CI 0.24 to 0.53, $P < 0.0001$).[17] It also found a significantly lower rate of parasitaemia at day 14 with chlorproguanil–dapsone compared with sulfadoxine–pyrimethamine (67/1480 [4.5%] with chlorproguanil–dapsone *v* 30/370 [8.1%] with sulfadoxine–pyrimethamine; RR 0.56, 95% CI 0.37 to 0.85, P value reported as significant). However, it found no significant difference in the proportion of people with fever (defined as temperature >37.5 °C) at day 14 between treatments (57/1480 [3.9%] with chlorproguanil–dapsone *v* 9/370 [2.4%] with sulfadoxine–pyrimethamine; RR 1.58, 95% CI 0.79 to 3.17). The second RCT identified by the review only reported rate of treatment failure at day 7.[18] **Versus amodiaquine:** We found no systematic review or RCTs comparing a 3 day regimen of chlorproguanil–dapsone (with 2.0 mg chlorproguanil) versus amodiaquine.

Harms: **Versus sulfadoxine–pyrimethamine:** The review found a wide range of adverse events in people taking chlorproguanil–dapsone or sulfadoxine–pyrimethamine, including vomiting, diarrhoea, anorexia, abdominal pain, pneumonia, progression to severe malaria, skin rash, red blood cell disorders (the most commonly reported adverse event overall), gastrointestinal disorders, and death.[16] It found no significant difference in rates of adverse events between treatments (727/1890 [38%] with chlorproguanil–dapsone *v* 222/789 [28%] with sulfadoxine–pyrimethamine; RR 0.97, 95% CI 0.87 to 1.09, P = 0.6). Both RCTs reported serious adverse events but found no significant difference in rates of serious adverse events between treatments (first RCT:[18] 30/410 [7%] with chlorproguanil–dapsone *v* 31/419 [7%] with sulfadoxine–pyrimethamine; RR 0.99, 95% CI 0.61 to 1.61; second RCT:[17] 16/1480 [1.1%] with chlorproguanil–dapsone *v* 4/370 [1.1%] with sulfadoxine–pyrimethamine; RR 1.00, 95% CI 0.34 to 2.97). The second RCT identified by the review listed safety among its primary outcomes and accordingly provided more data on adverse events than the other RCT.[17] It found that a significantly higher proportion of people had red blood cell disorders with chlorproguanil–dapsone compared with sulfadoxine–pyrimethamine (80/1480 [5.4%] with chlorproguanil–dapsone *v* 7/370 [1.9%] with sulfadoxine–pyrimethamine; RR 2.86, 95% CI 1.33 to 6.13). It also found a significantly higher mean level of methaemoglobin (reported as a percentage of total haemoglobin) at day 3 with chlorproguanil–dapsone compared with sulfadoxine–pyrimethamine (4.2%, 95% CI 3.8% to 4.6% in 301 people with chlorproguanil–dapsone *v* 0.4%, 95% CI 0.4% to 0.5% in 77 people with sulfadoxine–pyrimethamine; WMD 3.8%, 95% CI 3.4% to 4.2%). It found a higher proportion of people with clinically significant methaemoglobinaemia (defined as values > 10%) with chlorproguanil–dapsone compared with sulfadoxine–pyrimethamine, but this outcome was only evaluated at one site (Kenya) and the difference did not reach significance (RR 15.78, 95% CI 0.97 to 257.15). Anaemia, haemolysis, and haemolytic anaemia were slightly more frequent in people taking chlorproguanil–dapsone than in people taking sulfadoxine–pyrimethamine, although the differences did not reach significance (anaemia: 51/1480 [3.4%] with chlorproguanil–dapsone *v* 7/370 [1.9%] with sulfadoxine–pyrimethamine; RR 1.82, 95% CI 0.83 to 3.98; haemolysis: 6/1480 [0.4%] with chlorproguanil–dapsone *v* 0/370 [0%] with sulfadoxine–pyrimethamine; RR 3.26, 95% CI 0.18 to 57.68; haemolytic anaemia: 4/1480 [0.3%] with chlorproguanil–dapsone *v* 0/370 [0%] with sulfadoxine–pyrimethamine; RR 2.25, 95% CI 0.12 to 41.78). The first RCT found that 60/829 (7%) people developed severe malaria requiring admission to hospital, and reported one death.[18] It found no significant difference between the two treatments (RR 0.99, 95% CI 0.61 to 1.61). However, it found a significantly higher rate of adverse events leading to discontinuation of treatment with chlorproguanil–dapsone compared with sulfadoxine–pyrimethamine (RR 4.54, 95% CI 1.74 to 11.82). **Versus amodiaquine:** We found no systematic review or RCTs comparing a 3 day regimen of chlorproguanil–dapsone (with 2.0 mg chlorproguanil) versus amodiaquine.

Comment: **Versus sulfadoxine–pyrimethamine:** The second RCT identified by the systematic review defined serious adverse events as serious "Treatment Emergent Signs and Symptoms (TESS)".[17]

QUESTION **Are artemisinin combination treatments more effective than non-artemisinin treatments in people living in endemic areas?** New

OPTION **ARTESUNATE (3 DAYS) PLUS AMODIAQUINE** New

One systematic review found lower rates of parasitological failure at day 28 and gametocytaemia at day 7 with a 3 day regimen of artesunate plus amodiaquine compared with amodiaquine alone. It found no significant difference in serious adverse events between treatments. Amodiaquine is not used in South East Asia due to multidrug resistance.

Benefits: **Versus amodiaquine alone:** We found one systematic review (search date 2003, 3 RCTs in Africa, 936 people).[19] It found a significantly lower rate of parasitological failure**Ⓖ** at 28 days with a 3 day regimen of artesunate plus amodiaquine compared with amodiaquine alone (polymerase chain reaction**Ⓖ** unadjusted parasitological failure rate at day 28: 100/433 [23%] with artesunate plus amodiaquine *v* 169/437 [39%] with amodiaquine alone; OR 0.46, 95% CI 0.34 to 0.62, $P < 0.0001$). Similarly, it found that significantly lower proportion of people had gametocytaemia**Ⓖ** at day 7 with a 3 day regimen of artesunate plus amodiaquine compared with amodiaquine alone (13/385 [3%] with artesunate plus amodiaquine *v* 35/395 [9%] with amodiaquine alone; OR 0.36, 95% CI 0.15 to 0.85, $P < 0.0016$).

Harms: **Versus amodiaquine alone:** The review found similar rates of serious adverse events between the artesunate plus amodiaquine and amodiaquine alone.[19] One death occurred in the group taking amodiaquine alone but it was not associated with the drug.

Comment: Amodiaquine is not used in South East Asia due to multidrug resistance.

OPTION **ARTESUNATE (3 DAYS) PLUS SULFADOXINE–PYRIMETHAMINE** New

One systematic review found that artesunate plus sulfadoxine–pyrimethamine reduced parasitological failure rate at day 28 and gametocytaemia rate at day 7 compared with sulfadoxine–pyrimethamine alone. It found no significant difference in adverse events between treatments. One additional RCT found no significant difference in treatment failure rate at day 28, mean fever clearance time, and adverse events between treatments. However, it found that combination treatment reduced gametocytaemia in people with an absence of gametocytes at study onset compared with sulfadoxine–pyrimethamine alone. One RCT found that artesunate (3 days) plus sulfadoxine–pyrimethamine significantly increased polymerase chain reaction unadjusted parasitological failure rate at day 28 compared with amodiaquine plus sulfadoxine–pyrimethamine. It found no significant difference in polymerase chain reaction adjusted results between treatments. Sulfadoxine-pyrimethamine and amodiaquine are not used in South East Asia due to multidrug resistance.

Benefits: **Versus sulfadoxine–pyrimethamine alone:** We found one systematic review (search date 2003, 7 RCTs with 6 RCTs conducted in African children and 1 Peruvian RCT in children and adults, overall 3061 people)[19] and two additional RCTs.[20,21] The review (7 RCTs, 1852 people) found that artesunate plus sulfadoxine–pyrimethamine significantly reduced parasitological failure**Ⓖ** rate at day 28 compared with sulfadoxine–pyrimethamine alone (polymerase chain reaction [PCR**G**] unadjusted parasitological failure at day 28: 238/915 [26%] with artesunate plus sulfadoxine–pyrimethamine *v* 440/937 [47%] with sulfadoxine–pyrimethamine alone; OR 0.32, 95% CI 0.26 to 0.41, P < 0.0001). It also found that artesunate plus sulfadoxine–pyrimethamine significantly reduced the proportion of people with gametocytaemia**G** at day 7 (5 RCTs: 38/611 [6%] with artesunate plus sulfadoxine–pyrimethamine *v* 345/620 [56%] with sulfadoxine–pyrimethamine alone; OR 0.05, 95% CI 0.03 to 0.09, P < 0.0001). The first subsequent RCT (40 children in The Gambia) was a small pilot safety trial comparing combination treatment versus sulfadoxine–pyrimethamine alone.[20] It found that a lower proportion of children had positive smear at day 28 with combination treatment compared with sulfadoxine–pyrimethamine alone (PCR unadjusted rate of positive smear: 4/20 [20%] with artesunate plus sulfadoxine–pyrimethamine *v* 6/17 [35%] with sulfadoxine–pyrimethamine alone; PCR adjusted rate of positive smear [excluding untyped people]: 1/17 [6%] with artesunate plus sulfadoxine–pyrimethamine *v* 3/14 [21%] with sulfadoxine–pyrimethamine alone; P value not reported). One child in each group had gametocytaemia at enrolment. The RCT found that combination treatment reduced the proportion of children with gametocytaemia at some stage of the study compared with sulfadoxine–pyrimethamine alone although the difference did not reach significance (gametocytaemia adjusted for the number of blood films obtained for each child: 4/20 [20%] with artesunate plus sulfadoxine–pyrimethamine *v* 14/20 [70%] with sulfadoxine–pyrimethamine alone; OR 3.3, P = 0.057). Gametocytes appeared later and in higher density with sulfadoxine–pyrimethamine alone.[20] The second RCT (105 adults and children, Indonesia) found no significant difference in treatment failure**G** at day 28 with combination treatment (PCR unadjusted treatment failure at day 28: 5/48 [10%] with artesunate plus sulfadoxine–pyrimethamine *v* 11/50 [22%] with sulfadoxine–pyrimethamine alone; P = 0.12; PCR adjusted treatment failure at day 28: 2/45 [4%] with artesunate plus sulfadoxine–pyrimethamine *v* 7/46 [15%] with sulfadoxine–pyrimethamine alone; RR 0.29, 95% CI 0.06 to 1.33, P = 0.16).[21] It found a shorter mean fever clearance time with combination treatment compared with sulfadoxine–pyrimethamine alone although the difference did not reach significance (1.3 days with artesunate plus sulfadoxine–pyrimethamine *v* 1.7 days with sulfadoxine–pyrimethamine alone; P = 0.08). It also found that combination treatment significantly reduced mean parasite clearance time compared with sulfadoxine–pyrimethamine alone (1.4 days with artesunate plus sulfadoxine–pyrimethamine *v* 2.0 days with sulfadoxine–pyrimethamine alone; P < 0.0001). Although a greater proportion of people with combination treatment had gametocytaemia at study onset (7/47 [15%] with artesunate plus sulfadoxine–pyrimethamine *v* 2/46 [4%] with sulfadoxine–pyrimethamine alone, P value not reported), the RCT found that by days 7 and 14 combination treatment had reduced gametocytaemia to half the levels with sulfadoxine–pyrimethamine although the difference did not reach significance (day 7: RR 0.47, 95% CI 0.21 to 1.05; day 14: RR 0.48, 95% CI 0.21 to 1.09; P value not reported). In people with an absence of gametocytes at study onset, gametocytaemia at days 7 and 14 was significantly lower with combination treatment compared with sulfadoxine–pyrimethamine alone (day 7: RR 0.17, 95% CI 0.04 to 0.70; day 14: RR 0.18, 95% CI 0.04 to 0.77; P value not reported). **Versus amodiaquine plus sulfadoxine–pyrimethamine:** We found no systematic review but found one RCT (276 children aged

6–59 months, Uganda, 2001) comparing artesunate (3 days) plus sulfadoxine–pyrimethamine versus amodiaquine plus sulfadoxine–pyrimethamine.[15] It found that artesunate (3 days) plus sulfadoxine–pyrimethamine significantly increased parasitological failure at day 28 compared with amodiaquine plus sulfadoxine–pyrimethamine (PCR unadjusted treatment failure at day 28: 42/144 [29%] with artesunate (3 days) plus sulfadoxine–pyrimethamine *v* 22/132 [17%] with amodiaquine plus sulfadoxine–pyrimethamine; OR 0.49, 95% CI 0.27 to 0.87; P value not reported). However, it found no significant difference in treatment failure rates at day 28 between treatments, once new infections were excluded (PCR adjusted [including untyped] treatment failure at day 28: 17/132 [13%] with artesunate (3 days) plus sulfadoxine–pyrimethamine *v* 29/134 [22%] with amodiaquine plus sulfadoxine–pyrimethamine; OR 0.59, 95% CI 0.29 to 1.18, P = 0.14).

Harms: **Versus sulfadoxine–pyrimethamine alone:** The review found no significant difference in rates of serious adverse events between treatments (results tabulated by study, no statistical data reported).[19] One death occurred in each treatment group but neither of these was attributed to study medication by the authors. The pilot safety trial reported both drugs to be well tolerated.[20] It found no clinically significant adverse events in either group during the 28 days of follow up attributable to study medication. The second subsequent RCT found no significant difference in rates of "any adverse reaction" between treatments (RR 3.91, 95% CI 0.45 to 33.72, P = 0.37).[21] All reactions were mild and resolved without treatment. **Versus amodiaquine plus sulfadoxine–pyrimethamine:** The RCT gave no information on adverse events.[15]

Comment: Sulfadoxine–pyrimethamine and amodiquine are not used in South East Asia due to multidrug resistance.

OPTION ARTESUNATE (3 DAYS) PLUS MEFLOQUINE New

Two systematic reviews found that artesunate plus mefloquine reduced treatment failure at day 28 compared with mefloquine alone. Two additional RCTs found that combination treatment reduced the proportion of people with gametocytaemia at day 21 compared with mefloquine alone. The first review reported major adverse effects in both groups, including acute psychosis, anxiety, palpitations, and sleep disturbance. The second review found no significant difference in the rates of serious adverse events between treatments. The additional RCTs found no serious adverse events. In South East Asia artesunate plus mefloquinine is used due to multidrug resistance. In regions where other non-artimisinins are still effective, choosing artesunate plus mefloquinine involves a trade off between the higher cure associated with mefloquine and its adverse effects.

Benefits: **Versus mefloquine alone:** We found two systematic reviews (search date 1999, 10 RCTs, 2141 people[22]; search date 2003, 2 RCTs, 709 people[19]) and two additional RCTs.[23,24] The RCTs identified by the first systematic review used varying treatment regimens.[22] Seven of the 10 RCTs gave the same dose of mefloquine to both treatment groups within each study, whereas the remaining three studies increased the dose of mefloquine when it was given alone.[22] The first review found that a significantly higher proportion of people had parasite clearance at day 28 with artesunate plus mefloquine compared with mefloquine alone (OR 4.03, 95% CI 1.58 to 10.23). The difference remained significant if people lost to follow up were included as failures (no statistical data reported). The second review also found that artesunate plus mefloquine significantly reduced parasitological failure**G** at day 28 compared with mefloquine alone (2 RCTs, 709 people: polymerase chain reaction unadjusted: OR 0.09, 95% CI 0.05 to 0.18).[19] The two additional RCTs used a lower dose of mefloquine (15 mg/kg) compared with the one used in the studies included in the review (25 mg/kg).[23,24] The first additional RCT (115 adults and children, Peru) found no recurrence of parasitaemia at 28 days with either treatment (0/51 with artesunate plus mefloquine *v* 0/47 with mefloquine alone).[24] It also found that combination treatment significantly reduced the proportion of people with gametocytaemia**G** at days 3, 7, 14, and 21 compared with mefloquine alone (results presented graphically, P < 0.05). Among people with no gametocytaemia in their blood smears**G** on enrolment, the RCT found that combination treatment significantly reduced the proportion of people with gametocytaemia compared with mefloquine alone at day 3 (7.1% with artesunate plus mefloquine *v* 31.7% with mefloquine alone; P = 0.01), day 7 (0% with artesunate plus mefloquine *v* 26.8% with mefloquine alone; P = 0.001), and day 14 (0% with artesunate plus mefloquine *v* 17.1% with mefloquine alone; P = 0.005). The second additional RCT (149 adults and children, Bolivia) found no treatment failures**G** at day 28 with either treatment (0/70 with artesunate plus mefloquine *v* 0/73 with mefloquine alone).[23] On enrolment, the RCT found no significant difference in the proportion of people with gametocytaemia between treatments (33/73 [45.2%] with artesunate plus mefloquine *v* 29/70 [41.4%] with mefloquine alone). However, it found that combination treatment significantly reduced the proportion of people with gametocytaemia at days 7, 14, 21, and 28 compared with mefloquine alone (results presented graphically, P < 0.05). Among people with no gametocytaemia in their blood smears on enrolment, the RCT found that combination treatment significantly reduced the proportion of people with gametocytaemia compared with mefloquine alone at day 7 (55.5% with artesunate plus mefloquine *v* 100.0% with mefloquine alone; P = 0.009), at day 14 (27.8% with artesunate plus mefloquine *v* 83.3% with mefloquine alone; RR 4.33; 95% CI 1.18 to 15.86; P = 0.007), at day 21 (0% with artesunate plus mefloquine *v* 75.0% with mefloquine alone; RR 4.00, 95% CI 1.50 to 10.66, P < 0.0001), and at day 28 (0% with artesunate plus mefloquine *v* 41.7% with mefloquine alone; RR 1.71, 95% CI 1.06 to 2.77, P = 0.005)

Harms: **Versus mefloquine alone:** The first systematic review reported major adverse effects in both groups.[22] One RCT identified by the review reported that one person with mefloquine monotreatment suffered acute psychosis, recovering without additional treatment. Another RCT identified by the review reported that one person with artesunate plus mefloquine suffered acute psychosis, and another developed a depressive syndrome. Both resolved untreated without discontinuation of treatment. A third RCT identified by the review found that one person suffered anxiety, palpitations, and sleep disturbance 1 week after starting treatment with artesunate plus mefloquine, and one person with mefloquine suffered psychosis, delusions, and hallucinations requiring admission to hospital and sedation. The other review found no significant difference in the rates of serious adverse events between treatments.[19] Neither of the additional RCTs found serious adverse events.[23,24] Similarly, they found no new symptoms and no increase in the severity of pre-existing symptoms after treatment onset.

Comment: In South East Asia artesunate plus mefloquine is used due to multidrug resistance. In regions where other non-artemisinins are still effective, choosing artesunate plus mefloquine involves a trade off between the higher cure associated with mefloquine and its adverse effects.

OPTION ARTEMETHER–LUMEFANTRINE (6 DOSES) *New*

We found no RCTs comparing a 6 dose regimen of artemether–lumefantrine versus chloroquine, amodiaquine, sulfadoxine–pyrimethamine, or mefloquine.

Benefits: We found no systematic review and no RCTs comparing a 6 dose regimen of artemether–lumefantrine versus chloroquine, amodiaquine, sulfadoxine–pyrimethamine, or mefloquine.

Harms: We found no RCTs.

Comment: None.

OPTION ARTESUNATE (3 DAYS) PLUS CHLORPROGUANIL–DAPSONE *New*

We found no RCTs comparing a 3 day regimen of artesunate plus chlorproguanil–dapsone versus chlorproguanil–dapsone alone. Chloraproguanil-dapsone should not be used in South East Asia due to multidrug resistance.

Benefits: We found no systematic review and no RCTs comparing a 3 day regimen of artesunate plus chlorproguanil–dapsone versus chlorproguanil–dapsone alone.

Harms: We found no RCTs.

Comment: According to consensus opinion, chlorproguanil–dapsone should only be used in combination with artemisinin derivatives. Chlorproguanil–dapsone should not be used in South East Asia due to multidrug resistance.

QUESTION **Which artemisinin combination treatment is most effective in people living in endemic areas?** *New*

OPTION ARTEMETHER–LUMEFANTRINE (6 DOSES) *New*

One RCT found that six doses of artemether–lumefantrine given over 3 days increased treatment cure at 28 days compared with a 4 dose regimen. It found no serious adverse events and no adverse cardiovascular effects. One systematic review found no significant difference in parasitaemia at day 28 between six doses of artemether–lumefantrine and artesunate plus mefloquine. One RCT identified by the review found no significant difference in median parasite or fever clearance times between treatments. The review found no significant difference in mild to moderate or serious adverse events between treatments. One RCT found no significant difference in adequate clinical and parasitological response at day 14 between six doses of artemether–lumefantrine and artesunate plus amodiaquine. However, it found that six doses of artemether–lumefantrine reduced vomiting at days 1 and 2 compared with artesunate plus amodiaquine.

Benefits: **Versus artemether–lumefantrine (4 doses):** We found no systematic review but found one RCT comparing a 6 dose regimen versus a 4 dose regimen of artemether–lumefantrine.[25] The RCT (238 adults and children, Thailand) found a significantly higher rate of treatment cure at 28 days with the 6 dose regimen given over 3 days compared with the 4 dose regimen (polymerase chain reaction [PCR**G**] unadjusted treatment cure rate for intention to treat**G** population at day 28: 96/118 [81%], 95% CI 73.1% to 87.9% with 6 dose regimen *v* 85/120 [71%], 95% CI 61.8% to 78.8% with 4 dose regimen; $P < 0.001$; PCR adjusted treatment cure rate for evaluable population: 93/96 [97%],

95% CI 91.1% to 99.4% with 6 dose regimen *v* 85/102 [83%], 95% CI 74.7% to 90.0% with 4 dose regimen; P < 0.001). **Versus artesunate (3 days) plus mefloquine:** We found one systematic review (search date 2004, 2 RCTs, 419 people, Thailand).[26] The review found a higher proportion of people with parasitaemia at day 28 with artemether–lumefantrine compared with artesunate plus mefloquine although the pooled difference did not reach significance (PCR unadjusted parasitaemia rate: 11/289 [4%] with artemether–lumefantrine *v* 0/100 [0%] with artesunate plus mefloquine; RR 4.20, 95% CI 0.55 to 31.93, P = 0.2; PCR adjusted parasitaemia rate: 9/289 [3%] with artemether–lumefantrine *v* 0/100 [0%] with artesunate plus mefloquine; RR 3.50 95% CI 0.45 to 27.03, P = 0.2; see comment below). The first RCT identified by the review found no significant difference in median parasite clearance time between artemether–lumefantrine and artesunate plus mefloquine (29 hours, 95% CI 29 hours to 32 hours in 164 people with artemether–lumefantrine *v* 31 hours, 95% CI 26 hours to 31 hours in 55 people with artesunate plus mefloquine; P value not reported).[27] Similarly, it found no significant difference in median fever clearance time (29 hours, 95% CI 23 hours to 37 hours in 76 people with artemether–lumefantrine *v* 23 hours, 95% CI 15 hours to 30 hours in 29 people with mefloquine plus artesunate; P value not reported) or in median gametocyte clearance timeⒼ between treatments (72 hours, 95% CI 34 hours to 163 hours in 26 people with artemether–lumefantrine *v* 85 hours, 95% CI 46 hours to 160 hours in 10 people with mefloquine plus artesunate; P value not reported). The systematic review did not report results for any other outcomes from the second RCT. **Versus artesunate (3 days) plus amodiaquine:** We found no systematic review and no RCTs with a 28 day follow up period but found one RCT (295 children aged < 5 years, Burundi, 2001–2002) with a 14 day follow up period.[28] The RCT found no significant difference in the proportion of people with adequate clinical and parasitological responseⒼ at day 14 between treatments (140/141 [99.3%], 95% CI 97.9% to 100.0% with artemether–lumefantrine *v* 142/149 [95.3%], 95% CI 91.9% to 98.7% with artesunate plus amodiaquine; P value not reported).

Harms: **Versus artemether–lumefantrine (4 doses):** The RCT reported all adverse events to be mild or moderate in severity and possibly attributable to malaria.[25] It found no adverse cardiovascular effects. It found four serious adverse events but the authors did not consider these to be related to treatment. The RCT found no changes in QRS duration and PR interval during treatment in 66 people who had regular electrocardiographic monitoring. Similarly, it found no differences in mean and median QTc values between treatments. **Versus artesunate (3 days) plus mefloquine:** The systematic review found fewer mild to moderate adverse events with artemether–lumefantrine compared with artesunate plus mefloquine although the differences did not reach significance (nausea: 4/150 [3%] with artemether–lumefantrine *v* 6/50 [12%] with artesunate plus mefloquine; vomiting: 4/150 [3%] with artemether–lumefantrine *v* 5/50 [10%] with artesunate plus mefloquine; sleep disorders: 2/150 [1%] with artemether–lumefantrine *v* 8/50 [16%] with artesunate plus mefloquine; dizziness: 8/150 [5%] with artemether–lumefantrine *v* 18/50 [36%] with artesunate plus mefloquine; P values not reported).[26] It found no significant difference in the proportion of people with severe adverse events (1 person with each treatment). One person with artesunate plus mefloquine developed urticaria resulting in discontinuation of treatment, and one person with artemether–lumefantrine developed fever and coma. **Versus artesunate (3 days) plus amodiaquine:** The RCT found no significant difference in adverse events between treatments other than vomiting, which was significantly less frequent on days 1 and 2 with artemether–lumefantrine compared with artesunate plus amodiaquine (day 1: 5% with artemether–lumefantrine *v* 13% with artesunate plus amodiaquine; day 2: 1% with artemether–lumefantrine *v* 5% with artesunate plus amodiaquine; P values not reported).[28]

Comment: **Versus artesunate (3 days) plus mefloquine:** The results of the systematic review on rates of parasitological treatment failure**G** need to be treated with caution as the review reported significant heterogeneity between the RCTs and the pooled results were too imprecise to determine which treatment was more effective (first RCT:[27] RR 5.19, 95% CI 0.30 to 89.40; second RCT:[25] RR 3.20, 95% CI 0.18 to 58.34).[26] The review found a large overlap of confidence intervals for adverse events which makes it unlikely that a significant difference exists between treatments. However, the RCTs were too small to evaluate this outcome.

GLOSSARY

Adequate clinical and parasitological response According to the World Health Organization definition, absence of parasitaemia at day 28 irrespective of axillary temperature and without previously meeting any of the WHO criteria for early or late treatment failure, or late parasitological failure.[29]

Blood smear Blood taken for malaria microscopy.

Clinical failure Symptoms of malaria with parasitaemia on or before day 28.

Gametocytaemia Microscopic evidence of gametocytes in the blood.

Gametocyte clearance time Time to clearance of gametocytes from the blood after treatment.

Intention to treat A strategy for the analysis of RCTs which compares results for all people in the groups to which they were originally randomly assigned, irrespective of whether they completed the study or not.

Microscopy confirmed malaria Symptomatic people with malaria parasitaemia.

Parasitological conversion Clearance of parasitaemia within a specified time after treatment.

Parasitological failure Parasitaemia detected within a specified time after treatment.

Parasitological success Absence of parasitaemia within a specified time after treatment.

Polymerase chain reaction (PCR) adjusted treatment failure rate Parasitaemia on or by day 28 may be due to recrudescence of the original infection, or caused by a new infection. PCR adjusted values exclude parasitaemia caused by a new infection.

Rapid diagnostic tests Assist in the diagnosis of malaria by providing evidence of the presence of malaria parasites in human blood.

Total failure People presenting with clinical failure or with parasitaemia on day 28.

Treatment failure This term is used loosely in the literature, but generally means total failure, or failure (clinical or parasitological) within the period of follow up. The World Health Organization modified definitions of treatment failure in 2003 to include late parasitological failures.[29]

REFERENCES

1. Olliaro P, Mussano P. Amodiaquine for treating malaria. In: The Cochrane Library, Issue 2, 2003. Oxford: Update Software.
2. World Health Organization. WHO expert committee on malaria (twentieth report). *World Health Organ Tech Rep Ser* 2000;892:1–74 (available online at http://mosquito.who.int/docs/ecr20_toc.htm ; last accessed 16 February 2005).
3. Stepniewska K, Taylor WR, Mayxay M, et al. *In vivo* assessment of drug efficacy against *Plasmodium falciparum* malaria: duration of follow-up. *Antimicrob Agents Chemother* 2004;48:4271–4280.
4. McIntosh HM. Chloroquine or amodiaquine combined with sulfadoxine–pyrimethamine for treating uncomplicated malaria. In: The Cochrane Library, Issue 4, 2004. Chichester, UK: John Wiley & Sons Ltd. Search date 2001; primary sources The Cochrane Infectious Diseases Group trials register, the Cochrane Controlled Trials Register, Medline, Embase, Science Citation Index, African Index Medicus, and Lilacs plus contact with experts in the field and drug companies.
5. Blair S, Lopez ML, Pineros JG, et al. Therapeutic efficacy of 3 treatment protocols for non-complicated *Plasmodium falciparum* malaria, Antioquia, Colombia, 2002. *Biomedica* 2003;23:318–327. [In Spanish]
6. Ogwang S, Engl M, Vigl M, et al. Clinical and parasitological response of *Plasmodium falciparum* to chloroquine and sulfadoxine/pyrimethamine in rural Uganda. *Wien Klin Wochenschr* 2003;115(suppl):45–49.
7. Darlow B, Vrbova H, Gibney S, et al. Sulfadoxine–pyrimethamine for the treatment of

acute malaria in children in Papua New Guinea. I. *Plasmodium falciparum. Am J Trop Med Hyg* 1982;31:1–9.
8. 7. Bojang KA, Schneider G, Forck S, et al. A trial of Fansidar plus chloroquine or Fansidar alone for the treatment of uncomplicated malaria in Gambian children. *Trans R Soc Trop Med Hyg* 1998;92:73–76.
9. Schapira A, Schwalbach JF. Evaluation of four therapeutic regimens for falciparum malaria in Mozambique, 1986. *Bull World Health Organ* 1988;66:219–226.
10. Staedke SG, Kamya MR, Dorsey G, et al. Amodiaquine, sulfadoxine/pyrimethamine, and combination therapy for treatment of uncomplicated malaria in Kampala, Uganda: a randomised trial. *Lancet* 2001;358:368–374.
11. Dinis par DV, Schapira A. Comparative study of sulfadoxine–pyrimethamine and amodiaquine + sulfadoxine–pyrimethamine for the treatment of malaria caused by chloroquine-resistant *Plasmodium falciparum* in Maputo, Mozambique. *Bull Soc Path Ex* 1990;83:521–528. [In French]
12. Huang QL, Ouyang WC, Zhou JX, et al. Efficacy of amodiaquine, Fansidar and their combination in the treatment of chloroquine resistant falciparum malaria. *Zhongguo Ji Sheng Chong Xue Yu Ji Sheng Chong Bing Za Zhi* 1988;6:292–295. [In Chinese]
13. Basco LK, Same-Ekobo A, Ngane VF, et al. Therapeutic efficacy of sulfadoxine–pyrimethamine, amodiaquine and the sulfadoxine–pyrimethamine–amodiaquine combination against uncomplicated *Plasmodium falciparum* malaria in young children in Cameroon. *Bull World Health Organ* 2002;80:538–545.
14. Sowunmi A. A randomized comparison of chloroquine, amodiaquine and their combination with pyrimethamine–sulfadoxine in the treatment of acute, uncomplicated, *Plasmodium falciparum* malaria in children. *Ann Trop Med Parasitol* 2002;96:227–238.
15. Rwagacondo CE, Niyitegeka F, Sarushi J, et al. Efficacy of amodiaquine alone and combined with sulfadoxine–pyrimethamine and of sulfadoxine pyrimethamine combined with artesunate. *Am J Trop Med Hyg* 2003;68:743–747.
16. Bukirwa H, Garner P, Critchley J. Chlorproguanil–dapsone for treating uncomplicated malaria. In: The Cochrane Library, Issue 4, 2004. Chichester, UK: John Wiley & Sons, Ltd. Search date 2004; primary sources Cochrane Infectious Disease Group trials register, the Cochrane Controlled Trials Register, Medline, Embase, Science Citation Index, African Indewx Medicus and Lilacs, and contact with experts in the field and drug companies.
17. Alloueche A, Bailey W, Barton S, et al. Comparison of chlorproguanil–dapsone with sulfadoxine–pyrimethamine for the treatment of uncomplicated falciparum malaria in young African children: double-blind randomised controlled trial. *Lancet* 2004;363:1843–1848.
18. Sulo J, Chimpeni P, Hatcher J, et al. Chlorproguanil–dapsone versus sulfadoxine–pyrimethamine for sequential episodes of uncomplicated falciparum malaria in Kenya and Malawi: a randomised clinical trial. *Lancet* 2002;360:1136–1143.
19. Adjuik M, Babiker A, Garner P, et al. Artesunate combinations for treatment of malaria: meta-analysis. *Lancet* 2004;363:9–17. Search date 2003; primary sources WHO/TDR sponsored studies, Medline, Cochrane Controlled Trials Register, and contact with investigators of published trials.
20. Doherty JF, Sadiq AD, Bayo L, et al. A randomized safety and tolerability trial of artesunate plus sulfadoxine–pyrimethamine versus sulfadoxine–pyrimethamine alone for the treatment of uncomplicated malaria in Gambian children. *Trans R Soc Trop Med Hyg* 1999;93:543–546.
21. Tjitra E, Suprianto S, Currie BJ, et al. Therapy of uncomplicated falciparum malaria: a randomized trial comparing artesunate plus sulfadoxine–pyrimethamine versus sulfadoxine–pyrimethamine alone in Irian Jaya, Indonesia. *Am J Trop Med Hyg* 2001;65:309–317.
22. McIntosh HM, Olliaro P. Artemisinin derivatives for treating uncomplicated malaria. In: The Cochrane Library, Issue 4, 2004. Chichester, UK: John Wiley & Sons Ltd. Search date 1999; primary sources Cochrane Infectious Diseases Group trials register, Cochrane Controlled Trials Register, Medline, Embase, Science Citation Index, Lilacs, African Index Medicus; conference abstracts plus hand searches of reference lists of relevant articles and contact with organisations, researchers in the field and drug companies.
23. Avila JC, Villaroel R, Marquino W, et al. Efficacy of mefloquine and mefloquine–artesunate for the treatment of uncomplicated *Plasmodium falciparum* malaria in the Amazon region of Bolivia. *Trop Med Int Health* 2004;9:217–221.
24. Marquino W, Huilca M, Calampa C, et al. Efficacy of mefloquine and a mefloquine–artesunate combination therapy for the treatment of uncomplicated *Plasmodium falciparum* malaria in the Amazon Basin of Peru. *Am J of Trop Med Hyg* 2003;68:608–612.
25. Vugt MV, Wilairatana P, Gemperli B, et al. Efficacy of six doses of artemether–lumefantrine (benflumetol) in multidrug-resistant *Plasmodium falciparum* malaria. *Am J Trop Med Hyg* 1999;60:936–942.
26. Omari AA, Gamble C, Garner P. Artemether–lumefantrine for treating uncomplicated falciparum malaria. In: The Cochrane Library, Issue 4, 2004. Chichester, UK: John Wiley & Sons Ltd. Search date 2004, primary sources Cochrane Infectious Diseases Group trials register, the Cochrane Controlled Trials Register, Medline, Embase, Science Citation Index, African Index Medicus and Lilacs and contact with experts in the field and drug companies.
27. Lefevre G, Looareesuwan S, Treeprasertsuk S, et al. A clinical and pharmacokinetic trial of six doses of artemether–lumefantrine for multidrug-resistant *Plasmodium falciparum* malaria in Thailand. *Am J Trop Med Hyg* 2001;64:247–256.
28. Ndayiragije A, Niyungeko D, Karenzo J, et al. Efficacy of therapeutic combinations with artemisinin derivatives in the treatment of non complicated malaria in Burundi. *Trop Med Int Health* 2004;9:673–679. [In French]
29. World Health Organization. Assessment and monitoring of antimalarial drug efficacy for the treatment of uncomplicated malaria. 2003. http://mosquito.who.int/resistance.html (last accessed 16 February 2005).

David Taylor-Robinson
Liverpool School of Tropical Medicine, Liverpool, UK

Katharine Jones
Liverpool School of Tropical Medicine, Liverpool, UK

Paul Garner
Liverpool School of Tropical Medicine, Liverpool, UK

Competing interests: None declared.

TABLE 1 **RCTs comparing sulfadoxine-pyrimethamine plus amodiaquine versus sulfadoxine/pyrimethamine alone.**[4,13]

References/countries of origin	Outcome	Results
3 RCTs identified by the systematic review/2 in Africa, 1 in China[4]	Parasitological cure rate at day 28	**Overall difference:** RR 1.09, 95% CI 0.99 to 1.19; P = 0.07 (no significant difference)
1 RCT in Cameroon[13]	Adequate clinical response with negative smear at day 28	59/59 [100%] with sulfadoxine–pyrimethamine plus amodiaquine *v* 50/59 [85%] with sulfadoxine–pyrimethamine alone; P < 0.05
2 RCTs identified by the systematic review in Uganda and China[4]	Parasite clearance time (mean and standard deviation)	**Weighted mean difference:** +2.04 hours, 95% CI –4.13 hours to +8.21 hours; P = 0.5 (no significant difference)
1 RCT identified by the systematic review in China[4]	Fever clearance time	**Weighted mean difference in fever clearance time:** –30.40 hours, 95% CI –43.79 hours to –17.01 hours; P < 0.0001
1 RCT in Cameroon[13]		28.4 hours (95% CI 15.7 hours to 41.1 hours, range 13.7 hours to 70.2 hours) with sulfadoxine–pyrimethamine plus amodiaquine *v* 41.2 hours (95% CI 21.2 hours to 61.2 hours, range 14.7 hours to 94 hours) with sulfadoxine–pyrimethamine alone; P < 0.05

TABLE 2 RCTs comparing sulfadoxine-pyrimethamine plus amodiaquine versus amodiaquine alone.[4,13–15]

References/countries of origin	Outcome	Results
2 RCTs identified by the systematic review in China and Mozambique[4]	Parasitological cure rate at day 28	**Individual results:** China: 46/46 [100%] with combination treatment *v* 32/49 [65%] with amodiaquine alone; RR 1.53, 95% CI 1.25 to 1.88; Mozambique: 22/22 [100%] with combination treatment *v* 8/33 [24%] with amodiaquine alone; RR 4.13, 95% 2.26 to 7.54; **Combined relative risk:** RR 2.43, 95% CI 0.82 to 7.20 (no significant difference)
1 RCT in Nigeria[14]		75/75 [100%] with combination treatment *v* 81/82 [99%] with amodiaquine alone; P value not given (no significant difference)
1 RCT in Uganda[15]	Parasitological failure (non-PCR-corrected)	**PCR unadjusted failure rate:** 22/131[17%] with combination treatment *v* 24/103 [23%] with amodiaquine alone; **PCR adjusted (including untyped) failure rate:** 17/131 [13%] with combination treatment *v* 18/103 [17%] with amodiaquine alone Results reported as not significant
1 RCT in Cameroon[4]	Adequate clinical response with negative smear at day 28	59/59 [100%] with combination treatment *v* 51/59 [86%] with amodiaquine alone; $P < 0.05$
2 RCTs identified by the systematic review in China and Mozambique[4]	Mean parasite clearance time	**Weighted mean difference:** –5.96 hours, 95% CI –11.95 hours to +0.04 hours; $P = 0.05$ (slightly shorter with combination treatment)

TABLE 2 continued

References/countries of origin	Outcome	Results
1 RCT in Nigeria[14]		2.1 days (95% CI 1.4 days to 2.9 days, range 1 day to 4 days) with combination treatment *v* 2.6 days (95% CI 1.9 days to 3.3 days, range 1 days to 5 days) with amodiaquine alone; P < 0.0001 (shorter with combination treatment)
1 RCT identified by the systematic review in China[4]	Mean fever clearance time	**Weighted mean difference:** 5.00 hours, 95% CI –3.85 hours to 13.85 hours; P = 0.3 (slightly shorter with combination treatment but no significant difference)
1 RCT in Nigeria[14]		1.1 days (0.8 days to 1.4 days, range 1 day to 2 days) with combination treatment *v* 1.2 days (0.5 days to 1.9 days, range 1 day to 5 days) with amodiaquine alone; P value not given (no significant difference)
1 RCT in Cameroon[13]		28.4 hours (95% CI 15.7 hours to 41.1 hours, range 13.7 hours to 70.2 hours) with combination treatment *v* 27.6 hours (95% CI 15.4 hours to 29.8 hours; range 13.7 hours to 72.5 hours) with amodiaquine alone; P < 0.5 (shorter with combination treatment)

PCR, polymerase chain reaction.

TABLE 3 Overview of the number of RCTs for each treatment and comparison included in the review.

Treatment	Comparison	Number of systematic reviews (with number of relevant RCTs) reporting outcomes at 28 days	Number of additional RCTs reporting outcomes at 28 days	Number of systematic reviews (with number of relevant RCTs) reporting outcomes at less than 28 days only
Sulfadoxine–pyrimethamine plus chloroquine	Sulfadoxine–pyrimethamine	1 (0)		0 (2)
Sulfadoxine–pyrimethamine plus amodiaquine	Sulfadoxine–pyrimethamine	1 (3)	1	
	Amodiaquine	1 (3)	3	
Chlorproguanil–dapsone	Sulfadoxine–pyrimethamine	0 (0)		1 (2)
	Amodiaquine	0 (0)		
Artesunate (3 days) plus amodiaquine	Amodiaquine	1 (3)		
Artesunate (3 days) plus sulfadoxine–pyrimethamine	Sulfadoxine–pyrimethamine	1 (7)	2	
	Sulfadoxine–pyrimethamine plus amodiaquine	0 (1)		
Artesunate (3 days) plus mefloquine	Mefloquine	2 (12)	2	
Artesunate (3 days) plus chlorproguanil–dapsone	Chlorproguanil–dapsone	0 (0)		
Artemether–lumefantrine (6 doses)	Amodiaquine	0 (0)		
	Chloroquine	0 (0)		
	Sulfadoxine–pyrimethamine	0 (0)		
	Mefloquine	0 (0)		
	Artemether–lumefantrine (4 doses)	0 (1)		
	Artesunate (3 days) plus mefloquine	1 (2)		
	Artesunate (3 days) plus amodiaquine	0 (0)		1

TABLE 4 **Applying the evidence for local decision making - a pragmatic (but not evidence-based) framework.**

Clinical response to treatment will be influenced by the parasite (depending on whether it is completely, partially or not resistant to the antimalarial drug) and host immunity (depending on the intensity of exposure to malaria, and varying with age). One way of applying this chapter to clinical decision-making on antimalarial drugs for treating malaria in particular geographical regions, would be to use the following question-driven approach.

1. Does this drug have some effect on malaria parasites in vivo in this region? (if not, abandon this treatment option; if yes, proceed to the next question);
2. How does this drug compare with other drugs in general in terms of benefits and harms? (if considerably inferior, abandon this treatment option; if similar or better, proceed to the next question).
3. How does this drug perform in general when combined with other non-artemisinin antimalarial drugs? (if not better, use this treatment option as monotherapy; if better, combine with the other non-artemisinin antimalarial drug and proceed to the next question).
4. How does this drug/drug combination compare in general with other drug regimens containing an artemisinin derivative?
5. What cure rates have been achieved in this region with this drug/drug combination?
6. Consider other factors that might influence your decision: a) other benefits of this drug (for example, the potential public health benefit of artemisinin by slowing resistance spread; b) drug cost; c) drug availability; d) ease of implementation of change in the country.

Meningococcal disease

Search date May 2004

Jailson B Correia and C A Hart

QUESTIONS

INTERVENTIONS

PREVENTION IN CONTACTS AND CARRIERS

Likely to be beneficial

Antibiotics for throat carriage (reduce carriage, but unknown effect on risk of disease) 1013

Prophylactic antibiotics (sulfadiazine) in contacts* 1013

PRE-ADMISSION TREATMENT

Unknown effectiveness

Pre-admission parenteral penicillin in suspected cases* 1014

MENINGOCOCCAL MENINGITIS TREATMENT IN CHILDREN

Likely to be beneficial

Adding corticosteroids (reduced severe hearing loss in bacterial meningitis of any cause, but no difference in mortality and unknown effectiveness in meningococcal meningitis) . .1015

MENINGOCOCCAL MENINGITIS TREATMENT IN ADULTS

Likely to be beneficial

Adding corticosteroids (reduced mortality in bacterial meningitis of any cause, but unknown effectiveness in meningococcal meningitis) 1017

MENINGOCOCCAL SEPTICAEMIA TREATMENT IN CHILDREN

Unknown effectiveness

Adding corticosteroids 1018

MENINGOCOCCAL SEPTICAEMIA TREATMENT IN ADULTS

Unknown effectiveness

Adding corticosteroids 1019

To be covered in future updates

Hospital treatment of meningococcal disease

Vaccines (monovalent/multivalent, polysaccharide alone, or conjugate)

*Based on consensus or observational evidence. RCTs unlikely to be conducted.

See glossary Ⓖ

Key Messages

Prevention in contacts and carriers

- **Antibiotics for throat carriage (reduce carriage but unknown effectiveness on risk of disease)** RCTs found that antibiotics reduced throat carriage of meningococcus compared with placebo. We found no RCTs or observational evidence examining whether eradicating throat carriage of meningococcus reduces the risk of meningococcal disease.
- **Prophylactic antibiotics (sulfadiazine) in contacts*** We found no RCTs on the effects of prophylactic antibiotics on the incidence of meningococcal disease among contacts. One observational study found limited evidence that prophylactic sulfadiazine reduced the risk of meningococcal disease over 8 weeks compared with no prophylaxis. We found no evidence regarding which contacts should be treated.

Pre-admission treatment

- **Pre-admission parenteral penicillin in suspected cases*** We found no RCTs on the effects of pre-admission parenteral penicillin in suspected meningococcal disease in people of all ages. We found inconclusive evidence from observational studies on the benefit of pre-admission antibiotics. However, it is unlikely that RCTs on pre-admission antibiotics will be performed because of the unpredictably rapid course of disease in some people and the likely risks involved in delaying treatment, combined with a low risk of causing harm.

Meningococcal meningitis treatment in children

- **Adding corticosteroids (reduced severe hearing loss in bacterial meningitis of any cause, but no difference in mortality and unknown effectiveness in meningococcal meningitis)** We found no RCTs on adding corticosteroids specifically in children with meningococcal meningitis. One systematic review found no significant difference between adding corticosteroids and adding placebo in mortality in children with bacterial meningitis of any aetiology or in people of all ages with meningococcal meningitis. The review found that, compared with adding placebo, corticosteroids reduced severe hearing loss in children with bacterial meningitis of any aetiology, but it did not specifically assess the effect in children with meningococcal meningitis. The review found no significant difference between adding corticosteroids and adding placebo for short term or long term neurological sequelae in people of all ages with bacterial meningitis of any aetiology, but it did not separately assess the effect in children with meningococcal meningitis. Interpreting the results of available evidence on the use of corticosteroids in children with meningococcal meningitis demands caution, as age- and pathogen-specific evidence is scarce. In regions where the conjugate vaccine has been introduced, the incidence of *Haemophilus influenzae* type b (Hib) has fallen dramatically and the applicability of evidence from trials performed prior to this change in epidemiology is questionable. However, decisions on initial treatment such as adding corticosteroids almost always precede knowledge of the specific aetiology.

Meningococcal meningitis treatment in adults

- **Adding corticosteroids (reduced mortality in bacterial meningitis of any cause, but unknown effectiveness in meningococcal meningitis)** We found no RCTs on adding corticosteroids specifically in adults with meningococcal meningitis. One systematic review found that, compared with adding placebo, adding corticosteroids reduced mortality in adults with bacterial meningitis of any aetiology. Subgroup analysis for meningococcal meningitis found no significant difference in mortality with adding corticosteroids compared with adding placebo. The review found that, compared with adding placebo, adding corticosteroids reduced neurological sequelae in people with bacterial meningitis of any aetiology, but the difference did not quite reach significance. Subgroup analysis for meningococcal meningitis found no significant difference in neurological sequelae with adding corticosteroids compared with adding placebo. None of the RCTs included in the systematic review were powered to detect a significant effect of corticosteroid treatment in the subgroup of people with meningococcal meningitis, probably due to the lower rates of mortality and sequelae in this group. However, decisions on initial treatment with adding corticosteroids almost always precede knowledge of the specific aetiology.

Meningococcal septicaemia treatment in children

- **Adding corticosteroids** We found no RCTs on adding corticosteroids specifically in children with meningococcal septicaemia. Two RCTs found no significant difference in mortality between adding corticosteroids and adding placebo in children with severe sepsis and septic shock of any bacterial aetiology. It is questionable whether evidence from RCTs on severe sepsis and septic shock of any aetiology can be applied to children with meningococcal septicaemia.

Meningococcal septicaemia treatment in adults

- **Adding corticosteroids** We found no RCTs on adding corticosteroids specifically in adults with meningococcal septicaemia. One systematic review in adults with severe sepsis or septic shock of any aetiology found no significant difference in overall mortality at 28 days by adding corticosteroids to antibiotics or by adding high dose, short course corticosteroids compared with adding placebo, but that adding low dose, longer duration corticosteroids at doses of 300 mg or less of hydrocortisone or equivalent for 5 or more days reduced all cause mortality at 28 days compared with adding placebo. It is questionable whether evidence from RCTs on severe sepsis and septic shock of any aetiology can be applied to adults with meningococcal septicaemia.

*Based on consensus or observational evidence. RCTs unlikely to be conducted.

DEFINITION Meningococcal disease is any clinical condition caused by *Neisseria meningitidis* (the meningococcus) groups A, B, C, W135, or other serogroups. These conditions include purulent conjunctivitis, septic arthritis, meningitis, and septicaemia**G** with or without meningitis. In this chapter we cover meningococcal meningitis and meningococcal septicaemia with or without meningitis.

INCIDENCE/ PREVALENCE Meningococcal disease is sporadic in temperate countries, and is most commonly caused by group B or C meningococci. The annual incidence in Europe varies from fewer than 1 case/100 000 people in France, up to 4–5 cases/100 000 people in the UK and Spain, and in the USA it is 0.6–1.5 cases/100 000 people.[1,2] Occasional outbreaks occur among close family contacts**G**, secondary school pupils, military recruits, and students living in halls of residence. Sub-Saharan Africa has regular epidemics in countries lying in the expanded "meningitis belt", reaching 500 cases/100 000 people during epidemics, which are usually due to serogroup A, although recent outbreaks of serogroup W135 cause concern.[3–5] In sub-Saharan Africa, over 90% of cases present with meningitis alone.[3]

AETIOLOGY/ RISK FACTORS The meningococcus colonises and infects healthy people, and is transmitted by close contact, probably by exchange of upper respiratory tract secretions (see table 1, p 1022).[6–14] The risk of transmission is greatest during the first week of contact.[9] Risk factors include crowding and exposure to cigarette smoke.[15] In the UK, children younger than 2 years have the highest incidence of meningococcal disease, with a second peak between ages 15–24 years. There is currently an increased incidence of meningococcal disease among university students, especially among those in their first term and living in catered accommodation,[16] although we found no accurate numerical estimate of risk from close contact in, for example, halls of residence. Close contacts of an index case have a much higher risk of infection than do people in the general population.[9,12,13] The risk of epidemic spread is higher with groups A and C meningococci than with group B meningococci.[6–8,10] It is not known what makes a meningococcus virulent. Certain clones tend to predominate at different times and in different groups. Carriage of meningococcus in the throat has been reported in 10–15% of people; recent acquisition of a virulent meningococcus is more likely to be associated with invasive disease.

PROGNOSIS Mortality is highest in infants and adolescents, and is related to disease presentation and availability of therapeutic resources. In developed countries, case fatality rates have been around 19–25% for septicaemia, 10–12% for meningitis plus septicaemia, and less than 1% in meningitis alone, but an overall reduction in mortality was observed in recent years in people admitted to paediatric intensive care units.[17–21]

AIMS OF INTERVENTION To prevent disease in contacts; to prevent development of meningococcal disease and its complications, with minimal adverse effects.

OUTCOMES Rates of infection; rates of eradication of throat carriage; adverse effects of treatment; mortality; sequelae.

METHODS *Clinical Evidence* search and appraisal May 2004, including a search for observational studies. In addition, the authors drew from a collection of references from the pre-electronic data era and cross-references from relevant papers.

QUESTION What are the effects of interventions to prevent meningococcal disease in contacts and carriers?

OPTION PROPHYLACTIC ANTIBIOTICS IN CONTACTS

We found no RCTs on the effects of prophylactic antibiotics on the incidence of meningococcal disease among contacts. One observational study found limited evidence that prophylactic sulfadiazine reduced the risk of meningococcal disease over 8 weeks compared with no prophylaxis. We found no evidence regarding which contacts should be treated.

Benefits: We found no systematic review and no RCTs examining the effect of prophylactic antibiotics in people in contactⒼ with someone with meningococcal disease (see comment below). **Rifampicin:** We found no studies. **Phenoxymethylpenicillin:** We found one retrospective study, but the results of that study cannot be generalised beyond the sample tested.[22] **Sulfadiazine:** One cohort study of soldiers in temporary troop camps in the 1940s compared the incidence of meningococcal disease in camps where sulfadiazine (sulphadiazine) was given to everyone after a meningococcal outbreak versus the incidence in camps where no prophylaxis was given.[23] The study reported a higher incidence of meningococcal disease in soldiers not given prophylaxis (approximate figures 17/9500 [0.18%] *v* 2/7000 [0.03%] over 8 weeks, P value not reported).

Harms: **Rifampicin:** No excess adverse effects compared with placebo were found in RCTs on eradicating throat carriage of meningococcal disease.[24,25] However, rifampicin is known to cause various adverse effects, including turning urine and contact lenses orange, and inducing hepatic microsomal enzymes, potentially rendering oral contraception ineffective. Rifampicin prophylaxis may be associated with emergence of resistant strains.[26] **Sulfadiazine:** One in 10 soldiers experienced minor adverse events, including headache, dizziness, tinnitus, and nausea.[23]

Comment: RCTs addressing this question are unlikely to be performed because the intervention has few associated risks, whereas meningococcal disease has high associated risks. RCTs would also need to be large to find a difference in the incidence of meningococcal disease. In the sulfadiazine cohort study, the two infected people in the treatment group only became infected after leaving the camp.[23]

OPTION ANTIBIOTICS FOR THROAT CARRIAGE

RCTs found that antibiotics reduced throat carriage of meningococcus compared with placebo. We found no RCTs or observational evidence examining whether eradicating throat carriage of meningococcus reduces the risk of meningococcal disease.

Meningococcal disease

Benefits: We found no systematic review. **Incidence of disease:** We found no RCTs or observational studies that examined whether eradicating throat carriage**G** of meningococcus reduces the risk of meningococcal disease. **Throat carriage:** We found five placebo controlled RCTs that examined the effect of antibiotics on carriage of meningococcus in the throat (see table 2, p 1023).[24,25,27–29] All trials found that antibiotics (rifampicin, minocycline, or ciprofloxacin) achieved high rates of eradication (ranging from 90–97%), except one trial of rifampicin in students with heavy growth on culture, in which the rate of eradication was 73%.[24] Eradication rates on placebo ranged from 9–29%. We found seven RCTs that compared different antibiotic regimens (see table 3, p 1024).[30–36] One RCT conducted in the 1960s found that oral erythromycin was ineffective whereas intramuscular penicillin eradicated meningococcal carriage in 35% of carriers among army recruits during a group C meningococcal meningitis outbreak at a US army base.[30] Another RCT found that sulfamidine was ineffective whereas rifampicin eradicated meningococcal throat carriage in nearly 80% of carriers among household contacts in northern Nigeria.[32] Four RCTs found no significant difference between rifampicin and minocycline, ciprofloxacin, azithromycin, or intramuscular ceftriaxone in eradicating meningococcal throat carriage.[31,34–36] However, one RCT randomised households to different treatments and found that intramuscular ceftriaxone significantly increased eradication rates compared with rifampicin (see comment below).[33]

Harms: **Minocycline:** One RCT reported adverse effects (1 or more of nausea, anorexia, dizziness, and abdominal cramps) in 36% of participants.[31] **Rifampicin:** See harms of postexposure antibiotic prophylaxis, p 1013. **Ciprofloxacin:** Trials of single dose prophylactic regimens reported no more adverse effects than with comparators or placebo.[28,29,34] Ciprofloxacin is contraindicated in pregnancy and in children because animal studies have indicated a possibility of articular cartilage damage in developing joints.[37] **Ceftriaxone:** Two RCTs of ceftriaxone (given as a single intramuscular injection) found no significant adverse effects.[33,34] In another RCT, 12% of participants complained of headache.[35] **Azithromycin:** The RCT reported no serious or moderate adverse effects. It found no significant difference in the rate of adverse effects such as nausea, abdominal pain, and headache of short duration with azithromycin compared with rifampicin.[35]

Comment: There is consensus that eradicating meningococcal throat carriage is appropriate for preventing meningococcal disease. Due to the large number of participants required, it is unlikely that RCTs will be conducted on the efficacy of prophylactic antibiotics in preventing secondary community acquired meningococcal disease in household contacts**G**. **Ceftriaxone:** The fourth RCT used cluster randomisation, and therefore the results should be interpreted with caution.[33]

QUESTION What are the effects of interventions to treat suspected cases of meningococcal disease before admission to hospital?

OPTION PRE-ADMISSION PARENTERAL PENICILLIN

We found no RCTs on the effects of pre-admission parenteral penicillin in suspected meningococcal disease in people of all ages. We found inconclusive evidence from observational studies on the benefit of pre-admission antibiotics. However, it is unlikely that RCTs on pre-admission antibiotics will be performed because of the unpredictably rapid course of disease in some people and the likely risks involved in delaying treatment, combined with a low risk of causing harm.

Benefits: We found no systematic review or RCTs but found seven observational studies on the effect of pre-admission parenteral penicillin in suspected cases[G] of meningococcal disease (see table 4, p 1025).[38–44] We also found two reports of pooled data from three of the observational studies.[45,46] The first report (3 English observational studies,[38–40] 487 people) found that pre-admission parenteral antibiotics significantly reduced mortality compared with no pre-admission antibiotics (OR 2.61, 95% CI 1.04 to 7.18).[45] However, the second report (664 people; the same people in the English studies[38–40] plus partial data from a Danish cohort[47]) found no significant benefit with pre-admission parenteral antibiotics (outcomes not specified; OR 0.82, 95% CI 0.43 to 1.56).[46] Three observational studies found lower mortality rates with pre-admission parenteral antibiotics compared with no pre-admission antibiotics, although the difference between the two treatment groups in each study did not reach significance.[41,43,44] However, one study did not support this finding (mortality rate 9/77 [11.7%] with pre-admission parenteral penicillin *v* 26/402 [7%] with no pre-admission antibiotics; OR 1.9, 95% CI 0.9 to 4.3).[42]

Harms: It is difficult to differentiate people with early features of meningococcal disease from those with self limiting illnesses. According to more or less strict criteria for suspicion, between 28% and 89% of individuals receive parenteral penicillin unnecessarily.[48–51] One study of the harms of penicillin found that anaphylaxis occurred in about 0.04% of cases and that fatal anaphylaxis occurred in about 0.002% of cases.[52]

Comment: We found no studies about the relationship between early treatment with antibiotics and development of subsequent antibiotic resistance. Retrospective observational studies usually provide limited evidence for treatment interventions. In the case of pre-admission penicillin, no study was able to adjust adequately for clinical severity, stage of disease progression, or cointerventions such as earlier suspicion and referral (following media coverage and official recommendation). However, it is unlikely that RCTs on pre-admission antibiotics will be performed because of the unpredictably rapid course of disease in some people and the likely risks involved in delaying treatment, combined with a low risk of causing harm.

QUESTION What are the effects of treatments for meningococcal meningitis on admission in children?

OPTION ADDING CORTICOSTEROIDS

We found no RCTs on adding corticosteroids specifically in children with meningococcal meningitis. One systematic review found no significant difference between adding corticosteroids and adding placebo in mortality in children with bacterial meningitis of any aetiology or in people of all ages with meningococcal meningitis. The review found that, compared with adding placebo, corticosteroids reduced severe hearing loss in children with bacterial meningitis of any aetiology, but it did not specifically assess the effect in children with meningococcal meningitis. The review found no significant difference between adding corticosteroids and adding placebo for short term or long term neurological sequelae in people of all ages with bacterial meningitis of any aetiology, but it did not separately assess the effect in children with meningococcal meningitis. Interpreting the results of available evidence on the use of corticosteroids in children with meningococcal meningitis demands caution, as age- and pathogen-specific evidence is scarce. In regions where the conjugate vaccine has been introduced, the incidence of *Haemophilus influenzae* type b (Hib) has fallen dramatically and

the applicability of evidence from trials performed prior to this change in epidemiology is questionable. However, decisions on initial treatment such as adding corticosteroids almost always precede knowledge of the specific aetiology.

Benefits: We found no systematic review or RCTs on adding corticosteroids specifically in children with meningococcal meningitis**G**. We found one systematic review (search date 2002, 10 RCTs and 8 quasi-randomised studies, 4 trials including people over the age of 16 years) that compared adding corticosteroids to antibiotics versus adding placebo to antibiotics in people of all ages and bacterial meningitis of any aetiology for the outcomes of mortality, severe hearing loss, and neurological sequelae.[53] The systematic review performed subgroup analyses for two age groups (under 16 years and over 16 years) and for the causative organisms of bacterial meningitis. It found no significant difference between adding corticosteroids and adding placebo for mortality in children with bacterial meningitis of any aetiology (14 RCTs or quasi-randomised studies, 1478 children aged under 16 years; mortality: 46/746 [6.2%] with adding corticosteroids *v* 48/732 [6.6%] with placebo; RR 0.95, 95% CI 0.65 to 1.37).[53] A subgroup analysis in people with meningococcal meningitis found no significant difference between corticosteroids and placebo for the outcome of mortality in people of all ages (8 RCTs [2 RCTs included people aged over 16 years], 353 people, mortality: RR 0.61, 95% CI 0.23 to 1.64).[53] The review found that, compared with adding placebo, adding corticosteroids significantly reduced severe hearing loss in children with bacterial meningitis of any aetiology (12 RCTs, 1013 children aged under 16 years; severe hearing loss: 15/514 [2.9%] with corticosteroids *v* 49/499 [9.8%] with placebo; RR 0.31, 95% CI 0.18 to 0.54). The reduction in severe hearing loss remained significant when the causative agent, *Haemophilus influenzae*, was excluded from the analysis (10 RCTs, 394 children aged under 16 years; severe hearing loss: 6/191 [3.1%] with adding corticosteroids *v* 19/203 [9.4%] with controls; RR 0.42, 95% CI 0.20 to 0.89).[53] The review did not conduct a separate subgroup analysis for children less than 16 years of age for the outcome of neurological sequelae. It found no significant difference between adding corticosteroids and adding placebo for short term or long term neurological sequelae in people of all ages with bacterial meningitis of any aetiology (short term neurological sequelae: 8 RCTs [2 RCTs included people aged over 16 years], 482 people; RR 0.72, 95% CI 0.48 to 1.06; long term neurological sequelae: 10 RCTs [1 RCT included people aged over 16 years], 1163 people; RR 0.67, 95% CI 0.45 to 1.00).[53] The review defined hearing loss as severe when there was bilateral hearing loss of greater than 60 dB or requiring bilateral hearing aids, and defined neurological sequelae as focal neurological deficits other than hearing loss, such as epilepsy (not present before meningitis onset), severe ataxia, and severe memory or concentration disturbance. It defined short term neurological sequelae as those assessed between discharge and 6 weeks after hospital discharge and long term neurological sequelae as those assessed between 6 and 12 months after discharge.

Harms: The systematic review recorded adverse events (clinically evident gastrointestinal bleeding, pericarditis, reactive arthritis, herpes zoster, herpes simplex or fungal infections, persistent or secondary fever) as reported in 18 trials (1183 people, including 1008 children, all aetiologies).[53] It found no significant difference in their frequency between treatment groups (146/599 with corticosteroids *v* 131/584 with placebo; RR 1.06, 95% CI 0.88 to 1.27).

Comment: In clinical practice, when a child is brought to hospital with bacterial meningitis, clinical signs and a cloudy cerebrospinal fluid will direct the initiation of early treatment, as timing can affect prognosis, and the decision on whether to start corticosteroids almost always precedes knowledge of the specific aetiology. Interpreting the results of available evidence on the use of corticosteroids in the context of meningococcal meningitis in children demands caution, as age- and pathogen-specific evidence is scarce. In regions where the conjugate vaccine has been introduced, the incidence of *Haemophilus influenzae* type b (Hib) has fallen dramatically and the applicability of evidence from trials performed prior to this change in epidemiology is questionable. It is clinically relevant to group people with non-Hib meningitis together, but this strategy is not free of caveats because the different agents in this group may have different rates of death and sequelae and respond differently to corticosteroids.[53] We found one RCT comparing dexamethasone versus placebo in 598 Malawian children aged 2 months to 13 years with acute bacterial meningitis of all aetiologies, including 67 children with meningococcal meningitis. The RCT conducted subgroup analyses according to the causative agents of bacterial meningitis. In a subgroup analysis for the causative agent for meningococcal meningitis, *Neisseria meningitidis*, the RCT found no significant difference between dexamethasone and placebo for the outcomes of mortality or neurological sequelae including hearing loss (mortality: 1/32 [3%] with dexamethasone *v* 2/35 [6%] with placebo, P value reported as not significant; neurological sequelae including hearing loss: 5/30 [17%] with dexamethasone *v* 10/33 [30%] with placebo; RR 0.55, 95% CI 0.21 to 1.43, P = 0.33).[54] The results of this Malawian RCT may not be applicable in settings other than where there is late presentation, partial and inadequate treatment, or a high prevalence of HIV, anaemia, and malnutrition, all of which may considerably alter the results.[54]

QUESTION **What are the effects of treatments for meningococcal meningitis on admission in adults?**

OPTION **ADDING CORTICOSTEROIDS**

We found no RCTs on adding corticosteroids specifically in adults with meningococcal meningitis. One systematic review found that, compared with adding placebo, adding corticosteroids reduced mortality in adults with bacterial meningitis of any aetiology. Subgroup analysis for meningococcal meningitis found no significant difference in mortality with adding corticosteroids compared with adding placebo. The review found that, compared with adding placebo, adding corticosteroids reduced neurological sequelae in people with bacterial meningitis of any aetiology, but the difference did not quite reach significance. Subgroup analysis for meningococcal meningitis found no significant difference in neurological sequelae with adding corticosteroids compared with adding placebo. None of the RCTs included in the systematic review were powered to detect a significant effect of corticosteroid treatment in the subgroup of people with meningococcal meningitis, probably due to the lower rates of mortality and sequelae in this group. However, decisions on initial treatment with adding corticosteroids almost always precede knowledge of the specific aetiology.

Benefits: We found no systematic review or RCTs on adding corticosteroids specifically in adults with meningococcal meningitis**G**. We found one systematic review (search date 2003, 2 RCTs and 3 quasi-randomised studies, 623 people aged over 16 years with acute bacterial meningitis of any aetiology, including 232 people with meningococcal meningitis) comparing adding corticosteroids (dexamethasone in 4 trials; hydrocortisone in 1 RCT) versus adding placebo in people with bacterial meningitis of any aetiology for the outcomes of mortality and neurological sequelae.[55] The review found that, compared with adding placebo, adding corticosteroids significantly reduced mortality in adults with bacterial meningitis of any aetiology (mortality: 36/308 [12%] with dexamethasone *v* 69/315 [22%] with placebo; RR 0.60, 95% CI 0.40 to 0.81; P = 0.02). A subgroup analysis for meningococcal meningitis found no significant difference in mortality with adding corticosteroids compared with adding placebo (RR 0.9, 95% CI 0.3 to 2.1).[55] The review found that, compared with controls, adding corticosteroids reduced neurological sequelae in people with bacterial meningitis of any aetiology, but the difference did not quite reach significance (5 RCTs, 340 people aged over 16 years; neurological sequelae: 26/184 [14%] with dexamethasone *v* 35/156 [22%] with placebo; RR 0.60, 95% CI 0.40 to 1.00; P = 0.05). A subgroup analysis for meningococcal meningitis found no significant difference in neurological sequelae with adding corticosteroids compared with placebo (RR 0.5, 95% CI 0.1 to 1.7).[55]

Harms: The systematic review recorded data on adverse events in 391 patients, with clinically evident gastrointestinal bleeding occurring in 1% of cases in the corticosteroid group and in 4% in the placebo group.[55] It found no significant difference in the frequency of other adverse events (pericarditis, reactive arthritis, herpes zoster, herpes simplex or fungal infections, persistent or secondary fever) with corticosteroids compared with placebo (RR of any adverse event compared with placebo 1.0, 95% CI 0.5 to 2.0).

Comment: In clinical practice, when a person presents with bacterial meningitis, clinical signs and a cloudy cerebrospinal fluid will direct the initiation of early treatment, as timing can affect prognosis, and the decision on whether to start corticosteroids almost always precedes knowledge of the specific aetiology. None of the RCTs included in the systematic review were powered to detect a significant effect of corticosteroid treatment in the subgroup of people with meningococcal meningitis, probably as a result of the lower rates of mortality and sequelae in this group. One RCT identified by the review, involving various European centres, took 9 years to complete, but still failed to enrol enough patients with meningococcal meningitis to achieve significant results.[56]

QUESTION What are the effects of treatments for meningococcal septicaemia in children?

OPTION ADDING CORTICOSTEROIDS

We found no RCTs on the use of adding corticosteroids specifically in children with meningococcal septicaemia. Two RCTs found no significant difference in mortality between adding corticosteroids and adding placebo in children with severe sepsis and septic shock of any bacterial aetiology. It is questionable whether evidence from RCTs on severe sepsis and septic shock of any aetiology can be applied to children with meningococcal septicaemia.

Benefits: We found no systematic review or RCTs on the use of adding corticosteroids specifically in children with meningococcal septicaemia (see comment below).

Harms: We found no RCTs (see comment below).

Comment: We found one systematic review (search date 2003) in people of all ages with severe sepsis❻ or septic shock of any bacterial aetiology.[57] Two RCTs in children identified by the review found no significant difference in mortality between adding corticosteroids and placebo, but it is questionable whether evidence from RCTs on severe sepsis and septic shock of any aetiology can be applied to children with meningococcal septicaemia (mortality in the first RCT: 5/74 [6.8%] with adjunctive hydrocortisone *v* 4/61 [6.6%] with placebo, P value reported as not significant;[58] mortality in the second RCT: 6/36 [17%] with adjunctive dexamethasone *v* 4/36 [11%] with placebo; P = 0.73[59]).

QUESTION What are the effects of treatments for meningococcal septicaemia in adults?

OPTION ADDING CORTICOSTEROIDS

We found no RCTs on adding corticosteroids specifically in adults with meningococcal septicaemia. One systematic review in adults with severe sepsis or septic shock of any aetiology found no significant difference in overall mortality at 28 days by adding corticosteroids to antibiotics or by adding high dose, short course corticosteroids compared with adding placebo, but that adding low dose, longer duration corticosteroids at doses of 300 mg or less of hydrocortisone or equivalent for 5 or more days reduced all cause mortality at 28 days compared with adding placebo. It is questionable whether evidence from RCTs on severe sepsis and septic shock of any aetiology can be applied to adults with meningococcal septicaemia.

Benefits: We found no systematic review or RCTs on the use of adding corticosteroids specifically in adults with meningococcal septicaemia (see comment below).

Harms: We found no RCTs (see comment below).

Comment: We found one systematic review (search date 2003, 13 RCTs and 3 quasi-randomised trials, 2063 people, including 1856 adults, with severe sepsis❻ or septic shock of any bacterial aetiology) comparing adding corticosteroids (hydrocortisone, methylprednisolone, and dexamethasone) with two distinct dosing schemes — high dose, short course (>300 mg hydrocortisone or equivalent, for up to 5 days) and low dose, long course (300 mg hydrocortisone or less, for 5 days or more) — versus adding placebo.[57] Whether the results of the review can be extrapolated to the context of meningococcal septicaemia in adults remains unclear. The review found no significant difference in all cause mortality at 28 days with adding corticosteroids compared with placebo (351/1033 [34%] with adding corticosteroids *v* 329/989 [33%] with placebo; RR 0.92, 95% CI 0.75 to 1.14). Similarly, it found no significant difference in all cause mortality at 28 days with adding high dose, short course corticosteroids compared with placebo. However, it found that low dose, long course corticosteroids (5 RCTs, 465 adults) significantly reduced mortality at 28 days compared with placebo (all cause mortality at 28 days: 106/236 [45%] with adding corticosteroids given at low dose for 5 days or more *v* 129/229 [56%] with placebo; RR 0.80, 95% CI 0.67 to 0.95). The review found no significant difference in adverse events with adding corticosteroids compared with placebo (rate of gastrointestinal bleeding: 53/684 [8%] with adding corticosteroids *v* 43/637 [7%] with placebo; RR 1.16, 95% CI 0.82 to 1.65; rate of superinfections: 109/882 [12%] with adding corticosteroids *v* 107/823 [13%] with placebo; rate of hyperglycaemia: RR 1.22, 95% CI 0.84 to 1.78).[57]

GLOSSARY

Carrier Individual in whom *Neisseria meningitidis* can be retrieved from the nasopharynx by swabbing. Most carriers are asymptomatic and unaware of their carriage status
Contact Those recently exposed to an index case of meningococcal disease and who have a higher risk of developing the disease when compared with the general population (usually close, prolonged contact in the same household or direct contact with respiratory secretions).[60]
Meningitis (meningococcal) A case with clinical signs of meningitis (i.e. fever, headache, vomiting, nuchal rigidity) plus laboratory evidence of meningococcal infection, such as a positive blood or cerebrospinal fluid culture or polymerase chain reaction.[61]
Sepsis The systemic response to infection, manifested by two or more of the following: hyperthermia (or hypothermia), high heart rate, high respiratory rate (or low $PaCO_2$), high or low white blood cell count (or > 10% immature forms), although values are age dependent. Severe sepsis is associated with organ dysfunction, hypoperfusion, or hypotension. Septic shock is sepsis with hypotension, despite adequate fluid resuscitation, along with the presence of perfusion abnormalities.[62]
Septicaemia (meningococcal) A case with systemic signs and symptoms of infection (i.e. fever, malaise, patient "unwell") plus a skin rash, which can be purpuric (petechial, ecchymotic) or, less often, maculopapular. The laboratory provides evidence of meningococcal infection in the blood.
Suspected cases Cases with early clinical signs of meningitis, septicaemia, or both, where the healthcare worker (usually the general practitioner) suspects meningococcal aetiology.

REFERENCES

1. Hubert B, Caugant DA. Recent changes in meningococcal disease in Europe. *Euro Surveill* 1997;2:69–71.
2. Centers for Disease Control. Summary of notifiable diseases, United States, 1997. *MMWR Morb Mortal Wkly Rep* 1998;46: ii-vii 3–87
3. Hart CA, Cuevas LE. Meningococcal disease in Africa. *Ann Trop Med Parasitol* 1997;91:777–785.
4. Molesworth AM, Thomson MC, Connor SJ, et al. Where is the meningitis belt? Defining an area at risk of epidemic meningitis in Africa. *Trans R Soc Trop Med Hyg* 2002;96:242–249.
5. World Health Organization. Emergence of W135 meningococcal disease. Report of a WHO consultation, Geneva 17–18 September 2001. Geneva: World Health Organization; 2002. http://www.who.int/csr/resources/publications/meningitis/whocdscsrgar20021.pdf (last accessed 24 June 2003).
6. French MR. Epidemiological study of 383 cases of meningococcus meningitis in the city of Milwaukee, 1927–1928 and 1929. *Am J Public Health* 1931;21:130–137.
7. Pizzi M. A severe epidemic of meningococcus meningitis in 1941–1942, Chile. *Am J Public Health* 1944;34:231–239.
8. Lee WW. Epidemic meningitis in Indianapolis 1929–1930. *J Prev Med* 1931;5:203–210.
9. De Wals P, Herthoge L, Borlée-Grimée I, et al. Meningococcal disease in Belgium. Secondary attack rate among household, day-care nursery and pre-elementary school contacts. *J Infect* 1981;3(suppl 1):53–61.
10. Kaiser AB, Hennekens CH, Saslaw MS, et al. Seroepidemiology and chemoprophylaxis of disease due to sulphonamide resistant *Neisseria meningitidis* in a civilian population. *J Infect Dis* 1974;130:217–221.
11. Zangwill KM, Schuchat A, Riedo FX, et al. School-based clusters of meningococcal disease in the United States. *JAMA* 1997;277:389–395.
12. The Meningococcal Disease Surveillance Group. Meningococcal disease secondary attack rate and chemoprophylaxis in the United States. *JAMA* 1976;235:261–265.
13. Olcen P, Kjellander J, Danielson D, et al. Epidemiology of *Neisseria meningitidis*: prevalence and symptoms from the upper respiratory tract in family members to patients with meningococcal disease. *Scand J Infect Dis* 1981;13:105–109.
14. Hudson, PJ, Vogt PL, Heun EM, et al. Evidence for school transmission of *Neisseria meningitidis* during a Vermont outbreak. *Pediatr Infect Dis* 1986;5:213–217.
15. Stanwell-Smith RE, Stuart JM, Hughes AO, et al. Smoking, the environment and meningococcal disease: a case control study. *Epidemiol Infect* 1994;112:315–328.
16. Communicable Disease Surveillance Centre. Meningococcal disease in university students. *Commun Dis Rep CDR Wkly* 1998;8:49.
17. Andersen BM. Mortality in meningococcal infections. *Scand J Infect Dis* 1978;10:277–282.
18. Thomson APJ, Sills JA, Hart CA. Validation of the Glasgow meningococcal septicaemia prognostic score: a 10 year retrospective survey. *Crit Care Med* 1991;19:26–30.
19. Riordan FAI, Marzouk O, Thomson APJ, et al. The changing presentation of meningococcal disease. *Eur J Pediatr* 1995;154:472–474.
20. Booy R, Habibi P, Nadel S, et al. Reduction in case fatality rate from meningococcal disease associated with improved healthcare delivery. *Arch Dis Child* 2001;85:386–390.
21. Thorburn K, Baines P, Thomson A, et al. Mortality in severe meningococcal disease. *Arch Dis Child* 2001;85:382–385.
22. Hoiby EA, Moe PJ, Lystad A, et al. Phenoxymethyl-penicillin treatment of household contacts of meningococcal disease patients. *Antonie Van Leeuwenhoek* 1986;52:255–257.
23. Kuhns DW, Nelson CT, Feldman HA, et al. The prophylactic value of sulfadiazine in the control of meningococcic meningitis. *JAMA* 1943;123:335–339.
24. Deal WB, Sanders E. Efficacy of rifampicin in treatment of meningococcal carriers. *N Engl J Med* 1969;281:641–645.
25. Eickhoff TC. In vitro and in vivo studies of resistance to rifampicin in meningococci. *J Infect Dis* 1971;123:414–420.
26. Weidmer CE, Dunkel TB, Pettyjohn FS, et al. Effectiveness of rifampin in eradicating the meningococcal carrier state in a relatively closed population: emergence of resistant strains. *J Infect Dis* 1971;124:172–178.

27. Devine LF, Johnson DP, Hagerman CR, et al. The effect of minocycline on meningococcal nasopharyngeal carrier state in naval personnel. *Am J Epidemiol* 1971;93:337–345.
28. Renkonen OV, Sivonen A, Visakorpi R. Effect of ciproflaxacin on carrier rate of *Neisseria meningitidis* in army recruits in Finland. *Antimicrob Agents Chemother* 1987;31:962–963.
29. Dworzack DL, Sanders CC, Horowitz EA, et al. Evaluation of single dose ciprofloxacin in the eradication of *Neisseria meningitidis* from nasopharyngeal carriers. *Antimicrob Agents Chemother* 1988;32:1740–1741.
30. Artenstein MS, Lamson TH, Evans JR. Attempted prophylaxis against meningococcal infection using intramuscular penicillin. *Mil Med* 1967;132:1009–1011.
31. Guttler RB, Counts GW, Avent CK, et al. Effect of rifampicin and minocycline on meningococcal carrier rates. *J Infect Dis* 1971;124:199–205.
32. Blakebrough IS, Gilles HM. The effect of rifampicin on meningococcal carriage in family contacts in northern Nigeria. *J Infect* 1980;2:137–143.
33. Schwartz B, Al-Tobaiqi A, Al-Ruwais A, et al. Comparative efficacy of ceftriaxone and rifampicin in eradicating pharyngeal carriage of Group A *Neisseria meningitidis*. *Lancet* 1988;1:1239–1242.
34. Cuevas LE, Kazembe P, Mughogho GK, et al. Eradication of nasopharyngeal carriage of *Neisseria meningitidis* in children and adults in rural Africa: a comparison of ciprofloxacin and rifampicin. *J Infect Dis* 1995;171:728–731.
35. Girgis N, Sultan Y, Frenck RW Jr, et al. Azithromycin compared with rifampin for eradication of masopharyngeal colonization by *Neisseria meningitidis*. *Pediatr Infect Dis* J 1998;17:816–819.
36. Simmons G, Jones N, Calder L. Equivalence of ceftriaxone and rifampicin in eliminating nasopharyngeal carriage of serogroup B *Neisseria meningitidis*. *J Antimicrob Chemother* 2000;45:909–911.
37. Schulter G. Ciprofloxacin: a review of its potential toxicologic effects. *Am J Med* 1987(suppl 4A);82:91–93.
38. Strang JR, Pugh EJ. Meningococcal infections: reducing the case fatality rate by giving penicillin before admission to hospital. *BMJ* 1992;305:141–143.
39. Cartwright K, Reilly S, White D, et al. Early treatment with parenteral penicillin in meningococcal disease. *BMJ* 1992;305:143–147.
40. Gossain S, Constantine CE, Webberley JM. Early parenteral penicillin in meningococcal disease. *BMJ* 1992;305:523–524.
41. Woodward CM, Jessop EG, Wale MCJ. Early management of meningococcal disease. *Commun Dis Rep CDR Rev* 1995;5:R135–R137.
42. Nørg rd B, Sørensen HT, Jensen ES, et al. Pre-hospital parenteral antibiotic treatment of meningococcal disease and case fatality: a Danish population-based cohort study. *J Infect* 2002;45:144–151.
43. Jefferies C, Lennon D, Stewart J, et al. Meningococcal disease in Auckland, July 1992 – June 1994. *N Z Med J* 1999;112:115–117.
44. Jolly K, Stewart G. Epidemiology and diagnosis of meningitis: results of a five-year prospective, population-based study. *Commun Dis Public Health* 2001;4:124–129.
45. Cartwright K, Strang J, Gossain S, et al. Early treatment of meningococcal disease [letter]. *BMJ* 1992;305:774.
46. Sorensen HT, Steffensen FH, Schonheyder HC, et al. Clinical management of meningococcal disease. Prospective international registration of patients may be needed. *BMJ* 1998;316:1016–1017.
47. Sorensen HT, Moller-Petersen J, Krarup HB, et al. Early treatment of meningococcal disease. *BMJ* 1992;305:774.
48. Wells LC, Smith JC, Weston VC, et al. The child with a non-blanching rash: how likely is meningococcal disease? *Arch Dis Child* 2001;85:218–222.
49. Mandl KD, Stack AM, Fleisher GR. Incidence of bacteremia in infants and children with fever and petechiae. *J Pediatr* 1997;131:398–404.
50. Brogan PA, Raffles A. The management of fever and petechiae: making sense of rash decisions. *Arch Dis Child* 2000;83:506–507.
51. Nielsen HE, Andersen EA, Andersen J, et al. Diagnostic assessment of haemorrhagic rash and fever. *Arch Dis Child* 2001;85:160–165.
52. Idsoe O, Guthe T, Willcox RR, et al. Nature and extent of penicillin side-reactions, with particular reference to fatalities from anaphylactic shock. *Bull World Health Organ* 1968;38:159–188.
53. van de Beek D, de Gans J, McIntyre P, et al. Corticosteroids in acute bacterial meningitis (Cochrane Review). In: The Cochrane Library, Issue 1, 2004. Chichester, UK: John Wiley & Sons, Ltd. Search date 2002; primary sources Central, Medline, Embase, Healthline, Current Contents, reference lists of articles and trial authors.
54. Molyneux EM, Walsh AL, Forsyth H, et al. Dexamethasone treatment in childhood bacterial meningitis in Malawi: a randomised controlled trial. *Lancet* 2002;360:211–218.
55. van de Beek D, de Gans J, McIntyre P, et al. Steroids in adults with acute bacterial meningitis: a systematic review. *Lancet Infect Dis* 2004;4:139–143. Search date not stated, primary sources Central, Medline, Embase, Healthline, Current Contents, reference lists of articles, and trial authors.
56. de Gans J, van de Beek D. Dexamethasone in adults with bacterial meningitis. *N Engl J Med* 2002;347:1549–1556.
57. Annane D, Bellissant E, Bollaert P, et al. Corticosteroids for treating severe sepsis and septic shock (Cochrane Review). In: The Cochrane Library, Issue 1, 2004. Chichester, UK: John Wiley & Sons, Ltd. Search date 2003, primary sources Central, Medline, Embase, Lilacs, reference lists of articles, and trial authors.
58. Bennett IL, Finland M, Hamburger M, et al. The effectiveness of hydrocortisone in the management of severe infections. *JAMA* 1963;183:166
59. Slusher T, Gbadero D, Howard C, et al. Randomized, placebo-controlled, double blinded trial of dexamethasone in African children with sepsis. *Pediatr Infect Dis J* 1996;15:579–583.
60. Public Health Laboratory Service Meningococcus Forum. Guidelines for public health management of meningococcal disease in the UK. *Commun Dis Public Health* 2002;5:187–204.
61. Hackett SJ, Carrol ED, Guiver M, et al. Improved case confirmation in meningococcal disease with whole blood Taqman PCR. *Arch Dis Child* 2002;86:449–452.
62. Bone RC, Balk RA, Cerra FB, et al. Definitions for sepsis and organ failure and guidelines for the use of innovative therapies in sepsis. The ACCP/SCCM Consensus Conference Committee. American College of Chest Physicians/Society of Critical Care Medicine. *Chest* 1992;101:1644–1655.

Jailson B Correia
Dr
Instituto Materno Infantil de Pernambuco
Recife
Brazil

C A Hart
Professor
Department of Medical Microbiology and Genitourinary Medicine
University of Liverpool
Liverpool
UK

Competing interests: None declared.

TABLE 1 Risk of infection among contacts (see text, p 1012).

Group of meningococcus	Setting	Risk
A	Household contacts in Milwaukee, USA[6]	AR 1100/100 000; RR not possible to estimate
	General population in Santiago province, Chile	Attack rate in general population 23–262/100 000 (1941 and 1942)
	Household contacts in Chile[7]	Attack rate in household contacts 250/100 000 (0.25%) over both years
	General population in Indianapolis, USA[8]	AR 4500/100 000; RR not possible to estimate
B	Household contacts in Belgium[9]	RR 1245*
	Nursery schools[9]	RR 23*
	Day care centres[9]	RR 76*
C	Household contacts from two lower socioeconomic groups Dade County, Florida, USA[10]	Attack rate in two communities 13/100 000 population. Attack rate in household contacts 5/85 (582/100 000)
Unspecified	School based clusters in USA. Predominant meningococcal types: 13 clusters of Gp C, 7 Gp B, 1 Gp Y, 1 GpC/W135 (impossible to distinguish)[11]	RR 2.3*
	Household contacts from several states in USA, meningococcus types B and C predominantly[12]	RR 500–800*
	Household contact in Norway. Meningococcus types A, B, and C predominantly[13]	RR up to 4000*
	Schools in Vermont. Predominant meningococcus type C[14]	OR 14.1 (95% CI 1.6 to 127)

*Compared with the risk in the general population.

TABLE 2 Effect of antibiotics on throat carriage: results of placebo controlled RCTs (see text, p 1014).

Antibiotic	Group of meningococcus	Participants	Eradication: Treatment (%)	Eradication: Placebo (%)	RR (95% CI)
Rifampicin (oral)[24]	B, X, Z	30 students with heavy growth on culture	11/15 (73)	2/15 (13)	5.5 (1.5 to 21)
Rifampicin (oral)[25]	B, C, Y, Z29 E, W 135, NT	76 airforce recruits	36/38* (95)	3/22‡ (14)	7.0 (5.8 to 8.1)
Minocycline (oral)[27]	Predominantly Y (63%)	149 naval recruits	37/41 (90)†	14/48 (29)§	3.1 (2.6 to 3.6)
Ciprofloxacin (oral)[28]	Non-groupable (61%), B (17.5%)	120 army recruits in Finland	54/56 (97) 5 second samples missing	7/53 (13) 6 second samples missing or not a carrier	7.3 (6.5 to 8.1)
Ciprofloxacin (oral)[29]	B (41%), Z (33%)	46 healthy volunteers	22/23 (96) (1 did not adhere to treatment)	2/22 (9)	10.5 (8.9 to 12.1)

*9 lost to follow up. †37 either did not have meningococci prior to treatment or did not provide a full set of cultures. ‡7 lost to follow up. §23 either did not have meningococci prior to treatment or did not provide a full set of cultures.

TABLE 3 **Effects of antibiotics on throat carriage: results of comparative RCTs (see text, p 1014).**

Antibiotic	Group of meningococcus	Participants	Rate of eradication (%)	RR (95% CI)
Phenoxymethylpenicillin (im)[30]	C (49%), B (33%), NG (17%)	Adults	41/118 (35)	No data
Erythromycin (oral)[30]	C	Adults	0/7 (0)	
Rifampicin (oral)[32]	B + C (31%), NG (69%)	Adults	43/51 (84)	0.89 (0.76 to 1.02)
Minocycline (oral)[31]	B + C (31%), NG (69%)	Adults	36/38 (95)	Difference reported as not significant
Rifampicin (oral)[31]	A	Children	37/48 (77)	No data
Sulfadimidine (oral)[32]	A	Children	0/34 (0)	No data
Ceftriaxone (im)[33]	A	Adults and children	66/68 (97)	1.29 (1.10 to 1.49)
Rifampicin (oral)[33]	A	Adults and children	27/36 (75)	
Ceftriaxone (im)[34]	A	Adults and children	39/41 (95)	Difference reported as not significant
Ciprofloxacin (oral)[34]	A	Adults and children	70/79 (89)	
Rifampicin (oral)[34]	A	Adults and children	85/88 (97)	
Azithromycin (oral)[35]	B (63%), A (37%)	Adults	56/60 (93)	Difference reported as not significant
Rifampicin (oral)[35]	B (63%), A (37%)	Adults	56/59 (95)	
Ceftriaxone (im)[36]	B (54%), other serogroups (46%)	Adults and children	97/100 (97)	Difference reported as not significant
Rifampicin (oral)[36]	B (51%), other serogroups (49%)	Adults and children	78/82 (95.1)	

im, intramuscular.

TABLE 4 **Effects of early (pre-admission) parenteral penicillin: results of observational studies** (see text, p 1015).

Setting	Group of meningococcus	Participants	Parenteral penicillin (number of deaths/ number of people [%])		RR (95% CI)
			Given	Not given	
District general hospital in Darlington, UK (from 1986–1991)[38]	NR	46 people admitted to hospital with confirmed, probable, and possible MD, all age groups (52% < 5 years of age)	0/13 (0)	8/33 (24.3)	Incalculable
Three health districts in south-west England, UK (from 1982–1991)[39]	Mostly B and C	340* confirmed, probable, and possible cases of MD, all age groups (36% < 5 years of age)	5/93 (5.4)	22/246 (8.9)	RR 0.6 (0.23 to 1.54)
Worcester health district, England, UK (1986–1992)[40]	NR	102† confirmed, probable, and possible cases of MD; age distribution not reported	1/23 (4.4)	11/79 (13.9)	RR 0.31 (0.04 to 2.29)
District hospital in Wessex, England, UK (1990–1993)[41]	NR	68 cases of MD, all age groups (44% < 5 years of age)	0/13 (0)	3/55 (5.5)	Not calculated
Counties of North Jutland and Aarhus, Denmark‡[42]	Mostly B (56%) and C (22%)	479 cases of MD seen by GPs before admission to hospital. All age groups.	9/77 (11.7)	26/402 (6.5)	Adjusted OR 2.4 (95% CI 1.0 to 5.6)§
Hospitals in Auckland, New Zealand (1992–1997)[43]‡‡	Predominantly B	106 confirmed or probable cases of MD, all age groups.	1/24 (4.2)	2/42 (4.9)	RR 0.85 (0.08 to 8.93)
Health district in England, UK (from 1994–1998)[44]‡‡	Mostly B (53%) and C (30%)	258†† confirmed, probable, and possible cases of MD; all age groups (49% < 5 years of age)	2/72 (2.8)	16/186 (8.6)	RR 0.32 (0.08 to 1.37)

*Number of individuals seen by their general practitioners (GPs) before admission; in one fatal case, there was no information on previous antibiotic use. †A total of 109 patients had their records reviewed, but seven were excluded from analysis because they had received oral penicillin. ‡Two previous partial series of 177 and 302 cases from the Danish historical cohort were reported in 1992[45] and 1998,[46] respectively, showing similar trends of excess mortality in the treated group. §Adjusted OR, multivariate analysis. ††The paper also reports meningitis of other aetiologies. Only those regarded as meningococcal disease are described here. ‡‡The only prospective studies found. Others in the table are retrospective.
CI, confidence interval; MD, meningococcal disease; NR, not reported.

Postherpetic neuralgia

Search date January 2004

David Wareham

QUESTIONS

INTERVENTIONS

Key Messages

Preventing postherpetic neuralgia

- **Oral antiviral agents (aciclovir, famciclovir, valaciclovir, netivudine)** One systematic review found limited evidence from RCTs that aciclovir given for 7–10 days reduced pain at 1–3 months compared with placebo. One systematic review of one large RCT found that famciclovir reduced mean pain duration after acute herpes zoster compared with placebo. One RCT found that valaciclovir reduced the prevalence of postherpetic neuralgia at 6 months compared with aciclovir. One RCT found time to cessation of postherpetic neuralgia was reduced with aciclovir compared with netivudine. One RCT found no significant difference between valaciclovir and famciclovir in the resolution of postherpetic neuralgia. One systematic review of one RCT found no significant difference in pain between topical idoxuridine and oral aciclovir 1 month after rash healing. One systematic review found insufficient evidence from two RCTs about the effects of corticosteroids plus antiviral agents.
- **Tricyclic antidepressants (amitriptyline)** One RCT with weak methods provided insufficient evidence on the effects of amitriptyline in preventing postherpetic neuralgia.
- **Topical antiviral agents (idoxuridine) for pain at 6 months** One systematic review of heterogeneous poor quality RCTs found no significant difference in pain between topical idoxuridine and placebo at 6 months. One systematic review of one RCT found no significant difference in pain between topical idoxuridine and oral aciclovir 1 month after rash healing.
- **Corticosteroids** Systematic reviews found insufficient evidence from RCTs about the effects of corticosteroids alone on postherpetic neuralgia. One systematic review found insufficient evidence from two RCTs about the effects of corticosteroids plus antiviral agents. There is concern that corticosteroids may cause dissemination of herpes zoster.

Treating established postherpetic neuralgia

- **Gabapentin** Systematic reviews of two RCTs found that gabapentin reduced pain at 8 weeks compared with placebo.
- **Tricyclic antidepressants** One systematic review of three crossover RCTs found that tricyclic antidepressants increased pain relief in postherpetic neuralgia after 3–6 weeks compared with placebo.
- **Oral opioids (oxycodone, morphine, methadone, tramadol)** We found no RCTs examining effects of morphine or methadone in people with postherpetic neuralgia. One small crossover RCT found limited evidence that oral oxycodone reduced pain compared with placebo, but was associated with more adverse effects. One systematic review of one small RCT found limited evidence that tramadol reduced pain compared with clomipramine with or without levomepromazine after 6 weeks. One subsequent RCT found limited evidence that tramadol increased pain relief after 6 weeks compared with placebo.
- **Topical anaesthesia** We found insufficient evidence from three RCTs about the effects of lidocaine (lignocaine).
- **Topical counterirritants (capsaicin)** Two systematic reviews including the same two RCTs found limited evidence that the topical counterirritant capsaicin improved pain relief in postherpetic neuralgia compared with placebo. One subsequent RCT found no significant difference in pain between capsaicin and placebo. Capsaicin may cause painful skin reactions (including burning, stinging, and erythema).
- **Dextromethorphan** One systematic review of one small crossover RCT and one subsequent RCT found no evidence that dextromethorphan was more effective than placebo or lorazepam after 3–6 weeks, but found that dextromethorphan was associated with sedation and ataxia at high doses.

DEFINITION Postherpetic neuralgia is pain that sometimes follows resolution of acute herpes zoster and healing of the zoster rash. It can be severe, accompanied by itching, and follows the distribution of the original infection. Herpes zoster is caused by activation of latent varicella zoster virus (human herpes virus 3) in people who have been rendered partially immune by a previous attack of chickenpox. Herpes zoster infects the sensory ganglia and their areas of innervation. It is characterised by pain along the distribution of the affected nerve, and crops of clustered vesicles over the area.

INCIDENCE/ PREVALENCE In a UK general practice survey of 3600–3800 people, the annual incidence of herpes zoster was 3.4/1000.[1] Incidence varied with age. Herpes zoster was relatively uncommon in people under the age of 50 years (< 2/1000 a year), but rose to 5–7/1000 a year in people aged 50–79 years, and 11/1000 in people aged 80 years or older. In a population based study of 590 cases in Rochester, Minnesota, USA, the overall incidence was lower (1.5/1000) but there were similar increases in incidence with age.[2] Prevalence of postherpetic neuralgia depends on when it is measured after acute infection. There is no agreed time point for diagnosis.

AETIOLOGY/ RISK FACTORS The main risk factor for postherpetic neuralgia is increasing age. In a UK general practice study (involving 3600–3800 people, 321 cases of acute herpes zoster) there was little risk in those under the age of 50 years, but postherpetic neuralgia developed in over 20% of people who had had acute herpes zoster aged 60–65 years and in 34% of those aged over 80 years.[1] No other risk factor has been found to predict consistently which people with herpes zoster will experience continued pain. In a general practice study in Iceland (421 people followed for up to 7 years after an initial episode of herpes zoster), the risk of postherpetic neuralgia was 1.8% (95% CI 0.6% to 4.2%) for people under 60 years of age and the pain was mild in all cases.[2] The risk of severe pain after 3 months in people aged over 60 years was 1.7% (95% CI 0% to 6.2%).

PROGNOSIS About 2% of people with acute herpes zoster in the UK general practice survey had pain for more than 5 years.[1] Prevalence of pain falls as time elapses after the initial episode. Among 183 people aged over 60 years in the placebo arm of a UK trial, the prevalence of pain was 61% at 1 month, 24% at 3 months, and 13% at 6 months after acute infection.[3] In a more recent RCT, the prevalence of postherpetic pain in the placebo arm at 6 months was 35% in 72 people over 60 years of age.[4]

AIMS OF INTERVENTION To prevent or reduce postherpetic neuralgia by intervention during acute attack; to reduce the severity and duration of established postherpetic neuralgia, with minimal adverse effects of treatment.

OUTCOMES Prevalence of persistent pain 6 months after resolution of acute infection and healing of rash. We did not consider short term outcomes such as rash healing or pain reduction during the acute episode. In established postherpetic neuralgia it is difficult to assess the clinical significance of reported changes in "average pain"; therefore, we present data as dichotomous outcomes where possible (pain absent or greatly reduced, or pain persistent).

METHODS The initial search was part of two systematic reviews of treatments for acute herpes zoster and postherpetic neuralgia on the basis of comprehensive searches of published and unpublished studies to 1993.[5,6] The details of the searches are described in the published reports. This search was updated by a *Clinical Evidence* search and appraisal in January 2004. Where reliable meta-analyses from systematic reviews were available, they were taken to be the most accurate estimates of treatment effectiveness. In trials, the most common time point chosen for assessing the prevalence of persistent pain was 6 months, which we use in this review unless otherwise specified.

QUESTION **What are the effects of interventions during an acute attack of herpes zoster aimed at preventing postherpetic neuralgia?**

OPTION **ORAL ANTIVIRAL AGENTS (ACICLOVIR, FAMCICLOVIR, VALACICLOVIR, NETIVUDINE)**

One systematic review found limited evidence from RCTs that aciclovir given for 7–10 days reduced pain at 1–3 months compared with placebo. One systematic review of one large RCT found that famciclovir reduced mean pain duration after acute herpes zoster compared with placebo. One RCT found that valaciclovir reduced the prevalence of postherpetic neuralgia at 6 months compared with aciclovir. One RCT found time to cessation of postherpetic neuralgia was reduced with aciclovir compared with netivudine. One RCT found no significant difference between valaciclovir and famciclovir in the resolution of postherpetic neuralgia. One systematic review of one RCT found no significant difference in pain between topical idoxuridine and oral aciclovir 1 month after rash healing. One systematic review found insufficient evidence from two RCTs about the effects of corticosteroids plus antiviral agents.

Benefits: **Aciclovir versus placebo:** We found one systematic review (search date 1998).[7] It included results from 5 RCTs comparing aciclovir alone versus placebo. It found important heterogeneity among studies making it difficult to summarise results. Meta-analysis was not conducted. The first RCT (376 people) compared aciclovir (4 g/day for 7 days) versus placebo. It found no significant difference between aciclovir and placebo for pain at 3 or 6 months (at 3 months: AR for pain 24% in both groups; at 6 months AR 14% with aciclovir *v* 13% placebo; CI not reported in the review). The second RCT (187 people; aciclovir 4 g/day for 10 days) found that aciclovir significantly reduced pain compared with placebo at 1–3 months (AR for pain 4.2% with aciclovir *v* 16.7% with placebo; P = 0.012). However, it found no significant difference at 4–6 months (3.9% *v* 6.3%; CI not reported in the review). The third RCT (83 people; aciclovir 4 g/day for 7 days) found that aciclovir significantly reduced pain at 3 months (AR 10% *v* 40%; P = 0.0082). The fourth RCT (46 people; aciclovir 4 g/day for 10 days) found that aciclovir significantly reduced pain at 3 months (7% *v* 38%; P = 0.05), but the difference was not significant at 6 months (5% with aciclovir *v* 26% with placebo; P = 0.07). The fifth RCT (65 people; aciclovir 2 g/day for 10 days) found no significant difference in pain between aciclovir and placebo (time to outcome and AR not reported in the review). **Famciclovir versus**

placebo: We found one systematic review (search date 1998, 1 RCT, 419 people).[7] The multicentre RCT in the review compared two different doses of famciclovir in immunocompetent adults (age > 18 years) and defined duration of postherpetic neuralgia as time to pain resolution. It found that both doses of famciclovir significantly reduced the duration of pain after acute herpes zoster compared with placebo (median duration of pain with 500 mg [138 people] 63 days, with 750 mg [135 people] 61 days, with placebo [146 people] 119 days; lower dose *v* placebo P = 0.02, higher dose *v* placebo P = 0.005). **Aciclovir versus other antiviral agents:** We found one systematic review (search date 1998, 1 RCT, 1141 people).[7] The RCT in the review compared valaciclovir (a precursor of aciclovir) given three times daily for 7 or 14 days versus 7 days of aciclovir. When the results from the two valaciclovir regimens were combined, those treated with valaciclovir had a lower prevalence of pain at 6 months (AR 18.6% with valaciclovir *v* 25.7% with aciclovir; P = 0.02). We found one double blind RCT comparing netivudine versus aciclovir (511 people), which found no significant difference between groups in time to the first pain free period, but found a significantly shorter time to complete resolution of postherpetic neuralgia with aciclovir compared with netivudine (P = 0.007).[8] It found that the proportion of patients with persistent pain at 6 months was lower in people treated with aciclovir compared with netivudine (10% with aciclovir *v* 15% with netivudine; P value not reported).[8] **Addition of amitriptyline:** We found no systematic review or RCTs. **Valaciclovir versus famciclovir:** We found no systematic review. One RCT (597 immunocompetent people aged ≥ 50 years) compared valaciclovir (1 g 3 times daily) versus famciclovir (500 mg 3 times daily) started within 72 hours of appearance of the rash and given for 7 days.[9] It found no significant difference between groups in resolution of postherpetic neuralgia (HR 1.01, 95% CI 0.82 to 1.24). **Aciclovir versus topical idoxuridine:** See benefits of topical antiviral agents (idoxuridine), p 1029. **Aciclovir plus corticosteroids:** See benefits of corticosteroids, p 1030.

Harms: One previous systematic review (search date 1993) found that the most common adverse events reported with aciclovir were headache and nausea.[5] In placebo controlled trials, these effects occurred with similar frequency with treatment and placebo (headache 37% *v* 43%, nausea 13% *v* 14%). There were no major adverse events reported in the RCTs included in the systematic review.[5] In the RCTs, famciclovir, valaciclovir, and netivudine had similar safety profiles to aciclovir.[8,10,11] In the RCT comparing valaciclovir versus famciclovir the two drugs had similar safety profiles.[9]

Comment: We found no evidence on adherence to treatment, but it has been suggested that adherence to treatment may be better with the newer antiviral drugs because they are given one to three times daily compared with five times daily for aciclovir.

OPTION TOPICAL ANTIVIRAL AGENTS (IDOXURIDINE)

One systematic review of heterogeneous poor quality RCTs found no significant difference in pain between topical idoxuridine and placebo at 6 months. One systematic review of one RCT found no significant difference in pain between topical idoxuridine and oral aciclovir 1 month after rash healing.

Benefits: We found one systematic review (search date 1993, 4 RCTs, 431 people).[5] **Versus placebo:** Three included RCTs (242 people) compared topical idoxuridine versus placebo. Pooled results were not reported because of heterogeneity and poor quality of the trials. The review reported that two of the three studies found "beneficial effects" on pain reduction at 1 month (statistical analysis not reported, P value not reported), but none of the three RCTs found any significant difference at 6 months.[5] **Versus oral aciclovir:** The review[5] included one RCT (189 people)[12] that compared topical idoxuridine versus oral aciclovir. The review reported that the RCT found a non-significant trend towards fewer cases of postherpetic neuralgia in the idoxuridine group compared with aciclovir (pain 1 month after rash healing: 5% with topical idoxuridine *v* 13% with oral aciclovir; P value not reported).[5]

Harms: We found no reports of important adverse effects from idoxuridine. Application beneath dressings may be cumbersome.

Comment: None.

OPTION CORTICOSTEROIDS

Systematic reviews found insufficient evidence from RCTs about the effects of corticosteroids alone on postherpetic neuralgia. One systematic review found insufficient evidence from two RCTs about the effects of corticosteroids plus antiviral agents. There is concern that corticosteroids may cause dissemination of herpes zoster.

Benefits: **Corticosteroids alone:** We found two systematic reviews (search dates 1993[5] and 1998[7]). The earlier review (search date 1993) included RCTs of corticosteroids with conflicting results and concluded that it was not possible to assess the effect of corticosteroids.[5] The more recent review (search date 1998)[7] found similar results but identified one RCT subsequent to the earlier review.[14] This RCT is reported below. **Corticosteroids plus aciclovir:** We found one systematic review (search date 1998, 2 RCTs, 608 people).[7] The first identified RCT (400 people) randomised people into four active treatment groups: 7 days of aciclovir (101 people); 7 days of aciclovir plus 21 days of prednisone (99 people); 21 days of aciclovir (101 people); or 21 days of aciclovir plus prednisone (99 people).[13] It found no significant differences in relief of postherpetic neuralgia. The second RCT (208 people) had a factorial design, randomising people to 21 days of aciclovir plus prednisone (60 mg initially, tapered over 3 weeks), prednisone plus placebo, aciclovir plus placebo, or two placebos.[14] Although there was evidence of short term benefit from prednisone, there was no significant effect between groups on pain prevalence at 6 months after disease onset.

Harms: It is feared that corticosteroids might cause dissemination of herpes zoster. This effect was not reported in an RCT of prednisone in the earlier systematic review.[5] In the RCT of aciclovir plus prednisone, two people receiving prednisone plus aciclovir placebo and one receiving aciclovir plus prednisone placebo developed cutaneous dissemination of lesions (see harms of corticosteroids under rheumatoid arthritis, [Web only]).[14]

Comment: None.

OPTION TRICYCLIC ANTIDEPRESSANTS (AMITRIPTYLINE)

One RCT with weak methods provided insufficient evidence on the effects of amitriptyline in preventing postherpetic neuralgia.

Benefits: We found one systematic review (search date 1998, 1 RCT, 80 people).[7] The RCT in the review (80 people aged > 60 years) found that amitriptyline 25 mg taken within 48 hours of rash onset (prescribed with or without antiviral agents, at the practitioner's discretion) and continued for 90 days reduced the prevalence of postherpetic neuralgia at 6 months compared with placebo (pain free: 32/38 [84%] with amitriptyline with or without antiviral *v* 22/34 [65%] with placebo with or without antiviral; $P < 0.05$; see comment below).[4]

Harms: The RCT did not report adverse effects.[4] In another RCT, amitriptyline was associated with adverse anticholinergic effects such as dry mouth, sedation, and urinary difficulties.[5]

Comment: Interpretation of the RCT is complicated because practitioners were allowed to decide whether an antiviral agent was prescribed as well as amitriptyline.[4] Blinding may also have been inadequate.[7] The result was of borderline significance, and six people who had started treatment but had not completed a full course of amitriptyline or placebo were excluded from the analysis.[4]

QUESTION What are the effects of interventions to relieve established postherpetic neuralgia after the rash has healed?

OPTION TRICYCLIC ANTIDEPRESSANTS

One systematic review of three crossover RCTs found that tricyclic antidepressants increased pain relief in postherpetic neuralgia after 3–6 weeks compared with placebo.

Benefits: **Versus placebo:** We found two systematic reviews (search dates 1993[6] and 2000[15]). Three crossover RCTs (108 people) comparing tricyclic antidepressants versus placebo were common to both reviews. Two of these RCTs compared amitriptyline versus placebo. The other RCT compared desipramine versus placebo. The first review pooled results and found that tricyclic antidepressants taken for 3–6 weeks significantly improved pain relief from postherpetic neuralgia at the end of the treatment period compared with placebo (3 RCTs; OR 0.15, 95% CI 0.08 to 0.27; see comment below).[6] The more recent review did not pool results.[15] It found one subsequent RCT to the first review that compared amitriptyline alone; amitriptyline plus fluphenazine; fluphenazine alone; and placebo.[15] However, it did not report results for amitriptyline alone compared with placebo.

Harms: Tricyclic antidepressants are associated with anticholinergic adverse effects. In one RCT, amitriptyline increased the following adverse effects compared with placebo: dry mouth (AR 62% *v* 40%), sedation (AR 62% *v* 40%), and urinary difficulties (AR 12% *v* < 5%).[16] Syncope and heart block occurred in one person in a trial of desipramine in people with postherpetic neuralgia.[17]

Comment: The meta-analysis is based on post crossover results. The adverse effects of tricyclic antidepressants are dose related. Adverse effects may be less pronounced when treating postherpetic neuralgia rather than depression because lower doses are used. Treatments were not assessed for more than 8 weeks.

OPTION TOPICAL COUNTERIRRITANTS

Two systematic reviews including the same two RCTs found limited evidence that the topical counterirritant capsaicin improved pain relief in postherpetic neuralgia compared with placebo. One subsequent RCT found no significant difference in pain between capsaicin and placebo. Capsaicin may cause painful skin reactions (including burning, stinging, and erythema).

Benefits: We found two systematic reviews (search date 1993[6] and 2000[15]) and one subsequent RCT.[18] Both reviews identified the same two placebo controlled RCTs (see comment below). The first review found that capsaicin significantly improved pain relief compared with placebo (2 RCTs, 175 people; OR for complete or greatly reduced pain 0.29, 95% CI 0.16 to 0.54; see comment below).[6] The second review did not pool results, but reached the same conclusion. The subsequent RCT (31 people) found no significant difference in pain between capsaicin and placebo during 6 months (measured on visual analogue scale and by McGill's test; $P > 0.05$; see comment below).[18]

Harms: Reported local skin reactions included burning, stinging, and erythema.[6] These effects tended to subside with time and frequency of use.[19] In the subsequent RCT, 6 people had skin burning with capsaicin compared with none with placebo (P value not reported).[18]

Comment: The review noted the difficulty in blinding studies with capsaicin because of skin burning could have caused overestimation of benefit.[6] The first review also included one unpublished RCT (30 people) that found no significant difference in pain between capsaicin and placebo. It was excluded from the meta-analysis as when included, there was significant statistical heterogeneity between the RCTs, and clinically, it had used a weaker preparation of capsaicin, shorter treatment period, and different emollient vehicle.[6] The second review did not include the unpublished study.[15] In the subsequent RCT, 8 people did not complete the study (5 with capsaicin *v* 3 with placebo).[18]

OPTION TOPICAL ANAESTHESIA

We found insufficient evidence from three RCTs about the effects of lidocaine (lignocaine).

Benefits: We found one systematic review (search date 2000, 2 RCTs with evaluation period > 24 hours, 204 people)[15] and one additional RCT.[20] The first trial included in the review (unpublished, 171 people) found no significant difference in pain rated on a visual analogue scale between lidocaine patches and placebo after 3–4 weeks (reported as no significant difference, P value not provided).[15] The second RCT only recruited people who had responded to lidocaine patches (see comment below).[15] The additional RCT (35 people with pain present more than 1 month after healing of rash, and well defined area of painfully sensitive skin on torso or limbs) found that lidocaine patches significantly reduced average pain scores on a visual analogue scale over 12 hours compared with placebo.[20] However, it did not measure outcomes beyond 12 hours.

Harms: No systemic adverse effects were noted with lidocaine patches, and systemic absorption as determined by blood concentrations was minimal.[20]

Comment: One RCT included in the review only recruited people who had responded to lidocaine.[15] Results are therefore likely to be biased in favour of lidocaine. It found that lidocaine patches were more effective for pain relief than placebo.

OPTION GABAPENTIN

Systematic reviews of two RCTs found that gabapentin reduced pain in postherpetic neuralgia at 8 weeks compared with placebo.

Benefits: We found three systematic reviews (search date not reported,[21] search date 2002,[22] search date not reported[23]) that identified the same two multicentre RCTs.[24,25] The reviews did not pool data. Both included RCTs assessed pain using an 11 point Likert scale. The first RCT identified by the reviews (229 people who remained on tricyclic antidepressants or opiates during the trial) found that gabapentin significantly reduced the proportion of people reporting pain after 8 weeks of treatment (no pain: 16% with gabapentin *v* 8% with placebo; pain much or moderately reduced: 43% with gabapentin *v* 12% with placebo; P < 0.001).[25] The second RCT identified by the reviews (334 people) found that gabapentin (1800 mg/day or 2400 mg/day in 3 divided doses) significantly reduced mean daily pain scores at 7 weeks compared with placebo (pain reduction with gabapentin 1800 mg *v* placebo: –18.8%, 95% CI –10.9% to –26.8%; pain reduction with gabapentin 2400 mg *v* placebo: – 18.7%, 95% CI –10.7% to –26.7%).[24]

Harms: The first RCT included in the reviews found that gabapentin increased adverse effects compared with placebo (somnolence: 27% *v* 5%; dizziness: 24% *v* 5%; ataxia: 7% *v* 0%; peripheral oedema: 10% *v* 3%; infection: 8% *v* 3%; P values not reported).[25] It found similar withdrawal rates due to adverse effects between gabapentin and placebo (13.3% with gabapentin *v* 9.5% with placebo; P value not reported). The second RCT included in the reviews also found that gabapentin increased adverse effects compared with placebo (somnolence: 17% with 1800 mg *v* 20% with 2400 mg *v* 6% with placebo; dizziness: 31% *v* 33% *v* 10%; peripheral oedema: 5% *v* 11% *v* 0%; P values not reported).[24] This RCT found that gabapentin increased withdrawal rates due to adverse effect (13% with 1800 mg *v* 18% with 2400 mg *v* 6% with placebo; P value not reported).

Comment: None.

OPTION NARCOTIC ANALGESICS

We found no RCTs examining effects of morphine or methadone in people with postherpetic neuralgia. One small crossover RCT found limited evidence that oral oxycodone reduced pain compared with placebo, but was associated with more adverse effects. One systematic review of one small crossover RCT and one subsequent RCT found no evidence that dextromethorphan was more effective than placebo or lorazepam after 3–6 weeks, but found that dextromethorphan was associated with sedation and ataxia at high doses. One systematic review found limited evidence from one small RCT that tramadol reduced pain compared with clomipramine with or without levomepromazine after 6 weeks. One subsequent RCT found limited evidence that tramadol increased pain relief after 6 weeks compared with placebo.

Benefits: We found no RCTs examining the effects of morphine or methadone. We found one systematic review (search date 2000, 3 RCTs, 103 people),[15] and two subsequent RCTs studying different opiates.[26,27] The first RCT included in the review (a blinded crossover RCT; 50 people, 4 weeks on each treatment) found that oxycodone significantly improved pain measured on a visual analogue scale after 4 weeks compared with placebo, but the data were not converted into a dichotomous outcome (see comment below). However, it found that a significantly greater proportion of people preferred oxycodone to placebo (67% *v* 11%; P = 0.001).[15] A second, small, double blind crossover RCT (18 people) found no evidence of pain relief from 6 weeks' treatment with dextromethorphan (a codeine analogue) compared with placebo.[15] The third included RCT (35 people) compared tramadol versus clomipramine with or without levomepromazine.[15] It found that tramadol improved pain relief compared with other treatments (after 6 weeks, AR for "good or excellent" pain relief 60% with tramadol *v* 45% with control; RR, CI, and P values not reported in the review; see comment below). Drop out rates were high (approximately 40% in each group). The first subsequent crossover RCT (22 people) compared three treatments: dextromethorphan, memantine, and lorazepam.[26] It found no significant difference between dextromethorphan and lorazepam for pain score at 3 weeks (20 point pain Gracely score; mean difference between dextromethorphan and lorazepam −0.9, 95% CI −2.3 to +0.5). The second subsequent RCT (127 people) compared tramadol versus placebo.[27] The RCT found that tramadol significantly reduced mean pain intensity measured on a visual analogue scale compared with placebo after 6 weeks (pain intensity on visual analogue scale adjusted for mean pain at entry: 19.9 with tramadol *v* 28.5 with placebo; P = 0.0499), but found no significant difference between groups in mean pain assessed on a verbal rating scale after 6 weeks (P = 0.068).[27]

Harms: The review found that oxycodone produced adverse effects such as constipation, nausea, and sedation with greater frequency than placebo (76% *v* 49%; P = 0.0074).[15] High dose dextromethorphan produced sedation and ataxia, causing 5/18 (28%) people to stop treatment.[15] In the subsequent RCT comparing tramadol versus placebo, the percentage of people reporting at least one treatment associated adverse event were similar between groups (30% with tramadol *v* 32% with placebo) as were the total number of adverse events reported (31 with tramadol *v* 28 with placebo).[27]

Comment: The studies were small and in the tramadol study included in the systematic review,[15] results may have been biased by the co-intervention (levomepromazine). In the RCT comparing oxycodone versus placebo, 12/50 (24%) did not complete the study.

REFERENCES

1. Hope-Simpson RE. Postherpetic neuralgia. *J R Coll Gen Pract* 1975;25:571–575.
2. Ragozzino MW, Melton J III, Kurland LT, et al. Population based study of herpes zoster and its sequelae. *Medicine* 1982;61:310–316.
3. Mckendrick MW, McGill JI, Wood MJ. Lack of effect of aciclovir on postherpetic neuralgia. *BMJ* 1989;298:431.
4. Bowsher D. The effects of pre-emptive treatment of postherpetic neuralgia with amitriptyline: a randomised, double-blind, placebo-controlled trial. *J Pain Symptom Manage* 1997;13:327–331.
5. Lancaster T, Silagy C, Gray S. Primary care management of acute herpes zoster: systematic review of evidence from randomised controlled trials. *Br J Gen Pract* 1995;45:39–45. Search date 1993; primary sources Medline, hand searched primary care journals, references from books, specialists, and makers of drugs in identified trials for published and unpublished data.
6. Volmink J, Lancaster T, Gray S, et al. Treatments for postherpetic neuralgia — a systematic review of randomised controlled trials. *Fam Pract* 1996;13:84–91. Search date 1993; primary sources Medline and Embase.
7. Alper BS, Lewis R. Does treatment of acute herpes zoster prevent or shorten postherpetic neuralgia? A systematic review of the literature. *J Fam Pract* 2000;49:255–264. Search date 1998; primary sources Medline, Cochrane Controlled Trials Register, hand searched reference lists, and web based searches.
8. Soltz-Szots J, Tyring S, Andersen PL, et al. A randomised controlled trial of aciclovir versus netivudine for treatment of herpes zoster. International zoster study group. *J Antimicrob Chemother* 1998;41:549–556.
9. Tyring SK, Beutner KR, Tucker BA, et al. Antiviral therapy for herpes zoster: Randomised, controlled clinical trial of valaciclovir and famciclovir therapy in immunocompetent patients aged 50 years and older. *Arch Fam Med* 2000;9:863–869.
10. Tyring S, Barbarash RA, Nahlik JE, et al. Famciclovir for the treatment of acute herpes zoster: effects on acute disease and postherpetic neuralgia. A randomised, double-blind, placebo-controlled trial. Collaborative famciclovir herpes zoster study group. *Ann Intern Med* 1995;123:89–96.
11. Beutner KR, Friedman DJ, Forszpaniak C, et al. Valaciclovir compared with aciclovir for improved therapy for herpes zoster in immunocompetent adults. *Antimicrob Agents Chemother* 1995;39:1546–1553.
12. Aliaga A, Armijo M, Camacho F, et al. A topical solution of 40% idoxuridine in dimethyl sulfoxide compared to oral aciclovir in the treatment of herpes zoster. A double-blind multicenter clinical trial [in Spanish]. *Med Clin (Barc)* 1992;98:245–249.
13. Wood MJ, Johnson RW, McKendrick MW, et al. A randomised trial of aciclovir for 7 days or 21 days with and without prednisolone for treatment of acute herpes zoster. *N Engl J Med* 1994;330:896–900.
14. Whitley RJ, Weiss H, Gnann JW Jr, et al. Aciclovir with and without prednisone for the treatment of herpes zoster. A randomized, placebo-controlled trial. The National Institute of Allergy and Infectious Diseases Collaborative Antiviral Study Group. *Ann Intern Med* 1996;125:376–383.
15. Alper BS, Lewis PR. Treatment of postherpetic neuralgia: a systematic review of the literature. *J Fam Pract* 2002;51:121–128. Search date 2000; primary sources Medline, Cochrane Controlled Trials Register, Current Contents, and a manual search of reference lists, contact with authors, experts, and the FDA website.

16. Max MB, Schafer SC, Culnane M, et al. Amitriptyline, but not lorazepam, relieves postherpetic neuralgia. *Neurology* 1988;38:1427–1432.
17. Kishore-Kumar R, Max MB, Schafer SC, et al. Desipramine relieves postherpetic neuralgia. *Clin Pharmacol Ther* 1990;47:305–312.
18. Torre-Mollindo F, Ferna A, Barreira R, et al. Local capsaicin 0.025% in the management of postherpetic neuralgia. *Rev Soc Esp Dolor* 2001;8:468–475.
19. Bernstein JE, Korman NJ, Bickers DR, et al. Topical capsaicin treatment of chronic postherpetic neuralgia. *J Am Acad Dermatol* 1989;21:265–270.
20. Rowbotham MC, Davies PS, Verkempinck C, et al. Lidocaine patch: double-blind controlled study of a new treatment method for postherpetic neuralgia. *Pain* 1996;65:39–44.
21. Backonja, M and Glanzman, RL. Gabapentin dosing for neuropathic pain: evidence from randomized, placebo-controlled trials. *Clin Ther* 2003;25:81–104. Search date not stated; primary sources PubMed, Medline, manufacturer of gabapentin, and clinical trial web sites.
22. Singh D, Kennedy DH. The use of gabapentin for the treatment of postherpetic neuralgia. *Clin Ther* 2003;25:852–889. Search date 2002; primary sources Medline, Embase, Current Contents/Clinical Medicine, Cochrane Controlled Trials Register, Cochrane Database of Systematic Reviews, International Pharmaceutical Abstracts.
23. Stacey BR, Glanzman RL. Use of gabapentin for postherpetic neuralgia: results of two randomized, placebo-controlled studies. *Clin Ther* 2003;25:2597–2608. Search date not stated; primary source Medline.
24. Rice ASC, Maton S, Baronowski AP. Gabapentin in postherpetic neuralgia: A randomized, double blind, placebo controlled study. *Pain* 2001;94:215–224.
25. Rowbotham M, Harden N, Stacey B, et al. Gabapentin for the treatment of postherpetic neuralgia: a randomised controlled trial. *JAMA* 1998;280:1837–1842.
26. Sang CN, Booher S, Gilron I, et al. Dextromethorphan and memantine in painful diabetic neuropathy and postherpetic neuralgia: Efficacy and dose-response trials. *Anesthesiology* 2002;96:1053–1061.
27. Boureau F, Legallicier P, Kabir-Ahmadi, M. Tramadol in post-herpetic neuralgia: a randomized, double-blind, placebo-controlled trial. *Pain* 2003;104:323–331.

David Wareham
Clinical Training Fellow & Honorary SpR in Medical Microbiology
Queen Mary University of London & Barts & The London NHS Trust
London
UK

Competing interests: DW has received funding to attend an overseas infectious disease conference from Pfizer, the manufacturer of gabapentin.

We would like to acknowledge the previous contributors to this chapter, including Tim Lancaster and John Yaphe.

Tuberculosis

Search date August 2003

Paul Garner, Alison Holmes, and Lilia Ziganshina

QUESTIONS

INTERVENTIONS

See glossary Ⓖ

Key Messages

Preventing tuberculosis in high risk people without HIV infection

- **Isoniazid** One systematic review, in people without HIV infection at high risk of tuberculosis, found that, isoniazid prophylaxis for 6–12 months reduced the risk of active tuberculosis or extra-pulmonary tuberculosis compared with placebo. It also found that a short 6 month course was as effective as a 12 month course. One large RCT found that treatment with isoniazid significantly increased the risk of hepatotoxicity compared with placebo.

Treating newly diagnosed tuberculosis

- **Short course chemotherapy (as good as longer courses)** One RCT found that a 6 month regimen of rifampicin plus isoniazid improved relapse rate compared with isoniazid alone. One RCT found no evidence of a difference in relapse rates between short course regimens containing isoniazid (6 months) and longer term (8–9 months) chemotherapy in people with pulmonary tuberculosis. Three RCTs suggested that treatment with pyrazinamide speeds up sputum clearance after 2 months and improves risk of relapse compared with treatment without pyrazinamide.
- **Intermittent short course chemotherapy (as good as daily treatment)** Two RCTs in people with newly diagnosed tuberculosis found no significant difference in cure rates between daily and two or three times weekly short course chemotherapy regimens. However, the RCTs may have lacked power to exclude a clinically important difference.
- **Pyrazinamide** RCTs found that, in people with newly diagnosed tuberculosis, chemotherapy regimens containing pyrazinamide speed up sputum clearance in the first 2 months compared with other regimens, but have found limited evidence about effects on relapse rates.
- **Regimens containing quinolones** We found insufficient evidence about effects of regimens containing quinolones.
- **Chemotherapy for less than 6 months** One systematic review found limited evidence that reducing duration of treatment to less than 6 months significantly increased relapse rates compared with 12 months treatment.

Treating multidrug resistant tuberculosis

- **Comparative benefits of different regimens in multidrug resistant tuberculosis** We found no good evidence comparing different drug regimens for multidrug resistant tuberculosis.

Effects of low level laser therapy

- **Laser therapy** One systematic review found insufficient evidence about effects of low level laser therapy in people with tuberculosis.

Improving adherence and reattendance

- **Cash incentives** One systematic review has found that cash incentives improve attendance among people living in deprived circumstances compared with usual care. One subsequent RCT found that cash incentives improved treatment completion in intravenous drug users. Another subsequent RCT found no significant difference in treatment completion with immediate compared with deferred cash incentives.
- **Community health advisors** One RCT found that consultation with health advisors recruited from the community significantly increased the rate of treatment attendance compared with no consultation.
- **Defaulter actions** RCTs have found that intensive action (repeated home visits and reminder letters) improves completion of treatment compared with routine action (single reminder letter and home visit) for defaulters.
- **Health education by a nurse** One RCT found that health education by a nurse improved treatment completion compared with provision of an educational leaflet.

- **Direct observation treatment** One systematic review found no significant difference in cure rates between any direct observation treatment compared with self treatment. One large RCT, which allowed participants to choose their therapy supervisor, found that direct observative therapy significantly improved both cure rates and cure plus treatment completion rates combined, compared with self treatment. However, cointerventions factors may have contributed to better treatment adherence in this study.
- **Prompts and contracts to improve reattendance for Mantoux test reading** One RCT in healthy people found that telephone prompts to return for Mantoux test reading slightly increased the number of people who reattended compared with no prompts, but the difference was not significant. One RCT found that healthy people were more likely to reattend for Mantoux test reading after providing either a verbal or written commitment compared with no such commitment.
- **Health education by a doctor; prompts to adhere to treatment; sanctions for non-adherence; staff training** We found insufficient evidence on the effects of these interventions.

DEFINITION	Tuberculosis is caused by *Mycobacterium tuberculosis* and can affect many organs. Specific symptoms relate to site of infection and are generally accompanied by fever, sweats, and weight loss.
INCIDENCE/ PREVALENCE	About a third of the world's population is infected with *M tuberculosis*. The organism kills more people than any other infectious agent. The World Health Organization estimates that 95% of cases are in developing countries, and that 25% of avoidable deaths in developing countries are caused by tuberculosis.[1]
AETIOLOGY/ RISK FACTORS	Social factors include poverty, overcrowding, homelessness, and inadequate health services. Medical factors include HIV and immunosuppression.
PROGNOSIS	Prognosis varies widely and depends on treatment.[2]
AIMS OF INTERVENTION	To cure tuberculosis; eliminate risk of relapse; reduce infectivity; avoid emergence of drug resistance; and prevent death.
OUTCOMES	*M tuberculosis* in sputum (smear examination and culture), symptoms, weight, cure, relapse rates, attendance, completion of treatment.
METHODS	*Clinical Evidence* search and appraisal August 2003. Key words: tuberculosis, pulmonary, isoniazid, pyrazinamide, and rifampicin. We included all Cochrane systematic reviews and studies that were randomised or used alternate allocation, and had at least 1 year follow up after completion of treatment.

QUESTION What are the effects of interventions to prevent tuberculosis in high risk people without HIV infection?

OPTION ISONIAZID

One systematic review, in people without HIV infection at high risk of tuberculosis, found that, isoniazid prophylaxis for 6–12 months reduced the risk of active tuberculosis or extra-pulmonary tuberculosis compared with placebo. It also found that a short 6 month course was as effective as a 12 month course. One large RCT found that treatment with isoniazid increased the risk of hepatotoxicity compared with placebo.

Benefits: We found one systematic review (search date 2003; 11 RCTs: 73 375 people without HIV infection).[3] The review compared 6 to 12 month courses of isoniazid versus placebo in HIV negative people at increased risk of developing tuberculosis (people with previous pulmonary tuberculosis or positive skin tests; people with recent or remote contact with an active case of pulmonary tuberculosis; or people living in an area with a high incidence and prevalence of disease). It found that isoniazid significantly reduced the risk of active tuberculosis or extra-pulmonary tuberculosis compared with placebo (AR for active tuberculosis; 11 RCTs: 239/40 262 [0.6%] with isoniazid *v* 557/33 113 [1.7%] with placebo; RR 0.40, 95% CI 0.31 to 0.52; AR for extra-pulmonary tuberculosis; 4 RCTs: 9/22 379 [0.04%] with isoniazid *v* 28/22 257 [1.3%] with placebo). The review found no significant difference in active tuberculosis or extra-pulmonary tuberculosis between a 6 month and a 12 month course of isoniazid (AR for active tuberculosis; 1 RCT: 34/6965 [0.5%] with 6 months of isoniazid *v* 24/6919 [0.3%] with 12 months of isoniazid; RR 1.41, 95% CI 0.84 to 2.37). Isoniazid did not significantly reduce deaths from tuberculosis compared with placebo (2 RCTs: 3/16 318 [0.02%] with isoniazid *v* 10/9396 [0.1%]; RR 0.29, 95% CI 0.07 to 1.18).

Harms: The review found that hepatotoxicity was significantly more common in people receiving isoniazid compared with placebo (AR for hepatitis; 1 RCT: 77/13 884 [0.6%] with isoniazid *v* 7/6990 [0.1%] with placebo; RR 5.54, 95% CI 2.56 to 12.00). Other reported adverse effects of isoniazid therapy include mild and transient headache, nausea, and dizziness.

Comment: Even in the isoniazid group, the absolute risk of hepatotoxicity is still small.

QUESTION **What are the effects of different drug regimens in people with newly diagnosed pulmonary tuberculosis?**

OPTION **SHORT COURSE CHEMOTHERAPY**

One RCT found that a 6 month regimen of rifampicin plus isoniazid improved relapse rate compared with isoniazid alone. One RCT found no evidence of a difference in relapse rates between short course regimens containing isoniazid (6 months) and longer term (8–9 months) chemotherapy in people with pulmonary tuberculosis. Three RCTs suggested that treatment with pyrazinamide speeds up sputum clearance after 2 months and improves risk of relapse compared with treatment without pyrazinamide.

Benefits: We found no systematic review, but found four RCTs.[4–7] **Rifampicin in continuation phase:** We found one RCT (851 people).[4] It compared four daily short course chemotherapy regimens (three 6 months and one 8 months in duration). All four treatment arms had the same initial 2 month phase of streptomycin, isoniazid, rifampicin, and pyrazinamide. The continuation phase of the 6 month regimens was: isoniazid plus rifampicin; isoniazid plus pyrazinamide; or isoniazid alone. The continuation phase of the 8 month regimen was isoniazid alone. It found that bacteriological relapse was significantly reduced with isoniazid plus rifampicin compared with isoniazid alone at 6 months (relapse rate: 2% with rifampicin plus isoniazid *v* 9% with isoniazid alone; $P < 0.01$).[4] **Long versus short rifampicin regimens:** We found two RCTs (1295 people with untreated, culture/smear positive pulmonary tuberculosis), which compared 6 versus 8–9 months of chemotherapy.[4,5] Participants were followed up for at least 1 year after treatment was completed. The trials were performed in the UK and in east and central Africa, and used different combinations of isoniazid, rifampicin, ethambutol, streptomycin, and pyrazinamide for initial (first 2 months) and continuation treatment. Both RCTs found no significant difference in relapse rates between short and longer course chemotherapy regimens ($P > 0.1$). The first RCT (described above)[4] found no significant difference in relapse rate between 6 and 8 months continuation with isoniazid alone (relapse rate: 9% with isoniazid alone for 6 months *v* 3% with isoniazid alone for 8 months; $P > 0.1$). The second RCT compared an initial regimen of isoniazid, rifampicin, pyrazinamide plus either ethambutol or streptomycin for 6 months.[5] It found no difference in relapse rates between ethambutol and streptomycin (relapse rate: 4/127 [3.1%] with ethambutol v 2/119 [1.7%] with streptomycin). **Adding pyrazinamide:** We found 3 RCTs that compared chemotherapy regimens with or without pyrazinamide.[5–7] The first RCT (444 people) found that sputum conversion was faster with regimens containing pyrazinamide at 2 months (AR for negative cultures: 77% with pyrazinamide v 64% without pyrazinamide; $P < 0.01$).[5] The second RCT (833 people) compared four different 6 month regimens and found that bacterial relapse was significantly higher for those not receiving pyrazinamide in the 12 months after chemotherapy (12/160 [7.5%] v 8/625 [1.3%]; $P < 0.001$).[6] The third RCT (497 people) compared ongoing pyrazinamide versus no treatment.[7] It found that relapse at 18 months was more likely in those not receiving pyrazinamide, but the difference was not significant (3.1% with pyrazinamide v 1.0% with no pyrazinamide).

Harms: In the largest RCT, possible adverse reactions were reported in 24/851 people (3%), with six requiring modification of treatment.[4] Two people in the trial developed jaundice, one of whom died. **Pyrazinamide:** Adding pyrazinamide did not increase the risk of hepatitis (4% with pyrazinamide v 4% with no pyrazinamide).[5] However, mild adverse effects were more common, including arthralgia, skin rashes, flu-like symptoms, mild gastrointestinal disturbance, vestibular disturbance, peripheral neuropathy, and confusion. Arthralgia was the most common adverse effect, reported in about 1% of people on pyrazinamide, but was mild and never required modification of treatment.[4,5]

Comment: Short course chemotherapy may not be effective in people treated previously, because the organisms may have acquired drug resistance.

OPTION INTERMITTENT SHORT COURSE CHEMOTHERAPY

Two RCTs in people with newly diagnosed tuberculosis found no significant difference in cure rates between daily and two or three times weekly short course chemotherapy regimens. However, the RCTs may have lacked power to exclude a clinically important difference.

Benefits: We found one systematic review (search date 2001)[8] and one subsequent RCT (206 children).[9] The review found one RCT (399 people) that compared three times weekly versus daily chemotherapy for 6 months in people with newly diagnosed pulmonary tuberculosis. It found no significant difference in bacteriological cure rates (defined as negative sputum culture) or relapse rates between three times weekly versus daily chemotherapy 1 month after treatment was completed (bacteriological cure rate: 99.9% with 3 times weekly v 100% with daily; relapse rate: 5/186 [2.7%] with 3 times weekly v 1/192 [0.5%] with daily; RR 4.0, 95% CI 0.7 to 24.1).[8] The subsequent RCT compared twice weekly versus daily chemotherapy. It found no significant difference in cure rates between the two regimens (85/89 [95%] people with twice weekly v 114/117 [97%] people with daily; RR 0.98, 95% CI 0.84 to 1.02).[9]

Harms: Intermittent treatment has the potential to contribute to drug resistance, but this was not found in the studies.[8]

Comment: The RCTs had low event rates and were too small to exclude a clinically important effect difference between the dosing regimens. At least 12 cohort studies have found cure rates of 80–100% with three times weekly regimens taken over 6–9 months.[8]

OPTION CHEMOTHERAPY FOR LESS THAN 6 MONTHS

One systematic review found limited evidence that reducing duration of treatment to less than 6 months significantly increased relapse rates compared with 12 months treatment.

Benefits: We found one systematic review (search date 1999, 7 RCTs, 2248 outpatients with newly diagnosed pulmonary tuberculosis), which compared a variety of shorter (minimum 2 months) and longer (maximum 12 months) drug regimens.[10] The trials included people in India, Hong Kong, Singapore, and Germany. The review found that a 3 month regimen significantly increased relapse rates compared with a 12 month regimen (5 RCTs: RR 3.03, 95% CI 2.08 to 4.40). One of the RCTs found that people given a 2 month regimen were significantly less likely to change or discontinue drugs than those given a 12 month regimen (6/299 [2.0%] *v* 17/299 [5.7%]; RR 0.35; 95% CI 0.14 to 0.88).[10]

Harms: The review found similar rates of adverse events or toxicity with both shorter and longer regimens.

Comment: The treatments were given under optimal conditions. In clinical practice adherence is likely to be lower, so relapse rates associated with the shorter regimens are likely to be higher than those in clinical trials.

OPTION REGIMENS CONTAINING QUINOLONES

We found insufficient evidence about effects of regimens containing quinolones.

Benefits: We found no systematic review, but found two RCTs.[11,12] One RCT in Tanzania (200 people) compared a regimen containing a low dose of quinolone (750 mg/day ciprofloxacin) versus a regimen without a quinolone. It found that the quinolone regimen increased relapse rate, but the difference was not significant (RR of relapse at 6 months: 16.0, 95% CI 0.9 to 278.0).[11] The second RCT (160 people) compared a regimen containing ciprofloxacin versus a regimen without, and focused only on adverse effects (see harms below).[12]

Harms: Adverse effects, which were mild and responsive to symptomatic treatment, were similar in people taking quinolone regimens versus controls.[12]

Comment: Quinolones have good mycobactericidal activity *in vitro*. Some of the newer quinolones have greater antimycobacterial activity than ciprofloxacin.

QUESTION What are the effects of different drug regimens in people with multidrug resistant tuberculosis?

OPTION COMPARATIVE BENEFITS OF DIFFERENT REGIMENS IN MULTIDRUG RESISTANT TUBERCULOSIS

We found no RCTs comparing different drug regimens for multidrug resistant tuberculosis.

Benefits: We found no systematic review and no RCTs comparing different regimens in people with multidrug resistant tuberculosis.

Harms: We found no evidence.

Comment: Current clinical practice in multidrug resistant tuberculosis is to include at least three drugs to which the particular strain of tuberculosis is sensitive, using as many bactericidal agents as possible. People are observed directly and managed by a specialised clinician.

QUESTION What are the effects of low level laser therapy in people with tuberculosis?

OPTION LASER THERAPY

One systematic review found insufficient evidence about effects of low level laser therapy in people with tuberculosis.

Benefits: We found one systematic review (search date 2001, no RCTs; see comment below) and no subsequent RCTs.[13]

Harms: The systematic review did not provide reliable data on harms.

Comment: The systematic review found 29 observational studies, mainly from Russia and India.[13] It found no reliable evidence for a beneficial effect of low level laser therapy for people with tuberculosis, although a "range of positive effects" was reported.[13]

QUESTION Which interventions improve adherence to treatment?

OPTION STAFF TRAINING

We found insufficient evidence on the effects of staff training on adherence to treatment.

Benefits: We found one systematic review (search date 2000, 1 poorly randomised RCT; see comment below) comparing intensive staff supervision versus routine supervision at centres in Korea performing tuberculosis extension activities.[14] Centres were paired and randomised, and supervision was carried out by senior doctors. The review found that higher completion rates were achieved with intensive supervision (RR 1.2; CI not estimated because of cluster design).

Harms: None reported.

Comment: The trial used cluster randomisation, but the unit of analysis was the individual.

OPTION PROMPTS TO ADHERE TO TREATMENTS

We found no RCTs about the effects of prompts on adherence to treatment.

Benefits: We found one systematic review (search date 2000), which found no RCTs of prompts to return for treatment.[14]

Harms: None.

Comment: None.

OPTION DEFAULTER ACTIONS

One systematic review has found that intensive action (repeated home visits and reminder letters) improves completion of treatment compared with routine action (single reminder letter and home visit) for defaulters.

Benefits: We found one systematic review (search date 2000, 2 RCTs conducted in India).[14] The first included RCT (170 people randomised; 150 followed up) found that up to four home visits to defaulters**G** significantly improved completion of treatment compared with the routine policy of a reminder letter followed by one home visit (RR 1.32, 95% CI 1.02 to 1.71). The second RCT (200 people) found that up to two reminder letters significantly improved completion of treatment (RR 1.21, 95% CI 1.05 to 1.39), even in people who were illiterate.

Harms: None reported.

Comment: None.

OPTION CASH INCENTIVES

One systematic review has found that cash incentives improve attendance among people living in deprived circumstances compared with usual care. One subsequent RCT found that cash incentives improved treatment completion in intravenous drug users. Another subsequent RCT found no significant difference in treatment completion with immediate compared with deferred cash incentives.

Benefits: **Versus no cash incentive:** We found one systematic review (search date 2000, 2 RCTs conducted in the USA)[14] and one subsequent RCT.[15] The first included RCT (244 homeless men) found that a cash incentive ($5 [1992 US$]) significantly improved attendance at the first appointment compared with usual care (RR 1.6, 95% CI 1.3 to 2.0). The second RCT (248 migrants; 205 followed up) found that a cash incentive ($10 [1985 US$]) combined with health education significantly improved attendance in people on tuberculosis preventive therapy compared with usual care, but did not improve attendance in individuals with clinical disease (preventative therapy: RR 2.4, 95% CI 1.5 to 3.7; treatment: RR 1.07, 95% CI 0.97 to 1.19).[14] The subsequent RCT (163 drug users with positive tuberculin skin test) compared three groups: direct observation at a participant chosen site plus a cash incentive ($5 [1994–1997 US$]) per visit; direct observation at a designated site plus $5 a visit; and direct observation at a participant chosen site without a cash incentive. It found that both groups given cash incentives were significantly more likely to complete treatment compared with the group given no cash incentive (AR for treatment completion: 28/53 [53%] with chosen site plus cash *v* 2/55 [4%] with no cash incentive; OR 29.7, 95% CI 6.5 to 134.5; 33/55 [60%] with designated site plus cash *v* 2/55 [4%] with no cash incentive; OR 39.7, 95% CI 8.7 to 134.5).[15] **Immediate versus deferred cash incentive:** We found one RCT (300 intravenous drug users with latent tuberculosis), which compared three interventions: treatment with direct observation (see direct patient observation, p 1045) by a nurse; treatment with self administration plus peer counselling and education; and routine care. Participants in each group were further randomised to receive either an immediate versus a deferred cash incentive ($10 [1995–1997 US$]).[16] The immediate payment was given at the end of each month when people completed a routine assessment for adherence and drug toxicity. The deferred payment was given either after the 6 months' treatment period or when the person withdrew from the study. The RCT found no difference in treatment completion between immediate versus deferred payments (125/150 [83%] *v* 112/150 [75%]; P = 0.09).[16]

Harms: The RCTs did not assess adverse effects.

Comment: None.

OPTION HEALTH EDUCATION

One RCT found that health education by a nurse improved treatment completion compared with an educational leaflet alone, but found no evidence of benefit from health education by a doctor. One RCT in drug users found no significant effect of 5–10 minutes of health education on attendance rates for scheduled follow up.

Benefits: We found one systematic review (search date 2000, 2 RCTs conducted in the USA).[14] The first RCT (1004 people) identified by the review compared four methods of health education: telephoning by a nurse; visiting by a nurse; consultation by a clinic doctor; and provision of an educational leaflet. It found that nurse telephone call and nurse visit both significantly increased treatment completion compared with the leaflet alone (75/80 [94%] with nurse telephone call *v* 55/77 [71%] with leaflet; RR 1.30, 95% CI 1.18 to 1.37; 75/79 [95%] with nurse visit *v* 55/77 [71%] with leaflet; RR 1.33, 95% CI 1.20 to 1.38). However, it found no significant difference in treatment completion between consultation by the clinic doctor and the education leaflet alone (64/82 [78%] *v* 55/77 [71%]; RR 1.09, 95% CI 0.89 to 1.23). The second RCT (403 drug users) found that 5–10 minutes of health education had no significant effect on whether people kept a scheduled appointment compared with no targeted health education (RR 1.04, 95% CI 0.70 to 1.54).[14]

Harms: None measured.

Comment: Education is often part of a package of care that includes prompts and incentives, which makes it difficult to evaluate the independent effects of education.

OPTION SANCTIONS FOR NON-ADHERENCE

We found no RCTs on the effect of sanctions.

Benefits: We found one systematic review (search date 2000), which identified no RCTs of sanctions.[14]

Harms: The use of sanctions may be ethically dubious.

Comment: In New York (USA), incarcerating people who did not comply with treatment was thought to increase compliance with the Department of Health's community tuberculosis treatment programme.[17]

OPTION COMMUNITY HEALTH ADVISORS

One RCT found that consultation with health advisors recruited from the community significantly increased the rate of attendance for treatment compared with no consultation.

Benefits: We found one systematic review (search date 2000, 1 RCT).[14] The RCT (200 homeless people) found that consultation with health advisors recruited from the community significantly increased the rate of attendance for treatment compared with no consultation (62/83 [75%] *v* 42/79 [53%]; RR 1.4, 95% CI 1.1 to 1.8).

Harms: None reported.

Comment: None.

OPTION DIRECT OBSERVATION TREATMENT

One systematic review found no significant difference in cure rates between any direct observation treatment compared with self treatment. One large RCT, which allowed participants to choose their therapy observer, found that direct observation therapy significantly improved both cure rates and cure plus treatment completion rates combined, compared with self administration. However confounding factors may have contributed to better treatment adherence in this study.

Benefits: We found one systematic review (search date 2002, 6 RCTs, 1910 people).[18] **Versus self administered treatment**: The review found four RCTs that compared direct observation of people as they took their drugs (by a health professional, lay health worker, or family member) versus self administered treatment. Treatment for all studies was for 6 months, and cure was measured at the end of treatment (3 RCTs) or 1–2 months (1 RCT). The review found no significant difference in cure between any direct observation treatment compared with self treatment (4 RCTs; RR 1.06, 95% CI 0.98 to 1.14). When analysed by the person observing the treatment, there was no significant difference in cure and treatment completion rates combined between self administered treatment and treatment observed by either a health professional, lay health worker, or family member. However, one RCT (836 people), which allowed participants to choose their therapy observer, found that direct observation therapy significantly improved both cure rates and cure plus treatment completion rates combined, compared with self administration (cure: RR 1.13, 95% CI 1.04 to 1.24; cure and treatment completion combined: RR 1.11, 95% CI 1.03 to 1.18). However, cointerventions may have contributed to better treatment adherence in this study (see comments below).[18] The fifth RCT found no significant difference in treatment completion rate between direct observation at a participant chosen site compared with direct observation at a designated site, with or without cash incentives (see cash incentives, p 1043) at 12 months (RR 0.88; 95% CI 0.63 to 1.23).[15] The sixth RCT (300 intravenous drug users with latent tuberculosis) compared three interventions: treatment with direct observation by a nurse; treatment with self administration plus peer counselling and education; and routine care. Participants in each group were further randomised to receive either an immediate versus a deferred cash incentive ($10 [1995–1997 US$]) (see cash incentives, p 1043).[16] It found no significant difference between any direct observation therapy, with or without cash incentives, compared with self administration alone at 6 months (direct observation *v* self administration alone; RR 1.02, 95% CI 0.89 to 1.18).[18]

Harms: Potential harms include reduced cooperation between patient and doctor, removal of individual responsibility, detriment to long term sustainability of antituberculosis programmes, and increased burden on health services to the detriment of care for other diseases. None of these has been adequately investigated.

Comment: In the RCT in which people where given a choice of supervisor, cointerventions factors may have contributed to the positive findings.[18] Allocation concealment was inadequate, raising the possibility of selection bias. Furthermore, participants receiving direct observation therapy also received twice weekly home visits by health workers as part of the monitoring process which included tablet counting and urine testing for rifampicin. These cointerventions may have contributed to better adherence rates in this study. Numerous observational studies have evaluated interventions described as direct observation treatment, but all were packages of interventions that included specific investment in antituberculosis programmes, such as strengthened drug supplies; improved microscopy services; and numerous incentives, sanctions, and other co-interventions that were likely to influence adherence.[19,20]

QUESTION **Which interventions improve reattendance for Mantoux test reading?**

OPTION **PROMPTS AND CONTRACTS TO IMPROVE REATTENDANCE FOR MANTOUX TEST READING**

One RCT in healthy people found insufficient evidence on the effects of telephone prompts to return for Mantoux test reading. One RCT found that healthy people were more likely to return for Mantoux test reading after providing either a verbal or written commitment compared with no such commitment.

Benefits: **Prompts:** We found one systematic review (search date 2000, 1 RCT).[14] The RCT (701 healthy people) compared an automatic telephone message prompt to return for Mantoux reading versus no prompt. It found that people were slightly more likely to return for testing after prompting, but the difference was not significant (93% with prompting *v* 88% with no prompting; RR 1.05, 95% CI 1.00 to 1.10).[14] **Contracts:** We found no systematic review. One RCT (2053 healthy students in the USA) found that reattendance for Mantoux reading was significantly improved both by verbal and written commitments compared with no commitment (reattendance with verbal commitment: RR 1.10, 95% CI 1.03 to 1.18; reattendance with written commitment: RR 1.12, 95% CI 1.05 to 1.19).[21]

Harms: None reported.

Comment: None.

GLOSSARY

Defaulter actions Actions taken by health workers when people fail to attend for treatment of their tuberculosis.

REFERENCES

1. Global Tuberculosis Programme. *Treatment of tuberculosis*. Geneva: World Health Organization, 1997:WHO/TB/97.220.
2. Enarson D, Rouillon A. Epidemiological basis of tuberculosis control. In: Davis PD, ed. *Clinical tuberculosis*. 2nd ed. London: Chapman and Hall Medical, 1998.
3. Smieja MJ, Marchetti CA, Cook DJ, et al. Isoniazid for preventing tuberculosis in non-HIV infected persons (Cochrane Review). In: The Cochrane Library, Issue 4, 2003. Chichester, UK: John Wiley & Sons, Ltd.
4. East and Central African/British Medical Research Council Fifth Collaborative Study. Controlled clinical trial of 4 short-course regimens of chemotherapy (three 6-month and one 8-month) for pulmonary tuberculosis. *Tubercle* 1983;64:153–166.
5. British Thoracic Society. A controlled trial of 6 months chemotherapy in pulmonary tuberculosis, final report: results during the 36 months after the end of chemotherapy and beyond. *Br J Dis Chest* 1984;78:330–336.
6. Hong Kong Chest Service/British Medical Research Council. Controlled trial of four thrice weekly regimens and a daily regimen given for 6 months for pulmonary tuberculosis. *Lancet* 1981;1:171–174.
7. Farga V, Valenzuela P, Valenzuela MT, et al. Short-term chemotherapy of tuberculosis with 5-month regimens with and without pyrazinamide in the second phase (TA-82). *Rev Med Chil* 1986;114:701–705 [In Spanish].
8. Mwandumba HC, Squire SB. Fully intermittent dosing with drugs for tuberculosis in adults. In: The Cochrane Library, Issue 1, 2002. Oxford: Update Software. Search date 2001; primary sources Cochrane Infectious Diseases Group Trials Register, Cochrane Controlled Trials Register, Medline, Embase, reference lists of article, and researchers contacted for unpublished trials.
9. Naude JMTW, Donald PR, Huseey GD, et al. Twice weekly vs. daily chemotherapy for childhood tuberculosis. *Pediatr Infect Dis* 2000;19:405–410.
10. Gelband H. Regimens of less than six months treatment for TB. In: The Cochrane Library, Issue 1, 2002. Oxford: Update Software. Search date 1999; primary sources Medline, Cochrane Parasitic Diseases Trials Register, contact with researchers, and hand searches of reference lists.
11. Kennedy N, Berger L, Curran J, et al. Randomized controlled trial of a drug regimen that includes ciprofloxacin for the treatment of pulmonary tuberculosis. *Clin Infect Dis* 1996;22:827–833.
12. Kennedy N, Fox R, Uiso L, et al. Safety profile of ciprofloxacin during long-term therapy for pulmonary tuberculosis. *J Antimicrob Chemother* 1993:32:897–902.

13. Vlassov VV, Pechatnikov LM, MacLehose HG. Low level laser therapy for treating tuberculosis (Cochrane Review). In: The Cochrane Library, Issue 4, 2003. Chichester, UK: John Wiley & Sons, Ltd.
14. Volmink J, Garner P. Interventions for prompting adherence to tuberculosis treatment. In: The Cochrane Library, Issue 3, 2001. Oxford: Update Software. Search date 2000; primary sources Medline, Embase, Cochrane Controlled Trials Register 1998, Issue 3, Cochrane Collaboration Effective Professional Practice (CCEPP) Registry Trials, LILACS to 2000, hand searches of journals and reference lists, and contact with authors.
15. Malotte CK, Hollingshead JR, Larro M. Incentives vs. outreach workers for latent tuberculosis treatment in drug users. *Am J Prev Med* 2001;20:103–107.
16. Chaisson R, Barnes GL, Hackman JR, et al. A randomized, controlled trial of interventions to improve adherence to isoniazid therapy to prevent tuberculosis in injection drug users. *Am J Med* 2001;110:610–615.
17. Fujiwara PI, Larkin C, Frieden TR. Directly observed therapy in New York history, implementation, results and challenges. *Tuberculosis* 1997;18:135–148.
18. Volmink J, Garner P. Directly observed therapy for treating tuberculosis. In: The Cochrane Library, Issue 1, 2003. Oxford: Update Software. Search date 2002; primary sources, Cochrane Library, Medline, Embase, LILACS, hand searches of reference lists, and contact with experts in the field and relevant organisations.
19. Garner P. What makes DOT work? *Lancet* 1998;352:1326–1327.
20. Volmink J, Matchaba P, Garner P. Directly observed therapy and treatment adherence. *Lancet* 2000;355:1345–1350. Search date 1999; primary sources Medline, Embase, Cochrane Controlled Trials Register, and hand searches of reference lists.
21. Wurtele SK, Galanos AN, Roberts MC. Increasing return compliance in a tuberculosis detection drive. *J Behav Med* 1980;3:311–318.

Paul Garner
Professor
Liverpool School of Tropical Medicine
Liverpool
UK

Alison Holmes
Senior Lecturer
Hammersmith Hospital Imperial College
London
UK

Lilia Ziganshina
Professor
Department of Clinical Pharmacology and Pharmacotherapy, Kazan State Medical Academy
Kazan
Russia

Competing interests: None declared.

End stage renal disease

Search date October 2003

Yoshio N Hall and Glenn M Chertow

QUESTIONS

INTERVENTIONS

See glossary G

Key Messages

Peritoneal Dialysis

- **Icodextrin (reduces volume overload compared with 1.36% or 2.27% dextrose solutions)** Three RCTs in people receiving continuous ambulatory peritoneal dialysis found that 7.5% icodextrin solution for the long dwell increased ultrafiltration (fluid loss) compared with 1.36% or 2.27% dextrose solutions. Two of the RCTs found that 7.5% icodextrin reduced extracellular water or total body water compared with 1.36% or 2.27% dextrose solutions. One of the RCTs found that 7.5% icodextrin reduced left ventricular mass compared with 1.36% dextrose solution. However, one of the RCTs found no significant difference between 7.5% icodextrin solution and 3.86% dextrose solution in mean ultrafiltration during the long dwell.
- **Increased dose dialysis (no more effective than standard dose dialysis in reducing mortality)** One RCT found no significant difference in mortality between standard dose and increased dose peritoneal dialysis.

Haemodialysis

- **High membrane flux haemodialysis (no more effective than low membrane flux haemodialysis in reducing mortality)** One RCT found no significant difference in hospital admission for cardiac causes, or all cause mortality between high membrane flux and low membrane flux (with standard or increased dose haemodialysis).

- **Increased dose haemodialysis (no more effective than standard dose dialysis in reducing mortality)** One RCT found no significant difference in hospital admission for cardiac causes or all cause mortality between standard dose haemodialysis and increased dose haemodialysis (at high or low membrane flux).

Preventing complications

- **Sevelamer (reduces progression of coronary artery and aortic calcification compared with calcium salts)** One RCT found that sevelamer reduced the progression of coronary artery and aortic calcification compared with calcium salts at 52 weeks. It found similar mortality with sevelamer and calcium salts. One crossover RCT found no difference in reduction of serum phosphorus between sevelamer and calcium acetate. Both RCTs found that sevelamer reduced serum low density lipoprotein cholesterol levels and the incidence of hypercalcaemia compared with calcium salts.
- **Erythropoietin or darbepoetin** One RCT found no significant difference between darbepoetin α and recombinant human erythropoietin in maintenance of haemoglobin levels at 25–32 weeks. There is consensus based on observational studies that erythropoietin is effective for the treatment of anaemia in people with end stage renal disease.

DEFINITION End stage renal disease (ESRD) is defined as irreversible decline in a person's own kidney function, which is severe enough to be fatal in the absence of dialysisⒼ or transplantation. ESRD is included under stage 5 of the National Kidney Foundation Kidney Disease Outcomes Quality Initiative (K/DOQIⒼ) classification of chronic kidney disease (CKD), where it refers to individuals with an estimated glomerular filtration rate below 15 mL per minute per 1.73 m^2 body surface area, or those requiring dialysis irrespective of glomerular filtration rate.[1] The reduction or absence of kidney function leads to a host of maladaptive changes including fluid retention (extracellular volume overload), anaemia, disturbances of bone and mineral metabolism, dyslipidaemia, and protein energy malnutrition. **Fluid retention** in people with ESRD contributes significantly to the hypertension, ventricular dysfunction, and excess cardiovascular events observed in this population. **Anaemia** associated with CKD is normocytic and normochromic, and most commonly attributed to reduced erythropoietin synthesis by the affected kidneys. Additional factors such as iron deficiency from frequent phlebotomy, blood retention in the dialyser and tubing, and gastrointestinal bleeding; severe secondary hyperparathyroidism; acute and chronic inflammatory conditions (e.g. infection); and shortened red blood cell survival also contribute to the anaemia. **Disturbances of bone and mineral metabolism**, such as hyperparathyroidism, hyperphosphataemia, and hypo- or hypercalcaemia are common in people with CKD.[1] If untreated, these disturbances can cause pain, pruritus, anaemia, bone loss, and increased fracture risk, and can contribute to hypertension and cardiovascular disease.[2] **Dyslipidaemia** in people with CKD is characterised by high levels of very low density lipoprotein, low levels of high density lipoprotein, and elevated levels of modified low density lipoprotein, and is associated with increased cardiovascular risk.

INCIDENCE/ PREVALENCE The incidence and prevalence of ESRD continues to grow worldwide. According to data collected from 120 countries with dialysisⒼ programmes, at the end of 2001, about 1 479 000 people were receiving renal replacement therapy (RRTⒼ).[3] Among these individuals, 1 015 000 (69%) received haemodialysis and 126 000 (9%) received peritoneal dialysis, although an additional 338 000 (23%) were living with a kidney transplant.[3] Exact estimates of ESRD incidence and prevalence remain elusive, because international databases of renal registries exclude individuals with ESRD who do not receive RRT.[4] International comparisons of RRT pose similar challenges owing to differences in health care systems, government funding, acceptance of treatment, demographics, and access to care. Worldwide, the highest incidence and prevalence rates are reported from the US and Japan. According to the United States Renal Data System (USRDS) 2003 annual report, there were 93 327 new cases of ESRD in 2001, equivalent to an annual incidence of 336 cases per million population. The prevalence of ESRD in the US in 2002 was 406 081 (1403 cases/million population).[5] Similarly, according to reports published by the Japanese Society for Dialysis Therapy, 252 people per million population started dialysis in 2000. In 2001, there were 1721 people per million population in Japan receiving dialysis, the highest reported prevalence for industrialised nations.[6] In comparison, based on data pooled from the European Renal Association–European Dialysis and Transplant Association Registry and UK Renal Registry, the incidence of RRT in 2000 ranged from 89 cases per million population in Norway to 160 cases per million population in French and Belgium. The prevalence of RRT in 2000 ranged from about 300 cases per million population in Poland to 850 cases per million population in Belgium. In 2000, the Oceania region reported an annual incidence of ESRD of about 90 people per million population in Australia and 107 people per million population in New Zealand. The prevalence of ESRD in 2000 was similar for Australia and New Zealand, about 600 cases per million population.[4,7,8]

AETIOLOGY/ RISK FACTORS The amount of daily proteinuria remains one of the strongest predictors of progression to ESRD.[9–11] Hypertension is a strong independent risk for progression to ESRD, particularly in people with proteinuria.[11,12] Age is also a predictor for ESRD: people over 65 years old have a four to fivefold increase in risk of ESRD compared with people under 65 years old.[13] Additional risk factors for developing ESRD include a history of chronic renal insufficiency, diabetes mellitus, heroin abuse, tobacco or analgesic use, black race, lower socioeconomic status, and a family history of kidney disease.[14–20]

PROGNOSIS The overall prognosis of untreated ESRD remains poor. Most people with ESRD eventually die from complications of cardiovascular disease, infection, or if dialysisⒼ is not provided, progressive uraemia (hyperkalaemia, acidosis, malnutrition).[1,5,7,21] Exact mortality estimates, however, are unavailable as international renal registries omit individuals with ESRD who do not receive RRTⒼ.[4] Among people receiving RRT, cardiovascular disease is the leading cause of mortality, and accounts for over 40% of deaths in this population.[1,5,7] Extracellular volume overload and hypertension, common among people with CKD, are known predictors of left ventricular hypertrophy and cardiovascular mortality in this population.[22] Even after adjustment for age, gender, ethnicity, and the presence of diabetes, annual cardiovascular mortality remains roughly an order of magnitude higher in people with ESRD compared with the general population, particularly among younger individuals.[1,8]

AIMS OF INTERVENTION To prolong life; prevent uraemic complications such as hyperphosphataemia, dyslipidaemia, and anaemia; to reduce complications of cardiovascular disease (myocardial infarction, congestive heart failure, and stroke); to manage blood pressure and volume overload; and improve quality of life, with minimal adverse effects.

OUTCOMES Primary outcomes of interest include death; incidence of cardiovascular complications (myocardial infarction, congestive heart failure, and stroke); frequency and severity of uraemic complications; incidence and severity of dyslipidaemia; blood pressure; quality of life; and adverse effects of treatment.

METHODS *Clinical Evidence* search and appraisal October 2003. In addition, the authors conducted hand searches of the literature.

QUESTION What are the effects of different doses and osmotic agents for peritoneal dialysis? New

OPTION ICODEXTRIN New

Three RCTs in people receiving continuous ambulatory peritoneal dialysis found that 7.5% icodextrin solution for the long dwell increased ultrafiltration (fluid loss) compared with 1.36% or 2.27% dextrose solutions. Two of the RCTs found that 7.5% icodextrin reduced extracellular water or total body water compared with 1.36% or 2.27% dextrose solutions. One of the RCTs found that 7.5% icodextrin reduced left ventricular mass compared with 1.36% dextrose solution. However, one of the RCTs found no significant difference between 7.5% icodextrin solution and 3.86% dextrose solution in mean ultrafiltration during the long dwell.

Benefits: We found no systematic review. We found three RCTs that compared the effects of icodextrinⒼ (a glucose polymer) versus conventional dextrose solutions for the long dwellⒼ in people receiving continuous ambulatory peritoneal dialysisⒼ.[23–25] The first RCT (open label; 40 non-diabetic adults) found that 7.5% icodextrin reduced extracellular water**G** volume and left ventricular mass significantly more than dextrose solution 1.36% after 4 months (mean change in extracellular water volume: –1.7 L with icodextrin *v* +0.9 L with dextrose; P = 0.013; mean change in left ventricular mass: –12.9 g with icodextrin *v* +1 g with dextrose; P = 0.05).[23] Twenty four hour ultrafiltration**G** increased significantly in the icodextrin group, but not in the dextrose group at 4 months (24 hour ultrafiltration: 744 mL at baseline to 1670 mL at 4 months with icodextrin; P = 0.012; 907 mL at baseline to 1063 mL at 4 months with dextrose; P reported as not significant; between group comparison not reported).[23] The second RCT (double blind; 50 people with high solute transport characteristics on peritoneal equilibration testing**G**) found that 7.5% icodextrin significantly increased 24 hour ultrafiltration at 3 months compared with 2.27% dextrose (mean change in ultrafiltration from baseline: +87.9 mL with icodextrin *v* –311.1 mL with dextrose; P < 0.05). However, the increase in 24 hour ultrafiltration with icodextrin was not statistically significant at 6 months (mean change in ultrafiltration from baseline: +193.4 mL with icodextrin *v* –201.7 mL with dextrose; P > 0.1). Icodextrin significantly reduced body weight and total body water compared with dextrose at 3 and 6 months (mean body weight change from baseline displayed graphically, mean between group difference: 1.67 kg at 3 months; P = 0.026; 2.3 kg at 6 months; P = 0.036; mean total body water change from baseline displayed graphically, mean between group difference: 1.53 kg at 3 months; P = 0.003; 1.39 kg at 6 months; P = 0.036).[24] The third RCT (209 adults) randomised participants to either 7.5% icodextrin or dextrose for 6 months; the dextrose group was analysed according to the concentration of solution used for the overnight dwell**G** (1.36% or 3.86%, see comment below).[25] It found that icodextrin significantly increased mean ultrafiltration during 8 and 12 hour overnight dwells compared with 1.36% dextrose (8 hour dwell: 527 mL with icodextrin *v* 150 mL with 1.36% dextrose; P < 0.0001; 12 hour dwell: 561 mL with icodextrin *v* 101 mL with 1.36% dextrose; P < 0.0001). However, it found no significant difference between icodextrin and 3.86% dextrose in mean ultrafiltration during 8 or 12 hour dwells (8 hour dwell: 510 mL with icodextrin *v* 448 mL with 3.86% dextrose; P = 0.44; 12 hour dwell: 552 mL with icodextrin *v* 414 mL with 3.86% dextrose; P = 0.06).

Harms: In the first RCT one person in the icodextrin**G** group withdrew because of a hypersensitivity reaction (exfoliative dermatitis), which resolved after stopping icodextrin.[23] Two people in the dextrose group withdrew because of peritonitis, there were no withdrawals from the icodextrin group because of peritonitis (significance not reported). Technique failure was similar in the icodextrin and 1.36% dextrose solution groups (1 person in each group switched to haemodialysis). The second RCT reported that no icodextrin related adverse events were observed, and did not report on adverse events in the dextrose group.[24] The third RCT found that the number of major adverse events (primarily cardiovascular events) was similar in the icodextrin and dextrose groups (8 events with icodextrin *v* 6 events with dextrose; P value not reported).[25] The peritonitis rate was slightly higher in the icodextrin group than in the dextrose group, but this difference was not significant and may have been confounded by baseline differences between groups (7.7 episodes per 100 participant months with icodextrin *v* 6.3 episodes per 100 participant months with dextrose; P reported as not significant). The number of people withdrawing because of adverse events during treatment was higher in the icodextrin group, but the significance of this difference was not reported (8/106 [7.5%] with icodextrin *v* 6/103 [5.8%] with dextrose; P value not reported).

Comment: The third RCT had a high rate of withdrawal (34%; 39/106 [37%] from the icodextrin group *v* 32/103 [31%] from the dextrose group).[25] A large proportion of these withdrawals were attributed to either transplantation (16 people) or adverse events (15 people). Analysis was not by intention to treat, and the dextrose group was split into two subgroups for analysis, which may have reduced power and introduced confounding.

OPTION INCREASED DOSE DIALYSIS New

One RCT found no significant difference in mortality between standard dose and increased dose peritoneal dialysis.

Benefits: We found no systematic review. **Versus standard dose:** We found one RCT (multicentre design; 965 adults having continuous ambulatory peritoneal dialysis**G**) that compared standard dose dialysis**G** (4 daily exchanges using 2 L of standard peritoneal dialysis solution) versus increased dose dialysis (4–5 daily exchanges of 2.5–3.0 L to reach a target creatinine clearance of 60 L/week/1.73 m^2; see comment below).[26] It found no significant difference in overall mortality between increased dose dialysis and standard dose dialysis (results presented graphically; RR 1.00, 95% CI 0.80 to 1.24). Increased dose dialysis significantly reduced death from congestive heart failure or uraemia compared with standard dose dialysis (deaths from congestive heart failure: 5.7% with increased dose *v* 13.4% with standard dose; P < 0.05; deaths from uraemia 5.1% with increased dose *v* 12.2% with standard dose; P < 0.05). However, there was no significant difference between treatments in death from acute myocardial infarction (27.8% with increased dose *v* 22.4% with standard dose; P reported as not significant).

Harms: There was no significant difference between treatments in hospital admissions or peritonitis rates (hospital admissions per person per year: 1.17 with increased dose *v* 1.03 with standard dose; P = 0.17; peritonitis rates: 23.3 participant months per episode with increased dose *v* 24.4 participant months per episode with standard dose; P = 0.62). However, significantly more people receiving increased dose dialysis**G** withdrew from the study owing to discomfort from increased peritoneal volume compared with standard dose dialysis (study withdrawal: 17/481 [3.5%] with increased dose *v* 1/484 [0.2%] with standard dose; P < 0.001), although significantly more people receiving standard dose dialysis withdrew because of uraemia compared with people receiving increased dose dialysis (withdrawal because of uraemia: 0/481 [0%] with increased dose *v* 24/484 [5%] with standard dose; P < 0.0001). There was no significant difference between groups in generalised infections or stroke (data not reported).

Comment: In the increased dose group the initial dose of peritoneal dialysis**G** was calculated based on body surface area, and a maximum of two modifications in dialysis dose were allowed to achieve the clearance target.[26] Therefore some people ended up receiving more dialysis, and other less over the duration of the study. The mean peritoneal creatinine clearances**G** achieved over the entire duration of the study were 56.9 ± 0.48 L a week per 1.73 m^2 in the increased dose group compared with 46.1 ± 0.45 L a week per 1.73 m^2 in the standard dose group (P < 0.001). The RCT may have limited generalisability as participants were generally younger (mean age 47 years) and healthier than the general peritoneal dialysis population. For instance, only people with a peritoneal creatinine clearance of less than 60 L a week per 1.73 m^2 with or without residual renal function were eligible for inclusion in the trial, effectively excluding smaller individuals, and people with high peritoneal transport characteristics (i.e. those at the highest risk of death). Similarly, people with heart disease were also excluded (1 observational study found[27] the prevalence of a history of cardiovascular disease in people receiving continuous ambulatory peritoneal dialysis was about 34% in a Canadian cohort and 42% in a US cohort) and it is possible that the relative increase in mortality owing to heart failure in the control group compared with the intervention group might have been more striking if such people had been included in the study. Thus, the study may have selected for a population that was less dependent on peritoneal clearance of small solutes.[26,28]

QUESTION **What are the effects of different doses and membrane fluxes for haemodialysis?** New

OPTION **INCREASED DOSE OF HAEMODIALYSIS** New

One RCT found no significant difference in hospital admission for cardiac causes or all cause mortality between standard dose haemodialysis and increased dose haemodialysis (at high or low membrane flux).

Benefits: We found no systematic review. We found one multicentre RCT (1846 adults having maintenance haemodialysis).[29] It compared four treatments in a factorial design: standard dose dialysis**G** (equilibrated Kt/V**G** of 1.05); increased dose dialysis**G** (equilibrated Kt/V of 1.45); low membrane flux**G** dialysis; and high membrane flux dialysis. It found no significant difference in all cause mortality between increased dose dialysis and standard dose dialysis after a mean follow up of 4.5 years (AR 440/926 [47.5%] with standard dose dialysis *v* 431/920 [46.8%] with increased dose dialysis; adjusted RR 0.96, 95% CI 0.84 to 1.10; see comment below). It found no significant difference between groups in the risk of mortality because of cardiac causes (AR 169/926 [18.3%] with standard dose *v* 174/920 [18.9%] with increased dose dialysis; RR and CI displayed graphically). It found no significant difference between groups in the composite outcome of first admission to hospital owing to cardiac causes or mortality (AR 545/926 [58.9%] with standard dose dialysis *v* 534/920 [58.0%] with increased dose dialysis; adjusted RR 1.01, 95% CI 0.88 to 1.12; P = 0.91).

Harms: The RCT found no significant difference between increased dose and standard dose dialysis**G** in first admission to hospital owing to infection or death (557/926 [60%] with standard dose *v* 547/920 [59%] with increased dose dialysis; adjusted RR 1.03, 95% CI 0.91 to 1.14; P = 0.60).[29] It found no significant difference between groups in deaths because of infection (AR 99/926 [10.7%] with standard dose *v* 102/920 [11.1%] with increased dose dialysis; RR and CI displayed graphically).

Comment: The results of this RCT should be interpreted with caution owing to limitations in the 2 x 2 factorial design.[29] Specifically, the study did not purely compare increased dose versus standard dose dialysis**G**, but instead compared increased dose (pooling low and high flux) versus standard dose (pooling low and high flux). The RCT was powered to detect a 25% reduction in mortality between groups, smaller differences in clinical effect cannot be excluded. This RCT may have limited generalisability, because of the participants being younger (mean age 57.6 years), and an over-representation of African Americans compared with the general US dialysis population (62% African Americans *v* 37% general US dialysis population). African Americans are known to have improved survival on haemodialysis compared with age-matched white people.[30] The study also included people with a relatively long baseline time on dialysis (mean 3.7 years), effectively selecting for a fitter population that may not have benefited as much from an increase in dialysis dose or membrane flux**G**. This selection bias also raises the question of potential carryover effects in people previously treated with either a higher dialysis dose (baseline mean equilibrated Kt/V**G** 1.43 ± 0.21) or high flux membrane (baseline use 60.2%).[31]

OPTION HIGH MEMBRANE FLUX HAEMODIALYSIS New

One RCT found no significant difference in hospital admission for cardiac causes, or all cause mortality between high membrane flux and low membrane flux (with standard or increased dose haemodialysis).

Benefits: We found no systematic review. We found one multicentre RCT (1846 adults having maintenance haemodialysis; see comment below) which compared four treatments in a factorial design: low membrane flux**G**; high membrane flux**G**; standard dose dialysis**G**; and increased dose dialysis**G** (see benefits of different doses of haemodialysis, p 1052).[29] It found no significant difference in all cause mortality between high flux and low flux dialysis after a mean follow up of 4.5 years (AR 442/925 [47.8%] with low flux *v* 429/921 [46.6%] with high flux; adjusted RR 0.92, 95% CI 0.81 to 1.05). However, it found that high flux membrane dialysis significantly reduced the risk of mortality owing to cardiac causes compared with low flux dialysis (AR 187/925 [20.2%] with low flux *v* 156/921 [16.9%] with high flux; RR and CI presented graphically; $P < 0.05$). It found that high membrane flux reduced the risk of the combined outcome of first admission to hospital owing to cardiac causes or mortality compared with low membrane flux, but the difference did not reach significance (AR 550/925 [59.5%] with low flux *v* 529/921 [57.4%] with high flux; adjusted RR 1.10, 95% CI 0.99 to 1.20).[29]

Harms: The RCT found no significant difference between low flux and high flux dialysis**G** in the combined outcome of first admission to hospital owing to infection or death (AR 562/925 [60.8%] with low flux *v* 542/921 [58.8%] with high flux; RR and CI displayed graphically).[29] It found no significant difference between groups in risk of death from infection (11.2% with standard dose *v* 10.5% with high dose dialysis; RR and CI displayed graphically).

Comment: The results of this RCT should be interpreted with caution because of limitations in the 2 x 2 factorial design.[29] Specifically, the study did not purely compare high versus low flux, but instead compared high flux (pooling standard and increased dose) versus low flux (pooling standard and increased dose). See comment of increased doses of haemodialysis, p 1053.

QUESTION What are the effects of interventions aimed at preventing secondary complications? New

OPTION SEVELAMER New

One RCT found that sevelamer reduced the progression of coronary artery and aortic calcification compared with calcium salts at 52 weeks. It found similar mortality with sevelamer and calcium salts. One crossover RCT found no difference in reduction of serum phosphorus between sevelamer and calcium acetate. Both RCTs found that sevelamer reduced serum low density lipoprotein cholesterol levels and the incidence of hypercalcaemia compared with calcium salts.

Benefits: **Versus calcium:** We found two RCTs.[32,33] The first multicentre RCT (open label; 200 adults with end stage renal disease) compared sevelamer (a non-absorbed, non-calcium containing phosphate binder) versus calcium salts (calcium carbonate and calcium acetate) for 52 weeks.[32] It found that sevelamer significantly reduced the progression of coronary artery and aortic calcification (as measured by electron beam tomography) compared with calcium salts at 52 weeks (quantified using the Agatston score, a higher score indicates more severe calcification; mean score change from baseline in coronary artery calcification score: –46 with sevelamer *v* +151 with calcium salts; P = 0.04; mean score change from baseline in aortic calcification score: –532 with sevelamer *v* +185 with calcium salts; in participants with calcification scores ≥30 at baseline: median change in coronary artery calcification score: +6% with sevelamer *v* +25% with calcium salts; P = 0.02; in participants with calcification scores ≥30 at baseline: median change in aortic calcification score: +5% with sevelamer *v* +28% with calcium salts; P = 0.02). It also found that serum low density lipoprotein (LDL) cholesterol levels significantly decreased with sevelamer compared with calcium salts after 52 weeks (mean change in LDL cholesterol: –37 mg/dL with sevelamer *v* +1 mg/dL with calcium salts; P < 0.0001). It found similar mortality in both groups (AR 6/99 [6.1%] with sevelamer *v* 5/101 [5.0%] with calcium salts; significance not reported). The second RCT (open label, crossover trial with 2 week washout period; 83 adults on maintenance haemodialysis) compared sevelamer versus calcium acetate for 8 weeks.[33] The study did not present results before crossover. It found no significant difference between groups in reduction of serum phosphate from baseline at the end of treatment (mean reduction: 2.0 mg/dL with sevelamer *v* 2.1 mg/dL with calcium acetate; P = 0.71). In addition, serum LDL cholesterol levels decreased significantly more with sevelamer than with calcium acetate (mean change: –25.3 mg/dL with sevelamer *v* +4.1 mg/dL with calcium acetate; P < 0.0001).[33] **Versus aluminium:** We found no RCTs.

Harms: **Versus calcium:** The first RCT found that both sevelamer and calcium salts were well tolerated.[32] Significantly more people experienced at least one hypercalcaemic episode with calcium salts compared with sevelamer over 52 weeks (AR for hypercalcaemia: 17% with sevelamer *v* 43% with calcium salts; P = 0.0005). Serum bicarbonate concentrations were significantly higher in the calcium treated group (19.2 mEq/L with sevelamer *v* 22.1 mEq/L with calcium salts; P = 0.0003). There was no significant difference between groups in the risk of hospital admission and the number of days spent in hospital (AR for hospital admission: 37/99 [37.4%] with sevelamer *v* 48/101 [47.5%] with calcium salts; P = 0.15; total hospital days: 567 days with sevelamer *v* 980 days with calcium; P = 0.23).[32] The causes of hospital admission were not reported. The second RCT reported no serious adverse effects with either treatment.[33] There was no significant difference between groups in gastrointestinal complaints (34% with sevelamer *v* 28% with calcium acetate; P = 0.26). It found that serum alkaline phosphatase was significantly increased from baseline with sevelamer (from 87 U/L to 106 U/L; P < 0.0001) but not with calcium acetate (from 106 U/L to 96 U/L; P = 0.85). It was unclear whether this reflected effects on bile acid metabolism or bone turnover. No significant changes in the bone or liver subfractions of alkaline phosphatase were noted, and no adverse hepatic events were observed. The RCT found that significantly fewer people developed hypercalcaemia with sevelamer compared with calcium acetate (hypercalcaemia defined as serum calcium ≥11.0 mg/dL; AR 5% with sevelamer *v* 22% with calcium acetate; P = 0.0001).

During treatment with sevelamer, 18/80 (23%) people required an evening dose of calcium carbonate to maintain serum calcium concentrations, and 15/80 (18%) people developed hypocalcaemia (serum calcium < 8 mg/dL). **Versus aluminium:** We found no RCTs.

Comment: Traditional risk factors for coronary artery disease account for only a portion of the remarkable increase in cardiovascular mortality observed in people receiving dialysis**G**. Disorders of mineral metabolism (i.e. abnormalities of calcium, phosphorus, parathyroid hormone, and vitamin D) may play an important role in the accelerated atherosclerosis unique to the dialysis**G** population.[34] Several observational studies have shown a direct correlation between elevated levels of serum phosphorus and calcium, and higher coronary artery calcification scores and mortality in people receiving chronic haemodialysis.[35–37] In clinical practice, elevations in serum calcium and phosphorus often limit the use of conventional calcium salts and vitamin D analogues in controlling abnormalities of mineral metabolism seen in patients with end stage renal disease. Thus, recent attention has focused on the effects of non-calcium containing phosphate binders. Sevelamer is also known to act as a bile acid sequestrant. Hence, it is unclear whether the effects of sevelamer on serum LDL cholesterol contributed significantly to the beneficial effects on vascular calcification.[38] Further studies investigating the effects of sevelamer on all cause mortality and cardiovascular events are currently in process.

OPTION ERYTHROPOIETIN VERSUS DARBEPOETIN

New

One RCT found no significant difference between darbepoetin α and recombinant human erythropoietin in maintenance of haemoglobin levels at 25–32 weeks. There is consensus based on observational studies that erythropoietin is effective for the treatment of anaemia in people with end stage renal disease.

Benefits: We found one RCT in 522 people who were receiving haemodialysis or peritoneal dialysis**G**, and on stable recombinant human erythropoietin (rHuEPO) treatment (1–3 times/week).[39] It randomised people to either continued rHuEPO treatment, or to switching to darbepoetin α (received once every 2 weeks or once a week). It found no significant difference between darbepoetin and rHuEPO in maintenance of haemoglobin levels at 25–32 weeks (adjusted mean change from baseline: –0.03 g/dL with darbepoetin *v* –0.06 g/dL with rHuEPO; adjusted mean difference: 0.03 g/dL, 95% CI –0.16 g/dL to +0.21 g/dL).

Harms: The RCT found that adverse events were common, and occurred at a similar frequency with darbepoetin α and rHuEPO (AR for experiencing at least 1 adverse event: 96% with darbepoetin *v* 95% with rHuEPO; P value not reported).[39] There was no significant difference between treatments in six prespecified adverse events related to increasing haemoglobin in people with end stage renal disease (AR for events: hypertension 30% with darbepoetin *v* 28% with rHuEPO; vascular access thrombosis 10% *v* 9%; cerebrovascular disorder 2% *v* 1%; myocardial infarction 1% *v* 2%; seizures 2% *v* 2%; transient ischemic attack 0% *v* 1%; P ≥ 0.682 for all 6 outcomes). Pruritus was significantly more common with darbepoetin than with rHuEPO (14% with darbepoetin *v* 5% with rHuEPO; OR and CI presented graphically).

Comment: Since the introduction of rHuEPO in 1989, numerous studies have shown improvements in various physiologic and quality of life parameters (e.g. sexual, muscle, and cognitive function, regression of left ventricular hypertrophy, physical activity, etc) with the correction of anaemia in patients with chronic kidney disease.[1] Several observational studies have also shown that the survival of people receiving dialysis**G** declines as the haematocrit falls below a range of 30–33%.[40,41] One RCT comparing the effects of maintaining a normal haematocrit target (42%) versus low haematocrit target (30%) in people with end stage renal disease and clinically evident congestive heart failure or ischaemic heart disease found an overall higher mortality in the normal haematocrit group.[42] The optimal haemoglobin/haematocrit level in people with end stage renal disease, however, remains a source of ongoing debate. Based on collective data from observational trials and RCTs, the K/DOQI**G** Anemia Work Group recommends maintaining haemoglobin at 11–12 g/dL.[1] Additional prospective studies are needed to elucidate the relationship between anaemia and clinical outcomes in people with end stage renal disease further.

GLOSSARY

Automated peritoneal dialysis (APD) Form of peritoneal dialysis that involves the use of an automated cycler to perform nightly exchanges, typically supplemented with a long "daytime dwell" lasting 6–12 hours.[43]

Continuous ambulatory peritoneal dialysis (CAPD) Most common form of peritoneal dialysis worldwide that typically involves four daily 2.0–2.5 L exchanges of 4–8 hour duration (dwell) each.[26,43,44]

Dialysis Process by which the solute composition of a solution is altered by exposure to a second solution through a semipermeable membrane.[43]

Dialysis adequacy Most commonly measured by either the treatment related urea reduction ratio (URR) for haemodialysis or Kt/V for haemodialysis or peritoneal dialysis (see below).[43]

Dwell Terminology referring to the period of time in which the peritoneal dialysate is left in the peritoneal cavity to allow for solute exchange. The "**long dwell**" refers to the extended period of time (6–12 hours) each day during which an individual having peritoneal dialysis holds dialysate in the peritoneal cavity without performing an exchange.[43]

Extracellular fluid (ECF) The extracellular fluid represents about 25–45% of total body water, and is separated into intravascular and interstitial spaces. Expansion of the extracellular fluid volume occurs commonly in patients with end stage renal disease, and is associated with left ventricular hypertrophy and dysfunction.[23,24]

Extracellular water Surrogate for estimating extracellular fluid volume.[24]

High transporters Terminology referring to individuals who (by peritoneal equilibration test [PET]) achieve rapid and complete equilibration for creatinine and urea because of a relatively large effective peritoneal surface area or high intrinsic membrane permeability. In general, high transporters tend to have lower net ultrafiltration and higher dialysate protein losses compared with their low transport counterparts.[43]

Icodextrin Soluble glucose polymer derived from maltodextrin which was first introduced into clinical practice in the UK in 1994.[23–25]

Kidney Disease Outcomes Quality Initiative (K/DOQI) Initiative supported by the US National Kidney Foundation and designed by health care providers to offer evidence based practice guidelines for all stages of chronic kidney disease.[1]

Kt/V Dimensionless ratio representing fractional urea clearance (ratio of volume of fluid cleared of urea during a treatment to total body water. Many studies in dialysis adequacy still use Kt/V to reflect the amount of urea removal.[43]

Low transporters Terminology referring to individuals who have slower and less complete equilibration for creatinine and urea because of a relatively small effective peritoneal surface area or low intrinsic membrane permeability.[35]

Membrane flux Refers to the membrane pore characteristics of haemodialyzers. "High flux" dialysis membranes typically have pores of sufficient size to allow the passage of large molecules such as β2 microglobulin (molecular weight 11 800).[35]

Peritoneal creatinine clearance (pCrCl) Creatinine clearance attributed to the peritoneal dialysis prescription (as opposed to creatinine clearance from residual renal function) — typically measured in litres a week.[35]

Peritoneal equilibration test (PET) Method for measuring peritoneal transport characteristics which are important determinants of clearances (principally urea, creatinine, etc) in peritoneal dialysis.

Renal replacement therapy (RRT) General terminology that refers to the modalities for assisting or replacing kidney function, i.e. continuous and intermittent forms of haemodialysis, peritoneal dialysis, and kidney transplantation.[31]

Ultrafiltration Mechanism of solute transport across a semipermeable membrane (i.e. dialyser in haemodialysis, peritoneal membrane in peritoneal dialysis) — also known as convective transport. In clinical practice, the terminology "ultrafiltration" often refers to the amount of fluid (volume) removed during dialysis.[35]

REFERENCES

1. National Kidney Foundation. Kidney Disease Quality Outcomes Initiative (K/DOQI). http://www.kidney.org/professionals/kdoqi/guidelines.cfm (last accessed 8 February 2005).
2. Chertow GM. Slowing the progression of vascular calcification in hemodialysis. *J Am Soc Nephrol* 2003;14:S310–S314.
3. Moeller S, Gioberge S, Brown G. ESRD patients in 2001: global overview of patients, treatment modalities and development trends. *Nephrol Dial Transplant* 2002;17:2071–2076.
4. International Federation of Renal Registries website. http://www.ifrr.net (last accessed 8 February 2005).
5. United States Renal Data System. *USRDS 2003 annual data report: atlas of end-stage renal disease in the United States*. National Institutes of Health, National Institute of Diabetes and Digestive and Kidney Diseases, Bethesda, MD, 2003.
6. Nakai S, Shinzato T, Nagura Y, et al. An overview of regular dialysis treatment in Japan (as of 31 December 2001). *Ther Apher Dial* 2004;8:3–32.
7. UK Renal Registry website. http://www.renalreg.com (last accessed 8 February 2005)
8. Locatelli F, Pozzoni P, Del Vecchio L. Renal replacement therapy in patients with diabetes and end-stage renal disease. *J Am Soc Nephrol* 2004;15:S25–S29.
9. Buckalew VM Jr, Berg RL, Wang SR, et al. Prevalence of hypertension in 1,795 subjects with chronic renal disease: the modification of diet in renal disease study baseline cohort. Modification of Diet in Renal Disease Study Group. *Am J Kidney Dis* 1996;28:811–821.
10. Hovind P, Rossing P, Tarnow L, et al. Progression of diabetic nephropathy. *Kidney Int* 2001;59:702–709.
11. Peterson JC, Adler S, Burkart JM, et al. Blood pressure control, proteinuria, and the progression of renal disease. The Modification of Diet in Renal Disease Study. *Ann Intern Med* 1995;123:754–762.
12. Klag MJ, Whelton PK, Randall BL, et al. Blood pressure and end-stage renal disease in men. *N Engl J Med* 1996;334:13–18.
13. Ansell D, Feest T, Calvani M. *UK renal registry report 2002*. Bristol, UK, 2002.
14. Perneger TV, Klag MJ, Whelton PK. Recreational drug use: a neglected risk factor for end-stage renal disease. *Am J Kidney Dis* 2001;38:49–56.
15. Perneger TV, Whelton PK, Klag MJ. Race and end-stage renal disease. Socioeconomic status and access to health care as mediating factors. *Arch Intern Med* 1995;155:1201–1208.
16. Klag MJ, Whelton PK, Randall BL, et al. End-stage renal disease in African-American and white men. 16-year MRFIT findings. *JAMA* 1997;277:1293–1298.
17. Perneger TV, Whelton PK, Klag MJ. Risk of kidney failure associated with the use of acetaminophen, aspirin, and nonsteroidal antiinflammatory drugs. *N Engl J Med* 1994;331:1675–1679.
18. Brancati FL, Whelton PK, Randall BL, et al. Risk of end-stage renal disease in diabetes mellitus: a prospective cohort study of men screened for MRFIT. Multiple Risk Factor Intervention Trial. *JAMA* 1997;278:2069–2074.
19. Orth SR, Stockmann A, Conradt C, et al. Smoking as a risk factor for end-stage renal failure in men with primary renal disease. *Kidney Int* 1998;54:926–931.
20. Orth SR. Smoking and the kidney. *J Am Soc Nephrol* 2002;13:1663–1672.
21. Powe NR, Jaar B, Furth SL, et al. Septicemia in dialysis patients: incidence, risk factors, and prognosis. *Kidney Int* 1999;55:1081–1090.
22. Foley RN, Parfrey PS, Harnett JD, et al. Clinical and echocardiographic disease in patients starting end-stage renal disease therapy. *Kidney Int* 1995;47:186–192.
23. Konings CJ, Kooman JP, Schonck M, et al. Effect of icodextrin on volume status, blood pressure and echocardiographic parameters: a randomized study. *Kidney Int* 2003;63:1556–1563.
24. Davies SJ, Woodrow G, Donovan K, et al. Icodextrin improves the fluid status of peritoneal dialysis patients: results of a double-blind randomized controlled trial. *J Am Soc Nephrol* 2003;14:2338–2344.
25. Mistry CD, Gokal R, Peers E. A randomized multicenter clinical trial comparing isosmolar icodextrin with hyperosmolar glucose solutions in CAPD. MIDAS Study Group. Multicenter Investigation of Icodextrin in Ambulatory Peritoneal Dialysis. *Kidney Int* 1994;46:496–503.
26. Paniagua R, Amato D, Vonesh E, et al. Effects of increased peritoneal clearances on mortality rates in peritoneal dialysis: ADEMEX, a prospective, randomized, controlled trial. *J Am Soc Nephrol* 2002;13:1307–1320.
27. Churchill DN, Taylor DW, Keshaviah PR, for the CANUSA study group. Adequacy of dialysis and nutrition in continuous peritoneal dialysis: association with clinical outcomes. *J Am Soc Nephrol* 1996;7:198–207.
28. Churchill DN. The ADEMEX Study: make haste slowly. *J Am Soc Nephrol* 2002;13:1415–1418.
29. Eknoyan G, Beck GJ, Cheung AK, et al. Effect of dialysis dose and membrane flux in maintenance hemodialysis. *N Engl J Med* 2002;347:2010–2019.
30. Levin N, Greenwood R. Reflections on the HEMO study: the American viewpoint. *Nephrol Dial Transplant* 2003;18:1059–1060.
31. Locatelli F. Dose of dialysis, convection and haemodialysis patients outcome – what the HEMO study doesn't tell us: the European viewpoint. *Nephrol Dial Transplant* 2003;18:1061–1065.
32. Chertow GM, Burke SK, Raggi P. Sevelamer attenuates the progression of coronary and aortic calcification in hemodialysis patients. *Kidney Int* 2002;62:245–252.
33. Bleyer AJ, Burke SK, Dillon M, et al. A comparison of the calcium-free phosphate binder sevelamer hydrochloride with calcium acetate in the treatment of hyperphosphatemia in hemodialysis patients. *Am J Kidney Dis* 1999;33:694–701.
34. Block G, Port FK. Calcium phosphate metabolism and cardiovascular disease in patients with chronic kidney disease. *Semin Dial* 2003;16:140–147.
35. Lowrie EG, Lew NL. Death risk in hemodialysis patients: the predictive value of commonly measured

variables and an evaluation of death rate differences between facilities. *Am J Kidney Dis* 1990;15:458–482.
36. Block GA, Hulbert-Shearon TE, Levin NW, et al. Association of serum phosphorus and calcium x phosphate product with mortality risk in chronic hemodialysis patients: a national study. *Am J Kidney Dis* 1998;31:607–617.
37. Raggi P, Boulay A, Chasan-Taber S, et al. Cardiac calcification in adult hemodialysis patients. A link between end-stage renal disease and cardiovascular disease? *J Am Coll Cardiol* 2002;39:695–701.
38. Chertow GM. Slowing the progression of vascular calcification in hemodialysis. *J Am Soc Nephrol* 2003;14:S310–S314.
39. Vanrenterghem Y, Barany P, Mann JF, et al. Randomized trial of darbepoetin alfa for treatment of renal anemia at a reduced dose frequency compared with rHuEPO in dialysis patients. *Kidney Int* 2002;62:2167–2175.
40. Ma JZ, Ebben J, Xia H, et al. Hematocrit level and associated mortality in hemodialysis patients. *J Am Soc Nephrol* 1999;10:610–619.
41. Foley RN, Parfrey PS, Harnett JD, et al. The impact of anemia on cardiomyopathy, morbidity, and mortality in end-stage renal disease. *Am J Kidney Dis* 1996;28:53–61.
42. Besarab A, Bolton WK, Browne JK, et al. The effects of normal as compared with low hematocrit values in patients with cardiac disease who are receiving hemodialysis and epoetin. *N Engl J Med* 1998;339:584–590.
43. Daugirdas JT, Blake PG, Ing TS. *Handbook of dialysis*, third edition. Lippincott, Williams & Wilkins; 2001:25–35.
44. Bargman JM, Thorpe KE, Churchill DN; CANUSA Peritoneal Dialysis Study Group. Relative contribution of residual renal function and peritoneal clearance to adequacy of dialysis: a reanalysis of the CANUSA study. *J Am Soc Nephrol* 2001;12:2158–2162.

Yoshio Hall
Assistant Clinical Professor of Medicine
Division of Nephrology
Department of Medicine
University of California San Francisco
San Francisco General Hospital
San Francisco
California, USA

Glenn Chertow
Associate Professor of Medicine in Residence
Division of Nephrology
Department of Medicine
University of California San Francisco
UCSF/MT Xion Medical Center
San Francisco
California, USA

Competing interests: None declared.

Kidney stones

Search date March 2004

Robyn Webber, David Tolley, James Lingeman

QUESTIONS

INTERVENTIONS

To be covered in future updates

Flexible ureteroscopy

Laser lithotripsy using holmium:yttrium–aluminium–garnet (YAG) laser

Management of the acute phase (including pain management and rehydration)

Prevention of formation of new or recurrent kidney stones (metabolic kidney stones)

See glossary G

Key Messages

Asymptomatic kidney stones

- **Extracorporeal shockwave lithotripsy (ESWL) in people with asymptomatic renal or ureteric stones** One RCT found no significant difference in stone free rate at about 1 year between prophylactic extracorporeal shockwave lithotripsy and conservative treatment for people with asymptomatic renal stones less than 15 mm in diameter. However, it found limited evidence that more people required invasive procedures after conservative management. We found no RCTs on extracorporeal shockwave lithotripsy in people with larger renal stones or with ureteric stones.

- **Percutaneous nephrolithotomy (PCNL) in people with asymptomatic renal or ureteric stones** We found no RCTs on percutaneous nephrolithotomy in people with asymptomatic renal or ureteric stones.
- **Ureteroscopy in people with asymptomatic renal or ureteric stones** We found no RCTs on ureteroscopy in people with asymptomatic renal or ureteric stones.

Removal of renal stones

- **Extracorporeal shockwave lithotripsy (ESWL) in people with renal stones less than 20 mm** One RCT found that extracorporeal shockwave lithotripsy decreased the stone free rate at 3 months and increased the rate of treatment failure in people with symptomatic renal stones less than 30 mm in diameter compared with percutaneous nephrolithotomy. It found no significant difference in complication rate between extracorporeal shockwave lithotripsy and percutaneous nephrolithotomy, although complications were more frequent with percutaneous nephrolithotomy. We found no RCTs comparing extracorporeal shockwave lithotripsy with ureteroscopy or open nephrolithotomy in people with renal stones. There is consensus that extracorporeal shockwave lithotripsy is the first line treatment in people with renal stones less than 20mm in diameter as it is a less invasive intervention than percutaneous nephrolithotomy.
- **Percutaneous nephrolithotomy (PCNL) in people with renal stones** One RCT found that percutaneous nephrolithotomy increased the stone free rate at 3 months and reduced the rate of treatment failure in people with symptomatic renal stones less than 30 mm in diameter compared with extracorporeal shockwave lithotripsy. It found no significant differences in complication rates between percutaneous nephrolithotomy and extracorporeal shockwave lithotripsy, although complications were more frequent with percutaneous nephrolithotomy. We found no RCTs comparing percutaneous nephrolithotomy with conservative management, ureteroscopy, or open nephrolithotomy in people with renal stones.
- **Open nephrolithotomy in people with renal stones** We found no RCTs on open nephrolithotomy in people with renal stones.
- **Ureteroscopy in people with renal stones** We found no RCTs on ureteroscopy in people with renal stones.

Removal of ureteric stones

- **Extracorporeal shockwave lithotripsy (ESWL) in people with mid- and distal ureteric stones** Three RCTs found that overall stone free rates were lower and the time needed to become stone free longer in people with mid- and distal ureteric stones with extracorporeal shockwave lithotripsy compared with ureteroscopy. However, one RCT found no significant difference in stone free rates between treatments in people with distal ureteric stones of less than 15 mm. One RCT found a lower rate of treatment failure with extracorporeal shockwave lithotripsy compared with ureteroscopy. Three of the RCTs found a lower rate of severe complications with extracorporeal shockwave lithotripsy compared with ureteroscopy.
- **Ureteroscopy in people with mid- and distal ureteric stones** Three RCTs found that ureteroscopy increased overall stone free rate and decreased the time needed to become stone free in people with mid- and distal ureteric stones compared with extracorporeal shockwave lithotripsy. However, one RCT found no significant difference in stone free rates between treatments in people with distal ureteric stones of less than 15 mm. One RCT found a higher rate of treatment failure with ureteroscopy compared with extracorporeal shockwave lithotripsy. Three RCTs found a higher complication rate with ureteroscopy compared with extracorporeal shockwave lithotripsy.

- **Extracorporeal shockwave lithotripsy (ESWL) in people with proximal ureteric stones** We found no RCTs comparing extracorporeal shockwave lithotripsy versus ureteroscopy in people with proximal ureteric stones or comparing extracorporeal shockwave lithotripsy with conservative treatment or ureterolithotomy (open or laparoscopic) in people with ureteric stones.
- **Ureterolithotomy (open or laparoscopic) in people with ureteric stones** We found no RCTs on ureterolithotomy (open or laparoscopic) in people with ureteric stones.
- **Ureteroscopy in people with proximal ureteric stones** We found no RCTs comparing ureteroscopy versus extracorporeal shockwave lithotripsy in people with proximal ureteric stones or comparing ureteroscopy with conservative treatment, extracorporeal shockwave lithotripsy, or ureterolithotomy (open or laparoscopic) in people with ureteric stones.

DEFINITION **Nephrolithiasis** is the presence of stones within the kidney; **urolithiasis** is a more general term for stones anywhere within the urinary tract. A third of all kidney stones become clinically evident; typically causing pain, often severe in nature; renal angle tenderness; haematuria; or digestive symptoms (e.g. nausea, vomiting, or diarrhoea).[1] The onset of pain is usually sudden, typically felt in the loin, and radiating to the groin, and genitalia (scrotum or labia). People are typically restless, finding the pain excruciating and describing it as the worst pain ever experienced. Severe ureteric obstruction may cause hydronephrosis(G) or infection. Infection may also occur after invasive procedures for stone removal. Urolithiasis is usually categorised according to the anatomical location of the stones (i.e. renal calyces, renal pelvis, ureteric, bladder, and urethra). Ureteric urolithiasis is described further by stating in which portion (proximal, middle, or distal) the stone is situated. Kidney stones develop when crystals separate from the urine and aggregate within the kidney papillae, the renal pelvis, or the ureter. The most common type of stone contains varying amounts of calcium and oxalate, whereas "struvite" stones contain a mixture of magnesium, ammonium, and phosphate. Struvite stones are associated almost exclusively with infection with urease producing organisms, whilst calcium oxalate stones have several aetiologies. Rarer stones include those formed from uric acid, cysteine, and xanthine, although this list is not exhaustive. The aetiology and chemical composition of a stone may have some bearing on its diagnosis, management, and particularly on prevention of recurrence. Although the choices for surgical management in general remain the same for all types of stone disease, the recognition of a specific cause, such as recurrent infection with a urease producing organism for struvite stones, or cysteinuria for cysteine stones, will inform further management. Diagnosis is usually based on clinical history, supported by investigations with diagnostic imaging. Bleeding within the urinary tract may present with identical symptoms to kidney stones, particularly if there are blood clots present within the renal pelvis or ureter. Several other conditions may also mimic a renal colic and need to be considered for differential diagnosis. These include urinary tract infection (and indeed the two conditions may coexist), analgesic abuse (either renal damage from excessive ingestion of analgesics, or in people with a history of opiate abuse, who may feign a renal colic in an attempt to obtain opiate analgesia). Rarely, people with sickle cell disease may also present with severe abdominal pain, which needs to be distinguished from a renal colic. This chapter assesses the effects of treatments only for the removal of renal and ureteric stones. It excludes pregnant women, in whom some forms of diagnostic procedures and treatments for stone removal are contraindicated, and people with significant comorbidities (including severe cardiovascular and respiratory conditions) who may be at increased risk when having general anaesthesia.

INCIDENCE/ PREVALENCE The peak incidence for stone disease occurs at the ages of 20–40 years, although stones are seen in all age groups.[2] There is a male to female ratio of 3 : 1. Calcium oxalate stones, the most common variety, have a recurrence rate of 10% at 1 year, 35% at 5 years, and 50% at 5 years after the first episode of kidney stone disease in North America.

AETIOLOGY/ RISK FACTORS In many otherwise healthy people the aetiology is uncertain.[3] However, incidence is higher in people with hyperparathyroidism and people with disorders including small bowel dysfunction, urinary tract infection (in particular caused by urease producing organisms) and structural/anatomical abnormalities of the kidney and ureter (including obstruction of the pelviureteric junction, hydronephrotic renal pelvis or calyces, calyceal diverticulum, horseshoe kidney, ureterocele, vesicoureteral reflux, ureteric stricture, or medullary sponge kidney). Other conditions associated with the development of renal stones include gout (especially leading to uric acid calculi) and chronic metabolic acidosis (typically resulting in stones composed of calcium phosphate). Women with a history of surgical menopause are also at higher risk because of increased bone resorption, and urinary excretion of calcium. Drugs, including some decongestants, diuretics, and anticonvulsants are also associated with an increased risk of stone formation.

PROGNOSIS Most kidney stones pass within 48 hours with expectant treatment (including adequate fluid intake and analgesia). Others may take longer to pass and the observation period can be extended to 3–4 weeks where appropriate. Ureteric stones less than 5 mm in diameter will pass spontaneously in about 90% of people, compared with 50% of ureteric stones between 5 mm and 10 mm.[4] Expectant management is considered on a case to case basis, and only in people with stones which are asymptomatic or very small (although stone size may not correlate with symptom severity), or both, and in people with significant comorbidities (including severe cardiovascular and respiratory conditions, who may be at increased risk when having general anaesthesia), in whom the risks of treatment may outweigh the likely benefits. Stones may migrate regardless of treatment or after treatment for their removal, and may or may not present clinically once in the ureter. Stones blocking the urine flow may lead to hydronephrosis(G) and renal atrophy. They may also result in life threatening complications including urinary infection, perinephric abscess(G), or urosepsis. Some of these complications may cause kidney damage and compromised renal function.[5] Eventually, 10–20% of all kidney stones need treatment.

AIMS OF INTERVENTION To render people free of stones; to prevent the development of the complications of stone disease, with minimal adverse effects.

OUTCOMES Stone free rate (proportion of people becoming stone free, assessed radiologically); time to becoming stone free (duration of passing stone fragments); treatment failure (defined as no change in the stone, or the presence of large stone fragments, even if asymptomatic); complication rate of kidney stone disease (including sepsis, obstructive renal failure, hydronephrosis(G), and perinephric abscess(G)) complication rate of renal and ureteric surgery including renal and ureteric trauma, sepsis, haemorrhage, and death.

METHODS *Clinical Evidence* search and appraisal March 2004.

QUESTION What are the effects of treatments for stone removal in people with asymptomatic kidney stones? New

OPTION EXTRACORPOREAL SHOCKWAVE LITHOTRIPSY (ESWL) New

One RCT found no significant difference in stone free rate at about 1 year between prophylactic extracorporeal shockwave lithotripsy and conservative treatment for people with asymptomatic renal stones less than 15 mm in diameter. However, it found limited evidence that more people required invasive procedures after conservative management. We found no RCTs on extracorporeal shockwave lithotripsy in people with larger renal stones or with ureteric stones.

Benefits: **Versus conservative management (defined as observation, usually with serial imaging):** We found no systematic review but found one RCT (228 people with asymptomatic renal stones < 15 mm in diameter) comparing prophylactic extracorporeal shockwave lithotripsy [ESWL] versus conservative management.[6] People were followed annually for up to 5 years (mean follow up 2.2 years). At the "most recent" follow up (minimum 1 year of follow up, mean: 1.29 years with ESWL *v* 1.2 years with conservative management), the RCT found no significant difference in the stone free rate between ESWL and conservative management (28/101 [28%] with ESWL *v* 16/99 [17%] with conservative management; P = 0.06). It gave no results on outcomes at 5 years.

Versus percutaneous nephrolithotomy: We found no systematic review or RCTs comparing ESWL with percutaneous nephrolithotomy in people with asymptomatic kidney stones. **Versus ureteroscopy:** We found no systematic review or RCTs comparing ESWL with ureteroscopy in people with asymptomatic kidney stones.

Harms: **Versus conservative management:** The RCT found that during treatment with ESWL 35/98 (36%) people reported pain, 11/98 (12%) had nausea, though none vomited.[6] On simultaneous electrocardiograph recording, 9/98 (10%) people had bradycardia but none required treatment to be stopped or further intervention. Of the people undergoing ESWL, 3/98 (3%) were admitted to hospital with renal colic within 1 week of ESWL treatment and of the people with conservative management 20/115 (17%) required additional procedures. The RCT found that fewer people required invasive procedures after treatment with ESWL compared with conservative management (proportion of people requiring invasive procedures: 0/98 [0%] with ESWL *v* 8/115 [7%] with conservative management; P value not reported). **Versus percutaneous nephrolithotomy (PCNL) or ureteroscopy:** We found no RCTs.

Comment: None.

OPTION PERCUTANEOUS NEPHROLITHOTOMY (PCNL) New

We found no RCTs on percutaneous nephrolithotomy in people with asymptomatic renal or ureteric stones.

Benefits: **Versus conservative management:** We found no systematic review and no RCTs comparing percutaneous nephrolithotomy versus conservative management in people with asymptomatic kidney stones. **Versus extracorporeal shockwave lithotripsy:** We found no systematic review and no RCTs comparing percutaneous nephrolithotomy with extracorporeal shockwave lithotripsy in people with asymptomatic kidney stones. **Versus ureteroscopy:** We found no systematic review and no RCTs comparing percutaneous nephrolithotomy with ureteroscopy in people with asymptomatic kidney stones.

Harms: We found no RCTs.

Comment: None.

OPTION URETEROSCOPY New

We found no RCTs on ureteroscopy in people with asymptomatic renal or ureteric stones.

Benefits: We found no systematic review or RCTs comparing ureteroscopy with conservative management, extracorporeal shockwave lithotripsy, or percutaneous nephrolithotomy in people with asymptomatic kidney stones.

Harms: We found no RCTs.

Comment: None.

QUESTION What are the effects of treatments for the removal of symptomatic renal stones? New

OPTION EXTRACORPOREAL SHOCKWAVE LITHOTRIPSY New

One RCT found that extracorporeal shockwave lithotripsy decreased the stone free rate at 3 months and increased the rate of treatment failure in people with symptomatic renal stones less than 30 mm in diameter compared with

percutaneous nephrolithotomy. It found no significant difference in complication rate between extracorporeal shockwave lithotripsy and percutaneous nephrolithotomy, although complications were more frequent with percutaneous nephrolithotomy. We found no RCTs comparing extracorporeal shockwave lithotripsy with ureteroscopy or open nephrolithotomy in people with renal stones. There is consensus that extracorporeal shockwave lithotripsy is the first line treatment in people with renal stones less than 20mm in diameter as it is a less invasive intervention than percutaneous nephrolithotomy.

Benefits: **Versus percutaneous nephrolithotomy:** See benefits of percutaneous nephrolithotomy, p 1065. **Versus ureteroscopy:** We found no systematic review or RCTs comparing extracorporeal shockwave lithotripsy with ureteroscopy in people with renal stones. **Versus open nephrolithotomy:** We found no systematic review or RCTs comparing extracorporeal shockwave lithotripsy with open nephrolithotomy in people with renal stones.

Harms: **Versus percutaneous nephrolithotomy:** See harms of percutaneous nephrolithotomy, p 1066. **Versus ureteroscopy or open nephrolithotomy:** We found no RCTs.

Comment: The technology of the instrumentation for accessing and treating renal stones has advanced rapidly in recent years, making the findings of the reported RCTs, particularly with respect to the treatment of renal calculi that are not amenable to extracorporeal shockwave lithotripsy, difficult to apply to current practice. Further RCTs are required to evaluate these new modalities. There is consensus that extracorporeal shockwave lithotripsy is the first line treatment in people with renal stones less than 20mm in diameter as it is a less invasive intervention than percutaneous nephrolithotomy.

OPTION PERCUTANEOUS NEPHROLITHOTOMY New

One RCT found that percutaneous nephrolithotomy increased the stone free rate at 3 months and reduced the rate of treatment failure in people with symptomatic renal stones less than 30 mm in diameter compared with extracorporeal shockwave lithotripsy. It found no significant differences in complication rates between percutaneous nephrolithotomy and extracorporeal shockwave lithotripsy, although complications were more frequent with percutaneous nephrolithotomy. We found no RCTs comparing percutaneous nephrolithotomy with conservative management, ureteroscopy, or open nephrolithotomy in people with renal stones.

Benefits: **Versus conservative management:** We found no systematic review and no RCTs comparing percutaneous nephrolithotomy (PCNL) with conservative management. **Versus extracorporeal shockwave lithotripsy:** We found no systematic review but found one RCT (128 people with symptomatic renal calculi < 30 mm in size) comparing PCNL with extracorporeal shockwave lithotripsy (ESWL).[7] The RCT found that PCNL significantly increased the stone free rate at 3 months compared with ESWL (52/55 [95%] with PCNL *v* 19/52 [37%] with ESWL; $P < 0.001$). It found a lower rate of treatment failure with PCNL compared with ESWL (0/55 [0%] with PCNL *v* 9/64 [14%] with ESWL; 7/64 [11%] people subsequently had an invasive procedure; statistical data not reported). **Versus ureteroscopy:** We found no systematic review and no RCTs comparing PCNL with ureteroscopy in people with renal stones. **Versus open nephrolithotomy:** We found no systematic review and no RCTs comparing PCNL with open nephrolithotomy in people with renal stones.

Harms: **Versus conservative management:** We found no systematic review or RCTs. **Versus extracorporeal shockwave lithotripsy:** The RCT found no significant difference in the proportion of people with complications between percutaneous nephrolithotomy (PCNL) and extracorporeal shockwave lithotripsy (ESWL), although complications were more frequent with PCNL (13/57 [23%] with PCNL *v* 7/59 [12%] with ESWL; P = 0.087).[7] Severe complications with PCNL included ileus and perforation (3 people each); renal haematoma (2 people); and urinary tract infection, systemic sepsis, ureteric obstruction, haemorrhage requiring transfusion, and development of an arteriovenous fistula (1 person each). Complications with ESWL included renal colic and ureteric obstruction (2 people each); and urinary tract infection, renal haematoma, and steinstrasse**G** (1 one person each). **Versus ureteroscopy or open nephrolithotomy:** We found no systematic review or RCTs.

Comment: When comparing PCNL with ESWL, additional factors, such as stone size and location need to be taken into account. People with a larger stone burden are likely to take longer to pass stone fragments after ESWL. The RCT reported that stone removal from the lower pole using ESWL was particularly problematic for stones greater than 10 mm in diameter. Further RCTs are required to evaluate new modalities of accessing and treating renal stones which have been developed in recent years. Rapid advancements in this field make it difficult to apply the findings of the reported RCTs, particularly with respect to the treatment of renal stones that are not amenable to ESWL, to current practice.

OPTION URETEROSCOPY New

We found no RCTs on ureteroscopy in people with renal stones.

Benefits: We found no systematic review or RCTs comparing ureteroscopy with conservative management, extracorporeal shockwave lithotripsy, percutaneous nephrolithotomy, or open nephrolithotomy.

Harms: We found no RCTs.

Comment: None.

OPTION OPEN NEPHROLITHOTOMY New

We found no RCTs on open nephrolithotomy in people with renal stones.

Benefits: We found no systematic review or RCTs comparing open nephrolithotomy with conservative management, extracorporeal shockwave lithotripsy, percutaneous nephrolithotomy, or ureteroscopy in people with renal stones.

Harms: We found no RCTs.

Comment: In the Western world, open nephrolithotomy has been largely superseded by percutaneous nephrolithotomy and is performed only rarely, with people selected on a case by case basis.

QUESTION What are the effects of treatments for the removal of symptomatic ureteric stones? New

OPTION EXTRACORPOREAL SHOCKWAVE LITHOTRIPSY New

Three RCTs found that overall stone free rates were lower and the time needed to become stone free longer in people with mid- and distal ureteric stones with extracorporeal shockwave lithotripsy compared with ureteroscopy.

However, a fourth RCT found no significant difference in stone free rates between treatments (stone free rate of 91% in both cases) in people with distal ureteric stones of less than 15 mm. One RCT found a lower rate of treatment failure with extracorporeal shockwave lithotripsy compared with ureteroscopy. Three of the RCTs found a lower rate of severe complications with extracorporeal shockwave lithotripsy compared with ureteroscopy. We found no RCTs comparing extracorporeal shockwave lithotripsy versus ureteroscopy in people with proximal ureteric stones or comparing extracorporeal shockwave lithotripsy with conservative treatment or ureterolithotomy (open or laparoscopic) in people with ureteric stones.

Benefits: **Versus conservative management:** We found no systematic review or RCTs comparing extracorporeal shockwave lithotripsy with conservative management in people with ureteric stones. **Versus ureteroscopy:** See benefits of ureteroscopy, p 1067. **Versus ureterolithotomy (open or laparoscopic):** We found no systematic review or RCTs comparing extracorporeal shockwave lithotripsy with ureterolithotomy (open or laparoscopic) in people with ureteric stones.

Harms: **Versus conservative management:** We found no systematic review or RCTs. **Versus ureteroscopy:** See harms of ureteroscopy, p 1068. **Versus ureterolithotomy (open or laparoscopic):** We found no RCTs.

Comment: None.

OPTION URETEROSCOPY New

Three RCTs found that ureteroscopy increased overall stone free rate and decreased the time needed to become stone free in people with mid- and distal ureteric stones compared with extracorporeal shockwave lithotripsy. However, a fourth RCT found no significant difference in stone free rates between treatments (stone free rate of 91% in both cases) in people with distal ureteric stones of less than 15 mm. One RCT found a higher rate of treatment failure with ureteroscopy compared with extracorporeal shockwave lithotripsy. Three of the RCTs found a higher complication rate with ureteroscopy compared with extracorporeal shockwave lithotripsy. We found no RCTs comparing ureteroscopy versus extracorporeal shockwave lithotripsy in people with proximal ureteric stones or comparing ureteroscopy with conservative treatment, extracorporeal shockwave lithotripsy, or ureterolithotomy (open or laparoscopic) in people with ureteric stones.

Benefits: **Versus conservative management:** We found no systematic review or RCTs comparing ureteroscopy versus conservative management in people with ureteric stones. **Versus extracorporeal shockwave lithotripsy:** We found no systematic review but found four RCTs comparing ureteroscopy versus extracorporeal shockwave lithotripsy (ESWL) in people with ureteric stones.[8–11] The first RCT (156 people with mid- and distal ureteric stones of any size, symptoms not reported) found that ureteroscopy increased stone free rate at 3 months compared with ESWL (79/87 [91%] with ureteroscopy *v* 35/69 [51%] with ESWL; P value not reported).[8] It found a higher rate of treatment failure with ureteroscopy (13/87 [15%] with ureteroscopy [stones flushed up towards the kidney in 8 people, stones not reached or seen in 3 people, and technical problems in 2 people] *v* 2/69 [3%] with ESWL [stones not seen in 1 person, technical problems occurring in 1 person]; P value not reported). Similarly, the second RCT (80 people with radio-opaque**G** or symptomatic distal ureteric stones < 16 mm in diameter) found that ureteroscopy increased stone free rate on day 15 compared with ESWL (people with stones < 5 mm in diameter: 20/20 [100%] with ureteroscopy *v* 17/20 [85%] with ESWL; stones ≥ 5 mm in diameter: 20/20 [100%] with ureteroscopy *v* 18/20 [90%] with ESWL; P values not reported).[9] It also found that ureteroscopy significantly decreased the time to a stone free state compared with ESWL (stones < 5 mm in diameter, mean: 0.2 days (range 0 days to 1 day) with ureteroscopy *v* 10.8 days (range 1 day to 43 days) with ESWL; P < 0.005; stones ≥ 5 mm in diameter, mean: 3.7 days (range 0 days to 8.0 days) with ureteroscopy *v* 9.1 days (range 1.0 day to 43.0 days) with ESWL; P < 0.05). The third RCT (390 people with distal ureteric stones 5–21 mm in diameter, symptoms not reported) also found that ureteroscopy significantly increased stone free rate at days 7 and 28 compared with ESWL (day 7: 159/180 [88.3%] with ureteroscopy *v* 112/210 [53.3%] with ESWL; P < 0.05; day 28: 168/180 [93.3%] with ureteroscopy *v* 164/210 [78.1%] with ESWL; P < 0.05).[10] It gave no information on failure rates of treatments. However, the fourth RCT (64 people with distal ureteric stones < 15 mm in diameter, symptoms not reported) found no significant difference in stone free rates between the two groups at 3 weeks (29/32 [91%] with ureteroscopy *v* 29/32 [91%] with ESWL).[11] It gave no information on failure rates of treatments. **Versus ureterolithotomy:** We found no systematic review or RCTs comparing ureteroscopy versus ureterolithotomy (open or laparoscopic) in people with ureteric stones.

Harms: **Versus conservative management:** We found no systematic review or RCTs. **Versus extracorporeal shockwave lithotripsy:** We found four RCTs. The first RCT found higher intraoperative and postoperative complication rates with ureteroscopy compared with ESWL (intraoperative: 22/87 [25%] with ureteroscopy *v* 3/69 [4%] with ESWL; P value not reported; postoperative: 30/87 [35%] with ureteroscopy *v* 14/69 [20%] with ESWL; P value not reported).[8] Intraoperative complications with ureteroscopy included 9/87 (10%) people with ureteric perforation or damage to the ureter. Postoperative complications with ureteroscopy included haematuria (11 people); urinary tract infection (4 people); ureteric obstruction, renal colic, and pyrexia (3 people each); haematoma and pyelonephritis (2 people each); and systemic sepsis and urinoma (1 person each). Intraoperative bleeding occurred in one person with ESWL. Postoperative complications with ESWL included haematuria (8 people), renal colic (5 people), and ureteric obstruction (1 person). The second RCT found no complications with either treatment.[9] The third RCT found significantly more people with ureteric perforation at day 28 with ureteroscopy compared with ESWL (6/180 [3.3%] with ureteroscopy *v* 0/210 [0%] with ESWL; P < 0.05). It found no significant difference in the rates of postoperative infections or ureteric stricture between the two treatments.[10] It gave no information on failure rates of treatments. The fourth RCT found more people with complications after ureteroscopy compared with ESWL (8/32 [25%] with ureteroscopy *v* 3/32 [9%] with ESWL; P value not reported).[10] Complications with ureteroscopy included postoperative pain (3 people); acute retention of urine (2 people); and pulmonary embolus, pyrexia, and exacerbation of existing diabetes (1 person each). Complications with ESWL included admission to hospital for analgesia, acute retention of urine, and herniated intervertebral disk (although listed as having a complication of ESWL; 1 person each). **Versus ureterolithotomy (open or laparoscopic):** We found no systematic review or RCTs.

Comment: Ureteroscopic methods of fragmentation and removal of stones have advanced significantly in recent years.

OPTION URETEROLITHOTOMY (OPEN OR LAPAROSCOPIC) New

We found no RCTs on ureterolithotomy (open or laparoscopic) in people with ureteric stones.

Benefits: We found no systematic review or RCTs comparing ureterolithotomy (open or laparoscopic) with conservative management, extracorporeal shockwave lithotripsy, percutaneous nephrolithotomy, or ureteroscopy in people with ureteric stones.

Harms: We found no RCTs.

Comment: None.

GLOSSARY

Hydronephrosis Dilatation of the renal pelvis, with or without dilatation of the ureter, resulting from an obstruction within the renal tract.
Perinephric abscess Abscess lying within Gerota's fascia.
Radio-opaque calculus A stone which is visible on x-ray.
Steinstrasse A collection of stone fragments within the ureter. On x-ray, such collections have the appearance of a cobbled street, hence the term steinstrasse, in German meaning "street of stone".

REFERENCES

1. Glowacki LS, Beecroft ML, Cook RJ, et al. The natural history of asymptomatic urolithiasis. *J Urol* 1992;147:319–321.
2. Uribarri J, Oh MS, Carroll HJ. The first kidney stone. *Ann Intern Med* 1989;111:1006–1009.
3. Menon M, Parulkar BG, Drach GW. Urinary lithiasis: etiology, diagnosis and medical management. In: Walsh PC, Retik AB, Vaughan ED, et al, eds. *Campbells urology*. 7th edition. Philadelphia: WB Saunders Company, 1998.
4. Segura JW, Preminger GM, Assinos DG, et al. Ureteral Stones Clinical Guidelines Panel summary report on the management of ureteral calculi. *J Urol* 1997;158:1915–1921.
5. Blandy JP, Singh M. The case for a more aggressive approach to staghorn stones. *J Urol* 1976;115:505–506.
6. Keeley FX Jr, Tilling K, Elves A, et al. Preliminary results of a randomized controlled trial of prophylactic shock wave lithotripsy for small asymptomatic renal calyceal stones. *BJU Int* 2001;87:1–8.
7. Albala DM, Assimos DG, Clayman RV, et al. Lower pole I: a prospective randomized trial of extracorporeal shock wave lithotripsy and percutaneous nephrolithotomy for lower pole nephrolithiasis <en initial results. *J Urol* 2001;166:2072–2080. [Erratum in: *J Urol* 2002;167:1805]
8. Hendrikx AJ, Strijbos WE, de Knijff DW, et al. Treatment for extended-mid and distal ureteral stones: SWL or ureteroscopy? Results of a multicenter study. *J Endourol* 1999;13:727–733.
9. Peschel R, Janetschek G, Bartsch G. Extracorporeal shock wave lithotripsy versus ureteroscopy for distal ureteral calculi: a prospective randomized study. *J Urol* 1999;162:1909–1912.
10. Zeng GQ, Zhong WD, Cai YB, et al. Extracorporeal shock-wave versus pneumatic ureteroscopic lithotripsy in treatment of lower ureteral calculi. *Asian J Androl* 2002;4:303–305.
11. Pearle MS, Nadler R, Bercowsky E, et al. Prospective randomized trial comparing shock wave lithotripsy and ureteroscopy for management of distal ureteral calculi. *J Urol* 2001;166:1255–1260.

Robyn Webber
Consultant Urological Surgeon
Queen Margaret Hospital
Dunfermline
UK

David Tolley
Consultant Urological Surgeon
Western General Hospital
Edinburgh
UK

James Lingeman
Urologist
The Methodist Hospital
Indianapolis
Indiana, USA

Competing interests: None declared.

Renal failure (acute)

Search date April 2004

John A Kellum, Martine Leblanc, and Ramesh Venkataraman

QUESTIONS

INTERVENTIONS

To be covered in future updates

Endothelin receptor antagonists
Growth factors

See glossary G

Key Messages

Preventing acute renal failure

- **Low osmolality contrast media (reduced nephrotoxocity compared with standard media)** One systematic review found that low osmolality contrast media reduced nephrotoxicity in people with underlying renal failure needing contrast investigation compared with standard osmolality contrast media. One subsequent RCT found that non-ionic iso-osmolar contrast medium (iodixanol) reduced contrast media induced nephropathy compared with low osmolar non-ionic contrast medium (iohexol) in people with diabetes.

- **Acetylcysteine** One systematic review found that N-acetylcysteine plus hydration reduced contrast nephropathy (defined by an increase in serum creatinine) compared with hydration alone in people with chronic renal insufficiency who were having radiocontrast imaging studies. However, N-acetylcysteine may reduce serum creatinine independently of any effect on renal function, so conclusions about clinical efficacy should be interpreted with caution.
- **Fluids** One RCT of people having elective cardiac catheterisation found that intravenous sodium chloride hydration reduced acute renal failure compared with unrestricted oral fluids 48 hours after catheterisation. One RCT found that hydration with 0.9% sodium chloride infusion reduced contrast nephropathy compared with 0.45% sodium chloride. This effect was greater in women, people with diabetes, and people who received more than 250 mL of contrast. One RCT found inconclusive evidence on the effects of inpatient hydration regimens compared with outpatient hydration regimens.
- **Lipid formulations of amphotericin B (may cause less nephrotoxicity than standard formulations)** We found no RCTs. Lipid formulations of amphotericin B seem to cause less nephrotoxicity compared with standard formulations, but direct comparisons of long term safety are lacking.
- **Single dose aminoglycosides (as effective as multiple doses for treating infection, but with reduced nephrotoxicity)** One systematic review and one additional RCT compared single and multiple doses of aminoglycosides and found different results for nephrotoxicity. The systematic review, in people with fever and neutropenia receiving antibiotic treatment including aminoglycosides, found no significant difference in cure rates or nephrotoxicity between once daily compared with three times daily administration of the aminoglycoside. However, the RCT found that single doses of aminoglycosides reduced nephrotoxicity compared with multiple doses in people with fever and receiving antibiotic treatment including an aminoglycoside.
- **Fenoldopam** Five RCTs examined the role of fenoldopam in preventing acute renal failure. Although four small, poor quality, RCTs suggested that fenoldopam may improve renal perfusion and creatinine clearance compared with conventional care, the fifth and largest RCT, which focused on clinical outcomes in people having invasive cardiovascular procedures, found no evidence that it is more effective than conventional care for preventing acute renal failure. Fenoldopam may induce hypotension.
- **Mannitol** Small RCTs in people with traumatic rhabdomyolysis, or in people who had had coronary artery bypass, vascular, or biliary tract surgery, found that mannitol plus hydration did not reduce acute renal failure compared with hydration alone. One RCT found that mannitol increased the risk of acute renal failure compared with 0.45% sodium chloride infusion, but the difference was not significant.
- **Theophylline** One RCT in people with adequate hydration found that theophylline did not prevent contrast nephropathy compared with placebo. Three further RCTs, which did not report on the hydration status of participants, found mixed results. Two found that theophylline protected renal function compared with placebo and one found no significant difference. Another RCT found no significant reduction in renal impairment after elective coronary artery bypass surgery with theophylline compared with hydration alone but may have been underpowered to detect a clinically important difference.
- **Calcium channel blockers for early allograft dysfunction** One RCT found no significant difference between isradipine and placebo in preventing early allograft dysfunction in people receiving cadaveric or living renal transplant. One systematic review limited to people with cadaveric renal transplant found limited evidence from heterogeneous RCTs that calcium channel blockers given in the peri-operative period reduced post-transplant acute tubular necrosis, although it found no significant effect on graft loss, need for haemodialysis, or mortality. We found no RCTs assessing the effects of calcium channel blockers in preventing other forms of acute renal failure. Calcium channel blockers are associated with hypotension and bradycardia.

- **Dopamine** Two systematic reviews and one subsequent RCT found no significant difference between dopamine and placebo in the development of acute renal failure, the need for dialysis, or death. One RCT found insufficient evidence on the effects of combined dopamine and diltiazem in people having cardiac surgery. Dopamine is associated with serious adverse effects, such as extravasation necrosis, gangrene, and conduction abnormalities.
- **Loop diuretics** One systematic review and one subsequent RCT found that adding loop diuretics to fluids was not effective and may be harmful in preventing acute renal failure compared with fluids alone in people at high risk of acute renal failure.
- **Natriuretic peptides** One large RCT found no significant difference between natriuretic peptides and placebo in the prevention of acute renal failure induced by contrast media. Subgroup analysis in another large RCT found that atrial natriuretic peptide reduced dialysis free survival in non-oliguric people compared with placebo.

Treating acute renal failure

- **High dose continuous renal replacement therapy (reduced mortality compared with low dose)** One RCT found that high dose continuous renal replacement therapy (haemofiltration) reduced mortality compared with low dose continuous therapy. A small prospective study found that intensive (daily) intermittent haemodialysis reduced mortality in people with acute renal failure compared with conventional alternate day haemodialysis. A subsequent small three arm RCT found no significant difference in survival at 28 days between early, low dose haemofiltration; early, high dose haemofiltration; and late, low dose haemofiltration.
- **Combined diuretics and albumin** We found no RCTs on the effects of intravenous albumin supplementation plus loop diuretics in people with acute renal failure.
- **Continuous infusion of loop diuretics (compared with bolus injection)** We found no RCTs comparing continuous infusion versus bolus injection of loop diuretics in critically ill people with acute renal failure.
- **Continuous renal replacement therapy (compared with intermittent renal replacement therapy)** One systematic review found no significant difference between continuous and intermittent renal replacement therapy in mortality, renal death, or dialysis dependence in critically ill adults with acute renal failure.
- **Synthetic dialysis membranes (compared with cellulose based membranes)** Two systematic reviews provided inconclusive evidence of the effects of synthetic membranes on mortality in critically ill people with acute renal failure compared with cellulose based membranes.
- **Loop diuretics** Underpowered RCTs in people with oliguric renal failure found no significant difference between loop diuretics and placebo on renal recovery, the number of days spent on dialysis, or mortality. Loop diuretics have been associated with toxicity and low renal perfusion.
- **Dopamine** One systematic review found no significant difference in mortality or need for dialysis between dopamine and placebo. One additional RCT found that low dose dopamine did not reduce renal dysfunction compared with placebo. Dopamine has been associated with important adverse effects, including extravasation necrosis, gangrene, and conduction abnormalities.
- **Natriuretic peptides** RCTs found no significant difference between atrial natriuretic peptide, ularitide (urodilatin), and placebo in dialysis free survival in oliguric and non-oliguric people with acute renal failure. One of the RCTs found that atrial natriuretic peptide may reduce survival in non-oliguric people.

DEFINITION Acute renal failure is characterised by abrupt and sustained decline in glomerular filtration rate Ⓖ,[1] which leads to accumulation of urea and other chemicals in the blood. Most studies define it biochemically as a serum creatinine of 2–3 mg/dL (200–250 μmol/L), an elevation of more than 0.5 mg/dL (45 μmol/L) over a baseline creatinine below 2 mg/dL, or a twofold increase of baseline creatinine. A recent international, interdisciplinary, consensus panel has classified acute renal failure according to a change from baseline serum creatinine or urine output. The three level classification begins with "Risk", defined by either a 50% increase in serum creatinine or a urine output of less than 0.5 mL/kg/hour for at least 6 hours, and concludes with "Failure", defined by a threefold increase in serum creatinine or a urine output of less than 0.3 mL/kg/hour for 24 hours.[2] Acute renal failure is usually additionally classified according to the location of the predominant primary pathology (prerenal, intrarenal, and postrenal failure). Critically ill people are unstable and at imminent risk of death, which usually implies that they need to be in, or have been admitted to, the intensive care unit.

INCIDENCE/ PREVALENCE

Two prospective observational studies (2576 people) have found that established acute renal failure affects nearly 5% of people in hospital and as many as 15% of critically ill people, depending on the definitions used.[3,4]

AETIOLOGY/ RISK FACTORS

General risk factors: Risk factors for acute renal failure that are consistent across multiple causes include hypovolaemia; hypotension; sepsis; pre-existing renal, hepatic, or cardiac dysfunction; diabetes mellitus; and exposure to nephrotoxins (e.g. aminoglycosides, amphotericin, immunosuppressive agents, non-steroidal anti-inflammatory drugs, angiotensin converting enzyme inhibitors, iv contrast media) (see table 1, p 1092). **Risk factors/aetiology in critically ill people:** Isolated episodes of acute renal failure are rarely seen in critically ill people, but are usually part of multiple organ dysfunction syndromes**G**. Acute renal failure requiring dialysis is rarely seen in isolation (< 5% of people). The kidneys are often the first organs to fail.[9] In the perioperative setting, acute renal failure risk factors include prolonged aortic clamping, emergency rather than elective surgery, and use of higher volumes (> 100 mL) of intravenous contrast media. One study (3695 people) using multiple logistic regression identified the following independent risk factors: baseline creatinine clearance below 47 mL/minute (OR 1.20, 95% CI 1.12 to 1.30), diabetes (OR 5.5, 95% CI 1.4 to 21.0), and a marginal effect for doses of contrast media above 100 mL (OR 1.01, 95% CI 1.00 to 1.01). Mortality of people with acute renal failure requiring dialysis was 36% while in hospital.[5] Prerenal acute renal failure is caused by reduced blood flow to the kidney from renal artery disease, systematic hypotension, or maldistribution of blood flow. Intrarenal acute renal failure is caused by parenchymal injury (acute tubular necrosis, interstitial nephritis, embolic disease, glomerulonephritis, vasculitis, or small vessel disease). Postrenal acute renal failure is caused by urinary tract obstruction. Observational studies (in several hundred people from Europe, North America, and west Africa with acute renal failure) found a prerenal cause in 40–80%, an intrarenal cause in 10–50%, and a postrenal cause in the remaining 10%.[7,8,10–13] Prerenal acute renal failure is the most common type of acute renal failure in people who are critically ill,[7,14] but acute renal failure in this context is usually part of multisystem failure, and most frequently because of acute tubular necrosis resulting from ischaemic or nephrotoxic injury, or both.[15,16]

PROGNOSIS

One retrospective study (1347 people with acute renal failure) found that mortality was less than 15% in people with isolated acute renal failure.[17] One recent prospective study (> 700 people) found that, in people with acute renal failure, overall mortality and the need for dialysis were higher in an intensive care unit (ICU) than in a non-ICU setting, despite no significant difference between the groups in mean maximal serum creatinine (need for dialysis: 71% in ICU *v* 18% in non-ICU; $P < 0.001$; mortality: 72% in ICU *v* 32% in non-ICU; $P = 0.001$).[18] One large study (> 17 000 people admitted to Austrian ICUs) found that acute renal failure was associated with a greater than fourfold increase in mortality.[19] Even after controlling for underlying severity of illness, mortality was still significantly higher in people with acute renal failure (62.8% *v* 38.5%), suggesting that acute renal failure is independently responsible for increased mortality, even if dialysis is used. However, the exact mechanism that leads to increased risk of death is uncertain.

AIMS OF INTERVENTION

Prevention: To preserve renal function. **Treating critically ill people:** To prevent death; to prevent complications of acute renal failure (volume overload, acid–base disturbance, and electrolyte abnormalities); and to prevent the need for chronic dialysis, with minimum adverse effects.

OUTCOMES

Prevention: Rates of acute renal failure, nephrotoxicity**G**, or both. Surrogate outcomes were limited to measurements of biochemical evidence of organ function (serum creatinine or creatinine clearance) after the intervention. Surrogate markers such as urine output or renal blood flow were not considered as evidence of effectiveness. **Critically ill people:** Rate of death; rate of renal recovery; adverse effects of treatment. Extent of natriuresis is a proxy outcome.

METHODS

Clinical Evidence search and appraisal April 2004.

QUESTION What are the effects of interventions to prevent acute renal failure in people at high risk?

OPTION FLUIDS

One RCT of people having elective cardiac catheterisation found that intravenous sodium chloride hydration reduced acute renal failure compared with unrestricted oral fluids 48 hours after catheterisation. One RCT found that hydration with 0.9% sodium chloride infusion reduced contrast nephropathy compared with 0.45% sodium chloride. This effect was greater in women, people with diabetes, and people who received more than 250 mL of contrast. One RCT found inconclusive evidence on the effects of inpatient hydration regimens compared with outpatient hydration regimens.

Benefits: **Intravenous versus oral fluids:** We found one RCT (53 people having elective cardiac catheterisation with an iodine containing contrast agent) that compared intravenous sodium chloride hydration (0.9% sodium chloride for 24 hours at a rate of 1 mL/kg/hour begun 12 hours before catheterisation) versus unrestricted oral fluids.[20] It found that sodium chloride hydration significantly reduced acute renal failure compared with unrestricted oral fluids within 48 hours (acute renal failure defined as increase in serum creatinine by at least 44.2 μmol/L [0.5 mg/dL]: 1/27 [3.7%] with sodium chloride hydration *v* 9/26 [34.6%] with unrestricted fluids; RR 0.11, 95% CI 0.015 to 0.79). Older RCTs compared combinations of fluids (especially 0.45% sodium chloride infusion) versus other active treatments. Comparisons between outcomes in these trials and historical untreated controls are difficult to evaluate but suggest benefit from fluids.[21] In certain settings, such as traumatic rhabdomyolysis, early and aggressive fluid resuscitation has had dramatic benefits compared with historical controls.[6] **Comparison of intravenous fluids:** We found one RCT (1620 people who had coronary angiography), which compared effects of 0.9% sodium chloride infusion versus 0.45% sodium chloride in dextrose infusion on contrast nephropathy**G**.[22] Contrast nephropathy was defined as an increase in serum creatinine of more than 0.5 mg/dL (45 μmol/L) within 48 hours. The RCT found that hydration with 0.9% sodium chloride infusion significantly reduced contrast nephropathy compared with 0.45% sodium chloride in dextrose infusion (0.7% with 0.9% sodium chloride infusion *v* 2.0% with 0.45% sodium chloride infusion; $P = 0.04$). Three predefined subsets of people (women, people with diabetes, and people receiving > 250 mL of the contrast) benefited the most from 0.9% sodium chloride infusion hydration. **Inpatient versus outpatient hydration regimens:** We found one RCT (36 people), which compared an inpatient hydration regimen (0.45% sodium chloride solution at 75 mL/hour iv for 12 hours before and after cardiac catheterisation) with an outpatient hydration regimen (1 L of clear liquids over 10 hours followed by 6 hours of iv hydration beginning just before contrast exposure) for the prevention of radiocontrast induced renal dysfunction.[23] The predefined primary end point was maximal change in creatinine up to 48 hours after cardiac catheterisation. No significant differences were found in the maximal changes in serum creatinine between groups (0.21 ± 0.38 mg/dL [18±33μmol/L] for inpatients *v* 0.12 ± 0.23 mg/dL [11±20μmol/L] for outpatients; $P > 0.05$, no additional data reported). However, this study may be underpowered to rule out clinically important differences. The outpatient group also received more fluid volume.

Harms: The volumes of fluids recommended (e.g. 1 L) and the rates of infusion (generally < 500 mL/hour) have little potential for harm in most people. The RCT (53 people having non-emergency cardiac catheterisation) comparing sodium chloride hydration versus unrestricted oral fluids found no adverse effects with sodium chloride hydration.[20] No significant differences were found in cardiac or peripheral vascular complications between hydration with 0.9% sodium chloride and 0.45% sodium chloride plus dextrose (cardiac complications: 5.3% with 0.9% sodium chloride *v* 6.4% with 0.45% sodium chloride plus dextrose; P = 0.59; peripheral vascular complications: 1.6% with 0.9% sodium chloride *v* 1.5% with 0.45% sodium chloride plus dextrose; P = 0.93).[22] The RCT comparing inpatient and outpatient hydration regimens did not report harms data.[23]

Comment: Hypovolaemia is a significant risk factor for acute renal failure. The provision of adequate maintenance fluids is considered important in preventing acute renal failure. Additional fluid loading may be useful because it assures adequate intravascular volume. It also stimulates urine output, theoretically limiting renal exposure time to higher concentrations of nephrotoxins.

OPTION LOOP DIURETICS

One systematic review and one subsequent RCT found that adding loop diuretics to fluids was not effective and may be harmful in preventing acute renal failure compared with fluids alone in people at high risk of acute renal failure.

Benefits: We found one systematic review (search date 1997, 7 RCTs)[24] and one subsequent RCT,[25] which compared fluids alone versus diuretics plus fluids in people at risk of acute renal failure from various causes. The review found no evidence of improved survival, decreased incidence of acute renal failure, or need for dialysis associated with diuretics. The systematic review also assessed the efficacy of loop diuretics in the prevention of acute tubular necrosis (1 RCT, 121 people randomised to receive 1 mg/hour of furosemide or placebo immediately after major thoraco-abdominal or vascular surgery, and maintained during stay in the intensive care unit). It found no significant difference between furosemide and placebo in creatinine clearance. Both groups had significant reductions in creatinine clearance compared with baseline, but no differences were found between groups (reduction compared with baseline values: 83% with furosemide *v* 81% with placebo). The study did not address the use of loop diuretics given during the procedure.[26] The subsequent RCT (81 people after cardiac surgery) found that furosemide plus fluid significantly increased acute renal failure compared with 0.9% sodium chloride alone (6/41 [15%] with furosemide *v* 0/40 [0%] with sodium chloride; NNH 6, 95% CI 3 to 34).[25]

Harms: The systematic review and RCT did not report on adverse effects. [24] The subsequent RCT found that diuretics plus fluid significantly increased acute renal failure compared with fluids alone (see benefits above).[24,25]

Comment: None.

OPTION MANNITOL

Small RCTs in people with traumatic rhabdomyolysis, or in people who had had coronary artery bypass, vascular, or biliary tract surgery, found that mannitol plus hydration did not reduce acute renal failure compared with hydration alone. One RCT found that mannitol increased the risk of acute renal failure compared with 0.45% sodium chloride infusion, but the difference was not significant.

Benefits: We found no systematic review. Several small RCTs did not find a reduction in the incidence of acute renal failure with mannitol plus hydration over hydration alone in a variety of conditions, including coronary artery bypass surgery,[27] traumatic rhabdomyolysis,[28] and vascular,[29] and biliary tract surgery.[30] One trial comparing 0.45% sodium chloride, furosemide, and mannitol (78 people with chronic renal insufficiency who had a cardiac angiography, mean serum creatinine 2.1 ± 0.6 mg/dL [186 ± 53 μmol/L]) found that mannitol plus 0.45% sodium chloride increased acute renal failure (defined as an increase in serum creatinine ≥ 0.5 mg/dL [44 μmol/L] at 48 hours) compared with 0.45% sodium chloride alone, although the difference was not significant (AR 7/25 [28%] with mannitol *v* 3/28 [11%] with 0.45% sodium chloride; RR 2.61, 95% CI 0.76 to 9.03).[21]

Harms: The RCT did not report harms.

Comment: Mannitol is an intravascular volume expander and may also function as a free radical scavenger, as well as an osmotic diuretic. The trial addressing the effect of mannitol on renal function[21] provided a three way comparison showing significant differences among the three groups ($P < 0.05$). Although the same control group seems to have been used to compare both interventions, no adjustment was made for multiple comparisons.

OPTION DOPAMINE

Two systematic reviews and one subsequent RCT found no significant difference between dopamine and placebo in the development of acute renal failure, the need for dialysis, or death. One RCT found insufficient evidence on the effects of combined dopamine and diltiazem in people having cardiac surgery. Dopamine is associated with serious adverse effects, such as extravasation necrosis, gangrene, and conduction abnormalities.

Benefits: We found two systematic reviews[31,32] and one subsequent large RCT.[33] The first systematic review (search date 1999, 17 RCTs, 854 people) examined the effects of any dose of dopamine.[31] It was adequately powered and found no significant difference between dopamine and placebo in mortality, onset of acute renal failure, or need for dialysis (mortality: 11 RCTs, 508 people; 4.7% with dopamine *v* 5.6% with placebo; RR 0.83, 95% CI 0.39 to 1.77; onset of acute renal failure: 11 RCTs, 511 people; 15.3% with dopamine *v* 19.5% with placebo; RR 0.79, 95% CI 0.54 to 1.13; need for dialysis: 10 RCTs, 618 people; 13.9% with dopamine *v* 16.5% with placebo; RR 0.89, 95% CI 0.66 to 1.21). The second systematic review (search date 2000, 15 RCTs, 970 adults either with or at risk of acute renal insufficiency, see comments below) assessed the effects of low dose dopamine.[32] It was also adequately powered and found no significant difference between low dose dopamine (2–5 μg/kg/minute) and placebo in acute deterioration in renal function (defined as an increase in serum creatinine of > 25% from baseline; AR 31% with low dose dopamine *v* 33% with placebo; RR 1.01, 95% CI 0.79 to 1.28). The subsequent RCT (328 critically ill people with signs of sepsis) evaluated dopamine in early renal dysfunction**G**.[33] It found no significant difference between dopamine and placebo on the development of acute renal failure, the requirement for dialysis, intensive care unit length of stay, hospital length of stay, or mortality (acute renal failure: peak serum creatinine concentration during treatment was 2.7 ± 1.6 mg/dL [245 ± 144 μmol/L] with dopamine *v* 2.8 ± 1.6 mg/dL [249 ± 147 μmol/L] with placebo; P = 0.93; requirement for dialysis: 35/161 [22%] with dopamine *v* 40/163 [25%] with placebo; RR 0.89, 95% CI 0.58 to 1.30; intensive care unit length of stay: 13 ± 14 days with dopamine v 14 ± 15 days with placebo; P = 0.67; hospital length of stay: 29 ± 27 days with dopamine v 33 ± 39 days with placebo; P = 0.29; mortality: 69/161 [43%] with dopamine v 66/163 [40%] with placebo; RR 1.06, 95% CI 0.8 to 1.33).

Harms: The systematic reviews[31,32] and the subsequent RCT in people with sepsis[33] did not report on harms. Dopamine has known adverse effects, including extravasation necrosis, gangrene, tachycardia, headache, and conduction abnormalities.

Comment: Most of the studies examining effects of dopamine included people with early indications of renal dysfunction. The distinction between effects of dopamine for prevention and for treatment is, therefore, blurred. We have used the same studies to infer preventative and treatment effects. One RCT (60 people having coronary artery bypass grafting) compared four interventions: dopamine, diltiazem, dopamine plus diltiazem, and control (not specified). Drug administration (iv infusion rates 2 μg/kg/minute diltiazem and 2 μg/kg/minute dopamine) was initiated 24 hours before surgery and continued for 72 hours after surgery.[34] Creatinine clearance (primary end point) was significantly higher in the diltiazem plus dopamine group compared with the dopamine only, diltiazem only, and control groups 24 hours after surgery. However, this study was underpowered, and the hydration status of the people was not controlled. The increase in urine output associated with dopamine is often thought to be caused exclusively by the increase in renal blood flow and, therefore, it may be confused with evidence of benefit. However, dopamine also has a significant diuretic effect. The review comparing low dose dopamine versus placebo included people with normal renal function who were having elective vascular surgery, cardiac surgery, and liver transplantation; people with obstructive jaundice; people with diabetes; people receiving nephrotoxic drugs or having radiocontrast investigations; and people with renal insufficiency having cardiac surgery or receiving radiocontrast agents.[32]

OPTION DOPAMINE 1 RECEPTOR AGONISTS (FENOLDOPAM)

Five RCTs examined the role of fenoldopam in preventing acute renal failure. Although four small, poor quality, RCTs suggested that fenoldopam may improve renal perfusion and creatinine clearance compared with conventional care, the fifth and largest RCT, which focused on clinical outcomes in people having invasive cardiovascular procedures, found no evidence that it is more effective than conventional care for preventing acute renal failure. Fenoldopam may induce hypotension.

Benefits: We found five RCTs.[35–39] Four of the RCTs had weak methods; either they did not directly compare interventions between groups or did not assess clinical outcomes. The first RCT (31 people having elective coronary revascularisation) compared intravenous 0.1 μg/kg/minute fenoldopam versus placebo (not described, presumably 0.9% sodium chloride).[35] Mean creatinine clearance decreased in the placebo group from 107 ± 36 mL/minute to 71 ± 22 mL/minute ($P < 0.01$) for the 0–4 hour interval and from 107 ± 36 mL/minute to 79 ± 26 mL/minute ($P < 0.01$) for the 4–8 hour interval, but not the fenoldopam group after separation from cardiopulmonary bypass. However, the clinical importance of this end point is not clear, comparisons were made within rather than between groups, and this study was underpowered to assess relevant clinical outcomes, such as need for dialysis.[35] The second RCT[36] evaluated the role of fenoldopam in preventing acute renal failure after aortic surgery in 28 people having elective aortic surgery requiring infrarenal aortic cross-clamping. People were randomised to intravenous 0.1 μg/kg/minute fenoldopam or placebo (not described) before skin incision and until release of the aortic clamp. On application of the aortic cross-clamp, creatinine clearance decreased significantly in the placebo group (83 ± 20 mL/minute to 42 ± 29 mL/minute; $P < 0.01$) but not in the fenoldopam group. No comparisons were made between groups. This decrease persisted for at least 8 hours after release of the cross-clamp. Plasma creatinine concentration increased significantly from baseline on the first day after surgery in the placebo group (87 ± 12 mmol/L to 103 ± 28 mmol/L; $P < 0.01$) but not in the fenoldopam group. However, this study is small and the clinical importance of the end point studied is unclear. The third RCT[37] randomised 45 people with chronic renal insufficiency (defined as creatinine level 2.0–5.0 mg/dL [176–440 μmol/L]) and having contrast angiography to hydration plus 0.1 μg/kg/minute fenoldopam mesylate or hydration with 0.45% sodium chloride. The primary end point was change in renal plasma flow 1 hour after contrast infusion. The secondary end point was incidence of contrast nephropathy**G**, defined as a 0.5 mg/dL (44 μmol/L) or a 25% rise in serum creatinine at 48 hours. Fenoldopam plus hydration significantly increased renal plasma flow 1 hour after angiography compared with hydration alone (+15.8% with fenoldopam plus hydration *v* –33.2% with hydration alone; $P < 0.05$). Fenoldopam also produced a non-significant reduction in contrast nephropathy. Renal plasma flow is a surrogate outcome. Drugs that have been shown to improve renal plasma flow may not improve clinical outcomes (e.g. dopamine). The fourth small RCT (160 people with serum creatinine > 1.5 mg/dL [132 μmol/L] having cardiac surgery with cardiopulmonary bypass) compared low dose fenoldopam (0.1–0.3 μg/kg/minute during cardiopulmonary bypass and in the early postoperative period) versus conventional care.[38] It found that fenoldopam significantly reduced mechanical ventilation time and stay in intensive care unit compared with usual care (ventilation time: 4.7 hours with fenoldopam *v* 6.5 hours with usual care; $P < 0.01$; intensive care unit stay: 1.8 days with fenoldopam *v* 2.4 days with usual care; $P < 0.01$). It did not directly compare effects on renal function between treatments but found that, postoperatively, serum creatinine and creatinine clearance significantly improved from baseline with fenoldopam and significantly deteriorated from baseline with usual care ($P < 0.001$ for reduction in serum creatinine from baseline with fenoldopam *v* $P < 0.02$ for increase in serum creatinine from baseline with usual care; creatinine clearance improved from 51.34 mL/minute preoperatively to 67.14 mL/minute postoperatively with fenoldopam; $P < 0.001$ *v* deteriorated from 50.3 mL/minute to 44.9 mL/minute with usual care; $P < 0.02$). The RCT was confounded by differences between groups, including hydration status and intra-operative haemodynamic instability.[38] The fifth and largest RCT (double blind, multicentre, 315 people with creatinine clearance < 60 mL/minute having invasive cardiovascular procedures) compared intravenous fenoldopam mesylate (0.05 μg/kg/minute titrated to 0.10 μg/kg/minute) versus placebo.[39] All people were hydrated and treatment started 1 hour before angiography and continued for 12 hours. The outcome of incidence of contrast nephropathy was, defined as an increase of 25% or more in serum creatinine level within 96 hours after the procedure. The RCT found no significant difference between fenoldopam and placebo for contrast nephropathy or 30 day rates of death, dialysis, or readmission to hospital (contrast nephropathy: 33.6% with fenoldopam *v* 30.1% with placebo; RR 1.11, 95% CI 0.79 to 1.57; $P = 0.61$; death: 2.0% with fenoldopam *v* 3.8% with placebo; $P = 0.50$; dialysis: 2.6% with fenoldopam *v* 1.9% with placebo; $P = 0.72$); readmission to hospital: 17.6% with fenoldopam *v* 19.9% with placebo; $P = 0.66$).[39]

Harms: Only two of the five RCTs reported data on potential harm from fenoldopam.[37,39] One RCT (45 people) found that fenoldopam significantly lowered the mean arterial pressure within 30 minutes of the infusion and for the entire 4 hour infusion after angiography compared with sodium chloride.[37] The largest RCT found that fenoldopam significantly decreased blood pressure (P = 0.001) and increased heart rate (P = 0.01) compared with placebo (results presented graphically).[39] It found that fenoldopam treatment had to be stopped more often than placebo, most commonly for mild hypotension or tachycardia. It found no significant difference for the combined adverse effects outcome of death, dialysis, myocardial infarction, or readmission to hospital (23.4% with fenoldopam *v* 23.1% with placebo; P > 0.99).

Comment: None.

OPTION NATRIURETIC PEPTIDES

One large RCT found no significant difference between natriuretic peptides and placebo in the prevention of acute renal failure induced by contrast media. Subgroup analysis in another large RCT found that atrial natriuretic peptide reduced dialysis free survival in non-oliguric people compared with placebo.

Benefits: We found no systematic review, but found one large RCT (247 people) comparing three doses of atrial natriuretic peptide (0.01, 0.05, and 0.10 μg/kg/minute) versus placebo for preventing acute renal failure induced by contrast media.[42] It found a similar incidence of acute renal failure between groups (23% with 0.01 μg/kg/minute anaritide *v* 23% with 0.05 μg/kg/minute anaritide *v* 25% with 0.10 μg/kg/minute anaritide *v* 19% with placebo).

Harms: We found one RCT (504 people with early acute renal failure).[43] It found that atrial natriuretic peptide reduced rates of dialysis free survival in a subgroup of people (378 non-oliguric people) compared with placebo (dialysis free survival: 88/183 [48%] with atrial natriuretic peptide *v* 116/195 [59%] with placebo; RR 1.24, 95% CI 1.02 to 1.50; NNH 8, 95% CI 4 to 36).

Comment: Natriuretic peptides (atrial natriuretic peptide and urodilatin) have also been evaluated in the treatment of acute renal failure (see benefits of natriuretic peptides, p 1088).

OPTION THEOPHYLLINE

One RCT in people with adequate hydration found that theophylline did not prevent contrast nephropathy compared with placebo. Three further RCTs, which did not report on the hydration status of participants, found mixed results. Two found that theophylline protected renal function compared with placebo and one found no significant difference. Another RCT found no significant reduction in renal impairment after elective coronary artery bypass surgery with theophylline compared with hydration alone but may have been underpowered to detect a clinically important difference.

Benefits: **Contrast nephropathy:** We found four RCTs.[44–47] Only one of these RCTs reported that participants were receiving adequate intravenous hydration.[47] This RCT (80 people with pre-existent mild to moderate renal insufficiency, with glomerular filtration rate**G** preserved with hydration alone) found no significant difference in serum creatinine concentration and creatinine clearance between theophylline or with placebo. Two people (5.7%) in the theophylline group and one (3.4%) in the placebo group developed acute renal failure, defined as an increase in serum creatinine of at least 0.5 mg/dL (44 μmol/L).[47] In the other three RCTs, the hydration status of people receiving the radiocontrast agent was unclear.[44–46] The first RCT (39 people receiving 100 mL of non-ionic low osmolar contrast medium) found that glomerular filtration rates were unchanged with a pretreatment dose of 5 mg/kg of intravenous theophylline (75 ± 26 mL/minute/1.72 m^2 *v* 78 ± 33 mL/minute/1.72 m^2) but decreased modestly without pretreatment (88 ± 40 mL/minute/1.72 m^2 *v* 75 ± 32 mL/minute/1.72 m^2; $P < 0.01$).[44] The second RCT (58 people receiving 40 mL of high osmolar contrast medium) found that pretreatment with 165 mg theophylline abolished the decline in glomerular filtration rates seen with placebo (107.5 ± 3.6 mL/minute *v* 85.4 ± 3.8 mL/minute; $P < 0.001$). In people receiving placebo, radiocontrast agent induced a significant increase in plasma creatinine compared with baseline values (88.1 ± 2.7 μmol/L *v* 113.4 ± 4.7 μmol/L; $P < 0.001$). Theophylline prevented this increase (89.2 ± 3.1 μmol/L *v* 89.3 ± 3.5 μmol/L).[45] The third RCT (100 people with serum creatinine concentrations of ≥ 1.3 mg/dL [114 μmol/L], about to have coronary angiography) compared theophylline 200 mg versus placebo (0.9% sodium chloride).[46] It found that theophylline significantly reduced contrast nephropathy Ⓖ compared with placebo (AR for contrast nephropathy: 2/50 [4%] with theophylline *v* 10/50 [20%] with placebo; $P = 0.0138$). **After coronary artery bypass grafting:** We found one RCT (56 people with normal renal function), which compared theophylline (a bolus of 4 mg/kg and a subsequent continuous infusion of 0.25 mg/kg/hour for up to 96 hours) versus 0.9% sodium chloride for prevention of renal impairment after elective coronary artery bypass surgery.[48] It found no significant difference between theophylline and sodium chloride in rates of renal impairment, but the RCT may have been underpowered to detect clinically important differences (renal impairment, defined as an increase in serum creatinine of ≥ 0.4 mg/dL (35 μmol/L) from the baseline at day 5 after surgery: 5/28 [18%] with theophylline *v* 4/28 [14%] with sodium chloride; $P > 0.05$).

Harms: Theophylline has a narrow therapeutic index and known adverse effects (see harms of theophyllines under chronic obstructive pulmonary disease, p 1923). Harms were not reported in the above RCTs.[44–47]

Comment: We found no evidence of benefit from the use of theophylline in the prevention of renal failure in any setting.

OPTION CALCIUM CHANNEL BLOCKERS

One RCT found no significant difference between isradipine and placebo in preventing early allograft dysfunction in people receiving cadaveric or living renal transplant. One systematic review limited to people with cadaveric renal transplant found limited evidence from heterogeneous RCTs that calcium channel blockers given in the peri-operative period reduced post-transplant acute tubular necrosis, although it found no significant effect on graft loss, need for haemodialysis, or mortality. We found no RCTs assessing the effects of calcium channel blockers in preventing other forms of acute renal failure. Calcium channel blockers are associated with hypotension and bradycardia.

Benefits: **In people receiving live or cadaveric kidney transplant:** We found one RCT, which compared isradipine versus placebo after living and cadaveric renal transplants.[49] The RCT (210 people) found that isradipine significantly improved median serum creatinine levels at 3 months compared with placebo at 3 and 12 months (3 months: 185 μmol/L with isradipine *v* 220 μmol/L with placebo; $P = 0.002$; 12 months: 141 μmol/L with isradipine *v* 158 μmol/L with placebo; $P = 0.021$). However, it found no significant difference in the incidence or duration of graft dysfunction (graft dysfunction: 34/98 [35%] with isradipine *v* 44/112 [39%] with placebo; RR 1.13, 95% CI 0.79 to 1.62; duration of dysfunction: 9.1 days with isradipine *v* 9.3 days with placebo). **In people receiving cadaveric kidney transplant:** We found one systematic review (search date 2003, 9 RCTs, 445 people), which compared calcium channel blockers versus no calcium channel blocker after cadaveric kidney transplantation.[50] It included heterogeneous RCTs, in which any calcium channel blocker was given by any route pre- or immediately post-transplant, to recipient or donor, or added to the perfusate (see comments below).[50] Duration of follow up, where stated, ranged from 4 weeks to 4 years. None of the included studies mentioned loses to follow up. It found that calcium channel blockers in the peri-transplant period significantly decreased acute tubular necrosis (7 RCTs, 349 people: RR 0.57, 95% CI 0.40 to 0.82). However, it found no significant difference between treatments for graft loss, mortality, or requirement for haemodialysis postoperatively (graft loss, 6 RCTs, 347 people: RR 0.93, 95% CI 0.44 to 1.97; mortality, 5 RCTs, 284 people: RR 0.86, 95% CI: 0.16 to 4.66; haemodialysis, 4 RCTs: quantitative results not reported).

Harms: The systematic review found insufficient information to comment on adverse effects.[50] However, as a class, calcium channel blockers are associated with hypotension and bradycardia, as well as several less serious adverse effects. The incidence and nature of adverse effects varies between individual drugs (see harms of antihypertensive drug treatment?).

Comment: The systematic review (search date 2003[50]) did not include the RCT[49] that looked at effect of isradipine on renal function after renal transplantation, because it included living donors. This RCT is the biggest multicentre RCT to date. Moreover, implications of the conclusion of this systematic review are unclear because the studies pooled were heterogeneous. The studies differed in terms of drug used (diltiazem, nifedipine, gallopamil), dose, route, timing, recipient (transplant recipient or donor), and immunosuppression used after the transplant.

OPTION ACETYLCYSTEINE

One systematic review found that N-acetylcysteine plus hydration reduced contrast nephropathy (defined by an increase in serum creatinine) compared with hydration alone in people with chronic renal insufficiency who were having radiocontrast imaging studies. However, N-acetylcysteine may reduce serum creatinine independently of any effect on renal function, so conclusions about clinical efficacy should be interpreted with caution.

Benefits: We found one systematic review (search date 2003, 7 RCTs, 805 people with chronic renal insufficiency, proportion of diabetics 21–64%).[51] It compared N-acetylcysteine plus hydration versus hydration alone in people having radiocontrast imaging studies.[51] It found that acetylcysteine plus hydration significantly reduced contrast nephropathy**G** compared with hydration alone (RR 0.44, 95% CI 0.22 to 0.88). Significant statistical heterogeneity was found among studies. Four of the included RCTs found that acetylcysteine plus hydration significantly reduced contrast nephropathy compared with hydration alone, and the other three RCTs found no significant difference. The overall incidence of contrast nephropathy varied between 2% and 26% with acetylcysteine compared with 11% to 45% with control.

Harms: The systematic review did not report on harms of N-acetylcysteine.[51] However, N-acetylcysteine has been widely used to treat people with paracetamol (acetaminophen) overdose, and has virtually no toxicity at therapeutic levels (see harms of paracetamol poisoning, p 1758).

Comment: The primary outcome assessed in the RCTs included in the systematic review was contrast nephropathy**G** at 48 hours (defined as an increase in serum creatinine of 0.5 mg/dL [44 μmol/L] or > 25% from baseline after 48 hours).[51] The timing and dose of administration of N-acetylcysteine differed widely among included RCTs. One cohort study (50 healthy volunteers with normal renal function) found that N-acetylcysteine could independently decrease serum creatinine without any effect on glomerular filtration rate**G**.[52] The role of N-acetylcysteine to prevent acute renal failure therefore remains unclear.

OPTION SINGLE DOSE AMINOGLYCOSIDES

One systematic review and one additional RCT compared single and multiple doses of aminoglycosides and found different results for nephrotoxicity. The systematic review, in people with fever and neutropenia receiving antibiotic treatment including aminoglycosides, found no significant difference in cure rates or nephrotoxicity between once daily compared with three times daily administration of the aminoglycoside. However, the RCT found that single doses of aminoglycosides reduced nephrotoxicity compared with multiple doses in people with fever and receiving antibiotic treatment including an aminoglycoside.

Benefits: We found one systematic review[53] and one additional RCT.[54] The systematic review (search date 1995, 4 RCTs, 803 people with fever and neutropenia, not limited to people in intensive care units) found no significant difference between single and multiple doses of aminoglycosides in antimicrobial efficacy, clinical cure rates, and nephrotoxicity**G** (antimicrobial efficacy, 2 RCTs, 57 people: RR 1.00, 95% CI 0.86 to 1.16; clinical cure, 4 RCTs, 961 episodes: RR 0.97, 95% CI 0.91 to 1.05; nephrotoxicity, defined as increase in serum creatinine by > 35–45 μmol/L [about 0.5 mg/dL], 3 RCTs, 718 episodes: RR 0.78, 95% CI 0.31 to 1.94; see comment below).[53] The additional RCT (85 people with fever) compared a once daily dose of gentamicin versus three times daily doses of gentamicin.[54] It found that single dosing significantly reduced nephrotoxicity compared with multiple dosing (2/40 [5%] with single dosing *v* 11/45 [24%] with multiple dosing; RR 0.21, 95% CI 0.05 to 0.87; NNT 5, 95% CI 2 to 24).[54] Nephrotoxicity was defined as an increase in serum creatinine of 0.5 mg/dL (45 μmol/L) or more.

Harms: The review found no evidence of greater harm from once daily aminoglycoside dosing (see RR of nephrotoxicity**G** in benefits section above).[53]

Comment: The systematic review defined clinical cure according to the definitions used by investigators in the primary studies, which may have varied among studies.[53] The risk from aminoglycosides is highest in people with volume depletion; underlying renal, cardiac, or hepatic disease; or when combined with diuretics or other nephrotoxic agents**G**. Two studies included in the systematic review randomised episodes of infection, allowing for people to be included in more than one option in the study.[55]

OPTION LIPID FORMULATIONS OF AMPHOTERICIN B

We found no RCTs. Lipid formulations of amphotericin B seem to cause less nephrotoxicity compared with standard formulations, but direct comparisons of long term safety are lacking.

Benefits: We found no systematic review and no RCTs.

Harms: We found no evidence of greater harms from lipid formulations of amphotericin BⒼ. However, these formulations are still nephrotoxic and should be used with care.

Comment: A phase II trial of a lipid formulations of amphotericin BⒼ (556 people) found an incidence of renal toxicity (defined by any increase in serum creatinine) of 24% (*v* 60–80% with standard formulation of amphotericin B). People with baseline serum creatinine in excess of 2.5 mg/dL (221 μmol/L) on standard amphotericin B showed a significant decrease in serum creatinine when transferred to the lipid formulation ($P < 0.001$).[56] One trial found that simply infusing amphotericin B in a lipid solution designed for parenteral nutrition did not result in any benefit and may be associated with pulmonary adverse effects.[57] Fluid loading can be useful in reducing the risk of acute renal failure from all nephrotoxins. Considerable variability may exist between individual lipid formulations of amphotericin B in terms of efficacy and safety.

OPTION LOW OSMOLALITY CONTRAST MEDIA

One systematic review found that low osmolality contrast media reduced nephrotoxicity in people with underlying renal failure needing contrast investigation compared with standard osmolality contrast media. One subsequent RCT found that non-ionic iso-osmolar contrast medium (iodixanol) reduced contrast media induced nephropathy compared with low osmolar non-ionic contrast medium (iohexol) in people with diabetes.

Benefits: We found one systematic review (search date 1991, 31 RCTs, 5146 people)[55] comparing low osmolality contrast mediaⒼ versus standard contrast media and one subsequent RCT[58] that compared iso-osmolar contrast mediaⒼ versus low osmolar contrast media. The systematic review found no significant difference between low osmolality and standard contrast media in the development of acute renal failure or need for dialysis (these are rare events), but there was less nephrotoxicityⒼ with low osmolality contrast media, measured by serum creatinine. Subgroup analysis found that low osmolality contrast media significantly reduced the proportion of people with a rise in serum creatinine of 44 μg/L or more compared with standard contrast media in people with underlying renal failure. It found no significant difference between treatments for people without prior renal failure (prior underlying renal impairment, 8 RCTs, 1418 people: OR 0.50, 95% CI 0.36 to 0.68; no underlying renal impairment: 20 RCTs, 2865 people: OR 0.75, 95% CI 0.52 to 1.10). The subsequent RCT (129 people with diabetes mellitus treated with insulin or antidiabetic drugs and serum creatinine concentrations of 1.5–3.5 mg/dL [132–308 μmol/L]) compared non-ionic iso-osmolar contrast media (iodixanol) versus low osmolar (iohexol) contrast media in people having coronary or aortofemoral angiography.[58] It found that iso-osmolar contrast medium significantly reduced contrast medium induced nephropathy compared with low osmolar contrast medium (nephropathy, defined as an increase in serum creatinine > 0.5 mg/dL [44 μmol/L]: 2/64 [3%] with iso-osmolar contrast medium *v* 17/56 [26%] with low osmolar contrast medium; OR 0.09, 95% CI 0.02 to 0.40; see comment below). In the RCT, although both treatment groups received similar volumes of contrast media, both the volume of contrast media and the hydration regimens were not standardised.

Harms: The subsequent RCT found that iso-osmolar contrast medium reduced adverse events compared with low osmolar contrast media (13/67 [19%] with iso-osmolar contrast mediaⒼ *v* 29/67 [43%] with low osmolar contrast media; P value not reported).[58]

Comment: Acute renal failure induced by contrast media usually occurs in people with diabetic nephropathy (incidence nearly 50%, varies with the degree of baseline renal function). In the RCT comparing iso-osmolar versus low osmolar contrast media, the incidence of nephropathy with low osmolar contrast media (26%) was exceptionally high.[58]

QUESTION **What are the effects of treatments for critically ill people with acute renal failure?**

OPTION **CONTINUOUS RENAL REPLACEMENT THERAPY**

One systematic review found no significant difference between continuous and intermittent renal replacement therapy in mortality, renal death, or dialysis dependence in critically ill adults with acute renal failure.

Benefits: We found one systematic review (search date 2002, 6 RCTs, 624 critically ill adults with acute renal failure).[59] The systematic review compared continuous with intermittent renal haemodialysis. It found no significant difference between continuous and intermittent renal replacement therapy**G** in mortality, renal death, or dialysis dependence among survivors (mortality: RR 0.96, 95% CI 0.85 to 1.08; renal death: RR 1.02, 95% CI 0.89 to 1.17; dialysis dependence: RR 1.19, 95% CI 0.62 to 2.27).

Harms: Harms were not reported in the systematic review.[59] Heparin is often used with intermittent and continuous renal replacement therapy**G**, and may have adverse effects (see thromboembolism, p 194).[60] Hypotension is common with intermittent haemodialysis, whereas haemodynamic stability is better preserved with continuous renal replacement therapy.[61]

Comment: The evidence from the systematic review is insufficient to draw conclusions regarding the preferred mode of renal replacement for critically ill people with acute renal failure.[59] A prospective multicentre survey (587 people in 28 intensive care units) found no significant difference in survival between continuous and intermittent renal replacement therapy**G**.[62] Similarly, one RCT (1846 people with chronic rather than acute renal failure receiving chronic treatment with three times weekly sessions) found no survival benefit from increasing the dose of dialysis or from using a high flux membrane.[63] However, we found one earlier systematic review (search date 1998, 13 studies, 3 RCTs, 1400 critically ill people with acute renal failure),[64] which performed subgroup analysis, adjusting by baseline severity of illness, and found a survival benefit with continuous renal replacement therapy (mortality: RR 0.48, 95% CI 0.34 to 0.69). A secondary analysis in the review, including all studies and adjusting for study quality, found that continuous modalities significantly reduced mortality (RR 0.72, 95% CI 0.60 to 0.87).[64]

OPTION **HIGH DOSE CONTINUOUS RENAL REPLACEMENT THERAPY**

One RCT found that high dose continuous renal replacement therapy (haemofiltration) reduced mortality compared with low dose continuous therapy. A small prospective study found that intensive (daily) intermittent haemodialysis reduced mortality in people with acute renal failure compared with conventional alternate day haemodialysis. A subsequent small three arm RCT found no significant difference in survival at 28 days between early, low dose haemofiltration; early, high dose haemofiltration; and late, low dose haemofiltration.

Benefits: We found no systematic review but found two RCTs.[65,66] The first RCT (425 people) compared three doses of continuous replacement renal therapy (20, 35, and 45 mL/kg/hour of haemofiltration in postdilution).[65] Mortality was similar for the two high dose arms (60/139 [43%] with 35 mL/kg/hour *v* 59/140 [42%] with 45 mL/kg/hour), but was significantly higher in the low dose arm (86/146 [59%] with 20 mL/kg/hour). Survival time analysis was adjusted for three way comparison (combined RR 1.38, 95% CI 1.14 to 1.67; NNT 7, 95% CI 4 to 16). The second, three arm RCT (106 severely ill people with oliguric acute renal failure recruited from 2 different centres) compared early, high dose haemofiltration (72–96 L/day); early, low dose haemofiltration (24–36 L/day); or late, low dose haemofiltration (24–36 L/day).[66] It found no significant difference in survival at 28 days between groups, but the study had low power to detect differences. Haemofiltration was started at a mean of 7 hours after inclusion in the "early" groups and 42 hours after inclusion in the "late" group. No significant differences were found in survival at day 28 (26/35 [74%] with early, high dose *v* 24/35 [69%] with early, low dose *v* 27/37 [73%] with late, low dose; $P > 0.05$ for two way and three way comparisons).

Harms: We found no evidence that the higher dialysis dose was associated with increased adverse effects (such as haemodynamic instability, intolerance, or bleeding). In a prospective study on daily intermittent haemodialysis,[67] there was no evidence of increased morbidity compared with alternate day dialysis. In particular, hypotension was less common with daily treatment. No data on harms were found in the above RCTs.[65,66]

Comment: There is no standard method to compare dialysis dosage between continuous and intermittent renal replacement therapies**G**, but urea kinetic modelling predicts that the doses used in this study would be impossible to achieve without continuous renal replacement therapy.[68] In addition, the underlying mechanisms for solute removal are different, based on the type of treatment applied (convection with haemofiltration compared with diffusion with haemodialysis). This makes comparisons of elimination of diverse solutes difficult. However, a recent, small, prospective study (160 people) found that a higher dose of dialysis delivered as daily intermittent haemodialysis compared with alternate day haemodialysis sessions is associated with improved survival in people with acute renal failure (RR 0.59, 95% CI 0.39 to 91).[67] Although this study may have had low power to detect important differences and did not deliver the prescribed dialysis dose, it does support the concept that a dose–response relationship exists for dialysis in acute renal failure, and suggests that the traditional, end stage renal disease based dose recommendation may be too low.

OPTION SYNTHETIC DIALYSIS MEMBRANES

Two systematic reviews provided inconclusive evidence of the effects of synthetic membranes on mortality in critically ill people with acute renal failure compared with cellulose based membranes.

Benefits: We found two systematic reviews comparing synthetic and cellulose based**G** dialysis membranes in critically ill people with all cause acute renal failure.[69,70] The first systematic review (search date 2000, 7 RCTs and controlled clinical trials, 722 people) found no significant difference between synthetic membranes and cellulose based membranes in mortality among people with acute renal failure requiring in-centre haemodialysis. (RR 0.92, 95% CI 0.76 to 1.13).[69] Subgroup analysis revealed that synthetic membranes fared best against unsubstituted cellulose (RR 0.82, 95% CI 0.62 to 1.08), although the result was still not significant.[71] The second systematic review (search date 2000, 8 prospective trials providing survival data, data on recovery of renal function, or both, 867 people) found that synthetic membranes significantly increased survival rates (OR 1.37, 95% CI 1.02 to 1.83; P = 0.03) and showed a non-significant trend toward improved renal recovery (OR 1.23, 95% CI 0.90 to 1.68; P = 0.18).[70] A sensitivity analysis performed by stratifying studies according to the type of membrane used in the control group found that the mortality reduction observed with synthetic membranes was evident when compared with unsubstituted cellulose, but not when compared with modified cellulose.

Harms: Severe anaphylactoid reactions in people taking angiotensin converting enzyme inhibitors have been reported occasionally with certain synthetic biocompatible❻ membranes (exact frequency unknown).[71]

Comment: Many of the RCTs included in both systematic reviews had methodological limitations, and all studies were underpowered. Differences in effect on outcomes seem most easily demonstrable when synthetic membranes are compared with unsubstituted cellulose. Whether synthetic membranes are superior to modified cellulose (e.g. cellulose triacetate) remains controversial. However, no study has shown an advantage with any cellulose based❻ membrane over synthetic membranes, except that the former are generally less expensive.

OPTION DOPAMINE

One systematic review found no significant difference in mortality or need for dialysis between dopamine and placebo. One additional RCT found that low dose dopamine did not reduce renal dysfunction compared with placebo. Dopamine has been associated with important adverse effects, including extravasation necrosis, gangrene, and conduction abnormalities.

Benefits: We found one systematic review[31] and one additional RCT.[33] The systematic review (search date 1999, 58 trials, of which 17 were RCTs, 2149 people) found no significant difference between dopamine and placebo in mortality or need for dialysis (mortality, 11 trials, 508 people: 4.7% with dopamine *v* 5.6% with placebo; RR 0.83, 95% CI 0.39 to 1.77; need for dialysis, 10 trials, 618 people: 13.9% with dopamine *v* 16.5% with placebo; RR 0.89, 95% CI 0.66 to 1.21).[31] The additional RCT (multicentre, double blind, placebo controlled, 328 people with early renal dysfunction❻ defined as oliguria❻ or increase in serum creatinine) found no significant difference between low dose dopamine and placebo in mortality at discharge (69/161 [43%] with dopamine *v* 66/163 [41%] with placebo; RR 1.06, 95% CI 0.82 to 1.37).[33]

Harms: Dopamine has recognised adverse effects, including extravasation necrosis, gangrene, tachycardia, headache, and conduction abnormalities. The systematic review and the RCT reported no data on harms.[31,33]

Comment: Studies using dopamine to prevent renal failure or to ameliorate progression have found no benefit (see prevention of acute renal failure, p 1074). Studies evaluating the effectiveness of dopamine for the treatment of acute renal failure have focused on early renal dysfunction❻ and have often included people with normal renal function who were at risk of acute renal failure. The distinction between effects of dopamine for prevention and for treatment is, therefore, blurred, and we have used the same studies to infer preventative and treatment effects.

OPTION **LOOP DIURETICS**

Underpowered RCTs in people with oliguric renal failure found no significant difference between loop diuretics and placebo on renal recovery, the number of days spent on dialysis, or mortality. Loop diuretics have been associated with toxicity and low renal perfusion.

Benefits: We found no systematic review. We found two RCTs (66[72] and 58[73] people, some in intensive care units, proportion unknown) comparing intravenous furosemide versus placebo in people with oliguric acute renal failure of various causes. In the second RCT, all people received one dose of furosemide 1 g and were then randomised to continued treatment or placebo. Neither RCT found significant differences in renal recovery (first RCT: 19/33 [58%] with furosemide *v* 22/33 [67%] with placebo; RR 0.86, 95% CI 0.50 to 1.20;[72] second RCT: 10/28 [36%] with furosemide *v* 12/28 [43%] with placebo; RR 0.83, 95% CI 0.37 to 1.45)[73] or mortality. The RCTs lacked power to exclude a clinically important effect of loop diuretics on these outcomes.

Harms: Ototoxicity can occur with high doses of loop diuretics. No adverse effects were reported in the first RCT.[72] Deafness occurred in two people in the second RCT; both were randomised to furosemide. Hearing loss was permanent in one of these people.[73] Diuretics may reduce renal perfusion and add a prerenal component to the renal failure, but the frequency of this event is uncertain.[74] See harms of loop diuretics to prevent acute renal failure in people at high risk, p 1075.

Comment: None.

OPTION **CONTINUOUS INFUSION OF LOOP DIURETICS**

We found no RCTs comparing continuous infusion versus bolus injection of loop diuretics in critically ill people with acute renal failure.

Benefits: We found no systematic review and no RCTs comparing continuous infusion versus bolus injection of loop diuretics in critically ill people with acute renal failure.

Harms: One small crossover RCT (8 people with acute deterioration of chronic renal failure, mean creatinine clearance 0.28 mL/second) found that fewer people experienced myalgia when treated with continuous infusion than with bolus dosing of bumetanide (3/8 [38%] people with bolus dosing *v* 0/8 [0%] people with continuous infusion).[75]

Comment: The small crossover trial found that continuous infusion resulted in a net increase in sodium excretion over 24 hours (mean increase in sodium excretion 48 mmol/day, 95% CI 16 mmol/day to 60 mmol/day; $P = 0.01$).[75]

OPTION **INTRAVENOUS ALBUMIN SUPPLEMENTATION PLUS LOOP DIURETICS**

We found no RCTs on the effects of intravenous albumin supplementation plus loop diuretics in people with acute renal failure.

Benefits: We found no systematic review and no RCTs evaluating clinical outcomes in critically ill people with acute renal failure.

Harms: We found no RCTs in people with acute renal failure.

Comment: One systematic review (search date 2002, 30 RCTs, 1419 people, most without acute renal failure) found that albumin increased the risk of death in unselected critically ill people (mortality: 98/704 [14%] with albumin *v* 58/715 [8%] with control; RR 1.68, CI 1.26 to 2.23). All of the included trials were small and combined highly heterogeneous populations.[76] One crossover RCT (9 people with nephrotic syndrome) compared three interventions: furosemide alone, furosemide plus albumin, and albumin alone.[77] It found that furosemide was superior to albumin alone, and furosemide plus albumin resulted in the greatest urine and sodium excretion. The clinical significance of this finding is unclear.

OPTION NATRIURETIC PEPTIDES

RCTs found no significant difference between atrial natriuretic peptide, ularitide (urodilatin), and placebo in dialysis free survival in oliguric and non-oliguric people with acute renal failure. One of the RCTs found that atrial natriuretic peptide may reduce survival in non-oliguric people.

Benefits: We found no systematic review but found three RCTs.[43,78,79] One RCT (504 people) found no overall difference in dialysis free survival with atrial natriuretic peptide compared with placebo in people with acute renal failure.[43] Preplanned subgroup analysis suggested a possible benefit to people with oliguria**G**, and lower survival rates in non-oliguric people. However, one RCT (220 people)[78] in people with oliguric acute renal failure found no improvement in dialysis free survival with a 24 hour infusion of atrial natriuretic peptide compared with placebo. A third RCT compared ularitide ([urodilatin], a natriuretic peptide with fewer systemic haemodynamic effects) in a dose finding (5, 20, 40, or 80 ng/kg/minute ularitide), placebo controlled RCT (176 people). Ularitide did not reduce the requirement for dialysis (people who needed dialysis: 35% with 5 ng/kg/minute ularitide *v* 36% with 20 ng/kg/minute ularitide *v* 28% with 40 ng/kg/minute ularitide *v* 41% with 80 ng/kg/minute ularitide *v* 36% with placebo; P reported as non-significant, CI not reported).[79]

Harms: One RCT found that natriuretic peptide caused significant hypotension compared with placebo (95% with natriuretic peptide *v* 55% with placebo; $P < 0.01$). Also, atrial natriuretic peptide may be associated with a worse outcome in people with non-oliguric renal failure (dialysis free survival in 378 non-oliguric people was 48% with anaritide *v* 59% with placebo; $P = 0.03$).[78] See harms of natriuretic peptides, p 1079.

Comment: We found no evidence of significant improvement of acute renal failure with atrial natriuretic peptide.

GLOSSARY

Biocompatible Artificial materials can induce an inflammatory response. This response can be humoral (including complement) or cellular. Synthetic dialysis membranes seem to produce less of an inflammatory response *in vitro* and are classified as more "biocompatible". By contrast, cellulose based membranes (see below) seem to be less biocompatible (cause more inflammation). When cellulose based membranes are rendered semisynthetic by modifications or substitution of materials like acetate, they may be become more biocompatible. We found no standards by which this comparison can be made.

Cellulose based Dialysis membranes may be made from cellulose. "Unsubstituted" cellulose has not undergone modification to attempt to improve biocompatibility. Synthetic membranes do not use cellulose.

Continuous renal replacement therapy Any extracorporeal blood purification treatment intended to substitute for impaired renal function over an extended period of time and applied for, or aimed at being applied for, 24 hours a day.

Contrast nephropathy Intravenous radiocontrast increases serum creatinine in some people, particularly those with underlying kidney disease. Most studies define contrast nephropathy as a small change in serum creatinine (e.g. > 25% increase). It is not known whether agents that reduce the risk of contrast nephropathy also reduce the risk of acute renal failure.
Early allograft dysfunction Renal dysfunction that occurs after renal transplantation, and which is usually secondary to ischaemic injury.
Early renal dysfunction An acute derangement in renal function that is still evolving.
Glomerular filtration rate The rate of elaboration of protein free plasma filtrate (ultrafiltration) across the walls of the glomerular capillaries.
Intermittent renal replacement therapy Renal support that is not, nor intended to be, continuous; usually prescribed for a period of 12 hours or less.
Iso-osmolar contrast media Contrast media that are iso-osmolar compared with plasma, and therefore of lower osmolality than "low osmolality contrast media" (see below).
Lipid formulations of amphotericin B Complexes of amphotericin B and phospholipids or sterols. This reduces the toxicity of amphotericin B while preserving its antifungal activity.
Low osmolality contrast media Contrast media with osmolality between 600–800 mOsm/L.
Multiple organ dysfunction syndrome A syndrome of progressive organ failure, affecting one organ after another and believed to be the result of persistent or recurrent infection or inflammation.
Nephrotoxic agents Any agent that has the potential to produce nephrotoxicity.
Nephrotoxicity Renal parenchymal damage manifested by a decline in glomerular filtration rate, tubular dysfunction, or both.
Oliguria Urine output of less than 5 mL/kg daily.

REFERENCES

1. Nissenson AR. Acute renal failure: definition and pathogenesis. *Kidney Int Suppl* 1998;66:7–10.
2. Bellomo R, Ronco C, Kellum JA, et al. Acute renal failure – definition, outcome measures, animal models, fluid therapy and information technology needs: the Second International Consensus Conference of the Acute Dialysis Quality Initiative (ADQI) Group. *Crit Care* 2004;8:R204–R212.
3. Hou SH, Bushinsky DA, Wish JB, et al. Hospital-acquired renal insufficiency: a prospective study. *Am J Med* 1983;74:243–248.
4. Brivet FG, Kleinknecht DJ, Loirat P, et al. Acute renal failure in intensive care units — causes, outcomes and prognostic factors of hospital mortality: a prospective multicenter study. *Crit Care Med* 1996;24:192–198.
5. McCullough PA, Wolyn R, Rocher LL, et al. Acute renal failure after coronary intervention: incidence, risk factors, and relationship to mortality. *Am J Med* 1997;103:368–375.
6. Better OS, Stein JH. Early management of shock and prophylaxis of acute renal failure in traumatic rhabdomyolysis. *N Engl J Med* 1990;322:825–829.
7. Thadhani R, Pascual M, Bonventre JV. Acute renal failure. *N Engl J Med* 1996;334:1448–1460.
8. Kleinknecht D. Epidemiology in acute renal failure in France today. In: Biari D, Neild G, eds. *Acute renal failure in intensive therapy unit*. Berlin: Springer-Verlag, 1990:13–21.
9. Tran DD, Oe PL, De Fijter CWH, et al. Acute renal failure in patients with acute pancreatitis: prevalence, risk factors, and outcome. *Nephrol Dial Transplant* 1993;8:1079–1084.
10. Coar D. Obstructive nephropathy. *Del Med J* 1991;63:743–749.
11. Kaufman J, Dhakal M, Patel B, et al. Community acquired acute renal failure. *Am J Kidney Dis* 1991;17:191–198.
12. Bamgboye EL, Mabayoje MO, Odutala TA, et al. Acute renal failure at the Lagos University Teaching Hospital. *Ren Fail* 1993;15:77–80.
13. Nolan CR, Anderson RJ. Hospital-acquired acute renal failure. *J Am Soc Nephrol* 1998;9:710–718.
14. Cantarovich F, Bodin L. Functional acute renal failure. In: Cantarovich F, Rangoonwala B, Verho M, eds. *Progress in acute renal failure*. Paris: Hoechst Marion Roussel, 1998:55–65.
15. Brezis M, Rosen S. Hypoxia of the renal medulla. Its implication for disease. *N Engl J Med* 1995;332:647–655.
16. Bonventre JV. Mechanisms of ischemic acute renal failure. *Kidney Int* 1993;43:1160–1178.
17. Turney JH, Marshall DH, Brownjohn AM, et al. The evolution of acute renal failure, 1956–1988. *Q J Med* 1990;74:83–104.
18. Liano F, Junco E, Pascual J, et al. The spectrum of acute renal failure in the intensive care unit compared to that seen in other settings. The Madrid Acute Renal Failure Study Group. *Kidney Int Suppl* 1998;53:16–24.
19. Metnitz PG, Krenn CG, Steltzer H, et al. Effect of acute renal failure requiring renal replacement therapy on outcome in critically ill patients. *Crit Care Med* 2002;30:2051–2058.
20. Trivedi HS, Moore H, Nasr S, et al. A randomized prospective trial to assess the role of saline hydration on the development of contrast nephrotoxicity. *Nephron Clin Pract* 2003;93:C29–C34.
21. Solomon R, Werner C, Mann D, et al. Effects of saline, mannitol, and furosemide to prevent acute decreases in renal function induced by radiocontrast agents. *N Engl J Med* 1994;331:1416–1420.
22. Mueller C, Buerkle G, Buettner HJ, et al. Prevention of contrast media-associated nephropathy: randomized comparison of 2 hydration regimes in 1620 patients undergoing coronary angioplasty. *Arch Intern Med* 2002;162:329–336.
23. Taylor AJ, Hotchkiss D, Morse RW, et al. Preparation for angiography in renal dysfunction: a randomized trial of inpatient versus outpatient hydration protocols for cardiac catheterization in mild-to-moderate renal dysfunction. *Chest* 1998;114:1570–1574.
24. Kellum JA. The use of diuretics and dopamine in acute renal failure: a systematic review of the

evidence. *Crit Care* 1997;1:53–59. Search date 1997; primary sources Medline and hand searches of bibliographies of relevant articles.
25. Lassnigg A, Donner E, Grubhofer G, et al. Lack of renoprotective effects of dopamine and furosemide during cardiac surgery. *J Am Soc Nephrol* 2000;11:97–104.
26. Hager B, Betschart M, Krapf R. Effect of postoperative intravenous loop diuretic on renal function after major surgery. *Schweiz Med Wochenschr* 1996;126:666–673.
27. Ip-Yam PC, Murphy S, Baines M, et al. Renal function and proteinuria after cardiopulmonary bypass: the effects of temperature and mannitol. *Anesth Analg* 1994;78:842–847.
28. Homsi E, Barreiro MF, Orlando JM, et al. Prophylaxis of acute renal failure in patients with rhabdomyolysis. *Ren Fail* 1997;19:283–288.
29. Beall AC, Holman MR, Morris GC, et al. Mannitol-induced osmotic diuresis during vascular surgery. *Arch Surg* 1963;86:34–42.
30. Gubern JM, Sancho JJ, Simo J, et al. A randomized trial on the effect of mannitol on postoperative renal function in patients with obstructive jaundice. *Surgery* 1988;103:39–44.
31. Kellum JA, Decker JM. The use of dopamine in acute renal failure: a meta-analysis. *Crit Care Med* 2001;29:1526–1531. Search date 1999; primary sources Medline and bibliographies of review articles.
32. Marik PE. Low dose dopamine: a systematic review. *Intensive Care Med* 2002;28:877–883. Search date 2000; primary sources Medline and hand searches of bibliographies of relevant articles and reviews.
33. Bellomo R, Chapman M, Finfer S, et al. Low-dose dopamine in patients with early renal dysfunction: a placebo-controlled randomised trial. Australian and New Zealand Intensive Care Society (ANZICS) Clinical Trials Group. *Lancet* 2000;356:2139–2143.
34. Yavuz S, Ayabakan N, Goncu MT, et al. Effect of combined dopamine and diltiazem on renal function after cardiac surgery. *Med Sci Monit* 2002;8:PI45–PI50.
35. Halpenny M, Lakshmi S, O'Donnell A, et al. Fenoldopam: renal and splanchnic effects in patients undergoing coronary artery bypass grafting. *Anaesthesia* 2001;56:953–960.
36. Halpenny M, Rushe C, Breen P, et al. The effects of fenoldopam on renal function in patients undergoing elective aortic surgery. *Eur J Anaesthesiol* 2002;19:32–39.
37. Tumlin JA, Wang A, Murray PT, et al. Fenoldopam mesylate blocks reductions in renal plasma flow after radiocontrast dye infusion: a pilot trial in the prevention of contrast nephropathy. *Am Heart J* 2002;143:894–903.
38. Caimmi PP, Pagani L, Micalizzi E, et al. Fenoldopam for renal protection in patients undergoing cardiopulmonary bypass. *J Cardiothorac Vasc Anesth* 2003;17:491–494.
39. Stone GW, McCullough PA, Tumlin JA, et al. Fenoldopam mesylate for the prevention of contrast-induced nephropathy: a randomized controlled trial. *JAMA* 2003;290:2284–2291.
40. Chu VL, Cheng GW. Fenoldopam in the prevention of contrast media-induced acute renal failure. *Ann Pharmacother* 2001;35:1278–1282. Search date 2000; primary source Medline.
41. Mathur VS, Swan SK, Lambrecht LJ, et al. The effects of fenoldopam, a selective dopamine receptor agonist, on systemic and renal hemodynamics in normotensive subjects. *Crit Care Med* 1999;27:1832–1837.
42. Kurnik BR, Allgren RL, Genter FC, et al. Prospective study of atrial natriuretic peptide for the prevention of radiocontrast-induced nephropathy. *Am J Kidney Dis* 1998;31:674–680.
43. Allgren RL, Marbury TC, Rahman SN, et al. Anaritide in ATN. Auriculin anaritide ARF study group. *N Engl J Med* 1997;336:828–834.
44. Erley CM, Duda SH, Schlepckow S, et al. Adenosine antagonist theophylline prevents the reduction of glomerular filtration rate after contrast media application. *Kidney Int* 1994;45:1425–1431.
45. Kolonko A, Wiecek A, Kokot F. The nonselective adenosine antagonist theophylline does prevent renal dysfunction induced by radiographic contrast agents. *J Nephrol* 1998;11:151–156.
46. Huber W, Schipek C, Ilgmann K, et al. Effectiveness of theophylline prophylaxis of renal impairment after coronary angiography in patients with chronic renal insufficiency. *Am J Cardiol* 2003 15;91:1157–1162.
47. Erley CM, Duda SH, Rehfuss D, et al. Prevention of radiocontrast-media-induced nephropathy in patients with pre-existing renal insufficiency by hydration in combination with the adenosine antagonist theophylline. *Nephrol Dial Transplant* 1999;14:1146–1149.
48. Kramer BK, Preuner J, Ebenburger A, et al. Lack of renoprotective effect of theophylline during aortocoronary bypass surgery. *Nephrol Dial Transplant* 2002;17:910–915.
49. Van Riemsdijk IC, Mulder PG, De Fijter JW, et al. Addition of isradipine (lomir) results in a better renal function after kidney transplantation: a double-blind, randomized, placebo-controlled, multi-center study. *Transplantation* 2000;70:122–126.
50. Shilliday IR, Sherif M. Calcium channel blockers for preventing acute tubular necrosis in kidney transplant recipients. *The Cochrane Database Syst Rev* 2004; Issue 1.
51. Birck R, Krzossok S, Markowetz F, et al. Acetylcysteine for prevention of contrast nephropathy: meta-analysis. *Lancet* 2003; 362:598–603. Search date 2003; primary sources Medline, Web of Science, Cochrane Library, Current Contents Medizin, Pubmed, proceedings from major cardiology and nephrology meetings, and reference lists.
52. Hoffmann U, Fischereder M, Kruger B, et al. The value of N-acetylcysteine in the prevention of radiocontrast agent-induced nephropathy seems questionable. *J Am Soc Nephrol* 2004;15:407–410.
53. Hatala R, Dinh TT, Cook DJ. Single daily dosing of aminoglycosides in immunocompromised adults: a systematic review. *Clin Infect Dis* 1997;24:810–815. Search date 1995; primary sources Medline, hand searches of selected infectious diseases journals and bibliographies of relevant articles, and personal contact with primary investigators of selected studies.
54. Prins JM, Buller HR, Kuijper EJ, et al. Once versus thrice daily gentamicin in patients with serious infections. *Lancet* 1993;341:335–339.
55. Barrett BJ, Carlisle EJ. Metaanalysis of the relative nephrotoxicity of high- and low-osmolality iodinated contrast media. *Radiology* 1993;188:171–178. Search date 1991; primary sources Medline, Embase, hand searches of reference lists of selected articles, and personal contact with authors of selected primary studies and pharmaceutical companies manufacturing contrast media.
56. Walsh TJ, Hiemenz JW, Seibel NL, et al. Amphotericin B lipid complex for invasive fungal infections: analysis of safety and efficacy in 556 cases. *Clin Infect Dis* 1998;26:383–396.
57. Schoffski P, Freund M, Wunder R, et al. Safety and toxicity of amphotericin B in glucose 5% or intralipid 20% in neutropenic patients with pneumonia or fever of unknown origin: randomised study. *BMJ* 1998;317:379–384.
58. Aspelin P, Aubry P, Fransson SG, et al. Nephrotoxic effects in high-risk patients undergoing angiography. *N Engl J Med* 2003;348:491–499.
59. Tonelli M, Manns B, Feller-Kopman D. Acute renal failure in the intensive care unit: a systematic review of the impact of dialytic modality on mortality and renal recovery. *Am J Kidney Dis* 2002;40:875–885. Search date 2002; primary sources Medline, the Cochrane Library, DARE, abstracts of the major North American nephrology meetings, Science Citation Index, four major nephrology journals, three major critical care journals, and reference lists from identified studies and reviews articles.

60. Ronco C. Continuous renal replacement therapies for the treatment of acute renal failure in intensive care patients. *Clin Nephrol* 1993;40:187–198.
61. Heering P, Morgera S, Schmitz FJ, et al. Cytokine removal and cardiovascular hemodynamics in septic patients with continuous venovenous hemofiltration. *Intensive Care Med* 1997;23:288–296.
62. Guerin C, Girard R, Selli JM, et al. Intermittent versus continuous renal replacement therapy for acute renal failure in intensive care units: results from a multicenter prospective epidemiological survey. *Intensive Care Med* 2002;28:1411–1418.
63. Eknoyan G, Beck GJ, Cheung AK, et al. Hemodialysis (HEMO) Study Group: effect of dialysis dose and membrane flux in maintenance hemodialysis. *N Engl J Med* 2002;347:2010–2019.
64. Kellum JA, Angus DC, Johnson JP, et al. Continuous versus intermittent renal replacement therapy: a meta-analysis. *Intensive Care Med* 2002;28:29–37. Search date 1998; primary sources Medline, meeting abstracts, and bibliographies of review articles.
65. Ronco C, Bellomo R, Homel P, et al. Effects of different doses in continuous veno-venous haemofiltration on outcomes of acute renal failure: a prospective randomised trial. *Lancet* 2000;356:26–30.
66. Bouman CSC, Oudemans-van Straaten HM, Tijssen JGP, et al. Effects of early high-volume continuous venovenous hemofiltration on survival and recovery of renal function in intensive care patients with acute renal failure: a prospective, randomized trial. *Crit Care Med* 2002;30:2205–2211.
67. Schiffl H, Lang SM, Fischer R. Daily hemodialysis and the outcome of acute renal failure. *N Engl J Med* 2002;346:305–310.
68. Gotch FA, Sargent JA, Keen ML. Whither goest Kt/V? *Kidney Int* 2000;58(suppl 76):3–18.
69. Jaber BL, Lau J, Schmid CH, et al. Effect of biocompatibility of hemodialysis membranes on mortality in acute renal failure: a meta-analysis. *Clin Nephrol* 2002;57:274–282. Search date 2000; primary sources Medline, meeting abstracts, and bibliographies of review articles.
70. Subramanian S, Venkataraman R, Kellum JA. Influence of dialysis membrane on outcomes in acute renal failure: a meta-analysis. *Kidney Int* 2002;62:1819–1823. Search date 2000; primary sources Medline, meeting abstracts, and bibliographies of review articles.
71. Kammerl MC, Schaefer RM, Schweda F, et al. Extracorporal therapy with AN69 membranes in combination with ACE inhibition causing severe anaphylactoid reactions: still a current problem? *Clin Nephrol* 2000;53:486–488.
72. Kleinknecht D, Ganeval D, Gonzales-Duque LA, et al. Furosemide in acute oliguric renal failure. A controlled trial. *Nephron* 1976;17:51–58.
73. Brown CB, Ogg CS, Cameron JS. High dose furosemide in acute renal failure: a controlled trial. *Clin Nephrol* 1981;15:90–96.
74. Kellum JA. Use of diuretics in the acute care setting. *Kidney Int* 1998;53(suppl 66):67–70.
75. Rudy DW, Voelker JR, Greene PK, et al. Loop diuretics for chronic renal insufficiency: a continuous infusion is more efficacious than bolus therapy. *Ann Intern Med* 1991;115:360–366.
76. The Albumin Reviewers. Human albumin solution for resuscitation and volume expansion in critically ill patients. In: The Cochrane Library, Issue 1, 2004. Oxford: Update Software. Search date 2002; primary sources The Cochrane Injuries Group Register, the Cochrane Library, Medline, Embase, Bids, Index to Scientific and Technical Proceedings, hand searches of references, contact with authors and drug companies, and searches of the Medical Editor's Trial Amnesty.
77. Fliser D, Zurbruggen I, Mutschler E, et al. Coadministration of albumin and furosemide in patients with the nephrotic syndrome. *Kidney Int* 1999;55:629–634.
78. Lewis J, Salem M, Chertow GM, et al. Atrial natriuretic factor in oliguric acute renal failure. Anaritide Acute Renal Failure Study Group. *Am J Kidney Dis* 2000;36:767–774.
79. Meyer M, Pfarr E, Schirmer G, et al. Therapeutic use of natriuretic peptide ularitide in acute renal failure. *Ren Fail* 1999;21:85–100.

John Kellum
Associate Professor
Department of Critical Care Medicine
University of Pittsburgh
Pittsburgh
USA

Martine Leblanc
Assistant Professor of Nephrology and Critical Care
MaisonneuveRosemont Hospital University of Montreal
Montreal
Canada

Ramesh Venkataraman
Assistant Professor
Department of Critical Care Medicine
University of Pittsburgh
Pittsburgh
USA

Competing interests: JK has received compensation for lectures and consulting work for Gambro and Renal Tech. ML and RV: none declared.

Renal failure (acute)

TABLE 1 **Selected risk factors for acute renal failure (see text, p 1073).**

Risk factor	Incidence of ARF	Comments
Sepsis	Unknown	Sepsis seems to be a contributing factor in as many as 43% of ARF cases[5]
Aortic clamping	Approaches 100% when > 60 minutes[6]	Refers to cross-clamping (no flow) above the renal arteries
Rhabdomyolysis	16.5%[7]	None
Aminoglycosides	8–26%[8]	None
Amphotericin	88% with > 5 g total dose[9]	60% overall incidence of nephrotoxicity

Benign prostatic hyperplasia

Search date July 2003

Robyn Webber

QUESTIONS

INTERVENTIONS

See glossary Ⓖ

Key Messages

- **α Blockers** Systematic reviews have found that α blockers improve lower urinary tract symptom scores compared with placebo. Systematic reviews found limited evidence that different α blockers have similar effects. RCTs found limited evidence that α blockers improved symptom scores compared with the 5α reductase inhibitor finasteride. One RCT found no significant difference between tamsulosin and saw palmetto plant extracts in symptom scores or maximum flow rate after 1 year. Another RCT found limited evidence suggesting that α blockers were less effective than transurethral microwave thermotherapy in improving symptoms over 18 months. We found no RCTs comparing α blockers versus surgical treatment.
- **5α Reductase inhibitors** One systematic review and additional RCTs have found that 5α reductase inhibitors improve symptom scores and reduce complications compared with placebo. The review found that 5α reductase inhibitors were associated with more adverse events than placebo, including decreased libido, impotence, and ejaculatory dysfunction. RCTs found limited evidence that the 5α reductase inhibitor finasteride was less effective at improving symptom scores than α blockers. One systematic review found no significant difference in symptom scores between finasteride and saw palmetto plant extracts. We found no RCTs comparing 5α reductase inhibitors versus surgical treatment.
- **Saw palmetto plant extracts** One systematic review has found that saw palmetto plant extracts improve symptom scores compared with placebo. It found no significant difference in symptom scores between saw palmetto plant extracts and the α blocker tamsulosin or the 5α reductase inhibitor finasteride. One RCT found no significant difference in symptom scores between tamsulosin and tamsulosin plus saw palmetto plant extracts.
- **Transurethral microwave thermotherapy** RCTs found that transurethral microwave thermotherapy reduced symptom scores compared with sham treatment. We found limited evidence that thermotherapy was less effective in relieving short term symptoms than transurethral resection. One RCT found that transurethral microwave thermotherapy improved symptom scores over 18 months compared with α blockers.

- **Transurethral resection versus no surgery** RCTs found that transurethral resection reduced symptom scores more than watchful waiting, and did not increase the risk of erectile dysfunction or incontinence.
- **β-Sitosterol plant extract** One systematic review has found that β-sitosterol plant extract improves lower urinary tract symptom scores compared with placebo in the short term. We found no RCTs comparing β-sitosterol plant extract versus other treatments.
- ***Pygeum africanum*** One systematic review found limited evidence that *Pygeum africanum* increased peak urinary flow and reduced residual urine volume at 4–16 weeks compared with placebo. We found no RCTs comparing *Pygeum africanum* versus other treatments.
- **Rye grass pollen extract** One systematic review found limited evidence that rye grass pollen extract increased self rated improvement and reduced nocturia at 12–24 weeks compared with placebo. However, the review identified only two small RCTs, from which we were unable to draw reliable conclusions. We found no RCTs comparing rye grass pollen extract versus other treatments.
- **Transurethral resection versus less invasive surgical techniques** RCTs found no significant difference in symptom scores between transurethral resection and transurethral incision or between transurethral resection and electrical vaporisation. RCTs found limited evidence that transurethral resection improved symptom scores more than visual laser ablation but that transurethral resection may be associated with a higher risk of blood transfusion.
- **Transurethral resection versus transurethral needle ablation** One RCT found that transurethral resection reduced symptom scores compared with transurethral needle ablation after 1 year, although transurethral needle ablation caused fewer adverse effects.

DEFINITION Benign prostatic hyperplasia is defined histologically. Clinically, it is characterised by lower urinary tract symptoms (urinary frequency, urgency, a weak and intermittent stream, needing to strain, a sense of incomplete emptying, and nocturia) and can lead to complications, including acute urinary retention.

INCIDENCE/ PREVALENCE Estimates of the prevalence of symptomatic benign prostatic hyperplasia range from 10–30% for men in their early 70s, depending on how benign prostatic hyperplasia is defined.[1]

AETIOLOGY/ RISK FACTORS The mechanisms by which benign prostatic hyperplasia causes symptoms and complications are unclear, although bladder outlet obstruction is an important factor.[2] The best documented risk factors are increasing age and normal testicular function.[3]

PROGNOSIS Community and practice based studies suggest that men with lower urinary tract symptoms can expect slow progression of the symptoms.[4,5] However, symptoms can wax and wane without treatment. In men with symptoms of benign prostatic hyperplasia, rates of acute urinary retention range from 1–2% a year.[5–7]

AIMS OF INTERVENTION To reduce or alleviate lower urinary tract symptoms; to prevent complications; and to minimise adverse effects of treatment.

OUTCOMES Burden of lower urinary tract symptoms including peak urinary flow rate; residual urine volume, and rates of acute urinary retention and prostatectomy, self rated improvement; and adverse effects of treatment. Symptoms are measured using the validated International Prostate Symptom Score (IPSS), which includes seven questions measuring symptoms on an overall scale from 0–35, with higher scores representing more frequent symptoms.[8] RCTs reported in this chapter used a variety of symptom based assessment instruments, including the Boyarsky Symptom Score Ⓖ and the American Urological Association Symptom Index (AUASI) Ⓖ.

METHODS This review was originally based on ongoing Medline searches and prospective journal hand searches by the Patient Outcomes Research Team for Prostatic Diseases (Agency for Health Care Policy and Research grant number HS0839). *Clinical Evidence* search and appraisal July 2003.

QUESTION **What are the effects of medical treatments?**

OPTION **α BLOCKERS**

Systematic reviews have found that α blockers improve lower urinary tract symptom scores compared with placebo. Systematic reviews found limited evidence that different α blockers have similar effects. RCTs found limited evidence that α blockers improved symptom scores compared with the 5α reductase inhibitor finasteride. One RCT found no significant difference between tamsulosin and saw palmetto plant extracts in symptom scores or maximum flow rate after 1 year. Another RCT found limited evidence suggesting that α blockers were less effective than transurethral microwave thermotherapy in improving symptoms over 18 months. We found no RCTs comparing α blockers versus surgical treatment.

Benefits: **Versus placebo:** We found four systematic reviews[9–12] and three subsequent RCTs.[13–15] Two systematic reviews assessed any α blocker (search dates 1998, 21 RCTs;[9] and 1999, 24 RCTs[10]), one systematic review assessed tamsulosin (search date 2000, 6 RCTs[11]), and one systematic review assessed terazosin (search date 2001, 10 RCTs[12]). Most RCTs included in the first two reviews found a greater improvement in symptom scores with α blockers than with placebo, but overall results were not reported (results presented graphically or in tabular form).[9,10] The largest RCT (2084 men) identified by the reviews[11,12] compared terazosin at doses of up to 10 mg daily for 1 year versus placebo.[16] It found that terazosin significantly improved International Prostate Symptom Score (IPSS) compared with placebo (mean −7.6 points from baseline with terazosin *v* −3.7 with placebo; mean change, terazosin *v* placebo −3.9 points, 95% CI −5.5 points to −3.3 points).[16] One RCT (81 men) included in the first review[11] found that sustained release alfuzosin (5 mg twice daily) for 48 hours significantly increased the proportion of men who were able to pass urine after catheter removal in men catheterised for acute retention compared with placebo (22/40 [55%] with alfuzosin *v* 12/41 [29%] with placebo; OR 2.95, 95% CI 1.08 to 8.21).[17] The third review found that tamsulosin (0.4 or 0.8 mg/day) significantly improved symptom scores and peak urine flow compared with placebo (WMD for mean change in Boyarsky Symptom Score**Ⓖ** for 0.4 mg tamsulosin *v* placebo −1.1 points, 95% CI −1.49 points to −0.72 points; for 0.8 mg tamsulosin *v* placebo −1.6 points, 95% CI −2.3 points to −1.0 points; WMD for change in peak urine flow from baseline for 0.4 mg tamsulosin 1.1 mL/second, 95% CI 0.59 mL/second to 1.51 mL/second; for 0.8 mg tamsulosin 1.1 mL/second, 95% CI 0.65 mL/second to 1.48 mL/second).[11] The fourth review found that terazosin improved the Boyarsky Symptom Score and the American Urological Association Symptom Index (AUASI**Ⓖ**) at 4–52 weeks compared with placebo, but it did not assess the significance of the difference between groups (mean improvement in Boyarsky Symptom Score in 4 RCTs 37% with terazosin *v* 15% with placebo, P value not reported; mean improvement in AUASI in 2 RCTs 38% for terazosin *v* 17% for placebo, P value not reported).[12] It also found that terazosin improved peak urinary flow rates compared with placebo (improvement 23% with terazosin *v* 11% with placebo, P value not reported). The first subsequent RCT (795 men) compared three interventions: standard doxazosin, controlled released doxazosin, and placebo.[13] It found that more men had a reduction from baseline in IPSS of at least 30% with either formulation of doxazosin compared with placebo, but it did not report the significance of the difference between groups (74.7% with standard doxazosin *v* 73.5% with controlled release doxazosin *v* 53.5% with placebo; absolute figures and P value not reported). The second subsequent RCT (536 men) compared prolonged release alfuzosin 10 mg versus placebo, and prolonged release alfuzosin 15 mg versus placebo.[14] It found that alfuzosin 10 and 15 mg significantly improved symptom scores compared with placebo (mean change in IPSS from baseline at end point –3.6 points with alfuzosin 10 mg *v* –3.4 points with alfuzosin 15 mg *v* –1.6 points with placebo; alfuzosin 10 mg *v* placebo, P = 0.001; alfuzosin 15 mg *v* placebo, P = 0.004). It found no significant difference in symptom scores between 10 and 15 mg alfuzosin. The third subsequent RCT (1095 men) compared four interventions: standard doxazosin, finasteride, doxazosin plus finasteride, and placebo.[15] It found that doxazosin significantly improved total IPSS scores from baseline over 1 year compared with placebo (503 men: mean change –8.4 with doxazosin *v* –5.4 with placebo; P < 0.001). It also found that doxazosin significantly improved peak urinary flow rate (mean change +3.6 mL/second with doxazosin *v* +1.3 mL/second for placebo; P < 0.001).[15] **Versus each other:** We found two systematic reviews, one comparing tamsulosin versus other α blockers (search date 2000, 5 RCTs)[11] and one comparing terazosin versus other α blockers (search date 2001, 6 RCTs),[12] one additional RCT,[18] and two subsequent RCTs (reported in the same paper).[19] The first review did not pool results for comparisons between tamsulosin and all other α blockers combined.[11] It found no significant difference between tamsulosin 0.2 mg daily and terazosin 2–5 mg daily in IPSS and urine flow (4 RCTs; WMD for change in IPSS –0.72 points, 95% CI –2.54 points to +1.51 points; WMD for change in peak urine flow –0.26 mL/second, 95% CI –1.12 mL/second to +0.60 mL/second). It found no significant difference in symptoms between tamsulosin and alfuzosin or between tamsulosin and prazosin (tamsulosin *v* alfuzosin: 1 RCT; improvement in Boyarsky Symptom Score about 40% in each group; increase in peak urine flow about 16% in each group; tamsulosin *v* prazosin: 1 RCT; improvement in IPSS 26% with tamsulosin *v* 38% with prazosin; improvement in peak urine flow 15% with tamsulosin *v* 27% with prazosin, P values reported as non-significant, CI not reported). The second review found no significant difference between terazosin and tamsulosin in IPSS scores or peak urinary flow rates (3 RCTs; improvement in IPSS score 40% with terazosin *v* 41% with tamsulosin; WMD of IPSS score +0.72 points, 95% CI –1.51 points to +2.93 points; increase in peak flow 25% with terazosin *v* 29% with tamsulosin; WMD +0.26%, 95% CI –0.60% to +1.12%).[12] It found similar Boyarsky Symptom Scores for terazosin compared with doxazosin, and similar IPSS scores for terazosin and prazosin (terazosin *v* doxazosin: 1 RCT; improvement in Boyarsky Symptom Score 38–47% with terazosin *v* 42% with doxazosin, P value not reported; terazosin *v* prazosin: 1 RCT; improvement in IPPS score 39% with terazosin *v* 38% with prazosin; P value not reported). The additional RCT (103 people) found no significant difference in Boyarsky Symptom Score at 21 days between alfuzosin and prazosin (change in score: –2.6 with alfuzosin *v* – 2.8 with prazosin; P value not reported).[18] The results of the two subsequent RCTs (total 1475 men) were combined in a meta-analysis.[19] It found no significant difference between standard and controlled release doxazosin in IPSS improvement from baseline (–7.9 points with controlled release *v* –8.0 points with standard; adjusted mean difference –0.1 points, 95% CI –0.5 points to +0.3 points).[19] **Versus 5α reductase inhibitors:** We found one systematic review (search date 2001, 1 RCT, 1229 men)[12], and one additional[20] and two subsequent RCTs.[15,21] The RCT identified by the review[12] was poor quality (see comment below). It compared three interventions: terazosin, finasteride, and terazosin plus finasteride.[22] It found that terazosin significantly reduced AUASI score compared with finasteride (mean change in AUASI score –6.1 points with terazosin *v* –3.2 points with finasteride; WMD –2.80 points, 95% CI –3.88 points to –1.72

points; $P < 0.001$). There was no significant difference between finasteride plus terazosin and terazosin alone. The additional RCT (1051 men) compared alfuzosin versus finasteride versus both drugs combined over 6 months.[20] It found that alfuzosin significantly decreased the mean IPSS score from baseline compared with finasteride, and it found no significant difference between alfuzosin alone and alfuzosin plus finasteride.[20] The second subsequent RCT (1095 men) compared four interventions: standard doxazosin, finasteride, doxazosin plus finasteride, and placebo.[15] It found that both doxazosin and doxazosin plus finasteride significantly improved total IPSS and peak urinary flow rate over 1 year compared with finasteride alone (759 men; $P < 0.05$). The second subsequent RCT (205 men) compared tamsulosin versus finasteride.[21] It found that tamsulosin was significantly more effective than finasteride in improving IPSS score and mean peak urinary flow at 4 weeks (mean change in IPSS –3.5 with tamsulosin *v* –1.9 with finasteride; mean peak flow 1.0 mL/second with tamsulosin *v* +0.3 mL/second with finasteride; $P < 0.05$ for both outcomes) but found no significant difference in scores at 24 weeks (mean change in IPSS –6.9 with tamsulosin *v* –5.8 with finasteride; mean peak flow: +2.2 mL/second with tamsulosin *v* +2.2 mL/second with finasteride; P reported as non-significant, CI not reported for either outcome). **Versus transurethral microwave thermotherapy:** See benefits of transurethral microwave thermotherapy, p 1104. **Versus saw palmetto plant extracts:** See benefits of saw palmetto plant extracts, p 1105.

Harms: **Versus placebo:** The first systematic review found that withdrawals because of adverse events were similar with alfuzosin, tamsulosin (0.4 mg dose), and placebo (results presented graphically; CI not reported).[9] There was little observable difference in rates of dizziness between either alfuzosin or tamsulosin compared with placebo (results presented graphically; CI not reported). However, terazosin and doxazosin increased dizziness compared with placebo (results presented graphically; CI not reported). One non-systematic review of RCTs (3 RCTs, 830 people) suggested that both selective and less selective α blockers may be associated with abnormal ejaculation; the risk of abnormal ejaculation was significantly higher with tamsulosin than with placebo (4.5% with tamsulosin *v* 1.0% with placebo; $P = 0.042$).[23] Another systematic review found no significant difference between tamsulosin and placebo in withdrawal because of adverse events (4 RCTs; RR 1.08, 95% CI 0.72 to 1.62).[11] However, it found that tamsulosin significantly increased abnormal ejaculation, rhinitis, and dizziness compared with placebo (abnormal ejaculation: 4 RCTs; AR 10.8% with tamsulosin *v* < 1% with placebo; RR 17.0, 95% CI 2.5 to 114.0; rhinitis: 4 RCTs; AR 11.2% with tamsulosin *v* 6% with placebo; RR 1.84, 95% CI 1.24 to 2.72; dizziness: 5 RCTs; AR 11.9% with tamsulosin *v* 7.8% with placebo; RR 1.50, 95% CI 1.13 to 1.98). Another systematic review found that terazosin significantly increased dizziness, asthenia, and postural hypotension compared with placebo (dizziness: 6 RCTs; RR 2.43, 95% CI 1.82 to 3.25; asthenia: 5 RCTs; RR 2.24, 95% CI 1.68 to 3.00; postural hypotension: 4 RCTs; RR 5.27, 95% CI 5.27 to 10.72).[12] It found no significant difference in discontinuation rates between terazosin and placebo (10 RCTs: 27% with terazosin *v* 34% with placebo; RR 0.94, 95% CI 0.76 to 1.17). Discontinuations because of adverse events were significantly higher with terazosin compared with placebo (6 RCTs: 229/1817 [12.6%] with terazosin *v* 140/1607 [8.7%] with placebo; RR 1.50, 95% CI 1.23 to 1.83). **Versus each other:** We found three systematic reviews assessing harms.[9,11,12] The first review found no significant difference between tamsulosin and a less selective α blocker, alfuzosin (1 RCT; dizziness 7%, asthenia 2%, and postural hypotension 2% of men in each group).[9] The second review comparing tamsulosin versus other α blockers found that discontinuation of treatment due to adverse effects was less likely with tamsulosin 0.2 mg daily than with terazosin (4 RCTs; RR 0.15, 95% CI 0.04 to 0.57).[11] However, tamsulosin 0.4 or 0.2 mg daily was associated with greater all cause withdrawal from treatment than alfuzosin or prazosin, although the differences were not significant (tamsulosin *v* alfuzosin: 1 RCT; RR for withdrawal 1.46, 95% CI 0.66 to 3.25; tamsulosin *v* prazosin: 1 RCT; RR for withdrawal 2.87, 95% CI 0.65 to 12.65). The review found no significant difference between tamsulosin and alfuzosin in dizziness (1 RCT: AR 6.8% with tamsulosin *v* 7.3% with alfuzosin; RR 0.94, 95% CI 0.39 to 2.29), asthenia (1 RCT: AR 3% with tamsulosin *v* 1.6% with alfuzosin; RR 1.88, 95% CI 0.35 to 10.08), headache (1 RCT: AR 7.6% with tamsulosin *v* 3.2% with alfuzosin; RR 2.35, 95% CI 0.76 to 7.29). The review also found that risk of abnormal ejaculation increased with increasing dose of tamsulosin (0% with 0.2 mg/day; 18% with 0.8 mg/day; CI not reported). The third review found no significant difference in discontinuation rates between terazosin and either prazosin or doxazosin (terazosin *v* prazosin: 1 RCT; RR 3.93, CI 95% 0.92 to 16.72; terazosin *v* doxazosin: 1 RCT; RR 1.75, 95% CI 0.48 to 6.41).[12] The review found no significant difference between terazosin and alfuzosin in dizziness (1 RCT; 5.1% with terazosin *v* 0% with alfuzosin; RR 4.50, 95% CI 0.22 to 90.64). It found no significant difference in dizziness or headache between terazosin and doxazosin (dizziness: 1 RCT; 14.3% with terazosin *v* 4.5% with doxazosin; RR 3.14, 95% CI 0.35 to 27.88; headache: 1 RCT; 4.8% with terazosin *v* 4.5% with doxazosin; RR 1.05, 95% CI 0.07 to 15.69) but it may have lacked power to exclude a clinically important effect. **Versus 5α reductase inhibitors:** In the RCT identified by the review comparing terazosin versus finasteride, dizziness, generalised weakness, rhinitis, and postural hypotension were more common with terazosin than with finasteride (dizziness: 26% with terazosin *v* 8% with finasteride; generalised weakness: 14% with terazosin *v* 7% with finasteride; rhinitis: 7% with terazosin *v* 3% with finasteride; postural hypotension: 8% with terazosin *v* 2% with finasteride; significance not reported for any comparison), whereas sexual dysfunction was more common in men taking finasteride (impotence: 9% with finasteride *v* 6% with terazosin; significance not reported).[22] The other RCTs gave no information on adverse effects.[15,20,21] **Versus transurethral microwave thermotherapy:** See harms of transurethral microwave thermotherapy, p 1104. **Versus saw palmetto plant extracts:** See harms of saw palmetto plant extracts, p 1105.

Comment: Men with severe symptoms can expect the largest absolute fall in their symptom scores with medical treatment.[16,24] Prazosin, terazosin, and doxazosin lower blood pressure and may be used to treat both hypertension and benign prostatic hyperplasia.[25] The RCT included in the review that compared α blockers versus 5α reductase inhibitors is limited by its small sample size, low drug doses, and unclear methods of randomisation and blinding.[12]

OPTION 5α REDUCTASE INHIBITORS

One systematic review and additional RCTs have found that 5α reductase inhibitors improve symptom scores and reduce complications compared with placebo. The review found that 5α reductase inhibitors were associated with more adverse events than placebo, including decreased libido, impotence, and ejaculatory dysfunction. RCTs found limited evidence that the 5α reductase inhibitor finasteride was less effective at improving symptom scores than α blockers. One systematic review found no significant difference in symptom scores between finasteride and saw palmetto plant extracts. We found no RCTs comparing 5α reductase inhibitors versus surgical treatment.

Benefits: **Versus placebo:** We found one systematic review (search date 1999, 12 RCTs, 11 338 men),[10] one subsequent RCT (generating numerous publications)[7,26–29] and two additional RCTs.[15,30] Ten of the 12 RCTs included in the systematic review found that finasteride significantly reduced symptom scores compared with placebo.[10] The first RCT in the review (2902 men) found that 5 mg finasteride significantly improved symptom scores compared with placebo at 24 months (change in Boyarsky Symptom Score**G** –20% with finasteride *v* –13% with placebo; P < 0.001). The second RCT in the review (2112 men) found that 5 mg finasteride significantly improved symptom scores compared with placebo at 12 months (change in American Urological Association Symptom Index [AUASI**G**] score: –26% with finasteride *v* –20% with placebo; P < 0.01). The third RCT in the review (496 men) found that 5 mg finasteride significantly improved symptom scores compared with placebo at 12 months (change in Boyarsky Symptom Score: –20% with finasteride *v* –14% with placebo; P < 0.05). The fourth RCT in the review (472 men) found that 5 mg finasteride significantly improved symptom scores compared with placebo at 24 months (change in Boyarsky Symptom Score: –13% with finasteride *v* –4% with placebo; P < 0.01). The fifth RCT in the review (707 men) found that 5 mg finasteride significantly improved symptom scores compared with placebo at 24 months (change in Boyarsky Symptom Score: –15% with finasteride *v* +2% with placebo; P < 0.01). The sixth RCT in the review (895 men) found that 5 mg finasteride significantly improved symptom scores compared with placebo at 12 months (change in Boyarsky Symptom Score: –26% with finasteride *v* –10% with placebo; P < 0.05). The seventh RCT in the review (46 men) found that 5 mg finasteride significantly improved symptom scores compared with placebo at 6 months (change in AUASI score: –30% with finasteride *v* –12% with placebo; P < 0.05). The eighth RCT in the review (2760 men) found that 5 mg finasteride significantly improved symptom scores compared with placebo (change in AUASI scores: –17% with finasteride *v* –7% with placebo; P < 0.001). The ninth RCT in the review (99 men) found that 5 mg finasteride significantly improved symptom scores compared with placebo at 12 months (change in AUASI score: –30% with finasteride *v* –10% with placebo; P < 0.05). The 10th RCT in the review (182 men) found that 5 mg finasteride significantly improved symptom scores compared with placebo at 6 months (change in Boyarsky Symptom Score: –23% with finasteride *v* –9% with placebo; P = 0.05). The 11th RCT in the review (615 men) found no significant difference in symptom scores between 1–10 mg finasteride and placebo at 12 months (change in AUASI score: –20% with finasteride *v* –16% with placebo; P = 0.63). The 12th RCT in the review (52 men) found that finasteride improved symptom scores at 3 months compared with placebo but the significance of the difference between groups was not reported in the review (change in AUASI score: –21% with finasteride *v* –19% with placebo). The first subsequent RCT (3040 men) compared finasteride 5 mg daily versus placebo.[7] After 4 years, finasteride significantly reduced symptom scores compared with placebo (difference in symptom score –1.6 points, 95% CI –2.5 points to –0.7 points [range of score 0–34 points]). It also found that finasteride significantly reduced the risk of acute urinary retention and prostatectomy compared with placebo (urinary retention 6.6% with finasteride *v* 2.8% with placebo; NNT 26, 95% CI 22 to 38; prostatectomy 8.3% with finasteride *v* 4.2% with placebo; NNT 24, 95% CI 19 to 37). There was a greater effect among men with higher concentrations of prostate specific antigen at baseline (3.3–12.0 ng/mL), reflecting larger prostates (risk of either acute urinary retention or needing prostatectomy: 19.9% with placebo *v* 8.3% with finasteride; NNT 8, 95% CI 7 to 11).[27] The RCT also found that, after 4 years, finasteride produced a larger fall in International

Prostate Symptom Score compared with placebo. The fall was greater for men with prostate specific antigen levels greater than 1.3 ng/mL than for men with prostate specific antigen levels equal to or lower than 1.3 ng/mL.[26] The second subsequent RCT (1095 men) compared four interventions: finasteride, standard doxazosin, doxazosin plus finasteride, and placebo.[15] It found no significant difference between finasteride and placebo in International Prostate Symptom Score or peak urinary flow rate over 1 year (492 men; P reported as non-significant, CI not reported).[15] The third subsequent RCT (4325 men) compared dutasteride versus placebo.[30] It found that, compared with placebo, dutasteride significantly improved AUASI scores (–4.5 with dutasteride *v* –2.3 with placebo; $P < 0.001$), and peak urinary flow rate after 24 months (+2.2 mL/second with dutasteride *v* +0.6 mL/second with placebo; $P < 0.001$).[30] **Versus α blockers:** See benefits of α blockers, p 1095. **Versus saw palmetto plant extracts:** See benefits of saw palmetto plant extracts, p 1105.

Harms: **Versus placebo:** The systematic review found that finasteride increased adverse events in the first year compared with placebo.[10] The most common adverse events with finasteride in the first year were decreased libido, impotence, and ejaculatory dysfunction. The largest RCT (3168 men) found decreased libido, increased impotence, and increased ejaculatory dysfunction compared with placebo (decreased libido 4.0% *v* 2.8%; reported as non-significant; increased impotence 6.6% *v* 4.7%; reported as significant; ejaculatory dysfunction 2.1% *v* 0.6%; reported as significant; none of the P values reported). Another large RCT (2342 men) found decreased libido, increased impotence, and increased ejaculatory dysfunction compared with placebo (decreased libido 3.1% *v* 1.2%; reported as significant; impotence 6.8% *v* 3.2%; reported as significant; increased ejaculatory dysfunction 2.3% *v* 0.5%; reported as significant; none of the P values reported). The large subsequent 4 year RCT (3040 men) found that, after the first year of treatment, there was no significant difference in decreased libido (2.6% *v* 2.6%) or impotence (5.1% *v* 5.1%) between finasteride and placebo, but there was still a slightly greater rate of ejaculation disorder (0.2% *v* 0.1%; significance not tested).[7] Although finasteride reduced concentrations of prostate specific antigen by a mean of 50% (individual responses were highly variable), its use for up to 4 years did not change the rate of detection of prostate cancer compared with placebo.[7] The additional RCTs did not address harms. **Versus α blockers:** See harms of α blockers, p 1097. **Versus saw palmetto plant extracts:** See harms of saw palmetto plant extracts, p 1105.

Comment: We found two non-systematic reviews comparing finasteride versus placebo.[31,32] One of the non-systematic reviews (6 RCTs) found that finasteride significantly decreased symptom scores compared with placebo (difference in symptom score –0.9 points, 95% CI –1.2 points to –0.6 points [range of score 0–30 points]).[32] The benefit over placebo was greatest in men with larger prostates (≥ 40 g). The other non-systematic review (meta-analysis of 3 RCTs) found that finasteride reduced acute urinary retention requiring catheterisation after 2 years from 2.7% to 1.1%.[31] The meta-analysis also found that finasteride was significantly more effective than placebo in men with larger prostates at 1–2 years. However, the absolute difference in mean decrease of symptom score from baseline between men with the smallest and largest prostates was only about 1 point. The relative effectiveness of finasteride compared with placebo also seemed higher in men with slightly raised prostate specific antigen levels, and it is assumed that the higher prostate specific antigen is a proxy for a larger prostate.[26]

QUESTION What are the effects of surgical treatments?

OPTION TRANSURETHRAL RESECTION OF THE PROSTATE

RCTs found that transurethral resection of the prostate reduced symptom scores more than watchful waiting, and did not increase the risk of erectile dysfunction or incontinence. RCTs found no significant difference in symptom scores between transurethral resection and transurethral incision or between transurethral resection and electrical vaporisation. RCTs found limited evidence that transurethral resection improved symptom scores more than visual laser ablation but may be associated with a higher risk of blood transfusion.

Benefits: **Versus watchful waiting:** We found no systematic review. We found two RCTs comparing transurethral resection of the prostate (TURP) versus watchful waiting.[33,34] The first RCT (556 men with moderate symptoms of benign prostatic hyperplasia) found that TURP significantly improved symptom scores compared with watchful waiting (90% with TURP *v* 39% with watchful waiting; $P < 0.001$). After 5 years, the treatment failure rate was 10% with TURP compared with 21% with watchful waiting (NNT 9, 95% CI 7 to 17), and 36% of men assigned to watchful waiting had crossed over to surgery.[35] Treatment failure was defined as death, acute urinary retention, high residual urine volume, renal azotaemia, bladder stones, persistent incontinence, or a high symptom score. The major categories of treatment failure reduced by TURP were acute urinary retention, development of a large bladder residual (> 350 mL), and deterioration to a severe symptom level. The second RCT (223 men) had a shorter duration of follow up (7.5 months).[34] It found that TURP significantly improved the International Prostate Symptom Score (IPSS) compared with watchful waiting (difference in IPSS 10.4 points, 95% CI 8.5 points to 12.3 points). **Versus less invasive techniques:** We found four systematic reviews[36–39] and four subsequent RCTs.[40–43] The first systematic review (search date 1999, 9 RCTs) compared TURP versus transurethral incision.[36] Four of the included RCTs (243 men) examined symptom scores at 12 months and found no significant difference between TURP and transurethral incision (WMD +0.2 points, 95% CI –0.8 points to +1.1 points). The review found little good, long term evidence. The second systematic review (search date 1999, 5 RCTs) compared TURP versus visual laser ablation (4 RCTs, 331 men) or laser contact vaporisation (1 RCT, 28 men).[37] The review did not perform a meta-analysis. It found that TURP was more effective at reducing symptom score than visual laser ablation but increased the length of hospital stay. The largest RCT (151 men) identified by the second review found that TURP significantly improved symptom scores compared with ablation at 52 weeks (American Urological Association Symptom Index**G** mean score reduced from 18.2 to 5.1 with TURP *v* from 18.1 to 7.7 with laser ablation). The review found no significant difference between TURP and laser contact vaporisation in symptom scores or quality of life at 12 months' follow up. The third systematic review (search date 1999, 5 RCTs, 454 men) compared TURP versus electrical vaporisation.[38] It found no significant difference in symptom scores at 12–24 months between TURP and electrical vaporisation, although symptoms were improved more with electrical vaporisation (3 RCTs, figures reported as SMD +0.21, 95% CI –0.03 to +0.44). The fourth systematic review (search date 2002, 16 RCTs) compared TURP versus contact laser vaporisation (7 RCTs, 501 men) or visual laser ablation (8 RCTs, 864 men) or a hybrid laser technique (4 RCTs, 276 men).[39] For men undergoing contact laser vaporisation, the review analysed results separately for comparisons of TURP versus Nd:YAG or versus holmium laser resection. The review found no significant difference in symptom scores at 12 months between transurethral resection and Nd:YAG contact laser (2 RCTs; WMD +2.08 points, 95% CI –0.36 points to +4.51 points) or between TURP and holmium laser resection (5 RCTs; WMD +0.10 points, 95% CI –2.08 points to +1.88 points). It also found no significant difference in peak urinary flow at 12 months between TURP and Nd:YAG contact laser (4 RCTs; WMD 1.9 mL/second, 95% CI –0.21 mL/second to +4.02 mL/second). However, it found that holmium laser resection significantly reduced peak urinary flow rate at 12 months compared with TURP (1 RCT; WMD –4.8 mL/second, 95% CI –8.79 mL/second to –0.81 mL/second). It found similar reductions in symptoms scores at 12 months between TURP and visual laser ablation (mean decrease 63% with TURP *v* 59% with visual laser). The reported differences in significance between TURP and visual laser ablation varied depending on whether mean changes in symptom scores or mean scores at follow up had been recorded. If mean change in symptom scores was assessed, TURP was significantly less effective than visual laser ablation in reducing symptoms over 7–12 months (3 RCTs; WMD –2.5 points, 95% CI –4.24 points to –0.70 points). However, if mean symptom score at follow up was assessed there was no significant difference between TURP and visual laser ablation at 6 or 12 months (WMD 0.21 points, 95% CI –2.28 points to +2.70 points). The first subsequent RCT (98 men) found that TURP reduced surgical retreatment rates after 5 years compared with laser ablation (18/47 [38%] with visual laser ablation *v* 8/51 [16%] with TURP; P = 0.006).[40] The other subsequent RCTs compared TURP versus electrical vaporisation; all found similar improvements in symptoms between treatments.[41–43] The second subsequent RCT (100 men) found similar symptom scores at 3 months after treatment between TURP and electrical vaporisation (mean IPSS decreased from 21.6 points to 5.0 points with TURP *v* from 19.4 points to 4.0 points with vaporisation; CI and P value for direct comparison not reported).[41] The third subsequent RCT (185 men) also found similar improvements symptoms at 12 months (mean decrease in IPSS from baseline 12.8 points for TURP *v* 12.5 points for vaporisation; CI and P value not reported).[42] The fourth subsequent RCT (235 men) found no significant difference between TURP and electrical vaporisation after 6 months (mean change in IPSS from baseline: 20.9 to 6.9 with TURP *v* 20.7 to 8.5 with electrical vaporisation; mean increase in flow rate: 10.5 to 22.3 mL/second with TURP *v* 10.1 to 19.6 mL/second with electrical vaporisation; P > 0.12).[43] **Versus transurethral microwave therapy:** See benefits of transurethral microwave thermotherapy, p 1104. **Versus transurethral needle ablation:** See benefits of transurethral needle ablation, p 1104.

Harms: Analysis of administrative data found that mortality in the 30 days after TURP for benign prostatic hyperplasia ranged from 0.4% for men aged 65–69 years to 1.9% for men aged 80–84 years, and has fallen in recent years.[44] In one review of observational studies, TURP for benign prostatic hyperplasia was associated with immediate surgical complications in 12% of men, bleeding requiring intervention in 2%, erectile dysfunction in 14%, retrograde ejaculation in 74%, and incontinence in about 5%.[45–47] Analysis of claims data found a reoperation rate, implying need for retreatment, of about 1% a year.[44] However, in the only comparative trial, men randomised to prostatectomy did not seem to have a greater rate of erectile dysfunction or incontinence than did men assigned to watchful waiting.[33,35] One systematic review found that visual laser ablation was associated with a lower risk of blood transfusion than TURP but with a higher risk of urinary tract infection (blood transfusion: 0/145 [0%] with laser ablation *v* 15/146 [10%] with TURP;

RR 0.09, 95% CI 0.02 to 0.47; urinary tract infection: RR 3.85, 95% CI 1.87 to 7.94; absolute figures not reported).[37] The largest RCT found fewer cases of blood transfusion with visual laser ablation compared with TURP (0/76 [0%] with laser ablation v 12/75 [16%] with TURP). The third systematic review found that TURP and electrical vaporisation had similar risks of blood transfusion, irritative symptoms, and urinary tract infections, although confidence intervals were large.[38] However, electrical vaporisation was associated with a significant increase in the risk of urinary retention (17.1% with electrical vaporisation v 3.8% with TURP; RR 3.64, 95% CI 1.68 to 7.92; absolute figures not reported) compared with TURP. One RCT (150 men) in the review reported more transient stress urinary incontinence with electrical vaporisation than with TURP (13/70 [19%] with electrical vaporisation v 0/80 [0%] with TURP). Most of the RCTs included in the fourth systematic review did not comprehensively report adverse effects.[39] However, the review found that significantly more men undergoing TURP required blood transfusion (RR 25.0, 95% CI 5.9 to 100) and developed urethral strictures (RR 2.3, 95% CI 1.3 to 3.8) than men undergoing any laser procedure. It also found that urinary retention was significantly more common following treatment with any laser technique than treatment with TURP (RR 2.3, 95% CI 1.4 to 3.9), and that visual laser techniques had a higher incidence of dysuria (RR 3.6, 95% CI 1.0 to 13.1) and urinary tract infection (RR 2.2, 95% CI 1.0 to 4.9) than TURP.[39] One subsequent RCT (100 men) found that no-one having either TURP or electrical vaporisation required transfusion.[41] It also found no significant difference in rates of erectile dysfunction between the two groups (22% with TURP v 24% with vaporisation; P values and CI not reported). However, another subsequent RCT (185 men) found no significant difference between TURP and electrical vaporisation in rates of postoperative incontinence (6/92 [6.5%] with TURP v 5/93 [5.4%] with vaporisation; RR 1.2, 95% CI 0.4 to 3.8).[41] Rates of haemorrhage requiring blood transfusion and of urethral stricture were low in both groups and not significantly different (transfusion: 9/92 [9.8%] with TURP v 6/93 [6.5%] with vaporisation; RR 1.5, 95% CI 0.6 to 4.1; urethral stricture: 7/92 [7.6%] with TURP v 5/93 [5.4%] with vaporisation; RR 1.4, 95% CI 0.5 to 4.3). A further RCT (340 men) examined sexual function after TURP, laser prostatectomy, and conservative management.[48] It found that TURP reduced the proportions with erectile dysfunction, reduced pain or discomfort on ejaculation, and increased ejaculatory dysfunction compared with conservative management (erectile dysfunction OR 0.37, 95% CI 0.19 to 0.74; pain or discomfort on ejaculation OR 0.06, 95% CI 0.007 to 0.49; ejaculatory dysfunction OR 3.27, 95% CI 1.69 to 6.35).

Comment: Rapid changes in techniques and few controlled trials with adequate follow up make comparisons between TURP and newer surgical techniques difficult. The second review reported that RCTs comparing TURP versus laser ablation were limited generally by small sample size, brief follow up, and lack of blinding.[37] The third review comparing TURP versus electrical vaporisation found that none of the RCTs were blinded or analysed by intention to treat, but four out of five RCTs had less than 10% loss to follow up.[38]

OPTION TRANSURETHRAL MICROWAVE THERMOTHERAPY

RCTs found that transurethral microwave thermotherapy reduced symptom scores compared with sham treatment. We found limited evidence that thermotherapy was less effective in relieving short term symptoms than transurethral resection. One RCT found that transurethral microwave thermotherapy improved symptom scores over 18 months compared with α blockers.

Benefits: **Versus sham treatment:** We found no systematic review. We found three RCTs comparing transurethral microwave thermotherapy (TUMT) versus sham treatment.[49–51] In the largest RCT (220 men), TUMT improved the International Prostate Symptom Score (IPSS) significantly more than sham treatment (mean 5 points lower; $P < 0.05$).[49] In the second RCT (169 men), TUMT significantly improved IPSS more than sham treatment at 6 months ($P < 0.05$).[50] The third RCT (50 men) compared TUMT versus sham treatment. It found a greater reduction in Madsen symptom score (range 0–27, higher scores indicating worse symptoms) with TUMT compared with sham treatment (reduction in Madsen symptom score reduction 7.3 with TUMT *v* 3.9 with sham treatment; significance was not tested). **Versus transurethral resection of the prostate:** We found one systematic review[38] (search date 1999, 3 RCTs, 200 men) and one additional RCT comparing TUMT versus transurethral resection of the prostate (TURP).[52] In the systematic review, symptom improvement was significantly better with TURP in one RCT ($P < 0.05$) but not significantly different in the other two.[38] The additional RCT (147 men) found better symptomatic outcomes with TURP but the significance was not reported (IPSS improvement from baseline at 1 year: 60% with TUMT *v* 85% with TURP; CI not reported).[52] **Versus α blockers:** We found one RCT (103 men).[53,54] It found that TUMT significantly improved symptom scores at 6 and 18 months compared with terazosin (up to 10 mg/day; difference in IPSS at 18 months 35%; $P < 0.001$).

Harms: Adverse events associated with TUMT varied among trials, but included the need for catheterisation for more than 1 week (8% with TUMT *v* 2% with sham treatment),[50] persistent irritative symptoms (22% with TUMT *v* 8% with sham treatment),[49] haematuria (14% with TUMT *v* 1% with sham treatment),[49] and sexual dysfunction (mostly haematospermia and other ejaculatory abnormalities; 29% with TUMT *v* 1% with sham treatment).[49] In one RCT retrograde ejaculation was substantially less common after TUMT compared with TURP (27% with TUMT *v* 74% with TURP).[55] The RCT (103 men) comparing TUMT versus α blockers found more adverse events in the α blocker group over the first 6 months (17 events in 52 men with α blockers *v* 7 events in 51 men with TUMT; CI not reported).[53,54] With α blockers, the most common adverse effect was dizziness (7 cases) or asthenia (4 cases); in the TUMT group it was urinary tract infection (3 cases).

Comment: TUMT can be performed in an outpatient setting, and uses heat generated by a microwave antenna in the urethra to coagulate prostate tissue. The long term effects of TUMT have not been adequately evaluated in controlled studies. The systematic review reported that trials were limited by small sample size, short duration of follow up (maximum 30 months), and large loss to follow up.

OPTION TRANSURETHRAL NEEDLE ABLATION

One RCT found that transurethral resection reduced symptom scores compared with transurethral needle ablation after 1 year, although transurethral needle ablation caused fewer adverse effects.

Benefits: We found no systematic review. **Versus transurethral resection:** We found one RCT (121 men) comparing transurethral resection of the prostate (TURP) versus transurethral needle ablation (TUNA).[56] The mean International Prostate Symptom Score was significantly lower with TURP than TUNA at 1 year (11.1 points with TUNA *v* 8.3 points with TURP; $P = 0.04$).

Harms: Compared with TURP, TUNA was associated with less retrograde ejaculation (38% with TURP *v* 0% with TUNA) and bleeding (100% with TURP *v* 32% with TUNA).[56]

Comment: TUNA can be performed in an outpatient setting, and uses radiofrequency energy through two intraprostatic electrodes to generate heat to coagulate prostate tissue. Anaesthesia requirements vary in reported studies. The long term effects of treatment have not been adequately evaluated.

QUESTION What are the effects of herbal treatments?

OPTION SAW PALMETTO PLANT EXTRACTS

One systematic review has found that saw palmetto plant extracts improve symptom scores compared with placebo. It found no significant difference in symptom scores between saw palmetto plant extracts and the α blocker tamsulosin or the 5α reductase inhibitor finasteride. One RCT found no significant difference in symptom scores between tamsulosin and tamsulosin plus saw palmetto plant extracts.

Benefits: We found one systematic review that included all saw palmetto preparations (search date 1997, 18 RCTs, 2939 men)[57] and two subsequent RCTs.[58,59] **Versus placebo:** The systematic review found that more men reported self rated improvement with saw palmetto compared with placebo (6 relevant RCTs: RR 1.7, 95% CI 1.2 to 2.4).[57] It found a significant reduction in nocturia with saw palmetto compared with placebo (10 RCTs; WMD 0.76 episodes/night, 95% CI 0.32 to 1.21). **Versus α blockers:** We found one RCT (704 men).[58] It found no significant difference between tamsulosin and saw palmetto in International Prostate Symptom Score (IPSS) or peak flow rate at 12 months (increase in peak flow 1.8 mL/second with saw palmetto *v* 1.9 mL/second with tamsulosin).[58] **Versus 5α reductase inhibitors:** The systematic review (2 relevant RCTs, 1440 men) found no significant difference in IPSS between finasteride and saw palmetto (WMD +0.37 points, 95% CI –0.44 points to +1.19 points).[57] **Plus α blocker:** We found one RCT (352 patients).[59] It found no significant difference in symptom score between tamsulosin and tamsulosin plus saw palmetto (improvement in IPSS: 5.2 with tamsulosin *v* 6.0 with tamsulosin plus saw palmetto).

Harms: **Versus placebo:** The systematic review found significantly higher withdrawal rates with saw palmetto than with placebo (9% with saw palmetto *v* 7% with placebo; P = 0.02).[57] The risk of erectile dysfunction was similar with saw palmetto and placebo (1.1% with saw palmetto *v* 0.7% with placebo; P = 0.58). **Versus α blockers:** In one RCT comparing saw palmetto and tamsulosin, a similar proportion of men withdrew because of adverse events (7.7% with saw palmetto *v* 8.2% with tamsulosin).[58] The risk of ejaculatory disorder was significantly less with saw palmetto than with tamsulosin (2/349 [0.6%] with saw palmetto *v* 15/354 [4.2%] with tamsulosin; P = 0.001).[58] **Versus 5α reductase inhibitors:**The review found no significant difference in withdrawal rates between saw palmetto and finasteride (9% with saw palmetto *v* 11% with finasteride; P = 0.87).[57] Rates of erectile dysfunction were significantly lower with saw palmetto compared with finasteride (1.1% with saw palmetto *v* 4.9% with finasteride; P < 0.001).[57]

Comment: The RCTs included in the systematic reviews were short term and few used a validated symptom score. Different preparations, which may not be equivalent, are available directly to consumers without prescription in many countries.[57] The RCT comparing saw palmetto versus tamsulosin used a standardised preparation of saw palmetto.[58]

OPTION β-SITOSTEROL PLANT EXTRACT

One systematic review has found that β-sitosterol plant extract improves lower urinary tract symptom scores compared with placebo in the short term. We found no RCTs comparing β-sitosterol plant extract versus other treatments.

Benefits: **Versus placebo:** We found one systematic review (search date 1998, 4 RCTs, 519 men), which compared β-sitosterol versus placebo.[55] The review found that β-sitosterol significantly reduced the International Prostate Symptom Score (2 RCTs; WMD –4.9 points, 95% CI –6.3 points to –3.5 points) at 4–26 weeks. **Versus other treatments:** We found no RCTs.

Harms: **Versus placebo:** Gastrointestinal adverse effects were more common with β-sitosterol than with placebo (1.6% with β-sitosterol *v* 0% with placebo; CI not reported).[55] Impotence was also more common with β-sitosterol (0.5% β-sitosterol *v* 0% with placebo; CI not reported). Withdrawal rates were similar in both groups (7.8% with β-sitosterol *v* 8.0% with placebo; CI not reported).

Comment: The RCTs were limited by a short follow up period (maximum 26 weeks). Different preparations are available, which may be of variable content, making it difficult to generalise results.

OPTION RYE GRASS POLLEN EXTRACT

One systematic review found limited evidence that rye grass pollen extract increased self rated improvement and reduced nocturia at 12–24 weeks compared with placebo. However, the review identified only two small RCTs, from which we were unable to draw reliable conclusions. We found no RCTs comparing Rye grass pollen extract versus other treatments.

Benefits: **Versus placebo:** We found one systematic review (search date 1997, 2 RCTs, 163 men), which compared rye grass pollen extract versus placebo.[60] It found that pollen extract significantly increased self rated improvement and significantly reduced nocturia compared with placebo (proportion improved: 1 RCT, 60 men; 20/31 [65%] with pollen *v* 7/26 [27%] with placebo; RR 2.40, 95% CI 1.21 to 4.75; NNT 3, 95% CI 2 to 9; proportion with reduced nocturia: 2 RCTs; 50/79 [63%] with pollen *v* 23/74 [31%] with placebo; RR 2.05, 95% CI 1.41 to 3.99). However, the results should be interpreted with caution (see comment below). **Versus other treatments:** We found no RCTs.

Harms: The review found that nausea occurred in one man taking pollen extract (number in placebo group not stated).[60] Withdrawal rates were not significantly different (4.8% with pollen *v* 2.7% with placebo; P = 0.26).

Comment: Both RCTs were limited by small sample sizes and a short follow up period (12 and 24 weeks). Concealment of treatment allocation was unclear. The composition of the preparations was unknown, making it difficult to generalise results.

OPTION *PYGEUM AFRICANUM*

One systematic review found limited evidence that *Pygeum africanum* increased peak urinary flow and reduced residual urine volume at 4–16 weeks compared with placebo. We found no RCTs comparing Pygeum africanum versus other treatments.

Benefits: **Versus placebo:** We found one systematic review (search date 2000, 11 RCTs, 709 men) comparing *Pygeum africanum* versus placebo.[61] It found that *P africanum* significantly increased peak flow compared with placebo at 4–16 weeks (4 RCTs, 384 men; mean reduction 23% with *P africanum v* with placebo; WMD 2.5 mL/seconds, 95% CI 0.3 mL/seconds to 4.7 mL/seconds) and reduced residual urine volume by 24% (2 RCTs, 284 men; mean reduction 24% with *P africanum v* with placebo; WMD −13ml, 95% CI −23.3 mL to −3.0 mL).[61] These results should be interpreted with caution (see comment below). **Versus other treatments:** We found no RCTs.

Harms: The RCTs identified by the review gave little information on adverse effects.[61] The review found that adverse events in men taking *P africanum* were "generally mild and similar in frequency to placebo"; the most commonly reported adverse events associated with *P africanum* were gastrointestinal and were reported in 7 men in 5 RCTs (no further data reported).

Comment: The RCTs were limited by their short follow-up period (maximum 16 weeks). The designs of the RCTs and the composition of the preparations used varied, making it difficult to generalise results.

GLOSSARY

American Urological Association Symptom Index (AUASI) is a patient questionnaire that asks seven questions about the severity of symptoms (range 0–35). Mild symptoms score 0–7 points, moderate symptoms 8–19 points, and severe symptoms 20–35 points.

Boyarsky Symptom Score is a patient questionnaire that asks nine questions about severity of symptoms (range 0–27); no symptoms = 0, maximum severity = 27.

REFERENCES

1. Bosch JL, Hop WC, Kirkels WJ, et al. Natural history of benign prostatic hyperplasia: appropriate case definition and estimation of its prevalence in the community. *Urology* 1995;46(suppl A):34–40.
2. Barry MJ, Adolfsson J, Batista JE, et al. Committee 6: measuring the symptoms and health impact of benign prostatic hyperplasia and its treatments. In: Denis L, Griffiths K, Khoury S, et al, eds. *Fourth International Consultation on BPH, Proceedings.* Plymouth, UK: Health Publication Ltd, 1998:265–321.
3. Oishi K, Boyle P, Barry MJ, et al. Committee 1: Epidemiology and natural history of benign prostatic hyperplasia. In: Denis L, Griffiths K, Khoury S, et al, eds. *Fourth International Consultation on BPH, Proceedings.* Plymouth, UK: Health Publication Ltd, 1998:23–59.
4. Jacobsen SJ, Girman CJ, Guess HA, et al. Natural history of prostatism: longitudinal changes in voiding symptoms in community dwelling men. *J Urol* 1996;155:595–600.
5. Barry MJ, Fowler FJ, Bin L, et al. The natural history of patients with benign prostatic hyperplasia as diagnosed by North American urologists. *J Urol* 1997;157:10–15.
6. Jacobsen S, Jacobson D, Girman C, et al. Natural history of prostatism: risk factors for acute urinary retention. *J Urol* 1997;158:481–487.
7. McConnell J, Bruskewitz R, Walsh P, et al. The effect of finasteride on the risk of acute urinary retention and the need for surgical treatment among men with benign prostatic hyperplasia. *N Engl J Med* 1998;338:557–563.
8. Barry MJ, Fowler FJ Jr, O'Leary MP, et al. The American Urological Association symptom index for benign prostatic hyperplasia. *J Urol* 1992;148:1549–1557.
9. Djavan B, Marberger M. A meta-analysis on the efficacy and tolerability of α1-adrenoceptor antagonists in patients with lower urinary tract symptoms suggestive of benign prostatic obstruction. *Eur Urol* 1999;36:1–13. Search date 1998; primary source Medline.
10. Clifford GM, Farmer RDT. Medical therapy for benign prostatic hyperplasia: a review of the literature. *Eur Urol* 2000;38:2–19. Search date 1999; primary sources Medline, Embase, and the Cochrane Library.
11. Wilt TJ, MacDonald R, Nelson D. Tamsulosin for treating lower urinary tract symptoms compatible with benign prostatic obstruction: a systematic review of efficacy and adverse effects. *J Urol* 2002;167:177–183. Search date 2000; primary sources Medline, Embase, The Cochrane Library, Cochrane prostatic Disease and Urologic Malignancies Group Trial Register, and hand searched reference lists.
12. Wilt TJ, Howe W, MacDonald R. Terazosin for treating symptomatic benign prostatic obstruction: a systematic review of efficacy and adverse effects. *BJU Int* 2002;89:214–225. Search date: 2001; primary sources Medline, Embase, Cochrane Library, the Prostatic Diseases and Urological Malignancies Group specialised register, and reference lists from previous reviews.
13. Andersen M, Dahlstrand C, Hoye K. Double-blind trial of the efficacy and tolerability of doxazosin in the gastrointestinal therapeutic system, doxazosin standard, and placebo in patients with benign prostatic hyperplasia. *Eur Urol* 2000;38:400–409.
14. Roehrborn CG. Efficacy and safety of once-daily alfuzosin in the treatment of lower urinary tract symptoms and clinical benign prostatic hyperplasia: a randomized, placebo-controlled trial. *Urology* 2001;58:953–959.
15. Kirby RS, Roehrborn S, Boyle P, et al. Efficacy and tolerability of doxazosin and finasteride, alone or in combination, in treatment of symptomatic benign prostatic hyperplasia: the prospective European doxazosin and combination therapy (PREDICT) trial. *Urology* 2003;61:119–126.

16. Roehrborn CG, Oesterling JE, Auerbach S, et al. The Hytrin community assessment trial study: a one-year study of terazosin versus placebo in the treatment of men with symptomatic benign prostatic hyperplasia. *Urology* 1996;47:159–168.
17. McNeil SA, Daruwala PD, Mitchell IDC, et al. Sustained-release alfuzosin and trial without catheter after acute urinary retention: a prospective placebo-controlled trial. *BJU Int* 1999;84:622–627.
18. Buzelin JM, Herbert M, Blondin P, et al. Alpha-blocking treatment with alfuzosin in symptomatic benign prostatic hyperplasia: comparative study with prazosin. *Br J Urol* 1993;72:922–927.
19. Kirby RS, Andersen M, Gratzke P, et al. A combined analysis of double-blind trials of the efficacy and tolerability of doxazosin-gastrointestinal therapeutic system, doxazosin standard and placebo in patients with benign prostatic hyperplasia. *BJU Int* 2001;87:192–200.
20. Debruyne FMJ, Jardin A, Colloi D, et al. Sustained-release alfuzosin, finasteride and the combination of both in the treatment of benign prostatic hyperplasia. *Eur Urol* 1998;34:169–175.
21. Lee E. Comparison of tamsulosin and finasteride for lower urinary tract symptoms associated with benign prostatic hyperplasia in Korean patients. *J Int Med Res* 2002;30:584–590.
22. Lepor H, Williford WO, Barry MJ, et al. The efficacy of terazosin, finasteride, or both in benign prostatic hyperplasia. Veterans' Affairs cooperative studies benign prostatic hyperplasia study group. *N Engl J Med* 1996;335:533–539.
23. Hofner K, Claes H, De Reijke TM, et al. Tamsulosin 0.4 mg once daily: effect on sexual function in patients with lower urinary tract symptoms suggestive of benign prostatic obstruction. *Eur Urol* 1999;36:335–341.
24. Mobley D, Dias N, Levenstein M. Effects of doxazosin in patients with mild, intermediate, and severe benign prostatic hyperplasia. *Clin Ther* 1998;20:101–109.
25. Kaplan S, Kaplan N. Alpha-blockade: monotherapy for hypertension and benign prostatic hyperplasia. *Urology* 1996;48:541–550.
26. Roehrborn CG, Boyle P, Bergner D, et al. Serum prostate specific antigen and prostate volume predict long-term changes in symptoms and flow rate: results of a four-year, randomised trial comparing finasteride and placebo. *Urology* 1999:54;663–669.
27. Roehrborn CG, McConnell JD, Lieber M, et al. Serum prostate-specific antigen concentration is a powerful predictor of acute urinary retention and the need for surgery in men with clinical benign prostatic hyperplasia. *Urology* 1999;53:473–480.
28. Roehrborn CG, Bruskewitz R, Nickel GC, et al. Urinary retention in patients with BPH treated with finasteride or placebo over 4 years. *Eur Urol* 2000;37:528–536.
29. Kaplan S, Garvin D, Gilhooly P, et al. Impact of baseline symptom severity on future risk of benign prostatic hyperplasia-related outcomes and long-term response to finasteride. *Urology* 2000;56:610–616.
30. Roehrborn C, Boyle P, Nickel JC, et al. Efficacy and safety of a dual inhibitor of 5-alpha-reductase types 1 and 2 (Dutasteride) in men with benign prostatic hyperplasia. *Urology* 2003;60:434–441.
31. Andersen J, Nickel J, Marshall V, et al. Finasteride significantly reduces acute urinary retention and need for surgery in patients with symptomatic benign prostatic hyperplasia. *Urology* 1997;49:839–845.
32. Boyle P, Gould AL, Roehrborn CG. Prostate volume predicts outcome of treatment of benign prostatic hyperplasia with finasteride: meta-analysis of randomized clinical trials. *Urology* 1996;48:398–405.
33. Wasson J, Reda D, Bruskewitz R, et al. A comparison of transurethral surgery with watchful waiting for moderate symptoms of benign prostatic hyperplasia. *N Engl J Med* 1995;332:75–79.
34. Donovan JL, Peters T, Neal DE, et al. A randomized trial comparing transurethral resection of the prostate, laser therapy and conservative treatment of men with symptoms associated with benign prostatic enlargement: the ClasP study. *J Urol* 2000;164:65–70.
35. Flanigan RC, Reda DC, Wasson JH, et al. Five year outcome of surgical resection and watchful waiting for men with moderately symptomatic benign prostatic hyperplasia: a Department of Veterans' Affairs cooperative study. *J Urol* 1998;160:12–17.
36. Yang Q, Peters TJ, Donovan JL, et al. Transurethral incision compared with transurethral resection of the prostate for bladder outlet obstruction: a systematic review and meta-analysis of randomized controlled trials. *J Urol* 2001;165:1526–1532. Search date 1999; primary sources Medline, Embase, ISI, the Cochrane Library, and Cochrane Prostatic Diseases and Urologic Cancers Group Trial Register.
37. Wheelahan J, Scott NA, Cartmill R, et al. Minimally invasive laser techniques for prostatectomy: a systematic review. *BJU Int* 2000;86:805–815. Search date 1999; primary sources Medline, Embase, Current Contents, and the Cochrane Library.
38. Wheelahan J, Scott NA, Cartmill R, et al. Minimally invasive non-laser thermal techniques for prostatectomy: a systematic review. *BJU Int* 2000;86:977–988. Search date 1999; primary sources Medline, Embase, Current Contents, and the Cochrane Library.
39. Hoffman RM, MacDonald R, Slaton JW, et al. Laser prostatectomy versus transurethral resection for treating benign prostatic obstruction: a systematic review. *J Urol* 2003;169;210–215. Search date 2002; primary sources Medline, Cochrane Library, Prostatic Diseases and Urologic Cancers Group Registry, Science Citation Index and hand searches of reference lists of all identified articles and of *BJU International*, *The Journal of Urology* and *Urology* from 1998–2002.
40. McAllister WJ, Absalom MJ, Mir K, et al. Does endoscopic laser ablation of the prostate stand the test of time? Five-year test results from a multicentre randomised controlled trial of endoscopic laser ablation against transurethral resection of the prostate. *BJU Int* 2000;85:437–439.
41. Kupeli S, Yilmaz E, Soygur T, et al. Randomized study of transurethral resection of the prostate and combined transurethral resection and vaporization of the prostate as a therapeutic alternative in men with benign prostatic hyperplasia. *J Endourol* 2001;15:317–321.
42. Helke C, Manseck A, Hakenberg OW, et al. Is transurethral vaporesection of the prostate better than standard transurethral resection? *Eur Urol* 2001;39:551–557.
43. McAllister WJ, Karim O, Plail RO, et al. Transurethral electrovaporization of the prostate: is it any better than conventional transurethral resection of the prostate: *BJU Int* 2003;91:211–214.
44. Lu-Yao GL, Barry MJ, Chang CH, et al. Transurethral resection of the prostate among Medicare beneficiaries in the United States: time trends and outcomes. *Urology* 1994;44:692–698.
45. McConnell JD, Barry MJ, Bruskewitz RC, et al. *Direct treatment outcomes — complications. Benign prostatic hyperplasia: diagnosis and treatment.* Clinical Practice Guideline, Number 8. Rockville, Maryland: Agency for Health Care Policy and Research, Public Health Service, US Department of Health and Human Services, 1994:91–98.
46. McConnell JD, Barry MJ, Bruskewitz RC, et al. *Direct treatment outcomes — sexual dysfunction. Benign prostatic hyperplasia: diagnosis and treatment.* Clinical Practice Guideline, Number 8. Rockville, Maryland: Agency for Health Care Policy and Research, Public Health Service, US Department of Health and Human Services, 1994:99–103.
47. McConnell JD, Barry MJ, Bruskewitz RC, et al. *Direct treatment outcomes — urinary incontinence. Benign prostatic hyperplasia: diagnosis and treatment.* Clinical Practice Guideline, Number 8. Rockville, Maryland: Agency for Health Care Policy

and Research, Public Health Service, US Department of Health and Human Services, 1994:105–106.
48. Brookes ST, Donovan JL, Peters TJ, et al. Sexual dysfunction in men after treatment for lower urinary tract symptoms: evidence from randomized controlled trial. *BMJ* 2002;324:1059–1064.
49. Roehrborn C, Preminger G, Newhall P, et al. Microwave thermotherapy for benign prostatic hyperplasia with the Dornier Urowave: results of a randomized, double-blind, multicenter, sham-controlled trial. *Urology* 1998;51:19–28.
50. Larson T, Blute M, Bruskewitz R, et al. A high-efficiency microwave thermoablation system for the treatment of benign prostatic hyperplasia: results of a randomized, sham-controlled, prospective, double-blind, multicenter clinical trial. *Urology* 1998;51:731–742.
51. De la Rosette J, De Wildt M, Alivizatos G, et al. Transurethral microwave thermotherapy (TUMT) in benign prostatic hyperplasia: placebo versus TUMT. *Urology* 1994;44:58–63.
52. Francisca EA, D'Ancona FC, Meuleman EJ, et al. Sexual function following high energy microwave thermotherapy: results of a randomized controlled study comparing transurethral microwave thermotherapy to transurethral prostatic resection. *J Urol* 1999;161:486–490.
53. Djavan B, Roehrborn CG, Shariat S, et al. Prospective randomized comparison of high energy transurethral microwave thermotherapy versus alpha blocker treatment of patients with benign prostatic hyperplasia. *J Urol* 1999;161:139–143.
54. Djavan B, Seitz C, Roehrborn C, et al. Targeted transurethral microwave thermotherapy versus alpha-blockade in benign prostatic hyperplasia: outcomes at 18 months. *Urology* 2001;57:66–70.
55. Wilt TJ, Macdonald R, Ishani A. Beta-sitosterol for the treatment of benign prostatic hyperplasia: a systematic review. *BJU Int* 1999;83:976–983. Search date 1998; primary sources Medline, Embase, Phytodok, and the Cochrane Library.
56. Bruskewitz R, Issa M, Roehrborn C, et al. A prospective, randomized 1-year clinical trial comparing transurethral needle ablation to transurethral resection of the prostate for the treatment of symptomatic benign prostatic hyperplasia. *J Urol* 1998;159:1588–1594.
57. Wilt T, Ishani A, Stark G, et al. Serenoa repens for benign prostatic hyperplasia. In: The Cochrane Library, Issue 3, 2002. Oxford: Update Software. Search date 1997; primary sources Medline, Embase, Phytodok, and the Cochrane Library.
58. DeBruyne F, Koch G, Boyle P, et al. Comparison of a phytotherapeutic agent (Permixon) with an α blocker (Tamsulosin) in the treatment of benign prostatic hyperplasia: a 1-year randomized international study. *Eur Urol* 2002;41:497–507.
59. Glemain P, Coulange C, Billebaud T, et al. Tamsulosine avec ou sans Serenoa repens dans l'hypertrophie bénigne de la prostate: l'essai OCOS [in French]. *Prog Urol* 2002;12:395–403.
60. Macdonald R, Ishani A, Rutks I, et al. A systematic review of Cernilton for the treatment of benign prostatic hyperplasia. *BJU Int* 2000;85:836–841. Search date 1997; primary sources Embase and the Cochrane Library. Additional Medline search 1998.
61. Wilt T, Ishani A, MacDonald R, et al. Pygeum africanum for benign prostatic hyperplasia (Cochrane Review). In: The Cochrane Library, Issue 3, 2002. Oxford: Update Software. Search date 2000; primary sources Medline, Embase, Cochrane Library, Phytodok, hand searches of bibliographies, and contact with relevant manufacturers and researchers.

Robyn Webber
Consultant Urologist
Hairmyres Hospital
East Kilbride
Scotland

Competing interests: RW has been reimbursed by MSD, the manufacturers of finasteride, for attending several conferences. MB, none declared. CR has received a fee for consulting, speaking, research, and running educational programmes for MSD, GlaxoSmithKline, Sanofi-Synthélabo, and Urologix.

We would like to acknowledge the previous contributors of this chapter, including Michael Barry and Claus Roehrborn.

Chronic prostatitis

Search date July 2004

Thomas Jang and Anthony Schaeffer

QUESTIONS

INTERVENTIONS

See glossary G

Key Messages

Chronic bacterial prostatitis

- **α Blockers** We found no RCTs comparing α blockers versus placebo or no treatment. We found limited evidence from one RCT suggesting that adding α blockers to antimicrobials improved symptoms and reduced recurrence compared with antimicrobials alone.
- **Local injection of antimicrobials** We found no RCTs comparing local injection of antimicrobials with placebo or no treatment. One small RCT found that anal submucosal injection of amikacin improved symptom scores and bacterial eradication rates at 3 months compared with intramuscular amikacin.
- **Oral antimicrobial drugs** We found no RCTs comparing oral antimicrobial drugs versus placebo or no treatment. Two RCTs found no significant difference between ciprofloxacin and other quinolones (levofloxacin or lomefloxacin) in rates of clinical success or bacteriological cure at 6 months. Retrospective observational studies report cure rates of 0–88% depending on the drug used and the duration of treatment.
- **Radical prostatectomy** We found no RCTs on the effects of radical prostatectomy.
- **Transurethral resection** We found no RCTs on the effects of transurethral resection.

Chronic abacterial prostatitis

- **α Blockers** Two small RCTs identified by a systematic review and three small subsequent RCTs found limited evidence that α blockers improved quality of life and symptoms compared with placebo. The RCTs may have been too small to detect other clinically important differences.
- **5α reductase inhibitors** One RCT identified by a systematic review provided insufficient evidence about the effects of 5α reductase inhibitors compared with placebo in men with chronic abacterial prostatitis.

- **Allopurinol** One RCT identified by a systematic review provided insufficient evidence about the effects of allopurinol compared with placebo in men with chronic abacterial prostatitis.
- **Anti-inflammatory medications** One RCT identified by a systematic review provided insufficient evidence about the effects of anti-inflammatory medications compared with placebo or no treatment in men with chronic abacterial prostatitis.
- **Biofeedback** We found no RCTs on the effects of biofeedback.
- **Prostatic massage** We found no RCTs on the effects of prostatic massage.
- **Sitz baths** We found no RCTs on the effects of Sitz baths.
- **Transurethral microwave thermotherapy** One systematic review found limited evidence from one small RCT suggesting that transurethral microwave thermotherapy improved quality of life at 3 months and symptoms over 21 months compared with sham treatment. However, we were unable to draw reliable conclusions from this one small study.

DEFINITION **Chronic bacterial prostatitis** is characterised by a positive culture of expressed prostatic secretions. It may cause symptoms such as suprapubic, lower back, or perineal pain, or mild urgency, frequency, and dysuria, and may be associated with recurrent urinary tract infections. However, it may also be asymptomatic. **Chronic abacterial prostatitis**, or chronic pelvic pain syndrome (CPPS), is characterised by pelvic or perineal pain in the absence of pathogenic bacteria in expressed prostatic secretions. It is often associated with irritative and obstructive voiding symptoms including urgency, frequency, hesitancy, and poor interrupted flow. Symptoms can also include pain in the suprapubic region, lower back, penis, testes, or scrotum. Chronic abacterial prostatitis may be inflammatory (white cells present in prostatic secretions) or non-inflammatory (white cells absent in prostatic secretions).[1]

INCIDENCE/ PREVALENCE One community based study in the USA (58 955 visits by men ≥ 18 years to office based physicians) estimated that 9% of men have a diagnosis of chronic prostatitis at any one time.[2] Another study found that, of men with genitourinary symptoms, 8% presenting to urologists and 1% presenting to primary care physicians are diagnosed with chronic prostatitis.[3] Most cases of chronic prostatitis are abacterial. Acute bacterial prostatitis, although easy to diagnose, is rare.

AETIOLOGY/ RISK FACTORS Organisms commonly implicated in bacterial prostatitis include *Escherichia coli*, other Gram negative enterobacteriaceae, occasionally *Pseudomonas* species, and rarely Gram positive enterococci. The cause of abacterial prostatitis is unclear, although it has been suggested that it may be caused by undocumented infections with *Chlamydia trachomatis*,[4] *Ureaplasma urealyticum*,[5] *Mycoplasma hominis*,[6] and *Trichomonas vaginalis*.[7] Other factors might also be involved, including inflammation,[8] autoimmunity,[9] hormonal imbalances,[10] pelvic floor tension myalgia,[11] intra-prostatic urinary reflux,[12] and psychological disturbances.[13]

PROGNOSIS The natural history of untreated chronic bacterial and abacterial prostatitis remains ill-defined. Chronic bacterial prostatitis may cause recurrent urinary tract infections in men.[14] Furthermore, several investigators have reported an association between chronic bacterial prostatitis and infertility.[15] The sequelae of chronic abacterial prostatitis are similar to those of chronic bacterial prostatitis. Fertility may be decreased.[16] One study found that chronic abacterial prostatitis had an impact on quality of life similar to that from angina, Crohn's disease, or a previous myocardial infarction.[17]

AIMS OF INTERVENTION To relieve symptoms and eliminate infection where present, with minimum adverse effects.

OUTCOMES Symptom improvement (symptom scores, bother scores); quality of life; urodynamics; rates of bacteriological cure (clearance of previously documented organisms from prostatic secretions); adverse effects of treatment.

METHODS *Clinical Evidence* search and appraisal July 2004.

QUESTION **What are the effects of treatments for chronic bacterial prostatitis?**

OPTION **ORAL ANTIMICROBIAL DRUGS**

We found no RCTs comparing oral antimicrobial drugs versus placebo or no treatment. Two RCTs found no significant difference between ciprofloxacin and other quinolones (levofloxacin or lomefloxacin) in rates of clinical success or bacteriological cure at 6 months. Retrospective observational studies report cure rates of 0–88% depending on the drug used and the duration of treatment.

Benefits: **Versus placebo or no antimicrobials:** We found no systematic review or RCTs. **Oral antimicrobials versus each other:** We found no systematic review but found two RCTs.[18,19] The first RCT (182 men) compared lomefloxacin 400 mg daily versus ciprofloxacin 500 mg twice daily for 4 weeks.[18] It found no significant difference between lomefloxacin and ciprofloxacin in rates of clinical success or bacteriological cure after 6 months (clinical success: 61/93 [81.3%] with lomefloxacin *v* 64/89 [88.9%] with ciprofloxacin; difference –7.6%, 95% CI –23.6% to +6.0%; biological eradication: 49/93 [62.8%] with lomefloxacin *v* 54/89 [72.0%] with ciprofloxacin; difference –9.2%, 95% CI –26.0% to +6.0%). Clinical success was defined as clinical cure (baseline symptoms completely resolved) or improvement (symptoms improved but not completely resolved). The second RCT (377 men) compared levofloxacin 500 mg daily versus ciprofloxacin 500 mg twice daily for 28 days.[19] It found no significant difference between levofloxacin and ciprofloxacin in rates of clinical success or bacteriological cure after 6 months (clinical success defined as complete resolution of symptoms or clear improvement without need for additional antibiotics: 102/136 [75.0%] with levofloxacin *v* 91/125 [72.8%] with ciprofloxacin; difference –2.2%, 95% CI –13.3% to +8.9%; biological eradication: 102/136 [75.0%] with levofloxacin *v* 96/125 [76.8%] with ciprofloxacin; difference –1.8%, 95% CI –9.0% to +12.6%).

Harms: The first RCT comparing lomefloxacin with ciprofloxacin found that the most common adverse effects with both treatments were gastrointestinal disorders (5/93 [5%] with lomefloxacin *v* 8/89 [9%] with ciprofloxacin; P value not reported). Adverse effects caused the premature withdrawal of a similar proportion of men on both treatments (5/93 [5%] with lomefloxacin *v* 4/89 [4%] with ciprofloxacin).[18] The second RCT found similar proportions of men reporting at least one treatment related adverse event with ciprofloxacin and levofloxacin (87/197 [44%] with levofloxacin *v* 67/180 [37%] with ciprofloxacin; P value not reported).[19] It found that the most common adverse effects with both treatments were gastrointestinal events (19% with levofloxacin *v* 17% with ciprofloxacin; P value not reported).

Comment: We found data from an observational series about the cure rates of different antibiotics. These data do not compare antimicrobials versus placebo, no treatment, or other treatment. **Trimethoprim–sulfamethoxazole:** One non-systematic review identified eight retrospective case series in 1140 men with bacteriologically confirmed prostatitis treated with trimethoprim–sulfamethoxazole (sulphamethoxazole; 160 mg/800 mg twice daily for 10–140 days).[20] The studies reported cure rates of 0–71%. Over 30% of men were cured when treated for at least 90 days. The review did not report adverse effects. **Quinolones:** One review summarised three retrospective case series in 106 men treated with norfloxacin (400 mg twice daily for 10, 28, and 174 days).[21] The studies reported cure rates of 64–88%. We also found six retrospective case series in 141 men treated with ciprofloxacin (250–500 mg twice daily for 14–259 days), with cure rates of 60–75%. **Amoxicillin/clavulanic acid and clindamycin:** One case series included 50 men who were resistant to empirical treatment with quinolone. The expressed prostatic secretions from 24 of these men exhibited high colony counts of Gram positive and Gram negative anaerobic bacteria, either alone (18 men) or in combination with aerobic bacteria (6 men). After treatment with either amoxicillin (amoxycillin)/clavulanic acid or clindamycin for 3–6 weeks, all men had a decrease or total elimination of symptoms and no anaerobic bacteria were detected in prostatic secretions.[22] Higher cure rates with quinolones may be explained by greater penetration into the prostate.[23] We reviewed only studies that used standard methods to localise infection to the prostate.[24]

OPTION LOCAL INJECTION OF ANTIMICROBIALS

We found no RCTs comparing local injection of antimicrobials with placebo or no treatment. One small RCT found that anal submucosal injection of amikacin improved symptom scores and bacterial eradication rates at 3 months compared with intramuscular amikacin.

Benefits: We found no RCTs comparing local injection of antimicrobials versus placebo or no treatment. We found one small RCT (50 men with prostatic secretions sensitive to amikacin), which compared anal submucosal injection of amikacin 400 mg daily for 10 days versus intramuscular amikacin 400 mg daily for 10 days.[25] It found that anal submucosal injection of amikacin significantly improved NIH–CPSI**G** score and significantly increased bacteriological cure rates compared with intramuscular amikacin at 3 months (NIH–CPSI: 9.0 with submucosal injection *v* 22.5 with intramuscular injection; $P < 0.05$; negative bacterial culture: 28/30 [93%] with submucosal injection *v* 7/20 [35%] with intramuscular injection; $P < 0.05$).

Harms: The RCT comparing anal submucosal and intramuscular amikacin found no obvious adverse effects other than the passage of slightly blood stained faeces in 3/30 [10%] men after the first anal submucosal injection.[25] Infection is a theoretical risk of this invasive procedure.

Comment: One small cohort study (24 men with refractory chronic bacterial prostatitis) found that eradication of infection was eventually achieved after an unstated period in 15 men with gentamicin 160 mg plus cefazolin (cephazolin) 3 g injected directly into the prostate through the perineum.[26]

OPTION ALPHA BLOCKERS

We found no RCTs comparing α blockers versus placebo or no treatment. We found limited evidence from one RCT suggesting that adding α blockers to antimicrobials improved symptoms and reduced recurrence compared with antimicrobials alone.

Benefits: **Alpha blockers versus placebo:** We found no systematic review or RCTs comparing the α blocker, tamsulosin, versus placebo or no treatment. **Alpha blockers plus antimicrobials versus antimicrobials alone:** We found one RCT (64 men with bacterial prostatitis; mean age 48 years) comparing α blockers (either 1–2 mg/day terazosin, 2.5 mg/day terazosin, or 2.5 mg alfuzosin once or twice daily) plus antimicrobials versus antimicrobials alone.[27] It found that α blockers plus antimicrobials significantly increased symptomatic improvement and significantly reduced recurrence rates compared with antimicrobials alone (recurrence rates assessed by culture of expressed prostatic secretion; $P = 0.02$; no RR or CI reported; 5 people withdrew from treatment).

Harms: No adverse effects of α blockers were reported.[27]

Comment: None.

OPTION TRANSURETHRAL RESECTION

We found no RCTs on the effects of transurethral resection.

Benefits: We found no systematic review, RCTs, or prospective cohort studies.

Harms: One RCT in men with benign prostatic hypertrophy found no difference in the incidence of impotence or urinary incontinence with transurethral resection or watchful waiting.[28]

Comment: One retrospective study reported 40–50% cure rates in 50 men with chronic prostatitis treated with transurethral resection. However, proof of bacterial prostatitis was not obtained in many men.[29]

OPTION RADICAL PROSTATECTOMY

We found no RCTs on the effects of radical prostatectomy.

Benefits: We found no systematic review or RCTs.

Harms: Case series have found that radical prostatectomy can cause impotence (9–75% depending upon age)[30] and varying degrees of urinary stress incontinence.[31] Other potential harms include those associated with any open surgery.

Comment: We found one report of radical prostatectomy in two young men whose refractory bacterial prostatitis caused relapsing haemolytic crises.[32]

QUESTION What are the effects of treatments for chronic abacterial prostatitis?

OPTION ALPHA BLOCKERS

Two small RCTs identified by a systematic review and three small subsequent RCTs found limited evidence that α blockers improved quality of life and symptoms compared with placebo. The RCTs may have been too small to detect other clinically important differences.

Benefits: **Versus placebo:** We found one systematic review (search date 1999, 2 RCTs, 50 men)[33] and three subsequent RCTs.[34–36] The first RCT identified by the review (20 people) compared alfuzosin 2.5 mg three times daily versus placebo. It found that alfuzosin significantly improved maximal flow time from baseline compared with placebo (15.4–20.3 mL/second with alfuzosin *v* 13.9–15.6 mL/second with placebo; $P = 0.01$; RR not reported).[37] It found no significant difference in other outcomes (insufficient information was presented to assess comparative effects on symptom scores). The second RCT identified by the review (30 people) found that an α blocker (phenoxybenzamine 10 mg twice daily) significantly improved pain after prostatic massage🅖 compared with placebo at 6 weeks ($P < 0.05$).[33] The first subsequent RCT (86 men) compared terazosin (with dose escalation from 1–5 mg/day) versus placebo for 14 weeks.[34] It found that terazosin significantly improved quality of life and significantly reduced pain at 14 weeks compared with placebo [NIH–CPSI🅖] quality of life score 0–2: 24/43 [56%] with terazosin *v* 14/43 [33%] with placebo; P = 0.03; reduction NIH–CPSI pain score > 50% from baseline: 26/43 [60%] with terazosin *v* 16/43 [37%] with placebo; P = 0.03). It found no significant difference between terazosin and placebo in peak urinary flow rate or post-void residual urine (change in peak flow rate: 15.4–18.7 mL/second with terazosin *v* 18.1–19.7 mL/second with placebo; P value not reported; change in residual volume: 24.8–17.1 mL with terazosin *v* 20.6–16.0 mL with placebo; P value not reported).[34] The second subsequent RCT (70 men) compared three treatments for 6 months with follow up for a further 6 months: alfuzosin 5 mg twice daily, standard treatment (hot Sitz baths🅖 plus anti-inflammatory drugs), and placebo (see comment below).[35] However, men were only randomly allocated to alfuzosin and placebo, the 30 men who did not wish to be entered into the randomisation received standard treatment. The RCT found that alfuzosin improved symptoms and reduced pain after 6 months of treatment compared with placebo (change in total NIH–CPSI pain score from baseline: –9.9 with alfuzosin *v* –3.8 with placebo; change in NIH–CPSI pain score from baseline: –5.1 with alfuzosin *v* –1.1 with placebo; P values not reported). This effect was sustained at 12 months (6 months after treatment finished; change in NIH–CPSI total score from baseline: –3.5 with alfuzosin *v* –0.1 with placebo; P value not reported).[35] The third RCT (58 men < 55 years) compared tamsulosin versus placebo.[36] It found that tamsulosin significantly improved symptoms compared with placebo after 45 days (difference in change in NIH-CPSI scores from baseline –3.6, 95% CI –7.0 to –0.3; P = 0.04 in favour of tamsulosin). Subgroup analyses found that the relative benefit of tamsulosin was greater in men with more severe symptoms at baseline. **α Blockers versus each other:** We found no systematic review or RCTs.

Harms: The first RCT identified by the review reported a transient decrease in systolic blood pressure in four people and a slight decrease in libido in two people all treated with alfuzosin.[33] The first subsequent RCT found that terazosin significantly increased treatment related adverse effects compared with placebo (18/43 [42%] with terazosin *v* 9/43 [21%] with placebo; P = 0.04).[34] The most common adverse effects, dizziness and asthenia, were more common with terazosin (dizziness: 7/43 [16%] with terazosin *v* 2/43 [5%] with placebo; asthenia: 7/43 [16%] with terazosin *v* 3/43 [7%] with placebo; P values not reported). The second subsequent RCT found no withdrawals because of adverse effects with any treatment (alfuzosin, placebo, or standard treatment).[35] It reported that one man [5%] experienced heartburn and four men [21%] experienced decreased ejaculate volume with alfuzosin. The third RCT did not report on specific adverse effects.[36]

Comment: Two of the subsequent RCTs showed that duration of treatment is important to obtain maximum response. However, before definitive conclusions can be made, adequately powered studies with greater recruitment need to be performed.

OPTION 5 ALPHA REDUCTASE INHIBITORS

One RCT identified by a systematic review provided insufficient evidence about the effects of 5α reductase inhibitors compared with placebo in men with chronic abacterial prostatitis.

Benefits: We found one systematic review (search date 1999, 1 RCT, 41 men), which compared finasteride versus placebo.[33] The RCT found that, although symptom scores decreased significantly with finasteride after 1 year, there was no significant difference in pain between finasteride and placebo.[38] The RCT was small and had low power (31/41 [75%] of men were allocated to finasteride *v* 10/41 [25%] of men were allocated to placebo).

Harms: Three men treated with finasteride reported partial impotence compared with none in the placebo group.[38]

Comment: Finasteride is known to decrease prostate volume (as it did in this study; $P < 0.03$), but it is unclear how this relates to symptoms of prostatitis.[38]

OPTION ANTI-INFLAMMATORY MEDICATIONS

One RCT identified by a systematic review provided insufficient evidence about the effects of anti-inflammatory medications compared with placebo or no treatment in men with chronic abacterial prostatitis.

Benefits: We found one systematic review (search date 1999, 1 RCT, 30 men).[33] The RCT compared pentosan polysulfate sodium 100 mg twice daily versus placebo. Outcomes included symptom changes by physician rating, symptom score, and uroflowmetry. The RCT found no significant difference in either physician rated improvement or in local symptom scores at 3 months (physician rated improvement: 7/10 [70%] with pentosan polysulfate sodium *v* placebo 5/14 [36%] with placebo; RR 2.00, 95% CI 0.87 to 4.40; number of people reporting improvement in symptom score: 5/10 [50%] with pentosan polysulfate sodium *v* 6/14 [43%] with placebo; RR 1.2, 95% CI 0.5 to 2.8).[39] Six people were excluded from the analysis for non-compliance or having bacterial prostatitis (analysis was not intention to treat). The RCT may have been too small to rule out important clinical differences.

Harms: The RCT found that two men given pentosan polysulfate sodium reported diarrhoea.[33] No men treated with placebo developed gastrointestinal adverse symptoms.

Comment: "Physician rated improvement" is not an objective measurement. There was no significant difference between experimental and control groups with other, more objective and standardised, outcomes.

OPTION TRANSURETHRAL MICROWAVE THERMOTHERAPY

One systematic review found limited evidence from one small RCT suggesting that transurethral microwave thermotherapy improved quality of life at 3 months and symptoms over 21 months compared with sham treatment. However, we were unable to draw reliable conclusions from this one small study.

Benefits: We found one systematic review (search date 1999,[33] 1 double blind RCT,[40] 20 men). The RCT compared transurethral microwave thermotherapy versus sham treatment.[40] It found that thermotherapy significantly improved quality of life at 3 months compared with sham treatment (scale 0–10; quality of life improved from 4.4 to 3.0 with transurethral microwave thermotherapy *v* unchanged at 5.2 with sham treatment; $P < 0.05$). It found that thermotherapy significantly increased the proportion of men with improvement of a subjective global assessment by more than 50% over a mean of 21 months compared with sham treatment (7/10 [70%] with transurethral microwave thermotherapy *v* 1/10 [10%] with sham treatment; RR 7, 95% CI 1 to 47; NNT 2, 95% CI 2 to 6). The review found no good evidence on the effects of thermotherapy on cure or recurrence rate.

Harms: Four men complained of transient (resolved in 3 weeks) adverse reactions, including haematuria (2 men), urinary tract infection, impotence, urinary retention, urinary incontinence, and premature ejaculation (each occurring in 1 man).[40] However, the RCT did not report if the men with adverse events were treated with active treatment or sham treatment.

Comment: Thermotherapy caused persistent elevation of leucocytes in the prostatic fluid, which could indicate tissue damage.

OPTION ALLOPURINOL

One RCT identified by a systematic review provided insufficient evidence about the effects of allopurinol compared with placebo in men with chronic abacterial prostatitis.

Benefits: We found one systematic review (search date 2000,[41] 1 RCT,[42] 54 men). The RCT compared treatment with allopurinol 300 or 600 mg daily versus placebo. Thirty four men (63%) completed the study, which lasted 240 days. All recorded data were used in the analysis. The RCT found allopurinol significantly reduced the "degree of discomfort" score (pretreatment score = 0; score –1.1 with 300 and 600 mg allopurinol combined *v* –0.2 with placebo; P = 0.02).[42]

Harms: None of the men receiving allopurinol reported any significant adverse events, but the RCT did not explain what constitutes a significant adverse event; 55% of people on placebo and 68% of people on allopurinol completed the trial.[42]

Comment: The symptom score was not validated and the high withdrawal rate makes the results difficult to interpret.[42]

OPTION PROSTATIC MASSAGE

We found no RCTs on the effects of prostatic massage.

Benefits: We found no systematic review or RCTs.

Harms: We found no RCTs.

Comment: None.

OPTION SITZ BATHS

We found no RCTs on the effects of Sitz baths.

Benefits: We found no systematic review or RCTs.

Harms: We found no RCTs.

Comment: None.

OPTION BIOFEEDBACK

We found no RCTs on the effects of biofeedback.

Benefits: We found no systematic review or RCTs.

Harms: We found no RCTs.

Comment: None.

Chronic prostatitis

GLOSSARY

Biofeedback Training that helps people to consciously change the vital functions of the body, such as heart rate, which are normally controlled unconsciously.

NIH–CPSI (National Institute of Health–Chronic Prostatitis Symptom Index) Includes nine items across three domains: pain (4 items; 0–21); urinary symptoms (2 items; 0–10), and quality of life impact (3 items; 0–12). In all domains, higher scores indicate worse outcomes.

Prostatic massage Digital pressure applied to the prostate through the rectum.

Sitz bath A warm water bath taken in the sitting position. The water covers only the hips and buttocks.

Substantive changes

α Blockers One RCT added;[36] benefits and harms data enhanced. Categorisation unchanged.

REFERENCES

1. Nickel JC, Nyberg LM, Hennenfent M. Research guidelines for chronic prostatitis: consensus report from the first National Institutes of Health International Prostatitis Collaborative Network. *Urology* 1999;54:229–233.
2. Roberts RO, Lieber MM, Rhodes T, et al. Prevalence of a physician-assigned diagnosis of prostatitis: the Olmsted County study of urinary symptoms and health status among men. *Urology* 1998;51:578–584.
3. Collins MM, Stafford, RS, O'Leary MP, et al. How common is prostatitis? A national survey of physician visits. *J Urol* 1998;159:1224–1228.
4. Poletti F, Medici MC, Alinovi A, et al. Isolation of *Chlamydia trachomatis* from the prostatic cells in patients affected by nonacute abacterial prostatitis. *J Urol* 1985;134:691–693.
5. Weidner W, Brunner H, Krause W. Quantitative culture of *Ureaplasma urealyticum* in patients with chronic prostatitis or prostatosis. *J Urol* 1980;124:622–625.
6. Brunner H, Weidner W, Schiefer HG. Studies on the role of *Ureaplasma urealyticum* and *Mycoplasma hominis* in prostatitis. *J Infect Dis* 1983;147:807–813.
7. Skerk V, Schonwald S, Granic J, et al. Chronic prostatitis caused by *Trichomonas vaginalis* – diagnosis and treatment. *J Chemother* 2002;14:537–538.
8. Jang TL, Schaeffer AJ. The role of cytokines in prostatitis. *World J Urol* 2003;21:95–99. [Erratum in: *World J Urol* 2003;70:223.]
9. Alexander RB, Brady F, Ponniah S. Autoimmune prostatitis: evidence of T cell reactivity with normal prostatic proteins. *Urology* 1997;50:893–899.
10. Naslund MJ, Strandberg JD, Coffey DS. The role of androgens and estrogens in the pathogenesis of experimental nonbacterial prostatitis. *J Urol* 1988;140:1049–1053.
11. Nadler RB. Bladder training biofeedback and pelvic floor myalgia. *Urology* 2002;60:42–43.
12. Kirby RS, Lowe D, Bultitude MI, et al. Intra-prostatic urinary reflux: an aetiological factor in abacterial prostatitis. *Br J Urol* 1982;54:729–731.
13. de la Rosette JJ, Ruijgrok MC, Jeuken JM, et al. Personality variables involved in chronic prostatitis. *Urology* 1993;42:654–662.
14. Roberts RO, Lieber MM, Bostwick DG, et al. A review of clinical and pathological prostatitis syndromes. *Urology* 1997;49:809–821.
15. Giamarellou H, Tympanidis K, Bitos NA, et al. Infertility and chronic prostatitis. *Andrologia* 1984;16:417–422.
16. Leib Z, Bartoov B, Eltes F, et al. Reduced semen quality caused by chronic abacterial prostatitis: an enigma or reality? *Fertil Steril* 1994;61:1109–1116.
17. Wenninger K, Heiman JR, Rothman I, et al. Sickness impact of chronic nonbacterial prostatitis and its correlates. *J Urol* 1996;155:965–968.
18. Naber KG. Lomefloxacin versus ciprofloxacin in the treatment of chronic bacterial prostatitis. *Int J Antimicrob Agents* 2002;20:18–27.
19. Bundrick W, Heron SP, Ray P, et al. Levofloxacin versus ciprofloxacin in the treatment of chronic bacterial prostatitis: a randomized double-blind multicenter study. *Urology* 2003;62:537–541.
20. Hanus PM, Danzinger LH. Treatment of chronic bacterial prostatitis. *Clin Pharmacol* 1984;3:49–55.
21. Naber KG, Sorgel F, Kees F, et al. Norfloxacin concentration in prostatic adenoma tissue (patients) and in prostatic fluid in patients and volunteers. 15th International Congress of Chemotherapy, Landsberg. In: Weidner N, Madsen PO, Schiefer HG, eds. *Prostatitis: etiopathology, diagnosis and therapy*. New York: Springer Verlag, 1987.
22. Szoke I, Torok L, Dosa E, et al. The possible role of anaerobic bacteria in chronic prostatitis. *Int J Androl* 1998;21:163–168.
23. Cox CE. Ofloxacin in the management of complicated urinary tract infections, including prostatitis. *Am J Med* 1980;87(suppl 6c):61–68.
24. Meares EM, Stamey TA. Bacteriologic localization patterns in bacterial prostatitis and urethritis. *Invest Urol* 1968;5:492–518.
25. Hu WL, Zhong SZ, He HX. Treatment of chronic bacterial prostatitis with amikacin through anal submucosal injection. *Asian J Androl* 2002;4:163–167.
26. Baert L, Leonard A. Chronic bacterial prostatitis: 10 years of experience with local antibiotics. *J Urol* 1988;140:755–757.
27. Barbalias GA, Nikiforidis G, Liatsikos EN. Alpha-blockers for the treatment of chronic prostatitis in combination with antibiotics. *J Urol* 1998;159:883–887.
28. Wasson JH, Reda DJ, Bruskewitz RC, et al. A comparison of transurethral surgery with watchful waiting for moderate symptoms of benign prostatic hyperplasia. *N Engl J Med* 1995;332:75–79.
29. Smart CJ, Jenkins JD, Lloyd RS. The painful prostate. *Br J Urol* 1975;47:861–869.
30. Quinlan DM, Epstein JI, Carter BS, et al. Sexual function following radical prostatectomy: influence of preservation of neurovascular bundles. *J Urol* 1991;145:998–1002.
31. Steiner MS, Morton RA, Walsh PC. Impact of radical prostatectomy on urinary continence. *J Urol* 1991;145:512–515.
32. Davis BE, Weigel JW. Adenocarcinoma of the prostate discovered in 2 young patients following total prostatovesiculectomy for refractory prostatitis. *J Urol* 1990;144:744–745.
33. Collins M, MacDonald R, Wilt T. Diagnosis and treatment of chronic abacterial prostatitis: a systematic review. *Ann Intern Med* 2000;133:367–368. Search date 1999; primary sources Medline, The Cochrane Library, hand searches of bibliographies, and contact with an expert.

34. Cheah PY, Liong ML, Yuen KH, et al. Terazosin therapy for chronic prostatitis/chronic pelvic pain syndrome: a randomized, placebo controlled trial. *J Urol* 2003;169:592–596.
35. Mehik A, Alas P, Nickel JC, et al. Alfuzosin treatment for chronic prostatitis/chronic pelvic pain syndrome: a prospective, randomized, double-blind, placebo-controlled, pilot study. *Urology* 2003;62:425–429.
36. Nickel JC, Narayan P, McKay J, et al. Treatment of chronic prostatitis/chronic pelvic pain syndrome with tamsulosin: a randomized double blind trial. *J Urol* 2004;171:1594–1597.
37. de la Rosette JJ, Karthaus HF, van Kerrebroeck PE, et al. Research in "prostatitis syndromes": the use of alfuzosin (a new alpha 1-receptor-blocking agent) in patients mainly presenting with micturition complaints of an irritative nature and confirmed urodynamic abnormalities. *Eur Urol* 1992;22:222–227.
38. Leskinen M, Lukkarinen O, Marttila T. Effects of finasteride in patients with inflammatory chronic pelvic pain syndrome: a double-blind, placebo-controlled, pilot study. *Urology* 1999;53:502–505.
39. Wédren H. Effects of sodium pentosanpolysulphate on symptoms related to chronic non-bacterial prostatitis. *Scand J Urol Nephrol* 1987;21:81–88.
40. Nickel J, Sorensen R. Transurethral microwave thermotherapy for nonbacterial prostatitis: a randomized double-blind sham controlled study using new prostatitis specific assessment questionnaires. *J Urol* 1996;155:1950–1955.
41. McNaughton Collins M, MacDonald R, Wilt T. Interventions for chronic abacterial prostatitis. In: The Cochrane Library, Issue 2, 2004. Chichester, UK: John Wiley & Sons, Ltd. Search date 2000; primary sources Medline, The Cochrane Library, hand searches of bibliographies of identified articles and reviews, and contact with an expert.
42. Persson B, Ronquist G, Ekblom M. Ameliorative effect of allopurinol on nonbacterial prostatitis: a parallel double-blind controlled study. *J Urol* 1996;155:961–964.

Anthony Schaeffer
Professor and Chair
Department of Urology
Northwestern University Medical School
Chicago
USA

Thomas Jang
Department of Urology
Northwestern University Feinberg School of Medicine
Chicago
USA

Competing interests: None declared.

Erectile dysfunction

Search date August 2003

Robyn Webber

QUESTIONS

INTERVENTIONS

Key Messages

- **Intracavernosal alprostadil** One large RCT found that intracavernosal alprostadil increased the chances of a satisfactory erection compared with placebo. One small RCT found limited evidence that vacuum devices were as effective as intracavernosal alprostadil injection for rigidity but not for orgasm.
- **Intraurethral alprostadil** One large RCT (in men who had previously responded to alprostadil) found limited evidence that intraurethral alprostadil (prostaglandin E1) increased the chances of successful sexual intercourse and at least one orgasm over 3 months compared with placebo. About a third of men suffered penile ache. We found no direct comparisons of intraurethral alprostadil versus either intracavernosal alprostadil or oral drug treatments.
- **Sildenafil** One systematic review and 15 subsequent RCTs have found that sildenafil improves erections and increases rates of successful intercourse compared with placebo. Adverse effects, including headaches, flushing, and dyspepsia, are reported in up to a quarter of men. Deaths have been reported in men on concomitant treatment with oral nitrates.
- **Yohimbine** One systematic review found that yohimbine improves self reported sexual function and penile rigidity at 2–10 weeks compared with placebo. Transient adverse effects are reported in up to a third of men.
- **Topical alprostadil** Two quasi randomised trials found limited evidence that topical alprostadil increased the number of men with erections sufficient for intercourse compared with placebo but was commonly associated with skin irritation.
- **L-arginine** One small RCT found no significant difference in sexual function between L-arginine and placebo, but it may have been too small to exclude a clinically important difference.
- **Penile prostheses** We found no RCTs of penile prostheses in men with erectile dysfunction.
- **Trazodone** One small RCT found no significant difference in erections or libido with trazodone compared with placebo, but it may have been too small to exclude a clinically important difference.
- **Vacuum devices** Vacuum devices have not been adequately assessed in RCTs. One small RCT found limited evidence that they were as effective as intracavernosal alprostadil (prostaglandin E1) injections for rigidity but not for orgasm.

Clin Evid 2005;13:1120–1127.

DEFINITION Erectile dysfunction has largely replaced the term "impotence". It is defined as the persistent inability to obtain or maintain sufficient rigidity of the penis to allow satisfactory sexual performance.

INCIDENCE/ PREVALENCE We found little good epidemiological information, but one cross sectional study found that age is the variable most strongly associated with erectile dysfunction and that up to 30 million men in the USA may be affected.[1] Even among men in their 40s, nearly 40% report at least occasional difficulty obtaining or maintaining erection, whereas this approaches 70% in 70 year olds.

AETIOLOGY/ RISK FACTORS About 80% of cases of erectile dysfunction are believed to have an organic cause, the rest being psychogenic in origin. Risk factors include increasing age, smoking, and obesity. Erectile problems fall into three categories: failure to initiate; failure to fill, caused by insufficient arterial inflow into the penis to allow engorgement and tumescence because of vascular insufficiency; and failure to store because of veno-occlusive dysfunction. Erectile dysfunction is a recognised adverse effect of a wide variety of pharmaceutical agents.

PROGNOSIS We found no good evidence on prognosis in untreated organic erectile dysfunction.

AIMS OF INTERVENTION To restore satisfactory erections with minimal adverse effects.

OUTCOMES Patient and partner self reports of satisfaction and sexual function, objective tests of penile rigidity, and adverse effects of treatment.

METHODS *Clinical Evidence* search and appraisal August 2003.

QUESTION What are the effects of treatments?

OPTION YOHIMBINE

One systematic review found that yohimbine improves self reported sexual function and penile rigidity at 2–10 weeks compared with placebo. Transient adverse effects are reported in up to a third of men.

Benefits: **Versus placebo:** We found one systematic review (search date 1997, 7 RCTs, 11–100 men with erectile dysfunction, defined variously as organic, psychogenic, and of unknown cause) that compared yohimbine versus placebo.[2] Duration of treatment ranged from 2–10 weeks, and outcomes varied from self reported change in sexual function to objective tests of penile rigidity. The RCTs found positive responses in significantly more men who took yohimbine than in those who took placebo (34–73% *v* 9–45%; OR 3.85, 95% CI 2.22 to 6.67; absolute numbers not reported). One subsequent placebo controlled, crossover trial (22 men, randomisation not mentioned) that compared a single daily dose of yohimbine 100 mg for 30 days versus placebo found no significant difference between treatments in erectile function.[3]

Harms: The review found that adverse events were reported in 10–30% of men who received yohimbine compared with 5–16% with placebo (significance not reported) and were generally mild, including agitation, anxiety, headache, mild increase in blood pressure, increased urinary output, and gastrointestinal upset.[2] In the small subsequent trial, no men discontinued treatment.[3]

Comment: The endpoints in some of these trials were subjective and of questionable validity. The subsequent trial did not make clear whether it was randomised.[3]

OPTION SILDENAFIL

One systematic review and 15 subsequent RCTs found that sildenafil improved erections and increased rates of successful intercourse compared with placebo. Adverse effects, including headaches, flushing, and dyspepsia, were reported in up to a quarter of men. Deaths have been reported in men on concomitant treatment with oral nitrates.

Benefits: We found one systematic review (search date 2000, 27 RCTs)[4] and 15 subsequent RCTs.[5–19] **In men with any cause of erectile dysfunction:** The systematic review found that in trials that evaluated flexible "as needed" dosing (14 RCTs, 2283 men with any cause of erectile dysfunction), sildenafil significantly increased the proportion of men who experienced at least one episode of successful intercourse compared with placebo (2283 men: 83% with sildenafil *v* 45% with placebo; RR 1.8, 95% CI 1.7 to 1.9).[4] In trials that evaluated fixed doses of sildenafil (6 RCTs), efficacy was slightly higher on higher doses (> 50 mg) and lower on a low dose (< 25 mg). Eleven subsequent RCTs all found that sildenafil improved sexual function compared with placebo.[5–12,15,17,18] **In men with diabetes:** The systematic review included two RCTs restricted to men with diabetes and 14 trials (551 men with diabetes) that provided subgroup analysis in men with diabetes.[4] Based on subgroup analysis, the review found that sildenafil significantly increased successful erections and successful intercourse compared with placebo (AR for erections 63% with sildenafil *v* 19% with placebo; RR 3, 95% CI 2.5 to 3.7; AR for intercourse 44% with sildenafil *v* 16% with placebo; WMD 26.9, 95% CI 19.9 to 33.9). We found three subsequent RCTs. The first subsequent RCT (219 men) found that sildenafil (25–100 mg) improved participant rated erections and scores on questions 3 and 4 of the International Index of Erectile Dysfunction after 12 weeks (64.6% had improved erections with sildenafil *v* 10.5% with placebo; CI presented graphically; P < 0.0001; mean improvement in question 3 score 3.42 with sildenafil *v* 1.86 with placebo; mean improvement in question 4 score 3.35 with sildenafil *v* 1.84 with placebo; P < 0.0001 for both comparisons).[19] The second RCT (188 men) also found that sildenafil significantly improved scores on questions 3 and 4 of the International Index of Erectile Dysfunction compared with placebo after 12 weeks (mean question 3 score 3.61 with sildenafil *v* 2.71 with placebo; P = 0.001; mean question 4 score 3.25 with sildenafil *v* 2.19 with placebo; P = 0.001).[13] Sildenafil also increased the proportion of successful attempts at intercourse compared with placebo, although the result was of borderline significance (P = 0.051); it also increased global efficacy compared with placebo. The third subsequent RCT (112 men) found that sildenafil improved the capacity to obtain and maintain an erection as measured by questions 3 and 4 of the International Index of Erectile Dysfunction**G** compared with placebo (obtain erection: P < 0.0001 in favour of sildenafil; maintain an erection: P < 0.0001 in favour of sildenafil).[16] **In men with spinal cord injury:** The systematic review included two RCTs (203 men) restricted to men with spinal cord injury.[4] It found that sildenafil improved erections compared with placebo (AR for improved erections 83% with sildenafil *v* 12% with placebo; RR 7.2, 95% CI 4.7 to 10.9). **In men with prostate cancer:** We found one small RCT (60 men) in men with erectile dysfunction after external beam radiotherapy for prostate cancer.[14] It found that sildenafil significantly improved global efficacy and succesful intercourse compared with placebo after 6 weeks of treatment (AR for global efficacy 45% with sildenafil *v* 8% with placebo; P < 0.001; AR for successful intercourse 55% with sildenafil v 18% with placebo; P < 0.001).[14]

Harms: The systematic review found that in a subset of 14 flexible dose trials (3780 men), sildenafil significantly increased the risk of at least one adverse effect compared with placebo (AR for at least one adverse effect 48% with sildenafil *v* 36% with placebo; RR 1.4, 95% CI 1.3 to 1.6).[4] Adverse effects included headache (11% with sildenafil *v* 4% with placebo), flushing (12% *v* 2%), dyspepsia (5% *v* 1%), and visual disturbance (3% *v* 0.8%).[4] One RCT (236 men with any cause of erectile dysfunction) found that sildenafil was associated with facial flushing (25.2%), dizziness (6.7%), headache (5.9%), and palpitations (3.4%).[5] A second RCT found that headache, flushing, dyspepsia, and abnormal perception of colour or brightness were more common with sildenafil than placebo (20% *v* 6% for headache, 15% *v* 0% for dyspepsia, 15% *v* 1% for flushing, and 8% *v* 1% for abnormal vision).[6] A third RCT found similar results.[7] Another study reported specifically on adverse effects of sildenafil.[20] It summarised results from a series of RCTs (4274 men aged 19–87 years with erectile dysfunction because of a range of causes for > 6 months and a mean of 5 years). All men were treated for up to 6 months, and 2199 received further open label treatment for up to 1 year. It found more adverse events with sildenafil than with placebo, including headache (16% *v* 4%; significance not reported), flushing (10% *v* 1%; significance not reported), and dyspepsia (7% *v* 2%; significance not reported). Similar proportions in both groups discontinued treatment (about 2.4%).[20] An important contraindication to prescribing sildenafil is concomitant use of oral nitrates. This combination results in precipitous hypotension. One small RCT (105 men) evaluated the cardiovascular effects of sildenafil during exercise in men with coronary heart disease.[21] It found no effect on symptoms, presence, and extent of ischaemia induced by exercise. By 1999, about 60 deaths had been reported to the US Food and Drug Administration in men who had been prescribed sildenafil, but it is not known whether any of the deaths were directly attributable to the drug. Long term (> 1 year) safety of sildenafil is unknown. One of the RCTs in men with psychogenic or mixed aetiology erectile dysfunction found that adverse effects were mild and transient.[22] One small RCT (133 men) found sildenafil increased treatment related adverse events compared with placebo after 8 weeks (56.1% with sildenafil *v* 20.9% with placebo; P value not reported). The most common adverse events were flushing (21/66 [31.8%] with sildenafil *v* 3/67 [4.5%] with placebo; P value not reported), headache (15/66 [22.7%] with sildenafil *v* 6/67 [9.0%] with placebo; P value not reported), and abnormalities in colour vision (4/66 [6.1%] with sildenafil *v* 0/67 [0%] with placebo; P value not reported).[15] One RCT in men with diabetes (188 men) found that sildenafil increased adverse events compared with placebo (headache: 20% *v* 8%, flushing: 18% *v* 3%, and dyspepsia: 32% *v* 8%; significance not reported).[13] Another small RCT (60 men) reported similar results (headache 42% with sildenafil *v* 15% with placebo, P < 0.001; and dyspepsia: 32% *v* 8%, P < 0.001). It found no significant difference between sildenafil and placebo for other adverse effects, including myalgia, nasal congestion, visual disturbance, and dizziness.[14]

Comment: None.

OPTION L-ARGININE

One small RCT found no significant difference in sexual function between L-arginine and placebo, but it may have been too small to exclude a clinically important difference.

Benefits: We found no systematic review. We found one small RCT (50 men with erectile dysfunction) that compared high dose L-arginine (5 g/day given orally) versus placebo.[23] It found no significant difference in sexual function between L-arginine and placebo, although the power of the study was not adequate to rule out a clinically important difference (sexual function improved in 9/29 [31%] men with L-arginine v 2/17 [12%] with placebo; RR 2.6, 95% CI 0.6 to 10.8).

Harms: The trial reported decreases in systolic or diastolic blood pressure, or both, although this caused no systemic effects and required no drug interruptions. The trial found some "fluctuation in heart rate", which was described as clinically insignificant.[23]

Comment: Nausea, vomiting, diarrhoea, headache, flushing, and numbness have been reported after the administration of L-arginine, although none of the men in this study reported any such complaints.

OPTION TRAZODONE

One small RCT found no significant difference in erections or libido with trazodone compared with placebo, but it may have been too small to exclude a clinically important difference.

Benefits: We found no systematic review. One small crossover RCT (48 men with erectile dysfunction, washout period 3 weeks) compared trazodone versus placebo.[24] Men were treated with either trazodone (50 mg) or placebo at bedtime for 3 months. It found no evidence that trazodone improved erections or libido (improved erections reported by 19% with trazodone v 24% with placebo; CI and P value not reported, described as NS; improved libido reported by 35% with trazodone v 20% with placebo; CI and P value not reported, described as NS).

Harms: The trial reported drowsiness (31%), dry mouth (1%), and fatigue (19%) with trazodone. It did not report comparative rates of adverse effects for trazadone compared with placebo.[24]

Comment: None.

OPTION INTRAURETHRAL ALPROSTADIL

One large RCT (in men who had previously responded to alprostadil) found limited evidence that intraurethral alprostadil (prostaglandin E1) increased the chances of successful sexual intercourse and at least one orgasm over 3 months compared with placebo. About a third of men suffered penile ache. We found no direct comparisons of intraurethral alprostadil versus either intracavernosal alprostadil or oral drug treatments.

Benefits: We found no systematic review. We found one RCT (996 men aged 27–88 years who had previously responded to intraurethral alprostadil) that compared alprostadil versus placebo.[25] It found that those given alprostadil were more likely to report having successful sexual intercourse over 3 months (65% with alprostadil v 19% with placebo; $P < 0.001$) and at least one orgasm (64% with alprostadil v 24% with placebo; $P < 0.001$).

Harms: The most common adverse effect was mild to moderate penile ache, which occurred in about a third of men during clinic testing (36%). In total 36/1511 (2.4%) men withdrew from the trial because of this adverse effect.[25] We found no reports of priapism, penile fibrosis, or other serious adverse events.

Comment: The RCT preselected men who had a good response to alprostadil before randomisation. This would tend to increase the size of the effect compared with placebo.

OPTION INTRACAVERNOSAL ALPROSTADIL

One large RCT found that intracavernosal injection of alprostadil (prostaglandin E1) increased the chances of a satisfactory erection compared with placebo. We found no direct comparisons of intracavernosal alprostadil versus either intraurethral or oral drug treatments. One small RCT found limited evidence that vacuum devices were as effective as intracavernosal alprostadil injections for rigidity but not for orgasm.

Benefits: We found no systematic review. **Versus placebo:** We found one large multicentre trial (1128 men, of whom 300 were assigned randomly with all causes of erectile dysfunction; heavy smokers and men with uncontrolled hypertension or diabetes were excluded) that compared 2.5, 5, 10, or 20 μg alprostadil versus placebo.[26] Injections were given and outcome was assessed by an investigator or research nurse. None of the 59 men who received placebo had a response. Significant differences were seen in clinical evaluation with all the doses of alprostadil compared with placebo and a significant dose–response relation. **Versus vacuum devices:** One crossover RCT (50 men with erectile dysfunction, 44 of whom completed the study) compared intracavernosal self injections of alprostadil versus vacuum devices.[27] Outcome was assessed by a questionnaire given to men and their partners after 15 uses for each device, and couples were assessed for 18–24 months. No significant difference was noted in the ability to achieve an erection suitable for intercourse; however, the ability to attain orgasm was significantly better with alprostadil ($P < 0.05$). On a scale of 1 to 10, overall satisfaction was significantly better when using alprostadil both for men (6.5 with alprostadil *v* 5.4 with vacuum device; $P < 0.05$) and their partners (6.5 with alprostadil *v* 5.1 with vacuum device; $P < 0.05$). Younger men (< 60 years) and those with shorter duration of erectile dysfunction (< 12 months) favoured alprostadil ($P < 0.05$).

Harms: Penile pain was reported by a half of the men in the multicentre trial and priapism (prolonged erection for > 4 hours) by 1%.[26] No significant difference was noted in the frequency of adverse events between vacuum devices and alprostadil.[27]

Comment: Most men can be taught to inject themselves using small gauge needles. In the RCT that compared injections and vacuum devices, 80% of the 44 couples who completed the study were still using one or other treatment after 18–24 months.[27]

OPTION TOPICAL ALPROSTADIL

Two quasi randomised trials found limited evidence that topical alprostadil increased the number of men with erections sufficient for intercourse compared with placebo, but that it was associated commonly with skin irritation.

Benefits: We found no systematic review. We found two quasi randomised trials (see comment below).[28,29] The first, a single blind trial (48 men with erectile dysfunction because of organic, psychogenic, or mixed causes), compared topical alprostadil versus placebo.[28] Men were assigned in sequential order to either 0.5, 1, or 2.5 mg alprostadil gel (36 men) or placebo (12 men). One dose of alprostadil or placebo gel was applied to the glans and shaft of the penis and washed off after 3 hours. Alprostadil significantly increased the proportion of men who achieved an erection sufficient for intercourse compared with placebo (25/36 [69%] with alprostadil *v* 2/12 [17%] with placebo; RR 4.2, 95% CI 1.8 to 5.5; NNT 2, 95% CI 1 to 8). The second RCT (62 men) compared alprostadil topically applied only to the glans of the penis in a clinic setting versus placebo. Significantly more men reported an erection deemed sufficient for penetration with alprostadil compared with placebo (12/31 [39%] versus 2/29 [7%]; RR 5.6, 95% CI 1.4 to 23.0; NNT 3, 95% CI 2 to 9).[29]

Harms: Men who received alprostadil to the glans and shaft of the penis were more likely to have skin irritation than those who received placebo (100% on 0.5 mg dose *v* 67% on placebo; no P value reported). Irritation measured by mean irritation score (range 0–2) was more severe with alprostadil than with placebo (1.75 with 0.5 mg dose *v* 0.67 with placebo; $P < 0.0013$).[28] In the trial in which alprostadil was applied to the glans only, significantly greater erythema was reported with alprostadil than with placebo ($P < 0.001$; absolute figures not reported).[29] Severe erythema was reported by 3% of men.

Comment: Allocation of men in both trials was sequential and may mean that the groups were systematically different; the characteristics of each group were not reported.[28,29]

OPTION VACUUM DEVICES

Vacuum devices have not been adequately assessed in RCTs. One small RCT found limited evidence that they were as effective as intracavernosal alprostadil (prostaglandin E1) injections for rigidity but not for orgasm.

Benefits: **Versus placebo:** We found no systematic review and no RCTs. **Versus intracavernosal injections:** See benefits of intracavernosal alprostadil, p 1125.

Harms: We found insufficient evidence.

Comment: Vacuum devices may be less popular than injections because only the distal portion of the penis becomes firm, but they are presumed to be safe.[27]

OPTION PENILE PROSTHESES

We found no systematic reviews or RCTs of penile prostheses in men with erectile dysfunction. Use of penile prostheses is usually considered only after less invasive treatments have failed.

Benefits: We found no RCTs. Anecdotal evidence suggests that patient satisfaction may be high, but we found no good studies.

Harms: One recent study found the morbidity of penile prostheses to be 9% (surgical revision 7%, mechanical failure 2.5%). Infection rates were between 2% and 7%.[30]

Comment: Use of penile prostheses is usually considered only after less invasive treatments have failed.

GLOSSARY

International Index of Erectile Function: questions 3 and 4 The questions have been validated for assessing the effects of sildenafil on sexual function. The questions ask "over the past 4 weeks, when you have attempted sexual intercourse, how often were you able to penetrate (enter) your partner?", and "over the past 4 weeks, during sexual intercourse, how often were you able to maintain your erection after you have penetrated (entered) your partner?" Questions are answered on a six point scale.

REFERENCES

1. Feldman HA, Goldstein I, Dimitrios GH, et al. Impotence and its medical and psychosocial correlates: results of the Massachusetts male aging study. *J Urol* 1994;151:54–61.
2. Ernst E, Pittler MH. Yohimbine for erectile dysfunction: a systemic review and meta-analysis of randomized clinical trials. *J Urol* 1998;159:433–436. Search date 1997; primary sources Medline, Embase, The Cochrane Library, and hand searched references.
3. Teloken C, Rhoden EL, Sogari P, et al. Therapeutic effects of high dose yohimbine hydrochloride on organic erectile dysfunction. *J Urol* 1998;159:122–124.
4. Fink HA, MacDonald R, Rutks IR, et al. Sildenafil for male erectile dysfunction. A systematic review and meta-analysis. *Arch Intern Med* 2002;162:1349–1360. Search date 2000; primary sources Medline, Health-STAR, Current Contents, Cochrane Library, review of bibliographies of retrieved trials and review articles, and a hand search of urology journals and national meeting abstracts.
5. Chen KK, Hsieh JT, Huang ST, et al. ASSESS-3: a randomised, double-blind, flexible-dose clinical trial of the efficacy and safety of oral sildenafil in the treatment of men with erectile dysfunction in Taiwan. *Int J Impot Res* 2001;13:221–229.
6. Seidman SN, Roose SP, Menza MA, et al. Treatment of erectile dysfunction in men with depressive symptoms: results of a placebo-controlled trial with sildenafil citrate. *Am J Psychiatry* 2001;158:1623–1630.
7. Lewis R, Bennett CJ, Borkon WD, et al. Patient and partner satisfaction with Viagra (sildenafil citrate) treatment as determined by the Erectile Dysfunction Inventory of Treatment Satisfaction Questionnaire. *Urology* 2001;57:960–965.
8. Becher E, Tejada NA, Gomez R et al. Sildenafil citrate (Viagra) in the treatment of men with erectile dysfunction in southern Latin America: A double blind, randomized, placebo-controlled, parallel-group, multicenter, flexible-dose escalation study. *Int J Impot Res* 2002;14(suppl):33–41.
9. Glina S, Bertero E, Claro J, et al. Efficacy and safety of flexible dose oral sildenafil citrate (Viagra) in the treatment of erectile dysfunction in Brazilian and Mexican men. *Int J Impot Res* 2002;14(suppl): 27–32.
10. Gomez F, Davila H, Costa A, et al. Efficacy and safety of oral sildenafil citrate (Viagra) in the treatment of male erectile dysfunction in Colombia, Ecuador, and Venezuela: a double-blind, multicenter, placebo-controlled study. *Int J Impot Res* 2002;14(suppl):42–47.
11. Young JM, Bennett C, Gilhooly P, et al. Efficacy and safety of sildenafil citrate (Viagra) in black and Hispanic American men. *Urology* 2002;60(suppl 2B):39–48.
12. Levinson IP, Khalaf IM, Shaeer KZM, et al. Efficacy and safety of sildenafil citrate (Viagra) for the treatment of erectile dysfunction in men in Egypt and South Africa. *Int J Impot Res* 2003;15(suppl 1):S25–S29.
13. Stuckey BGA, Jadzinsky MN, Murphy LJ, et al. Sildenafil citrate for treatment of erectile dysfunction in men with type 1 diabetes. *Diabetes Care* 2003;26:279–284.
14. Incrocci L, Hop WCJ, Slob AK. Efficacy of sildenafil in an open-label study as a continuation of a double-blind study in the treatment of erectile dysfunction after radiotherapy for prostate cancer. *Urology* 2003;62:116–120.
15. Choi HK, Ahn TY, Kim JJ, et al. A double– blind, randomised, placebo–controlled, parallel group, multicentre, flexible–dose escalation study to assess the efficacy and safety of sildenafil administered as required to male outpatients with erectile dysfunction in Korea. *International Journal of Impotence Research* 2003;15:80–86.
16. Escobar–Jimenez F, et al. Efficacy and safety of sildenafil in men with type 2 diabetes mellitus and erectile dysfunction. *Med Clin (Barc)* 2002;119:121–124. (Spanish).
17. Kongkanand A, Ratana-Olarn K, Ruangdilokrat S, et al. The efficacy and safety of oral sildenafil in Thai men with erectile dysfunction: a randomized, double blind, placebo controlled, flexible-dose study. *Journal of the Medical Association of Thaliand* 2003;86:195–204.
18. Nurnberg HG, Hensley PL, Gelenberg AJ, et al. Treatment of antidepressant-associated sexual dysfunction with sildenafil. *JAMA* 2003;289:56–64.
19. Boulton AJ, Selam JL, Sweeney M, et al. Sildenafil citrate for the treatment of erectile dysfunction in men with Type II diabetes mellitus. *Diabetologia* 2001;44:1296–1301.
20. Morales A, Gingell C, Collins M, et al. Clinical safety of oral sildenafil citrate (Viagra) in the treatment of erectile dysfunction. *Int J Impot Res* 1998;10:69–74.
21. Arruda-Olson AM, Mahoney DW, Nehra DW et al. Cardiovascular effects of sildenafil during exercise in men with known or probable coronary artery disease: a randomized crossover trial. *JAMA* 2002; 287: 719–725.
22. Olsson AM, Speakman MJ, Dinsmore WW, et al. Sildenafil citrate (Viagra) is effective and well tolerated for treating erectile dysfunction of psychogenic or mixed aetiology. *Int J Clin Pract* 2000;54:561–566.
23. Chen J, Wollman Y, Chernichovsky T, et al. Effect of oral administration of high-dose nitric oxide donor L-arginine in men with organic erectile dysfunction: results of a double-blind randomized placebo-controlled study. *BJU Int* 1999;83:269–273.
24. Costabile RA, Spevak M. Oral trazodone is not effective therapy for erectile dysfunction: a double blind placebo-controlled trial. *J Urol* 1999;161:1819–1822.
25. Padma-Nathan H, Hellstrom WJ, Kaiser FE, et al, for the Medicated Urethral System for Erection (MUSE) Study Group. Treatment of men with erectile dysfunction with transurethral alprostadil. *N Engl J Med* 1997;336:1–7.
26. PGE1 Study Group. Prospective, multicenter trials of efficacy and safety of intracavernosal alprostadil (prostaglandin E1) sterile powder in men with erectile dysfunction. *N Engl J Med* 1996;334:873–877.
27. Soderdahl DW, Thrasher JB, Hansberry KL, et al. Intracavernosal drug induced erection therapy vs external vacuum device in the treatment of erectile dysfunction. *Br J Urol* 1997;79:952–957.
28. McVary KT, Polepalle S, Riggi S, et al. Topical prostaglandin E1 SEPA gel for the treatment of erectile dysfunction. *J Urol* 1999;162:726–730.
29. Goldstein I, Payton TR, Schechter PJ. A double blind placebo controlled efficacy and safety study of topical gel formulation of 1% alprostadil (Topiglan) for the in office treatment of erectile dysfunction. *Urology* 2001;57:301–305.
30. Goldstein I, Newman L, Baum N, et al. Safety and efficacy outcome of Mentor α 1 inflatable penile prosthesis implantation for impotence treatment. *J Urol* 1997;157:833–839.

Robyn Webber
Consultant Urological Surgeon
Hairmyres Hospital, East Kilbride, Scotland

Competing interests: The author has received funding from Pfizer to attend several educational meetings. *We would like to acknowledge the previous contributors of this chapter including Michael O'Leary and Bazian Ltd.*

Prostate cancer (non-metastatic)

Search date February 2003

Timothy Wilt

QUESTIONS

INTERVENTIONS

See glossary Ⓖ

Key Messages

Clinically localised prostate cancer

- **Radical prostatectomy** Two RCTs found no significant difference in death from any cause between radical prostatectomy and watchful waiting in men with clinically detected disease after median follow up of 6.2 and 23 years. The larger of the RCTs found that radical prostatectomy reduced death due to prostate cancer and metastases at 6 years compared with watchful waiting. Two small RCTs found that radical prostatectomy reduced the risk of treatment failure compared with external beam radiation. Radical prostatectomy carries the risks of major surgery and of sexual and urinary dysfunction.
- **Watchful waiting** Two RCTs found no significant difference in overall survival between watchful waiting and radical prostatectomy in men with clinically detected disease after median follow up of 6 and 23 years. The larger RCT found that radical prostatectomy reduced death rates due to prostate cancer and metastases at 6 years compared with watchful waiting. One RCT found that radical prostatectomy increased erectile dysfunction compared with watchful waiting but found no significant difference in quality of life after 12 months.

- **Androgen suppression** We found no RCTs of early androgen suppression on length or quality of life in men with asymptomatic, clinically localised prostate cancer. One RCT identified by a systematic review found limited evidence that oestrogen decreased prostate cancer related deaths compared with watchful waiting. It found no significant difference in overall survival. One preliminary report of three large ongoing RCTs in men with localised or locally advanced prostate cancer found that bicalutamide plus standard care reduced rates of radiological progression and bone metastases at 2–3 years compared with standard care alone. There was no significant difference between treatments in overall survival.
- **External beam radiation** We found no RCTs comparing external beam radiation versus watchful waiting. Two RCTs found that external beam radiation increased the risk of treatment failure compared with radical prostatectomy. Two small RCTs found no significant difference between conformal radiotherapy and conventional radiotherapy in overall survival or tumour control at 3–5 years. One systematic review found limited evidence that conformal radiotherapy with dose escalation reduced acute and late treatment related morbidity compared with conventional radiotherapy for men with T1 or T2 low or intermediate risk prostate cancer.
- **Androgen suppression in asymptomatic men with raised prostate specific antigen concentrations after early treatment; brachytherapy; cryosurgery** We found no RCTs on the effects of these interventions.

Locally advanced prostate cancer

- **Immediate androgen suppression after radical prostatectomy and pelvic lymphadenectomy in men with node positive prostate cancer (compared with radical prostatectomy and deferred androgen suppression)** One small RCT in men with node positive prostate cancer found that immediate androgen suppression compared with deferred androgen suppression after radical prostatectomy and pelvic lymphadenectomy reduced mortality over a median of 7 years' follow up.
- **Androgen suppression initiated at diagnosis** RCTs found no significant difference in overall survival between androgen suppression with bicalutamide and no androgen suppression in men with localised or locally advanced prostate cancer at 2–10 years. The RCTs found that bicalutamide reduced objective progression compared with no bicalutamide. One systematic review found that early androgen suppression increased survival at 10 years compared with deferred treatment in men with locally advanced prostate cancer but found no significant difference in survival at 5 years. One RCT found limited evidence that immediate androgen suppression reduced complications compared with deferred androgen suppression.
- **Early androgen suppression plus external beam radiation (compared with radiation and deferred androgen suppression)** RCTs found limited evidence that androgen suppression initiated at diagnosis plus external beam radiation improved long term survival compared with radiation alone or radiation plus deferred androgen suppression. One RCT found limited evidence that immediate androgen suppression reduced complications compared with deferred androgen suppression.

DEFINITION Prostatic cancer is staged according to two systems: the tumour, node, metastasis (TNM) classification system and the American urologic staging system (see table 1, p 1141). Non-metastatic prostate cancer can be divided into clinically localised disease and locally advanced disease. Clinically localised disease is prostate cancer thought, after clinical examination, to be confined to the prostate gland. Locally advanced disease is prostate cancer that has spread outside the capsule of the prostate gland but has not yet spread to other organs. Metastatic disease is prostate cancer that has spread outside the prostate gland to either local, regional, or systemic lymph nodes, seminal vesicles, or to other body organs (e.g. bone, liver, brain) and is not connected to the prostate gland. We consider clinically localised and locally advanced disease here. Metastatic disease is covered in a separate chapter (see prostate cancer [metastatic], [Web only]).

INCIDENCE/ PREVALENCE Prostate cancer is the sixth most common cancer in the world and the third most common cancer in men. In 2000, an estimated 513 000 new cases of prostate cancer were diagnosed and about 250 000 deaths were attributed to prostate cancers worldwide. Prostate cancer is uncommon under the age of 50 years. About 85% of men with prostate cancer are diagnosed after the age of 65 years.

Autopsy studies suggest that the prevalence of subclinical prostate cancer is high at all ages: 30% for men aged 30–39 years, 50% for men aged 50–59 years, and more than 75% for men older than 85 years. Incidence varies widely by ethnic group and around the world. The highest rates occur in men of black ethnic group living in the USA and the lowest among men living in China.[1]

AETIOLOGY/ RISK FACTORS Risk factors for prostate cancer include increasing age, family history of prostate cancer, black ethnic group, and possibly higher dietary consumption of fat and meat, low intake of lycopene (from tomato products), low intake of fruit, and high dietary calcium. In the USA, black men have about a 60% higher incidence than white men.[2] The prostate cancer incidence for black men living in the USA is about 90/100 000 in men aged less than 65 years and about 1300/100 000 in men aged 65–74 years. For white men, incidence is about 44/100 000 in men aged less than 65 years and 900/100 000 in men aged 65–74 years.[2]

PROGNOSIS The chance that men with well to moderately differentiated, palpable, clinically localised prostate cancer will remain free of symptomatic progression is 70% at 5 years and 40% at 10 years.[3] The risk of symptomatic disease progression is higher in men with poorly differentiated prostate cancer.[4] One retrospective analysis of a large surgical series in men with clinically localised prostate cancer found that the median time from the increase in prostate specific antigen (PSA) concentration to the development of metastatic disease was 8 years.[5] Time to PSA progression, PSA doubling time, and Gleason score(G) were predictive of the probability and time to development of metastatic disease. Once men developed metastatic disease, the median actuarial time to death was less than 5 years.[5] Morbidity from local or regional disease progression includes haematuria, bladder obstruction, and lower extremity oedema. The age adjusted prostate cancer specific mortality in the USA for all men aged 65 years and older has decreased by about 15% (244 deaths/100 000 to 207 deaths/100 000) from 1991–1997. The reasons for this are unclear, although inaccurate death certification, PSA screening, and earlier, more intensive treatment, including radical prostatectomy(G), radiotherapy, and androgen suppression(G), have been suggested. However, regions of the USA and Canada where PSA testing and early treatment are more common have similar prostate cancer mortality to regions with lower testing and early treatment rates.[6] Similarly, countries with low rates of PSA testing and treatment, such as the UK, have similar age adjusted prostate cancer mortality to countries with high rates of testing and treatment, such as the USA.[7]

AIMS OF INTERVENTION To prevent premature death and disability, and to minimise adverse effects of treatment.

OUTCOMES Survival; development of metastatic disease; development of symptomatic local or regional disease progression; time to progression; response in terms of symptoms and signs; quality of life; adverse effects of treatment. Where clinical outcomes are not available, surrogate outcomes have been used (PSA concentration; Gleason score for histological grade).

METHODS *Clinical Evidence* search and appraisal February 2003. Additional author search: Cochrane Library and Medline to 2001 for systematic reviews and RCTs, and using the search strategy of the Department of Veterans' Affairs Coordinating Center for the Cochrane Review Group on Prostatic Diseases.

QUESTION What are the effects of treatments for clinically localised prostate cancer?

OPTION WATCHFUL WAITING

Two RCTs found no significant difference in overall survival between watchful waiting and radical prostatectomy in men with clinically detected disease after median follow up of 6 and 23 years. One RCT found that radical prostatectomy reduced death due to prostate cancer and reduced metastases at 6 years compared with watchful waiting. One RCT found that radical prostatectomy increased erectile dysfunction compared with watchful waiting but found no significant difference in quality of life after 4 years.

Benefits: **Versus radical prostatectomy:** See benefits of radical prostatectomy, p 1131. **Versus early androgen suppression:** See benefits of androgen suppression, p 1135.

Harms: **Versus radical prostatectomy:** See harms of radical prostatectomy, p 1132. **Versus early androgen suppression:** See harms of androgen suppression, p 1135.

Comment: We found two large cohort studies, which found that, in men with clinically detected localised prostate cancer managed with watchful waiting, 15 year disease specific survival was 80% — ranging from 95% for well differentiated to 30% for poorly differentiated cancers.[10,11] However, most men with newly diagnosed prostate cancer are now detected by prostate specific antigen (PSA) testing. There is about a 10–15 year lead time between the detection of cancers by raised PSA concentrations and clinical detection by digital rectal examination or the development of symptoms.[12] This means that outcomes are likely to be similar in men with palpable tumours who are followed for 15 years and men whose tumours are detected because of raised PSA concentrations who are followed for 25–30 years (lead time bias). Therefore, compared with men with clinically detected prostate cancer, any benefit in men with PSA detected tumours (if it exists) is likely to be of smaller magnitude and require a longer period of time to occur. Until better information is available to guide treatment selection men have to weigh the potential but unproved risks and benefits of various treatment options. For example, men treated with watchful waiting may avoid the risks of surgery and may have similar overall survival and quality of life compared with men treated with other interventions. However, they do not have the opportunity to have their cancer removed or "definitively" treated with radiotherapy. This could potentially result in disease progression, disability, and premature death. Preliminary results from one RCT indicate that, on average, 25 men with clinically detected prostate cancer would need to be treated with surgery to prevent one death attributed to prostate cancer over a 6 year time period, without evidence that this would improve length or quality of life.[9] People should balance the potential risks and benefits of various treatment options.

OPTION RADICAL PROSTATECTOMY

Two RCTs found no significant difference in death from any cause between radical prostatectomy and watchful waiting in men with clinically detected disease after median follow up of 6.2 and 23 years. The larger of the RCTs found that radical prostatectomy reduced death due to prostate cancer and metastases at 6 years compared with watchful waiting. Two small RCTs found that that radical prostatectomy reduced the risk of treatment failure compared with external beam radiation. Radical prostatectomy carries the risks of major surgery and of sexual and urinary dysfunction.

Benefits: **Versus watchful waiting:** We found one systematic review (search date 2002, 2 RCTs) that compared radical prostatectomy**G** versus watchful waiting in men with clinically localised prostate cancer.[8] The first RCT in the review (142 men) found no significant difference in survival after median follow up of 23 years (range 19–27 years) between radical prostatectomy and watchful waiting (median survival 10.6 years with prostatectomy *v* 8 years with watchful waiting; CI not reported).[13] Analysis was not by intention to treat, treatment groups were not comparable at baseline for important prognostic factors, and the RCT is likely to have been too small to exclude a clinically important difference between groups. The second RCT in the review (695 men with newly diagnosed prostate cancer, clinical stage T1b, T1c, or T2) found that radical prostatectomy significantly reduced death due to prostate cancer after a median of 6.2 years follow up compared with watchful waiting.[9] There was no significant difference in overall death rates (death due to prostate cancer: 16/374 [4.6%] with surgery *v* 31/348 [8.9%] with watchful waiting; HR 0.50, 95% CI 0.27 to 0.91; distant metastases: HR 0.63, 95% CI 0.41 to 0.96; death from any cause: 53/347 [15.3%] with surgery *v* 62/348 [17.8%] with watchful waiting; HR 0.83, 95% CI 0.57 to 1.20). **Versus external beam radiation:** We found one systematic review (search date 2002, 1 RCT)[8] and one additional RCT.[14] The RCT in the review (95 men with either localised or locally advanced cancer) found that radical prostatectomy significantly increased prostate cancer specific survival after 5 years compared with external beam radiation (96.6% with prostatectomy *v* 84.6% with radiation, P = 0.02).[8] The additional RCT (106 men with clinically localised prostate cancer) found that radical prostatectomy significantly reduced treatment failure, primarily defined as a positive bone scan, compared with external beam radiation (4/41 [9.8%] treatment failures with prostatectomy *v* 17/56 [30.4%] with radiation; RR 0.32, 95% CI 0.12 to 0.88; NNT 5, 95% CI 3 to 25).[14]

Harms: One RCT (376 men with localised prostate cancer, 326 men followed up) compared self reported adverse effects and quality of life in men treated with radical prostatectomy and watchful waiting.[15] It found that radical prostatectomy increased erectile dysfunction and urinary leakage at 12 months or more after surgery compared with watchful waiting but reduced symptoms of urinary obstruction (erectile dysfunction: 80% with radical prostatectomy *v* 45% with watchful waiting; urinary leakage: 49% with surgery *v* 21% with watchful waiting; weak urinary stream: 28% with surgery *v* 44% with watchful waiting). The RCT found no significant difference between radical prostatectomy and watchful waiting in bowel function, anxiety, depression, wellbeing, or subjective quality of life (distress from bowel symptoms: 5/159 [3%] with surgery *v* 10/156 [6%] with watchful waiting; low or moderate psychological wellbeing: 35% with surgery *v* 36% with watchful waiting; low or moderate quality of life: 40% with surgery *v* 45% with watchful waiting). One systematic review found that 12 months after radical prostatectomy 20–70% of men reported reduced sexual function and 15–50% reported urinary problems.[8] Fatal complications have been reported in 0.5–1.0% of men treated with radical prostatectomy and may exceed 2% in men aged 75 years and older.[16] Nearly 8% of men older than 65 years suffered major cardiopulmonary complications within 30 days of operation. The incidence of other adverse effects of surgery was over 80% for sexual dysfunction, 30% for urinary incontinence requiring pads or clamps to control wetness, 18% for urethral stricture, 3% for total urinary incontinence, 5% for faecal incontinence, and 1% for bowel injury requiring surgical repair.[17–20]

Comment: Both RCTs of radical prostatectomy took place before the advent of tests for prostate specific antigen.[13,14] Radical prostatectomy may benefit selected groups of men with localised prostate cancer, particularly younger men with higher grade tumours, but the RCTs did not look for this effect. The available evidence suggests that in most men the benefits of radical prostatectomy in quality adjusted life expectancy are at best small and sensitive to individual preferences.[21] A non-randomised study examining a population based, self administered survey of men aged over 65 years in the USA found no differences in general health related quality of life between radical prostatectomy, radiation, or watchful waiting.[22] We are aware of two further ongoing trials comparing radical prostatectomy versus watchful waiting.[23,24] Any benefit of radical prostatectomy in men with prostate specific antigen detected tumours is likely to be of smaller magnitude and require a longer period of time to occur than clinically detected tumours. People should balance the potential risks and benefits of various treatment options.

OPTION EXTERNAL BEAM RADIATION

We found no RCTs comparing external beam radiation versus watchful waiting. Two RCTs found that external beam radiation increased the risk of treatment failure compared with radical prostatectomy. Two small RCTs found no significant difference between conformal radiotherapy and conventional radiotherapy in overall survival or tumour control at 3–5 years. One systematic review found limited evidence that conformal radiotherapy with dose escalation reduced acute and late treatment related morbidity compared with conventional radiotherapy for men with T1 or T2 low or intermediate risk prostate cancer.

Benefits: **Versus watchful waiting:** We found no RCTs. **Versus radical prostatectomy:** See benefits of radical prostatectomy, p 1131.[14] **Conformal versus conventional radiotherapy:** We found one systematic review (search date 2001, 1 RCT)[25] and one additional RCT that compared conformal radiotherapy🅖 versus conventional radiotherapy.[26] The RCT identified by the review (301 men with T1 or T2, low or intermediate risk prostate cancer) found no significant difference in overall survival at 5 years between conformal radiotherapy and conventional radiotherapy when used as sole treatment, but survival was greater with conformal treatment (69% with conventional *v* 79% with conformal, P = 0.06).[25] The additional RCT (225 men with non-metastatic prostate cancer T1–T4, N0, or M0) did not report on survival, but found no significant difference in tumour control (measured by prostate specific antigen [PSA] level) between treatments after a median follow up of 3.6 years.[26]

Harms: One systematic review (search date 2002) found that 20–40% of men with no prior erectile dysfunction who received external beam radiation developed dysfunction after 12–24 months.[8] One survey of men treated with external beam radiation found that 7% wore pads to control wetness, 23–32% were impotent, and 10% reported problems with bowel dysfunction.[27] Treatment related mortality was less than 0.5%.[17] External beam radiation requires that men return for daily outpatient treatment for up to 6 weeks. **Versus radical prostatectomy:** One systematic review (search date 2002, 1 meta-analysis of 40 non-randomised studies published before 1995) found that radiation increased the probability of retaining sexual function compared with radical prostatectomy (69% with radiotherapy *v* 42% with prostatectomy).[8] **Conventional versus conformal radiotherapy:** We found one systematic review (search date 2001, 3 RCTs reporting on toxicity).[25] Two of the three RCTs found that conformal radiotherapy (without an increase in dose) reduced acute toxicity compared with conventional radiotherapy. The third RCT found no significant difference in acute toxicity between conformal radiotherapy (with dose escalation) and conventional radiotherapy. Two of the three RCTs in the review reporting on chronic adverse effects (> 1 year after treatment) found no significant difference between an increased dose of conformal radiotherapy and conventional radiotherapy but the third RCT reporting on chronic adverse effects found that conventional radiotherapy significantly increased radiation induced proctitis and rectal bleeding compared with the same dose of conformal radiotherapy (proctitis ≥ grade 1 radiation and oncology grade 56% with conventional *v* 36% with conformal, P = 0.004; rectal bleeding ≥ grade 2 radiation and oncology grade 3% with conventional *v* 12% with conformal, P = 0.01).

Comment: Up to 30% of men with clinically localised prostate cancer treated with radiotherapy still have positive biopsies 2–3 years after treatment.[28] One retrospective, non-randomised, multicentre pooled analysis estimated overall survival at 5 years at 85%, disease specific survival at 95%, and freedom from biochemical failure (as defined by raised PSA) at 66%.[29] Estimated 5 year rates of no biochemical recurrence according to PSA concentrations before treatment and Gleason scores **G** ranged from 81% for pretreatment PSA less than 10 ng/mL to 29% for PSA of 20 ng/mL or more, and a Gleason score from 7–10.

OPTION BRACHYTHERAPY

A systematic review found no RCTs of brachytherapy in men with clinically localised prostate cancer.

Benefits: We found one systematic review (search date 2002), which identified no RCTs comparing brachytherapy **G** alone or in combination with other treatments (androgen suppression or radiation).[8]

Harms: The systematic review reported that 36% of men had some erectile dysfunction, 2–12% had some urinary symptoms (including urinary incontinence in 7%), and 18% had some bowel dysfunction 1 year after treatment.[8] However the review stated that these figures came from poor quality studies and should be interpreted with caution.

Comment: We found two older systematic reviews that have not been presented in the benefits section (search date 1999).[30,31] One systematic review[30] identified 13 case series and three cohort studies (2 retrospective, 1 prospective) and we found one additional retrospective cohort study.[32] The studies used proxy outcomes (evidence of disease measured by prostate specific antigen [PSA] testing).[30,32] Results varied considerably from one series to another and were highly dependent on tumour stage, grade, and pretreatment serum PSA levels. Results in men with T1 or T2 tumours, Gleason score **G** of 6 or lower, and serum PSA level of 10 ng/mL or less were similar to those from case series of people having a radical prostatectomy **G**. The additional cohort study (1872 men) found that in low risk men (stage T1c, stage T2, PSA concentration ≤ 10 ng/mL, and Gleason score ≤ 6) the chance of a high PSA concentration at 5 years was similar whether they were treated with radiation or brachytherapy implant (with or without preceding androgen suppression) or with radical prostatectomy.[32] Men at intermediate or high risk (Gleason score > 6 or PSA > 10 ng/mL) were more likely to have high PSA concentration at 5 years with brachytherapy than with radical prostatectomy (RR of high PSA in men at intermediate risk 3.1, 95% CI 1.5 to 6.1; RR in men at high risk 3.0, 95% CI 1.8 to 5.0).[32] RCTs comparing brachytherapy versus radical prostatectomy are ongoing (Wilt T, personal communication, 2000).

OPTION CRYOSURGERY

We found no RCTs of cryotherapy in men with clinically localised prostate cancer.

Benefits: We found no systematic review or RCTs.

Harms: Complications reported in case series include impotence (65%), transient scrotal oedema (10%), sloughed urethral tissue (3%), urethral stricture (1%), incontinence, urethrorectal fistula, and prostatic abscess (1%).[33]

Comment: One ongoing trial is comparing cryosurgery versus radiation (Wilt T, personal communication, 2000).

OPTION ANDROGEN SUPPRESSION

We found no RCTs of early androgen suppression on length or quality of life in men with asymptomatic, clinically localised prostate cancer. One RCT identified by a systematic review found limited evidence that oestrogen decreased prostate cancer related deaths compared with watchful waiting but it found no significant difference in overall survival. One preliminary report of three large ongoing RCTs in men with localised or locally advanced prostate cancer found that bicalutamide plus standard care reduced rates of radiological progression and bone metastases at 2–3 years compared with standard care alone but there was no significant difference between treatments in overall survival.

Benefits: We found no RCTs of primary treatment with early androgen suppression**G** in the absence of symptoms on length or quality of life in men with clinically localised prostate cancer. **Versus watchful waiting:** We found one systematic review (search date 2002, 1 RCT) in men with clinically localised prostate cancer.[8] The RCT identified by the review (285 men) compared three treatments: oestrogen, estramustine, and watchful waiting.[8] It found that oestrogen significantly reduced prostate cancer specific deaths compared with watchful waiting (prostate cancer related deaths: 12% with oestrogen *v* 28% with watchful waiting; P = 0.03). It found no significant difference between treatments in overall survival (overall survival: 47% with oestrogen *v* 40% with deferred treatment; P = 0.48). The RCT was methodologically flawed (see comment below). **Plus standard care versus standard care alone:** We found one preliminary report of three ongoing RCTs (8113 men with localised or locally advanced prostate cancer T1–T4, Nx/N, M0) comparing bicalutamide 150 mg daily plus standard care versus standard care alone.[1] Standard care included radical prostatectomy**G**, radiotherapy, and watchful waiting. The meta-analysis in the report found that bicalutamide plus standard care significantly reduced rates of radiological progression and bone metastases at 2–3 years compared with standard care alone (progression: 363/4052 [9.0%] with bicalutamide plus standard care *v* 595/4061 [14.7%] with standard care alone; HR 0.58, 95% CI 0.51 to 0.66; P < 0.0001; bone metastases: 214 events with bicalutamide plus standard care *v* 321 events with standard care alone; RR 0.67, 95% CI 0.56 to 0.79). There was no significant difference between treatments in overall survival (overall survival: HR 0.93, 95% CI 0.79 to 1.11).[1]

Harms: See harms of androgen suppression in men with locally advanced prostate cancer, p 1137. One preliminary report of three ongoing RCTs (8113 men with localised or locally advanced prostate cancer) found that bicalutamide plus standard care increased gynaecomastia, breast pain, asthenia, impotence, and hot flushes compared with standard care alone but the statistical significance of differences was not reported (gynaecomastia 66% with bicalutamide plus standard care *v* 8% with standard care alone; breast pain 73% with bicalutamide plus standard care *v* 7% with standard care alone; asthenia 10% with bicalutamide plus standard care *v* 7% with standard care alone; impotence 9% with bicalutamide plus standard care *v* 6% with standard care alone; hot flushes 9% with bicalutamide plus standard care v 5% with standard care alone).[1] The systematic review found that androgen deprivation treatment with luteinising hormone releasing hormone agonist reduced sexual function in 40–70% and led to breast swelling in 5–25%, and hot flushes in 50–60%.[8]

Comment: One RCT identified by the systematic review compared oestrogen with deferred treatment. It was not analysed on an intention to treat basis, 24% were excluded or withdrew, treatment groups were not comparable at baseline, and there was a high cardiovascular mortality in the oestrogen group.[8] We found one additional RCT, which is awaiting translation.[34]

QUESTION **In men who have received primary treatment and remain asymptomatic, should androgen suppression be offered when raised concentrations of prostate specific antigens are detected?**

OPTION **ANDROGEN SUPPRESSION IN ASYMPTOMATIC MEN WITH RAISED PROSTATE SPECIFIC ANTIGEN CONCENTRATIONS AFTER EARLY TREATMENT**

We found no RCTs of initiating androgen suppression when prostate specific antigen rises or persists after primary treatment.

Benefits: We found one systematic review (search date 1998), which identified no RCTs.[35]

Harms: See harms of androgen suppression in men with locally advanced prostate cancer, p 1137.

Comment: In the USA, clinicians often monitor blood concentrations of prostate specific antigen and offer androgen suppression**G** when these rise.[35] Consequently, more men with persistent disease are considered for androgen suppression and treatment is initiated earlier in the natural course of the disease. RCTs are needed to evaluate the effectiveness of this approach and of intermittent treatment, in which androgen suppression is initiated when prostate specific antigen rises after primary treatment and discontinued when the antigen concentrations return to the lowest level.[35]

QUESTION **What are the effects of treatments for locally advanced prostate cancer?**

OPTION **ANDROGEN SUPPRESSION**

RCTs found no significant difference in overall survival between androgen suppression with bicalutamide and no androgen suppression in men with localised or locally advanced prostate cancer after 2–10 years. The RCTs found that bicalutamide reduced radiological progression compared with no bicalutamide. One systematic review found that early androgen treatment increased survival at 10 years compared with deferred treatment in men with locally advanced prostate cancer. It found no significant difference in survival at 5 years. One RCT found limited evidence that immediate androgen suppression reduced complications compared with deferred androgen suppression.

Benefits: **Versus no androgen suppression:** We found one preliminary report of three ongoing RCTs[1] and one reanalysis of three RCTs performed between 1960 and 1975.[36] The three ongoing RCTs (8113 men with localised or locally advanced prostate cancer T1–T4, Nx/N, M0) compared bicalutamide 150 mg once daily plus standard care with standard care alone.[1] Standard care included radical prostatectomy**G**, radiotherapy, and watchful waiting. Meta-analysis found that bicalutamide plus standard care significantly reduced radiological progression and bone metastases after 2–3 years compared with standard care alone (progression: 363/4052 [9.0%] with bicalutamide plus standard care *v* 595/4061 [14.7%] with standard care alone; HR 0.58, 95% CI 0.51 to 0.66; P < 0.0001; bone metastases: 214 events with bicalutamide plus standard care *v* 321 events with standard care alone; RR 0.67, 95% CI 0.56 to 0.79). There was no significant difference between treatments in overall survival (overall survival: HR 0.93, 95% CI 0.79 to 1.11).[1] The three earlier RCTs (about 4000 men with all stages of newly diagnosed prostate cancer) compared androgen suppression**G** (diethylstilbestrol [stilboestrol], orchidectomy, or oestrogens) versus no initial treatment.[36] They found no significant difference in overall survival. Reanalysis of updated data (published 1988) from these RCTs provided limited evidence of a modest survival advantage with androgen suppression, particularly in younger people with more advanced disease.[36] **Immediate (initiated at diagnosis) versus deferred androgen suppression:** We found one systematic review (search date 2001, 4 RCTs, 2167 men with locally advanced prostate cancer).[37] All RCTs included in the review were conducted before prostate specific antigen testing was introduced. Each RCT used different methods of androgen suppression and had different requirements for initiation of treatment. It found no significant difference in overall survival at 1, 2, or 5 years with early compared with deferred androgen suppression (3 RCTs, 1307 men, at 1 year 88% with early *v* 86% with deferred; RR 1.04, 95% CI 0.99 to 1.09; at 2 years 73% with early *v* 71% with deferred; RR 1.05, 95% CI 0.97 to 1.12; at 5 years 44% with early *v* 37% with deferred; RR 1.08, 95% CI 0.96 to 1.22). However, it found that early treatment significantly increased survival at 10 years compared with deferred treatment (18% with early *v* 12% with deferred; OR 1.50, 95% CI 1.04 to 2.16). The most recent of the RCTs[38] identified by the review (938 men with stage C [locally advanced] or stage D [asymptomatic metastatic] disease) was not included in the meta-analysis (see comment below). It found that in men with stage C disease, immediate androgen suppression significantly improved survival compared with deferred treatment (survival benefit measured by survival curve; P = 0.02; CI not reported). The RCT found that in people with stage C disease, immediate androgen suppression was associated with a non-significant lower risk of major complications, such as pathological fractures compared with deferred treatment (3/256 [1.2%] with immediate *v* 6/244 [2.5%] with deferred; RR 0.48, 95% CI 0.12 to 1.90), ureteric obstruction (22/256 [8.6%] with immediate *v* 28/244 [11.5%] with deferred; RR 0.75, 95% CI 0.44 to 1.30), and extraskeletal metastases (17/256 [6.6%] with immediate *v* 26/244 [10.7%] with deferred; RR 0.62, 95% CI 0.35 to 1.10). Analysis including all participants found a significant reduction for combined results of pathological fracture and cord compression (RR 0.48, 95% CI 0.28 to 0.79). The RCT did not make clear the time interval over which outcomes were recorded, although this seemed to be at least 10 years.[38] One additional RCT in men with cancers of different stages found that bicalutamide significantly improved disease free progression at 2.6 years compared with placebo.[39] See benefits of androgen suppression under effects of treating clinically localised prostate cancer, p 1135.

Harms: Adverse events were not well reported in the review.[37] Earlier initiation of androgen suppression means longer exposure to adverse effects, which include osteoporosis, weight gain, hot flushes (10–60%), loss of muscle mass, gynaecomastia (5–10%), impotence (10–30%), and loss of libido (5–30%).[35] These adverse effects are particularly important in the treatment of men with long life expectancy or younger men with lower grade cancers. The review did not report on quality of life. See harms of androgen suppression under effects of treating clinically localised prostate cancer, p 1135.

Comment: The RCTs conducted in the 1960s and 1970s[35] included men who were older and had more advanced cancers than those in the more recent RCT.[38] The most recent RCT[38] will be included in the meta-analysis of the systematic review[37] in future updates of the Cochrane Library. RCTs are needed to evaluate the effectiveness of androgen suppression before surgery when disease extends beyond the capsule.

OPTION ANDROGEN SUPPRESSION PLUS EXTERNAL BEAM RADIATION VERSUS EXTERNAL BEAM RADIATION ALONE

RCTs found limited evidence that androgen suppression initiated at diagnosis plus external beam radiation improved long term survival compared with radiation alone or radiation plus deferred androgen suppression. One RCT found limited evidence that immediate androgen suppression reduced complications compared with deferred androgen suppression.

Benefits: We found one systematic review (search date 1998, 4 RCTs, 1565 men)[35] and one additional RCT.[40] The review compared early versus deferred androgen suppression**G** in men receiving external beam radiation.[35] Early androgen suppression was initiated at the same time as radiation treatment for locally advanced, or asymptomatic but clinically evident, metastatic prostate cancer, and was continued until the development of hormone refractory disease. The deferred group received radiation treatment alone, with androgen suppression initiated only in those in whom the disease progressed. The systematic review found that early androgen suppression significantly improved overall 5 year survival compared with deferred treatment (percentage surviving at 5 years 76.5% with early *v* 68.2% with deferred; ARR 8.3%; HR 0.63, 95% CI 0.48 to 0.83; NNT at 5 years 12).[35] Long term follow up of one of the RCTs included in the review (476 men, stages T2–T4, with or without pelvic lymph node involvement) found that more people survived with early androgen suppression at 8 years compared with deferred treatment, but the difference was not significant (53% with early *v* 44% with deferred; P = 0.1). There was a significant improvement in disease free survival (33% with early *v* 21% with deferred; P = 0.004) and in the incidence of distant metastases (34% with early *v* 45% with deferred; P = 0.04).[41] The additional RCT (277 men with advanced localised prostate cancer; T2–T4, M0, with and without nodal disease) compared three treatments: orchidectomy alone, radiotherapy alone, or radiotherapy in addition to orchidectomy.[40] It found no significant difference in overall survival or need for further treatment for local disease progression between the three treatment groups (data presented graphically; P value not reported), but it is likely to have been underpowered to detect a clinically important difference.

Harms: The review reported adverse effects of androgen suppression (see harms of androgen suppression for the treatment of men with locally advanced prostate cancer, p 1137).[35] In the additional RCT, adverse effects associated with radiotherapy included bowel symptoms (19%), urinary symptoms including transient frequency (8%), bowel and urinary complications (1%), rectal bleeding necessitating blood transfusion (2%), and radiation proctitis (1%), which was a contributory factor in two deaths. It found that the predominant adverse effect after orchidectomy was hot flushes (15%).[40]

Comment: We found no evidence from RCTs of external beam radiation alone in men with locally advanced prostate cancer.

OPTION ANDROGEN SUPPRESSION AFTER RADICAL PROSTATECTOMY AND PELVIC LYMPHADENECTOMY

One small RCT in men with node positive prostate cancer found that immediate androgen suppression compared with deferred androgen suppression after radical prostatectomy and pelvic lymphadenectomy reduced mortality over a median of 7 years' follow up.

Benefits: We found one RCT (98 men who had had a radical prostatectomy**G** and pelvic lymphadenectomy for nodal metastases) comparing immediate androgen suppression**G** (with either goserelin or bilateral orchidectomy) versus androgen suppression deferred until disease progression.[42] It found that androgen suppression significantly reduced mortality in the long term compared with watchful waiting (median follow up 7.1 years; mortality 7/47 [14.9%] with androgen suppression *v* 18/51 [35.3%] with watchful waiting; ARR 20.4%; RR 0.42, 95% CI 0.19 to 0.92; NNT 4, 95% CI 3 to 33), and resulted in a higher proportion of men with undetectable prostate specific antigen ($P < 0.001$).

Harms: The RCT found that, compared with deferred androgen suppression, immediate androgen suppression caused more haematological effects (15% with immediate *v* 4% with deferred), gastrointestinal effects (25% with immediate *v* 6% with deferred), non-specific genitourinary effects (48% with immediate *v* 12% with deferred), hot flushes (56% with immediate *v* 0% with deferred), and weight gain (18% with immediate *v* 2% with deferred).[42]

Comment: None.

GLOSSARY

Androgen suppression Monotherapy uses a single drug or surgical procedure for androgen suppression. Methods include orchidectomy (removal of both testes), diethylstilbestrol, luteinising hormone releasing hormone agonist injections, or non-steroidal antiandrogens. Combined androgen blockade uses the addition of a non-steroidal antiandrogen to standard androgen suppression monotherapy with orchidectomy, diethylstilbestrol, or luteinising hormone releasing hormone agonist injection.
Brachytherapy Radiotherapy where the sources of ionising radiation are radioactive implants, many of which are permanently inserted directly into the prostate gland.
Conformal radiotherapy Three dimensional radiotherapy planning systems and methods to match the radiation treatment to irregular tumour volumes.
Gleason score A number from 1–10 with 1 being the most well differentiated and 10 being the most poorly differentiated tumour or a histological examination.
Radical prostatectomy Surgical removal of the prostate with its capsule, seminal vesicles, ductus deferens, some pelvic fasciae, and sometimes pelvic lymph nodes; performed through either the retropubic or the perineal route.

REFERENCES

1. See WA, Wirth MP, McLeod DG et al. Bicalutamide as immediate therapy either alone or as adjuvant to standard care of patients with localized or locally advanced prostate cancer: first analysis of the early prostate cancer program. *J Urol* 2002;168:429–435.
2. Stanford JL, Stephenson RA, Coyle LM, et al. Prostate Cancer Trends 1973–1995, SEER Program, National Cancer Institute. NIH Pub. No. 99–4543. Bethesda, MD, 1999.
3. Adolfsson J, Steineck G, Hedund P. Deferred treatment of clinically localized low-grade prostate cancer: actual 10-year and projected 15-year follow-up of the Karolinska series. *Urology* 1997;50:722–726.
4. Johansson J-E, Holmberg L, Johansson S, et al. Fifteen-year survival in prostate cancer: prospective, population-based study in Sweden. *JAMA* 1997;277:467–471.
5. Pound CR, Partin AW, Eisenberger MA, et al. Natural history of progression after PSA elevation following radical prostatectomy. *JAMA* 1999;281:1591–1597.
6. Lu-Yao G, Albertsen PC, Stanford JL et al. Natural experiment examining impact of aggressive screening and treatment on prostate cancer mortality in two fixed cohorts from Seattle area and Connecticut. *BMJ* 2002;325:740.
7. Frankel S, Smith GD, Donovan J, et al. Screening for prostate cancer. *Lancet* 2003;361:1122–1128.

8. Harris RP, Lohr KN, Beck R, et al. *Screening for prostate cancer*. Systematic Evidence Review no. 16. Rockville, MD: Agency for Healthcare Research and Quality, 2001. Available online at http://www.ahrq.gov/clinic/serfiles.htm (last accessed 16 September 2003).
9. Holmberg L, Bill-Axelson A, Helgesen F et al. A randomized trial comparing radical prostatectomy with watchful waiting in early prostate cancer. *N Engl J Med* 2002;347:781–789.
10. Albertsen PC, Hanley JA, Gleason DF, et al. Competing risk analysis of men aged 55 to 74 years at diagnosis managed conservatively for clinically localized prostate cancer. *JAMA* 1998;280:975–980.
11. Lu-Yao GL, Yao S. Population-based study of long-term survival in patients with clinically localised prostate cancer. *Lancet* 1997;349:906–910.
12. Gann PH, Hennekens CH, Stampfer MJ. A prospective evaluation of plasma prostate-specific antigen for detection of prostatic cancer. *JAMA* 1995;273:289–294.
13. Iversen P, Madsen PO, Corle DK. Radical prostatectomy versus expectant treatment for early carcinoma of the prostate: 23 year follow-up of a prospective randomized study. *Scand J Urol Nephrol* 1995;172(suppl):65–72.
14. Paulson DF, Lin GH, Hinshaw W, et al. Radical surgery versus radiotherapy for adenocarcinoma of the prostate. *J Urol* 1982;128:502–504.
15. Steineck G, Helgesen Adolfsson J, et al. Quality of life after radical prostatectomy or watchful waiting. *N Engl J Med* 2002;347:790–796.
16. Lu-Yao GL, McLerran D, Wasson JH. An assessment of radical prostatectomy: time trends, geographic variation, and outcomes. *JAMA* 1993;269:2633–2636.
17. Middleton RG, Thompson IM, Austenfeld MS, et al. Prostate cancer clinical guidelines panel summary report on the management of clinically localized prostate cancer. *J Urol* 1995;154:2144–2148. Search date 1993; primary source Medline.
18. Anonymous. Screening for prostate cancer. *Ann Intern Med* 1997;126:480–484.
19. Fowler FJ, Barry MJ, Lu-Yao G, et al. Patient-reported complications and follow-up treatment after radical prostatectomy: the national Medicare experience 1988–1990 (updated June 1993). *Urology* 1993;42:622–629.
20. Bishoff JT, Motley G, Optenberg SA, et al. Incidence of fecal and urinary incontinence following radical perineal and retropubic prostatectomy in a national population. *J Urol* 1998;160:454–458.
21. Fleming C, Wasson J, Albertsen PC, et al. A decision analysis of alternative strategies for clinically localized prostate cancer. *JAMA* 1993;269:2650–2658.
22. Litwin MS, Hays RD, Fink A, et al. Quality-of-life outcomes in men treated for localized prostate cancer. *JAMA* 1995;273:129–135.
23. Wilt TJ, Brawer MK. The prostate cancer intervention versus observation trial. *Oncology* 1997;11:1133–1139.
24. Norlen BJ. Swedish randomized trial of radical prostatectomy versus watchful waiting. *Can J Oncol* 1994;4(suppl 1):38–42.
25. Brundage M, Lukka H, Crook J, et al. The use of conformal radiotherapy and the selection of radiation dose in T1 or T2 low or intermediate risk prostate cancer – a systematic review. *Radiother Oncol* 2002;64:239–250. Search date 2001; primary sources Medline, Cancerlit, proceedings of the *American Society of Clinical Oncology* and the *American Society for Therapeutic Radiology and Oncology*, personal files, and bibliographies of identified articles and reviews.
26. Dearnaley DP, Khoo VS, Norman AR, et al. Comparison of radiation side-effects of conformal and conventional radiotherapy in prostate cancer: a randomized trial. *Lancet* 1999;353:267–272.
27. Fowler FJ, Barry MJ, Lu-Yao G, et al. Outcomes of external beam radiation therapy for prostate cancer: a study of Medicare beneficiaries in three surveillance, epidemiology, and end results areas. *J Clin Oncol* 1996;14:2258–2265.
28. Crook J, Perry G, Robertson S, et al. Routine prostate biopsies: results for 225 patients. *Urology* 1995;45:624–632.
29. Shipley WU, Thames HD, Sandler HM, et al. Radiation therapy for clinically localized prostate cancer. A multi-institutional pooled analysis. *JAMA* 1999;281:1598–1604.
30. Crook J, Lukka H, Klotz L, et al. Systematic overview of the evidence for brachytherapy in clinically localized prostate cancer. *Can Med Assoc J* 2001;164:975–981. Search date 1999; primary sources Medline and Cancerlit.
31. Wills F, Hailey D. Brachytherapy for prostate cancer. Edmonton, AB, Canada: The Alberta Heritage Foundation for Medical Research. *Health Technol Assess* 1999:1–65. Search date 1999; primary sources The Cochrane Library, Medline, Healthstar, Cancerlit, Embase, Cinahl, hand searches of reference lists, and internet searches.
32. Talcott JA, Clark JC, Stark P, et al. Long term complications of brachytherapy for early prostate cancer. A survey of treated patients. American Society of Clinical Oncology Annual Meeting 1999; Abstract 1196.
33. Littrup PJ, Mody A, Sparschu RA. Prostate cryosurgery complications. *Semin Int Radiol* 1994;11:226–230.
34. Rauchenwald M. First results of the early prostate cancer program study. *J Urol Urogynakol* 2001;8:21–27.
35. Agency for Health Care Policy and Research. Relative effectiveness and cost-effectiveness of methods of androgen suppression in the treatment of advanced prostatic cancer. Summary. Rockville, MD: Agency for Health Care Policy and Research, 1999. (Evidence Report/Technology Assessment: No 4.) http://www.ahcpr.gov/clinic/epcsums/prossumm.htm (last accessed 10 July 2003). Search date 1998; primary sources Medline, Cancerlit, Embase, Current Contents, and Cochrane Library.
36. Byar DP, Corle DK. Hormone treatment for prostate cancer: results of the Veterans' Administration cooperative urologic research group studies. *NCI Monograph* 1988;7:165–170.
37. Nair B, Wilt T, MacDonald, R, et al. Early versus deferred androgen suppression in the treatment of advanced prostatic cancer. In: The Cochrane Library, Issue 2, 2002. Oxford: Update Software. Search date 2001; primary sources Medline, Embase, Cancerlit, Cochrane Library, VA Cochrane Prostate Disease register, and hand searches of bibliographies.
38. The Medical Research Council Prostate Cancer Working Party Investigators Group. Immediate versus deferred treatment for advanced prostatic cancer: initial results of the Medical Research Council trial. *Br J Urol* 1997;79:235–246.
39. Wirth M, Tyrrell C, Wallace M, et al. Bicalutamide (Casodex) 150 mg as immediate therapy in patients with localized or locally advanced prostate cancer significantly reduces the risk of disease progression. *Urology* 2001;58:146–150.
40. Fellows GJ, Clark PB, Beynon LL, et al. Treatment of advanced localised prostatic cancer by orchiectomy, radiotherapy, or combined treatment. *Br J Urol* 1992:70;304–309.
41. Pilepich M, Winter M, Madhu J, et al. Phase III Radiation Therapy Oncology Group (RTOG) trial 86–10 of androgen deprivation adjuvant to definitive radiotherapy in locally advanced carcinoma of the prostate. *Int J Radiat Oncol Biol Phys* 2001;50:1243–1252.
42. Messing EM, Manola J, Sarodsy M, et al. Immediate hormonal therapy compared with observation after radical prostatectomy and pelvic lymphadenectomy in men with node-positive prostate cancer. *N Engl J Med* 1999;341:1781–1789.

Prostate cancer (non-metastatic)

Timothy Wilt
Professor of Medicine
VA Coordinating Center for the Cochrane Review Group in Prostate Diseases and Urologic Malignancies and the Center for Chronic Diseases Outcomes Research
Minneapolis VA Hospital, Minneapolis, MN, USA

Competing interests: None declared.
We would like to acknowledge the previous contributors of this chapter, including Michael Brawer.

TABLE 1 **Prostatic cancer staging systems (see text, p 1129).**

Tumour, node, metastasis (TNM) classification system	
Tumour	
T0	Clinically unsuspected
T1	Clinically inapparent (not palpable or visible by imaging)
T2	Tumour confined within prostate
T3	Tumour outside capsule or extension into vesicle
T4	Tumour fixed to other tissue
Nodes	
N0	No evidence of involvement of regional nodes
N1	Involvement of regional nodes
Metastases	
M0	No evidence of distant metastases
M1	Evidence of distant metastases
American urologic staging system	
Stage A	No palpable tumour
Stage B	Tumour confined to the prostate gland
Stage C	Extracapsular extension
Stage D	Metastatic prostate cancer
Stage D1	Pelvic lymph node metastases
Stage D2	Distant metastases

Varicocele

Search date September 2004

Chandra Shekhar Biyani and Günter Janetschek

QUESTIONS

INTERVENTIONS

Key Messages

Treatments

- **Embolisation** We found no RCTs comparing embolisation with no treatment or sclerotherapy. Three RCTs provided insufficient evidence on the effects of embolisation for improving fertility in men with varicocele compared with ligation techniques. We found no evidence examining the effects of embolisation on pain or discomfort caused by varicocele.
- **Expectant management** One systematic review of poor quality, heterogeneous RCTs in couples with male factor subfertility found no consistent evidence of difference in pregnancy rate between expectant management and surgical ligation or sclerotherapy. The review found no RCTs comparing expectant management with embolisation. We found no evidence examining the effects of expectant management on pain or discomfort caused by varicocele.
- **Sclerotherapy** One RCT found no significant difference in pregnancy rate between sclerotherapy and no treatment. We found no evidence examining the effects of sclerotherapy on pain or discomfort caused by varicocele.
- **Surgical ligation** One systematic review and additional RCTs provided insufficient evidence on the effects of different surgical ligation techniques in pregnancy rate compared with no treatment, embolisation or each other. We found no RCTs comparing surgical ligation with sclerotherapy. We found no evidence examining the effects of ligation on pain or discomfort caused by varicocele.

DEFINITION Varicocele is a dilation of the pampiniform plexus of the spermatic cord. Severity is commonly graded as follows: **grade 0**, only demonstrable by technical investigation; **grade 1**, palpable or visible only on Valsalva manoeuvre (straining); **grade 2**, palpable but not visible when standing upright at room temperature; and **grade 3**, visible when standing upright at room temperature. Varicocele is unilateral and left sided in at least 85% of cases. In most of the remaining cases, the condition is bilateral. Unilateral right sided varicocele is rare. Many men who have a varicocele have no symptoms. Symptoms may include testicular ache or discomfort and distress about cosmetic appearance. The condition is widely believed to be associated with male factor infertility, which is the most common reason for referral for treatment. However, evidence for a causal relationship is sparse.[1]

INCIDENCE/ PREVALENCE We found few data on the prevalence of varicocele. Anecdotally, it has been estimated that about 10–15% of men and adolescent boys in the general population have varicocele.[1] One multicentre study found that, in couples with subfertility, the prevalence of varicocele in male partners was about 12%.[2] In men with abnormal semen analysis, the prevalence of varicocele was about 25%.

AETIOLOGY/ RISK FACTORS We found no reliable data on epidemiological risk factors for varicocele, such as a family history or environmental exposures. Anatomically, varicoceles are caused by dysfunction of the valves in the spermatic vein, which allows pooling of blood in the pampiniform plexus. This is more likely to occur in the left spermatic vein than in the right because of normal anatomical asymmetry.

PROGNOSIS Varicocele is believed to be associated with subfertility, although reliable evidence is sparse. The natural history of varicocele is unclear.

AIMS OF INTERVENTION To improve the rate of pregnancy in couples in which the male partner has varicocele and the woman has no identified fertility problems; to reduce pain and discomfort associated with varicocele, with minimal adverse effects.

OUTCOMES Where available, we have reported on spontaneous live birth rate (i.e. without assisted reproductive techniques such as in vitro fertilisation), spontaneous pregnancy rate, pain or discomfort (we found no scales that have been specifically validated for this condition), quality of life, and adverse effects of treatments. Non-clinical outcomes such as testicular temperature, blood flow, or sperm count were excluded.

METHODS *Clinical Evidence* search and appraisal September 2004. The authors also conducted an extensive search of Medline, the Indian Medlars Centre (http://medind.nic.in) using the word varicocele, and hand searches of the bibliographies of retrieved articles, published abstracts, and reviews. All relevant RCTs that were identified were reviewed.

QUESTION What are the effects of treatments in men with varicocele?

OPTION EXPECTANT MANAGEMENT (NO TREATMENT)

One systematic review of poor quality, heterogeneous RCTs in couples with male factor subfertility found no consistent evidence of difference in pregnancy rate between expectant management and surgical ligation or sclerotherapy. The review found no RCTs comparing expectant management with embolisation. We found no evidence examining the effects of expectant management on pain or discomfort caused by varicocele.

Benefits: We found no RCTs examining the effects of expectant management on pain or discomfort in people with varicocele. **Versus surgical ligation:** We found one systematic review (search date 2003, 4 RCTs; see comment below).[1] The review did not undertake an overall meta-analysis for this comparison. Only one of the identified RCTs found a significant difference in pregnancy rate between expectant management and surgical ligation. The first RCT included in the review (45 subfertile men with varicocele grade 1–3) found that surgical ligation of the spermatic vein using the Palomo technique**G** significantly improved pregnancy rate compared with no treatment after 12 months (15/25 [60%] with ligation *v* 2/20 [10%] with no treatment; OR 8.00, 95%

CI 2.41 to 26.55).[3] The second RCT included in the review (96 subfertile men with varicocele) found no significant difference in pregnancy rate between surgical ligation [Palomo technique] of one or both internal spermatic veins and no treatment after a mean of 53 months of follow up (4/51 [8%] with ligation *v* 8/45 [18%] with no treatment; OR 0.41, 95% CI 0.12 to 1.36).[4] The third RCT included in the review (92 subfertile men with varicocele) found no significant difference in pregnancy rate between high ligation of the internal spermatic vein(s) and no treatment after 12 months (3/45 [7%] with ligation *v* 4/40 [10%] with no treatment; OR 0.65, 95% CI 0.14 to 3.02).[5] The fourth RCT[6] identified by the review (68 men with low grade varicocele) reported no significant difference in rate of pregnancy between spermatic vein ligation (Palomo technique) and no treatment at 12 months (1/34 [3%] with vein ligation *v* 2/34 [6%] with no treatment; OR 0.50, 95%CI 0.05 to 1.96).[1] **Versus sclerotherapy:** We found one systematic review (search date 2003, 1 RCT, 67 men with varicocele who were childless for at least 12 months).[1] The RCT found no significant difference in pregnancy rate between sclerotherapy**G** and no treatment after 12 months (15.6% with sclerotherapy *v* 18.2% with no treatment; OR 0.88, 95% CI 0.18 to 4.06).[7] However, the study had important methodological weaknesses (see comment below). **Versus embolisation:** We found one systematic review (search date 2003), which found no RCTs. [1]

Harms: **Versus surgical ligation:** The systematic review (search date September 2003) did not report on harms.[1] The fourth RCT identified by the review reported no complications after surgery.[6] **Versus sclerotherapy:** The RCT did not report on harms.[7] **Versus embolisation:** See harms of embolisation, p 1146.

Comment: The systematic review described two RCTs that had more than two treatment arms.[1] One compared ligation (Palomo technique**G**), sclerotherapy**G**, embolisation**G**, and no treatment. The other compared ligation (Bernardi technique**G**), embolisation, and no treatment. We excluded these two studies because people were randomised in the treatment group, regardless of treatment technique, and therefore the effects of ligation or embolisation alone could not be assessed reliably.[1] We also found one RCT examining expectant management, which published preliminary results in abstract form only, and which will be considered for inclusion when it is published in full.[8] **Versus surgical ligation:** The systematic review found that the studies included were heterogeneous and of poor methodological quality.[1] The first RCT in the review is part of a large prospective WHO multicentre study, which started in 1984.[3] The full results of the multicentre study are awaited.[1] The third RCT in the review described a high ligation technique; it is not explicit that this was the Ivanissevich technique**G**.[5] None of the RCTs reported analysis on an intention to treat basis. **Versus sclerotherapy:** The RCT did not achieve the estimated sample size (460 men) needed for adequate power, recruiting only 67 men.[7] Out of these, 34 (51%) men did not return for follow up and it was assumed in the intention to treat analysis that their partners did not become pregnant.

OPTION SURGICAL LIGATION

One systematic review and additional RCTs provided insufficient evidence on the effects of different surgical ligation techniques in pregnancy rate compared with no treatment, embolisation or each other. We found no RCTs comparing surgical ligation with sclerotherapy. We found no evidence examining the effects of ligation on pain or discomfort caused by varicocele.

Benefits: We found no evidence examining the effects of surgical ligation on pain or discomfort caused by varicocele. **Versus no treatment:** See benefits of expectant management, p 1143. **Versus embolisation:** See benefits of embolisation, p 1145. **Versus sclerotherapy:** See benefits of sclerotherapy, p 1146. We found no RCTs. **Ligation techniques versus each other:** We found no systematic review. We found two RCTs.[9,10] The first RCT (137 infertile men with varicocele) compared the Ivanissevich technique of ligationⒼ, the Bernardi technique of ligationⒼ, and embolisationⒼ of the internal spermatic vein.[9] It found no significant difference in pregnancy rate between the Ivanissevich technique and the Bernardi technique at 18 months (13/34 [38%] with the Ivanissevich technique *v* 9/35 [26%] with the Bernardi technique; P value not reported). The second RCT (119 infertile men with varicocele) compared the Palomo technique of ligationⒼ the Bernardi technique of ligation, and transcatheter embolisation.[10] It found no significant difference in pregnancy rate between the ligation techniques after 2 years (29% with Palomo technique *v* 25% with Bernardi technique; P value not reported).

Harms: **Versus no treatment:** See harms of expectant management, p 1144. **Versus embolisation:** See harms of embolisation, p 1146. **Versus sclerotherapy:** See harms of sclerotherapy, p 1146. **Ligation techniques versus each other:** The first RCT did not report on harms.[9] The second RCT that compared high ligation, transinguinal ligation, and transcatheter embolisationⒼ reported two cases of pyrexia and flank tenderness in the embolisation group, and one case of wound infection in the ligation group.[10]

Comment: **Versus no treatment:** See comment under expectant management, p 1144.

OPTION EMBOLISATION

We found no RCTs comparing embolisation with no treatment or sclerotherapy. Three RCTs provided insufficient evidence on the effects of embolisation for improving fertility in men with varicocele compared with ligation techniques. We found no evidence examining the effects of embolisation on pain or discomfort caused by varicocele.

Benefits: We found no evidence examining the effects of embolisationⒼ on pain or discomfort owing to varicocele. **Versus no treatment:** See benefits of expectant management, p 1143. **Versus surgical ligation:** We found no systematic review. We found three RCTs.[9–11] The first RCT (107 men with primary infertility and 30 men with secondary infertility) compared the Ivanissevich technique of ligationⒼ, Bernardi technique of ligation, and embolisation.[9] It found that the Ivanissevich technique significantly increased the rate of pregnancy compared with embolisation (13/34 [38%] with the Ivanissevich technique *v* 9/35 [26%] with the Bernardi technique *v* 7/34 [21%] with embolisation; $P < 0.05$ between the Ivanissevich technique and embolisation; other P values not reported). The second RCT (119 men with primary and secondary infertility) compared the Palomo technique of ligationⒼ, Bernardi technique of ligationⒼ, and transcatheter embolisation.[10] It found no significant difference in pregnancy rate between the three treatment options after 2 years (29% with the Palomo technique *v* 25% with Bernardi technique *v* 28% with embolisation; P values not reported). The third RCT (71 infertile men) found no significant difference in pregnancy rate between surgical ligation and embolisation at 12 months (11/38 [29%] with ligation *v* 11/33 [33%] with embolisation; $P > 0.05$).[11] **Versus sclerotherapy:** We found no RCTs.

Harms: The first RCT that compared embolisation❻ with left internal sperm ligation reported some complications (3/51 [6%] with embolisation *v* 2/43 [5%] with the Palomo technique❻ *v* 2/43 [5%] with the Bernardi technique❻; P values not reported).[9] Left lower abdominal pain was the most common complaint in the embolisation group, and wound infection was the most common complaint in the ligation groups.

Comment: One systematic review described two RCTs that had more than two treatment arms.[1] One compared ligation (Palomo technique❻), sclerotherapy❻, embolisation❻, and no treatment. The other compared ligation (Bernardi technique❻), embolisation, and no treatment. We excluded these two studies because people were randomised in the treatment group, regardless of treatment technique, and therefore the effects of ligation or embolisation alone could not be assessed reliably.[1]

OPTION SCLEROTHERAPY

One RCT found no significant difference in pregnancy rate between sclerotherapy and no treatment. We found no evidence examining the effects of sclerotherapy on pain or discomfort caused by varicocele.

Benefits: We found no RCTs examining the effects of sclerotherapy❻ on pain or discomfort owing to varicocele. **Versus no treatment:** See benefits of expectant management, p 1143. **Versus surgical ligation or embolisation:** We found no RCTs.

Harms: **Versus no treatment:** The RCT comparing sclerotherapy❻ versus no treatment did not report on harms.[7] **Versus surgical ligation or embolisation:** We found no RCTs.

Comment: One systematic review described an RCT that had more than two treatment arms.[1] The RCT compared ligation (Palomo technique❻), [sclerotherapy❻], embolisation❻, and no treatment. We excluded this study because people were randomised in the treatment group, regardless of treatment technique, and therefore the effects of sclerotherapy alone could not be reliably assessed.

GLOSSARY

Bernardi technique of ligation The spermatic vein(s) are ligated close to the inguinal ring. Surgery is usually performed under general anaesthesia in an outpatient setting. Occasionally, the surgery is performed with a local anaesthetic.

Embolisation The left spermatic vein is catheterised via the left renal vein. Selective spermatic venography is then performed to demonstrate the venous anatomy. The vein is embolised by various liquids and materials, including coils (Gianturco or microcoils), detachable balloons, sclerosant agents (such as alcohol, sodium tetradecyl, or glue) or a combination. Transcatheter embolisation is performed as an outpatient procedure under intravenous sedation and analgesia.

Ivanissevich technique of ligation The spermatic vein(s) are ligated high, close to the iliac crest. Surgery is usually performed under general anaesthesia in an outpatient setting. Occasionally, the surgery is performed with a local anaesthetic.

Palomo technique of ligation The retroperitoneal internal spermatic vein(s) are ligated at the level of the anterior superior iliac spine. Surgery is usually performed under general anaesthesia in an outpatient setting. Occasionally, the surgery is performed with a local anaesthetic.

Sclerotherapy A sclerosing substance is injected into the spermatic vein to produce endothelial destruction resulting in occlusion owing to fibrosis. Sclerotherapy can be performed under local anaesthesia.

Substantive changes

One new systematic review found no new RCTs;[1] categorisation unchanged

REFERENCES

1. Evers JL, Collins JA. Surgery or embolisation for varicocele in subfertile men (Cochrane Review). In: The Cochrane Library, Issue 3, 2004. Chichester, UK: John Wiley & Sons Ltd. Search date 2003; primary sources Cochrane Menstrual Disorders and Subfertility Group's specialised register of controlled trials, Medline, hand searches of 22 specialist journals (first issue until 2004) and searches of references of identified studies.
2. World Health Organization. The influence of varicocele on parameters of fertility in a large group of men presenting to infertility clinics. *Fertil Steril* 1992;57:1289–1293.
3. Madgar I, Weissenberg R, Lunenfeld B, et al. Controlled trial of high spermatic vein ligation for varicocele in infertile men. *Fertil Steril* 1995;63:120–124.
4. Nilsson S, Edvinsson A, Nilsson B. Improvement of semen and pregnancy rate after ligation and division of the internal spermatic vein: fact or fiction? *Br J Urol* 1979;51:591–596.
5. Yamamoto M, Hibi H, Hirata Y, et al. Effect of varicocelectomy on sperm parameters and pregnancy rate in patients with subclinical varicocele: a randomized prospective controlled study. *J Urol* 1996;155:1636–1638.
6. Grasso M, Lania C, Castelli M, et al. Low-grade left varicocele in patients over 30 years old: the effect of spermatic vein ligation on fertility. *BJU Int* 2000;85:305–307.
7. Krause W, Müller HH, Schäfer H, et al. Does treatment of varicocele improve male fertility? Results of the "Deutsche Varikozelenstudie", a multicentre study of 14 collaborating centres. *Andrologia* 2002;34:164–171.
8. Dohle GR, Pierik F, Weber RF. Does varicocele repair result in more spontaneous pregnancies? A randomised prospective trial. *J Urol* 2003;169(suppl):408–409. [abstract 1525].
9. Yavetz H, Levy R, Papo L, et al. Efficacy of varicocele embolization versus ligation of the left internal spermatic vein for improvement of sperm quality. *Int J Androl* 1992;15:338–344.
10. Sayfan J, Soffer Y, Orda R. Varicocele treatment: prospective randomized trial of 3 methods. *J Urol* 1992;148:1447–1449.
11. Nieschlag E, Behre HM, Schlingheider A, et al. Surgical ligation vs angiographic embolization of the vena spermatica: a prospective randomized study for the treatment of varicocele-related infertility. *Andrologia* 1993;25:233–237.

Chandra Shekhar Biyani
Consultant Urological Surgeon
Pinderfields General Hospital
Wakefield
UK

Günter Janetschek
Professor of Urology
Elisabethinen
Linz
Austria

Competing interests: None declared.

Anorexia nervosa

Search date December 2003

Janet Treasure and Ulrike Schmidt

QUESTIONS

INTERVENTIONS

See glossary

Key Messages

Treatments

- **Inpatient versus outpatient treatment setting in anorexia nervosa** One small RCT found no significant difference between outpatient treatment and inpatient treatment for increasing weight and improving Morgan Russell scale global scores at 1, 2, and 5 years in people who did not need emergency intervention.
- **Psychotherapy** Small RCTs provided insufficient evidence to compare psychotherapy versus treatment as usual, dietary counselling, or each other.
- **Selective serotonin reuptake inhibitors** Three small RCTs provided insufficient evidence about the effects of selective serotonin reuptake inhibitors compared with placebo or no treatment in people with anorexia nervosa.
- **Zinc** One small RCT found limited evidence that zinc may improve daily body mass index gain compared with placebo in people managed in an inpatient setting. However, we were unable to draw reliable conclusions from this small study.
- **Cisapride** One small RCT found no significant difference between cisapride and placebo in weight gain at 8 weeks. Use of cisapride has been restricted in many countries because of concern about cardiac irregularities, including ventricular tachycardia, torsades de pointes, and sudden death.
- **Cyproheptadine** Two RCTs in inpatient settings found no significant difference between cyproheptadine and placebo in weight gain.
- **Neuroleptic drugs** We found no RCTs. The QT interval may be prolonged in people with anorexia nervosa, and many neuroleptic drugs (haloperidol, pimozide, sertindole, thioridazine, chlorpromazine, and others) also increase the QT interval. Prolongation of the QT interval may be associated with increased risk of ventricular tachycardia, torsades de pointes, and sudden death.

- **Tricyclic antidepressants** Two small RCTs found no evidence of benefit with amitriptyline compared with placebo. One RCT found that amitriptyline was associated with more adverse effects, such as drowsiness, dry mouth, and blurred vision. The QT interval may be prolonged in people with anorexia nervosa, and tricyclic antidepressants (amitriptyline, protriptyline, nortriptyline, doxepin, and maprotiline) also increase the QT interval. Prolongation of the QT interval may be associated with increased risk of ventricular tachycardia, torsades de pointes, and sudden death.

Prevent or treat complications

- **Oestrogen treatment** We found no RCTs on the effects of oestrogen treatment on fracture rates in people with anorexia nervosa. Two small RCTs found no significant difference between oestrogen and placebo or no treatment in bone mineral density in people with anorexia nervosa.

DEFINITION Anorexia nervosa is characterised by a refusal to maintain weight at or above a minimally normal weight (< 85% of expected weight for age and height, or body mass index Ⓖ < 17.5 kg/m^2), or a failure to show the expected weight gain during growth. In association with this, there is often an intense fear of gaining weight, preoccupation with weight, denial of the current low weight and its adverse impact on health, and amenorrhoea. Two subtypes of anorexia nervosa, binge–purge and restricting, have been defined.[1]

INCIDENCE/ PREVALENCE A mean incidence in the general population of 19/100 000 a year in females and 2/100 000 a year in males has been estimated from 12 cumulative studies.[2] The highest rate was in female teenagers (age 13–19 years), where there were 50.8 cases/100 000 a year. A large cohort study screened 4291 Swedish school children, aged 16 years, by weighing and subsequent interview, and found the prevalence of anorexia nervosa (defined using DSM-III and DSM-III-R criteria) to be 7/1000 for girls and 1/1000 for boys.[3] Little is known of the incidence or prevalence in Asia, South America, or Africa.

AETIOLOGY/ RISK FACTORS Anorexia nervosa has been related to family, biological, social, and cultural factors. Studies have found that anorexia nervosa is associated with a family history of anorexia nervosa (adjusted HR 11.4, 95% CI 1.1 to 89.0), bulimia nervosa (adjusted HR 3.5, 95% CI 1.1 to 14.0),[4] depression, generalised anxiety disorder, obsessive compulsive disorder, or obsessive compulsive personality disorder (adjusted RR 3.6, 95% CI 1.6 to 8.0).[5] A twin study suggested that anorexia nervosa may be related to genetic factors but it was unable to estimate reliably the contribution of non-shared environmental factors.[6] Specific aspects of childhood temperament thought to be related include perfectionism, negative self evaluation, and extreme compliance.[7] Perinatal factors include prematurity, particularly if the baby was small for gestational age (prematurity: OR 3.2, 95% CI 1.6 to 6.2; prematurity and small for gestational age: OR 5.7, 95% CI 1.1 to 28.7).[8]

PROGNOSIS One prospective study followed up 51 people with teenage-onset anorexia nervosa, about half of whom received no or minimal treatment (< 8 sessions). After 10 years, 14/51 people (27%) had a persistent eating disorder, three (6%) had ongoing anorexia nervosa, and six (12%) had experienced a period of bulimia nervosa. People with anorexia nervosa were significantly more likely to have an affective disorder than controls matched for sex, age, and school (lifetime risk of affective disorder 96% in people with anorexia *v* 23% in controls; ARI 73%, 95% CI 60% to 85%). Obsessive compulsive disorder was, similarly, significantly more likely in people with anorexia nervosa compared with controls (30% *v* 10%; ARI 20%, 95% CI 10% to 41%). However, in 35% of people with obsessive compulsive disorder and anorexia nervosa, obsessive compulsive disorder preceded the anorexia. About half of all participants continued to have poor psychosocial functioning at 10 years (assessed using the Morgan Russell scale Ⓖ and Global Assessment of Functioning Scale).[9] A summary of treatment studies (68 studies published between 1953 and 1989, 3104 people, length of follow up 1–33 years) found that 43% of people recover completely (range 7–86%), 36% improve (range 1–69%), 20% develop a chronic eating disorder (range 0–43%), and 5% die from anorexia nervosa (range 0–21%).[10] Favourable prognostic factors include an early age at onset and a short interval between onset of symptoms and the beginning of treatment. Unfavourable prognostic factors include vomiting, bulimia, profound weight loss, chronicity, and a history of premorbid developmental or clinical abnormalities. The all cause standardised mortality ratio of eating disorders (anorexia nervosa and bulimia nervosa) has been estimated at 538, about three times higher than that of other psychiatric illnesses.[11] The average annual mortality was 0.59% a year in females in ten eating disorder populations (1322 people) with a minimum follow up of 6 years.[12] The mortality was higher for people with lower weight and with older age at presentation. Young women with anorexia nervosa are at an increased risk of fractures later in life.[13]

AIMS OF INTERVENTION To restore physical health (weight within the normal range and no sequelae of starvation, e.g. regular menstruation, normal bone mass), normal patterns of eating and attitudes towards weight and shape, and no additional psychiatric comorbidity (e.g. depression, anxiety, obsessive compulsive disorder); to reduce the impact of the illness on social functioning and quality of life.

OUTCOMES The most widely used measure of outcome is the Morgan Russell scale,[14] which includes nutritional status, menstrual function, mental state, and sexual and social adjustment. Biological outcome criteria alone, such as weight (body mass index or in relation to matched population weight) and menstrual function are used infrequently as outcome measures. RCTs do not usually have sufficient power or long enough follow up periods to examine mortality. Other validated outcome measures include eating symptom measures.[15–18] Bone mineral density is included as a proxy outcome for fracture risk.

METHODS *Clinical Evidence* search and appraisal December 2003. The authors also performed hand searches of reference lists of identified reviews. To be included, an RCT had to include at least 30 people and follow up more than 75% of them. Results from each of the identified trials were extracted independently by the two reviewers. Any disagreements were discussed until a consensus was reached.

QUESTION **What are the effects of treatments in anorexia nervosa?**

OPTION **PSYCHOTHERAPY**

Small RCTs provided insufficient evidence to compare psychotherapy versus treatment as usual, dietary counselling, or each other.

Benefits: **Versus treatment as usual or dietary counselling:** We found one systematic review (4 small RCTs, 173 people, search date 2002).[19] The review did not conduct a meta analysis, and only three of the included RCTs met our inclusion criteria.[20–22] The three RCTs were of limited quality, and compared different types of psychotherapy**Ⓖ** versus dietary counselling**Ⓖ** or treatment as usual (see table A on web extra). All three RCTs were carried out in an outpatient setting in people with a late age of onset and long duration of illness. The largest RCT found significant improvements in weight gain for some types of psychotherapy compared with treatment as usual and for the proportion of people classified as recovered.[20] The second RCT found no difference in outcomes between the groups.[21] The third RCT found a significant improvement from baseline for cognitive therapy.[22] All people treated with dietary counselling either did not take up or withdrew from treatment and refused release of their results, making it impossible to compare the two groups. **Versus each other:** We found six small RCTs of limited quality that compared different types of psychotherapy. Three of these were undertaken in an outpatient setting in people with an early age of onset and short illness duration.[23–25] Two of the RCTs were carried out in an outpatient setting in people with a later age of onset and longer duration of illness.[20,26] One RCT included people with early and late onset anorexia nervosa and with long and short duration of illness (see table A on web extra).[27,28] None of the RCTs found an overall significant difference between different psychotherapies.

Harms: The acceptability of the treatment varied among RCTs. Failure to take up treatment ranged from 0–30% and withdrawal from treatment ranged from 0–70% among RCTs but this may have been caused by different methods of case ascertainment (see table A on web extra). The proportion of people admitted for inpatient treatmentⒼ also varied among RCTs, ranging from 0–36%. One death was attributed to anorexia nervosa in the control group in one outpatient RCT with a 1 year follow up.[20] Three deaths attributed to anorexia nervosa occurred in the 5 year follow up period of one inpatient based RCT.[28]

Comment: All the RCTs were small and had limited power to detect clinically important differences. The amount of therapeutic input varied considerably among and within the RCTs. There was variation in methods of recruitment, reporting of key results (e.g. withdrawal rates), and the description of participants' characteristics and selection. The people in the inpatient RCT covered a broad range of severity.[27] We found one systematic review (2 small RCTs, 32 people, search date 2002), which compared psychotherapies versus each other, although it used a narrower definition of psychotherapy than we have used in this topic.[19] Neither of the RCTs identified by the review met our inclusion criteria.

OPTION TRICYCLIC ANTIDEPRESSANTS

Two small RCTs found no evidence of benefit with amitriptyline compared with placebo. One RCT found that amitriptyline was associated with more adverse effects, such as drowsiness, dry mouth, and blurred vision. The QT interval may be prolonged in people with anorexia nervosa, and tricyclic antidepressants (amitriptyline, protriptyline, nortriptyline, doxepin, and maprotiline) also increase the QT interval. Prolongation of the QT interval may be associated with increased risk of ventricular tachycardia, torsades de pointes, and sudden death.

Benefits: We found no systematic review. We found two small RCTs.[29,30] The first RCT (43 people, 5 of them outpatients, with early onset and short duration anorexia nervosa, mean age 16.6 years, mean 27% below average weight, mean duration of anorexia nervosa 1.5 years) compared amitriptyline versus placebo.[29] Participants could also receive various kinds of psychotherapyⒼ. Eighteen people refused to participate and were used as a third comparison group. The RCT found no significant difference between the groups on any of the outcome scales measured at 5 weeks (> 50% improvement in global response 1/11 [9%] with amitriptyline *v* 1/14 [7%] with placebo; RR 1.2, 95% CI 0.1 to 16.7). The second RCT (72 women, mean age 20.6 years, mean 2.9 years' duration) compared amitriptyline (up to a maximum of 160 mg), cyproheptadine, and placebo.[30] It found no significant difference between amitriptyline and placebo for rate of weight gain.[30]

Harms: In the first RCT, adverse events more common with amitriptyline than placebo included increased perspiration (2/11 [18%] with amitriptyline *v* 0/14 [0%] with placebo), drowsiness (6/11 [55%] *v* 0/14 [0%]), dry mouth (4/11 [36%] *v* 2/14 [14%]), blurred vision (1/11 [9%] *v* 0/14 [0%]), urinary retention (1/11 [9%] *v* 0/14 [0%]), hypotension (2/11 [18%] *v* 0/14 [0%]), and leukopenia (1/11 [9%] *v* 0/14 [0%]).[29] Adverse events more common with placebo included palpitations (0/11 [0%] with amitriptyline *v* 1/14 [7%] with placebo) and dizziness (0/11 [0%] *v* 2/14 [14%]). The QT interval may be prolonged in people with anorexia nervosa,[31] and tricyclic antidepressants (amitriptyline, protriptyline, nortriptyline, doxepin, and maprotiline) also increase the QT interval.[32–34] In an observational study (495 people with mental illness and 101 healthy controls) an increased risk of prolonged QT interval was seen with tricyclic antidepressant use, adjusting for age and other drug use (adjusted OR 2.6, 95% CI 1.2 to 5.6).[35] General harms of tricyclic antidepressants are described in the section on depression (see depressive disorders, p 1238).

Comment: The RCTs were both of short duration. Prolongation of the QT interval may be associated with increased risk of ventricular tachycardia, torsades de pointes, and sudden death.[33,34] It is not clear if people in the second amitriptyline RCT also received psychotherapy.[30]

OPTION SELECTIVE SEROTONIN REUPTAKE INHIBITORS

Three small RCTs provided insufficient evidence about the effects of selective serotonin reuptake inhibitors compared with placebo or no treatment in people with anorexia nervosa.

Benefits: We found no systematic review. We found three small RCTs.[36–38] The first RCT (33 women; mean age 26.2 years; mean body mass index**G** 15.0 kg/m^2; mean duration of anorexia nervosa 8.0 years) compared fluoxetine 60 mg versus placebo for the duration (mean 36 days) of inpatient treatment, which included individual and group psychotherapy**G**.[36] There were two early withdrawals from the fluoxetine group. The RCT found no significant differences in weight gain, eating symptoms, or depressive symptoms between the groups. The second RCT (39 women, binge–purge type anorexia excluded, mean age about 22 years, mean duration of anorexia nervosa 4–7 years) compared fluoxetine (starting dosage 20 mg/day) with placebo for 1 year. All women had been discharged from hospital after weight gain (minimum weight restoration was to 75% of average body weight). Women were allowed additional psychotherapy. Women who had substantial and incapacitating symptoms were encouraged to withdraw from the study. Withdrawal rates were too high to draw reliable conclusions about effects, although the withdrawal rate was significantly lower with fluoxetine compared with placebo (6/16 [37%] with fluoxetine *v* 16/19 [84%] with placebo; RR 0.45, 95% CI 0.23 to 0.86).[37] The third RCT (52 adults with moderately severe restricting anorexia nervosa [body mass index 15.8 kg/m^2]) compared citalopram (10 mg/day increasing to 20 mg/day) versus waiting list control for 12 weeks before the start of standard integrated dietary and psychiatric treatment.[38] Reliability was limited because withdrawal rates were high (7/26 [29.5%] with citalopram *v* 6/26 [23.1%] with control). The RCT found no significant difference in weight gain between citalopram and control. It found that self reported depressive symptoms (and some additional measures of comorbidity) improved in the citalopram group only (change in weight from baseline to 12 weeks: from 43.5 kg to 46.5 kg with citalopram *v* from 42.5 kg to 43.9 kg with control; P value not reported; Beck Depression Inventory: 14.5 to 7.3 with citalopram *v* 12.7 to 12.3 with control; P value not reported).

Harms: General harms of selective serotonin reuptake inhibitors are described in the section on depression (see depressive disorders, p 1238). The RCT comparing citalopram with control did not report adverse effects or reasons for withdrawal.[38]

Comment: In the second RCT, four further women were excluded from the analysis. Three became aware of the treatment allocation and one stopped taking medication before the end of 30 days.[37]

OPTION NEUROLEPTIC DRUGS

We found no RCTs. The QT interval may be prolonged in people with anorexia nervosa, and many neuroleptic drugs (haloperidol, pimozide, sertindole, thioridazine, chlorpromazine, and others) also increase the QT interval. Prolongation of the QT interval may be associated with increased risk of ventricular tachycardia, torsades de pointes, and sudden death.

Benefits: We found no systematic review and no RCTs.

Harms: General harms of neuroleptic drugs are described in the section on schizophrenia (see schizophrenia, p 1338). The QT interval may be prolonged in people with anorexia nervosa,[31,32] and many neuroleptic drugs (haloperidol, pimozide, sertindole, thioridazine, chlorpromazine, and others) may also increase the QT interval.[33,34] An observational study (495 people with mental illness and 101 healthy controls) found an increased risk of prolonged QT interval with high and very high dose neuroleptic use after adjusting for age and other drug use (high dose: adjusted OR 3.4, 95% CI 1.2 to 10.1; very high dose: adjusted OR 5.6, 95% CI 1.6 to 19.3).[35]

Comment: Prolongation of the QT interval may be associated with an increased risk of ventricular tachycardia, torsades de pointes, and sudden death.[33,34]

OPTION ZINC

One small RCT found limited evidence that zinc may improve daily body mass index gain compared with placebo in people managed in an inpatient setting. However, we were unable to draw reliable conclusions from this small study.

Benefits: We found no systematic review. We found one RCT (54 people aged > 15 years, mean body mass index[G] 15.8 kg/m^2, mean duration of anorexia nervosa 3.7 years, admitted to two eating disorder units), which compared 100 mg zinc gluconate versus placebo.[39] All but three of the people had normal zinc levels before treatment. Treatment was continued until the individual had gained 10% of weight over the admission weight on two consecutive weeks. Ten people in the zinc group and nine in the placebo group did not complete the study. The RCT found that zinc significantly increased the daily rate of gain in body mass index compared with placebo (0.079 with zinc *v* 0.039 with placebo; P = 0.03).[39]

Harms: No harms were reported.

Comment: The rationale for zinc supplements in people with normal zinc levels is unclear.

OPTION CYPROHEPTADINE

Two RCTs in inpatient settings found no significant difference between cyproheptadine and placebo in weight gain.

Benefits: We found no systematic review. We found two small RCTs. The first RCT (81 women in 3 specialised inpatient units) compared cyproheptadine versus placebo, and behaviour therapy versus no behaviour therapy.[40] The effect of behaviour therapy was not reported. There were no significant differences in weight gain between the cyproheptadine and placebo groups. The second RCT (72 women, mean age 20.6 years, mean 77% of target weight, mean duration of anorexia 2.9 years, at two specialised inpatient units) compared amitriptyline versus cyproheptadine (up to a maximum of 32 mg) and versus placebo.[30] It found no significant difference between cyproheptadine and placebo for rate of weight gain.

Harms: No harms were reported in the first RCT.[40] In the second RCT, on both day 7 and day 21, placebo exceeded the amitriptyline group in number of physical adverse events rated moderate or severe. Adverse effects were less frequent with cyproheptadine. No one had to be withdrawn from the protocol because of adverse effects.[30]

Comment: Both RCTs were of short duration.

OPTION INPATIENT VERSUS OUTPATIENT TREATMENT SETTING IN ANOREXIA NERVOSA

One small RCT found no significant difference between outpatient treatment and inpatient treatment for increasing weight and improving Morgan Russell scale global scores at 1, 2, and 5 years in people who did not need emergency intervention.

Benefits: We found one systematic review (search date 1999) comparing inpatient treatment**G** versus outpatient care.[41] The review identified one RCT, which had a 5 year follow up.[42,43] Ninety people referred with anorexia nervosa (mean age 22 years, weight loss 26% of matched population mean weight, mean duration 3.2 years and not requiring emergency intervention) were randomised to four treatment groups: inpatient treatment, outpatient treatment (individual and family therapy**G**), outpatient group therapy, and assessment interview only. Assessors were not blind to treatment allocation. Adherence to allocated treatment (defined as accepting allocation and at least 1 attendance at a treatment group or individual treatment session) differed significantly among groups (adherence rates: inpatient treatment 18/30 [60%], outpatient treatment [individual and family therapy] 18/20 [90%], outpatient group psychotherapy**G** 17/20 [85%], and assessment interview only 20/20 [100%]). Treatment adherence differed significantly between outpatient and inpatient treatment (RR 1.5, 95% CI 1.1 to 2.0). Average acceptance of treatment also varied among groups (20 weeks' inpatient treatment, 9 outpatient sessions, and 5 group sessions). In the assessment interview only group, six people had no treatment of any kind in the first year and the others had treatment elsewhere (6 had inpatient treatment, 5 had outpatient hospital treatment, and 3 had at least weekly contact with their general practitioners). Six people in this group spent almost the entire year in treatment. There were no significant differences in mean weight or in the Morgan Russell scale**G** global scores among any of the four groups at 1, 2, and 5 years. The proportion of people with a good outcome with inpatient treatment was 5/29 (17%) at 2 years and 9/27 (33%) at 5 years; with outpatient treatment (individual and family therapy) 4/20 (20%) at 2 years and 8/17 (47%) at 5 years; with outpatient group psychotherapy 5/19 (26%) at 2 years and 10/19 (53%) at 5 years; and with assessment interview only 2/20 (10%) at 2 years and 6/19 (32%) at 5 years.

Harms: One person died from anorexia nervosa between the assessment and the start of outpatient group treatment, and one of the people allocated to inpatient treatment died from anorexia nervosa within 5 years.[42,43]

Comment: The systematic review[41] was unable to draw meaningful conclusions from numerous case series because participant characteristics, treatments, mortality, and outcomes varied widely. People admitted for inpatient treatment had a lower mean weight than those treated as outpatients. One subsequent observational study (355 people with anorexia nervosa; 169 of whom had bulimic type anorexia nervosa; mean age 25 years; mean duration of illness 5.7 years; 75% available for 2.5 years' follow up) found that people with a longer duration of illness had a higher likelihood of good outcome with longer duration of inpatient treatment.[44] People with a shorter duration of illness had a higher likelihood of good outcome with briefer inpatient treatment. Median duration of inpatient treatment was 11.6 weeks for anorexia nervosa and 10.6 weeks for bulimic type anorexia nervosa.

OPTION **CISAPRIDE**

One small RCT found no significant difference between cisapride and placebo in weight gain at 8 weeks. Use of cisapride has been restricted in many countries because of concern about cardiac irregularities, including ventricular tachycardia, torsades de pointes, and sudden death.

Benefits: We found no systematic review. We found one small RCT (34 inpatients aged 18–40 years at 2 hospitals; mean duration 2.7 years; body mass index**G** 15.1 kg/m^2) comparing cisapride 30 mg with placebo for 8 weeks.[45] The trial found no difference in weight gain (5.1 kg with cisapride *v* 5.7 kg with placebo; $P > 0.05$).

Harms: No adverse events were noted in this RCT. The QT interval in anorexia nervosa is prolonged even in the absence of medication. Therefore, cisapride, which may prolong the QT interval, is not recommended in anorexia nervosa. Use of cisapride has been restricted in many countries because of concern about cardiac irregularities, including ventricular tachycardia, torsades de pointes, and sudden death.[33,34]

Comment: Five people withdrew from the RCT and were not included in the analysis.

QUESTION **What are the effects of interventions to prevent or treat complications of anorexia nervosa?**

OPTION **OESTROGEN TREATMENT**

We found no RCTs on the effects of oestrogen treatment on fracture rates in people with anorexia nervosa. Two small RCTs found no significant difference between oestrogen and placebo or no treatment in bone mineral density in people with anorexia nervosa.

Benefits: We found no systematic review or RCTs which examined the effect of oestrogen treatment on fracture rates in people with anorexia. We found two RCTs which examined the effect of oestrogen treatment on bone mineral density (see comment).[46,47] The first RCT (48 women, mean age 23.7 years, mean duration of anorexia nervosa 4.0 years) compared hormone replacement therapy (conjugated oestrogens 0.625 mg on days 1–25 of each month plus medroxyprogesterone 5 mg on days 16–25) versus an oral contraceptive containing 35 µg ethinyl oestradiol versus no medication over 6 months.[46] All women maintained a calcium intake of 1500 mg using oral calcium carbonate. Spinal bone mineral density was measured at 6 monthly intervals. There was no significant difference in the final bone mineral density at follow up of 0.5–3.0 years. The second RCT (60 women aged 18–38 years, mean weight 44.7 kg; body mass index**G** 16.6 kg/m^2, duration of anorexia nervosa 2.3 years and with osteopenia at entry) compared four treatments: oral contraceptive alone (35 µg ethinyl oestradiol plus 0.4 mg norethindrone); placebo; recombinant human insulin-like growth factor-I alone; and oral contraceptive plus recombinant human insulin-like growth factor-I.[47] In addition, all women received calcium 1500 mg/day and vitamin D 400 IU/day. The RCT found no significant difference between oral contraceptives and placebo in bone mineral density at 9 months (hip density: $P = 0.071$; spine density: $P = 0.21$).

Harms: In the first RCT comparing hormone replacement therapy with the oral contraceptive pill and placebo, three women withdrew from the oestrogen treatment; two because of adverse effects, and one because she had left the country.[46] One woman who was in the control group was unwilling to return for further testing.

Anorexia nervosa

Comment: Improvements in bone mineral density may not reduce fracture risk.

GLOSSARY

Body mass index Weight (kg) divided by height (m) squared.
Dietary counselling Dieticians with experience of eating disorders discuss diet, mood, and daily behaviours.
Family therapy Treatment that includes members of the family of origin or the constituted family, and that addresses the eating disorder as a problem of family life.
Inpatient treatment This has been regarded as the standard approach to the management of anorexia nervosa.[48] One of the key components of inpatient treatment is refeeding, which is achieved through structured, supervised meals. Psychotherapy (of a variety of different types) and pharmacotherapy are included in many programmes.
Morgan Russell scale A widely used measure of outcome for anorexia nervosa that consists of two scores: an average outcome score and a general outcome score. The average outcome score is based on the outcome in five areas: nutritional status, menstrual function, mental state, sexual adjustment, and socioeconomic status.
Psychotherapy Different types of psychological treatments given individually or in groups are included here. These use psychodynamic, cognitive behavioural, or supportive techniques, or combinations of these.

REFERENCES

1. American Psychiatric Association. *Diagnostic and statistical manual of mental disorders (DSM-IV)*, 4th ed. Washington, DC: American Psychiatric Association, 1994.
2. Pawluck DE, Gorey KM. Secular trends in the incidence of anorexia nervosa: integrative review of population-based studies. *Int J Eat Disord* 1998;23:347–352.
3. Rastam M, Gillberg C, Garton M. Anorexia nervosa in a Swedish urban region. A population-based study. *Br J Psychiatry* 1989;155:642–646.
4. Strober M, Freeman R, Lampert C, et al. Controlled family study of anorexia nervosa and bulimia nervosa: evidence of shared liability and transmission of partial syndromes. *Am J Psychiatry* 2000;157:393–401.
5. Lilenfeld LR, Kaye WH, Greeno CG, et al. A controlled family study of anorexia nervosa and bulimia nervosa: psychiatric disorders in first-degree relatives and effects of proband comorbidity. *Arch Gen Psychiatry* 1998;55:603–610.
6. Wade TD, Bulik CM, Neale M, et al. Anorexia nervosa and major depression: shared genetic and environmental risk factors. *Am J Psychiatry* 2000;157:469–471.
7. Fairburn CG, Cooper Z, Doll HA, et al. Risk factors for anorexia nervosa: three integrated case-control comparisons. *Arch Gen Psychiatry* 1999;56:468–476.
8. Cnattingius S, Hultman CM, Dahl M, et al. Very preterm birth, birth trauma, and the risk of anorexia nervosa among girls. *Arch Gen Psychiatry* 1999;56:634–638.
9. Wentz E, Gillberg C, Gillberg IC, et al. Ten-year follow-up of adolescent-onset anorexia nervosa: psychiatric disorders and overall functioning scales. *J Child Psychol Psychiatry* 2001;42:613–622.
10. Steinhausen, H-C. The course and outcome of anorexia nervosa. In: Brownell K, Fairburn CG, eds. *Eating disorders and obesity: a comprehensive handbook*. New York, NY: Guilford Press, 1995:234–237.
11. Harri, EC, Barraclough B. Excess mortality of mental disorder. *Br J Psychiatry* 1998;173:11–53.
12. Nielsen S, Møller-Madsen S, Isager T, et al. Standardized mortality in eating disorders: a quantitative summary of previously published and new evidence. *J Psychosom Res* 1998;44:413–434.
13. Lucas A, Melton L, Crowson C, et al. Long term fracture risk among women with anorexia nervosa: a population-based cohort study. *Mayo Clin Proc* 1999;74:972–977.
14. Morgan HG, Russell GF. Value of family background and clinical features as predictors of long-term outcome in anorexia nervosa: four-year follow-up study of 41 patients. *Psychol Med* 1975;5:355–371.
15. Cooper Z, Fairburn CG. The Eating Disorders Examination. A semi-structured interview for the assessment of the specific psychopathology of eating disorders. *Int J Eat Disord* 1987;6:1–8.
16. Garner DM. *Eating Disorder Inventory-2 (EDI-2): professional manual*. Odessa, FL: Psychological Assessment Resources Inc, 1991.
17. Garner DM, Garfinkel PE. The eating attitudes test: an index of the symptoms of anorexia nervosa. *Psychol Med* 1979;9:273–279.
18. Henderson M, Freeman CPL. A self-rating scale for bulimia: the 'BITE'. *Br J Psychiatry* 1987;150:18–24.
19. Hay P, Bacaltchuk J, Claudino A, et al. Individual psychotherapy in the outpatient treatment of adults with anorexia nervosa (Cochrane Review). In: The Cochrane Library, Issue 1, 2004. Chichester, UK: John Wiley & Sons, Ltd. Search date 2002; primary sources Medline, Extramed, Embase, Psychlit, Current Contents, hand searches of *Int J Eat Disord*, and correspondence with researchers in the field.
20. Dare C, Eisler I, Russell G, et al. Psychological therapies for adult patients with anorexia nervosa: a randomised controlled trial of outpatient treatments. *Br J Psychiatry* 2001;178:216–221.
21. Hall A, Crisp AH. Brief psychotherapy in the treatment of anorexia nervosa. Outcome at one year. *Br J Psychiatry* 1987;151:185–191.
22. Serfaty MA. Cognitive therapy versus dietary counselling in the outpatient treatment of anorexia nervosa: effects of the treatment phase. *Eur Eat Dis Rev* 1999;7:334–350.
23. Eisler I, Dare C, Hodes M, et al. Family therapy for adolescent anorexia nervosa: the results of a controlled comparison of two family interventions. *J Child Psychol Psychiatry* 2000;41:727–736.
24. Robin AL, Siegel PT, Moye AW, et al. A controlled comparison of family versus individual therapy for adolescents with anorexia nervosa. *J Am Acad Child Adolesc Psychiatry* 1999;38:1482–1489.
25. Wallin U, Kronvall P, Majewski ML. Body awareness therapy in teenage anorexia nervosa: outcome after 2 years. *Eur Eat Dis Rev* 2000;8:19–30.
26. Treasure JL, Todd G, Brolly M, et al. A pilot study of a randomized trial of cognitive analytical therapy vs educational behavioral therapy for adult anorexia nervosa. *Behav Res Ther* 1995;33:363–367.
27. Russell GFM, Szmukler G, Dare C, et al. An evaluation of family therapy in anorexia nervosa and bulimia nervosa. *Arch Gen Psychiatry* 1987;44:1047–1056.

28. Eisler I, Dare C, Russell GFM, et al. Family and individual therapy in anorexia nervosa. A 5-year follow-up. *Arch Gen Psychiatry* 1997;54:1025–1030.
29. Biederman J, Herzog DB, Rivinus TM, et al. Amitriptyline in the treatment of anorexia nervosa: a double-blind, placebo-controlled study. *J Clin Psychopharmacol* 1985;5:10–16.
30. Halmi KA, Eckert E, LaDu TJ, et al. Anorexia nervosa. Treatment efficacy of cyproheptadine and amitriptyline. *Arch Gen Psychiatry* 1986;43:177–181.
31. Ackerman MJ. The long QT syndrome: ion channel diseases of the heart. *Mayo Clin Proc* 1998;73:250–269.
32. Becker A, Grinspoon SK, Klibanski A, et al. Current concepts: eating disorders. *N Engl J Med* 1999;340:1092–1098.
33. Yap Y, Camm J. Risk of torsades de pointes with non-cardiac drugs: doctors need to be aware that many drugs can cause QT prolongation. *BMJ* 2000;320:1158–1159.
34. Sheridan DJ. Drug-induced proarrhythmic effects: assessment of changes in QT interval. *Br J Clin Pharmacol* 2000;50:297–302.
35. Reilly JG, Ayis SA, Ferrier IN, et al. QTc interval abnormalities and psychotropic drug therapy in psychiatric patients. *Lancet* 2000;355:1048–1052.
36. Attia E, Haiman C, Walsh BT, et al. Does fluoxetine augment the inpatient treatment of anorexia nervosa? *Am J Psychiatry* 1998;155:548–551.
37. Kaye WH, Nagata T, Weltzin TE, et al. Double-blind placebo-controlled administration of fluoxetine in restricting- and restricting–purging-type anorexia nervosa. *Soc Biol Psych* 2001;49:644–652.
38. Fassino S, Leombruni P, Daga G, et al. Efficacy of citalopram in anorexia nervosa: a pilot study. *Eur Neuropsychopharmacol* 2002;12:453–459.
39. Birmingham CL, Goldner EM, Bakan R. Controlled trial of zinc supplementation in anorexia nervosa. *Int J Eat Disord* 1994;15:251–255.
40. Goldberg SC, Halmi KA, Eckert RC, et al. Cyproheptadine in anorexia nervosa. *Br J Psychiatry* 1979;134:67–70.
41. West Midlands Development and Evaluation Service. *In-patient versus out-patient care for eating disorders*. DPHE 1999 Report No 17. Birmingham: University of Birmingham, 1999. Search date 1999; primary sources Medline, Psychlit, The Cochrane Library, variety of internet sites, and hand searches of relevant editions of relevant journals and references from identified articles.
42. Crisp AH, Norton K, Gowers S, et al. A controlled study of the effect of therapies aimed at adolescent and family psychopathology in anorexia nervosa. *Br J Psychiatry* 1991;159:325–333.
43. Gowers S, Norton K, Halek C, et al. Outcome of outpatient psychotherapy in a random allocation treatment study of anorexia nervosa. *Int J Eat Disord* 1994;15:165–177.
44. Kåchele H for the study group MZ-ESS. Eine multizentrische studie zu aufwand und erfolg bei psychodynamischer therapie von eβstörungen. *Psychother Med Psychol (Stuttg)* 1999;49:100–108.
45. Szmukler GI, Young GP, Miller G, et al. A controlled trial of cisapride in anorexia nervosa. *Int J Eat Disord* 1995;17:347–357.
46. Klibanski A, Biller BMK, Schoenfeld DA, et al. The effects of estrogen administration on trabecular bone loss in young women with anorexia nervosa. *J Clin Endocrinol Metab* 1995;80:898–904.
47. Grinspoon S, Thomas L, Miller K, et al. Effects of recombinant human IGF-I and oral contraceptive administration on bone density in anorexia nervosa. *J Clin Endocrinol Metab* 2002;87:2883–2891.
48. American Psychiatric Association. Practice guideline for the treatment of patients with eating disorders (revision). *Am J Psychiatry* 2000;157(suppl 1):1–39.

Janet Treasure
Psychiatrist
Institute of Psychiatry
Kings College London
London
UK

Ulrike Schmidt
Psychiatrist
South London and Maudsley NHS Trust
London
UK

Competing interests: None declared.

Bipolar disorder

Search date August 2003

John Geddes

QUESTIONS

INTERVENTIONS

See glossary G

Key Messages

Treatments

- **Lithium** One RCT in people with bipolar type I disorder experiencing a manic episode identified by a systematic review found that lithium increased the proportion of people who responded after 3–4 weeks compared with placebo. One systematic review found that lithium increased the proportion of people who had remission of manic symptoms at 3 weeks compared with chlorpromazine. It found no significant difference in symptoms at 3–6 weeks between lithium and haloperidol, valproate, carbamazepine or clonazepam. One RCT identified by the systematic review found that lithium was less effective than risperidone in reducing manic symptoms at 4 weeks. RCTs found no significant difference in symptoms at 4 weeks between lithium and olanzapine or lamotrigine. Another RCT identified by a systematic review found that lithium plus olanzapine increased the proportion of people who responded at 3–6 weeks compared with placebo. Lithium can cause a range of adverse effects, including gastrointestinal disturbances, fine tremor, renal impairment, polydipsia, leucocytosis, weight gain, oedema, and hypothyroidism. The RCTs provided insufficient evidence about how the adverse effects of lithium compared with those of other antipsychotic drugs.

- **Olanzapine** One systematic review and one subsequent RCT in people with bipolar type I disorder found that olanzapine increased the proportion of people who responded at 3–6 weeks compared with placebo, both as monotherapy and in combination with lithium or valproate. One RCT found no significant difference in symptoms at 28 days between olanzapine and lithium. RCTs identified by a systematic review found that olanzapine was more effective in reducing symptoms than valproate, but was also more likely to cause adverse effects such as sedation and weight gain. The acceptability of olanzapine may be limited by weight gain.
- **Valproate** One systematic review in people with bipolar type I disorder experiencing a manic episode found that valproate increased the proportion of people who responded over 3 weeks compared with placebo but caused more dizziness. It found no significant difference in response rates at 1–6 weeks between valproate and lithium, haloperidol, or carbamazepine. It found that valproate was less effective in reducing manic symptoms than olanzapine, but was also less likely to cause adverse effects such as sedation and weight gain. One RCT identified by a systematic review found that valproate plus olanzapine increased the proportion of people who responded at 3–6 weeks compared with placebo.
- **Carbamazepine** RCTs in people with bipolar type I disorder experiencing a manic episode identified by a systematic review found no significant difference in manic symptoms at 4–6 weeks between carbamazepine and lithium or valproate. The review provided insufficient evidence to assess adverse effects of carbamazepine.
- **Clonazepam** We found no RCTs comparing clonazepam versus placebo in people with mania. RCTs in people with bipolar type I disorder experiencing a manic episode identified by a systematic review suggest that clonazepam may be as effective as lithium in improving manic symptoms at 1–4 weeks. The review provided insufficient evidence to assess adverse effects of clonazepam.
- **Haloperidol** We found no RCTs comparing haloperidol versus placebo in people with mania. RCTs in people with bipolar type I disorder experiencing a manic episode identified by a systematic review found no significant difference in manic symptoms at 1–3 weeks between haloperidol and lithium or valproate, although haloperidol was associated with more extrapyramidal adverse effects and sedation than valproate.
- **Risperidone** We found no RCTs comparing risperidone alone versus placebo. One RCT in people with mania taking lithium, valproate, or carbamazepine found no significant difference in symptoms between adding risperidone and placebo and found that adding risperidone increased extrapyramidal adverse effects. Another RCT in people with bipolar type I disorder experiencing a manic episode found that risperidone reduced manic symptoms at 4 weeks compared with lithium.
- **Ziprasidone** One RCT found that ziprasidone increased the proportion of people who responded at 3 weeks compared with placebo, but caused sedation, headaches, dizziness, and akathisia.
- **Chlorpromazine** One very small RCT in people with mania found limited evidence that chlorpromazine may improve manic symptoms over 7 weeks more than placebo or imipramine. One systematic review found that fewer people had remission of symptoms at 3 weeks with chlorpromazine than with lithium. The review and RCT provided insufficient evidence to assess adverse effects of chlorpromazine.
- **Gabapentin** One RCT in people with bipolar type I disorder experiencing a manic or mixed episode already taking lithium or valproate found that adding gabapentin was less effective in reducing manic symptoms over 10 months than placebo. Gabapentin was associated with somnolence, dizziness, diarrhoea, and memory loss.
- **Lamotrigine** We found no RCTs comparing lamotrigine versus placebo in people with mania. One RCT in people with bipolar type I disorder experiencing a manic episode identified by a systematic review found no significant difference in manic symptoms at 4 weeks between lamotrigine and lithium. The review provided insufficient evidence to assess adverse effects of lamotrigine.
- **Quetiapine** One RCT in adolescents found that quetiapine increased the proportion of people who responded at 6 weeks compared with placebo, but caused sedation.

- **Topiramate** One systematic review identified no RCTs of topiramate in people with mania.

Treating bipolar depression

- **Antidepressants** Systematic reviews found that antidepressants improved depressive symptoms at the end of the trial (unspecified) compared with placebo. They found no significant difference between selective serotonin reuptake inhibitors and tricyclic antidepressants in the proportion of people who responded, although people taking selective serotonin reuptake inhibitors were more likely to respond. The reviews and one subsequent RCT found no significant difference in symptoms between monoamine oxidase inhibitors and tricyclic antidepressants or between selective serotonin reuptake inhibitors and serotonin noradrenaline reuptake inhibitors. Antidepressants are associated with manic switching and the reviews and subsequent RCT suggested that tricyclic antidepressants are more likely to induce mania than selective serotonin reuptake inhibitors.
- **Lamotrigine** One RCT in people with bipolar type I disorder experiencing a depressive episode identified by a systematic review found that lamotrigine increased the proportion of people who responded over 7 weeks compared with placebo. Lamotrigine increased the proportion of people with headache compared with placebo.
- **Carbamazepine** One systematic review identified no RCTs of sufficient quality to assess carbamazepine in people with bipolar depression.
- **Lithium** One systematic review identified no RCTs of sufficient quality to assess lithium in people with bipolar depression.
- **Psychological treatments** We found no systematic review or RCTs of psychological treatments in people with bipolar depression.
- **Topiramate** One systematic review identified no RCTs of topiramate in people with bipolar depression. One subsequent RCT in people taking lithium or valproate found no significant difference in symptoms at 8 weeks between adding topiramate and adding bupropion. The RCT found that a third of people taking topiramate and a fifth of people taking bupropion withdrew because of adverse effects, including anxiety, increase or decrease in appetite, blurred vision, backache, headache, and nausea.
- **Valproate** We found no systematic review or RCTs of valproate in people with bipolar depression.

Preventing relapse

- **Lithium** Systematic reviews and subsequent RCTs found that lithium reduced relapse over 2 years compared with placebo. They found no significant difference in relapse between lithium and valproate, carbamazepine, or lamotrigine. RCTs found that more people had overall adverse effects (not specified) with lithium than with placebo, and that lithium may increase hypothyroidism. They found that lithium caused more polyuria, thirst, and diarrhoea than valproate but less sedation and infection. More people taking lithium than carbamazepine had adverse effects, including blurred vision, difficulty concentrating, thirst, hand tremor and muscle weakness, but more people taking carbamazepine had increased appetite. RCTs also found that fewer people taking lithium than lamotrigine had headaches.
- **Carbamazepine** We found no RCTs comparing carbamazepine versus placebo for preventing relapse. One systematic review and one subsequent RCT found no significant difference between carbamazepine and lithium in the proportion of people who relapsed over 1–3 years. The review and subsequent RCT found that carbamazepine was associated with fewer adverse effects than lithium.
- **Cognitive therapy** Two RCTs found that cognitive therapy reduced relapse over 6–12 months compared with usual care. Another RCT found no significant difference between cognitive therapy and usual care in the proportion of people who relapsed over 6 months, although fewer people receiving cognitive therapy relapsed. The RCT is likely to have been underpowered to detect a clinically important difference between treatments. The RCTs provided insufficient evidence to assess adverse effects of cognitive therapy.

- **Education to recognise symptoms of relapse** One RCT found limited evidence that an educational programme to recognise symptoms of relapse reduced manic relapse over 18 months, but that it may increase depressive episodes.
- **Lamotrigine (reduced relapse of bipolar depressive episodes)** Three RCTs found that lamotrigine reduced relapse compared with placebo. However, secondary analyses in two of the RCTs suggested that lamotrigine protected against depressive relapse, but not manic relapse. RCTs found no significant difference between lamotrigine and lithium in the proportion of people who relapsed and found that more people taking lamotrigine than lithium had headaches.
- **Valproate** One RCT identified by a systematic review found that valproate reduced relapse over 12 months compared with placebo. One systematic review found no significant difference between lithium and valproate in relapse over 12 months. The review found that valproate cause more sedation and infection than lithium but less polyuria, thirst, and diarrhoea.
- **Antidepressant drugs** One systematic review and one subsequent RCT provided insufficient evidence to assess antidepressants in preventing relapse of bipolar disorder.
- **Family focused psychoeducation** One RCT found that 21 sessions of family focused psychoeducation reduced relapse over 12 months compared with two family sessions plus crisis management. Another RCT found that family focused psychoeducation may reduce relapse compared with individual focused therapy. The RCTs gave no information on adverse effects.

DEFINITION Bipolar disorder (bipolar affective disorder, manic depressive disorder) is characterised by marked mood swings between mania (mood elevation) and bipolar depression that cause significant personal distress or social dysfunction, and are not caused by drugs or known physical disorders. **Bipolar type I disorder** is diagnosed when episodes of depression are interspersed with mania or mixed episodes. **Bipolar type II disorder** is diagnosed when depression is interspersed with less severe episodes of elevated mood that do not lead to dysfunction or disability (hypomania). Bipolar disorder has been subdivided in several further ways (see table 1, p 1181).[1]

INCIDENCE/ PREVALENCE One 1996 cross-national community based study (38 000 people) found lifetime prevalence rates of bipolar disorder ranging from 0.3% in Taiwan to 1.5% in New Zealand.[2] It found that men and women were at similar risk, and that the age at first onset ranged from 19–29 years (average of 6 years earlier than first onset of major depression).

AETIOLOGY/ RISK FACTORS The cause of bipolar disorder is uncertain, although family and twin studies suggest a genetic basis.[3] The lifetime risk of bipolar disorder is increased in first degree relatives of a person with bipolar disorder (40–70% for a monozygotic twin; 5–10% for other first degree relatives). If the first episode of mania occurs in an older adult, it may be secondary mania due to underlying medical or substance induced factors.[4]

PROGNOSIS Bipolar disorder is a recurring illness and one of the leading causes of worldwide disability, especially in the 15–44 year age group.[3] One 4 year inception cohort study (173 people treated for a first episode of mania or mixed affective disorder) found that 93% of people no longer met criteria for mania at 2 years (median time to recover from a syndrome 4.6 weeks), but that only 36% had recovered to premorbid function.[4] It found that 40% of people had a recurrent manic (20%) or depressive (20%) episode within 2 years of recovering from the first episode. A meta-analysis, comparing observed suicide expected rates of suicide in an age and sex matched sample of the general population, found that the lifetime prevalence of suicide was about 2%, or 15 times greater than expected, in people with bipolar disorder.[5]

AIMS OF INTERVENTION To alleviate mania and bipolar depressive symptoms; to prevent relapse Ⓖ and suicide; to optimise social and occupational functioning; and to improve quality of life, with minimal adverse effects of treatment.

OUTCOMES Level of symptoms on rating scales (completed by clinician, patient, or both); proportion of people with clinically important response to treatment; time to remission; quality of life scores; social and occupational functioning scores; relapse Ⓖ; hospital admission; rates of suicide; frequency of adverse effects; and clinical trial withdrawal rates. Commonly used instruments for assessing symptoms include the Young Mania Rating Scale, which rates 11 manic symptoms with a total score of 0–60; the Schedule for Affective Disorders Change Mania Sub Scale, which rates 18 manic items with a total score of 10–65; and the Hamilton Depression Rating Scale, which has both a 17 and a 21 item version. On these scales, a clinically important response to treatment is usually defined as a greater than 50% reduction in score from baseline.[6] A person is usually considered to be in remission if, at the end of trial, they score 12 or less on the Young Mania Rating Scale and 8 or less on the Hamilton Depression Rating Scale.[6] Quality of life is assessed by scales such as the SF-36, and social and occupational functioning on scales such as the Clinical Global Impression Scale.

METHODS *Clinical Evidence* search and appraisal August 2003.

QUESTION What are the effects of treatments in mania?

OPTION LITHIUM

One RCT in people with bipolar type I disorder experiencing a manic episode identified by a systematic review found that lithium increased the proportion of people who responded after 3–4 weeks compared with placebo. One systematic review found that lithium increased the proportion of people who had remission of manic symptoms at 3 weeks compared with chlorpromazine. It found no significant difference in symptoms at 3–6 weeks between lithium and haloperidol, valproate, carbamazepine or clonazepam. One RCT identified by the systematic review found that lithium was less effective than risperidone in reducing manic symptoms at 4 weeks. RCTs found no significant difference in symptoms at 4 weeks between lithium and olanzapine or lamotrigine. Another RCT identified by a systematic review found that lithium plus olanzapine increased the proportion of people who responded at 3–6 weeks compared with placebo. Lithium can cause a range of adverse effects, including gastrointestinal disturbances, fine tremor, renal impairment, polydipsia, leucocytosis, weight gain, oedema, and hypothyroidism. The RCTs provided insufficient evidence about how the adverse effects of lithium compared with those of other antipsychotic drugs.

Benefits: **Versus placebo:** We found one systematic review (search date 1999, 1 RCT, 179 people with bipolar type I disorder).[7] The RCT compared three treatments: lithium (36 people), valproate (69 people), and placebo (74 people). It found that lithium significantly increased the proportion of people who responded after 3–4 weeks compared with placebo (response defined as ≥50% improvement in mania score on the Schedule for Affective Disorders and Schizophrenia-Change [SADS-C]; 18/36 [50%] with lithium *v* 19/74 [27%] with placebo; RR 1.95, 95% CI 1.17 to 3.23; NNT 5, 95% CI 3 to 20). **Versus chlorpromazine:** We found one systematic review (search date 1999, 4 RCTs, 114 people with bipolar type I disorder).[7] It found that lithium significantly increased the proportion of people who had remission of symptoms at 3 weeks compared with chlorpromazine (remission not defined, 3 RCTs that assessed outcomes at 3 weeks: 23/57 [40%] with lithium *v* 7/57 [12%] with chlorpromazine; RR 1.96, 95% CI 1.02 to 3.77 [figures reported from table 5 in paper]; NNT 4, 95% CI 3 to 9). **Versus haloperidol:** We found one systematic review (search date 1999, 2 RCTs, 50 people with bipolar type I disorder).[7] It found no significant difference between haloperidol and lithium in symptom scores at 3 weeks (assessed by the Brief Psychiatric Rating Scale [BPRS]: effect size –2.14, 95% CI –6.57 to +2.30). **Versus risperidone:** We found one systematic review (search date 1999, 1 RCT, 54 people with bipolar type I disorder).[7] It found that risperidone was significantly more effective than lithium in improving symptom severity score at 4 weeks (assessed by BPRS: effect size –2.79, 95% CI

−4.22 to −1.36). **Versus olanzapine:** We found no systematic review but found one RCT (30 people with bipolar type I disorder).[8] It found no significant difference between lithium and olanzapine in Young Mania Rating Scale [YMRS] score at 28 days (13.2 with lithium *v* 10.2 with olanzapine; P = 0.315). **Versus valproate:** We found one systematic review (search date 2002, 3 RCTs, 158 people with bipolar type I disorder).[6] It found no significant difference between valproate and lithium in the proportion of people who failed to respond over 3–6 weeks (response defined as 50% reduction in mania score on the YMRS or the SADS-C; 45/97 [46%] with valproate *v* 26/61 [43%] with lithium; RR 1.05, 95% CI 0.74 to 1.50). **Versus carbamazepine:** We found one systematic review (search date 1999, 3 RCTs, 176 people with bipolar type I disorder).[7] The review could not perform a meta-analysis of all three RCTs because of differences in outcomes assessed. The first RCT (105 people) found no significant difference in the proportion of people who responded over 4 weeks between lithium and carbamazepine (15/54 [28%] with lithium *v* 14/51 [27%] with carbamazepine; RR 1.01, 95% CI 0.54 to 1.88). The other two RCTs (71 people) found no significant difference in global severity of symptoms over 4 weeks between lithium and carbamazepine (assessed by Clinical Global Impression [CGI] scores: effect size +0.44, 95% CI −0.78 to +1.67).[7] **Versus lamotrigine:** We found no systematic review but found one RCT (30 people with bipolar type I disorder).[9] It found no significant difference between lithium and lamotrigine in YMRS scores at 4 weeks (mean: 13.2 with lithium *v* 14.3 with lamotrigine; reported as non-significant; no further data reported). **Versus clonazepam:** We found one systematic review (search date 1999, 2 RCTs, 52 people with bipolar type I disorder).[7] The review could not perform a meta-analysis because the RCTs assessed different outcomes. The first RCT (12 people) found limited evidence that clonazepam improved some measures of mania more than lithium after 10 days of treatment (mean motor activity score: 1.8 with clonazepam *v* 2.8 with lithium; mean logorrhoea score assessing the rate of speech: 2.2 with clonazepam *v* 2.9 with lithium; CI not reported). The second RCT (40 people, open label) found no significant difference between lithium and clonazepam in symptom severity at 4 weeks assessed by BPRS (mean score: 6.27 with lithium *v* 7.79 with clonazepam) or global severity of symptoms assessed by CGI (mean score: 2.07 with lithium *v* 1.68 with clonazepam; reported as non-significant, CI not reported) after 4 weeks. **In combination with olanzapine:** See benefits of olanzapine, p 1167.

Harms: Lithium has a range of adverse effects, many of which are dose related and include gastrointestinal disturbances, fine tremor, renal impairment (particularly impaired urinary concentration and polyuria), polydipsia, leucocytosis, weight gain, oedema (may respond to dose reduction), and hypothyroidism. **Versus placebo:** The RCT identified by the review found that lithium significantly increased the proportion of people who had adverse effects compared with placebo (33/36 [92%] with lithium *v* 58/74 [78%] with placebo; RR 1.17, 95% CI 1.00 to 1.37; NNH 8, 95% CI 4 to 334).[7] Adverse effects were not specified. **Versus chlorpromazine:** The review provided inconclusive evidence on the proportion of people who had adverse effects with lithium compared with chlorpromazine.[7] Adverse effects were not specified. **Versus haloperidol:** The review gave no information on adverse effects.[7] **Versus risperidone:** The review gave no information on adverse effects.[7] **Versus olanzapine:** The RCT found no extrapyramidal adverse effects associated with lithium or olanzapine.[8] **Versus valproate:** The review found that valproate significantly reduced the proportion of people who had fever compared with lithium (1 RCT: 1/69 [1%] with valproate *v* 5/36 [14%] with lithium; RR 0.10, 95% CI 0.01 to 0.86). It found no significant difference in the rates of other adverse effects.[6]

Versus carbamazepine: The review found no significant difference in adverse effects between lithium and carbamazepine (2 RCTs: 27/73 [37%] with lithium *v* 35/66 [53%] with carbamazepine; RR 0.71, 95% CI 0.49 to 1.02).[7] Adverse effects were not specified. **Versus lamotrigine:** The RCT found "no significant adverse effects" between lithium and lamotrigine, but it is likely to have been too small to detect clinically important adverse effects.[9] One person taking lithium withdrew because of a seizure and one person taking lamotrigine withdrew because of aggravation of diabetes. **Versus clonazepam:** The review gave no information on adverse effects.[7] **In combination with olanzapine:** See harms of olanzapine, p 1167.

Comment: None.

OPTION VALPROATE

One systematic review in people with bipolar type I disorder experiencing a manic episode found that valproate increased the proportion of people who responded over 3 weeks compared with placebo but caused more dizziness. It found no significant difference in response rates at 1–6 weeks between valproate and lithium, haloperidol, or carbamazepine. It found that valproate was less effective in reducing manic symptoms than olanzapine, but was also less likely to cause adverse effects such as sedation and weight gain. One RCT identified by a systematic review found that valproate plus olanzapine increased the proportion of people who responded at 3–6 weeks compared with placebo.

Benefits: **Versus placebo:** We found one systematic review (search date 2002, 3 RCTs, 316 people with bipolar type I disorder).[6] It found that valproate significantly increased the proportion of people who responded over 3 weeks compared with placebo (response defined as 50% reduction in mania score on the Young Mania Rating Scale [YMRS] or the Schedule for Affective Disorders and Schizophrenia-Change [SADS-C]; proportion of people who failed to respond: 66/155 [42%] with valproate *v* 111/161 [69%] with placebo; RR of failing to respond 0.62, 95% CI 0.51 to 0.77).[6] **Versus lithium:** See benefits of lithium, p 1162. **Versus haloperidol:** We found one systematic review (search date 2002, 1 RCT, 36 people with bipolar type I disorder).[6] The RCT found no significant difference in the proportion of people who failed to respond over 6 days between valproate and haloperidol (11/21 [52%] with valproate *v* 10/15 [67%] with lithium; RR 0.79, 95% CI 0.46 to 1.35). **Versus olanzapine:** We found one systematic review (search date 2002, 2 RCTs, 363 people with bipolar type I disorder).[6] It found that people taking olanzapine had greater symptom reductions at the end of the trial (unspecified) than those taking valproate (symptoms assessed by the YMRS: WMD 2.81, 95% CI 0.83 to 4.79). One of the RCTs (251 people) found that olanzapine significantly increased the proportion of people who responded at the end of the trial (unspecified) compared with valproate (response defined as 50% reduction in YMRS; proportion of people who failed to respond: 77/123 [63%] with valproate *v* 57/125 [46%] with olanzapine; RR of failing to respond 1.27, 95% CI 0.99 to 1.62). **Versus carbamazepine:** We found one systematic review (2 RCTs, 59 people with bipolar type I disorder), which found no significant difference between valproate and carbamazepine in the proportion of people who failed to respond at 4–6 weeks (response defined with 50% reduction in mania score on the YMRS or SADS-C; 11/30 [37%] with valproate *v* 16/29 [55%] carbamazepine; RR 0.66, 95% CI 0.38 to 1.16).[6] **In combination with olanzapine:** See benefits of olanzapine, p 1167.

Harms: **Versus placebo:** The review found no significant difference between valproate and placebo in the proportion of people who withdrew from the trial because of adverse effects (9/158 [6%] with valproate *v* 5/163 [3%] with placebo; RR 1.95, 95% CI 0.66 to 5.71), but found that people taking valproate were significantly more likely to suffer from dizziness (13/138 [9%] with valproate *v* 4/141 [3%] with placebo; RR 3.17, 95% CI 1.13 to 8.88).[6] No other adverse effects were more commonly reported with valproate than with placebo. **Versus lithium:** See harms of lithium, p 1163. **Versus haloperidol:** The RCT found that, compared with haloperidol, valproate caused significantly fewer extrapyramidal adverse effects (0/21 [0%] with valproate *v* 8/15 [53%] with haloperidol; RR 0.04, 95% CI 0 to 0.69), dry mouth (1/21 [5%] with valproate *v* 3/15 [20%] with haloperidol; RR 0.24, 95% CI 0.03 to 2.07), and was less likely to cause sedation than haloperidol (1/21 [5%] with valproate *v* 4/15 [27%] with haloperidol; RR 0.18, 95% CI 0.02 to 1.44).[6] **Versus olanzapine:** The review found no significant difference between valproate and olanzapine in the proportion of people who withdrew because of adverse effects (1 RCT: 9/126 [7%] with valproate *v* 12/125 [10%] with olanzapine; RR 0.74, 95% CI 0.33 to 1.70) or had movement disorders (akathisia: WMD –0.02, 95% CI –0.27 to +0.23; abnormal involuntary movement: WMD –0.17, 95% CI –0.62 to +0.28).[6] It found that valproate caused significantly more nausea than olanzapine (1 RCT: 36/126 [28%] with valproate *v* 13/125 [10%] with olanzapine; RR 2.75, 95% CI 1.53 to 4.93), but caused less increased appetite (1 RCT: 3/126 [2%] with valproate *v* 15/125 [12%] with olanzapine; RR 0.20, 95% CI 0.06 to 0.67), less weight gain (WMD –2.14 kg, 95% CI –2.65 kg to –1.62 kg), dry mouth (8/126 [6%] with valproate *v* 42/125 [34%] with olanzapine; RR 0.19, 95% CI 0.09 to 0.39), and sedation (2 RCTs: 44/189 [23%] with valproate *v* 76/182 [42%] with olanzapine; RR 0.55, 95% CI 0.41 to 0.76). **Versus carbamazepine:** One RCT (28 people identified by the review) assessed adverse effects.[6] It found no significant difference in adverse effects between valproate and carbamazepine, but it is likely to have been underpowered to detect a clinically important difference. **In combination with olanzapine:** See harms of olanzapine, p 1167.

Comment: There are several formulations of valproic acid available, including sodium valproate, valpromide and valproate semisodium (divalproex). Valproate semisodium is the only preparation licensed for treatment of mania in the UK. In this chapter, we refer to the generic as valproate as this is the term in common usage.

OPTION CHLORPROMAZINE

One very small RCT in people with mania found limited evidence that chlorpromazine may improve manic symptoms over 7 weeks more than placebo or imipramine. One systematic review found that fewer people had remission of symptoms at 3 weeks with chlorpromazine than with lithium. The review and RCT provided insufficient evidence to assess adverse effects of chlorpromazine.

Benefits: **Versus placebo:** We found one non-systematic review, which identified one small RCT (13 people with mania) comparing three treatments: chlorpromazine, imipramine, and placebo.[10] It found that chlorpromazine significantly improved global outcome at 7 weeks compared with imipramine or placebo (assessed on a scale from –9 to +9 where +9 = improvement: +6.1 with chlorpromazine *v* +2.0 with imipramine *v* –2.8 with placebo; reported as significant; no further data reported). **Versus lithium:** See benefits of lithium, p 1162.

Harms: **Versus placebo:** The non-systematic review gave no information on adverse effects.[10] **Versus lithium:** See harms of lithium, p 1163.

Comment: The evidence for older antipsychotic drugs is sparse and there are currently no systematic reviews available. The drugs are, however, widely used in mania.

OPTION HALOPERIDOL

We found no RCTs comparing haloperidol versus placebo in people with mania. RCTs in people with bipolar type I disorder experiencing a manic episode identified by a systematic review found no significant difference in manic symptoms at 1–3 weeks between haloperidol and lithium or valproate, although haloperidol was associated with more extrapyramidal adverse effects and sedation than valproate.

Benefits: **Versus placebo:** We found no systematic review and no RCTs comparing haloperidol versus placebo. **Versus lithium:** See benefits of lithium, p 1162. **Versus valproate:** See benefits of valproate, p 1164.

Harms: **Versus placebo:** We found no RCTs. **Versus lithium:** See harms of lithium, p 1163. **Versus valproate:** See harms of valproate, p 1165.

Comment: The evidence for older antipsychotics is sparse and there are currently no systematic reviews available. The drugs are, however, widely used in mania.

OPTION RISPERIDONE

We found no RCTs comparing risperidone alone versus placebo. One RCT in people with mania taking lithium, valproate, or carbamazepine found no significant difference in symptoms between adding risperidone and placebo and found that adding risperidone increased extrapyramidal adverse effects. Another RCT in people with bipolar type I disorder experiencing a manic episode found that risperidone reduced manic symptoms at 4 weeks compared with lithium.

Benefits: **Versus placebo:** We found no RCTs. **Adding to lithium, valproate, or carbamazepine:** We found one RCT (151 inpatients with bipolar type I disorder, all taking lithium, valproate, or carbamazepine) that compared risperidone 1–6 mg daily versus placebo.[11] It found no significant difference between risperidone and placebo in manic symptoms at 4 weeks (mean difference in reduction on Young Mania Rating Scale score –3.10, 95% CI –7.60 to +0.54). **Versus lithium:** See benefits of lithium, p 1162.

Harms: **Versus placebo:** We found no RCTs. **Adding to lithium, valproate, or carbamazepine:** In the RCT, a similar proportion of people taking risperidone or placebo had adverse effects a (57% with risperidone *v* 51% with placebo).[11] People taking risperidone were twice as likely to suffer extrapyramidal adverse effects than those taking placebo (RR 2.67, 95% CI 1.15 to 6.33). **Versus lithium:** See harms of lithium, p 1163.

Comment: None.

OPTION OLANZAPINE

One systematic review and one subsequent RCT in people with bipolar type I disorder found that olanzapine increased the proportion of people who responded at 3–6 weeks compared with placebo, both as monotherapy and in combination with lithium or valproate. One RCT found no significant difference in symptoms at 28 days between olanzapine and lithium. RCTs identified by a

systematic review found that olanzapine was more effective in reducing symptoms than valproate, but was also more likely to cause adverse effects such as sedation and weight gain. The acceptability of olanzapine may be limited by weight gain.

Benefits: **Versus placebo:** We found one systematic review[12] and one subsequent RCT.[13] The review (search date 2002, 6 RCTs, 1422 people with bipolar type I disorder) found that olanzapine significantly increased the proportion of people who responded over 3–4 weeks compared with placebo (response defined as 50% reduction in mania score on the Young Mania Rating Scale; 2 RCTs; proportion who failed to respond: 56/125 [45%] with olanzapine *v* 89/129 [69%] with placebo; RR of failing to respond 0.64, 95% CI 0.52 to 0.81).[12] The subsequent RCT (201 people with bipolar type I disorder and agitation) compared 1– 3 intramuscular injections of olanzapine (10 mg /10 mg /5 mg), lorazepam (2 mg /2/ mg 1 mg) and placebo.[13] It found that olanzapine significantly increased the proportion of people who responded at 2 hours after the first injection compared with placebo (response defined as a ≥ 40% reduction in the Positive and Negative Syndrome Scale, Excited Component: at 2 hours: 81% with olanzapine *v* 44% with placebo; RR 1.85, 95% CI 1.40 to 2.67, NNT 3, 95% CI 2 to 4. The difference was not significant at 24 hours. **In combination with lithium or valproate:** The systematic review found that adding olanzapine to lithium or valproate significantly increased the proportion of people who responded at 6 weeks compared with placebo (1 RCT; proportion who failed to respond: 80/229 [35%] with olanzapine *v* 64/115 [56%] with placebo; RR of failing to respond 0.63, 95% CI 0.49 to 0.80).[12] **Versus lithium:** See benefits of lithium, p 1162. **Versus valproate:** See benefits of valproate, p 1164.

Harms: The review found that olanzapine, both as monotherapy and in combination with lithium or valproate, caused significantly more weight gain than placebo (3 RCTs, 581 people: WMD 2.27 kg, 95% CI 1.56 kg to 2.99 kg).[12] It found no significant difference in movement disorders between olanzapine and placebo (measured on the Barnes Akathisia Scale; 2 RCTs, 246 people: WMD –0.13, 95% CI –0.32 to +0.06), but found that olanzapine significantly increased somnolence (162/354 [46%] with olanzapine *v* 48/244 [20%] with placebo; RR 2.13, 95% CI 1.62 to 2.79), dry mouth (100/354 [28%] with olanzapine *v* 18/244 [7%] with placebo; RR 3.64, 95% CI 2.24 to 5.91), dizziness (54/354 [15%] with olanzapine *v* 16/244 [6%] with placebo; RR 2.37, 95% CI 1.39 to 4.04), muscle weakness (61/354 [17%] with olanzapine *v* 23/244 [9%] with placebo; RR 1.69, 95% CI 1.09 to 2.64), increased appetite (54/229 [23%] with olanzapine *v* 9/115 [8%] with placebo; RR 3.01, 95% CI 1.54 to 5.88), and speech disorder (15/229 [6%] with olanzapine *v* 1/115 [0.9%] with placebo; RR 7.53, 95% CI 1.01 to 56.32). **Versus lithium:** See harms of lithium, p 1163. **Versus valproate:** See harms of valproate, p 1165.

Comment: None.

OPTION ZIPRASIDONE

One RCT found that ziprasidone increased the proportion of people who responded at 3 weeks compared with placebo, but caused sedation, headaches, dizziness, and akathisia.

Benefits: **Versus placebo:** We found one RCT (201 people aged ≥ 18 years with bipolar type I disorder), which compared ziprasidone 80–160 mg daily versus placebo for 3 weeks.[14] It found that ziprasidone significantly increased the proportion of people who responded at 3 weeks compared with placebo (response defined as a ≥50% reduction in Young Mania Rating Scale score from baseline: 50% with ziprasidone *v* 35% with placebo; RR 1.45, 95% CI 1.02 to 2.13; NNT 6, 95% CI 3 to 128).

Harms: **Versus placebo:** The RCT found that, compared with placebo, more people taking ziprasidone had somnolence (37% with ziprasidone *v* 13% with placebo), headache (21% with ziprasidone *v* 19% with placebo), dizziness (22% with ziprasidone *v* 10% with placebo), and akathisia (11% with ziprasidone *v* 6% with placebo; CI not reported for any outcome).[14]

Comment: None.

OPTION QUETIAPINE

One RCT in adolescents found that quetiapine increased the proportion of people who responded at 6 weeks compared with placebo, but caused sedation.

Benefits: **Versus placebo:** We found one RCT (30 inpatients aged 12–18 years with bipolar type I disorder) comparing quetiapine up to 450 mg daily versus placebo for 6 weeks.[15] It found that quetiapine significantly increased the proportion of people who responded at 6 weeks compared with placebo (response defined as ≥50% reduction in score on the Young Mania Rating Scale: 87% with quetiapine *v* 53% with placebo; RR 1.63, 95% CI 1.01 to 2.94).

Harms: **Versus placebo:** The RCT found that quetiapine significantly increased the proportion of adolescents who experienced sedation compared with placebo (12/15 [80%] with quetiapine *v* 5/15 [33%] with placebo; P = 0.03).[15]

Comment: None.

OPTION CARBAMAZEPINE

RCTs in people with bipolar type I disorder experiencing a manic episode identified by a systematic review found no significant difference in manic symptoms at 4–6 weeks between carbamazepine and lithium or valproate. The review provided insufficient evidence to assess adverse effects of carbamazepine.

Benefits: **Versus placebo:** We found no systematic review or RCTs. **Versus lithium:** See benefits of lithium, p 1162. **Versus valproate:** See benefits of valproate, p 1164.

Harms: **Versus placebo:** We found no RCTs. **Versus lithium:** See harms of lithium, p 1163. **Versus valproate:** See harms of valproate, p 1165.

Comment: None.

OPTION CLONAZEPAM

We found no RCTs comparing clonazepam versus placebo in people with mania. RCTs in people with bipolar type I disorder experiencing a manic episode identified by a systematic review suggest that clonazepam may be as effective as lithium in improving manic symptoms at 1–4 weeks. The review provided insufficient evidence to assess adverse effects of clonazepam.

Benefits: **Versus placebo:** We found no systematic review or RCTs. **Versus lithium:** See benefits of lithium, p 1162.

Harms: **Versus placebo:** We found no RCTs. **Versus lithium:** See harms of lithium, p 1163.

Comment: None.

OPTION GABAPENTIN

One RCT in people with bipolar type I disorder experiencing a manic or mixed episode already taking lithium or valproate found that adding gabapentin was less effective in reducing manic symptoms over 10 months than placebo. Gabapentin was associated with somnolence, dizziness, diarrhoea, and memory loss.

Benefits: **Versus placebo:** We found one double blind RCT (117 people aged > 16 with bipolar type I disorder, all taking either valproate or lithium) comparing gabapentin 600–3600 mg daily versus placebo over 10 weeks.[16] It found that gabapentin reduced symptoms significantly less on the Young Mania Rating Scale than placebo (mean reduction: –6.5 with gabapentin *v* –9.9 with placebo; mean difference 3.34, 95% CI 0.32 to 6.35; P = 0.03).

Harms: **Versus placebo:** The RCT found that, compared with placebo, more people taking gabapentin had somnolence (24% with gabapentin *v* 12% with placebo), dizziness (19% with gabapentin *v* 5% with placebo), diarrhoea (16% with gabapentin *v* 12% with placebo), and memory loss (10% with gabapentin *v* 3% with placebo; CI not reported for any outcome).[16]

Comment: None.

OPTION LAMOTRIGINE

We found no RCTs comparing lamotrigine versus placebo in people with mania. One RCT in people with bipolar type I disorder experiencing a manic episode identified by a systematic review found no significant difference in manic symptoms at 4 weeks between lamotrigine and lithium. The review provided insufficient evidence to assess adverse effects of lamotrigine.

Benefits: **Versus placebo:** We found no systematic review or RCTs. **Versus lithium:** See benefits of lithium, p 1162.

Harms: **Versus placebo:** We found no RCTs. **Versus lithium:** See harms of lithium, p 1163.

Comment: None.

OPTION TOPIRAMATE

One systematic review identified no RCTs of topiramate in people with mania.

Benefits: **Versus placebo:** We found one systematic review (search date 2001), which identified no RCTs.[17]

Harms: **Versus placebo:** The review identified no RCTs in people with bipolar disorder.[17] It identified RCTs in people with epilepsy, which found that the most common adverse effects associated with topiramate were fatigue, dizziness, headache, abnormal thinking, confusion, somnolence, ataxia, impaired concentration, nystagmus, double vision, and anorexia.

Comment: None.

QUESTION **What are the effects of treatments in bipolar depression?**

OPTION **PSYCHOLOGICAL TREATMENTS**

We found no systematic review or RCTs of psychological treatments in people with bipolar depression.

Benefits: We found no systematic review or RCTs in people with bipolar depression (see comment below).

Harms: We found no RCTs.

Comment: We found no RCTs of psychological interventions in bipolar depression. It is unclear if it is reasonable to extrapolate from the evidence for treatments for unipolar depression. It is likely that specific interventions will have some effect, but RCTs are needed to estimate the size of any benefits and harms of these treatments. (See depressive disorders in adults, p 1238.)

OPTION **ANTIDEPRESSANTS**

Systematic reviews found that antidepressants improved depressive symptoms at the end of the trial (unspecified) compared with placebo. They found no significant difference between selective serotonin reuptake inhibitors and tricyclic antidepressants in the proportion of people who responded, although people taking selective serotonin reuptake inhibitors were more likely to respond. The reviews and one subsequent RCT found no significant difference in symptoms between monoamine oxidase inhibitors and tricyclic antidepressants or between selective serotonin reuptake inhibitors and serotonin noradrenaline reuptake inhibitors. Antidepressants are associated with manic switching and the reviews and subsequent RCT suggested that tricyclic antidepressants are more likely to induce mania than selective serotonin reuptake inhibitors.

Benefits: **Versus placebo:** We found one systematic review (search date not reported, 12 RCTs, 732 people with depressive disorder or mixed episode disorder with at least one previous episode of mania), published only as an abstract.[18] It found that people taking antidepressants (tricyclic antidepressants [TCAs], selective serotonin reuptake inhibitors [SSRIs], selective noradrenaline reuptake inhibitors [SNRIs], or monoamine oxidase inhibitors [MAOIs]) were significantly less likely to fail to respond to treatment at the end of the trial (unspecified) than people taking placebo (302 people: proportion who failed to respond: 87/180 [48%] with antidepressants *v* 92/122 [75%] with placebo; OR 0.30, 95% CI 0.18 to 0.48; NNT 4, 95% CI 3 to 7). **Versus each other:** We found two systematic reviews[18,19] and one subsequent RCT.[20] The first review (search date not reported, 12 RCTs, 732 people with depressive disorder or mixed episode disorder with at least one previous episode of mania) found no significant difference between SSRIs and TCAs in the proportion of people who responded to treatment at the end of the trial (unspecified), although people taking SSRIs were less likely to fail to respond (71 people: 31/65 [48%] with SSRIs *v* 44/69 [64%] with TCAs; OR 0.53, 95% CI 0.27 to 1.04).[18] It also found no significant difference in the proportion of people who responded at the end of the trial (unspecified) between MAOIs and TCAs (54/109 [49%] with MAOIs *v* 54/103 [52%] with TCAs; OR 0.89, 95% CI 0.52 to 1.52) or between SSRIs and SNRIs (19/34 [56%] with SSRIs *v* 21/35 [60%] with SNRIs; OR 0.85, 95% CI 0.33 to 2.17). The second review (search date 2000, 6 RCTs, 422 people with bipolar depression, 190 people with unipolar depression, about 25% taking lithium, carbamazepine, or valproate) also found similar responses to treatment among antidepressants, but did not quantify its conclusions.[19] The subsequent RCT (60 people with bipolar depression all taking mood stabilisers, primarily lithium, carbamazepine, or valproate) found no significant difference between venlafaxine and paroxetine in the proportion of people who responded at 6 weeks (13/30 [43%] with venlafaxine *v* 14/30 [47%] with paroxetine; RR 0.93; 95% CI 0.53 to 1.63).[20] **Versus adding lithium or valproate:** We found one small RCT (27 people with mania or bipolar depression receiving lithium or valproate), which compared the addition of paroxetine versus the addition of a second dose of lithium or valproate. It found no significant difference between groups in depressive or manic symptoms over 6 weeks (results presented graphically).[21]

Harms: Antidepressants are associated with manic switching**G**. **Versus each other:** The first review found that SSRIs were significantly less likely to induce mania than TCAs (OR 0.14, 95% CI 0.02 to 0.81).[18] The second review also concluded that tricyclic drugs were more likely to induce mania than other antidepressants, but did not quantify its conclusions.[19] The subsequent RCT found no significant difference between venlafaxine and paroxetine in the proportion of people who developed hypomania or mania, although more people taking venlafaxine experienced manic switching (4/13 [13%] with venlafaxine *v* 1/30 [3%] with paroxetine; RR 4.00, 95% CI 0.65 to 25.90).[20] The RCT may have been underpowered to detect a clinically important difference.

Comment: A systematic review of antidepressants in bipolar depression is in progress.[22] The evidence for treatment of unipolar depression (see depressive disorders in adults, p 1238) is believed to be applicable, although the efficacy of the treatments may be different, and specific adverse effects such as antidepressant induced mania should be considered.

OPTION LITHIUM

One systematic review identified no RCTs of sufficient quality to assess lithium in people with bipolar depression.

Benefits: We found one systematic review (search date 2000), which identified no RCTs of sufficient quality in people with bipolar depression.[19] The review identified one crossover trial in people with depression (52 people, 40 with bipolar depression).[19] Participants were randomised to 2 weeks of lithium and then crossed over to 6 days of placebo. The trial found that lithium improved symptoms in 32/40 (80%) people over 2 weeks, and that 12/32 (38%) of these relapsed when taking placebo. One crossover trial found limited evidence that lithium did not induce more manic switching**G** than placebo in bipolar depression.

Harms: We found no good RCTs.

Comment: None.

OPTION CARBAMAZEPINE

One systematic review identified no RCTs of sufficient quality to assess carbamazepine in people with bipolar depression.

Benefits: We found one systematic review (search date 2000), which identified no RCTs of sufficient quality in people with bipolar depression (see comment below).[19]

Harms: We found no good RCTs.

Comment: The review identified one crossover trial in people with depression (35 people, 24 with bipolar depression).[19] Participants were randomised to placebo before and after being crossed over to carbamazepine over 45 days. The trial found that carbamazepine improved symptoms in 62% of people over a mean 45 days. It found limited evidence that lithium did not induce more manic switching**G** than placebo in bipolar depression.

OPTION VALPROATE

We found no systematic review or RCTs of valproate in people with bipolar depression.

Benefits: We found no systematic review or RCTs of valproate in people with bipolar depression.

Harms: We found no RCTs.

Comment: None.

OPTION LAMOTRIGINE

One RCT in people with bipolar type I disorder experiencing a depressive episode identified by a systematic review found that lamotrigine increased the proportion of people who responded over 7 weeks compared with placebo. Lamotrigine increased the proportion of people with headache compared with placebo.

Benefits: We found one systematic review (search date 2000),[19] which identified one RCT (195 people aged 19–75 years with bipolar type I disorder experiencing a major depressive episode).[23] The RCT compared three treatments: lamotrigine 200 mg daily, lamotrigine 50 mg daily, and placebo.[23] It found no significant difference between lamotrigine and placebo in Hamilton Depression Rating Scale score over 7 weeks, but found that lamotrigine 200 mg daily significantly improved Montgomery–Asberg Depression Rating Scale score (mean reduction: –13.3 with lamotrigine *v* –7.8 with placebo; $P < 0.05$) and increased the proportion of people who responded to treatment (measured by Clinical Global Impression Scale scores: mean change: 2.6 with lamotrigine *v* 3.3 with placebo; $P < 0.05$).

Harms: The RCT found that significantly more people had headache with lamotrigine compared with placebo (20/63 [32%] with lamotrigine 200 mg *v* 11/65 [17%] with placebo; $P < 0.05$).[23]

Comment: None.

OPTION TOPIRAMATE

One systematic review identified no RCTs of topiramate in people with bipolar depression. One subsequent RCT in people taking lithium or valproate found no significant difference in symptoms at 8 weeks between adding topiramate and adding bupropion. The RCT found that a third of people taking topiramate and a fifth of people taking bupropion withdrew because of adverse effects, including anxiety, increase or decrease in appetite, blurred vision, backache, headache, and nausea.

Benefits: **Versus placebo:** We found one systematic review (search date 2001) that identified no RCTs.[17] **Versus bupropion:** We found one systematic review that identified no RCTs.[17] We found one subsequent RCT (36 people with bipolar depression, all taking lithium or valproate) comparing topiramate versus bupropion.[24] It found that both topiramate and bupropion significantly improved Clinical Global Impression scores from baseline at 8 weeks. It found no significant difference between treatments (P = 0.092; absolute numbers not reported).

Harms: **Versus placebo:** We found no RCTs.[17] **Versus bupropion:** The subsequent RCT found that 6/18 (33%) of people taking topiramate and 4/33 (22%) of people taking bupropion withdrew because of adverse effects, including anxiety, increase or decrease in appetite, blurred vision, backache, headache, and nausea (CI not reported).[24]

Comment: None.

QUESTION What are the effects of interventions to prevent relapse of mania or bipolar depression?

OPTION COGNITIVE THERAPY

Two RCTs found that cognitive therapy reduced relapse over 6–12 months compared with usual care. Another RCT found no significant difference between cognitive therapy and usual care in the proportion of people who relapsed over 6 months, although fewer people receiving cognitive therapy relapsed. The RCT is likely to have been underpowered to detect a clinically important difference between treatments. The RCTs provided insufficient evidence to assess adverse effects of cognitive therapy.

Benefits: We found no systematic review but found three RCTs.[25–27] In all three RCTs, cognitive therapy**G** was adapted for bipolar disorder and included advice on medication compliance, self monitoring of symptoms, establishing routine, and ensuring sufficient sleep to reduce risk of relapse**G**. The first RCT (42 outpatients aged ≥ 18 with bipolar type I disorder who had experienced ≥ 1 episode of mania/hypomania or bipolar depression in the preceding 2 years, most taking lithium alone or in combination with another mood stabiliser) compared cognitive therapy versus usual care for 6 months followed by cognitive therapy.[25] It found no significant difference between cognitive therapy and usual care in the proportion of people who relapsed over 6 months, although fewer people receiving cognitive therapy relapsed (1/21 [5%] with cognitive therapy *v* 2/21 [10%] with usual care; P = 0.06). The RCT is likely to have been underpowered to detect a clinically important difference. The second RCT (103 outpatients aged 18–70 years with bipolar type I disorder, not currently suffering from mania or bipolar depression, who had experienced ≥ 2 mood episodes in the preceding 2 years or 3 episodes in the preceding 5 years, all taking lithium, carbamazepine, or valproate sodium) compared cognitive therapy versus usual care for 1 year.[26] Cognitive therapy was given for 12–18 sessions over the first 6 months followed by two additional sessions in the following 6 months. The RCT found that cognitive therapy significantly reduced the proportion of people who relapsed over 12 months (21/48 [44%] with cognitive therapy *v* 36/48 [75%] with usual care; HR 0.40, 95% CI 0.21 to 0.74). The third RCT (25 outpatients aged 18–70 years with bipolar type I disorder, not currently suffering from mania or bipolar depression, who had experienced ≥ 2 mood episodes in the preceding 2 years or 3 episodes in the last 5 years) compared 12–20 sessions of cognitive therapy versus routine care for 6 months (see comment below).[27] It found that cognitive therapy significantly reduced relapse**G** over 6 months compared with usual care (RR 0.23, CI not reported; P < 0.001, absolute numbers not reported).

Harms: The first RCT found that there was one suicide in the people treated with cognitive therapy❻.[25]

Comment: None.

OPTION EDUCATION TO RECOGNISE SYMPTOMS OF RELAPSE

One RCT found limited evidence that an educational programme to recognise symptoms of relapse reduced manic relapse over 18 months, but that it may increase depressive episodes.

Benefits: We found no systematic review. We found one RCT (69 outpatients with bipolar disorder who had relapsed in the previous year) comparing an educational programme to recognise symptoms of relapse❻ versus treatment as usual over 18 months.[28] It found that people in the educational programme were significantly less likely to suffer a manic relapse❻ over 18 months compared with people receiving usual care (9/33 [27%] with educational programme *v* 20/35 [57%] with usual care; RR 0.48, 95% CI 0.25 to 0.86; NNT 4; 95% CI 2 to 16), but may have been more likely to suffer from a depressive episode (18/33 [55%] with educational programme *v* 13/35 [37%] with usual care; RR 1.47, 95% CI 0.87 to 2.54), although the difference was not significant. It found that, compared with usual care, the educational programme significantly improved social function from baseline at 18 months (measured on a 4 point scale assessing 8 areas of social activity where 0 = fair/good performance and 4 = inability to carry out function; mean difference in score 1.97, 95% CI 0.71 to 3.23).[28]

Harms: The RCT found that, compared with usual care, education may increase depressive relapse❻ (see benefits above).[28]

Comment: None.

OPTION FAMILY FOCUSED PSYCHOEDUCATION

One RCT found that 21 sessions of family focused psychoeducation reduced relapse over 12 months compared with two family sessions plus crisis management. Another RCT found that family focused psychoeducation may reduce relapse compared with individual focused therapy. The RCTs gave no information on adverse effects.

Benefits: We found no systematic review but found two RCTs.[29,30] The first RCT (101 people with bipolar disorder who had recently recovered from an acute episode recruited from inpatient and outpatient facilities, all taking antipsychotic drugs) compared 21 sessions of family focused psychoeducation versus two family sessions plus crisis management over 12 months.[29] Family focused psychoeducation involved education about the symptoms, causes, and treatment of bipolar disorder; education to recognise symptoms of relapse❻; preparation of a relapse prevention plan; and training in problem solving and communication skills. Crisis management involved emergency counselling sessions as needed, with a minimum of a monthly telephone call. The RCT found that family focused psychoeducation significantly reduced the proportion of people who relapsed over 12 months compared with family session plus crisis management (HR 1.47, CI not reported; P = 0.042).[29] The second RCT (53 people with bipolar type I disorder hospitalised after a manic episode, all taking lithium, valproate, carbamazepine, or a combination with or without antipsychotic or antidepressant drugs [not specified]) compared family focused psychoeducation versus individual focused therapy for 12 months' treatment.[30] It found no significant difference in the proportion of people who relapsed over 12 months treatment (46% with family focused psychoeducation v 52% with individual focused therapy; P = 0.11), although it found that family focused psychoeducation significantly reduced relapse rates over 1 year after treatment (28% with family focused psychoeducation v 60% with individual focused therapy; P < 0.05).

Harms: The RCTs gave no information on adverse effects.[29,30]

Comment: None.

OPTION LITHIUM

Systematic reviews and subsequent RCTs found that lithium reduced relapse over 2 years compared with placebo. They found no significant difference in relapse between lithium and valproate, carbamazepine, or lamotrigine. RCTs found that more people had overall adverse effects (not specified) with lithium than with placebo, and that lithium may increase hypothyroidism. They found that lithium caused more polyuria, thirst, and diarrhoea than valproate but less sedation and infection. More people taking lithium than carbamazepine had adverse effects, including blurred vision, difficulty concentrating, thirst, hand tremor and muscle weakness, but more people taking carbamazepine had increased appetite. RCTs also found that fewer people taking lithium than lamotrigine had headaches.

Benefits: **Versus placebo:** We found three systematic reviews in people with bipolar disorder, unipolar disorder, or mixed unipolar/bipolar disorder,[31–33] and two subsequent RCTs.[34,35] The first review (search date not reported, 9 RCTs, 825 people with bipolar or unipolar disorder) found that lithium reduced the risk of relapse**G** by 41% at up to 2 years compared with placebo (3 RCTs, 412 people with bipolar disorder: relapse**G** as defined in the trial [including hospital admission or requiring additional medication]: 73/202 [36%] with lithium v 128/210 [61%] with placebo; RR 0.59, 95% CI 0.48 to 0.73).[31] The review found no significant difference between lithium and placebo in the proportion of people with bipolar or unipolar disorder who committed suicide, but it is likely to have been underpowered to detect a clinically important difference (4 RCTs: 0/186 [0%] with lithium v 2/189 [1%] with placebo; RR 0.32, 95% CI 0.03 to 2.98). The second review (search date not reported, 15 RCTs, including 8 identified by the first review, 558 people with bipolar disorder) found that, in people with bipolar disorder, there was an average 48% decrease in the absolute risk of relapse by the end of the trial (unspecified) with lithium compared with placebo.[32] The third review (search date 2000, 3 RCTs identified by the first review, 19 observational studies) assessed the effect of long term lithium treatment on suicide rates.[33] It found that people with bipolar or unipolar disorder treated with lithium had lower suicide rates compared with untreated people (159 deaths per 100 000 patient years of treatment with lithium v 876 deaths per 100 000 patient years of treatment with no treatment; RR 8.85, 95% CI 4.12 to 19.1). Two subsequent RCTs (647 people aged ≥ 18 years with bipolar type I or type II disorder who had recently recovered from a manic or depressive/hypomanic episode and remained stable after an 8–16 week run in, during which they began taking lamotrigine and withdrew other psychotropic drugs), compared three treatments: lithium, lamotrigine, and placebo over 76 weeks.[34,35] Both RCTs found that, compared with placebo, lithium significantly increased the time to requirement of additional intervention for a manic or depressive episode (median time to additional medication: 24–42 weeks with lithium v 12–13 weeks with placebo; P = 0.05 in both RCTs). Secondary analyses in the RCTs suggested that lithium protected against manic but not depressive relapse. **Versus valproate:** We found one systematic review (search date not reported), which identified one RCT (372 people) comparing three treatments: lithium, valproate, and placebo.[36] It found no significant difference between lithium and valproate in relapse at 12 months (relapse defined as withdrawal due to episode of bipolar disorder: 12/187 [6%] with lithium *v* 9/91 [10%] with valproate; RR 0.8, 95% CI 0.5 to 1.2), but it is likely to have been too small to detect a clinically important difference. **Versus carbamazepine:** We found one systematic review[32] (search date not reported, 10 RCTs, 572 people with unipolar or bipolar disorder) and one subsequent RCT[37] comparing lithium versus carbamazepine. It found no significant difference between lithium and carbamazepine in the proportion of people who relapsed over 1–3 years (60% with lithium *v* 55% with carbamazepine; reported as non-significant; no further data reported; see comment below). The subsequent RCT (94 outpatients aged ≥18 years with bipolar disorder, who had experienced ≥2 mood episodes in the preceding 3 years) compared lithium (blood level 0.6–1.0 mmol/L) versus carbamazepine (blood level 6–10 mg/L) for 2 years of treatment.[37] It found no significant difference between lithium and carbamazepine in the proportion of people who relapsed over 2 years (relapse defined as developing an episode of mania or bipolar depression: 12/44 [27%] with lithium *v* 21/50 [42%] with carbamazepine; RR 1.54, 95% CI 0.88 to 2.78). A pre-planned subgroup analysis suggested that lithium was more effective in people who were randomised when euthymic. **Versus lamotrigine:** We found no systematic review but found two RCTs (638 people with bipolar type I or type II disorder who had recently recovered from a manic or depressive/hypomanic episode and remained stable after an 8–16 week run in, during which they began taking lamotrigine and withdrew other psychotropic drugs) comparing three treatments: lithium, lamotrigine, and placebo.[34,35] One of the RCTs was published only as an abstract.[35] The first RCT (175 people) found no significant difference between lithium and lamotrigine in the time to requirement of additional intervention for a mood episode compared (median time to additional medication: 24–42 weeks with lithium *v* 20–29 weeks with lamotrigine; $P > 0.05$).[34] Secondary analysis found no significant difference in manic relapse between lithium and lamotrigine, although fewer people taking lithium had manic relapse ($P = 0.092$).[34] Secondary analysis also found no significant difference in depressive relapse between lithium and lamotrigine ($P = 0.36$). The second RCT found similar results.[35]

Harms: **Versus placebo:** The first review found that significantly more people had overall adverse effects (not specified) with lithium than with placebo (160/233 [69%] with lithium *v* 112/225 [50%] with placebo; RR 1.4, 95% CI 1.2 to 1.6), and that lithium may increase hypothyroidism (7/158 [4%] with lithium *v* 0/152 [0%] with placebo; RR 5.1, 95% CI 0.9 to 27.7).[31] **Versus valproate:** The review found that valproate was significantly more likely than lithium to cause sedation (1 RCT: 78/187 [42%] with valproate *v* 24/91 [26%] with lithium; RR 1.6, 95% CI 1.1 to 2.3) and infection (type of infection not specified, 1 RCT: 51/187 [27%] with valproate *v* 12/91 [13%] with lithium; RR 2.1, 95% CI 1.2 to 3.7), but significantly less likely to cause polyuria (15/187 [8%] with valproate *v* 17/91 [19%] with lithium; RR 0.4, 95% CI 0.2 to 0.8), thirst (11/187 [6%] with valproate *v* 14/91 [15%] with lithium; RR 0.4, 95% CI 0.2 to 0.8), and possibly diarrhoea (65/187 [35%] with valproate *v* 42/91 [46%] with lithium; RR 0.75, 95% 0.6 to 1.0).[36] **Versus carbamazepine:** The review gave no information on adverse effects.[32] One RCT (144 people with bipolar disorder) identified by the review found that, although more people taking carbamazepine than taking lithium withdrew from the trials (9/70 [13%] with carbamazepine *v* 4/74 [5%] with lithium; reported as non-significant; no further data reported), a significantly higher proportion of people taking lithium compared with carbamazepine had "slight or moderate" adverse effects over 2.5 years (21% with carbamazepine *v* 61% with lithium; $P < 0.001$).[38] The subsequent RCT found that blurred vision, difficulty concentrating, thirst, hand tremor, and muscle weakness were more common with lithium than with carbamazepine.[37] Increased appetite was more common with carbamazepine. **Versus lamotrigine:** The first RCT found that lithium caused significantly fewer headaches than lamotrigine (4% with lithium *v* 20% with lamotrigine; $P = 0.02$) but more diarrhoea (28% with lithium *v* 5% with lamotrigine; $P = 0.002$).[34] The second RCT gave no information on adverse effects.[35]

Comment: **Versus carbamazepine:** The results of the review should be interpreted with caution as it combined trials of unipolar and bipolar disorder.[32]

OPTION VALPROATE

One RCT identified by a systematic review found that valproate reduced relapse over 12 months compared with placebo. One systematic review found no significant difference between lithium and valproate in relapse over 12 months. The review found that valproate cause more sedation and infection than lithium but less polyuria, thirst, and diarrhoea.

Benefits: **Versus placebo:** We found one systematic review (search date not reported, 1 RCT, 372 people with bipolar disorder) comparing three treatments: valproate, lithium, and placebo.[36] It found that valproate significantly reduced relapse❻ over 12 months compared with placebo (relapse❻ defined as withdrawal because of an episode of bipolar disorder: 45/187 [24%] with valproate *v* 36/94 [38%] with placebo; RR 0.6, 95% CI 0.4 to 0.9), but found no significant difference in time to relapse ($P = 0.33$; no further data reported). **Versus lithium:** See benefits of lithium, p 1171.

Harms: **Versus placebo:** The review found that valproate was significantly more likely than placebo to cause tremor (RR 3.2, 95% CI 1.9 to 5.6), weight gain (RR 2.9, 95% 1.3 to 6.2), alopecia (RR 2.4, 95% CI 1.1 to 5.7), and nausea (RR 1.4, 95% CI 1.0 to 1.9).[36] We also found one case control study (32 women aged 15–45 years with bipolar disorder), which found that 8/17 (47%) women taking valproate had current menstrual irregularities compared with 2/15 (13%) women not taking valproate.[39] **Versus lithium:** See harms of lithium, p 1176.

Comment: None.

OPTION CARBAMAZEPINE

We found no RCTs comparing carbamazepine versus placebo for preventing relapse. One systematic review and one subsequent RCT found no significant difference between carbamazepine and lithium in the proportion of people who relapsed over 1–3 years. The review and subsequent RCT found that carbamazepine was associated with fewer adverse effects than lithium.

Benefits: **Versus placebo:** We found no systematic review or RCTs comparing carbamazepine versus placebo in preventing relapse❻. **Versus lithium:** See benefits of lithium, p 1175.

Harms: **Versus placebo:** We found no RCTs. **Versus lithium:** See harms of lithium, p 1176.

Comment: A systematic review of the effects of carbamazepine in preventing relapse❻ is in progress.[40]

OPTION LAMOTRIGINE

Three RCTs found that lamotrigine reduced relapse compared with placebo. However, secondary analyses in two of the RCTs suggested that lamotrigine protected against depressive relapse, but not manic relapse. RCTs found no significant difference between lamotrigine and lithium in the proportion of people who relapsed and found that more people taking lamotrigine than lithium had headaches.

Benefits: **Versus placebo:** We found no systematic review but found three RCTs.[34,35,41] Two RCTs (647 people aged ≥ 18 years with bipolar type I or type II disorder who had recently recovered from a manic episode or depressive/hypomanic episode and remained stable after 8–16 weeks during which they began taking lamotrigine and withdrew other psychotropic drugs) compared three treatments over 76 weeks: lamotrigine, lithium, and placebo (see comment below).[34,35] Both RCTs found that, compared with placebo, lamotrigine significantly increased the time to requiring additional medication for a manic or bipolar depressive episode (median time to additional medication: 20–29 weeks with lamotrigine *v* 12–13 weeks with placebo; P = 0.05 in both RCTs).[34,35] Secondary analyses suggested that lamotrigine reduced depressive but not manic relapse**G**. The third RCT (182 people with rapid cycling bipolar disorder (see table 1, p 1181) found no significant difference between lamotrigine and placebo in the time to requiring additional medication (P = 0.177, results presented graphically).[41] **Versus lithium:** See benefits of lithium, p 1175.

Harms: **Versus placebo:** Two of the RCTs gave no information on adverse effects.[34,35] The third RCT found no significant difference between lamotrigine and placebo in the proportion of people who had adverse effects, including nausea and headache (67% with lamotrigine *v* 68% with placebo; reported as non-significant, CI not reported).[41] **Versus lithium:** See harms of lithium, p 1176.

Comment: The first RCT is published only as an abstract.[34]

OPTION ANTIDEPRESSANTS

One systematic review and one subsequent RCT provided insufficient evidence to assess antidepressants in preventing relapse of bipolar disorder.

Benefits: We found one systematic review (search date 2000; 4 RCTs, 258 people with bipolar type I or type II disorder) comparing tricyclic antidepressants versus placebo or lithium.[42] The review did not perform a meta-analysis or quantify its conclusions. It provided a narrative overview of the studies and found no clear evidence that tricyclic antidepressants reduce relapse**G** over 1–2 years compared with placebo. It suggested that tricyclic antidepressants may be less effective in preventing relapse**G** over 1–2 years than lithium.

Harms: The review suggested that antidepressants may induce mood instability or manic episodes.[42]

Comment: None.

GLOSSARY

Cognitive therapy Brief (20 sessions over 12–16 weeks) structured treatment aimed at changing the dysfunctional beliefs and negative automatic thoughts that characterise depressive disorders. It requires a highly trained therapist.

Manic switching involves onset of a manic episode shortly after treatment for a depressive episode. It may be more likely after treatment with antidepressants.

Relapse A return of symptoms to the extent that the disorder again meets criteria for the full syndromes. In practice, patients with bipolar disorder learn to recognise early warning signs and begin treatment before criteria are met. For this reason, relapse is often pragmatically defined as the need for drug treatment due to re-emergence of depressive or manic symptoms.

REFERENCES

1. Müller-Oerlinghausen B, Berghöfer A, Bauer M. Bipolar disorder. *Lancet* 2002;359:241–247.
2. Weissman MM, Bland RC, Canino GJ, et al. Cross-national epidemiology of major depression and bipolar disorder. *JAMA* 1996;276:293–299.
3. Murray CJ, Lopez AD. Global mortality, disability, and the contribution of risk factors: Global Burden of Disease Study. *Lancet* 1997;349:1436–1442.
4. Tohen M, Hennen J, Zarate C, et al. Harvard first episodes project: predictors of recovery and relapse. *Bipolar Disord* 2002;4:135–136.
5. Harris EC, Barraclough B. Suicide as an outcome for mental disorders. A meta-analysis. *Br J Psychiatry* 1997;170:205–208.
6. Macritchie K, Geddes JR, Scott J, et al. Valproate for acute mood episodes in bipolar disorder. In: The Cochrane Library, Issue 3, 2003. Oxford: Update Software. Search date 2002; primary sources Cochrane Collaboration Depression, Anxiety and Neurosis Review Group Controlled Trials Register; Cochrane Controlled Trials Register; hand searches of reference lists of relevant papers and textbooks; and personal contact with authors of trials, experts, and pharmaceutical companies.
7. Poolsup N, Li Wan Po A, de Oliveira IR. Systematic overview of lithium treatment in acute mania. *J Clin Pharm Ther* 2000;25:139–156. Search date 1999; primary sources Medline, Embase, Science Citation Index, the Cochrane Library, and hand searches of reference lists of identified RCTs and reviews.
8. Berk M, Ichim M, Brook S. Olanzapine compared to lithium in mania: a double-blind randomized controlled trial. *Int Clin Psychopharmacol* 1999;14:339–343.
9. Ichim L, Berk M, Brook S. Lamotrigine compared with lithium in mania: a double-blind randomized controlled trial. *Ann Clin Psychiatry* 2000;12:5–10.
10. McElroy SL, Keck PE. Pharmacologic agents for the treatment of acute bipolar mania. *Biol Psychiatry* 2000;48:539–557.
11. Yatham LN, Grossman F, Augustyns I, et al. Mood stabilisers plus risperidone or placebo in the treatment of acute mania. International double-blind, randomised controlled trials. *Br J Psychiatry* 2003;182:141–147. [Erratum in: *Br J Psychiatry* 2003;182:369]
12. Rendell JM, Gijsman HJ, Keck P, et al. Olanzapine alone or in combination for acute mania. In: The Cochrane Library, Issue 3, 2003. Oxford: Update Software. Search date 2002; primary sources The Cochrane Collaboration Depression, Anxiety and Neurosis Controlled Trials Register, The Cochrane Central Register of Controlled Trials, Embase, Medline, Cinahl, and Psychinfo.
13. Meehan K, Zhang F, David S, et al. A double-blind, randomized comparison of the efficacy and safety of intramuscular injections of olanzapine, lorazepam, or placebo in treating acutely agitated patients diagnosed with bipolar mania. *J Clin Psychopharmacol* 2001;21:389–397.
14. Keck PE, Versiani M, Potkin S, et al. Ziprasidone in the treatment of acute bipolar mania: a three-week, placebo-controlled, double-blind randomized trial. *Am J Psychiatry* 2003;160:741–748.
15. Delbello MP, Schwiers ML, Rosenberg HL, et al. A double-blind, randomized, placebo-controlled study of quetiapine as adjunctive treatment for adolescent mania. *J Am Acad Child Adolesc Psychiatry* 2002;41:1216–1223.
16. Pande AC, Crockatt JG, Janney CA, et al. Gabapentin in bipolar disorder: a placebo-controlled trial of adjunctive therapy. *Bipolar Disord* 2000;2:249–255.
17. Maidment ID. The use of topiramate in mood stabilization. *Ann Pharmacother* 2002;36:1277–1281. Search date 2001; primary sources Medline 1985–2001 and contact with the manufacturers of topiramate.
18. Gijsman HJ, Geddes JR, Rendell JM, et al. Systematic review of antidepressants for bipolar depression [abstract]. *J Psychopharmacol* 2001;15(suppl):A19. Search date not reported; primary sources Cochrane Collaboration Depression Anxiety and Neurosis Controlled Trials Register.
19. Nolen WA, Bloemkolk D. Treatment of bipolar depression: a review of the literature and a suggestion for an algorithm. *Neuropsychobiology* 2000;42:11–17. Search date 2000; primary sources Medline and hand searches of reference lists and recent congress abstracts books.
20. Vieta E, Martinez-Aran A, Goikolea JM, et al. A randomized trial comparing paroxetine and venlafaxine in the treatment of bipolar depressed patients taking mood stabilizers. *J Clin Psychiatry* 2002;63:508–512.
21. Young LT, Joffe RT, Robb JC, et al. Double-blind comparison of addition of a second mood stabilizer versus an antidepressant to an initial mood stabilizer for treatment of people with bipolar depression. *Am J Psychiatry* 2000;157:124–126.
22. Gijsman HJ, Rendell J, Geddes J, et al. Antidepressants for bipolar depression (protocol for a Cochrane Review). In: The Cochrane Library, Issue 3, 2003. Oxford: Update Software.
23. Calabrese JR, Bowden CL, Sachs GS, et al. A double-blind placebo controlled study of lamotrigine monotherapy in outpatients with bipolar 1 depression. *J Clin Psychiatry* 1999;60:79–88.
24. McIntyre RS, Mancini DA, McCann S, et al. Topiramate versus bupropion SR when added to mood stabilizer therapy for the depressive phase of bipolar disorder: a preliminary single-blind study. *Bipolar Disord* 2002;4:207–213.
25. Scott J, Garland A, Moorhead S. A pilot study of cognitive therapy in bipolar disorders. *Psychol Med* 2001;31:459–467.
26. Lam DH, Watkins ER, Hayward P, et al. A randomized controlled study of cognitive therapy for relapse prevention for bipolar affective disorder: outcome of the first year. *Arch Gen Psychiatry* 2003;60:145–152.
27. Lam DH, Bright J, Jones S, et al. Cognitive therapy for bipolar illness – a pilot study of relapse prevention. *Cognitive Ther Res* 2000;24:503–520.
28. Perry A, Tarrier N, Morriss R, et al. Randomised controlled trial of efficacy of teaching patients with bipolar disorder to identify early symptoms of relapse and obtain treatment. *BMJ* 1999;318:149–153.
29. Miklowitz DJ, Simoneau TL, George EL, et al. Family-focused treatment of bipolar disorder: 1-year effects of a psychoeducational program in conjunction with pharmacotherapy. *Biol Psychiatry* 2000;48:582–592.
30. Rea MM, Tompson MC, Miklowitz DJ, et al. Family-focused treatment versus individual treatment for bipolar disorder: results of a randomized clinical trial. *J Consult Clin Psychol* 2003;71:482–492.
31. Burgess S, Geddes J, Hawton K, et al. Lithium for maintenance treatment of mood disorders. In: The Cochrane Library, Issue 3, 2003. Oxford: Update Software. Search date not reported; primary sources Cochrane Collaboration Depression, Anxiety and Neurosis Review Group Specialised Register; Cochrane Controlled Trials Register; hand searches of reference lists of relevant papers, major textbooks of mood disorder, and the journals *Lithium* and

Lithium Therapy Monographs; and personal communication with authors, other experts in the field, and pharmaceutical companies.

32. Davis JM, Janicak PG, Hogan DM. Mood stabilizers in the prevention of recurrent affective disorders: a meta-analysis. *Acta Psychiatr Scand* 1999;100:406–417. Search date not reported; primary sources Medline, Psychlit, Pubmed, and hand searches of reference lists of identified studies and personal communication with colleagues.
33. Tondo L, Hennen J, Baldessarini RJ. Lower suicide risk with long-term lithium treatment in major affective illness: a meta-analysis. *Acta Psychiatrica Scand* 2001;104:163–172. Search date 2000; primary sources Medline, Current Contents, Psychlit, Pubmed, hand searches of reference lists of relevant publications and contents lists and/or indices of leading international psychiatric research journals, and personal communication with colleagues who have done research in the field.
34. Bowden CL, Calabrese JR, Sachs G, et al. A placebo-controlled 18-month trial of lamotrigine and lithium maintenance treatment in recently manic or hypomanic patients with bipolar 1 disorder. *Arch Gen Psychiatry* 2003;60:392–400.
35. Bowden CL, Calabrese JR, Baldwin D, et al. Lamotrigine delays mood episodes in recently depressed bipolar I patients. *Eur Neuropsychopharmacol* 2002;12:S216–S217.
36. Macritchie KAN, Geddes JR, Scott J, et al. Valproic acid, valproate and valproate semisodium in the maintenance treatment of bipolar disorder. In: The Cochrane Library, Issue 3, 2003. Oxford: Update Software. Search date not reported; primary sources Cochrane Collaboration Depression, Anxiety and Neurosis Review Group Specialised Register; Cochrane Controlled Trials Register; Embase; Medline; Lilacs; Psychlit; Psyndex; hand searches of reference lists of relevant papers, major textbooks on mood disorder, *Comprehensive Psychiatry*, and relevant conference proceedings; and personal communication with authors, other experts, and pharmaceutical companies.
37. Hartong EG, Moleman P, Hoogduin CA, et al. Prophylactic efficacy of lithium versus carbamazepine in treatment-naive bipolar patients. *J Clin Psychiatry* 2003;64:144–151.
38. Greil W, Ludwig–Mayerhofer W, Erazo N, et al. Lithium versus carbamazepine in the maintenance treatment of bipolar disorders: a randomised study. *J Affect Disord* 43:151–161.
39. O'Donovan C, Kusumaker V, Graves GR, et al. Menstrual abnormalities and polycystic ovary syndrome in women taking valproate for bipolar mood disorder. *J Clin Psychiatry* 2002;63:322–330.
40. Bandeira CA, Lima MS, Geddes J, et al. Carbamazepine for bipolar affective disorders (protocol for a Cochrane Review). In: The Cochrane Library, Issue 3, 2003. Oxford: Update Software.
41. Calabrese, JR Suppes, T, Bowden, CL, et al. A double-blind, placebo-controlled, prophylaxis study of lamotrigine in rapid-cycling bipolar disorder. Lamictal 614 Study Group. *J Clin Psychiatry* 2000;61:841–850.
42. Ghaemi SN, Lenox MS, Baldessarini RJ. Effectiveness and safety of long-term antidepressant treatment in bipolar disorder. *J Clin Psychiatry* 2001;62:565–569. Search date 2000; primary sources Medline, Healthstar, Current Contents, Psychinfo, and hand searches of bibliographies of identified reports and recent reviews.

John Geddes
Department of Psychiatry
University of Oxford
Oxford
UK

Competing interests: Sanofi-Synthelabo have donated supplies of Depakote and to the BALANCE trial of which JG in the principal investigator.

TABLE 1 **DSM-IV classification of bipolar disorders (see text, p 1161). Reprinted with permission from Elsevier (Mller-Oerlinghausen B, Berghfer A, Bauer M Bipolar Disorder Lancet 2002; 359: 241–47).[1]**

DSM IV Category	Criteria	Course specifiers and examples
Bipolar I disorder	One or more manic or mixed episodes, usually accompanied by one or more major depressive episodes	To describe current (or most recent episode): mild, moderate, severe without psychotic features; severe with psychotic features; in partial or full remission; with catatonic features; with postpartum onset
		To describe current (or most recent) major depressive episode: chronic; with melancholic features; with atypical features
		To describe pattern of episodes: with or without full interepisode recovery; with seasonal pattern; with rapid cycling (> 4 episodes in previous 12 months)
Bipolar II disorder	Recurrent major depressive episodes with one or more hypomanic (milder than manic) episodes	To describe current (or most recent episode): hypomanic; depressed
		To describe current (or most recent) major depressive episode and pattern of episodes: see bipolar I disorder
Cyclothymic disorder	Chronic (> 2 years), fluctuating mood disturbance involving numerous periods of mild hypomanic and depressive symptoms that do not meet criteria for a major depressive episode	Over 2 years any symptom free intervals last no longer than 2 months
Bipolar disorder (not otherwise specified)	Disorders with bipolar features that do not meet criteria for any specific bipolar disorder	Examples: very rapid cycling (over days); recurrent hypomanias without depressive symptoms; indeterminate whether primary or secondary (due to a general medical condition or substance abuse)

Bulimia nervosa

Search date August 2003

Phillipa J Hay and Josue Bacaltchuk

QUESTIONS

INTERVENTIONS

See glossary Ⓖ

Key Messages

Treatments for bulimia nervosa

- **Cognitive behavioural therapy for bulimia nervosa (CBT-BN)** One RCT found that CBT-BN improved remission rate, and reduced bulimic symptoms and depression compared with remaining on a waiting list. One RCT found no significant difference in remission of binge vomiting between guided self help CBT and CBT-BN after about 1 year. One RCT found no significant difference in remission rate or symptoms between cognitive behavioural therapy plus exposure response prevention and CBT-BN. One systematic review identified two RCTs, which found that interpersonal psychotherapy (IPT) was as effective as cognitive behavioural therapy for bulimia nervosa. One RCT found no significant difference between hypnobehavioural therapy (HBT) and CBT-BN for bulimia behavioural symptoms. One RCT found no clinically important difference in binge frequency between motivational enhancement therapy (MET) and CBT-BN. Two RCTs found no significant difference in remission or symptoms between CBT-BN and fluoxetine. Two RCTs comparing tricyclic antidepressants versus CBT-BN found mixed results. One found that imipramine improved remission compared with CBT-BN, and the other found no significant difference in remission rate between CBT-BN and desipramine. Two RCTs found no significant difference in remission rates or symptoms between CBT-BN and CBT-BN plus tricyclic antidepressants. Two RCTs found no significant difference in remission rates or symptoms between CBT-BN and CBT-BN plus fluoxetine.

Clin Evid 2005;13:1182–1199.

- **Combination treatment (antidepressants plus cognitive behavioural therapy as effective as either treatment alone)** Two RCTs found no significant difference in remission rates or symptoms between CBT-BN plus tricyclic antidepressants and CBT-BN or tricyclic antidepressants alone. Two RCTs found no significant difference in remission rates or symptoms between CBT-BN plus fluoxetine and CBT-BN or fluoxetine alone. One RCT found no significant difference in remission rates between unguided self help CBT plus fluoxetine and unguided self help CBT or fluoxetine alone.
- **Monoamine oxidase inhibitors** One systematic review identified three RCTs, which found that monoamine oxidase inhibitors improved remission rates compared with placebo.
- **Selective serotonin reuptake** inhibitors (evidence limited to fluoxetine) Three RCTs have found that fluoxetine 60 mg daily improves remission compared with placebo. Two RCTs found no significant difference in remission or symptoms between CBT-BN and fluoxetine. We found no RCTs of other serotonin reuptake inhibitors (fluvoxamine, paroxetine, sertraline, or citalopram).
- **Tricyclic antidepressants** One systematic review found that tricyclic antidepressants (desipramine and imipramine) improved bulimic symptoms and reduced binge eating compared with placebo. Two RCTs comparing tricyclic antidepressants versus CBT-BN found mixed results. One found that imipramine improved remission compared with CBT-BN, and the other found no significant difference in remission rate between CBT-BN and desipramine.
- **Cognitive orientation therapy** We found no RCTs of cognitive orientation therapy in people with bulimia nervosa.
- **Cognitive behavioural therapy plus exposure response prevention (CBT-ERP)** One RCT found no significant difference in vomiting frequency between CBT-ERP and waiting list, although it found that CBT-ERP improved depression scores compared with being on a waiting list. The RCT found no significant difference in remission rate or symptoms between CBT-ERP and CBT-BN.
- **Dialectical behavioural therapy** We found limited evidence from one small RCT that dialectical behavioural therapy improves bulimic symptoms compared with being on a waiting list.
- **Guided self help cognitive behavioural therapy** One RCT found no significant difference in behavioural symptoms between face to face or telephone guided self help and waiting list. One RCT found no significant difference in remission of binge vomiting between guided self help CBT and CBT-BN after about 1 year. One RCT found no significant difference in remission between unguided and guided self help CBT.
- **Hypnobehavioural therapy** One RCT found limited evidence that HBT improved abstinence from bingeing and purging compared with waiting list. The same RCT found no significant difference between HBT and CBT for bulimia behavioural symptoms.
- **Interpersonal psychotherapy** (as effective as cognitive behavioural therapy for bulimia nervosa) We found no RCTs comparing interpersonal psychotherapy versus no treatment, placebo, or waiting list control. One systematic review identified two RCTs, which found no significant difference in abstinence from binge eating between interpersonal psychotherapy and cognitive behavioural therapy for bulimia nervosa.
- **Motivational enhancement therapy** We found no RCTs comparing MET versus no treatment, placebo, or waiting list. One RCT found no clinically important difference in binge frequency between MET and CBT-BN.
- **Pure or unguided self help cognitive behavioural therapy** Two RCTs found no significant difference in remission or reduction in binge-purge frequency between pure or unguided self help CBT and waiting list. One RCT found no significant difference in remission between unguided and guided self help CBT. One RCT found no significant difference in remission between unguided self help CBT and fluoxetine alone or unguided self help CBT plus fluoxetine.
- **Mirtazapine; nefazodone; reboxetine; venlafaxine** We found no RCTs.

Discontinuing antidepressants in people with remission

- **Discontinuing fluoxetine** One RCT has found that continuing fluoxetine 60 mg daily is more effective than discontinuing fluoxetine and substituting placebo for maintaining a reduction in vomiting frequency in people who have responded well to an initial 8 week course of fluoxetine.

DEFINITION Bulimia nervosaⒼ is an intense preoccupation with body weight and shape, with regular episodes of uncontrolled overeating of large amounts of food (binge eatingⒼ) associated with use of extreme methods to counteract the feared effects of overeating. If a person also meets the diagnostic criteria for anorexia nervosa, then the diagnosis of anorexia nervosa takes precedence.[1] Bulimia nervosa can be difficult to identify because of extreme secrecy about binge eating and purgative behaviour. Weight may be normal but there is often a history of anorexia nervosa or restrictive dieting. Some people alternate between anorexia nervosa and bulimia nervosa. Some RCTs included people with subthreshold bulimia nervosa or a related eating disorder, binge eating disorder. Where possible, only results relevant to bulimia nervosa are reported in this review.

INCIDENCE/ PREVALENCE In community based studies, the prevalence of bulimia nervosa is between 0.5% and 1.0% in young women, with an even social class distribution.[2–4] About 90% of people diagnosed with bulimia nervosa are women. The numbers presenting with bulimia nervosa in industrialised countries increased during the decade that followed its recognition in the late 1970s and "a cohort effect" is reported in community surveys,[2,5,6] implying an increase in incidence. The prevalence of eating disorders such as bulimia nervosa is lower in non-industrialised populations,[7] and varies across ethnic groups. African-American women have a lower rate of restrictive dieting than white American women, but have a similar rate of recurrent binge eating.[8]

AETIOLOGY/ RISK FACTORS Young women from the developed world who restrict their dietary intake are at greatest risk of developing bulimia nervosa and other eating disorders. One community based case control study compared 102 people with bulimia nervosa with 204 healthy controls and found higher rates of the following in people with the eating disorder: obesity, mood disorder, sexual and physical abuse, parental obesity, substance misuse, low self esteem, perfectionism, disturbed family dynamics, parental weight/shape concern, and early menarche.[9] Compared with a control group of 102 women who had other psychiatric disorders, women with bulimia nervosa had higher rates of parental problems and obesity.[9]

PROGNOSIS A 10 year follow up study (50 people with bulimia nervosa from a placebo-controlled trial of mianserin treatment) found that 52% receiving placebo had fully recovered, and only 9% continued to experience full symptoms of bulimia nervosa.[10] A larger study (222 people from a trial of antidepressants and structured, intensive group psychotherapy) found that, after a mean follow up of 11.5 years, 11% still met criteria for bulimia nervosa, whereas 70% were in full or partial remissionⒼ.[11] Short term studies found similar results: about 50% of people made a full recovery, 30% made a partial recovery, and 20% continued to be symptomatic.[12] There are few consistent predictors of longer term outcome. Good prognosis has been associated with shorter illness duration, a younger age of onset, higher social class, and a family history of alcohol abuse.[10] Poor prognosis has been associated with a history of substance misuse,[13] premorbid and paternal obesity,[14] and, in some studies, personality disorder.[15–18] One study (102 women) of the natural course of bulimia nervosa found that 31% still had the disorder at 15 months and 15% at 5 years.[19] Only 28% received treatment during the follow up period. In an evaluation of response to cognitive behavioural therapyⒼ, early progress (by session 6) best predicted outcome.[20] A subsequent systematic review of the outcome literature found no consistent evidence to support early intervention and a better prognosis.[21]

AIMS OF INTERVENTION To reduce symptoms of bulimia nervosa; to improve general psychiatric symptoms; to improve social functioning and quality of life.

OUTCOMES Frequency of binge eating or bingeing, abstinence from binge eating or bingeing, frequency of behaviours to reduce weight and counter the effects of binge eating, severity of extreme weight and shape preoccupation, severity of general psychiatric symptoms, severity of depression, improvement in social and adaptive functioning, remission rates, relapse rates, and withdrawal rates.

METHODS *Clinical Evidence* search and appraisal August 2003 and hand searches of reference lists from identified reviews.

QUESTION What are the effects of treatments for bulimia nervosa in adults?

OPTION COGNITIVE BEHAVIOURAL THERAPY FOR BULIMIA NERVOSA

One RCT found that cognitive behavioural therapy for bulimia nervosa (CBT-BN) improved remission rate, and reduced bulimic symptoms and depression compared with remaining on a waiting list. One RCT found no significant difference in remission rate or symptoms between cognitive behavioural therapy plus exposure response prevention and CBT-BN. One RCT found no significant difference in remission of binge vomiting between guided self help CBT and CBT-BN after about 1 year. One systematic review identified two RCTs, which found that interpersonal psychotherapy was as effective as cognitive behavioural therapy for bulimia nervosa. One RCT found no significant difference between hypnobehavioural therapy and CBT-BN for bulimia behavioural symptoms. One RCT found no clinically important difference in binge frequency between motivational enhancement therapy and CBT-BN. Two RCTs found no significant difference in remission or symptoms between CBT-BN and fluoxetine. Two RCTs comparing tricyclic antidepressants versus CBT-BN found mixed results. One found that imipramine improved remission compared with CBT-BN, and the other found no significant difference in remission rate between CBT-BN and desipramine. Two RCTs found no significant difference in remission rates or symptoms between CBT-BN and CBT-BN plus tricyclic antidepressants. Two RCTs found no significant difference in remission rates or symptoms between CBT-BN and CBT-BN plus fluoxetine.

Benefits: We found one systematic review (search date 2002, 34 RCTs).[22] It included RCTs of other binge eating**G** disorders, although most studies were of people with bulimia nervosa**G** (18 RCTs in people with bulimia nervosa characterised by purging behaviour).[22] The review also reported data separately for bulimia nervosa. **Versus waiting list control:** The review identified one RCT (77 women with BN), which compared four groups: cognitive behavioural therapy for bulimia nervosa (CBT-BN)**G**; waiting list control; "self monitoring" only and cognitive behavioural therapy plus exposure response prevention**G** (CBT – ERP).[23] It found that CBT-BN increased binge eating remission**G** and improved bulimic symptoms and depression compared with waiting list control after 4 months' treatment (binge eating remission: 46% with CBT-BN *v* 5% with control; RR 0.58, 95% CI 0.39 to 0.86; bulimic symptoms SMD: –1.19, 95% CI –1.92 to –0.47; depression SMD: –1.43, 95% CI –2.18 to –0.67). **Versus cognitive behavioural therapy plus exposure response prevention (CBT-ERP):G**. See benefits of CBT-ERP, p 1186. **Versus pure self help CBT:G**. See benefits of pure or unguided CBT, p 1187. **Versus guided self help CBT:G**. See benefits of guided self help CBT, p 1188. **Versus cognitive orientation therapy:G**. See benefits of cognitive orientation therapy, p 1189. **Versus interpersonal psychotherapy:G**. See benefits of interpersonal psychotherapy, p 1189. **Versus hypnobehavioural therapy:G**. See benefits of HBT, p 1190. **Versus dialectical behavioural therapy:G**. See benefits of dialectical behavioural therapy, p 1190. **Versus motivational enhancement therapy:G**. See benefits of MET, p 1191. **Versus tricyclic antidepressants:** See benefits of tricyclic antidepressants, p 1192. **Versus fluoxetine:** See benefits of selective serotonin reuptake inhibitors, p 1191. **Versus other pharmacotherapy:** We found no RCTs comparing CBT versus monoamine oxidase inhibitors, mirtazapine, serotonin antagonists, or venlafaxine. **Versus combination treatment:** See benefits of combination treatment, p 1194.

Harms: The systematic review found that the RCTs did not report details of adverse effects.[22] It found no significant difference in completion rates between interventions, suggesting no major difference in acceptability. However, it could not exclude infrequent serious adverse effects.[22] An observational study found that group psychotherapy offered very soon after presentation was sometimes perceived as threatening.[10]

Comment: The systematic review[22] defined CBT as psychotherapy that uses the techniques and models specified by Wilson and Fairburn,[24] but it did not specify therapist expertise, the number of sessions, or their content (classical CBT-BN specifies 19 individual sessions over 20 weeks conducted by trained therapists and consists of specific structure and content[24]). Effect sizes for CBT were large, but over 50% of people were still binge eating at the end of treatment.[22] Further research is needed to evaluate the specific and non-specific effects of CBT and other psychotherapies, to explore individual characteristics (such as readiness to change) that may predict response, and to explore the long term effects of treatment. Waiting list or delayed treatment control groups are subject to bias because it is not possible to "blind" someone to their allocation. It is difficult to interpret the clinical importance of the statistically significant changes in depression scores. The quality of trials in the systematic review was variable (e.g. 57% were not blinded and sample sizes were often small).[22] Stricter inclusion criteria in the review removed previously included RCTs in people with binge eating disorders other than bulimia nervosa in supplementary analyses.[22] In these supplementary analyses of bulimia, only results comparing classical CBT-BN versus variants were included.[22] The RCT reported that 10/77 (12.9%) of people enrolled failed to complete treatment.[23] Results were not analysed on an intention-to-treat basis. Two further observational studies[25,26] found limited evidence that motivation and compliance factors may influence outcomes. One study [25] performed additional analyses of an RCT that compared CBT-BN versus interpersonal therapy (IPT).[27] It found that "stage of change" or psychological motivation and greater readiness to change was not related to non-completion, but was associated with a good outcome in those who completed IPT. The second study examined the effects of compliance on outcome in 62 people randomised to guided self help**G** or to full CBT for 16 weeks.[26] At 6 months' follow up, but not the end of treatment, binge eating abstinence rates were greater in those who had completed two or more of the CBT exercises (P = 0.04; CI not reported).

OPTION COGNITIVE BEHAVIOURAL THERAPY PLUS EXPOSURE RESPONSE THERAPY

One RCT found no significant difference in vomiting frequency between cognitive behavioural therapy plus exposure response therapy (CBT-ERP) and waiting list, although it found that CBT-ERP improved depression scores compared with being on a waiting list. The RCT found no significant difference in remission rate or symptoms between CBT-ERP and cognitive behavioural therapy for bulimia nervosa.

Benefits: **Versus waiting list:** We found one RCT (77 women with bulimia nervosa**G** characterised by purging behaviour), which compared four treatments: cognitive behavioural therapy for bulimia nervosa (CBT-BN)**G**; cognitive behavioural therapy plus exposure response prevention**G** (CBT-ERP) of vomiting; self monitoring of calorific intake and vomiting behaviour; and waiting list control.[23] It found no significant difference in vomiting frequency between CBT-ERP and waiting list control after 4 months of treatment (SMD from baseline in frequency of vomiting over 1 week: 6.4 with CBT-ERP *v* 0.2 with waiting list; P value not reported). However, the RCT found that CBT-ERP significantly improved depression scores compared with waiting list control (SMD from baseline in Beck Depression Inventory Score: 9.9 with CBT-ERP *v* 0.7 with waiting list; $P < 0.05$).[23] **Versus CBT-BN:** We found one systematic review (search date 2002; 4 RCTs, 193 people),[22] which identified one RCT (77 women; described above).[23] It found no significant difference between CBT-ERP and CBT-BN in binge eating remission rates, bulimic symptoms, or depression score at end of the 4 month period of treatment (binge eating remission: 46% with CBT-BN *v* 29% with CBT-ERP; RR 0.77, 95% CI 0.47 to 1.26; bulimic symptoms SMD: –0.35, 95% CI –1.03 to +0.34; depression SMD: –0.27, 95% CI –0.96 to +0.41). **Versus pharmacotherapy or combination treatment:** We found no RCTs.

Harms: **Versus waiting list:** The RCT did not report on harms.[23] However, it found no significant difference in withdrawal rate between CBT-ERP and waiting list control, although the confidence intervals were wide and the trial may have lacked power to detect an important difference (withdrawal rate: 23% with CBT-ERP *v* 5% with waiting list; RR 3.86, 95% CI 0.50 to 30.06). The RCT did not report on other harms. **Versus CBT alone:** The RCT identified by the review[22] similarly found no significant difference in withdrawal rates between CBT-ERP compared with CBT-BN.[23]

Comment: None.

OPTION PURE OR UNGUIDED SELF HELP COGNITIVE BEHAVIOURAL THERAPY

Two RCTs found no significant difference in remission or reduction in binge-purge frequency between pure or unguided self help cognitive behavioural therapy (CBT) and waiting list. One RCT found no significant difference in remission between unguided and guided self help CBT. One RCT found no significant difference in remission between unguided self help CBT and fluoxetine alone or unguided self help CBT plus fluoxetine.

Benefits: **Versus waiting list, no treatment, or placebo medication:** We found one systematic review (search date 2002),[22] which identified one RCT (85 women, 93% with purging bulimia nervosa; see comment below). The RCT compared two self help treatments (a specifically modified manual for bulimia nervosa [cognitive behavioural therapy [CBT] self help], and a non-specific manual on self assertion for women [non-specific self help]) versus waiting list control.[28] It found no significant difference in the proportion of women achieving a 50% reduction in binge eating or purging between either self help intervention and waiting list control after 8 weeks (AR for achieving a 50% reduction in binge eating or purging: 15/28 [53.6%] with CBT self help *v* 9/29 [31.0%] with waiting list; $P = 0.10$; 14/28 [50.0%] with non-specific self help *v* 9/29 [31.0%] with waiting list; $P = 0.08$). We found one additional RCT (91 women with bulimia nervosa), which compared four treatments: fluoxetine 60 mg daily alone; fluoxetine plus an unguided self help CBT manual; placebo plus an unguided self help CBT manual; and placebo alone. It found no significant difference in remission rates between unguided self help CBT manual plus placebo compared with placebo alone after 16 weeks (AR for remission: 5/22 [24%] with self help plus placebo *v* 2/22 [9%] with placebo; RR 2.50, 95% CI 0.54 to 11.54).[29] **Versus cognitive behavioural therapy for bulimia nervosa (CBT-BN):** We found no RCTs. **Versus guided self help CBT:** We found one systematic review (search date 2002),[22] which identified one RCT (71 people; 59% with bulimia nervosa; see comment below).[30] It compared four treatments: self help CBT with minimal guidance (participants received a brief explanation by a therapist of how to use the supplied self help manual); self help CBT with face to face guidance (participants received 4 guidance sessions over 4 months); self help CBT with telephone guidance (participants received the same guidance as the face to face group delivered over the telephone); and a waiting list control.[30] It found no significant difference in remission rates between self help with minimal guidance and face to face guided self help at 4 months (6% with self help *v* 10% with face to face guided self help; RR 0.63, 95% CI 0.11 to 3.48) and no significant difference in withdrawal rate (22% with self help *v* 23% with face to face guided self help; RR 0.94, 95% CI 0.37 to 2.36). **Versus fluoxetine:** We found one RCT (91 women), which compared four treatments: see above for details.[29] It found no significant difference in remission rate between placebo plus unguided self help CBT manual and fluoxetine alone after 16 weeks (AR for remission: 5/22 [24%] with placebo plus unguided self help CBT manual *v* 4/26 [16%] with fluoxetine alone; RR 1.48, 95% CI 0.45 to 4.84).[29] **Versus combination treatment:** See benefits of combination treatment, p 1194.

Harms: The RCTs did not report on harms.

Comment: **Versus waiting list, no treatment, or placebo:** The waiting list group had a significantly higher baseline frequency of purging compared with either of the two self help groups. Results should, therefore, be regarded with caution.[28] In trials with a drug treatment arm, people randomised to self help plus placebo were seen regularly by health professionals, so results may not generalise to self help, in which there is no contact with health professionals.

OPTION GUIDED SELF HELP COGNITIVE BEHAVIOURAL THERAPY

One RCT found no significant difference in behavioural symptoms between face to face or telephone guided self help cognitive behavioural therapy and waiting list. One RCT found no significant difference in remission of binge vomiting between guided self help cognitive behavioural therapy and cognitive behavioural therapy for bulimia nervosa after about 1 year. One RCT found no significant difference in remission between unguided and guided self help cognitive behavioural therapy.

Benefits: **Versus waiting list:** We found one RCT (121 people; 71 [59%] with bulimia nervosa**G**; see comment below), which compared four treatments: self help CBT manual with minimal guidance (participants received a brief explanation by a therapist of how to use the supplied self help manual); self help CBT manual with face to face guidance (participants received 4 guidance sessions over 4 months); self help CBT manual with telephone guidance (participants received the same guidance as the face to face group delivered over the telephone); and a waiting list control.[30] It found no significant difference in the proportion of people that improved (percentage change in key eating disorder behavioural symptoms) between either of the guidance groups compared with waiting list group after 4 months (proportion of people showing some improvement: 25% with minimal guidance *v* 50% with face to face guidance *v* 36% with telephone guidance *v* 19% with waiting list; P values not reported). **Versus cognitive behavioural therapy for bulimia nervosa (CBT-BN):** We found one RCT (62 people with DSM-IIIR bulimia nervosa), which compared 16 weekly sessions of CBT-BN**G** versus eight fortnightly sessions of a guided self help CBT**G**.[26,31] It found that CBT-BN increased remission**G** rate of binge vomiting compared with guided self help CBT at the end of treatment (AR 54.8% with CBT-BN *v* 12.9% with guided self help; P value not reported). However, after a mean follow up of 43 weeks from the end of treatment, it found no significant difference between treatments in remission of binge vomiting (AR 70.8% with CBT-BN *v* 60.9% with guided self help; ARR +10%, 95% CI –17% to +37%). **Versus pure self help:** See benefits of pure or unguided self help CBT, p 1187.

Harms: The RCTs did not report on harms.[26,30,31]

Comment: One RCT may have lacked power to detect clinically important effects.[30]

OPTION COGNITIVE ORIENTATION THERAPY

We found no RCTs of cognitive orientation therapy in people with bulimia nervosa.

Benefits: **Versus no treatment, placebo, or waiting list:** We found no RCTs that met our inclusion criteria. **Versus CBTⒼ; pharmacotherapy; or combination treatment:** We found no RCTs.

Harms: No harms were reported.

Comment: None.

OPTION INTERPERSONAL PSYCHOTHERAPY

We found no RCTs comparing interpersonal psychotherapy versus no treatment, placebo, or waiting list control. One systematic review identified two RCTs, which found no significant difference in abstinence from binge eating between interpersonal psychotherapy and cognitive behavioural therapy for bulimia nervosa.

Benefits: **Versus no treatment, placebo, or waiting list:** We found no RCTs. **Versus cognitive behavioural therapy for bulimia nervosa (CBT-BN):** We found one systematic review (search date 2002),[22] which identified two RCTs,[27,32] but did not pool results. The first RCT (220 people)[27] included in the review compared interpersonal psychotherapy (IPT)Ⓖ versus CBT-BNⒼ for bulimia nervosaⒼ that involved purging.[27] It found that CBT-BN significantly improved abstinence from binge eatingⒼ at the end of treatment (19 individual sessions conducted ≥ 20 weeks; intention to treat analysis; 29% with CBT-BN *v* 6% with IPT; $P < 0.01$). However, the difference was not significant at 4, 8, and 12 months of follow up, with improvement in both groups from baseline.[27] The second RCT (75 people, of whom 9 had non-purging bulimia nervosa), compared three treatments: 18 weeks of CBT-BN; behavioural therapy (a dismantled form of CBT); and IPT.[32] It found no significant difference among groups in binge eating frequency ($P = 0.36$) and cessation of binge episodes at the end of treatment (54% with IPT *v* 60% with CBT-BN using intention-to-treat comparison; RR calculated by systematic review 0.87, 95% CI 0.46 to 1.67). **Versus pharmacotherapy or combination treatment:** We found no RCTs.

Harms: The systematic review (search date 2002) found that the RCTs did not report details of adverse effects.[22] It found no significant difference in completion rates between interventions, suggesting no major difference in acceptability. However, it could not exclude infrequent serious adverse effects.[22] An observational study found that group psychotherapy offered very soon after presentation was sometimes perceived as threatening.[10]

Comment: None.

OPTION HYPNOBEHAVIOURAL THERAPY

One RCT found limited evidence that hypnobehavioural therapy improved abstinence from bingeing and purging in the short term compared with waiting list. The same RCT found no significant difference between hypnobehavioural therapy and cognitive behavioural therapy for bulimia behavioural symptoms.

Benefits: **Versus no treatment, placebo, or waiting list:** We found one RCT (78 women with bulimia nervosaⒼ; see comment below).[33] It compared three treatments: hypnobehavioural therapy (HBT)Ⓖ; cognitive behavioural therapy in bulimia nervosa (CBT-BN)Ⓖ; and waiting list control. It found that more people abstained from bingeing and purging after HBT compared with waiting list control in the week after treatment (AR for abstaining from bingeing: 43.0% with HBT *v* 4.5% with waiting list; P value not reported; AR for abstaining from purging: 33.3% with HBT *v* 4.5% with waiting list; P value not reported). **Versus CBT-BN:** We found one RCT (78 women with bulimia nervosa; see comment below).[33] It found that HBT was as effective as CBT-BN at increasing the proportion of people that abstained from bingeing and purging compared with waiting list control in the week after treatment (AR for abstaining from bingeing: 4.5% with waiting list *v* 50% with CBT-BN *v* 43% with HBT; P value not reported; AR for abstaining from purging: 4.5% with waiting list *v* 40% with CBT-BN *v* 33.3% with HBT; P value not reported). **Versus pharmacotherapy; combination treatment; or placebo:** We found no RCTs.

Harms: The RCT did not report on harms.[33]

Comment: The three treatment arms were not balanced at baseline. People in the CBT-BN group had had significantly longer duration of bulimic symptoms before study enrolment compared with people in the HBT group ($P < 0.05$).[33]

OPTION DIALECTICAL BEHAVIOURAL THERAPY

We found limited evidence from one small RCT that dialectical behavioural therapy improves bulimic symptoms compared with being on a waiting list.

Benefits: **Versus placebo, no treatment, or waiting list:** We found one RCT (31 people), which found that dialectical behavioural therapyⒼ significantly reduced bulimic symptom scores and dietary restraint scores compared with waiting list control over 20 weeks (bulimic symptom scores: SMD –1.35, 95% CI –2.17 to –0.53; dietary restraint scores: SMD –0.80, 95% CI –1.56 to –0.04).[34] However, it found no significant difference in depression scores between dialectical behavioural therapy and waiting list control (SMD –0.33, 95% CI –1.07 to +0.40).[34] **Versus cognitive behavioural therapy in bulimia nervosa (CBT-BN)Ⓖ; pharmacotherapy; or combination treatment:** We found no RCTs.

Harms: The RCT found no significant difference in treatment withdrawal rates between dialectical behavioural therapy and waiting list control (12.5% with dialectical behavioural therapy *v* 7% with waiting list; RR 1.88, 95% CI 0.19 to 18.6).[34]

Comment: None.

OPTION MOTIVATIONAL ENHANCEMENT THERAPY

We found no RCTs comparing motivational enhancement therapy versus no treatment, placebo, or waiting list. One RCT found no clinically important difference in binge frequency between motivational enhancement therapy and cognitive behavioural therapy in bulimia nervosa.

Benefits: **Versus no treatment, placebo, or waiting list:** We found no RCTs. **Versus cognitive behavioural therapy in bulimia nervosa (CBT-BN):** We found one RCT (125 people with bulimia nervosaⒼ), which compared four sessions of motivational enhancement therapyⒼ versus CBT-BNⒼ.[35] It found no significant difference between motivational enhancement therapy and CBT-BN in achieving a clinically significant reduction in binge frequency after 4 weeks (17/25 [68%] with CBT-BN *v* 23/43 [53%] with motivational enhancement therapy; RR 1.3, 95% CI 0.9 to 1.9). **Versus pharmacotherapy; other psychotherapy; or combination treatment:** We found no RCTs.

Harms: The RCT did not report on harms.[35]

Comment: None.

OPTION **SELECTIVE SEROTONIN REUPTAKE INHIBITORS (FLUOXETINE, FLUVOXAMINE, PAROXETINE, SERTRALINE, CITALOPRAM)**

Three RCTs have found that fluoxetine 60 mg daily improves remission compared with placebo. Two RCTs found no significant difference in remission or symptoms between cognitive behavioural therapy in bulimia nervosa and fluoxetine. We found no RCTs of other serotonin reuptake inhibitors (fluvoxamine, paroxetine, sertraline, or citalopram).

Benefits: **Versus placebo or no treatment:** We found one systematic review (search date 2001) comparing selective serotonin reuptake inhibitors (SSRIs) (all studies of fluoxetine 60 mg daily) versus placebo (see table 1, p 1199).[36] It found that fluoxetine non-significantly increased remissionⒼ and significantly increased the chance of clinical improvement and reduced non-completion rates compared with placebo (remission: 3 RCTs, 467 people; RR 0.89, 95% CI 0.76 to 1.03; clinical improvement [≥ 50% reduction in binge eatingⒼ episodes]; 3 RCTs, 706 people; RR 0.68, 95% CI 0.59 to 0.79; non-completion; 3 RCTs, 706 people; RR 0.82, 95% CI 0.68 to 0.99). However, it found no significant difference between fluoxetine and placebo for depression (1 RCT, 46 people; SMD –0.44, 95% CI –1.03 to +0.14). The review found no RCTs of other SSRIs, and we found no subsequent RCTs. **Versus cognitive behavioural therapy in bulimia nervosa (CBT-BN):** We found one systematic review (search date 2000,[37] 1 RCT,[38] 76 people) and one subsequent RCT (53 people).[39] We found one other trial comparing fluoxetine versus psychotherapy which is awaiting translation.[40] The RCT identified by the review found no significant differences between fluoxetine and binge eating remission rates, bulimic symptoms, or depression after 16 weeks (binge eating remission rate: 13% for both treatments; RR 0.99, 95% CI 0.80 to 1.24; mean bulimic symptoms: SMD +0.29, 95% CI –0.29 to +0.88; depression: SMD +0.10, 95% CI –0.47 to +0.67).[38] The subsequent RCT compared three treatments given for 4 months: group based CBT-BN, fluoxetine, and CBT-BN plus fluoxetine.[39] Completer analysis found no significant difference in abstinence from binge eating or self induced vomiting over the month preceding the end of treatment (abstinence from binge eating: 5/19 [26.3%] with CBT-BN *v* 2/16 [12.5%] with fluoxetine; RR 2.11, 95% CI 0.47 to 9.43; abstinence from self induced vomiting: 7/19 [36.8%] with CBT-BN *v* 1/16 [6.3%] with fluoxetine; RR 5.90, 95% CI 0.81 to 42.99).[39] **Versus other antidepressants:** We found no RCTs comparing SSRIs with other classes of antidepressants. **Versus combination treatment:** See benefits of combination treatment, p 1194. **Versus pure self help CBT:** We found no RCTs.

Harms: **Versus placebo:** The systematic review found that although significantly fewer people discontinued treatment with fluoxetine compared with placebo, there was no difference in treatment withdrawal because of adverse events (3 RCTs, 706 people; treatment withdrawal: 37% with fluoxetine *v* 40% with placebo; RR 0.82, 95% CI 0.68 to 0.99; treatment withdrawal because of adverse events: 3 RCTs, 706 people; RR 1.52, 95% CI 0.83 to 2.75).[36] **Versus CBT-BN:** The RCT[38] identified by the systematic review[37] found no significant difference in withdrawal rates between fluoxetine and CBT-BN (39% with fluoxetine *v* 33% with CBT-BN; RR 1.17, 95% CI 0.55 to 2.51). The subsequent RCT found no significant difference in withdrawals with fluoxetine compared with CBT-BN or combination treatment (42% with CBT-BN *v* 25% with fluoxetine; RR 1.68, 95% CI 0.62 to 4.57).

Comment: We found no consistent predictors of response to treatment.

OPTION MONOAMINE OXIDASE INHIBITORS

One systematic review identified three RCTs, which found that monoamine oxidase inhibitors improved remission rates compared with placebo.

Benefits: **Versus placebo or no treatment:** We found one systematic review (search date 2001 see table 1, p 1199).[36] It found that monoamine oxidase inhibitors significantly increased greater remission**G** rates compared with placebo, but found no significant difference in improvement in bulimic symptoms or depression scores (remission rates: 2 RCTs, 98 people; RR 0.81, 95% CI 0.68 to 0.96; improvement in bulimic symptoms: 3 RCTs, 138 people; SMD +0.22, 95% CI –0.94 to +1.37; depression scores: 4 RCTs, 156 people; SMD –0.14, 95% CI –0.50 to +0.22). **Versus other psychotherapy:** We found no RCTs. **Versus combination treatment:** See benefits of combination treatment, p 1194.

Harms: The systematic review found no difference in treatment withdrawal rates because of adverse events between monoamine oxidase inhibitors and placebo (3 RCTs, 15/88 [17%] with monoamine oxidase inhibitors *v* 7/87 [8%] with placebo, RR 2.06, 95% CI 0.45 to 9.53).[36]

Comment: None.

OPTION TRICYCLIC ANTIDEPRESSANTS

One systematic review found that tricyclic antidepressants (desipramine and imipramine) improved bulimic symptoms and reduced binge eating compared with placebo. Two RCTs comparing tricyclic antidepressants versus cognitive behavioural therapy in bulimia nervosa found mixed results. One found that imipramine improved remission compared with cognitive behavioural therapy in bulimia nervosa, and the other found no significant difference in remission rate between cognitive behavioural therapy in bulimia nervosa and desipramine.

Benefits: **Versus placebo:** We found one systematic review (search date 2001; 3 RCTs, 2 of desipramine, 1 of imipramine, 132 people)(see table 1, p 1199).[36] It found a significantly greater clinical improvement (a reduction of 50% or more in binge eating**G** episodes) and a significant improvement in bulimic symptoms with tricyclic antidepressants compared with placebo (clinical improvement: 2 RCTs, 44 people; RR 0.29, 95% CI 0.13 to 0.64; bulimic symptoms: 3 RCTs, 121 people: SMD –0.75, 95% CI –1.12 to –0.38). It also found no significant difference in either remission**G** rates or improvement of depressive symptoms between tricyclic antidepressants and placebo (remission rates: RR 0.90, 95% CI 0.79 to 1.04). **Versus cognitive behavioural therapy in bulimia nervosa (CBT-BN):** We found one systematic review (search date 2000),[37] which identified two RCTs meeting *Clinical*

Evidence criteria for inclusion.[41,42] The first RCT (140 people) compared three treatments: imipramine 200–300 mg daily; group based CBT-BN. It found that CBT-BN increased binge eating remission rate compared with imipramine at 10 weeks (binge eating remission rate: 50% with CBT-BN *v* 16% with imipramine; RR 1.67, 95% CI 1.17 to 2.38).[41] The second RCT (71 people) compared three treatments: desipramine (mean 167 mg daily); CBT-BN (16 weekly sessions with 2 follow up sessions), and CBT-BN plus desipramine.[42] It found no significant difference in binge eating remission rates or bulimic symptoms between desipramine and CBT-BN (remission rate: 42% with desipramine *v* 57% with CBT-BN; RR 1.34, 95% CI 0.69 to 2.62; bulimic symptoms: SMD –0.02, 95% CI –0.72 to +0.68). **Versus combination treatment:** See benefits of combination treatment, p 1194.

Harms: **Versus placebo:** The systematic review found that treatment withdrawal because of any cause was more likely with tricyclic antidepressants compared with placebo (6 RCTs, 2 of desipramine, 4 of imipramine; 277 people; 29% with tricyclic antidepressants *v* 14% with placebo; RR 1.93, 95% CI 1.15 to 3.25).[36] We found one RCT examining specific adverse effects. It found significant increases in reclining and standing blood pulse rate, lying systolic and diastolic blood pressure, and greater orthostatic effects on blood pressure with desipramine compared with placebo.[43] Cardiovascular changes were well tolerated and few people withdrew because of these effects. **Versus CBT-BN:** The first RCT found no significant difference in withdrawal rate between tricyclic antidepressants and CBT-BN, although confidence intervals were wide and an effect cannot be ruled out (RR 5.75, 95% CI 0.67 to 49.50).[41] The second RCT found that withdrawal rate was significantly higher with tricyclic antidepressants than with CBT-BN (43% with tricyclic antidepressants *v* 15% with CBT-BN; RR 2.9, 95% CI 1.22 to 6.89).[42] **Versus combination treatment:** See harms of combination treatment, p 1195.

Comment: We found no consistent predictors of response to treatment.

OPTION MIRTAZAPINE

We found no RCTs.

Benefits: We found no RCTs.

Harms: We found no RCTs.

Comment: Mirtazapine is a noradrenergic and specific serotonergic antidepressant.

OPTION REBOXETINE

We found no RCTs.

Benefits: We found no RCTs.

Harms: We found no RCTs.

Comment: Reboxetine is a noradrenergic antidepressant.

OPTION NEFAZODONE

We found no RCTs.

Benefits: We found no RCTs.

Harms: We found no RCTs.

Comment: Nefazodone is a noradrenergic and specific serotonergic antidepressant.

OPTION VENLAFAXINE

We found no RCTs.

Benefits: We found no RCTs.

Harms: We found no RCTs.

Comment: Venlafaxine is a serotonin and noradrenaline reuptake inhibitor.

OPTION COMBINATION TREATMENT

Two RCTs found no significant difference in remission rates or symptoms between cognitive behavioural therapy in bulimia nervosa (CBT-BN) plus tricyclic antidepressants and CBT-BN or tricyclic antidepressants alone. Two RCTs found no significant difference in remission rates or symptoms between CBT-BN plus fluoxetine and CBT-BN or fluoxetine alone. One RCT found no significant difference in remission rates between unguided self help CBT plus fluoxetine and unguided self help CBT alone or fluoxetine alone.

Benefits: **Cognitive behavioural therapy in bulimia nervosa (CBT-BN) plus tricyclic antidepressants versus tricyclic antidepressants alone:** We found one systematic review (search date 2000),[37] which identified two RCTs meeting *Clinical Evidence* inclusion criteria.[41,42] The first RCT (140 people) compared three treatments: imipramine 200–300 mg daily; group based CBT-BN. It found no significant difference in binge eating**Ⓖ** remission**Ⓖ** rates between combination treatment and tricyclic antidepressants alone (P value not reported).[41] The second RCT (71 people) compared three treatments: desipramine (mean 167 mg daily); CBT-BN (16 weekly sessions with 2 follow up sessions); and CBT-BN plus desipramine.[42] It similarly found no significant difference between combination treatment and tricyclic antidepressants alone in binge eating remission rates or bulimic symptoms at 24 weeks (remission rate: 42% with tricyclic antidepressants alone *v* 67% with combination treatment; RR 1.75, 95% CI 0.69 to 4.44; bulimic symptoms: SMD +0.10, 95% CI –0.70 to +0.90).[42] **CBT-BN plus tricyclic antidepressants versus CBT-BN alone:** We found one systematic review (search date 2000),[37] which identified two RCTs meeting *Clinical Evidence* inclusion criteria.[41,42] The first RCT (140 people) found no significant differences in binge eating remission**Ⓖ** rates between combination treatment and CBT-BN alone.[41] The second RCT (71 people) similarly found no significant difference between combination treatment and CBT-BN alone in binge eating remission rates or bulimic symptoms after 24 weeks (remission rate: 44% with CBT-BN *v* 67% with combination treatment; RR 1.70, 95% CI 0.71 to 4.07; bulimic symptoms: SMD +0.09, 95% CI –0.61 to +0.79).[42] **CBT-BN plus fluoxetine versus fluoxetine alone:** We found one systematic review (search date 2000,[37] 1 RCT,[38] 76 people) and one subsequent RCT (53 people).[39] The RCT identified by the review found no significant difference between combination treatment and fluoxetine alone in binge eating remission rates, bulimic symptoms, or depression scores (remission rate: 15% with fluoxetine *v* 21% with combination treatment; RR 1.10, 95% CI 0.86 to 1.40; bulimic symptoms: SMD +0.09, 95% CI –0.46 to +0.63; depression: SMD 0, 0.95% CI –0.55 to +0.54).[38] The subsequent RCT compared three treatments: group based CBT-BN; fluoxetine 60 mg daily; and CBT-BN plus fluoxetine.[39] Completer analysis found no significant difference in abstinence from binge eating or self induced vomiting for 1 month (abstinence from binge eating: 2/16 [12.5%] with fluoxetine *v* 3/18 [16.7%] with combination treatment; RR 1.05, 95% CI 0.80 to 1.30; abstinence from vomiting: 1/16 [6.3%] with fluoxetine *v* 1/18 [5.6%] with combination treatment; RR 0.99, 95% CI 0.84 to 1.18). **CBT-BN plus fluoxetine versus CBT-BN alone:** We found one systematic review (search date 2000,[37] 1 RCT,[38] 76 people) and one subsequent RCT (53 people).[39] The RCT identified by the review found no significant difference between combination treatment and CBT-BN alone in binge eating remission rates, bulimic symptoms, and depression score (12% with CBT-BN *v* 21% with combination treatment; RR 1.10, 96% CI 0.87 to 1.40; bulimic symptoms: SMD –0.09, 95% CI –0.74 to +0.36; depression: SMD –0.19, 95% CI –0.74 to +0.36).[38] The subsequent RCT compared three treatments: group based CBT-BN; fluoxetine 60 mg daily; and CBT-BN plus fluoxetine.[39] Completer analysis found no significant difference in abstinence from binge eating or self induced vomiting for 1 month (abstinence from binge eating: 5/19 [26.3%] with fluoxetine *v* 3/18 [16.7%] with combination treatment; RR 1.58, 95% CI 0.44 to 5.67; abstinence from vomiting: 7/19 [36.8%] with CBT-BN *v* 1/18 [5.6%] with combination treatment; RR 6.63, 95% CI 0.90 to 48.69). **Self help CBT plus fluoxetine versus fluoxetine alone:** We found one RCT (91 women with bulimia nervosa**G**), which compared four treatments: fluoxetine 60 mg daily alone; fluoxetine plus a self help CBT manual; placebo plus a self help manual; and placebo alone.[29] It found similar reductions in remission rates between self help CBT plus fluoxetine compared with fluoxetine alone (6/21 [26%] with self help CBT plus fluoxetine *v* 4/26 [16%] with fluoxetine; RR 1.86, 95% CI 0.60 to 5.73; data provided upon personal communication with author). **Self help CBT plus fluoxetine versus self help CBT alone:** We found one RCT (91 women with bulimia nervosa), which compared four treatments: fluoxetine 60 mg daily alone; fluoxetine plus a self help CBT manual; placebo plus a self help CBT manual; and placebo alone.[29] It found no significant difference in remission rates in last 2 weeks of treatment between combination treatment and self help CBT plus placebo (26% with combination treatment *v* 24% with self help CBT plus placebo).[29]

Harms: **CBT-BN plus tricyclic antidepressants versus tricyclic antidepressants alone:** The first RCT found that tricyclic antidepressants increased withdrawal rate compared with combination treatment, although the difference was not significant (43% with tricyclic antidepressants *v* 25% with combination treatment; RR 1.70, 95% CI 0.97 to 2.99).[41] The second RCT found no significant difference between combination treatment and tricyclic antidepressants alone in withdrawal (25% in both groups; RR 1.00, 95% CI 0.25 to 4.00).[42] **CBT-BN plus tricyclic antidepressants versus CBT-BN alone:** The first RCT found no significant difference in withdrawal rates between combination treatment and CBT-BN alone (15% with CBT-BN alone *v* 25% with combination treatment; RR 0.59, 95% CI 0.23 to 1.50).[41] The second RCT also found no significant difference in withdrawal rate between treatments (4% with CBT-BN *v* 25% with combination treatment; RR 0.17, 95% CI 0.02 to 1.50).[42] **CBT-BN plus fluoxetine versus fluoxetine alone:** The RCT identified by the review found no significant difference in withdrawal rates between combination treatment and fluoxetine alone (39% with fluoxetine *v* 55% with combination treatment; RR 0.71, 95% CI 0.39 to 1.30).[38] The subsequent RCT similarly found no significant difference in withdrawal rate between treatments.[39] **CBT-BN plus fluoxetine versus CBT-BN alone:** The RCT identified by the review found no significant difference in withdrawal rates between combination treatment and CBT-BN alone (33% with CBT-BN *v* 55% with combination treatment; RR 0.60, 95% CI 0.31 to 1.16).[38] The subsequent RCT similarly found no significant difference in withdrawal between treatments.[39] **Self help CBT plus fluoxetine versus fluoxetine alone:** The RCT did not report on harms. **Self help CBT plus fluoxetine versus self help CBT alone:** The RCT did not report on harms.

Comment: Modest effect sizes in these analyses may be clinically relevant, but the small number and size of trials limit conclusions.

QUESTION What are the effects of discontinuing treatment with antidepressants in people with remission?

OPTION ANTIDEPRESSANTS AS MAINTENANCE

One RCT has found that continuing fluoxetine 60 mg daily is more effective than placebo for maintaining a reduction in vomiting frequency in people who have responded well to an initial 8 week course of fluoxetine.

Benefits: We found one RCT (150 treatment responders [achieving a reduction of ≥ 50% from baseline in vomiting episodes in at least 1 of the preceding 2 weeks after an initial 8 weeks of fluoxetine]), which compared continued treatment with fluoxetine 60 mg daily versus placebo. It found that time to relapse (a return to baseline vomiting frequency for 2 consecutive weeks) was significantly prolonged with fluoxetine compared with placebo at one year (time to remission**G** not reported; $P < 0.02$).[44]

Harms: The RCT found no significant differences between fluoxetine and placebo in major adverse events, or in discontinuation because of relapse (AR for discontinuation because of relapse: 17/76 [22%] with fluoxetine *v* 22/74 [30%] with placebo).[44] However, rhinitis was more common with fluoxetine than with placebo (31.6% with fluoxetine *v* 16.2% with placebo; $P < 0.04$).

Comment: We found no RCTs assessing the effects of discontinuing treatment in people with complete abstinence from binging.

GLOSSARY

Binge eating Modified from DSM-IV.[1] Eating, in a discrete period (e.g. hours), a large amount of food, accompanied by a lack of control over eating during the episode.

Bulimia nervosa The American Psychiatric Association DSM-IV[1] criteria include recurrent episodes of binge eating; recurrent inappropriate compensatory behaviour to prevent weight gain; frequency of binge eating and inappropriate compensatory behaviour both, on average, at least twice a week for 3 months; self evaluation unduly influenced by body shape and weight; and disturbance occurring not exclusively during episodes of anorexia nervosa. Types of bulimia nervosa, modified from DSM-IV,[1] are purging: using self induced vomiting, laxatives, diuretics, or enemas; non-purging: fasting, exercise, but not vomiting or other abuse as for the purging type. However, many studies evaluate efficacy for samples that may include people with subthreshold bulimia nervosa or binge eating disorder. Where possible, only data of bulimia nervosa participants are reported in this review.

Cognitive behavioural therapy In bulimia nervosa a specific form of CBT (CBT-BN) has been developed[45] which uses three overlapping phases for 19 sessions over 20 weeks. Phase one aims to educate the person about bulimia nervosa. People are helped to increase regularity of eating, and resist urge to binge or purge. Phase two introduces procedures to reduce dietary restraint (e.g. broadening food choices). In addition, cognitive procedures supplemented by behavioural experiments are used to identify and correct dysfunctional attitudes and beliefs, and avoidance behaviours. Phase three is the maintenance phase. Relapse prevention strategies are used to prepare for possible future set backs.[24,45] While many studies have used variants of CBT for bulimia nervosa, for the purposes of this review only those that resemble CBT-BN are cited unless otherwise specified. In this topic, CBT-BN refers to all treatments that closely resemble CBT for bulimia nervosa.

Cognitive orientation therapy The cognitive orientation theory aims to generate a systematic procedure for exploring the meaning of a behaviour around themes, such as avoiding certain emotions. Therapy for modifying behaviour focuses on systematically changing beliefs related to themes, not beliefs referring directly to eating behaviour. No attempt is made to persuade the people that their beliefs are incorrect or maladaptive.[46]

Dialectical behavioural therapy A type of behavioural therapy that views emotional dysregulation as the core problem in bulimia nervosa, with binge eating and purging understood as attempts to influence, change, or control painful emotional states. People are taught a repertoire of skills to replace dysfunctional behaviours.[34]

Exposure therapy In bulimia nervosa this is a modification of the exposure and response prevention therapy developed for obsessive-compulsive disorder. It involves, for example, exposure to food, and then psychological prevention strategies to control weight behaviour, such as vomiting after eating until the urge or compulsion to vomit has receded.[47]

Guided self help cognitive behavioural therapy A modified form of cognitive behavioural therapy, in which a treatment manual is provided with support, usually from a non-professional or professional without specialist expertise in eating disorders. A good discussion of the development and types of self help can be found in Williams (2003).[48]

Hypnobehavioural psychotherapy Uses a combination of behavioural techniques, such as self monitoring, to change maladaptive eating disorders, and hypnotic techniques to reinforce and encourage behaviour change.

Interpersonal psychotherapy (IPT) In bulimia nervosa, this is a three phase treatment. Phase one analyses in detail the interpersonal context of the eating disorder. This leads to the formulation of an interpersonal problem area, which forms the focus of the second stage, which is aimed at helping the person make interpersonal changes. Phase three is devoted to the person's progress and an exploration of ways to handle future interpersonal difficulties. At no stage is attention paid to eating habits or body attitudes.[27]

Motivational enhancement therapy (MET) This is based on a model of change with focus on stages of change. Stages of change represent constellations of intentions and behaviours through which individuals pass as they move from having a problem to doing something to resolve it. People in "precontemplation" show no intention to change. People in "contemplation" acknowledge they have a problem and are thinking about change, but have not yet made a commitment to change. People in the third "action" stage are actively engaged in overcoming their problem, and people in "maintenance" work to prevent relapse. Transition from one stage to the next is sequential, but not linear. The aim of MET is to help people move from earlier stages into "action, utilising cognitive and emotional strategies". There is an emphasis on the therapeutic alliance. With precontemplators, the therapist explores perceived positive and negative aspects of their behaviours. Open-ended questions are used to elicit client expression, and reflective paraphrase is used to reinforce key points of motivation. During a session following structured assessment, most of the time is devoted to explaining feedback to the client. Later in MET, attention is devoted to developing and consolidating a change plan.[49]

Pure self help cognitive behavioural therapy A modified form of cognitive behavioural therapy, in which a treatment manual is provided for people to proceed with treatment on their own with no support (e.g. a book is mailed to the person). Unguided self help may be considered a variant of pure self help, where the self help is provided without guidance, but there is contact with treating professionals (e.g. if the participant is randomised to an arm of treatment that includes placebo or medication with the pure self help therapy). A good discussion of the development and types of self help can be found in Williams (2003).[48]

Remission Sustained abstinence (> 1 month) from binge eating.

Self psychology therapy This approaches bulimia nervosa as a specific case of the pathology of the self. The treated person cannot rely on people to fulfil their needs such as self esteem. They rely instead on a substance, food, to fulfil personal needs. Therapy progresses when the people move to rely on humans, starting with the therapist.[46]

REFERENCES

1. American Psychiatric Association. *Diagnostic and Statistical Manual of Mental Disorders.* 4th ed. Washington DC: American Psychiatric Press, 1994.
2. Bushnell JA, Wells JE, Hornblow AR, et al. Prevalence of three bulimic syndromes in the general population. *Psychol Med* 1990;20:671–680.
3. Garfinkel PE, Lin B, Goering P, et al. Bulimia nervosa in a Canadian community sample: prevalence, co-morbidity, early experiences and psychosocial functioning. *Am J Psychiatry* 1995;152:1052–1058.
4. Gard MCE, Freeman CP. The dismantling of a myth: a review of eating disorders and socioeconomic status. *Int J Eat Disord* 1996;20:1–12.
5. Hall A, Hay PJ. Eating disorder patient referrals from a population region 1977–1986. *Psychol Med* 1991;21:697–701.
6. Kendler KS, Maclean C, Neale M, et al. The genetic epidemiology of bulimia nervosa. *Am J Psychiatry* 1991;148:1627–1637.
7. Choudry IY, Mumford DB. A pilot study of eating disorders in Mirpur (Pakistan) using an Urdu version of the Eating Attitude Test. *Int J Eat Disord* 1992;11:243–251.
8. Striegel-Moore RH, Wifley DE, Caldwell MB, et al. Weight-related attitudes and behaviors of women who diet to lose weight: a comparison for black dieters and white dieters. *Obes Res* 1996;4:109–116.
9. Fairburn CG, Welch SL, Doll HA, et al. Risk factors for bulimia nervosa. A community-based case-control study. *Arch Gen Psychiatry* 1997;54:509–517.
10. Collings S, King M. Ten year follow-up of 50 patients with bulimia nervosa. *Br J Psychiatry* 1994;164:80–87.
11. Keel PK, Mitchell JE, Davis TL, et al. Long-term impact of treatment in women diagnosed with bulimia nervosa. *Int J Eat Disord* 2002;31:151–158.
12. Keel PK, Mitchell JE. Outcome in bulimia nervosa. *Am J Psychiatry* 1997;154:313–321.
13. Keel PK, Mitchell JE, Miller KB, et al. Long-term outcome of bulimia nervosa. *Arch Gen Psychiatry* 1999;56:63–69.
14. Fairburn CG, Norman PA, Welch SL, et al. A prospective study of outcome in bulimia nervosa and the long-term effects of three psychological treatments. *Arch Gen Psychiatry* 1995;52:304–312.
15. Coker S, Vize C, Wade T, et al. Patients with bulimia nervosa who fail to engage in cognitive behaviour therapy. *Int J Eat Disord* 1993;13:35–40.
16. Fahy TA, Russell GFM. Outcome and prognostic variables in bulimia. *Int J Eat Disord* 1993;14:135–146.
17. Rossiter EM, Agras WS, Telch CF, et al. Cluster B personality disorder characteristics predict outcome in the treatment of bulimia nervosa. *Int J Eat Disord* 1993;13:349–358.
18. Johnson C, Tobin DL, Dennis A. Differences in treatment outcome between borderline and nonborderline bulimics at 1-year follow-up. *Int J Eat Disord* 1990;9:617–627.
19. Fairburn C, Cooper Z, Doll H, et al. The natural course of bulimia nervosa and binge eating disorder in young women. *Arch Gen Psychiatry* 2000:57:659–665.
20. Agras WS, Crow SJ, Halmi KA, et al. Outcome predictors for the cognitive behavior treatment of bulimia nervosa: data from a multisite study. *Am J Psychiatry* 2000;157:1302–1308.
21. Reas DL, Schoemaker C, Zipfel S, et al. Prognostic value of duration of illness and early intervention in bulimia nervosa: a systematic review of the outcome literature. *Int J Eat Disord* 2001;30:1–10. Search date 1999; primary sources not reported.
22. Hay PJ, Bacaltchuk J. Psychotherapy for bulimia nervosa and binging. In: The Cochrane Library, Issue 1, 2003. Oxford: Update Software. Search date 2002; primary sources Medline, Extramed, Embase, Psychlit, Current Contents, Lilacs, Scisearch, Cochrane Controlled Trials Register 1997, Cochrane Collaboration Depression and Anxiety Trials Register, hand searches of *Int J Eat Disord* since its first issue, citation lists in identified studies and reviews, and personal contacts.
23. Agras WS, Schneider JA, Arnow B, et al. Cognitive-behavioral and response-prevention treatments for bulimia nervosa. *J Consult Clin Psychol* 1989;57:215–221.
24. Wilson GT, Fairburn CG. Treatments for eating disorders. In: Nathan PE, Gorman JM, eds. *A Guide to Treatments that Work.* New York: Oxford University Press, 1998:501–530.
25. Wolk SL, Devlin MJ. Stage of change as a predictor of response to psychotherapy for bulimia nervosa. *Int J Eat Disord* 2001;30:96–100.
26. Thiels C, Schmidt U, Troop N, et al. Compliance with a self-care manual in guided self-change for bulimia nervosa. *Eur Eat Disord Rev* 2001;9:115–122.
27. Agras WS, Walsh BT, Fairburn CG, et al. A multicenter comparison of cognitive-behavioral therapy and interpersonal psychotherapy. *Arch Gen Psychiatry* 2000;54:459–465.
28. Carter JC, Olmsted MP, Kaplan AS, et al. Self-help for bulimia nervosa: a randomized controlled trial. *Am J Psychiatry* 2003;160:973–978.
29. Mitchell JE, Fletcher L, Hanson K, et al. The relative efficacy of fluoxetine and manual-based self-help in the treatment of outpatients with bulimia nervosa. *J Clin Psychopharmacol* 2001;21:298–304.
30. Palmer RL, Birchall H, McGrain L, et al. Self-help for bulimic disorders: a randomised controlled trial comparing minimal guidance with face-to-face or telephone guidance. *Br J Psychiatry* 2002;181:230–235.
31. Thiels C, Schmidt U, Treasure J, et al. Guided self-change for bulimia nervosa incorporating use of a self-care manual. *Am J Psychiatry* 1998;155:947–953.
32. Fairburn CG, Jones R, Peveler RC, et al. Three psychological treatments for bulimia nervosa. A comparative trial. *Arch Gen Psychiatry* 1991;48:463–469.
33. Griffiths RA, Hadzi-Pavlovic D, Channon-Little L. A controlled evaluation of hypnobehavioural treatment for bulimia-nervosa: immediate pre-post-treatment effects. *Eur Eating Dis Rev* 1994;2:202–220.
34. Safer DL, Telch CF, Agras WS. Dialectical behavior therapy for bulimia nervosa. *Am J Psychiatry* 2001;158:632–634.
35. Treasure JL, Katzman M, Schmidt U, et al. Engagement and outcome in the treatment of bulimia nervosa: first phase of a sequential design comparing motivation enhancement therapy and cognitive behavioural therapy. *Behav Res Ther* 1999;37:405–418.
36. Bacaltchuk J, Hay P. Antidepressants versus placebo for people with bulimia nervosa. In: The Cochrane Library Issue 1, 2003. Oxford: Update Software. Search date 2001; primary sources Medline, Extramed, Embase, Psychlit, Current Contents, Lilacs, Scisearch, Cochrane Controlled Trials Register, Cochrane Collaboration Depression and Anxiety Trials Register, hand searches of citation lists in identified studies and reviews, and personal contacts.
37. Bacaltchuk J, Hay P. Antidepressants versus psychological treatments and their combination for people bulimia nervosa (Cochrane Review). In: The Cochrane Library Issue 1, 2003. Oxford: Update Software. Search date 2000; primary sources Medline, Extramed, Embase, Psychlit, Current Contents, Lilacs, Scisearch, Cochrane Controlled Trials Register, Cochrane Collaboration Depression and Anxiety Trials Register, hand searches of *Int J Eat*

Disord since its first issue, citation lists of identified studies and reviews, and personal contacts.
38. Goldbloom DS, Olmsted M, Davies R, et al. A randomized control trial of fluoxetine and cognitive behavioural therapy for bulimia nervosa: short-term outcome. *Behav Res Ther* 1997;35:803–811.
39. Jacobi C, Dahme B, Dittman R. Cognitive-behavioural, fluoxetine and combined treatment for bulimia nervosa: short- and long-term results. *Eur Eat Disord Rev* 2002;10:179–198.
40. Campanelli M. Cecinella confronto tra gli effetti della terapia farmacologica con fluoxetine e las psicoterapia nel trattamento della bulimia nervosa [in Italian]. *Minerva Psichiatr* 2002;43(suppl 1):1–24.
41. Mitchell JE, Pyle RL, Eckert ED, et al. A comparison study of antidepressants and structured intensive group psychotherapy in the treatment of bulimia nervosa. *Arch Gen Psychiatry* 1990;47:149–157.
42. Agras WS, Rossiter EM, Arnow B, et al. Pharmacologic and cognitive-behavioral treatment for bulimia nervosa: a controlled comparison. *Am J Psychiatry* 1992;149:82–87.
43. Walsh BT, Hadigan CM, Wong LM. Increased pulse and blood pressure associated with desipramine treatment of bulimia nervosa. *J Clin Psychopharmacol* 1992;12:163–168.
44. Romano SJ, Halmi KA, Sarkar NP, et al. A placebo-controlled study of fluoxetine in continued treatment of bulimia nervosa after successful acute fluoxetine treatment. *Am J Psychiatry* 2002;159:96–102.
45. Fairburn CG, Marcus MD, Wilson GT. Cognitive-behavioral therapy for binge eating and bulimia nervosa: a comprehensive treatment manual. In: Fairburn CG, Wilson GT, eds. *Binge Eating: Nature, Assessment, and Treatment*. New York: Guilford Press, 1993:361–404.
46. Bachar E, Latzer Y, Kreitler S, et al. Empirical comparison of two psychological therapies. Self psychology and cognitive orientation in the treatment of anorexia and bulimia. *J Psychother Pract Res* 1999;8:115–128.
47. Leitenberg H, Rosen J, Gross J, et al. Exposure plus response-prevention treatment of bulimia nervosa. *J Consult Clin Psychol* 1988;56:535–541.
48. Williams C. New technologies in self-help: another effective way to get better? *Eur Eat Disorders Rev* 2003;11:170–182.
49. Schmidt U, Treasure J, eds. *Clinician's Guide to Getting Better Bit(e) by Bit(e)*. Hove: Psychology Press, 1997.

Phillipa Hay
Psychiatrist
James Cook University, Townsville, Australia

Josue Bacaltchuk
Psychiatrist
Federal University of Sao Paulo, Sao Paulo, Brazil

Competing interests: PH has received reimbursement for attending symposia from Solvay Pharmaceuticals, Bristol-Myers Squibb, and Pfizer Pharmaceuticals, and for educational training of family doctors from Bristol-Myers Squibb, Pfizer Pharmaceuticals, and Lundbeck, and has been funded by Jansenn-Cilag to attend symposia. JB none declared.

TABLE 1 **Comparison of remission rates between active drug and placebo by class of antidepressant (see text, p 1191).[36]**

Class: drug(s)	Number of RCTs	Number of people	Absolute remission rates	RR (95% CI)
TCA: desipramine, imipramine	3	132	21% *v* 9%	0.90 (0.79 to 1.04)
SSRI: fluoxetine	3	467	81% *v* 89%	0.89 (0.76 to 1.03)
MAOI: phenylzine, isocarboxacid	2	98	24% *v* 6%	0.81 (0.68 to 0.96)

MAOI, monoamine oxidase inhibitor; SSRI, selective serotonin reuptake inhibitor; TCA, tricyclic antidepressant.

Deliberate self harm (and attempted suicide)

Search date October 2004

G Mustafa Soomro

QUESTIONS

INTERVENTIONS

Key Messages

- We found little RCT evidence for any intervention in people who have deliberately self harmed. Most RCTs and meta-analyses of small RCTs are likely to have been underpowered to detect clinically important differences between interventions.

Treating deliberate self harm

- **Continuity of care** One systematic review identified one RCT, which found limited evidence that follow up after hospital treatment with the same therapist may increase repetition of deliberate self harm compared with follow up with a different therapist over 3 months. However, the difference between groups may be explained by a higher level of risk factors for repetition in the group receiving follow up with the same therapist.
- **Dialectical behavioural therapy** One systematic review including one RCT found limited and equivocal evidence that dialectical behavioural therapy may reduce the proportion of people who repeat deliberate self harm over 12 months compared with usual care.
- **Emergency card** One systematic review found no significant difference in the proportion of people who repeated deliberate self harm over 12 months between emergency card (allowing emergency admission or contact with a doctor) and usual care.
- **Flupentixol depot injection** One systematic review including one small RCT found that flupentixol depot injection reduced the proportion of people who repeated deliberate self harm over 6 months compared with placebo. However, we were unable to draw reliable conclusions from this small study. Typical antipsychotics such as flupentixol are associated with a wide range of adverse effects.
- **Hospital admission** One systematic review found no significant difference between hospital admission and immediate discharge in the proportion of people who repeated deliberate self harm over 16 weeks.
- **Intensive outpatient follow up plus outreach** One systematic review found no significant difference in the proportion of people who repeated deliberate self harm over 4–12 months between intensive outpatient follow up plus outreach and usual care.

- **Manual assisted cognitive behavioural therapy** One RCT found no significant difference in repeat self harm rates at 1 year between manual assisted cognitive therapy and usual treatment (problem solving approaches, dynamic psychotherapy, short term counselling, or referral to a general practitioner or a voluntary group).
- **Mianserin** One systematic review provided insufficient evidence to assess mianserin.
- **Nurse led case management** One RCT found no significant difference between nurse led case management and usual care in the proportion of people who were admitted to emergency departments for episodes of deliberate self harm over 12 months.
- **Paroxetine** One systematic review, including one RCT in people who had previously deliberately self harmed, receiving concurrent psychotherapy, found no significant difference between paroxetine and placebo in the proportion of people who repeated self harm over 12 months. It found that paroxetine increased diarrhoea and tremor compared with placebo. Paroxetine, like other selective serotonin re-uptake inhibitors, has been linked to suicidal ideation. In clinical trials in children and adolescents with depression it showed higher rates of suicide related events. Abrupt withdrawal of SSRIs should be avoided. Withdrawal side-effects include headache, nausea, paraesthesia, dizziness and anxiety. Extrapyramidal reactions (including orofacial dystonias) and withdrawal syndrome have been reported more commonly with paroxetine than with other SSRIs.
- **Problem solving therapy** One systematic review of small RCTs found no significant difference between problem solving therapy and usual care in the proportion of people who repeated deliberate self harm over 6–12 months. A second systematic review found that problem solving therapy reduced symptoms of depression, anxiety, and hopelessness, and improved problems compared with usual care.
- **Psychodynamic interpersonal therapy** One RCT found that brief psychodynamic interpersonal therapy for 4 weeks reduced repetition of deliberate self harm, depression, and suicidal ideation over 6 months compared with usual care. However, we were unable to draw reliable conclusions from this single RCT.
- **Telephone contact** One RCT found no significant difference between telephone contact at 4 and 8 months and usual care in repetition of deliberate self harm, global functioning, and suicidal ideation over 12 months.
- **General practice based guidelines** One large cluster randomised trial comparing the use of general practitioner guidelines for management of deliberate self harm versus usual care found no significant difference in the proportion of people who repeated deliberate self harm over 12 months or in the time to repetition of self harm.

DEFINITION Deliberate self harm is an acute non-fatal act of self harm carried out deliberately in the form of an acute episode of behaviour by an individual with variable motivation.[1] The intention to end life may be absent or present to a variable degree. Other terms used to describe this phenomenon are "attempted suicide" and "parasuicide". For the purpose of this chapter the term deliberate self harm will be used throughout. Common methods of deliberate self harm include self cutting and self poisoning, such as overdosing on medicines. Some acts of deliberate self harm are characterised by high suicidal intent, meticulous planning (including precautions against being found out), and severe lethality of the method used. Other acts of deliberate self harm are characterised by no or low intention of suicide, lack of planning and concealing of the act, and low lethality of the method used. The related term of "suicide" is defined as an act with a fatal outcome that is deliberately initiated and performed by the person with the knowledge or expectation of its fatal outcome.[1] This review focuses on recent deliberate self harm, in all age groups, as the main presenting problem and excludes RCTs in which deliberate self harm is assessed as an outcome associated with other disorders, such as depression or borderline personality disorder. Deliberate self harm is not defined in the *Diagnostic and statistical manual of mental disorders* (DSM IV)[2] or the *International classification of mental and behavioural disorders* (ICD-10).[3]

INCIDENCE/ PREVALENCE Based on data from 16 European countries between 1989–1992, the lifetime prevalence of deliberate self harm in people treated in hospital and other medical facilities, including general practice settings, is estimated at about 3% for women and 2% for men.[4] Over the last 50 years there has been a rise in the incidence of deliberate self harm in the UK.[4] A reasonable current estimate is about 400/100 000 population a year.[5] In two community studies in the USA, 3–5% of responders said that they had made an attempt at deliberate self harm at some time.[6] Self poisoning using organophosphates is particularly common in developing countries.[7] A large hospital (catering for 900 000 people) in Sri Lanka reported 2559 adult hospital admissions and 41% occupancy of medical intensive care beds for deliberate self harm with organophosphates over 2 years.[8] An international survey using representative community samples of adults (aged 18–64 years) reported lifetime prevalence of self reported suicide attempts of 3.82% in Canada, 5.93% in Puerto Rico, 4.95% in France, 3.44% in West Germany, 0.72% in Lebanon, 0.75% in Taiwan, 3.2% in Korea, and 4.43% in New Zealand.[6]

AETIOLOGY/ RISK FACTORS Familial, biological, and psychosocial factors may contribute to deliberate self harm. Evidence for genetic factors includes a higher risk of familial suicide and greater concordance in monozygotic than dizygotic twins for deliberate self harm.[9] Evidence for biological factors includes reduced cerebrospinal fluid 5-hydroxyindole acetic acid levels and a blunted prolactin response to the fenfluramine challenge test, indicating a reduction in the function of serotonin in the central nervous system.[10] People who deliberately self harm and attempt suicide also show traits of impulsiveness and aggression, inflexible and impulsive cognitive style, and impaired decision making and problem solving.[11] Deliberate self harm is more likely to occur in women, young adults, and people who are single or divorced, of low education level, unemployed, disabled, or suffering from a psychiatric disorder,[12] particularly depression,[13] substance misuse,[14] borderline and antisocial personality disorders,[15] severe anxiety disorders,[16] and physical illness.[17]

PROGNOSIS Suicide is highest during the first year after deliberate self harm.[18] One systematic review found median rates of repetition of 16% (interquartile range [IQR] 12% to 25%) within the first year, 21% (IQR 12% to 30%) within 1–4 years, and 23% (IQR 11% to 32%) within 4 years or longer. It found median mortality from suicide after deliberate self harm of 1.8% (IQR 0.8% to 2.6%) within the first year, 3.0% (IQR 2.0% to 4.4%) within 1–4 years, 3.4% (IQR 2.5% to 6.0%) within 5–10 years, and 6.7% (IQR 5.0% to 11.0%) within 9 years or longer.[18] Repetition of deliberate self harm is more likely in people aged 25–49 years who are unemployed, divorced, from lower social class, or who suffer from substance misuse, depression, hopelessness, powerlessness, personality disorders, have unstable living conditions or live alone, have a criminal record, previous psychiatric treatment, a history of stressful traumatic life events, or a history of coming from a broken home or of family violence.[12] Factors associated with risk of suicide after deliberate self harm are aged over 45 years, male sex, being unemployed, retired, separated, divorced, or widowed, living alone, poor physical health, psychiatric disorder (particularly depression, alcoholism, schizophrenia, and sociopathic personality disorder), high suicidal intent in current episode including leaving a written note, violent method used in current episode, and history of previous deliberate self harm.[19]

AIMS OF INTERVENTION To reduce repetition of deliberate self harm; to reduce desire to self harm; to prevent suicide; and to improve social functioning and quality of life, with minimal adverse effects.

OUTCOMES Repetition of deliberate self harm, occurrence of suicide, admission to hospital, improvement in underlying psychiatric symptoms, improvement in coping, quality of life, and adverse effects. Some of the validated scales used for assessing psychiatric symptoms and deliberate self harm are: Symptom Checklist-90 (SCL-90), a self administered rating scale for assessing nine areas of psychopathology (somatisation, obsessive-compulsive, interpersonal sensitivity, depression, anxiety, hostility, phobic-anxiety, paranoid ideation, and psychoticism),[20–22] Beck Depression Inventory (a 21 item self administered Likert scale for measuring severity of depression),[23] Hospital Anxiety Depression Scale (a self administered 14 item Likert scale for measuring depression and anxiety),[24] Beck Scale for Suicidal Ideation (a 21 item self administered Likert scale covering thoughts and plans about suicide which aims at assessing the risk of a later suicide attempt),[25] Beck Hopelessness Scale (a 20 item true–false self administered scale which aims at assessing hopelessness about the future),[26] and Global Severity Index (GSI; a mean of all items in SCL-90).[21]

METHODS *Clinical Evidence* search and appraisal October 2004.

QUESTION **What are the effects of treatments for deliberate self harm and attempted suicide in adolescents and adults?**

OPTION **PAROXETINE**

One systematic review, including one RCT in people who had previously deliberately self harmed, receiving concurrent psychotherapy, found no significant difference between paroxetine and placebo in the proportion of people who repeated self harm over 12 months. It found that paroxetine increased diarrhoea and tremor compared with placebo. Paroxetine, like other selective serotonin re-uptake inhibitors, has been linked to suicidal ideation. In clinical trials in children and adolescents with depression it showed higher rates of suicide related events. Abrupt withdrawal of SSRIs should be avoided. Withdrawal side-effects include headache, nausea, paraesthesia, dizziness and anxiety. Extrapyramidal reactions (including orofacial dystonias) and withdrawal syndrome have been reported more commonly with paroxetine than with other SSRIs.

Benefits: We found one systematic review (search date 1999),[27] which identified one RCT[28] (91 outpatients aged >18 years who had previously been admitted to hospital for deliberate self harm, without current depression, receiving concurrent psychotherapy) comparing paroxetine 40 mg daily versus placebo for 12 months. It found no significant difference between paroxetine and placebo in the proportion of people repeating deliberate self harm over 12 months (15/46 [33%] with paroxetine *v* 21/45 [47%] with placebo; RR 0.70, 95% CI 0.40 to 1.18).

Harms: The one identified systematic review found that, compared with placebo, paroxetine significantly increased the proportion of people with diarrhoea (10/46 [22%] with paroxetine *v* 1/45 [2%] with placebo; $P = 0.007$), tremor (8/46 [17%] with paroxetine *v* 1/46 [2%] with control; $P = 0.03$), and delayed orgasm (9/46 [19%] with paroxetine *v* 0/45 [0%] with placebo; $P = 0.003$).[27] It also found that paroxetine was associated with large bruises in two people. Paroxetine, like other selective serotonin re-uptake inhibitors (SSRIs), has been linked to suicidal ideation. In clinical trials in children and adolescents with depression it showed higher rates of suicide related events.[29] Abrupt withdrawal of SSRIs should be avoided. Withdrawal effects include headache, nausea, paraesthesia, dizziness, and anxiety.[30] Extrapyramidal reactions (including orofacial dystonias) and withdrawal syndrome have been reported more commonly with paroxetine than with other SSRIs.[30]

Comment: The one identified systematic review did not report any other outcomes.[27] Many of the RCTs are sponsored by the manufacturer and sponsorship has been suggested as a potential factor influencing the outcome of RCTs.[31] Evidence of publication bias has been found in the RCTs of SSRIs and the efficacy and safety of these drugs is currently under review by the regulatory authorities in several countries.

OPTION **MIANSERIN**

One systematic review provided insufficient evidence to assess mianserin.

Benefits: We found one systematic review (search date 1999),[27] which identified two RCTs.[32,33] The first RCT (38 people with borderline or histrionic personality disorder and a history of deliberate self harm, admitted to hospital after an episode of self harm mean age 37.5 years) identified by the review found no significant difference between mianserin 30 mg daily and placebo in the proportion of people who repeated deliberate self harm over 6 months of treatment (8/17 [47%] with mianserin *v* 12/21 [57%] with placebo; RR 0.82, 95% CI 0.44 to 1.54). However, the study is likely to have been too small to detect a clinically important difference.[32] The second RCT (114 people admitted to hospital after deliberate self poisoning, history of deliberate self harm not reported aged 16–65 years) identified by the review compared mianserin 30–60 mg daily or nomifensine 75–150 mg daily versus placebo for 6 weeks' treatment (see comment below).[33] The RCT did not compare mianserin alone versus placebo. It found no significant difference between mianserin or nomifensine and placebo in the proportion of people who repeated deliberate self harm over 12 weeks (16/76 [21%] with mianserin or nomifensine *v* 5/38 [13%] with placebo; RR 1.60, 95% CI 0.63 to 4.04). However, the RCT is likely to have been too small to detect a clinically important difference.

Harms: The one identified systematic review[27] gave no information on adverse effects of mianserin. Nomifensine was withdrawn worldwide in the 1980s because of association with immune haemolytic anaemia.[34]

Comment: The identified systematic review did not report any other outcomes.[27]

OPTION FLUPENTIXOL DEPOT INJECTION

One systematic review including one small RCT found that flupentixol depot injection reduced the proportion of people who repeated deliberate self harm over 6 months compared with placebo. However, we were unable to draw reliable conclusions from this small study. Typical antipsychotics such as flupentixol are associated with a wide range of adverse effects.

Benefits: We found one systematic review (search date 1999), which identified one RCT (37 people aged 18–68 years with a history of deliberate self harm enrolled, 30 people completed, see comment below) comparing flupentixol decanoate (20 mg im once every 4 weeks) versus placebo for 6 months.[27] It found that flupentixol significantly reduced the proportion of people who repeated deliberate self harm over 6 months compared with placebo (3/14 [21%] with flupentixol *v* 12/16 [75%] with placebo; RR 0.29, 95% CI 0.10 to 0.81).

Harms: The systematic review gave no information on adverse effects (see comment below).[27] The identified RCT found that 2/18 (11%) of people taking flupentixol reported parkinsonian adverse effects at 1 month.[35]

Comment: In the RCT identified by the systematic review, withdrawal rates were 4/18 (22%) with flupentixol compared with 3/19 (16%) with placebo.[35] Reasons were not reported for any withdrawals with placebo or for two withdrawals with flupentixol. We found insufficient evidence about the adverse effects of flupentixol in people who have deliberately self harmed. Typical antipsychotics such as flupentixol are associated with a wide range of adverse effects.[36] The review did not investigate other outcomes.[27]

OPTION PROBLEM SOLVING THERAPY

One systematic review of small RCTs found no significant difference between problem solving therapy and usual care in the proportion of people who repeated deliberate self harm over 6–12 months. A second systematic review found that problem solving therapy reduced symptoms of depression, anxiety, and hopelessness, and improved problems compared with usual care.

Benefits: We found one systematic review (search date 1999)[27] that assessed the effects of problem solving therapy**G** on repetition of deliberate self harm and one systematic review (search date not reported)[37] that assessed the effects of problem solving therapy on depression, anxiety, and hopelessness. **Effects on rate of repetition of deliberate self harm:** The first review identified five RCTs (571 people aged > 15 years) comparing problem solving therapy versus usual care (standard care [from psychiatrist, community psychiatric nurse, or social worker], marital counselling, or general practitioner counselling).[27] Four of the RCTs were in people who had been admitted to hospital for deliberate self poisoning and included people with both a history of deliberate self harm and experiencing their first episode; one RCT was in people admitted to hospital after deliberate self harm who had self harmed at least once before in the previous year. The duration of interventions for four RCTs was 2–8 sessions, and for one RCT 3 months; follow up ranged from 6–12 months. The review found no significant difference between problem solving therapy and usual care in the proportion of people who repeated deliberate self harm over 6–12 months (45/290 [15%] with problem solving therapy *v* 54/281 [19%] with usual care; RR 0.77, 95% CI 0.55 to 1.08).[27] **Effects on psychiatric symptoms:** The second review[37] (6 RCTs, including all 5 identified by the first review[27]) found that, compared with usual care, problem solving therapy significantly reduced depression (assessed by Beck Depression Inventory and Hospital Anxiety Depression Scale, 4 RCTs, 158 people, SMD –0.36, 95% CI –0.61 to –0.11) and hopelessness (assessed by Beck Hopelessness Scale, 0-20 scale with 20 signifying the most hopelessness, 3 RCTs, 63 people; WMD –2.97, 95% CI –4.81 to –1.13), and "improved problems" (2 RCTs, 211 people; OR 2.31, 95% CI 1.29 to 4.13; see comment below).[37]

Harms: The two identified systematic reviews gave no information on adverse effects.[27,37]

Comment: The second of the two identified systematic reviews did not state how improvement in a problem was assessed.[37] Neither systematic review assessed other outcomes.[27,37]

OPTION DIALECTICAL BEHAVIOURAL THERAPY

One systematic review including one RCT found limited and equivocal evidence that dialectical behavioural therapy may reduce the proportion of people who repeat deliberate self harm over 12 months compared with usual care.

Benefits: We found one systematic review (search date 1999),[27] which identified one RCT (39 women aged 18–45 years with borderline personality disorder and a history of deliberate self harm who had self harmed in the previous 8 weeks) comparing dialectical behavioural therapy(G) versus usual care (alternative therapy referrals). It found that dialectical behavioural therapy significantly reduced the proportion of women who repeated deliberate self harm over 1 year compared with usual care (5/19 [26%] with dialectical behavioural therapy *v* 12/20 [60%] with usual care; OR 0.24, 95% CI 0.06 to 0.93; see comment below).[27]

Harms: The one identified systematic review gave no information on adverse effects.[27]

Comment: The results of the RCT included in the one identified systematic review are sensitive to the method of statistical calculation used; calculation of relative risk renders the difference between dialectical behavioural therapy(G) and usual care non-significant (RR 0.44, 95% CI 0.19 to 1.01).[27] The review did not assess other outcomes.

OPTION MANUAL ASSISTED COGNITIVE BEHAVIOURAL THERAPY

One RCT found no significant difference in repeat self harm rates at 1 year between manual assisted cognitive therapy and usual treatment (problem solving approaches, dynamic psychotherapy, short term counselling, or referral to a general practitioner or a voluntary group).

Benefits: We found no systematic review but we found one RCT (480 people mean age 32 years with recurrent deliberate self harm), which compared manual assisted cognitive behavioural therapy**G** versus treatment as usual.[38] Manual assisted cognitive behavioural therapy consisted of a 70 page booklet on cognitive therapy incorporating dialectical behavioural therapy**G** techniques plus up to seven sessions of cognitive behavioural therapy from a therapist during the first 3 months of the study. However, 90/239 (38%) people allocated to manual assisted cognitive therapy did not attend any sessions, so their treatment consisted of the booklet only. Usual treatment consisted of either problem solving approaches, dynamic psychotherapy, short term counselling, or referral to a general practitioner or voluntary group. It found no significant difference between treatments in the proportion of people with repeated deliberate self harm at 1 year (84/213 [39%] with manual assisted cognitive therapy *v* 99/217 [46%] with usual treatment; OR 0.78, 95% CI 0.53 to 1.14). It found no difference between the treatments at 12 months for quality of life or social functioning (difference in EuroQol Index: 0; CI and P value not reported; difference in Global Assessment of Functioning [Social subscale]: –1.7; CI and P value not reported).

Harms: The RCT identified gave no information on adverse effects.[38]

Comment: Further analysis of the data of the included RCT showed that 9/10 (90%) patients in the whole sample had some personality disturbance (42% of these with personality disorder).[38] Those with borderline personality disorder were most likely to repeat deliberate self harm episode quickly (mean 89 days for 25th percentile time to deliberate self harm event) and those with dissocial personality disorder were the slowest to repeat (equivalent mean 384 days).

OPTION CONTINUITY OF CARE

One systematic review identified one RCT, which found limited evidence that follow up after hospital treatment with the same therapist may increase repetition of deliberate self harm compared with follow up with a different therapist over 3 months. However, the difference between groups may be explained by a higher level of risk factors for repetition in the group receiving follow up with the same therapist.

Benefits: We found one systematic review (search date 1999),[27] which identified one RCT (141 people, age range not reported with a history of deliberate self harm who had been admitted to hospital for 3 day crisis intervention**G** after an episode of self harm) comparing follow up by the same therapist, who assessed them in hospital, versus follow up with a different therapist. All participants also received a "motivational interview**G**, letter, and assessment of motivation towards therapy". It found that follow up by the same therapist significantly increased the proportion of people who repeated deliberate self harm over 3 months compared with follow up with a different therapist (12/68 [18%] with same therapist *v* 4/73 [5%] with different therapist; RR 3.22, 95% CI 1.09 to 9.51; see comment below).

Harms: The one identified systematic review gave no information on adverse effects.[27]

Comment: The authors of the one identified systematic review commented that the increase in deliberate self harm in people who had continuity of care may have been because of a higher prevalence of unspecified risk factors for repetition in the same therapist group despite randomisation.[27] The review and RCTs did not assess other outcomes.

OPTION PSYCHODYNAMIC INTERPERSONAL THERAPY

One RCT found that brief psychodynamic interpersonal therapy for 4 weeks reduced repetition of deliberate self harm, depression, and suicidal ideation over 6 months compared with usual care. However, we were unable to draw reliable conclusions from this single RCT.

Benefits: We found no systematic review. We found one RCT (119 people aged 18–65 years admitted to hospital after deliberate self poisoning, 60% with a previous history of "deliberate self harm") that compared psychodynamic interpersonal therapy**G** versus usual care (referral to usual services) for 4 weeks.[39] It found that, compared with usual care, brief psychodynamic interpersonal therapy significantly reduced repetition of deliberate self harm at 6 months (5/58 [9%] with psychodynamic interpersonal therapy *v* 17/61 [28%] with usual care; P = 0.009). It also found that brief psychodynamic interpersonal therapy significantly reduced depression (measured by Beck Depression Inventory, mean difference in score with interpersonal therapy *v* usual care –5.0, 95% CI –9.7 to –0.3) and suicidal ideation (measured by Beck Scale for Suicidal Ideation, mean difference in score –4.9, 95% CI –8.2 to –1.6). Further analysis of the data using multiple regression showed that interpersonal psychotherapy was more effective in improving suicidal ideation (as measure by Beck Scale for Suicidal Ideation) in people with lower depression scores at baseline and no prior history of self harm (coefficient for baseline depression 0.256; P = 0.013; and coefficient for previous history of self harm –5.701; P = 0.016).

Harms: The RCT included in the identified systematic review gave no information on adverse effects.[39]

Comment: The RCT included in the identified systematic review did not assess other outcomes.[39]

OPTION INTENSIVE OUTPATIENT FOLLOW UP PLUS OUTREACH

One systematic review found no significant difference in the proportion of people who repeated deliberate self harm over 4–12 months between intensive outpatient follow up plus outreach and usual care.

Benefits: We found one systematic review (search date 1999, 6 RCTs, 1161 people aged > 15 years admitted to hospital after deliberate self harm, 30–100% with a previous history of deliberate self harm) comparing intensive outpatient follow up plus outreach versus usual care over 3–12 months.[27] The elements of intensive outpatient follow up plus outreach varied, but usually involved in-person or phone contact of the person in the community, including encouragement to attend health services. Usual care involved treatment by various professionals, not involving outreach. The RCTs found no significant difference between intensive outpatient follow up plus outreach and usual care in the proportion of people who repeated deliberate self harm over 4–12 months (92/580 [16%] with intensive intervention *v* 107/581 [18%] with usual care; RR 0.87, 95% CI 0.68 to 1.12).

Harms: The identified systematic review gave no information on adverse effects.[27]

Comment: The identified systematic review did not assess other outcomes.[27]

OPTION EMERGENCY CARD

One systematic review found no significant difference in the proportion of people who repeated deliberate self harm over 12 months between emergency card (allowing emergency admission or contact with a doctor) and usual care.

Benefits: We found one systematic review (search date 1999, 2 RCTs, 1 RCT in 212 adults admitted to hospital after their first episode of deliberate self harm, 1 RCT in 105 children and adolescents admitted to hospital after deliberate self harm, previous history of self harm not reported).[27] It compared an emergency card intervention (which involved giving a card to participants, indicating that a doctor was available and how to contact them or allowing readmission to a paediatric hospital ward) versus usual care (referral to and treatment from usual inpatient, outpatient, or primary care services as appropriate). It found no significant difference in the proportion of people who repeated deliberate self harm over 12 months between emergency card and usual care (8/148 [5%] with emergency card *v* 19/169 [11%] with usual care; RR 0.48, 95% CI 0.22 to 1.07; see comment below).

Harms: The review gave no information on adverse effects.[27]

Comment: The review pooled results from RCTs of heterogeneous populations (adults and children) to try to increase the power of its meta-analysis, but it may not be appropriate to pool results in such different groups.[27] The review did not assess other outcomes.

OPTION HOSPITAL ADMISSION

One systematic review found no significant difference between hospital admission and immediate discharge in the proportion of people who repeated deliberate self harm over 16 weeks.

Benefits: We found one systematic review (search date 1999),[27] which identified one RCT (77 people aged > 16 years). The RCT found no significant difference between hospital admission for a median of 17 hours and immediate discharge in the proportion of people who repeated deliberate self harm over 16 weeks (3/38 [8%] with hospital admission *v* 4/39 [10%] with immediate discharge; RR 0.77, 95% CI 0.18 to 3.21). However, it is likely to have lacked power to detect a clinically important difference.

Harms: The one identified systematic review gave no information on adverse effects.[27]

Comment: The one identified systematic review did not assess other outcomes.[27]

OPTION GENERAL PRACTICE BASED GUIDELINES

One large cluster randomised trial comparing the use of general practitioner guidelines for management of deliberate self harm versus usual care found no significant difference in the proportion of people who repeated deliberate self harm over 12 months or in the time to repetition of self harm.

Benefits: We found no systematic review. We found one cluster randomised trial (98 general practices randomised, 1932 people aged > 16 years who had attended hospital emergency departments after deliberate self harm, 11–14% with a recent recorded history of deliberate self harm).[40] It compared inviting people for consultation with their general practitioner, who followed guidelines for managing self harm versus usual care (provided by general practitioner or referral to mental health or other services as appropriate). It found no significant difference between use of guidelines and usual care in repetition of deliberate self harm (211/964 [22%] with guidelines *v* 189/968 [20%] with usual care; OR 1.17, 95% CI 0.94 to 1.47), mean repeat episodes per person (0.48 with guidelines *v* 0.37 with usual care; incident rate ratio 1.24, 95% CI 0.92 to 1.68), and mean days to first episode of self harm (105 with guidelines *v* 110 with usual care; HR 1.15, 95% CI 0.94 to 1.42).

Harms: The RCT included in the one identified systematic review gave no information on adverse effects.[40]

Comment: The RCT did not assess other outcomes.[40] The RCT stated that it did account for confounding effects of cluster randomisation in the analysis.

OPTION NURSE LED CASE MANAGEMENT

One RCT found no significant difference between nurse led case management and usual care in the proportion of people who were admitted to emergency departments for episodes of deliberate self harm over 12 months.

Benefits: We found no systematic review. We found one RCT (467 people aged > 19 years who had attended hospital emergency departments after deliberate self harm, 47% with a previous history of deliberate self harm) comparing nurse led case management**G** versus usual care (triage, psychiatric assessment, and inpatient care if appropriate) for 12 months.[41] It found no significant difference between groups in rates of readmission to hospital as a result of deliberate self harm over 12 months (19/220 [9%] with nurse led case management *v* 25/247 [10%] with usual care; OR 0.84, 95% CI 0.45 to 1.57).

Harms: The identified RCT gave no information on adverse effects.[41]

Comment: The RCT did not assess other outcomes.[41]

OPTION TELEPHONE CONTACT

One RCT found no significant difference between telephone contact at 4 and 8 months and usual care in repetition of deliberate self harm, global functioning, and suicidal ideation over 12 months.

Benefits: We found no systematic review. We found one RCT (216 people; mean age 41, admitted to hospital after deliberate self harm, 51–54% with a previous history of deliberate self harm), which compared telephone contact at 4 and 8 months aimed at increasing motivation versus usual care (undefined).[42] It found no significant difference between telephone contact and usual care in the proportion of people repeating deliberate self harm over 12 months (14/83 [17%] with telephone contact *v* 15/89 [17%] with usual care; reported as non-significant, CI not reported; results not intention to treat, 19% lost to follow up). It found similar rates in overall functioning between telephone contact and usual care (assessed by Global Assessment of Functioning Scale, mean score: 61.4 with telephone contact *v* 58.6 with usual care; CI not reported). It also found similar scores on the Scale for Suicidal Ideation (mean score: 5.8 with telephone contact *v* 4.0 with usual care; CI not reported) and on the Symptom Checklist-90 scale at 12 months (mean score: 0.82 with telephone contact group *v* 0.88 with usual care; CI not reported).

Harms: The RCT gave no information on adverse effects.[42]

Comment: None.

GLOSSARY

Case management Involves a case manager managing an individual's care including comprehensive assessment of their needs, development of individualised package of care, the arrangement of access to services, monitoring of quality of services provided, and long term flexible support.

Crisis intervention Involves short term help with current and acute difficult life events using variety of counselling, problem solving, and practical measures.

Dialectical behavioural therapy A multimodal cognitive behavioural therapy used particularly in the treatment of people with borderline personality disorder who repeatedly engage in deliberate self harm. It involves helping to replace extremes of emotions and behaviour with behaviour that is a moderate synthesis of extremes.

Manual assisted cognitive behavioural therapy Cognitive behavioural therapy assisted by a manual consisting of brief cognitive behavioural therapy and techniques from dialectical behavioural therapy.

Motivational interviewing Uses principles of motivational psychology and is aimed at helping people to change and engage in demanding treatments.

Problem solving therapy Uses a set of sequential steps in solving problems and aims at minimising negative emotion and maximising identification, evaluation, and implementation of optimal solutions.

Psychodynamic interpersonal therapy A psychotherapeutic intervention aimed at improving interpersonal problems using the model developed by Hobson.

REFERENCES

1. Gelder M, Mayou R, Cowen P. *Shorter Oxford textbook of psychiatry*. Oxford: Oxford University Press, 2001.
2. American Psychiatric Association. *Diagnostic and statistical manual of mental disorders*, 4th ed. Washington, DC: American Psychiatric Association, 1994.
3. World Health Organization. *The ICD-10 classification of mental and behavioural disorders*. Geneva: World Health Organization, 1992.
4. Schmidtke A, Bille-Brahe U, DeLeo D, et al. Attempted suicide Europe: rates, trends and sociodemographic characteristics of suicide attempters during the period 1989–1992. Results of the WHO/EURO Multicentre Study on Parasuicide. *Acta Psychiatr Scand* 1996;93:327–338.
5. The University of York. NHS Centre for Reviews and Dissemination. 1998. Deliberate self harm and attempted suicide. *Effective Health Care* 4:1–12.
6. Weissman MM, Bland RC, Canino GJ, et al. Prevalence of suicide ideation and suicide attempts in nine countries. *Psychol Med* 1999;29:9–17.
7. Eddleston M. Patterns and problems of deliberate self-poisoning in the developing world. *QJM* 2000;93:715–731.
8. Eddleston M, Sheriff MH, Hawton K. Deliberate self harm and attempted suicide in Sri Lanka: an overlooked tragedy in the developing world. *BMJ* 1998;317:133–135.
9. Roy A, Nielsen D, Rylander G, et al. Genetics of suicidal behaviour. In: Hawton K, van Heeringen K, eds. *International handbook of suicide and attempted suicide*. Chichester: Wiley, 2000: 209–221.
10. Traskman-Bendz L, Mann JJ. Biological aspects of suicidal behaviour. In: Hawton K, van Heeringen K, eds. *International handbook of suicide and attempted suicide*. Chichester: Wiley, 2000: 65–78.
11. Williams JMG, Pollock LR. The psychology of suicidal behaviour. In: Hawton K, van Heeringen K, eds. *International handbook of suicide and attempted suicide*. Chichester: Wiley, 2000:79–93.
12. Kerkhof AJFM. Attempted suicide: trends and patterns. In: Hawton K, van Heeringen K, eds. *International handbook of suicide and attempted suicide*. Chichester: Wiley, 2000: 49–64.
13. Lonnqvist JK. Psychiatric aspects of suicidal behaviour: depression. In: Hawton K, van Heeringen K, eds. *International handbook of suicide and attempted suicide*. Chichester: Wiley, 2000:107–120.
14. Murphy GE. Psychiatric aspects of suicidal behaviour: substance abuse. In: Hawton K, van Heeringen K, eds. *International handbook of suicide and attempted suicide*. Chichester: Wiley, 2000:135–146.
15. Linehan MM, Rizvi SL, Welch SS, et al. Psychiatric aspects of suicidal behaviour: personality disorder. In: Hawton K, van Heeringen K, eds. *International handbook of suicide and attempted suicide*. Chichester: Wiley, 2000:147–178.
16. Allgulander C. Psychiatric aspects of suicidal behaviour: anxiety disorders. In: Hawton K, van Heeringen K, eds. *International handbook of suicide and attempted suicide*. Chichester: Wiley, 2000:179–192.
17. Stenager EN, Stenager E. Physical illness and suicidal behaviour. In: Hawton K, van Heeringen K, eds. *International handbook of suicide and attempted suicide*. Chichester: Wiley, 2000:405–420.
18. Owens D, Horrocks J, House A. Fatal and non-fatal repetition of self-harm. Systematic review. *Br J Psychiatry* 2002;181:193–199.
19. Hawton K. Treatment of suicide attempters and prevention of suicide and attempted suicide. In:

Gelder MG, Lopez-Ibor JJ Jr, Andreasen NC, eds. *New Oxford textbook of psychiatry*. Oxford: Oxford University Press, 2000:1050–1059.
20. Bridges K, Goldberg D. Self-administered scales of neurotic symptoms. In: Thompson C, ed. *The instruments of psychiatric research*. London: Wiley, 1989:157–176.
21. Derogatis LR. Symptom Checklist-90-Revised (SCL-90-R). In: American Psychiatric Association, eds. *Handbook of psychiatric measures*. Washington, DC: American Psychiatric Association, 2000:81–84.
22. Thompson C. Anxiety. In: Thompson C, ed. *The instruments of psychiatric research*. London: Wiley, 1989:127–156.
23. Beck A, Steer A. Beck Depression Inventory (BDI). In: American Psychiatric Association, eds. *Handbook of psychiatric measures*. Washington, DC: American Psychiatric Association, 2000:519–523.
24. Snaith RP, Zigmond AS. Hospital Anxiety and Depression Scale (HADS). In: American Psychiatric Association, eds. *Handbook of psychiatric measures*. Washington, DC: American Psychiatric Association, 2000:547–548.
25. Beck A, Kovacs M, Weissman A. Beck Scale for Suicidal Ideation (BSS). In: American Psychiatric Association, eds. *Handbook of psychiatric measures*. Washington, DC: American Psychiatric Association, 2000:264–266.
26. Beck A, Weissman A, Lester D, et al. Beck Hopelessness Scale (BHS). In: American Psychiatric Association, eds. *Handbook of psychiatric measures*. Washington, DC: American Psychiatric Association, 2000:268–270.
27. Hawton K, Townsend E, Arensman E, et al. Psychosocial and pharmacological treatments for deliberate self harm and attempted suicide. In: The Cochrane Library, Issue 2, 2003. Oxford, Update Software. Search date 1999; primary sources Medline, Psychlit, Embase, Cochrane Controlled Trials Register, hand searches of 10 relevant journals, reference lists of relevant papers, and personal contact with trialists and other experts in the field.
28. Verkes RJ, Van der Mast RC, Hengeveld MW, et al. Reduction by paroxetine of suicidal behavior in patients with repeated suicide attempts but not major depression. *Am J Psychiatry* 1998;155:543–547.
29. Waechter F. Paroxetine must not be given to patients under 18. *BMJ* 2003;326:1282
30. British Medical Association and Royal Pharmaceutical Society of Great Britain. *British national formulary*. 48th ed. London: British Medical Association and Royal Pharmaceutical Society of Great Britain, 2004.
31. Stewart LA, Parmar MK. Bias in the analysis and reporting of randomized controlled trials. *Int J Technol Assess Health Care* 1996;12:264–275.
32. Montgomery SA, Roy D, Montgomery DB. The prevention of recurrent suicidal acts. *Br J Clin Pharmacol* 1983;15:183S–188S.
33. Hirsch SR, Walsh C, Draper R. Parasuicide: a review of treatment interventions. *J Affect Disord* 1982;4:299–311.
34. Lasser KE, Alan PD, Woolhandler SJ, et al. Timing of new black box warnings and withdrawals for prescription medications. *JAMA* 2002;287:2215–2220.
35. Montgomery SA, Montgomery DB, Jayanthi-Rani S, et al. Maintenance therapy in repeat suicidal behaviour: a placebo controlled trial. *Proceedings of the 10th International Congress for Suicide Prevention and Crisis Intervention*. Ottawa, Canada 1979:227–229.
36. British Medical Association and Royal Pharmaceutical Society of Great Britain. *British national formulary*. London: British Medical Association and Royal Pharmaceutical Society of Great Britain, 2002.
37. Townsend E, Hawton K, Altman DG, et al. The efficacy of problem-solving treatments after deliberate self-harm: meta-analysis of randomized controlled trials with respect to depression, hopelessness and improvement in problems. *Psychol Med* 2001;31:979–988. Search date not reported; primary sources Embase, Psychlit, Medline, Cochrane Controlled Trials Register, Cochrane Depression, Anxiety and Neurosis Review Group Trials Register, and hand searches of worldwide literature on deliberate self harm and attempted suicide.
38. Tyrer P, Thompson S, Schmidt U, et al. Randomized controlled trial of brief cognitive behaviour therapy versus treatment as usual in recurrent deliberate self-harm: the POPMACT study. *Psychol Med* 2003;33:969–976.
39. Guthrie E, Kapur N, Mackway-Jones K, et al. Randomised controlled trial of brief psychological intervention after deliberate self poisoning. *BMJ* 2001;323:135–138.
40. Bennewith O, Stocks N, Gunnell D, et al. General practice based intervention to prevent repeat episodes of deliberate self harm and attempted suicide: cluster randomised controlled trial. *BMJ* 2002;324:1254–1257.
41. Clarke T, Baker P, Watts CJ, et al. Self-harm in adults: a randomised controlled trial of nurse-led case management versus routine care only. *J Mental Health* 2002;11:167–176.
42. Cedereke M, Monti K, Ojehagen A. Telephone contact with patients in the year after a suicide attempt: does it affect treatment attendance and outcome? A randomised controlled study. *Eur Psychiatry* 2002;17:82–91.

G Mustafa Soomro
Honorary Research Fellow
Section of Community Psychiatry
St George's Hospital Medical School
London
UK

Competing interests: None declared.

Dementia

Search date February 2004

James Warner, Rob Butler, and Pradeep Arya

QUESTIONS

INTERVENTIONS

Key Messages

- People in RCTs of treatments for dementia are often not representative of people with dementia. Few RCTs are conducted in primary care and few are conducted in people with types of dementia other than Alzheimer's disease.

Cognitive symptoms

- **Donepezil** One systematic review in people with mild to moderate Alzheimer's disease and one subsequent RCT in people with moderate to severe Alzheimer's disease found that donepezil improved cognitive function and global clinical state at up to 52 weeks compared with placebo in people with mild to severe Alzheimer's disease. The review found no significant difference in patient rated quality of life at 12 or 24 weeks between donepezil and placebo. One large RCT identified by the review found that donepezil delayed the median time to "clinically evident functional decline" by 5 months compared with placebo. One open label RCT in people with mild to moderate Alzheimer's disease found no significant difference in cognitive function at 12 weeks between donepezil and rivastigmine, although fewer people taking donepezil withdrew from the trial for any cause. One RCT in people with Alzheimer's disease found no significant difference between donepezil and galantamine in cognitive function or adverse effects at 1 year. One systematic review in people with vascular dementia found that donepezil improved cognitive function compared with placebo at 24 weeks.

- **Galantamine** RCTs found that galantamine improved cognitive function and global clinical state over 6 months compared with placebo in people with Alzheimer's disease or vascular dementia. One RCT in people with Alzheimer's disease found no significant difference between galantamine and donepezil in cognitive function or adverse effects at 1 year.
- **Ginkgo biloba** RCTs found limited evidence that ginkgo biloba improved cognitive function over 24–26 weeks compared with placebo in people with Alzheimer's disease or vascular dementia. Preparations of gingo biloba available without prescription differ in terms of purity and concentrations of active ingredients compared with the high purity extract (EGb 761) used in most RCTs.
- **Memantine** Two RCTs identified by a systematic review found that memantine improved cognitive function at 12–28 weeks compared with placebo in people with mild to moderate vascular dementia. Subsequent RCTs found that memantine improved global clinical outcome and reduced care dependence at 12–28 weeks in people with more severe Alzheimer's disease or vascular dementia.
- **Reality orientation** One systematic review of small RCTs found that reality orientation improved cognitive function compared with no treatment in people with various types of dementia.
- **Physostigmine** One RCT in people with Alzheimer's disease found limited evidence that slow release physostigmine improved cognitive function over 12 weeks compared with placebo, but adverse effects, including nausea, vomiting, diarrhoea, dizziness, and stomach pain, were common.
- **Rivastigmine** One systematic review and one additional RCT found that rivastigmine improved cognitive function compared with placebo in people with Alzheimer's disease or Lewy body dementia, but adverse effects such as nausea, vomiting, and anorexia were common. Subgroup analysis from one RCT in people with Alzheimer's disease found limited evidence that people with vascular risk factors may respond better to rivastigmine than those without. One open label RCT in people with mild to moderate Alzheimer's disease found no significant difference in cognitive function at 12 weeks between rivastigmine and donepezil, although more people taking rivastigmine withdrew from the trial for any cause.
- **Tacrine** Two systematic reviews found limited evidence that tacrine improved cognitive function and global state at 3–36 weeks compared with placebo in people with Alzheimer's disease, but adverse effects, including nausea, vomiting, diarrhoea, anorexia, and abdominal pain, were common.
- **Lecithin** Small, poor RCTs identified by a systematic review provided insufficient evidence to assess lecithin in people with Alzheimer's disease.
- **Music therapy** Poor studies identified by a systematic review provided insufficient evidence to assess music therapy in people with dementia.
- **Nicotine** One systematic review found no RCTs of sufficient quality on the effects of nicotine in people with dementia.
- **Non-steroidal anti-inflammatory drugs** One RCT in people with Alzheimer's disease found no significant difference in cognitive function after 25 weeks' treatment with diclofenac plus misoprostol compared with placebo. Another RCT in people with Alzheimer's disease found insufficient evidence to compare indometacin versus placebo in people with Alzheimer's disease. A third RCT found no significant difference between naproxen or rofecoxib and placebo in cognitive function at 1 year.
- **Reminiscence therapy** One systematic review found insufficient evidence to assess reminiscence therapy in people with dementia.
- **Selegiline** One systematic review found that, in people with mild to moderate Alzheimer's disease, selegiline for 2–4 months improved cognitive function compared with placebo. It found no significant difference in global clinical state or activities of daily living. RCTs assessing outcomes beyond 4 months found no significant difference between selegiline and placebo.

- **Vitamin E** One RCT in people with moderate to severe Alzheimer's disease found limited evidence of no significant difference in cognitive function after 2 years' treatment with vitamin E compared with placebo. However, it found limited evidence that vitamin E reduced mortality, institutionalisation, loss of ability to perform activities of daily living, and the proportion of people who developed severe dementia.
- **Oestrogen** One systematic review found insufficient evidence that oestrogen with or without progestogen improved cognitive symptoms in postmenopausal women with dementia. However, there is concern that oestrogen treatment may increase the risk of developing breast cancer and cardiovascular events.

Behavioural and psychological symptoms

- **Carbamazepine** One RCT found that carbamazepine reduced agitation and aggression over 6 weeks compared with placebo in people with various types of dementia and behavioural and psychological symptoms.
- **Reality orientation** One systematic review of small RCTs found that reality orientation improved behaviour compared with no treatment in people with various types of dementia.
- **Haloperidol** One systematic review in people with various types of dementia plus behavioural and psychological symptoms found no significant difference in agitation at 6–16 weeks between haloperidol and placebo. However, it found that haloperidol may reduce aggression. It found that haloperidol increased the frequency and severity of extrapyramidal symptoms compared with placebo. Another systematic review in people with various types of dementia plus behavioural and psychological symptoms found limited evidence that haloperidol and risperidone were similarly effective in reducing agitation over 12 weeks but that haloperidol caused more frequent and more severe extrapyramidal symptoms. Two RCTs in people with agitated behaviour associated with dementia found no significant difference in agitation between trazodone and haloperidol, but may have been too small to exclude a clinically important difference.
- **Olanzapine** One RCT identified by a systematic review in nursing home residents with Alzheimer's disease or Lewy body dementia plus behavioural and psychological symptoms found that low and medium doses of olanzapine reduced agitation, hallucinations, and delusions over 6 weeks compared with placebo. Olanzapine has been associated with cerebrovascular adverse effects.
- **Risperidone** One systematic review and one subsequent RCT in people with various types of dementia, primarily Alzheimer's disease, all with behavioural and psychological symptoms, found that risperidone improved symptoms over 12 weeks compared with placebo. Another systematic review in people with various types of dementia plus aggressive behaviours found limited evidence that risperidone and haloperidol were similarly effective in reducing agitation over 12 weeks but that risperidone caused fewer and less severe extrapyramidal symptoms. Risperidone has been associated with cerebrovascular adverse events.
- **Sodium valproate** One RCT found limited evidence that sodium valproate reduced agitation over 6 weeks compared with placebo in people with dementia plus behavioural and psychological problems. Another RCT found no significant difference in aggressive behaviour over 8 weeks between sodium valproate and placebo.
- **Trazodone** We found no RCTs comparing trazodone versus placebo. One small RCT in people with agitated behaviour associated with dementia found no significant difference in agitation over 9 weeks between trazodone and haloperidol. Another small RCT in people with Alzheimer's disease and agitated behaviour found no significant difference in outcomes over 16 weeks among trazodone, haloperidol, behaviour management techniques, and placebo. The RCTs may have been underpowered to detect a clinically important difference.
- **Donepezil; galantamine** RCTs provided inconclusive evidence about the effects of donepezil or galantamine compared with placebo on behavioural and psychiatric symptoms in people with mild to moderate Alzheimer's disease.

DEFINITION **Dementia** is characterised by chronic, global, non-reversible impairment in cerebral function. It usually results in loss of memory (initially of recent events), loss of executive function (such as the ability to make decisions or sequence complex tasks), and changes in personality. **Alzheimer's disease** is a type of dementia characterised by an insidious onset and slow deterioration, and involves speech, motor, personality, and executive function impairment. It should be diagnosed after other systemic, psychiatric, and neurological causes of dementia have been excluded clinically and by laboratory investigation. **Vascular dementia** is multi-infarct dementia involving a stepwise deterioration in executive function with or without language and motor dysfunction occurring as a result of cerebral arterial occlusion. It usually occurs in the presence of vascular risk factors (diabetes, hypertension, and smoking). Characteristically, it has a more sudden onset and stepwise progression than Alzheimer's disease. **Lewy body dementia** is a type of dementia involving insidious impairment of executive function with Parkinsonism, visual hallucinations, fluctuating cognitive abilities, and increased risk of falls or autonomic failure.[1,2] Careful clinical examination of people with mild to moderate dementia and the use of established diagnostic criteria accurately identifies 70–90% of cases confirmed at postmortem.[3,4]

INCIDENCE/ PREVALENCE About 6% of people aged over 65 years and 30% of people aged over 90 years have some form of dementia.[5] Dementia is rare before the age of 60 years. Alzheimer's disease and vascular dementia (including mixed dementia) are each estimated to account for 35–50% of dementia, and Lewy body dementia is estimated to account for up to 20% of dementia in the elderly, varying with geographical, cultural, and racial factors.[1,5–9]

AETIOLOGY/ RISK FACTORS **Alzheimer's disease:** The cause of Alzheimer's disease is unclear. A key pathological process is deposition of abnormal amyloid in the central nervous system.[10] Most people with the relatively rare condition of early onset Alzheimer's disease (before age 60 years) show an autosomal dominant inheritance owing to mutations in presenelin or amyloid precursor protein genes. Several genes (*APP*, *PS-1*, and *PS-2*) have been identified. Later onset dementia is sometimes clustered in families, but specific gene mutations have not been identified. Head injury, Down's syndrome, and lower premorbid intellect may be risk factors for Alzheimer's disease. **Vascular dementia:** Vascular dementia is related to cardiovascular risk factors, such as smoking, hypertension, and diabetes. **Lewy body dementia:** The cause of Lewy body dementia is unknown. Brain acetylcholine activity is reduced in many forms of dementia, and the level of reduction correlates with cognitive impairment. Many treatments for Alzheimer's disease enhance cholinergic activity.[1,6]

PROGNOSIS **Alzheimer's disease:** Alzheimer's disease usually has an insidious onset with progressive reduction in cerebral function. Diagnosis is difficult in the early stages. Median life expectancy after diagnosis is 5–6 years.[11] **Vascular dementia:** We found no reliable data on prognosis. **Lewy body dementia:** People with Lewy body dementia have an average life expectancy of about 6 years after diagnosis.[5] Behavioural problems, depression, and psychotic symptoms are common in all types of dementia.[12,13] Eventually, most people with dementia find it difficult to perform simple tasks without help.

AIMS OF INTERVENTION To improve cognitive function (memory, orientation, attention, and concentration); to reduce behavioural and psychological symptoms (wandering, aggression, anxiety, depression, and psychosis); to improve quality of life for both the individual and carer, with minimum adverse effects.

OUTCOMES Primary outcomes are quality of life, time to institutionalisation or death, functional scores, and scales of cognitive function, global assessment of function and behavioural and psychological symptoms. Quality of life of the person with dementia or their carer and time to institutionalisation or death are rarely reported because of the short duration of most trials.[14] Functional scores include the Disability Assessment for Dementia (DAD), a 40 item scale assessing 10 domains of function,[15] and the Instrumental Activities of Daily Living Scale, maximum score 14 (lower scores indicate worse function).[16] **Cognitive symptoms and global assessment of function:** Quality of life of the person with dementia and their carer (rarely used in clinical trials). Comprehensive scales of cognitive function (e.g. Alzheimer's Disease Assessment Scale cognitive subscale [ADAS-cog], 70 point scale, lower scores indicate better function;[17] Mini Mental State Examination [MMSE], 30 point scale, lower scores indicate worse function;[18] Clinical Dementia Rating Scale [CDR], 3 point scale assessing six cognitive and functional parameters, higher scores indicate worse function;[14] Alzheimer's Disease Functional Assessment and Change Scale [ADFACS], 7 point scale, higher scores indicate worse function;[14] and Severe Impairment Battery, 100 point scale used in people with severe Alzheimer's disease, lower scores indicate worse function[19]). It has been suggested that ADAS-cog may be more sensitive than MMSE in assessing dementia, but neither scale directly reflects outcomes important to people with dementia or their carers. A 7 point change in the ADAS-cog has been regarded as clinically important. Measures of global state (e.g. Clinical Global Impression of Change [CGI-C] with caregiver input scale and Clinician's Interview Based Impression of Change-Plus [CIBIC-Plus], 7 point scale). **Behavioural and psychological symptoms:** Measures of psychiatric symptoms (e.g. Neuropsychiatric Inventory, 120 point scale, higher scores indicate greater difficulties; 12 item caregiver rated scale, maximum score 144, higher scores indicate greater difficulties; Dementia Mood Assessment Scale and Brief Psychiatric Rating Scale, higher scores indicate greater difficulties; Behave-AD scale, scores 0–75, higher scores indicate greater difficulties).

METHODS *Clinical Evidence* search and appraisal February 2004. Dementia is often considered to have two domains of symptoms: cognitive impairment and non-cognitive symptoms (behavioural and psychological symptoms). We have separated the evidence into these two domains because they are often therapeutic targets at different stages of dementia and many RCTs focus on one or other domain of symptoms. In many RCTs, missing data were managed using "last observation carried forward", which does not account for the tendency of people with dementia to deteriorate with time. These RCTs may overestimate the benefit derived from interventions, especially when there are higher withdrawal rates in the intervention arm compared with controls. We found few RCTs in people with types of dementia other than Alzheimer's disease and most trials were placebo controlled rather than comparative. We have not mentioned cross-comparisons within the option text unless any comparative RCTs were identified for that option.

QUESTION What are the effects of treatments on cognitive symptoms of dementia?

OPTION DONEPEZIL

One systematic review in people with mild to moderate Alzheimer's disease and one subsequent RCT in people with moderate to severe Alzheimer's disease found that donepezil improved cognitive function and global clinical state at up to 52 weeks compared with placebo in people with mild to severe Alzheimer's disease. The review found no significant difference in patient rated quality of life at 12 or 24 weeks between donepezil and placebo. One large RCT identified by the review found that donepezil delayed the median time to "clinically evident functional decline" by 5 months compared with placebo. One open label RCT in people with mild to moderate Alzheimer's disease found no significant difference in cognitive function at 12 weeks between donepezil and rivastigmine, although fewer people taking donepezil withdrew from the trial for any cause. One RCT in people with Alzheimer's disease found no significant difference between donepezil and galantamine in cognitive function or adverse effects at 1 year. One systematic review in people with vascular dementia found that donepezil improved cognitive function compared with placebo at 24 weeks.

Benefits: **Versus placebo in people with Alzheimer's disease:** We found one systematic review (search date 2003, 16 RCTs of 12, 24, and 52 weeks' duration, 4365 people with mild to moderate Alzheimer's disease)[20] and one subsequent RCT.[21] Nine RCTs identified by the review reported results using the Alzheimer's Disease Assessment Scale cognitive subscale (ADAS-cog) or the Clinician's Interview Based Impression of Change-Plus (CIBIC-Plus). The review found that donepezil 10 mg daily significantly improved cognitive function and global clinical state at 24 weeks compared with placebo (see table 1, p 1237). It found no significant difference in patient rated quality of life at 12 or 24 weeks (24 weeks: WMD +2.79, 95% CI –2.56 to +8.14).[20] One RCT (24 weeks, 290 people with more severe Alzheimer's disease aged

48–92 years, Mini Mental State Examination [MMSE] score 5–17) identified by the review compared donepezil 5–10 mg daily versus placebo.[26] It found that donepezil significantly improved CIBIC-Plus scores at 24 weeks compared with placebo (mean difference 0.54, CI not reported, results presented graphically; NNT 5, 95% CI 4 to 10 for improved or no change on CIBIC-Plus).[26] Another RCT (431 people with mild to moderate Alzheimer's disease aged 49–94 years, MMSE score 12–20) identified by the review compared donepezil 10 mg daily versus placebo for 1 year.[27] It found that donepezil delayed the median time to "clinically evident functional decline" by 5 months compared with placebo (median: 357 days with donepezil *v* 208 days with placebo; CI not reported). It found that a significantly higher proportion of people had no "clinically evident functional decline" at 1 year with donepezil compared with placebo (no functional decline: 123/207 [59%] with donepezil *v* 92/208 [44%] with placebo; NNT 7, 95% CI 5 to 17). The subsequent RCT (290 people living in the community with moderate to severe Alzheimer's dementia and MMSE score 5–17) found that donepezil (≤ 10 mg daily) slowed functional decline compared with placebo after 24 weeks of treatment (mean difference in Disability Assessment for Dementia 8.24; P = 0.0001).[21] **Versus rivastigmine in people with Alzheimer's disease:** We found no systematic review. We found one open label RCT (111 people with mild to moderate Alzheimer's disease, MMSE score 10–26) comparing donepezil 5–10 mg daily versus rivastigmine (1.5–6.0 mg twice daily). It found no significant difference in cognitive function at 12 weeks between donepezil and rivastigmine (assessed by clinicians blind to intervention; mean difference in ADAS-cog –0.15, 95% CI –1.47 to +1.71).[28] **Versus galantamine in people with Alzheimer's disease:** We found one single blind RCT (182 people with Alzheimer's disease, MMSE score 9–18), which compared donepezil (≤ 10 mg/day) versus galantamine (≤ 24 mg/day) for 52 weeks.[29] It found no significant differences between donepezil and galantamine in ADAS-cog scores or MMSE scores at the end of treatment (decline in ADAS-cog from baseline: 3.43 with donepezil *v* 2.22 with galantamine; decline in MMSE from baseline: 1.58 with donepezil *v* 0.52 with galantamine; P reported as non-significant for both outcomes).[29] **Versus placebo in people with vascular dementia:** We found one systematic review (search date 2003; 2 RCTs; 1219 people with vascular dementia).[30] It found that donepezil 5 or 10 mg daily improved cognitive function compared with placebo at 24 weeks (intent to treat analysis with last measurement carried forward: WMD in ADAS-cog for donepezil 10 mg *v* placebo: –2.17, 95% CI –2.93 to –1.37; WMD in ADAS-cog for donepezil 5 mg *v* placebo: –1.66, 95% CI –2.40 to –0.92).

Harms: Adverse effects common to all cholinesterase inhibitors include anorexia, nausea, vomiting, and diarrhoea. **Versus placebo in people with Alzheimer's disease:** The RCTs identified by the review found that donepezil was associated with nausea, vomiting, and diarrhoea, which tended to be mild and transient.[20] The review found no difference between donepezil and placebo in the proportion of people who withdrew for any cause (see table 1, p 1237).[20] Long term follow up of people taking donepezil (≤ 10 mg; open label extension) found that 86% experienced at least one adverse effect, often occurring later in the study. Common adverse events included agitation (24%), pain (20%), insomnia (11%), and diarrhoea (9%).[23] The subsequent RCT did not report on adverse effects.[21] **Versus rivastigmine in people with Alzheimer's disease:** The RCT found that fewer people had at least one adverse event with donepezil than with rivastigmine, but the difference was not significant (24/56 [43%] with donepezil *v* 32/55 [58%] with rivastigmine; RR 0.74, 95% CI 0.51 to 1.07). It found that, compared with rivastigmine, donepezil significantly reduced the proportion of people who withdrew from the trial for any cause (6/56 [11%] with donepezil *v* 17/55 [31%] with rivastigmine; RR 0.35, 95% CI 0.15 to 0.81; NNH 5, 95% CI 3 to 20).[28] **Versus galantamine in people with Alzheimer's disease:** The RCT found that rates of all adverse events, severe adverse events, and adverse events leading to withdrawal of medication were similar with donepezil and galantamine (all adverse events: 93.4% with donepezil *v* 90.7% with galantamine; severe adverse events: 19.8% with donepezil *v* 18.6% with galantamine; adverse events causing withdrawal: 13.2% with donepezil *v* 13.4% with galantamine; P values and CI not reported).[29] **Versus placebo in people with vascular dementia:** The systematic review found that donepezil 10 mg daily significantly increased the risk of adverse effects and withdrawal from treatment compared with placebo (adverse events: 91% with donepezil 10 mg *v* 88% with placebo; OR 1.95, 95% CI 1.20 to 3.15; withdrawal from treatment: 26% with donepezil 10 mg *v* 16% with placebo; OR 1.92, 95% CI 1.35 to 2.70).[30]

Comment: In the RCT identified by the review in people with moderate to severe dementia, "clinically evident functional decline" was defined as a decline of at least 1 point on the Alzheimer's Disease Functional Assessment and Change Scale (ADFACS) or an increase of at least 1 point on the Clinical Dementia Rating Scale.[27] An unblinded extension of one of the RCTs identified by the review observed 133 people taking donepezil 3–10 mg daily for up to 240 weeks.[23] It found that improved cognitive function compared with baseline was present for 38 weeks in people taking donepezil, and throughout the period of observation cognitive function remained above the level estimated had people not been treated. Donepezil is taken once daily; this is a potential advantage over other cholinesterase inhibitors for people with dementia. Improvement usually starts within 2–4 months of starting donepezil. Open label studies should be interpreted with caution but do suggest that the effect of continued treatment is sustained in the long term.[28] We found no RCTs of donepezil in people with Lewy body dementia.

OPTION GALANTAMINE

RCTs found that galantamine improved cognitive function and global clinical state over 6 months compared with placebo in people with Alzheimer's disease or vascular dementia. One RCT in people with Alzheimer's disease found no significant difference between donepezil and galantamine in cognitive function or adverse effects at 1 year.

Benefits: **Versus placebo:** We found one systematic review (search date 2002, 7 RCTs)[22] in people with mild to moderate Alzheimer's disease and one additional RCT[31] in people with vascular dementia (see comment below). The review found that, compared with placebo, galantamine (12 or 16 mg twice daily) significantly improved cognitive function (measured by Alzheimer's Disease Assessment Scale cognitive subscale [ADAS-cog] score) and improved global status (measured by Clinician's Interview Based Impression of Change-Plus [CIBIC-Plus] score) over 6 months (see table 1, p 1237). The additional RCT (592 people with vascular dementia or Alzheimer's disease plus cerebrovascular disease) compared galantamine 24 mg daily (396 people) versus placebo (196 people) for 6 months.[31] It found that galantamine significantly improved cognitive function from baseline at 6 months compared with placebo (4 point improvement in ADAS-cog: 35% with galantamine *v* 22% with placebo; NNT 8, 95% CI 5 to 17; absolute numbers not reported). It also found that galantamine significantly improved global clinical state at 6 months compared with placebo (CIBIC-Plus score "improved" or "no change": 74% with galantamine *v* 59% with placebo; NNT for "no change" 7, 95% CI 5 to 15).[31] **Versus donepezil:** See benefits of donepezil, p 1216.

Harms: Adverse effects common to all cholinesterase inhibitors include anorexia, nausea, vomiting, and diarrhoea. **Versus placebo:** The review found that galantamine 12–16 mg daily significantly increased the proportion of people who withdrew for any cause over 6 months compared with placebo (see table 1, p 1237). It also found that adverse effects were more frequent with higher doses of galantamine, including nausea (42% with galantamine 16 mg twice daily *v* 25% with placebo: OR 2.2, 95% CI 1.7 to 2.9) and vomiting (21% with galantamine 16 mg twice daily *v* 7% with placebo; OR 3.2, 95% CI 2.1 to 4.5). It also found that higher doses of galantamine increased the proportion of people who discontinued treatment because of adverse effects over 6 months (27% with galantamine 16 mg twice daily *v* 15% with galantamine 12 mg twice daily *v* 8% with placebo; 16 mg twice daily *v* placebo: OR 3.3, 95% CI 2.5 to 4.3).[22] The additional RCT comparing galantamine versus placebo in people with vascular dementia found that more people taking galantamine withdrew because of adverse effects (20% with galantamine *v* 8% with placebo; CI not reported).[31] **Versus donepezil:** See harms of donepezil, p 1217.

Comment: We found no RCTs of galantamine in people with Lewy body dementia.

OPTION RIVASTIGMINE

One systematic review and one additional RCT found that rivastigmine improved cognitive function in people with Alzheimer's disease or Lewy body dementia compared with placebo, but adverse effects such as nausea, vomiting, and anorexia were common. Subgroup analysis from one RCT in people with Alzheimer's disease found limited evidence that people with vascular risk factors may respond better to rivastigmine than those without. One open label RCT in people with mild to moderate Alzheimer's disease found no significant difference in cognitive function at 12 weeks between rivastigmine and donepezil, although more people taking rivastigmine withdrew from the trial for any cause.

Benefits: **Versus placebo:** We found one systematic review (search date 2000, 4 RCTs, 12 or 26 weeks' duration, 3370 people with mild to moderate Alzheimer's disease)[24] and one additional RCT[32] in people with Lewy body dementia (see comment below). The review found that rivastigmine (6–12 mg twice daily) produced small but significant improvements in cognitive function global clinical state over 26 weeks compared with placebo (see table 1, p 1237). A subgroup analysis of an RCT[33] identified by the review[24] (699 people with Alzheimer's disease) comparing rivastigmine 1–4 mg daily or 6–12 mg daily versus placebo over 26 weeks found that people with vascular risk factors responded better than those without (mean Alzheimer's Disease Assessment Scale cognitive subscale difference –2.3). The additional RCT (120 people with Lewy body dementia) found that rivastigmine (dose titrated to 6 mg twice daily) significantly improved a computerised psychometric measure of cognitive function at 20 weeks compared with placebo (intention to treat analysis; $P = 0.05$; no further data reported) and improved a global measure of behavioural function (NNT for at least 30% improvement on Neuropsychiatric Inventory score 3, 95% CI 2 to 6).[32] **Versus donepezil:** See benefits of donepezil, p 1216.

Harms: Adverse effects common to all cholinesterase inhibitors include anorexia, nausea, vomiting, and diarrhoea. **Versus placebo:** The systematic review in people with Alzheimer's disease found that rivastigmine increased the proportion of people who discontinued treatment for any cause compared with placebo (see table 1, p 1237).[24] The RCT in people with Lewy body dementia found that rivastigmine increased the proportion of people who had nausea compared with placebo (37% with rivastigmine *v* 22% with placebo), vomiting (25% with rivastigmine *v* 15% with placebo), anorexia (19% with rivastigmine *v* 10% with placebo), and somnolence (9% with rivastigmine *v* 5% with placebo; no further data reported).[32] **Versus donepezil:** See harms of donepezil, p 1217.

Comment: We found no RCTs of rivastigmine in people with vascular dementia.

OPTION PHYSOSTIGMINE

One RCT in people with Alzheimer's disease found limited evidence that slow release physostigmine improved cognitive function over 12 weeks compared with placebo but adverse effects, including nausea, vomiting, diarrhoea, dizziness, and stomach pain, were common.

Benefits: **Versus placebo:** We found one systematic review (search date 2000, 15 RCTs) comparing physostigmine versus placebo in people with mild to severe Alzheimer's disease (see comment below).[34] The RCTs differed widely in the preparations of physostigmine used, and most had weak reporting methods so the review could not perform a meta-analysis. Four were small trials of intravenous physostigmine, which did not report quantitative results. Seven were small trials (131 people, 6 crossover design) of standard oral preparation. The crossover trials did not provide results before crossover. One RCT (16 people) found no significant difference in cognition between oral physostigmine and placebo but it is likely to have been too small to exclude a clinically important difference. Four RCTs (1456 people) used controlled release preparations, but three of these reported results only for people who responded to physostigmine in a prestudy titration phase (see comment below). One RCT (170 people) found that slow release physostigmine 27 mg daily significantly improved cognition after 12 weeks compared with placebo (Alzheimer's Disease Assessment Scale cognitive subscale: WMD –2.0, 95% CI –3.6 to –0.5). It did not significantly improve activities of daily living or Clinician Based Impression of Change.

Harms: **Versus placebo:** Common adverse effects of physostigmine include nausea, vomiting, diarrhoea, dizziness, and stomach pain. In RCTs that randomised all people with Alzheimer's disease rather than selecting those who tolerated and responded to physostigmine, withdrawals were more common with physostigmine (234/358 [65%] with physostigmine *v* 31/117 [26%] with placebo; OR 4.80, 95% CI 3.17 to 7.33).[34]

Comment: We found no RCTs of physostigmine in people with Lewy body or vascular dementia. Physostigmine is a sympathomimetic drug and has a short half life. Screening out non-responders to a drug before the trial is likely to overestimate its effectiveness.

OPTION TACRINE

Two systematic reviews found limited evidence that tacrine improved cognitive function and global state at 3–36 weeks compared with placebo in people with Alzheimer's disease, but adverse effects, including nausea, vomiting, diarrhoea, anorexia, and abdominal pain, were common.

Benefits: **Versus placebo:** We found two systematic reviews comparing tacrine versus placebo in people with Alzheimer's disease (search date not reported, 12 RCTs, 1984 people;[35] search date 1997, 21 RCTs, including all 12 RCTs identified by the first review, 3555 people[36]). Various doses of tacrine were used in the RCTs, and the duration of treatment varied from 3–36 weeks. The first review found that, compared with placebo, tacrine significantly increased the proportion of people with overall clinical improvement (OR 1.58, 95% CI 1.18 to 2.11) and improved cognition (Mini Mental State Examination [MMSE] at 12 weeks: SMD 0.77, 95% CI 0.35 to 1.20; Alzheimer's Disease Assessment Scale cognitive subscale [ADAS-cog] at 12 weeks: SMD –2.70, 95% CI –2.78 to –1.36).[35] A subsequent subgroup analysis indicated that the five non-industry sponsored studies found no significant difference between tacrine and placebo, but most (6/7 [86%]) manufacturer supported studies found clinical benefit (1 RCT could not be located for inclusion in the subgroup analysis).[37] The second review assessed the methods and quality of tacrine RCTs and did not perform a meta-analysis.[36] It suggested that tacrine improved cognitive function in about 20% of people (improvement of 3–4 points in MMSE or ADAS-cog scores).

Harms: **Versus placebo:** The first review found that tacrine significantly increased the proportion of people who withdrew because of adverse effects, primarily elevated liver enzymes, compared with placebo (OR for withdrawal 3.6, 95% CI 2.8 to 4.7).[35] One RCT identified by the reviews found that tacrine 40–180 mg daily significantly increased withdrawals because of adverse events compared with placebo (265/479 [55%] with tacrine *v* 20/184 [11%] with placebo; RR 5.1, 95% CI 3.3 to 7.7; NNH 3, 95% CI 2 to 3), and that reversible elevation of liver enzymes occurred in 133/265 (50%) of people taking tacrine.[38] Common adverse events included nausea and vomiting (35% with 160 mg/day), diarrhoea (18%), anorexia (12%), and abdominal pain (9%).

Comment: The reviews suggested that the quality of tacrine RCTs was generally poor.[35,36] We found no RCTs of tacrine in people with Lewy body or vascular dementia.

OPTION LECITHIN

Small, poor RCTs identified by a systematic review provided insufficient evidence to assess lecithin in people with Alzheimer's disease.

Benefits: **Versus placebo:** We found one systematic review (search date 2002, 12 RCTs, 265 people with Alzheimer's disease, 21 with Parkinsonian dementia, 90 with subjective memory problems) comparing lecithin versus placebo (see comment below).[39] It found no significant difference between lecithin and placebo in cognition (1 RCT, 37 people; OR 0.91, 95% CI 0.25 to 3.34), functional performance (1 RCT, 30 people; WMD +0.76, 95% CI –0.91 to +2.43), or global impression (2 RCTs; 17/24 [71%] with lecithin *v* 12/28 [43%] with placebo; OR 3.01, 95% CI 0.92 to 9.81; see comment below).[39]

Harms: **Versus placebo:** The review found that adverse effects were more common with lecithin (14/34 [41%] with lecithin *v* 3/29 [10%] with placebo; OR 6.1, 95% CI 1.5 to 24.0).[39] The specific nature of the adverse effects was not stated.

Comment: One RCT (included in the systematic review) comparing lecithin versus placebo in people with minimal cognitive impairment found that some components of cognition were significantly better in the placebo group.[39] Most studies of lecithin were small and weak. Meta-analysis in the systematic review was hampered by diverse outcome criteria and it is likely that the meta-analyses were underpowered to detect a clinically important difference in outcomes. We found no RCTs of lecithin in people with Lewy body or vascular dementia.

OPTION NICOTINE

One systematic review found no RCTs of sufficient quality on the effects of nicotine in people with dementia.

Benefits: One systematic review (search date 2001) found no RCTs of sufficient quality.[40]

Harms: We found no RCTs.

Comment: None.

OPTION NON-STEROIDAL ANTI-INFLAMMATORY DRUGS

One RCT in people with Alzheimer's disease found no significant difference in cognitive function after 25 weeks' treatment with diclofenac plus misoprostol compared with placebo. Another RCT in people with Alzheimer's disease found insufficient evidence to compare indometacin versus placebo in people with Alzheimer's disease. A third RCT found no significant difference between naproxen or rofecoxib and placebo in cognitive function at 1 year.

Benefits: **Versus placebo:** We found three RCTs in people with Alzheimer's disease (see comment below).[41–43] The first RCT (41 people with Alzheimer's disease) found no significant difference in cognitive function after 25 weeks' treatment with diclofenac plus misoprostol compared with placebo (Alzheimer's Disease Assessment Scale cognitive subscale [ADAS-cog] score: mean difference +1.14, 95% CI –2.90 to +5.20) or global status (Clinician's Interview Based Impression of Change score: +0.24, 95% CI –0.26 to +0.74).[41] The second RCT (44 people with mild to moderate Alzheimer's disease) found that indometacin (indomethacin) (≤ 150 mg/day) for 6 months significantly improved cognitive function compared with placebo (assessed by averaging percentage changes in scores on Mini Mental State Examination scale, ADAS-cog, Boston Naming Test, and Token Test; mean increase 1.3% with indometacin *v* mean reduction 8.4% with placebo; results not intention to treat, 16/44 [36%] withdrew from the trial).[42] The third RCT (351 people with Alzheimer's disease) compared three treatments: rofecoxib 25 mg daily, naproxen 220 mg daily, and placebo.[43] It found no significant difference between treatments in change in ADAS-cog score at 1 year (mean change in ADAS-cog: –5.8 with naproxen *v* –7.6 with rofecoxib *v* –5.7 with placebo; P = 0.96 for naproxen *v* placebo; P = 0.09 for rofecoxib *v* placebo).[43]

Harms: See non-steroidal anti-inflammatory drugs, p 1. In one RCT, more people withdrew by week 25 with diclofenac plus misoprostol than with placebo (12/24 [50%] with diclofenac plus misoprostol *v* 2/17 [12%] with placebo).[41] No serious drug related adverse events were reported.[41] In the RCT of indometacin, 21% of people on indometacin withdrew because of gastrointestinal symptoms.[42] In the third RCT, fatigue, dizziness, and hypertension were more frequent with non-steroidal anti-inflammatory drugs (NSAIDs) than placebo (fatigue: 14% with naproxen *v* 15% with rofecoxib *v* 6% with placebo; P = 0.06 for naproxen *v* placebo; P = 0.05 for rofecoxib *v* placebo; dizziness: 12% with naproxen *v* 11% with rofecoxib *v* 5% with placebo; P = 0.06 for naproxen *v* placebo; P = 0.6 for rofecoxib *v* placebo; hypertension: 5% with naproxen *v* 7% with rofecoxib *v* 0% with placebo; P = 0.03 for naproxen *v* placebo; P = 0.004 for rofecoxib *v* placebo).[43] The RCT also found that serious adverse events (death, gastrointestinal bleeding or perforation, cerebrovascular events, subdural haematoma, or myocardial infarction) were more common with NSAIDs than placebo, although differences were reported to be not significantly different (number of serious adverse events: 25 with naproxen *v* 26 with rofecoxib *v* 15 with placebo; no further data reported; P value not reported).

Comment: We found one systematic review of aspirin for vascular dementia (search date 2000), which identified no RCTs.[44] Earlier versions of a systematic review of aspirin in vascular dementia included one RCT (70 people), which was subsequently removed because of inadequate quality, including a lack of placebo control.[44] We found no RCTs of NSAIDs in people with Lewy body dementia.

OPTION OESTROGEN (WITH OR WITHOUT PROGESTOGEN)

One systematic review found insufficient evidence that oestrogen with or without progestogen improved cognitive symptoms in postmenopausal women with dementia. However, there is concern that oestrogen treatment may increase the risk of developing breast cancer and cardiovascular events.

Benefits: **Versus placebo:** We found one systematic review (search date 2002; 5 RCTs, 210 postmenopausal women, all with Alzheimer's disease).[45] It performed many meta-analyses, examining different outcomes (including measures of cognitive function, memory, language, information processing, concentration, clinical impressions of change, and depression), for different types of oestrogen, at different doses, delivered by different routes and for different durations. Overall, it found no evidence of clinical benefit. After correction for multiple analyses, it found no significant difference in Mini Mental State Examination or Alzheimer's Disease Assessment Scale cognitive subscale scores between conjugated equine oestrogen 0.625 or 1.25 mg daily and placebo after 2 months (Mini Mental State Examination: uncorrected WMD 1.00, 95% CI 0.06 to 1.94; corrected P = 0.16; Alzheimer's Disease Assessment Scale cognitive subscale: WMD 0.38, 95% CI –1.20 to +1.96).

Harms: There is concern that oestrogen treatment may increase the risk of developing breast cancer and cardiovascular events (see harms of hormone replacement therapy under secondary prevention of ischaemic cardiac events, [Web only]).

Comment: Most RCTs in the review were small and heterogeneity may have distorted the results of the meta-analysis.[45] Most of the included RCTs examined effects of conjugated equine oestrogen, and results of the review may not extrapolate to other oestrogen preparations. More evidence is awaited from large, ongoing RCTs. The review found no RCTs of oestrogen in people with Lewy body or vascular dementia. A meta-analysis of 14 observational studies (5990 people, length of follow up not reported) found that hormone replacement therapy is associated with a lower risk of developing dementia (dementia in 13% with hormone replacement therapy *v* 21% with controls; RR 0.56, 95% CI 0.46 to 0.68).[46] Observational studies provide only indirect evidence; the observed association may be explained by confounders (e.g. educational level, lifestyle factors).

OPTION SELEGILINE

One systematic review found that, in people with mild to moderate Alzheimer's disease, selegiline for 2–4 months improved cognitive function compared with placebo. It found no significant difference in global clinical state or activities of daily living. RCTs assessing outcomes beyond 4 months found no significant difference between selegiline and placebo.

Benefits: **Versus placebo:** We found one systematic review (search date 2002, 17 RCTs) comparing selegiline versus placebo in people with mild to moderate Alzheimer's disease.[47] It found that, compared with placebo, selegiline 10 mg daily for 2–4 months significantly improved cognitive function (measured by various parameters: 11 RCTs, 866 people: WMD

2.40, 95% CI 0.06 to 4.74). It found no significant difference in global clinical state (5 RCTs, 275 people: WMD –0.03, 95% CI –0.13 to +0.07) or in activities of daily living (7 RCTs, 810 people: WMD –0.17, 95% CI –0.35 to 0). RCTs assessing outcomes beyond 4 months found no significant difference between selegiline and placebo.

Harms: **Versus placebo:** The RCTs identified by the review found a similar proportion of adverse effects (anxiety, agitation, dizziness, nausea, and dyspepsia) between selegiline and placebo.[47]

Comment: Many of the RCTs identified by the review were small and brief.[47] They used a variety of outcomes, making meta-analysis and comparison with other treatments difficult. Although selegiline may cause short term improvement, the improvement in cognition seems marginal and may not be of clinical importance. There is no evidence of long term benefit. We found no RCTs of selegiline in people with Lewy body or vascular dementia.

OPTION MEMANTINE

Two RCTs identified by a systematic review found that memantine improved cognitive function compared with placebo at 12–28 weeks in people with mild to moderate vascular dementia. Subsequent RCTs found that memantine improved global clinical outcome and reduced care dependence at 12–28 weeks in people with more severe Alzheimer's disease or vascular dementia.

Benefits: **Versus placebo:** We found one systematic review[48] and two subsequent RCTs[49,50] comparing memantine versus placebo. The review (search date 2002, 7 RCTs, 1532 people) did not meta-analyze many results because of differences in people included and in dose of memantine taken in the RCTs.[48] Two RCTs (154 people) included in the review were of poor quality and data are not reported here (see comment below).[52,53] The review identified two RCTs (900 people with mild to moderate vascular dementia, Mini Mental State Examination [MMSE] score 10–22). They found that, compared with placebo, memantine significantly improved cognitive function at 28 weeks (measured by Alzheimer's Disease Assessment Scale cognitive subscale [ADAS-cog]: WMD –2.19, 95% CI –3.16 to –1.21; results not intention to treat). They found no significant difference in global clinical state (measured by Gottsfries-Brane-Steen scale: 2 RCTs, 595 people; WMD –1.81, 95% CI –4.21 to +0.58). Subgroup analysis in one of the RCTs identified by the review suggested that the largest treatment effect occurred in people with baseline MMSE scores of less than 15 (mean difference 3.17 points; $P = 0.04$) and in people without cerebrovascular macrolesions (mean difference 2.29 points; $P = 0.002$).[51] The first subsequent RCT (166 people with Alzheimer's disease [49%] or vascular dementia [51%], MMSE < 10, Global Deterioration Scale stages 5–7) found that memantine 10 mg daily significantly increased the proportion of people with improved global clinical outcome at 12 weeks compared with placebo (measured by Clinical Global Impression of Change; 60/82 [73%] with memantine *v* 38/84 [45%] with placebo; RR 1.62, 95% CI 1.24 to 2.12; NNT 4, 95% CI 3 to 7). It also found that memantine significantly reduced care dependence compared with placebo (measured by a Behavioural Rating Scale for Geriatric Patients [BGP] care dependence subscore: mean difference 2.0 points; $P = 0.016$).[49] The second subsequent RCT (252 people with moderate to severe Alzheimer's disease) found that memantine 20 mg daily for 28 weeks significantly improved cognitive function compared with placebo (measured by the Severe Impairment Battery [SIB]; WMD 6.10, 95% CI 2.99 to 9.21), and activities of daily living (measured by the

Activities of Daily Living Scale: WMD 2.1, 95% CI 0.5 to 3.7; results not intention to treat; 71 [28%] people withdrew from the trial).[50] A resource utilisation analysis based on this RCT found that people taking memantine required significantly less caregiver time compared with people taking placebo (mean difference –52 hours/month, 95% CI –95 hours/month to –7 hours/month).[25]

Harms: The review found no significant difference between memantine and placebo in the proportion of people who had at least one adverse effect (2 RCTs; 351/460 [76%] with memantine *v* 327/440 [74%] with placebo; OR 1.11, 95% CI 0.82 to 1.51).[48] The subsequent RCTs also found that a similar proportion of people taking memantine and placebo had adverse effects.[25,50]

Comment: The methods of two memantine RCTs identified by the review were poor (follow up of 6 weeks, lack of blinding, unclear randomisation procedures, lack of intention to treat analysis, lack of ethics approval) and we have not reported the data here.[52,53] Memantine is a partial N-methyl-D-aspartate antagonist and has a different mechanism of action to cholinesterase inhibitors. Current evidence suggests it is well tolerated and may improve outcomes, especially in people with more severe dementia. However, it is difficult to compare memantine with cholinesterase inhibitors as most memantine RCTs are in people with more severe dementia and report different outcomes. Evidence for its use in mild to moderate dementia is inconclusive and more high quality trials are needed. We found no RCTs of memantine in people with Lewy body dementia.

OPTION GINKGO BILOBA

RCTs found limited evidence that ginkgo biloba improved cognitive function over 24–26 weeks compared with placebo in people with Alzheimer's disease or vascular dementia. Preparations of gingo biloba available without prescription differ in terms of purity and concentrations of active ingredients compared with the high purity extract (EGb 761) used in most RCTs.

Benefits: **Versus placebo:** We found one systematic review (search date 2002) comparing ginkgo biloba versus placebo in people with cognitive impairment, Alzheimer's disease, or vascular dementia (see comment below).[54] Trial duration ranged from 3–53 weeks, doses and preparations of ginkgo biloba varied widely, and diverse outcomes were assessed, making meta-analysis difficult.[54] The review included two large RCTs in people with Alzheimer's disease or vascular dementia. The first large RCT (216 people with mild to moderate Alzheimer's disease or vascular dementia) found that ginkgo biloba (≥ 200 mg/day) significantly increased the proportion of people who were rated as improved at 24 weeks (completer analysis: improvement in Clinician's Interview Based Impression of Change [criteria for improvement not defined] 57/79 [72%] with ginkgo biloba *v* 42/77 [55%] with placebo; RR 1.32, 95% CI 1.03 to 1.69).[54] The second large RCT (327 people, 236 people with Alzheimer's disease) had a high withdrawal rate (137/309 [44%] people withdrew).[55] However, it provided an intention to treat analysis. It found that, in people with Alzheimer's disease, ginkgo biloba significantly improved cognition (intention to treat analysis for people with Alzheimer's disease, change in Alzheimer's Disease Assessment Scale cognitive subscale [ADAS-cog] score: –1.7, 95% CI –3.1 to –0.20; NNT for 4 point change in ADAS-cog: 8, 95% CI 5 to 50) and caregiver assessed improvement over 26 weeks compared with placebo (change in Geriatric Evaluation by Relative's Rating Instrument score: –0.16, 95% CI –0.25 to –0.06). It found no significant difference in mean Clinician's Global Impression of Change score (change in score: +0.1, 95% CI –0.1 to +0.2).[55]

Harms: The review found no significant difference between ginkgo biloba and placebo in the proportion of people who had at least one adverse effect (adverse effects not specified; 5 RCTs, 1070 people; 117/591 [19.7%] with ginkgo biloba *v* 59/471 [12.5%] with placebo; RR 0.95, 95% CI 0.72 to 1.26).[54]

Comment: Many of the RCTs in the review included people with memory and cognitive impairment other than dementia so the results of the meta-analysis may not be fully generalisable to people with Alzheimer's disease or vascular dementia. We found no RCTs of ginkgo biloba in people with Lewy body dementia. Preparations of ginkgo biloba available without prescription differ in terms of purity and concentration of active ingredients compared with the high purity extract (EGb 761) used in most RCTs.

OPTION VITAMIN E

One RCT in people with moderate to severe Alzheimer's disease found limited evidence of no significant difference in cognitive function between vitamin E and placebo after 2 years' treatment. However, it found limited evidence that vitamin E reduced mortality, institutionalisation, loss of ability to perform activities of daily living, and the proportion of people who developed severe dementia.

Benefits: **Versus placebo:** We found one systematic review (search date 2000, 1 multicentre RCT, 169 people with moderate to severe Alzheimer's disease; see comment below).[56] The RCT compared four treatments: vitamin E (α-tocopherol; 2000 IU/day); selegiline; vitamin E plus selegiline; or placebo.[57] It found no significant difference in cognitive function with high dose vitamin E alone for 2 years compared with placebo (measured by the cognitive portion of the Alzheimer's Disease Assessment Scale, lower scores indicate worse function: mean reduction in score 8.3 with vitamin E *v* 6.7 with placebo; reported as non-significant; no further details reported; see comment below). It found that vitamin E significantly increased event free survival compared with placebo (defined as death, survival until institutionalisation, loss of ability to perform activities of daily living, or severe dementia [clinical dementia rating of 3]; OR 0.49, 95% CI 0.25 to 0.96).[57]

Harms: **Versus placebo:** The RCT found no significant difference in adverse effects between placebo and vitamin E.[57] Other studies found weak evidence of associations between high dose vitamin E and bowel irritation, headache, muscular weakness, visual complaints, vaginal bleeding, bruising, thrombophlebitis, deterioration of angina pectoris, worsening of diabetes, syncope, and dizziness.[58]

Comment: The groups in the RCT identified by the review were not matched evenly at baseline: the placebo group had a higher mean Mini Mental State Examination score, and these baseline scores were a significant predictor of outcome.[57] Attempts to correct for this imbalance suggested that vitamin E might increase mean survival, but the need for statistical adjustments weakens the strength of this conclusion. We found no RCTs of vitamin E in people with Lewy body or vascular dementia.

OPTION MUSIC THERAPY

Poor studies identified by a systematic review provided insufficient evidence to assess music therapy in people with dementia.

Benefits: **Versus control:** We found one systematic review of music therapy (G) (search date 1998, 21 studies, 336 people with various types of dementia).[59] It included studies with weak methods and found that music therapy significantly improved cognitive and behavioural outcomes compared with control interventions (mean effect size 0.79, 95% CI 0.62 to 0.95; see comment below). Significant effects were noted with different types of music therapy (active *v* passive, taped *v* live).

Harms: **Versus control:** The systematic review gave no information on harms.[59]

Comment: The primary studies lacked adequate controls, had potential for bias, used diverse interventions, and used inadequate outcome measures. Although one meta-analysis found significant benefits for music therapy on pooling the results of many studies, further high quality studies are needed to clarify whether the results are explained by a true effect or by bias. A previous Cochrane systematic review of music therapy has been withdrawn.[60]

OPTION REALITY ORIENTATION

One systematic review of small RCTs found that reality orientation improved cognitive function compared with no treatment in people with various types of dementia.

Benefits: **Versus no treatment:** We found one systematic review (search date 2000, 6 RCTs, 125 people with various types of dementia).[61] The RCTs compared reality orientation**G** versus no treatment and used different measures of cognition. The review found that reality orientation significantly improved cognitive function compared with no treatment (SMD –0.59, 95% CI –0.95 to –0.22). No separate analysis was done for specific types of dementia.

Harms: **Versus no treatment:** The RCTs gave no information on adverse effects.[61]

Comment: The RCTs did not use standardised interventions or outcomes.[61]

OPTION REMINISCENCE THERAPY

RCTs found insufficient evidence to assess reminiscence therapy in people with dementia.

Benefits: We found one systematic review of reminiscence therapy**G** (search date 2000, 2 RCTs, 42 people).[62] Analysis of pooled data was hindered by poor trial methods, diverse outcomes, and no separation of data for different types of dementia.

Harms: We found no RCTs.

Comment: None.

QUESTION What are the effects of treatments on behavioural and psychological symptoms of dementia?

OPTION HALOPERIDOL

One systematic review in people with various types of dementia plus behavioural and psychological symptoms found no significant difference in agitation at 6–16 weeks between haloperidol and placebo. However, it found that haloperidol may reduce aggression. It found that haloperidol increased the frequency and severity of extrapyramidal symptoms compared with placebo. Another systematic review in people with various types of dementia plus behavioural and psychological symptoms found limited evidence that

haloperidol and risperidone were similarly effective in reducing agitation over 12 weeks but that haloperidol caused more frequent and more severe extrapyramidal symptoms. Two RCTs in people with agitated behaviour associated with dementia found no significant difference in agitation between trazodone and haloperidol, but may have been too small to exclude a clinically important difference.

Benefits: **Versus placebo:** We found one systematic review (search date 2000, 5 RCTs) comparing haloperidol versus placebo in people with various types of dementia, including Alzheimer's disease and vascular dementia, all with behavioural and psychological symptoms.[63] It found no significant difference in agitation at 6–16 weeks between haloperidol and placebo (4 RCTs, 369 people; change in symptoms from baseline measured by the Cohen-Mansfield Agitation Inventory or the psychomotor score of the Behavioural Symptoms Scale for Dementia [BSSD]: WMD –0.45, 95% CI –1.43 to +0.53). However, it found that haloperidol significantly reduced aggression from baseline at 3–6 weeks compared with placebo (4 RCTs, 489 people; change in symptoms from baseline measured by Multidimensional Observation Scale for Elderly Subjects aggression subscore, Behave-AD scale, aggression subscore, or the physical aggression score of the BSSD: WMD –0.92, 95% CI –1.75 to –0.09).[63] **Versus risperidone:** We found one systematic review (search date 2002, 2 RCTs, 402 people with Alzheimer's disease, vascular dementia, or mixed dementia, all with behavioural and psychological symptoms) comparing haloperidol versus risperidone for 12 weeks.[64] The reviewers could not perform a meta-analysis because of differences in outcomes assessed and people included in the trials (outpatients and people in hospital). The first RCT (58 people) identified by the review found no significant difference in agitation over 12 weeks between haloperidol and risperidone (measured by Cohen-Mansfield Agitation Inventory and Behave-AD scale; reported as non-significant; no further data reported). The second RCT (344 people) identified by the review compared three interventions: haloperidol, risperidone, and placebo. It found that a similar proportion of people taking haloperidol or risperidone had improvements in agitation (63% with haloperidol *v* 54% with risperidone; CI not reported). **Versus trazodone:** See benefits of trazodone, p 1231.

Harms: **Versus placebo:** The review found that haloperidol (> 2 mg/day) significantly increased the proportion of people who had at least one extrapyramidal symptom or who withdrew because of adverse effects over 3–6 weeks (extrapyramidal symptom: OR 2.34, 95% CI 1.25 to 4.38; withdrawal: OR 2.99, 95% CI 1.26 to 7.10).[63] One study (2 year prospective, longitudinal, 71 people with dementia) found that the mean decline in cognitive scores in 16 people who took antipsychotics was twice that of people who did not (expanded Mini Mental State Examination: 21 with antipsychotics *v* 9 with no antipsychotics; $P = 0.002$).[65] **Versus risperidone:** The first RCT identified by the review did not compare adverse effects between haloperidol and risperidone directly. The second RCT found that haloperidol significantly increased frequency and severity of extrapyramidal symptoms compared with risperidone (frequency: 22% with haloperidol *v* 15% with risperidone; $P = 0.023$; severity: measured by Extrapyramidal Symptoms Rating Scale score: mean +1.6 with haloperidol *v* –0.3 with risperidone; $P < 0.05$).[64] **Versus trazodone:** See harms of trazodone, p 1231.

Comment: High response rates with placebo indicate that many behavioural problems resolve spontaneously in the short term. Most people with dementia are sensitive to adverse effects from antipsychotics, especially sedation and extrapyramidal symptoms. People with Lewy body dementia are particularly sensitive to these adverse effects,[66] suggesting that antipsychotics have a poor balance of benefits and harms in people with Lewy body dementia. More studies are needed to determine whether newer atypical antipsychotics have a better ratio of benefits to harms than older antipsychotics.

OPTION OLANZAPINE

One RCT identified by a systematic review in nursing home residents with Alzheimer's disease or Lewy body dementia plus behavioural and psychological symptoms found that low and medium doses of olanzapine reduced agitation, hallucinations, and delusions over 6 weeks compared with placebo. Olanzapine has been associated with cerebrovascular adverse effects.

Benefits: **Versus placebo:** We found one systematic review[64] (search date 2002), which identified one RCT[67] (double blind, 6 weeks' duration, 206 elderly US nursing home residents with Alzheimer's disease [177 people] or Lewy body dementia [29 people], all with psychotic or behavioural symptoms). The RCT compared olanzapine (given as a fixed dose of 5, 10, or 15 mg/day) versus placebo.[67] It found that agitation, hallucinations, and delusions were improved by the two lower doses but not by the highest dose of olanzapine compared with placebo (subscale of the Neuropsychiatric Inventory [nursing home version; higher scores indicate worse function]: –7.6 with olanzapine 5 mg *v* –6.1 with olanzapine 10 mg *v* –4.9 with olanzapine 15 mg *v* –3.7 with placebo; 5 mg *v* placebo, $P < 0.001$; 10 mg *v* placebo, $P = 0.006$; 15 mg *v* placebo, $P = 0.24$).

Harms: **Versus placebo:** The RCT found that olanzapine increased sedation (25% with olanzapine 5 mg *v* 26% with olanzapine 10 mg *v* 36% with olanzapine 15 mg *v* 6% with placebo) and gait disturbance (20% with olanzapine 5 mg *v* 14% with olanzapine 10 mg *v* 17% with olanzapine 15 mg *v* 2% with placebo) compared with placebo.[67]

Comment: See comment under haloperidol, p 1228. Following the suggestion of an association between olanzapine and cerebrovascular adverse events, the Food and Drug Administration in the USA and the Committee on Safety of Medicines in the UK have issued an alert that olanzapine has not been shown to be safe in people with psychosis associated with dementia.[68,69]

OPTION RISPERIDONE

One systematic review and one subsequent RCT in people with various types of dementia, primarily Alzheimer's disease, all with behavioural and psychological symptoms, found that risperidone improved symptoms over 12 weeks compared with placebo. Another systematic review in people with various types of dementia plus aggressive behaviours found limited evidence that risperidone and haloperidol were similarly effective in reducing agitation over 12 weeks but that risperidone caused fewer and less severe extrapyramidal symptoms. Risperidone has been associated with cerebrovascular adverse events.

Benefits: **Versus placebo:** We found one systematic review[64] and one subsequent RCT.[70] The review (search date 2002, 2 RCTs, 969 people with Alzheimer's disease [67–73%], vascular dementia, or mixed dementia, all with behavioural symptoms, 56–68% women) compared risperidone versus placebo for 12 weeks.[64] It found that risperidone modestly but significantly improved behavioural and psychological symptoms over 12 weeks compared with placebo (measured by Behave-AD scale:

mean difference with risperidone v placebo –1.80, 95% CI –3.22 to –0.38).[64] The subsequent RCT (167 people with Alzheimer's disease, vascular dementia, or mixed dementia, all with aggressive behaviours, mean age 83 years, 72% women) compared risperidone (mean 0.95 mg/day) versus placebo over 12 weeks.[70] It also found that risperidone significantly improved behavioural and psychological symptoms over 12 weeks compared with placebo (mean difference with risperidone v placebo measured by Behave-AD scale –4.50, 95% CI –6.45 to –2.46; measured by the Cohen-Mansfield Agitation Inventory aggression subscale –4.40, 95% CI –6.75 to –2.07). **Versus haloperidol:** See benefits of haloperidol, p 1228.

Harms: **Versus placebo:** The review found that risperidone was associated with increases in extrapyramidal symptoms, somnolence, and mild peripheral oedema (no further data reported).[64] Adverse effects increased with higher doses. Data from four RCTs (1230 elderly people with dementia) of risperidone suggested that risperidone was associated with an increase in cerebrovascular adverse events (including strokes and transient ischaemic attacks, some of which were fatal) compared with placebo (29/764 [4%] with risperidone v 7/466 [2%] with placebo; CI not reported; see comment below).[71] **Versus haloperidol:** See harms of haloperidol, p 1228.

Comment: See comment under haloperidol, p 1228. Following the suggestion of an association between risperidone and cerebrovascular adverse events, the Food and Drug Administration in the USA and the Committee on Safety of Medicines in the UK have issued an alert that risperidone has not been shown to be safe in people with psychosis associated with dementia.[68,69]

OPTION CARBAMAZEPINE

One RCT found that carbamazepine reduced agitation and aggression over 6 weeks compared with placebo in people with various types of dementia and behavioural and psychological symptoms.

Benefits: **Versus placebo:** We found no systematic review but found one RCT (single blind, 51 nursing home patients with agitation and Alzheimer's disease, vascular dementia, or mixed Alzheimer's disease and vascular dementia, 6 weeks' duration) comparing carbamazepine (individualised doses; modal dose 300 mg; mean serum level 5.3 μg/mL) versus placebo.[72] It found that carbamazepine significantly improved a measure of agitation and aggression (assessed by change in mean total Brief Psychiatric Rating Scale score: mean reduction 7.7 with carbamazepine v 0.9 with placebo; P = 0.03).

Harms: **Versus placebo:** The RCT found that adverse effects were significantly more common with carbamazepine than with placebo (16/27 [59%] with carbamazepine v 7/24 [29%] with placebo; P = 0.003). These were considered clinically important in two cases: one person with tics and one person with ataxia. Carbamazepine in the elderly may cause cardiac toxicity.[72] See also epilepsy, p 1588.

Comment: We found no RCTs of carbamazepine in people with Lewy body dementia.

OPTION SODIUM VALPROATE

One RCT found limited evidence that sodium valproate reduced agitation over 6 weeks compared with placebo in people with dementia plus behavioural and psychological problems. Another RCT found no significant difference in aggressive behaviour over 8 weeks between sodium valproate and placebo.

Benefits: **Versus placebo:** We found no systematic review but found two RCTs.[73,74] The first RCT (single blind, 56 people in nursing homes with Alzheimer's disease or vascular dementia, all with agitation) compared sodium valproate versus placebo for 6 weeks.[73] It found that when several covariates were taken into account, sodium valproate significantly improved agitation and aggression compared with placebo (measured by Brief Psychiatric Rating Scale score; P = 0.05 only after adjustment; see comment below) and a measure of global status (Clinical Global Impression rating: 68% with sodium valproate *v* 52% with placebo; P = 0.06). The second RCT (43 people with various types of dementia plus behavioural problems, crossover design) comparing sodium valproate 480 mg daily versus placebo for 3 weeks found no significant difference in aggressive behaviour over 8 weeks after crossover (mean change in Social Dysfunction and Aggression Scale-9 score: –0.72 with sodium valproate *v* –0.72 with placebo; P = 0.99).[74] The RCT did not report results before crossover.

Harms: **Versus placebo:** The first RCT found that adverse effects, generally rated as mild, were significantly more common with sodium valproate than with placebo (68% with sodium valproate *v* 33% with placebo; P = 0.003).[73] See also epilepsy, p 1588.

Comment: The need to perform adjustments for covariates in the first RCT weakens the findings.[73]

OPTION TRAZODONE

We found no RCTs comparing trazodone versus placebo. One small RCT in people with agitated behaviour associated with dementia found no significant difference in agitation over 9 weeks between trazodone and haloperidol. Another small RCT in people with Alzheimer's disease and agitated behaviour found no significant difference in outcomes over 16 weeks among trazodone, haloperidol, behaviour management techniques, and placebo. The RCTs may have been underpowered to detect a clinically important difference.

Benefits: **Versus placebo:** We found no RCTs. **Versus haloperidol:** We found no systematic review but found two RCTs.[75,76] The first RCT (double blind, 28 elderly people with agitated behaviour associated with Alzheimer's disease, vascular dementia, or mixed Alzheimer's disease and vascular dementia, 9 weeks' duration) compared trazodone 50–250 mg daily versus haloperidol 1–5 mg daily.[75] It found no significant difference in agitation between the groups, but the trial was too small to exclude a clinically important difference. The second RCT (double blind, 149 people with Alzheimer's disease and agitated behaviours, 16 weeks' duration) compared four treatments: haloperidol (mean dose 1.1 mg/day); trazodone (mean dose 200 mg/day); behaviour management techniques; or placebo.[76] It found no significant difference in outcome (Alzheimer's Disease Co-operative Study Clinical Global Impression of Change) between the four interventions, but it may have been too small to exclude a clinically important difference.

Harms: **Versus haloperidol:** In the first RCT, adverse effects were more common in the group treated with haloperidol than trazodone.[75] In the second RCT, no significant differences in adverse events were seen between the trazodone group and the placebo group.[76]

Comment: None.

OPTION DONEPEZIL

One RCT found that donepezil improved functional and behavioural symptoms at 24 weeks compared with placebo. Two RCTs found no significant difference in psychiatric symptoms at 6 months to 1 year between donepezil and placebo. Many of the people included in the RCTs did not have behavioural and psychological problems.

Benefits: **Versus placebo:** We found one systematic review (search date 2001)[77] and two additional RCTs.[26,78] The review did not report results for donepezil alone. It identified one RCT (286 people with mild to moderate Alzheimer's disease, Mini Mental State Examination [MMSE] score 10–26, at least 1 symptom on the Neuropsychiatric Inventory Score [NPI]) comparing donepezil (5 mg/day for 28 days, followed by 10 mg/day) versus placebo over 1 year.[79] It found no significant difference in psychiatric symptoms at 1 year (measured by NPI; reported as non-significant; no further data reported). The first additional RCT (208 people with mild to moderate Alzheimer's disease, at least 1 symptom on the Neuropsychiatric Inventory Score, Nursing Home version and living in a nursing home) found no significant difference in psychiatric symptoms after 24 weeks of treatment between donepezil and placebo (change in mean Neuropsychiatric Inventory Nursing Home version Q scores: –4.9 with donepezil *v* –2.3 with placebo; reported as non-significant; no further data reported).[78] The second additional RCT (290 people with moderate to severe Alzheimer's disease aged 48–92 years, MMSE score 5–17, Disability Assessment for Dementia score 2.5–100, at least 1 symptom on the NPI score) compared donepezil 5–10 mg daily versus placebo.[26] It found that donepezil significantly improved functional and behavioural symptoms at 24 weeks compared with placebo (Disability Assessment for Dementia score: mean difference 8.23; $P < 0.001$; NPI score: mean difference 5.64; $P < 0.0001$).

Harms: See harms of donepezil, p 1217.

Comment: Cholinesterase inhibitors improve cognitive function and are well tolerated in older people. Only one of the RCTs assessed behavioural and psychological problems as a primary outcome.[78] Many of the people included in the RCTs did not have behavioural and psychological problems.[26,78,79] Some people took sedatives, which may have affected the results.

OPTION GALANTAMINE

RCTs provided inconclusive evidence about the effects of galantamine compared with placebo on behavioural and psychiatric symptoms in people with mild to moderate Alzheimer's disease.

Benefits: **Versus placebo:** We found one systematic review (search date 2002), which identified two RCTs that assessed the effects of galantamine on behavioural and psychological symptoms.[22] A meta-analysis was not performed because of differences in length of follow up between the trials. Both trials used the Neuropsychiatric Inventory (NPI) scale. The first RCT (386 people with mild to moderate Alzheimer's disease; Mini Mental State Examination score 10–22) found no significant difference in psychiatric symptoms at 3 months between galantamine 12–16 mg twice daily and placebo (mean reduction in NPI score: –0.30 with galantamine *v* +0.50 with placebo; WMD –0.80, 95% CI –2.67 to +1.07). The second RCT (978 people with mild to moderate Alzheimer's disease; Mini Mental State Examination score 12–24) found that galantamine 16 mg daily significantly reduced psychiatric symptoms at 6 months compared with placebo (mean reduction in NPI score: –0.10 with galantamine *v* +2.00 with placebo; WMD –2.10, 95% CI –4.04 to –0.16). However, it found no significant difference with galantamine 8 or 24 mg daily.[22]

Harms: See harms of galantamine, p 1219.

Comment: Neither RCT assessed behavioural and psychological problems as a primary outcome.[22] Many of the people included in the RCTs did not have behavioural and psychological problems. Some people took sedatives, which may have affected the results.

OPTION REALITY ORIENTATION

One systematic review found that reality orientation improved behaviour compared with no treatment in people with various types of dementia.

Benefits: **Versus no treatment:** We found one systematic review (search date 2000, 6 RCTs, 125 people with various types of dementia).[61] It found that reality orientation**G** significantly improved behavioural symptoms compared with no treatment (SMD –0.66, 95% CI –1.27 to –0.05). No separate analysis was done for specific types of dementia.

Harms: **Versus no treatment:** The RCTs gave no information on adverse effects.[61]

Comment: The RCTs did not use standardised interventions or outcomes.[61]

GLOSSARY

Music therapy A process where a therapist uses active or passive musical experiences, and the relationships that develop through them, to promote health, either in an individual or group setting.

Reality orientation Involves presenting information that is designed to reorientate a person in time, place, or person. It may range in intensity from a board giving details of the day, date, and season, to staff reorienting a patient at each contact.

Reminiscence therapy Involves encouraging people to talk about the past in order to enable past experiences to be brought into consciousness. It relies on remote memory, which is relatively well preserved in mild to moderate dementia.

REFERENCES

1. van Duijn CM. Epidemiology of the dementia: recent developments and new approaches. *J Neurol Neurosurg Psychiatry* 1996;60:478–488.
2. McKeith IG, Galasko D, Kosaka K, et al. Consensus guidelines for the clinical and pathological diagnosis of dementia with Lewy bodies (DLB): report of the consortium on DLB International workshop. *Neurology* 1996;47:1113–1124.
3. Rasmusson DX, Brandt J, Steele C, et al. Accuracy of clinical diagnosis of Alzheimer disease and clinical features of patients with non-Alzheimer's disease neuropathology. *Alzheimer Dis Assoc Disord* 1996;10:180–188.
4. Verghese J, Crystal HA, Dickson DW, et al. Validity of clinical criteria for the diagnosis of dementia with Lewy bodies. *Neurology* 1999;53:1974–1982.
5. Lobo A, Launer LJ, Fratiglioni L, et al. Prevalence of dementia and major subtypes in Europe: a collaborative study of population-based cohorts. *Neurology* 2000;54:S4–S9.
6. Farrer L. Intercontinental epidemiology of Alzheimer's disease: a global approach to bad gene hunting. *JAMA* 2001;285:796–798.
7. Skoog I. A population-based study of dementia in 85 year olds. *N Engl J Med* 1993;328:153–158.
8. McKeith IG. Clinical Lewy body syndromes. *Ann N Y Acad Sci* 2000;920:1–8.
9. Inkeda M, Hokoishi K, Maki N, et al. Increased prevalence of vascular dementia in Japan: a community-based epidemiological study. *Neurology* 2001;57:839–844.
10. Hardy J. Molecular classification of Alzheimer's disease. *Lancet* 1991;1:1342–1343.
11. Corey-Bloom J. The natural history of Alzheimer's disease. In: O'Brien J, Ames D, Burns A, eds. Dementia 2nd ed. London: Arnold, 2000:405–415.
12. Eastwood R, Reisberg B. Mood and behaviour. In: Panisset M, Stern Y, Gauthier S, eds. *Clinical diagnosis and management of Alzheimer's disease*. 1st ed. London: Dunitz, 1996:175–189.
13. Mirea A, Cummings J. Neuropsychiatric aspects of dementia. In: O'Brien J, Ames D, Burns A, eds. *Dementia* 2nd ed. London: Arnold, 2000:61–79.
14. Burns A, Lawlor B, Craig S. Assessment scales in old age psychiatry. London: Martin Dunitz, 1998.
15. Gelinas I, Gauthier L, McIntyre M, et al. Development of a functional measure for persons with Alzheimer's disease: the Disability Assessment for Dementia. *Am J Occup Ther* 1999;53:471–481.
16. Lawton MP, Brody EM. Assessment of older people: self-maintaining and instrumental activities of daily living. *Gerontologist* 1969;9:179–186.
17. Rosen WG, Mohs RC, Davis KL. A new rating scale for Alzheimer's disease. *Am J Psychiatry* 1984;141:1356–1364.

18. Folstein MF, Folstein SE, McHugh PR. Mini Mental State: a practical method for grading the cognitive state of patients for the clinician. *J Psychiatr Res* 1975;12:189–198.
19. Schmitt FA, Ashford W, Ernesto C, et al. The severe impairment battery: concurrent validity and the assessment of longitudinal change in Alzheimer's disease. *Alzheimer Dis Assoc Disord* 1997;11:S51–S56.
20. Birks JS, Melzer D, Beppu H. Donepezil for mild and moderate Alzheimer's disease. In: The Cochrane Library, Issue 3, 2003. Oxford: Update Software. Search date 2003; primary sources Cochrane Dementia and Cognitive Impairment Group Specialized Register of Clinical Trials, Medline, Psychlit, Embase, the Donepezil Study Group, and Eisai Inc.
21. Feldman H, Gauthier S, Hecker J, et al. Efficacy of donepezil on maintenance of activities of daily living in patients with moderate to severe Alzheimer's disease and the effect on caregiver burden *J Am Geriatr Soc* 2003;51:737–744. [Erratum in: *J Am Geriatr Soc* 2003;51:1331].
22. Olin J, Schneider L, Olin J, et al. Galantamine for Alzheimer's disease. In: The Cochrane Library, Issue 3, 2003. Oxford: Update Software. Search date 2002; primary sources Cochrane Dementia Group Specialized Register of Clinical Trials, Cochrane Controlled Trials Register, Embase, Medline, Psychlit, Combined Health Information Database, National Research Register, Alzheimer's Disease Education and Referral Centre Clinical Database, Biomed (Biomedicine and Health), GlaxoWellcome Clinical Trials Register, National Institutes of Health Clinical Trials Databases, Current Controlled Trials, Dissertation Abstracts, Index to UK Theses, hand searches of reference lists, and additional information collected from an unpublished investigational brochure for galantamine.
23. Rogers SL, Doody RS, Pratt RD, et al. Long term efficacy and safety of donepezil in the treatment of Alzheimer's disease: final analysis of a US multicentre open-label study. *Eur Neuropsychopharmacol* 2000;10:195–203.
24. Birks J, Iakovidou V, Tsolaki M, et al. Rivastigmine for Alzheimer's disease. In: The Cochrane Library, Issue 3, 2003. Oxford: Update Software. Search date 2000; primary sources Cochrane Controlled Trials Register, Cochrane Dementia Group Specialized Register of Clinical Trials, Medline, Embase, Psychlit, Cinahl, and hand searches of geriatric and dementia journals and conference abstracts.
25. Wimo A, Winblad B, Stoffler A, et al. Resource utilisation and cost analysis of memantine in patients with moderate to severe Alzheimer's disease. *Pharmacoeconomics* 2003;21:327–340.
26. Feldman H, Gauthier S, Hecker J, et al. A 24-week, randomized, double blind study of donepezil in moderate to severe Alzheimer's disease. *Neurology* 2001;57:613–620.
27. Mohs, RC, Doody, RS, Morris, JC, et al, and Study Group. A 1-year, placebo-controlled preservation of function survival study of donepezil in AD patients. *Neurology* 2001;57:481–488.
28. Wilkinson DG, Passmore AP, Bullock R, et al. A multinational, randomised, 12-week, comparative study of donepezil and rivastigmine in patients with mild to moderate Alzheimer's disease. *Int J Clin Pract* 2002;56:441–446.
29. Wilcock G, Howe I, Coles H, et al. A long-term comparison of galantamine and donepezil in the treatment of Alzheimer's disease. *Drugs Aging* 2003;20:777–789.
30. Malouf R, Birks J. Donepezil for vascular cognitive impairment (Cochrane Review). In: The Cochrane Library, Issue 1, 2004. Chichester, UK: John Wiley & Sons, Ltd. Search date 2003; primary sources the Specialized Register of the Cochrane Dementia and Cognitive Improvement Group and unpublished trials were requested a drug company.
31. Erkinjuntti T, Kurz A, Gauthier S, et al. Efficacy of galantamine in probable vascular dementia and Alzheimer's disease combined with cerebrovascular disease: a randomised trial. *Lancet* 2002;359:1283–1290.
32. McKeith I, Del Ser T, Spano P, et al. Efficacy of rivastigmine in dementia with Lewy bodies: a randomised, double-blind, placebo-controlled international study. *Lancet* 2000;356:2031–2036.
33. Kumar V, Anand R, Messina J, et al. An efficacy and safety analysis of Exelon in Alzheimer's disease patients with concurrent vascular risk factors. *Eur J Neurol* 2000;7:159–169.
34. Coelho F, Filho JM, Birks J. Physostigmine for Alzheimer's disease. In: The Cochrane Library, Issue 3, 2003. Oxford: Update Software. Search date 2000; primary sources the Cochrane Dementia Group Specialized Register of Clinical Trials and pharmaceutical companies.
35. Qizilbash N, Whitehead A, Higgins J, et al. Cholinesterase inhibition for Alzheimer disease. *JAMA* 1998;280:1777–1782. Search date not reported; primary sources Cochrane Dementia Group Registry of Clinical Trials, contact with trial investigators, and Parke-Davis Pharmaceuticals.
36. Arrieta JR, Artalejo FR. Methodology, results and quality of clinical trials of tacrine in the treatment of Alzheimer's disease: a systematic review of the literature. *Age Ageing* 1998;27:161–179. Search date 1997; primary sources Cochrane Library and Medline.
37. Koepp R, Miles SH. Meta-analysis of tacrine for Alzheimer's disease: the influence of industry sponsors. *JAMA* 1999;281:2287–2288.
38. Knapp MJ, Knopman DS, Solomon PR, et al. A 30-week randomized controlled trial of high-dose tacrine in patients with Alzheimer's disease. The Tacrine Study Group. *JAMA* 1994;271:985–991.
39. Higgins JPT, Flicker L. Lecithin for dementia and cognitive impairment. In: The Cochrane Library, Issue 3, 2003. Oxford: Update Software. Search date 2002; primary sources Cochrane Dementia and Cognitive Impairment Group Specialized Register of Clinical Trials, Medline, Embase, Psychlit, ISI, Current Contents, and hand searches of reference lists and textbooks.
40. López-Arrieta JM, Rodr guez JL, Sanz F. Nicotine for Alzheimer's disease. In: The Cochrane Library, Issue 3, 2003. Oxford: Update Software. Search date 2001; primary source Cochrane Dementia Group Specialized Register of Clinical Trials.
41. Scharf S, Mander A, Ugoni A, et al. A double-blind, placebo-controlled trial of diclofenac/misoprostol in Alzheimer's disease. *Neurology* 1999;53:197–201.
42. Rogers J, Kirby LC, Hempleman SR, et al. Clinical trial of indomethacin in Alzheimer's disease. *Neurology* 1993;43:1609–1611.
43. Aisen PS, Schafer KA, Grundman M, et al. Effects of rofecoxib or naproxen vs placebo on Alzheimer disease progression: a randomized controlled trial. *JAMA* 2003;289:2819–2826.
44. Williams PS, Spector A, Orrell M, et al. Aspirin for vascular dementia. In: The Cochrane Library, Issue 3, 2003. Oxford: Update Software. Search date 2000; primary sources Medline, Cochrane Library Trials Register, Embase, Cinahl, Psychlit, Amed, Sigle, National Research Register, hand searches of reference lists, and contact with specialists.
45. Hogervorst E, Yaffe K, Richards M, et al. Hormone replacement therapy to maintain cognitive function in women with dementia (Cochrane Review). In: The Cochrane Library, Issue 1, 2004. Chichester, UK: John Wiley & Sons, Ltd. Search date 2002; primary sources Specialised Register of the Cochrane Dementia and Cognitive Impairment Group, Medline, Embase, PsychINFO, and Cinahl.
46. Hogervorst E, Williams J, Budge M, et al. The nature of the effect of female gonadal hormone replacement therapy on cognitive function in post-menopausal women: a meta-analysis. *Neuroscience* 2000;101:485–512. Search date 2000; primary sources Medline, Embase, Psychlit, and hand searches of reference lists.
47. Birks J, Flicker L. Selegiline for Alzheimer's disease. In: The Cochrane Library, Issue 3, 2003. Oxford:

Update Software. Search date 2002; primary source Cochrane Dementia and Cognitive Impairment Group Register of Clinical Trials.
48. Areosa Sastre A, Sherriff F. Memantine for dementia. In: The Cochrane Library, Issue 3, 2003. Oxford: Update Software. Search date 2002; primary sources Cochrane Dementia and Cognitive Improvement Group Specialised Trials Register.
49. Winblad B, Poritis N. Memantine in severe dementia: results of the M-Best study (benefit and efficacy in severely demented patients during treatment with memantine). *Int J Geriatr Psychiatry* 1999;14:135–146.
50. Reisberg B, Doody R, Stoffler A, et al. Memantine in moderate to severe Alzheimer's disease. *New Engl J Med* 2003;348:1333–1341.
51. Wilcock G, Mobius HJ, Stoffler A. A double-blind, placebo-controlled multicentre study of memantine in mild to moderate vascular dementia (MMM500). *Int Clin Psychopharmacol* 2002;17:297–305.
52. Gortelmeyer R, Erbler H. Memantine in the treatment of mild to moderate dementia syndrome. A double-blind placebo-controlled study. *Arzneimittelforschung/Drug Research* 1992;42:904–913.
53. Ditzler K. Efficacy and tolerability of memantine in patients with dementia syndrome. A double-blind, placebo controlled trial. *Arzneimittelforschung/Drug Research* 1991;41:773–780.
54. Birks J, Grimley Evans J, Van Dongen M. Ginkgo biloba for cognitive impairment and dementia In: The Cochrane Library, Issue 3, 2003. Oxford, Update Software. Search date 2002; primary source Cochrane Dementia and Cognitive Impairment Group Specialised Register of Controlled Clinical Trials.
55. Le Bars P, Katz MM, Berman N, et al. A placebo-controlled, double-blind, randomised trial of an extract of Ginkgo biloba for dementia. *JAMA* 1997;278:1327–1332.
56. Tabet N, Birks J, Grimley Evans J. Vitamin E for Alzheimer's disease. In: The Cochrane Library, Issue 3, 2003. Oxford: Update Software. Search date 2000; primary sources Cochrane Dementia and Cognitive Impairment Group Specialized Register of Clinical Trials
57. Sano M, Ernesto C, Thomas RG, et al. A controlled trial of selegiline, α-tocopherol, or both as treatment for Alzheimer's disease. *N Engl J Med* 1997;336:1216–1222.
58. Myers DG, Maloley PA, Weeks D. Safety of antioxidant vitamins. *Arch Intern Med* 1996;156:925–935.
59. Koger SM, Chaplin K, Brotons M. Is music therapy an effective intervention for dementia? A meta-analytic review of the literature. *J Music Ther* 1999;36:2–15. Search date 1998; primary sources Medline, Psychlit, and hand searches of reference lists.
60. Koger SM, Brotons M. Music therapy for dementia symptoms. In: Cochrane Library, Issue 3, 2003. Oxford: Update Software. Search date 2000; primary sources Medline, Cochrane Dementia and Cognitive Improvement Group Trials Register, Embase, Cinahl, and Psychlit.
61. Spector A, Orrell M, Davies S, et al. Reality orientation for dementia. In: The Cochrane Library, Issue 3, 2003. Oxford: Update Software. Search date 2000; primary sources Medline, Psychlit, Embase, Cochrane Database of Systematic Reviews, Omni, Bids, Dissertation Abstracts International, Sigle, plus internet searching of HealthWeb, Mental Health Infosources, American Psychiatric Association, Internet Mental Health, Mental Health Net, NHS Confederation, and hand searches of specialist journals.
62. Spector A, Orrell M. Reminiscence therapy for dementia. In: The Cochrane Library, Issue 3, 2003. Oxford: Update Software. Search date 2000; primary sources Cochrane Controlled Trials Register, Medline, Psychlit, Embase, Omni, Bids, Dissertation Abstracts International, Sigle, reference lists of relevant articles, internet sites, and hand searches of specialist journals.
63. Lonergan E, Luxenberg J, Colford J. Haloperidol for agitation in dementia. In: The Cochrane Library, Issue 3, 2003. Oxford: Update Software. Search date 2000; primary sources Cochrane Controlled Trials Register, Cochrane Dementia Group Specialized Register of Clinical Trials, Medline, Embase, Psychlit, Cinahl, and GlaxoWellcome Trials Database.
64. Pwee KH, Shukla VK, Hermann N, et al. Novel antipsychotics for agitation in dementia: a systematic review. Ottawa: Canadian Coordinating Office for Health Technology Assessment; 2003. Technology report No 36. Search date 2002; primary sources Medline, Embase, Psychinfo, Ageline, Biosis Previews, Pascal, Toxfile, Health Technology Assessment website and other relevant websites, hand searches of bibliographies and conference proceedings, and contact with experts in the field.
65. McShane R, Keene J, Gedling K, et al. Do neuroleptic drugs hasten cognitive decline in dementia? Prospective study with necropsy follow up. *BMJ* 1997;314:266–269.
66. McKeith IG. Dementia with Lewy Bodies. *Br J Psychiatry* 2002;180:144–147.
67. Street JS, Clark WS, Gannon KS, et al. Olanzapine treatment of psychotic and behavioural symptoms in patients with Alzheimer's disease in nursing care facilities: a double-blind, randomised, placebo-controlled trial. *Arch Gen Psychiatry* 2000;57:968–976.
68. Food and Drug Association. Medwatch. 2003 Safety Alert Risperdal (risperidone). Available online at http://www.fda.gov/medwatch/SAFETY/2003/risperdal.htm (last accessed 16 March 2004).
69. Atypical antipsychotic drugs and stroke. Committee on Safety of Medicines. Available online at http://www.mca.gov.uk (last accessed 17 March 2004).
70. Brodaty H, Ames D, Snowdon J, et al. A randomized placebo-controlled trial of risperidone for the treatment of aggression, agitation, and psychosis of dementia. *J Clin Psychiatry* 2003;64:134–143.
71. Wooltorton E. Risperidone (Risperdal): increased rate of cerebrovascular events in dementia trials. *CMAJ* 2002;167:1269–1270.
72. Tariot PN, Erb R, Podgorski CA, et al. Efficacy and tolerability of carbamazepine for agitation and aggression in dementia. *Am J Psychiatry* 1998;155:54–61.
73. Porsteinsson AOP, Tariot PN, Erb R, et al. Placebo-controlled study of divalproex sodium for agitation in dementia. *Am J Geriatr Psychiatry* 2001;9:58–66.
74. Sival RC, Haffmans PMJ, Jansen PAF, et al. Sodium valproate in the treatment of aggressive behaviour in patients with dementia — a randomised placebo controlled clinical trial. *Int J Geriatr Psychiatry* 2002;17:579–585.
75. Sultzer DL, Gray KF, Gunay I, et al. A double-blind comparison of trazodone and haloperidol for treatment of agitation in patients with dementia. *Am J Geriatr Psychiatry* 1997;5:60–69.
76. Teri L, Logsdon RG, Peskind E, et al. Treatment of agitation in AD: a randomised, placebo-controlled clinical trial. *Neurology* 2000;55:1271–1278.
77. Trinh NH, Hoblyn J, Mohanty S, et al. Efficacy of cholinesterase inhibitors in the treatment of neuropsychiatric symptoms and functional impairment in Alzheimer disease: a meta-analysis. *JAMA* 2003;289:210–216. Search date 2001; primary sources Medline, Dissertation Abstracts Online, Psychinfo, Biosis, Pubmed, Cochrane Controlled Trials Register, and hand searches of references of bibliographies and relevant articles.
78. Tariot PN, Cummings JL, Katz IR, et al. A randomized double blind placebo controlled study of the efficacy and safety of donepezil in patients with Alzheimer's disease in the nursing home setting. *J Am Geriatr Soc* 2001;49:1590–1599.
79. Winblad B, Engedal K, Soininen H, et al. A 1-year, randomized, placebo-controlled study of donepezil in patients with mild to moderate AD. *Neurology* 2001;57:489–495.

James Warner
Senior Lecturer/Consultant in Old Age Psychiatry
Imperial College
London
UK

Rob Butler
Honorary Clinical Lecturer in Psychiatry and Consultant in Old Age Psychiatry
University of Auckland and Waitemata Health
Auckland
New Zealand

Pradeep Arya
Specialist Registrar
St Mary's Higher Training Scheme
London
UK

Competing interests: JW has been reimbursed by Novartis, the manufacturer of rivastigmine, for conference attendance and has received speaker fees from Janssen Pharmaceuticals for educational events. RB has been reimbursed by Novartis for conference attendance. PA, none declared.

TABLE 1 Effects on cognitive symptoms of donepezil, galantamine, and rivastigmine compared with placebo.[20,22–25]

Drug	Dose (mg)	Duration (weeks)	Difference in ADAS-cog between treatment and placebo (CI)	NNT for at least 4 point change in ADAS-cog (CI)	OR for global improvement in Clinician Based Impression of Change	OR for all cause withdrawal	Ref
Donepezil	10 od	24	–2.9 (–3.7 to –2.2)	N/A	2.2 (1.5 to 3.1)	1.4 (1.0 to 1.8)	20
Galantamine	12 bd	24	–3.3 (–3.9 to –2.7)	5 (4 to 10)	1.8 (1.5 to 2.3)	1.7 (1.3 to 2.2)	22
	16 bd	24	–3.3 (–4.1 to –2.4)	7 (5 to 12)	1.7 (1.2 to 2.6)	2.09 (1.9 to 4.4)	
Rivastigmine	6–12 bd	28	–2.00 (–0.49 to –3.60)	17 (12 to 34)	1.5 (1.2 to 1.8)	2.4 (2.0 to 3.0)	24
Ginkgo biloba	120 od	52	–1.7 (–3.2 to –0.2 [completer analysis])	8 (5 to 50)	N/A	N/A	25

All results are intention to treat unless specified. ADAS-cog, Alzheimer's Disease Assessment Scale cognitive subscale; bd, twice daily; N/A, not available; od, once daily; ref, reference.

Depressive disorders

Search date April 2003

Rob Butler, Stuart Carney, Andrea Cipriani, John Geddes, Simon Hatcher, Jonathan Price, and Michael Von Korff

QUESTIONS

INTERVENTIONS

Key Messages

- **Mild to moderate depression** We found no reliable direct evidence that one type of treatment (drug or non-drug) is superior to another in improving symptoms of depression. However, we found strong evidence that some treatments are effective, whereas the effectiveness of others remains uncertain. **Severe depression** Of the interventions examined, prescription antidepressant drugs and electroconvulsive therapy are the only treatments for which there is good evidence of effectiveness in severe depressive disorders. We found no RCTs comparing drug and non-drug treatments in severe depressive disorders.

Interventions in mild to moderate, or severe depression

- **Prescription antidepressant drugs (tricyclic antidepressants [including low dose tricyclic antidepressants], selective serotonin reuptake inhibitors, monoamine oxidase inhibitors, reboxetine or venlafaxine) improved symptoms compared with placebo in mild to moderate and severe depression** Systematic reviews and subsequent RCTs in people aged 16 years or over in primary and secondary care found that prescription antidepressant drugs (tricyclic antidepressants [including low dose tricyclic antidepressants], selective serotonin reuptake inhibitors, monoamine oxidase inhibitors, reboxetine, or venlafaxine) were effective for treatment of all grades of depressive disorders compared with placebo. Two RCTs in people admitted to hospital with severe depression found that reboxetine increased the proportion of people who responded at 4–6 weeks compared with placebo. One RCT in people with major depressive disorder provided insufficient evidence to assess the effects of reboxetine compared with placebo on depressive symptoms, although it found that reboxetine improved social functioning over 8 weeks. One systematic review in people aged 55 years or over with all grades of depressive disorder found that tricyclic antidepressants, selective serotonin reuptake inhibitors, or monoamine oxidase inhibitors reduced the proportion of people who failed to recover over 26–49 days compared with placebo. The reviews gave little information on severe adverse effects of antidepressant drugs compared with placebo. Evidence of publication bias has been found in the RCTs of selective serotonin reuptake inhibitors and the efficacy and safety of these drugs is currently under review by the regulatory authorities in several countries.

- **Tricyclic antidepressants versus other prescription antidepressant drugs** Three systematic reviews found no significant difference in outcomes with different kinds of antidepressant drug (tricyclic antidepressants, selective serotonin reuptake inhibitors, or monoamine oxidase inhibitors). One systematic review found no significant difference between tricyclic antidepressants and venlafaxine in the proportion of people who responded over 1–12 months. Another systematic review suggested that tricyclic antidepressants were more effective than monoamine oxidase inhibitors in people with severe depressive disorders, but may be less effective in atypical depressive disorders with biological features such as increased sleep, and increased appetite. A third systematic review found that tricyclic antidepressants were associated with higher rates of adverse effects than selective serotonin reuptake inhibitors, but the difference was small. Two RCTs, primarily in people with severe depression, found no significant difference in symptoms at 4 weeks between desipramine or imipramine and reboxetine, but results were sensitive to outcome scales used. One systematic review found no significant difference between low dosage tricyclics and standard dosage tricyclics in the proportion of responders at 6–8 weeks.

- **Selective serotonin reuptake inhibitors and related drugs versus other prescription antidepressant drugs** Three systematic reviews found no significant difference in outcomes with different kinds of antidepressant drug (tricyclic antidepressants, selective serotonin reuptake inhibitors, or monoamine oxidase inhibitors), although one systematic review found that selective serotonin reuptake inhibitors were less effective than venlafaxine in increasing the proportion of people who responded. RCTs in people with major depression found similar response rates at 6 weeks between fluoxetine and reboxetine, but found that reboxetine may be slightly more effective in improving social functioning. One systematic review found that selective serotonin reuptake inhibitors were associated with fewer adverse effects than tricyclic antidepressants, but the difference was small. Another systematic review and one retrospective cohort study found no strong evidence that fluoxetine was associated with increased risk of suicide compared with tricyclic antidepressants or placebo. One RCT and observational data suggested that abrupt withdrawal of selective serotonin reuptake inhibitors was associated with symptoms including dizziness and rhinitis, and that these symptoms are more likely with drugs with a short half life, such as paroxetine. Evidence of publication bias has been found in the RCTs of selective serotonin reuptake inhibitors and the efficacy and safety of these drugs is currently under review by the regulatory authorities in several countries.
- **Monoamine oxidase inhibitors versus other prescription antidepressant drugs** Three systematic reviews found no significant difference in outcomes with different kinds of antidepressant drug (tricyclic antidepressants, selective serotonin reuptake inhibitors, or monoamine oxidase inhibitors). One systematic review found that monoamine oxidase inhibitors were less effective than tricyclic antidepressants in people with severe depressive disorders. However, the review found that monoamine oxidase inhibitors may be more effective in atypical depressive disorders with biological features such as increased sleep and increased appetite.
- **Venlafaxine versus other prescription antidepressant drugs** One systematic review found no significant difference between venlafaxine and tricyclic antidepressants in the proportion of people who responded over 1–12 months and found that venlafaxine increased the proportion of people who responded compared with selective serotonin reuptake inhibitors.
- **Cognitive therapy (in mild to moderate depression)** One systematic review in younger and older adults found that cognitive therapy improved symptoms compared with no treatment. Three systematic reviews in younger and older adults with mild to moderate depression found that psychological therapies (mainly interpersonal psychotherapy and cognitive therapy) increased the proportion of people who were in remission over 10–34 weeks compared with control (usual care, usual care plus pill placebo, or supportive therapy). These reviews did not report results for cognitive therapy alone compared with control. One systematic review found limited evidence that cognitive therapy was more effective than interpersonal therapy in improving recovery rates but this difference disappeared when low quality studies were excluded or if studies which relied on advertising or similar techniques to recruit people were excluded. One systematic review of poor

quality RCTs in people aged 55 years or over with mild to moderate depression found no significant difference in symptoms between psychological treatments (such as cognitive therapy or cognitive behavioural therapy) and no treatment. It also found no significant difference in symptoms between psychological treatments and similar but non-specific attention.

- **Electroconvulsive therapy (in moderate to severe depression)** One systematic review in people with moderate to severe depressive disorder, many of whom were inpatients, found that electroconvulsive therapy improved symptoms over 1–6 weeks' treatment compared with simulated electroconvulsive therapy or antidepressant drugs. The review found that bilateral electroconvulsive therapy improved symptoms compared with unilateral electroconvulsive therapy and that high dose electroconvulsive therapy was more effective than low dose. The degree of reported short term cognitive impairment seemed to be inversely related to treatment efficacy. Another systematic review provided insufficient evidence to assess electroconvulsive therapy in older adults. Because electroconvulsive therapy may be unacceptable to some people and, because it is a short term treatment, there is consensus that it should normally be reserved for people who cannot tolerate or have not responded to antidepressant drug treatment, although it may be useful when a rapid response is required.
- **Interpersonal psychotherapy (in mild to moderate depression)** Two systematic reviews in younger and older adults with mild to moderate depression found that both psychological therapies (mainly interpersonal psychotherapy and cognitive therapy) increased the proportion of people who were in remission over 10–34 weeks compared with control (usual care, usual care plus pill placebo, or supportive therapy). These reviews did not report results for interpersonal therapy alone compared with control. One RCT identified by a third review found that interpersonal therapy increased response rates compared with usual care. One systematic review found limited evidence that interpersonal therapy was less effective than cognitive therapy in improving recovery rates but this difference disappeared when low quality studies were excluded or if studies which relied on advertising or similar techniques to recruit people were excluded.
- **Combining prescription antidepressant drugs and psychological treatments (in mild to moderate and severe depression)** One non-systematic review of RCTs in people aged 18–80 years found that, in people with severe depression, adding antidepressant drug treatment to interpersonal psychotherapy or to cognitive therapy improved symptoms compared with either psychological treatment alone. The review found no significant difference in symptoms in people with mild to moderate depression. However, subsequent RCTs in younger and older adults with mild to moderate depression found that combining antidepressant drugs plus psychological treatments improved symptoms more than either antidepressant drugs or psychological treatments alone. One RCT in older adults with mild to moderate depression found that cognitive behavioural therapy plus desipramine improved symptoms more than desipramine alone.
- **Non-directive counselling (in mild to moderate depression)** One systematic review in people aged 18 years or over with recent onset psychological problems, including depression, found that brief, non-directive counselling in primary care reduced symptom scores in the short term (< 6 months) in people with mild to moderate depression compared with usual care. However, it found no significant difference in scores in the long term (> 6 months).
- **Problem solving therapy (in mild to moderate depression)** One systematic review in younger and older adults with mild to moderate depression in primary care found that psychological therapies (including problem solving therapy) improved outcomes compared with usual care. The review did not report results of problem solving therapy alone in people with moderate depression. It found no significant difference between problem solving therapy and usual care in symptoms at 6–11 weeks in people with mild depression or dysthymia. One large subsequent RCT

found that problem solving therapy increased the proportion of people who were not depressed at 6 months compared with usual care. However, it found no significant difference at 1 year. Another smaller RCT found no significant difference in symptoms at 8 or 26 weeks between problem solving therapy and usual care. RCTs found insufficient evidence to assess the relative efficacy of drug and non-drug treatment in severe depression.

- **Reboxetine versus other antidepressant drugs (in mild to moderate or severe depression)** Two RCTs, primarily in people with severe depression, found no significant difference in symptoms at 4 weeks between reboxetine and desipramine or imipramine, but results were sensitive to outcome scales used. RCTs in people with major depression found similar response rates at 6 weeks between reboxetine and fluoxetine, and found that reboxetine may slightly improve social functioning.
- **St John's Wort (in mild to moderate depression** Two systematic reviews and one subsequent RCT in people with mild to moderate depressive disorders found that St John's Wort (*Hypericum perforatum*) improved depressive symptoms over 4–12 weeks compared with placebo. However, two subsequent RCTs found no significant difference in symptoms at 8 weeks between St John's Wort and placebo. RCTs found no significant difference in symptoms between St John's Wort and prescription antidepressant drugs. The results of the RCTs should be interpreted with caution because many of the RCTs did not use standardised preparations of St John's Wort, and doses of antidepressant drugs varied. One subsequent RCT in people aged 18 years or over with major depressive disorder found no significant difference in depressive symptoms at 8 weeks between a standardised preparation of St John's Wort and sertraline, but it is likely to have been underpowered to detect a clinically important difference.
- **Befriending (in mild to moderate depression)** One small RCT provided insufficient evidence to assess befriending in people with mild to moderate depression.
- **Bibliotherapy (in mild to moderate depression)** One systematic review of RCTs in younger and older adults recruited by advertisement found limited evidence that bibliotherapy may reduce mild depressive symptoms compared with waiting list control or usual care. It is unclear whether people in the RCTs identified by the review are clinically representative of people with depressive disorders. Another RCT in people with depression found that bibliotherapy may improve symptoms over 2–6 months compared with antidepressant drugs.
- **Exercise (in mild to moderate depression)** One systematic review in younger and older adults found limited evidence from poor RCTs that exercise may improve symptoms compared with no treatment, and may be as effective as cognitive therapy. One poor RCT in older adults identified by the review found limited evidence that exercise may be as effective as antidepressant drugs in improving symptoms and may reduce relapse over 10 months.
- **Psychological treatments (cognitive therapy, interpersonal psychotherapy, non-directive counselling, and problem solving therapy) in severe depression** RCTs provided insufficient evidence to assess psychological treatments in severe depression.

Interventions in treatment resistant depression

- **Lithium augmentation** RCTs provided insufficient evidence to assess augmentation of prescription antidepressant drug treatment with lithium in younger and older adults with treatment resistant depression.
- **Pindolol augmentation** RCTs provided insufficient evidence to assess augmentation of prescription antidepressant drug treatment with pindolol in younger and older adults with treatment resistant depression.

Preventing relapse

- **Continuing prescription antidepressant drugs (reduced risk of relapse after recovery in people with mild to moderate depression)** One systematic review found that continuing prescription antidepressant drug treatment after recovery reduced the proportion of people who relapsed over 1–3 years compared with placebo. The effect of continuing antidepressants was independent of the underlying risk of relapse, the duration of treatment before randomisation, or the duration of previous antidepressant treatment. RCTs in people aged over 60 years found that continued treatment with dosulepin (dothiepin) or citalopram after recovery reduced the risk of relapse over 1–2 years compared with placebo, but may increase the risk of ischaemic heart disease.

- **Cognitive therapy (weak evidence that may reduce relapse over 1–2 years after stopping treatment in people with mild to moderate depression compared with antidepressant drugs)** One systematic review in younger and older adults with mild to moderate depression found limited evidence by combining relapse rates across different RCTs that cognitive therapy may reduce the risk of relapse over 1–2 years after stopping treatment compared with antidepressant drugs. One small RCT found that, in people with residual depressive symptoms after antidepressant drug treatment, cognitive therapy for 2 years after the initial depressive episode reduced relapse rates compared with continuing antidepressant drugs. We found no systematic review or RCTs specifically in older adults.
- **Relapse prevention programme (improved symptoms over 1 year after recovery in people with mild to moderate depression but no significant difference in relapse rates)** One large RCT in people who had recovered after 8 weeks of antidepressant treatment found that a relapse prevention programme improved depressive symptoms over 1 year compared with usual care. However, it found no significant difference in relapse rates.

Interventions to improve delivery of treatments

- **Care pathways (in mild to moderate depression)** One systematic review and four subsequent RCTs in people aged over 18 years with mild to moderate or major depression found that the effectiveness of treatment for depression (antidepressant drugs or cognitive behavioural therapy) may be improved by several care pathways, including collaborative working between primary care clinicians and psychiatrists, intensive patient education, case management, and telephone support. They also found that that clinical practice guidelines and educational strategies without other organisational processes improved neither detection nor outcome of depression compared with usual care. One RCT in people aged over 60 years with major depression, dysthymic depression, or both, treated in a variety of primary care clinics found that collaborative care was more effective than usual care in reducing depressive symptoms.

DEFINITION Depressive disorders are characterised by persistent low mood, loss of interest and enjoyment, and reduced energy. They often impair day to day functioning. Most of the RCTs assessed in this review classify depression using the Diagnostic and Statistical Manual of Mental Disorders (DSM-IV)[1] or the International Classification of Mental and Behavioural Disorders (ICD-10).[2] DSM-IV divides depression into major depressive disorder**G** or dysthymic disorder**G**. Major depressive disorder is characterised by one or more major depressive episodes (i.e. at least 2 weeks of depressed mood or loss of interest accompanied by at least 4 additional symptoms of depression). Dysthymic disorder is characterised by at least 2 years of depressed mood for more days than not, accompanied by additional symptoms that do not reach the criteria for major depressive disorder.[1] ICD-10 divides depression into mild to moderate or severe depressive episodes.[2] Mild to moderate depression**G** is characterised by depressive symptoms and some functional impairment. Treatment resistant depression is defined as an absence of clinical response to treatment with a tricyclic antidepressant at a minimum dose of 150 mg daily of imipramine (or equivalent drug) for 4–6 weeks.[3] Severe depression**G** is characterised by additional agitation or psychomotor retardation with marked somatic symptoms.[2] In this review, we use both DSM-IV and ICD-10 classifications, but treatments are considered to have been assessed in severe depression if the RCT included inpatients. **Older adults:** Older adults are generally defined as people aged 65 years or older. However, some of the RCTs of older people in this review included people aged 55 years or over. The presentation of depression in older adults may be atypical: low mood may be masked and anxiety or memory impairment may be the principal presenting symptoms.

Dementia should be considered in the differential diagnosis of depression in older adults.[4] This review does not cover intervention in women with postnatal depression (see postnatal depression, p 1796 or seasonal affective disorder.

INCIDENCE/ PREVALENCE Depressive disorders are common, with a prevalence of major depression between 5% and 10% of people seen in primary care settings.[5] Two to three times as many people may have depressive symptoms but do not meet DSM-IV criteria for major depression. Women are affected twice as often as men. Depressive disorders are the fourth most important cause of disability worldwide and they are expected to become the second most important cause by 2020.[6,7] **Older adults:** Between 10% and 15% of older people have depressive symptoms, although major depression is relatively rare in older adults.[8]

AETIOLOGY/ RISK FACTORS The causes are uncertain but include both childhood events and current psychosocial adversity.

PROGNOSIS About half of people suffering a first episode of major depressive disorder experience further symptoms in the next 10 years.[9] **Older adults:** One systematic review (search date 1996, 12 prospective cohort studies, 1268 people, mean age 60 years) found that the prognosis may be especially poor in elderly people with a chronic or relapsing course of depression.[10] Another systematic review (search date 1999, 23 prospective cohort studies in people aged ≥ 65 years, including 5 identified by the first review) found that depression in older people was associated with increased mortality (15 studies; pooled OR 1.73, 95% CI 1.53 to 1.95).[11]

AIMS OF INTERVENTION To improve mood, social and occupational functioning, and quality of life; to reduce morbidity and mortality; to prevent recurrence of depressive disorder; and to minimise adverse effects of treatment.

OUTCOMES Depressive symptoms rated by the depressed person and clinician; social functioning; occupational functioning; quality of life; admission to hospital; rates of self harm; relapse of depressive symptoms; rates of adverse events. RCTs often use continuous scales to measure depressive symptoms (such as the Hamilton Depression Rating Scale [HAM-D] and the Clinical Global Impression Scale [CGI]). A reduction in score of 50% or more on the HAM-D or a CGI score of 1 (very much improved) or 2 (much improved) is generally considered a clinically important response to treatment. Many RCTs express results in terms of effect size(G). **Older adults:** The HAM-D is not ideal for older people because it includes several somatic items that may be positive in older people who are not depressed. It has been the most widely used scale, although specific scales for elderly people (such as the Geriatric Depression Scale) avoid somatic items.

METHODS *Clinical Evidence* search and appraisal April 2003, including a search for data on depression in older adults. In this review, studies are included under the heading older adults if they specifically included people aged over 55 years.

QUESTION What are the effects of treatments in mild to moderate or severe depression?

OPTION PRESCRIPTION ANTIDEPRESSANT DRUGS VERSUS PLACEBO

Andrea Cipriani and John Geddes

Systematic reviews and subsequent RCTs in people aged 16 years or over in primary and secondary care found that prescription antidepressant drugs (tricyclic antidepressants [including low dose tricyclic antidepressants], selective serotonin reuptake inhibitors, monoamine oxidase inhibitors, or venlafaxine) were effective for treatment of all grades of depressive disorders compared with placebo. Two RCTs in people admitted to hospital with severe depression found that reboxetine increased the proportion of people who responded at 4–6 weeks compared with placebo. One RCT in people with major depressive disorder provided insufficient evidence to assess the effects of reboxetine compared with placebo on depressive symptoms, although it found that reboxetine improved social functioning over 8 weeks. One systematic review in people aged 55 years or over with all grades of depressive disorder found that tricyclic antidepressants, selective serotonin reuptake inhibitors, or monoamine oxidase inhibitors reduced the proportion of people who failed to recover over 26–49 days compared with placebo. The reviews gave little

information on severe adverse effects of antidepressant drugs compared with placebo. Evidence of publication bias has been found in the RCTs of selective serotonin reuptake inhibitors and the efficacy and safety of these drugs is currently under review by the regulatory authorities in several countries.

Benefits: We found five systematic reviews[12–16] and three subsequent RCTs.[17–19] All found that antidepressant drugs significantly improved depressive symptoms compared with placebo. The first review (search date 1995, 49 RCTs in people aged 18–70 years with mild to moderate or severe depressive disorders) included five RCTs in people admitted to hospital (probably with severe depressive disorders), 40 RCTs in a setting outside hospital, one in both settings, and three that did not specify the setting.[12] All RCTs identified by the review were of least 4 weeks' duration and included three way comparisons, including two antidepressant drugs (tricyclic antidepressants [TCAs], selective serotonin reuptake inhibitors [SSRIs], or monoamine oxidase inhibitors [MAOIs]) and placebo. The review only included RCTs that measured improvement in depressive symptoms using validated scales such as the Hamilton Depression Rating Scale (HAM-D) and Montgomery-Asberg Depression Rating Scale. It found that, on average, 69% of people taking placebo had worse outcomes over a mean of 6 weeks than the average person taking antidepressant drugs (mean effect size 0.5 for change in score with antidepressant drugs *v* placebo; see comment below).[12] The second review (search date 2000, 35 RCTs, none included in the first review, 2013 people aged ≥ 18 years with all grades of depression, some with a physical illness) compared low dose (75–100 mg/day) TCAs (amitriptyline, clomipramine, doxepin, dosulepin [dothiepin], imipramine, lofepramine, trimipramine) versus placebo.[15] It found that low dose TCAs significantly increased the proportion of people who responded at 4 weeks and at 3–12 months compared with placebo (response defined as ≥ 50% reduction in symptoms measured on a validated scale; at 4 weeks: 274/603 [45%] with TCAs *v* 159/557 [28%] with placebo; RR 1.65, 95% CI 1.36 to 2.00; at 3–12 months: 40/76 [53%] with TCAs *v* 18/77 [23%] with placebo; RR 2.14, 95% CI 1.41 to 3.26; results not intention to treat). The significant difference in response rates between low dosage TCAs and placebo was not maintained when an intention to treat analysis based on the worst case scenario was performed. The third review (search date 1998, 150 RCTs, ≥ 16 000 people with major depression, see comment below) compared newer antidepressants (SSRIs [43 RCTs], MAOIs, or venlafaxine) versus placebo for at least 6 weeks.[16] Response was defined as a 50% reduction in depression rating scale score or a Clinical Global Impression Scale (CGI) score of 1 (very much improved) or 2 (much improved). The review found that newer depressants significantly increased the proportion of people who responded compared with placebo (51% with newer antidepressants *v* 31% with placebo; RR 1.6, 95% CI 1.5 to 1.7). The third review[16] also performed a separate analysis of results for people in primary care.[20] It found that results remained significant; the average response rate was 63% for newer agents, 35% for placebo, and 60% for TCAs (RR for SSRIs versus placebo 1.6, 95% CI 1.2 to 2.1). The fourth review (search date 1997, 15 RCTs, none included in the other reviews, some comparing two antidepressants *v* placebo, 1871 people aged ≥ 18 years) compared antidepressant and other drugs (TCAs [5 RCTs], SSRIs [4 RCTs], MAOIs [3 RCTs], other [2 RCTs]) versus placebo in people with dysthymia (chronic mild depressive disorders).[13] It found that antidepressant or other drugs significantly increased the proportion of people who responded to treatment over 4–12 weeks compared with placebo (response defined as a 50% reduction in HAM-D score or scoring 1 or 2 on item 2 of the CGI score; RR 1.9, 95% CI 1.6 to 2.3; NNT 4, 95% CI 3 to 5). The fifth review (search date 1998, 18 RCTs, none included in the first or second reviews, 838 people aged > 18 years with depression and a physical illness [e.g. cancer, cardiovascular disorders, diabetes]) found that antidepressant drugs (TCAs, SSRIs, or MAOIs) significantly reduced the proportion of people who failed to recover over 4–12 weeks compared with placebo (177/366 [48%] with antidepressant *v* 229/325 [70%] with placebo; RR 0.68, 95% CI 0.60 to 0.77; NNT 4, 95% CI 3 to 7).[14] People taking antidepressant drugs were significantly more likely to withdraw from the study for any cause than those taking placebo (NNH 10, 95% CI 5 to 43). We found three subsequent RCTs of reboxetine.[17–19] The first RCT (56 people aged 18–65 years admitted to hospital, probably with severe depressive disorders, mean HAM-D score > 35) compared reboxetine (6 mg daily for 1 day increasing to 10 mg over 3 days) versus placebo for 6 weeks' treatment.[17] It found that reboxetine significantly increased the proportion of people who responded at 6 weeks compared with placebo (response defined as ≥ 50% reduction in HAM-D score: 74% with reboxetine *v* 20% with placebo; P < 0.001). The second RCT (258 people aged 18–65 years admitted to hospital with severe depression**Ⓖ**) compared three interventions: reboxetine 4–8 mg daily (84 people), desipramine 100–200 mg daily (89 people), and placebo (84 people).[18] It found that reboxetine at any dose significantly increased the proportion of people who responded over 4 weeks compared with placebo (response defined as ≥ 50% reduction on continuous rating scale assessed by HAM-D: 60% with reboxetine *v* 35% with placebo; assessed by CGI score: 51% with reboxetine *v* 22% with placebo; P < 0.05 for response on either scale with reboxetine *v* placebo). The third RCT (381 people aged 18–65 years with major depressive disorder**Ⓖ** without psychotic features) assessed the effects of reboxetine 8–10 mg daily, paroxetine 20–40 mg daily, and placebo on social functioning.[19] It found that reboxetine significantly improved mean Social Adaptation Self Evaluation Scale score at 8 weeks compared with placebo (35.3 with reboxetine *v* 27.2 with placebo; P < 0.05). **In older adults:** We found one systematic review (search date 2000, 17 RCTs, 1326 people aged ≥ 55 years with mild to moderate or severe depression) comparing antidepressant drugs versus placebo.[21] It found that TCAs, SSRIs, or MAOIs significantly reduced the proportion of people who failed to recover over 4–7 weeks compared with placebo (125/245 [51%] with TCAs *v* 167/223 [75%] with placebo: RR 0.68, 95% CI 0.59 to 0.78, NNT 4, 95% CI 4 to 5; 261/365 [72%] with SSRIs *v* 310/372 [83%] with placebo: RR 0.86, 95% CI 0.79 to 0.93, NNT 9, 95% CI 9 to 10; 34/58 [59%] with MAOIs *v* 57/63 [90%] with placebo: RR 0.64, 95% CI 0.50 to 0.81, NNT 4, 95% CI 3 to 4).[21]

Harms: The first review gave no information on adverse effects.[12] The second review found that people taking low dose TCAs were 111% (95% CI 35% to 228%) more likely than people taking placebo to withdraw because of adverse effects.[15] However, it found no significant difference between low dose TCAs and placebo in the proportion of people who withdrew for any cause (RR 1.08, 95% CI 0.93 to 1.26). People taking low dosage TCAs were 63% (95% CI 36% to 95%) more likely to experience at least one adverse effect than people taking placebo. The third review found that significantly more people taking SSRIs than placebo withdrew because of adverse effects (ARR 5.5%, 95% CI 3.4% to 7.6%).[16] The review gave no information on adverse effects of MAOIs, TCAs, or venlafaxine compared with placebo. The fourth review found that, compared with placebo, TCAs significantly increased the proportion of people who had constipation (2 RCTs, 78/239 [33%] with TCAs *v* 27/244 [11%] with placebo; RR 2.95, 95% CI 1.97 to 4.41), dizziness (59/239 [25%] with TCAs *v* 32/244 [13%] with placebo; RR 1.89, 95% CI 1.28 to 2.79), and dry mouth (163/239 [68%] with TCAs *v* 45/244 [18%] with placebo; RR 3.70, 95% CI 2.80 to 4.88).[13] It found that, compared with placebo, SSRIs significantly increased the proportion of people who had sweating (2 RCT, 41/311 [13%] with TCAs *v* 12/308 [4%] with placebo; RR 3.40, 95% CI 1.81 to 6.36), sexual dysfunction (22/153 [14%] *v* 9/156 [6%]; RR 2.49, 95% CI 1.18 to 5.23), insomnia (68/292 [23%] *v* 48/292 [16%]; RR 1.42, 95% CI 1.02 to 1.98), and dry mouth (52/292 [18%] with TCAs *v* 34/292 [12%] with placebo; RR 1.56, 95% CI 1.05 to 2.31). The review found insufficient evidence from one RCT to compare the adverse effects of MAOIs versus placebo.[13] The fifth review gave no information on adverse effects.[14] The first subsequent RCT found that, compared with placebo, more people taking reboxetine had dry mouth (16/28 [57%] with reboxetine *v* 6/28 [21%] with placebo), insomnia (7/28 [25%] *v* 0/28 [0%]), blurred vision (5/28 [18%] *v* 1/28 [4%]), sweating (5/28 [18%] *v* 0/28 [0%]), constipation (4/28 [14%] *v* 2/28 [7%]), vomiting (4/28 [14%] *v* 1/28 [4%]), tremor (4/28 [14%] *v* 3/28 [11%]), hypotension (3/28 [11%] *v* 0/28 [0%]), decreased appetite (3/28 [11%] *v* 0/28 [0%]), and sexual disturbance (3/28 [11%] with reboxetine *v* 1/28 [4%] with placebo); but fewer people had headache (2/28 [7%] with reboxetine *v* 5/28 [18%] with placebo; CI not reported for any outcomes).[17] The second subsequent RCT found that, compared with placebo, significantly more people taking reboxetine had urinary hesitancy (11% with reboxetine *v* 1% with placebo; reported as significant, CI not reported).[18] The third subsequent RCT gave no information on adverse effects.[19] **In older adults:** We found no specific evidence on adverse effects in older adults.

Comment: Many of the RCTs were sponsored by the manufacturer and sponsorship has been suggested as a potential factor influencing the outcome of RCTs.[22] Evidence of publication bias has been found in the RCTs of SSRIs and the efficacy and safety of these drugs is currently under review by the regulatory authorities in several countries. For mild to moderate depression**G**, most RCTs were short term and focused exclusively on improvement in depressive symptoms. Longer term RCTs that could provide more data on the sustainability of benefits and the potential adverse effects are lacking. Although effects on depressive symptoms are clear, effects on functional status and health related quality of life outcomes are not well described. Most RCTs analyzed results using "last observation carried forward": this method may bias the estimate of treatment efficacy. A "pure" intention to treat analysis, following participants for the whole trial duration even if they withdraw would be more conservative and would replicate what happens in clinical practice. The first review found that results were sensitive to the diagnostic criteria used; the mean effect size for antidepressant drugs was 0.5 in those RCTs in which depressive disorders were diagnosed according to standard criteria (mainly *Diagnostic and statistical manual of mental disorders*, 3rd edition, revised) and 0.4 in those RCTs that did not use objective diagnostic criteria.[12] The third review[16] forms part of a larger review of 315 RCTs in people with depression and we were unable to obtain the full reference list; it is therefore unclear whether it contains RCTs assessed in the other reviews. **In older adults:** The systematic review comparing antidepressant drugs versus placebo in older people was limited by the diversity of populations included and by the brevity of the RCTs.[14] The reviewers recommended at least 6 weeks of antidepressant treatment in elderly people to achieve optimal effect. Metabolic and physical changes with age mean that older people may be more prone to adverse effects such as falls. Because older people often take more medications, they may be at greater risk of drug interactions.

OPTION TRICYCLIC ANTIDEPRESSANTS VERSUS OTHER PRESCRIPTION ANTIDEPRESSANT DRUGS

Andrea Cipriani and John Geddes

Three systematic reviews found no significant difference in outcomes with different kinds of antidepressant drug (tricyclic antidepressants, selective serotonin reuptake inhibitors, or monoamine oxidase inhibitors). One systematic review found no significant difference between tricyclic antidepressants and venlafaxine in the proportion of people who responded over 1–12 months. Another systematic review suggested that tricyclic antidepressants were more effective than monoamine oxidase inhibitors in people with severe depressive disorders, but may be less effective in atypical depressive disorders with biological features such as increased sleep, and increased appetite. A third systematic review found that tricyclic antidepressants were associated with higher rates of adverse effects than selective serotonin reuptake inhibitors, but the difference was small. Two RCTs, primarily in people with severe depression, found no significant difference in symptoms at 4 weeks between desipramine or imipramine and reboxetine, but results were sensitive to outcome scales used. One systematic review found no significant difference between low dosage tricyclics and standard dosage tricyclics in the proportion of responders at 6–8 weeks.

Benefits: **Versus selective serotonin reuptake inhibitors:** See benefits of selective serotonin reuptake inhibitors, p 1249. **Versus monoamine oxidase inhibitors:** See benefits of monoamine oxidase inhibitors, p 1252. **Versus reboxetine:** See benefits of reboxetine, p 1253. **Low dose tricyclic antidepressants versus standard dose tricyclic antidepressants:** We found one systematic review (search date 2000, 6 RCTs, 551 people) that found no significant difference between low dosage tricyclic antidepressants (TCAs) and standard dosage TCAs in the proportion of responders at 6–8 weeks (RR 1.11, 95% CI 0.76 to 1.61).[15] It is likely that these RCTs were designed to show equivalence between treatments rather than superiority of one over another so the clinical relevance of this result is unclear. **Tricyclic antidepressants plus benzodiazepines versus tricyclic antidepressants alone:** We found one systematic review (search date 1999, 9 RCTs, 679 people aged 18–73 years with major depression) comparing combination treatment with antidepressant drugs (primarily TCAs) plus benzodiazepines versus antidepressant drugs alone.[23] It found that combination treatment was significantly more likely to produce a response within 1 week compared with antidepressant drugs alone (RR of > 50% reduction on symptom rating scale 1.64, 95% CI 1.19 to 2.27), although this difference was not apparent at 6 weeks.

Harms: **Versus selective serotonin reuptake inhibitors:** See harms of selective serotonin reuptake inhibitors, p 1250. **Versus monoamine oxidase inhibitors:** See harms of monoamine oxidase inhibitors, p 1252. **Versus reboxetine:** See harms of reboxetine, p 1253. **Low dose tricyclic antidepressants versus standard dose tricyclic antidepressants:** The review found that people taking low dose TCAs were 55% (95% CI 24% to 73%) less likely than people taking standard dose TCAs to withdraw because of adverse effects.[15] However, it found no significant difference between low dose and standard dose TCAs in the proportion of people who withdrew for any cause (RR 0.95, 95% CI 0.75 to 1.20). **Tricyclic antidepressants plus benzodiazepines versus tricyclic antidepressants alone:** The review found that TCAs plus benzodiazepines significantly reduced the proportion of people who withdrew from the trial because of adverse effects compared with antidepressants alone (23/342 [7%] with TCAs plus benzodiazepines *v*

46/337 [14%] with TCAs alone; RR 0.53, 95% CI 0.32 to 0.86).[23] **During pregnancy:** One systematic review (search date 1999) assessing the risk of fetal harm of antidepressant drugs (TCAs and selective serotonin reuptake inhibitors) in pregnancy found four small prospective studies published since 1993.[24] It found no evidence of increased risk, although the risk of adverse effects cannot be excluded. Decreased birth weights of infants exposed to fluoxetine during the third trimester were identified in one study, and direct drug effects and withdrawal syndromes were identified in some neonates. See harms of tricyclic antidepressants in postnatal depression, p 1796.

Comment: See comment of prescription antidepressant drugs versus placebo option, p 1247.

OPTION SELECTIVE SEROTONIN REUPTAKE INHIBITORS VERSUS OTHER PRESCRIPTION ANTIDEPRESSANT DRUGS

Andrea Cipriani and John Geddes

Three systematic reviews found no significant difference in outcomes with different kinds of antidepressant drug (tricyclic antidepressants, selective serotonin reuptake inhibitors, or monoamine oxidase inhibitors), although one systematic review found that selective serotonin reuptake inhibitors were less effective than venlafaxine in increasing the proportion of people who responded. RCTs in people with major depression found similar response rates at 6 weeks between fluoxetine and reboxetine, but found that reboxetine may be slightly more effective in improving social functioning. One systematic review found that selective serotonin reuptake inhibitors were associated with fewer adverse effects than tricyclic antidepressants, but the difference was small. Another systematic review and one retrospective cohort study found no strong evidence that fluoxetine was associated with increased risk of suicide compared with tricyclic antidepressants or placebo. One RCT and observational data suggested that abrupt withdrawal of selective serotonin reuptake inhibitors was associated with symptoms including dizziness and rhinitis, and that these symptoms are more likely with drugs with a short half life, such as paroxetine. Evidence of publication bias has been found in the RCTs of selective serotonin reuptake inhibitors and the efficacy and safety of these drugs is currently under review by the regulatory authorities in several countries.

Benefits: **Versus tricyclic antidepressants:** We found three systematic reviews[16,25,26] and one subsequent RCT[27] in people with mild to moderate or severe depression**G** comparing selective serotonin reuptake inhibitors [SSRIs] versus tricyclic antidepressants (TCAs). The reviews found no significant difference in overall effectiveness between TCAs and SSRIs.[16,25,26] The first review (search date 1999, 63 RCTs, 6767 people) found no significant difference in overall symptoms between SSRIs and TCAs (mean effect size**G** +0.03, 95% CI –0.02 to +0.09).[25] The second review (search date 1997, 95 RCTs, 10 533 people aged 18–80 years) found that SSRIs may be slightly more acceptable overall than TCAs, as measured by the number of people who withdrew from clinical trials for any cause (RR of withdrawal 0.88, 95% CI 0.83 to 0.93; NNH 26, 95% CI 18 to 46).[26] The third review (search date 1998, 150 RCTs, ≥ 16 000 people with major depression; see comment below) compared newer antidepressants (SSRIs [43 RCTs], MAOIs, and venlafaxine) versus TCAs for at least 6 weeks.[16] Response was defined as a 50% reduction in depression rating scale score or a Clinical Global Impression Scale score of 1 (very much improved) or 2 (much improved). The review found no significant difference between newer antidepressants and TCAs in the proportion of people who responded (54% with newer antidepressants *v* 54% with placebo; RR 1.00, 95% CI 0.97 to 1.06). The results were similar when the analysis was restricted to RCTs conducted in primary care.[20] The subsequent RCT (152 people with major depression) found no significant difference in adherence over 12 weeks between dosulepin (dothiepin) and fluoxetine.[27] However, the RCT is likely to have been underpowered to detect a clinically important difference between treatments. **Versus venlafaxine:** See benefits of venlafaxine, p 1252. **Versus reboxetine:** See benefits of reboxetine, p 1253. **Selective serotonin reuptake inhibitors plus benzodiazepines versus selective serotonin reuptake inhibitors alone:** We found one RCT (50 people aged 18–70 years with moderate to severe depression for at least 1 month and a HAM-D score of 18–26) comparing fluoxetine 20–40 mg daily plus clonazepam 0.5–1 mg daily for 18 weeks versus fluoxetine plus placebo.[28] It found no significant difference between fluoxetine plus clonazepam and fluoxetine alone in the proportion of people who responded at 6 weeks (response defined as Clinical Global Impression Scale score of 1 [very much improved] or 2 [much improved]: 76% with fluoxetine plus clonazepam *v* 56% with fluoxetine alone; reported as non-significant, CI not reported). The RCT is likely to have been underpowered to detect a clinically important difference in outcomes.

Harms: **Common adverse events with selective serotonin reuptake inhibitors versus tricyclic antidepressants:** One systematic review (search date 1996) compared adverse events with SSRIs versus TCAs in people aged 18 years or over with all severities of depression (see table 1, p 1273).[29] It found that about twice as many people taking TCAs compared with SSRIs had dry mouth, constipation, and dizziness but that slightly more people taking SSRIs had nausea, diarrhoea, anxiety, agitation, insomnia, nervousness, and headache. **Suicide with selective serotonin reuptake inhibitors versus tricyclic antidepressants:** One systematic review (search date not reported, 17 RCTs completed by December 1989, 3065 people with depressive disorders aged 12–90 years) compared three interventions: fluoxetine, a TCA, or placebo.[30] It found no significant difference in the rate of suicidal acts between groups (0.3% with fluoxetine *v* 0.4% with TCAs *v* 0.2% with placebo). It found that development of suicidal ideation was significantly less frequent in the fluoxetine group (1% with fluoxetine *v* 3% with placebo; P = 0.04; 1% with fluoxetine *v* 4% with TCAs; P = 0.001). One historical cohort study followed 172 598 people who had at least one prescription for one of 10 antidepressant drugs during the study period in general practice in the UK.[31] It found that the risk of suicide was higher in people who received fluoxetine (19/10 000 person years, 95% CI 9/10 000 person years to 34/10 000 person years) than in those receiving dosulepin (RR of suicide *v* dosulepin 2.1, 95% CI 1.1 to 4.1). In a nested case controlled subgroup analysis in people with no history of suicidal behaviour or previous antidepressant prescription, the risk remained the same, although the confidence interval broadened to make the result non-significant (RR 2.1, 95% CI 0.6 to 7.9). Although the apparent association may be because of residual confounding, there remains uncertainty about the possible association between fluoxetine and suicide. However, any absolute increase in risk is unlikely to be large. **Adverse effects with different selective serotonin reuptake inhibitors:** One large cohort study of people receiving four different SSRIs (fluvoxamine [983 people], fluoxetine [692 people], sertraline [734 people], and paroxetine [13 741 people]) in primary care in the UK found that reports of common adverse events (nausea/vomiting, malaise/lassitude, dizziness, and headache/migraine) varied between SSRIs (fluvoxamine 78/1000 participant months; fluoxetine 23/1000 participant months; RR *v* fluvoxamine 0.29, 95% CI 0.27 to 0.32; paroxetine 28/1000 participant months; RR *v* fluvoxamine 0.35, 95% CI 0.33 to 0.37; sertraline 21/1000 participant months; RR *v* fluvoxamine 0.26, 95% CI 0.25 to 0.28).[32] Only 52% of people responded to the questionnaire, although this response rate was similar for all four drugs. A study of spontaneous reports to the UK Committee on Safety of Medicines found similar safety profiles among the same four SSRIs.[33] **Withdrawal effects with selective serotonin reuptake inhibitors:** We found one RCT in people aged 18 years or over (average 30–40 years) comparing abrupt discontinuation of fluoxetine (96 people) versus continued treatment (299 people) in people who had been taking the drug for 12 weeks.[34] It found that abrupt discontinuation was associated with increased dizziness (7% with abrupt discontinuation *v* 1% with continued treatment), dysmenorrhoea (3% with abrupt discontinuation *v* 0% with continued treatment), rhinitis (10% with abrupt discontinuation *v* 3% with continued treatment), and somnolence (4% with abrupt discontinuation *v* 0% with continued treatment). However, there was a high withdrawal rate in this RCT because of the return of symptoms of depression (39%), so these may be underestimates of the true rate of withdrawal symptoms. Between 1987 and 1995 the rate of spontaneous reports of suspected withdrawal reactions per million defined daily doses to the World Health Organization Collaborating Centre for International Drug Monitoring was higher for paroxetine than for sertraline and fluoxetine.[35] The most common withdrawal effects were dizziness, nausea, paraesthesia, headache, and vertigo. **Adverse events with selective serotonin reuptake inhibitors versus venlafaxine:** See harms of venlafaxine, p 1252. **Versus reboxetine:** See harms of reboxetine, p 1253. **Adverse events with selective serotonin reuptake inhibitors plus benzodiazepines:** The RCT found that 30% of people taking fluoxetine plus clonazepam had decreased appetite.[28] It also found that 28% of people taking fluoxetine alone had headache and 24% had sleep disturbance.

Comment: The second review forms part of a larger review of 315 RCTs in people with depression and we were unable to obtain the full reference list; it is therefore unclear whether it contains RCTs assessed in the other reviews.[16] We found one systematic review (search date 2000, 103 RCTs) that assessed the effects of fluoxetine dose on outcomes in RCTs comparing fluoxetine versus tricyclic, heterocyclic and related antidepressants, SSRIs, and newer antidepressants in people with depression.[36] The review found that the weighted rate of fluoxetine responders was higher in RCTs where fluoxetine was the experimental drug (70%) compared with RCTs where fluoxetine was the control drug (58%), possibly reflecting the use of higher doses of fluoxetine in RCTs where fluoxetine was the experimental drug. The review did not assess the proportion of responders with other antidepressants and did not adjust for possible confounders. See comment of prescription antidepressant drugs versus placebo option, p 1247.

OPTION MONOAMINE OXIDASE INHIBITORS VERSUS OTHER PRESCRIPTION ANTIDEPRESSANT DRUGS

Andrea Cipriani and John Geddes

Three systematic reviews found no significant difference in outcomes with different kinds of antidepressant drug (tricyclic antidepressants, selective serotonin reuptake inhibitors, or monoamine oxidase inhibitors). One systematic review found that monoamine oxidase inhibitors were less effective than tricyclic antidepressants in people with severe depressive disorders. However, the review found that monoamine oxidase inhibitors may be more effective in atypical depressive disorders with biological features such as increased sleep and increased appetite.

Benefits: **Versus tricyclic antidepressants:** We found two systematic reviews.[16,37] The first review (search date 1998, 150 RCTs, ≥16 000 people with major depression) found no significant difference in overall effectiveness between tricyclic antidepressants (TCAs) and newer antidepressants including monoamine oxidase inhibitors (MAOIs; see benefits of selective serotonin reuptake inhibitors, p 1249).[16] The second review (search date not reported, 55 RCTs) compared MAOIs versus TCAs in people aged 18–80 years with mild to moderate or severe depression.[37] It found that MAOIs were less effective than TCAs in people with severe depressive disorders. However, the review found that MAOIs may be more effective in atypical depressive disorders (depressive disorders with reversed biological features, e.g. increased sleep, increased appetite, mood reactivity, and rejection sensitivity).

Harms: **Versus tricyclic antidepressants:** The first review gave no information on adverse effects.[16] The second review found that MAOIs were associated with a similar level of overall adverse effects as were TCAs.[37] Adverse effects associated with MAOIs included hypotension, dizziness, mydriasis, piloerection, oedema, tremor, anorgasmia, and insomnia.

Comment: See comment of prescription antidepressant drugs versus placebo option, p 1247.

OPTION VENLAFAXINE VERSUS OTHER PRESCRIPTION ANTIDEPRESSANT DRUGS

Andrea Cipriani and John Geddes

One systematic review found no significant difference between venlafaxine and tricyclic antidepressants in the proportion of people who responded over 1–12 months and found that venlafaxine increased the proportion of people who responded compared with selective serotonin reuptake inhibitors.

Benefits: **Versus tricyclic antidepressants:** We found one systematic review (search date 2000, 8 RCTs, 1356 people with mild to moderate depression**G**) comparing venlafaxine versus tricyclic antidepressants (TCAs).[38] It found no significant difference between venlafaxine and TCAs in the proportion of people who responded over 1 month to 1 year (response defined as ≥50% reduction on continuous rating scale: OR 1.29, 95% CI 0.89 to 1.85; absolute numbers not reported). **Versus selective serotonin reuptake inhibitors:** We found one systematic review (search date 2000, 20 RCTs, 3844 people with mild to moderate depression) comparing venlafaxine versus selective serotonin reuptake inhibitors.[38] It found that venlafaxine significantly increased the proportion of people who responded over 1 month to 1 year compared with selective serotonin reuptake inhibitors (response defined as ≥50% reduction on continuous rating scale: RR 1.26, 95% CI 1.02 to 1.58).

Harms: **Versus tricyclic antidepressants or selective serotonin reuptake inhibitors:** The review gave no information on adverse effects.[38]

Comment: See comment of prescription antidepressant drugs versus placebo option, p 1247.

OPTION REBOXETINE VERSUS OTHER PRESCRIPTION ANTIDEPRESSANT DRUGS

Andrea Cipriani and John Geddes

Two RCTs, primarily in people with severe depression, found no significant difference in symptoms at 4 weeks between reboxetine and desipramine or imipramine, but results were sensitive to outcome scales used. RCTs in people with major depression found similar response rates at 6 weeks between reboxetine and fluoxetine, and found that reboxetine may slightly improve social functioning.

Benefits: **Versus tricyclic antidepressants:** We found no systematic review, but found two RCTs.[18,39] The first RCT (258 people aged 18–65 years admitted to hospital with severe depression**G**) compared three interventions: reboxetine 4–8 mg daily (84 people), desipramine 100–200 mg daily (89 people), and placebo (84 people). It found no significant difference between reboxetine and desipramine in the proportion of people who responded over 4 weeks if response was assessed by HAM-D scores (response defined as ≥ 50% reduction in HAM-D score: 60% with reboxetine *v* 48% with desipramine; P reported as non-significant, CI not reported). However, it found that reboxetine significantly increased the proportion of people who responded if response was assessed by Clinical Global Impression Scale (CGI) score (response defined as ≥ 50% reduction in CGI: 51% with reboxetine *v* 33% with desipramine; $P < 0.05$). This difference in results when assessed by different scales makes it difficult to assess the clinical importance of the difference in outcomes between reboxetine and desipramine. The second RCT (256 people aged 18–65 years with moderate to severe depression, 80% receiving reboxetine and 72% receiving imipramine with severe depression) compared reboxetine 8–10 mg daily versus imipramine 150 –200 mg daily for 6 weeks.[39] It found that reboxetine significantly improved symptoms at 6 weeks measured by HAM-D score (mean reduction: 15.8 points with reboxetine *v* 14.3 points with imipramine group; mean difference –1.5, 95% CI –1.0 to –4.0) and increased the proportion of people who responded compared with imipramine (response defined as ≥ 50% reduction in HAM-D: 68.5% with reboxetine *v* 56.2% with imipramine; difference 12.3%, 95% CI 0.3% to 24.3%). However, it found no significant difference in Montgomery-Asberg Depression Rating Scale score at 6 weeks (mean reduction: 5.9 with reboxetine *v* 6.0 with imipramine; reported as non-significant, CI not reported). However, it found that reboxetine significantly This makes the results difficult to interpret. **Versus selective serotonin reuptake inhibitors:** We found no systematic review, but found two RCTs.[19,40] The first RCT (168 people aged 18–65 years with major depressive disorder**G** without psychotic features) compared reboxetine 8–10 mg daily versus fluoxetine 20–40 mg daily.[40] It found that a similar proportion of people responded over 6 weeks with reboxetine and fluoxetine (response defined as CGI score of 1 [very much improved] or 2 [much improved]: 78% with reboxetine *v* 76% with fluoxetine; CI not reported). The second RCT (381 people aged 18–65 years with major depressive disorder without psychotic features) assessed the effects of reboxetine 8–10 mg daily, paroxetine 20–40 mg daily, and placebo on social functioning.[19] It found that reboxetine significantly improved mean Social Adaptation Self Evaluation Scale score at 8 weeks compared with fluoxetine (35.3 with reboxetine *v* 31.9 with fluoxetine; $P < 0.05$). The clinical importance of this difference in scores is unclear.

Harms: **Versus tricyclic antidepressants:** The first RCT found that more people taking reboxetine had urinary hesitancy compared with people taking desipramine, although the difference was not significant (11%

with reboxetine *v* 5% with desipramine). However, it found that significantly more people taking desipramine had dry mouth (21% with desipramine *v* 13% with reboxetine), and blurred vision (17% with desipramine *v* 4% with reboxetine; reported as significant, CI not reported).[18] In the second RCT, 81.5% of people taking reboxetine and 81.7% of people taking imipramine had at least one adverse effect.[39] The RCT found that more people taking reboxetine than imipramine had headache, urinary hesitancy, and nausea, but more people taking imipramine had dry mouth, hypotension, insomnia, tachycardia, somnolence, and tremor (CI not reported for any outcome). **Versus selective serotonin reuptake inhibitors:** The first RCT found no significant difference between reboxetine and fluoxetine in the proportion of people who had at least one adverse effect (67.1% with reboxetine *v* 67.4% with fluoxetine; P = 0.307).[40] Adverse events experienced more frequently by people taking reboxetine were dry mouth (34% with reboxetine *v* 9 % with fluoxetine), constipation (21% with reboxetine *v* 7% with fluoxetine), hypotension (19% with reboxetine *v* 8% with fluoxetine), urinary hesitancy (13% with reboxetine *v* 1% with fluoxetine), and paraesthesia (6% with reboxetine *v* 1% with fluoxetine). Adverse effects experienced more frequently by people taking fluoxetine were agitation, nervousness, or anxiety (4% with reboxetine *v* 11% with fluoxetine) and diarrhoea (1% with reboxetine *v* 7% with fluoxetine). The second RCT gave no information on adverse effects.[19]

Comment: **Versus tricyclic antidepressants:** In the RCTs comparing reboxetine, a tricyclic antidepressant, and placebo in people with severe depression,[18,39] the high response rates to tricyclic antidepressants and the low response rates to placebo (20% in one RCT and 35% in the other) contrast with those of a previous study using imipramine and amitriptyline. This suggested that response rates to these antidepressants were lower in people with severe depression than in people with mild to moderate depression**G** (proportion of people defined as good responders 39% with severe depression *v* 67% with mild to moderate depression).[41]

OPTION ST JOHN'S WORT (*HYPERICUM PERFORATUM*)

Andrea Cipriani and John Geddes

Two systematic reviews and one subsequent RCT in people with mild to moderate depressive disorders found that St John's Wort (*H perforatum*) improved depressive symptoms over 4–12 weeks compared with placebo. However, two subsequent RCTs found no significant difference in symptoms at 8 weeks between St John's Wort and placebo. RCTs found no significant difference in symptoms between St John's Wort and prescription antidepressant drugs. The results of the RCTs should be interpreted with caution because many of the RCTs did not use standardised preparations of St John's Wort, and doses of antidepressant drugs varied. One subsequent RCT in people aged over 18 years with major depressive disorder found no significant difference in depressive symptoms at 8 weeks between a standardised preparation of St John's Wort and sertraline, but it is likely to have been underpowered to detect a clinically important difference.

Benefits: **Versus placebo:** We found two systematic reviews[42,43] and three subsequent RCTs.[44–46] Both reviews and one of the subsequent RCTs found that St John's Wort significantly improved symptoms compared with placebo. The first review (search date 1998, 14 RCTs, 1168 people aged > 18 years with mild to moderate depression**G**) compared single preparations of St John's Wort versus placebo.[42] It found that *H perforatum* preparations significantly increased the proportion of people who responded over 4–12 weeks compared with placebo (response defined as a Hamilton Depression Rating Scale (HAM-D) score of < 10 or < 50% reduction in score from baseline; 267/465 [57%] with *H perforatum v* 122/485 [25%] with placebo; RR 2.47, 95% CI 1.69 to 3.61). The second review (search date 2000, 14 RCTs, including 9 RCTs identified by the first review, 2776 people with mild to moderate depression) also found that St John's Wort significantly increased the proportion of people who responded over 4–8 weeks compared with placebo (14 RCTs, 390/690 [57%] with *H perforatum v* 184/646 [28%] with placebo; RR 1.98, 95% CI 1.49 to 2.62).[43] These results did not change when only RCTs that met stricter methodological criteria were combined (6 RCTs: 153/257 [60%] with *H perforatum v* 79/232 [34%] with placebo; RR 1.77, 95% CI 1.16 to 2.70). The review did not state how response was defined. The first subsequent RCT (340 people aged > 18 years with major depressive disorder**G** defined as a total score of ≥ 20 on the HAM-D) compared three interventions: St John's Wort (standardised extract, hypericin 0.12–0.28%, 900–1500 mg daily), sertraline 50–100 mg daily, or placebo.[44] It found no significant difference in the proportion of people who responded at 8 weeks between St John's Wort and placebo (response defined as Clinical Global Impression Scale score of 1 [very much improved] or 2 [much improved] or a HAM-D score of < 8: 24% with St John's Wort *v* 32% with placebo; P = 0.21). The RCT is likely to have been underpowered to detect a clinically important difference between groups.[44] The second subsequent RCT (200 people aged > 18 years with single episode or recurrent major depressive disorder without psychotic features for 4 weeks to 2 years, with a HAM-D score of ≥ 20) compared St John's Wort (standardised extract, composition not specified, 900–1200 mg daily) versus placebo for 8 weeks.[45] It found no significant difference in the proportion of people who responded at 8 weeks (response defined as ≥ 50% reduction in HAM-D score from baseline: 26/98 [26%] with St John's Wort *v* 19/102 [19%] with placebo; P = 0.15). The third subsequent RCT (375 people aged 18–65 years with major depressive disorder for at least 2 weeks, with a HAM-D score of 18–25) compared St John's Wort (extract WS5570, a standardised preparation containing 3–6% hyperforin plus 0.12–0.28% hypericin, 900 mg daily) versus placebo for 6 weeks.[46] It found that St John's Wort significantly increased the proportion of people who responded compared with placebo (response defined as ≥ 50% reduction in HAM-D from baseline: 98/186 [53%] with St John's Wort *v* 80/189 [42%] with placebo; P < 0.05). **Versus tricyclic antidepressants:** We found two systematic reviews.[42,43] The first review (search date 1998, 7 RCTs, 1123 people) compared St John's Wort (single preparations of hypericum [5 RCTs] or combinations of hypericum plus valeriana [2 RCTs]) versus tricyclic antidepressant (TCAs).[42] It found no significant difference in the proportion of people who responded between St John's Wort and TCAs (177/352 [50%] with single preparations *v* 176/339 [52%] with TCAs; RR 1.01, 95% CI 0.87 to 1.16; 88/130 [68%] with combinations *v* 66/132 [50%] with TCAs; RR 1.52, 95% CI 0.78 to 2.94). The second review (search date 2000, 6 RCTs, including 3 RCTs identified by the first review, 1394 people with mild to moderate depression) also found no significant difference in depressive symptoms over 4–6 weeks between St John's Wort and other antidepressants (422/694 [61%] with St John's Wort *v* 423/700 [60%] with other antidepressants; RR 1.00, 95% CI 0.91 to 1.11). These results did not change when only RCTs that met stricter methodological treatment were combined (4 RCTs: 260/440 [59%] with St John's Wort *v* 261/468 [56%] with other antidepressants; RR 1.04, 95% CI 0.94 to 1.15). **Versus selective serotonin reuptake inhibitors:** We found no systematic review but found one RCT (340 people aged > 18 years with major depressive disorder defined as a total score of ≥ 20 on the HAM-D) that compared three interventions: St John's Wort (standardised extract, hypericin

0.12–0.28%, 900–1500 mg daily), sertraline 50–100 mg daily, or placebo.[44] It found no significant difference in the proportion of people who responded at 8 weeks between St John's Wort and sertraline (response defined as Clinical Global Impression Scale score of 1 [very much improved] or 2 [much improved] or a HAM-D score of < 8: 24% with St John's Wort *v* 25% with sertraline; reported as non-significant, CI not reported). The RCT is likely to have been underpowered to detect a clinically important difference between groups.[44] **Older adults:** We found no systematic review or RCTs specifically in older adults.

Harms: Interactions between St John's Wort and antidepressant drugs have been reported, and, because it induces the cytochrome P-450 system, hypericum can also reduce plasma levels or efficacy of various conventional drugs.[47] **Versus placebo or tricyclic antidepressant drugs:** We found three systematic reviews assessing adverse effects of St John's Wort.[42,43,48] The first review (search date 1998) found that adverse events were poorly reported in the trials.[42] Adverse effects were reported by 26% of people taking St John's Wort compared with 45% of people taking TCAs or sedative drugs (RR 0.57, 95% CI 0.47 to 0.69), and by 15% of people taking combinations of hypericum plus valeriana compared with 27% taking amitriptyline or desipramine (RR 0.49, 95% CI 0.23 to 1.04). The second review (search date 2000) found no significant difference in the proportion of people who had adverse effects (including gastrointestinal effects, headaches, restlessness, and fatigue) between St John's Wort and placebo (43/236 [18%] with St John's Wort *v* 29/177 [16%] with placebo; RR 1.04, 95% CI 0.68 to 1.58), and found that St John's Wort significantly reduced the proportion of people with adverse effects compared with TCAs or SSRIs (62/157 [39%] *v* 105/167 [63%]; RR 0.59, 95% CI 0.52 to 0.71).[43] The third review (search date 1997) included RCTs and observational surveillance studies conducted after the marketing of St John's Wort.[48] It found that the most common adverse effects of St John's Wort in the included studies were gastrointestinal symptoms, dizziness/confusion, tiredness/sedation, and dry mouth, although all occurred less frequently with St John's Wort than with TCAs or sedative drugs. Findings from observational studies were consistent with these results. Photosensitivity is theoretically possible; however, only two cases were reported. The first subsequent RCT found that significantly more people taking St John's Wort compared with placebo had diarrhoea, nausea, anorgasmia, forgetfulness, frequent urination, sweating, and swelling ($P < 0.05$ for all outcomes).[44] The second subsequent RCT found that St John's Wort significantly increased headaches compared with placebo (39/95 [41%] with St John's Wort *v* 25/100 [25%] with placebo; $P = 0.02$).[45] The third subsequent RCT found that a similar proportion of people had adverse effects with St John's Wort compared with placebo (57/186 [31%] with St John's Wort *v* 70/189 [37%] with placebo; CI not reported).[46]

Comment: The results of the systematic reviews must be interpreted with caution because the preparations and doses of *H perforatum* and types and doses of antidepressant drugs varied widely.[42,43] RCTs are needed using standardised preparations.

OPTION ELECTROCONVULSIVE THERAPY

Stuart Carney, Rob Butler, and John Geddes

One systematic review in people with moderate to severe depressive disorder, many of whom were inpatients, found that electroconvulsive therapy [ECT] improved symptoms over 1–6 weeks' treatment compared with simulated electroconvulsive therapy or antidepressant drugs. The review found that bilateral ECT improved symptoms compared with unilateral ECT and that high

dose ECT was more effective than low dose. The degree of reported short term cognitive impairment seemed to be inversely related to treatment efficacy. Another systematic review provided insufficient evidence to assess electroconvulsive therapy in older adults. Because ECT may be unacceptable to some people and, because it is a short term treatment, there is consensus that it should normally be reserved for people who cannot tolerate or have not responded to antidepressant drug treatment, although it may be useful when a rapid response is required.

Benefits: We found one systematic review (search date 2001) of electroconvulsive therapy (ECT) in younger and older adults with moderate to severe depression**G**, primarily inpatients.[49] The review used change in symptoms on a continuous scale as the primary outcome measure (see comment below). **Versus simulated ECT:** The review found that ECT significantly improved symptoms compared with simulated ECT at the end of 1–6 weeks' treatment (6 RCTs, 256 people; mean difference in Hamilton Depression [HAM-D] Rating Scale score 9.7, 95% CI 5.7 to 13.5 with ECT *v* simulated ECT). **Versus prescription antidepressant drugs:** The review found that ECT significantly improved symptoms compared with antidepressant drugs (tricyclic antidepressants, monoamine oxidase inhibitors, selective serotonin reuptake inhibitors, phenelzine, and trytophan) over 3–12 weeks (18 RCTs, 1144 people, mean difference in HAM-D Rating Scale score 5.2, 95% CI 1.4 to 8.9). **Different regimens:** The review found that bilateral ECT improved symptoms compared with unilateral ECT (22 RCTs, 1408 people, mean difference in HAM-D score 3.6, 95% CI: 2.2 to 5.2). High dose ECT also significantly improved symptoms compared with low dose (7 RCTs, 342 people, mean difference in HAM-D score 4.1, 95% CI 2.4 to 5.9). The review found no significant difference in outcomes between twice weekly treatment and three times weekly or between brief pulse waveform and sine wave. **Older adults:** We found one systematic review (search date 2000), which identified three RCTs (83 people aged 57–87 years), all of which were of poor quality in that methods of randomisation and assessment of outcomes were unclear.[50] The review stated that no firm conclusions could be drawn about the effects of ECT in older adults.

Harms: The review could not perform a meta-analysis assessing effects on cognitive function because cognitive function was inconsistently assessed.[49] **Versus simulated ECT:** One RCT identified by the review suggested that ECT was more likely to impair cognitive functioning immediately after treatment than simulated ECT, but found no significant difference in cognitive functioning at 6 months. **Versus prescription antidepressant drugs:** One RCT identified by the review found that ECT was more likely to impair cognitive functioning immediately after treatment than antidepressant drug treatment and another RCT found no significant difference in cognitive function. The RCTs are likely to have been underpowered to detect a clinically important difference. The review found that significantly more people taking antidepressant drugs compared with ECT withdrew from treatment (OR 0.41, 95% CI: 0.12 to 0.88). **Different regimens:** Bilateral ECT and high dose ECT were more likely to result in short term cognitive impairment than unilateral ECT and low dose ECT. Data on long term cognitive functioning were limited. **Older adults:** The RCTs identified by the review provided no reliable information on adverse effects.[50]

Comment: To aid interpretation of results, the reviewers calculated standardised weighted mean differences and translated them into mean differences in symptoms on the HAM-D.[49] Many of the RCTs included in the systematic review were small and old. There was substantial clinical heterogeneity among participants (diagnostic criteria used, severity of depression, inpatients and outpatients, previous treatments) and the modes of treatment compared (electrode placement, dose, waveform, frequency of administration, duration of treatment) but the review did not formally assess statistical heterogeneity. Because ECT may be unacceptable to some people and, because it is a short term treatment, there is consensus that it should normally be reserved for people who cannot tolerate or have not responded to antidepressant drug treatment, although it may be useful when a rapid response is required.

OPTION COGNITIVE THERAPY

Simon Hatcher

One systematic review in younger and older adults has found that cognitive therapy improves symptoms compared with no treatment. Three systematic reviews in younger and older adults with mild to moderate depression found that psychological therapies (mainly interpersonal psychotherapy and cognitive therapy) increased the proportion of people who were in remission over 10–34 weeks compared with control (usual care, usual care plus pill placebo, or supportive therapy). These reviews did not report results for cognitive therapy alone compared with control. One systematic review found limited evidence that cognitive therapy was more effective than interpersonal therapy in improving recovery rates but this difference disappeared when low quality studies were excluded or if studies which relied on advertising or similar techniques to recruit people were excluded. One systematic review of poor RCTs in people aged over 55 years with mild to moderate depression found no significant difference in symptoms between psychological treatments (such as cognitive therapy or cognitive behavioural therapy) and no treatment. It also found no significant difference in symptoms between psychological treatments and similar but non-specific attention. RCTs found insufficient evidence to assess the relative efficacy of drug and non-drug treatment in severe depression.

Benefits: We found four systematic reviews (see table 2, p 1274).[51–54] All of the reviews found that cognitive therapy❻ improved symptoms compared with usual care. RCTs found insufficient evidence to assess the relative efficacy of drug and non-drug treatment in severe depression❻ (see comment below). **Older adults:** We found one systematic review of pharmacological and psychological treatments (search date 1995, 14 RCTs of psychological therapies, 587 people, age > 55 years in an outpatient or community setting).[58] It found four RCTs that compared cognitive or behavioural therapy versus no treatment. It found that, combined, cognitive, or behavioural therapy significantly improved symptoms compared with no treatment (mean difference in the Hamilton Depression Rating Scale score –7.3, 95% CI –10.1 to –4.4). It found three RCTs that compared psychodynamic or interpersonal psychotherapy❻ versus no treatment. Combined, it found no significant difference between psychodynamic or interpersonal psychotherapy and no treatment (reported as non-significant, CI not reported).[58]

Harms: Three of the reviews gave no information on adverse effects.[51,52,54] One review stated that reporting of adverse effects in the RCTs it identified was poor, therefore, it could not draw any conclusions about adverse effects of psychological therapies.[53] **Older adults:** The review gave no information on adverse effects.[58]

Comment: Large RCTs are needed in more representative people in a range of clinical settings, including primary care. Because of varying exclusion criteria, the generalisability of the studies is questionable (see table 2, p 1274). Other factors to be considered when psychological treatments are compared with drug treatment include whether serum concentrations of drugs reach therapeutic concentrations, whether changes in medication are allowed (reflecting standard clinical practice), and whether studies reflect the natural course of depressive disorders. It is difficult to conduct studies of psychological treatments for severe depression because of the ethics surrounding withholding a proven treatment (prescription antidepressant drugs) in a group of people at risk of self harm or neglect.[59]

OPTION INTERPERSONAL PSYCHOTHERAPY

Simon Hatcher

Two systematic reviews in younger and older adults with mild to moderate depression found that psychological therapies (mainly interpersonal psychotherapy and cognitive therapy) increased the proportion of people who were in remission over 10–34 weeks compared with control (usual care, usual care plus pill placebo, or supportive therapy). These reviews did not report results for interpersonal therapy alone compared with control. One RCT identified by a third review found that interpersonal therapy increased response rates compared with usual care. One systematic review found limited evidence that interpersonal therapy was less effective than cognitive therapy in improving recovery rates but this difference disappeared when low quality studies were excluded or if studies which relied on advertising or similar techniques to recruit people were excluded. RCTs found insufficient evidence to assess the relative efficacy of drug and non-drug treatment in severe depression.

Benefits: We found three systematic reviews, which found that interpersonal psychotherapy**G** improved symptoms compared with usual care (see table 2, p 1274).[52–54] RCTs found insufficient evidence to assess the relative efficacy of drug and non-drug treatment in severe depression**G** (see comment below). **In older adults:** See benefits of cognitive therapy in psychological treatments option, p 1258.

Harms: Two of the reviews gave no information on adverse effects.[52,54] One review stated that reporting of adverse effects in the RCTs it identified was poor, therefore, it could not draw any conclusions about adverse effects of psychological therapies.[53]

Comment: See comment of cognitive therapy, p 1266.

OPTION NON-DIRECTIVE COUNSELLING

Simon Hatcher

One systematic review in people aged over 18 years with recent onset psychological problems, including depression, found that brief, non-directive counselling in primary care reduced symptom scores in the short term (< 6 months) in people with mild to moderate depression compared with usual care. However, it found no significant difference in scores in the long term (> 6 months). RCTs found insufficient evidence to assess the relative efficacy of drug and non-drug treatment in severe depression.

Benefits: We found one systematic review, which suggested that brief non-directive counselling**G** may improve symptoms over 6 months, although the improvement may not be maintained in the longer term (see table 2, p 1274).[55] RCTs found insufficient evidence to assess the relative efficacy of drug and non-drug treatment in severe depression**G** (see comment below). **In older adults:** We found no RCTs specifically in older adults.

Harms: The systematic review gave no information on adverse effects.[55]

Comment: See comment of cognitive therapy, p 1266.

OPTION PROBLEM SOLVING THERAPY

Simon Hatcher

One systematic review in younger and older adults with mild to moderate depression in primary care found that psychological therapies (including problem solving therapy) improved outcomes compared with usual care. The review did not report results of problem solving therapy alone in people with moderate depression. It found no significant difference between problem solving therapy and usual care in symptoms in people with mild depression or dysthymia. One large subsequent RCT found that problem solving therapy increased the proportion of people who were not depressed at 6 months compared with usual care. However, it found no significant difference at 1 year. Another smaller RCT found no significant difference in symptoms at 8 or 26 weeks between problem solving therapy and usual care. RCTs found insufficient evidence to assess the relative efficacy of drug and non-drug treatment in severe depression.

Benefits: We found one systematic review of psychological therapies, including problem solving therapy**G**,[54] one subsequent[56] and one additional RCT.[57] They provided inconclusive evidence about the effects of problem solving therapy (see table 2, p 1274). RCTs found insufficient evidence to assess the relative efficacy of drug and non-drug treatment in severe depression**G** (see comment below). **In older adults:** We found no RCTs specifically in older adults.

Harms: The review[54] and RCTs[56,57] gave no information on adverse effects.

Comment: See comment of cognitive therapy, p 1266.

OPTION COMBINING PSYCHOLOGICAL TREATMENTS AND ANTIDEPRESSANT DRUGS

Simon Hatcher

One non-systematic review of RCTs in people aged 18–80 years found that, in people with severe depression, adding antidepressant drug treatment to interpersonal psychotherapy or to cognitive therapy improved symptoms compared with either psychological treatment alone. The review found no significant difference in symptoms in people with mild to moderate depression. However, subsequent RCTs in younger and older adults with mild to moderate depression found that combining antidepressant drugs plus psychological treatments improved symptoms more than either antidepressant drugs or psychological treatments alone. One RCT in older adults with mild to moderate depression found that cognitive behavioural therapy plus desipramine improved symptoms more than desipramine alone.

Benefits: We found no systematic review, but found one non-systematic review[59] and three subsequent RCTs.[60–62] The non-systematic review (6 RCTs, 595 people aged 18–80 years with major depression) found that, in more severe depressive disorders, antidepressant drugs plus interpersonal psychotherapy**G** or plus cognitive therapy**G** significantly increased the proportion of people who responded after 16 weeks of treatment compared with interpersonal psychotherapy or cognitive therapy alone (response defined as 4 weeks with Hamilton Depression Rating Scale [HAM-D] score < 7; $P = 0.001$).[59] It found no advantage in combining antidepressant drugs and specific psychological treatments in mild to moderate depressive disorders ($P = 0.10$). The first subsequent RCT (681 adults with chronic major depressive disorder, mean age 43 years) compared three interventions: nefazodone alone, cognitive behavioural therapy**G** alone, or nefazodone plus cognitive behavioural therapy.[60] It found that combined treatment significantly improved the proportion of people with a clinical response compared with either treatment alone (defined as at least 50% reduction in HAM-D score and a score of ≤ 15; 152/226 [67%] with combined treatment *v* 92/220 [42%] with nefazodone alone *v* 90/226 [40%] with psychotherapy alone; combined treatment *v* either single intervention; P < 0.001; NNT 5, 95% CI 3 to 6). The second subsequent RCT (167 people with a major depressive episode) compared antidepressant drugs (fluoxetine, amitriptyline, or moclobemide) plus short term psychodynamic supportive psychotherapy**G** versus antidepressant drugs alone (see comment below).[61] It found that combined treatment significantly increased the proportion of people who had improved after 24 weeks compared with antidepressant drugs (improvement defined as HAM-D score of ≤ 7, Clinical Global Impression Scale score of 1 or 2, Symptom Checklist-90 or Quality of Life Depression Scale score of at least 1 standard deviation from baseline; mean success rate 59% with combined treatment *v* 41% with antidepressants; NNT 5, 95% CI 3 to 11). The third subsequent RCT (707 people aged 18–74 years with dysthymia with or without previous major depressive disorder) compared three treatments: sertraline alone, sertraline plus interpersonal psychotherapy, and interpersonal psychotherapy alone.[62] It found no significant difference between sertraline alone and sertraline plus interpersonal therapy in the proportion of people who responded at 6 months. However, it found that both interventions increased response rates compared with interpersonal psychotherapy alone (response defined as 40% improvement on the Montgomery-Asberg Depression Rating Scale: 60% with sertraline alone *v* 58% with sertraline plus interpersonal psychotherapy *v* 47% with interpersonal psychotherapy alone; P = 0.02 for sertraline or sertraline plus interpersonal psychotherapy *v* interpersonal psychotherapy alone). Similar results were found after a further 18 months' follow up. **Older adults:** We found one RCT (102 people aged > 60 years with major depressive disorder) that compared three interventions: desipramine plus cognitive behavioural therapy, desipramine alone, or cognitive behavioural therapy alone.[63] It found that all three groups showed a significant reduction in symptoms from baseline as assessed using the HAM-D after 16–20 weeks of treatment (reduction: 0.20 with desipramine *v* 0.36 with cognitive behavioural therapy *v* 0.41 with combined treatments; P < 0.05 for all comparisons). It found that combined treatment significantly improved symptoms over 16–20 weeks compared with desipramine alone (P < 0.05). It found no significant difference between combined treatment and cognitive behavioural therapy alone (reported as non-significant, CI not reported). It found no significant difference among groups in the proportion of people who withdrew for any cause (34% with desipramine *v* 23% with cognitive behavioural therapy *v* 33% with combined treatments; P = 0.52).

Harms: The non-systematic review[59] and RCTs[60–63] gave no information on adverse effects.

Comment: A systematic review is needed to address this treatment option. In the second subsequent RCT, 38/167 (23%) people initially randomised refused the proposed treatment: 27/84 (32%) of people offered antidepressant drugs and 11/83 (13%) of people offered combined treatment.[61] This makes the results of the RCT very difficult to interpret.

OPTION BEFRIENDING

Simon Hatcher

One small RCT provided insufficient evidence to assess befriending in people with mild to moderate depression.

Benefits: We found one small RCT (86 women with chronic depression, aged > 18 years, primarily aged 25–40 years) compared befriending**G** versus waiting list control.[64] Initial identification was by postal screening of women registered with, but not attending, primary care and probably with only mild depression. The RCT found that befriending significantly increased the proportion of women with remission of symptoms at 13 months compared with waiting list control (65% with befriending v 39% with control; $P < 0.05$; NNT 4, 95% CI 2 to 18). **Older adults:** We found no systematic review or RCTs specifically in older adults.

Harms: The RCT gave no information on adverse effects.[64]

Comment: In the RCT, 14% of women in the befriending group and 12% of women in the waiting list control group were taking antidepressant drugs.[64] Fewer than half of the women screened by post were interested in befriending as a treatment option.

OPTION BIBLIOTHERAPY

Simon Hatcher

One systematic review of RCTs in younger and older adults recruited by advertisement found limited evidence that bibliotherapy may reduce mild depressive symptoms compared with waiting list control or usual care. It is unclear whether people in the RCTs identified by the review are clinically representative of people with depressive disorders. Another RCT in people with depression found that bibliotherapy may improve symptoms over 2–6 months compared with antidepressant drugs.

Benefits: **Younger and older adults:** We found two systematic reviews (search date not reported[65] and search date 1999[66]). The first review identified six small short term RCTs comparing bibliotherapy**G** versus waiting list control in 273 people (described as adults in 4 RCTs and elderly in 2 RCTs; no age range reported) recruited by advertisement through the media and probably with only mild depression (see comment below).[65] The mean bibliotherapy was 0.82 (95% CI 0.50 to 1.15). This means that 79% of people in the waiting list control group had a worse outcome than the average person in the bibliotherapy group. The second review identified eight randomised and non-randomised trials in younger and older people, but only one of them included people with depression.[66] This RCT found that, compared with antidepressant drugs, bibliotherapy significantly improved symptoms of anxiety over 4 weeks as assessed using the Hamilton Depression Rating Scale. However, it found no significant difference in symptoms of depression at 4 or 12 weeks. **Older adults:** We found no systematic review or RCTs specifically in older adults.

Harms: The reviews gave no information on adverse effects.[65,66]

Comment: The review did not clearly describe the characteristics of the people in the RCTs it identified, and it is unclear whether people were receiving interventions in addition to bibliotherapy.[65] Further RCTs are needed in clinically representative groups.

OPTION EXERCISE

Simon Hatcher

One systematic review in younger and older adults found limited evidence from poor RCTs that exercise may improve symptoms compared with no treatment, and may be as effective as cognitive therapy. One poor RCT in older adults identified by the review found limited evidence that exercise may be as effective as antidepressant drugs in improving symptoms and may reduce relapse over 10 months.

Benefits: We found one systematic review (search date 1999, 14 RCTs, 851 people).[67] It found limited evidence that exercise may improve symptoms compared with no treatment and that exercise may be as effective as cognitive therapy**G**. However, it suggested that these results were inconclusive because of methodological problems in all RCTs included; randomisation was adequately concealed in only three RCTs, intention to treat analysis was undertaken in only two, and assessment of outcome was blinded in only RCT. **Older adults:** The systematic review[67] identified one RCT (156 people with major depression, aged 50–77 years) comparing aerobic exercise, sertraline hydrochloride (a selective serotonin reuptake inhibitor), and combined treatment for 16 weeks.[68] It found no significant difference among groups in the proportion of people who recovered (those no longer meeting criteria for depression or with a Hamilton Depression Rating Scale score < 8: 60% with exercise *v* 69% with sertraline *v* 66% with combined treatment). A 10 month follow up of this RCT found significantly lower relapse rates with exercise than with antidepressant drugs (30% with exercise *v* 52% with sertraline *v* 55% with combined treatment; P = 0.28 for exercise *v* either treatment).[69] However, about half of the people in the medication group engaged in exercise during follow up, making it difficult to draw firm conclusions. The clinical importance of the observed difference at 10 months remains unclear.

Harms: The review gave no information about adverse effects.[67]

Comment: There is a need for a well designed RCT of the effects of exercise in people with all grades of depression assessing clinical outcomes over an adequate time period.

QUESTION What are the effects of interventions in treatment resistant depression?

Rob Butler

OPTION AUGMENTING PRESCRIPTION ANTIDEPRESSANT DRUG TREATMENT WITH LITHIUM

RCTs provided insufficient evidence to assess augmentation of prescription antidepressant drug treatment with lithium in younger and older adults with treatment resistant depression.

Benefits: We found one systematic review[70] and one subsequent RCT.[71] The systematic review (search date 2000, 2 RCTs, 50 people aged 18–75 years with major depression who had not responded to a minimum of 4 weeks of imipramine or equivalent) compared lithium augmentation**G** versus placebo augmentation. It found that lithium augmentation significantly increased the proportion of people who responded over 2 weeks compared with placebo (11/26 [42%] with lithium *v* 4/24 [17%] with placebo; absolute risk difference 25%, 95% CI 2% to 49%; RR not reported). The subsequent RCT (35 people with major depression who had failed to respond to at least 1 earlier trial of antidepressants during the current episode of depression or to 6 weeks' treatment with nortriptyline) compared lithium augmentation versus placebo augmentation.[71] It found no significant difference between lithium augmentation and placebo in the proportion of people who responded over 6 weeks (response defined as ≥ 50% reduction in the HAM-D-17 scores: 2/18 [11%] with lithium *v* 3/17 [18%] with placebo; reported as non-significant, CI not reported).

Harms: The systematic review[70] and subsequent RCT[71] gave no information on adverse effects. For further details about the harms of lithium, see the topic on bipolar disorder, p 1158.

Comment: The review[70] and subsequent RCT[71] are likely to have been underpowered to detect a clinically important difference in outcomes.

OPTION AUGMENTING PRESCRIPTION ANTIDEPRESSANT DRUG TREATMENT WITH PINDOLOL

RCTs provided insufficient evidence to assess augmentation of prescription antidepressant drug treatment with pindolol in younger and older adults with treatment resistant depression.

Benefits: We found one systematic review (search date 2000), which identified three RCTs (106 people aged 18–75 years with major depression who had not responded to a minimum of 4 weeks of imipramine or equivalent) comparing pindolol augmentationⒼ versus placebo augmentation.[70] It found no significant difference in the proportion of people who responded over 1–8 weeks between pindolol augmentation and placebo (10/53 [19%] with pindolol augmentation *v* 6/53 [11%] with placebo; absolute risk difference +8%, 95% CI –6 to +21%; RR not reported). The meta-analysis is likely to have been underpowered to detect a clinically important difference between interventions.

Harms: The systematic review gave no information on adverse effects.[70]

Comment: None.

QUESTION Which interventions reduce relapse rates?

OPTION CONTINUING PRESCRIPTION ANTIDEPRESSANT DRUG TREATMENT

Stuart Carney, Rob Butler and John Geddes

One systematic review found that continuing prescription antidepressant drug treatment after recovery reduced the proportion of people who relapsed over 1–3 years compared with placebo. The effect of continuing antidepressants was independent of the underlying risk of relapse, the duration of treatment before randomisation, or the duration of previous antidepressant treatment. RCTs in people aged over 60 years found that continued treatment with dosulepin (dothiepin) or citalopram after recovery reduced the risk of relapse over 1–2 years compared with placebo, but may increase the risk of ischaemic heart disease.

Benefits: We identified one systematic review (search date 2000, 31 RCTs, 4410 people with first episode or recurrent depression) comparing continuation treatment with prescription antidepressant drugs versus placebo over 12 months in people who had responded to antidepressant treatment over the previous 1 month to 3 years.[72] The review found that, overall, continuing antidepressant drugs in people who had responded to them significantly reduced the proportion of people who relapsed compared with placebo (465/2527 [18%] with continuing antidepressants *v* 1031/2505 [41%] with placebo; OR 0.30, 95% CI 0.22 to 0.38). The review found that, in people who had responded to antidepressants after 2 months' treatment, the number needed to treat by continuing antidepressants to prevent one additional relapse over 6 months was 6 (95% CI: 5 to 8), to prevent relapse over 12 months 5 (95% CI 4 to 6), and over 24–36 months 4 (95% CI 3 to 7). The review found that relapse was most likely to occur in the first 12 months after discontinuation of antidepressants (relapse over 12 months: 19% with continuing antidepressants v 60% with placebo), but the benefits of continuing were apparent for up to 36 months (relapse over 24–36 months: 10% with continuing antidepressants v 29% with placebo). **Older adults:** We found two RCTs.[73,74] The first RCT (69 people aged > 60 years with mild to moderate or severe depression**G** who had recovered sufficiently and consented to enter a 2 year trial of continuation treatment**G**), which compared dosulepin (dothiepin) versus placebo.[73] It found that dosulepin significantly reduced the risk of relapse over 2 years after recovery compared with placebo (RR 0.45, 95% CI 0.22 to 0.96). The second RCT (121 people aged > 64 years with major depression who had responded to citalopram 20–40 mg for 8 weeks and who continued to receive the dose they had responded to for a further 16 weeks) compared citalopram versus placebo for 48 weeks or more.[74] It found that citalopram significantly reduced the proportion of people who relapsed after recovery over 48 weeks compared with placebo (19/60 [32%] with citalopram v 41/61 [67%] with placebo; HR 0.32, 95% CI 0.19 to 0.56).

Harms: Adverse effects seem to be similar to those reported in trials of acute treatment.[72] The review found that significantly more people continuing prescription antidepressant drugs withdrew from the trials compared with people taking placebo (18% with antidepressants v 15% with placebo; OR 1.30, 95% CI 1.07 to 1.59). Six people continuing antidepressant drugs committed suicide (5/767 [0.7%] taking maprotiline and 1/185 [0.5%] taking sertraline) compared with one person taking placebo (OR 5.96; 95% CI: 0.72 to 49.47). **Older adults:** The first RCT gave no information on adverse effects.[73] However, a case control study found that, after adjustment for confounding factors and the use of other antidepressants, people who had taken dosulepin were significantly more likely to develop ischaemic heart disease than those who had not (OR 1.67, 95% CI 1.17 to 2.36).[75] The second RCT found that, compared with placebo, continuing citalopram significantly increased sweating (4/60 [7%] with citalopram v 3/61 [5%] with placebo), tremor (3/60 [5%] with citalopram v 0/61 [0%] with placebo), and fatigue (10/60 [17%] with citalopram v 6/61 [10%] with placebo; reported as significant for all outcomes, CI not reported).[74]

Comment: None.

OPTION COGNITIVE THERAPY

Simon Hatcher

One systematic review in younger and older adults with mild to moderate depression found limited evidence by combining relapse rates across different RCTs that cognitive therapy may reduce the risk of relapse over 1–2 years after stopping treatment compared with antidepressant drugs. One small RCT found that, in people with residual depressive symptoms after antidepressant drug treatment, cognitive therapy for 2 years after the initial depressive episode reduced relapse rates compared with continuing antidepressant drugs. We found no systematic review or RCTs specifically in older adults.

Benefits: **Versus antidepressant drugs:** We found one systematic review (search date not reported) comparing cognitive therapy**G** versus antidepressant drugs in people with mainly mild to moderate depressive disorders.[51] The review identified eight small RCTs (261 people, mean age 39.3 years) that assessed long term (1–2 year) relapse rates after treatment had stopped. Relapse was defined as a return of depressive symptoms (Beck Depression Inventory Score > 16) at 6–9 months after a 2 month remission. It found limited evidence by combining relapse rates across different RCTs that, overall, 30% of people treated with cognitive therapy relapsed compared with 60% of those treated with either antidepressant drugs or antidepressant drugs plus cognitive therapy. We also found one RCT (40 people) comparing cognitive therapy versus usual care (antidepressant drugs) in people who had largely responded to antidepressant drugs but had some residual depressive symptoms.[76] It found that, at 2 years, fewer people relapsed with continued cognitive therapy than with antidepressant drugs. **Older adults:** We found no systematic review or RCTs specifically in older adults.

Harms: See harms of antidepressant drugs, p 1246.

Comment: The review did not present information on the proportion of people who recovered and continued to remain well after 2 years.[51] The largest RCT identified by the review found that only a fifth of people remained well over 18 months' follow up, and that there were no significant differences between interpersonal psychotherapy**G**, cognitive therapy, or drug treatment.[51] Further large scale comparative studies are needed of the long term effectiveness of treatments in people with all severities of depressive disorders.

OPTION RELAPSE PREVENTION PROGRAMME

Jonathan Price

One large RCT in people who had recovered after 8 weeks of antidepressant treatment found that a relapse prevention programme improved depressive symptoms over 1 year compared with usual care. However, it found no significant difference in relapse rates.

Benefits: We found one systematic review,[77] which identified one RCT.[78] The RCT (386 people aged > 18 years with recurrent major depression or dysthymia who had largely recovered after 8 weeks of antidepressant treatment) compared a relapse prevention programme (2 primary care visits and 3 telephone calls) versus usual care for 1 year.[78] It found that relapse prevention significantly improved depressive symptoms over 1 year compared with usual care (results presented graphically; P = 0.04). However, it found no significant difference in relapse rates (35% in both groups). **Older adults:** We found no systematic review or RCTs specifically in older adults.

Harms: The RCT gave no information on adverse effects.[78]

Comment: None.

QUESTION What are the effects of interventions to improve delivery of treatments?

OPTION CARE PATHWAYS

Rob Butler, Jonathan Price, and Michael Von Korff

One systematic review and four subsequent RCTs in people aged over 18 years with mild to moderate or major depression found that the effectiveness of treatment for depression (antidepressant drugs or cognitive behavioural therapy) may be improved by several care pathways, including collaborative working between primary care clinicians and psychiatrists, intensive patient education, case management, and telephone support. They also found that that clinical practice guidelines and educational strategies without other organisational processes improved neither detection nor outcome of

depression compared with usual care. One RCT in people aged over 60 years with major depression, dysthymic depression, or both, treated in a variety of primary care clinics found that collaborative care was more effective than usual care in reducing depressive symptoms.

Benefits: We found one systematic review (search date 2002, 27 RCTs, total number of people not reported),[77] four subsequent RCTs,[79–82] and one extended follow up of an RCT included in the review.[83] Most of the interventions in the RCTs included in the review consisted of two or more components delivered in people with mild to moderate depression**G**.[77] Individual components of care pathways included patient education; shared case management**G** between primary care physician, psychiatrist, and psychologist (collaborative care); provision of written or audiovisual materials for people with depression; active follow up**G**; active response to results of follow up**G**; group psychoeducation; patient checklists; clinician education or care guidelines for clinicians; use of patient centred, motivational approaches**G**, and pharmacy feedback. The review did not perform any meta-analyses. It was unable to determine which individual components of care pathways were effective. However, it suggested that care pathways that included elements of nurse delivered case management, clinician education, and collaborative working improved outcomes compared with usual care. It also suggested that care guidelines for clinicians did not improve outcomes unless they were accompanied by interventions such as case management. An extended follow up of an RCT included in the review compared continuing case management delivered by nurses between 7 and 24 months after starting treatment for major depression versus usual care. It found that, at 24 months, AR for remission was significantly greater in the continuing case management group than the usual care group (74% with continuing case management *v* 41% with usual care; ARR 33%, 95% CI 7% to 46%).[83] The first subsequent RCT (240 women aged 30–60 years with major depressive disorder) compared collaborative care versus usual care.[79] Collaborative care involved a health worker (nurse or social worker) who lead nine sessions of group psychoeducation, monitored adherence to antidepressant drugs, and carried out regular follow up to refer the person to their primary care physician if symptoms worsened or adjust antidepressant drug treatment.[79] The RCT found that collaborative care significantly increased the proportion of people who responded over 6 months (response defined as Hamilton Depression Rating Scale score < 8; 73/104 [70%] with collaborative care *v* 32/107 [30%] with usual care; OR 5.52, 95% CI 3.06 to 9.95; NNT 3, 95% CI 2 to 4).The second subsequent RCT (354 people aged 40–70 years with major depression or dysthymia) compared collaborative care versus usual care.[80] Collaborative care involved a team (including a clinical psychologist, psychiatrist, social worker, and an assistant) who met to develop a treatment plan and conduct 6 and 12 week evaluations of each person. Usual care involved co-ordination of care by the primary care provider alone. The RCT found that people receiving collaborative care had a significantly greater reduction in symptoms from baseline at 3 months compared with people receiving usual care (mean reduction in Symptom Checklist 20 [SCL-20] scores: 0.34 with collaborative care *v* 0.14 with usual care; P < 0.025). However, it found no significant difference in symptoms at 9 months (0.41 with collaborative care *v* 0.25 with usual care; P = 0.17).[80] The third subsequent RCT (1356 people with major depressive disorder or dysthymia, 1073 with co-morbid medical conditions) compared treatment quality improvement programmes versus usual care.[81] The treatment quality improvement programmes involved a nurse specialised in care of people with depression who provided education and case management, individual or group cognitive therapy**G** of each person with depression, and education of primary care providers. The RCT found that, in people with comorbid medical conditions, treatment quality improvement programmes significantly reduced the proportion of people who remained depressed at 12 months compared with usual care (depression defined by major depressive disorder criteria: 45% with quality improvement *v* 55% with usual care; P = 0.01). In people without comorbid medical conditions, it found no significant difference between treatment quality improvement and usual care in the proportion of people who remained depressed, although fewer people receiving quality improvement remained depressed (29% with quality improvement *v* 38% with usual care; P = 0.17). The fourth subsequent RCT (199 people with major depression, 39% Spanish speaking, all with low income) compared 12 sessions of group cognitive behavioural therapy**G** (CBT) plus case management versus CBT alone over 6 months.[82] It reported results for Spanish and English speakers separately, having found a significant effect of language on outcome, but did not report combined results. It found that more Spanish speaking people had improved symptoms at 4 and 6 months with case management plus CBT compared with CBT alone (mean Beck Depression Inventory Score at 6 months: 19 with CBT plus case management *v* 22 with CBT alone; CI not reported). It found no significant difference in symptoms at 6 months in English speaking people (mean Beck Depression Inventory Score at 6 months: 18 with CBT plus case management *v* 25 with CBT alone; reported as non-significant, CI not reported). **Older adults:** We found one RCT (1801 people aged ≥ 60 years with major depressive disorder) compared collaborative care versus usual care.[84] Collaborative care involved a depression care manager (nurse or psychologist) who offered education, assisted in preparing a treatment plan, and either managed the person's antidepressant regimen alongside their primary care physician or gave 6–8 session of problem solving therapy**G** for each person. Eighty per cent of people received antidepressants and 30% received problem solving therapy. The RCT found that, compared with usual care (including antidepressant drugs), the addition of collaborative care significantly increased the proportion of people who responded over 12 months (response defined as ≥ 50% reduction in depressive symptoms on the Symptom Checklist-90: 398/889 [45%] with collaborative care *v* 167/870 [19%] with usual care; OR 3.45, 95% CI 2.71 to 4.38).[84]

Harms: The review and subsequent RCTs gave no information about adverse effects.[77,79–82,84]

Comment: None.

GLOSSARY

Active follow up involves intensive follow up to assess adherence to the prescribed treatment, whether symptoms are improving, and whether any adverse effects are tolerable. Patient checklists may be used, which include details of depression symptom scores, early warning signs of depression, and adherence to antidepressant medication. Alternatively, follow up may be face to face, or by telephone.

Active response to results of follow up involves proactively adjusting the treatment plan if a person with depression is not improving, is not adhering to treatment, or is having intolerable adverse effects. These adjustments may include changing the medicine or its dose, adding another form of treatment, or obtaining a specialist psychiatric opinion.

Augmentation involves adding a medication to enhance the effects of another.

Befriending involves a person who is not depressed meeting the person with depression to talk and socialise for at least 1 hour a week, acting as a friend.

Bibliotherapy Advising people to read written material such as *Feeling good: the new mood therapy* by David Burns (New York: New American Library, 1980).

Brief, non-directive counselling Helping people to express feelings and clarify thoughts and difficulties; therapists suggest alternative understandings and do not give direct advice but try to encourage people to solve their own problems.

Case management involves assigning a care manager to each person with depression, who co-ordinates the package of augmented care. The care manager may be a medical staff member, a practice nurse, a clinical psychologist, or a graduate mental health worker.

Cognitive behavioural therapy Brief (20 sessions over 12–16 weeks) structured treatment, incorporating elements of cognitive therapy and behavioural therapy. Behavioural therapy is based on learning theory and concentrates on changing behaviour. It requires a highly trained therapist.

Cognitive therapy Brief (20 sessions over 12–16 weeks) structured treatment aimed at changing the dysfunctional beliefs and negative automatic thoughts that characterise depressive disorders. It requires a highly trained therapist.

Continuation treatment Continuation of treatment after successful resolution of a depressive episode to prevent relapse.

Dysthymic disorder Characterised by at least 2 years of depressed mood for more days than not, accompanied by additional symptoms that do not reach the criteria for major depressive disorder.

Effect size This expresses the degree of overlap between the range of scores in the control and experimental groups. The effect size can be used to estimate the proportion of people in the control group who had a poorer outcome than the average person in the experimental group; a proportion of 50% or less indicates that the treatment has no effect.

Interpersonal psychotherapy Standardised form of individual brief psychotherapy (usually 12–16 weekly sessions) primarily intended for outpatients with unipolar depressive disorders without psychotic features. It focuses on improving the person's interpersonal functioning and identifying the problems associated with the onset of the depressive episode.

Major depressive disorder Characterised by one or more major depressive episodes (i.e. at least 2 weeks of depressed mood or loss of interest accompanied by at least 4 additional symptoms of depression).

Mild to moderate depression Characterised by depressive symptoms and some functional impairment.

Problem solving therapy Consists of three stages: (1) identifying the main problems for the person, (2) generating solutions, and (3) trying out the solutions. Potentially briefer and simpler than cognitive therapy and may be feasible in primary care.

Psychodynamic supportive psychotherapy Aims to facilitate change by detecting and resolving underlying psychological conflicts. The treatment aims to be less challenging by incorporating supportive elements.

Severe depression Characterised by agitation or psychomotor retardation in addition to depressive symptoms and functional impairment with marked somatic symptoms. Treatments are considered to have been assessed in severe depression if the RCT included inpatients.

Use of patient centred, motivational approaches involves encouraging people to actively participate in their own care. Booklets or videos may be made available for patients and carers, which deliver information about the illness, its prognosis, its treatment, and simple cognitive and behavioural self treatment approaches. One or more professionals may deliver group teaching sessions on depression and how to recover.

REFERENCES

1. American Psychiatric Association. *Diagnostic and statistical manual of mental disorders*, 4th ed. Washington, DC: American Psychiatric Association, 1994.
2. World Health Organization. *The ICD-10 classification of mental and behavioural disorders*. Geneva: World Health Organization, 1992.
3. World Psychiatric Association. Symposium on therapy resistant depression. *Pharmacother Bull* 1974;21:705–706.
4. Rosenstein, Leslie D. Differential diagnosis of the major progressive dementias and depression in middle and late adulthood: a summary of the literature of the early 1990s. *Neuropsychol Rev* 1998;8:109–167.
5. Katon W, Schulberg H. Epidemiology of depression in primary care. *Gen Hosp Psychiatry* 1992;14:237–247.
6. Murray CJ, Lopez AD. Regional patterns of disability-free life expectancy and disability-adjusted life expectancy: global burden of disease study. *Lancet* 1997;349:1347–1352.
7. Murray CJ, Lopez AD. Alternative projections of mortality and disability by cause 1990–2020: global burden of disease study. *Lancet* 1997;349:1498–1504.

8. Beekman AT, Copeland JR, Prince MJ. Review of community prevalence of depression in later life. *Br J Psychiatry* 1999;174:307–311.
9. Judd LL, Akiskal HS, Maser JD, et al. A prospective 12 year study of subsyndromal and syndromal depressive symptoms in unipolar major depressive disorders. *Arch Gen Psychiatry* 1988;55:694–700.
10. Cole MG, Bellavance F, Mansour A. Prognosis of depression in elderly community and primary care populations: a systematic review and meta-analysis. *Am J Psychiatry* 1999;156:1182–1189. Search date 1996; primary sources Medline 1981–1996, Psychinfo 1984–1996, and hand searches of the bibliographies of relevant articles.
11. Saz P, Dewey ME. Depression, depressive symptoms and mortality in persons aged 65 and older living in the community: a systematic review of the literature. *Int J Geriatr Psychiatry* 2001;16:622–630. Search date 1999; primary sources Embase, Medline, personal files, and hand searches of reference lists.
12. Joffe R, Sokolov S, Streiner D. Antidepressant treatment of depression: a meta-analysis. *Can J Psychiatry* 1996;41:613–616. Search date 1995; primary source Medline.
13. Lima MS, Moncrieff J. Drugs versus placebo for dysthymia. In: The Cochrane Library, Issue 2, 2003. Oxford: Update Software. Search date 1997; primary sources Biological Abstracts, Medline, Psychlit, Embase, Lilacs, The Cochrane Library, personal communication, conference abstracts, unpublished trials from the pharmaceutical industry, and book chapters on the treatment of depression.
14. Gill D, Hatcher S. Antidepressants for depression in medical illness. In: The Cochrane Library, Issue 2, 2003. Oxford: Update Software. Search date 1998; primary sources Medline, Cochrane Library Trials Register, Cochrane Depression and Neurosis Group Trials Register, and hand searches of two journals and reference lists.
15. Furukawa TA, McGuire H, Barbui C. Meta-analysis of effects and side effects of low dosage tricyclic antidepressants in depression: systematic review. *BMJ* 2002;325:991–999. Search date 2000; primary sources Cochrane Collaboration Depression, Anxiety and Neurosis Controlled Trials Register, Medline, Embase, Cinahl, Psychinfo, Psychindex, Lilacs, and hand searches.
16. Williams JW, Mulrow CD, Chiquette E, et al. A systematic review of newer pharmacotherapies for depression in adults: evidence report summary: clinical guidelines, Part 2. *Ann Intern Med* 2000;132:743–756. Search date 1998; primary sources Cochrane Collaboration Depression, Anxiety and Neurosis Group's Specialized Registry of Clinical Trials, Medline, Embase, Psychlit, Lilacs, Psychindex, Sigle, Cinahl, Biological Abstracts, The Cochrane Library, hand searches, contacts with pharmaceutical companies, and consultation with experts.
17. Versiani M, Amin M, Chouinard G. Double-blind, placebo-controlled study with reboxetine in inpatients with severe major depressive disorder. *J Clin Psychopharmacol* 2000;20:28–34.
18. Ban TA, Gaszner P, Aguglia E, et al. Clinical efficacy of reboxetine: a comparative study with desipramine, with methodological considerations. *Human Psychopharmacol* 1998;13:S29–S39.
19. Dubini A, Bosc M, Polin V. Noradrenaline-selective versus serotonin-selective antidepressant therapy: differential effects on social functioning. *J Psychopharmacol* 1997;11:S17–S23.
20. Mulrow CD, Williams JW, Chiqueete E, et al. Efficacy of newer medications for treating depression in primary care patients. *Am Med J* 2000;108:54–64. Search date 1998; primary sources Cochrane Depression Anxiety and Neurosis Group Specialised Register of Clinical Trials, hand searches of trials and 46 pertinent meta-analyses, and consultation with experts.
21. Wilson K, Mottram P, Sivanranthan A, et al. Antidepressants versus placebo for the depressed elderly. In: The Cochrane Library, Issue 2, 2003. Oxford: Update Software. Search date 2000; primary sources Psychlit, Medline, Embase, Cinahl, Cochrane Controlled Trials register, Cochrane CollaborationDepression, Anxiety and Neurosis Controlled Trials Register, and hand searches.
22. Stewart LA, Parmar MK. Bias in the analysis and reporting of randomized controlled trials. *Int J Technol Assess Health Care* 1996;12:264–275.
23. Furukawa TA, Streiner DL, Young LT. Antidepressant and benzodiazepine for major depression. In: The Cochrane Library, Issue 2, 2003. Oxford: Update Software. Search date 1999; primary sources Medline, Embase, International Pharmaceutical Abstracts, Biological Abstracts, Lilacs, Psychlit, The Cochrane Library, Cochrane Depression, Anxiety and Neurosis Group Trial Register, Scisearch, hand searches of reference lists, and personal contacts.
24. Wisner KL, Gelenberg AJ, Leonard H, et al. Pharmacologic treatment of depression during pregnancy. *JAMA* 1999;282:1264–1269. Search date 1999; primary sources Medline, Healthstar, hand searches of bibliographies of review articles, and discussions with investigators in the field.
25. Geddes JR, Freemantle N, Mason J, et al. Selective serotonin reuptake inhibitors (SSRIs) for depression. In: The Cochrane Library, Issue 2, 2003. Oxford: Update Software. Search date 1999; primary sources Medline, Embase, Cochrane Group Register of Controlled Trials, hand searches of reference lists of all located studies, and contact with manufacturers.
26. Anderson IM. Selective serotonin reuptake inhibitors versus tricyclic antidepressants: a meta-analysis of efficacy and tolerability. *J Affect Disord* 2000;58:19–36. Search date 1997; primary sources Medline, and hand searches of reference lists of meta-analyses and reviews.
27. Thompson C, Peveler RC, Stephenson D, et al. Compliance with antidepressant medication in the treatment of major depressive disorder in primary care: a randomized comparison of fluoxetine and a tricyclic antidepressant. *Am J Psychiatry* 2000;157:338–343.
28. Smith WT, Londborg PD, Glaudin V, et al. Is extended clonazepam cotherapy of fluoxetine effective for outpatients with major depression? *J Affect Disord* 2002;70:251–259.
29. Trindade E, Menon D. *Selective serotonin reuptake inhibitors (SSRIs) for major depression. Part I. Evaluation of the clinical literature*. Ottawa: Canadian Coordinating Office for Health Technology Assessment, 1997 August Report 3E. *Evidence-based Mental Health* 1998;1:50. Search date 1996; primary sources Medline, Embase, Psychinfo, International Pharmaceutical Abstracts, Pascal, Health Planning and Administration, Mental Health Abstracts, Pharmacoeconomics and Outcomes News, Current Contents databases, scanning bibliographies of retrieved articles, hand searches of journals, and contact with researchers.
30. Beasley CM Jr, Dornseif BE, Bosomworth JC, et al. Fluoxetine and suicide: a meta-analysis of controlled trials of treatment for depression. *BMJ* 1991;303:685–692. Search date not reported, but included trials that had been completed/analysed by December 1989; primary sources not given in detail but based on clinical report form data from trials and data from the Drug Experience Network Database.
31. Jick SS, Dean AD, Jick H. Antidepressants and suicide. *BMJ* 1995;310:215–218.
32. Mackay FJ, Dunn NR, Wilton LV, et al. A comparison of fluvoxamine, fluoxetine, sertraline and paroxetine examined by observational cohort studies. *Pharmacoepidemiol Drug Safety* 1997;6:235–246.
33. Price JS, Waller PC, Wood SM, et al. A comparison of the post marketing safety of four selective serotonin reuptake inhibitors including the investigation of symptoms occurring on withdrawal. *Br J Clin Pharmacol* 1996;42:757–763.
34. Zajecka J, Fawcett J, Amsterdam J, et al. Safety of abrupt discontinuation of fluoxetine: a randomised, placebo controlled study. *J Clin Psychopharmacol* 1998;18:193–197.

35. Stahl MM, Lindquist M, Pettersson M, et al. Withdrawal reactions with selective serotonin reuptake inhibitors as reported to the WHO system. *Eur J Clin Pharmacol* 1997;53:163–169.
36. Barbui C, Hotopf M, Garattini S. Fluoxetine dose and outcome in antidepressant drug trials. *Eur J Clin Pharmacol* 2002;58:379–386. Search date 2000; primary sources Cochrane Collaboration Depression, Anxiety and Neurosis Controlled Trials Register, Cochrane Controlled Trials Register, Medline, and Embase.
37. Thase ME, Trivedi MH, Rush AJ. MAOIs in the contemporary treatment of depression. *Neuropsychopharmacology* 1995;12:185–219. Search date not reported; primary sources Medline and Psychological Abstracts.
38. Smith D, Dempster C, Glanville J, et al. Efficacy and tolerability of venlafaxine compared with selective serotonin reuptake inhibitors and other antidepressants: a meta-analysis. *Br J Psychiatry* 2002;180:396–404. Search date 2000; primary sources an existing database (Eccles et al, 2000), Medline, Embase, Biosis, Psychlit, National research Register, Healthstar, Sigle, Cochrane Database of Systematic Reviews, Dare, Cochrane Controlled Trials Register and Current Controlled Trials, hand searches, and contacts with authors and study sponsors for unpublished data.
39. Berzewski H, Van Moffaert M, Gagiano CA. Efficacy and tolerability of reboxetine compared with imipramine in a double-blind study in patients suffering from major depressive episodes. *Eur Neuropsychopharmacol* 1997;7:S37–S47.
40. Massana J, Moller HJ, Burrows GD, et al. Reboxetine: a double-blind comparison with fluoxetine in major depressive disorder. *Int Clin Psychopharmacol* 1999;14:73–80.
41. Kocsis JH, Croughan JL, Katz MM, et al. Response to treatment with antidepressants of patients with severe or moderate nonpsychotic depression and of patients with psychotic depression. *Am J Psychiatry* 1990;147:621–624.
42. Linde K, Mulrow CD. St John's Wort for depression. In: The Cochrane Library, Issue 2, 2003. Oxford: Update Software. Search date 1998; primary sources Medline, Embase, Psychlit, Psychindex, specialised databases: Cochrane Complementary Medicine Field, Cochrane Depression and Neurosis CRG, Phytodok, hand searches of references of pertinent articles, and contact with manufacturers and researchers.
43. Whiskey A, Werneke U, Taylor D. A systematic review and meta-analysis of *Hypericum perforatum* in depression: a comprehensive clinical review. *Int Clin Psychopharmacol* 2001;16:239–252. Search date 2000; primary sources (in English or German) Medline, Embase, and hand searches of references of primary studies.
44. Davidson JRT, Gadde KM, Fairbank JA. Effect of *Hypericum perforatum* (St John's Wort) in major depressive disorder: a randomized controlled trial. *JAMA* 2002;287:1807–1814.
45. Shelton RC, Keller MB, Gelenberg A, et al. Effectiveness of St. John's wort in major depression: a randomized controlled trial. *JAMA* 2001;285:1978–1986.
46. Lecrubier Y, Clerc G, Didi R, et al. Efficacy of St. John's wort extract WS 5570 in major depression: a double-blind, placebo-controlled trial. *Am J Psychiatry* 2002;159:1361–1366.
47. De Smet P. Drug therapy: herbal remedies. *New Engl J Med* 2002;347:2046–2056.
48. Ernst E, Rand JI, Barnes J, et al. Adverse effects profile of the herbal antidepressant St. John's Wort (*Hypericum perforatum L*). *Eur J Clin Pharmacol* 1998;54:589–594. Search date 1997; primary sources Amed, The Cochrane Library 1997 Issue 2, Embase, Medline, hand searches of reference lists, contact with WHO Collaborating Centre for International Drug Monitoring, UK Committee on Safety of Medicines, and German Bundesinstitut für Arzneimittel und Medizinproducte plus 12 German manufacturers of hypericum products.
49. UK ECT Review Group. The efficacy and safety of electroconvulsive therapy in depressive disorders: a systematic review and meta-analysis. *Lancet* 2003;361:799–808.
50. Van der Wurff FB, Stek ML, Hoogendijk WL, et al. Electroconvulsive therapy for the depressed elderly. In: The Cochrane Library, Issue 2, 2003. Oxford: Update Software. Search date 2000, primary sources Cochrane Collaboration Depression, Anxiety and Neurosis Controlled Trials Register, Medline, Embase, Biological Abstracts, Cinahl, Lilacs, Psychlit, and hand searches of reference lists of relevant papers and of *Journal of ECT* and the *Journal of Geriatric Psychiatry*.
51. Gloaguen V, Cottraux J, Cucherat M, et al. A meta-analysis of the effects of cognitive therapy in depressed people 1998. *J Affect Disord* 1998;49:59–72. Search date not reported; primary sources Medline, Embase, references in books and papers, previous reviews and meta-analyses, abstracts from congress presentations, and preprints sent by authors.
52. Casacalenda N, Perry JC, Looper K. Remission in major depressive disorder: a comparison of pharmacotherapy, psychotherapy, and control conditions. *Am J Psychiatry* 2002;159:1354–1360.
53. Churchill R, Hunot V, Corney R et al. A systematic review of controlled trials of the effectiveness and cost-effectiveness of brief psychological treatments for depression. *Health Technol Assess* 2001;5:1–173. Search date not reported; primary sources Medline, Psychinfo, Embase, Science Scisearch, Social Scisearch, and Cochrane Collaboration Controlled Trials Register.
54. van Schaik DJ, van Marwijk HW, van der Windt DA, et al. Effectiveness of psychotherapy for depressive disorder in primary care. A systematic review. *Tijdschrift voor Psychiatrie* 2002;44:609–619. [In Dutch]
55. Bower P, Rowland N, Hardy R. The clinical effectiveness of counselling in primary care: a systematic review and meta-analysis. *Psychol Med* 2003:33:203–215. An update of the Bower et al Cochrane Review; 7 RCTs, 824 patients; search date not reported.
56. Dowrick C, Dunn G, Ayuso-Mateos JL, et al. Problem solving treatment and group psychoeducation for depression: multicentre randomised controlled trial. *BMJ* 2000;321:1450–1454.
57. Mynors-Wallis L, Davies I, Gray A, et al. A randomised controlled trial and cost analysis of problem-solving treatment for emotional disorders given by community nurses in primary care. *Br J Psychiatry* 1997;170:113–119.
58. McCusker J, Cole M, Keller E, et al. Effectiveness of treatments of depression in older ambulatory people. *Arch Intern Med* 1998;158:705–712. Search date 1995; primary sources Medline, Psychinfo, and hand searches of references.
59. Thase ME, Greenhouse JB, Frank E, et al. Treatment of major depression with psychotherapy or psychotherapy–pharmacotherapy combinations. *Arch Gen Psychiatry* 1997;54:1009–1015. Pooled results of six research protocols conducted in 1982–1992 at the Mental Health Clinical Research Center, University of Pittsburgh School of Medicine.
60. Keller MB, McCullough JP, Klein DN, et al. A comparison of nefazodone, the cognitive behavioral-analysis system of psychotherapy, and their combination for the treatment of chronic depression. *N Engl J Med* 2000;342:1462–1470.
61. De Jonghe F, Kool S, van Aalst G, Dekker J, Peen J. Combining psychotherapy and antidepressants in the treatment of depression. *J Affect Disord* 2001;64:217–229.
62. Browne G, Steiner M, Roberts J, et al. Sertraline and/or interpersonal psychotherapy for patients with dysthymic disorder in primary care: 6-month comparison with longitudinal 2-year follow-up of effectiveness and costs. *J Affect Disord* 2002;68:317–330.
63. Thompson LW, Coon DW, Gallagher-Thompson D, et al. Comparison of desipramine and cognitive

behavioural therapy in the treatment of elderly outpatients with mild-to-moderate depression. *Am J Geriatr Psychiatry* 2001;9:225–240.
64. Harris T, Brown GW, Robinson R. Befriending as an intervention for chronic depression among women in an inner city: randomised controlled trial. *Br J Psychiatry* 1999;174:219–224.
65. Cuijpers P. Bibliotherapy in unipolar depression: a meta-analysis. *J Behav Ther Exp Psychiatry* 1997;28:139–147. Search date not reported; primary sources Psychlit, Psychinfo, and Medline.
66. Bower P, Richards D, Lovell K. The clinical and cost-effectiveness of self-help treatments for anxiety and depressive disorders in primary care: a systematic review. *Br J Gen Pract* 2001;51:838–845. Search date 1999; primary sources Psychinfo, Medline, Embase, Cinahl, The Cochrane Library, Counselling in Primary Care Counsel.lit database, National Research Register, personal contact with researchers, and hand searches of reference lists and two journals.
67. Lawlor DA, Hopker SW. The effectiveness of exercise as an intervention in the management of depression: systematic review and meta-regression analysis of randomised controlled trials. *BMJ* 2001;322:763–767. Search date 1999; primary sources Medline, Embase, Sports Discus, Psychlit, The Cochrane Library, and hand searches of reference lists and nine journals.
68. Blumenthal JA, Babyak MA, Moore KA, et al. Effects of exercise training on older people with major depression. *Arch Intern Med* 1999;159:2349–2356.
69. Babyak M, Blumenthal JA, Herman S, et al. Exercise treatment for major depression: maintenance of therapeutic benefit at 10 months. *Psychosom Med* 2000;62:633–638.
70. Stimpson N, Agrawal N, Lewis G. Randomised controlled trials investigating pharmacological and psychological interventions for treatment-refractory depression. Systematic review. *Br J Psychiatry* 2002;181:284–294.
71. Nierenberg AA, Papakostas GI, Petersen T, et al. Lithium augmentation of nortriptyline for subjects resistant to multiple antidepressants. *J Clin Psychopharmacol* 2003;23:92–95.
72. Geddes JG, Carney SM, Davies C, et al. Relapse prevention with antidepressant drug treatment in depressive disorders: a systematic review. *Lancet* 2003;361:653–661.
73. Old Age Depression Interest Group. How long should the elderly take antidepressants? A double-blind placebo-controlled study of continuation/prophylaxis therapy with dothiepin. *Br J Psychiatry* 1993;162:175–182.
74. Klysner R, Bent-Hansen J, Hansen HL, et al. Efficacy of citalopram in the prevention of recurrent depression in elderly patients: placebo-controlled study of maintenance therapy. *Br J Psychiatry* 2002:181:29–35.
75. Hippisley-Cox J, Pringle M, Hammersley V, et al. Antidepressants as risk factor for ischaemic heart disease: case-control study in primary care. *BMJ* 2001;323:666–669.
76. Fava GA, Rafanelli C, Grandi S, et al. Prevention of recurrent depression with cognitive behavioral therapy: preliminary findings. *Arch Gen Psychiatry* 1998;55:816–820.
77. The University of York. NHS Centre for Reviews and Dissemination. Improving the recognition and management of depression in primary care. *Effective Health Care* 2002;7:1–12.
78. Katon W, Rutter C, Ludman EJ, et al. A randomized trial of relapse prevention of depression in primary care. *Arch Gen Psychiatry* 2001;58:241–247.
79. Araya R, Rojas G, Fritsch R, et al. Treating depression in primary care in low-income women in Santiago, Chile: a randomised controlled trial. *Lancet* 2003;361:995–1000.
80. Hedrick SC, Chaney EF, Felker B, et al. Effectiveness of collaborative care depression treatment in Veterans' Affairs primary care. *J Gen Intern Med* 2003;18:9–16.
81. Koike AK, Unutzer J, Wells KB Improving the care for depression in patients with comorbid medical illness. *Am J Psychiatry* 2002;159:1738–1745. [Erratum in: *Am J Psychiatry* 2003;160:204]
82. Miranda J, Azocar F, Organista KC, et al. Treatment of depression among impoverished primary care patients from ethnic minority groups. *Psychiatr Serv* 2003;54:219–225.
83. Rost K, Nutting P, Smith JL, et al. Managing depression as a chronic disease: a randomised trial of ongoing treatment in primary care. *BMJ* 2002;325:934–937.
84. Unutzer J, Katon W, Callahan CM, et al. Collaborative care management of late-life depression in the primary care setting: a randomized controlled trial. *JAMA* 2002:288:2836–2845.

John Geddes
Professor of Epidemiological Psychiatry
University of Oxford
Oxford
UK

Rob Butler
Clinical Lecturer in Psychiatry/Consultant in
Old Age Psychiatry
University of Auckland and Waitemata
Health

Simon Hatcher
Senior Lecturer in Psychiatry/Honorary
Consultant in Liaison Psychiatry
University of Auckland
Auckland
New Zealand

Andrea Cipriani
Specialist Registrar
University of Verona
Verona
Italy

Jonathan Price
Clinical Tutor in Psychiatry
University of Oxford

Stuart Carney
Clinical Lecturer in Psychiatry
University of Oxford
Oxford
UK

Michael Von Korff
Associate Director and Senior Investigator
Center for Health Studies, Group Health
Cooperative
Seattle
USA

Competing interests: RB has been reimbursed by Novartis for attending a conference. JG and SH none declared.

We would like to acknowledge the previous contributors of this chapter, including James Warner.

TABLE 1 **Adverse events (% of people) with selective serotonin reuptake inhibitors versus tricyclic antidepressant drugs (see text, p 1246).[29]**

Adverse effects	SSRI event rates (%)	TCA event rates (%)
Dry mouth	21	55
Constipation	10	22
Dizziness	13	23
Nausea	22	12
Diarrhoea	13	5
Anxiety	13	7
Agitation	14	8
Insomnia	12	7
Nervousness	15	11
Headache	17	14

SSRI, selective serotonin reuptake inhibitors; TCA, tricyclic antidepressants.

TABLE 2 **Effects of specific psychological treatments for depressive disorders (see benefits of cognitive therapy, interpersonal psychotherapy, non-directive counselling, and problem solving therapy, p 1258).**

Intervention	Evidence	Benefits	Disadvantages
CT	4 SRs of psychological therapies including CT.[51–54]		Requires extensive training. Limited availability. CT in primary care suggest limited acceptability to some people.
	1 SR (search date not reported, 48 RCTs of psychological therapies, 2765 people, mean age 39.3 years). RCTs mainly in outpatients in secondary care; therefore, probably with mild to moderate depression; people with psychotic or bipolar symptoms were excluded. 20 RCTs compared CT versus placebo or waiting list control and 17 compared CT versus antidepressant drugs.[51]	79% of people receiving placebo were more symptomatic than the average person receiving CT ($P < 0.0001$).[51] 65% of people receiving CT were less symptomatic than the average person treated with antidepressants ($P < 0.0001$).	
	1 SR (6 RCTs, 2 included in the first SR, 883 people with major depression without psychotic features, mean age 30–40 years, 3 RCTs in psychiatric outpatients and 3 RCTs in primary care) comparing 3 interventions: psychotherapy (mainly CT [2 RCTs] and IFT [3 RCTs]), and antidepressant drugs (TCAs or phenelzine), and control (pill placebo or antidepressant plus usual care or supportive therapy) for an average of 16 weeks.[52]	Psychotherapy significantly increased proportion of people in remission over 10–34 weeks compared with control (46.3% with psychotherapy *v* 24.4% with control; $P < 0.0001$). Remission defined as score of 6 or 7 on HAM-D. About 50% of control group withdrew from treatment compared with 22% receiving psychotherapy.[52] No results reported for CT alone.	

TABLE 2 continued

Intervention	Evidence	Benefits	Disadvantages
	1 SR (search date not reported, 63 RCTs and controlled clinical trials, 23 RCTs included in the first or second reviews, of brief psychological therapies (≤ 20 sessions) in people aged 16–65 years with mild to moderate depression. 43 studies in university psychology departments, 13 in psychiatry outpatient clinics, and 7 in primary care. 13 RCTs (886 people) compared psychological therapies versus usual care. 16 RCTs (1024 people) compared CT versus IPT, brief psychodynamic therapy, or supportive therapy.[53]	All psychological therapies significantly increased proportion of people who recovered compared with usual care (13 RCTs, 886 people: recovery defined as score < 10 on Beck Depression Inventory Score or < 10 on HAM-D: OR 3.0, 95% CI 2.4 to 4.0).[53] CT increased proportion of people who recovered compared with usual care (12 RCTs, 654 people; OR 3.42, 95% CI 1.98 to 5.93). CT better than IPT, brief psychodynamic therapy, or supportive therapy at producing recovery (17 RCTs: 262/491 [53%] with CT *v* 196/333 [59%] with IPT, brief psychodynamic therapy, or supportive therapy; OR 2.4, 95% CI 1.4 to 4.2), but this difference disappeared when low quality studies were excluded or if studies which relied on advertising or similar techniques to recruit people were excluded.[53]	
	1 SR of psychological therapies in people with mild to moderate depression in primary care (search date not reported, 10 RCTs, 2 of CT, 1 CT plus non-directive counselling, 1 IPT, and 2 non-directive counselling, 2 included in the previous reviews[51–53]).[54]	All psychological therapies slightly but significantly better than usual care (5 RCTs, 623 people; SMD 0.31, 95% CI 0.12 to 0.50; no other statistical assessment reported). No significant difference between psychological therapies and antidepressants (7 RCTs, 882 people; SMD –0.08, 95% CI –0.21 to –0.05). No results reported for CT alone.	
IPT	3 SRs of psychological therapies including IPT.[52–54]	Two SRs did not report outcomes for IPT alone.[52,54] See CT above. In the third SR, IPT increased the proportion of people who recovered compared with usual care (1 RCT, 185 people; OR 3.45, 95% CI 1.91 to 6.51.[53] See above for IPT *v* CT.	Requires extensive training. Limited availability.

TABLE 2 continued

Intervention	Evidence	Benefits	Disadvantages
Non-directive counselling	1 SR (search date not reported, 7 RCTs, people ≥ 18 years with recent onset psychological problems, including depression, in UK primary care) compared counselling *v* standard physician care.[55]	Counselling *v* standard care significantly improved symptoms at 1–6 months (6 RCTs, 741 people; SMD –0.28, 95% CI –0.43 to –0.13), but no significant difference in the long term (4 RCTs, 447 people, > 6 months; SMD –0.07, 95% CI –0.26 to +0.12).[55] Over 1–6 months, 36% of people receiving counselling showed reliable and clinically important change compared with 23% receiving usual care.	
PS therapy	1 SR (search date not reported, 4 RCTs of PS therapy).[54]	No analysis of PS therapy alone in people with moderate depression.[54] See CT above. No significant difference between PS therapy and placebo pill in people with mild depression or dysthymia (2 RCTs, 439 people; reported as non-significant, CI not reported).[54] PS *v* control significantly increased the proportion of people who were not depressed at 6 months, but no significant difference at 1 year.[56]	Requires some training. Limited availability.
	1 subsequent RCT (452 people aged 18–65 years with mild to moderate depression or adjustment disorders derived from a general population sample following a survey, probably with mild to moderate depression) compared PS, group treatment, and control.[56] 1 additional RCT (70 people aged 18–65 years in primary care with emotional disorders of at least 1 month) compared PS with usual care from GP.[57]	No significant difference between PS and usual care in symptoms at 8 or 26 weeks (mean Clinical Interview Schedule score at 8 weeks: 12.4 with PS *v* 10.5 with usual care; at 26 weeks: 9.3 with PS *v* 7.2 with usual care; reported as non-significant, CI not reported).[57]	

CT, cognitive therapy; HAM-D, Hamilton Depression Rating Scale; IPT, interpersonal psychotherapy; PS, problem solving; TCA, tricyclic antidepressant.

Generalised anxiety disorder

Search date February 2004

Christopher Gale and Mark Oakley-Browne

QUESTIONS

INTERVENTIONS

Key Messages

- **Antidepressants (imipramine, opipramol, paroxetine, and venlafaxine)** One systematic review found that antidepressants (imipramine, paroxetine, and venlafaxine) improved symptoms over 4–28 weeks compared with placebo. One subsequent RCT found that paroxetine increased response rates compared with placebo. One RCT found no significant difference in response rates between venlafaxine and placebo at 24 weeks. One RCT found that opipramol increased response rate after 28 days compared with placebo. RCTs found no significant difference among these antidepressants or between antidepressants and benzodiazepines or buspirone. RCTs and observational studies have found that antidepressants are associated with sedation, dizziness, nausea, falls, and sexual dysfunction.
- **Buspirone** RCTs found that buspirone improved symptoms over 4–9 weeks compared with placebo. RCTs found no significant difference in symptoms over 6–8 weeks between buspirone and antidepressants, diazepam, or hydroxyzine, but the studies may have lacked power to detect clinically important differences among treatments.
- **Cognitive behavioural therapy** Two systematic reviews and three subsequent RCTs found that cognitive behavioural therapy (using a combination of interventions, such as exposure, relaxation, and cognitive restructuring) improved anxiety and depression over 4–12 weeks compared with waiting list control, anxiety management alone, relaxation alone, or non-directive psychotherapy. Three subsequent RCTs found no significant difference in symptoms at 13 weeks, 6 months, or 24 months between cognitive therapy and applied relaxation.
- **Hydroxyzine** Three RCTs comparing hydroxyzine versus placebo found different results. Two RCTs found that, compared with placebo, hydroxyzine improved symptoms of anxiety at 4 or 12 weeks, but a third RCT found no significant difference in the proportion of people with improved symptoms of anxiety at 5 weeks. One of the RCTs found that hydroxyzine increased somnolence and headaches compared with placebo. One RCT found no significant difference between hydroxyzine and bromazepam in the proportion of people who responded after 6 weeks. Another RCT found no significant difference between hydroxyzine and buspirone in the proportion of people who responded after 4 weeks.

- **Benzodiazepines** One systematic review and one subsequent RCT found that benzodiazepines reduced symptoms over 2–9 weeks compared with placebo. RCTs found no significant difference in symptoms over 3–8 weeks between alprazolam and bromazepam or mexazolam, or between benzodiazepines and buspirone, hydroxyzine, abecarnil, or antidepressants. RCTs and observational studies found that benzodiazepines increased the risk of dependence, sedation, industrial accidents, and road traffic accidents. If used in late pregnancy or while breast feeding, benzodiazepines may cause adverse effects in neonates. One systematic review of poor quality RCTs provided insufficient evidence to assess long term treatment with benzodiazepines.
- **Kava** One systematic review in people with a variety of anxiety disorders, including generalised anxiety disorder, found that kava reduced symptoms of anxiety over 1–24 weeks compared with placebo. It is unclear whether results of the review can be extrapolated to people with generalised anxiety disorder. Observational evidence suggests that kava may be associated with hepatotoxicity.
- **Trifluoperazine** One large RCT found that trifluoperazine reduced anxiety after 4 weeks compared with placebo, but caused more drowsiness, extrapyramidal reactions, and other movement disorders.
- **Abecarnil** One RCT found limited evidence that low dose abecarnil improved symptoms compared with placebo. Another RCT found no significant difference in symptoms at 6 weeks between abecarnil and placebo or diazepam. Both RCTs found that abecarnil increased drowsiness compared with placebo.
- **Applied relaxation** We found no RCTs comparing applied relaxation versus placebo or no treatment. Three RCTs found no significant difference in symptoms at 13 weeks, 6 months, or 24 months between applied relaxation and cognitive behavioural therapy.
- **β Blockers** We found no RCTs on the effects of β blockers in people with generalised anxiety disorder.

DEFINITION Generalised anxiety disorder (GAD) is defined as excessive worry and tension about every day events and problems, on most days, for at least 6 months, to the point where the person experiences distress or has marked difficulty in performing day to day tasks.[1] It may be characterised by the following symptoms and signs: increased motor tension (fatigability, trembling, restlessness, and muscle tension); autonomic hyperactivity (shortness of breath, rapid heart rate, dry mouth, cold hands, and dizziness); and increased vigilance and scanning (feeling keyed up, increased startling, and impaired concentration), but not panic attacks.[1] One non-systematic review of epidemiological and clinical studies found marked reduction in quality of life and psychosocial functioning in people with anxiety disorders (including GAD).[2] It also found that people with GAD had low overall life satisfaction and some impairment in ability to fulfil roles, social tasks, or both.[2]

INCIDENCE/ PREVALENCE One overview of observational studies found that the prevalence of GAD among adults in the community was 1.5–3.0%.[3] It found that 3–5% of adults had had GAD in the past year and 4–7% had had GAD during their lives. The US National Comorbidity Survey found that over 90% of people diagnosed with GAD had a comorbid diagnosis, including dysthymia (22%), depression (39–69%), somatisation, other anxiety disorders, bipolar disorder, or substance abuse.[4] The Harvard–Brown Anxiety Research Program also found that only 30/180 people (17%) had GAD alone.[5] Subgroup analysis suggested that 46/122 people (38%) with GAD had comorbid personality disorder.[6] A systematic review of the comorbidity of eating disorders and anxiety disorders (search date 2001, 2 observational studies, 55 people) found a lifetime prevalence of GAD among people with anorexia nervosa of 24% in one study and 31% in the other.[7] The lifetime prevalence of GAD in the control group of one of the studies (44 people) was 2%. The reliability of the measures used to diagnose GAD in epidemiological studies is unsatisfactory.[8,9] One US study, with explicit diagnostic criteria (DSM-III-R), estimated that 5% of people will develop GAD at some time during their lives.[9] A recent cohort study of people with depressive and anxiety disorders found that 49% of people initially diagnosed with GAD retained this diagnosis over 2 years.[10] The incidence of GAD in men is half the incidence in women[11] and is lower in older people.[12] A non-systematic review (20 observational studies in younger and older adults) suggested that autonomic arousal to stressful tasks was decreased in older people, and that older people became accustomed to stressful tasks more quickly than younger people.[13]

AETIOLOGY/ RISK FACTORS GAD is believed to be associated with an increase in the number of minor stressors, independent of demographic factors,[14,15] but this finding is also common in people with other diagnoses.[10] One non-systematic review (5 case control studies) of psychological sequelae to civilian trauma found that rates of GAD reported in four of the five studies were significantly increased compared with a control population (rate ratio 3.3, 95% CI 2.0 to 5.5).[16] One systematic review (search date 1997) of cross-sectional studies found that bullying (or peer victimisation) was associated with a significant increase in the incidence of GAD (effect size 0.21, CI not reported).[17] Genetic factors are also implicated. One systematic review (search date not reported, 2 family studies, 45 index cases, 225 first degree relatives) found a significant association between GAD in the index cases and in their first degree relatives (OR 6.1, 95% CI 2.5 to 14.9).[18] The review also identified three twin studies (13 305 people), which estimated that 32% (95% CI 24% to 39%) of the variance in liability to GAD was explained by genetic factors.

PROGNOSIS One systematic review found that 25% of adults with GAD will be in full remission after 2 years, and 38% will have a remission after 5 years.[3] The Harvard–Brown anxiety research program reported 5 year follow up of 167 people with GAD.[19] In this period, the weighted probability for full remission was 38% and for at least partial remission was 47%; the probability of relapse from full remission was 27% and relapse from partial remission was 39%.

AIMS OF INTERVENTION To reduce symptoms of anxiety; to minimise disruption of day to day functioning; and to improve quality of life, with minimum adverse effects.

OUTCOMES Severity of symptoms and effects on quality of life, as measured by symptom scores on continuous rating scales, usually the Hamilton Anxiety Scale, State–Trait Anxiety Inventory, or Clinical Global Impression Scale. Other continuous scales include the Penn State Worry Questionnaire and the GAD Severity Scale. Most RCTs define a 20% reduction in symptoms scores on the relevant scale as a clinical response. Where numbers needed to treat are given, these represent the number of people requiring treatment within a given time period (usually 6–12 weeks) for one additional person to achieve a certain improvement in symptom score. The method for obtaining numbers needed to treat was not standardised across studies. Some RCTs defined a reduction by, for example, 20 points in the Hamilton Anxiety Scale as a clinical response; others defined a clinical response as a reduction by, for example, 50% of the premorbid score. The authors have not attempted to standardise methods, but instead have used the response rates reported in each study to calculate numbers needed to treat. Similarly, the authors have calculated numbers needed to harm from original trial data.

METHODS *Clinical Evidence* search and appraisal February 2004. Recent changes in diagnostic classification make it hard to compare older studies with more recent ones. In the earlier classification system (DSM-III-R), the diagnosis was made only in the absence of other psychiatric disorders. In current systems (DSM-IV and ICD-10), GAD can be diagnosed in the presence of any comorbid condition.

QUESTION What are the effects of treatments?

OPTION COGNITIVE BEHAVIOURAL THERAPY

Two systematic reviews and three subsequent RCTs found that cognitive behavioural therapy (using a combination of interventions such as exposure, relaxation, and cognitive restructuring) improved anxiety and depression over 4–12 weeks compared with waiting list control, anxiety management alone, relaxation alone, or non-directive psychotherapy. Three subsequent RCTs found no significant difference in symptoms at 13 weeks, 6 months, or 24 months between cognitive therapy and applied relaxation.

Benefits: We found two systematic reviews[20,21] and six subsequent RCTs[22–27] comparing cognitive behavioural therapy**G** versus waiting list control (no treatment) or versus other psychotherapies in people with generalised anxiety disorder (GAD) (see table 1, p 1291). The first systematic review (search date 1996) found that cognitive behavioural therapy significantly improved symptoms over 4–12 weeks compared with control (waiting list, anxiety management alone, relaxation alone, or non-directive psychotherapy).[20] The second systematic review (search date not reported) found that cognitive behavioural therapy or analytical psychotherapy**G** improved symptoms compared with waiting list control.[21] The first subsequent RCT (75 people) found no significant difference between cognitive therapy and a discussion group in the proportion of people who no longer met the criteria for GAD immediately after treatment.[24] The second subsequent RCT (80 people) found that cognitive therapy significantly increased the proportion of people who responded immediately after treatment compared with minimal contact.[23] The third subsequent RCT (36 people) found no significant difference between cognitive therapy and applied relaxation**G** in the proportion of people who responded after 13 weeks.[22] The fourth subsequent RCT (76 people) found no significant difference between cognitive therapy, applied relaxation, and a combination of these methods in the proportion of people in each group who no longer met criteria for GAD immediately after treatment and at 24 months.[23] The fifth subsequent RCT (45 people) found no significant difference between cognitive therapy and applied relaxation in the proportion of people who responded at 6 months.[26] The sixth subsequent RCT (52 people) found that cognitive therapy significantly improved scores on the Penn State Worry Questionnaire and the Beck Anxiety Inventory compared with waiting list control at the end of 14 weeks of treatment.[27]

Harms: The reviews and subsequent RCTs gave no information on harms.[20–28]

Comment: A third systematic review (search date 1998, 6 RCTs comparing cognitive therapy versus a variety of other psychological treatments, 404 people) did not compare treatments directly.[29] It reanalysed the raw data from individual RCTs to calculate the proportion of people who experienced a clinically important improvement in symptoms after treatment and maintained that improvement for 6 months. It found limited evidence that more people who had individual cognitive therapy maintained recovery after 6 months than people who had other psychological treatments, with the exception of applied relaxation (proportion of people who maintained improvement: 41% with individual cognitive therapy, 19% with non-directive treatment, 18% with group cognitive therapy, 12% with group behaviour therapy, 18% with individual behaviour therapy, 0% with analytical psychotherapy, and 52% with applied relaxation; P values not reported).[29] Many of the RCTs were small and were not analysed on an intention to treat basis.

OPTION APPLIED RELAXATION

We found no RCTs comparing applied relaxation with placebo or no treatment. Three RCTs found no significant difference in symptoms at 13 weeks, 6 months, or 24 months between applied relaxation and cognitive therapy.

Benefits: **Versus placebo or no treatment:** We found no systematic review or RCTs. **Versus other psychological treatments:** See benefits of cognitive therapy, p 1280.

Harms: **Versus other psychological treatments:** See harms of cognitive therapy, p 1280.

Comment: We found one systematic review (search date 1998, 6 RCTs, 404 people) comparing applied relaxation**G** versus a variety of other psychological treatments, which did not compare treatments directly (see comment under cognitive behavioural therapy, p 1280).[29]

OPTION BENZODIAZEPINES

One systematic review and one subsequent RCT found that benzodiazepines reduced symptoms over 2–9 weeks compared with placebo. RCTs found no significant difference in symptoms over 3–8 weeks between alprazolam and bromazepam or mexazolam, or between benzodiazepines and buspirone, hydroxyzine, abecarnil, or antidepressants. RCTs and observational studies found that benzodiazepines increased the risk of dependence, sedation, industrial accidents, and road traffic accidents. If used in late pregnancy or while breast feeding, benzodiazepines may cause adverse effects in neonates. One systematic review of poor quality RCTs provided insufficient evidence to assess long term treatment with benzodiazepines.

Benefits: **Versus placebo:** We found one systematic review (search date 1996, 17 RCTs, 2044 people)[20] and one subsequent RCT.[29] The review found that benzodiazepines significantly improved symptoms over 2–9 weeks compared with placebo (pooled mean effect size 0.70; CI not reported).[20] The subsequent RCT (310 people) compared three interventions: diazepam (15–35 mg/day), abecarnil (7.5–17.5 mg/day), and placebo.[30] It found that diazepam significantly increased the proportion of people with moderate improvement on the Clinical Global Impression (CGI) scores at 6 weeks compared with placebo (73% with diazepam *v* 56% with placebo; $P < 0.01$).[30] **Versus each other:** The systematic review did not compare different benzodiazepines directly.[20] We found two RCTs.[31,32] The first RCT (121 people) compared sustained release alprazolam versus bromazepam.[31] It found no significant difference in Hamilton Anxiety Scale scores or CGI scores over 5 weeks between alprazolam and bromazepam (reported as non-significant, results presented graphically).[31] The second RCT (64 people) comparing mexazolam versus alprazolam found no significant difference in the proportion of people who had "highly improved" or "moderately improved" CGI scores at 3 weeks (98% with "highly improved" *v* 87% with "moderately improved"; $P > 0.05$; absolute numbers presented graphically).[32] **Long term treatment:** We found one systematic review (search date 1998, 8 RCTs, any benzodiazepine medication, > 2 months' duration).[33] It found that the weak methods of the RCTs prevented firm conclusions being made.[33] **Versus buspirone:** See benefits of buspirone, p 1282. **Versus hydroxyzine:** See benefits of hydroxyzine, p 1283. **Versus abecarnil:** See benefits of abecarnil, p 1284. **Versus antidepressants:** See benefits of antidepressants, p 1285.

Harms: **Versus placebo:** The review gave no information on harms.[20] The subsequent RCT found that, compared with placebo, both diazepam and abecarnil significantly increased drowsiness (52% with diazepam *v* 47% with abecarnil *v* 14% with placebo; $P < 0.05$ for either drug *v* placebo) and dizziness (11% with diazepam *v* 16% with abecarnil *v* 3% with placebo; $P < 0.05$ for either drug *v* placebo).[30] **Dependence and sedation:** One non-systematic review of the harms of benzodiazepines found that rebound anxiety on withdrawal has been reported in 15–30% of people.[34] It also found that there is a high risk of substance abuse and dependence with benzodiazepines. Benzodiazepines have been found to cause impairment in attention, concentration, and short term memory. One RCT identified by the review found an increased rate of drowsiness (71% with diazepam *v* 13% with placebo; $P = 0.001$) and dizziness (29% with diazepam *v* 11% with placebo; $P = 0.001$).[20] Sedation can interfere with concomitant psychotherapy. **Memory:** Thirty one people with agoraphobia/panic disorder in an RCT comparing alprazolam versus placebo for 8 weeks were reviewed after 3.5 years.[35] Five people were still taking benzodiazepines and had significant impairment in memory tasks. There was no clear difference in memory performance between those who had been in the placebo group and those who had been given alprazolam but were no longer taking the drug.[35] **Road traffic accidents:** We found one systematic review (search date 1997) examining the relation between benzodiazepines and road traffic accidents.[36] In the case control studies, the odds ratio for death or emergency medical treatment in those who had taken benzodiazepines compared with those who had not taken them was 1.45–2.40. The odds ratio increased with higher doses and more recent intake. In the police and emergency ward studies, benzodiazepine use was a factor in 1–65% of accidents (usually 5–10%). In two studies in which people had blood alcohol concentrations under the legal limit, benzodiazepines were found in 43% and 65% of people. For drivers over 65 years of age, the risk of being involved in reported road traffic accidents was higher if they had taken longer acting and larger quantities of benzodiazepines. These results are from case control studies and are, therefore, subject to confounding. **Pregnancy and breast feeding:** One systematic review (search date 1997) of 23 case series and reports found no association between cleft lip and palate and benzodiazepines in the first trimester of pregnancy.[37] However, case reports in one non-systematic review suggested that benzodiazepines taken in late pregnancy may be associated with neonatal hypotonia and withdrawal syndrome.[38] Benzodiazepines are secreted in breast milk, and there have been reports of sedation and hypothermia in infants.[39] **Other:** One non-systematic industry funded review (8 RCTs) comparing benzodiazepines versus placebo or buspirone found that recent use of benzodiazepines limited the effectiveness of buspirone in people with generalised anxiety disorder.[39]

Comment: All of the RCTs assessing benzodiazepines were short term (at most 12 weeks).[20,30,31]

OPTION BUSPIRONE

RCTs found that buspirone improved symptoms over 4–9 weeks compared with placebo. RCTs found no significant difference in symptoms over 6–8 weeks between buspirone and antidepressants, diazepam, or hydroxyzine, but the studies may have lacked power to detect clinically important differences among treatments.

Benefits: **Versus placebo:** We found one systematic review (search date 1996, 9 RCTs)[20] and two subsequent RCTs.[40,41] The systematic review found that buspirone significantly improved symptoms over 4–9 weeks compared with placebo (pooled mean effect size 0.39; CI not reported, withdrawal rate 17%).[20] The first subsequent RCT (162 people) comparing buspirone versus placebo found similar results (55% with buspirone *v* 35% with placebo; $P < 0.05$).[40] The second subsequent RCT (365 people) compared four interventions: buspirone (30 mg/day), venlafaxine (75 mg/day), venlafaxine (150 mg/day), and placebo over 8 weeks (see also benefits of antidepressants, p 1285).[41] It found that, compared with placebo, buspirone significantly increased the proportion of people who responded after 8 weeks of treatment (response defined as score of 1 or 2) on the Clinical Global Impression Scale; 52/95 [55%] with buspirone *v* 38/98 [39%] with placebo; $P = 0.03$).[41] **Versus benzodiazepines:** The systematic review[20] found one large RCT (240 people), which compared three interventions: buspirone, diazepam, and placebo.[42] It found that a similar proportion of people responded over 6 weeks with buspirone compared with diazepam (response defined as ≥ 40% reduction in Hamilton Anxiety Scale score; 54% with buspirone v 61% with diazepam; P values not reported). **Versus antidepressants:** See benefits of antidepressants, p 1285. **Versus hydroxyzine:** See benefits of hydroxyzine, p 1283.

Harms: The systematic review gave no information on harms.[20] The first subsequent RCT found that, compared with placebo, buspirone significantly increased the proportion of people with nausea (27/80 [34%] with buspirone v 11/82 [13%] with placebo; RR 2.5, 95% CI 1.3 to 4.7; NNH 5, 95% CI 4 to 14), dizziness (51/80 [64%] with buspirone v 10/82 [12%] with placebo; RR 5.2, 95% CI 2.9 to 9.6; NNH 2, 95% CI 2 to 3), and somnolence (15/80 [19%] with buspirone v 6/82 [7%] with placebo; RR 2.6, 95% CI 1.0 to 6.3; NNH 9, 95% CI 5 to 104).[40] Diazepam was associated with more fatigue and weakness compared with buspirone, but less headache and dizziness.[42] **Pregnancy and breast feeding:** We found no evidence on the effects of buspirone during pregnancy or breast feeding.

Comment: We found one non-systematic review (8 RCTs, 520 people) that was sponsored by pharmaceutical companies and had been included in regulatory submissions for buspirone.[43] It found that buspirone significantly increased the proportion of people "much or very much improved" as rated by their physician compared with placebo (54% with buspirone v 28% with placebo; P ≤ 0.001). Another non-systematic industry funded review (8 RCTs) comparing benzodiazepines versus placebo or buspirone found that recent use of benzodiazepines limited the effectiveness of buspirone in people with generalised anxiety disorder.[39]

OPTION HYDROXYZINE

Three RCTs comparing hydroxyzine versus placebo found different results. Two RCTs found that, compared with placebo, hydroxyzine improved symptoms of anxiety at 4 or 12 weeks, but a third RCT found no significant difference in the proportion of people with improved symptoms of anxiety at 5 weeks. One of the RCTs found that hydroxyzine increased somnolence and headaches compared with placebo. One RCT found no significant difference between hydroxyzine and bromazepam in the proportion of people who responded after 6 weeks. Another RCT found no significant difference between hydroxyzine and buspirone in the proportion of people who responded after 4 weeks.

Benefits: **Versus placebo:** We found one non-systematic review (2 RCTs, 354 people)[44] that was conducted as part of an RCT protocol and one additional RCT.[45] The first RCT (110 people) identified by the review found that hydroxyzine (50 mg/day) significantly improved Clinical Global Impression Scale scores after 4 weeks compared with placebo (mean improvement 1.53 with hydroxyzine v 0.95 with placebo; P < 0.02).[44] The second RCT (244 people entered, 213 people analysed) identified by the review compared three interventions, hydroxyzine, buspirone, and placebo, for 28 days, followed by placebo in all groups for 7 days. It found no significant difference between hydroxyzine 50 mg/day and placebo in the proportion of people with a Hamilton Anxiety Scale (HAM-A) score reduction of 50% or greater at 35 days (30/71 [42%] with hydroxyzine v 20/70 [29%] with placebo; RR 1.50, 95% CI 0.93 to 2.23; analysis not by intention to treat).[44] The additional RCT (369 people) also compared three interventions, hydroxyzine, bromazepam, and placebo, for 12 weeks, followed by placebo in all groups for 1 week.[45] It found that, compared with placebo, hydroxyzine significantly increased the proportion of people who responded at 42 days (response defined as ≥ 50% reduction in HAM-A scores from baseline; P = 0.022; absolute numbers presented graphically). **Versus**

benzodiazepines: The additional RCT found no significant difference in the proportion of people who responded at 42 days between hydroxyzine and bromazepam (response defined as a HAM-A score reduction of ≥50%; reported as non-significant, no further data provided).[45] **Versus buspirone:** The second RCT identified by the non-systematic review also found no significant difference between hydroxyzine and buspirone in the proportion of people who responded at 28 days (response defined as HAM-A score reduction of ≥ 50%: 30/71 [42%] with hydroxyzine *v* 26/72 [36%] with buspirone; RR 1.20, 95% CI 0.78 to 1.80).[44]

Harms: **Versus placebo:** The second RCT (244 people) identified by the review found that, compared with placebo, more people taking hydroxyzine had somnolence (AR 10% with hydroxyzine *v* 0% with placebo) and headaches (AR 6% with hydroxyzine *v* 1% with placebo).[44] Overall adverse effects were reported in 40% of people taking hydroxyzine and 28% taking placebo.

Comment: None.

OPTION ABECARNIL

One RCT found limited evidence that low dose abecarnil improved symptoms compared with placebo. Another RCT found no significant difference in symptoms at 6 weeks between abecarnil and placebo or diazepam. Both RCTs found that abecarnil increased drowsiness compared with placebo.

Benefits: We found no systematic review, but found two multicentre RCTs of abecarnil (an anxiolytic).[30,46] The first RCT (129 people) compared 3 weeks of treatment with abecarnil in three separate dose regimens (3–9, 7.5–15, and 15–30 mg/day) versus placebo.[46] Within each group the dose was escalated from the minimum to the maximum over the length of the trial. It found that lower doses of abecarnil (3–9 mg/day) significantly improved symptoms compared with placebo (outcome 50% reduction in Hamilton Anxiety Scale score; 19/31 [61%] with abecarnil *v* 8/26 [31%] with placebo; RR 1.99, 95% CI 1.05 to 3.78), but found no significant difference in symptoms between higher doses of abecarnil and placebo. Results were not calculated by intention to treat (12/34 [35%] people withdrew with abecarnil 15–30 mg/day *v* 4/35 [11%] with abecarnil 7.5–15 mg/day *v* 1/32 [3%] with abecarnil 3–9 mg/day *v* 2/28 [7%] with placebo).[46] The second RCT (310 people) compared three interventions: abecarnil (7.5–17.5 mg/day), diazepam (15–35 mg/day), and placebo.[30] It found no significant difference between abecarnil and placebo or diazepam in the proportion of people with moderate improvement on the Clinical Global Impression scores at 6 weeks (AR for moderate improvement 62% with abecarnil *v* 56% with placebo *v* 73% with diazepam; reported as non-significant; P values not reported).[30]

Harms: The first RCT found that abecarnil (3–9 mg/day) was associated with fatigue (4/32 [13%] with abecarnil *v* 0/28 [0%] with placebo), equilibrium loss (2/32 [6%] with abecarnil *v* 0/28 [0%] with placebo), and drowsiness (10/32 [31%] with abecarnil *v* 4/28 [14%] with placebo). Higher doses were associated with more adverse effects (62% of people taking abecarnil 15–30 mg experienced at least 1 adverse effect *v* 51% of people taking abecarnil 7.5–15 mg *v* 22% with abecarnil 3–9 mg *v* 21% with placebo).[46]

Comment: None.

OPTION ANTIDEPRESSANTS

One systematic review found that antidepressants (imipramine, paroxetine, and venlafaxine) improved symptoms over 4–28 weeks compared with placebo. One subsequent RCT found that paroxetine increased response rates compared with placebo. One RCT found no significant difference in response rates between venlafaxine and placebo at 24 weeks. One RCT found that opipramol increased response rate after 28 days compared with placebo. RCTs found no significant difference among these antidepressants or between antidepressants and benzodiazepines or buspirone. RCTs and observational studies have found that antidepressants are associated with sedation, dizziness, nausea, falls, and sexual dysfunction.

Benefits: **Versus placebo:** We found one systematic review (search date 2002, 8 RCTs, 2058 people[47]), two subsequent RCTs,[48,49] and one additional RCT (see table 2, p 1294).[50] The systematic review found that antidepressants (imipramine, paroxetine, and venlafaxine) significantly increased the proportion of people who responded at 8–28 weeks compared with placebo.[47] It also found that each antidepressant significantly increased response rates compared with placebo. The first subsequent RCT found that paroxetine (20 or 40 mg/day) significantly increased response rates compared with placebo.[48] The second subsequent RCT (244 people) found no significant difference between venlafaxine and placebo in response or remission at 24 weeks (see table 2, p 1294).[49] The additional RCT found that opipramol significantly increased response rate after 28 days compared with placebo (see table 2, p 1294).[50] **Versus each other:** The systematic review[47] identified one RCT (56 people), which found no significant difference between paroxetine and imipramine in the proportion of people who responded over 8 weeks of treatment (see table 2, p 1294). **Versus benzodiazepines:** The systematic review[47] identified two RCTs[51,52] and we found one additional RCT (see table 2, p 1294).[50] The first RCT identified by the review found similar improvements with imipramine, trazodone, diazepam, and placebo, but did not directly compare the significance of differences between groups.[51] The second RCT identified by the review found that paroxetine and imipramine significantly improved anxiety after 8 weeks compared with 2'-chlordesmethyldiazepam.[52] The additional RCT found no significant difference between opipramol and alprazolam at 28 days (see table 2, p 1294).[50] **Versus buspirone:** One RCT identified by the review found similar response rates between venlafaxine and buspirone at 8 weeks (see table 2, p 1294).[41]

Harms: **Withdrawals:** The review found no significant difference between antidepressants and placebo in the proportion of people who withdrew for any cause (403/1273 [31%] with antidepressants *v* 240/678 [35%] with placebo; RR 0.95, 95% CI 0.73 to 1.24).[47] A survival analysis of the two RCTs of venlafaxine (767 people) identified by the review[47] found no significant difference between venlafaxine and placebo in the proportion of people who withdrew because of adverse effects over 6 months (36/253 [14%] with venlafaxine *v* 91/514 [18%] with placebo; RR 1.24, 95% CI 0.87 to 1.77.[53] **Common adverse events:** The review found that people taking venlafaxine were more likely to report nausea, dry mouth, insomnia, constipation, flatulence, anorexia, somnolence, and sexual dysfunction than people taking placebo.[47] One RCT found sedation, confusion, dry mouth, and constipation with both imipramine and trazodone.[51] RCTs reported nausea, somnolence, dry mouth, sweating, constipation, anorexia, and sexual dysfunction with venlafaxine (nausea: 31% with venlafaxine *v* 9.9% with placebo; sweating: 13.1% with venlafaxine *v* 1.7% with placebo, P not reported).[49]

Most of the adverse effects (apart from dizziness and sexual dysfunction) decreased over 6 months in those who continued to take the medication. There have been case reports of nausea in people taking paroxetine.[52] **Adverse effects when discontinuing treatment:** Abrupt discontinuation of selective serotonin reuptake inhibitors has been associated with adverse effects including dizziness, headache, nausea, vomiting, diarrhoea, movement disorders, insomnia, irritability, visual disturbance, lethargy, anorexia, and lowered mood. One RCT (120 people receiving maintenance selective serotonin reuptake inhibitors for depression) found that significantly more people had adverse effects when discontinuing paroxetine or sertraline compared with people discontinuing fluoxetine (60% with paroxetine *v* 66% with sertraline *v* 16% taking fluoxetine; $P < 0.01$ for paroxetine or sertraline *v* fluoxetine).[54] **Overdose:** In a series of 239 coroner directed necropsies from 1970–1989, tricyclic antidepressants were considered to be a causal factor in 12% of deaths and hypnosedatives (primarily benzodiazepines and excluding barbiturates) in 8% of deaths.[55] **Accidental poisoning:** Tricyclic antidepressants are a major cause of accidental poisoning.[56] A study estimated that there was one death for every 44 children admitted to hospital after ingestion of tricyclic antidepressants.[57] **Hyponatraemia:** One case series reported 736 incidents of hyponatraemia in people taking selective serotonin reuptake inhibitors; 83% of episodes were in hospital inpatients aged over 65 years.[58] It is not possible to establish causation from this type of data. **Falls:** One retrospective cohort study (2428 elderly residents of nursing homes) found an increased risk of falls in new users of antidepressants (665 people taking tricyclic antidepressants; adjusted RR 2.0, 95% CI 1.8 to 2.2; 612 people taking selective serotonin reuptake inhibitors; adjusted RR 1.8, 95% CI 1.6 to 2.0; and 304 people taking trazodone; adjusted RR 1.2, 95% CI 1.0 to 1.4).[59] The increased rate of falls persisted through the first 180 days of treatment and beyond. One case control study (8239 people aged ≥ 66 years, treated in hospital for hip fracture) found an increased risk of hip fracture in those taking antidepressants (adjusted OR, selective serotonin reuptake inhibitors 2.4, 95% CI 2.0 to 2.7; secondary amine tricyclic antidepressants such as nortriptyline 2.2, 95% CI 1.8 to 2.8; and tertiary amine tricyclic antidepressants such as amitriptyline 1.5, 95% CI 1.3 to 1.7).[60] This study could not control for confounding factors; people taking antidepressants may be at increased risk of hip fracture for other reasons. **In pregnancy:** We found no reports of harmful effects in pregnancy. One case control study found no evidence that imipramine or fluoxetine increased the rate of malformations in pregnancy.[61] **Sexual dysfunction:** A survey (1022 people mostly suffering from depression; 610 women) of people using antidepressants with acceptable sexual function before antidepressant treatment has reported the incidence of sexual dysfunction (decreased desire, delayed ejaculation, and anorgasmia) to be 71% with paroxetine, 67% with venlafaxine, and 63% with fluvoxamine.[62]

Comment: None.

OPTION ANTIPSYCHOTIC DRUGS

One large RCT found that trifluoperazine reduced anxiety after 4 weeks compared with placebo, but caused more drowsiness, extrapyramidal reactions, and other movement disorders.

Benefits: We found no systematic review. We found 1 RCT (415 people) comparing 4 weeks of trifluoperazine treatment (2–6 mg/day) versus placebo.[63] It found that trifluoperazine significantly reduced the total score on the Hamilton Anxiety Scale compared with placebo (difference 14 points; $P < 0.001$).

Harms: The RCT reported more cases of drowsiness (43% with trifluoperazine *v* 25% with placebo) and extrapyramidal reactions and movement disorders (17% with trifluoperazine *v* 8% with placebo) with trifluoperazine compared with placebo.[63] A cohort study found that in the longer term, rates of tardive dyskinesia are increased if trifluoperazine treatment is frequently interrupted.[64]

Comment: None.

OPTION β BLOCKERS

We found no RCTs on the effects of β blockers in people with generalised anxiety disorder.

Benefits: We found no systematic review or RCTs.

Harms: We found no RCTs.

Comment: None.

OPTION KAVA

One systematic review in people with a variety of anxiety disorders, including generalised anxiety disorder, found that kava reduced symptoms of anxiety over 1–24 weeks compared with placebo. It is unclear whether the results of the review can be extrapolated to people with generalised anxiety disorder. Observational evidence suggests that kava may be associated with hepatotoxicity.

Benefits: **Versus placebo:** We found one systematic review (search date 2002, 11 RCTs, 645 people with a variety of anxiety disorders, including generalised anxiety disorder, preoperative anxiety, and climacteric).[65] It found that kava significantly improved Hamilton Anxiety Scale scores over 1–24 weeks compared with placebo (6 RCTs, 345 people: WMD 4.97, 95% CI 1.14 to 8.81).

Harms: The review gave little information on adverse effects.[65] Eight RCTs identified by the review found that kava was associated with adverse effects, including stomach complaints, restlessness, drowsiness, tremor, headache, and tiredness.[65] We found one systematic review (search date 2000, 30 studies including 9 clinical trials) assessing adverse effects associated with kava.[66] Adverse effects in the clinical trials were gastrointestinal symptoms, tiredness, restlessness, tremor, and headache. Post-marketing surveillance (4049 adults taking 150 mg/day kava extract) found an adverse reaction rate of 1.5% (61/4094). Case reports included five cases of dermatological reactions, four cases of acute dyskinesias, nine cases of liver damage, and one case of myoglobulinuria (the incidence of these adverse effects was not reported).[66] One case was found where kava may have interacted with alprazolam, leading to a decreased level of consciousness.[66]

Comment: It is unclear whether the results of the review can be extrapolated to people with generalised anxiety disorder, as we were unable to ascertain how many people in the RCTs included in the review had generalised anxiety disorder.[65] The review found that, although research about kava has been published in languages other than English, there was a trend for positive results to be published in English and negative results in other languages, and that this could lead to a bias when extracting data.[65] There have been concerns that kava may cause liver damage.[67]

GLOSSARY

Applied relaxation A technique involving training in relaxation techniques and self monitoring of symptoms without challenging beliefs.

Cognitive behavioural therapy Brief (20 sessions over 12–16 weeks) structured treatment incorporating elements of cognitive therapy and behavioural therapy. Covers a variety of techniques. *Behavioural therapy* is based on learning theory and concentrates on changing behaviour. *Cognitive therapy* is aimed at identifying anxiety associated thoughts and beliefs, changing over monitoring of physical symptoms, and minimising the catastrophising that characterises generalised anxiety disorder. This is combined with relaxation, exercise, and testing the validity of beliefs in real life situations. *Cognitive restructuring* involves systematic challenging of thought processes and underlying assumptions related to the symptoms. *Exposure* entails being confronted (through visualisation, image, or the stimulus) with an anxiogenic stimulus in a repetitive and prolonged manner. *Relaxation* involves practising techniques that lead to muscular or bodily relaxation. *Systematic desensitisation* is a type of exposure. Anxiety management training is a structured therapy involving education about anxiety, relaxation training, and exposure to anxiogenic stimuli; however, it does not include cognitive restructuring.

Analytical psychotherapy A semi-structured therapy involving exploration of previous events in relation to an underlying theory around emotional states, generally based on one of the psychoanalytical theories.

REFERENCES

1. American Psychiatric Association. *Diagnostic and statistical manual of mental disorders*, 4th ed. Washington, DC: American Psychiatric Association, 1994.
2. Mendlowicz MV, Stein MB. Quality of life in individuals with anxiety disorders. *Am J Psychiatry* 2000;157:669–682.
3. Kessler RD Wittchen HU. Patterns and correlates of generalized anxiety disorder in community samples. *J Clin Psychiatry* 2002;63(suppl 8):4–10.
4. Stein D. Comorbidity in generalised anxiety disorder: impact and implications. *J Clin Psychiatry* 2001;62(suppl 11):29–34 [review].
5. Goldenberg IM, White K, Yonkers K, et al. The infrequency of "pure culture" diagnoses among the anxiety disorders. *J Clin Psychiatry* 1996;57:528–533.
6. Dyck IR, Phillips KA, Warshaw MG, et al. Patterns of personality pathology in patients with generalized anxiety disorder, panic disorder with and without agoraphobia, and social phobia. *J Personal Disord* 2001;15:60–71.
7. Godart NT, Flament MF, Perdereau F, et al. Comorbidity between eating disorders and anxiety disorders: a review. *Int J Eat Disord* 2002;32:253–270. Search date 2001; primary source Medline.
8. Judd LL, Kessler RC, Paulus MP, et al. Comorbidity as a fundamental feature of generalised anxiety disorders: results from the National Comorbidity Study (NCS). *Acta Psychiatr Scand* 1998;98(suppl 393):6–11.
9. Andrews G, Peters L, Guzman AM, et al. A comparison of two structured diagnostic interviews: CIDI and SCAN. *Aust N Z J Psychiatry* 1995;29:124–132.
10. Kessler RC, McGonagle KA, Zhao S, et al. Lifetime and 12-month prevalence of DSM-III-R psychiatric disorders in the United States: results from the national comorbidity survey. *Arch Gen Psychiatry* 1994;51:8–19.
11. Seivewright N, Tyrer P, Ferguson B, et al. Longitudinal study of the influence of life events and personality status on diagnostic change in three neurotic disorders. *Depress Anxiety* 2000;11:105–113.
12. Pigott T. Gender differences in the epidemiology and treatment of anxiety disorders. *J Clin Psychiatry* 1999;60(suppl 18):4–15.
13. Jorm AF. Does old age reduce the risk of anxiety and depression? A review of epidemiological studies across the adult life span. *Psychol Med* 2000;30:11–22.
14. Lau AW, Edelstein BA, Larkin KT. Psychophysiological arousal in older adults: a critical review. *Clin Psychol Rev* 2001;21:609–630 [review].
15. Brantley PJ, Mehan DJ Jr, Ames SC, et al. Minor stressors and generalised anxiety disorders among low income patients attending primary care clinics. *J Nerv Ment Dis* 1999;187:435–440.
16. Brown ES, Fulton MK, Wilkeson A, et al. The psychiatric sequelae of civilian trauma. *Comp Psychiatry* 2000;41:19–23.
17. Hawker DSJ, Boulton MJ. Twenty years' research on peer victimisation and psychosocial maladjustment: a meta-analytic review of cross-sectional studies. *J Child Psychol Psychiatr* 2000;41:441–445. Search date 1997; primary sources Psychlit, Social Science Citation Index, OCLC Firstsearch, hand searches of relevant journals, bibliographies, reviews, reference lists of relevant articles, and book chapters, and personal contact with authors.
18. Hettema JM, Neale MC, Kendler KS. A review and meta-analysis of the genetic epidemiology of anxiety disorders. *Am J Psychiatry* 2001;158:1568–1578. Search date not reported; primary source Medline.
19. Yonkers KA, Dyck IR, Warshaw M, et al. Factors predicting the clinical course of generalised anxiety disorder. *Br J Psychiatry* 2000;176:544–549.
20. Gould RA, Otto MW, Pollack MH, et al. Cognitive behavioral and pharmacological treatment of generalized anxiety disorder: a preliminary meta-analysis. *Behav Ther* 1997;28:285–305. Search date 1996; primary sources Psychlit, Medline, examination of reference lists, and unpublished articles presented at national conferences.
21. Westen D, Morrison K. A multidimensional meta-analysis of treatments for depression, panic and generalized anxiety disorder: an empirical examination of the status of empirically supported therapies. *J Consult Clin Psychol* 2001;69:875–889. Search date not reported but only included studies published 1990–1999; primary source hand searches of 10 journals and psychological abstracts.
22. Ost L, Breitholts E. Applied relaxation vs. cognitive therapy in the treatment of generalized anxiety disorder. *Behav Res Ther* 2000;38:777–790.
23. Borkovec TD, Newman MG, Pincus AL. A component analysis of cognitive-behavioural therapy for

generalized anxiety disorder and the role of interpersonal process. *J Consult Clin Psychol* 2002;70:288–298.

24. Stanley MA, Beck JG, Novy DM, et al. Cognitive-behavioural treatment of late-life generalized anxiety disorder. *J Consult Clin Psychol* 2003;71:309–319.
25. Wetherall JL, Gatx M, Craske MG. Treatment of generalized anxiety disorder in older adults. *J Consult Clin Psychol* 2003;71:31–40.
26. Arntz A. Cognitive therapy versus applied relaxation as treatment for generalized anxiety disorder. *Behav Res Ther* 2003;41:633–646.
27. Dugas MJ, Ladouceur R, Leger E, et al. Group cognitive-behavioral therapy for generalized anxiety disorder: treatment outcome and long-term follow-up. *J Consult Clin Psychol* 2003;71:821–825.
28. Barrowclough C, King P, Russell E, et al. A randomized trial of effectiveness of cognitive-behavioural therapy and supportive counselling for anxiety disorders in older adults. *J Consult Clin Psychol* 2001;69:756–762.
29. Fisher PL, Durham RC. Recovery rates in generalized anxiety disorder following psychological therapy: an analysis of clinically significant change in the STAI-T across outcome studies since 1990. *Psychol Med* 1999;29:1425–1434. Search date 1998; primary sources Medline, Psychlit, and Cochrane Controlled Trials Register.
30. Rickels K, DeMartinis N, Aufdembrinke B. A double-blind, placebo controlled trial of abecarnil and diazepam in the treatment of patients with generalized anxiety disorder. *J Clin Psychopharmacol* 2000;20:12–18.
31. Figueira ML. Alprazolam SR in the treatment of generalised anxiety: a multicentre controlled study with bromazepam. *Hum Psychother* 1999;14:171–177.
32. Vaz-Serra A, Figuerra L, Bessa-Peixoto A, et al. Mexazolam and alprazolam in the treatment of generalized anxiety disorder. *Clin Drug Invest* 2001;21:257–263.
33. Mahe V, Balogh A. Long-term pharmacological treatment of generalized anxiety disorder. *Int Clin Psychopharmacol* 2000;15:99–105. Search date 1998; primary sources Medline, Biosis, and Embase.
34. Tyrer P. Current problems with the benzodiazepines. In: Wheatly D, ed. *The anxiolytic jungle: where next?* Chichester: Wiley, 1990:23–47.
35. Kilic C, Curran HV, Noshirvani H, et al. Long-term effects of alprazolam on memory: a 3.5 year follow-up of agoraphobia/panic patients. *Psychol Med* 1999;29:225–231.
36. Thomas RE. Benzodiazepine use and motor vehicle accidents. Systematic review of reported association. *Can Fam Physician* 1998;44:799–808. Search date 1997; primary source Medline.
37. Dolovich LR, Addis A, Regis Vaillancourt JD, et al. Benzodiazepine use in pregnancy and major malformations of oral cleft: meta-analysis of cohort and case-control studies. *BMJ* 1998;317:839–843. Search date 1997; primary sources Medline, Embase, Reprotox, and references of included studies and review articles.
38. Bernstein JG. *Handbook of drug therapy in psychiatry*, 3rd ed. St Louis, MO: Mosby Year Book, 1995:401.
39. DeMartinis N, Rynn M, Rickels K, et al. Prior benzodiazepine use and buspirone response in the treatment of generalized anxiety disorder. *J Clin Psychiatry* 2000;61:91–94.
40. Sramek JJ, Transman M, Suri A, et al. Efficacy of buspirone in generalized anxiety disorder with coexisting mild depressive symptoms. *J Clin Psychiatry* 1996;57:287–291.
41. Davidson JR, DuPont RL, Hedges D, et al. Efficacy, safety and tolerability of venlafaxine extended release and buspirone in outpatients with generalised anxiety disorder. *J Clin Psychiatry* 1999;60:528–535.
42. Rickels K, Weisman K, Norstad N, et al. Buspirone and diazepam in anxiety: a controlled study. *J Clin Psychiatry* 1982;12:81–86.
43. Gammans RE, Stringfellow JC, Hvisdos AJ, et al. Use of buspirone in patients with generalized anxiety disorder and coexisting depressive symptoms: a meta-analysis of eight randomized, controlled trials. *Pharmacopsychiatry* 1992;25:193–201.
44. Lader M, Anxiolytic effect of hydroxyzine: a double-blind trial versus placebo and buspirone. *Hum Psychopharmacol Clin Exp* 1999;14:S94–S102.
45. Llorca PM, Spadone C, Sol O, et al. Efficacy and safety of hydroxyzine in the treatment of generalized anxiety disorder: a 3-month double-blind study. *J Clin Psychiatry* 2002;63:1020–1027.
46. Ballenger JC, McDonald S, Noyes R, et al. The first double-blind, placebo-controlled trial of a partial benzodiazepine agonist, abecarnil (ZK 112–119) in generalised anxiety disorder. *Adv Biochem Psychopharmacol* 1992;47:431–447.
47. Kapczinski F, Schmitt R, Lima MS. Antidepressants for generalized anxiety disorder. In: The Cochrane Library, Issue 2, 2003. Oxford: Update Software. Search date 2002; primary sources CCDAN and CSG Controlled Trials Register, Medline, Lilacs, reference searching, personal communication, conference abstracts, pharmaceutical industry, and book chapters on the treatment of generalised anxiety disorder.
48. Rickels K, Zaninelli R, McCafferty J, et al. Paroxetine treatment of generalized anxiety disorder: a double-blind, placebo-controlled study. *Am J Psychiatry* 2003;160:749–756.
49. Lenox-Smith AJ, Reynolds A. A double-blind, randomised, placebo controlled study of venlafaxine XL in patients with generalised anxiety disorder in primary care. *Br J Gen Pract* 2003;53:772–777.
50. Moller HJ, Volz HP, Reimann IW, et al. Opipramol for the treatment of generalised anxiety disorder: a placebo-controlled trial including an alprazolam-treated group. *J Clin Psychopharmacol* 2001;21:51–65.
51. Rickels K, Downing R, Schweizer E, et al. Antidepressants for the treatment of generalised anxiety disorder: a placebo-controlled comparison of imipramine, trazodone and diazepam. *Arch Gen Psychiatry* 1993;50:884–895.
52. Rocca P, Fonzo V, Scotta M, et al. Paroxetine efficacy in the treatment of generalized anxiety disorder. *Acta Psychiatr Scand* 1997;95:444–450.
53. Montgomery SA, Mahe V, Haudiquet V, et al. Effectiveness of venlafaxine, extended release formulation, in the short-term and long-term treatment of generalized anxiety disorder: results of a survival analysis. *J Clin Psychopharmacol* 2002;22:561–567.
54. Rosenbaum JF, Fava M, Hoog SL, et al. Selective serotonin reuptake inhibitor discontinuation syndrome: a randomized clinical trial. *Biol Psychiatry* 1998;44:77–87.
55. Dukes PD, Robinson GM, Thomson KJ, et al. Wellington coroner autopsy cases 1970–89: acute deaths due to drugs, alcohol and poisons. *N Z Med J* 1992;105:25–27. [Erratum in *N Z Med J* 1992;105:135.]
56. Kerr GW, McGuffie AC, Wilkie S. Tricyclic antidepressant overdose: a review. *Emerg Med J* 2001;18:236–241.
57. Pearn J, Nixon J, Ansford A, et al. Accidental poisoning in childhood: five year urban population study with 15 year analysis of fatality. *BMJ* 1984;288:44–46.
58. Liu BA, Mittmann N, Knowles SR, et al. Hyponatremia and the syndrome of inappropriate secretion of antidiuretic hormone associated with the use of selective serotonin reuptake inhibitors: a review of spontaneous reports. *Can Med Assoc J* 1995;155:519–527. [Erratum in *Can Med Assoc J* 1996;155:1043.]
59. Thapa PB, Gideon P, Cost TW, et al. Antidepressants and the risk of falls among nursing home residents. *N Engl J Med* 1998;339:875–882.

60. Liu B, Anderson G, Mittmann N, et al. Use of selective serotonin-reuptake inhibitors of tricyclic antidepressants and risk of hip fractures in elderly people. *Lancet* 1998;351:1303–1307.
61. Kulin NA, Pastuszak A, Koren G. Are the new SSRIs safe for pregnant women? *Can Fam Physician* 1998;44;2081–2083.
62. Montejo AL, Llorca G, Izquierdo JA, et al. Incidence of sexual dysfunction associated with antidepressant agents: a prospective multicentre study of 1022 outpatients. *J Clin Psychiatry* 2000;62(suppl 3):10–21.
63. Mendels J, Krajewski TF, Huffer V, et al. Effective short-term treatment of generalized anxiety with trifluoperazine. *J Clin Psychiatry* 1986;47:170–174.
64. Van Harten PN, Hoek HW, Matroos GE, et al. Intermittent neuroleptic treatment and risk of tardive dyskinesia: Curacao Extrapyramidal Syndromes study III. *Am J Psychiatry* 1998;155:565–567.
65. Pittler MH, Ernst E. Kava extract for treating anxiety. In: The Cochrane Library, Issue 2, 2003. Oxford: Update Software. Search date 2002; primary sources Medline, Embase, Biosis, Amed, Ciscom, Cochrane Library, hand searches of references, personal files, and contact with manufacturers of kava preparations and experts.
66. Stevensin C, Huntley A, Ernst E. A systematic review of the safety of Kava extract in the treatment of anxiety. *Drug Saf* 2002;25;251–256. Search date 2000; primary sources Medline, Embase, Amed, Cochrane Library, reference lists, departmental files, contact with colleagues in herbal medicine, World Health Organization, US Food and Drug Administration, UK Committee on Safety of Medicines, German Bundesinstitut für Arzneimittel und Medizinprodukte, and 10 manufacturers of kava preparations.
67. National Center for Complimentary and Alternative Medicine. Consumer Advisory. Kava linked to liver damage. Internet 2003 [cited February 10]; http://www.nccam.nih.gov/health/alerts/kava/index.htm (last accessed 20 October 2003).
68. Rocca P, Fonzo V, Scotta M, et al. Paroxetine efficacy in the treatment of generalized anxiety disorder. Acta Psychiatr Scand 1997;95:444–450.

Christopher Gale
Consultant Psychiatrist, Clinical Senior Lecturer
Faculty of Medicine and Health Sciences
University of Auckland
Auckland
New Zealand

Mark Oakley-Browne
Professor of Rural Psychiatry
University of Monash
Victoria
Australia

Competing interests: CG has been paid by Eli Lilly, the manufacturer of Prozac (fluoxetine), and by Janssen to attend symposia. MOB has been paid by GlaxoSmithKline, the manufacturer of Aropax (paroxetine) for contributing to educational sessions for general practitioners. MOB has also been reimbursed by Pfizer for attending a conference.

TABLE 1 Studies examining effects of cognitive behavioural therapy (see text, p 1280).

Reference and study design	Population	Intervention	Results
20 Systematic review (search date 1996)	13 RCTs, 722 people aged 18–60 years, 60% women.	Cognitive behavioural therapy (which involved, alone or in combination, cognitive restructuring, relaxation, exposure, and systematic desensitisation) *v* control (remaining on a waiting list, anxiety management alone, relaxation alone, and non-directive psychotherapy)	Cognitive behavioural therapy significantly improved symptoms over 4–12 weeks compared with control (effect size for anxiety 0.70, 95% CI 0.57 to 0.83 and for depression 0.77, 95% CI 0.64 to 0.90; dichotomous data not reported)
21 Systematic review (search date not reported)	5 RCTs, 313 people aged 18–60 years. Included three RCTs identified by the first review.[20]	Cognitive behavioural therapy (including relaxation, cognitive therapy, behavioural therapy, and anxiety management training, alone or in combination) or analytical psychotherapy Versus waiting list control	Cognitive behavioural therapy improved symptoms compared with waiting list control (median effect size 0.9; CI not reported)
25 RCT	75 people aged > 55 years	Cognitive therapy versus attending a discussion group on worrying topics versus waiting list control Duration: 12 weeks	Either cognitive therapy or a discussion group significantly increased the proportion of people who no longer met criteria for generalised anxiety disorder (GAD) immediately after treatment compared with waiting list control (people without GAD: 54% with cognitive therapy *v* 50% with discussion group *v* 13% with control; $P < 0.01$ for either treatment *v* control; absolute numbers not reported). It found no significant difference between cognitive therapy and a discussion group in the proportion of people who no longer met criteria for GAD immediately after treatment ($P = 0.78$) or at 6 months (72% with cognitive therapy *v* 53% with discussion group; $P = 0.23$)

TABLE 1 continued

Reference and study design	Population	Intervention	Results
24 RCT	80 people aged > 60 years	Cognitive therapy versus minimal contact involving one telephone call a week (see comment below). Duration: 15 weeks Comment: the control group received minimal contact rather than usual care without cognitive behavioural therapy; this may have overestimated the effect of cognitive therapy.	Symptoms were assessed by Hamilton Anxiety Scale, State-Trait Anxiety Inventory, Penn State Worry Questionnaire, and GAD Severity Scale. Cognitive therapy significantly increased the proportion of people who responded immediately after treatment compared with minimal contact (response defined as a 20% reduction in symptoms on 3 of the 4 assessment scales: 13/29 [45%] with cognitive therapy *v* 3/35 [8%] with minimal contact; RR 5.2, 95% CI 1.6 to 16.5; NNT 3, 95% CI 2 to 8)
22 RCT	36 people aged 18–60 years	Cognitive therapy versus applied relaxation Duration: 12 weekly sessions	No significant difference between 12 weekly sessions of cognitive therapy and applied relaxation in the proportion of people who responded after 13 weeks (response defined as improvement to score 3 or 4 on Cognitive Global Impression Scale: 10/18 [56%] with cognitive therapy *v* 8/15 [53%] with applied relaxation; RR 1.04, 95% CI 0.55 to 1.95)
23 RCT	76 people, mean age 37 years, 69 people completed	Cognitive therapy versus applied relaxation versus a combination of these methods Duration: 15 weekly sessions	Similar proportions of people in each group no longer met criteria for GAD immediately after treatment and at 24 months (people without GAD at follow up: 8.7% in each group immediately after treatment; 14.3% with cognitive therapy *v* 19.1% with applied relaxation *v* 19.1% with combination of treatments at 24 months; P value not reported)

TABLE 1 continued

Reference and study design	Population	Intervention	Results
26 RCT	45 people aged 17–70 years	Cognitive therapy versus applied relaxation Duration: 12 weeks	No significant difference between cognitive therapy and applied relaxation in the proportion of people who responded at 6 months (response defined as a score of ≤ 46 on the State-Trait Anxiety Inventory: 55% with cognitive therapy *v* 53.3% with applied relaxation; results not analysed by intention to treat; reported as non-significant; absolute numbers not reported)
27 RCT	52 people on stable medication, mean age 41 years, average duration of GAD 17 years.	Group cognitive therapy (14 2-hour group sessions, 4–6 people per group) versus waiting list control treatment in which people were contacted by phone every 3 weeks and offered active treatment after 6 months. Duration: 14 weeks	Cognitive therapy significantly improved scores on the Penn State Worry Questionnaire (PSWQ) and the Beck Anxiety Inventory (BAI); at the end of treatment, change in scores from baseline, PSWQ: 6.36 to 3.40 with therapy *v* 5.82 to 5.30 with control; BAI: 18.48 to 8.04 with therapy *v* 16.30 to 15.63 with control, $P < 0.05$ for both group/time interactions)

TABLE 2 **Studies examining effects of antidepressants (see text, p 1285).**

Reference and study design	Population	Intervention	Results
47 Systematic review (search date 2002)	8 RCTs, 2058 people	Antidepressants (imipramine, paroxetine, and venlafaxine) versus placebo Each individual antidepressant compared with placebo Duration: 8 to 28 weeks	Antidepressants (imipramine, paroxetine, and venlafaxine) significantly increased response rates at 8–28 weeks compared with placebo (4 RCTs, proportion of people who failed to respond 277/606 [46%] with antidepressants *v* 280/449 [62%] with placebo; RR of not responding 0.70, 95% CI 0.62 to 0.79; NNT 6, 95% CI 5 to 9). Imipramine significantly increased response rates compared with placebo (1 RCT; RR 0.67, 95% CI 0.50 to 0.91; NNT 4, 95% CI 3 to 14). Venlafaxine significantly increased response rates compared with placebo (2 RCTs; RR 0.68, 95% CI 0.46 to 0.99; NNT 5, 95% CI 4 to 9). Paroxetine significantly increased response rates compared with placebo (1 RCT; RR 0.72, 95% CI 0.56 to 0.92; NNT 7, 95% CI 4 to 25)
48	565 people	Paroxetine (20 or 40 mg/day) versus placebo Duration: 8 weeks	Response defined as Clinical Global Impression [CGI] scores ≤ 2 Paroxetine (20 or 40 mg/day) significantly increased response rates compared with placebo (paroxetine 20 mg/day: 116/188 [62%] *v* 82/180 [45%]; RR 1.36, 95% CI 1.11 to 1.64; NNT 6, 95% CI 4 to 13; paroxetine 40 mg/day: 134/197 [68%] *v* 82/180 [45%]; RR 1.49, 95% CI 1.24 to 1.79; NNT 4, 95% CI 3 to 6)

TABLE 2 continued

Reference and study design	Population	Intervention	Results
50	318 people	Opipramol (a tricyclic antidepressant with minimal serotonin reuptake blocking properties) versus alprazolam versus placebo Duration: 28 days	Opipramol significantly increased response rate after 28 days compared with placebo (response defined as CGI scale score of < 2; 63/100 [63%] with opipramol *v* 50/107 [47%] with placebo; RR 1.35, 95% CI 1.05 to 1.69; NNT 7; 95% CI 1 to 26)
49	244 people with GAD and depression from general practice	Venlafaxine (sustained release 75–150 mg per day) versus placebo Duration: 24 weeks	Response defined as a 50% reduction in HAM-A and remission defined as HAM-A score of < 7. It found no significant difference between venlafaxine and placebo in response or remission rates at 24 weeks (response: 52.5% with venlafaxine *v* 48.4% with placebo, P = 0.68; remission: 27.9% with venlafaxine *v* 18.9% with placebo, P = 0.11). Venlafaxine significantly increased CGI at 24 weeks compared with placebo (CGI score 1 or 2 meaning much or very much improved: 65% with venlafaxine *v* 46% with placebo, P = 0.003)
68 identified by systematic review[47]	56 people	Paroxetine versus imipramine Duration: 8 weeks.	No significant difference between paroxetine and imipramine in the proportion of people who responded over 8 weeks of treatment (proportion who failed to respond 3/36 [8%] with paroxetine *v* 2/30 [7%] with imipramine; RR of failing to respond 1.73, 95% CI 0.31 to 9.57)
51 identified by systematic review[47]	230 people	Variable doses of four interventions: imipramine versus trazodone versus diazepam versus placebo Duration: 8 weeks	Similar improvements among groups in participant assessed global improvement after 8 weeks of treatment (results not analysed by intention to treat; 73% of people improved with imipramine *v* 67% with trazodone *v* 66% with diazepam). The RCT did not directly compare the significance of differences between groups

TABLE 2 continued

Reference and study design	Population	Intervention	Results
52 identified by systematic review[47]	81 people	Paroxetine versus Imipramine versus 2–chlordesmethyldiazepam Duration: 8 weeks	Paroxetine and imipramine significantly improved anxiety after 8 weeks compared with 2'-chlordesmethyldiazepam (mean Hamilton Anxiety Scale score: 11.1 with paroxetine *v* 10.8 with imipramine *v* 12.9 with 2'-chlordesmethyldiazepam; P = 0.05 for either comparison *v* 2'-chlordesmethyldiazepam)
50	307 people	Opipramol versus alprazolam Duration: 28 days	No significant difference between opipramol and alprazolam in response rate over 28 days (63/100 [63%] with opipramol *v* 67/105 [64%] with alprazolam; RR 1.01, 95% CI 0.79 to 1.25)
41 identified by systematic review[47]	365 people	Venlafaxine (75 or 150 mg/day) versus buspirone (30 mg/day) versus placebo	Similar response rates between venlafaxine and buspirone after 8 weeks of treatment (response defined as CGI score of 1 or 2; 54/87 [62%] with venlafaxine 75 mg *v* 44/89 [49%] with venlafaxine 150 mg *v* 52/95 [55%] with buspirone; P values not reported)

Obsessive compulsive disorder

Search date September 2003

G Mustafa Soomro

QUESTIONS

INTERVENTIONS

See glossary G

Key Messages

Initial treatment

- **Behavioural therapy** We found no RCTs comparing behavioural therapy versus no treatment. One systematic review and subsequent RCTs have found that behavioural therapy improves symptoms compared with relaxation. The review and one subsequent RCT found no significant difference in symptoms over 4–16 weeks between behavioural therapy and cognitive therapy. One subsequent RCT found limited evidence that group behavioural therapy improved symptoms after 12 weeks compared with group cognitive behavioural therapy.
- **Cognitive or cognitive behavioural therapy** We found no RCTs comparing cognitive therapy versus no treatment. One RCT found that cognitive behavioural group therapy improved symptoms and quality of life compared with no treatment after 12 weeks. One systematic review and one subsequent RCT found no significant difference in symptoms over 4–16 weeks between behavioural therapy and cognitive therapy. Another subsequent RCT found limited evidence that group behavioural therapy improved symptoms over 12 weeks compared with group cognitive behavioural therapy.

- **Serotonin reuptake inhibitors (citalopram, clomipramine, fluoxetine, fluvoxamine, paroxetine, sertraline)** RCTs have found that selective and non-selective serotonin reuptake inhibitors (citalopram, clomipramine, fluoxetine, fluvoxamine, paroxetine) improve symptoms compared with placebo. Two systematic reviews found inconsistent results about the effects of sertraline compared with placebo. RCTs have found that selective and non-selective serotonin reuptake inhibitors (citalopram, clomipramine, fluoxetine, fluvoxamine, paroxetine, sertraline) improve symptoms compared with tricyclic antidepressants or monoamine oxidase inhibitors. RCTs have found no consistent evidence of a difference in efficacy among serotonin reuptake inhibitors, but have found that the non-selective serotonin reuptake inhibitor clomipramine is associated with more adverse effects than selective serotonin reuptake inhibitors.
- **Behavioural or cognitive therapy plus serotonin reuptake inhibitors (compared with behavioural or cognitive therapy alone)** RCTs provided insufficient evidence to assess the effects of adding serotonin reuptake inhibitors to behavioural or cognitive therapy.
- **Electroconvulsive therapy** We found no RCTs of electroconvulsive therapy in people with obsessive compulsive disorder.
- **Venlafaxine** One RCT provided insufficient evidence to compare venlafaxine versus clomipramine.

Maintenance treatment

- **Optimum duration of treatment with serotonin reuptake inhibitors** RCTs provided insufficient evidence to define the optimum duration of treatment with serotonin reuptake inhibitors.

In people who do not respond to selective and non-selective serotonin reuptake inhibitors

- **Addition of antipsychotics in people who have not responded to serotonin reuptake inhibitors** Three small RCTs in people unresponsive to serotonin reuptake inhibitors found that the addition of antipsychotics improved symptoms compared with placebo.

DEFINITION Obsessive compulsive disorder involves obsessions, compulsions, or both, that are not caused by drugs or a physical disorder, and which cause significant personal distress or social dysfunction.[1,2] The disorder may have a chronic or an episodic course Ⓖ. **Obsessions** are recurrent and persistent ideas, images, or impulses that cause pronounced anxiety and that the person perceives to be self produced. **Compulsions** are repetitive behaviours or mental acts performed in response to obsessions or according to certain rules, which are aimed at reducing distress or preventing certain imagined dreaded events. People with obsessive compulsive disorder may have insight into their condition, in that obsessions and compulsions are usually recognised and resisted. There are minor differences in the criteria for obsessive compulsive disorder between the third, revised third, and fourth editions of the *Diagnostic and Statistical Manual* (DSM-III, DSM-III-R, and DSM-IV)[1] and *The ICD-10 Classification of Mental and Behavioural Disorders*.[2]

INCIDENCE/ PREVALENCE One national, community based survey of obsessive compulsive disorder in the UK (1993, 10 000 people) found that 1% of men and 1.5% of women reported symptoms in the past month.[3] An epidemiological catchment area (ECA) survey carried out in the USA in 1984 (about 10 000 people) found age and sex standardised annual prevalence of obsessive compulsive disorder in people aged 26–64 years of 1.3%, and lifetime prevalence of 2.3%.[4] Subsequent cross national surveys using methodology comparable to ECA found age and sex standardised annual and lifetime prevalence in people aged 26–64 years as follows: Canada (survey size about 2200 people), annual prevalence 1.4% (SE 0.25), and lifetime prevalence 2.3% (SE 0.32); Puerto Rico (survey size about 1200 people), annual prevalence 1.8% (SE 0.39), and lifetime prevalence 2.5% (SE 0.46); Germany (survey size 4811 people), annual prevalence 1.6% (SE 0.57), and lifetime prevalence 2.1% (SE 0.66); Taiwan (survey size about 7400 people), annual prevalence 0.4% (SE 0.07), and lifetime prevalence 0.7% (SE

0.10); Korea (survey size about 4000 people), annual prevalence 1.1% (SE 0.10), and lifetime prevalence 1.9% (SE 0.20); and New Zealand (survey size about 1200 people), annual prevalence 1.1% (SE 0.31), and lifetime prevalence 2.2% (SE 0.42).[4]

AETIOLOGY/ RISK FACTORS The cause of obsessive compulsive disorder is uncertain. Behavioural, cognitive, genetic, and neurobiological factors have been implicated.[5–11] Risk factors include a family history of obsessive compulsive disorder, being single (which could be a consequence of the disorder), and belonging to a higher socioeconomic class.[12] Other risk factors include cocaine abuse, female sex, not being in paid employment, past history of alcohol dependence, affective disorder, and phobic disorder.[4]

PROGNOSIS One study (144 people followed for a mean of 47 years) found that an episodic course of obsessive compulsive disorder was more common during the initial years (about 1–9 years), but a chronic course was more common afterwards.[13] Over time, the study found that 39–48% of people had symptomatic improvement. A 1 year prospective cohort study found that 46% of people had an episodic course and 54% had a chronic course.[14]

AIMS OF INTERVENTION To improve symptoms, and to reduce the impact of illness on social functioning and quality of life, with minimal adverse effects of treatment.

OUTCOMES Severity of symptoms; social functioning; and adverse effects of treatment. Commonly used instruments for measuring symptoms include the Hamilton Anxiety Rating scale; the Hamilton Depression Rating scale; and the Yale-Brown Obsessive Compulsive Scale, which is observer rated and well validated. It rates severity of both obsessions and compulsions across five dimensions (time spent, interference with functioning, distress, resistance, and control), each on a five point scale from 0–4 (0 means that the dimension is absent and 4 means that the dimension is present to extremely severe degree). The total score range of obsessions and compulsions combined is 0–40 (the higher the score the more severe the condition).[15–17] Most trials use a 25% reduction in Yale-Brown scale scores from baseline as indicative of clinically important improvement, but some studies use a 35% reduction.[17]

METHODS *Clinical Evidence* search and appraisal September 2003.

QUESTION **What are the effects of initial treatments in adults?**

OPTION **SEROTONIN REUPTAKE INHIBITORS (CITALOPRAM, CLOMIPRAMINE, FLUOXETINE, FLUVOXAMINE, PAROXETINE, SERTRALINE)**

RCTs have found that selective and non-selective serotonin reuptake inhibitors (citalopram, clomipramine, fluoxetine, fluvoxamine, paroxetine) improve symptoms compared with placebo. Two systematic reviews found inconsistent results about the effects of sertraline compared with placebo. RCTs have found that selective and non-selective serotonin reuptake inhibitors (citalopram, clomipramine, fluoxetine, fluvoxamine, paroxetine, sertraline) improve symptoms compared with tricyclic antidepressants or monoamine oxidase inhibitors. One RCT found no significant difference in symptoms between clomipramine and venlafaxine, but it is likely to have been underpowered to detect a clinically important difference. RCTs have found no consistent evidence of a difference in efficacy among serotonin reuptake inhibitors, but have found that the non-selective serotonin reuptake inhibitor clomipramine is associated with more adverse effects than selective serotonin reuptake inhibitors.

Benefits: **Versus placebo:** We found two systematic reviews (search dates 1994[18] and not reported[19]) and three subsequent RCTs.[20–22] The two systematic reviews and three subsequent RCTs found that selective or non-selective serotonin reuptake inhibitors (citalopram, clomipramine, fluoxetine, fluvoxamine, paroxetine) significantly improved symptoms compared with placebo (see comment below).[18–22] One of the reviews found that sertraline significantly improved symptoms compared with placebo,[18] and the other review found no significant difference in symptoms (see table 1, p 1310).[19] **Versus each other:** We found two systematic reviews[18,19] and five subsequent RCTs.[23–27] All found no significant difference in symptoms between different selective and non-selective serotonin reuptake inhibitors.[18,19,23–27] The first review (search date 1994, 85 people, 3 RCTs) found no significant difference in symptoms among clomipramine, fluoxetine and fluvoxamine (SMD –0.04, 95% CI –0.43 to +0.35).[18] The second review (search date not reported) found no significant difference in symptoms between clomipramine and fluvoxamine (4 RCTs, including 2 RCTs from the first review; change in Yale-Brown scale score; SMD +1.23, 95% CI –1.11 to +3.56).[19] It also found no significant difference in symptoms between clomipramine and fluoxetine (1 RCT, not included in the first review, 55 people; change in Yale-Brown scale score; SMD +1.40, 95% CI –5.74 to +2.94) or clomipramine and paroxetine (1 RCT not included in the first review, 300 people; change in Yale-Brown scale score; SMD 0.00, 95% CI –1.94 to +1.94).[19] The first subsequent RCT (170 people) found that sertraline significantly improved symptoms compared with clomipramine (8% greater mean reduction in Yale-Brown scale score, $P = 0.036$; see comment below).[23] The second subsequent RCT (133 people) found no significant difference in symptoms between clomipramine and fluvoxamine (change in Yale-Brown scale score, 12.6 with clomipramine *v* 12.3 with fluvoxamine; reported as non-significant, no further data reported).[24] The third subsequent RCT (227 people, double blind) found no significant difference between clomipramine (150–300 mg) and fluvoxamine (150–300 mg) in severity of symptoms after 10 weeks (mean reduction in Yale-Brown scale score about 12 in both groups; P value not reported; proportion of people achieving at least 35% reduction in Yale-Brown scale score 65% with clomipramine *v* 62% with fluvoxamine, reported as non-significant).[25] The fourth subsequent RCT (150 people) compared sertraline (50–200 mg) versus fluoxetine (20–80 mg).[26] It found similar symptom severity at 24 weeks between sertraline and fluoxetine (reduction in Yale-Brown scale score 9.6 with sertraline *v* 9.7 with fluoxetine, CI not reported). The fifth subsequent RCT (30 people, observer blinded) compared three interventions: fluvoxamine, paroxetine, and citalopram.[27] It found no significant difference in symptoms among drugs, but was too small to exclude a clinically important difference. **Versus tricyclic antidepressants and monoamine oxidase inhibitors:** We found one systematic review[18] and two subsequent RCTs.[28,29] These found that serotonin reuptake inhibitors significantly improved symptoms compared with tricyclic antidepressants or monoamine oxidase inhibitors. The systematic review (search date 1994, 7 RCTs, 147 people with obsessive compulsive disorder, including 67 children/adolescents) found that, compared with tricyclic antidepressants (desipramine, imipramine, nortripytyline) or monoamine oxidase inhibitors (clorgiline, phenelzine), clomipramine significantly improved symptoms (SMD 0.65, 95% CI 0.36 to 0.92).[18] The first subsequent RCT (54 people) compared three interventions: fluoxetine, phenelzine (a monoamine oxidase inhibitor), and placebo.[28] It found that fluoxetine significantly improved symptoms over 10 weeks compared with phenelzine or placebo (mean reduction in Yale-Brown scale score 2.8 with fluoxetine *v* 1.7 with phenelzine *v* 0.2 with placebo; $P < 0.05$ for fluoxetine *v* either comparator). The second subsequent RCT (164 people with concurrent obsessive compulsive disorder and major depressive disorder) found that sertraline significantly increased the proportion of people who had a clinically important reduction in obsessive compulsive symptoms compared with desipramine (> 40% improvement on Yale-Brown scale, 38/79 [48%] with sertraline *v* 26/85 [31%] with desipramine; $P = 0.01$) and significantly increased the proportion of people with remission of depressive symptoms (< 7 on Hamilton Depression Rating Scale, 39/79 [49%] with sertraline *v* 30/85 [35%] with desipramine; $P = 0.04$).[29] **Versus venlafaxine:** We found one RCT (73 people), which compared clomipramine (150–225 mg daily, 47 people) versus venlafaxine (225–350 mg daily, 26 people).[30] It found no significant difference in response at 12 weeks between clomipramine and venlafaxine (response defined as ≥ 35% reduction in Yale-Brown scale score and Clinical Global Impression Scale score of ≥ 2, 9/25 [36%] *v* 20/40 [50%]; RR 1.39, 95% CI 0.76 to 2.55). **Versus behavioural therapy:** We found one systematic review (search date 1997, number of studies and people not reported).[31] It found no significant difference in symptoms among serotonin reuptake inhibitors, behavioural therapy**Ⓖ**, and placebo, but these conclusions must be treated with caution as the review made indirect comparisons of effect sizes (standardised mean differences).[31] **Plus behavioural or cognitive therapy:** See behavioural or cognitive therapy plus serotonin reuptake inhibitors, p 1305.

Harms: **Versus placebo:** One systematic review (search date 1995, 16 RCTs) found that serotonin reuptake inhibitors significantly increased overall adverse effects (unspecified) compared with placebo (RRI *v* placebo: 54% with clomipramine, 11% with fluoxetine, 19% with fluvoxamine, and 27% with sertraline).[32] The other systematic reviews gave no information on adverse effects.[18,19] The first subsequent RCT found that fluoxetine significantly increased tremor ($P < 0.001$), dry mouth ($P < 0.001$), and nausea ($P < 0.01$) compared with placebo (absolute numbers presented graphically).[20] The second subsequent RCT found that citalopram significantly increased nausea, insomnia, fatigue, sweating, dry mouth, and ejaculatory failure compared with placebo ($P < 0.05$).[21] The third subsequent RCT (253 people) found that more people withdrew because of adverse effects with controlled release fluvoxamine than with placebo (20% with fluvoxamine *v* 7% with placebo; P value not reported).[22] Compared with placebo, fluvoxamine increased insomnia (35% with fluvoxamine *v* 20% with placebo), somnolence (27% *v* 11%), asthenia (25% *v* 8%, nausea (34% *v* 13%), diarrhoea (18% *v* 8%), anorexia (13% *v* 5%), and decreased libido (7% *v* 3%). **Versus each other:** The systematic reviews gave no information on adverse effects.[18,19] Three subsequent RCTs found that clomipramine increased adverse effects compared with selective serotonin reuptake inhibitors,[23–25] and one subsequent RCT[26] found no significant difference in adverse effects between the selective serotonin reuptake inhibitors sertraline and fluoxetine. The first subsequent RCT (170 people) found that significantly more people withdrew because of adverse effects with clomipramine than with sertraline ($P < 0.05$).[23] Clomipramine was associated with dry mouth, nausea, tremor, anxiety, and constipation, whereas sertraline was associated with nausea and diarrhoea. The second subsequent RCT (133 people) found that clomipramine significantly increased dry mouth (38% *v* 10%) and constipation (26% *v* 10%) compared with fluvoxamine ($P < 0.05$).[24] The third subsequent RCT comparing clomipramine versus fluvoxamine (227 people) found that more people stopped clomipramine prematurely (16% withdrew with clomipramine *v* 8% with fluvoxamine; CI not reported), and found that clomipramine significantly increased the proportion of people who had anticholinergic adverse effects (dry mouth 43% with clomipramine *v* 10% with fluvoxamine; constipation 25% *v* 9%; tremor 22% *v* 9%; and dizziness 18% *v* 7%; $P = 0.05$ for frequency of all anticholinergic adverse effects with clomipramine *v* fluvoxamine).[25] The fourth subsequent RCT found no significant difference in adverse effects between sertraline and fluoxetine.[26] The fifth subsequent RCT gave no information on adverse effects.[27] One systematic review (search date 1997) of controlled and uncontrolled studies found that the withdrawal rate because of adverse effects was 11% with clomipramine, 10% with fluoxetine, 13% with fluvoxamine, 9% with sertraline, and 11% with paroxetine.[31] One non-systematic review of three prospective cohort studies and five surveys found that fluoxetine during pregnancy did not increase the risk of spontaneous abortion or major malformation (numerical values not provided).[33] The review included one prospective cohort study (174 people) and three surveys that found similar outcomes with other selective serotonin reuptake inhibitors (sertraline, paroxetine, and fluvoxamine). One prospective cohort study of 55 preschool children exposed to fluoxetine *in utero* found no significant difference from unexposed children in global IQ, language, or behaviour. It included no information on long term harms for the other selective serotonin reuptake inhibitors. The non-systematic review of effects in pregnancy did not describe how articles were selected.[33] **Versus tricyclic antidepressants and monoamine oxidase inhibitors:** The systematic review gave no information on adverse effects.[18] The second subsequent RCT (164 people) found that significantly more people discontinued treatment because of adverse effects with desipramine than with sertraline (26% *v* 10%; P = 0.009).[29] One systematic review comparing the harms of selective serotonin reuptake inhibitors versus tricyclic antidepressants found that selective serotonin reuptake inhibitors were associated with fewer anticholinergic adverse effects but more nausea, diarrhoea, anxiety, agitation, insomnia, and headache.[34] **Versus venlafaxine:** The RCT (73 people) found that significantly more people had overall adverse effects with clomipramine than with venlafaxine (43/47 [92%] with clomipramine *v* 16/26 [62%] with venlafaxine; P = 0.002).[30] It found that, compared with venlafaxine, clomipramine significantly increased the proportion of people who had dry mouth (16/47 [34%] with clomipramine *v* 3/26 [12%] with venlafaxine; P = 0.036) and constipation (17/47 [36%] *v* 2/26 [8%]; P = 0.008).

Comment: One of the reviews found that sertraline was more effective than placebo,[18] whereas the other did not.[19] This may have been due to different methods of meta analysis. The reviews found heterogeneity in the selection of participants and duration of treatment in the RCTs identified; the first review[18] found that this heterogeneity reached significance in RCTs comparing clomipramine versus placebo. Two RCTs comparing clomipramine versus placebo in the first review included 73 children, but the review did not analyse these RCTs separately.[18] Some RCTs identified by the reviews included people with depression associated with obsessive compulsive disorder. The first systematic review performed a subgroup analysis in people with obsessive compulsive disorder without depression and found that, compared with placebo, clomipramine improved symptoms of obsessive compulsive disorder in people without depression (5 RCTs, 594 people, standardised mean differences 1.37, 95% CI 1.19 to 1.55).[18] This suggests that the effect of serotonin reuptake inhibitors on obsessive compulsive symptoms is independent of their effect on symptoms of depression. In the first subsequent RCT comparing sertraline versus clomipramine, people taking clomipramine received very low doses (median 90 mg/day). This makes the results of the RCT difficult to interpret. **Factors predicting outcome:** Four RCTs found that people who did not respond to serotonin reuptake inhibitors had younger age of onset, longer duration of the condition, higher frequency of symptoms, coexisting personality disorders, and a greater likelihood of previous hospital admission. Predictors of good response were older age of onset, history of remissions, no previous drug treatment, more severe obsessive compulsive disorder, and either high or low score on the Hamilton Depression Rating

Scale.[35–38] Two cohort studies of people with obsessive compulsive disorder found that poor response to serotonin reuptake inhibitors was predicted by concomitant schizotypal personality disorder, by tic disorder**G**, and also by severe obsessive compulsive disorder with cleaning rituals (OR 4.9, 95% CI 1.1 to 21.2).[39,40]

OPTION BEHAVIOURAL THERAPY

We found no RCTs comparing behavioural therapy versus no treatment. One systematic review and subsequent RCTs have found that behavioural therapy improves symptoms compared with relaxation. The review and one subsequent RCT found no significant difference in symptoms over 4–16 weeks between behavioural therapy and cognitive therapy. Another subsequent RCT found limited evidence that group behavioural therapy may improve symptoms over 12 weeks compared with group cognitive behavioural therapy.

Benefits: **Versus no treatment:** We found no systematic review or RCTs. **Versus relaxation:** We found one systematic review (search date 1995, 2 RCTs, 121 people), which found that behavioural therapy**G** significantly improved symptoms over 4–16 weeks of treatment compared with relaxation (standardised mean differences 1.18, CI not reported; $P < 0.01$).[32] One subsequent RCT (218 people with DSM-IV obsessive compulsive disorder, 49% of whom were also taking a serotonin reuptake inhibitor) compared three treatments: behavioural therapy guided by a computer, behavioural therapy guided by a clinician, and relaxation.[41] It found that both types of behavioural therapy significantly improved Yale-Brown scale score after 10 weeks of treatment compared with relaxation (mean reduction 5.6 with computer guided behavioural therapy *v* 8.0 with clinician guided behavioural therapy *v* 1.7 with relaxation; $P = 0.001$ for relaxation *v* either type of behavioural therapy; $P = 0.035$ for clinician guided *v* computer guided behavioural therapy; analysis not by intention to treat).[41] **Versus cognitive or cognitive behavioural therapy:** We found one systematic review[32] and two subsequent RCTs.[42,43] The systematic review (search date 1995, 4 RCTs, 92 people) found no significant difference in symptoms over 4–16 weeks between behavioural therapy and cognitive therapy**G** (SMD –0.19; reported as $P > 0.05$, no further data reported).[32] The first subsequent RCT (76 people) found no significant difference between group behavioural therapy (exposure with response prevention) and group cognitive behavioural therapy in recovery (defined as ≥ 6 point Yale-Brown scale score reduction and score ≤ 12) immediately after 12 weeks of treatment (AR 12/32 [38%] with behavioural therapy *v* 5/31 [16%] with cognitive behavioural therapy; $P = 0.09$), but found that behavioural therapy significantly improved recovery at 3 months follow up compared with cognitive behavioural therapy (AR 14/31 [45%] with behavioural therapy *v* 4/31 [13%] with cognitive behavioural therapy; $P = 0.01$; analysis not by intention to treat). The second subsequent RCT (63 people) found no significant difference between behavioural therapy and cognitive therapy in the proportion of people achieving at least 25% improvement in Yale-Brown scale score after 16 weeks of treatment (OR 0.7, 95% CI 0.2 to 2.0).[43] **Versus serotonin reuptake inhibitors:** See benefits of serotonin reuptake inhibitors, p 1299. **Plus serotonin reuptake inhibitors:** See behavioural therapy or cognitive therapy plus serotonin reuptake inhibitors, p 1305.

Harms: We found no evidence from RCTs or cohort studies of adverse effects from behavioural therapy. Case reports have described unbearable and unacceptable anxiety in some people receiving behavioural therapy.

Comment: **Factors predicting outcome:** We found two RCTs of behavioural therapy (total 96 people, duration 2.5 months and 32 weeks) and two retrospective cohort studies (total 346 people, duration 1 year and 11 weeks), which assessed factors predicting outcome.[44–47] These found that poorer outcome was predicted by initial severity, depression, longer duration, poorer motivation, and dissatisfaction with the therapeutic relationship. Good outcome was predicted by early adherence to exposure homework**G**, employment, living with one's family, no previous treatment, having fear of contamination, overt ritualistic behaviour, and absence of depression.[44–46] Good outcome for women was predicted by having a co-therapist (someone, usually related to the woman concerned, who is enlisted to help with treatment outside regular treatment sessions; OR 19.5, 95% CI 2.7 to 139).[47] Two systematic reviews of drug, behavioural, cognitive, and combination treatments for obsessive compulsive disorder are being prepared. **Maintenance of improvement:** A prospective follow up (20 people with obsessive compulsive disorder, specific diagnostic criteria not provided) after a 6 month RCT of behavioural therapy found that 79% maintained improvement in obsessive compulsive symptoms at 2 years follow up.[48] A prospective non-inception cohort study of behavioural therapy in 21 people with obsessive compulsive disorder (specific diagnostic criteria not provided) found that, after 2 weeks of treatment, 68–79% maintained complete or much improvement in symptoms at 3 months follow up.[49] In both RCTs, some people received additional behavioural therapy during follow up.

OPTION COGNITIVE OR COGNITIVE BEHAVIOURAL THERAPY

We found no RCTs comparing cognitive therapy versus no treatment. One RCT found that cognitive behavioural group therapy improved symptoms and quality of life compared with no treatment after 12 weeks. One systematic review and one subsequent RCT found no significant difference in symptoms over 4–16 weeks between behavioural therapy and cognitive therapy. Another subsequent RCT found limited evidence that group behavioural therapy improved symptoms over 12 weeks compared with group cognitive behavioural therapy.

Benefits: **Versus no treatment:** We found one RCT (47 people with DSM-IV obsessive compulsive disorder, 45% of whom were also taking a serotonin reuptake inhibitor), which compared cognitive behavioural group therapy versus no therapy.[50] It found that cognitive behavioural group therapy significantly increased the proportion of people achieving at least 35% improvement in Yale-Brown scale score after 12 weeks treatment, and significantly improved quality of life compared with no treatment (16/23 [69.6%] with cognitive behavioural group therapy *v* 1/24 [4.2%] with no treatment; OR 16.7, 95% CI 2.2 to 115.9; mean reduction in Yale-Brown scale score 11.6 with cognitive behavioural group therapy *v* 1.5 with no treatment, P value not reported; difference in quality of life: $P < 0.04$ in favour of cognitive behavioural therapy).[50] **Versus behavioural therapy:** See behavioural therapy, p 1303. **Plus serotonin reuptake inhibitors:** See behavioural therapy or cognitive therapy plus serotonin reuptake inhibitors, p 1305.

Harms: **Versus no treatment:** The RCT reported that one person withdrew from the treatment group owing to to severe anxiety during response prevention and exposure homework**G** exercises.[50]

Comment: None.

OPTION BEHAVIOURAL OR COGNITIVE THERAPY PLUS SEROTONIN REUPTAKE INHIBITORS

RCTs provided insufficient evidence to assess the effects of adding serotonin reuptake inhibitors to behavioural or cognitive therapy.

Benefits: We found one systematic review[31] and two subsequent RCTs.[51,52] The systematic review (search date 1997, 77 studies, number of people not reported) did not make direct comparisons between treatments.[31] It included all types of study with the exception of case control studies. In indirect comparisons, it found similar reductions in symptoms with behavioural therapy alone versus placebo, behavioural therapy plus serotonin reuptake inhibitors (clomipramine, fluoxetine, fluvoxamine, paroxetine, or sertraline) versus placebo, and serotonin reuptake inhibitors alone versus placebo. One subsequent RCT (99 people in an outpatient setting) compared four interventions: behavioural therapy, cognitive therapy❻, behavioural therapy plus fluvoxamine (a selective serotonin reuptake inhibitor), and cognitive therapy plus fluvoxamine. It found no significant difference among interventions in symptoms after 16 weeks of treatment (mean reduction in Yale-Brown scale score 17.1 with behavioural therapy *v* 13.5 with cognitive therapy *v* 12.6 with behavioural therapy plus fluvoxamine *v* 15.6 with cognitive therapy plus fluvoxamine, reported as non-significant, no further data reported).[51] Another subsequent RCT (49 people in a hospital setting) found that behavioural therapy plus fluvoxamine significantly increased the proportion of people with improved symptoms after 9 weeks of treatment compared with behavioural therapy plus pill placebo (number of people with > 35% reduction of Yale-Brown scale score 21/24 [88%] *v* 15/25 [60%]; RR 1.46, 95% CI 1.02 to 2.08).[52]

Harms: We found no evidence from RCTs or cohort studies of adverse effects from behavioural therapy. Case reports have described unbearable and unacceptable anxiety in some people receiving behavioural therapy. See harms of serotonin reuptake inhibitors, p 1301. See harms of cognitive therapy, p 1304.

Comment: None.

OPTION ELECTROCONVULSIVE THERAPY

We found no RCTs of electroconvulsive therapy in people with obsessive compulsive disorder.

Benefits: We found no systematic review or RCTs.

Harms: We found no RCTs.

Comment: People with obsessive compulsive disorder who also have depression may be treated with electroconvulsive therapy. The evidence for the effects of electroconvulsive therapy in depression is summarised elsewhere in *Clinical Evidence* (see depressive disorders in adults, p 1238).

QUESTION What are the best forms of maintenance treatment in adults?

OPTION OPTIMUM DURATION OF MAINTENANCE TREATMENT WITH SEROTONIN REUPTAKE INHIBITORS

RCTs provided insufficient evidence to define the optimum duration of treatment with serotonin reuptake inhibitors.

Benefits: Most RCTs lasted only 10–12 weeks.[53] We found two RCTs that assessed maintenance of serotonin reuptake inhibitors for 1 year in people who had responded to treatment.[54,55] The first RCT (70 people who had responded to a 20 week course of fluoxetine) found no significant difference between maintenance of fluoxetine and replacement by placebo for 1 year in relapse rate over 1 year (21% with fluoxetine *v* 32% with placebo; P = 0.137).[54] The second RCT compared sertraline versus placebo in 223 people with obsessive compulsive disorder, who had all previously responded to 1 year's treatment with sertraline (response defined as at least 25% reduction in Yale-Brown scale score from baseline).[55] People continuing on sertraline were prescribed their previous dose (mean 183 mg). The RCT found that, compared with placebo, sertraline significantly reduced the proportion of people who withdrew because of relapse or insufficient clinical response over 24 weeks (9% with sertraline *v* 24% with placebo; P = 0.006). It found that sertraline reduced the proportion of people who had worsening of symptoms compared with placebo (12% with sertraline *v* 35% with placebo; P = 0.001), but found no significant difference in relapse rate over 24 weeks (2.7% with sertraline *v* 4.4% with placebo; P = 0.34).[55]

Harms: The first RCT found no significant difference between fluoxetine and placebo in overall adverse effects (reported as non-significant, adverse effects not specified, absolute numbers and CI not reported) or in the proportion of people who withdrew from the trial for any cause over 52 weeks (16/36 [44%] with fluoxetine *v* 23/35 [66%] with placebo; P = 0.072).[54] The second RCT found that upper respiratory infection, headache, and malaise were reported in ≥ 10% of people taking sertraline, and that people taking placebo had dizziness and depression (no further data reported).[55] It found that fewer people taking sertraline withdrew because of adverse effects than people taking placebo (5/109 [5%] with sertraline *v* 12/114 [11%] with placebo; P value not reported).

Comment: One prospective, 1 year study found further improvement after a 40 week open label extension of the study, with continuing adverse effects.[56] One observational study found that 16/18 (89%) of people relapsed within 7 weeks of replacing clomipramine with placebo treatment.[57]

QUESTION What are the effects of treatments in adults who have not responded to initial treatment with serotonin reuptake inhibitors?

OPTION ADDITION OF ANTIPSYCHOTICS TO SEROTONIN REUPTAKE INHIBITORS

Three small RCTs in people unresponsive to serotonin reuptake inhibitors found that the addition of antipsychotics improved symptoms compared with placebo.

Benefits: We found no systematic review, but found three small RCTs that assessed combined antipsychotics and serotonin reuptake inhibitors in people who did not respond to serotonin reuptake inhibitors alone.[58–60] The first RCT (34 people with obsessive compulsive disorder who had not responded to 8 weeks of treatment with fluvoxamine) compared fluvoxamine (a selective serotonin reuptake inhibitor) plus haloperidol (an antipsychotic; maximum dose of haloperidol 10 mg/day) versus fluvoxamine plus placebo.[58] It found that fluvoxamine plus haloperidol significantly increased the proportion of people who met two out of three different response criteria compared with fluvoxamine plus placebo

(11/17 [65%] *v* 0/17 [0%]; NNT 2, 95% CI 2 to 3; P < 0.0002). The second RCT (36 people with obsessive compulsive disorder who did not respond to 12 weeks of treatment with a serotonin reuptake inhibitor) found that, compared with addition of placebo, addition of 6 weeks of risperidone (an antipsychotic) to the prior serotonin reuptake inhibitor significantly improved symptoms of obsessive compulsive disorder (reduction in the Yale-Brown scale score 36% *v* 9%; P = 0.001), depression (reduction in the Hamilton Depression Rating Scale 35% *v* 20%; P = 0.002), and anxiety (reduction in the Hamilton Anxiety Rating Scale 31% *v* 12%; P = 0.007).[59] People taking risperidone were more likely to have met two of the response criteria (8/18 [44%] with serotonin reuptake inhibitor plus risperidone *v* 0/15 [0%] with serotonin reuptake inhibitor plus placebo; NNT 2, 95% CI 2 to 3; P < 0.005). The third RCT (27 people who did not respond to 3 months of treatment with fluoxetine, fluvoxamine, or clomipramine in an open label trial) compared a serotonin reuptake inhibitor plus quetiapine (an atypical antipsychotic 50–200 mg daily) versus a serotonin reuptake inhibitor plus placebo for 8 weeks.[60] People received the same serotonin reuptake inhibitors in the RCT as they had in the open label phase of the study. The RCT found that a serotonin reuptake inhibitor plus quetiapine significantly increased the proportion of people who responded compared with a serotonin reuptake inhibitor plus placebo (response defined as 30% or greater reduction in the Yale-Brown scale score; 10/14 [71%] with a serotonin reuptake inhibitor plus quetiapine *v* 0/14 [0%] with a serotonin reuptake inhibitor plus placebo; P < 0.0001).

Harms: Extrapyramidal adverse effects are common with haloperidol, which can also cause prolactinaemia. The RCT of serotonin reuptake inhibitors plus risperidone found that sedation, restlessness, increased appetite, dry mouth, or tinnitus were experienced by at least 10% of people taking serotonin reuptake inhibitors plus risperidone, and that blurred vision, excessive perspiration, headache, increased appetite, lightheadedness, restlessness, and sedation were experienced by at least 10% of people taking placebo.[59] Risperidone is commonly associated with hypotension and prolactinaemia. The RCT of serotonin reuptake inhibitors plus quetiapine found that people taking a serotonin reuptake inhibitor plus quetiapine had nausea (6/14), sedation (3/14), and dizziness (1/14), and people taking a serotonin reuptake inhibitor plus placebo had sedation (2/13), headache (1/13), and nervousness (1/13).[60]

Comment: None.

GLOSSARY

Behavioural therapy Consists of exposure to the anxiety provoking stimuli and prevention of ritualistic behaviour (engaging in compulsions).

Chronic obsessive compulsive disorder Continuous course without periods of remission since first onset.

Cognitive therapy Aims to correct distorted thoughts (such as exaggerated sense of harm and personal responsibility) by Socratic questioning, logical reasoning, and hypothesis testing.

Episodic obsessive compulsive disorder Episodic course with periods of remission since first onset.

Exposure homework Tasks involving contact with anxiety provoking situations to be carried out outside regular psychotherapy sessions.

Schizotypal personality disorder Characterised by discomfort in close relationships, cognitive and perceptual distortions, and eccentric behaviour.

Tic disorder Characterised by motor tics, vocal tics, or both.

REFERENCES

1. American Psychiatric Association. *Diagnostic and statistical manual of mental disorders,* 4th ed. Washington, DC: APA, 1994:669–673.
2. World Health Organization. *The ICD-10 classification of mental and behavioural disorders*. Geneva: World Health Organization, 1992.
3. Bebbington PE. Epidemiology of obsessive–compulsive disorder. *Br J Psychiatry* 1998;35(suppl.):2–6.
4. Horwath E, Weissman MM. The epidemiology and cross-national presentation of obsessive-compulsive disorder. *Psychiatr Clin North Am* 2000;23:493–507.
5. Baer L, Minichiello WE. Behavior therapy for obsessive–compulsive disorder. In: Jenike MA, Baer L, Minichiello WE, eds. *Obsessive–compulsive disorders*. St Louis: Mosby, 1998: 337–367.
6. Steketee GS, Frost RO, Rheaume J, et al. Cognitive theory and treatment of obsessive–compulsive disorder. In: Jenike MA, Baer L, Minichiello WE, eds. *Obsessive–compulsive disorders*. St Louis: Mosby, 1998: 368–399.
7. Alsobrook JP, Pauls DL. The genetics of obsessive–compulsive disorder. In: Jenike MA, Baer L, Minichiello WE, eds. *Obsessive–compulsive disorders*. St Louis: Mosby, 1998:276–288.
8. Rauch SL, Whalen PJ, Dougherty D, et al. Neurobiologic models of obsessive compulsive disorder. In: Jenike MA, Baer L, Minichiello WE, eds. *Obsessive–compulsive disorders*. St Louis: Mosby, 1998: 222–253.
9. Delgado PL, Moreno FA. Different roles for serotonin in anti-obsessional drug action and the pathophysiology of obsessive–compulsive disorder. *Br J Psychiatry* 1998;35(suppl.):21–25.
10. Saxena S, Brody AL, Schwartz JM, et al. Neuroimaging and frontal–subcortical circuitry in obsessive–compulsive disorder. *Br J Psychiatry* 1998;35(suppl.):26–37.
11. Rauch SL, Baxter LR Jr. Neuroimaging in obsessive–compulsive disorder and related disorders. In: Jenike MA, Baer L, Minichiello WE, eds. *Obsessive–compulsive disorders*. St Louis: Mosby, 1998:289–317.
12. Yaryura-Tobias JA, Neziroglu FA. *Obsessive-compulsive disorder spectrum*. Washington, DC: American Psychiatric Press, Inc., 1997.
13. Skoog G, Skoog I. A 40-year follow up of patients with obsessive–compulsive disorder. *Arch Gen Psychiatry* 1999;56:121–127.
14. Ravizza L, Maina G, Bogetto F. Episodic and chronic obsessive–compulsive disorder. *Depress Anxiety* 1997;6:154–158.
15. Goodman WK, Price LH, Rasmussen SA, et al. The Yale-Brown obsessive compulsive scale. I. Development, use, and reliability. *Arch Gen Psychiatry* 1989;46:1006–1011.
16. Goodman WK, Price LH, Rasmussen SA, et al. The Yale-Brown obsessive compulsive scale. II. Validity. *Arch Gen Psychiatry* 1989;46:1012–1016.
17. Goodman WK, Price LH. Rating scales for obsessive–compulsive disorder. In: Jenike MA, Baer L, Minichiello WE, eds. *Obsessive–compulsive disorders*. St Louis: Mosby, 1998:97–117.
18. Piccinelli M, Pini S, Bellantuono C, et al. Efficacy of drug treatment in obsessive–compulsive disorder. A meta-analytic review. *Br J Psychiatry* 1995;166:424–443. Search dates 1994; primary sources Medline and Excerpta Medica-Psychiatry.
19. Ackerman DL, Greenland S. Multivariate meta-analysis of controlled drug studies for obsessive-compulsive disorder. *J Clin Psychopharmacol* 2002;22:309–317. Search date not reported; primary sources Medline, Psycinfo, and hand searches of bibliographies of published reviews and previous meta-analyses.
20. Tollefson GD, Rampey AH, Potvin JH, et al. A multicenter investigation of fixed-dose fluoxetine in the treatment of obsessive–compulsive disorder. *Arch Gen Psychiatry* 1994;51:559–567.
21. Montgomery SA, Kasper S, Stein DJ, et al. Citalopram 20 mg, 40 mg and 60 mg are all effective and well tolerated compared with placebo in obsessive-compulsive disorder. *Int Clin Psychopharmacol* 2001;16:75–86.
22. Hollander E, Koran LM, Goodman WK, et al. A double-blind, placebo-controlled study of the efficacy and safety of controlled-release fluvoxamine in patients with obsessive-compulsive disorder. *J Clin Psychiatry* 2003;64:640–647.
23. Bisserbe JC, Lane RM, Flament MF. A double blind comparison of sertraline and clomipramine in outpatients with obsessive–compulsive disorder. *Eur Psychiatry* 1997;12:82–93.
24. Mundo E, Maina G, Uslenghi C. Multicentre, double-blind, comparison of fluvoxamine and clomipramine in the treatment of obsessive–compulsive disorder. *Int Clin Psychopharmacol* 2000;15:69–76.
25. Mundo E, Rouillon F, Figuera L, et al. Fluvoxamine in obsessive-compulsive disorder: Similar efficacy but superior tolerability in comparison with clomipramine. *Hum Psychopharmacol* 2001;16:461–468.
26. Bergeron R, Ravindran AV, Chaput Y, et al. Sertraline and fluoxetine treatment of obsessive-compulsive disorder: Results of a double-blind, 6-month treatment study. *J Clin Psychopharmacol* 2002;22:148–154.
27. Mundo E, Bianchi L, Bellodi L. Efficacy of fluvoxamine, paroxetine, and citalopram in the treatment of obsessive–compulsive disorder: a single-blind study. *J Clin Psychopharmacol* 1997;17:267–271.
28. Jenike MA, Baer L, Minichiello WE, et al. Placebo-controlled trial of fluoxetine and phenelzine for obsessive–compulsive disorder. *Am J Psychiatry* 1997;154:1261–1264.
29. Hoehn-Saric R, Ninan P, Black DW, et al. Multicenter double-blind comparison of sertraline and desipramine for concurrent obsessive–compulsive and major depressive disorders. *Arch Gen Psychiatry* 2000;57:76–82.
30. Albert U, Aguglia E, Maina G, et al. Venlafaxine versus clomipramine in the treatment of obsessive-compulsive disorder: a preliminary single-blind, 12-week, controlled study. *J Clin Psychiatry* 2002;63:1004–1009.
31. Kobak KA, Greist JH, Jefferson JW, et al. Behavioral versus pharmacological treatments of obsessive compulsive disorder: a meta-analysis. *Psychopharmacology (Berl)* 1998;136:205–216. Search date 1997; primary sources Medline, PsycINFO, Dissertations, and Abstracts International databases.
32. Abramowitz JS. Effectiveness of psychological and pharmacological treatments for obsessive–compulsive disorder: a quantitative review. *J Consult Clin Psychol* 1997;65:44–52. Search date 1995; primary sources Medline and PsycLIT.
33. Goldstein DJ, Sundell K. A review of safety of selective serotonin reuptake inhibitors during pregnancy. *Hum Psychopharmacol Clin Exp* 1999;14:319–324.
34. Trindade E, Menon D. Selective serotonin reuptake inhibitors differ from tricyclic antidepressants in adverse events [abstract]. Selective serotonin reuptake inhibitors for major depression. Part 1. Evaluation of clinical literature. Ottawa: Canadian Coordinating Office for Health Technology Assessment, August 1997 Report 3E. *Evid Based Ment Health* 1998;1:50.
35. Ravizza L, Barzega G, Bellino S, et al. Predictors of drug treatment response in obsessive–compulsive disorder. *J Clin Psychiatry* 1995;56:368–373.
36. Cavedini P, Erzegovesi S, Ronchi P, et al. Predictive value of obsessive–compulsive personality disorder in antiobsessional pharmacological treatment. *Eur Neuropsychopharmacol* 1997;7:45–49.

37. Ackerman DL, Greenland S, Bystritsky A. Clinical characteristics of response to fluoxetine treatment of obsessive–compulsive disorder. *J Clin Psychopharmacol* 1998;18:185–192.
38. Ackerman DL, Greenland S, Bystritsky A, et al. Predictors of treatment response in obsessive–compulsive disorder: multivariate analyses from a multicenter trial of clomipramine. *J Clin Psychopharmacol* 1994;14:247–254.
39. Mundo E, Erzegovesi S, Bellodi L. Follow up of obsessive–compulsive patients treated with proserotonergic agents [letter]. *J Clin Psychopharmacol* 1995;15:288–289.
40. Alarcon RD, Libb JW, Spitler D. A predictive study of obsessive–compulsive disorder response to clomipramine. *J Clin Psychopharmacol* 1993;13:210–213.
41. Greist JH, Marks IM, Baer L, et al. Behavior therapy for obsessive-compulsive disorder guided by a computer or by a clinician compared with relaxation as a control. *J Clin Psychiatry* 2002;63:138–145.
42. McLean PD, Whittal ML, Thordarson DS, et al. Cognitive versus behavior therapy in the group treatment of obsessive-compulsive disorder. *J Consult Clin Psychol* 2001;69:205–214.
43. Cottraux J, Note I, Yao SN, et al. A randomized controlled trial of cognitive therapy versus intensive behavior therapy in obsessive compulsive disorder. *Psychother Psychosom* 2001;70:288–297.
44. Keijsers GP, Hoogduin CA, Schaap CP. Predictors of treatment outcome in the behavioural treatment of obsessive–compulsive disorder. *Br J Psychiatry* 1994;165:781–786.
45. De Araujo LA, Ito LM, Marks IM. Early compliance and other factors predicting outcome of exposure for obsessive–compulsive disorder. *Br J Psychiatry* 1996;169:747–752.
46. Buchanan AW, Meng KS, Marks IM. What predicts improvement and compliance during the behavioral treatment of obsessive compulsive disorder? *Anxiety* 1996;2:22–27.
47. Castle DJ, Deale A, Marks IM, et al. Obsessive–compulsive disorder: prediction of outcome from behavioural psychotherapy. *Acta Psychiatr Scand* 1994;89:393–398.
48. Marks IM, Hodgson R, Rachman S. Treatment of chronic obsessive–compulsive neurosis by in-vivo exposure. A two-year follow up and issues in treatment. *Br J Psychiatry* 1975;127:349–364.
49. Foa EB, Goldstein A. Continuous exposure and complete response prevention in obsessive–compulsive neurosis. *Behav Ther* 1978;9:821–829.
50. Cordioli AV, Heldt E, Bochi DB, et al. Cognitive–behavioral group therapy in obsessive-compulsive disorder: A randomized clinical trial. *Psychother Psychosom* 2003;72:211–216.
51. van Balkom AJ, de Haan E, van Oppen P, et al. Cognitive and behavioral therapies alone versus in combination with fluvoxamine in the treatment of obsessive compulsive disorder. *J Nerv Ment Dis* 1998;186:492–499.
52. Hohagen F, Winkelmann G, Rasche-Ruchle H, et al. Combination of behaviour therapy with fluvoxamine in comparison with behaviour therapy and placebo. Results of a multicentre study. *Br J Psychiatry* 1998;35(suppl):71–78.
53. Rauch SL, Jenike MA. Pharmacological treatment of obsessive compulsive disorder. In: Nathan PE, Gorman JM, eds. *Treatments that work*. New York: Oxford University Press, 1998:359–376.
54. Romano S, Goodman W, Tamura R, et al. Long-term treatment of obsessive-compulsive disorder after an acute response: a comparison of fluoxetine versus placebo. *J Clin Psychopharmacol* 2001;21:46–52.
55. Koran LM, Hackett E, Rubin A, et al. Efficacy of sertraline in the long-term treatment of obsessive-compulsive disorder. *Am J Psychiatry* 2002;159:88–95.
56. Rasmussen S, Hackett E, DuBoff E, et al. A 2-year study of sertraline in the treatment of obsessive–compulsive disorder. *Int Clin Psychopharmacol* 1997;12:309–316.
57. Pato MT, Zohar-Kadouch R, Zohar J, et al. Return of symptoms after discontinuation of clomipramine in patients with obsessive–compulsive disorder. *Am J Psychiatry* 1988;145:1521–1525.
58. McDougle CJ, Goodman WK, Leckman JF, et al. Haloperidol addition in fluvoxamine-refractory obsessive-compulsive disorder. A double-blind, placebo-controlled study in patients with and without tics. *Arch Gen Psychiatry* 1994;51:302–308.
59. McDougle CJ, Epperson CN, Pelton GH, et al. A double-blind, placebo-controlled study of risperidone addition in serotonin reuptake inhibitor-refractory obsessive-compulsive disorder. *Arch Gen Psychiatry* 2000;57:794–801.
60. Atmaca M, Kuloglu M, Tezcan E, et al. Quetiapine augmentation in patients with treatment resistant obsessive-compulsive disorder: a single-blind, placebo-controlled study. Int Clin Psychopharmacol 2002;17:115–119.

G Mustafa Soomro
Honorary Research Fellow
Section of Community Psychiatry, St George's Hospital Medical School
London
UK

Competing interests: None declared.

TABLE 1 **Serotonin reuptake inhibitors (clomipramine, citalopram, fluoxetine, fluvoxamine, paroxetine, sertraline) versus placebo (see text, p 1299).**

Intervention and reference	Study design	Symptom improvement
Citalopram**		
21	RCT (401 people)	AR 57% with citalopram 20 mg v 52% with 40 mg v 65% with 60 mg v 37% with placebo; NNT for 20 mg citalopram v placebo 5, 95% CI 3 to 14
Clomipramine*¶		
18	SR (9 RCTs; 668 people)	SMD 1.31 (95% CI 1.15 to 1.47)
19	SR (7 RCTs; 808 people)	SMD –8.19 (95% CI –10.53 to –5.85)
Fluoxetine†¶		
18	SR (1 RCT; 287 people)	SMD 0.57 (95% CI 0.33 to 0.81)
19	SR (3 RCTs; 329 people)	SMD –1.61 (95% CI –2.18 to –1.04)
20	RCT (350 people)	Mean reduction in score 4.6 with fluoxetine 20 mg, 5.5 with 40 mg, 6.5 with 60 mg v 0.9 with placebo ($P < 0.001$ for all doses v placebo)
Fluvoxamine‡		
18	SR	SMD 0.57 (95% CI 0.37 to 0.77)
19	SR	SMD –4.84 (95% CI –7.78 to –1.83) (measured as a change in raw score of Yale Brown)
22	RCT (253 people)	Mean reduction in score 8.5 with fluvoxamine controlled release 100–300 mg v 5.6 with placebo ($P = 0.001$)
Paroxetine¶		
19	SR (1 RCT; 300 people)	SMD –3.00 (95% CI –4.91 to –1.09)
Sertraline§¶		
18	SR (3 RCTs; 270 people)	SMD 0.52 (95% CI 0.27 to 0.77)
19	SR (4 RCTs; 598 people)	SMD –2.57 (95% CI –6.13 to +1.20 [NS])

*The total number of different RCTs identified was 11; †the total number of different RCTs identified was 5; ‡the total number of different RCTs identified was 6; §the total number of different RCTs identified was 4; ¶symptoms assessed by Yale-Brown scale score; ** 25% reduction in Yale-Brown score. NS, non-significant.

Panic disorder

Search date September 2003

Shailesh Kumar and Mark Oakley-Browne

QUESTIONS

INTERVENTIONS

To be covered in future updates
Aerobic exercise
Bibliotherapy
Clonidine
Cognitive behavioural therapy
Psychotherapies

See glossary Ⓖ

Key Messages

- **Selective serotonin reuptake inhibitors** Systematic reviews and one additional RCT have found that selective serotonin reuptake inhibitors improve symptoms in panic disorder compared with placebo. One subsequent RCT found that discontinuation of sertraline in people with a good response increased exacerbation of symptoms. A second subsequent RCT found that paroxetine plus cognitive behavioural therapy improved symptoms compared with placebo plus cognitive behavioural therapy.
- **Tricyclic antidepressants (imipramine)** One systematic review, one subsequent RCT, and one additional RCT have found that imipramine improves symptoms compared with placebo. One subsequent RCT found that imipramine reduced relapse rates over 12 months.
- **Benzodiazepines** One systematic review and one additional RCT have found that alprazolam reduces the number of panic attacks and improves symptoms compared with placebo. However, benzodiazepines are associated with a wide range of adverse effects, both during and after treatment.
- **Buspirone** We found insufficient evidence to assess the effects of buspirone.
- **Monoamine oxidase inhibitors** We found no RCTs on the effects of monoamine oxidase inhibitors.

DEFINITION A panic attack is a period in which there is sudden onset of intense apprehension, fearfulness, or terror often associated with feelings of impending doom. Panic disorder occurs when there are recurrent, unpredictable attacks followed by at least 1 month of persistent concern about having another panic attack, worry about the possible implications or consequences of the panic attacks, or a significant behavioural change related to the attacks.[1] The term panic disorder excludes panic attacks attributable to the direct physiological effects of a general medical condition, a substance, or another mental disorder. Panic disorder is sometimes categorised as being with or without agoraphobia.[1] Alternative categorisations focus on phobic anxiety disorders and specify agoraphobia with or without panic disorder.[2]

INCIDENCE/PREVALENCE Panic disorder often starts at around 20 years of age (between late adolescence and the mid-30s).[3] Lifetime prevalence is 1–3%, and panic disorder is more common in women than in men.[4] An Australian community study found 1 month prevalence rates for panic disorder (with or without agoraphobia) of 0.4% using International Classification of Diseases (ICD)-10 diagnostic criteria, and of 0.5% using Diagnostic and Statistical Manual (DSM)-IV diagnostic criteria.[5]

AETIOLOGY/RISK FACTORS Stressful life events tend to precede the onset of panic disorder,[6,7] although a negative interpretation of these events in addition to their occurrence has been suggested as an important causal factor.[8] Panic disorder is associated with major depression,[9] social phobia, generalised anxiety disorder, obsessive compulsive disorder,[10] and a substantial risk of drug and alcohol abuse.[11] It is also associated with avoidant, histrionic, and dependent personality disorders.[10]

PROGNOSIS The severity of symptoms in people with panic disorder fluctuates considerably, and patients commonly experience periods of no attacks, or only mild attacks with few symptoms. There is often a long delay between the initial onset of symptoms and presentation for treatment. Recurrent attacks may continue for several years, especially if associated with agoraphobia. Reduced social or occupational functioning varies among people with panic disorder and is worse in people with associated agoraphobia. Panic disorder is also associated with an increased rate of attempted, but unsuccessful, suicide.[12] One study analysing data from RCTs and systematic reviews found that co-existence of anxiety and depressive features adversely affected treatment response at 12 years compared with treatment of panic disorder alone.[13]

AIMS OF INTERVENTION To reduce the severity and frequency of panic attacks, phobic avoidance, and anticipatory anxiety; to improve social and occupational functioning, with minimal adverse effects of treatment.

OUTCOMES Measures of panic attacks, agoraphobia, and associated disability (self reported and clinician rated, before and after treatment, and longer term) using general or specific scales for panic disorder (e.g. the panic and agoraphobia scale, the mobility inventory for agoraphobia).

METHODS *Clinical Evidence* search and appraisal September 2003. Studies with follow up periods of less than 6 months were excluded.

QUESTION What are the effects of drug treatments for panic disorder?

OPTION TRICYCLIC ANTIDEPRESSANTS

One systematic review, one subsequent RCT, and one additional RCT have found that imipramine improves symptoms in people with panic disorder compared with placebo. One subsequent RCT found that imipramine reduced relapse rates after 12 months in people with panic disorder compared with placebo.

Benefits: We found one systematic review (search date not reported, 27 RCTs, 2348 people),[14] one additional RCT,[15] and two subsequent RCTs.[16,17] The systematic review compared imipramine, selective serotonin reuptake inhibitors (SSRIs; paroxetine, fluvoxamine, zimelidine, and clomipramine; see comment below), and alprazolam verssu placebo and versus each other (see benefits of SSRIs, p 1314 and benzodiazepines, p 1315).[14] It found that imipramine significantly increased the proportion of people judged to have improved compared with placebo (P < 0.0001; see comment below). The additional RCT (181 people with panic disorder with or without agoraphobia) compared three treatments: oral imipramine (maximum dose 225 mg; see comment below), oral alprazolam (maximum dose 10 mg; see comment below), and placebo (see benefits of benzodiazepines, p 1315).[15] It found that imipramine reduced the number of panic attacks after 8 months compared with placebo (results presented graphically, significance not calculated). The first subsequent RCT (56 adults with panic disorder and agoraphobia in stable remission after 24 weeks' treatment with oral imipramine) comparing oral imipramine 2.25 mg/kg daily versus placebo found that significantly fewer people taking imipramine relapsed after 12 months (see comment below; 1/29 [3%] with imipramine *v* 10/27 [37%] with placebo; RR 0.09, 95% CI 0.01 to 0.68; NNT 5, 95% CI 3 to 14).[16] The second subsequent RCT (312 people) compared five groups: oral imipramine (maximum dose 300 mg/day; see comment below), cognitive behavioural therapy**G**, placebo, cognitive behavioural therapy plus oral imipramine (maximum dose 300 mg/day; see comment below), and cognitive behavioural therapy plus placebo.[17] It found that imipramine significantly increased the proportion of people judged to have responded (using the panic disorder severity scale) compared with placebo after 6 months (response rate: 38% with imipramine *v* 13% with placebo; absolute numbers not provided; P = 0.02).

Harms: Adverse effects associated with imipramine treatment included blurred vision, tachycardia, palpitations, blood pressure changes, insomnia, nervousness, malaise, dizziness, headache, nausea, vomiting, and reduced appetite (see harms of prescription antidepressant drugs under depressive disorders, p 1238).[15,18]

Comment: The review included clomipramine as an SSRI. This drug is also often described as a tricyclic antidepressant.[14] The review used improvement as an outcome measure without a clear definition of this term. In the additional RCT and the second subsequent RCT, flexible dosing was used according to tolerance and therapeutic need.[15,17] In the subsequent RCT comparing imipramine versus placebo, relapse rate was not clearly defined.[16] **Short term effects:** We found one systematic review (search date 1999, 43 studies including 34 RCTs, 2367 people, drop-out rate 24%, analysis based on completers) that compared the short term efficacy of SSRIs (fluoxetine, fluvoxamine, paroxetine, citalopram, and sertraline) versus tricyclic antidepressants (imipramine, desipramine, nortryptiline, and clomipramine) and analysed effect size within treatment group rather than within studies.[19] It found no significant difference between treatments in the proportion of people who were free of panic attacks at 6–10 weeks, but found that tricyclic antidepressants significantly increased drop-out rates (free of panic attacks: 60% with tricyclic antidepressants *v* 55% with SSRIs, P value not reported; drop-outs: 31% with tricyclic antidepressants *v* 18% with SSRIs, P < 0.001).

OPTION SELECTIVE SEROTONIN REUPTAKE INHIBITORS

Systematic reviews and one additional RCT have found that selective serotonin reuptake inhibitors improve symptoms compared with placebo in panic disorder. One subsequent RCT found that discontinuation of sertraline in people with a good response increased exacerbation of symptoms. A second subsequent RCT found that paroxetine plus cognitive behavioural therapy improved symptoms compared with placebo plus cognitive behavioural therapy.

Benefits: **Versus placebo:** We found two systematic reviews (see benefits of tricyclic antidepressants, p 1312 and benzodiazepines, p 1315),[14,20] one additional RCT,[21] and two subsequent RCTs.[22,23] The first systematic review (search date not reported, 27 RCTs, 2348 people) found that selective serotonin reuptake inhibitors (SSRIs; paroxetine, fluvoxamine, zimelidine, and clomipramine; see comment below) significantly increased the proportion of people who improved compared with placebo ($P < 0.0001$; see comment below).[14] The second systematic review (search date not reported, 12 RCTs, 1741 people) only reported combined results as an effect size against placebo (effect size 0.55), and did not report statistical significance.[20] The additional RCT (279 people) compared five groups: oral citalopram 10 or 15 mg daily, oral citalopram 20 or 30 mg daily, oral citalopram 40 or 60 mg daily, oral clomipramine 60 or 90 mg daily, and placebo.[21] It found that citalopram (at all doses) significantly increased the proportion of people who responded (defined as no panic attacks and either no episodic increases in anxiety or only slight increases in anxiety precipitated by definite events or activities) compared with placebo after 12 months (citalopram 10 or 15 mg/day *v* placebo, $P = 0.05$; citalopram 20 or 30 mg/day *v* placebo, $P = 0.001$; citalopram 40 or 60 mg/day *v* placebo, $P = 0.003$; results presented graphically). The first subsequent RCT (182 people who had responded to open label sertraline for 52 weeks) compared double blind placebo (discontinuation of sertraline) versus sertraline for 28 weeks.[22] It found that significantly more people on placebo had exacerbation of symptoms (33% with placebo *v* 13% with sertraline; $P = 0.005$; CI not reported). The second subsequent RCT (43 people with panic disorder with or without agoraphobia who had been unsuccessfully treated with 15 sessions of manual guided cognitive behavioural therapy [CBT**G**] alone) compared paroxetine 40 mg plus CBT versus placebo plus CBT (see comment below).[23] Success was defined as no panic attacks for a 2 week period or achieving cut-off scores or lower on panic disorder scales. It found that combined treatment significantly increased success compared with placebo plus CBT (12/19 [63%] with combined treatment *v* 5/19 [26%] with placebo plus CBT; RR 2.4, 95% CI 1.1 to 5.6; NNT 3, 95% CI 2 to 21).

Harms: The additional RCT reported that harms associated with citalopram included headache, tremor, dry mouth, and somnolence (see harms of prescription antidepressant drugs under depressive disorders, p 1238).[21] The first subsequent RCT found the highest incidence of adverse events with sertraline in the first 12 weeks of the study, and tolerability seemed to improve with time.[22] The most common adverse events over the 52 week trial period were headache, malaise, insomnia, upper respiratory infection, diarrhoea, nausea, and dizziness. The second subsequent RCT did not report on adverse events.[23]

Comment: The first review included clomipramine as an SSRI, although this drug is often described as a tricyclic antidepressant.[14] It also included the SSRI zimelidine, which is rarely used these days. In addition, the review used improvement as an outcome measure, without defining this term clearly. In the additional RCT, only 28/54 (52%) completed the trial; analysis was by intention to treat and people who withdrew from the trial were counted as treatment failures.[21] The RCT used flexible dosing according to tolerance and therapeutic need. SSRIs can cause initial increased anxiety, which can exacerbate a tendency to focus on internal sensations and to avoid situations that trigger these sensations (catastrophise somatic sensations). Education about this event is likely to improve adherence with medication. The second systematic review found that smaller RCTs were associated with larger effect sizes, suggesting the possibility of publication bias.[20] The second subsequent RCT only used 8 weeks of medication as opposed to a more common 12

weeks, it only used clinician rated outcomes, and most people in both the placebo and paroxetine groups guessed correctly which treatment they had been allocated (62% with placebo v 79% with paroxetine).[23]
Tricyclic antidepressants versus selective serotonin reuptake inhibitors: See comment under tricyclic antidepressants, p 1313.

OPTION MONOAMINE OXIDASE INHIBITORS

We found no RCTs on the effects of monoamine oxidase inhibitors in panic disorder.

Benefits: We found no systematic review and no RCTs.

Harms: We found no evidence of harms associated specifically with the use of monoamine oxidase inhibitors in the long term treatment of panic disorder.

Comment: Our search strategy excluded studies with follow up of less than 6 months.

OPTION BUSPIRONE

We found insufficient evidence to assess the effects of buspirone in people with panic disorder.

Benefits: We found no systematic review but found two RCTs.[24,25] The first RCT (48 people) compared oral buspirone (maximum 60 mg/day) plus (CBTⒼ) versus placebo plus CBT for 16 weeks.[24] It found that oral buspirone plus CBT significantly improved self rated panic and agoraphobia scores after 1 year (using a 90 point symptom scale where each symptom was graded from 0 = not present to 4 = severe; $P = 0.03$; absolute numbers not reported).[24] The second RCT (41 people with panic disorder and agoraphobia) compared 16 weeks of oral buspirone 30 mg daily plus CBT versus 16 weeks of placebo plus CBT.[25] It found no significant difference in the proportion of people who had a reduction of at least 50% in their agoraphobic symptoms after 68 weeks (44% with buspirone plus CBT v 68% with placebo plus CBT; absolute numbers of people not provided).

Harms: The RCTs did not report harms (see harms of buspirone under generalised anxiety disorder, p 1277).

Comment: The first RCT used a flexible dosing regimen with maximum dose adjustment according to tolerance and therapeutic need.[24]

OPTION BENZODIAZEPINES

One systematic review and one additional RCT have found that alprazolam reduces the number of panic attacks and improves symptoms compared with placebo. However, benzodiazepines are associated with a wide range of adverse effects, both during and after treatment.

Benefits: We found one systematic review (search date not reported, 27 RCTs, 2348 people; see benefits of tricyclic antidepressants, p 1312 and selective serotonin reuptake inhibitors, p 1314)[14] and one additional RCT.[15] The review found that alprazolam significantly increased the proportion of people judged to have improved compared with placebo ($P < 0.0001$; see comment below).[14] The additional RCT (181 people with panic disorder with or without agoraphobia) compared three treatments: oral alprazolam (maximum 10 mg/day; see comment below), oral imipramine (maximum 225 mg/day; see comment below), and placebo (see benefits of tricyclic antidepressants, p 1312 and selective serotonin reuptake inhibitors, p 1314).[15] It found that alprazolam was associated with fewer panic attacks after 8 months compared with placebo (results presented graphically; significance not calculated).

Harms: The systematic review did not report harms.[14] Adverse effects associated with alprazolam include sedation, insomnia, memory lapses, nervousness, irritability, dry mouth, tremor, impaired coordination, constipation, urinary retention, altered libido, and altered appetite (see harms of benzodiazepines under generalised anxiety disorder, p 1281).[15] We found one non-systematic review of the effects of benzodiazepines in anxiety disorder in people with a history of substance abuse or dependence.[26] The review reported that the mortality of long term benzodiazepine users was no higher than that of matched controls. It reported that the most pronounced adverse effects followed sudden withdrawal and included tinnitus, paraesthesia, vision disturbance, depersonalisation, seizures, withdrawal psychosis, and persistent discontinuation syndrome.

Comment: The review used improvement as an outcome measure without clearly defining this term.[14] The additional RCT used flexible dosing according to tolerance and therapeutic need.[15] Many RCTs of psychological and pharmacological treatments (even those not involving benzodiazepines) allowed people to receive small amounts of anxiolytic drugs during the study because benzodiazepine abuse is quite prevalent in people who suffer from panic disorder.

GLOSSARY

Cognitive behavioural therapy (CBT) Brief structured treatment using relaxation and exposure procedures, and aimed at changing dysfunctional beliefs and negative automatic thoughts (typically 20 sessions over 12–16 weeks).

REFERENCES

1. American Psychiatric Association. *Diagnostic and statistical manual of mental disorders*, 4th ed. Washington, DC: American Psychiatric Association, 1994.
2. World Health Organization. *The ICD-10 classification of mental and behavioural disorders*. Geneva: World Health Organization, 1992.
3. Robins LN, Regier DA, eds. *Psychiatric disorders in America: the epidemiologic catchment area study*. New York, NY: Free Press, 1991.
4. Weissman MM, Bland MB, Canino GJ, et al. The cross-national epidemiology of panic disorder. *Arch Gen Psychiatry* 1997;54:305–309.
5. Andrews G, Henderson S, Hall W. Prevalence, comorbidity, disability and service utilisation. Overview of the Australian National Mental Health Survey. *Br J Psychiatry* 2001;178:145–153.
6. Last CG, Barlow DH, O'Brien GT. Precipitants of agoraphobia: role of stressful life events. *Psychol Rep* 1984;54:567–570.
7. De Loof C, Zandbergen H, Lousberg T, et al. The role of life events in the onset of panic disorder. *Behav Res Ther* 1989;27:461–463.
8. Rapee RM, Mattick RP, Murrell E. Impact of life events on subjects with panic disorder and on comparison subjects. *Am J Psychiatry* 1990;147:640–644.
9. Hirschfield RMA. Panic disorder: diagnosis, epidemiology and clinical course. *J Clin Psychiatry* 1996;57:3–8.
10. Andrews G, Creamer M, Crino R, et al. *The treatment of anxiety disorders*. Cambridge: Cambridge University Press, 1994.
11. Page AC, Andrews G. Do specific anxiety disorders show specific drug problems? *Aust N Z J Psychiatry* 1996;30:410–414.
12. Gorman JM, Coplan JD. Comorbidity of depression and panic disorder. *J Clin Psychiatry* 1996;57:34–41.
13. Tyrer P, Seivewright H, Simmonds S, et al. Prospective studies of cothymia (mixed anxiety-depression): how do they inform clinical practice? *Eur Arch Psychiatry Clin Neurosci* 2001;251:II53–II56.
14. Boyer W. Serotonin uptake inhibitors are superior to imipramine and alprazolam in alleviating panic attacks: a meta-analysis. *Int Clin Psychopharmacol* 1995;10:45–49. Search date not reported; primary sources Medline, Embase, Psychlit, and sponsoring agencies of two trials contacted for supplementary statistical information.
15. Curtis GC, Massana J, Udina C, et al. Maintenance drug therapy of panic disorder. *J Psychiatr Res* 1993;27:127–142.
16. Mavissakalian MR, Perel JM. Long-term maintenance and discontinuation of imipramine therapy in panic disorder with agoraphobia. *Arch Gen Psychiatry* 1999;56:821–827.
17. Barlow DH, Gorman J, Shear MK, et al. Cognitive-behavioral therapy, imipramine, or their combination for panic disorder: a randomized controlled trial. *JAMA* 2000;283:2529–2536.
18. Cassano GB, Toni C, Petracca A, et al. Adverse effects associated with the short-term treatment of panic disorder with imipramine, alprazolam or placebo. *Eur Neuropsychopharmacol* 1994;4:47–53.
19. Bakker A, van Balkom AJLM, Spinhoven P. SSRIs vs TCAs in the treatment of panic disorder: a meta-analysis. *Acta Psychiatr Scand* 2002;106:163–167. Search date 1999; primary sources Medline, Embase, PsychInfo, and hand searches of reference lists of articles obtained.

20. Otto M, Tuby K, Gould R, et al. An effect-size analysis of the relative efficacy and tolerability of serotonin selective reuptake inhibitors for panic disorder. *Am J Psychiatry* 2001;158:1989–1992. Search date not reported; primary sources Medline, Psychlit, and hand searches of references.
21. Lepola UM, Wade AG, Leinonen EV, et al. A controlled, prospective, 1-year trial of citalopram in the treatment of panic disorder. *J Clin Psychiatry* 1998;59:528–534.
22. Rapaport M, Wolkow R, Rubin A, et al. Sertraline treatment of panic disorder: results of a long term study. *Acta Psych Scand* 2001;104:289–298.
23. Kampman M, Keijsers GP, Hoogduin CA, et al. A randomized, double-blind, placebo-controlled study of the effects of adjunctive paroxetine in panic disorder patients unsuccessfully treated with cognitive-behavioral therapy alone. *J Clin Psychiatry* 2002;63:772–777.
24. Bouvard M, Mollard E, Guerin J, et al. Study and course of the psychological profile in 77 patients expressing panic disorder with agoraphobia after cognitive behaviour therapy with or without buspirone. *Psychother Psychosom* 1997;66:27–32.
25. Cottraux J, Note ID, Cungi C, et al. A controlled study of cognitive behaviour therapy with buspirone or placebo in panic disorder with agoraphobia. *Br J Psychiatry* 1995;167:635–641.
26. Posternak M, Mueller T. Assessing the risks and benefits of benzodiazepines for anxiety disorders in patients with a history of substance abuse or dependence. *Am J Addict* 2001;10:48–68.

Shailesh Kumar
Division of Psychiatry Auckland Medical School
Auckland
New Zealand

Mark Oakley-Browne
Professor of Rural Psychiatry
Monash University
Gippsland, Victoria
Australia

Competing interests: SK was reimbursed by Eli-Lilly, the manufacturers of Prozac (fluoxetine), for attending several conferences. MOB has been paid by GlaxoSmithKline for contributing to educational sessions for general practitioners. The programme topic was "the recognition and management of generalised anxiety disorder". MOB has received reimbursement from Pfizer for attending a symposium.

Post-traumatic stress disorder

Search date January 2004

Jonathan Bisson

QUESTIONS

INTERVENTIONS

See glossary G

Key Messages

Preventive interventions

- **Multiple session cognitive behavioural therapy in people with acute stress disorder** Two small RCTs in people with acute stress disorder after a traumatic event (accident or non-sexual assault) found that five sessions of cognitive behavioural therapy reduced the proportion of people with post-traumatic stress disorder after 6 months compared with supportive counselling.
- **Hydrocortisone** One small RCT in people in intensive care with septic shock provided insufficient evidence to assess hydrocortisone in preventing post-traumatic stress disorder.
- **Multiple session cognitive behavioural therapy in all people exposed to a traumatic event** One RCT found that four sessions of cognitive behavioural therapy in people with psychological distress following physical injury reduced post-traumatic stress symptoms at 13 months compared with no psychological intervention. However, it found no significant difference in the proportion of people meeting the

DSM-IV diagnostic criteria for post-traumatic stress disorder. One RCT in bus drivers who had been attacked in the past 5 months found that cognitive behavioural therapy improved measures of anxiety and intrusive symptoms at 6 months compared with standard care. However, it found no significant difference in measures of depression or avoidance symptoms. One RCT provided insufficient evidence to assess cognitive behavioural therapy plus educational techniques in preventing post-traumatic stress disorder in road traffic accident survivors. Another small RCT provided insufficient evidence to compare memory structuring versus supportive listening in road traffic accident survivors.

- **Multiple session collaborative trauma support** Two RCTs provided insufficient evidence to assess multiple session collaborative trauma support interventions involving emotional, social, and practical support in people exposed to a traumatic event in the past 24 hours to 1 week.
- **Multiple session education** We found no systematic review or RCTs assessing effects of multiple session education alone. One RCT provided insufficient evidence to assess educational techniques plus cognitive behavioural therapy in preventing post-traumatic stress disorder in road traffic accident survivors.
- **Propranolol** One small RCT provided insufficient evidence to assess propranolol in preventing post-traumatic stress disorder in people with early symptoms of post-traumatic stress disorder after a traumatic event.
- **Single session group debriefing** We found no RCTs comparing single session group debriefing with no debriefing. One RCT found that early group debriefing (within 10 hours of the traumatic event) reduced post-traumatic stress disorder compared with delayed group debriefing (after 48 hours).
- **Temazepam** One small RCT provided insufficient evidence to assess temazepam in preventing post-traumatic stress disorder in people with acute stress disorder or early symptoms of post-traumatic stress disorder after road traffic accident, industrial accident, or non-sexual assault.
- **Single session individual debriefing** One systematic review of RCTs in people who had been exposed to a traumatic event in the previous month found no significant difference between a single session of individual psychological debriefing and no debriefing in the incidence of post-traumatic stress disorder at 3 months or 1 year.
- **Supportive counselling** Two RCTs in people with acute stress disorder after a traumatic event (road traffic accident or non-sexual assault) found that supportive counselling was less effective than five sessions of cognitive behavioural therapy in reducing the proportion of people with post-traumatic stress disorder after 6 months.

Treatments

- **Cognitive behavioural therapy** RCTs found that cognitive behavioural therapy improved post-traumatic stress disorder symptoms, anxiety, and depression immediately after treatment and at up to 1 year compared with no treatment or supportive counselling. RCTs provided no consistent evidence of a difference in symptoms between cognitive behavioural therapy and eye movement desensitisation and reprocessing.
- **Eye movement desensitisation and reprocessing** RCTs found that eye movement desensitisation and reprocessing improved symptoms compared with no treatment, but provided no consistent evidence of a difference in symptoms between eye movement desensitisation and reprocessing and cognitive behavioural therapy.
- **Fluoxetine** One RCT found that fluoxetine improved symptoms compared with placebo at 3 months. One small RCT found no significant difference between fluoxetine and placebo in response rate at 3 months, but is likely to have been underpowered to detect a clinically important difference.
- **Paroxetine** Two RCTs found that paroxetine improved response rate compared with placebo at 3 months. One smaller RCT found no significant difference between paroxetine and placebo in response rate at 3 months, but may have been underpowered to detect a clinically important difference.

- **Sertraline** Three RCTs found that sertraline reduced symptoms at 3–7 months compared with placebo. Two small RCTs found no significant difference between sertraline and placebo in symptoms at up to 3 months, but were likely to be underpowered to detect a clinically important difference between groups. One RCT provided insufficient evidence to compare sertraline with nefazodone.
- **Affect management** We found insufficient evidence about the effects of this intervention in improving symptoms.
- **Benzodiazepines** One systematic review identified no RCTs of sufficient quality in people with post-traumatic stress disorder.
- **Brofaromine** We found insufficient evidence about the effects of this intervention in improving symptoms
- **Carbamazepine** We found no RCTs of carbamazepine in people with post-traumatic stress disorder.
- **Drama therapy** We found insufficient evidence about the effects of this intervention in improving symptoms.
- **Eclectic psychotherapy** We found insufficient evidence about the effects of this intervention in improving symptoms.
- **Group therapy** We found insufficient evidence about the effects of this intervention in improving symptoms.
- **Hypnotherapy** We found insufficient evidence about the effects of this intervention in improving symptoms.
- **Inpatient treatment programmes** We found insufficient evidence about the effects of this intervention in improving symptoms.
- **Internet based psychotherapy** We found insufficient evidence about the effects of this intervention in improving symptoms.
- **Lamotrigine** One RCT provided insufficient evidence to assess lamotrigine in people with post-traumatic stress disorder.
- **Mirtazapine** We found insufficient evidence about the effects of this intervention in improving symptoms.
- **Nefazodone** We found insufficient evidence about the effects of this intervention in improving symptoms.
- **Olanzapine** We found no good quality RCTs that assessed olanzapine in people with post-traumatic stress disorder.
- **Phenelzine** We found insufficient evidence about the effects of this intervention in improving symptoms
- **Propranolol** We found no RCTs of propranolol in people with post-traumatic stress disorder.
- **Psychodynamic psychotherapy** We found insufficient evidence about the effects of this intervention in improving symptoms.
- **Risperidone** We found no RCTs of risperidone in people with post-traumatic stress disorder.
- **Supportive psychotherapy** We found insufficient evidence about the effects of this intervention in improving symptoms.
- **Tricyclic antidepressants** RCTs provided insufficient evidence to assess imipramine or amitriptyline in people with post-traumatic stress disorder.

DEFINITION **Post-traumatic stress disorder (PTSD)** can occur after any major traumatic event. Symptoms include upsetting thoughts and nightmares about the traumatic event, avoidance behaviour, numbing of general responsiveness, increased irritability, and hypervigilance.[1] To fulfil the *Diagnostic and statistical manual of mental disorders* (DSM-IV) criteria for PTSD, an individual must have been exposed to a traumatic event; have at least one re-experiencing, three avoidance, and two hyperarousal phenomena; have had the symptoms for at least 1 month; and the symptoms must cause clinically important distress or reduced day to day functioning.[1] People with sub-syndromal PTSD Ⓖ have all the criteria for PTSD except one of the re-experiencing, avoidance, or hyperarousal phenomena. **Acute stress disorder** occurs within the first month after a major traumatic event and requires the presence of symptoms for at least 2 days. It is similar to PTSD but dissociative symptomsⒼ are required to make the diagnosis. Treatments for PTSD may have similar effects, regardless of the traumatic event that precipitated PTSD. However, great caution should be applied when generalising from one type of trauma to another.

INCIDENCE/ PREVALENCE One large cross-sectional study in the USA found that 1/10 (10%) women and 1/20 (5%) men experience PTSD at some stage in their lives.[2]

AETIOLOGY/ RISK FACTORS Risk factors include major trauma, such as rape, a history of psychiatric disorders, acute distress and depression after the trauma, lack of social support, and personality factors.[3]

PROGNOSIS One large cross-sectional study in the USA found that over a third of people with previous PTSD continued to satisfy the criteria for PTSD 6 years after initial diagnosis.[2] However, cross-sectional studies provide weak evidence about prognosis.

AIMS OF INTERVENTION To reduce initial distress after a traumatic event; to prevent PTSD and other psychiatric disorders; to reduce levels of distress in the long term; to improve function and quality of life; with minimal adverse effects.

OUTCOMES Presence or absence of PTSD and severity of symptoms assessed by continuous measures. Continuous measures for assessing changes in symptoms include Impact of Event Scale (range 0–75), Post-traumatic Stress Diagnostic Scale (range 0–51), Clinician Administered PTSD Scale, Trauma Symptom Checklist 40 (range 0–160), Post-traumatic Stress Disorder Checklist, and Clinical Global Impression Scale (a composite measure of symptoms and everyday functioning; range very much worse–very much improved). Symptoms assessed include anxiety, depression, intrusion, and avoidance. Changes in continuous measures are often expressed as effect sizes. It is difficult to interpret effect sizes in terms of clinical importance. Some categorise effect sizes of less than 0.5 as small, 0.5–0.8 as medium, and greater than 0.8 as large.

METHODS *Clinical Evidence* search and appraisal January 2004.

QUESTION What are the effects of preventive interventions?

OPTION SINGLE SESSION DEBRIEFING

One systematic review of RCTs in people who had been exposed to a traumatic event in the past month found no significant difference between a single session of individual psychological debriefing and no debriefing in the incidence of post-traumatic stress disorder at 3 months or 1 year. We found no RCTs comparing single session group debriefing with no debriefing. One RCT found that early group debriefing (within 10 hours of the traumatic event) reduced post-traumatic stress disorder compared with delayed group debriefing (after 48 hours).

Benefits: We found one systematic review (search date 2000, 11 RCTs, 1759 people)[4] and one subsequent RCT[5] comparing early (within 1 month) single session interventions ("debriefing") versus no intervention. The RCTs in the review used single session individual psychological debriefingⒼ or similar techniques after traumatic events. The review found no significant difference between single session individual debriefing and no debriefing in the risk of post-traumatic stress disorder at 3 months and 1 year, although the risk of post-traumatic stress disorder was non-significantly higher in people receiving debriefing (OR at 3 months: 1.1, 95% CI 0.6 to 2.5; OR at 12 months: 2.0, 95% CI 0.9 to 4.5).[4] The review found no RCTs comparing group debriefing with no debriefing.[4] The subsequent RCT (77 people who had been robbed) compared early group debriefing (within 10 hours) versus delayed group debriefing (after 48 hours).[5] It found that early debriefing significantly reduced symptom severity measured on the Post-traumatic Stress Diagnostic Scale at 2 weeks compared with delayed debriefing (mean score 6.94 with early debriefing *v* 33.10 with delayed debriefing; $P < 0.001$).

Harms: Two RCTs included in the systematic review found an increased risk of subsequent psychological problems in people receiving the intervention.[4] However, initial traumatic exposure had been higher in these people.

Comment: The systematic review of single session debriefing found that the overall quality of RCTs was poor.[4] Problems included lack of blinding, failure to state loss to follow up, lack of intention to treat analysis, and high withdrawal rates.

OPTION MULTIPLE SESSION COGNITIVE BEHAVIOURAL THERAPY

One RCT found that four sessions of cognitive behavioural therapy in people with psychological distress following physical injury reduced post-traumatic stress symptoms at 13 months compared with no psychological intervention. However, it found no significant difference in the proportion of people meeting the DSM-IV diagnostic criteria for post-traumatic stress disorder. One RCT in bus drivers who had been attacked in the past 5 months found that cognitive behavioural therapy improved measures of anxiety and intrusive symptoms at 6 months compared with standard care. However, it found no significant difference in measures of depression or avoidance symptoms. One RCT provided insufficient evidence to assess cognitive behavioural therapy plus educational techniques in preventing post-traumatic stress disorder in road traffic accident survivors. Another small RCT provided insufficient evidence to compare memory structuring with supportive listening in road traffic accident survivors. Two small RCTs in people with acute stress disorder after a traumatic event (road traffic accident or non-sexual assault) found that five sessions of cognitive behavioural therapy reduced the proportion of people with post-traumatic stress disorder after 6 months compared with supportive counselling.

Benefits: **Versus no treatment or standard care:** We found no systematic review. We found two RCTs.[6,7] The first RCT (132 bus drivers who had been attacked in the past few days) compared 1–6 sessions of cognitive behavioural therapy**G** versus standard care.[6] It found that cognitive behavioural therapy significantly improved measures of anxiety and intrusive symptoms at 6 months compared with standard care, but found no significant difference in measures of depression or avoidance symptoms.[6] The second RCT (152 people with psychological distress following physical injury, 116 followed up at 13 months), compared four sessions of cognitive behavioural therapy between 5 and 10 weeks after the injury versus no psychological intervention.[7] It found that therapy reduced the proportion of people meeting DSM-IV criteria for post-traumatic stress disorder (PTSD) at 13 months compared with no therapy, but the reduction was not statistically significant (10/61 [16%] with therapy *v* 15/55 [27%] with no therapy; RR 0.6, 95% CI 0.3 to 1.5; analysis by intention to treat). It found that therapy significantly reduced PTSD symptoms compared with no therapy at 13 months (Impact of Event Scale; mean score reduction: 20.7 with therapy *v* 11.2 with no therapy; adjusted mean difference 8.4, 95% CI 2.4 to 14.4).[7] **Cognitive behavioural therapy plus education versus no treatment:** We found one RCT (151 people who had been involved in a road traffic accident in the past month) that compared 3–6 sessions of cognitive behavioural therapy plus educational techniques versus no psychological intervention (see comment below).[8] The RCT found that people in the treatment group had a significantly higher baseline risk of PTSD compared with the no intervention group, which makes the results difficult to interpret. The RCT found no significant difference between groups in rates of PTSD at 6 months. **Versus supportive counselling:** We found two RCTs.[9,10] The first RCT (24 people with acute stress disorder 2 weeks after a road traffic accident or industrial accident) compared five sessions of cognitive behavioural therapy versus five sessions of supportive counselling**G**.[9] It found that cognitive behavioural therapy significantly reduced the proportion of people who met diagnostic criteria for PTSD immediately after treatment compared with supportive counselling and at 6 months (post-treatment: AR 8% with cognitive behavioural therapy *v* 83% with supportive counselling; $P < 0.001$; 6 months: AR 17% with cognitive behavioural therapy *v* 67% with supportive counselling; $P < 0.05$). The second RCT (45 people with acute stress disorder 2 weeks after a road traffic accident or non-sexual assault) compared three treatments: five 90 minute sessions of prolonged exposure (see glossary under CBT**G**) therapy alone; prolonged exposure therapy plus anxiety management**G**; or supportive counselling.[10] It found that, immediately after completion of treatment, both prolonged exposure alone and prolonged exposure plus anxiety management significantly reduced rates of PTSD compared with supportive counselling (measured by Clinician Administered PTSD Scale: AR 2/14 [14%] with prolonged exposure *v* 3/15 [20%] with prolonged exposure plus anxiety management *v* 9/16 [56%] with supportive counselling; $P < 0.05$ for either group *v* supportive counselling). The differences remained significant at 6 months' follow up (AR 2/13 [15%] with prolonged exposure *v* 3/13 [23%] with anxiety management *v* 10/15 [67%] with supportive counselling; $P < 0.05$ for each group *v* supportive counselling). **Memory structuring versus supportive listening:** We found one RCT (17 survivors of a road traffic accident in the past 24–48 hours) comparing two sessions of memory structuring**G** versus supportive listening (see glossary under CBT**G**).[11] It found that memory structuring significantly reduced mean scores on the Post-traumatic Stress Diagnostic Scale at 3 months compared with supportive listening (mean score: 8.1 with memory structuring *v* 18.5 with supportive listening; $P < 0.05$).[11]

Harms: The RCTs gave no information on adverse effects.[6–11]

Comment: The overall quality of RCTs was poor.[6–11] Problems included lack of blinding, failure to state loss to follow up, and lack of intention to treat analysis despite high withdrawal rates. The RCT comparing cognitive behavioural therapy**G** plus educational techniques versus no psychological intervention included multiple types of intervention (help, information, support, and reality testing/confrontation) in the treatment group.[8]

OPTION MULTIPLE SESSION COLLABORATIVE TRAUMA SUPPORT

Two RCTs provided insufficient evidence to assess multiple session collaborative trauma support interventions involving emotional, social, and practical support in people exposed to a traumatic event in the past 24 hours to 1 week.

Benefits: We found no systematic review but found two RCTs.[12,13] The first RCT (70 people who had been admitted to hospital after a road traffic accident in the past week) compared three treatments: a multiple session collaborative trauma support**G** intervention (emotional, practical, and social support for 2–10 hours in the first 3 months); immediate review (a single debriefing intervention); and no intervention.[12] It found that multiple session collaborative trauma support significantly reduced the risk of a poor outcome (based on Traumatic Neurosis Symptoms) compared with immediate review, although both interventions reduced the risk of a poor outcome compared with no intervention (AR for a poor outcome: 30% with multiple session collaborative trauma support *v* 60% with immediate review *v* 87% with no intervention; ARR for multiple session collaborative trauma support *v* no intervention 57%; NNT 2; ARR for immediate review *v* no intervention 27%, NNT 4; CI not reported; $P < 0.001$ for either intervention group *v* no intervention; $P < 0.05$ for comparison between the intervention groups). The second RCT (34 survivors of road traffic accidents or assault in the past 24 hours) compared a 4 month multiple session collaborative trauma support intervention (emotional, practical, and social support from a trauma support specialist) versus no intervention.[13] After 4 months, the risk of developing post-traumatic stress disorder was lower with multiple session collaborative trauma support than with no intervention, but the difference was not significant (AR for post-traumatic stress disorder assessed by Post-traumatic Stress Disorder Checklist: 17% with multiple session collaborative trauma support *v* 43% with no intervention; CI not reported; $P > 0.1$). The RCT might have lacked power to exclude a clinically important difference in outcomes.

Harms: The RCTs gave no information on adverse effects.[12,13]

Comment: The overall quality of RCTs was poor.[12,13] Problems included lack of blinding, failure to state loss to follow up, and lack of intention to treat analysis despite high withdrawal rates.

OPTION MULTIPLE SESSION EDUCATION

We found no systematic review or RCTs assessing effects of multiple session education alone. One RCT provided insufficient evidence to assess educational techniques plus cognitive behavioural therapy in preventing post-traumatic stress disorder in road traffic accident survivors.

Benefits: **Multiple session education alone:** We found no systematic review or RCTs. **Multiple session education plus cognitive behavioural therapy:** See benefits of multiple session cognitive behavioural therapy❻, p 1322.

Harms: **Multiple session education alone:** We found no systematic review or RCTs. **Multiple session education plus cognitive behavioural therapy:** See harms of multiple session cognitive behavioural therapy, p 1323.

Comment: None.

OPTION SUPPORTIVE COUNSELLING

Two RCTs in people with acute stress disorder after a traumatic event (road traffic accident or non-sexual assault) found that supportive counselling was less effective than five sessions of cognitive behavioural therapy in reducing the proportion of people with post-traumatic stress disorder after 6 months.

Benefits: **Versus no treatment:** We found no systematic review or RCTs comparing supportive counselling❻ versus no treatment. **Versus cognitive behavioural therapy:** See benefits of cognitive behavioural therapy❻, p 1322.

Harms: **Versus no treatment:** We found no RCTs. **Versus cognitive behavioural therapy:** See harms of cognitive behavioural therapy, p 1323.

Comment: None.

OPTION HYDROCORTISONE

One small RCT in people in intensive care with septic shock provided insufficient evidence to assess hydrocortisone in preventing post-traumatic stress disorder.

Benefits: We found no systematic review but found one small RCT (20 people in an intensive care unit with septic shock) comparing intravenous hydrocortisone versus saline.[14] It found that hydrocortisone significantly reduced the proportion of people with post-traumatic stress disorder at 31 months compared with saline (assessed by Structured Clinical Interview using DSM-IV criteria for post-traumatic stress disorder: 1/9 [11%] with hydrocortisone *v* 7/11 [64%] with placebo; RR 0.07, 95% CI 0.01 to 0.80). The results of this RCT may not be generalisable to people with non-septic shock induced trauma.

Harms: The RCT gave no information on adverse effects.[14]

Comment: None.

OPTION PROPRANOLOL

One small RCT provided insufficient evidence to assess propranolol in preventing post-traumatic stress disorder in people with early symptoms of post-traumatic stress disorder after a traumatic event.

Benefits: We found no systematic review but found one RCT (41 people with early symptoms of post-traumatic stress disorder 6 hours after a traumatic event) comparing propranolol 40 mg four times daily versus placebo for 10 days.[15] It found no significant difference between propranolol and placebo in the proportion of people with post-traumatic stress disorder at 1 month (measured by Clinician Administered PTSD Scale: 2/11 [18%] with propranolol *v* 6/20 [30%] with placebo; RR 0.52, 95% CI 0.09 to 3.16) or 3 months (1/11 [9%] with propranolol *v* 2/15 [13%] with placebo; RR 0.65, 95% CI 0.05 to 8.23; results were not by intention to treat).

Harms: The RCT gave no information on adverse effects.[15]

Comment: The RCT had a high withdrawal rate, and results were not intention to treat, which makes them difficult to interpret.[15]

OPTION TEMAZEPAM

One small RCT provided insufficient evidence to assess temazepam in preventing post-traumatic stress disorder in people with acute stress disorder or early symptoms of post-traumatic stress disorder after road traffic accident, industrial accident, or non-sexual assault.

Benefits: We found no systematic review but found one RCT (22 people with post-traumatic stress disorder symptoms and sleep initiation difficulties a mean 14 days after a road traffic accident, industrial accident, or non-sexual assault, 7 with acute stress disorder) comparing temazepam 30 mg daily for 5 days followed by 15 mg daily for 2 days versus placebo.[16] It found no significant difference in the proportion of people with post-traumatic stress disorder at 6 weeks (assessed by Structured Clinical Interview using DSM-IV criteria for post-traumatic stress disorder: 6/11 [54%] with temazepam *v* 3/11 [27%] with placebo; RR 3.2,

95% CI 0.54 to 18.98). It found that temazepam significantly improved sleep after one night compared with placebo (P < 0.04), but found similar total sleep patterns after 1 week (P value not reported). The RCT is likely to have been underpowered to detect clinically important differences in outcomes.

Harms: The RCT gave no information on adverse effects.[16]

Comment: The RCT was published as a letter to the editor.[16]

QUESTION What are the effects of treatments?

OPTION COGNITIVE BEHAVIOURAL THERAPY

RCTs found that cognitive behavioural therapy improved post-traumatic stress disorder symptoms, anxiety, and depression immediately after treatment and at up to 1 year compared with no treatment or supportive counselling. RCTs provided no consistent evidence of a difference in symptoms between cognitive behavioural therapy and eye movement desensitisation and reprocessing.

Benefits: **Versus supportive counselling or no treatment:** We found one systematic review (search date not reported)[17] and nine subsequent RCTs of cognitive behavioural therapy**G**.[18–26] The review compared a range of specific psychological treatments versus supportive counselling**G** or no treatment.[17] It identified 17 RCTs (690 people), including six RCTs (232 people) of cognitive behavioural therapy. All RCTs identified by the review found that psychological treatments were associated with a greater improvement immediately after treatment (using a composite score of post-traumatic stress disorder [PTSD] symptoms, anxiety, and depression) compared with supportive counselling**G** or no treatment (17 RCTs, 690 people: overall effect size immediately after treatment 0.54, 95% CI 0.39 to 0.68). The difference was still evident at 1 year (overall effect size from 12 RCTs with long term follow up 0.53, 95% CI 0.37 to 0.69). The first subsequent RCT (87 people) compared exposure, cognitive therapy, or both, versus relaxation treatment**G**.[18] It found that all cognitive behavioural therapies reduced symptoms of PTSD more than relaxation treatment, immediately after treatment and at 3 months (53 people evaluated; no intention to treat analysis performed). The second subsequent RCT (72 people) found no significant difference in symptoms at 1 year between 16 1-hour sessions of imaginal exposure therapy (see glossary under CBT**G**) and cognitive therapy (results not intention to treat; 54 people analysed; effect size 0.88 with imaginal exposure therapy**G** *v* 1.06 with cognitive therapy; reported as non-significant). It found that overall 21/54 (39%) of people continued to suffer from PTSD at 1 year.[19] The third subsequent RCT (168 female victims of sexual assault or childhood sexual abuse with PTSD and chronic nightmares) compared three sessions of imagery rehearsal therapy**G** versus no treatment over 5 weeks.[20] It found that imagery rehearsal therapy significantly improved PTSD symptoms at 3 or 6 months compared with no treatment (AR for symptoms improving by at least 1 level of clinical severity 65% with imagery rehearsal *v* 31% with no treatment; ARR 34%; NNT 3, CI not reported; P < 0.001). The fourth subsequent RCT (171 female victims of sexual assault) compared three treatments: cognitive processing therapy**G**; prolonged exposure (see glossary under CBT**G**); or minimal attention (telephone call every 2 weeks) for 6 weeks.[21] It found that, immediately after treatment, both cognitive processing therapy and prolonged exposure significantly reduced rates of PTSD compared with minimal attention (AR of not having PTSD assessed by several measures, including Clinician Administered PTSD Scale: 33/62 [53%] with cognitive processing *v* 33/62 [53%] with prolonged exposure *v* 1/45 [2%] with minimal attention; P < 0.001 for either intervention *v* placebo). The fifth subsequent RCT (78 people with PTSD or severe sub-syndromal PTSD❻ 6 months after a road traffic accident) compared three interventions: 8–12 sessions of cognitive behavioural therapy; 8–12 sessions of supportive psychotherapy❻; and waiting list control.[22] It found that, immediately after treatment, cognitive behavioural therapy significantly increased the proportion of people who responded compared with supportive psychotherapy or waiting list control (20/27 [74%] with cognitive behavioural therapy *v* 14/27 [52%] with supportive psychotherapy *v* 4/24 [17%] with waiting list control; P < 0.05 for cognitive behavioural therapy *v* either comparison). These results were maintained at 3 months' follow up. The sixth RCT (85 motor vehicle accident survivors with PTSD, 79 followed up at 9 months) compared three treatments started 4 months after the accident: up to 12 weekly sessions of cognitive therapy; a self help booklet; and repeated assessments.[23] All participants had failed to recover after a 3 week self monitoring period. The RCT found that cognitive therapy significantly reduced the proportion of people with PTSD at 9 months compared with the booklet and repeated assessment (intention to treat analysis: 3/28 [11%] with cognitive therapy *v* 17/28 [61%] with self help booklet *v* 16/29 [55%] with repeated assessment; OR for cognitive therapy *v* booklet: 12.9, 95% CI 3.1 to 53.1; OR for therapy *v* assessment: 10.3, 95% CI 2.5 to 41.7). The seventh RCT (58 people with PTSD after civilian trauma, 45 people completed treatment) compared three treatments: imaginal exposure alone; imaginal exposure plus cognitive restructuring; and supportive counselling.[24] Sessions were conducted weekly for 8 weeks and involved homework. It found that combined imaginal exposure and cognitive therapy reduced the proportion of people meeting criteria for PTSD at 6 months compared with supportive counselling but there was no significant difference between combined therapy and imaginal exposure alone (intention to treat analysis, 40% with combined treatment *v* 78% with counselling; P < 0.05; 40% with combined therapy *v* 50% with imaginal exposure alone; P = 0.07). The eighth RCT (37 women with PTSD and a history of experiencing domestic violence, 32 analysed post-treatment) compared cognitive trauma therapy (8–11 sessions) with a waiting list control.[25] It found that cognitive therapy reduced the proportion of women meeting PTSD criteria after treatment (1/18 [5%] with therapy *v* 14/14 [100%] with waiting list; P value not reported). The ninth RCT (105 people with PTSD referred from general practice or psychiatrists, 72 included in analysis) compared three treatments over 10 weeks: eye movement desensitisation and reprocessing❻; exposure plus cognitive restructuring; and waiting list control.[26] The RCT assessed clinically significant change, defined as an improvement in Impact of Event Scale score of more than two standard deviations from levels before treatment. It found that exposure plus cognitive restructuring significantly increased the proportion of people with clinically significant improvement after treatment compared with the waiting list control (9/21 [43%] with exposure plus cognitive restructuring *v* 1/24 [4%] with waiting list control; P < 0.001).[26] **Versus eye movement desensitisation and reprocessing:** (See benefits of eye movement desensitisation and reprocessing, p 1328).

Harms: The systematic review[17] and subsequent RCTs[18–26] gave no information on adverse effects. Overall, cognitive behavioural therapy❻ seems well tolerated. However, there have been case reports of worsening symptoms in some people receiving imaginal flooding (see glossary under CBT❻), leading to calls for caution when evaluating people for treatment.[27]

Comment: None.

OPTION EYE MOVEMENT DESENSITISATION AND REPROCESSING

RCTs found that eye movement desensitisation and reprocessing improved symptoms compared with no treatment, but provided no consistent evidence of a difference in symptoms between eye movement desensitisation and reprocessing and cognitive behavioural therapy.

Benefits: **Versus no treatment or waiting list:** We found one systematic review (search date 2000, 9 RCTs, number of people not reported)[28] and one subsequent RCT.[26] The review found that eye movement desensitisation and reprocessing (EMDR**G**) was significantly more effective than no treatment in reducing symptoms of post-traumatic stress disorder (PTSD) (effect size 0.39, CI not reported; $P < 0.05$; see comment below). The subsequent RCT (105 people with PTSD referred from general practice or psychiatrists, 72 included in analysis) compared three treatments over 10 weeks: EMDR; exposure plus cognitive restructuring; and wait list control.[26] The RCT assessed clinically significant change defined as improvement in Impact of Event Scale score of more than two standard deviations. It found that EMDR significantly increased the proportion of people with clinically significant improvement after treatment compared with the waiting list control (17/27 [63%] with EMDR *v* 1/24 [4%] with waiting list control; $P < 0.001$).[26]
Versus cognitive behavioural therapy: We found one systematic review[28] and four subsequent RCTs.[26,29–31] The review found no significant difference between EMDR and cognitive behavioural therapy**G** or between EMDR with eye movements and EMDR without eye movements (effect size for EMDR *v* cognitive behavioural therapy –0.44, CI not reported; reported as non-significant; effect size for EMDR with *v* without eye movement: 0.22, CI not reported; reported as non-significant; see comment below).[28] The first subsequent RCT (24 people with PTSD) found no significant difference between stress inoculation (see glossary under CBT**G**) training plus prolonged exposure and EMDR in the proportion of people with PTSD immediately after 8–12 weeks' treatment or at 3 months (after treatment, assessed by structured interview: 9/12 [75%] with stress inoculation training plus prolonged exposure *v* 10/12 [83%] with EMDR; RR 0.60, 95% CI 0.08 to 4.45; 3 months: 10/12 [83%] in each group; RR 1.00, 95% CI 0.12 to 8.56).[29] The second subsequent RCT (22 people with PTSD, mainly after rape or other crime, who completed at least one active treatment session after 3 preparatory sessions) compared EMDR with prolonged exposure therapy.[30] The RCT defined "cure" as a 70% reduction in PTSD symptoms. People treated with prolonged exposure had higher Beck Depression Inventory scores at baseline, which makes results difficult to interpret. It found that three sessions of EMDR significantly increased cure rates compared with three sessions of prolonged exposure (7/10 [70%] with EMDR *v* 2/12 [17%] with prolonged exposure therapy; $P = 0.021$). People who were not cured after three sessions were offered an additional three sessions of the allocated therapy. Analysis after this extension phase found that 3–6 sessions of EMDR significantly increased cure rates compared with 3–6 sessions with prolonged exposure therapy (9/10 [90%] with EMDR *v* 4/12 [33%] with prolonged exposure; $P = 0.021$).[30] The third subsequent RCT (105 people with PTSD) compared three treatments over 10 weeks: EMDR; exposure plus cognitive restructuring; and waiting list control.[26] It found no significant difference between EMDR and exposure plus cognitive restructuring in the proportion of people with clinically significant change after treatment (clinically significant change in Impact of Event Scale score: 17/27 [63%] with EMDR *v* 9/21[43%] with exposure; P reported as not significant).[26] The fourth RCT (60 survivors of different traumatic events,

97% of whom had PTSD, 45 people completed) compared eight sessions of three treatments: EMDR; exposure therapy; and relaxation training.[31] At 3 months, it found that EMDR increased the proportion of people no longer meeting PTSD criteria compared with relaxation and decreased the proportion of people no longer meeting PTSD criteria compared with exposure, but neither difference was significant (53% with EMDR *v* 30% with relaxation *v* 82% with exposure; $P > 0.05$ for each comparison with exposure).[31]

Harms: The systematic review[28] and two of the subsequent RCTs[26,29] gave no information on adverse effects. In one RCT, 2/12 [17%] people treated with prolonged exposure therapy reported that talking about the trauma was too stressful, and withdrew from treatment.[30] One RCT (60 people) found that none of the people receiving EMDR**G** or exposure experienced a worsening of their symptoms, although one person receiving relaxation had a worsening of symptoms.[31]

Comment: The review did not report duration of treatment or state when the outcome of improvement in symptoms was measured.[28]

OPTION OTHER PSYCHOLOGICAL TREATMENTS

RCTs provided insufficient evidence to assess affect management, eclectic psychotherapy, group therapy, internet based psychotherapy, psychodynamic psychotherapy, or hypnotherapy. We found no RCTs on drama therapy, inpatient treatment, or supportive psychotherapy programmes.

Benefits: **Affect management:** We found no systematic review but found one RCT (48 women) comparing 15 weeks of affect management**G** treatment (in addition to drug treatment) versus waiting list control.[32] It found that affect management improved post-traumatic stress disorder (PTSD) symptoms compared with waiting list control (assessed by the Davidson Trauma Scale: mean 45.8 with affect management *v* 73.1 with waiting list control; $P = 0.02$) and dissociative symptoms**G** from baseline (assessed by the Dissociative Experiences Scale: mean 11.9 with affect management *v* 25.2 with waiting list control; $P = 0.02$). **Eclectic psychotherapy:** We found no systematic review but found one RCT (42 police officers) comparing brief eclectic psychotherapy (combining components of cognitive behavioural therapy**G** and psychodynamic psychotherapy**G**) versus waiting list control over 16 sessions of treatment.[33] It found that eclectic psychotherapy significantly reduced the proportion of people with PTSD immediately after treatment and at 3 months (AR for PTSD assessed by Structured Clinical Interview using DSM-IV criteria for PTSD: 9% with eclectic psychotherapy *v* 50% with waiting list control; $P < 0.01$; 3 months: AR 4% with eclectic psychotherapy *v* 65% with waiting list control; $P < 0.01$). **Group therapy:** We found no systematic review but found two RCTs.[34,35] The first RCT (55 female survivors of childhood sexual abuse with PTSD) compared three treatments: trauma focused group therapy**G**; present focused group therapy**G**; or waiting list control.[34] Group therapy was undertaken in 90 minute sessions for 24 weeks. The RCT found that either type of group therapy significantly improved symptoms of dissociation and sexual abuse trauma ($P < 0.05$ for both outcomes) compared with waiting list control. It found no significant difference in overall symptoms (symptoms assessed using the Trauma Symptom Checklist 40; mean difference in score: 8.1 with group therapy *v* 3.8 with waiting list control; reported as non-significant; no further data reported). The RCT prospectively defined three groups, but combined results for both active treatment groups in its analysis. This makes the results difficult to interpret. It is likely to have been underpowered to detect a clinically important difference in outcomes. The second RCT (360 Vietnam veterans with PTSD, most with history of mood or substance use disorder, 325 included in analysis) compared 30 weeks of trauma focused group psychotherapy versus present focused group psychotherapy.[35] It found no significant difference between treatments in mean PTSD symptom score at 1 year (72.8 with trauma focused therapy *v* 74.8 with present focused therapy; P value not reported). **Internet based psychotherapy:** We found no systematic review but found one RCT (25 people) that compared internet based psychotherapy❻ versus waiting list control for 5 weeks.[36] It found that, at 5 weeks, internet based psychotherapy significantly improved intrusive symptom score from baseline compared with waiting list control (mean reduction: 11.0 with internet based psychotherapy *v* 3.6 with waiting list control; $P < 0.04$) and reduced avoidance score (mean reduction: 9.6 with internet based psychotherapy *v* 2.9 with waiting list control; $P < 0.03$). **Psychodynamic psychotherapy:** We found one systematic review (search date not reported)[17] which identified one RCT.[37] The RCT (112 people) compared four interventions: psychodynamic psychotherapy; trauma desensitisation; hypnotherapy❻; and waiting list control. It found that psychodynamic therapy improved intrusion and avoidance symptom score significantly more than waiting list control at 4 months (improvement in intrusion/avoidance score from baseline: 19.3 with psychodynamic therapy *v* 4.6 with control; $P < 0.05$).[37] **Hypnotherapy:** We found one systematic review (search date not reported)[17] which identified one four arm RCT (see benefits of psychodynamic psychotherapy, above).[37] The RCT (112 people) found that hypnotherapy improved intrusion and avoidance symptom score significantly more than waiting list control at 4 months (improvement in intrusion/avoidance score from baseline: 19.1 with hypnotherapy *v* 4.6 with control; $P < 0.05$).[37] **Drama therapy; inpatient treatment programmes; supportive psychotherapy:** We found no RCTs on drama therapy❻, inpatient treatment programmes❻, or supportive psychotherapy❻.

Harms: The systematic review[17] and RCTs[32–37] gave no information on adverse effects.

Comment: None.

OPTION SELECTIVE SEROTONIN REUPTAKE INHIBITORS AND RELATED ANTIDEPRESSANTS

Three RCTs found that sertraline reduced symptoms at 3–7 months compared with placebo. Two small RCTs found no significant difference between sertraline and placebo in symptoms at up to 3 months, but were likely to be underpowered to detect a clinically important difference between groups. Two RCTs found that paroxetine improved response rate compared with placebo at 3 months. One smaller RCT found no significant difference between paroxetine and placebo in response rate at 3 months, but may have been underpowered to detect a clinically important difference. One RCT found that fluoxetine improved symptoms compared with placebo at 3 months. One small RCT found no significant difference between fluoxetine and placebo in response rate at 3 months, but is likely to have been underpowered to detect a clinically important difference. RCTs provided insufficient evidence to compare mirtazapine with placebo or sertraline with nefazodone.

Benefits: **Versus placebo:** We found one systematic review (search date 1999)[38] and seven subsequent RCTs (3 evaluating sertraline,[39–41] 2 evaluating paroxetine,[42,43] 1 evaluating fluoxetine,[44] and 1 evaluating mirtazapine[45]). The review identified four RCTs (375 people) comparing selective serotonin reuptake inhibitors versus placebo that used the Clinical Global Impression Scale change item or close equivalent as the primary outcome measure.[38] Response was defined as a Clinical Global Impression Scale score of 1 (very much improved) or 2 (much improved). The first RCT identified by the review (187 people) found that sertraline significantly increased the proportion of people who responded after 3 months (OR for non-response 0.44, 95% CI 0.24 to 0.78). The second small RCT identified by the review (51 people) found no significant difference in the proportion of responders between sertraline and placebo at 3 months (OR for non-response 0.44, 95% CI 0.12 to 1.60). However, this RCT is likely to have lacked power to detect a clinically significant difference between groups. One RCT identified by the review (280 people) found no significant difference between paroxetine and placebo in the proportion of people who responded after 3 months (OR for non-response 0.64, 95% CI 0.40 to 1.02) and another small RCT (53 people) found no significant difference between fluoxetine and placebo in the proportion of people who responded after 3 months (OR for non-response 0.30, 95% CI 0.09 to 1.02),[38] but these RCTs may have lacked power to detect a clinically important difference. Five of the subsequent placebo controlled RCTs found improved symptoms with selective serotonin reuptake inhibitors. The first subsequent RCT (208 people) found that sertraline 50–200 mg daily significantly improved symptoms at 12 weeks compared with placebo (mean reduction in post-traumatic stress disorder [PTSD] symptom score on the Clinician Administered PTSD Scale: –33.0 with sertraline *v* –26.2 with placebo; P = 0.04).[39] The second subsequent RCT (96 people who had previously responded to sertraline for acute treatment of PTSD) found that sertraline significantly reduced PTSD relapse after 28 weeks compared with placebo (AR: 5% with sertraline *v* 26% with placebo; ARR 21%; NNT 5; CI not reported; P < 0.02).[40] The third subsequent RCT (42 veteran male soldiers) found no significant difference between sertraline 50–200 mg daily and placebo in symptoms of PTSD after 10 weeks of treatment (mean reduction in Clinician Administered PTSD Scale score: –18.7 with sertraline *v* –13.5 with placebo; P = 0.53; see comment below).[41] The fourth subsequent RCT (307 people) found that paroxetine 20–50 mg daily significantly increased response rate at 12 weeks compared with placebo (response defined as "very much improved" or "much improved" on the Clinical Global Impression Scale; AR: 59% with paroxetine *v* 38% with control; ARR 21%; NNT 5; CI not reported; P = 0.008).[42] The fifth subsequent RCT (551 people) found that paroxetine 20 or 40 mg daily significantly improved response rate (using the same definition) at 12 weeks compared with placebo (AR for response: 62% with 20 mg paroxetine *v* 54% with 40 mg paroxetine *v* 37% with placebo; P < 0.001 for both paroxetine groups compared with placebo).[43] The sixth subsequent RCT (301 people, mainly male soldiers) found that fluoxetine 50–80 mg daily significantly improved symptoms compared with placebo after 12 weeks' treatment (mean reduction in Clinician Administered PTSD Scale score: –34.6 with fluoxetine *v* –29.6 with placebo; P = 0.021).[44] The clinical importance of this difference in symptoms is unclear. The seventh subsequent RCT (29 people with PTSD) compared mirtazapine 45 mg daily versus placebo for 8 weeks' treatment.[45] It found that mirtazapine significantly improved response compared with placebo at 8 weeks (response defined as an "improved" or "much improved" score on the short PTSD rating interview: 11/17 [65%] with mirtazapine *v* 2/9 [22%] with placebo; P = 0.04; analysis not by intention to treat). However, results of this RCT should be interpreted with caution as people allocated to mirtazapine had less severe symptoms at baseline, and there was a withdrawal rate (31%). **Versus each other:** We found one RCT comparing sertraline 50–100 mg daily versus nefazodone 200–400 mg daily.[46] It found no significant difference in symptoms at 5 months (mean total eight item PTSD scale [TOP-8] score: 5.23 with sertraline v 4.35 with nefazodone; P = 0.36). However, the results of this RCT should be interpreted with caution because, despite randomisation, people taking sertraline had significantly higher baseline TOP-8 scores than people taking nefazodone.

Harms: The systematic review gave no information on adverse effects, although it found no significant difference between antidepressants and placebo in the proportion of people who withdrew for any cause (7 RCTs; 712 people; RR 0.85, 95% CI 0.63 to 1.14).[38] The first subsequent RCT found that, compared with placebo, sertraline significantly increased insomnia (35% with sertraline v 22% with placebo; P = 0.04), diarrhoea (28% with sertraline v 11% with placebo; P = 0.003), and nausea (23% with sertraline v 11% with placebo; P = 0.03), and decreased appetite (12% with sertraline v 1% with placebo; P = 0.001).[39] The fourth subsequent RCT comparing paroxetine versus placebo found that adverse effects with an incidence of at least 10% and twice that of placebo were nausea (19.2% with paroxetine v 8.3% with placebo), somnolence (17.2% with paroxetine v 3.8% with placebo), dry mouth (13.9% with paroxetine v 4.5% with placebo), asthenia (13.2% with paroxetine v 5.2% with placebo), and abnormal ejaculation (11.8% with paroxetine v 3.7% with placebo).[42] In the seventh subsequent RCT three people taking mirtazapine withdrew because of adverse effects, including sedation, panic attacks, increased anxiety and irritability.[45] Three people taking placebo withdrew because of pain, or lack of efficacy. The RCT found that significantly more people taking placebo had palpitations (3/9 [33%] with placebo v 0/17 [0%] with mirtazapine; P = 0.03) and more people taking mirtazapine had increased appetite and weight gain (increased appetite: 6/17 [35%] with mirtazapine v 1/9 [11%] with placebo; weight gain: 3/17 [18%] with mirtazapine v 1/9 [11%] with placebo; P value not reported for either comparison). A further RCT (65 people) assessing the harms of fluoxetine in people with PTSD found that fluoxetine was associated with significantly higher rates of nausea, diarrhoea, and thirst compared with placebo ($P < 0.05$ for all outcomes).[47] Known adverse effects of selective serotonin reuptake inhibitors include nausea and headache (see harms of prescription antidepressant drugs under depressive disorders, p 1246).

Comment: The veteran soldiers in the third subsequent RCT evaluating sertraline had higher baseline Clinician Administered PTSD Scale scores (mean baseline score 94.3) than people in the other RCTs of sertraline (mean baseline score about 74); this may explain the lack of significant improvement in symptoms between sertraline and placebo.[41]

OPTION TRICYCLIC ANTIDEPRESSANTS

RCTs provided insufficient evidence to assess imipramine or amitriptyline in people with post-traumatic stress disorder.

Benefits: We found one systematic review (search date 1999) of antidepressant drugs for post-traumatic stress disorder.[38] The review identified two RCTs (81 people) comparing tricyclic antidepressants versus placebo that used the Clinical Global Impression Scale change item or close equivalent as the primary outcome measure.[38] One RCT (41 people) identified by the review found that the proportion of non-responders at 2 months was significantly lower with imipramine than with placebo (response defined as Clinical Global Impression Scale score of 1 [very much improved] or 2 [much improved]; OR 0.21, 95% CI 0.05 to 0.78). The other RCT (40 people) identified by the review found no significant difference between amitriptyline and placebo in the proportion of people who responded after 2 months (OR 0.41, 95% CI 0.12 to 1.42).[38]

Harms: The systematic review gave no information on adverse effects, although it found no significant difference between antidepressants and placebo in the proportion of people who withdrew for any cause (7 RCTs; 712 people; RR 0.85, 95% CI 0.63 to 1.14).[38] Known adverse effects of tricyclic antidepressants include anticholinergic effects (see harms of prescription antidepressant drugs under depressive disorders, p 1246).

Comment: None.

OPTION MONOAMINE OXIDASE INHIBITORS

RCTs provided insufficient evidence to assess brofaromine or phenelzine in people with post-traumatic stress disorder.

Benefits: We found one systematic review (search date 1999) of antidepressant drugs for post-traumatic stress disorder.[38] The review identified three RCTs (247 people) comparing monoamine oxidase inhibitors versus placebo that used the Clinical Global Impression Scale change item or close equivalent as the primary outcome measure.[38] Two RCTs found no significant difference between brofaromine and placebo in the proportion of non-responders at 14 weeks (response defined as Clinical Global Impression Scale of 1 [very much improved] or 2 [much improved]; first RCT (114 people): OR 0.94, 95% CI 0.45 to 1.99; second RCT (64 people): OR 0.40, 95% CI 0.15 to 1.08). One RCT (37 people) found that phenelzine significantly increased the proportion of responders at 2 months compared with placebo (OR 0.21, 95% CI 0.06 to 0.73).[38]

Harms: The systematic review gave no information on adverse effects, although it found no significant difference between antidepressants and placebo in the proportion of people who withdrew for any cause (7 RCTs; 712 people; RR 0.85, 95% CI 0.63 to 1.14).[38] Known adverse effects of monoamine oxidase inhibitors include possible hypertensive crisis. Monoamine oxidase inhibitors may also require a need for dietary restriction (see harms of prescription antidepressant drugs under depressive disorders, p 1246).

Comment: None.

OPTION CARBAMAZEPINE

We found no RCTs of carbamazepine in people with post-traumatic stress disorder.

Benefits: We found no systematic review or RCTs.

Harms: We found no RCTs.

Comment: None.

OPTION RISPERIDONE

We found no RCTs of risperidone in people with post-traumatic stress disorder.

Benefits: We found no systematic review or RCTs.

Harms: We found no RCTs.

Comment: None.

OPTION LAMOTRIGINE

One RCT provided insufficient evidence to assess lamotrigine in people with post-traumatic stress disorder.

Benefits: We found one systematic review (search date 1999),[38] which identified one small RCT (14 people) comparing lamotrigine versus placebo that used the Clinical Global Impression Scale change item or close equivalent as the primary outcome measure. The RCT found no significant difference between lamotrigine and placebo in the proportion of non-responders at 2 months (response defined as Clinical Global Impression Scale score of 1 [very much improved] or 2 [much improved]; OR 0.39, 95% CI 0.04 to 3.71). However, it is likely to have been underpowered to detect a clinically important difference between groups.

Harms: The systematic review gave no information on adverse effects, although it found no significant difference between antidepressants and placebo in the proportion of people who withdrew for any cause (7 RCTs; 712 people; RR 0.85, 95% CI 0.63 to 1.14).[38]

Comment: None.

OPTION BENZODIAZEPINES

One systematic review identified no RCTs of sufficient quality in people with post-traumatic stress disorder.

Benefits: We found one systematic review (search date 1999), which identified no RCTs of sufficient quality.[38]

Harms: We found no RCTs.

Comment: None.

OPTION PROPRANOLOL

We found no RCTs of propranolol in people with post-traumatic stress disorder.

Benefits: We found no systematic review or RCTs.

Harms: We found no RCTs.

Comment: None.

OPTION OLANZAPINE

We found no good quality RCTs that assessed olanzapine in people with post-traumatic stress disorder.

Benefits: We found no systematic review and no reliable RCTs (see comment below).

Harms: We found no RCTs.

Comment: We found one small RCT (15 people with post-traumatic stress disorder, of whom 4 withdrew), which did not meet *Clinical Evidence* inclusion criteria because of small sample size and high withdrawal rate.[48]

GLOSSARY

Affect management A type of group treatment focusing on regulation of mood.

Anxiety management Involves teaching techniques to reduce anxiety levels. Examples include muscular relaxation in which individuals are taught to alternatively tense and relax specific muscle groups and breathing retraining to avoid overbreathing.

Cognitive behavioural therapy Covers a variety of techniques. *Imaginal exposure* entails exposure to a detailed account or image of what happened. *Real life exposure* involves confronting real life situations that have become associated with the trauma and cause fear and distress. *Cognitive therapy* entails challenging distorted thoughts about the trauma, the self, and the world. *Imaginal flooding* involves the intense reliving of the traumatic experience. *Memory structuring* involves listening to and clarifying the individual's narrative and structuring it for them to repeat to friends and family. *Prolonged exposure* entails repeated exposure to memories of the trauma, and to non-dangerous real life situations that are avoided because of trauma related fear. *Stress inoculation* entails instruction in coping skills and some cognitive techniques such as restructuring. *Supportive listening* involves actively listening to the individual's narrative and clarifying factual, sensory, and affective details.

Cognitive processing therapy Includes elements of cognitive therapy and writing and reading about the traumatic event.

Dissociative symptoms Involve a disruption to memory or perception of the environment, e.g. an inability to recall details of a traumatic event that cannot be accounted for by ordinary forgetfulness or an organic cause such as head injury.

Drama therapy Entails using drama as a form of expression and communication.

Eye movement desensitisation and reprocessing (EMDR) Entails asking the person to focus on the traumatic event, a negative cognition associated with it, and the associated emotions.[49] The person is then asked to follow the therapist's finger as it moves from side to side.

Hypnotherapy Entails hypnosis to allow people to work through the traumatic event.

Imagery rehearsal therapy Involves encouraging participants to practice pleasant imagery exercises and employ cognitive behavioural tools to deal with unpleasant images.

Inpatient treatment programmes Individuals receive a planned package of care, usually as a group, as inpatients. The programmes can include various techniques, including cognitive behavioural therapy, group therapy, and medication.

Internet based psychotherapy A protocol driven treatment delivered through the internet, which includes psychoeducation and cognitive reappraisal. For further information, see http://www.interapy.com/Public2/.

Multiple session collaborative trauma support Entails counselling, liaison, and coordination of care after discharge.

Present focused group therapy A group intervention that involves identifying and modifying patterns of behaviour that have arisen from their past traumatic experience.

Psychodynamic psychotherapy Entails analysis of defence mechanisms, interpretations, and pre-trauma experiences.

Psychological debriefing A technique that entails detailed consideration of the traumatic event and the normalisation of psychological reactions.

Relaxation treatment A technique involving imagination of relaxing situations to induce muscular and mental relaxation.

Sub-syndromal PTSD This term is sometimes used to describe individuals with traumatic stress symptoms who would not fulfil the full DSM-IV or ICD-10 criteria for a diagnosis of post-traumatic stress disorder.

Supportive counselling A non-directive intervention dealing with current issues rather than the trauma itself.

Supportive psychotherapy A non-directive intervention that involves helping an individual to explore their thoughts, feelings, and behaviour with the aim of achieving clearer understanding of self and the ability to cope with situations more effectively.

Trauma focused group therapy A group intervention that involves reconstructing a past traumatic event, identifying and modifying negative self images associated with it, and integrating memories of the event into the individual's conscious awareness of self and others.

REFERENCES

1. American Psychiatric Association. *Diagnostic and statistical manual of mental disorders*. 4th ed. Washington: APA, 1994.
2. Kessler RC, Sonnega A, Bromet E, et al. Posttraumatic stress disorder in the national comorbidity survey. *Arch Gen Psychiatry* 1995;52:1048–1060.
3. O'Brien S. *Traumatic events and mental health*. Cambridge: Cambridge University Press, 1998.
4. Rose S, Bisson J, Wessely S. Psychological debriefing for preventing post traumatic stress disorder (PTSD). In: The Cochrane Library, Issue 1, 2004. Chichester, UK: John Wiley & Sons, Ltd. Search date 2000; primary sources Medline, Embase, Psychlit, Pilots, Biosis, Pascal, Occupational Safety and Health, Sociofile, Cinahl, Psychinfo, Psyndex, Sigle, Lilacs, Cochrane Controlled Clinical Trials, National Research Register, hand searches of *Journal of Traumatic Stress*, and contact with leading researchers.
5. Campfield KM, Hills AM. Effect of timing of critical incident stress debriefing (CISD) on posttraumatic symptoms. *J Trauma Stress* 2001;14:327–340.

6. Brom D, Kleber RJ, Hofman MC. Victims of traffic accidents: incidence and prevention of post-traumatic stress disorder. *J Clin Psychol* 1993;49:131–140.
7. Bisson JI, Shepherd JP, Joy D, et al. Early cognitive-behavioural therapy for post-traumatic stress symptoms after physical injury. Randomised controlled trial. *Br J Psychiatry* 2004;184:63–69.
8. Andre C, Lelord F, Legeron P, et al. Controlled study of outcomes after 6 months to early intervention of bus driver victims of aggression. *Encephale* 1997;23:65–71. [In French]
9. Bryant RA, Harvey AG, Basten C, et al. Treatment of acute stress disorder: a comparison of cognitive behavioural therapy and supportive counselling. *J Consult Clin Psychol* 1998;66:862–866.
10. Bryant RA, Sackville T, Dang ST, et al. Treating acute stress disorder: an evaluation of cognitive behavior therapy and supportive counselling techniques. *Am J Psychiatry* 1999;156:1780–1786.
11. Gidron Y, Gal R, Freedman S, et al. Translating research findings to PTSD prevention: results of a randomised controlled pilot study. *J Trauma Stress* 2001;14:773–780.
12. Bordow S, Porritt D. An experimental evaluation of crisis intervention. *Soc Sci Med* 1979;13A:251–256.
13. Zatzick DF, Roy-Byrne P, Russo JE, et al. Collaborative interventions for physically injured trauma survivors: a pilot randomized effectiveness trial. *Gen Hosp Psychiatry* 2001;23:114–123.
14. Schelling G, Briegel J, Roozendaal B, et al. The effect of stress doses of hydrocortisone during septic shock on posttraumatic stress disorder in survivors. *Biol Psychiatry* 2001;50:978–985.
15. Pitman RK, Sanders KM, Zusman RM, et al. Pilot study of secondary prevention of posttraumatic stress disorder with propranolol. *Biol Psychiatry* 2002;51:189–192.
16. Mellman TA, Bustamante V, David D, et al. Hypnotic medication in the aftermath of trauma. *J Clin Psychiatry* 2002;63:1183–1184.
17. Sherman JJ. Effects of psychotherapeutic treatments for PTSD: a meta-analysis of controlled clinical trials. *J Trauma Stress* 1998;11:413–436. Search date not reported; primary sources Psychlit, Eric, Medline, Cinahl, Dissertation Abstracts, and Pilots Traumatic Stress Database.
18. Marks I, Lovell K, Noshirvani H, et al. Treatment of posttraumatic stress disorder by exposure and/or cognitive restructuring: a controlled study. *Arch Gen Psychiatry* 1998;55:317–325.
19. Tarrier N, Sommerfield C, Pilgrim H, et al. Cognitive therapy or imaginal exposure in the treatment of post-traumatic stress disorder. *Br J Psychiatry* 1999;175:571–575.
20. Krakow B, Hollifield M, Johnston L, et al. Imagery rehearsal therapy for chronic nightmares in sexual assault survivors with posttraumatic stress disorder: a randomized controlled trial. *JAMA* 2001;286:537–545.
21. Resick A, Nishith P, Weaver TL, et al. A comparison of cognitive-processing therapy with prolonged exposure and a waiting condition for the treatment of chronic posttraumatic stress disorder in female rape victims. *J Consult Clin Psychol* 2002;70:867–879.
22. Blanchard EB, Hickling EJ, Devineni T, et al. A controlled evaluation of cognitive behavioral therapy for posttraumatic stress in motor vehicle accident survivors. *Behav Res Ther* 2003;41:79–96.
23. Ehlers A, Clarke DM, Hackmann A, et al. A randomized controlled trial of cognitive therapy, a self-help booklet, and repeated assessments as early interventions for posttraumatic stress disorder. *Arch Gen Psychiatry* 2003;60:1024–1032.
24. Bryant RA, Moulds ML, Guthrie RM, et al. Imaginal exposure alone and imaginal exposure with cognitive restructuring in treatment of posttraumatic stress disorder. *J Consult Clin Psychol* 2003;71:706–712.
25. Kubany ES, Hill EE, Owens JA. Cognitive trauma therapy for battered women with PTSD: preliminary findings. *J Trauma Stress* 2003;16:81–91.
26. Power K, McGoldrick T, Brown K, et al. A controlled comparison of eye movement desensitization and reprocessing versus exposure plus cognitive restructuring versus waiting list in the treatment of post-traumatic stress disorder. *Clin Psychol Psychotherapy* 2002;9:299–318.
27. Pitman RK, Altman B, Greenwald E, et al. Psychiatric complications during flooding therapy for posttraumatic stress disorder. *J Clin Psychiatry* 1991;52:17–20.
28. Davidson PR, Parker KC. Eye movement desensitisation and reprocessing (EMDR): a meta-analysis. *J Consult Clin Psychol* 2001;69:305–316. Medline and Psychinfo searched from 1988 to April 2000, and Current Contents searched from 1997 to March 2000, plus reference lists from articles found in these searches.
29. Lee C, Gavriel H, Drummond, et al. Treatment of PTSD: stress inoculation training with prolonged exposure compared to EMDR. *J Clin Psychol* 2002;58:1071–1089.
30. Ironson G, Freund B, Strauss JL, et al. Comparison of two treatments for traumatic stress: a community-based study of EMDR and prolonged exposure. *J Clin Psychol* 2002;58:113–128.
31. Taylor S, Thordarson DS, Maxfield L, et al. Comparative efficacy, speed, and adverse effects of three PTSD treatments: exposure therapy, EMDR, and relaxation training. *J Consult Clin Psychol* 2003;71:330–338.
32. Zlotnick C, Shea T, Rosen K, et al. An affect-management group for women with posttraumatic stress disorder and histories of childhood sexual abuse. *J Trauma Stress* 1997;10:425–436.
33. Gersons BPR, Carlier IVE, Lamberts RD, et al. Randomised clinical trial of brief eclectic psychotherapy for police officers with posttraumatic stress disorder. *J Trauma Stress* 2000;13:333–348.
34. Classen C, Koopman C, Nevill-Manning K, et al. A preliminary report comparing trauma-focused and present-focused group therapy against a wait-listed condition among childhood sexual abuse survivors with PTSD. *J Aggress Maltreat Trauma* 2001;4:265–288.
35. Schnurr PP, Friedman MJ, Foy DW, et al. Randomized trial of trauma-focused group therapy for posttraumatic stress disorder: results from a department of veterans affairs cooperative study. *Arch Gen Psychiatry* 2003;60:481–489.
36. Lange A, Van de Ven JP, Schrieken B, et al. Interapy: treatment of posttraumatic stress through the Internet: a controlled trial. *J Behav Ther Exp Psychiatry* 2001;32:73–90.
37. Brom D, Kleber RJ, Defares PB. Brief psychotherapy of posttraumatic stress disorders. *J Consult Clin Psychol* 1989;57:607–612.
38. Stein DJ, Zungu-Dirwayi N, Van der Linden GJ, et al. Pharmacotherapy for posttraumatic stress disorder. In: The Cochrane Library, Issue 1, 2004. Chichester, UK: John Wiley & Sons, Ltd. Search date 1999; primary sources Medline; Psychlit; Pilots Traumatic Stress Database; Dissertation Abstracts; trials register of the Cochrane Depression, Anxiety and Neurosis Controlled Group; hand searches of reference lists; and personal contact with post-traumatic stress disorder researchers and pharmaceutical companies.
39. Davidson JR, Rothbaum BO, van der Kolk BA, et al. Multicenter, double blind comparison of sertraline and placebo in the treatment of posttraumatic stress disorder. *Arch Gen Psychiatry* 2001;58:485–492.
40. Davidson J, Pearlstein T, Londborg P, et al. Efficacy of sertraline in preventing relapse of posttraumatic stress disorder: results of a 28-week double-blind, placebo-controlled study. *Am J Psychiatry* 2001;158:1974–1981.
41. Zohar J, Amital D, Miodownik C. Double-blind placebo-controlled pilot study of sertraline in military veterans with posttraumatic stress disorder. *J Clin Psychopharmacol* 2002;22:190–195.
42. Tucker P, Zaninelli R, Yehuda R, et al. Paroxetine in the treatment of chronic posttraumatic stress

disorder: results of a placebo-controlled, flexible-dosage trial. *J Clin Psychiatry* 2001;62:860–868.
43. Marshall RD, Beebe KL, Oldham M, et al. Efficacy and safety of paroxetine treatment for chronic PTSD: a fixed-dose, placebo-controlled study. *Am J Psychiatry* 2001;158:1982–1988.
44. Martenyi F, Brown EB, Zhang H, et al. Fluoxetine versus placebo in posttraumatic stress disorder. *J Clin Psychiatry* 2002;63:199–206.
45. Davidson JRT, Weisler RH, Butterfield MI, et al. Mirtazapine vs. placebo in posttraumatic stress disorder: a pilot trial. *Biol Psychiatry* 2003;53:188–191.
46. Saygin MZ, Sungur MZ, Sabol EU, et al. Nefazodone versus sertraline in treatment of posttraumatic stress disorder. *Bull Clin Psychopharmacol* 2002;12:1–5.
47. Barnett SD, Tharwani HM, Hertzberg MA, et al. Tolerability of fluoxetine in posttraumatic stress disorder. *Prog Neuropsychopharmacol Biol Psychiatry* 2002;26:363–367.
48. Butterfield MI, Becker ME, Connor KM, et al. Olanzapine in the treatment of post-traumatic stress disorder: a pilot study. *Int Clin Psychopharmacol* 2001;16:197–203.
49. Shapiro F. Eye movement desensitisation: a new treatment for post-traumatic stress disorder. *J Behav Ther Exp Psychiatry* 1989;20:211–217.

Jonathan Bisson
Consultant Liaison Psychiatrist
Cardiff and Vale NHS Trust
Cardiff
UK

Competing interests: None declared.

Schizophrenia

Search date April 2004

Zia Nadeem, Andrew McIntosh, and Stephen Lawrie

QUESTIONS

INTERVENTIONS

To be covered in future updates

Augmentation of antipsychotic treatment
Effects of early intervention
Treating depression in schizophrenia
Treating acute behavioural disturbance

*These drugs are beneficial in schizophrenia but all have important harms, which may include parkinsonism, dystonia, cholinergic effects, and weight gain.

See glossary G

Key Messages

- Most evidence is from systematic reviews of RCTs that report disparate outcomes. There is a need for larger RCTs, over longer periods, with well designed end points, including standardised, validated symptom scales. No intervention has been found to reduce negative symptoms consistently.

Drug treatment for positive and negative symptoms

- **Amisulpride** Two systematic reviews found that amisulpride improved symptoms more than standard antipsychotic drugs. One review found that extrapyramidal adverse effects were less likely with amisulpride than with standard antipsychotic drugs. One RCT found no significant difference in symptoms between amisulpride and olanzapine. One systematic review found no significant difference in symptoms between amisulpride and risperidone.
- **Chlorpromazine** One systematic review found that, compared with placebo, chlorpromazine reduced the proportion of people with no improvement or with worse severity of illness at 6 months on a psychiatrist rated scale. The review found that, compared with placebo, chlorpromazine caused more adverse effects, such as sedation, acute dystonia, and parkinsonism.
- **Clozapine** One systematic review found that clozapine improved symptoms over 4–10 weeks compared with standard antipsychotic drugs (predominantly haloperidol and chlorpromazine) and was less likely to lead to antipsychotic induced movement disorders. RCTs provided insufficient evidence to compare clozapine versus other, newer antipsychotic drugs. RCTs found that clozapine may be associated with blood dyscrasias.
- **Depot bromperidol decanoate** One systematic review of three small RCTs found no significant difference between depot bromperidol decanoate and haloperidol or fluphenazine decanoate in the proportion of people who needed additional medication, left the trial early, or had movement disorders over 6–12 months. The review may have lacked power to detect a clinically important difference.
- **Depot haloperidol decanoate** One small RCT identified by a systematic review found no significant difference between depot haloperidol decanoate and oral haloperidol in global clinical state at 4 months, but it may have been too small to exclude a clinically important difference. Haloperidol is associated with acute dystonia, akathisia, and parkinsonism.
- **Haloperidol** One systematic review found that haloperidol increased physician rated global improvement at 6 and 24 weeks compared with placebo, but was associated with acute dystonia, akathisia, and parkinsonism.
- **Olanzapine** One systematic review found no significant difference in psychotic symptoms between olanzapine and standard antipsychotic drugs. The review and one subsequent RCT found that olanzapine was associated with fewer extrapyramidal adverse effects than standard antipsychotic drugs. RCTs found no clear difference in symptoms or adverse effects between olanzapine, amisulpride, risperidone, and clozapine.
- **Pimozide** One systematic review found no significant difference between pimozide and standard antipsychotic drugs in global clinical impression, and found that pimozide decreased sedation but increased tremor. It found no overall difference in cardiovascular adverse effects such as rise or fall in blood pressure or dizziness between pimozide and standard antipsychotic drugs. Pimozide has been associated with sudden cardiac death at doses above 20 mg daily.
- **Risperidone** One large systematic review found that risperidone improved symptoms more than standard antipsychotic drugs (mainly haloperidol). One small additional RCT found no significant difference between risperidone and haloperidol in responders over 8 weeks. One systematic review found that risperidone decreased extrapyramidal side effects and the need for antiparkinsonian medication, but increased weight gain, compared with standard antipsychotic drugs. Systematic reviews found no significant difference in symptoms between risperidone and other new antipsychotic drugs (olanzapine, sulpiride, and clozapine).

- **Thioridazine** One systematic review found that thioridazine improved global mental state compared with placebo over 3–12 months.
- **Zotepine** One systematic review found weak evidence that zotepine increased the proportion of people with a clinically important improvement in symptoms compared with standard antipsychotic drugs, and reduced akasthesia, dystonia, and rigidity. This finding was not robust because removal of a single RCT from the analysis meant that the difference between zotepine and standard antipsychotic drugs was no longer significant.
- **Loxapine; molindone; quetiapine; sulpiride; ziprasidone** Systematic reviews found no significant difference between these newer antipsychotic drugs and standard antipsychotic drugs in symptom improvement, and that they have different profiles of adverse effects.
- **Perazine** One weak RCT found no significant difference in global clinical impression over 28 days between perazine and haloperidol. Two small RCTs provided insufficient evidence to compare perazine versus zotepine, and one small RCT found no significant difference in mental state at 28 days between perazine and amisulpride. Three RCTs found no significant difference in extrapyramidal effects over 28 days between perazine and zotepine or amisulpride.

Interventions to reduce relapse rates

- **Continuation of antipsychotic drugs for at least 6 months after an acute episode** Systematic reviews found that continuing antipsychotic drugs for at least 6 months after an acute episode reduced relapse rates compared with no treatment or placebo. Eight systematic reviews found no significant difference in relapse rates among antipsychotic drugs. One systematic review found that clozapine reduced relapse rates over 12 weeks compared with standard antipsychotic drugs. Another review found that fewer people taking depot zuclopenthixol decanoate relapsed over 12 weeks to 1 year compared with people taking other depot preparations. A third review found that bromperidol increased the proportion of people who relapsed compared with haloperidol or fluphenazine. One additional RCT found that risperidone reduced relapse over 2.2 years compared with haloperidol.
- **Multiple session family interventions** One systematic review found that multiple session family interventions reduced relapse rates at 12 months compared with usual care, single session family interventions, or psychoeducational interventions.
- **Psychoeducational interventions** One systematic review found that psychoeducation reduced relapse rates at 9–18 months compared with usual care.
- **Cognitive behavioural therapy** Limited evidence from a systematic review of two RCTs found no significant difference in relapse rates between cognitive behavioural therapy plus standard care and standard care alone.
- **Social skills training** One systematic review of small RCTs provided insufficient evidence to assess the effect of social skills training on relapse rates.

Treatments in people resistant to standard treatment

- **Clozapine (compared with standard antipsychotic drugs)** One systematic review in people resistant to standard antipsychotic drugs found that clozapine improved symptoms after 12 weeks and after 2 years compared with standard antipsychotic drugs. One systematic review found no significant difference in symptoms between clozapine and other new antipsychotic drugs in people resistant to standard antipsychotic drugs.
- **Olanzapine** Small RCTs identified by a systematic review found no significant difference in psychotic symptoms over 8 weeks between olanzapine and chlorpromazine or between olanzapine and clozapine.

Interventions to improve adherence to antipsychotic medication

- **Behavioural therapy** One small RCT found limited evidence that behavioural interventions improved adherence to antipsychotic medication compared with usual treatment. Two RCTs found limited evidence that behavioural interventions improved adherence more than psychoeducational therapy.

- **Compliance therapy** Two RCTs found limited evidence that compliance therapy increased adherence to antipsychotic drugs at 6 and 18 months compared with supportive or non-specific counselling.
- **Psychoeducational interventions** One systematic review found limited evidence that psychoeducational interventions improved adherence to antipsychotic medication compared with usual care. Two RCTs found limited evidence that psychoeducational interventions improved adherence less than behavioural therapy.
- **Multiple session family interventions** One systematic review found that "compliance with medication" over 9–24 months was higher in people who received multiple family interventions compared with usual care, single family interventions, or psychoeducational interventions, but the difference was not statistically significant.

DEFINITION Schizophrenia is characterised by the positive symptoms**G** of auditory hallucinations, delusions, and thought disorder, and by the negative symptoms**G** of demotivation, self neglect, and reduced emotion.[1] People are defined as being resistant to standard antipsychotic drugs if, over the preceding 5 years, they have not had a clinically important improvement in symptoms after 2–3 regimens of treatment with standard antipsychotic drugs for at least 6 weeks (from at least 2 classes at doses equivalent to or greater than 1000 mg/day chlorpromazine) and they have had no period of good functioning.[2,3] About 30% (10–45%) of people with schizophrenia meet these criteria.[3]

INCIDENCE/ PREVALENCE Onset of symptoms typically occurs in early adult life (average age 25 years) and is earlier in men than in women.[4,5] Prevalence worldwide is 2–4/1000. One in 100 people will develop schizophrenia in their lifetime.

AETIOLOGY/ RISK FACTORS Risk factors include a family history (although no major genes have been identified), obstetric complications, developmental difficulties, central nervous system infections in childhood, cannabis use, and acute life events.[4] The precise contributions of these factors and ways in which they may interact are unclear.

PROGNOSIS About three quarters of people suffer recurrent relapse and continued disability, although the proportion of people who improved significantly increased after the mid-1950s (mean 48.5% from 1956–1985 *v* 35.4% from 1895–1956).[6] Outcome may be worse in people with insidious onset and delayed initial treatment, social isolation, or a strong family history; in people living in industrialised countries; in men; and in people who misuse drugs.[5] Drug treatment is generally successful in treating positive symptoms, but up to a third of people derive little benefit, and negative symptoms are notoriously difficult to treat. About half of people with schizophrenia do not adhere to treatment in the short term. The figure is even higher in the longer term.[7]

AIMS OF INTERVENTION To relieve symptoms and to improve quality of life, with minimal adverse effects of treatment.

OUTCOMES Severity of positive and negative symptoms; global clinical improvement; global clinical impression (a composite measure of symptoms and everyday functioning); rate of relapse; adherence to treatment; adverse effects of treatment. Some systematic reviews calculate effect sizes in order to meta-analyse primary studies that use different outcome measures. Effect size is a difficult measure to interpret clinically, so we have given lower priority to analyses that use this measure.

METHODS *Clinical Evidence* search and appraisal April 2004. Most RCTs were small, short term, with high withdrawal rates, and employed many different outcome measures.[8] There were a large number of good systematic reviews. Therefore, if possible, we focused primarily on systematic reviews and included only the outcomes that we thought were the most clinically relevant. Because each treatment is associated with different benefits and harms, we used estimates of global effectiveness if they were available. We searched for placebo controlled RCTs of standard antipsychotic medication and comparative RCTs of newer antipsychotic drugs.

QUESTION What are the effects of drug treatments for positive and negative symptoms?

OPTION CHLORPROMAZINE

One systematic review found that, compared with placebo, chlorpromazine reduced the proportion of people with no improvement or worse severity of illness at 6 months on a psychiatrist rated scale. The review found that, compared with placebo, chlorpromazine caused more adverse effects, such as sedation, acute dystonia, and parkinsonism.

Benefits: **Versus placebo:** We found one systematic review (search date 2002, 50 RCTs, 4968 people, mean dose 574 mg/day, range 25–2400 mg/day).[9] It found that chlorpromazine significantly reduced the proportion of people who had no improvement on a psychiatrist rated global impression scale at 6 months compared with placebo and significantly reduced the proportion of people who had worse severity of illness on a psychiatrist rated scale at 1 week to 6 months (failure to improve: 13 RCTs, 1121 people; RR 0.76, 95% CI 0.67 to 0.87; NNT 7, 95% CI 5 to 10; marked or worse illness severity: 5 RCTs, 778 people; 323/493 [66%] with chlorpromazine *v* 231/285 [81%] with placebo; RR 0.67, 95% CI 0.51 to 0.88; NNT 6, 95% CI 5 to 11).

Harms: **Versus placebo:** The systematic review (search date 2002) found that, compared with placebo, chlorpromazine significantly increased sedation, acute dystonia**G**, parkinsonism, weight gain, skin photosensitivity, dizziness caused by hypotension, dry mouth, and constipation compared with placebo (sedation: RR 2.6, 95% CI 1.9 to 3.7; NNH 5, 95% CI 4 to 6; acute dystonia: RR 3.4, 95% CI 1.4 to 8.0; NNH 22, 95% CI 15 to 46; parkinsonism: RR 2.6, 95% CI 1.2 to 5.4; NNH 10, 95% CI 8 to 16; weight gain: RR 4.4, 95% CI 2.1 to 9.3; NNH 3, 95% CI 2 to 5; skin photosensitivity: RR 5.2, 95% CI 3 to 10; NNH 7, 95% CI 6 to 10; dizziness caused by hypotension: RR 2.1, 95% CI 1.5 to 2.8; NNH 10, 95% CI 8 to 15; dry mouth: RR 4.3, 95% CI 2.2 to 8.4; NNH 13, 95% CI 10 to 22; and constipation: RR 2.0, 95% CI 1.3 to 3.2; NNH 22, 95% CI 13 to 75).[9] Chlorpromazine was also associated with increased blood dyscrasias, although the difference did not reach significance (RR 2.0, 95% CI 0.7 to 6.0). We found no long term data on the risk of tardive dyskinesia or the rare but potentially fatal neuroleptic malignant syndrome. Despite the frequent adverse effects, the review found that people taking chlorpromazine were more likely to stay in RCTs in both the short and the medium term than people taking placebo.

Comment: The review did not categorise symptoms as positive or negative because this information was rarely available from included RCTs.[9] It found significant heterogeneity among RCTs, but found that the analysis of global improvement over 9 weeks to 6 months remained significant after removal of the heterogeneous RCTs (11 RCTs, 1083 people: RR 0.81, 95% CI 0.7 to 0.9; NNT 8, 95% CI 6 to 10).

OPTION HALOPERIDOL

One systematic review found that haloperidol increased psychiatrist rated global improvement at 6 and 24 weeks compared with placebo, but was associated with acute dystonia, akathisia, and parkinsonism.

Benefits: **Versus placebo:** We found one systematic review (search date 1998, 20 RCTs, 1001 people).[10] It found that haloperidol (over a wide range of doses) significantly increased psychiatrist rated global improvement at 6 and 24 weeks compared with placebo (6 weeks: 3 RCTs, 159 people; 61/88 [69%] with haloperidol *v* 23/71 [32%] with placebo; RR 2.3, 95% CI 1.7 to 3.3; NNT 3, 95% CI 2 to 5; 24 weeks: 8 RCTs; 72/163 [44%] *v* 21/150 [14%]; RR 3.5, 95% CI 2.3 to 5.6; NNT 3, 95% CI 3 to 5).

Harms: **Versus placebo:** The systematic review found that haloperidol significantly increased the risk of acute dystonia**G**, akathisia, and parkinsonism compared with placebo (dystonia: 2 RCTs; RR 4.7, 95% CI 1.7 to 44.0; NNH 5, 95% CI 3 to 9; akathisia**G** 3 RCTs; RR 6.5, 95% CI 1.5 to 28.0; NNH 6, 95% CI 4 to 14; parkinsonism: 4 RCTs; RR 8.9, 95% CI 2.6 to 31.0; NNH 3, 95% CI 2 to 5).[10] People taking haloperidol were significantly more likely to be treated with anticholinergic drugs than people taking placebo (4 RCTs; RR 4.9, 95% CI 1.01 to 24.00; NNH 2, 95% CI 1 to 3).

Comment: The median size of RCTs in the review was 38 people, but the quality of the RCTs was higher than average for schizophrenia trials.[10] Although the dose range was very wide, most RCTs used 4–20 mg daily and adjusted dose according to need. The review found evidence of publication bias for the 6–24 month global outcome ratings.[10]

OPTION THIORIDAZINE

One systematic review found that thioridazine improved global mental state compared with placebo over 3–12 months.

Benefits: **Versus placebo:** We found one systematic review (search date 1999, 11 RCTs, 560 people).[11] It found that thioridazine significantly reduced the proportion of people who were "no better or worse" in global clinical impression at 3–12 months compared with placebo (5 RCTs; 27/84 [32%] with thioridazine *v* 57/81 [70%] with placebo; RR 0.5, 95% CI 0.37 to 0.68; NNT 3, 95% CI 3 to 5).

Harms: **Versus placebo:** The review found no significant difference in adverse effects between thioridazine and placebo, but may have lacked power to detect a clinically important difference.[11]

Comment: None.

OPTION DEPOT BROMPERIDOL DECANOATE

One systematic review of three small RCTs found no significant difference between depot bromperidol decanoate and haloperidol or fluphenazine decanoate in the proportion of people who needed additional medication, left the trial early, or had movement disorders over 6–12 months. The review may have lacked power to detect a clinically important difference.

Benefits: **Versus standard antipsychotic drugs:** One systematic review (search date 1999, 3 RCTs, 97 people) found no significant difference between depot bromperidol and haloperidol or fluphenazine decanoate in the proportion of people who needed additional antipsychotic drugs or benzodiazepines over 6–12 months or who left the trial early (additional antipsychotic drugs: 10/33 [30%] with bromperidol *v* 6/34 [18%] with haloperidol or fluphenazine; RR 1.72, 95% CI 0.70 to 4.24; additional benzodiazepines: 19/48 [39%] with bromperidol *v* 18/49 [37%] with haloperidol or fluphenazine; RR 1.08, 95% CI 0.68 to 1.70; left trial early: 10/48 [21%] with bromperidol *v* 5/49 [10%] with haloperidol or fluphenazine; RR 1.92, 95% CI 0.80 to 4.60).[12]

Harms: **Versus standard antipsychotic drugs:** The review found no significant difference in movement disorders over 6–12 months between bromperidol and haloperidol or fluphenazine (2 RCTs; 16/38 [42%] with bromperidol *v* 22/39 [56%] with haloperidol or fluphenazine; RR 0.74, 95% CI 0.47 to 1.17).[12]

Comment: None.

OPTION DEPOT HALOPERIDOL DECANOATE

One small RCT identified by a systematic review found no significant difference between depot haloperidol decanoate and oral haloperidol in global clinical state at 4 months, but it may have been too small to exclude a clinically important difference. Haloperidol is associated with acute dystonia, akathisia, and parkinsonism.

Benefits: **Versus standard antipsychotic drugs:** We found one systematic review (search date 1998) that identified one small RCT (22 people) comparing depot haloperidol versus oral haloperidol.[13] It found no significant difference in the proportion of people with "no improvement" in global clinical impression at 4 months (8/11 [73%] with depot haloperidol *v* 9/11 [82%] with oral haloperidol; RR of no improvement 0.89, 95% CI 0.56 to 1.40). The RCT may have been too small to detect a clinically important difference.

Harms: **Versus standard antipsychotic drugs:** The RCT found no significant difference between depot and oral haloperidol in the proportion of people who needed anticholinergic drugs for movement disorders (3/11 [27%] with depot haloperidol *v* 1/11 [9%] with oral haloperidol; RR 3.00, 95% CI 0.37 to 24.58).[13] See also harms of haloperidol, p 1343.

Comment: Depot injection is believed to ensure adherence, but we found no evidence from RCTs to support this.

OPTION CLOZAPINE

One systematic review found that clozapine improved symptoms over 4–10 weeks compared with standard antipsychotic drugs (predominantly haloperidol and chlorpromazine) and was less likely to lead to antipsychotic induced movement disorders. RCTs provided insufficient evidence to compare clozapine versus other, newer antipsychotic drugs. RCTs found that clozapine may be associated with blood dyscrasias.

Benefits: **Versus standard antipsychotic drugs:** We found one systematic review (search date 1999, 31 RCTs, 2589 people), which compared clozapine versus standard antipsychotic drugs, such as chlorpromazine and haloperidol.[14] It found that clozapine significantly reduced the proportion of people with no clinical improvement over 4–10 weeks compared with standard antipsychotic drugs (14 RCTs; 267/561 [48%] with clozapine *v* 377/570 [66%] with standard antipsychotic drugs; RR of no important improvement 0.75, 95% CI 0.66 to 0.84; NNT 6, 95% CI 5 to 7). The review found that, despite the requirement for regular blood tests, significantly fewer people withdrew from treatment with clozapine over 7–24 months compared with standard antipsychotic drugs (111/750 [15%] with clozapine *v* 140/763 [18%] with standard antipsychotic drugs; RR 0.76, 95% CI 0.66 to 0.92). **Versus olanzapine:** We found one systematic review (search date 2002, 3 RCTs, 397 people)[15] and one subsequent

RCT.[16] The systematic review found no significant difference between olanzapine and clozapine in symptoms (effect size estimated using the Positive and Negative Syndrome Scale, the Brief Psychiatric Rating Scale, and the Clinical Global Rating: 0.089, 95% CI –0.34 to +0.52).[15] The subsequent RCT (890 people with schizophrenia at high risk of suicide because of previous attempts of current suicidal ideation, 27% refractory to previous treatment) found that clozapine (mean daily dose 274 mg) significantly reduced suicidal behaviour compared with olanzapine (mean daily dose 16.6 mg) over 2 years (suicide attempts or hospitalisation to prevent suicide: HR 0.76, 95% CI 0.58 to 0.97; worsening on the Clinical Global Scale of Suicide Severity: HR 0.78, 95% CI 0.61 to 0.99).[16] **Versus risperidone:** We found one systematic review (search date 2002, 7 RCTs, 836 people).[15] It found no significant difference between risperidone and clozapine in symptoms (effect size, estimated using Positive and Negative Syndrome Scale, the Brief Psychiatric Rating Scale, or the Clinical Global Rating: –0.109, 95% CI –0.31 to +0.01).[15]

Harms: **Versus standard antipsychotic drugs:** The systematic review (search date 1999) found that, compared with standard antipsychotic drugs, clozapine was significantly more likely to cause hypersalivation, increased temperature, and sedation but that it was less likely to cause dry mouth and extrapyramidal adverse effects (hypersalivation: 351/699 [50%] with clozapine *v* 161/720 [22%] with standard antipsychotic drugs; RR 2.23, 95% CI 1.95 to 2.57; NNH 3, 95% CI 3 to 4; increased temperature: 129/560 [23%] with clozapine *v* 86/587 [15%] with standard antipsychotic drugs; RR 1.57, 95% CI 1.27 to 1.98; NNH 11, 95% CI 7 to 25; sedation: 392/751 [52%] with clozapine *v* 332/776 [43%] with standard antipsychotic drugs; RR 1.23, 95% CI 1.13 to 1.34; NNH 10, 95% CI 6 to 22; dry mouth: 40/397 [10%] with clozapine *v* 111/402 [28%] with standard antipsychotic drugs; RR 0.36, 95% CI 0.26 to 0.51; NNT 6, 95% CI 4 to 8; extrapyramidal adverse effects: 202/614 [33%] with clozapine *v* 304/621 [49%] with standard antipsychotic drugs; RR 0.67, 95% CI 0.58 to 0.77; NNT 6, 95% CI 5 to 9).[14] A large case series found leucopenia in 3% of 99 502 people taking clozapine over 5 years.[17] However, it found that monitoring white cell (neutrophil) counts was associated with a lower rate of cases of agranulocytosis and deaths in people taking clozapine (agranulocytosis: 382 *v* 995; AR 0.38% *v* 1%; deaths: 12 *v* 149).[17] The review found that clozapine significantly increased blood problems, including leucopenia and neutropenia, compared with standard antipsychotic drugs (24/637 [4%] with clozapine *v* 12/656 [2%] with standard antipsychotic drugs; RR 1.85, 95% CI 0.99 to 3.47).[14] **Versus olanzapine:** The review did not report on harms.[15] The subsequent RCT found no significant difference in overall adverse effects between clozapine and olanzapine over 2 years (no data presented).[16] It found that clozapine significantly increased salivary hypersecretion, somnolence, nausea, and dizziness compared with olanzapine (salivary hypersecretion: 48% *v* 6%; $P < 0.001$; somnolence: 46% *v* 25%; $P < 0.001$; nausea: 17% *v* 10%; $P = 0.003$; dizziness: 27% *v* 12%; $P < 0.001$). It found that olanzapine significantly increased weight gain compared with clozapine (AR for weight gain: 31% *v* 56%; $P < 0.001$). **Versus risperidone:** The review did not report on harms.[15]

Comment: Some of the benefits of clozapine were more apparent in the long term, depending on which drug was used for comparison in the RCTs.

OPTION AMISULPRIDE

Two systematic reviews found that amisulpride improved symptoms more than standard antipsychotic drugs. One review found that extrapyramidal adverse effects were less likely with amisulpride than with standard antipsychotic drugs. One RCT found no significant difference in symptoms between amisulpride and olanzapine. One systematic review found no significant difference in symptoms between amisulpride and risperidone.

Benefits: **Versus standard antipsychotic drugs:** We found two systematic reviews.[15,18] The first systematic review (search date 2000, 14 RCTs, 1701 people) compared amisulpride versus standard antipsychotic drugs (haloperidol, flupentixol).[18] It found that amisulpride significantly reduced the proportion of people who were less than "much improved" in global clinical impression compared with standard antipsychotic drugs (4 RCTs, 651 people; 107/324 [33%] with amisulpride *v* 163/327 [50%] with standard antipsychotic drugs; RR of failing to improve 0.66, 95% CI 0.55 to 0.80; NNT 6, 95% CI 5 to 11). It also found that amisulpride significantly reduced the proportion of people who left the study early (14 RCTs; 282/881 [32%] with amisulpride *v* 242/631 [38%] with standard antipsychotic drugs; RR 0.72, 95% CI 0.62 to 0.83; NNT 9, 95% CI 7 to 16). The second systematic review (search date 2002, 12 RCTs, 1494 people) found that amisulpride significantly reduced symptoms compared with standard antipsychotic drugs (effect size, estimated using Positive and Negative Syndrome Scale, the Brief Psychiatric Rating Scale, or the Clinical Global Rating: 0.286, 95% CI 0.16 to 0.41).[15] **Versus olanzapine:** We found no systematic review but found one RCT (377 people) comparing amisulpride versus olanzapine for 2 months.[19] It found no significant difference in symptoms at 2 months, assessed by the Brief Psychiatric Rating Scale score (mean reduction 17.6 with amisulpride *v* 16.3 with olanzapine; reported as non-significant; CI not reported). **Versus risperidone:** We found one systematic review (search date 2002, 2 RCTs, 472 people).[15] It found no significant difference between amisulpride and risperidone (effect size estimated using the Positive and Negative Syndrome Scale, the Brief Psychiatric Rating Scale, or the Clinical Global Rating: –0.102, 95% CI –1.27 to +1.07).

Harms: **Versus standard antipsychotic drugs:** The first review found that, compared with standard antipsychotic drugs, amisulpride significantly reduced the proportion of people who had at least one adverse effect (6 RCTs; 261/373 [70%] with amisulpride *v* 308/378 [81%] with standard antipsychotic drugs; RR 0.85, 95% CI 0.79 to 0.92; NNT 9, 95% CI 6 to 17).[18] It also found that amisulpride significantly reduced the proportion of people with at least one extrapyramidal symptom (7 RCTs; 161/383 [42%] with amisulpride *v* 234/388 [60%] with standard antipsychotic drugs; RR 0.68, 95% CI 0.60 to 0.79; NNT 5, 95% CI 4 to 8). The second review did not report on harms.[15] **Versus olanzapine:** The RCT found that significantly fewer people had clinically important weight gain (more than 7% total body weight) with amisulpride than with olanzapine (27/189 [14%] with amisulpride *v* 48/188 [25%] with olanzapine; P = 0.007).[19] **Versus risperidone:** The systematic review (search date 2002) did not report adverse effects.[15]

Comment: None.

OPTION LOXAPINE

One systematic review found no significant difference between loxapine and standard antipsychotic drugs in global improvement or adverse effects.

Benefits: **Versus standard antipsychotic drugs:** We found one systematic review (search date 1999, 22 RCTs, 1073 people), which compared loxapine (dose range 25–250 mg/day) versus standard antipsychotic drugs, primarily chlorpromazine.[20] It found no significant difference in clinical global improvement between loxapine and standard antipsychotic drugs (9 RCTs; 59/206 [29%] with loxapine *v* 65/205 [32%] with standard antipsychotic drugs; RR of no improvement 0.82, 95% CI 0.52 to 1.31).

Harms: The review found no significant difference in adverse effects between loxapine and standard antipsychotic drugs (11 RCTs; 164/255 [64%] with loxapine *v* 166/251 [66%] with standard antipsychotic drugs; RR 0.90, 95% CI 0.57 to 1.41).[20]

Comment: All of the RCTs identified by the review were conducted in the USA or India, and none lasted longer than 12 weeks.[20]

OPTION MOLINDONE

One systematic review found no significant difference in global clinical improvement or in the proportion of people who had adverse effects over 4–12 weeks between molindone and standard antipsychotic drugs.

Benefits: **Versus standard antipsychotic drugs:** We found one systematic review (search date 1999, 9 RCTs, 4 CCTs, 150 people) comparing molindone versus standard antipsychotic drugs, primarily haloperidol or chlorpromazine.[21] It found no significant difference between molindone and standard antipsychotic drugs in global clinical improvement over 4–12 weeks, as assessed by a physician (4 RCTs; 25/84 [29.8%] with molindone *v* 20/66 [30.3%] with standard antipsychotic drugs; RR of no improvement 1.10, 95% CI 0.68 to 1.78).

Harms: **Versus standard antipsychotic drugs:** The review found no significant difference between molindone and standard antipsychotic drugs in movement disorders (rigidity, tremor, akasthesia, use of antiparkinsonian medication) or in the proportion of people who had adverse effects (2 RCTs, 1 CCT; 24/42 [57%] with molindone *v* 25/42 [59%] with standard antipsychotic drugs; RR 0.96, 95% CI 0.73 to 1.27).[21] One RCT identified by the review found that significantly more people taking molindone compared with standard antipsychotic drugs experienced confusion (9/14 [64%] with molindone *v* 6/30 [20%] with standard antipsychotic drugs; RR 3.21, 95% CI 1.42 to 7.26). The review also found that significantly more people had weight loss with molindone than with standard antipsychotic drugs (2 RCTs; 12/30 [40%] with molindone *v* 4/30 [13%] with standard antipsychotic drugs; RR 2.78, 95% CI 1.10 to 6.99) and that fewer people had weight gain with molindone than with standard antipsychotic drugs (2 RCTs; 4/30 [13%] with molindone *v* 11/30 [37%] with standard antipsychotic drugs; RR 0.39, 95% CI 0.95 to 1.00).

Comment: None.

OPTION OLANZAPINE

One systematic review found no significant difference in psychotic symptoms between olanzapine and standard antipsychotic drugs. The review and one subsequent RCT found that olanzapine was associated with fewer extrapyramidal adverse effects than standard antipsychotic drugs. RCTs found no clear difference in symptoms or adverse effects between olanzapine, amisulpride, risperidone, and clozapine.

Benefits: **Versus standard antipsychotic drugs:** We found one systematic review (search date 1999, 15 RCTs, 3282 people),[22] and one subsequent RCT[23], which compared olanzapine versus standard antipsychotic drugs, usually haloperidol.[22] It found no significant difference in people with persisting psychotic symptoms over 6–8 weeks between olanzapine (2.5–25 mg/day) and standard antipsychotic drugs (4 RCTs; 1056/1926 [55%] with olanzapine *v* 596/852 [70%] with standard antipsychotic drugs; RR for no important response [defined as a 40% reduction on any scale] 0.90, 95% CI 0.76 to 1.06). The subsequent RCT only examined harms of olanzapine versus standard haloperidol (see harms section).[23] **Versus clozapine:** See benefits of clozapine, p 1344. **Versus amisulpride:** See benefits of amisulpride, p 1346. **Versus risperidone:** We found one systematic review[24] and one subsequent RCT.[25] The review (search date 1999, 3 RCTs) found that olanzapine improved mean Positive and Negative Syndrome Scale scores at 28–30 weeks compared with risperidone, although it found no significant difference at 54 weeks (28–30 weeks, 2 RCTs, 392 people; WMD 7.5 points, 95% CI 2.9 to 12.0 on a scale of 210 points; 54 weeks, 1 RCT, 435 people; WMD 6.1, 95% CI 1.9 to 10.3).[24] Olanzapine significantly reduced withdrawals for any cause at 28–30 weeks compared with risperidone (2 RCTs; 85/204 [42%] with olanzapine *v* 109/200 [54%] with risperidone; RR 0.76, 95% CI 0.62 to 0.94).[24] The subsequent RCT (377 people) found no significant difference between olanzapine and risperidone in the proportion of people who responded at 8 weeks (response defined as a $< 20\%$ reduction in Positive and Negative Syndrome Scale score: 48% with olanzapine *v* 51% with risperidone; reported as non-significant; no further data provided).[25]

Harms: **Versus standard antipsychotic drugs:** The review found no significant difference between olanzapine and standard antipsychotic drugs in the proportion of people who withdrew from the trial for any cause at 4–8 weeks (9 RCTs; 744/2068 [36%] with olanzapine *v* 464/952 [49%] with standard antipsychotic drugs; RR 0.85, 95% CI 0.65 to 1.10) or at 1 year (4 RCTs; 1577/1905 [83%] *v* 748/833 [90%]; RR 0.90, 95% CI 0.75 to 1.08).[22] It found that, compared with standard antipsychotic drugs, olanzapine significantly reduced the proportion of people who required anticholinergic drugs for extrapyramidal adverse effects and caused significantly less nausea and drowsiness (anticholinergic drugs: 293/1884 [15%] with olanzapine *v* 401/810 [49%] with standard antipsychotic drugs; RR 0.26, 95% CI 0.17 to 0.40; nausea: 174/1576 [11%] with olanzapine *v* 117/771 [15%] with standard antipsychotic drugs; RR 0.74, 95% CI 0.59 to 0.92; NNT 25, 95% CI 14 to 85; vomiting: 97/1336 [7%] with olanzapine *v* 81/660 [12%] with standard antipsychotic drugs; RR 0.59, 95% CI 0.45 to 0.78; NNT 20, 95% CI 12 to 46; drowsiness: 443/1576 [28%] with olanzapine *v* 268/771 [34%] with standard antipsychotic drugs; RR 0.82, 95% CI 0.72 to 0.92; NNT 15, 95% CI 9 to 38). Olanzapine was associated with a significantly greater increase in appetite and weight gain (increase in appetite: 1 RCT; 343/1336 [26%] with olanzapine *v* 103/660 [16%] with standard antipsychotic drugs; RR 1.65, 95% CI 1.35 to 2.01; NNH 10, 95% CI 7 to 15).[22] We found one subsequent RCT (182 people, 80% in hospital at baseline, 174 people in analysis), which compared extrapyramidal symptoms over 8 weeks between olanzepine (5 mg/day increased to a maximum of 15 mg/day) and haloperidol (4 mg/day increased to a maximum of 12 mg/day).[23] It found that olanzapine significantly reduced extrapyramidal symptoms compared with haloperidol (mean change in Drug Induced Extrapyramidal Symptoms Scale total score from baseline: –0.50 with olanzapine *v* +1.5 with haloperidol; $P < 0.001$). It found that olanzepine significantly reduced withdrawal due to adverse events compared with haloperidol (8.9% with olanzepine *v* 26.2% with haloperidol; $P = 0.003$). **Versus clozapine:** See harms of clozapine, p 1345. **Versus amisulpride:** See harms of amisulpride, p 1346. **Versus risperidone:** The review found that olanzapine was associated with significantly fewer extrapyramidal adverse effects compared with risperidone (1 RCT; 32/172 [19%] with olanzapine *v* 52/167 [31%] with risperidone; RR 0.60, 95% CI 0.41 to 0.88; NNT 8, 95% CI 5 to 28), less parkinsonism (1 RCT; 22/172 [13%] with olanzapine *v* 37/167 [22%] with risperidone; RR 0.58, 95% CI 0.37 to 0.94; NNT 11, 95% CI 6 to 77), and less need for antiparkinsonian medication (1 RCT; 34/172 [20%] with olanzapine *v* 55/167 [33%] with risperidone; RR 0.60, 95% CI 0.41 to 0.87; NNT 8, 95% CI 4 to 25).[24] People taking olanzapine had greater weight gain, but the difference was not significant either at 28–30 weeks (2 RCTs; WMD +2.86, 95% CI –0.68 to +6.34) or at 54 weeks (WMD +3.56, 95% CI –0.20 to +6.90). The subsequent RCT found no significant difference between olanzapine and risperidone in severity of extrapyramidal adverse effects, need for anticholinergics, or withdrawals from the trial.[25] Fewer people on risperidone experienced clinically important weight gain (AR for ≥ 7% weight gain 27.3% with olanzapine *v* 11.6% with risperidone).

Comment: **Versus standard antipsychotic drugs:** The results of the review is dominated by one large multicentre RCT reported by drug company employees.[22] Benefits seem to be highest at a dose of 15 mg daily, and higher doses may be associated with more harms. Results depended on the statistical test used, and their reliability may be compromised by heterogeneity.

OPTION PERAZINE

One weak RCT found no significant difference in global clinical impression over 28 days between perazine and haloperidol. Two small RCTs provided insufficient evidence to compare perazine versus zotepine, and one small RCT found no significant difference in mental state at 28 days between perazine and amisulpride. Three RCTs found no significant difference in extrapyramidal effects over 28 days between perazine and zotepine or amisulpride.

Benefits: **Versus standard antipsychotic drugs:** We found one systematic review (search date 2001, 2 RCTs, 71 people) comparing perazine versus haloperidol.[26] It could not perform a meta-analysis because of poor reporting in one of the RCTs. One of the RCTs (32 people) found no significant difference between perazine and haloperidol in the proportion of people who were "no better or worse" in global clinical impression at 28 days (8/17 [47%] with perazine *v* 6/15 [60%] with haloperidol; RR 1.18, 95% CI 0.53 to 2.62). **Versus other new antipsychotic drugs:** The review identified two RCTs comparing perazine versus zotepine.[26] It could not perform a meta-analysis because of methodological differences between the RCTs. The first RCT (34 people) found that perazine was significantly less effective than zotepine in improving symptoms, as assessed by the mean Brief Psychiatric Rating Scale score at 28 days (WMD 7.9, 95% CI 1.1 to 14.7). The second RCT (40 people), which used a different method to calculate mean Brief Psychiatric Rating Scale score, found that perazine was significantly more effective than zotepine in improving symptoms at the end of the trial (trial duration not specified: WMD –0.4, 95% –0.7 to –0.1). One RCT identified by the review found no significant difference between perazine and amisulpride in the proportion of people whose mental state was "no better or worse" at 28 days (4/15 [27%] with perazine *v* 3/15 [20%] with amisulpride; RR 1.33, 95% CI 0.36 to 4.97).[26]

Harms: **Versus standard antipsychotic drugs:** The review gave no information about the adverse effects of perazine compared with haloperidol.[26] **Versus other new antipsychotic drugs:** The review (3 RCTs) found no significant difference between perazine and zotepine or amisulpride in the risk of akathesia (3/56 [5%] with perazine *v* 10/55 [18%] with zotepine or amisulpride; RR 0.30, 95% CI 0.09 to 1.00), dyskinesia (1/56 [2%] with perazine *v* 3/55 [5%] with zotepine or amisulpride; RR 0.42, 95% CI 0.06 to 2.74), or parkinsonism (10/41 [24%] with perazine *v* 8/40 [20%] with zotepine or amisulpride; RR 1.22, 95% CI 0.54 to 2.78) over 28 days.[26]

Comment: None.

OPTION PIMOZIDE

One systematic review found no significant difference between pimozide and standard antipsychotic drugs in global clinical impression, and found that pimozide decreased sedation but increased tremor. It found no overall difference in cardiovascular adverse effects such as rise or fall in blood pressure or dizziness between pimozide and standard antipsychotic drugs. Pimozide has been associated with sudden cardiac death at doses above 20 mg daily.

Benefits: **Versus standard antipsychotic drugs:** We found one systematic review (search date 1999) comparing pimozide (mean dose 7.5 mg/ day, range 1–75 mg/day) versus standard antipsychotic drugs, including chlorpromazine, haloperidol, fluphenazine, and carpipramine.[27] It found no significant difference in the proportion of people reporting no improvement or worsening of global clinical impression between pimozide and standard antipsychotic drugs at 1–3 months (3 RCTs; 18/50 [36%] with pimozide *v* 22/50 [44%] with standard antipsychotic drugs; RR 0.82, 95% CI 0.52 to 1.29) or at 4–6 months (6 RCTs; 57/104 [55%] with pimozide *v* 55/102 [54%] with standard antipsychotic drugs; RR 1.01, 95% CI 0.80 to 1.28).

Harms: **Versus standard antipsychotic drugs:** The review found that, over 1–3 months, pimozide caused significantly less sedation than standard antipsychotic drugs but that it was more likely to cause tremor (sedation: 53/117 [45%] with pimozide *v* 68/115 [59%] with standard antipsychotic drugs; RR 0.77, 95% CI 0.61 to 0.98; NNT 7, 95% CI 4 to 61; tremor: 43/97 [44%] with pimozide *v* 27/95 [28%] with standard antipsychotic drugs; RR 1.57, 95 CI 1.07 to 2.29; NNH 6, 95% CI 3 to 44).[27] It found similar cardiovascular symptoms such as rise or fall in blood pressure and dizziness between pimozide and standard antipsychotic drugs. There was little usable ECG data. One RCT in the review found no significant difference in ECG changes between pimozide and standard antipsychotic drugs, but it may have been too small to detect a clinically important difference (2/28 [7%] with pimozide *v* 3/28 [11%] with standard antipsychotic drugs; RR 0.67, 95% CI 0.1 to 3.7).

Comment: Sudden death has been reported in a number of people taking pimozide at doses over 20 mg daily, but we found no evidence from RCTs that pimozide is more likely to cause sudden death than other antipsychotic drugs.[27] The manufacturer recommends periodic ECG monitoring in all people taking more than 16 mg daily pimozide, and avoidance of other drugs known to prolong the QT interval on an ECG or cause electrolyte disturbances (other antipsychotic drugs, antihistamines, antidepressants, and diuretics).

OPTION QUETIAPINE

One systematic review found no significant difference in mental state between quetiapine and standard antipsychotic drugs (mainly haloperidol), but found that quetiapine reduced akathisia, parkinsonism, and the proportion of people who left the trial early.

Benefits: **Versus standard antipsychotic drugs:** We found one systematic review (search date 2000, 7 RCTs), which compared quetiapine (50–800 mg/day) versus standard antipsychotic drugs (usually haloperidol).[28] It found no significant difference in mental state over 6 weeks between quetiapine and standard antipsychotic drugs (Brief Psychiatric Rating Scale or Positive and Negative Syndrome Scale score not improved, 4 RCTs; 367/723 [51%] with quetiapine *v* 283/524 [54%] with standard antipsychotic drugs; RR 0.91, 95% CI 0.73 to 1.13).

Harms: **Versus standard antipsychotic drugs:** The review found that, compared with standard antipsychotic drugs, quetiapine significantly reduced withdrawals from treatment at 6 weeks due to any cause, dystonia, akathisia**Ⓖ**, and parkinsonism, but it found that quetiapine significantly increased dry mouth (withdrawals from treatment: 6 RCTs; 334/913 [36.5%] with quetiapine *v* 254/711 [35.7%] with standard antipsychotic drugs; RR 0.86, 95% CI 0.75 to 0.98; dystonia: 3 RCTs; 4/580 [0.69%] with quetiapine *v* 19/379 [5%] with standard antipsychotic drugs; RR 0.24, 95% CI 0.04 to 0.49; akathisia: 3 RCTs; 19/580 [3%] with quetiapine *v* 68/379 [18%] with standard antipsychotic drugs; RR 0.24, 95% CI 0.15 to 0.38; parkinsonism: 2 RCTs; 31/479 [6%] with quetiapine *v* 92/279 [33%] with standard antipsychotic drugs; RR 0.22, 95% CI 0.15 to 0.33; dry mouth: 2 RCTs; 31/322 [10%] with quetiapine *v* 11/327 [3%] with standard antipsychotic drugs; RR 2.85, 95% CI 1.46 to 5.57).[28]

Comment: The RCTs in the review had substantial withdrawal rates and did not conduct intention to treat analyses.[28]

OPTION RISPERIDONE

One large systematic review found that risperidone improved symptoms more than standard antipsychotic drugs (mainly haloperidol). One small additional RCT found no significant difference between risperidone and haloperidol in responders over 8 weeks. One systematic review found that risperidone decreased extrapyramidal side effects and the need for antiparkinsonian medication, but increased weight gain compared with standard antipsychotic drugs. Systematic reviews found no significant difference in symptoms between risperidone and other new antipsychotic drugs (olanzapine, sulpiride, and clozapine).

Benefits: **Versus standard antipsychotic drugs:** We found one systematic review (search date 2002, 22 RCTs, 3799 people)[15] and one additional RCT.[29] The systematic review found that risperidone significantly reduced symptoms compared with standard antipsychotic drugs that included haloperidol (predominantly), perphenazine, and zuclopenthixol (effect size, estimated using the Positive and Negative Syndrome Scale, Brief Psychiatric Rating Scale, and Clinical Global Rating: 0.252, 95% CI 0.18 to 0.33).[15] The additional RCT (99 people) compared a range of doses of risperidone versus haloperidol.[29] It found no significant difference in the proportion of people who responded over 8 weeks (response defined as ≥ 20% reduction in Positive and Negative Syndrome Scale; reported as non-significant; results presented graphically).[29] **Versus olanzapine:** See benefits of olanzapine, p 1348. **Versus amisulpride:** See benefits of amisulpride, p 1346. **Versus clozapine:** See benefits of clozapine, p 1344.

Harms: **Versus standard antipsychotic drugs:** The systematic review reported in the benefits section did not report on harms.[15] We found one other systematic review (search date 2002), which did describe harms.[30] It found no significant difference between risperidone and standard antipsychotic drugs in the proportion of people who withdrew from treatment because of adverse effects (11 RCTs; 142/1619 [9%] with risperidone v 70/624 [11.2%] with standard antipsychotic drugs; RR 0.82, 95% CI 0.61 to 1.09).[30] It found that risperidone significantly reduced extrapyramidal effects and the need for administration of antiparkinsonian medication compared with standard antipsyschotic drugs (extrapyramidal effects: 10 RCTs; 384/1937 [20%] with risperidone v 289/765 [38%] with standard antipsychotic drugs; RR 0.63, 95% CI 0.56 to 0.71; antiparkinsonian medication: 11 RCTs; 461/1856 [25%] with risperidone v 289/668 [43%] with standard antipsychotic drugs; RR 0.66, 95% CI 0.58 to 0.74). However, it found that risperidone significantly increased the proportion of people with weight gain compared with standard antipsychotic drugs (4 RCTs; 420/1320 [32%] with risperidone v 71/388 [18%] with standard antipsychotic drugs; RR 1.55, 95% CI 1.25 to 1.93). The additional RCT found no significant difference in the rate of overall adverse effects between risperidone and haloperidol.[29] **Versus olanzapine:** See harms of olanzapine, p 1348 **Versus amisulpride:** See harms of amisulpride, p 1346. **Versus clozapine:** See harms of clozapine, p 1345.

Comment: None.

OPTION SULPIRIDE

One systematic review found no significant difference in global clinical impression over 4–10 weeks between sulpiride and standard antipsychotic drugs. The review found that the use of antiparkinsonian drugs over 4–10 weeks was less frequent with sulpiride compared with standard antipsychotic drugs.

Benefits: **Versus standard antipsychotic drugs:** One systematic review (search date 1998, 7 RCTs, 366 people) found no significant difference in the proportion of people who had no improvement in global clinical impression over 4–10 weeks between sulpiride and standard antipsychotic drugs, usually haloperidol chlorpromazine, or perphenazine (74/248 [30%] with sulpiride v 96/266 [36%] with standard antipsychotic drugs; RR of no important improvement 0.82, 95% CI 0.64 to 1.05).[31]

Harms: **Versus standard antipsychotic drugs:** The review found that the use of antiparkinsonian drugs over 4–10 weeks was significantly less frequent with sulpiride compared with standard antipsychotic drugs (84/253 [33%] v 115/258 [44%]; RR 0.73, 95% CI 0.59 to 0.90).[31]

Comment: The review stated that the other two RCTs it identified reported improvement in mental state with sulpiride compared with placebo, but that no raw data could be obtained because of poor reporting in the RCTs.[31] Observational evidence and clinical experience suggest that sulpiride may be associated with galactorrhoea, but RCT data did not quantify the risk.[32]

OPTION ZIPRASIDONE

One systematic review found no significant difference in symptoms between ziprasidone and standard antipsychotic drugs (mainly haloperidol). One earlier systematic review found that ziprasidone reduced akathisia and acute dystonia but increased nausea and vomiting compared with haloperidol.

Benefits: **Versus standard antipsychotic drugs:** We found one systematic review (search date 2002, 4 RCTs, 1335 people, see comment below).[15] It found no significant difference in symptoms between ziprasidone and standard antipsychotic drugs (mainly haloperidol and also chlorpromazine; effect size, estimated using the Positive and Negative Syndrome Scale, the Brief Psychiatric Rating Scale, and the Clinical Global Rating: –0.038, 95% CI –0.15 to +0.08).[15]

Harms: **Versus standard antipsychotic drugs:** We found two systematic reviews.[15,33] The more recent review (search date 2002) did not report on harms.[15] The earlier review (search date 1999, 4 RCTs, 690 people) found no clear difference in overall adverse effects between ziprasidone and haloperidol.[33] It found that ziprasidone was significantly less likely to cause akathisia and acute dystonia**G** over 1 week and akathisia over 28 weeks compared with haloperidol (akathisia over 1 week: 2 RCTs; 19/296 [6%] with ziprasidone *v* 27/142 [19%] with haloperidol; RR 0.34, 95% CI 0.20 to 0.59; NNH 8, 95% CI 5 to 18; akathisia over 28 weeks: 1 RCT; 7/148 [5%] with ziprasidone *v* 25/153 [16%] with haloperidol; RR 0.3, 95% CI 0.1 to 0.7; NNH 9, 95% CI 5 to 21; acute dystonia over 1 week: 2 RCTs; 13/296 [4%] with ziprasidone *v* 15/142 [10%] with haloperidol; RR 0.42, 95% CI 0.20 to 0.85; NNH 16, 95% CI 9 to 166). Ziprasidone was associated with significantly more nausea and vomiting both over 1 and 28 weeks (1 week: 59/206 [29%] with ziprasidone *v* 8/100 [8%] with haloperidol; RR 3.58, 95% CI 1.78 to 7.20; NNH 5, 95% CI 4 to 8; 28 weeks: 1 RCT; 31/148 [21%] with ziprasidone *v* 15/153 [10%] with haloperidol; RR 2.14, 95% CI 1.20 to 3.79; NNH 9, 95% CI 5 to 33).

Comment: The duration of RCTs in the more recent systematic review was less than 24 weeks.[15]

OPTION ZOTEPINE

One systematic review found weak evidence that zotepine increased the proportion of people with a clinically important improvement in symptoms compared with standard antipsychotic drugs, and reduced akasthesia, dystonia, and rigidity. This finding was not robust because removal of a single RCT from the analysis meant that the difference between zotepine and standard antipsychotic drugs was no longer significant.

Benefits: **Versus standard antipsychotic drugs:** We found one systematic review (search date 1999, 8 RCTs, 356 people) comparing zotepine (75–450 mg/day) versus standard antipsychotic drugs, usually haloperidol.[34] It found that zotepine was significantly more likely than standard antipsychotic drugs to bring about "clinically important improvement" at 4–12 weeks, as defined by a prestated cut off point on the Brief Psychiatric Rating Scale (4 RCTs; 89/179 [50%] with zotepine *v* 62/177 [35%] with standard antipsychotic drugs; RR 1.25, 95% CI 1.1 to 1.4; NNT 7, 95% CI 4 to 22; see comment below).

Harms: The review found that, compared with standard antipsychotic drugs, zotepine caused significantly less akathisia (67/199 [34%] with zotepine *v* 91/197 [46%] with standard antipsychotic drugs; RR 0.73, 95% CI 0.58 to 0.93; NNT 8, 95% CI 5 to 34), dystonia**G** (7/35 [20%] with zotepine *v* 15/35 [43%] with standard antipsychotic drugs; RR 0.47, 95% CI 0.24 to 0.93; NNT 4, 95% CI 2 to 56), and rigidity (19/83 [23%] with zotepine *v* 30/81 [37%] with standard antipsychotic drugs; RR 0.63, 95% CI 0.40 to 0.98; NNT 7, 95% CI 4 to 360).[34] Two RCTs found abnormal ECG results in people taking zotepine, but few additional details were given.

Comment: All but one RCT identified by the earlier review were of ≤ 12 weeks' duration and all were conducted in Europe.[34] Only one RCT included in the review found zotepine to be significantly more effective than standard antipsychotic drugs for clinically important improvement, and removal of this RCT from the meta-analysis rendered the results non-significant.

QUESTION Which interventions reduce relapse rates?

OPTION CONTINUED TREATMENT WITH ANTIPSYCHOTIC DRUGS

Systematic reviews found that continuing antipsychotic drugs for at least 6 months after an acute episode reduced relapse rates compared with no treatment or placebo. Eight systematic reviews found no significant difference in relapse rates among antipsychotic drugs. One systematic review found that clozapine reduced relapse rates over 12 weeks compared with standard antipsychotic drugs. Another review found that fewer people taking depot zuclopenthixol decanoate relapsed over 12 weeks to 1 year compared with people taking other depot preparations. A third review found that bromperidol increased the proportion of people who relapsed compared with haloperidol or fluphenazine. One additional RCT found that risperidone reduced relapse over 2.2 years compared with haloperidol.

Benefits: **Versus no treatment or placebo:** We found two systematic reviews.[9,10] The first review (search date 2002, 5 RCTs) found that continuing chlorpromazine significantly reduced relapse rates over 6–24 months compared with placebo (3 RCTs; 106/264 [40%] with chlorpromazine *v* 176/248 [71%] with placebo; RR 0.57, 95% CI 0.48 to 0.67; NNT 3, 95% CI 3 to 4).[9] The second review (search date 2000, 2 RCTs, 70 people currently in remission) compared haloperidol versus placebo over 1 year.[10] It found that haloperidol significantly reduced relapse over 1 year compared with placebo (32/47 [68%] with haloperidol *v* 23/23 [100%] with placebo; RR 0.67, 95% CI 0.54 to 0.83; NNT 4, 95% CI 2 to 7). **Choice of drug:** We found 11 systematic reviews[12–14,22,27,35-40] and one additional RCT[41] evaluating the effects of newer versus older antipsychotic drugs, newer antipsychotic drugs versus each other, and oral versus intramuscular administration of antipsychotics on relapse rates (see table 1, p 1364). Eight reviews found no significant difference between antipsychotic drugs in relapse rates,[13,22,27,35–39] but in two of the reviews[22,27] the number of people studied was too small to rule out a clinically important difference. A ninth review (search date 1999) found that clozapine significantly reduced relapse rates over 12 weeks compared with standard antipsychotic drugs (19 RCTs; RR 0.6, 95% CI 0.5 to 0.8).[14] A tenth review (search date 1998) found that significantly fewer people taking depot zuclopenthixol decanoate relapsed over 12 weeks to 1 year compared with people taking other depot preparations (3 RCTs; 296 people: RR 0.7, 95% CI 0.6 to 1.0; NNT 9, 95% CI 5 to 53).[40] An eleventh review (search date 2003) found that bromperidol significantly increased the proportion of people who relapsed compared with haloperidol or fluphenazine (2 RCTs; 67 people; RR 3.92, 95% CI 1.05 to 14.6; NNH 5, 95% CI 3 to 28).[12] The additional RCT (365 people) found that risperidone significantly reduced relapse over 2.2 years compared with haloperidol (NNT 5, 95% CI 4 to 10).[41]

Harms: **Versus no treatment or placebo:** The reviews gave no information on adverse effects of continuing treatment with antipsychotic drugs.[9,10] **Choice of drug:** The review comparing different depot antipsychotic drugs found that the annual incidence of tardive dyskinesia was 5%.[40]

Comment: Some clinicians use depot antipsychotic drugs in selected people to ensure adherence to medication. We found no evidence from RCTs to support this practice.

OPTION COGNITIVE BEHAVIOURAL THERAPY

Limited evidence from a systematic review of two RCTs found no significant difference in relapse rates between cognitive behavioural therapy plus standard care and standard care alone.

Benefits: We found one systematic review (search date 2001, 2 RCTs, 123 people) comparing the effects of cognitive behavioural therapy plus standard care versus standard care alone on relapse rates.[42] Both RCTs identified by the review incorporated challenging key beliefs, problem solving, and enhancement of coping. The review found no significant difference between cognitive behavioural therapy plus standard care and standard care alone in relapse or readmission to hospital over 10 weeks or over 9–24 months (10 weeks: 1 RCT; 0/33 [0%] with cognitive behavioural therapy plus standard care *v* 4/28 [14%] with standard care alone; RR 0.09, 95% CI 0.01 to 1.69; 9–24 months: 2 RCTs; 36/63 [57%] with cognitive behavioural therapy plus standard care *v* 31/60 [52%] with standard care alone; RR 1.13, 95% CI 0.82 to 1.56).[42]

Harms: The systematic review gave no information on harms.[42]

Comment: None.

OPTION FAMILY INTERVENTIONS

One systematic review found that multiple session family interventions reduced relapse rates at 12 months compared with usual care, single session family interventions, or psychoeducational interventions.

Benefits: We found one systematic review (search date 1999) that compared multiple family interventions versus usual care, single family interventions, or psychoeducational interventions.[43] Family interventions consisted mainly of education about the illness and training in problem solving over at least six weekly sessions. The review found that multiple family interventions significantly reduced relapse rates at 12 months compared with other interventions (11 RCTs, 729 people; OR 0.52, 95% CI 0.31 to 0.89; absolute numbers not provided). On average, eight families would have to be treated to avoid one additional relapse (and likely hospitalisation) at 12 months in the family member with schizophrenia (NNT 8, 95% CI 6 to 18).[43]

Harms: The review gave no information on harms.[43]

Comment: These results may overestimate the effect of family interventions because of the difficulty of blinding people and investigators.[43] Although no harms were reported, illness education could possibly have adverse consequences on morale and outlook. The mechanism for the effects of family intervention remains unclear. It is thought to work by reducing "expressed emotion" (hostility and criticism) in relatives of people with schizophrenia. The time consuming nature of this intervention, which must normally take place at evenings or weekends, can limit its availability. It cannot be applied to people who have little contact with home based carers.

OPTION PSYCHOEDUCATIONAL INTERVENTIONS

One systematic review found that psychoeducation reduced relapse rates at 9–18 months compared with usual care.

Benefits: **Versus usual treatment:** We found one systematic review (search date 2002), which identified one RCT of a brief individual intervention (10 sessions or less), six RCTs of brief group psychoeducational interventions, and four RCTs of standard length group psychoeducational interventions (11 sessions or more).[44] It found that standard length group psychoeducational interventions were significantly more effective than usual care in preventing relapse without readmission over 9–18 months (2 RCTs; 14/57 [24%] with psychoeducation *v* 24/57 [42%] with usual care; RR 0.58, 95% CI 0.34 to 0.99). It also found that brief group psychoeducational interventions were significantly more effective than usual care in preventing relapse or readmission over 1 year (5 RCTs; 153/326 [47%] with psychoeducation *v* 162/296 [55%] with usual care; RR 0.85, 95% CI 0.74 to 0.98; NNT 12, CI 6 to 83). The review found that any form of psychoeducation significantly reduced relapse with or without readmission to hospital over 9–18 months compared with usual care (6 RCTs; 176/383 [46%] with psychoeducation *v* 192/337 [57%] with usual care; RR 0.78, 95% CI 0.62 to 0.98; NNT 9, 95% CI 6 to 22; see comment below).

Harms: The systematic review gave no information on harms.[44]

Comment: The systematic review found few good RCTs.[44] There was significant heterogeneity of both interventions and outcomes.

OPTION SOCIAL SKILLS TRAINING

One systematic review of small RCTs provided insufficient evidence to assess the effect of social skills training on relapse rates.

Benefits: We found one systematic review (search date 1999), which identified nine RCTs (471 people) comparing the effect of social skills training versus standard care or psychoeducational interventions on relapse rates.[45] It found no significant difference in relapse rates over 1 year of treatment between social skills training and other interventions but found that social skills training reduced relapse over 2 years of treatment (social skills *v* other interventions, 4 RCTs, 125 people; OR 0.74, 95% CI 0.43 to 1.29; absolute numbers not provided; change in relapse with social skills, 2 RCTs, 264 people; OR 3.03, 95% CI 1.11 to 8.33; absolute numbers not provided).

Harms: The review gave no information on harms.[45]

Comment: None.

QUESTION Which interventions are effective in people who are resistant to standard antipsychotic drugs?

OPTION INTERVENTIONS IN PEOPLE WHO ARE RESISTANT TO STANDARD ANTIPSYCHOTIC DRUGS

One systematic review in people resistant to standard antipsychotic drugs found that clozapine improved symptoms after 12 weeks and after 2 years compared with standard antipsychotic drugs. One systematic review found no significant difference in symptoms between clozapine and other new antipsychotic drugs in people resistant to standard antipsychotic drugs. One small RCT identified by a systematic review found no significant difference in psychotic symptoms over 8 weeks between olanzapine and chlorpromazine.

Benefits: **Clozapine versus standard antipsychotic drugs:** We found one systematic review (search date 1999, 6 RCTs) comparing clozapine versus standard antipsychotic drugs in people who were resistant to standard treatment.[14] It found that, compared with standard antipsychotic drugs, clozapine significantly increased the proportion of people who improved at 6–12 weeks and at 12–24 months (6–12 weeks: 4 RCTs, 370 people; RR for no improvement compared with standard antipsychotic drugs 0.7, 95% CI 0.6 to 0.8; 12–24 months: 2 RCTs, 648 people; RR 0.8, 95% CI 0.6 to 1.0). It found no difference in relapse rates at 12 weeks. **Clozapine versus other new antipsychotic drugs:** We found one systematic review (search date 1989, 8 RCTs, 5 in people with treatment resistant schizophrenia, 595 people), which compared clozapine versus olanzapine, risperidone, and zotepine.[46] It found no significant difference between clozapine and other new antipsychotic drugs in global clinical impression (Clinical Global Impression [CGI] score: WMD –0.09, 95% CI –0.34 to +0.15) or mental state (Brief Psychiatric Rating Scale or Positive and Negative Syndrome Scale < 20% improved: 83/173 [48%] with clozapine *v* 81/178 [45%] with olanzapine or risperidone; RR 1.05, 95% CI 0.84 to 1.32). However, the number of people studied was too small to rule out a clinically important difference. **Olanzapine versus standard antipsychotic drugs:** One systematic review (search date 1999, 1 RCT, 84 people) found no significant difference in persistence of psychotic symptoms over 8 weeks between olanzapine (25 mg/day) and chlorpromazine (no important response defined as a < 20% reduction on the CGI scale; AR for no important response: 39/42 [93%] with olanzapine *v* 42/42 [100%]; RR 0.93, 95% CI 0.85 to 1.01).[22] The RCT is likely to have been too small to exclude a clinically important difference. **Olanzapine versus other new antipsychotic drugs:** We found one systematic review (search date 1999, 1 RCT, 180 people) comparing olanzapine versus clozapine, which found no significant difference in psychotic symptoms over 8 weeks (45/90 [50%] with olanzapine *v* 55/90 [61%] with clozapine; RR for no important response [defined as a 40% reduction on the CGI scale] 0.82, 95% CI 0.63 to 1.07).[22] The RCT is likely to have been too small to exclude a clinically important difference. **Other interventions:** We found no RCTs examining the effects of other interventions in people resistant to standard treatment.

Harms: **Clozapine versus standard antipsychotic drugs:** See harms of clozapine, p 1345. **Clozapine versus other new antipsychotic drugs:** The review found that, compared with other new antipsychotic drugs (mainly olanzapine and risperidone), clozapine was significantly less likely to cause extrapyramidal adverse effects (305 people; RR 0.3, 95% CI 0.1 to 0.6; NNT 6, 95% CI 4 to 9).[46] It also found that clozapine may be less likely to cause dry mouth and more likely to cause fatigue, nausea, dizziness, hypersalivation, and hypersomnia than other new antipsychotic drugs, but these findings were from one or at most two RCTs. It found that people taking clozapine tended to be more satisfied with their treatment than those taking other new antipsychotic drugs, but also tended to withdraw from RCTs more often. It found no significant difference in rates of blood dyscrasias between clozapine and other new antipsychotic drugs, but the number of people studied was too small (558) to rule out a clinically important difference.[46]

Comment: Some RCTs in the reviews included people who were partial responders to neuroleptic drugs and people unable to take some neuroleptic medications because of adverse effects.[14,22,46] The reviews did not specify the duration of treatment resistant illness of the participants in the RCTs. RCTs are under way to clarify the mode of action of cognitive behavioural therapy and establish its effects in people who are resistant to standard treatments.

QUESTION Which interventions improve adherence to antipsychotic medication?

OPTION BEHAVIOURAL THERAPY

One small RCT found limited evidence that behavioural interventions improved adherence to antipsychotic medication compared with usual treatment. Two RCTs found limited evidence that behavioural interventions improved adherence more than psychoeducational therapy.

Benefits: We found no systematic review. **Versus usual treatment:** We found one RCT (36 men).[47] The behavioural training method comprised being told the importance of adhering to antipsychotic medication and instructions on how to take medication. Each participant was given a self monitoring spiral calendar, which featured a dated slip of paper for each dose of antipsychotic drug. Adherence was estimated by pill counts (see comment below). After 3 months, fewer people had high pill adherence after usual treatment compared with behaviour therapy (figures not provided). **Versus psychoeducational therapy:** See benefits of psychoeducational interventions, p 1359.

Harms: None reported.

Comment: Assessing adherence by pill count has potential confounders, in that people may throw pills away.[47]

OPTION COMPLIANCE THERAPY

Two RCTs found limited evidence that compliance therapy increased adherence to antipsychotic drugs at 6 and 18 months compared with supportive or non-specific counselling.

Benefits: We found no systematic review, but found two RCTs.[48,49] The first RCT (47 people with acute psychoses, most of whom fulfilled criteria for schizophrenia or had been admitted with the first episode of a psychotic illness) compared compliance therapy**G** versus supportive counselling.[48] It found that, compared with counselling, compliance therapy significantly increased the proportion of people with improved adherence at 4–6 weeks and at 6 months (improved adherence defined as a score ≥ 5 on a scale from 1–7, where 1 is complete refusal and 7 active participation, ready acceptance, and taking some responsibility for adhering to antipsychotic medication; 4–6 weeks: OR 6.3, 95% CI 1.6 to 24.6; 6 months: OR 5.2, 95% CI 1.5 to 18.3; absolute numbers not provided; see comment below).[48] The second RCT (74 people with acute psychoses, most of whom fulfilled criteria for schizophrenia and had been admitted to hospital with relapse of symptoms) found that compliance therapy significantly improved compliance over 18 months, measured on a 7 point scale of medication adherence compared with non-specific counselling (mean difference 1.4, 95% CI 0.9 to 1.6).[49]

Harms: The RCTs gave no information on harms.[48,49]

Comment: Other trials have examined the potential benefits of compliance therapy but either did not employ a standardised measure of adherence or did not assess adherence in a blind fashion. In the first RCT, about a third of each group did not complete the RCT, and missing data are estimated from the mean scores in each group.[48]

OPTION FAMILY INTERVENTIONS

One systematic review found that "compliance with medication" over 9–24 months was higher in people who received multiple family interventions compared with usual care, single family interventions, or psychoeducational interventions, but the difference was not statistically significant.

Benefits: We found one systematic review (search date 1999), which compared multiple family interventions versus usual care, single family interventions, or psychoeducational interventions.[43] Family interventions consisted mainly of education about the illness and training in problem solving over at least six weekly sessions. The review found that "compliance with medication" over 9–24 months was higher in people who received multiple family interventions compared with other interventions, but the difference did not quite reach significance (5 RCTs, 393 people; OR 0.63, 95% CI 0.40 to 1.01; no further data provided).[43]

Harms: The review gave no information on harms.[43]

Comment: Although no harms were reported, illness education could possibly have adverse consequences on morale and outlook. The mechanism for the effects of family intervention remains unclear. It is thought to work by reducing "expressed emotion" (hostility and criticism) in relatives of people with schizophrenia. The time consuming nature of this intervention, which must normally take place at evenings or weekends, can limit its availability. It cannot be applied to people who have little contact with home based carers.

OPTION PSYCHOEDUCATIONAL INTERVENTIONS

One systematic review found limited evidence that psychoeducational interventions improved adherence to antipsychotic medication compared with usual care. Two RCTs found limited evidence that psychoeducational interventions improved adherence less than behavioural therapy.

Benefits: **Versus usual treatment:** We found one systematic review (search date 2002), which identified four RCTs that assessed adherence with medication.[44] The RCTs compared individual or group psychoeducational intervention**G** of either standard length (11 sessions or more) or brief length (10 sessions or less) versus usual care. The first RCT (67 people) found no significant difference in adherence between brief individual psychoeducation and usual care, measured on a continuous scale of medication compliance. The second RCT (82 people) found no significant difference in adherence over 18 months between standard length group interventions and usual care. However, two further RCTs identified by the review comparing brief group psychoeducational interventions versus control suggested that psychoeducation was more effective in improving adherence. The third RCT (236 people) found that a brief group psychoeducational intervention significantly improved adherence compared with control (measured on a continuous scale of "medication concordance"; WMD –0.4, 95% CI –0.6 to –0.2). The fourth RCT (46 people) comparing a brief psychoeducational intervention versus usual care found limited evidence that psychoeducational interventions may improve adherence over 1 year (mean number of non-compliant episodes 0.38 with psychoeducation *v* 1.14 with usual care).[44] **Versus behavioural therapy:** We found two RCTs.[47,50] The first RCT (36 men) compared three interventions: psychoeducation, behavioural therapy, or usual treatment.[47] The behavioural training method comprised being told the importance of complying with antipsychotic medication and instructions on how to take medication. Each participant was given a self monitoring spiral calendar, which featured a dated slip of paper for each dose of antipsychotic drug. Adherence was estimated by pill counts (see comment below). The RCT found that, after 3 months, fewer people had high pill adherence after psychoeducation compared with behavioural therapy, but the difference was not significant (3/11 [27%] with psychoeducation *v* 8/11 [72%] with behavioural therapy had pill adherence scores of 80% measured by pill counts; RR of high pill adherence score 0.37, 95% CI 0.13 to 1.05). The RCT is likely to have been too small to detect a clinically important difference.[47] The second RCT (39 people) compared a psychoeducational intervention, a behavioural intervention given individually, and a behavioural intervention involving the person with schizophrenia and their family.[50] The individual behavioural intervention consisted of specific written guidelines, and oral instructions given to people to use a pill box consisting of 28 compartments for every medication occasion during a week. The behavioural intervention, when given to the individual and their family, contained additional instructions for the family members to compliment the person with schizophrenia for taking their prescribed medication. The primary outcome measure was pill count at 2 months (see comment below). The RCT found that medication adherence was significantly more likely with behavioural interventions than with psychoeducation (> 90% adherence at 2 months: 25/26 [96%] with behavioural interventions *v* 6/13 [46%] with psychoeducation; RR 2.08, 95% CI 1.15 to 3.77; NNT 2, 95% CI 2 to 5).

Harms: None reported.

Comment: Assessing adherence by pill count has potential confounders, in that people may throw pills away.[47,50] Each psychoeducational intervention varied in the protocol used and few employed the same outcome measurements.

GLOSSARY

Compliance therapy A treatment based on cognitive behavioural therapy and motivational interviewing techniques with a view to improving adherence to medication.

Negative symptoms This generally refers to qualities that are abnormal by their absence (e.g. loss of drive, motivation, and self care).

Positive symptoms This refers to symptoms that characterise the onset or relapse of schizophrenia, usually hallucinations and delusions, but sometimes including thought disorder.

Psychoeducational intervention Intervention programmes aimed at the education of a person with psychiatric disorder in subject areas that serve the goals of treatment and rehabilitation. The terms "patient education", "patient teaching", and "patient instruction" have also been used for this process.

Dystonia A slow movement or extended spasm in a group of muscles. It can be generalised or focal. Wry neck or writer's cramps are examples of focal dystonias.

Akathisia A sense of "inner restlessness", which is a subjective sensation of restlessness that has a strong component of motor restlessness (the person cannot keep physically still and maintain a static posture for an extended period of time).

REFERENCES

1. Andreasen NC. Symptoms, signs and diagnosis of schizophrenia. *Lancet* 1995;346:477–481.
2. Kane JM, Honigfeld G, Singer J, et al. Clozapine for the treatment-resistant schizophrenic. *Arch Gen Psychiatry* 1988;45:789–796.
3. Meltzer HY. Treatment-resistant schizophrenia: the role of clozapine. *Curr Med Res Opin* 1997;14:1–20.
4. Cannon M, Jones P. Neuroepidemiology: schizophrenia. *J Neurol Neurosurg Psychiatry* 1996;61:604–613.
5. Jablensky A, Sartorius N, Ernberg G, et al. Schizophrenia: manifestations, incidence and course in different cultures. A World Health Organization ten-country study. *Psychol Med* 1992; monograph supplement 20:1–97.
6. Hegarty JD, Baldessarini RJ, Tohen M, et al. One hundred years of schizophrenia: a meta-analysis of the outcome literature. *Am J Psychiatry* 1994;151:1409–1416.
7. Johnstone EC. Schizophrenia: problems in clinical practice. *Lancet* 1993;341:536–538.
8. Thornley B, Adams C. Content and quality of 2000 controlled trials in schizophrenia over 50 years. *BMJ* 1998;317:1181–1184. Search date 1997; primary sources hand searching of conference proceedings,

Biological Abstracts, Cinahl, The Cochrane Library, Embase, Lilacs, Psychlit, Psyindex, Medline, and Sociofile.

9. Thornley B, Adams CE, Awad G. Chlorpromazine versus placebo for those with schizophrenia. In: The Cochrane Library, Issue 3, 2004. Chichester, UK: John Wiley & Sons, Ltd. Search date 2002; primary sources Biological Abstracts, Embase, Medline, Psychlit, SciSearch, The Cochrane Library, Cochrane Schizophrenia Group's Register, hand searches of reference lists, and personal contact with pharmaceutical companies and authors of trials.
10. Joy CB, Adams CE, Lawrie SM. Haloperidol versus placebo for schizophrenia. In: The Cochrane Library, Issue 3, 2004. Chichester, UK: John Wiley & Sons, Ltd. Search date 2000; primary sources Biological Abstracts, Cinahl, The Cochrane Schizophrenia Group's Register, Embase, Medline, Psychlit, SciSearch, hand searches of references, and contact with authors of trials and pharmaceutical companies.
11. Sultana A, Reilly J, Fenton M. Thioridazine for schizophrenia. In: The Cochrane Library, Issue 3, 2004. Chichester, UK: John Wiley & Sons, Ltd. Search date 1999; primary sources Biological Abstracts, Cinahl, The Cochrane Library, The Cochrane Schizophrenia Group's Register, Embase, Medline, Psychlit, Sociofile, reference lists, pharmaceutical companies, and authors of trials.
12. Quraishi S, David A, Adams CE. Depot bromperidol decanoate for schizophrenia. In: The Cochrane Library, Issue 3, 2004. Chichester, UK: John Wiley & Sons, Ltd. Search date 2003; primary sources Biological Abstracts, The Cochrane Library, Cochrane Schizophrenia Group's Register, Embase, Medline, Psychlit, hand searches of reference lists, and personal contact with Janssen Cilag.
13. Quraishi S, David A. Depot haloperidol decanoate for schizophrenia. In: The Cochrane Library, Issue 3, 2004. Chichester, UK: John Wiley & Sons, Ltd. Search date 1998; primary sources Biological Abstracts, Embase, Medline, Psychlit, SciSearch, The Cochrane Library, reference lists, authors of studies, and pharmaceutical companies.
14. Wahlbeck K, Cheine M, Essali MA. Clozapine versus typical neuroleptic medication for schizophrenia. In: The Cochrane Library, Issue 3, 2004. Chichester, UK: John Wiley & Sons, Ltd. Search date 1999; primary sources Biological Abstracts, Cochrane Schizophrenia Group's Register, The Cochrane Library, Embase, Lilacs, Medline, Psychlit, SciSearch, Science Citation Index, hand searches of reference lists, and personal communication with pharmaceutical companies.
15. Davis JM, Chen N, Click ID. Meta-analysis of the efficacy second-generation antipsychotics. *Arch Gen Psychiatry* 2003;60:553–564. Search date 2002; primary sources Medline, International Abstracts, Cinahl, Psychinfo, Cochrane database of systematic reviews, reference lists, US Food and Administration website, poster presentations, conference proceedings and manuscripts submitted for publication, and contact with researchers and manufacturers.
16. Meltzer HY, Alphs L, Green AI, et al. Clozapine treatment for suicidality in schizophrenia. International Suicide Prevention Trial (InterSePT). *Arch Gen Psychiatry* 2003;60:82–91.
17. Honigfeld G, Arellano F, Sethi J, et al. Reducing clozapine-related morbidity and mortality: five years of experience of the clozaril national registry. *J Clin Psychiatry* 1998;59(suppl 3):3–7.
18. Mota Neto JIS, Lima MS, Soares BGO. Amisulpride for schizophrenia. In: The Cochrane Library, Issue 3, 2004. Chichester, UK: John Wiley & Sons, Ltd. Search date 2000; primary sources Biological Abstracts Cinahl, The Cochrane Library, The Cochrane Schizophrenia Group's Register, Embase, Lilacs, Medline, Psychlit, Science Citation Index, hand searches of reference lists, and personal contact with the manufacturer of amisulpride.
19. Martin S, Ljo H, Peuskens J, et al. A double blind, randomised comparative trial of amisulpiride versus olanzapine in the treatment of schizophrenia: short term results at two months. *Curr Med Res Opin* 2002;18:355–362.
20. Fenton M, Murphy B, Wood J, et al. Loxapine for schizophrenia. In: The Cochrane Library, Issue 3, 2004. Chichester, UK: John Wiley & Sons, Ltd. Search date 1999; primary sources Biological Abstracts, The Cochrane Library, The Cochrane Schizophrenia Group's Register, Embase, Lilacs, Psyindex, Psychlit, and hand searches of reference lists.
21. Bagnall AM, Fenton M, Lewis R, et al. Molindone for schizophrenia and severe mental illness. In: The Cochrane Library, Issue 3, 2004. Chichester, UK: John Wiley & Sons, Ltd. Search date 1999; primary sources Biological Abstracts, The Cochrane Library, The Cochrane Schizophrenia Group's Register, Cinahl, Embase, Psychlit, pharmaceutical databases, hand searches of reference lists, and personal contact with authors of trials.
22. Duggan L, Fenton M, Dardennes RM, et al. Olanzapine for schizophrenia. In: The Cochrane Library, Issue 3, 2004. Chichester, UK: John Wiley & Sons, Ltd. Search date 1999; primary sources Biological Abstracts, Embase, Medline, Psychlit, The Cochrane Library, hand searches of reference lists and conference abstracts, and personal communication with pharmaceutical companies and authors of trials.
23. Inada T, Yagi G, Miura S. Extrapyramidal symptom profiles in Japanese patients with schizophrenia treated with olanzapine or haloperidol. *Schizophr Res* 2002;57:227–238.
24. Gilbody SM, Bagnall AM, Duggan L, et al. Risperidone versus other atypical antipsychotic medication for schizophrenia. In: The Cochrane Library, Issue 3, 2004. Chichester, UK: John Wiley & Sons, Ltd. Search date 1999; primary sources Biological Abstracts, The Cochrane Library, The Cochrane Schizophrenia Group's Register, Embase, Medline, Lilacs, Psyindex, Psychlit, pharmaceutical databases on the Dialog Corporation Datastar and Dialog services, hand search of reference lists, and contact with pharmaceutical companies and authors of trials.
25. Conley RR, Mahmoud R. A randomized double-blind study of risperidone and olanzapine in the treatment of schizophrenia or schizoaffective disorder. *Am J Psychiatry* 2001;158:765–774.
26. Leucht S, Hartung B. Perazine for schizophrenia. In: The Cochrane Library, Issue 3, 2004. Chichester, UK: John Wiley & Sons, Ltd. Search date 2001; primary sources The Cochrane Schizophrenia Group's register (January 2001), Biological Abstracts, CINAHL, The Cochrane Library, Embase, Medline, Psychlit, Lilacs, Psyindex, Sociological Abstracts, Sociofile, hand searches of reference lists, and personal contact with pharmaceutical companies and authors.
27. Sultana A, McMonagle T. Pimozide for schizophrenia or related psychoses. In: The Cochrane Library, Issue 3, 2004. Chichester, UK: John Wiley & Sons, Ltd. Search date 1999; primary sources Biological Abstracts, The Cochrane Schizophrenia Group's Register, Embase, Janssen-Cilag UK's register of studies, Medline, hand searches of reference lists, and personal contact with pharmaceutical companies.
28. Srisurapanont M, Disayavanish C, Taimkaew K. Quetiapine for schizophrenia. In: The Cochrane Library, Issue 3, 2004. Chichester, UK: John Wiley & Sons, Ltd. Search date 2000; primary sources Biological Abstracts, Embase, Medline, Psychlit, The Cochrane Library, Cinahl, Sigle, Sociofile, hand searches of journals, and personal communication with authors of studies and pharmaceutical companies.
29. Lopez Ibor JJ, Ayuso JL, Gutierrez M, et al. Risperidone in the treatment of chronic schizophrenia: multicenter study comparative to haloperidol. *Actas Luso Esp Neurol Psiquiatr Cienc Afines* 1996;24:165–172.

30. Hunter RH, Joy CE, Kebbedy E, et al. Risperidone versus typical antipsychotic medication for schizophrenia. In: The Cochrane Library, Issue 3, 2004. Chichester, UK: John Wiley & Sons, Ltd. Search date 2002; primary sources Biological Abstracts, The Cochrane Trials Register, Embase, Medline, Psychlit, hand searches of reference lists, and personal communication with pharmaceutical companies.
31. Soares BGO, Fenton M, Chue P. Sulpiride for schizophrenia. In: The Cochrane Library, Issue 3, 2004. Chichester, UK: John Wiley & Sons, Ltd. Search date 1998; primary sources Biological Abstracts, Cinahl, Cochrane Schizophrenia Group's Register, The Cochrane Library, Embase, Medline, Psychlit, Sigle, and Sociofile.
32. Harnryd C, Bjerkenstedt L, Bjork K, et al. Clinical evaluation of sulpiride in schizophrenic patients — a double-blind comparison with chlorpromazine. *Acta Psych Scand* 1984;311:7–30.
33. Bagnall AM, Lewis RA, Leitner ML, et al. Ziprasidone for schizophrenia and severe mental illness. In: The Cochrane Library, Issue 3, 2004. Chichester, UK: John Wiley & Sons, Ltd. Search date 1999; primary sources Biological Abstracts, The Cochrane Library, The Cochrane Schizophrenia Group's Register, Embase, Lilacs, Psyindex, Psychlit, pharmaceutical databases, hand searches of reference lists, and personal contact with authors of trials.
34. Fenton M, Morris F, De Silva P, et al. Zotepine for schizophrenia. In: The Cochrane Library, Issue 3, 2004. Chichester, UK: John Wiley & Sons, Ltd. Search date 1999; primary sources Biological Abstracts, The Cochrane Library, The Cochrane Schizophrenia Group's Register, Embase, Dialog Corporation Datastar service, Medline, Psychlit, hand searches of reference lists, and personal contact with pharmaceutical companies and authors of trials.
35. Quraishi S, David A. Depot pipothiazine palmitate and undeclynate for schizophrenia. In: The Cochrane Library, Issue 3, 2004. Chichester, UK: John Wiley & Sons, Ltd. Search date 1998; primary sources Biological Abstracts, The Cochrane Library, The Cochrane Schizophrenia Group's Register, Embase, Medline, Psychlit, hand searches of reference lists, and personal communication with pharmaceutical companies.
36. Adams CE, Eisenbruch M. Depot fluphenazine versus oral fluphenazine for those with schizophrenia. In: The Cochrane Library, Issue 1, 2004. Oxford: Update Software. Search date 1999; primary sources Biological Abstracts, The Cochrane Library, The Cochrane Schizophrenia Group's Register, Embase, Medline, Psychlit, Science Citation Index, hand searches of reference lists, and personal communication with pharmaceutical companies.
37. David A, Adams CE, Quraishi SN. Depot flupenthixol decanoate for schizophrenia or similar psychotic disorders. In: The Cochrane Library, Issue 3, 2004. Chichester, UK: John Wiley & Sons, Ltd. Search date 1998; primary sources Biological Abstracts, The Cochrane Library, The Cochrane Schizophrenia Group's Register, Embase, Medline, Psychlit, SciSearch, references, and personal communication with pharmaceutical companies and authors of trials.
38. Quraishi S, David A. Depot fluspirilene for schizophrenia. In: The Cochrane Library, Issue 3, 2004. Chichester, UK: John Wiley & Sons, Ltd. Search date 1998; primary sources Biological Abstracts, The Cochrane Library, The Cochrane Schizophrenia Group's Register, Embase, Medline, Psychlit, and hand searches of reference lists.
39. Quraishi S, David A. Depot perphenazine decanoate and enanthate for schizophrenia. In: The Cochrane Library, Issue 3, 2004. Chichester, UK: John Wiley & Sons, Ltd. Search date 1998; primary sources Biological Abstracts, The Cochrane Library, The Cochrane Schizophrenia Group's Register, Embase, Medline, Psychlit, hand searches of reference lists, and personal communication with pharmaceutical companies.
40. Coutinho E, Fenton M, Quraishi S. Zuclopenthixol decanoate for schizophrenia and other serious mental illnesses. In: The Cochrane Library, Issue 3, 2004. Chichester, UK: John Wiley & Sons, Ltd. Search date 1998; primary sources Biological Abstracts, Cinhal, The Cochrane Library, The Cochrane Schizophrenia Group's Register, Embase, Medline, and Psychlit. References of all eligible studies were searched for further trials. The manufacturer of zuclopenthixol was contacted.
41. Csernansky JG, Mahmoud R, Brenner R; The Risperidone-USA-79 Study Group. A comparison of risperidone and haloperidol for the prevention of relapse in patients with schizophrenia. *New Engl J Med* 2002;346:16–22.
42. Cormac I, Jones C, Campbell C. Cognitive behavioural therapy for schizophrenia. In: The Cochrane Library, Issue 3, 2004. Chichester, UK: John Wiley & Sons, Ltd. Search date 2001; primary sources Biological Abstracts, The Cochrane Schizophrenia Group's Register, Cinahl, The Cochrane Library, Medline, Embase, Psychlit, Sigle, Sociofile, reference lists of articles, and personal communication with authors of trials.
43. Pilling S, Bebbington P, Kuipers E, et al. Psychological treatments in schizophrenia: I. Meta-analysis of family interventions and cognitive behaviour therapy. *Psychol Med* 2002;32:763–782.
44. Pekkala E, Merinder L. Psychoeducation for schizophrenia. In: The Cochrane Library, Issue 3, 2004. Chichester, UK: John Wiley & Sons, Ltd. Search date 2002; primary sources Cinahl, The Cochrane Library, The Cochrane Schizophrenia Group's Register, Embase, Medline, Psychlit, Sociofile, hand searched reference lists, and personal contact with authors.
45. Pilling S, Bebbington P, Kuipers E, et al. Psychological treatments in schizophrenia: II. Meta-analysis of randomised controlled trials of social skills training and cognitive remediation. *Psychol Med* 2002;32:783–791.
46. Tuunainen A, Gilbody SM. Newer atypical antipsychotic medication versus clozapine for schizophrenia. In: The Cochrane Library, Issue 3, 2004. Chichester, UK: John Wiley & Sons, Ltd. Search date 1999; primary sources Biological Abstracts, The Cochrane Schizophrenia Group's Register, The Cochrane Library, Embase, Lilacs, Medline, Psychlit, hand searches of reference lists, and personal contact with pharmaceutical companies and authors of trials.
47. Boczkowski JA, Zeichner A, DeSanto N. Neuroleptic compliance among chronic schizophrenic outpeople: an intervention outcome report. *J Consult Clin Psychol* 1985;53:666–671.
48. Kemp R, Kirov G, Everitt B, et al. Randomised controlled trial of compliance therapy. 18-month follow-up. *Br J Psychiatry* 1998;172:413–419.
49. Kemp R, Hayward P, Applewhaite G, et al. Compliance therapy in psychotic people: randomised controlled trial. *BMJ* 1996;312:345–349.
50. Azrin NH, Teichner G. Evaluation of an instructional program for improving medication compliance for chronically mentally ill outpatients. *Behav Res Ther* 1998;36:849–861.

Zia Nadeem
Research Fellow
Department of Psychiatry
Edinburgh
UK

Andrew McIntosh
Lecturer in Psychiatry
Department of Psychiatry
Edinburgh
UK

Stephen Lawrie
Senior Clinical Research Fellow and
Honorary Consultant Psychiatrist
University of Edinburgh
Edinburgh
UK

Competing interests: SL has been paid for speaking about critical appraisal by employees of the manufacturers of olanzapine, quetiapine, risperidone, and ziprasidone, and has been paid to speak about the management of schizophrenia by employees of the manufacturers of amisulpiride, olanzapine, risperidone, and clozapine. AM and ZN none declared.

TABLE 1 **Continued treatment with antipsychotic drugs: choice of drugs (see text, p 1354).**

Review	Search date	Number of RCTs	Comparisons	Results	Main Conclusion
39	1995	6	Oral *v* depot fluphenazine	Relapse: OR 0.95, 95% CI 0.46 to 2.00	No significant difference
13	1998	7	Haloperidol decanoate *v* other depots	Clinical Global Impression: OR 0.14, 95% CI 0.04 to 0.55; NNT 2, 95% CI 1 to 5 Relapse: OR 1.25, 95% CI 0.65 to 2.42 Side effects: OR 1.85, 95% CI 0.161 to 5.60	No significant difference
40	1999	8	Flupenthixol decanoate *v* other depots	Relapse: OR 1.6, 95% CI 0.7 to 1.9 Withdrawal: OR 1, 95% CI 0.6 to 1.7	No significant difference
38	1999	7	Pipotiazine (pipothiazine) palmitate *v* other depots	Global improvement: OR 0.5, 95% CI 0.05 to 5.0 BPRS: OR 1.2, 95% CI 0.05 to 5.00 Withdrawal: OR 1.5, 95% CI 0.9 to 2.3 Side effects: OR 0.5, 95% CI 0.2 to 1.1	No significant difference
38	1999	2	Pipotiazine (pipothiazine) palmitate *v* oral antipsychotics	Relapse: OR 1.7, 95% CI 0.7 to 4.0 Withdrawal: OR 1, 95% CI 0.4 to 2.3 Side effects: OR 0.6, 95% CI 0.3 to 1.4	No significant difference
41	1999	1	Fluspirilene decanoate *v* oral chlorpromazine	Relapse: OR 1, 95% CI 0.1 to 7.7 Withdrawal: OR 1, 95% CI 0.1 to 7.7 Side effects: Significantly more people on fluspiriline needed anticholinergic drugs; OR 5.4, 95% CI 1.1 to 27; NNT 4, 95% CI 0.22 to 10	No significant difference
41	1999	3	Fluspirilene decanoate *v* other depots	Global improvements: OR 0.38, 95% CI 0.08 to 1.8 Relapse: OR 0.4, 95% CI 0.15 to 1.2 Withdrawal: OR 1.5, 95% CI 0.15 to 1.2 Side effects: Significantly fewer with fluspirilene; OR 0.4, 95% CI 0.2 to 0.8	No significant difference

TABLE 1 continued

Review	Search date	Number of RCTs	Comparisons	Results	Main Conclusion
42	1999	1	Perphenazine enanthate *v* clopenthixol decanoate	Global improvement: OR 1.3, 95% CI 0.7 to 2.4 Relapse: OR 1.5, 95% CI 0.8 to 2.8 Withdrawal: OR 1.5, 95% CI 0.8 to 28 Side effects: Significantly more people on perphenazine needed anticholinergic drugs; OR 3.6, 95% CI 1.2 to 10.0	No significant difference
29	2000	11	Pimozide *v* standard antipsychotics	Global improvement: RR 1.2, 95% CI 0.6 to 2.6 Relapse: RR 0.9, 95% CI 0.4 to 2.0 Withdrawal: RR 1.1, 95% CI 0.6 to 2.0 Side effects: RR 1.5, 95% CI 1.1 to 2.3; NNH 6, 95% CI 3 to 44	No significant difference
23	1999	1	Olanzapine *v* standard antipsychotics	Global improvement: RR 0.9, 95% CI 0.76 to 1.06 Relapse: RR 0.94, 95% CI 0.9 to 1.0 BPRS: WMD –2.8, 95% CI –8.4 to +2.8 Negative symptoms: WMD –1.7, 95% CI –2.4 to –1.1	No significant difference
43	1998	3	Zuclopenthixol decanoate *v* other depots	Relapse: Significantly reduced with zuclopenthixol; OR 0.54, 95% CI 0.3 to 0.9; NNT 8, 95% CI 5 to 53	People taking zuclopenthixol had lower relapse rates over 12 weeks to 1 year
14	1999	19	Clozapine *v* standard antipsychotics	Relapse: Significantly reduced with clozapine; OR 0.6, 95% CI 0.4 to 0.8; NNT 20, 95% CI 17 to 38 Global improvement: OR 0.4, 95% CI 0.2 to 0.6; NNT 5, 95% CI 4 to 8 Negative symptoms: SMD 0.7, 95% CI 0.5 to 0.8	Relapse rates up to 12 weeks were lower with clozapine
12	1999	2	Bromperidol *v* haloperidol or fluphenazine	Relapse: Significantly reduced with haloperidol or fluphenazine; OR 3.92, 95% CI 1.05 to 11.60	Relapse rates over 6–12 months were lower with haloperidol or fluphenazine

Ankle sprain

Search date March 2004

Peter Struijs and Gino Kerkhoffs

QUESTIONS

INTERVENTIONS

See glossary G

Key Messages

Treating ankle sprain

- **Functional treatment (early mobilisation with use of an external support)** One systematic review and one subsequent RCT found limited evidence that functional treatment reduced the risk of the ankle giving way compared with minimal treatment. One systematic review and one subsequent RCT found that, compared with immobilisation, functional treatment improved symptoms and functional outcomes at short (< 6 weeks), intermediate (6 weeks to 1 year), or long term (> 1 year) follow up. However, effects were found to be less marked at long term follow up, or if only results from high quality trials were analysed. One systematic review and one subsequent RCT provided insufficient evidence to compare functional treatment versus surgery. One systematic review and three additional RCTs provided insufficient evidence to compare different functional treatments.
- **Immobilisation** There is consensus that immobilisation is more effective than no treatment; however one systematic review and one subsequent RCT found that, compared with functional treatment, immobilisation was associated with less improvement in symptoms and functional outcomes at either short (< 6 weeks), intermediate (6 weeks to 1 year), or long term (> 1 year) follow up. Effects were less marked at long term follow up, or if only results from high quality trials were analysed. One systematic review found no significant difference between immobilisation and surgery in pain, swelling, recurrence, or subjective instability. However, the review found that compared with immobilisation, surgery improved stability and increased the proportion of people able to return to sports. One systematic review found insufficient evidence to compare immobilisation versus physiotherapy.
- **Surgery** One systematic review found no significant difference between surgery and immobilisation in pain, swelling, recurrence, or subjective instability. However, the review found that surgery increased the proportion of people able to return to sports and increased ankle stability compared with immobilisation. Other systematic reviews and one subsequent RCT provided insufficient evidence to compare surgery versus functional treatment or conservative treatment (including both immobilisation and functional treatment).

- **Diathermy** One systematic review found insufficient evidence on the effects of diathermy compared with placebo on walking ability and reduction in swelling.
- **Homeopathic ointment** One small RCT found limited evidence that homeopathic ointment improved outcome based on a "composite criteria of treatment success" compared with placebo.
- **Cold treatment** One RCT found no significant difference in symptoms between cold pack placement and placebo (simulated treatment). One RCT found no significant difference between ice treatment plus physiotherapy and physiotherapy alone. One RCT found less oedema with cold pack placement compared with heat or a contrast bath at 3–5 days after injury.
- **Ultrasound** One systematic review found no significant difference between ultrasound and sham ultrasound in the general improvement of symptoms or the ability to walk or bear weight at 7 days. Three RCTs found no significant difference between ultrasound and other treatments.

DEFINITION Ankle sprain is an injury of the lateral ligament complex of the ankle joint. The injury is graded on the basis of severity.[1–5] Grade I is a mild stretching of the ligament complex without joint instability; grade II is a partial rupture of the ligament complex with mild instability of the joint (such as isolated rupture of the anterior talofibular ligament); and grade III involves complete rupture of the ligament complex with instability of the joint. Practically, this gradation may be considered as purely theoretical, because it has no therapeutic or prognostic consequences.[6] Unless otherwise stated, studies included in this topic did not specify the grades of injury included, or included a wide range of grades.

INCIDENCE/ PREVALENCE Ankle sprain is a common problem in acute medical care, occurring at a rate of about one injury per 10 000 people a day.[7] Injuries of the lateral ligament complex of the ankle form a quarter of all sports injuries.[7]

AETIOLOGY/ RISK FACTORS The usual mechanism of injury is inversion and adduction (usually referred to as supination) of the plantar flexed foot. Predisposing factors are a history of ankle sprains and specific malalignment, like crus varum(G) and pes cavo-varus(G).

PROGNOSIS Some sports (e.g. basketball, football/soccer, and volleyball) are associated with a particularly high incidence of ankle injuries. Pain is the most frequent residual problem, often localised on the medial side of the ankle.[4] Other residual complaints include mechanical instability, intermittent swelling, and stiffness. People with more extensive cartilage damage have a higher incidence of residual complaints.[4] Long term cartilage damage can lead to degenerative changes, especially if there is persistent or recurrent instability. Every further sprain has the potential to add new damage.

AIMS OF INTERVENTION To reduce swelling and pain; to restore the stability of the ankle joint.

OUTCOMES Return to pre-injury level of sports; return to pre-injury level of work; pain; swelling; subjective instability; objective instability; recurrent injury; ankle mobility; complications; patient satisfaction.

METHODS *Clinical Evidence* search and appraisal March 2004.

QUESTION What are the effects of treatment strategies for acute ankle ligament ruptures?

OPTION IMMOBILISATION

There is consensus that immobilisation is more effective than no treatment; however one systematic review and one subsequent RCT found that, compared with functional treatment, immobilisation was associated with less improvement in symptoms and functional outcomes at either short (< 6 weeks), intermediate (6 weeks to 1 year), or long term (> 1 year) follow up. Effects were less marked at long term follow up, or if only results from high quality trials were analysed. One systematic review found no significant difference between immobilisation and surgery in pain, swelling, recurrence,

or subjective instability. However, the review found that compared with immobilisation, surgery improved stability and increased the proportion of people able to return to sports. One systematic review found insufficient evidence to compare immobilisation versus physiotherapy.

Benefits: **Versus functional treatment:** We found one systematic review (search date 2001, 21 RCTs, 2184 people)[8] and one subsequent RCT.[9] The systematic review included any inpatient, outpatient, or home based intervention programme consisting of immobilisation**G** with or without a plaster cast.[8] It included any trials comparing immobilisation versus either another type or duration of immobilisation or a functional treatment**G** for injuries to the lateral ligament complex of the ankle and it reported outcomes at short, intermediate, or long term follow up (see comment below). The review analysed a variety of different forms of functional treatment, including strapping, bracing, use of an orthosis, tubigrips, bandages, elastic bandages, and special shoes for at least 5 weeks. It found that functional treatment significantly improved seven outcomes measured at different follow up times compared with immobilisation. At short term follow up, it found that functional treatment significantly reduced the proportion of people with persistent swelling compared with immobilisation (3 RCTs; RR 1.7, 95% CI 1.2 to 2.6) and significantly decreased the proportion of people not returning to work (2 RCTs; RR 5.75, 95% CI 1.01 to 32.71). At intermediate term follow up, it found that immobilisation significantly increased objective instability, as assessed with stress x ray, compared with functional treatment (1 RCT; WMD 2.6°, 95% CI 1.2° to 4.0°) and found that significantly more people were satisfied with functional treatment compared with immobilisation (2 RCTs; RR 4.2, 95% CI 1.1 to 16.1). At long term follow up, it found that functional treatment significantly decreased the proportion of people not returning to sports compared with immobilisation (5 RCTs; RR 1.9, 95% CI 1.2 to 2.9), the time taken to return to work (6 RCTs; WMD 8.2 days, 95% CI 6.3 days to 10.2 days), and the time taken to return to sports (3 RCTs; WMD 4.9 days, 95% CI 1.5 days to 8.3 days). At longer term follow up, differences in outcomes for persistent swelling, objective instability, proportion of people not returning to work, and patient satisfaction were no longer significant. A subgroup analysis using only 11 "high quality" RCTs (defined as scoring ≥50% on a recognised quality evaluation tool) found that functional treatment significantly reduced the time taken to return to work compared with immobilisation (2 RCTs; WMD 12.9 days, 95% CI 7.1 days to 18.7 days).[8,10] The subsequent RCT (121 semiprofessional sports people with acute grade III lateral ankle ligament) compared 3 weeks of functional treatment (strapping plus early controlled mobilisation) versus immobilisation in a plaster cast.[9] It found that functional treatment significantly reduced time taken to return to normal physical training and reduced pain, swelling, and subjective instability compared with immobilisation at 3 months (mean time to return to normal training: 5.4 weeks with functional treatment *v* 6.3 weeks with immobilisation; $P = 0.02$; pain: 35% with functional treatment *v* 61% with immobilisation; $P = 0.008$); swelling: 16% with functional treatment *v* 49% with immobilisation; $P < 0.01$; subjective instability: 22% with functional treatment *v* 54% with immobilisation; $P = 0.001$; CI for differences in outcomes not reported). However, the RCT found no significant differences between treatments for pain, swelling, or subjective instability at 12 months ($P \geq 0.3$ for all comparisons).[9] **Versus surgery:** We found one systematic review (search date 2000, 12 RCTs, 1516 people) which compared surgery (anatomic reconstruction**G**) versus immobilisation alone for acute injuries to the lateral ligament complex of the ankle (see comment below).[6] It found that surgery significantly reduced the proportion of people who did not return to sports compared with immobilisation (3 RCTs; RR 0.48, 95% CI 0.31 to 0.76) and who had objective instability (6 RCTs; RR 0.35, 95% CI 0.21 to 0.60). It found no significant difference between surgery and immobilisation in recurrence (8 RCTs; RR 0.86, 95% CI 0.63 to 1.18), pain (8 RCTs; RR 0.64, 95% CI 0.33 to 1.23), subjective instability (8 RCTs; RR 0.77, 95% CI 0.43 to 1.37), or swelling (9 RCTs; RR 0.67, 95% CI 0.38 to 1.18). **Versus physiotherapy:** We found one systematic review (search date 2000, 1 RCT, 165 people). The review was unable to calculate outcomes because of insufficient data.[6] **Different forms of immobilisation:** We found one systematic review (search date 2000, 2 RCTs, 229 people).[6] The first RCT identified by the review found that a semirigid cast for 4 weeks significantly reduced the time taken to return to work compared with a rigid cast (WMD 3.80 days, 95% CI 1.16 days to 6.44 days).[6] It found no significant difference in pain, swelling, or objective instability at short term follow up (RR for pain 2.10, 95% CI 0.69 to 6.35; RR for swelling 1.59, 95% CI 0.80 to 3.17; RR for objective instability 0.60, 95% CI 0.12 to 3.00). The review was unable to calculate outcomes from the second RCT.

Harms: Two RCTs found fewer cases of deep venous thrombosis after cast immobilisation**G** than after surgery (deep venous thrombosis: 2/47 [4%] after cast immobilisation *v* 3/34 [9%] after surgery; 0/33 [0%] after cast immobilisation *v* 1/32 [3%] after surgery).[6,11] One RCT identified by a systematic review found an equal risk of deep vein thrombosis in both groups (1/50 [2%] after cast immobilisation *v* 1/50 [2%] after surgery).[6] Other RCTs did not specifically address harms. Other known harms of immobilisation include pain and impairment in activities of daily living.[11] The systematic review[8] and one RCT did not report on harms.[9]

Comment: There is a consensus that immobilisation**G** is more effective in the treatment of ankle sprain than no treatment. **Versus functional treatment:** In the systematic review, follow up periods for outcome measures were categorised as short term (within 6 weeks of randomisation), intermediate term (6 weeks to 1 year), or long term (1–2 years after treatment).[8] The review excluded trials that focused on the treatment of chronic instability or post-surgical treatment unless such injuries occurred in under 10% of the whole study population. The subsequent study included only semiprofessional sports people so the results may not be applicable to the general population.[9] **Versus surgery:** The systematic review noted that all included RCTs had methodological flaws, and there was insufficient evidence to determine the relative effectiveness of surgical and conservative treatment (see comment under surgery, p 1372).[6]

OPTION FUNCTIONAL TREATMENT (EARLY MOBILISATION WITH USE OF AN EXTERNAL SUPPORT)

One systematic review and one subsequent RCT found limited evidence that functional treatment reduced the risk of the ankle giving way compared with minimal treatment. One systematic review and one subsequent RCT found that, compared with immobilisation, functional treatment improved symptoms and functional outcomes at short (< 6 weeks), intermediate (6 weeks to 1 year), or long term (> 1 year) follow up. However, effects were found to be less marked at long term follow up, or if only results from high quality trials were analysed. One systematic review and one subsequent RCT provided insufficient evidence to compare functional treatment versus surgery. One systematic review and three additional RCTs provided insufficient evidence to compare different functional treatments.

Benefits: **Versus minimal treatment:** We found one systematic review (search date 1998, 3 RCTs, 214 people)[12] and one subsequent RCT.[13] The review compared functional treatment**G** versus a minimal treatment policy. It found that functional treatment significantly reduced the risk of the ankle giving way (RR 0.34, 95% CI 0.17 to 0.71).[12] The review found no significant difference between treatments in the proportion of people with residual pain (RR 0.53, 95% CI 0.27 to 1.02).[12] The subsequent RCT (30 people with subacute or chronic ankle sprain without gross mechanical instability) compared the mortise separation adjustment**G** versus detuned ultrasound.[13] It found that mobilisation significantly reduced pain, increased ankle range of motion, and improved ankle function at 1 month (results presented graphically). **Versus immobilisation:** See benefits of immobilisation, p 1368. **Versus surgery:** We found one systematic review (search date 2000, 9 RCTs, 1347 people)[6] and one subsequent RCT,[14] which compared surgery (tenodesis**G** or anatomic reconstruction**G**) versus functional treatment alone (see comment below). The review found no significant difference between surgery and functional treatment in return to sports (2 RCTs; RR 0.6, 95% CI 0.3 to 1.3), recurrence (5 RCTs; RR 1.2, 95% CI 0.8 to 1.8), pain (5 RCTs; RR 1.0, 95% CI 0.7 to 1.6), subjective instability (5 RCTs; RR 0.9, 95% CI 0.7 to 1.3), objective instability (4 RCTs; RR 0.6, 95% CI 0.3 to 1.2), and swelling (5 RCTs; RR 0.9, 95% CI 0.6 to 1.5; see comment below).[6] The subsequent RCT (370 people with rupture of at least 1 lateral ankle ligament) compared functional treatment with surgery (anatomic reconstruction).[14] Functional treatment consisted of a non-weight bearing cast for 5 days followed by elastic bandaging or taping for 6 weeks. People in both groups received a standard rehabilitation programme. The RCT found that functional treatment was less effective than surgery for residual pain, subjective instability, and recurrent sprains after 6–11 years' follow up (317 people analysed; pain: 25% with functional treatment *v* 16% with surgery, RR 1.56, 95% CI 1.00 to 2.44; subjective instability: 32% with functional treatment *v* 20% with surgery, RR 1.61, 95% CI 1.09 to 2.38; recurrent sprains: 34% with functional treatment *v* 22% with surgery, RR 1.51, 95% CI 1.06 to 2.22). **Versus different types of functional treatment:** We found one systematic review (search date 2001, 9 RCTs, 892 people)[15] and three additional RCTs.[16–18] The review compared different types of functional treatment (elastic bandage, tape, lace-up ankle support, and semirigid ankle support) in people with an acute injury to the lateral ligament complex of the ankle.[15] It reported outcomes at short, intermediate, and long term follow up (see comment below). At short term follow up, it found that lace-up ankle support significantly reduced persistent swelling compared with semirigid ankle support (1 RCT; RR 4.2, 95% CI 1.3 to 14.0), elastic bandage (1 RCT; RR 5.5, 95% CI 1.7 to 17.8), and tape (1 RCT; RR 4.1, 95% CI 1.2 to 13.7). A semirigid ankle support significantly reduced the proportion of people with subjective instability compared with an elastic bandage (1 RCT; RR 8.00, 95% CI 1.03 to 62.07).[15] It found no significant differences between different types of functional treatments at intermediate or long term follow up. It found that a semirigid ankle support significantly reduced the time taken to return to work (2 RCTs; WMD 4.2 days, 95% CI 2.4 days to 6.0 days) and the time taken to return to sports (1 RCT; WMD 9.6 days, 95% CI 6.3 days to 12.8 days) compared with an elastic bandage. It found no other significant differences in outcomes between treatments (see comment below).[15] The first additional RCT (61 people without previous fractures in the ankle joint or clinically demonstrable ankle instability; mean follow up of 230 days) found that elastic bandage plus proprioceptis training reduced the risk of recurrent sprains compared with elastic bandage alone (RR 0.46, 95% CI 0.20 to 1.00).[16] Thirteen people withdrew from the RCT and were not included in the analysis. The remaining two additional RCTs found no significant differences in outcomes between treatments.[17,18] The second RCT (116 people with all grades of ankle sprain) compared a semirigid device versus tape and found no significant difference between treatments in the proportion of people with recurrent sprains (4% with semirigid device *v* 0% with tape).[17] The third RCT (119 people not requiring surgery, treated within 24 hours of injury) compared two types of tape treatment and found no significant differences between treatment groups in pain, swelling, or range of movement 5–7 days after treatment (AR for pain: 8% *v* 5%; swelling: 58% *v* 47%; limited range of movement: 36% *v* 47%).[18]

Harms: Allergic reactions and skin problems have been recorded with tape.[19] Two RCTs identified by a systematic review which compared different functional treatments**G**, found that tape treatment was associated with significantly more complications compared with elastic bandage (0/104 [0%] with elastic bandage *v* 8/104 [8%] with tape; RR 0.11, 95% CI 0.01 to 0.86).[15] Most of these complications were skin problems (absolute numbers with skin problems not reported). The other review[6] and RCTs[14,17,18] described did not examine harms.

Comment: **Versus surgery:** The review noted that all included RCTs had methodological flaws, and there was insufficient evidence to determine the relative effectiveness of surgical and conservative treatment (see comment under surgery, p 1372).[6] **Different types of functional treatment:** The systematic review reported follow up periods for outcome measures as short term (< 6 weeks of treatment), intermediate term (6 weeks to 1 year), or long term (1–2 years after treatment).[15] It noted that definitive conclusions were hampered by the variety of treatments used and the inconsistency of reported follow up times, and no definite conclusions concerning the optimal functional treatment**G** strategy could be drawn.[15]

OPTION SURGERY

One systematic review found no significant difference between surgery and immobilisation in pain, swelling, recurrence, or subjective instability. However, the review found that surgery increased the proportion of people able to return to sports and increased ankle stability compared with immobilisation. Other systematic reviews and one subsequent RCT provided insufficient evidence to compare surgery versus functional treatment or conservative treatment (including both immobilisation and functional treatment).

Benefits: **Versus immobilisation:** See benefits of immobilisation, p 1368. **Versus functional treatment:** See benefits of functional treatment, p 1369. **Versus conservative (immobilisation and functional) treatment:** We found one systematic review (search date 2000, 17 RCTs, 1950 people) which compared surgery (anatomical reconstruction and tenodesis**G**) versus conservative treatment including both immobilisation**G** and functional treatments**G** for acute injuries to the lateral ligament complex of the ankle.[6] Significant results were often not robust to sensitivity analysis (see comment below). When data from one quasi-randomised trial were excluded, the review found that surgery significantly decreased the proportion of people with objective instability compared with conservative treatment (4 RCTs; RR 0.4, 95% CI 0.2 to 0.7). It also found that surgery significantly increased the proportion of people with ankle stiffness compared with conservative treatment (2 RCTs; RR 1.9, 95% CI 1.2 to 3.1). It found no significant difference between groups in recurrence (10 RCTs; RR 0.96, 95% CI 0.70 to 1.20), pain on activity (8 RCTs; RR 0.9, 95% CI 0.7 to 1.2), swelling (9 RCTs; RR 0.83, 95% CI 0.60 to 1.10), or people not returning to sports (3 RCTs; RR 0.7, 95% CI 0.4 to 1.2; see comment below).[6]

Harms: Neurological injuries, infections, bleeding, osteoarthritis, and death are known harms of surgery.[11,20,21] Two RCTs found fewer cases of deep venous thrombosis after cast immobilisation**G** compared with surgery (deep venous thrombosis: 2/47 [4%] with cast immobilisation *v* 3/34 [9%] with surgery; 0/33 [0%] with cast immobilisation *v* 1/32 [3%] with surgery).[6,11] One RCT found an equal occurrence of deep vein thrombosis in both groups (1/50 [2%] with cast immobilisation *v* 1/50 [2%] with surgery).[6] Other RCTs found dysaesthesia**G** in 4–12% of people after surgery.[22–27] Wound necrosis after surgery was reported in two RCTs (2/73 [3%] with surgery;[25] 3/45 [7%] with surgery[26]). Tenderness of the scar was reported in six RCTs after surgical intervention, occurring in 2–19% of people.[23,24,27–30]

Comment: The systematic review comparing surgery versus conservative treatment noted that all RCTs had methodological flaws.[6] Data for pooling for individual outcomes were available for a maximum of 11 trials, and quality assessment ranged from six to 13 out of a possible 22 using a recognised quality evaluation tool.[6] Included trials were often heterogeneous, and significant results were often sensitive to the method of analysis used (random or fixed effects meta-analysis) or when data from quasi-randomised trials were excluded. The review concluded that "there is insufficient evidence available from randomised controlled trials to determine the relative effectiveness of surgical and conservative treatment for acute injuries of the lateral ligament complex of the ankle."[6]

OPTION ULTRASOUND

One systematic review found no significant difference between ultrasound and sham ultrasound in the general improvement of symptoms or the ability to walk or bear weight at 7 days. Three RCTs found no significant difference between ultrasound and other treatments.

Benefits: **Versus placebo:** We found one systematic review (search date 2001; see comment below) which compared ultrasound versus sham ultrasound treatment.[31] It found no significant difference in general improvement of symptoms between ultrasound and sham ultrasound at 7 days (3 RCTs; 121/169 [72%] with ultrasound *v* 116/172 [68%] with sham ultrasound; RR 1.04, 95% CI 0.92 to 1.17).[31] It also found no significant difference in functional disability (the ability to walk or bear weight) between ultrasound and sham ultrasound at 7 days (2 RCTs; 69/95 [73%] with ultrasound *v* 61/92 [66%] with sham ultrasound; RR 1.09, 95% CI 0.92 to 1.30).[31] **Versus other treatments:** We found one systematic review (search date 2001, 3 RCTs, 360 people; see comment below) which compared ultrasound versus other treatment modalities.[31] The first RCT (220 people) identified by the review compared ultrasound plus felbinac gel, sham ultrasound plus felbinac gel, and ultrasound plus placebo gel over 1 week. It found no significant differences between treatments in the proportion of people with moderate or marked (investigator assessed) improvement in pain at 7 days (67/75 [89%] with ultrasound plus felbinac gel *v* 57/72 [79%] with sham ultrasound *v* 61/73 [84%] with ultrasound plus placebo gel; ARR for ultrasound plus felbinac gel *v* sham ultrasound: +10%, 95% CI –2% to +22%; ARR for ultrasound plus placebo gel *v* sham ultrasound: +5%, 95% CI –8% to +18%; ability to bear full weight: 60/75 [80%] with ultrasound plus felbinac gel *v* 53/72 [74%] with sham ultrasound *v* 56/73 [77%] with ultrasound plus placebo gel; ARR for ultrasound plus felbinac gel *v* sham ultrasound: +6%, 95% CI –7% to +20%; ARR for ultrasound plus placebo gel *v* sham ultrasound: 3%, 95% CI –11% to 17%; moderate or marked improvement of general severity: 65/75 [87%] with ultrasound plus felbinac gel *v* 61/72 [85%] with sham ultrasound *v* 61/73[84%] with ultrasound plus placebo gel; ARR for ultrasound plus felbinac gel *v* sham ultrasound: +2%, 95% CI –9% to +13%; ARR ultrasound plus placebo gel *v* sham ultrasound: –1%, 95%

CI –13 to +11%). The second RCT identified by the review (60 people) compared ultrasound versus electrotherapy or sham ultrasound. It found no significant difference between treatments in the proportion of people with swelling, ability to walk, or who were free of pain at 7 days (RR for swelling: 13/20 [65%] with ultrasound *v* 17/20 [85%] with electrotherapy *v* 8/20 [40%] with sham ultrasound; ARR for swelling with ultrasound *v* electrotherapy: –20%, 95% CI –46% to +6%; ARR for ultrasound *v* sham ultrasound: +25%, 95% CI –5% to +55%; RR for ability to walk: 9/20 [45%] with ultrasound *v* 14/20 [70%] with electrotherapy *v* 8/20 [40%] with sham ultrasound; ARR for ability to walk with ultrasound *v* electrotherapy: –25%, 95% CI –55% to +5%; ARR for ultrasound *v* sham ultrasound: +5%, 95% CI –26% to +36%; RR for pain: 15/20 [75%] with ultrasound *v* 18/20 [90%] with electrotherapy *v* 11/20 [55%] with sham ultrasound; ARR for absence of pain with ultrasound *v* electrotherapy: –15%, 95% CI –38% to +8%; ARR for ultrasound *v* sham ultrasound: +20%, 95% CI –9% to +49%).[31] The third RCT (80 people) compared ultrasound versus immobilisation**G** with Elastoplast over 2 weeks' follow up. It found no significant difference in the proportion of people who recovered with ultrasound compared with immobilisation after 7 days (46% with ultrasound *v* 27% with immobilisation; ARR +19%, 95% CI –2% to +40%).[31] However, after 14 days, it found a significant difference in the proportion of people who recovered with ultrasound compared with immobilisation (86% with ultrasound *v* 59% with immobilisation; ARR 27%, 95% CI 8% to 46%).[31]

Harms: Two RCTs included in the systematic review addressed adverse reactions.[32,33] The first RCT found no adverse reactions.[32] The second RCT found that 8/73 (11%) of people treated with ultrasound plus placebo gel reported 11 non-serious adverse reactions, including gastrointestinal events and skin reactions.[33] One person was withdrawn from the RCT because of skin reactions.[33]

Comment: In the review, the quality of four of the included RCTs was described as "modest" and one as "good".[31] The review reported RCTs in which one or more of pain, swelling, and functional disability because of an acute ankle sprain were present, and in which at least one group was treated with active ultrasound treatment. All the RCTs included follow up of less than 4 weeks.

OPTION COLD TREATMENT

One RCT found no significant difference in symptoms between cold pack placement and placebo (simulated treatment). One RCT found no significant difference between ice treatment plus physiotherapy and physiotherapy alone. One RCT found less oedema with cold pack placement compared with heat or a contrast bath at 3–5 days after injury.

Benefits: **Versus placebo:** We found one systematic review (search date 1994, 1 RCT, 143 people) which compared cryotherapy versus placebo (simulated treatment).[34] The RCT found no significant difference between treatments (P value reported as not significant).[35] **Versus different treatments:** We found one systematic review (search date 1994, 2 RCTs) which compared different cold treatments.[34] The first RCT (30 people) identified by the review compared ice treatment plus physiotherapy versus no ice plus physiotherapy. It found no significant difference between treatments (P value reported as not significant).[36] The second RCT (30 people) identified by the review found significantly less oedema with a cold pack compared with heat or a contrast bath (see comment below) at 3–5 days after injury ($P < 0.05$).[37]

Harms: None of the RCTs addressed harms from cold pack placement.

Comment: The systematic review was narrative in character and no data were pooled.[34] The systematic review did not report the grade of injuries. In the second RCT identified by the systematic review which compared cold compared with heat or a contrast bath, the injured ankle in the contrast bath group was submerged in warm water for 3 minutes and then in cold water for 1 minute. This was continued until the ankle had been given five heat and four cold treatments beginning and ending with heat.[37]

OPTION DIATHERMY

One systematic review found insufficient evidence on the effects of diathermy compared with placebo on walking ability and reduction in swelling.

Benefits: **Versus placebo:** We found one systematic review (search date 1994, 5 RCTs).[34] The review included a range of severity of ankle sprains but excluded the most severe injuries (avulsion and osteochondral fractures). The first RCT identified by the review (300 people with time from injury to treatment of ≤ 4 days) compared two forms of pulsating short wave treatment versus placebo.[38] The RCT found that high frequency electromagnetic pulsing significantly improved walking ability more quickly compared with placebo ($P < 0.01$). It found no significant difference in walking ability between low frequency electromagnetic pulsing and placebo. However, low frequency pulsing significantly reduced swelling compared with placebo. There was no significant difference in swelling between the high frequency group compared with placebo (change in circumference of ankle: 4.5 mm with high frequency *v* 5.0 mm with low frequency *v* 2.6 mm with placebo; $P < 0.01$ for low frequency *v* placebo). The second RCT (50 people) found that pulsating short wave diathermy**G** significantly reduced oedema compared with placebo ($P < 0.01$).[39] The third RCT (73 people) found no significant difference between treatments for pain, oedema, or range of motion compared with placebo (results presented graphically).[40] The fourth RCT (37 people) found no significant difference between treatments (for pain, oedema, or range of motion) compared with placebo.[41] The fifth RCT (30 people) found no significant differences between treatments for (pain, oedema, or range of motion) compared with placebo.[42] The grades of injuries were not clearly described in these RCTs and results were not pooled.

Harms: No harms were reported.

Comment: None.

OPTION HOMEOPATHIC OINTMENT

One small RCT found limited evidence that homeopathic ointment improved outcome based on a "composite criteria of treatment success" compared with placebo.

Benefits: **Versus placebo:** We found one systematic review (search date 1998, 69 people with acute ankle sprains; see comment below),[43] which included one RCT.[44] The RCT found that people treated with a homeopathic ointment had a significantly better outcome based on a "composite criteria of treatment success" compared with people treated with placebo ($P = 0.028$; no further data reported).[43] The number of people initially randomised in the RCT and losses to follow up were not reported.

Harms: Harms were not addressed in the review.

Comment: None.

GLOSSARY

Anatomic reconstruction Surgical reconstruction of lateral ankle ligament complex through suturing of the ligaments.

Crus varum Varus of the lower leg (O-leg).

Diathermy Warming body tissues using electromagnetic radiation, electric current, or ultrasonic waves for the reduction of inflammatory response, oedema, and pain.

Dysaesthesia Decreased sensitivity of the skin for stimuli.

Functional treatment Involves dorsal and plantar flexion exercises of the ankle joint. The main differences between functional treatment strategies are the types of external device applied for treatment. The supports can be divided according to rigidity into elastic bandage, tape, lace-up ankle support, and semirigid ankle support. Functional treatment may involve strapping, bracing, use of an orthosis, tubigrips, bandages, elastic bandages, and the use of special shoes. Propriocepsis training (to enhance joint stability) may also be involved in this regimen.

Immobilisation Limiting the mobility of a joint complex to zero degrees with the use of a plaster cast or soft cast, thus fully immobilising the ankle joint.

Mortise separation adjustment An adjustment technique involving special manual manipulation of the foot and ankle.[13]

Pes cavo-varus Severe high arched, varus foot.

Tenodesis Surgical reconstruction of lateral ankle ligament complex using tendon graft.

REFERENCES

1. Bernett P, Schirmann A. Acute sporting injuries of the ankle joint. *Unfallheilkunde* 1979;82:155–160. [In German]
2. Lassiter TE, Malone TR, Garret WE. Injuries to the lateral ligaments of the ankle. *Orthop Clin North Am* 1989;20:629–640.
3. Marti RK. Bagatelletsels van de voet. 56–61. 1982. Capita selecta, *Reuma Wereldwijd*.
4. Van Dijk CN, Bossuyt PM, Marti RK. Medial ankle pain after lateral ligament rupture. *J Bone Joint Surg Br* 1996;78:562–567.
5. Watson-Jones R. *Fractures and joint injuries*. London: Churchill Livingstone, 1976.
6. Kerkhoffs GMMJ, Handoll HHG, de Bie R, et al. Surgical versus conservative treatment for acute injuries of the lateral ligament complex of the ankle in adults (Cochrane Review). In: The Cochrane Library, Issue 1, 2004. Chichester, UK: John Wiley & Sons, Ltd. Search date 2001; primary sources Cochrane Musculoskeletal Injuries Group specialised register, Cochrane Controlled Trials Register, Medline, Embase, Biosis, Current Contents, hand searches of reference lists of articles, and personal contact with organisations and researchers in the field.
7. Katcherian DA. Treatment of Freiberg's disease. *Orthop Clin North Am* 1994;25:69–81.
8. Kerkhoffs GMMJ, Rowe BH, Assendelft WJJ, et al. Immobilisation and functional treatment for acute lateral ankle ligament injuries in adults (Cochrane Review). In: The Cochrane Library, Issue 1, 2004. Chichester, UK: John Wiley & Sons, Ltd. Search date 2001; primary sources Cochrane Musculoskeletal Injuries Group specialised register, Cochrane Controlled Trials Register, Medline, Embase, hand searches of reference lists of articles, and personal contact with organisations (Medical Departments of the Dutch Defence Forces and the Royal Dutch Football Association) and researchers in the field.
9. Ardevol J, Bolibar I, Belda V, et al. Treatment of complete rupture of the lateral ligaments of the ankle: a randomized clinical trial comparing cast immobilization with functional treatment. *Knee Surg Sports Traumatol Arthrosc* 2002;10:371–377.
10. Verhagen AP, de Vet HC, de Bie RA, et al. The Delphi list: a criteria list for quality assessment of randomized clinical trials for conducting systematic reviews developed by Delphi consensus. *J Clin Epidemiol* 1998; 51:1235–1241.
11. Korkala O, Rusanen M, Jokipii P, et al. A prospective study of the treatment of severe tears of the lateral ligament of the ankle. *Int Orthop* 1987;11:13–17.
12. Pijnenburg AC, Van Dijk CN, Bossuyt PM, et al. Treatment of ruptures of the lateral ankle ligaments: a meta-analysis. *J Bone Joint Surg Am* 2000;82:761–773. Search date 1998; primary sources Cochrane, Medline, Embase, hand searches of references from the published reviews, and personal contact with authors.
13. Pellow JE, Brantingham JW. The efficacy of adjusting the ankle in the treatment of subacute and chronic grade I and grade II ankle inversion sprains. *J Manipulative Physiol Ther* 2001;24:17–24.
14. Pijnenburg ACM, Bogaard K, Krips R, et al. Operative and functional treatment of rupture of the lateral ligament of the ankle. A randomised, prospective trial. *J Bone Joint Surg Br* 2003;85:525–530.
15. Kerkhoffs GMMJ, Struijs PAA, Marti RK, et al. Different functional treatment strategies for acute lateral ankle ligament injuries in adults (Cochrane Review). In: The Cochrane Library, Issue 1, 2004. Chichester, UK: John Wiley & Sons. Search date 2001; primary sources Cochrane Musculoskeletal Injuries Group specialised register, Cochrane Controlled Trials Register, Medline, Embase, Biosis, Current Contents, hand searches of reference lists of articles, and personal contact with organisations (Medical Departments of the Dutch Defence Forces and the Royal Dutch Football Association) and researchers in the field.
16. Wester JU, Jespersen SM, Nielsen KD, et al. Wobble board training after partial sprains of the lateral ligaments of the ankle: a prospective randomized study. *J Orthop Sports Phys Ther* 1996;23:332–336.
17. Johannes EJ, Sukul DM, Spruit PJ, et al. Controlled trial of a semi-rigid bandage ("Scotchrap") in patients with ankle ligament lesions. *Curr Med Res Opin* 1993;13:154–162.
18. Viljakka T, Rokkanen P. The treatment of ankle sprain by bandaging and antiphlogistic drugs. *Ann Chir Gynaecol* 1983;72:66–70.
19. Zeegers AVCM. Supination injury of the ankle joint [thesis]. Utrecht: University of Utrecht, The Netherlands, 1995.
20. Biegler M, Lang A, Ritter J. Comparative study on the effectiveness of early functional treatment using special shoes following surgery of ruptures of fibular ligaments. *Unfallchirurg* 1985;88:113–117. [In German]

21. Sommer HM, Schreiber H. Early functional conservative therapy of fresh fibular capsular ligament rupture from the socioeconomic viewpoint. *Sportverletz Sportschaden* 1993;7:40–46. [In German]
22. Zwipp H, Hoffmann R, Thermann H, et al. Rupture of the ankle ligaments. *Int Orthop* 1991;15:245–249.
23. Evans GA, Hardcastle P, Frenyo AD. Acute rupture of the lateral ligament of the ankle. To suture or not to suture? *J Bone Joint Surg Br* 1984;66:209–212.
24. Delfosse P, Lafontaine D, Hardy D, et al. Rupture of the ankle ligaments: to repair or not to repair? Preliminary results of a randomized study [abstract]. 6th Congress of the European Society of Sports Traumatology, Knee Surgery and Arthroscopy 1994;S66.
25. Povacz P, Salzburg F, Unger SF, et al. A randomized, prospective study of operative and non-operative treatment of injuries of the fibular collateral ligaments of the ankle. *J Bone Joint Surg Am* 1998;80:345–351.
26. Prins JG. Diagnosis and treatment of injury to the lateral ligament of the ankle: a comparative clinical study. *Acta Chir Scand Suppl* 1978;486:3–139.
27. Brostrom L. Sprained ankles V. Treatment and prognosis in recent ligament ruptures. *Acta Chir Scand* 1966;132:537–550.
28. Niedermann A, Andersen A, Bryde Andersen S, et al. Rupture of the lateral ligaments of the ankle: operation or plaster cast? *Acta Orthop Scand* 1981;52:579–587.
29. Klein J, Schreckenberger C, Roddecker K, et al. Operative or conservative treatment of recent rupture of the fibular ligament in the ankle. A randomized clinical trial. *Unfallchirurg* 1988;91:154–160. [In German]
30. Van den Hoogenband CR, Van Moppes FI. Diagnostic and therapeutic aspects of inversion trauma of the ankle joint [thesis]. Maastricht: University of Maastricht, 1982.
31. Van der Windt DAWM, Van der Heijden GJMG, Van den Berg SGM, et al. Ultrasound therapy for acute ankle sprains (Cochrane Review). In: The Cochrane Library, Issue 2, 2003. Oxford: Update Software. Search date 2001; primary sources Cochrane Musculoskeletal Injuries Group specialised register, Cochrane Controlled Trials Register, Cochrane Rehabilitation and Related Therapies Field database, Medline, Embase, Cinahl, PEDro — the Physiotherapy Evidence Database, hand searches of reference lists of articles, and personal contact with colleagues.
32. Nyanzi CS, Langridge J, Heyworth JR, et al. Randomized controlled study of ultrasound therapy in the management of acute lateral ligament sprains of the ankle joint. *Clin Rehabil* 1999;13:16–22.
33. Oakland C. A comparison of the efficacy of the topical NSAID felbinac and ultrasound in the treatment of acute ankle injuries. *Br J Clin Res* 1993;4:89–96.
34. Ogilvie-Harris DJ, Gilbart M. Treatment modalities for soft tissue injuries of the ankle: a critical review. *Clin J Sport Med* 1995;5:175–186. Search date 1994; primary sources Medline and Excerpta Medica.
35. Sloan JP, Hain R, Pownall R. Clinical benefits of early cold therapy in accident and emergency following ankle sprain. *Arch Emerg Med* 1989;6:1–6.
36. Laba E, Roestenburg M. Clinical evaluation of ice therapy for acute ankle sprain injuries. *NZ J Physiother* 1989;17:7–9.
37. Cote DJ, Prentice WEJ, Hooker DN, et al. Comparison of three treatment procedures for minimizing ankle sprain swelling. *Physical Ther* 1988;68:1072–1076.
38. Pasila M, Visuri T, Sundholm A. Pulsating shortwave diathermy: value in treatment of recent ankle and foot sprains. *Arch Phys Med Rehabil* 1978;59:383–386.
39. Pennington GM, Danley DL, Sumko MH, et al. Pulsed, non-thermal, high-frequency electromagnetic energy (DIAPULSE) in the treatment of grade I and grade II ankle sprains. *Mil Med* 1993;158:101–104.
40. Barker AT, Barlow PS, Porter J, et al. A double-blind clinical trial of low power pulsed shortwave therapy in the treatment of a soft tissue injury. *Physiotherapy* 1985;71:500–504.
41. McGill SN. The effects of pulsed shortwave therapy on lateral ligament sprain of the ankle. *NZ J Physiother* 1988;16:21–24.
42. Michlovitz S, Smith W, Watkins M. Ice and high voltage pulsed stimulation in treatment of acute lateral ankle sprains. *J Orthop Sports Phys Ther* 1988;9:301–304.
43. Cucherat M, Haugh MC, Gooch M, et al. Evidence of clinical efficacy of homeopathy: a meta-analysis of clinical trials. *Eur J Clin Pharmacol* 2000;56:27–33. Search date 1998; primary sources Medline; Embase; Biosis; Psychinfo; Cinahl; British Library Stock Alert Service; Sigle; Amed; hand searches of homeopathy journals, conference abstracts, references provided by colleagues, and reference lists of selected papers; and personal contact with pharmaceutical companies.
44. Zell R, Connert WD, Mau J, et al. Treatment of acute sprains of the ankle joint. Double-blind study assessing the effectiveness of a homeopathic ointment preparation. *Fortschr Med* 1988;106:96–100. [In German]

Peter Struijs
Resident surgery, Ferik Hendrikplontsoen 74–2
Amsterdam
Netherlands

Gino Kerkhoffs
Academic Medical Center
Amsterdam
The Netherlands

Competing interests: None declared.

Bunions

Search date June 2004

Jill Ferrari

QUESTIONS

INTERVENTIONS

Key Messages

Conservative treatments

- **Night splints** One systematic review found no reliable RCTs comparing night splints with any other or no treatment.
- **Orthoses to treat hallux valgus in adults** One RCT in adults found that, orthoses reduced pain compared with no treatment at 6 months but not at 1 year and that orthoses were less effective at improving outcomes than chevron osteotomy.
- **Antipronatory orthoses in children** One RCT in children found that antipronatory orthoses increased deterioration in metatarsophalangeal joint angles after 3 years compared with no treatment, although the difference was not statistically significant.

Surgical treatments

- **Chevron osteotomy (more effective than no treatment or orthoses but insufficient evidence to compare with other metatarsal osteotomies)** One systematic review found conflicting evidence on the effects of chevron osteotomy compared with other metatarsal osteotomies. One RCT found that chevron osteotomy improved outcomes compared with orthoses or no treatment after 1 year.

- **Chevron osteotomy plus Akin osteotomy** One systematic review identified one small RCT comparing chevron osteotomy plus Akin osteotomy and Akin osteotomy plus distal soft tissue reconstruction, which found no significant difference in outcomes between treatments at 1 year. However, this trial may have lacked power to detect a clinically significant difference.
- **Chevron osteotomy plus adductor tenotomy** One systematic review found no evidence that adductor tenotomy plus chevron osteotomy improved outcomes compared with chevron osteotomy alone.
- **Different methods of bone fixation (standard fixation, absorbable pin fixation, screw fixation plus early weight bearing, suture fixation plus delayed weight bearing)** One small RCT identified by a systematic review found no significant difference between standard fixation and absorbable pin fixation in clinical or radiological outcomes; however, it may have lacked power to detect a clinically significant difference. A second small RCT identified by the review found that screw fixation plus early weight bearing reduced time to return to work and social activity compared with suture fixation and later weight bearing, but found no significant difference in radiological outcomes.
- **Keller's arthroplasty** We found no RCTs comparing Keller's arthroplasty versus no treatment. One systematic review found insufficient evidence from limited RCTs on the effects of Keller's arthroplasty compared with other types of operation.

Postoperative care

- **Continuous passive motion** One systematic review provided insufficient evidence on the effects of continuous passive motion.
- **Early weight bearing** One systematic review provided insufficient evidence on the effects of early weight bearing.
- **Slipper casts** One systematic review provided insufficient evidence on the effects of plaster slipper casts.

DEFINITION **Hallux valgus** is a deformity of the great toe, whereby the hallux (great toe) moves towards the second toe, overlying it in severe cases. This abduction (movement away from the midline of the body) is usually accompanied by some rotation of the toe so that the nail is facing the midline of the body (valgus rotation). With the deformity, the metatarsal head becomes more prominent and the metatarsal is said to be in an adducted position as it moves towards the midline of the body.[1] Radiological criteria for hallux valgus vary, but a commonly accepted criterion is to measure the angle formed between the metatarsal and the abducted hallux. This is called the metatarsophalangeal joint angle or hallux abductus angle and it is considered abnormal when it is greater than 14.5°.[2] **Bunion** is the lay term used to describe a prominent and often inflamed metatarsal head and overlying bursa. Symptoms include pain, limitation in walking, and problems with wearing normal shoes.

INCIDENCE/PREVALENCE The prevalence of hallux valgus varies in different populations. In a recent study of 6000 UK school children aged 9–10 years, 2.5% had clinical evidence of hallux valgus, and 2% met both clinical and radiological criteria for hallux valgus. An earlier study found hallux valgus in 48% of adults.[2] Differences in prevalence may result from different methods of measurement, varying age groups, or different diagnostic criteria (e.g. metatarsal joint angle > 10° or > 15°).[3]

AETIOLOGY/RISK FACTORS Nearly all population studies have found that hallux valgus is more common in women. Footwear may contribute to the deformity, but studies comparing people who wear shoes with those who do not have found contradictory results. Hypermobility of the first ray(G) and excessive foot pronation are associated with hallux valgus.[4]

PROGNOSIS We found no studies that looked at the progression of hallux valgus. While progression of deformity and symptoms is rapid in some people, others remain asymptomatic. One study found that hallux valgus is often unilateral initially, but usually progresses to bilateral deformity.[2]

AIMS OF INTERVENTION To reduce symptoms and deformity, with minimum adverse effects.

OUTCOMES Hallux abductus/metatarsophalangeal joint angle; intermetatarsal joint angle; range of motion of the first metatarsophalangeal joint (the total range of both dorsiflexion and plantarflexion); incidence of complications such as infection; reoperation; non-union; avascular necrosis; pain; general satisfaction and satisfaction with appearance; requirement for specialist or extra-width footwear; proportion of people with mobility problems; time to healing; development of transfer lesionsⒼ; and adverse effects of treatment.

METHODS *Clinical Evidence* search and appraisal June 2004. An electronic search using a strategy developed by the Cochrane Musculoskeletal Injuries Group was undertaken to October 2003 and a hand search of podiatry journals to October 2003.

QUESTION What are the effects of conservative treatments?

OPTION ORTHOSES

One RCT in children found that antipronatory orthoses increased deterioration in metatarsophalangeal joint angles after 3 years compared with no treatment, although the difference was not statistically significant. One RCT in adults with hallux valgus found that orthoses reduced pain compared with no treatment at 6 months but not at 1 year and that orthoses were less effective at improving outcomes than chevron osteotomy.

Benefits: We found one systematic review (search date 2003).[5] It identified two RCTs.[2,6] **In children:** The first RCT compared antipronatory orthosesⒼ versus no treatment in 122 children aged 9–10 years (13% of whom were boys) with metatarsophalangeal joint angles greater than 14.5° in one or both feet (see comment below).[2] On the basis of a clinical examination, 150 children were selected for x ray examination, and 122 of these children (13% of whom were boys) who were found to have metatarsophalangeal joint angles greater than 14.5° in one or both feet were subsequently included in the trial (see comment below). The RCT found that the metatarsophalangeal joint angles deteriorated both with orthoses and with no treatment, and found that the deterioration was greater in children treated with orthoses, although this difference was not significant after 3 years (analysis not by intention to treat; no direct statistical comparisons reported).[2] **In adults:** The second RCT (209 adults) compared three treatments: chevron osteotomyⒼ, orthoses, and no treatment (see benefits of chevron osteotomy, p 1381).[6] The RCT found that orthoses significantly reduced pain intensity after 6 months compared with no treatment (pain intensity on visual analogue scale with range 0 [no pain] to 100 [unbearable pain]; pain score: 36 with orthoses *v* 45 with no treatment; difference adjusted for baseline characteristics: –14, 95% CI –22 to –6), but found no significant difference in pain intensity after 12 months (mean pain score: 40 with orthoses *v* 40 with no treatment; difference adjusted for baseline characteristics: –6, 95% CI –15 to +3). The RCT also found that orthoses significantly improved "global assessment" (not further defined in the paper) compared with no treatment but found no significant difference in satisfaction or functional assessment scores (American Orthopoedic Foot and Ankle Score [AOFASⒼ]) after 12 months (proportion with improved global assessment: 46% with orthoses *v* 24% with no treatment; RR adjusted for baseline characteristics: 0.38, 95% CI 0.18 to 0.78; satisfaction on visual analogue scale with range 0 [totally unsatisfied] to 100 [totally satisfied]: 70 with orthoses *v* 61 with no treatment; difference adjusted for baseline characteristics: +9, 95% CI –1 to +20; AOFAS: 64 with orthosis *v* 66 with no treatment; difference adjusted for baseline characteristics: 0, 95% CI –4 to +5). It also found no significant difference between orthoses and no treatment in the duration of the pain, ability to work, and cosmetic disturbance.[6] For a description of the results of the comparison of orthoses versus chevron osteotomy in this RCT (see benefits of chevron osteotomy, p 1381).

Harms: The RCT in children did not report on harms.[2] The RCT in adults reported no complications with orthoses (see harms of chevron osteotomy, p 1381).

Comment: The use of antipronatory orthoses**G** in children is questionable because earlier studies have found that hallux valgus in children is not related to pronation but arises from positional changes in the first ray**G**.[7] The first RCT reported that 29/122 (25%) children (mainly from the control group) were lost to follow up.[2]

OPTION NIGHT SPLINTS

One systematic review found no reliable RCTs comparing night splints with any other or no treatment.

Benefits: We found one systematic review (search date 2003), which identified no RCTs that met *Clinical Evidence* inclusion criteria.

Harms: We found no RCTs.

Comment: None.

QUESTION What are the effects of surgery?

OPTION KELLER'S ARTHROPLASTY

We found no RCTs comparing Keller's arthroplasty versus no treatment. One systematic review found insufficient evidence from limited RCTs on the effects of Keller's arthroplasty compared with other types of operation.

Benefits: We found one systematic review (search date 2003, 3 relevant RCTs; see comment below).[5] **Versus no treatment:** The review included no RCTs. **Versus distal osteotomy:** The review included one RCT (33 people) comparing distal metatarsal osteotomy versus Keller's arthroplasty**G**.[8] The RCT found that osteotomy significantly improved both intermetatarsal angle and range of movement compared with Keller's arthroplasty but found no significant difference in proportion with unresolved pain or dissatisfaction after 3 years (intermetatarsal angle: 12.0° with Keller's arthroplasty *v* 7.0° with distal osteotomy; difference: –5.0°, 95% CI –8.9° to –1.1°; reduction in range of movement: 14.0° with Keller's arthroplasty *v* 1.0° with distal osteotomy; difference: 13.0°, 95% CI 5.0° to 21.1°; proportion with unresolved pain: 4/14 [29%] with Keller's arthroplasty *v* 4/15 [27%] with distal osteotomy; OR 0.91, 95% CI 0.18 to 4.64; proportion dissatisfied: 4/14 [29%] with Keller's arthroplasty *v* 4/15 [27%] with distal osteotomy; OR 0.91, 95% CI 0.18 to 4.64). **Versus arthrodesis:** The second RCT included in the review (100 people) found that Keller's arthroplasty significantly reduced the proportion of people with reduced mobility compared with arthrodesis**G**, but found no significant difference in the proportion with unresolved pain or dissatisfaction after 2 years (proportion with reduced mobility: 4/44 [9%] with Keller's arthroplasty *v* 11/37 [30%] with arthrodesis; OR 0.24, 95% CI 0.07 to 0.82; proportion with unresolved pain: 5/44 [11%] with Keller's osteotomy *v* 4/37 [11%] with osteotomy; OR 1.05, 95% CI 0.26 to 4.35; proportion dissatisfied: 11/44 [25%] with Keller's osteotomy *v* 10/37 [27%] with arthrodesis; OR 0.90, 95% CI 0.33 to 2.44).[9] **Plus joint distraction:** The third RCT (35 people) included in the review found that a Kirschner wire**G** to distract the joint during healing after Keller's arthroplasty significantly improved subjective assessment scores for symptoms after a minimum of 1 year compared with Keller's arthroplasty with no wire (assessment scale of 1 = constant pain to 4 = no symptoms; no actual scores provided; $P < 0.05$), but found no significant difference in the hallux abductus angle, pain, or movement after a minimum of 1 year (hallux valgus angle: 21° for both groups, no P value reported; no data reported for pain or movement).[10]

Harms: Reduced toe function has been described after Keller's procedure.[5] The systematic review reported high levels of patient dissatisfaction (up to 29%) in most trials.[5] **Versus arthrodesis:** The RCT did not present complete data for complications, but reported that cock-up deformity**G** was more common in the Keller's group (25/44 people) than the arthrodesis group (11/37), although this difference was not significant.[9] **Versus distal osteotomy:** The RCT found no significant difference in the incidence of postoperative superficial wound infections between groups (3/14 in the Keller's group *v* 1/15 in the osteotomy group; OR 3.85, 95% CI 0.35 to 50.00).[8] **Plus joint distraction:** In the RCT examining the effects of joint distraction**G** after Keller's arthrodesis, one participant in each group had delayed wound healing.[10]

Comment: Both the RCT comparing Keller's arthroplasty versus arthrodesis and the RCT looking at the effects of joint distraction included people with hallux rigidus. Most of the people included in the review having surgery were under 50 years of age and were followed up for no more than 3 years.[5] Longer term outcomes remain unclear. The RCTs reported results for numbers of feet, and did not always report standard deviations of the results. The systematic review analysed the results by numbers of people.[5]

OPTION CHEVRON OSTEOTOMY

One systematic review found conflicting evidence on the effects of chevron osteotomy compared with other metatarsal osteotomies. One RCT found that chevron osteotomy improved outcomes compared with orthoses or no treatment after 1 year. One systematic review found no evidence that adductor tenotomy plus chevron osteotomy improved outcomes compared with chevron osteotomy alone. One systematic review identified one small RCT comparing chevron osteotomy plus Akin osteotomy and Akin osteotomy plus distal soft tissue reconstruction, which found no significant difference in outcomes between treatments at 1 year. However, this trial may have lacked power to detect a clinically significant difference.

Benefits: **Versus no treatment or versus orthoses:** We found one systematic review (search date 2003, 1 RCT,[6] 209 people).[6] The RCT compared three treatments: chevron osteotomy**G**, orthoses, and no treatment (see benefits of orthoses, p 1379).[6] It found that chevron osteotomy significantly reduced pain intensity and significantly improved cosmetic appearance and functional status compared with no treatment at 1 year (mean pain intensity on a visual analogue scale from 0 [no pain] to 100 [unbearable pain]: 23 with chevron osteotomy *v* 40 with no treatment; difference adjusted for baseline characteristics: –19, 95% CI –28 to –10; mean cosmetic appearance on a 7 point scale ranging from 0 [no cosmetic disturbance] to 6 [maximal cosmetic disturbance]: 1.9 with chevron osteotomy *v* 2.8 with no treatment; difference adjusted for baseline characteristics: –1.2, 95% CI –1.8 to –0.6; mean functional status [AOFAS**G**]: 75 with chevron osteotomy *v* 66 with no treatment; difference adjusted for baseline characteristics: 11, 95% CI 7 to

16). It found no significant difference in the ability to work after 1 year (ability to work on a visual analogue scale from 0 [total inability to work] to 100 [maximal working ability]: 89 with chevron osteotomy *v* 83 with no treatment; difference adjusted for baseline characteristics: +4, 95% CI –3 to +11). The RCT also found that chevron osteotomy significantly reduced pain intensity and significantly improved cosmetic appearance and functional status compared with orthoses, but found no significant difference in the ability to work after 1 year (pain intensity on a visual analogue score ranging from 0 [no pain] to 100 [unbearable pain]: 23 with chevron osteotomy *v* 40 with orthosis; difference adjusted for baseline characteristics: –14, 95% CI –22 to –5; cosmetic appearance on a 7 point scale ranging from 0 [no cosmetic disturbance] to 6 [maximal cosmetic disturbance]: 1.9 with chevron osteotomy *v* 2.6 with orthosis; difference adjusted for baseline characteristics: –1.4, 95% CI –2.1 to –0.8; functional status [AOFAS]: 75 with chevron osteotomy *v* 64 with orthosis; difference adjusted for baseline characteristics: 11, 95% CI 7 to 15; ability to work on a visual analogue scale from 0 [total inability to work] to 100 [maximal working ability]: 89 with chevron osteotomy *v* 81 with orthosis; difference adjusted for baseline characteristics: 6, 95% CI 0 to 13). **Proximal chevron osteotomy versus other types of proximal osteotomy:** We found one systematic review (search date 2003, 1 RCT that met *Clinical Evidence* inclusion criteria, 66 people).[5] The RCT (66 people) included in the review found no significant difference between proximal chevron osteotomy and proximal crescentic osteotomy**G** in the hallux abductus angle, intermetatarsal angle, transfer lesions**G**, or functional assessment score (AOFAS) after 22 months.[11] It found that proximal chevron osteotomy significantly reduced healing time compared with proximal crescentic osteotomy ($P < 0.001$) and significantly reduced postoperative dorsiflexion at the healed site ($P = 0.005$). **Distal chevron osteotomy versus proximal osteotomy:** We found one systematic review (search date 2003, 1 RCT, 68 people).[5] The RCT found that distal chevron osteotomy significantly improved the hallux abductus and intermetatarsal angle compared with proximal osteotomy. It found no significant difference in the proportion of participants experiencing pain, dissatisfaction with treatment, problems with footwear, or mobility between proximal osteotomy and distal chevron osteotomy after 2 years (OR for remaining in pain: 0.55, 95% CI 0.13 to 2.42; AR for dissatisfaction with outcome: 33% with both treatments; OR 0.99, 95% CI 0.36 to 2.75; OR for needing specialist footwear: 0.38, 95% CI 0.04 to 3.83; OR for reduced mobility: 0.38, 95% CI 0.04 to 3.83; all ORs for proximal osteotomy *v* chevron osteotomy).[12] Proximal osteotomy significantly improved hallux abductus angle and intermetatarsal angle compared with distal chevron osteotomy at 2 years (hallux abductus angle: 25.0° with chevron osteotomy *v* 20.0° with proximal osteotomy; difference: 5.0°, 95% CI 0.5° to 9.5°; intermetatarsal angle: 13.0° with chevron osteotomy *v* 10.0° with proximal osteotomy; difference: 3.0°, 95% CI 1.0° to 5.0°). **Distal chevron osteotomy versus other types of distal osteotomy:** We found one systematic review (search date 2003, 1 RCT, 51 people).[5] The RCT found that Wilson osteotomy**G** significantly improved the hallux abductus angle compared with chevron osteotomy but found no significant difference in problems with footwear or mobility after 38 months (hallux abductus angle: 25.7° with chevron osteotomy *v* 13.3° with Wilson osteotomy; difference: +12.4°, 95% CI +7.5° to +17.5°; footwear problems: 8/24 [33%] with chevron osteotomy *v* 3/26 [12%] with Wilson osteotomy; OR 3.85, 95% CI 0.87 to 16.67; limited walking: 5/24 [21%] with chevron osteotomy *v* 4/26 [15%] with Wilson osteotomy; OR 1.45, 95% CI 0.34 to 6.25).[13] **Plus adductor tenotomy:** We found one systematic review (search date 2003, 1 relevant RCT, 84 people).[5] The RCT included in the review found no significant difference in hallux abductus angle, range of motion, pain, patient satisfaction, people requiring special footwear, and mobility between chevron osteotomy plus adductor tenotomy and chevron osteotomy alone (final hallux abductus angle: 20.2° with chevron osteotomy plus adductor tenotomy *v* 23.5° with chevron osteotomy alone; mean difference: –3.3°, 95% CI –8.63° to +2.03°; range of motion: 69° with chevron osteotomy plus adductor tenotomy *v* 67° with chevron osteotomy alone; mean difference: +2°, 95% CI –2.7° to +6.73°; people remaining in pain: 8/38 [21%] with chevron osteotomy plus adductor tenotomy *v* 6/46 [13%] with chevron osteotomy alone; OR 1.78, 95% CI 0.56 to 5.67; people remaining dissatisfied: 10/38 [26%] with chevron osteotomy plus adductor tenotomy *v* 7/46 [15%] with chevron osteotomy alone; OR 1.99, 95% CI 0.68 to 5.87; people requiring special footwear: 2/38 [5%] with chevron osteotomy plus adductor tenotomy *v* 7/46 [15%] with chevron osteotomy alone; OR 0.31, 95% CI 0.06 to 1.59; people with reduced mobility: 1/38 [3%] with chevron osteotomy plus adductor tenotomy *v* 1/46 [2%] with chevron osteotomy alone; OR 1.22, 95% CI 0.07 to 20.12).[14] **Plus Akin osteotomy:** We found one systematic review (search date 2003, 1 RCT, 23 people; see comment below).[5] The RCT compared Akin osteotomy**G** plus chevron osteotomy versus Akin osteotomy plus distal soft tissue reconstruction (DSTR**G**).[15] It found no significant difference in hallux abductus angle, intermetatarsal angle, or range of toe motion between the two treatment options after a minimum of 1 year (hallux abductus angle: 12.5° with chevron osteotomy plus Akin osteotomy *v* 17° with DSTR plus Akin osteotomy; mean difference: +4.5°, 95% CI –5.77° to +14.72°; intermetatarsal angle: 7° with chevron osteotomy plus Akin osteotomy *v* 10° with DSTR plus Akin osteotomy; mean difference: +3°, 95% CI –1.45° to +7.45°; range of toe motion: mean difference: –3°, 95% CI –12.07° to +6.07°). However, this trial may have lacked power to detect a clinically important significant difference.

Harms: Complications were reported by most of the RCTs. **Versus no treatment or versus orthoses:** The RCT comparing chevron osteotomy**G**, orthoses, and no treatment reported complications in 4/71 (6%) people undergoing chevron osteotomy (complications consisted of one wound infection, one stress fracture, one episode of nerve damage, and one recurrence of deformity).[6] The RCT reported no complications associated with orthoses. **Versus other metatarsal osteotomies:** The RCT comparing proximal crescentic osteotomy**G** versus proximal chevron osteotomy found one case of delayed wound healing in the chevron group and two cases in the proximal osteotomy group. Eight further people experienced complications, although the authors did not state which group they belonged to.[11] The RCT comparing proximal osteotomy and chevron osteotomy reported one wound infection and two stress fractures in people undergoing chevron osteotomy and 11 complications in people undergoing proximal osteotomy, consisting mostly of pain in other areas of the forefoot (metatarsalgia).[12] The RCT comparing Wilson osteotomy**G** versus chevron osteotomy found no significant difference in the proportion with complications (11/26 [42%] with Wilson osteotomy *v* 9/24 [38%] with chevron osteotomy; RR 1.30, 95% CI 0.57 to 2.24).[13] Complications included swelling, over correction, slow healing, and recurrence of bunion. Transfer pain**G** and lesions**G** were recurring problems in both groups. The RCT found that although Wilson osteotomy resulted in a significantly shortened metatarsal compared with chevron osteotomy ($P = 0.02$), with metatarsal dorsiflexion in 20% of people, this change in position did not correlate with development of new corns, callous, or pain. **Plus adductor tenotomy:** In the RCT that compared chevron osteotomy plus adductor tenotomy versus chevron osteotomy alone, about 25% of both groups remained dissatisfied during follow up.[14] This may be related to greater postoperative reduction in the circumference of the ball of the foot; the RCT found that the ball circumference of dissatisfied people was significantly greater than that of satisfied people (P = 0.005). **Plus Akin osteotomy:** The RCT reported two complications with Akin osteotomy plus chevron osteotomy (one non-union and one where a transfer lesion developed, resulting in further surgery) and one complication with Akin osteotomy plus distal soft tissue reconstruction (nerve damage in the great toe).[15]

Comment: None of the RCTs included long term follow up. The RCT comparing chevron osteotomy**G** plus Akin osteotomy**G** with Akin osteotomy plus distal soft tissue reconstruction**G** was poorly randomised and seems to comprise a subset of data from a larger RCT.[15]

OPTION DIFFERENT METHODS OF BONE FIXATION

One small RCT identified by a systematic review found no significant difference between standard fixation and absorbable pin fixation in clinical or radiological outcomes; however, it may have lacked power to detect a clinically significant difference. A second small RCT identified by the review found that screw fixation plus early weight bearing reduced time to return to work and social activity compared with suture fixation and later weight bearing, but found no significant difference in radiological outcomes.

Benefits: We found one systematic review (search date 2003, 2 RCTs, 58 people).[5] Both trials compared different methods of bone fixation after Mitchell's osteotomy**G**.[16,17] The first RCT (28 people, 39 feet; see comment below) found no significant difference between a standard method of fixation and absorbable pin fixation in clinical or radiological outcomes after a mean follow up of 11 months (range 2–24 months; range of movement: 61.2° with standard fixation *v* 69.2° with absorbable pin fixation; mean difference: +8.0°, 95% CI –7.3° to +23.6°; people remaining in pain on walking: 1/17 [5.9%] with standard fixation *v* 2/21 [9.5%] absorbable pin fixation; P = 0.58; people with marked walking limitation: 1/17 [5.9%] with standard fixation *v* 1/21 [4.8%] with absorbable pin fixation; P = 0.24; people dissatisfied with cosmetic appearance: 1/17 [5.9%] with standard fixation *v* 3/21 [14.3%] with absorbable pin fixation; P = 0.38; radiological outcomes: hallux abductus angle: 15.8° with standard fixation *v* 18.2° with absorbable pin fixation; mean difference: +2.40°, 95% CI –4.81° to +9.61°; intermetatarsal angle: 9.1° with standard fixation *v* 9.4° with absorbable pin fixation; mean difference: +0.3°, 95% CI –1.77° to +2.37°).[16] The second RCT (30 people) compared screw fixation followed by early weight bearing in a plaster shoe versus vicryl suture fixation followed by 6 weeks of non-weight bearing in a plaster boot.[17] It found that screw fixation followed by early weight bearing in a plaster shoe significantly reduced time taken to return to social activities and time taken to return to work, but found no significant difference in radiological outcomes after 6 months (social activities: mean 2.9 weeks with screw fixation *v* 5.7 weeks with suture fixation; P < 0.001; work: mean 4.9 weeks with screw fixation *v* 8.7 weeks with suture fixation; P < 0.001; radiological: hallux abductus angle 10.8° with suture fixation *v* 12° with screw fixation; mean difference: +1.2°, 95% CI –2.35° to +4.75°; intermetatarsal angle: 9.1° with suture fixation *v* 10.7° with screw fixation; mean difference: +1.6°, 95% CI –0.56° to +3.76°).[17]

Harms: The first RCT (28 people, 39 feet) reported more complications with standard compared with pin fixation, although the difference was not significant (14/17 [82%] feet *v* 16/22 [73%] feet; RR 1.13, 95% CI 0.81 to 1.59).[16] Complications included recurrence of deformity (3/17 [18%] feet *v* 2/22 [9%] feet), problems primarily resulting in pain

(5/17 [29%] feet *v* 6/22 [27%] feet), and continued swelling (3/17 [18%] feet *v* 0/22 [0%] feet). In the RCT (30 people) of screw fixation compared with suture fixation, 2/15 (13%) people had the screw removed because of pain.[17] The RCT reported that superficial infection occurred in three people overall (2 with screw fixation *v* 1 with suture fixation) and also found that fixation followed by early weight bearing in a plaster shoe significantly increased metatarsophalangeal joint stiffness after both 3 and 6 months.

Comment: Applicability of the results from the first RCT may be limited, as people were used as the unit of randomisation and feet as the unit of statistical analysis.[16] In addition, the first RCT was small and may have lacked power to detect clinically significant differences between treatments.

QUESTION What are the effects of postoperative care?

OPTION CONTINUOUS PASSIVE MOTION

One systematic review provided insufficient evidence on the effects of continuous passive motion.

Benefits: We found one systematic review (search date 2003, 1 relevant RCT, 39 people).[5] The RCT included in the review found no significant difference in the range of motion or time taken to return to normal footwear between continuous passive motion plus physiotherapy and physiotherapy alone (range of motion: 9.3° with continuous passive motion plus physiotherapy *v* 2.6° with physiotherapy alone; mean difference: −6.7°, 95% CI −13.6° to +0.3°; time to return to normal footwear: no AR provided; $P < 0.01$).

Harms: No complications were reported by the RCT.[5]

Comment: None.

OPTION EARLY WEIGHT BEARING

One systematic review provided insufficient evidence on the effects of early weight bearing.

Benefits: We found one systematic review (search date 2003, 1 relevant RCT, 56 people).[5] The RCT compared early weight bearing (initial weight bearing in a cast from 2–4 weeks after the operation) with late weight bearing (initial weight bearing 4 weeks after the operation).[5] It found no significant difference in rates of non-union at the site of arthrodesis**G** (1/29 [3%] with early weight bearing *v* 2/27 [7%] with late weight bearing; RR 0.46, 95% CI 0.05 to 4.85).

Harms: See benefits above.

Comment: The only outcome assessed by the RCT was non-union at the site of arthrodesis.[5]

OPTION SLIPPER CASTS

One systematic review provided insufficient evidence on the effects of plaster slipper casts.

Benefits: We found one systematic review (search date 2003, 2 RCTs, 106 people).[5] The first RCT (54 feet) compared a plaster slipper cast versus a crepe bandage after a Wilson osteotomy**G**.[18] Cast and dressings were changed 12 days after surgery and then kept on for a further 4 weeks.

The RCT found no significant difference between the plaster slipper and the crepe bandage in pain at 3 months, or time to return to normal activities (pain measured on a visual analogue scale: higher score = more painful, lower score = less painful, scale endpoints not stated; pain at 3 months: 1.5 with plaster slipper *v* 1.6 with crepe bandage; time to return to normal activities: 6.2 weeks with plaster slipper *v* 6.6 weeks with crepe bandage; P values not stated for either comparison). The second RCT (52 feet) compared a plaster slipper versus a crepe bandage after first metatarsophalangeal joint fusion.[19] Casts and dressings were changed 12 days after surgery and then kept on for a further 4 weeks. It found no significant difference between the plaster slipper and the crepe bandage in improvement in hallux valgus angle at 6 weeks postoperatively (mean change in hallux valgus angle: –13.4° with plaster slipper *v* –12.8° with crepe bandage; P value not reported).

Harms: The first RCT found that one failed union occurred with crepe bandaging and that two people receiving plaster slipper cast treatment developed superficial wound infections.[18] The second RCT found three failed corrections, four non-unions, and two wound infections in the plaster slipper group and one failed correction, one non-union, and two wound infections in the crepe bandage group.[19]

Comment: Both RCTs were small and may have lacked power to detect clinically significant differences between the groups.[18,19]

GLOSSARY

Akin osteotomy A procedure involving resection of the medial prominence of the first metatarsal head and a medial wedge osteotomy of the proximal phalanx of the great toe.

Antipronatory orthoses Insoles designed to reduce the amount of in-roll or flattening of the foot when walking.

AOFAS score American Orthopaedic Foot and Ankle Society functional assessment score, ranging from 0 to 100, higher scores indicating better functional ability.

Arthrodesis The joint between adjoining bones is removed by fusing the bone ends together. No movement can then occur at the joint.

Chevron osteotomy A v-shaped wedge of bone is removed from the distal end of the metatarsal shaft, allowing the metatarsal head to be realigned on the shaft. The wedge can be removed either at the distal (distal chevron osteotomy) or proximal (proximal chevron osteotomy) end of the bone.

Cock-up deformity Inability to place pulp of the great toe on the ground with the foot weight bearing.

Distal soft tissue reconstruction A procedure involving the release of various ligaments, the capsule, and tendons around the first metatarsophalangeal joint.

First ray The first metatarsal and medial cuneiform function as a single unit called the first ray.

Joint distraction Operation in which the bone ends are held apart after the operation so that fusion of the bone ends does not occur.

Keller's arthroplasty A procedure involving removal of the medial side of the metatarsal head and straight resection of the base of the proximal phalanx.

Kirschner wire A thin but rigid wire that is used to fix bone fragments. It is passed through drilled channels in the bone (sometimes called a K-wire).

Mitchell's osteotomy A form of distal metatarsal osteotomy, whereby an incomplete osteotomy is performed perpendicular to the long axis of the bone. The distal portion is moved laterally and fixed in position. This results in shortening of the bone.

Proximal crescentic osteotomy A curved cut is made across the base of the metatarsal shaft. The distal portion of bone is slid across the proximal end of bone and fixed into a corrected position.

Transfer lesions Areas of corns or callus that develop when the weight bearing forces are transferred from one area of the foot to another.

Transfer pain Refers to pain that occurs in another area of the foot after surgery. It usually occurs in the second/third metatarsal heads after the surgeon has altered the first metatarsal head.

Wilson osteotomy A double oblique cut is made in the distal portion of the metatarsal shaft and the metatarsal head is slid into a corrected position.

REFERENCES

1. Dykyj D. Pathological anatomy of hallux abducto valgus. *Clin Podiatr Med Surg* 1989;6:1–15.
2. Kilmartin TE, Barrington RL, Wallace WA. A controlled prospective trial of a foot orthosis for juvenile hallux valgus. *J Bone Joint Surg Br* 1994;76:210–214.
3. Morris JB, Brash LF, Hird MD. Chiropodial survey of geriatric and psychiatric hospital in-patients – Angus District. *Chiropodist* 1980;April:128–139.
4. LaPorta G, Melillo T, Olinsky D. X-ray evaluation of hallux abducto valgus deformity. *J Am Podiatr Med Assoc* 1974;64:544–566.
5. Ferrari J, Higgins JPT, Prior TD. Interventions for treating hallux valgus (abductovalgus) and bunions. In: The Cochrane Library, Issue 3, 2004. Chichester, UK: John Wiley & Sons, Ltd. Search date 2003; primary sources Medline, Embase, Cinahl, Amed, Cochrane Controlled Trials Register, Cochrane Musculoskeletal Injuries Trials Register, bibliographies of identified trials, and hand searches of podiatry journals.
6. Torkki M, Malmivaara A, Seitsalo S, et al. Surgery vs orthosis vs watchful waiting for hallux valgus. A randomized controlled trial. *JAMA* 2001;285:2474–2480.
7. Kilmartin TE, Wallace WA, Hill TW. First metatarsal position in juvenile hallux abductovalgus — a significant clinical measurement? *Br J Podiatr Med* 1991;3:43–45.
8. Turnbull T, Grange W. A comparison of Keller's arthroplasty and distal metatarsal osteotomy in the treatment of adult hallux valgus. *J Bone Joint Surg Br* 1986;68:132–137.
9. O'Doherty PD, Lowrie IG, Magnussen PA, et al. The management of the painful first metatarsophalangeal joint in the older patient. Arthrodesis or Keller's arthroplasty? *J Bone Joint Surgery Br* 1990;72:839–842.
10. Sherman KP, Douglas DL, Benson MK. Keller's arthroplasty: is distraction useful? A prospective trial. *J Bone Joint Surgery Br* 1984;66:765–769.
11. Easley ME, Kiebzak GM, Davis WH, et al. Prospective, randomized comparison of proximal crescentric and proximal chevron osteotomies for correction of hallux valgus deformity. *Foot Ankle Int* 1996;17:307–316.
12. Resch S, Stenstrom A, Jonsson K, et al. Results after chevron osteotomy and proximal osteotomy for hallux valgus: a prospective, randomised study. *Foot* 1993;3:99–104.
13. Klosok IK, Pring DJ, Jessop JH, et al. Chevron or Wilson metatarsal osteotomy for hallux valgus. A prospective randomised trial. *J Bone Joint Surg Br* 1993;75:825–829.
14. Resch S, Stenstrom A, Reynisson K, et al. Chevron osteotomy for hallux valgus not improved by additional adductor tenotomy. A prospective, randomised study of 84 patients. *Acta Orthop Scand* 1994;65:541–544.
15. Basile A, Battaglia A, Campi A. Comparison of chevron–Akin osteotomy and distal soft tissue reconstruction–Akin osteotomy for correction of mild hallux valgus. *Foot Ankle Surg* 2000;6:155–163.
16. Prior TD, Grace DL, MacLean JB, et al. Correction of hallux abductovalgus by Mitchell's osteotomy: comparing standard fixation methods with absorbable polydioxanone pins. *Foot* 1997;7:121–125.
17. Calder JDF, Hollingdale JP, Pearse MF. Screw versus suture fixation of Mitchell's osteotomy. A prospective randomised study. *J Bone Joint Surg Br* 1999;81:621–624.
18. Meek RMD, Anderson EG. Plaster slipper versus crepe bandage after Wilson's osteotomy for hallux valgus. *Foot* 1999;9:138–141.
19. Meek RMD, Anderson EG. Plaster slipper versus crepe bandage after first metatarsophalangeal joint fusion. *Foot Ankle Surg* 1998;4:213–217.

Jill Ferrari
School of Health and Bioscience
University of East London
London
UK

Competing interests: None declared.

Carpal tunnel syndrome

Search date January 2004

Nigel Ashworth

QUESTIONS

INTERVENTIONS

See glossary Ⓖ

Key Messages

Drug treatment

- **Local corticosteroid injection (short term)** Two small RCTs found that local corticosteroid injection (methylprednisone, hydrocortisone) improved symptoms after 4–6 weeks compared with placebo or no treatment. One small RCT found that local betamethasone injection improved symptoms after 1 month compared with betamethasone injection into the deltoid. One small RCT found no significant difference between local methylprednisone injection and oral prednisone in symptoms after 2 weeks, but found that local methylprednisone injection improved symptoms after 8 and 12 weeks.
- **Oral corticosteroids (short term)** Three small RCTs found that oral prednisone improved symptoms after 2 weeks, and two of the three RCTs found the improvement was maintained at 4–8 weeks. We found no RCTs that measured the effects of oral corticosteroids on symptoms in the longer term. One small RCT found no significant difference in symptoms at 2 weeks between local methylprednisone injection and oral prednisone, but found that local methylprednisone injection improved symptoms after 8 and 12 weeks. One RCT found that oral prednisone reduced symptoms compared with a non-steroidal anti-inflammatory drug (tenoxicam) and with a diuretic (trichlormethiazide) after 4 weeks.

- **Non-steroidal anti-inflammatory drugs** One small RCT found no significant difference between tenoxicam and placebo in symptoms after 2 or 4 weeks. However, the RCT may have lacked power to detect a clinically important difference One RCT found that oral prednisone reduced symptoms compared with a non-steroidal anti-inflammatory drug (tenoxicam) after 4 weeks. One RCT found no significant difference in symptoms between a diuretic (trichlormethiazide) and a non-steroidal anti-inflammatory drug (tenoxicam) at 4 weeks.
- **Pyridoxine** One small RCT found a similar improvement in symptoms with pyridoxine compared with placebo or no treatment after 10 weeks. The RCT may have been too small to detect a clinically important difference between treatments. One small RCT found no significant difference between pyridoxine and placebo in nocturnal pain, numbness, or tingling after 12 weeks.
- **Local corticosteroid injection (long term); oral corticosteroids (long term)** We found no RCTs on the effects of these interventions.
- **Diuretics** One small RCT found no significant difference between trichlormethiazide and placebo in symptoms after 2 or 4 weeks. One RCT found no significant difference between bendrofluazide and placebo in the proportion of people with no improvement in symptoms after 4 weeks. One RCT found no significant difference in symptoms between a diuretic (trichlormethiazide) and a non-steroidal anti-inflammatory drug (tenoxicam) at 4 weeks. One RCT found that oral prednisone reduced symptoms compared with a diuretic (trichlormethiazide) after 4 weeks.

Non-drug treatment

- **Nerve and tendon gliding exercises** One small RCT found no significant difference between nerve and tendon gliding exercises plus neutral angle wrist splint and neutral angle wrist splint alone in symptom severity or function 8 weeks after the end of 4 weeks of treatment.
- **Therapeutic ultrasound** One RCT found that ultrasound increased the proportion of wrists with satisfactory improvement or complete remission of symptoms after 6 months compared with placebo. One RCT found no significant difference in symptom severity between high or low intensity ultrasound compared with placebo after 2 weeks.
- **Wrist splints** One RCT found that a nocturnal hand brace improved symptoms after 2 and 4 weeks compared with no treatment. One small RCT found no significant difference in symptoms after 2 weeks between neutral angle compared with 20° extension wrist splinting. One small RCT found no significant difference in symptoms at 6 weeks between full time compared with night time only neutral angle wrist splinting.

Surgical treatment

- **Endoscopic carpal tunnel release versus open carpal tunnel release** One systematic review and subsequent RCTs found no consistent difference in symptoms up to 12 months after surgery or time taken to return to work between endoscopic and open carpal tunnel release. Harms resulting from endoscopic and open carpal tunnel release vary between RCTs. One systematic review and two RCTs comparing the interventions suggests that endoscopic carpal tunnel release may cause more transient nerve problems, whereas open carpal tunnel release may cause more wound problems.
- **Surgery versus placebo or non-surgical intervention** We found no RCTs comparing surgery with placebo. One small RCT identified by a systematic review and one subsequent RCT found that surgery increased symptom resolution compared with splinting at 12–15 months. One systematic review and five subsequent RCTs provided no clear evidence of a difference in symptoms or time taken to return to work between endoscopic and open carpal tunnel release up to 12 months after the operation. Harms resulting from endoscopic and open carpal tunnel release vary among RCTs. One systematic review and two RCTs comparing the interventions suggests that endoscopic carpal tunnel release may cause more transient nerve problems, whereas open carpal tunnel release may cause more wound problems.

- **Internal neurolysis in conjunction with open carpal tunnel release** RCTs identified by a systematic review found no significant difference in symptoms between open carpal tunnel release alone and open carpal tunnel release plus internal neurolysis in symptoms.

Postoperative treatment

- **Wrist splints after carpal tunnel release surgery** Two RCTs in people after carpal tunnel release surgery found no significant difference between wrist splinting and no splinting in grip strength or in the proportion of people who considered themselves "cured" at 2–4 weeks. A third RCT found that splinting increased pain at 1 month and the time to return to work compared with no splinting.

DEFINITION Carpal tunnel syndrome is a neuropathy caused by compression of the median nerve within the carpal tunnel.[1] Classical symptoms of carpal tunnel syndrome include numbness, tingling, burning, or pain in at least two of the three digits supplied by the median nerve (i.e. the thumb, index, and middle fingers).[2] The American Academy of Neurology has described diagnostic criteria Ⓖ that rely on a combination of symptoms and physical examination findings.[3] Other diagnostic criteria include results from electrophysiological studies.[2]

INCIDENCE/ PREVALENCE A general population survey in Rochester, Minnesota, found the age adjusted incidence of carpal tunnel syndrome to be 105 (95% CI 99 to 112) cases per 100 000 person years.[4,5] Age adjusted incidence rates were 52 (95% CI 45 to 59) cases for men and 149 (95% CI 138 to 159) cases for women per 100 000 person years. The study found incidence rates increased from 88 (95% CI 75 to 101) cases per 100 000 person years in 1961–1965 to 125 (95% CI 112 to 138) cases per 100 000 person years in 1976–1980. Incidence rates of carpal tunnel syndrome increased with age for men, whereas for women they peaked between the ages of 45–54 years. A general population survey in the Netherlands found prevalence to be 1% for men and 7% for women.[6] A more comprehensive study in southern Sweden found the general population prevalence for carpal tunnel syndrome was 3% (95% CI 2% to 3%).[7] As in other studies, the overall prevalence in women was higher than in men (male to female ratio 1 : 1.4); however, among older people, the prevalence in women was almost four times that in men (age group 65–74 years: men 1%, 95% CI 0% to 4%; women 5%, 95% CI 3% to 8%).

AETIOLOGY/ RISK FACTORS Most cases of carpal tunnel syndrome have no easily identifiable cause (idiopathic).[4] Secondary causes of carpal tunnel syndrome include the following: space occupying lesions (tumours, hypertrophic synovial tissue, fracture callus, and osteophytes); metabolic and physiological (pregnancy, hypothyroidism, rheumatoid arthritis); infections; neuropathies (associated with diabetes mellitus or alcoholism); and familial disorders.[4] One case control study found that risk factors in the general population included repetitive activities requiring wrist extension or flexion, obesity, very rapid dieting, shorter height, hysterectomy without oopherectomy, and recent menopause.[8]

PROGNOSIS One observational study (carpal tunnel syndrome defined by symptoms and electrophysiological study results) found that 34% of people with idiopathic carpal tunnel syndrome without treatment had complete resolution of symptoms (remission) within 6 months of diagnosis.[9] Remission rates were higher for younger age groups, for women versus men, and for pregnant versus non-pregnant women. A more recent observational study of untreated idiopathic carpal tunnel syndrome also demonstrated that symptoms may spontaneously resolve in some people. The main positive prognostic indicators were short duration of symptoms and young age, whereas bilateral symptoms and a positive Phalen's test were indicators of a poorer prognosis.[10]

AIMS OF INTERVENTION To improve symptoms and reduce the physical signs of carpal tunnel syndrome; to prevent progression and loss of hand function secondary to carpal tunnel syndrome; to minimise loss of time from work.

OUTCOMES Clinical improvement of symptoms and reduction in physical signs; hand function; time to return to work.

METHODS *Clinical Evidence* search and appraisal January 2004.

QUESTION What are the effects of drug treatment?

OPTION ORAL CORTICOSTEROIDS

Three small RCTs found that oral prednisone improved symptoms after 2 weeks, and two of the three RCTs found the improvement was maintained at 4–8 weeks. We found no RCTs that measured the effects of oral corticosteroids on symptoms in the longer term. One small RCT found no significant difference in symptoms at 2 weeks between local methylprednisone injection and oral prednisone, but found that local methylprednisone injection improved symptoms after 8 and 12 weeks. One RCT found that oral prednisone reduced symptoms compared with a non-steroidal anti-inflammatory drug (tenoxicam) and with a diuretic (trichlormethiazide) after 4 weeks.

Benefits: **Versus placebo:** We found one systematic review (search date 2000, 2 RCTs) and one subsequent RCT.[11,12] The systematic review did not pool data.[11] The first RCT (15 people) included in the review compared oral prednisone (20 mg daily for the first wk followed by 10 mg daily for the second wk) versus placebo.[13] The RCT found that prednisone significantly improved symptoms based on the mean Global Symptom Score (GSS) compared with placebo at 2 weeks, but significance was not maintained at 4 or 8 weeks (results presented graphically; CI not provided). The second RCT (91 people) included in the review compared four treatments: oral prednisone (20 mg daily for 2 wks followed by 10 mg daily for another 2 wks); an oral slow release non-steroidal anti-inflammatory drug (tenoxicam 20 mg daily); an oral diuretic (trichlormethiazide 2 mg daily); and placebo (see comment below).[14] It found that prednisone (26 people) significantly reduced the mean GSS after 2 and 4 weeks compared with placebo (23 people) (2 weeks: difference in mean GSS −6.6, 95% CI −10.4 to −2.8; 4 weeks: −10.8, 95% CI −15.0 to −6.7). The subsequent RCT (36 people) found that oral prednisone (25 mg daily for 10 days) significantly reduced the median GSS at 2 and 8 weeks compared with placebo (difference in median GSS, 2 weeks: −6, 95% CI −11 to −1; 8 weeks: −6, 95% CI −11 to 0).[12] **Versus injected corticosteroids:** We found one systematic review,[15] which included one RCT (60 people)[16] comparing a single local corticosteroid injection (methylprednisone 15 mg) plus oral placebo versus oral corticosteroid (prednisone 25 mg daily for 10 days) plus placebo injection. The RCT found no significant difference in the mean GSS between local methylprednisone injection and oral prednisone after 2 weeks, but found a significant improvement with local methylprednisone injection after 8 and after 12 weeks (2 weeks: WMD −4.2, 95% CI −8.7 to +0.3; 8 weeks: WMD −7.2, 95% CI −11.5 to −2.9; 12 weeks: WMD −7.0, 95% CI −11.6 to −2.4).[15] **Versus NSAIDs:** We found one RCT (91 people; described above), which compared four treatments: oral prednisone; oral non-steroidal anti-inflammatory drug (tenoxicam); oral diuretic (trichlormethiazide 2 mg daily) and placebo (see comment below).[14] It found that prednisone significantly reduced mean GSS compared with tenoxicam at 4 weeks (27.9 to 10.0 with prednisone *v* 29.7 to 24.0 with tenoxicam). **Versus diuretics:** (See benefits of diuretics, p 1393).

Harms: **Versus placebo:** In the first RCT included in the review, three people in each group reported adverse effects, although none of these people discontinued their treatment.[13] Adverse effects with prednisone included mild hyperglycaemia in one person with diabetes, nausea, abdominal discomfort, constipation, and altered taste sensation. Symptoms in the placebo group included nausea, abdominal discomfort, constipation, insomnia, headache, dysuria, and burning nostrils. The second RCT included in the review found that adverse effects included nausea and epigastric pain (nausea: 3/23 [13%] of people with prednisone *v* 1/16 [6%] of people with placebo; epigastric pain: 2/23 [9%] *v* 2/16 [12%]).[14] The subsequent RCT did not report adverse events.[12] **Versus injected corticosteroids:** The RCT reported nine adverse effects (out of 30 people) in people receiving oral prednisone plus saline injection: bloating (2 people), insomnia (2 people), polyphagia (3 people), and injection pain (2 people). Two people receiving corticosteroid injections had injection pain.[16] Common adverse effects with oral corticosteroids include nausea, anxiety, acne, menstrual irregularities, insomnia, headaches, and mood swings. More serious adverse reactions include peptic ulcer, steroid psychosis, osteoporosis, and adrenal insufficiency.[17] **Versus NSAIDs:** The RCT reported no major adverse effects.[14] However, nausea and epigastric pain were more common with tenoxicam than with oral prednisone (nausea: 3/18 [17%] with tenoxicam *v* 3/23 [13%] with prednisone; epigastric pain: 3/18 [17%] with tenoxicam *v* 2/23 [9%] with prednisone; P values not reported). **Versus diuretics:** See harms of diuretics, p 1393.

Comment: The RCT comparing oral prednisone with placebo reported that 18/91 (20%) people did not complete the trial, although analysis of data was not by intention to treat.[14]

OPTION NON-STEROIDAL ANTI-INFLAMMATORY DRUGS

One small RCT found no significant difference between tenoxicam and placebo in symptoms after 2 or 4 weeks. One RCT found that oral prednisone reduced symptoms compared with a non-steroidal anti-inflammatory drug (tenoxicam) after 4 weeks. One RCT found no significant difference in symptoms between a diuretic (trichlormethiazide) and a non-steroidal anti-inflammatory drug (tenoxicam) at 4 weeks.

Benefits: **Versus placebo:** We found one systematic review (search date 2000),[11] which included one RCT.[14] The RCT (91 people) compared four treatments: prednisone; an oral slow release non-steroidal anti-inflammatory drug (NSAID) (tenoxicam 20 mg daily for 4 wks); trichlormethiazide; and placebo (see the benefits and comment under oral corticosteroids, p 1391).[14] It found no significant difference between tenoxicam (18 people) and placebo (16 people) in mean Global Symptom Score**G** after 2 or 4 weeks (difference in mean Global Symptom Score, 2 weeks: +3.1, 95% CI −1.4 to +7.6; 4 weeks: +3.2, 95% CI −1.7 to +8.1). **Versus oral corticosteroids:** See benefits of oral corticosteroids, p 1391. **Versus diuretics:** See benefits of diuretics, p 1393.

Harms: Versus placebo: The RCT reported no major side effects.[14] The RCT found that tenoxicam increased nausea and epigastric pain (nausea: 3/18 [17%] of people with tenoxicam *v* 1/16 [6%] of people with placebo; epigastric pain: 3/18 [17%] *v* 2/16 [12%]; P values not reported).[14] **Versus oral corticosteroids:** See benefits of oral corticosteroids, p 1391. **Versus diuretics:** See benefits of diuretics, p 1393.

Comment: None.

OPTION DIURETICS

One small RCT found no significant difference between trichlormethiazide and placebo in symptoms after 2 or 4 weeks. One RCT found no significant difference between bendrofluazide and placebo in the proportion of people with no improvement in symptoms after 4 weeks. One RCT found no significant

difference in symptoms between a diuretic (trichlormethiazide) and a non-steroidal anti-inflammatory drug (tenoxicam) at 4 weeks. One RCT found that oral prednisone reduced symptoms compared with a diuretic (trichlormethiazide) after 4 weeks.

Benefits: **Versus placebo:** We found one systematic review (search date 2000),[11] which included two RCTs.[14,18] The review did not pool data. The first RCT (91 people) included in the review compared four treatments: prednisone; a non-steroidal anti-inflammatory drug; an oral diuretic (trichlormethiazide 2 mg daily for 4 wks); and placebo (see benefits and comment under oral corticosteroids, p 1391).[14] It found no significant difference between trichlormethiazide (16 people) and placebo (16 people) in mean Global Symptom ScoreⒼ after either 2 or 4 weeks (difference in mean Global Symptom Score, 2 weeks: +0.7, 95% CI –3.0 to +4.4; 4 weeks: +0.8, –3.2 to +4.8).[14] The second RCT (48 people) included in the review compared bendrofluazide 5 mg daily for 4 weeks versus placebo.[18] It found no significant difference between bendrofluazide and placebo in the proportion of people with "no improvement in symptoms at all" after 4 weeks (no improvement at all: 54% of people with bendrofluazide *v* 50% of people with placebo; difference +4%, 95% CI –18% to +25%; see comment below).[11] **Versus NSAIDs:** We found one RCT (91 people; described above).[14] It found no significant difference in GSS between trichlormethiazide and tenoxicam at 4 weeks (GSS changed from 26.0 at baseline to 21.6 at 4 weeks with trichlormethiazide *v* 29.7 to 24.0 with tenoxicam). **Versus oral corticosteroids:** We found one RCT (91 people; described above).[14] It found that prednisone significantly reduced mean GSS compared with trichlormethiazide after 4 weeks (change in GSS: 27.9 to 10.0 with prednisone *v* 26.0 to 21.6 with trichlormethiazide).

Harms: **Versus placebo:** The first RCT found similar rates of epigastric pain with trichlormethiazide and placebo (2/16 [12%] with diuretic *v* 2/16 [12%] with placebo.[14] The second RCT reported one person "felt unwell in a non-specific way" on bendrofluazide and was withdrawn from the study.[18] **Versus NSAIDs:** The RCT found that nausea and epigastric pain were less common with trichlormethiazide than with tenoxicam (nausea: 0/16 people with trichlormethiazide *v* 3/18 [17%] with tenoxicam; epigastric pain: 2/16 [13%] with trichlormethiazide *v* 3/18 [17%] with tenoxicam; P values not reported).[14] **Versus oral corticosteroids:** The RCT found that nausea was less common with trichlormethiazide than with prednisone, although epigastric pain was more common with trichlormethiazide than with prednisone (nausea: 0/16 with trichlormethiazide *v* 3/23 [13%] with prednisone; epigastric pain: 2/16 [13%] with trichlormethiazide *v* 2/23 [9%] with prednisone).[14]

Comment: The RCT comparing bendrofluazide versus placebo used a numerical score from 0 to 5 to assess the degree of improvement in symptoms reported by people (0 = no improvement at all; 5 = full recovery).[18]

OPTION PYRIDOXINE

One small RCT found a similar improvement in symptoms with pyridoxine compared with placebo or no treatment after 10 weeks. The RCT may have been too small to detect a clinically important difference between treatments. One small RCT found no significant difference between pyridoxine and placebo in nocturnal pain, numbness, or tingling after 12 weeks.

Benefits: We found one systematic review (search date 2000),[11] which included two RCTs.[19,20] The review did not pool data.[11] The first RCT (15 people) included in the review compared oral pyridoxine (200 mg daily); placebo (dextrose pill); and no treatment.[20] The RCT found similar rates of improvement in symptoms between pyridoxine and placebo or no treatment after 10 weeks (symptoms improved: 3/6 [50%] with pyridoxine *v* 4/5 [80%] with placebo *v* 3/4 [75%] with no treatment; no statistical analysis reported; see comment below).[20] The second RCT (35 people) included in the review found no significant difference between oral pyridoxine (200 mg daily) and placebo in nocturnal pain, numbness, or tingling after 12 weeks (reported as not significant; P values not provided).[19]

Harms: Neither RCT reported harms.[19,20] Common adverse reactions associated with pyridoxine include numbness, paraesthesia, and an unsteady gait.[17]

Comment: The first RCT did not specify which symptoms were assessed nor how changes were scored.[20] The RCT may have been too small to detect a clinically important difference between treatments.[20] The second RCT used an unvalidated 4-point questionnaire with discrete numerical scoring of symptom severity (0 = no symptoms; 4 = severe symptoms).[19]

OPTION LOCAL CORTICOSTEROID INJECTION

Two small RCTs found that local corticosteroid injection (methylprednisone, hydrocortisone) improved symptoms after 4–6 weeks compared with placebo or no treatment. One small RCT found that local betamethasone injection improved symptoms after 1 month compared with betamethasone injection into the deltoid. One small RCT found no significant difference between local methylprednisone injection and oral prednisone in symptoms after 2 weeks, but found that local methylprednisone injection improved symptoms after 8 and 12 weeks.

Benefits: **Versus placebo or no treatment:** We found one systematic review (search date 2002, 1 RCT, 60 people)[15] and one additional RCT.[21] The RCT identified by the review (60 people) found that local methylprednisone injection (40 mg) significantly improved symptom severity after 1 month compared with placebo injection (clinical improvement: 23/30 [77%] with methylprednisone injection *v* 6/30 [20%] with placebo injection; RR 3.8, 95% CI 1.82 to 8.05; see comment below).[22] The additional RCT (84 people) compared three treatments: local injection of low dose hydrocortisone (25 mg); local injection of high dose hydrocortisone (100 mg); and no injection.[21] It found that both doses of hydrocortisone significantly increased the proportion of people with improved symptoms at 6 weeks compared with no injection (see comment below; 21/32 [66%] with low dose hydrocortisone *v* 1/20 [5%] with no injection; RR 13.1, 95% CI 1.9 to 90.1; NNT 2, 95% CI 2 to 3; 20/32 [63%] with high dose hydrocortisone *v* 1/20 [5%] with no injection; RR 12.5, 95% CI 1.8 to 86.0; NNT 2, 95% CI 2 to 4). The RCT found no significant difference between high and low dose hydrocortisone in the proportion of people with improvement at 6 weeks (21/32 [66%] with low dose hydrocortisone *v* 20/32 [63%] with high dose hydrocortisone; RR 1.0, 95% CI 0.7 to 1.5). **Versus systemic steroids:** The systematic review included two RCTs.[16,23] The first RCT included in the review (37 people) compared local injection of betamethasone (1.5 mg) plus placebo (saline) injection into the deltoid muscle versus local placebo injection plus betamethasone (1.5 mg) injection into the deltoid muscle.[23] It found that local betamethasone injection significantly improved symptom severity after 1 month compared with systemic injection (clinical improvement: 9/18 [50%] with local injection *v* 3/19 [16%] with systemic injection; RR 3.17, 95% CI 1.02 to 9.87; see comment below). The second RCT included in the review compared a single local corticosteroid injection plus oral placebo versus oral corticosteroid plus placebo injection.[16] See benefits of oral corticosteroids, p 1391.

Harms: The systematic review did not report adverse events.[15] The RCT comparing local corticosteroid injection with oral corticosteroid reported nine side effects with oral prednisone plus placebo injection: bloating (2 people), insomnia (2 people), polyphagia (3 people), and injection pain (2 people).[16] The RCT reported two people had injection pain in the local corticosteroid injection group. Known serious adverse effects of local corticosteroid injection into the carpal tunnel include tendon rupture and injection into the median nerve.[24]

Comment: Two RCTs included in the systematic review only defined clinical outcomes loosely using a subjective ordinal ranking scale, and neither RCT specified the magnitude of symptomatic improvement or the changes in specific symptoms.[22,23] The RCT comparing hydrocortisone injection with placebo reported the number of people who scored their symptoms as "better" or "much better", but these terms were not quantified and changes in individual symptoms were not described.[21]

QUESTION What are the effects of non-drug treatment?

OPTION WRIST SPLINTS

One RCT found that a nocturnal hand brace improved symptoms after 2 and 4 weeks compared with no treatment. One small RCT found no significant difference in symptoms after 2 weeks between neutral angle compared with 20° extension wrist splinting. One small RCT found no significant difference in symptoms at 6 weeks between full time compared with night time only neutral angle wrist splinting.

Benefits: **Versus no treatment:** We found one RCT (83 people), which compared a nocturnal hand brace worn for 4 weeks versus no treatment.[25] It found that the hand brace significantly improved symptoms at 2 or 4 weeks compared with no treatment (symptoms assessed using Boston Carpal Tunnel Symptom Questionnaire, 2 weeks: –1.03, 95% CI –1.98 to –0.08; 4 weeks: –1.07, 95% CI –2.01 to –0.13). **Versus other treatments:** We found no RCTs. **Versus different splinting regimens:** We found one systematic review (search date 1997, 1 RCT)[26] and one subsequent RCT.[27] The RCT in the review (59 people, 90 wrists) compared neutral angle wrist splinting versus wrist splinting in 20° extension (see comment below).[28] It found no significant difference after 2 weeks' follow up in the proportion of people reporting some degree of improvement in their symptoms (40/45 [89%] with neutral angle splinting *v* 38/45 [84%] with extension splinting; RR 1.1, 95% CI 0.9 to 1.2). The subsequent RCT (24 people) compared full time (day and night) wear of neutral angle wrist splints versus night time only wear. It found no significant difference after 6 weeks in mean symptom severity score (see comment below; difference in mean symptom severity score +0.1, 95% CI –0.3 to +0.5).[27]

Harms: In the RCT comparing nocturnal hand brace to no treatment, four people in the hand brace group experienced transient paraesthesias after the hand brace was removed.[25] Harms were not reported by the other RCTs.

Comment: The RCT in the systematic review graded improvement in symptoms as "none", "some", "a lot", or "complete"; however, individual symptoms and the method for grading changes in symptoms were not described.[28]

The subsequent RCT used a validated numerical scale to assess changes in symptom severity.[27] The use of a night time splint was complete or nearly complete in 85% of people allocated to night time splinting only, but 23% of the people reported limited additional daytime use. Complete or nearly complete daytime wear was reported by only 27% of people allocated to full time wear. More men than women were included in the trial than would have been expected from the usual sex distribution of carpal tunnel syndrome.

OPTION NERVE AND TENDON GLIDING EXERCISES

One small RCT found no significant difference between nerve and tendon gliding exercises plus neutral angle wrist splint and neutral angle wrist splint alone in symptom severity or function 8 weeks after the end of 4 weeks of treatment.

Benefits: We found no systematic review but found one RCT.[29] The RCT (28 people, 36 wrists) compared nerve gliding and tendon gliding exercises**G** plus a custom made neutral angle wrist splint versus a wrist splint alone. The nerve and tendon gliding exercises were undertaken five times per day for 4 weeks, and people were instructed to wear the neutral angle wrist splints all night and during the day as much as possible for 4 weeks. The RCT found no significant difference between nerve and tendon gliding exercises plus neutral angle wrist splint and neutral angle wrist splint alone in mean Symptom Severity score ($P = 0.2$) or mean Functional Status score ($P = 0.5$) at 8 weeks after the end of the treatment (see comment below).[29] The RCT found that exercise significantly improved pinch strength compared with wrist splint alone ($P = 0.026$,) but found no significant difference in other physical examination parameters (grip strength, Phalen's sign, or Tinel's sign; see comment below).

Harms: The RCT did not report adverse events.[29]

Comment: The Symptom Severity Scale has 11 items concerning pain, nocturnal symptoms, numbness, tingling, and weakness; the Functional Status Scale measures eight items, including difficulty in writing, buttoning clothes, opening jars, holding a book, gripping a telephone handle, household chores, carrying of grocery bags, bathing, and dressing.[29] Phalen's sign was performed by full flexion of the wrist for 60 seconds with the test recorded positive if paresthesia was experienced in at least one of three radial digits.[29] Tinel's sign was performed by percussing the median nerve at the wrist, with the test recorded positive if paresthesia was experienced in at least one of three radial digits.[29]

OPTION THERAPEUTIC ULTRASOUND

One RCT found that ultrasound increased the proportion of wrists with satisfactory improvement or complete remission of symptoms after 6 months compared with placebo. One RCT found no significant difference in symptom severity between high or low intensity ultrasound compared with placebo after 2 weeks.

Benefits: **Versus placebo:** We found one systematic review (search date 2000),[11] which included two RCTs.[30,31] The review did not pool data.[11] The first RCT (45 people, 90 wrists) included in the review compared ultrasound (15 min, 5 times weekly for 2 wks followed by twice weekly for 5 wks at an intensity of 1.0 W/cm^2) versus placebo.[31] The dominant wrist was randomly allocated to ultrasound or placebo and the contralateral wrist was allocated to the other treatment. The RCT found that ultrasound treatment significantly increased the proportion of wrists with satisfactory improvement or complete remission of symptoms at 6 months (22/30 [73%] wrists with ultrasound *v* 6/30 [20%] wrists with placebo; RR 3.7, 95% CI 1.7 to 7.7; NNT 2, 95% CI 2 to 4; see comment below).[31] The second RCT (18 women, 30 wrists) included in the review compared three treatments: low intensity ultrasound (0.8 W/cm^2); high intensity ultrasound (1.5 W/cm^2); and placebo.[30] Each treatment was performed for 5 minutes, five times a week for 2 weeks. The RCT found no significant difference between low and high intensity ultrasound treatments or between either ultrasound treatment and placebo in mean symptom severity graded on a visual analogue scale at 2 weeks (mean difference with high intensity ultrasound *v* placebo –1.1, 95% CI –3.0 to +0.9; mean difference with low intensity ultrasound *v* placebo –0.4, 95% CI –2.5 to +1.6; mean difference with high intensity ultrasound *v* low intensity ultrasound –0.7, 95% CI –2.4 to +0.9).[30]

Harms: The first RCT reported that ultrasound non-significantly reduced nerve conduction velocity compared with placebo.[30] The second RCT included in the review reported that there were no adverse effects with ultrasound.[31]

Comment: In the first RCT, 15/45 (33%) people did not complete the trial, and analysis of data was not by intention to treat.[31] The RCT used "satisfactory improvement" and "complete remission" as outcome measures, although these terms were not clearly defined.

QUESTION **What are the effects of surgical treatment?**

OPTION **SURGERY**

We found no RCTs comparing surgery with placebo. One small RCT identified by a systematic review, and one subsequent RCT, found that surgery increased symptom resolution compared with splinting at 12–15 months. One systematic review and five subsequent RCTs provided no clear evidence of a difference in symptoms or time taken to return to work between endoscopic and open carpal tunnel release up to 12 months after the operation. Harms resulting from endoscopic and open carpal tunnel release vary among RCTs. One systematic review and two RCTs comparing the interventions suggests that endoscopic carpal tunnel release may cause more transient nerve problems, whereas open carpal tunnel release may cause more wound problems.

Benefits: **Surgery versus placebo or non-surgical intervention:** We found no RCTs comparing surgery versus placebo. We found one systematic review (search date 2002, 1 RCT), which compared any type of surgery with any non-surgical intervention and one subsequent RCT.[32,33] The small RCT identified by the review (22 women, symptoms ranging from 1 month to 20 years) compared open surgical section of the anterior carpal ligament versus splinting of the hand, wrist, and arm for 1 month.[32] It found that surgery significantly increased the proportion of people with clinical improvement after 1 year compared with splinting (clinical improvement: 10/11 [91%] with surgery *v* 2/11 [18%] with splinting; RR 5, 95% CI 1.4 to 17.8; see comment below).[32] The subsequent larger RCT (176 people, including 143 women, symptoms for 16–104 weeks) compared open carpal tunnel surgery with splinting of the wrist for at least 6 months.[33] It found that surgery significantly increased success rates (defined as completely recovered or much improved on a 6 point scale) compared with splinting at 3, 12, and 18 months (3 months: 62/78 [80%] with surgery *v* 46/86 [54%] with splinting, $P < 0.001$; 12 months: 67/73 [92%] with surgery *v* 60/83 [72%] with splinting, $P = 0.002$; 18 months: 61/68 [90%] with surgery *v* 59/79 [75%] with splinting, $P = 0.02$). By 18 months, 41% of the people allocated to splinting had undergone surgery. **Endoscopic versus open carpal tunnel release:** We found one systematic review (search date 2000, 7 RCTs, 739 people; see comment below)[34] and five subsequent RCTs.[35–39] The systematic review included three "high quality" RCTs and four "low quality" RCTs comparing endoscopic carpal tunnel release versus open carpal tunnel release.[34] It found no significant difference in symptoms after 3 months between endoscopic and open carpal tunnel release (3 RCTs, reported as improvement in paraesthesia, numbness in 99% with endoscopic carpal tunnel release *v* 98% with open carpal tunnel release after 12 wks, difference +1%, 95% CI –3 to +5% in 1 RCT; reported as "no significant difference" in pain after 3 months in 1 RCT; reported as "no significant difference" in symptom severity score after 3 months in 1 RCT; P values not provided).[34] The review found no significant difference in pain between endoscopic and open carpal tunnel release after 6 months and 12 months (1 RCT, reported as "no significant difference"; P value not provided).[34] Seven RCTs identified by the review assessed time taken to return to work or activities and found different results. Four RCTs found that endoscopic release significantly decreased the time taken to return to work, activities of daily living, or both, compared with open carpal tunnel release, and three RCTs found no significant difference (time decreased: endoscopic carpal tunnel release *v* open carpal tunnel release: reported as median 14 days *v* 28 days, P < 0.05 in 1 RCT; mean 24 days *v* 42 days, P < 0.05 in 1 RCT; mean 14 days *v* 39 days, P < 0.05 in 1 RCT; mean 20 days *v* 30 days, P < 0.05 in 1 RCT; No difference in time, endoscopic carpal tunnel release *v* open carpal tunnel release: reported as mean 17 days *v* 19 days, "no significant difference" in 1 RCT; reported as more than 4 wks absence from work 16% *v* 13%, difference 3%, 95% CI –7% to +4% in 1 RCT; reported as time to return to work 17 days *v* 17 days, "no significant difference" in 1 RCT; P value not provided).[34] The first subsequent small RCT (26 men) found that endoscopic release improved tingling sensations and severity of night time numbness at 2 weeks compared with open carpel tunnel release, but found no significant difference at 4 weeks (P values not provided).[36] It found that endoscopic release significantly improved the severity of night time hand or wrist pain after 4 weeks compared with open carpal tunnel release (P value not provided).[36] The second subsequent RCT (25 people with bilateral carpal tunnel syndrome) randomly assigned one wrist to undergo endoscopic release, at which time the contralateral wrist on the same person was assigned to undergo open release.[35] All operations in the RCT were carried out by the same surgeon. The RCT found no significant difference between endoscopic and open carpal tunnel release in hand function, grip strength, or sensation assessed at 6, 12, 26, or 52 weeks after the operation (reported as not significant; results presented graphically; P value not provided).[35] The RCT found no significant difference between endoscopic and open carpal tunnel release in people's satisfaction with either procedure assessed over the same period (reported as not significant; results presented graphically; P value not provided).[35] The third subsequent RCT (123 people, 91 randomised to endoscopic and 32 to open surgery) found no significant difference between endoscopic and open carpel tunnel in symptom severity after 12 weeks (Symptom Severity Scale: 1.8 with endoscopic *v* 2 with open; P not reported).[37] It found that open surgery significantly decreased the secondary outcomes of grip strength and pain at 1 and 6 weeks but not at 12 weeks (grip strength in kg: 15, 26, 27 with endoscopic surgery *v* 11, 19 and 27 with open surgery; P not reported; mean McGill pain scores: 13, 12 and 8 with endoscopic surgery *v* 26, 22 and 12 at 1, 6 and 12 weeks with open surgery; P not reported).[37] It found no significant difference between treatments in time to return to work (no data presented). The fourth subsequent RCT (30 people with bilateral carpal tunnel syndrome randomised either to endoscopic or limited open carpel tunnel release on the dominant hand with the other hand having the alternative technique) found no significant difference between endoscopic and open surgery in symptoms or function at 1 year (complete resolution of symptoms: 17/30 [57%] hands with endoscopic *v* 19/30 [63%] hands with open surgery; minimal residual symptoms: 33% *v* 27%; no change or partial relief: 10% *v* 6.7%; P not reported).[38] It found that open surgery significantly reduced pain at 2 and 4 weeks, but found no significant difference after 8 weeks (1 to 10 point VAS, 2 weeks: 2.5 with open *v* 3.3 with endoscopic; P = 0.004; 4 weeks: 1.5 with open *v* 2.5 with endoscopic; P = 0.008). The fifth subsequent RCT (123 people, 150 hands) found no significant differences between endoscopic and open surgery in pain, function, or symptoms (anterior carpal tenderness from 11 for painless to 55 for severe pain: 22 with endoscopic *v* 24 with open; P = 0.18; Levine functional score from 8 for no impact to 40 for no activities possible: 109 with endoscopic *v* 108 with open; P = 0.98; Levine symptom score from 11 for asymptomatic to 55 for severe symptoms: 120 with endoscopic *v* 119 with open; P = 0.70).[39] It found that, for the 85 people in employment at baseline, endoscopic surgery significantly reduced time to return to work compared with open surgery (time off work: 18 days with endoscopic *v* 26 days with open; difference 8 days, 95% CI 2 to 13 days). During surgery, 9/74 [12%] of hands randomised to endoscopic surgery were converted to open surgery. Data were analysed on an intention to treat basis.

Harms: **Surgery versus placebo or non surgical intervention:** The subsequent RCT found that many people reported adverse effects during 18 months' follow up, but that most were mild and did not last long (any adverse effect: 58/87 [67%] with surgery *v* 46/89% [52%] with splinting [41% underwent surgery in the follow up period and were analysed in the splinting group]; P not reported).[33] It found that one person [1%] developed reflex sympathetic dystrophy after surgery. The review did not report on harms.[32] **Endoscopic versus open carpal tunnel release:** All seven RCTs included in the systematic review reported complications.[34] For endoscopic carpal tunnel release, complications included partial transection of superficial palmar arch (1/84 hands), digital nerve contusion (1/84 hands), ulnar nerve neurapraxia**G** (1/84 hands), wound haematoma (1/84 hands), conversion to the open procedure (3/79 hands), transient neurapraxia (1/25 people), transient numbness on radial side of ring finger (3/16 hands), ulnar nerve paraesthesia (1/53 hands), incomplete release (1/53 hands), increased numbness in fingertips (1/87 people), subcutaneous heamatoma (1/20 hands), loss of strength and mobility in wrist (1/20 hands), and algodystrophy (1/54 hands). For open carpal tunnel release, complications included painful hypertrophic scar [1/22 peoples], reflex sympathetic dystrophy (1/22 people), prolonged wound secretion (1/16 hands), wound infection (1/52 hands), scar tethering (1/52 hands), scar hypertrophy (5/52 hands), loss of strength (2/20 hands), and swollen/stiff fingers (1/20 hands). The systematic review stated "it seems that endoscopic carpal tunnel release gives more transient nerve problems (e.g. neurapraxia, numbness, paraesthesia) and open carpal tunnel release more wound problems (e.g. infection, hypertrophic scar, scar tenderness)".[34] One subsequent RCT reported persisting wound pain (1 wrist) with endoscopic release, and persisting symptoms and signs of carpal tunnel syndrome (1 wrist), superficial sensory nerve injury (1 wrist), and persisting wound pain (1 wrist) with open release.[35]The third subsequent RCT found no serious complications after either type of surgery, although, within 4 years, 5% of the endoscopic surgery treated group had to have repeat surgery compared with none who initially received open surgery.[37] The fourth subsequent RCT found no serious complications (wound infections, haematomas, neurovascular, or tendon injury) with either endoscopic or limited open carpel tunnel release.[38] It found that a similar proportion of people developed trigger fingers that responded to conservative treatment after both types of surgery (3/30 [10%] with both). The fifth subsequent RCT (150 hands) found no permanent neurovascular injury after either open or endoscopic surgery.[39] It found that one person [1.3%] needed reoperation because of incomplete release of the flexor retinaculum after each type of surgery. Other adverse effects included wound infection (one person in each treatment group), hyperaesthesia over the scar (1 person after open surgery), and transient index finger numbness (1 person after endoscopic surgery). Harms resulting from endoscopic and open carpal tunnel release vary between RCTs, although rates of complications for both procedures are generally low.[36,40–46]

Comment: **Surgery versus placebo or non surgical intervention:** The RCT identified by the review was not blinded, there was no information on baseline clinical and electrophysiological status of the two groups, and the method of randomisation was not described.[32] The larger subsequent RCT was of much better quality, and followed participants for up to 18 months.[33] **Endoscopic versus open carpal tunnel release:** Meta-analysis in the systematic review was not undertaken, as the data could not be pooled.[34] Endoscopic release techniques vary between RCTs, which may account for some of the variation in complication rates.[47]

OPTION INTERNAL NEUROLYSIS IN CONJUNCTION WITH OPEN CARPAL TUNNEL RELEASE

RCTs identified by a systematic review found no significant difference in symptoms between open carpal tunnel release alone and open carpal tunnel release plus internal neurolysis in symptoms.

Benefits: We found one systematic review (search date 2001), which did not pool results from RCTs only.[48] The review identified three RCTs that compared open carpal tunnel release alone versus open carpal tunnel release plus internal neurolysis**G**[49–51] and three trials (one RCT; two quasi-randomised trials) that compared surgery plus epineurectomy versus surgery alone.[52–54] The terms "epineurectomy" and "neurolysis" were used interchangeably in the review (see comment below). However, it is likely that in these studies, quite different surgical procedures may have been undertaken, which might lead to considerable heterogeneity in the results. The first three RCTs found no significant difference between open carpal tunnel release alone and open carpal tunnel release plus internal neurolysis**G**.[49–51] The first RCT (59 people, 63 wrists) found no significant difference between treatments in the proportion of people reporting relief from all or most of their symptoms after 12 months (28/32 [88%] with open carpal tunnel release alone *v* 25/31 [81%] with open carpal tunnel release plus internal neurolysis; RR 1.1, 95% CI 0.9 to 1.3).[49] The second RCT (48 people, 48 wrists) found no significant difference between treatments in the proportion of people who reported complete relief of symptoms after 6 months (23/24 [96%] with open carpal tunnel release alone *v* 23/24 [96%] with open carpal tunnel release plus internal neurolysis; RR 1.0, 95% CI 0.9 to 1.1).[51] The third RCT (41 people, 47 wrists with severe carpal tunnel syndrome; see comment below) found no significant difference after 3 months between treatments in the proportion of wrists with a good (resolution of pain, improvement in sensory deficit, and no surgical complications) or excellent (resolution of pain, resolution of sensory deficit, and no surgical complications) clinical response (15/23 [65%] wrists with open carpal tunnel release alone *v* 16/24 [67%] wrists with open carpal tunnel release plus internal neurolysis; RR 1.0, 95% CI 0.6 to 1.5).[50] The remaining three trials (randomised or quasi-randomised) found no significant difference between surgery plus epineurectomy versus surgery alone.[52–54] The fourth RCT (44 people, 50 hands) found no significant difference in the proportion of people who were symptom free at 2 years (15/25 [60%] with surgery plus epineurectomy *v* 14/25 [56%] with surgery alone, P > 0.05).[52] The fifth trial (75 people, quasi-randomised; see comment below) found no significant difference in pain or numbness at 1 year among people having these symptoms preoperatively (pain free: 42/42 [100%] with epineurectomy *v* 19/25 [76%] with no epineurectomy; no numbness: 38/47 [81%] with epineurectomy *v* 15/24 [63%] with no epineurectomy; P not reported).[53] The sixth trial (quasi-randomised; 36 people entered, 23 people analysed for telephone survey, see comment below) found no significant difference in the proportion of people who were improved at 30 months or in the time to return to work (improved: 14/15 [93%] with epineurectomy *v* 8/8 [100%] with no epineurectomy; P not reported; median time to return to work: 59 days *v* 53 days, P not reported).

Harms: The first and second RCTs did not report harms.[49,51] The third RCT (41 people, 47 wrists) found no significant difference between treatments in the proportion of wrists with persistent incisional pain, which was the most common complication reported in the trial (3/23 [13%] of wrists with open carpal tunnel release alone *v* 4/24 [17%] of wrists with open carpal tunnel release plus internal neurolysis; RR 0.8, 95% CI 0.2 to 3.1).[50] Other complications included 4% (1/24) wrists with hand swelling, 4% (1/24) wrists with adhesive capsulitis**G** in the open carpal tunnel release plus internal neurolysis group, and 4% (1/23) wrists with causalgia in the open carpal tunnel release alone group. The fourth, fifth and sixth trials did not report harms.[52–54]

Comment: The fifth and sixth RCTs used quasi-random methods of treatment allocation (even or odd hospital number[53] and birthdate[54]). The terms epineurectomy and neurolysis were used interchangeably in the review, and yet both may refer to different surgical procedures. This may result in considerable heterogeneity between studies, and questions the validity of combining the results in a meta-analysis.

QUESTION What are the effects of postoperative treatment?

OPTION WRIST SPLINTS AFTER CARPAL TUNNEL RELEASE SURGERY

Two RCTs in people after carpal tunnel release surgery found no significant difference between wrist splinting and no splinting in grip strength or in the proportion of people who considered themselves "cured" at 2–4 weeks. A third RCT found that splinting increased pain at 1 month and the time to return to work compared with no splinting.

Benefits: **Versus unrestricted range of motion:** We found no systematic review. We found three RCTs.[55–57] The first RCT (74 people, 82 wrists) compared rigid wrist splinting for 4 weeks after surgery versus no splinting plus advice to mobilise the affected wrist or wrists.[55] It found no significant difference between treatments in median grip strength (as a percentage of median preoperative grip strength: unsplinted 78%, 95% CI 70% to 86% *v* splinted 76%, 95% CI, 71% to 85%). The second RCT (47 people, 51 wrists) compared rigid wrist splinting for 2 weeks after surgery versus no splinting.[56] It found no significant difference in the proportion of people who considered themselves "cured" at follow up (see comment below; 12/26 [46%] with splinting *v* 8/17 [47%] with no splinting; RR 1.0, 95% CI 0.5 to 1.9). The third RCT (50 people, 50 wrists) compared rigid wrist splinting for 2 weeks after surgery versus no splinting.[56] It found that the average number of days taken to return to work was significantly lower in the unsplinted group (17 days with no splinting *v* 27 days with splinting; P = 0.005; RR and CI not provided). **Versus bulky dressings:** We found one systematic review (search date 1997) comparing wrist splinting versus bulky dressings after carpal tunnel decompression.[26] It found no RCTs.

Harms: The first RCT found no significant difference between treatments in the proportion of people reporting scar pain after 6 months (6/37 [16%] with splinting *v* 6/44 [14%] with no splinting; RR 1.2, 95% CI 0.4 to 3.4).[55] The second RCT reported complications for one person in the unsplinted group who had persistent symptoms and required reoperation.[56] The third RCT found that splinting significantly increased pillar pain❻ and scar tenderness at 1 month, but found no significant difference between treatments in pain at 3 or 6 months after surgery (pillar pain: P = 0.02; scar tenderness: P = 0.04; pain: data not reported).[57]

Comment: In the second RCT, although the term "cured" was used as an outcome measure, its meaning was not defined in the context of the trial, and the length of follow up was not specified.[55] The RCT found that 7/47 (15%) people were lost to follow up. Analysis of data was not by intention to treat. The RCTs were too small to exclude the possibility of a clinically important increase in the risk of some complications (e.g. transient ulnar nerve injury) with splinting compared with no splinting.

GLOSSARY

Adhesive capsulitis A condition in which the joint capsule becomes contracted and thickened causing restriction in the range of movement.

American Academy of Neurology diagnostic criteria[3] The likelihood of carpal tunnel syndrome increases with the number of standard symptoms and provocative factors. Symptoms include dull aching discomfort in the hand, forearm or upper arm; paraesthesia in the hand; weakness or clumsiness of the hand; dry skin, swelling, or colour changes in the hand; or occurrence of any of these symptoms in the distribution of the median nerve. Provocative factors include sleep, sustained arm or hand positions, or repetitive actions of the hand or wrist. Relieving factors include changes in hand posture and shaking the hand. Physical examination may be normal, or symptoms may be elicited by tapping or direct pressure over the median nerve at the wrist or with forced flexion or extension of the wrist. Physical signs include sensory loss in the median nerve distribution; weakness or atrophy in the thenar muscles; and dry skin on the thumb, index, or middle fingers. Electromyography and nerve conduction studies can confirm, but not exclude, the diagnosis of carpal tunnel syndrome.

Global Symptom Score The numerical sum of five common carpal tunnel syndrome symptoms (pain, numbness, paresthesia, weakness/clumsiness, and nocturnal wakening), which are each rated from 0 (no symptoms) to 10 (severe symptoms).[13,14]

Internal neurolysis Decompression within the nerve accomplished by performing an epineurotomy and then dividing the nerve into multiple fascicular groups.[50]

Nerve gliding exercises Exercise therapy directed at restoring and maximising excursion of the median nerve through the carpal tunnel.[58]

Pillar pain Pain at the radial or ulnar border of the carpal tunnel.

Tendon gliding exercises Exercise therapy directed at restoring and maximising excursion of the finger flexor tendons through the carpal tunnel.[58]

Ulnar neurapraxia Failure of nerve conduction of the ulnar nerve, usually reversible, due to metabolic or microstructural abnormalities without disruption of the axon.

REFERENCES

1. Rozmaryn LM. Carpal tunnel syndrome: a comprehensive review. *Curr Opin Orthop* 1997;8:33–43.
2. Rempel D, Evanoff B, Amadio PC, et al. Consensus criteria for the classification of carpal tunnel syndrome in epidemiologic studies. *Am J Public Health* 1998;88:1447–1451.

3. Anonymous. Practice parameter for carpal tunnel syndrome (summary statement). Report of the Quality Standards Subcommittee of the American Academy of Neurology. *Neurology* 1993;43:2406–2409.
4. von Schroeder H, Botte MJ. Carpal tunnel syndrome. *Hand Clin* 1996;12:643–655.
5. Stevens JC, Sun S, Beard CM, et al. Carpal tunnel syndrome in Rochester, Minnesota, 1961 to 1980. *Neurology* 1988;38:134–138.
6. Dumitru D. *Textbook of electrodiagnostic medicine.* Hanley and Belfus, eds. Philadelphia: Mosby Publications, 1995.
7. Atroshi I, Gummesson C, Johnsson R, et al. Prevalence of carpal tunnel syndrome in a general population. *JAMA* 1999;282:153–158.
8. De Krom MCTF, Kester A, Knipschild P, et al. Risk factors for carpal tunnel syndrome. *Am J Epidemiol* 1990;132:1102–1110.
9. Fatami T, Kobayashi A, Utika T, et al. Carpal tunnel syndrome; its natural history. *Hand Surgery* 1997;2:129–130.
10. Padua L, Padua R, Aprile I, et al. Multiperspective follow-up of untreated carpal tunnel syndrome. A multicenter study. *Neurology* 2001;56:1459–1466.
11. Gerritsen AAM, de Krom MCTFM, Struijs MA, et al. Conservative treatment options for carpal tunnel syndrome: a systematic review of randomised controlled trials. *J Neurol* 2002;249:272–280. Search date 2000; primary sources Medline, Embase, Cochrane Controlled Trials Register, and hand searched references.
12. Hiu ACF, Wong SM, Wong KS, et al. Oral steroid in the treatment of carpal tunnel syndrome. *Ann Rheum Dis* 2001;60:813–814.
13. Herskovitz S, Berger AR, Lipton RB. Low-dose, short-term oral prednisone in the treatment of carpal tunnel syndrome. *Neurology* 1995;45:1923–1925.
14. Chang MH, Chiang HT, Lee SS, et al. Oral drug of choice in carpal tunnel syndrome. *Neurology* 1998;51:390–393.
15. Marshall S, Tardif G, Ashworth N. Local corticosteroid injection for carpal tunnel syndrome. In: Cochrane Library, Issue 4, 2002. Oxford: Update Software. Search date 2002; primary sources Cochrane Neuromuscular Disease Group Register, Medline, Embase, and Cinahl. No company sponsorship declared.
16. Wong SM, Hui ACF, Tang A, et al. Local vs systemic corticosteroids in the treatment of carpal tunnel syndrome. *Neurology* 2001;56:1565–1567.
17. Canadian Pharmacists Association. *Compendium of Pharmaceuticals and Specialties 2000.* Ottawa: Canadian Pharmacists Association, 2000.
18. Pal B, Mangion P, Hossain MA, et al. Should diuretics be prescribed for idiopathic carpal tunnel syndrome? Results of a controlled trial. *Clin Rehab* 1988;2:299–301.
19. Spooner GR, Desai HB, Angel JF, et al. Using pyridoxine to treat carpal tunnel syndrome. Randomized control trial. *Can Fam Physician* 1993;39:2122–2127.
20. Stransky M, Rubin A, Lava NS, et al. Treatment of carpal tunnel syndrome with vitamin B6: a double-blind study. *South Med J* 1989;82:841–842.
21. O'Gradaigh D, Merry P. Corticosteroid injection for the treatment of carpal tunnel syndrome. *Ann Rheum Dis* 2000;59:918–919.
22. Dammers JW, Veering MM, Vermeulen M, et al. Injection with methylprednisolone proximal to the carpal tunnel: randomized double blind trial. *BMJ* 1999;319:884–886.
23. Ozdogan H, Yazici H. The efficacy of local steroid injections in idiopathic carpal tunnel syndrome: a double-blind study. *Br J Rheumatol* 1984;23:272–275.
24. Babu SR, Britton JM. The role of steroid injection in the management of carpal tunnel syndrome. *J Orthop Rheumatol* 1994;7:59–60.
25. Manente G, Torrieri F, Di Blasio F, et al. An innovative hand brace for carpal tunnel syndrome: a randomised controlled trial. *Muscle Nerve* 2001;24:1020–1025.
26. Feuerstein M, Burrell LM, Miller VI, et al. Clinical management of carpal tunnel syndrome: a 12-year review of outcomes. *Am J Ind Med* 1999;35:232–245. Search date 1997; primary sources Medline, Cinahl, Psychlit, and Nioshtic. No company sponsorship declared.
27. Walker WC, Metzler M, Cifu DX, et al. Neutral wrist splinting in carpal tunnel syndrome: a comparison of night-only versus full-time wear instructions. *Arch Phys Med Rehabil* 2000;81:424–429.
28. Burke TD, Burke MM, Stewart GW, et al. Splinting for carpal tunnel syndrome: In search of the optimal angle. *Arch Phys Med Rehabil* 1994;75:1241–1244.
29. Akalin E, El O, Peker O, et al. Treatment of carpal tunnel syndrome with nerve and tendon gliding exercises. *Am J Phys Med Rehabil* 2002;81:108–113.
30. Oztas O, Turan B, Bora I, et al. Ultrasound therapy effect in carpal tunnel syndrome. *Arch Phys Med Rehabil* 1998;79:1540–1544.
31. Ebenbichler GR, Resch KL, Nicolakis P, et al. Ultrasound treatment for treating the carpal tunnel syndrome: randomised "sham" controlled trial. *BMJ* 1998;316:731–735.
32. Verdugo RJ, Salinas RS, Castillo J, Cea JG. Surgical versus non–surgical treatment for carpal tunnel syndrome. In: The Cochrane Library, Issue 1, 2003. Oxford: Update Software. Search date 2002; primary sources Medline, Embase, Lilacs, hand searched references, and contact with authors.
33. Gerritsen AA, de Vet HC, Scholten RJ, et al. Splinting versus surgery in the treatment of carpal tunnel syndrome. *JAMA* 2002;288:1245–1251.
34. Gerritsen AA, Uitdehaag BMJ, van Geldere D, et al. Systematic review of randomised clinical trials of surgical treatment for carpal tunnel syndrome. *Br J Surg* 2001;88:1285–1295. Search date 2000; primary sources Medline, Embase, the Cochrane Controlled Trials Register, reference lists of retrieved studies.
35. Ferdinand RD, MacLean JGB. Endoscopic versus open carpal tunnel release in bilateral carpal tunnel syndrome. A prospective, randomised, blinded assessment. *J Bone Joint Surg* 2002;84–B:375–379.
36. Mackenzie DJ, Hainer R, Wheatley MJ. Early recovery after endoscopic vs. short-incision open carpal tunnel release. *Ann Plastic Surg* 2000;44:601–604.
37. MacDermid JC, Richards RS, Roth JH, et al. Endoscopic versus open carpal tunnel release: a randomized trial. *J Hand Surg* 2003;28A:475–480.
38. Wong KC, Hung LK, Ho PC, Wong JMW. Carpal tunnel release: a prospective, randomized study of endoscopic versus limited-open methods. *J Bone Joint Surg Br* 2003;85B:863–868.
39. Saw NL, Jones S, Shepstone L, et al. Early outcome and cost-effectiveness of endoscopic versus open carpal tunnel release: A randomized prospective trial. *J Hand Surg* 2003;28B:5:444–449.
40. Hoefnagels WAJ, Van Kleef JGF, Mastenbroek GGA, et al. Surgical treatment of the carpal tunnel syndrome: Endoscopic or classical (open) surgery? A prospective randomised study. *Ned Tijdschr Geneeskd* 1997;141:878–882.
41. Benedetti RB, Sennwald G. Endoscopic decompression of the median nerve by the technique of Agee: A prospective study in comparison with the open decompression. *Handchir Mikrochir Plast Chir* 1996;28:151–155.
42. Stark B, Engkvist-Lofmark C. Carpal tunnel syndrome. Endoscopic release or conventional surgery. *Handchir Mikrochir Plast Chir* 1996;28:128–132.
43. Herren DB. Complications after endoscopic carpal tunnel decompression. *Z Unfallchir Versicherungsmed* 1994;87:120–127.
44. Brown RA, Gelberman RH, Seiler III, et al. Carpal tunnel release. A prospective, randomized assessment of open and endoscopic methods. *J Bone Joint Surg Am* 1993;75:1265–1275.
45. Erdmann MWH. Endoscopic carpal tunnel decompression. *J Hand Surg* 1994;19:5–13.

46. Agee JM, McCarroll J, Tortosa RD, et al. Endoscopic release of the carpal tunnel: a randomized prospective multicenter study. *J Hand Surg* 1992;17:987–995.
47. Jimenez DF, Gibbs SR, Clapper AT. Endoscopic treatment of carpal tunnel syndrome: a critical review [see comments]. *J Neurosurg* 1998;88:817–826. Search date 1997; primary sources not stated.
48. Chapell R, Coates V, Turkelson C. Poor outcome for neural surgery (epineurotomy or neurolysis) for carpal tunnel syndrome compared with carpal tunnel release alone: a meta-analysis of global outcomes. *Plast Reconstr Surg* 2003;112:983–990.
49. Mackinnon SE, McCabe S, Murray JF, et al. Internal neurolysis fails to improve the results of primary carpal tunnel decompression. *J Hand Surg Am* 1991;16:211–218.
50. Lowry WE Jr, Follender AB. Interfascicular neurolysis in the severe carpal tunnel syndrome. A prospective, randomized, double-blind, controlled study. *Clin Orthop* 1988;227:251–254.
51. Holmgren-Larsson H, Leszniewski W, Linden U et al. Internal neurolysis or ligament division only in carpal tunnel syndrome — results of a randomized study. *Acta Neurochir (Wien)* 1985;74:118–121.
52. Leinberry CF, Hammond NL, Siegfried JW. The role of epineurotomy in the operative treatment of carpal tunnel syndrome. *J Bone Joint Surg Am* 1997;79:555–557.
53. Blair WF, Goetz DD, Ross MA, et al. Carpal tunnel release with and without epineurotomy: a comparative prospective trial. *J Hand Surg Am* 1996;21:655–661.
54. Foulkes GD, Atkinson RE, Beuchel C, Doyle JR, Singer DI. Outcome following epineurotomy in carpal tunnel syndrome: a prospective, randomized clinical trial. *J Hand Surg Am* 1994;19:539–547.
55. Finsen V, Andersen K, Russwurm H. No advantage from splinting the wrist after open carpal tunnel release. A randomized study of 82 wrists. *Acta Orthop Scand* 1999;70:288–292.
56. Bury TF, Akelman E, Weiss AP. Prospective, randomized trial of splinting after carpal tunnel release. *Ann Plastic Surg* 1995;35:19–22.
57. Cook AC, Szabo RM, Birkholz SW, et al. Early mobilization following carpal tunnel release. A prospective randomized study. *J Hand Surg Br* 1995;20:228–230.
58. Rozmaryn LM, Dovelle S, Rothman ER, et al. Nerve and tendon gliding exercises and the conservative management of carpal tunnel syndrome. *J Hand Ther* 1998;11:171–179.

Nigel Ashworth
Associate Professor
University of Alberta
Edmonton
Canada

Competing interests: None declared.

Chronic fatigue syndrome

Search date November 2003

Steven Reid, Trudie Chalder, Anthony Cleare, Matthew Hotopf, and Simon Wessely

QUESTIONS

INTERVENTIONS

Key Messages

- **Cognitive behavioural therapy** One systematic review found that cognitive behavioural therapy administered by highly skilled therapists in specialist centres improved quality of life and physical functioning compared with standard medical care or relaxation therapy. One additional multicentre RCT found that cognitive behavioural therapy administered by less experienced therapists may also be effective compared with guided support groups or no interventions.
- **Graded aerobic exercise** RCTs found that a graded aerobic exercise programme improved measures of fatigue and physical functioning compared with flexibility and relaxation training or general advice. One RCT found that an educational package to encourage graded exercise improved measures of physical functioning, fatigue, mood, and sleep at 1 year compared with written information alone.
- **Dietary supplements** One small RCT found no significant difference between a nutritional supplement (containing multivitamins, minerals, and coenzymes) and placebo in fatigue severity or functional impairment at 10 weeks.
- **Evening primrose oil** One small RCT found no significant difference between evening primrose oil and placebo in depression scores at 3 months.
- **Magnesium (intramuscular)** One small RCT found that intramuscular magnesium injections improved symptoms at 6 weeks compared with placebo. However, we were unable to draw reliable conclusions from this small study.
- **Antidepressants; corticosteroids; oral nicotinamide adenine dinucleotide** RCTs provided insufficient evidence about the effects of these interventions in people with chronic fatigue syndrome.
- **Immunotherapy** Small RCTs provided limited evidence that immunoglobulin G modestly improved physical functioning and fatigue at 3–6 months compared with placebo, but it was associated with considerable adverse effects. Small RCTs provided insufficient evidence on the effects of interferon alfa or aciclovir compared with placebo. One RCT found that staphylococcus toxoid improved symptoms at six months compared with placebo, although it is associated with local reaction and could cause anaphylaxis.
- **Prolonged rest** We found no RCTs on the effects of prolonged rest. Indirect observational evidence in healthy volunteers and in people recovering from a viral illness suggests that prolonged rest may perpetuate or worsen fatigue and symptoms.

Chronic fatigue syndrome

DEFINITION Chronic fatigue syndrome (CFS) is characterised by severe, disabling fatigue and other symptoms, including musculoskeletal pain, sleep disturbance, impaired concentration, and headaches. Two widely used definitions of CFS, from the US Centers for Disease Control and Prevention (CDC, current criteria issued in 1994, which superseded CDC criteria issued in 1988)[1] and from Oxford, UK,[2] were developed as operational criteria for research (see table 1, p 1418). There are important differences between these definitions. The UK criteria insist upon the presence of mental fatigue, whereas the US criteria include a requirement for several physical symptoms, reflecting the belief that CFS has an underlying immunological or infective pathology.

INCIDENCE/ PREVALENCE Community and primary care based studies have reported the prevalence of CFS to be up to 3%, depending on the criteria used.[3,4] Systematic population surveys have found similar prevalences of CFS in people of different socioeconomic status and in all ethnic groups.[4,5]

AETIOLOGY/ RISK FACTORS The cause of CFS is poorly understood. Women are at higher risk than men (RR 1.3–1.7 depending on diagnostic criteria used).[6]

PROGNOSIS Studies have focused on people attending specialist clinics. A systematic review of studies of prognosis (search date 1996) found that children with CFS had better outcomes than adults: 54–94% of children showed definite improvement (after up to 6 years' follow up), whereas 20–50% of adults showed some improvement in the medium term and only 6% returned to premorbid levels of functioning.[7] Despite the considerable burden of morbidity associated with CFS, we found no evidence of increased mortality. The systematic review found that outcome was influenced by the presence of psychiatric disorders (depression and anxiety) and beliefs about causation and treatment.[7]

AIMS OF INTERVENTION To reduce levels of fatigue and associated symptoms, to increase levels of activity, and to improve quality of life.

OUTCOMES Severity of symptoms and their effects on physical function and quality of life. These outcomes are measured in several different ways: the medical outcomes survey short form general health survey (SF-36),[8] a rating scale measuring limitation of physical functioning caused by ill health (score range 0–100, where 0 = limited in all activities and 100 = able to carry out vigorous activities); the Karnofsky scale,[9] a modified questionnaire originally developed for the rating of quality of life in people undergoing chemotherapy for malignancy, where 0 = death and 100 = no evidence of disease; the Beck Depression Inventory,[10] a checklist for quantifying depressive symptoms (score range 0–63, where a score of 20 or more is usually considered clinically significant depression); the Hospital Anxiety and Depression scale (HADs;[11] consists of 2 subscales, each with score range 0–21, where a score of 11 or more is considered clinically significant); the Sickness Impact Profile,[12] a measure of the influence of symptoms on social and physical functioning; the Chalder fatigue scale,[13] a rating scale measuring subjective fatigue (score range 0–11, where scores ≥ 4 = excessive fatigue); the Abbreviated Fatigue Questionnaire,[14] a rating scale of subjective bodily fatigue (score range 4–28, where a lower score indicates a higher degree of fatigue); the clinical global impression scale,[15] a validated measure of overall change compared with baseline at study onset, with seven possible scores from "very much worse" (score 7) to "very much better" (score 1); the Checklist Individual Strength fatigue subscale (score range 8 [no fatigue at all] to 56 [maximally fatigued])[16]; the Nottingham health profile,[17] with questions in six categories: energy, pain perception, sleep patterns, sense of social isolation, emotional reactions, and physical mobility (maximum weighted score 100 [all listed complaints present], and minimum 0 [none of listed complaints present]); and self reported severity of symptoms and levels of activity.

METHODS *Clinical Evidence* search and appraisal November 2003.

QUESTION **What are the effects of treatments?**

OPTION **ANTIDEPRESSANTS**

RCTs provided insufficient evidence about the effects of antidepressants in people with chronic fatigue syndrome.

Benefits: We found one systematic review (search date 2000), which did not report quantified results.[18] **Fluoxetine:** The review[18] identified two RCTs.[19,20] The first RCT (107 depressed and non-depressed people with chronic fatigue syndrome [CFS], Oxford criteria) compared fluoxetine versus placebo for 8 weeks.[19] It found that fluoxetine significantly improved the Beck Depression Inventory compared with placebo (mean difference between fluoxetine and placebo in improvement in Beck Depression Inventory –0.19, 95% CI –0.35 to –0.02), but the difference is small and therefore may not be clinically important. It found no significant difference between fluoxetine and placebo in fatigue severity (mean difference between fluoxetine and placebo on the fatigue subscale of Checklist Individual Strength: –0.16, 95% CI –0.64 to +0.31).[21] The second RCT (136 people with CFS, Oxford criteria) compared four groups: fluoxetine plus graded exercise; drug placebo plus graded exercise; fluoxetine plus general advice to exercise; and drug placebo plus general advice to exercise. It found no significant difference between the groups using fluoxetine and the groups using drug placebo in the level of fatigue, although modest improvements in measures of depression were seen at 12 weeks in people using fluoxetine (HADs mean change 1.1, 95% CI 0.03 to 2.2).[11,20] **Phenelzine:** The review[18] identified one RCT.[22] The RCT (30 people with CFS, CDC 1988 criteria) compared phenelzine versus placebo, using a modified Karnofsky scale and other outcome measures (including functional status questionnaire, profile of mood states, Centres for Epidemiological Study of Depression fatigue severity scale, and symptom severity checklist).[22] This study concluded that there was a pattern of improvement across several measures with phenelzine compared with placebo at 6 weeks (significance tests for individual measures not carried out). **Moclobemide:** The review[18] identified one RCT.[23] The RCT (90 people with CFS, Australian criteria, similar to CDC criteria) compared moclobemide (450–600 mg daily) versus placebo. It found that at 6 weeks moclobemide was associated with a non-significant increase in subjectively reported global improvement (moclobemide 24/47 [51%] *v* placebo 14/43 [33%]; OR 2.16, 95% CI 0.9 to 5.1), and a non-significant improvement in the clinician rated Karnofsky scale.[23] **Sertraline versus clomipramine:** We found one RCT (40 people with CFS), which found no significant difference between sertraline and clomipramine.[24]

Harms: **Fluoxetine:** The first RCT assessed the symptoms separately (which could be attributed to either CFS or to known adverse effects of fluoxetine) before starting treatment, after 2 weeks, after 6 weeks, and at the end of treatment (week 8). It found that fluoxetine significantly increased complaints of tremor and perspiration compared with placebo at 8 weeks (tremor: $P = 0.006$; perspiration: $P = 0.008$).[19] It found no significant difference between fluoxetine and placebo at 2 and 6 weeks. It found that fluoxetine was associated with increased withdrawal due to adverse effects compared with placebo (9/54 [17%] with fluoxetine *v* 2/53 [4%] with placebo; P value not reported). The second RCT also found increased withdrawal rates with fluoxetine (24/68 people [36%] with fluoxetine withdrew *v* 16/69 people [24%] with placebo; P value not reported).[20] **Phenelzine:** Three of 15 people (20%) who took phenelzine withdrew because of adverse effects compared with none who took placebo.[22] **Sertraline versus clomipramine:** The RCT provided no information on adverse effects.[24]

Comment: Clinical trials were performed in specialist clinics. **Fluoxetine:** The first RCT[19] used a shorter duration of treatment and studied people with a longer duration of illness compared with the second RCT.[20]

OPTION CORTICOSTEROIDS

RCTs found insufficient evidence about the effects of corticosteroids compared with placebo in people with chronic fatigue syndrome.

Benefits: We found one systematic review (search date 2000), which did not report quantified results.[18] **Fludrocortisone:** The review[18] identified two RCTs.[25,26] The first RCT (100 people with neurally mediated hypotension and chronic fatigue syndrome [CFS], CDC criteria) compared fludrocortisone (titrated to 0.1 mg daily) versus placebo for 9 weeks.[25] It found no significant difference on a self rated 100 point global scale of "wellness" (AR for improvement of ≥ 15 points: 14% with fludrocortisone *v* 10% with placebo; P = 0.76; raw data not reported).[25] The second randomised crossover trial (25 people, CDC criteria) measured change in symptom severity (visual analogue scale of symptoms from 0–10 corresponding to "no problem" to "could not be worse") and functional status (using the SF-36) for 6 weeks.[26] It found no significant difference between fludrocortisone and placebo in symptom severity or functional status. **Hydrocortisone:** The review[18] identified two RCTs.[27,28] The first RCT (65 people with CFS, CDC 1988 criteria) compared hydrocortisone (25–35 mg daily) versus placebo for 12 weeks.[27] It found that hydrocortisone significantly improved "wellness" on a self rated 100 point scale (AR for improvement of ≥ 5 points: 53% with hydrocortisone *v* 29% with placebo; P = 0.04). Other self rating scales did not show significant benefit with hydrocortisone (change in score from baseline: Beck Depression Inventory: hydrocortisone –2.1 *v* placebo –0.4, P = 0.17; activity scale: hydrocortisone 0.3 *v* placebo 0.7, P = 0.32; Sickness Impact Profile: hydrocortisone –2.5 *v* placebo –2.2; P = 0.85). The second RCT (32 people with CFS, Oxford criteria, crossover design) compared a lower dose of hydrocortisone (5 or 10 mg daily) versus placebo for 1 month.[28] It found that hydrocortisone improved fatigue compared with placebo at one month (participant assessed 11 item scale, overall score range 0–33, higher score indicates greater fatigue; mean pre-crossover score change from baseline: –6.7 with hydocortisone v –2.4 with placebo; P value not reported, see comment below). **Hydrocortisone plus fludrocortisone:** We found one RCT (100 people with CFS, CDC criteria, crossover design, see comment below), which compared a combination of hydrocortisone (5 mg daily) and fludrocortisone (50 μg daily) versus placebo for three months.[29] It found no significant difference in measures of subjective fatigue at 3 months (visual analogue scale from 0 = no fatigue to 10 = severe fatigue: mean score 6.6 with corticosteroids v 6.7 with placebo, P = 0.76; Abbreviated Fatigue Questionnaire: mean score 8 with corticosteroids v 7 with placebo, P = 0.69; pre-crossover results not presented, no washout period between treatments, see comment below).

Harms: **Fludrocortisone:** In the first RCT, fludrocortisone increased withdrawal rates due to adverse events compared with placebo (12/50 [24%] *v* 4/50 [8%]; RR 3, 95% CI 1.04 to 8.67; NNT 6, 95% CI 3 to 8).[25] Three people receiving fludrocortisone withdrew from the second RCT because of worsening CFS symptoms (fatigue, headache, or insomnia).[26] **Hydrocortisone:** The first RCT found that 12 people (40%) taking higher dose hydrocortisone (25–35 mg daily) experienced adrenal suppression (assessed by measuring cortisol levels).[27] The second RCT reported minor adverse effects in up to 10% of participants taking lower dose hydrocortisone (5 or 10 mg daily).[28] Three people on hydrocortisone had exacerbation of acne and nervousness, and one person on placebo had an episode of fainting. **Hydrocortisone plus fludrocortisone:** Two participants withdrew from the RCT because of concerns about the effect of corticosteroids, and one due to adverse effects (acne and weight gain).[29]

Comment: The results of the crossover RCTs should be interpreted with caution as it is possible that treatment effects may persist after crossover. The RCTs used different reasons for their choice of active treatment. The use of fludrocortisone, a mineralocorticoid, was based on the hypothesis that CFS is associated with neurally mediated hypotension.[30] The use of hydrocortisone, a glucocorticoid, in the other RCTs was based on evidence of underactivity of the hypothalamic–pituitary–adrenocortical axis in some people with CFS.[31] One crossover RCT found that although fatigue decreased with low dose hydrocortisone, fatigue increased within 28 days of crossover into the placebo group.[28] Therefore, any benefit from low dose hydrocortisone may be short lived, while higher doses are associated with adverse effects.

OPTION ORAL NICOTINAMIDE ADENINE DINUCLEOTIDE

One small RCT provided insufficient evidence about the effects of oral nicotinamide adenine dinucleotide compared with placebo in people with chronic fatigue syndrome.

Benefits: We found one systematic review (search date 2000), which did not report quantified results.[18] It identified one poor quality randomised crossover trial (35 people with chronic fatigue syndrome, CDC criteria), which compared nicotinamide adenine dinucleotide (10 mg daily) versus placebo for 4 weeks.[32] Of the 35 people, two were excluded from the analysis for non-compliance and seven were excluded for using psychotropic drugs. The RCT found that nicotinamide adenine dinucleotide significantly improved symptom scores compared with placebo (measured on a self devised 50 item symptom rating scale; AR for 10% improvement: 8/26 people [30%] with nicotinamide adenine dinucleotide *v* 2/26 people [8%] with placebo; $P < 0.05$, analysis not by intention to treat, see comment below).

Harms: Minor adverse effects (loss of appetite, dyspepsia, and flatulence) were reported on active treatment but did not lead to cessation of treatment.[32]

Comment: The RCT had a number of problems with its methods, including the use of inappropriate statistical analyses, the inappropriate exclusion of people from the analysis, and lack of numerical data preventing independent analysis of the published results.[33]

OPTION GRADED AEROBIC EXERCISE

RCTs found that a graded aerobic exercise programme improved measures of fatigue and physical functioning compared with flexibility training and relaxation training or general advice. One RCT found that an educational package to encourage graded exercise improved measures of physical functioning, fatigue, mood, and sleep at 1 year compared with written information alone.

Benefits: We found one systematic review (search date 2000), which did not report quantified results.[18] **Graded aerobic exercise:** The review identified two RCTs.[20,34] The first RCT (66 people with chronic fatigue syndrome [CFS], Oxford criteria) compared graded aerobic exercise (active intervention) versus flexibility and relaxation training (control intervention) over 12 weeks.[34] All participants undertook individual weekly sessions supervised by an exercise physiologist. The aerobic exercise group built up their level of activity to 30 minutes of exercise a day (walking, cycling, swimming up to a maximum oxygen consumption of 60% of V_{O2}max). People in the flexibility and relaxation training group were taught stretching and relaxation techniques (maximum 30 minutes daily, 5 days/week) and were specifically told to avoid any extra physical activities. The RCT found that graded aerobic exercise significantly increased reports of feeling "much better" or "very much better" compared with the control intervention (clinical global impression scale: 52% with exercise *v* 27% with control, $P = 0.04$). It also found that graded aerobic exercise significantly decreased physical fatigue and improved physical functioning compared with control (mean change in Chalder fatigue score: –8.4 with exercise *v* –3.1 with control, $P = 0.004$; mean change in SF-36 physical function score: 20.5 with exercise *v* 8.0 with control, $P = 0.01$). The second RCT (136 people with CFS, Oxford criteria) compared four groups (graded aerobic exercise plus fluoxetine; graded aerobic exercise plus drug placebo; general advice plus fluoxetine; general advice plus drug placebo) over 24 weeks.[20] The graded exercise groups were given specific advice to undertake preferred aerobic exercise (such as walking, jogging, swimming, or cycling) for 20 minutes three times a week up to an energy expenditure of 75% of V_{O2}max. People in the general advice groups were not given any specific advice on frequency, intensity, or duration of aerobic activity that they should be undertaking. The RCT found that graded exercise with or without fluoxetine reduced fatigue at 26 weeks compared with general advice with or without fluoxetine (Chalder fatigue scale < 4: 12/67 [18%] with graded exercise *v* 4/69 [6%] with advice; RR 3.1, 95% CI 1.05 to 9.1; NNT 9, 95% CI 5 to 91). **Educational intervention:** The review[18] identified one RCT (148 people with CFS, Oxford criteria).[35] The RCT compared three types of educational interventions to encourage graded exercise versus written information only (control group).[35] All participants in the three educational intervention groups received a minimum intervention consisting of two treatment sessions, two telephone follow ups, and an educational package that provided an explanation of symptoms and encouraged home based exercise. One group received the minimum intervention only, one group received seven additional follow up telephone calls, and another received seven additional face to face sessions over 4 months. People in the written information group received advice and an information booklet that encouraged graded activity but gave no explanation for the symptoms. The RCT found no significant difference between the educational interventions. The RCT found that the educational interventions improved physical functioning, fatigue, mood, sleep, and disability (self reported) compared with written information only at 1 year (mean for 3 educational intervention groups *v* written information, SF-36 physical function subscale: ≥ 25 or an increase of ≥ 10, 1 year after randomisation, 69% *v* 6%, $P < 0.001$; Chalder fatigue scale: 3 *v* 10, $P < 0.001$; HADs: depression 4 *v* 10, $P < 0.001$; anxiety 7 *v* 10, $P < 0.01$).

Harms: None of the RCTs reported data on adverse effects, and we found no evidence that exercise is harmful in people with chronic fatigue syndrome. The second graded aerobic exercise RCT found no significant difference in withdrawal rates between graded exercise alone and no exercise (25/68 [37%] with exercise *v* 15/69 [22%] without exercise; RR 1.7, 95% CI 0.98 to 2.9).[20] The reasons for the withdrawals from the graded exercise groups were not reported.

Comment: Experience suggests that symptoms of chronic fatigue syndrome may be exacerbated by overly ambitious or overly hasty attempts at exercise.

OPTION **PROLONGED REST**

We found no RCTs on the effects of prolonged rest. Indirect observational evidence in healthy volunteers and in people recovering from a viral illness suggests that prolonged rest may perpetuate or worsen fatigue and symptoms.

Benefits: We found no systematic review or RCTs of prolonged rest in people with chronic fatigue syndrome.

Harms: We found no direct evidence of harmful effects of rest in people with chronic fatigue syndrome. We found observational evidence, which suggested that prolonged inactivity may perpetuate or worsen fatigue and is associated with symptoms in both healthy volunteers[36] and people recovering from viral illness.[37]

Comment: It is not clear that evidence from people recovering from viral illness can be extrapolated to people with chronic fatigue syndrome.

OPTION **DIETARY SUPPLEMENTS**

One small RCT found no significant difference between a nutritional supplement (containing multivitamins, minerals, and coenzymes) and placebo in fatigue severity or functional impairment at 10 weeks.

Benefits: We found one RCT (53 people who fulfilled CDC criteria for chronic fatigue syndrome with high fatigue severity and high disability scores; duration of illness ranged from 2 to 12 years) that compared a polynutrient supplement (containing several vitamins, minerals, and coenzymes, taken twice daily) versus placebo for 10 weeks.[38] It found no significant difference between treatments in fatigue severity or functional impairment (change in Checklist Individual Strength fatigue subscale from baseline to 10 weeks: 51.4 to 48.6 with supplements *v* 51.3 to 48.2 with placebo; difference +2.16, 95% CI –4.30 to +4.39; Sickness Impact Profile score < 750 at 10 weeks: 4% with supplements *v* 12% with placebo; P value not reported).

Harms: Three people (11%) on active treatment withdrew because of nausea.[38]

Comment: The RCT may have been too small to detect a clinically important difference between groups.[38]

OPTION **MAGNESIUM (INTRAMUSCULAR)**

One small RCT found that intramuscular magnesium injections improved symptoms at 6 weeks compared with placebo. However, we were unable to draw reliable conclusions from this small study.

Benefits: We found one systematic review (search date 2000), which did not report quantified results.[18] The review identified one RCT (32 people with chronic fatigue syndrome, but not magnesium deficiency; see comment below), which compared weekly intramuscular injections of magnesium sulphate 50% versus placebo injections (water) for 6 weeks.[39] It found that magnesium improved overall benefit, Nottingham Health Profile energy, pain, and emotional reaction subscale scores compared with placebo (AR for reporting overall benefit: 12/15 [80%] with magnesium *v* 3/17 [18%] with placebo; RR 4.5, 95% CI 1.6 to 13.1; NNT 2, 95% CI 2 to 4; Nottingham Health Profile mean change in score from baseline for magnesium *v* placebo: energy subscale –51.04 *v* –4.5, P = 0.002; pain subscale –19.63 *v* +2.7, P = 0.001; emotional reaction subscale –33.3 *v* +7.4, P = 0.013; score decrease represents improvement).

Harms: The RCT reported no adverse effects.

Comment: In the RCT, plasma and whole blood magnesium were normal and only the red blood cell concentrations of magnesium were slightly lower than the normal range.[39] Three subsequent case control studies have not found a deficiency of magnesium in people with chronic fatigue syndrome.[40–42] In these three studies, magnesium was in the normal range and no different from controls without chronic fatigue syndrome. However, none of the studies state how the normal range was established, so it is difficult to say if they are equivalent.

OPTION EVENING PRIMROSE OIL

One small RCT found no significant difference between evening primrose oil and placebo in depression scores at 3 months.

Benefits: We found one systematic review (search date 2000), which did not report quantified results.[18] The review identified one RCT (50 people with chronic fatigue syndrome, Oxford criteria), which compared evening primrose oil (4 g daily) with placebo for 3 months.[43] It found no significant difference between treatments in depression scores (Beck Depression Inventory), physical symptoms, or participant assessment (participant assessment at 3 months: 46% reported improvement with placebo *v* 29% with evening primrose oil; $P = 0.09$; RR and CIs not reported)

Harms: The RCT reported no adverse effects.

Comment: We found one RCT (63 people) that compared evening primrose oil (4 g daily) versus placebo in people with a diagnosis of postviral fatigue syndrome.[44] This diagnosis was made on the basis of overwhelming fatigue, myalgia, and depression, which had been present for at least 1 year, and all had been preceded by a febrile illness. At 3 months, 85% (33/39) of people on active treatment reported improvement compared with 17% (4/24) on placebo — a significant benefit ($P < 0.0001$). The difference in outcome may be partly explained by participant selection: the study in people with chronic fatigue syndrome used currently accepted diagnostic criteria.[43] Also, whereas the RCT in people with postviral fatigue syndrome used liquid paraffin as a placebo,[44] the chronic fatigue syndrome RCT used sunflower oil, which is better tolerated and less likely to affect the placebo response adversely.[43]

OPTION IMMUNOTHERAPY

Small RCTs provided limited evidence that immunoglobulin G modestly improved physical functioning and fatigue at 3–6 months compared with placebo, but it was associated with considerable adverse effects. Small RCTs provided insufficient evidence on the effects of interferon alfa or aciclovir compared with placebo. One RCT found that staphylococcus toxoid improved symptoms at six months compared with placebo, although it is associated with local reaction and could cause anaphylaxis.

Benefits: We found one systematic review (search date 2000), which did not report quantified results.[18] **Immunoglobulin G:** The review identified four relevant RCTs comparing immunoglobulin G versus placebo for 6 months.[45–48] The first RCT (30 people with chronic fatigue syndrome [CFS], CDC 1988 criteria) compared monthly intravenous injections of immunoglobulin G (1 g/kg) versus placebo (albumin).[45] After 6 months, no significant differences were found in measures of fatigue (self reported symptom severity) or in physical and social functioning (SF-36). It found that placebo significantly improved social function compared with immunoglobulin G (dichotomous figures and P value not reported). The second RCT (49 people with CFS, Australian criteria, similar to CDC criteria) compared monthly intravenous immunoglobulin G (2 g/kg) with intravenous placebo (a maltose solution) for 3 months.[46] It found that immunoglobulin G significantly increased the proportion of people with physician rated improvement in symptoms and disability compared with placebo 3 months after the completion of treatment (10/23 [44%] with immunoglobulin G *v* 3/26 [11%] with placebo; $P = 0.03$). The third RCT (99 adults with CFS, Australian criteria, similar to CDC criteria) compared low, medium, and high doses of immunoglobulin G (0.5, 1, or 2 g/kg) versus placebo (albumin).[47] It found no significant difference between groups in improvement in Karnofsky performance score or quality of life scores on visual analogue scales at 6 months (improvement in median Karnofsky score: 2.5 with low dose *v* 10 with medium dose *v* 5 with high dose *v* 7.5 with placebo, $P > 0.13$; quality of life: $P > 0.09$, scores not reported). The fourth RCT (71 adolescents aged 11–18 years with CFS, CDC criteria) compared immunoglobulin G (1 g/kg) versus placebo (a solution of maltose plus albumin).[48] Three infusions were given 1 month apart. The RCT found that immunoglobulin G significantly improved mean functional outcome (assessed using the mean of clinician ratings from four areas of the participants' activities) compared with placebo at 6 months (AR for improvement of ≥25%: 52% [26/36] with immunoglobin G *v* 31% [15/34] with placebo; RR 1.6, 95% CI 1.1 to 2.5). **Other treatments:** We found one systematic review (search date 2000)[18] and one subsequent RCT.[49] The review identified two RCTs comparing interferon alfa versus placebo.[50,51] The first RCT (30 people with CFS, Oxford criteria) identified by the review only found treatment benefit on subgroup analysis of people with isolated natural killer cell dysfunction.[50] The second randomised crossover trial (20 people with CFS) identified by the review did not present results in a manner that allowed clear interpretation of treatment effect.[51] Other RCTs in the review found no significant difference between placebo and acyclovir,[52] dialysable leucocyte extract (in a factorial design with cognitive behavioural therapy; see benefits of cognitive behavioural therapy, p 1414),[53] or terfenadine.[54] The subsequent RCT (100 women who met both the American Cancer Society criteria for fibromyalgia and the CDC criteria for CFS and had functional impairment > 6 months) compared weekly subcutaneous injections of staphylococcus toxoid (dose increased weekly from 0.1 to 1.0 mL, followed by 1.0 mL doses every 4 weeks) versus placebo.[49] It found that staphylococcus toxoid significantly improved the clinical global impression of change scale at 26 weeks compared with placebo (AR for "minimally improved", "much improved" or "very much improved": 65% [32/49] with toxoid *v* 18% [9/49] with placebo; $P < 0.001$).

Harms: **Immunoglobulin G:** In the first RCT, adverse effects judged to be worse than pretreatment symptoms in either group included gastrointestinal complaints (18 people), headaches (23 people), arthralgia (6 people), and worsening fatigue.[45] Of these symptoms, only headaches differed significantly between the groups (14/15 [93%] with immunoglobulin G *v* 9/15 [60%] with placebo). Three participants from each group had major adverse effects. Adverse events by treatment group were only reported for headache. **Other treatments:** In the RCT comparing interferon alfa versus placebo 15% (2/13) of the people taking active treatment developed neutropenia.[50] The RCT comparing staphylococcus toxoid with placebo found no significant difference between groups in reported adverse effects, excluding local reactions (13/49 [26%] with toxoid v 7/49 [14%] with placebo, P = 0.14).[49] All those receiving the toxoid had a local reaction at the injection site.

Comment: **Immunoglobulin G:** The first two RCTs differed in that the second used twice the dose of immunoglobulin G, did not require participants to fulfil the operational criteria (similar but not identical to US Centers for Disease Control and Prevention criteria) for chronic fatigue syndrome, and made no assessments of them during the study, instead waiting until 3 months after completion.[46] **Other treatments:** Terfenadine, particularly at high blood concentrations, is associated with rare hazardous cardiac arrhythmias.[55] The RCT that compared staphylococcus toxoid with placebo only included women who also had a diagnosis of fibromyalgia.[49]

OPTION COGNITIVE BEHAVIOURAL THERAPY

One systematic review found that cognitive behavioural therapy administered by highly skilled therapists in specialist centres improved quality of life and physical functioning compared with standard medical care or relaxation therapy. One additional multicentre RCT found that cognitive behavioural therapy administered by less experienced therapists may also be effective compared with guided support groups or no interventions.

Benefits: We found two systematic reviews (search dates 1998[56] and 2000[18]). The first review[56] identified three RCTs that met the reviewers' inclusion criteria (all participants fulfilled accepted diagnostic criteria for chronic fatigue syndrome (CFS) and the trials used adequate randomisation and controls).[53,57,58] The second review[18] identified one additional RCT that met inclusion criteria, but the review did not report quantified results.[59] The first RCT (90 people with CFS, Australian criteria, similar to CDC criteria) identified by the reviews evaluated cognitive behavioural therapy (CBT) and immunological therapy (dialysable leucocyte extract, DLE) using a factorial design.[53] The four treatment arms were CBT plus DLE; CBT plus placebo (saline); standard care plus DLE; and standard care plus placebo (saline). Cognitive behavioural therapy was given every 2 weeks for six sessions of 30–60 minutes each, and people were encouraged to exercise at home and feel less helpless. The trial found no significant difference in quality of life measures (Karnofsky scale and symptom report on a visual analogue scale) between pooled CBT groups and pooled standard care groups (P value not reported). The second RCT (60 people with CFS, Oxford criteria) identified by the reviews compared CBT versus normal general practice care in people attending a secondary care centre.[58] It found that CBT significantly improved quality of life (Karnofsky scale) at 12 months compared with standard medical care (final score > 80: 22/30 [73%] with CBT v 8/30 [27%] with placebo; RR 2.75, 95% CI 1.54 to 5.32; NNT 3, 95% CI 2 to 5). The active treatment consisted of a cognitive behavioural assessment, followed by 16 weekly sessions of behavioural experiments, problem solving activity, and re-evaluation of thoughts and beliefs that inhibited a return to normal functioning. The third RCT (60 people with CFS, CDC diagnostic criteria in people attending a secondary care centre) identified by the reviews compared CBT with relaxation therapy.[57] It found that CBT significantly improved physical functioning compared with relaxation therapy (improvement based on predefined absolute or relative increases in the SF-36 score: 19/30 [63%] with CBT v 5/30 [17%] with relaxation; RR 3.70, 95% CI 2.37 to 6.31; NNT 3, 95% CI 1 to 7). Improvement continued over 6–12 months' follow up. Cognitive behavioural therapy was given in 13 weekly sessions. A 5 year follow up study of 53 (88%) of the original participants found that more people rated themselves as "much improved" or "very much improved" with CBT compared with relaxation therapy (17/25 [68%] with CBT *v* 10/28 [36%] with relaxation therapy; RR 1.9, 95% CI 1.1 to 3.4; NNT 4, 95% CI 2 to 19).[60] More people treated with CBT met the authors' criteria for complete recovery at 5 years, but the difference was not significant (17/31 [55%] with CBT *v* 7/22 [32%] with relaxation therapy; RR 1.7, 95% CI 0.9 to 3.4). The additional multicentre RCT identified by the second review (278 people with CFS, CDC criteria) compared CBT, guided support groups, or no intervention.[59] The CBT consisted of 16 sessions over 8 months administered by 13 therapists with no previous experience of treating CFS. The guided support groups were similar to CBT in terms of treatment schedule, with the participants receiving non-directive support from a social worker. At 8 months' follow up, the RCT found that more people in the CBT group met the criteria for clinical improvement in fatigue severity (Checklist Individual Strength) and self reported improvement in fatigue compared with the guided support and no treatment groups (improved fatigue severity: CBT *v* support group, 27/83 [33%] with CBT *v* 10/80 [13%], RR 2.6, 95% CI 1.3 to 5.0; CBT *v* no intervention 27/83 [33%] *v* 8/62 [13%], RR 2.5, 95% CI 1.2 to 5.2; self reported improvement: CBT *v* support group 42/74 [57%] *v* 12/71 [17%], RR 3.4, 95% CI 1.9 to 5.8; CBT *v* no intervention 42/74 [57%] *v* 23/78 [30%], RR 1.9, 95% CI 1.3 to 2.9; analysis not by intention to treat; see comment below).

Harms: No harmful effects were reported.

Comment: The effectiveness of CBT for CFS outside of specialist settings has been questioned. The results of the multicentre RCT[59] suggest that cognitive behavioural therapy may be effective when administered by less experienced therapists with adequate supervision. The trial had a high withdrawal rate (25% after 8 months), especially in the CBT and guided support groups. Although the presented confidence intervals are not adjusted for multiple comparisons, the results would remain significant after any reasonable adjustment. The authors commented that the results were similar after intention to treat analysis, but these results were not presented.[59] A randomised trial that comparing CBT and non-directive counselling found that both interventions were of benefit in the management of people who consulted their family doctor because of fatigue symptoms.[61] In this study, 28% of the sample conformed to CDC criteria for CFS.

REFERENCES

1. Fukuda K, Straus S, Hickie I, et al. The chronic fatigue syndrome: a comprehensive approach to its definition and study. *Ann Intern Med* 1994;121:953–959.
2. Sharpe M, Archard LC, Banatvala JE. A report — chronic fatigue syndrome: guidelines for research. *J R Soc Med* 1991;84:118–121.
3. Wessely S, Chalder T, Hirsch S, et al. The prevalence and morbidity of chronic fatigue and chronic fatigue syndrome: a prospective primary care study. *Am J Public Health* 1997;87:1449–1455.
4. Steele L, Dobbins JG, Fukuda K, et al. The epidemiology of chronic fatigue in San Francisco. *Am J Med* 1998;105(suppl 3A):83–90.
5. Lawrie SM, Pelosi AJ. Chronic fatigue syndrome in the community: prevalence and associations. *Br J Psychiatry* 1995;166:793–797.
6. Wessely S. The epidemiology of chronic fatigue syndrome. *Epidemiol Rev* 1995;17:139–151.
7. Joyce J, Hotopf M, Wessely S. The prognosis of chronic fatigue and chronic fatigue syndrome: a systematic review. *QJM* 1997;90:223–233. Search date 1996; primary sources Medline, Embase, Current Contents, and Psychlit.
8. Stewart AD, Hays RD, Ware JE. The MOS short-form general health survey. *Med Care* 1988;26:724–732.
9. Karnofsky DA, Burchenal JH, MacLeod CM. *The clinical evaluation of chemotherapeutic agents in cancer.* New York: Columbia University Press; 1949:191–206.
10. Beck AT, Ward CH, Mendelson M, et al. An inventory for measuring depression. *Arch Gen Psychiatry* 1961;4:561–571.
11. Zigmond AS, Snaith RP. The Hospital Anxiety and Depression Scale (HAD). *Acta Psychiatr Scand* 1983;67:361–370.
12. Bergner M, Bobbit RA, Carter WB, et al. The sickness impact profile: development and final revision of a health status measure. *Med Care* 1981;19:787–805.
13. Chalder T, Berelowitz C, Pawlikowska T. Development of a fatigue scale. *J Psychosom Res* 1993;37:147–154.
14. Alberts M, Smets EM, Vercoulen JH, et al. Abbreviated fatigue questionnaire: a practical tool in the classification of fatigue. *Ned Tijdschr Geneeskd* 1997;141:1526–1530. [In Dutch]

15. Guy W. *ECDEU assessment manual for psychopharmacology*. Rockville: National Institute of Mental Health, 1976:218–222.
16. Vercoulen JH, Swanink CM, Fennis JF, et al. Dimensional assessment of chronic fatigue syndrome. *J Psychosom Res* 1994;38:383–392.
17. Hunt SM, McEwen J, McKenna SP. Measuring health status: a new tool for clinicians and epidemiologists. *J Roy Coll Gen Prac* 1985,35:185–188.
18. Whiting P, Bagnall A-M, Sowden A, et al. Interventions for the treatment and management of chronic fatigue syndrome: A systematic review. *JAMA* 2001;286:1360–1368. Search date 2000; primary sources Medline, Embase, Psychlit, ERIC, Current Contents, Internet searches, bibliographies from the retrieved references, individuals and organisations through a website dedicated to the review, and members of advisory panels.
19. Vercoulen J, Swanink C, Zitman F. Randomised, double-blind, placebo-controlled study of fluoxetine in chronic fatigue syndrome. *Lancet* 1996;347:858–861.
20. Wearden AJ, Morriss RK, Mullis R, et al. Randomised, double-blind, placebo controlled treatment trial of fluoxetine and a graded exercise programme for chronic fatigue syndrome. *Br J Psychiatry* 1998;172:485–490.
21. Vercoulen JHMM, Swanink CMA, Galama JMD, et al. Dimensional assessment of chronic fatigue syndrome. *J Psychosom Res* 1994;38:383–392.
22. Natelson BH, Cheu J, Pareja J, et al. Randomised, double blind, controlled placebo-phase in trial of low dose phenelzine in the chronic fatigue syndrome. *Psychopharmacology* 1996;124:226–230.
23. Hickie IB, Wilson AJ, Murray Wright J, et al. A randomized, double-blind, placebo-controlled trial of moclobemide in patients with chronic fatigue syndrome. *J Clin Psychiatry* 2000;61:643–648.
24. Behan PO, Hannifah H. 5-HT reuptake inhibitors in CFS. *J Immunol Immunopharmacol* 1995;15:66–69.
25. Rowe PC, Calkins H, DeBusk K, et al. Fludrocortisone acetate to treat neurally mediated hypotension in chronic fatigue syndrome. *JAMA* 2001;285:52–59.
26. Peterson PK, Pheley A, Schroeppel J, et al. A preliminary placebo-controlled crossover trial of fludrocortisone for chronic fatigue syndrome. *Arch Intern Med* 1998;158:908–914.
27. McKenzie R, O'Fallon A, Dale J, et al. Low-dose hydrocortisone for treatment of chronic fatigue syndrome. *JAMA* 1998;280:1061–1066.
28. Cleare AJ, Heap E, Malhi G, et al. Low-dose hydrocortisone in chronic fatigue syndrome: a randomised crossover trial. *Lancet* 1999;353:455–458.
29. Blockmans D, Persoons P, Van Houdenhove B, et al. Combination therapy with hydrocortisone and fludrocortisone does not improve symptoms in chronic fatigue syndrome: a randomized, placebo-controlled, double-blind, crossover study. *Am J Med* 2003;114:736–741.
30. Bou-Holaigah I, Rowe P, Kan J, et al. The relationship between neurally mediated hypotension and the chronic fatigue syndrome. *JAMA* 1995;274:961–967.
31. Demitrack M, Dale J, Straus S, et al. Evidence for impaired activation of the hypothalamic-pituitary-adrenal axis in patients with chronic fatigue syndrome. *J Clin Endocrinol Metab* 1991;73:1224–1234.
32. Forsyth LM, Preuss HG, MacDowell AL, et al. Therapeutic effects of oral NADH on the symptoms of patients with chronic fatigue syndrome. *Ann Allergy Asthma Immunol* 1999;82:185–191.
33. Colquhoun D, Senn S. Re: Therapeutic effects of oral NADH on the symptoms of patients with chronic fatigue syndrome. *Ann Allergy Asthma Immunol* 2000;84:639–640.
34. Fulcher KY, White PD. A randomised controlled trial of graded exercise therapy in patients with the chronic fatigue syndrome. *BMJ* 1997;314:1647–1652.
35. Powell P, Bentall RP, Nye FJ, et al. Randomised controlled trial of patient education to encourage graded exercise in chronic fatigue syndrome. *BMJ* 2001;322:387–390.
36. Sandler H, Vernikos J. *Inactivity: physiological effects*. London: Academic Press, 1986.
37. Dalrymple W. Infectious mononucleosis: 2. Relation of bed rest and activity to prognosis. *Postgrad Med* 1961;35:345–349.
38. Brouwers FM, van der Werf S, Bleijenberg G, et al. The effect of a polynutrient supplement on fatigue and physical activity of patients with chronic fatigue syndrome: a double-blind randomized controlled trial. *QJM* 2002;95:677–683.
39. Cox IM, Campbell MJ, Dowson D. Red blood cell magnesium and chronic fatigue syndrome. *Lancet* 1991;337:757–760.
40. Clague JE, Edwards RHT, Jackson MJ. Intravenous magnesium loading in chronic fatigue syndrome. *Lancet* 1992;340:124–125.
41. Hinds G, Bell NP, McMaster D, et al. Normal red cell magnesium concentrations and magnesium loading tests in patients with chronic fatigue syndrome. *Ann Clin Biochem* 1994;31:459–461.
42. Swanink CM, Vercoulen JH, Bleijenberg G, et al. Chronic fatigue syndrome: a clinical and laboratory study with a well matched control group. *J Intern Med* 1995;237:499–506.
43. Warren G, McKendrick M, Peet M. The role of essential fatty acids in chronic fatigue syndrome. *Acta Neurol Scand* 1999;99:112–116.
44. Behan PO, Behan WMH, Horrobin D. Effect of high doses of essential fatty acids on the postviral fatigue syndrome. *Acta Neurol Scand* 1990;82:209–216.
45. Peterson PK, Shepard J, Macres M, et al. A controlled trial of intravenous immunoglobulin G in chronic fatigue syndrome. *Am J Med* 1990;89:554–560.
46. Lloyd A, Hickie I, Wakefield D, et al. A double-blind, placebo-controlled trial of intravenous immunoglobulin therapy in patients with chronic fatigue syndrome. *Am J Med* 1990;89:561–568.
47. Vollmer-Conna U, Hickie I, Hadzi-Pavlovic D, et al. Intravenous immunoglobulin is ineffective in the treatment of patients with chronic fatigue syndrome. *Am J Med* 1997;103:38–43.
48. Rowe KS. Double-blind randomized controlled trial to assess the efficacy of intravenous gammaglobulin for the management of chronic fatigue syndrome in adolescents. *J Psychiatr Res* 1997;31:133–147.
49. Zachrisson O, Regland B, Jahreskog M, et al. Treatment with staphylococcus toxoid in fibromyalgia/chronic fatigue syndrome – a randomised controlled trial. *Eur J Pain* 2002;6:455–466.
50. See DM, Tilles JG. Alpha interferon treatment of patients with chronic fatigue syndrome. *Immunol Invest* 1996;25:153–164.
51. Brook M, Bannister B, Weir W. Interferon-alpha therapy for patients with chronic fatigue syndrome. *J Infect Dis* 1993;168:791–792.
52. Straus SE, Dale JK, Tobi M, et al. Acyclovir treatment of the chronic fatigue syndrome. Lack of efficacy in a placebo-controlled trial. *N Engl J Med* 1988;319:1692–1698.
53. Lloyd A, Hickie I, Boughton R, et al. Immunologic and psychological therapy for patients with chronic fatigue syndrome. *Am J Med* 1993;94:197–203.
54. Steinberg P, McNutt BE, Marshall P, et al. Double-blind placebo-controlled study of efficacy of oral terfenadine in the treatment of chronic fatigue syndrome. *J Allergy Clin Immunol* 1996;97:119–126.
55. Medicines Control Agency (UK). *Current Problems in Pharmacovigilance*, Volume 23, September 1997.
56. Price JR, Couper J. Cognitive behaviour therapy for chronic fatigue syndrome in adults. In: The Cochrane Library, Issue 4, 2003. Chicester, UK: John Wiley & Sons, Ltd. Search date 1998; primary sources Medline, Embase, Biological Abstracts, Sigle, Index to Theses of Great Britain and Ireland, Index to Scientific and Technical Proceedings, Science

Citation Index, Trials Register of the Depression, Anxiety and Neurosis Group, citation lists, and personal contacts.

57. Deale A, Chalder T, Marks I, et al. Cognitive behaviour therapy for chronic fatigue syndrome: a randomized controlled trial. *Am J Psychiatry* 1997;154:408–414.
58. Sharpe M, Hawton K, Simkin S, et al. Cognitive behaviour therapy for chronic fatigue syndrome: a randomized controlled trial. *BMJ* 1996;312:22–26.
59. Prins JB, Bleijenberg G, Bazelmans E, et al. Cognitive behaviour therapy for chronic fatigue syndrome: a multicentre randomised controlled trial. *Lancet* 2001;357:841–847.
60. Deale A, Husain K, Chalder T, et al. Long-term outcome of cognitive behaviour therapy versus relaxation therapy for chronic fatigue syndrome: a 5-year follow-up study. *Am J Psychiatry* 2001;158:2038–2042.
61. Ridsdale L, Godfrey E, Chalder T, et al. Chronic fatigue in general practice: is counselling as good as cognitive behaviour therapy? A UK randomised trial. *Br J Gen Pract* 2001;51:19–24.

Steven Reid
Consultant Liaison Psychiatrist
St Mary's Hospital
London
UK

Trudie Chalder
Professor of Cognitive Behavioural Psychotherapy
Department of Psychological Medicine
Weston Education Centre
London
UK

Anthony Cleare
Senior Lecturer
Institute of Psychiatry
Maudsley Hospital
London
UK

Matthew Hotopf
Reader of Psychological Medicine
Institute of Psychiatry
Weston Education Centre
London
UK

Simon Wessely
Professor of Epidemiological and Liaison Psychiatry
Guy's, King's and St Thomas' School of
Medicine and Institute of Psychiatry
London
UK

Competing interests: None declared.

TABLE 1 Diagnostic criteria for chronic fatigue syndrome (see text, p 1406).

CDC 1994[1]	Oxford, UK[2]
Clinically evaluated, medically unexplained fatigue of at least 6 months' duration that is:	Severe, disabling fatigue of at least 6 months' duration that:
– of new onset	– affects both physical and mental functioning
– not a result of ongoing exertion	– was present for more than 50% of the time
– not substantially alleviated by rest	
– a substantial reduction in previous levels of activity	
The occurrence of four or more of the following symptoms:	Other symptoms, particularly myalgia, sleep, and mood disturbance, may be present.
– subjective memory impairment	
– tender lymph nodes	
– muscle pain	
– joint pain	
– headache	
– unrefreshing sleep	
– postexertional malaise (> 24 hours)	
Exclusion criteria	
– Active, unresolved, or suspected disease likely to cause fatigue	– Active, unresolved, or suspect disease likely to cause fatigue
– Psychotic, melancholic, or bipolar depression (but not uncomplicated major depression)	– Psychotic, melancholic, or bipolar depression (but not uncomplicated major depression)
– Psychotic disorders	– Psychotic disorders
– Dementia	– Dementia
– Anorexia or bulimia nervosa	– Anorexia or bulimia nervosa
– Alcohol or other substance misuse	
– Severe obesity	

CDC, US Centers for Disease Control and Prevention.

Fracture prevention in postmenopausal women

Search date January 2004

Olivier Bruyere, John Edwards, and Jean-Yves Reginster

QUESTIONS

INTERVENTIONS

Key Messages

Prevention of fractures

- **Alendronate** Two systematic reviews in postmenopausal women found that alendronate reduced vertebral and non-vertebral fractures compared with placebo at 1–4 years.
- **Parathyroid hormone** One RCT in women with prior vertebral fractures found that parathyroid hormone reduced the proportion of women with vertebral and non-vertebral fractures compared with placebo. Another RCT in women with osteoporosis found that parathyroid hormone plus oestrogen reduced vertebral fractures compared with oestrogen alone after 3 years.
- **Raloxifene** One large RCT in postmenopausal women with osteoporosis found that raloxifene reduced vertebral fractures compared with placebo, but no significant difference was found in non-vertebral fractures. We found no RCTs examining the effects of other selective oestrogen receptor modulators.
- **Risedronate** One systematic review in postmenopausal women found that compared with control (placebo, calcium, or calcium plus vitamin D) risedronate reduced vertebral and non-vertebral fractures at 4 years.
- **Calcitonin** One systematic review in postmenopausal women found that calcitonin reduced vertebral fractures compared with placebo at 1–5 years after treatment, but found no significant difference between calcitonin and placebo in non-vertebral fractures.
- **Calcium plus vitamin D** One large RCT in women aged 69–106 years living in nursing homes found that calcium plus vitamin D3 reduced hip fractures and all non-vertebral fractures over 18 months to 3 years compared with placebo. One smaller RCT in women and men aged 65 years or older found that calcium plus

vitamin D3 reduced non-vertebral fractures at 3 years compared with placebo, but found no significant difference in hip fractures. Another smaller RCT in postmenopausal women found no significant difference between calcium plus vitamin D3 and placebo in hip fractures after 2 years. The two smaller RCTs may have lacked power to detect clinically important differences.

- **Etidronate** One systematic review in postmenopausal women found that etidronate reduced vertebral fractures compared with control (placebo, calcium, or calcium plus vitamin D) over 2 years, but found no significant difference in non-vertebral fractures.
- **Vitamin D analogue (calcitriol)** One systematic review found limited evidence from two small RCTs in postmenopausal women that calcitriol reduced vertebral fractures over 3 years compared with placebo.
- **Environmental manipulation** We found no systematic review and no RCTs assessing environmental manipulation alone.
- **Exercise** Three RCTs found no significant difference in falls resulting in fracture at 8 months to 1 year between exercise (advice to walk briskly three times weekly, balance and strength exercises plus walking, or low-intensity exercise plus incontinence care) and control. One small RCT in postmenopausal women found no significant difference between a 2 year back strengthening exercise programme and usual care in vertebral fractures over 10 years.
- **Hip protectors** One systematic review in elderly community dwelling or nursing home residents found no significant difference in hip fractures at 6 months to 2 years between hip protectors and no protectors in RCTs where individuals were randomised. However, the review found that hip protectors reduced fractures at 11–19 months in RCTs that used cluster analysis. The systematic review found no significant difference in pelvic fractures at 6 months to 2 years between hip protectors and no hip protectors in RCTs where individuals were randomised, but in RCTs with cluster analysis, the review found that hip protectors were associated with a reduction in pelvic fractures at 11–19 months. The review found no significant difference between hip protectors and no hip protectors in the rate of other fractures.
- **Calcium alone** One systematic review in postmenopausal women found no significant difference between calcium supplementation and placebo in vertebral or non-vertebral fractures at 1.5–4 years.
- **Vitamin D alone** One large RCT in postmenopausal women and two large RCTs in postmenopausal women and elderly men provided no evidence of a difference between vitamin D3 and placebo in hip, vertebral, and non-vertebral fractures after 2–5 years.
- **Hormone replacement therapy** We found insufficient evidence of benefit, but reliable evidence of harm. One systematic review in postmenopausal women found that hormone replacement therapy reduced vertebral fractures compared with control. However, another systematic review and two subsequent RCTs in postmenopausal women found no significant difference in vertebral fractures. Two systematic reviews and two subsequent RCTs provided insufficient evidence about the effects of hormone replacement therapy on non-vertebral fractures. One large RCT of oestrogen plus progestin versus placebo for primary prevention of coronary heart disease in healthy postmenopausal women was stopped because hormonal treatment increased risks of invasive breast cancer, coronary events, stroke, and pulmonary embolism.

DEFINITION This topic covers interventions to prevent fractures in postmenopausal women. Fractures may be symptomatic or asymptomatic. A fracture is a break or disruption of bone or cartilage. Symptoms and signs may include immobility, pain, tenderness, numbness, bruising, joint deformity, joint swelling, limb deformity, and limb shortening.[1] Diagnosis is usually based on a typical clinical picture combined with results from an appropriate imaging technique. Usually, in trials dealing with osteoporosis, menopause is considered to be present 12 months after the last menstruation.

INCIDENCE/ PREVALENCE	The lifetime risk of fracture in white women is 20% for the spine, 15% for the wrist, and 18% for the hip.[2] The incidence of postmenopausal fracture increases with age.[3] One observational study found that age specific incidence rates for postmenopausal fracture of the hip increased exponentially beyond the age of 50 years.[4]
AETIOLOGY/ RISK FACTORS	Fractures usually arise from trauma. General risk factors include those associated with increased risks of falling (such as ataxia, drug and alcohol intake, loose carpets), age, osteoporosis, bony metastases, and other bone disorders. Postmenopausal women are at increased risk of fracture because of hormone related bone loss. Risk factors for fractures in postmenopausal women include increasing age; low body mass index; time since menopause; alcohol consumption; smoking; some endocrine diseases, such as hyperparathyroidism or thyroid disease; and steroid use, among others.
PROGNOSIS	Fractures may result in pain, short or long term disability, haemorrhage, thromboembolic disease (see thromboembolism, p 194), shock, and death. Vertebral fractures are associated with pain, physical impairment, muscular atrophy, changes in body shape, loss of physical function, and lower quality of life.[5] About 20% of women die in the first year after a hip fracture, representing an increase in mortality of 12–20% compared with women of similar age and no hip fracture. Half of elderly women who had been independent become partly dependent after hip fracture. A third become totally dependent.
AIMS OF INTERVENTION	To prevent fractures, with minimal adverse effects from treatment.
OUTCOMES	Incidence of hip, wrist, non-vertebral, and vertebral fractures (we have not reported intermediate outcomes such as bone mineral density data).
METHODS	*Clinical Evidence* search and appraisal January 2004. We also hand searched journals of bone diseases and carried out manual searches using the bibliographies of review articles published after 1985. Some of the RCTs identified provide results generalised to fracture per person per year overall fractures. These results provide an idea of the group effect of an intervention, but not of its effects on the incidence of fracture in an individual. Data on multiple fractures in one person clearly differ from data on multiple people experiencing a single fracture. Regulatory authorities and scientific groups have recommended that the results of studies evaluating new interventions are expressed in terms of the proportion of people experiencing new fractures.[6] This topic examines fracture prevention in postmenopausal women. However, we have included RCTs undertaken in people outside this group (men, premenopausal women) in some sections, as results from these trials may be generalisable to postmenopausal women.

QUESTION What are the effects of treatments to prevent fractures in postmenopausal women?

OPTION BISPHOSPHONATES

Olivier Bruyere and Jean-Yves Reginster

Two systematic reviews in postmenopausal women found that alendronate reduced vertebral and non-vertebral fractures compared with placebo at 1–4 years. One systematic review in postmenopausal women found that etidronate reduced vertebral fractures compared with control (placebo, calcium, or calcium plus vitamin D) over 2 years, but found no significant difference in non-vertebral fractures. One systematic review in postmenopausal women found that risedronate reduced vertebral and non-vertebral fractures compared with control (placebo, calcium, or calcium plus vitamin D) at 4 years.

Benefits: **Alendronate:** We found two systematic reviews.[7,8] The first systematic review (search date 1999, 11 RCTs, 12 855 postmenopausal women) included RCTs that randomised postmenopausal women to alendronate or placebo and had a follow up of at least 1 year.[7] It found that alendronate (≥ 5 mg) significantly reduced vertebral fractures compared with placebo (8 RCTs, 9360 women; RR 0.52, 95% CI 0.43 to 0.65). It also found that alendronate (≥ 10 mg) significantly reduced non-vertebral fractures compared with placebo (6 RCTs, 3723 women; RR 0.51, 95% CI 0.38 to 0.69). The review did not state how fractures were diagnosed. The second systematic review (search date 1998, 7 RCTs, 10 287 postmenopausal women aged 39–85 years) found that, compared with placebo, alendronate significantly reduced vertebral fractures (fractures confirmed radiologically; 4 RCTs; RR 0.54, 95% CI 0.45 to 0.66) and non-vertebral fractures (6 RCTs; RR 0.81, 95% CI 0.72 to 0.92).[8] It found that fewer people had hip fractures over 1–4 years, but the difference was not significant (3 RCTs; RR 0.64, 95% CI 0.40 to 1.01; results presented graphically). **Etidronate:** We found one systematic review (search date 1998, 13 RCTs, 1010 postmenopausal women) comparing etidronate versus placebo, calcium, or calcium plus vitamin D.[9] It found that etidronate (intermittent cyclic administration of 400 mg/day for 14–20 days followed by calcium and/or vitamin D) significantly reduced vertebral fractures over 2 years compared with control (9 RCTs; 32/538 [6%] *v* 54/538 [10%]; RR 0.60, 95% CI 0.41 to 0.88), but found no significant difference in non-vertebral fractures (7 RCTs; 48/433 [11%] *v* 49/434 [11%]; RR 0.98, 95% CI 0.68 to 1.42). The review did not describe clearly how fractures were diagnosed. **Risedronate:** We found one systematic review (search date 2001, 8 RCTs), which compared risedronate versus control (placebo, calcium, or calcium plus vitamin D).[10] It found that risedronate (2.5 or 5 mg) significantly reduced vertebral and non-vertebral fractures compared with control at 4 years (vertebral fractures, 5 RCTs, 2604 postmenopausal women: RR 0.64, 95% CI 0.52 to 0.77; non-vertebral fractures, 7 RCTs, 12 958 postmenopausal women: RR 0.73, 95% CI 0.61 to 0.87). The review did not describe clearly how fractures were diagnosed.

Harms: **Alendronate:** Observational evidence suggests that oral alendronate is associated with oesophageal erosions and ulcerative oesophagitis. However, one RCT[11] identified by the second review[8] (in which people took alendronate with 180–240 mL water on rising in the morning and remained upright for at least 30 minutes after swallowing the tablet and until they had eaten something) found no significant difference in oesophagitis with alendronate compared with placebo. **Risedronate:** One systematic review (search date 2001) found no significant difference between risedronate (2.5 or 5 mg) and control in withdrawal due to any adverse effect or gastrointestinal effects, or in abdominal pain (withdrawal due to any adverse effect, 8 RCTs, 13 998 postmenopausal women: RR 0.94, 95% CI 0.84 to 1.06; withdrawal due to gastrointestinal effects, 4 RCTs, 12 313 women: RR 0.97, 95% CI 0.91 to 1.04; abdominal pain, 5 RCTs, 12 835 women: RR 0.93, 95% CI 0.83 to 1.05).[10] One observational study found limited evidence suggesting that the gastrointestinal safety of risedronate seems to be in the same range as alendronate.[12]

Comment: **Risedronate:** The systematic review (search date 2001) noted that all of the included RCTs analysed data on an intention to treat basis, but that 5 RCTs had withdrawal rates greater than 25%. However, the authors noted that the magnitude of the treatment effect was unrelated to loss to follow up.[10]

OPTION CALCIUM ALONE

Olivier Bruyere and Jean-Yves Reginster

One systematic review in postmenopausal women found no significant difference between calcium supplementation and placebo in vertebral or non-vertebral fractures at 1.5–4 years.

Benefits: **Calcium versus placebo:** We found one systematic review (search date 1998, 15 RCTs, 1806 postmenopausal women; see comment below).[13] It found no significant difference between calcium (600–2000 mg) and placebo in vertebral or non-vertebral fractures at 1.5–4 years (vertebral fractures, 5 RCTs, 576 women: RR 0.79, 95% CI 0.54 to 1.09; non-vertebral fractures, 2 RCTs, 222 women: RR 0.86, 95% CI 0.43 to 1.72).[13] It noted that the two RCTs reporting non-vertebral fractures had very few events, and that the pooled confidence intervals were wide (absolute numbers not reported).

Harms: The systematic review (search date 2001) did not report any data on harms.[13]

Comment: The systematic review (search date 2001) found that 13 of the 15 RCTs had withdrawal rates of 5–20% and two RCTs had losses greater than 20%.[13]

OPTION VITAMIN D ALONE

Olivier Bruyere and Jean-Yves Reginster

One large RCT in postmenopausal women and two large RCTs in postmenopausal women and elderly men provided no evidence of a difference between vitamin D3 and placebo in hip, vertebral, and non-vertebral fractures after 2–5 years.

Benefits: **Vitamin D3 versus placebo:** We found one systematic review (search date 2000, 1 RCT)[14] and two subsequent RCTs.[15,16] The RCT identified by the review (2578 people [1916 women and 662 men], aged 70 years or older, living at home; see comment below) found no significant difference between vitamin D3 and placebo in hip fracture (confirmed by clinical assessment and x ray films; 58/1284 [4.5%] *v* 48/1280 [3.7%]; RR 1.20, 95% CI 0.83 to 1.75), or any non-vertebral fracture over 3 years (135/1284 [11%] *v* 122/1280 [10%]; RR 1.10, 95% CI 0.87 to 1.39).[14] The first subsequent RCT (1144 people resident in nursing homes; mean age 85 years; 75% women) found no significant difference between vitamin D3 (10 μg/day) and placebo in hip fracture or any non-vertebral fracture (fractures confirmed by hospital discharge letter or x ray film) after 2 years' treatment (hip fracture: 50/569 [8.8%] with vitamin D *v* 47/575 [8.2%] with placebo; RR 1.09, 95% CI 0.73 to 1.63; non-vertebral fracture: 69/569 [12.1%] with vitamin D *v* 76/575 [13.2%] with placebo; RR 0.92, 95% CI 0.66 to 1.27).[15] The second subsequent RCT (2686 people; 2037 men and 649 women; aged 65–85 years) reported separate results for men and women in the trial.[16] In women, it found no significant difference between vitamin D3 and placebo in first fractures at any site after 5 years (42/326 [13%] with vitamin D3 *v* 58/323 [18%] with placebo; RR 0.68, 95% CI 0.46 to 1.01). In women, it also found no significant difference between vitamin D3 and placebo in first hip fractures after 5 years (10/326 [3%] with vitamin D3 *v* 10/323 [3%] with placebo; RR 0.98, 95% CI 0.41 to 2.36) or vertebral fractures (4/326 [1%] with vitamin D3 *v* 6/323 [2%] with placebo; RR 0.65, 95% CI 0.18 to 2.3).

Harms: **Vitamin D3 or vitamin D analogue (calcitriol) versus placebo or calcium:** One systematic review found that vitamin D or vitamin D analogues compared with placebo or calcium increased hypercalcaemia (5 RCTs, 1009 people; 22/498 [4.4%] with vitamin D or vitamin D analogues *v* 18/511 [3.5%] with placebo or calcium; RR 1.71, 95% CI 1.01 to 2.89).[14]

Comment: Although some RCTs included both men and women at risk of hip fracture, it is likely that the results are generalisable to postmenopausal women.[14,15]

OPTION CALCIUM PLUS VITAMIN D

Olivier Bruyere and Jean-Yves Reginster

One large RCT in women aged 69–106 years living in nursing homes found that calcium plus vitamin D3 reduced hip fractures and all non-vertebral fractures over 18 months to 3 years compared with placebo. One smaller RCT in women and men aged 65 years or older found that calcium plus vitamin D3 reduced non-vertebral fractures at 3 years compared with placebo, but found no significant difference in hip fractures. Another smaller RCT in postmenopausal women found no significant difference between calcium plus vitamin D3 and placebo in hip fractures after 2 years. The two smaller RCTs may have lacked power to detect clinically important differences.

Benefits: **Calcium plus vitamin D3 versus placebo:** We found one systematic review (search date 2000, 2 RCTs, 3715 people)[14] and one subsequent RCT.[17] The first RCT identified by the review (3270 mobile elderly women, aged 69–106 years, living in nursing homes) found that, compared with placebo, calcium plus vitamin D3 significantly reduced hip fractures (80/1387 [6%] with calcium plus vitamin D3 *v* 110/1403 [8%] with placebo; RR 0.74, 95% CI 0.60 to 0.91) and all non-vertebral fractures (160/1387 [11%] with calcium plus vitamin D3 *v* 215/1403 [15%] with placebo; RR 0.75, 95% CI 0.62 to 0.91) over 18 months. This difference remained significant after 3 years of treatment (hip fractures: 137/1176 [12%] with calcium plus vitamin D3 *v* 178/1127 [16%] with placebo; RR 0.74, 95% CI 0.60 to 0.91; all non-vertebral fractures: 255/1176 [22%] with calcium plus vitamin D3 *v* 308/1127 [27%] with placebo; RR 0.72, 95% CI 0.60 to 0.84). The review did not state how fractures were diagnosed.[14] The second RCT identified by the review (246 women and 199 men, aged 65 years or older, living at home; see comment below) found no significant difference between calcium plus vitamin D3 and placebo in hip fractures over 3 years (0/187 [0%] *v* 1/202 [0.5%]; RR 0.36, 95% CI 0.01 to 8.78), but was underpowered to exclude a clinically important difference. It found that calcium plus vitamin D reduced overall non-vertebral fractures compared with placebo (11/187 [6%] with calcium plus vitamin D *v* 26/202 [13%] with placebo; RR 0.46, 95% CI 0.23 to 0.90). Fractures were diagnosed by self report, interview, and validation from case records.[14] The subsequent RCT (583 women in institutional care, mean age 85 years, range 64–99 years) found no significant difference between calcium plus vitamin D3 and placebo in hip fracture at 2 years (27/393 [6.9%] with calcium plus vitamin D *v* 21/190 [11.1%] with placebo; RR 0.59, 95% CI 0.33 to 1.04).[17]

Harms: **Vitamin D3 or vitamin D analogue (calcitriol) versus placebo or calcium:** See harms of vitamin D, p 1423.

Comment: Although some RCTs included both men and women at risk of hip fracture, it is likely that the results are generalisable to postmenopausal women.[14,15]

OPTION VITAMIN D ANALOGUES (CALCITRIOL)

Olivier Bruyere and Jean-Yves Reginster

One systematic review found limited evidence from two small RCTs in postmenopausal women that calcitriol reduced vertebral fractures over 3 years compared with placebo.

Benefits: **Vitamin D analogue (calcitriol) versus placebo:** One systematic review[14] identified two small RCTs (68 women aged ≥ 54 years) comparing calcitriol (1,25-dihydroxy vitamin D) versus placebo. It found that calcitriol significantly reduced new vertebral fractures over 3 years compared with placebo (fractures confirmed radiologically; 8/34 [23%] with calcitriol *v* 17/34 [50%] with placebo; RR 0.49, 95% CI 0.25 to 0.95).

Harms: **Vitamin D3 or vitamin D analogue (calcitriol) versus placebo or calcium:** See harms of vitamin D, p 1423.

Comment: None.

OPTION CALCITONIN

Olivier Bruyere and Jean-Yves Reginster

One systematic review in postmenopausal women found that calcitonin reduced vertebral fractures compared with placebo at 1–5 years after treatment, but found no significant difference between calcitonin and placebo in non-vertebral fractures.

Benefits: We found one systematic review in postmenopausal women.[18] The systematic review (search date 2000, 30 RCTs, 3993 postmenopausal women) included trials of at least 1 year's duration, which compared calcitonin versus placebo or calcium and/or vitamin D in postmenopausal women.[18] It found that calcitonin significantly reduced vertebral fractures compared with placebo 1–5 years after treatment (4 RCTs, 1404 women; RR 0.46, 95% CI 0.25 to 0.87; see comment below). It found no significant difference between calcitonin and placebo in non-vertebral fractures (3 RCTs, 1481 women; RR 0.52, 95% CI 0.22 to 1.23).

Harms: The systematic review found that the relative risk for headache from one included RCT was 0.57 (95% CI 0.34 to 0.93) and that for climacteric symptoms from another included RCT was 0.20 (95% CI 0.05 to 0.77).[18] It noted that, in general, included trials were poor in their reporting of adverse events.

Comment: The systematic review suggested caution in interpreting the magnitude of the effect of calcitonin in the pooled estimates.[18] The pooled estimate for vertebral fractures was based on three small RCTs and a fourth larger RCT, with a large variability in results between them. Losses to follow up were 18.7%, 21%, 45%, and 59.3% in the four RCTs.[18] Similar issues were raised in the pooled estimate for non-vertebral fractures.[18] We found a second systematic review (search date 1996, 14 RCTs [7 RCTs in perimenopausal women with crush fractures or osteoporosis, 7 RCTs in men and women with osteoporosis or taking corticosteroids], 1309 people, exact proportions of women and men not specified; see comment below) compared calcitonin (salcatonin) versus placebo, no treatment, calcium, or calcium plus vitamin D.[19] It included three RCTs identified by the first systematic review. It found that fewer people developed vertebral or non-vertebral fractures with calcitonin compared with no calcitonin, but the difference was not significant (vertebral fractures: 166/1190 [14%] people with calcitonin *v* 96/554 [17%] with no calcitonin; RR 0.80, 95% CI 0.64 to 1.01; non-vertebral fractures: RR 0.48, 95% CI 0.20 to 1.15; no further data reported). The review did not state how fractures were diagnosed. The second systematic review commented that its conclusions are limited because many of the RCTs identified did not report the occurrence of fractures, were not double blinded, and only two of the RCTs identified were of over 2 years' duration.[19] The second systematic review gave no information on harms.[19]

OPTION HORMONE REPLACEMENT THERAPY

Olivier Bruyere and Jean-Yves Reginster

We found insufficient evidence of benefit, but reliable evidence of harm. One systematic review in postmenopausal women found that hormone replacement therapy reduced vertebral fractures compared with control. However, another systematic review and two subsequent RCTs in postmenopausal women found no significant difference in vertebral fractures. Two systematic reviews and two subsequent RCTs provided insufficient evidence about the effects of hormone replacement therapy on non-vertebral fractures. One large RCT of oestrogen plus progestin versus placebo for primary prevention of coronary heart disease in healthy postmenopausal women was stopped because hormonal treatment increased risks of invasive breast cancer, coronary events, stroke, and pulmonary embolism.

Benefits: **Vertebral fractures:** We found two systematic reviews[28,29] and two subsequent RCTs.[30,31] The first systematic review (search date 2001, 22 RCTs, mean age 48–73 years) included RCTs of postmenopausal women who were healthy, or who also had coronary artery disease, a vertebral fracture, or established osteoporosis.[28] It included RCTs that compared hormone replacement therapy (HRT) with placebo, calcium with or without vitamin D, or no treatment, with a follow up of at least 1 year. It found that HRT significantly reduced the incidence of vertebral fractures compared with control (13 RCTs; 42/3507 [1.2%] with HRT *v* 63/3216 [2%] with control; RR 0.67, 95% CI 0.45 to 0.98). The second systematic review (search date 1999, 57 RCTs, including 8 RCTs identified by the first review) included RCTs that evaluated fracture rates in postmenopausal women.[29] It excluded three RCTs included in the first systematic review[28] on methodological grounds.[29] The HRT could be given in conjunction with a calcium and vitamin D supplement, provided that the comparison group received the same supplement, and that the follow up was for at least 1 year. It found no significant difference between HRT and control in the incidence of vertebral fractures (5 RCTs, 3385 women; RR 0.66, 95% CI 0.41 to 1.07). The first subsequent RCT (16 608 postmenopausal women, aged 50–79 years) found that HRT (oestrogen plus progestin) significantly reduced vertebral fractures compared with placebo (HR 0.66, 95% CI 0.44 to 0.98).[30] However, after adjustment for multiple statistical testing as outlined in the monitoring plan, the difference between groups was no longer significant (HR 0.66, 95% CI 0.32 to 1.34). The second subsequent RCT (191 postmenopausal women) compared nylestriol–levonorgestrel versus placebo for 1 year.[31] It found no vertebral fractures in either treatment group. However, this study is likely to have been underpowered to detect any clinically important differences between treatment groups. **Non-vertebral fractures:** We found two systematic reviews[29,32] and two subsequent RCTs[30,33] comparing HRT versus placebo, no treatment, calcium, or calcium plus vitamin D. The first review (search date 2000, 22 RCTs, 8774 women) found that HRT compared with placebo, no treatment, calcium, or calcium plus vitamin D significantly reduced the proportion of women with non-vertebral fractures after 1–10 years' follow up (258/4929 [5%] *v* 307/3845 [8%]; RR 0.73, 95% CI 0.56 to 0.94).[32] This reduction remained significant in women taking HRT who had a mean age younger than 60 years (14 RCTs; RR 0.67, 95% CI 0.46 to 0.98; no further data provided). When RCTs in women with a mean age of 60 years or older were analysed, the review found no significant difference in non-vertebral fractures between HRT and placebo (8 RCTs; RR 0.88, 95% CI 0.71 to 1.08; no further data provided).[32] The second review (search date 1999) found no significant difference between HRT and control in non-vertebral fractures (6 RCTs, 5383 postmenopausal women;

RR 0.87, 95% CI 0.71 to 1.08).[29] The first subsequent RCT (2763 postmenopausal women, aged < 80 years) found no significant difference between HRT and placebo in hip fractures (fractures confirmed radiologically; 14/1380 [1.0%] with HRT v 13/1383 [0.9%] with placebo; RR 1.1, 95% CI 0.5 to 2.3) or wrist fractures (29/1380 [2.1%] with HRT v 29/1383 [2.0%] with placebo; RR 1.0, 95% CI 0.6 to 1.7), but it may have been too small to exclude a clinically important difference because the outcomes of interest were rare.[33] In this RCT, prevention of fractures was a secondary outcome, the primary outcome was the secondary prevention of coronary heart disease.[33] The second subsequent RCT (16 608 healthy postmenopausal women, aged 50–79 years) compared HRT (oestrogen plus progestin) versus placebo.[30] The primary outcome assessed in the RCT was incidence of coronary heart disease in healthy postmenopausal women but it also assessed fracture rate. It found that HRT significantly reduced hip fractures after a mean 5.2 years' follow up compared with placebo (fractures confirmed radiologically; 44/8506 [0.52%] with HRT v 62/8102 [0.77%] with placebo; RR of hip fracture 0.66, 95% CI 0.45 to 0.98). However, after adjustment for multiple significance testing as specified in the monitoring plan, the difference was no longer significant (RR 0.66, 95% CI 0.33 to 1.33).

Harms: In one of the RCTs[34] identified by the second review[32] assessing non-vertebral fractures, 96/464 women (21%) withdrew from the trial, and more women withdrew from the HRT groups than from the non-HRT groups (72/232 [31%] from HRT group v 24/232 [10%] from non-HRT group; RR 3.0, 95% CI 2.0 to 4.6). The most common reasons cited for withdrawal were menstrual disorders and headache. The subsequent RCT comparing oestrogen plus progestin versus placebo as a primary prevention strategy for coronary heart disease in healthy postmenopausal women was stopped after 5.2 years' follow up because of increased risk of invasive breast cancer, coronary events, stroke, and pulmonary embolism among women receiving HRT compared with placebo (invasive breast cancer: 166/8506 [2.0%] with HRT v 124/8102 [1.5%] with placebo; RR 1.3, 95% CI 1.0 to 1.6; coronary events: 164/8506 [1.9%] with HRT v 122/8102 [1.5%] with placebo; RR 1.3, 95% CI 1.0 to 1.6; stroke: 127/8506 [1.5%] with HRT v 85/8102 [1.1%] with placebo; RR 1.4, 95% CI 1.1 to 1.9; pulmonary embolism: 70/8506 [0.8%] with HRT v 31/8102 [0.4%] with placebo; RR 2.1, 95% CI 1.4 to 3.3).[30] See also HRT under secondary prevention of ischaemic cardiac events (web only).

Comment: In the second RCT identified by the review assessing non-vertebral fractures,[32] the use of multiple treatment groups without the correct statistical analyses limits the validity of the study results.[34] In addition to the RCTs described, we found many observational studies with conflicting results.[2–41] One non-systematic review of 11 observational studies found a reduced risk of hip fracture in women taking oestrogen compared with non-users.[2] A prospective cohort study (9704 women, aged ≥ 65 years) found a significant reduction in radiologically confirmed hip fractures with oral oestrogen only in women who started HRT within 5 years of menopause and who used it continuously thereafter.[38] Other observational studies found similar fracture rates with HRT compared with no HRT.[42] We found no observational studies that detected an increased risk of fracture with HRT. Several observational studies found that only 8–20% of women continued HRT for at least 3 years.[43,44]

OPTION PARATHYROID HORMONE New

Olivier Bruyere and Jean-Yves Reginster

One RCT in women with prior vertebral fractures found that parathyroid hormone reduced the proportion of women with vertebral and non-vertebral fractures compared with placebo. Another RCT in women with osteoporosis found that parathyroid hormone plus oestrogen reduced vertebral fractures compared with oestrogen alone after 3 years.

Benefits: **Vertebral fractures:** We found two RCTs. The first RCT (1637 women with prior vertebral fractures) found that both 20 µg and 40 µg of parathyroid hormone significantly reduced the proportion of women with vertebral fractures compared with placebo after a mean of 21 months (AR: 22/444 [5%] with 20 µg *v* 19/434 [4%] with 40 µg *v* 64/448 [14%] with placebo; RR for 20 µg *v* placebo 0.35, 95% CI 0.22 to 0.55; RR for 40 µg *v* placebo 0.31, 95% CI 0.19 to 0.50).[45] The second RCT (34 women with osteoporosis taking hormone replacement therapy) found that parathyroid hormone plus oestrogen significantly reduced the proportion of women with vertebral fractures (diagnosed as a 15% reduction in vertebral height) compared with oestrogen alone after 3 years (2/17 [12%] with parathyroid hormone plus oestrogen *v* 7/17 [41%] with oestrogen alone; P = 0.04).[46] **Non-vertebral fractures:** We found one RCT (1637 women with prior vertebral fractures), which found that both 20 µg and 40 µg of parathyroid hormone significantly reduced the proportion of women with new non-vertebral fractures compared with placebo after a mean of 21 months (AR: 34/541[6%] with 20 µg *v* 32/552 [6%] with 40 µg *v* 53/544 [10%] with placebo; P = 0.04 for 20 µg *v* placebo; P = 0.02 for 40 µg *v* placebo).[45]

Harms: The first RCT found that parathyroid hormone 40 µg/day increased the proportion of women who experienced transitory nausea and headache compared with placebo (nausea: 18% with 40 µg/day parathyroid hormone *v* 8% with placebo; P < 0.001; headache: 13% with 40 µg/day parathyroid hormone *v* 8% with placebo; P = 0.01).[45] Two women in the second RCT were reported to have withdrawn due to parathyroid hormone treatment. The first of these was due to increased back pain, the second due to the development of subcutaneous nodules at injection sites. There were no withdrawals in the oestrogen alone group.[46]

Comment: An intention to treat analysis was not conducted for vertebral fractures in the first RCT, as not all women had adequate radiographic evidence.[45] Both RCTs used parathyroid hormone (1–34).[45,46] Women in the second RCT were not blinded to treatment.[46]

OPTION SELECTIVE OESTROGEN RECEPTOR MODULATORS New

Olivier Bruyere and Jean-Yves Reginster

One large RCT in postmenopausal women with osteoporosis found that raloxifene reduced vertebral fractures compared with placebo, but no significant difference was found in non-vertebral fractures. We found no RCTs examining the effects of other selective oestrogen receptor modulators.

Benefits: **Vertebral fractures:** We found one large RCT (7705 postmenopausal women with osteoporosis, aged 31–80 years), which found that 60 mg/day and 120 mg/day of raloxifene significantly reduced the proportion of women with vertebral fractures compared with placebo after 36 months (6.6% with 60 mg/day *v* 5.4% with 120 mg/day *v* 10.1% with placebo; RR for 60 mg/day *v* placebo 0.7, 95% CI 0.5 to 0.8; RR for raloxifene 120 mg/day *v* placebo 0.6, 95% CI 0.4 to 0.7).[22] The proportion of women with fractures remained significantly lower after 4 years (RR for

60 mg/day *v* placebo 0.64, 95% CI 0.53 to 0.76; RR for raloxifene 120 mg/day *v* placebo 0.57, 95% CI 0.48 to 0.69).[47] We found no RCTs examining the effects of other selective oestrogen receptor modulators. **Non-vertebral fractures:** We found one RCT (7705 postmenopausal women with osteoporosis aged 31–80 years), which found no significant difference in the proportion of women with non-vertebral fractures between 60 mg/day and 120 mg/day of raloxifene and placebo after 36 months (8.5% with combined raloxifene results *v* 9.3% with placebo; RR 0.9, 95% CI 0.8 to 1.1).[22] The difference remained non-significant after 4 years (10.7% with combined raloxifene results *v* 11.5% with placebo; RR 0.93, 95% CI 0.81 to 1.06 with raloxifene).[47] We found no RCTs examining the effects of other selective oestrogen receptor modulators.

Harms: The RCT found that raloxifene significantly increased the risk of venous thromboembolic events compared with placebo (1.0% with 60 mg/day *v* 1.0% with 120 mg/day *v* 0.3% with placebo; RR for placebo *v* combined raloxifene 3.1, 95% CI 1.5 to 6.2).[22]

Comment: None.

OPTION ENVIRONMENTAL MANIPULATION

John Edwards

We found no systematic review and no RCTs assessing environmental manipulation alone.

Benefits: We found no systematic review and no RCTs assessing fracture risk with environmental manipulation**G** alone.

Harms: We found no systematic review and no RCTs assessing fracture risk with environmental manipulation**G** alone.

Comment: We found one RCT (674 men and women, aged > 70 years) comparing health visitor care (aimed at assessing nutritional deficiencies, reducing smoking and alcohol intake, improving muscle tone and fitness, assessing medical conditions and use of medication, and improving home environment, such as lighting) versus control (not specified).[20] It found no significant difference between health visitor care and control in new fractures over 4 years (16/350 [4.5%] with health visitor care *v* 14/324 [4.3%] with control; RR 1.06, 95% CI 0.52 to 2.13). The RCT did not state how fractures were diagnosed and gave no information on harms.[20] Although the RCT included both men and women at risk of hip fracture, it is likely that the results are generalisable to postmenopausal women.[20] We found two further RCTs assessing different multifactorial interventions (including an environmental manipulation component — see comment for hip protectors, p 1431).[21,22]

OPTION EXERCISE

John Edwards

Three RCTs found no significant difference in falls resulting in fracture at 8 months to 1 year between exercise (advice to walk briskly three times weekly, balance and strength exercises plus walking, or low-intensity exercise plus incontinence care) and control. One small RCT in postmenopausal women found no significant difference between a 2 year back strengthening exercise programme and usual care in vertebral fractures over 10 years.

Benefits: We found one systematic review (search date 2003,[23] 3 RCTs comparing exercise alone versus control in preventing falls resulting in fracture) and one additional RCT (excluded from the systematic review, as it does not report on falls outcomes).[24] The review did not perform a meta-analysis because of the heterogeneity of methods and interventions among trials.[23] The first RCT identified by the review (165 postmenopausal women living in the community who had fractured an upper limb in the previous 2 years) compared advice to walk briskly for up to 40 minutes three times weekly versus advice to carry out upper limb exercises. It found no significant difference between groups in falls resulting in fracture after 1 year (2/81 [2%] with brisk walking *v* 3/84 [4%] with upper limb exercises; RR 0.69, 95% CI 0.12 to 4.03). The second RCT identified by the review (77 women and 22 men, aged > 65 years, living in the community; see comment below) compared a home based exercise programme (balance and strength exercises plus walking) versus no exercise programme for 14 weeks. It found no significant difference between groups in falls resulting in fracture over 44 weeks (1/45 [2%] with exercise *v* 0/48 [0%] with no exercise; RR 3.20, 95% CI 0.13 to 76.48). The third RCT (162 women and 78 men, aged > 75 years; see comment below) found no significant difference in falls resulting in fracture over 1 year with a home exercise programme (balance and strength exercises plus walking) compared with usual care (2/121 [2%] with home exercise *v* 7/119 [6%] with usual care; RR 0.28, 95% CI 0.06 to 1.33). The additional RCT excluded from the systematic review (65 postmenopausal women) compared a programme of back muscle strengthening exercises versus usual care for 2 years.[24] It found no significant difference in vertebral fractures at 10 years between strengthening exercises and usual care (fractures confirmed radiologically; 3/27 [11.1%] with exercise *v* 7/23 [30.4%] with usual care; P = 0.85).

Harms: One of the RCTs found that brisk walking significantly increased the number of falls compared with control (15.0/100 person years, 95% CI 1.4/100 person years to 29.0/100 person years — see methods, p 1421).[23] This result should be interpreted with caution, as reporting of falls is subject to recall bias.

Comment: Most of the RCTs identified by the review examined falls rather than fractures as the main outcome of interest.[23] A fourth RCT identified by the review (190 incontinent men and women, all elderly, with multiple pathology and resident in nursing homes) compared exercise plus incontinence management versus usual care over 8 months.[25] It found no significant difference between treatments in falls resulting in fracture at 8 months (4/92 [4%] with exercise and incontinence management *v* 1/98 [1%] with usual care; RR 4.26, 95% CI 0.49 to 37.42). The review did not state how fractures were diagnosed in the RCTs.[23] We found two further RCTs assessing a multifactorial intervention (including an exercise component — see comment of hip protectors, p 1431).[21,22]

OPTION HIP PROTECTORS

John Edwards

One systematic review in elderly community dwelling or nursing home residents found no significant difference in hip fractures at 6 months to 2 years between hip protectors and no protectors in RCTs where individuals were randomised. However, the review found that hip protectors reduced fractures at 11–19 months in RCTs that used cluster analysis. The systematic review found no significant difference in pelvic fractures at 6 months to 2 years between hip protectors and no hip protectors in RCTs where individuals were randomised, but in RCTs with cluster analysis, the review found that hip protectors were associated with a reduction in pelvic fractures at 11–19 months. The review found no significant difference between hip protectors and no hip protectors in the rate of other fractures.

Benefits: **Hip fractures:** We found one systematic review (search date 2003, 13 RCTs, 6849 people, predominantly women; see comment below), which compared the effect of hip protectors versus no hip protectors on hip fractures.[26] The review did not pool all the RCTs in a meta-analysis because some of the RCTs used cluster randomisation and others randomised individuals. In the RCTs that randomised individuals, the review found no significant difference in fracture rate between hip protectors and no hip protectors at 6 months to 2 years (7 RCTs, 2392 people, > 75% women in 6 RCTs and proportion of women not reported in 1 RCT; AR 64/1306 [5%] with hip protectors *v* 64/1086 [6%] with no hip protectors; RR 0.94, 95% CI 0.67 to 1.31). Analysis subdivided by location (community dwelling or nursing/residential care) demonstrated no significant difference in fracture rate between intervention or control groups in either setting (community dwelling, 2 RCTs, 966 people: RR 1.11, 95% CI 0.65 to 1.90; nursing home/residential care, 5 RCTs, 1426 people: RR 0.83, 95% CI 0.54 to 1.29). Separate meta-analysis of the cluster randomised trials found that hip fractures were significantly reduced in the hip protector intervention clusters at 11–19 months (5 RCTs, 4316 people, ≥ 70% women in 4 RCTs and proportion of women not stated in the other RCT; AR 47/1749 [3%] with hip protectors *v* 165/2567 [6%] with no hip protectors; RR 0.40, 95% CI 0.29 to 0.55). The review did not state how fractures were diagnosed.[26] **Pelvic fractures:** The systematic review (search date 2003) identified 10 RCTs.[26] The proportion of women, where reported, varied from 70% to 100% (one RCT did not report any details; see comment below). Meta-analysis of RCTs randomising individuals found no significant difference in pelvic fractures at 6 months to 2 years between hip protectors and control (6 RCTs, 16/1266 [1.3%] with hip protectors *v* 13/1055 [1.2%] with no hip protectors; RR 1.15, 95% CI 0.58 to 2.31). Meta-analysis of cluster randomised RCTs found a significant reduction in pelvic fractures at 11–19 months in the intervention clusters (4 RCTs, 3/1447 [0.2%] with hip protectors *v* 17/2125 [0.8%] with no hip protectors; RR 0.31, 95% CI 0.10 to 0.99). The other RCTs did not report pelvic fracture outcomes. **Other fractures:** We found one systematic review (search date 2003, 10 RCTs).[26] In the RCTs identified by the review, the proportion of women varied from 70% to 100% (not reported in 1 RCT); see comment below. Meta-analysis of RCTs randomising individuals found no significant difference in non-hip, non-pelvic fractures between intervention and control groups (6 RCTs: 63/1266 [5%] with hip protectors *v* 56/1055 [5%] with no hip protectors; RR 1.06, 95% CI 0.75 to 1.50). Meta-analysis of the four cluster randomised RCTs showed no significant difference between treatments in non-hip, non-pelvic fractures in the intervention clusters (78/1447 [5%] with hip protectors *v* 119/2125 [6%] with no hip protectors; RR 0.93, 95% CI 0.70 to 1.24).

Harms: The systematic review (search date 2003) found that "no important adverse effects of the hip protectors were reported".[26]

Comment: Much of the evidence is taken from RCTs that included both men and women at risk of hip fracture. However, it is likely that the results are generalisable to postmenopausal women.[21,26] The systematic review (search date 2003) found that compliance with hip protectors was poor, particularly in the long term (rates ranged from 24–70% among 7 RCTs).[26] Two additional RCTs were excluded from the review, as they examined multifaceted interventions that included hip protectors, rather than hip protectors alone.[21,27] The first additional RCT was a cluster randomised trial (439 men and women resident in institutional care, aged ≥ 65 years, 72% women).[21] It compared a multifactorial intervention (including staff education, environmental manipulation**G**, exercise, walking aids, drug regimen reviews, and hip protectors for those considered at higher risk) versus usual care for 34 weeks. It found that the multifactorial intervention significantly reduced hip fractures over 34 weeks compared with usual care (3/188 [1.6%] with active intervention *v* 12/196 [6.1%] with usual care; RR 0.26, 95% CI 0.07 to 0.91). The RCT did not state how hip fractures were diagnosed. It was not clear which components of the intervention were responsible for reported effects. The second additional RCT was also cluster randomised (981 nursing home residents, mean age 85 years, 79% women).[27] It compared environmental modification and modification of nursing care plus, optionally, staff training and feedback, information and education of residents, exercise, and hip protectors versus control (usual care). It found no significant difference in hip fractures at 1 year between intervention and control groups but it may have been too small to exclude a clinically important difference (17/509 [3%] with intervention *v* 15/472 [3%] with usual care; RR 1.05, 95% CI 0.53 to 2.08).[27] The RCT did not state how hip fractures were diagnosed.

GLOSSARY

Environmental manipulation This involves the restructuring of a person's environment to remove hazards and reduce the risk of falling or of a fall resulting in fracture.

Substantive changes

Biphosphonates One systematic review added;[10] categorisation unchanged.
Calcium One systematic review added;[13] categorisation unchanged.
Hormone replacement therapy New RCT added;[31] categorisation unchanged.
Hip protectors Updated systematic review added;[26] categorisation changed to Unknown effectiveness from Likely to be beneficial, in view of conflicting evidence from individually randomised and cluster randomised RCTs.

REFERENCES

1. Cooper C. The crippling consequences of fracture and their impact on quality of life. *Am J Med* 1997;103:12–19.
2. Grady D, Rubin S, Petitti D, et al. Hormone therapy to prevent disease and prolong life in postmenopausal women. *Ann Intern Med* 1992;117:1016–1037.
3. Riggs BL, Melton LJ. Involutional osteoporosis. *N Engl J Med* 1986;314:1676–1686.
4. Kiel DP, Felson DT, Andresson JJ, et al. Hip fracture and the use of estrogens in postmenopausal women. *N Engl J Med* 1987;317:1169–1174.
5. Leidig-Bruckner G, Minne HW, Schlaich C, et al. Clinical grading of spinal osteoporosis: quality of life components and spinal deformity in women with chronic low back pain and women with vertebral osteoporosis. *J Bone Miner Res* 1997;12:663–675.
6. Reginster JY, Jones EA, Kaufman JM, et al (on behalf of the GREES). Recommendations for the registration of new chemical entities used in the prevention and treatment of osteoporosis. *Calcif Tissue Int* 1995;57:247–250.
7. Cranney A, Wells G, Willan A, et al. II. Meta-analysis of alendronate for the treatment of postmenopausal women. *Endocr Rev* 2002;23:508–516. Search date 1999; primary sources Medline, Embase, Current Contents, the Cochrane Controlled trials registry, citations of relevant articles, and the proceedings of international meetings.
8. Arboleya LR, Morales A, Fiter J. Effect of alendronate on bone mineral density and incidence of fractures in postmenopausal women with osteoporosis. A meta-analysis of published studies. *Med Clin* 2000;114:79–84. Search date 1998; primary sources Medline and Embase.
9. Cranney A, Welch V, Adachi JD, et al. Etidronate for treating and preventing postmenopausal osteoporosis. In: The Cochrane Library, Issue 4, 2003. Oxford: Update Software. Search date 1998; primary sources Medline, Healthstar, Embase, Current Contents, hand searches of conference abstracts, citations of relevant articles, the proceedings of international osteoporosis meetings, and contact with osteoporosis investigators to identify additional studies, primary authors, and pharmaceutical industry sources for unpublished data.
10. Cranney A, Waldegger L, Zytaruk N, et al. Risedronate for the prevention and treatment of postmenopausal osteoporosis. The Cochrane Library, Issue 4, 2003. Chichester, UK: John Wiley & Sons, Ltd. Search date 2001; Primary sources Cochrane Controlled Trials Register, Medline, Current Contents, hand searching of relevant journals and conference proceedings, and contact with experts and pharmaceutical companies.
11. Black DM, Cummings SR, Karpf DB, et al. Randomised trial of the effect of alendronate on the risk of fracture in women with existing vertebral fractures. *Lancet* 1996;348:1535–1541.
12. Lanza F, Schwartz H, Sahba B, et al. An endoscopic comparison of the effects of alendronate and risedronate on upper gastrointestinal mucosae. *Am J Gastroenterol* 2000;95:3112–3117.
13. Shea B, Wells G, Cranney A, et al. Calcium supplementation on bone loss in postmenopausal women. The Cochrane Library, Issue 4, 2003. Chichester, UK: John Wiley & Sons, Ltd. Search date 2001; Primary sources Cochrane Controlled Trials Register, Medline, Embase, reference lists, and conference proceedings.
14. Gillespie WJ, Avenell A, Henry DA, et al. Vitamin D and vitamin D analogues for preventing fractures associated with involutional and post-menopausal osteoporosis. In: The Cochrane Library, Issue 4, 2003. Oxford: Update Software. Search date 2000; primary sources Medline, Embase, Cinahl, Lilacs, Cabnar, Biosis, Healthstar, Current Contents, The Cochrane Database of Systematic Reviews, the

Cochrane Musculoskeletal Injuries Group trials register, and bibliographies of identified trials and reviews.
15. Meyer HE, Smedshaug GB, Kvaavik E, et al. Can vitamin D supplementation reduce the risk of fracture in the elderly? A randomized controlled trial. *J Bone Miner Res* 2002;17:709–715.
16. Trivedi DP, Doll R, Khaw KT. Effect of four monthly oral vitamin D3 (cholecalciferol) supplementation on fractures and mortality in men and women living in the community: randomised double blind controlled trial. *BMJ* 2003;326:469–472.
17. Chapuy MC, Pamphile R, Paris E, et al. Combined calcium and vitamin D3 supplementation in elderly women: confirmation of reversal of secondary hyperparathyroidism and hip fracture risk: the Decalyos II study. *Osteoporos Int* 2002;13:257–264.
18. Cranney A, Tugwell P, Zytaruk N, et al. VI. Meta-analysis of calcitonin for the treatment of postmenopausal osteoporosis. *Endocr Rev* 2002;23:540–551. Search date 2000; primary sources Medline, Embase, citations of relevant articles, proceedings of international osteoporosis meetings, and contact with osteoporosis investigators and primary authors.
19. Kanis JA, McCloskey EV. Effect of calcitonin on vertebral and other fractures. *QJM* 1999;92:143–149. Search date 1996; primary sources Medline, conference proceedings, and reference lists of various review articles and books.
20. Vetter NJ, Lewis PA, Ford D. Can health visitors prevent fractures in elderly people? *BMJ* 1992;304:888–890.
21. Jensen J, Lundin-Olsen L, Nyberg L, et al. Fall and injury prevention in older people living in residential care facilities. *Ann Intern Med* 2002;136:733–741.
22. Ettinger B, Black DM, Mitlak BH, et al. Reduction of vertebral fracture risk in postmenopausal women with osteoporosis treated with raloxifene. Results from a 3-year randomized clinical trial. *JAMA* 1999;282:637–645.
23. Gillespie LD, Gillespie WJ, Robertson MC, et al. Interventions for preventing falls in elderly people. In: The Cochrane Library, Issue 4, 2003. Chichester, UK John Wiley & Sons, Ltd. Search date 2003; primary sources Cochrane Musculoskeletal Group specialised register, Cochrane Controlled Trials Register, Medline, Embase, Cinahl, The National Research Register, Current Controlled Trials, reference lists of articles, and contact with researchers in the field.
24. Sinaki M, Itol E, Wahner HW. Stronger back muscles reduce the incidence of vertebral fractures: a prospective 10 year follow-up of postmenopausal women. *Bone* 2002;30:836–841.
25. Schnelle JF, Alessi CA, Simmons SF. Translating clinical records into practice. A randomised controlled trial of exercise and incontinence care with nursing home residents. *J Am Geriatr Soc* 2002;50:1476–1483.
26. Parker MJ, Gillespie LD, Gillespie WJ. Hip protectors for preventing hip fractures in the elderly. In: The Cochrane Library, Issue 4, 2003. Chichester, UK John Wiley & Sons, Ltd. Oxford. Search date 2003; primary sources the Cochrane Musculoskeletal Injuries Group specialised register, Cochrane Controlled Trials Register, Medline, Embase, Cinahl, and reference lists of relevant articles.
27. Becker C, Kron M, Lindemann U. Effectiveness of a multifaceted intervention on falls in nursing home residents. *J Am Geriatr Soc* 2003;51:306–313.
28. Torgerson DJ, Bell-Syer SEM. Hormone replacement therapy and prevention of vertebral fractures: a meta-analysis of randomised trials. *BMC Musculoskelet Disord* 2001;2:7. Search date 2001; primary sources Medline, Embase, Science Citation Index, Cochrane Controlled Trials Register, reference lists of systematic reviews, and contact with authors, researchers in the field, and pharmaceutical companies.
29. Wells G, Tugwell P, Shea B, et al. V. Meta-analysis of the efficacy of hormone replacement therapy in treating and preventing osteoporosis in postmenopausal women. *Endocr Rev* 2002;23:529–539. Search date 1999; primary sources Medline, Embase, the Cochrane Controlled Register, citations of relevant articles, proceedings of international meetings, and contact with osteoporosis investigators and primary authors.
30. Writing group for the Women's Health Initiative Investigators. Risk and benefits of estrogen plus progestin in healthy postmenopausal women. Principal results from the Women's Health Initiative randomized controlled trial. *JAMA* 2002;288:321–333.
31. Liao EY, Luo XH, Deng XG, et al. The effect of low dose nylestriol–levonorgestrel replacement therapy on bone mineral density in women with post menopausal osteoporosis. *Endocr Res* 2003;29:217–226.
32. Torgerson DJ, Bell-Syer SEM. Hormone replacement therapy and prevention of nonvertebral fractures. A meta-analysis of randomized trials. *JAMA* 2001;285:2891–2897. Search date 2000; primary sources Medline, Embase, Science Citation Index, Cochrane Controlled Trials Register, reference lists of systematic reviews, and contact with authors, researchers in the field, and pharmaceutical companies.
33. Cauley JA, Black DM, Barrett-Connor, et al. Effects of hormone replacement therapy on clinical fractures and height loss: the heart and estrogen/progestin replacement study (HERS). *Am J Med* 2001;110:442–450.
34. Komulainen M, Kröger H, Tuppurainen M, et al. HRT and vitamin D in prevention of non-vertebral fractures in postmenopausal women; a 5 year randomized trial. *Maturitas* 1998;31:45–54.
35. Ettinger B, Genant H, Cann C. Long-term estrogen replacement therapy prevents bone loss and fractures. *Ann Intern Med* 1985;102:319–324.
36. Maxim P, Ettinger B, Spitalny M. Fracture protection provided by long-term estrogen treatment. pharmaceutical companies *Osteoporos Int* 1995;5:23–29.
37. Kanis J, Johnell O, Gullberg B, et al. Evidence for efficacy of drugs affecting bone metabolism in preventing hip fracture. *BMJ* 1992;305:1124–1128.
38. Cauley J, Seeley D, Ensrud K, et al. Estrogen replacement therapy and fractures in older women. *Ann Intern Med* 1995;122:9–16.
39. Michaëlsson K, Baron J, Farahmand B, et al. Hormone replacement therapy and risk of hip fracture: population based case-control study. *BMJ* 1998;316:1858–1863.
40. Michaëlsson K, Baron J, Johnell O, et al. Variation in the efficacy of hormone replacement therapy in the prevention of hip fracture. *Osteoporos Int* 1998;8:540–546.
41. Nguyen T, Jones G, Sambrook N, et al. Effects of estrogen exposure and reproductive factors on bone mineral density and osteoporotic fractures. *J Clin Endocrin Metab* 1995;80:2709–2714.
42. Kiel D, Baron J, Anderson J, et al. Smoking eliminates the protective effect of oral estrogens on the risk for hip fracture among women. *Ann Intern Med* 1992;116:716–721.
43. Ettinger B, Li D, Lein R. Continuation of postmenopausal hormone replacement therapy: comparison of cyclic versus continuous combined schedules. *Menopause* 1996;3:185–189.
44. Groeneveld F, Bareman F, Barentsen R, et al. Duration of hormonal replacement therapy in general practice: a follow up study. *Maturitas* 1998;29:125–131.
45. Neer RM, Arnaud CD, Zanchetta JR, et al. Effect of parathyroid hormone (1–34) on fractures and bone mineral density in postmenopausal women with osteoporosis. *N Engl J Med* 2001;344:1434–1441.

46. Lindsay R, Nieves J, Formica C, et al. Randomised controlled study of effect of parathyroid hormone on vertebral-bone mass and fracture incidence among postmenopausal women on oestrogen with osteoporosis. *Lancet* 1997;350:550–555.

47. Delmas PD, Ensrud KE, Adachi JD, et al. Efficacy of raloxifene on vertebral fracture risk reduction in postmenopausal women with osteoporosis: four-year results from a randomized clinical trial. *J Clin Endocrinol Metab* 2002;87:3609–3617.

Olivier Bruyere
Research Fellow
WHO Collaborating Center for Public Health Aspects of Osteoarticular Disease
Liege
Belgium

John Edwards
General Practitioner
Wolstanton Medical Centre
Newcastle-under-Lyme
UK

Jean-Yves Reginster
Professor of Epidemiology and Public Health
Bone and Cartilage Metabolism Unit
University of Liege
Liege
Belgium

Competing interests: OB and JE none declared. JR has participated in several preclinical and clinical trials, reviewed and consulted scientific documentation, has been an author of publications, and has chaired and spoken at scientific meetings for the following companies: Asahi, Bayer, Boehringer Ingelheim, Chiesi, Eli Lilly, Hoechst-Marion-Roussel, Hologic, Hybritech, Igea, Johnson & Johnson, Merck Sharp & Dohme, Negma, Organon, Pfizer, Pharmascience, Procter & Gamble Pharmaceuticals, Rotta Research, Sanofi, Servier, SmithKline Beecham, Teva, Therabel, Tosse, Byk, UCB, and Will Pharma.

Gout

Search date June 2004

Martin Underwood

QUESTIONS

INTERVENTIONS

Key Messages

Treatment

- **Colchicine (oral)** One small RCT provided limited evidence that colchicine improved pain in people with gout. However, we were unable to draw reliable conclusions from this small RCT. The high incidence of adverse effects in people taking colchicine precludes its use as routine treatment.
- **Corticosteroids** We found no RCTs on the effects of intra-articular, parenteral, or oral corticosteroids in people with gout.
- **Non-steroidal anti-inflammatory drugs** One small RCT provided limited evidence that tenoxicam reduced short term pain and tenderness in people with gout compared with placebo. However, this study was too small to provide reliable conclusions. We found no RCTs comparing other non-steroidal anti-inflammatory drugs with placebo in people with gout. Five RCTs found no significant difference in effectiveness between different non-steroidal anti-inflammatory drugs. However, these RCTs may have lacked power to detect clinically relevant differences. Two equivalence studies found no difference in pain between etoricoxib and indometacin, but found that indometacin was associated with more adverse effects. The adverse effects of non-steroidal anti-inflammatory drugs include gastrointestinal ulceration and haemorrhage, and for at least some COX-2 inhibitors, increased cardiovascular risk.

Prevention of recurrence

- **Advice to lose weight** We found no RCTs on the effects of advice to lose weight to prevent attacks of gout in people with prior episodes.
- **Advice to reduce alcohol intake** We found no RCTs on the effects of advice to reduce alcohol intake to prevent attacks of gout in people with prior episodes.
- **Advice to reduce dietary intake of purines** We found no RCTs on the effects of advice to reduce dietary intake of purines to prevent attacks of gout in people with prior episodes.
- **Allopurinol** We found no RCTs on the effects of allopurinol to prevent attacks of gout in people with prior episodes.

- **Benzbromarone** We found no RCTs on the effects of benzbromarone to prevent attacks of gout in people with prior episodes.
- **Colchicine** We found no RCTs on the effects of colchicine in preventing attacks of gout in people with prior episodes.
- **Probenecid** We found no RCTs on the effects of probenecid to prevent attacks of gout in people with prior episodes.
- **Sulphinpyrazone** We found no RCTs on the effects of sulphinpyrazone to prevent attacks of gout in people with prior episodes.

DEFINITION Gout is a syndrome caused by deposition of urate crystals.[1] It typically presents as an acute monoarthritis of rapid onset. The first metatarsophalangeal joint is the most commonly affected joint (podagra). Gout also affects other joints: joints in the foot, ankle, knee, wrist, finger, and elbow are the most frequently affected. Crystal deposits (tophi) may develop around hands, feet, elbows, and ears. Diagnosis is usually made clinically. The American College of Rheumatology (ACR) criteria for diagnosing gout are as follows: (1) characteristic urate crystals in joint fluid; (2) a tophus proved to contain urate crystals; or (3) the presence of six or more defined clinical laboratory and x ray phenomena (see table 1, p 1442).[2] We have included studies of people meeting the ACR criteria, studies in which the diagnosis was made clinically, and studies that used other criteria.

INCIDENCE/ PREVALENCE Gout is more common in older people and men.[3] In people aged 65–74 years in the UK, the prevalence is about 50/1000 in men and about 9/1000 in women.[4] The annual incidence of gout in people aged over 50 years in the USA is 1.6/1000 for men and 0.3/1000 for women.[5] One 12 year longitudinal study of 47 150 male health professionals with no previous history of gout estimated that annual incidence of gout ranged from 1/1000 for those aged 40–44 years to 1.8/1000 for those aged 55–64 years.[6] Gout may be more common in some non-white ethnic groups.[3] A pooled analysis of two cohort studies of former medical students found the annual incidence of gout to be 3.1/1000 in black men and 1.8/1000 in white men.[7] After correcting for the higher prevalence of hypertension among black men, which is a risk factor for gout, the relative risk of gout in black men compared with white men was 1.30 (95% CI 0.77 to 2.19).

AETIOLOGY/ RISK FACTORS Urate crystals form when serum urate concentration exceeds 0.42 mmol/L.[8] Serum urate concentration is the principal risk factor for a first attack of gout,[9] although 40% of people have normal serum urate concentration during an attack of gout.[8,10–12] A cohort study of 2046 men followed for about 15 years found that the annual incidence is about 0.4% in men with a urate concentration of 0.42–0.47 mmol/L, rising to 4.3% when serum urate concentration is 0.45–0.59 mmol/L.[13] A 5 year longitudinal study of 223 asymptomatic men with hyperuricaemia estimated 5 year cumulative incidence of gout to be 10.8% for those with baseline serum urate of 0.42–0.47 mmol/L, 27.7% for baseline urate 0.48–0.53 mmol/L, and 61.1% for baseline urate levels of 0.54 mmol/L or more.[9] The study found that a 0.6 mmol/L difference in baseline serum urate increased the odds of an attack of gout by a factor of 1.8 (OR adjusted for other risk factors for gout: 1.84, 95% CI 1.24 to 2.72). One 12 year longitudinal study (47 150 male health professionals with no history of gout)[6,14] estimated that the relative risk of gout from one additional daily serving of different foods (weekly for seafood) was: meat 1.21 (95% CI 1.04 to1.41), seafood (fish, lobster, and shellfish) 1.07 (95% CI 1.01 to 1.12), purine rich vegetables 0.97 (95% CI 0.79 to 1.19), low fat dairy products 0.79 (95% CI 0.71 to 0.87), and high fat dairy products 0.99 (95% CI 0.89 to 1.10).[6] Alcohol consumption of greater than 14.9 g daily significantly increased the risk of gout compared with no alcohol consumption (compared with no alcohol consumption: RR for 15.0 g/day to 29.9 g/day: 1.49, 95% CI 1.14 to 1.94; RR for 30.0 g/day to 49.9 g/day: 1.96, 95% CI 1.48 to 2.60; RR for ≥ 50 g/day: 2.53, 95% CI 1.73 to 3.70).[14] The longitudinal study also estimated the relative risk of an additional serving of beer (355 mL, 12.8 g alcohol), wine (118 mL, 11.0 g alcohol), and spirits (44 mL, 14.0 g alcohol). It found that an extra daily serving of beer or spirits was significantly associated with gout, but an extra daily serving of wine was not (RR for 355 mL/day beer: 1.49, 95% CI 1.32 to 1.70; RR for 44 mL/day spirits: 1.15, 95% CI 1.04 to 1.28; RR for 118 mL/day wine: 1.04, 95% CI 0.88 to 1.22). Other suggested risk factors for gout include obesity, insulin resistance, dyslipidaemia, hypertension, and cardiovascular disorders.[15,16]

PROGNOSIS We found few reliable data about prognosis or complications of gout. One study found that 3/11 (27%) people with untreated gout of the first metatarsophalangeal joint experienced spontaneous resolution after 7 days.[17] A case series of 614 people with gout who had not had treatment to reduce urate levels, and could recall the interval between first and second attacks, reported recurrence rates of 62% after 1 year, 78% after 2 years, and 84% after 3 years.[18] An analysis of two prospective cohort studies of 371 black and 1181 white male former medical students followed up for about 30 years found no significant difference in risk of coronary heart disease in men who had developed gout compared with men who had not (RR 0.85, 95% CI 0.40 to 1.81).[19]

AIMS OF INTERVENTION **For treating gout:** to reduce the severity and duration of pain and loss of function, with minimal adverse effects of treatment. **For preventing recurrence:** to reduce the frequency and severity of recurrent attacks, and minimise the adverse effects of interventions.

OUTCOMES **For treating gout:** severity of symptoms (pain scores, proportion of people with improved symptoms), adverse effects of treatment. **For preventing recurrence (over 6 months):** number of recurrent episodes a year, severity of recurrent episodes a year, adverse effects of treatment.

METHODS *Clinical Evidence* search and appraisal June 2004. Only papers with 6 months or longer of follow up were included for prevention of recurrent gout. We excluded studies that were non-randomised, had 10 or fewer people in each treatment arm, had more than 20% loss to follow up, were crossover trials that did not present results before crossover, were not fully published (e.g. abstracts of conference proceedings, which could not be appraised for quality), or which reported only non-clinical outcomes such as serum urate levels.

QUESTION What are the effects of treatments for acute gout?

OPTION NON-STEROIDAL ANTI-INFLAMMATORY DRUGS

One small RCT provided limited evidence that tenoxicam reduced short term pain and tenderness in people with gout compared with placebo. However, this study was too small to provide reliable conclusions. We found no RCTs comparing other non-steroidal anti-inflammatory drugs with placebo in people with gout. Five RCTs found no significant difference in effectiveness between different non-steroidal anti-inflammatory drugs. However, these RCTs may have lacked power to detect clinically relevant differences. Two equivalence studies found no difference in pain between etoricoxib and indometacin, but found that indometacin was associated with more adverse effects. The adverse effects of non-steroidal anti-inflammatory drugs include gastrointestinal ulceration and haemorrhage, and for at least some COX-2 inhibitors, increased cardiovascular risk.

Benefits: We found no systematic review. **Versus placebo:** We found one RCT (30 people aged 21–70 years with gout of the knee, ankle, wrist, big toe, or elbow), which compared tenoxicam (40 mg once daily) with placebo.[20] Tenoxicam significantly increased the proportion of people showing at least a 50% reduction in pain and tenderness compared with placebo after 1 day (pain and tenderness assessed on a four point scale: "disappeared", "improved by ≥ 50%", "unchanged or improved by < 50%", or "increased"; AR for "pain improved by ≥ 50%": 10/15 [67%] with tenoxicam *v* 4/15 [26%] with placebo; $P < 0.05$; AR for "tenderness improved by ≥ 50%": 6/15 [40%] with tenoxicam *v* 1/15 [7%] with placebo; $P < 0.05$; AR for "pain on mobilisation improved ≥ 50%": 4/15 [27%] with tenoxicam *v* 1/15 [7%] with placebo; $P < 0.05$). However, it found no significant difference between tenoxicam and placebo in physician rated efficacy after 4 days (physician rated efficacy "good or excellent": 7/15 [47%] with tenoxicam *v* 4/15 [26%] with placebo; P value not reported).[20] **Versus each other:** We found seven RCTs comparing different non-steroidal anti-inflammatory drugs (NSAIDs) versus each other. Two RCTs were designed as equivalence studies.[21,22] They found no significant difference between etoricoxib and indometacin in effect on pain. The remaining five RCTs found no significant difference in effectiveness between different NSAIDs. However they may have lacked power to show differences (see table 2, p 1443).[23–27]

Harms: The harms of NSAIDs are considered in detail elsewhere in *Clinical Evidence* and include gastrointestinal ulceration and haemorrhage, and for at least some COX-2 inhibitors, increased cardiovascular risk (see non-steroidal anti-inflammatory drugs, p 1525). **Versus each other:** (see table 2 for harms, p 1443).

Comment: **Versus placebo:** The RCT comparing tenoxicam versus placebo conducted multiple significance tests and no adjustment was reported for this.[20] **Versus each other:** Phenylbutazone and indometacin were established as treatments for gout based on uncontrolled studies. Only the comparisons between etoricoxib and indometacin were powered to show equivalence in efficacy between the two compounds tested.[20,22] Etoricoxib, a selective inhibitor of cyclo-oxygenase-2, may be a useful alternative to conventional NSAIDs for people at high risk of gastrointestinal adverse effects. We found five RCTs that compared phenylbutazone with other NSAIDs. These have not been considered further because phenylbutazone for gout has been restricted in many countries because it can cause aplastic anaemia and other serious adverse effects.[28] We found one RCT (62 people), which compared meloxicam and diclofenac with rofecoxib.[29] However, the RCT was not designed to compare meloxicam with diclofenac directly. This study also excluded people who had previously not responded to NSAIDS. Investigators, but not trial participants, were blinded. Analysis was not intention to treat, and results were not corrected for multiple analysis. Rofecoxib has been withdrawn worldwide because of cardiovascular adverse effects. We have, therefore, excluded this study.

OPTION CORTICOSTEROIDS

We found no RCTs on the effects of intra-articular, parenteral, or oral corticosteroids in people with gout.

Benefits: We found no systematic review or RCTs.

Harms: We found insufficient evidence in people with gout. Potential harms of oral corticosteroids are covered elsewhere in *Clinical Evidence* (see asthma, p 1891).

Comment: None.

OPTION COLCHICINE (ORAL)

One small RCT provided limited evidence that colchicine improved pain in people with gout. However, we were unable to draw reliable conclusions from this small RCT. The high incidence of adverse effects in people taking colchicine precludes its use as routine treatment.

Benefits: We found no systematic review. **Versus placebo:** We found one small RCT (43 hospital inpatients with acute gout confirmed by synovial fluid examination, aged 55–91 years, 40/43 men), which compared colchicine (1 mg followed by 0.5 mg every 2 hours as tolerated or until complete response) versus placebo.[30] It found that colchicine significantly reduced pain compared with placebo after 48 hours (pain assessed on a 10 cm visual analogue scale; proportion with ≥ 50% improvement in pain: 73% with colchicine *v* 36% with placebo; $P < 0.05$).

Harms: The RCT found that all people taking colchicine experienced diarrhoea, vomiting, or both, within about 24 hours; 5/21 [24%] people taking placebo developed nausea (P value not reported).[30] The 50% improvement in pain occurred before diarrhoea and vomiting in 9/22 (40%), after the onset of diarrhoea and vomiting in 12/22 (55%), and at the same time in 1/22 (5%) people.

Comment: Colchicine has been used since antiquity to treat gout. A large number of observational studies support its use. Although it may be efficacious, narrow benefit to toxicity ratio limits its use in people with gout.[31]

QUESTION What are the effects of treatments to prevent gout in people with prior acute episodes?

OPTION COLCHICINE

We found no RCTs on the effects of colchicine in preventing attacks of gout in people with prior episodes.

Benefits: We found no systematic review or RCTs.

Harms: We found no RCTs.

Comment: None.

OPTION ADVICE TO LOSE WEIGHT

We found no RCTs on the effects of advice to lose weight to prevent attacks of gout in people with prior episodes.

Benefits: We found no systematic review or RCTs.

Harms: We found no RCTs.

Comment: None.

OPTION ADVICE TO REDUCE ALCOHOL INTAKE

We found no RCTs on the effects of advice to reduce alcohol intake to prevent attacks of gout in people with prior episodes.

Benefits: We found no systematic review or RCTs.

Harms: We found no RCTs.

Comment: A large 12 year longitudinal study (47 150 male health professionals with no history of gout) found that increased intake of beer or spirits significantly increased the incidence of gout. However, it found no significant increase in incidence of gout with increased intake of wine (see aetiology, p 1436).[14]

OPTION ADVICE TO REDUCE DIETARY INTAKE OF PURINES

We found no RCTs on the effects of advice to reduce dietary intake of purines to prevent attacks of gout in people with prior episodes.

Benefits: We found no systematic review or RCTs.

Harms: We found no RCTs.

Comment: A large longitudinal study (47 150 male health professionals with no history of gout) found that increased intake of meat or seafood significantly increased the incidence of gout. However, increased intake of purine rich vegetables did not significantly affect the incidence of gout. It also found that an increased intake of low fat dairy produce significantly reduced the incidence of gout (see aetiology, p 1436).[6]

OPTION ALLOPURINOL

We found no RCTs on the effects of allopurinol to prevent attacks of gout in people with prior episodes.

Benefits: We found no systematic review or RCTs.

Harms: We found no RCTs.

Comment: We found one quasi-randomised trial (37 men with a history of gout, aged 27–78 years), which compared probenecid 1–2 g daily versus allopurinol 300–600 mg daily.[32] Both groups took prophylactic colchicine during the first few months of treatment. Treatment allocation was by the last digit of the hospital number. The trial found no significant difference between probenecid and allopurinol for recurrence after a mean follow up of 18.6 months (recurrence free: 8/17 [47%] with probenecid *v* 9/20 [45%]; P value not reported). However, results may have been biased by non-random treatment allocation and because five people allocated to probenecid received sulphinpyrazone instead. Many experts believe that allopurinol should not normally be started during an attack of gout.

OPTION PROBENECID

We found no RCTs on the effects of probenecid to prevent attacks of gout in people with prior episodes.

Benefits: We found no systematic review or RCTs (see comment below).

Harms: We found no RCTs.

Comment: We found one quasi-randomised trial (37 men with a history of gout, aged 27–78 years), which compared probenecid 1–2 g daily versus allopurinol 300–600 mg daily.[32] See comment under allopurinol for details, p 1440.

OPTION SULPHINPYRAZONE

We found no RCTs on the effects of sulphinpyrazone to prevent attacks of gout in people with prior episodes.

Benefits: We found no systematic review or RCTs.

Harms: We found no RCTs.

Comment: None.

OPTION BENZBROMARONE

We found no RCTs on the effects of benzbromarone to prevent attacks of gout in people with prior episodes.

Benefits: We found no systematic review or RCTs.

Harms: We found no RCTs.

Comment: None.

Substantive changes

Non-steroidal anti-inflammatory drugs One RCT added.[22] Benefits and harms data enhanced. Categorisation unchanged.

REFERENCES

1. Emmerson BT. The management of gout. *N Engl J Med* 1996;334:445–451.
2. Wallace SL, Robinson H, Masi AT, et al. Preliminary criteria for the classification of the acute arthritis of primary gout. *Arthritis Rheum* 1977;20:895–900.
3. Kim KY, Schumacher HR, Hunsche E, et al. A literature review of the epidemiology and treatment of acute gout. *Clin Ther* 2003;25:1593–1616.
4. Harris CM, Lloyd DC, Lewis J. The prevalence and prophylaxis of gout in England. *J Clin Epidemiol* 1995;48:1153–1158.
5. Abbott RD, Brand FN, Kannel WB, et al. Gout and coronary heart disease: the Framingham Study. *J Clin Epidemiol* 1988;41:237–242.
6. Choi HK, Atkinson K, Karlson EW, et al. Purine-rich foods, dairy and protein intake, and the risk of gout in men. *N Engl J Med* 2004;350:1093–1103.
7. Hochberg MC, Thomas J, Thomas DJ, et al. Racial differences in the incidence of gout. The role of hypertension. *Arthritis Rheum* 1995;38:628–632.
8. McGill NW. Gout and other crystal-associated arthropathies. *Baillieres Best Pract Res Clin Rheumatol* 2000;14:445–460.
9. Lin KC, Lin HY, Chou P. The interaction between uric acid level and other risk factors on the development of gout among asymptomatic hyperuricemic men in a prospective study. *J Rheumatol* 2000;27:1501–1505.
10. Schlesinger N, Baker DG, Schumacher HR Jr. Serum urate during bouts of acute gouty arthritis. *J Rheumatol* 1997;24:2265–2266.
11. Logan JA, Morrison E, McGill PE. Serum uric acid in acute gout. *Ann Rheum Dis* 1997;56:696–697.
12. Stewart OJ, Silman AJ. Review of UK data on the rheumatic diseases – 4. Gout. *Br J Rheumatol* 1990;29:485–488.
13. Campion EW, Glynn RJ, DeLabry LO. Asymptomatic hyperuricemia. Risks and consequences in the Normative Aging Study. *Am J Med* 1987;82:421–426.
14. Choi HK, Atkinson K, Karlson EW, et al. Alcohol intake and risk of incident gout in men: a prospective study. *Lancet* 2004;363:1277–1281.
15. Culleton BF. Uric acid and cardiovascular disease: a renal-cardiac relationship? *Curr Opin Nephrol Hypertens* 2001;10:371–375.
16. Bryan, E. Are gout and increased uric acid levels risk factors for cardiac disease? Centre for Clinical Effectiveness, Monash University. 2002. http://www.med.monash.edu/healthservices/cce/evidence/pdf/b/805.pdf (last accessed 5 January 2005).
17. Bellamy N, Downie WW, Buchanan WW. Observations on spontaneous improvement in patients with podagra: implications for therapeutic trials of non-steroidal anti-inflammatory drugs. *Br J Clin Pharmacol* 1987;24:33–36.
18. Yu TF, Gutman AB. Efficacy of colchicine prophylaxis in gout. *Ann Intern Med* 1961;55:179–192.
19. Gelber AC, Klag MJ, Mead LA, et al. Gout and risk for subsequent coronary heart disease. The Meharry-Hopkins Study. *Arch Intern Med* 1997;157:1436–1440.
20. Garcia de la Torre I. Double-blind parallel study comparing tenoxicam and placebo in acute gouty arthritis. *Invet Med Int* 1987;14:92–97. [In Spanish]
21. Schumacher HR Jr, Boice JA, Daikh DI, et al. Randomised double blind trial of etoricoxib and indometacin in treatment of acute gouty arthritis. *BMJ* 2002;324:1488–1492.
22. Rubin BR, Burton R, Navarra S, et al. Efficacy and safety profile of treatment with etoricoxib 120 mg once daily compared with indomethacin 50 mg three times daily in acute gout: a randomized controlled trial. *Arthritis Rheum* 2004;50:598–606.
23. Fraser RC, Davis RH, Walker FS. Comparative trial of azapropazone and indomethacin plus allopurinol in acute gout and hyperuricaemia. *J R Coll Gen Pract* 1987;37:409–411.
24. Maccagno A, Di Giorgio E, Romanowicz A. Effectiveness of etodolac ("Lodine") compared with naproxen in patients with acute gout. *Curr Med Res Opin* 1991;12:423–429.
25. Lederman R. A double-blind comparison of Etodolac (Lodine™) and high doses of naproxen in the treatment of acute gout. *Adv Ther* 1990;7:344–354.
26. Altman RD, Honig S, Levin JM, et al. Ketoprofen versus indomethacin in patients with acute gouty arthritis: a multicenter, double blind comparative study. *J Rheumatol* 1988;15:1422–1426.
27. Lomen PL, Turner LF, Lamborn KR, et al. Flurbiprofen in the treatment of acute gout. A comparison with indomethacin. *Am J Med* 1986;80:134–139.
28. Non-steroidal anti-inflammatory drugs. In: Royal Pharmaceutical Society of Great Britain, eds. *British national formulary.* Wallingford: Pharmaceutical Press, 2003:478–506.
29. Cheng TT, Lai HM, Chiu CK, et al. A single-blind, randomized, controlled trial to assess the efficacy and tolerability of rofecoxib, diclofenac sodium, and meloxicam in patients with acute gouty arthritis. *Clin Ther* 2004;26:399–406.
30. Ahern MJ, Reid C, Gordon TP, et al. Does colchicine work? The results of the first controlled study in acute gout. *Aust N Z J Med* 1987;17:301–304.
31. Schlesinger N, Schumacher HR Jr. Gout: can management be improved? *Curr Opin Rheumatol* 2001;13:240–244.
32. Scott JT. Comparison of allopurinol and probenecid. *Ann Rheum Dis* 1966;25:623–626.

Martin Underwood
Professor of General Practice
Institute of Community Health Sciences, Barts and the London, Queen Mary's School of Medicine and Dentistry, Queen Mary, University of London, London, UK

Competing interests: MU has received speaker fees from Pfizer, the manufacturers of valdecoxib and celecoxib and from Menarini Pharmaceuticals, the manufacturers of ketoprofen and dexketoprofen. His salary was provided by NHS Research and Development. MU is a current or recent applicant on research projects funded in excess of £100,000 by NHS Health Technology Assessment Programme, Arthritis Research Campaign and UK Medical Research Council.

TABLE 1	American College of Rheumatology criteria for acute gout (people must fulfill six or more criteria; see text, p 1436).[2]
1	More than one attack of acute arthritis
2	Maximum inflammation developed within 1 day
3	Monoarthritis attack
4	Redness observed over joints
5	First metatarsophalangeal joint painful or swollen
6	Unilateral first metatarsophalangeal joint attack
7	Unilateral tarsal joint attack
8	Tophus (proved or suspected)
9	Hyperuricaemia
10	Asymmetric swelling within a joint on x ray film
11	Subcortical cysts without erosions on x ray film
12	Monosodium urate monohydrate microcrystals in joint fluid during an attack
13	Joint culture negative for organism during attack

TABLE 2 **RCTs comparing NSAIDs versus each other in people with gout (see text, p 1437).**

Comparison	Population	Outcomes	Results	Adverse events
Indometacin (50 mg 3 times/day) *v* etoricoxib (120 mg/day). Equivalence study[22]	189 people, gout < 48 hours, who had previously responded to NSAIDS, 93% male, mean age 52 years	Pain measured on Likert scale over days 2–5: 0 = no pain to 4 = extreme pain; Equivalence pre-specified as a difference of no more than ± 0.5	Difference: –0.08, 95% CI –0.29 to +0.13	People reporting ≥ 1 adverse events: 45/103 [44%] with etoricoxib *v* 49/86 [57%] with indometacin; P = 0.08 Drug related adverse events: 17/103 [17%] with etoricoxib *v* 32/86 [37%] with indometacin; P = 0.002*
Indometacin (50 mg 3 times/day) *v* etoricoxib (120 mg/day). Equivalence study[21]	150 men, gout < 24 hours, mean age 49 years	Pain measured on Likert scale over days 2–5: 0 = no pain to 4 = extreme pain; Equivalence pre-specified as a difference of no more than ± 0.5	Difference: +0.11, 95% CI –0.14 to +0.35	Proportion with adverse events: 17/75 [23%] with etoricoxib *v* 35/75 [47%] with indometacin; P = 0.003
Indometacin (200 mg for 1 day in divided doses followed by a reducing regimen for 28 days) *v* azapropazone (600 mg 3 times daily for 4 days followed by 600 mg twice daily for 28 days)[20]	93 people	Proportion of people who reported that the treatment "suited them" after 4 days	35/47 [74%] with indometacin *v* 40/46 [87%] with azapropazone; P value reported as not significant	Study reported no differences in important adverse event rates

TABLE 2 continued

Comparison	Population	Outcomes	Results	Adverse events
Etodolac (300 mg twice daily) *v* naproxen (500 mg twice daily)[21]	61 people, 18–75 years	Mean pain scores assessed on a scale 0–5 (higher scores indicating worse pain) after 2, 4, and 7 days	Day 2: 2.6 with etodolac *v* 2.8 with naproxen; P value reported as not significant; Day 4: 1.8 with etodolac *v* 2.0 with naproxen; P value reported as not significant; Day 7: 1.4 with etodolac *v* 1.4 with naproxen; P value reported as not significant	The study reported no important adverse events
Etodolac (300 mg twice daily) *v* naproxen (500 mg twice daily)[22]	60 people, 18–75 years	Pain assessed on a five point rating scale: 1 = no pain to 5 = very severe pain after 1, 2, 4, and 7 days	The study reported there was no significant difference in pain between etodolac and naproxen after 1, 2, 4, and 7 days; results presented graphically, no AR or P values reported	The study reported no important adverse events
Indometacin (up to 225 mg for 1 day in divided doses followed by 50 mg 3 times daily) *v* ketoprofen (450 mg in divided doses for 1 day followed by 100 mg 3 times daily)[23]	59 people, gout < 48 hours, 35–88 years	Mean pain scores assessed on a four point scale: 0 = no pain to 3 = severe pain after 2, 5, or 8 days	Day 2: 0.9 with indometacin *v* 1.1 with ketoprofen; P value reported as not significant; Day 5: 0.8 with indometacin *v* 1.3 with ketoprofen; P value reported as not significant; Day 8: 0.3 with indometacin *v* 0.4 with ketoprofen; P value reported as not significant	No differences in important adverse event rates were found
Indometacin (50 mg 4 times daily for 4 days followed by 25 mg 4 times daily for 5 days) *v* flurbiprofen (100 mg 4 times daily for 1 day followed by 50 mg 4 times daily for 5 days)[24]	29 people	Proportion of people with improved pain at rest after 2 days	11/12 [92%] with indometacin *v* 11/12 [92%] with flurbiprofen; P value not reported	No differences in important adverse event rates were found

NSAID, non-steroidal anti–inflammatory drug; *the RCT did not define serious and drug related adverse events.

Herniated lumbar disc

Search date May 2004

Jo Jordan, Tamara Shawver Morgan, and James Weinstein

QUESTIONS

INTERVENTIONS

See glossary G

Key Messages

Drug treatments

- **Analgesics** We found no systematic review or RCTs on the use of analgesics for treatment of people with symptomatic herniated lumbar discs.
- **Antidepressants** We found no systematic review or RCTs on the use of antidepressants for treatment of people with symptomatic herniated lumbar discs.
- **Muscle relaxants** We found no systematic review or RCTs on the use of muscle relaxants for treatment of people with symptomatic herniated lumbar discs.
- **Epidural corticosteroid injections** One systematic review found limited evidence that epidural corticosteroid injections increased global improvement compared with placebo. However, one subsequent RCT found no significant difference between epidural corticosteroid injections plus conservative treatment and conservative treatment alone in pain, mobility, or people returning to work at 6 months. Another subsequent RCT found no significant difference between epidural corticosteroid injection and control injection in pain, disability, or self rated improvement after 35 days.
- **Non-steroidal anti-inflammatory drugs** One systematic review found no significant difference in overall improvement between non-steroidal anti-inflammatory drugs and placebo in people with sciatica caused by disc herniation.

Non-drug treatments

- **Spinal manipulation** One RCT identified by a systematic review in people with sciatica caused by disc herniation found that spinal manipulation increased self perceived improvement after 2 weeks compared with a placebo of infrequent infrared heat. Another RCT identified by the review, comparing spinal manipulation, manual traction, exercise, and corsets, found no significant difference among groups in self perceived improvement after 1 month. One subsequent RCT found that spinal manipulation increased the proportion of people with improved symptoms compared with traction. Concerns exist regarding possible further herniation from spinal manipulation in people who are surgical candidates.
- **Acupuncture** One systematic review found insufficient evidence on the effects of acupuncture in people with herniated lumbar discs.
- **Advice to stay active** One systematic review of conservative treatments for sciatica caused by lumbar disc herniation found no RCTs on advice to stay active.
- **Exercise therapy** One systematic review of one RCT found no significant difference in global improvement between isometric exercise and manual traction in people with sciatica caused by disc herniation.
- **Heat or ice** One systematic review identified no RCTs of heat or ice for sciatica caused by lumbar disc herniation.
- **Massage** One systematic review identified no RCTs of massage in people with symptomatic lumbar disc herniation.
- **Bed rest** One systematic review of conservative treatment found no RCTs on bed rest in people with symptomatic herniated discs. One subsequent RCT in people with sciatica found no significant difference between bed rest and watchful waiting for 2 weeks in people's perceived improvement, mean pain scores, mean disability scores, or mean satisfaction scores after 12 weeks.

Surgery

- **Microdiscectomy (as effective as standard discectomy)** We found no RCTs comparing microdiscectomy versus conservative treatment. Three RCTs found no significant difference in clinical outcomes between microdiscectomy and standard discectomy. One RCT found no significant difference in satisfaction or pain between video-assisted arthroscopic microdiscectomy and standard discectomy at about 30 months, although postoperative recovery was slower with standard discectomy. We found insufficient evidence on the effects of automated percutaneous discectomy compared with microdiscectomy.
- **Standard discectomy (short term benefit)** One RCT found that standard discectomy increased self reported improvement at 1 year, but not at 4 and 10 years, compared with conservative treatment (physiotherapy). Three RCTs found no significant difference in clinical outcomes between standard discectomy and microdiscectomy. Adverse effects were similar with both procedures. One RCT found no significant difference in satisfaction or pain between standard discectomy and video-assisted arthroscopic microdiscectomy at about 30 months, although postoperative recovery was slower with standard discectomy.
- **Automated percutaneous discectomy** We found no RCTs comparing automated percutaneous discectomy versus either conservative treatment or standard discectomy. We found insufficient evidence on the clinical effects of automated percutaneous discectomy compared with microdiscectomy.
- **Laser discectomy** We found no systematic review or RCTs on the use of laser discectomy for treatment of people with symptomatic herniated lumbar discs.

DEFINITION Herniated lumbar disc is a displacement of disc material (nucleus pulposus or annulus fibrosis) beyond the intervertebral disc space.[1] The diagnosis can be confirmed by radiological examination; however, magnetic resonance imaging findings of herniated disc are not always accompanied by clinical symptoms.[2,3] This review covers treatment of people who have clinical symptoms relating to confirmed or suspected disc herniation. It does not include treatment of people with spinal cord compression or people with cauda equina syndrome Ⓖ, which requires emergency intervention. The management of non-specific acute low back pain, p 1465 and chronic low back pain, p 1479 are covered elsewhere in *Clinical Evidence*.

INCIDENCE/ PREVALENCE The prevalence of symptomatic herniated lumbar disc is about 1–3% in Finland and Italy, depending on age and sex.[4] The highest prevalence is among people aged 30–50 years,[5] with a male to female ratio of 2 : 1.[6] In people aged between 25 and 55 years, about 95% of herniated discs occur at the lower lumbar spine (L4–L5 level); disc herniation above this level is more common in people over 55 years of age.[7,8]

AETIOLOGY/ RISK FACTORS Radiographical evidence of disc herniation does not reliably predict low back pain in the future or correlate with symptoms; 19–27% of people without symptoms have disc herniation on imaging.[2,9] Risk factors for disc herniation include smoking (OR 1.7, 95% CI 1.0 to 2.5), weight bearing sports (e.g. weight lifting, hammer throw etc), and certain work activities such as repeated lifting. Driving motor vehicles is also associated with increased risk (OR 1.7, 95% CI 0.2 to 2.7).[6,10,11] This may be because the resonant frequency of the spine is similar to that of certain vehicles.

PROGNOSIS The natural history of disc herniation is difficult to determine because most people take some form of treatment for their back pain, and a formal diagnosis is not always made.[6] Clinical improvement is usual in most people, and only about 10% of people still have sufficient pain after 6 weeks to consider surgery. Sequential magnetic resonance images have shown that the herniated portion of the disc tends to regress over time, with partial to complete resolution after 6 months in two thirds of people.[12]

AIMS OF INTERVENTION To relieve pain; increase mobility and function; and improve quality of life.

OUTCOMES **Primary outcomes:** pain, function, or mobility; individuals' perceived overall improvement; quality of life; and adverse effects of treatment. **Secondary outcomes:** return to work; use of analgesia; and duration of hospital admission.

METHODS *Clinical Evidence* search and appraisal May 2004. The authors searched Amed and the Physiotherapy Evidence Database (PEDro) in January 2003.

QUESTION What are the effects of drug treatments?

OPTION NON-STEROIDAL ANTI-INFLAMMATORY DRUGS

One systematic review found no significant difference in overall improvement between non-steroidal anti-inflammatory drugs and placebo in people with sciatica caused by disc herniation.

Benefits: **Versus placebo:** We found one systematic review (search date 1998, 3 RCTs, 321 people) of medical treatments for sciatica caused by disc herniation.[13] The RCTs compared non-steroidal anti-inflammatory drugs (NSAIDs) (piroxicam 40 mg/day for 2 days or 20 mg/day for 12 days; indometacin [indomethacin] 75–100 mg 3 times daily; phenylbutazone 1200 mg/day for 3 days or 600 mg/day for 2 days) versus placebo. The review found no significant difference between NSAIDs and placebo in global improvement after 5–30 days (pooled AR for improvement in pain: 80/172 [46.5%] with NSAIDs *v* 57/149 [38.3%] with placebo; OR for global improvement 0.99, 95% CI 0.60 to 1.70; see comment below).

Harms: The systematic review did not report the adverse effects of NSAIDs. NSAIDs may cause gastrointestinal complications (see non-steroidal anti-inflammatory drugs topic, p 1525).

Comment: The absolute numbers in the RCTs relate to the outcomes of improvement in pain (3 RCTs) and return to work (1 RCT).[13] However, the meta-analysis used the outcome measure of global improvement. The relationship between these measures is unclear.

OPTION ANALGESICS

We found no systematic review or RCTs on the use of analgesics for treatment of people with symptomatic herniated lumbar discs.

Benefits: We found no systematic review or RCTs.

Harms: We found no RCTs.

Comment: None.

OPTION ANTIDEPRESSANTS

We found no systematic review or RCTs on the use of antidepressants for treatment of people with symptomatic herniated lumbar discs.

Benefits: We found no systematic review or RCTs.

Harms: We found no RCTs.

Comment: None.

OPTION MUSCLE RELAXANTS

We found no systematic review or RCTs on the use of muscle relaxants for treatment of people with symptomatic herniated lumbar discs.

Benefits: We found no systematic review or RCTs.

Harms: We found no RCTs.

Comment: None.

OPTION EPIDURAL CORTICOSTEROID INJECTIONS

One systematic review found limited evidence that epidural corticosteroid injections increased global improvement compared with placebo. However, one subsequent RCT found no significant difference between epidural corticosteroid injections plus conservative treatment and conservative treatment alone in pain, mobility, or people returning to work at 6 months. Another subsequent RCT found no significant difference between epidural corticosteroid injection and control injection in pain, disability, or self rated improvement after 35 days.

Benefits: We found one systematic review (search date 1998, 4 RCTs of epidural corticosteroid, 265 people)[13] of medical treatments for sciatica caused by disc herniation and two subsequent RCTs.[14,15] The review compared four different doses of epidural corticosteroid injections (8 mL methylprednisolone 80 mg; 2 mL methylprednisolone 80 mg; 10 mL methylprednisolone 80 mg; and 2 mL methylprednisolone acetate 80 mg) versus placebo (saline or lidocaine [lignocaine] 2 mL) after follow up periods of 2, 21, and 30 days.[13] The review found limited evidence that epidural corticosteroid increased the proportion of people with self perceived global improvement (which was not defined) compared with placebo. The result was of borderline significance (73/160 [45.6%] with steroid *v* 56/172 [32.5%] with placebo; OR 2.2, 95% CI 1.0 to 4.7). The first subsequent RCT (36 people with disc herniation confirmed by magnetic resonance imaging) compared epidural corticosteroid (3 injections of methylprednisolone 100 mg in 10 mL bupivacaine 0.25% during the first 14 days in hospital) plus conservative non-operative treatment versus conservative treatment alone.[14] Conservative treatment involved initial bed rest and analgesia followed by graded rehabilitation (hydrotherapy, electroanalgesia, postural exercise classes) followed by physiotherapy. It found no significant difference between groups in mean pain scores at 6 weeks and 6 months measured on a visual analogue scale (at 6 months: 32.9 [range 0–85.0] with corticosteroids *v* 39.2 [range 0–100.0] with conservative treatment). It found no significant difference in mean mobility scores (Hannover Functional Ability Questionnaire: 61.8 [range 25.0–88.0] with corticosteroids *v* 57.2 [range 13.0–100.0] with conservative treatment), in the proportion of people who had back surgery (2/17 [12%] with corticosteroids *v* 4/19 [21%] with conservative treatment; RR 0.56, 95% CI 0.09 to 2.17), or in people returning to work within 6 months (15/17 [88%] with corticosteroids *v* 14/19 [74%] with conservative treatment; RR 1.19, 95% CI 0.75 to 1.33).[14] The second subsequent double blind RCT (85 people with sciatica caused by herniated disc) compared epidural corticosteroid injections (2 mL prednisolone acetate at 2 day intervals for a total of 3 injections) versus control (2 mL isotonic saline).[15] It found no significant difference between groups in self rated success of treatment after 35 days (people rating improvement as "recovery" or "marked improvement": 21/43 [49%] with corticosteroid *v* 20/42 [48%] with control; P = 0.91). The RCT also found no significant difference between corticosteroid injection and control injection in pain scores after 35 days (mean change from baseline measured by unspecified visual analogue scale: –30.3 mm with corticosteroid *v* –25.2 mm with control; treatment effect –5.1, 95% CI –18.7 to +8.4) or disability/function (Roland-Morris Index score, mean change from baseline: –5.3 with corticosteroid *v* –3.2 with control; treatment effect –2.1, 95% CI –5.0 to +0.8).[15]

Harms: No serious adverse effects were reported in the RCTs included in the systematic review, although 26 people complained of transient headache or transient increase in sciatic pain.[13] The first subsequent RCT did not report adverse effects of epidural injections.[14] The second subsequent RCT reported that clinically significant adverse effects occurred in 2/43 (5%) people in the corticosteroid group and 3/42 (7%) people in the control group (P = 0.676).[15] It reported that headache occurred in two people in each group, and thoracic pain occurred in one person with control.

Comment: None.

QUESTION **What are the effects of non-drug treatments?**

OPTION **BED REST**

One systematic review of conservative treatment found no RCTs on bed rest in people with symptomatic herniated discs. One subsequent RCT in people with sciatica found no significant difference between bed rest and watchful waiting for 2 weeks in people's perceived improvement, mean pain scores, mean disability scores, or mean satisfaction scores after 12 weeks.

Benefits: We found one systematic review[13] and one subsequent RCT.[16] The systematic review (search date 1998) of conservative treatments for sciatica caused by disc herniation identified no RCTs of bed rest for treatment of people with symptomatic herniated discs.[13] The subsequent RCT (183 people with sciatica, intensity sufficient to justify 2 weeks of bed rest as treatment) compared bed rest at home (instructed to stay in the supine or lateral recumbent position with 1 pillow under the head) versus a control of watchful waiting (advised to be up and about whenever possible) for 2 weeks.[16] Most people had nerve root compression on magnetic resonance imaging (109 people out of 161 people who had magnetic resonance imaging performed). It found no significant difference between bed rest and control in people's perceived improvement (87% with bed rest v 87% with control; OR 1.0, 95% CI 0.4 to 2.9; based on regression analysis; see comment below), mean pain scores (McGill Pain Questionnaire: 8 with bed rest v 7 with control; difference –0.6, 95% CI –3.3 to +2.1; based on regression analysis), mean disability scores (revised Roland Disability Scale: 15.2 with bed rest v 15.7 with control; difference –0.5, 95% CI –2.6 to +1.6; based on regression analysis), or mean satisfaction scores (7 with bed rest v 8 with control; difference –0.1, 95% CI –0.6 to +0.3; based on regression analysis) after 12 weeks.

Harms: The subsequent RCT did not report on harms of bed rest.[16]

Comment: The regression analysis in the RCT adjusted odds ratios and differences between treatments for several variables including baseline differences in age, sex, presence or absence of paresis, disease duration, and people's history with respect to sciatica, among others.[16] We found one further systematic review (search date 1996) of bed rest and advice to stay active in people with acute low back pain that found three RCTs that included people with sciatica or radiating pain.[17] However, no further details were given in the review on the proportion of people in these RCTs with herniated discs. The review concluded that there was little evidence on bed rest specifically for herniated lumbar discs, although the RCTs they did find questioned the efficacy of bed rest for sciatica.[17]

OPTION ADVICE TO STAY ACTIVE

One systematic review of conservative treatments for sciatica caused by lumbar disc herniation found no RCTs on advice to stay active.

Benefits: We found one systematic review (search date 1998) of conservative treatments for sciatica caused by disc herniation, which found no RCTs of advice to stay active.[13] We found no subsequent RCTs.

Harms: We found no RCTs.

Comment: None.

OPTION MASSAGE

One systematic review identified no RCTs of massage in people with symptomatic lumbar disc herniation.

Benefits: We found one systematic review (search date 1998) of conservative treatments for sciatica caused by disc herniation, which found no RCTs of massage.[13] We found no subsequent RCTs.

Harms: We found no systematic review or RCTs.

Comment: None.

OPTION HEAT OR ICE

One systematic review identified no RCTs of heat or ice for sciatica caused by lumbar disc herniation.

Benefits: We found one systematic review (search date 1998) of conservative treatments for sciatica caused by disc herniation, which identified no RCTs on the use of heat or ice for herniated lumbar discs.[13] We found no subsequent RCTs.

Harms: We found no systematic review or RCTs.

Comment: None.

OPTION SPINAL MANIPULATION

One RCT identified by a systematic review in people with sciatica caused by disc herniation found that spinal manipulation increased self perceived improvement after 2 weeks compared with a placebo of infrequent infrared heat. Another RCT identified by the review, comparing spinal manipulation, manual traction, exercise, and corsets, found no significant difference among groups in self perceived improvement after 1 month. One subsequent RCT found that spinal manipulation increased the proportion of people with improved symptoms compared with traction. Concerns exist regarding possible further herniation from spinal manipulation in people who are surgical candidates.

Benefits: We found two systematic reviews[13,18] and one subsequent RCT.[19] The first systematic review (search date 1998), which did not perform meta-analysis, identified two RCTs of spinal manipulation for sciatica caused by disc herniation.[13] The second systematic review (search date not reported) identified no RCTs.[18] The first RCT (207 people) included in the first review compared spinal manipulation (every day if necessary) versus placebo (infrared heat 3 times weekly).[13] It found that spinal manipulation increased overall self perceived improvement at 2 weeks compared with placebo (98/123 [80%] with spinal manipulation *v* 56/84 [67%] with placebo; RR 1.19, 95% CI 1.01 to 1.32; NNT 8, 95% CI 5 to 109).[13] The second included RCT (322 people) compared four interventions: spinal manipulation, manual traction, exercise, and corsets, in a factorial design.[13] It found no significant difference among treatments in overall self perceived improvement after 28 days (quantified results not reported). The subsequent RCT (112 people with symptomatic herniated lumbar disc) compared pulling and turning manipulation versus traction.[19] It found that significantly more people were "improved" (absence of lumbar pain, improvement in lumbar functional movement) or "cured" (absence of lumbar pain, straight leg raising of $> 70°$, ability to return to work) with spinal manipulation compared with traction (54/62 [87%] with spinal manipulation *v* 33/50 [66%] with traction; RR 1.32, 95% CI 1.06 to 1.65; NNT 5, 95% CI 4 to 16; timescale not reported).

Harms: The first systematic review did not report adverse effects.[13] The second systematic review identified one review of 135 case reports of serious complications after spinal manipulation published between 1950 and 1980.[18] However, the frequency of these effects was not certain. The case review attributed these complications to cervical manipulation, misdiagnosis, presence of coagulation dyscrasias, presence of herniated nucleus pulposus, or improper techniques. The subsequent RCT found that two out of 60 people receiving traction had syncope; no adverse effects were reported in people receiving manipulation.[19] We found a third systematic review (search date 2001, 5 prospective observational studies).[20] The largest study included in the review (4712 treatments in 1058 people having both cervical and lumbar spinal manipulations) found that the most common reaction was local discomfort (53%), followed by headache (12%), tiredness (11%), radiating discomfort (10%), dizziness (5%), nausea (4%), hot skin (2%), and other complaints (2%). The incidence of serious adverse effects is reported as rare, and is estimated from published case series and reports to occur in one in 1–2 million treatments. The most common of these serious effects were cerebrovascular accidents (the total proportion of people having manipulations was not reported and the rate of this adverse effect cannot be estimated). However, it is difficult to assess whether such events are directly related to treatment.

Comment: In the third review, which examined risks, the percentages include both cervical and lumbar spinal manipulations, which may overestimate the effect of lumbar spinal manipulations.[20] The authors of the review advise caution in interpreting these results, as they are speculative and based on assumptions about the numbers of manipulations performed and unreported cases. More reliable data are needed on the incidence of specific risks. It is unclear whether the populations studied in the RCTs cited included people who were surgical candidates for disc herniation. Concerns exist regarding possible further herniation from spinal manipulation in people who are surgical candidates.

OPTION EXERCISE THERAPY

One systematic review of one RCT found no significant difference in global improvement between isometric exercise and manual traction in people with sciatica caused by disc herniation.

Benefits: We found one systematic review (search date 1998) of conservative treatments for sciatica caused by disc herniation.[13] The review included one RCT (50 people) that compared isometric exercise versus manual traction (both for 5–7 days; see comment below). The review found no significant difference between groups in a global measure of improvement (reported as no significant difference, absolute numbers and P value not reported; see comment below). We found no subsequent RCTs.

Harms: The review did not report on harms of exercise.[13]

Comment: The review did not report further details of treatment regimens. The global measure of improvement was not further defined.[13]

OPTION ACUPUNCTURE

One systematic review found insufficient evidence on the effects of acupuncture in people with herniated lumbar discs.

Benefits: We found one systematic review (search date 1998) in people with back and neck pain, which identified one small RCT of acupuncture in people with sciatica.[21] The RCT (30 people with acute sciatica; see comment below) compared acupuncture at electronically detected non-traditional points versus sham acupuncture. The review reported that the RCT found that acupuncture significantly improved three outcomes compared with sham acupuncture and reported that the RCT concluded that there was an overall benefit of acupuncture.[21] However, the review disagreed with the RCT's overall conclusion of benefit stating that it only found a significant difference between groups in three out of 12 outcome measures, and that there was no significant difference between acupuncture and sham acupuncture in pain intensity at rest, the most clinically relevant outcome, after 5 days (absolute numbers and P value not reported).[21] The review found one RCT in people with neck and lumbar pain (see comment below).

Harms: No adverse effects from the two RCTs were reported in the systematic review.[21]

Comment: In the RCT of people with acute sciatica, the acute sciatica may not have been caused by disc herniation.[21] The review also included one small crossover RCT (42 people, radicular and pseudo radicular cervical and lumbar pain owing to stenosis, herniated disc, or both) that compared laser acupuncture at traditional points versus sham laser acupuncture. The review found no significant difference between groups in reduction of pain intensity after 24 hours, although pain was significantly improved in the laser acupuncture group at 15 minutes, 1 hour, and 6 hours compared with control. The sample sizes in both RCTs included in the review were small and provide little evidence of the effectiveness of acupuncture specifically in people with herniated lumbar disc.

QUESTION What are the effects of surgery?

OPTION STANDARD DISCECTOMY

One RCT found that standard discectomy increased self reported improvement at 1 year, but not at 4 and 10 years, compared with conservative treatment (physiotherapy). Three RCTs found no significant difference in clinical outcomes between standard discectomy and microdiscectomy. Adverse effects were similar with both procedures. One RCT found no significant difference in satisfaction or pain between standard discectomy and video-assisted arthroscopic microdiscectomy at about 30 months, although post-operative recovery was slower with standard discectomy.

Benefits: **Versus conservative treatment:** We found two systematic reviews (search dates 1999[22] and not reported[23]) which included the same RCT (126 people with symptomatic L5/S1 disc herniation)[24] comparing standard discectomy**G** versus conservative treatment (6 weeks of physiotherapy). Each person assessed and graded their improvement in terms of pain and function into four categories: "good" (completely satisfied), "fair", "poor", and "bad" (completely incapacitated for work because of pain). The RCT found that discectomy significantly increased the proportion of people reporting their improvement as "good" after 1 year compared with conservative treatment (intention to treat analysis: 39/60 [65.0%] with surgery *v* 24/66 [36.4%] with conservative treatment; RR 1.79, 95% CI 1.30 to 2.18; NNT 3, 95% CI 2 to 9). However, at 4 and 10 years, there was no significant difference in the same outcome (at 4 years, AR for "good" improvement: 40/60 [66.7%] with surgery *v* 34/66 [51.5%] with conservative treatment; RR 1.29, 95% CI 0.96 to 1.56; at 10 years: 35/60 [58.3%] with surgery *v* 37/66 [56.1%] with conservative treatment; RR 1.04, 95% CI 0.73 to 1.32).
Versus microdiscectomy: One systematic review (search date 1999)[22] identified three RCTs (219 people) comparing standard discectomy versus microdiscectomy**G**. It did not perform a meta-analysis because outcomes were not comparable. The first RCT in the review (60 people with lumbar disc herniation) found no significant difference between standard discectomy and microdiscectomy in the proportion of people who rated their operative outcome as "good", "almost recovered", or "totally recovered" at 1 year (intention to treat analysis: 26/30 [87%] with standard discectomy *v* 24/30 [80%] with microdiscectomy; RR 1.08, 95% CI 0.78 to 1.20).[25] It found no difference between treatments in the change in preoperative and postoperative pain scores (visual analogue scale; P value not reported) or in the duration of time taken to return to work (both 10 weeks). The second RCT in the review (79 people with lumbar disc herniation) found no significant difference between microdiscectomy and standard discectomy in pain in the legs or back (visual analogue scale, not specified) or in analgesia use at any

point during the 6 week follow up (absolute numbers not reported).[26] The third RCT (80 people) found that clinical outcomes and duration of sick leave were similar at 15 months, but the review did not provide further details.[22] **Versus video-assisted arthroscopic microdiscectomy:** See benefits of microdiscectomy, p 1454.

Harms: **Versus conservative treatment:** The RCT included in both systematic reviews did not report on complications of standard discectomyⒼ.[24] **Versus microdiscectomy:** One systematic review reported that there was no significant difference between standard discectomy and microdiscectomyⒼ in perioperative bleeding, duration of stay, or scar tissue (numbers not reported).[22] The first RCT included in the review reported one person in each group with a nerve root tear and, of the people having microdiscectomy, one had a dural leak and one had suspected discitis.[25] The second RCT included in the review did not report on the complications of either procedure.[26] Complication rates were reported inconsistently in studies, making it difficult to combine results to produce overall rates. Rates of complications for all types of discectomy have been compiled (see table 1, p 1458).[23]

Comment: The RCT comparing standard discectomyⒼ versus conservative treatment had considerable crossover between the two treatment groups.[24] Of 66 people randomised to receive conservative treatment, 17 received surgery; of 60 people randomised to receive surgery, one refused the operation.[24] The results presented above are based on an intention to treat analysis. One systematic review of published reports (search date not reported) found 99 cases of vascular complications after lumbar disc surgery since 1965.[27] Reported risk factors for vascular complications included: previous disc or abdominal surgery leaving adhesions; chronic disc pathology from disruption or degeneration of anterior annulus fibrosus and anterior longitudinal ligament or peridiscal fibrosis; improper positioning of the patient; retroperitoneal vessels and operated disc in close proximity; and vertebral anomalies, such as hypertrophic spurs compressing vessels during operation. The systematic review did not state out of how many operations the 99 complications arose from, therefore we can not estimate the incidence of adverse vascular events from discectomy.[27]

OPTION MICRODISCECTOMY

We found no RCTs comparing microdiscectomy versus conservative treatment. Three RCTs found no significant difference in clinical outcomes between microdiscectomy and standard discectomy. One RCT found no significant difference in satisfaction or pain between video-assisted arthroscopic microdiscectomy and standard discectomy at about 30 months, although postoperative recovery was slower with standard discectomy. We found insufficient evidence on the effects of automated percutaneous discectomy compared with microdiscectomy.

Benefits: We found no systematic review. **Versus conservative treatment:** We found no RCTs. **Versus standard discectomy:** See benefits of standard discectomy, p 1453. **Video-assisted arthroscopic microdiscectomy versus standard discectomy:** We found one RCT (60 people with proved lumbar disc herniation and associated radiculopathy after failed conservative treatment).[28] It found no significant difference between video-assisted arthroscopic discectomy and standard discectomyⒼ in the proportion of people who were "very satisfied" on a 4 point satisfaction scale after about 31 months (22/30 [73%] with microdiscectomyⒼ *v* 20/30 [67%] with standard discectomy; RR 1.10, 95% CI 0.71 to 1.34). There was also no significant difference in mean pain score (visual analogue scale from 0 [no pain] to

10 [severe and incapacitating pain]: 1.2 with microdiscectomy *v* 1.9 with standard discectomy). However, the mean duration of postoperative recovery was almost twice as long with open surgery as with microdiscectomy (27 days with microdiscectomy *v* 49 days with standard discectomy; P value not reported). **Versus automated percutaneous discectomy:** See benefits of automated percutaneous discectomy, p 1455.

Harms: **Video-assisted arthroscopic microdiscectomy versus open discectomy:** The RCT reported that one person having open discectomy had leakage of spinal fluid from the dural sac 2 weeks after the operation.[28] No other postoperative complications or neurovascular injuries were observed in either the standard discectomy**G** or the microdiscectomy**G** groups. Complication rates were reported inconsistently in studies, making it difficult to combine results to produce overall rates. Rates of complications for all types of discectomy have been compiled (see table 1, p 1458).[23]

Comment: None.

OPTION AUTOMATED PERCUTANEOUS DISCECTOMY

We found no RCTs comparing automated percutaneous discectomy versus either conservative treatment or standard discectomy. We found insufficient evidence on the clinical effects of automated percutaneous discectomy compared with microdiscectomy.

Benefits: **Versus conservative treatment:** We found no systematic review or RCTs. **Versus standard discectomy:** One systematic review (search date not reported) identified no RCTs comparing automated percutaneous discectomy (APD**G**) versus standard discectomy**G**.[23] **Versus microdiscectomy:** One systematic review (search date 1999) identified two RCTs that were not directly comparable because there were differences in the equipment used.[22] One RCT (71 people with radiographical confirmation of disc herniation) was stopped prematurely, after an interim analysis at 6 months found that APD was associated with significantly lower success rate than microdiscectomy**G** (overall outcome was classified as "success" or "failure" by the clinician and a masked observer [details not reported]: 9/31 [29%] with APD *v* 32/40 [80%] with microdiscectomy; $P < 0.001$).[29] However, the other RCT (40 people with radiographical confirmation of disc herniation) reported similar improvements in the composite clinical score with APD and microdiscectomy (scale 0–10, including back and leg pain, and sensory and motor deficit) at 2 years (preoperative scores: 4.55 with APD *v* 4.20 with microdiscectomy; scores at 2 years: 8.23 with APD *v* 7.67 with microdiscectomy).[30] More people in the APD group rated their surgical outcomes as "excellent" or "good" than did those in the microdiscectomy group 2 years after surgery (14/20 [70%] with APD *v* 11/20 [55%] with microdiscectomy; $P = 0.33$).

Harms: The systematic review found that re-operations for recurrent or persistent disc herniations at the same level as the initial operations were reported more frequently with APD**G** compared with either microdiscectomy**G** or standard discectomy**G** (APD 83%, 95% CI 76% to 88% *v* microdiscectomy 64%, 95% CI 48% to 78% *v* standard discectomy 49%, 95% CI 38% to 60%).[23] The first RCT did not report adverse effects.[29] The second RCT reported that no complications had occurred with APD, but did not comment on whether there had been any complications in the microdiscectomy group.[30] The mean duration of recovery after surgery was longer in people who had microdiscectomy compared with those who had APD (mean weeks of postoperative recovery [range]: 22.9 weeks [4 weeks to 1 year] with microdiscectomy v 7.7 weeks [1–26 weeks] with APD). Complication rates were reported inconsistently in studies, making it difficult to combine results to produce overall rates. Rates of complications for all types of discectomy have been compiled (see table 1, p 1458).[23]

Comment: None.

OPTION LASER DISCECTOMY

We found no systematic review or RCTs on the use of laser discectomy for treatment of people with symptomatic herniated lumbar discs.

Benefits: Three systematic reviews (search dates 1999,[22] not reported,[23] and 2000[31]) found no RCTs on the effectiveness of laser discectomy**G**.

Harms: We found no RCTs.

Comment: None.

GLOSSARY

Automated percutaneous discectomy Techniques using minimal skin incisions (generally several, all < 3–5 mm) to allow small instruments to be inserted, using radiography to visualise these instruments, and using extensions for the surgeon to reach the operative site without having to dissect tissues.

Cauda equina A collection of spinal roots descending from the lower part of the spinal cord, which occupy the vertebral canal below the spinal cord.

Cauda equina syndrome Compression of the cauda equina causing symptoms, including changes in perineal sensation (saddle anaesthesia), and loss of sphincter control.

Laser discectomy The surgeon places a laser through a delivery device that has been directed under radiographic control to the disc, and removes the disc material using the laser. It uses many of the same techniques used in automated percutaneous discectomy.

Microdiscectomy Removal of protruding disc material, using an operating microscope to guide surgery.

Standard discectomy Surgical removal, in part or whole, of an intervertebral disc, generally with loop magnification (i.e. eyepieces).

REFERENCES

1. Fardon DF, Milette PC. Nomenclature and classification of lumbar disc pathology: recommendations of the Combined Task Forces of the North American Spine Society, American Society of Spine Radiology, and American Society of Neuroradiology. *Spine* 2001;26:E93–E113.
2. Boden SD. The use of radiographic imaging studies in the evaluation of patients who have degenerative disorders of the lumbar spine. *J Bone Joint Surg Am* 1996;78:114–125.
3. Borenstein DG, O'Mara JW Jr, Boden SD, et al. The value of magnetic resonance imaging of the lumbar spine to predict low-back pain in asymptomatic subjects. *J Bone Joint Surg Am* 2001;83-A(9):1306–1311.
4. Andersson G. Epidemiology of spinal disorders. In: Frymoyer JW, Ducker TB, Hadler NM, et al, eds. *The adult spine: principles and practice*. New York, NY: Raven Press, 1997:93–141.
5. Heliovaara M. *Epidemiology of sciatica and herniated lumbar intervertebral disc*. Helsinki, Finland: The Social Insurance Institution, 1988.
6. Postacchini F, Cinotti G. Etiopathogenesis. In: Postacchini F, ed. *Lumbar disc herniation*. New York: Springer-Verlag, 1999.
7. Friberg S, Hirsch C. Anatomical and clinical studies on lumbar disc degeneration. *Acta Orthop Scand* 1949;19:222–242.
8. Schultz A, Andersson G, Ortengren R, et al. Loads on the lumbar spine. *J Bone Joint Surg Am* 1982;64:713–720.
9. Jensen MC, Brant-Zawadzki MN, Obuchowski N, et al. Magnetic resonance imaging of the lumbar spine in people without back pain. *N Engl J Med* 1994;331:69–73.
10. Kelsey JL, Githens P, O'Connor T, et al. Acute prolapsed lumbar intervertebral disc: an epidemiologic study with special reference to driving automobiles and cigarette smoking. *Spine* 1984;9:608–613.
11. Pedrini-Mille A, Weinstein JN, Found ME, et al. Stimulation of dorsal root ganglia and degradation of rabbit annulus fibrosus. *Spine* 1990;15:1252–1256.
12. Deyo RA, Weinstein JN. Low back pain. *N Engl J Med* 2001;344:365–370.
13. Vroomen PC, de Krom MC, Slofstra PD, et al. Conservative treatment of sciatica: a systematic review. *J Spinal Disord* 2000;13:463–469. Search date 1998; primary sources Medline and Embase/Excerpta Medica.
14. Buchner M, Zeifang F, Brocai DR, et al. Epidural corticosteroid injection in the conservative management of sciatica. *Clin Orthop* 2000;375:149–156.

15. Valat JP, Giraudeau B, Rozenberg S, et al. Epidural corticosteroid injections for sciatica: a randomised, double blind, controlled clinical trial. *Ann Rheum Dis* 2003;62:639–643.
16. Vroomen PC, de Krom MC, Wilmink JT, et al. Lack of effectiveness of bed rest for sciatica. *N Engl J Med* 1999;340:418–423.
17. Waddell G, Feder G, Lewis M. Systematic reviews of bed rest and advice to stay active for acute low back pain. *Br J Gen Prac* 1997;47:647–652. Search date April 1996; primary sources Medline and Embase, checked abstracts of all back pain RCTs, citation tracking by hand and using ISI Science and Social Sciences Citation indices, consulted experts and researchers.
18. Shekelle PG, Adams AH, Chassin MR, et al. Spinal manipulation for low-back pain. *Ann Intern Med* 1992;117:590–598. Search date not reported; primary sources Medline and Index Medicus 1952 onwards, reference lists, and consulted experts.
19. Liu J, Zhang S. Treatment of protrusion of lumbar intervertebral disc by pulling and turning manipulations. *J Tradit Chin Med* 2000;20:195–197.
20. Stevinson C, Ernst E. Risks associated with spinal manipulation. *Am J Med* 2002;112:566–570. Search date 2001; primary sources Medline, Embase, The Cochrane Library, authors' files, consulted experts, and reference lists.
21. Smith LA, Oldman AD, McQuay HJ, et al. Teasing apart quality and validity in systematic reviews: an example from acupuncture trials in chronic neck and back pain. *Pain* 2000;86:119–132. Search date 1998; primary sources Medline, Embase, Cinahl, Psychlit, Pubmed, The Cochrane Library, Oxford Pain Relief Database, and reference lists.
22. Gibson JN, Grant IC, Waddell G. Surgery for lumbar disc prolapse. In: The Cochrane Library, Issue 2, 2004. Chichester, UK: John Wiley & Sons, Ltd. Search date 1999; primary sources Medline, Embase, Biosis, dissertation abstracts, Index to UK Theses, Cochrane Controlled Trials Register, reference lists, personal bibliographies, and hand searches of *Spine* 1975–1997.
23. Hoffman RM, Wheeler KJ, Deyo RA. Surgery for herniated lumbar discs: a literature synthesis. *J Gen Intern Med* 1993;8:487–496. Search date not reported; primary sources Medline, reference lists, book bibliographies, and colleagues' files.
24. Weber H. Lumbar disc herniation: a controlled, prospective study with ten years of observation. *Spine* 1983;8:131–140.
25. Tullberg T, Isacson J, Weidenhielm L. Does microscopic removal of lumber disc herniation lead to better results than the standard procedure? Results of a one-year randomized study. *Spine* 1993;18:24–27.
26. Henriksen L, Schmidt V, Eskesen V, et al. A controlled study of microsurgery versus standard lumbar discectomy. *Br J Neurosurg* 1996;10:289–293.
27. Papadoulas S, Konstantinou D, Kourea HP, et al. Vascular injury complicating lumbar disc surgery. A systematic review. *Eur J Vasc Endovasc Surg* 2002;24:189–195. Search date not reported; primary source Medline 1965 onwards.
28. Hermantin FU, Peters T, Quartararo L, et al. A prospective, randomized study comparing the results of open discectomy with those of video-assisted arthroscopic microdiscectomy. *J Bone Joint Surg Am* 1999;81:958–965.
29. Chatterjee S, Foy PM, Findlay GF. Report of a controlled clinical trial comparing automated percutaneous lumbar discectomy and microdiscectomy in the treatment of contained lumbar disc herniation. *Spine* 1995;20:734–738.
30. Mayer HM, Brock M. Percutaneous endoscopic discectomy: surgical technique and preliminary results compared to microdiscectomy. *J Neurosurg* 1993;78:216–225.
31. Boult M, Fraser RD, Jones N, et al. Percutaneous endoscopic laser discectomy. *Aust N Z J Surg* 2000;70:475–479. Search date 2000; primary sources Medline, Current Contents, Embase, and The Cochrane Library.

Jo Jordon
Research assistant: Systematic Reviews
Primary Care Sciences Research Centre
Keele University
Keele, Staffordshire
UK

Tamara Shawver Morgan
Research Associate
Dartmouth Medical School
Hanover, NH
USA

James Weinstein
Chair of Orthopaedics, Dartmouth Medical School; Director, The Spine Center and the Center for Shared Decision-Making, Dartmouth-Hitchcock Medical Center; Co-Director, Dartmouth Clinical Trials Center
Dartmouth Medical School
Hanover, NH
USA

Competing interests: None declared.

TABLE 1 Reported complications from surgical procedures (see text, p 1454).[23]

Complications	Standard discectomy		Microdiscectomy		Percutaneous discectomy	
	Mean (% [95% CI])	Studies (n)*	Mean (% [95% CI])	Studies (n)*	Mean (% [95% CI])	Studies (n)*
Operative mortality	0.15 (0.09–0.24)	25	0.06 (0.01–0.42)	8	–	3
Total wound infections	1.97 (1.97–2.93)	25	1.77 (0.92–3.37)	16	–	2
Deep wound infections	0.34 (0.23–0.50)	17	0.06 (0.01–0.23)	8	–	2
Discitis	1.39 (0.97–2.01)	25	0.67 (0.44–1.02)	20	1.43 (0.42–4.78)	8
Dural tear	3.65 (1.99–6.65)	17	3.67 (2.03–6.58)	16	0.00	2
Total nerve root injuries	3.45 (2.21–5.36)	8	0.84 (0.24–2.92)	12	0.30 (0.11–0.79)	6
Permanent nerve root injuries	0.78 (0.42–1.45)	10	0.06 (0.00–0.26)	8	–	6
Thrombophlebitis	1.55 (0.78–1.30)	13	0.82 (0.49–1.35)	4	Not reported	0
Pulmonary emboli	0.56 (0.29–1.07)	14	0.44 (0.20–0.98)	5	Not reported	0
Meningitis	0.30 (0.15–0.60)	5	Not reported	0	Not reported	0
Cauda equina syndrome	0.22 (0.13–0.39)	3	Not reported	0	Not reported	0
Psoas haematoma	Not reported	0	Not reported	0	4.65 (1.17–15.5)	5
Transfusions	0.70 (0.19–2.58)	6	0.17 (0.08–0.39)	11	Not reported	0

*81 studies were included; 2 RCTs, 7 non-randomised controlled trials, 10 case control studies and 62 case series.

Leg cramps

Search date February 2004

Gavin Young

QUESTIONS

INTERVENTIONS

Key Messages

Idiopathic leg cramps

- **Quinine** One systematic review has found that quinine reduces the frequency of nocturnal leg cramp attacks compared with placebo over 4 weeks. We found no evidence about the optimal dose of quinine or length of treatment.
- **Quinine plus theophylline** One small RCT found limited evidence that quinine plus theophylline reduced the number of nights affected by leg cramps compared with quinine alone over 2 weeks.
- **Analgesics; antiepileptic drugs; compression hosiery** We found no RCTs on the effects of these interventions on idiopathic leg cramps.
- **Vitamin E** One small RCT found no significant difference between vitamin E and placebo in the number of nights disturbed by leg cramps.

Leg cramps in pregnancy

- **Magnesium salts** One systematic review identified one small RCT in pregnant women, which found that magnesium tablets (primarily magnesium lactate, magnesium citrate) reduced leg cramps compared with placebo after 3 weeks.
- **Calcium salts** One systematic review identified two RCTs that compared calcium versus vitamin C or no treatment. The RCTs found different results.
- **Multivitamins and mineral supplements** One systematic review identified one small RCT in pregnant women, which found no significant difference between a multivitamin plus mineral tablet and placebo in leg cramps in the ninth month of pregnancy.
- **Sodium chloride** One systematic review found insufficient evidence about the effects of sodium chloride on leg cramps in pregnancy.

Leg cramps

DEFINITION	Leg cramps are involuntary, localised, and usually painful skeletal muscle contractions, which commonly affect calf muscles. Leg cramps typically occur at night and usually last only seconds to minutes. Leg cramps may be idiopathic (of unknown cause) or related to a definable process or condition such as pregnancy, renal dialysis, or venous insufficiency.
INCIDENCE/ PREVALENCE	Leg cramps are common and their incidence increases with age. About half of people attending a general medicine clinic have had leg cramps within 1 month of their visit, and over two thirds of people over 50 years of age have experienced leg cramps.[1]
AETIOLOGY/ RISK FACTORS	Very little is known about the causes of leg cramps. Risk factors include pregnancy, exercise, salt depletion, renal dialysis, electrolyte imbalances, peripheral vascular disease (both venous and arterial), peripheral nerve injury, polyneuropathies, motor neuron disease, muscle diseases, and certain drugs. Other causes of acute calf pain include trauma, deep venous thrombosis (see thromboembolism, p 194), and ruptured Baker's cyst.
PROGNOSIS	Leg cramps may cause severe pain and sleep disturbance.
AIMS OF INTERVENTION	To reduce the frequency and severity of attacks of cramp, with minimal adverse effects of treatment.
OUTCOMES	Frequency, duration, and severity of attacks; number of disturbed nights.
METHODS	*Clinical Evidence* search and appraisal February 2004.

QUESTION What are the effects of treatments for idiopathic leg cramps?

OPTION COMPRESSION HOSIERY

We found no RCTs on the effects of compression hosiery in people with idiopathic leg cramps.

Benefits: We found no systematic review or RCTs.

Harms: We found no evidence on harms related to compression hosiery in people with idiopathic leg cramps. For information on adverse effects of compression hosiery in the prevention and treatments of leg ulcers, see venous leg ulcers, p 2507.

Comment: None.

OPTION QUININE

One systematic review has found that quinine reduces the frequency of nocturnal leg cramps compared with placebo over 4 weeks. We found no evidence about the optimal dose of quinine or length of treatment.

Benefits: We found one systematic review (search date 1997, 8 RCTs, 659 people).[2] Meta-analysis of individual patient data found that quinine significantly reduced the frequency of nocturnal leg cramps compared with placebo over a 4 week period (ARR 3.6 cramps/month with quinine *v* placebo, 95% CI 2.15 to 5.05; RR 0.21, 95% CI 0.12 to 0.30).

Harms: Adverse effects of quinine include headache, digestive disorders, tinnitus, fever, blurred vision, dizziness, and pruritus.[2] In the systematic review, tinnitus was significantly more common with quinine than placebo (AR for tinnitus 20/659 [3.0%] with quinine *v* 7/659 [1.1%] with placebo; RR 2.86, 95% CI 1.22 to 6.71; NNH 50, 95% CI 27 to 230). Elevated quinine levels may cause cinchonism, a syndrome caused by derivatives of cinchona bark. This usually presents with nausea, vomiting, headache, tinnitus, deafness, vertigo, and visual disturbance.[3]

Comment: The systematic review excluded two RCTs because of a lack of individual patient data. Both of these RCTs found that quinine reduced leg cramps compared with placebo. We found no evidence about the optimal dose of quinine or length of treatment.

OPTION QUININE PLUS THEOPHYLLINE

One small RCT found limited evidence that quinine plus theophylline reduced nocturnal leg cramps compared with quinine alone over 2 weeks.

Benefits: We found no systematic review. We found one single blind RCT (164 people), which compared quinine plus theophylline versus quinine alone for 2 weeks.[4] Baseline frequencies of leg cramp were measured for 1 week before randomisation, when all people received placebo. Among 126 people who completed at least 4 days' treatment in the 2 week period, quinine plus theophylline was rated as "good" or "very good" significantly more often than quinine alone or placebo (34/39 [87%] with quinine plus theophylline *v* 28/45 [62%] with quinine *v* 17/42 [40%] with placebo; $P < 0.001$ for quinine plus theophylline *v* either comparison; see comment below). After 2 weeks of treatment, theophylline plus quinine significantly reduced the mean number of nights affected by cramp compared with quinine alone (from 4.7 nights to 1.1 nights with theophylline plus quinine *v* from 4.8 nights to 2.2 nights with quinine alone; $P = 0.009$).

Harms: Six people reported adverse effects while taking placebo in the week before randomisation (nausea and vomiting in 2 people, nausea, heartburn, depression, bitter aftertaste). Three people reported adverse effects with quinine (nausea and vomiting, bloating and tenesmus, and nausea alone), resulting in two people withdrawing from the study. Four people had adverse effects with quinine plus theophylline (fall in blood pressure and dizziness, nausea in 2 cases, palpitations and tinnitus) and all four withdrew from the study.

Comment: The results of the RCT should be treated with caution, as it did not specify criteria to categorise outcomes as "good" or "very good" and pooled the results only for people who received treatment for at least 4 out of 14 days (126 people out of 164 enrolled) without using an intention to treat analysis.

OPTION VITAMIN E

One small RCT found no significant difference between vitamin E and placebo in the frequency of nights disturbed by leg cramps.

Benefits: We found no systematic review. We found one crossover RCT (27 men), which compared vitamin E versus placebo.[5] It found no significant difference between treatments in the median number of nights with leg cramps (14 nights with vitamin E *v* 15 nights with placebo; $P > 0.05$).

Harms: Adverse effects were reported as similar in the vitamin E and placebo groups, but no details were provided.[5]

Comment: None.

OPTION ANALGESICS

We found no RCTs on the effects of analgesics on idiopathic leg cramps.

Benefits: We found no systematic review or RCTs.

Harms: We found no RCTs.

Comment: None.

OPTION ANTIEPILEPTIC DRUGS

We found no RCTs on the effects of antiepileptic drugs on idiopathic leg cramps.

Benefits: We found no systematic review or RCTs.

Harms: Harms associated with the use of antiepileptic drugs are well described (see epilepsy, p 1588).

Comment: None.

QUESTION What are the effects of treatments for leg cramps in pregnancy?

OPTION MAGNESIUM SALTS

One systematic review identified one small RCT in pregnant women, which found that magnesium tablets (primarily magnesium lactate, magnesium citrate) reduced leg cramps compared with placebo after 3 weeks.

Benefits: We found one systematic review (search date 2001,[6] 1 RCT,[7] 73 pregnant women 22–36 weeks' gestation), which compared chewable magnesium tablets (magnesium lactate, magnesium citrate) versus chewable placebo tablets (sorbitol, fructose–dextrose) given for 3 weeks. The review found that magnesium significantly reduced the proportion of women reporting leg cramps compared with placebo after 3 weeks' treatment (AR for persistence 23/34 [68%] with magnesium *v* 33/35 [94%] with placebo; OR 0.18, 95% CI 0.05 to 0.60; see comment below).[6] The RCT found that magnesium decreased the proportion of women who rated themselves "unchanged" or "worse" compared with placebo ("unchanged": 7/34 [21%] with magnesium *v* 16/35 [46%] with placebo; "worse": 0/34 [0%] with magnesium *v* 5/35 [14%] with placebo).[7]

Harms: Adverse effects (mainly slight nausea) were described as infrequent in both groups.[6] One woman in the placebo group discontinued treatment because of severe nausea.[6]

Comment: The RCT did not describe the method of randomisation, and symptoms were assessed after 3 weeks of treatment with no further follow up.[6]

OPTION MULTIVITAMINS AND MINERAL SUPPLEMENTS

One systematic review identified one small RCT in pregnant women, which found no significant difference between multivitamin plus mineral tablet and placebo in leg cramps in the ninth month of pregnancy.

Benefits: We found one systematic review (search date 2001,[6] 1 RCT,[8] 62 pregnant women), which compared a multivitamin plus mineral tablet (containing 12 different ingredients; see comment below) versus placebo. Supplements were given from 3 months' gestation. The review found no significant difference between multivitamin plus mineral and placebo in the proportion of women reporting leg cramps in the ninth month of pregnancy (AR for persistence 2/11 [18%] with multivitamin plus mineral *v* 10/18 [56%] with placebo; OR 0.23, 95% CI 0.05 to 1.01).[6]

Harms: The RCT found that 4% of women had adverse effects (nausea, vomiting, diarrhoea), but did not make clear how many of these women were taking an active treatment.[8]

Comment: This small RCT was primarily undertaken to examine the effects of a multivitamin plus mineral supplement on zinc and copper levels during pregnancy.[8] In total, 29/62 (48%) of women were assessed for cramp at 9 months' gestation.[6] The high dropout rate is not explained. The supplement contained: zinc gluconate, copper gluconate, iron gluconate, magnesium lactate, chromium chloride, ascorbic acid, thiamine nitrate, riboflavin (riboflavine), pyridoxal chlorhydrate, folic acid, cyanocobalamin, and α-tocopheral acetate.[6]

OPTION SODIUM CHLORIDE

One systematic review found insufficient evidence about the effects of sodium chloride in pregnant women with leg cramps.

Benefits: We found one systematic review (search date 2001, no RCTs),[6] which identified one controlled clinical trial[9] published in 1947 (see comment below).

Harms: We found no RCTs.

Comment: The controlled clinical trial was of poor quality. Initially, sodium chloride and calcium lactate were given to alternate participants.[9] It was then decided, based on the difference between the results of the two treatments, to also use two further control groups (saccharin and no treatment).[9] The dose of sodium chloride changed during the course of the study.[6]

OPTION CALCIUM SALTS

One systematic review identified two RCTs that compared calcium versus vitamin C or no treatment. The RCTs found different results.

Benefits: We found one systematic review (search date 2001),[6] which included two RCTs[10,11] and one controlled clinical trial, which was of poor quality (see comment under sodium chloride, p 1463). The first RCT (42 pregnant women) found that calcium (calcium gluconate, lactate, and carbonate) significantly improved leg cramps compared with no treatment (AR for lack of improvement in cramps 2/21 [10%] with calcium *v* 18/21 [86%] with no treatment; OR 0.05, 95% CI 0.02 to 0.17).[6] The second RCT (60 pregnant women) found no significant difference in leg cramps with calcium (calcium gluconate, lactate, and carbonate) compared with vitamin C (AR for lack of improvement in cramps 11/30 [37%] with calcium *v* 8/30 [27%] with vitamin C; OR 1.58, 95% CI 0.54 to 4.63; see comment below).[6]

Harms: The RCTs did not report harms.[6]

Comment: There was a marked difference in the response of the control group in the two included RCTs. In the first RCT, 18/21 (86%) women with no treatment had no improvement in cramps.[10] In the second RCT, 8/30 (27%) women with vitamin C had no improvement.[11]

REFERENCES

1. Hall AJ. Cramp and salt balance in ordinary life. *Lancet* 1947;3:231–233.
2. Man-Son-Hing M, Wells G, Lau A. Quinine for nocturnal leg cramps: a meta-analysis including unpublished data. *J Gen Intern Med* 1998;13:600–606. Search date 1997; primary sources Medline, Embase, Current Contents, and contact with authorities.
3. McGee SR. Muscle cramps. *Arch Intern Med* 1990;150:511–518.
4. Gorlich HD, Gablez VE, Steinberg HW. Treatment of recurrent nocturnal leg cramps. A multicentric

double blind, placebo controlled comparison between the combination of quinine and theophylline ethylene diamine and quinine. *Arzneimittelforschung* 1991;41:167–175.

5. Connolly PS, Shirley EA, Wasson JH, et al. Treatment of nocturnal leg cramps: a crossover trial of quinine vs vitamin E. *Arch Intern Med* 1992;152:1877–1880.
6. Young GL, Jewell D. Interventions for leg cramps in pregnancy (Cochrane Review). In: The Cochrane Library, Issue 2, 2003. Oxford: Update Software. Search date 2001; primary sources Cochrane Pregnancy and Childbirth Group trials register.
7. Dahle LO, Berg G, Hammar M, et al. The effect of oral magnesium substitution on pregnancy-induced leg cramps. *Am J Obstet Gynecol* 1995;173:175–180.
8. Thauvin E, Fusselier M, Arnaud J, et al. Effects of a multivitamin mineral supplement on zinc and copper status during pregnancy. *Biol Trace Elem Res* 1992;32:405–414.
9. Robinson M. Cramps in pregnancy. *J Obstet Gynaecol Br Commonw* 1947;54:826–829.
10. Hammar M, Larsson L, Tegler L. Calcium treatment of leg cramps in pregnancy. *Acta Obstet Gynecol Scand* 1981;60:345–347.
11. Hammar M, Berg G, Solheim F, et al. Calcium and magnesium status in pregnant women. A comparison between treatment with calcium and vitamin C in pregnant women with leg cramps. *Int J Vitam Nutr Res* 1987;57:179–183.

Gavin Young
General Practitioner
Temple Sowerby Surgery
Penrith
UK

Competing interests: None declared.

Low back pain (acute)

Search date October 2003

Maurits van Tulder and Bart Koes

QUESTIONS

INTERVENTIONS

See glossary Ⓖ

Key Messages

Oral drug treatments

- **Non-steroidal anti-inflammatory drugs (NSAIDs)** One systematic review found that NSAIDs increased overall improvement after 1 week and reduced the proportion of people requiring additional analgesics compared with placebo. One systematic review and additional RCTs found no significant difference among NSAIDs or between NSAIDs and other drug treatments (paracetamol, opioids, muscle relaxants, NSAIDs plus muscle relaxants) in pain relief. One systematic review found insufficient evidence about effects of NSAIDs compared with non-drug treatments.
- **Muscle relaxants** One systematic review found that benzodiazepine and non-benzodiazepine muscle relaxants reduced pain and improved overall clinical assessment compared with placebo, but found no significant difference among muscle relaxants. The review found that muscle relaxants were commonly associated with adverse effects, particularly drowsiness, dizziness, and nausea.

- **Analgesics (paracetamol, opioids)** Three small RCTs identified by a sytematic review found no significant difference in symptoms or return to work between an opioid analgesic, paracetamol, and an NSAID. One small RCT identified by the review found that electroacupuncture reduced pain compared with paracetamol. Another RCT identified by the review found that ultrasound improved pain relief compared with analgesics.
- **Colchicine** One RCT found insufficient evidence on the effects of colchicine.

Local injections

- **Epidural steroid injections** One systematic review identified one small RCT, which found no significant difference between epidural steroids and epidural saline, epidural bupivacaine, or dry needling in the proportion of people cured or improved.

Non-drug treatments

- **Advice to stay active** One systematic review and one subsequent RCT found that advice to stay active reduced sick leave and chronic disability compared with no advice or traditional medical treatment (analgesics as required, advice to rest, and "let pain be your guide"). One RCT identified by a systematic review and one subsequent RCT found that advice to stay active reduced sick leave compared with advice to rest in bed, but found mixed results for function and pain.
- **Behavioural therapy** One RCT identified by a systematic review found that cognitive behavioural therapy reduced acute low back pain and disability after 9–12 months compared with traditional care.
- **Multidisciplinary treatment programmes (for subacute low back pain)** One systematic review in people with subacute low back pain found limited evidence that multidisciplinary treatment, including a workplace visit, reduced sick leave compared with usual care.
- **Spinal manipulation** (in the short term) One systematic review found that spinal manipulation slightly reduced pain within 6 weeks compared with sham treatment, but found no significant difference in functional outcomes. The review found no significant difference in pain or functional outcomes between spinal manipulative therapy and general practitioner care, physical therapy, exercises, or back school.
- **Acupuncture** We found no RCTs of acupuncture specifically in people with acute low back pain.
- **Back schools** One systematic review found limited evidence from one RCT that back schools increased rates of recovery and reduced sick leave compared with control in the short term. The review found no consistent difference in outcomes between back school and physiotherapy, and found limited evidence from one RCT that a single session of back school exercise increased pain and sick leave compared with ongoing McKenzie exercises.
- **Massage** One RCT identified by a systematic review found insufficient evidence about the effects of massage compared with spinal manipulation or electrical stimulation.
- **Multidisciplinary treatment programmes (for acute low back pain)** We found no RCTs on the effect of multidisciplinary treatment programmes.
- **Traction** Two RCTs identified by systematic reviews found different results on the effects of traction. One RCT found that traction increased overall improvement compared with bed rest plus corset at 1 and 3 weeks but not at 3 months. The second RCT found no significant difference in overall improvement between traction and infrared treatment after 2 weeks.
- **Electromyographic biofeedback; lumbar supports; temperature treatments (short wave diathermy, ultrasound, ice, heat); transcutaneous electrical nerve stimulation** We found insufficient evidence on the effects of these interventions.
- **Back exercises** Systematic reviews and additional RCTs found either no significant difference in pain or disability between back exercises and conservative or inactive treatments, or found that back exercises increased pain or disability.

- **Bed rest** One systematic review found no evidence that bed rest is better, but found limited evidence that it could be worse than no treatment, advice to stay active, back exercises, physiotherapy, spinal manipulation, or non-steroidal anti-inflammatory drugs. One systematic review found that adverse effects of bed rest included joint stiffness, muscle wasting, loss of bone mineral density, pressure sores, and venous thromboembolism.

DEFINITION Low back pain is pain, muscle tension, or stiffness localised below the costal margin and above the inferior gluteal folds, with or without leg pain (sciatica**G**),[1] and is defined as acute when it persists for less than 12 weeks.[2] Non-specific low back pain is low back pain not attributed to a recognisable pathology (such as infection, tumour, osteoporosis, rheumatoid arthritis, fracture, or inflammation).[1] This review excludes acute low back pain with symptoms or signs at presentation that suggest a specific underlying condition. People with sciatica (lumbosacral radicular syndrome) and herniated discs are also excluded. Unless otherwise stated, people included in this review have acute back pain (i.e. of less than 12 weeks' duration).

INCIDENCE/ PREVALENCE Over 70% of people in developed countries will experience low back pain at some time in their lives.[3] Each year, 15–45% of adults suffer low back pain, and 1/20 (5%) people present to a health care professional with a new episode. Low back pain is most common between the ages of 35–55 years.[3] About 30% of European workers reported that their work caused low back pain. Prevalence rates from different countries range from 13% to 44%. About 70% of people with sick leave due to low back pain return to work within 1 week, and 90% return within 2 months. However, the longer the period of sick leave, the less likely return to work becomes. Less than half of people with low back pain who have been off work for 6 months will return to work.[3,4]

AETIOLOGY/ RISK FACTORS Symptoms, pathology, and radiological appearances are poorly correlated. Pain is non-specific in about 85% of people. About 4% of people with low back pain in primary care have compression fractures and about 1% have a tumour. The prevalence of prolapsed intervertebral disc is about 1–3%.[3] Ankylosing spondylitis and spinal infections are less common.[5] Risk factors for the development of back pain include heavy physical work, frequent bending, twisting, lifting, and prolonged static postures. Psychosocial risk factors include anxiety, depression, and mental stress at work.[3,6]

PROGNOSIS Acute low back pain is usually self limiting (90% of people recover within 6 weeks), although 2–7% develop chronic pain. Acute low back pain has a high recurrence rate with symptoms recurring, to a lesser degree, in 50–80% of people within a year.[7]

AIMS OF INTERVENTION To relieve pain; to improve function; to develop coping strategies for pain, with minimal adverse effects from treatment; and to prevent the development of chronic back pain (see definition under low back pain, p 1479).[2,8]

OUTCOMES Pain intensity (visual analogue or numerical rating scale); overall improvement (self reported or observed); back pain specific functional status (such as Roland Morris questionnaire, Oswestry questionnaire); impact on employment (days of sick leave, number of people returned to work); medication use; intervention specific outcomes (such as coping and pain behaviour for behavioural treatment, strength and flexibility for exercise, depression for antidepressants, and muscle spasm for muscle relaxants and electromyographic biofeedback**G**).

METHODS *Clinical Evidence* search and appraisal October 2003. In addition, the authors searched Medline (1966 to October 2003), Embase (1980 to October 2003), and Psychlit (1984 to October 2003), using the search strategy recommended by the Cochrane Back Review Group.[9] Most earlier RCTs of treatments for low back pain were small (< 50 people/intervention group; range 9–169 people/ intervention group), short term (mostly < 6 months' follow up), and of low overall quality. Problems included lack of power, no description of randomisation procedure, incomplete analysis with failure to account for people who withdrew from trials, and lack of blinding.[10] The quality of many recent RCTs is higher.

QUESTION **What are the effects of oral drug treatments?**

OPTION **ANALGESICS (PARACETAMOL, OPIOIDS)**

Three small RCTs identified by a sytematic review found no significant difference in symptoms or return to work between an opioid analgesic, paracetamol, and a non-steroidal anti-inflammatory drug. One small RCT identified by the review found that electroacupuncture reduced pain compared with paracetamol. Another RCT identified by the review found that ultrasound improves pain relief compared with analgesics.

Benefits: We found one systematic review (search date 1998; 6 RCTs; no statistical pooling of data provided).[11] Versus **placebo:** The review identified no RCTs.[11] **Versus non-steroidal anti-inflammatory drugs:** The review identified three small RCTs, none of which found a significant difference in clinical outcome between paracetamol or opioid analgesics and non-steroidal anti-inflammatory drugs.[11] The first RCT (48 people) found that, after 10 weeks, 54% of people taking paracetamol were symptom free, compared with 67% taking ibuprofen. The second RCT (45 people) found that return to work was similar among treatments (mean number of days until return to full activity: 5.7 with paracetamol, 6.5 with phenylbutazone, 5.7 with aspirin). The third RCT (60 people) identified by the review found that pain was similar among treatments (mean daily pain index on a 4 point scale: 1.7 with paracetamol, 1.4 with aspirin, 1.5 with indomethacin, 1.4 with mefenamic acid, 1.4 with phenylbutazone, and 1.7 on dextropropoxyphene). **Versus non-drug treatments:** The review identified one RCT (40 people), which found that electroacupuncture**G** increased pain relief compared with paracetamol after 6 weeks (pain scores on a 100 point visual analogue scale: 54.4 at baseline and 13.7 at 6 weeks with paracetamol v 52.7 and 3.3 with electroacupuncture).[11] The review identified a second RCT (73 people), which found that ultrasound treatment significantly increased the proportion of people who were pain free after 4 weeks compared with analgesics.[11]

Harms: See paracetamol (acetaminophen) poisoning, p 1756. RCTs have found adverse effects (constipation and drowsiness) with analgesics in about 50% of people. One earlier systematic review (search date 1995) found that combinations of paracetamol plus weak opioids increased the risk of adverse effects compared with paracetamol alone (15 single dose studies; OR 1.1, 95% CI 0.8 to 1.5; 3 multiple dose studies; OR 2.5, 95% CI 1.5 to 4.2).[12]

Comment: None.

OPTION **COLCHICINE**

One RCT found insufficient evidence on the effects of colchicine.

Benefits: We found one systematic review (search date not reported, 1 RCT, 27 people), which found no significant difference in pain intensity after 1, 2, 4, 6 and 12 weeks between oral colchicine and placebo, although the RCT identified by the review was too small to rule out a clinically important difference.[2]

Harms: The review reported gastrointestinal irritation in about 75% of people taking colchicines and in 27% of those taking placebo.[2] Other adverse effects included skin problems, chemical cellulitis, and agranulocytosis.[13]

Comment: The review identified two further RCTs, which did not distinguish between acute and chronic low back pain.[2]

OPTION MUSCLE RELAXANTS

One systematic review found that benzodiazepine and non-benzodiazepine muscle relaxants reduced pain and improved overall clinical assessment compared with placebo, but found no significant difference among muscle relaxants. The review found that muscle relaxants were commonly associated with adverse effects, particularly drowsiness, dizziness and nausea.

Benefits: Benzodiazepines versus placebo: We found one systematic review (search date 2001),[14] which identified one poor quality RCT (68 people).[15] The RCT found that intramuscular diazepam followed by oral diazepam for 5 days significantly reduced pain and increased the rate of overall improvement compared with placebo (overall effect rated good or very good: 21/33 [64%] with diazepam v 6/35 [17%] with placebo; P value not reported in the review; pain results not reported in the review). However, treatment groups were not comparable at baseline. Non-benzodiazepines versus placebo: The review identified nine RCTs comparing non-benzodiazepines (tizanidine, cyclobenzaprine, carisoprodol, baclofen, orphenadrine) versus placebo.[14] Meta-analysis of RCTs with adequate data found that oral non-benzodiazepines (cyclobenzaprine, tizanidine, and orphenadrine) significantly reduced pain and improved global assessment after 2–4 days (presence of pain: 4 RCTs, 294 people; RR 0.80, 95% CI 0.71 to 0.89; global assessment at 24 days: 4 RCTs, 222 people; RR 0.49, 95% CI 0.25 to 0.95). Versus each other: We found one systematic review (search date 2001),[14] which identified three RCTs. The RCTs found no important differences in effect among muscle relaxants (cyclobenzaprine, carisoprodol, diazepam, and tizanidine), although the results were not pooled in the review. The first RCT (80 people) found that carisoprodol significantly increased overall improvement compared with diazepam but found no significant difference in pain at 7 days (improvement rated as very good or excellent; 70% with carisoprodol v 45% with diazepam; pain on 100 mm visual analogue scale: 58 mm with carisoprodol v 48 mm with diazepam; P values not reported in the review).[16] The second RCT (78 people) found no significant difference between carisoprodol and cylcobenzaprine in pain or overall improvement after 8 days (pain on 100 mm visual analogue scale: 30 mm with carisoprodol v 28 mm with cylcobenzaprine; overall improvement good or excellent: 70% with carisoprodol v 70% with cylcobenzaprine; P values not reported in review).[17] The third RCT (30 people with acute back pain, 20% with concomitant acute neck pain) was small and found no significant difference between diazepam and tizanidine in pain or function at 7 days (pain relief: 77.4% with tizanidine v 48% with diazepam; improvement in daily activities: 87% with tizanidine v 93% with diazepam; P values not reported in review).[18]

Harms: The review found that muscle relaxants (both benzodiazepines and non-benzodiazepines) significantly increased adverse effects, particularly central nervous system effects, compared with placebo (all adverse effects: 8 RCTs, 724 people; RR 1.50, 95% CI 1.14 to 1.98; nervous system effects: 8 RCTs, 724 people; RR 2.04, 95% CI 1.23 to 3.37).[14] The most common adverse effects were drowsiness, dizziness, and nausea.

Comment: None.

OPTION NON-STEROIDAL ANTI-INFLAMMATORY DRUGS

One systematic review found that non-steroidal anti-inflammatory drugs (NSAIDs) increased overall improvement after 1 week and reduced the proportion of people requiring additional analgesics compared with placebo. One systematic review and additional RCTs found no significant difference among NSAIDs or between NSAIDs and other drug treatments (paracetamol, opioids, muscle relaxants, NSAIDs plus muscle relaxants) in pain relief. One systematic review found insufficient evidence about effects of NSAIDs compared with non-drug treatments.

Benefits: We found one systematic review (search date 1998, 45 RCTs, statistical pooling only for NSAIDs *v* placebo)[11] and three additional RCTs.[19–21] **NSAIDs versus placebo:** We found one systematic review (search date 1998, 9 RCTs).[11] The review found that NSAIDs significantly increased the proportion of people experiencing global improvement and reduced the proportion of people requiring additional analgesics compared with placebo after 1 week (global improvement; 6 RCTs, 535 people: OR 2.0, 95% CI 1.4 to 3.0; additional analgesia; 3 RCTs, 537 people: OR 1.55, 95% CI 1.09 to 2.21).[11] **Versus each other:** We found one systematic review (search date 1998; 18 RCTs, 1982 people)[11] and one subsequent RCT.[19] The review found no significant difference among NSAIDs in outcomes.[11] The subsequent RCT (104 people) found that nimesulide improved functional status compared with ibuprofen, but found no significant difference in pain relief after 10 days.[19] **Versus paracetamol:** See benefits of analgesics (paracetamol, opioids), p 1468. **Versus muscle relaxants or opioid analgesics:** We found one systematic review (search date 1998, 5 RCTs, 399 people), which found no significant difference between NSAIDs and muscle relaxants or opioids in pain relief or overall improvement.[11] **Versus non-drug treatments:** We found one systematic review (search date 1998, 3 RCTs, 461 people).[11] Two included RCTs provided inconclusive evidence about effects of NSAIDs and bed rest. The first RCT (110 people) found that NSAIDs significantly improved combined score on pain, disability, and range of movement compared with bed rest. The second RCT (241 people) found no significant difference between treatments in range of movement, and did not examine effects on pain or function. Two included RCTs (354 people) comparing NSAIDs versus physiotherapy or spinal manipulation found no significant difference in pain relief or improvement in mobility. **Versus NSAIDs plus adjuvant treatment:** The review identified three RCTs (232 people), which found no significant difference between NSAIDs alone and NSAIDs plus muscle relaxants in outcomes.[11] One RCT identified by the review[11] and one additional RCT[21] found no significant difference between NSAIDs and NSAIDs plus vitamin B in pain relief, although one of the RCTs found that NSAIDs alone significantly reduced the proportion of people returning to work after 1 week compared with NSAIDs plus vitamin B combinations (78% of people with combination treatment *v* 35% with NSAIDs alone).

Harms: NSAIDs may cause gastrointestinal complications (see non-steroidal anti-inflammatory drugs, p 1525). One systematic review of harms of NSAIDs found that ibuprofen and diclofenac had the lowest gastrointestinal complication rate, mainly because of the low doses used in practice (pooled OR for adverse effects v placebo 1.30, 95% CI 0.91 to 1.80).[22]

Comment: None.

QUESTION **What are the effects of local injections?**

OPTION **EPIDURAL STEROID INJECTIONS**

One systematic review identified one small RCT, which found no significant difference between epidural steroids and epidural saline, epidural bupivacaine, or dry needling in the proportion of people cured or improved.

Benefits: We found one systematic review (search date 1998, 1 RCT).[23] The RCT (63 people) compared four treatments: epidural steroids, epidural saline, epidural bupivacaine, and dry needling. It found no significant difference between any of the treatments in the proportion of people improved or cured.

Harms: The RCT found that adverse effects were infrequent and included headache, fever, subdural penetration, and, more rarely, epidural abscess and respiratory depression.[23]

Comment: None.

QUESTION **What are the effects of non-drug treatments?**

OPTION **ADVICE TO STAY ACTIVE**

One systematic review and one subsequent RCT found that advice to stay active reduced sick leave and chronic disability compared with no advice or traditional medical treatment (analgesics as required, advice to rest, and "let pain be your guide"). One RCT identified by a systematic review and one subsequent RCT found that advice to stay active reduced sick leave compared with advice to rest in bed, but found mixed results for function and pain.

Benefits: Versus no advice or traditional medical treatment: We found one systematic review (search date not reported, 6 RCTs, 1957 people)[24] and one subsequent RCT.[25] The review compared advice to stay active with or without other treatments versus those other treatments alone and found that advice to stay active significantly reduced sick leave and reduced chronic disability compared with traditional medical treatment (analgesics as required, advice to rest, and "let pain be your guide") up to 1 year.[24] The subsequent RCT (457 people) found that advice to stay active significantly increased return to work compared with no advice after 3, 6, and 12 months (at 3 months: AR 52% with advice v 36% with no advice; at 6 months: 61% v 45%; at 12 months: 86% v 56%).[25] Versus bed rest: We found one systematic review (search date 1998, 1 RCT, 186 people with acute back pain or sciatica[G], no statistical pooling of data; see comments)[26] and one subsequent RCT.[27] The review found that advice to stay active significantly improved functional status and reduced sick leave after 3 weeks compared with advice to rest in bed for 2 days (1 RCT, 186 people; weighted mean improvement in Oswestry questionnaire score for advice to remain active *v* bed rest 4.4, 95% CI 0.6 to 8.2; weighted mean reduction in days of sick leave for advice to remain active *v* bed rest 4.5 days, 95% CI 1.4 days to 7.6 days). However, it found no significant difference in pain intensity between groups after 3 weeks. The subsequent RCT (278 people) found no significant differences in pain intensity and functional disability between advice to stay active and bed rest after 1 month (intensity of pain measured on visual analogue scale [0 = no pain and 100 = extreme unbearable pain]: 10.2 mm with advice *v* 13.7 mm with bed rest; difference +3.5 mm; 97.5% CI −2.6 mm to +0.5 mm; functional disability measured on the Eifel index [a French version of the

Roland–Morris questionnaire; range 0–24]; at 1 month: 2.47 with advice v 3.3 with bed rest; difference –0.82, 99% CI –2.55 to +0.50). However, it found that advice to stay active significantly reduced sick leave compared with bed rest up to day 5 (52% with advice to stay active v 86% with bed rest; $P < 0.0001$).[27]

Harms: The reviews and subsequent RCT did not report harms.[24,26,27]

Comment: Limitations in methods preclude meaningful quantification of effect sizes. Advice to stay active was provided either as a single treatment or in combination with other interventions such as back schools**G**, a graded activity programme, or behavioural counselling. The two lower quality RCTs included in the review of advice to stay active versus bed rest were reported to have moderate to high risk of bias.[26] The first did not measure pain at follow up. The second found that 48 hours of strict bed rest significantly improved pain compared with advice to stay active (time to outcome and further details not reported in the review).

OPTION BACK SCHOOLS

One systematic review found limited evidence from one RCT that back schools increased rates of recovery and reduced sick leave compared with control in the short term. The review found no consistent difference in outcomes between back school and physiotherapy, and found limited evidence from one RCT that a single session of back school exercises increased pain and sick leave compared with ongoing McKenzie exercises.

Benefits: We found one systematic review (search date 1997, 2 RCTs, no statistical pooling of data provided).[28] The first included RCT (217 people) found that back schools**G** significantly increased recovery and reduced sick leave compared with control (mean days until recovery: 14.8 with back schools v 28.7 with control; median days of absence from work: 20.5 with back schools v 26.5 with control). The RCT also found that back schools significantly reduced sick leave compared with physiotherapy, but found no significant difference in recovery between back school and physiotherapy (median days of absence from work 20.5 with back school v 26.5 with physiotherapy). The second included RCT (100 people) found that ongoing McKenzie exercises**G** significantly reduced pain and sick leave compared with one 45 minute session of back school for up to 5 years (no data reported for pain; median days of sick leave 11.9 with exercises v 21.6 with back school; AR for any sick leave between 1 and 5 years: 24/47 with exercises v 32/42 with back school).

Harms: The review did not report harms.[28]

Comment: None.

OPTION BED REST

One systematic review found no evidence that bed rest is better, but found limited evidence that it could be worse than no treatment, advice to stay active, back exercises, physiotherapy, spinal manipulation, or non-steroidal anti-inflammatory drugs. One systematic review found that adverse effects of bed rest included joint stiffness, muscle wasting, loss of bone mineral density, pressure sores, and venous thromboembolism.

Benefits: We found one systematic review (search date 1999, 9 RCTs;[29] no statistical pooling provided). **Versus no treatment:** The review identified five RCTs (663 people), which compared bed rest versus no treatment and found either no significant difference between treatments or that no treatment improved outcomes compared with bed rest.[29] **Versus different lengths of bed rest:** The review identified two RCTs (254 people), which found no significant difference in outcomes with 7 days versus 2–4 days of bed rest.[29] Versus advice to stay active: See benefits of advice to stay active, p 1471. **Versus other interventions:** The review identified five RCTs (921 people), which compared bed rest versus other interventions (back exercises, physiotherapy, spinal manipulation, or non-steroidal anti-inflammatory drugs).[29] They found either no significant difference in outcomes (pain, recovery rate, time to return to daily activities, and sick leave) or an improvement in outcomes with the comparative interventions.

Harms: One previous systematic review assessed harms.[24] It found that adverse effects of bed rest included joint stiffness, muscle wasting, loss of bone mineral density, pressure sores, and venous thromboembolism (see thromboembolism, p 194).

Comment: None.

OPTION BEHAVIOURAL THERAPY

One RCT identified by a systematic review found that cognitive behavioural therapy reduced acute low back pain and disability after 9–12 months compared with traditional care.

Benefits: We found one systematic review (search date 1995, 1 RCT, 107 people).[10] The RCT identified by the review found that cognitive behavioural therapy**G** reduced pain and perceived disability after 9–12 months compared with traditional care (analgesics plus back exercises until pain had subsided).

Harms: The review did not report on harms.[10]

Comment: None.

OPTION ELECTROMYOGRAPHIC BIOFEEDBACK

We found no RCTs on the effects of electromyographic biofeedback.

Benefits: We found no systematic reviews or RCTs of electromyographic biofeedback in people with acute low back pain.

Harms: We found no evidence on harms.

Comment: None.

OPTION BACK EXERCISES

Systematic reviews and additional RCTs found either no significant difference in pain or disability between back exercises and conservative or inactive treatments, or found that back exercises increased pain or disability.

Benefits: We found one systematic review (search date 1999;[30] no statistical pooling of data provided) and two additional RCTs.[31,32] The review identified eight RCTs (1149 people), which compared specific back exercises (flexion, extension, aerobic, or strengthening programmes such as McKenzie exercises**G**) versus other conservative treatments (usual care by general practitioner, continuation of ordinary activities, bed rest, manipulation, non-steroidal anti-inflammatory drugs, mini back school, or short wave diathermy).[30] Seven of these RCTs found either no difference between treatments or that back exercises increased pain intensity and disability. The eighth RCT found that back exercises improved pain and return to work compared with a mini back school. The review identified four RCTs (888 people) comparing back exercises versus inactive treatments (bed rest, educational booklet, and placebo ultrasound). It found no significant difference between back exercises and inactive treatment in pain relief, global improvement, or functional status. The first additional RCT (66 people) found that endurance training back exercises significantly increased improvement in functioning and pain relief after 3 weeks compared with no treatment, but found no significant difference in functioning or pain after 6 weeks (data were presented graphically).[31] The second additional RCT (41 people) found no significant difference between advice, minimal bed rest, or analgesics versus the same treatment plus specific, localised exercise of the multifidus muscle in pain and disability.[32]

Harms: The review and additional RCTs did not report harms.[30–32]

Comment: None.

OPTION LUMBAR SUPPORTS

We found no RCTs on the effects of lumbar supports.

Benefits: We found no systematic reviews or RCTs specifically in people with acute low back pain.

Harms: Harms associated with prolonged lumbar support use include decreased strength of the trunk musculature, a false sense of security, heat, skin irritation, and general discomfort.[2]

Comment: None.

OPTION MULTIDISCIPLINARY TREATMENT PROGRAMMES

We found no RCTs in people with acute low back pain. However, one systematic review in people with subacute low back pain found limited evidence that multidisciplinary treatment, including a workplace visit, reduced sick leave compared with usual care.

Benefits: We found no RCTs specifically in people with acute back pain. We found one systematic review (search date 1998, 2 RCTs, 233 people with subacute low back pain, duration > 4 weeks and < 3 months), which found that multidisciplinary treatment**G**, including a workplace visit, significantly reduced sick leave compared with usual care (time to return to work: 10 weeks with multidisciplinary treatment v 15 weeks with usual care in one RCT; RR for return to work rate 2.4, 95% CI 1.2 to 4.9 in the other RCT).[33]

Harms: The review did not report harms.[33]

Comment: None.

OPTION TEMPERATURE TREATMENTS (SHORT WAVE DIATHERMY, ULTRASOUND, ICE, AND HEAT)

Two systematic reviews identified no RCTs on the effects of temperature treatments.

Benefits: We found two systematic reviews (search date not reported[2] and 1992[34]), which found no RCTs.

Harms: The reviews did not report harms.[2,34]

Comment: None.

OPTION MASSAGE

One RCT identified by a systematic review found insufficient evidence about the effects of massage compared with spinal manipulation or electrical stimulation.

Benefits: We found one systematic review (search date 2001, 1 RCT).[35] It identified one RCT (90 people), which compared massage**G** versus spinal manipulation or electrical stimulation and found no significant difference in pain relief, functional status, or mobility.[35]

Harms: The review gave no information on harms.[35]

Comment: None.

OPTION SPINAL MANIPULATION

One systematic review found that spinal manipulation slightly reduced pain within 6 weeks compared with sham treatment, but found no significant difference in functional outcomes. The review found no significant differences in pain or functional outcomes between spinal manipulative therapy and general practitioner care, physical therapy, exercises, or back school.

Benefits: We found one systematic review (search date 2000, 29 RCTs).[36] **Versus placebo or sham treatment:** The review found that spinal manipulative therapy significantly reduced pain in the short term (< 6 weeks) compared with sham therapy, but found no significant difference in the longer term (short term difference in pain on 100 mm visual analogue scale: 10 mm, 95% CI 2 mm to 17 mm).[36] It found that spinal manipulation reduced disability in the short term compared with sham therapy but the difference was not statistically significant (difference in disability on Roland Disability questionnaire: 2.8 mm, 95% CI –0.1 mm to +5.6 mm). There was no significant difference in disability in the longer term (data not reported). **Versus other treatments:** The review found no significant difference between spinal manipulative therapy and general practitioner care, physical therapy, exercises, or back school (results presented graphically).[36]

Harms: The systematic review (search date 2000) did not report on harms.[36] A second systematic review assessed harms of spinal manipulation.[37] In RCTs identified by the review that used a trained therapist to select people and perform spinal manipulation, the risk of serious complications was low (estimated risk: vertebrobasilar strokes 1/20 000–1/1 000 000 people; cauda equina syndrome < 1/1 000 000 people).

Comment: Current guidelines do not advise spinal manipulation in people with severe or progressive neurological deficit.[2,13]

OPTION TRACTION

Two RCTs identified by systematic reviews found different results on the effects of traction. One RCT found that traction increased overall improvement compared with bed rest plus corset at 1 and 3 weeks but not at 3 months. The second RCT found no significant difference in overall improvement between traction and infrared treatment after 2 weeks.

Benefits: We found three systematic reviews (search dates 1995[8,10] and 1992[38]). The reviews identified two RCTs solely in people with acute low back pain (225 people), which compared traction versus bed rest plus corset or infrared treatment and found different results. The first RCT (82 people) found that traction significantly increased overall improvement compared with bed rest plus corset after 1 and 3 weeks but not after 3 months (AR for improvement after 1 week: 17/41 [41%] with traction v 2/41 [5%] with bed rest and corset; after 3 weeks: 20/41 [49%] v 8/41 [20%]; after 3 months: 19/41 [46%] v 24/41 [59%]).[39] The second RCT (143 people) found no significant difference in overall improvement after 2 weeks between traction and infrared treatment (AR for improvement at 2 weeks: 40/77 [52%] with traction v 27/54 [50%] with infrared).[40]

Harms: The reviews did not report on harms.[8,10,38] Potential adverse effects of traction include debilitation, loss of muscle tone, bone demineralisation, and thrombophlebitis.[2]

Comment: Of 16 RCTs identified by the reviews, 14 RCTs did not distinguish between acute and chronic low back pain, included only chronic low back pain, or included people with back pain of specific cause.[8,10,38,41,42]

OPTION TRANSCUTANEOUS ELECTRICAL NERVE STIMULATION

We found no RCTs about effects of transcutaneous electrical nerve stimulation in people with acute back pain.

Benefits: We found no systematic reviews or RCTs specifically in people with acute low back pain.

Harms: We found no RCTs in people with acute low back pain.

Comment: None.

OPTION ACUPUNCTURE

We found no RCTs of acupuncture specifically in people with acute low back pain.

Benefits: We found two systematic reviews (search dates 1996; see comment below), which found no RCTs of acupuncture[G] in people with acute low back pain.[43,44]

Harms: One systematic review (search date 1996) found that serious, rare, adverse effects included infections (HIV, hepatitis, bacterial endocarditis) and visceral trauma (pneumothorax, cardiac tamponade).[45]

Comment: Three RCTs identified by the systematic reviews combined acute and chronic low back pain and two RCTs did not specify the duration of symptoms.[43,44] One RCT included people with back and neck pain.

GLOSSARY

Acupuncture Needle puncture of the skin at traditional "meridian" acupuncture points. Modern acupuncturists also use non-meridian points and trigger points (tender sites occurring in the most painful areas). The needles may be stimulated manually or electrically. Placebo acupuncture is needling of traditionally unimportant sites or non-stimulation of the needles once placed.

Back school Traditionally, this is a series of group education sessions on low back pain. Sessions are usually supervised by a physiotherapist or physician and often include information on an exercise programme.

Cognitive behavioural therapy This aims to identify and modify people's understanding of their pain and disability using cognitive restructuring techniques (such as imagery and attention diversion) or by modifying maladaptive thoughts, feelings, and beliefs.

Electromyographic biofeedback A person receives external feedback of their own electromyogram (using visual or auditory scales), and uses this to learn how to control the electromyogram and hence the tension within their own muscles. Electromyogram biofeedback for low back pain aims to relax the paraspinal muscles.

Massage Massage is manipulation of soft tissues (i.e. muscle and fascia) using the hands or a mechanical device, to promote circulation and relaxation of muscle spasm or tension. Different types of soft tissue massage include Shiatsu, Swedish, friction, trigger point, or neuromuscular massage.
McKenzie exercises Extension exercises that use self generated stresses and forces to centralise pain from the legs and buttocks to the lower back. This method emphasises self care.
Multidisciplinary treatment Intensive physical and psychosocial training by a team (e.g. a physician, physiotherapist, psychologist, social worker, and occupational therapist). Training is usually given in groups and does not involve passive physiotherapy.
Sciatica Pain that radiates from the back into the buttock or leg and may also be used to describe pain anywhere along the course of the sciatic nerve.

REFERENCES

1. Van der Heijden GJMG, Bouter LM, Terpstra-Lindeman E. De effectiviteit van tractie bij lage rugklachten. De resultaten van een pilotstudy. *Ned T Fysiotherapie* 1991;101:37–43.
2. Bigos S, Bowyer O, Braen G, et al. Acute low back problems in adults. Clinical Practice Guideline no. 14. AHCPR Publication No. 95–0642. Rockville MD: Agency for Health Care Policy and Research, Public Health Service, US, Department of Health and Human Services, December 1994. Search date not reported; primary sources The Quebec Task Force on Spinal Disorders Review to 1984, search carried out by National Library of Medicine from 1984, and references from expert panel.
3. Andersson GBJ. The epidemiology of spinal disorders. In: Frymoyer JW, ed. *The adult spine: principles and practice*. 2nd ed. New York: Raven Press, 1997:93–141.
4. Waddell G. *The back pain revolution*. Edinburgh: Churchill Livingstone; 1998.
5. Deyo RA, Rainville J, Kent DL. What can the history and physical examination tell us about low back pain? *JAMA* 1992;268:760–765.
6. Bongers PM, de Winter CR, Kompier MA, et al. Psychosocial factors at work and musculoskeletal disease. *Scand J Work Environ Health* 1993;19:297–312.
7. Frymoyer JW. Back pain and sciatica. *N Engl J Med* 1988;318:291–300.
8. Evans G, Richards S. *Low back pain: an evaluation of therapeutic interventions.* Bristol: Health Care Evaluation Unit, University of Bristol, 1996. Search date 1995; primary sources Medline, Embase, A-Med, Psychlit, and hand searches of references.
9. Van Tulder MW, Assendelft WJJ, Koes BW, et al, and the Editorial Board of the Cochrane Collaboration Back Review Group. Method guidelines for systematic reviews in the Cochrane Collaboration back review group for spinal disorders. *Spine* 1997;22:2323–2330.
10. Van Tulder MW, Koes BW, Bouter LM. Conservative treatment of acute and chronic nonspecific low back pain: a systematic review of randomized controlled trials of the most common interventions. *Spine* 1997;22:2128–2156. Search date 1995; primary sources Medline, Embase, Psychlit, and hand searches of references.
11. Van Tulder MW, Scholten RJPM, Koes BW, et al. Non-steroidal anti-inflammatory drugs (NSAIDs) for non-specific low back pain. In: The Cochrane Library, Issue 3, 2004. Oxford: Update Software. Search date 1998; primary sources Medline, Embase, Cochrane Controlled Trials Register, and hand searches of references.
12. De Craen AJM, Di Giulio G, Lampe-Schoenmaeckers AJEM, et al. Analgesic efficacy and safety of paracetamol–codeine combinations versus paracetamol alone: a systematic review. *BMJ* 1996;313:321–325. Search date 1995; primary sources Medline, Embase, International Pharmaceutical Abstracts, Biosis, contact with pharmaceutical companies, and hand searches of references.
13. Waddell G, Feder G, McIntosh A, et al. *Low back pain evidence review.* London: Royal College of General Practitioners, 1999. Search date 1999; primary sources Medline, Embase, Science Citation Index, Social Sciences Citation Index, correspondence with experts and researchers, and hand searches of references.
14. van Tulder MW, Touray T, Furlan AD, et al. Muscle relaxants for non-specific low back pain. In The Cochrane Library. Issue 4, 2003. Chicester, UK; John Wiley & Sons Ltd. Search date 2001; primary sources Medline, Embase, Cochrane Library, and reference lists.
15. Moll W. Therapy of acute lumbovertebral syndromes through optimal muscle relaxation using diazepam. Results of a double-blind study on 68 cases [In German]. *Med Welt* 1973;24:1747–1751.
16. Boyles W, Glassman, Soyka J. Management of acute musculokeletal conditions: thoracolumbar strain or sprain. Double-blind evaluation comparing the efficacy and safety of carisoprodol with diazepam. *Today's Ther Trends* 1983;1:1–16.
17. Rollings H. Management of acute musculoskeletal conditions – thoracolumbar strain or sprain: a double-blind evaluation comparing the efficacy and safety of carisoprodol with cyclobenzaprine hydrochloride. *Curr Ther Res* l983;34:917–928.
18. Hennies O. A new skeletal muscle relaxant (DS 103–282) compared to diazepam in the treatment of muscle spasm of local origin. *Int Med Res* 1981;9:62–68.
19. Pohjolainen T, Jekunen A, Autio L, et al. Treatment of acute low back pain with the COX-2 selective anti-inflammatory drug nimesulide: results of a randomised, double-blind comparative trial versus ibuprofen. *Spine* 2000;25:1579–1585.
20. Laws D. Double blind parallel group investigation in general practice of the efficacy and tolerability of acemetacin, in comparison with diclofenac, in patients suffering with acute low back pain. *Br J Clin Res* 1994;5:55–64.
21. Bruggemann G, Koehler CO, Koch EM. Results of a double-blind study of diclofenac + vitamin B1, B6, B12 versus diclofenac in patients with acute pain of the lumbar vertebrae: a multicenter study. *Klinische Wochenschrift* 1990;68:116–120.
22. Henry D, Lim LLY, Rodriguez LAG, et al. Variability in risk of gastrointestinal complications with individual non-steroidal anti-inflammatory drugs: results of a collaborative meta-analysis. *BMJ* 1996;312:1563–1566. Search date 1994; primary sources Medline, contact with study authors, and hand searches of references.
23. Koes BW, Scholten RJPM, Mens JMA, et al. Epidural steroid injections for low back pain and sciatica: an updated systematic review of randomized clinical trials. *Pain Digest* 1999;9:241–247. Search date 1998; primary sources Medline and hand searches of relevant publications.
24. Waddell G, Feder G, Lewis M. Systematic reviews of bed rest and advice to stay active for acute low back pain. *Br J Gen Pract* 1997;47:647–652. Search date not reported; primary sources Medline,

contacted recently published authors and pharmaceutical companies, and hand searches of references.
25. Hagen EM, Eriksen HR, Ursin H. Does early intervention with a light mobilization program reduce long-term sick leave for low back pain? *Spine* 2000;25:1973–1976.
26. Hilde G, Hagen KB, Jamtvedt G, et al. Advice to stay active as a single treatment for low back pain and sciatica (Cochrane Review). In: The Cochrane Library, Issue 3, 2004. Oxford: Update Software. Search date 1998; primary sources Medline, Embase, Sport, Cochrane Controlled Trials Register, Musculoskeletal Group's trials register, and Scisearch.
27. Rozenberg S, Delval C, Rezvani Y, et al. Bed rest or normal activity for patients with acute low back pain: a randomized controlled trial. *Spine* 2002;27:1487–1493.
28. Van Tulder MW, Esmail R, Bombardier C, et al. Back schools for non-specific low back pain. In: The Cochrane Library, Issue 3, 2004. Oxford: Update Software. Search date 1998; primary sources Medline, Embase, and hand searches of references.
29. Hagen KB, Hilde G, Jamtvedt G, et al. Bed rest for acute low back pain and sciatica (Cochrane Review). In: The Cochrane Library, Issue 3, 2004. Oxford: Update Software. Search date 1999; primary sources Cochrane Musculoskeletal Group's trials register, Cochrane Controlled Trials Register, Cochrane Library, Medline, Embase, Sport, Scisearch, and hand searches of reference lists and personal contact with the authors of included articles.
30. van Tulder MW, Malmivaara A, Esmail R, et al. Exercise therapy for non-specific low back pain. In: The Cochrane Library, Issue 3, 2004. Oxford: Update Software. Search date 1999; primary sources Medline, Psychlit, Cochrane Controlled Trials Register, Embase, and hand searches of reference lists.
31. Chok B, Lee R, Latimer J, et al. Endurance training of the trunk extensor muscles in people with subacute low back pain. *Phys Ther* 1999;79:1032–1042.
32. Hides JA, Richardson CA, Jull GA. Multifidus muscle recovery is not automatic after resolution of acute first episode low back pain. *Spine* 1996;21:2763–2769.
33. Karjalainen K, Malmivaara A, van Tulder M, et al. Multidisciplinary biopsychosocial rehabilitation for subacute low back pain among working age adults. In: The Cochrane Library, Issue 3, 2004. Oxford: Update Software. Search date 2002; primary sources Medline, Embase, Psychlit, Cochrane Register of Controlled Clinical Trials, Science Citation Index, hand searches of reference lists, and personal contact with experts.
34. Gam AN, Johannsen F. Ultrasound therapy in musculoskeletal disorders: a meta-analysis. *Pain* 1995;63:85–91. Search date 1992; primary sources Index Medicus, Medline, and hand searches of references.
35. Furlan AD, Brosseau L, Imamura M, et al. Massage for low back pain. In: The Cochrane Library, Issue 3, 2004. Oxford: Update Software. Search date 2001; primary sources Medline, Embase, Cochrane Controlled Trials Register, Healthstar, Cinahl, Dissertation Abstracts, hand searches of references, and contact with content experts and massage associations.
36. Assendelft WJJ, Morton SC, Yu EI, et al. Spinal manipulative therapy for low back pain: a meta-analysis of effectiveness relative to other therapies. *Ann Intern Med* 2003;138:871–881.
37. Assendelft WJJ, Bouter LM, Knipschild PG. Complications of spinal manipulation: a comprehensive review of the literature. *J Fam Pract* 1996;42:475–480.
38. Van der Heijden GJMG, Beurskens AJHM, Koes BW, et al. The efficacy of traction for back and neck pain: a systematic, blinded review of randomized clinical trial methods. *Phys Ther* 1995;75:93–104. Search date 1992; primary sources Medline, Embase, Index to Chiropractic Literature, Physiotherapy Index, and hand searches of non-indexed journals.
39. Larsson U, Chöler U, Lidström A, et al. Auto-traction for treatment of lumbago-sciatica. *Acta Orthop Scand* 1980;51:791–798.
40. Mathews JA, Mills SB, Jenkins VM, et al. Back pain and sciatica: controlled trials of manipulation, traction, sclerosant and epidural injections. *Br J Rheumatol* 1987;26:416–423.
41. Ljunggren E, Weber H, Larssen S. Autotraction versus manual traction in patients with prolapsed lumbar intervertebral discs. *Scand J Rehabil Med* 1984;16:117–124.
42. Werners R, Pynsent PB, Bulstrode CJK. Randomized trial comparing interferential therapy with motorized lumbar traction and massage in the management of low back pain in a primary care setting. *Spine* 1999;24:1579–1584.
43. Ernst E, White AR. Acupuncture for back pain. A meta-analysis of randomized controlled trials. *Arch Intern Med* 1998;158:2235–2241. Search date 1996; primary sources Medline, Cochrane Controlled Trials Register, Ciscom, contacted authors and experts, and hand searches of references.
44. Van Tulder MW, Cherkin DC, Berman B, et al. Acupuncture in low back pain. In: The Cochrane Library, Issue 3, 2004. Oxford: Update Software. Search date 1997; primary sources Medline, Embase, Cochrane Complementary Medicine Field trials register, Cochrane Controlled Trials Register, Science Citation Index, and hand searches of references.
45. Ernst E, White A. Life-threatening adverse reactions after acupuncture? A systematic review. *Pain* 1997;71:123–126. Search date 1996; primary sources Medline, Ciscom, other specialised databases, contacted experts, and hand searches of references.

Maurits van Tulder
Institute for Research in Extramural Medicine
Vrije Universiteit Medical Centre
Amsterdam
The Netherlands

Bart Koes
Department of General Practice Erasmus University
Rotterdam
The Netherlands

Competing interests: None declared.

Low back pain (chronic)

Search date October 2003

Maurits van Tulder and Bart Koes

QUESTIONS

INTERVENTIONS

See glossary G

Key Messages

Oral drug treatments

- **Analgesics** One RCT found that tramadol (an opioid) decreased pain and increased function at 7 weeks compared with placebo. One RCT found that a combination of tramadol and paracetamol (acetaminophen) decreased pain and increased function at 3 months compared with placebo. One RCT found no significant difference between paracetamol and diflusinal in the proportion of people who rated the treatment as good or excellent. One RCT found no significant difference in pain relief between a parenteral non-steroidal anti-inflammatory drug and a parenteral opioid analgesic.
- **Antidepressants** One systematic review found that antidepressants decreased pain compared with placebo, but found no consistent difference in function. One RCT found that maproteline increased pain relief compared with paroxetine. Four additional RCTs found no significant difference in depression between antidepressants and placebo, and two additional RCTs found that antidepressants improved depression in people with chronic low back pain.
- **Non-steroidal anti-inflammatory drugs** One small RCT found that naproxen reduced pain compared with placebo. One systematic review and one subsequent RCT found no significant differences in symptoms between different non-steroidal anti-inflammatory drugs. One RCT identified by the review found no significant

difference between diflunisal and paracetamol in the proportion of people who rated the treatment as good or excellent. One RCT found no significant difference in pain relief between a parenteral non-steroidal anti-inflammatory drug and a parenteral opioid analgesic. Two RCTs found that COX 2 inhibitors decreased pain and improved function at 4–12 weeks compared with placebo, but effects were small.

- **Muscle relaxants** Two RCTs identified by a systematic review found that tetrazepam reduced pain and increased overall improvement after 10–14 days compared with placebo. Two RCTs identified by a systematic review found that non-benzodiazepines (flupirtine and tolperisone) increased overall improvement at 7–21 days, but found no significant difference for pain. Adverse effects of muscle relaxants include dizziness and drowsiness.

Injection therapy

- **Epidural steroid injections** We found no systematic reviews or RCTs in people with chronic back pain who did not have sciatica.
- **Local injections** One systematic review found no significant difference between local injections (local anaesthetic and corticosteroids) and placebo in short term pain relief.
- **Facet joint injections** One RCT identified by a systematic review found no significant difference in pain relief and disability between corticosteroid and saline injections after 1 and after 3 months. Adverse effects include infection, haemorrhage, chemical meningitis. and neurological damage.

Non-drug treatments

- **Multidisciplinary treatment programmes** One systematic review has found that intensive multidisciplinary biopsychosocial rehabilitation with functional restoration reduced pain and improved function compared with inpatient or outpatient non-multidisciplinary treatments or usual care. The review found no significant difference between less intensive multidisciplinary treatments and non-multidisciplinary treatment or usual care in pain or function.
- **Back schools** One systematic review and one subsequent RCT found limited evidence that back schools reduced pain and disability compared with inactive treatments (waiting list control, placebo gel, or written advice) or no treatment within 6 months, although results suggested that benefits may not persist in the longer term. Three RCTs identified by the review compared back schools with other treatments and found mixed results.
- **Behavioural therapy** One systematic review found that behavioural therapy reduced pain and improved functional status and behavioural outcomes compared with no treatment, placebo, or waiting list control. The review and one subsequent RCT provided no evidence of a difference in functional status, pain, or behavioural outcomes between different types of behavioural therapy. The review found insufficient evidence to compare behavioural therapy with other treatments.
- **Exercise** RCTs found insufficient evidence on the effects of different types of exercise, or exercise compared with other treatments.
- **Physical conditioning (cognitive behavioural approach plus physical training)** Two RCTs identified by a systematic review found that physical conditioning programmes (consisting of a cognitive behavioural approach plus physical training) reduced sick days overall but not the risk of being off work at 12 months compared with general practitioner care.
- **Spinal manipulative therapy** One systematic review found that spinal manipulative therapy reduced pain in the short and long term and improved short term function compared with sham manipulation, but found no significant difference in long term function (> 6 weeks). The systematic review found no significant difference in pain or function between spinal manipulative therapy and general practitioner care, physical therapy, exercises, or back school. Two subsequent RCTs compared spinal manipulation with exercise and found that spinal manipulation reduced pain at 6–12 months, but found different results for function. One of the RCTs found that spinal manipulation increased return to work at 12 months compared with exercise therapy.

- **Acupuncture** Two systematic reviews and two subsequent RCTs found insufficient evidence about the effects of acupuncture compared with placebo or no treatment. One systematic review and one subsequent RCT found limited evidence that acupuncture reduced pain intensity and increased overall improvement compared with transcutaneous electrical nerve stimulation.
- **Electromyographic biofeedback** One systematic review found no significant difference in pain relief or functional status between electromyographic biofeedback and placebo or waiting list control, but found insufficient evidence on the effects of electromyographic biofeedback compared with other treatments.
- **Lumbar supports** We found insufficient evidence on the effects of lumbar supports.
- **Massage** One systematic review found insufficient evidence about effects of massage compared with inactive treatments or other treatments.
- **Transcutaneous electrical nerve stimulation** One systematic review found no significant difference in pain relief between transcutaneous electrical nerve stimulation and sham stimulation.
- **Traction** One systematic review and two additional RCTs found no significant difference between traction and placebo or between traction plus massage and interferential treatment in pain relief or functional status.

DEFINITION Low back pain is pain, muscle tension, or stiffness localised below the costal margin and above the inferior gluteal folds, with or without leg pain (sciatica**G**),[1] and is defined as chronic when it persists for 12 weeks or more (see definition of low back pain and sciatica [acute], p 1465).[2] Non-specific low back pain is low back pain not attributed to a recognisable pathology (such as infection, tumour, osteoporosis, rheumatoid arthritis, fracture, or inflammation).[1] This review excludes low back pain with symptoms or signs at presentation that suggest a specific underlying condition. People with sciatica (lumbosacral radicular syndrome) or pain due to herniated discs are also excluded.

INCIDENCE/ PREVALENCE Over 70% of people in developed countries will experience low back pain at some time in their lives.[3] Each year, 15–45% of adults suffer low back pain, and 1/20 people present to hospital with a new episode. About 2–7% of patients with acute low back pain will go on to become chronic. Low back pain is most common between the ages of 35–55 years.[3]

AETIOLOGY/ RISK FACTORS Symptoms, pathology, and radiological appearances are poorly correlated. Pain is non-specific in about 85% of people. About 4% of people with low back pain in primary care have compression fractures and about 1% have a tumour. The prevalence of prolapsed intervertebral disc among people with low back pain in primary care is about 1–3%. [3] Ankylosing spondylitis and spinal infections are less common.[4] This chapter only covers non-specific chronic low back pain. Risk factors for the development of non-specific low back pain include heavy physical work, frequent bending, twisting, lifting, and prolonged static postures. Psychosocial risk factors include anxiety, depression, and mental stress at work.[3,5] Having a previous history of low back pain and a longer duration of the present episode are significant risk factors for chronicity. A recently published systematic review of prospective cohort studies found that some psychological factors (distress, depressive mood, and somatisation) are associated with an increased risk of chronic low back pain.[6] Individual and workplace factors have also been reported to be associated with the transition to chronic low back pain.[7]

PROGNOSIS Generally, the clinical course of an episode of low back pain seems to be favourable, and most pain will resolve within 2 weeks. Back pain among people in a primary care setting typically has a recurrent course characterised by variation and change, rather than an acute, self limiting course.[8] Most people with back pain have experienced a previous episode, and acute attacks often occur as exacerbations of chronic low back pain. In general, recurrences will occur more frequently and be more severe if people have had frequent or long lasting low back pain complaints in the past. The course of sick leave due to low back pain is similarly favourable. One study reported that 67% of patients with sick leave due to low back pain returned to work within a week, and 90% within 2 months. However, the longer the period of sick leave, the less likely the return to work becomes. Less than 50% of people with low back pain who have been off work for 6 months will return to work. After 2 years of work absenteeism, the chance of returning to work is almost zero.[9]

AIMS OF INTERVENTION To relieve pain; to improve function; to develop coping strategies for pain, with minimal adverse effects from treatment.[2,10]

OUTCOMES Pain intensity (visual analogue or numerical rating scale); overall improvement (self reported or observed); back pain specific functional status (such as Roland Morris questionnaire, Oswestry questionnaire); impact on employment (days of sick leave, number of people returned to work); medication use; intervention specific outcomes (such as coping and pain behaviour for behavioural treatment, strength, and flexibility for exercise, depression [in people with depression and low back pain] for antidepressants, and muscle spasm for muscle relaxants and electromyographic biofeedback(G)).

METHODS *Clinical Evidence* search and appraisal October 2003. The authors also searched Medline (1966 to December 2003), Embase (1980 to December 2003), and Psychlit (1984 to December 2003), using the search strategy recommended by the Cochrane Back Review Group.[11] Most of the earlier RCTs of treatments for low back pain were small (< 50 people/intervention group; range 9–169), short term (mostly < 6 months' follow up), and of low overall quality. Problems included lack of power, no description of randomisation procedure, incomplete analysis with failure to account for people who withdrew from trials, and lack of blinding.[12] The quality of the methods used by many recent RCTs is higher.

QUESTION What are the effects of oral drug treatments?

OPTION ANALGESICS (PARACETAMOL, OPIOIDS)

One RCT found that tramadol (an opioid) decreased pain and increased function at 7 weeks compared with placebo. One RCT found that a combination of tramadol and paracetamol (acetaminophen) decreased pain and increased function at 3 months compared with placebo. One RCT found no significant difference between paracetamol and diflusinal in the proportion of people who rated the treatment as good or excellent. One RCT found no significant difference in pain relief between a parenteral non-steroidal anti-inflammatory drug and a parenteral opioid analgesic.

Benefits: **Analgesics versus placebo:** We found no systematic reviews but we found two RCTs.[13,14] The first RCT (254 people) found that tramadol (an opioid) significantly decreased pain and significantly improved functional status at 7 weeks compared with placebo (pain on a 10 cm visual analogue scale: 3.5 with tramadol *v* 5.1 with placebo; function using 0–24 point Roland Morris Disability Scale: 8.8 with tramadol *v* 10.2 with placebo).[13] The second RCT (318 people) found that a combination of tramadol plus paracetamol (acetaminophen) significantly decreased pain and significantly improved function compared with placebo at 3 months (pain score at baseline and 3 months on 100 mm visual analogue scale, 311 people: 71.1–44.4 mm with combination *v* 68.8–52.3 mm with placebo; $P = 0.015$ for difference in final values; change in function on Roland Morris Disability Questionnaire, 297 people: −4.1 with combination *v* −2.6 with placebo; $P = 0.023$).[14]
Analgesics versus non-steroidal anti-inflammatory drugs: See non-steroidal anti-inflammatory drugs, p 1525.

Harms: RCTs found adverse effects (constipation and drowsiness) with analgesics in about 50% of people.[2,15] The RCT comparing tramadol plus paracetamol (acetaminophen) versus placebo found that combination treatment increased discontinuation because of adverse effects and significantly increased nausea, somnolence and constipation compared with placebo (discontinuation: 18.6% *v* 5.7%, P not reported; nausea: 13% *v* 3.2%, $P = 0.001$; somnolence: 12.4% *v* 1.3%, $P < 0.001$; constipation: 11.2% *v* 5.1%, $P = 0.003$).[14] One systematic review (search date 1995) in people with pain of different types compared combinations of paracetamol plus weak opioids versus paracetamol alone.[15] It found that combination treatment increased the risk of adverse effects in multiple dose studies (single dose studies OR 1.1, 95% CI 0.8 to 1.5; multiple dose studies OR 2.5, 95% CI 1.5 to 4.2).

Comment: None.

OPTION ANTIDEPRESSANTS

One systematic review found that antidepressants decreased pain compared with placebo, but found no consistent difference in function. One RCT found that maproteline increased pain relief compared with paroxetine. Four additional RCTs found no significant difference in depression between antidepressants and placebo, and two additional RCTs found that antidepressants improved depression in people with chronic low back pain.

Benefits: **Versus placebo:** We found one systematic review (search date 2000; 9 RCTs, 504 people)[16] and six additional RCTs (2 RCTs in people with low back pain and depression; 2 RCTs in people with low back pain without depression; 2 RCTs did not report whether people were depressed).[17–22] The review found that antidepressants significantly increased pain relief compared with placebo but found no significant difference in functioning (pain: SMD 0.41, 95% CI 0.22 to 0.61; function: SMD +0.24, 95% CI –0.21 to +0.69).[16] The six additional RCTs compared an antidepressant (imipramine, amitriptyline, trazodone, nortriptyline, doxepin, maprotiline, paroxetine, or clomipramine) versus placebo and reported on depression. Four RCTs found no significant difference in depression, although two RCTs[18,20] found that antidepressants significantly reduced depression compared with placebo. **Versus each other:** We found one systematic review (search date 2000; 1 RCT[21], 67 people).[16] The included RCT found that maprotiline significantly increased pain relief compared with paroxetine (mean decrease on 0–20 scale: 5.41 with maprotiline *v* 2.34 with paroxetine).[21]

Harms: Adverse effects of antidepressants include dry mouth, drowsiness, constipation, urinary retention, orthostatic hypotension, and mania.[2] One RCT found that the prevalence of dry mouth, insomnia, sedation, and orthostatic symptoms was 60–80% with tricyclic antidepressants.[17] However, rates were only slightly lower in the placebo group and none of the differences were significant.

Comment: None.

OPTION MUSCLE RELAXANTS

Two RCTs identified by a systematic review found that tetrazepam reduced pain and increased overall improvement after 10–14 days compared with placebo. Two RCTs identified by a systematic review found that non-benzodiazepines (flupirtine and tolperisone) increased overall improvement after 7–21 days but found no significant difference for pain. Adverse effects of muscle relaxants include dizziness and drowsiness.

Benefits: We found one systematic review (search date 2001, 5 RCTs).[23] **Benzodiazepines versus placebo:** The review (2 RCTs, 222 people) found that 50 mg tetrazepam three times daily significantly reduced pain and significantly increased overall improvement after 8–14 days compared with placebo (pain: RR 0.71, 95% CI 0.54 to 0.93; no overall improvement: RR 0.63, 95% CI 0.42 to 0.97).[23] **Non-benzodiazepines versus placebo:** The review identified three RCTs, which compared non-benzodiazepines (flupirtine, tolperisone, cyclobenzaprine) versus placebo, and found different results.[23] The first

RCT identified by the review (107 people) found that flupirtine reduced pain at 7 days compared with placebo, but the difference was not statistically significant (AR for reduction in pain intensity by 2 categories on 5 point scale: 54.3% with flupirtine v 33.4% with placebo).[24] However, it found that flupirtine significantly improved overall assessment by physician compared with placebo at 7 days (physician rating "very good", "good" or "satisfactory": 84.8% with flupirtine v 54.3% with placebo). The second RCT identified by the review (112 people) found that tolperisone 100 mg three times daily significantly increased the proportion of people reporting improvement at 21 days compared with placebo, but found no significant difference between treatments in pain.[25] The third RCT identified by the review (76 people) did not assess pain, global improvement, or function.[26]

Harms: The review found that central nervous system adverse effects of muscle relaxants (most commonly drowsiness or dizziness) were consistently reported with all benzodiazepines and non-benzodiazepines (rates of adverse effects were not reported in the review).[23]

Comment: None.

OPTION NON-STEROIDAL ANTI-INFLAMMATORY DRUGS

One small RCT found that naproxen reduced pain compared with placebo. One systematic review and one subsequent RCT found no significant differences in symptoms between different non-steroidal anti-inflammatory drugs. One RCT identified by the review found no significant difference between diflunisal and paracetamol in the proportion of people who rated the treatment as good or excellent. One RCT found no significant difference in pain relief between a parenteral non-steroidal anti-inflammatory drug and a parenteral opioid analgesic. Two RCTs found that COX 2 inhibitors decreased pain and improved function at 4–12 weeks compared with placebo, but effects were small.

Benefits: **NSAIDs versus placebo:** We found one systematic review (search date 1998).[27] One small RCT (37 people) identified by the review found that naproxen but not diflunisal significantly increased pain relief compared with placebo (data presented graphically).[27] **NSAIDs versus each other:** We found one systematic review (search date 1998; 4 RCTs, 453 people)[27] and one subsequent RCT.[28] All four RCTs identified by the review found no significant difference between different non-steroidal anti-inflammatory drugs for symptoms.[27] The subsequent RCT (196 people) found no significant difference between nimesulide and diclofenac in pain or functional status.[28] **NSAIDs versus analgesics:** We found one systematic review (search date 1998; 2 RCTs, 184 people).[27] The first RCT (29 people) identified by the review found no significant difference between diflunisal and paracetamol in the proportion of people rating their treatment as good or excellent at 4 weeks (10/16 [62%] v 4/12 [33%]).[27] However, the study may have lacked power to exclude a clinically important difference. The second RCT (155 people) identified by the review found no significant difference in pain relief between a parenteral non-steroidal anti-inflammatory drug and a parenteral opioid.[27] **COX 2 inhibitors versus placebo:** We found no systematic review, but found two RCTs.[29,30] Both RCTs found that COX 2 inhibitors decreased pain and improved function compared with placebo, but effects were small. The first RCT (319 people) found that etoricoxib 60 mg and 90 mg significantly decreased pain and improved functioning compared with placebo at 12 weeks (reduction in pain compared with placebo on 100 mm visual analogue scale: 12.9 mm for 60 mg etoricoxib and 10.3 mm for 90 mg etoricoxib, both $P \leq 0.001$; improvement in function compared with placebo on Roland Morris Disability Score [on a scale from 0–24 points]: 2.42 with 60 mg etoricoxib, $P \leq 0.001$ and 2.06 with 90 mg etoricoxib, $P \leq 0.01$).[29] The second RCT (690 people) found that rofecoxib 25 mg and 50 mg significantly decreased pain and improved function compared with placebo at 4 weeks (improvement in pain compared with placebo on 100 mm visual analogue scale: 13.5 mm with 25 mg rofecoxib and 13.8 mm with 50 mg rofecoxib; $P < 0.001$; improvement compared with placebo in function on Roland Morris Disability Score [0–24 points]: 2.2 with 25 mg rofecoxib and 2.3 with 50 mg refecoxib; $P < 0.001$).[30]

Harms: Non-steroidal anti-inflammatory drugs may cause gastrointestinal complications (see non-steroidal anti-inflammatory drugs, p 1525). Some RCTs in people with acute and chronic back pain have found that ibuprofen and diclofenac have the lowest gastrointestinal complication rate mainly because of the low doses used in practice (pooled OR for adverse effects *v* placebo 1.30, 95% CI 0.91 to 1.80).[2,31,32] The first subsequent RCT found that nimesulide has a similar rate of gastrointestinal adverse effects to diclofenac.[28] The third subsequent RCT found no significant difference between etoricoxib (60 mg and 90 mg) and placebo in overall adverse effects or headache, nausea, or diarrhoea at 12 weeks (overall: 46.8% with placebo *v* 58.3% with 60 mg etoricoxib *v* 52.3% with 90 mg etoricoxib; headache: 5.5% with placebo *v* 11.7% with 60 mg etoricoxib *v* 5.6% with 90 mg etoricoxib; nausea: 2.8% with placebo *v* 5.8% with 60 mg etoricoxib *v* 7.5% with 90 mg etoricoxib; diarrhoea: 1.8% with placebo *v* 3.9% with 60 mg etoricoxib *v* 8.4% with 90 mg etoricoxib).[29] The fourth subsequent RCT found no significant difference between rofecoxib (25 mg and 50 mg) and placebo in overall adverse effects at 4 weeks (40.8% with placebo *v* 48.1% with 25 mg rofecoxib *v* 46.4% with 50 mg rofecoxib).[30] It found that the most common adverse effects were headache and diarrhoea (headache: 10.1% with placebo *v* 8.2% with 25 mg rofecoxib *v* and 6.6% with 50 mg rofecoxib; diarrhoea: 3.5% with placebo *v* 7.3% with 25 mg rofecoxib *v* 4.8% with 50 mg rofecoxib).[30]

Comment: None.

QUESTION What are the effects of injection therapy?

OPTION EPIDURAL STEROID INJECTIONS

We found no systematic reviews or RCTs in people with chronic back pain who did not have sciatica.

Benefits: **Versus placebo:** We found one systematic review (search date 1996, 4 RCTs, 302 people) comparing epidural steroid injections versus placebo.[33] However, all identified RCTs included people with sciatica**G**, which is not discussed in this topic. We found no subsequent RCTs.

Harms: We found no RCTs.

Comment: None.

OPTION FACET JOINT INJECTIONS

One RCT identified by a systematic review found no significant difference in pain relief and disability between corticosteroid and saline injections after 1 and 3 months. Adverse effects include infection, haemorrhage, chemical meningitis. and neurological damage.

Benefits: We found one systematic review (search date 1996, 1 RCT, 101 people with chronic back pain and without sciatica**G**; see comment below).[33] The RCT found no significant difference in pain relief and disability between corticosteroid and saline injections after 1 and 3 months (1 month: RR 0.89, 95% CI 0.65 to 1.21; 3 months: RR 0.90, 95% CI 0.69 to 1.17).

Harms: The review found that adverse effects included pain at injection site, infection, haemorrhage, neurological damage, and chemical meningitis.[33]

Comment: Two other RCTs identified by the review[33] did not distinguish between acute and chronic pain, involved people with sciatica, and so these RCTs have not been included.

OPTION LOCAL INJECTIONS

One systematic review found no significant difference between local injections (local anaesthetic and corticosteroids) and placebo in short term pain relief.

Benefits: We found one systematic review (search date 1996, 4 RCTs, 200 people).[33] It found no significant difference between local injection therapy (local anaesthetic and corticosteroids) and placebo in short term pain relief (3 RCTs; 137 people; RR 0.80, 95% CI 0.40 to 1.59).

Harms: The review found that potential harms included nerve or other tissue damage, infection, and haemorrhage.[2]

Comment: One study included in the review compared local injection plus forceful manipulation with light manipulation plus placebo injection, and was not included.

QUESTION What are the effects of non-drug treatments?

OPTION BACK SCHOOLS

One systematic review and one subsequent RCT found limited evidence that back schools reduced pain and disability compared with inactive treatments (waiting list control, placebo gel, or written advice) or no treatment within 6 months, although results suggested that benefits may not persist in the longer term. Three RCTs identified by the review compared back schools with other treatments and found mixed results.

Benefits: We found one systematic review[34] (search date 1997, 8 RCTs in people with chronic back pain) and one subsequent RCT.[35] RCTs identified by the review used back schools**G** interventions of variable intensity.[34] The review did not pool data from the studies (see table 1, p 1498). **Versus no treatment or inactive control treatments:** Results from six RCTs identified by the review provided limited evidence that back schools improved pain and disability compared with inactive treatments (placebo gel, waiting list, written information) in the short term (6 months or less), but suggested that benefits did not persist in the longer term (see table 1, p 1498).[36–38,41–43] The subsequent RCT (104 male construction workers with chronic low back pain) found that back schools significantly increased overall improvement compared with no treatment after 8 weeks and 6 months (8 weeks: AR for reduced or no back pain: 71% with back school *v* 14% with no treatment pain; 6 months 43% with back school *v* 14% with no treatment; P value not reported).[35] **Versus other treatments:** Three RCTs identified by the review compared back school versus other active treatments (spinal manipulation, non-steroidal anti-inflammatory drugs, physiotherapy, callisthenics, and exercise) and found different results (see table 1, p 1498).[38–40] The first RCT found that back school reduced pain compared with exercise at 16 weeks.[40] The second RCT found that callisthenics significantly reduced the duration of low back pain compared with back school.[39] The third RCT found that back school improved pain at 2 and 6 months compared with controls, which included spinal manipulation, non-steroidal anti-inflammatory drugs, and physiotherapy in a subgroup of people with chronic pain.[38]

Harms: The review and subsequent RCT did not report on harms.[34,35]

Comment: We found another more recent systematic review (search date 2000, 18 RCTs), which combined randomised and non-randomised studies, compared back schools, no treatment, and other active treatments in the same meta-analysis, and did not take the methods of the studies into account.[44] This systematic review found that back schools significantly increased pain relief after 3 months compared with no treatment or any other treatment, but found no significant difference in outcomes in the long term.[44]

OPTION BEHAVIOURAL THERAPY

One systematic review found that behavioural therapy reduced pain and improved functional status and behavioural outcomes compared with no treatment, placebo, or waiting list control. The review and one subsequent RCT provided no evidence of a difference in functional status, pain, or behavioural outcomes between different types of behavioural therapy. The review found insufficient evidence to compare behavioural therapy with other treatments.

Benefits: We found one systematic review[45] (search date 1999; 20 RCTs) and one subsequent RCT.[46] **Versus placebo, no treatment, or waiting list control:** The review (7 RCTs, 419 people) found that behavioural therapy significantly reduced pain intensity and behavioural outcomes (e.g. pain behaviour, cognitive errors, perceived or observed levels of tension, anxiety, depression) compared with no treatment, placebo, or waiting list control (pain: SMD 0.62, 95% CI 0.25 to 0.98; behavioural outcomes: SMD 0.40, 95% CI 0.10 to 0.70).[45] It found that behavioural therapy increased function but the difference was not statistically significant (SMD +0.35, 95% CI –0.04 to +0.74). **Different types of behavioural therapy versus each other:** The review identified nine RCTs (308 people), which found no statistically significant difference between different types of behavioural therapy (cognitive behavioural therapy, operant behavioural treatments, and respondent behavioural treatment**G**) in functional status, pain, or behavioural outcomes (including anxiety, depression, pain behaviour, and coping).[45] The subsequent RCT (84 people recently on sick leave with low back pain) compared problem solving therapy versus group education.[46] All participants also received behavioural graded activity**G**. The RCT found that problem solving therapy significantly reduced total sick leave compared with group education between 6 months and 1 year after treatment (8.3 days at baseline to 18.5 days with problem solving *v* 10.4 days at baseline to 37.9 days with group education; $P < 0.05$).[46] However, at baseline, people in the problem solving group had fewer days sick leave and fewer had returned to work than people allocated to group education. Results of the RCT may, therefore, be confounded by these factors, and not due to difference in relative effectiveness of the treatments. The RCT found no significant difference between problem solving therapy and group education in return to work rates at 1 year (return to normal work: 8.9% at baseline to 75% at 6 months and 85.4% at 12 months with problem solving *v* 20.5% at baseline to 70.3% at 6 months and

62.9% at 12 months with group education; P value not reported). **Versus other treatments:** Two RCTs (202 people) identified by the review found that behavioural therapy significantly increased the proportion of people who had returned to work after 12 weeks compared with traditional care (rest, analgesics, or physiotherapy) or back exercises, but found no significant difference in pain or depression after 6 months or 12 months (no statistical pooling of data).[45] Six RCTs (343 people) identified by the review comparing behavioural therapy plus other treatments (physiotherapy and back education, multidisciplinary treatment❻ programmes, inpatient pain management programmes, and back exercises) found that behavioural therapy plus the other treatments significantly improved functional status in the short term compared with other treatments alone, but found no significant difference in pain or behavioural outcomes (no statistical pooling of data).[45]

Harms: The review did not report on harms.[45]

Comment: None.

OPTION ELECTROMYOGRAPHIC BIOFEEDBACK

One systematic review found no significant difference in pain relief or functional status between electromyographic biofeedback and placebo or waiting list control, but found insufficient evidence on the effects of electromyographic biofeedback compared with other treatments.

Benefits: We found one systematic review (search date 1995, 5 RCTs, 168 people, no statistical pooling of data).[12] **Versus placebo or waiting list control:** Three RCTs (102 people) identified by the review found no significant difference between electromyographic biofeedback❻ and placebo or waiting list control in pain relief or functional status.[12] **Versus other treatments:** Two RCTs (40 people) identified by the review found different results with electromyographic biofeedback compared with progressive relaxation training in pain reduction.[12] One RCT (30 people) identified by the review found no significant difference between rehabilitation programmes plus biofeedback and biofeedback alone in pain or range of movement.[12]

Harms: The review did not report on harms.[12]

Comment: None.

OPTION EXERCISE

RCTs found insufficient evidence on the effects of different types of exercise, or exercise compared with other treatments.

Benefits: **Versus inactive treatment:** We found one systematic review (search date 1999; 6 RCTs, 587 people)[47] and one additional small RCT.[48] The RCTs identified by the review compared exercise versus inactive treatments (hot packs plus rest, semi-hot packs plus sham traction, waiting list control, transcutaneous electrical nerve stimulation [TENS], sham TENS, detuned ultrasound, or short wave diathermy).[47] Three of these RCTs found that exercise significantly increased overall improvement, whereas the remaining three RCTs found no significant difference in overall improvement. The additional small RCT (59 people) found that active rehabilitation consisting of 24 exercise sessions during 12 weeks significantly improved pain intensity and functional disability compared with inactive treatments.[48] **Versus other treatments:** We found one systematic review[47] (search date 1999; 9 RCTs, 1020 people), three additional RCTs (four publications),[49–52] and one subsequent RCT.[53]

Three high quality RCTs identified by the review found no significant difference between exercise and conventional physiotherapy in pain, functional status, overall improvement, or return to work. The first additional RCT found that exercise (as part of a combined physiotherapy programme) significantly improved pain, functional status, and return to work compared with usual care by the general practitioner.[52] The second additional RCT (132 people) found that exercise with or without psychological pain management did not significantly reduce sick leave, but was significantly less effective at improving pain and functioning compared with a multidisciplinary programme after 4 and 24 months (after 4 months: median days of sick leave 13 with exercise *v* 122 with exercise plus psychosocial pain management *v* 25 with multidisciplinary programme; after 24 months: 11 with exercise *v* 37 with exercise plus psychosocial pain management *v* 2.5 with multidisciplinary programme).[49,50] The third additional RCT (190 people) found no significant difference between exercise and massage**G** in pain and disability 4 weeks after the end of treatment (data for comparison not reported).[51] The small subsequent RCT (49 people) compared 16 sessions of manual therapy (spinal manipulation, specific mobilisation, and stretching) versus exercise therapy for 8 weeks.[53] It found that manual therapy significantly decreased pain and increased functioning and return to work compared with exercise therapy at 1 year (pain on 0–100 mm visual analogue scale: 21 mm with manual *v* 35 mm with exercise; $P < 0.01$; function on 0–45 point Oswestry Low Back Pain Disability Questionnaire score: 17 with manual *v* 26 with exercise; $P < 0.01$; partly or fully sick listed: 19.5% with manual *v* 59% with exercise; $P < 0.01$).[53] **Versus each other:** We found two RCTs (five publications).[54–58] The first RCT (148 people) found no significant difference between active physiotherapy, muscle reconditioning with training devices, and low impact aerobics in pain intensity after 6 months and 1 year, but found that muscle reconditioning and also aerobic exercises reduced disability after 6 and 12 months compared with active physiotherapy, but differences were very small (disability on Roland Morris Disability Scale: 6.7 *v* 6.3 *v* 6.8; 12 months: 5.7 *v* 5.4 *v* 7.7).[55–58] The second RCT found that a combined exercise and motivation programme significantly reduced pain and significantly improved disability after 4 and 12 months compared with exercises alone (pain on 110 mm VAS, 4 months: 32.7 mm with combination *v* 39.8 mm with exercise alone; $P = 0.026$; 12 months: 26.4 mm with combination *v* 41.9 mm with exercise alone; $P = 0.006$; disability on Greenough and Fraser scale [scale of results 0–75], 4 months: 57.2 with combination *v* 51.0 with exercise alone; $P = 0.004$; 12 months: 58.9 with combination *v* 50.9 with exercise alone; $P = 0.004$).[54] **Extension exercises (including McKenzie exercisesG):** We found one systematic review (search date 1999; 3 RCTs, 153 people), which compared extension versus flexion back exercises.[47] Two of the identified RCTs found no significant difference in pain intensity, and the third RCT found that extension exercises significantly reduced global improvement compared with flexion exercises. A subsequent RCT (60 patients) found no significant difference between extension exercises and whole body vibration exercises in pain intensity (VAS scale 0–10) and disability (Pain Disability Index 0–70, where 0 = no limitation and 70 = most severe limitation) during 12 weeks of treatment and after 6 months (pain intensity: data not shown; change in pain disability index: from 20.3 at baseline to 10.5 after treatment with extension *v* 20.7 at baseline to 11.6 after treatment with vibration).[59] **Strengthening exercises:** We found one systematic review (search date 1999; 9 RCTs, 899 people), which found no significant difference between strengthening exercises and other types of exercise in outcomes, and found conflicting evidence on strengthening exercises compared with inactive treatment.[47]

Postural exercises (Mensendieck/Cesar): We found two RCTs (three publications).[60–62] The first RCT (77 people who had just finished treatment for their last episode of back pain) found that a Mensendieck exercise**G** group treatment for 13 weeks significantly reduced recurrences of back pain compared with usual care, but found no significant differences in sick leave, pain, or functioning after 1 and 3 years (recurrence: 58% *v* 77%).[61,62] The second RCT (222 people) found that Cesar therapy**G** significantly increased overall improvement after 3 and 6 months compared with usual care by the general practitioner, but found no statistically significant difference after 1 year (3 months: 80% *v* 47%; 6 months: 78% *v* 51%; 1 year: 61% *v* 66%).[60] **Group exercises:** We found one RCT (109 people).[51] It found no significant differences between individual and group exercises in pain and disability 4 weeks after the end of treatment (P = 0.55 for difference in pain and disability).

Harms: The reviews and RCTs did not report on harms.[47,48,50,51,53–58,60–62]

Comment: None.

OPTION LUMBAR SUPPORTS

We found insufficient evidence on the effects of lumbar supports.

Benefits: We found one systematic review (search date 1999, 1 RCT).[63] The small RCT (19 people) identified by the review found that a lumbar corset plus a synthetic support improved symptom severity and functional disability compared with lumbar corset without synthetic support, but data were poorly reported.[63] No RCT compared lumbar supports with placebo, no treatment, or other treatments for chronic low back pain.

Harms: The review did not report on harms.[63] Harms associated with prolonged lumbar support use include decreased strength of the trunk musculature, a false sense of security, heat, skin irritation, and general discomfort.

Comment: Five RCTs (1200 people) identified by the review did not differentiate between acute and chronic pain.[63]

OPTION MULTIDISCIPLINARY TREATMENT PROGRAMMES

One systematic review found that intensive multidisciplinary biopsychosocial rehabilitation with functional restoration reduced pain and improved function compared with inpatient or outpatient non-multidisciplinary treatments or usual care. The review found no significant difference between less intensive multidisciplinary treatments and non-multidisciplinary treatment or usual care in pain or function.

Benefits: We found one systematic review (search date 1998, 10 RCTs, 1964 people, no statistical pooling), which compared multidisciplinary treatment**G** versus a control treatment.[64] The review found that intensive (more than 100 hours of therapy) multidisciplinary biopsychosocial rehabilitation with functional restoration significantly reduced pain and improved function compared with inpatient or outpatient non-multidisciplinary treatments or usual care.[64] The review found no statistically significant difference between less intensive outpatient multidisciplinary treatments and non-multidisciplinary outpatient treatment or usual care in pain or function.[64]

Harms: The review did not report on harms.[64]

Comment: We found one RCT (195 people), which compared three treatments: extensive multidisciplinary treatment, light multidisciplinary treatment, and usual care.[65] There was no overall analysis according to treatment allocation. However, subgroup analysis found that men returned to work more quickly with light multidisciplinary treatment (one sessions of 4 hours) than with usual care. It found no significant differences between extensive multidisciplinary treatment (6 hour sessions, 5 days per week, 4 weeks) and usual care in men and no significant differences between any two interventions in women.[65]

OPTION PHYSICAL CONDITIONING PROGRAMMES

Two RCTs identified by a systematic review found that physical conditioning programmes (consisting of a cognitive behavioural approach plus physical training) reduced sick days overall but not the risk of being off work at 12 months compared with general practitioner care.

Benefits: We found one systematic review of physical conditioning programmes compared with other treatments in adults with work disability related to back pain (search date 2000, 16 relevant RCTs).[66] The programmes were heterogeneous, all involving a cognitive behavioural approach plus a range of types of physical training (including aerobics, muscle strength and endurance training, and co-ordination training) given by a physiotherapist or a multidisciplinary team. The interventions varied in length from one session only to 1 hour per week for 18 months, most lasting between 3 and 6 weeks. **Versus general practitioner care:** The review found that physical conditioning programmes reduced the number of sick days compared with general practitioner advice or care after 12 months (2 RCTs, 160 people, average reduction in sick days: 45, 95% CI 3 to 88). There was no significant difference between physical conditioning programmes and general practitioner advice or care in the proportion of people off work at 12 months (physical conditioning *v* general practitioner care: OR 0.8, 95% CI 0.58 to 1.09).[66]

Harms: The review did not report on harms.[66]

Comment: None.

OPTION MASSAGE

One systematic review found insufficient evidence about effects of massage compared with inactive treatments or other treatments.

Benefits: We found one systematic review (search date 2001; 9 RCTs, 891 people; no statistical pooling of data; see comment below).[67] The review included one RCT (107 people), which found that massage**G** combined with exercises and education significantly reduced pain and improved functioning compared with soft tissue manipulation, remedial exercise and posture education, and inactive treatment (sham laser) after treatment (pain, mean McGill pain questionnaire PPI 0.44 with massage *v* 1.04 with soft tissue manipulation *v* 1.64 with remedial exercise and positive eduction *v* 1.65 with inactive treatment; function, mean Roland Morris score 2.36 *v* 3.44 *v* 6.82 *v* 6.85). Results after 1 month were similar. However, this RCT included people with back pain of between 1 week and 8 months duration (mean duration 3 months). Seven RCTs included in the review compared massage with other treatments and found conflicting results.

Harms: The review did not report on harms.[67]

Comment: Problems with control group selection in the included RCTs limit the usefulness of their results.[67]

OPTION SPINAL MANIPULATIVE THERAPY

One systematic review found that spinal manipulative therapy reduced pain in the short and long term and improved short term function compared with sham manipulation, but found no significant difference in function after more than 6 weeks. The systematic review found no significant difference in pain or function between spinal manipulative therapy and general practitioner care, physical therapy, exercises, or back school. Two subsequent RCTs compared spinal manipulation with exercise and found that spinal manipulation reduced pain at 6–12 months, but found different results for function. One of the RCTs found that spinal manipulation increased return to work at 12 months compared with exercise therapy.

Benefits: We found one systematic review (search date 2001, 14 RCTs, 1596 people),[68] and two subsequent RCTs.[53,69] The review found that spinal manipulative therapy reduced pain in the short (< 6 weeks) and long term (> 6 weeks) compared with sham manipulation, and improved function in the short term (3 RCTs, 229 people; mean score improvement between groups in short term on 100 mm VAS: 10 mm; 95% CI 3 to 17 mm; in long term: 19 mm; 95% CI 3 to 35 mm; mean improvement between groups in function on Roland Morris Scale: 3.3; 95% CI 0.6 to 6.0).[68] The review found no significant difference in short or long term pain or long term function between spinal manipulative therapy and general practitioner care (4 RCTs, 428 people), physical therapy, exercise (2 RCTs, 361 people), or back school**G** (3 RCTs, 238 people).[68] Data were presented graphically in the review. The review found that spinal manipulative therapy reduced pain and improved function in the short term compared with therapies judged to be ineffective or harmful (traction, bed rest, home care topical gel, no treatment, diathermy, or minimal massage**G**; improvement in pain on VAS: 4 mm; 95% CI 0 to 8; improvement in function on Roland Morris Scale: 2.6 points, 95% CI 0.5 points to 4.8 points). The first subsequent RCT (49 people sick listed > 8 weeks) compared spinal manipulative therapy with exercise therapy in a course of 16 treatments over 2 months.[53] It found that spinal manipulation significantly decreased pain and increased functioning and return to work at 12 months compared with exercise therapy (pain on a 0–100 mm VAS scale: 21 mm with manipulation *v* 35 mm with exercise, $P < 0.01$; disability on the 0–50 point Oswestry Disability Index: 17 with manipulation *v* 26 with exercise, $P < 0.01$; partly or fully sick listed: 19% with manipulation *v* 59% with exercise, RR 0.31, 95% CI 0.11 to 0.78).[53] The second subsequent RCT (91 people, 66 assessed at 6 months) compared three treatments: osteopathic manipulation; sham manipulation; and no treatment control.[69] Manipulation was carried out in seven sessions over 5 months. It found that spinal manipulation therapy and sham manipulation significantly reduced pain at 6 months compared with no treatment, but found no significant difference in function (pain on 10 cm VAS: results presented graphically, $P = 0.02$ for both comparisons; no values for function using Roland Morris Disability scores).[69]

Harms: In the RCTs identified by the review that used a trained therapist to select people and perform spinal manipulation, the risk of serious complications was low (estimated risks: vertebrobasilar strokes 1/20 000 to 1/1 000 000 people; cauda equina syndrome < 1/1 000 000 people).[68] Neither of the subsequent RCTs assessed harms.[53,69]

Comment: Current guidelines do not advise spinal manipulation in people with severe or progressive neurological deficit.[2,70]

OPTION TRACTION

One systematic review and two additional RCTs found no significant difference between traction and placebo or between traction plus massage and interferential treatment in pain relief or functional status.

Benefits: We found one systematic review (search date 1995, 1 RCT)[10] and two additional RCTs.[71,72] Two RCTs (176 people) found no significant difference between traction and placebo in global improvement, pain relief, or functional status after 5–9 weeks.[10,72] The second additional RCT (152 people) found no significant difference between lumbar traction plus massage and interferential treatment**G** in pain relief or improvement of disability 3 weeks and 4 months after the end of treatment.[71]

Harms: The review and additional RCTs did not report on harms.[10,71,72] Potential adverse effects include debilitation, loss of muscle tone, bone demineralisation, and thrombophlebitis.[2]

Comment: None.

OPTION TRANSCUTANEOUS ELECTRICAL NERVE STIMULATION

One systematic review found no significant difference in pain relief between transcutaneous electrical nerve stimulation and sham stimulation.

Benefits: We found one systematic review (search date 2000, 5 RCTs, 421 people).[73] It found no significant difference between transcutaneous electrical nerve stimulation and sham stimulation in pain measured using a visual analogue scale (3 RCTs, 171 people; pooled standardised mean difference –0.21, 95% CI –0.51 to +0.1).[73]

Harms: The review did not report on harms.[73]

Comment: None.

OPTION ACUPUNCTURE

Two systematic reviews and two subsequent RCTs found insufficient evidence about the effects of acupuncture compared with placebo or no treatment. One systematic review and one subsequent RCT found limited evidence that acupuncture reduced pain intensity and increased overall improvement compared with transcutaneous electrical nerve stimulation.

Benefits: We found two systematic reviews (search dates 1996, 12 RCTs; see comment below)[74,75] and three subsequent RCTs.[76–78] The reviews identified seven RCTs (380 people) comparing acupuncture**G** versus no treatment, placebo acupuncture, waiting list control, or transcutaneous electrical nerve stimulation (TENS).[74,75] One review found no significant difference between acupuncture and placebo acupuncture or no treatment in clinical outcomes. This review concluded that the methodological quality of the trials was very poor and did not warrant any firm conclusions.[75] The second review found that acupuncture increased overall improvement compared with control interventions but found no significant difference between acupuncture and placebo acupuncture in pain and functioning (versus controls: OR 2.3, 95% CI 1.3 to 4.1; versus placebo: OR 1.4, 95% CI 0.8 to 2.3).[74] The first subsequent RCT (60 people) found that acupuncture significantly reduced pain intensity and the number of analgesic tablets consumed a week compared with TENS (median pain intensity on a 200 mm visual analogue scale: 140 at baseline and 60 at follow up with acupuncture *v* 101 at baseline and 63 at follow up with TENS; mean weekly analgesic tablet consumption 28 at baseline and 14 at follow up with acupuncture *v* 42 at baseline and

24 at follow up with TENS). However, at baseline, people in the acupuncture group had a higher pain score and used fewer tablets than people allocated to TENS. Results of the RCT may, therefore, be confounded by these factors, and not due to difference in relative effectiveness of the treatments.[76] The second RCT (50 people) compared three treatments: manual acupuncture, electroacupuncture, and mock TENS (placebo).[77] It found that manual and electroacupuncture significantly increased overall clinical improvement after 1 month compared with placebo (judged subjectively by investigator blinded to treatment allocation; 16/34 [47%] with acupuncture *v* 2/16 [13%] with placebo, $P < 0.05$; CI not reported). The third RCT (131 people) compared three treatments: acupuncture, sham acupuncture, and no treatment.[78] It found that acupuncture significantly reduced pain intensity and disability after 3 months, and disability after 9 months compared with no treatment. It found no significant difference between acupuncture and sham acupuncture for pain intensity and disability 9 months after the end of treatment (improvement in 10 cm visual analogue pain score 1.7 for acupuncture *v* 1.8 for sham acupuncture and 0.9 for no treatment; improvement in 70 point pain disability index 9.0 for acupuncture *v* 8.5 for sham acupuncture and 2.3 for no treatment).

Harms: One systematic review found that serious and rare adverse effects included infections (HIV, hepatitis, bacterial endocarditis) and visceral trauma (pneumothorax, cardiac tamponade).[75]

Comment: Three RCTs identified by the systematic reviews combined acute and chronic low back pain, and two RCTs did not specify the duration of symptoms.[74,75] One RCT identified by the reviews included people with back and neck pain.[74,75]

GLOSSARY

Acupuncture Acupuncture is needle puncture of the skin at traditional "meridian" acupuncture points. Modern acupuncturists also use non-meridian points and trigger points (tender sites occurring in the most painful areas). The needles may be stimulated manually or electrically. Placebo acupuncture is needling of traditionally unimportant sites or non-stimulation of the needles once placed.

Back school Back school techniques vary widely, but essentially consist of repeated sessions of instruction about anatomy and function of the back and isometric exercises to strengthen the back.

Behavioural graded activity Graded activity is an operant behavioural treatment that aims to increase activity levels by means of quota systems. The training includes registration of baseline levels during the first 2 weeks, a treatment contract, positive reinforcement for activity increments, and a workplace visit.

Cesar therapy Cesar therapy is based on the hypothesis that there is an association between postural and movement deficiencies and back pain. The treatment aims to initiate a learning process aimed at correction of postural and movement deficiencies.

Cognitive behavioural therapy Cognitive behavioural therapy aims to identify and modify peoples understanding of their pain and disability using cognitive restructuring techniques (such as imagery and attention diversion) or by modifying maladaptive thoughts, feelings, and beliefs.

Electromyographic biofeedback With electromyographic biofeedback, a person receives external feedback of their own electromyogram (using visual or auditory scales), and uses this to learn how to control the electromyogram and hence the tension within their own muscles. Electromyogram biofeedback for low back pain aims to relax the paraspinal muscles.

Interferential therapy Interferential therapy is a low frequency current treatment that uses two medium frequency currents which "interfere" with each other to produce a beat frequency that the body recognises as a low frequency energy source. It is used as treatment for disorders in which inflammation is supposed to be a problem, such as back pain, osteoarthritis, rheumatoid arthritis, muscular pain/strain, and sports injuries.

Massage Massage is manipulation of soft tissues (i.e. muscle and fascia) using the hands or a mechanical device, to promote circulation and relaxation of muscle spasm or tension. Different types of soft tissue massage include Shiatsu, Swedish, friction, trigger point, or neuromuscular massage.
McKenzie exercises McKenzie exercises use self generated stresses and forces to centralise pain from the legs and buttocks to the lower back. This method emphasises self care.
Mensendieck therapy The Mensendieck approach combines postural exercises and education, emphasising "learning by doing". It is based on the assumption that human beings, through insight and guidance, can take responsibility for their own health and thus avoid the consequences of functional disability. Mensendieck therapy has been used for decades in the Netherlands and Scandinavia.
Multidisciplinary treatment Multidisciplinary treatment is intensive physical and psychosocial training by a team (e.g. a physician, physiotherapist, psychologist, social worker, and occupational therapist). Training is usually given in groups and does not involve passive physiotherapy.
Operant behavioural treatments Operant behavioural treatments include positive reinforcement of healthy behaviours and consequent withdrawal of attention from pain behaviours, time contingent instead of pain contingent pain management, and spouse involvement, while undergoing a programme aimed at increasing exercise tolerance towards a preset goal.
Respondent behavioural treatment Respondent behavioural treatment aims to modify physiological responses directly (e.g. reducing muscle tension by explaining the relation between tension and pain, and using relaxation techniques).
Sciatica Pain that radiates from the back into the buttock or leg and is most commonly caused by prolapse of an intervertebral disk; the term may also be used to describe pain anywhere along the course of the sciatic nerve.

REFERENCES

1. Van der Heijden GJMG, Bouter LM, Terpstra-Lindeman E. De effectiviteit van tractie bij lage rugklachten. De resultaten van een pilotstudy. *Ned T Fysiotherapie* 1991;101:37–43.
2. Bigos S, Bowyer O, Braen G, et al. *Acute low back problems in adults*. Clinical Practice Guideline no. 14. AHCPR Publication No. 95–0642. Rockville MD: Agency for Health Care Policy and Research, Public Health Service, US, Department of Health and Human Services. December 1994. Search date not stated; primary sources The Quebec Task Force on Spinal Disorders Review to 1984, search carried out by National Library of Medicine from 1984, and references from expert panel.
3. Andersson GBJ. The epidemiology of spinal disorders. In: Frymoyer JW, ed. *The adult spine: principles and practice*. 2nd ed. New York: Raven Press, 1997:93–141.
4. Deyo RA, Rainville J, Kent DL. What can the history and physical examination tell us about low back pain? *JAMA* 1992;268:760–765.
5. Bongers PM, de Winter CR, Kompier MA, et al. Psychosocial factors at work and musculoskeletal disease. *Scand J Work Environ Health* 1993;19:297–312.
6. Pincus T, Burton AK, Vogel S, et al. A systematic review of psychological factors as predictors of chronicity/disability in prospective cohorts of low back pain. *Spine* 2002;27:E109–E120.
7. Fransen M, Woodward M, Norton R, et al. Risk factors associated with the transition from acute to chronic occupational back pain. *Spine* 2002;27:92–98.
8. Von Korff M, Saunders K. The course of back pain in primary care. *Spine* 1996;21:2833–2837.
9. Waddell G. The clinical course of low back pain. In: *The back pain revolution*. Edinburgh: Churchill Livingstone, 1998:103–117.
10. Evans G, Richards S. *Low back pain: an evaluation of therapeutic interventions*. Bristol: Health Care Evaluation Unit, University of Bristol, 1996. Search date 1995; primary sources Medline, Embase, A-Med, Psychlit, and hand searches of references.
11. Van Tulder MW, Assendelft WJJ, Koes BW, et al. Method guidelines for systematic reviews in the Cochrane Collaboration Back Review Group for spinal disorders. *Spine* 1997;22:2323–2330.
12. Van Tulder MW, Koes BW, Bouter LM. Conservative treatment of acute and chronic nonspecific low back pain: a systematic review of randomized controlled trials of the most common interventions. *Spine* 1997;22:2128–2156. Search date 1995; primary sources Medline, Embase, Psychlit, and hand searches of references.
13. Schnitzer TJ, Gray WL, Paster RZ, et al. Efficacy of tramadol in treatment of chronic low back pain. *J Rheumatol* 2000;27:772–778.
14. Ruoff GE, Rosenthal N, Jordan D, et al. Tramadol/acetaminophen combination tabelts for the treatment of chronic lower back pain: a multicenter, randomized, double-blind, placebo-controlled ourpatient study. *Clin Ther* 2003;23:1123–41.
15. De Craen AJM, Di Giulio G, Lampe-Schoenmaeckers AJEM, et al. Analgesic efficacy and safety of paracetamol–codeine combinations versus paracetamol alone: a systematic review. *BMJ* 1996;313:321–325. Search date 1995; primary sources Medline, Embase, International Pharmaceutical Abstracts, Biosis, contact with pharmaceutical companies, and hand searches of references.
16. Salerno SM, Browning R, Jackson JL. The effect of antidepressant treatment in chronic back pain: a meta-analysis. *Arch Intern Med* 2002;162:19–24. Search date 2000; primary sources Medline, Psychlit, Cinahl, Embase, Aidsline, Healthstar, Cancerlit, Cochrane Library, Micromedex, Federal Research in Progress databases, and reference lists of articles.
17. Atkinson JH, Slater MA, Williams RA, et al. A placebo-controlled randomized clinical trial of nortriptyline for chronic low back pain. *Pain* 1998;76:287–296.
18. Hameroff SR, Cork RC, Scherer K, et al. Doxepin effects on chronic pain, depression and plasma opioids. *J Clin Psychiatry* 1982;43:22–27.

19. Hameroff SR, Weiss JL, Lerman JC, et al. Doxepin's effects on chronic pain and depression: a controlled study. *J Clin Psychiatry* 1984;45:47–52.
20. Treves R, Montane de la Roque P, Dumond JJ, et al. Prospective study of the analgesic action of clomipramine versus placebo in refractory low back pain and sciatica (68 cases) [In French]. *Rev Rhum Mal Osteoartic* 1991;58:549–552.
21. Atkinson JH, Slater MA, Wahlgren DR, et al. Effects of noradrenergic and serotonergic antidepressants on chronic low back pain intensity. *Pain* 1999;83:137–145.
22. Dickens C, Jayson M, Sutton C, et al. The relationship between pain and depression in a trial using paroxetine in sufferers of chronic low back pain. *Psychosomatics* 2000;41:490–499.
23. Van Tulder MW, Touray T, Furlan AD, *et al*. Muscle relaxants for non-specific low back pain: a systematic review within the framework of the Cochrane Collaboration. *Spine* 2003;17:1978–1992. Search date: 2001; primary sources Medline, Embase, Cochrane Library and reference lists.
24. Worz R, Bolten W, Heller J, et al. Flupirtin im vergleich zu chlormezanon und placebo bei chronische muskuloskelettalen ruckenschmerzcn [In German]. *Fortschr Ther* 1996;114:3–6.
25. Pratzel HG, Alken RG, Ramm S. Efficacy and tolerance of repeated oral doses of tolperisone hydrochloride in the treatment of painful reflex muscle spasm: results of a prospective placebo-controlled double-blind trial. *Pain* 996;67:417–425.
26. Basmajian J. Cyclobenzaprine hydrochloride effect on skeletal muscle spasm in the lumbar region and neck: two double–blind controlled clinical and laboratory studies. *Arch Phys Med Rehabil* 1978;59:58–63.
27. Van Tulder MW, Scholten RJPM, Koes BW, et al. Non-steroidal anti-inflammatory drugs for low back pain. In: The Cochrane Library, Issue 2, 2002. Oxford: Update Software. Search date 1998; primary sources Medline, Embase, Cochrane Controlled Trials Register, and hand searches of reference lists from relevant papers.
28. Famaey JP, Bruhwyler J, Vandekerckhove K, et al. Open controlled randomised multicenter comparison of nimesulide and diclofenac in the treatment of subacute and chronic low back pain. *J Drug Assess* 1998;1:349–368.
29. Birbara CA, Puopolo AD, Munoz DR, et al. Treatment of chronic low back pain with etoricoxib, a new cyclo-oxygenase-2 selective inhibitor: improvement in pain and disability: a randomised, placebo-controlled, 3-month trial. *J Pain* 2003;4:307–315.
30. Katz N, Ju WD, Krupa DA, et al. Efficacy and safety of rofecoxib in patients with chronic low back pain: results from two 4-week, randomised, placebo-controlled, parallel-group. Double-blind trials. *Spine* 2003;28:851–859.
31. Waddell G, Feder G, McIntosh A, et al. *Low back pain evidence review.* London: Royal College of General Practitioners, 1996. Search date 1996; primary sources Medline, Embase, Science Citation Index, Social Sciences Citation Index, correspondence with experts and researchers, and hand searches of references.
32. Watts RW, Silagy CA. A meta-analysis on the efficacy of epidural corticosteroids in the treatment of sciatica. *Anaesth Intensive Care* 1995;23:564–569. Search date not stated; primary sources Medline, hand searches from published reviews and clinical trials, and personal contact with published authors in the field and the pharmaceutical manufacturer.
33. Nelemans PJ, de Bie RA, de Vet HCW, et al. Injection therapy for subacute and chronic benign low back pain. In: The Cochrane Library, Issue 3, 2002. Oxford: Update Software. Search date 1996; primary sources Medline, Embase, and hand searches of reference lists.
34. Van Tulder MW, Esmail R, Bombardier C, et al. Back schools for non-specific low back pain. In: The Cochrane Library, Issue 1, 2003. Oxford: Update Software. Search date 1997; primary sources Medline, Embase, and hand searches of references.
35. Dalichau S, Scheele K, Perrey RM, et al. Ultraschallgestützte Haltungs-und Bewegungsanalyse der Lendenwirbelsaüle zum Nachweis der Wirksamkeit einer Rückenschule [In German]. *Zentralbl Arbeitsmed* 1999;49:148–156.
36. Keijsers JFEM, Groenman NH, Gerards FM, et al. A back school in the Netherlands: evaluating the results. *Patient Educ Couns* 1989;14:31–44.
37. Linton SJ, Bradley LA, Jensen I, et al. The secondary prevention of low back pain: a controlled study with follow-up. *Pain* 1989;36:197–207.
38. Postacchini F, Facchini M, Palieri P. Efficacy of various forms of conservative treatment in low-back pain. A comparative study. *Neuro-Orthopedics* 1988;6:28–35.
39. Donchin M, Woolf O, Kaplan L, et al. Secondary prevention of low–back pain. A clinical trial. *Spine* 1990;15:1317–1320.
40. Klaber Moffett JA, Chase SM, Portek I, et al. A controlled prospective study to evaluate the effectiveness of a back school in the relief of chronic low–back pain. *Spine* 1986;11:120–122.
41. Harkapaa K, Jarvikoski A, Mellin G, et al. A controlled study on the outcome of inpatient and outpatient treatment for low-back pain. Part I. *Scand J Rehab Med* 1989;21:81–89.
42. Hurri H. The Swedish back school in chronic low–back pain. Part I. Benefits. *Scand J Rehab Med* 1989;21:33–40.
43. Keijsers JFME, Steenbakkers WHL, Meertens RM, et al. The efficacy of the back school: a randomized trial. *Arthritis Care Res* 1990;3:204–209.
44. Maier-Riehle B, Härter M. The effects of back schools: a meta-analysis. *Int J Rehab Res* 2001;24:199–206. Search date 2000; primary sources Medline, Psychlit, Psyindex, and hand searches of reference lists from relevant publications.
45. Van Tulder MW, Ostelo R, Vlaeyen JWS, et al. Behavioural treatment for chronic low back pain. In: The Cochrane Library, Issue 3, 2002. Oxford: Update Software. Search date 1999; primary sources Medline, Psychlit, Cochrane Controlled Trials Register, Embase, and hand searches of reference lists.
46. Van den Hout JHC, Vlaeyen JWS, Heuts PHTG, et al. Secondary prevention of work-related disability in non-specific low back pain: does problem-solving therapy help? A randomised clinical trial. *Clin J Pain* 2003;19:87–96.
47. Van Tulder MW, Malmivaara A, Esmail R, et al. Exercise therapy for non-specific low back pain. In: The Cochrane Library, Issue 3, 2002. Oxford: Update Software. Search date 1999; primary sources Medline, Psychlit, Cochrane Controlled Trials Register, Embase, and hand searches of reference lists.
48. Kankaanpaa M, Taimela S, Airaksinen O, et al. The efficacy of active rehabilitation in chronic low back pain. Effect on pain intensity, self-experienced disability, and lumbar fatigability. *Spine* 1999;24:1034–1042.
49. Bendix AF, Bendix T, Ostenfeld S, et al. Active treatment programs for patients with chronic low back pain: a prospective, randomized, observer-blinded study. *Eur Spine J* 1995;4:148–152.
50. Bendix AF, Bendix T, Labriola M, et al. Functional restoration for chronic low back pain: two-year follow-up of two randomized clinical trials. *Spine* 1998;23:717–725.
51. Franke A, Gebauer S, Franke K, et al. Acupuncture massage vs Swedish massage and individual exercise vs group exercise in low back pain sufferers–a randomized controlled clinical trial in a 2 x 2 factorial design [In German]. *Forsch Komplementarmed Klass Naturheilkd* 2000;7:286–293.
52. Moseley, L. Combined physiotherapy and education is efficacious for chronic low back pain. *Aust J Physiother* 2002;48:297–302.
53. Aure OF, Nilsen JH, Vasseljen O. Manual therapy and exercise therapy in patients with chronic low back pain: a randomised, controlled trial with 1-year follow-up. *Spine* 2003;28:525–532.
54. Friedrich M, Gittler G, Halberstadt Y, et al. Combined exercise and motivation program: effect on the compliance and level of disability of patients with chronic low back pain: a randomized controlled trial. *Arch Phys Med Rehabil* 1998;79:475–487.

55. Mannion AF, Muntener M, Taimela S, et al. A randomized clinical trial of three active therapies for chronic low back pain. *Spine* 1999;24:2435–2448.
56. Mannion AF, Muntener M, Taimela S, et al. Comparison of three active therapies for chronic low back pain: results of a randomized clinical trial with one-year follow-up. *Rheumatology* 2001;40:772–778.
57. Mannion AF, Junge A, Taimela S, et al. Active therapy for chronic low back pain: part 3. Factors influencing self-rated disability and its change following therapy. *Spine* 2001;26:920–929.
58. Mannion AF, Taimela S, Muntener M, et al. Active therapy for chronic low back pain part 1. Effects on back muscle activation, fatigability, and strength. *Spine* 2001;26:897–908.
59. Rittweger J, Just K, Kautzsch K, et al. Treatment of chronic lower back pain with lumbar extension and whole-body vibration exercise: a randomized controlled trial. *Spine* 2002;27:1829–1834.
60. Hildebrandt VH, Proper KI, van den Berg R, et al. Cesar therapy is temporarily more effective in patients with chronic low back pain than the standard treatment by family practitioner: randomized, controlled and blinded clinical trial with 1 year follow-up [In Dutch]. *Nederlands Tijdschrift voor Geneeskunde* 2000;144:2258–2264.
61. Soukup MG, Glomsrod B, Lonn JH, et al. The effect of a Mensendieck exercise program as secondary prophylaxis for recurrent low back pain. A randomized, controlled trial with 12-month follow-up. *Spine* 1999;24:1585–1591.
62. Soukup MG, Lonn J, Glomsrod B, et al. Exercises and education as secondary prevention for recurrent low back pain. *Physiother Res Int* 2001;6:27–39.
63. Van Tulder MW, Jellema P, van Poppel MNM, et al. Lumbar supports for prevention and treatment of low back pain. In: The Cochrane Library, Issue 1, 2003. Oxford: Update Software. Search date 1999; primary sources Medline, Cinahl, Current Contents, Cochrane Controlled Trials Register, Embase, Science Citation Index, and hand searches of reference lists.
64. Guzman J, Esmail R, Karjalainen K, et al. Multidisciplinary rehabilitation for chronic low back pain: systematic review. *BMJ* 2001;322:1511–1516. Search date 1998; primary sources Medline, Embase, Psychlit, Cinahl, Healthstar, Cochrane Library, citation tracking, and personal contact with content experts.
65. Skouen JS, Grasdal AL, Haldorsen EMH, et al. Relative cost-effectiveness of extensive and light multidisciplinary treatment programs versus treatment as usual for patients with chronic low back pain on long-term sick leave. *Spine* 2002;27:901–910.
66. Schonstein E, Kenny DT, Keating J, et al. Work conditioning, work hardening and functional restoration for workers with back and neck pain. In: The Cochrane Library, Issue 1, 2003. Oxford: Update Software. Search date 2000; primary sources Medline, Embase, Cinahl, Biomedical Collection I to IV; Psychinfo, Pedro, Cochrane Controlled Trials Register, hand searches of reference lists of identified studies, and personal communication with the Cochrane Collaboration Back Group and domain experts.
67. Furlan AD, Brosseau L, Welch V, et al. Massage for low back pain. In: The Cochrane Library, Issue 1, 2003. Oxford: Update Software. Search date 2001; primary sources Medline, Embase, Cochrane Controlled Trials Register, Healthstar, Cinahl, Dissertation Abstracts, and hand searches of reference lists and contact with content experts and massage associations.
68. Assendelft WJJ, Morton SC, Yu EI, et al. Spinal manipulative therapy for low back pain: a meta-analysis of effectiveness relative to other therapies. *Ann Intern Med* 2003;138:71–81. Search date 2001; primary sources Medline, Embase, Cinahl, Cochrane Controlled Trials Register, reviews and reference lists.
69. Liccardione JC, Stoll ST, Fulda KG, et al. Osteopathic manipulative treatment for chronic low back pain: a randomised controlled trial. *Spine* 2003;28:1355–1362.
70. Shekelle PG, Adams AH, Chassin MR, et al. Spinal manipulation for low back pain. *Ann Intern Med* 1992;117:590–598. Search date not stated; primary sources Medline, Index Medicus, contact with experts, and hand searches of references.
71. Werners R, Pynsent PB, Bulstrode CJK. Randomized trial comparing interferential therapy with motorized lumbar traction and massage in the management of low back pain in a primary care setting. *Spine* 1999;24:1579–1584
72. Ljunggren E, Weber H, Larssen S. Autotraction versus manual traction in patients with prolapsed lumbar intervertebral discs. *Scand J Rehabil Med* 1984;16:117–124.
73. Milne S, Welch V, Brosseau L, et al. Transcutaneous electrical nerve stimulation (TENS) for chronic low back pain. In: The Cochrane Library, Issue 1, 2003. Oxford: Update Software. Search date 2000; primary sources Medline, Embase, Pedro, Cochrane Controlled Trials Register, hand searches of bibliographic references, reference lists, Current Contents, abstracts in specialised journals, conference proceedings, and personal contact with co-ordinating offices of the trials registries of the Cochrane Field of Physical and Related Therapies and Cochrane Musculoskeletal Group and content experts.
74. Ernst E, White AR. Acupuncture for back pain. A meta-analysis of randomized controlled trials. *Arch Intern Med* 1998;158:2235–2241. Search date 1996; primary sources Medline, Cochrane Controlled Trials Register, Ciscom, contacted authors and experts, and hand searches of references.
75. Van Tulder MW, Cherkin DC, Berman B, et al. Acupuncture in low back pain. In: The Cochrane Library, Issue 1, 2003. Oxford: Update Software. Search date 1996; primary sources Medline, Embase, Cochrane Complementary Medicine Field trials register, Cochrane Controlled Trials Register, Science Citation Index, and hand searches of references.
76. Grant DJ, Bishop-Miller J, Winchester DM, et al. A randomized comparative trial of acupuncture versus transcutaneous electrical nerve stimulation for chronic back pain in the elderly. *Pain* 1999;82:9–13.
77. Carlsson CPO, Sjölund BH. Acupuncture for chronic low back pain: a randomized placebo-controlled study with long-term follow-up. *Clin J Pain* 2001;17:296–305.
78. Leibing E, Leonhardt U, Köster G, et al. Acupuncture treatment of chronic low back pain — a randomized, blinded, placebo-controlled trial with 9-month follow-up. *Pain* 2002;96:189–196.

Maurits van Tulder
Institute for Research in Extramural Medicine
VU University Medical Centre, Amsterdam, The Netherlands

Bart Koes
Department of General Practice, Erasmus University, Rotterdam, The Netherlands

Competing interests: None declared.

TABLE 1 RCTs of back schools in people with chronic back pain included in a systematic review[33] (see text, p 1486).

Ref	Participants	Interventions	Results
36	40 people with back pain > 6 months duration	Maastricht back school (7 sessions of 2.5 hours plus refresher at 8 weeks) v waiting list control	10 drop outs. No significant difference for most outcomes measured after the programme (e.g. pain on VAS: 28.9 with back school v 31.9 with control, P not reported in review).
37	66 nurses who had been sick listed for back pain in previous 2 years	Back school (5 weeks in back clinic, 8 hours per day) + individual physical therapy programmes + behaviour therapy v waiting list control	Back school significantly reduced pain at 6 weeks and 6 months compared with waiting list control (data presented graphically; P not reported in review)
38	239 people with continuous back pain > 2 months duration or an acute-on-chronic episode of back pain	Back school based on Canadian Back Education Unit (four 1 hour sessions over 1 week) v spinal manipulation by chiropractor daily for 1 week, then twice weekly for 6 weeks v non-steroidal anti-inflammatory drug for 15–20 days; physiotherapy; light massage; electrical stimulation, and diathermy daily for 3 weeks v physiotherapy; light massage; electrical stimulation, and diathermy daily for 3 weeks v placebo gel twice daily for 2 weeks	Back school improved pain and disability compared with other interventions at 2 and 6 months (combined pain disability and spinal mobility score at 2 months: 4.6 with back school v 2.6 with spinal manipulation v 2.2 with NSAIDs v 4.2 with physiotherapy v 1.2 with placebo; 6 months: 8.9 with back school v 4.3 with manipulation v 4.0 with NSAIDs v 6.0 with physiotherapy v 2.0 with placebo; details of scoring system not reported in review; P not reported in review).

TABLE 1 continued

Ref	Participants	Interventions	Results
39	142 hospital employees	Back school (4 sessions, 90 minutes each over 2 weeks with further session at 2 months) *v* callisthenics (45 minutes sessions twice weekly for 3 months) *v* waiting list control	Callisthenics reduced duration of low back pain compared with back school and waiting list control at 1 year (7.3 months with back school v 4.5 months with callisthenics *v* 7.4 months with waiting list control; P not reported in review).
40	92 people with and without leg pain	Swedish back school (3 sessions on anatomy, body mechanics, ergonomic counselling and exercises *v* exercises alone	Back school reduced pain and improved function compared with exercises alone at 16 weeks (data presented graphically; P not reported in review).
41	476 people with reduced physical capacity and sick leave in previous 2 years	Inpatient back school (3 weeks rehabilitation with modified Swedish back school, exercises, relaxation, heat, massage) *v* outpatient back school (15 sessions over 2 months with modified Swedish back school, exercises, relaxation, heat, massage) *v* written and oral advice on back exercises and ergonomics	Back school (inpatient and outpatient) significantly reduced pain and disability compared with no back school at 3 months, but no significant difference at 2.5 years (data presented graphically; P values not reported in review).
42	204 women	Back school (six 60 minute education and exercise sessions over 3 weeks with refresher sessions at 6 months) *v* written information about back school	Back school significantly reduced pain and disability compared with written information at 6 months, but no significant difference at 1 year (data presented graphically).

TABLE 1 continued

Ref	Participants	Interventions	Results
43	90 people, mean duration of back pain 7.5 years	Maastricht back school, education, skills programme (7 sessions of 2.5 hours each plus refresher at 6 months) v waiting list control	No significant difference between back school and control in pain and function at 2 and 6 months (pain on VAS, 2 months: 5.4 with back school v 5.2 with control; 6 months: 5.4 with back school v 4.6 with control, P not reported in review; data for function not reported in review).
35	104 male construction workers	Back school v no treatment	8 weeks: AR for reduced or no back pain: 71% with back school v 14% with no treatment pain; 6 months 43% with back school v 14% with no treatment; P value not reported.

NSAIDS, non-steroidal anti-inflammatory drugs; Ref, reference; VAS, visual analogue scale.

Neck pain

Search date May 2004

Allan Binder

QUESTIONS

INTERVENTIONS

See glossary G

Key Messages

- The evidence about the effects of individual interventions for neck pain is often contradictory because of the poor quality of the RCTs, the tendency for interventions to be given in combination, and for RCTs to be conducted in diverse groups. This lack of consistency in study design makes it difficult to isolate which intervention may be of use in which type of neck pain.

Uncomplicated neck pain

- **Exercise** Systematic reviews and subsequent RCTs, primarily in people with chronic uncomplicated neck pain, found that strengthening exercise or active physical treatment including exercise reduced pain compared with usual care including drug treatment, stress management, or no specific exercise programme. RCTs identified by several systematic reviews provided insufficient evidence about the effects of exercise compared with traction. The reviews identified one RCT in people with chronic neck pain that compared low technology strengthening exercises plus manipulation, high technology strengthening exercises, and manipulation alone. It found that low technology strengthening exercises plus manipulation improved participant satisfaction, objective strength, and range of movement at 11 weeks compared with manipulation alone. At 1 and 2 years it found that both low technology strengthening exercises plus manipulation and high technology strengthening exercises improved pain and patient satisfaction compared with manipulation alone. The 2 year follow up was in a subset of participants only. Another RCT identified by a systematic review found no significant difference in pain after treatment or at 12 months among exercise, manipulation, or mobilisation. A third RCT found that exercise was less effective in improving pain than mobilisation in people with neck pain for over 2 weeks.

- **Manipulation** One systematic review found no significant difference in symptoms between manipulation and usual care in people with subacute or chronic neck or back pain. The meta-analysis performed by the review may have been underpowered to detect a clinically important difference. One RCT found limited evidence that manipulation may be more effective in reducing pain at 1 year than less active physical treatment (massage, pulsed electrical field treatment, and slight traction). We found one RCT in people with chronic neck pain that compared manipulation plus low technology strengthening exercises, high technology strengthening exercises, and manipulation alone. It found that manipulation plus low technology strengthening exercises improved pain and objective range of movement at 11 weeks compared with manipulation alone. At 1 and 2 years it found that both manipulation plus low technology strengthening exercises and high technology strengthening exercises improved pain and patient satisfaction compared with manipulation alone. The 2 year follow up was in a subset of participants only. Two RCTs provided insufficient evidence to compare manipulation versus mobilisation in people with uncomplicated neck pain.
- **Manipulation plus exercise** One RCT in people with chronic neck pain found that manipulation plus strengthening exercise improved pain and objective range of movement at 11 weeks compared with either treatment alone. At 1 and 2 years the difference in outcomes remained significant with manipulation plus strengthening exercise compared with manipulation alone but not compared with exercise alone. The 2 year follow up was in a subset of participants only.
- **Mobilisation** One RCT found that mobilisation improved symptoms compared with usual care (drug treatment) or exercise in people with neck pain for over 2 weeks. Another RCT identified by several systematic reviews found no significant difference in pain after treatment or at 12 months among mobilisation, manipulation, or exercise. A third RCT identified by several systematic reviews found limited evidence that manual treatment (mobilisation or manipulation) may be more effective in reducing pain at 1 year than less active physical treatment. Two RCTs provided insufficient evidence to compare mobilisation versus manipulation in people with uncomplicated neck pain. Weak RCTs, some identified by systematic reviews, provided insufficient evidence to compare mobilisation versus acupuncture or transcutaneous electrical nerve stimulation in people with uncomplicated neck pain.
- **Acupuncture** Systematic reviews of weak RCTs provided insufficient evidence about the effects of acupuncture compared with a range of other treatments, including sham acupuncture, sham transcutaneous electrical nerve simulation, diazepam, traction, short wave diathermy, and mobilisation in people with acute or chronic uncomplicated neck pain.
- **Biofeedback** Three systematic reviews identified no RCTs of biofeedback in people with uncomplicated neck pain.

- **Drug treatments (analgesics, non-steroidal anti-inflammatory drugs, antidepressants, or muscle relaxants)** We found insufficient evidence on the effects of analgesics, non-steroidal anti-inflammatory drugs, antidepressants, or muscle relaxants for neck pain, although they are widely used. Several drugs used to treat neck pain are associated with well documented adverse effects.
- **Heat or cold** Two systematic reviews identified no RCTs of sufficient quality of heat or cold in people with uncomplicated neck pain. One large RCT of people with chronic neck and back pain found that heat combined with other physical treatment was less effective in improving outcomes than manipulation or mobilisation.
- **Multimodal treatment** One RCT identified by a systematic review provided insufficient evidence to assess multimodal treatment in people with uncomplicated neck pain.
- **Pulsed electromagnetic field treatment** One RCT identified by several systematic reviews provided insufficient evidence to compare pulsed electromagnetic field treatment versus sham treatment in people with uncomplicated neck pain. RCTs in people with chronic neck and back pain identified by another systematic review found that pulsed electromagnetic field treatment combined with other physical treatments was less effective in improving outcomes than manipulation or mobilisation.
- **Soft collars and special pillows** We found no RCTs of sufficient quality on the effects of soft collars or special pillows in people with uncomplicated neck pain.
- **Spray and stretch** One RCT identified by several systematic reviews provided insufficient evidence about the effects of spray and stretch in people with uncomplicated neck pain.
- **Traction** Systematic reviews in people with acute or chronic neck pain provided insufficient evidence about the effects of traction compared with a range of other physical treatments, including sham traction, placebo tablets, exercise, acupuncture, heat, collar, and analgesics. Systematic reviews identified no RCTs of sufficient quality comparing traction versus manipulation or mobilisation.
- **Transcutaneous electrical nerve stimulation** Five systematic reviews identified no RCTs of sufficient quality of transcutaneous electrical nerve stimulation in people with uncomplicated neck pain.
- **Patient education** Two RCTs in people with chronic neck, back, or shoulder pain found no significant difference among patient education (individual advice, pamphlets, or group instruction) with or without analgesics and no treatment, stress management, and cognitive behavioural therapy.

Acute whiplash

- **Early mobilisation** Four RCTs identified by several systematic reviews provided limited evidence that early mobilisation reduced pain compared with immobilisation or rest plus a collar.
- **Early return to normal activity** One RCT in people with acute whiplash identified by one systematic review provided limited evidence that advice to "act as usual" plus anti-inflammatory drugs improved some symptoms (including pain during daily activities, neck stiffness, memory, concentration, and headache) at 6 months compared with immobilisation plus 14 days' sick leave. It found no significant difference in neck range or sick leave and found that a similar proportion of people had severe neck pain.
- **Multimodal treatment** One RCT identified by a systematic review found that multimodal treatment reduced pain at 1 and 6 months compared with physical treatments.
- **Drug treatments (analgesics, non-steroidal anti-inflammatory drugs, antidepressant drugs, or muscle relaxants** Two systematic reviews identified no RCTs of drug treatments in people with acute whiplash injury.
- **Exercise** One RCT found no significant difference between two home exercise programmes in pain or disability.

- **Pulsed electromagnetic field treatment** One small RCT identified by two systematic reviews found limited evidence that electromagnetic field treatment reduced pain after 4 weeks but not after 3 months compared with sham treatment.

Chronic whiplash

- **Percutaneous radiofrequency neurotomy** One RCT identified by a systematic review found limited evidence that percutaneous radiofrequency neurotomy reduced pain after 27 weeks compared with sham treatment in people with chronic whiplash injury.
- **Multimodal treatment** One small RCT found no difference between multimodal treatment and physical treatments in disability, pain, or range of movement at the end of treatment or at 3 months but it may have been too small to detect a clinically important difference.
- **Physical treatments** One small RCT found no significant difference between physical treatments alone and multimodal treatment in disability, pain, or range of movement at the end of treatment or at 3 months but it may have been too small to detect a clinically important difference.

Neck pain with radiculopathy

- **Drug treatments (epidural steroid injections, analgesics, non-steroidal anti-inflammatory drugs, or muscle relaxants)** We found no RCTs examining the effects of analgesics, non-steroidal anti-inflammatory drugs, or muscle relaxants in people with neck pain with radiculopathy. Two RCTs found limited evidence that cervical steroid epidural injections may improve pain from baseline in people with chronic neck pain with or without radiculopathy.
- **Surgery versus conservative treatment** One RCT found no significant difference in pain at 1 year between surgery and conservative treatment in people with neck pain with radiculopathy.

DEFINITION In this chapter we have differentiated uncomplicated neck pain from whiplash, although many studies, particularly in people with chronic pain (duration > 3 months), do not specify which types of people are included. Most studies of acute pain (duration < 3 months) are confined to whiplash. Uncomplicated neck pain is defined as pain with a postural or mechanical basis, often called cervical spondylosis. It does not include pain associated with fibromyalgia. Uncomplicated neck pain may include some people with a traumatic basis for their symptoms, but not people for whom pain is specifically stated to have followed sudden acceleration — deceleration injuries to the neck, that is, whiplash. Whiplash is commonly seen in road traffic accidents or sports injuries. It is not accompanied by radiographic abnormalities or clinical signs of nerve root damage. Neck pain often occurs in combination with limited movement and poorly defined neurological symptoms affecting the upper limbs. The pain can be severe and intractable, and can occur with radiculopathy or myelopathy. We have included under radiculopathy those studies involving people with predominantly radicular symptoms arising in the cervical spine.

INCIDENCE/ PREVALENCE About two thirds of people will experience neck pain at some time in their lives.[1,2] Prevalence is highest in middle age. In the UK about 15% of hospital based physiotherapy and in Canada 30% of chiropractic referrals are for neck pain.[3,4] In the Netherlands neck pain contributes up to 2% of general practitioner consultations.[5]

AETIOLOGY/ RISK FACTORS The aetiology of uncomplicated neck pain is unclear. Most uncomplicated neck pain is associated with poor posture, anxiety and depression, neck strain, occupational injuries, or sporting injuries. With chronic pain, mechanical and degenerative factors (often referred to as cervical spondylosis) are more likely. Some neck pain results from soft tissue trauma, most typically seen in whiplash injuries. Rarely, disc prolapse and inflammatory, infective, or malignant conditions affect the cervical spine and present with neck pain with or without neurological features.

PROGNOSIS Neck pain usually resolves within days or weeks but can recur or become chronic. In some industries, neck related disorders account for as much time off work as low back pain (see low back pain and sciatica [acute], p 1465).[6] The proportion of people in whom neck pain becomes chronic depends on the cause but is thought to be about 10%,[1] similar to low back pain. Neck pain causes severe disability in 5% of affected people.[2] Whiplash injuries are more likely to cause disability than neck pain because of other causes; up to 40% of sufferers reported symptoms even after 15 years' follow up.[7] Factors associated with a poorer outcome after whiplash are not well defined.[8] The incidence of chronic disability after whiplash varies among countries, although reasons for this variation are unclear.[9]

AIMS OF INTERVENTION To recover from acute episode within 4 weeks; to maintain activities of daily living and reduce absenteeism from work; to prevent development of long term symptoms; to improve symptoms.

OUTCOMES Pain; range of movement; function; return to work; level of disability (Neck Disability Index Ⓖ); adverse effects of treatment.[10]

METHODS *Clinical Evidence* search and appraisal May 2004. We also searched the following databases: Chirolars (now called Mantis) for English language articles from 1966 to November 1999; Bioethicsline (1973–1997); Cumulative Index to Nursing and Allied Health (Cinahl) (1982–1997); and Current Contents (1994–1997). Criteria for assessment of RCTs were based on the 100 point Koes/Assendelft scale, which assesses study population, interventions, effects, data presentation, and analysis.[11] In the question on uncomplicated neck pain, we have excluded RCTs if they had fewer than 30 people per treatment arm or if they scored less than 40 on the assessment scale, unless they were of injection treatments. We have included smaller, weaker RCTs in the questions on acute and chronic whiplash because of the paucity of evidence in these people.

QUESTION What are the effects of treatments for people with uncomplicated neck pain without severe neurological deficit?

OPTION EXERCISE

Systematic reviews and subsequent RCTs, primarily in people with chronic uncomplicated neck pain, found that strengthening exercise or active physical treatment including exercise reduced pain compared with usual care including drug treatment, stress management, or no specific exercise programme. RCTs identified by several systematic reviews provided insufficient evidence about the effects of exercise compared with traction. The reviews identified one RCT in people with chronic neck pain that compared low technology strengthening exercises plus manipulation, high technology strengthening exercises, and manipulation alone. It found that low technology strengthening exercises plus manipulation improved participant satisfaction, objective strength, and range of movement at 11 weeks compared with manipulation alone. At 1 and 2 years it found that both low technology strengthening exercises plus manipulation and high technology strengthening exercises improved pain and patient satisfaction compared with manipulation alone. The 2 year follow up was in a subset of participants only. Another RCT identified by a systematic review found no significant difference in pain after treatment or at 12 months among exercise, manipulation, or mobilisation. A third RCT found that exercise was less effective in improving pain than mobilisation in people with neck pain for over 2 weeks.

Benefits: We found four systematic reviews (search dates 1993,[12] 1995,[13] 2000,[14] 2001[15]), which between them identified two RCTs (3 published papers) of sufficient quality.[16–18] We also found three subsequent RCTs (4 published papers).[19–22] None of the reviews could perform a meta-analysis because of heterogeneity among the trials in types of exercise and comparisons assessed. **Proprioceptive and strengthening exercise versus usual care (analgesics, non-steroidal anti-inflammatory drugs, or muscle relaxants):** The reviews identified one RCT.[16] The RCT (60 people with chronic neck pain, 37% with radiographic evidence of osteoarthritis) found that a proprioceptive and strengthening exercise programme significantly reduced pain at 10 weeks compared with usual care (pain measured on a 100 mm visual analogue scale [0 mm = no pain; 100 mm = unbearable pain: −21.8 with exercise v −4.3 with usual care; P < 0.004).[16] The exercise programme involved 15 individual exercise sessions aimed at improving eye–neck coordination through passive and active movements of the head whilst maintaining gaze on a fixed or slow mobile target. **Endurance or strengthening (isometric) exercise versus no specific exercise programme:** The reviews identified no RCTs but we found one subsequent RCT.[19] The subsequent RCT (180 female office workers with chronic neck pain) compared a programme of specific "endurance" (dynamic) or "strength" (isometric) exercises carried out three times a week for 1 year versus no specific exercise programme.[19] All participants were encouraged to undertake simple aerobic and stretching exercises. The RCT found that endurance and strength exercises significantly improved neck pain after 12 months of treatment compared with control (pain assessed on a 100 mm visual analogue scale; median improvement in pain score: 40 with strength exercise v 35 with endurance exercise v 16 with control; P < 0.001 for exercise groups v control). Strength and endurance exercises also significantly improved disability after 12 months compared with control (median improvement in Neck Disability Index**G**: 9 with strength exercise v 8 with endurance exercise v 3 with control; P < 0.001).[19] **Exercise (strength training, endurance training, or coordination exercises) versus stress management:** The reviews identified one RCT (2 published papers).[17,18] The RCT (103 women with work related neck pain for ≥ 1 year) compared three exercise regimens (strength training, endurance training, or coordination exercises) versus stress management over 10 weeks.[17,18] It found that any type of exercise significantly reduced pain compared with stress management after 10–12 weeks (P < 0.05). It found no significant difference in outcomes among any of the exercise programmes. It also found no significant difference in neck pain among the four groups after 3 years' follow up (AR for neck pain: 47% with strength training v 50% with endurance training v 58% with coordination exercises v 39% with stress management; reported as non-significant, no individual P values reported for exercise v stress management or exercise regimens versus each other). **Exercise (dynamic muscle training) versus relaxation training or advice to continue with ordinary activity:** The reviews identified no RCTs but we found one subsequent RCT.[22] The subsequent RCT (393 women office workers with neck pain for ≥ 12 weeks) compared three interventions for 12 weeks: dynamic muscle training, relaxation training, and advice to continue with ordinary activities. The main outcome measures were pain (measured on a scale from 0–10 where 0 = no pain and 10 = unbearable pain) and neck disability (measured on a scale from 0–80, based on 8 questions about pain) at 3, 6, and 12 months. Subjective work ability, range of movement, and depression were also assessed. The RCT found no significant difference in outcomes between exercise and control at any follow up assessment (for example, pain at 12 months: 3.1 with exercise v 3.2 with control; WMD +0.5, 95% CI −0.1 to +1.0; neck disability at 12 months: 19 with exercise v 17 with control; WMD −0.1, 95% CI −3.0 to +3.1; see comment below).[22] There was also no significant difference in outcomes among treatment groups at any time. In this RCT, the average the number of 30 minute training sessions completed by participants over 12 weeks for both treatment groups was only 40% of the maximum available; this low uptake might have been insufficient to have an effect. **Exercise (strengthening isometric) versus traction or no treatment:** The reviews identified no RCTs of sufficient quality. **Exercise versus manual treatment (manipulation or mobilisation); exercise plus manipulation; exercise combined**

with other physical treatments versus manipulation or mobilisation: See benefits of manipulation, p 1510. **Exercise versus mobilisation:** See benefits of mobilisation, p 1513. **Exercise versus multimodal treatment:** See benefits of multimodal treatment, p 1514.

Harms: We found no good data on harms. The incidence of serious adverse events seems to be low for all physical treatments considered.

Comment: None.

OPTION TRACTION

Systematic reviews in people with acute or chronic neck pain provided insufficient evidence about the effects of traction compared with a range of other physical treatments, including sham traction, placebo tablets, exercise, acupuncture, heat, collar, and analgesics. Systematic reviews identified no RCTs of sufficient quality comparing traction versus manipulation or mobilisation.

Benefits: We found three systematic reviews (search dates 1992,[23] 1993,[12] 1995[13]), which between them identified two RCTs[24,25] of sufficient quality comparing traction versus sham traction, placebo tablets, exercise, acupuncture, heat, collar, and analgesics. The RCTs found no consistent difference in pain between traction and any of the other interventions. **Traction versus sham traction:** The reviews identified one RCT.[24] The RCT (100 people with chronic neck pain, most with cervical spondylosis) found no significant difference between 4 weeks' traction and sham traction in pain, sleep disturbance, social dysfunction, and activities of daily living either directly after treatment or at 3 months (pain measured on a visual analogue from 0–10 where 0 = no pain: 2.78 with traction *v* 3.29 with placebo; reported as non-significant, CI not reported).[24] **Traction versus positioning, instruction in posture, neck collar, placebo tablets, or untuned short wave diathermy:** The reviews identified one RCT.[25] The RCT (493 people with acute or chronic neck pain, 57% having first occurrence of pain, 19% having ≥ 5 previous occurrences) compared six interventions: traction (combined with gentle exercise and heat as determined by a physiotherapist), positioning, instruction in posture, neck collar, placebo tablets, and untuned short wave diathermy.[25] All participants received analgesics. The RCT found no significant difference among groups in the proportion of people who physicians assessed as "cured" (21% with traction *v* 23% with positioning *v* 24% with collar *v* 12% with placebo tablets *v* 21% with untuned diathermy; reported as non-significant, CI not reported). It also found no significant difference in pain or the need for further treatment among groups at 6 months (reported as non-significant, CI not reported). **Traction versus acupuncture:** See benefits of acupucture, p 1509. **Traction versus exercise:** See benefits of exercise, p 1505. **Traction combined with other physical treatment versus mobilisation:** See benefits of mobilisation, p 1513.

Harms: We found no good data on harms. The incidence of serious adverse events seems to be low for all physical treatments considered.

Comment: None.

OPTION PULSED ELECTROMAGNETIC FIELD TREATMENT

One RCT identified by several systematic reviews provided insufficient evidence to compare pulsed electromagnetic field treatment versus sham treatment in people with uncomplicated neck pain. RCTs in people with

chronic neck and back pain identified by another systematic review found that pulsed electromagnetic field treatment combined with other physical treatments was less effective in improving outcomes than manipulation or mobilisation.

Benefits: We found two systematic reviews (search date 1993,[12] 1995[13]), which between them identified one RCT of sufficient quality comparing pulsed electromagnetic field treatment versus sham pulsed electromagnetic field treatment in people with chronic neck pain.[26] The RCT (81 people with neck pain and radiographic evidence of cervical osteoarthritis and 86 people with osteoarthritis of the knee; all of whom had symptoms for at least 1 year; see comment below) identified by the reviews compared true versus sham pulsed electromagnetic field treatment.[26] Although randomisation was properly conducted in the RCT, baseline characteristics of treated and placebo groups were, by chance, different. People allocated to active treatment had higher pain scores, more tenderness, and more difficulty with the activities of daily living than the placebo group. The analysis in the RCT was based on changes from the baseline value, and it is not known how much of the observed effect was caused by bias introduced by the baseline differences. Subgroup analysis in people with chronic neck pain found that pulsed electromagnetic field treatment significantly reduced pain ($P < 0.04$) and pain on passive motion compared with sham pulsed electromagnetic field treatment ($P = 0.03$). The RCT found no significant difference between pulsed electromagnetic field treatment and sham pulsed electromagnetic field treatment in difficulty with activities of daily living, tenderness, self assessment of improvement, or physicians' global assessment after 18 episodes of treatment. However, it found that active compared with sham pulsed electromagnetic field treatment significantly increased the proportion of people who had improved in at least three of six variables (pain, pain on passive motion, activities of daily living, tenderness, self assessed improvement, physicians' global assessment; 57/82 [70%] with active treatment *v* 37/82 [45%] with sham treatment; RR 1.54, 95% CI 1.21 to 1.80; NNT 4, 95% CI 3 to 11). This benefit was sustained up to 1 month (see comment below).[26] **Pulsed electromagnetic field treatment combined with other physical treatment versus manipulation or mobilisation:** See benefits of manipulation, p 1510.

Harms: We found no good data on harms. The incidence of serious adverse events seems to be low for all physical treatments considered.

Comment: Although one poor quality RCT suggested a slight benefit for pulsed electromagnetic field treatment, this treatment is not widely available in clinical practice.

OPTION ACUPUNCTURE

Systematic reviews of weak RCTs provided insufficient evidence about the effects of acupuncture compared with a range of other treatments, including sham acupuncture, sham transcutaneous electrical nerve simulation, diazepam, traction, short wave diathermy, and mobilisation in people with acute or chronic uncomplicated neck pain.

Benefits: We found four systematic reviews (search dates 1993,[12] 1995,[13] 1998[28,29]), which between them identified 14 RCTs comparing needle or laser acupuncture versus different control procedures (sham acupuncture, sham transcutaneous electrical nerve simulation, diazepam, traction, short wave diathermy, and mobilisation Ⓖ) in people with acute or chronic neck pain. None of the reviews performed a meta-analysis. The RCTs identified by the reviews found no consistent differences between acupuncture and other treatments.

Harms: We found no good data on harms. The incidence of serious adverse events seems to be low for all physical treatments considered.

Comment: None.

OPTION TRANSCUTANEOUS ELECTRICAL NERVE STIMULATION

Five systematic reviews identified no RCTs of sufficient quality of transcutaneous electrical nerve stimulation in people with uncomplicated neck pain.

Benefits: **Transcutaneous electrical nerve stimulation versus mobilisation or neck collar:** We found five systematic reviews (search dates 1990,[11] 1993,[12] 1995,[13,27] 2000[14]), which identified no RCTs of sufficient quality.

Harms: We found no RCTs.

Comment: None.

OPTION HEAT OR COLD

Two systematic reviews identified no RCTs of sufficient quality of heat or cold in people with uncomplicated neck pain. One large RCT of people with chronic neck and back pain found that heat combined with other physical treatment was less effective in improving outcomes than manipulation or mobilisation.

Benefits: We found two systematic reviews (search dates 1993,[12] 1995[13]), which identified no RCTs of sufficient quality. **Heat combined with other physical treatment versus manipulation or mobilisation:** See benefits of manipulation, p 1510.

Harms: We found no good data on harms. The incidence of serious adverse events seems to be low for all physical treatments considered.

Comment: None.

OPTION BIOFEEDBACK

Three systematic reviews identified no RCTs of biofeedback in people with uncomplicated neck pain.

Benefits: We found three systematic reviews (search dates 1990,[11] 1993,[12] 1995[13]), which identified no RCTs of biofeedback in people with uncomplicated neck pain.

Harms: We found no RCTs.

Comment: None.

OPTION SPRAY AND STRETCH

One RCT identified by several systematic reviews provided insufficient evidence about the effects of spray and stretch in people with uncomplicated neck pain.

Benefits: We found two systematic reviews (search dates 1990,[11] 1993[12]), which identified one RCT (74 people with neck pain) comparing spray and stretch versus placebo. It found no significant difference between treatments in pain after 5 treatments (SMD +0.1, 95% CI –0.6 to +0.8).[12]

Harms: We found no good data on harms. The incidence of serious adverse events seems to be low for all physical treatments considered.

Comment: None.

OPTION MANIPULATION

One systematic review found no significant difference in symptoms between manipulation and usual care in people with subacute or chronic neck or back pain. The meta-analysis performed by the review may have been underpowered to detect a clinically important difference. One RCT identified by several systematic reviews found limited evidence that manual treatment (manipulation or mobilisation) may be more effective in reducing pain at 1 year than less active physical treatment. Another RCT identified by the reviews found no significant difference in pain after treatment or at 12 months among exercise, manipulation, or mobilisation. The reviews identified one RCT in people with chronic neck pain that compared manipulation plus low technology strengthening exercises, high technology strengthening exercises, and manipulation alone. It found that manipulation plus low technology strengthening exercises improved participant satisfaction, objective strength, and movement at 11 weeks compared with manipulation alone. At 1 and 2 years it found that both manipulation plus low technology strengthening exercises and high technology strengthening exercises improved pain and patient satisfaction compared with manipulation alone. The 2 year follow up was in a subset of participants only. Another RCT identified by a systematic review found no significant difference in pain after treatment or at 6 months among manipulation, mobilisation, or exercise. Two RCTs provided insufficient evidence to compare manipulation versus mobilisation in people with uncomplicated neck pain.

Benefits: We found six systematic reviews (search dates 1990,[11] 1993,[12] 1995,[13,27] 2002,[30] and 2003[31]) which between them identified six RCTs (7 published reports).[32–38] comparing manipulationⒼ versus other treatments including mobilisationⒼ, one of which had three arms and combined data comparing manipulation and mobilisation versus other treatments. We also found one additional RCT.[39] One systematic review performed a meta-analysis that found no significant difference between manipulation and usual care or drug treatment but individual RCTs identified by several reviews found that manipulation or mobilisation improved symptoms compared with a variety of other physical treatments. Two RCTs provided insufficient evidence to compare manipulation versus mobilisation. **Manipulation versus diazepam, anti-inflammatory drugs, or usual care:** One of the reviews[27] performed a meta-analysis (3 RCTs,[34–36] 155 people with subacute or chronic pain, primarily chronic neck pain but people in 1 of the RCTs[34] had chronic neck and back pain) comparing manipulation versus diazepam, anti-inflammatory drugs, or usual care. It found no significant difference in improvement in pain at 3 weeks between manipulation and other treatments although all treatments improved pain (difference on a 100 mm visual analogue scale between manipulation and other treatments: +12.6 mm, 95% CI –0.15 mm to +25.5 mm).[27] The meta-analysis may have been underpowered to detect a clinically important difference. One of the RCTs included in the meta-analysis compared four treatment groups (see below); the meta-analysis included data only from the manipulation and the usual care treatment arms.[34] **Manipulation or mobilisation versus other physical treatments (exercises plus massage with or without heat, pulsed electromagnetic field treatment, ultrasound, or shortwave diathermy), usual care, or placebo:** The reviews identified one RCT.[34] The RCT (256 people with chronic neck and back pain, 48 with chronic neck and back pain, 64 having chronic neck pain alone) identified by the reviews compared four treatment groups: manual treatment (mobilisation, manipulation, or both); physical treatments (consisting of exercises plus massage with or without heat, pulsed electromagnetic field treatment, ultrasound, or shortwave diathermy; treatment at the discretion of the physiotherapist); usual care (analgesics, advice, home exercise, and bed rest); and placebo (detuned shortwave diathermy or detuned ultrasound).[34] It found that manual treatment (mobilisation or manipulation) significantly improved outcomes after 12 months compared with all of the other treatments (statistical analysis specifically for people with neck pain was not reported). However, it was not possible to compare directly the effects of mobilisation with manipulation, and more people received manipulation. **Manipulation or mobilisation versus exercise:** The reviews identified one RCT.[33] The RCT (119 people with neck pain for ≥3 months) compared three treatments: mobilisation, manipulation, and intensive exercise training.[33] It found no significant difference in pain among groups by the end of treatment (P = 0.44) or after 12 months, although pain score improved from baseline in all groups (median pain score on a 30 point scale improved from 13 to 6 with manipulation *v* from 12 to 6 with intensive training or mobilisation). **Manipulation plus strengthening exercises versus either treatment alone:** The reviews identified one RCT.[32] The RCT (191 people with chronic neck pain who received training about a home exercise programme and were able to use proprietary medication) compared three treatments: low technology exercises plus manipulation (combined treatment), high technology MedX exercises, and manipulation alone.[32] Low technology exercises involved a short aerobic warm up followed by supervised progressive strengthening exercises for the neck and upper body. High technology exercises involved one to one sessions of stretching and upper body strengthening using the MedX cervical extension rotation machines plus aerobic exercise using a stationary bicycle. The duration of each treatment episode was the same (1 hour). The RCT found that combined treatment significantly improved participant satisfaction (P = 0.03), objective strength, and range of movement (P < 0.05 for both outcomes) compared with manipulation alone after 11 weeks. The RCT also found that both combined treatment and high technology strengthening exercises significantly improved pain (P = 0.02) and patient satisfaction (P = 0.002) compared with manipulation alone after 1 year, although it found no significant difference among treatments in health status, neck disability, or medication use. The 2 year follow up to this RCT[32] (data available for 145/191 [76%] of original participants who completed the 11 week treatment period) found that combined treatment or high technology strengthening exercises significantly improved participant rated pain compared with manipulation alone (P = 0.04).[38] It found that combined treatment significantly improved patient satisfaction at 2 years compared with either other treatment (P < 0.001 for combined treatment *v* manipulation alone; P = 0.02 for combined treatment *v* high technology exercises).[38] The two year follow up found no significant differences in neck disability and general health status among the three groups. **Manipulation versus mobilisation:** The reviews identified one RCT[37] and we found one additional RCT.[39] The RCT (100 people with acute or chronic neck pain) identified by the reviews compared a single manipulation treatment versus a single mobilisation treatment.[37] It found no significant difference between treatments in immediate improvement in pain (85% with manipulation *v* 69% with mobilisation; RR of improvement in pain 1.23; CI not reported; P = 0.16 after adjusting for pretreatment differences between groups). It also found that people in the manipulation group had improved range of movement, but the result was not significant (5.1° with manipulation *v* 3.9° with mobilisation; P = 0.5).[37] The additional RCT (336 people with acute or chronic neck pain) found no significant difference between manipulation and mobilisation in average pain, severe pain (average and severe pain measured on a 0–10 point index: 0 = no pain; 10 = unbearable pain), and neck disability scores (Neck Disability Index**G** measured on a 0–50 point index: 0 = no disability; 50 = most severe disability) between a variable number of chiropractic mobilisations and a variable number of manipulations after 6 months (severe pain difference from manipulation *v* mobilisation: –0.02 points; 95% CI –0.69 points to +0.65 points; average pain from manipulation *v* mobilisation: +0.01 points; 95% CI –0.52 points to +0.54 points; difference in neck disability scores: +0.46 points; 95% CI –0.89 points to +1.82 points).[39] In this RCT, only 336/960 (35%) eligible people agreed to participate.[39] This may reduce the external validity of the study.

Harms: **Manipulation:** The estimated risk from case reports of cerebrovascular accident is 1–3/million manipulations**G**,[40] and estimated risk of all serious adverse effects (such as death or disc herniation) is 5–10/10 million manipulations.[27] **Manipulation versus diazepam, anti-inflammatory drugs, or usual care:** One RCT found that two people, both receiving manipulation, reported "new discomfort in their necks".[35] The other two RCTs gave no information on adverse effects.[34,36] **Manipulation or mobilisation versus exercise:** The RCT gave no information on adverse effects.[33] **Manipulation plus strengthening exercises versus either treatment alone:** The RCT found no significant difference in adverse effects among manipulation plus exercises, manipulation alone, and exercise alone (P = 0.49), although 6–10 people in each group had increased neck pain or headache after treatment.[32] **Manipulation versus mobilisation:** The RCT found that 5% of people receiving manipulation and 6% receiving mobilisation**G** had worse pain after treatment.[37] The additional RCT[39] (336 people with acute or chronic neck pain) carried out a follow up questionnaire[41] of adverse effects at 2 weeks. It found that 30% of the 280 people who responded reported at least one minor adverse effect such as increased pain or headache associated with manipulation or mobilisation.[41] The questionnaire found that people receiving manipulation had more adverse effects compared with people receiving mobilisation, although the difference was not significant (adjusted OR 1.44, 95% CI 0.85 to 2.43; absolute numbers not reported). It also found that people who reported adverse events were less satisfied with their care and less likely to achieve meaningful improvement in pain and disability, although again the difference was not significant.[41]

Comment: We found one systematic review (search date 2002) examining mobilisation**G** and manipulation**G** for mechanical neck disorders.[42] It included people with many types of neck pain, including uncomplicated pain, whiplash, and neck pain with radiculopathy, and reported that trials were clinically heterogeneous. However, it did not provide a subgroup analysis in people with uncomplicated neck pain. When assessing any type of neck pain, it found the best evidence of efficacy for interventions that included mobilisation or manipulation plus exercise[31] when compared with any other treatments.

OPTION MOBILISATION

One RCT found that mobilisation improved symptoms compared with usual care (drug treatment) or exercise in people with neck pain for over 2 weeks. Another RCT identified by several systematic reviews found no significant difference in pain after treatment or at 12 months among mobilisation, manipulation, or exercise. A third RCT identified by several systematic reviews found limited evidence that manual treatment (mobilisation or manipulation)

may be more effective in reducing pain at 1 year than less active physical treatment. Two RCTs provided insufficient evidence to compare mobilisation versus manipulation in people with uncomplicated neck pain. Weak RCTs, some identified by systematic reviews, provided insufficient evidence to compare mobilisation versus acupuncture or transcutaneous electrical nerve stimulation in people with uncomplicated neck pain.

Benefits: We found six systematic reviews (search dates 1990,[11] 1993,[12] 1995,[13,27] 2002,[30] and 2003[31]) which between them identified five RCTs[33,34,36,37,39] of sufficient quality comparing mobilisation**Ⓖ** versus other treatments including manipulation**Ⓖ**, one of which had three arms and combined data comparing mobilisation and manipulation versus other treatments. We also found one additional RCT (published in 2 reports),[20,21] and four systematic reviews (search dates 1993,[12] 1995,[13] 1998[28,29]) of acupuncture that included RCTs comparing mobilisation versus acupuncture. The RCTs identified by the reviews found that mobilisation improved symptoms compared with a variety of control procedures. Two RCTs provided insufficient evidence to compare mobilisation versus manipulation. **Mobilisation versus exercise or usual care:** The reviews identified no RCTs but we found one additional RCT[20] (183 people with neck pain for > 2 weeks) which compared three 6 week courses of treatment: mobilisation, exercise, or usual care (analgesics, education, and counselling). It found that mobilisation slightly but significantly improved treatment "success" at 7 weeks compared with exercise or usual care (AR for "success": 68.3% with mobilisation *v* 50.8% with exercise [ARI 17.5%, 95% CI 0.1% to 34.8%] *v* 35.9% with usual care [ARI 32%, 95% CI 16% to 49%]). Treatment success was assessed by participant rating on a 6 point scale from "much worse" to "completely recovered". "Success" was defined as "much improved" or "completely recovered". The RCT found no significant difference in the "success" rate at 7 weeks between exercise and usual care (ARI +14.9%, 95% CI –2.4% to +32.3%).[20] Long term follow up of this RCT found that mobilisation significantly increased "success" rate compared with other treatments at 26 weeks, but not at 1 year (no figures reported for "success" at 26 weeks; AR for "success" at 1 year: 71.7% with mobilisation *v* 62.7% with active exercise [ARI +9.0%, 95% CI –7.9% to +25.8%] *v* 56.3 with usual care [ARI +15.4%, 95% CI –1.3% to +32.1%]).[21] **Mobilisation or manipulation versus other physical treatments (exercises plus massage with or without heat, pulsed electromagnetic field treatment, ultrasound, or shortwave diathermy), usual care, or placebo:** See benefits of manipulation, p 1510. **Mobilisation or manipulation versus exercise; mobilisation versus manipulation:** See benefits of manipulation, p 1510. **Mobilisation versus acupuncture:** See benefits of acupuncture, p 1509. **Mobilisation versus transcutaneous electrical nerve stimulation or neck collar:** See benefits of transcutaneous electrical nerve stimulation, p 1508.

Harms: **Mobilisation versus exercise or usual care:** The RCT found that more people receiving mobilisation**Ⓖ** than exercise or usual care had an increase in neck pain that lasted more than 2 days (18% with mobilisation *v* 7% with exercise *v* 5% with usual care; significance of difference among groups not assessed).[20] It found that more people receiving mobilisation or exercise compared with usual care had headache and arm pain/paraesthesia (headache: 28% with mobilisation *v* 32% with active exercise *v* 6% with usual care; arm pain: 13% with mobilisation *v* 12% with exercise *v* 6% with usual care; significance of difference among groups not assessed). **Mobilisation versus manipulation:** See harms of manipulation, p 1512.

Comment: The incidence of serious adverse events seems to be low for all physical treatments considered. We found one systematic review (search date 2002) examining mobilisation**G** and manipulation**G** for mechanical neck disorders.[42] It included people with many types of neck pain, including uncomplicated pain, whiplash, and neck pain with radiculopathy, and reported that trials were clinically heterogeneous. However, it did not provide a subgroup analysis in people with uncomplicated neck pain. When assessing any type of neck pain, it found the best evidence of efficacy for interventions that included mobilisation or manipulation plus exercise[32] when compared with any other treatments.

OPTION MULTIMODAL TREATMENT

One RCT identified by a systematic review provided insufficient evidence to assess multimodal treatment in people with uncomplicated neck pain.

Benefits: We found one systematic review[43] (search date 2002, 1 RCT[44]) of multimodal treatment**G** in people with chronic neck pain. **Multimodal treatment versus exercise plus behavioural modification:** The review identified one RCT comparing two types of multimodal treatment.[44] The RCT (66 people with chronic neck and shoulder pain) identified by the review compared exercise plus behavioural modification (including patient education lectures and advice, with a psychologist acting as an advisor to other staff) versus exercise plus cognitive behavioural therapy (with cognitive behavioural therapy administered directly by a psychologist). It found no significant difference in pain or time off work after 6 months between interventions (proportion with improved pain: 32% with multimodal cognitive behavioural therapy *v* 26% with exercise plus behavioural modification, reported as non-significant, P value not reported; time off work: $P = 0.822$; absolute results presented graphically).[44]

Harms: **Multimodal treatment versus exercise plus behavioural modification:** The RCT gave no information on adverse effects.[44]

Comment: None.

OPTION PATIENT EDUCATION

Two RCTs in people with chronic neck, back, or shoulder pain found no significant difference among patient education (individual advice, pamphlets, or group instruction) with or without analgesics and no treatment, stress management, and cognitive behavioural therapy.

Benefits: We found two RCTs.[45,46] The first RCT (243 people with neck and back pain) compared three interventions: an educational pamphlet, a more extensive information programme, and cognitive behavioural therapy (6 sessions).[45] The duration of pain was unspecified but recruitment into the trial was based on self perception that participants were "at risk of developing a chronic problem". The RCT found no significant difference among treatments in pain (worst pain on 0–10 on an Outcome Evaluation Questionnaire: 6.1 with a pamphlet *v* 6.5 with information programme *v* 5.7 with cognitive behavioural therapy; reported as non-significant, P value not reported). Post hoc analysis suggested that cognitive behavioural therapy significantly reduced time off work compared with an educational pamphlet (AR for sick leave of > 30 days in 6 months: 1% with cognitive behavioural therapy *v* 10% with educational pamphlets; $P < 0.05$). The second RCT (282 nursing aides with neck, shoulder, or back pain in the preceding 12 months) compared three interventions: an individualised education and exercise programme, stress management, and no intervention.[46] The RCT found no significant difference in pain among the groups immediately after treatment, or at 12 and 18 months (people with improved pain at 12 months: 8/41 [20%] with individualised education *v* 19/57 [33%] with stress management *v* 18/57 [32%] with no intervention).[46]

Harms: The RCTs gave no information on adverse effects.[45,46]

Comment: None.

OPTION SOFT COLLARS AND SPECIAL PILLOWS

We found no RCTs of sufficient quality on the effects of soft collars or special pillows in people with uncomplicated neck pain.

Benefits: **Soft collars or special pillows:** We found no systematic review or RCTs of sufficient quality.

Harms: We found no RCTs.

Comment: None.

OPTION DRUG TREATMENTS (ANALGESICS, NON-STEROIDAL ANTI-INFLAMMATORY DRUGS, ANTIDEPRESSANTS, OR MUSCLE RELAXANTS)

We found insufficient evidence on the effects of analgesics, non-steroidal anti-inflammatory drugs, antidepressants, or muscle relaxants for neck pain, although they are widely used. Several drugs used to treat neck pain are associated with well documented adverse effects.

Benefits: We found one systematic review (search date 1993[12]) and one subsequent RCT.[47] **Simple analgesics (paracetamol, opioids) and oral non-steroidal anti-inflammatory drugs:** The review found no RCTs. **Antidepressants:** The review found no RCTs in people with uncomplicated neck pain (see comment below). **Muscle relaxants and benzodiazepines:** We found no systematic review or RCTs solely in people with neck pain. We found one systematic review (2 RCTs, 159 people with chronic neck or back pain with acute spasm), which compared three treatments: cyclobenzaprine, diazepam, and placebo.[12] Both RCTs identified by the review found that cyclobenzaprine significantly improved symptoms compared with diazepam and placebo after 2 weeks ($P < 0.05$ in each study), but measured and follow up pain data could not be extracted.[48,49] Applicability of results may be limited in people with uncomplicated neck pain because people with other musculoskeletal disorders were included in the studies. The subsequent RCT (157 people with chronic neck pain) found that eperisone significantly improved pain control compared with placebo after 6 weeks ($P < 0.05$).[47]

Harms: **Simple analgesics (paracetamol and opioids):** We found no reports of harm from simple analgesics. **Oral non-steroidal anti-inflammatory drugs:** See harms of non-steroidal anti-inflammatory drugs, p 1525. One systematic review found no direct comparisons of harms of manipulationⒼ and non-steroidal anti-inflammatory drugs.[40] Calculations based on indirect comparisons found that the risk of a harm with non-steroidal anti-inflammatory drugs was considerably greater than for manipulationⒼ. **Antidepressants:** The review found no RCTs (see harms of antidepressants under generalised anxiety disorder, p 1277). **Muscle relaxants and benzodiazepines:** The RCTs found minor adverse effects, including weakness, dizziness, drowsiness, and gastrointestinal problems occurring in 4% of people treated with muscle relaxants.[12,47] (see harms of benzodiazepines under generalised anxiety disorder, p 1277).

Comment: Applicability of results in people with uncomplicated neck pain may be limited, because many of the RCTs included people with other musculoskeletal disorders, including back pain and acute whiplash.

QUESTION **What are the effects of treatments for acute whiplash injury?**

OPTION **EARLY MOBILISATION**

Four RCTs identified by several systematic reviews provided limited evidence that early mobilisation reduced pain compared with immobilisation or rest plus a collar.

Benefits: **Early mobilisation (including exercises) versus immobilisation or less active treatment:** We found two systematic reviews (search dates 1993[8] and 2003[50]) which between them identified four RCTs.[51–54] The first RCT (61 people with acute whiplash) identified by the reviews compared two treatments: early mobilisation**G** (including Maitland joint mobilisation plus home exercises) versus immobilisation in a collar plus rest for 14 days followed by gradual mobilisation.[51] All participants received analgesics. It found that early mobilisation significantly increased pain relief and improved range of movement after 4 and 8 weeks compared with immobilisation plus less active treatment ($P < 0.01$). The second RCT (247 people with acute whiplash) identified by the reviews compared three interventions: advice on early mobilisation, physical treatments (heat and cold, pulsed electromagnetic field treatment, hydrotherapy, traction, or active and passive repetitive movements), or rest for 7–14 days followed by gentle mobilisation.[52] All participants were given a soft collar and analgesics. Follow up at 2 years of 167 people responding to a questionnaire found that advice on early mobilisation significantly reduced the proportion of people who still had symptoms compared with physical treatments or rest (11/48 [23%] with advice on early mobilisation *v* 22/54 [44%] with physical treatments *v* 12/26 [46%] with rest; $P = 0.02$ for early mobilisation *v* other treatments). The difference remained significant when the 44 people who were not reviewed were assumed to have the same rate of continuing symptoms as the people who rested. The third RCT (97 people with acute whiplash) identified by the reviews found that mobilisation (home exercises based on McKenzie**G** principles) significantly improved pain compared with rest plus a neck collar ($P < 0.001$), but only if mobilisation was started immediately after injury.[53] If mobilisation was delayed by more than 96 hours, there was no significant difference between treatments after 6 months. However, follow up of this RCT found that, at 3 years, mobilisation significantly reduced pain and sick leave ($P < 0.05$) compared with rest plus a neck collar, even if it was delayed for 2 weeks, although only people who had received active intervention within 96 hours had a total cervical range similar to matched controls.[55] The fourth RCT (97 people with acute whiplash) identified by the reviews found early benefits in pain relief and movement with early mobilisation compared with immobilisation in a collar (proportion with neck pain at 6 weeks: 11% with mobilisation *v* 62% with collar; neck stiffness: 2% with mobilisation *v* 38% with collar), but similar pain relief after 12 weeks (proportion with neck pain: 2% with mobilisation *v* 16% with collar).[54] The RCT did not assess the significance of the difference between groups.

Harms: The reviews and RCTs did not consistently report adverse effects.[8,50–54]

Comment: The management of acute whiplash injury remains controversial and needs further investigation. The second review compared active interventions versus no treatment, active versus passive treatments, and active treatments versus each other.[50] It found limited evidence that active and passive interventions seemed more effective than no treatment, but less convincing evidence about the effects of active interventions compared with passive ones. It could no longer justify the conclusion of the previous version of the review that "rest makes rusty". We found one systematic review (search date 2002) examining mobilisation**G** and manipulation**G** for mechanical neck disorders.[42] It included people with many types of neck pain, including uncomplicated pain, whiplash, and neck pain with radiculopathy, and reported that trials were clinically heterogeneous. However, it did not provide a subgroup analysis in people with whiplash. When assessing any type of neck pain, it found the best evidence of efficacy for interventions that included mobilisation or manipulation plus exercise[32] when compared with any other treatments.

OPTION EARLY RETURN TO NORMAL ACTIVITY

One RCT in people with acute whiplash identified by one systematic review provided limited evidence that advice to "act as usual" plus anti-inflammatory drugs improved some symptoms (including pain during daily activities, neck stiffness, memory, concentration, and headache) at 6 months compared with immobilisation plus 14 days' sick leave. It found no significant difference in neck range or sick leave and found that a similar proportion of people had severe neck pain.

Benefits: We found one systematic review (search date 2003),[50] which identified one RCT[56] comparing early return to normal activity versus immobilisation plus rest. The RCT (201 people presenting to an emergency department with acute whiplash) compared advice to "act as usual" plus non-steroidal anti-inflammatory drugs (NSAIDs) versus immobilisation plus 14 days' sick leave plus NSAIDs.[56] It found that advice to "act as usual" plus NSAIDs significantly improved some symptoms (including pain during daily activities, neck stiffness, memory, concentration, and headache; $P < 0.05$ for all outcomes) after 6 months compared with immobilisation plus 14 days' sick leave plus NSAIDs. It found no significant difference between treatments in neck range or length of sick leave (reported as non-significant for both outcomes, P value not reported). The RCT also found that a similar proportion of people had severe symptoms of neck pain after 6 months (proportion of people with severe symptoms defined as > 3 on a scale from 0–5: 11% with advice to "act as usual" *v* 15% with immobilisation).

Harms: The systematic review[50] and RCT[56] gave no information on adverse effects.

Comment: The management of acute whiplash injury remains controversial and needs further investigation. The review compared active interventions versus no treatment, active versus passive treatments, and active treatments versus each other.[50] It found limited evidence that active and passive interventions seemed more effective than no treatment, but less convincing evidence about the effects of active interventions compared with passive ones. It could no longer justify the conclusion of the previous version of the review that "rest makes rusty".

OPTION EXERCISE

One RCT found no significant difference between two home exercise programmes in pain or disability.

Benefits: We found two systematic reviews (search dates 2001[15] and 2003[50]), both of which identified the same single RCT.[57] The RCT (59 people with acute whiplash) compared two home exercise regimens: a regular exercise regimen versus the same exercise regimen plus instructions to perform an isometric exercise at least three times daily.[57] It found no significant difference between treatments in disability or pain after 3 or 6 months (at 6 months: disability measured by Pain Disability Index scale 0–70: mean 15.1 with regular exercise *v* 15.8 with additional isometric exercise; pain measured on a visual analogue scale from 0–10: 2.0 with regular exercise *v* 1.8 with additional isometric; P value reported as non-significant for both outcomes, CI not reported).

Harms: The systematic reviews[15,50] and RCT[57] gave no information on adverse effects.

Comment: Only the 40% of people most severely affected by whiplash were included in the RCT comparing home exercise programmes, which may have led to a poorer outcome than that seen in practice.[57] The management of acute whiplash injury remains controversial and needs further investigation. The second review compared active interventions versus no treatment, active versus passive treatments, and active treatments versus each other.[50] It found limited evidence that active and passive interventions seemed more effective than no treatment, but less convincing evidence about the effects of active interventions compared with passive ones. It could no longer justify the conclusion of the previous version of the review that "rest makes rusty".

OPTION PULSED ELECTROMAGNETIC FIELD TREATMENT

One small RCT identified by two systematic reviews found limited evidence that electromagnetic field treatment reduced pain after 4 weeks but not after 3 months compared with sham treatment.

Benefits: We found two systematic reviews (search dates 1993,[8] 2003[50]), both of which identified the same single RCT.[58] The RCT (40 people with acute whiplash who all received analgesia and a neck collar) compared pulsed electromagnetic field treatment versus sham pulsing electromagnetic field treatment.[58] It found that electromagnetic field treatment significantly reduced pain compared with sham treatment after 4 weeks ($P < 0.05$), but not after 3 months (reported as non-significant, P value not reported; absolute results for both outcomes presented graphically).

Harms: The RCT gave no information on adverse effects.[58]

Comment: The management of acute whiplash injury remains controversial and needs further investigation.

OPTION MULTIMODAL TREATMENT

One RCT identified by a systematic review found that multimodal treatment reduced pain at 1 and 6 months compared with physical treatments.

Benefits: We found one systematic review[50] (search date 2003, 1 RCT,[59] 60 people with whiplash as a result of a road traffic accident in the previous 2 months) that compared multimodal treatment **G** (postural training, psychological support, eye fixation exercises, and manual treatment) versus physical treatments (electrical treatment, sonic treatment, ultrasound, and transcutaneous electrical nerve stimulation).[59] It found that multimodal treatment significantly reduced pain by the end of treatment ($P < 0.05$) and after 1 and 6 months ($P < 0.001$) compared with physical treatments. The RCT also found that multimodal treatment reduced the time taken to return to work.

Harms: The systematic review[50] and RCT[59] gave no information on adverse effects.

Comment: None.

OPTION **DRUG TREATMENTS (ANALGESICS, NON-STEROIDAL ANTI-INFLAMMATORY DRUGS, ANTIDEPRESSANT DRUGS, OR MUSCLE RELAXANTS**

Two systematic reviews identified no RCTs of drug treatments in people with acute whiplash injury.

Benefits: We found two systematic reviews (search date 1993,[8] 2003[50]), which identified no RCTs.

Harms: We found no RCTs.

Comment: None.

QUESTION **What are the effects of treatments for chronic whiplash injury?**

OPTION **PERCUTANEOUS RADIOFREQUENCY NEUROTOMY**

One RCT identified by a systematic review found limited evidence that percutaneous radiofrequency neurotomy reduced pain after 27 weeks compared with sham treatment in people with chronic whiplash injury.

Benefits: **Percutaneous radiofrequency neurotomy versus sham treatment:** We found one systematic review[60] of percutaneous radiofrequency neurotomy for neck pain (search date 2002; 1 RCT;[61] 24 people). The RCT identified by the review found that neurotomy significantly increased the proportion of people who were free from pain compared with sham treatment after 27 weeks (58% with active treatment *v* 8% with sham treatment; ARR 50%, 95% CI 3% to 85%; NNT 2, 95% CI 1 to 29), and that neurotomy significantly increased the median time taken for more than half of the pain to return (263 days with radiofrequency neurotomy *v* 8 days with sham treatment; $P = 0.04$).[61]

Harms: The RCT gave no information on adverse effects.[61]

Comment: Few RCTs have considered treatment for chronic whiplash and many people with whiplash are included in general RCTs of chronic mechanical neck pain.

OPTION **MULTIMODAL TREATMENT**

One small RCT found no difference between multimodal treatment and physical treatments in disability, pain, or range of movement at the end of treatment or at 3 months but it may have been too small to detect a clinically important difference.

Benefits: **Multimodal treatment versus physical treatment:** We found one RCT (33 people with chronic whiplash), which compared physical treatments alone versus multimodal treatment**G** (see comment below).[62] It found no significant difference between treatments in disability, pain, or range of movement at the end of treatment or at 3 months. However, significantly more people treated with multimodal treatment were satisfied with pain control at the end of treatment and their ability to perform activities at 3 months ($P < 0.05$).

Harms: The RCT gave no information on adverse effects.[62]

Comment: Few RCTs have considered treatment for chronic whiplash and many people with whiplash are included in general RCTs of chronic mechanical neck pain. Limitations of this RCT include its small size, and the difference in time spent with the therapist in the two groups.[62]

OPTION PHYSICAL TREATMENTS

One small RCT found no significant difference between physical treatments alone and multimodal treatment in disability, pain, or range of movement at the end of treatment or at 3 months but it may have been too small to detect a clinically important difference.

Benefits: **Physical treatments versus multimodal treatment:** See benefits of multimodal treatment, p 1519.

Harms: The RCT gave no information on adverse effects.[62]

Comment: See comment of multimodal treatment, p 1520.

QUESTION What are the effects of treatments for neck pain with radiculopathy?

OPTION SURGERY VERSUS CONSERVATIVE TREATMENT

One RCT found no significant difference in pain at 1 year between surgery and conservative treatment in people with neck pain with radiculopathy.

Benefits: We found one systematic review (search date 1998,[63] 1 RCT[64]). The RCT included in the review (81 people with severe radicular symptoms for at least 3 months; outcome assessors not blinded; see comment below) compared three interventions: surgery, physical treatments, and immobilisation in a neck collar.[64] It found no significant difference among treatments in symptoms after 1 year (mean pain on a 100 mm visual analogue scale at 12 months: 30 mm with surgery *v* 39 mm with physical treatments *v* 35 mm with collar; P value reported as non-significant, CI not reported).

Harms: The RCT gave no information on adverse effects.[64]

Comment: In the RCT, the number of people with prolapsed intervertebral disc was not reported.[64] The RCT reported that people who did not improve between 3 months and 12 months were given additional treatments: one person in the physical treatment group and five in the collar group had surgery; eight people in the surgery group had a second operation; and 12 people in the surgery group and 11 in the collar group received physical treatments. The RCT also assessed emotional state and reported that, when assessing all participants in the trial, 41% of people had a high anxiety score and 31% of people had a high depression score, which correlated with pain intensity after but not before treatment.[65] At 1 year, 19% of people in the trial were depressed, which suggests that treatment should aim to improve both physical and psychological symptoms.[65] Conservative treatment needs further assessment, particularly in people considered to be poor risk candidates for surgery.

OPTION DRUG TREATMENTS (EPIDURAL STEROID INJECTIONS, ANALGESICS, NON-STEROIDAL ANTI-INFLAMMATORY DRUGS, OR MUSCLE RELAXANTS)

We found no RCTs examining the effects of analgesics, non-steroidal anti-inflammatory drugs, or muscle relaxants in people with neck pain with radiculopathy. Two RCTs found limited evidence that cervical steroid epidural injections may improve pain from baseline in people with chronic neck pain with or without radiculopathy.

Benefits: **Periradicular, cervical epidural steroid injections, or both:** We found one systematic review[66] (search date 2003, 2 RCTs,[67,68] 76 people with neck pain with radiculopathy). The first RCT (52 people with chronic cervical brachialgia) identified by the review compared cervical epidural steroid plus lidocaine injection versus steroid plus lidocaine injections into the posterior neck muscles.[67] It found that more people receiving cervical epidural steroid injections had reduced pain at 1 year than people receiving steroids injections to the posterior neck muscles (68% with epidural *v* 12% with control; significance of difference between groups not reported in review[66]). The second RCT (24 people with neck pain with radiculopathy for > 1 year) found similar success rates over 1 year between epidural steroid (triamcinolone) plus lidocaine, and epidural steroid (triamcinolone) plus lidocaine plus morphine (78.5% with epidural steroid plus lidocaine *v* 80% with epidural steroid plus lidocaine plus morphine; significance of difference from baseline within group and difference between groups not reported in review). **Simple analgesics (paracetamol and opioids) and oral non-steroidal anti-inflammatory drugs; antidepressants; muscle relaxants and benzodiazepines:** We found no systematic review or RCTs.

Harms: **Periradicular, cervical epidural steroid injections, or both:** The review reported occasional complications, such as infection or abscess formation after cervical epidural injection.[66]

Comment: None.

GLOSSARY

Manipulation A manual treatment involving the use of short or long lever high velocity thrusts directed at one or more of the cervical spine joints that does not involve anaesthesia or instrumentation. Manual treatment is usually performed by chiropractors or osteopaths.

McKenzie treatment A type of mobilisation consisting of a comprehensive mechanical evaluation to assess the effect of repetitive movements, static positioning, or both, on the patient's symptoms. This mechanical diagnosis is meant to enable the physiotherapist to prescribe a series of individualised exercises. The emphasis is on active patient involvement, with the aim of minimising the number of visits to the clinic. For people with more difficult mechanical problems, a certified McKenzie physiotherapist can provide advanced hands on techniques until the person is able to perform the prescribed exercises alone.

Mobilisation Any manual treatment to improve joint function that does not involve high velocity movement, anaesthesia, or instrumentation. Usually performed by physiotherapists.

Multimodal treatment includes a physical or mechanical treatment plus psychotherapy such as cognitive behavioural therapy. Usually performed by physiotherapists and psychologists working together. In this review, multimodal treatment does not include the use of combinations of physical and mechanical treatments, although some reviews and RCTs use this definition.

Neck Disability Index (NDI) is a 10 item self report measure. Items pertain to pain intensity, personal care, lifting, reading, headaches, concentration, work, driving, sleeping, and recreation. Each item is rated on a 6 point scale (0–5), so the NDI scores vary from 0–50. The results are recalculated and expressed on a scale ranging from 0% (no disability) to 100% (maximum disability).

Substantive changes

This chapter has been restructured into more individual interventions in order to better isolate, where possible, which interventions could be of use in different types of neck pain.

Exercise for uncomplicated neck pain One subsequent RCT added;[22] categorisation unchanged.

Manipulation for uncomplicated neck pain Two systematic reviews added;[30,31] categorisation unchanged.

Manipulation versus mobilisation for uncomplicated neck pain One follow up questionnaire added;[41] categorisation unchanged.

Mobilisation for uncomplicated neck pain Two systematic reviews added;[30,31] categorisation unchanged.

Drug treatments for neck pain with radiculopathy One systematic review added;[66] categorisation unchanged.

Early mobilisation for acute whiplash injury One follow up of an RCT added;[55] categorisation unchanged.

REFERENCES

1. Måkelå M, Heliövaara M, Sievers K, et al. Prevalence, determinants, and consequences of chronic neck pain in Finland. *Am J Epidemiol* 1991;134:1356–1367.
2. Cote P, Cassidy D, Carroll L. The Saskatchewan health and back pain survey: the prevalence of neck pain and related disability in Saskatchewan adults. *Spine* 1998;23:1689–1698.
3. Hackett GI, Hudson MF, Wylie JB, et al. Evaluation of the efficacy and acceptability to patients of a physiotherapist working in a health centre. *BMJ* 1987;294:24–26.
4. Waalen D, White P, Waalen J. Demographic and clinical characteristics of chiropractic patients: a 5-year study of patients treated at the Canadian Memorial Chiropractic College. *J Can Chiropract Assoc* 1994;38:75–82.
5. Lamberts H, Brouwer H, Groen AJM, et al. The traditional model in practice. *Huisart Wet* 1987;30:105–113. [In Dutch]
6. Kvarnstrom S. Occurrence of musculoskeletal disorders in a manufacturing industry with special attention to occupational shoulder disorders. *Scand J Rehabil Med Suppl* 1983;8:1–114.
7. Squires B, Gargan MF, Bannister GC. Soft-tissue injuries of the cervical spine: 15 year follow-up. *J Bone Joint Surg Br* 1996;78:955–957.
8. Spitzer WO, Skovron ML, Salmi LR, et al. Scientific monograph of the Quebec Task Force on whiplash-associated disorders: redefining "whiplash" and its management. *Spine* 1995;20(suppl 8):1–73. Search date 1993; primary sources Medline, TRIS, NTIS, personal contacts, and Task Force reference lists. [Erratum in *Spine* 1995;20:2372]
9. Ferrari R, Russell AS. Epidemiology of whiplash: an international dilemma. *Ann Rheum Dis* 1999;58:1–5.
10. Vernon H, Mior S. The neck disability index: a study of reliability and validity. *J Manipulative Physiol Ther* 1991;14:409–415.
11. Koes BW, Assendelft WJ, Van der Heijden GJ, et al. Spinal manipulation and mobilisation for back and neck pain: a blinded review. *BMJ* 1991;303:1298–1303. Search date 1990; primary source Medline.
12. Aker PD, Gross AR, Goldsmith CH, et al. Conservative management of mechanical neck pain: systematic overview and meta-analysis. *BMJ* 1996;313:1291–1296. Search date 1993; primary sources Medlars, Embase, Cinahl, and Chirolars.
13. Kjellman GV, Skargren EI, Oberg BE. A critical analysis of randomised clinical trials on neck pain and treatment efficacy. A review of the literature. *Scand J Rehabil Med* 1999;31:139–152. Search date 1995; primary sources Medline, Cinahl, and hand searches of reference lists.
14. Philadelphia Panel. Evidence-based clinical practice guidelines on selected rehabilitation interventions for neck pain. *Phys Ther* 2001;81:1701–1717. Search date 2000; primary sources Medline, Embase, Current Contents, Cinahl, Cochrane Controlled Trials Register, Cochrane Field of Rehabilitation and Related Therapies, Cochrane Musculoskeletal Group, and Pedro.
15. Sarig-Bahat, H. Evidence for exercise therapy in mechanical neck disorders. *Man Ther* 2003;8:10–20. Search date 2001; primary sources Amed, Cinahl, Embase, SportsDiscus, and Pedro.
16. Revel M, Minguet M, Gregory P, et al. Changes in cervicocephalic kinesthesia after a proprioceptive rehabilitation program in patients with neck pain: a randomised controlled study. *Arch Phys Med Rehabil* 1994;75:895–899.
17. Waling K, Sundelin G, Ahlgren C, et al. Perceived pain before and after three exercise programs — a controlled clinical trial of women with work-related trapezius myalgia. *Pain* 2000;85:201–207.
18. Waling K, Jaörvholm B, Sundelin G. Effects of training on female trapezius myalgia: an intervention study with a 3-year follow-up period. *Spine* 2002;27:789–796.
19. Ylinen J, Takala E, Nykanen M, et al. Active neck muscle training in the treatment of chronic neck pain in women: a randomized controlled trial. *JAMA* 2003;289:2509–2516.
20. Hoving J, Koes B, de Vet H, et al. Manual therapy, physical therapy, or continued care by a general practitioner for patients with neck pain. A randomized, controlled trial. *Ann Intern Med* 2002;136:713–722.
21. Korthals-de Bos I, Hoving J, Van Tulder, M, et al. Cost effectiveness of physiotherapy, manual therapy, and general practitioner care for neck pain: economic evaluation alongside a randomised controlled trial. *BMJ* 2003;326:911–914.
22. Viljanen M, Malmivaara A, Uitti J, et al. Effectiveness of dynamic muscle training, relaxation training, or ordinary activity for chronic neck pain: randomised controlled trial. *BMJ* 2003;327:475–477.
23. Van der Heijden GJ, Beurskens AJ, Koes BW, et al. The efficacy of traction for back and neck pain: a systematic, blinded review of randomized clinical trial methods. *Phys Ther* 1995;75:93–104. Search date 1992; primary sources Medline, Embase, Index to Chiropractic Literature, and Physiotherapy Index.

24. Klaber Moffett JA, Hughes GI, Griffiths P. An investigation of the effects of cervical traction. Part 1: Clinical effectiveness. *Clin Rehabil* 1990;4:205–211.
25. British Association of Physical Medicine. Pain in the neck and arm: a multicentre trial of the effects of physiotherapy. *BMJ* 1966;5426:253–258.
26. Trock DH, Bollet AJ, Markoll R. The effect of pulsed electromagnetic fields in the treatment of osteoarthritis of the knee and cervical spine. Report of randomized double-blind placebo controlled trials. *J Rheumatol* 1994;21:1903–1911.
27. Hurwitz EL, Aker PD, Adams AH, et al. Manipulation and mobilization of the cervical spine: a systematic review of the literature. *Spine* 1996;21:1746–1760. Search date 1995; primary sources Medline, Embase, Chirolars, and Cinahl.
28. White AR, Ernst E. A systematic review of randomized controlled trials of acupuncture for neck pain. *Rheumatology* 1999;38:143–147. Search date 1998; primary sources Medline, Embase, Cochrane Library, and CISCOM (a database specialising in complementary medicine).
29. Smith LA, Oldman AD, McQuay HJ, et al. Teasing apart quality and validity in systematic reviews: an example from acupuncture trials in chronic neck and back pain. *Pain* 2000;86:119–132. Search date 1998; primary sources: Cochrane Controlled Trials Register. Medline, Embase, Cinahl, Psychlit, Oxford Pain Relief Database, and hand searches of reference lists.
30. Ernst E. Chiropractic spinal manipulation for neck pain: a systematic review. *J Pain* 2003;4:417–421. Search date 2002; Medline, Embase, Ciscom, Amed, and Cochrane Library. [Comment]
31. Oduneye F. Spinal manipulation for chronic neck pain. In Bazian Ltd (Ed) *STEER: Succinct and Timely Evaluated Reviews* 2004; 4(4). Bazian Ltd and Wessex Institute for Health Research and Development, University of Southampton. Search date 2003; primary sources Medline, Embase, Cochrane Library, *Clinical Evidence*, Centre for Reviews and Dissemination Databases, University of York.
32. Bronfort G, Evans R, Nelson B, et al. A randomized clinical trial of exercise and spinal manipulation for patients with chronic neck pain. *Spine* 2001;26:788–797.
33. Jordan A, Bendix T, Nielsen H, et al. Intensive training, physiotherapy, or manipulation for patients with chronic neck pain. A prospective, single-blinded, randomized clinical trial. *Spine* 1998;23:311–319.
34. Koes BW, Bouter LM, Van Mameren H, et al. Randomised clinical trial of manipulative therapy and physiotherapy for persistent back and neck complaints: results of one year follow up. *BMJ* 1992;304:601–605.
35. Sloop PR, Smith DS, Goldenberg E, et al. Manipulation for chronic neck pain: a double-blind controlled study. *Spine* 1982;7:532–535.
36. Howe DH, Newcombe RG, Wade MT. Manipulation of the cervical spine: a pilot study. *J R Coll Gen Pract* 1983;33:574–579.
37. Cassidy JD, Lopes AA, Yong-Hing K. The immediate effect of manipulation versus mobilization on pain and range of motion in the cervical spine: a randomised controlled trial. *J Manipulative Physiol Ther* 1992;15:570–575.
38. Evans R, Bronfort G, Nelson B, et al. Two-year follow-up of a randomized clinical trial of spinal manipulation and two types of exercise for patients with chronic neck pain. *Spine* 2002;27:2383–2389.
39. Hurwitz EL, Morgenstern H, Harber P, et al. A randomized trial of chiropractic manipulation and mobilization for patients with neck pain: clinical outcomes from the UCLA neck-pain study. *Am J Public Health* 2002;92:1634–1641.
40. Dabbs V, Lauretti WJ. A risk assessment of cervical manipulation vs NSAIDS for the treatment of neck pain. *J Manipulative Physiol Ther* 1995;18:530–536.
41. Hurwitz EL, Morgenstern H, Vassilaki M, et al. Adverse reactions to chiropractic treatment and their effects on satisfaction and clinical outcomes among patients enrolled in the UCLA Neck Pain Study. *J Manipulative Physiol Ther* 2004;27:16–25.
42. Gross AK, Hoving JL, Haines TA et al. Cervical overview group. Manipulation and mobilisation for mechanical neck disorders (Cochrane review). In: The Cochrane Library, Issue 1, 2004. Chichester, UK: John Wiley & Sons Ltd. Search date 2002; primary sources Cochrane Controlled Trials Register, Medline, Embase, Mantis, Cinahl, and ICL.
43. Karjalainen K, Malmivaara A, Van Tulder M, et al. Multidisciplinary biopsychosocial rehabilitation for neck and shoulder pain among working age adults (Cochrane Review). In: The Cochrane Library, Issue 2, 2004. Chichester, UK: John Wiley & Sons, Ltd. Search date 2002; primary sources Cochrane Register of Medline, Psychlit, Embase, and Cochrane.
44. Jensen I, Nygren A, Gamberale F, et al. The role of the psychologist in multidisciplinary treatments for chronic neck and shoulder pain: a controlled cost-effectiveness study. *Scand J Rehabil Med* 1995;27:19–26.
45. Linton SJ, Andersson T. Can chronic disability be prevented? A randomized trial of a cognitive-behaviour intervention and two forms of information for patients with spinal pain. *Spine* 2000:25:2825–2831.
46. Horneij E, Hemborg B, Jensen I, et al. No significant differences between intervention programmes on neck, shoulder and low back pain: a prospective randomized study among home-care personnel. *J Rehabil Med* 2001;33:170–176.
47. Bose K. The efficacy and safety of eperisone in patients with cervical spondylosis: results of a randomised double-blind placebo-controlled trial. *Methods Find Exp Clin Pharmacol* 1999;21:209–213.
48. Basmajian JV. Cyclobenzaprine hydrochloride effect on skeletal muscle spasm in the lumbar region and neck: two double-blind controlled clinical and laboratory studies. *Arch Phys Med Rehabil* 1978;59:58–63.
49. Bercel NA. Cyclobenzaprine in the treatment of skeletal muscle spasm in osteoarthritis of the cervical and lumbar spine. *Curr Ther Res* 1977;22:462–468.
50. Verhagen AP, Scholten-Peeters GG, de Bie RA, et al. Conservative treatment for whiplash (Cochrane Review). In: The Cochrane Library, Issue 1, 2004. Chichester, UK: John Wiley & Sons, Ltd. Search date 2003; primary sources Medline, Embase, Cinahl, Psychlit, Pedro and the database of the Dutch Institute of Allied Health Professions.
51. Mealy K, Brennan H, Fenelon GC. Early mobilisation of acute whiplash injuries. *BMJ* 1986;292:656–657.
52. McKinney LA. Early mobilisation and outcome in acute sprains of the neck. *BMJ* 1989;299:1006–1008.
53. Rosenfeld M, Gunnarsson R, Borenstein P. Early intervention in whiplash-associated disorders: a comparison of two treatment protocols. *Spine* 2000;25:1782–1787.
54. Bonk AD, Ferrari R, Giebel GD, et al. Prospective, randomized, controlled study of activity versus collar, and the natural history for whiplash injury, in Germany. *J Musculoskel Pain* 2000;8:123–132.
55. Rosenfeld M, Seferiadis A, Carlsson J, et al. Active intervention in patients with whiplash-associated disorders improves long-term prognosis: a randomized controlled clinical trial. *Spine* 2003;28:2491–2498.
56. Borchgrevink GE, Kaasa A, McDonagh D, et al. Acute treatment of whiplash neck sprain injuries: a randomised trial of treatment during the first 14 days after a car accident. *Spine* 1998;23:25–31.
57. Söderlund A, Olerud C, Lindberg P. Acute whiplash-associated disorders (WAD): the effects of early mobilization and prognostic factors in long-term symptomatology. *Clin Rehab* 2000;14:457–467.
58. Foley-Nolan D, Moore K, Codd M, et al. Low energy high frequency pulsed electromagnetic therapy for

acute whiplash injuries. A double blind randomised controlled study. *Scand J Rehabil Med* 1992;24:51–59.

59. Provinciali L, Baroni M, Illuminati L, et al. Multimodal treatment to prevent the late whiplash syndrome. *Scand J Rehabil Med* 1996;28:105–111.
60. Niemisto L, Kalso E, Malmivaara A, et al. Radiofrequency denervation for neck and back pain (Cochrane Review). In: The Cochrane Library Issue 2, 2004, Chichester, UK. John Wiley & son Ltd. Search date 2002; primary sources Cochrane Controlled Trials Register, Medline, Psychlit, and Embase.
61. Lord SM, Barnsley L, Wallis BJ, et al. Percutaneous radio-frequency neurotomy for chronic cervical zygapophyseal-joint pain. *N Engl J Med* 1996;335:1721–1726.
62. Söderlund A, Lindberg P. Cognitive behavioural components in physiotherapy management of chronic whiplash associated disorders (WAD) — a randomised group study. *Physiother Theory Pract* 2001;17:229–238.
63. Fouyas IP, Statham PF, Sandercock PA, et al. Surgery for cervical radiculomyelopathy (Cochrane Review). In: The Cochrane Library, Issue 2, 2004, Chichester, UK. John Wiley & Son Ltd. Search date 1998; primary sources Medline, Embase, and Cochrane Controlled Trials Register.
64. Persson LC, Carlsson CA, Carlsson JY. Long-lasting cervical radicular pain managed with surgery, physiotherapy, or a cervical collar: a prospective randomised study. *Spine* 1997;22:751–758.
65. Persson LCG, Lilja A. Pain, coping, emotional state and physical function in patients with chronic radicular neck pain. A comparison between patients treated with surgery, physiotherapy or neck collar — a blinded, prospective randomized study. *Disabil Rehabil* 2001;23:325–335.
66. Boswell MV, Hansen HC, Trescot AM, Hirsch J. A. Epidural steroids in the management of chronic spinal pain and radiculopathy. *Pain Physician* 2003;6:319–334. Search date 2003; primary sources Medline, Embase, systematic reviews, and narrative reviews.
67. Stav A, Ovadia L, Sternberg A, et al. Cervical epidural steroid injection for cervicobrachialgia. *Acta Anaesthesiol Scand* 1993;37:562–566.
68. Castagnera L, Maurette P, Pointillart V, et al. Long-term results of cervical epidural steroid injection with and without morphine in chronic cervical radicular pain. *Pain* 1994;58:239–243.

Allan Binder
Consultant Rheumatologist
Lister Hospital
Stevenage
UK

Competing interests: None declared.

Non-steroidal anti-inflammatory drugs

Search date January 2004

Peter C Gøtzsche

QUESTIONS

INTERVENTIONS

See glossary Ⓖ

Key Messages

Differences between non-steroidal anti-inflammatory drugs (NSAIDs)

- **Choice between different NSAIDs** Systematic reviews found no important differences in efficacy between different NSAIDs. Cyclo-oxygenase-2 (COX 2) inhibitors reduce gastroscopically diagnosed ulcers compared with other NSAIDs, but the reduction in clinical effects was less marked, and COX 2 inhibitors may increase the risk of myocardial infarction.
- **NSAIDs in increased doses** Systematic reviews found that benefits of NSAIDs increased towards a maximum value at high doses. Recommended doses are close to creating the maximum benefit. In contrast, three systematic reviews found no ceiling for adverse effects, which increased in an approximately linear fashion with dose.

Preventing gastrointestinal adverse effects

- **H_2 blockers in people who cannot avoid NSAIDs** One systematic review in people who had taken NSAIDs for 3 months found that H_2 blockers reduced endoscopically diagnosed gastric and duodenal ulcers compared with placebo. One weak RCT found limited evidence that misoprostol reduced the number of people with NSAID induced gastric ulcers compared with 300 mg daily ranitidine.
- **Omeprazole in people who cannot avoid NSAIDs** One systematic review in people who had taken NSAIDs for at least 3 months found that omeprazole reduced endoscopically diagnosed gastric and duodenal ulcers compared with placebo.

- **Misoprostol in people who cannot avoid NSAIDs** One systematic review in people who had taken NSAIDs for at least 3 months found that misoprostol reduced gastric or duodenal ulcers compared with placebo. However, RCTs found that misoprostol increased clinical gastrointestinal adverse events, such as diarrhoea and abdominal pain, compared with placebo. One RCT found no significant difference in the number of people taking NSAIDs and with proven gastric ulceration or erosion in successful response to treatment with misoprostol compared with omeprazole.

Topical NSAIDs

- **Topical NSAIDs in acute and chronic pain conditions** One systematic review in people with acute and chronic pain conditions found that topical NSAIDs reduced pain compared with placebo.
- **Topical versus systemic NSAIDs or alternative analgesics** One systematic review found no high quality RCTs of topical NSAIDs compared with oral forms of the same NSAID, or with paracetamol.

DEFINITION Non-steroidal anti-inflammatory drugs (NSAIDs) have anti-inflammatory, analgesic, and antipyretic effects, and inhibit platelet aggregation. The drugs have no documented effect on the course of musculoskeletal diseases, such as osteoarthritis, (Web only).

INCIDENCE/PREVALENCE NSAIDs are widely used. Almost 10% of people in the Netherlands used a non-aspirin NSAID in 1987, and the overall use was 11 defined daily doses Ⓖ per 1000 population per day.[1] In Australia in 1994, overall use was 35 defined daily doses per 1000 population per day, with 36% of the people receiving NSAIDs for osteoarthritis, 42% for sprain and strain or low back pain, and 4% for rheumatoid arthritis; 35% were aged over 60 years.[2]

AIMS OF INTERVENTION To reduce symptoms in rheumatic disorders; to avoid severe gastrointestinal adverse effects.

OUTCOMES **Primary outcomes:** pain intensity; personal preference for one drug over another; global efficacy; clinically significant gastrointestinal complications. **Secondary outcomes:** number of tender joints; perforation; gastrointestinal haemorrhage; dyspepsia; and ulcer detected by routine endoscopy; other adverse effects.

METHODS *Clinical Evidence* search and appraisal January 2004. More than 100 systematic reviews and thousands of RCTs have compared various NSAIDs. Many RCTs are unpublished or published in sources that are not indexed in publicly available databases. The quality of the RCTs is variable and bias is common, both in the design and analysis of the RCTs, to such an extent that one systematic review identified false significant findings favouring new drugs over control drugs in 6% of RCTs.[3] We included only large RCTs that provided clinically important information not already covered in the systematic reviews. We have favoured systematic reviews that have not been sponsored or authored by industry, as bias in such reviews has been repeatedly demonstrated, but may be difficult to detect.[4] For example, it is easy to seemingly follow the rules for systematic reviews and yet adopt inclusion and exclusion criteria that omit inconvenient studies.

QUESTION Are there any important differences between available non-steroidal anti-inflammatory drugs (NSAIDs)?

OPTION DIFFERENCES BETWEEN AVAILABLE NSAIDS

Systematic reviews found no important differences in efficacy between different NSAIDs. Cyclo-oxygenase-2 (COX 2) inhibitors reduce gastroscopically diagnosed ulcers compared with other NSAIDs, but the reduction in clinical effects was less marked, and COX 2 inhibitors may increase the risk of myocardial infarction. Systematic reviews found that

benefits of NSAIDs increased towards a maximum value at high doses. Recommended doses are close to creating the maximum benefit. In contrast, three systematic reviews found no ceiling for adverse effects, which increased in an approximately linear fashion with dose.

Benefits: **Indometacin (indomethacin) versus newer NSAIDs:** We found one systematic review (search date 1985, 37 crossover RCTs, 1416 people with rheumatoid arthritis), which compared indometacin (indomethacin) with 10 newer NSAIDs for a median of 2 weeks with each drug.[5] Four of the RCTs included a placebo period and one RCT compared four drugs. It found that 5% more people (95% CI 0% to 10%) preferred the newer NSAID to indometacin. **COX 2 inhibitors versus older NSAIDs:** We found two systematic reviews.[6,7] Both found that COX 2 inhibitors were no more effective for clinical outcomes than older NSAIDs. **Other comparisons of NSAIDs:** We found five other systematic reviews comparing different NSAIDs.[8–12] The first of these systematic reviews (search date 1988, 88 RCTs each comparing 2 NSAIDs, 6440 people with rheumatoid arthritis) found no significant differences in the number of tender joints improved between 17 different NSAIDs.[8] The second and third reviews (search dates 1994[9] and 1996[10]) found no clear differences between various NSAIDs used to treat osteoarthritis of the hip (39 RCTs)[9] or the knee (16 RCTs; see NSAIDs under osteoarthritis, [Web only]).[10] The fourth and fifth systematic reviews were of people with acute musculoskeletal syndromes and identified generally poor quality RCTs.[11,12] The fourth review (search date 1998, 17 RCTs for shoulder pain) was inconclusive.[12] The fifth systematic review (search date 1993, 84 RCTs, 32 025 people with soft tissue injuries of the ankle) was unable to pool data.[11] **Dose response relation:** We found three systematic reviews.[13,14,8] The first review (search date 1985; 19 RCTs in which participants were randomised to more than 1 dose of 9 different NSAIDs) found a dose response relation that saturated at high doses.[13] This and the second systematic review (search date 1992, 1545 people)[14] found that the recommended dosages were close to providing a ceiling effect.[13,14] The third of these reviews (115 RCTs) found no significant differences between various doses of drugs;[8] 10/21 RCTs of ibuprofen had used a daily dosage of 1200 mg or less.[8]

Harms: **Indometacin (indomethacin) versus newer NSAIDs:** The systematic review that compared indometacin with newer NSAIDs[5] did not report on harms separately, but combined benefits and harms in one overall outcome that was patient preference. **COX 2 inhibitors versus older NSAIDs:** We found two systematic reviews in people with rheumatoid arthritis, one prespecified meta-analysis in people with osteoarthritis, and one systematic review assessing the risk of cardiovascular events associated with selective COX 2 inhibitors.[6,7,15,16] Overall, they found that COX 2 inhibitors reduced endoscopically detected upper gastrointestinal ulcers compared with other NSAIDs, although effects on clinical gastrointestinal adverse effects were less marked, and there was some evidence that COX-2 inhibitors may increase cardiovascular risk compared with other NSAIDs. **Other comparisons of NSAIDs:** The systematic reviews did not report useful data on harms.[8–12] **Dose response relation:** Four systematic reviews (search dates 1992[14,17]; 1994[18], and 2001[19]) found no ceiling effect for adverse effects, and found that the incidence of adverse effects increased in an approximately linear fashion with dose.

Comment: Important differences in adverse effects seem to exist between different NSAIDs. In contrast, the beneficial effects of NSAIDs seem similar. People's preferences for particular drugs have not been replicated and could, therefore, be because of chance or natural fluctuations in disease activity.[20,21] The evidence suggests that if the NSAID is unsatisfactory, switching to another NSAID will not solve the problem.[20,21] Likewise, doubling the dose of an NSAID leads to only a small increase in effect, which may not be clinically relevant. In acute musculoskeletal problems, it is doubtful whether NSAIDs have any clinically relevant anti-inflammatory effect; we found no large double blind RCT comparing an NSAID with paracetamol. Paracetamol has been studied in osteoarthritis, where it had much the same effect as naproxen (see simple analgesics v NSAIDs under osteoarthritis, p 000). One RCT identified by the review of celecoxib (the CLASS study), which compared the gastrointestinal toxicity of celecoxib versus ibuprofen and diclofenac, has been criticised because the publication differs from the trial protocol in objectives, primary outcomes, statistical analysis, and trial duration.[6]

QUESTION **What are the effects of co-treatments to reduce the risk of gastrointestinal adverse effects of non-steroidal anti-inflammatory drugs (NSAIDs)?**

OPTION **CO-TREATMENTS TO REDUCE THE RISK OF GASTROINTESTINAL ADVERSE EFFECTS OF NSAIDS**

One systematic review in people who had taken NSAIDs for 3 months found that H_2 blockers misoprostol and omeprazole reduced endoscopically diagnosed gastric and duodenal ulcers compared with placebo. One systematic review in people who had taken NSAIDs for at least 3 months has found that misoprostol reduces gastric or duodenal ulcers compared with placebo. One weak RCT found limited evidence that misoprostol reduced the number of people with NSAID induced gastric ulcers compared with 300 mg of ranitidine daily. However, RCTs found that misoprostol increased clinical gastrointestinal adverse events, such as diarrhoea and abdominal pain, compared with placebo. One RCT found that omeprazole was more effective than ranitidine in achieving remission of gastric ulcers after 6 months.

Benefits: We found one systematic review.[22] **Misoprostol versus placebo:** The systematic review (search date 2002) included people who had received NSAIDs for at least 3 months.[22] Eleven RCTs (3641 people) assessed endoscopically diagnosed ulcers and found that misoprostol (all doses from 400 to 800 μg per day combined) significantly reduced endoscopically confirmed ulcers compared with placebo after at least 3 months (gastric ulcer: RR 0.26, 95% CI 0.17 to 0.39; duodenal ulcer: RR 0.47, 95% CI 0.33 to 0.69). Indirect comparisons of different RCTs suggested a dose response relationship for gastric ulcers in the dose range 400 to 800 μg (misoprostol 400 μg: RR 0.42, 95% CI 0.28 to 0.67; misprostol 800 μg: RR 0.17, 95% CI 0.11 to 0.24; difference between 400 and 800 μg; P = 0.006). Only one RCT (8843 people with rheumatoid arthritis, mean age 68 years, all treated with NSAIDs) presented clinically relevant outcomes.[23] It found that misoprostol 800 μg significantly reduced gastrointestinal events (perforation, gastric outlet obstruction, or bleeding detected by clinical symptoms or investigation) compared with placebo at 6 months (25/4404 [0.6%] with misoprostol *v* 42/4439 [1.0%] with placebo; ARR 0.4%; NNT 265, 95% CI 133 to 6965).[23] The NNT would drop as higher risk patients are considered. **H_2 blockers versus placebo:** The systematic review identified five RCTs (1005 people who had received NSAIDs for at least 3 months) comparing H_2 blockers with placebo.[22] It found that standard doses of H_2 blockers significantly reduced endoscopic ulcers at 3 months or longer (48/494 [10%] with H_2 blockers *v* 75/487 [15%] with placebo; RR 0.63, 95% CI 0.45 to 0.88) **Omeprazole versus placebo:** The systematic review identified three RCTs (774 people who had received NSAIDs for at least 3 months comparing omeprazole with placebo).[22] It found that omeprazole reduced the development of ulcers detected by endoscopy compared with placebo (ARR 13%, 95% CI 8% to 18% for gastric ulcer; ARR 9%, 95% CI 5% to 12% for duodenal ulcer). **Misoprostol versus proton pump inhibitor:** The systematic review identified two RCTs comparing misoprostol with proton pump inhibitors.[22] The first RCT in the review (935 people treated with NSAIDs who had ulcers or more than 10 erosions at endoscopy) compared misoprostol (200 µg four times daily) with omeprazole (20 mg or 40 mg daily) once daily.[24] Treatment success was defined as fewer than five erosions at each site, no ulcers, and not more than mild dyspepsia.[24] It found no significant difference in treatment success between misoprostol and omeprazole at 8 weeks (71% with misoprostol *v* 76% with omeprazole 20 mg *v* 75% with omeprazole 40 mg). The second RCT in the review (537 people, long term NSAID users with endoscopically confirmed gastric ulcer) compared four treatments: misoprostol (200 µg four times daily); two different doses of lansoprazole (15 mg and 30 mg) once daily, and placebo. It found that misoprostol significantly increased the length of time to recurrence compared with the other treatments (time to gastric ulcer: misoprostol *v* placebo, $P < 0.001$; misoprostol *v* lansoprazole 15 mg, $P = 0.01$; misoprostol *v* lansoprazole 30 mg, $P = 0.04$; AR of being free of gastric ulcer at 12 weeks: 93% with misoprostol *v* 51% with placebo *v* 80% with lansoprazole 15 mg *v* 82% with lansoprazole 30 mg).[25] **Omeprazole versus H_2 blockers:** In a similarly designed RCT (541 people), treatment was successful in 80% given omeprazole (20 mg), 79% given omeprazole (40 mg), and 63% given ranitidine (300 mg daily).[26] The estimated proportions in remission after 6 months were 72% with omeprazole (20 mg) and 59% with ranitidine (300 mg) (ARR for omeprazole *v* ranitidine 13%, 95% CI 4% to 22%; NNT 8). **Misoprostol versus H_2 blockers:** The systematic review identified one RCT comparing misoprostol (800 µg) with ranitidine (300 mg daily).[22] In the RCT (538 people with NSAID related upper gastrointestinal pain without endoscopic evidence of ulcers), one third of the people were excluded from analysis because of problems with adherence and missing endoscopic examinations.[27] It found that misoprostol significantly reduced the number of people with gastric ulcers at least 3 mm in diameter at 8 weeks compared with ranitidine (1% with misoprostol *v* 6% with ranitidine; ARR 5% for misoprostol *v* ranitidine, 95% CI 2% to 9%; NNT 20). It found no significant difference in the number of people with duodenal ulcers (1% with both drugs).[27]

Harms: **Misoprostol versus placebo:** In one of the large RCTs, significantly more people receiving misoprostol than placebo withdrew from the study because of adverse events, primarily diarrhoea and abdominal pain (1210/4404 [27%] *v* 896/4439 [20%]; ARI 7%; RR 1.36, 95% CI 1.26 to 1.47; NNH 14, 95% CI 12 to 19).[23] There was no significant difference in the number of deaths (17/4404 [0.4%] deaths in the misoprostol group *v* 21/4439 [0.5%] in the placebo group; ARR 0.1%; RR 0.82, 95% CI 0.43 to 1.55). One person on placebo died as a direct result of gastrointestinal toxicity. **Omeprazole versus H_2 blockers:** Few adverse events were reported in the RCT comparing omeprazole with ranitidine. Treatment discontinuations (all causes) occurred in 10% of people taking omeprazole (20 mg), 10% taking omeprazole (40 mg), and 14% taking ranitidine; significance not reported.[26] **Misoprostol versus H_2 blockers:** In the largest RCT comparing misoprostol versus ranitidine, adverse events (mostly gastrointestinal) occurred in 77% of people taking misoprostol and 66% taking ranitidine, with withdrawal rates of 13% on misoprostol and 7% on ranitidine (ARR for withdrawal ranitidine *v* misoprostol 6%, 95% CI 1% to 11%; NNT 17).[27]

Comment: The clinical relevance of results for gastrointestinal ulceration is doubtful. The only RCT that used clinically relevant outcomes found little difference between active drug and placebo, except for people at high risk.[23] The rate of ulcers was more than 10 times higher in the studies where the investigators looked for them with regular endoscopy than in earlier RCTs of NSAIDs.[28] These ulcers were sometimes defined as endoscopic lesions with a size of only 3 mm, sometimes as any lesion of an unequivocal depth, and sometimes no definition was provided at all.

QUESTION **What are the effects of topical non-steroidal anti-inflammatory drugs (NSAIDs)?**

OPTION **TOPICAL NSAIDS**

One systematic review in people with acute and chronic pain conditions found that topical NSAIDs reduced pain compared with placebo. One systematic review found no high quality RCTs of topical compared with oral forms of the same NSAID, or with paracetamol.

Benefits: We found one systematic review (search date 1996, 86 RCTs, 10 160 people) and one additional RCT.[29,30] **Versus placebo:** The review, partly sponsored by two manufacturers, performed separate subgroup analyses in people with acute and chronic conditions. The review identified 37 RCTs in about 2000 people with acute pain conditions (soft tissue trauma, strains and sprains). Most of these RCTs were small. Meta-analysis of all seven RCTs with more than 80 people per group found that topical NSAIDs were more effective than placebo (RR for "good outcome" defined by patient global judgement; pain on movement; spontaneous pain; and physician global judgement was 1.6, 95% CI 1.3 to 1.9; NNT 5, 95% CI 4 to 6). In people with chronic pain conditions (osteoarthritis, tendinitis; 12 RCTs in about 1000 people), meta-analysis found that topical NSAIDs were more effective than placebo (RR for "good outcome" defined by patient global judgement; pain on movement; spontaneous pain; and physician global judgement was 2.0, 95% CI 1.5 to 2.7; NNT 4, 95% CI 3 to 4). The additional RCT (116 people with osteoarthritis of the hip or knee) compared copper salicylate gel with placebo applied to the forearm.[30] It found no significant difference in the proportion of people reporting good effect (term not defined but measured on a four-point ranking scale, with very good, good, fair, and poor: 22% with copper salicylate gel *v* 21% with placebo). **Versus oral NSAIDs:** Five RCTs in the systematic review compared topical with oral NSAIDs, but they all had inadequate design and power.[29] We found no high quality RCT comparing the same NSAID given orally and topically. **Versus paracetamol:** We found no RCTs.

Harms: **Versus placebo:** In the systematic review, local adverse effects occurred in 3% of people in both groups and systemic adverse events in 1%.[29] In the additional RCT, more people receiving copper salicylate gel reported adverse reactions, most commonly skin reactions (any adverse event 48/58 [83%] with copper salicylate gel *v* 29/56 [52%] with placebo; RR 1.6, 95% CI 1.2 to 2.1; NNH 4, 95% CI 3 to 7), and more people withdrew from the RCT because of these reactions (10/58 [17%] *v* 1/58 [2%]; ARR 13%; RR 10, 95% CI 1 to 76; NNH 6, 95% CI 3 to 20).[30] **Versus topical NSAIDs:** We found no reliable RCT comparing the same drug in topical and oral formulations. **Versus paracetamol:** We found no RCTs.

Comment: Sample size bias hampers the interpretation of the available RCTs. We found no high quality RCTs comparing topical versus systemic administration of the same NSAID, and no RCTs comparing a topical NSAID with paracetamol.

GLOSSARY

Defined daily dose The assumed average daily dose for the main indication of a specified drug. The defined daily dose per 1000 population per day is an estimate of the proportion of that population receiving treatment with that drug.

REFERENCES

1. Leufkens HG, Ameling CB, Hekster YA, et al. Utilization patterns of non-steroidal anti-inflammatory drugs in an open Dutch population. *Pharm Weekbl Sci* 1990;12:97–103.
2. McManus P, Primrose JG, Henry DA, et al. Pattern of non-steroidal anti-inflammatory drug use in Australia 1990–1994. A report from the drug utilization sub-committee of the pharmaceutical benefits advisory committee. *Med J Aust* 1996;164:589–592.
3. Gøtzsche PC. Methodology and overt and hidden bias in reports of 196 double-blind trials of nonsteroidal anti-inflammatory drugs in rheumatoid arthritis (published erratum appears in *Control Clin Trials* 1989;10:356). *Control Clin Trials* 1989;10:31–56. Search date 1985; primary source Medline.
4. Smith GD, Matthias E. Meta-analysis: unresolved issues and future developments. *BMJ* 1998;316:221–225.
5. Gøtzsche PC. Patients' preference in indomethacin trials: an overview. *Lancet* 1989;i:88–91. Search date 1985; primary sources Medline, personal contact with companies that marketed proprietary products, and hand searched reference lists of collected articles.
6. Garner S, Fidan D, Frankish R, et al. Celecoxib for rheumatoid arthritis . In: The Cochrane Library, Issue 3, 2004. Oxford: Update Software. Search date 2002; primary sources Medline, Embase, Cochrane Database of Systematic Reviews, Cochrane Controlled Trials Register, National Research Register, NHS Economic Evaluation Database, Health Technology Assessment Database, and personal contact with experts.
7. Garner S, Fidan D, Frankish R, et al. Rofecoxib for rheumatoid arthritis. In: The Cochrane Library, Issue 3, 2004. Oxford: Update Software. Search date 2002; primary sources Medline, Embase, Cochrane Database of Systematic Reviews, Cochrane Controlled Trials Register, National Research Register, NHS Economic Evaluation Database, Health Technology Assessment database, the manufacturers.
8. Gøtzsche PC. Meta-analysis of NSAIDs: contribution of drugs, doses, trial designs, and meta-analytic techniques. *Scand J Rheumatol* 1993;22:255–260. Search date 1988; primary source Medline.
9. Towheed T, Shea B, Wells G, et al. Analgesia and non-aspirin, non-steroidal anti-inflammatory drugs in osteoarthritis of the hip. In: The Cochrane Library, Issue 3, 2004. Oxford: Update Software. Search date 1994; primary sources Cochrane Controlled Trials Register, Medline, and hand searched references.
10. Watson MC, Brookes ST, Kirwan JR, et al. Non-aspirin, non-steroidal anti-inflammatory drugs for treating osteoarthritis of the knee. In: The Cochrane Library, Issue 3, 2004. Oxford: Update Software. Search date 1996; primary sources Medline and Embase.
11. Ogilvie Harris DJ, Gilbart M. Treatment modalities for soft tissue injuries of the ankle: a critical review. *Clin J Sport Med* 1995;5:175–186. Search date 1993; primary sources Medline and Embase.
12. Green S, Buchbinder R, Glazier R, et al. Interventions for shoulder pain. In: The Cochrane Library, Issue 3, 2004. Oxford: Update Software. Search date 1998; primary sources Cochrane Musculoskeletal Group Trials Register, Cochrane Controlled Trials Register, Medline, Embase, Cinahl, and Science Citation Index.
13. Gøtzsche PC. Review of dose-response studies of NSAIDs in rheumatoid arthritis. *Dan Med Bull* 1989;36:395–399. Search date 1985; primary sources Medline, hand searches of reference lists, and contact with companies marketing proproctary preparations.
14. Eisenberg E, Berkey CS, Carr DB, et al. Efficacy and safety of nonsteroidal antiinflammatory drugs for cancer pain: a meta-analysis. *J Clin Oncol* 1994;12:2756–2765. Search date 1992; primary source Medline.
15. Langman MJ, Jensen DM, Watson DG, et al. Adverse upper gastrointestinal effects of rofecoxib compared with NSAIDs. *JAMA* 1999;282:1929–1933.
16. Mukherjee D, Nissen SE, Topol EJ. Risk of cardiovascular events associated with selective COX-2 inhibitors. *JAMA* 2001;286:954–959. Search date 2001; primary sources Medline, the internet, and review of relevant submissions to the US Food and Drug Administration by pharmaceutical companies.
17. Cappelleri JC, Lau J, Kupelnick B, et al. Efficacy and safety of different aspirin dosages on vascular diseases in high-risk patients. A metaregression analysis. *Online J Curr Clin Trials* 1995;Doc No 174. Search date 1992; primary sources Medline and Current Contents.
18. Henry D, Lim LL, Garcia Rodriguez LA, et al. Variability in risk of gastrointestinal complications with individual non-steroidal anti-inflammatory drugs: results of a collaborative meta-analysis. *BMJ* 1996;312:1563–1566. Search date 1994; primary source Medline.
19. Henry D, McGettigan P. Epidemiology overview of gastrointestinal and renal toxicity of NSAIDs. *Int J Clin Pract* 2003;135(suppl):43–49. Search date 2001; primary sources Medline, Embase, Cochrane Library, HealthSTAR, CINAHL, IDIS; reference lists and handsearches.
20. Huskisson EC, Woolf DL, Balme HW, et al. Four new anti-inflammatory drugs: responses and variations. *BMJ* 1976;i:1048–1049.
21. Cooperating Clinics Committee of the American Rheumatism Association. A seven-day variability study of 499 patients with peripheral rheumatoid arthritis. *Arthritis Rheum* 1965;8:302–334.
22. Rostom A, Dube C, Wells G, Tugwell P, Welch V, Jolicoeur E, McGowan J. Prevention of NSAID-induced gastroduodenal ulcers. In: The Cochrane Library, Issue 3, 2004. Oxford: Update Software. Oxford: Update Software. Search date 2002; primary sources Medline, Current Contents, Embase, Cochrane Controlled Trials Register, hand searched conference proceedings, and personal contact with experts and companies.
23. Silverstein FE, Graham DY, Senior JR, et al. Misoprostol reduces serious gastrointestinal complications in patients with rheumatoid arthritis receiving nonsteroidal anti-inflammatory drugs. A randomized, double-blind, placebo-controlled trial. *Ann Intern Med* 1995;123:241–249.
24. Hawkey CJ, Karrasch JA, Szczepanski L, et al. Omeprazole compared with misoprostol for ulcers associated with nonsteroidal antiinflammatory drugs. Omeprazole versus misoprostol for NSAID-induced ulcer management (OMNIUM) study group. *N Engl J Med* 1998;338:727–734.
25. Graham DY, Agrawal NM, Campbell DR, et al. Ulcer prevention in long-term users of nonsteroidal antiinflamatory drugs: results of a double-blind, randomized, multicentre, active- and placebo-controlled study of misoprostol and lansoprazole. *Arch Intern Med* 2002;162:169–175.
26. Yeomans ND, Tulassay Z, Juhasz L, et al. A comparison of omeprazole with ranitidine for ulcers associated with nonsteroidal antiinflammatory drugs.

Acid suppression trial: ranitidine versus omeprazole for NSAID associated ulcer treatment (ASTRONAUT) study group. *N Engl J Med* 1998;338:719–726.
27. Raskin JB, White RH, Jaszewski R, et al. Misoprostol and ranitidine in the prevention of NSAID-induced ulcers: a prospective, double-blind, multicenter study. *Am J Gastroenterol* 1996;91:223–227.
28. Chalmers TC, Berrier J, Hewitt P, et al. Meta-analysis of randomized controlled trials as a method of estimating rare complications of non-steroidal anti-inflammatory drug therapy. *Aliment Pharmacol Ther* 1988;2(suppl 1):9–26. Search date not stated; primary source Medline.
29. Moore RA, Tramer MR, Carroll D, et al. Quantitative systematic review of topically applied non-steroidal anti-inflammatory drugs. *BMJ* 1998;316:333–338. Search date 1996; primary sources Medline, Embase, Oxford Pain Relief Database 1950–1994, contact with pharmaceutical companies, and hand searched references.
30. Shackel NA, Day RO, Kellett B, et al. Copper-salicylate gel for pain relief in osteoarthritis: a randomised controlled trial. *Med J Aust* 1997;167:134–136.

Peter C Gøtzsche
Director
The Nordic Cochrane Centre
Copenhagen
Denmark

Competing interests: None declared.

Plantar heel pain and fasciitis

Search date August 2004

Fay Crawford

QUESTIONS

INTERVENTIONS

Key Messages

Treatments

- **Casted orthoses (custom made insoles)** One systematic review found no RCTs comparing the effects of casted orthoses versus placebo or no treatment. One RCT found no significant difference in pain between heel pad plus orthoses and corticosteroid injection plus local anaesthesia plus non-steroidal anti-inflammatory drugs. One RCT found that orthoses plus heel pads reduced pain compared with heel pads plus paracetamol at 8 weeks. One RCT found that heel pads plus stretching reduced pain compared with custom made orthoses plus stretching at 8 weeks. One RCT found that stretching plus heel pad (silicone insert, rubber insert, or felt insert) improved symptoms compared with stretching alone at 8 weeks. One RCT found no significant difference in pain between orthoses plus stretching (Achilles tendon stretching and plantar fascia stretching) and stretching alone after 8 weeks. One RCT provided insufficient evidence to compare orthoses versus night splints.
- **Corticosteroid injection (in the short term)** One systematic review identified no RCTs comparing short term effects of corticosteroid injections versus placebo, orthoses, heel pads, analgesic medication, or corticosteroid injection plus local anaesthesia. Observational studies found a high rate of plantar fascia rupture and other complications associated with corticosteroid injections, which may lead to chronic disability in some people.
- **Corticosteroid injection plus local anaesthetic injection in the short term (with or without non-steroidal anti-inflammatory drugs or heel pads)** One systematic review identified no RCTs comparing short term effects of corticosteroid injections plus local anaesthesia versus placebo or no treatment. RCTs provided insufficient evidence about clinically important short term effects of corticosteroids

plus local anaesthesia (alone or combined with non-steroidal anti-inflammatory drugs or heel pads) compared with other treatments. Observational studies found a high rate of plantar fascia rupture and other complications associated with corticosteroid injections, which may lead to chronic disability in some people.

- **Extracorporeal shock wave therapy** One systematic review and four subsequent RCTs of extracorporeal shock wave therapy in people with heel pain found insufficient evidence to assess the effect on pain of extracorporeal shock wave therapy compared with placebo. Two RCTs found limited evidence that high dose extracorporeal shock wave therapy reduced pressure pain and walking pain scores compared with low dose therapy. However, the clinical importance of these effects is unclear.
- **Heel pads and heel cups** One systematic review found no RCTs on the effects of heel pads and heel cups compared with placebo, no treatment, or corticosteroid injection. One RCT found no significant difference in pain relief between heel pads and heel pads plus corticosteroid injection. One RCT provided insufficient evidence about clinically important effects of heel pads compared with corticosteroids plus local anaesthesia (alone or combined with non-steroidal anti-inflammatory drugs or heel pads). One RCT found that stretching plus heel pad (silicone insert, rubber insert, or felt insert) improved symptoms compared with stretching alone at 8 weeks. One RCT found that heel pads plus stretching reduced pain compared with custom made orthoses plus stretching at 8 weeks. One RCT found that heel pads plus orthoses reduced pain compared with heel pads plus paracetamol at 8 weeks.
- **Lasers** One small RCT identified by a systematic review found no significant difference between laser treatment and placebo.
- **Local anaesthetic injection** One systematic review identified no RCTs comparing local anaesthesia versus placebo or no treatment. One RCT found that combining local anaesthetic with a corticosteroid injection compared with local anaesthetic injection alone slightly improved pain score at 1 month. However, it found no significant difference in pain thereafter. The clinical importance of this result is unclear.
- **Night splints plus non-steroidal anti-inflammatory drugs** One RCT found no significant difference in pain between a night splint plus non-steroidal anti-inflammatory drugs and non-steroidal anti-inflammatory drugs alone after 3 months. There was insufficient evidence from one RCT comparing night splints versus orthoses.
- **Stretching exercises** One systematic review identified no RCTs comparing stretching exercises versus no treatment in people with heel pain. One RCT found no significant difference in pain between stretching alone (Achilles tendon stretching and plantar fascia stretching) and stretching plus orthoses after 8 weeks. One RCT found that stretching plus heel pad (silicone insert, rubber insert, or felt insert) improved symptoms compared with stretching alone at 8 weeks. One RCT found no significant difference in pain between sustained and intermittent Achilles tendon stretching exercises. One RCT found that plantar fascia stretching plus heel pad was more effective at reducing morning heel pain than Achilles tendon stretching plus heel pad.
- **Surgery** One systematic review found no RCTs of surgery for heel pain.
- **Ultrasound** One small RCT identified by a systematic review found no significant difference in pain between ultrasound and sham ultrasound.
- **Corticosteroid injection in the medium to long term (with or without heel pad)** One systematic review identified no RCTs comparing medium to long term effects of corticosteroid injections versus placebo, orthoses, heel pads, analgesic medication, or corticosteroid injection plus local anaesthesia. One small RCT provided insufficient evidence about the long term effects of corticosteroid injection plus heel pad compared with placebo plus heel pad. Observational studies found a high rate of plantar fascia rupture and other complications associated with corticosteroid injections, which may lead to chronic disability in some people.

- **Corticosteroid injection plus local anaesthetic injection in the medium to long term (with or without non-steroidal anti-inflammatory drugs or heel pads)** One systematic review identified no RCTs comparing medium to long term effects of corticosteroid injections plus local anaesthesia versus placebo or no treatment. RCTs identified by the review provided insufficient evidence about clinically important long term effects of corticosteroids plus local anaesthesia (alone or combined with non-steroidal anti-inflammatory drugs or heel pads) compared with other treatments. Observational studies have found a high rate of plantar fascia rupture and other complications associated with corticosteroid injections, which may lead to chronic disability in some people.

DEFINITION	Plantar heel pain is soreness or tenderness of the heel that is restricted to the sole of the foot. It often radiates from the central part of the heel pad**G** or the medial tubercle of the calcaneum, but may extend along the plantar fascia into the medial longitudinal arch of the foot. Severity may range from an irritation at the origin of the plantar fascia, which is noticeable on rising after rest, to an incapacitating pain. This review excludes clinically evident underlying disorders, for example, infection, calcaneal fracture, and calcaneal nerve entrapment, which may be distinguished clinically — a calcaneal fracture may present after trauma, and calcaneal nerve entrapment gives rise to shooting pains and feelings of "pins and needles" on the medial aspect of the heel.
INCIDENCE/ PREVALENCE	The incidence and prevalence of plantar heel pain is uncertain. Plantar heel pain primarily affects those in mid to late life.[1]
AETIOLOGY/ RISK FACTORS	Unknown.
PROGNOSIS	One systematic review found that almost all of the included trials reported an improvement in discomfort regardless of the intervention received (including placebo), suggesting that the condition is at least partially self limiting.[1] A telephone survey of 100 people treated conservatively (average follow up 47 months) found that 82 people had resolution of symptoms, 15 had continued symptoms but no limitations of activity or work, and three had persistent bilateral symptoms that limited activity or changed work status.[2] Thirty one people said that they would have seriously considered surgical treatment at the time that medical attention was sought.
AIMS OF INTERVENTION	To reduce pain and immobility, with minimal adverse effects.
OUTCOMES	Pain reduction (often measured using visual analogue scales); walking distance.
METHODS	*Clinical Evidence* search and appraisal August 2004.

QUESTION **What are the effects of treatments for plantar heel pain?**

OPTION **CORTICOSTEROID INJECTIONS**

One systematic review identified no RCTs comparing short or long term effects of corticosteroid injections versus placebo, orthoses, heel pads, analgesic medication, or corticosteroid injection plus local anaesthesia. One small RCT provided insufficient evidence about the long term effects of corticosteroid injection plus heel pad compared with placebo plus heel pad. Observational studies found a high rate of plantar fascia rupture and other complications associated with corticosteroid injections, which may lead to chronic disability in some people.

Benefits: **Versus placebo or no treatment:** We found one systematic review (search date 2002), which found no RCTs.[1] **Corticosteroid injection plus heel pad versus placebo plus heel pad:** We found one systematic review (search date 2002, 1 RCT).[1] The RCT (19 people [22 heels] with recalcitrant heel pain but not arthritis) found no significant difference in the proportion of heels with no pain relief between corticosteroid (hydrocortisone acetate 25 mg) injection plus heel pad**G** and saline injection plus heel pad 6–18 months after the injection (3/13 [23%]

heels with hydrocortisone *v* 4/9 [44%] heels with placebo; RR 0.52, 95% CI 0.15 to 1.79).[1] However, the study may have lacked power to detect clinically important differences between treatments. **Versus orthoses:** We found one systematic review (search date 2002), which found no RCTs.[1] **Versus pads:** We found one systematic review (search date 2002), which found no RCTs.[1] **Versus analgesic medication alone:** We found one systematic review (search date 2002), which found no RCTs.[1] **Corticosteroid injection plus local anaesthesia:** We found one systematic review (search date 2002), which found no RCTs.[1]

Harms: The RCT identified by the review gave no information on harms.[1] Corticosteroid injections can be painful. Complications observed from local corticosteroid injection throughout the body include infection, subcutaneous fat atrophy, skin pigmentation changes, fascial rupture, peripheral nerve injury, and muscle damage, among others.[3] Observational studies have reported rupture of the plantar fascia in people receiving corticosteroid injections.[4,5] One study reported a 10% incidence of rupture among 122 injected heels.[5] A second study examined 37 people with a presumptive diagnosis of plantar fascia rupture, all of whom had had plantar fasciitis and had previously been treated with corticosteroid injection.[4] Their history revealed that in 13/37 (35%) people the rupture had been a sudden event, whereas in the remainder it seemed to be gradual. The study reported that most had resolution of symptoms, but this often took 6–12 months to occur.[4] Rupture may relieve the original heel pain, but may cause arch and mid-foot strain, lateral plantar nerve dysfunction, stress fracture, deformity, and swelling, all of which may persist.

Comment: The evidence from observational studies does not allow us to say with certainty whether plantar fascia rupture is caused by corticosteroid injection, or whether it is coincidental. It is also difficult to define the clinical importance of rupture of the plantar fascia from the evidence provided by observational studies. Plantar fascia rupture is not necessarily a harmful phenomenon as it may be clinically silent in some people.

OPTION LOCAL ANAESTHETIC INJECTION

One systematic review identified no RCTs comparing local anaesthesia versus placebo or no treatment. One RCT found that combining local anaesthetic with a corticosteroid injection compared with local anaesthetic injection alone slightly improved pain score at 1 month. However, it found no significant difference in pain thereafter. The clinical importance of this result is unclear.

Benefits: **Versus placebo or no treatment:** We found one systematic review (search date 2002), which found no RCTs.[1] **Versus corticosteroids plus local anaesthetic:** See benefits of corticosteroids plus local anaesthesia, p 1537.

Harms: See harms of corticosteroid injections plus local anaesthetic, p 1538.

Comment: Epinephrine (adrenaline) is not recommended in local anaesthetics for procedures that involve the appendages because of the risk of ischaemic necrosis.[6]

OPTION CORTICOSTEROID INJECTIONS PLUS LOCAL ANAESTHESIA

One systematic review identified no RCTs comparing corticosteroid injections plus local anaesthesia versus placebo or no treatment. RCTs identified by the review provided insufficient evidence about clinically important effects of corticosteroids plus local anaesthesia (alone or combined with non-steroidal

anti-inflammatory drugs or heel pads) compared with other treatments. Observational studies found a high rate of plantar fascia rupture and other complications associated with corticosteroid injections, which may lead to chronic disability in some people.

Benefits: **Versus placebo or no treatment:** We found one systematic review (search date 2002), which found no RCTs.[1] **Versus corticosteroid alone:** We found one systematic review (search date 2002), which found no RCTs.[1] **Versus local anaesthetic alone:** We found one systematic review (search date 2002, 1 RCT).[1] The RCT (91 people [106 heels, randomisation by heel]) compared a single injection of 1 mL prednisolone acetate 25 mg/mL plus 1 mL lidocaine hydrochloride 2% versus 2 mL lidocaine hydrochloride 2% alone. It found that the combined injection slightly improved pain score at 1 month, although the clinical importance of this result is unclear (10 cm visual analogue scale: mean difference –0.8 cm, 95% CI –1.5 cm to –0.2 cm). However, it found no significant difference in pain thereafter (3 months: mean difference +0.1 cm, 95% CI –1.2 cm to +1.3 cm; 6 months: +0.5 cm, 95% CI –0.8 cm to +1.7 cm).[7] **Versus heel pad:** We found one systematic review (search date 2002, 2 RCTs).[1] The first RCT (80 people) included people with pain on the plantar aspect of the heel, but excluded people taking anti-inflammatory medication; people who had had a corticosteroid injection during the past 6 months; people with rheumatoid arthritis; and people with pain that radiated along the plantar fascia more distally.[8] It compared three treatments: a heel pad**G** alone; a corticosteroid plus local anaethestic injection alone (triamcinolone hexacetonide 20 mg plus 2% lidocaine [lignocaine]), and injection plus heel pad (an "anti-pronatory insole"). Analysis was not by intention to treat, and four people (5%) were lost to follow up. The RCT found that corticosteroid plus local anaesthetic injection significantly improved pain compared with heel pads at 1 month (100 mm visual analogue scale: mean difference –45 mm, 95% CI –59 mm to –31 mm). At 24 weeks, there was greater mean pain reduction with the injection alone compared with the heel pad alone, but the difference was not significant (85% with injection alone *v* 75% with heel pad alone). The second RCT (17 people) identified by the review compared triamcinolone 20 mg plus 2% lidocaine injection versus heel pad (prefabricated silicone type).[9] Although more people improved after treatment with the heel pad at 12 weeks (33% with injection *v* 66% with heel pad), the difference in pain was not significant at 1, 2, or 12 weeks. **Versus corticosteroid plus local anaesthetic plus heel pad:** We found one systematic review (search date 2002, 1 RCT, 80 people).[1] The RCT (for details of RCT see versus heel pad above) found that corticosteroid injection plus local anaesthesia alone significantly improved pain compared with the combined injection plus a heel pad after 1 month, although the clinical importance of these results is unclear (100 mm visual analogue scale: mean difference 16.0 mm, 95% CI 0.7 mm to 31.2 mm).[8] At 24 weeks, people treated with heel pad plus injection had less pain compared with injection alone, but the difference was reported as non-significant (94% with heel pad plus injection *v* 85% with injection alone; $P > 0.05$). **Plus heel pad versus heel pad alone:** We found one systematic review (search date 2002, 1 RCT, 80 people).[1] The RCT (for details of RCT see versus heel pad above) found that corticosteroid injection plus local anaesthesia plus heel pad significantly reduced pain compared with heel pad alone at 4 and 12 weeks (100 mm visual analogue scale: mean difference at 4 weeks –29 mm, 95% CI –44 mm to –14 mm), but not at 24 weeks (mean difference –10.7 mm, 95% CI –25.5 mm to +4.1 mm; AR for pain reduction: 94% with injection plus heel pad *v* 75% with heel pad alone).[8] However, the clinical importance of these results is unclear. **Plus non-steroidal anti-inflammatory drugs versus heel pad plus**

paracetamol: We found one systematic review (search date 2002, 1 RCT, 103 people).[1] It compared three interventions: three injections of corticosteroid plus local anaesthetic into the heel plus non-steroidal anti-inflammatory drugs (anti-inflammatory treatment); heel pads plus paracetamol (acetaminophen) as required (accommodative treatment); and a heel pad before fitting of casted (custom made) orthoses**G** (mechanical treatment). Treatment in the anti-inflammatory group consisted of etodolac 600 mg and 0.5 mL dexamethasone sodium phosphate 4 mg/mL plus 1 mL of 0.5% bupivacaine hydrochloride without adrenaline (epinephrine).[10] If there was no response, 0.2 mL of dexamethasone acetate 16 mg/mL injection was added cumulatively to the second (2nd week) and third (4th week) injections. Analysis was not by intention to treat and 18 people (17.5%) were lost to follow up. The RCT found no significant difference between injection plus anti-inflammatory drugs and heel pads at 3 months (10 cm visual analogue scale: mean difference –1.2 cm, 95% CI –2.8 cm to +0.4 cm). **Plus non-steroidal anti-inflammatory drugs versus heel pad plus orthoses:** We found one systematic review (search date 2002, 1 RCT, 103 people).[1] The RCT (for details of RCT see plus non-steroidal anti-inflammatory drugs versus heel pad plus paracetamol above) found that both anti-inflammatory treatment (corticosteroid injection plus local anaesthesia plus non-steroidal anti-inflammatory drugs) and mechanical treatment (heel pad plus orthoses) improved pain at 3 months, but the difference was not significant (10 cm visual analogue scale: mean difference –1.0 cm, 95% CI –2.5 cm to +0.5 cm).[10]

Harms: In the RCT identified in the review,[1] participants' heels were injected through the medial aspect of the heel pad**G**.[7] Half of the 106 randomised heels were given a tibial nerve block and half received local injection only. The RCT found no significant difference between these groups in pain at time of injection.[7] The other RCTs did not report on harms. See also harms of corticosteroid injections, p 1536.

Comment: The RCTs had many flaws (lack of intention to treat analysis, lack of power, high withdrawal rates, and lack of placebo control). Limitations of the available evidence make the use of corticosteroid injections in heel pain difficult to categorise in terms of benefits and harms. Heterogeneity of interventions prevented data pooling. A survey of UK rheumatologists found that corticosteroid injections are the most common treatment of heel pain and are used by 98% of UK rheumatologists (Crawford F, personal communication, 2000), confirming the results of similar surveys.[3] We found evidence from two observational studies of high rates of moderately severe harms from this treatment (see harms of corticosteroid injections, p 1536). This is also consistent with evidence about harms of corticosteroid injections in other areas.[3] These harms are particularly relevant because the evidence of benefit is poor, and spontaneous resolution of symptoms is common.

OPTION STRETCHING EXERCISES

One systematic review identified no RCTs comparing stretching exercises versus no treatment in people with heel pain. One RCT found no significant difference in pain between stretching alone (Achilles tendon stretching and plantar fascia stretching) and stretching plus orthoses after 8 weeks. One RCT found that stretching plus heel pad (silicone insert, rubber insert, or felt insert) improved symptoms compared with stretching alone at 8 weeks. One RCT found no significant difference in pain between sustained and intermittent Achilles tendon stretching exercises. One RCT found that plantar fascia stretching plus heel pad was more effective at reducing morning heel pain than Achilles tendon stretching plus heel pad.

Benefits: **Versus no treatment:** We found one systematic review (search date 2002), which found no RCTs.[1] **Versus orthoses plus stretching exercises:** We found one systematic review (search date 2002, 1 RCT, 236 people).[1] The RCT compared four treatments: stretching exercises alone (Achilles tendon stretching**G** and plantar fascia stretching**G** for 10 minutes twice daily); casted (custom made) orthoses**G** plus stretching exercises; and three types of heel pad**G** (prefabricated shoe inserts made from either silicone or felt) plus stretching exercises.[11] It found no significant difference in pain improvement at 8 weeks between stretching alone and orthoses plus stretching (100 mm visual analogue scale: difference −3.2 mm, 95% CI −17.4 mm to +11.0 mm; see comment below).[11] **Versus heel pad plus stretching:** We found one systematic review (search date 2002, 1 RCT).[1] The RCT (for details of RCT see versus orthoses plus stretching exercises above) compared four treatments.[11] It found that stretching plus heel pad (silicone insert, rubber insert, or felt insert) significantly improved symptoms compared with stretching alone at 8 weeks (95% with silicone insert *v* 88% with rubber insert *v* 81% with felt insert *v* 72% with stretching alone; results combined for all materials; P = 0.022).[11] **Sustained versus intermittent Achilles tendon stretching:** We found one RCT (94 people [122 heels]).[12] It found no significant difference in foot and ankle pain scores between sustained Achilles tendon stretching (performed for 3 minutes, 3 times daily for at least 4 months) and intermittent Achilles tendon stretching (5 x 20 second repetitions performed in 2 daily sessions after 4 months; pain score not further described; P = 0.31).[12] **Plantar fascia stretching plus heel pad versus Achilles tendon stretching plus heel pad:** We found one RCT (101 people with chronic proximal plantar fasciitis for at least 10 months), which found that plantar fascia stretching (held for a count of 10 and repeated 3 times daily) plus prefabricated full length heel pads (soft insoles) reduced first step pain after rest compared with Achilles tendon stretching (held for a count of 10 and repeated 3 times daily) plus prefabricated full length soft insoles after 8 weeks (WMD in first step pain after rest: −17.9, 95% CI −19.8 to −15.9). The RCT did not report on adherence to either intervention.[13]

Harms: The RCTs did not report on harms.[11–13]

Comment: Subgroup analysis in the RCT with five treatment arms found that, among people who stood for more than 8 hours daily, a greater reduction in pain was achieved with stretching alone than with customised orthoses plus stretching exercises.[11] It found no significant difference in people who stood for less than 8 hours daily. This hypothesis requires testing as the primary outcome in an RCT. Only half of the people in this subgroup analysis responded to the pain questionnaire.

OPTION CASTED ORTHOSES (CUSTOM MADE INSOLES)

One systematic review found no RCTs comparing the effects of casted orthoses versus placebo or no treatment. One RCT found no significant difference in pain between heel pad plus orthoses and corticosteroid injection plus local anaesthesia plus non-steroidal anti-inflammatory drugs. One RCT found that orthoses plus heel pads reduced pain compared with heel pads plus paracetamol at 8 weeks. One RCT found that heel pads plus stretching reduced pain compared with custom made orthoses plus stretching at 8 weeks. One RCT found that stretching plus heel pad (silicone insert, rubber insert, or felt insert) improved symptoms compared with stretching alone at 8 weeks. One RCT found no significant difference in pain between orthoses plus stretching (Achilles tendon stretching and plantar fascia stretching) and stretching alone after 8 weeks. One RCT provided insufficient evidence to compare orthoses versus night splints.

Benefits: **Versus placebo or no treatment:** We found one systematic review (search date 2002), which found no RCTs.[1] **Orthoses plus heel pad versus steroid plus local anaesthesia injections plus non-steroidal anti-inflammatory drugs:** See benefits of corticosteroid injections plus local anaesthesia, p 1537. **Orthoses plus heel pad versus heel pad plus pain medication:** We found one systematic review (search date 2002, 1 RCT, 103 people).[1] The RCT compared three interventions: three injections of corticosteroid plus local anaesthetic into the heel plus non-steroidal anti-inflammatory drugs (anti-inflammatory treatment); heel pad**G** (viscoelastic) plus paracetamol (acetaminophen) as required (accommodative treatment); and a heel pad for 4 weeks before a casted (custom made) orthosis**G** was fitted (mechanical treatment). Analysis was not by intention to treat and 18 people (17.5%) were lost to follow up. It found that heel pad plus orthoses significantly reduced pain compared with heel pad plus paracetamol at 3 months (10 cm visual analogue scale: difference –2.2 cm, 95% CI –3.8 cm to –0.5 cm).[10] **Orthoses plus stretching exercises versus heel pad plus stretching exercises:** We found one systematic review (search date 2002, 1 RCT, 236 people).[1] The RCT compared four treatments: stretching exercises alone; (Achilles tendon stretching**G** and plantar fascia stretching**G** (for 10 minutes twice daily); custom made orthoses plus stretching exercises; and three different types of heel pads (prefabricated shoe inserts) made from silicone or felt, plus stretching exercises. It found that heel pads plus stretching significantly reduced pain compared with custom made orthoses plus stretching at 8 weeks (results combined for all materials; $P = 0.007$).[11] **Orthoses plus stretching exercises versus stretching exercises alone:** See benefits of stretching exercises, p 1539. **Versus night splints:** We found one systematic review (search date 2002, 1 RCT, 255 people).[1] The RCT compared custom made orthoses versus night splints. The results were difficult to interpret because there was a large difference in withdrawals between the groups (26% with night splints *v* 7% with orthoses), and we were not able to report intention to treat analysis.[14]

Harms: None of the RCTs reported on harms.

Comment: We found one RCT comparing heel pads**G** versus casted (custom made) orthoses**G**.[15] However, there was a significant difference in mean weight between the groups at baseline (8.6 kg) and weight was associated with severity of heel pain. This makes the results difficult to interpret.

OPTION HEEL PADS AND HEEL CUPS

One systematic review found no RCTs on the effects of heel pads and heel cups compared with placebo, no treatment, or corticosteroid injection. One RCT found no significant difference in pain relief between heel pads and heel pads plus corticosteroid injection. One RCT provided insufficient evidence about clinically important effects of heel pads compared with corticosteroids plus local anaesthesia (alone or combined with non-steroidal anti-inflammatory drugs or heel pads). One RCT found that stretching plus heel pad (silicone insert, rubber insert, or felt insert) improved symptoms compared with stretching alone at 8 weeks. One RCT found that heel pads plus stretching reduced pain compared with custom made orthoses plus stretching at 8 weeks. One RCT found that heel pads plus orthoses reduced pain compared with heel pads plus paracetamol at 8 weeks.

Benefits: **Versus placebo or no treatment:** We found one systematic review (search date 2002), which found no RCTs.[1] **Versus corticosteroid injection:** We found one systematic review (search date 2002), which found no RCTs.[1] **Versus heel pad plus corticosteroid injection:** See benefits of corticosteroid injections, p 1535. **Versus corticosteroid injections plus local anaesthesia:** See benefits of corticosteroid injections plus local anaesthesia, p 1537. **Heel pad plus pain medication versus corticosteroid injection plus local anaesthesia plus non-steroidal anti-inflammatory drugs:** See benefits of corticosteroids plus local anaesthesia, p 1537. **Heel pad plus stretching exercises versus stretching exercises alone:** See benefits of stretching exercises, p 1539. **Heel pad plus stretching exercises versus orthoses plus stretching exercises:** See benefits of casted orthoses (custom made insoles), p 1540. **Heel pad plus orthoses versus heel pad plus pain medication:** See benefits of casted orthoses (custom made insoles), p 1540. **Heel pad plus orthoses versus corticosteroid injection plus local anaesthesia plus non-steroidal anti-inflammatory drugs:** See benefits of corticosteroids plus local anaesthesia, p 1537. **Heel pad plus corticosteroid injection plus local anaesthetic versus corticosteroid plus local anaesthetic:** See benefits of corticosteroids plus local anaesthesia, p 1537.

Harms: None of the RCTs reported harms.

Comment: Heel cups**G** and heel pads**G** can be made from several different materials, but rubber, viscoelastic, and silicone can be bought as prefabricated shoe inserts. Podiatrists or orthotists sometimes use felt and foam to construct heel pads. We found one additional RCT comparing heel pads versus orthoses but the results were difficult to interpret. See comment of casted orthoses (custom made insoles), p 1540.[15]

OPTION EXTRACORPOREAL SHOCK WAVE THERAPY

One systematic review and four subsequent RCTs of extracorporeal shock wave therapy in people with heel pain found insufficient evidence to assess the effect on pain of extracorporeal shock wave therapy compared with placebo. Two RCTs found limited evidence that high dose extracorporeal shock wave therapy reduced pressure pain and walking pain scores compared with low dose therapy. However, the clinical importance of these effects is unclear.

Benefits: **Versus placebo:** We found one systematic review[1] (search date 2002, 4 RCTs[20–25]) and four subsequent RCTs[16–19] comparing extracorporeal shock wave therapy (ESWT**G**) versus placebo or sham treatment (see table 1, p 1545). The RCTs provided insufficient reliable evidence to assess clinical effects of ESWT. **Different doses:** We found one systematic review (search date 2002, 2 RCTs).[1] The first RCT (50 people) identified by the review compared three 500 impulses of ESWT versus three 100 impulses (both at intensity 0.08 mJ/mm^2) in people with recalcitrant heel pain.[22] It found no significant difference in pain on pressure at 6 weeks (10 cm visual analogue scale: mean difference –0.4 cm, 95% CI –2.0 cm to +1.2 cm) or at 12 weeks (mean difference –1.4 cm, 95% CI –3.0 cm to +0.2 cm). It also found no significant difference in walking pain at 6 weeks (mean difference –0.8 cm, 95% CI –2.4 cm to +0.7 cm) or at 12 weeks (mean difference –0.9 cm, 95% CI –2.5 cm to +0.7 cm). Walking pain scores at 12 months suggested a marginal long term benefit from higher doses of ESWT (10 cm visual analogue scale: mean difference –2.0 cm, 95% CI –3.7 cm to –0.2 cm). The second RCT (119 people with recalcitrant heel pain) compared 1000 impulses of 0.08 mJ/mm^2 versus 10 impulses. All treatments were given three times at weekly intervals. It found greater improvements in pressure pain between weeks 0–12 with the higher dose (100 mm visual analogue scale: mean difference –47 mm, 95% CI –54 mm to –40 mm).[23]

Harms: ESWT🅖 without local anaesthetic can be painful. One RCT reported a sensation of heat and numbness or bruising in two people receiving ESWT, and a burning sensation in the heel and ankle in one person receiving placebo.[24] One RCT reported significantly more adverse effects with ESWT than with sham treatment (OR 2.26, 95% CI 1.02 to 5.18).[16] Adverse effects included skin reddening, pain and local swelling, and, less frequently, dizziness, sleep disturbance, haematoma, nausea, and hair loss.

Comment: Availability of ESWT🅖 is limited. Pain associated with ESWT and differences in procedures suggest that the single blinding in the first placebo controlled RCT was probably not maintained.[1] One large RCT reported a large increase in the number of people not using pain medications with ESWT (measured as any use between weeks 10 and 12: 70% with ESWT *v* 35% with sham treatment).[25] A long term follow up of one RCT (78/119 [66%] of the people enrolled) found significantly less pain on manual pressure with high dose compared with low dose ESWT at 5 years (100 mm visual analogue scale: mean difference –20 mm, 95% CI –28 mm to –11 mm). However, there are potential confounding effects from additional treatments received by unresponsive people in both groups.[23]

OPTION SURGERY

One systematic review found no RCTs of surgery for heel pain.

Benefits: We found one systematic review (search date 2002), which identified no RCTs of surgery for heel pain.[1]

Harms: We found one systematic review (search date 2002), which identified no RCTs of surgery for heel pain.[1]

Comment: The systematic review identified many observational studies of surgery for chronically painful heels.[1] One of the largest observational studies (76 people) compared postoperative complication rates after endoscopic fasciotomy compared with traditional plantar fasciotomy.[26] It found that serious complications (recurrent pain, neuritis, and infection) were less common in people treated with endoscopic fasciotomy compared with traditional surgery (serious incidents per procedure: 11/66 [17%] with endoscopic fasciotomy *v* 9/26 [35%] with traditional surgery).

OPTION LASERS

One small RCT identified by a systematic review found no significant difference between laser treatment and placebo.

Benefits: **Versus placebo:** We found one systematic review (search date 2002, 1 RCT, 32 people). The RCT included people with pain of at least 1 month's duration; tenderness to pressure at the origin of the plantar fascia; pain at the mid-anterior inferior border of the calcaneus; and sharp shooting, localised, or both, inferior foot pain made worse with activity or on rising in the morning).[1] It compared low intensity laser treatment (30 mW continuous wave diode laser) versus placebo (treatment with a disabled laser) and found no evidence of a significant effect (data not reported).

Harms: The RCT reported that 96% of people had no adverse effects, with 4% reporting a "mild sensation" during or after treatment.[1]

Comment: None.

OPTION ULTRASOUND

One small RCT identified by a systematic review found no significant difference in pain between ultrasound and sham ultrasound.

Benefits: **Versus placebo:** We found one systematic review (search date 2002), which identified one small RCT (19 people, 7 with bilateral heel pain).[1] It compared ultrasound (8 treatments in 4 weeks; dose 0.5 W/cm^2, pulsed 1:4, 3 MHz for 8 minutes) versus the same number of applications of sham ultrasound (only the timer on the machine was activated). Inclusion criteria were pain radiating from the medial tubercle of the calcaneum in response to both pressure and weight bearing first thing in the morning. It found no significant difference in pain between ultrasound and sham ultrasound (10 cm visual analogue scale; mean difference +0.1 cm, 95% CI –1.8 cm to +2.1 cm).[1]

Harms: The RCT did not assess harms.[1]

Comment: None.

OPTION NIGHT SPLINTS

One RCT found no significant difference in pain between a night splint plus non-steroidal anti-inflammatory drugs and non-steroidal anti-inflammatory drugs alone after 3 months. There was insufficient evidence from one RCT comparing night splints versus orthoses.

Benefits: **Night splint plus non-steroidal anti-inflammatory drugs versus non-steroidal anti-inflammatory drugs alone:** We found one systematic review (search date 2002, 1 RCT).[1] The RCT (116 people with recalcitrant heel pain) compared treatment with a night splint that dorsiflexed the ankle joint by 5°, worn nightly for 3 months, versus no night splint. All participants received ankle dorsiflexion exercises and a non-steroidal anti-inflammatory drug (piroxicam 20 mg/day for 30 days). The RCT found no significant difference in pain between night splinting and no splinting (RR 1.0, 95% CI 0.8 to 1.3).[27] **Versus orthoses:** See benefits of casted orthoses (custom made insoles), p 1540.

Harms: The RCTs did not assess harms.[1]

Comment: The first RCT only studied the most symptomatic foot in people with bilateral complaints, because of potential inconvenience and poor compliance from wearing two night splints simultaneously.[1]

GLOSSARY

Achilles tendon stretching A stretch achieved by hanging the heel from a step while keeping the knee straight or by leaning into the wall from a standing position with the affected leg placed behind the other leg. For people with flat foot arches, the stretch is achieved by hanging the heel from a step and inverting the foot.

Casted orthoses Made from polyurethane or similar material to a negative cast of a person's foot.

Extracorporeal shock wave therapy (ESWT) Shock waves are pulsed acoustic waves that dissipate mechanical energy at the interface of two substances with different acoustic impedance.

Heel cups Prefabricated rubber heel cups (firmer than viscoelastic heel pads) that extend up the sides of the heel and enclose the fibro fatty heel pad.

Heel pads Prefabricated viscoelastic heel pads made of malleable material. Heel pads can also be constructed from semicompressed felt, sponge, rubber, and silicone.

Plantar fascia stretching A stretch achieved by crossing the affected leg over the other leg from a seated position, placing the fingers of the affected side across the base of the toes (distal to the metatarsal phalangeal joints), and pulling the toes back until a stretch in the arch of the foot can be felt.

REFERENCES

1. Crawford F, Thomson C. Interventions for treating plantar heel pain (Cochrane Review). In: The Cochrane Library, Issue 3, 2004. Chichester, UK: John Wiley & Sons, Ltd. Search date 2002; primary sources Medline, Embase, the Cochrane Library, hand searches of four podiatry journals to 1998 plus contact with UK schools of podiatry to identify dissertations on the management of heel pain, and investigators in the field to identify unpublished data or research in progress.
2. Wolgin M, Cook C, Graham C, et al. Conservative treatment of plantar heel pain: long term follow up. *Foot Ankle Int* 1994;15:97–102.
3. Fadale PD, Wiggins MD. Corticosteroid injections: their use and abuse. *J Am Acad Orthop Surg* 1994;2:133–140.
4. Sellman JR. Plantar fascial rupture associated with corticosteroid injection. *Foot Ankle Int* 1994;15:376–381.
5. Acevedo JI, Beskin JL. Complications of plantar fascial rupture associated with steroid injection. *Foot Ankle Int* 1998;19:91–97.
6. McCauley WA, Gerace RV, Scilley C. Treatment of accidental digital injection of epinephrine. *Ann Emerg Med* 1991;6:665–668.
7. Crawford F, Atkins D, Young P, et al. Steroid injection for heel pain: evidence of short term effectiveness. A randomised controlled trial. *Rheumatology* 1999;38:974–977.
8. Kriss S. Heel pain: an investigation into its etiology and management [thesis]. London: University of Westminster, 1990.
9. Black AJ. A preliminary study of the comparative effects of steroid injection versus orthosis (Viscoheel sofspot) on plantar fasciitis [dissertation]. Belfast: Queen's University, 1996.
10. Lynch DM, Goforth WP, Martin JE, et al. Conservative treatment of plantar fasciitis. A prospective study. *J Am Podiatr Assoc* 1998;88:375–380.
11. Pfeffer G, Bacchetti P, Deland J, et al. Comparison of custom and prefabricated orthoses in the initial treatment of proximal plantar fasciitis. *Foot Ankle Int* 1999;20:214–221.
12. Porter D, Barrill E, Oneacre K, et al. The effects of duration and frequency of Achilles tendon stretching on dorsiflexion and outcome in painful heel syndrome: a randomized, blinded, controlled study. *Foot Ankle Int* 2002;23:619–624.
13. DiGiovanni BF, Nawoczenski DA, Lintal ME, et al. Tissue-specific plantar fascia stretching exercises enhances outcomes in patients with chronic heel pain. *J Bone Joint Surg* 2003;85A:1270–1277.
14. Martin J, Hosch J, Goforth W, et al. Mechanical treatment of plantar fasciitis. A prospective study. *J Am Podiatr Med Assoc* 2001;91:55–62.
15. Turlik M, Donatelli T, Veremis M. A comparison of shoe inserts in relieving mechanical heel pain. *Foot* 1999;9:84–87.
16. Haake M, Buch M, Scvhoellener C, et al. Extracorporeal shock wave therapy for plantar fasciitis: randomized controlled multicentred trial. *BMJ* 2003;327:75.
17. Rompe J, Decking J, Schollner C, et al. Shockwave application for chronic plantar fasciitis in running athletes. *Am J Sports Med* 2003;31:268–275.
18. Buch M, Knorr U, Fleming L, et al. Extracorporeal shock wave therapy in the treatment of symptomatic heel spur — a review. *Orthopade* 2002;31:637–644.
19. Abt T, Hopfenmukker W, Mellerowicz H. Shock wave therapy for recalcitrant plantar fasciitis with heel spur: a prospective randomized placebo-controlled double-blind study. *Z Orthop* 2002;140:548–554. [In German]
20. Speed CA, Nichols D, Wies J, et al. Extracorporeal shock wave therapy for plantar fasciitis. A double blind randomised controlled trial. *J Orthop Res* 2003;21:937–940.
21. Rompe JD, Hopf C, Nafe B, Burger R. Low-energy extracorporeal shock wave therapy for painful heel: a prospective controlled single blind study. *Arch Orthop Trauma Surg* 1996;115:75–79.
22. Krischeck O, Rompe JD, Herbsthrofer B, et al. Symptomatic low-energy shockwave therapy in heel pain and radiologically detected plantar heel spur. *Z Orthop Ihre Grenzgeb* 1998;136:169–174. [In German]
23. Rompe JD, Kulmer K, Riehle HM, et al. Effectiveness of low-energy extracorporeal shockwaves for chronic plantar fasciitis. *Foot Ankle Surg* 1996;2:215–221.
24. Buchbinder R, Ptasnik R, Gordon J, et al. Ultrasound-guided extra corporeal shock wave therapy for plantar fasciitis. A randomized controlled trial. *JAMA* 2002;288:1364–1372.
25. Odgen J, Alvarex R, Levitt R, et al. Shock wave therapy for chronic proximal plantar fasciitis. *Clin Orthop Related Res* 2001;1:47–59.
26. Kinley S, Frascone S, Calderone D, et al. Endoscopic plantar fasciotomy versus traditional heel spur surgery: a prospective study. *J Foot Ankle Surg* 1993;32:595–603.
27. Probe RA, Baca M, Adams R, et al. Night splint treatment for plantar fasciitis. *Clin Orthop* 1999;368:191–195.

Fay Crawford
Senior Research Fellow
Dental Health Services Research Unit
Dundee
UK

Competing interests: None declared.

TABLE 1 **Reported complications from surgical procedures (see text, p 1539).[23]**

Ref	Number of people	ESWT regimen	Results
16	272	3 x 4000 impulses; 0.08 mJ/mm^2 every 2 weeks	No significant difference between ESWT and placebo in morning pain or pressure pain at 6 or 12 weeks (WMD at 6 weeks: +0.03, 95% CI –0.45 to +1.05; WMD at 12 weeks: –0.50, 95% CI –1.30 to +0.30)
17	45	6300 impulses; 0.16 mJ/mm^2; 4 Hz; weekly for 3 weeks	ESWT significantly reduced morning pain compared with placebo at 6 months (WMD in pain scores on 10 point scale: –2.6, 95% CI –3.7 to –1.4)
18	150	Single treatment of 300 impulses of incremental strength, followed by 3500 impulses; 0.36 mJ/mm^2; 240 Hz	No significant difference in pain between ESWT and placebo at 3 months (WMD on 10 point VAS: –0.70, 95% CI –1.66 to +0.26)
19	32	1000 impulses; 0.8 mJ/mm^2	ESWT significantly reduced pain at rest compared with placebo at 48 weeks (mean score on 10 cm VAS [0 cm = no pain, 10 cm = maximal pain]: 0.7 cm with ESWT v 1.8 cm with placebo; P = 0.01) ESWT improved exercise tolerance (with footwear) compared with placebo at 48 weeks (AR for ability to walk for > 60 minutes: 15/17 [88%] with ESWT v 8/15 [53%] with placebo; significance not reported)
20	88	1500 impulses; 0.12 mJ/mm^2	No significant difference in pain scores between ESWT and placebo at 6 months (mean reduction from baseline on 100 mm VAS: 39 mm with ESWT v 41 mm with sham; P value reported as not significant)
21	36 (6 people withdrew from trial; analysis not intention to treat)	1000 impulses; 0.06 mJ/mm^2	ESWT significantly improved pain and pain-free walking compared with placebo at 6 weeks ($P < 0.005$)
24	166	1000 impulses; 0.08 mJ/mm^2 weekly for 3 weeks	No significant difference in pain between ESWT and placebo at 12 weeks (mean difference in score on 100 mm VAS: ESWT v placebo: +0.6 mm, 95% CI –10.3 mm to +11.5 mm)
25	260	1500 impulses; 18 kV	No significant difference between ESWT and placebo in improvement of pain from baseline by > 50% and by > 4 cm on 10 cm VAS (71/119 [60%] with ESWT v 56/116 [48%] with sham treatment; RR 1.24, 95% CI 0.97 to 1.57; results recalculated by *Clinical Evidence*)

ESWT, extracorporeal shock wave therapy; VAS, visual analogue scale.

Raynaud's phenomenon (primary)

Search date October 2004

Janet Pope

QUESTIONS

INTERVENTIONS

Key Messages

Treatments

- **Nifedipine** Six RCTs found that nifedipine reduced the frequency and severity of attacks over 4–12 weeks compared with placebo, and was rated by participants as more effective than placebo in improving overall symptoms. The RCTs found that nifedipine was associated with higher rates of adverse effects compared with placebo, including flushing, headache, oedema, and tachycardia.
- **Amlodipine** We found no satisfactory RCTs of the effects of amlodipine.
- **Diltiazem** We found no satisfactory RCTs of the effects of diltiazem.
- **Exercise** We found no satisfactory RCTs of the effects of exercise.
- **Inositol nicotinate** Two RCTs provided insufficient evidence to assess inositol nicotinate.
- **Keeping warm** We found no satisfactory RCTs of the effects of keeping warm.
- **Moxisylyte (thymoxamine)** We found no satisfactory RCTs of the effects of moxisylyte (thymoxamine).
- **Naftidrofuryl oxalate** One RCT found that, compared with placebo, naftidrofuryl oxalate reduced the duration and intensity of Raynaud's attacks over 2 months and reduced the impact of attacks on daily activities. However, we were unable to draw reliable conclusions from this single study.
- **Nicardipine** One RCT found that nicardipine decreased the frequency of Raynaud's attacks over 8 weeks after crossover compared with placebo, but found no significant difference in the severity of attacks. Another RCT found no significant difference in frequency, severity, or duration of attacks with nicardipine compared with placebo, but it is likely to have been too small to detect a clinically important difference in outcomes.
- **Prazosin** One small crossover RCT found limited evidence that prazosin reduced the number and duration of attacks over 6 weeks after crossover compared with placebo, but found no significant difference in the severity of attacks. However, we were unable to draw reliable conclusion from this single study.

Clin Evid 2005;13:1546–1554.

DEFINITION Raynaud's phenomenon is episodic vasospasm of the peripheral arteries, causing pallor followed by cyanosis and redness with pain and sometimes paraesthesia, and, rarely, ulceration of the fingers and toes (and in some cases of the ears or nose). Primary or idiopathic Raynaud's phenomenon (Raynaud's disease) occurs without an underlying disease. Secondary Raynaud's phenomenon (Raynaud's syndrome) occurs in association with an underlying disease — usually connective tissue disorders such as scleroderma, systemic lupus erythematosus, rheumatoid arthritis, or polymyositis. This review excludes secondary Raynaud's phenomenon.

INCIDENCE/ PREVALENCE The prevalence of primary Raynaud's phenomenon varies by gender, country, and exposure to workplace vibration. One large US cohort study (4182 people) found symptoms in 9.6% of women and 8.1% of men, of whom 81% had primary Raynaud's phenomenon.[1] Smaller cohort studies in Spain have estimated the prevalence of Raynaud's phenomenon to be 3.7–4.0%, of which 90% is primary Raynaud's phenomenon.[2,3] One cohort study in Japan (332 men, 731 women) found symptoms of primary Raynaud's phenomenon in 3.4% of women and 3.0% of men.[4]

AETIOLOGY/ RISK FACTORS The cause of primary Raynaud's phenomenon is unknown.[5] There is evidence for genetic predisposition,[6,7] most likely in those people with early onset Raynaud's phenomenon (aged < 40 years).[8] One prospective observational study (424 people with Raynaud's phenomenon) found that 73% of sufferers first developed symptoms before age 40 years.[8] Women are more at risk than men (OR 3.0, 95% CI 1.2 to 7.8, in 1 US case control study [235 people]).[9] The other known risk factor is occupational exposure to vibration from tools (symptoms developed in about 8% with exposure *v* 2.7% with no exposure in 2 cohorts from Japan).[10,11] People who are obese may be less at risk.[9] Symptoms are often worsened by cold or emotion.

PROGNOSIS Attacks may last from several minutes to a few hours. One systematic review (search date 1996, 10 prospective observational studies, 639 people with primary Raynaud's phenomenon) found that 13% of long term sufferers later manifested an underlying disorder such as scleroderma.[12]

AIMS OF INTERVENTION To reduce the number and severity of attacks; to prevent tissue damage; to minimise adverse effects of treatment.

OUTCOMES Frequency and severity of symptoms (as assessed by patient diary); severity assessed by visual analogue scales, Likert scales, or the Raynaud's Condition Score;[13] rates, size, and healing of digital ulceration.

METHODS *Clinical Evidence* search and appraisal October 2004. We searched for any RCTs comparing amlodipine, diltiazem, inositol nicotinate, moxisylyte, naftidrofuryl oxalate, nicardipine, nifedipine, or prazosin versus placebo or versus each other in people with primary Raynaud's and included all RCTs of sufficient quality. Many RCTs included people with both primary and secondary Raynaud's phenomenon. We excluded RCTs in which less than 50% of people had primary Raynaud's phenomenon or where the type of Raynaud's was unclear. We also excluded RCTs in which attacks were experimentally induced (e.g. by dipping the hands in cold water) or which did not assess clinical outcomes. Some RCTs compared changes in symptoms from baseline within each treatment group rather than directly comparing outcomes between treatment groups. These have been described in the comment sections.

QUESTION What are the effects of treatments for primary Raynaud's phenomenon?

OPTION NIFEDIPINE

Six RCTs found that nifedipine reduced the frequency and severity of attacks over 4–12 weeks compared with placebo, and was rated by participants as more effective than placebo in improving overall symptoms. The RCTs found that nifedipine was associated with higher rates of adverse effects compared with placebo, including flushing, headache, oedema, and tachycardia.

Benefits: **Versus placebo:** We found six RCTs comparing nifedipine versus placebo (457 people, 451 with primary Raynaud's phenomenon, 2 parallel, 4 crossover trials) (see table 1, p 1553).[14–19] All RCTs found that nifedipine significantly reduced the mean frequency of attacks over 4–12 weeks compared with placebo.[14–19] One RCT found that nifedipine reduced the mean grade of the most severe attack over 4 weeks compared with placebo,[18] but another RCT found no significant difference in the mean severity of attacks over 6 weeks.[15] Three RCTs found that a significantly higher proportion of people rated nifedipine as more effective than placebo in improving overall symptoms.[14,15,19]

Harms: Five RCTs found higher rates of adverse effects with nifedipine.[14–17,19] The first RCT found that significantly more people taking nifedipine compared with placebo had oedema (24% with nifedipine *v* 0% with placebo; $P < 0.01$) or flushing (8% with nifedipine *v* 0% with placebo; $P < 0.01$).[14] Two people taking nifedipine had tachycardia. The second RCT found that 10/22 (45%) people taking nifedipine 10 mg, 16/22 (72%) people taking nifedipine 20 mg, and 6/22 (27%) people taking placebo had adverse effects (CI not reported).[15] The third RCT found no significant difference between nifedipine and placebo in the overall incidence of adverse effects, but found that nifedipine significantly increased the risk of palpitations (7/18 [38.8%] with nifedipine *v* 1/18 [5.5%] with placebo; $P < 0.05$).[16] The fourth RCT found that significantly more people had adverse effects, including headaches, flushing, and ankle swelling over 8 weeks after crossover with nifedipine compared with placebo (14/23 [61%] with nifedipine *v* 2/23 [9%] with placebo; $P = 0.05$).[17] The fifth RCT found that 16/21 (76%) people had adverse effects with nifedipine, but did not report adverse effects with placebo.[18] The sixth RCT (34 people) found that more people had adverse effects, including flushing, headache, and oedema, with nifedipine over 12 weeks after crossover compared with placebo (26/34 [76%] with nifedipine *v* 5/34 [15%] with placebo; P value not reported).[19]

Comment: One of the RCTs included six people with secondary Raynaud's phenomenon.[19]

OPTION NICARDIPINE

One RCT found that nicardipine decreased the frequency of Raynaud's attacks over 8 weeks after crossover compared with placebo, but found no significant difference in the severity of attacks. Another RCT found no significant difference in frequency, severity, or duration of attacks with nicardipine compared with placebo, but it is likely to have been too small to detect a clinically important difference in outcomes.

Benefits: We found two RCTs.[20,21] The first RCT (69 people with primary Raynaud's, crossover design, outcomes assessed after crossover; see comment below) found that nicardipine significantly decreased the frequency of attacks over 8 weeks compared with placebo (attacks/week: 4.9 with nicardipine *v* 5.8 with placebo; mean difference 0.9, 95% CI 0 to 2.2; $P = 0.02$) and reduced overall disability (measured on a visual analogue scale of 10 cm where 0 represented no disability; mean 2.6 with nicardipine *v* 3.3 with placebo; $P = 0.018$), but found no significant difference in the severity of attacks (measured on a scale of 1–4 where 1 represented mild and 4 highly severe; 1.36 with nicardipine *v* 1.55 with placebo; mean difference in severity 0.2, 95% CI 0 to 0.4; P reported as non-significant; no further data reported).[20] The second RCT (25 people, 16 with primary Raynaud's phenomenon, crossover design, outcomes assessed after crossover; see comment below) found no significant difference in frequency, severity, or duration of attacks at 6 weeks between nicardipine 30 mg twice daily and placebo (analysis in 16 people with primary Raynaud's; mean frequency 4.4 attacks/day with nicardipine *v* 4.4 attacks/day with placebo; mean severity of attacks on a 10 point scale where 0 represented no pain; 3.5 with nicardipine *v* 3.7 with placebo; mean duration of attacks 13 minutes with nicardipine *v* 11 minutes with placebo; reported as non-significant for all outcomes; no further data reported).[21] The RCT is likely to have been too small to detect a clinically important difference in outcomes.

Harms: The first RCT found that 7/69 (10%) people withdrew from the trial because of adverse effects: five people while taking nicardipine and two while taking placebo.[20] In the second RCT, three people withdrew because of adverse effects (including flushing, headache, and palpitations), two while taking nicardipine, and one while taking placebo.[21]

Comment: The second RCT included nine people with secondary Raynaud's phenomenon.[21] The results of the crossover trials should be viewed with caution as no precrossover results were available and results may not allow for confounding factors such as inadequate washout and the naturally variable course of Raynaud's phenomenon.[20,21]

OPTION AMLODIPINE

We found no satisfactory RCTs of the effects of amlodipine.

Benefits: We found no RCTs that provided between group comparisons of amlodipine versus placebo (see comment below).

Harms: We found no satisfactory RCTs (see comment below).

Comment: We found one RCT that presented within group comparisons of changes in outcomes from baseline (24 people, 15 with primary Raynaud's phenomenon, crossover design, outcomes assessed after crossover).[22] It found that amlodipine significantly reduced the number of acute attacks a week from baseline at 7 weeks (from 11.8 attacks/week at baseline to 8.6 attacks/week after treatment; $P < 0.001$) and reduced the severity of attacks from baseline (from a discomfort score of 7.8 at baseline to 5.1 after treatment). However, the RCT did not assess the significance of the difference in frequency and severity of attacks between groups. It found that amlodipine was associated with ankle oedema (55% of people taking amlodipine *v* 0% of people taking placebo), flushing, and headaches compared with placebo (10–20% with amlodipine *v* 0% with placebo).[22] The RCT included people with secondary Raynaud's phenomenon, so results may not be applicable in people with primary Raynaud's phenomenon.

OPTION DILTIAZEM

We found no satisfactory RCTs of the effects of diltiazem.

Benefits: We found no satisfactory RCTs (see comment below).

Harms: We found no satisfactory RCTs (see comment below).

Comment: One crossover RCT (30 people, 19 with primary Raynaud's phenomenon, outcomes assessed after crossover) found that diltiazem significantly reduced the number of attacks compared with placebo (mean reduction in attacks from baseline 22.9/month with diltiazem *v* 4.6/month with placebo; $P = 0.01$) and reduced duration of attacks (mean reduction from baseline 444 minutes/month with diltiazem *v* 160 minutes/month with placebo; $P < 0.01$) over 8 weeks.[23] The results of this RCT should be interpreted with caution as it reported comparisons from baseline, thus removing the benefits of randomisation, and the results are not intention to treat (8/30 [27%] withdrew from the trial). Two people withdrew from the trial because of adverse effects (rash or headache) while taking diltiazem. The RCT included people with secondary Raynaud's phenomenon, so results may not be fully applicable in people with primary Raynaud's phenomenon.

OPTION NAFTIDROFURYL OXALATE

One RCT found that, compared with placebo, naftidrofuryl oxalate reduced the duration and intensity of Raynaud's attacks over 2 months and reduced the impact of attacks on daily activities. However, we were unable to draw reliable conclusions from this single study.

Benefits: We found one RCT (102 people, 87 with primary Raynaud's phenomenon) comparing naftidrofuryl oxalate 600 mg daily versus placebo for 2 months.[24] It found that, over 2 months, naftidrofuryl oxalate significantly reduced the duration of attacks ($P < 0.05$), intensity of attacks ($P < 0.001$), and reduced the impact of attacks on daily activities compared with placebo ($P < 0.05$) over 2 months.[24]

Harms: The RCT found no adverse effects associated with naftidrofuryl oxalate.[24]

Comment: The RCT included people with secondary Raynaud's phenomenon, so results may not be applicable in people with primary Raynaud's phenomenon.[24]

OPTION INOSITOL NICOTINATE

Two RCTs provided insufficient evidence to assess inositol nicotinate.

Benefits: We found two RCTs.[25,26] The first RCT (23 people with primary Raynaud's phenomenon) compared inositol nicotinate (4 g daily) versus placebo for 84 days during the winter.[25] It found that, compared with placebo, people taking inositol nicotinate had fewer and shorter attacks over 84 days, but the difference was not significant (P reported as non-significant; no further data reported). The RCT is likely to have been too small to detect a clinically important difference.[25] The second RCT (65 people, 54 with primary Raynaud's phenomenon) found that, compared with placebo, more people taking inositol nicotinate 2 g twice daily improved over 12 weeks (as measured by a 5 point scale from 0 [no problem] to 5 [very severe]), but the difference was not significant (19/34 [56%] people scored 0–1 with inositol *v* 11/33 [33%] with placebo; RR 1.58, 95% CI 0.90 to 2.76; calculated from data in the paper; see comment below).[26]

Harms: The first RCT found no adverse effects associated with inositol nicotinate.[25] In the second RCT, three people taking inositol nicotinate withdrew from the trial because of gastrointestinal disturbance or dizziness compared with one person taking placebo.[26]

Comment: The second RCT included people with secondary Raynaud's phenomenon, so results may not be fully applicable in people with primary Raynaud's phenomenon.[26]

OPTION PRAZOSIN

One small crossover RCT found limited evidence that prazosin reduced the number and duration of attacks over 6 weeks after crossover compared with placebo, but found no significant difference in the severity of attacks. However, we were unable to draw reliable conclusion from this single study.

Benefits: We found one RCT (24 people, 14 with primary Raynaud's phenomenon, crossover design, outcomes assessed after crossover; see comment below) comparing prazosin (1 mg twice daily) versus placebo.[27] It found that, compared with placebo, prazosin significantly reduced the mean number of attacks over 6 weeks after crossover (attacks/day; 2.5 with prazosin *v* 4.1 with placebo; P = 0.003) and reduced duration of attacks (21.9 minutes with prazosin *v* 29.9 minutes with placebo; P = 0.02), but found no difference in the severity of attacks (measured on a 10 point scale where 0 represented no pain; 4.1 with prazosin *v* 4.8 with placebo; P = 0.11).

Harms: The RCT found that 50% of people taking prazosin had adverse effects, including dizziness and palpitations, compared with 29% of people taking placebo.[27]

Comment: The results of the RCT should be viewed with caution as no precrossover results were available and results may not allow for confounding factors such as inadequate washout and the naturally variable course of Raynaud's phenomenon.[27] The RCT included people with secondary Raynaud's phenomenon, so results may not be fully applicable in people with primary Raynaud's phenomenon.

OPTION MOXISYLYTE (THYMOXAMINE)

We found no satisfactory RCTs of the effects of moxisylyte (thymoxamine).

Benefits: We found no RCTs of moxisylyte that assessed clinical outcomes.

Harms: We found no satisfactory RCTs.

Comment: None.

OPTION KEEPING WARM

We found no satisfactory RCTs of the effects of keeping warm.

Benefits: We found no RCTs of keeping warm that met our inclusion criteria.

Harms: We found no RCTs.

Comment: None.

OPTION EXERCISE

We found no satisfactory RCTs of the effects of exercise.

Benefits: We found no RCTs.

Harms: We found no RCTs.

Comment: None.

REFERENCES

1. Brand FN, Larson MG, Kannel WB, et al. The occurrence of Raynaud's phenomenon in a general population: the Framingham Study. *Vasc Med* 1997;2:296–301.
2. Rodriguez Garcia JL, Sabin Ruiz J. [Raynaud's phenomenon.] *Rev Clin Esp* 1989;184:311–321.
3. Riera G, Vilardell M, Vaque J, et al. Prevalence of Raynaud's phenomenon in a healthy Spanish population. *J Rheumatol* 1993;20:66–69.
4. Inaba R, Maeda M, Fujita S, et al. Prevalence of Raynaud's phenomenon and specific clinical signs related to progressive systemic sclerosis in the general population of Japan. *Int J Dermatol* 1993;32:652–655.
5. Wigley FM. Raynaud's phenomenon. *Curr Opin Rheumatol* 1993;5:773–784.
6. Smyth AE, Hughes AE, Bruce IN, et al. A case-control study of candidate vasoactive mediator genes in primary Raynaud's phenomenon. *Rheumatology (Oxford)* 1999;38:1094–1098.
7. Freedman RR, Mayes MD. Familial aggregation of primary Raynaud's disease. *Arthritis Rheum* 1996;39:1189–1191.
8. Planchon B, Pistorius Ma, Beurrier P, et al. Primary Raynaud's phenomenon. Age of onset and pathogenesis in a prospective study of 424 patients. *Angiology* 1994;45:677–686.

9. Keil JE, Maricq HR, Weinrich MC, et al. Demographic, social and clinical correlates of Raynaud phenomenon. *Int J Epidemiol* 1991;20:221–224.
10. Komura Y, Yoshida H, Nagata C, et al. Differences in the prevalences of Raynaud's phenomenon in general; populations living in a mountain area and in a plain area. [in Japanese] *Nippon Koshu Eisei Zasshi* 1992;39:421–427.
11. Mirbod SM, Inaba R, Iwata H. A study on the vibration-dose limit for Japanese workers exposed to hand-arm vibration. *Ind Health* 1992;30:1–22.
12. Spencer-Green G. Outcomes in primary Raynaud phenomenon: a meta-analysis of the frequency, rates, and predictors of transition to secondary diseases. *Arch Intern Med* 1998;158:595–600. Search date 1996; primary sources Medline and hand searches of bibliographies of articles retrieved.
13. Merkel PA, Herlyn K, Martin RW, et al. Measuring disease activity and functional status in patients with scleroderma and Raynaud's phenomenon. *Arthritis Rheum* 2002;46:2410–2420.
14. Raynaud's Treatment Study Investigators. Comparison of sustained-release nifedipine and temperature biofeedback for treatment of primary Raynaud phenomenon. Results from a randomized clinical trial with 1-year follow-up. *Arch Intern Med* 2000;160:1101–1108.
15. Challenor VF, Waller DG, Hayward RA, et al. Vibrotactile sensation and response to nifedipine dose titration in primary Raynaud's phenomenon. Angiology 1989;40:122–128.
16. Sarkozi J, Bookman AA, Mahon W, et al. Nifedipine in the treatment of idiopathic Raynaud's syndrome. *J Rheumatol* 1986;13:331–336.
17. Corbin DO, Wood DA, Macintyre CC, et al. A randomized double blind cross-over trial of nifedipine in the treatment of primary Raynaud's phenomenon. *Eur Heart J* 1986;7:165–170.
18. Gjorup T, Kelbaek H, Hartling OJ, et al. Controlled double-blind trial of the clinical effect of nifedipine in the treatment of idiopathic Raynaud's phenomenon. *Am Heart J* 1986;111:742–745.
19. Waller DG, Challenor VF, Francis DA, et al. Clinical and rheological effects of nifedipine in Raynaud's phenomenon. *Br J Clin Pharmacol* 1986;22:449–454.
20. French Cooperative Multicenter Group for Raynaud Phenomenon. Controlled multicenter double-blind trial of nicardipine in the treatment of primary Raynaud phenomenon. *Am Heart J* 1991;122:352–355.
21. Wollershiem H, Thien T. Double-blind placebo-controlled crossover study of oral nicardipine in the treatment of Raynaud's phenomenon. *J Cardiovasc Pharmacol* 1991;18:813–818.
22. La Civita L, Pitaro N, Rossi M, et al. Amlodipine in the treatment of Raynaud's phenomenon. A double-blind placebo-controlled crossover study. *Clin Drug Invest* 1997;13:126–131.
23. Rhedda A, McCans J, Willan AR, et al. A double blind controlled crossover randomized trial of diltiazem in Raynaud's phenomenon. *J Rheumatol* 1985;12:724–727.
24. Davinroy M, Mosnier M. Double-blind clinical-evaluation of naftidrofuryl in Raynaud's phenomenon. *Sem Hop Paris* 1993;69:1322–1326. [In French]
25. Sunderland GT, Belch JJF, Sturrock RD, et al. A double blind randomised placebo controlled trial of Hexopal in primary Raynaud's disease. *Clin Rheumatol* 1988;7:46–49.
26. Murphy R. The effect of inositol nicotinate (Hexopal) in patients with Raynaud phenomenon — a placebo-controlled study. *Clin Trials J* 1985;22:521–529.
27. Wollershiem H, Thien T, Fennis J, et al. Double-blind, placebo-controlled study of prazosin in Raynaud's phenomenon. *Clin Pharmacol Ther* 1986;40:219–225.

Janet Pope
Rheumatologist
St Joseph's Health Care
London, Ontario
Canada

Competing interests: None declared.

TABLE 1 **RCTs comparing nifedipine versus placebo in people with primary Raynaud's phenomenon (see text, p 1547).[14–19]**

Ref	Intervention	Number of people	RCT design	Time to outcome (weeks)	Results	Comment
14	Nifedipine (30 mg/day for 2 weeks, adjusted to daily, twice daily, or depending on adverse effects) *v* placebo, biofeedback, or sham biofeedback for 1 year	313 people with primary Raynaud's	Parallel	56	**Frequency of attacks:** mean attacks/day 0.07 with nifedipine *v* 0.21 with placebo; P < 0.001 **Subjective assessment:** 51/70 (73%) people rated themselves as "improved" with nifedipine *v* 54/164 (33%) with placebo; P < 0.001	**Frequency:** attacks defined as the person reporting a Raynaud's episode at least 30 minutes after a previously recorded diary entry and indicating a corresponding code consistent with a true Raynaud's attack **Subjective assessment:** results not intention to treat; withdrawals not stated
15	Nifedipine (10 mg twice daily for 3 weeks, then 20 mg twice daily for 3 weeks) *v* placebo	22 people with primary Raynaud's	Crossover	6	**Frequency of attacks:** mean attacks/week 4.4 with nifedipine *v* 7.3 with placebo; P < 0.01 **Severity of attacks:** mean severity 1.7 with nifedipine *v* 1.9 with placebo; P reported as non-significant **Subjective assessment:** 12/22 (54%) people rated nifedipine *v* placebo as more effective; P < 0.01	**Severity:** measured on a scale of 1–3, where 1 represented mild, 2 moderate, and 3 severe attack **Subjective assessment:** measured on a 5 point scale
16	Nifedipine (10 mg 3 times daily increased to 20 mg 3 times daily after 5 weeks if no improvement) *v* placebo for 10 weeks	39 people with primary Raynaud's	Parallel	10	**Frequency of attacks:** mean reduction in frequency of attacks/week 48% with nifedipine *v* 25% with placebo; P < 0.05	No direct comparison of nifedipine *v* placebo; results are based on comparing changes in outcomes in each group before and after treatment

TABLE 1 continued

Ref	Intervention	Number of people	RCT design	Time to outcome (weeks)	Results	Comment
17	Nifedipine (5 mg 3 times daily for 1 week followed by 10 mg 3 times daily for 1 week and 15 mg 3 times daily for 2 weeks) *v* placebo	23 women with primary Raynaud's	Crossover	8	**Frequency of attacks:** median number of attacks/week in final 2 weeks of treatment after crossover 2.3 with nifedipine *v* 5.0 with placebo; $P < 0.01$	No precrossover results available*
18	Nifedipine (20 mg twice daily for 1 week followed by 40 mg twice daily for 1 week if no adverse effects, *v* placebo	26 people with primary Raynaud's	Crossover	4	**Frequency of attacks:** mean number of attacks/day after crossover: range 0–3.64 with nifedipine v 0.57–5.71 with placebo; $P < 0.01$ **Severity of attacks:** mean grade of the most severe attack: range 0–7.00 with nifedipine *v* 1.00–8.14 with placebo; $P < 0.01$	**Severity:** measured on a scale of 0–10 where 0 represented minimum and 10 maximum severity. No precrossover results available*
19	Nifedipine (20 mg twice daily for 8 weeks) *v* placebo (2 weeks washout between each 4 weeks of treatment)	34 people; 28 with primary Raynaud's	Crossover	12	**Frequency of attacks:** mean number of attacks/week after crossover 7.5 with nifedipine *v* 10.0 with placebo; $P < 0.001$ **Subjective assessment:** 20/29 (69%) rated nifedipine *v* placebo as more effective; $P < 0.001$	**Subjective assessment:** measured on a 5 point scale. No precrossover results available.* Included people with secondary Raynaud's phenomenon, so results may not be fully applicable in people with primary Raynaud's phenomenon

*Results after crossover may not allow for confounding factors such as inadequate washout and the naturally variable course of Raynaud's phenomenon.
Ref, reference.

Shoulder pain

Search date June 2003

Cathy Speed and Brian Hazleman

QUESTIONS

INTERVENTIONS

Key Messages

- Shoulder pain is not a specific diagnosis. Well designed, double blind RCTs of specific interventions in specific shoulder disorders are needed. Systematic reviews have found RCTs mostly with poor methods, and pronounced heterogeneity of study populations and outcome measures. We found insufficient evidence on the effects of most interventions in people with non-specific shoulder pain.
- **Laser treatment** One systematic review found three small RCTs. Two of the RCTs found that laser improved pain after 2–3 weeks compared with placebo, and one RCT found no significant difference at 8 weeks between treatments, although it may have lacked power to detect a difference. One additional RCT found that laser significantly increased recovery rates at 1 month compared with placebo.
- **Physiotherapy (manual treatment and exercises)** One RCT in people with mixed shoulder disorders found that physiotherapy improved function at 4 weeks compared with no treatment. One RCT in people with rotator cuff disease found that a supervised exercise regimen plus advice on pain management improved pain and function compared with no exercise regimen at 6 months and 2.5 years. One RCT in people with adhesive capsulitis found that intra-articular steroids improved pain and function at 6 weeks compared with physiotherapy, although the magnitude of effect declined by 12 months.
- **Surgical arthoscopic decompression/forced manipulation** One RCT found that arthroscopic decompression by experienced surgeons followed by physiotherapy improved pain and function compared with sham laser but not compared with supervised exercises at 6 months and 2.5 years. One small RCT found that forced manipulation plus intra-articular hydrocortisone injection increased recovery rate at 3 months compared with intra-articular hydrocortisone injection alone.

- **Arthroscopic laser subacromial decompression** One systematic review found no RCTs on arthroscopic subacromial decompression.
- **Electrical stimulation** Three small RCTs provided insufficient evidence about the effects of electrical stimulation in people with shoulder pain.
- **Extracorporeal shock wave therapy** Small and limited RCTs provided insufficient evidence about the effects of extracorporeal shock wave therapy compared with sham treatment or no treatment in people with non-calcifying rotator cuff tendinosis and chronic supraspinatus tendinosis. There was limited evidence of benefit in people with calcific tendinitis.
- **Ice** One small RCT provided insufficient evidence about the effects of ice.
- **Intra-articular corticosteroid injection** We found inconclusive evidence about the effects of intra-articular steroids, with or without local anaesthetic or physiotherapy, compared with placebo or physiotherapy alone in people with shoulder pain.
- **Intra-articular guanethidine** We found no systematic review or RCTs of intra-articular guanethidine in people with non-arthritic shoulder pain.
- **Multidisciplinary biopsychosocial rehabilitation** One systematic review found no good quality RCTs of multidisciplinary biopsychosocial rehabilitation in people with shoulder pain.
- **Oral corticosteroids** Two small RCTs found no evidence of reduced pain or improved abduction with oral corticosteroids compared with placebo or no treatment at 4–8 months. Adverse effects of corticosteroids are well documented (see asthma, p 1891).
- **Oral non-steroidal anti-inflammatory drugs** One systematic review and one additional RCT provided insufficient evidence to draw reliable conclusions about the effects of oral non-steroidal anti-inflammatory drugs compared with placebo in people with non-specific shoulder pain.
- **Phonophoresis** We found no RCTs solely in people with shoulder pain.
- **Subacromial corticosteroid injection** We found no RCTs comparing subacromial injection of steroids versus placebo. Three small RCTs in people with rotator cuff tendinitis and one small RCT in people with subacromial impingement provided insufficient evidence to compare the clinical effects of corticosteroid plus lidocaine versus lidocaine alone. One RCT found no significant difference between subacromial steroid plus lidocaine and physiotherapy in terms of diability or successful outcome at 6 months in people attending their general practitioner because of a new episode of unilateral shoulder pain, but found that steroid injection increased the need for repeat consultation or other interverntions.
- **Transdermal glyceryl trinitrate** We found no reliable RCTs.
- **Ultrasound** One RCT identified by a systematic review found that ultrasound significantly improved pain and quality of life at the end of treatment (6 weeks) in people with calcific tendinitis, but found no significant difference at 9 months. Four other RCTs identified by the review found no significant difference between ultrasound and sham ultrasound, but may have been too small to detect a clinically important difference.
- **Paracetamol or opiates; topical or intra-articular non-steroidal anti-inflammatory drugs** We found no RCTs about these interventions.

DEFINITION Shoulder pain arises in or around the shoulder from the glenohumeral, acromioclavicular, sternoclavicular, "subacromial", and scapulothoracic articulations, and surrounding soft tissues. Regardless of the disorder, pain is the most common reason for consulting a practitioner. In adhesive capsulitis (frozen shoulder), pain is associated with pronounced restriction of movement. For most shoulder disorders, diagnosis is based on clinical features, with imaging studies playing a role in some people. Post-stroke shoulder pain is not addressed in this chapter.

INCIDENCE/ PREVALENCE Each year in primary care in the UK, about 1% of adults aged over 45 years present with a new episode of shoulder pain.[1] Prevalence is uncertain, with estimates from 4–20%.[2–6] One community survey (392 people) found a 1 month prevalence of shoulder pain of 34%.[7] A second community survey (644 people aged ≥ 70 years) reported a point prevalence of 21%, with a higher frequency in women than men

(25% *v* 17%).[8] Seventy per cent of cases involved the rotator cuff. One survey of 134 people in a community based rheumatology clinic found that 65% of cases were rotator cuff lesions; 11% were caused by localised tenderness in the pericapsular musculature; 10% acromioclavicular joint pain; 3% glenohumeral joint arthritis; and 5% were referred pain from the neck.[9] One survey found that, in adults, the annual incidence of frozen shoulder was about 2%, with those aged 40–70 years most commonly affected.[10] The age distribution of specific shoulder disorders in the community is unknown.

AETIOLOGY/ RISK FACTORS Rotator cuff disorders are associated with excessive overloading, instability of the glenohumeral and acromioclavicular joints, muscle imbalance, adverse anatomical features (narrow coracoacromial arch and a hooked acromion), cuff degeneration with ageing, ischaemia, and musculoskeletal diseases that result in wasting of the cuff muscles.[11–14] Risk factors for frozen shoulder include female sex, older age, shoulder trauma, surgery, diabetes, cardiorespiratory disorders, cerebrovascular events, thyroid disease, and hemiplegia.[10,15,16] Arthritis of the glenohumeral joint can occur in numerous forms, including primary and secondary osteoarthritis, rheumatoid arthritis, and crystal arthritides.[11]

PROGNOSIS One survey in an elderly community found that most people with shoulder pain were still affected 3 years after the initial survey.[17] One prospective cohort study of 122 adults in primary care found that 25% of people with shoulder pain reported previous episodes and 49% reported full recovery at 18 months' follow up.[18]

AIMS OF INTERVENTION To reduce pain and to improve range of movement and function, with minimal adverse effects.

OUTCOMES Pain scores (overall score, on activity, at night, at rest, during the day, analgesia count); range of movement measures; assessment of overall severity (self assessed or by blinded assessor); functional score; global improvement scores (self assessed or by blinded assessor); tenderness; strength; stiffness; and adverse effects of treatment. The shoulder pain and disability index (SPADI)Ⓖ is a validated shoulder related pain and disability questionnaire.[19–24] Other validated participant rated disability scores have been developed.[20]

METHODS *Clinical Evidence* search and appraisal June 2003. We found some articles that were not published in English; these articles are being translated and, if appropriate, will be included in future updates.

QUESTION What are the effects of treatments?

OPTION ORAL NON-STEROIDAL ANTI-INFLAMMATORY DRUGS

One systematic review and one additional RCT provided insufficient evidence to draw reliable conclusions about the effects of oral non-steroidal anti-inflammatory drugs compared with placebo in people with non-specific shoulder pain.

Benefits: **Versus placebo:** We found one systematic review (search date 1998, 4 small RCTs, 151 people with shoulder pain for more than 72 hours)[25] and one additional RCT.[26] The review pooled results from RCTs that reported sufficient data (90 people with rotator cuff tendinitis) and found no significant reduction in pain and no significant improvement in abduction between oral non-steroidal anti-inflammatory drugs (NSAIDs — diclofenac, naproxen) and placebo after 4 weeks (pain: visual analogue scale, WMD +3%, 95% CI –19% to +25% where positive values represent deterioration; abduction: WMD +26°, 95% CI –9° to +61° where positive values represent improvement).[27,28] The additional RCT (69 people with acute shoulder pain of less than 96 hours' duration) found that oral flurbiprofen (300 mg daily) improved pain relief judged by the investigator compared with placebo at 14 days (global assessment by investigator: 30/35 [86%] improved with NSAID *v* 19/32 [59%] with placebo; ARR 26%, CI 5% to 46%; NNT 4, 95% CI 3 to 20).[26]

Harms: Withdrawal because of adverse events occurred in less than 10% of people in non-randomised comparative studies, but in up to 20% of people in RCTs. Adverse events were mostly gastrointestinal symptoms, skin rash, headache, or dizziness. The review found no evidence that the incidence or nature of adverse effects varied among NSAIDs (naproxen, diclofenac, flurbiprofen, indometacin [indomethacin], etodolac, ibuprofen, fentiazac, phenylbutazone, piroxicam). We found no systematic review of the adverse effects of cyclo-oxygenase type II selective agents in people with shoulder pain (see differences between NSAIDs under the NSAIDs topic, p 1525).

Comment: Evidence about the effects of NSAIDs in shoulder disorders is limited by the lack of standardised approaches: diverse disorders have been considered under the universal term shoulder pain, different types of NSAIDs were used, and outcome measures and follow up periods vary among RCTs. In addition, pain is a symptom, and so relying on investigator rated pain may not be valid.

OPTION TOPICAL NON-STEROIDAL ANTI-INFLAMMATORY DRUGS

We found no RCTs about the effects of topical non-steroidal anti-inflammatory drugs in people with shoulder pain.

Benefits: We found no systematic review or RCTs of topical non-steroidal anti-inflammatory drugs specifically in people with shoulder pain.

Harms: We found no systematic review or RCTs specifically in people with shoulder pain.

Comment: See topical non-steroidal anti-inflammatory drugs under osteoarthritis, (web only).

OPTION INTRA-ARTICULAR NON-STEROIDAL ANTI-INFLAMMATORY DRUGS

We found no systematic review or RCTs evaluating intra-articular injection of non-steroidal anti-inflammatory drugs.

Benefits: We found no systematic review or RCTs evaluating intra-articular injection of non-steroidal anti-inflammatory drugs.

Harms: We found no RCTs.

Comment: None.

OPTION PARACETAMOL OR OPIATES

We found no RCTs evaluating paracetamol or opiates in people with shoulder pain.

Benefits: We found no systematic review or RCTs evaluating paracetamol or opiates in people with shoulder pain.

Harms: We found no RCTs.

Comment: None.

OPTION SUBACROMIAL CORTICOSTEROID INJECTIONS

We found no RCTs comparing subacromial injection of steroids versus placebo. Three small RCTs in people with rotator cuff tendinitis and one small RCT in people with subacromial impingement provided insufficient evidence to compare clinical effects of corticosteroid plus lidocaine with lidocaine alone.

One RCT found no significant difference between subacromial steroid plus lidocaine and physiotherapy in terms of disability or successful outcome at 6 months in people attending their general practitioner because of a new episode of unilateral shoulder pain, but found that steroid injection increased the need for repeat consultation or other intervention.

Benefits: **Versus placebo:** We found no RCTs. **Plus lidocaine versus lidocaine alone:** We found one systematic review (search date 2002, 4 RCTs).[29] The first RCT identified by the review (50 people with rotator cuff tendinitis) compared three treatments: subacromial triamcinolone plus lidocaine (1 mL of 80 mg/mL triamcinolone plus 2 mL of 0.5% lidocaine); subacromial lidocaine (3 mL of 0.5%); and oral diclofenac plus subacromial lidocaine (diclofenac 50 mg 3 times daily plus 3 mL of 0.5% lidocaine). It found that subacromial triamcinolone plus lidocaine significantly increased clinical response rates at 4 weeks compared with lidocaine alone, but it found no significant difference in pain (clinical response defined as improvement in a combination of overall pain severity score, range of active abduction, and limitation of function: 70% for triamcinolone plus lidocaine *v* 0% for lidocaine alone; $P < 0.001$; reduction in pain: WMD +7%, 95% CI −33% to +47%). The second RCT identified by the review (55 people with rotator cuff tendinitis) found no significant difference between subacromial methylprednisolone (40 mg) plus lidocaine (1 mL of 1%) and lidocaine alone for pain or remission rate at 12 weeks (pain using visual analogue scale 0–30: median pain improved by 8 points with active treatment *v* 8 points with placebo; P value not reported; remission defined as score of 0 on pain, active abduction, flexion, and external rotation: 32% in remission with corticosteroids *v* 26% with placebo; P value not reported). The third RCT in the review (published in abstract form only; 52 people with rotator cuff tendinitis or partial tear, of whom results for 41 people reported) found no significant difference between lidocaine (4 mL of 2%) plus betamethasone (1 mL with 6 mg) and lidocaine (5 mL of 2%) alone for clinical response at 6 months (response rate, measured by American Shoulder and Elbow Surgeons criteria: $P = 0.77$; no further data reported). The fourth RCT in the review (40 people with subacromial impingement who received physiotherapy) found that triamcinolone acetonide (2 mL with 40 mg) plus lidocaine (4 mL of 1%) significantly reduced pain compared with lidocaine alone (6 mL of 1%), but found no significant difference in activities of daily living after a mean follow up of about 30 weeks (moderate or severe pain: 3/19 [16%] with corticosteroid plus lidocaine v 15/21 [71%] with lidocaine alone; P value not reported). Loss to follow up was not clear, and it was not clear whether analysis was by intention to treat. The timing of follow up ranged from 12–55 weeks. **Combined intra-articular and subacromial corticosteroid injections:** We found one systematic review (search date 2002, 2 RCTs).[29] The first RCT (100 people with pain or tenderness over supraspinatus during preceding 3 months) compared four treatments: intra-articular plus subacromial triamcinolone plus lidocaine plus oral naproxen; intra-articular plus subacromial triamcinolone plus lidocaine; intra-articular plus subacromial lidocaine plus oral naproxen; and placebo (intra-articular plus subacromial lidocaine).[28] It found that intra-articular plus subacromial triamcinolone plus lidocaine increased remission rates compared with placebo at 4 weeks (remission defined as a perfect score in active abduction, pain, and limitation of function: 28% for triamcinolone *v* 8% for placebo; P value not reported).[28] The second RCT in the review (42 people with adhesive capsulitis and night pain) compared four treatments: subacromial plus intra-articular steroid; mobilisation; ice therapy; and no treatment. It found no significant difference between treatment groups at 6 months (no data reported).[30] **Plus lidocaine versus physiotherapy:** We found one RCT (207 people attending general practitioner with new episode of unilateral shoulder pain).[31] It found no significant difference between subacromial methylprednisolone (40 mg) plus lidocaine (4 mL of 1%) and physiotherapy (8 sessions over 6 weeks) in disability or successful outcome at 6 months (disability, measured on validated shoulder disability questionnaire from 0 [no disability] to 23 [severe disability]: mean difference 1.4, 95% CI –0.2 to +3.0; successful outcome defined as 50% drop in disability score from baseline: 53% with injection v 60% with physiotherapy; difference 7%, 95% CI –6.8% to +20.4%). It found that steroid injection significantly increased the combined outcome of repeat consultation or other intervention for shoulder pain compared with physiotherapy (57% v 40%; difference 17%, 95% CI 4% to 31%).

Harms: The first RCT included in the review (50 people with rotator cuff tendinitis) found no adverse effects with subacromial corticosteroid plus lidocaine compared with lidocaine alone, apart from mild discomfort.[27] Another RCT (50 people with rotator cuff tendinitis receiving treatments of interest) found a similar adverse event rate with subacromial plus intra-articular corticosteroid injection and with placebo (3/25 [12%, mild gastrointestinal symptoms; pityriasis rosea 2 days after the injection; increased frequency of urination] with corticosteroid injection v 3/25 [12%, mild gastrointestinal symptoms; diarrhoea; vasovagal reaction] with placebo).[28]

Comment: Range of movement is not a satisfactory surrogate measure of function. We found no evidence on the accuracy of placement of subacromial injections.

OPTION INTRA-ARTICULAR CORTICOSTEROID INJECTIONS

We found inconclusive evidence about the effects of intra-articular steroids, with or without local anaesthetic or physiotherapy, compared with placebo or physiotherapy alone in people with shoulder pain.

Benefits: **Versus placebo:** We found no systematic review, but we found one RCT.[32] The RCT (93 people with adhesive capsulitis) compared four treatments: intra-articular steroid injection (40 mg triamcinalone hexacetonide under fluoroscopic control) plus physiotherapy; steroid injection alone; saline injection plus physiotherapy; and saline injection alone.[32] It found that intra-articular steroids (with or without physiotherapy) significantly improved pain and disability at 6 weeks compared with placebo, but found no significant difference at 12 months (improvement in SPADI**G** score at 6 weeks: 46.5 with steroid plus physiotherapy v 36.7 with steroid alone v 18.9 with placebo; P = 0.0004 for both steroid treatments v placebo; 12 months: 48.3 with steroid plus physiotherapy v 50.1 with steroid alone v 47.2 with placebo; P value not reported). **Plus lidocaine (lignocaine) versus lidocaine alone:** We found one systematic review (search date 2002, 2 RCTs).[29] The first RCT identified by the review (48 people with frozen shoulder) compared four treatments: intra-articular methylprednisolone plus lidocaine; intra-articular lidocaine; intra-bursal methylprednisolone plus lidocaine; and intra-bursal lidocaine.[33] It found no significant difference between intra-articular methylprednisolone plus lidocaine and lidocaine alone in pain score or shoulder motion at 24 weeks (pain on 6 point pain scale [0 = no pain; 5 = most severe]: improvement of about 1 in point both groups [absolute score about 3 in both groups]; P > 0.05; shoulder motion: improvement of about 50° in both groups [absolute range of movement about 350° in both groups]; P > 0.05).[33] The second RCT in the review (60 people with rotator cuff lesions, 12 in each treatment group) compared five treatments: tolmetin plus methyl prednisolone plus lidocaine; methyl prednisolone plus lidocaine; acupuncture; ultrasound; and placebo. It found no significant difference between intra-articular injection and placebo in pain or treatment success at 4 weeks (pain on a 100 mm visual analogue scale: 29.2 mm with intra-articular injection *v* 22.0 mm with placebo; P value not reported). These two RCTs may have been too small to detect a clinically important difference. **Combined intra-articular and subacromial corticosteroid injections versus placebo:** See sub-acromial corticosteroid injection, p 1559. **Versus physiotherapy:** The systematic review identified one RCT and we found one subsequent RCT.[29,32] The RCT identified by the review (109 people with adhesive capsulitis) compared up to three injections of 40 mg intra-articular triamcinalone acetonide versus 12 physiotherapy sessions over 6 weeks.[34] It found that steroid injection significantly increased success rates at 7 weeks compared with physiotherapy, but the difference in severity score was less significant at 52 weeks (success defined as complete recovery or much improved at 7 weeks: 40/52 [77%] with steroids v 26/56 [46%] with physiotherapy; RR 1.66, 95% CI 1.21 to 2.28; mean improvement in severity score at 52 weeks: 70 with steroids v 59 with physiotherapy; difference 11, 95% CI 1 to 23). The subsequent RCT (93 people with adhesive capsulitis) compared four treatments: 40 mg intra-articular triamcinalone hexacetonide under fluoroscopic control plus physiotherapy; steroid injection alone; saline injection plus physiotherapy; and saline injection alone.[32] It found that steroid alone significantly improved pain and disability at 6 weeks compared with physiotherapy alone, but found no significant difference at 12 months (improvement in SPADI score at 6 weeks: 36.7 with steroid alone v 22.2 with physiotherapy alone; $P < 0.05$; 12 months: 50.1 with steroid alone v 45.5 with physiotherapy alone; P value not reported).

Harms: Intra-articular injections are rarely associated with infection (estimated at 1/14 000 to 1/50 000 injections).[35,36] An acute self limited synovitis was reported in up to 2% of people. Prevalence of tendon rupture, including rupture of the bicipital tendon and rotator cuff, was reported in less than 1% of people after local injection of corticosteroids.[35] Subcutaneous fat necrosis or skin atrophy was found in less than 1%. Corticosteroid arthropathy and osteonecrosis were rare (< 0.8%) and seem to affect mostly weight bearing joints.[27] One RCT identified by the systematic review[29] compared corticosteroid injection versus physiotherapy in painful stiff shoulders, and reported that corticosteroids were associated with more facial flushing (9/52 [17%] people treated with corticosteroid injections *v* 1/56 [2%] treated with physiotherapy) and more new menstrual irregularities (6/52 [12%] people treated with local corticosteroid injections *v* 0/56 [0%] after physiotherapy).[34] The RCT comparing steroid with and without physiotherapy versus placebo did not report harms.[32]

Comment: Few RCTs of interventions in shoulder pain used high quality methods. One case control study found that clinical outcome correlated with accuracy of injection.[37] Another case control study found that only 10% of intra-articular injections were placed correctly even by experienced operators.[38] Confirmation of injection accuracy can be obtained with fluoroscopy or ultrasound. **Different doses:** We found one RCT (57 people with frozen shoulder).[39] It found that higher dose (40 mg) compared with lower dose (10 mg) triamcinolone injection significantly reduced pain after 6 weeks (change on 100 mm visual analogue scale: 31 mm with low dose *v* 49 mm with high dose; CI not reported; $P < 0.01$), movement restriction, and self rated functional impairment (change on 4 point ordinal scale: 0.7 with low dose *v* 1.3 with high dose; CI not reported; $P = 0.03$), but did not significantly improve sleep disturbance. The RCT found no significant difference in any outcome after 6 months.

OPTION ORAL CORTICOSTEROIDS

Two small RCTs found no evidence of reduced pain or improved abduction with oral corticosteroids compared with placebo. Adverse effects of corticosteroids are well documented.

Benefits: **Versus placebo:** We found no systematic review but found one RCT (32 people with frozen shoulder), which compared oral corticosteroids (cortisone acetate, 200 mg a day for first 3 days, 100 mg up to day 14, then 12.5 mg every 2 days up to 4 weeks) versus placebo.[40] It found no evidence that oral corticosteroids reduced pain more than placebo after 18 weeks, but inter-group comparisons were not reported (mean improvement of 4 point rating scale [0 = no pain, 3 = severe pain]: from 1.4 at baseline to 0.5 with oral corticosteroids *v* 1.4 at baseline to 0.6 with placebo; P values not reported).[40] **Plus home exercise versus home exercise alone:** We found one small RCT (40 people with frozen shoulder).[41] People in both groups also took non-salicylate analgesics and diazepam (5 mg) at night as needed. It found no significant difference between oral corticosteroids (10 mg for 4 weeks and 5 mg for a further 2 weeks) plus advice on home pendular excercises and advice alone for pain at 8 months (no figures available).[41]

Harms: Adverse effect of corticosteroids are well documented (see asthma, p 1891). One RCT (40 people with frozen shoulder) reported mild indigestion in two people, which settled after reducing the dose of oral corticosteroids below 10 mg.[41] No other adverse events were reported. The other RCT did not report adverse events.[40]

Comment: None.

OPTION PHYSIOTHERAPY (MANUAL TREATMENT AND EXERCISES)

One RCT in people with mixed shoulder disorders found that physiotherapy improved function at 4 weeks compared with no treatment. One RCT in people with rotator cuff disease found that a supervised exercise regimen plus advice on pain management improved pain and function compared with no exercise regimen at 6 months and 2.5 years. One RCT in people with adhesive capsulitis found that intra-articular steroids improved pain and function at 6 weeks compared with physiotherapy, although the magnitude of effect declined by 12 months.

Benefits: **Versus placebo or no treatment:** We found one systematic review (search date 2002, 3 RCTs).[42] The first RCT identified by the review (66 people with mixed shoulder disorders) found that physiotherapy plus home exercises significantly increased recovery and improved function at 4 weeks compared with no treatment (recovery RR 7.74, 95% CI 1.97 to 30.32; improved function RR 1.53, 95% CI 0.98 to 2.39).[43] The second RCT identified by the review (125 people with rotator cuff disease) compared three treatments: exercise supervised by an experienced physiotherapist plus home exercises plus pain management; arthroscopic decompression plus physiotherapy; and sham laser over 6 weeks.[44] It found that physiotherapy significantly improved Neer score**G** compared with sham laser at 6 months (median Neer score 86 with physiotherapy *v* 66 with sham laser: $P < 0.001$). Long term follow up of 110 participants from the RCT found that physiotherapy significantly increased success rate compared with sham laser at 2.5 years (success defined as Neer score > 80: 27/44 [61%] with physiotherapy *v* 7/28 [25%] with sham laser; $P < 0.01$).[45] The third small RCT identified by the review (42 people with adhesive capsulitis and night pain) compared four treatments: subacromial plus intra-articular steroid; Maitland mobilisation❻ ; ice therapy; and no treatment. It found no significant difference in pain or range of motion between treatment groups at 3 months (no data reported). The RCT may have lacked power to detect a clinically important difference.[30] **Versus surgical arthoscopic decompression:** See surgery, p 1568. **Versus intra-articular corticosteroids:** See intra-articular corticosteroids, p 1560.

Harms: One RCT comparing physiotherapy versus corticosteroid injection in people with painful stiff shoulders found frequent adverse effects in both groups (32/57 [56%] with physiotherapy *v* 30/57 [53%] with corticosteroid injection). After physiotherapy, these effects lasted longer than 2 days in 13% of people.[34] Fever during treatment was found in 1% of people and local skin irritation in 2% of people; 4% of people reported tingling, radiation of pain down the arm, or slight swelling after treatment.

Comment: Studies on the effects of physiotherapy in shoulder disorders are limited by the lack of standardised approaches. Diverse disorders are considered under the universal term shoulder pain, diverse forms of physiotherapy have been evaluated, and outcome measures and follow up periods vary.

OPTION ULTRASOUND

One RCT identified by a systematic review found that ultrasound significantly improved pain and quality of life at the end of treatment (6 weeks) in people with calcific tendinitis but found no significant difference at 9 months. Four other RCTs identified by the review found no significant difference between ultrasound and sham ultrasound but may have been too small to detect a clinically important difference.

Benefits: **Versus placebo or no treatment:** We found one systematic review (search date 2002, 5 RCTs).[42] The review included studies in people with different clinical conditions.[42] The first RCT in the review (180 people with either pain over deltoid on movement or reduced range of shoulder movement, who had failed to respond to 6 sessions of exercise) compared five treatments: pulsed ultrasound; dummy ultrasound; bipolar interferential electrotherapy; dummy electrotherapy; and dummy electrotherapy plus dummy ultrasound.[46] It assessed recovery using a 7 point Likert scale scored from "very large improvement, including recovery" to "very much worse". It found no significant difference in the proportion rating themselves as "very large improvement" between ultrasound and either no treatment or dummy ultrasound at 6 weeks (26% with ultrasound *v* 19% with dummy ultrasound; difference 7%, 95% CI −7% to +20%; 26% with ultrasound *v* 20% with no treatment; difference 6%, 95% CI −16% to +17%). Similarly, it found no significant difference between ultrasound and control for functional status, pain, or range of movement after 12 months. The second RCT in the review (randomised 70 shoulders in 63 people with calcific tendinitis) compared pulsed ultrasound (frequency 890 Hz; intensity 2.5 W/cm^2; pulsed mode 1 : 4) versus sham treatment over the area of calcification.[47] The first 15 treatments were given daily (5 times weekly) and the remainder three times weekly for 3 weeks. The treating therapist was blind to treatment allocation. Nine people (9 shoulders) did not complete the treatment: three in the ultrasound group and six in the sham group, two in the latter because of pain. The RCT found that ultrasound significantly improved pain and quality of life at the end of treatment (6 weeks) but found no significant difference at 9 months (6 weeks: mean improvement in 15 point pain score was 6.4 with ultrasound *v* 1.6 with sham; $P < 0.001$; mean improvement in 10 point quality of life score was 2.6 with ultrasound *v* 0.4 with sham; P = 0.002; 9 months: mean improvement in 15 point pain score 5.7 points with ultrasound *v* 4.0 points with sham; P = 0.23; mean improvement in 10 point quality of life score 2.4 with ultrasound *v* 1.9 with sham; P = 0.52).[47] The third RCT in the review (60 people with rotator cuff lesions) compared five treatments: ultrasound (no details reported); tolmetin plus methyl prednisolone plus lidocaine; methyl prednisolone plus lidocaine; acupuncture; and placebo. It found no significant difference between ultrasound and placebo in pain or treatment success at 4 weeks, although the study may have lacked power to detect clinically important differences (mean pain score on a 100 mm visual analogue scale from baseline to 4 weeks: 48.2 to 41.2 with ultrasound *v* 52.2 to 22.0 with placebo; P value not reported).[48] The fourth RCT in the review (20 people with shoulder pain and limited movement for > 1 month) found similar proportions of people with either minimal or no pain after 4 weeks between ultrasound (1 MHz, 1.2 W/cm^2 , for 6 minutes) compared with sham ultrasound, although the study may have lacked power to detect clinically important effects (7/11 [64%] with ultrasound *v* 4/9 [44%] with placebo; P value not reported).[49] The fifth RCT in the review (61 people with rotator cuff disease without tear) found no significant difference between pulsed ultrasound (1.0 MHz, on : off ratio 1 : 4, intensity 1.0 W/cm^2, 10 minutes) and placebo in pain or function after 12 months (difference in pain scored using index from 1 to 5, no further details: 0.1, 95% CI –0.1 to +0.3; difference in function using Activities of Daily Living index scored from 2 to 10, no further details: –0.2, 95% CI –0.5 to +0.1).[50]

Harms: None of the RCTs included in the review assessed harms of ultrasound.[42]

Comment: In most RCTs, with the exception of the most recent (second RCT in the review[47]), there was considerable heterogeneity of the groups, interventions, and follow up duration among the RCTs. It is not clear whether ultrasound machines were always adequately calibrated before use.

OPTION LASER TREATMENT

One systematic review found three small RCTs. Two of the RCTs found that laser improved pain in rotator cuff tendinitis after 2–3 weeks compared with placebo, and one RCT found no significant difference at 8 weeks between treatments, although it may have lacked power to detect a difference. One additional RCT found that laser significantly increased recovery rates at 1 month compared with placebo.

Benefits: **Versus placebo:** We found one systematic review[42] (search date 2002, 4 RCTs) and one additional RCT.[51] The first RCT in the review (35 people with rotator cuff tendinitis) found no significant difference between continuous irradiation laser and dummy laser (10 minute sessions, twice weekly for 8 weeks) for pain or abduction at 8 weeks (pain on 10 cm visual analogue scale: improved by 3.6 cm with laser *v* 1.2 cm with placebo; P = 0.34; range of movement improved by 36° with laser *v* 29° with placebo; P = 0.23).[52] The second RCT in the review (20 people with rotator cuff tendinitis) compared three treatments: low level infrared laser (5 minutes 3 times weekly for 2 weeks); sham laser; and naproxen. It found that laser significantly reduced pain after 2 weeks compared with sham laser (pain score difference on 10 cm visual analogue scale 2.5%, 95% CI 2.0% to 3.0%).[53] The third RCT in the review (24 people with supraspinatus tendinitis) found that low level laser (9 treatments over a 3 week period) significantly improved pain at 3 weeks compared with dummy laser (pain improved: 80% with laser *v* 20% with dummy laser; P < 0.05).[54] A fourth RCT in the review (40 people with shoulder periarthritis) compared 15 laser treatments with sham laser and is awaiting translation.[55] The additional RCT (91 people with rotator cuff tendinitis) found that laser significantly increased recovery rates at 1 month compared with placebo (42/47 [89%] *v* 18/44 [41%]; ARR 48%, 95% CI 31% to 65%).[51]

Harms: None of the RCTs included in the review assessed harms of laser therapy.[42]

Comment: The quality of studies on the effects of laser treatment in shoulder disorders is limited by the lack of standardised approaches.

OPTION ELECTRICAL STIMULATION

Three small RCTs provided insufficient evidence about the effects of electrical stimulation in people with shoulder pain.

Benefits: **Versus placebo:** We found one systematic review (search date 2002, 3 RCTs).[42] The first RCT in the review (180 people with pain over deltoid or reduced movement not improved by 6 exercise sessions) compared electrical stimulation (bipolar interferential electrical stimulation) with dummy electrical stimulation, and compared pulsed ultrasound with dummy ultrasound in a blinded two by two factorial design (see benefits of ultrasound, p 1563). It found no significant difference in the proportion of people who reported a "large improvement" at 6 weeks (AR 17/73 [23%] with electrical stimulation *v* 16/72 [22%] with control; ARR +1%, 95% CI –13% to +15%). The second RCT in the review (60 people with symptomatic calcific tendinitis) found that pulsed electromagnetic field significantly improved calcific tendinitis at 6 weeks compared with sham treatment (see comment). The third RCT in the review (29 people with rotator cuff tendinitis not cured by corticosteroid injection) compared electrical stimulation induced by pulsed electromagnetic fields (5–9 hours/day for 4 weeks) versus placebo, but it did not report on clinical improvement or resolution.

Harms: The review provided no evidence on harms.

Comment: The quality of studies on the effects of electrical treatments in shoulder disorders is limited by the lack of standardised approaches. We found no good evidence that different forms of electrical stimulation produce different effects. Further details of the outcomes in the second RCT in the review should be available when this RCT is translated.[56]

OPTION ICE

One small RCT provided insufficient evidence about the effects of ice.

Benefits: We found one small RCT (42 people with adhesive capsulitis and night pain), which compared four treatments: subacromial plus intra-articular steroid; mobilisation**G**; ice therapy; and no treatment. It found no significant difference in pain or range of motion between treatment groups at 3 months (no data reported).[30] However, the study may have lacked power to detect clinically important effects of treatment.

Harms: The RCT provided no evidence on harms.

Comment: None.

OPTION INTRA-ARTICULAR GUANETHIDINE

We found no systematic review or RCTs of intra-articular guanethidine in people with non-arthritic shoulder pain.

Benefits: We found no systematic review or RCTs of intra-articular guanethidine in people with non-arthritic shoulder pain (see comment below).

Harms: We found no RCTs.

Comment: We found one RCT (18 people with resistant shoulder pain, including 6 people with rheumatoid arthritis, 5 with osteoarthritis, 5 with frozen shoulder, 1 with rotator cuff tendinitis, and 1 with psoriatic arthritis) comparing intra-articular guanethidine versus intra-articular saline.[57] It found that guanethidine significantly reduced pain compared with placebo after 8 weeks but found no significant difference in the range of movement (pain improvement on a 10 cm visual analogue scale: 36% with guanethidine *v* 16% with placebo; P < 0.05; range of abduction 53° at baseline and 52° at 8 weeks with guanethidine *v* 57° at baseline and 56° at 8 weeks with placebo; CI not reported).

OPTION TRANSDERMAL GLYCERYL TRINITRATE

We found no reliable RCTs.

Benefits: We found no systematic review but found one small RCT (20 people with supraspinatus tendinitis), which compared local transdermal glyceryl trinitrate with placebo.[58] The RCT did not report direct comparisons between the treatment and placebo groups (see comment below).

Harms: Headaches were reported in 20% of the treatment group 24 hours after the treatment was started (no comparative figures available).[58]

Comment: The RCT[58] found that glyceryl trinitrate significantly reduced pain at 24 hours compared with baseline (mean pain intensities with active treatment measured on a 0–10 analogue scale: 7.1 at baseline; 4.5 at 24 hours, P < 0.001; 2.0 at 48 hours, P < 0.001). Changes in the placebo group were not reported. Relief was maintained after 15 days (figures not available). Mean duration of pain was also significantly reduced with active treatment (figures not available). Mean mobility (assessor rated 4 point scale) significantly improved with active treatment (2.0 at baseline *v* 0.1 at 5 days; P < 0.0001), but not with placebo (1.2 at baseline *v* 1.2 at 15 days). The significance figures quoted are not direct comparisons. Significance figures for treatment versus placebo were not stated.

OPTION PHONOPHORESIS

We found no RCTs solely in people with shoulder pain.

Benefits: **Versus placebo or sham phonophoresis:** We found no RCTs solely in people with shoulder pain (see comment below). **Versus other treatment:** We found no RCTs.

Harms: Adverse effects were not reported.

Comment: One RCT (24 people, 13 with rotator cuff tendinitis, 1 with biceps tendinitis, 1 triceps tendinitis, 9 with knee tendinitis) compared active phonophoresis(G) using topical dexamethasone, lidocaine (lignocaine), and aqueous gel with placebo phonophoresis using aqueous gel only (5 sessions over 5–10 days).[59] It found no significant difference in perceived pain (visual analogue scale [0 cm = no pain, 10 cm = extreme pain]; pain changed from 2.4 cm to 1.3 cm with active treatment *v* from 2.6 cm to 1.5 cm with placebo; not significant, P value not reported). It found no significant effect for tenderness (localised force needed to elicit pain: 198 g, 95% CI 164 g to 235 g at session 1 to 204 g, 95% CI 170 g to 238 g at session 5 with active phonophoresis v 196 g, 95% CI 153 g to 235 g at session 1 to 249 g, 95% CI 221 g to 275 g at session 5 with placebo phonophoresis).

OPTION EXTRACORPOREAL SHOCK WAVE THERAPY

Small and limited RCTs provided insufficient evidence about the effects of extracorporeal shock wave therapy compared with sham treatment or no treatment in people with non-calcifying rotator cuff tendinosis and chronic suprapinatus tendinosis. There was limited evidence of benefit in people with calcific tendinitis.

Benefits: We found no systematic review but found three RCTs.[60–62] The first RCT (115 people with calcific tendinitis) compared three different extracorporeal shock wave therapy regimens (low energy treatment in a single session v a single high energy session v 2 high energy sessions 1 week apart) versus no treatment.[60] It found that high energy treatment increased subjective improvement of pain compared with low energy treatment or placebo at 3 months (81 people analysed; AR for improvement 14/20 [70%] with 2 high energy sessions v 12/20 [60%] with 1 high energy session v 6/21 [29%] with low energy treatment v 0/20 [0%] with placebo; NNT 2 for high energy treatment compared with placebo, 95% CI 1 to 21 for single session and 1–14 for 2 session treatment). It also found that high energy treatment significantly improved a combined measure of pain and function in activities of daily living compared with placebo (the Constant score difference; $P < 0.0001$). However, results should be interpreted with caution because of the high drop out rate and lack of an intention to treat analysis. The second RCT (74 people with chronic non-calcifying rotator cuff tendinitis) found no significant difference between extracorporeal shock wave therapy (1500 pulses at 0.12 mJ/mm) and sham treatment (3 sessions at monthly intervals) in shoulder pain or night pain at 3 or 6 months (improvement of 50% from baseline for shock wave therapy versus sham at 3 months on SPAD index**G**: OR 1.760, 95% CI 0.081 to 0.710; night pain OR 0.94, 95% CI 0.65 to 1.36).[61] The RCT may have lacked power to exclude clinically important effects. The third RCT (40 people with chronic suprapinatus tendinosis, 38 analysed) found no significant difference between extracorporeal shock wave therapy (6000 pulses at 0.11 mJ/mm) and sham treatment (2 sessions weekly for 3 weeks) in function or pain at 12 weeks (difference treatment v control: pain at rest on 10 point visual analogue scale +1.4, 95% CI –1.0 to +3.9; pain during activity on 10 point scale: +2.5, 95% CI –0.81 to +3.33).[62] The RCT may have lacked power to exclude clinically important effects.

Harms: High intensity extracorporeal shock wave therapy can be painful during treatment. Small haematomas were reported in the first RCT, but the incidence was not stated and they could have been related to subcutaneous infiltration of local anaesthetic before treatment.[60]

Comment: The first RCT found no significant difference between two sessions and a single session of extracorporeal shock wave therapy for continued pain (91 people analysed; 23/49 [47%] with 2 sessions v 23/42 [55%] with 1 session; RR of continued pain 0.85, 95% CI 0.50 to 1.23).[60] The mechanism of action of extracorporeal shock wave therapy remains unclear. There was radiological disappearance or disintegration of calcium deposits in a significantly greater proportion of people who received high energy treatment than placebo; 77% of those receiving two sessions of treatment had radiological disappearance or disintegration of calcium deposits after 6 months compared with 47% who had one session (P = 0.05).[60] Technical factors and the dosing regimen of shockwave administration are likely to be important to clinical outcome.

OPTION SURGICAL ARTHROSCOPIC DECOMPRESSION/FORCED MANIPULATION

One RCT found that arthroscopic decompression by experienced surgeons followed by physiotherapy improved pain and function compared with sham laser, but not compared with supervised exercises at 6 months and 2.5 years. One small RCT found that forced manipulation plus intra-articular hydrocortisone injection increased recovery rate at 3 months compared with intra-articular hydrocortisone injection alone.

Benefits: **Versus placebo:** We found one RCT (125 people with rotator cuff disease), which compared three treatments: arthroscopic decompression by experienced surgeons plus physiotherapy; exercise supervised by experienced physiotherapist plus home exercises plus pain management; and sham laser for 6 weeks.[44] It found that surgery significantly improved Neer score**G** compared with sham laser at 6 months (median Neer score 87 with surgery *v* 66 with sham laser; P < 0.001). Long term follow up of 110 people in the RCT found that surgery significantly increased success rate compared with sham laser at 2.5 years (success defined as Neer score > 80: 27/44 [61%] with physiotherapy *v* 7/28 [25%] with sham laser; P < 0.01).[45] **Versus physiotherapy:** The same RCT (125 people with rotator cuff disease) found no significant difference in Neer score between arthroscopic decompression and supervised exercises at 6 months (median Neer score 87 with surgery *v* 86 with exercises, difference 4.0; 95% CI –2 to +11).[44] Long term follow up of 110 people found no significant difference in success rates at 2.5 years (success defined as Neer score > 80: 26/38 [68%] with physiotherapy *v* 7/28 [25%] with sham laser; P < 0.01).[45] **Forced manipulation plus intra-articular hydrocortisone injection versus intra-articular hydrocortisone injection alone:** We found one RCT (30 people with frozen shoulder).[63] It found that forced manipulation under sedation plus intra-articular hydrocortisone injection alone increased recovery rates compared with intra-articular hydrocortisone injection at 3 months (recovery defined as no disability: 7/15 [47%] with forced manipulations *v* 2/15 [13%] with control; ARI 33%, 95% CI 1% to 65%).[63]

Harms: The RCTs did not report adverse effects.[44,63]

Comment: None.

OPTION MULTIDISCIPLINARY BIOPSYCHOSOCIAL REHABILITATION

One systematic review found no good quality RCTs in people with shoulder pain of multidisciplinary biopsychosocial rehabilitation.

Benefits: We found one systematic review (search date 2002).[64] If found no good quality RCTs solely in people with shoulder pain of multidisciplinary biopsychosocial rehabilitation**G** compared with usual treatment (see comment below).

Harms: The review found no reliable RCTs.[64]

Comment: The systematic review found one low quality RCT (70 people aged 20–55 years) in people with chronic neck and shoulder pain.[64] Co-interventions were not avoided, blinding of therapists was not specified, analysis was not by intention to treat, and treatment groups were dissimilar at baseline. It found no significant difference for multidisciplinary biopsychosocial rehabilitation versus usual treatment. The rehabilitation combined physiotherapy with psychological, behavioural, and educational interventions.

OPTION ARTHROSCOPIC LASER SUBACROMIAL DECOMPRESSION

One systematic review found no RCTs about arthroscopic subacromial decompression with a holmium:YAG laser.

Benefits: We found one systematic review (search date 2000) of arthroscopic subacromial decompression with holmium: YAG laser for people with shoulder pain due to impingement syndrome.[65] It identified no RCTs.

Harms: We found no RCTs.

Comment: None.

GLOSSARY

Interferential electrical stimulation Typically a high frequency current (4000 Hz) amplitude modulated at a lower frequency (60–100 Hz) given in bursts of 4 seconds and repeated for up to 15 minutes.

Maitland mobilisation A graded system of manipulations and exercises intended to increase mobility of specific joints.

Multidisciplinary biopsychosocial rehabilitation Combined physical, social, and psychological rehabilitation.

Phonophoresis The application of topical medication followed by ultrasound to the same area; the theory being that the ultrasound energy drives the medication through the skin.

Shoulder pain and disability index (SPADI) A self administered instrument for measuring pain (5 items) and disability (8 items).

Neer score Assesses pain during the past week, clinical testing of shoulder function, active range of movement, and anatomical or radiological examination. Scores range from 0–100 points.

REFERENCES

1. Royal College of General Practitioners; Office of Populations, Censuses and Surveys. Third National Morbidity Survey in General Practice, 1980–1981; Department of Health and Social Security, series MB5 No 1. London: HMSO.
2. Bergunnud H, Lindgarde F, Nilsson B, et al. Shoulder pain in middle age. *Clin Orthop* 1988;231:234–238.
3. McCormack RR, Inman RD, Wells A, et al. Prevalence of tendinitis and related disorders of the upper extremity in a manufacturing workforce. *J Rheumatol* 1990;17:958–964.
4. Allander E. Prevalence, incidence and remission rates of some common rheumatic diseases or syndromes. *Scand J Rheumatol* 1974;3:145–153.
5. Badley EM, Tennant A. Changing profile of joint disorders with age: findings from a postal survey of the population of Calderdale, West Yorkshire, UK. *Ann Rheum Dis* 1992;51:366–371.
6. Andersson HI, Ejlertsson G, Leden I, et al. Chronic pain in a geographically defined general population: studies of differences in age, gender, social class and pain localisation. *Clin J Pain* 1993;9:174–182.
7. Pope DP, Croft PR, Pritchard CM, et al. The frequency of restricted range of movement in individuals with self-reported shoulder pain: results from a population-based survey. *Br J Rheumatol* 1996:35;1137–1141.
8. Chard M, Hazleman R, Hazleman BL, et al. Shoulder disorders in the elderly: a community survey. *Arthritis Rheum* 1991;34:766–769.
9. Vecchio-P, Kavanagh R, Hazleman BL, et al. Shoulder pain in a community-based rheumatology clinic. *Br J Rheumatol* 1995;34:440–442.
10. Lundberg B. The frozen shoulder. *Acta Orthop Scand* 1969:suppl 119.
11. Riordan J, Dieppe PA. Arthritis of the glenohumeral joint. *Baillieres Clin Rheumatol* 1989;3:607–626.
12. Bonutti PM, Hawkins RJ. Rotator cuff disorders. *Baillieres Clin Rheumatol* 1989;3:535–550.
13. Jobe FW, Kvitne RS. Shoulder pain in the overhand or throwing athlete: the relationship of anterior instability and rotator cuff impingement. *Orthop Rev* 1989;18:963–975.
14. Soslowsky LJ, An CH, Johnston SP, et al. Geometric and mechanical properties of the coracoacromial ligament and their relationship to rotator cuff disease. *Clin Orthop* 1994;304:10–17.
15. Nash P, Hazleman BL. Frozen shoulder. *Baillieres Clin Rheumatol* 1989;3:551–566.
16. Wohlgethan JR. Frozen shoulder in hyperthyroidism. *Arthritis Rheum* 1987;30:936–939.
17. Vecchio PC, Kavanagh RT, Hazleman BL, et al. Community survey of shoulder disorders in the elderly to assess the natural history and effects of treatment. *Ann Rheumatol Dis* 1995;54:152–154.
18. Croft P, Pope D, Silman A. The clinical course of shoulder pain: prospective cohort study in primary care. *BMJ* 1996;313:601–602.
19. Roach KE, Budiman-Mak E, Songsiridej N, et al. Development of a shoulder pain and disability index. *Arthritis Care Res* 1991;4:143–149.

20. Croft P, Pope D, Zonca M, et al. Measurement of shoulder related disability: results of a validation study. *Ann Rheum Dis* 1994;53:525–528.
21. Beaton DE, Richards RR. Measuring function of the shoulder. A cross-sectional comparison of five questionnaires. *J Bone Joint Surg Am* 1996;78;882–890.
22. Gerber C. Integrated scoring systems for the functional assessment of the shoulder. In: Matsen III FA, Fu EH, Hawkins RJ, eds. *The shoulder: a balance of mobility and stability.* Rosemont, Illinois, US: The American Academy of Orthopaedic Surgeons, 1993:531–550.
23. Richards RR, An KN, Bigliani LU, et al. A standardised method for the assessment of shoulder function. *J Shoulder Elbow Surg* 1994;3:347–352.
24. L'Insalata JC, Warren RF, Cohen SF, et al. A self-administered questionnaire for assessment of symptoms and function of the shoulder. *J Bone Joint Surg* 1997;79:738–748.
25. Green S, Buchbinder R, Glazier R, et al. Interventions for shoulder pain. In: The Cochrane Library, Issue 2, 2003. Oxford: Update Software. Search date 1998; primary sources Cochrane Musculoskeletal Group trials register, Cochrane Controlled Trials Register, Medline, Embase, Cinahl, and Science Citation Index, and hand searches of major textbooks, bibliographies of relevant literature, the fugitive literature, and the subject indices of relevant journals.
26. Mena HR, Lomen PL, Turner LF, et al. Treatment of acute shoulder syndrome with flurbiprofen. *Am J Med* 1986;80:141–144.
27. Adejabo AO, Nash P, Hazleman BL. A prospective blind dummy placebo controlled study comparing triamcinolone hexacetonide injection with oral diclofenac 50 mg tds in patients with rotator cuff tendinitis. *J Rheumatol* 1990;17:1207–1210.
28. Petri M, Dobrow R, Neiman R, et al. Randomised double blind, placebo controlled study of the treatment of the painful shoulder. *Arthritis Rheum* 1987;30:1040–1045
29. Buchbinder R, Green S, Youd JM.Corticosteroid injections for shoulder pain. In: The Cochrane Library, Issue 2, 2003. Oxford: Update Software. Search date 2002; primary sources Medline, Embase, Cinahl, Central Science Citation Index, and reference lists.
30. Bulgen D, Binder A, Hazleman B, et al. Frozen shoulder: prospective clinical study with an evaluation of three treatment regimes. *Ann Rheum Dis* 1984;43:353–360.
31. Hay EM, Thomas E, Paterson SM, et al. A pragmatic randomised controlled trial of local corticosteroid injection and physiotherapy for the treatment of new episodes of unilateral shoulder pain in primary care. *Ann Rheum Dis* 2003;62:394–399.
32. Carette S, Moffet H, Tardif J, et al. Intraarticular corticosteroids, supervised physiotherapy, or a combination of the two in the treatment of adhesive capsulitis of the shoulder: a placebo-controlled trial. *Arthritis Rheum* 2003;48:829–838.
33. Rizk T, Pinals R, Talaiver A. Corticosteroid injections in adhesive capsulitis: investigation of their value and site. *Arch Phys Med* 1991;72:20–22.
34. Van der Windt DA, Koes BW, Deville W, et al. Effectiveness of corticosteroid injections versus physiotherapy for treatment of painful stiff shoulder in primary care: randomised trial. *BMJ* 1998;317:1292–1296.
35. Gray RG, Gottlieb NL. Intra-articular corticosteroids. An updated assessment. *Clin Orth* 1983;177:235–263.
36. Hollander JL. The use of intra-articular hydrocortisone, its analogues, and its higher esters in arthritis. *Md Med J* 1970;61:511.
37. Eustace JA, Brophy DP, Gibney RP, et al. Comparison of the accuracy of steroid placement with clinical outcome in patients with shoulder symptoms. *Ann Rheum Dis* 1997;56:59–63.
38. Jones A, Regan M, Ledingham J, et al. Importance of placement of intra-articular steroid injections. *BMJ* 1993;307:1329–1330.
39. De Jong BA, Dahmen R, Hogeweg JA, et al. Intra-articular triamcinolone acetonide injection in patients with capsulitis of the shoulder: a comparative study of two dose regimens. *Clin Rehabil* 1998;12:211–215.
40. Blockey N, Wright J. Oral cortisone therapy in periarthritis of the shoulder. *BMJ* 1954;i:1455–1457.
41. Binder A, Hazleman BL, Parr G, et al. A controlled study of oral prednisolone in frozen shoulder. *Br J Rheumatol* 1986;25:288–292.
42. Green S, Buchbinder R, Hetrick S. Physiotherapy interventions for shoulder pain. In: The Cochrane Library, Issue 2, 2003. Oxford: Update Software. Search date 2002; primary sources Medline, Embase, the Cochrane Clinical Trails Register, Cinahl, previous reviews, Science Citation Index.
43. Ginn KA, Herbert RD, Khouw W, Lee R. A randomized, controlled trials of a treatment for shoulder pain. *Phys Ther* 1997;77:802–811.
44. Brox J, Staff P, Ljunggren A, Brevik J. Arthroscopic surgery compared with supervised exercises in patients with rotator cuff disease](stage II impingement syndrome). *BMJ* 1993;307:899– 903.
45. Brox JI, Gjengedal E, Uppheim G, et al. Arthroscopic surgery versus supervised exercises in patients with rotator cuff disease (stage II impingement syndrome): a prospective, randomised, controlled study in 125 patients with a 2 1/2 year follow-up. *J Shoulder Elbow Surg* 1999;8:102–111.
46. Van der Heijden GJMG, Leffers P, Wolters PJMC, et al. No effect of bipolar interferential electrotherapy and pulsed ultrasound for soft tissue shoulder disorders: a randomised controlled trial. *Ann Rheum Dis* 1999;58:530–540.
47. Ebenbichler GR, Erdogmus CB, Resch KL, et al. Ultrasound therapy for calcific tendinitis of the shoulder. *N Engl J Med* 1999;340:1533–1588.
48. Berry H, Fernandes L, Bloom B, Clark RJ, et al. Clinical study comparing acupuncture, physiotherapy, injection and oral anti-inflammatory treatment in shoulder lesions. *Curr Med Res Opin* 1980;7:121–126.
49. Downing D, Weinstein A. Ultrasound therapy of subacromial bursitis. *Phys Ther* 1986;66:194–199.
50. Nykanen M. Pulsed ultrasound treatment of the painful shoulder: a randomised, double-blind, placebo-controlled study. *Scand J Rehabil Med* 1995;27:105–108.
51. Gudmundssen J, Vikne J. Laser treatment for epicondylitis humeri and rotator cuff syndrome. *Nord Tidskr Idrettsmed* 1987;2:6–15.
52. Vecchio P, Cave C, King V, et al. A double blind study of the effectiveness of low level laser treatment of rotator cuff tendinitis. *Br J Rheumatol* 1993;32:740–742
53. England S, Farrell A, Coppock J, et al. Low laser therapy of shoulder tendinitis. *Scand J Rheumatol* 1989;18:427–443.
54. Saunders L. The efficacy of low level laser therapy in supraspinatus tendinitis. *Clin Rehabil* 1995;9:126–134.
55. Taverna E, Parrini M, Cabitza P. Laser therapy in the treatment of some bone and joint pathology. [Laserterapia IR versus placebo nel trattamento di alcune patologie a carcio dell'apparato locomotore] *Minerva Ortop Traumatol* 1990;41:631–636.
56. Dal Conte G, Rivoltini P, Combi F. [Trattamento della periartrite calcarea di spalla con campi magnetici pulsanti: studio controllato]. *Riabilitazione* 1990;23:27–33.
57. Gado I, Emery P. Intra-articular guanethidine injection for resistant shoulder pain: a preliminary double blind study of a novel approach. *Ann Rheum Dis* 1996;55:199–201.
58. Berrazueta JR, Losada A, Poveda J, et al. Successful treatment of shoulder pain syndrome due to supraspinatus tendinitis with transdermal nitroglycerin. A double blind study. *Pain* 1996;66:63–67.

59. Penderghest CE, Kimura IF, Gulick DT. Double-blind clinical efficacy study of pulsed phonophoresis on perceived pain associated with symptomatic tendinitis. *J Sport Rehabil* 1998;7:9–19.
60. Loew M, Daecke W, Kusnierczak D, et al. Shock-wave therapy is effective for chronic calcifying tendinitis of the shoulder. *J Bone Joint Surg Br* 1999;81:863–867.
61. Speed CA, Richards C, Nichols D, et al. Extracorporeal shock-wave therapy for tendinitis of the rotator cuff. A double-blind, randomised, controlled trial. *J Bone Joint Surg* 2002;84:509–512.
62. Schmitt J, Haake M, Tosche A, et al. Low-energy extracorporeal shock-wave treatment for tendinitis of the supraspinatus. *J Bone Joint Surg* 2001;83:873–876.
63. Thomas D, Williams R, Smith D. The frozen shoulder. A review of manipulative treatment. *Rheumatol Rehabil* 1980;19:173–179.
64. Karjalainen K, Malmivaara A, van Tulder M, et al. Multidisciplinary biopsychosocial rehabilitation for neck and shoulder pain among working age adults. In: The Cochrane Library, Issue 2, 2003. Oxford: Update Software. Search date 2002; primary sources Medline, Embase, Cochrane Library, Medic (Finnish medical database), Science Citation Index, and hand searches of reference lists and contact with 24 experts in the field of rehabilitation.
65. Boult M, Wicks M, Watson DI, et al. Arthroscopic Subacromial Decompression with a holmium : YAG laser: review of the literature. *ANZ J Surg* 2001;71:172–177. Search date 2000; primary sources Medline, Embase, Current Contents, and The Cochrane Library.

Cathy Speed
Rheumatologist/Director of Sports and Exercise Medicine Unit

Brian Hazleman
Senior Consultant
Addenbrooke's Hospital
Cambridge
UK

Competing interests: None declared.

Tennis elbow

Search date April 2003

Willem Assendelft, Sally Green, Rachelle Buchbinder, Peter Struijs, and Nynke Smidt

QUESTIONS

INTERVENTIONS

Key Messages

- **Topical non-steroidal anti-inflammatory drugs for short term pain relief** One systematic review has found that topical non-steroidal anti-inflammatory drugs improve pain in the short term compared with placebo. Minor adverse effects have been reported. We found no RCTs comparing oral versus topical non-steroidal anti-inflammatory drugs.
- **Oral non-steroidal anti-inflammatory drugs for short term pain relief** One systematic review found limited evidence that an oral non-steroidal anti-inflammatory drug reduced pain and improved function compared with placebo in the short term, although we found limited evidence that it was less effective than corticosteroid injection in the short term.
- **Corticosteroid injections** One systematic review and subsequent RCTs of corticosteroid injections found limited evidence of a short term improvement in symptoms with steroid injections compared with placebo, a local anaesthetic, orthoses (elbow strapping), physiotherapy, or oral non-steroidal anti-inflammatory drugs. We found no good evidence on long term effects of corticosteroids compared with placebo, local anaesthetic, physiotherapy (mobilisation plus massage) or elbow strapping, and found limited evidence that corticosteroid injection was less effective than physiotherapy or oral non-steroidal anti-inflammatory drugs in the long term.
- **Acupuncture** We found insufficient evidence from small, methodologically weak RCTs about effects of needle acupuncture, laser acupuncture, or electro-acupuncture) in people with tennis elbow.
- **Exercise and mobilisation** One small RCT identified by a systematic review found limited evidence that exercise reduced symptoms at 8 weeks compared with ultrasound plus friction massage. However, we were unable to draw reliable conclusions from this small study.

Clin Evid 2005;13:1572–1581.

- **Non-steroidal anti-inflammatory drugs for longer term pain relief** We found insufficient evidence to assess the longer term effects of oral or topical non-steroidal anti-inflammatory drugs, although one RCT found that oral non-steroidal anti-inflammatory drugs were more effective than corticosteroid injections in the long term.
- **Orthoses** One systematic review found insufficient evidence about the effects of orthoses (braces) compared with placebo or physiotherapy. It found limited evidence of a short term improvement in symptoms compared with corticosteroid infections.
- **Surgery** One systematic review found no RCTs of surgical treatment.
- **Extracorporeal shock wave therapy** One systematic review and one subsequent RCT found no significant difference in symptoms between extracorporeal shock wave therapy and sham treatment at 3 months.

DEFINITION Tennis elbow has many analogous terms, including lateral elbow pain, lateral epicondylitis, rowing elbow, tendonitis of the common extensor origin, and peritendinitis of the elbow. Tennis elbow is characterised by pain and tenderness over the lateral epicondyle of the humerus and pain on resisted dorsiflexion of the wrist, middle finger, or both. For the purposes of this review, tennis elbow is restricted to lateral elbow pain or lateral epicondylitis.

INCIDENCE/ PREVALENCE Lateral elbow pain is common (population prevalence 1–3%).[1] Peak incidence is at 40–50 years of age, and for women of 42–46 years of age the incidence increases to 10%.[2,3] The incidence of lateral elbow pain in general practice is 4–7/1000 people a year.[3–5]

AETIOLOGY/ RISK FACTORS Tennis elbow is considered to be an overload injury, typically after minor and often unrecognised trauma of the extensor muscles of the forearm. Despite the title tennis elbow, tennis is a direct cause in only 5% of those with lateral epicondylitis.[6]

PROGNOSIS Although lateral elbow pain is generally self limiting, in a minority of people symptoms persist for 18 months to 2 years and in some cases for much longer.[7] The cost is therefore high, both in terms of lost productivity and healthcare use. In a general practice trial of an expectant waiting policy, 80% of the people with elbow pain of already greater than 4 weeks' duration had recovered after 1 year.[8]

AIMS OF INTERVENTION To reduce lateral elbow pain and improve function, with minimal adverse effects.

OUTCOMES Pain at rest, with activities and resisted movements (visual analogue scale or Likert scale); function (validated disability questionnaire, includes 30 point Disabilities of the Arm, Shoulder, and Hand questionnaire, or visual analogue scale or Likert scale); quality of life (validated questionnaire); grip strength (dynamometer); return to work, normal activities, or both; overall participant reported improvement; adverse effects (participant or researcher report); Roles–Maudsley subjective pain score where 1 = excellent, no pain, full movement, full activity; 2 = good, occasional discomfort, full movement and full activity; 3 = fair, some discomfort after prolonged activity; and 4 = poor, pain limiting activities.

METHODS *Clinical Evidence* search and appraisal April 2003. We included all RCTs and quasi-RCTs of any of the listed interventions in (1) people older than 16 years of age with (2) lateral elbow pain for greater than 3 weeks' duration and (3) no history of significant trauma or systemic inflammatory conditions such as rheumatoid arthritis. We included trials in people with various soft tissue diseases and pain due to tendinitis at all sites, provided that the lateral elbow pain results were presented separately or that greater than 90% of people had lateral elbow pain.

QUESTION What are the effects of treatments?

OPTION ACUPUNCTURE

Sally E Green and Rachelle Buchbinder

We found insufficient evidence from small, methodologically weak RCTs about effects of needle acupuncture, laser acupuncture, or electro-acupuncture in people with tennis elbow.

Benefits: **Versus placebo** We found one systematic review (search date 2001, 4 RCTs, 239 people with tennis elbow defined as lateral elbow pain aggravated by wrist and finger dorsiflexion)[9] and one subsequent RCT.[10] None of the RCTs evaluated the effects of acupuncture on quality of life or return to work. The review found that there were important problems with the methodology of the included trials (particularly small populations, uncertain allocation concealment, and substantial loss to follow up) and clinical differences between trials. Results could not be combined in a meta-analysis. The first RCT (48 people) comparing needle acupuncture with sham acupuncture (with needles not inserted) found that acupuncture significantly increased the duration of pain relief and significantly increased the proportion of people with at least 50% reduction in pain after one treatment (duration of pain relief: WMD 18.8 hours, 95% CI 10.1 hours to 27.5 hours; pain reduction: 19/24 [79%] with acupuncture *v* 6/24 [25%] with sham treatment; RR 3.2, 95% CI 1.5 to 6.5; see comment below).[11] The second RCT found that needle acupuncture significantly increased the proportion of people with a self reported good or excellent result compared with sham treatment (22/44 [50%] with needle acupuncture *v* 8/38 [21%] with sham treatment; RR 2.4, 95% CI 1.2 to 4.7) after 10 treatments.[12] However, it found no significant difference in the longer term (after 3 or 12 months). The third RCT found no significant difference between laser acupuncture and sham treatment in the proportion of participants reporting no improvement or worsening of symptoms (after 10 sessions: 6/23 [26.1%] with laser *v* 5/26 [19.2%] with sham treatment; RR 1.36, 95% CI 0.48 to 3.86; at 3 months: 2/22 [9.1%] with laser *v* 6/25[24%] with sham treatment; RR 0.38, 95% CI 0.09 to 1.69; after 12 months: 1/18 [5.6%] *v* 0/21 [0%] with sham treatment; RR 3.47, 95% CI 0.15 to 80.36).[9] The fourth RCT found no significant difference in cure rate (definition of cure not reported) between vitamin B12 injection plus acupuncture and vitamin B12 injection alone (risk of cure with B12 injection alone: RR 0.44, 95% CI 0.15 to 1.29).[9] The subsequent RCT (45 people) compared 10 treatments of acupuncture with sham acupuncture.[10] It found significantly greater reductions in pain intensity and functional impairment with acupuncture compared with sham treatment at 2 weeks (on 30 mm visual analogue scale pain improved by 8.43 with acupuncture *v* 4.89 with sham treatment, $P < 0.05$; Disabilities of the Arm, Shoulder, and Hand questionnaire improved by 23.70 with acupuncture *v* 8.54 with sham treatment, $P < 0.05$). **Manual versus electro-acupuncture:** We found one small RCT (20 people) comparing manual versus electro-acupuncture and assessed pain immediately following a course of six treatments over 2 weeks.[13] It found that electro-acupuncture significantly reduced pain compared with manual acupuncture (pain scored on 10 cm visual analogue scale; pain reduction: 50% with electro-acupuncture *v* 32% with manual acupuncture, $P < 0.001$). We found no RCT on the effect of acupuncture on quality of life, strength, or return to work.

Harms: Long term follow up of one RCT[10] found that one person (1/45) withdrew due to pain from acupuncture.[14] It found no other adverse events. The other RCTs did not report on harms.

Comment: **Versus placebo:** Although statistically significant, an increase of 18 hours in pain relief after needle acupuncture may not be clinically important.[9]

OPTION ORTHOSES (BRACES)

Willem JJ Assendelft and Peter AA Struijs

One systematic review found insufficient evidence about the effects of orthoses (braces) compared with placebo or physiotherapy. It found limited evidence of a short term improvement in symptoms compared with corticosteroid injections.

Benefits: We found one systematic review (search date 1999).[15] Results were not pooled because of considerable heterogeneity among trials. **Versus placebo or no treatment:** The review identified no RCTs.[15] We found no subsequent RCTs. **Versus corticosteroid injections:** The review found two RCTs comparing orthoses versus corticosteroid injections.[15] The first RCT (16 people) compared an orthotic device versus corticosteroid injections. It found no significant difference in short term improvement in pain (improvement: 27.1 with corticosteroid *v* 13.6 with orthotic device; 100 mm visual analogue score difference +13.5, 95% CI –4.6 to +31.6).[15] The second RCT (70 people, 4 treatment groups) found that corticosteroid injection significantly increased the proportion of people having a good or excellent self reported outcome at 2 weeks compared with a splint or elbow band but found no significant difference at 6 or 12 months (2 weeks: AR 34/37 [92%] pooled results for splint and elbow band group *v* 6/19 [32%] with injection; RR 2.9, 95% CI 1.8 to 5.7; 6 months: 19/37 [51%] *v* 14/19 [74%]; RR 0.7, 95% CI 0.46 to 1.05; 12 months: 22/37 [59%] *v* 13/19 [68%]; RR 0.9, 95% CI 0.6 to 1.03).[15] **Versus physiotherapies:** The review found one RCT (84 people) comparing an elbow support versus an unspecified physical therapy.[15] It found no significant difference in short term self reported satisfaction (23/49 [47%] with elbow support *v* 16/35 [46%] with unspecified physical therapy; RR 1.03, 95% CI 0.64 to 1.64). This study provided insufficient information to assess pain improvement. It also had a withdrawal rate of 30%. **Versus non-steroidal anti-inflammatory cream:** The review found one RCT (17 people) comparing a non-steroidal anti-inflammatory cream (details of cream not reported in review) versus an elbow strap.[15] It found greater short term pain reduction with the cream (WMD [scale not specified] 0.38, 95% CI 0.02 to 0.70).

Harms: The review did not report on harms.[15]

Comment: The review reported that validity scores for the RCTs ranged from low to medium.[15] The review identified three RCTs comparing adding an orthotic device to corticosteroid injections or ultrasound. All three RCTs reported only short term results and there were insufficient data or the power of the study was too low to indicate the effect of orthoses.

OPTION CORTICOSTEROID INJECTIONS

Willem JJ Assendelft and Nynke Smidt

One systematic review and subsequent RCTs of corticosteroid injections found limited evidence of a short term improvement in symptoms with steroid injections compared with placebo, a local anaesthetic, orthoses (elbow strapping), physiotherapy, or oral non-steroidal anti-inflammatory drugs. We found no good evidence on long term effects of corticosteroids compared with placebo, local anaesthetic, physiotherapy(mobilisation plus massage), or elbow strapping, and found limited evidence that corticosteroid injection was less effective than physiotherapy or oral non-steroidal anti-inflammatory drugs in the long term.

Benefits: We found one systematic review (search date 1999)[16] and two subsequent RCTs.[17,18] None of the RCTs evaluated the effects of corticosteroid injections on quality of life or return to work. **Versus placebo or no**

treatment: The review identified two RCTs comparing corticosteroid injection (1 mL methylprednisolone acetate) versus injection of saline solution. The first RCT (29 people in smallest group; see comment below) found that corticosteroid significantly increased short term global improvement compared with saline injection (timescale not further specified; RR 0.11, 95% CI 0.04 to 0.33). The RCT did not measure pain or grip strength. The second RCT (10 people in smallest group) found no significant difference in short term pain, global improvement, or grip strength. The first subsequent RCT (39 people with symptoms > 4 weeks) compared corticosteroid injection versus a control injection.[17] All people received rehabilitation. It found that corticosteroid injection significantly improved pain compared with control from 8 weeks to 6 months (improvement on 100 point visual analogue scale: 24.3 with steroid injection *v* 8.9 with control injection; P = 0.04; CI not reported). It found no significant difference in other pain outcomes or grip strength. The second subsequent RCT (59 people in smallest group) compared corticosteroid injection with no treatment and with physiotherapy.[18] It found corticosteroid injection significantly improved mean "main complaint" and functional disability at 3 and 6 weeks compared with no treatment (at 6 weeks, mean difference in "main complaint" 24%, 95% CI 14% to 35%). It found no significant difference at 12, 26, and 52 weeks (at 52 weeks, mean difference in "main complaint" –9%, 95% CI –19% to +2%). **Versus local anaesthetic:** The review identified three RCTs comparing corticosteroid injections versus local anaesthetic alone.[16] Two RCTs (18 and 35 people in smallest groups) found greater global improvement in the short term (4 weeks; follow up not stated) with corticosteroid injections (1 mL hydrocortisone acetate 25 mg and 1 mL methylprednisolone acetate 10 mg), but data could not be pooled because of heterogeneity. The third RCT (7 people in smallest group) reported only medium term results. It found no significant difference in global improvement at 9–17 weeks (chance of not getting a good outcome: RR 0.97, 95% CI 0.41 to 2.32). **Versus orthoses:** See benefits of orthoses, p 1575. **Versus physiotherapies:** The review identified two RCTs comparing corticosteroid injections (1 mL triamcinolone acetate 1% plus 1 mL lidocaine [lignocaine]) versus physiotherapies,[16] and we found one additional RCT.[18] The first RCT identified by the review (53 people in smallest group) found that friction massage and a manipulation technique significantly reduced the chance of overall improvement compared with steroid injection (overall improvement: RR 0.45, 95% CI 0.29 to 0.69). It found no significant difference in any outcome at 52 weeks. The review was unable to report measured results for the second RCT (12 people in smallest group). The additional RCT (59 people in smallest group) compared a corticosteroid injection with no treatment and with physiotherapy consisting of nine sessions of ultrasound, deep friction massage, and an exercise programme over 6 weeks (see versus placebo or no treatment above).[18] It found that corticosteroid injection significantly improved the "main complaint" and functional disability at 3 and 6 weeks compared with physiotherapy (at 6 weeks, mean difference in "main complaint" 20%, 95% CI 10% to 31%). However, there was no significant difference at 12 weeks, and at 26 and 52 weeks physiotherapy significantly improved the "main complaint" compared with corticosteroid injection (at 52 weeks, mean difference in "main complaint" 15%, 95% CI 5% to 25%). **Versus non-steroidal anti-inflammatory drugs:** See oral non-steroidal anti-inflammatory drugs versus corticosteroid injections, p 1577.

Harms: The review (8 RCTs) found no significant difference in adverse events between corticosteroid injections and control interventions (including facial flushes, post-injection pain, and local skin atrophy).[16] However, the review did not report P values.

Comment: The review provided the number of people in the smallest group for each trial rather than the total number of people in the trial. The review found that in the longer term there was a high rate of improvement in all groups.[16] It found that in general the quality of the methodology of the RCTs was poor to modest. The corticosteroid suspensions used in these trials were methylprednisolone (2 RCTs), triamcinolone (4 RCTs), betamethasone (2 RCTs), hydrocortisone (5 RCTs), and dexamethasone (1 RCT). In one RCT, two different substances were used. The RCTs with longer term results for corticosteroid compared with non-steroidal anti-inflammatory drugs and with physiotherapy suggested that a steroid injection improved outcomes in the short term but increased recurrences in the medium term.

OPTION NON-STEROIDAL ANTI-INFLAMMATORY DRUGS

Sally E Green and Rachelle Buchbinder

One systematic review has found that topical non-steroidal anti-inflammatory drugs improve symptoms in the short term compared with placebo. Minor adverse effects have been reported. The review found limited evidence that oral non-steroidal anti-inflammatory drugs improved symptoms in the short term compared with placebo, although we also found limited evidence that it was less effective than corticosteroid injection in the short term. We found insufficient evidence to assess the longer term effects of non-steroidal anti-inflammatory drugs compared with placebo, although one RCT found that oral non-steroidal anti-inflammatory drugs were more effective than corticosteroid injections in the long term. We found no RCTs comparing oral versus topical non-steroidal anti-inflammatory drugs.

Benefits: We found one systematic review (search date 2001)[19] and no subsequent RCTs. None of the RCTs in the review evaluated the effect of non-steroidal anti-inflammatory drugs (NSAIDs) on return to work or quality of life. **Topical NSAIDs versus placebo:** The review found that topical NSAIDs significantly improved pain at up to 4 weeks compared with placebo and significantly reduced participant opinion of no benefit (3 RCTs, 130 people; pain: WMD –1.88, 95% CI –2.54 to –1.21; scale 0 [no pain] to 10 [maximum pain]; no benefit: 2 RCTs; RR 0.39, 95% CI 0.23 to 0.66).[19] Inclusion of unblinded trials did not significantly change the results. It found no significant differences between topical NSAIDs and placebo for grip strength (reported as non-significant, further data not reported) or range of motion (RR for limitation of movement 1.01, 95% CI 0.80 to 1.28). It found that NSAIDs significantly improved the doctor's opinion of effect on pain and in tenderness with placebo (pain: WMD –1.88, 95% CI –2.54 to –1.21; scale 0 [no pain] to 10 [maximum pain]; RR for tenderness 0.83, 95% CI 0.70 to 0.99). The topical NSAIDs used were diclofenac (2 RCTs) and benzydamine (1 RCT). **Oral NSAIDs versus placebo:** The review found two RCTs.[19] The RCTs were not pooled because one reported means and standard deviations and the other medians and ranges. One RCT found limited evidence that diclofenac improved short term pain and function compared with placebo but did not assess long term results (WMD –13.9, 95% CI –23.2 to –4.6 on 100 point scale). The second RCT found no significant difference in pain over 28 days, 6 months, or 1 year or for function at 6 months or 1 year (median [range] pain score, 28 days: 4 [2–6] with naproxen *v* 3.5 [2–6] with placebo; 6 months: 1 [0–3] with NSAIDs *v* 1 [0–2.2] with placebo; 12 months: 0 [0–2] with NSAIDs *v* 0 [0–2] with placebo; function at 6 months: 0 [0–2.75] with NSAIDs *v* 0.5 [0–2] with placebo; at 12 months: 1 [0–1] with NSAIDs *v* 0 [0–0] with placebo). **Oral NSAIDs versus corticosteroid injection:** The review found three RCTs.[19] Only two RCTs were included in the meta-analysis because of incomplete reporting of results. The first of these RCTs compared 20 mg methylprednisolone plus lidocaine versus 500 mg naproxen, and the second compared 6 mg betamethasone plus prilocaine plus placebo tablets versus 500 mg naproxen (initial high dose, then 250 mg). Meta-analysis of self reported perception of benefit found a significant difference in favour of injection at 4 weeks (RR of participant perceived benefit of injection 3.06, 95% CI 1.55 to 6.06). One RCT was not included in the meta-analysis because of skewed data; it found less functional limitation at 4 weeks in the injection group (median [range] 0 [0–2] with injection *v* 3 [1–5] with NSAIDs). The greater benefit of injection compared with naproxen was only found in the short term. The largest RCT (53 people in smallest group) found significantly greater improvement in pain at 26 weeks with an NSAID (RR 1.71, 95% CI 1.17 to 2.51). It found no significant difference in grip strength and results were not reported for global improvement.

Harms: **Topical NSAIDs:** One RCT identified by the review found that topical NSAIDs significantly increased any adverse event compared with placebo (RR 2.26, 95% CI 1.04 to 4.94).[20] Adverse effects were mild and no one was withdrawn from the study. Adverse effects reported in the published trials were foul breath and minor skin irritation. **Oral NSAIDs:** One trial of oral NSAIDs found an increased risk of abdominal pain and diarrhoea (pain: RR 3.17, 95% CI 1.35 to 7.41; diarrhoea: RR 1.92, 95% CI 1.08 to 3.14). One systematic review (search date 1994, 12 RCTs of NSAIDs in a variety of disorders)[21] found that the overall relative risk of complications from oral NSAIDs was 3.0–5.0. Adverse effects were predominantly gastrointestinal. See important differences between available NSAIDs in the NSAIDs chapter, p 1525.

Comment: Both topical and oral NSAIDs may provide short term relief of pain in tennis elbow, although topical NSAIDs may be associated with fewer adverse effects. Further placebo controlled and comparative trials of oral compared with topical NSAIDs would help to clarify the effects of NSAIDs in the treatment of tennis elbow. Few trials used intention to treat analysis, and the sample size of most was small (populations range from 18–128 people for trials included in the meta-analysis).[19]

OPTION EXERCISE AND MOBILISATION

Willem JJ Assendelft and Nynke Smidt

One small RCT identified by a systematic review found limited evidence that exercise reduced symptoms at 8 weeks compared with ultrasound plus friction massage. However, we were unable to draw reliable conclusions from this small study. We found no RCTs of mobilisation.

Benefits: We found one systematic review (search date 1999, 1 RCT, 19 people).[22] The small RCT found that exercise significantly improved symptoms at 8 weeks compared with ultrasound plus friction massage (SMD –0.95, 95% CI –1.64 to –0.26). Four other RCTs were either of poor validity or provided insufficient data on relevant outcome measures. We found no RCTs of mobilisation.

Harms: No harms were described in the systematic review.[22]

Comment: None.

OPTION EXTRACORPOREAL SHOCK WAVE THERAPY

Rachelle Buchbinder and Sally E Green

One systematic review and one subsequent RCT found no significant difference in symptoms between extracorporeal shock wave therapy and sham treatment at 3 months.

Benefits: **Versus placebo:** We found one systematic review (search date 2001, 2 RCTs, 286 people)[23] and one subsequent RCT comparing extracorporeal shock wave therapy (ESWT) versus placebo.[24] Both RCTs identified by the review had similar study populations (mean age 41.9–46.9 years, slightly more women) with chronic symptoms (mean duration 21.9–27.6 months) who had not improved on at least 6 months of conservative treatment, including non-steroidal anti-inflammatory drugs, injections, brace or taping, casting, and physiotherapy. The frequency, doses, and technique of ESWT application were similar in both trials. The first RCT in the review used 1000 impulses of 0.08 mJ/mm^2 of ESWT at weekly intervals for 3 weeks.[23] The second RCT in the review used "low energy" ESWT with 2000 pulses under local anaesthesia (3 mL mepivacaine 1%) at weekly intervals for 3 weeks using device dependent energy flux density (ED+) between 0.07 and 0.09 mJ/mm^2.[23] The review found no significant difference in treatment failure (defined as Roles–Maudsley subjective pain score of 4) between ESWT and placebo at 6 weeks and at 1 year (6 weeks: RR 0.40, 95% CI, 0.08 to 1.91; 1 year: RR 0.44, 95% CI 0.09 to 2.17). After 6 weeks, it found no significant improvement in pain at rest, pain with resisted wrist extension, or pain with resisted middle finger extension (pain scored out of 100 points; pain at rest: WMD −11.4, 95% CI −26.1 to +3.3; pain with resisted wrist extension: WMD −16.2, 95% CI −47.8 to +15.4; pain with resisted middle finger extension: WMD −20.5, 95% CI −56.6 to +15.6). At 12 and 24 weeks, it found no significant difference between treatments in pain at 12 to 24 weeks (pain scored out of 100 points; improvement in pain at rest: WMD −14.7, 95% CI −35.4 to +6.1; pain with resisted wrist extension: WMD −14.70, 95% CI −43.4 to +14.0; pain with resisted middle finger extension: WMD −21.1, 95% CI −58.3 to +16.1). The effect of ESWT on function, quality of life, and return to work was not reported. The effect of ESWT on grip strength was reported in both trials but the results were difficult to interpret in one RCT. The other RCT found no difference in improvement in grip strength between groups at 6 weeks, 12 weeks, or 1 year. The subsequent RCT (75 people) found no significant difference between ESWT (1500 pulses at 0.18 mJ/mm^2 at weekly intervals for 3 weeks) and sham treatment in pain at 3 months (50% or greater improvement in pain measured on 10 mm visual analogue scale: 14/40 [35%] with ESWT *v* 12/35 [34%] with sham; RR 1.3, 95% CI 0.75 to 2.4).[24]

Harms: One RCT in the review did not report adverse events.[23] The other RCT in the review reported significantly more adverse effects in the EWST group compared with placebo (OR 4.3, 95% CI 2.9 to 6.3). However, there were no treatment discontinuations or dosage adjustments related to adverse effects. The most frequently reported adverse effects in the ESWT treated group were transitory reddening of the skin (21.1% with ESWT *v* 4.7% with placebo); pains (4.8% with ESWT *v* 1.7% with placebo); and petechiae, bleeding, or haematomas (4.5% with ESWT *v* 1.7% with placebo). Migraine occurred in four people and syncope in three people after ESWT, compared with no people treated with placebo. No significant adverse effects were reported in the subsequent RCT.[24]

Comment: The two RCTs in the review found conflicting results.[23] When data from both trials were pooled, the benefits observed in the first trial were no longer apparent. This RCT, which found a significant improvement, had uncertain allocation concealment and no analysis of early withdrawals (15/115 [13%]).

OPTION SURGERY

Rachelle Buchbinder and Sally E Green

One systematic review found no RCTs of surgical treatment.

Benefits: We found one systematic review (search date 2001), which identified no RCTs.[25] We found no subsequent RCTs.

Harms: We found no RCTs.

Comment: Various open and percutaneous operations for lateral elbow pain have been described based upon the surgeon's concept of the pathological entity. The most commonly described surgical procedures involve excision of abnormal tissue (comprising microscopic degeneration, rupture, or both, and immature reparative tissue) within the origin of extensor carpi radialis brevis, release of the extensor carpi radialis brevis from the lateral epicondyle region, or both. Additional procedures include release of the anterior capsule, removal of inflamed synovial folds, resection of a third of the orbicular ligament, debridement of articular damage, release of the posterior interosseous nerve, denervation of the lateral epicondyle, denervation of the radiohumeral joint, and excision of a radiohumeral bursa.[26–38]

REFERENCES

1. Allander E. Prevalence, incidence and remission rates of some common rheumatic diseases and syndromes. *Scand J Rheumatol* 1974;3:145–153.
2. Chard MD, Hazleman BL. Tennis elbow — a reappraisal. *Br J Rheumatol* 1989;28:186–190.
3. Verhaar J. Tennis elbow: anatomical, epidemiological and therapeutic aspects. *Int Orthop* 1994;18:263–267.
4. Hamilton P. The prevalence of humeral epicondylitis: a survey in general practice. *J R Coll Gen Pract* 1986;36:464–465.
5. Kivi P. The etiology and conservative treatment of lateral epicondylitis. *Scand J Rehabil Med* 1983;15:37–41.
6. Murtagh J. Tennis elbow. *Aust Fam Physician* 1988;17:90–91,94–95.
7. Hudak P, Cole D, Haines T. Understanding prognosis to improve rehabilitation: the example of lateral elbow pain. *Arch Phys Rehabil* 1996;77:568–593.
8. Smidt N, van der Windt DAWM, Assendelft WJJ, et al. Corticosteroid injections for lateral epicondylitis are superior to physiotherapy and a wait and see policy at short-term follow-up, but inferior at long-term follow-up: results from a randomised controlled trial. *Lancet* 2002;359:657–662.
9. Green S, Buchbinder R, Barnsley L, et al. Acupuncture for lateral elbow pain. In: The Cochrane Library, Issue 3, 2002. Oxford: Update Software. Search date 2001; primary sources Medline, Cinahl, Embase, Scisearch, Cochrane Controlled Trials Register, and Cochrane Musculoskeletal Review Group Specialised Trial Database.
10. Fink M, Wolkenstein E, Karst M, et al. Acupuncture in chronic epicondylitis: a randomized controlled trial. *Rheumatology* 2002;41:205–209.
11. Molsberger A, Hille E. The analgesic effect of acupuncture in chronic tennis elbow pain. *Br J Rheumatol* 1994;33:1162–1165.
12. Haker E, Lundberg T. Acupuncture treatment in epicondylalgia: a comparative study of two acupuncture techniques. *Clin J Pain* 1990;6:221–226.
13. Tsui P, Leung MCP. Comparison of the effectiveness between manual acupuncture and electroacupuncture on patients with tennis elbow. *Acupunct Electrother Res* 2002;27:107–117.
14. Fink M, Wolkenstein E, Luennemann M, et al. Chronic epicondylitis: effect of real and sham acupuncture treatment. A randomized controlled patient- and examiner-blinded long-term trial. *Forsch Komplementarmed Klass Naturheilkd* 2002;9:210–215.
15. Struijs PAA, Smidt N, Arola H, et al. Orthotic devices for the treatment of tennis elbow. In: The Cochrane Library, Issue 3, 2002. Oxford: Update Software. Search date 1999; primary sources Medline, Embase, Cinahl, Cochrane Controlled Trials Register, Current Contents, hand searches of reference lists from all retrieved articles, and personal contact with subject experts.
16. Smidt N, Assendelft WJJ, van der Windt DAWM, et al. Corticosteroid injections for lateral epicondylitis: a systematic review. *Pain* 2002;96:23–40. Search date 1999; primary sources Medline, Embase, Cinahl, Cochrane Controlled Trials Register, Current Contents, Cochrane Rehabilitation and Related Therapies Field Trials Register, and hand searches of references from retrieved articles.
17. Newcomber K, Laskowski E, Idank D, et al. Corticosteroid injection in early treatment of lateral epicondylitis. *Clin J Sport Med* 2001;11:214–222.
18. Smidt N, van der Windt D, Assendelft W, et al. Corticosteroid injections, physiotherapy, or a wait-and-see policy for lateral epicondylitis: a randomised controlled trial. *Lancet* 2002;359:657–662.
19. Green S, Buchbinder R, Barnsley L, et al. Non-steroidal anti-inflammatory drugs (NSAIDs) for treating lateral elbow pain in adults. In: The Cochrane Library, Issue 3, 2002. Oxford: Update Software. Search date 2001; primary sources Medline, Cinahl, Embase, Scisearch, Cochrane Musculoskeletal Review Group Specialised Trials Register, and Cochrane Controlled Trials Register.
20. Percy E, Carson J. The use of DMSO in tennis elbow and rotator cuff tendonitis: a double blind study. *Med Sci Sports Exerc* 1981;13:215–219.
21. Rodriguez LAG. Nonsteroidal antiinflammatory drugs, ulcers and risk: a collaborative meta-analysis. *Semin Arthritis Rheum* 1997;26:16–20. Search date 1994; primary sources Medline, hand searches of bibliographies of previous meta-analyses, and personal contact with authors of relevant studies.
22. Smidt N. Chapter 2. In: Smidt N. *Conservative treatments for tennis elbow in primary care* [thesis]. Wasenlngen: Ponsen and Looijen BV, 2001. Search date 1999; primary sources Medline, Embase, Cinahl, Cochrane Controlled Trials Register, Current Contents, Cochrane Rehabilitation and Related Therapies Field Trials Register, and hand searches of references from retrieved articles.
23. Buchbinder R, Green S, White M, et al. Shock wave therapy for lateral elbow pain. In: The Cochrane Library, Issue 3, 2002. Oxford: Update Software. Search date 2001; primary sources of Medline, Cinahl, Embase, Scisearch, Cochrane Controlled Trials Registrar, and Cochrane Musculoskeletal Review Group Specialised Trials Database.
24. Speed C, Nichols D, Richards C, et al. Extracorporeal shock wave therapy for lateral epicondylitis — a double blind randomized controlled trial. *J Orthop Res* 2002;20:895–898.
25. Buchbinder R, Green S, Bell S, et al. Surgery for lateral elbow pain. In: The Cochrane Library, Issue 3,

2002. Oxford: Update Software. Search date 2001; primary sources Medline, Cinahl, Embase, Scisearch, Cochrane Controlled Trials Registrar, and Cochrane Musculoskeletal Review Group Specialised Trials Database.
26. Bosworth DM. Surgical treatment of tennis elbow. A follow-up study. *J Bone Joint Surg Am* 1965;47:1533–1536.
27. Boyd HB, McLeod HC Jr. Tennis elbow. *J Bone Joint Surg Am* 1973;55:1183–1187.
28. Calvert PT, Macpherson IS, Allum RL, et al. Simple lateral release in treatment of tennis elbow. *J R Soc Med* 1985;78:912–915.
29. Coonrad RW, Hooper WR. Tennis elbow: its course, natural history, conservative and surgical management. *J Bone Joint Surg Am* 1973;55:1177–1182.
30. Friden J, Lieber R. Physiological consequences of surgical lengthening of extensor carpi radialis brevis muscle–tendon junction for tennis elbow. *J Hand Surg Am* 1994;19A:269–274.
31. Goldberg EJ, Abraham E, Siegel I. The surgical treatment of chronic lateral humeral epicondylitis by common extensor release. *Clin Orthop* 1988;233:208–212.
32. Kaplan EB. Treatment of tennis elbow (epicondylitis) by denervation. *J Bone Joint Surg Am* 1959;41:147–151.
33. Nirschl RP, Pettrone FA. The surgical treatment of lateral epicondylitis. *J Bone Joint Surg Am* 1979;61:832–839.
34. Posch JN, Goldberg VM, Larrey R. Extensor fasciotomy for tennis elbow: a long term follow-up study. *Clin Orthop* 1978;135:179–182.
35. Verhaar J, Walenkamp G, Kester A, et al. Lateral extensor release for tennis elbow. A prospective long-term follow-up study. *J Bone Joint Surg Am* 1993;75:1034–1043.
36. Wilhelm A. Tennis elbow: treatment of resistant cases by denervation. *J Hand Surg Br* 1996;21:523–533.
37. Wittenberg RH, Schaal S, Muhr G. Surgical treatment of persistent elbow epicondylitis. *Clin Orthop* 1992;278:73–80.
38. Yerger B, Turner T. Percutaneous extensor tenotomy for chronic tennis elbow. *Orthopedics* 1985;8:1261–1263.

Willem Assendelft
Head of Department of Guideline Development and Research Policy
Dutch College of General Practitioners
Utrecht
The Netherlands

Sally Green
Senior Lecturer
Institute of Health Services Research
Monash University
Melbourne
Australia

Rachelle Buchbinder
Director
Department of Clinical Epidemiology
Cabrini Hospital and Monash University
Department of Epidemiology and Preventive Medicine
Melbourne
Australia

Peter Struijs
Academic Medical Center
Amsterdam
The Netherlands

Nynke Smidt
Institute for Research in Extramural Medicine
Amsterdam
The Netherlands

Competing interests: The authors of this piece are the authors of the Cochrane Reviews from which most of the evidence is drawn. WA has supervised and PS has conducted a trial sponsored by Bauerfeind, a manufacturer of orthoses. RB, SG, and NS none declared.

Altitude sickness

Search date January 2004

David Murdoch

QUESTIONS

INTERVENTIONS

*Although we found no RCTs on the effects of these interventions, there is a general consensus that they are effective

Key Messages

Prevention

- **Acetazolamide** One systematic review and one subsequent RCT found that acetazolamide reduced the incidence of acute mountain sickness compared with placebo. The review found that acetazolamide caused polyuria and/or paraesthesia in over a third of people. We found no RCTs of sufficient quality comparing acetazolamide versus dexamethasone.
- **Dexamethasone** One systematic review and further RCTs found that dexamethasone was more effective than placebo for preventing acute mountain sickness. However, the review found that adverse effects (including depression) occurred in a quarter of people on withdrawal of dexamethasone. We found no RCTs of sufficient quality comparing dexamethasone versus acetazolamide.
- **Slow ascent (or acclimatisation)** We found no RCTs evaluating different rates of ascent or acclimatisation. One non-randomised trial, observational studies, and consensus opinion suggest that slower ascent reduces the risk of acute mountain sickness compared with more rapid ascent.

Treatment

- **Descent compared with resting at the same altitude** We found no RCTs on the effects of descent compared with resting at the same altitude in people with acute mountain sickness. Consensus opinion suggests that people with acute mountain sickness should descend if possible. However, we found no RCTs examining the effects of different distances of descent, or about the balance of risks and benefits in people who might find it difficult to descend.
- **Dexamethasone** One small RCT in climbers with symptoms and signs of acute mountain sickness found that dexamethasone reduced mean acute mountain sickness scores compared with placebo.

Clin Evid 2005;13:1582–1587.

- **Acetazolamide** We found no RCTs of sufficient quality on the effects of acetazolamide compared with placebo for treating people with acute mountain sickness.

DEFINITION Altitude sickness (or high altitude illness) includes acute mountain sickness, high altitude pulmonary oedema, and high altitude cerebral oedema. Acute mountain sickness typically occurs at altitudes greater than 2500 metres (about 8000 feet) and is characterised by the development of some or all of the symptoms of headache, weakness, fatigue, listlessness, nausea, insomnia, and suppressed appetite. Symptoms may take days to develop or may occur within hours, depending on the rate of ascent and the altitude attained. More severe forms of altitude sickness have been identified. High altitude pulmonary oedema is characterised by symptoms and signs typical of pulmonary oedema, such as shortness of breath, coughing, and production of frothy or blood stained sputum. High altitude cerebral oedema is characterised by confusion, ataxia, and decreasing conscious level. This review covers only acute mountain sickness.

INCIDENCE/ PREVALENCE The incidence of acute mountain sickness increases with absolute height attained and with the rate of ascent. One survey in Taiwan (93 people ascending above 3000 metres) found that 27% of people experienced acute mountain sickness.[1] One survey in the Himalayas (278 unacclimatised hikers at 4243 metres) found that 53% of people developed acute mountain sickness.[2] One survey in the Swiss Alps (466 climbers at 4 altitudes between 2850 metres and 4559 metres) found the prevalence of two or more symptoms of acute mountain sickness to be 9% of people at 2850 metres; 13% of people at 3050 metres; 34% of people at 3650 metres; and 53% of people at 4559 metres.[3]

AETIOLOGY/ RISK FACTORS The Himalayan study identified the rate of ascent and absolute height attained as the only risk factors.[2] It found no evidence of a difference in risk between men and women, or that previous episodes of altitude experience, load carried, or recent respiratory infections affected risk. However, the study was too small to exclude these as risk factors or to quantify risks reliably. One systematic review of RCTs (search date 1999) comparing prophylactic agents versus placebo found that, among people receiving placebo, the incidence of acute mountain sickness was higher with a faster rate of ascent (54% of people at a mean ascent rate of 91 metres/hour; 73% at a mean ascent rate of 1268 metres/hour; 89% at a simulated ascent rate in a hypobaric chamber of 1647 metres/hour).[4] One survey in Switzerland (827 mountaineers ascending to 4559 metres) examined the effects of susceptibility, pre-exposure, and ascent rate on acute mountain sickness.[5] In this study, pre-exposure was defined as having spent more than 4 days above 3000 metres in the preceding 2 months, and slow ascent was defined as ascending in more than 3 days. It found that in susceptible people (who had previously had acute mountain sickness at high altitude) the prevalence of acute mountain sickness was 58% with rapid ascent and no pre-exposure, 29% with pre-exposure only, 33% with slow ascent only, and 7% with both pre-exposure and slow ascent.[5] In non-susceptible people, the corresponding values were 31%, 16%, 11%, and 4%. The overall odds ratio for developing acute mountain sickness in susceptible compared with non-susceptible people was 2.9, 95% CI 2.1 to 4.1.[5]

PROGNOSIS We found no reliable data on prognosis. It is widely held that if no further ascent is attempted, the symptoms of acute mountain sickness tend to resolve over a few days. We found no reliable data about long term sequelae in people whose symptoms have completely resolved.

AIMS OF INTERVENTION To prevent acute mountain sickness; to achieve rapid resolution of acute mountain sickness, with minimal adverse effects.

OUTCOMES **Prevention:** Incidence of acute mountain sickness, incidence of individual symptoms. **Treatment:** Clinical resolution of acute mountain sickness, resolution of individual symptoms.

METHODS *Clinical Evidence* search and appraisal January 2004. We excluded RCTs with fewer than 10 people in each treatment arm, and crossover trials that did not report pre-crossover results. We excluded RCTs if rates of ascent and absolute altitude were different between treatment groups. We excluded individual RCTs that examined effects of simulated altitude in hypobaric chambers. However, one systematic review (search date 1999, 18 RCTs) included three RCTs that simulated altitude in this way.[4] We have not adjusted its meta-analysis to exclude these studies.

QUESTION What are the effects of interventions to prevent acute mountain sickness?

OPTION SLOW ASCENT (OR ACCLIMATISATION)

We found no RCTs evaluating different rates of ascent or acclimatisation. One non-randomised trial, observational studies, and consensus opinion suggest that slower ascent reduces the risk of acute mountain sickness compared with more rapid ascent.

Benefits: We found no RCTs (see comment below).

Harms: We found no RCTs. Slow ascent is, in itself, unlikely to be harmful.

Comment: We found one non-randomised controlled trial (60 male soldiers without previous high altitude exposure) comparing faster versus slower ascent to an altitude of 3500 metres.[6] Faster ascent was achieved by flying people to the target altitude (ascent time 1 hour) and slower ascent by driving them (ascent time 4 days). The trial found that slower ascent reduced the risk of any symptom of acute mountain sickness compared with faster ascent ("one symptom or another": 51% with slower ascent *v* 84% with faster ascent; P value not reported). Observational data suggest that faster ascent is a risk factor for acute mountain sickness (see aetiology/risk factors, p 1583).[4] Consensus opinion suggests that slower ascent helps to prevent acute mountain sickness.

OPTION ACETAZOLAMIDE

One systematic review and one subsequent RCT found that acetazolamide reduced the incidence of acute mountain sickness compared with placebo. The review found that acetazolamide caused polyuria and/or paraesthesia in over a third of people. We found no RCTs of sufficient quality comparing acetazolamide versus dexamethasone.

Benefits: **Versus placebo:** We found one systematic review (search date 1999, 9 RCTs, 295 people)[4] and one subsequent RCT.[7] The systematic review compared acetazolamide (500 mg or 750 mg daily) versus placebo at altitudes above 4000 metres.[4] It found that acetazolamide significantly increased the proportion of people who remained free of acute mountain sickness compared with placebo (AR for freedom from acute mountain sickness: 67% of people with acetazolamide *v* 42% with placebo; RR 1.58, 95% CI 1.27 to 1.96; see comment below). The subsequent RCT (197 trekkers in Nepal) compared acetazolamide (125 mg twice daily) versus placebo at altitudes between 4243 and 4937 metres.[7] It found that acetazolamide significantly reduced the incidence of acute mountain sickness compared with placebo (acute mountain sickness: 20/81 [25%] with placebo v 9/74 [12%] with acetazolamide; $P = 0.043$; see comment below).[7] **Versus dexamethasone:** We found no systematic reviews or RCTs of sufficient quality.

Harms: The review found that polyuria and paraesthesia were significantly more common with acetazolamide compared with placebo (AR for polyuria: 33% with acetazolamide *v* 6% with placebo; RR 4.24, 95% CI 1.92 to 9.37; AR for paraesthesia: 43% with acetazolamide *v* 10% with placebo; RR 4.02, 95% CI 1.71 to 9.43).[4] The review reported that the adverse effects with acetazolamide were of "minor severity": the term "minor" was not further defined.[4] The subsequent RCT found that paraesthesia was significantly more common with acetazolamide compared with placebo (3.7% with placebo v 48.6% with acetazolamide; $P < 0.001$).[7]

Comment: The review undertook subgroup analysis for different doses of acetazolamide.[4] It found that acetazolamide 750 mg was significantly more effective than placebo, but it found no significant difference between acetazolamide 500 mg and placebo (AR for freedom from acute mountain sickness: 66% of people with acetazolamide 750 mg *v* 32% with placebo; RR 2.18, 95% CI 1.52 to 3.15; AR for freedom from acute mountain sickness: 68% of people with acetazolamide 500 mg *v* 54% with placebo; RR 1.22, 95% CI 0.93 to 1.59). However, the analysis comparing 500 mg acetazolamide versus placebo may have lacked power to exclude clinically important effects. Ascent rates varied among RCTs, and the lack of effect of acetazolamide 500 mg versus placebo may be due to lower ascent rates in RCTs included in the analysis at that dosage. The subsequent RCT found that acetazolamide 125 mg twice daily was significantly more effective than placebo.[7] In the subsequent RCT, 42/197 (21%) people were lost to follow up, with a similar distribution in both groups (21.4% with placebo v 21.3% with acetazolamide; P = 0.99).

OPTION DEXAMETHASONE

One systematic review and further RCTs found that dexamethasone was more effective than placebo for preventing acute mountain sickness. However, the review found that adverse effects (including depression) occurred in a quarter of people on withdrawal of dexamethasone. We found no RCTs of sufficient quality comparing dexamethasone versus acetazolamide.

Benefits: **Versus placebo:** We found one systematic review,[4] two additional RCTs (reported in one publication),[8] and one subsequent RCT.[9] The systematic review (search date 1999, 8 RCTs, 161 people) compared dexamethasone (8, 12, or 16 mg daily) versus placebo at altitudes above 4000 metres.[4] It found that dexamethasone significantly increased the proportion of people who were free of acute mountain sickness compared with placebo (AR for freedom from acute mountain sickness: 62% with dexamethasone *v* 26% with placebo; RR 2.50, 95% CI 1.71 to 3.66). The two additional RCTs were excluded from the review because they compared dexamethasone versus placebo at altitudes below 4000 metres.[8] Both RCTs were undertaken in health professionals aged 18 to 65 years, who normally lived at altitudes less than 450 metres, and who were participating in continuing medical education programmes in the Rocky Mountains. The first additional RCT (73 people, altitude 2700 metres) found that dexamethasone (4 mg every 6 hours for a total of 6 doses) significantly reduced the incidence of acute mountain sickness compared with placebo (3/38 [8%] developed acute mountain sickness with dexamethasone *v* 14/35 [40%] with placebo; ARR 32%, 95% CI 14% to 50%; RR 0.20, 95% CI 0.06 to 0.65).[8] The second additional RCT (50 people, altitude 2050 metres) found no significant difference in the incidence of acute mountain sickness between dexamethasone (4 mg every 6 hours for a total of 6 doses) and placebo (5/25 [20%] with dexamethasone *v* 4/25 [16%] with placebo; ARI +4%, 95% CI −17% to +25%; RR 1.25, 95% CI 0.62 to 1.78; see comment below).[8] The subsequent RCT (50 men, aged 19–24 years, normally resident at sea level) compared five different treatments (3 different dosages of prednisolone, dexamethasone, and placebo).[9] One arm (10 men) compared dexamethasone 0.5 mg daily versus placebo.[9] Acute mountain sickness was assessed using a scoring system based on symptoms and clinical assessment. People in the RCT were airlifted to an altitude of 3450 metres. The RCT found that dexamethasone significantly reduced the mean acute mountain sickness score after 2 days compared with placebo ($P < 0.001$, results presented graphically, further details not reported). **Versus acetazolamide:** We found no systematic reviews or RCTs of sufficient quality.

Harms: The review reported that adverse effects, mainly depression, occurred on withdrawal of dexamethasone.[4] The review found that withdrawal of dexamethasone significantly increased the incidence of all adverse effects compared with placebo (adverse reactions on withdrawal: 27% of people with dexamethasone *v* 0% with placebo; RR 4.45, 95% CI 1.08 to 18.3). The severity of depression was not reported.[4]

Comment: In the RCT conducted at 2050 metres, event rates were low in both groups, probably because of the relatively low altitude.[8] The study may therefore have lacked power to detect clinically important differences between dexamethasone and placebo.

QUESTION What are the effects of treatments for acute mountain sickness?

OPTION ACETAZOLAMIDE

We found no RCTs of sufficient quality on the effects of acetazolamide compared with placebo for treating people with acute mountain sickness.

Benefits: We found no systematic reviews or RCTs of sufficient quality (see comment below).

Harms: We found no RCTs of sufficient quality (see comment below). See harms of acetazolamide in prevention, p 1584.

Comment: We found one small RCT (12 climbers in Alaska with established acute mountain sickness, at an altitude of 4200 metres) comparing acetazolamide versus placebo.[10] Acute mountain sickness was assessed using a recognised symptom scoring system (defined as a score of 2 or greater on a symptom severity scale of 1 to 3, where 3 was the most severe). One person was assigned (non-randomly) to placebo because of drug allergy. It found that acetazolamide significantly improved symptoms of acute mountain sickness after 24 hours compared with placebo (acute mountain sickness: 1/6 [17%] with acetazolamide v 6/6 [100%] with placebo; P = 0.015). The RCT stated that "no significant side effects of acetazolamide were reported".[10]

OPTION DEXAMETHASONE

One small RCT in climbers with symptoms and signs of acute mountain sickness found that dexamethasone reduced mean acute mountain sickness scores compared with placebo.

Benefits: We found no systematic review. We found one RCT (35 climbers arriving at an alpine hut with symptoms of acute mountain sickness, at an altitude of 4559 metres) comparing dexamethasone (8 mg initially, then 4 mg after 6 and 12 hours) versus placebo without concurrent descent in either group.[11] Acute mountain sickness was assessed using a scoring system based on symptoms and clinical assessment (score 0 to 14, where 14 was the most severe). The RCT found that after treatment for 12 hours at the same altitude, dexamethasone improved mean symptoms scores significantly more than placebo (improvement in mean score: 4.1 with dexamethasone *v* 0.4 with placebo; difference between groups 3.7, 95% CI 2.2 to 5.3).

Harms: The RCT did not report on harms.[11] See harms of dexamethasone in prevention, p 1586.

Comment: None.

OPTION **DESCENT COMPARED WITH RESTING AT THE SAME ALTITUDE**

We found no RCTs on the effects of descent compared with resting at the same altitude in people with acute mountain sickness. Consensus opinion suggests that people with acute mountain sickness should descend if possible. However, we found no RCTs examining the effects of different distances of descent, or about the balance of risks and benefits in people who might find it difficult to descend.

Benefits: We found no systematic reviews or RCTs.

Harms: We found no RCTs.

Comment: Consensus opinion suggests that people with acute mountain sickness should descend if possible. However, we found no RCTs examining the effects of different distances of descent, or about the balance of risks and benefits in people who might find it difficult to descend (for example, due to symptoms of acute mountain sickness or unrelated injury).

REFERENCES

1. Kao WF, Kuo CC, Hsu TF, et al. Acute mountain sickness in Jade Mountain climbers of Taiwan. *Aviat Space Environ Med* 2002;73:359–362.
2. Hackett PH, Rennie D. The incidence, importance, and prophylaxis of acute mountain sickness. *Lancet* 1976;2:1149–1155.
3. Maggiorini M, Buhler B, Walter M, et al. Prevalence of acute mountain sickness in the Swiss Alps. *BMJ* 1990;301:853–855.
4. Dumont L, Mardirosoff C, Tramer MR. Efficacy and harm of pharmacological prevention of acute mountain sickness: quantitative systematic review. *BMJ* 2000;321:267–272. Search date 1999; primary sources Medline, Embase, Cochrane Library, and the high altitude bibliography website.
5. Schneider M, Bernasch D, Weymann J, et al. Acute mountain sickness: influence of susceptibility, preexposure, and ascent rate. *Med Sci Sports Exerc* 2002;34:1886–1891.
6. Purkayastha SS, Ray US, Arora BS, et al. Acclimatization at high altitude in gradual and acute induction. *J Appl Physiol* 1995;79:487–492.
7. Basnyat B, Gertsch JH, Johnson EW, et al. Efficacy of low-dose acetazolamide (125 mg BID) for the prophylaxis of acute mountain sickness: a prospective, double-blind, randomized, placebo-controlled trial. *High Alt Med Biol* 2003;4:45–52.
8. Montgomery AB, Luce JM, Michael P, et al. Effects of dexamethasone on the incidence of acute mountain sickness at two intermediate altitudes. *JAMA* 1989;261:734–736.
9. Basu M, Sawhney RC, Kumar S, et al. Glucocorticoids as prophylaxis against acute mountain sickness. *Clin Endocrinol* 2002;57:761–767.
10. Grissom CK, Roach RC, Sarnquist FH, et al. Acetazolamide in the treatment of acute mountain sickness: clinical efficacy and effect on gas exchange. *Ann Intern Med* 1992;116:461–465.
11. Ferrazzini G, Maggiorini M, Kriemler S, et al. Successful treatment of acute mountain sickness with dexamethasone. *BMJ* 1987;294:1381–1383.

David Murdoch
Professor
Christchurch School of Medicine and Health Sciences, University of Otago
Christchurch
New Zealand

Competing interests: None declared.

We would like to acknowledge the previous contributors of this chapter, including Bazian Ltd.

Epilepsy

Search date November 2003

Anthony Marson and Sridharan Ramaratnam

QUESTIONS

INTERVENTIONS

*Categorisation based on consensus. See glossary Ⓖ

Key Messages

Treatment of single seizures

- **Antiepileptic drugs after a single seizure** RCTs found that treatment of a single seizure with antiepileptic drugs reduced seizure recurrence at 2 years compared with no treatment. However, we found no evidence that treatment alters long term prognosis. Long term antiepileptic drug treatment is potentially harmful.

Partial epilepsy: monotherapy

- **Antiepileptic monotherapy in partial epilepsy*** We found no placebo controlled RCTs of the main antiepileptic drugs (carbamazepine, phenobarbital, phenytoin, sodium valproate) used as monotherapy in people with partial epilepsy, but widespread consensus holds that these drugs are effective. Systematic reviews found no reliable evidence on which to base a choice among drugs in terms of seizure control. Systematic reviews found that phenobarbital was more likely to be withdrawn than phenytoin or carbamazepine.

Generalised epilepsy: monotherapy

- **Antiepileptic monotherapy in generalised epilepsy*** We found no placebo controlled trials of the main antiepileptic drugs (carbamazepine, phenobarbital, phenytoin, sodium valproate), but widespread consensus holds that these drugs are effective. Systematic reviews found insufficient evidence on which to base a choice among these drugs in terms of seizure control.

Drug-resistant partial epilepsy

- **Addition of second line drugs (gabapentin, levetiracetam, lamotrigine, oxcarbazepine, tiagabine, topiramate, vigabatrin, or zonisamide) for drug resistant partial epilepsy** Systematic reviews in people with drug resistant partial epilepsy found that adding gabapentin, levetiracetam, lamotrigine, oxcarbazepine, tiagabine, topiramate, vigabatrin, or zonisamide to usual treatment reduced seizure frequency compared with adding placebo. The reviews found that adding any of the drugs increased the frequency of adverse effects compared with adding placebo. We found no good evidence from RCTs on which to base a choice among drugs.

Drug withdrawal and relapse during remission

- **Antiepileptic drug withdrawal for people in remission** One RCT in people who had been seizure free for at least 2 years found that further seizures were more likely if people stopped treatment than if they continued antiepileptic medication. Clinical predictors of relapse after drug withdrawal included age, seizure type, number of antiepileptic drugs being taken, whether seizures had occurred since antiepileptic drugs were started, and the period of remission before drug withdrawal.

Behavioural and psychological treatment: epilepsy

- **Educational programmes** One RCT found that a 2 day educational programme reduced seizure frequency at 6 months compared with waiting list control. However, it found no significant difference in health related quality of life. RCTs found that educational packages improved knowledge and understanding of epilepsy, adjustment to epilepsy, and psychosocial functioning compared with control.
- **Biofeedback** One systematic review provided insufficient evidence about the effects of electroencephalographic biofeedback.
- **Cognitive behavioural therapy** Two small RCTs provided insufficient evidence about the effects of cognitive behavioural therapy in people with epilepsy.
- **Family counselling** One small RCT with methodological weaknesses provided insufficient evidence about the effects of family counselling.
- **Relaxation plus behavioural modification therapy** One systematic review provided insufficient evidence about the effects of combined relaxation and behavioural modification treatment on seizures.

- **Relaxation therapy** Systematic reviews provided insufficient evidence on the effects of relaxation therapy in people with epilepsy.
- **Yoga** One systematic review provided insufficient evidence about effects of yoga in people with epilepsy.

Surgery for drug-resistant temporal lobe epilepsy

- **Temporal lobectomy*** One RCT identified by a systematic review found that temporal lobectomy improved seizure control and quality of life after 1 year compared with continued medical treatment in people with poorly controlled temporal lobe epilepsy. There is consensus that temporal lobectomy is beneficial for people with drug resistant temporal lobe epilepsy.
- **Amygdalohippocampectomy*** We found no systematic review and no RCTs that examined the effect of amygdalohippocampectomy for people with drug resistant temporal lobe epilepsy. However, there is consensus that amygdalohippocampectomy is likely to be beneficial for people with drug resistant temporal lobe epilepsy.
- **Lesionectomy** We found no systematic review and no RCTs that examined the effects of lesionectomy in people with drug resistant temporal lobe epilepsy thought to be caused by a known cerebral lesion.

*Categorisation based on consensus.

DEFINITION Epilepsy is a group of disorders rather than a single disease. Seizures can be classified by type as partial (categorised as simple partial Ⓖ, complex partial Ⓖ, and secondary generalised tonic clonic Ⓖ seizures), or generalised (categorised as generalised tonic clonic, absence Ⓖ, myoclonic Ⓖ, tonic Ⓖ, and atonic Ⓖ seizures).[1]

INCIDENCE/ PREVALENCE Epilepsy is common, with an estimated prevalence in the developed world of 5–10/1000, and an annual incidence of 50/100 000 people.[2] About 3% of people will be given a diagnosis of epilepsy at some time in their lives.[3]

AETIOLOGY/ RISK FACTORS Epilepsy can also be classified by cause.[1] Idiopathic generalised epilepsies (such as juvenile myoclonic Ⓖ epilepsy or childhood absence Ⓖ epilepsy) are largely genetic. Symptomatic epilepsies result from a known cerebral abnormality; for example, temporal lobe epilepsy may result from a congenital defect, mesial temporal sclerosis, or a tumour. Cryptogenic epilepsies are those that cannot be classified as idiopathic or symptomatic and in which no causative factor has been identified, but is suspected.

PROGNOSIS For most people with epilepsy the prognosis is good. About 70% go into remission, defined as being seizure free for 5 years on or off treatment. This leaves 20–30% who develop chronic epilepsy, which is often treated with multiple antiepileptic drugs.[4] About 60% of untreated people have no further seizures in the 2 years after their first seizure.[5]

AIMS OF INTERVENTION To reduce the risk of subsequent seizures and to improve the prognosis of the seizure disorder; in people in remission, to withdraw antiepileptic drugs without causing seizure recurrence; to minimise adverse effects of treatment.

OUTCOMES **For treatment after a single seizure:** time to subsequent seizures, time to achieve remission, proportion of people achieving remission. **For treatment of newly diagnosed epilepsy:** retention on allocated treatment or time to withdrawal of allocated treatment, time to remission, time to first seizure after treatment. **For treatment of drug resistant epilepsy:** percentage reduction in seizure frequency, proportion of responders (response defined as ≥ 50% reduction in seizure frequency). **For drug withdrawal:** time to seizure recurrence. **Improvement in quality of life:** reduction in anxiety, depression, and fear of seizures; coping or adjustment to epilepsy (assessed by validated measures).

METHODS *Clinical Evidence* search and appraisal November 2003.

QUESTION Should single seizures be treated?

OPTION ANTIEPILEPTIC DRUGS AFTER A SINGLE SEIZURE

RCTs found that treatment of a single seizure with antiepileptic drugs reduced seizure recurrence at 2 years compared with no treatment. However, we found no evidence that treatment alters long term prognosis. Long term antiepileptic drug treatment is potentially harmful.

Benefits: We found no systematic review. We found three RCTs, the largest of which (419 people, 42% women, 28% aged ≤ 16 years, 66% aged 16–60 years, 6% aged ≥ 60 years) compared immediate treatment after a first unprovoked seizure versus no immediate treatment.[6] People were randomised within 7 days of their first tonic clonic seizure**G**. Longer term follow up of the RCT found that there were half as many second seizures with immediate treatment compared with no treatment at 2 years (HR 0.36, 95% CI 0.24 to 0.53).[7] However, it found no significant difference in the proportion of people achieving a 2 year remission in seizures (AR: 60% with immediate treatment *v* 68% with no treatment; RR 0.82, 95% CI 0.64 to 1.03; RR adjusted for time of starting treatment 0.96, 95% CI 0.77 to 1.22).[7]

Harms: The RCT gave no information on adverse effects of antiepileptic drugs.[6,7] However, these are well known and include idiosyncratic reactions, teratogenesis, and cognitive effects.

Comment: The RCT was too small to rule out the possibility that treating a first seizure alters the long term prognosis of epilepsy.[6,7] One systematic review of prospective observational studies (search date not reported, about 2500 people, 30% receiving treatment) concluded that, within 2 years of their first seizure, 40% (95% CI 37% to 43%) of people have further seizures.[5]

QUESTION What are the effects of monotherapy in newly diagnosed partial epilepsy?

OPTION ANTIEPILEPTIC MONOTHERAPY IN NEWLY DIAGNOSED PARTIAL EPILEPSY

We found no placebo controlled RCTs of the main antiepileptic drugs (carbamazepine, phenobarbital, phenytoin, sodium valproate) used as monotherapy in people with partial epilepsy, but widespread consensus holds that these drugs are effective. Systematic reviews found no reliable evidence on which to base a choice among drugs in terms of seizure control. Systematic reviews found that phenobarbital was more likely to be withdrawn than phenytoin or carbamazepine.

Benefits: We found no systematic review or RCTs comparing antiepileptic drugs versus placebo or no treatment (see comment below). We found five systematic reviews that compared antiepileptic drugs versus each other.[8–12] **Sodium valproate versus carbamazepine:** The first systematic review (search date 2003, 5 RCTs, 1265 people, of whom 830 had partial epilepsy and 395 had generalised epilepsy, aged 3–83 years, follow up < 5 years) compared sodium valproate versus carbamazepine.[8] The systematic review included a meta-analysis of the subgroup of people with partial epilepsy (with results expressed as HRs; HR > 1 for an event that is more likely with sodium valproate). It found no significant difference for treatment withdrawal between sodium valproate and carbamazepine (HR 1.00, 95% CI 0.79 to 1.26). Sodium valproate decreased 12 month remission compared with carbamazepine and significantly increased risk of first seizure (remission: HR 0.82, 95% CI 0.67 to 1.00; first seizure: HR 1.22, 95% CI 1.04 to 1.44). A test for statistical interaction was performed and was significant for time to first seizure but not for time to 12 month remission. These subgroup analyses must therefore be treated with caution. **Sodium valproate versus phenytoin:** The second systematic review (search date 2003, 5 RCTs, 250 people with partial epilepsy and 395 with generalised epilepsy, aged 3–95 years, follow up < 5 years) compared sodium valproate versus phenytoin.[9] It included a meta-analysis in people with partial epilepsy (with results expressed as HRs; HR > 1 for an event that is more likely with phenytoin). It found no significant difference in treatment withdrawal, 12 month remission, or first seizure (treatment withdrawal: HR 1.23, 95% CI 0.77 to 1.98; 12 month remission: HR 1.02, 95% CI 0.68 to 1.54; first seizure: HR 0.81, 95% CI 0.59 to 1.10). **Phenobarbital versus phenytoin:** The third systematic review (search date 2002, 3 RCTs, 599 people with partial or generalised epilepsy, aged 3–77 years) compared phenobarbital versus phenytoin.[10] Results were expressed as hazard ratios (HR > 1 for an event more likely with phenobarbital), but it did not undertake subgroup analyses for people with partial or generalised epilepsy. Overall, it found no significant difference in 12 month remission or first seizure (12 month remission: HR 0.93, 95% CI 0.70 to 1.23; first seizure: HR 0.84, 95% CI 0.68 to 1.05). It found that treatment withdrawal was greater with phenobarbital than with phenytoin, presumably because it was less well tolerated (HR 1.62, 95% CI 1.22 to 2.14). **Carbamazepine versus phenobarbital:** The fourth systematic review (search date 2002, 4 RCTs, 680 people, of whom 523 had partial epilepsy) compared carbamazepine versus phenobarbital.[11] Results were expressed as hazard ratios (HR > 1 for an event more likely on phenobarbital). For people with partial epilepsy it found that phenobarbital was significantly more likely to be withdrawn than carbamazepine (HR 1.60, 95% CI 1.18 to 2.17). It found no significant difference in remission during the next 12 months (HR 1.03, 95% CI 0.72 to 1.49). However, it found that phenobarbital significantly increased time to first seizure compared with carbamazepine (HR 0.71, 95% CI 0.55 to 0.91). **Carbamazepine versus phenytoin:** The fifth systematic review (search date 2003, 3 RCTs, 552 adults and children, of whom 431 had partial epilepsy) compared carbamazepine versus phenytoin.[12] The review did not present results separately for people with partial epilepsy (see comment below).

Harms: Two RCTs found similar prevalence of adverse effects with carbamazepine and sodium valproate.[13,14] Rashes occurred more often with carbamazepine than with sodium valproate (11.0% *v* 1.7%; P < 0.05: 6.3% *v* 3.4%; NS). Weight gain was more common with sodium valproate (12.0% *v* 1.1%; P < 0.05: 10.0% *v* 3.9%; NS), usually after at least 3 months of treatment. Other adverse events with carbamazepine included dizziness (6.7% *v* 2.9%; NS: 6.3% *v* 0.8%; P < 0.05), headaches (6.1% *v* 3.4%), ataxia (2.2% *v* 0%), somnolence (20.0% *v* 9.3%; P < 0.05), fatigue (10.0% *v* 5.1%; NS), diplopia (3.9% *v* 0%; NS), and insomnia (3.9% *v* 0%; NS). Other drug related adverse events with sodium valproate were tremor (5.2% *v* 1.7%; NS), alopecia (2.9% *v* 0.6%; NS: 4.2% *v* 1.6%; NS), and appetite increase (2.3% *v* 0%; NS: 9.3% *v* 0%; P < 0.01). Treatment was withdrawn because of adverse events in 9% of people taking sodium valproate compared with 18% taking carbamazepine (18 people *v* 15 people).[13,14]

Comment: Placebo controlled trials of these drugs would now be considered unethical. The meta-analysis provides weak evidence in support of the consensus view to use carbamazepine as the drug of choice in people with partial epilepsy.[8] The systematic review comparing carbamazepine versus phenytoin did not present results separately for people with generalised epilepsy and people with partial epilepsy.[12] Overall, however, it found no significant difference between carbamazepine and phenytoin for treatment withdrawal, first seizure, or 12 month remission (treatment withdrawal: HR 0.97, 95% CI 0.74 to 1.28; first seizure: HR 0.91, 95% CI 0.74 to 1.12; time to 12 month remission: HR 1.00, 95% CI 0.78 to 1.29).

QUESTION What are the effects of monotherapy in newly diagnosed generalised epilepsy?

OPTION ANTIEPILEPTIC MONOTHERAPY IN NEWLY DIAGNOSED GENERALISED EPILEPSY

We found no placebo controlled trials of the main antiepileptic drugs (carbamazepine, phenobarbital, phenytoin, sodium valproate), but widespread consensus holds that these drugs are effective. Systematic reviews found insufficient evidence on which to base a choice among these drugs in terms of seizure control.

Benefits: **Versus placebo:** We found no systematic review or RCTs comparing antiepileptic drugs versus placebo. We found four systematic reviews that compared different antiepileptic drugs.[8,9,11,12] The first two reviews were of RCTs that recruited people if they had generalised onset tonic clonic seizures**G** with or without other generalised seizure types (e.g. absence**G** or myoclonus).[8,9] **Carbamazepine versus sodium valproate:** The first systematic review compared carbamazepine versus sodium valproate (search date 2003, 5 RCTs, 4 of the RCTs included 395 people with generalised epilepsy, aged 3–79 years, follow up < 5 years).[8] Results were expressed as hazard ratios (HR > 1 indicates that an event is more likely with sodium valproate). A meta-analysis of the generalised epilepsy subgroup found no significant difference between sodium valproate and carbamazepine for treatment withdrawal (HR 0.89, 95% CI 0.62 to 1.29), 12 month remission (HR 0.96, 95% CI 0.75 to 1.24), or first seizure (HR 0.86, 95% CI 0.68 to 1.09; see comment below). **Phenytoin versus sodium valproate:** The second systematic review compared phenytoin and sodium valproate (search date 2003, 5 RCTs, 395 people aged 3–95 years with generalised epilepsy).[9] Results were expressed as hazard ratios (HR > 1 indicates that an event is more likely with phenytoin). A meta-analysis of the generalised epilepsy subgroup found no significant difference between sodium valproate and phenytoin for time to treatment withdrawal, 12 month remission, or first seizure (treatment withdrawal: HR 0.98, 95% CI 0.60 to 1.58; 12 month remission: HR 1.06, 95% CI 0.71 to 1.57; first seizure: HR 1.03, 95% CI 0.77 to 1.39; see comment below). **Carbamazepine versus phenobarbital:** The third systematic review (search date 2002, 4 RCTs, 680 people, of whom 157 had generalised epilepsy) compared carbamazepine versus phenobarbital.[11] Subgroup analysis in people with a generalised epilepsy found no significant differences for first seizure, 12 month remission, or treatment withdrawal (first seizure: HR 0.61, 95% CI 0.36 to 1.03; 12 month remission: HR 0.61, 95% CI 0.36 to 1.03; treatment withdrawal: HR 1.78, 95% CI 0.87 to 3.62). **Carbamazepine versus phenytoin:** The fourth systematic review (search 2003, 3 RCTs, 552 people, of whom 121 had generalised epilepsy) compared carbamazepine versus phenytoin.[12] It did not present results separately for people with generalised epilepsy (see comment under effects of monotherapy in newly diagnosed partial epilepsy, p 1592).

Harms: See harms under effects of monotherapy in newly diagnosed partial epilepsy, p 1591.

Comment: Although no difference was found in the systematic reviews between sodium valproate and either carbamazepine or phenytoin, the confidence intervals are wide and these results do not establish equivalence of sodium valproate and carbamazepine or phenytoin.[8,9] Also, the age distribution of people classified as having generalised epilepsy suggests errors in the classification of epilepsy type. Failure of the RCTs to document generalised seizures other than tonic clonic seizures(G) is an important limitation. The meta-analysis does not provide evidence to support or refute the use of sodium valproate for people with generalised tonic clonic seizures as part of generalised epilepsy.

QUESTION **Does the addition of second line drugs benefit people with drug resistant partial epilepsy?**

OPTION **ADDITION OF SECOND LINE DRUGS IN PEOPLE WITH DRUG RESISTANT PARTIAL EPILEPSY**

Systematic reviews in people with drug resistant partial epilepsy found that adding gabapentin, levetiracetam, lamotrigine, oxcarbazepine, tiagabine, topiramate, vigabatrin, or zonisamide to usual treatment reduced seizure frequency compared with adding placebo. The reviews found that adding any of the drugs increased the frequency of adverse effects compared with adding placebo. We found no good evidence from RCTs on which to base a choice among drugs.

Benefits: We found eight systematic reviews that compared the addition of active drugs versus placebo in people who had not responded to usual drug treatment.[15–22] **Gabapentin versus placebo:** One systematic review (search date 2003, 5 RCTs, 997 people) found that adding gabapentin to usual treatment significantly reduced seizure frequency compared with adding placebo and that efficacy increased with increasing dose (see table 1, p 1605).[15] **Levetiracetam versus placebo:** One systematic review (search date 2002, 4 RCTs, 1023 people) found that adding levetiracetam to usual treatment significantly reduced seizure frequency compared with adding placebo (see table 2, p 1606).[16] **Lamotrigine versus placebo:** One systematic review (search date 2003, 11 RCTs, 1243 people) found that adding lamotrigine to usual treatment significantly reduced seizure frequency compared with adding placebo (see table 2, p 1606).[17] **Oxcarbazepine versus placebo:** One systematic review (search date 2002, 2 RCTs, 961 adults and children) found that adding oxcarbazepine to usual treatment significantly reduced seizure frequency compared with adding placebo (see table 2, p 1606).[18] **Tiagabine versus placebo:** One systematic review (search date 2003, 3 RCTs, 769 people) found that adding tiagabine to usual treatment significantly reduced seizure frequency compared with adding placebo (see table 2, p 1606).[22] **Topiramate versus placebo:** One systematic review (search date 2002, 9 RCTs, 1049 people) found that adding topiramate to usual treatment significantly reduced seizure frequency compared with adding placebo (see table 1, p 1605).[20] **Vigabatrin versus placebo:** One systematic review (search date 1995, 4 RCTs, 495 people) found that adding vigabatrin to usual treatment significantly reduced seizure frequency compared with adding placebo (see table 1, p 1605).[19] **Zonisamide versus placebo:** One systematic review (search date 2003, 3 RCTs, 499 people) found that adding zonisamide to usual treatment significantly reduced seizure frequency compared with adding placebo (see table 2, p 1606).[21]

Harms: Adverse effects and treatment withdrawal were more frequent with additional treatment than with placebo (see table 1, p 1605 and table 2, p 1606).[15,20] Lamotrigine is associated with a rash, which may be avoided by slower titration of the drug. Vigabatrin causes concentric visual field abnormalities in about 40% of people, which are probably irreversible.[23]

Comment: Few RCTs have compared second line drugs directly with each other. Because of the irreversible visual field abnormalities associated with vigabatrin, the consensus view among neurologists is not to recommend this drug.

QUESTION Which people in remission from seizures are at risk of relapse on withdrawal of drug treatment?

OPTION ANTIEPILEPTIC DRUG WITHDRAWAL FOR PEOPLE IN REMISSION

One RCT in people who had been seizure free for at least 2 years found that further seizures were more likely if people stopped treatment than if they continued antiepileptic medication. Clinical predictors of relapse after drug withdrawal included age, seizure type, number of antiepileptic drugs being taken, whether seizures had occurred since antiepileptic drugs were started, and the period of remission before drug withdrawal.

Benefits: One large RCT (1013 people who had been seizure free for > 2 years) compared continued antiepileptic treatment with slow antiepileptic drug withdrawal.[24,25] At 2 years, 78% of people who continued treatment remained seizure free compared with 59% in the withdrawal group. There were no significant differences in psychosocial outcomes between groups. Risk reductions with 95% confidence intervals for the main factors predicting recurrence of seizures are tabulated (see table 3, p 1607).[24]

Harms: Sixteen people died during the trial, 10 in the continued treatment group and six in the withdrawal group.[25] Only two deaths were attributed to epilepsy, and both of these occurred in people randomised to continued treatment.

Comment: One systematic review of observational studies (search date not reported) found that, at 2 years, 29% (95% CI 24% to 34%) of people in remission from all types of epilepsy would relapse if antiepileptic drugs were withdrawn.[26] People with a seizure recurrence were less likely to be in paid employment at 2 years.[24,25]

QUESTION What are the effects of behavioural and psychological treatments for people with epilepsy?

OPTION RELAXATION THERAPY

Systematic reviews provided insufficient evidence on the effects of relaxation therapy in people with epilepsy.

Benefits: **Seizure frequency:** We found one systematic review (search date 2003,[27] 3 small unblinded controlled trials,[28–30] 50 people, including 32 women). The trials used weak methods (see comment below). Two of the studies found a non-significant reduction in seizure frequency with relaxation therapy**G** compared with no relaxation therapy, and one study found a significantly reduced seizure frequency. The weak methods preclude reliable conclusions.

Harms: The RCTs gave no information on adverse effects.[28–30]

Comment: All three trials used weak methods.[28–30] The treatment allocation methods were strict alternation,[30] alternation in blocks of five,[29] or were not reported.[28] The baseline seizure frequency varied considerably among the allocated groups in all of the trials. In one trial, two people in the treatment group had new antiepileptic medication added during the study period and one of these had a greater than 50% reduction in seizure frequency; another person discontinued antiepileptic medication.[29] Antiepileptic drug treatment was also adjusted during the trial, making it difficult to conclude whether the observed results were because of changes in drug treatment or because of the intervention. The trial duration and follow up was short. The possibility of publication bias cannot be excluded. The effects of relaxation therapy❻ remain unclear.

OPTION YOGA

One systematic review provided insufficient evidence about effects of yoga in people with epilepsy.

Benefits: **Seizure frequency:** We found one systematic review (search date 2002,[31] 1 quasi-randomised trial,[32] 32 people). The trial compared sahaja yoga (10 people) versus control (sham yoga 10 people, no intervention 12 people). It found that yoga reduced seizure frequency compared with control but it used weak methods, which precludes reliable conclusions.

Harms: The trial gave no information on adverse effects.[32]

Comment: The baseline seizure frequency and duration varied among the groups, making results difficult to interpret.[32]

OPTION BIOFEEDBACK

One systematic review provided insufficient evidence about the effects of electroencephalographic biofeedback.

Benefits: **Seizure frequency:** We found one systematic review (search date 2003,[27] 1 controlled trial,[33] 24 people with uncontrolled epilepsy) of electroencephalographic biofeedback❻ compared with control treatment. The trial compared three treatments: EEG biofeedback, sham (non-contingent) feedback, and no intervention (8 people in each group). It found a significant reduction in seizure frequency compared with the baseline frequency in people given biofeedback (median seizure reduction with biofeedback 61%; $P < 0.005$ *v* baseline; see comment below).

Harms: The trial gave no information on harms.[33]

Comment: The RCT did not provide data about seizure frequency in the control group.[33] We were therefore unable to compare the electroencephalographic biofeedback❻ and control groups. The RCT did not report the proportion of people who had greater than 50% reduction in seizure frequency. The study was not blinded and the randomisation method is not clear. The duration of follow up was only 6 weeks. The evidence is insufficient to draw reliable conclusions about the effects of EEG biofeedback.

OPTION COGNITIVE BEHAVIOURAL THERAPY

Two small RCTs provided insufficient evidence about the effects of cognitive behavioural therapy in people with epilepsy.

Benefits: **Seizure frequency:** We found one systematic review (search date 2003)[27] that found one RCT (30 people)[34] comparing cognitive behavioural therapy**G** versus control treatment. The RCT found no significant difference between cognitive behavioural therapy and control treatment in seizure frequency, but the RCT was too small to exclude a clinically important difference. **Psychosocial functioning:** The RCT included in the review found no significant differences between cognitive behavioural therapy and control treatments in various psychological scales, such as the Washington Psycho Social Inventory**G**, the Minnesota Multiphasic Personality Inventory**G**, and the Beck Depression Inventory**G**.[34] Another RCT (15 people with epilepsy and depression) found that cognitive behavioural therapy significantly reduced depression and self reported anxiety or anger, and significantly increased involvement in social activities compared with control treatment.[35] The RCT did not report seizure frequencies, or specify the intervention given to controls or the concomitant antidepressant treatment.

Harms: The trial gave no information on harms.[34]

Comment: The method of randomisation concealment is not known for these small RCTs.[34,35] Publication bias cannot be excluded. The evidence is insufficient to define the effects of cognitive behavioural therapy**G** in people with epilepsy.

OPTION EDUCATIONAL PROGRAMMES

One RCT found that a 2 day educational programme reduced seizure frequency at 6 months compared with waiting list control. However, it found no significant difference in health related quality of life. RCTs found that educational packages improved knowledge and understanding of epilepsy, adjustment to epilepsy, and psychosocial functioning compared with control.

Benefits: We found one systematic review (search date 2003,[27] 3 RCTs[36–38] and one quasi-randomised trial[39]). **Seizure frequency:** One RCT in the review (242 people) reported on seizure frequency.[38] It found that a 2 day educational programme significantly reduced seizure frequency at 6 months compared with waiting list control (proportion of people with at least 2 point reduction in seizure frequency on a 6 point scale [0 = no seizures in last 6 months, 5 = ≥ 1 seizure daily]: 19.0% with education *v* 7.2% with control; P value not reported).[38] However, the clinical importance of this effect is unclear. **Psychosocial functioning:** The review identified four RCTs assessing psychological functioning.[36–39] The first RCT included in the review (100 adults with epilepsy) found that a specific 2 day educational programme significantly improved responses to a 50 item true/false questionnaire compared with control intervention (overall understanding of epilepsy, significant decrease in fear of seizures, significant decrease in hazardous medical self management) and significantly improved compliance with current medication (shown by serum antiepileptic drug levels).[36] The second RCT included in the review (252 children with epilepsy aged 7–14 years) found that a child centred, family focused educational programme significantly improved questionnaire responses compared with control intervention (knowledge about what to do during a seizure, purpose of the electroencephalographic**G** examination, and minimal restriction in activities), increased the proportion of children likely to participate in normal activities, improved perceived academic and social competencies of the children, and reduced the anxiety of parents (see comment below).[37] The third RCT in the review that also reported seizure frequency found that a 2 day educational programme had no significant effect on SF-36 questionnaire scores**G** 6 months after the programme compared with waiting list control (SF-36**G** mental health component score: 43.7 with educational package *v* 42.5 with control; P value not reported; SF-36 physical component score: 50.4 with educational package *v* 52.0 with control; P value not reported).[38] Scales validated using the study population revealed significant improvement in epilepsy knowledge and coping with epilepsy. The quasi-randomised trial in the review (30 adults) compared a 2 day modular didactic psychoeducational programme on adjustment to epilepsy, stigma, psychoneurotic traits, depression, and knowledge about epilepsy versus waiting list control.[39] It found that the educational programme significantly improved depression and neurotic disorders at 2 months compared with control (change in depression measured using Beck Depression Inventory**G** scores: from 15.0 at baseline to 1.5 with psychoeducational programme *v* 15.1 at baseline to 10.0 with control; $P < 0.0001$; neurotic disorders assessed using change in Crown Crisp Experiential Index**G** scores: from 36.4 at baseline to 7.3 with psychoeducational programme *v* 35.6 at baseline to 34.1 with control; $P < 0.0001$).[39]

Harms: None reported.

Comment: All the RCTs had weak methods.[36–38] In one RCT, randomisation was by random number assignment, but only a proportion of medical records were available to the authors (65% in the psychoeducational programme group *v* 47% in the control group).[36] In the second RCT the method of randomisation was not reported.[37] A minority of the people in the first RCT actively participated in the interventions (23/50 [46%] in the psychoeducational programme group *v* 20/50 [40%] in the control group) or completed the study (20/50 [40%] in the psychoeducational programme group *v* 18/50 [36%] in the control group).[36] In the third RCT, the method of randomisation was not reported, and among 383 people randomised 242 (113 in the psychoeducational programme group and 119 in control group) completed the study.[38] In the fourth RCT, randomisation was by alternate allocation.[39]

OPTION RELAXATION PLUS BEHAVIOURAL MODIFICATION THERAPY

One systematic review provided insufficient evidence about the effects of combined relaxation and behavioural modification treatment on seizures.

Benefits: **Seizure frequency:** We found one systematic review (search date 2003)[27] that identified two RCTs comparing relaxation plus behavioural modification therapy versus control.[40,41] The first small RCT (18 children with uncontrolled epilepsy) compared three interventions for 6 weeks: behavioural modification (broad spectrum behavioural modification programme, which included teaching of symptom discrimination, relaxation, and countermeasure techniques to interrupt and abort seizures during early cues of the onset of a seizure); attention control (non-directive discussion around and experience of seizures, other people's reactions to seizures, and current problems); and control (usual care).[40] Both active treatments were given in six 1 hour sessions. It found that behaviour modification significantly reduced the median seizure index (the product of the seizure frequency and the seizure duration in seconds) compared with baseline after 1 year and that the median seizure index was increased compared with baseline in the control groups after 1 year. Long term follow up of the RCT found that behaviour modification significantly reduced the median seizure index after 8 years.[42] The RCT did not report actual values for these observations, so comparison of groups is not possible. The second RCT (150 adults with uncontrolled epilepsy) compared Jacobson's muscle relaxation plus behavioural therapy versus control treatment.[41] It reported separately the mean seizure frequencies for each seizure type but did not specify the number in each category. It reported separately the mean seizure frequencies for those people with fewer than 20 seizures and those with more than 20 seizures per month at baseline. We were unable to analyze these results in a meaningful way. **Psychological outcomes:** The second RCT found that relaxation plus behavioural modification therapy significantly improved anxiety (Spielberger's self assessment questionnaire for trait and state anxiety; $P < 0.01$), and home, health, social, and emotional adjustment compared with control (assessed by adjustment inventory; P values not reported).[41]

Harms: The RCTs gave no information on harms.[40,41]

Comment: The randomisation method was not reported for one study and was by alternate allocation in the other. The seizure index reported in one study is not an ideal outcome measure.[40] One of the RCTs recruited only 18 children and the groups would not be expected to be balanced for baseline characteristics.[40] It is possible that the results of the psychological interventions on psychosocial functioning may depend on the baseline personality of the persons included in the study, and their education and intelligence.

OPTION FAMILY COUNSELLING

One small RCT with methodological weaknesses provided insufficient evidence about the effects of family counselling.

Benefits: We found no systematic review but found one small RCT (36 people with epilepsy and job loss) that compared three interventions: family therapy (no detailed description but it seems that the family was present for discussion of problems for a mean of 7.8 sessions); one family session (in which information about the seizure profile was given); and usual care (vocational assistance in obtaining a job with no follow up other than site visit).[43] It did not report seizure frequencies, but found a significantly improved psychosocial inventory score with family therapy (Washington Psycho Social Inventory G, 27 completers: improved perceived acceptance by family, emotional adjustment, interpersonal adjustment, adjustment to seizures, and overall psychosocial function). It found a trend toward improvement in job stability.

Harms: The study did not report harms.[43]

Comment: The method of concealment of randomisation was not described in the RCT.[43] Nine of the 36 people did not complete the study and withdrawal was uneven across the groups (2 with family therapy, 6 with 1 family session, 1 with no intervention). The available evidence is insufficient to define the effects of family counselling.

QUESTION What are the effects of surgery in people with drug resistant temporal lobe epilepsy? New

OPTION TEMPORAL LOBECTOMY New

Sridharan Ramaratnam

One RCT identified by a systematic review found that temporal lobectomy improved seizure control and quality of life after 1 year compared with continued medical treatment in people with poorly controlled temporal lobe epilepsy. There is consensus that temporal lobectomy is beneficial for people with drug resistant temporal lobe epilepsy.

Benefits: **Seizure outcome:** We found one systematic review (search date 2001, 1 RCT, 80 people with poorly controlled temporal lobe epilepsy).[44] The RCT compared temporal lobectomy**G** versus medical treatment for 1 year.[45] After 1 year, it found that temporal lobectomy significantly increased the proportion of people who were completely free of seizures and the proportion who were free of seizures with or without auras compared with medical treatment (seizure free: 38.0% with surgery *v* 2.5% with control; NNT 3, 95% CI 2 to 5; seizure free with or without auras: 58.0% with surgery *v* 7.5% with control; NNT 2, 95% CI 2 to 3).[45] **Quality of life:** We found one systematic review (search date 2001, 1 RCT, 80 people with poorly controlled temporal lobe epilepsy).[44] The RCT found that surgery improved quality of life at 1 year compared with medical treatment (Quality of Life in Epilepsy Inventory-89, range 0 to maximum quality of 100: 73.8 with surgery *v* 64.3 with medical treatment; $P < 0.001$ after adjusting for baseline differences).[45] **Employment status:** We found one systematic review (search date 2001, 1 RCT, 80 people with poorly controlled temporal lobe epilepsy).[44] The RCT identified by the review found that surgery increased the proportion of people who were employed or attending school at 1 year compared with medical treatment, but the increase was not significant (56.4% with surgery *v* 38.5% with medical treatment; $P = 0.11$).[45]

Harms: **Mortality:** The RCT identified by the review[44] found no deaths at 1 year after surgery and one death, of unknown cause, with medical treatment.[45] **Other adverse effects:** The RCT found that neurological adverse effects were more common with surgery than with medical treatment at 1 year (4/40 [10%] with surgery [1 small thalamic infarct causing thigh dysaesthesia, 1 infected wound, 2 people with decline in verbal memory affecting occupation for 1 year] *v* 0/40 with medical treatment; P value not reported).[45] It found that 22/40 (55%) people had asymptomatic superior subquadrantic visual field defects after surgery. The RCT found similar rates of depression with surgical and medical treatment (18% with surgery *v* 20% with medical treatment; P value not reported).[45] **Psychosis:** The RCT found transient psychosis in one person (1/40 [2.5%]) in each treatment group.[45]

Comment: There is consensus that temporal lobectomy**G** is beneficial for people with drug resistant temporal lobe epilepsy.

OPTION AMYGDALOHIPPOCAMPECTOMY New

Sridharan Ramaratnam

We found no systematic review and no RCTs that examined the effect of amygdalohippocampectomy for people with drug resistant temporal lobe epilepsy. However, there is consensus that amygdalohippocampectomy is likely to be beneficial for people with drug resistant temporal lobe epilepsy.

Benefits: We found no systematic review and no RCTs that examined the effect of amygdalohippocampectomy**G** for people with drug resistant temporal lobe epilepsy.

Harms: We found no systematic review and no RCTs.

Comment: There is consensus that amygdalohippocampectomy**G** is likely to be beneficial for people with drug resistant temporal lobe epilepsy.

OPTION LESIONECTOMY New

Sridharan Ramaratnam

We found no systematic review and no RCTs that examined the effects of lesionectomy in people with drug resistant temporal lobe epilepsy thought to be caused by a known cerebral lesion.

Benefits: We found no systematic review and no RCTs on the effects of lesionectomy**G** in people with drug resistant temporal lobe epilepsy thought to be caused by a known cerebral lesion.

Harms: We found no systematic review and no RCTs.

Comment: We found one systematic review of observational studies (search date 2001, 8 studies, 131 people with lesions).[44] It found that between 1 and 4 years 63% of the 131 people who had lesionectomy**G** were free of disabling seizures. Surgical removal of tumours and vascular lesions may be indicated to prevent bleeding, herniation, or paralysis.

GLOSSARY

Absence seizure Previously known as "petit mal". Brief episodes of unconsciousness with vacant staring, sometimes with fluttering of the eyelids, as if "daydreaming". People with absence seizure do not fall to the ground and generally have a rapid recovery. The condition is rare in adults.

Atonic seizure Momentary loss of limb muscle tone causing sudden falling to the ground or drooping of the head.

Beck Depression Inventory Standardised scale to assess depression. This instrument consists of 21 items to assess the intensity of depression. Each item is a list of four statements (rated 0, 1, 2, or 3) arranged in increasing severity about a particular symptom of depression. The range of scores possible are 0 = least severe depression to 63 = most severe depression. Recommended for people 13–80 years of age. Scores more than 12 or 13 indicate presence of depression.

Cognitive behavioural therapy A broad category of interventions designed to identify and control stress and minimise its effects, often by using intellectual experience to correct damaging thoughts and behaviour.

Complex partial seizure Consciousness is impaired and memory of the episode is distorted, but the person may not collapse. The person may exhibit automatic behaviours ("automatisms", such as chewing, scratching the head, undressing). Complex partial seizures can spread to the rest of the brain to become a secondary generalised tonic clonic seizure (see below). The electrical abnormality commonly starts in the temporal lobes.

Crown Crisp Experiential Index Formerly known as Middlesex Hospital Questionnaire (MHQ) is a self reported questionnaire providing information on psychoneurotic traits. It has 48 items with an overall score for neuroticism with further subscores for free floating anxiety, phobic anxiety, obsessionality, somatic anxiety, depression, and hysterical anxiety. A higher score indicates more overall neurotic disorder.

Electroencephalographic (EEG) biofeedback A technique of making EEG activity apparent to a person, who is then taught to produce certain EEG waves that are believed to increase the threshold for seizures.

Lesionectomy Excision of a lesion consisting of a small area of abnormality (such as focal scar, vascular malformation, or tumour) in the brain where seizures originate.

Minnesota Multiphasic Personality Inventory (MMPI) A battery of standardised tests to assess personality (psychopathology).

Myoclonic seizure Sudden, symmetrical, shock like limb movements with or without loss of consciousness.

Relaxation therapy Techniques to train people to control muscle tension.

Selective amygdalohippocampectomy Removal of the amygdala and hippocampus only.

SF-36 score A scale that assesses health related quality of life across eight domains: limitations in physical activities (physical component); limitations in social activities; limitations in usual role activities because of physical problems; pain; psychological distress and wellbeing (mental health component); limitations in usual role activities because of emotional problems; energy and fatigue; and general health perceptions.

Simple partial seizure Electrical activity confined to one localised part of the brain causing symptoms and signs that depend on the part of the brain affected. The person remains conscious and fully aware.

Temporal lobectomy surgery Removal of the lesion or epileptogenic area responsible for the development of complex partial seizures, which are most common seizures associated with temporal lobe epilepsy. An en bloc anterior temporal lobectomy is a standardised operative procedure in which 4.5–5.0 cm of the anterior lateral temporal lobe neocortex is removed along with the amygdala, the anterior aspect of the parahippocampal gyrus, and the hippocampus in the medial portion of the temporal lobe.

Tonic clonic seizure Also known as a convulsion or "grand mal" attack. The person will become stiff (tonic) and collapse, and have generalised jerking (clonic) movements. Breathing might stop and the bladder might empty. Generalised jerking movements lasting typically for a few minutes are followed by relaxation and deep unconsciousness, before the person slowly comes round. People are often tired and confused, and may remember nothing. Tonic clonic seizures may follow simple partial or complex partial seizures (see above), where they are classified as secondary generalised tonic clonic seizures. Tonic clonic seizures occurring without warning and in the context of generalised epilepsy are classified as generalised tonic clonic seizures.

Tonic seizure Stiffening of the whole body with or without loss of consciousness.

Washington Psycho Social Inventory (WPSI) A standardised battery of tests to assess adjustment in various spheres (measure of psychosocial difficulties) in people with epilepsy.

Substantive changes

Educational programmes Updated review[27] with one new RCT.[39] Categorisation unchanged.

REFERENCES

1. Commission on classification and terminology of the international league against epilepsy. Proposal for revised classification of epilepsies and epileptic syndromes. *Epilepsia* 1989;30:389–399.
2. Hauser AW, Annegers JF, Kurland LT. Incidence of epilepsy and unprovoked seizures in Rochester, Minnesota 1935–84. *Epilepsia* 1993;34:453–468.
3. Hauser WA, Kurland LT. The epidemiology of epilepsy in Rochester, Minnesota, 1935 through 1967. *Epilepsia* 1975;16:1–66.
4. Cockerell OC, Johnson AL, Sander JW, et al. Remission of epilepsy: results from the national general practice study of epilepsy. *Lancet* 1995;346:140–144.
5. Berg AT, Shinnar S. The risk of seizure recurrence following a first unprovoked seizure: a quantitative review. *Neurology* 1991;41:965–972. Search date not reported; primary sources Cumulated Index Medicus, and bibliographies of relevant papers.
6. First Seizure Trial Group (FIRST Group). Randomized clinical trial on the efficacy of antiepileptic drugs in reducing the risk of relapse after a first unprovoked tonic clonic seizure. *Neurology* 1993;43:478–483.
7. Musicco M, Beghi E, Solari A, et al, for the FIRST Group. Treatment of first tonic clonic seizure does not improve the prognosis of epilepsy. *Neurology* 1997;49:991–998.
8. Marson AG, Williamson PR, Hutton JL, et al. on behalf of the Epilepsy Monotherapy Trialists. Carbamazepine versus valproate monotherapy for epilepsy. In: The Cochrane Library, Issue 4, 2003. Chichester, UK: John Wiley & Sons, Ltd. Search date 2003; primary sources Medline, Cochrane Library, Cochrane Epilepsy Group Trials Register, and personal contact with the drug manufacturers and investigators of the relevant trials found.
9. Tudur Smith C, Marson AG, Williamson PR. Phenytoin versus valproate monotherapy for partial onset seizures and generalized onset tonic-clonic seizures. In: The Cochrane Library, Issue 4, 2003. Chichester, UK: John Wiley & Sons, Ltd. Search date 2003; primary sources Cochrane Epilepsy Group trial register; Medline; hand searches of the journals *Epilepsia*, *Epilepsy Research*, and *Acta Neurologica Scandinavica*; and personal contact with the drug manufacturers and original investigators of relevant trials.
10. Taylor S, Tudur Smith C, Williamson PR, et al. Phenobarbitone versus phenytoin monotherapy for partial onset seizures and generalized onset tonic-clonic seizures. In: The Cochrane Library, Issue 4, 2003. Chichester, UK: John Wiley & Sons, Ltd. Search date 2002; primary sources Medline; Cochrane Controlled Trials Register; hand searches of the journals *Epilepsia*, *Epilepsy Research*, and *Acta Neurologica Scandinavica*; and personal contact with the pharmaceutical industry and researchers in the field.
11. Tudur Smith C, Marson AG, Williamson PR. Carbamazepine versus phenobarbitone monotherapy for epilepsy (Cochrane Review). In: The Cochrane Library, Issue 4, 2003. Chichester, UK: John Wiley & Sons, Ltd. Search date 2002; primary sources Cochrane Epilepsy Group trial register, Cochrane Controlled Trials Register, Medline, Embase, hand searches, and personal contact with trial investigators and manufacturers of carbamazepine.
12. Tudur Smith C, Marson AG, Clough HE, et al. Carbamazepine versus phenytoin monotherapy for epilepsy (Cochrane Review). In: The Cochrane Library, Issue 4, 2003. Chichester, UK: John Wiley & Sons, Ltd. Search date 2003; primary sources Cochrane Epilepsy Group trial register, Cochrane Controlled Trials Register, Medline, Embase, hand searches, and personal contact with trial investigators and manufacturers of carbamazepine.
13. Mattson RH, Cramer JA, Collins JF. A comparison of valproate with carbamazepine for the treatment of complex partial seizures and secondarily generalized tonic-clonic seizures in adults. The Department of Veterans Affairs Epilepsy Cooperative Study No. 264 Group. *N Engl J Med* 1992;10:327:765–771.
14. Richens A, Davidson DL, Cartlidge NE, et al. A multicentre comparative trial of sodium valproate and carbamazepine in adult onset epilepsy: adult EPITEG collaborative group. *J Neurol Neurosurg Psychiatry* 1994;57:682–687.
15. Marson AG, Kadir ZA, Hutton JL, et al. Gabapentin add-on for drug-resistant partial epilepsy. In: The Cochrane Library, Issue 4, 2003. Chichester, UK: John Wiley & Sons, Ltd. Search date 2003; primary sources Cochrane Epilepsy Group trials register, Cochrane Controlled Trials Register, hand searches of reference lists of articles, and personal contact with the manufacturers of gabapentin and experts in the field.
16. Chaisewikul R, Privitera MD, Hutton JL, et al. Levetiracetam add-on for drug-resistant localization related (partial) epilepsy. In: The Cochrane Library, Issue 4, 2003. Chichester, UK: John Wiley & Sons,

Ltd. Search date 2002; primary sources Cochrane Epilepsy Group trials register, Cochrane Controlled Trials Register, and personal contact with the manufacturers of levetiracetam and experts in the field.
17. Ramaratnam S, Marson AG, Baker GA. Lamotrigine add-on for drug-resistant partial epilepsy. In: The Cochrane Library, Issue 4, 2003. Chichester, UK: John Wiley & Sons, Ltd. Search date 2003; primary sources Cochrane Epilepsy Group trials register, Cochrane Controlled Trials Register, Medline, hand searches of reference lists of articles, and personal contact with the manufacturers of lamotrigine.
18. Castillo S, Schmidt DB, White S. Oxcarbazepine add-on for drug-resistant partial epilepsy. In: The Cochrane Library, Issue 4, 2003. Chichester, UK: John Wiley & Sons, Ltd. Search date 2002; primary sources Cochrane Epilepsy Group trials register, Cochrane Controlled Trials Register, Medline, hand searches of reference lists of articles, and personal contact with the manufacturers of oxcarbazepine and experts in the field.
19. Marson AG, Kadir ZA, Hutton JL, et al. The new antiepileptic drugs: a systematic review of their efficacy and tolerability. *Epilepsia* 1997;38:859–880. Search date 1995; primary sources Medline, hand searches of key journals, and contact with pharmaceutical companies.
20. Jette NJ, Marson AG, Hutton JL. Topiramate add-on for drug-resistant partial epilepsy. In: The Cochrane Library, Issue 4, 2003. Chichester, UK: John Wiley & Sons, Ltd. Search date 2002; primary sources Cochrane Epilepsy Group specialized register, Cochrane Controlled Trials Register, and personal contact with the manufacturers of topiramate and experts in the field.
21. Chadwick DW, Marson AG. Zonisamide add-on for drug-resistant partial epilepsy. In: The Cochrane Library, Issue 4, 2003. Chichester, UK: John Wiley & Sons, Ltd. Search date 2003; primary sources Cochrane Epilepsy Group trial register, Cochrane Controlled Trials Register, and personal contact with the manufacturers/licensees of zonisamide and experts in the field.
22. Pereira J, Marson AG, Hutton JL. Tiagabine add-on for drug-resistant partial epilepsy. In: The Cochrane Library, Issue 4, 2003. Chichester, UK: John Wiley & Sons, Ltd. Search date 2003; primary sources Cochrane Epilepsy Group trials register, Cochrane Controlled Trials Register, Medline, and personal contact with the manufacturers of tiagabine and experts in the field.
23. Kalviainen R, Nousiainen I, Mantyjarvi M, et al. Vigabatrin, a gabaergic antiepileptic drug, causes concentric visual field defects. *Neurology* 1999;53:922–926.
24. Medical Research Council Antiepileptic Drug Withdrawal Study Group. Prognostic index for recurrence of seizures after remission of epilepsy. *BMJ* 1993;306:1374–1378.
25. Medical Research Council Antiepileptic Drug Withdrawal Study Group. Randomised study of antiepileptic drug withdrawal in patients in remission. *Lancet* 1991;337:1175–1180.
26. Berg AT, Shinnar S. Relapse following discontinuation of antiepileptic drugs. *Neurology* 1994;44:601–608. Search date not reported; primary sources Index Medicus and bibliographies of relevant papers.
27. Ramaratnam S, Baker GA, Goldstein L. Psychological treatments for epilepsy. In: The Cochrane Library, Issue 4, 2003. Chichester, UK: John Wiley & Sons, Ltd. Search date 2003; primary sources Cochrane Epilepsy Group trial register, Cochrane Controlled Trials Register, Medline, and hand searches of reference lists from identified publications.
28. Dahl J, Melin L, Lund L. Effects of a contingent relaxation treatment program on adults with refractory epileptic seizures. *Epilepsia* 1987;28:125–132.
29. Puskarich CA, Whitman S, Dell J, et al. Controlled examination of effects of progressive relaxation training on seizure reduction. *Epilepsia* 1992;33:675–680.
30. Rousseau A, Hermann B, Whitman S. Effects of progressive relaxation on epilepsy: analysis of a series of cases. *Psychol Rep* 1985;57:1203–1212.
31. Ramaratnam S, Sridharan K. Yoga for epilepsy. In: The Cochrane Library, Issue 4, 2003. Chichester, UK: John Wiley & Sons, Ltd. Search date 2002; primary sources Cochrane Epilepsy Group trial register, Cochrane Controlled Trials Register, Medline, Registries of the Research Council for Complimentary Medicine, hand searches of references of identified studies, and personal contact with experts in the field.
32. Panjwani U, Selvamurthy W, Singh SH, et al. Effect of sahaja yoga practice on seizure control and EEG changes in patients of epilepsy. *Ind J Med Res* 1996;103:165–172.
33. Lantz DL, Sterman MB. Neuropsychological assessment of subjects with uncontrolled epilepsy: effects of EEG feedback training. *Epilepsia* 1988;29:163–171.
34. Tan SY Bruni J. Cognitive behavior therapy with adult patients with epilepsy: a controlled outcome study. *Epilepsia* 1986;27:225–233.
35. Davis GR, Armstrong HE Jr, Donovan DM, et al. Cognitive-behavioral treatment of depressed affect among epileptics: preliminary findings. *J Clin Psychol* 1984;40:930–935.
36. Helgeson DC, Mittan R, Tan SY, et al. Sepulveda epilepsy education: the efficacy of a psychoeducational treatment program in treating medical and psychosocial aspects of epilepsy. *Epilepsia* 1990;31:75–82.
37. Lewis MA, Salas I, De La Sota A, et al. Randomized trial of a program to enhance the competencies of children with epilepsy. *Epilepsia* 1990;31:101–109.
38. May TW, Pifflin M. The efficacy of an educations treatment program for patients with epilepsy (MOSES): results of a controlled, randomized study. *Epilepsia* 2002;43:539–549.
39. Olley BO, Osinowo HO, Brieger WR. Psycho-educational therapy among Nigerian adult patients with epilepsy: a controlled outcome study. *Patient Educ Couns* 2001;42:25–33.
40. Dahl J, Melin L, Brorson LO, et al. Effects of a broad-spectrum behavior modification treatment program on children with refractory epileptic seizures. *Epilepsia* 1985;26:303–309.
41. Sultana SM. *A study on the psychological factors and the effect of psychological treatment in intractable epilepsy*. PhD Thesis, University of Madras, India 1987.
42. Dahl J, Brorson LO, Melin L. Effects of a broad-spectrum behavioral medicine treatment program on children with refractory epileptic seizures: an 8-year follow-up. *Epilepsia* 1992;33:98–102.
43. Earl WL. Job stability and family counseling. *Epilepsia* 1986;27:215–219.
44. Engel J Jr, Wiebe S, French J, et al. Practice parameter: temporal lobe and localized neocortical resections for epilepsy: report of the Quality Standards Subcommittee of the American Academy of Neurology, in association with the American Epilepsy Society and the American Association of Neurological Surgeons. *Neurology* 2003;60:538–547. Search date 2001; primary sources Medline and Current Contents. [Erratum in: *Neurology* 2003;60:1396].
45. Wiebe S, Blume WT, Girvin JP, et al. A randomized, controlled trial of surgery for temporal lobe epilepsy. *N Engl J Med* 2001;345:311–318.

Anthony Marson
Lecturer in Neurology
University of Liverpool
Liverpool
UK

Sridharan Ramaratnam
Senior Consultant Neurologist
Apollo Hospitals
Chennai (Madras)
India

Competing interests: AM has been paid for speaking at meetings by Johnson & Johnson, manufacturers of topiramate, and by Janssen-Cilag, Sanofi, and GlaxoSmithKline for attending conferences. SR has received hospitality from the following pharmaceutical companies: Sun Pharmaceuticals (India) and Novartis (India) for attending conferences and from GlaxoSmithKline for writing a case report. SR was also involved in several of the systematic reviews referenced in this topic.

TABLE 1 **Effects of additional drug treatment in people not responding to usual treatment: results of systematic reviews (see text, p 1594).**

Drug	Daily dose (mg)	Percentage responding (95% CI)*	RR treatment withdrawal (95% CI)	RR adverse effects with CI (95% unless otherwise stated)	Comment
Gabapentin	**Adults only**				
	Placebo	9.9 (7.2 to 13.5)	1.4 (0.8 to 2.5)	Dizziness 2.25 (1.3 to 4)	5 RCTs (1 in children, 4 in adults)
	600	14.4 (12.0 to 17.3)		Fatigue 2.25 (1.1 to 4.6)	Efficacy increased with increasing dose. No plateauing of response, so doses tested may not have been optimal
	900	17.3 (14.6 to 20.3)		Somnolence 2.04 (1.2 to 3.4)	
	1200	20.6 (17.1 to 24.6)			
	1800	28.5 (21.5 to 36.7)			
	Adults and children		**Adults and children**	**Adults and children**	
	600–1800	RR 1.81 (1.32 to 2.49)	1.04 (0.71 to 1.52)	Dizziness 2.19 (1.24 to 3.89)	
				Fatigue 2.30 (1.11 to 4.75)	
				Somnolence 1.91 (1.20 to 3.05)	
Topiramate	Placebo 200	11.7 (8.7 to 15.7)	2.06 (1.38 to 3.08)	Ataxia 1.95 (99% CI 1.04 to 3.65)	9 RCTs
	400–1000	26.8 (15.8 to 41.3)		Dizziness 1.55 (99% CI 1.07 to 2.24)	
		46.5 (42.5 to 50.5)		Fatigue 2.21 (99% CI 1.42 to 3.45)	
				Somnolence 2.26 (99% CI 1.48 to 3.46)	
				Difficulty thinking 5.54 (99% CI 2.34 to 13.12)	
Vigabatrin (adults)	Placebo	13.8 (9.7 to 19.2)	2.95 (1.25 to 7.00)	No adverse effects significantly more frequent but 40% develop concentric visual field abnormalities[23]	3 RCTs
	1000 or 2000	22.8 (14.5 to 34.9)			
	3000 or 6000	45.9 (39.5 to 52.5)			

Results show percentage responding at particular daily doses, but results for treatment withdrawal and adverse effects are calculated for all doses.
*50% reduction in seizure frequency.

TABLE 2 **Effects of additional drug treatment in people not responding to usual treatment: results of systematic reviews (see text, p 1594).**

Drug	Daily dose (mg)	Percentage responding (95% CI)*	RR treatment withdrawal (95% CI)	RR adverse effects (95% CI)	Comment
Levetiracetam (adults)	1000–3000	3.78 (2.62 to 5.44)	1.21 (0.88 to 1.66)	Dizziness 2.50 (1.16 to 5.41) Infection 1.76 (1.03 to 3.02)	4 RCTs. Results of regression models with CI (95% unless otherwise stated) do not provide reliable estimates for a response to individual doses.
Lamotrigine (adults)	200–500	2.32 (1.67 to 3.23)	1.10 (0.81 to 1.50)	Ataxia 3.23 (1.93 to 5.42) Diplopia 3.47 (1.91 to 6.31) Dizziness 2.05 (1.52 to 2.78) Nausea 1.76 (1.18 to 2.64)	11 RCTs
Oxcarbazepine (adults and children)	600–2400	2.51 (1.88 to 3.33)	1.72 (1.35 to 2.18)	Ataxia 3.54 (1.75 to 7.13) Dizziness 2.87 (1.82 to 4.52) Fatigue 1.81 (1.00 to 3.29) Nausea 3.09 (1.74 to 5.49) Somnolence 2.36 (1.54 to 3.62) Diplopia 7.25 (3.12 to 16.80)	2 RCTs
Tiagabine	16–56	RR 3.67 (2.30 to 5.86)	1.81 (1.25 to 2.62)	Dizziness 1.69 (99% CI 1.13 to 2.51)	3 RCTs. Results of regression models do not provide accurate estimates for a response to individual doses
Zonisamide	400	2.46 (1.61 to 3.76)	1.64 (1.02 to 2.62)	Ataxia 4.50 (99% CI 1.05 to 19.22) Somnolence 1.91 (99% CI 1.08 to 3.38) Aggitation/irritability 2.37 (99% CI 1.00 to 5.64) Anorexia 3.00 (99% CI 1.31 to 6.88)	3 RCTs

*>50% reduction in seizure frequency. All results are calculated for all doses.

TABLE 3 **Relative risks of seizure recurrence within 2 years of treatment withdrawal, according to prognostic variable (see text, p 1595).[24,25]**

Prognostic variable	RR (95% CI) of seizure recurrence within 2 years
Age < 16 years	1.8 (1.3 to 2.4)
Tonic clonic seizures	1.6 (1.1 to 2.2)
Myoclonus	1.8 (1.1 to 3.0)
Treatment with more than one antiepileptic drug	1.9 (1.4 to 2.4)
Seizures since antiepileptic drugs were started	1.6 (1.2 to 2.1)
Any electroencephalographic abnormality	1.3 (1.0 to 1.8)

Risk of recurrence also declined as the seizure free period increased, but in a complex manner.

Essential tremor

Search date March 2004

Joaquim Ferreira and Cristina Sampaio

QUESTIONS

INTERVENTIONS

Key Messages

- We found few RCTs that assessed long term effects of drug treatments for essential tremor.

Drug treatment

- **Propranolol** Small RCTs found that propranolol for up to 1 month improved clinical scores, tremor amplitude, and self evaluation of severity at up to 6 weeks compared with placebo. One RCT comparing propranolol versus clonidine found that the initial improvement in tremor from baseline was similar with both drugs and was maintained throughout follow up for 1 year. RCTs provided insufficient evidence to compare propranolol versus other β blockers.
- **Topiramate (improved tremor scores after 2 weeks' treatment but associated with appetite suppression, weight loss, and paraesthesia)** One RCT found limited evidence that topiramate improved observer rated tremor score after 2 weeks' treatment compared with placebo but was associated with adverse effects, including appetite suppression, weight loss, and paraesthesia. The clinical importance of the difference in tremor score is uncertain. We found no RCTs addressing long term outcomes.

Clin Evid 2005;13:1608–1621.

- **Botulinum A toxin–haemagglutinin complex (improves clinical rating scales at 4–12 weeks but associated with hand weakness)** Two RCTs in people with essential hand tremor found that botulinum A toxin–haemagglutinin complex improved clinical rating scales at 4–12 weeks. They found no consistent improvement in motor tasks or functional disability. Hand weakness, which is dose dependent and transient, is a frequent adverse effect. We found no RCTs addressing long term outcomes.
- **Phenobarbital (improved tremor at 5 weeks but associated with depression and cognitive adverse effects)** One small RCT found that phenobarbital improved tremor at 5 weeks compared with placebo. However, another two RCTs found no significant difference in tremor scores at 4–5 weeks between phenobarbital and placebo. Phenobarbital is associated with depression and cognitive and behavioural adverse effects.
- **Primidone (improved tremor and function at 5 weeks compared with placebo and at 1 year compared with baseline but associated with depression and cognitive adverse effects)** Three small, short term RCTs found limited evidence that primidone improved tremor and functional ability over 4–10 weeks compared with placebo. One RCT comparing different doses of primidone found that it improved tremor from baseline at 1 year with no significant difference in outcome between groups. Primidone is associated with depression and cognitive and behavioural adverse effects.
- **Benzodiazepines** Two small short term RCTs found weak evidence that alprazolam may improve tremor and function at 2–4 weeks compared with placebo. However, we were unable to draw reliable conclusions about effects. One very small RCT provided insufficient evidence to compare clonazepam versus placebo. Adverse effects with benzodiazepines, including dependency, sedation and cognitive and behavioural effects, have been well described for other conditions (see panic disorder, p 1311).
- **Calcium channel blockers (dihydropyridine)** Poor quality RCTs provided insufficient evidence to compare the dihydropyridine calcium channel blockers nicardipine and nimodipine versus placebo.
- **Carbonic anhydrase inhibitors** Small RCTs provided insufficient evidence to assess methazolamide or acetazolamide in people with essential tremor. We found no RCTs addressing long term outcomes.
- **Clonidine** One RCT found no significant difference between clonidine and placebo in essential hand tremor. However, the study lacked power to rule out a clinically important difference. Another RCT comparing clonidine versus propranolol found that the initial improvement in tremor from baseline was similar with both drugs and was maintained throughout follow up for 1 year.
- **Flunarizine** One small RCT found weak evidence that flunarizine reduced the symptoms of essential hand tremor after 1 months' treatment compared with placebo.
- **Gabapentin** Small RCTs provided insufficient evidence to compare gabapentin versus placebo. We found no RCTs addressing long term outcomes.
- **Isoniazid** One RCT found no significant difference between isoniazid and placebo in essential hand tremor, but it may have lacked power to detect a clinically important difference. We found no RCTs addressing long term outcomes.
- **β Blockers other than propranolol (atenolol, metoprolol, nadolol, pindolol, and sotalol)** Three small RCTs found weak evidence that atenolol or sotalol improved symptoms and self evaluated measures of tremor at 5 days to 4 weeks compared with placebo. One small RCT found no significant difference in symptoms between metoprolol and placebo and another small RCT found that pindolol worsened tremor amplitude compared with placebo. A third very small RCT provided insufficient evidence to compare nadolol versus placebo. RCTs provided insufficient evidence to compare other β blockers versus propranolol.
- **Mirtazapine** One RCT in people taking antitremor drugs such as propranolol, found no significant difference in tremor between adding mirtazapine and placebo and found that adverse effects were frequent.

DEFINITION	Tremor is a rhythmic, mechanical oscillation of at least one body region. The term essential tremor is used when there is either a persistent bilateral tremor of hands and forearms, or an isolated tremor of the head without abnormal posturing, and when there is no evidence that the tremor arises from another identifiable cause. The diagnosis is not made if there are abnormal neurological signs; known causes of enhanced physiological tremor; a history or signs of psychogenic tremor; sudden change in severity; primary orthostatic tremor; isolated voice tremor; isolated position specific or task specific tremors; and isolated tongue, chin, or leg tremor.[1]
INCIDENCE/ PREVALENCE	Essential tremor is one of the most common movement disorders throughout the world, with a prevalence of 0.4–3.9% in the general population.[2]
AETIOLOGY/ RISK FACTORS	Essential tremor is sometimes inherited with an autosomal dominant pattern. About 40% of people with essential tremor have no family history. Alcohol ingestion provides symptomatic benefit in 50–70% of people.[3]
PROGNOSIS	Essential tremor is a persistent and progressive condition. It usually begins during early adulthood and the severity of the tremor increases slowly. Only a small proportion of people with essential tremor seek medical advice, but the proportion in different surveys varies from 0.5–11%.[2] Most people with essential tremor are only mildly affected. However, most of the people who seek medical care are disabled to some extent, and most are socially handicapped by the tremor.[3] A quarter of people receiving medical care for the tremor change jobs or retire because of essential tremor induced disability.[4,5]
AIMS OF INTERVENTION	To reduce tremor; to minimise disability and social embarrassment; to improve quality of life, with minimal adverse effects from treatment.
OUTCOMES	Severity of symptoms and disability measured by clinical rating scales or patient self evaluation. Clinical rating scales are often composite scores that grade tremor amplitude in each body segment in specific postures or tasks. Few scales have been formally validated. In the more recent trials, the Fahn-Tolosa-Marin clinical evaluation scale,[6] which addresses the impairment and the disability domains of tremor, has become the preferred scale. Accelerometer recordings**G** are reported in many trials but they are proxy outcomes that have been included in this review only when clinical outcomes were not available.
METHODS	*Clinical Evidence* search and appraisal March 2004. We excluded single dose studies and RCTs lasting under 1 week. We included small RCTs because of the paucity of evidence in this population.

QUESTION What are the effects of drug treatments in people with essential tremor of the hand?

OPTION PROPRANOLOL

Small RCTs found that propranolol for up to 1 month improved clinical scores, tremor amplitude, and self evaluation of severity at up to 6 weeks compared with placebo. One RCT comparing propranolol versus clonidine found that the initial improvement in tremor from baseline was similar with both drugs and was maintained throughout follow up for 1 year. RCTs provided insufficient evidence to compare propranolol versus other β blockers.

Benefits: We found no systematic review. **Versus placebo:** We found 12 small (10–24 people), brief (2–4 weeks' treatment, up to 6 weeks follow up) RCTs, many of which had a crossover design.[7–18] Four RCTs compared three interventions: propranolol, metoprolol, and placebo in one RCT;[11] propranolol, atenolol, and placebo in a second;[17] propranolol, pindolol, and placebo in a third;[16] and propranolol, nicardipine, and placebo in a fourth.[18] One RCT compared four interventions: propranolol, atenolol, sotalol, and placebo, each for 2 weeks' treatment.[13] Nine RCTs evaluated clinical outcomes, including self evaluation of severity,[7–9,11-15,18] the other three assessed accelerometer readings**G**.[10,16,17] All RCTs found that propranolol improved symptoms compared with placebo ($P < 0.05$). Four of the RCTs found that, compared with placebo, propranolol 60–160 mg daily significantly increased the proportion of people categorised as "responders".[7–9,15] The precise definition of responder varied among the RCTs, but the results were similar (AR after crossover: 22/23 [96%] with propranolol v 5/23 [22%] with placebo; ARR 69%, 95% CI 49% to 89%;[7] ARR 80%, 95% CI 69% to 91%;[8] ARR 64%, 95% CI 33% to 95%, NNT 2, 95% CI 2 to 4;[9] AR 10/16 [63%] with propranolol v 5/16 [31%] with placebo; ARR 32%, 95% CI 17% to 47%, NNT 4, 95% CI 2 to 6[15]). **Versus beta-blockers other than propranolol:** See benefits of beta blockers other than propranolol, p 1612. **Versus clonidine:** We found one RCT (186 people) comparing propranolol 250 mg daily versus clonidine 0.45 mg daily for 1 year.[19] The trial was designed to test equivalence between the drugs. The RCT found that both propranolol and clonidine significantly reduced tremor from baseline at 3 months and 1 year (mean score on the Fahn-Tolosa-Marin Clinical evaluation scale for tremor [maximum score 144] at 3 months: 22.6 with propranolol v 24.4 with clonidine; P = 0.0004 for propranolol v baseline, P = 0.04 for clonidine v baseline; at 1 year: 19.4 with propranolol v 29.3 with clonidine; P = 0.001 for propranolol v baseline, P = 0.002 for clonidine v baseline). It found no significant difference in mean scores over 1 year between propranolol and clonidine (P = 0.4).

Harms: **Versus placebo:** Withdrawals (mainly because of fatigue and bradycardia) were uncommon (e.g. 1/10 [10%] people in 1 RCT).[9] Depression, diarrhoea, breathlessness, sedation, blurred vision, and sexual problems were each reported in fewer than 5% of people taking propranolol. **Versus beta-blockers other than propranolol:** See harms of beta blockers other than propranolol, p 1613. **Versus clonidine:** In the RCT, seven people taking propranolol withdrew, mainly because of lack of efficacy and 22 people taking clonidine withdrew because of adverse effects.[19] The RCT found that propranolol significantly increased the proportion of people who had hypotension (58% with propranolol v 15% with clonidine), depression (37% with propranolol v 9% with clonidine), and body coldness (43% with propranolol v 13% with clonidine). Clonidine increased dry mouth (27% of people with propranolol v 74% with clonidine), sleepiness (34% with propranolol v 56% with clonidine), and dizziness (28% with propranolol v 50% with clonidine; P < 0.05 for all outcomes).

Comment: We found no placebo controlled RCTs addressing long term outcomes. All trials were analyzed as "on treatment" rather than by intention to treat, and this may have biased results. Accelerometry**G** is a proxy outcome that was reported in several RCTs. All accelerometry results were in favour of propranolol, but there is an inconsistent relationship between accelerometry and clinical measures of effectiveness. People with congestive heart failure, second degree heart block, asthma, severe allergy, and insulin dependent diabetes were generally excluded from the RCTs. All but one of the studies were small. The possibility of publication bias has not been excluded. The RCT comparing propranolol versus clonidine for 1 year is the only source of double blind data about long term outcomes of propranolol.[19] This is a well designed trial but the absence of the placebo arm is problematic because propranolol has never been studied under double blind conditions for more than 6 weeks. It is worth noting that the population in the RCT was non-Caucasian and had mostly mild to moderate essential tremor at baseline.

OPTION β **BLOCKERS OTHER THAN PROPRANOLOL**

Three small RCTs found weak evidence that atenolol or sotalol improved symptoms and self evaluated measures of tremor at 5 days to 4 weeks compared with placebo. One small RCT found no significant difference in symptoms between metoprolol and placebo and another small RCT found that pindolol worsened tremor amplitude compared with placebo. A third very small RCT provided insufficient evidence to compare nadolol versus placebo. RCTs provided insufficient evidence to compare other β blockers versus propranolol.

Benefits: We found no systematic review. **Versus placebo:** We found six small (9–24 people) brief (5 days to 4 weeks) RCTs comparing different β blockers (sotalol, atenolol, metoprolol, nadolol, and pindolol) versus placebo.[12,13,16,17,20,21] Three of these RCTs compared three interventions: propranolol, metoprolol, and placebo in one RCT;[12] propranolol, pindolol, and placebo in a second;[16] and propranolol, atenolol, and placebo in a third.[17] One RCT compared four interventions: propranolol, atenolol, sotalol, and placebo, each for 2 weeks' treatment.[13] Two RCTs selected participants known to be responders or non-responders to propranolol.[13,20] The first RCT (16 people, crossover design) reported three outcomes: a composite clinical score, self evaluation, and accelerometer records**G**.[12] It found no significant difference between metoprolol 150–300 mg daily and placebo in any outcomes (reported as non-significant, CI not reported). The second RCT (9 people, crossover design) found that both sotalol and atenolol significantly reduced symptom scores compared with placebo (mean score: 6.8 with sotalol *v* 8.1 with atenolol *v* 10.7 with placebo; $P < 0.01$ with sotalol, $P < 0.02$ with atenolol).[13] The third RCT (24 people, crossover design) found that people taking pindolol 120 mg daily had significantly worse tremor amplitude accelerometer recordings ($P < 0.05$) compared with people taking placebo.[16] It found no significant difference between pindolol and placebo in tremor frequency (reported as non-significant, CI not reported). The fourth RCT (24 people, crossover design) found that atenolol significantly improved tremor intensity measured by accelerometer readings compared with placebo (P 0.001).[17] The fifth RCT (10 people) comparing nadolol versus placebo found significant results at 4 weeks only with a subgroup analysis in six people who had previously responded to propranolol.[20] The sixth RCT (24 people) found that sotalol significantly improved self evaluated measures of tremor compared with placebo ($P < 0.05$).[21] **Versus propranolol:** We found no systematic review but found four small (16–24 people)[12,13,16,17] and one large (175 people)[22] crossover RCTs. The first RCT (16 people) found that, compared with metoprolol 150 mg daily, propranolol 120 mg daily significantly improved clinical scores ($P < 0.05$) and self assessment ($P < 0.01$).[12] It also found that propranolol 240 mg significantly improved self assessment ($P < 0.05$) compared with metoprolol 300 mg. The second RCT (9 people, crossover design) found no significant difference in symptom scores between sotalol and propranolol but found that atenolol was significantly less effective than propranolol (mean score: 6.8 with sotalol *v* 8.1 with atenolol *v* 6.6 with propranolol; $P > 0.01$ for sotalol *v* propranolol, $P < 0.05$ for atenolol *v* propranolol).[13] The second RCT (24 people) found that pindolol 30 mg daily significantly ($P < 0.005$) worsened tremor amplitude measured by accelerometer readings compared with propranolol 120 mg daily.[16] The third RCT (24 people) found no significant difference between atenolol and propranolol in tremor intensity measured by accelerometer readings (reported as non-significant, CI not reported), but more people preferred propranolol to atenolol (12/24 [50%] with propranolol *v* 1/24 [4%] with atenolol; CI not reported).[17] The fourth RCT (175 people) compared arotinolol 10–30 mg daily versus propranolol 40–160 mg daily for 18 weeks.[22] Participants received each drug for 6 weeks, receiving escalating doses of the drug every 2 weeks, with a washout period of 2 weeks before crossover to the next drug. Analysis was by intention to treat and the analysis was adjusted to allow for crossover effects. The RCT found no significant difference in self reported disability scale score between arotinolol and propranolol over 8–14 weeks (scores from dose based direct comparisons: 9.78 with arotinolol 10 mg *v* 10.12 with propranolol 40 mg; 9.18 with arotinolol 20 mg *v* 9.82 with propranolol 80 mg; 8.90 with arotinolol 30 mg *v* 9.38 with propranolol 80 mg; reported as non-significant; P values not reported). It also found no significant difference in motor task performance score (8.63 with arotinolol 10 mg *v* 8.35 with propranolol 40 mg; 7.93 with arotinolol 20 mg *v* 9.82 with propranolol 80 mg; 7.52 with arotinolol 30 mg *v* 7.65 with propranolol 80 mg; reported as non-significant, P values not reported).

Harms: **Versus placebo:** Two RCTs found that similar proportions of people taking metoprolol, atenolol, or placebo had adverse effects, including breathlessness, palpitations, dizziness, tiredness, headache, and nausea.[12,17] One RCT gave no information on adverse effects,[16] and three RCTs suggested that no-one taking metoprolol, sotalol, atenolol,[13,21] or nadolol[20] had adverse effects. **Versus propranolol:** The first RCT found that similar proportions of people taking metoprolol or propranolol had adverse effects, including tiredness, headache, and breathlessness.[12] The second RCT gave no information on adverse effects.[16] The third RCT found that similar proportions of people taking atenolol or propranolol had adverse effects, including tiredness, dizziness, and nausea.[17] The fourth RCT found no significant difference between arotinolol and propranolol in the proportion of people who had adverse effects during treatment (10/175 [6%] with arotinolol *v* 13/175 [7%] with propranolol; $P = 0.52$).[22] Among these, one person taking propranolol was withdrawn from treatment because of severe bradycardia. The most frequently reported adverse effects (occurring in > 1% of people) were gastrointestinal discomfort (dyspepsia, diarrhoea, gastric upset), bradycardia, headache, dizziness, sleep disturbance, and skin rash.

Comment: People with congestive heart failure, second degree heart block, asthma, severe allergy, and insulin dependent diabetes were generally excluded from the RCTs. We found no RCTs addressing long term outcomes.

OPTION BARBITURATES

Three small, short term RCTs found limited evidence that primidone improved tremor and functional ability over 4–10 weeks compared with placebo. One RCT comparing different doses of primidone found that it improved tremor from baseline at 1 year with no significant difference in outcome between groups. One small RCT found that phenobarbital improved tremor at 5 weeks compared with placebo. However, another two RCTs found no significant difference in tremor scores at 4–5 weeks between phenobarbital and placebo. Phenobarbital and primidone are associated with depression and cognitive and behavioural adverse effects. We found no RCTs of phenobarbital that addressed long term outcomes.

Benefits: We found no systematic review. **Primidone versus placebo:** We found three crossover RCTs.[23–24] All were small (8–22 people) and brief (2–5 weeks' treatment). The first RCT (16 people) compared three interventions: primidone (up to 750 mg/day), phenobarbital (phenobarbitone) (up to 150 mg/day), and placebo.[23] It found that primidone significantly improved a clinical score and self evaluation of tremor at 5 weeks after crossover compared with placebo ($P < 0.05$). The second RCT (22 people) also found that, at 10 weeks after crossover, primidone (up to 750 mg/day) significantly improved hand tremor measured by clinical scores (P < 0.02), functional tests (P < 0.01), and self evaluation (P < 0.01) compared with placebo. The results of this trial should be interpreted with caution as no intention to treat analysis was performed and only 16/22 (73%) people completed the trial.[24] The third RCT (22 people) compared four interventions: primidone (up to 750 mg/day, mean dose 402 mg), alprazolam, acetazolamide, and placebo for 4 weeks' treatment with a 2 week washout between treatments.[25] It found that primidone improved function compared with placebo at 4 weeks before crossover (observer rated score based on ability to write, feed, and function socially [0 = normal, 11 = unable to keep pencil on paper, needs help to feed, and no social activity]: 5.2 with primidone *v* 7.8 with placebo). The RCT did not assess the significance of the difference between primidone and placebo. **Different doses of primidone:** We found one RCT (113 people, 87 completers) that compared primidone 250 mg daily versus primidone 750 mg daily for 1 year.[27] The trial was designed to test equivalence between doses. The RCT found no significant difference between primidone at either dose in tremor at 1 year (mean score on the Fahn-Tlosa-Marin clinical evaluation scale [maximum score 144]: 19 with primidone 250 mg *v* 26.3 with primidone 750 mg; P < 0.06). It found that both doses significantly improved tremor from baseline (P < 0.0001 for either dose *v* baseline). **Pentobarbital versus placebo:** We found three small, short term, crossover RCTs.[14,23,26] The first RCT (17 people) compared three interventions: phenobarbital (1.25 mg/kg/day), propranolol (1.7 mg/kg/day), and placebo.[14] It found no significant difference in a clinical tremor score or functional tests at 4 weeks between phenobarbital and placebo. The results of this trial should be interpreted with caution as no intention to treat analysis was performed and only 12/17 (70%) people completed the trial.[14] The second RCT (16 people) compared three interventions: phenobarbital, primidone, and placebo.[23] It found no significant difference in clinical score and self evaluation of tremor at 5 weeks between phenobarbital and placebo (reported as non-significant, CI not reported).[23] The third RCT (12 people) found that, compared with placebo, phenobarbital 120 mg daily significantly improved accelerometer recordings**G** (P < 0.01) and a symptom rating scale (P < 0.05) after 5 weeks. It found no significant difference in handwriting tests or self evaluation of tremor.[26] It found that phenobarbital significantly increased the proportion of people who responded compared with placebo (response defined as decrease in tremor score measured by accelerometer of ≥ 15%: 11/11 [100%] with phenobarbital *v* 6/11 [55%] with placebo; ARR 45%, 95% CI 15% to 75%; NNT 3, 95% CI 2 to 7).[26]

Harms: **Primidone:** In one RCT, 5/22 (23%) people taking primidone withdrew because of adverse effects (first dose acute toxic reaction, sedation, daytime sleepiness, tiredness, and depression).[24] In another RCT, 8/24 (33%) people receiving primidone discontinued treatment because of adverse effects, including nausea, ataxia, dizziness, or confusion.[25] **Different doses of primidone:** The RCT found that primidone at either dose was associated with somnolence (33% of people in both groups), dizziness and instability (19.5%), nausea (14%), non-specific cephalic discomfort (27.5%), and generalised discomfort (8%).[27] Fifteen people withdraw because of adverse events, 13 of them taking high dose primidone. **Barbiturates:** Both primidone (metabolised to phenobarbital) and phenobarbital are associated with depression and cognitive and behavioural effects (particularly in children, elderly people, and people with neuropsychiatric problems). See epilepsy, p 1588.

Comment: The RCTs were short term, small, and many randomised people did not complete the trials. The only RCT that addressed long term outcomes is the trial that compared different doses of primidone.[27] Equivalence trials are difficult to interpret in the absence of previous placebo controlled trials. Nevertheless this was a well designed trial and the reported effect size is similar to the one seen in the RCT comparing propranolol versus clonidine.[19]

OPTION BENZODIAZEPINES

Two small short term RCTs found weak evidence that alprazolam may improve tremor and function at 2–4 weeks compared with placebo. However, we were unable to draw reliable conclusions about effects. One very small RCT provided insufficient evidence to compare clonazepam versus placebo. Adverse effects with benzodiazepines, including dependency, sedation and cognitive and behavioural effects, have been well described for other conditions (see panic disorder, p 1311).

Benefits: We found no systematic review. **Alprazolam versus placebo:** We found two RCTs.[25,28] The first RCT (22 people) compared four interventions: alprazolam (up to 1.5 mg/day, mean dose 0.75 mg), acetazolamide, primidone, and placebo.[25] It found that alprazolam improved function compared with placebo after 4 weeks (observer rated score based on ability to write, feed, and function socially [0 = normal, 11 = unable to keep pencil on paper, needs help to feed, and no social activity]: 6.0 with alprazolam *v* 7.8 with placebo; P value not reported). The second RCT (24 people) did not directly compare alprazolam (up to 3 mg/day) versus placebo, rather it assessed changes from baseline within each group. It found that alprazolam improved observer rated global impression from baseline at 2 weeks compared with placebo, but found no significant difference in clinical scores, functional tests, or self evaluation of tremor.[28] **Clonazepam versus placebo:** We found one RCT (15 people), which found no significant difference between clonazepam and placebo in any outcome.[29] However, nine people withdrew during an open run-in period with clonazepam, so only six entered the double blind phase; the trial is therefore likely to have been underpowered to detect a clinically important difference in outcomes.

Harms: We found no data addressing harms of benzodiazepines specifically in populations with essential tremor. Adverse effects with benzodiazepines, including dependency, sedation, and cognitive and behavioural effects, have been well described for other conditions (see panic disorder, p 1311).

Comment: We found no RCTs addressing long term outcomes.

OPTION CARBONIC ANHYDRASE INHIBITORS

Small RCTs provided insufficient evidence to assess methazolamide or acetazolamide in people with essential tremor. We found no RCTs addressing long term outcomes.

Benefits: We found no systematic review. **Methazolamide versus placebo:** We found one crossover RCT (25 people), which found no significant difference between methazolamide (up to 300 mg/day) and placebo in clinical score, functional tasks, or self evaluation (7/18 [39%] improved with methazolamide *v* 4/18 [22%] with placebo; ARR +16%, 95% CI –15% to +45%; see comment below).[30] **Acetazolamide versus placebo:** We found one RCT (22 people) comparing acetazolamide (up to 750 mg/day, mean dose 562 mg) versus alprazolam versus primidone versus placebo.[25] It found no significant difference in function at

4 weeks between acetazolamide and placebo, although more people taking acetazolamide had improved function (observer rated score based on ability to write, feed, and function socially [0 = normal, 11 = unable to keep pencil on paper, needs help to feed, and no social activity]; 7.3 with acetazolamide v 7.8 with placebo; P = 0.81).

Harms: **Methazolamide versus placebo:** The RCT gave no information on adverse effects.[30] **Acetazolamide versus placebo:** In the RCT, 3/19 (16%) people receiving acetazolamide complained of tolerable paraesthesias.[25]

Comment: In the first RCT, the results were analyzed on treatment rather than by intention to treat.[30] Seven people withdrew from the trial. We found no RCTs addressing long term outcomes.

OPTION CALCIUM CHANNEL BLOCKERS (DIHYDROPYRIDINE)

Poor quality RCTs provided insufficient evidence to compare the dihydropyridine calcium channel blockers nicardipine and nimodipine versus placebo.

Benefits: We found no systematic review. **Nicardipine versus placebo:** We found two crossover RCTs.[18,31] The first RCT (11 people) found no significant difference in accelerometer recordings(G) after 1 month between nicardipine and placebo.[31] No clinical outcomes were assessed. The second RCT (14 people) compared three interventions: nicardipine (1 mg/kg/day), propranolol 160 mg daily, and placebo for 1 month.[18] It found that nicardipine improved a symptom score at 1 month compared with placebo (CI not reported). **Nimodipine versus placebo:** We found one crossover RCT (15 people), which found no significant difference in clinical scores after 2 weeks' treatment between nimodipine 90 mg daily and placebo (ARR +20%, 95% CI –15% to +55%).[32]

Harms: Nicardipine and nimodipine can provoke or aggravate heart failure. They are associated with dizziness, flushing, peripheral oedema, lethargy, headache, and fatigue. Adverse gastrointestinal effects (nausea/vomiting, loss of appetite, constipation, weight gain, thirst, indigestion, or altered taste) are reported by 1–3% of people. Abnormalities of laboratory tests (liver function tests) have been observed, usually within 1–8 weeks after starting treatment.

Comment: The possibility of publication bias has not been excluded. The evidence is too weak to assess the role of calcium channel blockers in essential hand tremor. We found no RCTs addressing long term outcomes.

OPTION FLUNARIZINE

One small RCT found weak evidence that flunarizine reduced the symptoms of essential hand tremor after 1 months' treatment compared with placebo.

Benefits: We found no systematic review. **Versus placebo:** We found one crossover RCT (17 people), which found that flunarizine 10 mg daily significantly improved clinical scores and tremor amplitude after 1 month of treatment compared with placebo (P = 0.0006).[33] Most of the people who completed the RCT were considered improved with flunarizine (13/15 [87%]), but the number improving with placebo was not reported.

Harms: Observational studies suggest that flunarizine is associated with adverse neuropsychiatric effects, and with the development of parkinsonism and other movement disorders.[34–37]

Comment: The RCT was small and brief. The evidence is inconclusive. We found no RCTs addressing long term outcomes.

OPTION CLONIDINE

One RCT found no significant difference between clonidine and placebo in essential hand tremor. However, the study lacked power to rule out a clinically important difference. Another RCT comparing clonidine versus propranolol found that the initial improvement in tremor from baseline was similar with both drugs and was maintained throughout follow up for 1 year.

Benefits: We found no systematic review. **Versus placebo:** One crossover RCT (10 people) found no significant difference in the proportion of people who improved between clonidine (up to 0.6 mg/day) and placebo (1/10 [10%] with clonidine *v* 1/10 [10%] with placebo).[38] **Versus propranolol:** See benefits of propranolol, p 1610.

Harms: **Versus placebo:** The RCT gave no information on adverse effects.[38] Clonidine has been associated in other studies with sedation, lethargy, drowsiness, constipation, dry mouth, headache, dizziness, fatigue, and weakness. **Versus propranolol:** See harms of propranolol, p 1611.

Comment: None.

OPTION ISONIAZID

One RCT found no significant difference between isoniazid and placebo in essential hand tremor, but it may have lacked power to detect a clinically important difference. We found no RCTs addressing long term outcomes.

Benefits: We found no systematic review. **Versus placebo:** One brief, crossover RCT (15 people, 11 with essential tremor) comparing isoniazid (up to 1200 mg/day) versus placebo found similar clinical scores and accelerometer recordings**G** between treatments no quantitative data reported.[39]

Harms: One person in the RCT withdrew from the trial because of dizziness and one had to discontinue medication because of hepatotoxicity.[39] In other studies, isoniazid has been associated with hepatotoxicity and peripheral neuropathy.

Comment: We found no RCTs addressing long term outcomes.

OPTION GABAPENTIN

Small RCTs provided insufficient evidence to compare gabapentin versus placebo. We found no RCTs addressing long term outcomes.

Benefits: We found no systematic review. **Versus placebo:** We found three small crossover RCTs (16–25 people).[15,40,41] The first RCT (16 people) compared three interventions: gabapentin (up to 1200 mg/day), propranolol (up to 120 mg/day), and placebo. It found that, compared with placebo, gabapentin significantly improved response rate (10/16 [63%] responded with gabapentin *v* 5/16 [31%] with placebo; ARR 32%, 95% CI 17% to 47%; NNT 4, 95% CI 2 to 6), clinical scores ($P < 0.05$), disability ($P < 0.01$), self evaluation ($P < 0.006$), and accelerometer recordings**G** ($P < 0.05$) at 2 weeks before crossover.[15] The second RCT (20 people) compared gabapentin 1800 mg daily versus placebo for 2 weeks' treatment. It found no significant difference in clinical scores, activities of daily living, or self evaluation at 6 weeks after crossover (reported as non-significant, CI not reported).[40] The third RCT (25 people) compared three interventions: gabapentin 1800 mg daily, gabapentin 3600 mg daily, and placebo. It found that, compared with placebo, gabapentin (at either dose) significantly improved participants' global assessments ($P < 0.05$), water pouring scores ($P < 0.05$), and scores of activities of daily living ($P < 0.005$). It found no significant difference between gabapentin and placebo in accelerometry scores, spirographs, or investigator global impression scores.[41] The RCT also found no significant difference between high and low doses of gabapentin in the 20 people who completed the trial.

Harms: The RCTs reported fatigue, drowsiness, nausea, dizziness, and decreased libido in people taking gabapentin.[15,40,41] See epilepsy, p 1588.

Comment: The results of the three RCTs differ. It is unclear whether the difference arose by chance or whether confounding variables, such as prior use of antitremor medications, baseline severity, or assessment rating scales, explain the difference. We found no RCTs addressing long term outcomes.

OPTION BOTULINUM A TOXIN–HAEMAGGLUTININ COMPLEX

Two RCTs in people with essential hand tremor found that botulinum A toxin–haemagglutinin complex improved clinical rating scales at 4–12 weeks. They found no consistent improvement in motor tasks or functional disability. Hand weakness, which is dose dependent and transient, is a frequent adverse effect. We found no RCTs addressing long term outcomes.

Benefits: We found no systematic review. **Versus placebo:** We found two RCTs.[42,43] The first RCT (25 people with essential hand tremor unresponsive to "optimal medical therapy"; see comment below) compared botulinum A toxin–haemagglutinin complex versus placebo.[42] Botulinum toxin 50 U was injected in forearm muscles and repeated if necessary after 1 month (100 U). The RCT found that botulinum toxin significantly increased the proportion of people who responded to the first injection compared with placebo (12/13 [92%] with botulinum toxin *v* 1/12 [8%] with placebo; $P < 0.001$). After 4 weeks, mild to moderate improvement was significantly more likely with botulinum toxin (75% with botulinum toxin *v* 27% with placebo; ARR 48%, 95% CI 30% to 66%; NNT 3, 95% CI 2 to 4). It also found that botulinum toxin significantly improved clinical scores compared with placebo ($P < 0.05$), but found no significant difference in functional tests and accelerometer recordings🅖. The second RCT (133 people with essential tremor of the hand by the Tremor Investigation Group criteria, 16 weeks' follow up) compared three interventions: single injections of low dose botulinum A toxin–haemagglutinin complex (50 U), high dose botulinum A toxin–haemagglutinin complex (100 U), and placebo into the wrist flexors and extensors.[43] It found that botulinum toxin type A at either dose significantly improved postural tremor on clinical rating scales was after 12 weeks ($P = 0.004$ with low dose, $P = 0.0003$ with high dose). It found no significant difference between botulinum toxin at either dose in kinetic tremor, motor task performance, or functional disability.[43]

Harms: The main adverse effect of botulinum A toxin–haemagglutinin complex is dose dependent transient hand weakness.

Comment: The first RCT stated that participants were unresponsive to "optimal medical therapy" but did not state what this involved.[42] We found no RCTs addressing long term outcomes.

OPTION TOPIRAMATE

One RCT found limited evidence that topiramate improved observer rated tremor score after 2 weeks' treatment compared with placebo but was associated with adverse effects, including appetite suppression, weight loss, and paraesthesia. The clinical importance of the difference in tremor score is uncertain. We found no RCTs addressing long term outcomes.

Benefits: We found no systematic review. **Versus placebo:** We found one crossover RCT (24 people with tremor of hand, head, or voice), which compared topiramate (400 mg/day or maximum tolerated dose; mean dose 333 mg/day) versus placebo for 2 weeks' treatment with a 2 week washout between treatments.[44] It found that topiramate significantly improved observer rated tremor score at 6 weeks after crossover compared with placebo (tremor score improvement: 0.88 with topiramate *v* 0.15 with placebo; $P = 0.015$).

Harms: Nine out of the 24 (38%) people withdrew from the RCT; six because of adverse effects (5 with topiramate, 1 with placebo).[44] The most common adverse effects with topiramate were appetite suppression, weight loss, and paraesthesia (see epilepsy, p 1588).

Comment: The RCT did not report tremor scores specifically for the hand.[44] However, 23 of the 24 participants had hand tremor and only four patients also had tremor in other locations. The primary outcome of observer rated tremor was assessed by a non-validated scale developed by Fahn, et al.[6] The clinical relevance of the difference is uncertain. We found no RCTs addressing long term outcomes.

OPTION MIRTAZAPINE New

One RCT in people taking antitremor drugs such as propranolol, found no significant difference in tremor between adding mirtazapine and placebo and found that adverse effects were frequent.

Benefits: We found no systematic review. **Versus placebo:** We found one crossover RCT (17 people, 13 of whom were receiving other drug treatments including propranolol and primidone) comparing adding mirtazapine versus placebo.[45] Participants received mirtazapine or placebo 15 mg daily for 1 week with weekly dose escalation to reach the target dose of 45 mg daily. This dose was maintained for 2 weeks. There was a minimum washout period of 14 days before crossover. The RCT did not report results before crossover. The RCT found no significant difference between mirtazapine and placebo in tremor at 6 weeks (tremor measured by questions 1–10 on the Fahn-Tolosa-Marin Tremor Rating Scale: mean 9.5 with both treatments, reported as non-significant, P value not reported, significance set at $P < 0.01$ by the authors of the RCT).

Harms: Adverse effects were more common in people taking mirtazapine and included drowsiness, confusion, dry mouth, weight gain, polyuria, itching, nausea, gait and balance problems, blurred vision, and bad taste; three people withdrew because of adverse effects when taking mirtazapine 15 mg daily.[45] The RCT did not assess the significance of the difference between groups.

Comment: The RCT is small but it seems sufficient to show that a beneficial effect of mirtazapine is unlikely and there are adverse reactions associated with taking the drug.[45]

GLOSSARY

Accelerometer recording Recording of the movements from a body segment to allow measurement of frequency, amplitude, or intensity of a tremor. Intensity of tremor is a measure of the overall magnitude of movement; it often refers to the product of the amplitude of tremor multiplied by its frequency.

Substantive changes

Propranolol One RCT comparing propranolol versus clonidine added.[19] Data on long term outcomes enhanced. Categorisation of propranolol and clonidine unchanged.
β blockers other than propranolol One RCT added.[22] Categorisation unchanged.
Barbiturates One RCT added.[27] Data on long term outcomes enhanced. Categorisation unchanged.

REFERENCES

1. Deuschl G, Bain P, Brin M, et al. Consensus statement of the Movement Disorder Society on Tremor. *Mov Disord* 1998;13(suppl 3):2–23.
2. Louis ED, Ottman R, Hauser WA. How common is the most common adult movement disorder? Estimates the prevalence of essential tremor throughout the world. *Mov Disord* 1988;13:803–808.
3. Auff E, Doppelbauer A, Fertl E. Essential tremor: functional disability vs. subjective impairment. *J Neural Transm Suppl* 1991;33:105–110.
4. Koller WC, Busenbark K, Miner K. The relationship of essential tremor to other movement disorders: report on 678 patients. Essential Tremor Study Group. *Ann Neurol* 1994;35:717–723.
5. Bain PG, Findley LJ, Thompson PD, et al. A study of hereditary essential tremor. *Brain* 1994;117:805–824.
6. Fahn SE, Tolosa E, Marin C. Clinical rating scale for tremor. In: Jankovic J, Tolosa E, eds. *Parkinson's disease and movement disorders*, 2nd ed. Baltimore: Williams & Wilkins, 1988:225–234.
7. Winkler GF, Young RR. Efficacy of chronic propranolol therapy in action tremors of the familial, senile or essential varieties. *N Engl J Med* 1974;290:984–988.
8. Tolosa ES, Loewenson RB. Essential tremor: treatment with propranolol. *Neurology* 1975;25:1041–1044.
9. Morgan MH, Hewer RL, Cooper R. Effect of the beta adrenergic blocking agent propranolol on essential tremor. *J Neurol Neurosurg Psychiatry* 1973;36:618–624.
10. Calzetti S, Findley LJ, Perucca E, et al. The response of essential tremor to propranolol evaluation of clinical variables governing its efficacy on prolonged administration. *J Neurol Neurosurg Psychiatry* 1983;46:393–398.
11. Cleeves L, Findley LJ. Propranolol and propranolol-LA in essential tremor: a double blind comparative study. *J Neurol Neurosurg Psychiatry* 1988;51:379–384.
12. Calzetti S, Findley LJ, Perucca E, et al. Controlled study of metoprolol and propranolol during prolonged administration in people with essential tremor. *J Neurol Neurosurg Psychiatry* 1982;45:893–897.
13. Jefferson D, Jenner P, Marsden CD. Beta-adrenoreceptor antagonists in essential tremor. *J Neurol Neurosurg Psychiatry* 1979;42:904–909.
14. Baruzzi A, Procaccianti G, Martinelli P, et al. Phenobarbitone and propranolol in essential tremor: a double-blind controlled clinical trial. *Neurology* 1983;33:296–300.
15. Gironell A, Kulisevsky J, Barbanoj M, et al. A randomised placebo-controlled comparative trial of gabapentin and propranolol in essential tremor. *Arch Neurol* 1999;56:475–480.
16. Teravainen H, Larsen A, Fogelholm R. Comparison between the effects of pindolol and propranolol on essential tremor. *Neurology* 1977;27:439–442.
17. Larsen TA, Teravainen H, Calne DB. Atenolol vs. propranolol in essential tremor. A controlled, quantitative study. *Acta Neurol Scand* 1982;66:547–554.
18. Jimenez-Jimenez FJ, Garcia-Ruiz PJ, Cabrera-Valdivia F. Nicardipine versus propranolol in essential tremor. *Acta Neurol (Napoli)* 1994;16:184–188.
19. Serrano-Duenas M. Clonidine versus propranolol in the treatment of essential tremor. A double-blind trial with a one-year follow-up. *Neurologia* 2003;18:248–254. [In Spanish]
20. Koller WC. Nadolol in essential tremor. *Neurology* 1983;33:1076–1077.
21. Leigh PN, Jefferson D, Twomey A, et al. Beta-adrenoreceptor mechanisms in essential tremor; a double-blind placebo controlled trial of metoprolol, sotalol and atenolol. *J Neurol Neurosurg Psychiatry* 1983;46:710–715.
22. Lee KS, Kim JS, Kim JW, et al. A multicenter randomized crossover multiple-dose comparison study of arotinolol and propranolol in essential tremor. *Parkinsonism Relat Disord* 2003;9:341–347.
23. Sasso E, Perucca E, Calzetti S. Double-blind comparison of primidone and phenobarbitone in essential tremor. *Neurology* 1988;38:808–810.
24. Findley LJ, Cleeves L, Calzetti S. Primidone in essential tremor of the hands and head: a double-blind controlled clinical study. *J Neurol Neurosurg Psychiatry* 1985;48:911–915.
25. Gunal DI, Afsar N, Bekiroglu N, et al. New alternative agents in essential tremor therapy: double-blind placebo-controlled study of alprazolam and acetazolamide. *Neurol Sci* 2000;21:315–317.
26. Findley LJ, Cleeves L. Phenobarbitone in essential tremor. *Neurology* 1985;35:1784–1787.
27. Serrano-Duenas M. Use of primidone in low doses (250 mg/day) versus high doses (750 mg/day) in the management of essential tremor. Double-blind comparative study with one-year follow-up. *Parkinsonism Relat Disord* 2003;10:29–33.
28. Huber SJ, Paulson GW. Efficacy of alprazolam for essential tremor. *Neurology* 1988;38:241–243.
29. Thompson C, Lang A, Parkes JD, et al. A double-blind trial of clonazepam in benign essential tremor. *Clin Neuropharmacol* 1984;7:83–88.
30. Busenbark K, Pahwa R, Hubble J, et al. Double-blind controlled study of methazolamide in treatment of essential tremor. *Neurology* 1993;43:1045–1047.
31. Garcia-Ruiz PJ, Garcia-de-Yebenes-Prous J, Jimenez-Jimenez J. Effect of nicardipine on essential tremor: brief report. *Clin Neuropharmacol* 1993;16:456–459.
32. Biary N, Bahou Y, Sofi MA, et al. The effect of nimodipine on essential tremor. *Neurology* 1995;45:1523–1525.
33. Biary N, Deeb S, Langenberg P. The effect of flunarizine in essential tremor. *Neurology* 1991;41:311–312.

34. Micheli FE, Pardal MM, Giannaula R, et al. Movement disorders and depression due to flunarizine and cinnarizine. *Mov Disord* 1989;4:139–146.
35. Capella D, Laporte JR, Castel JM, et al. Parkinsonism, tremor, and depression induced by cinnarizine and flunarizine. *BMJ* 1988;297:722–723.
36. Chouza C, Scaramelli A, Caamano JL, et al. Parkinsonism, tardive dyskinesia, akathisia and depression induced by flunarizine. *Lancet* 1986;1:1303–1304.
37. Micheli F, Pardal MF, Gatto M. Flunarizine and cinnarizine induced extrapyramidal reactions. *Neurology* 1987;37:881–884.
38. Koller W, Herbster G, Cone S. Clonidine in the treatment of essential tremor. *Mov Disord* 1986;4:235–237.
39. Hallett M, Ravitis J, Dubinsky RM, et al. A double-blind trial of isoniazid for essential tremor and other action tremors. *Mov Disord* 1991;6:253–256.
40. Pahwa R, Lyons K, Hubble JP, et al. Double-blind controlled trial of gabapentin in essential tremor. *Mov Disord* 1998;13:465–467.
41. Ondo W, Hunter C, Vuong KD, et al. Gabapentin for essential tremor: a multiple-dose, double-blind, placebo-controlled trial. *Mov Disord* 2000;15:678–682.
42. Jankovic J, Schwartz K, Clemence W, et al. A randomised, double-blind, placebo-controlled study to evaluate botulinum toxin type A in essential hand tremor. *Mov Disord* 1996;11:250–256.
43. Brin MF, Lyons KE, Doucette J, et al. A randomized, double masked, controlled trial of botulinum toxin type A in essential hand tremor. *Neurology* 2001;56:1523–1528.
44. Connor G. A double-blind placebo-controlled trial of topiramate treatment for essential tremor. *Neurology* 2002;59:132–134.
45. Pahwa R, Lyons KE. Mirtazapine in essential tremor: a double-blind, placebo-controlled pilot study. *Mov Disord* 2003;18:584–587.

Joaquim Ferreira
Neurologist
School of Medicine
University of Lisbon
Lisbon
Portugal

Cristina Sampaio
Assistant Professor
School of Medicine
University of Lisbon
Lisbon
Portugal

Competing interests: CS has accepted reimbursement for attending symposia, fees for speaking, fees for organising education, and funds for a member of staff from Allergan (Botox) and IPSEN (Dysport). JF has been paid by Allergen (Botox) and IPSEN (Dysport) for running educational programmes. JF declares involvement in the design and conduct of multiple clinical trials testing antiparkinsonian, antidystonic, and antiepileptic drugs developed by multiple companies. He declares no previous or present participation in trials in the field of tremor.

Migraine headache

Search date August 2003

Luis E Morillo

QUESTIONS

INTERVENTIONS

Key Messages

- **Eletriptan** One systematic review and subsequent RCTs have found that eletriptan increases headache relief at 2 hours compared with placebo. One systematic review and subsequent RCTs have found that eletriptan 40 and 80 mg increases headache relief at 2 hours compared with sumatriptan 50 and 100 mg. One RCT found that eletriptan 40 and 80 mg increased headache relief at 2 hours compared with ergotamine plus caffeine.
- **Ibuprofen** Five RCTs have found that ibuprofen improves migraine symptoms compared with placebo.
- **Naratriptan** One systematic review and subsequent RCTs have found that naratriptan increases headache relief at 2 hours compared with placebo. One systematic review has found that sumatriptan 100 mg increases headache relief at 2 hours compared with naratriptan 2.5 mg. However, one subsequent RCT found no significant difference in headache recurrence. One RCT found no significant difference between naratriptan 2.5 mg and zolmitriptan 2.5 mg in headache relief at 4 hours. One RCT identified by a systematic review found that naratriptal reduced headache relief at 2 hours compared with rizatriptan.
- **Rizatriptan** One systematic review and subsequent RCTs have found that rizatriptan improves headache relief compared with placebo. Two RCTs found no significant difference between rizatriptan and zolmitriptan in headache relief at 2 hours. One RCT identified by a systematic review found that rizatriptan increased headache relief at 2 hours compared with naratriptan. One RCT found that rizatriptan increased headache relief and reduced nausea and vomiting at 2 hours compared with ergotamine plus caffeine.
- **Salicylates** RCTs have found that oral or intravenous salicylates (alone or in combination with metoclopramide, paracetamol, or caffeine) increase headache relief compared with placebo. One RCT found no significant difference between aspirin and paracetamol plus codeine in headache relief. One RCT found no significant difference between aspirin plus metoclopramide and sumatriptan in headache relief. One RCT found that oral lysine acetylsalicylate plus metoclopramide increased headache relief and reduced nausea and vomiting at 2 hours compared with ergotamine plus caffeine. One RCT found no significant difference in headache relief between aspirin plus metoclopramide and zolmitriptan.

- **Sumatriptan** Systematic reviews and subsequent RCTs have found that subcutaneous, oral, or intranasal sumatriptan increases headache relief compared with placebo. RCTs found no significant difference in headache relief between sumatriptan and aspirin plus metoclopramide, tolfenamic acid, or zolmitriptan. RCTs have found that oral or nasal sumatriptan increase headache relief compared with oral or nasal ergotamine. One systematic review has found that sumatriptan 100 mg increases headache relief at 2 hours compared with naratriptan 2.5 mg. However, one subsequent RCT found no significant difference in headache recurrence. One systematic review and subsequent RCTs have found that eletriptan 40 and 80 mg increases headache relief at 2 hours compared with sumatriptan 50 and 100 mg.
- **Zolmitriptan** One systematic review and two subsequent RCTs have found that oral zolmitriptan increases headache relief compared with placebo. One systematic review and two subsequent RCTs found no significant difference between zolmitriptan and sumatriptan in headache relief. One RCT found no significant difference in headache relief between aspirin plus metoclopramide and zolmitriptan. One RCT found no significant difference between naratriptan 2.5 mg and zolmitriptan 2.5 mg in headache relief at 4 hours.
- **Diclofenac** RCTs have found that oral or intramuscular diclofenac improves headache symptoms compared with placebo. One RCT found that intramuscular diclofenac improved migraine symptoms compared with intramuscular paracetamol.
- **Ergotamine** One systematic review found limited evidence from four RCTs that ergotamine (with or without caffeine) improved headache relief compared with placebo. One overview of harms suggested that ergotamine increased nausea and vomiting compared with placebo. RCTs have found that ergotamine (or its derivatives, with or without caffeine and cyclizine) is less effective for migraine symptoms than sumatriptan. They found limited evidence that it was less effective than naproxen. RCTs found that thalergotarine plus caffeine reduced headache relief and increase nausea and vomiting at 2 hours compared with oral lysine acetylsalicylate plus metoclopramide and rizatriptan.
- **Naproxen** Three small RCTs found that naproxen reduced migraine symptoms compared with placebo. Two RCTs found that naproxen reduced symptoms compared with ergotamine (with or without caffeine plus cyclizine). However, one further RCT found no significant difference between naproxen and ergotamine in pain relief after 1 hour.
- **Tolfenamic acid** RCTs found limited evidence that tolfenamic acid improved duration and severity of headache compared with placebo. RCTs found no significant difference in symptom relief between tolfenamic acid and sumatriptan or paracetamol.

DEFINITION Migraine is a primary headache disorder manifesting as recurring attacks usually lasting for 4–72 hours and involving pain of moderate to severe intensity, often with nausea, sometimes vomiting, and/or sensitivity to light, sound, and other sensory stimuli. The 1988 International Headache Society criteria Ⓖ include separate criteria for migraine with and migraine without associated aura.[1] Unless stated otherwise, RCTs used International Headache Society criteria for migraine with or without aura.

INCIDENCE/ PREVALENCE Migraine is common worldwide. Prevalence has been reported to be 5–25% in women and 2–10% in men. Overall, the highest incidence for migraine without aura has been reported between the ages of 10 and 11 years (10/1000 person years). The peak incidence of migraine without aura in males is between ages 10 and 11 years (10/1000 person years) and in females between ages 14 and 17 years (19/1000 person years).[2] The incidence of migraine with aura peaks in males at age 5 years (7/1000 person years) and in females at age 12–13 years (14/1000 person years).[2] Female prevalence of migraine with or without aura has a declining trend after age 45–50 years.

AETIOLOGY/ RISK FACTORS Data from independent representative samples from Canada,[3,4] the USA,[5,6] several countries in Latin America,[7] and several countries in Europe,[8–11] Hong Kong,[12] and Japan[13] show a female to male predominance and a peak in middle aged women. Migraine has been reported to be 50% more likely in people with a family history of migraine.[14]

PROGNOSIS	Acute migraine is self limiting and only rarely results in permanent neurological complications. Chronic recurrent migraine may cause disability through pain, and may affect daily functioning and quality of life.
AIMS OF INTERVENTION	To reduce frequency of migraine, intensity of accompanying symptoms, and duration of headache, with minimal adverse effects.
OUTCOMES	Headache relief or being pain free Ⓖ at different times after medication. Pain relief at specific post-dose times. In this review, headache relief is reported at 2 hours unless otherwise stated. Some RCTs include the need for rescue medication and headache recurrence Ⓖ as outcome measures.
METHODS	*Clinical Evidence* search and appraisal August 2003.

QUESTION What are the effects of drug treatments for acute migraine?

OPTION SALICYLATES

RCTs have found that oral or intravenous salicylates (alone or in combination with metoclopramide, paracetamol, or caffeine) increase headache relief compared with placebo. One RCT found no significant difference between aspirin and paracetamol plus codeine in headache relief. One RCT found no significant difference between aspirin plus metoclopramide and sumatriptan in headache relief. One RCT found that oral lysine acetylsalicylate plus metoclopramide increased headache relief and reduced nausea and vomiting at 2 hours compared with ergotamine plus caffeine. One RCT found no significant difference in headache relief between aspirin plus metoclopramide and zolmitriptan.

Benefits: We found no systematic review but found 12 RCTs.[15–26] **Oral lysine acetylsalicylate (L-ASA):** One RCT (266 people, 475 migraine attacks) found that oral L-ASA 1620 mg plus metoclopramide 10 mg significantly increased headache relief Ⓖ compared with placebo (AR 56% with L-ASA *v* 28% with placebo; RR 2.0, 95% CI 1.6 to 2.5).[15] A second RCT compared three treatments: oral L-ASA 1620 mg plus metoclopramide 10 mg, oral sumatriptan 100 mg, and placebo.[16] It found that L-ASA plus metoclopramide significantly increased headache relief compared with placebo (AR 57% with L-ASA *v* 24% with placebo; RR 2.4, 95% CI 1.7 to 3.3). The difference between active treatment groups was not significant (AR 57% with L-ASA *v* 54% with sumatriptan; P = 0.50). **Intravenous L-ASA:** One RCT (278 people) compared three treatments: L-ASA 1800 mg intravenously, sumatriptan 6 mg subcutaneously, and placebo.[17] It found that both L-ASA and sumatriptan significantly increased headache relief compared with placebo, and that sumatriptan significantly increased headache relief compared with L-ASA (AR 74% with L-ASA *v* 91% with sumatriptan *v* 24% with placebo; RR for L-ASA *v* placebo 3.1, 95% CI 1.8 to 5.4; RR for L-ASA *v* sumatriptan 0.8, 95% CI 0.7 to 0.9). A second, smaller, crossover RCT (112 attacks in 56 people) compared L-ASA 1000 mg intravenously versus ergotamine 0.5 mg subcutaneously.[18] It found no significant difference between groups in pain intensity score on a visual analogue scale. **Effervescent aspirin:** One crossover RCT (120 people) compared effervescent aspirin 650 mg with and without metoclopramide 10 mg versus placebo.[19] At 2 hours aspirin with or without metoclopramide reduced headache significantly more than placebo (P < 0.001). A second RCT (374 people) compared effervescent aspirin 1000 mg versus placebo.[20] It found that aspirin significantly increased headache relief compared with placebo (AR 55% with aspirin *v* 37% with placebo; RR 1.5, 95% CI 1.2 to 1.9). **Dispersible aspirin:** One crossover RCT (101 people with migraine, 73 of whom received both treatments) compared mouth dispersible aspirin 900 mg versus placebo in two consecutive attacks.[21] It found that aspirin significantly increased headache relief at 2 hours compared with placebo, and significantly reduced need for rescue medication**G** (AR for headache relief 48% with aspirin *v* 19% with placebo; P = 0.0005; difference in need for rescue medication: P < 0.01). **Other combinations:** One large RCT (1357 people with non-disabling migraine) compared oral paracetamol 250 mg plus aspirin 250 mg plus caffeine 65 mg versus placebo.[22] Combination treatment improved headache relief compared with placebo (AR 59% with combination *v* 33% with placebo; RR 1.8, 95% CI 1.6 to 2.1). A second, crossover RCT (198 people treated for 3 consecutive migraine attacks) found no significant difference in headache relief between aspirin 1000 mg orally and paracetamol 400 mg plus codeine 25 mg.[23] However, both improved headache relief compared with placebo (P = 0.0003 with aspirin and P = 0.0002 with paracetamol plus codeine). **Aspirin versus sumatriptan:** One RCT (358 people) found no significant difference between oral aspirin 900 mg plus metoclopramide 10 mg and oral sumatriptan 100 mg in headache relief at 2 hours (AR 45% with aspirin plus metoclopramide *v* 56% with sumatriptan; P = 0.078).[24] **Aspirin versus tolfenamic acid:** See benefits of tolfenamic acid, p 1628. **Aspirin versus zolmitriptan:** See benefits of zolmitriptan, p 1637. **Aspirin versus ergotamine:** See benefits of ergotamine, p 1629.

Harms: One RCT reported adverse effects related to L-ASA in 2%, to sumatriptan in 15%, and to placebo in 2% of people treated.[17] In this trial, severe harms were related to L-ASA in 3%, to sumatriptan in 5%, and to placebo in 2% of people treated. Another trial reported premature withdrawal of treatment in 1% with L-ASA, 3% with sumatriptan, and 2% with placebo.[16] The most frequently reported harms for L-ASA were somnolence, abdominal pain, nausea or vomiting, fatigue, and headache. The RCT comparing the combination of paracetamol, aspirin, and caffeine versus placebo reported no serious adverse effects.[22] **Versus zolmitriptan:** See harms of zolmitriptan, p 1638. **Versus ergotamine:** See harms of ergotamine, p 1630.

Comment: None.

OPTION DICLOFENAC

RCTs have found that oral or intramuscular diclofenac improves headache symptoms compared with placebo. One RCT found that intramuscular diclofenac improved migraine symptoms compared with intramuscular paracetamol.

Benefits: We found no systematic review. **Versus placebo:** We found three RCTs of oral diclofenac[27,28,30] and one RCT of intramuscular diclofenac.[29] The first RCT (170 people) found that diclofenac improved treatment success compared with placebo (success defined at 2 hours as a visual analogue scale score < 10 mm or headache duration of < 2 hours without need for rescue medication**G** within this period: AR 27% with diclofenac *v* 19% with placebo; RR 1.5, 95% CI 1.0 to 2.2).[27] The second RCT (72 people) found that diclofenac 50 or 100 mg significantly increased headache relief**G** compared with placebo (AR 39% with 50 mg *v* 44% with 100 mg *v* 22% with placebo; RR diclofenac 50 mg *v* placebo 1.8, 95% CI 1.0 to 3.1; RR diclofenac 100 mg *v* placebo 1.9, 95% CI 1.1 to 3.3).[28] The RCT found no significant difference between 50 mg and 100 mg doses of diclofenac. However, it found that diclofenac 100 mg significantly reduced need for rescue medication compared with placebo (AR 37% with diclofenac *v* 58% with placebo; RR 0.64, 95% CI 0.44 to 0.93). The third RCT (120 people with migraine with or without aura) compared intramuscular diclofenac

75 mg versus placebo.[29] At 1 hour, it found that diclofenac improved headache relief and reduced need for rescue medication compared with placebo in people with and without aura (headache relief in people without aura: AR 43.3% with diclofenac *v* 16.7% with placebo; P < 0.01; headache relief in people with aura: AR 50% with diclofenac *v* 13.3% with placebo; P < 0.01; rescue medication in people without aura: 20% with diclofenac *v* 50% with placebo; P < 0.05; rescue medication in people with aura: 11% with diclofenac *v* 42% with placebo; P < 0.05). The fourth RCT (156 people meeting International Headache Society criteria**G** for migraine with or without aura) compared three treatments: diclofenac potassium 50 or 100 mg, oral sumatriptan 100 mg, and placebo.[30] The trial found that diclofenac significantly reduced headache pain (measured on a visual analogue scale) at 2 hours compared with placebo (P < 0.001). **Versus sumatriptan:** The RCT comparing diclofenac, sumatriptan, and placebo found no significant difference between either dose of diclofenac and sumatriptan.[30] **Versus paracetamol:** One RCT (86 people) compared intramuscular diclofenac 75 mg versus intramuscular paracetamol in people with paroxysmal headaches accompanied by at least two of the following features: unilateral pain, nausea, visual and limb symptoms, and positive family history.[31] The trial found that diclofenac increased the proportion of people with partial relief of overall migraine symptoms (intensity and duration) within 35 minutes compared with paracetamol (AR 89% with diclofenac *v* 17% with paracetamol; RR 4.9, 95% CI 2.5 to 9.8).

Harms: In one RCT (72 people), 33% of people reported one or more adverse effects during one or more attacks.[28] Most adverse effects were rated as mild or moderate (gastrointestinal complaints were the most common, followed by tiredness and fatigue), but 12% of people rated adverse experiences as severe. In another RCT (170 people), 14% of people reported at least one adverse effect, with gastrointestinal effects being the most common (50%).[27] Only three people withdrew because of gastrointestinal symptoms. See non-steroidal anti-inflammatory drugs, p 1525.

Comment: None.

OPTION IBUPROFEN

Five RCTs have found that ibuprofen improves migraine symptoms compared with placebo.

Benefits: **Versus placebo:** We found no systematic review but found five RCTs comparing ibuprofen versus placebo.[32–36] The first RCT (729 people) found that oral ibuprofen (400 and 600 mg in gel formulation) significantly improved headache relief**G** compared with placebo (AR 72% with 400 mg *v* 72% with 600 mg *v* 50% with placebo; ibuprofen 400 mg *v* placebo RR 1.4, 95% CI 1.2 to 1.7; ibuprofen 600 mg *v* placebo RR 1.4, 95% CI 1.2 to 1.7).[32] It found no significant difference in the need for rescue medication**G**. The second RCT (25 people, 146 migraines) found that ibuprofen significantly improved migraine index**G** (25 with ibuprofen *v* 46 with placebo; P = 0.0014) and reduced the need for rescue medication 4 hours after treatment (26% with ibuprofen *v* 56% with placebo; P = 0.007) compared with placebo.[33] The third RCT (40 people with common and classic migraine, 345 migraines) compared ibuprofen 800–1200 mg orally versus placebo.[34] The trial found that significantly more attacks were rated as mild with ibuprofen compared with placebo (P < 0.001) and significantly fewer attacks were rated as moderate (P < 0.05) or severe (P < 0.05). It also found that ibuprofen reduced the need for rescue medication compared with placebo (AR 22% with ibuprofen *v* 81% with placebo; RR 0.27, 95% CI 0.20 to 0.36). One RCT (660 people with headache intensity**G** not requiring bed rest or inhibiting daily activities in more than 50% of attacks) compared ibuprofen 200 or 400 mg versus placebo with a follow up of 6 hours.[35] It found that ibuprofen significantly increased headache relief at 2 hours compared with placebo (AR 41.7% with ibuprofen 400 mg *v* 40.8% with ibuprofen 200 mg *v* 28.1% with placebo; P = 0.006 for both doses *v* placebo). The fifth RCT (40 people) compared an ibuprofen arginine preparation (400 mg orally) versus placebo.[36] It found that more people taking ibuprofen arginine versus placebo achieved "considerable" or "complete" relief within 2 hours (51% with ibuprofen *v* 7% with placebo; P < 0.01). Fewer people taking ibuprofen arginine received rescue medication (31% with ibuprofen *v* 48% with placebo) but no statistical analysis was performed.

Harms: One RCT did not report adverse effects.[34] Another RCT reported pain and stomach discomfort in 12% of people on treatment, which was not considered serious.[33] Another reported no significant difference in adverse events among treatment groups, and no serious adverse events.[35] See non-steroidal anti-inflammatory drugs, p 1525.

Comment: None.

OPTION NAPROXEN

Three small RCTs found that naproxen reduced migraine symptoms compared with placebo. Two RCTs found that naproxen reduced symptoms compared with ergotamine (with or without caffeine plus cyclizine). However, one further RCT found no significant difference between naproxen and ergotamine in pain relief after 1 hour.

Benefits: We found no systematic review. **Versus placebo:** We found one crossover RCT (37 people with classic or common migraine) comparing oral naproxen 750–1250 mg versus placebo.[37] It found that naproxen significantly reduced headache intensity**G** (P = 0.047). However, it found no significant difference in need for rescue medication**G** (absolute numbers not reported; P = 0.13). A second crossover RCT (40 people with common or classic migraine) comparing naproxen 750–1000 mg versus placebo found that naproxen reduced overall pain intensity (rated as mild, moderate, or severe; P = 0.011; time of evaluation not reported).[38] The need for rescue medication after 2 hours was also significantly lower for naproxen (AR 47% with naproxen *v* 72% with placebo; P = 0.002; insufficient data for calculation of RR). A third RCT compared three treatments: naproxen, ergotamine (plus caffeine plus cyclizine), and placebo.[39] It found that naproxen significantly increased pain relief compared with ergotamine at 1 hour after the first dose (P = 0.032). **Versus ergotamine:** We found three RCTs, which compared oral naproxen 750–1750 mg versus ergotamine 2–4 mg alone or with caffeine 91.5 mg plus cyclizine chlorhydrate 50 mg.[39–41] The first RCT (114 people) found that naproxen significantly reduced migraine intensity (rated as mild, moderate, severe, or incapacitating) compared with ergotamine plus caffeine plus cyclizine (P = 0.014). However, it found no significant difference in need for rescue medication.[39] The second RCT (37 people with classic or common migraine) compared naproxen versus ergotamine.[40] In this trial, 47% of people were reported to have terminated the study prematurely. The trial found that naproxen significantly reduced migraine intensity (rated as none, mild, moderate, or severe) compared with ergotamine (P = 0.04). However, it found no significant difference in need for rescue medication (23% with naproxen v 29% with ergotamine). The third RCT (41 people) compared three treatments: naproxen, ergotamine, and placebo.[41] It found no significant difference in pain relief at 1 hour after the first dose between naproxen and ergotamine (P = 0.65).

Harms: In one RCT, adverse effects were reported in 5/32 (16%) people taking naproxen; four had stomach pain and dyspepsia, and one withdrew from the trial because of severe stomach pain.[37] One RCT comparing naproxen versus ergotamine found that vomiting was more frequent with ergotamine (10% with naproxen v 34% with ergotamine; P = 0.0083), and more people taking ergotamine withdrew because of severe symptoms (diarrhoea, vomiting, dizziness, nausea, shivering, and sweating) compared with those taking naproxen (2% with naproxen v 8% with ergotamine).[41] In another RCT, more people taking naproxen versus ergotamine discontinued medication (6/19 [32%] with naproxen v 2/17 [12%] with ergotamine).[40] One RCT found that more people taking ergotamine versus naproxen had severe adverse effects (1/48 [2%] with naproxen v 8/48 [17%] with ergotamine), and two people taking ergotamine withdrew from the study.[52] See non-steroidal anti-inflammatory drugs, p 1525.

Comment: None of the RCTs used the International Headache Society criteria**G** to identify cases.

OPTION **TOLFENAMIC ACID**

RCTs found limited evidence that tolfenamic acid improved duration and severity of headache compared with placebo. RCTs found no significant difference in symptom relief between tolfenamic acid and sumatriptan or paracetamol.

Benefits: We found no systematic review. **Versus placebo or sumatriptan:** One RCT (141 people, 289 migraine attacks) compared three treatments: tolfenamic acid 200 mg, sumatriptan 100 mg, and placebo.[42] The trial found that tolfenamic acid significantly increased headache relief**G** compared with placebo (AR 77% with tolfenamic acid v 29% with placebo; RR 2.6, 95% CI 1.5 to 4.2). However, it found no significant difference between tolfenamic acid and sumatriptan. The use of rescue medication**G** was not significantly different between any of the three arms. **Versus placebo or aspirin or ergotamine:** One crossover RCT (20 women with common or classic migraine, 160 migraines) compared tolfenamic acid 200 mg, aspirin 500 mg, and ergotamine 1 mg versus placebo.[43] The RCT found that tolfenamic acid significantly reduced the duration of attacks compared with placebo (P < 0.001; time of evaluation not reported). The mean duration of attack was shortest with tolfenamic acid compared with the other treatments, but this was not significantly shorter than the mean duration of attack with the other drugs combined (P values not reported). The need for rescue medication after 2 hours was not significantly different. **Versus paracetamol:** One RCT (149 people with common or classic migraine) compared tolfenamic acid 400 mg versus paracetamol 1000 mg.[44] It found no significant difference between treatments in headache intensity**G**, adverse effects, strength, effect duration, or need for additional medication after 3 hours. **Combination preparations:** One crossover RCT (49 people with common or classic migraine, 482 migraines) compared tolfenamic acid alone or in combination with either caffeine or metoclopramide versus placebo.[45] The trial found that tolfenamic acid, either alone or in combination, significantly reduced headache intensity (measured on a scale of no, slight, moderate, or severe symptoms) compared with placebo. All combinations of tolfenamic acid significantly reduced the need for rescue medication compared with placebo ($P < 0.01$).

Harms: In one RCT comparing tolfenamic acid versus sumatriptan, the frequency of adverse effects was similar (30% *v* 41%).[41] See non-steroidal anti-inflammatory drugs, p 1525.

Comment: None.

OPTION ERGOTAMINE

One systematic review found limited evidence from four RCTs that ergotamine (with or without caffeine) improved headache relief compared with placebo. One overview of harms suggested that ergotamine increased nausea and vomiting compared with placebo. RCTs have found that ergotamine (or its derivatives, with or without caffeine and cyclizine) is less effective for migraine symptoms than sumatriptan. They found limited evidence that it was less effective than naproxen. RCTs found that ergotamine plus caffeine reduced headache relief and increased nausea and vomiting at 2 hours compared with oral lysine acetylsalicylate plus metoclopramide and rizatriptan.

Benefits: **Versus placebo:** We found one systematic review (search date 1991, 7 RCTs, 588 people).[46] Ergotamine was given orally at doses between 1 and 6 mg. Ergotamine was given alone in three RCTs, combined with caffeine in three RCTs, and combined with alkaloids and barbiturates in one RCT. The RCT of ergotamine plus alkaloids plus barbiturates was not evaluable. None of the trials used International Headache Society criteria**G** for participant inclusion, and defined responders according to a variety of 3 point to 10 point scales. Two RCTs identified by the review found that ergotamine alone significantly increased headache relief**G** compared with placebo ($P < 0.01$ in 1 RCT; reported as "significant" in the other RCT; P value not reported) and one RCT found that ergotamine alone significantly reduced the duration of attacks compared with placebo ($P < 0.001$). Two RCTs identified by the review found a similar use of rescue medication**G** with ergotamine alone and with placebo (P value not reported; no further data reported). Two RCTs identified by the review measuring nausea or vomiting associated with migraine found similar results with ergotamine alone and placebo (P value not reported). One RCT identified by the review found that ergotamine plus caffeine significantly increased headache relief (reported as "significant"; P value not reported) compared with placebo, but another RCT found no significant difference (P value not reported). The RCTs comparing ergotamine plus caffeine versus placebo did not assess duration of attack. Two RCTs identified by the review found that ergotamine plus caffeine significantly reduced need for rescue medication ($P < 0.05$ in 1 RCT; reported as "significant" in the other, P value not reported). Two RCTs identified by the review measuring nausea or vomiting found that placebo reduced these symptoms compared with ergotamine plus caffeine (no statistical analysis reported). **Versus sumatriptan:** One RCT (580 people) compared oral ergotamine 2 mg plus oral caffeine 100 mg with oral sumatriptan 100 mg.[47] The trial found that ergotamine plus caffeine significantly reduced headache relief compared with sumatriptan (AR 48% with ergotamine plus caffeine *v* 66% with sumatriptan; RR 0.73, 95% CI 0.62 to 0.85; $P < 0.001$). Significantly more people required rescue medication with ergotamine plus caffeine than with sumatriptan (AR 44% with ergotamine plus caffeine *v* 24% with sumatriptan; RR 1.82, 95% CI 1.38 to 2.39). A second RCT (crossover design; 368 people treating 2 attacks) compared dihydroergotamine nasal spray (1 or 2 mg) with sumatriptan nasal spray (20 mg).[48] It found that sumatriptan significantly increased headache relief at 1 and 2 hours, and significantly reduced nausea at 1 hour compared with dihydroergotamine (headache relief at 1 hour: 53% with sumatriptan *v* 41% with dihydroergotamine; $P < 0.001$; headache relief at 2 hours: $P = 0.003$; relief of nausea at 1 hour: 64% with sumatriptan *v* 40% with dihydroergotamine; $P = 0.006$). However, the RCT found no significant differences between treatments with respect to relief from vomiting, photophobia, or phonophobia. **Versus eletriptan:** See benefits of eletriptan, p 1631. **Versus rizatriptan:** See benefits of rizatriptan, p 1634. **Plus metoclopramide:** One RCT (24 women with common or classic migraine, 176 migraines) found no significant difference between ergotamine alone and ergotamine plus metoclopramide in headache intensity**G** (measured on a 3 point scale as more than usual, usual, or less than usual) or need for rescue medication.[49] **Versus naproxen:** See benefits of naproxen, p 1627. **Plus caffeine versus salicylates:** One RCT (250 people randomised, 227 in efficacy analysis) found that lysine acetylsalicylate (L-ASA) 1620 mg plus metoclopramide 10 mg significantly increased headache relief compared with ergotamine 2 mg plus caffeine 200 mg (86/112 [77%] with L-ASA plus metoclopramide *v* 70/115 [61%] with ergotamine plus caffeine; $P = 0.01$).[25] It found that L-ASA plus metoclopramide significantly reduced nausea and vomiting compared with ergotamine plus caffeine after 2 hours (people free from nausea or vomiting: 73/112 [65%] with L-ASA plus metoclopramide *v* 46/115 [40%] with ergotamine plus caffeine; $P = 0.001$).

Harms: **Versus placebo:** In the systematic review comparing ergotamine versus placebo, two RCTs measuring nausea and vomiting found that ergotamine alone increased nausea and vomiting compared with placebo (no statistical analysis reported), and two RCTs found that ergotamine plus caffeine increased nausea and vomiting compared with placebo (no statistical analysis conducted).[46] We found one overview of the safety of dihydroergotamine mesylate (DHE) and ergotamine tartrate.[50] This overview identified two trials (24 and 311 people), which found that adverse effects with intramuscular DHE occurred in fewer than 10% of people (with leg cramps and pain at the injection site being most common) and that harms resolved within 1 hour. Three RCTs in the overview found that nausea and vomiting were the most common adverse effects, which subsided within 15 minutes. In another open trial (300 people), 32% of people taking DHE complained of nausea. Post-marketing surveillance studies have reported ischaemic complications, nausea, vomiting, seizures, cardiac and non-cardiac vascular disorders such as vasospasm and infarction, liver abnormalities, leg pain, chest pain, hypertensive crisis, injection site reactions, head and shoulder pain, and paraesthesia. Treatment related phenomena were reported in fewer than 4% of people receiving intranasal DHE. A bitter or unpleasant taste was reported by 2%. Dizziness and muscle pain were reported by less than 1%. Discontinuation of treatment occurred in 1% of people included in the RCTs. Worsening of baseline nausea or vomiting was suggested in 5/7 RCTs comparing acute administration of ergotamine tartrate versus placebo. Single case reports of less common adverse effects include abdominal discomfort, numbness or tingling of fingers or toes, ischaemic complications, swollen fingers, and leg cramps. With chronic use in excessive doses, ischaemic neuropathy, anorectal ulcers following suppository use, habituation, and overuse headaches have been reported.[50] **Versus sumatriptan:** In the RCT comparing sumatriptan versus dihydroergotamine nasal sprays, the incidence of adverse events was similar (about 10%) in both treatment groups after the first dose. The most common were disturbance of taste after sumatriptan, and nasal or sinus symptoms such as congestion, irritation, and rhinitis after dihydroergotamine. These were reported as being mild and self limiting.[48] **Plus caffeine versus salicylates:** One RCT found no significant difference in the proportion of people reporting at least one adverse event between L-ASA 1620 mg plus metoclopramide 10 mg and ergotamine 2 mg plus caffeine 200 mg (17% with L-ASA plus metoclopramide *v* 23% with ergotamine plus caffeine).[25] It found that the most common adverse events with the L-ASA regimen were somnolence (3.2%), dizziness (1.6%), and dry mouth (1.6%) and that abdominal pain (6.65), malaise (3.3%), anxiety (2.5%), and nervousness (1.7%) were the most common adverse events with the ergotamine regimen.

Comment: None.

OPTION ELETRIPTAN

One systematic review and subsequent RCTs have found that eletriptan increases headache relief at 2 hours compared with placebo. One systematic review and subsequent RCTs have found that eletriptan 40 and 80 mg increases headache relief at 2 hours compared with sumatriptan 50 and 100 mg. One RCT has found that eletriptan 40 and 80 mg increases headache relief at 2 hours compared with ergotamine plus caffeine.

Benefits: **Versus placebo:** We found one systematic review (search date 2000, 8 RCTs, 5370 people)[51] and six subsequent RCTs.[52–57] The review found that all doses of eletriptan significantly increased headache relief**G** compared with placebo at 2 hours (eletriptan 20 mg, 499 people; eletriptan 40 mg, 1870 people; eletriptan 80 mg, 1393 people; total placebo groups 1113 people; AR for 20 mg: 48.9%; for 40 mg: 60.2%; for 80 mg: 65.8%; AR for placebo about 25%; ARR for 80 mg *v* placebo 42%, 95% CI 36% to 48%; for 40 mg *v* placebo 35.2%, 95% CI 29.8% to 40.7%). All six subsequent RCTs found that eletriptan significantly improved headache relief compared with placebo (See table A on web extra).[52–57] **Versus sumatriptan:** We found one systematic review[51] and two subsequent RCTs.[52,54] The review (search date 2000, 2 RCTs) found that eletriptan 40 and 80 mg significantly increased headache relief at 2 hours compared with sumatriptan 100 mg. It found no significant difference between eletriptan 20 mg and sumatriptan 100 mg (ARI for complete headache relief: eletriptan 80 mg: 18%, 95% CI 9% to 26%; eletriptan 40 mg: 11%, 95% CI 2% to 19%; eletriptan 20 mg: –1%, 95% CI –13% to +12%).[51] It found that eletriptan 40 and 80 mg significantly increased headache relief at 2 hours compared with sumatriptan 50 mg (ARI for eletriptan 80 mg: 15%, 95% CI 8% to 23%; eletriptan 40 mg: 10%, 95% CI 3% to 18%). The first subsequent RCT (1008 people) compared two doses of eletriptan (40 and 80 mg), two doses of sumatriptan (50 and 100 mg), and placebo.[52] It found that both doses of eletriptan significantly increased headache relief compared with sumatriptan at 2 hours (AR 108/169 [64%] with eletriptan 40 mg *v* 107/160 [67%] with eletriptan 80 mg *v* 88/176 [50%] with sumatriptan 50 mg *v* 85/160 [53%] with sumatriptan 100 mg; $P < 0.01$ for either dose eletriptan *v* sumatriptan 50 mg; $P < 0.05$ for either dose eletriptan *v* sumatriptan 100 mg). The second subsequent RCT (2072 people) compared three treatments: eletriptan 40 mg, sumatriptan 100 mg, and placebo.[54] It found that that eletriptan 40 mg significantly increased headache relief compared with sumatriptan 100 mg at 2 hours (67% with eletriptan *v* 59% with sumatriptan; $P < 0.001$). It found that eletriptan significantly reduced nausea compared with sumatriptan 100 mg at 2 hours (nausea absent: 74% with eletriptan *v* 67% with sumatriptan; $P < 0.01$). **Versus ergotamine plus caffeine:** We found one RCT (733 people treated included in the systematic review[51]) that compared two doses of eletriptan (40 and 80 mg), ergotamine plus caffeine, and placebo. It found that both doses of eletriptan significantly increased headache relief and reduced nausea at 2 hours compared with ergotamine plus caffeine (headache relief: 111/206 [54%] with eletriptan 40 mg *v* 142/209 [68%] with eletriptan 80 mg *v* 65/197 [33%] with ergotamine plus caffeine; $P < 0.05$; nausea: results presented graphically; $P \leq 0.0001$ for both comparisons).[51]

Harms: **Versus placebo:** We found one systematic review (search date 2000)[51] and four subsequent RCTs[54–57] that reported harms. The review found that higher doses of eletriptan 40 and 80 mg significantly increased any adverse event and central nervous system (CNS) adverse events**G** compared with placebo. It found no significant difference in adverse event rates with eletriptan 20 mg (ARI compared with placebo for any adverse event: 20 mg +1.9%, 95% CI –15.5% to +19.3%; 40 mg 7.3%, 95% CI 2.7% to 11.8%; 80 mg 18.9%, 95% CI 11.2% to 26.6%; CNS events: 20 mg +2.6%, 95% CI –6.6% to +11.7%; 40 mg 7.5%, 95% CI 4.5% to 10.6%; 80 mg 14.6%, 95% CI 10.2% to 19.0%). It found that 80 mg eletriptan significantly increased chest symptoms compared with placebo. It found no significant difference with 40 and 20 mg eletriptan (ARR compared with placebo, 20 mg –0.3%, 95% CI –3.1% to +2.6%; 40 mg +0.9%, 95% CI –0.2% to +2.0%; 80 mg 2.6%, 95% CI 0.6% to 4.5%).[51] The first subsequent RCT (2072 people analysed) found similar rates of adverse events between eletriptan 40 and 80 mg and placebo (about 30% in each group, P value not reported).[54] The second subsequent RCT (309 people analysed) found that eletriptan 20, 40, and 80 mg increased adverse events compared with placebo (16.3% with eletriptan 20 mg *v* 62.5% with eletriptan 40 mg *v* 45.5% with eletriptan 80 mg *v* 15.5% with placebo; P value not reported).[55] The most common adverse events were asthenia, nausea, and somnolence (asthenia: 1.3% with eletriptan 20 mg *v* 2.5% with eletriptan 40 mg *v* 11.7% with eletriptan 80 mg *v* 1.2% with placebo; nausea: 3.8% with eletriptan 20 mg *v* 7.5% with eletriptan 40 mg *v* 10.4% with eletriptan 80 mg *v* 2.4% with placebo; somnolence: 6.3% with eletriptan 20 mg *v* 10.0% with eletriptan 40 mg *v* 16.9% with eletriptan 80 mg *v* 3.6% with placebo, P value not reported).The third subsequent RCT found that eletriptan 40 and 80 mg increased nausea, chest symptoms, and asthenia compared with placebo (nausea: 5% with eletriptan 40 mg *v* 11% with eletriptan 80 mg *v* 8% with placebo; chest symptoms: 4% with eletriptan 40 mg *v* 5% with eletriptan 80 mg *v* 0% with placebo; asthenia: 5% with eletriptan 40 mg *v* 12% with eletriptan 80 mg *v* 2% with placebo, P value not reported).[56] The fourth subsequent RCT found that the most common adverse event was somnolence (2.8% with eletriptan 20 mg *v* 7.1% with eletriptan 40 mg *v* 8.7% with eletriptan 80 mg *v* 4.5% with placebo, P value not reported).[57] Other common adverse events with higher doses of eletriptan were asthenia and dizziness (asthenia: 3.1% with eletriptan 20 mg *v* 3.4% with eletriptan 40 mg *v* 7.1% with eletriptan 80 mg *v* 2.7% with placebo; dizziness: 2.8% with eletriptan 20 mg *v* 5.1% with eletriptan 40 mg *v* 6.1% with eletriptan 80 mg *v* 3.1% with placebo, P value not reported). **Versus sumatriptan:** The systematic review (search date 2000, 2 RCTs) found no significant difference between eletriptan 40 mg and sumatriptan 100 mg in adverse events or CNS related events (ARI, any event: 0%, 95% CI –11% to +11%; CNS events: –3%, 95% CI –13% to +8%).[51] It found that sumatriptan 50 mg significantly reduced adverse events and CNS related events compared with eletriptan 40 mg (ARR, any event: 8%, 95% CI 1% to 15%; CNS events: 8%, 95% CI 2% to 13%).[51] One subsequent RCT found similar rates of adverse events with eletriptan 40 mg and with sumatriptan 100 mg (31% with eletriptan *v* 37% with sumatriptan).[54] **Versus ergotamine plus caffeine:** One RCT (733 people treated) that compared two doses of eletriptan (40 and 80 mg), ergotamine 1 mg plus caffeine 100 mg, and placebo found that the most common adverse events were nausea and asthenia (nausea: 5% with eletriptan 40 mg *v* 10% with eletriptan 80 mg *v* 7% with ergotamine plus caffeine; asthenia: 4% with eletriptan 40 mg *v* 10% with eletriptan 80 mg *v* 3% with ergotamine plus caffeine, P value not reported).[51]

Comment: None.

OPTION NARATRIPTAN

One systematic review and subsequent RCTs have found that naratriptan increases headache relief at 2 hours compared with placebo. One systematic review has found that sumatriptan 100 mg increases headache relief at 2 hours compared with naratriptan 2.5 mg. However, one subsequent RCT found no significant difference in headache recurrence. One RCT found no significant difference between naratriptan 2.5 mg and zolmitriptan 2.5 mg in headache relief at 4 hours. One RCT identified by a systematic review found that naratriptan reduced headache relief at 2 hours compared with rizatriptan.

Benefits: **Versus placebo:** We found one systematic review (search date 2000, 5 RCTs, 1077 people)[51] and two subsequent RCTs.[58,59] The review found that naratriptan significantly increased headache relief**Ⓖ** compared with placebo (ARI 22.2%, 95% CI 16.9% to 27.5%).[51] The first subsequent RCT (643 people) found that naratriptan 2.5 mg or sumatriptan 100 mg significantly increased headache relief at 4 hours compared with placebo (AR 63% with naratriptan *v* 80% with sumatriptan *v* 31% with placebo; $P < 0.05$ for either drug compared with placebo).[58] In the second subsequent RCT a subgroup of 206 people with a poor response to sumatriptan 50 mg in a first attack were randomised 1 week later to either naratriptan 2.5 mg orally or placebo.[59] Naratriptan significantly increased headache relief at 2 hours (AR 25% with naratriptan *v* 10% with placebo; RR 2.5, 95% CI 1.3 to 4.7) and at 4 hours (AR 41% with naratriptan *v* 19% with placebo; RR 2.2, 95% CI 1.4 to 3.5) compared with placebo. **Versus sumatriptan:** We found one systematic review (search date 2000, 2 RCTs, 480 people)[51] and one subsequent RCT.[60] The review found that sumatriptan 100 mg significantly increased headache relief at 4 hours compared with naratriptan 2.5 mg (AR not reported; ARI: 8%, 95% CI 0% to 16%).[51] The subsequent RCT comparing naratriptan 2.5 mg orally with sumatriptan 100 mg orally found no significant difference in headache recurrence**Ⓖ**.[60] **Versus zolmitriptan:** We found one systematic review (search date 2000, 1 RCT, 179 people).[51] It found no significant difference between naratriptan 2.5 mg and zolmitriptan 2.5 mg in headache relief at 4 hours (difference: +1%, 95% CI –15% to +17%). **Versus rizatriptan:** See benefits of rizatriptan, p 1634.

Harms: **Versus placebo:** The systematic review found no significant difference in overall adverse events, central nervous system (CNS) adverse events, and chest related adverse events**Ⓖ** between naratriptan 2.5 mg and placebo (ARI for naratriptan *v* placebo; any event: +2.4%, 95% CI –2.2% to +7.0%; CNS events: +1.9%, 95% CI –12.2% to +5.0%; chest symptoms: +0.4%, 95% CI –0.8% to +1.6).[51] One subsequent RCT found similar adverse effects with naratriptan 2.5 mg orally and placebo (21% with naratriptan *v* 23% with placebo; significance not reported).[58] **Versus sumatriptan:** The systematic review (search date 2000, 2 RCTs) found that sumatriptan 100 mg significantly increased adverse events compared with naratriptan 2.5 mg (difference: 11.3%,

95% CI 1% to 22.5%).[51] **Versus zolmitriptan:** The systematic review (search date 2000, 1 RCT) found that naratriptan 2.5 mg significantly reduced adverse events compared with zolmitriptan 2.5 mg (difference: −23%, 95% CI −37% to −8%).[51] **Versus rizatriptan:** See harms of rizatriptan, p 1634.

Comment: Naratriptan or a different triptan in a second attack may be beneficial in people responding poorly to sumatriptan in a first attack, but this requires confirmation in further RCTs.

OPTION RIZATRIPTAN

One systematic review and subsequent RCTs have found that rizatriptan improves headache relief compared with placebo. Two RCTs found no significant difference between rizatriptan and zolmitriptan in headache relief at 2 hours. One RCT identified by a systematic review found that rizatriptan increased headache relief at 2 hours compared with naratriptan. One RCT found that rizatriptan increased headache relief and reduced nausea and vomiting at 2 hours compared with ergotamine plus caffeine.

Benefits: **Versus placebo:** We found one systematic review (search date 2000, 12 RCTs, 6395 people)[51] and one subsequent RCT.[61] The systematic review found that rizatriptan significantly increased headache relief**G** at 2 hours compared with placebo (AR: 62.4% with rizatriptan 5 mg *v* 68.6% with rizatriptan 10 mg *v* about 34% with placebo; ARI compared with placebo presented graphically: about 28% with rizatriptan 5 mg *v* 35% with rizatriptan 10 mg). The subsequent RCT (727 people) compared three treatments: rizatriptan 10 mg, zolmitriptan 2.5 mg, and placebo.[61] It found that rizatriptan significantly increased headache relief compared with placebo (AR 71% with rizatriptan *v* 30% with placebo; $P < 0.05$).[61] **Versus zolmitriptan:** We found one systematic review (search date 2000, 1 RCT, 435 people)[51] and one subsequent RCT.[61] The systematic review found no significant difference between rizatriptan 10 mg and zolmitriptan 2.5 mg in headache relief at 2 hours (difference: +4%, 95% CI −4% to +11%).[51] The subsequent RCT (727 people) comparing rizatriptan 10 mg, zolmitriptan 2.5 mg, and placebo found no significant difference between rizatriptan and zolmitriptan in headache relief (AR 71% with rizatriptan *v* 67% with zolmitriptan; $P = 0.23$).[61] **Versus naratriptan:** One systematic review (search date 2000; 1 RCT 522 people) found that rizatriptan 10 mg significantly increased headache relief at 2 hours compared with naratriptan 2.5 mg (ARI 20%, 95% CI 11% to 30%).[51] **Versus ergotamine:** One RCT (439 people) compared oral rizatriptan 10 mg with ergotamine 2 mg plus caffeine 100 mg for the first migraine attack with the other treatment for a second attack.[62] It found that rizatriptan significantly increased headache relief and reduced nausea and vomiting at 2 hours compared with ergotamine plus caffeine (headache relief: 75.9% with rizatriptan *v* 47.3% with ergotamine plus caffeine; $P \leq 0.001$; no nausea: 82.7% with rizatriptan *v* 56.2% with ergotamine plus caffeine; $P \leq 0.001$; no vomiting: 96.2% with rizatriptan *v* 89.5% with ergotamine plus caffeine; $P \leq 0.001$).

Harms: **Versus placebo:** We found one meta-analysis (search date 2000, 1963 people given rizatriptan 5 mg, 2783 people given rizatriptan 10 mg, and 1649 given placebo) that used individual patient data from published and unpublished RCTs.[51] It found that rizatriptan (5 and 10 mg) significantly increased overall and chest related adverse events**G** compared with placebo (placebo subtracted events: any event 7.9%, 95% CI 4.7% to 11.1% with rizatriptan 5 mg and 13.5%, 95% CI 10.6% to 16.3% with 10 mg rizatriptan; CNS events: 6.1%, 95% CI 3.2% to 9.0% with rizatriptan 5 mg and 9.4%, 95% CI 7.2% to 11.6%

with rizatriptan 10 mg).[51] It found no significant difference in chest related adverse events between rizatriptan 5 mg and placebo but found that rizatriptan 10 mg significantly increased chest related adverse events compared with placebo (placebo subtracted chest symptoms: +0.9%, 95% CI –0.04 to +1.8 with rizatriptan 5 mg and 1.5%, 95% CI 0.8% to 2.3% with rizatriptan 10 mg). **Versus zolmitriptan:** The meta-analysis (search date 2000, 1 RCT) found no significant difference in adverse events between rizatriptan 10 mg and zolmitriptan 2.5 mg (difference: –8%, 95% CI –15% to 0%).[51] **Versus naratriptan:** The meta-analysis (search date 2000, 1 RCT) found that rizatriptan 10 mg significantly increased adverse events compared with naratriptan 2.5 mg (difference: 10%, 95% CI 1% to 19%).[51] **Versus ergotamine:** One RCT comparing rizatriptan 10 mg with ergotamine 2 mg plus caffeine 100 mg found no significant difference in adverse events (35.4% with rizatriptan *v* 34.5% with ergotamine plus caffeine).[62] The most common adverse events were dizziness, nausea, and somnolence (dizziness: 6.7% with rizatriptan *v* 5.3% with ergotamine; nausea: 4.2% with rizatriptan *v* 8.5% with ergotamine; somnolence: 5.5% with rizatriptan *v* 2.3% with ergotamine, P values not reported).

Comment: None.

OPTION SUMATRIPTAN

Systematic reviews and subsequent RCTs have found that subcutaneous, oral, or intranasal sumatriptan increases headache relief compared with placebo. RCTs found no significant difference in headache relief between sumatriptan and aspirin plus metoclopramide, tolfenamic acid, or zolmitriptan. RCTs have found that oral or nasal sumatriptan increases headache relief compared with oral or nasal ergotamine. One systematic review has found that sumatriptan 100 mg increases headache relief at 2 hours compared with naratriptan 2.5 mg. However, one subsequent RCT found no significant difference in headache recurrence. One systematic review and subsequent RCTs have found that eletriptan 40 and 80 mg increases headache relief at 2 hours compared with sumatriptan 50 and 100 mg.

Benefits: **Subcutaneous sumatriptan:** We found one systematic review (search date 1997),[63] one additional RCT,[64] and one subsequent RCT.[65] The review found that subcutaneous sumatriptan 6 mg significantly increased headache relief**G** at 1 hour compared with placebo (12 RCTs, 3127 people; 69% with sumatriptan *v* 19% with placebo; RR 3.7, 95% CI 3.3 to 4.2).[63] One additional crossover RCT (246 people with up to 12 migraines) comparing subcutaneous sumatriptan 6 mg with usual headache treatment (49% combinations, 24% ergotamine, 19% non-steroidal anti-inflammatory drugs, and 7% dihydroergotamine) found that sumatriptan significantly improved headache relief (78% with sumatriptan *v* 34% with usual treatment; P < 0.001).[64] The subsequent RCT (200 people consisting of 50 white people and 150 non-white people) compared headache relief across multiple attacks.[65] It analysed results by ethnic group. It found that subcutaneous sumatriptan 6 mg significantly increased headache relief in non-white people and white people (non-white: 87% with sumatriptan *v* 37% with placebo; white: 87% with sumatriptan *v* 19% with placebo; sumatriptan *v* placebo P < 0.001 in either ethnic group). **Oral sumatriptan:** We found one systematic review (search date 2000, 11 RCTs, 3185 people),[51] one additional RCT[66] and two subsequent RCTs.[52,54] The review found that sumatriptan significantly increased headache relief at 2 hours compared with placebo (AR 56.0% with sumatriptan 25 mg *v* 62.7% with sumatriptan 50 mg *v* 59.0% with sumatriptan 100 mg *v* about 30% with placebo; ARI about 25% with sumatriptan 25 mg [presented graphically] *v* about 33% with sumatriptan 50 mg [presented graphically] v 29%, 95% CI 26% to 34% with sumatriptan 100 mg).[51] The additional RCT (495 people) found that oral sumatriptan 50 mg significantly increased the proportion of people with headache relief after 4 hours in people with one attack compared with placebo (62% with sumatriptan v 32% with placebo; $P < 0.001$).[66] The first subsequent RCT (1008 people randomised, 774 people treated) compared two doses of eletriptan (40 and 80 mg), two doses of sumatriptan (50 and 100 mg), and placebo.[52] At 2 hours it found that both doses of sumatriptan significantly increased headache relief compared with placebo (50% with sumatriptan 50 mg v 53% with sumatriptan 100 mg v 31% with placebo; $P < 0.01$ for either dose of sumatriptan v placebo). The second subsequent RCT (2072 people) compared three treatments: eletriptan 40 mg, sumatriptan 100 mg, and placebo.[54] It found that that sumatriptan 100 mg significantly increased headache relief at 2 hours compared with placebo (59% with sumatriptan 100 mg v 26% with placebo; $P < 0.0001$). It found that sumatriptan 100 mg significantly reduced nausea at 2 hours compared with placebo (nausea absent: 67% with sumatriptan 100 mg v 57% with placebo; $P < 0.001$). **Intranasal sumatriptan:** We found one review (search date 1997)[63] and three additional RCTs.[67–69] The review found that intranasal sumatriptan 20 mg significantly increased headache relief compared with placebo (6 RCTs, 1420 people; 61% with sumatriptan v 30% with placebo; RR 2.1, 95% CI 1.8 to 2.4).[63] The three additional RCTs (2475 people) found that intranasal sumatriptan significantly increased headache relief compared with placebo (60–64% with sumatriptan v 25–35% with placebo).[67–69] **Versus aspirin plus metoclopramide:** See benefits of salicylates, p 1624. **Versus tolfenamic acid:** See benefits of tolfenamic acid, p 1628. **Versus ergotamine:** See benefits of ergotamine, p 1629. **Versus naratriptan:** See benefits of naratriptan, p 1633. **Versus zolmitriptan:** See benefits of zolmitriptan, p 1637. **Versus eletriptan:** See benefits of eletriptan, p 1631. **Versus ergotamine derivatives:** See benefits of ergotamine, p 1629.

Harms: **Subcutaneous sumatriptan:** In one systematic review (search date 1997), 7/12 RCTs found that adverse effects were more common with subcutaneous sumatriptan 6 mg than with placebo (65% with sumatriptan v 32% with placebo; OR 4, 95% CI 3 to 5).[63] The subsequent RCT found that subcutaneous sumatriptan increased adverse events compared with placebo in both non-white and white people (non-white: 63% with sumatriptan v 30% with placebo; white: 63% with sumatriptan v 23% with placebo; P value not reported).[65] It found nine serious adverse events with sumatriptan compared with none with placebo (no details reported and number exposed was not clear). **Oral sumatriptan versus placebo:** The systematic review found that sumatriptan 25, 50, and 100 mg) significantly increased overall adverse events compared with placebo (ARI: any event 4.4%, 95% CI 0.1% to 8.8% with sumatriptan 25 mg; 7.8%, 95% CI 2.6% to 13.1% with sumatriptan 50 mg; and 13.2%, 95% CI 8.6% to 17.8% with sumatriptan 100 mg).[51] It found that the two higher doses of sumatriptan (50 and 100 mg) significantly increased central nervous system (CNS) adverse events and chest related adverse events[G] compared with placebo. However, it found no significant difference between low dose sumatriptan 25 mg and placebo (ARI; CNS events: +1.7%, 95% CI –1.2% to +4.7% with sumatriptan 25 mg; 3.7%, 95% CI 1.0% to 6.5% with sumatriptan 50 mg; 6.3%, 95% CI 3.2% to 9.5% with sumatriptan 100 mg; chest related events: +0.8%, 95% CI –1.0%

to +2.6% with sumatriptan 25 mg; 1.9%, 95% CI 0.4% to 3.3% with sumatriptan 50 mg; 1.7%, 95% CI 0.8% to 2.5% with sumatriptan 100 mg). One subsequent RCT found similar rates of adverse effects between sumatriptan and placebo (37% with sumatriptan *v* 34% with placebo, P value not reported).[54]

Comment: There is a consensus that sumatriptan should not be used in people with ischaemic heart disease or concomitantly with ergotamine.

OPTION ZOLMITRIPTAN

One systematic review and two subsequent RCTs have found that oral zolmitriptan increases headache relief compared with placebo. One systematic review and two subsequent RCTs found no significant difference between zolmitriptan and sumatriptan in headache relief. One RCT found no significant difference in headache relief between aspirin plus metoclopramide and zolmitriptan. One RCT found no significant difference between naratriptan 2.5 mg and zolmitriptan 2.5 mg in headache relief at 4 hours.

Benefits: **Versus placebo:** We found one systematic review (search date 2000, 9 RCTs , 4641 people)[51] and two subsequent RCTs.[70,71] The systematic review found that zolmitriptan significantly increased headache relief**G** at 2 hours compared with placebo (AR: 63.5% with zolmitriptan 2.5 mg *v* 62.8% with zolmitriptan 5 mg *v* about 30% with placebo; ARI: about 30% with zolmitriptan 2.5 mg *v* about 33% with zolmitriptan 5 mg; results presented graphically). The first subsequent RCT (289 people, 229 in analysis) compared three doses of zolmitriptan (1, 2.5, and 5 mg) versus placebo.[70] It found that zolmitriptan 2.5 mg significantly increased headache relief at 2 hours compared with placebo (53.3% with zolmitriptan 1 mg; 55.6% with zolmitriptan 2.5 mg; 65.4% with zolmitriptan 5 mg; 37.5% with placebo; P = 0.032 for zolmitriptan 2.5 mg *v* placebo, other P values not reported; analysis not by intention to treat). The open label second subsequent RCT (470 people) found that orally dispersible zolmitriptan 2.5 mg significantly increased headache relief at 2 hours compared with placebo (63% with zolmitriptan *v* 22% with placebo; OR 6.1, 95% CI 4.0 to 9.3).[71] It found that zolmitriptan reduced nausea at 2 hours compared with placebo, but the statistical significance was not reported (no nausea: 52% with zolmitriptan *v* 32% with placebo). **Versus sumatriptan:** We found one systematic review (search date 2000, 3 RCTs)[51] and two subsequent RCTs.[72,73] The review found no significant difference between zolmitriptan 2.5 and 5 mg and sumatriptan 25, 50, and 100 mg in headache relief at 2 hours (ARR for sumatriptan 100 mg *v* zolmitriptan 5 mg: +1%, 95% CI –4% to +6%; sumatriptan 50 mg *v* zolmitriptan 2.5 mg: +2%, 95% CI –6% to +9%; sumatriptan 50 mg *v* zolmitriptan 5 mg: +1%, 95% CI –4% to +6%; sumatriptan 25 mg *v* zolmitriptan 2.5 mg: –8%, 95% CI –16% to 0%; sumatriptan 25 mg *v* zolmitriptan 5 mg: –7%, 95% CI –15% to 0%).[51] In the first subsequent RCT (1522 people), up to six consecutive attacks were treated with zolmitriptan 2.5 mg (500 people, 2671 attacks), zolmitriptan 5 mg (514 people, 2744 attacks), or sumatriptan 50 mg (508 people, 2693 attacks).[72] The RCT found no significant difference among groups for headache relief at 2 hours (AR 62.9% with zolmitriptan 2.5 mg *v* 65.7% with zolmitriptan 5 mg zolmitriptan *v* 66.6% with sumatriptan 50 mg). The second subsequent RCT (1445 people) compared zolmitriptan 2.5–5 mg versus sumatriptan 25–50 mg.[73] The trial found no significant difference in headache relief between treatments at any dose. **Versus salicylates:** One RCT (666 people) found no significant difference between aspirin 900 mg plus metoclopramide 10 mg and zolmitriptan 2.5 mg in headache relief at 2 hours over three migraine attacks. However, it found that zolmitriptan significantly increased the proportion of people who were pain free**G** at 2 hours (headache relief: 32.9% with salicylates *v* 33.4% with zolmitriptan; OR 1.06, 95% CI 0.77 to 1.47; pain free: 10.7% with zolmitriptan *v* 5.3% with salicylates; OR 2.19, 95% CI 1.23 to 4.03).[26] It found that rates of nausea were similar with both treatments but the statistical significance was not reported (about 30% in each group). **Stratified care versus step care:** One open label RCT (835 people) randomised people into three arms.[74] The first arm, named "stratified care", randomised people with low disability scores to aspirin 800–1000 mg plus metoclopramide 10 mg, and people with higher disability scores to zolmitriptan 2.5 mg. The second arm, named "step care", involved treating initial attacks with aspirin plus metoclopramide and then switching to zolmitriptan 2.5 mg for the remaining two to three attacks. The third arm involved "step care within attacks", whereby all attacks were initially treated with aspirin plus metoclopramide, and non-responders were given zolmitriptan after 2 hours. It found that stratified care significantly increased the proportion of people with headache relief compared with either of the step care groups (AR 53% with stratified care *v* 40% with step care *v* 36% with step care within attacks; RR stratified care *v* step care 1.3, 95% CI 1.1 to 1.7; stratified care *v* step care within attacks 1.4, 95% CI 1.2 to 1.7). **Versus naratriptan:** See benefits of naratriptan, p 1633.

Harms: **Versus placebo:** The systematic review found that zolmitriptan 2.5 and 5 mg significantly increased overall adverse events, central nervous system (CNS) adverse events, and chest related adverse events**G** compared with placebo (ARI compared with placebo; any adverse event: 15.9%, 95% CI 9.6% to 22.1% with 2.5 mg *v* 24.5%, 95% CI 15.3% to 33.5% with 5 mg; CNS events: 9.9%, 95% CI 4.3% to 15.5% with 2.5 mg *v* 11.5%, 95% CI 6.1% to 16.8% with 5 mg; chest related events: 2.0%, 95% CI 0.7% to 3.3% with 2.5 mg *v* 2.9%, 95% CI 1.2% to 4.6% with 5 mg).[51] The first subsequent RCT (289 Japanese people) found that zolmitriptan 5 mg increased asthenia, hypoaesthesia, and abdominal pain compared with placebo (asthenia: 7.0% with zolmitriptan 5 mg *v* 1.6% with 2.5 mg *v* 1.7% with placebo; hypoaesthesia: 7.0% with zolmitriptan 5 mg *v* 1.6% with 2.5 mg *v* 0% with placebo; abdominal pain: 7.0% with zolmitriptan 5 mg *v* 1.6% with 2.5 mg *v* 1.7% with placebo, P values not reported).[70] The open label second subsequent RCT found that zolmitriptan increased asthenia, throat tightness, and somnolence compared with placebo (asthenia: 3.5% with zolmitriptan *v* 1.3% with placebo; throat tightness: 2.6% with zolmitriptan *v* 0% with placebo; somnolence: 3.0% with zolmitriptan *v* 1.7% with placebo, P values not reported).[71] **Versus sumatriptan:** The systematic review (search date 2000, 3 RCTs) found no significant difference in adverse events between zolmitriptan 5 mg and sumatriptan 50 or 100 mg (ARI for zolmitriptan 5 mg *v* sumatriptan 100 mg: –2%, 95% CI –8% to +4%; zolmitriptan 2.5 mg *v* sumatriptan 50 mg: 4%, 95% CI 0% to 8%; zolmitriptan 5 mg *v* sumatriptan 50 mg: –2%, 95% CI –6% to +2%).[51] However, it found that sumatriptan 25 mg significantly reduced adverse events compared with zolmitriptan 5 mg (ARR: 12%, 95% CI 6% to 18%). The first subsequent RCT comparing zolmitriptan 2.5 and 5 mg with sumatriptan 50 mg found no significant difference in adverse events.[72] **Versus salicylates:** One RCT found that zolmitriptan increased adverse events compared with salicylates plus metoclopramide but found no difference between treatments in withdrawals due to adverse events (adverse events: 40.8% with zolmitriptan *v* 29.1% with salicylates plus metoclopramide, P value not reported; withdrawal due to adverse events: 0.9% with zolmitriptan *v* 1.5% with salicylates plus metoclopramide, P value not reported).[26] It found that zolmitriptan increased paraesthesia (4.3% with zolmitriptan *v* 1.5% with salicylates plus metoclopramide), dizziness (2.8% with zolmitriptan *v* 0.6% with salicylates plus metoclopramide), and tightness (3.7% with zolmitriptan v 0.6% with salicylates plus metoclopramide) and that salicylates plus metoclopramide increased abdominal pain (2.8% with zolmitriptan v 5.0% with salicylates plus metoclopramide) and diarrhoea (1.2% with zolmitriptan v 2.1% with salicylates plus metoclopramide).

Comment: None.

GLOSSARY

Central nervous system (CNS) adverse events Events associated with triptans, including asthenia, abnormal dreams, agitation, aphasia, ataxia, confusion, dizziness, somnolence, speech disorders, abnormal thinking, tremor, vertigo, and other focal neurological symptoms.

Chest related adverse events Events associated with triptans, including chest pressure, chest pain, radiating pain to the arms, other chest discomfort, heavy arms, shortness of breath, palpitations, and anxiety.

Headache intensity Mild: normal activity allowed. Moderate: disturbing, but not prohibiting normal activity; bed rest not necessary. Severe: normal activity discontinued; bed rest may be necessary.

Headache recurrence In responders, change in headache intensity (see above) from mild/none to moderate/severe within 24 hours of study medication initial dose.

Headache relief Change in headache intensity (see above) score from severe/moderate to mild/none.

International Headache Society criteria (1988) *Migraine without aura (common migraine)* is defined as five or more headache attacks lasting for 4–72 hours with accompanying symptoms of either nausea/vomiting and/or phonophobia and photophobia. Pain should comply with at least two of the following four characteristics: unilateral, throbbing, moderate to severe intensity, and increase with physical activity. For *migraine with aura (classic migraine)*, two or more headache attacks are required that comply with three of the following four characteristics: one or more fully reversible aura symptom indicating focal cerebral cortical and/or brainstem dysfunction; at least one aura symptom developing gradually over more than 4 minutes or two or more symptoms occurring in succession; no aura symptom should last more than 1 hour; and headache follows aura with a pain free (see below) interval of less than 60 minutes. In both migraine with and without aura, secondary causes of headache should be excluded; if any structural damage is found, then it should not explain headache characteristics. Less stringent criteria for migraine without aura can be used. In clinical practice, the so called borderline migraine can be diagnosed when one of the above criteria is not met. International Headache Society criteria were not developed with the intention of identifying potential responders to different medications.

Major and minor adverse effect A major adverse effect is defined as death, serious illness, or any adverse effect of sufficient severity to cause withdrawal from the study. A minor adverse effect is defined as any adverse effect that does not fulfil the criteria for a major harm.

Migraine index Pain scale for migraine resulting from duration times intensity of migraine where intensity is classified as 0 = none, 1 = mild, 2 = moderate, and 3 = severe.

Pain free Change in headache intensity (see above) score from severe/moderate to none.

Rescue medication Additional medications different to study medication permitted in non-responders, usually limited to the habitual medications a person uses to treat their migraine headache.

REFERENCES

1. Headache Classification Committee of the International Headache Society. Classification and diagnostic criteria for headache disorders, cranial neuralgias and face pain. *Cephalalgia* 1988;8:12–96.
2. Stewart W, Linet M, Celentano D, et al. Age and sex specific incidence rates of migraine with and without visual aura. *Am J Epidemiol* 1991;134:1111–1120.
3. O'Brien B, Goerre R, Streiner D. Prevalence of migraine headache in Canada: a population based survey. *Int J Epidemiol* 1994;23:1020–1026.
4. Pryse-Phillips W, Findlay H, Tugwell P, et al. A Canadian population survey on the clinical, epidemiological and societal impact of migraine and tension type headache. *Can J Neurol Sci* 1992;19:333–339.

5. Stewart W, Lipton R, Celentano D, et al. Prevalence of migraine headache in the United States. *JAMA* 1992;267:64–69.
6. Kryst S, Scherl E. A population based survey of social and personal impact of headache. *Headache* 1994;34:344–350.
7. Morillo L, Sanin L, Takeuchi Y, et al. Headache in Latin America: a multination population-based survey. *Neurology* 2001;56(suppl 3):A454.
8. Bank J, Marton S. Hungarian migraine epidemiology. *Headache* 2000;40:164–169.
9. Henry P, Michel P, Brochet B, et al. A nationwide survey of migraine in France: prevalence and clinical features. *Cephalalgia* 1992;12:229–237.
10. Rasmussen B, Jensen R, Schroll, et al. Epidemiology of headache in a general population: a prevalence study. *J Clin Epidemiol* 1991;44:1147–1157.
11. Steiner T, Stewart W, Kolodner K, et al. Epidemiology of migraine in England. *Cephalalgia* 1999;19:305.
12. Cheung RTF. Prevalence of migraine, tension type headache and other headaches in Hong Kong. *Headache* 2000;40:473–479.
13. Sakai F, Igarashi H. Prevalence of migraine in Japan: a nationwide survey. *Cephalalgia* 1997;17:15–22.
14. Stewart W, Staffa J, Lipton R, et al. Familial risk of migraine: a population based study. *Ann Neurol* 1997;41:166–172.
15. Chabriat H, Joire J, Danchot J, et al. Combined oral lysine acetylsalicylate and metoclopramide in the acute treatment of migraine: a multicentre double-blind placebo-controlled study. *Cephalalgia* 2001;14:297–300.
16. Tfelt-Hansen P, Henry P, Mulder L, et al. The effectiveness of combined oral lysine acetylsalicylate and metoclopramide compared with oral sumatriptan for migraine. *Lancet* 1995;346:923–926.
17. Deiner H. Efficacy and safety of intravenous acetylsalicylic acid lysinate compared to subcutaneous sumatriptan and parenteral placebo in the acute treatment of migraine: a double-blind, double-dummy, randomized, multicenter, parallel group study. The ASASUMAMIG Study Group. *Cephalalgia* 1999;19:581–588.
18. Limmroth V, May A, Diener H. Lysine-acetylsalicylic acid in acute migraine attacks. *Eur Neurol* 1999;41:88–93.
19. Tfelt-Hansen P, Olesen J. Effervescent metoclopramide and aspirin (Migravess) versus effervescent aspirin or placebo for migraine attacks: a double-blind study. *Cephalalgia* 1984;4:107–111.
20. Lange R, Schwarz JA, Hohn M. Acetylsalicylic acid effervescent 1000 mg (aspirin) in acute migraine attacks; a multicentre, randomized, double-blind, single dose, placebo-controlled parallel group study. *Cephalalgia* 2000;20:663–667.
21. MacGregor EA, Dowson A, Davies PTG. Mouth-dispersible aspirin in the treatment of migraine: a placebo-controlled study. *Headache* 2002;42:249–259.
22. Lipton R, Stewart W, Ryan RJ, et al. Efficacy and safety of paracetamol, aspirin, and caffeine in alleviating migraine headache pain: three double-blind, randomized, placebo-controlled trials. *Arch Neurol* 1998;55:210–217.
23. Boureau F, Joubert JM, Lasserre V, et al. Double-blind comparison of an acetaminophen 400 mg-codeine 25 mg combination versus aspirin 1000 mg and placebo in acute migraine attack. *Cephalalgia* 1994;14:156–161.
24. The Oral Sumatriptan and Aspirin plus Metoclopramide Comparative Study Group. A study to compare oral sumatriptan with oral aspirin plus metoclopramide in the acute treatment of migraine. *Eur Neurol* 1992;32:177–184.
25. Titus F, Escamilla C, da Costa Palmeira MM, ET AL. A double-blind comparison of lysine acetylsalicylate plus metoclopramide vs ergotamine plus caffeine in migraine effects on nausea, vomiting and headache symptoms. *Clin Drug Invest* 2001;21:87–94.
26. Geraud G, Compagnon A, Rossi A. Zolmitriptan versus a combination of acetylsalicylic acid and metoclopramide in the acute oral treatment of migraine: a double-blind, randomised, three-attack study. *Eur Neurol* 2002;47:88–98.
27. Massiou H, Serrurier D, Lasserre O, et al. Effectiveness of oral diclofenac in the acute treatment of common migraine attacks: a double-blind study versus placebo. *Cephalalgia* 1991;11:59–63.
28. Dahlof C, Bjorkman R. Diclofenac-K (50 and 100 mg) and placebo in the acute treatment of migraine. *Cephalalgia* 1993;13:117–123.
29. Bigal ME, Bordini CA, Speciali JG. Intramuscular diclofenac in the acute treatment of migraine: a double-blind placebo controlled study. *Arq Neuropsiquiatr* 2002;60:410–415. [In Portuguese]
30. The Diclofenac-K/Sumatriptan Migraine Study Group. Acute treatment of migraine attacks: efficacy and safety of nonsteroidal anti-inflammatory drug, diclofenac-potassium in comparison to oral sumatriptan and placebo. *Cephalalgia* 1999;19:232–240.
31. Karachalios G, Fotiadou A, Chrisikos N, et al. Treatment of acute migraine attack with diclofenac sodium: a double blind study. *Headache* 1992;32:98–100.
32. Kellstein D, Lipton R, Geetha R, et al. Evaluation of a novel solubilized formulation of ibuprofen in the treatment of migraine headache: a randomized, double-blind, placebo-controlled, dose-ranging study. *Cephalalgia* 2000;20:233–243.
33. Kloster R, Nestvold K, Vilming S. A double-blind study of ibuprofen versus placebo in the treatment of acute migraine attacks. *Cephalalgia* 1992;12:169–171.
34. Havanka-Kanniainen H. Treatment of acute migraine attack: ibuprofen and placebo compared. *Headache* 1989;29:507–509.
35. Codispoti JR, Prior MJ, Fu M, et al. Efficacy of non-prescription doses of ibuprofen in treating migraine headache. A randomized clinical trial. *Headache* 2001;41:665–679.
36. Sandrini G, Franchini S, Lanfranchi S, et al. Effectiveness of ibuprofen-arginine in the treatment of acute migraine attacks. *Int J Clin Pharmacol Res* 1998;18:145–150.
37. Andersson P, Hinge H, Johansen O, et al. Double-blind study of naproxen v placebo in the treatment of acute migraine attacks. *Cephalalgia* 1989;9:29–32.
38. Nestvold K, Kloster R, Partinen M, et al. Treatment of acute migraine attack: naproxen and placebo compared. *Cephalalgia* 1985;5:115–119.
39. Pradalier A, Rancurel G, Dordain G, et al. Acute migraine attack therapy: comparison of naproxen sodium and an ergotamine tartrate compound. *Cephalalgia* 1985;5:107–112.
40. Treves T, Streiffler M, Korczyn A. Naproxen sodium versus ergotamine tartrate in the treatment of acute migraine attacks. *Headache* 1992;32:280–282.
41. Sargent J, Baumel B, Peters K, et al. Aborting a migraine attack: naproxen v ergotamine plus caffeine. *Headache* 1988;28:263–266.
42. Myllyla V, Havanka H, Herrala L, et al. Tolfenamic acid rapid release versus sumatriptan in the acute treatment of migraine: comparable effect in a double-blind, randomized, controlled, parallel-group study. *Headache* 1998;38:201–207.
43. Hakkarainen H, Vapaatalo H, Gothoni G, et al. Tolfenamic acid is as effective as ergotamine during migraine attacks. *Lancet* 1979;2:326–328.
44. Norrelund N, Christiansen L, Plantener S. Tolfenamic acid versus paracetamol in migraine attacks. A double-blind study in general practice. *Ugeskr Laeger* 1989;151:2436–2438.
45. Tokola R, Kangasniemi P, Neuvonen P, et al. Tolfenamic acid, metoclopramide, caffeine and their combinations in the treatment of migraine attacks. *Cephalalgia* 1984;4:253–263.
46. Dahlof C. Placebo-controlled clinical trials with ergotamine in the acute treatment of migraine. *Cephalalgia* 1993;13:166–171. Search date 1991; primary sources Medline, Embase, and hand searches of reference lists.

47. Multinational Oral Sumatriptan Cafergot Comparative Study Group. A randomized, double-blind comparison of sumatriptan and Cafergot in the acute treatment of migraine. *Eur Neurol* 1991;31:314–322.
48. Bourea F, Kappos L, Schoenen J, et al. A clinical comparison of sumatriptan nasal spray and dihydroergotamine nasal spray in the acute treatment of migraine. *Int J Clin Pract* 2000;54:281–286.
49. Hakkarainen H. Ergotamine vs. metoclopramide vs. their combination in acute migraine attacks. *Headache* 1982;22:10–12.
50. Lipton R. Ergotamine tartrate and dihydroergotamine mesylate: safety profiles. *Headache* 1997;37:S33–S41.
51. Ferrari MD, Goadsby PJ, Roon KI, et al. Triptans (serotonin, 5-HT_1 B/1D agonists) in migraine: detailed results and methods of a meta-analysis of 53 trials. *Cephalalgia* 2002;22:633–658. Search date: 2000; primary sources five pharmaceutical companies and systematic review of literature (no details). [Erratum in: *Cephalalgia* 2003;23:71]
52. Sandrini G, Farkkila M, Gurgess G, et al. Eletriptan versus sumatriptan: a double-blind, multiple migraine attack study. *Neurology* 2002;59:1210–1217.
53. Stark R, Dahlos C, Haughie S, et al. Efficacy, safety and tolerability of oral eletriptan in the acute treatment of migraine: results of a phase III, multicentre, placebo controlled study across three attacks. *Cephalalgia* 2002;22:23–32.
54. Mathew NT, Schoenen J, Winner P, et al. Comparative efficacy of eletriptan 40 mg versus sumatriptan 100 mg. *Headache* 2003;43:214–222.
55. Eletriptan Steering Committee in Japan. Efficacy and safety of eletriptan 20 mg, 40 mg and 80 mg in Japanese migraineurs. *Cephalalgia* 2002;22:416–423.
56. Färkkilä M, Olesen J, Dahlöf C, et al. Eletriptan for the treatment of migraine in patients with previous poor response or tolerance to oral sumatriptan. *Cephalalgia* 2003;23:463–471.
57. Sheftell F, Ryan R, Pitman V. Efficacy, safety, and tolerability of oral eletriptan for treatment of acute migraine: a multicenter, double-blind, placebo-controlled study conducted in the United States. *Headache* 2003;43:202–213.
58. Havanka H, Dahlof C, Pop P, et al. Efficacy of naratriptan tablets in the acute treatment of migraine: a dose-ranging study. *Clin Ther* 2000;22:970–980.
59. Stark S, Spierings E, McNeal S, et al. Naratriptan efficacy in migraineurs who respond poorly to oral sumatriptan. *Headache* 2000;40:513–520.
60. Gobel H, Winter P, Boswell D, et al. Comparison of naratriptan and sumatriptan in recurrence-prone migraine patients. *Clin Ther* 2000;22:981–989.
61. Pascual J, Vega P, Deiner H-C, et al. Comparison of rizatriptan 10 mg vs. zolmitriptan 2.5 mg in the acute treatment of migraine. *Cephalalgia* 2000;20:455–461.
62. Christie S, Gobel H, Mateos V, et al. Crossover comparison of efficacy and preference for rizatriptan 10 mg versus ergotamine/caffeine in migraine. *Eur Neurol* 2003;49:20–29.
63. Tfelt-Hansen P. Efficacy and harms of subcutaneous, oral, and intranasal sumatriptan used for migraine treatment: a systematic review based on number needed to treat. *Cephalalgia* 2001;18:532–538. Search date 1997; primary sources Medline and hand searches of *Arch Neurol*, *Neurology*, *Headache*, and *Cephalalgia* from 1990.
64. Boureau F, Chazot G, Emile J, et al. Comparison of subcutaneous sumatriptan with usual acute treatments for migraine. French Sumatriptan Study Group. *Eur Neurol* 1995;35:264–269.
65. Burke-Ramirez P, Asgharnejad M, Webster C, et al. Efficacy and tolerability of subcutaneous sumatriptan for acute migraine: a comparison between ethnic groups. *Headache* 2001;41:873–882.
66. Savani N, Brautaset NJ, Reunanen M, et al. A double-blind placebo-controlled study assessing the efficacy and tolerability of 50 mg sumatriptan tablets in the acute treatment of migraine. Sumatriptan Tablets S2CM07 Study Group. *Int J Clin Pract Suppl* 1999;105:7–15.
67. Peikert A, Becker WJ, Ashford EA, et al. Sumatriptan nasal spray: a dose-ranging study in the acute treatment of migraine. *Eur J Neurol* 1999;6:43–49.
68. Diamond S, Elkind A, Jackson RT, et al. Multiple-attack efficacy and tolerability of sumatriptan nasal spray in the treatment of migraine. *Arch Fam Med* 1998;7:234–240.
69. Ryan R, Elkind A, Baker CC, et al. Sumatriptan nasal spray for the acute treatment of migraine. Results of two clinical studies. *Neurology* 1997;49:1225–1230.
70. Sakai F, Iwata M, Tashiro K, et al. Zolmitriptan is effective and well tolerated in Japanese patients with migraine: a dose–response study. *Cephalalgia* 2002;22:376–383.
71. Dowson AJ, MacGregor EA, Purdy RA, et al. Zolmitriptan orally disintegrating tablet is effective in the acute treatment of migraine. *Cephalalgia* 2002;22:101–106.
72. Gruffyd-Jones K, Kies B, Middleton A, et al. Zolmitriptan versus sumatriptan for the acute oral treatment of migraine: a randomized, double-blind, international study. *Eur J Neurol* 2001;8:237–245.
73. Gallagher R, Dennidh G, Spierings E, et al. A comparative trial of zolmitriptan and sumatriptan for the acute oral treatment of migraine. *Headache* 2000;40:119–128.
74. Lipton RB, Stewart WF, Stone AM, et al. Stratified care vs step care strategies for migraine: the Disability in Strategies of Care (DISC) study: a randomized trial. *JAMA* 2000;284:2599–2605.

Luis E Morillo
Associate Professor
Javeriana University Faculty of Medicine
Department of Neurosciences, Neurology
Unit and Clinical Epidemiology and
Biostatistics Unit
Bogota
Colombia

Competing interests: LEM has received travel and grant support from the pharmaceutical companies involved in the manufacturing of some of the drugs discussed.

Multiple sclerosis

Search date November 2003

Mike Boggild and Helen Ford

QUESTIONS

INTERVENTIONS

Key Messages

- We found no evidence from RCTs that any treatment alters long term outcome in multiple sclerosis.

Reducing relapse rates and disability

- **Glatiramer acetate** One RCT in people with relapsing and remitting multiple sclerosis found that glatiramer acetate reduced relapse rates over 2 years compared with placebo but found no effect on disability. We found no good quality RCTs in people with secondary progressive multiple sclerosis.

- **Interferon beta** Two RCTs in people experiencing a first demyelinating event found that interferon beta-1a decreased the risk of conversion to clinically definite multiple sclerosis over 2–3 years compared with placebo. One systematic review in people with active relapsing remitting multiple sclerosis found limited evidence that interferon beta-1a/b reduced exacerbations and disease progression over 2 years compared with placebo. One subsequent RCT in people with relapsing remitting multiple sclerosis found that interferon beta-1b reduced the proportion of people with relapse over 2 years compared with interferon beta-1a. Three RCTs provided insufficient evidence to assess the effects of interferon beta on disease progression in people with secondary progressive multiple sclerosis.
- **Azathioprine** One systematic review in people with relapsing and remitting or progressive multiple sclerosis comparing azathioprine versus placebo or no treatment found a modest reduction in relapse rates over 2 years but no evidence of a difference in disability. However, we were unable to draw reliable conclusions because of clinical heterogeneity among the included RCTs.
- **Intravenous immunoglobulin** One RCT in people with relapsing and remitting multiple sclerosis found that intravenous immunoglobulin reduced disability over 2 years compared with placebo. However, the clinical importance of this reduction is unclear. We found no good quality RCTs in people with secondary progressive multiple sclerosis.
- **Methotrexate** One small RCT provided insufficient evidence to assess the effects of methotrexate in reducing relapse rates and disability in people with multiple sclerosis.
- **Mitoxantrone** One RCT in people with worsening, relapsing, remitting, or progressive multiple sclerosis found that mitoxantrone reduced progression of disability over 2 years compared with placebo. One small RCT in people with active multiple sclerosis found limited evidence that mitoxantrone plus methylprednisolone reduced relapse over 6 months compared with methylprednisolone alone. However, mitoxantrone is associated with leukopenia, menstrual disorders, and arrhythmia.

Treating acute relapses

- **Corticosteroids (methylprednisolone or corticotrophin)** One systematic review in people with multiple sclerosis requiring treatment for acute exacerbations found that corticosteroids (methylprednisolone or corticotrophin) improved symptoms compared with placebo within the first 5 weeks of treatment. The optimal dose, route, and duration of treatment are unclear.
- **Plasma exchange** One small RCT provided insufficient evidence to assess plasma exchange in people with acute relapses of multiple sclerosis.

Treating fatigue

- **Amantadine** Four poor quality RCTs identified by two systematic reviews provided insufficient evidence to assess amantadine in people with multiple sclerosis related fatigue.
- **Behaviour modification** We found no RCTs on the effects of behavioural modification treatment in people with multiple sclerosis related fatigue.
- **Exercise** Two weak RCTs provided insufficient evidence to assess exercise in people with multiple sclerosis related fatigue.
- **Pemoline** Two poor quality RCTs identified by a systematic review provided insufficient evidence to assess the effects of pemoline compared with placebo on multiple sclerosis related fatigue.

Treating spasticity

- **Botulinum toxin** One small RCT provided insufficient evidence about the effects of botulinum toxin on functional outcomes in people with spasticity due to multiple sclerosis.
- **Intrathecal baclofen** One small crossover RCT provided insufficient evidence to assess functional effects of intrathecal baclofen in people with spasticity due to multiple sclerosis.

Multiple sclerosis

- **Oral drug treatments** One systematic review provided insufficient evidence about the effects of oral baclofen, dantrolene, or tizanidine on functional outcomes in people with spasticity due to multiple sclerosis.
- **Physiotherapy** Two small RCTs provided insufficient evidence to assess physiotherapy in people with spasticity due to multiple sclerosis. One of the RCTs found limited evidence that twice weekly hospital or home based physiotherapy for 8 weeks briefly improved mobility compared with no physiotherapy. The other, in people with progressive multiple sclerosis, found no significant difference between early versus delayed physiotherapy in mobility or activities of daily living.

Multidisciplinary care

- **Inpatient rehabilitation** Two small RCTs provided insufficient evidence to assess inpatient rehabilitation in people with multiple sclerosis. Both RCTs found short term functional benefit but no reduction in neurological impairment. Longer term effects are uncertain.
- **Outpatient rehabilitation** Two small RCTs provided insufficient evidence to assess outpatient rehabilitation in people with multiple sclerosis.

DEFINITION	Multiple sclerosis is a chronic inflammatory disease of the central nervous system. Diagnosis requires evidence of lesions that are separated in both time and space, and the exclusion of other inflammatory, structural, or hereditary conditions that might give a similar clinical picture. The disease takes three main forms: relapsing and remitting multiple sclerosis, characterised by episodes of neurological dysfunction interspersed with periods of stability; primary progressive multiple sclerosis, in which progressive neurological disability occurs from the outset; and secondary progressive multiple sclerosis, in which progressive neurological disability occurs later in the course of the disease.
INCIDENCE/ PREVALENCE	Prevalence varies with geography and racial group; it is highest in white populations in temperate regions.[1] In Europe and North America, prevalence is 1/800 people, with an annual incidence of 2–10/100 000, making multiple sclerosis the most common cause of neurological disability in young adults. Age of onset is broad, peaking between 20 and 40 years.[2]
AETIOLOGY/ RISK FACTORS	The cause remains unclear, although current evidence suggests that multiple sclerosis is an autoimmune disorder of the central nervous system resulting from an environmental stimulus in genetically susceptible individuals. Multiple sclerosis is currently regarded as a single disorder with clinical variants, but there is some evidence that it may consist of several related disorders with distinct immunological, pathological, and genetic features.[1,3]
PROGNOSIS	In 90% of people, early disease is relapsing and remitting. Although some people follow a relatively benign course over many years, most develop secondary progressive disease, usually 6–10 years after onset. In 10% of people, initial disease is primary progressive. Apart from a minority of people with "aggressive" multiple sclerosis, life expectancy is not greatly affected and the disease course is often of more than 30 years' duration.
AIMS OF INTERVENTION	To prevent or delay disability; to improve function; to alleviate symptoms of spasticity; to prevent complications (contractures, pressure sores); to optimise quality of life.
OUTCOMES	Neurological disability, spasticity, fatigue, general health, relapse rate, and quality of life. **Neurological disability:** In clinical trials, disability in multiple sclerosis is usually measured using the disease specific Expanded Disability Status Scale, which ranges from 0 (no disability) to 10 (death from multiple sclerosis) in half point increments.[4] Lower scores (0–4) reflect specific neurological impairments and disability; higher scores reflect reducing levels of mobility (4–7) and upper limb and bulbar function (7–9.5). The scale is non-linear and has been criticised for indicating change poorly, for emphasising neurological examination and mobility, and for failing to reflect other disabilities (e.g. fatigue, sexual disability). Some timed outcomes include ambulation (time taken to walk a specified short distance), the nine-hole peg test (time taken to place some pegs into holes in a block), and the box and block test (time taken to transfer blocks between boxes). **Sustained disease progression:** This is reported when an increase in disability from either disease progression or incomplete recovery from relapse is sustained for 3 or 6 months. A relapse that resolves within this time period constitutes

non-sustained progression. **Spasticity:** A variety of clinical measures are used, the most common being the Ashworth Scale, which scores muscle tone on a scale of 0–4, with 0 representing normal tone and 4 severe spasticity. For the purposes of this review, the Ashworth Scale was considered to represent an appropriate clinical outcome and was selected over other outcome measures for spasticity (e.g. neurophysiological measures, examination ratings) that represent proxy clinical outcomes. **General health:** Attempts have been made to customise generic health status scales, but these scales have not been widely used.[5]

METHODS *Clinical Evidence* search and appraisal November 2003. We included only trials focusing on clinical outcomes (disability, relapses, and symptoms).

QUESTION **What are the effects of interventions aimed at reducing relapse rates and disability?**

OPTION **INTERFERON BETA**

Two RCTs in people experiencing a first demyelinating event found that interferon beta-1a decreased the risk of conversion to clinically definite multiple sclerosis over 2–3 years compared with placebo. One systematic review in people with active relapsing remitting multiple sclerosis found limited evidence that interferon beta-1a/b reduced exacerbations and disease progression over 2 years compared with placebo. One subsequent RCT in people with relapsing remitting multiple sclerosis found that interferon beta-1b reduced the proportion of people with relapse over 2 years compared with interferon beta-1a. Three RCTs provided insufficient evidence to assess the effects of interferon beta on disease progression in people with secondary progressive multiple sclerosis.

Benefits: **First demyelinating event:** We found two RCTs comparing interferon beta-1a versus placebo in people experiencing a first demyelinating event with evidence of subclinical demyelination on magnetic resonance imaging of the brain.[6,7] Both RCTs found that interferon beta-1a significantly reduced the risk of a second clinical event and, therefore, of conversion to a definite diagnosis of multiple sclerosis. The first RCT (383 people) found that interferon beta-1a significantly decreased the risk of conversion to clinically definite multiple sclerosis after 3 years compared with placebo (cumulative probability of conversion to clinically definite multiple sclerosis: 35% with interferon beta-1a *v* 50% with placebo; HR 0.56, 95% CI 0.38 to 0.81).[6] The second RCT (308 people) found that interferon beta-1a significantly decreased the proportion of people with clinically definite multiple sclerosis after 2 years compared with placebo (52/154 [34%] with interferon beta-1a *v* 69/154 [45%] with placebo; OR 0.61, 95% CI 0.37 to 0.99).[7] **Relapsing and remitting multiple sclerosis:** We found one systematic review (search date 2000, 1215 people), which identified seven RCTs comparing interferon beta-1a/b versus placebo in people with active relapsing remitting multiple sclerosis (2 relapses in previous 2 or 3 years).[8] The review found that, over 2 years, interferon significantly reduced the risk of exacerbations and disease progression compared with placebo (3 RCTs, 919 people, RR for exacerbation 0.80, 95% CI 0.73 to 0.88; RR for disease progression, defined as 1 point progression on the Expanded Disability Status Scale sustained over 3 or 6 months 0.69, 95% CI 0.55 to 0.87). The review found that results for exacerbation or disease progression were not significant if a sensitivity analysis assumed that all people lost to follow up had exacerbation or experienced disease progression (worst case scenario).[8] One subsequent RCT (188 people with relapsing remitting multiple sclerosis) compared interferon beta-1b (250 μg given on alternate days) versus interferon beta-1a (30 μg given once weekly).[9] Over 2 years, the proportion of people remaining relapse free was significantly higher with interferon beta-1b given on alternate days than with interferon beta-1a given once a week (relapse free: 49/96 [51%] with interferon beta-1b *v* 33/92 [36%] with interferon beta-1a; RR of relapse 0.76, 95% CI 0.59 to 0.99). Analysis was by intention to treat but investigators were not blinded to treatment allocation. **Secondary progressive multiple sclerosis:** We found three RCTs.[10–12] The first RCT (718 people) compared interferon beta-1b (8 MIU on alternate days) versus placebo in people with secondary progressive multiple sclerosis and an Expanded Disability Status Scale score of 3.0–6.5.[10] After a median of 30 months' follow up, the RCT found that, compared with placebo, interferon delayed sustained progression of disability (measured by the Expanded Disability Status Scale) by 9–12 months, significantly reduced risk of progression, and reduced the risk of being wheelchair bound (OR for confirmed progression 0.65, 95% CI 0.52 to 0.83; NNT to prevent 1 additional person becoming wheelchair bound 13, 95% CI 8 to 49). The treatment effect was apparent in people of all levels of baseline disability. However, a large number of people in each group withdrew from the trial (27% placebo and 25% interferon), and no data on quality of life were reported. The second RCT (618 people) compared subcutaneous interferon beta-1a (22 or 44 μg, 3 times weekly) versus placebo.[11] It found no significant difference in confirmed progression of disability, although interferon reduced risk of relapse compared with placebo (HR for progression of disability 0.83, 95% CI 0.65 to 1.07; AR for relapse in 1 year 50% with interferon *v* 71% with placebo; $P < 0.001$). The third RCT (436 people) found no significant difference in Expanded Disability Status Scale score after 2 years between interferon beta (60 μg once weekly) and placebo.[12] However, Expanded Disability Status Scale was a secondary outcome measure. The RCT also found that interferon beta reduced progression after 2 years compared with placebo (progression measured by Multiple Sclerosis Functional Composite score comprising a 25-foot timed walk, nine-hole peg test, and the paced auditory serial addition test; difference between groups $P = 0.033$). However, this outcome has not been assessed in other RCTs and its clinical importance is uncertain.

Harms: The RCTs did not report any serious adverse effects.[10,13–15] Mild to moderate effects included early flu-like symptoms (50% of people) and, rarely, leukopenia and asymptomatic elevation in transaminases. Injection site reactions occurred with subcutaneous administration in 80% of people. The RCT comparing interferon beta-1b versus interferon beta-1a found that most adverse events (flu-like syndrome, fever, fatigue, increased liver enzymes) were most frequent during the first months of treatment and reduced in frequency after the first 6 months.[9] Frequency of adverse events was similar in both groups. However, local skin reactions occurred more frequently in the interferon beta-1b group, with one case of skin necrosis that caused treatment withdrawal.[9]

Comment: None.

OPTION GLATIRAMER ACETATE

One RCT in people with relapsing and remitting multiple sclerosis found that glatiramer acetate reduced relapse rates over 2 years compared with placebo but found no effect on disability. We found no good quality RCTs in people with secondary progressive multiple sclerosis.

Benefits: We found no systematic review. **Relapsing and remitting multiple sclerosis:** We found one RCT (251 people, Expanded Disability Status Scale score 0–5) comparing glatiramer acetate versus placebo.[16] The

RCT found that glatiramer acetate (copolymer 1) 20 mg daily significantly reduced relapse rates over 2 years compared with placebo (mean relapse rate over 24 months: 1.19 with glatiramer acetate *v* 1.68 with placebo; ARR 29%; P = 0.007). It found no significant effect on disability. **Secondary progressive multiple sclerosis:** We found no good quality RCTs.

Harms: The RCT found that a self limiting allergic type reaction (flushing, chest tightness, and anxiety) lasting up to 30 minutes was reported by 15% of people taking glatiramer acetate on at least one occasion (maximum 7 reactions).[16]

Comment: None.

OPTION INTRAVENOUS IMMUNOGLOBULIN

One RCT in people with relapsing and remitting multiple sclerosis found that intravenous immunoglobulin reduced disability over 2 years compared with placebo. However, the clinical importance of this reduction is unclear. We found no good quality RCTs in people with secondary progressive multiple sclerosis.

Benefits: We found no systematic review. **Relapsing and remitting multiple sclerosis:** We found one RCT (150 people with relapsing and remitting multiple sclerosis) comparing intravenous immunoglobulin 0.2 g/kg monthly versus placebo.[17] Treatment was for a maximum of 2 years, but average duration was 21 months. The RCT found that intravenous immunoglobulin significantly improved the level of disability from baseline at 2 years compared with placebo (change in Expanded Disability Status Scale score –0.23, 95% CI –0.43 to –0.03 *v* +0.12 with placebo; P = 0.008; see comment below).[17] The RCT did not report time to development of sustained progression of disability. **Secondary progressive multiple sclerosis:** We found no RCTs meeting our quality criteria.

Harms: The RCT found that four people receiving intravenous immunoglobulin withdrew because of adverse effects (skin rash) compared with one person taking placebo.[17] However, higher doses of intravenous immunoglobulin have been associated with aseptic meningitis and other systemic reactions.[18]

Comment: The reduction in disability score with intravenous immunoglobulin was modest. The clinical importance of this small effect is unclear.

OPTION AZATHIOPRINE

One systematic review in people with relapsing and remitting or progressive multiple sclerosis comparing azathioprine versus placebo or no treatment found a modest reduction in relapse rates over 2 years but no evidence of a difference in disability. However, we were unable to draw reliable conclusions because of clinical heterogeneity among the included RCTs.

Benefits: We found one systematic review of azathioprine (search date 1989, 7 RCTs, 793 people with relapsing and remitting multiple sclerosis or progressive multiple sclerosis; see comment below).[19] It found that azathioprine significantly reduced the relapse rate at 2 years compared with placebo or no treatment (5 RCTs; OR of remaining relapse free 2.04, 95% CI 1.42 to 2.93) and reduced disability scores but the difference did not quite reach significance (4 RCTs; Expanded Disability Status Scale mean score difference –0.22, 95% CI –0.43 to +0.003).

Harms: The review found that about 10% of people were unable to tolerate therapeutic doses of azathioprine.[19] Well documented adverse effects include hepatotoxicity and bone marrow suppression.[19] There are concerns about long term cancer risk.[20] In one large RCT identified by the review, 21% of people on azathioprine withdrew after 1 year compared with 12% on placebo.[20]

Comment: The methods used in the multiple sclerosis trials have improved, making it hard to compare older RCTs with more recent ones. Trials in the systematic review included people with different categories of multiple sclerosis and used different definitions of relapse.[21] We were therefore unable to draw reliable conclusions about the effects of azathioprine.

OPTION METHOTREXATE

One small RCT provided insufficient evidence to assess the effects of methotrexate in reducing relapse rates and disability in people with multiple sclerosis.

Benefits: We found no systematic review. We found one RCT (60 people with primary or secondary progressive multiple sclerosis) comparing low dose methotrexate (7.5 mg weekly) versus placebo.[22] The RCT found that methotrexate significantly reduced the risk of progression compared with placebo (ARR 31%; P = 0.01), defined by a composite outcome measure, including Expanded Disability Status Scale, ambulation, nine-hole peg test, and box and block test. However, the clinical importance of these results is unclear (see comment below).

Harms: No major toxicity was reported in the RCT, but as bone marrow suppression and hepatotoxicity can occur with low dose methotrexate, regular monitoring is advised.[22]

Comment: The findings of the RCT mainly reflected changes in upper limb function.[22] RCTs of other drugs have not used composite outcome measures, which makes comparisons difficult. Relative risks for treatment failure were not reported.

OPTION MITOXANTRONE

One RCT in people with worsening, relapsing, remitting, or progressive multiple sclerosis found that mitoxantrone reduced progression of disability over 2 years compared with placebo. One small RCT in people with active multiple sclerosis found limited evidence that mitoxantrone plus methylprednisolone reduced relapse over 6 months compared with methylprednisolone alone. However, mitoxantrone is associated with leukopenia, menstrual disorders, and arrhythmia.

Benefits: We found no systematic review. We found two RCTs.[23,24] The first RCT studied 194 people with worsening, relapsing, remitting, or secondary progressive multiple sclerosis and an Expanded Disability Status Scale score of 3.0–6.0.[23] It compared mitoxantrone (5 mg/m^2 or 12 mg/m^2 intravenously every 3 months) versus placebo for 24 months. It found that the higher dose of mitoxantrone significantly improved disability after 24 months compared with placebo (mean change in the Expanded Disability Status Scale score from baseline: –0.13 with 12 mg/m^2 mitoxantrone *v* 0.23 with placebo; difference between groups 0.24, 95% CI 0.04 to 0.44). The RCT reported that lower dose mitoxantrone also significantly improved disability compared with placebo (P = 0.01; no further data reported). A second, smaller open label RCT (42 people with active multiple sclerosis) compared monthly intravenous mitoxantrone (20 mg) plus methylprednisolone (1 g) versus methylprednisolone alone.[24] It found that, compared with methylprednisolone alone, mitoxantrone plus methylprednisolone significantly reduced disease activity after 6 months (as assessed by appearance on magnetic resonance imaging) and significantly lowered annual clinical relapse rates (mitoxantrone plus methylprednisolone 0.7 *v* methylprednisolone alone 3.0; $P < 0.01$).[24]

Harms: The major risk is dose related cardiotoxicity, but this is rare at the doses used in multiple sclerosis (see comment below). Leukopenia, nausea, and amenorrhoea are commonly reported.[25] The RCT comparing higher and lower dose mitoxantrone versus placebo found that nausea, alopecia, urinary tract infection, menstrual disorder, leukopenia, and arrhythmia were more common with the higher dose of mitoxantrone than with placebo (nausea: 20% with placebo *v* 76% with higher dose mitoxantrone; alopecia: 31% *v* 61%; urinary tract infection: 13% *v* 32%; menstrual disorder: 26% *v* 61%; leukopenia: 0% *v* 19%; arrhythmia: 8% *v* 18%).[23]

Comment: One retrospective case series of 1378 people with multiple sclerosis treated with mitroxantrone reported two cases of cardiotoxicity[26] and one case of acute leukaemia.[27]

QUESTION What are the effects of treatments for acute relapse?

OPTION CORTICOSTEROIDS

One systematic review in people with multiple sclerosis requiring treatment for acute exacerbations found that corticosteroids (methylprednisolone or corticotrophin) improved symptoms compared with placebo within the first 5 weeks of treatment. The optimal dose, route, and duration of treatment are unclear.

Benefits: We found one systematic review (search date 1999, 377 people with multiple sclerosis requiring treatment for acute exacerbations, 4 RCTs of methylprednisolone, 2 RCTs of corticotrophin *v* placebo).[28] The systematic review found that, compared with placebo, methylprednisolone or corticotrophin significantly reduced the proportion of people whose symptoms were worse or unimproved within 5 weeks of treatment (5 RCTs; worse or unimproved within 5 weeks from randomisation: 63/175 [36%] with methylprednisolone or corticotrophin *v* 94/155 [60%] with placebo; OR 0.37, 95% CI 0.24 to 0.57). A small subgroup analysis using an indirect comparison suggested no difference between 5 days and 15 days of treatment with methylprednisolone.[28] One of the included RCTs (51 people) found no significant difference between oral methylprednisolone and placebo in the prevention of new relapses or in disability after 1 year (proportion who relapsed: 17/26 [65%] with methylprednisolone *v* 13/25 [52%] with placebo; RR 1.26, 95% CI 0.79 to 2.01).

Harms: The review found that gastrointestinal symptoms occurred more often in people taking oral high dose methylprednisolone than in people taking placebo (38% *v* 8%; CI not reported).[28] It also found that psychic disorders (insomnia, elevated mood, "psychosis", or dysphonia) were more common in people receiving oral high dose methylprednisolone than in people receiving placebo, although the difference was not significant (11/50 [22%] *v* 5/44 [11%]; RR 1.87, 95% CI 0.77 to 4.55).[28] Weight gain and oedema were more frequent in people receiving corticotrophin than in people receiving placebo (absolute numbers and CI not reported).[28]

Comment: None.

OPTION PLASMA EXCHANGE

One small RCT provided insufficient evidence to assess plasma exchange in people with acute relapses of multiple sclerosis.

Benefits: We found no systematic review. We found one small, double blind, crossover RCT (22 people) comparing plasma exchange versus sham treatment in people with acute relapses of multiple sclerosis (12 people) or other demyelinating disease (10 people; see comment below).[29] Analysing pre-crossover results, the RCT found a non-significant increase in moderate or greater improvement in neurological disability in people receiving plasma exchange compared with sham treatment (before crossover: 5/11 [46%] with plasma exchange *v* 1/11 [9%] with sham treatment; P = 0.0743).[29]

Harms: The RCT reported no serious adverse effects.[29]

Comment: At the time of randomisation, all 22 people had failed to respond to standard doses of intravenous corticosteroids and were within 3 months of onset of the acute deficit.[29]

QUESTION What are the effects of treatments for fatigue?

OPTION AMANTADINE

Four poor quality RCTs identified by two systematic reviews provided insufficient evidence to assess amantadine in people with multiple sclerosis related fatigue.

Benefits: We found two systematic reviews (search date 1999[30]; search date 2002[31]). Both reviews found one parallel and three crossover RCTs (236 people with multiple sclerosis; see comment below) comparing amantadine versus placebo for 1–6 weeks. Both found limited evidence favouring amantadine compared with placebo and found important methodological weaknesses in the included RCTs (see comment below).[30,31] The parallel RCT (82 people) identified by the reviews found that, compared with placebo, amantadine significantly improved fatigue at 6 weeks as measured by "MS-specific Fatigue Scale" (P < 0.05).[30] The RCT found that amantadine significantly increased the proportion of people who "preferred treatment 2 weeks after end of trial" but analysed results only in people who had expressed a preference. However, the reviews performed an analysis by intention to treat and found no significant difference in the proportion of people who "preferred treatment 2 weeks after end of trial" (15/39 [38%] with amantadine *v* 13/43 [30%] with placebo; RR 1.3, 95% CI 0.7 to 2.3).[30] The RCT found no significant difference in "preferred treatment at the end of trial", "Fatigue Severity Scale", or "Rand Index of Vitality" (reported as non-significant, CI not reported).[30] The three crossover RCTs identified by the reviews found different results with different measures of fatigue. The first RCT found that amantadine significantly improved fatigue measured by "effects on most affected activity VAS [visual analogue scale]", "effects on activities of daily living", "response over previous period", and "preferred treatment" (P < 0.05), but not by "effects on fatigue VAS".[30] The second RCT found that amantadine significantly improved fatigue measured by "preferred treatment" (P < 0.05); and the third RCT found that amantadine significantly improved fatigue measured by "preferred treatment" (P < 0.05), but did not improve fatigue measured by daily ratings on a point scale from 1–5 (reported as non-significant, no further data reported).[30]

Harms: Both reviews reported that a similar proportion of people talking amantadine and placebo had adverse effects, including sleep disturbance, nightmares, anxiety, headaches, and nausea (40% with amantadine *v* 35% with placebo; CI not reported).[31]

Comment: Both reviews reached the same conclusions and reported the same absolute data but the second review[31] did not report details regarding the significance of the differences between groups, and therefore we have reported full results from the first review only.[30] The RCTs used a variety of methods to assess fatigue, and the significance of the results was sensitive to the scales or measures used.[30,31] Both systematic reviews stated that all of the RCTs were open to bias arising from lack of clarity about the randomisation methods, blinding, incompleteness of follow up, lack of analysis by intention to treat, and difficulties with interpretation of crossover RCTs. There was insufficient evidence about the effects of amantadine on quality of life in people with multiple sclerosis.

OPTION PEMOLINE

Two poor quality RCTs identified by a systematic review provided insufficient evidence to assess the effects of pemoline compared with placebo on multiple sclerosis related fatigue.

Benefits: We found one systematic review (search date 1999).[30] It found one parallel and one crossover RCT (126 people with multiple sclerosis). The parallel RCT found no significant difference between pemoline and placebo in the self reporting of fatigue at 6 weeks (measured using the Fatigue Severity Scale, P = 0.394; measured using the MS-specific Fatigue Scale, P = 0.394) The crossover RCT found that more people taking pemoline than taking placebo had excellent or good relief from fatigue at 10 weeks (19/41 [46%] with pemoline *v* 8/41 [20%] with placebo; CI not reported).

Harms: The review found more reports of adverse effects (sleep disturbance, nausea, mood change, palpitations, irritability, insomnia, anorexia) with pemoline than with placebo.[30]

Comment: The RCTs used a variety of methods to assess fatigue.[30] The systematic review stated that all the RCTs were open to bias (arising from lack of clarity about the randomisation methods, blinding, incompleteness of follow up, and difficulties with interpretation of crossover RCTs).[30]

OPTION BEHAVIOURAL MODIFICATION TREATMENT

We found no RCTs on the effects of behavioural modification treatment in people with multiple sclerosis related fatigue.

Benefits: We found no systematic review or RCTs.

Harms: We found no RCTs.

Comment: None.

OPTION EXERCISE

Two weak RCTs provided insufficient evidence to assess exercise in people with multiple sclerosis related fatigue.

Benefits: We found no systematic review, but found two RCTs (see comment below).[32,33] The first RCT (46 people, Expanded Disability Status Scale score 0–6) compared 15 weeks of aerobic training versus no exercise.[32]

Using a scale that measures mental and physical fatigue, the RCT found a significant reduction in fatigue from baseline at 10 weeks within the exercise group ($P < 0.05$) but not at 15 weeks after completion of the exercise programme. A different scale that measured only physical fatigue remained unchanged from baseline in both groups of people. The RCT found significant improvements from baseline in other measures of emotional behaviour and quality of life within the exercise group (Profile of Mood States depression and anger score, Sickness Impact profile scores; $P < 0.05$). The second RCT (26 people with clinically definite multiple sclerosis taking part in an inpatient rehabilitation programme, Expanded Disability Status Scale score 1–6.5) compared adding aerobic exercise training (five supervised training sessions/week for 3–4 weeks) to the usual rehabilitation programme versus the usual rehabilitation programme alone.[33] It found no significant change in fatigue from baseline in either group ($P = 0.09$ with exercise, P reported as non-significant with inpatient rehabilitation alone).

Harms: The first RCT gave no information on adverse effects.[32] The second additional RCT found that aerobic exercise was associated with symptom exacerbation (increased spasticity, paraesthesia, vertigo) in 6% of people.[33]

Comment: People with moderate disability or severe fatigue may have difficulty adhering to an aerobic exercise programme. The results of the RCTs should be interpreted with caution because they did not compare groups directly.[32,33] Their results were expressed as changes from baseline within each group before and after intervention using a recognised fatigue severity scale.

QUESTION What are the effects of treatments for spasticity?

OPTION PHYSIOTHERAPY

Two small RCTs provided insufficient evidence to assess physiotherapy in people with spasticity due to multiple sclerosis. One of the RCTs found limited evidence that twice weekly hospital or home based physiotherapy for 8 weeks briefly improved mobility compared with no physiotherapy. The other, in people with progressive multiple sclerosis, found no significant difference between early and delayed physiotherapy in mobility or activities of daily living.

Benefits: We found no systematic review but found two RCTs.[34,35] The first RCT (40 people, single blind crossover) compared hospital based or home based physiotherapy (45 minutes, twice weekly for 8 weeks) versus no physiotherapy.[34] It found that, compared with no physiotherapy, either hospital or home physiotherapy significantly improved mobility assessed 1 week after treatment (hospital physiotherapy *v* no physiotherapy: Rivermead mobility index increased by 1.4 units, 95% CI 0.6 units to 2.1 units, $P < 0.001$; home physiotherapy *v* no physiotherapy: Rivermead mobility index increased by 1.5 units, 95% CI 0.7 units to 2.2 units, $P < 0.001$). The treatment effect was short lived, being largely lost 8 weeks after treatment. The second RCT (45 people with progressive multiple sclerosis, open label) compared early versus delayed physiotherapy (9 weeks of inpatient treatment).[35] It found no significant difference in mobility (timed walk, $P = 0.073$; Rivermead mobility index, $P = 0.054$) or activities of daily living (measured by Barthel Activities of Daily Living, $P = 0.770$). It found that treated people reported significantly reduced mobility related stress ($P < 0.001$).

Harms: The RCTs gave no information on adverse effects.[34,35]

Comment: None.

OPTION ORAL DRUG TREATMENT

One systematic review provided insufficient evidence about the effects of oral baclofen, dantrolene, or tizanidine on functional outcomes in people with spasticity due to multiple sclerosis.

Benefits: We found one systematic review (search date 2003, 39 RCTs of duration > 7 days).[36] Of the included RCTs, only 15 used an appropriate outcome measure for assessing spasticity (the Ashworth Scale). **Oral baclofen versus placebo:** The systematic review[36] identified one crossover RCT (30 people)[37] comparing four interventions: stretching exercises plus placebo, stretching exercises plus baclofen 20 mg, baclofen alone, and placebo alone that used the Ashworth Scale for 10 weeks.[37] It found no significant difference in spasticity between baclofen alone or baclofen plus exercise and placebo ($P = 0.105$ for combined treatment *v* placebo, P value not reported for baclofen alone *v* placebo). **Oral dantrolene versus placebo:** The review found no RCTs that used a validated outcome measure such as the Ashworth Scale.[36] **Oral tizanidine versus placebo:** The review[36] identified two RCTs[38,39] that used the Ashworth Scale. The first RCT (220 people) found no significant difference in muscle tone as assessed by Ashworth Scale score ($P = 0.46$) but found that tizanidine 2–36 mg daily for 12 weeks' treatment significantly reduced self reported clonus and spasm ($P = 0.05$).[38] The second RCT (187 people) found that tizanidine 24–36 mg daily significantly reduced Ashworth Scale scores compared with placebo (proportion of people with improvement of ≥1 point: 71% with tizanidine *v* 50% with placebo; $P < 0.005$). The clinical relevance of this result is unclear because many muscle groups were assessed. **Oral baclofen versus oral tizanidine:** The review identified three RCTs comparing baclofen versus tizanidine that used the Ashworth Scale.[36] The RCTs found no significant difference in spasticity, spasms, or clonus between baclofen and tizanidine (no further data reported).

Harms: **Oral baclofen versus placebo:** The RCT identified by the review[36] gave no information on adverse effects.[37] **Oral tizanidine versus placebo:** The first RCT identified by the review found that tizanidine significantly increased asthenia, dry mouth, somnolence, and dizziness compared with placebo ($P < 0.001$ for all outcomes *v* placebo).[38] **Oral baclofen versus oral tizanidine:** Comparative RCTs of baclofen and tizanidine found similar levels of adverse effects (including muscle weakness, sedation, and dry mouth).[36] One non-systematic review suggested that tizanidine may be less likely than baclofen to cause muscle weakness.[40]

Comment: The review concluded that the absolute and comparative efficacy of antispasmodic drugs in multiple sclerosis is poorly documented.[36] The major difficulty in planning and designing future RCTs is the lack of a functionally relevant, well validated measure of spasticity.

OPTION INTRATHECAL BACLOFEN

One small crossover RCT provided insufficient evidence to assess functional effects of intrathecal baclofen in people with spasticity due to multiple sclerosis.

Benefits: We found no systematic review. We found one small crossover RCT comparing intrathecal baclofen versus intrathecal saline (19 non-ambulant people with multiple sclerosis or spinal cord injury and with spasticity resistant to oral baclofen).[41] It found that baclofen significantly reduced spasticity and spasm frequency (see comment below). Mean Ashworth Scale scores in all participants fell from 4.0 at baseline to 1.2 after 3 days of treatment ($P < 0.0001$), with scores for all people improving from baseline.[41]

Harms: The RCT conducted an open label extension and found no adverse effects associated with intrathecal baclofen over a mean 19.2 months' follow up.[41] Potential problems include pump failure, infection, and, rarely, baclofen overdose.

Comment: The results of the RCT should be interpreted with caution because it did not directly compare groups, presenting only changes from baseline, it did not report results before crossover, and it included people with spinal cord injury.[41] We found no evidence about intrathecal baclofen in ambulant people.

OPTION BOTULINUM TOXIN

One small RCT provided insufficient evidence about the effects of botulinum toxin on functional outcomes in people with spasticity due to multiple sclerosis.

Benefits: We found no systematic review but found one RCT.[42] The RCT (74 people) compared three different doses of intramuscular botulinum toxin (500, 1000, and 1500 units) versus placebo for the treatment of hip adductor spasticity in multiple sclerosis. It did not examine functional outcomes. The RCT found that the 1500 unit dose (17 people) compared with placebo (16 people) significantly improved maximum distance between the knees at 4 weeks ($P = 0.02$).[42] The 1000 unit (20 people) and 1500 unit (17 people) doses improved median hygiene scores from baseline at 4 weeks.

Harms: Botulinum toxin can cause local weakness. Adverse events were reported in 55% of people with botulinum toxin compared with 63% of people with placebo.[42] The most frequent were hypertonia (22% of people with botulinum toxin *v* 25% of people with placebo), weakness of non-injected muscles (14% *v* 6%), fatigue (7% *v* 13%), urinary tract infection (5% *v* 19%), headache (5% *v* 13%), micturition frequency (5% *v* 13%), back pain (5% *v* 0%), and diarrhoea (5% *v* 0%).[42] Twice as many adverse events were reported by the 1500 unit group (mean 2.7/person) compared with the 500 unit group (mean 1.1/person) and the 1000 unit group (mean 1.2/person).[42] Six people had serious adverse events (2 with botulinum toxin, 4 with placebo). The events (hospital admissions with diarrhoea, multiple infections, bowel spasticity, gastroparesis, pulmonary embolism, and blocked catheter) were considered to be unrelated to the study medication.[42]

Comment: None.

QUESTION What are the effects of multidisciplinary management?

OPTION INPATIENT REHABILITATION

Two small RCTs provided insufficient evidence to assess inpatient rehabilitation in people with multiple sclerosis. Both RCTs found short term functional benefit but no reduction in neurological impairment. Longer term effects are uncertain.

Benefits: We found no systematic review but found two RCTs.[43,44] The first RCT compared brief inpatient rehabilitation (average 25 days) versus waiting list control in 66 people with progressive multiple sclerosis who were selected as "good candidates" for rehabilitation.[43] It found that rehabilitation significantly improved disability at 6 weeks assessed by the functional independence measure compared with waiting list control ($P < 0.001$) and the London Handicap Scale ($P < 0.01$), despite unchanged levels of neurological impairment (Expanded Disability Status Scale). Benefit persisted for up to 9 months. The second RCT compared 3 weeks of inpatient rehabilitation versus exercises at home in 50 ambulant people with multiple sclerosis (Expanded Disability Status Scale score 3–7).[44] The RCT found that, compared with exercises at home, inpatient rehabilitation significantly improved disability over 3 weeks' treatment, assessed by the functional independence measure ($P < 0.004$), which persisted at 9 but not at 15 weeks' follow up.

Harms: The RCTs gave no information on adverse effects.[43,44]

Comment: None.

OPTION OUTPATIENT REHABILITATION

Two small RCTs provided insufficient evidence to assess outpatient rehabilitation in people with multiple sclerosis.

Benefits: We found no systematic review but found one RCT[45] and one controlled clinical trial.[46] The RCT (111 people with progressive multiple sclerosis) compared a 6 week individualised outpatient rehabilitation programme versus no treatment.[45] It found that outpatient rehabilitation significantly improved disability at 12 weeks compared with no treatment (improvement of ≥2 steps in the Functional Independence Measure: 32/58 [55%] *v* 4/53 [8%]; $P < 0.0001$). It found no significant difference in impairment (improvement of half a step in the Expanded Disability Status Scale 5/58 [9%] *v* 4/53 [7.5%], reported as non-significant, CI not reported). The controlled clinical trial (46 people with progressive multiple sclerosis) compared outpatient rehabilitation (5 hours/week for 1 year) versus remaining on the waiting list (no treatment).[46] It found that rehabilitation reduced the frequency of fatigue (effect size –0.27) and multiple sclerosis symptoms (effect size –0.32) compared with no treatment, despite no significant change in neurological impairment in either group.

Harms: The RCT and controlled clinical trial gave no information on adverse effects.[45,46]

Comment: RCTs are needed that record effects on disability and quality of life as well as impairment.

REFERENCES

1. Compston A. Genetic epidemiology of multiple sclerosis. *J Neurol Neurosurg Psychiatry* 1997;62:553–561.
2. Weinshenker BG, Bass B, Rice GPA, et al. The natural history of multiple sclerosis: a geographically based study. 1. Clinical course and disability. *Brain* 1989;112:133–146.
3. Lucchinetti CF, Bruck W, Rodriguez M, et al. Distinct patterns of multiple sclerosis pathology indicates heterogeneity in pathogenesis. *Brain Pathol* 1996;6:259–274.
4. Kurtzke JF. Rating neurological impairment in multiple sclerosis: an Expanded Disability Status Scale (EDSS). *Neurology* 1983;33:1444–1452.
5. Vickrey BG, Hays RD, Genovese BJ, et al. Comparison of a generic to disease-targeted health-related quality-of-life measures for multiple sclerosis. *J Clin Epidemiol* 1997;50:557–569.
6. Jacobs LD, Beck RW, Simon JH, et al. Intramuscular interferon beta-1a therapy initiated during a first demyelinating event in multiple sclerosis. *N Engl J Med* 2000;343:898–904.
7. Comi G, Fillipi M, Barkhof F, et al. Effect of early interferon treatment on conversion to definite multiple sclerosis: a randomised study. *Lancet* 2001;357:1576–1582.
8. Rice GA, Incorvaia B, Munari L, et al. Interferon in relapsing-remitting multiple sclerosis. In: The Cochrane Library, Issue 3, 2004. Chichester, UK: John Wiley & Sons, Ltd. Search date 2000; primary sources Medline, Embase, hand searches of reference lists, and personal contact with researchers and pharmaceutical companies.
9. Durelli L, Verdun E, Barbero P, et al. Every-other-day interferon beta-1b versus once weekly interferon beta-1a for multiple sclerosis: results of a 2 year prospective randomised multicentre study (INCOMIN). *Lancet* 2002;359:1453–1460.
10. Kappos L, Polman C, Pozzilli C, et al. Placebo-controlled multicentre randomised trial of interferon beta-1b in treatment of secondary progressive multiple sclerosis. *Lancet* 1998;352:1491–1497.
11. King J, McLeod J, Gonsette RE, et al. Randomised controlled trial of interferon beta-1a in secondary progressive MS: clinical results. *Neurology* 2001;56:1496–1504.
12. Cohen JA, Cutter GR, Fischer JS, et al. Benefit of interferon beta-1a on MSFC progression in secondary progressive MS. *Neurology* 2002;59:679–687.

13. Ebers GC, Rice G, Lesaux J, et al. Randomised double-blind placebo-controlled study of interferon beta-1a in relapsing/remitting multiple sclerosis. *Lancet* 1998;352:1498–1504.
14. Duquette P, Girard M, Despault L, et al. Interferon beta-1b is effective in relapsing–remitting multiple sclerosis. Clinical results of a multicenter, randomised, double-blind, placebo-controlled trial. *Neurology* 1993;43:655–661.
15. Jacobs LD, Cookfair DL, Rudick RA, et al. Intramuscular interferon beta-1a for disease progression in relapsing multiple sclerosis. *Ann Neurol* 1996;39:285–294.
16. Johnson KP, Brooks BR, Cohen JA, et al. Copolymer-1 reduces relapse rate and improves disability in relapsing-remitting multiple sclerosis: results of a Phase III multicenter, double-blind, placebo-controlled trial. *Neurology* 1995;45:1268–1276.
17. Fazekas F, Deisenhammer F, Strasser-Fuchs S, et al. Randomised placebo-controlled trial of monthly intravenous immunoglobulin therapy in relapsing–remitting multiple sclerosis. *Lancet* 1997;349:589–593.
18. Stangel M, Hartung HP, Marx P, et al. Side-effects of high-dose intravenous immunoglobulins. *Clin Neuropharmacol* 1997;20:385–393.
19. Yudkin PL, Ellison GW, Ghezzi A, et al. Overview of azathioprine treatment in multiple sclerosis. *Lancet* 1991;338:1051–1055. Search date 1989; primary sources Medline and hand searches of references.
20. Confavreux C, Saddier P, Grimaud J, et al. Risk of cancer from azathioprine therapy in multiple sclerosis: a case-control study. *Neurology* 1996;46:1607–1612.
21. Hughes RAC. Double-masked trial of azathioprine in multiple-sclerosis. *Lancet* 1988;2:179–183.
22. Goodkin DE, Rudick RA, VanderBrug Medendorp S, et al. Low-dose (7.5 mg) oral methotrexate reduces the rate of progression in chronic progressive multiple sclerosis. *Ann Neurol* 1995;37:30–40.
23. Hartung H, Gonsette R, Konig N, et al. Mitoxantrone in progressive multiple sclerosis: a placebo-controlled, double blind, randomised, multicentre trial. *Lancet* 2002;360:2018–2025.
24. Edan G, Miller D, Clanet M, et al. Therapeutic effect of mitoxantrone combined with methylprednisolone in multiple sclerosis: a randomised multicentre study of active disease using MRI and clinical criteria. *J Neurol Neurosurg Psychiatry* 1997;62:112–118.
25. MacDonald M, Posner LE, Dukart G, et al. A review of the acute and chronic toxicity of mitoxantrone. *Future Trends Chemother* 1985;6:443–450.
26. Ghalie RG, Edan G, Laurent M, et al. Cardiac adverse events associated with mitoxantrone (novantrone) therapy in patients with MS. *Neurology* 2002;59:909–913.
27. Ghalie RG, Mauch E, Edan G, et al. A study of therapy-related acute leukaemia after Mitoxantrone therapy for multiple sclerosis. *Mult Scler* 2002;8:441–445.
28. Filippini G, Brusaferri F, Sibley WA, et al. Corticosteroids or ACTH for acute exacerbations in multiple sclerosis. In: The Cochrane Library, Issue 4, 2003. Chichester, UK: John Wiley & Sons, Ltd. Search date 1999; primary sources Medline, Cochrane Controlled Trials Register, hand searches of reference lists, main neurology journals, conference abstracts, dissertations, and personal contact with researchers and manufacturers.
29. Weinshenker BG, O'Brien PC, Petterson TM, et al. A randomised trial of plasma exchange in acute central nervous system inflammatory demyelinating disease. *Neurology* 1999;46:878–886.
30. Branas P, Jordan R, Fry-Smith A, et al. Treatments for fatigue in multiple sclerosis: a rapid and systematic review. The National Coordinating Centre for Health Technology Assessment (NCCHTA). 13665278. *Health Technol Assess* 2000;4:27:1–73. Search date 1999; primary sources Medline, Embase, hand searches of reference lists, and personal contact with experts.
31. Taus C, Giuliani G, Pucci E, et al. Amantadine for fatigue in multiple sclerosis (Cochrane review). In: The Cochrane Library, Issue 3, 2004. Chichester, UK: John Wiley & Sons, Ltd. Search date 2002, primary sources Medline, Embase, hand searches of bibliographies of relevant articles and relevant journals, and personal contact with drug companies and researchers in the field.
32. Petajan JH, Gappmaier E, White AT, et al. Impact of aerobic training on fitness and quality of life in multiple sclerosis. *Ann Neurol* 1996;39:432–441.
33. Mostert S, Kesselring J. Effects of a short-term exercise training program on aerobic fitness, fatigue, health perception and activity level of subjects with multiple sclerosis. *Mult Scler* 2002;8:161–168.
34. Wiles CM, Newcombe RG, Fuller KJ, et al. Controlled randomised crossover trial of the effects of physiotherapy on mobility in chronic multiple sclerosis. *J Neurol Neurosurg Psychiatry* 2001;70:174–179.
35. Fuller KJ, Dawson K, Wiles CM. Physiotherapy in chronic multiple sclerosis: a controlled trial. *Clin Rehabil* 1996;10:195–204.
36. Shakespeare DT, Young CA, Boggild M. Anti-spasticity agents for multiple sclerosis (Cochrane Review). In: The Cochrane Library, Issue 4, 2003. Chichester, UK: John Wiley & Sons, Ltd. Search date 2003; primary sources Medline, Cochrane Controlled Trials Register, Cochrane MS Review Group Specialised Trial Registry, National Health Service National Research Register, Medical Research Council Clinical Trials Directory, hand searches of reference lists, main neurology journals, conference abstracts, dissertations, and personal contact with researchers and manufacturers.
37. Brar S, Smith MB, Nelson LM, et al. Evaluation of treatment protocols on minimal to moderate spasticity in multiple sclerosis. *Arch Phys Med Rehabil* 1991;72:186–189.
38. Smith C, Birnbaum G, Carter JL, et al. Tizanidine treatment of spasticity caused by multiple sclerosis: results of a double-blind, placebo-controlled trial. *Neurology* 1994;44:34–42.
39. Barnes MP, Bates D, Corston RN, et al. A double-blind, placebo-controlled trial of tizanidine in the treatment of spasticity caused by multiple sclerosis. *Neurology* 1994;44:S70–S78.
40. Groves L, Shellenberger MK, Davis CS. Tizanidine treatment of spasticity: a meta-analysis of controlled, double-blind, comparative studies with baclofen and diazepam. *Adv Ther* 1998;15:241–251. Search date not stated; primary source records of Sandoz (now Novartis).
41. Penn RD, Savoy SM, Corcos D, et al. Intrathecal baclofen for severe spinal spasticity. *N Engl J Med* 1989;320:1517–1521.
42. Hyman N, Barnes M, Bhakta B, et al. Botulinum toxin (Dysport) treatment of hip adductor spasticity in multiple sclerosis: a prospective, randomised, double-blind, placebo controlled, dose ranging study. *J Neurol Neurosurg Psychiatry* 2000;68:707–712.
43. Freeman JA, Langdon DW, Hobart JC, et al. The impact of inpatient rehabilitation on progressive multiple sclerosis. *Ann Neurol* 1997;42:236–244.
44. Solari A, Fillipini G, Gasco P, et al. Physical rehabilitation has a positive effect on disability in multiple sclerosis patients. *Neurology* 1999;52:57–62.
45. Patti F, Ciancio MR, Cacopardo M, et al. Effects of a short outpatient rehabilitation treatment on disability of multiple sclerosis: a randomised controlled trial. *J Neurol* 2003;250:861–866.
46. Di Fabio RP, Soderberg J, Choi T, et al. Extended outpatient rehabilitation: its influence on symptom frequency, fatigue and functional status for persons with progressive multiple sclerosis. *Arch Phys Med Rehabil* 1998;79:141–146.

Multiple sclerosis

Mike Boggild
Consultant Neurologist
The Walton Centre for Neurology and Neurosurgery
Liverpool
UK

Helen Ford
Consultant Neurologist
St James's University Hospital
Leeds
UK

Competing interests: MB has received financial support for attending scientific meetings from Biogen, Serono Pharmaceuticals, and Teva Pharmaceuticals, and has organised educational sessions for Serono. HF has received financial support for attending scientific meetings by Serono Pharmaceuticals, Schering and Biogen.

Parkinson's disease

Search date May 2004

Carl Clarke and A Peter Moore

QUESTIONS

INTERVENTIONS

To be covered in future updates

Catechol-*O*-methyltransferase inhibitors

*We have used the term "levodopa" to refer to a combination of levodopa and a peripheral decarboxylase inhibitor.

See glossary G

Key Messages

Drugs in early Parkinson's

- **Selegiline** RCTs found that selegiline improved the symptoms of Parkinson's disease and delayed the need for levodopa compared with placebo. One of the RCTs found limited evidence of increased mortality in people treated with selegiline.

- **Dopamine agonists (reduced dyskinesia and motor fluctuations compared with levodopa*, but were associated with increased treatment withdrawal and poorer motor scores)** One systematic review and one subsequent RCT (published only as an abstract) found that dopamine agonist monotherapy reduced the incidence of dyskinesias and motor complications compared with levodopa monotherapy. However, the subsequent RCT found that dopamine agonist monotherapy was associated with poorer motor scores than levodopa monotherapy, and an increased risk of treatment withdrawal. There is consensus that levodopa improves motor function, but that dyskinesias and fluctuations in motor response are related to long term levodopa treatment and are irreversible.
- **Dopamine agonists plus levodopa* (reduced dyskinesia compared with levodopa alone, but increased disability)** One systematic review and subsequent RCTs found that dopamine agonists plus levodopa reduced dyskinesia compared with levodopa alone. However, some of the RCTs found that levodopa alone improved motor impairments and disability compared with dopamine agonists plus levodopa. One subsequent RCT found no significant difference between lisuride (lysuride) plus levodopa and levodopa alone in motor complications at 5 years. One RCT found that pramipexole plus rescue levodopa increased somnolence and hallucinations compared with levodopa alone. There is consensus that levodopa improves motor function, but that dyskinesias and fluctuations in motor response are related to long term levodopa treatment and are irreversible.
- **Levodopa* (more effective at improving motor scores but increased dyskinesia and motor fluctuations compared with dopamine agonists)** We found no placebo controlled RCTs, although experience suggests that levodopa improves motor function, but that dyskinesias and fluctuations in motor response are related to long term levodopa treatment and are irreversible.
- **Modified release levodopa* (no more effective than immediate release levodopa)** Two RCTs in people with early Parkinson's disease found no significant difference between modified and immediate release levodopa in dyskinesia, motor fluctuations, and motor impairment after 5 years. The first RCT found no significant difference between UPDRS activities of daily living score at five years. The second RCT found that modified release co-careldopa improved the activities of daily living score and was better tolerated than immediate release co-careldopa.

Levodopa plus dopamine agonist

- **Adding a dopamine agonist to levodopa*** Systematic reviews found that in people with response fluctuations to levodopa, certain dopamine agonists reduced "off" time, improved motor impairment and activities of daily living, and reduced levodopa dose, but increased dopaminergic adverse effects and dyskinesia.

Surgery in later Parkinson's

- **Pallidal surgery** One systematic review found that unilateral pallidotomy improved motor examination and activities of daily living compared with medical treatment. There is a high incidence of adverse effects with pallidotomy. One RCT found insufficient evidence to assess the effects of pallidotomy compared with those of deep brain stimulation. We found no RCTs comparing pallidal deep brain stimulation versus medical treatment. Three RCTs found insufficient evidence to assess the effects of pallidal deep brain stimulation compared with those of subthalamic deep brain stimulation. Adverse effects are probably less frequent with pallidal deep brain stimulation than with pallidotomy.
- **Subthalamic surgery** One systematic review found no RCTs comparing subthalamic deep brain stimulation versus medical treatment. One small RCT comparing subthalamic deep brain stimulation versus pallidal deep brain stimulation found no significant difference in motor scores.
- **Thalamic surgery** Systematic reviews identified no RCTs comparing thalamic surgery versus medical treatment. One RCT found that thalamic deep brain stimulation improved functional status and caused fewer adverse effects compared with thalamotomy. Case series found that, in 14–23% of people, thalamotomy was associated with permanent complications, including speech disturbance, apraxia, or death.

Rehabilitation

- **Occupational therapy** One systematic review provided insufficient evidence to assess the effects of occupational therapy in later Parkinson's disease.
- **Physiotherapy** Two systematic reviews and a subsequent small crossover RCT found insufficient evidence of the effects of physiotherapy in Parkinson's disease.
- **Speech and language therapy for speech disturbance** One systematic review provided insufficient evidence to assess the effects of speech and language therapy for speech disturbance in later Parkinson's disease.
- **Swallowing therapy for dysphagia** We found no RCTs of swallowing therapy for dysphagia.

DEFINITION Idiopathic Parkinson's disease is an age related neurodegenerative disorder, which is associated with a combination of asymmetrical bradykinesia, hypokinesia, and rigidity, sometimes combined with rest tremor and postural changes. Clinical diagnostic criteria have a sensitivity of 80% and a specificity of 30% (likelihood ratio +ve test 1.14, –ve test 0.67) compared with the gold standard of diagnosis at autopsy.[1] The primary pathology is progressive loss of cells that produce the neurotransmitter dopamine from the substantia nigra in the brainstem. Treatment aims to replace or compensate for the lost dopamine. A good response to treatment supports, but does not confirm, the diagnosis. Several other catecholaminergic neurotransmitter systems are also affected in Parkinson's disease. There is no consistent definition of early and late stage Parkinson's disease. In this chapter we consider people with early stage disease to be those who have not yet developed motor complications associated with long term levodopa treatment (such as dyskinesias**G** and motor fluctuations**G**, also known as "on/off" fluctuations). Late stage Parkinson's disease is taken to mean that motor complications of long term levodopa treatment are present.

INCIDENCE/ PREVALENCE Parkinson's disease occurs worldwide with equal incidence in both sexes. In 5–10% of people who develop Parkinson's disease, the condition appears before the age of 40 years (young onset), and the mean age of onset is about 65 years. Overall age adjusted prevalence is 1% worldwide and 1.6% in Europe, rising from 0.6% at age 60–64 years to 3.5% at age 85–89 years.[2,3]

AETIOLOGY/ RISK FACTORS The cause is unknown. Parkinson's disease may represent different conditions with a final common pathway. People may be affected differently by a combination of genetic and environmental factors (viruses, toxins, 1-methyl-4-phenyl-1,2,3,6-tetrahydropyridine, well water, vitamin E, and smoking).[4–7] First degree relatives of affected people may have twice the risk of developing Parkinson's disease (17% chance of developing the condition in their lifetime) compared with people in the general population.[8–10] However, purely genetic varieties probably affect a small minority of people with Parkinson's disease.[11,12] The parkin gene on chromosome 6 may be associated with Parkinson's disease in families with at least one member with young onset Parkinson's disease, and multiple genetic factors, including the tau gene on chromosome 17q21, may be involved in idiopathic late onset disease.[13,14]

PROGNOSIS Parkinson's disease is currently incurable. Disability is progressive and associated with increased mortality (RR of death compared with matched control populations ranges from 1.6–3.0).[15] Treatment can reduce symptoms and slow progression but it rarely achieves complete control. The question of whether treatment reduces mortality remains controversial.[16] Levodopa seemed to reduce mortality in the UK for 5 years after its introduction, before a "catch up" effect was noted and overall mortality rose toward previous levels. This suggested a limited prolongation of life.[17] An Australian cohort study followed 130 people treated for 10 years.[18] The standardised mortality ratio was 1.58 ($P < 0.001$). At 10 years, 25% had been admitted to a nursing home and only four were still employed. The mean duration of disease until death was 9.1 years. In a similar Italian cohort study conducted over 8 years, the relative risk of death for affected people compared with healthy controls was 2.3 (95% CI 1.60 to 3.39).[19] Age at initial census date was the main predictor of outcome (for people aged < 75 years: RR of death 1.80, 95% CI 1.04 to 3.11; for people aged > 75 years: RR of death 5.61, 95% CI 2.13 to 14.80).

AIMS OF INTERVENTION To improve symptoms and quality of life; to slow disease progression; to limit short and long term adverse effects of treatment, such as motor fluctuations**G**.

OUTCOMES Disease severity; severity of drug induced symptoms or signs; rate of progression of symptoms; need for levodopa or other treatment; adverse effects of treatment;

withdrawals from treatment; and quality of life measures. There are no universal scales, but commonly used scales are the Unified Parkinson's Disease Rating Score (UPDRS**G**), the Hoehn and Yahr**G** disability staging scale, the Webster scale**G**, the Core Assessment Programme for Intracerebral Transplantation,[20,21] the Parkinson's Disease Quality of Life questionnaire,[22] and the Parkinson's Disease questionnaire 39.[23]

METHODS *Clinical Evidence* search and appraisal May 2004. Unless stated otherwise, we have used the term "levodopa" to refer to a combination of levodopa and a peripheral dopa decarboxylase inhibitor.

QUESTION **What are the effects of drug treatments in people with early stage Parkinson's disease?**

OPTION **SELEGILINE**

RCTs found that selegiline improved the symptoms of Parkinson's disease and delayed the need for levodopa compared with placebo. One of the RCTs found limited evidence of increased mortality in people treated with selegiline.

Benefits: **Selegiline versus placebo:** We found no systematic review but found nine RCTs comparing selegiline versus placebo in people with early Parkinson's disease.[24–32] The first RCT (54 people) found that selegiline significantly delayed the need for levodopa compared with placebo (549 days to levodopa with selegiline *v* 312 days to levodopa with placebo; $P < 0.002$).[24] The second RCT (800 people) found that selegiline significantly delayed the need for levodopa compared with placebo for 9 months (HR 0.50 for requiring levodopa in each time period, 95% CI 0.41 to 0.62).[25] The third RCT (101 people newly diagnosed with Parkinson's disease) found that selegiline significantly reduced the deterioration in total Unified Parkinson's Disease Rating Scale (UPDRS**G**) score after 12 months of treatment and 2 months of washout compared with placebo (mean increase in total UPDRS score [a higher score denotes greater disability]: 0.4 with selegiline *v* 5.8 with placebo, $P < 0.001$).[26] The fourth RCT (782 people) found no significant difference between selegiline and placebo in disability after 4 years (Hoehn and Yahr scale**G**: data not presented; North Western University disability scale**G**: results presented graphically; modified 12 item Webster rating scale**G** [0 = normal; 3 = maximum disturbance]: adjusted difference in score 0.51, 95% CI –0.89 to +1.19, $P = 0.95$).[27] The fifth RCT (116 people) found that selegiline significantly reduced the proportion of people who needed an increase in levodopa of 50% or more compared with placebo over a 5 year period (proportion needing increased dose: 50% with selegiline *v* 74% with placebo, $P = 0.03$).[28] The sixth RCT (163 people) found that selegiline significantly improved motor function after 5 years compared with placebo (UPDRS 3 motor score [a higher score denotes greater disability]: 16.6 with selegiline *v* 23.8 with placebo, $P < 0.01$).[29] The seventh RCT (157 people) found that selegiline significantly delayed the need for levodopa compared with placebo (time to levodopa: 12.7 months with selegiline *v* 8.6 months with placebo; $P = 0.028$).[30] The eighth RCT (93 people) found that selegiline significantly improved overall function (determined by total UPDRS score) and motor function scores (UPDRS 3) compared with placebo, but found no significant difference in activities of daily living scores (UPDRS 2) at 3 months (improvement in total UPDRS score: 11.3 with selegiline *v* 5.6 with placebo, $P = 0.008$; improvement in UPDRS 3 motor score: 7.0 with selegiline *v* 1.7 with placebo, $P = 0.03$; improvement in UPDRS 2 activities of daily living score: 3.1 with selegiline *v* 2.3 with placebo, $P = 0.08$).[31] The final RCT (44 people) found that selegiline significantly delayed the need to start levodopa compared with placebo (median time to levodopa: 545 days with selegiline *v* 372 days with placebo; P = 0.03).[32] **Selegiline versus other drugs:** We found no systematic review but found one RCT (475 people), which compared selegiline versus levodopa, bromocriptine, and lisuride. All four drugs improved functional ability, but improvement was significantly lower with selegiline than with the other drugs after a mean of 2 months (mean improvement in UPDRS 2 activities of daily living score: 1.4 with selegiline *v* 2.5 with levodopa *v* 1.9 with bromocriptine *v* 2.6 with lisuride; P = 0.03) for selegiline *v* all other treatments.[33] It found no significant difference between selegiline and the other treatments in improving motor function scores (mean improvement in UPDRS 3 motor score: 2.4 with selegiline *v* 3.4 with levodopa *v* 2.3 with bromocriptine *v* 3.2 with lisuride; P value not reported).[33] The RCT did not report separate statistical differences for selegiline compared with each of the other drugs, so the clinical importance of the results is unclear.

Harms: **Selegiline versus placebo:** One non-systematic review (5 RCTs, 589 people) found no significant difference between selegiline and placebo in mortality at 2.5–4.0 years (15% with selegiline *v* 6% with placebo; HR 1.02, 95% CI 0.44 to 2.37).[34] Extended follow up of one large RCT[25] found no significant difference between selegiline and placebo in mortality at 35 months (no further data reported).[35] Another RCT found that selegiline versus placebo significantly increased mortality at interim analysis after 5.6 years' follow up (HR 1.57, 95% CI 1.07 to 2.31).[27] Consequently, the selegiline arm of the trial was terminated early. Updated analysis (including blinded assessment of cause specific mortality) found that the increase in mortality did not quite reach significance (HR 1.30, 95% CI 0.99 to 1.72).[36,37] **Selegiline versus other drugs:** One retrospective observational study in 12 621 people who had taken an antiparkinsonian drug (excluding those also taking antipsychotic drugs) found increased mortality in people prescribed selegiline, but the increase was of borderline significance (ARI 11%, 95% CI 0% to 23%).[38]

Comment: One RCT (163 people) found that there was no deterioration in symptoms on withdrawal of selegiline after 5 years, whereas there had been an initial wash in beneficial effect when selegiline was started. This suggests that the initial symptomatic effect of selegiline had disappeared after 5 years' therapy.[29] Other studies of early selegiline treatment were either too small or too short to reach a conclusion regarding either the efficacy or safety of selegiline.[34] A systematic review and a large RCT are under way (Clarke C, personal communication, 2005).

OPTION MODIFIED RELEASE LEVODOPA (COMPARED WITH IMMEDIATE RELEASE LEVODOPA)

Two RCTs in people with early Parkinson's disease found no significant difference between modified and immediate release levodopa in dyskinesia, motor fluctuations, and motor impairment after 5 years. The first RCT found no significant difference between UPDRS activities of daily living score at five years. The second RCT found that modified release co-careldopa improved the activities of daily living score and was better tolerated than immediate release co-careldopa.

Benefits: **Modified release levodopa versus immediate release levodopa:** We found no systematic review but found two RCTs.[39,40] The first RCT (134 people with early Parkinson's disease) compared modified release versus immediate release co-beneldopa and found no significant difference at 5 years in the incidence of dyskinesia**G** (41% with modified release levodopa *v* 34% with immediate release levodopa; RR 1.21, 95% CI 0.59 to 1.92). It also found no significant difference in the incidence of motor fluctuations**G** (59% with modified release *v* 57% with immediate release; RR 1.03, 95% CI 0.60 to 1.39), motor impairment (reported as non-significant, data not presented), or activities of daily living (Unified Parkinson's Disease Rating Scale (UPDRS**G**) total scores: data presented graphically, P = 0.53).[39] The second RCT (618 people with early Parkinson's disease) compared modified release versus immediate release co-careldopa. It found no significant difference in dyskinesia or motor fluctuations measured by diary data at 5 years, but found that modified release co-careldopa significantly improved UPDRS 2 activities of daily living compared with immediate release co-careldopa (combined incidence of dyskinesia or motor fluctuations: 22% with modified release co-careldopa *v* 21% with immediate release co-careldopa, reported as non-significant, P value not reported; mean improvement in UPDRS 2 activities of daily living score at 5 years: +0.8 with modified release co-careldopa *v* –0.2 with immediate release co-careldopa, P = 0.03).[40]

Harms: The second RCT found that immediate release co-careldopa significantly increased withdrawals because of nausea compared with modified release co-careldopa (figures not provided, P = 0.007).[40]

Comment: The first RCT had a high withdrawal rate (withdrawal: 42% with immediate release *v* 54% with modified release; analyses were per protocol).[39]

OPTION DOPAMINE AGONISTS VERSUS LEVODOPA IN EARLY DISEASE

One systematic review and one subsequent RCT (published only as an abstract) found that dopamine agonist monotherapy reduced the incidence of dyskinesias and motor complications compared with levodopa monotherapy. However, the subsequent RCT found that dopamine agonist monotherapy was associated with poorer motor scores than levodopa monotherapy, and an increased risk of treatment withdrawal. There is consensus that levodopa improves motor function, but that dyskinesias and fluctuations in motor response are related to long term levodopa treatment and are irreversible.

Benefits: **Dopamine agonists versus levodopa:** We found one systematic review (search date 1999, 6 RCTs, 1170 people)[41] and one subsequent RCT (published only as an abstract).[42] The review compared bromocriptine versus levodopa.[41] It found limited evidence that bromocriptine delayed motor complications and dyskinesias**G** compared with levodopa (data presented graphically), and that, compared with bromocriptine, levodopa reduced motor impairment during the first year of therapy. It found no significant difference between groups for disability (data presented graphically). The subsequent RCT (294 people) found that pergolide significantly reduced the proportion of people experiencing one or more motor complications at 3 years compared with levodopa (16% with pergolide *v* 33% with levodopa, P<0.004), but the Unified Parkinson's Disease Rating Scale**G** motor scores were worse in the pergolide group.[42]

Harms: **Dopamine agonists versus levodopa:** The systematic review comparing bromocriptine versus levodopa identified three RCTs that reported on the incidence of side effects.[41] The first RCT reported nausea in 12/24 (50%) people with levodopa compared with 7/23 (30%) with bromocriptine, the second RCT found that one person in each group experienced hallucinations, and the third RCT found more nausea and hallucinations in those people taking levodopa (further details not given). None of these adverse effects led to withdrawal from the trial. The largest RCT identified by the review found that significantly more people in the bromocriptine group withdrew for all causes than people taking levodopa (RR 2.81, 95% CI 2.20 to 3.58). The RCT comparing pergolide versus levodopa found that significantly more people in the pergolide group withdrew from treatment (18% with pergolide *v* 10% with levodopa, $P < 0.05$).[42]

Comment: There is consensus that levodopa improves motor function, but that dyskinesias**G** and fluctuations in motor response are related to long term levodopa treatment and are irreversible. A large UK based RCT is examining quality of life and health economic outcomes of agonist monotherapy in people likely to develop motor complications (Clarke C, personal communication, 2005). A multicentre North American study is investigating the effect of levodopa on dopaminergic cell death.[43]

OPTION DOPAMINE AGONISTS PLUS RESCUE LEVODOPA VERSUS LEVODOPA ALONE IN EARLY DISEASE

One systematic review and subsequent RCTs found that dopamine agonists plus levodopa reduced dyskinesia compared with levodopa alone. However, some of the RCTs found that levodopa alone improved motor impairments and disability compared with dopamine agonists plus levodopa. One subsequent RCT found no significant difference between lisuride (lysuride) plus levodopa and levodopa alone in motor complications at 5 years. One RCT found that pramipexole plus rescue levodopa increased somnolence and hallucinations compared with levodopa alone. There is consensus that levodopa improves motor function, but that dyskinesias and fluctuations in motor response are related to long term levodopa treatment and are irreversible.

Benefits: We found one systematic review (search date 2000, 5 RCTs, 803 people)[44] and five additional RCTs.[45–49] The review compared bromocriptine plus levodopa versus levodopa alone and found no evidence of consistent differences in occurrence and severity of motor complications, motor impairment, and disability scores (data presented graphically).[44] The first additional RCT (268 people) found that ropinirole plus rescue levodopa significantly reduced the proportion of people developing dyskinesias**G** compared with levodopa alone after 5 years (dyskinesias: 20% with ropinirole plus rescue levodopa *v* 45% with levodopa alone; RR 0.44, 95% CI 0.31 to 0.64).[45] It found no significant difference in disability after 5 years measured by Unified Parkinson's Disease Rating Scale (UPDRS) activities of daily living scores (deterioration in UPDRS**G** activities of daily living score: 1.6 with ropinirole plus rescue levodopa *v* 0.0 with levodopa; adjusted difference 1.53, 95% CI –0.14 to +3.22, $P = 0.08$). It also found that levodopa alone was more effective in increasing motor scores than ropinirole alone (mean improvement in UPDRS II motor score: 0.8 with ropinirole plus levodopa *v* 4.8 with levodopa; adjusted treatment difference 4.48 points, 95% CI 1.25 points to 7.72 points, $P = 0.008$).[45] The second additional RCT (301 people) found that pramipexole plus rescue levodopa significantly reduced the risk of motor complications compared with levodopa alone at 2 years (AR for motor complications: 28% with pramipexole plus rescue levodopa *v* 51% with levodopa alone; HR 0.45, 95% CI 0.30 to 0.66).[46] Improvements in UPDRS motor and activities of daily living scores were significantly greater in the levodopa alone group (mean improvement in motor score: 3.4 with pramipexole plus rescue levodopa *v* 7.3 with levodopa alone, difference in treatments –3.9, 95% CI –5.7 to –2.1, $P < 0.001$; mean improvement in UPDRS activities of daily living score: 1.1 with pramipexole plus rescue levodopa *v* 2.2 with levodopa alone, difference in treatments –1.4, 95% CI –2.2 to –0.5, $P = 0.001$). The third additional RCT (419 people, published as an abstract) compared cabergoline plus rescue levodopa versus levodopa alone.[47] It found that cabergoline significantly reduced motor complications compared with levodopa at 5 years (22% with cabergoline *v* 34% with levodopa, $P < 0.05$), but activities of daily living scores were worse with cabergoline. The fourth additional RCT (90 people, unblinded) comparing lisuride plus rescue levodopa versus levodopa alone found fewer motor complications in the lisuride group after 4 years, although UPDRS motor and activities of daily living scores were worse in those treated with lisuride alone.[48] The fifth additional RCT (82 people, double blinded for first year and subsequently unblinded) found no significant difference between lisuride plus levodopa and levodopa alone in increased motor complications after 5 years (UPDRS 4 score deterioration: 0.47 with levodopa alone *v* 0.41 with levodopa plus lisuride; P reported as non-significant).[49]

Harms: The review found no significant difference between bromocriptine plus levodopa and levodopa alone in occurrence of adverse effects and withdrawal (hallucinations and disorientation, 5 RCTs, 727 people: 51/361 (14%) with bromocriptine plus levodopa *v* 62/366 (17%) with levodopa alone, OR 0.81, 95% CI 0.54 to 1.22; nausea, 5 RCTs, 733 people: OR 1.05, 95% CI 0.74 to 1.48; orthosis, 4 RCTs, 199 people: OR 0.92, 95% CI 0.13 to 6.69; withdrawal, 5 RCTs, 730 people: OR 0.71, 95% CI 0.52 to 0.98).[44] The first additional RCT found that adverse effects, including nausea, vomiting, dizziness, confusion, hallucinations, and delusions, were similar in both treatment groups, although the incidence of hallucinations was higher with ropinirole (hallucinations: 31/179 [17%] with ropinirole *v* 5/89 [6%] with levodopa, P value not reported).[45] The second additional RCT found that pramipexole plus levodopa significantly increased somnolence and hallucinations compared with levodopa alone (somnolence: 49/151 [32%] with pramipexole plus rescue levodopa *v* 26/150 [17%] with levodopa alone, $P < 0.01$; hallucinations: 14/151 [9%] with pramipexole plus rescue levodopa *v* 5/150 [3%] with levodopa alone, $P < 0.05$).[46]

Comment: There is consensus that levodopa improves motor function, but that dyskinesias**G** and fluctuations in motor response are related to long term levodopa treatment and are irreversible. The subsequent RCTs with 5 years of follow up had withdrawal rates of about 50%.[45,47,49] In the fourth additional RCT, the levodopa doses used were low.[48] We found no direct comparisons of individual dopamine agonists in people with early stage Parkinson's disease. See comment under dopamine agonists versus levodopa in early disease, p 1664.

QUESTION **What are the effects of adding a dopamine agonist in people with motor complications from levodopa?**

OPTION **ADDING A DOPAMINE AGONIST TO LEVODOPA**

Systematic reviews found that in people with response fluctuations to levodopa, certain dopamine agonists reduced "off" time, improved motor impairment and activities of daily living, and reduced levodopa dose, but increased dopaminergic adverse effects and dyskinesia.

Benefits: **Adjuvant dopamine agonist versus placebo:** We found six systematic reviews and one subsequent RCT.[50–56] The first review (search date not reported, 7 RCTs, 396 people with later Parkinson's disease taking levodopa) compared adjuvant bromocriptine versus placebo.[50] Heterogeneity in trial design and outcomes made it impossible to draw reliable conclusions. The second review (search date not reported) comparing lisuride versus placebo identified no RCTs.[51] The third review (search date 1998, 1 RCT, 376 people with Parkinson's disease taking levodopa) found that pergolide significantly reduced daily "off" time🅖 over 24 weeks compared with placebo (mean difference in "off" time: 1.6 hours/day; P < 0.001), significantly reduced daily levodopa dose (mean reduction in dose: 235 mg/day with pergolide *v* 51 mg/day with placebo, P < 0.001), and improved motor function and activities of daily living scores (Modified Columbia rating scale🅖 motor score: 46.6 with pergolide *v* 22.3 with placebo, P < 0.001; Modified Columbia rating scale activities of daily living score: 9.7 with pergolide *v* 2.8 with placebo, P < 0.001).[52] The fourth review (search date not reported, 4 RCTs, 669 people with later Parkinson's disease taking levodopa) found that, compared with placebo, pramipexole significantly reduced daily "off" time (WMD 1.8 hours, 95% CI 1.2 hours to 2.3 hours), reduced levodopa dose (WMD 115 mg, 95% CI 87 mg to 143 mg), and improved activities of daily living scores (data presented graphically).[53] The fifth review (search date not reported, 1 RCT, 149 people with Parkinson's disease taking levodopa) compared ropinirole versus placebo.[54] It found insufficient evidence to fully compare ropinirole versus placebo, although it found that ropinirole significantly reduced the required dose of levodopa (WMD 180 mg, 95% CI 106 mg to 253 mg). Complete information on motor impairment and disability was not available. The sixth review (search date not reported) identified three RCTs (268 people with Parkinson's disease taking levodopa). It found no significant difference between cabergoline and placebo in "off" time (2 RCTs, 61 people, WMD +1.14 hours, 95% CI –0.06 hours to +2.33 hours) but found that cabergoline significantly reduced the required dose of levodopa (1 RCT, 188 people, mean levodopa dose reduction: 175 mg with cabergoline v 25.5 mg with placebo; WMD 150 mg, 95% CI 94 mg to 205 mg).[55] There was limited evidence of small but significant benefits in Unified Parkinson's Disease Rating Score (UPDRS🅖) activities of daily living and motor scores with cabergoline (activities of daily living score: data presented graphically; motor scores, 2 RCTs: data presented graphically). The subsequent RCT (313 people) found that pramipexole significantly improved UPDRS🅖 activities of daily living and motor scores compared with placebo (improvement in activities of daily living score: 3.98 with pramipexole *v* 2.03 with placebo, P < 0.001; motor score improvement: 11.75 with pramipexole *v* 5.55 with placebo, P < 0.001) but did not report on "off" time and levodopa dose changes.[56] **Adjuvant dopamine agonists versus each other:** We found five systematic reviews and one subsequent RCT.[56–61] The first systematic review (search date not reported) identified one RCT (20 people with Parkinson's disease taking levodopa) comparing lisuride versus bromocriptine. The RCT found no significant difference in motor fluctuations🅖 (data not presented) or in the Columbia University Rating Scale after 12 weeks (Columbia Rating Scale improvement in mean total score: 20.8. with lisuride *v* 16.2 with bromocriptine; no P value or CI reported).[57] However, follow up may have been too short and the study too small to detect clinically important differences. The second systematic review (search date 1997, 3 RCTs, 293 people with Parkinson's disease taking levodopa) compared pergolide versus bromocriptine.[58] It found that pergolide significantly increased the proportion of people with "marked or moderate improvement" compared with bromocriptine, as measured using a seven point clinician's global assessment scale, but it found no significant difference in reduction in levodopa dose after 8–12 weeks (clinician's global assessment scale, "marked or moderate improvement", 2 RCTs, 305 people: AR 43% with pergolide *v* 30% with bromocriptine; RR 1.45, 95% CI 1.08 to 1.95; difference in reduction in levodopa dose, 3 RCTs: WMD +3 mg/day,

95% CI –4 mg/day to +10 mg/day). Two of the RCTs found that pergolide significantly improved motor impairment compared with bromocriptine (data presented graphically). The third systematic review (search date not reported, 1 RCT, 163 people with Parkinson's disease taking levodopa) compared pramipexole versus bromocriptine.[59] It found that pramipexole reduced "off" time compared with bromocriptine (mean "off" time reduction, 1 RCT, 152 people: 2.6 with pramipexole *v* 1.2 with bromocriptine; WMD 1.4 hours/day, 95% CI 0.0 hours/day to 2.8 hours/day). There were similar UPDRS scores and dyskinesias**G** (no quantitative data provided; no P value or CI reported). The fourth systematic review (search date not reported, 3 RCTs, 482 people with Parkinson's disease taking levodopa) compared ropinirole versus bromocriptine.[60] It found that ropinirole improved "off" time and levodopa dose reduction compared with bromocriptine after 8–25 weeks, but these differences were not significant ("off" time reduction, 2 RCTs, 201 people: WMD +0.8 hours/day, 95% CI –0.1 hours/day to +1.7 hours/day; difference in levodopa dose reduction, 2 RCTs, 203 people: +50 mg/day, 95% CI –49 mg/day to +150 mg/day). It found no significant difference in motor impairments and disability ratings (clinician global impression scale "much" or ("very much" improved, 2 RCTs, 332 people: OR 1.36, 95% CI 0.87 to 2.13; UPDRS motor scores: data presented graphically). The fifth systematic review (search date not reported, 5 RCTs, 1071 people with Parkinson's disease taking levodopa) compared cabergoline versus bromocriptine.[61] Cabergoline improved "off" time compared with bromocriptine after 12–36 weeks, but the difference was not significant ("off" time, 4 RCTs, 612 people: WMD +0.3 hours/day, 95% CI –0.1 hours/day to +0.7 hours/day). Four of the RCTs found no significant difference in motor scores or activities of daily living scores (data presented graphically). Four RCTs found no significant difference in levodopa dose reduction (levodopa dose reduction, 4 RCTs, 909 people: WMD: 6.00, 95% CI –21.8 to +33.8). The subsequent RCT compared pramipexole versus bromocriptine versus placebo. It found no significant difference in UPDRS activities of daily living and motor scores between pramipexole and bromocriptine but was under powered to detect differences between the two (improvement in UPDRS 2 activities of daily living score: 4.0 with pramipexole *v* 3.3 with bromocriptine, P = 0.18; improvement in UPDRS 3 motor score: 11.8 with pramipexole *v* 10.0 with bromocriptine; P = 0.38).[56]

Harms: **Adjuvant dopamine agonist versus placebo:** Six systematic reviews and one subsequent RCT found that agonist treatment significantly increased dopaminergic adverse effects**G** compared with placebo.[50–56] In particular, dyskinesia**G** was significantly increased with pergolide (OR 4.6, 95% CI 3.1 to 7.0), pramipexole (OR 2.1, 95% CI 1.5 to 2.9), and ropinirole (OR 2.9, 95% CI 1.4 to 6.2).[52–54] Withdrawal from treatment was significantly lower with pramipexole than with placebo (OR 0.64, 95% CI 0.44 to 0.93) but not with pergolide, ropinirole, or cabergoline (all cause withdrawals; pramipexole, 4 RCTs, 669 people: OR 0.64, 95% CI 0.44 to 0.93; pergolide, 1 RCT, 376 people: OR 0.88, 95% CI 0.51 to 1.51; ropinirole, 1 RCT, 149 people: OR 0.52, 95% CI 0.24 to 1.09; cabergoline, 3 RCTs, 268 people: OR 0.58, CI not stated, P = 0.13).[52,54,55] **Adjuvant dopamine agonists versus each other:** The four systematic reviews found no significant difference in adverse events between pergolide and bromocriptine, or between pramipexole and bromocriptine,[56,58,59] but nausea was significantly less frequent with ropinirole compared with bromocriptine (OR 0.5, 95% CI 0.3 to 0.8).[60] Dyskinesias and confusion were reported as adverse events more commonly with cabergoline than with bromocriptine, but there was no significant difference in the frequency of other dopaminergic adverse events (dyskinesia: OR 1.6, 95% CI 1.1 to 2.4; confusion: OR 2.0, 95% CI 1.1 to 3.8).[61] We found no studies that directly compared other dopamine agonists.

Comment: None.

QUESTION **What are the effects of surgery in people with later Parkinson's disease?**

OPTION **PALLIDAL SURGERY**

One systematic review found that unilateral pallidotomy improved motor examination and activities of daily living compared with medical treatment. There is a high incidence of adverse effects with pallidotomy. One RCT found insufficient evidence to assess the effects of pallidotomy compared with those of deep brain stimulation. We found no RCTs comparing pallidal deep brain stimulation versus medical treatment. Three RCTs found insufficient evidence to assess the effects of pallidal deep brain stimulation compared with those of subthalamic deep brain stimulation. Adverse effects are probably less frequent with pallidal deep brain stimulation than with pallidotomy.

Benefits: **Pallidotomy versus medical treatment:** We found one systematic review (search date 1999, 2 RCTs), which evaluated mainly unilateral posteroventral pallidotomy**G** in people with later stage Parkinson's disease.[62] The first RCT in the review was initially published as an abstract.[63] The subsequent full report found that pallidotomy significantly improved total Unified Parkinson's Disease Rating Scale (UPDRS**G**) scores compared with medical therapy at 6 months (mean UPDRS score improvement: +25.5 with pallidotomy *v* –3.8 with medical therapy, P < 0.0001).[64] It also found that, compared with medical therapy, pallidotomy significantly improved the "off" phase outcomes for contralateral tremor, bradykinesia, contralateral rigidity, gait, postural, motor fluctuations**G**, dyskinesias**G**, and "off" time**G** (mean improvement from baseline scores, contralateral tremor: 0.7 with pallidotomy *v* 0.1 with medical therapy, P = 0.0007; bradykinesia: 0.8 with pallidotomy *v* ±0.0 with medical therapy, P = 0.004; contralateral rigidity: 2.0 with pallidotomy *v* 0.1 with medical therapy, P = 0.0003; gait: 0.8 with pallidotomy *v* ±0.0 with medical therapy, P = 0.0002; postural stability: +0.6 with pallidotomy *v* –0.3 with medical therapy, P = 0.002; motor fluctuations: +1.38 with pallidotomy *v* –0.02 with medical therapy, P < 0.0001; dyskinesias: +1.8 with pallidotomy *v* –0.1 with medical therapy, P < 0.0001).[64] The second RCT in the systematic review (37 people) compared unilateral pallidotomy versus medical treatment.[65] It found that at 6 months pallidotomy significantly improved "off" phase assessment for UPDRS 3 motor examination, Barthel index**G** activities of daily living, UPDRS II activities of daily living, and Schwab and England scale**G**, but not pain ratings (UPDRS III motor score median improvement: +15 with pallidotomy *v* –2 with medical therapy, P = 0.0004; Barthel index activities of daily living median improvement in score [scale of 0–20; an increase denotes greater functional independence]: +2.5 with pallidotomy *v* –0.5 with medical treatment, P = 0.004; UPDRS 2 median improvement: +7 with pallidotomy *v* –2 with medical treatment, P = 0.002; Schwab and England scale median improvement: +15 with pallidotomy *v* –5 with medical treatment, P = 0.0009; pain score on a 100 mm visual analogue scale: decreased from 27 mm to 14 mm with pallidotomy *v* increased from 15 mm to 22 mm with medical treatment, P = 0.13, CIs not reported).[65] **Pallidotomy versus pallidal deep brain stimulation:** We found one systematic review (search date 2000, 1 RCT).[66] The RCT (13 people) in the systematic review found no significant difference between pallidotomy and deep brain stimulation**G** for symptoms, activities of daily living, and adverse effects over 3 months, but may have been too small to detect clinically important differences.[67] **Pallidal deep brain stimulation versus medical treatment:** We found one systematic review (search date 2000), which identified no RCTs comparing pallidal deep brain stimulation versus medical treatment.[66] We found no subsequent RCTs. **Pallidal deep brain stimulation versus subthalamic deep brain stimulation:** We found two RCTs comparing bilateral pallidal deep brain stimulation versus bilateral subthalamic deep brain stimulation.[1,68] The first RCT (10 people) found no difference in motor scores after 12 months (UPDRS 3 improvement scores: 39% with pallidal stimulation *v* 44% with subthalamic stimulation, P value and CI not reported), but may lacked power to detect clinically important differences.[68] The second RCT (32 people, published only as an abstract) found no significant difference between the groups at 1 year, except reduction of dyskinesia was significantly greater with pallidal stimulation (reduction in dyskinesia score: 63% for pallidal stimulation *v* 14% for subthalamic nucleus stimulation, P = 0.049).[1] **Pallidotomy versus subthalamic deep brain stimulation:** One RCT (34 people) compared unilateral pallidotomy versus bilateral subthalamic deep brain stimulation.[69] It found that unilateral pallidotomy was less effective than bilateral subthalamic stimulation in improving parkinsonian symptoms (median improvement in UPDRS scores after 6 months: 7 with unilateral pallidotomy *v* 19 with bilateral subthalamic deep brain stimulation, P = 0.002; improvement in "on" phase UPDRS motor score: 1 for unilateral pallidotomy *v* 7 for bilateral subthalamic stimulation, P = 0.02; dyskinesias duration score: unchanged with unilateral pallidotomy *v* improved by 1 point with bilateral subthalamic stimulation, P = 0.004). However, there was no significant difference in severity of dyskinesia, P = 0.7).

Harms: **Pallidotomy versus medical treatment:** In the systematic review,[62] the full report of the first RCT (36 people),[63] comparing pallidotomy**G** versus medical treatment, found that 2/18 (11%) people receiving pallidotomy had seizures and 1/18 (6%) had subcortical haemorrhage and transient speech impairment.[64] In the second RCT (35 people), comparing pallidotomy versus medical treatment, 6/19 (31.5%) people who had unilateral pallidotomy had adverse effects persisting for 6 months after surgery, including dysarthria, dysphasia, facial paresis, and urinary incontinence (further data not reported).[65] We found two RCTs assessing neuropsychological, cognitive, or behavioural effects of pallidotomy versus medical treatment.[70,71] The first RCT (35 people) found that left sided, but not right sided, pallidotomy reduced verbal fluency (deterioration in category fluency: 8.7 after left pallidotomy, 3.1 after right pallidotomy, P = 0.04, Kruskal–Wallis test; change in Controlled Oral Word Association Test**G** letter fluency [negative score = deterioration]: –8.0 after left pallidotomy, +2.6 after right pallidotomy, P = 0.01, Kruskal–Wallis test).[70] The second RCT (33 people) found subtle changes on measures of frontal lobe function after 6 months in people with unilateral pallidotomy, and that surgery, particularly left sided surgery, reduced letter fluency compared with medical management at 3 months (actual figures not reported, P = 0.011).[71] One systematic review of case series (search date 1998) found that the incidence of permanent adverse effects of unilateral pallidotomy was 4–46%, with a risk of a serious complication (including death) of 3–10%.[72] Another systematic review of case series (search date 1998) estimated a 10–15% incidence of persistent adverse effects with unilateral pallidotomy.[73] **Pallidotomy versus pallidal deep**

brain stimulation: One systematic review (1 RCT, 13 people) found that side effects and surgery complications occurred in 6/13 [38%] patients and were mild, transient, and unrelated to optic tract injury (adverse effects: 3/16 [19%] with pallidotomy *v* 3/16 [19%] with pallidal deep brain stimulation).[67] One RCT (6 people) compared bilateral pallidotomy versus unilateral pallidotomy plus contralateral pallidal deep brain stimulation**G**.[74] It found that all three people with bilateral pallidotomy experienced severe adverse effects. This led to discontinuation of the study. **Pallidal deep brain stimulation versus medical treatment:** We found one systematic review (search date 2000), which identified no RCTs comparing pallidal deep brain stimulation versus medical treatment.[66] We found no subsequent RCTs. **Pallidal deep brain stimulation versus subthalamic deep brain stimulation** We found two RCTs comparing bilateral pallidal deep brain stimulation versus bilateral subthalamic deep brain stimulation.[1,68] The first RCT (10 people) found no serious intraoperative or perioperative complications in either group, but postoperative complications in both groups included paresthesia, balance impairment, dysarthria, dysphagia, hypomania, and unintentional switching off of stimulators by external electromagnetic fields (data not reported).[68] **Pallidotomy versus subthalamic nucleus deep brain stimulation** One RCT (34 people) compared unilateral pallidotomy versus bilateral subthalamic nucleus deep brain stimulation.[69] It found that adverse effects included one suicide in the pallidotomy group and emotional instability in the subthalamic nucleus deep brain stimulation group (emotional instability: 0/14 [0%] with unilateral pallidal deep brain stimulation *v* 6/20 [30%] with bilateral subthalamic nucleus deep brain stimulation; P values not reported).

Comment: One cohort study found that the improvements seen after unilateral pallidotomy**G** were maintained for 12 months.[75] One recent non-systematic review and consensus statement suggested that gait, balance disorders, and hypophonia were less responsive to surgery than other features of parkinsonism (no further data reported).[76] Transplants and implants of dopaminergic tissue remain experimental. Uncontrolled studies and limited RCT information suggest that adverse effects may be more frequent after lesioning procedures than deep brain stimulation**G** and are more likely to be permanent. Bilateral lesioning is likely to carry a high risk of adverse axial effects**G**. In general, complication rates decline as surgeons develop experience in performing pallidotomy.[76] Some surgeons propose that if bilateral procedures are required, then deep brain stimulation rather than lesioning should be carried out on one side of the brain. Adverse effects linked with deep brain stimulation include haemorrhage, lead displacement, visual deficit, speech, motor or sensory disturbances, psychosis, confusion, and disorientation. Eventually, equipment or battery replacement may be needed, which will require further surgery.

OPTION THALAMIC SURGERY

Systematic reviews identified no RCTs comparing thalamic surgery versus medical treatment. One RCT found that thalamic deep brain stimulation improved functional status and caused fewer adverse effects compared with thalamotomy. Case series found that, in 14–23% of people, thalamotomy was associated with permanent complications, including speech disturbance, apraxia, or death.

Benefits: **Thalamotomy versus medical treatment:** We found two systematic reviews (search dates 1999[62] and 1998[73]), which identified no RCTs of thalamotomy versus medical treatment for Parkinson's disease (see comment below). **Thalamic deep brain stimulation versus medical**

treatment: We found one systematic review (search date 2000).[66] It found no RCTs of thalamic deep brain stimulation**G** versus medical treatment. **Thalamotomy versus thalamic deep brain stimulation:** We found one systematic review (search date 2000).[66] It identified one RCT (68 people with tremor, 45 of whom had Parkinson's disease), which compared thalamotomy versus thalamic deep brain stimulation.[77] Subgroup analysis in people with Parkinson's disease found that thalamic deep brain stimulation significantly improved functional status after 6 months compared with thalamotomy (outcome assessed using Frenchay Activities Index: 0 = worst score, 60 = best score; improvement in score: 5.5 with deep brain stimulation *v* 0.8 with thalamotomy, 95% CI for between group difference 1.2 to 8.0).

Harms: **Thalamotomy versus medical treatment:** Case series included in the second systematic review found that thalamotomy was associated with reversible complications (lasting < 3 months) in 36–61% of people and permanent complications, including speech disturbance, apraxia, or death, in 14–23%.[73] Bilateral thalamotomy carries a high risk of speech disturbance.[73] **Thalamic deep brain stimulation versus medical treatment:** The systematic review did not identify any RCTs.[66] **Thalamotomy versus thalamic deep brain stimulation:** We found one systematic review (search date 2000).[66] One RCT found that adverse effects including somnolence, cognitive deterioration, dysarthria, weakness, and ataxia were significantly less common with deep brain stimulation**G** than with thalamotomy after 6 months (AR 47% with thalamotomy *v* 18% with deep brain stimulation, P = 0.02).[77]

Comment: The reviews found limited evidence from case series that thalamic surgery may not be as useful as pallidal or subthalamic surgery**G** for parkinsonian features other than tremor.[62,73] The second systematic review did not describe fully the case series it identified, focusing on results from "key studies".[73] See comment under pallidal surgery, p 1670.

OPTION SUBTHALAMIC SURGERY

One systematic review found no RCTs comparing subthalamic deep brain stimulation versus medical treatment. One small RCT comparing subthalamic deep brain stimulation versus pallidal deep brain stimulation found no significant difference in motor scores.

Benefits: **Subthalamic deep brain stimulation versus medical treatment:** We found one systematic review (search date 2000), which identified no RCTs comparing subthalamic deep brain stimulation**G** versus medical treatment.[66] We found no subsequent RCTs. **Subthalamic deep brain stimulation versus pallidal deep brain stimulation:** See benefits of pallidal surgery, p 1668.

Harms: **Subthalamic deep brain stimulation versus medical treatment:** We found one systematic review (search date 2000), which identified no RCTs comparing subthalamic deep brain stimulation**G** versus medical treatment.[66] We found no subsequent RCTs. **Subthalamic deep brain stimulation versus pallidal deep brain stimulation:** See comment under pallidal surgery, p 1670.

Comment: Larger and longer term RCTs are needed to compare the effects of pallidal versus subthalamic stimulation. A large RCT comparing quality of life and costs of subthalamic or pallidal lesioning and deep brain stimulation**G** surgery versus best medical treatment is currently under way in the UK (Clarke C, personal communication, 2002).

QUESTION **What are the effects of rehabilitation treatments in people with Parkinson's disease?**

OPTION **PHYSIOTHERAPY**

Two systematic reviews and a subsequent small crossover RCT found insufficient evidence of the effects of physiotherapy in Parkinson's disease.

Benefits: We found two systematic reviews and one crossover subsequent RCT.[78–80] The first review (search date 2000, 11 RCTs, 280 people with early or late stage Parkinson's disease) compared physiotherapy versus no treatment or versus inactive physiotherapy.[78] The review was unable to draw conclusions on the effects of physiotherapy in Parkinson's disease because of the small numbers of people, methodological flaws, different types of physiotherapy used, and the wide variety of outcome measures in the RCTs. The second systematic review (search date 1999, 8 RCTs included in the first review, 4 quasi-randomised studies) compared physiotherapy versus no treatment or versus other treatment (occupational therapy, regular exercises, non-specified psychological treatment).[79] It also found that methodological flaws of trials and trial heterogeneity made it difficult to draw conclusions on the effects of physiotherapy. The subsequent crossover RCT (17 people with early Parkinson's disease) found that speed dependent treadmill training (STTⒼ) and limited progressive treadmill training (LTTⒼ) were more effective than conventional gait training (CGTⒼ) or a control intervention in improving speed and stride length.[80] However, these results must be viewed with caution, as the numbers in the study were small, the intervention lasted only one day, and no washout period was included.

Harms: The systematic reviews and subsequent RCT gave no information on adverse effects.[78–80]

Comment: Further, larger, well designed RCTs are required.

OPTION **OCCUPATIONAL THERAPY**

One systematic review provided insufficient evidence to assess the effects of occupational therapy in later Parkinson's disease.

Benefits: We found one systematic review (search date 2000, 2 RCTs, 84 people with early stage or late stage Parkinson's disease).[81] One RCT in the review compared occupational therapy versus no treatment, and the other RCT compared occupational therapy plus physiotherapy versus physiotherapy alone. The review was unable to draw conclusions on the effects of occupational therapy because of the small number of people in the RCTs, methodological flaws, trial heterogeneity, and the variety of outcome measures used.[81]

Harms: The RCTs in the review gave no information on adverse effects.[81]

Comment: Further, larger, well designed RCTs are required.

OPTION **SPEECH AND LANGUAGE THERAPY FOR SPEECH DISTURBANCE**

One systematic review provided insufficient evidence to assess the effects of speech and language therapy for speech disturbance in later Parkinson's disease.

Benefits: We found one systematic review (search date 2000, 3 RCTs, 63 people), which compared speech and language therapy versus no treatment for speech disturbance.[82] It was unable to draw conclusions on the effects of speech and language therapy because of the small number of people, methodological flaws, and the variety of outcome measures used in the RCTs.

Harms: The RCTs in the review gave no information on adverse effects.[82]

Comment: Further, larger, well designed RCTs are required.

OPTION SWALLOWING THERAPY FOR DYSPHAGIA

We found no RCTs of swallowing therapy for dysphagia.

Benefits: We found one systematic review (search date 2000) of swallowing therapy for dysphagia, which did not identify any RCTs.[83]

Harms: We found one systematic review (search date 2000) of swallowing therapy for dysphagia, which did not identify any RCTs.[83]

Comment: None.

GLOSSARY

Axial effects Changes affecting axial body sections, such as head and trunk, rather than the limbs.

Barthel index Assessment of functional ability to perform activities of daily living, using 14 different items and a scale of 0–20; a higher score denotes greater functional independence.

Columbia University Rating Scale Assessment of motor impairment and activities of daily living against 13 items, using a five point scale for each to give a total score between 0 = normal to 65 = maximum disability.

Conventional gait training (CGT) Physiotherapeutic gait therapy based on the latest description of the principles of the proprioceptive neuromuscular facilitation and Bobath concepts.

Controlled Oral Word Association Test (COWAT) Most frequently used for assessing verbal fluency and the ease with which a person can think of words that begin with a specific letter; a higher score denotes greater verbal fluency. Different forms of this procedure exist.

Dopaminergic adverse effects Include dyskinesia, hallucinations, and psychosis.

Dyskinesias Abnormal or involuntary writhing or jerky movements distinct from tremor.

Hoehn and Yahr scale Five stage disability scale: stage one = least severe; stage five = most severe. This rating system has been largely supplanted by the Unified Parkinson's Disease Rating Scale, which is much more complicated.

Limited progressive treadmill training (LTT) The patient's maximum overground walking speed is determined before the first training session. Training speed is increased over a number of sessions by a percentage of the maximum initial walking speed.

Modified 12 item Webster rating scale Assessment of severity of disease and clinical impairment against 12 items using a scale of 0 = normal to 3 = maximum impairment: bradykinesia, rigidity, posture, upper extremity swing, gait, tremor at rest, facies, seborrhoea, speech, self care, balance, and rising from a chair.

Motor fluctuations Fluctuations in motor symptoms, such as bradykinesia, rigidity, and tremor, during a day. Motor fluctuations are sometimes called "on/off" fluctuations.

North Western University disability scale Measurement of six functions overall: four items measured on a 10 point scale (walk, clothing, toilet, word; 0 = maximum disturbance; 10 = normal, for example for walk: "never moves " (0–3), "sometimes moves" (4–6), "always moves" (7–10); two items (food, meal) measured on a progressing five point scale.

"Off" time Periods when treatment is not working. "On" time is the period when treatment is working. "On/off" fluctuations are sometimes known as motor fluctuations.

Pallidal, thalamic or sub-thalamic deep brain stimulation Focal electrical brain stimulation through a stereotactically implanted wire.

Pallidotomy Making a permanent surgical lesion, usually thermally or electrically, in the globus pallidum.
Response fluctuations Fluctuations in a person's overall response to treatment during a day.
Schwab and England scale Assessment of functional disability on a scale of **0%** = vegetative to **100%** = completely independent (able to do all chores without slowness, difficulty, or impairment).
The patient's maximum overground walking speed is determined before the first training session. After a warm up, the belt speed is increased, in communication with the patient, to the highest speed at which the patient can walk safely and without stumbling. At each subsequent training session, the treadmill is set (after a short warm up) to the last achieved maximum speed from the previous session.
Subthalamic surgery Includes subthalamotomy, in which a lesion is made in the subthalamic nucleus, or subthalamic deep brain stimulation, in which a stimulator is placed in the subthalamic nucleus.
Unified Parkinson's Disease Rating Scale (UPDRS) A scale used to measure the severity of Parkinson's disease. A higher score denotes greater disability. It has six parts: mentation, behaviour, and mood (UPDRS 1); activities of daily living (UPDRS 2); motor examination (UPDRS 3); complications of treatment (UPDRS 4); a global disability staging score (UPDRS 5); and a global activities of daily living score (UPDRS 6).
Webster rating scale Assessment of severity of disease and clinical impairment against 10 items using a scale of 0 = normal to 3 = maximum impairment: bradykinesia, rigidity, posture, upper extremity swing, gait, tremor at rest, facies, seborrhoea, speech, and self care.

Substantive changes

Adding a dopamine agonist to levodopa One RCT added; [56] categorisation unchanged.
Pallidal surgery Two RCTs added;[1,69] categorisation unchanged.
Physiotherapy One RCT added;[80] categorisation unchanged.

REFERENCES

1. Marks W, Chadwick W, Ostrem J, Starr P. A prospective, randomized trial of globus pallidus vs. subthalamic nucleus deep brain stimulation for Parkinson's disease. *Mov Disord* 2004;19:S318–S319.
2. Zhang Z, Roman G. Worldwide occurrence of Parkinson's disease: an updated review. *Neuroepidemiology* 1993;12:195–208.
3. De Rijk MC, Tzourio C, Breteler MMB, et al. Prevalence of parkinsonism and Parkinson's disease in Europe: the EUROPARKINSON collaborative study. *J Neurol Neurosurg Psychiatry* 1997;62:10–15.
4. Ben-Shlomo Y. How far are we in understanding the cause of Parkinson's disease? *J Neurol Neurosurg Psychiatry* 1996;61:4–16.
5. De Rijk M, Breteler M, den Breeilnen J, et al. Dietary antioxidants and Parkinson's disease: the Rotterdam study. *Arch Neurol* 1997;54:762–765.
6. Hellenbrand W, Seidler A, Robra B, et al. Smoking and Parkinson's disease: a case-control study in Germany. *Int J Epidemiol* 1997;26:328–339.
7. Tzourio C, Rocca W, Breteler M, et al. Smoking and Parkinson's disease: an age-dependent risk effect? *Neurology* 1997;49:1267–1272.
8. Marder K, Tang M, Mejia H, et al. Risk of Parkinson's disease among first degree relatives: a community based study. *Neurology* 1996;47:155–160.
9. Jarman P, Wood N. Parkinson's disease genetics comes of age. *BMJ* 1999;318:1641–1642.
10. Lazzarini A, Myers R, Zimmerman T, et al. A clinical genetic study of Parkinson's disease: evidence for dominant transmission. *Neurology* 1994;44:499–506.
11. Gasser T, Müller-Myhsok B, Wszolek Z, et al. A susceptibility locus for Parkinson's disease maps to chromosome 2p13. *Nat Genet* 1998;18:262–265.
12. Tanner C, Ottman R, Goldman S, et al. Parkinson's disease in twins. An etiologic study. *JAMA* 1999;281:341–346.
13. Scott WK, Nance MA, Watts RL, et al. Complete genomic screen in Parkinson disease: evidence for multiple genes. *JAMA* 2001;286:2239–2244.
14. Martin ER, Scott WK, Nance MA, et al. Association of single-nucleotide polymorphisms of the tau gene with late-onset Parkinson disease. *JAMA* 2001;286:2245–2250.
15. Parkinson Study Group. Mortality in DATATOP: a multicenter trial in early Parkinson's disease. *Ann Neurol* 1998;43:318–325.
16. Rajput A, Uitti J, Offord K. Timely levodopa (LD) administration prolongs survival in Parkinson's disease. *Parkinson Relat Disord* 1997;3:159–165.
17. Clarke CE. Does levodopa therapy delay death in Parkinson's disease? A review of the evidence. *Mov Disord* 1995;10:250–256.
18. Hely MA, Morris JGL, Traficante R, et al. The Sydney multicentre study of Parkinson's disease: progression and mortality at 10 years. *J Neurol Neurosurg Psychiatry* 1999;67:300–307.
19. Morgante L, Salemi G, Meneghini F, et al. Parkinson disease survival. A population-based study. *Arch Neurol* 2000;57:507–512.
20. Fahn S, Elton L, for the UPDRS Development Committee. Unified Parkinson's disease rating scale. In: Fahn S, Marsden C, Calne D, et al, eds. *Recent developments in Parkinson's disease*, Vol. 2. Florham Park: Macmillan Healthcare Information, 1987:153–163.
21. Langston JW, Widner H, Goetz CG, et al. Core Assessment Program for Intracerebral Transplantations (CAPIT). *Mov Disord* 1992;7:2–13.
22. De Boer A, Wijker W, Speelman J, et al. Quality of life in people with Parkinson's disease: development of a questionnaire. *J Neurol Neurosurg Psychiatry* 1996;61:70–74.
23. Peto V, Jenkinson C, Fitzpatrick R, et al. The development and validation of a short measure of

functioning and well being for individuals with Parkinson's disease. *Qual Life Res* 1995;4:241–248.
24. Tetrud JW, Langston JW. The effect of deprenyl (selegiline) on the natural history of Parkinson's disease. *Science* 1989;245:519–522.
25. The Parkinson's Disease Study Group. Effects of tocopherol and deprenyl on the progression of disability in early Parkinson's disease. *N Engl J Med* 1993;328:176–183.
26. Olanow CW, Hauser RA, Gauger L, et al. The effect of deprenyl and levodopa on the progression of Parkinson's disease. *Ann Neurol* 1995;38:771–777.
27. Lees AJ, for the Parkinson's Disease Research Group of the United Kingdom. Comparison of therapeutic effects and mortality data of levodopa and levodopa combined with selegiline in people with early, mild Parkinson's disease. *BMJ* 1995;311:1602–1607.
28. Przuntek H, Conrad B, Dichgans J, et al. SELEDO: a 5-year long-term trial on the effect of selegiline in early Parkinsonian patients treated with levodopa. *Eur J Neurol* 1999;6:141–150.
29. Larson JP, Boas J, Erdal JE, et al. Does selegiline modify the progression of early Parkinson's disease? Results from a five-year study. *Eur J Neurol* 1999;6:539–547.
30. Palhagen S, Heinonen E, Hagglund J, et al. Selegiline delays the onset of disability in *de novo* parkinsonian patients. *Neurology* 1998;51:520–525.
31. Allain H, Pollack P, Neukirch H, et al. Symptomatic effect of selegiline in *de novo* parkinsonian patients. *Mov Disord* 1993;8:S36–S40.
32. Myllala V, Sotaniemi K, Hakulinen P, et al. Selegiline as the primary treatment of Parkinson's disease-a long term double-blind study. *Acta Neurol Scand* 1997;95:211–218.
33. The Italian Parkinson Study Group. A multicenter Italian randomised study on early treatment of Parkinson disease: comparison of L-dopa, L-deprenyl and dopaminoagonists. Study design and short term results. *Italian J Neurol Sci* 1992;13:735–739.
34. Olanow CW, Myllyla V, Sotaniemi K, et al. Effect of selegiline on mortality in people with Parkinson's disease: a meta-analysis. *Neurology* 1998;51:825–830.
35. Parkinson Study Group. Impact of deprenyl and tocopherol treatment for Parkinson's disease in DATATOP people requiring levodopa. *Ann Neurol* 1996;39:37–45.
36. Ben-Shlomo Y, Churchyard A, Head J, et al. Investigation by Parkinson's Disease Research Group of United Kingdom into excess mortality seen with combined levodopa and selegiline treatment in people with early, mild Parkinson's disease: further results of randomised trial and confidential inquiry. *BMJ* 1998;316:1191–1196.
37. Counsell C. Effect of adding selegiline to levodopa in early, mild Parkinson's disease. *BMJ* 1998;17:1586.
38. Thorogood M, Armstrong B, Nichols T, et al. Mortality in people taking selegiline: observational study. *BMJ* 1998;317:252–254.
39. Dupont E, Andersen A, Boas J, et al. Sustained-release Madopar HBS compared with standard Madopar in the long-term treatment of *de novo* Parkinsonian patients. *Acta Neurol Scand* 1996;93:14–20.
40. Block G, Liss C, Reines S, et al. Comparison of immediate release and controlled release carbidopa/levodopa in Parkinson's disease. *Eur Neurol* 1997;37:23–27.
41. Ramaker C, van Hilten JJ. Bromocriptine versus levodopa in early Parkinson's disease. In: The Cochrane Library, Issue 3, 2003. Oxford: Update Software. Search date 1999; primary sources Cochrane Movement Disorders Group Specialised Register, Cochrane Controlled Trials Register, Medline, Embase, pharmaceutical companies, experts for unpublished studies, and hand searches of references and selected neurology journals.
42. Oertel WH. Pergolide versus levodopa monotherapy (PELMOPET). *Mov Disord* 2000;15(suppl 3):4.
43. Fahn S. Parkinson's disease, the effect of levodopa and the ELLDOPA trial. *Arch Neurol* 1999;56:529–535.
44. Ramaker C, van Hilten JJ. Bromocriptine/levodopa combined versus levodopa alone for early Parkinson's disease (Cochrane Review). In: The Cochrane Library, Issue 3, 2003. Oxford :Update Software. Search date 2000; primary sources Cochrane Movement Disorders Group Specialised Register, Cochrane Controlled Trials Register, Medline, Embase, pharmaceutical companies, experts for unpublished studies, and hand searches of references and selected neurology journals.
45. Rascol O, Brooks D, Korczyn A, et al. A five-year study of the incidence of dyskinesia in people with early Parkinson's disease who were treated with ropinirole or levodopa. *N Engl J Med* 2000;342:1484–1491.
46. Parkinson Study Group. Pramipexole versus levodopa as initial treatment for Parkinson's disease. *JAMA* 2000;284:1931–1938.
47. Rinne U. A 5-year double-blind study with cabergoline versus levodopa in the treatment of early Parkinson's disease. *Parkinsonism Relat Disord* 1999;5(suppl):84.
48. Rinne U. Lisuride, a dopamine agonist in the treatment of early Parkinson's disease. *Neurology* 1989;39:336–339.
49. Allain H, Destee A, Petit H, et al. Five-year follow-up of early lisuride and levodopa combination therapy versus levodopa monotherapy in de novo Parkinson's disease. *Eur Neurol* 2000;44:22–30.
50. van Hilten JJ, Ramaker C, van de Beek WJT, et al. Bromocriptine for levodopa-induced motor complications in Parkinson's disease. In: The Cochrane Library, Issue 3, 2003. Oxford: Update Software. Search date not reported; primary sources Cochrane Controlled Trials Register, Medline, Scisearch, pharmaceutical companies, experts for unpublished studies, and hand searches of references.
51. Clarke CE, Speller JM. Lisuride for levodopa-induced complications in Parkinson's disease. In: The Cochrane Library, Issue 3, 2003. Oxford: Update Software. Search date not reported; primary sources Medline, Embase, Cochrane Controlled Trials Register, pharmaceutical companies, and hand searches of references.
52. Clarke CE, Speller JM. Pergolide for levodopa-induced complications in Parkinson's disease. In: The Cochrane Library, Issue 3, 2003. Oxford: Update Software. Search date 1998; primary sources Medline, Embase, Cochrane Controlled Trials Register, pharmaceutical companies, and hand searches of references.
53. Clarke CE, Speller JM, Clarke JA. Pramipexole for levodopa-induced complications in Parkinson's disease. In: The Cochrane Library, Issue 3, 2003. Oxford: Update Software. Search date not reported; primary sources Cochrane Movement Disorders Group Specialised Register, Cochrane Controlled Trials Register, Medline, Embase, pharmaceutical companies, experts for unpublished studies, and hand searches of references and selected neurology journals.
54. Clarke CE, Deane KHO. Ropinirole for levodopa-induced complications in Parkinson's disease. In: The Cochrane Library, Issue 3, 2003. Oxford: Update Software. Search date not reported; primary sources Cochrane Movement Disorders Group Specialised Register, Cochrane Controlled Trials Register, Medline, Embase, pharmaceutical companies, experts for unpublished studies, and hand searches of references and selected neurology journals.
55. Clarke CE, Deane KH. Cabergoline for levodopa-induced complications in Parkinson's disease. In: The Cochrane Library, Issue 3, 2003. Oxford: Update Software. Search date not reported; primary sources Medline, Embase, Cochrane Controlled Trials Register, hand searches of references and selected neurology journals, and contact with Pharmacia Upjohn.

56. Mizuno Y, Yanagisawa N, Kuno S, et al., Japanese Pramipexole Study Group. Randomized, double-blind study of pramipexole with placebo and bromocriptine in advanced Parkinson's disease. *Mov Disord* 2003;18:1149–1156.
57. Clarke CE, Speller JM. Lisuride versus bromocriptine for levodopa-induced complications in Parkinson's disease. In: The Cochrane Library, Issue 3, 2003. Oxford: Update Software. Search date not reported; primary sources Medline, Embase, Cochrane Controlled Trials Register, hand searches of the neurology literature, reference lists of identified studies, and contact with pharmaceutical companies.
58. Clarke CE, Speller JM. Pergolide versus bromocriptine for levodopa-induced motor complications in Parkinson's disease. In: The Cochrane Library, Issue 3, 2003. Oxford: Update Software. Search date 1997; primary sources Medline, Embase, Cochrane Controlled Trials Register, pharmaceuticals companies, and hand searches of references.
59. Clarke CE, Speller JM, Clarke JA. Pramipexole versus bromocriptine for levodopa-induced complications in Parkinson's disease. In: The Cochrane Library, Issue 3, 2003. Oxford: Update Software. Search date not reported; primary sources Cochrane Movement Disorders Group Specialised Register, Cochrane Controlled Trials Register, Medline, Embase, pharmaceutical companies, experts for unpublished studies, and hand searches of references and selected neurology journals.
60. Clarke CE, Deane KHO. Ropinirole versus bromocriptine for levodopa-induced complications in Parkinson's disease. In: The Cochrane Library, Issue 3, 2003. Oxford: Update Software. Search date not reported; primary sources Cochrane Movement Disorders Group Specialised Register, Cochrane Controlled Trials Register, Medline, Embase, pharmaceutical companies, experts for unpublished studies, and hand searches of references and selected neurology journals.
61. Clarke CE, Deane KD. Cabergoline versus bromocriptine for levodopa-induced complications in Parkinson's disease. In: The Cochrane Library, Issue 3, 2003. Oxford: Update Software. Search date not reported; primary sources Cochrane Movement Disorders Group Specialised Register, Cochrane Controlled Trials Register, Medline, Embase, pharmaceutical companies, experts for unpublished studies, and hand searches of references and selected neurology journals.
62. Development and Evaluation Committee. Report 105. *Pallidotomy, thalotomy and deep brain stimulation for severe Parkinson's disease*. Southampton: Wessex Institute for Health Research and Development, 1999. Search date 1999; primary sources Cochrane Library, Health Technology Assessment database, Medline, Science Citation Index, Biosis, Embase, Index to Scientific and Technical Proceedings, Inspec, and Best Evidence.
63. Vitek J, Bakay R, Freeman A, et al. Randomised clinical trial of pallidotomy for Parkinson's disease. *Neurology* 1998;50(suppl 4):A80.
64. Vitek JL, Bakay RA, Freeman A, et al. Randomized trial of pallidotomy versus medical therapy for Parkinson's disease. *Ann Neurol* 2003;53:558–569.
65. De Bie R, de Haan R, Nijssen P, et al. Unilateral pallidotomy in Parkinson's disease: a randomised, single-blind, multicentre trial. *Lancet* 1999;354:1665–1669.
66. Medical Services Advisory Committee. Deep brain stimulation for Parkinson's disease. Australian Department of Health and Ageing, Canberra, 2001. Search date 2000; primary sources Cochrane library, Medline, Psycinfo, Cinahl, Current Contents, PreMedline, Healthstar, Trip, and Australasian Medical Index.
67. Merello M, Nouzeilles MI, Kuzis G, et al. Unilateral radiofrequency lesion versus electrostimulation of posteroventral pallidum: a prospective randomized comparison. *Mov Disord* 1999;14:50–56.
68. Esselink R, Bie de R, de Haan R, et al. Unilateral pallidotomy versus bilateral subthalamic nucleus stimulation in PD: A randomized trial. *Neurology* 2004;62:201–207.
69. Burchiel K, Anderson V, Favre J, et al. Comparison of pallidal and subthalamic nucleus deep brain stimulation for advanced Parkinson's disease: results of a randomized, blinded pilot study. *Neurosurgery* 1999;45:1375–1384.
70. Schmand B, de Bie R, Koning-Haanstra M, et al. Unilateral pallidotomy in PD. A controlled study of cognitive and behavioural effects. *Neurology* 2000;54:1058–1064.
71. Green J, McDonald W, Vitek J, et al. Neuropsychological and psychiatric sequelae of pallidotomy for PD. Clinical trial findings. *Neurology* 2002;58:858–865.
72. Gregory R. Posteroventral pallidotomy for advanced Parkinson's disease: a systematic review. *Neurol Rev Int* 1999;3:8–12. Search date 1998; primary sources not stated.
73. Hallett M, Litvan I. The Task Force on Surgery for Parkinson's Disease. Evaluation of surgery for Parkinson's disease. A report of the Therapeutics and Technology Assessment Subcommittee of the American Academy of Neurology. *Neurology* 1999;53:1910–1921. Search date 1998; primary sources Medline, Embase, Biosis.
74. Merello M, Starkstein S, Nouzeilles M, et al. Bilateral pallidotomy for treatment of Parkinson's disease induced corticobulbar syndrome and psychic akinesia avoidable by globus pallidus lesion combined with contralateral stimulation. *J Neurol Neurosurg Psychiatry* 2001;71:611–614.
75. De Bie R, Schuurman P, Bosch D, et al. Outcome of unilateral pallidotomy in advanced Parkinson's disease: cohort study of 32 patients. *J Neurol Neurosurg Psychiatry* 2001;71:375–382.
76. Bronstein JM, DeSalles A, DeLong MR. Stereotactic pallidotomy in the treatment of Parkinson's disease. *Arch Neurol* 1999;56:1064–1069.
77. Schuurman P, Bosch D, Bossuyt P, et al. A comparison of continuous thalamic stimulation and thalamotomy for suppression of severe tremor. *N Engl J Med* 2000;342:461–468.
78. Deane KHO, Jones D, Playford ED, et al. Physiotherapy versus placebo or no intervention in Parkinson's disease. In: The Cochrane Library. Issue 3, 2003. Oxford: Update Software. Search date 2000; primary sources Medline, Embase, Cinahl, Isi-Sci, Amed, Mantis, Rehabdata, Rehadat, Gerolit, Pascal, Lilacs, MedCarib, Jicst-EPlus, Aim, IMEMR, Sigle, ISI-ISTP, Dissabs, Conference Papers Index, Aslib Index to Theses, Cochrane Library, the CentreWatch Clinical Trials listing service, the metaRegister of Controlled Trials, ClinicalTrials.gov, Crisp, Pedro, Niddr and NRR, and hand searches of references.
79. de Goede CJ, Keus SH, Kwakkel G, et al. The effects of physical therapy in Parkinson's disease: a research synthesis. *Arch Phys Med Rehab* 2001;2:509–515. Search date 1999; primary sources Medline, Cinahl, and hand searches of references.
80. Pohl M, Rockstroh G, Ruckriem S, et al. Immediate effects of speed-dependent treadmill training on gait parameters in early Parkinson's disease. *Arch Phys Med Rehab* 2003;84:1760–1766.
81. Deane KHO, Ellis-Hill C, Playford ED, et al. Occupational therapy for Parkinson's disease. In: The Cochrane Library. Issue 3, 2003. Oxford: Update Software. Search date 2000; primary sources Medline, Embase, Cinahl, Isi-Sci, Amed, Mantis, Rehabdata, Rehadat, Gerolit, Pascal, Lilacs, MedCarib, Jicst-EPlus, Aim, IMEMR, Sigle, ISI-ISTP, Dissabs, Conference Papers Index, Aslib Index to Theses, Cochrane Library, the CentreWatch Clinical Trials listing service, the metaRegister of Controlled Trials, ClinicalTrials.gov, Crisp, Pedro, Niddr and NRR, and hand searches of references.
82. Deane KHO, Whurr R, Playford ED, et al. Speech and language therapy versus placebo or no intervention for dysarthria in Parkinson's disease. In: The

Cochrane Library Issue 3, 2003. Oxford: Update Software. Search date 2000; primary sources Medline, Embase, Cinahl, Isi-Sci, Amed, Mantis, Rehabdata, Rehadat, Gerolit, Pascal, Lilacs, MedCarib, Jicst-EPlus, Aim, IMEMR, Sigle, ISI-ISTP, Dissabs, Conference Papers Index, Aslib Index to Theses, Cochrane Library, the CentreWatch Clinical Trials listing service, the metaRegister of Controlled Trials, ClinicalTrials.gov, Crisp, Pedro, Niddr and NRR, and hand searches of references.

83. Deane KHO, Whurr R, Clarke CE, et al. Non-pharmacological therapies for dysphagia in Parkinson's disease. In: The Cochrane Library Issue 3, 2003. Oxford: Update Software. Search date 2000; Primary sources Medline, Embase, Cinahl, Isi-Sci, Amed, Mantis, Rehabdata, Rehadat, Gerolit, Pascal, Lilacs, MedCarib, Jicst-EPlus, Aim, IMEMR, Sigle, ISI-ISTP, Dissabs, Conference Papers Index, Aslib Index to Theses, Cochrane Library, the CentreWatch Clinical Trials listing service, the metaRegister of Controlled Trials, ClinicalTrials.gov, Crisp, Pedro, Niddr and NRR, and hand searches of references.

Carl Clarke
Reader in Clinical Neurology
University of Birmingham
Birmingham
UK

A Peter Moore
Senior Lecturer in Neurology
University of Liverpool
Liverpool
UK

Competing interests: APM has been reimbursed by various manufacturers for attending and speaking at conferences, and for consulting. CC has been paid by various manufacturers of the drugs dealt with above for speaking at meetings and attending conferences.

Trigeminal neuralgia

Search date November 2003

Joanna M Zakrzewska and Benjamin C Lopez

QUESTIONS

INTERVENTIONS

Key Messages

- **Carbamazepine** One systematic review of three crossover RCTs found that carbamazepine increased pain relief compared with placebo, but also increased adverse effects (drowsiness, dizziness, constipation, and ataxia). One small RCT provided insufficient evidence to compare tizanidine versus carbamazepine. One RCT found that carbamazepine was less effective than pimozide in reducing pain over 8 weeks, but was associated with fewer adverse effects (including hand tremors, memory impairment, and involuntary movements). One systematic review identified one RCT of tocainide versus carbamazepine that was of insufficient quality.
- **Pimozide** One RCT found that pimozide reduced pain over 8 weeks compared with carbamazepine, but increased adverse effects (including hand tremors, memory impairment, and involuntary movements). Cardiac toxicity and sudden death have been reported with pimozide.
- **Combined streptomycin and lidocaine nerve block** Small RCTs provided insufficient evidence about the effects of nerve block using streptomycin plus lidocaine compared with nerve block using lidocaine alone.
- **Proparacaine eye drops** One RCT found no significant difference in pain at 30 days between placebo and a single application of proparacaine hydrochloride eye drops to the eye on the same side as the pain.
- **Tocainide** One systematic review found one RCT of tocainide versus carbamazepine, which was of insufficient quality. The use of tocainide is limited by considerable harms (including serious haematological effects).

Clin Evid 2005;13:1678–1686.

- **Baclofen; lamotrigine; other drugs (phenytoin, clonazepam, sodium valproate, gabapentin, mexiletine, oxcarbazepine, topiramate); peripheral laser treatment; stereotactic radiosurgery; tizanidine** We found insufficient evidence about the effects of these interventions.
- **Cryotherapy of peripheral nerves; nerve block; peripheral acupuncture; peripheral injection of alcohol; peripheral injection of phenol; peripheral neurectomy; peripheral radiofrequency thermocoagulation** We found no RCTs about the effects of these interventions.

DEFINITION Trigeminal neuralgia is a characteristic pain in the distribution of one or more branches of the fifth cranial nerve. The diagnosis is made on the history alone, based on characteristic features of the pain.[1–3] It occurs in paroxysms with each pain, lasting a few seconds to 2 minutes. The frequency of paroxysms is highly variable, ranging from hundreds of attacks a day to long periods of remission that can last years. Between paroxysms, the person is asymptomatic. The pain is severe and described as intense, sharp, superficial, stabbing, shooting, like an electric shock. In any individual, the pain has the same character in different attacks. It is triggered by light touch in a specific area or by eating, talking, washing the face, or cleaning the teeth. Other causes of facial pain may need to be excluded.[1–3] In trigeminal neuralgia the neurological examination is usually normal.[1–3]

INCIDENCE/ PREVALENCE Most evidence about the incidence and prevalence of trigeminal neuralgia is from the USA.[4] The annual incidence (when age adjusted to 1980 age distribution of the USA) is 5.9/100 000 women and 3.4/100 000 men. The incidence tends to be slightly higher in women at all ages. The incidence increases with age. In men aged over 80 years the incidence is 45.2/100 000.[5] Other published surveys are small. One questionnaire survey of neurological disease in a single French village found one person with trigeminal neuralgia among 993 people.[6]

AETIOLOGY/ RISK FACTORS The cause of trigeminal neuralgia remains unclear.[7,8] It is more common in people with multiple sclerosis (RR 20.0, 95% CI 4.1 to 59.0).[5] Hypertension is a risk factor in women (RR 2.1, 95% CI 1.2 to 3.4) but the evidence is less clear for men (RR 1.53, 95% CI 0.30 to 4.50).[5] A study in the USA found that people with trigeminal neuralgia smoked less, consumed less alcohol, had fewer tonsillectomies, and were less likely than matched controls to be Jewish or an immigrant.[9]

PROGNOSIS One study found no reduction of 10 year survival with trigeminal neuralgia.[10] We found no evidence about the natural history of trigeminal neuralgia. The illness is characterised by recurrences and remissions. Many people have periods of remission with no pain for months or years.[8] Anecdotal reports suggest that in many people it becomes more severe and less responsive to treatment with time.[11] Most people with trigeminal neuralgia are initially managed medically, and a proportion eventually have a surgical procedure.[8] We found no good evidence about the proportion of people who require surgical treatment for pain control. Anecdotal evidence indicates that pain relief is better after surgery than with medical treatment.[8,11]

AIMS OF INTERVENTION To relieve pain with minimal adverse effects.

OUTCOMES Pain frequency and severity scores; measures of psychological distress; ability to perform normal activities; adverse effects.

METHODS *Clinical Evidence* search and appraisal November 2003. Author (JMZ) performed an additional hand search of her own bibliography.

QUESTION What are the effects of treatments on trigeminal neuralgia?

OPTION CARBAMAZEPINE

One systematic review of three crossover RCTs found that carbamazepine increased pain relief compared with placebo, but also increased adverse effects (drowsiness, dizziness, constipation, and ataxia). One small RCT provided insufficient evidence to compare tizanidine versus carbamazepine. One RCT found that carbamazepine was less effective than pimozide in

reducing pain over 8 weeks, but was associated with fewer adverse effects (including hand tremors, memory impairment, and involuntary movements). One systematic review identified one RCT of tocainide versus carbamazepine that was of insufficient quality.

Benefits: **Versus placebo:** We found one systematic review (search date 1999, 3 crossover RCTs, 161 people with trigeminal neuralgia), which found that carbamazepine (for 5 days to 2 weeks) significantly increased the proportion of people having a "good" or "excellent" response compared with placebo (57% with carbamazepine *v* 18% with placebo; OR 4.8, 95% CI 3.4 to 6.9; NNT 3, 95% CI 2 to 4).[12] **Versus tizanidine:** See benefits of tizanidine, p 1680. **Versus pimozide:** See benefits of pimozide, p 1681. **Versus tocainide:** See benefits of tocainide, p 1681.

Harms: The review found that carbamazepine significantly increased adverse effects (drowsiness, dizziness, constipation, and ataxia) compared with placebo (NNH 3, 95% CI 2 to 7).[12] Another systematic review (search date 1994) found that significantly more people withdrew from the RCTs because of adverse effects with carbamazepine compared with placebo (NNH for withdrawal 24, 95% CI 14 to 112).[13] Other adverse effects described in observational studies include rashes, leucopenia, and abnormal liver function tests.[14]

Comment: The RCTs used a crossover design, and one RCT[15] used multiple crossovers so that each individual was counted more than once when calculating the estimates of effectiveness in the systematic review.[12,13] The RCTs included in the systematic review were small and short term. All of the RCTs used simple measures for pain outcomes and no quality of life measures. Diagnostic criteria were not clearly stated. Previous treatment and duration of pain varied considerably. Long term effects of carbamazepine have been assessed only in open trials. We found one report (143 people with trigeminal neuralgia followed for up to 16 years) on the long term benefits of carbamazepine.[16] Initially carbamazepine was successful in 99 (69%) participants, but by 5–16 years only 31 (22%) participants were still finding carbamazepine effective and 63 (44%) required additional or alternative treatment.

OPTION TIZANIDINE

One systematic review of one small RCT provided insufficient evidence to compare tizanidine versus carbamazepine.

Benefits: **Versus placebo:** We found no RCTs. **Versus carbamazepine:** We found one systematic review (search date 1999, 1 double blind RCT,[17] 12 people).[12] It found that similar proportions of people rated tizanidine (≤ 18 mg/day) and carbamazepine (≤ 900 mg/day) as having "very good" efficacy (analysis not by intention to treat; 1/5 [20%] people with tizanidine *v* 4/6 [67%] with carbamazepine; P value not reported).

Harms: No adverse effects were reported but two people withdrew because of inadequate pain control.[12]

Comment: The RCT was too small to establish or exclude clinically important effects.

OPTION PIMOZIDE

One RCT found that pimozide reduced pain over 8 weeks compared with carbamazepine, but increased adverse effects (including hand tremors, memory impairment, and involuntary movements). Cardiac toxicity and sudden death have been reported with pimozide.

Benefits: **Versus placebo:** We found no RCTs. **Versus carbamazepine:** We found one systematic review (search date 1999)[12] that identified one double blind crossover RCT[18] comparing pimozide versus carbamazepine in 48 people with trigeminal neuralgia that was refractory to other medical treatment. Precrossover results found that significantly more people achieved a large reduction in pain severity with 8 weeks of pimozide treatment compared with carbamazepine (total pain score reduction: absolute results presented graphically, $P < 0.001$).[18]

Harms: The RCT found that pimozide significantly increased adverse effects compared with carbamazepine (40/48 [83%] with pimozide *v* 22/48 [46%] with carbamazepine; OR 7.8, 95% CI 3.7 to 20.0).[12] Adverse effects included hand tremors, memory impairment, and involuntary movements. The use of pimozide is restricted by its cardiac toxicity and by reports of sudden death.[14,19]

Comment: This was a well conducted multicentre trial using a variety of outcome measures. The crossover design limits interpretation of the results.

OPTION TOCAINIDE

One systematic review identified one RCT of tocainide versus carbamazepine that was of insufficient quality. The use of tocainide is limited by considerable harms (including serious haematological effects).

Benefits: **Versus placebo:** We found no RCTs. **Versus carbamazepine:** We found one systematic review (search date 1999, 1 RCT,[20] 12 people with trigeminal neuralgia).[12] The double blind, crossover RCT had weak methods and did not report precrossover results (see comment below).

Harms: The RCT reported that one person withdrew because of a skin rash and three people had other adverse effects.[20] The use of tocainide is limited by considerable harms (including severe haematological effects).[14,21]

Comment: In the RCT, combined analysis of precrossover and postcrossover results found that people taking tocainide had a similar reduction in pain measured by a visual analogue scale compared with carbamazepine (figures directly comparing tocainide *v* carbamazepine not reported).[20] The available evidence is poor, but provides no support for the use of tocainide in trigeminal neuralgia.

OPTION LAMOTRIGINE

One systematic review of one small RCT provided insufficient evidence to compare lamotrigine versus placebo in people with trigeminal neuralgia.

Benefits: **Versus placebo:** We found one systematic review (search date 1999)[12] that identified one small crossover RCT (14 people)[22] comparing lamotrigine versus placebo. However, the RCT did not report precrossover results for global improvement (see comment below).

Harms: In the RCT, adverse effects with lamotrigine included dizziness, constipation, nausea, and drowsiness. It may also cause serious skin rash and allergic reactions. The total number of people reporting adverse effects was the same as with placebo (7/14 [50%] with lamotrigine *v* 7/14 [50%] with placebo).[22]

Comment: The RCT (double blind crossover, 14 people with refractory trigeminal neuralgia using either carbamazepine or phenytoin) found that adding lamotrigine in addition to the current medication increased the proportion of people who improved after 2 weeks of treatment compared with placebo (postcrossover results: 10/13 [77%] with lamotrigine v 8/14 [57%] with placebo; ARI +20%, 95% CI –16% to +55%).[22] This RCT was a small study and lamotrigine was used in addition to existing treatment. The crossover design and short period of treatment limits interpretation.

OPTION BACLOFEN

We found no RCTs of sufficient quality of baclofen compared with placebo or other active drugs.

Benefits: **Versus placebo:** We found no RCTs of sufficient quality (see comment below). **Versus other active drugs:** We found no RCTs of sufficient quality (see comment below).

Harms: Baclofen is associated with transient sedation and loss of muscle tone. Abrupt discontinuation may cause seizures and hallucinations. One small, poor quality trial comparing racemic (standard) baclofen versus L-baclofen reported dizziness, confusion, or lethargy (6/15 [40%] v 1/15 [7%]; ARI 33%, 95% CI 3% to 64%; see comment below).[23]

Comment: **Versus placebo:** We found one controlled trial (double blind, crossover, 10 people, 4 using carbamazepine or phenytoin, not clearly randomised).[24] Postcrossover analysis found that baclofen in addition to pre-existing treatment increased the proportion of people with relief of pain after treatment for 2 weeks compared with placebo (7/10 [70%] with baclofen v 1/10 [10%] with placebo).[24] **Racemic versus L-baclofen:** We found one trial (double blind crossover, 15 people, not clearly randomised) that compared racemic (standard) baclofen versus L-baclofen over 2 weeks.[23] It found no significant difference in response rates between racemic baclofen and L-baclofen (9/15 [60%] with L-baclofen v 6/15 [40%] with racemic baclofen; ARI +20%, 95% CI –16% to +56%). Some people included in the study were also taking other treatments, making interpretation difficult.

OPTION PROPARACAINE HYDROCHLORIDE EYE DROPS

One RCT found no significant difference in pain at 30 days between placebo and a single application of proparacaine hydrochloride eye drops to the eye on the same side as the pain.

Benefits: **Versus placebo:** We found no systematic review but found one double blind RCT (47 people with trigeminal neuralgia) of proparacaine hydrochloride eye drops versus placebo eye drops instilled for 20 minutes on the same side as the trigeminal neuralgia on one occasion only.[25] It found no significant reduction of pain after 3, 10, and 30 days (at 30 days: 6/25 [24%] improved with proparacaine v 5/22 [23%] with placebo; ARI +1.3%, 95% CI –23% to +26%).

Harms: The RCT gave no information on adverse effects.

Comment: None.

OPTION OTHER DRUGS

We found no systematic review and no RCTs of sufficient quality about effects of the antiepileptic drugs phenytoin, clonazepam, sodium valproate, gabapentin, oxcarbazepine, or topiramate and the antiarrhythmic drug mexiletine in people with trigeminal neuralgia.

Benefits: We found no systematic review and no RCTs of sufficient quality examining the effects of the antiepileptic drugs phenytoin, clonazepam, sodium valproate, gabapentin, oxcarbazepine, or topiramate and the antiarrhythmic drug mexiletine in people with trigeminal neuralgia (see comment below).

Harms: For harms of phenytoin, sodium valproate, gabapentin, oxcarbazepine, and topiramate see harms of antiepileptic drugs under epilepsy, p 1588. Harms of mexiletine include dizziness, nausea, vomiting, confusion, and tremor.[26] The crossover RCT (see comment below) reported adverse effects with topiramate included irritability and diarrhoea (in 2 people) and fatigue/sedation, hyperactivity, nausea, abdominal cramps, lightheadedness, and cognitive impairment (in 1 person each).[27]

Comment: We found one small double blind crossover RCT (3 people with trigeminal neuralgia) that compared 12 weeks of topiramate (25 mg/day titrated up to 600 mg/day) versus placebo.[27] Titration was by weekly telephone assessment of symptoms. Washout period between crossover was 2 weeks. The trial found that topiramate reduced pain (on a 10 point scale) compared with placebo in all three people (P = 0.04).[27] However, the trial was at high risk of detecting effects by chance. An extended confirmatory study in which two people continued to take medication for three 8 week segments (4 weeks of placebo and 4 weeks of topiramate assigned in random order) found no significant pain reduction with topiramate compared with placebo.[27] Concurrent medications continued during the study included carbamazepine and baclofen in one person, clonazepam and tricyclic antidepressants in one person, and carbamazepine and gabapentin in one person.[27]

OPTION CRYOTHERAPY OF PERIPHERAL NERVES

We found no RCTs on the effects of cryotherapy⊕ in people with trigeminal neuralgia.

Benefits: We found no RCTs.

Harms: We found no RCTs.

Comment: We found many articles that reported studies of limited reliability, duplicated data, or included people with different types of pain.

OPTION NERVE BLOCK

We found no RCTs comparing nerve block versus placebo or no treatment. Small RCTs provided insufficient evidence about the effects of nerve block using streptomycin plus lidocaine compared with nerve block using lidocaine alone.

Benefits: **Nerve block versus placebo or no treatment:** We found no systematic review and no RCTs. **Local anaesthetic versus streptomycin plus local anaesthetic:** We found two RCTs comparing injections of streptomycin 1 g plus lidocaine (2 mL of 2% solution) versus lidocaine injections alone (1 injection weekly for 5 weeks).[28,29] The first RCT included 18 people with trigeminal neuralgia who had previously responded poorly to lidocaine injection alone (≤ 24 hours' pain relief from lidocaine alone). One person who did not gain pain relief from allocated treatment was excluded (see comment below). One week after the final injection, combined streptomycin plus lidocaine improved the chance of being pain free compared with lidocaine alone (AR for being pain free: 89% with combined injection *v* 38% with lidocaine alone; ARR 51%, CI not reported, P = 0.04). After 30 months the RCT found no significant difference between treatments (AR for being pain free: 33% with combined injection *v* 25% with lidocaine alone; ARR 8%, CI not reported, P = 0.38).[28] The second RCT compared weekly injections of streptomycin 1 g plus lidocaine (3 mL of 2% solution) versus lidocaine alone for 5 weeks in a crossover design involving 20 people with idiopathic or traumatic trigeminal neuralgia. It found no significant short term differences between the groups in severity or frequency of pain as assessed after crossover by a variety of clinical tests such as a visual analogue scale and from pain diaries.[29]

Harms: Some people (2/20 [10%]) found the injections painful and some refused to have further injections.[29] No sensory changes or other adverse effects were reported.

Comment: Neither trial reported the method of randomisation. Reliability of results in the first RCT may have been limited by selection bias[28] and the second RCT had short term follow up[29] (see benefits above). Streptomycin was used on the assumption that it causes a long term peripheral nerve block.

OPTION PERIPHERAL INJECTIONS OF ALCOHOL

We found no RCTs on the effects of injecting peripheral nerves with alcohol in people with trigeminal neuralgia.

Benefits: We found no RCTs.

Harms: We found no RCTs.

Comment: None.

OPTION PERIPHERAL NEURECTOMY

We found no RCTs on the effects of peripheral neurectomy in people with trigeminal neuralgia.

Benefits: We found no RCTs.

Harms: We found no RCTs.

Comment: None.

OPTION PERIPHERAL RADIOFREQUENCY THERMOCOAGULATION

We found no RCTs on the effects of peripheral radiofrequency thermocoagulation in people with trigeminal neuralgia.

Benefits: We found no RCTs.

Harms: We found no RCTs.

Comment: None.

OPTION STEREOTACTIC RADIOSURGERY

Three systematic reviews found no RCTs comparing stereotactic radiosurgery versus placebo or versus other treatments. One weak RCT provided insufficient evidence to compare different radiosurgery regimens.

Benefits: Three systematic reviews found no RCTs comparing stereotactic radiosurgery versus placebo or versus other treatments.[30–32] We found one weak RCT comparing different radiosurgery regimens (see comment below).[33]

Harms: One RCT comparing two different radiosurgery regimens reported numbness (8/43 [19%] with 2 isocentres *v* 3/44 [7%] with 1 isocentre), mild paraesthesia (5/43 [12%] with 2 isocentres *v* 4/44 [9%] with 1 isocentre), and severe paraesthesia (1/43 [2%] with 2 isocentres *v* 0/44 [0%] with 1 isocentre; see comment below).[33]

Comment: One RCT (87 people with trigeminal neuralgia) compared radiosurgery using either one isocentre or two isocentres, the latter regimen to treat a longer length of the trigeminal nerve.[33] It found similar rates of maximal pain control (no pain with or without drugs: 29/44 [66%] with 1 isocentre *v* 28/43 [65%] with 2 isocentres) and pain control at final follow up (no pain with or without drugs: 20/44 [45%] with 1 isocentre *v* 23/43 [53%] with 2 isocentres).[33] The median follow up was 26 months (range 1–36 months).[33] People in the RCT took additional pain medication which was not specified. It reported more complications in the two isocentres group (see harms above), but pain outcomes were similar in both groups.[33] Typically, pain relief with radiosurgery is not immediate.

OPTION PERIPHERAL INJECTION OF PHENOL

We found no RCTs on the effects of peripheral nerve injection with phenol in people with trigeminal neuralgia.

Benefits: We found no RCTs.

Harms: We found no RCTs.

Comment: None.

OPTION PERIPHERAL ACUPUNCTURE

We found no RCTs on the effects of peripheral acupuncture in people with trigeminal neuralgia.

Benefits: We found no RCTs.

Harms: We found no RCTs.

Comment: None.

OPTION PERIPHERAL LASER TREATMENT

We found no RCTs of sufficient quality of peripheral laser treatment⊕ in people with trigeminal neuralgia.

Benefits: We found no RCTs of sufficient quality (see comment below).

Harms: We found no RCTs of sufficient quality.

Comment: We found one RCT (35 people with trigeminal neuralgia) comparing helium neon laser (3 treatments/week for 10 weeks, 1 mW, 632.5 nm, 20 Hz applied for 20 seconds on skin overlying the trigger nerve and 30 seconds on painful areas of the face) versus sham treatment with apparatus that emitted no light.[34] The trial did not compare the two groups directly. However, it found that mean pain score significantly improved from baseline at weeks 6 and 7 with laser, but did not change significantly from baseline for any week with sham treatment. This analysis has limited reliability.

GLOSSARY

Cryotherapy After surgical exposure of the trigger nerve, three freeze–thaw cycles are applied under local anaesthesia and sedation as necessary.
Peripheral laser treatment Laser irradiation of skin overlying the trigger nerve.

REFERENCES

1. Classification Subcommittee of the International Headache Society. The international classification of headache disorders. *Cephalalgia* 2004;24(suppl 1):1–160.
2. Katusic S, Williams DB, Beard CM, et al. Epidemiology and clinical features of idiopathic trigeminal neuralgia and glossopharyngeal neuralgia: similarities and differences, Rochester, Minnesota, 1945–1984. *Neuroepidemiology* 1991;10:276–281.
3. Zakrzewska JM. Diagnosis and differential diagnosis of trigeminal neuralgia. *Clin J Pain* 2002;18:14–21.

4. Zakrzewska JM, Hamlyn PJ. Facial pain. In: Crombie IKCPR, Linton SJ, LeResche L, et al, eds. *Epidemiology of pain*. Seattle: IASP, 1999:171–202.
5. Katusic S, Beard CM, Bergstralh E, et al. Incidence and clinical features of trigeminal neuralgia, Rochester, Minnesota, 1945–1984. *Ann Neurol* 1990;27:89–95.
6. Munoz M, Dumas M, Boutros-Toni F, et al. A neuro-epidemiologic survey in a Limousin town. *Rev Neurol (Paris)* 1988;144:266–271.
7. Devor M, Amir R, Rappaprot ZH. Pathophysiology of trigeminal neuralgia: the ignition hypothesis. *Clin J Pain* 2002;18:4–13.
8. Zakrzewska JM. Trigeminal neuralgia. In: Zakrzewska JM, Harrison SD, eds. *Assessment and management of orofacial pain*, 1st ed. Amsterdam: Elsevier Sciences; 2002:267–370.
9. Rothman KJ, Monson RR. Epidemiology of trigeminal neuralgia. *J Chronic Dis* 1973;26:3–12.
10. Rothman KJ, Monson RR. Survival in trigeminal neuralgia. *J Chronic Dis* 1973;26:303–309.
11. Zakrzewska JM, Patsalos PN. Long term cohort study comparing medical (oxcarbazepine) and surgical management of infractable trigeminal neuralgia. *Pain* 2002; 95:259–266.
12. Wiffen P, Collins S, McQuay H, et al. Anticonvulsant drugs for acute and chronic pain. In: The Cochrane Library, Issue 1, 2003. Oxford: Update Software. Search date 1999; primary sources Medline, Embase, Sigle, Cochrane Controlled Trials Register, and hand searches of 40 medical journals and published reports.
13. McQuay H, Carroll D, Jadad AR, et al. Anticonvulsant drugs for management of pain: a systematic review. *BMJ* 1995;311:1047–1052. Search date 1994; primary sources Medline and hand searches of 40 medical journals, reference lists, and published reports.
14. Sweetman SC (Ed). *Martindale: the complete drug reference*. 33rd ed. London: Pharmaceutical Press, 2002.
15. Campbell FG, Graham JG, Zilkha KJ. Clinical trial of carbamazepine (Tegretol) in trigeminal neuralgia. *J Neurol Neurosurg Psychiatry* 1966;29:265–267.
16. Taylor JC, Brauer S, Espir MLE. Long-term treatment of trigeminal neuralgia with carbamazepine. *Postgrad Med J* 1981;57:16–18.
17. Vilming ST, Lyberg T, Latase X. Tizanidine in the management of trigeminal neuralgia. *Cephalalgia* 1986;6:181–182.
18. Lechin F, van der Dijs B, Lechin ME, et al. Pimozide therapy for trigeminal neuralgia. *Arch Neurol* 1989;46:960–963.
19. Committee on Safety of Medicines/Medicines Control Agency. Cardiac arrhythmias with pimozide (Orap). *Current Problems* 1995;21:2.
20. Lindstrom P, Lindblom V. The analgesic effect of tocainide in trigeminal neuralgia. *Pain* 1987;28:45–50.
21. Denaro CP, Benowitz NL. Poisoning due to class 1B antiarrhythmic drugs. Lignocaine, mexiletine and tocainide. *Med Toxicol Adverse Drug Exp* 1989;4:412–428.
22. Zakrzewska JM, Chaudhry Z, Patton DW, et al. Lamotrigine in refractory trigeminal neuralgia: results from a double-blind placebo controlled crossover study. *Pain* 1997;73:223–230.
23. Fromm GH, Terrence CF. Comparison of L-baclofen and racemic baclofen in trigeminal neuralgia. *Neurology* 1987;37:1725–1728.
24. Fromm GH, Terrence CF, Chattha AS. Baclofen in the treatment of trigeminal neuralgia: double-blind study and long-term follow-up. *Ann Neurol* 1984;15:240–244.
25. Kondziolka D, Lemley T, Kestle JR, et al. The effect of single-application topical ophthalmic anesthesia in patients with trigeminal neuralgia. A randomized double-blind placebo-controlled trial. *J Neurosurg* 1994;80:993–997.
26. Wooten JM, Earnest J, Reyes J. Review of common adverse effects of selected antiarrhythmic drugs. *Crit Care Nurs Q* 2000;22:23–38.
27. Gilron I, Booher SL, Rowan JS, et al. Topiramate in trigeminal neuralgia: a randomized, placebo-controlled multiple crossover pilot study. *Clin Neuropharmacol* 2001;24:109–112
28. Stajcic Z, Juniper RP, Todorovic L. Peripheral streptomycin/lidocaine injections versus lidocaine alone in the treatment of idiopathic trigeminal neuralgia. A double blind controlled trial. *J Craniomaxillofac Surg* 1990;18:243–246.
29. Bittar GT, Graff-Radford SB. The effects of streptomycin/lidocaine block on trigeminal neuralgia: a double blind crossover placebo controlled study. *Headache* 1993;33:155–160.
30. Lopez BC, Hamlyn PJ, Zakrzewska JM. Systematic review of ablative neurosurgical techniques for the treatment of trigeminal neuralgia. *Neurosurgery* 2004;54:973–982.
31. Lopez BC, Hamlyn PJ, Zakrzewska JM. Stereotactic radiosurgery for primary trigeminal neuralgia: state of the evidence and recommendations for future reports. *J Neurol Neurosurg Psychiatry* 2004;75:1019–1024.
32. Lim JNW, Ayiku L. The clinical efficacy and safety of stereotactic radiosurgery (gamma knife) in the treatment of trigeminal neuralgia. 2004 (http://www.nice.org.uk/pdf/ip/173systematicreview.pdf).
33. Flickinger JC, Pollock BE, Kondziolka D, *et al.* Does increased nerve length within the treatment volume improve trigeminal neuralgia radiosurgery? A prospective double-blind, randomized study. *Int J Radiation Oncology Biol Phys* 2001;51:449–54.
34. Walker JB, Akhanjee LK, Cooney MM, et al. Laser therapy for pain of trigeminal neuralgia. *Clin J Pain* 1988;3:183–187.

Joanna M Zakrzewska
Professor
Barts and the London Queen Mary's School of Medicine and Dentistry
London
UK

Benjamin C Lopez
Mr
Department of Neurosurgery
Barts and the London NHS Trust
London
UK

Competing interests: JMZ has been reimbursed by GlaxoWellcome (manufacturer of lamotrigine) for attending a conference and for conducting the lamotrigine RCT. BCL none declared.

Aphthous ulcers (recurrent)

Search date April 2004

Stephen Porter and Crispian Scully CBE

QUESTIONS

INTERVENTIONS

To be covered in future updates

Barrier techniques
Laser
Low intensity ultrasound
Novel toothpastes
Other drug treatments

See glossary G

Key Messages

Treatment

- **Chlorhexidine** RCTs found that chlorhexidine gluconate mouth rinses reduced the severity of each episode of ulceration, but did not affect the incidence of ulceration. Limited evidence from one RCT suggested that 0.2% chlorhexidine gel may reduce the incidence and duration of ulceration compared with a control preparation. RCTs found that chlorhexidine reduced the mean severity of pain compared with an inert preparation.
- **Topical corticosteroids** Small RCTs found that topical corticosteroids reduced the number of ulcer days compared with control preparations. RCTs found no consistent effect of topical corticosteroids on the incidence of new ulcers compared with control preparations. They found weak evidence that topical corticosteroids may reduce the duration and pain of ulcers and hasten pain relief without causing notable local or systemic adverse effects.
- **Hexitidine** Limited evidence from RCTs found no significant difference in any of the reported outcomes between hexitidine mouthwash or a proprietary antibacterial mouthwash and control mouthwashes.

Aphthous ulcers (recurrent)

DEFINITION	Recurrent aphthous ulcers are superficial and rounded, painful mouth ulcers usually occurring in recurrent bouts at intervals of a few days to a few months.[1]
INCIDENCE/ PREVALENCE	The point prevalence of recurrent aphthous ulcers in Swedish adults has been reported as 2%.[1] Prevalence may be 5–10% in some groups of children. Up to 66% of young adults give a history consistent with recurrent aphthous ulceration.
AETIOLOGY/ RISK FACTORS	The causes of aphthous ulcers remain unknown. Associations with haematinic deficiency, infections, gluten sensitive enteropathy, food sensitivities, and psychological stress have rarely been confirmed. Similar ulcers are seen in Behçet's syndrome. Local physical trauma may initiate ulcers in susceptible people. Recurrent aphthous ulcers are uncommon on keratinised oral mucosal surfaces, and the frequency of recurrent aphthous ulcers may fall if people cease any tobacco smoking habit.
PROGNOSIS	About 80% of people with recurrent aphthous ulcers develop a few ulcers smaller than 1 cm in diameter that heal within 5–14 days without scarring (the pattern known as minor aphthous ulceration). The episodes recur typically after an interval of 1–4 months. One in 10 people with recurrent ulceration may have multiple minute ulcers (herpetiform ulceration). Likewise, one in 10 sufferers has a more severe form (major aphthous ulceration), with lesions larger than 1 cm that may recur after a shorter interval and can cause scarring. Most of the trials in this review have focused upon the treatment of minor aphthous ulceration.
AIMS OF INTERVENTION	To reduce the severity of the episode and the incidence, duration, and pain of ulceration with minimal adverse effects.
OUTCOMES	**Ulcer day index:** The sum of the number of ulcers each day over a period, usually 4–8 weeks, which indicates the severity of the episode and reflects the mean prevalence and duration of ulcers; number of ulcer free days during a specified period; **incidence of new ulcers:** number of new ulcers appearing within a specified period, usually 4–8 weeks; **duration of ulceration:** mean duration of individual ulcers (difficult to determine because of uncertainty in detecting the point of complete resolution); **severity of pain:** symptom score based on subjective pain severity recorded in categories on a questionnaire (e.g. from 0–3, ranging from no pain to severe pain) or on a 10 cm visual analogue scale; **user preference:** preference of people for one treatment over another. The **diameter of lesions** is a proxy measure of the clinical severity of an episode of ulceration.
METHODS	*Clinical Evidence* search and appraisal April 2004.

QUESTION **What are the effects of treatments for recurrent aphthous ulcers?**

OPTION **TOPICAL CORTICOSTEROIDS**

Small RCTs found that topical corticosteroids reduced the number of ulcer days compared with control preparations. RCTs found no consistent effect of topical corticosteroids on the incidence of new ulcers compared with control preparations. They found weak evidence that topical corticosteroids may reduce the duration and pain of ulcers and hasten pain relief without causing notable local or systemic adverse effects.

Benefits: We found no systematic review but found nine RCTs that reported clinical outcomes in people with recurrent aphthous ulcers (see table 1, p 1692).[2–9] Overall, one RCT found larger effect sizes than the others.[2] **Ulcer days index:** We found four RCTs reporting data on the number of ulcer days.[2,4,5,7] They found that topical corticosteroids reduced the number of ulcer days compared with control, although the reduction was significant in only two of the RCTs. **Incidence of new ulcers:** Five crossover RCTs (102 people) reported inconsistent effects on the incidence of new ulcers.[2,4,5,8] One RCT found no effect on reducing frequency of ulcer recurrence during follow up in either treatment or control groups.[8] **Duration of ulceration:** We found six RCTs reporting data on ulcer duration, three of which had a crossover design.[3,4,6–9] Four RCTs reported the mean duration of ulcers with topical corticosteroids compared with control preparations but found no evidence of a consistent effect.[3,4,7,9] One RCT found that topical corticosteroids significantly increased the proportion of people who had mean ulcer duration ≤ 6 days compared with control preparations.[6] One RCT found that topical corticosteroids significantly reduced the total number of ulcer days compared with control preparations.[8] **Severity of pain:** Four RCTs, three of which had a crossover design, reported on severity of pain with topical corticosteroids versus control, but all presented their results in different ways.[6–9] One RCT found that topical corticosteroids significantly increased the proportion of people with pain relief compared with a control preparation.[6] The first crossover RCT found that topical corticosteroids reduced symptom scores compared with a control preparation, but the difference was not significant.[7] The second crossover RCT found that topical corticosteroids significantly increased the proportion of people with reduced pain severity compared with a control preparation.[8] The third crossover RCT found that the pain score fell with time in both treatment and control groups (see comment below), but the rate of fall was significantly faster when using topical corticosteroids ($P < 0.0001$).[9] **User preference:** Three crossover RCTs found that more users preferred topical corticosteroids than control preparations, however, no significance data was presented.[4–7]

Harms: In five of the nine RCTs, no adverse effects were found.[2,3,6–8] One RCT reported adrenal suppression in one man using betamethasone disodium phosphate.[5] However, limited studies of adrenal function found no evidence that 0.05% fluocinonide in adhesive paste and betamethasone-17-valerate mouth rinse caused adrenal suppression.[8,10] Two RCTs gave no information on adverse effects.[4,9]

Comment: The trials differed in many ways: selection of people, type of topical corticosteroid and formulation used, control preparation used (although this was usually a base without topical steroid), duration of treatment, reported outcomes, and design (double or single blind, parallel group or crossover, presence and length of washout period). In one crossover RCT, the pain score fell during the course of the trial irrespective of the treatment received.[9] The study did not make clear if the effect of crossover sequence had been allowed for. Withdrawal rates were high. Most people in the trials had more severe ulceration than the average person with recurrent aphthous ulceration.

OPTION CHLORHEXIDINE AND SIMILAR AGENTS

RCTs found that chlorhexidine gluconate mouth rinses reduced the severity of each episode of ulceration, but did not affect the incidence of ulceration. Limited evidence from one RCT suggested that 0.2% chlorhexidine gel may reduce the incidence and duration of ulceration compared with a control preparation. RCTs found that chlorhexidine reduced the mean severity of pain compared with an inert preparation. Limited evidence from RCTs found no significant difference in any of the reported outcomes between hexitidine mouthwash or a proprietary antibacterial mouthwash and control mouthwashes.

Benefits: We found no systematic review but found five RCTs (203 people with recurrent aphthous ulceration) comparing chlorhexidine gluconate or similar preparations versus inactive control preparations (see table 1, p 1692).[11–15] Four of the RCTs used a crossover design with a randomised sequence comparing a control preparation versus 1% chlorhexidine gel,[11] 0.2% chlorhexidine gel,[12] 0.2% chlorhexidine mouthwash,[13] or 0.1% hexetidine mouthwash.[14] One RCT compared a proprietary antibacterial rinse with a hydroalcoholic control.[15] **Ulcer days index:** Three RCTs reported the ulcer days index.[12–14] Two RCTs found that chlorhexidine significantly reduced the ulcer day index compared with a control preparation.[12,13] One of these RCTs found that chlorhexidine significantly increased the number of ulcer free days per 6 weeks of treatment compared with an inert preparation.[13] A third RCT found that hexitidine had no significant effect on the ulcer day index compared with a control preparation.[14] **Incidence of ulceration:** All five RCTs reported the number of ulcers, defined as either the total number of ulcers or the number of new ulcers with each treatment per week.[11–15] Only one RCT, using 0.2% chlorhexidine gel, found that active treatment significantly reduced the number of new ulcers (see comment below).[12] **Duration of ulceration:** The mean duration of individual ulcers was reported in four of the RCTs.[11,13–15] The mean duration of individual ulcers was reduced by active treatment in all four RCTs, but the difference was significant in only one RCT, using 1% chlorhexidine gel,[11] and the mean difference was less than 1 day in the others. Three RCTs found that the number of ulcers fell during the course of the study, irrespective of the treatment received (see comment below).[13–15] **Severity of pain:** All five RCTs reported on pain severity scores.[11–15] Two RCTs found that chlorhexidine significantly reduced the mean severity of pain compared with an inert preparation.[11,12] One RCT which compared a proprietary antibacterial mouthwash versus the alcohol containing control preparation found no significant difference in pain severity between the treatment groups, but found a large improvement in clinical outcomes in both groups compared with baseline levels (see comment below).[15] **User preference:** One crossover RCT found no significant difference in user preference between 0.1% hexetidine mouthwash and control mouthwash, but found that many more people preferred the treatment received second.[14]

Harms: One RCT found that chlorhexidine had a bitter taste and was associated with brown staining of teeth and tongue and with nausea.[12] In one RCT, one person reported a severe inflammation of the gums during the treatment with 0.1% hexitidine mouthwash.[14] Three RCTs gave no information on adverse events.[11,13,15]

Comment: Four of the RCTs used a crossover design and reported high withdrawal rates. A consistent observation was that outcomes improved during the course of the trials irrespective of the treatment received. One of the crossover studies did not make it clear if reported results took account of the effect of confounding factors such as inadequate washout period and different loss to follow up in the two treatment periods (data were available from only 12/26 people who were recruited).[12] The parallel group trial had fewer withdrawals: 106 people with recurrent aphthous ulceration were recruited and 96 completed the study.[15] Analysis was not by intention to treat and the method of randomisation was not specified. People recruited to the trials might not be typical of the average person with recurrent aphthous ulceration.

REFERENCES

1. Porter SR, Scully C, Pedersen A. Recurrent aphthous stomatitis. *Crit Rev Oral Biol Med* 1998;9:306–321.
2. Cooke BED, Armitage P. Recurrent Mikulicz's aphthae treatment with topical hydrocortisone hemisuccinate sodium. *BMJ* 1960;1:764–766.
3. McFall WT Jr. Effect of flurandrenolone on oral aphthae. *J Periodontol* 1968;39:364–365.
4. Browne RM, Fox EC, Anderson RJ. Topical triamcinolone acetonide in recurrent aphthous stomatitis. *Lancet* 1968;1:565–567.
5. MacPhee IT, Sircus W, Farmer ED, et al. Use of steroids in treatment of aphthous ulceration. *BMJ* 1968;2:147–149.
6. Merchant HW, Gangarosa LP, Glassman AB, et al. Betamethasone-17-benzoate in the treatment of recurrent aphthous ulcers. *Oral Surg Oral Med Oral Pathol* 1978;45:870–875.
7. Pimlott SJ, Walker DM. A controlled clinical trial of the efficacy of topically applied fluocinonide in the treatment of recurrent aphthous ulceration. *Br Dent J* 1983;154:174–177.
8. Thompson AC, Nolan A, Lamey P-J. Minor aphthous oral ulceration: a double-blind cross-over study of beclomethasone diproprionate aerosol spray. *Scot Med J* 1989;34:531–532.
9. Miles DA, Bricker SL, Razmus TF, et al. Triamcinolone acetonide versus chlorhexidine for treatment of recurrent stomatitis. *Oral Surg Oral Med Oral Pathol* 1993;75:397–402.

10. Lehner T, Lyne C. Adrenal function during topical oral corticosteroid treatment. *BMJ* 1969;4:138–141.
11. Addy M, Carpenter R, Roberts WR. Management of recurrent aphthous ulceration — a trial of chlorhexidine gluconate gel. *Br Dent J* 1976;141:118–120.
12. Addy M. Hibitane in the treatment of recurrent aphthous ulceration. *J Clin Periodontol* 1977;4:108–116.
13. Hunter L, Addy M. Chlorhexidine gluconate mouthwash in the management of minor aphthous stomatitis. *Br Dent J* 1987;162:106–110.
14. Chadwick B, Addy M, Walker DM. Hexetidine mouthrinse in the management of minor aphthous ulceration and as an adjunct to oral hygiene. *Br Dent J* 1991;171:83–87.
15. Meiller TF, Kutcher MJ, Overholser CD, et al. Effect of an antimicrobial mouthrinse on recurrent aphthous ulcerations. *Oral Surg Oral Med Oral Pathol* 1991;72:425–429.

Stephen Porter
Professor and Head of Department
Eastman Dental Institute
for Oral Health Care Sciences UCL
University of London
London
UK

Crispian Scully CBE
Dean and Director of Studies
Eastman Dental Institute
for Oral Health Care Sciences UCL, and
International Centres for Excellence in
Dentistry and Research
University of London
London
UK

Competing interests: None declared.

TABLE 1 **Effects of treatments on different outcomes: results of RCTs (see text, p 1688).**

Intervention	Outcomes	Ref	Participants	Treatment duration (weeks)	Results		Effect (%)* (significance)
					Treatment	Control	
Topical cortisteriods versus inert preparations							
	Ulcer day index (definition see below)	2	17	8	26.3	65.9	–60% (P < 0.01)
		4	26	8	58.3	71.3	–18% (NS)
		5 main	25	4	24.0	30.7	–22% (NS)
		7		6	48.3	70.6	–32 (P <0.05)
	Incidence of new ulcers	2	17	8	0.51	1.15	–55% (P 0.05)
		4	26	8	0.84	0.94	–11% (NS)
	Number of new ulcers/week	5 pilot	8	4	2.07	1.85	+12% (NS)
		5 main	31†	4	0.73	0.82	–11% (NS)
		5	20	6	1.27	1.92	+6% (NS)
	Effect on reducing frequency of ulcer recurrence during follow-up	8	15	26	no effect	no effect	not given
	Duration of ulceration						
	Mean number of days of ulcer duration	3	50	UCH	6.00	6.00	0% (NS)
		4	26	8	8.07	8.94	–10% (NS)
		7	20	6	4.93	7.83	–37% (P < 0.001)
		9	19	12	5.93	5.92	0% (NS)
	Proportion of people with ulcer duration <6 days	6	63	UCH	23/33	14/30	P < 0.05
	Proportion of people with the total number of ulcer days reduced by preparation	8	15	4	13/15	not given	P < 0.001

TABLE 1 continued

Intervention	Outcomes	Ref	Participants	Treatment duration (weeks)	Results: Treatment	Results: Control	Effect (%)* (significance)
	Severity of pain						
	Proportion of people with pain relief	6	63	UCH	29/33	18/30	P < 0.01
	Average pain severity score during ulcer days	7	20	6	2.77	3.54	NS
	Proportion of people with reduced pain severity	8	15	4	11/15	not given	P < 0.05
	User preference						
	Proportion of people receiving both forms of treatment preferring active treatment	4	26	8	113/26		N/A
		6	17	UCH	10/13		N/A
		7	20	6	18/20		N/A
	Adverse effects	2	17	8	None found	None found	
		5	31	4	1**	Not given	
		6	63	UCH	None found	None found	
		7	20	6	None found	None found	
		8	15	4	None found	None found	
Topical antibacterial versus inert preparations	**Severity of episode**						
	Ulcer day index (definition see below)	11	12	5	9.5	17.0	P < 0.05
		12	38	6	42.8	52.3	P < 0.05
		13	37	6	79.7	65.7	NS
	Number of ulcer free days	12	38	6	22.9	17.5	P < 0.02

TABLE 0 continued

TABLE 1 continued

Intervention	Outcomes	Ref	Participants	Treatment duration (weeks)	Results		Effect (%)* (significance)
					Treatment	Control	
	Incidence of ulceration						
	Number of new ulcers/week	10	20	5	1.04	1.4	NS
		11	12	5	0.60	1.02	P < 0.05
		12	38	6	1.26	1.38	NS
		13	37	6	1.48	1.39	NS
		14	96	26	0.09	0.13	NS
	Duration of ulceration						
	Mean number of days of ulcer duration	10	20	5	4.8	7.80	P < 0.01
		12	38	6	5.02	5.78	NS
		13	37	6	6.64	6.80	NS
	Median fall in days of ulcer duration from start to end of trial	14	96	26	2.42	1.58	NS
			26				
	Severity of pain						
	Mean pain severity score	10	20	5	0.93	1.22	P < 0.05
	Mean total pain severity score	11	12	5	appr. 49 (graph)	appr. 24 (graph)	P < 0.05
		12	38	6	16.31	16.35	NS
		13	37	6	16.9	17.8	NS
	Adverse effects	11	12	5	Bitter taste, tooth staining	Not given	Not given
		13	37	6	1/37***	0/37	Not given

*Defined as difference between outcome measures for control and treatment, expressed as a fraction of the control. ** One case adrenal suppression in one person using beta methasone disocium phosphate. *** One case of severe gum inflammation in one person using 0.1% hexitidine mouthwash. †Each participant received one treatment for 4 weeks, a blank month, then another treatment with another drug. The trial compared an inert base, two local steroids and two other preparations. The steroids and with the inert base. NS, not significant; ref, reference. N/A Not applicable; UCH: Until complete

Burning mouth syndrome

Search date January 2004

John Buchanan and Joanna Zakrzewska

QUESTIONS

INTERVENTIONS

Key Messages

- **Cognitive behavioural therapy** One small RCT found that cognitive behavioural therapy reduced symptom intensity in people with resistant burning mouth syndrome after 6 months compared with placebo treatment.
- **Antidepressants; benzydamine hydrochloride** We found insufficient evidence on the effects of these interventions.
- **Dietary supplements** We found insufficient evidence from three small methodologically flawed RCTs to draw reliable conclusions about the effects of alphalipoic acid in people with burning mouth syndrome. We found no RCTs evaluating other vitamin or coenzyme supplements.
- **Hormone replacement therapy in postmenopausal women** We found limited evidence from one small methodologically flawed RCT that tibolone improved symptoms compared with oryzanol plus vitamin E at 6 months.

DEFINITION	Burning mouth syndrome is a psychogenic or idiopathic burning discomfort or pain affecting people with clinically normal oral mucosa in whom a medical or dental cause has been excluded.[1–3] Terms previously used to describe what is now called burning mouth syndrome include glossodynia, glossopyrosis, stomatodynia, stomatopyrosis, sore tongue, and oral dysaesthesia.[4] A survey of 669 men and 758 women randomly selected from 48 500 people aged between 20 and 69 years found that people with burning mouth also have subjective dryness (66%), take some form of medication (64%), report other systemic illnesses (57%), and have altered taste (11%).[5] Many studies of people with symptoms of burning mouth do not distinguish those with burning mouth syndrome (i.e. idiopathic disease) from those with other conditions (such as vitamin B deficiency), making results unreliable. Local and systemic factors (such as infections, allergies, ill fitting dentures,[6] hypersensitivity reactions,[7] and hormone and vitamin deficiencies[8–10]) may cause the symptom of burning mouth and should be excluded before diagnosing burning mouth syndrome.
INCIDENCE/ PREVALENCE	Burning mouth syndrome mainly affects women,[11–13] particularly after the menopause, when its prevalence may be 18–33%.[14] One recent study in Sweden found a prevalence of 4% for the symptom of burning mouth without clinical abnormality of the oral mucosa (11/669 [2%] men, mean age 59 years; 42/758 [6%] women, mean age 57 years), with the highest prevalence (12%) in women aged 60–69 years.[5] Reported prevalence in general populations varies from 1%[15] to 15%.[11] Incidence and prevalence vary according to diagnostic criteria,[4] and many studies included people with the symptom of burning mouth rather than with burning mouth syndrome as defined above.
AETIOLOGY/ RISK FACTORS	The cause is unknown, and we found no good aetiological studies. Possible causal factors include hormonal disturbances associated with the menopause,[12–14] psychogenic factors (including anxiety, depression, stress, life events, personality disorders, and phobia of cancer),[6,16,17] and neuropathy in so-called supertasters Ⓖ.[18]
PROGNOSIS	We found no prospective cohort studies or other reliable evidence describing the natural history of burning mouth syndrome.[19] We found anecdotal reports of at least partial spontaneous remission in about half of people with burning mouth syndrome within 6–7 years.[16]
AIMS OF INTERVENTION	To alleviate symptoms, with minimal adverse effects.
OUTCOMES	Self reported relief of symptoms (burning mouth, altered taste, dry mouth); incidence and severity of anxiety and depression; quality of life using a validated ordinal scale.
METHODS	*Clinical Evidence* search and appraisal January 2004.

QUESTION What are the effects of treatments?

OPTION COGNITIVE BEHAVIOURAL THERAPY

One small RCT found that cognitive behavioural therapy reduced symptom intensity in people with resistant burning mouth syndrome after 6 months compared with placebo treatment.

Benefits: We found one systematic review (search date 2000, 1 RCT, 30 people).[20] The small RCT identified by the review (30 people with resistant burning mouth syndrome) compared cognitive behavioural therapy (12–15 sessions of 1 hour/week) versus a control group who received similar attention but without the cognitive behavioural therapy sessions. It found that cognitive behavioural therapy significantly reduced the intensity of symptoms at 6 months (measured on a visual analogue scale ranging from 1 = endurable to 7 = unendurable; mean pretreatment score: 5.0 with cognitive behavioural therapy *v* 4.3 with placebo; mean score change at 6 months: –3.6 with cognitive behavioural therapy *v* +0.4 with placebo; P < 0.001; AR for being symptom free at 6 months: 4/15 [27%] with cognitive behavioural therapy *v* 0/15 [0%] with placebo; significance not reported).[20]

Harms: The RCT provided no information on adverse effects.[20]

Comment: The trial was small and individual characteristics of the two groups were not described; therefore, the groups may not have been comparable. The visual analogue scale for assessing oral burning was not validated.[20]

OPTION HORMONE REPLACEMENT THERAPY IN POSTMENOPAUSAL WOMEN

We found limited evidence from one small methodologically flawed RCT that tibolone improved symptoms compared with oryzanol plus vitamin E at 6 months.

Benefits: We found one systematic review (search date 2000), which identified no RCTs of sufficient quality.[20] We found one subsequent RCT (56 postmenopausal women), which compared oral tibolone (2.5 mg/day) versus oryzanol (30 mg 3 times daily; see comment below) plus vitamin E (100 mg 3 times daily). The study had several methodological flaws (see comment below).[21] It found that tibolone significantly improved symptoms compared with oryzanol plus vitamin E at 3 and 6 months (AR for improvement at 3 months: 84.6% with tibolone *v* 13.3 % with oryzanol plus vitamin E; $P < 0.005$; AR for improvement at 6 months: 88.5% with tibolone *v* 16.7% with oryzanol plus vitamin E; $P < 0.005$).

Harms: Adverse effects of hormone replacement therapy are well documented (see oestrogens under menopausal symptoms, p 2392).

Comment: Oryzanol is a product mainly derived from rice bran oil and is used as a food supplement. We found three non-randomised intervention studies with no clear diagnostic criteria or outcome measures.[22–24] The subsequent RCT (which was reported in Chinese) has a number of design weaknesses, which suggests that the results need to be interpreted with caution.[21] It gives no clear definition of burning mouth syndrome; it does not specify the method of randomisation; the study was not blinded; the scale used for assessing improvement of symptoms was not validated; and there were important differences between the groups at baseline.

OPTION DIETARY SUPPLEMENTS

We found insufficient evidence from three small methodologically flawed RCTs to draw reliable conclusions about the effects of alphalipoic acid in people with burning mouth syndrome. We found no RCTs evaluating other vitamin or coenzyme supplements.

Benefits: We found one systematic review (search date 2000, 1 RCT, 42 people)[20] and two subsequent RCTs.[25,26] All three RCTs evaluated outcomes on a five point scale (symptoms "worsening", "unchanged", "slight improvement", "decided improvement", or "resolution"). The RCT included in the review compared alphalipoic acid (600 mg/day for 20 days, followed by 200 mg/day for 10 days) versus placebo.[20] It found that alphalipoic acid significantly improved symptoms compared with placebo (AR for "slight improvement" or "decided improvement": 16/21 [76%] with alphalipoic acid *v* 3/14 [21%] with placebo; RR 3.6, 95% CI 1.6 to 7.7; NNT 2, 95% CI 1 to 3; follow up period unclear). The first subsequent RCT (60 people) found that alphalipoic acid (200 mg 3 times daily) significantly improved symptoms after 2 months compared with placebo (AR for "slight improvement", "decided improvement", or "resolution": 29/30 [97%] with alphalipoic acid *v* 12/30 [40%] with placebo; $P < 0.0001$).[25] The second subsequent RCT (80 people) compared alphalipoic acid (200 mg 3 times daily), lactoperoxidase mouth rinse (5–6 times daily), bethanecol (5 mg 3 times daily), and placebo.[26] It found that alphalipoic acid increased the proportion of people reporting improvement on the symptom scale at 60 days compared with the three other treatment options (18/20 [90%] with alphalipoic acid *v* 2/20 [10%] with bethanecol *v* 0/20 [0%] with lactoperoxidase *v* 0/20 [0%] with placebo; it is unclear to what comparison the reported P value of < 0.0001 refers).

Harms: In the second subsequent RCT, four people in the alphalipoic acid arm reported heartburn, which settled with ranitidine. Four people taking bethanecol experienced adverse events, including nausea, dizziness, cold perspiration, or abdominal pain.[26]

Comment: The three RCTs of alphalipoic acid were performed by the same group at overlapping time periods.[20,25,26] Therefore, we could not exclude the possibility that duplicate data may have been reported. Two of the trials were not clearly reported as being blinded. Unblinded assessment of subjective outcomes should be interpreted with caution.

OPTION ANTIDEPRESSANTS

We found insufficient evidence on the effects of antidepressants in people with burning mouth syndrome.

Benefits: We found one systematic review (search date 2000, 2 RCTs, 290 people of whom 114 had burning mouth syndrome)[20] and one small subsequent RCT.[27] **Clomipramine and mianserin:** The review identified one short term RCT (253 people with chronic idiopathic pain syndrome, including 77 people with burning mouth syndrome) comparing clomipramine, mianserin, and placebo (see comment below).[20] The study had a number of significant methodological flaws (see comment below). It found no significant difference in improvement in pain between the three treatments over 6 weeks (analysis not by intention to treat; improvement defined as a 50% reduction in pain scores on a visual analogue scale and the Clinical Global Impression Scale; results displayed graphically; P = 0.11). **Trazodone:** The review identified one double blind RCT (37 women with burning mouth syndrome) comparing trazodone (200 mg/day) versus placebo.[20] It found no significant difference in pain or related symptoms between trazodone and placebo measured on a visual analogue scale (0 mm = best score and 100 mm = worst score) at 8 weeks (–4.8 mm, 95% CI –20.3 mm to +10.7 mm). **Selective serotonin reuptake inhibitors versus amisulpride:** We found one small RCT (76 people), which found similar reduction in pain score (pain assessed by 10 point visual analogue scale, higher scores indicating more severe pain) with sertraline (50 mg/day), paroxetine (20 mg/day), and amisulpride (50 mg/day) at 8 weeks (mean score reduction: 4.4 with sertraline *v* 3.7 with paroxetine *v* 4 with amisulpride; P value not reported).[27] However, the study may have lacked power to detect clinically important differences among treatments and lacked a placebo comparison.

Harms: **Clomipramine and mianserin:** Adverse effects of clomipramine, mianserin, and other antidepressants are documented elsewhere (see depressive disorders, p 1238). **Trazodone:** The RCT found that adverse effects caused 7/18 (39%) people taking trazodone to withdraw from the trial compared with 2/19 (10%) taking placebo.[20] Significantly more people given trazodone experienced dizziness and drowsiness compared with placebo (dizziness: 11/18 with trazodone *v* 1/19 with placebo, P < 0.001; drowsiness: 9/18 with trazodone *v* 2/19 with placebo, P < 0.05). **Selective serotonin reuptake inhibitors versus amisulpride:** The RCT reported no serious adverse effects in any treatment group.[27]

Comment: The trial of clomipramine and mianserin versus placebo included in the systematic review was too small to exclude an effect of treatment, did not use adequate diagnostic criteria, was of short duration, and had limited follow up.[20] In addition, the review was not able to identify how many people with burning mouth syndrome were allocated to each treatment group. Therefore, this study does not provide sufficient evidence to determine the role of antidepressants in treating burning mouth syndrome. Although the trial of trazodone versus placebo was well conducted and used several pertinent outcome measures, including psychological ones, it was too small and brief to detect clinically important effects.[20] In the RCT comparing selective serotonin reuptake inhibitors versus amisulpride, 34 people had a concurrent psychiatric diagnosis.[27] The widespread use of antidepressants in burning mouth syndrome may be because of their effects on neuropathic pain,[28] and the association of burning mouth syndrome with generalised anxiety disorder, depression, and adverse life events.[29]

OPTION BENZYDAMINE HYDROCHLORIDE

We found insufficient evidence on the effects of benzydamine hydrochloride in burning mouth syndrome.

Benefits: We found one systematic review (search date 2000).[20] It found one small RCT (30 people with burning mouth syndrome) comparing benzydamine hydrochloride oral rinse (15 mL of 0.15% for 1 minute 3 times daily for 4 weeks), placebo, and no treatment. It found no significant difference in improvement in symptoms between groups at 4 weeks (AR for improvement: 10% with benzydamine hydrochloride *v* 20% with placebo *v* 10% with no therapy; P value not reported). However, the trial was too small to exclude a clinically important difference.[20]

Harms: No adverse effects were reported.

Comment: Inclusion criteria were well defined. The trial was incompletely blinded because the third group received no treatment.

GLOSSARY

Supertaster Persons who have the highest density of fungiform papillae, which are responsible for taste, on the anterior tongue and taste 6–n–propylthiouracil as intensely bitter.

REFERENCES

1. Fox H. Burning tongue glossodynia. *N Y State J Med* 1935;35:881–884.
2. Zakrzewska JM. The burning mouth syndrome remains an enigma. *Pain* 1995;62:253–257.
3. Van der Waal I. *The burning mouth syndrome*. 1st ed. Copenhagen: Munksgaard, 1990.
4. Merksey H, Bogduk N, eds. *Classification of chronic pain*. 2nd ed. Seattle: International Association for the Study of Pain Press, 1994.
5. Bergdahl M, Bergdahl J. Burning mouth syndrome: prevalence and associated factors. *J Oral Pathol Med* 1999;28:350–354.
6. Grushka M, Sessle BJ. Burning mouth syndrome. *Dent Clin North Am* 1991;35:171–184.
7. Bergdahl J, Anneroth G, Anneroth I. Clinical study of patients with burning mouth. *Scand J Dent Res* 1994;102:299–305.
8. Maragou P, Ivanyi L. Serum zinc levels in patients with burning mouth syndrome. *Oral Surg Oral Med Oral Pathol Oral Radiol Endod* 1991;71:447–450.
9. Lamey PJ, Allam BF. Vitamin status of patients with burning mouth syndrome and the response to replacement therapy. *Br Dent J* 1986;168:81–84.
10. Hugoson A, Thorstensson B. Vitamin B status and response to replacement therapy in patients with burning mouth syndrome. *Acta Odontol Scand* 1991;49:367–375.
11. Tammiala-Salonen T, Hiidenkarii T, Parvinen T. Burning mouth in a Finnish adult population. *Community Dent Oral Epidemiol* 1993;21:67–71.
12. Basker RM, Sturdee DW, Davenport JC. Patients with burning mouths. A clinical investigation of causative factors, including the climacteric and diabetes. *Br Dent J* 1978;145:9–16.
13. Grushka M. Clinical features of burning mouth syndrome. *Oral Surg Oral Med Oral Pathol Oral Radiol Endod* 1987;63:30–36.
14. Wardrop RW, Hailes J, Burger H, et al. Oral discomfort at the menopause. *Oral Surg Oral Med Oral Pathol Oral Radiol Endod* 1989;67:535–540.
15. Lipton JA, Ship JA, Larach-Robinson D. Estimated prevalence and distribution of reported orofacial pain in the United States. *J Am Dent Assoc* 1993;124:115–121.
16. Rojo L, Silvestre FJ, Bagan JV, et al. Psychiatric morbidity in burning mouth syndrome. Psychiatric interview versus depression and anxiety scales. *Oral Surg Oral Med Oral Pathol Oral Radiol Endod* 1993;75:308–311.

17. Lamey PJ, Lamb AB. The usefulness of the HAD scale in assessing anxiety in patients with burning mouth syndrome. *Oral Surg Oral Med Oral Pathol Oral Radiol Endod* 1989;67:390–392.
18. Bartoshuk LM, Grushka M, Duffy VB, et al. Burning mouth syndrome: damage to CN VII and pain phantoms in CN V. *Chem Senses* 1999;24:609.
19. Zakrzewska JM, Hamlyn PJ. Facial pain. In: Crombie IK, Croft PR, Linton SJ, et al, eds. *Epidemiology of pain*. Seattle: International Association for the Study of Pain Press, 1999:177–202.
20. Zakrzewska JM, Glenny AM, Forsell H. Interventions for the treatment of burning mouth syndrome. In: The Cochrane Library, Issue 2, 2003. Oxford: Update Software. Search date 2000; primary sources Medline, Embase, The Cochrane Library, and The Cochrane Oral Health Group's Specialised Register.
21. Peng JY,Wu YF, Han WN, et al. Clinical efficacy of burning mouth syndrome treated by livial. *Bull Hunan Med Univ* 2001,26:157–158.
22. Pisanty S, Rafaely B, Polshuk WZ. The effects of steroid hormones on buccal mucosa of menopausal women. *Oral Surg Oral Med Oral Pathol Oral Radiol Endod* 1975;40:346–353.
23. Ferguson MM, Carter J, Boyle P, et al. Oral complaints related to climacteric symptoms in oophorectomized women. *J R Soc Med* 1981;74:492–497.
24. Forabosco A, Crisculo M, Coukos G, et al. Efficacy of hormone replacement therapy in postmenopausal women with oral discomfort. *Oral Surg Oral Med Oral Pathol Oral Radiol Endod* 1992;73:570–574.
25. Femiano F, Scully C. Burning mouth syndrome (BMS): double blind controlled study of alpha-lipoic acid (thioctic acid) therapy. *J Oral Pathol Med* 2002:31:267–269.
26. Femiano F. Burning mouth syndrome (BMS): an open trial of comparative efficacy of alpha-lipoic acid (thioctic acid) with other therapies. *Minerva Stomatol* 2002;51:405–409.
27. Maina G, Vitalucci A, Gandolfo S, et al. Comparative efficacy of SSRIs and amisulpiride in burning mouth syndrome: A single–blind study. *J Clin Psychiatry* 2002;63:38–43.
28. McQuay HJ, Tramer M, Nye BA, et al. A systematic review of antidepressants in neuropathic pain. *Pain* 1996;68:217–227.
29. Bogetto F, Maina G, Ferro G, et al. Psychiatric comorbidity in patients with burning mouth syndrome. *Psychosom Med* 1998;60:378–385.

John Buchanan
Specialist Registrar/Honorary Lecturer in Oral Medicine
The Eastman Dental Institute for Dental Health Care Sciences
University College London
London
UK

Joanna Zakrzewska
Professor of Pain in Relation to Oral Medicine
St Bartholomew's and the London Queen Mary's School of Medicine and Dentistry
London
UK

Competing interests: None declared.

Candidiasis (oropharyngeal)

Search date June 2004

Caroline Pankhurst

QUESTIONS

INTERVENTIONS

To be covered in future updates

Prevention and treatment in neonates

Treatment of systemic candidiasis

Key Messages

Immunosuppressed adults

- **Antifungal prophylaxis with absorbed or partially absorbed antifungal drugs in people undergoing cancer treatments** One systematic review and one subsequent RCT found that absorbed antifungal drugs (ketoconazole, itraconazole, fluconazole) reduced the risk of oropharyngeal candidiasis compared with placebo or no drug treatment, or compared with unabsorbed antifungals (nystatin alone, nystatin plus chlorhexidine, amphotericin B alone, or amphotericin B combined with nystatin, norfloxacin, natamycin, thymostimulin, or chlorhexidine). The review also found that partially absorbed antifungal drugs (miconazole, clotrimazole) reduced the risk of oropharyngeal candidiasis compared with placebo or no drug treatment. The review found no significant difference in the risk of oropharyngeal candidiasis between unabsorbed drugs and placebo. However, there was significant heterogeneity among studies. The review found no significant difference in adverse events between absorbed antifungal drugs and placebo.
- **Antifungal prophylaxis in people receiving tissue transplants** Two small RCTs in people with liver transplant found no significant difference in the risk of oropharyngeal candidiasis between nystatin and fluconazole or clotrimazole. However, the trials may have lacked power to detect clinically important differences. We found insufficient evidence from two RCTs about the effects of prophylactic chlorhexidine mouth rinse with or without nystatin compared with placebo in people receiving bone marrow transplant.
- **Antifungal treatment in people undergoing chemotherapy, radiotherapy, or both treatments for cancer** One systematic review and one subsequent RCT found insufficient evidence about the clinical effects of antifungals compared with placebo for treating oropharyngeal candidiasis in people undergoing chemotherapy or radiotherapy, or about the effects of different antifungal agents or doses in people with oropharyngeal candidiasis receiving radiotherapy or chemotherapy.

Infants and children

- **Antifungal treatment with miconazole or fluconazole in immunocompetent and immunocompromised infants and children (more effective than nystatin)** RCTs found that miconazole and fluconazole increased clinical cure of oropharyngeal candidiasis compared with nystatin in immunocompetent and immunocompromised infants and children.
- **Antifungal prophylaxis with fluconazole in immunocompromised infants and children (more effective than oral nystatin or amphotericin B)** One large RCT in immunocompromised infants and children found that fluconazole reduced the incidence of oropharyngeal candidiasis compared with oral nystatin, amphotericin B, or both.

In diabetes

- **Treatments in people with diabetes mellitus** We found no systematic review or RCTs assessing preventive interventions or treatments for oropharyngeal candidiasis in people with diabetes.

Dentures

- **Antifungal treatment for denture stomatitis** We found insufficient evidence from small RCTs to compare effects of antifungal agents versus placebo or versus each other for treating oropharyngeal candidiasis in people who wear dentures.
- **Denture hygiene** We found insufficient evidence from three RCTs, two of which were underpowered, to assess clinical effects on oropharyngeal candidiasis of mouth rinses, disinfectants, denture soaks, denture scrubbing, and microwave irradiation of dentures. Microwave treatment is not suitable for all dentures.

Prevention/treatment in HIV

- **Antifungal prophylaxis with fluconazole, itraconazole or nystatin in people with advanced HIV disease** RCTs in people with HIV infection found that daily or weekly antifungal prophylaxis with fluconazole, itraconazole, or nystatin reduced incidence and relapse of oropharyngeal candidiasis compared with placebo. One large RCT found that fluconazole reduced recurrence of oropharyngeal candidiasis compared with clotrimazole.
- **Oral suspension of systemically absorbed azoles in people with HIV infection** RCTs found that topical preparations of itraconazole, fluconazole, miconazole nitrate, and clotrimazole effectively treated oropharyngeal candidiasis in people with HIV infection. One RCT found that fluconazole reduced symptoms and signs of oropharyngeal candidiasis compared with topical nystatin.

Reducing drug resistance

- **Continuous prophylaxis versus intermittent treatment in people with HIV infection and acute episodes of oropharyngeal candidiasis (in preventing antifungal resistance)** One RCT in people with HIV infection and acute episodes of oropharyngeal candidiasis found no significant difference between continuous antifungal prophylaxis with fluconazole and intermittent antifungal treatment with fluconazole in terms of the emergence of antifungal resistance.

DEFINITION Oropharyngeal candidiasis is an opportunistic mucosal infection caused, in most cases, by *Candida albicans*. The four main types of oropharyngeal candidiasis are: (1) pseudomembranous (thrush), consisting of white discrete plaques on an erythematous background, on the buccal mucosa, throat, tongue, or gingivae; (2) erythematous, consisting of smooth red patches on the hard or soft palate, dorsum of tongue, or buccal mucosa; (3) hyperplastic, consisting of white, firmly adherent patches or plaques, usually bilaterally distributed on the buccal mucosa; and (4) denture induced stomatitis, presenting as either a smooth or granular erythema confined to the denture bearing area of the hard palate and often associated with an angular cheilitis.[1] Symptoms vary, ranging from none to a sore and painful mouth with a burning tongue and altered taste. Oropharyngeal candidiasis can impair speech, nutritional intake, and quality of life.

INCIDENCE/PREVALENCE *Candida* species are commensals in the gastrointestinal tract. Transmission occurs directly between infected people or on fomites (objects that can harbour pathogenic organisms). *Candida* is found in the mouth of 31–60% of healthy people.[2] Denture stomatitis associated with *Candida* is prevalent in 65% of denture wearers.[2] Oropharyngeal candidiasis affects 15–60% of people with haematological or oncological malignancies during periods of immunosuppression.[3] Oropharyngeal candidiasis occurs in 7–48% of people with HIV infection and in over 90% of those with advanced disease. In severely immunosuppressed people, relapse rates are high (30–50%) and relapse usually occurs within 14 days of stopping treatment.[4]

AETIOLOGY/RISK FACTORS Risk factors associated with symptomatic oropharyngeal candidiasis include local or systemic immunosuppression, haematological disorders, broad spectrum antibiotic use, inhaled or systemic steroids, xerostomia, diabetes, and wearing dentures, obturators, or orthodontic appliances.[1,5] The same strain may persist for months or years in the absence of infection. In people with HIV infection, there is no direct correlation between the number of organisms and the presence of clinical disease. Symptomatic oropharyngeal candidiasis associated with *in vitro* resistance to fluconazole occurs in 5% of people with advanced HIV disease.[6] Resistance to azole antifungals is associated with severe immunosuppression ($\leq$ 50 CD4 cells/mm^3), more episodes treated with antifungal drugs, and longer median duration of systemic azole treatment.[7]

PROGNOSIS In most people, untreated candidiasis persists for months or years unless associated risk factors are treated or eliminated. In neonates, spontaneous cure of oropharyngeal candidiasis usually occurs after 3–8 weeks.

AIMS OF INTERVENTION To resolve signs and symptoms of oropharyngeal candidiasis; to prevent or delay relapse in immunocompromised people; and to minimise drug induced resistance, with minimum adverse effects.

OUTCOMES Resolution of signs and symptoms; clinical cure; rate of recurrence on the basis of scoring of signs and symptoms. Many RCTs report the results of mycological culture but, whenever possible, this review does not use these intermediate outcomes because the relation between the clinical and mycological culture findings is uncertain.

METHODS *Clinical Evidence* search and appraisal June 2004, including a search for observational studies on dental hygiene. This was supplemented by a search of the author's library, selecting publications in English language from 1975–2004. We included only systematic reviews and RCTs that specified oropharyngeal candidiasis in the protocol design and outcome measurements. RCTs dealing with oesophagitis and invasive, systemic candidal infections were excluded.

QUESTION What are the effects of interventions to prevent and treat oropharyngeal candidiasis in adults receiving treatment causing immunosuppression?

OPTION ANTIFUNGAL PROPHYLAXIS IN PEOPLE RECEIVING CANCER TREATMENTS

One systematic review and one subsequent RCT found that absorbed antifungal drugs (ketoconazole, itraconazole, fluconazole) reduced the risk of oropharyngeal candidiasis compared with placebo or no drug treatment, or compared with unabsorbed antifungals (nystatin alone, nystatin plus chlorhexidine, amphotericin B alone, or amphotericin B combined with nystatin, norfloxacin, natamycin, thymostimulin, or chlorhexidine). The review also found that partially absorbed antifungal drugs (miconazole, clotrimazole) reduced the risk of oropharyngeal candidiasis compared with placebo or no drug treatment. The review found no significant difference in the risk of oropharyngeal candidiasis between unabsorbed drugs and placebo. However, there was significant heterogeneity among studies. The review found no significant difference in adverse events between absorbed antifungal drugs and placebo.

Benefits: We found one systematic review (search date 2001, 27 RCTs, 4137 people receiving chemotherapy or radiotherapy for cancer)[8] and one subsequent RCT that compared oral and topical antifungal prophylaxis versus placebo, no treatment, or each other.[9] The drugs were categorised by degree of absorption from the gastrointestinal tract. **Absorbed antifungals versus placebo:** The review found that absorbed antifungal drugs (ketoconazole, itraconazole, fluconazole) significantly reduced the risk of oral candidiasis compared with placebo or no drug treatment (7 RCTs: 1153 people; RR 0.45, 95% CI 0.32 to 0.64).[8] **Partially absorbed antifungals versus placebo:** The review found that partially absorbed antifungal drugs (miconazole, clotrimazole) significantly reduced the risk of oral candidiasis compared with placebo or no drug treatment (4 RCTs: 292 people; RR 0.13, 95% CI 0.06 to 0.27).[8] **Unabsorbed antifungals versus placebo:** The review found no significant difference in the risk of oral candidiasis between unabsorbed drugs (nystatin alone, nystatin plus chlorhexidine, amphotericin B alone, or amphotericin B combined with nystatin, norfloxacin, natamycin, thymostimulin, or chlorhexidine) and placebo (8 RCTs: 382 people; RR 0.68, 95% CI 0.46 to 1.02).[8] However, the review found significant heterogeneity in the included studies of these drugs ($P < 0.001$). **Absorbed versus unabsorbed antifungals:** The review found that absorbed antifungal drugs reduced the risk of oral candidiasis compared with unabsorbed antifungal drugs (7 RCTs: 2014 people; RR 0.40, 95% CI 0.21 to 0.76).[8] The subsequent RCT (106 adults with haematological malignancies and neutropenia) compared itraconazole solution (5 mg/kg twice daily) versus unabsorbed amphotericin B solution (1000 mg three times daily; treatments given until neutropenia had resolved).[9] It found that itraconazole solution significantly reduced *Candida* colonisation and infection compared with amphotericin B solution during neutropenia (*Candida* colonisation rate in the rectum: 19.6% with itraconazole *v* 38.9% with amphotericin B; P < 0.05; *Candida* colonisation rate in the oropharynx: 19.6% with itraconazole *v* 40.6% with amphotericin B; P < 0.05; fungal infection rate: 3.8% with itraconazole *v* 14.8% with amphotericin B; P < 0.05).

Harms: The systematic review found no significant difference in adverse effects between absorbed antifungal drugs and placebo (62/437 [14%] with absorbed antifungals *v* 52/434 [12%] with placebo; RR 1.18, 95% CI 0.84 to 1.66). The most common adverse effects were abdominal pain, nausea, vomiting, and rash.[8] The subsequent RCT did not report on harms.[9]

Comment: The subsequent RCT did not achieve its desired power, which would have required 80 participants in each treatment group.

OPTION **ANTIFUNGAL PROPHYLAXIS IN ADULTS WHO HAVE RECEIVED TISSUE TRANSPLANTS**

Two small RCTs in people with liver transplant found no significant difference in the risk of oropharyngeal candidiasis between nystatin and fluconazole or clotrimazole. However, the trials may have lacked power to detect clinically important differences. We found insufficient evidence from two RCTs about the effects of prophylactic chlorhexidine mouth rinse with or without nystatin compared with placebo in people receiving bone marrow transplant.

Benefits: **In people receiving liver transplant:** We found no systematic review. We found two small RCTs in people with liver transplant comparing the abilities of different antifungal agents to prevent oropharyngeal candidiasis.[10,11] The first RCT (143 people) found similar rates of oropharyngeal candidiasis between fluconazole and nystatin at 28 days (rate of oropharyngeal candidiasis: 8/76 [11%] with fluconazole *v* 14/67 [21%] with nystatin; P value not reported).[10] The second RCT (34 people) found similar rates of oropharyngeal candidiasis between clotrimazole and nystatin during hospital stay after transplantation (rate of oropharyngeal candidiasis: 1/17 [6%] with clotrimazole *v* 1/17 [6%] with nystatin; P value not reported).[11] However, the RCTs may have lacked power to detect clinically important differences. **In people receiving bone marrow transplant:** We found no systematic review. We found two RCTs in people with neutropenia who had received bone marrow transplants.[12,13] The first RCT (51 people) found that chlorhexidine significantly reduced the risk of oropharyngeal candidiasis compared with placebo at 60 days (2/24 [8%] with chlorhexidine *v* 15/27 [56%] with placebo; ARR 47%, 95% CI 24% to 54%; RR 0.15, 95% CI 0.03 to 0.57; NNT 2, 95% CI 2 to 4).[12] The second RCT (86 adults with leukaemia and bone marrow transplant) found similar rates of development of oropharyngeal candidiasis between rinses containing saline alone, chlorhexidine alone, nystatin alone, or nystatin plus chlorhexidine (no statistical analysis available).[13]

Harms: There was no increased hepatotoxicity, cyclosporin interaction, or emergence of clinically relevant resistant strains reported in people receiving antifungal prophylaxis after liver transplantation.[10] The other three RCTs did not report on adverse effects.[11–13]

Comment: The RCTs of chlorhexidine found conflicting results about its effect on oropharyngeal candidiasis and mucositis,[12,13] but the second RCT had four parallel arms and was not powered to detect a clinically important difference.[13]

OPTION **ANTIFUNGAL TREATMENT IN PEOPLE RECEIVING CHEMOTHERAPY AND RADIOTHERAPY**

One systematic review and one subsequent RCT found insufficient evidence about the clinical effects of antifungals compared with placebo for treating oropharyngeal candidiasis in people undergoing chemotherapy or radiotherapy, or about the effects of different antifungal agents or doses in people with oropharyngeal candidiasis receiving radiotherapy or chemotherapy.

Benefits: We found one systematic review (search date 2003, 8 RCTs, 418 people with cancer receiving chemotherapy, radiotherapy, or both)[14] and one subsequent RCT that compared antifungal treatment of oral candidiasis versus placebo or another active intervention.[15] **Antifungals versus placebo:** The systematic review included one small RCT that met *Clinical Evidence* inclusion criteria.[14] The RCT (56 people) found that ketoconazole significantly decreased oral candidiasis compared with placebo at 14 days (persistence of oral candidiasis: 10/36 [28%] people with ketoconazole *v* 16/20 [80%] people with placebo; RR 0.35, 95% CI 0.20 to 0.61). **Versus different dosages:** One RCT (52 people) included in the review found no significant difference in clinically assessed cure of oral candidiasis between a 50 mg troche of clotrimazole and 10 mg clotrimazole (persistence of oral candidiasis: 1/26 [4%] with clotrimazole 50 mg *v* 1/26 [4%] with clotrimazole 10 mg; RR 1.00, 95% CI 0.07 to 15.15).[14] The timing of outcome measurement was unclear. **Absorbed antifungals versus each other:** The systematic review found no significant difference in clinically assessed cure rates between different absorbed antifungals (2 RCTs; persistence of oral candidiasis: 6/46 [13%] with fluconazole *v* 8/44 [18%] with ketoconazole/itraconazole; RR 0.72, 95% CI 0.27 to 1.88).[14] **Absorbed versus non-absorbed antifungals:** The review found three RCTs comparing absorbed versus non-absorbed antifungals.[14] There was significant heterogeneity among the RCTs (P = 0.01). One RCT found that fluconazole significantly improved clinical cure rates compared with nystatin. One RCT found no significant difference between ketoconazole and nystatin in clinical or mycological cure rates. One RCT found fluconazole significantly improved cure rates when assessed clinically compared with amphotericin B.[14] Pooling the results of the three RCTs, the review found no significant difference between absorbed and non-absorbed drugs in clinical cure rates (3 RCTs; persistence of oral candidiasis: 16/105 [15%] with fluconazole/ketoconazole *v* 35/102 [34%] with amphotericin/nystatin; RR 0.50, 95% CI 0.11 to 2.27; random effects model). However, given the heterogeneity of the included studies, these results may not be robust. We found one subsequent RCT (268 people with head and neck cancer, 243 evaluated), which compared fluconazole oral suspension 50 mg once daily versus amphotericin B oral suspension 0.5 mg three times daily for 7–14 days.[15] It found no significant difference in rates of clinical cure of oral candidiasis between fluconazole and amphotericin (clinical cure: 26/123 [21%] with fluconazole *v* 17/120 [14%] with amphotericin B).

Harms: The systematic review and subsequent RCT did not report on harms.[14,15]

Comment: In assessing outcomes, the review noted that few RCTs described the clinical criteria used.[14] The review concluded that there were insufficient trials to make strong recommendations for patient care, and that there was a need for further well designed, placebo controlled trials to assess the effectiveness of old and new interventions for treating oral candidiasis.[14]

QUESTION What are the effects of interventions to prevent and treat oropharyngeal candidiasis in infants and children?

OPTION ANTIFUNGAL PREVENTION IN IMMUNOCOMPROMISED INFANTS AND CHILDREN

One large RCT in immunocompromised infants and children found that fluconazole reduced the incidence of oropharyngeal candidiasis compared with oral nystatin, amphotericin B, or both.

Benefits: We found no systematic review. We found no placebo controlled RCTs. We found one large, open label, multicentre RCT (502 immunocompromised infants and children aged 6 months to 17 years about to undergo initial or repeat courses of chemotherapy or radiotherapy for haematological or oncological malignancies).[3] It found that fluconazole significantly reduced the incidence of oropharyngeal candidiasis compared with oral polyenes (nystatin, oral amphotericin B, or both) (3/236 [1%] with fluconazole *v* 15/249 [6%] with oral polyenes; RR 0.21, 95% CI 0.06 to 0.72; NNT 21, 95% CI 18 to 58). Eighteen of the children from the multicentre RCT[3] were enrolled in a second, small RCT (50 children in total), which compared fluconazole versus oral nystatin for preventing oropharyngeal candidiasis.[16] The RCT found no significant difference in the incidence of oral candidiasis (2/25 [8%] with fluconazole *v* 3/25 [12%] with nystatin; P = 0.63). However, inclusion of pre-treated children may have biased results, and the study may have lacked power to detect clinically important differences.

Harms: In the first RCT, adverse events caused 8/245 (3%) children on fluconazole to withdraw compared with 3/257 (1%) on oral polyenes.[3] In the second RCT no children were withdrawn from the study, but three children treated with fluconazole reported nausea and abdominal discomfort and one reported pruritus.[16]

Comment: None.

OPTION ANTIFUNGAL TREATMENT IN CHILDREN

RCTs found that miconazole and fluconazole increased clinical cure of oropharyngeal candidiasis compared with nystatin in immunocompetent and immunocompromised infants and children.

Benefits: **Immunocompetent infants and children:** We found no systematic review. We found no placebo controlled RCTs. We found two RCTs in immunocompetent infants with oropharyngeal candidiasis, which compared miconazole gel, nystatin suspension, and nystatin gel.[17,18] We found one RCT, which compared fluconazole versus nystatin.[19] Both RCTs comparing miconazole versus nystatin found that miconazole significantly increased the rate of clinical cure. The larger RCT (183 infants age < 1 year with signs of oropharyngeal candidiasis) found that miconazole gel had a significantly increased cure rate compared with nystatin (at day 5: cure rate 83/98 [85%] with miconazole gel 25 mg 4 times daily *v* 18/85 [21%] with nystatin suspension 100 000 U 4 times daily; P < 0.0001; at day 12: 97/98 [99%] with miconazole *v* 46/85 [54%] with nystatin; P < 0.0001).[17] The smaller RCT (95 infants, mean age 5 months, range 2–17 months with clinical oral thrush) found that miconazole gel significantly increased clinical cure at 14 days compared with two brands of nystatin gel preparation (P = 0.0032 and P = 0.00068).[18] One RCT (47 infants aged 1–12 months with clinical signs of oral candidiasis and culture positive for *Candida* species) compared nystatin oral suspension 100 000 IU/mL four times daily for

10 days versus fluconazole suspension 3 mg/kg once daily for 7 days.[19] It found that fluconazole significantly increased clinical cure compared with nystatin (36 infants evaluated; clinical cure: 15/15 [100%] with fluconazole v 6/19 [32%] with nystatin; P < 0.0001).[19] **Immunocompromised infants and children:** We found no systematic review. We found no placebo controlled RCTs. We found one multicentre RCT (32 centres, 182 immunocompromised infants and children aged 5 months to 14 years), which compared fluconazole suspension 3 mg/kg versus nystatin 400 000 U four times daily for 14 days.[20] It found that fluconazole significantly increased clinical cure rate compared with nystatin (78/86 [91%] with fluconazole v 37/73 [51%] with nystatin; RR 1.8, 95% CI 1.6 to 1.9; NNT 2, 95% CI 2 to 3).[20] In subgroup analyses of children with HIV infection, fluconazole significantly increased clinical cure compared with nystatin (clinical cure: 28/35 [80%] with fluconazole v 6/29 [21%] with nystatin; P < 0.001), and for children with malignancy (clinical cure: 49/50 [98%] with fluconazole v 30/42 [71%] with nystatin; P = 0.001). Clinical relapse rates after 2 weeks were similar (18% with fluconazole v 24% with nystatin).

Harms: **Immunocompetent infants and children:** The most common adverse events with both miconazole and nystatin were vomiting and, more rarely, diarrhoea, affecting less than 4.5% of infants.[17,18] **Immunocompromised infants and children:** Adverse events caused 2/94 (2%) children on fluconazole to withdraw versus 0/88 (0%) children on nystatin (P = 0.04).[20]

Comment: **Immunocompetent infants and children:** The RCTs were not blinded nor placebo controlled.[17–19] There is potential for observer bias, but the clinical results were corroborated by mycological findings, which were blinded.[17] The larger RCT was carried out in 26 general practices,[17] and so it is representative of the context in which most otherwise healthy infants with oropharyngeal candidiasis would be treated, especially regarding adherence and cure rate. **Immunocompromised infants and children:** Participants included in the RCT were immunocompromised for different reasons: 64 had HIV infection, 92 had a malignancy, and 26 were receiving immunosuppressive treatment.[20]

QUESTION What are the effects of interventions to prevent and treat oropharyngeal candidiasis in people with diabetes?

OPTION ANTIFUNGAL DRUGS

We found no systematic review or RCTs assessing preventive interventions or treatments for oropharyngeal candidiasis in people with diabetes.

Benefits: We found no systematic review or RCTs.

Harms: We found no RCTs.

Comment: None.

QUESTION What are the effects of interventions for oropharyngeal candidiasis in people with dentures?

OPTION ANTIFUNGAL DRUGS

We found insufficient evidence from small RCTs to compare effects of antifungal agents versus placebo or versus each other for treating oropharyngeal candidiasis in people who wear dentures.

Benefits: **Versus placebo:** We found no systematic review. We found three small RCTs comparing topical oral antifungals versus placebo for the treatment of denture stomatitis.[21–23] The first small RCT (46 people) found that topical oral polyenes (nystatin, amphotericin B) significantly improved clinical cure of denture stomatitis after 4 weeks of treatment compared with placebo (nystatin *v* placebo, $P \le 0.05$; amphotericin B *v* placebo, $P \le 0.01$).[21] The second small RCT (36 people) found no significant difference in the resolution of palatal symptoms between miconazole dental lacquer (applied to the fit surface of an upper denture as a single application) and a placebo lacquer at 14 days (symptom resolution: 54% with lacquer *v* 23% with placebo; RR 2.40, 95% CI 0.89 to 3.80).[22] The third small RCT (38 people) found that fluconazole significantly increased clinical improvement or cure rates compared with placebo at 2 and 4 weeks (at 2 weeks: 10/19 [53%] with fluconazole *v* 0/18 [0%] with placebo; $P < 0.001$; at 4 weeks: 5/19 [26%] with fluconazole *v* 0/19 [0%] with placebo; $P < 0.02$).[23] **Different antifungal treatments:** We found no systematic review. We found two RCTs.[24,25] The first small RCT (29 people) found similar rates of clinical cure rate between fluconazole 50 mg daily for 14 days and amphotericin B lozenges plus denture cream for 28 days (84% with fluconazole *v* 90% with amphotericin B; P value not reported).[24] Clinical relapse was common in both groups at 12 weeks. The second RCT (multicentre; 305 elderly people, 176 with dentures) found similar rates of clinical cure between fluconazole 50 mg and amphotericin B 0.5 g. Wearing dentures did not affect the response to antifungal treatment (clinical cure rate: 151/176 [86%] of denture wearers *v* 102/124 [82%] of non-denture wearers; P value not reported).[25] **Different modes of administration:** We found no systematic review. Two RCTs (41 people[26] and 33 people[27]) compared a single application of miconazole dental lacquer versus miconazole gel 2% applied to the denture four times daily. Neither RCT found a significant difference in palatal erythema (largest RCT, 14 days after treatment: 13/20 [65%] with lacquer *v* 16/21 [76%] with gel; RR of erythema with lacquer *v* gel: 0.85, 95% CI 0.42 to 1.20).[26,27]

Harms: None of the trials exclusively enrolling people with dentures were large enough to report reliably on adverse effects. In the large RCT of elderly people, 6/150 (4%) in the fluconazole arm and 0/155 (0%) in the amphotericin arm experienced adverse events, including diarrhoea, buccal bitterness, aggravation of pre-existing renal dysfunction (1 person, withdrawn from RCT), and increased liver transaminases (1 person, not withdrawn).[25]

Comment: Co-interventions included professional cleaning of the dentures at the start of the study, combined with advice on denture hygiene and advice not to wear the dentures while asleep at night. Because the fit surface of the denture may act as a reservoir of primary and recurrent infection, this cleaning and advice may explain the high clinical cure rate in the placebo groups. The RCTs comparing different antifungals were not sufficiently powered to detect clinically important differences between treatments.

OPTION DENTURE HYGIENE

We found insufficient evidence from three RCTs, two of which were underpowered, to assess clinical effects on oropharyngeal candidiasis of mouth rinses, disinfectants, denture soaks, denture scrubbing, and microwave irradiation of dentures. Microwave treatment is not suitable for all dentures.

Benefits: We found no systematic review, but found three RCTs.[28–30] The first small crossover RCT (43 people aged 35–73 years) compared daily soaking of dentures in disinfectant (potassium persulphate 1%) versus placebo (water, peppermint, dye) for 4 weeks.[28] The results provided for the outcome of stomatitis were difficult to interpret and therefore no firm conclusions can be drawn. The second RCT (78 people with mild to moderate denture stomatitis) compared three treatments: mouth rinsing three times daily plus denture soaking once daily, using an antimicrobial mouth rinse; the same procedure, using a control mouth rinse; and weekly relining of the fit surface of the denture (to improve retention and reduce denture trauma) for 4 weeks.[29] It found that the antimicrobial mouth rinse significantly reduced symptoms of denture stomatitis compared with control mouth rinse ($P < 0.01$; absolute numbers not reported). The third, small RCT (34 people in long term care with acrylic dentures and a positive test for *C albicans*) compared microwave treatment (dentures scrubbed with antibacterial soap and water and then microwaved individually for 1 minute at 850 W on days 1, 5, and 10) versus control treatment (dentures soaked in 0.2% chlorhexidine solution overnight for 14 days and scrubbed with antibacterial soap and water on days 1, 5, and 10).[30] Both groups also received the same course of topical antifungal medication (nystatin lozenges daily for 14 days). The RCT found no significant difference between treatments in the rates of dentures recolonised with *C albicans* after 3 months, although it may have lacked power to detect a clinically important difference (RR 0.64, 95% CI 0.38 to 1.06). It found that microwave treatment significantly decreased the proportion of people with infection of the oral mucosa on cytological smear after 3 months compared with control dental soak (RR 0.25, 95% CI 0.06 to 0.59).[30]

Harms: The first two RCTs did not report on adverse effects.[28,29] In the microwave RCT, exposure time was decided arbitrarily.[30] In the RCT, exposure to microwave at 850 W for 90 seconds seemed to damage the denture material.[30] The RCT noted that microwave treatment may damage complete dentures that have been relined, repaired, or both by producing a bubble (pocketing) in the acrylic material, and porcelain teeth with metal retaining pins may cause the microwave to spark and scorch the denture material.[30] It noted microwave treatment was not suitable for all dentures and should be used with caution.[30] Microwave treatment cannot be used for chrome dentures or dentures with metal clasps.

Comment: We found no RCTs evaluating the effect of removing dentures at night on preventing denture stomatitis. Two observational studies found a correlation between the prevalence of denture stomatitis and an unhealthy lifestyle (a global measure including dietary habits, physical activity, alcohol consumption, and smoking), wearing dentures at night, and poor oral hygiene.[31,32]

QUESTION What are the effects of interventions to prevent and treat oropharyngeal candidiasis in people with HIV infection?

OPTION CONTINUOUS ANTIFUNGAL PROPHYLAXIS

RCTs in people with HIV infection found that daily or weekly antifungal prophylaxis with fluconazole, itraconazole, or nystatin reduced incidence and relapse of oropharyngeal candidiasis compared with placebo. One large RCT found that fluconazole reduced recurrence of oropharyngeal candidiasis compared with clotrimazole.

Benefits: We found one systematic review (search date 2000).[33] The review was narrative in character and no data were pooled. We found 10 RCTs using different prophylaxis protocols with follow up of 3–29 months.[34–43] All RCTs enrolled people with AIDS, AIDS related complex, or CD4 cell counts less than or equal to 300 cells/mm^3. **Fluconazole versus placebo:** We found six RCTs that used daily or weekly regimens.[34,35,37–39,44] All six RCTs found that fluconazole reduced oropharyngeal candidiasis compared with placebo. The first RCT (24 people) found that fluconazole 150 mg weekly reduced clinical relapse compared with placebo during 6 months of prophylaxis (relapse: 4/9 [44%] with fluconazole *v* 5/5 [100%] with placebo; P value not provided).[34] The second RCT (323 women with HIV infection) compared fluconazole 200 mg weekly versus placebo and found similar results; fluconazole significantly reduced the risk of recurrent oropharyngeal candidiasis over 29 months (RR 0.50, 95% CI 0.33 to 0.74).[35] The third RCT (84 people) found that fluconazole significantly reduced relapse compared with placebo (73 people; median time to relapse: 168 days with fluconazole *v* 37 days with placebo; $P < 0.0001$; relapse rate: 13/31 [42%] with fluconazole *v* 25/26 [96%] with placebo).[37] The fourth RCT (60 people) found that fluconazole 50 or 100 mg reduced relapse compared with no treatment at 137–215 days (58 people evaluated; rate of relapse: 11% with fluconazole 50 mg *v* 21% with fluconazole 100 mg *v* 95% with no treatment; significance not assessed).[38] The fifth small RCT (25 people with 1–4 previous episodes of thrush, but none at baseline) found that fluconazole significantly reduced oral candidiasis compared with placebo at 12 weeks (0/12 [0%] with fluconazole *v* 8/13 [62%] with placebo; $P = 0.002$).[39] The sixth RCT (143 people) found that fluconazole reduced relapse compared with placebo (median time to relapse: 175 days with fluconazole *v* 35 days with placebo; $P < 0.00001$; freedom from relapse at 37 months: 26/67 [39%] with fluconazole *v* 7/71 [10%] with placebo).[44] **Itraconazole versus placebo:** We found three RCTs.[41–43] All found that intraconazole significantly reduced relapse or the incidence of oral candidiasis. The first RCT (70 people) found that daily prophylaxis with itraconazole 200 mg for 24 weeks significantly reduced relapse rate (5/24 [21%] with itraconazole *v* 14/20 [70%] with placebo; ARR 49%, 95% CI 19% to 64%; NNT 2, 95% CI 2 to 5) and increased the time to relapse (median time to relapse: 10.4 weeks with itraconazole *v* 8.0 weeks with placebo; $P = 0.001$).[41] The second RCT (374 people) compared itraconazole 200 mg daily versus placebo.[42] The primary study end point was time to development of deep fungal infections. The study was terminated because of inadequate power (see comment below). The mean duration of study treatment was 448 days with itraconazole and 386 days with placebo. The RCT found that itraconazole significantly reduced the incidence of oral candidiasis and significantly prolonged the time to development of oral candidiasis compared with placebo (oral candidiasis: RR 0.33, CI not provided; $P < 0.001$, logistic regression; time to development of oral candidiasis: 508 days with itraconazole *v* 413 days with placebo; $P < 0.001$, log rank test; see comment below).[42] The third RCT (129 people) compared itraconazole 200 mg daily versus placebo.[43] The duration of follow up was 6–104 weeks in the itraconazole group and 5–104 weeks in the placebo group. The RCT found that itraconazole significantly reduced the proportion of people with two or more episodes of oral candidiasis compared with placebo (6/63 [10%] with itraconazole *v* 15/66 [23%] with placebo; $P = 0.04$).[43] **Nystatin versus placebo:** One RCT (128 men) found that prophylaxis with one or two nystatin 200 000 U pastilles once daily over 20 weeks significantly delayed the onset of oropharyngeal candidiasis compared with placebo (HR 0.59, 95% CI 0.40 to 0.82; $P < 0.001$).[36] **Fluconazole versus clotrimazole:** One large RCT (428 people from 29 sites) that compared fluconazole

200 mg daily and clotrimazole 10 mg five times daily over 35 months found that fluconazole significantly reduced the recurrence of oropharyngeal candidiasis (5.7 episodes/100 person years with fluconazole *v* 38.1 episodes/100 person years with clotrimazole; $P \leq 0.001$).[40]

Harms: In one RCT comparing two different daily doses of fluconazole versus no treatment, one person stopped fluconazole because of an allergic rash.[38] One RCT found no significant difference in adverse effects between fluconazole and placebo (10/12 [83%] with fluconazole *v* 9/13 [69%] with placebo; $P = 0.6$).[39] One RCT comparing itraconazole and placebo found that 95% (177/187) of people with itraconazole and 95% (178/187) with placebo reported adverse effects, the most frequent being gastrointestinal.[42] Most were classified as mild or moderate. Severe adverse events were reported by 38% of people with itraconazole and 36% of people with placebo. However, most adverse events were not considered to be related to study medication but, rather, related to HIV disease.[42] Study medication was withdrawn in 20% of people with itraconazole and 23% of people with placebo predominantly because of nausea and abdominal pain.[42] One RCT comparing itraconazole versus placebo reported that the most frequent adverse effects were skin rashes (16/63 [25%] with itraconazole *v* 15/66 [23%] with placebo), mild anaemia (4/63 [6%] with itraconazole *v* 5/66 [8%] with placebo), and diarrhoea (3/63 [5%] with itraconazole *v* 5/66 [8%] with placebo).[43] One person discontinued treatment with itraconazole because of a skin rash, and concerns about hepatotoxicity resulted in treatment being discontinued in two people (1 with itraconazole and 1 with placebo). There was one case of Stevens–Johnson syndrome in a person also taking trimethoprim–sulfamethoxazole.[43] One RCT found no significant difference in the rate of microbial resistance between fluconazole and placebo over 37 months (8/67 [12%] with fluconazole *v* 4/71 [6%] with placebo group; $P = 0.20$).[44] In the other RCTs, the most commonly reported adverse effects were gastrointestinal symptoms, rash, and headache, but data on adverse events were not presented in all of the RCTs. Concomitant medication and severe underlying disease may have confounded attribution of adverse events.

Comment: Many of the RCTs were small and not blinded, and most did not adjust for confounding factors such as antiretroviral treatment and other established risk factors for oropharyngeal candidiasis. No RCTs used quality of life scores. The optimal dosage schedule and frequency of administration of preventative treatment have not been established. We found no RCTs comparing weekly versus daily regimens of antifungal drugs. We found one RCT that compared two different doses of fluconazole.[38] It found no significant difference between 50 and 100 mg daily doses of fluconazole (oropharyngeal candidiasis: 2/18 [11%] with 50 mg *v* 4/19 [21%] with 100 mg; RR 0.53, 95% CI 0.09 to 2.09).[38] Subgroup analysis in the RCT comparing fluconazole versus placebo found that people with a history of oropharyngeal candidiasis had an absolute benefit of treatment with weekly fluconazole that was higher than in those with no history of infection (ARR 25.6/100 person years for those with previous infection *v* ARR 11.2/100 person years for those with no history of infection).[35] In the RCT comparing itraconazole versus placebo, too few deep fungal infections occurred to assess accurately the impact of itraconazole prophylaxis, and on the basis of statistical advice the study was terminated.[42] Discontinuation rates were high and 145/187 (78%) of people with itraconazole versus 154/187 (82%) with placebo did not complete 2 years of medication.[42] Reasons for discontinuation were as follows: withdrawal of consent (33 people with itraconazole *v* 46 with placebo); adverse events (31 with itraconazole *v* 29 with placebo); loss to follow up (17 with itraconazole *v* 11 with placebo); use of disallowed medication (15 with itraconazole v 3 with placebo); reaching of a study end point (5 with itraconazole v 11 with placebo); death (5 with itraconazole v 8 with placebo); elevated liver function test (2 with itraconazole v 3 with placebo); pregnancy (0 with itraconazole v 1 with placebo); and other (37 with itraconazole v 42 with placebo).[42] The extended time interval to relapse with itraconazole may reflect the introduction of highly active antiretroviral treatment.[42]

OPTION TOPICAL ANTIFUNGAL TREATMENT

RCTs found that topical preparations of itraconazole, fluconazole, miconazole nitrate, and clotrimazole effectively treated oropharyngeal candidiasis in people with HIV infection. One RCT found that fluconazole reduced symptoms and signs of oropharyngeal candidiasis compared with topical nystatin.

Benefits: We found one systematic review (search date 2000)[33] and two subsequent RCTs.[45,46] The review was narrative in character and no data were pooled. In all, we identified six RCTs comparing topical (suspensions or pastilles) versus orally absorbed antifungals for treatment of oropharyngeal candidiasis in people with HIV infection, which included four RCTs identified by the review and two subsequent RCTs.[45–50] Four RCTs found that itraconazole oral solution 100 or 200 mg used in a swish and swallow mode was as effective as topical fluconazole 100 mg once daily for 14 days or topical clotrimazole 10 mg five times daily.[47–50] Three of these RCTs achieved clinical response rates of over 90%.[47–49] The fifth RCT comparing fluconazole 100 mg daily versus nystatin liquid for 14 days found that fluconazole significantly increased complete resolution of signs and symptoms of oropharyngeal candidiasis (60/69 [87%] with fluconazole v 36/69 [52%] with nystatin liquid; ARI 35%, 95% CI 22% to 42%; RR 1.67, 95% CI 1.42 to 1.80; NNT 3, 95% CI 2 to 5).[45] The sixth RCT (357 HIV positive adults with oropharyngeal candidiasis) compared topical miconazole nitrate (10 mg once daily slow release mucoadhesive buccal tablet) versus ketoconazole (400 mg once daily).[46] It found no significant difference between treatments in clinical cure rates at 7 or 14 days (day 7: 87% with miconazole nitrate v 90% with ketoconazole; ARI –3.0%, 90% CI –9.0% to +3.0%; day 14: 92% with miconazole nitrate v 96% with ketoconazole; ARI –4.0%, 90% CI –7.6% to +0.5%; see comment below).

Harms: The most frequently reported adverse effects were gastrointestinal symptoms (nausea, diarrhoea, and vomiting). Altered taste, dry mouth, headache, and rashes were also recorded.[45–49] In two RCTs there were no withdrawals because of adverse effects.[46,50] On the basis of data from five RCTs (861 people), in which adverse events were considered to be drug induced and resulted in withdrawal from the study, adverse events were reported with fluconazole (4 people), itraconazole (14 people), clotrimazole (12 people), and nystatin (1 person).[45,47–50] The RCT of miconazole nitrate versus ketoconazole found similar rates of adverse effects between the two groups, with the exception of vomiting (rate of vomiting: 1% with miconazole nitrate v 8% with ketoconazole; P value not reported).[46]

Comment: Once daily dosing is likely to increase adherence to treatment. Non-adherence was reported with clotrimazole because of the inconvenience of taking multiple doses. The sixth RCT[46] described a 90% confidence interval, which is more likely to show a statistical similarity between treatments than the conventional 95% confidence interval.

QUESTION **Which treatments reduce the risk of acquiring resistance to antifungal drugs?**

OPTION **CONTINUOUS ANTIFUNGAL PROPHYLAXIS VERSUS INTERMITTENT ANTIFUNGAL TREATMENT**

One RCT in people with HIV infection and acute episodes of oropharyngeal candidiasis found no significant difference between continuous antifungal prophylaxis with fluconazole and intermittent antifungal treatment with fluconazole in terms of the emergence of antifungal resistance.

Benefits: We found no systematic review. We found one RCT comparing the effects of continuous prophylaxis with fluconazole versus intermittent treatment with fluconazole 200 mg daily on the development of acquired resistance in people with HIV infection and evidence of active oropharyngeal candidiasis over a mean follow up of 11 months.[51] Antifungal sensitivity testing followed the National Committee for Clinical Laboratory Standards guidelines.[52] The RCT found that continuous prophylaxis with fluconazole reduced median annual relapse rates compared with intermittent treatment (0 episodes/year with continuous prophylaxis *v* 4.1 episodes/year with intermittent treatment; $P \leq 0.001$). It also found that antifungal resistance developed in more people on continuous prophylaxis than on intermittent treatment, but the difference was not significant (9/16 [56%] with continuous *v* 13/28 [46%] with intermittent; $P = 0.75$).[51]

Harms: No adverse reactions were reported in the RCT.[52]

Comment: Optimal treatment regimens to reduce the risk of acquiring resistance have not been evaluated adequately. In a prospective observational study of protease inhibitor treatment, 93 people with HIV and with a history of recurrent oropharyngeal candidiasis were followed up for 1 year. Oropharyngeal candidiasis was diagnosed in 2/30 (7%) people given protease inhibitors and 23/63 (37%) given other treatment ($P \leq 0.001$; CI not provided).[53] Immunomodulating antiretroviral treatments (e.g. highly active antiretroviral treatment), by reducing the number of recurrences of oropharyngeal candidiasis, act indirectly as antifungal sparing agents, thereby reducing exposure to antifungals and the potential risk of resistance.

Substantive changes

Antifungal prophylaxis in people receiving cancer treatments One RCT added;[9] benefits data enhanced and categorisation unchanged.
Topical antifungal treatment One RCT added;[46] benefits and harms data enhanced and categorisation unchanged.

REFERENCES

1. Ellepola ANB, Samaranayake LP. Antimycotic agents in oral candidosis: an overview: 1. Clinical variants. *Dent Update* 2000;27:111–116.
2. Webb BC, Thomas CJ, Willcox MD, et al. Candida-associated denture stomatitis. Aetiology and management: a review. Part 3. Treatment of oral candidosis. *Aust Dent J* 1998;43:244–249.
3. Ninane JA. Multicentre study of fluconazole versus oral polyenes in the prevention of fungal infection in children with hematological or oncological malignancies. Multicentre study group. *Eur J Clin Microbiol Infect Dis* 1994;13:330–337.
4. Philips P, Zemcov J, Mahmood W, et al. Itraconazole cyclodextrin solution for fluconazole-refractory oropharyngeal candidiasis in AIDS: correlation of clinical response with *in vitro* susceptibility. *AIDS* 1996;10:1369–1376.
5. Wilson J. The aetiology, diagnosis and management of denture stomatitis. *B Dental J* 1998;185:380–384.
6. Rex JH, Rinald MG, Pfaler MA. Resistance of Candida species to fluconazole. *Antimicrob Agents Chemother* 1995;39:1–8.
7. Maenza JR, Keruly JC, Moore RD, et al. Risk factors for fluconazole-resistant candidiasis in human immuno-deficiency virus-infected patients. *J Infect Dis* 1996;173:219–225.
8. Worthington HV, Clarkson JE, Eden OB. Interventions for preventing oral candidiasis for patients with cancer receiving treatment. In: The Cochrane Library, Issue 2, 2004. Chichester, UK: John Wiley & Sons, Ltd. Search date 2001; Primary sources Medline, Embase, Cinahl, Cancerlit, the Cochrane Controlled Trials Register, and the Cochrane Oral Health Group Specialist Register.

9. Lass-Flöri C, Gunsilius E, Gastl G, et al. Fungal colonization in neutropenic patients: a randomised study comparing itraconazole solution and amphotericin B solution. *Ann Hematol* 2003;82:565–569.
10. Lumbreras C, Cuervas-Mons V, Jara P, et al. Randomized trial of fluconazole versus nystatin for the prophylaxis of Candida infection following liver transplantation. *J Infect Dis* 1996;174:583–588.
11. Ruskin JD, Wood RP, Bailey MR, et al. Comparative trial of oral clotrimazole and nystatin for oropharyngeal candidiasis prophylaxis in orthotopic liver transplant patients. *Oral Surg Oral Med Oral Pathol Oral Radiol Endod* 1992;74:567–571.
12. Ferretti GA, Ash RC, Brown AT, et al. Control of oral mucositis and candidiasis in marrow transplantation: a prospective, double-blind trial of chlorhexidine digluconate oral rinse. *Bone Marrow Transplant* 1988;3:483–493.
13. Epstein JB, Vickars L, Spinelli J, et al. Efficacy of chlorhexidine and nystatin rinses in prevention of oral complications in leukemia and bone marrow transplantation. *Oral Surg Oral Med Oral Pathol Oral Radiol Endod* 1992;73:682–689.
14. Clarkson JE, Worthington HV, Eden OB. Interventions for treating oral candidiasis for patients with cancer receiving treatment. In: The Cochrane library, Issue 2, 2004. Chichester, UK: John Wiley & Sons, Ltd. Search date August 2003; primary sources Cochrane Oral Health Group Specialised Register, Cochrane Controlled Trials Register, Medline, and Embase. Reference lists from relevant articles were searched and the authors of eligible trials were contacted to identify trials.
15. Lefebvre JL, Domenge C. A comparative study of the efficacy and safety of fluconazole oral suspension and amphotericin B oral suspension in cancer patients with mucositis. *Oral Oncol* 2002;38:337–342.
16. Groll AH, Just-Nuebling G, Kurz M, et al. Fluconazole versus nystatin in the prevention of Candida infections in children and adolescents undergoing remission induction or consolidation chemotherapy for cancer. *J Antimicrob Chemother* 1997;40:855–862.
17. Hoppe J, Burr R, Ebeling H, et al. Treatment of oropharyngeal candidiasis in immunocompetent infants: a randomized multicenter study of miconazole gel vs. nystatin suspension. *Pediatr Infect Dis J* 1997;16:288–293.
18. Hoppe JE, Hahn H. Randomized comparison of two nystatin oral gels with miconazole oral gel for treatment of oral thrush in infants. Antimycotics study group. *Infection* 1996;24:136–139.
19. Goins RA, Ascher D, Waecker N, et al. Comparison of fluconazole and nystatin oral suspensions for treatment of oral candidiasis in infants. *Pediatr Infect Dis J* 2002;21:1165–1167.
20. Flynn PM, Cunningham CK, Kerkering T, et al. Oropharyngeal candidiasis in immunocompromised children: a randomized, multicenter study of orally administered fluconazole suspension versus nystatin. The multicenter fluconazole study group. *J Pediatr* 1995;127:322–328.
21. Nairn RI. Nystatin and amphotericin B in the treatment of denture-related candidiasis. *Oral Surg Oral Med Oral Pathol Oral Radiol Endod* 1975;40:68–75.
22. Konsberg R, Axell T. Treatment of Candida-infected denture stomatitis with a miconazole lacquer. *Oral Surg Oral Med Oral Pathol Oral Radiol Endod* 1994;78:306–311.
23. Budtz-Jorgensen E, Holmstrup P, Krogh P. Fluconazole in the treatment of Candida-associated denture stomatitis. *Antimicrob Agents Chemother* 1988;32:1859–1863.
24. Bissell V, Felix DH, Wray D. Comparative trial of fluconazole and amphotericin B in the treatment of denture stomatitis. *Oral Surg Oral Med Oral Pathol Oral Radiol Endod* 1993;76:35–39.
25. Taillandier J, Esnault Y, Alemanni M, and the multicentre study group. A comparison of fluconazole oral suspension and amphotericin B oral suspension in older patients with oropharyngeal candidosis. *Age Ageing* 2000;29:117–123.
26. Budtz-Jorgensen E, Carlino P. A miconazole lacquer in the treatment of Candida-associated denture stomatitis. *Mycoses* 1994;37:131–135.
27. Parvinen T, Kokko J, Yli-Urpo A. Miconazole lacquer compared with gel in treatment of denture stomatitis. *Scand J Dental Res* 1994;102:361–366.
28. Mahonen K, Virtanen K, Larmas M. The effect of prosthesis disinfection on salivary microbial levels. *J Oral Rehabil* 1998;25:304–310.
29. DePaola LG, Minah GE, Elias SA, et al. Clinical and microbial evaluation of treatment regimens to reduce denture stomatitis. *Int J Prosthodont* 1990;3:369–374.
30. Banting DW, Hill SA. Microwave disinfection of dentures for the treatment of oral candidiasis. *Spec Care Dentist* 2001;21:4–8.
31. Sakki TK, Knuuttila ML, Laara E, et al. The association of yeasts and denture stomatitis with behavioral and biologic factors. *Oral Surg Oral Med Oral Pathol Oral Radiol Endod* 1997;84:624–629.
32. Fenlon MR, Sherriff M, Walter JD. Factors associated with the presence of denture related stomatitis in complete denture wearers: a preliminary investigation. *Eur J Prosthodont Restor Dent* 1998;6:145–147.
33. Patton LL, Bonito AJ, Shugars DA. A systematic review of the effectiveness of antifungal drugs for the prevention and treatment of oropharyngeal candidiasis in HIV positive patients. *Oral Surg Oral Med Oral Pathol Oral Radiol Endod* 2001;92:170–179. Search date 2000; primary sources Medline, Embase, and the Cochrane Library, and a manual check of reference lists of review articles.
34. Leen CLS, Dunbar EM, Ellis ME, et al. Once-weekly fluconazole to prevent recurrence of oropharyngeal candidiasis in patients with AIDS and AIDS-related complex: a double-blind placebo controlled study. *J Infect* 1990;21:55–60.
35. Schuman P, Capps L, Peng G, et al. Weekly fluconazole for the prevention of mucosal candidiasis in women with HIV infection. A randomized, double-blind, placebo-controlled trial. Terry Beirn community programs for clinical research on AIDS. *Ann Intern Med* 1997;126:689–696.
36. MacPhail LA, Hilton JF, Dodd CL, et al. Prophylaxis with nystatin pastilles for HIV-associated oral candidiasis. *J Acquir Immune Defic Syndr* 1996;12:470–476.
37. Marriott DJE, Jones PD, Hoy JF, et al. Fluconazole once a week as secondary prophylaxis against oropharyngeal candidiasis in HIV-infected patients. A double-blind placebo-controlled study. *Med J Aust* 1993;158:312–316.
38. Just-Nubling G, Gentschew G, Meissner K, et al. Fluconazole prophylaxis of recurrent oral candidiasis in HIV-positive patients. *Eur J Clin Microbiol Infect Dis* 1991;10:917–921.
39. Stevens DA, Greene SI, Lang OS. Thrush can be prevented in patients with acquired immunodeficiency syndrome and the acquired immunodeficiency syndrome-related complex. Randomized, double-blind, placebo-controlled study of 100 mg oral fluconazole daily. *Arch Intern Med* 1991;151:2458–2464.
40. Powderly WG, Finklestein DM, Feinberg J, et al. A randomised trial comparing fluconazole with clotrimazole troches for the prevention of fungal infection in patients with advanced human immunodeficiency virus infection. *N Engl J Med* 1995;332:700–705.
41. Smith D, Midgley J, Gazzard B. A randomised, double-blind study of itraconazole versus placebo in the treatment and prevention of oral or oesophageal candidosis in patients with HIV infection. *Int J Clin Pract* 1999;53:349–352.
42. Smith DE, Bell J, Johnson M, et al. A randomized, doubled-blind, placebo-controlled study of itraconazole capsules for the prevention of deep

fungal infections in immunodeficient patients with HIV infection. *HIV Medicine* 2001;2:78–83.

43. Chariyalertsak S, Supparatpinyo K, Sirisanthana, T, et al. A controlled trial of itraconazole as primary prophylaxis for systemic fungal infections in patients with advanced human immunodeficiency virus infection in Thailand. *Clin Infect Dis* 2002;34:277–284.
44. Pagani JL, Chave JP, Casjka C, et al. Efficacy, tolerability and development of resistance in HIV-positive patients treated with fluconazole for secondary prevention of oropharyngeal candidiasis: a randomized, double-blind, placebo-controlled trial. *J Antimicrob Chemother* 2002;50:231–240.
45. Pons V, Greenspan D, Lozada-Nur F, et al. Oropharyngeal candidiasis in patients with AIDS: randomized comparison of fluconazole versus nystatin oral suspensions. *Clin Infect Dis* 1997;24:1204–1207.
46. van Roey J, Haxaire M, Kamya M, et al. Comparative efficacy of topical therapy with a slow-release mucoadhesive buccal tablet containing miconazole nitrate versus systemic therapy with ketaconazole in HIV-positive patients with oropharyngeal candidiasis. *J Acquir Immune Defic Syndr* 2004;35:144–150.
47. Graybill JR, Vazquez J, Darouiche RO, et al. Randomized trial of itraconazole oral solution for oropharyngeal candidiasis in HIV/AIDS patients. *Am J Med* 1998;104:33–39.
48. Phillips P, De Beule K, Frechette G, et al. A double-blind comparison of itraconazole oral solution and fluconazole capsules for the treatment of oropharyngeal candidiasis in patients with AIDS. *Clin Infect Dis* 1998;26:1368–1373.
49. Murray PA, Koletar SL, Mallegol I, et al. Itraconazole oral solution versus clotrimazole troches for the treatment of oropharyngeal candidiasis in immunocompromised patients. *Clin Ther* 1997;19:471–480.
50. Linpiyawan R, Jittreprasert K, Sivayathorn A. Clinical trial: clotrimazole troche vs. itraconazole oral solution in the treatment of oral candidosis in AIDS patients. *Int J Dermatol* 2000;39:859–861.
51. Revankar SG, Kirkpatrick WR, McAtee RK, et al. A randomized trial of continuous or intermittent therapy with fluconazole for oropharyngeal candidiasis in HIV-infected patients: clinical outcomes and development of fluconazole resistance. *Am J Med* 1998;105:7–11.
52. National Committee for Clinical Laboratory Standards. Reference method for broth dilution antifungal susceptibility testing of yeasts: approved standard. Wayne, Penn: NCCLS, 1997 (document M27-A).
53. Cauda R, Tacconelli E, Tumbarello M, et al. Role of protease inhibitors in preventing recurrent oral candidiasis in patients with HIV infections: a prospective case control study. *J Acquir Immune Defic Syndr* 1999;21:20–25.

Caroline Pankhurst
Guy's, King's College, and St Thomas's Dental Institute
London
UK

Competing interests: None declared.

Halitosis

Search date December 2003

Bazian Ltd

QUESTIONS

INTERVENTIONS

See glossary

Key Messages

- **Regular-use mouthwash** Two RCTs found that regular use of a mouthwash (one mouthwash containing cetylpyridinium chloride plus chlorhexidine plus zinc lactate; the other mouthwash containing cetylpyridinium chloride) reduced breath odour at 2–4 weeks compared with placebo.
- **Single-use mouthwash (short term benefit only)** Four small RCTs found limited evidence that single-use mouthwash reduced odour unpleasantness and odour intensity between 1–8 hours after use compared with distilled water, saline rinse, or no treatment. One of these RCTs found no significant difference between single-use mouthwash and distilled water in odour unpleasantness or odour intensity after 24 hours.
- **Artificial saliva; sugar free chewing gums; tongue cleaning, brushing, or scraping; zinc toothpastes** We found no RCTs on the effects of these interventions.

Halitosis

DEFINITION Halitosis is an unpleasant odour emitted from the mouth. It may be caused by oral conditions including poor oral hygiene and periodontal disease or extraoral conditions such as chronic sinusitis and bronchiectasis.[1,2] In this chapter, we deal only with physiological halitosis, that is, confirmed persistent bad breath in the absence of systemic, periodontal, or gum disease. We have excluded halitosis due to underlying disease, which would require disease specific treatment, pseudo-halitosis (in people who believe they have bad breath but whose breath is not considered malodourous by others), and artificially induced halitosis (e.g. in studies requiring people to stop brushing their teeth). This topic is only applicable, therefore, to people in whom underlying causes have been ruled out, and in whom pseudo-halitosis has been excluded. There is no consensus regarding duration of bad breath for diagnosis of halitosis, although the standard organoleptic test**G** for bad breath involves smelling the breath on at least two or three different days.[1]

INCIDENCE/ PREVALENCE We found no reliable estimate of prevalence, although several studies report the population prevalence of halitosis (physiological or because of underlying disease) to be about 50%.[1,3–5] One cross-sectional study of 491 people found that about 5% of people with halitosis have pseudo-halitosis and about 40% of people with halitosis have physiological bad breath not due to underlying disease.[6] We found no reliable data about age or sex distribution of physiological halitosis.

AETIOLOGY/ RISK FACTORS We found no reliable data about risk factors for physiological bad breath. Mass spectrometric and gas chromatographic analysis of expelled air from the mouth of people with any type of halitosis have shown that the main malodourants are volatile sulphur compounds including hydrogen sulphide, methyl mercaptan, and dimethyl suphide.[7,8]

PROGNOSIS We found no evidence on the prognosis of halitosis.

AIMS OF INTERVENTION To improve social functioning; to reduce embarrassment; to reduce odour with minimum adverse effects.

OUTCOMES Organoleptic test scores, other odour scales, quality of life scores, embarrassment scores, and social functioning scores. We excluded non-clinical outcomes such as gas chromatography and spectroscopy results and concentrations of compounds in exhaled air.

METHODS *Clinical Evidence* search and appraisal December 2003.

QUESTION **What are the effects of treatments in people with physiological halitosis?**

OPTION TONGUE CLEANING, BRUSHING, OR SCRAPING

We found no RCTs on the effects of tongue cleaning, brushing, or scraping.

Benefits: We found no systematic review or RCTs.

Harms: We found no RCTs.

Comment: None.

OPTION MOUTHWASHES (CONTAINING ZINC, CHLORHEXIDINE, HYDROGEN PEROXIDE, OR OTHER ANTIMICROBIAL AGENTS)

Two RCTs found that regular use of a mouthwash (one mouthwash containing cetylpyridinium chloride plus chlorhexidine plus zinc lactate; the other mouthwash containing cetylpyridinium chloride) reduced breath odour at 2–4 weeks compared with placebo. Four small RCTs found limited evidence that single-use mouthwash reduced odour unpleasantness and odour intensity between 1–8 hours after use compared with distilled water, saline rinse, or no treatment. One of these RCTs found no significant difference between single-use mouthwash and distilled water in odour unpleasantness or odour intensity after 24 hours.

Benefits: **Regular-use:** We found two RCTs.[9,10] The first RCT (40 people) compared an active treatment mouthwash (containing chlorhexidine plus cetylpyridinium chloride plus zinc lactate) versus a placebo mouthwash.[9] The mouthwashes were used twice daily for 2 weeks, and breath odour was assessed on a scale from 0 (no halitosis) to 5 (offensive halitosis) by one trained examiner. The active treatment mouthwash significantly reduced breath odour compared with placebo mouthwash after 2 weeks (mean odour score change from baseline: –1.3 with active treatment *v* –0.2 with placebo; P < 0.005).[9] The second RCT (99 people) compared four mouthwashes used twice daily for 4 weeks: one containing essential oils; one containing cetylpyridinium chloride; one containing chlorine dioxide plus zinc; and a placebo mouthwash (composition not stated).[10] Two experienced examiners assessed breath odour on a scale from 0 (no odour) to 5 (extremely foul odour). The RCT found that only the cetylpyridinium chloride containing mouthwash significantly reduced breath odour compared with placebo mouthwash after 4 weeks, but found no significant difference between the three active treatment mouthwashes (mean score change from baseline after 4 weeks: –0.41 with cetylpyridinium chloride containing mouthwash *v* +0.06 with chlorine dioxide plus zinc containing mouthwash *v* 0 with essential oil containing mouthwash *v* +0.16 with placebo mouthwash; cetylpyridinium chloride containing mouthwash *v* placebo, P < 0.05; two other active mouthwashes *v* placebo, P value reported as not significant; cetylpyridinium chloride containing mouthwash *v* two other active mouthwashes, P value reported as not significant). **Single-use:** We found four small RCTs that compared single-use mouthwash versus control or no treatment.[2,10–12] The first two RCTs compared single-use 0.1% chlorine dioxide containing mouthwash versus distilled water in healthy adults with confirmed oral malodour.[2,11] In both RCTs, three examiners scored unpleasant breath odour on a scale from +3 (very pleasant/fresh) to –3 (very unpleasant/stale) and odour intensity from 0 (no odour) to 4 (very strong odour). The first RCT (31 people) found that chlorine dioxide containing mouthwash significantly reduced odour unpleasantness score and odour intensity score at 2, 4, and 8 hours after treatment compared with distilled water (odour unpleasantness, baseline to 8 hours: –1.25 to –0.63 with chlorine dioxide containing mouthwash *v* –1.40 to –1.29 with distilled water, P < 0.01; odour intensity, baseline to 8 hours: 1.27 to 0.63 with chlorine dioxide containing mouthwash *v* 1.42 to 1.29 with distilled water, P < 0.01).[2] It found no significant difference in odour unpleasantness or intensity between groups at 24, 48, 72, and 96 hours. The second RCT (12 people, crossover design, 96 hour washout period between treatments) found that chlorine dioxide containing mouthwash significantly reduced odour unpleasantness score at 0.5, 1, 2, and 4 hours after treatment and odour intensity score at 2 and 4 hours after treatment compared with distilled water (odour unpleasantness, baseline to 4 hours: –1.25 to –0.61 with chlorine dioxide containing mouthwash *v* –1.06 to –1.08 with distilled water, P < 0.01; odour intensity, baseline to 4 hours: 1.14 to 0.81 with chlorine dioxide containing mouthwash *v* 1.11 to 1.19 with distilled water, P = 0.03).[11] The third RCT (62 people) compared three treatments: test mouthwash (see comment below), saline rinse, and no treatment.[12] Three trained examiners rated breath odour from 0 (low odour) to 3 (high odour). It found that the test mouthwash significantly reduced odour compared with saline rinse and no treatment at 1, 2, and 3 hours (baseline to 3 hours: 1.63 to 1.03 with test mouthwash *v* 1.51 to 1.72 with saline rinse *v* 1.63 to 1.88 with no treatment; P < 0.05 for test mouthwash *v* saline rinse or no treatment). The fourth RCT (99 people) compared the regular use of three active treatment mouthwashes versus placebo mouthwash, but also reported results after a single use (see benefits of regular-use mouthwash above).[10] The RCT found that at 4 hours after single use, only the cetylpyridinium chloride containing mouthwash significantly reduced breath odour compared with placebo mouthwash, and that this mouthwash significantly reduced breath odour compared with the two other active treatment mouthwashes (mean odour score change from baseline to 4 hours: –0.94 with cetylpyridinium chloride containing mouthwash *v* –0.52 with chlorine dioxide plus zinc containing mouthwash *v* –0.42 with essential oils containing mouthwash *v* –0.22 with placebo mouthwash; cetylpyridinium chloride containing mouthwash *v* other active treatments or placebo, $P < 0.05$; other active treatments *v* placebo, P value reported as not significant).

Harms: **Regular-use:** The first RCT reported that people in the active treatment group (mouthwash containing chlorhexidine plus cetylpyridinium chloride plus zinc lactate) had significantly more tongue discolouration than people using placebo mouthwash after 2 weeks (assessed using the Winkel tongue discolouration index [measured in 6 tongue areas, range 0 = no discolouration to 12 = severe discolouration]; mean score change from baseline: +2.8 with active treatment *v* +0.3 with placebo; P = 0.002).[9] There was no significant difference in tooth staining between groups. In the second RCT, 13 people reported adverse effects such as lip blisters, localised gingival oedema, and sores (figures not reported by treatment group).[10] The RCT reported "it was determined that these adverse events were unlikely to be related to the product usage". **Single-use:** The first three RCTs did not report harms.[2,11,12] The fourth RCT did not separately report on harms after a single use (see harms of regular-use mouthwash above).[10]

Comment: **Regular-use:** In the second RCT, four people were excluded or withdrew after randomisation, and analysis of results was not by intention to treat.[10] **Single-use:** The first two RCTs of chlorine dioxide containing mouthwash were conducted by the same research group.[2,11] The third RCT did not report details of the composition of the mouthwash used.[12]

OPTION SUGAR FREE CHEWING GUMS

We found no RCTs on the effects of sugar free chewing gum.

Benefits: We found no systematic review and no RCTs.

Harms: We found no RCTs.

Comment: None.

OPTION ZINC TOOTHPASTES

We found no RCTs on the effects of zinc toothpaste.

Benefits: We found no systematic review and no RCTs.

Harms: We found no RCTs.

Comment: None.

OPTION ARTIFICIAL SALIVA

We found no RCTs on the effects of artificial saliva.

Benefits: We found no systematic review and no RCTs.

Harms: We found no RCTs.

Comment: None.

GLOSSARY

Organoleptic test scores These are assigned by one or more examiners who sniff the person's exhaled breath on two or three different days. People having this examination should not have had antibiotics in the previous 3 weeks and should have refrained from eating garlic or onions and spicy foods for 48 hours and refrained from usual oral hygiene and smoking for the previous 12 hours.[1] Scoring systems vary among studies.

REFERENCES

1. Yaegaki K, Coil JM. Examination, classification, and treatment of halitosis; clinical perspectives. *J Can Dent Assoc* 2000;66:257–261.
2. Frascella J, Gilbert RD, Fernandez P, et al. Efficacy of a chlorine dioxide-containing mouthrinse in oral malodor. *Compend Contin Educ Dent* 2000;21:241–254.
3. Meningaud JP, Bado F, Favre E, et al. Halitosis in 1999 [in French]. *Rev Stomatol Chir Maxillofac* 1999;100:240–244.
4. Bollen CM, Rompen EH, Demanez JP. Halitosis: a multidisciplinary problem [in French]. *Rev Med Liege* 1999;54:32–36.
5. Tomas Carmona I, Limeres Posse J, Diz Dios P, et al. Extraoral etiology of halitosis. *Med Oral* 2001;6:40–47.
6. Delanghe G, Bollen C, van Steenberghe D, et al. Halitosis, foetor ex ore [in Dutch]. *Ned Tijdschr Tandheelkd* 1998;105:314–317.
7. Tonzetich J. Direct gas chromatographic analysis of sulphur compounds in mouth air in man. *Arch Oral Biol* 1971;16:587–597.
8. Kleinberg I, Westbay G. Oral malodor. *Crit Rev Oral Biol Med* 1990;1:247–259.
9. Winkel EG, Roldan S, Van Winkelhoff AJ, et al. Clinical effects of a new mouthrinse containing chlorhexidine, cetylpyridinium chloride and zinc-lactate on oral halitosis. A dual-center, double-blind placebo-controlled study. *J Clin Periodontol* 2003;30:300–306.
10. Borden LC, Chaves ES, Bowman JP, et al. The effect of four mouthrinses on oral malodor. *Compend Contin Educ Dent* 2002;23:531–546.
11. Frascella J, Gilbert R, Fernandez P. Odor reduction potential of a chlorine dioxide mouthrinse. *J Clin Dent* 1998;9:39–42.
12. Schmidt NF, Tarbet WJ. The effect of oral rinses on organoleptic mouth odor ratings and levels of volatile sulfur compounds. *Oral Surg Oral Med Oral Pathol* 1978;45:876–883.

Bazian Ltd
London
UK

Competing interests: None declared.

Impacted wisdom teeth

Search date August 2004

Marco Esposito

QUESTIONS

INTERVENTIONS

Key Messages

Impacted wisdom teeth extraction

- **Prophylactic extraction** One RCT identified by a systematic review found no evidence that prophylactic extraction of asymptomatic impacted wisdom teeth improved outcomes compared with no extraction. Removal of lower wisdom teeth causes permanent numbness of the lower lip or tongue in about 2% of people.

DEFINITION	Wisdom teeth are third molars that develop in almost all adults and generally erupt between the ages of 18 and 24 years, although there is a wide variation in the age of eruption. In some people, the teeth become partially or completely impacted below the gum line because of lack of space, obstruction, or abnormal position. Impacted wisdom teeth may be diagnosed because of pain and swelling or incidentally by routine dental radiography.
INCIDENCE/ PREVALENCE	Third molar impaction is common. Over 72% of Swedish people aged 20–30 years have at least one impacted lower third molar.[1] The surgical removal of impacted third molars (symptomatic and asymptomatic) is the most common procedure performed by oral and maxillofacial surgeons. It is performed on about 4/1000 people a year in England and Wales, making it one of the top 10 inpatient and day case procedures.[2–4] Up to 90% of people on oral and maxillofacial surgery hospital waiting lists are awaiting removal of wisdom teeth.[3]
AETIOLOGY/ RISK FACTORS	Retention and impaction of wisdom teeth may be more common than it was previously because the modern diet tends to be softer than in the past.[5]
PROGNOSIS	Impacted wisdom teeth can cause pain, swelling, and infection, and may destroy adjacent teeth and bone. The removal of diseased and symptomatic wisdom teeth alleviates pain and suffering and improves oral health and function. We found no good evidence on untreated prognosis in people with asymptomatic impacted wisdom teeth.
AIMS OF INTERVENTION	To prevent harms and maximise benefits of wisdom teeth removal.
OUTCOMES	Pain; rates of infection; oral health and function; serious complications of intervention, including permanent or prolonged paraesthesia or anaesthesia of the lingual or inferior alveolar nerves, fracture of the mandible or the maxillary tuberosity, and oro-antral communication.
METHODS	*Clinical Evidence* search and appraisal August 2004.

QUESTION Should asymptomatic and disease-free impacted wisdom teeth be removed prophylactically?

OPTION EXTRACTION OF ASYMPTOMATIC IMPACTED WISDOM TEETH

One RCT identified by a systematic review found no evidence that prophylactic extraction of asymptomatic impacted wisdom teeth improved outcomes compared with no extraction. Removal of lower wisdom teeth causes permanent numbness of the lower lip or tongue in about 2% of people.

Benefits: We found one systematic review evaluating people with unerupted or impacted third molars (search date 1999, 2 RCTs, 1 published as abstract only, see comments below).[6] The systematic review was subsequently updated (search date 2003) but no further RCTs were identified.[7] The first RCT identified by the review (164 people with asymptomatic impacted wisdom teeth) compared the effects of early third molar extraction on late crowding of the lower incisors versus no extraction of third molars.[8] It found no clinically important difference between treatments. However, there was a large loss to follow up in the RCT, which limits reliability (77 [47%] people followed up, for an average of 66 months).

Harms: Pain and swelling are almost universal after removal of impacted wisdom teeth.[9,10] The removal of the lower wisdom teeth carries the risk of damage to the inferior alveolar nerve (injured in 1–8% of people[11,12] with permanent damage in up to 1% of people[13]) and to the lingual nerve (permanently injured in up to 1% of people).[14] The risks seem to be greater with greater depth of impaction. The risks are the same whether the wisdom tooth is symptomatic or asymptomatic. Observational studies found limited evidence that complications associated with the removal of wisdom teeth are more frequent when operators are less experienced, and in older people with deeply impacted teeth.[15–20]

Comment: Implementing RCTs to answer this question is difficult. Evidence is, therefore, largely of inferior quality. Thousands of participants, and decades of follow up, would be required to provide enough power, because disease events are rare in previously normal wisdom teeth. Preliminary results (abstract only) from the second RCT identified by the review suggested that no extraction could improve outcomes such as functional health status and reduce harms.[6] However, more participants and longer follow up times are needed to investigate this preliminary conclusion. We found one treatment guideline based on available non-RCT evidence (search date 2000; 8 clinical studies of different designs; number of participants not reported), which evaluated management of unerupted and impacted wisdom teeth.[21] It suggested that extraction is not advisable in people with deeply impacted wisdom teeth who have no history of pertinent local or systemic pathology. However, the guidelines suggested that removal of disease-free wisdom teeth in people without symptoms may be beneficial in the presence of caries in the adjacent second molar, which cannot be properly treated without the removal of the wisdom teeth. Extraction may also be beneficial in the presence of periodontal pockets distally to the second molar; and in case of resorption of the distal root of the second molar if it seems to be caused by the wisdom tooth.

REFERENCES

1. Hugoson A, Kugelberg CF. The prevalence of third molars in a Swedish population. An epidemiological study. *Community Dent Health* 1988;5:121–138.
2. Mercier P, Precious D. Risks and benefits of removal of impacted third molars. *Int J Oral Maxillofac Surg* 1992;21:17–27.
3. Shepherd JP, Brickley M. Surgical removal of third molars. *BMJ* 1994;309:620–621.
4. Worrall SF, Riden K, Corrigan AM. UK National Third Molar project: the initial report. *Br J Oral Maxillofac Surg* 1998;36:14–18.
5. Silvestri AR Jr, Singh I. The unresolved problem of the third molar: would people be better off without it? [Comment] *J Am Dent Assoc* 2003;134:450–455.
6. Song F, O'Meara S, Wilson P, et al. The effectiveness and cost-effectiveness of prophylactic removal of wisdom teeth. *Health Technol Assess* 2000;4:1–55. Search date 1999; primary sources Medline, Embase, Science Citation Index, Cochrane Controlled Trials Register, National Research Register, Database of Reviews of Effectiveness, hand searches of paper sources, web-based resources, and contact with relevant organisations and professional bodies.
7. Berge TG, Espeland LV, Klock K, et al. Prophylactic removal of wisdom teeth. Norwegian Health Services Research Centre (NHSRC) 2003 (SMM-Report 10/2003). URL: http://nhscrd.york.ac.uk/online/hta/20031252.htm (last visited 14 October 2004). Search date from 1999 to May 2003; primary sources the Cochrane Controlled Trial Register, DARE, HTA Database, Medline, Embase, National Guideline Clearinghouse, PRODIGY Guidance, NICE, SIGN (Scottish Intercollegiate Guidelines Network), OHE Economic Evaluations Database, NHS Economic Evaluation Database, and hand searches of paper sources and web-based resources.
8. Harradine N, Pearson M, Toth B. The effect of extraction of third molars on late lower incisor crowding: a randomised controlled trial. *Br J Orthodont* 1998;25:117–122.
9. Bramley P. Sense about wisdoms? *J R Soc Med* 1981;74:867–868.
10. Capuzzi P, Montebugnoli L, Vaccaro MA. Extraction of impacted third molars. *Oral Surg Oral Med Oral Pathol Oral Radiol Endod* 1994;77:341–343.
11. Schultze-Mosgau S, Reich RH. Assessment of inferior alveolar and lingual nerve disturbances after dentoalveolar surgery, and recovery of sensitivity. *Int J Oral Maxillofac Surg* 1993;22:214–217.
12. Rood JP. Permanent damage to inferior alveolar nerves during the removal of impacted mandibular third molars: comparison of two methods of bone removal. *Br Dent J* 1992;172:108–110.
13. Blackburn CW, Bramley PA. Lingual nerve damage associated with removal of lower third molars. *Br Dent J* 1989;167:103–107.
14. Robinson PP, Smith KG. Lingual nerve damage during lower third molar removal: a comparison of two surgical methods. *Br Dent J* 1996;180:456–461.
15. Sisk AL, Hammer WB, Shelton DW, et al. Complications following removal of impacted third molars: the role of the experience of the surgeon. *J Oral Maxillofac Surg* 1986;44:855–859.
16. Larsen PE. Alveolar osteitis after surgical removal of impacted mandibular third molars. Identification of the patient at risk. *Oral Surg Oral Med Oral Pathol* 1992;73:393–397.
17. Christiaens I, Reychler H. Complications after third molar extractions: retrospective analysis of 1,213 teeth. *Rev Stomatolo Chir Maxillofac* 2002;103:269–274. [In French]
18. Chiapasco M, Crescentini M, Romanoni G. Germectomy or delayed removal of mandibular impacted third molars: the relationship between age

and incidence of complications. *J Oral Maxillofac Surg* 1995;53:418–422; discussion 422–433.
19. Osborn TP, Frederickson G, Small IA, et al. A prospective study of complications related to mandibular third molar surgery. *J Oral Maxillofac Surg* 1985;43:767–769.
20. Bruce RA, Frederickson GC, Small GS. Age of patients and morbidity associated with mandibular third molar surgery. *J Am Dent Assoc* 1980;101:240–245.
21. Management of unerupted and impacted third molar teeth. SIGN (Scottish Intercollegiate Guidelines Network) publication no 43, 2000. Initial search date 1997 updated before 2000; primary sources Medline and Embase for English language papers.

Marco Esposito
DDS, PhD, Associate Professor
Department of Biomaterials and
Department of Prosthetic Dentistry/Dental
Material Sciences
The Sahlgrenska Academy at
Göteborg University
Göteborg
Sweden

Competing interests: None declared.

The following previous contributors of this topic would also like to be acknowledged: Stephen Worrall.

Postoperative pulmonary infections

Search date March 2004

Andrew Smith

QUESTIONS

INTERVENTIONS

See glossary G

Key Messages

- **Regional anaesthesia for surgery** One systematic review found that spinal or epidural anaesthesia (alone or in combination with general anaesthesia) reduced postoperative pneumonia compared with general anaesthesia alone.
- **Postoperative chest physiotherapy (deep breathing exercises)** One systematic review and one subsequent RCT found that deep breathing exercises reduced postoperative pulmonary infections compared with control. One RCT found no significant difference between physiotherapy plus deep breathing exercises and physiotherapy alone in postoperative pulmonary complications. We were unable to draw conclusions from one small RCT comparing deep breathing and coughing exercises (with or without intensive physiotherapy) versus no physiotherapy.
- **Postoperative chest physiotherapy (incentive spirometry and intermittent positive pressure breathing)** Two RCTs found that incentive spirometry reduced pulmonary complications compared with control. One RCT found that intermittent positive pressure breathing reduced postoperative pulmonary complications compared with control.
- **Advice to stop smoking preoperatively** We found no RCTs about the effects of preoperative advice to stop cigarette smoking on postoperative pulmonary infections. Two observational studies found that people who smoked were more likely to develop postoperative pulmonary complications of all kinds than those who did not. One study suggested that people who had stopped smoking 6 months prior to surgery reverted to the risk of those who had never smoked.

DEFINITION A working diagnosis of postoperative pulmonary infection may be based on three or more new findings from: cough, phlegm, shortness of breath, chest pain, temperature above 38 °C, and pulse rate above 100 a minute.[1] In this chapter, we are dealing strictly with pneumonia that is regarded to be a complication of the operation. We examine a selection of pre-, intra-, and postoperative techniques to reduce the risk of this complication. In this chapter, the diagnosis of pneumonia implies consolidation observed in a chest radiograph.[2]

INCIDENCE/ PREVALENCE Reported morbidity for chest complications depends on how carefully they are investigated. One study found blood gas and chest radiograph abnormalities in about 50% of people after open cholecystectomy.[3] However, fewer than 20% of these had abnormal clinical signs and only 10% had a clinically significant chest infection. Another study estimated the incidence of pneumonia as 20%.[4] Another used a similarly strict definition and found the incidence to be 23%.[5]

AETIOLOGY/ RISK FACTORS Risk factors include increasing age (> 50 years), cigarette smoking, obesity, thoracic or upper abdominal operations, and pre-existing lung disease.[6] One multivariate analysis did not confirm the association with cigarette smoking, but suggested that longer preoperative hospital stay and higher grading on the American Society of Anesthesiologists' physical status scale (> 2) increased the risk of postoperative pulmonary complications.[5] Depression of the immune system may also contribute.[7]

PROGNOSIS In one large systematic review (search date 1997, 141 RCTs, 9559 people), 10% of people with postoperative pneumonia died.[8] If systemic sepsis ensues, mortality is likely to be substantial.[9] Pneumonia delays recovery from surgery and poor tissue oxygenation may contribute to delayed wound healing.

AIMS OF INTERVENTION To prevent the development of postoperative pulmonary infection; to minimise postoperative pain; to reduce mortality; to minimise adverse effects of treatment.

OUTCOMES Rates of clinically diagnosed postoperative pulmonary infection (as in the definition above); pain, measured using a variety of pain scales. Postoperative pulmonary complications are a commonly used outcome, but this combines pulmonary infections with other adverse outcomes. Where possible, we have reported on postoperative pulmonary infections in favour of pulmonary complications.

METHODS *Clinical Evidence* search and appraisal March 2004, including a search for observational studies on preoperative advice to stop smoking.

QUESTION What are the effects of preventive interventions?

OPTION ADVICE TO STOP SMOKING PREOPERATIVELY

We found no RCTs about the effects of preoperative advice to stop cigarette smoking on postoperative pulmonary infections. Two observational studies found that people who smoked were more likely to develop pulmonary complications of all kinds than those who did not. One study suggested that people who had stopped smoking 6 months prior to surgery reverted to the risk of those who had never smoked.

Benefits: We found one systematic review (search date 2001), which identified no RCTs.[10] We found no subsequent RCTs.

Harms: We found no RCTs.

Comment: One prospective observational study (200 people having coronary artery bypass surgery) found that smokers were more likely than non-smokers to develop postoperative pulmonary complications of all types.[11] People who had stopped smoking 6 months preoperatively reverted to the risk of those who had never smoked. A benefit was seen only in people who had stopped smoking for 2 months or more. A later prospective cohort study (410 people having a variety of elective procedures) found that current smokers were more likely to have postoperative pneumonia than those who had never smoked, but the differences were not tested statistically.[12] For all postoperative pulmonary complications, the odds ratio for developing complications for current smokers compared with those who had never smoked was 5.5 (95% CI 1.2 to 14.8). One multivariate analysis of postoperative pulmonary infections did not confirm the association with cigarette smoking.[5]

OPTION REGIONAL ANAESTHESIA

One systematic review found that spinal or epidural anaesthesia (alone or in combination with general anaesthesia) reduced postoperative pneumonia compared with general anaesthesia alone.

Benefits: We found one systematic review (search date 1997, 28 RCTs), which compared intraoperative neuraxial blockade**G** (with or without general anaesthesia) versus no neuraxial blockade (primarily general anaesthesia plus systemic analgesia).[8] It found that neuraxial blockade significantly reduced postoperative pneumonia compared with general anaesthesia (149/4871 [3%] with neuraxial blockade *v* 238/4688 [5%] with general anaesthesia; ARR 2%; RR 0.60, 95% CI 0.49 to 0.74; NNT 50, 95% CI 36 to 82).[8] The review found some evidence that the risk of developing pneumonia may be lower after thoracic epidural anaesthesia than after lumbar epidural or spinal anaesthesia.

Harms: The review did not report on adverse effects of the anaesthetic agents or techniques.[8] We found one large prospective French cohort study (30 413 epidural anaesthetics) of the incidence of harms from epidural analgesia.[13] This study estimated the frequency of cardiac arrest (usually owing to inadvertent intravascular injection of local anaesthetic) as 1/10 000; seizures (usually the same cause) as 1.3/10 000; neurological injury as 2/10 000; radiculopathy as 1.6/10 000; and paraplegia as 0.3/10 000.[13] There were no deaths attributable to epidural analgesia. In a large US case series (1297 people receiving epidurals), 0.4% of people were judged to need naloxone to reverse the adverse effects of epidural opioids on breathing.[14] One case series reported three cases in which epidural analgesia was thought to contribute to the development of postoperative pressure sores.[15] Inadvertent dural puncture with the epidural needle can cause headache (frequency increases with gauge of needle).[16] Effective pain relief can delay recognition of surgical complications, such as anastomotic breakdown, peritonitis, or compartment compression syndrome of the legs.

Comment: The review sought aggregated benefit for all types of intraoperative neuraxial blockade compared with no neuraxial blockade and had more power.[8] One sensitivity analysis suggested that the overall benefits of regional anaesthesia in reducing all types of postoperative complications held for all types of surgery studied. The overall benefit of regional anaesthesia seemed independent of whether it was combined with general anaesthesia.

OPTION POSTOPERATIVE CHEST PHYSIOTHERAPY

One systematic review and one subsequent RCT found that deep breathing exercises reduced postoperative pulmonary infections compared with control. One RCT found no significant difference between physiotherapy plus deep breathing exercises and physiotherapy alone in postoperative pulmonary complications. We were unable to draw conclusions from one small RCT comparing deep breathing and coughing exercises (with or without intensive physiotherapy) versus no physiotherapy. Two RCTs found that incentive spirometry reduced pulmonary complications compared with control. One RCT found that intermittent positive pressure breathing reduced postoperative pulmonary complications compared with control.

Benefits: **Incentive spirometry:** We found two systematic reviews (search date 1992;[17] search date 2000[18]). The reviews identified the same two RCTs comparing incentive spirometry**G** versus control (details of control not stated in the reviews), but only the first review performed a meta-analysis.[17] It found that incentive spirometry significantly reduced the risk of postoperative pulmonary complications compared with control (212 people; OR 0.44, 95% CI 0.18 to 0.99; absolute numbers not reported). **Deep breathing/coughing exercises:** We found two systematic reviews (search date 1992;[17] search date 2003[19]). The first review[17] identified four RCTs (564 people) comparing deep breathing exercises**G** versus control (details of control not reported in the review); the second review[19] identified two further RCTs in people who had undergone cardiac surgery,[20,21] and we found one additional RCT.[22] The first review found that deep breathing exercises significantly reduced pulmonary complications compared with control, but there was significant heterogeneity between trials (OR 0.43, 95% CI 0.27 to 0.63; absolute number not reported). One of the four RCTs (60 people) used an outcome measure that could not in itself diagnose pulmonary infection. Of the two RCTs identified by the second review,[19] the first (120 people having coronary artery surgery) compared two physiotherapy groups with no treatment.[20] It found low rates of chest infections in all groups (1/40 [2.5%] with no physiotherapy *v* 4/40 [10%] with instruction to perform deep breathing and coughing exercises *v* 1/40 [2.5%] with instruction to perform deep breathing and coughing exercises and more intensive attention from the physiotherapist). The RCT did not report formal statistical analysis because of the small number of complications. The second RCT identified by the review (230 people, 198 completed) compared physiotherapy plus deep breathing exercises versus physiotherapy without deep breathing exercises.[21] It found no significant difference between treatments in postoperative pulmonary complications (intention to treat analysis: 5/115 [4.3%] with deep breathing *v* 3/115 [2.6%] with no deep breathing, P = 0.42). The additional RCT (368 people having major abdominal surgery) compared instruction to perform deep breathing exercises versus no physiotherapy instruction.[22] Additional resistance training was given to people in the treatment group at high risk (defined as aged > 50 years or with 1 of the following: smoker or ex-smoker for < 12 months, body mass index > 30, pulmonary disease needing daily medication, or other coexisting medical condition). The RCT found that, in all people having surgery, deep breathing exercises significantly reduced the risk of developing pneumonia compared with control (1/172 [0.6%] with deep breathing *v* 13/192 [6.8%] with control; RR 0.09, 95% CI 0.01 to 0.65; NNT 16, 95% CI 10 to 39). The relative risk of developing pneumonia in people at high risk was not given. **Intermittent positive pressure breathing:** We found one systematic review (search date 1992[17]), which identified one RCT[1] (172 people) comparing four interventions: intermittent positive pressure breathing**G**; incentive spirometry; deep breathing exercises; and no treatment. It found that intermittent positive pressure breathing significantly reduced pulmonary complications compared with no treatment (10/45 [22%] with intermittent positive pressure breathing *v* 21/44 [48%] with no treatment; RR 0.5, 95% CI 0.2 to 0.9; NNT 4, 95% CI 3 to 18).[1]

Harms: Two reviews gave no information on adverse effects.[17,18] The third review found four trials that provided data on adverse effects.[19] It found gastric distension in 2–10% of people and nausea in 0–12%, but did not state which treatments these results applied to.

Comment: Some RCTs in the earliest review distinguished between people at low and high risk of pulmonary complications.[17] Individual RCTs in low risk people often did not find the benefits of physiotherapy that were seen when all RCTs were pooled. The RCT[20] identified by the most recent review and the additional RCT[22] were conducted in people at lower risk of pulmonary infection. The earliest review assessed study validity by two independent assessors using the following criteria: reproducibility of patient population and surgical procedure; comparability of groups; clear description of experimental manoeuvre; presence of control group; clear description of outcome measures; random allocation with blinding; withdrawals listed; prior estimate of study power; and some measure of test of compliance with treatment.[17]

GLOSSARY

The following three modalities of physiotherapy all count as methods to increase lung volume. Increasing lung volume is thought to cause a reduction in airways resistance and an improvement in ventilation:[23]

Deep breathing The person is instructed to breathe in deeply, comfortably, and slowly through the nose, and then sigh out through the mouth. Optimum conditions to ensure that deep breaths reach poorly ventilated dependent regions include accurate positioning, ensuring that the person is comfortable and relaxed, avoiding distractions, and allowing the person to get their breath back after turning to avoid breathlessness.

Incentive spirometry The flow and volume achieved by a controlled and sustained deep breaths can be encouraged by an incentive spirometer, which gives the person visual feedback on their performance. The same effect can theoretically be obtained without the device, but the incentive of using a tangible object may increase inhaled volume and produce more controlled flow.

Intermittent positive pressure breathing Assisted breathing with a pressure cycled ventilator triggered into inspiration by the user and allowing passive expiration. The user begins to inhale through the machine, which senses the breath and augments it by delivering gas to the user. When a preset pressure is reached, the machine stops delivering gas and allows the user to breathe out. In most devices, the inspiratory sensitivity, flow rate, and pressure can be varied to suit the user's needs, but some devices adjust the sensitivity and flow automatically.

Neuraxial blockade Involves spinal or epidural anaesthesia.

REFERENCES

1. Celli BR, Rodriguez KS, Snider GL. A controlled trial of intermittent positive pressure breathing, incentive spirometry, and deep breathing exercises in preventing pulmonary complications after abdominal surgery. *Am Rev Respir Dis* 1984;130:12–15.
2. Hall JC, Tarala RA, Tapper J, et al. Prevention of respiratory complications after abdominal surgery: a randomised clinical trial. *BMJ* 1996;312:148–152.
3. Wirén FE, Janson L, Hellekant C. Respiratory complications after upper abdominal surgery. *Acta Chir Scand* 1981;147:623–627.
4. Garibaldi RA, Britt MR, Coleman ML, et al. Risk factors for postoperative pneumonia. *Am J Med* 1981;70:677–680.
5. Hall JC, Tarala RA, Hall JL, et al. A multivariate analysis of the risk of pulmonary complications after laparotomy. *Chest* 1991;99:923–927.
6. Christensen EF, Schultz P, Jensen OV, et al. Postoperative pulmonary complications and lung function in high-risk patients: a comparison of three physiotherapy regimens after upper abdominal surgery in general anaesthesia. *Acta Anaesthesiol Scand* 1991;35:97–104.
7. Sabiston DC Jr, ed. *Textbook of surgery: the biological basis of modern surgical practice, 15th ed.* Philadelphia: WB Saunders, 1997:345.
8. Rodgers A, Walker N, Schug S, et al. Reduction of postoperative mortality and morbidity with epidural or spinal anaesthesia: results from overview of randomised trials. *BMJ* 2000;321:1493–1497. Search date 1997; primary sources Medline, Embase, Current Contents, the Cochrane Library, hand searches of reference lists from all identified papers and of selected conference proceedings, and personal contact with authors.
9. Miller G, Ellis ME. Hospital-acquired pneumonia. In: Ellis M, ed. *Infectious diseases of the respiratory tract.* Cambridge: Cambridge University Press, 1998.
10. Møller A, Villebro N, Pedersen T. Interventions for preoperative smoking cessation. In: The Cochrane Library, Issue 3, 2004. Oxford: Update Software. Search date 2001: primary sources Medline, Embase, Cinahl, and Cochrane Controlled trials register.
11. Warner MA, Offord KP, Warner ME, et al. Role of preoperative cessation of smoking and other factors in postoperative pulmonary complications: a blinded prospective study of coronary artery bypass patients. *Mayo Clin Proc* 1989;64:609–616.
12. Bluman LG, Mosca L, Newman N, et al. Preoperative smoking habits and postoperative pulmonary complications. *Chest* 1998;113:148–152.
13. Auroy Y, Narchi P, Messiah A, et al. Serious complications related to regional anesthesia. *Anesthesiology* 1997;87:479–486.
14. Scott DA, Beilby DSN, McClymont C. Postoperative analgesia using epidural infusions of fentanyl with bupivacaine. *Anesthesiology* 1995;83:727–737.
15. Shah JL. Postoperative pressure sores after epidural anaesthesia. *BMJ* 2000;321:941–942.
16. Bromage PR. *Epidural analgesia.* Philadelphia: WB Saunders, 1978.
17. Thomas JA, McIntosh JM. Are incentive spirometry, intermittent positive pressure breathing and deep breathing exercises effective in the prevention of postoperative pulmonary complications after upper abdominal surgery? A systematic overview and meta-analysis. *Phys Ther* 1994;74:3–16. Search date 1992; primary sources Medline, Cinahl, and hand searches of reference lists from relevant

articles and reference lists, and unpublished abstracts from a Consensus Exercise on Physical Therapy for the Surgical Patient 1989.
18. Overend TJ, Anderson C, Lucy, SD, et al. The effect of incentive spirometry on postoperative pulmonary complications: a systematic review. *Chest* 2001;120:971–978. Search date 2000; primary sources Medline, Cinahl, Healthstar, and Current Contents databases, and hand searches of reference lists from relevant articles.
19. Pasquina P, Tramer MR, Walder B. Prophylactic respiratory physiotherapy after cardiac surgery: systematic review *BMJ* 2003;327:1379–84. Search date 2003; primary sources Medline, Embase, Cinahl, and Cochrane controlled trials register, and hand searches of reference lists from relevant articles.
20. Stiller K, Montarello J, Wallace M, et al. Efficacy of breathing and coughing exercises in the prevention of pulmonary complications after coronary artery surgery. *Chest* 1994;105:741–747.
21. Brasher PA, McClelland KH, Denehy L, et al. Does removal of deep breathing exercises from a physiotherapy program including pre-operative education and early mobilization after cardiac surgery alter patient outcomes? *Aust J Physiother* 2003;49:165–173.
22. Fagevik-Olsen M, Hahn I, Nordgren S, et al. Randomized controlled trial of prophylactic chest physiotherapy in major abdominal surgery. *Br J Surg* 1997;84:1535–1538.
23. Hough A. *Physiotherapy in respiratory care: a problem-solving approach, 3rd ed.* London: Chapman and Hall, 2001.

Andrew Smith
Department of Anaesthesia Royal
Lancaster Infirmary
Lancaster
UK

Competing interests: None declared.

Carbon monoxide poisoning (acute)

Search date August 2004

Nicholas Phin

QUESTIONS

INTERVENTIONS

*Categorisation is based on consensus and physiological studies

See glossary G

Key Messages

- Many cases of mild to moderate carbon monoxide poisoning are probably misdiagnosed. A history of known exposure to carbon monoxide and the presence of clinical signs and symptoms should not be ignored even if the percentage carboxyhaemoglobin is low or within the normal range.
- In cases of suspected carbon monoxide poisoning, the immediate and essential actions are to remove the person from the source of carbon monoxide and to give oxygen, preferably 100%, through a non-re-breather mask.
- In a hospital setting, any decision to use hyperbaric oxygen needs to be based on the clinical history, percentage carboxyhaemoglobin, condition of the person, and feasibility of safe transportation to a hyperbaric facility.

Oxygen treatments

- **Oxygen 100% via non-re-breather mask (compared with air)*** We found no systematic review, RCTs, or analytical observational studies comparing oxygen 100% by non-re-breather mask versus air for clinically relevant outcomes of interest. Such an RCT in people with suspected acute carbon monoxide poisoning would be considered unethical. One retrospective chart review in people with various levels of severity of acute carbon monoxide poisoning receiving oxygen 100% either by non-re-breather mask or by ventilation if intubated in a tertiary teaching hospital setting found that oxygen 100% reduced carboxyhaemoglobin half life. We found no systematic review or RCTs for other clinical outcomes of interest in people with acute carbon monoxide poisoning. Based on physiological studies, the benefits of oxygen 100% by non-re-breather mask in the emergency situation are universally accepted but there is still considerable debate about the optimum duration of treatment in secondary or tertiary care settings.
- **Hyperbaric oxygen 100% at 2-3 ATA (compared with normobaric oxygen 100% in moderate to severe poisoning)** One RCT in people with moderate to severe acute carbon monoxide poisoning found limited evidence that, compared with normobaric oxygen 100%, hyperbaric oxygen 100% delivered within 24 hours of presentation at pressures of 2–3 atmospheres reduced cognitive sequelae at 6 weeks. However, it is unclear which the types of people will benefit, the optimum

treatment regime, and how long after exposure the treatment has an effect. The size of the effect derived from hyperbaric oxygen treatment may be highly sensitive to the pressure at which the oxygen is delivered, the number of treatment sessions, and the oxygen content of control treatments.

- **Oxygen 28% (compared with air)*** We found no systematic review, RCTs, or analytical observational studies comparing 28% normobaric oxygen versus air in people with carbon monoxide poisoning for clinically relevant outcomes of interest. It may be considered unethical to conduct analytical studies. Oxygen 28% will affect carboxyhaemoglobin levels but may not be as effective as higher concentrations of oxygen for reducing carboxyhaemoglobin half life. UK paramedics routinely use oxygen 28% so that individuals who may be dependent on their hypoxic drive are not adversely affected.
- **Hyperbaric oxygen 100% (compared with oxygen 100% in mild poisoning)** We found no systematic review or RCTs only in people with mild carbon monoxide poisoning. Two RCTs in people with mild to moderate acute carbon monoxide poisoning found insufficient evidence to draw conclusions about the effects of hyperbaric oxygen versus oxygen 100% via non-re-breather mask for prevention of delayed neurological complications. We found no systematic review or RCTs for other clinical outcomes of interest.

*Categorisation is based on consensus and physiological studies

---

DEFINITION Carbon monoxide is an odourless, colourless gas and poisoning causes hypoxia, cell damage, and death.[1,2] **Diagnosis of carbon monoxide poisoning:** Exposure to carbon monoxide is measured either directly from blood samples and expressed as a percentage of carboxyhaemoglobin or indirectly using the carbon monoxide in expired breath. Percentage carboxyhaemoglobin is the most frequently used biomarker of carbon monoxide exposure. Although the diagnosis of carbon monoxide poisoning can be confirmed by detecting elevated levels of blood carboxyhaemoglobin levels, the presence of clinical signs and symptoms after known exposure to carbon monoxide should not be ignored. The signs and symptoms of carbon monoxide poisoning are mainly associated with the brain and heart which are most sensitive to hypoxia. The symptoms of carbon monoxide poisoning are non-specific and varied and include headache, fatigue,[3] malaise, "trouble thinking", confusion, nausea, dizziness, visual disturbances, chest pain, shortness of breath, loss of consciousness, and seizures.[4–6] In people suffering from coexisting morbidities, symptoms such as shortness of breath or chest pain may be more evident. The classical signs of carbon monoxide, described as cherry-red lips, peripheral cyanosis, and retinal haemorrhages, are in reality rarely seen.[7] **Interpretation of carboxyhaemoglobin levels:** Non-smokers living away from urban areas have carboxyhaemoglobin levels of between 0.4% and 1.0% reflecting endogenous carbon monoxide production whereas levels of up to 5% may be considered normal in a busy urban or industrial setting.[8] Smokers are exposed to increased levels of carbon monoxide in cigarettes and otherwise healthy heavy smokers can tolerate levels of carboxyhaemoglobin of up 15%.[9] The use of percentage carboxyhaemoglobin as a measure of severity of carbon monoxide poisoning or to predict treatment options is limited because carboxyhaemoglobin levels are affected by the removal from the source of carbon monoxide and any oxygen treatment given before measurement of percentage carboxyhaemoglobin. In addition, people with co-morbidities that make them more sensitive to the hypoxia associated with carbon monoxide can present with symptoms of poisoning at carboxyhaemoglobin levels that are either low or within the normal range.[10] Attempts have been made in the literature to equate symptoms and signs to different carboxyhaemoglobin levels[11] but it is accepted that carboxyhaemoglobin levels in an acutely poisoned person only roughly correlate with the clinical signs and symptoms, especially those relating to neurological function.[12] Earlier studies attempted to differentiate between smokers and non- smokers. Attempts have also been made in the literature to divide carbon monoxide poisoning into mild, moderate, and severe based on percentage carboxyhaemoglobin levels and clinical symptoms,[13] but there is no clear clinical consensus or agreement on this issue. The degree of poisoning has been described in the literature as *mild carbon monoxide poisoning:* a carboxyhaemoglobin level of greater than 10% without clinical signs or symptoms of carbon monoxide poisoning; *moderate carbon monoxide poisoning:* a carboxyhaemoglobin level of greater than 10% and less than 20–25% with minor clinical signs and symptoms of poisoning such as headache, lethargy or fatigue; and *severe carbon monoxide poisoning:* a carboxyhaemoglobin level of greater than 20–25%, loss of consciousness and confusion or signs of cardiac ischaemia, or both. **Population:** For the purpose of this review, we have included adults presenting to health care professionals with suspected carbon monoxide poisoning. Although there is as yet no clear consensus on this issue, most studies examining carbon monoxide poisoning and its management use a carboxyhaemoglobin level of 10% or more or the presence of clinical signs and symptoms after known exposure to carbon monoxide to be indicative of acute carbon monoxide poisoning. Unless otherwise stated this is the definition of acute carbon monoxide poisoning that has been used throughout this chapter. Where appropriate, the terms mild, moderate, or severe have been used to reflect the descriptions of populations in individual studies.

INCIDENCE/ PREVALENCE

Carbon monoxide poisoning is considered to be one of the leading causes of death and injury worldwide and a major public health problem.[14] In 2000, there were 521 deaths where carbon monoxide was the recorded cause of death (ICD 9 – E986) in England and Wales[15] compared with 1363 deaths recorded in 1985;[16] a trend that has also been observed in the US.[17] Of the 521 deaths attributed to carbon monoxide poisoning, 148 were accidental and the remaining 373 the result of suicide or self inflicted injury. Poisoning by carbon monoxide is almost certainly underdiagnosed because of the varied ways in which it can present and it has been estimated in the US that there are over 40 000 emergency department visits a year; many presenting with a flu-like illness.[18] In 2003, there were 534 recorded medical episodes in English hospitals involving people suffering from the toxic effects of carbon monoxide.[19] This may be a substantial underestimate if the US experience reflects the true morbidity associated with carbon monoxide poisoning. Studies in the US have shown that the incidence of accidental carbon monoxide poisoning peaks during the winter months,[20,21] and is associated with increased use of indoor heating and petrol powered generators and reduced external ventilation. This seasonal rise in numbers coincides with the annual increase in influenza notifications and given the similarity in symptoms many cases of mild carbon monoxide poisoning are probably misdiagnosed.

AETIOLOGY/ RISK FACTORS

People at high risk: People who are most at risk from carbon monoxide poisoning include those with coronary heart disease, vascular disease, or anaemia; pregnant women and their fetus; infants; and the elderly. In people with coronary heart disease, experimentally induced blood carboxyhaemoglobin levels of 4.5% shorten the period of exercise before the onset of anginal pain and the duration of pain is prolonged.[22–24] In people with anaemia the oxygen carrying capacity of the blood is already compromised and therefore they will be more sensitive to carbon monoxide.[25] The elderly are at risk because of existing co-morbidities such as heart disease or respiratory disease and because of a reduced compensatory response to hypoxic situations. During pregnancy, a woman's oxygen carrying capacity is reduced because of an increased endogenous carbon monoxide production and additional endogenous carbon monoxide from the developing fetus leading to an increased carboxyhaemoglobin concentration.[26] A higher ventilation rate during pregnancy will lead to increased uptake of carbon monoxide at any given carbon monoxide concentration.[27] The fetus is also at risk and there have been occasional fetal deaths in non-fatal maternal exposures.[26,28,29] In the developing fetus, oxygen is released at a lower oxygen partial pressure and fetal haemoglobin binds with carbon monoxide more quickly compared with adults. Carbon monoxide may be a teratogen where there is a significant increase in maternal carboxyhaemoglobin or where there is moderate to severe maternal toxicity.[30] Infants may be more susceptible to the effect of carbon monoxide because of their greater oxygen consumption in relation to adults and their response and symptoms are more variable. There are recorded instances of children travelling in the same car and having varying symptoms with similar carboxyhaemoglobin levels or widely varying carboxyhaemoglobin levels with similar carbon monoxide exposure.[31] **Sources of carbon monoxide:** Carbon monoxide is produced by the incomplete combustion of carbon containing fuel, such as gas (domestic or bottled), charcoal, coke, oil, and wood. Gas stoves, fires, and boilers; gas powered water heaters; car exhaust fumes; charcoal barbeques; paraffin heaters; solid fuel powered stoves; boilers; and room heaters that are faulty or inadequately ventilated are all potential sources. A sometimes overlooked source of carbon monoxide is methylene chloride in some paint strippers and sprays. Methylene chloride is readily absorbed through the skin and lungs and once in the liver, is converted to carbon monoxide. Methylene chloride is stored in body tissues and released gradually; the carbon monoxide elimination half life in people exposed to methylene chloride is more than twice that of inhaled carbon monoxide. Natural background levels of carbon monoxide in the outdoor environment range from 0.01–0.23 mg/m^3 (0.009–.0.2 ppm)[32] but in urban traffic in the UK the 8 hour mean concentrations are higher at about 20 mg/m^3 (17.5 ppm);[33] exposure to this level for prolonged periods could result in a carboxyhaemoglobin level of about 3%.

PROGNOSIS The data regarding prognosis in carbon monoxide poisoning are inconclusive and contradictory. However, there is general agreement that outcome and prognosis are related to the level of carbon monoxide that a person is exposed to, the duration of exposure, and the presence of underlying risk factors.[33] A poor outcome is predicted by lengthy carbon monoxide exposure, loss of consciousness, and advancing age. In addition, hypotension and cardiac arrest independently predict permanent disability and death. After acute carbon monoxide poisoning the organs most sensitive to hypoxia will be most affected; i.e. the brain and the heart. Pre-existing co-morbidities that affect these organs will to an extent influence the clinical presentation and the prognosis; an individual with pre-existing heart disease may present with myocardial ischaemia that could lead to infarction and death. The prognosis for people resuscitated after experiencing cardiac arrest with carbon monoxide poisoning is poor. In a small retrospective study,[34] 18 people with carboxyhaemoglobin levels of 31.7 ± 11.0% given hyperbaric oxygen Ⓖ after resuscitation after cardiac arrest all died. The effects on the brain are more subtle given that different sections of the brain are more sensitive to hypoxic insults either as a consequence of reduced oxygen delivery or by direct effects on intracellular metabolism.[35] Therefore, in addition to the acute neurological sequelae leading to loss of consciousness, coma and death, neurological sequelae such as poor concentration and memory problems may be apparent in people recovering from carbon monoxide poisoning (persistent neurological sequelae) or develop after a period of apparent normality (delayed neurological sequelae). Delayed neurological sequelae develop between 2 days to 240 days after exposure and are reported to affect 10–32% of people recovering from carbon monoxide poisoning.[36,37] Symptoms include cognitive changes, personality changes, incontinence, psychosis, and Parkinsonism.[38] Fortunately 50–75% of people recover within 1 year.[39]

AIMS OF INTERVENTION To reduce mortality, normalise carboxyhaemoglobin levels, alleviate symptoms, reduce the incidence of delayed neuropsychological sequelae, and reduce cardiovascular morbidity.

OUTCOMES Improve conscious levels and cardiovascular parameters; limit neurological sequelae; reduce mortality, hyperoxic seizures, barotrauma associated with hyperbaric oxygen Ⓖ, and serum carboxyhaemoglobin levels.

METHODS *Clinical Evidence* search and appraisal August 2004. Studies and trials were considered in a hierarchical manner with systematic reviews of RCTs being considered as most robust evidence and anecdote the least robust. In the event of no systematic reviews or RCTs being available, observational study data were considered but only included where it was considered unethical or impractical to conduct an RCT. Studies where the population consisted wholly of children or adolescents have been excluded.

QUESTION **What are the effects of oxygen treatments for acute carbon monoxide poisoning?** New

OPTION **OXYGEN 28%** New

We found no systematic review, RCTs, or analytical observational studies comparing 28% normobaric oxygen versus air in people with carbon monoxide poisoning for clinically relevant outcomes of interest. It may be considered unethical to conduct analytical studies. Oxygen 28% will affect carboxyhaemoglobin levels but may not be as effective as higher concentrations of oxygen for reducing carboxyhaemoglobin half life. UK paramedics routinely use oxygen 28% so that individuals who may be dependent on their hypoxic drive are not adversely affected.

Benefits: **Oxygen 28% versus air:** We found no systematic review, RCTs, or analytical observational studies comparing normobaric oxygen**G** 28% versus air for clinically relevant outcomes of interest. An RCT comparing normobaric oxygen 28% versus air in people with suspected acute carbon monoxide poisoning may be considered unethical. There is consensus that there will be an increased benefit with normobaric oxygen 28% compared with air.

Harms: **Oxygen 28% versus air:** We found no systematic review, RCTs, or analytical observational studies comparing normobaric oxygen**G** 28% versus air in people with acute carbon monoxide poisoning for clinically relevant outcomes of interest.

Comment: Based on physiological studies, UK paramedics use normobaric oxygen**G** 28% so that individuals who may be dependent on their hypoxic drive are not adversely affected. Normobaric oxygen 28% will affect carboxyhaemoglobin levels but may not be as effective as higher concentrations of oxygen for reducing carboxyhaemoglobin half life.

OPTION OXYGEN 100% VIA NON-RE-BREATHER MASK New

We found no systematic review, RCTs, or analytical observational studies comparing oxygen 100% by non-re-breather mask versus air for clinically relevant outcomes of interest. Such an RCT in people with suspected acute carbon monoxide poisoning would be considered unethical. One retrospective chart review in people with various levels of severity of acute carbon monoxide poisoning receiving oxygen 100% either by non-re-breather mask or by ventilation if intubated in a tertiary teaching hospital setting found that oxygen 100% reduced carboxyhaemoglobin half life. We found no systematic review or RCTs for other clinical outcomes of interest in people with acute carbon monoxide poisoning. Based on physiological studies, the benefits of oxygen 100% by non-re-breather mask in the emergency situation are universally accepted but there is still considerable debate about the optimum duration of treatment in secondary or tertiary care settings.

Benefits: The maximum concentration of oxygen that can be delivered with a re-breather mask, regardless of the oxygen flow, is just under 50% In order to get as high an inspired oxygen concentration as possible a non-re-breather mask**G** is needed. **Oxygen 100% via non-re-breather mask versus air:** We found no systematic review, RCTs, or analytical observational studies comparing 100% normobaric oxygen**G** via tight fitting non-re-breather mask versus air in people with suspected acute carbon monoxide poisoning for clinically relevant outcomes of interest. Such an RCT would be considered unethical. We found one retrospective chart review of 93 people with various levels of severity of acute carbon monoxide poisoning receiving normobaric oxygen 100% either by non-re-breather mask or by ventilation if intubated in a tertiary teaching hospital setting.[40] The study found that oxygen 100% delivered by non-re-breather mask or endotracheal tube reduced carboxyhaemoglobin half life to 74 ± 25 minutes (mean ± 1 standard deviation) with a range from 26 minutes to 148 minutes. In young healthy volunteers breathing air at sea level the half life of carboxyhaemoglobin is 320 minutes (range: 128 minutes to 409 minutes). Administration of oxygen 100% at 1 atmosphere reduces the half life to 80 minutes.[41] **Duration of treatment:** We found no systematic review, RCTs, or cohort studies that indicated the optimal duration of treatment.

Harms: **Oxygen 100% via non-re-breather mask versus air:** Oxygen toxicity is not usually seen in oxygen concentrations of less than 50%; the maximum concentration that the commonly used re-breather masks on maximum flow can achieve. The first signs of toxicity can appear after

10 hours of exposure to oxygen at concentrations greater than 50% with increasing incidence of signs and symptoms with increasing duration of exposure. Oxygen toxicity can present as either central nervous system toxicity (the Bert Effect) or pulmonary toxicity (the Smith Effect). Pulmonary toxicity can include a progressive decrease in vital capacity, tightness in the chest, discomfort, coughing, congestion, increased depth of respiration, rapid panting or asthma-like attacks, and a cog wheel like breathing. CNS toxicity, such as hyperoxic seizures, is usually only seen when high concentrations of hyperbaric oxygen are used. Cardiovascular effects may include bradycardia and peripheral vasoconstriction. Bilateral progressive constriction of visual acuity has been found after breathing pure oxygen for 4.5 hours at normal atmospheric pressures.[42,43] **Duration of treatment:** We found no systematic review, RCTs, or cohort studies that indicated the optimal duration of treatment.

Comment: Based on physiological studies, the benefits of normobaric oxygen🅖 100% via non-re-breather mask🅖 in the emergency situation and in the field are universally accepted but there is still considerable debate about what is the optimum duration of treatment in secondary or tertiary care setting. Further clinical research on the optimum duration of exposure to oxygen 100% is needed. In the absence of such studies, it has been suggested[44] that people with mild carbon monoxide poisoning (see definition, p 1733) should receive normobaric oxygen 100% for no less than 6 hours' duration. In moderate to severe carbon monoxide poisoning (see definition, p 1733) oxygen 100% is usually given until the carboxyhaemoglobin is within normal parameters, i.e. less than 5% and any signs and symptoms of carbon monoxide toxicity have completely resolved.

OPTION HYPERBARIC OXYGEN New

We found no systematic review or RCTs only in people with mild carbon monoxide poisoning. Two RCTs in people with mild to moderate carbon monoxide poisoning found insufficient evidence to compare the effects of hyperbaric oxygen with oxygen 100% via non-re-breather mask. One RCT found no significant difference between hyperbaric oxygen 100% compared with oxygen 100% via non-re-breather mask in the proportion of people who did not develop neurological symptoms at 4 weeks. Another RCT found that, compared with oxygen 100% by via non-re-breather mask, hyperbaric oxygen 100% reduced the proportion of people developing neurological symptoms at 4 weeks. It is difficult to draw any firm conclusions from these two RCTs because the first RCT did not use validated neurophysiological tests, the second RCT used a vague definition of delayed neurological symptoms and neither study was blind. These are important limitations as neurophysiological changes would be subtle and slight in people with mild to moderate carbon monoxide poisoning. One RCT in people with moderate to severe acute carbon monoxide poisoning found limited evidence that, compared with normobaric oxygen 100%, hyperbaric oxygen 100% delivered within 24 hours of presentation at pressures of 2–3 atmospheres reduced cognitive sequelae at 6 weeks. However, it is unclear which the types of people will benefit, the optimum treatment regime, and how long after exposure the treatment has an effect. The size of the effect derived from hyperbaric oxygen treatment may be highly sensitive to the pressure at which the oxygen is delivered, the number of treatment sessions, and the oxygen content of control treatments. One RCT in people with all levels of carbon monoxide poisoning but including a high proportion (73%) of people with severe carbon monoxide poisoning found no significant difference between 3 day continuous normobaric oxygen 100% and 3 day continuous normobaric oxygen 100% interspersed with sessions of hyperbaric oxygen in the incidence of persistent neurological sequelae in people with all levels of carbon monoxide poisoning. The use of oxygen 100%

for 3 days or more is not a widely used treatment for carbon monoxide poisoning as high doses of oxygen can cause adverse effects. We found no systematic reviews or RCTs for other clinical outcomes of interest.

Benefits: We found three systematic reviews (search dates 1999,[45,46] 2002[47]) all of which identified the same six RCTs. The reviews came to different conclusions regarding the possible benefit of hyperbaric oxygen**G**. Only one of the reviews performed a meta-analysis, which we have not reported because of the heterogeneity of the study populations and regimens.[46] Out of the six RCTs identified in the systematic reviews, we have excluded two RCTs because one RCT provided only an interim analysis[48] and the other RCT was published only as an abstract, was small (26 people), had a questionable surrogate outcome (electroencephalogram abnormalities and a reduced cerebral blood flow reactivity to acetazolamide), and was not blinded.[49] We have reported below the four remaining RCTs.[50–53] **Hyperbaric oxygen 100% versus normobaric oxygen 100% in mild poisoning:** We found no systematic review or RCTs only in people with mild carbon monoxide poisoning. We found two RCTs comparing hyperbaric oxygen 100% versus oxygen 100% via non-re-breather mask**G** in people with mild to moderate carbon monoxide poisoning.[50,51] The first RCT found no significant difference with hyperbaric oxygen 100% at 2 ATA**G** for 2 hours plus 4 hours of normobaric oxygen**G** compared with oxygen 100% via non-re-breather mask for 6 hours in the proportion of people with mild to moderate acute carbon monoxide poisoning who did not develop neurological symptoms at 4 weeks (1 RCT, 307 people fitting the definition of mild to moderate acute carbon monoxide poisoning; absence of neurological symptoms at 4 weeks: 108/159 [67.9%] with hyperbaric oxygen 100% *v* 98/148 [66.2%] with oxygen 100% via non-re-breather mask; OR and CI not reported; $P = 0.75$).[50] However, this RCT has important limitations that influence the conclusions that can be drawn from the results because any neurophysiological changes would be subtle and slight in people with mild to moderate carbon monoxide poisoning. In this RCT, acute carbon monoxide poisoning was defined as carboxyhaemoglobin levels of 5% or more in non-smokers or 10% or more in smokers and no impairment of consciousness and recovery was defined as the absence of neurological signs and symptoms of carbon monoxide poisoning. However the study was not blind and no validated neurophysiological tests were used. Self administered patient questionnaires were used without any apparent standardisation of the testing for neurological symptoms such as "impaired vision" and "difficulty in concentrating" thus allowing an unknown degree of subjectivity and inter observer variation. The follow up was 89.7% at 4 weeks (343 people entered with 36 lost to follow up). This RCT also included a group of more severely poisoned people in whom one session of hyperbaric oxygen was compared with two, but this aspect is not included in this review. The second RCT[51] found that, compared with oxygen 100% by non-re-breather mask given until all symptoms resolved, hyperbaric oxygen 100% at 2.8 ATA for 30 minutes followed by 2.0 ATA for 90 minutes significantly reduced the proportion of people developing neurological symptoms at 4 weeks (1 RCT, 60 people with mild to moderate carbon monoxide poisoning; neurological symptoms at 4 weeks: 0/30 [0%] with hyperbaric oxygen 100% *v* 7/30 [23%] with normobaric oxygen 100%; difference between groups 23.0%, 95% CI 8.2% to 38.4%; $P < 0.05$). Treatment was given within 6 hours of the people being removed from the source of carbon monoxide. However, this RCT has important limitations that influence the conclusions that can be drawn from the results because any neurophysiological changes would be subtle and slight in people with mild to moderate carbon monoxide poisoning. In this RCT, acute carbon monoxide poisoning was defined as a history of acute exposure to combustion products, an increased carboxyhaemoglobin level not explained by a smoking history, and the presence of symptoms consistent with carbon monoxide poisoning. People were excluded if there was a history of loss of consciousness or cardiac compromise or they declined to participate. However the study was not blind and the definition of delayed neurological symptoms was vague. Delayed neurological sequelae was defined as a recurrence of original symptoms or development of new symptoms considered to be typical of the delayed neurological syndrome, plus deterioration in one or more of six neuropsychological tests, at 4 weeks. A control group of eight people had neuropsychological testing to see if repeated screening improved scores. The value of including and comparing with a control group of eight people is questionable. We found no systematic review or RCTs for other clinical outcomes of interest. **Hyperbaric oxygen 100% versus normobaric oxygen 100% in moderate to severe poisoning:** We found two RCTs.[52–54] One RCT found that, compared with one 150 minute session of 100% normobaric oxygen followed by two 120 minute sessions of normobaric air, one 150 minute session of 100% oxygen at 3 ATA followed by two 120 minute sessions of 100% oxygen at 2 ATA significantly reduced cognitive sequelae at 6 weeks (cognitive sequelae at 6 weeks: 19/76 [25%] with hyperbaric oxygen *v* 35/76 [46%] with normobaric oxygen; unadjusted odds ratio 0.39, 95% CI 0.20 to 0.78; P = 0.007).[52,53] The trial was stopped after the third of four interim analyses because hyperbaric oxygen was judged to be efficacious (P < 0.01). The results of the analysis of the incidence of cognitive sequelae at 6 and 12 months was presented but neither the raw figures nor the follow up rates were reported and so these have not been included here. A potential weakness of this RCT is that although all participants received normobaric oxygen 100% for a mean duration of 4.5 hours (± 2.2 hours in the normobaric group *v* ± 2.6 hours in the hyperbaric group) before entering the study and the levels of carboxyhaemoglobin were below 5% and not significantly different, only one session of normobaric oxygen 100% was given to people in the normobaric oxygen arm. Supplemental oxygen was given, if necessary, after treatment to maintain the arterial oxygen saturation at a level higher that 90% but it was not reported how frequently this occurred. This information would have indicated the effectiveness of one session of normobaric oxygen. In this RCT acute carbon monoxide poisoning was defined as a documented exposure to carbon monoxide (carboxyhaemoglobin greater than 10% or elevated ambient carbon monoxide) or an obvious exposure to carbon monoxide and symptoms consistent with carbon monoxide poisoning. People were excluded if 24 hours had elapsed since the exposure to carbon monoxide had ended; they were moribund, pregnant, under 16 years of age; or informed consent could not be obtained. The primary outcome was the incidence of neurological sequelae, as measured by six neuropsychological tests at 6 weeks. Neurological sequelae were considered present if any T score was more than two standard deviations below the mean; if two or more tests were one standard deviation below the mean; if the people difficulties with memory, attention, or concentration and one T score was more than one standard deviation below the mean. The second RCT was in people with all levels of carbon monoxide poisoning but included a high proportion (73%) of people with severe carbon monoxide poisoning.[54] The RCT found no significant difference between 3 day continuous normobaric oxygen 100% and 3 day continuous normobaric oxygen 100% interspersed with sessions of hyperbaric oxygen in the incidence of persistent neurological sequelae in people with all levels of carbon monoxide poisoning (1 RCT, 191 people including 139 people with severe CO poisoning; persistent neurological sequelae after treatment hyperbaric oxygen *v* normobaric oxygen: OR 1.7, 95% CI 0.8 to 4.0; P = 0.19). It found an increase in persistent neurological sequelae on completion of treatment in people with severe carbon monoxide poisoning who had received hyperbaric oxygen (139 people; persistent neurological sequelae after treatment hyperbaric oxygen *v* normobaric oxygen: OR 3.6, 95% CI 1.1 to 11.9; P = 0.03). However the use of oxygen 100% for 3 days or more is not a widely used treatment for carbon monoxide poisoning as high doses of oxygen can cause adverse effects.[54] Overall the Mini-mental scores **G** were high and showed little change at the end of treatment, this is surprising given that 102 of the participants were in coma and 36 were being ventilated at initial assessment. There is a possibility that bias may have been introduced. The RCT used cluster randomisation for participants presenting simultaneously with the risk of introducing bias by assigning people with similar baseline characteristics to one type of treatment. The design of this trial was double blind for participants and assessors by using sham hyperbaric sessions, but not to the hyperbaric technicians and nursing staff.

Harms: Two systematic reviews did not include the harms associated with hyperbaric oxygen**G** treatment in their assessments of costs and benefits.[46,47] The third systematic review included a list of the possible harms associated with hyperbaric treatment (similar to those listed below) but did not include these in an overall assessment of the costs and benefits.[45] **Hyperbaric oxygen 100% versus normobaric oxygen 100% in mild poisoning:** One RCT reported that in the group considered in this review, 6/170 (3.5%) people receiving one session of hyperbaric treatment reported anxiety and 1/170 (0.6%) experienced barotrauma.[50] One RCT did not report any harms associated with hyperbaric oxygen treatment.[51] **Hyperbaric oxygen 100% versus normobaric oxygen 100% in moderate to severe poisoning:** One RCT reported that at least one session of hyperbaric treatment was stopped prematurely in 7/76 (9.2%) people because of anxiety, 1/76 (1.3%) because of tympanic membrane rupture, 1/76 (1.3%) because of cough, and 4/76 (5.3%) because of difficulty in equalising middle ear pressure.[52,53] It should be noted that there was no consistency in the pressures and durations of hyperbaric treatment used in the RCTs listed above. One RCT reported that treatment was stopped early in 7/104 (6.7%) people because of ear barotraumas, 1/104 (1.0%) because of oxygen toxicity (convulsions), and 1/104 (1.0%) because of severe claustrophobia in people given hyperbaric treatment.[54] In addition, 1/87 (1.1%) people given sham hyperbaric treatment developed severe claustrophobia. The most common fatal complication of hyperbaric oxygen treatment is fire; from 1927 to 1996 there were 35 hyperbaric fires with 77 fatalities.[55] Since then there has been a fire in a chamber in Milan in 1997 that killed 10 patients and one nurse. Other problems include claustrophobia, barotraumas (including rupture of the tympanic membrane), sinus damage, pneumothorax, and gas emboli. The risk of pneumothorax is high in those people that have received external cardiac massage. Oxygen 100% when used at greater than atmospheric pressure can have toxic effects and produce a variety of symptoms that increase in severity with the duration of treatment. It is generally accepted that hyperbaric oxygen 100% delivered at 3 atmospheres for less than 120 minutes is safe. Respiratory effects are similar to those seen in oxygen toxicity at 1 ATA**G**. The primary difference is that the duration of exposure before symptoms appear is shorter. They include tightness in the chest; discomfort; coughing; congestion; oedema; atelectasis (partial or complete collapse of the lung); increased depth of respiration, rapid panting, asthma-like attacks, or apnoea on inspiration. Cardiovascular effects include bradycardia, hyperthermia or hypothermia, and peripheral vasoconstriction. Central nervous system toxicity is seen primarily in hyperbaric oxygen treatment where pressures of 3 ATA or more are used for periods in excess of 2 hours. Signs and symptoms include mood changes, dizziness, slowing of mental processes, paraesthesia, fasciculation of the lips and face, muscular twitching, visual and auditory hallucinations progressing to vertigo, nausea, and convulsions. The incidence of hyperoxic convulsions is estimated to be about 1.3/10 000.[56] At increased atmospheric pressures, vision may be affected with reversible myopia and mydriasis.

Comment: From a purely physiological perspective, it has been demonstrated and is universally accepted, that hyperbaric oxygen 100% reduces the half-life of carboxyhaemoglobin significantly.[57] The question is whether there is any worthwhile clinical effect in terms of prognosis or outcome. The size of the effect derived from hyperbaric oxygen**G** treatment may be highly sensitive to the pressure at which the oxygen is delivered, the number of treatment sessions, and the oxygen content of control treatments. Although there seems to be evidence of benefit from 100% hyperbaric oxygen in moderate to severe carbon monoxide poisoning, further research is needed to address these important clinical questions. These include the optimal duration of treatment, the optimum pressure within the chamber, the duration after presentation when treatment may be effective, the types of people who will benefit from treatment, and whether hyperbaric treatment is indicated in mild carbon monoxide poisoning. Most people will need to be transported to a hyperbaric centre and the numbers available are limited. In making a decision about whether hyperbaric treatment is need the effects of a long ambulance trip and associated risks need to be considered. The possibility of using an inflatable portable hyperbaric chamber (a modified Gamow bag used to treat altitude sickness) to treat carbon monoxide poisoning has been explored in a small (10 people) study.[58] The results suggested that the 1.58 ATA**G** pressures used to treat experimentally induced elevated carboxyhaemoglobin levels in the study may increase the rate at which carbon monoxide dissociates from carboxyhaemoglobin and field studies of a device capable of delivering higher pressures are currently being tested. If successful, this device may prove to be a possible treatment option for those centres situated some distance from a hyperbaric chamber.

GLOSSARY

ATA An abbreviation of atmospheres absolute used to describe atmospheric pressure; one ATA is about roughly equivalent to sea level atmospheric pressure.

Hyperbaric oxygen Oxygen supplied at a barometric pressure greater than that a sea level; usually 2–3 atmospheres. This is delivered in single or multiple occupancy hyperbaric chambers.

Mini-mental score A score derived from the Folstein Mini Mental State Examination. This examination is used to evaluate dementia and consists of a series of questions and tasks to assess a patient's orientation, attention, calculation, language, visuospatial, executive, and short-term memory abilities. The cut off for dementia is a score of less than 24 out of a possible 30.

Non-re-breather mask Usually, a tight fitting mask fitted with an oxygen reservoir bag and a one way valve that remains open during inspiration; the mask will allow oxygen concentrations of 80–100% to be delivered in a situation where high levels of inspired oxygen are required.

Normobaric oxygen Oxygen supplied at a barometric pressure equivalent to sea level pressure.

REFERENCES

1. Stewart RD. The effect of carbon monoxide on humans. *J Occup Med* 1976;18:304–309.
2. Piantadosi CA. Carbon monoxide poisoning. *Undersea Hyperb Med* 2004;31:167–177.
3. Kirkpatrick JN. Occult carbon monoxide poisoning. *West J Med* 1987;146:52–56.
4. Burney RE, Wu SC, Nemiroff MJ. Mass carbon monoxide poisoning: clinical effects and results of the treatment of 184 victims. *Ann Emerg Med* 1982;11:394–399.
5. Hampson NB, Kramer CC, Dunford RG, et al. Carbon monoxide poisoning from indoor burning of charcoal briquettes. *JAMA* 1994;271:52–53.

6. Miller RL, Toal BF, Foscue K, et al. Unintentional carbon monoxide poisonings in residential settings — Conneticut, November 1993–March 1994. *MMWR Morb Mortal Wkly Rep* 1995;44:765–767.
7. Hardy KR, Thom SR. Pathophysiology and treatment of carbon monoxide poisoning. *J Toxicol Clin Toxicol* 1994;32:613–629.
8. Stewart RD, Baretta ED, Platte LR, et al. Carboxyhemoglobin levels in American blood donors. *JAMA* 1974;229:1187–1195.
9. *Indoor air quality in the home (2): carbon monoxide* (Assessment A5). Institute for Environment and Health, Leicester, 1998.
10. Coburn RF, Forster RE, Kane PB. Considerations of the physiological variables that determine the blood carboxyhemoglobin concentration in man. *J Clin Invest* 1965;44:1899 –1910.
11. Reisdorff EJ, Wiegenstein JG. Carbon monoxide poisoning. In: Tintinalli JE, Krome RL, Ruiz E. *Emergency medicine: a comprehensive study guide*. 3rd edition. New York: McGraw Hill; 1992:704.
12. Chale S. Carbon monoxide poisoning. In: Viccellio P, ed. *Handbook of medical toxicology*. 1st edition. New York: Little, Brown and Company. 1993;639–647.
13. Ilano AL, Raffin TA. Management of carbon monoxide poisoning. *Chest* 1990;97:165–169.
14. Raub JA, Mathieu-Nolf M, Hampson NB, et al. Carbon monoxide poisoning – a public health perspective. *Toxicology* 2000;145:1–14.
15. Office of National Statistics. http://www.statistics.gov.uk/STATBASE/xsdataset.asp?More=Y
16. *Mortality statistics 1985 – cause*. Series DH2, ICD code 986. Office of Population, Censuses and Surveys. London HMSO, 1987.
17. Cobb N, Etzel RA. Unintentional carbon monoxide-related deaths in the United States, 1979 through 1988. *JAMA* 1991;266:659–663.
18. Hampson NB. Emergency department visits for carbon monoxide poisoning in the Pacific Northwest. *J Emerg Med* 1998;16:695–698.
19. Hospital Episode Statistics 2002/03. Department of Health.
20. Anon. Deaths from motor-vehicle-related unintentional carbon monoxide poisoning – Colorado, 1996, New Mexico, 1980–1995, and United States, 1979–1992. *MMWR Morb Mortal Wkly Rep* 1996;45:1029–1032.
21. Anon. Carbon monoxide poisoning at a indoor ice arena and bingo hall – Seattle, 1996. *MMWR Morb Mortal Wkly Rep* 1996;45:265–267.
22. Anderson EW, Andelman RJ, Strauch JM, et al. Effect of low-level carbon monoxide exposure on onset and duration of angina pectoris. A study of ten patients with ischemic heart disease. *Ann Intern Med* 1973;79:46–50.
23. Kleinman MT, Davidson DM, Vandagriff RB, et al. Effects of short-term exposure to carbon monoxide in subjects with coronary artery disease. *Arch Environ Health* 1989;44:361–369.
24. Allred EN, Bleecker ER, Chaitman BR, et al. Short-term effects of carbon monoxide exposure on the exercise performance of subjects with coronary artery disease. *N Engl J Med* 1989;321:1426–1432. [Erratum in: *N Engl J Med* 1990;322:1019]
25. Coburn RF, Williams WL, Kahn SB. Endogenous carbon monoxide production in patients with haemolytic anaemia. *J Clin Invest* 1966;45:460–8.
26. Longo LD. The biological effects of carbon monoxide on the pregnant woman, fetus and newborn infant. *Am J Obstet Gynaecol* 1977;129:69–103.
27. Marx CM, Pope JF, Blumer JL. Developmental toxicology. In: Haddad LM, Winchester JY, eds. *Clinical management of poisoning and drug overdose*. Philadelphia, WB Saunders, 1990.
28. Farrow J, Davis GJ, Roy TM, et al. Fetal death due to nonlethal maternal carbon monoxide poisoning. *J Forensic Sci* 1990;35:1448–1452.
29. Cramer CR. Fetal death due to accidental maternal carbon monoxide poisoning. *J Toxicol Clin Toxicol* 1982;19:297–301.
30. Norman CA, Halton DM. Is carbon monoxide a workplace teratogen? A review and evaluation of the literature. *Ann Occup Hyg* 1990;34:335–347.
31. Sanchez R, Fosarelli P, Felt B, et al. Carbon monoxide poisoning due to automobile exposure: disparity between carboxy hemoglobin levels and symptoms of victims. *Pediatrics* 1988;82:663–665.
32. WHO. *Air quality guidelines for Europe*. Copenhagen, Denmark; WHO Regional Office for Europe, 1994.
33. Department of the Environment Expert Panel on Air Quality Standards. Carbon monoxide. London. HMSO, 1994.
34. Hampson NB, Zmaeff JL. Outcome of patients experiencing cardiac arrest with carbon monoxide poisoning treated with hyperbaric oxygen. *Ann Emerg Med* 2001;38:36–41.
35. Roos RAC. Neurological complications of carbon monoxide intoxication. In: Vinken PJ, Bruyn GW, eds. *Intoxications of the nervous system*. Amsterdam, Elsevier Science, 1994;31–38.
36. Gorman DF, Clayton D, Gilligan JE, et al. A longitudinal study of 100 consecutive admissions for carbon monoxide poisoning to the Royal Adelaide Hospital. *Anaesth Intensive Care* 1992;20:311–316.
37. Norris CR, Trench JM, Hook R. Delayed carbon monoxide encephalopathy: clinical and research implications. *J Clin Psychiatry* 1982;43:294–295.
38. Choi IS. Parkinsonism after carbon monoxide poisoning. *Eur Neurol* 2002;48:30–33.
39. Choi IS. Delayed neurologic sequelae in carbon monoxide intoxication. *Arch Neurol* 1983;40:433–435.
40. Weaver LK, Howe S, Hopkins R, et al. Carboxyhemoglobin half-life in carbon monoxide-poisoned patients treated with 100% oxygen at atmospheric pressure. *Chest* 2000;117:801–808.
41. Petersen JE, Stewart RD. Absorption and elimination of carbon monoxide by inactive young men. *Arch Environ Health* 1970;21:165–171.
42. Balentine JD. *Pathology of oxygen toxicity*. New York: Academic Press, 1982.
43. Edwards C, Lowry C, Pennefarther J. Oxygen toxicity. In: Edwards C, Lowry C, Pennefarther J, eds. *Diving and subaquatic medicine*. Oxford: Butterworth Heineman, 1992:241–256.
44. Schienkestel CD, Jones K, Myles PS, et al. Where to now with carbon monoxide poisoning? *Emerg Med Australas* 2004;16:151–154.
45. Saunders P. Hyperbaric oxygen therapy in the management of carbon monoxide poisoning, osteoradionecrosis, burns, skin grafts and crush injury. Birmingham: University of Birmingham, Department of Public Health and Epidemiology, 2000:1–52.
46. Juurlink DN, Stanbrook MB, McGuigan MA. Hyperbaric oxygen for carbon monoxide poisoning (Cochrane Review). In: The Cochrane Library, Issue 3, 2004, Chichester, UK: John Wiley & Sons, Ltd. Search date: 2001; primary sources Medline, Embase, the Controlled Trials Register of the Cochrane Collaboration, supplemented by a manual review of bibliographies of identified articles and discussion with recognized content experts.
47. Dent THS. Hyperbaric oxygen therapy for carbon monoxide poisoning. In: Bazian Ltd (Ed) STEER: Succinct and Timely Evaluated Evidence Reviews 2002; 2 (13). Wessex Institute for health research & Development, University of Southampton. http://www.signpoststeer.org
48. Mathieu D, Wattel F, Mathieu Nolf M, et al. Interim analysis – controlled clinical trial of hyperbaric oxygen in acute carbon monoxide (CO) poisoning. *Undersea Hyperb Med* 1996;23(suppl):7–8.
49. Ducasse JL, Celsis P, Marc-Vergnes JP. Non-comatose patients with acute carbon monoxide poisoning: hyperbaric or normobaric oxygenation? *Undersea Hyperb Med* 1995;22:9–15.

50. Raphael JC, Elkharrat D, Jars-Guincestre MC, et al. Trial of normobaric and hyperbaric oxygen for acute carbon monoxide intoxication. *Lancet* 1989;2:414–419.
51. Thom SR, Taber RL, Mendiguren II, et al. Delayed neuropsychologic sequelae after carbon monoxide poisoning: prevention by treatment with hyperbaric oxygen. *Ann Emerg Med* 1995;25:474–480.
52. Weaver LK, Hopkins RO, Chan KJ, et al. Hyperbaric oxygen for acute carbon monoxide poisoning. *New Engl J Med* 2002;347:1057–1067.
53. Weaver LK, Hopkins RO, Larson Lohr V, et al. Double blind, controlled, prospective, randomized clinical trial (RCT) in patients with acute carbon monoxide (CO) poisoning: outcome of patients treated with normobaric oxygen or hyperbaric oxygen (HBO_2) – an interim report. *Undersea Hyperb Med* 1995;22(suppl):1.
54. Scheinskestel CD, Bailey M, Myles PS, et al. Hyperbaric or normobaric oxygen for acute carbon monoxide poisoning: a randomised controlled clinical trial. *Med J Aust* 1999;170:203–210.
55. Sheffield P, Desautels DA. Hyperbaric and hypobaric chamber fires: a 73-year analysis. *Undersea Hyperb Med* 1997;24:153–164.
56. Beer MH, Berkow R, eds. Adverse effects of hyperbaric oxygen. In: *Merck manual of diagnosis and therapy*. Section 21, Chapter 299.
57. Pace N, Strajman E, Walker EL. Acceleration of carbon monoxide elimination in man by high pressure oxygen. *Science* 1950;III:652–654.
58. Jay GD, Tetz DJ, Hartigan CF, et al. Portable hyperbaric oxygen therapy in the emergency department with the modified Gamow bag. *Ann Emerg Med* 1995;26:707–711.

Nicholas Phin
Health Protection Agency
Microbiology laboratory
Cheshire and Merseyside Health
Protection Unit
Chester
UK

Competing interests: None declared.

Organophosphorus poisoning (acute)

Search date September 2004

Michael Eddleston, Surjit Singh, and Nick Buckley

QUESTIONS

INTERVENTIONS

*Based on consensus, RCTs would be considered unethical

See glossary G

Key Messages

Treatments

- **Atropine*** Atropine is considered the mainstay of treatment, and many case series have found that it reverses the early muscarinic effects of acute organophosphorus poisoning. We found no RCTs comparing atropine versus placebo but it would now be considered unethical to perform such an RCT. One small RCT found no significant difference in mortality or ventilation rates between atropine and glycopyrronium bromide, but it may have lacked power to detect clinically important differences.
- **Benzodiazepines to control organophosphorus induced seizures*** Diazepam is considered standard treatment for organophosphorus induced seizures. We found no RCTs comparing diazepam or other benzodiazepines versus placebo or another anticonvulsant. It would now be considered unethical to perform an RCT comparing benzodiazepines versus placebo in people with seizures.
- **Glycopyrronium bromide (glycopyrrolate)*** We found no RCTs comparing glycopyrronium bromide (glycopyrrolate) versus placebo, but it is unlikely that such a trial would be considered ethical unless glycopyrronium bromide and placebo were administered in addition to atropine. One small RCT found no significant difference in mortality or ventilation rates between glycopyrronium bromide and atropine, but it may have lacked power to detect clinically important differences. Glycopyrronium bromide has been used instead of atropine because it is thought to have fewer adverse effects on the central nervous system.
- **Washing the poisoned person and removing contaminated clothes*** We found no RCTs or observational studies of sufficient quality that evaluated washing the poisoned person and removing contaminated clothes. However, this appears to be an obvious way to reduce further dermal and mucocutaneous exposure and is widely

recommended. An RCT would therefore be considered unethical. Healthcare workers should ensure that washing does not distract them from other treatment priorities and they should also protect themselves through the use of gloves, aprons, and eye protection, with careful disposal of contaminated equipment and clothes.

- **Activated charcoal (single or multiple dose)** We found no systematic review, RCTs, or observational studies of sufficient quality evaluating activated charcoal, in either single or multiple dose regimens, in people with acute organophosphorus poisoning.
- **Gastric lavage** We found no RCTs or observational studies of sufficient quality evaluating gastric lavage in people with acute organophosphorus poisoning. Adverse effects are common when gastric lavage is performed in physically restrained, non-consenting patients without careful control of the airway. If the patient cannot be sedated and intubated, the risk of harm due to aspiration is likely to outweigh its potential benefits.
- **Milk or other home remedy immediately after ingestion** We found no RCTs or observational studies of sufficient quality that assessed giving a "home remedy" soon after the ingestion.
- **N-methyl-D-aspartate receptor antagonists** We found no RCTs or observational studies of sufficient quality evaluating n-methyl-D-aspartate receptor antagonists in people with acute organophosphorus poisoning.
- **Organophosphorus hydrolases** We found no RCTs or observational studies of sufficient quality evaluating organophosphorus hydrolases in people with acute organophosphorus poisoning.
- **Oximes** One systematic review provided insufficient evidence to assess oximes in people with acute organophosphorus poisoning.
- **Sodium bicarbonate** We found no RCTs or observational studies of sufficient quality evaluating sodium bicarbonate in acute organophosphorus poisoning.
- **α_2 Adrenergic receptor agonists (clonidine)** We found no RCTs or observational studies of sufficient quality evaluating clonidine in people with acute organophosphorus poisoning.
- **Cathartics** We found no RCTs or observational studies of sufficient quality evaluating cathartics in people with acute organophosphorus poisoning. Organophosphorus poisoning itself causes diarrhoea, which may lead to electrolyte imbalance. This may be exacerbated by cathartics, suggesting that the risk of harm may outweigh its potential benefits.
- **Ipecacuanha (ipecac)** We found no RCTs or observational studies of sufficient quality evaluating ipecacuanha (ipecac) in people with acute organophosphorus poisoning. Clinical consensus suggests that the risk of harm, although not quantified, probably outweighs any potential benefits.

DEFINITION Acute organophosphorus poisoning occurs after dermal, respiratory, or oral exposure to either low volatility pesticides (e.g. chlorpyrifos, dimethoate) or high volatility nerve gases (e.g. sarin, tabun). Inhibition of acetylcholinesterase**G** at synapses results in accumulation of acetylcholine and over-activation of acetylcholine receptors at the neuromuscular junction and in the autonomic and central nervous systems.[1] Early clinical features reflect involvement of the parasympathetic system: bronchorrhoea, miosis, salivation, lachrymation, defecation, urination, and hypotension. Features indicating involvement of the neuromuscular junction (muscle weakness and fasciculations) and central nervous system (seizures [with nerve gases], coma, respiratory failure) are also common at this stage. An intermediate syndrome has been described (cranial nerve palsies and proximal muscle weakness with preserved distal muscle power after resolution of early cholinergic symptoms), but its definition, pathophysiology, and incidence are still unclear. A late motor or motor/sensory peripheral neuropathy may also develop after recovery from acute poisoning with some organophosphorus compounds.[1]

INCIDENCE/ PREVALENCE Most cases occur in the developing world following occupational or deliberate exposure to organophosphorus pesticides.[2] Although data are sparse, organophosphates appear to be the most important cause of death from deliberate self poisoning worldwide.[3] For example, in Sri Lanka, about 10 000 to 20 000 admissions to hospital for organophosphorus poisoning occur each year. Of these, about 10% die. In most cases, the poisoning is intentional.[4] Case fatality rates across the developing world are commonly greater than 20%.[3] In Central America, occupational poisoning is more common than intentional poisoning, and deaths are fewer.[5] Extrapolating from limited data, the World Health Organization has estimated that each year more than 200 000 people worldwide die from pesticide poisoning,[6] but these figures are old and widely contested.[2] Most deaths occur in Asia, and organophosphorus pesticides probably cause at least 50% of cases.[3] Deaths from organophosphorus nerve gases occurred during the Iran–Iraq war.[7] Military or terrorist action with these chemical weapons remains possible. Twelve people died in a terrorist attack in Tokyo and probably thousands died in Iran after military use.

AETIOLOGY/ RISK FACTORS The widespread accessibility of pesticides in rural parts of the developing world makes them easy options for acts of self harm.[3] Occupational exposure is usually due to insufficient or inappropriate protective equipment.[2]

PROGNOSIS There are no validated scoring systems for categorising severity or predicting outcome, although many have been proposed. The highly variable natural history and difficulty in determining ingested dose make predicting outcome for an individual inaccurate and potentially hazardous, because people admitted in good condition can deteriorate rapidly and require intubation and mechanical ventilation. Prognosis in acute self poisoning is likely to depend on dose and toxicity of the ingested organophosphorus (e.g. neurotoxicity potential, half life, rate of ageing whether activation to the toxic compound is required [pro-poison], and whether dimethylated or diethylated [see comment under oximes, p 1751]).[8] Prognosis in occupational exposure is better because the dose is normally smaller and the route is dermal.

AIMS OF INTERVENTION To prevent mortality; to reduce rates of intubation (with or without ventilation), pneumonia, the intermediate syndrome (see definition above), and delayed polyneuropathy; and to reduce the duration of ventilation and intensive care.

OUTCOMES Mortality; rates of intubation, pneumonia, the intermediate syndrome, delayed polyneuropathy; and duration of ventilation or intensive care.

METHODS *Clinical Evidence* search and appraisal September 2004. The contributors also searched Medline, Embase, and Cochrane databases; hand searched toxicological and Indian journals (search date June 2004); and contacted experts in the field to identify unpublished studies.

QUESTION **What are the effects of treatments for acute organophosphorus poisoning?**

OPTION **MILK OR OTHER HOME REMEDY SOON AFTER ORAL ORGANOPHOSPHORUS EXPOSURE**

We found no RCTs or observational studies of sufficient quality that assessed giving a "home remedy" soon after the ingestion.

Benefits: We found no systematic review, RCTs, or observational studies of sufficient quality.

Harms: We found no systematic review, RCTs, or observational studies of sufficient quality assessing adverse effects.

Comment: The lay practice of giving a "home remedy" soon after ingestion, before bringing the poisoned person to hospital, is common in many parts of the world. Problems may occur when large volumes of fluid are given "to dilute the poison" or to make the person vomit. Gastric emptying of a fluid is proportional to volume. It is therefore believed that increasing the volume of fluid in the stomach increases the rate of emptying into the small bowel where the pesticide is absorbed. Giving fluids therefore risks speeding the onset of poisoning and causing respiratory arrest before the patient arrives at a healthcare facility. In contrast, a small volume, highly lipid home remedy (such as raw eggs) may slow gastric emptying and delay the onset of poisoning and respiratory failure until the patient has reached a healthcare facility.

OPTION WASHING THE POISONED PERSON AND REMOVING CONTAMINATED CLOTHES

We found no RCTs or observational studies of sufficient quality that evaluated washing the poisoned person and removing contaminated clothes. However, this appears to be an obvious way to reduce further dermal and mucocutaneous exposure and is widely recommended. An RCT would therefore be considered unethical. Healthcare workers should ensure that washing does not distract them from other treatment priorities and they should also protect themselves through the use of gloves, aprons, and eye protection, with careful disposal of contaminated equipment and clothes.

Benefits: We found no systematic review, RCTs, or observational studies of sufficient quality.

Harms: We found no systematic review, RCTs, or observational studies of sufficient quality. No important adverse effects are envisaged, unless washing the poisoned person distracts healthcare workers from other priorities, such as resuscitation and careful observation for deterioration.

Comment: Absorption of organophosphorus compounds through the skin varies, according to the volatility of the organophosphorus, its solvent, and the temperature and hydration of the skin.[9] Absorption of pesticides seems to be low, with studies of malathion, chlorpyrifos, and diazinon suggesting that less than 5% is absorbed and excreted in the urine.[10–12] However, washing appears to be an obvious way to reduce further dermal and mucocutaneous exposure and is widely recommended. An RCT would therefore be considered unethical. Healthcare workers should protect themselves through the use of gloves, aprons, and eye protection, with careful disposal of contaminated equipment and clothes.

OPTION IPECACUANHA (IPECAC)

We found no RCTs or observational studies of sufficient quality evaluating ipecacuanha (ipecac) in people with acute organophosphorus poisoning. Clinical consensus suggests that the risk of harm, although not quantified, probably outweighs any potential benefits.

Benefits: We found no systematic review, RCTs, or observational studies of sufficient quality.

Harms: We found no systematic review, RCTs, or observational studies of sufficient quality assessing the adverse effects of ipecacuanha in people with acute organophosphorus poisoning, and no large, high quality RCTs comparing ipecacuanha versus placebo in any form of poisoning that might have allowed calculation for rates of adverse effects. Adverse effects of ipecacuanha may include aspiration, diarrhoea, ileus, dysrhythmias during vomiting, dystonia from treatment of vomiting, and haematemesis from vomiting.[13] Use of ipecacuanha in acute organophosphorus poisoning may be particularly hazardous because most organophosphorus compounds are dissolved in aromatic hydrocarbons, which cause serious harm if aspirated (see comment).[13]

Comment: One non-systematic review identified no studies examining the effects of ipecacuanha specifically in people with organophosphorus poisoning.[13] In people with other forms of poisoning, it found no evidence of benefit.[13] Administration of ipecacuanha may delay administration of activated charcoal and specific treatment for organophosphorus poisoning, in addition to increasing the risk of aspiration.

OPTION CATHARTICS

We found no RCTs or observational studies of sufficient quality evaluating cathartics in people with acute organophosphorus poisoning. Organophosphorus poisoning itself causes diarrhoea, which may lead to electrolyte imbalance. This may be exacerbated by cathartics, suggesting that the risk of harm may outweigh its potential benefits.

Benefits: We found no systematic review, RCTs, or observational studies of sufficient quality.

Harms: We found no systematic review, RCTs, or observational studies of sufficient quality. Recognised complications include electrolyte imbalance and dehydration.

Comment: Cathartics have been used to treat organophosphorus poisoning because they speed the passage of poisons out of the gastrointestinal tract.[14] Reduced transit time reduces the absorption of poison. One non-systematic review identified no studies examining the effects of cathartics specifically in people with organophosphorus poisoning.[14] In people with other forms of poisoning, it found no evidence of benefit.[14] Organophosphorus poisoning itself causes diarrhoea. This can lead to electrolyte imbalance, which may be exacerbated by cathartics.

OPTION GASTRIC LAVAGE

We found no RCTs or observational studies of sufficient quality evaluating gastric lavage in people with acute organophosphorus poisoning. Adverse effects are common when gastric lavage is performed in physically restrained, non-consenting patients without careful control of the airway. If the patient cannot be sedated and intubated, the risk of harm due to aspiration is likely to outweigh its potential benefits.

Benefits: We found no systematic review, RCTs, or observational studies of sufficient quality.

Harms: We found no systematic review, RCTs, or observational studies of sufficient quality assessing the adverse effects of gastric lavage in people with acute organophosphorus poisoning, and no large, high quality RCTs comparing gastric lavage versus placebo in any form of poisoning that might allow calculation of rates of adverse effects. Adverse effects of gastric lavage may include aspiration, hypoxia, laryngeal spasm, and oesophageal perforation.[15] Adverse effects are common when gastric lavage is performed in physically restrained, non-consenting people without careful control of the airway.

Comment: One non-systematic review identified no studies examining the effects of gastric lavage specifically in people with organophosphorus poisoning.[15] In people with other forms of poisoning, it found no evidence of benefit.[15] Gastric lavage may delay administration of activated charcoal and specific treatment for organophosphorus poisoning. It is unclear how long organophosphorus pesticides remain in the stomach after ingestion. If studies indicate that a substantial proportion of organophosphorus remains in the stomach on admission to hospital, it may be appropriate to conduct an RCT to assess gastric lavage after protection of the airway.

OPTION ACTIVATED CHARCOAL (SINGLE OR MULTIPLE DOSE)

We found no systematic review, RCTs, or observational studies of sufficient quality evaluating activated charcoal, in either single or multiple dose regimens, in people with acute organophosphorus poisoning.

Benefits: We found no systematic review, RCTs, or observational studies of sufficient quality.

Harms: We found no systematic review, RCTs, or cohort studies evaluating adverse effects in people with acute organophosphorus poisoning receiving activated charcoal, and no large, high quality RCTs comparing activated charcoal versus placebo in any form that might allow calculation of rates of adverse effects. Adverse effects of activated charcoal may include aspiration, pneumonia, vomiting, diarrhoea, constipation, ileus, and reduced absorption of oral medication.[16–18] A large retrospective case series (878 people treated with multiple dose activated charcoal) suggests that rates of adverse events with multiple dose regimens (> 2 doses) are likely to be low (significant pulmonary aspiration in 6/878 [0.6%], 95% CI 0.1% to 1.1%).[19]

Comment: **Single dose regimens:** Animal studies indicate that activated charcoal can bind to organophosphorus pesticides.[20] However, one non-systematic review found no human studies examining the effects of single dose activated charcoal specifically in people with organophosphorus poisoning.[16] In people with other forms of poisoning, it found no evidence of benefit.[16] **Multiple dose regimens:** We found no studies of multiple dose activated charcoal in people with organophosphorus poisoning.[17] One non-systematic review found no human studies examining the effects of multiple dose activated charcoal specifically in people with organophosphorus poisoning.[17] In people with other forms of poisoning, it found no evidence of benefit.[17] Activated charcoal may reduce the efficacy of treatments given by mouth. A large RCT comparing single or multiple dose activated charcoal versus placebo in acute organophosphorus pesticide poisoning started in Sri Lanka in 2002; the findings should be reported in 2005.[21]

OPTION ATROPINE

Atropine is considered the mainstay of treatment, and many case series have found that it reverses the early muscarinic effects of acute organophosphorus poisoning. We found no RCTs comparing atropine versus placebo but it would now be considered unethical to perform such an RCT. One small RCT found no significant difference in mortality or ventilation rates between atropine and glycopyrronium bromide, but it may have lacked power to detect clinically important differences.

Benefits: **Versus placebo:** We found no systematic review, RCTs, or cohort studies (see comment below). Many case series have found that atropine reverses the early muscarinic effects of acute organophosphorus poisoning.[22] **Versus glycopyrronium bromide:** See benefits of glycopyrronium bromide, p 1750.

Harms: We found no systematic review, RCTs, or observational studies of sufficient quality assessing adverse effects in people with acute organophosphorus poisoning receiving atropine. Excessive treatment with atropine results in toxicity, characterised by confusion and tachycardia.[22] In hypoxic people, supplemental oxygen may reduce toxicity caused by tachycardia.

Comment: Atropine competes with excess acetylcholine at muscarinic acetylcholine receptors. We found no RCTs, but consensus holds that its effectiveness is now beyond question, so it would be unethical to perform an RCT comparing atropine versus placebo. **Dosage and administration:** The optimum dose of atropine has not been determined.[23] It varies among poisoned people because of variation in the dose taken and possibly because of coadministration of an oxime (oximes have been proposed to have anticholinergic action at high dose; see oximes, p 1751).[24] The first doses are given as boluses to reverse the muscarinic signs. Current recommendations are then to set up an atropine infusion.[24] Recent RCTs from India on the use of oximes have used an infusion of atropine sufficient to keep the pupils at mid-point, heart rate greater than 100 beats a minute, normal bowel sounds, clear lungs, and no bronchorrhoea.[25–28] The atropine dose regimen has not been compared with other regimens with different end points of atropinisation**G**.

OPTION GLYCOPYRRONIUM BROMIDE (GLYCOPYRROLATE)

We found no RCTs comparing glycopyrronium bromide (glycopyrrolate) versus placebo, but it is unlikely that such a trial would be considered ethical unless glycopyrronium bromide and placebo were administered in addition to atropine. One small RCT found no significant difference in mortality or ventilation rates between glycopyrronium bromide and atropine, but it may have lacked power to detect clinically important differences. Glycopyrronium bromide has been used instead of atropine because it is thought to have fewer adverse effects on the central nervous system.

Benefits: **Versus placebo:** We found no systematic review or RCTs comparing glycopyrronium bromide versus placebo (see comment below) **Versus atropine:** We found one small RCT (39 people) comparing glycopyrronium bromide versus atropine.[29] It found no significant difference between atropine and glycopyrronium bromide in death rates, need for ventilation, or respiratory infection (death rates: AR 1/22 [5%] with atropine *v* 2/17 [12%] with glycopyrronium; RR 0.39, 95% CI 0.04 to 3.91; need for ventilation: AR 8/22 [36%] with atropine *v* 6/17 [35%] with glycopyrronium; RR 1.03, 95% CI 0.44 to 2.41; respiratory infection: AR 12/22 [55%] with atropine *v* 5/17 [29%] with glycopyrronium; RR 1.86, 95% CI 0.81 to 4.25). The study may have lacked power to detect clinically important differences in mortality, ventilation, or intermediate syndrome.

Harms: We found no systematic review, RCTs, or observational studies of sufficient quality assessing adverse effects in people with acute organophosphorus poisoning receiving glycopyrronium bromide. Treatment with glycopyrronium bromide may result in peripheral anticholinergic effects such as tachycardia, dry mouth, and ileus.[30] When these symptoms arise, treatment is defined as excessive.

Comment: It is unlikely that an RCT comparing glycopyrronium bromide versus placebo would be considered ethical unless glycopyrronium bromide and placebo were administered in addition to atropine. Glycopyrronium bromide has similar effects to atropine in humans, but is more selective for peripheral cholinergic synapses, resulting in less tachycardia and confusion than occur with atropine.[30] Animal studies have found that glycopyrronium bromide is less effective than atropine at controlling bradycardia and central nervous system complications of organophosphorus poisoning. It is not widely used and is more expensive. We found no large RCT comparing atropine versus glycopyrronium bromide. In some regions, glycopyrronium bromide is combined with atropine to limit the central stimulation produced by atropine.

OPTION OXIMES

One systematic review provided insufficient evidence to assess oximes in people with acute organophosphorus poisoning.

Benefits: We found one systematic review[31] (search date 2002) of oximes in organophosphorus poisoned people, which identified two RCTS (182 people) of pralidoxime (reported in four publications).[25–28] Neither of the RCTs found any benefit of pralidoxime. The first RCT found that an infusion of 12 g pralidoxime (no loading dose, administered over 4 days) increased mortality, intermediate syndrome, and the need for ventilation compared with a bolus of 1 g pralidoxime. However, confidence intervals were wide, and the difference was not significant (mortality: AR 8/36 [22%] with 12 g pralidoxime v 5/36 [14%] with 1 g pralidoxime; OR 1.77, 95% CI 0.52 to 6.0; intermediate syndrome 20/36 [56%] with 12 g pralidoxime v 13/36 [36%] with 1 g pralidoxime; OR not reported; requirement for ventilation 24/36 [67%] with 12 g pralidoxime v 17/36 [47%] with 1 g pralidoxime; OR 2.04, 95% CI 0.78 to 5.3).[25,26] The second RCT (110 people) found that an infusion of 12 g pralidoxime over 3 days increased mortality, intermediate syndrome, and requirement for ventilation compared with placebo (mortality: AR 16/55 [29%] with pralidoxime v 3/55 [5%] with placebo; RR 5.3, 95% CI 1.7 to 17.3; intermediate syndrome: 36/55 [65%] with pralidoxime v 19/55 [35%] with placebo; RR 1.9, 95% CI 1.3 to 2.9; requirement for ventilation: 36/55 [67%] with pralidoxime v 22/55 [40%] with placebo; RR 1.7, 95% CI 1.1 to 2.4).[27,28]

Harms: Neither RCT reported the incidence of adverse effects in people with acute organophosphorus poisoning receiving oximes.[25–28] Adverse effects of oximes include hypertension, cardiac dysrhythmias (including cardiac arrest with rapid administration), headache, blurred vision, dizziness, and epigastric discomfort.[32] Such adverse effects with pralidoxime have been reported only with either rapid administration or doses greater than 30 mg/kg bolus. It may be difficult to distinguish these adverse effects from the effects of organophosphorus. In one observational clinical study of a different oxime (obidoxime), a high dose regimen (8 mg/kg bolus, then 2 mg/kg/hour infusion) produced hepatitis in 3/12 people.[7] Two of six deaths were due to liver failure. The use of pralidoxime in eight people in the same study (dose 30 mg/kg bolus, then 8 mg/kg/hour infusion) did not produce hepatitis. A more recently developed oxime (HI-6) has also been used in humans, with no reported adverse effects.[33] We found no human studies that assessed the harms of giving oximes for carbamate poisoning (which presents with a similar cholinergic crisis but has a better prognosis).[1]

Comment: Oximes (such as pralidoxime, obidoxime, and HI-6) reactivate acetylcholinesterases**G** inhibited by organophosphorus poisoning.[8,24] Reactivation is limited by ageing**G** of the acetylcholinesterases and high concentrations of pesticides. Ageing of acetylcholinesterases takes longer with diethyl organophosphorus compounds than with dimethyl organophosphorus compounds. Oximes may therefore be effective if given within about 120 hours for diethyl organophosphorus poisoning and 12 hours for dimethyl organophosphorus poisoning. Treatment may be beneficial if continued for as long as the person is symptomatic because it may take several days for the pesticide concentration to drop below the point at which the rate of reactivation surpasses reinhibition.[8] Both RCTs[26,28] used doses of pralidoxime that are different from the regimen currently recommended by the World Health Organization (at least 30 mg/kg bolus, then 8 mg/kg/hour iv infusion). The reporting of the methods was poor, and baseline differences in the second RCT suggested that more severely poisoned people might have been randomised to the intervention arm.[31] Post hoc analysis of the first RCT suggested that people receiving pralidoxime 1 g in the first 12 hours may be less likely to develop the intermediate syndrome than those receiving less than 1 g in the first 12 hours (29% v 51%; RR 0.58, 95% CI 0.27 to 1.26).[25] Studies in poisoned people indicate that oximes can reactivate acetylcholinesterase but have not been able to prove clinical benefit.[34] In vitro studies have also revealed mechanisms whereby oximes may be detrimental.[35] A large RCT was started in Sri Lanka in 2004, and the findings are expected to be reported in 2007.[36]

OPTION ORGANOPHOSPHORUS HYDROLASES

We found no RCTs or observational studies of sufficient quality evaluating organophosphorus hydrolases in people with acute organophosphorus poisoning.

Benefits: We found no systematic review, RCTs, or observational studies of sufficient quality.

Harms: We found no systematic review, RCTs, or observational studies of sufficient quality assessing adverse effects.

Comment: Oxime efficacy is normally limited by the presence of high pesticide concentrations, which reinhibit acetylcholinesterases**G** that have been reactivated by the oximes.[31] A method of rapidly reducing pesticide concentrations could potentially allow oximes to be more effective. Animal studies have found that organophosphorus hydrolases (such as mammalian paraoxanase or the bacterial hydrolase isolated from *Pseudomonas* species) cleave organophosphorus compounds, lowering blood and tissue concentrations of organophosphorus.[37,38] These may prove beneficial for managing people with either pesticide or nerve gas organophosphorus poisoning.

OPTION SODIUM BICARBONATE

We found no RCTs or observational studies of sufficient quality evaluating sodium bicarbonate in acute organophosphorus poisoning.

Benefits: We found no systematic review, RCTs, or observational studies of sufficient quality.

Harms: We found no systematic review, RCTs, or observational studies of sufficient quality assessing adverse effects in people with acute organophosphorus poisoning receiving sodium bicarbonate. Dose dependent adverse effects of sodium bicarbonate may include sodium and fluid overload and decreased oxygen delivery.[39]

Comment: Animal studies suggest that increasing the pH with sodium bicarbonate reduces mortality.[40,41] This effect is independent of correction of acidosis because it is seen in animals that are not acidotic. Studies conducted in Brazil[41] and Iran[42] have claimed good results in uncontrolled studies. The mechanism of action of sodium bicarbonate in organophosphorus poisoning is unknown. However, it is unclear whether the limited increase in pH that is possible in vivo is sufficient to make a significant difference in organophosphorus hydrolysis rates. A Cochrane review is now underway.[43]

OPTION BENZODIAZEPINES

Diazepam is considered standard treatment for organophosphorus induced seizures. We found no RCTs comparing diazepam or other benzodiazepines versus placebo or another anticonvulsant. It would now be considered unethical to perform an RCT comparing benzodiazepines versus placebo in people with seizures.

Benefits: We found no systematic review, RCTs, or cohort studies. Many case series have reported that diazepam controls seizures in acute organophosphorus poisoning.[44,45]

Harms: We found no systematic review, RCTs, or observational studies of sufficient quality assessing adverse effects rates in people with acute organophosphorus poisoning receiving diazepam. Excessive treatment with diazepam may result in respiratory depression requiring intubation and ventilation. However, this is also a direct complication of organophosphorus poisoning, and it is difficult to distinguish between the two.[44]

Comment: Benzodiazepines such as diazepam, lorazepam, and midazolam are widely used for treating organophosphorus induced seizures. However, the seizures are believed to be started by excess acetylcholine in the brain following inhibition of acetylcholinesterase**G**, with subsequent disruption of other neurotransmitter systems such as glutamate and catecholamine. Benzodiazepines work at γ-aminobutyric acid receptors. Other treatments may therefore be beneficial. Sufficient atropinisation**G** may help to manage organophosphorus induced seizures. Routine use of benzodiazepines before any seizure occurs has support from animal models, but we found no studies in humans.[46]

OPTION α_2 ADRENERGIC RECEPTOR AGONISTS (CLONIDINE)

We found no RCTs or observational studies of sufficient quality evaluating clonidine in people with acute organophosphorus poisoning.

Benefits: We found no systematic review, RCTs, or observational studies of sufficient quality.

Harms: We found no systematic review, RCTs, or observational studies of sufficient quality assessing adverse effects in people with acute organophosphorus poisoning receiving clonidine. Adverse effects of clonidine may include sedation, hypotension, bradycardia, and (with prolonged use) rebound hypertension.[47]

Comment: Clonidine inhibits the release of acetylcholine from cholinergic neurones and has α_2 adrenergic agonist effects. Animal studies have found that pretreatment with clonidine improves survival after organophosphorus poisoning; combination with atropine was more than additive.[48] This treatment has not yet been studied in organophosphorus poisoning in humans.

OPTION N-METHYL-D-ASPARTATE RECEPTOR ANTAGONISTS

We found no RCTs or observational studies of sufficient quality evaluating n-methyl-D-aspartate receptor antagonists in people with acute organophosphorus poisoning.

Benefits: We found no systematic review, RCTs, or observational studies of sufficient quality.

Organophosphorus poisoning (acute)

Harms: We found no systematic review, RCTs, or cohort studies of adverse effects in people with acute organophosphorus poisoning receiving N-methyl-D-aspartate (NMDA) receptor antagonists. A dose ranging clinical study found that adverse effects of NMDA receptor antagonists include dizziness, vomiting, nausea, stupor, agitation, and hallucinations.[49]

Comment: Primate studies have found that treating organophosphorus poisoning with NMDA receptor antagonists, such as gacyclidine, improves clinical recovery, reduces neural death, and improves electroencephalogram activity.[50]

GLOSSARY

Acetylcholinesterase An enzyme that cleaves acetylcholine.

Ageing Esterases (such as acetylcholinesterase and neurotoxic target esterase) are inhibited by organophosphorus through phosphorylation. Inhibited acetylcholinesterase reactivates spontaneously at very slow rates; oximes speed up this reaction. However, phosphorylated acetylcholinesterase may lose an alkyl side chain non-enzymatically, leaving a hydroxyl group in its place ("ageing"). Regeneration is then no longer possible.

Atropinisation Administering atropine until it reaches sufficiently high blood levels to suppress cholinergic signs clinically.

Pro-poisons Some organophosphorus pesticides require activation in vivo to become toxic.

Rates of ageing The rate depends on the identity of the alkyl side chains on each organophosphorus. Those with two methyl groups will age faster than those with two ethyl groups and thus become unresponsive to oximes at an earlier time point.

REFERENCES

1. Lotti M. Clinical toxicology of anticholinesterase agents in humans. In:Krieger RI, Doull J, eds. *Handbook of Pesticide toxicology*. San Diego: Academic press, 2001:1043–1085.
2. Karalliedde L, Eddleston M, Murray V. The global picture of organophosphate insecticide poisoning. In: Karalliedde L, Feldman F, Henry J, et al, eds. *Organophosphates and health*. London: Imperial Press, 2001:432–471.
3. Eddleston M. Patterns and problems of deliberate self-poisoning in the developing world. *Q J Med* 2000;93:715–731.
4. Roberts D, Karunarathna A, Buckley N, et al. Influence of pesticide regulation on acute poisoning deaths in Sri Lanka. *Bull WHO* 2003, 81: 789–798.
5. Wesseling C, McConnell R, Partanen T, et al. Agricultural pesticide use in developing countries: health effects and research needs. *Int J Health Serv* 1997;27:273–308.
6. World Health Organization in collaboration with the United Nations Environment Programme. *Public health impact of pesticides used in agriculture*. Geneva: World Health Organization, 1990.
7. Balali-Mood M, Shariat M. Treatment of organophosphate poisoning. Experience of nerve agents and acute pesticide poisoning on the effects of oximes. *J Physiol Paris* 1998;92:375–378.
8. Eyer P. The role of oximes in the management of organophosphorus pesticide poisoning. *Toxicol Rev* 2003; 22:165–190.
9. Riviere JE, Chang SK. Transdermal penetration and metabolism of organophosphate insecticides. In: Chambers JE, Levi PE, eds. *Organophosphates: chemistry, fate and effects*. San Diego: Academic Press, 1992:241–253.
10. Wester RC, Sedik L, Melendres J, et al. Percutaneous absorption of diazinon in humans. *Food Chem Toxicol* 1993;31:569–572.
11. Krieger RI, Dinoff TM. Malathion deposition, metabolite clearance, and cholinesterase status of date dusters and harvesters in California. *Arch Environ Contam Toxicol* 2000;38:546–553.
12. Griffin P, Mason H, Heywood K, et al. Oral and dermal absorption of chlorpyrifos: a human volunteer study. *Occup Environ Med* 1999;56:10–13.
13. American Academy of Clinical Toxicology, European Association of Poison Centres and Clinical Toxicologists. Position statement: ipecac syrup. *J Toxicol Clin Toxicol* 1997;35:699–709.
14. American Academy of Clinical Toxicology and European Association of Poison Centres and Clinical Toxicologists. Position statement: cathartics. *J Toxicol Clin Toxicol* 1997;35:743–752.
15. American Academy of Clinical Toxicology, European Association of Poison Centres and Clinical Toxicologists. Position statement: gastric lavage. *J Toxicol Clin Toxicol* 1997;35:711–719.
16. American Academy of Clinical Toxicology, European Association of Poison Centres and Clinical Toxicologists. Position statement: single-dose activated charcoal. *J Toxicol Clin Toxicol* 1997;35:721–741.
17. American Academy of Clinical Toxicology, European Association of Poison Centres and Clinical Toxicologists. Position statement and practice guidelines on the use of multi-dose activated charcoal in the treatment of acute poisoning. *J Toxicol Clin Toxicol* 1999;37:731–751.
18. Mauro LS, Nawarskas JJ, Mauro VF. Misadventures with activated charcoal and recommendations for safe use. *Ann Pharmacother* 1994;28:915–924.
19. Dorrington CL, Johnson DW, Brant R, et al. The frequency of complications associated with the use of multiple-dose activated charcoal. *Ann Emerg Med* 2003;41:370–377.
20. Tuncok Y, Gelal A, Apaydin S, et al. Prevention of oral dichlorvos toxicity by different activated charcoal products in mice. *Ann Emerg Med* 1995;25:353–355.
21. University of Oxford. Acute organophosphate pesticide poisoning in Sri Lanka — management, complications and pharmacogenetics. ISRCTN02920054 allocated July 2002. http://www.controlled-trials.com/isrctn/trial/02920054/0/02920054.html (last accessed 28 January 2004).
22. Heath AJW, Meredith T. Atropine in the management of anticholinesterase poisoning. In: Ballantyne B,

Marrs TC, eds. *Clinical and experimental toxicology of organophosphates and carbamates*. Oxford: Butterworth Heinemann, 1992:543–554.

23. Eddleston M, Buckley N, Checketts H, et al. Speed of initial atropinisation in significant organophosphorus pesticide poisoning — a systematic comparison of recommended regimens. *J Toxicol Clin Toxicol* 2004;42:865–875.
24. Johnson MK, Jacobsen D, Meredith TJ, et al. Evaluation of antidotes for poisoning by organophosphorus pesticides. *Emerg Med* 2000;12:22–37.
25. Samuel J, Thomas K, Jeyaseelan L, et al. Incidence of intermediate syndrome in organophosphorus poisoning. *J Assoc Physic India* 1995;43:321–323.
26. Samuel J, Peter JV, Thomas K, et al. Evaluation of two treatment regimens of pralidoxime (1gm single bolus dose vs 12gm infusion) in the management of organophosphorus poisoning. *J Assoc Physicians India* 1996;44:529–531.
27. Cherian AM, Jeyaseelan L, Peter JV, et al. *Effectiveness of pralidoxime in the treatment of organophosphorus poisoning — a randomised, double-blind, placebo-controlled clinical trial*. INCLEN Monograph series on Critical International Health Issues No. 7, 1997.
28. Cherian AM, Peter JV, Samuel J, et al. Effectiveness of P2AM (PAM — pralidoxime) in the treatment of organophosphorus poisoning. A randomised, double-blind, placebo-controlled trial. *J Assoc Physicians India* 1997;45:22–24.
29. Bardin PG, van Eeden SF. Organophosphate poisoning: grading the severity and comparing treatment between atropine and glycopyrrolate. *Crit Care Med* 1990;18:956–960.
30. Ali-Melkkila T, Kanto J, Iisalo E. Pharmacokinetics and related pharmacodynamics of anticholinergic drugs. *Acta Anaesthesiol Scand* 1993;37:633–642.
31. Eddleston M, Szinicz L, Eyer P, et al. Oximes in acute organophosphorus pesticide poisoning: a systematic review of clinical trials. *Q J Med* 2002;95:275–283. Search date 2002; primary sources Medline, Embase, The Cochrane Library, checking of reference lists, contact with experts, and a web search using Google.
32. Bismuth C, Inns RH, Marrs TC. Efficacy, toxicity and clinical uses of oximes in anticholinesterase poisoning. In: Ballantyne B, Marrs TC, eds. *Clinical and experimental toxicology of organophosphates and carbamates*. Oxford: Butterworth Heinemann, 1992:555–577.
33. Kusic R, Jovanovic D, Randjelovic S, et al. HI-6 in man: efficacy of the oxime in poisoning by organophosphorus insecticides. *Hum Exp Toxicol* 1991;10:113–118.
34. Worek F, Backer M, Thiermann H, et al. Reappraisal of indications and limitations of oxime therapy in organophosphate poisoning. *Hum Exp Toxicol* 1997;16:466–472.
35. Worek F, Eyer P, Kiderlen D, et al. Effect of human plasma on the reactivation of sarin-inhibited human erythrocyte acetylcholinesterase. *Arch Toxicol* 2000;74:21–26.
36. University of Oxford. Acute organophosphate pesticide poisoning in Sri Lanka — management, complications and pharmacogenetics. ISRCTN55264358 allocated July 2002. http://www.controlled-trials.com/isrctn/trial/20/0/55264358.html (last accessed 27 January 2004).
37. Sogorb MA, Vilanova E, Carrera V. Future applications of phosphotriesterases in the prophylaxis and treatment of organophosporus insecticide and nerve agent poisonings. *Toxicol Lett* 2004;151:219–233.
38. Raushel FM. Bacterial detoxification of organophosphate nerve agents. *Curr Opin Microbiol* 2002;5:288–295.
39. Forsythe SM, Schmidt GA. Sodium bicarbonate for the treatment of lactic acidosis. *Chest* 2000;117:260–267.
40. Cordoba D, Cadavid S, Angulo D, et al. Organophosphate poisoning: modifications in acid base equilibrium and use of sodium bicarbonate as an aid in the treatment of toxicity in dogs. *Vet Hum Toxicol* 1983;25:1–3.
41. Wong A, Sandron CA, Magalhaes AS, et al. Comparative efficacy of pralidoxime vs sodium bicarbonate in rats and humans severely poisoned with O-P pesticide. *J Toxicol Clin Toxicol* 2000;38:554–555.
42. Balali-Mood M, Ayati MH, Ali-Akbarian H. Effects of high doses of sodium bicarbonate in acute organophosphate pesticide poisoning [abstract]. *J Toxicol Clin Toxicol* 2003;41:383.
43. Roberts DM, Buckley NA. Alkalinisation for treating organophosphorus pesticide poisoning. Cochrane Database of Systematic Reviews. In press protocol 2005.
44. Sellstrom A. Anticonvulsants in anticholinesterase poisoning. In: Ballantyne B, Marrs TC, eds. *Clinical and experimental toxicology of organophosphates and carbamates*. Oxford: Butterworth Heinemann, 1992:578–586.
45. Marrs TC. Diazepam in the treatment of organophosphorus ester pesticide poisoning. *Toxicol Rev* 2003; 22:75–81.
46. Murphy MR, Blick DW, Dunn MA, et al. Diazepam as a treatment for nerve agent poisoning in primates. *Aviat Space Environ Med* 1993;64:110–115.
47. van Zwieten PA. Centrally acting antihypertensive drugs. Present and future. *Clin Exp Hypertens* 1999;21:859–873.
48. Liu WF. A symptomatological assessment of organophosphate-induced lethality in mice: comparison of atropine and clonidine protection. *Toxicol Lett* 1991;56:19–32.
49. Lees KR, Dyker AG, Sharma A, et al. Tolerability of the low-affinity, use-dependent NMDA antagonist AR-R15896AR in stroke patients: a dose-ranging study. *Stroke* 2001;32:466–472.
50. Lallement G, Baubichon D, Clarencon D, et al. Review of the value of gacyclidine (GK-11) as adjuvant medication to conventional treatments of organophosphate poisoning: primate experiments mimicking various scenarios of military or terrorist attack by soman. *Neurotoxicology* 1999;20:675–684.

Michael Eddleston
Centre for Tropical Medicine
University of Oxford
Oxford
UK

Surjit Singh
Department of Internal Medicine
Postgraduate Institute of Medical Education and Research
Chandigarh
India

Nick Buckley
Department of Clinical Pharmacology and Toxicology
Canberra Hospital
Canberra
Australia

Competing interests: None declared.

Paracetamol (acetaminophen) poisoning

Search date March 2004

Nick Buckley and Michael Eddleston

QUESTIONS

INTERVENTIONS

Key Messages

- **Acetylcysteine** One systematic review found one RCT in people with established paracetamol induced liver failure. It found that acetylcysteine reduced mortality after 21 days compared with placebo. One observational study found that people given early treatment with acetylcysteine were less likely to develop liver damage than untreated historical controls. We found no RCTs comparing acetylcysteine versus methionine.
- **Methionine** One small RCT identified by a systematic review found no significant difference in mortality between methionine and supportive care, although it lacked power to detect a clinically important difference. It found limited evidence that methionine reduced hepatotoxicity compared with supportive care. We found no RCTs comparing methionine versus acetylcysteine.
- **Activated charcoal (single or multiple dose)** One systematic review found no evidence on the effects of activated charcoal, whether in single or multiple dose regimens, in people poisoned by paracetamol. One large case series found that clinically significant complications of multiple dose activated charcoal were rare.
- **Gastric lavage** One systematic review found no RCTs examining the effects of gastric lavage in paracetamol poisoning.
- **Ipecacuanha** One systematic review found no RCTs examining the effects of ipecacuanha in paracetamol poisoning.

DEFINITION Paracetamol poisoning occurs as a result of either accidental or intentional overdose with paracetamol (acetaminophen).

INCIDENCE/ PREVALENCE Paracetamol is the most common drug used for self poisoning in the UK.[1] It is also a common means of self poisoning in the rest of Europe, North America, and Australasia. An estimated 41 200 cases of poisoning with products containing paracetamol occurred in 1989–1990 in England and Wales, with a mortality of 0.40% (95% CI 0.38% to 0.46%). Overdoses owing to paracetamol alone result in an estimated 150–200 deaths and 15–20 liver transplants each year in England and Wales. More recent studies suggest that paracetamol poisoning is at least as common now in the UK, although there is limited evidence that there have been modest reductions in large overdoses, liver transplants, and deaths since packaging restrictions were instituted in 1998.[2]

AETIOLOGY/ RISK FACTORS Most cases in the UK are impulsive acts of self harm in young people.[1,3] In one study of 80 people who had overdosed with paracetamol, 42 had obtained the tablets for the specific purpose of taking an overdose and 33 had obtained them less than 1 hour before the act.[3]

PROGNOSIS People with blood paracetamol concentrations above the standard treatment line (defined in the UK as a line joining 200 mg/L at 4 hours and 30 mg/L at 15 hours on a semilogarithmic plot) have a poor prognosis without treatment (see figure 1, p 1762).[4–6] In one study of 57 untreated people with blood concentrations above this line, 33 developed severe liver damage and three died.[5] People with a history of chronic alcohol misuse, use of enzyme inducing drugs, eating disorders, or multiple paracetamol overdoses may be at risk of liver damage with blood concentrations below this line.[7] In the USA, a lower line is used as an indication for treatment, but we found no data relating this line to prognostic outcomes.[8] **Dose effect:** The dose ingested also indicates the risk of hepatotoxicity. People ingesting less than 125 mg/kg had no significant hepatotoxicity, with a sharp dose dependent rise for higher doses.[9] The threshold for toxicity after acute ingestion may be higher in children, where a single dose of less than 200 mg/kg has not been reported to lead to death and rarely causes hepatotoxicity.[10] For people who present later than 24 hours or an unknown time after ingestion, several other prognostic indicators have been proposed, including prothrombin time and abnormal liver function tests.[11,12] These have not been validated prospectively.

AIMS OF INTERVENTION To prevent liver failure, liver transplantation, or death, with minimal adverse effects.

OUTCOMES Mortality, hepatotoxicity (most commonly defined by the objective criterion of blood aspartate aminotransferase > 1000 U/L), liver failure, or liver transplantation.

METHODS *Clinical Evidence* search and appraisal March 2004, including a search for observational studies. The authors also searched Current Awareness in Clinical Toxicology (http://www.npis.org/cact/cact.htm) and contacted experts in the field to identify unpublished studies.

QUESTION What are the effects of treatments for acute paracetamol poisoning?

OPTION ACETYLCYSTEINE

One systematic review found one RCT in people with established paracetamol induced liver failure. It found that acetylcysteine reduced mortality after 21 days compared with placebo. One observational study found that people given early treatment with acetylcysteine were less likely to develop liver damage than untreated historical controls. We found no RCTs comparing acetylcysteine versus methionine.

Benefits: Versus placebo: We found one systematic review (search date 2001, 1 RCT, 50 people with established paracetamol induced liver failure), which compared intravenous acetylcysteine (150 mg/kg over 15 minutes, 50 mg/kg over 4 hours, and then 100 mg/kg diluted in 5% dextrose over 16 hours, continued until death or recovery) versus a placebo infusion of 5% dextrose.[13] It found that, after 21 days, acetylcysteine significantly reduced mortality compared with placebo (mortality: 13/25 [52%] with acetylcysteine *v* 20/25 [80%] with placebo; RR 0.65, 95% CI 0.43 to 0.99; NNT 4, 95% CI 2 to 16). **Versus methionine:** See benefits of methionine, p 1760.

Harms: Versus placebo: The systematic review found no evidence that quantified harms from acetylcysteine,[13] and the included RCT did not specifically assess adverse outcomes and none were noted.[14] Six case series found that the incidence of adverse effects from intravenous acetylcysteine was 4–23%.[15–20] These were predominantly rash, urticaria, and occasionally more serious anaphylactoid reactions occurring with the initial "loading" dose. In most or all cases, adverse effects responded to temporary stopping of infusions and symptomatic treatment, and did not recur when treatment recommenced. Three deaths have been reported, two followed a 10-fold miscalculation of the dose of acetylcysteine and the other occurred in a person with severe asthma.[21,22] Adverse reactions seem to be more common in people with asthma and those who have non-toxic paracetamol concentrations.[17] Vomiting is common after oral acetylcysteine and occurred in 63% of people in one series, despite previous administration of metoclopramide.[18] Oral acetylcysteine can also cause hypersensitivity and anaphylactoid reactions.[23] **Versus methionine:** See harms of methionine, p 1760.

Comment: In the RCT, allocation was concealed but treatment was not blinded.[14] There were differences between the groups in prognostic variables (prothrombin time, coma grade) and other treatments, but a possible confounding effect could not be assessed adequately because of the small size of the study. One observational study evaluated the effects of intravenous acetylcysteine in people presenting early to hospital.[5] It found that people treated within 10 hours of ingestion were less likely to develop liver damage than were untreated historical controls (1/62 [2%] with treated people *v* 33/57 [58%] with untreated people). As a result, subsequent RCTs were considered unethical. A systematic review of numerous case series found evidence that acetylcysteine is beneficial in paracetamol poisoning.[15] For both oral and intravenous acetylcysteine, overall hepatotoxicity was worse if treatment was delayed beyond 8–10 hours (1% in those treated within 8 hours *v* 46% in those treated after 16 hours).[5,15] We found no RCTs of different regimens and no evidence of a difference between oral and intravenous routes of administration.[15] The optimal dose, route, and duration of treatment is unknown. Two recent observational studies comparing different protocols for intravenous[24] and oral[25] acetylcysteine did not find marked differences in outcomes.

OPTION ACTIVATED CHARCOAL (SINGLE OR MULTIPLE DOSE)

One systematic review found no evidence on the effects of activated charcoal, whether in single or multiple dose regimens, in people poisoned by paracetamol. One large case series found that clinically significant complications of multiple dose activated charcoal were rare.

Benefits: We found one systematic review (search date 2001), which found no RCTs that examined clinical outcomes after paracetamol poisoning.[13]

Harms: The systematic review found no large study of complications in people poisoned by paracetamol who received single doses of activated charcoal.[13] Reported harms may include aspiration pneumonia, vomiting, diarrhoea, constipation, ileus, and interference with regular medications.[26] One large retrospective case series (878 people treated with multiple dose activated charcoal) suggested that rates of clinically significant adverse events with multiple dose regimens are likely to be low (significant pulmonary aspiration in 6/878 [0.6%], 95% CI 0.1% to 1.1%).[27]

Comment: **Single dose regimens:** The systematic review included simulated overdose studies in volunteers, and found that activated charcoal given within 2 hours of paracetamol ingestion decreased absorption by a variable amount and that this amount diminished with time.[13] One cohort study in 450 consecutive people who had taken ≥ 10 g of paracetamol found that those who had been given activated charcoal were significantly less likely to have high risk blood paracetamol concentrations than those who had not been given activated charcoal (OR 0.36, 95% CI 0.23 to 0.58).[4] The effect was seen only in those treated within 2 hours, and the study was not large enough to assess the effect of many potential confounders.[4] One non-systematic review of activated charcoal in all forms of poisoning found no evidence that activated charcoal improved outcome in poisoned people.[28] **Multiple dose regimens:** The review found no studies of simulated overdose that evaluated multiple dose regimens in paracetamol poisoning.[13] One non-systematic review of case series and reports of multiple dose regimens in all forms of poisoning found no evidence that multiple dose regimens improved outcomes in poisoned people.[29] The rapid absorption and short half life of paracetamol suggest that a beneficial effect is unlikely.

OPTION GASTRIC LAVAGE

One systematic review found no RCTs examining the effects of gastric lavage in paracetamol poisoning.

Benefits: We found one systematic review (search date 2001), which found no RCTs or cohort studies that reported clinical outcomes.[13]

Harms: The systematic review found no large study of complications in people poisoned by paracetamol who received gastric lavage.[13] One RCT (876 people with acute oral overdose of a variety of drugs) compared gastric emptying (ipecacuanha induced [209 people] or gastric lavage [220 people]) plus charcoal versus charcoal alone.[30] It found no significant difference in complications between gastric emptying plus charcoal and charcoal alone (13% with gastric emptying *v* 8% with no emptying; P = 0.43).[30] The RCT did not analyse harms data separately for gastric lavage or ipecacuanha. Harms with any method of gastric emptying plus charcoal included aspiration (17/459), diarrhoea (3 people), ileus (3 people), arrhythmia during vomiting (2 people), dystonia from metoclopramide given for vomiting (1 person), and haematemesis (2 people). These harms results may not generalise to gastric lavage, since about 50% of people were treated with ipecacuanha.

Comment: The systematic review included studies of simulated overdose in human volunteers, and found that gastric lavage carried out within 1 hour removed a variable number of paracetamol tablets and that the number diminished with time.[13] One cohort study (described previously) (see comment under activated charcoal, p 1759) found that those given activated charcoal were significantly less likely to have high risk blood paracetamol concentrations than those who were not given activated charcoal (OR 0.36, 95% CI 0.23 to 0.58).[4] The addition of gastric lavage to activated charcoal regimens did not decrease the risk further (OR 1.12, 95% CI 0.57 to 2.20).[4] One non-systematic review of gastric lavage in all forms of poisoning found no evidence that gastric lavage improved outcome in poisoned people.[31]

OPTION IPECACUANHA

One systematic review found no RCTs examining the effects of ipecacuanha in paracetamol poisoning.

Benefits: We found one systematic review (search date 2001), which found no evidence of clinical effects of ipecacuanha in paracetamol poisoning.[13]

Harms: The systematic review found no studies that quantified harms from ipecacuanha in paracetamol poisoning.[13] We found one RCT (876 people with overdose of different drugs), which compared gastric emptying (ipecacuanha or gastric lavage) plus charcoal versus charcoal alone.[30] However, the RCT did not analyse the effects of ipecacuanha separately (see harms of gastric lavage, p 1759).

Comment: Human simulated overdose studies suggest that ipecacuanha given within 1 hour could reduce paracetamol absorption but no studies have shown a change in clinical outcome.[26] One non-systematic review of ipecacuanha in all forms of poisoning found no evidence that ipecacuanha improved outcome in poisoned people.[26] Administration of ipecacuanha may delay the administration of activated charcoal and oral antidotes.

OPTION METHIONINE

One small RCT identified by a systematic review found no significant difference in mortality between methionine and supportive care, although it may have lacked power to detect a clinically important difference. It found limited evidence that methionine reduced hepatotoxicity compared with supportive care. We found no RCTs comparing methionine versus acetylcysteine.

Benefits: **Versus supportive care:** We found one systematic review (search date 2001, 1 RCT, 40 people with blood concentrations of paracetamol above the UK standard treatment line [see figure 1, p 1762]), which compared oral methionine (2.5 g 4 hourly for 4 doses), intravenous mercaptamine (formerly named cysteamine, 3.6 g over 20 hours), and supportive care.[13] The RCT found no significant effect on mortality (0 deaths with methionine *v* 1 with supportive care).[32] Only 27 people had a liver biopsy. Fewer people suffered grade III hepatic necrosis with methionine than with supportive care (0/9 [0%] with methionine *v* 6/10 [60%] with supportive care) or had peak aspartate aminotransferase greater than 1000 U (1/13 [8%] with methionine *v* 8/13 [62%] with supportive care; RR 0.13, 95% CI 0.02 to 0.86; NNT 2, 95% CI 2 to 6). **Versus acetylcysteine:** We found one systematic review (search date 2003), which identified no RCTs.[33]

Harms: Neither systematic review addressed harms from methionine.[13,33] No serious adverse effects associated with treatment were reported in the included RCT, but vomiting after administration of methionine occurred in 8/13 people (62%).[32] The incidence of adverse effects in the control group was not reported.

Comment: **Versus supportive care:** Interpretation of liver biopsy results from the RCT was difficult, as not all people were tested and an intention to treat analysis was not possible.[32]

REFERENCES

1. Gunnell D, Hawton K, Murray V, et al. Use of paracetamol for suicide and non-fatal poisoning in the UK and France: are restrictions on availability justified? *J Epidemiol Community Health* 1997;51:175–179.
2. Camidge DR, Wood RJ, Bateman DN. The epidemiology of self-poisoning in the UK. *Br J Clin Pharmacol* 2003;56:613–619.
3. Hawton K, Ware C, Mistry H, et al. Paracetamol self-poisoning. Characteristics, prevention and harm reduction. *Br J Psychiatry* 1996;168:43–48.

4. Buckley NA, Whyte IM, O'Connell DL, et al. Activated charcoal reduces the need for *N*-acetylcysteine treatment after acetaminophen (paracetamol) overdose. *J Toxicol Clin Toxicol* 1999;37:753–757.
5. Prescott LF, Illingworth RN, Critchley JAJH, et al. Intravenous *N*-acetylcysteine: the treatment of choice for paracetamol poisoning. *BMJ* 1979;2:1097–1100.
6. Rumack BH, Matthew H. Acetaminophen poisoning and toxicity. *Pediatrics* 1975;55:871–876.
7. Vale JA, Proudfoot AT. Paracetamol (acetaminophen) poisoning. *Lancet* 1995;346:547–552.
8. Smilkstein MJ, Knapp GL, Kulig KW, et al. Efficacy of oral *N*-acetylcysteine in the treatment of acetaminophen overdose. Analysis of the National Multicentre Study (1976–1985). *N Engl J Med* 1988;319:1557–1562.
9. Prescott LF. Paracetamol overdosage. Pharmacological considerations and clinical management. *Drugs* 1983;25:290–314.
10. Caravati EM. Unintentional acetaminophen ingestion in children and the potential for hepatotoxicity. *J Toxicol Clin Toxicol* 2000;38:291–296.
11. Schiodt FV, Ott P, Christensen E, et al. The value of plasma acetaminophen half-life in antidote-treated acetaminophen overdosage. *Clin Pharmacol Ther* 2002;71:221–225.
12. James LP, Wells E, Beard RH, et al. Predictors of outcome after acetaminophen poisoning in children and adolescents. *J Pediatr* 2002;140:522–526.
13. Brok J, Buckley N, Gluud C. Interventions for paracetamol (acetaminophen) overdoses. In: The Cochrane Library, Issue 3, 2004. Chichester, UK: John Wiley & Sons, Ltd. Search date 2001; primary sources Cochrane Hepato-Biliary Group Controlled Trials Register, Cochrane Controlled Trials Register, Medline, Embase, and hand searching of reference lists from RCTs, textbooks, review articles and meta-analyses, and personal contact with authors of relevant RCTs.
14. Keays R, Harrison PM, Wendon JA, et al. Intravenous acetylcysteine in paracetamol induced fulminant hepatic failure: a prospective controlled trial. *BMJ* 1991;303:1026–1029.
15. Buckley NA, Whyte IM, O'Connell DL, et al. Oral or intravenous *N*-acetylcysteine: which is the treatment of choice for acetaminophen (paracetamol) poisoning? *J Toxicol Clin Toxicol* 1999;37:759–767.
16. Chan TY, Critchley JA. Adverse reactions to intravenous *N*-acetylcysteine in Chinese patients with paracetamol (acetaminophen) poisoning. *Hum Exp Toxicol* 1994;13:542–544.
17. Schmidt LE, Dalhoff K. Risk factors in the development of adverse reactions to *N*-acetylcysteine in patients with paracetamol poisoning. *Br J Clin Pharmacol* 2001;51:87–91.
18. Wright RO, Anderson AC, Lesko SL, et al. Effect of metoclopramide dose on preventing emesis after oral administration of *N*-acetylcysteine for acetaminophen overdose. *J Toxicol Clin Toxicol* 1999;37:35–42.
19. Sanaei-Zadeh H, Taghaddosinejad F, Jalali N, et al. Adverse effects of intravenous N-acetylcysteine. *Clin Drug Invest* 2003;23;129–133.
20. Kao LW, Kirk MA, Furbee RB, et al. What is the rate of adverse events after oral N-acetylcysteine administered by the intravenous route to patients with suspected acetaminophen poisoning? *Ann Emerg Med* 2003;42:741–750.
21. Mant TG, Tempowski JH, Volans GN, et al. Adverse reactions to acetylcysteine and effects of overdose. *BMJ* 1984;289:217–219.
22. Appelboam AV, Dargan PI, Jones AL, et al. Fatal anaphylactoid reaction to *N*-acetylcysteine: caution in asthmatics. *J Toxicol Clin Toxicol* 2002;40:366–367.
23. Perry HE, Shannon MW. Efficacy of oral versus intravenous *N*-acetylcysteine in acetaminophen overdose: results of an open-label, clinical trial. *J Pediatr* 1998;132:149–152.
24. Dougherty T, Greene T, Roberts JR. Acetaminophen overdose: comparison between continuous and intermittent intravenous *N*-acetylcysteine 48-hour protocols. *Ann Emerg Med* 2000;36:S83.
25. Woo OF, Mueller PD, Olson KR, et al. Shorter duration of oral *N*-acetylcysteine therapy for acute acetaminophen overdose. *Ann Emerg Med* 2000;35:363–368.
26. Krenzelok EP, McGuigan M, Lheur P. Position statement: ipecac syrup. American Academy of Clinical Toxicology and European Association of Poisons Centres and Clinical Toxicologists. *J Toxicol Clin Toxicol* 1997;35:699–709.
27. Dorrington CL, Johnson DW, Brant R. The frequency of complications associated with the use of multiple-dose activated charcoal. *Ann Emerg Med* 2003;41:370–377.
28. Chyka PA, Seger D. Position statement: single-dose activated charcoal. American Academy of Clinical Toxicology; European Association of Poisons Centres and Clinical Toxicologists. *J Toxicol Clin Toxicol* 1997;35:721–741.
29. American Academy of Clinical Toxicology, European Association of Poison Centres, and Clinical Toxicologists. Position statement and practice guidelines on the use of multi-dose activated charcoal in the treatment of acute poisoning. *J Toxicol Clin Toxicol* 1999;37:731–751.
30. Pond SM, Lewis-Driver DJ, Williams GM, et al. Gastric emptying in acute overdose: a prospective randomised controlled trial. *Med J Aust* 1995;163:345–349.
31. Vale JA. Position statement: gastric lavage. American Academy of Clinical Toxicology, European Association of Poisons Centres, and Clinical Toxicologists. *J Toxicol Clin Toxicol* 1997;35:711–719.
32. Hamlyn AN, Lesna M, Record CO, et al. Methionine and cysteamine in paracetamol (acetaminophen) overdose, prospective controlled trial of early therapy. *J Int Med Res* 1981;9:226–231.
33. Alsalim W, Fadel M. Oral methionine compared with intravenous n-acetyl cysteine for paracetamol overdose. *Emerg Med J* 2003;20:366–367. Search date 2003; primary source Medline.

Nick Buckley
Consultant Clinical Pharmacologist and Toxicologist
Canberra Hospital
Canberra
Australia

Michael Eddleston
Wellcome Trust Career Development Fellow
Centre for Tropical Medicine University of Oxford
Oxford
UK

Competing interests: None declared.

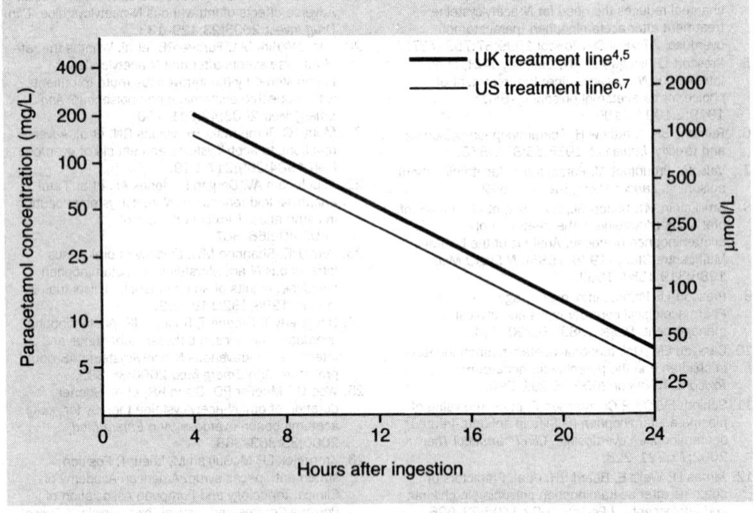

FIGURE 1 **Nomograms used to determine acetylcysteine or methionine treatment, based on the blood concentrations between 4 hours and 24 hours after ingestion of paracetamol. Published with permission (see text, p 1757).[4]**

Ectopic pregnancy

Search date April 2003

Bazian Ltd

QUESTIONS

INTERVENTIONS

See glossary Ⓖ

Key Messages

- **Choice between open and laparoscopic salpingostomy** One systematic review found that, compared with laparoscopic salpingostomy, open salpingostomy increased rates of elimination of tubal pregnancy. It found no significant difference in rates of subsequent intrauterine pregnancy or repeat ectopic pregnancy, but perioperative blood loss was higher with open salpingostomy.
- **Methotrexate (oral)** One small RCT identified by a systematic review found no significant difference between oral methotrexate 2.5 mg daily for 5 days and expectant management in the need for laparoscopy for persistent adnexal mass within 3 months.
- **Methotrexate (intramuscular, multiple or single dose)** One RCT identified by a systematic review found no significant difference in rates of elimination of tubal pregnancy, tubal preservation, spontaneous intrauterine pregnancy, or repeat ectopic pregnancy at 18 months between multiple dose intramuscular methotrexate (1 mg/kg on days 1, 2, 4, and 6) plus folic acid compared with laparoscopic salpingostomy. The same RCT found that multiple dose methotrexate decreased health related quality of life compared with laparoscopic salpingostomy. One systematic review found higher rates of persistent ectopic pregnancy and lower rates of elimination of tubal pregnancy with single dose intramuscular methotrexate 1 mg/kg or 50 mg/m^2 compared with laparoscopic salpingostomy.
- **Salpingostomy** We found no RCTs comparing salpingostomy with expectant management. One RCT identified by a systematic review found no significant difference in rates of elimination of tubal pregnancy, tubal preservation, spontaneous intrauterine pregnancy, or repeat ectopic pregnancy at 18 months between multiple dose intramuscular methotrexate (1 mg/kg on days 1, 2, 4, and 6) plus folic acid compared with laparoscopic salpingostomy. The same RCT found that multiple dose methotrexate decreased health related quality of life compared with laparoscopic salpingostomy. One systematic review found higher rates of persistent ectopic pregnancy and lower rates of elimination of tubal pregnancy with single dose intramuscular methotrexate 1 mg/kg or 50 mg/m^2 compared with laparoscopic salpingostomy.
- **Fimbrial expression, salpingectomy, salpingo-oophorectomy** We found no systematic review or RCTs that evaluated these interventions.

DEFINITION In ectopic pregnancy, the fertilised ovum implants on a surface other than the uterine endometrium. Almost all ectopic pregnancies implant in the fallopian tubes. Ectopic pregnancies are detected by clinical suspicion and serial measurement of serum human chorionic gonadotrophin (hCG) or ultrasound.[1] Spontaneous resolution occurs only in selected cases: in women with a small adnexal mass on transvaginal sonography, decreasing hCG levels, and only minor symptoms.[2,3] **Population:** This chapter covers management in women with non-ruptured, tubal ectopic pregnancy only. Typically, this group would consist of women with small tubal pregnancies confirmed ultrasonographically or based on serial hCG levels. We have excluded women with an acute presentation of ectopic pregnancy (such as peritonism, or with evidence of rupture or bleeding).

INCIDENCE/ PREVALENCE Small studies suggest that 1–2% of reported pregnancies are ectopic.[4,5] A recent large study attempted to estimate the proportion of ectopic pregnancies in the USA using national data sets, but found that data were too flawed to provide an accurate estimate of the incidence.[6]

AETIOLOGY/ RISK FACTORS A recent large case-control study suggested that the main risk factors for ectopic pregnancy were history of pelvic infection (OR 3.4, 95% CI 2.4 to 5.0) and smoking (OR 3.9, 95% CI 2.6 to 5.9).[7] Other risk factors were age, previous spontaneous abortion, history of infertility, and previous use of an intrauterine contraceptive device.[7] Earlier studies have found that previous ectopic pregnancy, previous tubal surgery including tubal sterilisation, documented tubal pathology, intrauterine contraceptive device, previous genital infections, smoking and *in utero* diethylstilbestrol exposure were associated with ectopic pregnancy.[8–10] The risk of ectopic pregnancy varies with method of tubal sterilisation. Women sterilised by bipolar tubal coagulation before the age of 30 years were found to have a risk of ectopic pregnancy 27 times greater than women who had postpartum partial salpingectomy Ⓖ.[9]

PROGNOSIS Risks of ectopic pregnancy include tubal rupture, life-threatening bleeding, and subsequent infertility. The combination of transvaginal ultrasound and hCG measurements allow the condition to be diagnosed earlier now than previously. Consequently, mortality has fallen over time in the developed world from 35.5 deaths per 10 000 cases to 3.8 deaths per 10 000 cases between 1970 and 1989 in the USA and from 16 deaths per 10 000 cases to three deaths per 10 000 pregnancies between 1973 and 1993 in the UK.[3] However, mortality remains high in poorer countries: 100–300 deaths per 10 000 cases in one African survey.[11] Evaluating expectant management Ⓖ to assess prognosis is difficult because of ethical concerns about exposing women to undue risk of acute complications, which may also have medico-legal implications.[12] However, expectant management has been suggested as a feasible option in women at low risk of acute complications (such as asymptomatic women and women with small adnexal masses and decreasing hCG levels), and in the presence of close monitoring. A recent non-systematic review found rates of spontaneous resolution with expectant management to range from 46–65%.[3] One prospective cohort study (118 women) found that rates of spontaneous resolution varied with hCG level from 98% where hCG concentrations were less than 200 mIU/mL to 25% for hCG concentration greater than 2000 mIU/mL.[2] However, no factors have yet been found that reliably predict tubal rupture or bleeding.[3]

AIMS OF INTERVENTION To prevent tubal rupture; reduce maternal death; increase chances of future intrauterine pregnancy; and minimise adverse effects of treatments.

OUTCOMES Maternal mortality, tubal rupture, persistence or elimination of ectopic pregnancy (measured by ultrasound or by serial hCG levels); recurrence rate; long term spontaneous live birth rate (i.e. without subsequent intervention for infertility); quality of life; acute clinical complications of treatment (e.g. haemorrhage, infection); long term fertility; and complications of surgery, such as bleeding, hysterectomy, and transfusion.

METHODS *Clinical Evidence* search and appraisal April 2003.

QUESTION What are the effects of treatments for non-ruptured tubal pregnancy?

OPTION FIMBRIAL EXPRESSION

We found no systematic review or RCTs that evaluated fimbrial expression.

Benefits: We found no systematic review or RCTs that compared fimbrial expression**G** with either expectant management**G** or other treatment.

Harms: We found no systematic review or RCTs.

Comment: It may not be ethically feasible to compares surgical management versus expectant management in an RCT (see prognosis, p 1764).

OPTION SALPINGECTOMY

We found no systematic review or RCTs that evaluated salpingectomy.

Benefits: We found no systematic review or RCTs that compared salpingectomy**G** with either expectant management**G** or other treatment.

Harms: We found no systematic review or RCTs.

Comment: It may not be ethically feasible to compare surgical management versus expectant management in an RCT (see prognosis, p 1764).

OPTION SALPINGO-OOPHORECTOMY

We found no systematic review or RCTs that evaluated salpingo-oophorectomy.

Benefits: We found no systematic review or RCTs that compared salpingo-oophorectomy**G** with either expectant management**G** or other treatment.

Harms: We found no systematic review or RCTs.

Comment: It may not be ethically feasible to compare surgical management versus expectant management in an RCT (see prognosis, p 1764).

OPTION SALPINGOSTOMY (OPEN OR LAPAROSCOPIC)

We found no RCTs comparing salpingostomy with expectant management. One systematic review found that, compared with laparoscopic salpingostomy, open salpingostomy increased rates of elimination of tubal pregnancy. It found no significant difference in rates of subsequent intrauterine pregnancy or repeat ectopic pregnancy, but perioperative blood loss was higher with open salpingostomy. One RCT identified by the review found no significant difference between laparoscopic salpingostomy and intramuscular methotrexate (multiple dose, 1 mg/kg on days 1, 2, 4, and 6) plus folic acid in terms of rate of elimination of tubal pregnancy, tubal preservation, spontaneous intrauterine pregnancy, or repeat ectopic pregnancy at 18 months. The same RCT found that multiple dose methotrexate decreased health related quality of life compared with laparoscopic salpingostomy.

Benefits: **Versus expectant management:** We found no systematic review or RCTs. **Open versus laparoscopic salpingostomy:** We found one systematic review (search date not reported), which identified three RCTs.[1] The review found that, compared with laparoscopic salpingostomy, open salpingostomy significantly increased rates of elimination of tubal pregnancies. It found no significant difference in rates of persistent ectopic pregnancy (3 RCTs, 228 with small unruptured tubal pregnancy; elimination of tubal pregnancy: RR 1.11, 95% CI 1.03 to 1.20; persistent ectopic pregnancy: RR 0.28, 95% CI 0.05 to 1.58). The review also found no significant difference between open and laparoscopic salpingostomy in rates of subsequent intrauterine pregnancy or repeat ectopic pregnancy among 145 women trying to conceive (3 RCTs, 145 women trying to conceive; rates of subsequent intrauterine pregnancy: RR 0.83, 95% CI 0.66 to 1.14; repeat ectopic pregnancy: RR 2.33, 95% CI 0.83 to 6.70). The review did not distinguish between spontaneous pregnancy and pregnancy after *in vitro* fertilisation. **Laparoscopic salpingostomy versus systemic methotrexate:** See benefits of systemic methotrexate, p 1766.

Harms: **Versus expectant management:** We found no systematic review or RCTs. **Open versus laparoscopic salpingostomy:** The review found that laparoscopic salpingostomy reduced perioperative blood loss compared with open salpingostomy (blood loss varied among studies: 62–79 mL with laparoscopic salpingostomy *v* 115–195 mL with open salpingostomy).[1] One RCT included in the review (60 women) found intraoperative complications in 2/30 women (both haematosalpinx) with laparoscopy compared with no complications with laparotomy.[13] Other complications in this RCT included wound infection in 2/30 with laparotomy and 1/30 with postoperative fever with each type of surgery. **Laparoscopic salpingostomy versus systemic methotrexate:** See harms of systemic methotrexate, p 1767.

Comment: It may not be ethically feasible to compare surgical management with expectant management in an RCT (see prognosis, p 1764).

OPTION SYSTEMIC METHOTREXATE

One small RCT identified by a systematic review found no significant difference between oral methotrexate 2.5 mg daily for 5 days and expectant management in the need for laparoscopy for persistent adnexal mass within 3 months. The review found higher rates of persistent ectopic pregnancy and lower rates of elimination of tubal pregnancy with single dose intramuscular methotrexate 1 mg/kg or 50 mg/m^2 compared with laparoscopic salpingostomy. One RCT identified by the review found no significant difference in rates of elimination of tubal pregnancy plus tubal preservation, spontaneous intrauterine pregnancy, or repeat ectopic pregnancy at 18 months between multiple dose intramuscular methotrexate (1 mg/kg on days 1, 2, 4, and 6) plus folic acid compared with laparoscopic salpingostomy. The same RCT found that multiple dose methotrexate decreased health related quality of life compared with laparoscopic salpingostomy.

Benefits: We found one systematic review (search date not reported).[1] **Oral methotrexate versus expectant management:** The review identified one RCT, which found no significant difference between oral methotrexate 2.5 mg daily for 5 days and expectant management🅖 in the need for laparoscopy within 3 months (1 RCT, 60 women with ectopic pregnancy < 4 cm and serum human chorionic gonadotrophin concentration < 5000 IU/L, mean age 31 years; need for laparoscopy within 3 months: 77% with each treatment [absolute numbers not provided]; RR 1.00, 95% CI 0.76 to 1.30).[12] The RCT did not report results on subsequent fertility. In the RCT, laparoscopy was performed if the adnexal mass remained visible on transvaginal ultrasonography and human chorionic gonadotrophin concentration was less than 1.0 IU/L. **Single dose intramuscular methotrexate versus laparoscopic salpingostomy:** The review found significantly higher rates of persistent ectopic pregnancy🅖 and lower rates of elimination of tubal pregnancy with single dose intramuscular methotrexate 1 mg/kg or 50 mg/m^2 compared with laparoscopic salpingostomy (3 RCTs, 207 women, haemodynamically stable with a small unruptured pregnancy, persistent ectopic pregnancy: RR 3.6, 95% CI 1.7 to 8.0; elimination of tubal pregnancy: RR 0.83, 95% CI 0.71 to 0.97).[1] The review found no significant difference between treatments in subsequent intrauterine pregnancies or repeat ectopic pregnancy (intrauterine pregnancy: RR 0.99, 95% CI 0.55 to 1.80; repeat ectopic pregnancy: RR 0.27, 95% CI 0.02 to 4.50). One RCT (62 women) identified by the review found that single dose intramuscular methotrexate significantly increased physical function compared with laparoscopic salpingostomy ($P < 0.01$) but found no significant difference in psychological functioning.[14] **Multiple dose intramuscular methotrexate versus laparoscopic salpingostomy:** The review identified one RCT, which found no significant difference in rates of elimination of tubal pregnancy plus tubal preservation, spontaneous intrauterine pregnancy, or repeat ectopic pregnancy at 18 months between multiple dose methotrexate (1 mg/kg on days 1, 2, 4, and 6) plus folic acid compared with laparoscopic salpingostomy (1 RCT, 100 women, elimination of tubal pregnancy plus tubal preservation: RR 1.20, 95% CI 0.93 to 1.40; spontaneous intrauterine pregnancy in 74 women trying to conceive: 12/34 [35%] with methotrexate *v* 16/40 [40%] with laparoscopic salpingostomy; RR 0.89, 95% CI 0.42 to 1.90; repeat ectopic pregnancy: RR 0.77, 95% CI 0.17 to 3.40).[15]

Harms: **Oral methotrexate versus expectant management:** The RCT identified by the review[1] did not report on harms.[12] **Single dose intramuscular methotrexate versus laparoscopic salpingostomy:** The review did not report on adverse events for this comparison.[1] **Multiple dose intramuscular methotrexate versus laparoscopic salpingostomy:** The RCT (100 women) identified by the review[1] found that, compared with laparoscopic salpingostomy, multiple dose methotrexate significantly decreased health related quality of life (physical functioning, role functioning, social functioning, energy, pain, physical symptoms, overall quality of life, and depression; $P < 0.05$).[1]

Comment: **Oral methotrexate versus expectant management:** In the RCT, 23% of women in both treatment groups required surgical management but no details were given in the report of the RCT.[12] **Higher versus lower single dose intramuscular methotrexate:** The review identified one RCT which was published as an abstract only.[16] The RCT found no significant difference in rates of elimination of tubal pregnancy or persistent ectopic pregnancy between 25 and 50 mg/m^2 of intramuscular methotrexate (40 women, elimination of tubal pregnancy: RR 1.30, 95% CI 0.75 to 2.10; persistent ectopic pregnancy: RR 0.75, 0.27 to 2.00).[16]

GLOSSARY

Expectant management A "watch and wait" policy of observation only, involving no immediate intervention to eliminate the ectopic pregnancy. Intervention is indicated if the condition deteriorates or fails to resolve spontaneously.

Fimbrial expression In fimbrial expression (also known as tubal milking) the tubal pregnancy is milked out of the end of the fallopian tube.

Persistent ectopic pregnancy In persistent ectopic pregnancy some of the tissue from the pregnancy remains in the tube and resumes growing.

Salpingectomy In salpingectomy the fallopian tube is surgically removed.

Salpingo-oophorectomy In salpingo-oophorectomy the ovary and the fallopian tube are both surgically removed.

Salpingostomy In salpingostomy (open or laparoscopic), the surgeon makes an incision in the fallopian tube and removes the tubal pregnancy.

REFERENCES

1. Hajenius PJ, Mol BW, Bossuyt PM, et al. Interventions for tubal pregnancy. In: The Cochrane Library, Issue 1, 2003. Oxford: Update Software. Search date not reported; primary sources The Cochrane Library Menstrual Disorders and Subfertility Group trials register and Medline.
2. Korhonen J, Stenman UH, Ylostalo P. Serum human chorionic gonadotrophin dynamics during spontaneous resolution of ectopic pregnancy. *Fertil Steril* 1994;61:632–636.
3. Sau AK, Auld BJ, Mita S. Current status of management of ectopic pregnancy. *Gynaecol Endosc* 1999;8:73–79.
4. Khaleeque F, Siddiqui RI, Jafarey SN. Ectopic pregnancies: a three year study. *J Pak Med Assoc* 2001;51:240–243.
5. Centres for Disease Control. Ectopic pregnancies — United States, 1988–1989. *MMWR Morb Mortal Wkly Rep* 1992;41:591–594.
6. Zane SB, Kieke BA Jr, Kendrick JS, et al. Surveillance in a time of changing health care practices: estimating ectopic pregnancy incidence in the United States. *Matern Child Health J* 2002;6:227–236.
7. Bouyer J, Coste J, Shojaei T, et al. Risk factors for ectopic pregnancy: a comprehensive analysis based on a large case-control, population-based study in France. *Am J Epidemiol* 2003;157:185–194.
8. Ankum WM, Mol BW, Van der Veen F, et al. Risk factors for ectopic pregnancy: a meta-analysis. *Fertil Steril* 1996;65:1093–1099. Search date 1994; primary source Medline, and hand searches of 10 gynaecological journals, five epidemiological journals, and reference lists of identified studies.
9. Peterson H, Xia Z, Hughes JH, et al. The risk of ectopic pregnancy after tubal sterilization. *New Engl J Med* 1997;336:762–767. Search date 1994; primary source Medline.
10. Xiong X, Buekens P, Wollast E. IUD use and the risk of ectopic pregnancy: a meta-analysis of case-control studies. *Contraception* 1995;52:23–34.
11. Goyaux N, Leke R, Keita N, et al. Ectopic pregnancy in African developing countries. *Acta Obstet Gynecol Scand* 2003;82:305–312.
12. Korhonen J, Stenman UH, Ylostalo P. Low-dose oral methotrexate with expectant management of ectopic pregnancy. *Obstet Gynaecol* 1996;88:775–778.
13. Vermesh M, Silva PD, Rosen GF, et al. Management of unruptured ectopic gestation by linear salpingostomy: a prospective randomized clinical trial of laparoscopy versus laparotomy. *Obstet Gynaecol* 1989;73:400–404.
14. Sowter MC, Farquhar CM, Petrie KJ, et al. A randomised trial comparing single dose systemic methotrexate and laparoscopic surgery for the treatment of unruptured ectopic pregnancy. *Br J Obstet Gynaecol* 2001;108:192–203.
15. Hajenius PJ, Engelsbel S, Mol BW, et al. Randomised trial of systemic methotrexate versus laparoscopic salpingostomy in tubal pregnancy. *Lancet* 1997;350:774–779.
16. Yalcinkaya TM, Brown SE, Thomas DW, et al. A comparison of 25 mg/m^2 and 50 mg/m^2 dose of methotrexate for the treatment of ectopic pregnancy. Abstract of the scientific oral and poster sessions of the American Society for Reproductive Medicine, Boston, USA, 1996:0-027.

Bazian Ltd
London
UK

Competing interests: None declared.

Nausea and vomiting in pregnancy

Search date July 2003

Richmal Oates-Whitehead

QUESTIONS

INTERVENTIONS

See glossary Ⓖ

Key Messages

Nausea and vomiting in pregnancy

- **Ginger** Three RCTs and one randomised crossover trial found that ginger reduced nausea and vomiting in early pregnancy. One further RCT found that ginger reduced nausea and dry retching, but had no effect on episodes of vomiting.
- **Acupressure** One systematic review of small RCTs found limited evidence that P6 acupressure reduced self reported morning sickness compared with sham acupressure or no intervention. Three subsequent RCTs and two randomised crossover trials found that P6 acupressure reduced the duration, but not necessarily the intensity, of nausea and vomiting.
- **Antihistamines (H_1 antagonists)** Two systematic reviews found limited evidence that antihistamines reduced nausea and vomiting, with no evidence of teratogenicity.
- **Cyanocobalamin (vitamin B_{12})** One systematic review has found that cyanocobalamin reduces vomiting episodes compared with placebo.
- **Pyridoxine (vitamin B_6)** Two systematic reviews found limited evidence that pyridoxine reduced nausea but found no evidence of an effect on vomiting.
- **Acupuncture** One RCT found that acupuncture reduced nausea and retching compared with no acupuncture, with no evidence of adverse effects. However, an improvement was also found with sham acupuncture compared with no treatment. A second smaller RCT found no significant difference in nausea between acupuncture and sham acupuncture.
- **Dietary interventions (other than ginger)** We found no RCTs of dietary interventions (other than ginger).

- **Phenothiazines** One systematic review found limited evidence that phenothiazines reduced the proportion of women with nausea and vomiting. However, the results were not conclusive. The review found no evidence of teratogenicity.

Hyperemesis gravidarum

- **Acupuncture** One small randomised, crossover RCT found a faster reduction in nausea, as measured on a visual analogue scale, after active PC6 acupuncture compared with sham acupuncture. Episodes of vomiting were also reduced. However, we were unable to draw reliable conclusions from this study.
- **Corticosteroids** One small RCT found no significant improvement in persistent vomiting or readmission to hospital after 1 week of treatment with prednisolone compared with placebo. One small RCT found no significant improvement in persistence of vomiting but found that prednisolone reduced admission to hospital compared with promethazine.
- **Corticotropins** One small RCT found no significant difference in nausea and vomiting between intramuscular corticotropin (adrenocorticotrophic hormone [ACTH]) and placebo.
- **Diazepam** One RCT provided insufficient evidence to assess the effects of diazepam in women with hyperemesis gravidarum.
- **Dietary interventions (other than ginger)** One small crossover RCT found no significant difference in nausea and vomiting after 3 weeks of dietary supplementation with carob seed flour compared with placebo.
- **Ginger** One small RCT provided insufficient evidence to assess the effects of ginger in hyperemesis gravidarum.
- **Ondansetron** One small RCT provided insufficient evidence to assess the effects of ondansetron in hyperemesis gravidarum.

DEFINITION **Nausea and vomiting** are both common in early pregnancy. Although often called "morning sickness", nausea and vomiting can occur at any time of the day and may be constant.[1] Symptoms usually start between 4 and 7 weeks' gestation (one study found this to be the case in 70% of affected women)[2] and stop by 16 weeks in about 90% of women.[1–3] One study found that fewer than 10% of affected women suffer nausea and/or vomiting before the first missed period.[3] Most women do not require treatment. However, persistent vomiting and severe nausea can progress to hyperemesis if the woman is unable to maintain adequate hydration, fluid and electrolyte balance, and nutrition. **Hyperemesis gravidarum** is a diagnosis of exclusion, characterised by prolonged and severe nausea and vomiting, dehydration, and weight loss.[1] Laboratory investigation may show ketosis, hyponatraemia, hypokalaemia, hypouricaemia, metabolic hypochloraemic alkalosis(G), and ketonuria.

INCIDENCE/ PREVALENCE Nausea affects about 70% and vomiting about 60% of pregnant women.[1] The true incidence of hyperemesis gravidarum is not known. It has been documented to range from 3 to 20 per thousand pregnancies. However, most authors report an incidence of 1 in 200.[2]

AETIOLOGY/ RISK FACTORS The causes of nausea and vomiting in pregnancy are unknown. One theory, that they are caused by the rise in human chorionic gonadotrophin concentration, is compatible with the natural history of the condition, its severity in pregnancies affected by hydatidiform mole(G), and its good prognosis (see prognosis below).[4] The aetiology of hyperemesis gravidarum is also uncertain. Again, endocrine and psychological factors are suspected, but evidence is inconclusive.[4]

PROGNOSIS One systematic review (search date 1988) found that nausea and vomiting were associated with a reduced risk of miscarriage (6 studies, 14 564 women; OR 0.36, 95% CI 0.32 to 0.42) but found no association with perinatal mortality.[5] Nausea and vomiting and hyperemesis usually improve over the course of pregnancy, but in one cross sectional observational study 13% of women reported that nausea and vomiting persisted beyond 20 weeks' gestation.[6]

AIMS OF INTERVENTION To reduce the incidence and severity of nausea and vomiting in early pregnancy; to reduce the incidence and severity of hyperemesis gravidarum; to minimise adverse effects of treatment and possible teratogenic effects on the fetus.

OUTCOMES Persistence, severity, or both, of nausea and vomiting episodes as measured on validated scales; maternal mortality; rates of admission and readmission to hospital and duration of hospital stay; incidence and severity of adverse effects of treatment; and incidence of teratogenic effects of treatments on the fetus.

METHODS *Clinical Evidence* search and appraisal July 2003. The author also performed additional searches of the Cochrane Library Issue 2, 2003, Medline, Embase, and Cinahl in April 2003.

QUESTION What are the effects of treatment for nausea and vomiting in early pregnancy?

OPTION ACUPRESSURE

One systematic review of small RCTs has found limited evidence that P6 acupressure reduces self reported morning sickness compared with sham acupressure or no treatment. Three subsequent RCTs and two randomised crossover trials found that P6 acupressure reduced the duration, but not necessarily the intensity, of nausea and vomiting.

Benefits: We found one systematic review (search date 2001, 4 RCTs, 661 women),[7] three subsequent RCTs,[8–10] one additional RCT (excluded because it was small and of poor quality),[11] and two randomised crossover trials.[12,13] The review found that, compared with placebo or sham treatment, acupressure significantly reduced the proportion of women reporting morning sickness (2 RCTs, 404 women; OR 0.35, 95% CI 0.23 to 0.54; see comment below).[7] However, the authors commented that the odds ratio may be an overestimate as the two trials that could not be included in the summary calculation[14,15] found no evidence of effect and one of these RCTs had the highest completion rate of all four trials (92%).[15] The first subsequent RCT (97 women, 8–12 weeks' gestation) found that, compared with a sham acupressure wristband, 4 day administration of acupressure wristband significantly reduced the duration of nausea and vomiting (WMD 1.89 hours/12 hour cycle, 95% CI 0.33 hours/12 hour cycle to 3.45 hours/12 hour cycle), but did not reduce the intensity (measured with a non-graded visual analogue scale ranging from zero to five; WMD +0.25 units, 95% CI −0.12 units to +0.62 units).[8] The second RCT (138 women randomised at 13 weeks of gestation, 110 women analysed) found that acupressure administered via a wristband to the P6 point reduced the frequency and severity of nausea compared with a sham acupressure wristband (data were not provided in a way that allowed further statistical calculation).[9] The third RCT (60 women, with mean gestational ages of 9.8 weeks in the P6 group, 9.6 weeks in the placebo group, and 10.8 weeks for those receiving no treatment) compared acupressure administered via a wristband to the P6 point for 14 days versus sham acupressure and no treatment.[10] On day one, a significant improvement in nausea scores was found with both acupressure and sham acupressure compared with no treatment (acupressure: WMD −2.4 average degree of nausea score, 95% CI −3.78 to −1.02; sham acupressure: WMD −2.00 average degree of nausea score, 95% CI −3.30 to −0.70). By day 6, the significant improvement with acupressure compared with no treatment remained (WMD −2.0, 95% CI −3.37 to −0.63) and there was a trend towards improvement with acupressure compared with sham acupressure (WMD −1.4, 95% CI −2.89 to +0.09; P = 0.07). By day 14, the significant improvement with both acupressure and sham acupressure compared with no treatment was still evident (acupressure: WMD −2.3 average degree of nausea score, 95% CI −3.79 to −0.81; sham acupressure: WMD −1.70 average degree of nausea score, 95% CI −3.25 to −0.15). There was no significant difference between any of the groups in episodes of vomiting at the end of the 14 day treatment. The randomised crossover RCTs (both with 23 women randomised at 16 and 14 weeks of gestation, respectively, 15 [65%] women analysed) found a significant improvement in the severity of nausea with P6 acupressure measured with a 10 cm visual analogue scale compared with sham acupuncture (first study: WMD 1.69 cm, 95% CI 0.32 cm to 3.06 cm; second study provided insufficient data).[12,13]

Harms: None reported.

Comment: Conducting high quality trials in this area is difficult because nausea and vomiting tend to resolve spontaneously and interventions are difficult to mask and to control with credible placebos. The trial with the largest sample size[16] was subsequently described in a paper that questioned the reliability of the randomisation.[17] The type of acupressure differed in the two RCTs included in the summary calculation in the systematic review.[7] In the first included RCT, P6 acupressure was applied as a band applying pressure to the P6 point. Placebo treatment comprised a similar band with the point blunted, not exerting pressure on the P6 point. Each type of band was put on each wrist in sequence. Data for meta-analysis were taken from the third phase, when one group received active treatment to both wrists and the other placebo treatment to both wrists, for 72 hours. In the second RCT included in the review, acupressure to the P6 point was compared with pressure applied to a point close to the right elbow (sham acupressure), both for 5 minutes every 4 hours on four successive mornings. A control group without treatment was asked only to complete a record form.[7]

OPTION ACUPUNCTURE

One RCT found that acupuncture reduced nausea and retching compared with no acupuncture, with no evidence of adverse effects. However, an improvement was also found with sham acupuncture compared with no treatment. A second smaller RCT found no significant difference in nausea between acupuncture and sham acupuncture.

Benefits: We found no systematic review but found two RCTs.[18,19] The first RCT (593 women with nausea and vomiting in early pregnancy) compared weekly traditional acupuncture for 4 weeks versus PC6 acupuncture**G**, sham acupuncture, or no acupuncture.[18] Rates of vomiting did not differ significantly between groups. However, significantly more women receiving traditional, PC6, or sham acupuncture reported improvement in nausea compared with women receiving no acupuncture (see comment below). The improvement compared with no acupuncture was noted after 1 week of treatment with traditional acupuncture (13/135 [10%] with acupuncture *v* 4/127 [3%] with no acupuncture; RR 0.93, 95% CI 0.88 to 0.99; NNT 15, CI not reported), after 2 weeks in women receiving PC6 acupuncture ($P < 0.05$), and after 3 weeks in women receiving sham acupuncture ($P < 0.01$). Women receiving PC6 and sham acupuncture also reported significantly less dry retching compared with no acupuncture ($P < 0.001$). The second RCT (55 women, 6–10 weeks' gestation) found no significant difference in nausea between multisite acupuncture and sham acupuncture ($P = 0.9$).[19]

Harms: A follow up study of the first RCT[18] found no differences between study groups in perinatal outcome, congenital abnormalities, pregnancy complications, or other infant outcomes.[20]

Comment: In the first RCT, the significant improvement in all groups receiving an intervention (traditional acupuncture, PC6 acupuncture, and sham acupuncture) makes it difficult to establish whether the results were influenced by a placebo effect.[18]

OPTION ANTIHISTAMINES (H_1 ANTAGONISTS)

Two systematic reviews found limited evidence that antihistamines reduced nausea and vomiting, with no evidence of teratogenicity.

Benefits: We found two systematic reviews.[7,21] The more recent systematic review (search date 2001, 12 RCTs, 1505 women) found that, compared with placebo, antihistamines as a group significantly reduced nausea (timeframes not specified; OR 0.17, 95% CI 0.13 to 0.21).[7] The earlier systematic review (search date 1998, 7 RCTs, 1190 women) found that H_1 antagonist antihistamines significantly reduced treatment failure (RR 0.34, 95% CI 0.27 to 0.43).[21] However, the conclusions need to be interpreted with care because significant heterogeneity was found between studies.[21]

Harms: The earlier review included 24 controlled studies in > 200 000 women treated between 1960 and 1991.[21] It found no significant increase in teratogenicity with antihistamines (RR 0.76, 95% CI 0.60 to 0.94). The more recent review included three RCTs that gathered evidence on harms from 179 women.[7] It found that antihistamines significantly increased drowsiness (23/94 [24%] with antihistamines *v* 9/85 [11%] with placebo; RR 2.3, 95% CI 1.1 to 4.7; NNH 7, 95% CI 3 to 32).

Comment: The trials identified by the reviews were old and did not provide details on randomisation or concealment strategies.[7,21] The more recent review combined results from trials in which different antihistamines (e.g. buclizine, dimenhydrinate, doxylamine, hydroxyzine, meclozine) were compared with placebo.[7] The earlier review found important heterogeneity in the meta-analysis, which may be attributed to the variety of drugs included.[21] A preparation combining doxylamine plus dicycloverine plus pyridoxine assessed in the reviews was found to reduce nausea and vomiting. However, this preparation was withdrawn from the market in several countries after publication of papers suggesting teratogenicity, although such claims have subsequently been refuted.

OPTION CYANOCOBALAMIN (VITAMIN B_{12})

One systematic review has found that cyanocobalamin reduces vomiting episodes compared with placebo.

Benefits: We found one systematic review (search date 1998, 2 RCTs, 1018 women).[21] It found that cyanocobalamin (oral vitamin B_{12}) significantly reduced vomiting episodes compared with placebo (timeframes not specified; RR 0.49, 95% CI 0.28 to 0.86).[21]

Harms: The review searched for controlled trials addressing potential teratogenicity of cyanocobalamin and found no evidence of this.[21]

Comment: The conclusions of the review are mostly based on one RCT, which accounted for 1000 women and used a daily dose of a multivitamin compound that contained 4 μg cyanocobalamin in each tablet.[22] The smaller RCT used a dose of cyanocobalamin of 25 μg orally twice daily for 7 days (Jewell D, personal communication, 2001). It is believed that the combination of cyanocobalamin plus folic acid may prevent neural tube defects.

OPTION DIETARY INTERVENTIONS (OTHER THAN GINGER)

We found no RCTs of dietary interventions (other than ginger).

Benefits: We found no systematic review or RCTs.

Harms: We found no systematic review or RCTs.

Comment: None.

OPTION GINGER

Three RCTs and one randomised crossover trial found that ginger reduced nausea and vomiting in early pregnancy. One further RCT found that ginger reduced nausea and dry retching, but had no effect on episodes of vomiting.

Benefits: We found no systematic review. We found three RCTs[23–25] and one randomised crossover trial[26] examining the use of ginger as an antiemetic in early pregnancy. The first RCT (70 women of < 17 weeks gestation) compared 250 mg of ginger in oral capsules taken four times daily versus placebo.[23] It found that ginger significantly reduced the proportion of women with vomiting after 4 days compared with placebo (12/32 [38%] with ginger *v* 23/35 [66%] with placebo; RR 0.57, 95% CI 0.34 to 0.95; NNT 4, 95% CI 2 to 12), and significantly reduced symptoms (non-specifically described) after 7 days (28/32 [88%] with ginger *v* 10/35 [29%] with placebo; RR 0.18, 95% CI 0.07 to 0.45; NNT 2, CI not reported). The second RCT (26 women with gestational age < 13 weeks) compared 15 ml of ginger syrup containing 250 mg of ginger taken four times daily versus placebo.[24] After 6 days, significantly more women had stopped vomiting with ginger (8/12 [67%] with ginger *v* 2/10 [20%] with placebo; RR 0.42, 95% CI 0.18 to 0.98; NNT 2, CI not reported). The third RCT (120 women with gestational age ranging between 5.5 weeks and 18 weeks compared 125 mg of ginger in oral capsules taken four times daily for four days versus placebo.[25] It found that ginger significantly reduced nausea severity scores over each of the 4 treatment days (reported as significant, results presented graphically). It also significantly reduced dry retching, but only on the first 2 days of treatment (reported as significant, no further data reported). Ginger had no significant effect on episodes of vomiting (reported as non-significant, no further data reported). The randomised crossover trial (30 women) compared 250 mg of ginger in oral capsules taken four times daily for 4 days versus placebo.[26] It found that ginger significantly reduced nausea and vomiting severity scores compared with placebo (P = 0.035).

Harms: The first RCT found no significant difference in spontaneous abortions between ginger and placebo (1/32 [3%] with ginger *v* 3/38 [8%] with placebo; P = 0.4), but the sample size may have been too small to rule out a clinically important difference.[23] The third RCT found that the most serious adverse effect was heartburn and reflux (no data available to establish a comparison between groups).[25]

Comment: Ginger used for the first RCT[23] and the randomised crossover trial[26] was derived from fresh ginger roots and given in capsules. The authors of the RCT warn that different presentations of ginger may have a different magnitude of effects. The active ingredient that improves nausea and vomiting has not been isolated.[23]

OPTION PHENOTHIAZINES

One systematic review found limited evidence that phenothiazines reduced the proportion of women with nausea and vomiting. However, the results were not conclusive. The review found no evidence of teratogenicity.

Benefits: We found one systematic review (search date 1998, 3 RCTs, 398 women).[21] It found that, compared with placebo, phenothiazines significantly reduced the proportion of women with nausea or vomiting (timeframes not specified; RR 0.31, 95% CI 0.24 to 0.42). One of the RCTs recruited women after the first trimester of pregnancy. After excluding this RCT, the results favouring phenothiazines remained significant. The review found that phenothiazines significantly reduced treatment failure compared with placebo (definition not reported; 26/145 [18%] with phenothiazines *v* 89/139 [64%] with placebo; RR 0.28, 95% CI 0.19 to 0.41; NNT 3, 95% CI 2 to 3).

Harms: The review assessed harms, gathering evidence from seven controlled observational trials (78 440 women), which found no evidence of teratogenicity (RR 1.00, 95% CI 0.84 to 1.18).[21] However, harms associated with different phenothiazines vary, making it difficult to interpret a summary analysis.

Comment: The trials identified by the review were old and lacked sufficient information to appraise the quality of randomisation or allocation concealment. Only two RCTs provided support for the review's conclusions and the analysis in the review combined results for different phenothiazines. It should therefore be viewed with caution.

OPTION PYRIDOXINE (VITAMIN B_6)

Two systematic reviews of pyridoxine found limited evidence that pyridoxine reduced nausea but found no evidence of an effect on vomiting. One review found no evidence of teratogenicity.

Benefits: We found two systematic reviews.[7,21] The first review (search date 1998, 3 RCTs, 949 women) found that pyridoxine had similar "failure rates" compared with placebo (3 RCTs, 949 women; RR 0.97, 95% CI 0.78 to 1.20; see comment below).[21] However, pyridoxine significantly improved nausea scores (2 RCTs, 395 women; WMD 0.92, 95% CI 0.44 to 1.40). The second systematic review (search date 2001, 2 RCTs, 392 women) compared pyridoxine versus placebo or no treatment.[7] It found that pyridoxine did not significantly reduce vomiting (timeframes not specified; OR 0.91, 95% CI 0.60 to 1.38) but significantly reduced nausea (change in a 10 cm visual analogue scale; WMD 0.9 cm, 95% CI 0.4 cm to 1.4 cm).

Harms: The first review searched for evidence on harms (search date 1998, 1 cohort study, 1369 women).[21] It found no significant increase in major fetal malformations attributable to pyridoxine (RR 1.05, 95% CI 0.60 to 1.84).[21]

Comment: The first review[21] included one RCT in which the nature of randomisation was unclear.[7] The remaining two RCTs were included in both reviews.[7,21] "Failure rates" were defined in various subjective ways and included failure to achieve resolution or a clinically important improvement in symptoms.[21]

QUESTION What are the effects of treatments for hyperemesis gravidarum?

OPTION ACUPUNCTURE

One small randomised crossover RCT found a faster reduction in nausea, as measured on a visual analogue scale, after active PC6 acupuncture compared with sham acupuncture. Episodes of vomiting were also reduced. However, we were unable to draw reliable conclusions from this study.

Nausea and vomiting in pregnancy

Benefits: We found no systematic review or RCTs. We found one crossover RCT (50 women admitted to hospital with vomiting and gestational age range between 6 and 16 weeks, comparing PC6 acupuncture versus sham acupuncture.[27] PC6 acupuncture was applied 5 mm beneath the skin at days 1, 2, 5, and 6 and evaluated at the eighth day, while sham acupuncture was applied 1–2 mm beneath the skin on the lateral side of the forearm. Both interventions were given three times daily for 30 minutes.[27] All women were vomiting on the day of randomisation. The RCT found that women receiving acupuncture had a significantly faster resolution of nausea than women receiving sham acupuncture (P = 0.032). No significant differences were found between groups with regard to food intake and the need for intravenous fluids.[27]

Harms: No adverse effects were reported.

Comment: The placebo treatment (sham acupuncture) used in the RCT was superficial acupuncture on an area away from a "real" acupuncture point. Needles were inserted only 1–2 mm into the skin. The authors of the RCT state that this kind of stimulation minimises the specific effects of acupuncture.[27] However, it may not be an entirely inert placebo, as some sensory stimulation does occur.

OPTION CORTICOTROPINS

One small RCT found no significant difference in nausea and vomiting between intramuscular corticotropin (adrenocorticotrophic hormone [ACTH]) and placebo.

Benefits: We found two systematic reviews of corticotropins in hyperemesis gravidarum, which identified the same single RCT (search dates 1998[21] and 2001;[7] 1 RCT, 32 women whose gestational ages and severity of hyperemesis were not described). The RCT compared 0.5 mg of intramuscular corticotropin versus placebo.[28] It found no significant difference between intramuscular corticotropin and placebo in nausea relief scores (measured on a scale ranging from 15 denoting a lack of nausea to 20 denoting the worst possible hyperemesis; WMD +0.6 mean relief score, 95% CI –1.65 to +2.85). There was no significant difference between groups in the time from starting treatment to stopping vomiting, and all women stopped vomiting while in hospital. Women remained at hospital for at least 10 days. There was no significant difference between groups in the number of readmissions to hospital.

Harms: The systematic reviews reported no adverse effects.[7,21]

Comment: None.

OPTION CORTICOSTEROIDS

One small RCT found no significant improvement in persistent vomiting or readmission to hospital after 1 week of treatment with prednisolone compared with placebo. One small RCT found no significant improvement in persistence of vomiting but found that prednisolone reduced admission to hospital compared with promethazine.

Benefits: We found two systematic reviews and one subsequent RCT.[7,21,29] The two reviews identified the same single RCT (search dates 1998[21] and 2001[7]; 1 RCT, 40 women). **Versus placebo:** The subsequent RCT (25 women with severe hyperemesis, mean gestational age of 10.6 weeks for prednisolone and 8.3 weeks for placebo) compared oral prednisolone 20 mg twice daily versus placebo for 1 week.[29] Oral prednisolone had no significant effect on persistent vomiting (5/12 [42%] with prednisolone *v* 7/12 [58%] with placebo; RR 1.4 95% CI 0.6 to

3.2) or on subsequent readmission to hospital (5/12 [42%] with prednisolone *v* 8/12 [67%] with placebo; RR 1.6, 95% CI 0.7 to 3.5). **Versus promethazine:** The RCT identified by the reviews compared oral methylprednisolone versus promethazine (40 women admitted to hospital at < 16 weeks' gestation).[30] It found that methylprednisolone had no significant effect on persistence of vomiting compared with promethazine (OR 1.56, 95% CI 0.25 to 9.94). However, there was a reduction in rates of subsequent admission to hospital (0/17 [0%] with methylprednisolone *v* 5/18 [28%] with promethazine; OR 0.11, 95% CI 0.02 to 0.71).

Harms: The first review also included controlled observational studies (8 studies, 109 602 women) and found no evidence of teratogenicity (RR 1.24, 95% CI 0.97 to 1.60).[21]

Comment: The rates of spontaneous resolution of symptoms in control groups were high. The possible benefit (based on a single small trial)[30] of methylprednisolone in preventing subsequent admission to hospital must be balanced against possible adverse effects of steroids given in the first trimester of pregnancy. The subsequent RCT was too small to rule out a clinically important effect.[29]

OPTION DIAZEPAM

One RCT provided insufficient evidence to assess the effects of diazepam in women with hyperemesis gravidarum.

Benefits: We found one systematic review (search date 2001, 1 RCT, 50 women admitted to hospital)[7] comparing intravenous fluids containing a multivitamin preparation with or without diazepam 20 mg daily. After symptoms settled, women were randomised to receive oral diazepam 5 mg twice daily for 1 week or placebo. The trial found no significant difference in persistence of vomiting after 2 days of treatment (assessment not clearly specified; OR 0.64, 95% CI 0.10 to 4.19), but reported a difference in rates of readmission to hospital (4% with diazepam *v* 27% with placebo; detailed figures not reported).[7]

Harms: The trial did not report on adverse effects or acceptability of treatment.

Comment: The trial was too small to draw reliable conclusions. The rate of resolution in the control group was high and the effects of the vitamins used in the RCT are unknown.

OPTION DIETARY INTERVENTIONS (OTHER THAN GINGER)

One small crossover RCT found no significant difference in nausea and vomiting after 3 weeks of dietary supplementation with carob seed flour compared with placebo.

Benefits: We found no systematic review. We found one crossover RCT (43 women), which compared 1 g daily of a powder containing 96.5% carob seed flour plus 3.5% calcium lactate versus placebo for 3 weeks.[31] It found no significant difference in relief of vomiting (subjective improvement: 20/34 [59%] with carob seed flour *v* 18/36 [50%] with placebo; RR 1.18, 95% CI 0.82 to 1.70].[31]

Harms: The RCT found no adverse effects.[31]

Comment: The trial was conducted in 1966. It is unclear whether the composition of carob seed flour now commercially available will be the same as was used in the trial.[31]

OPTION GINGER

One small RCT provided insufficient evidence on the effects of ginger.

Benefits: We found one systematic review (search date 2001, 1 crossover RCT, 27 women), which compared ginger 250 mg in oral capsules taken four times daily versus placebo.[7] After 4 days of treatment the RCT found no improvement in a hyperemesis score that evaluated the degree of nausea, vomiting, and weight loss (WMD +3.15, 95% CI –0.92 to +7.22).

Harms: The RCT found no adverse effects.

Comment: The trial reported results before crossover but it was too small to allow reliable conclusions.

OPTION ONDANSETRON

One small RCT provided evidence to assess the effects of ondansetron in hyperemesis gravidarum.

Benefits: **Versus placebo:** We found no systematic review or RCTs. **Versus promethazine:** We found one systematic review (search date 2001, 1 RCT, 27 women admitted to hospital).[7] The RCT compared ondansetron 10 mg versus promethazine 50 mg, both given by 50 mL solution over 30 minutes. Subsequent doses were given as needed every 8 hours until the woman was able to eat a bland diet. The RCT found no significant difference in persistence of vomiting between ondansetron and promethazine (2/15 [13%] with ondansetron *v* 3/12 [25%] with promethazine; OR 0.33, 95% CI 0.04 to 2.60).[7]

Harms: The RCT gave no information on adverse effects.[7]

Comment: The RCT was too small to draw reliable conclusions.[7]

GLOSSARY

Acupressure Pressure applied to a specific point of the body. It does not require needles and can be administered by patients themselves. Commercial products available include an elastic band to fit around the wrist with a plastic disc to apply pressure at the P6 point.
Hydatidiform mole A condition in which there is abnormal cystic development of the placenta. The uterus is often large for the duration of pregnancy and there may be vaginal bleeding, lack of fetal movement and fetal heart sounds, and severe nausea and vomiting. Rarer, but important, complications include haemorrhage, intrauterine infection, raised blood pressure, and persistent gestational trophoblastic disease, which may infiltrate local tissues or metastasise to distant sites.
Metabolic hypochloraemic alkalosis Excess base alkali in the body fluids caused by chloride loss.
P6 acupressure Pressure is applied at the P6 (Neiguan) point on the volar aspect of the wrist.
PC6 acupuncture The needle is applied at the PC6 point located near to the wrist crease.

REFERENCES

1. Nelson-Piercy C. Treatment of nausea and vomiting in pregnancy. When should it be treated and what can be safely taken? *Drug Saf* 1998;19:155–164.
2. Eliakim R, Abulafia O, Sherer DM. Hyperemesis gravidarum: a current review. *Am J Perinatol* 2000;17:207–218.
3. Gadsby R, Barnie-Adshead AM, Jagger C. A prospective study of nausea and vomiting during pregnancy. *Br J Gen Pract* 1993;43:245–248.
4. Baron TH, Ramirez B, Richter JE. Gastrointestinal motility disorders during pregnancy. *Ann Intern Med* 1993;118:366–375.
5. Weigel MM, Weigel RM. Nausea and vomiting of early pregnancy and pregnancy outcome. A meta-analytical review. *Br J Obstet Gynaecol* 1989;96:1312–1318. Search date 1988; primary sources Medline and hand searches of references cited in identified articles.

6. Whitehead SA, Andrews PLR, Chamberlain GVP. Characterisation of nausea and vomiting in early pregnancy: a survey of 1000 women. *J Obstet Gynaecol* 1992;12:364–369.
7. Jewell D, Young G. Interventions for nausea and vomiting in early pregnancy. In: The Cochrane Library, Issue 3, 2001. Oxford: Update Software. Search date 2001; primary sources Cochrane Pregnancy and Childbirth Group Trials Register and the Cochrane Controlled Trials Register.
8. Norheim AJ, Pedersen EJ, Fønnebø V, et al. Acupressure treatment of morning sickness in pregnancy: a randomised, double-blind, placebo-controlled study. *Scand J Prim Health Care* 2001;19:43–47.
9. Steele NM, French J, Gatherer-Boyles J, et al. Effect of acupressure by Sea-Bands on nausea and vomiting of pregnancy. *J Obstet Gynecol Neonatal Nurs* 2001;30:61–70.
10. Werntoft E, Dykes A-K. Effect of acupressure on nausea and vomiting during pregnancy: a randomised controlled, pilot study. *J Reprod Med* 2001;46:835 839.
11. Stone CL. Acupressure wristbands for the nausea of pregnancy. *Nurse Pract* 1993;18:15.
12. Bayreuther J, Lewith GT, Pickering R. A double-blind cross-over study to evaluate the effectiveness of acupressure at pericardium 6 (P6) in the treatment of early morning sickness (EMS). *Complement Ther Med* 1994;2:70–76.
13. Evans AT, Samuels SN, Marshall C, et al. Suppression of pregnancy-induced nausea and vomiting with sensory afferent stimulation. *J Reprod Med* 1993;38:603–606.
14. Belluomini J, Litt RC, Lee KA, et al. Acupressure for nausea and vomiting of pregnancy: a randomized, blinded study. *Obstet Gynecol* 1994;84:245–248.
15. O'Brien B, Relyea MJ, Taerum T. Efficacy of P6 acupressure in the treatment of nausea and vomiting during pregnancy. *Am J Obstet Gynecol* 1996;174:708–715.
16. Dundee JW, Sourial FBR, Ghaly RG, et al. P6 acupressure reduces morning sickness. *J R Soc Med* 1988;81:456–457.
17. Dundee J, McMillan C. Some problems encountered in the scientific evaluation of acupuncture emesis. *Acupunct Med* 1992;10:2–8.
18. Smith C, Crowther C, Beilby J. Pregnancy outcome following women's participation in a randomised controlled trial of acupuncture to treat nausea and vomiting in early pregnancy. *Complement Ther Med* 2002;10:78–83.
19. Knight B, Mudge C, Openshaw S, et al. Effect of acupuncture on nausea of pregnancy: a randomized, controlled trial. *Obstet Gynecol* 2001;97:184–188.
20. Smith C, Crowther C, Beilby J. Pregnancy outcome following women's participation in a randomised controlled trial of acupuncture to treat nausea and vomiting in early pregnancy. *Complement Ther Med* 2002;10:78–83
21. Mazzotta P, Magee LA. A risk–benefit assessment of pharmacological and nonpharmacological treatments for nausea and vomiting of pregnancy. *Drugs* 2000;59:781–800. Search date 1998; primary sources Medline, Pregnancy and Childbirth Module of the Cochrane Database of Systematic Reviews, hand searches of bibliographies of retrieved papers, standard toxicology text (Drugs in Pregnancy and Lactation), and personal contact with pharmaceutical companies, researchers, and clinicians in the fields of pharmacology, toxicology, obstetrics, and paediatrics.
22. Czeizel AE, Dudas I, Fritz G, et al. The effect of periconceptional multivitamin-mineral supplementation on vertigo, nausea and vomiting in the first trimester of pregnancy. *Arch Gynecol Obstet* 1992;251:181–185.
23. Vutyavanich T, Kraisarin T, Ruangsri R. Ginger for nausea and vomiting in pregnancy: randomized, double-masked, placebo-controlled trial. *Obstet Gynaecol* 97;2001:577–582.
24. Keating A, Chez RA. Ginger syrup as an antiemetic in early pregnancy. *Altern Ther Health Med* 2002;8:89–91.
25. Willetts K, Ekangaki A, Eden J. Effect of a ginger extract on pregnancy-induced nausea: a randomised controlled trial. *Aust N Z J Obstet Gynaecol* 2003;43:139–144.
26. Fischer-Rasmussen W, Kjaer SK, Dahl C, et al. Ginger treatment of hyperemesis gravidarum. *Eur J Obstet Gynecol Reprod Biol* 1990;38:19–24.
27. Carlsson CP, Axemo P, Bodin A, et al. Manual acupuncture reduces hyperemesis gravidarum: a placebo-controlled, randomized, single-blind, crossover study. *J Pain Symptom Manage* 2000;20:273–279.
28. Ylikorkala O, Kauppila A, Ollanketo ML. Intramuscular ACTH or placebo in the treatment of hyperemesis gravidarum. *Acta Obstet Gynecol Scand* 1979;58:453–455.
29. Nelson-Piercy C, Fayers P, de Swiet M. Randomised, double-blind, placebo-controlled trial of corticosteroids for the treatment of hyperemesis gravidarum. *Br J Obstet Gynaecol* 2001;108:9–15.
30. Safari HR, Fassett MJ, Souter IC, et al. The efficacy of methylprednisolone in the treatment of hypermesis gravidarum: a randomized, double-blind, controlled study. *Am J Obstet Gynecol* 1998;179:921–924.
31. General Practitioner's Research Group. Hyperemesis treated with a pharmacologically inert compound. *Practitioner* 1966;196:711–714.

Richmal Oates-Whitehead
Clinical Editor/Editor Cochrane Heart Group
BMJ Knowledge
BMA House
London
UK

Competing interests: None declared.

Perineal care

Search date April 2004

Chris Kettle

QUESTIONS

INTERVENTIONS

THIRD AND FOURTH DEGREE TEARS

Unknown effectiveness

To be covered in future updates

Postnatal interventions to reduce morbidity associated with perineal trauma

Third trimester and intrapartum perineal massage

Water births

See glossaryⒼ

Key Messages

Intrapartum surgical interventions

- **Restrictive use of episiotomy (reduces risk of posterior trauma compared with routine use)** One systematic review found that restricting episiotomy to specific fetal and maternal indications reduced the rates of posterior perineal trauma, need for suturing, and healing complications compared with routine use, but increased the rates of anterior vaginal and labial trauma, which carries minimal morbidity.
- **Vacuum extraction (less perineal trauma than with forceps but newborns have increased risk of cephalhaematoma)** One systematic review and subsequent RCTs found that vacuum extraction reduced the rate of severe perineal trauma compared with forceps delivery, but increased the incidence of neonatal cephalhaematoma and retinal haemorrhage.
- **Midline episiotomy incision (associated with higher risk of third or fourth degree tears compared with mediolateral incision)** We found no evidence that midline episiotomy incision improved perineal pain or wound dehiscence compared with mediolateral incision. Limited evidence from one quasi-randomised trial suggested that midline incision may increase the risk of third and fourth degree tears compared with mediolateral incision.
- **Epidural anaesthesia (increases instrumental delivery, which is associated with increased rates of perineal trauma)** One systematic review found no direct evidence about the effects of epidural compared with other forms of anaesthesia on rates of perineal trauma. However, RCTs identified by the review found that epidural anaesthesia maintained beyond the first stage of labour compared with epidural restricted to the first stage of labour increased the risk of instrumental delivery, which in turn is associated with an increased risk of perineal trauma.

Intrapartum non-surgical interventions

- **Continuous support during labour (reduces operative vaginal birth compared with usual care)** One systematic review found that providing continuous support for women during childbirth reduced the rate of operative vaginal birth (vacuum extraction or forceps) compared with usual care. It found no significant difference in the overall rates of episiotomy or perineal trauma (defined as episiotomy or laceration requiring suturing).
- **Upright versus supine or lithotomy position during delivery (fewer episiotomies but more second degree tears than supine or lithotomy positions)** One systematic review found that any upright position for delivery marginally reduced episiotomies compared with supine or lithotomy positions but this was offset by an increase in second degree tears. Rates of assisted vaginal delivery were slightly reduced in the upright group.
- **"Hands poised" versus "hands on" method of delivery (increases pain and need for manual delivery of placenta, no significant difference in rate of perineal trauma, and reduces episiotomy rate)** One multicentre RCT and one quasi-randomised trial found that the "hands poised" method (not touching the baby's head or supporting the mother's perineum) reduced episiotomy rates

compared with the conventional "hands on" method (applying pressure to the baby's head during delivery and supporting the mother's perineum). The RCT found no evidence of an effect on the risk of perineal trauma, but found that the "hands poised" group had an increased risk of requiring manual removal of the placenta and higher rates of short term perineal pain.

- **Passive descent in the second stage of labour** One RCT comparing passive fetal descent versus immediate active pushing found no significant difference in perineal trauma.
- **Sustained breath holding (Valsalva) method of pushing** One systematic review of two poor quality controlled clinical trials found no significant difference in the extent or rate of perineal trauma between sustained breath holding (Valsalva) and spontaneous exhalatory methods of pushing during the second stage of labour.

First and second degree tears

- **Absorbable synthetic sutures for perineal repair of first and second degree tears and episiotomies (reduced short term pain compared with catgut sutures)** One systematic review found that absorbable synthetic sutures reduced pain at up to 10 days after birth compared with catgut sutures. One subsequent RCT, however, found no significant difference in perineal pain at 3 days, although it may have lacked power to detect a clinically important effect. The systematic review and the subsequent RCT found no significant difference between absorbable synthetic sutures and catgut sutures in pain or dyspareunia at 3 months, but one RCT with 12 months' follow up, which was included in the review, found lower rates of dyspareunia with absorbable synthetic sutures. RCTs found no significant difference between rapidly absorbed and standard synthetic sutures in overall perineal pain, pain on sitting, or dyspareunia. RCTs also found reduced perineal pain on walking and a reduction in suture material removal with rapidly absorbed synthetic sutures.
- **Continuous subcutaneous technique of perineal skin closure of first and second degree tears and episiotomies (reduced short term pain compared with interrupted sutures)** One systematic review found that continuous subcuticular sutures for perineal skin reduced short term pain compared with interrupted sutures, but found no significant difference in perineal pain or dyspareunia at 3 months postpartum. One RCT found that a loose continuous technique for repair of all layers reduced short term perineal pain and suture removal compared with interrupted sutures up to 3 months postpartum.
- **Non-suturing of perineal skin in first and second degree tears and episiotomies (reduces dyspareunia)** One large RCT found no significant difference between leaving the perineal skin unsutured compared with conventional suturing in pain at 10 days after birth. A second RCT found that non-suturing reduced pain for up to 3 months after delivery. Both RCTs found that non-suturing of the perineal skin reduced dyspareunia at 3 months after birth.
- **Non-suturing of muscle and skin in first and second degree perineal tears (poorer wound healing than with suturing)** Two small RCTs found no significant difference in short term perineal pain between non-suturing and suturing of first and second degree tears. One of the RCTs found no significant difference in healing between groups but the second RCT found that a greater proportion of women in the non-sutured group had poorer wound healing at 6 weeks after birth.

Third and fourth degree tears

- **Different methods and materials for repair of third and fourth degree tears** One small RCT comparing the overlap method versus the end-to-end method for primary repair of third degree obstetric tears found no significant difference in perineal discomfort and a non-significant reduction in the rate of reported faecal urgency and anal incontinence with the overlap technique compared with the end-to-end method.

DEFINITION Perineal trauma is any damage to the genitalia during childbirth that occurs spontaneously or intentionally by surgical incision (episiotomy). Anterior perineal trauma is injury to the labia, anterior vagina, urethra, or clitoris, and is usually associated with little morbidity. Posterior perineal trauma is any injury to the posterior vaginal wall, perineal muscles, or anal sphincter. First degree spontaneous tears involve only skin; second degree tears involve perineal muscles; third degree tears partially or completely disrupt the anal sphincter; and fourth degree tears completely disrupt the external and internal anal sphincter and epithelium.[1]

INCIDENCE/ PREVALENCE Over 85% of women having a vaginal birth sustain some form of perineal trauma,[2] and 60–70% receive stitches — equivalent to 400 000 women a year in the UK in 1997.[2,3] There are wide variations in rates of episiotomy: 8% in the Netherlands, 14% in England, 50% in the USA, and 99% in east European countries.[4–6] Sutured spontaneous tears are reported in about a third of women in the USA[6] and the UK,[7] but this is probably an underestimate because of inconsistency of reporting and classification of perineal trauma. The incidence of anal sphincter tears varies between 0.5% in the UK, 2.5% in Denmark, and 7% in Canada.[8]

AETIOLOGY/ RISK FACTORS Perineal trauma occurs during spontaneous or assisted vaginal delivery and is usually more extensive after the first vaginal delivery.[1] Associated risk factors also include increased fetal size, mode of delivery, and malpresentation and malposition of the fetus. Other maternal factors that may increase the extent and degree of trauma are ethnicity (white people are probably at greater risk than black people), older age, abnormal collagen synthesis, and poor nutritional state.[9] Clinicians' practices or preferences in terms of intrapartum interventions may influence the severity and rate of perineal trauma (e.g. use of ventouse *v* forceps).

PROGNOSIS Perineal trauma affects women's physical, psychological, and social wellbeing in the immediate postnatal period as well as the long term. It can also disrupt breast feeding, family life, and sexual relations. In the UK, about 23–42% of women will continue to have pain and discomfort for 10–12 days postpartum, and 7–10% of women will continue to have long term pain (3–18 months after delivery);[2,3,10] 23% of women will experience superficial dyspareunia at 3 months; 3–10% will report faecal incontinence;[11,12] and up to 24% will have urinary problems.[2,3] Complications depend on the severity of perineal trauma and on the effectiveness of treatment.

AIMS OF INTERVENTION To reduce the rate and severity of trauma; to improve the short and long term maternal morbidity associated with perineal injury and repair.

OUTCOMES Quality of life; incidence and severity of perineal trauma; rates of episiotomy, assisted vaginal delivery (indirectly associated with an increased risk of episiotomy and perineal trauma especially with forceps delivery); psychological trauma; short and long term perineal pain; blood loss; infection; wound dehiscence; superficial dyspareunia; stress incontinence; faecal incontinence; adverse effects of treatment.

METHODS *Clinical Evidence* search and appraisal April 2004.

QUESTION What are the effects of intrapartum surgical interventions on rates of perineal trauma?

OPTION RESTRICTIVE VERSUS ROUTINE USE OF EPISIOTOMY

One systematic review found that restricting episiotomy to specific fetal and maternal indications reduced the rates of posterior perineal trauma, need for suturing, and healing complications compared with routine use, but increased the rates of anterior vaginal and labial trauma, which carries minimal morbidity.

Benefits: We found one systematic review (search date not reported, 6 RCTs, 4850 women) comparing restricted versus routine episiotomy.[13] In the routine episiotomy group 1752/2409 (73%) women had an episiotomy compared with 673/2441 (28%) women in the restricted group. The review found that restricted use of episiotomy was associated with significantly lower rates of posterior perineal trauma, less perineal pain at discharge from hospital, less suturing, and fewer healing complications compared with routine use of episiotomy (posterior perineal trauma, 4 RCTs, 2079 women: 744/1039 [72%] with restricted *v* 849/1040 [82%] with routine; RR 0.88, 95% CI 0.84 to 0.92; NNT 10,

95% CI 8 to 16; perineal pain at discharge from hospital, 1 RCT, 2422 women: 371/1207 [31%] with restricted v 516/1215 [42%] with routine; RR 0.72, 95% CI 0.65 to 0.81; NNT 9, 95% CI 7 to 12; suturing, 5 RCTs, 4133 women: 1327/2080 [64%] with restricted v 1768/2053 [86%] with routine; RR 0.74, 95% CI 0.71 to 0.77; NNT 4, 95% CI 4 to 5; healing complications, 1 RCT, 1119 women: 114/555 [21%] with restricted v 168/564 [30%] with routine; RR 0.69, 95% CI 0.56 to 0.85; NNT 11, 95% CI 7 to 23). The review found no significant difference between groups in overall rates of severe vaginal or perineal trauma, dyspareunia within 3 months or dyspareunia in the next 3 years, or urinary incontinence at 3 months (severe vaginal or perineal trauma, 3 RCTs, 4284 women: 87/2155 [4.0%] with restricted v 77/2129 [3.6%] with routine; RR 1.11, 95% CI 0.83 to 1.50; dyspareunia within 3 months, 1 RCT, 895 women: 96/438 [22%] with restricted v 82/457 [18%] with routine; RR 1.22, 95% CI 0.94 to 1.59; dyspareunia in the next 3 years, 1 RCT, 674 women: 52/329 [16%] with restricted v 45/345 [13%] with routine; RR 1.21, 95% CI 0.84 to 1.75; and urinary incontinence at 3 months, 2 RCTs, 1569 women: 140/775 [18%] with restricted v 147/794 [19%] with routine; RR 0.98, 95% CI 0.79 to 1.20).[13]

Harms: We found no reports of serious adverse effects associated with restricted use of episiotomy apart from higher rates of anterior perineal trauma, which carries minimal morbidity (4 RCTs, 4342 women; 425/2144 [20%] with restricted v 243/2198 [11%] with routine; RR 1.79, 95% CI 1.55 to 2.07; NNH 11, 95% CI 9 to 16).[13]

Comment: The six RCTs included in the review varied in quality. The method of randomisation was not clear in one trial. All trials performed intention to treat analysis. The trials took place in the UK, Canada, and Argentina. The types of episiotomy performed were mediolateral in five of the trials and midline in the sixth.

OPTION MIDLINE VERSUS MEDIOLATERAL EPISIOTOMY INCISION

We found no evidence that midline episiotomy incision improved perineal pain or wound dehiscence compared with mediolateral incision. Limited evidence from one quasi-randomised trial suggested that midline incision may increase the risk of third and fourth degree tears compared with mediolateral incision.

Benefits: We found no systematic review comparing mediolateral versus midline episiotomy incisions. We found one quasi-randomised trial (407 primigravidas, 24% withdrawals)[14] and one abstract (no detailed data)[15] comparing midline versus mediolateral episiotomies. These were of poor quality and found no evidence of a difference in perineal pain or wound dehiscence. Women who had had a midline episiotomy experienced significantly less perineal bruising and resumed sexual intercourse earlier.

Harms: The quasi-randomised trial found that midline episiotomies significantly increased the risk of third or fourth degree tears (39/163 [24%] with midline episiotomy v 22/244 [9%] with mediolateral episiotomy; RR 2.7, 95% CI 1.6 to 4.3; NNH 6, 95% CI 4 to 13).[14] However, these results have to be approached with care because the study limitations compromise their validity. Two retrospective cohort studies, including 5376 primiparous and 341 multiparous women, also found that midline episiotomies were associated with a fourfold increased risk of third and fourth degree tears after allowing for multiple confounders (CI not reported).[16,17]

Comment: It is claimed that midline incision is easier to repair and that it is associated with less blood loss, better healing, less pain, and earlier resumption of sexual intercourse. We found no reliable evidence to support these claims. One of the trials had an increased risk of selection bias because of quasi-random treatment allocation and because analysis was not by intention to treat.[14] The other trial did not describe the method of treatment allocation.[15]

OPTION EPIDURAL ANAESTHESIA

One systematic review found no direct evidence about the effects of epidural compared with other forms of anaesthesia on rates of perineal trauma. However, RCTs identified by the review found that epidural anaesthesia maintained beyond the first stage of labour compared with epidural restricted to the first stage of labour increased the risk of instrumental delivery, which in turn is associated with an increased risk of perineal trauma.

Benefits: We found one systematic review (search date not reported, 11 RCTs comparing epidural anaesthesia *v* other forms of analgesia, 3157 women).[18] The RCTs did not report the incidence of perineal trauma. Six RCTs (1252 women) reported rates of instrumental delivery when the epidural block was maintained beyond the first stage of labour. The review found that epidurals significantly increased the risk of instrumental delivery compared with non-epidural (6 RCTs: 168/628 [26.8%] with epidural analgesia *v* 102/624 [16.3%] with non-epidural analgesia; OR 2.03, 95% CI 1.51 to 2.73).[18] Two RCTs (131 women) reported rates of instrumental delivery when the epidural block was restricted to the first stage of labour. The review found no significant difference in the risk of instrumental delivery between epidural analgesia compared with non-epidural analgesia (2 RCTs: 18/67 [27%] with epidural analgesia *v* 14/64 [22%] with non-epidural analgesia; OR 1.30, 95% CI 0.59 to 2.88).

Harms: Analysis of observational evidence found that epidural block was associated with an increased incidence of chronic backache, chronic headache, bladder problems, tingling and numbness, and "sensory confusion".[19]

Comment: The quality of the trials was variable in that the methods of randomisation in five of the trials included in the systematic review were not clearly described.

OPTION VACUUM EXTRACTION VERSUS FORCEPS

One systematic review and subsequent RCTs found that vacuum extraction reduced the rate of severe perineal trauma compared with forceps delivery, but increased the incidence of neonatal cephalhaematoma and retinal haemorrhage.

Benefits: We found one systematic review[20] and three subsequent RCTs.[21–23] The systematic review (search date 1999, 10 RCTs comparing vacuum extraction versus forceps delivery, 2885 women) found that women allocated to vacuum extraction rather than forceps were significantly less likely to suffer severe perineal injury and severe perineal pain at 24 hours (severe perineal injury, 7 RCTs, 2582 women: 127/1296 [10%] with vacuum *v* 261/1286 [20%] with forceps; RR 0.46, 95% CI 0.38 to 0.56; NNT 10, 95% CI 8 to 12; severe perineal pain, 1 RCT, 495 women: 21/247 [9%] with vacuum *v* 37/248 [15%] with forceps; RR 0.57, 95% CI 0.34 to 0.94; NNT 16, 95% CI 10 to 119).[20] The subsequent RCTs found that fewer women had severe perineal trauma[21,22] and third degree tears[23] with vacuum extraction compared with forceps delivery, but the difference was not significant (perineal trauma: 2/70 [2.8%] with vacuum *v* 4/70 [5.7%] with forceps; RR 0.50, 95% CI 0.10 to 2.64[21] and 2/204 [1.0%] with vacuum *v* 4/238 [1.7%] with forceps; RR 0.58, 95% CI 0.19 to 3.15;[22] third degree tear: 5/69 [7%] with vacuum *v* 10/61 [16%] with forceps; RR 0.44, 95% CI 0.16 to 1.22[23]). The third subsequent RCT found that vacuum extraction significantly reduced the proportion of women complaining of altered faecal continence compared with forceps at 3 months after birth (intention to treat analysis: 23/69 [33%] with vacuum *v* 36/61 [59%] with forceps; RR 0.35, 95% CI 0.17 to 0.71).[23]

Harms: The systematic review and two of the subsequent RCTs found that babies delivered by vacuum extraction were at higher risk of cephalhaematoma (systematic review:[20] 6 RCTs, 1966 women: 98/995 [10%] with vacuum *v* 40/971 [4%] with forceps; RR 2.34, 95% CI 1.64 to 3.35; NNH 17, 95% CI 10 to 35; first subsequent RCT:[21] 6/70 [8.6%] with vacuum *v* 2/70 [2.8%] with forceps; RR 3.0, 95% CI 0.63 to 14.36; second subsequent RCT:[22] 12/204 [5.9%] with vacuum *v* 2/238 [0.8%] with forceps; RR 7.00, 95% CI 1.59 to 30.91). The systematic review also found that vacuum extraction was associated with significantly higher rates of retinal haemorrhage and failed delivery with the selected instrument than forceps (retinal haemorrhage, 5 RCTs, 445 women: 109/224 [49%] with vacuum *v* 74/221 [34%] with forceps; RR 1.46, 95% CI 1.17 to 1.83; NNH 7, 95% CI 4 to 17; failed delivery with selected instrument, 9 RCTs, 2849 women: 166/1436 [12%] with vacuum *v* 102/1413 [7%] with forceps; RR 1.60, 95% CI 1.27 to 2.02; NNH 23, 95% CI 14 to 51).[20]

Comment: The trials in the systematic review varied in quality, some using quasi-random treatment allocation.[20] None of the trials attempted to "blind" the allocated intervention during the postnatal assessments. The trials took place in different countries (UK, USA, South Africa, Denmark, Sweden, and Greece), and the procedures in the studies were comparable to everyday practice when an assisted delivery is required. Although some studies were performed in teaching hospitals, they were pragmatic, with wide inclusion criteria. The evidence is likely to be generalisable. The subsequent RCTs were carried out in teaching hospitals in Mexico,[21] Sri Lanka,[22] and Ireland.[23] One of the trials had an additional control group of 70 women having a spontaneous vaginal delivery.[21] The most recent RCT failed to reach adequate power to detect a 20% difference between vacuum and forceps in morbidity.[23]

QUESTION What are the effects of intrapartum non-surgical interventions on the rates of perineal trauma?

OPTION CONTINUOUS SUPPORT DURING LABOUR

One systematic review found that providing continuous support❻ for women during childbirth reduced the rate of operative vaginal birth (vacuum extraction or forceps) compared with usual care. It found no significant difference in the overall rates of episiotomy or perineal trauma (defined as episiotomy or laceration requiring suturing).

Benefits: We found one systematic review (search date 2003, 15 RCTs, ≥ 12 791 women) comparing continuous❻, one to one intrapartum support from a professional nurse, midwife, or lay person with usual care.[24] It found that continuous support❻ significantly reduced operative vaginal birth compared with usual care (14 RCTs, 12 757 women; 1039/6344 [16%] with continuous support *v* 1159/6413 [18%] with usual care;

RR 0.89, 95% CI 0.83 to 0.96). The review found no significant difference in the overall rate of episiotomy or perineal trauma (episiotomy, 1 RCT, 6915 women: 894/3454 [25.9%] with continuous support *v* 919/3461 [26.5%] with usual care; RR 0.97, 95% CI 0.90 to 1.05); perineal trauma, 2 RCTs, 7328 women: 1996/3663 [54%] with continuous support *v* 2026/3665 [55%] with usual care; RR 0.99, 95% CI 0.95 to 1.03).[24]

Harms: We found no evidence of harmful effects. The trials in the review examined a wide range of outcomes, but none revealed harmful effects.[24]

Comment: The trials in the systematic review were of reasonable quality, with one trial using a central computerised randomisation service, 12 using sealed opaque envelopes, and two using methods that were centrally controlled, but not concealed for treatment allocation.[24] Although the experimental intervention was always described as one to one support, the experience, relationship to the labouring woman, timing, and duration of support varied between trials. The pragmatic trials took place in a wide variety of settings (Australia, Belgium, Botswana, Canada, Finland, France, Greece, Guatemala, Mexico, South Africa, and the USA).

OPTION UPRIGHT POSITION DURING DELIVERY

One systematic review found that any upright position for delivery marginally reduced episiotomies compared with supine or lithotomy positions but this was offset by an increase in second degree tears. Rates of assisted vaginal delivery were slightly reduced in the upright group.

Benefits: We found one systematic review (search date 2003, 19 RCTs, 5764 women) comparing any upright position for delivery (birthing chairs, stools, cushions, and squatting) versus supine or lithotomy positions.[25] It found that the upright position significantly reduced the episiotomy rate compared with supine or lithotomy positions but this was offset by an increase in second degree tears (episiotomy, 12 RCTs, 4081 women: 742/2039 [36.4%] in upright position *v* 870/2042 [42.6%] in supine or lithotomy position; RR 0.84, 95% CI 0.79 to 0.91; NNH 17, 95% CI 12 to 35; second degree tears: 11 RCTs, 4492 women: 405/2225 [18.2%] in upright position *v* 352/2267 [15.5%] in supine or lithotomy position; RR 1.23, 95% CI 1.09 to 1.39; NNH 40, 95% CI 20 to 574). There was a marginal but significant reduction in assisted vaginal deliveries in the upright group and no significant difference in rates of third and fourth degree tears (assisted vaginal delivery, 18 RCTs, 5506 women: 277/2737 [10%] in upright position *v* 326/2769 [12%] in supine or lithotomy position; RR 0.84, 95% CI 0.73 to 0.98; third and fourth degree tears, 4 RCTs, 1478 women: 5/719 [0.7%] in upright position *v* 6/759 [0.8%] in supine or lithotomy position; RR 0.91, 95% CI 0.31 to 2.68).[25]

Harms: The review found that women delivering in the upright position were slightly more at risk of blood loss estimated to be greater than 500 ml and there was a non-significant increase in blood transfusion (blood loss > 500 ml, 11 RCTs, 4542 women: 160/2256 [7%] in upright position *v* 96/2286 [4%] in supine or lithotomy position; RR 1.68, 95% CI 1.32 to 2.15; NNH 36, 95% CI 21 to 82; blood transfusion, 2 RCTs, 1747 women: 14/891 [2%] in upright position *v* 8/856 [1%] in supine or lithotomy position; RR 1.66, 95% CI 0.70 to 3.94).[25]

Comment: The findings of this systematic review should be interpreted with caution because of the variable qualities of the trials and diversity of the treatment interventions (squatting, kneeling, Gardosi cushion**G**, birthing chair).[25] The reviewers state that the main outcome measures may have been affected because of participants being excluded from some of the trials after randomisation, and several women allocated to deliver in the upright position had difficulty complying. Further, well designed trials are needed, with particular attention given to methodological and clinical heterogeneity, observer bias, intention to treat analysis, and standardised objective measurements of blood loss.

OPTION ALTERNATIVE METHODS OF BEARING DOWN (PUSHING)

One systematic review of two poor quality controlled clinical trials found no significant difference in the extent or rate of perineal trauma between sustained breath holding (Valsalva) and spontaneous exhalatory methods of pushing during the second stage of labour. One additional RCT comparing passive fetal descent❻ with immediate active pushing also found no significant difference in the rates of perineal trauma.

Benefits: **Sustained breath holding (valsalva) method of pushing:** We found one systematic review (search date 1993, 5 trials, of which 2 were known to be RCTs, 471 women) comparing bearing down by sustained breath holding (Valsalva) versus exhalatory or spontaneous pushing.[26] Only two of the trials provided data on perineal trauma requiring suturing, and they found no significant difference between the two interventions (2 RCTs, 338 women; 57/172 [33%] with sustained Valsalva *v* 66/166 [40%] with exhalatory bearing down; RR 0.83, 95% CI 0.61 to 1.10). **Passive descent in the second stage of labour:** We found one additional RCT (252 women) which compared passive fetal descent❻ versus active pushing from the start of the second stage of labour.[27] It found no significant difference between bearing down methods for rates of perineal laceration or instrumental delivery (laceration rate in primiparous women: 46.9% with passive descent❻ *v* 46.2% with active pushing; P = 0.94; laceration rate in multiparous women: 36.4% with passive descent *v* 33.3% with active pushing; P = 0.73; rate of instrumental delivery in primiparous women: 22.6% with passive descent *v* 29.7% with active pushing; P = 0.36; rate of instrumental delivery in multiparous women: 3.1% with passive descent *v* 12.7% with active pushing; P = 0.078; CI not reported).

Harms: It is unclear whether the rate of adverse perineal outcomes is affected by different types of bearing down during the second stage of labour.

Comment: The review included published and unpublished trials.[26] Three of the trials were small and of poor quality. Two of these trials found reduced rates of perineal trauma in the spontaneous bearing down group, but this was not supported by data from the two subsequent, more robust controlled trials.

OPTION "HANDS POISED" VERSUS "HANDS ON"

One multicentre RCT and one quasi-randomised trial found that the "hands poised" method (not touching the baby's head or supporting the mother's perineum) reduced episiotomy rates compared with the conventional "hands on" method (applying pressure to the baby's head during delivery and supporting the mother's perineum). The RCT found no evidence of an effect on the risk of perineal trauma, but found that the "hands poised" group had an increased risk of requiring manual removal of the placenta and higher rates of short term perineal pain.

Benefits: We found no systematic review. We found one randomised and one quasi-randomised trial comparing the "hands poised" versus the "hands on" method of delivery.[2,28] Both trials found that the "hands poised" method of delivery reduced episiotomy rates compared with the "hands on" method. The RCT (5471 women) found that the "hands poised" method significantly reduced the episiotomy rate compared with the "hands on" method (280/2740 [10%] with "hands poised" *v* 351/2731 [13%] with "hands on"; RR 0.79, 95% CI 0.65 to 0.96; NNT 38, 95% CI 23 to 106).[2] It found no significant difference between methods in the risk of perineal trauma requiring suturing or in third and fourth degree tears (suturing required: 1636/2740 [60%] with "hands poised" *v* 1605/2731 [59%] with "hands on"; RR 1.02, 95% CI 0.97 to 1.06; third and fourth degree tears: 40/2740 [1.5%] with "hands poised" *v* 31/2731 [1.2%] with "hands on"; RR 1.3, 95% CI 0.81 to 2.05). The quasi-randomised trial (1161 women) found that the "hands poised" method significantly reduced episiotomy rates and third degree tears (episiotomy: 51/502 [10%] with "hands poised" *v* 103/574 [18%] with "hands on"; RR 0.57, 95% CI 0.41 to 0.78; third degree tears: 5/502 [1.0%] with "hands poised" *v* 16/574 [2.8%] with "hands on"; RR 0.36, 95% CI 0.13 to 0.97).[28] There was no significant difference in the rate of first and second degree perineal trauma (175/502 [35%] with "hands poised" *v* 171/574 [30%] with "hands on"; RR 1.17, 95% CI 0.98 to 1.39).

Harms: The RCT found that the "hands poised" method significantly increased the risk of requiring manual removal of the placenta and significantly increased perineal pain 10 days after delivery (manual removal: 71/2740 [2.6%] with "hands poised" *v* 42/2731 [1.5%] with "hands on"; RR 1.69, 95% CI 1.16 to 2.46; NNH 95, 95% CI 45 to 417; perineal pain: 910/2669 [34%] with "hands poised" *v* 823/2647 [31%] with "hands on"; RR 1.10, 95% CI 1.02 to 1.19; NNH 33, 95% CI 18 to 212).[2]

Comment: The RCT was a large robust multicentre pragmatic trial carried out in the UK and the results are likely to be generalisable.[2] The quasi-randomised trial, carried out in the University Hospital of Vienna, used alternate allocation based on the date of delivery: even days allocated to "hands on", odd days to "hands poised". Data were missing for 45 women in the "hands poised" group and 40 in the "hands on" group.[28]

QUESTION **What are the effects of different methods and materials for primary repair of first and second degree tears and episiotomies?**

OPTION **NON-SUTURING**

Non-suturing of muscle and skin in first and second degree perineal tears (poorer wound healing than with suturing). Two small RCTs found no significant difference in short term perineal pain between non-suturing and suturing of first and second degree tears. One of the RCTs found no significant difference in healing between groups but the second RCT found that a greater proportion of women in the non-sutured group had poorer wound healing at 6 weeks after birth. Non-suturing of perineal skin in first and second degree tears and episiotomies (reduces dyspareunia) One large RCT found no significant difference between leaving the perineal skin unsutured compared with conventional suturing in pain at 10 days after birth. A second RCT found that non-suturing reduced pain for up to 3 months after delivery. Both RCTs found that non-suturing of the perineal skin reduced dyspareunia at 3 months after birth.

Benefits: We found no systematic review. **Non-suturing of perineal muscle and skin:** We found two small RCTs comparing non-suturing versus suturing of first and second degree tears.[29,30] Results from the first small RCT (78 primiparous women in Sweden) should be interpreted with caution (see comment below).[29] It found no significant difference between suturing and non-suturing in rates of a "burning sensation" and soreness at 2–3 days after birth, although women not having suturing reported higher rates for both outcomes (burning sensation: 9/40 [23%] in non-sutured *v* 4/38 [11%] in sutured; RR 0.47, 95% CI 0.16 to 1.39; soreness: 3/40 [8%] in non-sutured *v* 1/38 [3%] in sutured; RR 0.35, 95% CI 0.04 to 3.23). It found no significant difference in healing at 2–3 days and 8 weeks after birth (see comment below).[29] The second RCT (74 primiparous women in Scotland) found no significant difference in McGill pain scores at 10 days and 6 weeks between the non-sutured and sutured groups (P = 0.8 at both 10 days and 6 weeks), but found that wound healing was significantly poorer with non-suturing at up to 6 weeks after delivery (proportion of women with a closed tear: 16/36 [44%] in non-sutured *v* 26/31 [84%] in sutured; RR 0.53, 95% CI 0.36 to 0.79).[30] **Non-suturing of perineal skin alone:** We found two RCTs that compared leaving the perineal skin unsutured but apposed (the vagina and perineal muscle were sutured) versus a conventional repair in which all three layers were sutured.[31,32] The RCTs found different results for perineal pain. The first RCT (1780 primiparous and multiparous women with first and second degree tears or episiotomies after spontaneous or assisted vaginal delivery in a single UK centre) found no significant difference in the proportion of women reporting perineal pain at 10 days after birth (221/886 [25%] with skin unsutured *v* 244/885 [28%] with skin sutured; RR 0.91, 95% CI 0.77 to 1.06).[31] The second RCT was a multicentre trial carried out in Nigeria (823 women who sustained a second degree tear or episiotomy).[32] It found that leaving the perineal skin unsutured significantly reduced the proportion of women with perineal pain at 48 hours, 14 days, 6 weeks, and 3 months after delivery (48 hours: 237/417 [57%] with skin unsutured *v* 265/406 [65%] with skin sutured; RR 0.87, 95% CI 0.78 to 0.97; 14 days: 93/417 [22%] with skin unsutured *v* 117/406 [29%] with skin sutured; RR 0.77, 95% CI 0.61 to 0.98; 6 weeks: 41/417 [10%] with skin unsutured *v* 62/406 [15%] with skin sutured; RR 0.64, 95% CI 0.44 to 0.93; 3 months: 4/417 [1%] with skin unsutured *v* 21/406 [5%] with skin sutured; RR 0.19, 95% CI 0.06 to 0.54). Both RCTs found that leaving the perineal skin unsutured significantly reduced superficial dyspareunia at 3 months after birth (first RCT:[31] 128/828 [16%] with skin unsutured *v* 162/836 [19%] with skin sutured; RR 0.80, 95% CI 0.64 to 0.99; NNT 26, 95% CI 14 to 345; second RCT:[32] 26/417 [6%] with skin unsutured *v* 49/406 [12%] with skin sutured; RR 0.52, 95% CI 0.33 to 0.81).

Harms: **Non-suturing of perineal muscle and skin:** See benefits above. No additional harms were reported in the two identified RCTs.[29,30] **Non-suturing of perineal skin alone:** See benefits above. The two RCTs found that leaving the perineal skin unsutured but apposed increased rates of wound gaping at 48 hours compared with suturing (203/885 [23%] with skin unsutured *v* 40/889 [4%] with skin sutured; RR 5.10, 95% CI 3.68 to 7.06[31] and 107/417 [26%] with skin unsutured *v* 21/406 [5%] with skin sutured; RR 4.96, 95% CI 3.17 to 7.76[32]). One RCT found that non-suturing of the skin increased wound gaping at 10 days[31] but the second RCT found no significant differences in wound gaping at 14 days after birth (10 days: 227/886 [26%] with skin unsutured *v* 145/885 [16%] with skin sutured; RR 1.56, 95% CI 1.30 to 1.88;[31] 14 days: 86/417 [21%] with skin unsutured *v* 67/406 [17%] with skin sutured; RR 1.25, 95% CI 0.94 to 1.67;[32] longer term results were not reported in the second RCT[32]). The second RCT judged wounds as gaping if the edges were more than 0.5 cm apart.[32] One RCT found no significant differences in wound breakdown at 14 days (13/417 [3%] with skin unsutured *v* 10/406 [2%] with skin sutured; RR 1.27, 95% CI 0.56 to 2.85).[32]

Comment: **Non-suturing of perineal muscle and skin:** Results from one of the small RCTs comparing non-suturing versus suturing must be interpreted with caution because the study limitations compromise the validity of these results.[29] It is unclear how healing was defined and assessed, and the study had an insufficient sample size to rule out clinically important differences. This is suggested by the broad confidence intervals in the presence of a big difference in rates between the study groups. The second small RCT evaluating non-suturing versus suturing was of reasonable methodological quality and used sealed opaque envelopes to allocate treatment. It was acknowledged that it was impossible to blind assessors to the allocated treatment and that this may have biased results.[30] **Non-suturing of perineal skin alone:** The two RCTs evaluating non-suturing of perineal skin were pragmatic studies, and the results are likely to be generalisable.[31,32] The subsequent RCT recruited 1077 women into the trial but only 823 of these responded up to 3 months after birth and were included in the analysis.[32]

OPTION ABSORBABLE SUTURES

One systematic review found that absorbable synthetic sutures reduced pain at up to 10 days after birth compared with catgut sutures. One subsequent RCT, however, found no significant difference in perineal pain at 3 days, although it may have lacked power to detect a clinically important effect. The systematic review and the subsequent RCT found no significant difference between absorbable synthetic sutures and catgut sutures in pain or dyspareunia at 3 months, but one RCT with 12 months' follow up, which was included in the review, found lower rates of dyspareunia with absorbable synthetic sutures. RCTs found no significant difference between rapidly absorbed and standard synthetic sutures in overall perineal pain, pain on sitting, or dyspareunia. RCTs also found reduced perineal pain on walking and a reduction in suture material removal with rapidly absorbed synthetic sutures.

Benefits: **Absorbable synthetic sutures versus catgut:** We found one systematic review (search date 1999, 8 RCTs conducted in Europe and the USA, 3681 primiparous and multiparous women)[33] and one subsequent RCT carried out in Australia (391 women who sustained a first or second degree tear or episiotomy after a spontaneous vaginal delivery)[34] that compared absorbable synthetic (standard polyglactin 910 or polyglycolic acid) versus catgut suture material for perineal repair. The systematic review found that absorbable synthetic material significantly reduced analgesia use up to 10 days (analgesic use: 5 RCTs, 2820 women; AR 262/1422 [18%] with absorbable synthetic *v* 338/1398 [24%] with catgut; RR 0.74, 95% CI 0.65 to 0.85; NNT 18, 95% CI 13 to 35).[33] At 3 months, there was no significant difference in perineal pain or dyspareunia between absorbable synthetic sutures and catgut (perineal pain, 2 RCTs; AR: 92/1061 [9%] with absorbable synthetic *v* 112/1068 [11%] with chromic catgut; RR 0.86, 95% CI 0.64 to 1.08; dyspareunia, 3 RCTs; AR: 171/1086 [16%] with absorbable synthetic *v* 180/1089 [17%] with chromic catgut; RR 0.95, 95% CI 0.79 to 1.15). At 12 months after birth (1 RCT, 793 women),[35] rates of dyspareunia were lower with absorbable synthetic sutures than with chromic catgut (AR 30/395 [8%] with absorbable synthetic *v* 51/398 [13%] with chromic catgut; RR 0.59, 95% CI 0.39 to 0.91; NNT 20, 95% CI 11 to 106).[36] The subsequent RCT found no significant difference in perineal pain at 3 days or at 3 months between absorbable synthetic sutures and catgut, although it may have lacked power to detect clinically important effects (perineal pain at 3 days: 112/187 [60%] with absorbable synthetic *v* 124/188 [66%] with chromic catgut; RR 0.91, 95% CI 0.78 to 1.06; perineal pain at 3 months: 17/167 [10%] with absorbable synthetic v 14/174 [8%] with chromic catgut; RR 1.26, 95% CI 0.64 to 2.48).[34] The RCT found no significant difference between absorbable sutures and catgut in dyspareunia at 3 and 6 months and perineal pain at 6 months, although rates were higher with absorbable sutures (dyspareunia at 3 months: 35/132 [27%] with absorbable synthetic v 27/144 [19%] with chromic catgut; RR 1.41, 95% CI 0.91 to 2.20; perineal pain at 6 months: 9/158 [6%] with absorbable synthetic v 5/159 [3%] with chromic catgut; RR 1.81, 95% CI 0.62 to 5.28; dyspareunia at 6 months: 24/148 [16%] with absorbable synthetic v 19/147 [13%] with chromic catgut; RR 1.25, 95% CI 0.72 to 2.19).[34] **Different types of absorbable synthetic suture:** We found no systematic review. We found three RCTs comparing rapidly absorbed polyglactin 910 versus standard polyglactin 910 (153 women in Northern Ireland;[37] 308 primiparous women in Demark;[38] 1542 women in the UK[39]). The first RCT did not report data in a format that was suitable for inclusion here.[37] The other two RCTs both found that rapidly absorbed sutures significantly reduced pain on walking in the 2 weeks postpartum compared with standard sutures (AR: 46/138 [33.3%] with rapidly absorbed v 65/134 [48.5%] with standard; RR 0.69, 95% CI 0.51 to 0.92;[38] AR: 259/769 [33.7%] with rapidly absorbed v 314/770 [40.8%] with standard; RR 0.83, 95% CI 0.73 to 0.94[39]). It found no significant difference in overall perineal pain, pain on sitting, or dyspareunia between rapidly absorbed and standard sutures. Rapidly absorbed sutures were removed significantly less frequently than standard sutures during the 3 months postpartum (22/769 [2.7%] with rapidly absorbed v 98/770 [12.7%] with standard; RR 0.23, 95% CI 0.14 to 0.35).[39]

Harms: **Absorbable synthetic sutures versus catgut:** The systematic review[33] found that suture removal was significantly more common in the absorbable synthetic group than in the catgut group up to 3 months after birth (2 RCTs, 2129 women: 191/1061 [18%] with absorbable synthetic v 108/1068 [10%] with chromic catgut; RR 1.78, 95% CI 1.44 to 2.20; NNH 13, 95% CI 8 to 22).[29,36] The subsequent RCT found that more people repaired with absorbable synthetic material reported problems with their sutures at 6 weeks compared with people repaired with catgut, although the difference was not significant (8/184 [4.4%] with absorbable synthetic v 3/184 [1.6%] with chromic catgut; OR 2.61, 95% CI 0.59 to 12.41).[34] **Different types of absorbable synthetic suture:** Suture removal was significantly less frequent in the rapidly absorbed polyglactin 910 group than in the standard polyglactin 910 group (22/769 [3%] with rapidly absorbed polyglactin v 98/770 [13%] with standard polyglactin; OR 0.26, 95% CI 0.18 to 0.37).[39]

Comment: **Absorbable synthetic sutures versus catgut:** The trials in the systematic review varied in quality and in operator skills and training. It was not possible to "blind" outcome assessment because of the obvious differences in method and materials used. Most of the trials used "intention to treat" as the method of analysis. The subsequent RCT used sealed opaque envelopes for treatment allocation and analysis was by intention to treat.[34] It was not possible to blind operators to allocated treatments because of obvious differences in suture materials. Follow up was by face to face interview until participants were discharged from hospital and then by telephone interview. The RCT was powered to detect a reduction in short term pain from 60% to 45%. **Different types of absorbable synthetic suture:** The RCT comparing different types of absorbable sutures also compared continuous versus interrupted sutures for all layers (see continuous sutures, p 1793).[39] Suture materials were produced by the manufactures in an identical form in order to "blind" allocated treatments from the participants, operators, and assessors. It was a large, robust trial, and its results are likely to be generalisable.[39]

OPTION **CONTINUOUS SUTURES**

One systematic review found that continuous subcuticular sutures for perineal skin reduced short term pain compared with interrupted sutures, but found no significant difference in perineal pain or dyspareunia at 3 months postpartum. One RCT found that a loose continuous technique for repair of all layers reduced short term perineal pain and suture removal compared with interrupted sutures up to 3 months postpartum.

Benefits: **For repair of perineal skin:** We found one systematic review that compared continuous subcuticular with interrupted sutures inserted close to the perineal skin to appose the perineal skin (search date 1999, 4 RCTs conducted in Europe and the UK, 1864 primiparous and multiparous women).[40] It found that continuous sutures significantly reduced the proportion of women with pain at up to 10 days compared with interrupted sutures (3 RCTs, 1588 women: 160/789 [20%] with continuous *v* 218/799 [27%] with interrupted; RR 0.75, 95% CI 0.63 to 0.89; NNT 14, 95% CI 10 to 34). It found no significant difference in the proportion of women with pain at 3 months (1 RCT, 961 women: 58/465 [13%] with continuous *v* 51/451 [11%] with interrupted; RR 1.10, 95% CI 0.77 to 1.57).[40] **For repair of all layers:** We found no systematic review. We found one RCT (1542 women with second degree tears or episiotomy in the UK) comparing a loose continuous suture for all layers with interrupted sutures.[39] It found that continuous sutures reduced the proportion of women with pain at 10 days: 204/770 [26.5%] with continuous *v* 338/769 [44.0%] with interrupted; OR 0.47, 95% CI 0.38 to 0.58). It found no significant difference in the proportion of women with pain at 3 months (70/751 [9%] with continuous *v* 95/741 [13%] with interrupted; OR 0.70, 95% CI 0.54 to 1.47) or at 12 months (31/700 [4%] with continuous *v* 47/689 [7%] with interrupted; OR 0.64, 95% CI 0.35 to 1.16). It found no significant difference in rates of local dyspareunia at 3 or 12 months (at 3 months: 98/581 [17%] with continuous *v* 102/593 [17%] with interrupted; OR 0.98, 95% CI 0.72 to 1.33; at 12 months: 94/658 [14%] with continuous *v* 91/667 [14%] with interrupted; OR 1.05, 95% CI 0.77 to 1.43).[39]

Harms: **For repair of perineal skin:** The RCT found that suture removal was significantly more common up to 3 months in the interrupted suture group than in the continuous group (166/451 [37%] with interrupted v 121/465 [26%] with continuous; RR 1.41 95% CI 1.16 to 1.72).[40] **For repair of all layers:** The RCT found that suture removal was significantly more common up to 3 months postpartum in the interrupted suture group than in the continuous group (96/769 [12%] with interrupted v 24/770 [3%] with continuous; RR 4.01, 95% CI 2.59 to 6.19).[39]

Comment: The RCT comparing continuous with interrupted sutures for all layers also compared different types of absorbable sutures (see absorbable sutures, p 1791). It was a large, robust trial, and its results are likely to be generalisable.[39]

QUESTION **What are the effects of different methods and materials for primary repair of third and fourth degree tears?**

OPTION **DIFFERENT METHODS AND MATERIALS FOR REPAIR OF THIRD AND FOURTH DEGREE TEARS**

One small RCT comparing the overlap method versus the end-to-end method for primary repair of third degree obstetric tears found no significant difference in perineal discomfort and a non-significant reduction in the rate of reported faecal urgency and anal incontinence with the overlap technique compared with the end-to-end method.

Benefits: We found no systematic review. We found one small RCT (112 primiparous women in Ireland) comparing overlap**G** versus end-to-end**G** approximation for primary repair of third degree obstetric anal sphincter tears.[41] It found no significant difference in perineal discomfort, faecal urgency, or faecal incontinence (perineal discomfort: 20/55 [36%] with overlap *v* 22/57 [39%] with end-to-end; RR 0.94, 95% CI 0.58 to 1.52; faecal urgency: 11/55 [20%] with overlap *v* 17/57 [30%] with end-to-end; RR 0.67, 95% CI 0.35 to 1.30; faecal incontinence: 2/55 [4%] with overlap *v* 5/57 [9%] with end-to-end; RR 0.42, 95% CI 0.08 to 2.05).

Harms: The RCT assessed the presence of residual defects of the anal sphincter with ultrasound and found no significant difference between groups. Two thirds (74/112 [66.0%]) of women had a residual full thickness defect in the external anal sphincter ultrasound after primary repair at 3 months postpartum (34/55 [62.0%] with overlap**G** *v* 40/57 [70.0%] with end-to-end**G**; RR 0.88, 95% CI 0.67 to 1.15). No other harms were reported and the clinical significance of this finding is unclear.

Comment: A pilot study for an RCT comparing the overlap**G** with the end-to-end**G** method for repair of third and fourth degree obstetric anal sphincter tears should be published later this year (Fernando R, personal communication, 2004).

GLOSSARY

Continuous support during labour The presence of a companion (lay person or health care worker) who provides continuous social support for the woman during the intrapartum period; social support may include advice, information, assistance, or emotional support.

End-to-end technique for primary repair of third degree obstetric anal sphincter tears involves the torn ends of the external anal sphincter being juxtaposed with interrupted sutures.

Gardosi cushion An obstetric aid used during the second stage of labour, which allows most of the woman's weight to rest on her thighs instead of her feet, while being in a squatting position.

Overlap technique for primary repair of third degree obstetric anal sphincter tears involves the torn ends of the external anal sphincter being overlapped and sutured with interrupted stitches.

Passive fetal descent An alternative method of bearing down, involving a period of rest to allow passive descent of the fetus before active pushing.

REFERENCES

1. Sultan AH, Kamm MA, Bartram CI, et al. Perineal damage at delivery. *Contemp Rev Obstet Gynaecol* 1994;6:18–24.
2. McCandlish R, Bowler U, van Asten H, et al. A randomised controlled trial of care of the perineum during second stage of normal labour. *Br J Obstet Gynaecol* 1998;105:1262–1272.
3. Sleep J, Grant A, Garcia J, et al. West Berkshire perineal management trial. *BMJ* 1984;298:587–690.
4. Wagner M. *Pursuing the birth machine: the search for appropriate technology*. Camperdown: ACE Graphics, 1994;165–174.
5. Statistical Bulletin–NHS Maternity Statistics, England: 2001–2002. London: Department of Health, 2003.
6. Graves EJ, Kozak LJ. National hospital discharge survey: annual summary, 1996. *Vital Health Stat* 13. 1999;(140):i–iv,1–46.
7. Audit Commission. *First class delivery: improving maternity services in England and Wales*. London: Audit Commission Publications, 1997.
8. Sultan AH, Monga AK, Kumar D, et al. Primary repair of anal sphincter using the overlap technique. *Br J Obstet Gynaecol* 1999;106:318–323.
9. Renfrew MJ, Hannah W, Albers L, et al. Practices that minimize trauma to the genital tract in childbirth: a systematic review of the literature. *Birth* 1998;25:143–160. Search date 1997; primary sources Cochrane Database of Systematic Reviews, Medline, Cinahl, Miriad, Midirs, Index Medicus, and hand searches of current textbooks of obstetrics, midwifery, and nursing.
10. Glazener CMA, Abdalla M, Stroud P, et al. Postnatal maternal morbidity: extent, causes, prevention and treatment. *Br J Obstet Gynaecol* 1995;102:286–287.
11. Sleep J, Grant A. Pelvic floor exercises in postnatal care. *Br J Midwifery* 1987;3:158–164.
12. Sultan AH, Kamm MA, Hudson CN. Anal sphincter disruption during vaginal delivery. *N Engl J Med* 1993;329:1905–1911.
13. Carroli G, Belizan J. Episiotomy for vaginal birth (Cochrane Review). In: The Cochrane Library, Issue 1, 2004. Chichester, UK: John Wiley & Sons, Ltd. Search date not reported; primary sources Cochrane Pregnancy and Childbirth Group Trials Register.
14. Coats PM, Chan KK, Wilkins M, et al. A comparison between midline and mediolateral episiotomies. *Br J Obstet Gynaecol* 1989;87:408–412.

15. Werner CH, Schuler W, Meskendahl I. Midline episiotomy versus mediolateral episiotomy: a randomised prospective study. *Int J Gynaecol Obstet* Proceedings of 13th World Congress of Gynaecology and Obstetrics (FIGO), Singapore 1991; Book 1:33.
16. Shiono P, Klebanof MD, Carey JC. Midline episiotomies: more harm than good? *Obstet Gynaecol* 1990;75:756–770.
17. Klein MC, Gauthier MD, Robbins JM, et al. Relationship of episiotomy to perineal trauma and morbidity, sexual function, and pelvic floor relaxation. *Am J Obstet Gynecol* 1994;17:591–598.
18. Howell CJ. Epidural versus non-epidural analgesia for pain relief in labour (Review). In: The Cochrane Library, Issue 1, 2004. Chichester, UK: John Wiley & Sons, Ltd. Search date not reported; primary source Cochrane Pregnancy and Childbirth Group Specialised Register of Controlled Trials.
19. Howell CJ, Chalmers I. A review of prospectively controlled comparisons of epidural with non-epidural forms of pain relief during labour. *Int J Obstet Anaesth* 1992;1:93–110.
20. Johanson RB, Menon BKV. Vacuum extraction versus forceps for assisted vaginal delivery (Cochrane Review). In: The Cochrane Library, Issue 1, 2004. Chichester, UK: John Wiley & Sons, Ltd. Search date 1999; primary source Cochrane Pregnancy and Childbirth Group Trials Register
21. Pliego Perez AR, Moncada Navarro O, Neri Ruz ES, et al. Comparative assessment of efficacy and safety of assisted vaginal delivery with forceps and with vacuum extractor. *Ginecol Obstet Mex* 2000;68:453–459. [In Spanish]
22. Weerasekera DS, Premaratne S. A randomised prospective trial of the obstetric forceps versus vacuum extraction using defined criteria. *J Obstet Gynaecol* 2002;22:344–345.
23. Fitzpatrick M, Behan M, O'Connell PR, et al. Randomised clinical trial to assess anal sphincter function following forceps or vacuum assisted vaginal delivery. *Br J Obstet Gynaecol* 2003;110:424–429.
24. Hodnett ED, Gates S, Hofmeyr GJ, et al. Continuous support for women during childbirth (Cochrane Review). In: The Cochrane Library, Issue 1, 2004. Chichester, UK: John Wiley & Sons, Ltd. Search date 2003; primary sources Cochrane Pregnancy and Childbirth Group Trials Register, Central, and Cochrane Controlled Trials Register.
25. Gupta JK, Hofmeyr GJ. Position for women during second stage of labour (Cochrane Review). In: The Cochrane Library, Issue 2, 2004. Chichester, UK: John Wiley & Sons, Ltd. Search date 2003; primary sources Cochrane Pregnancy and Childbirth Group Trials Register and personal contact with authors of published and unpublished trials.
26. Nikodem VC. Sustained (Valsalva) vs exhalatory bearing down in 2nd stage of labour. In: Enkin MW, Keirse MJ, Renfrew MJ, et al, eds. *Pregnancy and childbirth module*. In: The Cochrane Library, Issue 1, 1994. Oxford: Update Software. Search date 1993; primary sources Cochrane Pregnancy and Childbirth Database, Medline, and hand searches of specialist journals and conference proceedings.
27. Hansen SL, Clark SL, Foster JC. Active pushing versus passive fetal descent in the second stage of labor: a randomized controlled trial. *Obstet Gynecol* 2002;99:29–34.
28. Mayerhofer K, Bodner-Adler B, Bodner K, et al. Traditional care of the perineum during birth. A prospective, randomized, multicenter study of 1,076 women. *J Reprod Med* 2002;47:477–482.
29. Lundquist M, Olsson A, Nissen E, et al. Is it necessary to suture all lacerations after a vaginal delivery? *Birth* 2000;27:79–85.
30. Fleming EM, Hagen S, Niven C. Does perineal suturing make a difference? The SUNS trial. *Br J Obstet Gynaecol* 2003;110: 684–689.
31. Gordon B, Mackrodt C, Fern E, et al. The Ipswich Childbirth study: 1. A randomised evaluation of two stage after birth perineal repair leaving the skin unsutured. *Br J Obstet Gynaecol* 1998;105:435–440.
32. Oboro VO, Tabowei TO, Loto OM, et al. A multicentre evaluation of the two-layer repair of after birth perineal trauma. *J Obstet Gynaecol* 2003;1:5–8.
33. Kettle C, Johanson RB. Absorbable synthetic versus catgut suture material for perineal repair (Cochrane Review). In: The Cochrane Library, Issue 1, 2004. Chichester, UK: John Wiley & Sons, Ltd. Search date 1999; primary source Cochrane Pregnancy and Childbirth Group Trials Register.
34. Upton A, Roberts CL, Ryan M, et al. A randomised trial, conducted by midwives, of perineal repairs comparing a polyglycolic suture material and chromic catgut. *Midwifery* 2002;18:223–229.
35. Mackrodt C, Gordon B, Fern E, et al. The Ipswich Childbirth study: 2. A randomised comparison of polyglactin 910 with chromic catgut for after birth perineal repair. *Br J Obstet Gynaecol* 1998;105:441–445.
36. Grant A, Gordon B, Mackrodt C, et al. The Ipswich Childbirth study: one year follow up of alternative methods used in perineal repair. *Br J Obstet Gynaecol* 2001;108:34–40.
37. McElhinney BR, Glenn DRJ, Harper MA. Episiotomy repair: Vicryl versus Vicryl rapide. *Ulster Med J* 2000;69:27–29.
38. Gemynthe A, Langhoff-Roos J, Sahl S, et al. New Vicryl formulation: an improved method of perineal repair? *Br J Midwifery* 1996;4:230–234.
39. Kettle C, Hills RK, Jones P, et al. Continuous versus interrupted perineal repair with standard or rapidly absorbed sutures after spontaneous vaginal birth: a randomised controlled trial. *Lancet* 2002;359:2217–2223.
40. Kettle C, Johanson RB. Continuous versus interrupted sutures for perineal repair (Cochrane Review). In: The Cochrane Library, Issue 1, 2004. Chichester, UK: John Wiley & Sons, Ltd. Search date 1999; primary source Cochrane Pregnancy and Childbirth Group Specialised Register of Controlled Trials.
41. Fitzpatrick M, Fynes M, Behan M, et al. A randomized clinical trial comparing primary overlap with approximation repair of third-degree obstetric tears. *Am J Obstet Gynecol* 2000;183:1220–1224.

Chris Kettle
Clinical Midwife Specialist
University Hospital of North Staffordshire (NHS Trust)
Stoke-on-Trent
UK

Competing interests: The author was the recipient of a fellowship from the Iolanthe Midwifery Research Trust, which provided funding to enable her to carry out a randomised controlled trial of perineal repair after childbirthThe Methods or Materials Study (MOMS). The Iolanthe Midwifery Research Trust and Ethicon Ltd, UK (manufacturers of suture material) provided funding for employment of a part time data management clerk for the trial. The author has received a Smith & Nephew Fellowship 20012002, to provide funding to allow her to complete her research (MOMS) and PhD thesis.

We would like to acknowledge the previous contributors of this chapter, including Bazian Ltd.

Postnatal depression

Search date January 2004

Louise Howard

QUESTIONS

INTERVENTIONS

Covered elsewhere in *Clinical Evidence*

Depressive disorders, p 1238

See glossary

Key Messages

- **Antidepressants (fluoxetine)** Limited evidence from one small RCT suggested that fluoxetine may improve postnatal depression at 4 and 12 weeks compared with placebo. The RCT had problems with recruitment and a high drop out rate, and it excluded breastfeeding women. We found no RCTs that satisfactorily compared fluoxetine with psychological treatment. We found no RCTs on the effects of other antidepressants in women with postnatal depression, and no RCTs that satisfactorily compared other antidepressants with psychological treatments.
- **Cognitive behavioural therapy (individual)** One RCT found limited evidence that individual cognitive behavioural therapy and ideal standard care both improved depressive symptoms, but that there was no significant difference between the two interventions. Limited evidence from one RCT suggested that individual cognitive behavioural therapy may improve postnatal depression in the short term (immediately after treatment) compared with routine primary care. The RCT found no clear longer term benefits (9 months to 5 years postpartum) from individual cognitive behavioural therapy compared with routine primary care, non-directive counselling, or psychodynamic therapy.
- **Interpersonal psychotherapy** One RCT found that interpersonal psychotherapy improved postnatal depression compared with waiting list controls at 12 weeks.
- **Non-directive counselling** Limited evidence from two RCTs suggests that, in the short term (immediately after treatment), non-directive counselling may improve postnatal depression compared with routine primary care. The one RCT with follow up beyond 12 weeks found no clear longer term benefits (from 9 months to 5 years postpartum) from non-directive counselling compared with routine primary care, individual cognitive behavioural therapy, or psychodynamic therapy.
- **Psychodynamic therapy** Limited evidence from one RCT suggests that psychodynamic therapy may improve postnatal depression in the short term (immediately after treatment) compared with routine primary care. The RCT found no clear longer term benefits (9 months to 5 years postpartum) from psychodynamic therapy compared with routine primary care, non-directive counselling, or cognitive behavioural therapy.

Clin Evid 2005;13:1796–1809.

- **Antidepressants other than fluoxetine** We found no RCTs on the effects of antidepressants in women with postnatal depression, and no RCTs that satisfactorily compared antidepressants other than fluoxetine versus psychological treatments.
- **Cognitive behavioural therapy (group)** One small RCT in women with a high level of depressive symptoms on screening found that group cognitive behavioural therapy improved symptoms at 6 months compared with routine primary care.
- **Hormones** Limited evidence from one small RCT in women with severe postnatal depression suggests that oestrogen treatment may improve postnatal depression at 3 and 6 months compared with placebo.
- **Light therapy** We found no RCTs evaluating light therapy.
- **Mother–infant interaction coaching** One small RCT found that mother–infant interaction coaching had no significant effect on maternal depression scores compared with usual treatment, but it improved maternal responsiveness to the infant within 10 weeks of starting treatment.
- **Psychoeducation with partner** One small RCT found that psychoeducation with partner reduced patients' depression scores and partners' psychiatric morbidity at 10 weeks compared with psychoeducation without partner.
- **Telephone based peer support (mother to mother)** One small RCT found that telephone based peer support reduced depression scores after 8 weeks compared with usual treatment.

DEFINITION Postnatal depression (PND) is broadly defined as non-psychotic depression occurring during the first 6 months postpartum. Puerperal mental disorders have only recently been categorised separately in psychiatric classifications, but both the International Classification of Diseases (ICD-10)[1] and the Diagnostic and Statistical Manual of mental disorders, fourth edition (DSM-IV) (see table 1, p 1809) require certain qualifications to be met that limit their use: ICD-10 categorises mental disorders that occur postpartum as puerperal, but only if they cannot otherwise be classified, and DSM-IV allows "postpartum onset" to be specified for mood disorders starting within 4 weeks' postpartum.[2] In clinical practice and research, the broader definition above is often used, because whether or not PND is truly distinct from depression in general, depression in the postpartum period raises treatment issues for the nursing mother and has implications for the developing infant (see prognosis below). The symptoms are similar to symptoms of depression at other times of life, but in addition to low mood, sleep disturbance, change in appetite, diurnal variation in mood, poor concentration, and irritability, women with PND also experience guilt about their inability to look after their new baby. In many countries, health visitors screen for PND using the Edinburgh Postnatal Depression Scale**G**,[3,4] which elicits depressive symptoms.

INCIDENCE/ PREVALENCE The prevalence of depression in women postpartum is similar to that found in women generally. However, the incidence of depression in the first month after childbirth is three times the average monthly incidence in non-childbearing women.[5] Studies across different cultures have shown a consistent incidence of postnatal depression (PND) (10–15%),[6] with higher rates in teenage mothers. A meta-analysis of studies mainly based in the developed world found the incidence of postnatal depression to be 12–13%.[7]

AETIOLOGY/ RISK FACTORS Three systematic reviews have identified the following risk factors for postnatal depression: past history of any psychopathology (including history of previous postnatal depression), low social support, poor marital relationship, and recent life events.[7–9]

PROGNOSIS Most episodes of PND resolve spontaneously within 3–6 months,[10] but about one in four affected mothers are still depressed on the child's first birthday.[11] In the developed world, suicide is now the main cause of maternal deaths in the first year postpartum,[12] but the suicide rate is lower at this time than in age matched non-postpartum women.[13] PND is also associated with reduced likelihood of secure attachment,[14] deficits in maternal–infant interactions,[15] and impaired cognitive and emotional development of the child, particularly in boys living in areas of socioeconomic deprivation.[15–17] These associations remain significant even after controlling for subsequent episodes of depression in the mother.

AIMS OF INTERVENTION To improve symptoms, quality of life, mother–infant interaction, with minimal adverse effects on mother and child.

OUTCOMES Symptom scores (e.g. the Edinburgh Postnatal Depression Scale❻[3,4]) and other scales used in studies of depression at other times in life (see depressive disorders, p 1238), quality of life, mother–infant interaction (rated using questionnaires or observer rated videos), effect on marital/family relationship (rated using questionnaires), and rates of suicide.

METHODS *Clinical Evidence* search and appraisal January 2004. We searched Medline (1996 to date), Embase (1980 to date), the Cochrane Library 2003, Issue 4, and two independent critical appraisers appraised the results. We included only RCTs with a minimum of 6 weeks' follow up. We included non-blinded studies as it can be difficult to blind patients and assessors to psychological interventions.

QUESTION What are the effects of treatments?

OPTION ANTIDEPRESSANTS

Limited evidence from one small RCT suggested that fluoxetine may improve postnatal depression at 4 and 12 weeks compared with placebo. The RCT had problems with recruitment and a high drop out rate, and it excluded breastfeeding women. We found no RCTs that satisfactorily compared fluoxetine with psychological treatment. We found no RCTs on the effects of other antidepressants in women with postnatal depression, and no RCTs that satisfactorily compared other antidepressants with psychological treatments.

Benefits: We found three systematic reviews (search dates 1998,[18] 1999,[19] and 2000[20]). All three reviews found the same single RCT[21] (87 women recruited from community based screening, 51 with a major and 36 with a minor depressive episode defined by research diagnostic criteria[22]). This trial conducted a four way comparison: fluoxetine 20 mg plus one session (the assessment session) of cognitive behavioural counselling❻, fluoxetine 20 mg plus six sessions of cognitive behavioural counselling, placebo plus one session of cognitive behavioural counselling, and placebo plus six sessions of cognitive behavioural counselling. Outcomes were assessed at 4 and 12 weeks using the Clinical Interview Schedule (revised)❻,[23] the Edinburgh Postnatal Depression Scale❻,[3,4] and the Hamilton Depression Scale❻,[24] using an intention to treat analysis. The trial had several weaknesses (see comment below). Fluoxetine significantly reduced revised Clinical Interview Schedule scores at 4 and 12 weeks compared with placebo (percentage difference of geometric mean scores between fluoxetine and placebo at 4 weeks: 37.1%, 95% CI 5.7% to 58.0%; at 12 weeks: 40.7%, 95% CI 10.9% to 60.6%). The trial did not report on infant outcomes.

Harms: **Effects on the infant:** The RCT excluded breastfeeding mothers and did not report on adverse effects on the infant.[21] We found some evidence of short term adverse effects in case reports and case series of infants whose mothers were using antidepressants while breastfeeding. One review of 95 case reports and small case series on the use of psychotropic medications during breastfeeding found one case of respiratory depression in a nursing infant whose mother was treated with doxepin, which resolved 24 hours after discontinuation of breastfeeding.[25] The review also identified 10 cases of adverse effects in 190 nursing infants whose mothers were treated with fluoxetine. Six infants had unconfirmed and unspecified adverse effects that resolved spontaneously. Three infants were reported to have colic. One infant had an episode of transient seizure-like activity at 3 weeks of age, and episodes of unresponsiveness at 4 months of age, with one episode of peripheral cyanosis at 5.5 months of age. The results of neurological monitoring were within normal limits up to 1 year of age. The review found no adverse effects in the infants of breastfeeding mothers taking other tricyclic antidepressants. A review of three controlled follow up studies of antidepressants used during breastfeeding (79 infants) found no infant developmental abnormalities with tricyclics or sertraline.[26] We found no good evidence on long term risks to the developing child from maternal use of antidepressants. **Effects on the mother:** The RCT reported no suicides in the 12 week follow up period.[21] See harms of antidepressants in the chapter on depressive disorders, p 1238.

Comment: The RCT had several weaknesses.[21] Most of the women who were approached (101/188 [54%]) refused to participate, most commonly because of reluctance to take antidepressants. A further 26/87 (30%) of the participants dropped out after randomisation. However, the authors performed an appropriate intention to treat analysis. The design of the trial does not allow comparison between fluoxetine and cognitive behavioural counselling, as all the women received one session of cognitive behavioural counselling.

OPTION HORMONES

Limited evidence from one small RCT in women with severe postnatal depression suggests that oestrogen treatment may improve postnatal depression at 3 and 6 months compared with placebo.

Benefits: We found two systematic reviews (search dates 2000[20] and 2001[27]), both of which found the same single RCT[28] (61 women with major depression beginning within 3 months postpartum who, at enrolment, were < 18 months postpartum, recruited from outpatient clinics, general practitioners, and self referrals). Women were excluded if they were breastfeeding, had a medical history that would contraindicate oestrogen therapy, or had changed psychotropic medication in the previous 6 weeks. The RCT compared oestrogen treatment (oestradiol skin patches for 6 months plus additional dydrogesterone tablets for 12 days each month) versus placebo (patches and tablets). After 3 and 6 months, the women taking oestrogen had significantly lower Edinburgh Postnatal Depression Scale❻ scores than those taking placebo (WMD at 3 months –3.20, 95% CI –5.97 to –0.43; at 6 months –4.38, 95% CI –1.89 to –6.87). The trial did not report on infant outcomes.

Harms: **Effects on the infant:** The RCT did not report on adverse effects on the infant.[28] **Effects on the mother:** Endometrial curettage at the end of treatment showed endometrial changes (details not reported) in three women in the treatment group, which had resolved by follow up at 9 months.[28] One woman in the oestrogen group, who had been admitted to a psychiatric ward soon after the start of the study because of her worsening mental state, committed suicide. However, her clinical consultant had stopped the oestrogen treatment soon after admission. For harms of oestrogen treatment see also menopausal symptoms, p 2392.

Comment: None.

OPTION LIGHT THERAPY

We found no RCTs evaluating light therapy.

Benefits: We found one systematic review (search date 2000, no RCTs)[20] and no subsequent RCTs.

Harms: We found no good information on adverse effects of light therapy.

Comment: Case studies of two women with postnatal depression found a drop in depression scores with 4 weeks of daily light therapy.[29]

OPTION NON-DIRECTIVE COUNSELLING

Limited evidence from two RCTs suggests that, in the short term (immediately after treatment), non-directive counselling may improve postnatal depression compared with routine primary care. The one RCT with follow up beyond 12 weeks found no clear longer term benefits (from 9 months to 5 years postpartum) from non-directive counselling compared with routine primary care, individual cognitive behavioural therapy, or psychodynamic therapy.

Benefits: We found three systematic reviews (search dates 1997,[30] 2000,[20] and 2001[31]), all of which found the same single RCT.[32] We also found one subsequent RCT.[33,34] The RCT identified by all three reviews (55 women with depression defined by research diagnostic criteria[21] recruited from the community up to 13 weeks postpartum) compared non-directive counselling**G** delivered by trained health visitors (subsequently termed "active listening visits") for 8 weeks with routine primary care.[32] The subsequent larger RCT (193 women with major depression [DSM-III-R][2] recruited from the community within 8 weeks' postpartum) had several methodological flaws (see comment below). It compared non-directive counselling, psychodynamic therapy**G**, individual cognitive behavioural therapy**G**, and routine primary care conducted in the women's homes by trained therapists on a weekly basis from 8 to 18 weeks' postpartum.[33,34] Outcomes, assessed at 4.5 months, 9 months, 18 months, and 5 years postpartum, were as follows: the proportion of women with a diagnosis of depression, using the Structured Clinical Interview**G** for DSM-III-R Diagnoses (SCID) adjusted for mean baseline SCID scores; depression scores, using the Edinburgh Postnatal Depression Scale**G**; at 4.5 months: mother–infant interactions, using rated videotapes; maternal management of the infant and problems in mother and infant relationship, both using a checklist; at 18 months: infant emotional and behavioural problems, using a modified Behavioural Screening Questionnaire**G** with maternal reports; infant attachment, using Ainsworth Strange Situation Procedure**G**; and infant cognitive development, using the Mental Development Index of the Bayley Scales of Infant Development**G**; at 5 years: child emotional and behavioural difficulties, using maternal reports on the Rutter A[2] Scale**G**; teacher reports, using the Preschool Behaviour Checklist**G**; and child cognitive development, using the McCarthy Scales**G**. **Versus routine primary care:** The first, smaller RCT found that, after an average of 5 weeks' treatment, non-directive counselling significantly reduced the number of women who were categorised as depressed compared with routine primary care (69% with non-directive counselling *v* 38% with routine primary care; difference 31.7%, 95% CI 5% to 58%; P = 0.03).[32] The subsequent, larger RCT found that, immediately after treatment (at 4.5 months' postpartum), non-directive counselling increased (though not significantly) the proportion of women without depression compared with routine primary care (26/48 [54%] with non-directive counselling *v* 20/50 [40%] with routine primary care; RR 1.38, 95% CI 0.82 to 1.89).[33,34] It also found that non-directive counselling significantly reduced depression scores compared with routine primary care (mean EPDS score adjusted for mean centred baseline EPDS scores: 9.9 with non-directive counselling *v* 11.3 with routine primary care; treatment effect for non-directive counselling: –2.1, 95% CI –3.8 to –0.3; P = 0.02). It also found that non-directive counselling significantly reduced the proportion of women with mother–infant relationship difficulties compared with routine primary care (proportion of women reporting problems, adjusted for relationship problems before treatment: 53% [23/43] with non-directive counselling *v* 74% [26/35] with routine primary care; RR 0.63, 95% CI 0.32 to 0.97). After controlling for baseline differences between groups, there were no significant differences between non-directive counselling and routine primary care in terms of behavioural management problems (P = 0.77), nor in terms of maternal sensitivity in mother–infant interactions (P = 0.14), except for women with high social adversity, among whom non-directive counselling significantly improved maternal sensitivity (P = 0.04). In the longer term (at 9 months, 18 months, and 5 years postpartum), there were no significant differences in any outcomes except for some evidence that non-directive counselling improved infant emotional and behavioural problems compared with routine primary care at 18 months postpartum (P = 0.001). However, this outcome relied solely on maternal reports (see comment below). **Versus cognitive behavioural therapy (individual):** The RCT[33,34] found no significant difference between non-directive counselling and individual cognitive behavioural therapy for any outcomes immediately after treatment or in the longer term. There was some evidence that non-directive counselling improved infant emotional and behavioural problems compared with cognitive behavioural therapy at 18 months postpartum. However, this outcome relied solely on maternal reports (see comment below). **Versus psychodynamic therapy:** The RCT[33,34] found no significant difference between non-directive counselling and psychodynamic therapy for any outcomes immediately after treatment or in the longer term. There was some evidence that non-directive counselling improved infant emotional and behavioural problems compared with psychodynamic therapy at 18 months postpartum. However, this outcome relied solely on maternal reports (see comment below). **Versus antidepressants:** We found no RCTs comparing non-directive counselling versus antidepressants.

Harms: None reported.

Comment: The subsequent, larger RCT[33,34] had several methodological flaws. It was underpowered to detect differences between treatment groups, and there was no adjustment for multiple comparisons. More women in the routine primary care group had experienced social adversity compared with the treatment groups (35% in the routine primary care group *v* 30% in the non-directive counselling group *v* 24% in the cognitive behavioural therapy group *v* 10% in psychodynamic therapy group), and this was not controlled for in some analyses. Ten per cent of the women who were randomised did not complete the trial. More women dropped out of the non-directive counselling and psychodynamic therapy groups (6 from the non-directive counselling group *v* 8 from the psychodynamic therapy group *v* 1 from the cognitive therapy group *v* 4 from the routine primary care group). Reasons for non-completion were not investigated, and the authors did not perform an intention to treat analysis. Women who did not complete therapy were younger (P = 0.004) and more likely to be single or separated (P = 0.05). The infant outcomes that showed a beneficial effect of treatment (i.e. fewer mother–infant relationship problems at 4.5 months and fewer emotional and behavioural problems at 18 months) relied solely on maternal reports.

OPTION COGNITIVE BEHAVIOURAL THERAPY (INDIVIDUAL)

One RCT provided limited evidence that individual cognitive behavioural therapy and ideal standard care both improved depressive symptoms, but that there was no significant difference between the two interventions. Limited evidence from one RCT suggested that individual cognitive behavioural therapy may improve postnatal depression in the short term (immediately after treatment) compared with routine primary care. The RCT found no clear longer term benefits (9 months to 5 years postpartum) from individual cognitive behavioural therapy compared with routine primary care, non-directive counselling, or psychodynamic therapy.

Benefits: We found no systematic review. We found two RCTs.[33-35] The first RCT (37 women, 32% major depression, 68% minor depression, recruited from the community) compared modified cognitive behavioural therapy (CBT)Ⓖ delivered by specifically trained early childhood nurses once a week for 6 weeks versus ideal standard care (weekly 20–60 minute appointments for mothercraft advice and non-specific support delivered by early childhood nurses who had not received specific training).[35] For a description of the second RCT and a comment on its methodology see non-directive counselling, p 1800.[33,34] **Versus ideal standard care:** The first RCT found that individual CBT and ideal standard care were both effective in improving depressive symptoms immediately and at 6 months after treatment, but there was no significant difference between the two interventions (Edinburgh Postnatal Depression [EPDS] mean score: 15.9 pretreatment CBT group *v* 13.7 with ideal standard care, P = 0.03; 8.1 post intervention CBT *v* 6.5 with ideal standard care, P value not reported, reported as not significant; 6.2 at 6 months with CBT *v* 7.7 with ideal standard care, P value not reported, reported as not significant)[35] (see comment below). **Versus routine primary care:** The second RCT found that immediately after treatment (at 4.5 months postpartum), individual CBT increased (though not significantly) the proportion of women without depression compared with routine primary care (57% [24/42] with CBT *v* 40% [20/50] with routine primary care; RR 1.50, 95% CI 0.92 to 1.98).[33,34] It also found that individual CBT significantly reduced depression scores compared with routine primary care (mean EPDS score: 9.2 with CBT *v* 11.3 with routine primary care; treatment effect for CBT –2.7, 95% CI –4.5 to –0.9; P = 0.003). It also found that individual CBT significantly reduced the proportion of women with mother–infant relationship difficulties compared with routine primary care (proportion of women reporting problems, adjusted for relationship problems before treatment: 39% [16/41] with CBT *v* 74% [26/35] with routine primary care; RR 0.46, 95% CI 0.2 to 0.81).[33,34] After controlling for baseline differences between groups, there were no significant differences between CBT and routine primary care in terms of behavioural management problems (P = 0.60), nor in terms of mother–infant interactions (results presented graphically; P value not reported). In the medium to longer term (at 9 months, 18 months, and 5 years postpartum), there were no significant differences in any outcome, except for infant emotional and behavioural problems, for which CBT achieved significant improvement at 18 months postpartum compared with routine primary care (P = 0.06). However, this outcome relied solely on maternal reports (see comment under non-directive counselling, p 1801).**Versus non-directive counselling:** See benefits of non-directive counselling, p 1800. **Versus psychodynamic therapy:** The second RCT found no significant difference between CBT and psychodynamic counselling for any outcomes.[33,34] **Versus antidepressants:** We found no satisfactory RCTs comparing CBT versus antidepressants.

Harms: None reported.

Comment: The first RCT was probably underpowered to compare modified CBT versus ideal standard care effectively. There was a trend towards CBT being more effective. Adjusting for baseline EPDS (which was higher in the CBT group) in a multivariate analysis had no impact on results at any time point.[35] For a comment on the methodology of the second RCT, see comment under non-directive counselling, p 1801.[33,34]

OPTION COGNITIVE BEHAVIOURAL THERAPY (GROUP)

One small RCT in women with a high level of depressive symptoms on screening found that group cognitive behavioural therapy improved symptoms at 6 months compared with routine primary care.

Benefits: We found no systematic review but found one RCT (45 women < 1 year postpartum, recruited from the community with the Edinburgh Postnatal Depression Scale [EPDS] > 12, but no confirmation of diagnosis of postnatal depression by diagnostic interview, block randomised).[36] The RCT compared group cognitive behavioural therapy❻, including education and relaxation, given by two health visitors for 2 hours each week for 8 weeks, versus routine primary care. At 6 months, group cognitive therapy significantly improved depression scores (proportion of women scoring < 13 on the EPDS: 65% [15/23] with group cognitive therapy *v* 36% [8/22] with routine primary care; P = 0.05). The RCT did not report on outcomes in infants.

Harms: None reported.

Comment: The RCT's criteria for inclusion (EPDS > 12) and response to treatment (EPDS < 13) meant that a small change in EPDS would count as a response to treatment.

OPTION PSYCHOEDUCATION WITH PARTNER

One small RCT found that psychoeducation with partner reduced patients' depression scores and partners' psychiatric morbidity at 10 weeks compared with psychoeducation without partner.

Benefits: We found one systematic review[20] (search date 2000, 1 RCT,[37] 29 women < 12 months postpartum, referred to hospital with major depression of postpartum onset). All women in the RCT attended seven clinic visits for assessment of mood, adjustment of medication, and psychoeducation❻. The women in the intervention group brought their partners to four of the visits. The RCT found significantly lower depression scores in the group attending with their partners at 10 weeks' follow up (mean Edinburgh Postnatal Depression Scale [EPDS] 8.6 with partner *v* 14.7 without partner; P = 0.01). It also found significantly lower psychological morbidity in partners who attended clinics (mean General Health Questionnaire score 18.4 in partners who attended *v* 43 in the control group; P = 0.01). The RCT did not report on outcomes in infants.

Harms: None reported

Comment: Women taking psychotropic medication were included and no adjustment was made for any potential confounding effect of medication.

OPTION INTERPERSONAL PSYCHOTHERAPY

One RCT found that interpersonal psychotherapy improved postnatal depression compared with waiting list controls at 12 weeks.

Benefits: We found one systematic review (search date 2000, 1 RCT).[20] The RCT[38] (120 women recruited from the community with major depression [DSM-IV criteria and > 11 on the Hamilton Depression Rating Scale; HDRS][24] for an average duration of 7 months) found that interpersonal psychotherapy❻, performed by experienced psychotherapists for 1 hour once a week for 12 weeks, significantly increased the proportion of women recovering from depression compared with remaining on a waiting list (proportion of women recovering, defined as

HDRS < 7: 31% [19/60] with interpersonal psychotherapy v 15% [9/60] with control; RR 2.11, 95% CI 1.04 to 4.28). There were also significant improvements in social adjustments (mean score on the Social Adjustment Scale-Self Report [SAS-SR][39]: 1.93 with interpersonal psychotherapy v 2.35 with waiting list control; P < 0.001). Subscales of the SAS-SR showed significant improvements in relationship with spouse (P < 0.001), relationship with children older than 2 years (P < 0.05), relationship with immediate family (P = 0.002), and relationship with friends (P = 0.003; absolute numbers not reported). The Postpartum Adjustment Questionnaire❻[40] also showed a significant effect of interpersonal psychotherapy (mean reduction 0.30 with interpersonal pyschotherapy v 0.12 with waiting list control; P = 0.001). There were no significant differences between groups for the Dyadic Adjustment Scale❻, a specific measure of adjustment in relationship with partner.[41] The RCT did not report on outcomes in infants.

Harms: No harms reported.

Comment: The RCT had problems with recruitment (132 women declined to participate), but achieved an 80% follow up (withdrawal rate 20% in the treatment group v 15% among controls; P = 0.47). There were no significant clinical or demographic differences between women who dropped out and women who stayed in the study.

OPTION PSYCHODYNAMIC THERAPY

Limited evidence from one RCT suggests that psychodynamic therapy may improve postnatal depression in the short term (immediately after treatment) compared with routine primary care. The RCT found no clear longer term benefits (9 months to 5 years postpartum) from psychodynamic therapy compared with routine primary care, non-directive counselling, or cognitive behavioural therapy.

Benefits: We found no systematic review but found one RCT (193 women with major depression [DSM-III-R][2] recruited from the community within 8 weeks postpartum).[33,34] For a description of the RCT and a comment on its methodological flaws, see non-directive counselling, p 1800. **Versus routine primary care:** The RCT found that immediately after therapy (at 4.5 months postpartum), psychodynamic therapy❻ significantly increased the proportion of women without depression compared with routine primary care (71% [32/45] with psychodynamic therapy v 40% [20/50] with routine primary care; RR 1.89, 95% CI 1.33 to 2.33).[33,34] It also found that psychodynamic therapy significantly reduced depression scores compared with routine primary care (mean Edinburgh Postnatal Depression Scores [EPDS]: 8.9 with psychodynamic therapy v 11.3 with routine primary care; treatment effect for psychodynamic therapy –2.6, 95% CI –4.4 to –0.9; P = 0.003). It also found that psychodynamic therapy significantly reduced the proportion of women with mother–infant relationship difficulties compared with routine primary care (proportion of women reporting problems, adjusted for relationship problems before treatment: 47% [20/43] with psychodynamic therapy v 74% [26/35] with routine primary care; RR 0.57, 95% CI 0.28 to 0.92). After controlling for baseline differences between groups, there were no significant differences between psychodynamic therapy and routine primary care in behavioural management problems or mother–infant interactions. In the longer term (at 9 months, 18 months, and 5 years postpartum), there were no significant differences for any outcomes except for infant emotional and behavioural problems, for which psychodynamic therapy achieved significant improvement at 18 months postpartum (P = 0.03) compared with routine primary care.

However, this outcome relied solely on maternal reports (see comment under non-directive counselling, p 1801). **Versus non-directive counselling:** See benefits of non-directive counselling, p 1800. **Versus cognitive behavioural therapy:** See benefits of cognitive behavioural therapy (individual), p 1802. **Versus antidepressants:** We found no satisfactory RCTs comparing psychodynamic therapy versus antidepressants.

Harms: None reported.

Comment: For comments on the RCT's methodology see comment under non-directive counselling, p 1801.[33,34]

OPTION MOTHER–INFANT INTERACTION COACHING

One small RCT found that mother–infant interaction coaching had no significant effect on maternal depression scores compared with usual treatment, but it improved maternal responsiveness to the infant within 10 weeks of starting treatment.

Benefits: We found no systematic review but found one RCT (122 women recruited from the community with Edinburgh Postnatal Depression Scale > 10 at 4–8 weeks postpartum).[42] This compared interaction coaching**G** using, a variable number of 15 minute sessions depending on the needs of the mother and infant, versus treatment as usual. After 6 to 10 weeks, there was no significant difference in depression scores between treatment and control groups. However, there was a significant difference in maternal responsiveness in Dyadic Mutuality Code**G** scores,[43,44] based on videotaped mother–infant interactions rated by a researcher blind to randomisation status (mean score at 6 weeks: 9.73 with interaction coaching *v* 8.77 with usual treatment; P = 0.02; mean at 10 weeks: 9.55 with interaction coaching *v* 8.80 with usual treatment; P = 0.03). Baseline scores were not significantly different in the two groups. The RCT did not investigate infant outcomes.

Harms: None reported.

Comment: Additional psychiatric treatment for depression was given to women if required.

OPTION TELEPHONE BASED PEER SUPPORT (MOTHER TO MOTHER)

One small RCT found that telephone based peer support reduced depression scores after 8 weeks compared with usual treatment.

Benefits: We found no systematic review but found one RCT (42 women recruited from the community identifed as high risk for postnatal depression with Edinburgh Postnatal Depression Scale [EPDS] > 9 at 8 weeks' postpartum) comparing individually tailored mother to mother telephone based support, using trained lay volunteers with a personal history of postnatal depression, versus treatment as usual.[45] It found that telephone support significantly reduced depression scores after 8 weeks compared with usual care (proportion of women with EPDS > 12: 15% [3/20] with telephone support *v* 52% [11/21] with usual care; OR 6.23, 95% CI 1.40 to 27.8; P = 0.01). The RCT did not investigate infant outcomes.

Harms: None reported.

Comment: The acceptance rate for enrolment into the trial was 67%. Over a third of peer volunteers (38%) referred a mother to a professional health service, and this was not controlled for in the analysis.

GLOSSARY

Ainsworth Strange Situation Procedure is a laboratory procedure used to assess infant attachment style. The procedure consists of pre-specified episodes of parental separation and return. The infant's behaviour upon the parent's return is the basis for classifying the infant into attachment categories (e.g secure and insecure).

Behavioural Screening Questionnaire is a maternal interview that examines infant difficulties, such as sleep disturbance, feeding problems, separation problems, and excessive temper tantrums. It has been found to distinguish between infants of mothers with and without depression.

Clinical Interview Schedule - Revised (CIS-R) is a semi-structured interview covering non-psychotic symptoms particularly those associated with depression and anxiety.

Cognitive behavioural counselling is derived from cognitive behavioural therapy, and is designed to be delivered by professionals such as health visitors who are not specialists in mental health. It is sometimes known as CREST because it incorporates Child care advice, Reassurance, Enjoyment, Support from others, and Targets.

Cognitive behavioural therapy (CBT) uses a range of techniques including examination and challenging of unhelpful thoughts, help with changing behaviours, and examination of underlying dysfunctional assumptions.

Dyadic Adjustment Scale is a specific self report measure of adjustment in relationship with partner. The four subscales are Dyadic Satisfaction, Dyadic Consensus, Dyadic Cohesion, and Affectional Expression.

Dyadic Mutuality Code (DMC) Scores are based on live or videotaped observations of face-to-face interactions between mother and infant. The DMC shows the level of responsiveness in the maternal-infant relationship where responsiveness is defined as the mother's ability to accommodate to her infant's behaviour and to give it meaning through regulation of her own behavioural responses. The DMC contains six key components of responsive interactions: mutual attention, positive affect, turn-taking, maternal pauses, infant clarity of cues, and maternal sensitivity.

The Edinburgh Postnatal Depression Scale (EPDS) was designed as a screening questionnaire to identify possible depression in a clinical or research setting. The EPDS has a high sensitivity (95%) and specificity (93%) for postnatal depression, and is used by many health visitors and in many clinical research studies of postnatal depression.

Group cognitive behavioural therapy In the trial described here, it consisted of weekly meetings run by health visitors in primary care. It included education, provision of information on postnatal depression, strategies for coping with difficult childcare situations and eliciting social support, use of cognitive behavioural techniques to tackle women's erroneous cognitions about motherhood, and strategies for coping with anxiety, such as the use of relaxation.

Hamilton Depression Rating Scale is a rating scale that provides a measure of depressive symptoms.

Interaction coaching for at risk parents and their infants is a six key element intervention strategy designed to strengthen the early parent–infant relationship. This includes teaching the mother to identify the infant's behavioural cues and to tailor responses to match the infant's preferences by demonstrating ways to modulate the use of pauses, imitation, sequences, and combinations of facial expressions, voice, and touch.

Interpersonal psychotherapy places the depression in an interpersonal context, reviews the patient's current and past interpersonal relationships, and relates problematic aspects of these relationships to the patient's depression.

McCarthy Scales of Children's Abilities is a general measure of children's cognitive development.

The Mental Development Index of the Bayley Scales of Infant Development provides information about the child's language development and problem solving skills.

Non-directive counselling provides women with the opportunity to air their feelings about any current concerns, such as marital problems or financial difficulties, as well as problems they might raise about their infant.

Postpartum Adjustment Questionnaire is a specific self report measure of postpartum adjustment, with subscales measuring work in the home, relationship with spouse, relationships with children other than the baby, relationships with friends, work outside of the home, relationships with other family members and, relationship with the new baby.

Preschool Behaviour Checklist is a questionnaire completed by preschool and reception class teachers to identify significant child behaviour problems.

Psychodynamic therapy is therapy in which an understanding of the mother's representation of her infant and her relationship with her infant is promoted by exploring aspects of the mother's own early attachment history.

Psychoeducation consists of education about the psychological disorder the patient is suffering from, in addition to monitoring and treatment of the patient's mental disorder.

Rutter A^2 Scale is a reliable and well validated questionnaire completed by the mother, which identifies clinically significant child behaviour problems at 5 years.

Social Adjustment Scale-Self Report is a questionnaire with subscales measuring work in the home, work outside of the home, relationship with spouse, relationship with children older than 2 years, relationship with immediate family, and relationships with friends.

Structured Clinical Interview for DSM-III-R (SCID) is a structured interview to generate an operationalised diagnosis that would fulfil DSM III-R criteria.

REFERENCES

1. World Health Organization. *Tenth Revision of the International Classification of Diseases and Related Health Problems. Clinical Descriptions and Diagnostic Guidelines*. Geneva: WHO, 1992.
2. American Psychiatric Association. *Diagnostic and Statistical Manual of Mental Disorders, fourth edition*. New York: American Psychiatric Association, 1994.
3. Murray L, Carothers AD. The validation of the Edinburgh Post-natal Depression Scale on a community sample. *Br J Psychiatry* 1990;157:288–290.
4. Cox JL, Holden JM, Sagovsky R. Detection of postnatal depression. Development of the 10-item Edinburgh Postnatal Depression Scale. *Br J Psychiatry* 1987;150:782–786.
5. Cox JL, Murray D, Chapman G. A controlled study of the onset, duration and prevalence of postnatal depression. *Br J Psychiatry* 1993;163:27–31.
6. Kumar R. Postnatal mental illness: a transcultural perspective. *Soc Psychiatry Psychiatr Epidemiol* 1994;29:250–264.
7. O'Hara MW, Swain AM. Rates and risks of postpartum depression: a meta-analysis. *Int Rev Psychiatry* 1996;8:37–54.
8. Beck CT. A meta-analysis of predictors of postpartum depression. *Nurs Res* 1996;45:297–303.
9. Wilson LM, Reid AJ, Midmer DK, et al. Antenatal psychosocial risk factors associated with adverse postnatal family outcomes. *CMAJ* 1996;154:785–799.
10. Cooper PJ, Murray L. Course and recurrence of postnatal depression. Evidence for the specificity of the diagnostic concept. *Br J Psychiatry* 1995;166:191–195.
11. Kumar R, Robson KM. A prospective study of emotional disorders in childbearing women. *Br J Psychiatry* 1984;144:35–47.
12. *The fifth report of the Confidential Enquiries into Maternal Deaths in the United Kingdom*. London: Royal College of Obstetricians and Gynaecologists, 2001.
13. Appleby L. Suicide during pregnancy and in the first postnatal year. *BMJ* 1991;302:137–140.
14. Martins C, Gaffan EA. Effects of early maternal depression on patterns of infant–mother attachment: a meta-analytic investigation. *J Child Psychol Psychiatry* 2000;41:737–746.
15. Murray L, Cooper PJ. The impact of postpartum depression on child development. *Int Rev Psychiatry* 1996;8:55–63.
16. Carter AS, Garrity-Rokous EF, Chazan-Cohen R, et al. Maternal depression and comorbidity: Predicting early parenting, attachment security, and toddler social-emotional problems and competencies. *J Am Acad Child Adolesc Psychiatry* 2001;40:18–26.
17. Hay DF, Pawlby S, Sharp D, et al. Intellectual problems shown by 11-year-old children whose mothers had postnatal depression. *J Child Psychol Psychiatry* 2001;42:871–889.
18. Mulrow C, Williams J, Trivedi M, et al. Treatment of depression — newer pharmacotherapies. *Psychopharm Bull* 1998;34:409–795. Search date 1998.
19. Hoffbrand S, Howard LM, Crawley H. Antidepressant drug treatment for postnatal depression. In: The Cochrane Library, Issue 2, 2001. Oxford: Update Software. Search date 1999; primary sources the Cochrane Depression, Anxiety and Neurosis Group's Specialised Register of Controlled Trials, Cochrane Library Controlled Trials Register, Cochrane Pregnancy and Childbirth Group's Specialised Register, Medline, Science Citation Index, MIDIRS Midwifery Database, UK National Research Register, HSRProj, Current Controlled Trials website, search of reference lists and book bibliographies, and contact with pharmaceutical companies, experts and organisations.
20. Boath E, Henshaw C. The treatment of postnatal depression: a comprehensive literature overview. *J Reprod Infant Psychol* 2001;19:215–248. Search date 2000; primary sources Medline, PsychLit, Sociofile, CINAHL, COPAC, published books held by BL, hand search, reference checking and search of Marce Society conference proceedings and abstracts.
21. Appleby L, Warner R, Whitton A, et al. A controlled study of fluoxetine and cognitive-behavioural counselling in the treatment of postnatal depression. *BMJ* 1997;314:932–936.
22. Spitzer RL, Endicott J, Robins E. Research diagnostic criteria: rationale and reliability. *Arch Gen Psychiatry* 1978;35:773–782.
23. Lewis G, Pelosi AJ, Arya R, et al. Measuring psychiatric disorder in the community: a standardised assessment for use by lay interviewers. *Psychol Med* 1992;22:465–486.
24. Hamilton M. Hamilton depression scale. In: Guy W, ed. *ECDEU assessment manual for psychopharmacology, revised edition*. Rockville MD: U.S. National Institute of Mental Health Psychopharmacology Research Branch, 1976:179–192.
25. Burt VK, Suri R, Altshuler L, et al. The use of psychotropic medications during breast-feeding. *Am J Psychiatry* 2001;158:1001–1009.

26. Austin M, Mitchell P. Use of psychotropic medications in breastfeeding women: acute and prophylactic treatment. *Aust N Z J Psychiatry* 1998;32:778–784.
27. Lawrie TA, Herxheimer A, Dalton K. Oestrogens and progestogens for preventing and treating postnatal depression. In: The Cochrane Library, Issue 2, 2003. Oxford: Update Software. Search date 2001; primary sources Cochrane Pregnancy and Childbirth Group's Specialised Register of Controlled Trials, Cochrane Controlled Trials Register, reference list check.
28. Gregoire AJP, Kumar R, Everitt B, et al. Transdermal oestrogen for treatment of severe postnatal depression. *Lancet* 1996;347:930–933.
29. Corral M, Kuan A, Kostaras D. Bright light therapy's effect on postpartum depression. *Am J Psychiatry* 2000;157:303–304.
30. Elkan R, Kendrick D, Hewitt M, et al. The effectiveness of domiciliary health visiting: a systematic review of international studies and a selective review of the British literature. *Health Technol Assess* 2000;4:1–339. Search date 1997; primary sources Medline, CINAHL, EMBASE, the internet, the Cochrane Library, index to theses, hand search of *Health Visitor*, reference list check, and contact with key individuals and organisations.
31. Ray KL, Hodnett ED. Caregiver support for postpartum depression. In: The Cochrane Library, Issue 2, 2003. Oxford: Update Software. Search date 2001; primary source Cochrane Pregnancy and Childbirth Group trials register.
32. Holden JM, Sagovsky R, Crawley H. Counselling in a general practice setting: controlled study of health visitor intervention in treatment of postnatal depression. *BMJ* 1989;298:223–226.
33. Cooper PJ, Murray L, Wilson A, et al. Controlled trial of the short and long-term effect of psychological treatment of postpartum depression. I. Impact on maternal mood. *Br J Psychiatry* 2003;182:412–419.
34. Murray L, Cooper PJ, Wilson A, et al. Controlled trial of the short and long-term effect of psychological treatment of postpartum depression: 2: Impact on the mother–child relationship and child outcome. *Br J Psychiatry* 2003;182:420–427.
35. Prendergast J, Austin M-P. Early childhood nurse-delivered cognitive behavioural counselling for postnatal depression. *Australas Psychiatry* 2001;9:255–259.
36. Honey K, Bennet P, Morgan M. A brief psycho-educational group intervention for postnatal depression. *Br J Clin Psychol* 2002;41:405–409.
37. Misri S, Kostaras X, Fox D, et al. The impact of partner support in the treatment of postnatal depression. *Can J Psychiatry* 2000;45:554–558.
38. O'Hara MW, Stuart S, Gorman, L, et al. Efficacy of interpersonal psychotherapy for postpartum depression. *Arch Gen Psychiatry* 2000;57:1039–1045.
39. Weissman MM, Bothwell S. Assessment of social adjustment by patient self-report. *Arch Gen Psychiatry* 1976;33:1111–1115.
40. O'Hara MW, Hoffman JG, Phillips LHC, et al. Adjustment in childbearing women: the Postpartum Adjustment Questionnaire. *Psychol Assess* 1992;4:160–169.
41. Spanier GB. Measuring dyadic adjustment: new scales for assessing the quality of marriage and similar dyads. *J Marriage Fam* 1976;38:15–28.
42. Horowitz JA, Bell M, Trybulski J, et al. Promoting responsiveness between mothers with depressive symptoms and their infants. *J Nurs Scholarsh* 2001;33:323–329.
43. Censullo M, Bowler R, Lester B, et al. Development of an instrument to measure infant–adult synchrony. *Nurs Res* 1987;36:244–248.
44. Censullo M. *Dyadic mutuality code manual*. Wellesley MA: Wellesley College Center for Research on Women, 1991.
45. Dennis C. The effect of peer support on postpartum depression: a pilot randomized controlled trial. *Can J Psychiatry* 2003;48:115–124.

Louise Howard
Senior Lecturer
Health Services Research Department
Institute of Psychiatry
London
UK

Competing interests: None declared.

TABLE 1 **Diagnostic criteria for postnatal depression (see text, p 1797).**

Psychiatric classification	Criteria for postnatal depression
International Classification of Diseases Version 10, World Health Organization	Depressed mood for most of the day Loss of interest or pleasure in normally pleasurable activities such as playing with the baby Tiredness, decreased energy and fatigue Additionally, any four of the following should be present: Loss of confidence and self esteem Feelings of guilt and blaming oneself Recurrent thoughts of suicide or death, including that of the child Difficulty in concentration Agitation or lethargy Sleep disturbance Appetite disturbance
DSM IV - Postpartum onset specifier	*Onset of depressive episode must be within 4 weeks postpartum* Symptoms do not differ from symptoms in non-postpartum mood episodes and may include: Fluctuations in mood Preoccupation with infant wellbeing Severe anxiety Panic attacks Fearfulness of being alone with infant

Pre-eclampsia and hypertension

Search date December 2003

Lelia Duley

QUESTIONS

INTERVENTIONS

To be covered in future updates

Interventions in women with pre-existing hypertension
Treatment for postpartum hypertension

*Consensus opinion is that women with severe hypertension during pregnancy should have antihypertensive treatment. Placebo controlled trials would therefore be unethical.

See glossary G

Key Messages

Prevention

- **Antiplatelet drugs** One systematic review and one subsequent RCT found that, in women considered at risk of pre-eclampsia, antiplatelet drugs (mainly aspirin) reduced the risk of pre-eclampsia, death of the baby, and delivery before 37 weeks compared with placebo or no treatment. The RCTs found no significant difference in other important outcomes. The systematic review found no evidence that aspirin increased the risk of bleeding in mother or baby compared with placebo.
- **Calcium supplementation** One systematic review found that calcium supplementation (mainly 2 g/day) reduced the risk of pre-eclampsia and reduced the risk of having a baby with birth weight under 2500 g compared with placebo. It found no significant difference between calcium supplements and placebo on the risk of caesarean section, preterm delivery, or stillbirth or death of the baby before discharge from hospital.
- **Antioxidants** Two RCTs found limited evidence that antioxidants (vitamins C plus E or lycopene) reduced the risk of pre-eclampsia compared with placebo. The RCTs provided insufficient evidence on other clinically important outcomes.
- **Magnesium supplementation** One systematic review found insufficient evidence about the effects of magnesium supplements on the risk of pre-eclampsia or its complications.
- **Other pharmacological agents (atenolol or nitrates)** We found two small RCTs; one compared atenolol versus placebo and the other compared glyceryl trinitrate patches versus placebo. Both RCTs were too small to allow any reliable conclusions to be drawn.
- **Salt restriction** Limited evidence from one systematic review found no significant difference in the risk of pre-eclampsia with a low salt diet compared with a normal diet.
- **Fish oil and/or evening primrose oil** We found six RCTs of fish oil and/or evening primrose oil, which were too small to allow reliable conclusions to be drawn.

Treatments for women who develop mild–moderate hypertension during pregnancy

- **Antihypertensive drugs for mild to moderate hypertension** Two systematic reviews have found that antihypertensive agents may halve the risk of severe hypertension but the effects of antihypertensive agents on other important outcomes are unclear. Systematic reviews found that angiotensin converting enzyme inhibitors used in pregnancy were associated with fetal renal failure, and found that β blockers increased the risk of the baby being small for its gestational age. It remains unclear whether treatment of mild to moderate hypertension during pregnancy is worthwhile with any antihypertensive agent compared with no treatment.
- **Bed rest/hospital admission** We found insufficient evidence about hospital admission or bed rest compared with outpatient or day care or normal activities in hospital.

Treatment for women who develop severe pre-eclampsia or very high blood pressure during pregnancy

- **Prophylactic magnesium sulphate in severe pre-eclampsia** One systematic review found that prophylactic magnesium sulphate halved the risk of eclampsia compared with placebo in women with severe pre-eclampsia. It found that magnesium sulphate reduced maternal mortality compared with placebo, although differences between groups did not reach significance. The review found no significant difference between magnesium sulphate and placebo on the risk of stillbirth or neonatal death in babies born to women with severe pre-eclampsia. The review also found that magnesium sulphate reduced the risk of eclampsia compared with phenytoin or nimodipine. A quarter of women given magnesium sulphate reported side effects (mainly flushing) compared with 5% of those given placebo. The review found insufficient evidence about the effects of diazepam compared with magnesium sulphate in women with severe pre-eclampsia.

- **Antihypertensive drugs for very high blood pressure** Consensus opinion is that women with severe hypertension during pregnancy should have antihypertensive treatment. Placebo trials would therefore be unethical. One systematic review and one subsequent RCT in women with blood pressures high enough to merit immediate treatment found that all of the included antihypertensives reduced blood pressure, but found no evidence of a difference in the control of blood pressure by various antihypertensive drugs. The studies were too small to draw any further conclusions about the relative effects of different agents. Ketanserin and diazoxide may be associated with more adverse effects than hydralazine and labetalol, respectively.
- **Interventionist obstetric management for severe early onset pre-eclampsia** One systematic review based on two small RCTs found no evidence that interventionist obstetric management reduced stillbirth or perinatal death rates compared with expectant management in babies born to mothers with severe early onset pre-eclampsia. However, it found that interventionist management increased rates of admission to neonatal intensive care and increased the risk of necrotising enterocolitis and respiratory distress in the baby compared with expectant management. The review found insufficient evidence about the effects of interventionist compared with expectant management in the mother.
- **Antioxidants in severe pre-eclampsia** One RCT found insufficient evidence about the effects of a combination of vitamin E plus vitamin C plus allopurinol compared with placebo.
- **Choice of analgesia during labour with severe pre-eclampsia** One RCT in women with severe pre-eclampsia found that epidural analgesia during labour reduced mean pain scores compared with patient controlled analgesia given intravenously, but the clinical importance of the difference was unclear.
- **Plasma volume expansion in severe pre-eclampsia** One systematic review comparing plasma volume expansion versus no expansion found insufficient evidence to draw reliable conclusions.

Anticonvulsant treatment in women with eclampsia

- **Magnesium sulphate for eclampsia (better and safer than other anticonvulsants)** Systematic reviews found that magnesium sulphate reduced the risk of further fits in women with eclampsia compared with phenytoin, diazepam, or lytic cocktail. One systematic review found that magnesium sulphate reduced the risk of maternal death compared with diazepam. Two other systematic reviews found lower maternal death rates with magnesium sulphate compared with phenytoin or lytic cocktail, although differences between groups did not reach significance.

DEFINITION Hypertension during pregnancy may be associated with one of several conditions. **Pregnancy induced hypertension** is a rise in blood pressure, without proteinuria, during the second half of pregnancy. **Pre-eclampsia** is a multisystem disorder, unique to pregnancy, which is usually associated with raised blood pressure and proteinuria. It rarely presents before 20 weeks' gestation. **Eclampsia** is one or more convulsions in association with the syndrome of pre-eclampsia. **Pre-existing hypertension** (not covered in this chapter) is known hypertension before pregnancy or raised blood pressure before 20 weeks' gestation. It may be essential hypertension or, less commonly, secondary to underlying disease.[1]

INCIDENCE/ PREVALENCE Pregnancy induced hypertension affects 10% of pregnancies, and pre-eclampsia complicates 2–8% of pregnancies.[2] Eclampsia occurs in about 1/2000 deliveries in developed countries.[3] In developing countries, estimates of the incidence of eclampsia vary from 1/100–1/1700.[4,5]

AETIOLOGY/ RISK FACTORS The cause of pre-eclampsia is unknown. It is likely to be multifactorial, and may result from deficient placental implantation during the first half of pregnancy.[6]

Pre-eclampsia is more common among women likely to have a large placenta, such as those with multiple pregnancy, and among women with medical conditions associated with microvascular disease, such as diabetes, hypertension, and collagen vascular disease.[7,8] Other risk factors include genetic susceptibility, increased parity, and older maternal age.[9] Cigarette smoking seems to be associated with a lower risk of pre-eclampsia, but this potential benefit is outweighed by an increase in adverse outcomes such as low birth weight, placental abruption, and perinatal death.[10]

PROGNOSIS The outcome of pregnancy in women with pregnancy induced hypertension alone is at least as good as that for normotensive pregnancies.[7,11] However, once pre-eclampsia develops, morbidity and mortality rise for both mother and child. For example, perinatal mortality for women with severe pre-eclampsia is double that for normotensive women.[7] Perinatal outcome is worse with early gestational hypertension.[7,9,11] Perinatal mortality also increases in women with severe essential hypertension.[12]

AIMS OF INTERVENTION To delay or prevent the development of pre-eclampsia and eclampsia, and to improve outcomes for women and their children. Once pre-eclampsia has occurred, to minimise morbidity and mortality for women and their children, and to ensure that health service resources are used appropriately.

OUTCOMES **For the woman:** Rates of pre-eclampsia (proteinuria and hypertension), eclampsia, death, severe morbidity (such as renal failure, coagulopathy, cardiac failure, liver failure, and stroke), placental abruption, and caesarean section; use of resources (such as dialysis, ventilation, admission to intensive care, or length of stay); adverse effects of treatment. **For the child:** Rates of death, intrauterine growth restriction, prematurity, and severe morbidity (such as intraventricular haemorrhage, respiratory distress syndrome, or asphyxia); measures of infant and child development (such as cerebral palsy or significant learning disability); use of resources (such as admission to special care nursery, ventilation, length of stay in hospital, and special needs in the community); adverse effects of treatment.

METHODS *Clinical Evidence* search and appraisal December 2003 and author search of the register of trials held by the Cochrane Pregnancy and Childbirth Group June 2002.

QUESTION What are the effects of preventive interventions in women at risk of pre-eclampsia?

OPTION ANTIPLATELET DRUGS

One systematic review and one subsequent RCT found that, in women considered at risk of pre-eclampsia, antiplatelet drugs (mainly aspirin) reduced the risk of pre-eclampsia, death of the baby, and delivery before 37 weeks compared with placebo or no treatment. The RCTs found no significant difference in other important outcomes. The systematic review found no evidence that aspirin increased the risk of bleeding in mother or baby compared with placebo.

Benefits: We found one systematic review[13] of antiplatelet agents (search date 1999, 39 RCTs, 30 563 women) and three subsequent RCTs.[14–16] **Versus placebo/no antiplatelet drug:** The systematic review found that, in women considered at risk of pre-eclampsia, antiplatelet agents significantly reduced pre-eclampsia compared with control (32 RCTs: 975/14 743 women [6.6%] with antiplatelet *v* 1142/14 588 women [7.8%] with no antiplatelet; RR 0.85, 95% CI 0.78 to 0.92; NNT 89, 95% CI 59 to 167), premature delivery before 37 completed weeks (23 RCTs: 2447/14 169 women [17.3%] with antiplatelet *v* 2621/14 099 [18.6%] with no antiplatelet; RR 0.92, 95% CI 0.88 to 0.97; NNT 72, 95% CI 44 to 200), and baby deaths (30 RCTs: 383/15 091 women [2.5%] with antiplatelet *v* 439/15 002 [2.9%] with no antiplatelet; RR 0.86, 95% CI 0.75 to 0.98; NNT 250, 95% CI 95 to > 10 000).[13] There were no clear effects on other important outcomes. There was no effect of starting treatment before 20 weeks, and no significant difference in the relative risk reduction between women at high and low risk for pre-eclampsia and its complications. The benefit was greatest for women given more than 75 mg aspirin daily. We found three subsequent RCTs (3944 women).[14–16] One RCT reported aspirin significantly reduced the incidence of pre-eclampsia compared with placebo,[14] whereas two RCTs found no significant difference between groups.[15,16] However, overall, the three RCTs had results consistent with those of the systematic review in that the 95% confidence intervals for outcomes reported by these three RCTs overlapped with those for relevant outcomes within the systematic review. **Versus each other:** Trials comparing one antiplatelet agent versus another were too small to allow reliable conclusions to be drawn.[13]

Harms: The systematic review found no evidence that aspirin increased the risk of bleeding for mother or baby.[13] Two studies followed up children of mothers enrolled in trials comparing aspirin versus placebo for 12–18 months.[17,18] They found no significant difference between aspirin and placebo for hospital visits for congenital malformations, motor deficit, developmental delay, respiratory problems, or bleeding problems; height or weight below the third centile; or bleeding rates in children of treated mothers.

Comment: Almost all RCTs used low dose aspirin 50–75 mg daily and most were placebo controlled. The RCTs included women with a variety of risk factors, including a history of previous early onset disease, diabetes, or chronic hypertension, and were conducted in different countries in the developed and developing world. The number needed to treat values cannot be applied directly to different populations of women; the values stated represent estimates for women with a risk of pre-eclampsia that is an average over all the participants in the RCTs. The absolute benefit was higher (and the NNT lower) in women at higher risk of pre-eclampsia.

OPTION CALCIUM SUPPLEMENTATION

One systematic review found that calcium supplementation (mainly 2 g/day) reduced the risk of pre-eclampsia and reduced the risk of having a baby with birth weight under 2500 g compared with placebo. It found no significant difference between calcium supplements and placebo on the risk of caesarean section, preterm delivery, or stillbirth or death of the baby before discharge from hospital.

Benefits: **Versus placebo:** We found one systematic review of calcium supplementation (search date 2001, 11 RCTs, 7203 women; see comment below).[19] It found that calcium (mainly 2 g/day) significantly reduced the risk of pre-eclampsia compared with placebo (11 RCTs: 197/3427 [6%] with calcium supplementation *v* 294/3452 [9%] with placebo; RR 0.68, 95% CI 0.57 to 0.81; NNT 38, 95% CI 26 to 67). Subgroup analysis found that the greatest effect was in women with low dietary calcium (27/907 [3%] with calcium supplementation *v* 90/935 [10%] with placebo for low dietary calcium compared with 169/2505 [7%] with calcium supplementation *v* 197/2517 [8%] with placebo for normal dietary calcium). It found that calcium supplementation significantly reduced the risk of having a baby with birth weight under 2500 g (234/3230 [7.2%] with calcium supplementation *v* 283/3261 [8.7%] with placebo; RR 0.83, 95% CI 0.71 to 0.98; NNT 67, 95% CI 36 to 1000). It found no significant difference between calcium supplements and placebo on the risk of caesarean delivery, preterm delivery, or stillbirth or death of the baby before discharge from hospital. **Calcium plus evening primrose oil versus placebo:** One small trial (48 women) did not provide sufficient evidence for reliable conclusions to be drawn.[20]

Harms: After follow up of 518 children to 7 years of age, the review found no harms associated with maternal calcium supplements.[19]

Comment: Most trials in the systematic review were of good quality and included a wide range of women. They were conducted largely in the USA and South America. They included mainly women at low risk with adequate dietary calcium, so the proportion of women in the category who would benefit most from calcium supplementation was small. Several studies reported that adherence to treatment was between 60–90%.[19] The proportion of women taking 90–100% of all allocated treatment was low (20% in 1 study).[19]

OPTION OTHER DIETARY CHANGE

We found insufficient evidence from six small RCTs about effects on pre-eclampsia or preterm birth of fish oil, evening primrose oil, or both, compared with either placebo or each other. Limited evidence from one systematic review found no significant difference in the risk of pre-eclampsia with a low salt diet compared with a normal diet. One systematic review found insufficient evidence about the effects of magnesium supplements on the risk of pre-eclampsia or its complications. Two RCTs found limited evidence that antioxidants (vitamin C plus E or lycopene) reduced the risk of pre-eclampsia compared with placebo. The RCTs of antioxidants provided insufficient evidence on other clinically important outcomes. One small RCT found that supplementation with protein, fish oil, and calcium, plus rest in the left lateral position, reduced the risk of pre-eclampsia compared with iron supplementation.

Benefits: **Fish oil and/or evening primrose oil:** We found no systematic review. We found six RCTs of fish oil and/or evening primrose oil that were too small to draw reliable conclusions.[21–26] **Protein, fish oil, and calcium, plus rest in left lateral position:** We found one RCT (74 women with a positive roll over test**G** at 28–29 weeks).[27] It compared protein 25 mg, fish oil 300 mg, and calcium 300 mg three times a week plus 15 minutes rest in the left lateral position twice daily versus ferrous sulphate 105 mg three times a week. It found that the multiple supplements reduced pre-eclampsia compared with iron supplementation (2/37 [5%] with multiple supplements *v* 16/37 [46%] with iron suplementation; RR 0.12, 95% CI 0.03 to 0.51; NNT 3, 95% CI 2 to 6). It was too small for reliable conclusions on other outcomes. **Salt restriction:** We found one systematic review (search date 1999, 2 RCTs, 600 women) comparing reduced salt with normal dietary salt.[28] It found no significant difference for rates of pre-eclampsia, although the trials may have lacked power to detect clinically important effects (RR 1.11, 95% CI 0.46 to 2.66). **Magnesium:** We found one systematic review (search date 2001, 2 RCTs, 474 women) reporting pre-eclampsia.[29] The RCTs were too small for reliable conclusions. **Antioxidants:** We found one RCT (283 high risk women), which found that vitamin C 1000 mg daily plus vitamin E 400 IU daily significantly reduced pre-eclampsia compared with placebo (11/141 [8%] with vitamins *v* 24/142 [17%] with placebo; RR 0.46, 95% CI 0.24 to 0.91; NNT 11, 95% CI 8 to 61).[30] Another RCT (251 primigravida women) found that lycopene 4 mg daily significantly reduced the risk of pre-eclampsia compared with placebo (10/116 [8.6%] with lycopene *v* 24/135 [17.7%] with placebo; RR 0.48, 95% CI 0.24 to 0.97).[31] The two RCTs were too small to provide reliable evidence about effects on other more substantive clinical outcomes.[30,31]

Harms: **Fish oil and/or evening primrose oil:** One RCT (533 women) found no significant difference between fish oil and olive oil or no supplement for rates of post-term delivery (RR 1.19, 95% CI 0.73 to 1.93) and post-partum haemorrhage (RR 1.21, 95% CI 0.76 to 1.92).[32] These outcomes were not reported in the other smaller studies. Vomiting was more commonly reported in the oil treated groups, but numbers were not provided.[25] No other adverse events were reported. **Reduced salt:** We found no evidence of harmful effects in the trials.[28] **Magnesium:** There was no significant difference between the groups in the number of reported adverse effects (RR 0.84, 95% CI 0.65 to 1.08).[29] **Antioxidents:** We found little evidence about the safety of vitamins C and E or of lycopene at the doses used in these RCTs.[30,31]

Comment: The fish oil RCTs may have been difficult to blind because of the distinctive taste of fish oil. One study found that olive oil provided better masking than a no oil placebo.[32] The trials of salt restriction were conducted in the Netherlands, where advice to restrict salt intake during pregnancy has been routine for many years. Such advice is no longer widespread elsewhere. An updated systematic review of fish oil for prevention of pre-eclampsia will be available soon.[33]

OPTION OTHER PHARMACOLOGICAL AGENTS

We found two small RCTs. One compared atenolol with placebo and the other compared glyceryl trinitrate patches with placebo. Both RCTs were too small to allow any reliable conclusions to be drawn.

Benefits: **Atenolol:** We found one small RCT (68 women without hypertension selected because they had a cardiac output > 7.4 L/minute), which found no significant reduction in the risk of pre-eclampsia with atenolol 100 mg daily (1/28 [4%] with atenolol *v* 5/28 [18%] with placebo; RR 0.20, 95% CI 0.02 to 1.60).[34] **Glyceryl trinitrate:** One small RCT (40 women) found no significant difference between glyceryl trinitrate patches and placebo (RR 1.13, 95% CI 0.35 to 3.60), but the confidence interval was wide.[35]

Harms: The RCT comparing atenolol with placebo found that mean birth weight was significantly lower with atenolol for a subgroup of primiparous women (mean difference 440 g; P = 0.02).[34]

Comment: Although the possible benefits of atenolol for prevention of pre-eclampsia remain unclear, the reduction in birth weight may be real. Concerns about the possible harmful effects of atenolol on fetal growth and development have been discussed for some time (see harms of antihypertensive agents, p 1818).[36,37]

QUESTION What are the effects of interventions in women who develop mild–moderate hypertension during pregnancy?

OPTION BED REST/HOSPITAL ADMISSION

We found insufficient evidence about hospital admission or bed rest compared with outpatient or day care.

Benefits: **Versus no hospital admission:** We found two systematic reviews of hospital admission.[38,39] The first systematic review (search date 1993, 3 trials, 408 women) compared hospital admission versus outpatient clinic assessment for non-proteinuric hypertension and found no significant difference for any major outcome.[38] The second systematic review (search date 1993, 2 RCTs, 145 women with proteinuric hypertension) compared bed rest in hospital versus normal ambulation in hospital, but the trials were too small for any reliable conclusions.[39] **Versus antenatal day care units:** We found one systematic review (search date 2001, 1 RCT, 54 women).[40] The RCT was too small for reliable conclusions.

Harms: It has been suggested that hospital admission increases the risk of venous stasis, thromboembolic disease, or infection, but we found no evidence in this context. In the trial of antenatal day care, women preferred not to be admitted to hospital. We found no evidence from the other trials about the views of women and their families.

Comment: Trials of hospital admission and bed rest in hospital were conducted before widespread introduction of day care assessment units. Women with hypertension during pregnancy are now often seen in day care units, but only one small trial has compared day care assessment versus assessment in an outpatient clinic. An updated systematic review of bed rest with or without hospitalisation is in preparation.[41]

OPTION ANTIHYPERTENSIVE AGENTS

Two systematic reviews have found evidence that antihypertensive agents may halve the risk of severe hypertension but the effects of antihypertensive agents on other important outcomes are unclear. Systematic reviews found that angiotensin converting enzyme inhibitors used in pregnancy are associated with fetal renal failure, and found that β blockers may increase the risk of the baby being small for gestational age. It remains unclear whether treatment of mild to moderate hypertension during pregnancy is worthwhile with any antihypertensive agent compared with no treatment.

Benefits: We found two systematic reviews[42,43] and two small subsequent RCTs.[44,45] The first systematic review (search date 2000, 40 RCTs, > 3797 women with mild to moderate hypertension) included studies that compared any antihypertensive drug versus placebo or versus another antihypertensive drug.[42] The second systematic review (search date 2002, 29 RCTs, 2500 women with mild to moderate hypertension) included only studies that compared β blockers versus no antihypertensive drug or versus another antihypertensive drug.[43] **Versus placebo or no antihypertensive drug:** The first review found that antihypertensive drugs significantly reduced the risk of developing severe hypertension compared with no antihypertensive drugs but found no significant difference between groups for pre-eclampsia and perinatal death (severe hypertension, 17 RCTs: RR 0.52, 95% CI 0.41 to 0.64; NNT 12, 95% CI 9 to 17; pre-eclampsia: RR 0.99, 95% CI 0.84 to 1.18; perinatal death: RR 0.71, 95% CI 0.46 to 1.09).[42] The second review found that β blockers significantly reduced the development of severe hypertension compared with no β blockers (11 RCTs, 1128 women: RR 0.37, 95% CI 0.26 to 0.53).[43] The review found insufficient evidence for other maternal outcomes. The first subsequent small RCT (70 primigravidae) also found that antihypertensive treatment significantly reduced the risk of developing severe hypertension compared with no treatment (3/34 [8.8%] with antihypertensive *v* 18/36 [50%] with no treatment).[44] **Versus other antihypertensive agents:** Neither systematic review found any clear difference among any of these drugs for the risk of developing severe hypertension or pre-eclampsia.[42,43] The first review found that methyldopa may increase the risk of the baby dying compared with other antihypertensive agents but the RCTs were small and used weak methods, so that the difference may have arisen because of random error or bias (baby death, 14 RCTs: RR 0.49, 95% CI 0.24 to 0.99).[42] The second small subsequent RCT (33 women) comparing alternative antihypertensive drugs found no significant differences in the risk of pre-eclampsia.[45]

Harms: The antihypertensive agents included in the systematic reviews[42,43] seem to be well tolerated during pregnancy, but adverse effects have not been reported in many RCTs. All antihypertensive drugs cross the placenta, but few trials reported possible adverse effects for the baby. The second review found β blockers significantly increased the baby's risk of being small for its gestational age (13 RCTs, 854 women: RR 1.34, 95% CI 1.01 to 1.79).[43] Meta regression within a systematic review suggested that lowering blood pressure for women with mild or moderate hypertension may increase the risk of having a baby that is small for its gestational age.[46] One systematic review (search date 1999, 13 small RCTs in women with pre-existing chronic hypertension) found that angiotensin converting enzyme inhibitors used in the second or third trimester are associated with fetal renal failure.[47,48]

Comment: The RCTs were too small to exclude beneficial effects of antihypertensive agents. The trials had problems with their methods. Many were not placebo controlled, and few attempted to blind blood pressure measurement. Many important outcomes were reported by only a few studies. We found little evidence about adherence to treatment. One systematic review found that the effects of antihypertensive agents in women with pre-existing chronic hypertension were similar to those described above for women with pregnancy induced hypertension. The review did not establish or exclude benefit from treatment.[47,48]

QUESTION What are the effects of interventions in women who develop severe pre-eclampsia or very high blood pressure during pregnancy?

OPTION ANTIHYPERTENSIVE DRUGS FOR VERY HIGH BLOOD PRESSURE

Consensus opinion is that women with severe hypertension during pregnancy should have antihypertensive treatment. Placebo trials would therefore be unethical. One systematic review and one subsequent RCT in women with blood pressures high enough to merit immediate treatment found that all of the included antihypertensives reduced blood pressure, but found no evidence of a difference in the control of blood pressure by various antihypertensive drugs. The studies were too small to draw any further conclusions about the relative effects of different agents. Ketanserin and diazoxide may be associated with more adverse effects than hydralazine and labetalol, respectively.

Benefits: We found one systematic review (search date 2002, 20 RCTs, 1637 women)[49] and one small subsequent RCT.[50] The review compared many antihypertensives (such as labetalol, nifedipine, methyldopa, diazoxide, prostacyclin, urapidil, magnesium sulphate, prazosin, nimodipine, and ketanserin) mainly versus hydralazine.[49] It found that all the antihypertensives reduced blood pressure, but there was no significant evidence that one drug was better than another. The subsequent RCT (126 women) compared nifedipine 8 mg sublingually versus hydralazine (5 mg iv followed by further doses of 10 mg).[50] It found that nifedipine significantly delayed development of hypertensive crisis compared with hydralazine (median time to hypertensive crisis 3.1 hours with nifedipine *v* 2.1 hours with hydralazine; P = 0.005).

Harms: The use of ketanserin is associated with more persistent hypertension than hydralazine (RR 8.44, 95% CI 2.05 to 34.70), and labetalol is associated with less hypotension requiring treatment than diazoxide (RR 0.06, 95% CI 0 to 0.99).[49] Hypotension may compromise fetoplacental blood flow. Few RCTs reported adverse effects, and frequency varied from 5–50%. Antihypertensive drugs cross the placenta, but we found little evidence about effects on the baby.

Comment: Consensus opinion is that women with severe hypertension during pregnancy should have antihypertensive treatment. Placebo trials would therefore be unethical. Women in these studies had blood pressures high enough to merit immediate treatment, and many also had proteinuria or "severe pre-eclampsia". The trials were small and reported few outcomes other than control of blood pressure. In most trials, there was no blinding after trial entry. One small RCT (60 women with severe hypertension) found no significant difference in treatment success between intravenous labetalol and nicardipine given over 1 hour (blood pressure decreased by 20%: 63% with labetalol *v* 70% with nicardipine, P = 0.58).[51]

OPTION PLASMA VOLUME EXPANSION

One systematic review comparing plasma volume expansion versus no expansion found insufficient evidence to draw reliable conclusions.

Benefits: We found one systematic review (search date 2000, 3 RCTs, 61 women; see comment below)[52] evaluating colloid solutions compared with placebo or no infusion. The RCTs were too small for reliable conclusions but suggest that plasma volume expansion is not beneficial.[52]

Harms: RCTs found no significant difference between plasma volume expansion and either placebo or no infusion in the risk of caesarean section or in the need for additional treatment (caesarean section: RR 1.5, 95% CI 0.8 to 2.9; additional treatment: RR 1.5, 95% CI 0.7 to 3.1).[52]

Comment: In one RCT included in the review, all women had severe pre-eclampsia; in the other two RCTs some women did not have proteinuria at trial entry and those with severe hypertension were excluded.[52] These three RCTs all used a colloid rather than crystalloid solution. Two systematic reviews (search dates 2002[53] and 1999[54]) of plasma volume expansion in critically ill men and non-pregnant women have found an increased mortality with albumin (a colloid) when compared with either no expansion or crystalloid.

OPTION ANTIOXIDANTS

One RCT found insufficient evidence about the effects of a combination of vitamin E plus vitamin C plus allopurinol compared with placebo.

Benefits: We found no systematic review. We found one RCT (56 women with severe pre-eclampsia at 24–32 weeks' gestation) comparing vitamin E plus vitamin C plus allopurinol versus placebo.[55] It was too small for reliable conclusions to be drawn.

Harms: We found insufficient evidence for reliable conclusions.

Comment: None.

OPTION PROPHYLACTIC ANTICONVULSANTS FOR WOMEN WITH SEVERE PRE-ECLAMPSIA

One systematic review found that prophylactic magnesium sulphate halved the risk of eclampsia compared with placebo in women with severe pre-eclampsia. It found that magnesium sulphate reduced maternal mortality compared with placebo, although differences between groups did not reach significance. The review found no significant difference between magnesium sulphate and placebo on the risk of stillbirth or neonatal death in babies born to women with severe pre-eclampsia. The review also found that magnesium sulphate reduced the risk of eclampsia compared with phenytoin or

nimodipine. A quarter of women given magnesium sulphate reported side effects (mainly flushing) compared with 5% of those given placebo. The review found insufficient evidence about the effects of diazepam compared with magnesium sulphate in women with severe pre-eclampsia.

Benefits: We found one systematic review (search date 2002, 13 RCTs, 15 558 women).[56] **Magnesium sulphate versus placebo or no anticonvulsant:** In this review, six RCTs (11 444 women) compared magnesium sulphate versus placebo. Prophylactic magnesium sulphate significantly reduced the risk of eclampsia compared with placebo (43/5722 [0.8%] with magnesium sulphate *v* 107/5722 [1.9%] with placebo; RR 0.41, 95% CI 0.29 to 0.58; NNT 100, 95% CI 50 to 100). Magnesium sulphate also reduced maternal mortality compared with placebo, although the results were not statistically significant (2 RCTs; 11/5400 [0.2%] with magnesium sulphate *v* 21/5395 [0.4%] with placebo; RR 0.54, 95% CI 0.26 to 1.10). For women randomised before delivery, there was no significant difference in the risk of stillbirth or neonatal death (3 RCTs; 634/5003 [13%] with magnesium sulphate *v* 611/4958 [12%] with placebo; RR 1.04, 95% CI 0.93 to 1.15).[56] **Magnesium sulphate versus phenytoin, nimodipine, or diazepam:** Two RCTs (2241 women) included in the review found that magnesium sulphate significantly reduced the risk of eclampsia compared with phenytoin (0/1109 [0%] with magnesium sulphate *v* 10/1132 [0.8%] with phenytoin; RR 0.05, 95% CI 0.00 to 0.84).[56] Another RCT (1650 women) found that magnesium sulphate significantly reduced the risk of eclampsia compared with nimodipine (7/831 [0.8%] with magnesium sulphate *v* 21/819 [2.6%] with nimodipine; RR 0.33, 95% CI 0.14 to 0.77).[56] There was insufficient evidence for reliable conclusions about magnesium sulphate compared with diazepam (2 RCTs, 66 women).[56]

Harms: One large placebo controlled trial in the review reported adverse effects in detail.[57] In this RCT, a quarter of women experienced side effects with magnesium sulphate (1201/4999 [24%] with magnesium sulphate *v* 228/4993 [5%] with placebo).[57] Specific effects included flushing (2 RCTs; 1032/5066 [20%] with magnesium sulphate *v* 110/5061 [2%] with placebo).[56] Respiratory depression was rare (2 RCTs; 52/5344 [1%] with magnesium sulphate *v* 26/5333 [0.5%] with placebo).[56] Magnesium sulphate slightly increased the risk of caesarean section compared with placebo (2528/5082 [50%] with magnesium sulphate *v* 2370/5026 [47%] with placebo; RR 1.05, 95% CI 1.01 to 1.10; NNH 34, 95% CI 25 to 100). The review found that, compared with phenytoin, magnesium sulphate was also associated with an increased risk of caesarean section (RR 1.21, 95% CI 1.05 to 1.41; NNH 21, 95% CI 12 to 83).[56] Compared with nimodipine, magnesium sulphate was associated with an increase in respiratory problems (11/831 [1%] with magnesium sulphate *v* 3/819 [0.4%] with nimodipine; RR 3.61, 95% CI 1.01 to 12.91).[56] One small RCT evaluated magnesium sulphate for preventing and treating preterm labour in women who did not have pre-eclampsia. It found an increase in infant mortality for babies born to these women. Many of the infants had very low birth weight (< 1500 g).[58]

Comment: Most of the data in these trials refer to women with relatively severe pre-eclampsia. One small study recruited only women with mild pre-eclampsia. Long term follow up of women and children in one large RCT that compared magnesium sulphate versus placebo is continuing.[57] Weak evidence from two case control studies suggested that magnesium sulphate may be associated with a decreased risk of cerebral palsy in babies weighing less than 1500 g.[59,60] This hypothesis has been tested in a large RCT.[61] The RCT found that magnesium sulphate was associated with a non-significant reduction in the composite outcome of death or cerebral palsy compared with placebo (123/629 [20%] with magnesium sulphate *v* 149/626 [24%] with placebo; RR 0.83, 95% CI 0.66 to 1.03).[61]

OPTION — INTERVENTIONIST OBSTETRIC MANAGEMENT FOR SEVERE EARLY ONSET PRE-ECLAMPSIA

One systematic review based on two small RCTs found no evidence that interventionist obstetric management reduced stillbirth or perinatal death rates compared with expectant management in babies born to mothers with severe early onset pre-eclampsia. However, it found that interventionist management increased rates of admission to neonatal intensive care and increased the risk of necrotising enterocolitis and respiratory distress in the baby compared with expectant management. The review found insufficient evidence about the effects of interventionist compared with expectant management in the mother.

Benefits: We found one systematic review (search date 2002, 2 RCTs, 133 women at 28–34 weeks' gestation), which compared a policy of early elective delivery by induction or caesarean section depending on individual obstetric circumstances (interventionist management) versus a policy of delayed delivery to allow more time for fetal maturation (expectant management) in women with severe pre-eclampsia.[62] It found that, for the baby, there was no significant difference in rates of stillbirth or death after delivery for interventionist management compared with expectant care (RR of death or stillbirth for interventional *v* expectant care 1.50, 95% CI 0.42 to 5.41). Babies of mothers in the interventionist management group were less likely to be small for gestational age than those in the expectant group (RR for interventionist *v* expectant management 0.36, 95% CI 0.14 to 0.90). The review found insufficient evidence about effects on maternal outcomes.

Harms: The review found that interventionist management increased risks of respiratory distress syndrome, necrotising enterocolitis, and rate of admission to neonatal intensive care in babies born to mothers with severe pre-eclampsia (respiratory distress syndrome: 34/66 [52%] babies with interventionist management *v* 15/67 [22%] with expectant care; RR 2.30, 95% CI 1.39 to 3.81; necrotising colitis: RR 5.5, 95% CI 1.04 to 29.56; admission to neonatal intensive care: RR 1.32, 95% CI 1.13 to 1.55).[62] We found insufficient evidence for reliable conclusions about effects of expectant management on maternal morbidity.

Comment: None.

OPTION — CHOICE OF ANALGESIA DURING LABOUR

One RCT in women with severe pre-eclampsia found that epidural analgesia during labour reduced pain scores compared with patient controlled analgesia given intravenously, but the clinical importance of the difference was not clear.

Benefits: We found one RCT (105 women with severe pre-eclampsia) comparing patient controlled analgesia given intravenously versus epidural analgesia.[63] It found that epidural analgesia significantly reduced mean pain scores but the clinical importance of the difference is unclear. The trial was too small for a reliable conclusion about other outcomes. We found no RCTs of other forms of intrapartum analgesia for this group of women.

Harms: Women allocated an epidural were more likely to have hypotension requiring intravenous ephedrine (5/56 [9%] with epidural v 0/60 [0%] with patient controlled analgesia).[63] Neonatal naloxone was more likely to be given after patient controlled analgesia given intravenously (31/60 [54%] with patient controlled analgesia given intravenously v 5/56 [9%] with epidural analgesia; RR 5.71, 95% CI 2.39 to 13.60; NNH 3, 95% CI 2 to 4). The trial was too small for reliable conclusions about other outcomes.

Comment: The drug used for patient controlled analgesia was not reported.

QUESTION What is the best choice of anticonvulsant for women with eclampsia?

OPTION ANTICONVULSANTS FOR WOMEN WITH ECLAMPSIA

Systematic reviews found that magnesium sulphate reduced the risk of further fits in women with eclampsia compared with phenytoin, diazepam, or lytic cocktail. One systematic review found that magnesium sulphate reduced the risk of maternal death compared with diazepam. Two other systematic reviews found lower maternal death rates with magnesium sulphate compared with phenytoin or lytic cocktail, although differences between groups did not reach significance.

Benefits: **Magnesium sulphate versus diazepam:** We found one systematic review (search date 2002, 7 RCTs, 1441 women).[64] It found that magnesium sulphate significantly reduced both maternal mortality and further fits compared with diazepam (maternal death: 6 RCTs; 26/677 [3.8%] with magnesium sulphate v 42/659 [6.4%] with diazepam; RR 0.59, 95% CI 0.37 to 0.94; further fits: 7 RCTs; 71/737 [10%] v 162/704 [23%]; RR 0.44, 95% CI 0.34 to 0.57). It found no significant differences in any other outcomes for the mother. For the babies, it found that magnesium sulphate significantly reduced the proportion of babies with Apgar scores less than seven at 5 minutes compared with diazepam (2 RCTs; 69/309 [22%] with magnesium sulphate v 90/288 [31%] with diazepam; RR 0.72, 95% CI 0.55 to 0.94) and significantly reduced the proportion of babies with a length of stay in special care baby unit more than 7 days compared with diazepam (3 RCTs; 42/329 [13%] with magnesium sulphate v 59/302 [20%] with diazepam; RR 0.66, 95% CI 0.46 to 0.95).[64] **Magnesium sulphate versus phenytoin:** We found one systematic review (search date 2002, 6 RCTs, 897 women).[65] It found that, compared with phenytoin, magnesium sulphate significantly reduced the risk of further fits (5 RCTs; 25/448 [6%] with magnesium sulphate v 83/447 [19%] with phenytoin; RR 0.31, 95% CI 0.20 to 0.47); pneumonia (1 RCT, 775 women; RR 0.44, 95% CI 0.24 to 0.79); requirement for ventilation (1 RCT, 775 women; RR 0.66, 95% CI 0.49 to 0.90); and admission to intensive care unit (1 RCT, 775 women; RR 0.67, 95% CI 0.50 to 0.89).[65] It also found that magnesium sulphate significantly reduced the proportion of babies with the composite outcome of dying or staying in a special baby care unit for more than 7 days compared with phenytoin (1 RCT, 643 babies; RR 0.77, 95% CI 0.63 to 0.95). The lower maternal death rate with magnesium sulphate compared with phenytoin was not significant, but the confidence interval was wide and a clinically important effect could not be excluded (2 RCTs; 10/399 [2.5%] with magnesium sulphate v 20/398 [5.0%] with phenytoin; RR 0.50, 95% CI 0.24 to 1.05).[65] **Magnesium sulphate versus lytic cocktail:** We found one systematic review (search date 2000, 2 RCTs, 199 women).[66] Magnesium sulphate compared with lytic cocktail Ⓖ significantly reduced further fits, pneumonia, respiratory depression, and fetal or infant death (further fits: 4/96 [4%] with magnesium sulphate *v* 49/102 [48%] with lytic cocktail; RR 0.09, 95% CI 0.03 to 0.24; pneumonia: 1/51 [2%] with magnesium sulphate *v* 11/57 [19%] with lytic cocktail; RR 0.08, 95% CI 0.02 to 0.42; respiratory depression: 0/96 [0%] with magnesium sulphate *v* 8/102 [8%] with lytic cocktail; RR 0.12, 95% CI 0.02 to 0.91; fetal or infant death: 14/89 [16%] with magnesium sulphate *v* 30/88 [34%] with lytic cocktail; RR 0.45, 95% CI 0.26 to 0.79). There was a non-significant reduction in maternal deaths (1/96 [1%] with magnesium sulphate *v* 6/102 [6%] with lytic cocktail; RR 0.25, 95% CI 0.04 to 1.43).

Harms: We found no good evidence from RCTs about harms. Clinical experience suggests that magnesium sulphate is safer than phenytoin for both the woman and her baby, and considerably safer than lytic cocktail.

Comment: Most information about the comparisons with diazepam and phenytoin comes from one large multicentre trial, in which adherence to treatment was 99%. The lytic cocktail trials included women with antepartum or postpartum eclampsia.

GLOSSARY

Lytic cocktail A mixture of pethidine, chlorpromazine, and promethazine.

Roll over test A test in which a woman lies on her left side for 15 minutes after which blood pressure is recorded. She then rolls into the supine position and, after 5 minutes, blood pressure is measured again. A rise in diastolic blood pressure in the supine position of more than 20 mm Hg is defined as abnormal. The value of this test has been questioned.

REFERENCES

1. Gifford RW, August P, Chesley LC, et al. National high blood pressure education program working group report on high blood pressure in pregnancy. *Am J Obstet Gynecol* 1990;163(5 Pt 1):1691–1712.
2. WHO international collaborative study of hypertensive disorders of pregnancy. Geographic variation in the incidence of hypertension in pregnancy. *Am J Obstet Gynecol* 1988;158:80–83.
3. Douglas K, Redman C. Eclampsia in the United Kingdom. *BMJ* 1994;309:1395–1400.
4. Crowther CA. Eclampsia at Harare maternity hospital. An epidemiological study. *S Afr Med J* 1985;68:927–929.
5. Bergström S, Povey G, Songane F, et al. Seasonal incidence of eclampsia and its relationship to meteorological data in Mozambique. *J Perinat Med* 1992;20:153–158.
6. Roberts JM, Redman CWG. Pre-eclampsia: more than pregnancy-induced hypertension. *Lancet* 1993;341:1447–1451.
7. Taylor DJ. The epidemiology of hypertension during pregnancy. In: Rubin PC, ed. *Hypertension in pregnancy*. Amsterdam: Elsevier Science, 1988: 223–240.
8. Sibai BM, Caritis S, Hauth J. Risks of preeclampsia and adverse neonatal outcomes among women with pregestational diabetes mellitus. National Institute of Child Health and Human Development Network of Maternal-Fetal Medicine Units. *Am J Obstet Gynecol* 2000;182:364–369.
9. MacGillivray I. *Pre-eclampsia. The hypertensive disease of pregnancy*. London: WB Saunders, 1983.
10. Conde-Agudelo A, Althabe F, Belizan JM, et al. Cigarette smoking during pregnancy and risk of preeclampsia: a systematic review. *Am J Obstet Gynecol* 1999;181:1026–1035. Search date 1998; primary sources Medline, Embase, Popline, Cinahl, Lilacs, and hand searches of proceedings of international meetings on pre-eclampsia and reference lists of retrieved articles.
11. Chamberlain GVP, Philip E, Howlett B, et al. *British births*. London: Heinemann, 1970.
12. Sibai B, Lindheimer M, Hauth J, et al. Risk factors for preeclampsia, abruptio placentae, and adverse neonatal outcomes among women with chronic hypertension. *N Engl J Med* 1998;339:667–671.
13. Knight M, Duley L, Henderson-Smart DJ, et al. Antiplatelet agents for preventing and treating pre-eclampsia. In: The Cochrane Library, Issue 4, 2003. Oxford: Update Software. Search date 1999; primary sources Cochrane Pregnancy and Childbirth Group Trials Register and conference proceedings.
14. Vainio M, Kujansuu E, Iso-Mustajarvi M, et al. Low dose acetylsalicylic acid in prevention of pregnancy-induced hypertension and intrauterine growth retardation in women with bilateral uterine artery notches. *Br J Obstet Gynaecol* 2002;109:161–167.
15. Subtil D, Goeusse P, Puech F, et al. Aspirin (100 mg) used for prevention of pre-eclampsia in nulliparous women: the Essai Regional Aspirine Mere-Enfant study (Part 1). *Br J Obstet Gynaecol* 2003;110:475–484.
16. Yu CK, Papageorghiou AT, Parra M, et al. Randomized controlled trial using low-dose aspirin in the prevention of pre-eclampsia in women with abnormal uterine artery Doppler at 23 weeks' gestation. *Ultrasound Obstet Gynecol* 2003;22:233–239.
17. Grant A, Farrell B, Heineman J, et al. Low dose aspirin in pregnancy and early childhood development: follow up of the collaborative low dose aspirin study in pregnancy. *Br J Obstet Gynaecol* 1995;102:861–868.
18. Parazzini F, Bortolus R, Chatenoud L, et al. Follow-up of children in the Italian study of aspirin in pregnancy. *Lancet* 1994;343:1235.
19. Atallah AN, Hofmeyr GJ, Duley L. Calcium supplementation during pregnancy for preventing hypertensive disorders and related problems. In: The Cochrane Library, Issue 4, 2003. Oxford: Update Software. Search date 2001; primary source Cochrane Pregnancy and Childbirth Group Trials Register.
20. Herrera JA, Arevalo-Herrera M, Herrera S. Prevention of pre-eclampsia by linoleic acid and calcium supplementation: a randomized controlled trial. *Obstet Gynecol* 1998;91:585–590.

21. Salvig JD, Olsen SF, Secher NJ. Effects of fish oil supplementation in late pregnancy on blood pressure: a randomised controlled trial. *Br J Obstet Gynaecol* 1996;103:529–533.
22. Onwude JL, Lilford RJ, Hjartardottir H, et al. A randomised double blind placebo controlled trial of fish oil in high risk pregnancy. *Br J Obstet Gynaecol* 1995;102:95–100.
23. Bulstra-Ramakers MTE, Huisjes HJ, Visser GHA. The effects of 3 g eicosapentaenoic acid daily on recurrence of intrauterine growth retardation and pregnancy induced hypertension. *Br J Obstet Gynaecol* 1995;102:123–126.
24. Laivuori H, Hovatta O, Viinikka L, et al. Dietary supplementation with primrose oil or fish oil does not change urinary excretion of prostacyclin and thromboxane metabolites in pre-eclamptic women. *Prostaglandins Leukot Essent Fatty Acids* 1993;49:691–694.
25. D'Almeida A, Carter JP, Anatol A, et al. Effects of a combination of evening primrose oil (gamma linolenic acid) and fish oil (eicosapentaenoic + docahexaenoic acid) versus magnesium, and versus placebo in preventing pre-eclampsia. *Women Health* 1992;19:117–131.
26. Moodley J, Norman RJ. Attempts at dietary alteration of prostaglandin pathways in the management of pre-eclampsia. *Prostaglandins Leukot Essent Fatty Acids* 1989;37:145–147.
27. Herrera JA. Nutritional factors and rest reduce pregnancy-induced hypertension and pre-eclampsia in positive roll-over test primigravidas. *Int J Gynaecol Obstet* 1993;41:31–35.
28. Duley L, Henderson-Smart D. Reduced salt intake compared to normal dietary salt, or high intake, in pregnancy. In: The Cochrane Library, Issue 4, 2003. Oxford: Update Software. Search date 1999; primary source Cochrane Pregnancy and Childbirth Group Trials Register.
29. Makrides M, Crowther CA. Magnesium supplementation in pregnancy. In: The Cochrane Library, Issue 4, 2003. Oxford: Update Software. Search date 2001; primary source Cochrane Pregnancy and Childbirth Group Trials Register.
30. Chappell LC, Seed PT, Briley AL, et al. Effect of antioxidants on the occurrence of pre-eclampsia in women at increased risk: a randomised trial. *Lancet* 1999;354:810–816.
31. Sharma JB, Kumar A, Kumar A, et al. Effect of lycopene on pre-eclampsia and intra-uterine growth retardation in primigravidas. *Int J Gynecol Obstet* 2003;81:257–262.
32. Olsen SF, Sorensen JD, Secher NJ, et al. Randomised controlled trial of effect of fish oil supplementation on pregnancy duration. *Lancet* 1992;339:1003–1007.
33. Makrides M, Duley L, Olsen SF. Fish oil and other prostaglandin precursor supplementation during pregnancy for reducing pre-eclampsia, preterm birth, low birth weight and intrauterine growth restriction (protocol for a Cochrane Review). In: The Cochrane Library, Issue 4, 2003. Oxford: Update Software.
34. Easterling TR, Brateng D, Schucker B, et al. Prevention of preeclampsia: a randomized trial of atenolol in hyperdynamic patients before onset of hypertension. *Obstet Gynecol* 1999;93:725–733.
35. Lees C, Valensise H, Black R, et al. The efficacy and fetal-maternal cardiovascular effects of transdermal glycerol trinitrate in the prophylaxis of pre-eclampsia and its complications: a randomized double blind placebo controlled trial. *Ultrasound Obstet Gynaecol* 1998;12:334–338.
36. Butters L, Kennedy S, Rubin PC. Atenolol in essential hypertension during pregnancy. *BMJ* 1990;301:587–589.
37. Churchill D, Bayliss H, Beevers G. Fetal growth restriction. *Lancet* 1999;355:1366–1367.
38. Duley L. Hospitalisation for non-proteinuric pregnancy hypertension. In: Keirse MJNC, Renfrew MJ, Neilson JP, et al, eds. *Pregnancy and childbirth module*. In: The Cochrane Library, Issue 2, 1995. Oxford: Update Software. Search date 1993; primary source Cochrane Pregnancy and Childbirth Group Trials Register.
39. Duley L. Strict bed rest for proteinuric hypertension in pregnancy. In: Keirse MJNC, Renfrew MJ, Neilson JP, et al, eds. *Pregnancy and childbirth module*. In: The Cochrane Library, Issue 4, 1995. Oxford: Update Software. Search date 1993; primary source Cochrane Pregnancy and Childbirth Group Trials Register.
40. Kröner C, Turnbull D, Wilkinson C. Antenatal day care units versus hospital admission for women with complicated pregnancy. In: The Cochrane Library, Issue 4, 2003. Oxford: Update Software. Search date 2001; primary sources Cochrane Pregnancy and Childbirth Group Trials Register, Cochrane Controlled Trials Register, Cinahl, Current Contents, and conference proceedings.
41. Abalos E, Carroli G. Bed rest with or without hospitalisation for hypertension during pregnancy (protocol for a Cochrane Review). In: The Cochrane Library, Issue 4, 2003. Oxford: Update Software.
42. Abalos E, Duley L, Steyn DW, et al. Antihypertensive drug therapy for mild to moderate hypertension during pregnancy. In: The Cochrane Library, Issue 4, 2003. Oxford: Update Software. Search date 2000; primary sources Cochrane Pregnancy and Childbirth Group Trials Register, Cochrane Controlled Trials Register, Medline, and Embase.
43. Magee LA, Duley L. Oral beta-blockers for mild to moderate hypertension during pregnancy. In: The Cochrane Library, Issue 4, 2003. Oxford: Update Software. Search date 2002; primary sources Cochrane Pregnancy and Childbirth Group Trial Register, Medline, and hand searches of reference lists.
44. Elhassan EM, Mirghani OA, Habour AB, et al. Methyldopa versus no drug treatment in the management of mild pre-eclampsia. *East Afr Med J* 2002;79:172–175.
45. Rudnicki M, Frolich A, Pilsgaard K, et al. Comparison of magnesium and methyldopa for the control of blood pressure in pregnancies complicated with hypertension. *Gynecol Obstet Invest* 2000;49:231–235.
46. Von Dadelszen P, Ornstein MP, Bull SB, et al. Fall in mean arterial pressure and fetal growth restriction in pregnancy hypertension: a meta-analysis. *Lancet* 2000;355:87–92. Search date 1997; primary sources Medline, Embase, hand searches of reference lists, *Hypertension and Pregnancy* 1992–1997, and a standard toxicology text.
47. Ferrer RL, Sibai BM, Mulrow CD, et al. Management of mild chronic hypertension during pregnancy: a review. *Obstet Gynecol* 2000;96:849–860. Search date 1999; primary sources 16 electronic databases, textbook references, and contact with experts.
48. Mulrow CD, Chiquette E, Ferrer RL, et al. Management of chronic hypertension during pregnancy. Evidence Report/Technology Assessment No 14 (prepared by the San Antonio Evidence-based Practice Center based at the University of Texas Health Science Center at San Antonio under Contract No 290–97-0012). AHRQ Publication No 00-E011. Rockville, MD: Agency for Healthcare Research and Quality. August 2000. Search date 1999; primary sources 16 electronic databases, textbook references, and experts. Http://www.ahrq.gov/clinic/epcsums/pregsum.htm.
49. Duley L, Henderson-Smart DJ. Drugs for treatment of very high blood pressure during pregnancy. In: The Cochrane Library, Issue 4, 2003. Oxford: Update Software. Search date 2002; primary source Cochrane Pregnancy and Childbirth Group Trials Register.
50. Aali BS, Nejad SS. Nifedipine or hydralazine as a first-line agent to control hypertension in severe preeclampsia. *Acta Obstet Gynecol Scand* 2002;81:25–30.
51. Elatrous S, Nouira S, Ouanes Besbes L, et al. Short-term treatment of severe hypertension of

pregnancy: prospective comparison of nicardipine and labetalol. *Intensive Care Med* 2002;28:1281–1286.

52. Duley L, Williams J, Henderson-Smart DJ. Plasma volume expansion for treatment of pre-eclampsia. In: The Cochrane Library, Issue 4, 2003. Oxford: Update Software. Search date 2000; primary source Cochrane Pregnancy and Childbirth Group Trials Register.
53. The Albumin Reviewers (Alderson P, Bunn F, Li Wan Po L, et al). Human albumin solution for resuscitation and volume expansion in critically ill patients. In: The Cochrane Library, Issue 4, 2003. Oxford: Update Software. Search date 2002; primary sources Cochrane Injuries Group Trials Register, Cochrane Controlled Trials Register, Medline, Embase, Bids Scientific and Technical Proceedings, hand searches of reference lists of trials and review articles, and personal contact with authors of identified trials.
54. Alderson P, Schierhout G, Roberts I, et al. Colloids versus crystalloids for fluid resuscitation in critically ill patients. In: The Cochrane Library, Issue 4, 2003. Oxford: Update Software. Search date 1999; primary sources Cochrane Clinical Trials Register, Medline, Embase, Bids Index to Scientific and Technical Proceedings, and reference lists of trials and review articles.
55. Gülmezoglu AM, Hofmeyr GJ, Oosthuizen MMJ. Antioxidants in the treatment of severe preeclampsia: a randomized explanatory study. *Br J Obstet Gynaecol* 1997;104:689–696.
56. Duley L, Gülmezoglu AM, Henderson-Smart D. Magnesium sulphate and other anticonvulsants for women with pre-eclampsia. In: The Cochrane Library Issue 4, 2003. Oxford: Update Software. Search date 2002; primary source Cochrane Pregnancy and Childbirth Group Trials Register.
57. The Magpie Trial Collaborative Group. Do women with pre-eclampsia, and their babies, benefit from magnesium sulphate? The Magpie Trial: a randomised placebo-controlled trial. *Lancet* 2002;359:1877–1890.
58. Mittendorf R, Covert R, Boman J, et al. Is tocolytic magnesium sulphate associated with increased total paediatric mortality? *Lancet* 1997;350:1517–1518.
59. Nelson K, Grether JK. Can magnesium sulfate reduce the risk of cerebral palsy in very low birthweight infants? *Pediatrics* 1995;95:263–269.
60. Schendel DE, Berg CJ, Yeargin-Allsopp M, et al. Prenatal magnesium sulfate exposure and the risk of cerebral palsy or mental retardation among very low-birth-weight children aged 3 to 5 years. *JAMA* 1996;276:1805–1810.
61. Crowther CA, Hiller JE, Doyle LW, et al. Effect of magnesium sulfate given for neuroprotection before preterm birth. A randomized controlled trial. *JAMA* 2003;290:2669–2676.
62. Churchill D, Duley L. Interventionist versus expectant care for severe pre-eclampsia before term (Cochrane Review). In: The Cochrane Library, Issue 4, 2003. Oxford: Update Software. Search date 2002; primary sources Cochrane Pregnancy and Childbirth Group Trials Register and Cochrane Controlled Trials Register.
63. Head BB, Owen J, Vincent Jr RD, et al. A randomized trial of intrapartum analgesia in women with severe preeclampsia. *Obstet Gynecol* 2002;99:452–457.
64. Duley L, Henderson-Smart D. Magnesium sulphate versus diazepam for eclampsia. In: The Cochrane Library, Issue 4, 2003. Oxford: Update Software. Search date 2002; primary source Cochrane Pregnancy and Childbirth Group Trials Register.
65. Duley L, Henderson-Smart D. Magnesium sulphate versus phenytoin for eclampsia. In: The Cochrane Library, Issue 4, 2003. Oxford: Update Software. Search date 2002; primary source Cochrane Pregnancy and Childbirth Group Trials Register.
66. Duley L, Gulmezoglu AM. Magnesium sulphate versus lytic cocktail for eclampsia. In: The Cochrane Library, Issue 4, 2003. Oxford: Update Software. Search date 2000; primary sources Cochrane Pregnancy and Childbirth Group Trials Register and Cochrane Controlled Trials Register.

Lelia Duley
Obstetric Epidemiologist
Institute of Health Sciences
Oxford
UK

Competing interests: None declared.

Preterm birth

Search date September 2003

Bridgette Byrne and John J Morrison

QUESTIONS

INTERVENTIONS

Clin Evid 2005;13:1826–1843.

To be covered in future updates
Effects of repeated doses of antenatal corticosteroid
Uterine activity monitoring for singleton and multiple pregnancies in prevention of preterm birth

Covered elsewhere in *Clinical Evidence*
Antibiotic treatment of bacterial vaginosis to prevent preterm birth: see bacterial vaginosis, p 1968

See glossary G

Key Messages

Prevention

- **Prophylactic cervical cerclage for women at risk of cervical incompetence where cervical changes have not been identified** Systematic reviews identified five RCTs that found different results for women where cervical changes have not been identified. One large RCT found that cervical cerclage at 9–29 weeks reduced delivery before 33 weeks' gestation in women with a previous preterm delivery or previous cervical surgery, but doubled the risk of puerperal pyrexia compared with no cerclage. The other four smaller RCTs found no significant difference in preterm delivery before 34 weeks between cerclage at 10–30 weeks and no cerclage in women with a variety of risk factors for preterm delivery.
- **Prophylactic cervical cerclage for women at risk of cervical incompetence where cervical changes have been identified** Two RCTs identified by a systematic review found different results for women where cervical changes were present. One RCT found no significant difference in delivery before 34 weeks. The other small RCT found that cerclage plus bed rest reduced delivery before 34 weeks compared with bed rest alone. Neither RCT found a significant difference in perinatal death between cerclage plus bed rest and bed rest alone.
- **Enhanced antenatal care programmes for socially deprived population groups/high risk groups** RCTs carried out in a range of countries found no significant difference between enhanced antenatal care and usual care in reducing the risk of preterm delivery.

Improving outcome after preterm rupture

- **Antibiotic treatment for premature rupture of the membranes (prolongs gestation and may reduce infection, but unknown effect on perinatal mortality)** One systematic review in women with premature rupture of membranes has found that antibiotics prolong pregnancy and reduce the risk of neonatal morbidity, such as neonatal infection, requirement for treatment with oxygen, and abnormal cerebral ultrasound, compared with placebo. It found that co-amoxiclav (amoxycillin plus clavulanic acid) increased the risk of neonatal necrotising enterocolitis compared with placebo.
- **Amnioinfusion for preterm rupture of the membranes** One systematic review found insufficient evidence from one RCT about the effects of amnioinfusion compared with no amnioinfusion in improving neonatal outcomes after preterm rupture of the membranes.

Stopping Contractions

- **Calcium channel blockers** We found no systematic review or RCTs comparing calcium channel blockers versus placebo. One systematic review has found that calcium channel blockers significantly reduce deliveries within 48 hours, neonatal morbidity, and withdrawals caused by maternal adverse effects compared with other tocolytics (mainly β agonists).
- **Oxytocin receptor antagonists (atosiban)** One systematic review identified two RCTs that compared atosiban with placebo and found different results. The larger RCT found that atosiban prolonged pregnancy compared with placebo but found that atosiban appeared to increase fetal deaths below 28 weeks' gestation. The other RCT found that atosiban increased delivery within 48 hours.

- **Prostaglandin inhibitors (indometacin)** One systematic review found limited evidence that indometacin reduced delivery within 48 hours and 7 days and delivery before 37 weeks' gestation compared with placebo. However, it found no significant difference between indometacin and placebo or no treatment in perinatal mortality, respiratory distress syndrome, bronchopulmonary dysplasia, necrotising enterocolitis, neonatal sepsis, or low birth weight. The review may have lacked power to detect a clinically important effect.
- **Magnesium sulphate** One systematic review found no significant difference between magnesium sulphate and placebo in delivery before 36 weeks; perinatal mortality or respiratory distress syndrome. A second systematic review found no significant difference between magnesium sulphate and other tocolytics (betamimetics, calcium channel blockers, prostaglandin synthetase inhibitors, nitroglycerine, alcohol and dextrose infusion) in delivery within 48 hours, although results were heterogeneous.
- **Betamimetics** One systematic review has found no significant difference between β_2 agonists and placebo or no treatment in perinatal mortality, respiratory distress syndrome or birth weight less than 2500 g. It found that β_2 agonists increased maternal adverse effects such as chest pain, palpitations, dyspnoea, tremor, nausea, vomiting, headache, hyperglycaemia, hypokalaemia compared with placebo or no treatment.

Elective *v* selective caesarean delivery

- **Elective rather than selective caesarean delivery in preterm labour** One systematic review has found that elective caesarean delivery increases maternal morbidity compared with selective caesarean delivery, and found no significant difference in neonatal morbidity or mortality. The RCTs may have been underpowered to detect a clinically important neonatal benefit.

Improving outcome in preterm delivery

- **Antenatal corticosteroids** One systematic review found that antenatal corticosteroids significantly reduced respiratory distress syndrome, intraventricular haemorrhage, and neonatal mortality compared with placebo or no treatment.
- **Antibiotic treatment for preterm labour with intact membranes** One systematic review found that antibiotics do not prolong pregnancy and do not reduce perinatal mortality compared with placebo, but they do reduce the incidence of maternal infection.
- **Thyrotropin releasing hormone plus corticosteroids before preterm delivery** One systematic review in women at risk of preterm birth has found no significant difference between thyrotropin releasing hormone plus corticosteroids and corticosteroids alone in improving neonatal outcomes. Thyrotropin releasing hormone plus corticosteroids increased maternal and fetal adverse events compared with corticosteroids alone.

DEFINITION Preterm or premature birth is defined by the World Health Organization as delivery of an infant before 37 completed weeks of gestation.[1] There is no set lower limit to this definition, but 23–24 weeks' gestation is widely accepted,[1] which approximates to an average fetal weight of 500 g.

INCIDENCE/ PREVALENCE Preterm birth occurs in about 5–10% of all births in developed countries,[2–4] but in recent years the incidence seems to have increased in some countries, particularly the USA.[5] We found little reliable evidence for incidence (using the definition of premature birth given above) in less developed countries. The rate in northwestern Ethiopia has been reported to vary between 11–22% depending on the age group of mothers studied, and is highest in teenage mothers.[6]

AETIOLOGY/ RISK FACTORS About 30% of preterm births are unexplained and spontaneous.[4,7,8] The two strongest risk factors for idiopathic preterm labourⒼ are low socioeconomic status and previous preterm delivery. Multiple pregnancy accounts for about another 30% of cases.[4,7] Other known risk factors include genital tract infection, preterm rupture of the membranesⒼ, antepartum haemorrhage, cervical incompetence, and congenital uterine abnormalities, which collectively account for about 20–25% of cases. The remaining cases (15–20%) are attributed to elective preterm delivery secondary to hypertensive disorders of pregnancy, intrauterine fetal growth restriction, congenital abnormalities, trauma and medical disorders of pregnancy.[4,5,7,8]

PROGNOSIS Preterm labour usually results in preterm birth. One systematic review (search date not reported), which compared tocolysis versus placebo, found that about 27% of preterm labours resolved spontaneously and about 70% progressed to preterm delivery.[9] Observational studies have found that one preterm birth significantly raises the risk of another in a subsequent pregnancy.[10]

AIMS OF INTERVENTION To prevent preterm birth; to prolong the interval between threatened preterm labour and delivery; to optimise the condition of the fetus in preparation for delivery in order to improve neonatal outcome; to minimise maternal morbidity.

OUTCOMES Perinatal Ⓖ mortality, neonatal mortality, and morbidity (incidence of respiratory distress syndrome, intraventricular haemorrhage, necrotising enterocolitis, neonatal sepsis, and neonatal convulsions); maternal adverse effects. Proxy outcomes include duration of pregnancy, number of hours or days between onset of labour and delivery, and incidence of preterm delivery.

METHODS *Clinical Evidence* search and appraisal September 2003.

QUESTION What are the effects of preventive interventions in women at high risk of preterm delivery?

OPTION ENHANCED ANTENATAL CARE FOR SOCIALLY DEPRIVED POPULATION GROUPS/HIGH RISK GROUPS

RCTs carried out in a range of countries found no significant difference between enhanced antenatal care and usual care in reducing the risk of preterm delivery.

Benefits: We found no systematic review. We found 11 RCTs.[11–21] All of the RCTs (carried out in Europe, USA, and Latin America; number of high risk women ranging from 150 to 2200) found no significant difference between enhanced antenatal care Ⓖ and usual antenatal care in reducing preterm birth (see table 1, p 1843).

Harms: The RCTs gave no information on adverse effects.[11–21]

Comment: The definition of enhanced antenatal care varied.[11–21] Examples of enhanced antenatal care include increased number of antenatal visits, a bed rest programme including rest periods three times daily, home visits by midwives, fortnightly social worker counselling sessions, nutritional education, peer group education, and counselling by a psychologist.

OPTION PROPHYLACTIC CERVICAL CERCLAGE IN WOMEN AT RISK OF CERVICAL INCOMPETENCE

Systematic reviews identified five RCTs that found different results for women where cervical changes have not been identified. One large RCT found that cerclage at 9–29 weeks reduced delivery before 33 weeks' gestation in women with a previous preterm delivery or previous cervical surgery, but doubled the risk of puerperal pyrexia compared with no cerclage. The other four smaller RCTs found no significant difference in preterm delivery before 34 weeks between cerclage at 10–30 weeks and no cerclage in women with a variety of risk factors for preterm delivery. Two RCTs identified by a systematic review found different results for women where cervical changes were present. One RCT found no significant difference in delivery before 34 weeks.

The other small RCT found that cerclage plus bed rest reduced delivery before 34 weeks compared with bed rest alone. Neither RCT found a significant difference in perinatal death between cerclage plus bed rest and bed rest alone.

Benefits: **When cervical changes have not been identified:** We found one systematic review (search date 2002, 5 RCTs).[22] The review did not pool data from these RCTs. The first RCT identified by the review (1292 women, 71% with a history of preterm delivery and 11% with previous cervical surgery, obstetricians were uncertain whether to advise cervical cerclage**G**) found that cerclage at 9 to 29 weeks significantly reduced delivery before 33 weeks' gestation but found no significant difference in the rate of deliveries occurring between weeks 33 and 36 (before 33 weeks: 83/647 [13%] with cerclage *v* 110/645 [17%] with no cerclage; RR 0.75, 95% CI 0.57 to 0.98; NNT 24, 95% CI 14 to 275).[23] The second RCT identified by the review (194 women with 2 to 4 previous preterm deliveries or 1 or more second trimester losses) found no significant difference in delivery before 34 weeks' gestation between cerclage at 15 to 21 weeks and no cerclage (12/96 [13%] with cerclage *v* 10/98 [10%] with no cerclage; OR 1.29, 95% CI 0.53 to 3.15).[24] The third RCT identified by the review (506 women judged to be at moderate risk of preterm labour**G** due to previous live pregnancy at 29 to 36 weeks, previous preterm labour, or late miscarriage) found no significant difference in delivery before 34 weeks' gestation between cerclage at 10 to 28 weeks and no cerclage (14/268 [1.5%] with cerclage *v* 1/238 [0.4%] with no cerclage; OR 0.88, 95% CI 0.36 to 2.16).[25] The fourth RCT identified by the review (50 women with twin pregnancies after induction of ovulation, excluding women with cervical insufficiency) found no significant difference in delivery before 34 weeks' gestation between cerclage at 13 weeks and no cerclage (6/25 [24%] with cerclage *v* 5/25 [20%] with no cerclage; OR 1.26, 95% CI 0.33 to 4.84).[26] The fifth RCT identified by the review (71% of women had previous first or second trimester miscarriage, 29% previous preterm birth, number of women not stated in review) found no significant difference in delivery before 34 weeks' gestation between cerclage at 21–30 weeks and no cerclage (OR 0.70, 95% CI 0.33 to 1.48).[27]

When cervical changes are present: We found one systematic review (search date 2002, 2 RCTs, 148 women) of cervical cerclage when cervical change has been detected by transvaginal ultrasound.[28] It found significant heterogeneity between RCTs for delivery before 34 weeks ($P = 0.03$).[28] The first RCT identified by the review (35 women with cervical length < 25 mm and gestational age < 27 weeks) found that cerclage plus bed rest significantly reduced delivery before 34 weeks compared with bed rest alone (0/19 [0%] with cerclage plus bed rest *v* 7/16 [44%] with bed rest alone; NNT 3, 95% CI 2 to 5; $P = 0.002$). It found no significant difference in neonatal survival between cerclage plus bed rest and bed rest alone (19/19 [100%] with cerclage plus bed rest *v* 13/16 [81%] with bed rest alone; ARR +0.19, 95% CI –0.02 to +0.43).[29] The second RCT identified by the review (113 women between 16 and 24 weeks of gestation and distal cervix < 2.5 cm or membrane prolapse into endocervical canal at least 25% of cervical length) found no significant difference between cerclage plus bed rest and with bed rest alone in delivery before 34 weeks, perinatal**G** death, placental abruption, or chorioamnionitis (delivery < 34 weeks: 35% with cerclage plus bed rest *v* 36% with bed rest alone; $P = 0.80$; perinatal death: 13% with cerclage plus bed rest *v* 12% with bed rest alone; $P = 0.90$; placental abruption: 11% with cerclage plus bed rest *v* 14% with bed rest alone; $P = 0.80$; chorioamnionitis: 20% with cerclage plus bed rest *v* 10% with bed rest alone; $P = 0.20$).[30]

Harms: **When cervical changes have not been identified:** The first RCT identified by the review (1292 women) addressing prophylactic use of cerclage found that insertion of cervical sutures doubled the risk of puerperal pyrexia compared with no sutures (24/415 [6%] with cerclage *v* 11/405 [3%] with no cerclage; RR 2.13, 95% CI 1.06 to 4.15; NNH 33, 95% CI 12 to 607).[23] Information about puerperal pyrexia was collected only after 360 women had already been recruited to the trial. It was defined as a temperature of greater than 38 °C but uterine infection was mentioned as a possible cause of the pyrexia in only 13/24 (54%) in the cerclage group and 6/11 (55%) in the non-cerclage groups. The second smaller RCT identified by the review (194 women) found that cervical cerclage increased puerperal pyrexia but the increase was not statistically significant (10% with cerclage *v* 3% with no cerclage; P = 0.07).[24] **When cervical changes are present:** The systematic review (search date 2002) found no significant difference between cerclage and no cerclage in maternal infection (2 RCTs, 148 women: RR 0.78, 95% CI 0.39 to 1.56).[28] One RCT identified by the review found no significant difference between cerclage and no cerclage in chorioamnionitis (20% with cerclage *v* 10.3% with no cerclage; P = 0.2).[30]

Comment: Both systematic reviews presented results from meta-analyses using data from all included RCTs.[22,28] The authors of the second review considered that, although no significant statistical heterogeneity was found, pooling was inappropriate in view of the difference in the characteristics and quality of the RCTs. Timing of suturing ranged from 13 to 30 weeks.[22] The RCTs included women with twin or singleton pregnancies; women with previous second trimester miscarriage or preterm delivery; previous cervical surgery; premature rupture of membranes before 32 weeks; women with second trimester dilation of internal os on ultrasonography; and women with primary or secondary infertility after induced ovulation. The second review found that overall, cervical cerclage significantly reduced spontaneous preterm birth before 34 weeks compared with no cerclage, but found no significant difference between treatments for preterm delivery before 37 weeks (before 34 weeks, 7 RCTs: OR 0.75, 95% CI 0.59 to 0.96; before 37 weeks, 6 RCTs: OR 0.86, 95% CI 0.71 to 1.05).[22] The first review found that overall, cervical cerclage significantly reduced spontaneous preterm birth before 32 weeks compared with no cerclage but found no significant difference between treatments for preterm delivery before 37 weeks (before 32 weeks, 3 RCTs, 770 women: RR 1.29, 95% CI 0.67 to 2.49; before 37 weeks: 4 RCTs, 2062 women: RR 1.04, 95% CI 0.99 to 1.10).[28] The two RCTs that examined cervical cerclage in the mid-trimester with documented cervical change differed in terms of patient selection and methodology.[29,30] Broad confidence intervals suggest that sample size may have been insufficient to rule out clinically important differences in neonatal mortality.

QUESTION **What are the effects of interventions to improve outcome after preterm rupture of the membranes?**

OPTION **ANTIBIOTIC TREATMENT FOR PRETERM RUPTURE OF THE MEMBRANES**

One systematic review in women with premature rupture of membranes has found that antibiotics prolong pregnancy and reduce the risk of neonatal morbidity, such as neonatal infection, requirement for treatment with oxygen, and abnormal cerebral ultrasound, compared with placebo. It found that co-amoxiclav (amoxycillin plus clavulanic acid) increased the risk of neonatal necrotising enterocolitis compared with placebo.

Benefits: One systematic review (search date 2003, 19 RCTs, > 6000 women with rupture of membranes before 37 weeks' gestation) found that antibiotics (including erythromycin, co-amoxiclav, benzylpenicillin, ampicillin, piperacillin, or clindamycin) significantly reduced the proportion of babies born within 48 hours and within 7 days following preterm premature rupture of the membranes**G** compared with placebo (within 48 hours: RR 0.71, 95% CI 0.58 to 0.87; within 7 days: RR 0.80, CI 0.71 to 0.90).[31] It found that antibiotics significantly reduced neonatal infection, requirement for supplementary oxygen and abnormal cerebral ultrasound compared with placebo but found no significant difference between treatments in perinatal**G** mortality (neonatal infection: RR 0.68, CI 0.53 to 0.87; requirement for supplementary oxygen: RR 0.88, 95% CI 0.81 to 0.96; abnormal cerebral ultrasound: RR 0.82, 95% CI 0.68 to 0.98). **Penicillins (excluding co-amoxiclav):** The review found that any penicillin (except co-amoxiclav) significantly reduced the proportion of babies born within 48 hours and within 7 days compared with placebo (< 48 hours, 3 RCTS, 220 babies: RR 0.41, 95% CI 0.25 to 0.66; < 7 days, 3 RCTs, 220 babies: RR 0.68, 95% CI 0.56 to 0.82).[31] It found that penicillin significantly reduced neonatal infection and major cerebral abnormality on ultrasound before discharge (neonatal infection, 4 RCTs, 416 babies: RR 0.33, 95% CI 0.14 to 0.81; major cerebral abnormality, 3 RCTs, 267 babies: RR 0.49, 95% CI 0.25 to 0.97). **Co-amoxiclav**: The review found that co-amoxiclav significantly reduced the proportion of babies born within 48 hours and within 7 days compared with placebo (< 48 hours, 1 RCT, 2430 babies: 0.75, 95% CI 0.67 to 0.84; < 7 days, 1 RCT, 2430 babies: RR 0.91, 95% CI 0.85 to 0.97).[31] **Erythromycin:** The review found that erythromycin significantly reduced the proportion of babies born within 48 hours (2 RCTs, 2635 babies: RR 0.84, 95% CI 0.76 to 0.93).[31]

Harms: **Co-amoxiclav**: The review (search date 2003) found that co-amoxiclav significantly increased the proportion of babies with necrotising enterocolitis compared with placebo (2 RCTs, 2492 babies: RR 4.60, 95% CI 1.98 to 10.72).[31]

Comment: Most of the RCTs in the review did not include antenatal administration of steroids but 77% of the women in one large RCT received steroids.[32] All but one of the RCTs in the review gave data on the percentage of withdrawals, which was always less than 20%.[31]

OPTION — AMNIOINFUSION FOR PRETERM RUPTURE OF THE MEMBRANES

One systematic review found insufficient evidence from one RCT about the effects of amnioinfusion compared with no amnioinfusion in improving neonatal outcomes after preterm rupture of the membranes.

Benefits: We found one systematic review (search date 2001, 1 RCT, 66 women) comparing amnioinfusion**G** with no amnioinfusion.[33] It found no significant difference between amnioinfusion and no amnioinfusion in rates of caesarean section, low Apgar scores**G**, neonatal mortality, or endometritis.

Harms: No adverse effects were reported in the RCT identified by the review.[33]

Comment: The RCT was too small to detect clinically important changes in some of the outcomes (rates of caesarean section, neonatal mortality, and infectious morbidity) and had shortcomings in methods used (unspecified method of random assignment of women; blinding of treatment not possible).[33]

QUESTION What are the effects of treatments to stop contractions in preterm labour?

OPTION BETAMIMETICS

One systematic review has found no significant difference between β_2 agonists and placebo or no treatment in perinatal mortality, respiratory distress syndrome or birth weight less than 2500 g. It found that β_2 agonists increased maternal adverse effects such as chest pain, palpitations, dyspnoea, tremor, nausea, vomiting, headache, hyperglycaemia, hypokalaemia compared with placebo or no treatment.

Benefits: We found one systematic review (search date 1998, 8 RCTs).[34] The systematic review found no significant difference between β_2 agonists and placebo or no treatment in perinatal🅖 mortality, respiratory distress syndrome or birth weight less than 2500 g (perinatal mortality: 62/682 [9%] with β_2 agonists *v* 48/604 [8%] with placebo or no treatment; OR 1.08, 95% CI 0.72 to 1.62; respiratory distress syndrome, 6 RCTs: 117/639 [18%] with β_2 agonists *v* 140/565 [25%] with placebo or no treatment; OR 0.76, 95% CI 0.57 to 1.01; birth weight less than 2500 g, 5 RCTs: 332/601 [55%] with β_2 agonists *v* 332/525 [63%] with placebo or no treatment; OR 0.79, 95% CI 0.61 to 1.01).[34] It found no significant difference between treatments in patent ductus arteriosus, necrotising enterocolitis, intraventricular haemorrhage, seizures, hypoglycaemia, or neonatal sepsis.[34]

Harms: The systematic review found that β_2 agonists significantly increased maternal adverse effects, such as chest pain, palpitations, dyspnoea, tremor, nausea, vomiting, headache, hyperglycaemia, or hypokalaemia compared with placebo or no treatment (chest pain, 2 RCTs: 39/406 [10%] with β_2 agonists *v* 3/408 [1%] with placebo or no treatment; OR 6.2, 95% CI 3.3 to 11.5), palpitations, 3 RCTs: 200/420 [48%] with β_2 agonists *v* 19/423 [4%] with placebo or no treatment; OR 10.2, 95% CI 7.4 to 13.9; dyspnoea, 2 RCTs: 55/406 [14%] with β_2 agonists *v* 4/408 [1%] with placebo or no treatment; OR 6.6, 95% CI 3.9 to 11.2; tremor, 1 RCT: 138/352 [39%] with β_2 agonists *v* 13/356 [4%] with placebo or no treatment; OR 8.3, 95% CI 5.8 to 11.9; nausea, 1 RCT: 72/352 [20%] with β_2 agonists *v* 42/356 [12%] with placebo or no treatment; OR 1.9, 95% CI 1.3 to 2.8; vomiting, 2 RCTs: 48/366 [13%] with β_2 agonists *v* 29/371 [8%] with placebo or no treatment; OR 1.8, 95% CI 1.1 to 2.9; headache, 2 RCTs: 84/366 [23%] with β_2 agonists *v* 22/371 [6%] with placebo or no treatment; OR 4.0, 95% CI 2.6 to 6.0; hyperglycaemia, 1 RCT: 106/352 [30%] with β_2 agonists *v* 37/356 [10%] with placebo or no treatment; OR 3.4, 95% CI 2.4 to 4.9; hypokalaemia, 1 RCT: 138/352 [39%] with β_2 agonists *v* 23/356 [6%] with placebo or no treatment; OR 6.4, 95% CI 4.5 to 9.1).[34] Frequently, these adverse effects necessitated discontinuation of treatment (3 RCTs: 25/88 [28%] with β_2 agonists *v* 0/86 [0%] with placebo or no treatment; OR 11.5, 95% CI 4.8 to 27.5).

Comment: None.

OPTION CALCIUM CHANNEL BLOCKERS

We found no systematic review or RCTs comparing calcium channel blockers versus placebo. One systematic review has found that calcium channel blockers significantly reduce deliveries within 48 hours, neonatal morbidity, and withdrawals caused by maternal adverse effects compared with other tocolytics (mainly β agonists).

Benefits: **Versus placebo:** We found no systematic review or RCTs comparing calcium channel blockers versus placebo. **Versus other tocolytics:** We found one systematic review (search date 2002, 12 RCTs, 1029 women) comparing calcium channel blockers (nifedipine and nicardipine in 2 RCTs) versus other tocolytics**G** (10 RCTs *v* ritodrine; 1 RCT each *v* salbutamol and magnesium sulphate) for preterm labour**G** (between 20 and 36 weeks).[35] The review found that calcium channel blockers significantly reduced delivery within 48 hours and 7 days and reduced delivery before 34 weeks compared with other tocolytics (delivery within 48 hours, 9 RCTs, 761 women: 74/383 [19%] with calcium channel blocker *v* 87/378 [23%] with other tocolytics; RR 0.8, 95% CI 0.61 to 1.0; delivery within 7 days, 4 RCTs, 453 women: 71/229 [31%] with calcium channel blocker *v* 86/224 [38%] with other tocolytics; RR 0.76, 95% CI 0.60 to 0.97; delivery before 34 weeks, 6 RCTs, 619 women: 107/311 [34%] with calcium channel blocker *v* 122/308 [40%] with other tocolytics; RR 0.83, 95% CI 0.69 to 0.99). It found that calcium channel blockers significantly reduced neonatal morbidity including respiratory distress syndrome, necrotising enterocolitis, and intraventricular haemorrhage (respiratory distress syndrome, 9 RCTs, 763 newborns: 48/386 [12%] with calcium channel blocker *v* 72/377 [19%] with other tocolytics; RR 0.63, 0.46 to 0.88; necrotising enterocolitis, 3 RCTs, 323 newborns: 1/166 [1%] with calcium channel blocker *v* 8/157 [5%] with other tocolytics; RR 0.21, 95% CI 0.05 to 0.96; intraventricular haemorrhage, 3 RCTs, 340 newborns: 19/173 [11%] with calcium channel blocker *v* 31/167 [19%] with other tocolytics; RR 0.59, 95% CI 0.36 to 0.98). No significant differences were found in perinatal mortality (10 RCTs, 810 newborns: 13/400 [3%] with calcium channel blocker *v* 7/410 [2%] with other tocolytics; RR 1.65, 95% CI 0.74 to 3.64).

Harms: **Versus other tocolytics:** The systematic review (search date 1998) found that calcium channel blockers significantly reduced discontinuation because of adverse effects compared with other tocolytics (10 RCTs, 833 women: 1/419 [0.2%] with calcium channel blocker *v* 29/414 [7.0%] with other tocolytics; RR 0.14, 95% CI 0.05 to 0.36).[35] The systematic review did not report specific adverse effects of calcium channel blockers.

Comment: None.

OPTION MAGNESIUM SULPHATE

One systematic review found no significant difference between magnesium sulphate and placebo in delivery before 36 weeks; perinatal mortality or respiratory distress syndrome. A second systematic review found no significant difference between magnesium sulphate and other tocolytics (betamimetics, calcium channel blockers, prostaglandin synthetase inhibitors, nitroglycerine, alcohol and dextrose infusion) in delivery within 48 hours, although results were heterogeneous.

Benefits: **Versus placebo:** One systematic review (search date 1998, 4 RCTs) found no significant difference between magnesium sulphate and placebo or no treatment in delivery before 36 weeks (2 RCTs, 191 women: 61/92 [66%] with magnesium sulphate *v* 74/99 [75%] with placebo or no treatment; OR 0.67, 95% CI 0.36 to 1.26).[34] It found no significant difference between magnesium sulphate and placebo or no treatment for perinatal**G** mortality or respiratory distress syndrome (perinatal mortality: 11/169 [6.5%] with magnesium sulphate *v* 7/182 [3.8%] with placebo or no treatment; OR 1.83, 95% CI 0.70 to 4.77; respiratory distress syndrome, 3 RCTs: 22/139 [16%] with magnesium sulphate *v* 22/153 [14%] with placebo or no treatment; OR 1.19, 95%

CI 0.61 to 2.31).[34] It also found no significant difference between magnesium sulphate and placebo or no treatment in birth weight less than 2500 g, patent ductus arteriosus, necrotising enterocolitis, intraventricular haemorrhage, seizures, hypoglycaemia, or neonatal sepsis. The number of newborns assessed for these outcomes was small. **Versus other tocolytics:** A second systematic review (search date 2002) compared magnesium sulphate versus placebo, no treatment, and other tocolytics**G** (betamimetics, calcium channel blockers, prostaglandin synthetase inhibitors, nitroglycerine, alcohol and dextrose infusion).[36] The studies included in the review comparing magnesium sulphate versus placebo, no treatment, or sedation were the same as those included in the initial review except for the addition of a study that compared magnesium sulphate versus barbiturate and bed rest.[37] The review found no significant difference between magnesium sulphate and other treatment in delivery within 48 hours, although significant statistical heterogeneity was found (11 RCTs, 881 women: RR 0.85, 95% CI 0.58 to 1.25).

Harms: **Versus placebo:** The systematic review found that magnesium sulphate significantly increased discontinuation of treatment compared with placebo or no treatment (3 RCTs: 10/137 [7%] with magnesium sulphate *v* 0/144 [0%] with placebo or no treatment; OR 8.36, 95% CI 2.36 to 29.61).[34] **Versus other tocolytics:** The second systematic review found that the magnesium sulphate significantly increased fetal, neonatal, and infant mortality (7 RCTs, 727 babies: 18/340 [5%] with magnesium sulphate *v* 6/387 [2%] with other tocolytics; RR 2.82, 95% CI 1.20 to 6.62).[36]

Comment: None.

OPTION OXYTOCIN RECEPTOR ANTAGONISTS (ATOSIBAN)

One systematic review identified two RCTs that compared atosiban with placebo and found different results. The larger RCT found that atosiban prolonged pregnancy compared with placebo but found that atosiban appeared to increase fetal deaths below 28 weeks' gestation. The other RCT found that atosiban increased delivery within 48 hours.

Benefits: **Versus placebo:** We found one systematic review (search date 1998, 2 RCTs).[34] The first RCT identified by the systematic review (120 women at 20–36 weeks' gestation, with more than 4 contractions/hour and with no cervical changes, 114 deliveries) found that atosiban (300 μg/minute for 2 hours) increased delivery within 48 hours, but the statistical significance was not reported (5/56 [8.9%] with atosiban *v* 2/56 [3.6%] with placebo; P value not reported).[38] The second RCT identified by the review was identified as an abstract. The later full publication of this RCT (501 women with preterm labour**G** diagnosed by uterine contractions and cervical changes, at 20 to 33 weeks) found that atosiban significantly increased the proportion women undelivered without use of an alternative tocolytic**G** at 24 and 48 hours and 7 days (24 hours: 73% with atosiban *v* 58% with placebo; OR 1.93, 95% CI 1.30 to 2.86; 48 hours: 67% with atosiban *v* 36% with placebo; OR 1.62, 95% CI 1.10 to 2.37; 7 days: 62% with atosiban *v* 49% with placebo; OR 1.70, 95% CI 1.17 to 2.46).[39] It found no significant difference between atosiban and placebo in the median time to delivery (25.6 days with atosiban *v* 21.0 days with placebo; P value not reported). For pregnancies over 28 weeks' gestation (424 pregnancies), it found that atosiban significantly prolonged pregnancy for up to 24 hours, 48 hours, and up to 7 days compared with placebo (delay up to 24 hours: 150/203 [74%] with atosiban *v* 128/221 [58%] with placebo; RR 1.28, 95% CI 1.11 to 1.47; NNT 7, 95% CI 4 to 15; delay 48 hours: 140/203 [69%] with atosiban v 122/221 [55%] with placebo; RR 1.25, 95% CI 1.08 to 1.45; NNT 8, 95% CI 5 to 23; delay up to 7 days: 131/203 [65%] with atosiban v 105/220 [48%] with placebo; RR 1.35, 95% CI 1.14 to 1.60; NNT 6, 95% CI 4 to 14).[39]

Harms: The systematic review found increased nausea with atosiban compared with placebo or no treatment but found no significant difference in vomiting (nausea, 2 RCTs: 33/306 [11%] with atosiban v 15/307 [5%] with placebo or no treatment; OR 2.3, 95% CI 1.3 to 4.1; vomiting, 2 RCTs: 10/306 [3%] with atosiban v 13/307 [4%] with placebo or no treatment; OR 0.8, 95% CI 0.3 to 1.8).[34] Atosiban significantly reduced chest pain and dyspnoea (chest pain, 2 RCTs: 3/306 [1%] with atosiban v 13/307 [4%] with placebo or no treatment; OR 0.3, 95% CI 0.1 to 0.8; dyspnoea, 1 RCT: 1/250 [0.4%] with atosiban v 7/251 [3%] with placebo or no treatment; OR 0.22, 95% CI 0.05 to 0.89) compared with placebo or no treatment). The subsequent full report of one of the included RCTs found that atosiban significantly increased injection site reactions after prolonged use and significantly increased withdrawal owing to adverse effects (injection site reaction: 110/250 [44%] with atosiban v 58/251 [23%] with placebo; RR 1.90, 95% CI 1.46 to 2.48; NNH 4, 95% CI 3 to 7; withdrawal: 16% with atosiban v 4% with placebo).[39] It found that atosiban increased infant death compared with placebo (13/288 [4.5%] with atosiban v 5/295 [1.7%] with placebo; P value not reported).[39] Analysis by gestational age at admission found that most of the mortality with atosiban occurred in pregnancies less than 26 weeks' gestation (mortality in pregnancies < 26 weeks: 10/27 [37%] with atosiban v 0/16 [0%] with placebo; see comment below; 26–28 weeks: 0/26 [0%] with atosiban v 1/26 [4%] with placebo; 28–32 weeks: 2/126 [2%] with atosiban v 2/125 [2%] with placebo; ≥ 32 weeks: 1/109 [1%] with atosiban v 2/128 [2%] with placebo).[39]

Comment: In the first RCT identified by the systematic review, infusions were halted in two people (one in each treatment group) and these people were not included in the analysis.[38] Tocolytic rescue with ritodrine was used in the second RCT comparing atosiban versus placebo.[39] In this RCT, 24/246 (10%) women randomised to receive atosiban and 13/255 (5%) women randomised to receive placebo were recruited at less than 26 weeks' gestation. This may have contributed to a higher incidence of fetal mortality at less than 26 weeks' gestation in the atosiban group.

OPTION PROSTAGLANDIN INHIBITORS (INDOMETACIN)

One systematic review found limited evidence that indometacin reduced delivery within 48 hours and 7 days and delivery before 37 weeks' gestation compared with placebo. However, it found no significant difference between indometacin and placebo or no treatment in perinatal mortality, respiratory distress syndrome, bronchopulmonary dysplasia, necrotising enterocolitis, neonatal sepsis, or low birth weight. The review may have lacked power to detect a clinically important effect.

Benefits: We found one systematic review comparing indometacin versus placebo (search date 1998, 3 RCTs, 100 women).[34] It found that indometacin significantly reduced delivery within 48 hours, 7 days and delivery before 37 weeks compared with placebo but the number of women studied was small (within 48 hours, 2 RCTs: 4/34 [12%] with indometacin v 22/36 [61%] with placebo; OR 0.12, 95% CI 0.05 to 0.32; within 7 days, 1 RCT: 3/18 [17%] with indometacin v 15/18 [83%] with placebo; OR 0.07, 0.02 to 0.27; before 37 weeks, 1 RCT: 3/18 [17%] with indometacin v 14/18 [78%] with placebo; OR 0.09, 95% CI 0.03 to 0.24). It found no significant difference between indometacin and placebo or no treatment in perinatal❻ mortality, respiratory distress syndrome, bronchopulmonary dysplasia, necrotising enterocolitis, neonatal sepsis, or low birth weight.[34] The number of newborns assessed for these outcomes may be too small to exclude a clinically important difference.

Harms: The systematic review found that indometacin significantly increased the incidence of postpartum haemorrhage compared with placebo or no treatment but found no significant difference in nausea or chorioamnionitis (haemorrhage, 1 RCT: 7/16 [44%] with indometacin *v* 2/18 [11%] with placebo or no treatment; OR 5.1, 95% CI 1.1 to 22.9; nausea, 1 RCT: 2/18 [11%] with indometacin *v* 0/18 [0%] with placebo or no treatment; OR 7.8, 95% CI 0.5 to 130.5; chorioamnionitis, 1 RCT: 2/15 [13%] with indometacin *v* 0/15 with placebo or no treatment; OR 7.9, 95% CI 0.5 to 133.3).[34] The number of women assessed for these outcomes may be too small to exclude a clinically important difference.

Comment: None.

QUESTION **What are the effects of elective compared with selective caesarean delivery for women in preterm labour?**

OPTION **ELECTIVE VERSUS SELECTIVE CAESAREAN DELIVERY**

One systematic review has found that elective caesarean delivery increases maternal morbidity compared with selective caesarean delivery, and found no significant difference in neonatal morbidity or mortality. The RCTs may have been underpowered to detect a clinically important neonatal benefit.

Benefits: We found one systematic review (search date not reported, 6 RCTs, 122 women).[40] It found no significant difference in neonatal morbidity and mortality between elective caesarean❻ delivery and selective caesarean❻ delivery (low Apgar score❻ at 5 minutes: OR 0.68, 95% CI 0.29 to 1.60; need for neonatal intubation: OR 0.58, 95% CI 0.26 to 1.31; intracranial haemorrhage: OR 0.86, 95% CI 0.20 to 3.67; perinatal❻ death: OR 0.32, 95% CI 0.07 to 1.36).

Harms: The review found that major maternal complications were reported in 7/84 (8%) women, all after caesarean delivery, although one of these women was allocated to expectant management.[40] Maternal complications were therefore significantly higher in women allocated to elective caesarean compared with selective caesarean delivery (4 RCTs, 84 women: AR 6/44 [14%] with elective caesarean delivery *v* 1/40 [3%] with selective caesarean delivery; OR 6.18, 95% CI 1.27 to 30.10). Elective caesarean delivery may occasionally result in unnecessary preterm delivery; two women allocated to the selective delivery group did not deliver until some weeks after entry to one trial.

Comment: The confidence intervals in the systematic review suggest that RCTs were underpowered and no meaningful conclusions can be drawn on the neonatal effects of elective caesarean section.[40] The fetus presented by the breech in three of the studies. About a sixth of each group delivered by an alternative route, but the analysis was by intention to treat. Sample size of trials was small and most of the trials were terminated because of recruitment difficulties.

QUESTION **What are the effects of interventions to improve outcome in preterm delivery?**

OPTION **ANTENATAL CORTICOSTEROIDS BEFORE PRETERM DELIVERY**

One systematic review found that antenatal corticosteroids significantly reduced respiratory distress syndrome, intraventricular haemorrhage, and neonatal mortality compared with placebo or no treatment.

Benefits: We found one systematic review (search date 1996, 18 RCTs, > 3700 babies) in women experiencing anticipated preterm delivery (elective or after spontaneous onset of preterm labour**G**) that compared corticosteroids (betamethasone, dexamethasone, or hydrocortisone) versus placebo or no treatment.[41] The review found that antenatal corticosteroids significantly reduced respiratory distress syndrome compared with placebo or no treatment (18 RCTs, 3735 neonates: 292/1885 [15%] with corticosteroids *v* 439/1850 [24%] with placebo or no treatment; OR 0.52, 95% CI 0.44 to 0.62). Three RCTs (48 neonates) identified by the review found no significant difference between antenatal corticosteroids and placebo or no treatment in respiratory distress syndrome in neonates delivered before 28 weeks' gestation (7/17 [41%] with corticosteroids *v* 18/31 [58%] with placebo or no treatment; OR 0.64, 95% CI 0.16 to 2.50). Six RCTs identified by the review (349 neonates) found no significant difference between antenatal corticosteroids and placebo or no treatment in respiratory distress syndrome in babies delivered within less than 24 hours of initial treatment (45/176 [26%] with corticosteroids *v* 57/173 [33%] with placebo or no treatment; OR 0.70, 95% CI 0.43 to 1.16). One RCT (42 neonates) identified by the review found no significant difference between antenatal corticosteroids and placebo or no treatment in respiratory distress syndrome in babies delivered within less than 48 hours of initial treatment (3/23 [13%] with corticosteroids *v* 6/19 [32%] with placebo or no treatment; OR 0.34, 95% CI 0.08 to 1.47). The review found that both betamethasone and dexamethasone significantly reduced respiratory distress, but hydrocortisone did not (data not reported in the review). The small numbers of evaluable neonates from twin pregnancies did not allow a confident statement about the effects in multiple pregnancy. Antenatal corticosteroids significantly reduced neonatal mortality and intraventricular haemorrhage (neonatal mortality, 14 RCTs: 129/1770 [7%] with corticosteroids *v* 204/1747 [12%] with placebo or no treatment; OR 0.60, 95% CI 0.48 to 0.75; intraventricular haemorrhage (diagnosed at autopsy: 7/446 [1.6%] with corticosteroids *v* 23/417 [5.5%] with placebo or no treatment; OR 0.29, 95% CI 0.14 to 0.61; intraventricular haemorrhage diagnosed by ultrasound: 47/300 [16%] with corticosteroids *v* 77/296 [26%] with placebo or no treatment; OR 0.48, 95% CI 0.32 to 0.72). It found no significant difference between antenatal corticosteroids and placebo in necrotising enterocolitis or chronic lung disease (necrotising enterocolitis: 17/587 [3%] with corticosteroids *v* 27/567 [5%] with placebo or no treatment; OR 0.59, 95% CI 0.32 to 1.09; chronic lung disease: 38/204 [19%] with corticosteroids *v* 25/207 [12%] with placebo or no treatment; OR 1.57, 95% CI 0.87 to 2.84).[41]

Harms: The RCTs in the review found no strong evidence of any adverse effects of corticosteroids.[41] Subgroup analysis in one RCT in the review suggested that corticosteroids may be associated with death in hypertensive women, but no deaths in hypertensive women were observed in the other three RCTs in the review for which data were available.

Comment: The absence of a significant beneficial effect of corticosteroids on respiratory distress syndrome at less than 28 weeks' gestation may be because of the small numbers available for analysis at this gestation.[41] No RCTs in the review addressed the potentially harmful effects of repeated doses of antenatal corticosteroids, or whether one form of corticosteroid was more harmful than another, as a retrospective cohort study (883 babies delivered between 24 and 31 weeks' gestation) suggests.[42]

OPTION THYROTROPIN RELEASING HORMONE PLUS CORTICOSTEROIDS BEFORE PRETERM DELIVERY

One systematic review in women at risk of preterm birth has found no significant difference between thyrotropin releasing hormone plus corticosteroids and corticosteroids alone in improving neonatal outcomes. Thyrotropin releasing hormone plus corticosteroids increased maternal and fetal adverse events compared with corticosteroids alone.

Benefits: We found one systematic review (search date 1999, 11 RCTs, > 4500 women at risk of preterm birth) that compared thyrotropin releasing hormone (TRH) plus steroids with steroids alone.[43] It found no significant difference between TRH plus steroids and steroids alone in gestational age at delivery, respiratory distress syndrome, periventricular or intraventricular haemorrhage, necrotising enterocolitis or death prior to hospital discharge (mean gestational age of 32 weeks in both groups; respiratory distress syndrome: 676/1832 [37%] with TRH plus steroids *v* 640/1837 [35%] with steroids alone; RR 1.06, 95% CI 0.97 to 1.16; periventricular or intraventricular haemorrhage: 282/1819 [16%] with TRH plus steroids *v* 262/1826 [14%] with steroids alone; RR 1.08, 95% CI 0.93 to 1.26; necrotising enterocolitis: 56/1555 [4%] with TRH plus steroids *v* 61/1548 [4%] with steroids alone; RR 0.91, 95% CI 0.64 to 1.30; death prior to hospital discharge: 185/1842 [10%] with TRH plus steroids *v* 177/1852 [9%] with steroids alone; RR 1.05, 95% CI 0.86 to 1.27).

Harms: The review found that TRH plus steroid significantly increased the risk of low Apgar score**G** at 5 minutes and increased the requirement for assisted ventilation compared with steroids alone (low Apgar; OR 1.80, 95% CI 1.14 to 1.92; assisted ventilation: OR 1.16, CI 1.02 to 1.29).[43] One RCT included in the review found that TRH plus steroids significantly increased motor delay, motor impairment, sensory impairment, and social delay after 12 months compared with steroids alone (motor delay: RR 1.31, 95% CI 1.09 to 1.56; motor impairment: RR 1.51, 95% CI 1.02 to 2.24; sensory impairment: RR 1.97, 95% CI 1.10 to 3.53; social delay: RR 1.25, 95% CI 1.03 to 1.51).[43] TRH plus steroids significantly increased maternal blood pressure compared with steroids alone (1 RCT: risk of an increase of 25 mm Hg in systolic blood pressure; 36/506 [7%] with TRH plus steroids *v* 20/505 [4%] with steroids alone; RR 1.80, 95% CI 1.05 to 3.06; risk of an increase of 15 mm Hg in diastolic blood pressure; 115/506 [23%] with TRH plus steroids *v* 71/505 [14%] with steroids alone; RR 1.62, 95% CI 1.24 to 2.12). The review also found that TRH plus steroids significantly increased other maternal adverse effects including nausea, vomiting, light-headedness, urgency of micturition and facial flushing compared with steroid alone (nausea: 3 RCTs: 303/1175 [26%] with TRH plus steroids *v* 77/1195 [6%] with steroids alone; RR 3.92, 95% CI 3.13 to 4.90; vomiting: 1 RCT: 40/506 [8%] with TRH plus steroids *v* 17/505 [3%] with steroids alone; RR 2.35, 95% CI 1.35 to 4.09; light-headedness: 1 RCT: 139/506 [27%] with TRH plus steroids *v* 80/505 [16%] with steroids alone;

RR 1.73, 95% CI 1.36 to 2.20; urgency of micturition (1 RCT: 115/506 [23%] with TRH plus steroids v 48/505 [10%] with steroids alone; RR 2.39, 95% CI 1.75 to 3.27; facial flushing: 3 RCTs: 397/1252 [32%] with TRH plus steroids v 149/1271 [12%] with steroids alone; RR 2.67, 95% CI 2.26 to 3.16).[43]

Comment: TRH regimens varied in the RCTs identified by the review.[43] Seven of the RCTs analysed by intention to treat.

OPTION ANTIBIOTIC TREATMENT FOR PRETERM LABOUR WITH INTACT MEMBRANES

One systematic review found that antibiotics do not prolong pregnancy and do not reduce perinatal mortality compared with placebo, but they do reduce the incidence of maternal infection.

Benefits: We found one systematic review (search date 2002, 11 RCTs) comparing single or combined antibiotics with placebo or no antibiotic in women in preterm labour**G** and with intact membranes.[44] It found no significant difference between antibiotics and no antibiotic in delivery within 48 hours or within 7 days (4 RCTs, 6800 women: 509/4959 [10%] with antibiotics v 183/1841 [10%] without antibiotics; OR 1.04, 95% CI 0.89 to 1.23; within 7 days: 7 RCTs, 6957 women: 813/5044 [16%] with antibiotics v 337/1913 [18%] without antibiotics; OR 0.98, 95% CI 0.87 to 1.10). It found no significant difference between treatments in neonatal morbidity, respiratory distress syndrome, necrotising enterocolitis, intraventricular haemorrhage or perinatal**G** mortality (respiratory distress syndrome, 8 RCTs, 7104 newborns: 460/5112 [9%] with antibiotics v 194/1992 [10%] without antibiotics; RR 0.99, 95% CI 0.84 to 1.16; necrotising enterocolitis, 6 RCTs, 6880 newborns: 62/5004 [1.2%] with antibiotics v 25/1876 [1.3%] without antibiotics; RR 1.06, 95% CI 0.64 to 1.73; intraventricular haemorrhage, 4 RCTs, 6717 newborns: 59/4921 [1.2%] with antibiotics v 30/1796 [1.7%] without antibiotics; RR 0.76, 95% CI 0.48 to 1.19; perinatal mortality, 9 RCTs, 7208 newborns: 140/5166 [2.7%] with antibiotics v 42/2042 [2.1%] without antibiotics; RR 1.22, 95% CI 0.88 to 1.70). It found that antibiotics significantly reduced maternal infection, namely chorioamnionitis and endometritis compared with no antibiotics (9 RCTs, 7242 women: 456/5185 [9%] with antibiotics v 230/2057 [11%] without antibiotics; RR 0.74, 95% CI 0.64 to 0.87). It found that β-lactams either alone or in combination with a macrolide significantly reduced chorioamnionitis and endometritis (β-lactams alone, 3 RCTs: 144/1635 [9%] with β-lactams v 70/621 [11.3%] with no antibiotics; RR 0.75, 95% CI 0.56 to 0.98; β-lactam plus macrolide, 4 RCTs: 165/1790 [9%] with β-lactam plus macrolide v 97/773 [13%] with no antibiotics; RR 0.75, 95% CI 0.59 to 0.95). It found no significant difference between either a macrolide alone or antibiotics used to treat anaerobic bacteria compared with no antibiotic (macrolide alone, 2 RCTs: 157/1653 [9%] with macrolide v 64/569 [11%] with no antibiotics; RR 0.81, 95% CI 0.62 to 1.07; antibiotics used to treat anaerobic bacteria, 3 RCTs: 5/155 [3%] with antianaerobic antibiotic v 6/139 [4%] with no antibiotic; RR 0.76, 95% CI 0.25 to 2.34).

Harms: There was a trend but not a statistically significant increase in neonatal deaths in the group receiving antibiotics (7 RCTs, 6877 newborns: 99/5005 [2.0%] with antibiotics v 24/1872 [1.3%] with no antibiotics; RR 1.52, 95% CI 0.99 to 2.34).[44]

Comment: The ORACLE trial[45] dominated the review[44] because it was six times larger than all of the previous RCTs. It differed from the other RCTs because the diagnosis of preterm labour was made by each clinician (as distinct from the other studies, which used similar definitions of preterm labour including uterine contractions and cervical dilatation) and it was one of only two trials in the review in which antibiotics were administered orally and some women were recruited after 34 weeks. Tocolysis was used in 9 of the 11 RCTs (56% in the ORACLE RCT) and 30–90% of women received corticosteroids.[44,45] Maternal chorioamnionitis and endometritis is reduced by the prescription of prophylactic β-lactam antibiotics but approximately 88% of women with threatened preterm birth and intact membranes would receive antibiotics unnecessarily for an infection that is easily diagnosed and treated.

GLOSSARY

Amnioinfusion Infusion of physiological saline or Ringer's lactate through a catheter transabdominally or transcervically into the amniotic cavity.
Apgar score Clinical scoring method that assesses neonatal heart rate, respirations, tone, colour, and reflexes immediately after delivery.
Cervical cerclage Insertion of a cervical suture, using non-absorbable suture material, circumferentially around the cervix. May be done transvaginally or transabdominally.
Elective caesarean section When the operation is done at a pre-selected time before the onset of labour, usually after 38 weeks' gestation.
Enhanced antenatal care Includes various programmes of increased medical, midwifery, psychological, social, and nutritional support during pregnancy.
Perinatal Refers to the period after 24 weeks' gestation and includes the first 7 days of postnatal life for the neonate.
Preterm labour Onset of labour (regular uterine contractions with cervical effacement and dilatation) in the preterm period.
Preterm rupture of membranes Leakage of amniotic fluid from the amniotic cavity during the preterm period owing to rupture of the fetal membranes.
Selective caesarean section When the operation is done after the onset of labour.
Tocolytics Pharmacological agents that inhibit uterine contractions.

REFERENCES

1. Morrison JJ, Rennie JM. Clinical, scientific and ethical aspects of fetal and neonatal care at extremely preterm periods of gestation. *Br J Obstet Gynaecol* 1997;104:1341–1350.
2. Rush RW, Keirse MJNC, Howat P, et al. Contribution of preterm delivery to perinatal mortality. *BMJ* 1976;2:965–968.
3. Creasy RK. Preterm birth prevention: where are we? *Am J Obstet Gynecol* 1993;168:1223–1230.
4. Burke C, Morrison JJ. Perinatal factors and preterm delivery in an Irish obstetric population. *J Perinat Med* 2000;28:49–53.
5. Goldenberg RL, Rouse DJ. Prevention of premature birth. *N Engl J Med* 1998;339:313–320.
6. Kumbi S, Isehak A. Obstetric outcome of teenage pregnancy in northwestern Ethiopia. *East Afr Med J* 1999;76:138–140.
7. Iannucci TA, Tomich PG, Gianopoulos JG. Etiology and outcome of extremely low-birth-weight infants. *Am J Obstet Gynecol* 1996;174:1896–1902.
8. Main DM, Gabbe SG, Richardson D, et al. Can preterm deliveries be prevented? *Am J Obstet Gynecol* 1985;151:892–898.
9. King JF, Grant A, Keisre MJNC, et al. β Mimetics in preterm labour: an overview of the randomised controlled trials. *Br J Obstet Gynaecol* 1988;95:211–222. Search date not reported; primary sources Oxford Database of Perinatal Trials, hand searches of reference lists, and personal contacts.
10. Keirse MJNC, Rush RW, Anderson AB, et al. Risk of preterm delivery and/or abortion. *Br J Obstet Gynaecol* 1978;85:81–85.
11. Spencer B, Thomas H, Morris J. A randomized controlled trial of the provision of a social support service during pregnancy; the South Manchester Family Worker project. *Br J Obstet Gynaecol* 1989;96:281–288.
12. Mueller-Heubach E, Reddick D, Barrett B, et al. Preterm birth prevention: evaluation of a prospective controlled randomized trial. *Am J Obstet Gynecol* 1989;160:1172–1178.
13. Goldenberg R, Davis R, Copper R, et al. The Alabama birth prevention project. *Obstet Gynecol* 1990;75:933–939.
14. Blondel B, Breart G, Glado J, et al. Evaluation of the home-visiting system for women with threatened preterm labour. Results of a randomized controlled trial. *Eur J Obstet Gynaecol Reprod Biol* 1990;34:47–58.
15. Villar J, Farnot U, Barros F, et al. A randomized trial of psychosocial support during high-risk pregnancies. *N Engl J Med* 1992;327:1266–1271.
16. Collaborative Group on Preterm Birth Prevention. Multicenter randomized controlled trial of a preterm birth prevention program. *Am J Obstet Gynecol* 1993;169:352–366.
17. Moore ML, Meis PJ, Ernest JM, et al. A randomized trial of nurse intervention to reduce preterm and low birth weight births. *Obstet Gynecol* 1998;91:656–661.
18. Olds DL, Henderson CR Jr, Tatelbaum R, et al. Improving the delivery of prenatal care and outcomes of pregnancy: a randomized trial of nurse home visitation. *Pediatrics* 1986;77:16–28.
19. Koniak-Griffin D, Anderson NL, Verzemnieks I, et al. A public health nursing early intervention program for adolescent mothers: outcomes from pregnancy through 6 weeks postpartum. *Nursing Res* 2000;49:130–138.
20. Heins HC, Nance NW, McCarthy BJ, et al. A randomised trial of nurse–midwifery prenatal care to reduce low birth weight. *Obstet Gynecol* 1990;75:341–345.
21. Klerman LV, Ramey SL, Goldenberg RL, et al. A randomised controlled trial of augmented prenatal

care for multiple-risk Medicaid eligible African American women. *Am J Public Health* 2001;91:105–111.

22. Bachmann LM, Coomarasamy A, Honest H, et al. Elective cervical cerclage for prevention of preterm birth: a systematic review. *Acta Obstet Gynecol Scand* 2003;82:9–404. Search date 2002; primary sources Medline, Embase, Cochrane Library, Science Citation Index, reference lists, and reviews.
23. MRC/RCOG Working party on cervical cerclage. Final report of the Medical Research Council/Royal College of Obstetricians and Gynaecologists multicentre randomised trial of cervical cerclage. *Br J Obstet Gynaecol* 1993;100:516–523.
24. Rush RW, Isaacs S, McPherson K, et al. A randomised controlled trial of cervical cerlage in women at high risk of spontaneous preterm delivery. *Br J Obstet Gynaecol* 1984;91:724–730.
25. Lazar P, Gueguen S, Dreyfus J, et al. Mulitcentred controlled trials of cervical cerclage in women at moderate risk of preterm delivery. *Br J Obstet Gynaecol* 1984;91:731–735.
26. Dor J, Shalev J, Mashiach S, et al. Elective cervical suture of twin pregnancies diagnosed ultrasonically in the first trimester following induced ovulation. *Gynecol Obstet Invest* 1982;13:55–60.
27. Szeverenyi M, Chalmels J, Grant A, et al. Surgical cerclage in the treatment of cervical incompetence during pregnancy (determining the legitimacy of the procedure). *Orv Hetil* 1992;133:1823–1826.
28. Drakeley AJ, Roberts D, Alfirevic Z. Cervical stitch (cerclage) for preventing pregnancy loss in women. In: The Cochrane Library, Issue 4, 2003. Chichester, UK: John Wiley & Sons, Ltd. Search date 2002; primary sources Cochrane Pregnancy and Childbirth Group Trials Register, congress proceedings of International and European Society meetings of feto-maternal medicine, recurrent miscarriage and reproductive medicine, and contact with researchers.
29. Althuisius SM, Dekker GA, Hummel P, et al. Final results of the Cervical Incompetence Prevention Randomised Cerclage Trial (CIPRACT): therapeutic cerclage with bed rest versus bed rest alone. *Am J Obstet Gynecol* 2001;185:1106 –1112.
30. Rust OA, Atlas RO, Reed J, et al. Revisiting the short cervix detected by transvaginal ultrasound in the second trimester: why cerclage therapy may not help. *Am J Obstet Gynecol* 2001;185:1098–1105.
31. Kenyon S, Boulvain M. Antibiotics for preterm premature rupture of membranes. In: The Cochrane Library, Issue 4, 2003. Chichester, UK: John Wiley & Sons, Ltd. Search date 2003; primary source Cochrane Pregnancy Childbirth Group Trials Register.
32. Kenyon SL, Taylor DJ, Tarnow-Mordi W. Broad-spectrum antibiotics for preterm, prelabour rupture of fetal membranes: the ORACLE I randomised trial. *Lancet* 2001;357:979–988.
33. Hofmeyr GJ. Amnioinfusion for preterm rupture of membranes. In: The Cochrane Library, Issue 4, 2003. Chichester, UK: John Wiley & Sons, Ltd. Search date 2001; primary sources Cochrane Pregnancy and Childbirth Group Trials Register and Cochrane Register of Controlled Trials.
34. Gyetvai K, Hannah ME, Hodnett ED, et al. Tocolytics for preterm labor: a systematic review. *Obstet Gynecol* 1999;94:869–877. Search date 1998; primary sources Medline and Cochrane Register of Controlled Trials.
35. King JF, Flenady VJ, Papatsonis DNM et al. Calcium channel blockers for inhibiting preterm labour. In; The Cochrane Library, Issue 4, 2003. Chichester, UK: John Wiley & Sons, Ltd. Search date 2002; primary sources Cochrane Controlled Trials Register, Medline, Embase, Current Contents, hand searched relevant references, and contact with experts.
36. Crowther CA, Hiller JE, Doyle LW. Magnesium sulphate for preventing preterm birth in threatened preterm labour. In: The Cochrane Library, Issue 4, 2002. Oxford: Update Software. Search date 2002.
37. Ma L. Magnesium sulfate in prevention of preterm labour (translation). *Chung Hua I Hsueh Tsa Chih Taipei* 1992;72:158–161.
38. Goodwin TM, Paul R, Silver H, et al. The effect of the oxytocin antagonist atosiban on preterm uterine activity in the human. *Am J Obstet Gynecol* 1994;170:474–478.
39. Romero R, Sibai BM, Sanchez-Ramos L, et al. An oxytocin receptor antagonist (atosiban) in the treatment of preterm labor: a randomized, double-blind, placebo-controlled trial with tocolytic rescue. *Am J Obstet Gynecol* 2000;182;1173–1183.
40. Grant A, Penn ZJ, Steer PJ. Elective or selective caesarean delivery of the small baby? A systematic review of the controlled trials. *Br J Obstet Gynaecol* 1996;103:1197–1200. Search date not reported; primary sources not reported.
41. Crowley P. Prophylactic corticosteroids for preterm birth. In: The Cochrane Library, Issue 4, 2003. Chichester, UK: John Wiley & Sons, Ltd. Search date 1996; primary sources Cochrane Pregnancy and Childbirth Group Trials Register.
42. Baud O, Foix-L'Helias L, Kaminski M, et al. Antenatal glucocorticoid treatment and cystic periventricular leukomalacia in very premature infants. *N Engl J Med* 1999;341:1190–1196.
43. Crowther CA, Alfirevic Z, Haslam RR. Prenatal thyrotropin-releasing hormone (TRH) for preterm birth. In: The Cochrane Library, Issue 4, 2003. Chichester, UK: John Wiley & Sons, Ltd. Search date 1999; primary sources Cochrane Pregnancy and Childbirth Group Trials Register.
44. King J, Flenady V. Prophylactic antibiotic for inhibiting preterm labour with intact membranes. In: The Cochrane Library, Issue 4, 2003. Chichester, UK: John Wiley & Sons, Ltd. Search date 2002; primary sources Cochrane Pregnancy and Childbirth Group Trials Register, personal contacts, and hand searches of reference lists.
45. Kenyon SL, Taylor DJ, Tarnow-Mordi W. Broad-spectrum antibiotics for spontaneous preterm labour: the ORACLE II randomised trial. *Lancet* 2001;357:989–994.

Bridgette Byrne
Senior Lecturer in Obstetrics and Gynaecology
Royal College of Surgeons of Ireland
Coombe Women's Hospital, Dublin, Ireland

John J Morrison
Professor of Obstetrics and Gynaecology
Clinical Science Institute
University College Hospital, Galway, Ireland

Competing interests: None declared.

TABLE 1 Summary of RCTs addressing enhanced care on preterm birth rates compared with usual care (see text, p 1829).

Outcome	Absolute risks: Antibiotic	Absolute risks: Control	ARR (95% CI)	OR (95% CI)	NNT (95% CI)
Born within 48 hours of rupture	140/513 (27%)	207/545 (38%)	11% (6% to 16%)	0.6 (0.46 to 0.77)	9 (6 to 17)
Born within 7 days of rupture	283/483 (59%)	364/508 (72%)	14% (8% to 21%)	0.54 (0.41 to 0.70)	7 (5 to 13)
Chorio–amnionitis	122/736 (17%)	188/763 (25%)	8% (4% to 11%)	0.61 (0.47 to 0.79)	12 (9 to 24)
Neonatal infection	86/775 (11%)	127/799 (16%)	5% (2% to 8%)	0.62 (0.45 to 0.86)	18 (12 to 52)
Perinatal death	50/700 (7%)	53/732 (7%)	0.1% (–3% to +2%)	0.98 (0.66 to 1.47)	ND
Necrotising enterocolitis	43/611 (7%)	48/644 (7.5%)	0.4% (–2.9% to +2.7%)	0.93 (0.61 to 1.44)	ND

ND, no data.

Bronchitis (acute)

Search date July 2004

Peter Wark

QUESTIONS

INTERVENTIONS

TREATMENTS

Trade off between benefits and harms

Unknown effectiveness

Covered elsewhere in *Clinical Evidence*

Asthma
Asthma and other wheezing disorders of childhood
Chronic obstructive pulmonary disease
Upper respiratory tract infection

See glossary

Key Messages

Treatments

- **Antibiotics** One systematic review and one subsequent RCT found that antibiotics (doxycycline, erythromycin and sulphamethoxazole-trimethoprim) modestly reduced cough at 1–2 weeks compared with placebo. However, they found no significant difference in quality of life or impairment in normal activity compared with placebo. We found no RCTs comparing amoxicillin (amoxycillin) versus placebo. RCTs found no significant difference in clinical improvement or cure between amoxicillin and roxithromycin or cefuroxime. RCTs found no significant difference between azithromycin and clarithromycin, among different cephalosporins, or between cefuroxime and amoxicillin plus clavulanic acid. Antibiotics increased the risk of adverse events such as nausea, vomiting, rash, headache, and vaginitis compared with placebo. Two RCTs found that adverse effects were less common with cefuroxime than with amoxicillin plus clavulanic acid. Widespread antibiotic use may lead to bacterial resistance to antibiotics.
- **Antihistamines** One RCT found insufficient evidence about the effects of antihistamines compared with placebo in people with acute bronchitis.
- **Antitussives** RCTs found no significant difference in cough severity between codeine or dextromethorphan and placebo in children or adults with acute bronchitis. The RCTs may have been too small to detect a clinically important difference. We found limited evidence from one RCT that moguisteine modestly reduced cough severity compared with placebo in adults, but was associated with more adverse gastrointestinal effects.
- **Expectorants** We found no RCTs about the effects of expectorants in people with acute bronchitis.
- **β_2 Agonists** One systematic review found no significant difference in cough or ability to return to work between β_2 agonists (inhaled or oral) and placebo in people with acute bronchitis. It found limited evidence from one small RCT that β_2 agonists reduced cough compared with erythromycin. The review found that β_2 agonists were more frequently associated with shaking and tremor in adults than placebo.

Clin Evid 2005;13:1844–1852.

DEFINITION Acute bronchitis is transient inflammation of the trachea and major bronchi. Clinically, it is diagnosed on the basis of cough and occasionally sputum, dyspnoea, and wheeze. This review is limited to episodes of acute bronchitis in people (smokers and non-smokers) with no pre-existing respiratory disease such as a pre-existing diagnosis of asthma or chronic bronchitis, evidence of fixed airflow obstruction, or both, and excluding those with clinical or radiographic evidence of pneumonia. However, using a clinical definition for acute bronchitis implies that people with conditions such as transient/mild asthma or mild chronic obstructive pulmonary disease may have been recruited to some of the reported studies.

INCIDENCE/ PREVALENCE Acute bronchitis affects 44/1000 adults (> 16 years old) a year, with 82% of episodes occurring in autumn or winter.[1] One survey found that acute bronchitis was the fifth most common reason to present to a general practitioner in Australia.[2]

AETIOLOGY/ RISK FACTORS Infection is believed to be the trigger for acute bronchitis. However, pathogens have been identified in fewer than 55% of people.[1] Community studies that attempted to isolate pathogens from the sputum of people with acute bronchitis found viruses in 8–23%, typical bacteria (*Streptococcus pneumoniae*, *Haemophilus influenzae*, *Moraxella catarrhalis*) in 45%, and atypical bacteria (*Mycobacterium pneumoniae*, *Chlamydia pneumoniae*, *Bordetella pertussis*) in 0–25%.[1,3,4] It is unclear whether smoking affects the risk for developing acute bronchitis.

PROGNOSIS Acute bronchitis is regarded as a mild self limiting illness but there are few data on prognosis and rates of complications such as chronic cough or progression to chronic bronchitis or pneumonia. One prospective longitudinal study reviewed 653 previously well adults who presented to suburban general practices over a 12 month period with symptoms of acute lower respiratory tract infection.[1] It found that within the first month of the illness 20% of people re-presented to their general practitioner with persistent or recurrent symptoms. One prospective study of 138 previously well adults found that 34% had symptoms consistent with either chronic bronchitis or asthma 3 years after initial presentation with acute bronchitis.[5] It is also unclear whether acute bronchitis plays a causal role in the progression to chronic bronchitis or is simply a marker of predisposition to chronic lung disease. Although smoking has been identified as the most important risk factor for chronic bronchitis,[6,7] it is unclear whether the inflammatory effects of cigarette smoke and infection causing acute bronchitis have additive effects in leading to chronic inflammatory airway changes.

AIMS OF INTERVENTION To improve symptoms associated with acute bronchitis; to reduce complications, with minimal adverse effects.

OUTCOMES Duration of symptoms, particularly cough, sputum production, and fever; quality of life scores; adverse effects of treatment; complications, especially chronic cough, pneumonia, and chronic bronchitis.

METHODS *Clinical Evidence* search and appraisal July 2004. We included people of any age or sex with acute bronchitis. We excluded trials conducted in people who had chronic respiratory disease or other acute respiratory diseases. We excluded non-systematic reviews, non-randomised trials, and RCTs of less than 4 days' treatment duration.

QUESTION What are the effects of treatments for acute bronchitis in people without chronic respiratory disease?

OPTION ANTIBIOTICS

One systematic review and one subsequent RCT found that antibiotics (doxycycline, erythromycin and sulphamethoxazole-trimethoprim) modestly reduced cough at 1–2 weeks compared with placebo. However, they found no significant difference in quality of life or impairment in normal activity compared with placebo. We found no RCTs comparing amoxicillin (amoxycillin) versus placebo. RCTs found no significant difference in clinical improvement or cure between amoxicillin and roxithromycin or cefuroxime. RCTs found no significant difference between azithromycin and clarithromycin, among different cephalosporins, or between cefuroxime and amoxicillin plus

clavulanic acid. Antibiotics increased the risk of adverse events such as nausea, vomiting, rash, headache, and vaginitis compared with placebo. Two RCTs found that adverse effects were less common with cefuroxime than with amoxicillin plus clavulanic acid. Widespread antibiotic use may lead to bacterial resistance to antibiotics.

Benefits: **Any antibiotic versus placebo:** We found one systematic review, which compared antibiotics versus placebo (search date 2000, 9 RCTs; 750 people aged 8 to > 65 years and included smokers, but excluded people with chronic bronchitis).[8] Acute bronchitis was defined by cough, sputum production, or physician diagnosis. The antibiotics used were doxycycline (4 RCTs), erythromycin (4 RCTs), and sulphamethoxazole plus trimethoprim (1 RCT). The review found that antibiotics significantly reduced the proportion of people with cough after 1–2 weeks and mean number of days with reported cough compared with placebo (people with cough, 4 RCTs: 47/143 [33%] with antibiotics *v* 67/132 [51%] with placebo; RR 0.64, 95% CI 0.49 to 0.85; WMD in number of days with cough, 5 RCTs: –0.58 days, 95% CI –1.16 days to –0.009 days). However, it found no significant difference between antibiotics and placebo in night time cough or productive cough after 1–2 weeks, or for days of impaired activity (night time cough, 3 RCTs: RR for antibiotics *v* placebo 0.76, 95% CI 0.45 to 1.30; productive cough, 7 RCTs: RR for antibiotics *v* placebo 0.97, 95% CI 0.82 to 1.16; WMD in days of impaired activity, 5 RCTs: –0.48 days, 95% CI –0.96 days to +0.01 days).[8] For analyses of specific types of antibiotic versus placebo, see below. **Amoxicillin versus placebo:** We found no RCTs comparing amoxicillin versus placebo. **Macrolides versus placebo:** We found one systematic review (search date 2000, 4 RCTs)[8] and one subsequent RCT.[9] In the review, participants were aged 8 to 65 years and over and included smokers, but excluded people with chronic bronchitis. Acute bronchitis was defined by cough, sputum production, or physician diagnosis. One RCT identified by the review (91 people aged ≥ 8 years) which compared erythromycin versus placebo found a significant reduction in the mean number of days of impaired activities with erythromycin compared with placebo (see web extra table A).[10] However, none of the four RCTs included in the review found significant differences between treatment and control groups in the number of people with cough, night time cough, productive cough, limitation in work/activities, or abnormal lung examination; the proportion of people who had not improved clinically at follow up; and the mean number of days of cough, productive cough, or feeling ill (see web extra table A).[8,10–12] The subsequent RCT (220 adults with a clinical diagnosis of acute bronchitis and no history of chronic lung disease) compared azithromycin versus vitamin C (as a placebo) for 5 days.[9] It found no significant difference between azithromycin and vitamin C in quality of life after 8 days (acute bronchitis specific health related quality of life score, ranging from 0 [not troubled at all] to 6 [extremely troubled]: 0.9 with azithromycin *v* 0.9 with vitamin C; difference adjusted for baseline score +0.03, 95% CI –0.2 to +0.26).[9] **Tetracyclines versus placebo:** We found one systematic review, which compared doxycycline versus placebo (search date 2000, 4 RCTs).[8] Participants were aged 8 to 65 years and over and included smokers, but excluded people with chronic bronchitis).[8] Acute bronchitis was defined by cough, sputum production, or physician diagnosis (see web extra table A).[8] Two of the RCTs identified by the review found that doxycycline significantly reduced the number of people with cough at follow up compared with placebo.[11,12] One RCT found that doxycycline significantly reduced the mean number of days of cough compared with placebo.[11] None of the RCTs found significant effects of doxycycline on the number of people with productive cough, night time cough, limitation in work/activities, abnormal lung examination; the proportion of people who had not improved clinically at follow up; or the mean number of days with productive cough, productive cough, or feeling ill compared with placebo.[8] **Amoxicillin versus cephalosporins:** We found one RCT (296 adults with clinically diagnosed acute bronchitis and no pre-existing lung disease) comparing amoxicillin 250 mg three times daily versus cefuroxime 250 mg twice daily for 7 days.[13] It found no significant difference in clinical cure rates between amoxicillin and cefuroxime at 72 hours post-treatment (123/153 [80%] with amoxicillin *v* 109/143 [76%] with cefuroxime; P = 0.8). **Amoxicillin versus macrolides:** We found one RCT (196 adults with clinically diagnosed acute bronchitis and no pre-existing lung disease) comparing amoxicillin 500 mg three times daily versus roxithromycin 150 mg once daily for 10 days.[14] It found no significant difference between amoxicillin and roxithromycin in the proportion with physician assessed improvement or cure (89/96 [93%] with roxithromycin *v* 88/96 [92%] with amoxicillin; P = 0.8). **Macrolides versus each other:** We found one RCT (214 adults with clinically diagnosed acute bronchitis and no pre-existing lung disease) comparing azithromycin 500 mg once daily for 2 days then 250 mg once daily for 3 days versus clarithromycin 250 mg once daily for 5 days.[15] It found no significant difference between azithromycin and clarithromycin in clinical cure rates or relapse rates after 6–7 days (cure rate: 55/103 [53%] with azithromycin *v* 70/108 [65%] with clarithromycin; P = 0.4; relapse rate: 2/95 [2.1%] with azithromycin *v* 1/101 [1.0%] with clarithromycin; P = 0.5). **Cephalosporins versus each other:** We found two RCTs.[16,17] The first RCT (465 children < 12 years old with clinically diagnosed acute bronchitis and no pre-existing lung disease) compared cefuroxime 250 mg twice daily versus cefixime 400 mg once daily for 10 days.[16] It found no significant difference in clinical outcome between cefuroxime and cefixime after 14 days (proportion with satisfactory clinical outcome, as assessed by the treating general practitioner: 130/148 [88%] with cefuroxime *v* 217/238 [91%] with cefixime; P = 0.8). It was not clear how "satisfactory clinical outcome" was defined. The second RCT (196 elderly people with clinically diagnosed acute purulent bronchitis and no pre-existing lung disease) comparing cefuroxime 250 mg twice daily versus cefpodoxime 200 mg twice daily for 5 days found no significant difference in physician rated satisfactory clinical response between cefuroxime and cefpodoxime after 10 days (86/95 [91%] with cefuroxime *v* 87/92 [95%] with cefpodoxime; P = 0.76).[17] It was not clear how "satisfactory clinical outcome" was defined. **Cephalosporins versus amoxicillin plus clavulanic acid:** We found two RCTs.[18,19] The first RCT (312 adults with clinically diagnosed acute bronchitis and no pre-existing lung disease) compared cefuroxime 250 mg twice daily versus amoxicillin 875 mg plus clavulanic acid 125 mg twice daily for 5 days.[18] It found no significant difference between cefuroxime and amoxicillin plus clavulanic acid in self reported clinical improvement at 10–14 days (114/133 [86%] with cefuroxime *v* 128/142 [90%] with amoxicillin plus clavulanic acid; P = 0.27). The second RCT (537 people aged ≥ 12 years with clinically diagnosed acute bronchitis and no pre-existing lung disease) compared cefuroxime 250 mg twice daily for 5 days versus cefuroxime 250 mg twice daily for 10 days versus amoxicillin 500 mg plus clavulanic acid 125 mg three times daily for 10 days.[19] It found no significant difference between the groups in cure rates 1–3 days after completing treatment (84/177 [47%] with cefuroxime for 5 days *v* 100/177 [56%] with cefuroxime for 10 days *v* 116/183 [63%] with amoxicillin plus clavulanic acid; cefuroxime for 5 days *v* cefuroxime for 10 days, P = 0.41; cefuroxime for 5 days *v* amoxicillin plus clavulanic acid, P = 0.91; cefuroxime for 10 days *v* amoxicillin plus clavulanic acid, P = 0.45).

Harms: **Antibiotics versus placebo:** In the systematic review, adverse events were significantly more common with antibiotics compared with placebo (7 RCTs, adverse events: 60/327 [18%] antibiotics *v* 38/316 [12%] with placebo; RR 1.48; 95% CI 1.02 to 2.14).[8] Adverse events included nausea, vomiting, headache, skin rash, and vaginitis. **Amoxicillin versus placebo:** We found no RCTs. **Macrolides versus placebo:** One RCT included in the review found that significantly more people had adverse effects with erythromycin compared with placebo (18/49 [37%] with erythromycin *v* 6/42 [14%] with placebo; RR 2.57, 95% CI 1.12 to 5.88) (see web extra table A).[10] The other three RCTs included in the review found no significant difference in adverse effects between erythromycin and placebo.[8] **Tetracyclines versus placebo:** Two RCTs included in the review found no significant difference in adverse effects between doxycycline and placebo (see web extra table A).[8] The other two RCTs included in the review gave no information on adverse effects. **Amoxicillin versus cephalosporins:** The RCT did not report on adverse events.[13] **Amoxicillin versus macrolides:** The RCT gave no information on adverse effects.[14] **Macrolides versus each other:** The RCT found no significant difference between azithromycin and clarithromycin in adverse effects (17/105 [16%] with azithromycin *v* 13/109 [12%] with clarithromycin; $P = 0.56$).[15] **Cephalosporins versus each other:** The RCT comparing cefuroxime with cefixime did not report on adverse events.[16] The RCT comparing cefuroxime with cefpodoxime found that the rate of adverse events was similar with cefuroxime and cefpodoxime (4/95 [4.2%] with cefuroxime *v* 6/92 [6.5%] with cefpodoxime; CI not reported).[17] Most of the adverse events were gastrointestinal. **Cephalosporins versus amoxicillin plus clavulanic acid:** The first RCT found that cefuroxime was associated with fewer adverse effects than was amoxicillin plus clavulanic acid (16/133 [12%] with cefuroxime *v* 45/142 [32%] with amoxicillin plus clavulanic acid; $P = 0.001$).[18] Most of the adverse effects were gastrointestinal. The second RCT found that a significantly lower proportion of people had gastrointestinal symptoms with cefuroxime than with amoxicillin plus clavulanic acid (24/157 [15%] with cefuroxime for 5 days *v* 48/130 [37%] with amoxicillin plus clavulanic acid; $P < 0.01$).[19]

Comment: Physicians may be more likely to prescribe antibiotics for smokers with acute bronchitis than for non-smokers (90% in smokers *v* 75% in non-smokers; $P < 0.05$).[20] Seven of the trials in the systematic review found that smoking status did not affect response to antibiotics.[8] All trials mentioned above diagnosed acute bronchitis on clinical grounds and commenced treatment independently of sputum culture results. As shown above, there is no evidence that extended spectrum antibiotics are more effective than amoxicillin or doxycycline. Therefore, their use does not seem justified, particularly as widespread antibiotic use in acute bronchitis may lead to bacterial resistance.[21]

OPTION ANTITUSSIVES

RCTs found no significant difference in cough severity between codeine or dextromethorphan and placebo in children or adults with acute bronchitis. The RCTs may have been too small to detect a clinically important difference. We found limited evidence from one RCT that moguisteine modestly reduced cough severity compared with placebo in adults, but was associated with more adverse gastrointestinal effects.

Benefits: **In children:** We found two systematic reviews (search dates 2000, see comment below).[22,23] The first review compared non-prescription medications versus placebo in children with acute cough. It identified one RCT (57 children) that met our inclusion criteria.[24] The RCT compared three treatments: dextromethorphan 15 mg once daily, codeine 10 mg once daily, and placebo at bedtime for 3 nights.[24] It found no significant difference between treatments in mean cough score after 3 days (reduction in mean cough score [range 0–4, higher score indicating more severe cough]: 2.1 with dextromethorphan *v* 2.2 with codeine *v* 2.2 with placebo; dextromethorphan *v* placebo, P = 0.4; codeine *v* placebo, P = 0.7).[24] The second systematic review identified one additional RCT (75 children with acute bronchitis or acute cough).[25] The RCT compared three treatments: dextromethorphan (7.5 mg once daily for children < 7 years and 15 mg once daily for children ≥ 7 years), dextromethorphan plus salbutamol (albuterol) (1 mg once daily for children < 7 years and 2 mg once daily for children ≥ 7 years), and placebo once daily for 3 days. It found no significance difference in cough symptoms with dextromethorphan compared with placebo (mean cough score day 1: 1.30 with dextromethorphan *v* 1.44 with placebo; day 2: 0.93 with dextromethorphan *v* 1.06 with placebo; day 3: 0.60 with dextromethorphan *v* 0.76 with placebo; differences reported as non-significant for all days) or general condition (mean general condition score day 1: 1.0 with dextromethorphan *v* 1.4 with placebo; day 2: 1.48 with dextromethorphan *v* 1.64 with placebo; day 3: 2.0 with dextromethorphan *v* 2.08 with placebo; difference reported as non-significant for all days) on either of the 3 treatment days.[25] More than half of the people reported some or marked relief from the medication (16/24 [66%] with dextromethorphan *v* 19/26 [73%] with placebo) but the differences between the groups were not significant. **In adults:** We found one systematic review (search date 2000, 2 RCTs meeting our inclusion criteria, see comment below).[22,26,27] The first RCT identified by the review (81 adults) compared codeine 30 mg four times daily with placebo for 4 days.[26] It found no significant difference between codeine and placebo in mean cough severity score (higher score indicates worse cough, scale end points unclear) over a 5 day period (mean cough severity score: 17.2 with codeine *v* 18.0 with placebo; P = 0.5). The second RCT (108 adults) compared moguisteine 200 mg three times daily for 5 days versus placebo.[27] It found that moguisteine modestly reduced cough severity score compared with placebo (mean difference in cough score on a scale of 0–9 [higher score indicating more severe cough]: 0.5; P < 0.05).

Harms: **In children:** No additional adverse events were recorded with treatment compared with placebo (the event rates for each group were not reported).[24] The RCT identified by the second review found a low incidence of serious adverse effects in all treatment groups and no significant difference between the dextromethorphan and placebo groups (children with serious adverse effects: 3/24 [13%] with dextromethorphan *v* 1/26 [4%] with placebo; difference reported as non-significant).[25] **In adults:** The first RCT identified by the systematic review gave no information on adverse effects.[26] The second RCT found that moguisteine increased nausea, vomiting, and abdominal pain compared with placebo (13/58 [22%] with moguisteine *v* 5/58 [9%] with placebo; P < 0.05).[27]

Comment: Two of the five RCTs identified by the first systematic review were excluded because treatment duration was less than 4 days.[22] The first systematic review stated that it examined the effects of treatments in people with “upper respiratory tract infection” rather than “acute bronchitis”.[22] However, the clinical criteria used to define this population were consistent with the definition of acute bronchitis used in this topic. Moguisteine is available without prescription only in the UK.

OPTION β_2 AGONISTS

One systematic review found no significant difference in cough or ability to return to work between β_2 agonists (inhaled or oral) and placebo in people with acute bronchitis. It found limited evidence from one small RCT that β_2 agonists reduced cough compared with erythromycin. The review found that β_2 agonists were more frequently associated with shaking and tremor in adults than placebo.

Benefits: We found one systematic review (search date 2000; 2 RCTs in 109 children and 5 RCTs in 418 adults, both smokers and non-smokers, with acute bronchitis or acute cough).[23] People with pre-existing lung disease, with another acute respiratory disorder, or aged under 24 months were excluded. Four of the RCTs included in the systematic review compared an oral β_2 agonist (salbutamol [albuterol]) versus placebo. Three RCTs compared inhaled β_2 agonists (salbutamol and fenoterol) versus placebo. Two RCTs had more than two study arms.[23,28] Results from children and adults were analysed separately. **Versus placebo:** The review found no significant difference between inhaled or oral β_2 agonists and placebo in the proportion of children or adults with cough after 7 days (1 RCT, 59 children: 11/30 [37%] with β_2 agonists *v* 12/29 [41%] with placebo; RR 0.89, 95% CI 0.47 to 1.65; 3 RCTs, 110 adults: RR 0.86, 95% CI 0.63 to 1.18). Similarly, it found no significant difference between β_2 agonists and placebo in the proportion of adults unable to work after 4 days of treatment (2 RCTs, 149 adults: RR for β_2 agonists *v* placebo 0.82, 95% CI 0.28 to 2.34). **Versus antibiotics:** The systematic review[23] identified one small RCT which compared inhaled β_2 agonists versus oral erythromycin for 7 days.[29] It found that β_2 agonists significantly reduced the proportion of adults with cough after 7 days compared with erythromycin (7/17 [41%] with inhaled β_2 agonists *v* 15/17 [88%] with erythromycin; RR 0.47, 95% CI 0.26 to 0.85).

Harms: **Versus placebo:** The systematic review found that in children, shaking and tremor were more frequently associated with β_2 agonists compared with placebo, although the difference was not significant (2 RCTs, 108 children: 6/55 [11%] with β_2 agonists *v* 0/53 [0%] with placebo; RR undefined).[23] In adults, a significantly larger proportion of people reported shaking and tremor with β_2 agonists (both oral and inhaled) compared with placebo (3 RCTs, 211 adults: 58/105 [55%] with β_2 agonists *v* 12/106 [11%] with placebo; OR 7.94, 95% CI 1.17 to 53.94). **Versus antibiotics:** One RCT identified by the review found that tremor and shaking were more frequently associated with β_2 agonists compared with erythromycin (6/17 [35%] with β_2 agonists *v* 0/17 [0%] with erythromycin; RR 13.0, 95% CI 0.8 to 214.0), although the difference was not significant.[23,29] The RCT found no significant difference between β_2 agonists and erythromycin in other adverse effects (2/23 [8.7%] with β_2 agonists *v* 2/23 [8.7%] with erythromycin; RR 1.00, 95% CI 0.15 to 1.51).

Comment: None.

OPTION EXPECTORANTS

We found no RCTs about the effects of expectorants in people with acute bronchitis.

Benefits: We found one systematic review (search date 2000) of non-prescription medications for acute cough in people with acute bronchitis, which found no RCTs evaluating the effect of expectorants in people with acute bronchitis.[22] We found no subsequent RCTs.

Harms: We found no RCTs.

Comment: The systematic review stated that it examined the effects of treatments in people with "upper respiratory tract infection" rather than "acute bronchitis".[22] However, the clinical criteria used to define this population were consistent with the definition of acute bronchitis used in this topic.

OPTION ANTIHISTAMINES

One RCT found insufficient evidence about the effects of antihistamines compared with placebo in people with acute bronchitis.

Benefits: We found one systematic review of non-prescription medications in people with acute bronchitis (search date 2000).[22] The review identified one RCT (100 adult non-smokers) that met our inclusion criteria.[30] It compared terfenadine 100 mg twice daily versus placebo for 4 or 5 days. It found no significant difference in mean cough score between terfenadine and placebo at day 4 (mean cough score [range 0–3, higher scores indicating worse cough]: 0.80 with terfenadine *v* 0.65 with placebo; P = 0.35).

Harms: The RCT reported a low incidence of adverse events but did not specify these.[30]

Comment: The systematic review stated that it examined the effects of treatments in people with "upper respiratory tract infection" rather than "acute bronchitis".[22] However, the clinical criteria used to define this population were consistent with the definition of acute bronchitis used in this topic.

REFERENCES

1. Macfarlane J, Holmes W, Gard P, et al. Prospective study of the incidence, aetiology and outcome of adult lower respiratory tract illness in the community. *Thorax* 2001;56:109–114.
2. Meza RA. The management of acute bronchitis in general practice results from the Australian morbidity and treatment survey. *Aust Fam Physician* 1994;23:1550–1553.
3. Boldy DAR, Skidmore SJ, Ayres JG. Acute bronchitis in the community: clinical features, infective factors, changes in pulmonary function and bronchial reactivity to histamine. *Respir Med* 1990;84:377–385.
4. Grayston JT, Aldous MB, Easton A, et al. Evidence that *Chlamydia pneumoniae* causes pneumonia and bronchitis. *J Infect Dis* 1993;168:1231–1235.
5. Jonsson JS, Gislason T, Gislason D, et al. Acute bronchitis and clinical outcome three years later: prospective cohort study. *Thorax* 1998;317:1433.
6. Whittemore AS, Perlin SA, DiCiccio Y. Chronic obstructive pulmonary disease in lifelong nonsmokers: results from NHANES. *Am J Public Health* 1995;85:702–706.
7. Brunekreef B, Fischer P, Remijn B, et al. Indoor air pollution and its effects on pulmonary function of adult non-smoking women: III passive smoking and pulmonary function. *Int J Epidemiol* 1985;14:227–230.
8. Smucny J, Fahey T, Becker L, et al. Antibiotics for acute bronchitis. In: The Cochrane Library, Issue 1, 2003. Oxford: Update Software. Search date 2000; primary sources Medline, Embase, Scisearch, Cochrane controlled trials register, hand searches of reference lists, and contact with study authors and drug manufacturers.
9. Evans AT, Husain S, Durairaj L, et al. Azithromycin for acute bronchitis: a randomised, double blind, controlled trial. *Lancet* 2002;359:1648–1654.
10. King DE, Williams WC, Bishop L, et al. Effectiveness of erythromycin in the treatment of acute bronchitis. *J Fam Pract* 1996;42:601–605.
11. Verheij TJ, Hermans J, Mulder JD. Effects of doxycycline in patients with acute cough and purulent sputum: a double blind placebo controlled trial. *Br J Gen Pract* 1994;44:400–404.
12. Williamson HA. A randomised, controlled trial of doxycycline in the treatment of acute bronchitis. *J Fam Pract* 1984;19:481–486.
13. Shah SH, Shah IS, Turnbull G, et al. Cefuroxime axetil in the treatment of bronchitis: comparison with amoxicillin in a multicentre study in general practice patients. *Br J Clin Pract* 1994;48:185–189.
14. Hopstaken RM, Nelemans P, Stobberingh EE, et al. Is roxithromycin better than amoxicillin in the treatment of acute lower respiratory tract infections in primary care? A double blind randomised controlled trial. *J Fam Pract* 2002;51:329–336.
15. Vincken W, Yernault JC. Efficacy and tolerability of clarithromycin versus azithromycin in the short course treatment of acute bronchitis. *Drug Invest* 1993:3;170–175.
16. Arthur M, McAdoo M, Guerra J, et al. Clinical comparison of cefuroxime axetil with cefixime in the treatment of acute bronchitis. *Am J Ther* 1996;3:622–629.
17. Camus P, Beraud A, Phillip-Joet F, et al. Five days treatment of acute purulent bronchitis in the elderly with cefpodoxime proxetil. *Med Maladies Infect* 1994;24:681–685
18. Henry DC, Ruoff GE, Noonan M, et al. Comparison of the efficacy and tolerability of short-course cefuroxime axetil and amoxicillin clavulanic acid in the treatment of secondary bacterial infections of acute bronchitis. *Clin Drug Invest* 1999;18:335–344.
19. Henry DC, Ruoff GE, Noonan M, et al. Effectiveness of short course therapy (5 days) with cefuroxime

axetil in treatment of secondary bacterial infections of acute bronchitis. *Antimicrob Agents Chemother* 1995;39:2528–2534.
20. Oeffinger KC, Snell LM, Foster BM, et al. Treatment of acute bronchitis in adults. A national survey of family physicians. *J Fam Pract* 1998;46:469–475.
21. Wise R, Hart T, Cars O, et al. Antimicrobial resistance is a major threat to public health [Editorial]. *BMJ* 1998;317:609–610.
22. Schroeder K, Fahey T. Over the counter medications for acute cough in children and adults in ambulatory settings. In: The Cochrane Library, Issue 1, 2003. Oxford: Update Software. Search date 2000; primary sources Cochrane library, Medline, Embase, UK Dept Health National Research Register, and contact with study authors and pharmaceutical companies.
23. Smucny J, Flynn C, Becker L, et al. Beta2 agonists for acute bronchitis. In: The Cochrane Library, Issue 1, 2003. Oxford: Update Software. Search date 2000; primary sources Cochrane library, Medline, Embase, conference proceedings, and Science Citation Index.
24. Taylor JA, Novack AH, Almquist JR, et al. Efficacy of cough suppressants in children. *J Pediatr* 1993;122:799–802.
25. Korppi M, Laurikainen K, Pietikainen M, et al. Antitussives in the treatment of acute transient cough in children. *Acta Pediatr Scand* 1991;80:969–971.
26. Eccles R, Morris S, Jawad M. Lack of effect of codeine in the treatment of cough associated with acute upper respiratory tract infection. *J Clin Pharmacol Ther* 1992;17:175–180.
27. Adams R, Hosie J, James I, et al. Antitussive activity and tolerability of moguisteine in patients with acute cough: a randomised double blind placebo controlled study. *Adv Ther* 1993;10:263–271.
28. Tukiainen J, Karttunen P, Silvasti M, et al. The treatment of acute transient cough: a placebo-controlled comparison of dextromethorphan and dextromethorphan-beta 2-sympathomimetic combination. *Eur J Respir Dis* 1986;69:95–99.
29. Hueston W. A comparison of albuterol and erythromycin for the treatment of acute bronchitis. *J Fam Pract* 1991;33:476–480.
30. Berkowitz RB, Tinkelman DG. Evaluation of oral terfenadine for treatment of the common cold. *Ann Allergy* 1991;67:593–597.

Peter Wark
Consultant Respiratory Physician
Brooke Laboratories
University of Southampton
Southampton
UK

Competing interests: None declared.

Common cold

Search date May 2004

Bruce Arroll

QUESTIONS

INTERVENTIONS

Key Messages

Treatments

- **Antihistamines (may improve runny nose and sneezing, no significant difference in overall symptoms)** One systematic review found that chlorpheniramine or doxylaminine reduced runny nose and sneezing after 2 days compared with placebo in people with common cold, but the clinical benefit was small. Another review, that assessed a wide variety of antihistamines, found no significant difference in overall cold symptoms at 1–10 days between antihistamines and placebo and found that first generation antihistamines increased adverse effects, including sedation.
- **Decongestants (norephedrine, oxymetazoline, or pseudoephedrine) provided short term (3–10 hour) relief of congestive symptoms** One systematic review found that, compared with placebo, decongestants (norephedrine, oxymetazoline, or pseudoephedrine) reduced nasal congestion over 3–10 hours after a single dose in people with common cold. The review identified no RCTs of other decongestants. One case control study found weak evidence that phenylpropanolamine may increase the risk of haemorrhagic stroke.
- **Analgesics or anti-inflammatory drugs** We found no RCTs of analgesics or anti-inflammatory drugs in people with common cold.
- **Decongestants (insufficient evidence to assess longer term [> 10 hours] effects on congestive symptoms)** One systematic review provided insufficient evidence to assess the effects of longer use of decongestants in people with colds.
- **Echinacea** Systematic reviews found limited evidence that some preparations of echinacea may improve cold symptoms compared with placebo, but we found insufficient evidence about the effects of any specific product. Two subsequent RCTs, one in adults and one in children, found no significant difference between echinacea and placebo in severity or duration of cold symptoms.

- **Steam inhalation** One systematic review provided insufficient evidence to assess steam inhalation in people with common cold.
- **Vitamin C** One systematic review found limited evidence from quasi-randomised and controlled trials that vitamin C slightly reduced the duration of cold symptoms compared with placebo. However, the beneficial effect was small.
- **Zinc (intranasal gel or lozenges)** One systematic review found limited evidence that zinc gluconate or acetate lozenges may reduce duration of cold symptoms at 7 days compared with placebo. Another review found no significant difference in duration of symptoms. Both reviews found that symptoms were unchanged at 3 or 5 days. Two RCTs found that zinc intranasal gel reduced the mean duration of cold symptoms compared with placebo. A third RCT found no significant difference in overall symptom duration between intranasal zinc and placebo.
- **Antibiotics** Systematic reviews and one additional RCT found no significant difference between antibiotics and placebo in cure or general improvement at 6–14 days in people with colds. The additional RCT found that, in a subgroup of people (20%) with nasopharyngeal culture positive *H influenzae*, *M catarrhalis*, or *S pneumonia*, antibiotics increased recovery at 5 days compared with placebo. However, we have no methods currently of easily identifying such people at first consultation.

DEFINITION Common colds are defined as upper respiratory tract infections that affect the predominantly nasal part of the respiratory mucosa. Since upper respiratory tract infections can affect any part of the mucosa, it is often arbitrary whether an upper respiratory tract infection is called a "cold" or "sore throat" ("pharyngitis" or "tonsillitis"), "sinusitis", "acute otitis media", or "bronchitis" (see figure 1 in sore throat, p 1876). Sometimes all areas (simultaneously or at different times) are affected in one illness. Symptoms include sneezing, rhinorrhoea (runny nose), headache, and general malaise. In addition to nasal symptoms, half of sufferers experience sore throat and 40% experience cough.[1] This review does not include treatments for people with acute sinusitis (see acute sinusitis, p 646), acute bronchitis, (see acute bronchitis, p 1844), or sore throat (see sore throat, p 1876).

INCIDENCE/ PREVALENCE Upper respiratory tract infections, nasal congestion, throat complaints, and cough are responsible for 11% of general practice consultations in Australia.[2] Each year, children suffer about five such infections and adults two to three infections.[2–4] One cross-sectional study in Norwegian children aged 4–5 years found that 48% experienced more than two common colds annually.[5]

AETIOLOGY/ RISK FACTORS Transmission of common cold infection is mostly through hand to hand contact with subsequent passage to the nostrils or eyes rather than, as commonly perceived, through droplets in the air.[1] The organisms for common colds are mainly viruses (typically rhinovirus, but also coronavirus and respiratory syncytial virus, or metapneumovirus and others). For many colds, no infecting organism can be identified.

PROGNOSIS Common colds are usually short-lived, lasting a few days, with a few lingering symptoms lasting longer, especially cough. Symptoms peak within 1–3 days and generally clear by 1 week, although cough often persists.[1] Although they cause no mortality or serious morbidity, common colds are responsible for considerable discomfort, lost work, and medical costs.

AIMS OF INTERVENTION To relieve symptoms, shorten the illness, or reduce complications, to reduce infectivity to others, with minimal adverse effects from treatments.

OUTCOMES Cure rate; duration of symptoms; time away from work or school; incidence of complications; adverse effects of treatment.

METHODS *Clinical Evidence* search and appraisal May 2004. Where possible, we have excluded RCTs undertaken solely in people with experimentally induced colds, although meta-analyses in some systematic reviews do include such RCTs. We have also excluded RCTs that only assessed the outcome of bacteriological clearance. We performed a broad search for RCTs of any decongestant, analgesic or anti-inflammatory in people with common cold and included any RCTs of sufficient quality.

QUESTION **What are the effects of treatments?**

OPTION **VITAMIN C**

One systematic review found limited evidence from quasi-randomised and controlled trials that vitamin C slightly reduced the duration of cold symptoms compared with placebo. However, the beneficial effect was small.

Benefits: **Versus placebo:** We found one systematic review (search date not reported, 13 RCTs, 17 quasi-randomised or controlled trials identified by two previous systematic reviews[6,7]) that compared vitamin C 1 g or more daily versus placebo for naturally acquired colds.[8] It found that vitamin C reduced the duration of symptoms by about half a day compared with placebo (17 trials, 9365 people; WMD 0.44 days/cold episode, 95% CI 0.23 days/cold episode to 0.64 days/cold episode) representing about 15% fewer symptomatic days per episode.

Harms: The systematic review found no adverse effects associated with vitamin C.[8]

Comment: The RCTs identified by the review had high withdrawal rates (30–40%).[8] The beneficial effect reported in the review was small.

OPTION **ZINC**

One systematic review found limited evidence that zinc gluconate or acetate lozenges may reduce duration of cold symptoms at 7 days compared with placebo. Another review found no significant difference in duration of symptoms. Both reviews found that symptoms were unchanged at 3 or 5 days. Two RCTs found that zinc intranasal gel reduced the mean duration of cold symptoms compared with placebo. A third RCT found no significant difference in overall symptom duration between intranasal zinc and placebo.

Benefits: **Zinc lozenges versus placebo:** We found two systematic reviews (search date 1997, 7 RCTs;[9] search date 1998, 8 RCTs[10]) comparing zinc lozenges (gluconate or acetate) versus placebo for the treatment of naturally acquired colds. The reviews had different inclusion criteria. Both reviews found that symptoms were unchanged at 3 and 5 days. The first review (7 RCTs, including 2 RCTs excluded from the second review because they were in people with experimentally induced colds, 681 people with naturally acquired colds, 73 people with experimentally induced colds) found that zinc lozenges significantly reduced continuing symptoms at 7 days compared with placebo (random effects model: 14/93 [15%] with zinc *v* 46/94 [49%] with placebo; RR 0.31, 95% CI 0.18 to 0.52).[9] However, the second review (8 RCTs, including 3 RCTs included in the first review and 1 RCT excluded from the first review on methodological grounds, all in people with naturally acquired colds) found no significant difference between zinc lozenges and placebo in continuing symptoms at 7 days (OR 0.52, 95% CI 0.25 to 1.20; absolute results presented graphically).[10] The results at 7 days were statistically heterogeneous, which may be because the RCTs retrieved by the reviews used different zinc formulations, were undertaken in people with different types of virus, or because of other unknown factors. **Zinc intranasal gel versus placebo:** We found three RCTs comparing intranasal zinc versus placebo.[11–13] The first RCT (213 people with naturally acquired colds of < 24 hours' duration) found that intranasal zinc significantly reduced overall symptom duration compared with placebo (mean duration: 2.3 days with intranasal zinc *v* 9.0 days with placebo; $P < 0.05$).[11] The second RCT (80 people with naturally acquired colds) also found that intranasal zinc significantly reduced the duration of cold symptoms compared with placebo (median duration of symptoms: 4.3 days with intranasal zinc *v* 6.0 days with placebo; P = 0.002).[12] The third RCT (160 people with naturally acquired colds of < 24 hours' duration) found no significant difference in overall symptom duration between intranasal zinc and placebo (mean duration 7 days for each group; P = 0.45).[13]

Harms: **Zinc lozenges:** The first review stated that, in some of the RCTs, a higher proportion of people had nausea, altered taste, dry mouth, abdominal pain, and headache with zinc lozenges than with placebo, but did not state whether the difference was significant.[9] The second review gave no information on adverse effects.[10] **Zinc intranasal gel:** The first RCT found that a similar proportion of people experienced a tingling or burning sensation with zinc intranasal gel compared with placebo (45/108 [42%] with zinc *v* 39/105 [37%] with placebo; CI not reported).[11] The second RCT found no significant difference between zinc intranasal gel and placebo in the proportion of people who had one or more adverse effect, although almost twice as many people taking zinc had one or more adverse effect (12/40 [30%] with intranasal gel *v* 5/38 [14%] with placebo; P = 0.10).[12] The third RCT found a similar proportion of people had adverse effects, including nausea, mouth or nasal irritation, abdominal pain, or headache with zinc intranasal gel compared with placebo (any adverse effect: 41/81 [51%] with zinc *v* 40/78 [52%] with placebo).[13]

Comment: None.

OPTION ECHINACEA

Systematic reviews found limited evidence that some preparations of echinacea may improve cold symptoms compared with placebo, but we found insufficient evidence about the effects of any specific product. Two subsequent RCTs, one in adults and one in children, found no significant difference between echinacea and placebo in severity or duration of cold symptoms.

Benefits: **Versus placebo:** We found two systematic reviews (search date 1998, 8 RCTs, 2109 people with naturally acquired colds;[14] search date 1999, 5 RCTs, including 3 RCTs identified by the first review [15]) and two subsequent RCTs[16,17] comparing a variety of echinacea preparations versus placebo (see comment below). Results were not combined because of trial heterogeneity. Five of the RCTs found that echinacea was significantly more effective than placebo in reducing duration of illness, runny nose, or overall symptom score. One RCT published only as an abstract found that echinacea significantly improved symptoms compared with placebo only in a predefined subgroup of people who had been treated in an early phase of the infection. Two RCTs found no significant difference in symptoms between echinacea and placebo, although in one of these RCTs baseline severity of illness was higher in people taking echinacea.[14] Quantitative results about effects on symptoms could be extracted for only two RCTs for duration of illness, three RCTs for runny nose, and five RCTs for a summary symptom score. The second review also found that RCTs were heterogeneous and of poor quality and it reached the same conclusions as the first review.[15] The first subsequent RCT (128 people aged 18–65 years with naturally acquired colds) found that people taking echinacea 10 times a day had similar total daily symptom scores over 7 days than people taking placebo (mean symptom score: 16.3 with echinacea *v* 19.9 with placebo; P value not reported).[16] The echinacea preparation contained various parts of the *Echinacea purpurea* plant. The second RCT (524 children aged 2–11 years who had 707 colds) found no significant difference between echinacea and placebo in severity of symptoms (measured by the sum of daily symptom scores, range 1–12: median 33 days in both groups; P = 0.69). It also found no significant difference in duration of symptoms between echinacea and placebo (median 9 days in both groups; P = 0.89).[17] The echinacea preparation contained dried press juice from the *Echinacea purpurea* herb.

Harms: Three of the RCTs reported adverse effects, usually gastrointestinal adverse effects, headache, or dizziness in people taking echinacea.[14,15] Adverse effects were generally infrequent and there were similar rates in people taking echinacea and placebo. The first subsequent RCT found that echinacea and placebo were associated with a similar incidence of gastrointestinal adverse effects (nausea, heartburn, and constipation: 13% with echinacea *v* 11% with placebo) and other adverse effects (itching, burning, and numbness: 13% with echinacea *v* 11% with placebo; P value not reported for any outcome).[16] The second subsequent RCT found that echinacea significantly increased the proportion of children who had rash compared with placebo (7% with echinacea *v* 3% with placebo; P = 0.008).[17] Outside the trials, anaphylaxis has been reported with echinacea.[18]

Comment: Echinacea is not a single product. There are more than 200 different preparations based on different plants, different parts of the plant (roots, herbs, whole plant), and different methods of extraction. The weakness of trial methods and differences in interventions make it difficult to draw conclusions about effectiveness. Large RCTs may be difficult because echinacea is not patentable and each producer controls a small share of the market. The authors of the systematic review received personal information about several unpublished studies that they were not able to include.

OPTION STEAM INHALATION

One systematic review provided insufficient evidence to assess steam inhalation in people with common cold.

Benefits: **Versus sham inhalation:** We found one systematic review (search date 2003, 6 RCTs, 319 people: 4 RCTs in people with naturally acquired colds, 2 in people with experimentally induced colds), comparing steam inhalation at 40–47 °C versus sham inhalation (air at ≥ 30 °C).[19] The review could not perform a meta-analysis of all of the RCTs because of heterogeneity in populations, methods used to assess symptoms, and poor reporting in some of the RCTs (see comment below). Pooling of data from two RCTs (146 people with naturally or experimentally induced acquired colds) that used similar methods of assessing symptoms found limited evidence that, compared with sham inhalation, steam inhalation significantly reduced the proportion of people with symptoms immediately after steam inhalation in one RCT and at 4 days in the other (29/77 [38%] with steam *v* 46/69 [68%] with sham; RR 0.56, 95% CI 0.40 to 0.79; see comment below). Another RCT (20 people with experimentally induced colds) identified by the review that used a different method of assessing symptoms found no significant difference between steam and sham inhalation in the proportion of people with improved symptoms at the end of treatment (no improvement in symptom score: 23/45 [51%] with steam *v* 26/39 [67%] with sham; RR 0.77, 95% CI 0.53 to 1.10), but may have been too small to exclude a clinically important difference.[19]

Harms: The RCTs identified by the review found no evidence of adverse effects.[19] There may be a danger from spilling hot water and from nosocomial infections related to humidifier units.

Comment: The review stated that the RCTs used different symptom score indexes but did not specify which indices were used.[19] It is unclear whether sham inhalation is a valid control.

OPTION DECONGESTANTS

One systematic review found that, compared with placebo, decongestants (norephedrine, oxymetazoline, or pseudoephedrine) reduced nasal congestion over 3–10 hours after a single dose in people with common cold, but found insufficient evidence to assess the effects of longer use of decongestants. The review identified no RCTs of other decongestants. One case control study found weak evidence that phenylpropanolamine may increase the risk of haemorrhagic stroke.

Benefits: **Versus placebo:** We found one systematic review (search date 1999, 4 RCTs, 246 adults with naturally acquired colds).[20] It found that, compared with placebo, a single dose of nasal decongestant (norephedrine, oxymetazoline, or pseudoephedrine) moderately but significantly reduced nasal congestion over 3–10 hours (3 RCTs, 155 adults; congestion measured on a scale from 0–1: WMD –0.13, 95% CI –0.19 to –0.06). It found no good evidence on the effects of repeated use over several days. The review identified no RCTs of other decongestants.

Harms: Information about harms was not sought actively or reported in the RCTs identified by the review.[20] The review identified no RCTs of phenylpropanolamine. One case control study compared the use of cold preparations containing phenylpropanolamine among 702 people with a history of haemorrhagic stroke versus 1376 control people with no history of stroke. The study found a non-significant trend towards increased haemorrhage stroke with phenylpropanolamine (RR 1.50, 95% CI 0.85 to 2.65).[21] However, the study was too small to make definitive conclusions.

Comment: The review found no RCTs in children.

OPTION ANTIHISTAMINES

One systematic review found that chlorpheniramine or doxylaminine reduced runny nose and sneezing after 2 days compared with placebo in people with common cold, but the clinical benefit was small. Another review, that assessed a wide variety of antihistamines, found no significant difference in overall cold symptoms at 1–10 days between antihistamines and placebo and found that first generation antihistamines increased adverse effects, including sedation.

Benefits: **Versus placebo:** We found two systematic reviews.[22,23] The first review (search date not reported, 9 RCTs, 1757 adults, 7 RCTs in adults with naturally acquired colds, 2 RCTs in adults with experimentally induced colds) included previously unpublished individual patient data comparing antihistamines versus placebo.[22] It found that antihistamines reduced the symptoms of runny nose and sneezing for the first 2 days of colds. The effects were small. On a severity scale ranging from 0 (no symptoms) to 3 or 4 (severe symptoms), antihistamines reduced the score by about 0.25 (95% CI 0.10 to 0.40; results presented graphically) for runny nose on days 1 and 2, 0.15 (95% CI 0 to 0.30) for sneezing on day 1, and 0.30 (95% CI 0.15 to 0.45) for sneezing on day 2. The second review (search date 2003, 32 RCTs, 8228 adults and children with naturally acquired colds, 702 with experimentally induced colds) compared antihistamines alone or antihistamines in combination with another treatment, usually decongestants, versus placebo (see comment below).[23] The review found no significant difference in overall symptoms at 1–10 days between antihistamines alone and placebo (proportion recovered at 1–2 days, 5 RCTs: 998/1825 [55%] with antihistamines alone *v* 892/1667 [54%] with placebo; RR 0.99, 95% CI 0.93 to 1.05; at 3–5 days, 3 RCTs: RR 1.03, 95% CI 0.92 to 1.16; at 8–10 days, 4 RCTs: RR 0.95, 95% CI 0.83 to 1.09).

Harms: Harms were not actively looked for in the RCTs identified by the first review.[22] The second review found that antihistamines were associated with sedation, dizziness, dry mouth, and headache.[23] It found that first generation antihistamines significantly increased the proportion of people who had one or more adverse effect, particularly sedation (9 RCTs: RR 1.20, 95% CI 1.03 to 1.40). It found no significant difference in the proportion of people who had one or more adverse effect between non-sedating antihistamines and placebo (3 RCTs: RR 1.10, 95% CI 0.55 to 2.18). Some non-sedating antihistamines are associated with arrhythmias and adverse interactions with other drugs.

Comment: The RCTs identified by the second review assessed a wide variety of antihistamines, including cetirizine, chlorpheniramine, clemastine, doxylamine succinate, loratidine, promethazine hydrochloride, and terfenidine.[23] Decongestants used in combination with antihistamines included phenypropanolamine and pseudoephedrine.

OPTION ANALGESICS OR ANTI-INFLAMMATORY DRUGS

We found no RCTs of analgesics or anti-inflammatory drugs in people with common cold.

Benefits: We found no systematic review or RCTs in people with common cold.

Harms: We found no RCTs.

Comment: None.

OPTION ANTIBIOTICS

Systematic reviews and one additional RCT found no significant difference between antibiotics and placebo in cure or general improvement at 6–14 days in people with colds. The additional RCT found that, in a subgroup of people (20%) with nasopharyngeal culture positive *H influenzae*, *M catarrhalis*, or *S pneumonia*, antibiotics increased recovery at 5 days compared with placebo. However, we have no methods currently of easily identifying such people at first consultation.

Benefits: **Versus placebo:** We found two systematic reviews[24,25] and one additional RCT.[26] The first review (search date 2001, 9 RCTs, 2249 people aged 2 months to 79 years with naturally acquired colds) found no significant difference between antibiotics and placebo in general improvement or cure at 7 days (6 RCTs: 168/664 [25%] with antibiotics *v* 170/483 [35%] with placebo; RR 0.89, 95% CI 0.77 to 1.04).[24] The second review (search date not reported, 12 RCTs including 4 RCTs identified by the first review and 8 RCTs excluded from the first review for methodological reasons, 1699 children with naturally acquired colds who had symptoms in the previous 2 weeks) found no significant difference between antibiotics and placebo in the proportion of children with worse or unchanged clinical outcome at 6–14 days (6 RCTs with adequate data: 309/835 [37%] with antibiotics *v* 280/647 [43%] with placebo; RR 1.01, 95% CI 0.90 to 1.13; figures reported from table in paper; see comment below), or with complications or progression (5 RCTs: 38/549 [6.9%] with antibiotics *v* 28/293 [9.5%] with placebo; RR 0.71, 95% CI 0.45 to 1.12).[25] The additional RCT (314 adults with naturally acquired colds for 1–30 days; < 7 days in 85% of people) comparing amoxicillin/clavulanic acid (co-amoxiclav) (375 mg 3 times daily) versus placebo found no overall difference in "cure" rates at 5 days (P value not reported).[26] However, a predefined subgroup analysis found that in the 61 people (20%) who were found to have positive nasopharyngeal cultures for *H influenzae*, *M catarrhalis*, or *S pneumoniae* there was a significant difference in recovery at 5 days (27% with co-amoxiclav *v* 4% with placebo; P = 0.001). If such people could be identified at first consultation, then treating four of these people with antibiotic rather than placebo would result in an average of one more recovery at 5 days (NNT 4, CI not reported). However, we have no methods currently of easily identifying these people at first consultation.

Harms: Adverse effects such as nausea, vomiting, headache, rash, or vaginitis were more common in people taking antibiotics than placebo.[24,25] For example, one review of antibiotics in people with bronchitis found one extra adverse effect for every 16 people treated.[27] We found no evidence of the size of the risk of antibiotic resistance or pseudomembranous colitis.

Comment: The relative risk (RR 1.01, 95% CI 0.90 to 1.13) surrounding clinical outcome reported by the second review does not match the absolute results reported; we have quoted it directly from the paper.[25] Because most common colds are viral, the potential benefit from antibiotics is limited. Until rapid identification of those people likely to benefit is possible, the modest effects seen in trials must be weighed against the adverse effects of antibiotics, costs, and potential for inducing antibiotic resistance.

REFERENCES

1. Lauber B. The common cold. *J Gen Intern Med* 1996;11:229–236.
2. Fry J, Sandler G. Common diseases. Their nature prevalence and care. Dordrecht, The Netherlands: Kluwer Academic, 1993.
3. Tupasi TE, de Leon LE, Lupisan S, et al. Patterns of acute respiratory tract infection in children: a longitudinal study in a depressed community in Metro Manila. *Rev Infect Dis* 1990;12:S940–S949.
4. Cruz JR, Pareja G, de Fernandez A, et al. Epidemiology of acute respiratory tract infections among Guatemalan ambulatory preschool children. *Rev Infect Dis* 1990;12:1029S–1034S.
5. Kvaerner KJ, Nafstad P, Jaakkola JJ. Upper respiratory morbidity in preschool children: a cross-sectional study. *Arch Otolaryngol Head Neck Surg* 2000;126:1201–1206.
6. Kleijnen J, Ter Riet G, Knipschild PG. Vitamin C and the common cold: review of a megadoses literature. *Ned Tijdschr Geneeskd* 1989;133:1532–1535. Search date 1998; primary sources Medline and hand searches of references. [In Dutch]
7. Hemila H. Vitamin C and the common cold. *Br J Nutr* 1992;67:3–16. Search date and primary sources not reported.
8. Douglas RM, Chalker EB, Treacy B. Vitamin C for preventing and treating the common cold. In: The Cochrane Library, Issue 2, 2004. Chichester, UK: John Wiley & Sons, Ltd. Search date not reported; primary sources reviews by Kleijnen, et al.[6] and Hemila.[7]
9. Marshall I. Zinc for the common cold. In: The Cochrane Library, Issue 2, 2004. Chichester, UK: John Wiley & Sons, Ltd. Search date 1997; primary sources Medline, Embase, the Cochrane Library, and hand searches of journals.
10. Jackson JL, Lesho E, Peterson C. Zinc and the common cold: a meta-analysis revisited. J Nutrition 2000;130(Suppl):1512S–1515S. Search date 1998; primary sources Medline, National Institute of Health database of funded studies, the Cochrane Randomised Clinical Trial database, and relevant papers.
11. Hirt M, Nobel S, Barron E. Zinc nasal gel for the treatment of common cold symptoms: a double-blind, placebo-controlled trial. *Ear Nose Throat J* 2000;79:778–782.
12. Mossad SB. Effect of zincum gluconicum nasal gel on the duration and symptom severity of the common cold in otherwise healthy adults. *QJM* 2003;96:35–43.
13. Belongia EA, Berg R, Liu K. A randomized trial of zinc nasal spray for the treatment of upper respiratory illness in adults. *Am J Med* 2001;111:103–108.
14. Melchart D, Linde K, Fischer P, et al. Echinacea for preventing and treating the common cold. In: The Cochrane Library, Issue 2, 2004. Chichester, UK: John Wiley & Sons, Ltd. Search date 1998; primary sources Medline, Embase, database of the Cochrane Acute Respiratory Infections Group, database of the Cochrane Field Complementary Medicine, Phytodok, bibliographies of existing reviews, and personal communications.
15. Giles JT, Palat CT III, Chien SH, et al. Evaluation of echinacea for treatment of the common cold. Pharmacotherapy 2000;20:690–697. Search date 1999; primary sources Medline, International Pharmaceutical Abstracts, Cambridge Scientific Abstracts Biological Sciences, Alt-Health Watch, Embase, and references from published articles.
16. Goel V, Lovlin R, Barton R, et al. Efficacy of a standardized echinacea preparation (Echinilin) for the treatment of the common cold: a randomized, double-blind, placebo-controlled trial. *J Clin Pharm Ther* 2004;29:75–83.
17. Taylor JA, Weber W, Standish L, et al. Efficacy and safety of echinacea in treating upper respiratory tract infections in children: a randomized controlled trial. *JAMA* 2003;290:2824–2830.
18. Mullins RJ. Echinacea associated anaphylaxis. *Med J Aust* 1998;168:170–171.
19. Singh M. Heated, humidified air for the common cold. In: The Cochrane Library, Issue 2, 2004. Chichester, UK: John Wiley & Sons, Ltd. Search date 2003, primary sources Cochrane Central Register of Controlled Trials (CENTRAL), The Cochrane Library, Medline, Embase, and Current Contents (past five

years) plus hand searches of review articles, and personal contact with manufacturers for any unpublished data.

20. Taverner D, Bickford L, Draper M. Nasal decongestants for the common cold. In: The Cochrane Library, Issue 2, 2004. Chichester, UK: John Wiley & Sons, Ltd. Search date 1999; primary sources Medline, Embase, Current Contents, Cochrane Acute Respiratory Infectious Group's trials register, hand searches of reference lists, and personal contacts with known investigators and pharmaceutical companies.
21. Kernan WN, Viscoli CM, Brass LM, et al. Phenylpropanolamine and the risk of hemorrhagic stroke. *N Engl J Med* 2000;343:1826–1832.
22. D'Agostino RB Sr, Weintraub M, Russell HK, et al. The effectiveness of antihistamines in reducing the severity of runny nose and sneezing: a meta-analysis. *Clin Pharmacol Ther* 1998;64:579–596. Search date not reported; primary sources Medline and FDA unpublished clinical trials.
23. De Sutter AIM, Lemiengre M, Campbell H, et al. Antihistamines for the common cold. In: The Cochrane Library, Issue 2, 2004. Chichester, UK: John Wiley & Sons, Ltd. Search date 2003; primary sources Cochrane Acute Respiratory Infections Group Specialized Register, Embase to December 2002; Cochrane Central Register of Controlled Trials (CENTRAL) and Medline to February, plus hand searches of references in identified papers, requests for further articles at a major international conference on Acute Respiratory Infections (1997), and personal contact with experts and pharmaceutical companies.
24. Arroll B, Kenealy T. Antibiotics for the common cold and acute purulent rhinitis. In: The Cochrane Library, Issue 2, 2004. Chichester, UK: John Wiley & Sons, Ltd. Search date 2001; primary sources Cochrane Controlled Trials Register, Medline, Embase, Family Medicine database, reference lists in articles, and principal investigators.
25. Fahey T, Stocks N, Thomas T. Systematic review of the treatment of upper respiratory tract infection. *Arch Dis Child* 1998;79:225–230. Search date not reported; primary sources Medline, Embase, Science Citation Index, Cochrane Controlled Trials Register, authors of published RCTs, drug manufacturers, and hand searches of references.
26. Kaiser L, Lew D, Hirschel B, et al. Effects of antibiotic treatment in the subset of common-cold patients who have bacteria in nasopharyngeal secretions. *Lancet* 1996;347:1507–1510.
27. Smucny J, Fahey T, Becker L, et al. Antibiotics for acute bronchitis. In: The Cochrane Library, Issue 2, 2004. Chichester, UK: John Wiley & Sons, Ltd. Search date 2000; primary sources Medline, Embase, Science Citation Index (1989–1996), and hand searches of reference lists of relevant trials, textbooks, and review articles.

Bruce Arroll
Associate Professor
Department of General Practice and Primary Health Care
University of Auckland
Auckland
New Zealand

Competing interests: None declared.

Community acquired pneumonia

Search date April 2004

Mark Loeb

QUESTIONS

INTERVENTIONS

Key Messages

Prevention

- **Influenza vaccine (in elderly people)** We found no RCTs that assessed the effects of influenza vaccine in preventing community acquired pneumonia. Observational studies suggest that influenza vaccine may reduce the incidence of pneumonia and may reduce mortality in the elderly.

- **Pneumococcal vaccine (for all cause pneumonia and mortality in immunocompetent adults)** One systematic review found no significant difference in pneumonia rates or all cause mortality between pneumococcal vaccination and no pneumococcal vaccination in immunocompetent adults. The review found some evidence that pneumococcal vaccine may reduce definitive pneumococcal infection compared with no vaccination in immunocompetent adults.

Treatments (outpatients)

- **Antibiotics (amoxicillin, cephalosporins, macrolides, penicillin, quinolones) in outpatient settings** One systematic review that evaluated different oral antibiotics in outpatient settings has found clinical cure or improvement in over 90% of people regardless of antibiotic taken. Another systematic review found limited evidence that azithromycin reduced clinical failures over 6–21 days compared with other macrolides, cephalosporins, or penicillin. A third systematic review and a subsequent RCT found no significant difference in clinical cure or improvement between quinolones and amoxicillin, cephalosporins, or macrolides. One RCT found no significant difference between oral telithromycin and oral clarithromycin in clinical cure rates. Most trials were designed to show equivalence between treatments rather than superiority of one antibiotic over another.

Treatments (hospital)

- **Antibiotics (amoxicillin, cephalosporins, macrolides, penicillin, quinolones) in hospital** RCTs that compared different oral or intravenous antibiotics in people admitted to hospital found clinical cure or improvement in 73–96% of people. Four RCTs found no significant difference in clinical cure or improvement among different antibiotics. Two RCTs found that quinolones may increase clinical cure compared with co-amoxiclav (amoxicillin plus clavulanic acid) or cephalosporins. However, most trials were small and were designed to show equivalence between treatments rather than superiority of one antibiotic over another.
- **Early mobilisation** One RCT in people receiving antibiotics and usual medical care found that early mobilisation plus bottle blowing physiotherapy plus encouragement to sit up regularly and take deep breaths reduced mean hospital stay compared with early mobilisation alone. It found no significant difference in duration of fever. One RCT found that early mobilisation reduced hospital stay compared with usual care.
- **Intravenous antibiotics in immunocompetent people in hospital without life threatening illness (compared with oral antibiotics)** One systematic review found no significant difference for clinical cure rates or mortality between oral and intravenous antibiotics in people hospitalised with non-severe community acquired pneumonia. One RCT found that inpatient regimens consisting of staged intravenous and oral antibiotic therapy reduced hospital stay compared with regimens consisting of intravenous antibiotics alone.

Treatments (intensive care)

- **Prompt administration of antibiotics in people admitted to intensive care with community acquired pneumonia (improved outcomes compared with delayed antibiotic treatment)** We found no systematic review and no RCTs comparing prompt versus delayed antibiotic treatment. Two retrospective studies found that prompt administration of antibiotics improved survival. It would probably be unethical to perform an RCT of delayed antibiotic treatment.
- **Different combinations of antibiotics in intensive care settings** We found no RCTs that compared one combination of antibiotics versus another in intensive care units.

Guidelines

- **Guidelines for treating pneumonia (for clinical outcomes)** One systematic review found no significant difference in clinical outcomes between usual care and a guideline based management strategy that incorporated early switch from intravenous to oral antibiotics and early discharge (or both). One subsequent RCT found no significant difference in clinical outcomes between a guideline plus a multifaceted implementation strategy and the issued guideline alone.

Community acquired pneumonia

DEFINITION Community acquired pneumonia is pneumonia contracted in the community rather than in hospital. It is defined by clinical symptoms (such as cough, sputum production, and pleuritic chest pain) and signs (such as fever, tachypnoea, and rales), with radiological confirmation.

INCIDENCE/ PREVALENCE In the northern hemisphere, community acquired pneumonia affects about 12/1000 people a year, particularly during winter and at the extremes of age (incidence: < 1 year old 30–50/1000 per year; 15–45 years 1–5/1000 per year; 60–70 years 10–20/1000 per year; 71–85 years 50/1000 per year).[1–6]

AETIOLOGY/ RISK FACTORS More than 100 microorganisms have been implicated in community acquired pneumonia, but most cases are caused by *Streptococcus pneumoniae* (see table 1, p 1875).[4–7] Smoking is probably an important risk factor.[8] One large cohort study conducted in Finland (4175 people aged ≥ 60 years) suggested that risk factors for pneumonia in the elderly included alcoholism (RR 9.0, 95% CI 5.1 to 16.2), bronchial asthma (RR 4.2, 95% CI 3.3 to 5.4), immunosuppression (RR 3.1, 95% CI 1.9 to 5.1), lung disease (RR 3.0, 95% CI 2.3 to 3.9), heart disease (RR 1.9, 95% CI 1.7 to 2.3), institutionalisation (RR 1.8, 95% CI 1.4 to 2.4), and increasing age (≥ 70 years *v* 60–69 years; RR 1.5, 95% CI 1.3 to 1.7).[9]

PROGNOSIS Severity varies from mild to life threatening illness within days of the onset of symptoms. One systematic review of prognosis studies for community acquired pneumonia (search date 1995, 33 148 people) found overall mortality to be 13.7%, ranging from 5.1% for ambulant people to 36.5% for people who required intensive care.[10] The following prognostic factors were significantly associated with mortality: male sex (OR 1.3, 95% CI 1.2 to 1.4); pleuritic chest pain (OR 0.5, 95% CI 0.3 to 0.8, i.e. lower mortality); hypothermia (OR 5.0, 95% CI 2.4 to 10.4); systolic hypotension (OR 4.8, 95% CI 2.8 to 8.3); tachypnoea (OR 2.9, 95% CI 1.7 to 4.9); diabetes mellitus (OR 1.3, 95% CI 1.1 to 1.5); neoplastic disease (OR 2.8, 95% CI 2.4 to 3.1); neurological disease (OR 4.6, 95% CI 2.3 to 8.9); bacteraemia (OR 2.8, 95% CI 2.3 to 3.6); leucopenia (OR 2.5, 95% CI 1.6 to 3.7); and multilobar radiographic pulmonary infiltrates (OR 3.1, 95% CI 1.9 to 5.1).

AIMS OF INTERVENTION **Prevention:** To prevent onset of pneumonia. **Treatment:** To cure infection clinically, to reduce mortality, to alleviate symptoms, to enable return to normal activities, and to prevent recurrence, while minimising adverse effects of treatments.

OUTCOMES **Prevention:** Incidence of pneumonia, adverse effects of vaccination. **Treatment:** Clinical cure, variably defined but usually defined as return to premorbid health status or complete absence of symptoms such as fever, chills, cough, dyspnoea, or sputum production; improvement (relief of symptoms); admission to hospital; complications (empyema, endocarditis, lung abscess); death; adverse effects of antibiotics.

METHODS *Clinical Evidence* search and appraisal April 2004.

QUESTION What are the effects of preventive interventions?

OPTION INFLUENZA VACCINE

We found no RCTs that assessed the effects of influenza vaccine in preventing community acquired pneumonia. Observational studies suggest that influenza vaccine may reduce the incidence of pneumonia and may reduce mortality in the elderly.

Benefits: We found no systematic review or RCTs (see comment below).

Harms: We found no RCTs (see comment below).

Comment: We found one systematic review of cohort studies (search date not reported, 20 studies) that compared influenza vaccine versus no vaccine.[11] It found that influenza vaccine significantly reduced the incidence of pneumonia and significantly reduced mortality (incidence: 24 774 people; ARR 53%, 95% CI 35% to 66%; mortality: 29 928 people; ARR 68%, 95% CI 56% to 76%). Timescales were not reported for any outcomes. Analysis of an administrative database (≥ 25 000 people aged ≥ 64 years) suggested that influenza vaccination reduced the rate of admission to hospital in people with pneumonia or influenza by 48–57% ($P < 0.01$).[12] We found one systematic review (search date 2000,[13] 1 RCT[14]) and two additional RCTs (3 publications) that assessed the effects of influenza vaccine in preventing influenza and reducing mortality.[15–17] **Effects in vaccinated people:** The RCT (> 1800 people aged ≥ 60 years) identified by the review[13] compared split virion vaccine versus saline solution.[14] It found that vaccine significantly reduced the incidence of clinical influenza at 5 months compared with placebo (AR 17/927 [1.8%] with vaccine *v* 31/911 [3.4%] with placebo; RR 0.53, 95% CI 0.39 to 0.73). The first additional RCT (523 elderly residents of nursing homes) compared parenteral trivalent inactivated vaccine plus intranasal live attenuated cold adapted vaccine versus parenteral trivalent inactivated vaccine alone.[15] It found that inactivated vaccine plus live attenuated vaccine significantly reduced the incidence of influenza A compared with inactivated vaccine alone (9/162 [5.5%] with inactivated vaccine plus live attenuated vaccine *v* 24/169 [14.2%] with inactivated vaccine alone; RR 0.39, 95% CI 0.18 to 0.81; NNT 12, 95% CI 9 to 38). A reduction in rates of influenza does not necessarily imply a reduction in rates of pneumonia. However, in people with influenza, death is usually caused by pneumonia. Therefore, interventions that reduce influenza mortality exert their effects by reducing pneumonia rates. The second additional RCT (2 publications) found that adverse effects included pain and tenderness at the site of injection.[16,17] Influenza-vaccination programs for the seasons of 1992-1993 and 1993-1994 were associated with 1 to 2 additional cases of the Guillain-Barré syndrome per 1 million vaccinated persons.[18]

OPTION PNEUMOCOCCAL VACCINE

One systematic review found no significant difference in pneumonia rates or all cause mortality between pneumococcal vaccination and no pneumococcal vaccination in immunocompetent adults. The review found some evidence that pneumococcal vaccine may reduce definitive pneumococcal infection compared with no vaccination in immunocompetent adults.

Benefits: We found one systematic review (search date 2003, 14 RCTs, > 75 000 adults aged ≥ 16 years), which compared pneumococcal vaccination versus no vaccination.[19] Studies were conducted in a variety of countries between 1937 and 1995. The review excluded studies of people who were HIV positive. It found no significant difference between vaccination and no vaccination for all cause pneumonia or all cause mortality, but significant heterogeneity was found for both meta-analyses (see comment below; all cause pneumonia: 14 RCTs; OR 0.77, 95% CI 0.58 to 1.02; all cause mortality: 11 RCTs; OR 0.90, 95% CI 0.76 to 1.07). It found that pneumococcal vaccine significantly reduced definitive pneumococcal pneumonia compared with no vaccination, but significant heterogeneity was found and results were sensitive to the removal of one older poorer quality RCT (see comment below; 8 RCTs: 0.13% with vaccination *v* 0.54% with no vaccination; OR 0.28, 95% CI 0.15 to 0.52).

Harms: The systematic review found few RCTs that gave information on adverse effects.[19] One RCT in the review found that pneumococcal vaccination was associated with erythema and induration compared with no vaccination. Another RCT in the review found that pneumococcal vaccination increased sore arm, swollen arm, and fever compared with no vaccination.

Comment: Several of the RCTs included in the systematic review reported incomplete data and clarification of data was not possible due to the age of some RCTs.[19] In the review the heterogeneity for all cause mortality and definitive pneumococcal pneumonia appeared to be partly explained by inclusion of one older poorer quality RCT. After omitting this RCT, the review found no significant difference between treatments for all cause mortality or definitive pneumococcal pneumonia (all cause mortality: 10 RCTs; OR 0.95, 95% CI 0.90 to 1.01; definitive pneumococcal pneumonia: 13 RCTs; 2.8% with vaccination *v* 3.9% with no vaccination; OR 0.84, 95% CI 0.65 to 1.08). The systematic review also examined non-randomised studies. Pooling of five case–control studies found that vaccination significantly reduced invasive pneumococcal disease (OR 0.47, 95% CI 0.37 to 0.59). The fact that older studies examined vaccines with different valencies also may explain some of the heterogeneity. The more recent studies in the review were consistent in providing no evidence of efficacy of the vaccine against pneumonia.

QUESTION What are the effects of interventions in outpatient settings?

OPTION ANTIBIOTICS

One systematic review that evaluated different oral antibiotics in outpatient settings has found clinical cure or improvement in over 90% of people regardless of antibiotic taken. Another systematic review found limited evidence that azithromycin reduced clinical failures over 6–21 days compared with other macrolides, cephalosporins, or penicillin. A third systematic review and a subsequent RCT found no significant difference in clinical cure or improvement between quinolones and amoxicillin, cephalosporins, or macrolides. One RCT found no significant difference between oral telithromycin and oral clarithromycin in clinical cure rates. Most trials were designed to show equivalence between treatments rather than superiority of one antibiotic over another.

Benefits: We found three systematic reviews[20–22] and two subsequent RCTs.[23,24] The first systematic review (search date not reported, 9 RCTs, 1164 people) compared different oral antibiotics in outpatient settings.[20] The antibiotics evaluated were amoxicillin (amoxycillin) with and without clavulanate, macrolides, cephalosporins, and quinolones. The review did not perform a meta-analysis that directly compared antibiotics. Clinical cure or improvement was reported in more than 90% of people regardless of antibiotic taken (no further data reported). **Azithromycin versus other macrolides, cephalosporins, or penicillins:** The second systematic review (search date 2000, 18 RCTs, 2 of which were included in the first review, 1664 people) found that, compared with other macrolides (clarithromycin, erythromycin, or roxithromycin; 13 RCTs), cephalosporins (cefaclor, 2 RCTs), or penicillins (co-amoxiclav [amoxicillin plus clavulanic acid] or penicillin; 3 RCTs), azithromycin significantly reduced clinical failures over 6–21 days (56/928 [6%] with azithromycin *v* 72/736 [10%] with other oral antibiotics; OR 0.63, 95% CI 0.42 to 0.95).[21] These results should be interpreted with caution because most of the RCTs were not blinded. **Quinolones versus amoxicillin, macrolides, or cephalosporins:** The third systematic review (search date 1999, 8 RCTs, none of which were included in the first or second review, 3131 people) found no significant difference in clinical success (cure or improvement) between quinolones (gatifloxacin, levofloxacin, moxifloxacin, sparfloxacin, and trovafloxacin) and high dose amoxicillin, cefaclor, cefpodoxime, ceftriaxone, ceftriaxone plus clarithromycin, cefuroxime axetil, clarithromycin, co-amoxiclav, erythromycin, or roxithromycin (ARR +1.7%, 95% CI –1.4% to +4.8%;

no further data reported).[22] One subsequent RCT (299 people) compared oral clarithromycin 1000 mg daily versus oral levofloxacin 500 mg daily.[23] It found no significant difference in clinical cure rates at 7 days between oral clarithromycin and levofloxacin (113/128 [88%] with clarithromycin *v* 107/124 [86%] with levofloxacin; RR 1.02, 95% CI 0.93 to 1.12). **Ketolides versus macrolides:** The second subsequent RCT (493 adults, 318 adults in per protocol analysis) compared a 10 day course of oral telithromycin 800 mg daily versus a 10 day course of oral clarithromycin 500 mg daily.[24] It found no significant difference in rates of clinical cure after 17 days of follow up (cure defined as return to pre-infection state or improvement without additional antibiotics: 143/162 [88%] with telithromycin *v* 138/156 [89%] with clarithromycin; RR 1.0, 95% CI 0.92 to 1.08).

Harms: The first and third reviews gave no information on adverse effects.[20,22] The second review found that azithromycin significantly reduced withdrawals because of adverse effects compared with co-amoxiclav (no further data reported).[21] It also found limited evidence from indirect comparisons that withdrawals because of adverse effects were lower with azithromycin than with clarithromycin, erythromycin, or cefaclor. The first subsequent RCT found no significant difference in the proportion of people who had adverse effects (primarily diarrhoea, nausea, and headache) with clarithromycin compared with levofloxacin (26% with clarithromycin *v* 20% with levofloxacin; reported as non-significant; CI not reported), although clarithromycin significantly increased taste disturbance (20/156 [13%] with clarithromycin *v* 1/143 [0.7%] with levofloxacin; $P < 0.001$).[23] The second subsequent RCT found that telithromycin increased adverse effects compared with clarithromycin, but the statistical significance of this finding was not reported (57% with telithromycin *v* 49% with clarithromycin).[24] The most common adverse effects were gastrointestinal (68% with telithromycin *v* 48% with clarithromycin). Antibiotics can cause allergic reactions (including anaphylaxis), rash, gastrointestinal intolerance (nausea, vomiting, and diarrhoea), vaginal or oral candidiasis, and *Clostridium difficile* diarrhoea (including pseudomembranous colitis). The frequency of adverse effects varies with the antibiotic used.

Comment: Most trials were designed to show equivalence between treatments rather than superiority of one antibiotic over another.

QUESTION What are the effects of treatments in people admitted to hospital?

OPTION ANTIBIOTICS

RCTs that compared different oral or intravenous antibiotics in people admitted to hospital found clinical cure or improvement in 73–96% of people. Four RCTs found no significant difference in clinical cure or improvement among different antibiotics. Two RCTs found that quinolones may increase clinical cure compared with co-amoxiclav (amoxicillin plus clavulanic acid) or cephalosporins. However, most trials were small and were designed to show equivalence between treatments rather than superiority of one antibiotic over another.

Benefits: **Cephalosporins versus penicillin:** We found no systematic review. We found several RCTs that were too small, too old, or both, to be reliable given the changing sensitivity of organisms to antibiotics. One RCT (378 people) compared intravenous co-amoxiclav (amoxicillin plus clavulanic acid) followed by oral co-amoxiclav versus intravenous ceftriaxone followed by intramuscular ceftriaxone.[25] People in both groups also received intravenous erythromycin as decided by their physician (17/184 [9%] people taking co-amoxiclav and 25/194 [13%] people taking ceftriaxone). It found no significant difference in clinical cure at long term follow up, which was not specified (136/184 [73.9%] with co-amoxiclav *v* 144/194 [74.2%] with ceftriaxone; RR 0.99, 95% CI 0.88 to 1.12). **Quinolones versus high dose amoxicillin:** We found no systematic review. We found two multicentre double blind RCTs.[26,27] The first RCT (329 people in hospital in France, South Africa, or Switzerland) compared sparfloxacin 400 mg on day 1 followed by 200 mg once daily versus amoxicillin 1000 mg three times daily.[26] It found no significant difference in clinical cure at 14–21 days (133/159 [84%] with sparfloxacin *v* 144/170 [85%] with amoxicillin; RR 0.99, 95% CI 0.87 to 1.07). It found that fewer people treated with sparfloxacin discontinued the drug at days 3, 4, or 5 because of a lack of response compared with ampicillin, but the difference did not reach significance (3/126 [2%] with sparfloxacin *v* 11/140 [8%] with amoxicillin; RR 0.30, 95% CI 0.08 to 1.05). The second RCT (411 people with suspected pneumococcal pneumonia, 285 of whom were admitted to hospital) compared oral moxifloxacin 400 mg once daily versus oral amoxicillin 1000 mg three times daily.[27] It found no significant difference in clinical cure or improvement at 3–4 weeks after the end of 5–7 days' treatment (154/200 [77.0%] with moxifloxacin *v* 164/208 [78.8%] with amoxicillin; RR 0.97, 95% CI 0.86 to 1.07). **Quinolones versus amoxicillin plus clavulanic acid (co-amoxiclav):** We found no systematic review. We found one multicentre RCT (628 people) that compared moxifloxacin 400 mg once daily (iv followed by oral) versus amoxicillin plus clavulanic acid (co-amoxiclav) 1.2 g intravenously followed by 625 mg orally three times daily with or without clarithromycin for 7–14 days.[28] It found that moxifloxacin significantly increased the clinical cure rate at 5–7 days after treatment compared with co-amoxiclav (225/241 [93%] with moxifloxacin *v* 204/239 [85%] with co-amoxiclav; P = 0.004).[28] **Quinolones versus cephalosporins:** We found no systematic review. We found one unblinded RCT (590 people, 280 of whom had been admitted to hospital) that compared oral or intravenous levofloxacin, or both, versus intravenous ceftriaxone or oral cefuroxime axetil, or both.[29] It found that levofloxacin significantly increased the proportion of people clinically cured or improved at 5–7 days compared with cephalosporins (96% with levofloxacin *v* 90% with cephalosporins; reported as significant; CI not reported). **Quinolones versus macrolides plus cephalosporins:** We found no systematic review. We found one multicentre open label RCT (236 people) that compared levofloxacin 500 mg daily (orally or iv) versus intravenous azithromycin 500 mg plus intravenous ceftriaxone 1 g for 2 days followed by an optional transition to oral azithromycin 500 mg.[30] It found no significant difference in clinical cure between groups (100/115 [87%] with levofloxacin *v* 97/121 [80%] with azithromycin plus ceftriaxone; RR 1.08, 95% CI 0.97 to 1.21).

Harms: Also see harms of option on treatments (outpatients), p 1864. **Cephalosporins versus penicillin:** The RCT gave no information on adverse effects.[25] **Quinolones versus high dose amoxicillin:** The first RCT found that fewer people had gastrointestinal disturbances with sparfloxacin compared with amoxicillin (19 with amoxicillin *v* 10 with sparfloxacin; CI not reported).[26] Four people (2.5%) taking sparfloxacin withdrew because of adverse effects compared with two people (1.2%) taking amoxicillin (P value not reported). The second RCT found no significant difference in gastrointestinal adverse effects with moxifloxacin compared with amoxicillin (56/200 [28%] with moxifloxacin *v* 42/208 [20%] with amoxicillin; RR 1.39, 95% CI 0.98 to 1.97).[27] **Quinolones versus amoxicillin plus clavulanic acid (co-amoxiclav):** The RCT found similar rates of overall adverse effects (primarily nausea and diarrhoea) between moxifloxacin and co-amoxiclav (39% in both groups; CI not reported).[28] **Quinolones versus cephalosporins:** The RCT found that a similar proportion of people had gastrointestinal adverse effects (primarily nausea and diarrhoea) with levofloxacin compared with cephalosporins (5.8% levofloxacin *v* 8.5% with cephalosporins; absolute numbers and CI not reported).[29] **Quinolones versus macrolides plus cephalosporins:** The RCT found no significant difference in overall adverse event rates (primarily gastrointestinal adverse effects) between levofloxacin and azithromycin plus ceftriaxone (6/113 [5%] with levofloxacin *v* 11/118 [9%] with azithromycin; RR 0.57, 95% CI 0.22 to 1.49).[30]

Comment: Most trials were small and were designed to show equivalence between treatments rather than superiority of one antibiotic over another. Although detection of penicillin resistant and multidrug resistant *S pneumoniae* is commonly reported, it is difficult to enrol people with this infection in randomised studies. One study was carried out in areas with high prevalence of penicillin resistant *S pneumoniae*.[26] It found that 8/135 (6.9%) isolates tested were resistant to penicillin, but none showed high level resistance as measured by the minimum inhibitory concentration of penicillin (where pneumococcal strains with minimum inhibitory concentration ≥ 2 μg are termed highly resistant).[31] The trials in uncomplicated pneumonia may not apply to people with comorbidities such as meningitis.[31] There are also concerns about macrolide resistant *S pneumoniae*, but, so far, treatment failure in ambulatory people with community acquired pneumonia is uncommon.[32] In the RCT that compared levofloxacin versus cephalosporins the route of administration was decided by the doctor, and it is unclear whether all participants who received intravenous antibiotics were admitted to hospital.[29] We found one retrospective review (12 945 people ≥ 65 years old in hospital with community acquired pneumonia).[33] It found that initial treatment with a second generation cephalosporin (cefuroxime) plus a macrolide (azithromycin, clarithromycin, or erythromycin), a non-pseudomonal third generation cephalosporin (ceftriaxone, cefotaxime, ceftizoxime) plus a macrolide, or a fluoroquinolone (ciprofloxacin, ofloxacin) reduced mortality at 30 days compared with initial treatment with a β-lactam/β-lactamase inhibitor (ampicillin plus sulbactam, ticarcillin plus clavulanic acid, piperacillin plus tazobactam) plus a macrolide, or an aminoglycoside plus another antimicrobial agent.[33] One retrospective cohort study found that people infected with penicillin resistant compared with non-penicillin resistant *S pneumoniae* were at greater risk of death in hospital (RR 2.1, 95% CI 1.0 to 4.3) and suppurative complications (RR 4.5, 95% CI 1.0 to 19.3).[34] From national surveillance data, penicillin resistant pneumonia was associated with significantly higher mortality after the first 4 days in hospital than non-penicillin resistant pneumonia.[35] These results should be interpreted with caution, however, because they may not account for confounding factors.

OPTION INTRAVENOUS ANTIBIOTICS

One systematic review found no significant difference for clinical cure rates or mortality between oral and intravenous antibiotics in people hospitalised with non-severe community acquired pneumonia. One RCT found that inpatient regimens consisting of staged intravenous and oral antibiotic therapy reduced hospital stay compared with regimens consisting of intravenous antibiotics alone.

Benefits: We found one systematic review (search date 2003, 7 RCTs, 1366 people)[36] that compared oral versus intravenous antibiotics in people admitted to hospital with non life-threatening community acquired pneumonia, and one RCT that assessed different durations of treatment with intravenous antibiotics.[37] The systematic review found no significant difference between oral and intravenous antibiotics in clinical success or mortality (clinical success: 261/290 [90%] with oral *v* 220/255 [86%] iv; RR 1.07, 95% CI 0.98 to 1.16; mortality: 8/292 [3%] with oral *v* 14/299 [5%] with iv; RR 0.61, 95% CI 0.26 to 1.4).[36] The RCT (73 people, no intention to treat analysis) that assessed different durations of treatment with intravenous antibiotics compared 2 days of intravenous cefuroxime followed by 8 days of oral cefuroxime (group 1); 5 days of oral cefuroxime followed by 5 days of intravenous cefuroxime (group 2); and 10 days of intravenous cefuroxime (group 3).[37] People were excluded if they had empyema, septic shock, or respiratory failure. It found no significant difference among groups in the proportion of people with clinical cure after 28 days (18/20 [90%] in group 1 *v* 17/20 [85%] in group 2 *v* 16/17 [94%] in group 3; reported as non-significant, no further data reported). However, it found that people in group 1 had a significantly shorter hospital stay compared with people in either of the other groups (6 days with group 1 *v* 8 days with group 2 *v* 11 days with group 3; reported as significant; CI not reported).[37]

Harms: The systematic review and RCT gave no information on adverse effects.[36,37]

Comment: Intravenous antibiotics are used in people who cannot take oral medication because of severe nausea or vomiting. A follow up study (96 people admitted to hospital with community acquired pneumonia) found clinical cure of pneumonia at 30 days in people who were switched from intravenous to oral antibiotics when they had been afebrile for 8 hours, symptoms of cough and shortness of breath were improving, white blood cell counts were returning to normal, and they could tolerate oral medication.[38]

OPTION EARLY MOBILISATION

One RCT in people receiving antibiotics and usual medical care found that early mobilisation plus bottle blowing physiotherapy plus encouragement to sit up regularly and take deep breaths reduced mean hospital stay compared with early mobilisation alone. It found no significant difference in duration of fever. One RCT found that early mobilisation reduced hospital stay compared with usual care.

Benefits: We found no systematic review. We found two RCTs.[39,40] The first RCT (145 people in hospital with community acquired pneumonia) compared three interventions: early mobilisation alone, early mobilisation plus encouragement to sit up 10 times a day and take 20 deep breaths, and early mobilisation plus encouragement to sit up 10 times a day and blow bubbles through a plastic tube for 20 breaths into a bottle containing 10 cm of water (bottle blowing).[39] Participants concurrently received benzylpenicillin or phenoxymethylpenicillin and usual medical care independently of the study interventions. The RCT found that bottle blowing plus early mobilisation plus encouragement significantly reduced mean hospital stay compared with early mobilisation alone (3.9 days with bottle blowing plus early mobilisation plus encouragement *v* 5.3 days with early mobilisation alone; P = 0.01). It found no significant difference among groups in duration of fever (2.3 days with early mobilisation alone *v* 1.7 days with encouragement to take deep breaths *v* 1.6 days with bottle blowing; P = 0.28 for all groups *v* each other). The second RCT (459 people) compared early mobilisation alone versus usual care.[40] It found that early mobilisation reduced mean duration of hospital stay compared with usual care (5.8 days with early mobilisation *v* 6.9 days with usual care; absolute difference 1.1 days, 95% CI 0.0 to 2.2 days).

Harms: The RCTs gave no information on adverse effects.[39,40]

Comment: None.

QUESTION **What are the effects of treatments in people with community acquired pneumonia receiving intensive care?**

OPTION **DIFFERENT COMBINATIONS OF ANTIBIOTICS**

We found no RCTs that compared one combination of antibiotics versus another in intensive care units.

Benefits: We found no systematic review and no RCTs that compared one combination of antibiotics versus another in intensive care units (see comment below).

Harms: We found no RCTs.

Comment: Use of a combination of antibiotics is regarded as current best practice for ventilator related pneumonia. Choice of antibiotics varies, depending on local guidelines.

OPTION **PROMPT VERSUS DELAYED ANTIBIOTIC TREATMENT**

We found no systematic review and no RCTs comparing prompt versus delayed antibiotic treatment. Two retrospective studies found that prompt administration of antibiotics improved survival. It would probably be unethical to perform an RCT of delayed antibiotic treatment.

Benefits: We found no systematic review and no RCTs (see comment below). One multicentre retrospective review (medical records of ≥ 14 000 people aged ≥ 65 years admitted to acute [emergency] care hospitals in the USA who were severely ill with community acquired pneumonia) found that antibiotics given within 8 hours of admission to hospital were associated with lower 30 day mortality (OR 0.85, 95% CI 0.75 to 0.96).[41] The review did not specify whether oral or intravenous antibiotics were given. Another retrospective study (39 people with serologically confirmed Legionnaires' disease and clinically diagnosed community acquired pneumonia) examined outcome and time to start of treatment.[42] For the 10 people who died, the median delay between diagnosis of pneumonia and start of intravenous erythromycin was 5 days (range 1–10 days), and for those who survived it was 1 day (range 1–5 days; $P < 0.001$).

Harms: The retrospective studies gave no information on harms.[41,42]

Comment: It would probably be regarded as unethical to perform an RCT of delayed antibiotic treatment.

QUESTION **What are the effects of guidelines on the treatment of community acquired pneumonia?**

OPTION **GUIDELINES**

One systematic review found no significant difference in clinical outcomes between usual care and a guideline based management strategy that incorporated early switch from intravenous to oral antibiotics and early discharge (or both). One subsequent RCT found no significant difference in clinical outcomes between a guideline plus a multifaceted implementation strategy and the issued guideline alone.

Benefits: We found one systematic review (search date 2000, 3 RCTs, 7 cohort studies).[43] The systematic review compared a guideline incorporating early switch from intravenous to oral antibiotics or early discharge, or both, versus usual care. It found no significant difference between treatments in therapeutic success (not defined), readmission to hospital, admission to intensive care unit, complications, mortality, or any adverse outcome (no further data reported). It also found no significant difference between guideline and usual care in mean length of hospital stay (mean 6.0 days with guideline *v* 7.6 days with usual care; $P = 0.05$). We found one subsequent RCT (608 people), which compared a practice guideline implemented with a multifaceted intervention versus a practice guideline alone.[44] It found no significant difference in the time to discontinuation of intravenous antibiotic therapy or in duration of hospital stay (time to stopping intravenous antibiotics: HR 1.23, 95% CI 1.00 to 1.52; $P = 0.11$; length of hospital stay: HR 1.16, 95% CI 0.97 to 1.38; $P = 0.11$).

Harms: The review found no significant difference in "any adverse outcome" (not specified) between guideline and usual care (no further data reported).[43]

Comment: None.

Substantive changes

Pneumococcal vaccine One systematic review added;[19] categorisation changed to Unlikely to be beneficial.
Antibiotics (outpatients) One RCT added;[24] categorisation unchanged.
Intravenous antibiotics (compared with oral antibiotics) One systematic review added;[36] categorisation unchanged.
Early mobilisation One RCT added;[40] categorisation changed to Likely to be beneficial.
Guidelines One RCT added;[44] categorisation unchanged.

REFERENCES

1. Foy HM, Cooney MK, Allan I, et al. Rates of pneumonia during influenza epidemics in Seattle, 1964–1975. *JAMA* 1979;241:253–258.
2. Murphy TF, Henderson FW, Clyde WA, et al. Pneumonia: an 11 year study in a pediatric practice. *Am J Epidemiol* 1981;113:12–21.
3. McConnochie KM, Hall CB, Barker WH. Lower respiratory tract illness in the first two years of life: epidemiologic patterns and costs in a suburban pediatric practice. *Am J Public Health* 1988;78:34–39.
4. Porath A, Schlaeffer F, Lieberman D. The epidemiology of community-acquired pneumonia among hospitalized adults. *J Infect* 1997;34:41–48.
5. Jokinen C, Heiskanen L, Juvonen H, et al. Incidence of community-acquired pneumonia in the population of four municipalities in eastern Finland. *Am J Epidemiol* 1993;137:977–988.
6. Houston MS, Silverstein MD, Suman VJ. Risk factors for 30-day mortality in elderly patients with lower respiratory tract infection. *Arch Intern Med* 1997;157:2190–2195.
7. Bartlett JG, Mundy LM. Community-acquired pneumonia. *N Engl J Med* 1995;333:1618–1624.
8. Almirall J, Gonzalez CA, Balanco X, et al. Proportion of community-acquired pneumonia attributable to tobacco smoking. *Chest* 1999;116:375–379.
9. Koivula I, Sten M, Makela PH. Risk factors for pneumonia in the elderly. *Am J Med* 1994;96:313–320.
10. Fine MJ, Smith MA, Carson CA, et al. Prognosis and outcomes of patients with community-acquired pneumonia: a meta-analysis. *JAMA* 1995;274:134–141. Search date 1995; primary sources Medline and hand searches of reference lists.
11. Gross PA, Hermogenes AW, Sacks HS, et al. The efficacy of influenza vaccine in elderly persons: a

meta-analysis and review of the literature. *Ann Intern Med* 1995;123:518–527. Search date not reported; primary source Medline.
12. Nichol KL, Margolis KL, Wuorenma J, et al. The efficacy and cost effectiveness of vaccination against influenza among elderly persons living in the community. *N Engl J Med* 1994;331:778–784.
13. Vu T, Farish S, Jenkins M, et al. A meta-analysis of influenza vaccine in persons aged 65 years and over living in the community. *Vaccine* 2002;20:1831–1836. Search date 2000; primary sources Medline, Biosis, Firstsearch, Bandolier, Cochrane Library, Current Contents, Effectiveness Matters, Derwent Drug File, American College of Physicians Journal Club, Database of Abstracts of Effectiveness, FluNet, CDC Influenza Home Page, Influenza Bibliography, several government Internet sites, hand searches of reference lists, and contact with prominent researchers in the field.
14. Govaert TM, Thijs CT, Masurel N, et al. The efficacy of influenza vaccination in elderly individuals: a randomized double-blind placebo-controlled trial. *JAMA* 1994;272:1661–1665.
15. Treanor JJ, Mattison HR, Dumyati G, et al. Protective efficacy of combined live intranasal and inactivated influenza A virus vaccines in the elderly. *Ann Intern Med* 1992;117:625–633.
16. Potter J, Stott DJ, Roberts MA, et al. Influenza vaccination of health care workers in long-term-care hospitals reduces the mortality of elderly patients. *J Infect Dis* 1997;175:1–6.
17. Carmen WF, Elder AG, Wallace LA, et al. Effects of influenza vaccination of health-care workers on mortality of elderly people in long-term care: a randomized controlled trial. *Lancet* 2000;355:93–97.
18. Lasky T, Terracciano GJ, Magder L, et al. The Guillain-Barré syndrome and the 1992-1993 and 1993-1994 influenza vaccines. *N Engl J Med* 1998;339:1797-1802.
19. Dear K, Holden J, Andrews R, et al. Vaccines for preventing pneumococcal infection in adults (Cochrane Review). In: The Cochrane Library, Issue 3, 2004. Chichester, UK: John Wiley & Sons, Ltd. Search date 2003; primary sources Cochrane Central Register of Controlled Trails, Medline, Embase, bibliographies, and contact with vaccine manufacturers and lead authors of newly identified studies.
20. Pomilla PV, Brown RB. Outpatient treatment of community-acquired pneumonia in adults. *Arch Intern Med* 1994;154:1793–1802. Search date not reported; primary source Medline.
21. Contopoulos-Ioannidis DG, Ioannidis JPA, Chew P, et al. Meta-analysis of randomized controlled trials on the comparative efficacy and safety of azithromycin against other antibiotics for lower respiratory tract infections. *J Antimicrob Chemother* 2001;48:691–703. Search date 2000; primary sources Embase, Medline, and Cochrane Controlled Trials Registry.
22. Metge CJ, Vercaigne L, Carrie A, et al. The new fluoroquinolones in community-acquired pneumonia: clinical and economic perspectives. Technology overview no 5. Ottawa: Canadian Coordinating Office for Health Technology Assessment, 2001. Search date 1999; primary sources Medline and Embase.
23. Gotfried MH, Dattani D, Riffer E, et al. A controlled, double-blind, multicenter study comparing clarithromycin extended-release tablets and levofloxacin tablets in the treatment of community-acquired pneumonia. *Clin Ther* 2002;24:736–751.
24. Dunbar LM, Hassman J, Tellier G. Efficacy and tolerability of once-daily oral telithromycin compared with clarithromycin for the treatment of community-acquired pneumonia in adults. *Clin Ther* 2004;26:48–62.
25. Roson B, Carratala J, Tubau F, et al. Usefulness of betalactam therapy for community-acquired pneumonia in the era of drug-resistant *Streptococcus pneumoniae*: a randomized study of amoxicillin-clavulanate and ceftriaxone. *Microb Drug Resist* 2001;7:85–96.
26. Aubier M, Verster R, Regamey C, et al and the Sparfloxacin European Study Group. Once-daily sparfloxacin versus high-dosage amoxicillin in the treatment of community-acquired, suspected pneumococcal pneumonia in adults. *Clin Infect Dis* 1998;26:1312–1320.
27. Petitpretz P, Arvis P, Marel M, et al. Oral moxifloxacin vs high-dosage amoxicillin in the treatment of mild-to-moderate, community-acquired, suspected pneumococcal pneumonia in adults. *Chest* 2001;119:185–195.
28. Finch R, Schurmann D, Collins O, et al. Randomized controlled trial of sequential intravenous (i.v.) and oral moxifloxacin compared with sequential i.v. and oral co-amoxiclav with or without clarithromycin in patients with community-acquired pneumonia requiring initial parenteral treatment. *Antimicrob Agents Chemother* 2002;46:1746–1754.
29. File TM Jr, Segreti J, Dunbar L, et al. A multicenter, randomized study comparing the efficacy and safety of intravenous and/or oral levofloxacin versus ceftriaxone and/or cefuroxime axetil in treatment of adults with community-acquired pneumonia. *Antimicrob Agents Chemother* 1997;41:1965–1972.
30. Frank E, Liu J, Kinasewitz G, et al. A multicenter, open-label, randomized comparison of levofloxacin and azithromycin plus ceftriaxone in hospitalized adults with moderate to severe community-acquired pneumonia. *Clin Ther* 2002;24:1292–1308.
31. Friedland IR, McCracken GH Jr. Management of infections caused by antibiotic-resistant *Streptococcus pneumoniae*. *N Engl J Med* 1994;331:377–382.
32. Siegel RE. The significance of serum vs. tissue levels of antibiotics in the treatment of penicillin-resistant *Streptococcus pneumoniae* and community-acquired pneumonia. Are we looking in the wrong place? *Chest* 1999;116:535–538.
33. Gleason PP, Meehan TP, Fine JM, et al. Associations between initial antimicrobial therapy and medical outcomes for hospitalized elderly patients with pneumonia. *Arch Intern Med* 1999;159:2562–2572.
34. Metlay JP, Hofmann J, Cetron MS, et al. Impact of penicillin susceptibility on medical outcomes for adult patients with bacteremic pneumococcal pneumonia. *Clin Infect Dis* 2000;30:520–528.
35. Faikin DR, Schuchat A, Kolczak M, et al. Mortality from invasive pneumococcal pneumonia in the era of antibiotic resistance, 1995–1997. *Am J Public Health* 2000;90:223–229.
36. Marras TK, Nopmaneejumruslers C, Chan CK. Efficacy of exclusively oral antibiotic therapy in patients hospitalized with nonsevere community-acquired pneumonia: a retrospective study and meta-analysis. *Am J Med* 2004;116:385–393. Search date 2003; primary sources Medline, PreMedline, Embase, American College of Physicians Journal Club, Cochrane Controlled Trials Register, Cochrane Database of Systematic Reviews, DARE and bibliographies of relevant studies and reviews.
37. Siegel RE, Halperin NA, Almenoff PL, et al. A prospective randomized study of inpatient IV antibiotics for community-acquired pneumonia: the optimal duration of therapy. *Chest* 1996;110:965–971.
38. Ramirez JA, Ahkee S. Early switch from intravenous antimicrobials to oral clarithromycin in patients with community acquired pneumonia. *Infect Med* 1997;14:319–323.
39. Bjorkqvist M, Wiberg B, Bodin L, et al. Bottle-blowing in hospital-treated patients with community-acquired pneumonia. *Scand J Infect Dis* 1997;29:77–82.
40. Mundy L, Leet TL, Darst K, et al. Early mobilization of patients hospitalized with community-acquired pneumonia. *Chest* 2003;124:883–889.

41. Meehan TP, Fine MJ, Krumholz HM, et al. Quality of care, process, and outcomes in elderly patients with pneumonia. *JAMA* 1997;278:2080–2084.
42. Heath CH, Grove DI, Looke DFM. Delay in appropriate therapy of Legionella pneumonia associated with increased mortality. *Eur J Clin Microbiol Infect Dis* 1966;15:286–290.
43. Rhew DC, Tu GS, Ofman J, et al. Early switch and early discharge strategies in patients with community-acquired pneumonia: a meta-analysis. *Arch Intern Med* 2001;161:722–727. Search date 2000; primary sources Medline, Healthstar, Embase, Cochrane Library, and Best Evidence.
44. Fine MJ, Stone RA, Lave JR, et al. Implementation of an evidence-based guideline to reduce duration of intravenous antibiotic and length of stay for patients hospitalized with community-acquired pneumonia: a randomized controlled trial. *Am J Med* 2003;115:343–351.

Mark Loeb
Associate Professor
Departments of Pathology & Molecular Medicine and Clinical Epidemiology & Biostatistics
McMaster University
Hamilton
Canada

Competing interests: The author has received research grants from Bayer and Aventis and has attended conferences sponsored by Janssen Ortho and Aventis.

We would like to acknowledge the previous contributors of this chapter, including Thomas Marrie.

TABLE 1 **Causes of community acquired pneumonia (see text, p 1864).**

	USA (% of participants)*	UK (% of participants)†	Susceptibility (laboratory results)‡
Streptococcus pneumoniae	20–60	60–75	25% penicillin resistant, sensitive to quinolones
Haemophilus influenzae	3–10	4–5	30% ampicillin resistant, sensitive to cephalosporins or co-amoxiclav
Staphylococcus aureus	3–5	1–5	Methicillin resistant *S aureus* rare as cause of community acquired pneumonia
Chlamydia pneumoniae	4–6	ND	Sensitive to macrolides, tetracyclines, quinolones
Mycoplasma pneumoniae	1–6	5–18	Sensitive to macrolides, tetracyclines, quinolones
Legionella pneumophila	2–8	2–5	Sensitive to macrolides, tetracyclines, quinolones
Gram negative bacilli	3–10	Rare	
Aspiration	6–10	ND	
Viruses	2–15	8–16	

*Pooled data from 15 published reports from North America;[7] †data from British Thoracic Society;[7] ‡susceptibility data from recent studies. ND, no data.

Sore throat

Search date May 2004

Chris Del Mar and Paul Glasziou

QUESTIONS

INTERVENTIONS

Key Messages

Treatment

- **Non-steroidal anti-inflammatory drugs** RCTs identified by a systematic review found that non-steroidal anti-inflammatory drugs reduced sore throat symptoms both over ≤ 24 hours and at 2–5 days compared with placebo. The range of benefit was 25–75% over ≤ 24 hours, and 33–93% at 2–5 days. Non-steroidal anti-inflammatory drugs are associated with gastrointestinal and renal adverse effects.
- **Paracetamol** Two RCTs identified by a systematic review found that a single dose of paracetamol reduced acute sore throat pain at 2–3 hours compared with placebo. Another RCT identified by the review found that paracetamol three times daily reduced sore throat pain at 2 days compared with placebo. We found no RCTs of other analgesics in people with sore throat.
- **Antibiotics** One systematic review found that antibiotics reduced the proportion of people with sore throat, fever, and headache at 3 days compared with placebo. The review found limited evidence from indirect comparisons that the absolute and relative reduction in sore throat symptoms at 3 days was greater in people with positive throat swabs for *Streptococcus* than in people with negative swabs. It gave no information on adverse effects. We found no RCTs that assessed the effects of antibiotics in reducing the severity of sore throat symptoms. Antibiotics may increase the risk of nausea, vomiting, rash, headache, and vaginitis. Widespread antibiotic use may lead to bacterial resistance to antibiotics.
- **Corticosteroids** One RCT in children and adolescents with moderate to severe sore throat infection found that oral dexamethasone reduced throat pain at 24 hours compared with placebo, and reduced the duration of pain. Another RCT in people with severe sore throat infection identified by a systematic review found that adding corticosteroids to antibiotics reduced the proportion of people with sore throat pain

Clin Evid 2005;13:1876–1883.

at 24 hours compared with adding placebo. It found more limited evidence that adding corticosteroids to antibiotics also reduced the duration of pain. The RCTs provided insufficient evidence to assess adverse effects of corticosteroids in people with sore throat. However, data from systematic reviews in people with other disorders suggest that corticosteroids may be associated with serious adverse effects, although this may be only after long term use.

- **Probiotics** RCTs suggested that super-colonisation with *Streptococcus* isolated from healthy individuals apparently resistant to infections from *Streptococcus* may reduce recurrent sore throat over 2–3 months compared with placebo. However, at present, super-colonisation with *Streptococcus* is available only experimentally. We found no RCTs of other probiotics.

Preventing complications

- **Antibiotics** One systematic review found that antibiotics reduced suppurative and non-suppurative complications of β haemolytic streptococcal pharyngitis compared with placebo. However, in industrialised countries, non-suppurative complications are extremely rare. Widespread antibiotic use may lead to bacterial resistance to antibiotics.

DEFINITION Sore throat is an acute upper respiratory tract infection that affects the respiratory mucosa of the throat. Since infections can affect any part of the mucosa, it is often arbitrary whether an acute upper respiratory tract infection is called "sore throat" ("pharyngitis" or "tonsillitis"), "common cold", "sinusitis", "otitis media", or "bronchitis" (see figure 1, p 1883). Sometimes, all areas are affected (simultaneously or at different times) in one illness. In this chapter, we aim to cover people whose principal presenting symptom is sore throat. This may be associated with headache, fever, and general malaise. Suppurative complications include acute otitis media (most commonly), acute sinusitis, and peritonsillar abscess (quinsy). Non-suppurative complications include acute rheumatic fever and acute glomerulonephritis.

INCIDENCE/ PREVALENCE There is little seasonal fluctuation in sore throat. About 10% of the Australian population present to primary healthcare services annually with an upper respiratory tract infection consisting predominantly of sore throat.[1] This reflects about one fifth of the overall annual incidence.[1] However, it is difficult to distinguish between the different types of upper respiratory tract infection.[2]

AETIOLOGY/ RISK FACTORS The causative organisms of sore throat may be bacteria (*Streptococcus*, most commonly Group A β haemolytic, although sometimes others: *Haemophilus influenzae*, *Moraxella catarrhalis*, and others) or viruses (typically rhinovirus, but also coronavirus, respiratory syncytial virus, metapneumovirus, Ebstein–Barr, and others). It is difficult to distinguish bacterial from viral infections clinically. Some features are thought to predict the probability of the infection being caused by *Streptococcus* (fever > 38.5 °C; exudate on the tonsils; anterior neck lymphadenopathy; absence of cough).[3] Sore throat can be caused by processes other than primary infections, including gastro-oesophageal reflux, physical or chemical irritation (from nasogastric tubes or smoke, for example), and occasionally hay fever. However, we do not consider causes other than primary infection here.

PROGNOSIS Sore throat infections usually last a few days, with a few symptoms lasting longer, especially cough.[4] The untreated symptoms of sore throat disappear by 3 days in about 40% of people and untreated fevers in about 85%. By 1 week, 85% of people are symptom free. This natural history is similar in *Streptococcus* positive, negative, and untested patients.

AIMS OF INTERVENTION To relieve symptoms and to prevent suppurative and non-suppurative complications of sore throat.

OUTCOMES Reduction in severity and duration of symptoms (sore throat pain, general malaise, headache, fever); reduction in suppurative complications (acute otitis media, acute sinusitis, and quinsy) and non-suppurative complications (acute rheumatic fever, acute glomerulonephritis); time off work or school; patient satisfaction; healthcare utilisation.

METHODS *Clinical Evidence* search and appraisal May 2004. We excluded RCTs that only provided data about bacteriological studies of the throat, because bacteriological cure is not a clinically useful outcome for spontaneously remitting illness.

QUESTION **What are the effects of interventions to reduce symptoms of acute infective sore throat?**

OPTION **ANALGESICS**

Two RCTs identified by a systematic review found that a single dose of paracetamol reduced acute sore throat pain at 2–3 hours compared with placebo. Another RCT identified by the review found that paracetamol three times daily reduced sore throat pain at 2 days compared with placebo. We found no RCTs of other analgesics in people with sore throat.

Benefits: We found one systematic review (search date 1999, 3 RCTs, 312 people with acute sore throat for ≤ 4 days, severity unclear) comparing paracetamol (acetaminophen) versus placebo.[5] All of the RCTs found that paracetamol significantly reduced sore throat pain compared with placebo. Two RCTs (81 adults, 77 children) found that a single dose of paracetamol significantly reduced sore throat pain at 2–3 hours compared with placebo (50% greater reduction than placebo in 1 RCT; $P < 0.01$; 31% greater reduction than placebo in the other; $P < 0.05$). The third RCT (154 children) found that paracetamol three times daily significantly reduced sore throat symptoms after 2 days (34% greater reduction than placebo; $P < 0.01$). It is unclear how pain was assessed in the RCTs. We found no RCTs of other analgesics.

Harms: The review gave no information on adverse effects.[5]

Comment: An update of the review[5] is under way.[6]

OPTION **ANTIBIOTICS**

One systematic review found that antibiotics reduced the proportion of people with sore throat, fever, and headache at 3 days compared with placebo. The review found limited evidence from indirect comparisons that the absolute and relative reduction in sore throat symptoms at 3 days was greater in people with positive throat swabs for *Streptococcus* than in people with negative swabs. It gave no information on adverse effects. We found no RCTs that assessed the effects of antibiotics in reducing the severity of sore throat symptoms. Antibiotics may increase the risk of nausea, vomiting, rash, headache, and vaginitis. Widespread antibiotic use may lead to bacterial resistance to antibiotics.

Benefits: We found one systematic review (search date 2003, 26 randomised or quasi-randomised trials, 12 669 people with sore throat, severity unclear).[4] It found that, compared with placebo, antibiotics slightly but significantly reduced the proportion of people with symptoms of sore throat at 3 days compared with placebo (14 trials; 930/1966 [47%] with antibiotics *v* 993/1499 [66%] with placebo; RR 0.41, 95% CI 0.36 to 0.48; NNT 3, 95% CI 2 to 3). This represents an average shortening of symptoms by about 1 day. The reduction in symptoms of sore throat remained significant at 6–8 days (12 trials; 226/1739 [13%] with antibiotics *v* 199/1079 [18%] with placebo; RR 0.61, 95% CI 0.52 to 0.73; NNT at 7 days 14, 95% CI 6 to 20), an average shortening of 16 hours. The review also found that antibiotics significantly reduced the proportion of people with fever at 3 days compared with placebo (7 trials; 87/712 [12%] with antibiotics *v* 114/622 [23%] with placebo; RR 0.69, 95% CI 0.53 to 0.88; NNT 21, 95% CI 14 to 54) and reduced headache at 3 days (3 trials; 152/545 [28%] with antibiotics *v* 117/366 [32%] with placebo; RR 0.79, 95% CI 0.65 to 0.96; NNT 15, 95% CI 9 to 78). The review found limited evidence from indirect comparisons that, in people with throat swabs positive for *Streptococcus*, the absolute and relative reduction in sore throat symptoms at 3 days was greater than in people with negative swabs (positive swabs: 10 trials; 432/1020 [42%] with antibiotics *v* 516/723 [71%] with placebo; RR 0.56, 95% CI 0.51 to 0.61; NNT 3, 95% CI 3 to 4; negative swabs: 5 trials; 222/411 [54%] with antibiotics *v* 192/265 [73%] with placebo; RR 0.76, 95% CI 0.68 to 0.86; NNT 6, 95% CI 4 to 10). We found no systematic review or RCTs that assessed severity of sore throat symptoms.

Harms: The systematic review gave no information on adverse effects. However, data from systematic reviews in people with other disorders suggested that antibiotics were associated with nausea, vomiting, headache, skin rash, and vaginitis (see acute bronchitis, p 1844, and acute otitis media in children, p 227).

Comment: Widespread antibiotic use may lead to bacterial resistance to antibiotics (see acute bronchitis, p 1844).

OPTION NON-STEROIDAL ANTI-INFLAMMATORY DRUGS

RCTs identified by a systematic review found that non-steroidal anti-inflammatory drugs reduced sore throat symptoms both over ≤ 24 hours and at 2–5 days compared with placebo. The range of benefit was 25–75% over ≤ 24 hours, and 33–93% at 2–5 days. Non-steroidal anti-inflammatory drugs are associated with gastrointestinal and renal adverse effects.

Benefits: We found one systematic review (search date 1999, 12 RCTs, 114 people with acute sore throat for ≤ 5 days, severity unclear) comparing non-steroidal anti-inflammatory drugs (NSAIDs) versus placebo.[5] The review did not perform a meta-analysis. Seven RCTs (493 people) identified by the review assessed the effects of NSAIDs (including 1 RCT of aspirin) over 24 hours or less. All of the RCTs found that NSAIDs significantly reduced throat pain compared with placebo. The range of significant improvements in throat pain compared with placebo ranged from 25–75% ($P < 0.05$ in all RCTs). Six RCTs (697 people) identified by the review assessed the effects of NSAIDs over more than 24 hours. All of the RCTs found that NSAIDs significantly reduced symptoms (primarily throat pain) over 2–5 days. The range of significant improvements in symptoms compared with placebo ranged from 33–93% ($P < 0.05$ in all RCTs). It is unclear how pain was assessed in the RCTs.[5]

Harms: The review gave no information on adverse effects.[5] However, data from systematic reviews in people with other disorders suggested that NSAIDs were associated with gastrointestinal and renal adverse effects (see NSAID chapter, p 1525).

Comment: An update of the review[5] is under way.[6]

OPTION CORTICOSTEROIDS

One RCT in children and adolescents with moderate to severe sore throat infection found that oral dexamethasone reduced throat pain at 24 hours compared with placebo, and reduced the duration of pain. Another RCT in people with severe sore throat infection identified by a systematic review found that adding corticosteroids to antibiotics reduced the proportion of people with sore throat pain at 24 hours compared with adding placebo. It found more limited evidence that adding corticosteroids to antibiotics also reduced the duration of pain. The RCTs provided insufficient evidence to

assess adverse effects of corticosteroids in people with sore throat. However, data from systematic reviews in people with other disorders suggest that corticosteroids may be associated with serious adverse effects, although this may be only after long term use.

Benefits: We found one systematic review (search date 1999, 1 RCT) and one subsequent RCT.[5,7] **Versus placebo:** The review identified no RCTs of corticosteroids alone in people with sore throat.[5] The subsequent RCT (98 children and adolescents aged 5–18 years with moderate to severe sore throat infection defined as the presence of odynophagia/dysphagia associated with a McGrath Pain Face Scale of F or higher (happy [A]–sad [I]) compared oral corticosteroid (dexamethasone 10 mg) versus placebo over 24 hours.[7] It was reported only in an abstract. It found that dexamethasone significantly reduced the duration of throat pain compared with placebo (time to being pain free 9.8 hours with dexamethasone *v* 15.8 with placebo; $P < 0.02$) and significantly increased the proportion of people who were completely pain free at 48 hours (proportion with McGrath Pain Face Scale of A or B: 32/40 [80%] with dexamethasone *v* 27/46 [59%] with placebo; $P = 0.03$). **Plus antibiotics versus antibiotics alone:** The review[5] identified one RCT (51 adults with severe sore throat infection) comparing adding corticosteroid injection (dexamethasone 10 mg) to antibiotics versus adding placebo over 24 hours.[8] It found that adding dexamethasone significantly reduced sore throat pain at 24 hours (mean improvement in pain measured on a visual analogue scale from 0–30: 1.8 with adding dexamethasone *v* 1.2 with adding placebo; $P < 0.05$). It also found limited evidence that adding dexamethasone significantly reduced the duration of throat pain compared with placebo (completer analysis in 50% of people followed up for 7 days; mean time to being pain free reduced from 35 hours to 15 hours; $P < 0.02$).

Harms: The RCT found no adverse effects associated with oral dexamethasone, but may have been too small to detect clinically important adverse effects. **In combination with antibiotics:** The review gave no information on adverse effects.[5] However, data from systematic reviews in people with other disorders suggests that antibiotics may be associated with serious adverse effects, although this may be only after long term use. Potential harms of oral corticosteroids are covered elsewhere in *Clinical Evidence* (see asthma, p 1891).

Comment: More RCTs are needed. An update of the review[5] is under way.[6]

OPTION PROBIOTICS

RCTs suggested that super-colonisation with *Streptococcus* isolated from healthy individuals apparently resistant to infections from *Streptococcus* may reduce recurrent sore throat over 2–3 months compared with placebo. However, at present, super-colonisation with *Streptococcus* is available only experimentally. We found no RCTs of other probiotics.

Benefits: We found one systematic review[5] (search date 1999, 2 RCTs[9,10]) and one subsequent RCT[11] comparing super-colonisation with *Streptococcus* grown from a child resistant to infections from *Streptococcus* versus placebo (see comment below). We found no RCTs of other probiotics. The first RCT (36 people aged 5–40 years with culture confirmed recurrence of sore throat, all taking antibiotics) identified by the review found that super-colonisation with *Streptococcus* significantly reduced the proportion of people who had recurrence of streptococcal sore throat over 3 months compared with placebo (1/17 [6%] with super-colonisation *v* 11/19 [59%] with placebo; $P < 0.001$).[9] The second RCT

(130 people aged 3–59 years with culture confirmed recurrence of sore throat, all taking antibiotics) identified by the review found no significant difference between super-colonisation with *Streptococcus* and placebo in the proportion of people who had recurrence of streptococcal sore throat over 8 weeks compared with placebo, although fewer people using bacterial spray with *Streptococcus* had recurrence (22% with super-colonisation *v* 38% with placebo; P = 0.064).[10] The subsequent RCT (342 people, all treated with antibiotics) found that super-colonisation with *Streptococcus* significantly reduced recurrence over a mean of 3 months compared with placebo (proportion with recurrent sore throat: 36/189 [19%] with super-colonisation *v* 28/93 [30%] with placebo; P = 0.04).[11]

Harms: Both RCTs found no adverse effects associated with *Streptococcus* bacteriological spray.[9,11]

Comment: Super-colonisation with *Streptococcus* isolated from healthy individuals apparently resistant to infections from *Streptococcus* is available only experimentally. An update of the review[5] is under way.[6]

QUESTION What are the effects of interventions to prevent complications of acute infective sore throat?

OPTION ANTIBIOTICS

One systematic review found that antibiotics reduced suppurative and non-suppurative complications of β haemolytic streptococcal pharyngitis compared with placebo. However, in industrialised countries, non-suppurative complications are extremely rare. Widespread antibiotic use may lead to bacterial resistance to antibiotics.

Benefits: We found one systematic review (search date 2003, 26 randomised or quasi-randomised trials, 12 669 people with sore throat, severity unclear) comparing antibiotics versus placebo to prevent complications of sore throat infection.[4] **Acute otitis media:** The review found that antibiotics significantly reduced acute otitis media at 14 days compared with placebo, although it was a rare complication in the trials identified (11 trials; 11/2325 [0.5%] with antibiotics *v* 28/1435 [2.0%] with placebo; RR 0.26, 95% CI 0.14 to 0.49; NNT 71, 95% CI 60 to 107).[4] **Acute rheumatic fever:** It found that antibiotics significantly reduced the proportion of people who had developed acute rheumatic fever at 2 months compared with placebo (16 trials; 37/5656 [0.7%] with antibiotics *v* 74/4445 [1.8%] with placebo; RR 0.29, 95% CI 0.18 to 0.44; NNT 77, 95% CI 67 to 98; see comment below).[4] The incidence of acute rheumatic fever has declined with time. The 111 cases of acute rheumatic fever assessed by the review all occurred in 10 trials undertaken between 1950 and 1961; there were no cases in the remaining five trials undertaken between 1987 and 2000. **Acute glomerulonephritis:** There were too few people who had acute glomerulonephritis to detect any possible protective effect of antibiotics in 11 trials (5147 people: 0/2927 [0%] with antibiotics *v* 2/2220 [0.1%] with placebo; RR 0.22, 95% CI 0.02 to 2.02; see comment below). **Acute sinusitis:** The review found no significant difference in the proportion of people who had developed acute sinusitis at 14 days between antibiotics and placebo, but there may have been too few events to detect a clinically important difference (8 trials; 4/1545 [0.3%] with antibiotics *v* 4/842 [0.5%] with placebo; RR 0.53, 95% CI 0.18 to 1.55). **Peritonsillar abscess (quinsy):** The review found that antibiotics significantly reduced peritonsillar abscess at 2 months compared with placebo (6 trials; 2/1438 [0.1%] with antibiotics *v* 23/995 [2.3%] with placebo; RR 0.14, 95% CI 0.05 to 0.39; NNT 50, 95% CI 46 to 71).

Harms: The systematic review gave no information on adverse effects. However, data from systematic reviews in people with other disorders suggested that antibiotics were associated with nausea, vomiting, headache, skin rash, and vaginitis (see acute bronchitis topic, p 1844, and acute otitis media in children, p 227).

Comment: Acute rheumatic fever and acute glomerulonephritis associated with sore throat infection may be related to host antibodies to *Streptococcus* cross-reacting with host tissue in the heart and kidney. See also comment on antibiotics under treatments for sore throat, p 1879. Widespread antibiotic use may lead to bacterial resistance to antibiotics (see acute bronchitis, p 1844).

REFERENCES

1. Del Mar C, Pincus D. Incidence patterns of respiratory illness in Queensland estimated from sentinel general practice. *Aust Fam Physician* 1995;24:625–9,32.
2. Benediktsdottir B. Upper airway infections in preschool children — frequency and risk factors. *Scand J Prim Health Care* 1993;11:197–201.
3. Dagnelie CF, Bartelink ML, van der Graaf Y, et al. Towards a better diagnosis of throat infections (with group A beta-hemolytic streptococcus) in general practice. *Br J Gen Pract* 1998;48:59–62.
4. Del Mar CB, Glasziou PP, Spinks AB. Antibiotics for sore throat. In: The Cochrane Library, Issue 3, 2004. Chichester, UK: John Wiley & Sons, Ltd. Search date 2003; primary sources Medline, Cochrane Library, and hand searches of reference lists of relevant articles.
5. Thomas M, Del Mar C, Glaziou P. How effective are treatments other than antibiotics for acute sore throat? *Br J Gen Pract* 2000;50:817–820. Search date 1999; primary sources Medline and Cochrane Controlled Trials Registry.
6. Francis D, Del Mar C, Thomas M, et al. Non-antibiotic treatments for sore throat (Protocol for a Cochrane Review). In: The Cochrane Library, Issue 3, 2004. Chichester, UK: John Wiley & Sons, Ltd.
7. Olympia R., Khine H, and Avner J. The effectiveness of oral dexamethasone in the treatment of moderate to severe pharyngitis in children and young adults. *Acad Emerg Med* 2003;10:434.
8. O'Brien JF, Meade JL, and Falk JL. Dexamethasone as adjuvant therapy for severe acute pharyngitis. *Ann Emerg Med* 1993;22:212–215.
9. Roos K, Holm SE, Grahn E, et al. Alpha-streptococci as supplementary treatment of recurrent streptococcal tonsillitis: a randomized placebo-controlled study. *Scand J Infect Dis* 1993;25:31–35.
10. Roos K, Holm SE, Grahn-Hakansson E, et al. Recolonization with selected alpha-streptococci for prophylaxis of recurrent streptococcal pharyngotonsillitis — a randomized placebo-controlled multicentre study. *Scand J Infect Dis* 1996;28:459–462.
11. Falck G, Grahn-Hakansson E, Holm SE, et al. Tolerance and efficacy of interfering α streptococci in recurrence of streptococcal pharyngotonsillitis: a placebo-controlled study. *Acta Otolaryngol* 1999;119:944–948.

Chris Del Mar
Dean of Health Science and Medicine
Bond University
Gold Coast
Australia

Paul Glasziou
Director: Centre for Evidence-based Practice
Oxford University
Oxford
UK

Competing interests: The authors wrote several of the systematic reviews from which material for this topic was drawn.

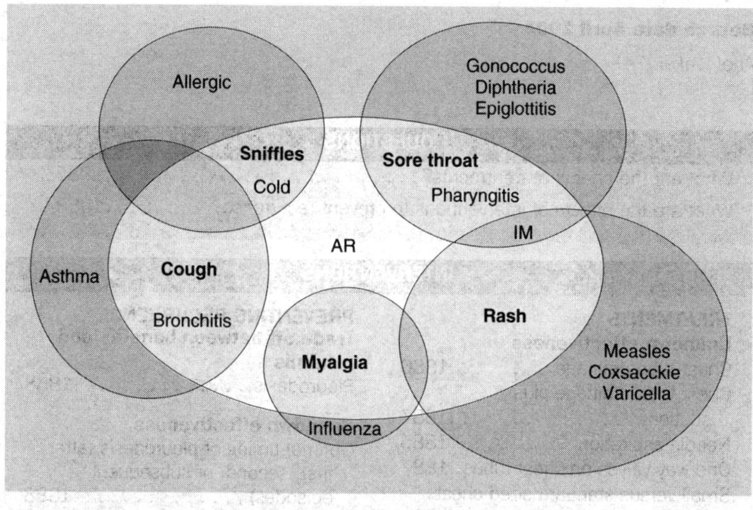

FIGURE 1 Confusion and overlap in the classification of acute respiratory infections

Spontaneous pneumothorax

Search date April 2004

Abel Wakai

QUESTIONS

INTERVENTIONS

See glossary G

Key Messages

- We found insufficient evidence to determine whether any intervention is more effective than no intervention for spontaneous pneumothorax.

Treatments

- **Chest tube drainage** We found no RCTs comparing chest tube drainage versus observation. RCTs provided insufficient evidence to compare chest tube drainage versus needle aspiration or chest tube drainage plus suction.
- **Chest tube drainage plus suction** One RCT and one controlled clinical trial found no significant difference in rate of resolution of pneumothorax whether chest tube drainage bottles were connected to suction or not. However, both trials were too small to rule out a clinically important difference.
- **Needle aspiration** Four RCTs provided insufficient evidence to compare needle aspiration versus observation or chest tube drainage.
- **One way valves on chest tubes** One RCT found no significant difference in rate of resolution between one way valves and drainage bottles with underwater seals, but it is likely to have been too small to detect a clinically important difference. It found that people treated with one way valves used less analgesia and were less likely to be admitted to hospital than people treated with drainage bottles.
- **Small versus standard sized chest tubes** We found no RCTs assessing small or standard sized tubes for chest drainage.

Preventing recurrence

- **Pleurodesis** Two RCTs found that adding chemical pleurodesis to chest tube drainage reduced the rate of recurrence of spontaneous pneumothorax compared with chest tube drainage alone. One of the RCTs found that chemical pleurodesis injection was intensely painful. The RCTs found no significant difference in length of hospital stay. One RCT found that thoracoscopic surgery with talcum powder instillation reduced the rate of recurrence at 5 years compared with chest tube drainage. Two RCTs provided insufficient evidence to compare video assisted thoracoscopic surgery versus thoracotomy. We found no RCTs comparing chemical versus surgical pleurodesis.

Clin Evid 2005;13:1884–1890.

- **Optimal timing of pleurodesis (after first, second, or subsequent episodes)** We found no RCTs or high quality cohort studies assessing whether pleurodesis should take place after the first, second, or subsequent episodes of spontaneous pneumothorax.

DEFINITION A pneumothorax is air in the pleural space. A spontaneous pneumothorax occurs when there is no provoking factor, such as trauma, surgery, or diagnostic intervention. It implies a leak of air from the lung parenchyma through the visceral pleura into the pleural space. This review does not include people with tension pneumothorax.

INCIDENCE/ PREVALENCE In a survey in Minnesota, USA, the incidence of spontaneous pneumothorax was 7/100 000 for men and 1/100 000 for women.[1] In England and Wales, the overall rate of people consulting with pneumothorax (in both primary and secondary care combined) is 24/100 000 a year for men and 9.8/100 000 a year for women.[2] The overall annual incidence of emergency hospital admissions for pneumothorax in England and Wales is 16.7/100 000 for men and 5.8/100 000 for women.[2] Smoking increases the likelihood of spontaneous pneumothorax by 22 times for men and eight times for women.[3] A dose–response relationship was observed.[3]

AETIOLOGY/ RISK FACTORS Spontaneous pneumothorax can be primary (typically in young fit people and thought to be because of a congenital abnormality of the visceral pleura) or secondary (caused by underlying lung disease, typically occurring in older people with emphysema or pulmonary fibrosis).

PROGNOSIS Death from spontaneous pneumothorax is rare. Morbidity with pain and shortness of breath is common. Published recurrence rates vary. One cohort study in Denmark found that, after a first episode of primary spontaneous pneumothorax, 23% of people suffered a recurrence within 5 years, most within 1 year.[4] Recurrence rates had been thought to increase substantially after the first recurrence, but one retrospective case control study (147 military personnel) found that 28% of men with a first primary spontaneous pneumothorax had a recurrence; 23% of the 28% had a second recurrence; and 14% of that 23% had a third recurrence, giving a total recurrence rate of 35%.[5]

AIMS OF INTERVENTION To reduce morbidity; to restore normal function as quickly as possible; to prevent recurrence and mortality, with minimum adverse effects.

OUTCOMES Successful resolution of spontaneous pneumothorax after a stated period; time to full expansion of the lung; duration of hospital stay; time off work; harmful effects of treatments (pain, surgical emphysema, wound, and pleural space infection); and rate of recurrence.

METHODS *Clinical Evidence* search and appraisal April 2004. Most of the literature consisted of uncontrolled case series.

QUESTION What are the effects of treatments?

OPTION NEEDLE ASPIRATION

Four RCTs provided insufficient evidence to compare needle aspiration versus observation or chest tube drainage.

Benefits: **Versus observation:** We found no systematic review. We found one RCT (21 people), which found faster resolution with needle aspiration compared with observation (time to full expansion: 1.6 weeks in 8 people successfully treated with needle aspiration *v* 3.2 weeks in 10 people treated conservatively).[6] However, two people randomised to needle aspiration required a chest tube. The RCT did not assess the significance of the difference between groups. **Versus chest tube drainage:** We found no systematic review but found three RCTs.[7-9] The first RCT (73 people) found that fewer people had immediate resolution of pneumothorax with needle aspiration compared with chest tube drainage (28/35 [80%] with needle aspiration *v* 38/38 [100%] with chest tube drainage). The people who did not have successful resolution of pneumothorax with needle aspiration were subsequently treated with chest tube drainage.[7] It found that, on average, people receiving needle aspiration spent significantly fewer days in hospital than people receiving chest tube drainage (3.2 days with needle aspiration v 5.3 days with chest tube drainage; P = 0.005).[7] It found no significant difference in the rate of recurrence at 1 year (5/30 [17%] with needle aspiration v 10/35 [29%] with chest tube drainage; ARR +12%, 95% CI –9% to +32%; RR 0.58, 95% CI 0.22 to 1.52). The second RCT (61 people) found that, at 24 hours, pneumothorax resolved in significantly fewer people with needle aspiration compared with chest tube drainage (22/33 [67%] with needle aspiration v 26/28 [93%] with chest tube drainage; ARR 26%, 95% CI 6% to 47%; RR of failure to resolve 0.72, 95% CI 0.55 to 0.93).[8] It found no significant difference in the rate of recurrence at 3 months (6/33 [18%] with needle aspiration v 7/28 [25%] with chest tube drainage; ARR +7%, 95% CI –14% to +28%; RR 0.73, 95% CI 0.28 to 1.92). The RCT was not designed to find a difference in duration of hospital stay because chest tube drainage was done on admission, whereas in most people needle aspiration was performed after 3 days of observation in hospital. The third RCT (60 people) found no significant difference between needle aspiration and chest tube drainage in immediate resolution rates (16/27 [59%] with needle aspiration v 21/33 [64%] with chest tube drainage; P = 0.9).[9] Resolution was defined for needle aspiration as complete or nearly complete lung expansion after manual aspiration, and for chest tube drainage as complete lung expansion and chest tube removal within 72 hours. It also found no significant difference between needle aspiration and chest tube drainage in mean hospital stay (3.5 days with needle aspiration v 4.5 days with chest tube drainage; P = 0.2) or recurrence rate at 1 year (7/26 [26%] with needle aspiration v 9/33 [27%] with chest tube drainage; P = 0.9). The RCT is likely to have been too small to detect a clinically important difference in outcomes.

Harms: **Versus observation:** The RCT gave no information on adverse effects.[6] **Versus chest tube drainage:** The first RCT found that people treated with needle aspiration had significantly less pain on daily pain scores during their hospital stay (mean score: 0.7 with needle aspiration v 1.5 with chest tube; P < 0.001).[7] The second RCT found no significant difference in pain or dyspnoea between needle aspiration and chest tube drainage (reported as non-significant; results presented graphically).[8] The third RCT did not assess pain.[9]

Comment: The RCT comparing needle aspiration versus observation was published as a letter.[6] A large case series undertaken in the 1960s reported that 88/119 (74%) people presenting to an outpatient chest clinic with spontaneous pneumothorax were managed successfully without intervention or hospital admission.[10] However, the current clinical relevance of this case series is unclear. A systematic review comparing chest tube drainage versus needle aspiration is underway.[11]

OPTION CHEST TUBE DRAINAGE

We found no RCTs comparing chest tube drainage versus observation. RCTs provided insufficient evidence to compare chest tube drainage versus needle aspiration or chest tube drainage plus section. We found no RCTs assessing small or standard sized tubes for chest drainage.

Benefits: **Versus observation:** We found no systematic review. We found no RCTs. **Versus needle aspiration:** See benefits of needle aspiration, p 1885. **Small versus standard sized chest tubes:** We found no systematic review. We found no RCTs (see comment below). **Versus chest tube drainage plus suction:** See benefits of chest tube drainage plus suction, p 1887.

Harms: **Versus needle aspiration:** See harms of needle aspiration, p 1886. **Small versus standard sized chest tubes:** We found no RCTs (see comment below). **Versus chest tube drainage plus suction:** See harms of chest tube drainage plus suction, p 1888.

Comment: **Small versus standard sized chest tubes:** Small gauge chest tubes are usually easier to insert. One non-randomised trial (44 people) compared small gauge catheters (8 French gauge**G**) versus standard chest tubes.[12] It found no significant difference in duration of drainage between groups (5 days *v* 6 days; reported as non-significant, no further data reported). In people with large pneumothoraces (> 50% lung volume), successful resolution was significantly more likely with standard chest tubes than small gauge (100% with standard tubes *v* 57% with small tubes; $P < 0.05$). No such difference was found in people with small (< 50%) pneumothoraces. The trial found that conventional chest tubes significantly increased the risk of subcutaneous emphysema (9/23 [39%] with conventional tubes *v* 0/21 [0%] with small tubes; $P < 0.05$) and pain compared with small gauge catheters.[12]

OPTION ONE WAY VALVES ON CHEST TUBES

One RCT found no significant difference in rate of resolution between one way valves and drainage bottles with underwater seals, but it is likely to have been too small to detect a clinically important difference. It found that people treated with one way valves used less analgesia and were less likely to be admitted to hospital than people treated with drainage bottles.

Benefits: We found no systematic review. We found one RCT (30 people with spontaneous pneumothorax and respiratory distress).[13] The RCT compared a chest tube (13 French gauge**G**) connected to a one way valve versus a chest tube (14 French gauge) connected to a drainage bottle with an underwater seal. It found no significant difference between groups in rate of resolution at 48 hours (complete or nearly complete expansion: 15/17 [88%] with one way valve *v* 11/13 [85%] with drainage bottle; RR 1.04, 95% CI 0.78 to 1.39). It found that one way valves significantly reduced hospital admissions compared with drainage bottles (5/17 [29%] with one way valve *v* 13/13 [100%] with drainage bottle; RR 0.29, 95% CI 0.14 to 0.61).[13] It found that significantly fewer people treated with a one way valve required analgesia (5/17 [29%] with one way valve *v* 10/13 [77%] with drainage bottle; RR 0.38, 95% CI 0.17 to 0.85).[13]

Harms: The RCT found no significant difference in rates of complications between one way valves and drainage bottles with underwater seals (need for a second drain: 3/17 [18%] with one way valve *v* 1/13 [8%] with drainage bottle; skin emphysema: 3/17 [18%] with one way valve *v* 3/13 [23%] with drainage bottle; reported as non-significant, no further data reported).[13]

Comment: None.

OPTION CHEST TUBE DRAINAGE PLUS SUCTION

One RCT and one controlled clinical trial found no significant difference in rate of resolution of pneumothorax whether chest tube drainage bottles were connected to suction or not. However, both trials were too small to rule out a clinically important difference.

Benefits: **Versus chest tube drainage alone:** We found no systematic review, but found one RCT (53 people, 23 with primary spontaneous pneumothorax and 30 with secondary)[14] and one controlled clinical trial (40 people)[15] comparing chest tube drainage using an underwater seal only versus drainage plus suction. The RCT found no significant difference between chest tube drainage plus suction and chest tube drainage alone in the proportion of people with full lung expansion at 10 days (13/23 [57%] with suction *v* 15/30 [50%] without suction; ARI +7%, 95% CI –21% to +34%; RR 1.13, 95% CI 0.68 to 1.88), but is likely to have been too small to exclude a clinically important difference. Suction pressures ranged from 8–20 cm H_2O.[14] The controlled clinical trial assigned people to chest tube drainage plus suction or chest tube drainage alone by alternate allocation.[15] It also found no significant difference in time taken for lung expansion between adding low pressure suction to chest drainage and chest drainage alone (mean: 5.2 days with suction *v* 6.2 days with no suction; reported as non-significant, CI not reported). The trial did not state whether spontaneous pneumothorax was primary or secondary, or what suction pressure was applied.

Harms: The RCT[14] and controlled clinical trial[15] gave no information on adverse effects.

Comment: None.

QUESTION **What are the effects of interventions to prevent recurrence?**

OPTION **PLEURODESIS**

Two RCTs found that adding chemical pleurodesis to chest tube drainage reduced the rate of recurrence of spontaneous pneumothorax compared with chest tube drainage alone. One of the RCTs found that chemical pleurodesis injection was intensely painful. The RCTs found no significant difference in length of hospital stay. One RCT found that thoracoscopic surgery with talcum powder instillation reduced the rate of recurrence at 5 years compared with chest tube drainage. Two RCTs provided insufficient evidence to compare video assisted thoracoscopic surgery versus thoracotomy. We found no RCTs comparing chemical versus surgical pleurodesis. We found no RCTs or high quality cohort studies assessing whether pleurodesis should take place after the first, second, or subsequent episodes of spontaneous pneumothorax.

Benefits: **Adding chemical pleurodesis to chest tube drainage versus chest tube drainage alone:** We found no systematic review. We found two RCTs.[16,17] The first RCT (unblinded, 229 men with pneumothorax successfully treated by chest tube; mean age 54 years; 55% with chronic obstructive pulmonary disease) found that adding intrapleural instillation of tetracycline significantly reduced recurrence rates over 30 months compared with chest tube alone (26/104 [25%] with tetracycline *v* 44/108 [41%] with chest tube alone; RR 0.61, 95% CI 0.41 to 0.92).[16] It found no significant difference between groups in length of hospital stay (5 days with tetracycline *v* 7 days with chest tube alone) or 5 year mortality (40/113 [35%] with tetracycline *v* 42/116 [36%] with chest tube alone; RR 0.98, 95% CI 0.62 to 1.38). The second RCT (96 people treated with chest tube drainage) compared three groups: no further treatment, tetracycline pleurodesis**G**, and talcum powder pleurodesis.[17] Mean follow up was 4.6 years. It found that either type of chemical pleurodesis significantly reduced the pneumothorax recurrence rate over 4.6 years compared with no treatment (2/24 [8%] with talcum powder pleurodesis *v* 3/23 [13%] with tetracycline pleurodesis *v* 9/25 [36%] with no treatment; ARR of recurrence with either form of pleurodesis 25%, 95% CI 6% to 45%). It found no significant difference in mean hospital stay (mean 7 days with tetracycline *v* 6 days with talcum powder or with chest tube alone; reported as non-significant, no further data reported). **Thoracoscopic surgery with talc instillation**

versus chest tube drainage: We found no systematic review. We found one multicentre RCT (108 people with large primary spontaneous pneumothorax or primary spontaneous pneumothorax that had failed aspiration) that compared thoracoscopic surgery with talcum powder instillation versus chest tube drainage.[18] It found that thoracoscopic surgery plus talcum powder instillation significantly reduced the recurrence rate at 5 years compared with chest tube drainage (3/59 [5%] with surgery v 16/47 [34%] with chest tube drainage; P < 0.01). It found similar length of hospital stay (mean: 8.0 days with surgery v 7.4 days with drainage; no further data reported). **Video assisted thoracoscopic surgery versus thoracotomy:** We found no systematic review. We found two RCTs.[19,20] The first RCT (60 people with primary spontaneous pneumothorax, either first recurrence or non-resolving first episode) compared video assisted thoracoscopic surgery versus thoracotomy.[19] It found no significant difference between video assisted thoracoscopic surgery and thoracotomy in recurrence rates after 3 years (3/30 [10%] with video assisted surgery v 0/30 [0%] with thoracotomy; ARR +10%, 95% CI –1% to +21%). It found that video assisted surgery significantly reduced the use of analgesia and hospital stay compared with thoracotomy (mean hospital stay: 6.5 days with video assisted surgery v 10.7 days with thoracotomy; P < 0.0001). The second RCT (60 people, 30 with primary pneumothorax, 30 with secondary, either with recurrence or an air leak persisting for > 5 days) compared video assisted thoracoscopic surgery versus thoracotomy.[20] It found no significant difference between video assisted thorascopic surgery and thoracotomy in use of analgesia or hospital stay (mean hospital stay: 4 days with video assisted surgery v 5 days with thoracotomy; reported as non-significant, CI not reported). It also found no significant difference in recurrence rate at 15 months (2/15 [13%] with video assisted surgery v 1/15 [7%] with thoracotomy; reported as non-significant, CI not reported). The RCT is likely to have been too small to detect a clinically important difference. **Chemical versus surgical pleurodesis:** We found no systematic review or RCTs. **Optimal timing of pleurodesis:** We found no systematic review. We found no RCTs or high quality cohort studies comparing pleurodesis undertaken at different times (after the first, second, or subsequent episodes of spontaneous pneumothorax; see comment below).

Harms: **Adding chemical pleurodesis to chest tube drainage versus chest tube drainage alone:** In the first RCT, 61/105 (58%) people reported intense chest pain on injection of tetracycline.[16] The second RCT found that similar proportions of people reported pain with chemical pleurodesis**G** compared with chest tube alone (17/33 [52%] with tetracycline v 14/29 [48%] with talc v 18/34 [53%] with chest tube alone; no further data reported).[17] **Thoracoscopic surgery with talc instillation versus chest tube drainage:** The RCT did not establish a protocol for analgesia; four centres gave postoperative systemic opioids and three did not.[18] It found that thoracoscopic surgery modestly but significantly increased pain during the first 3 days compared with chest tube drainage (results presented graphically). It found no significant difference in pain between groups when people received systemic opioids. **Video assisted thoracoscopic surgery versus thoracotomy:** The first RCT gave no information on adverse effects.[19] The second RCT reported that three people with secondary spontaneous pneumothorax died, one receiving video assisted thorascopic surgery and two receiving thoracotomy, one of whom had previously had unsuccessful video assisted thoracoscopic surgery.[20] **Chemical versus surgical pleurodesis:** We found no RCTs. **Optimal timing of pleurodesis:** We found no RCTs or high quality cohort studies.

Comment: One observational study suggested that the 5 year recurrence rate after a first pneumothorax is about 28%, so there may be little reason to perform pleurodesis**G** after the first episode of pneumothorax.[5] There has been a consensus that pleurodesis is warranted after the second or third episode of pneumothorax. Even though the probability of success with pleurodesis is high, clinicians will have to weigh the likelihood of recurrence against the morbidity associated with the procedure. Chemical pleurodesis may be appropriate for people unfit or unwilling to have surgery.

GLOSSARY

French gauge A measure of the size of a catheter or drainage tube defined (in France by JFB Charrière in 1842) to be the outside diameter of the tube in units of 1/3 mm. A 12 French gauge tube has an outer diameter of 4 mm. Sometimes the French gauge is called the Charrière (Ch) gauge.

Pleurodesis The instillation of substances (sclerosants) into the pleural space leading to a sterile inflammatory reaction with formation of dense adhesions. It may be performed non-operatively through a chest tube or thoracoscope (chemical pleurodesis) or operatively (surgical pleurodesis).

REFERENCES

1. Melton LJ, Hepper NG, Offord KP. Incidence of spontaneous pneumothorax in Olmsted County, Minnesota: 1950 to 1974. *Am Rev Respir Dis* 1979;120:1379–1382.
2. Gupta D, Hansell A, Nichols T, et al. Epidemiology of pneumothorax in England. *Thorax* 2000;55:666–671.
3. Bense L, Eklung G, Wiman LG. Smoking and the increased risk of contracting spontaneous pneumothorax. *Chest* 1987;92:1009–1012.
4. Lippert HL, Lund O, Blegvad S, et al. Independent risk factors for cumulative recurrence rate after first spontaneous pneumothorax. *Eur Respir J* 1991;4:324–331.
5. Voge VM, Anthracite R. Spontaneous pneumothorax in the USAF aircrew population: a retrospective study. *Aviat Space Environ Med* 1986;57:939–949.
6. Flint K, Al-Hillawi AH, Johnson NM. Conservative management of spontaneous pneumothorax. *Lancet* 1984;1:687–688.
7. Harvey J, Prescott RJ. Simple aspiration versus intercostal tube drainage for spontaneous pneumothorax in patients with normal lungs. British Thoracic Society Research Committee. *BMJ* 1994;309:1338–1339.
8. Andrivet P, Djedaini K, Teboul JL, et al. Spontaneous pneumothorax. Comparison of thoracic drainage vs immediate or delayed needle aspiration. *Chest* 1995;108:335–339.
9. Noppen M, Alexander P, Driesen P, et al. Manual aspiration versus chest tube drainage in first episodes of primary spontaneous pneumothorax: a multicenter, prospective, randomized pilot study. *Am J Respir Crit Care Med* 2002;165:1240–1244.
10. Stradling P, Poole G. Conservative management of spontaneous pneumothorax. *Thorax* 1966;21:145–149.
11. Wakai, A, O'Sullivan RG, Deasy C, et al. Simple aspiration versus intercostal tube drainage for primary spontaneous pneumothorax in adults (protocol for a Cochrane review). In: The Cochrane Library, Issue 4, 2003. Chichester, UK: John Wiley & Sons, Ltd.
12. Kang YJ, Koh HG, Shin JW, et al. The effect of 8 French catheter and chest tube on the treatment of spontaneous pneumothorax. *Tuber Respir Dis* 1996;43:410–419.
13. Roggla M, Wagner A, Brunner C, et al. The management of pneumothorax with the thoracic vent versus conventional intercostal tube drainage. *Wien Klin Wochenschr* 1996;108:330–333.
14. So SY, Yu DYC. Catheter drainage of spontaneous pneumothorax: suction or no suction, early or late removal? *Thorax* 1982;37:46–48.
15. Sharma TN, Agnihotri SP, Jain NK, et al. Intercostal tube thoracostomy in pneumothorax: factors influencing re-expansion of lung. *Indian J Chest Dis Allied Sci* 1988;30:32–35.
16. Light RW, O'Hara VS, Moritz TE, et al. Intrapleural tetracycline for the prevention of recurrent spontaneous pneumothorax. Results of a Department of Veterans Affairs cooperative study. *JAMA* 1990;264:2224–2230.
17. Almind M, Lange P, Viskum K. Spontaneous pneumothorax: comparison of simple drainage, talc pleurodesis, and tetracycline pleurodesis. *Thorax* 1989;44:627–630.
18. Tschopp J-M, Boutin C, Astoul P, et al. Talcage by medical thoracoscopy for primary spontaneous pneumothorax is more cost-effective than drainage: a randomised study. *Eur Respir J* 2002;20:1003–1009.
19. Ayed AK, Al-Din HJ. Video-assisted thoracoscopy versus thoracotomy for primary spontaneous pneumothorax: a randomized controlled trial. *Med Principles Pract* 2000;9:113–118.
20. Waller DA, Forty J, Morritt GN. Video-assisted thoracoscopic surgery versus thoracotomy for spontaneous pneumothorax. *Ann Thorac Surg* 1994;58:372–376.

Abel Wakai
Specialist Registrar in Emergency Medicine
St James' Hospital, Dublin, Ireland

Competing interests: Abel Wakai is the co-author of an ongoing systematic review, presently published as a protocol for a cochrane review, that is referenced in this chapter.

We would like to acknowledge the previous contributors of this chapter, including John Cunnington.

Asthma

Search date May 2003

Rodolfo J Dennis, Ivan Solarte, and J Mark FitzGerald

QUESTIONS

INTERVENTIONS

To be covered in future updates
Allergen avoidance
Oral β_2 agonists

Covered elsewhere in *Clinical Evidence*
Asthma and other wheezing disorders of childhood, p 239

*Categorisation based on consensus. RCTs are unlikely to be conducted.
See glossary Ⓖ

Key Messages

In people with chronic asthma

- **Adding long acting inhaled β_2 agonists in people with mild, persistent asthma that is poorly controlled by inhaled corticosteroids** One systematic review and three additional RCTs have found that adding regular doses of long acting inhaled β_2 agonists improves lung function and symptoms and reduces rescue medication compared with increasing the dose of inhaled corticosteroids. However, one further RCT found that increasing inhaled corticosteroid dose reduced exacerbations compared with adding long acting inhaled β_2 agonists. We found insufficient evidence about effects of adding long acting inhaled β_2 agonists on mortality.
- **Adding long acting inhaled β_2 agonists to inhaled corticosteroids in poorly controlled mild to moderate, persistent asthma (for symptom control)** RCTs have found that, in people with asthma that is poorly controlled with inhaled corticosteroids, adding regular long acting inhaled β_2 agonists improves symptoms and lung function compared with adding placebo or a leukotriene antagonist. We found insufficient evidence about effects of adding long acting inhaled β_2 agonists on mortality.
- **Low dose, inhaled corticosteroids in mild, persistent asthma** Systematic reviews and RCTs have found that, in people with mild, persistent asthma, low doses of inhaled corticosteroids improve symptoms and lung function compared with placebo or regular inhaled β_2 agonists.
- **Short acting inhaled β_2 agonists as needed for symptom relief (as effective as regular use) in mild to moderate, persistent asthma** One systematic review and one subsequent RCT found no significant difference between regular and as needed short acting inhaled β_2 agonists for clinically important outcomes.
- **Adding leukotriene antagonists in people with mild to moderate, persistent asthma (likely to be better than adding no treatment, but no clear evidence of benefit over adding inhaled corticosteroids)** RCTs in people taking β_2 agonists alone have found that leukotriene antagonists reduce asthma symptoms and β_2 agonist use compared with placebo. One systematic review and three out of nine subsequent RCTs have found that adding leukotriene antagonists increases exacerbations, reduces lung function, and are less effective for symptom control compared with inhaled corticosteroids. The other six RCTs found no significant difference between adding leukotriene antagonists and adding corticosteroids. Two RCTs have found that an inhaled corticosteroid plus a long acting β_2 agonist improved symptoms, lung function, and exacerbations compared with a leukotriene antagonist at 12 weeks.
- **Adding theophylline in people with mild to moderate, persistent asthma poorly controlled by inhaled corticosteroids** One RCT has found that adding theophylline improves peak expiratory flow rate compared with continuing low dose corticosteroids plus placebo after 6 months in people with mild to moderate, persistent asthma that was poorly controlled with inhaled corticosteroids alone. One small RCT found no significant difference in lung function or symptoms between theophylline and formoterol (a long acting β agonist) or between theophylline and zafirlukast (a leukotriene antagonist) after 3 months.

- **Adding leukotriene antagonists plus inhaled corticosteroids in people with mild to moderate, persistent asthma** One systematic review in people taking inhaled corticosteroids found no significant difference between leukotriene antagonists and placebo for exacerbation rates at 4–16 weeks. However, one subsequent RCT in people taking a stable dose of budesonide found that adding montelukast increased asthma free days and decreased nocturnal waking compared with placebo at 16 weeks. One RCT in people taking inhaled corticosteroids found no significant difference between adding montelukast and doubling budesonide in peak expiratory flow rate, daytime symptoms, nocturnal wakening, days with asthma exacerbations, and quality of life.

In people with acute exacerbations of asthma

- **Inhaled corticosteroids for acute asthma (better than placebo)** One systematic review has found that inhaled corticosteroids given in the emergency department reduces hospital admission rates in adults compared with placebo. One systematic review and one subsequent RCT found no significant difference in relapse rates following emergency department discharge between oral and inhaled steroids at 7–10 days. One systematic review found no significant difference in relapse rates between inhaled plus oral corticosteroids and oral corticosteroids alone up to 24 days.
- **Inhaled plus oral corticosteroids for acute asthma (as effective as oral corticosteroid alone)** One systematic review found no significant difference in relapse rates for inhaled plus oral corticosteroid compared with oral corticosteroids up to 24 days.
- **Ipratropium bromide added to β_2 agonists for acute exacerbations** Two systematic reviews and one subsequent RCT have found that ipratropium bromide plus salbutamol improves lung function compared with salbutamol alone and is likely to reduce hospital admission in people with severe acute asthma.
- **Short courses of systemic corticosteroids for acute exacerbations** Two systematic reviews and one subsequent RCT have found that early treatment with systemic corticosteroids reduce admission and relapse rates compared with placebo in people with acute asthma. One systematic review and one small subsequent RCT found no significant difference between oral and inhaled steroids after emergency department discharge in relapse rates at 7–10 days in adults with acute asthma.
- **Spacer devices for delivering inhaled medications from pressurised metered dose inhalers in acute asthma (as good as nebulisers)** One systematic review in people with acute, but not life threatening exacerbations of asthma found no significant difference between β_2 agonists delivered by spacer device compared with nebulisers in rates of hospital admission, time spent in the emergency department, peak expiratory flow rate, or forced expiratory volume in 1 second.
- **Education about acute asthma** One systematic review and one subsequent RCT provided evidence that education to facilitate self management of asthma in adults reduced hospital admission, unscheduled visits to the doctor, and days off work compared with usual care. One subsequent RCT provided insufficient evidence about effects of asthma education on quality of life or social functioning at 6 months.
- **Magnesium sulphate for people with severe acute asthma** We found limited evidence from one systematic review and two subsequent RCTs that intravenous magnesium improved lung function compared with placebo in people with severe acute asthma. One systematic review and three subsequent RCTs found no significant difference between intravenous magnesium sulphate and placebo for hospital admission rates.
- **Mechanical ventilation for people with severe acute asthma** We found no RCTs comparing mechanical ventilation with or without inhaled β_2 agonists versus no mechanical ventilation in people with severe acute asthma. Evidence from cohort studies support its use, although observational studies suggest that ventilation is associated with a high level of morbidity.
- **Oxygen supplementation for acute asthma** We found no systematic review or RCTs of oxygen in acute asthma. However, consensus opinion and pathophysiology suggest that its role is vital in acute asthma.

- **Specialist care for acute exacerbations (more effective than generalist care)** One systematic review found limited evidence that specialist care improved outcomes in people with acute asthma compared with generalist care.
- **Continuous nebulised short acting β_2 agonists for acute asthma (no more effective than intermittent nebulised short acting β_2 agonists)** One systematic review and one subsequent RCT found no significant difference in admission rate between continuous and intermittent nebulised short acting β_2 agonists for hospital admission rates in adults. The subsequent RCT also found no significant difference between continuous and intermittent nebulised short acting β_2 agonists in lung function.
- **Helium–oxygen mixture for acute asthma** One systematic review found no significant difference between helium–oxygen mixture and air or oxygen in pulmonary function tests at 60 minutes for adults and children.
- **Intravenous short acting β_2 agonists for acute asthma (no more effective than nebulised short acting β_2 agonists)** One systematic review found that intravenous delivery of short acting β_2 agonists was no more effective than nebulised delivery in improving peak expiratory flow rate at 60 minutes.

DEFINITION Asthma is characterised by variable airflow obstruction and airway hyperresponsiveness. Symptoms include dyspnoea, cough, chest tightness, and wheezing. The normal diurnal variation of peak expiratory flow rate(G) is increased in people with asthma (see table 1, p 1917). **Chronic asthma** is defined here as asthma requiring maintenance treatment. Asthma is classified differently in the USA and UK (see table 1, p 1917). Where necessary, the text specifies the system of classification used.[1,2] **Acute asthma** is defined here as an exacerbation of underlying asthma requiring urgent treatment.

INCIDENCE/ PREVALENCE Reported prevalence of asthma is increasing worldwide. About 10% of people have suffered an attack of asthma.[3–5] Epidemiological studies have also found marked variations in prevalence in different countries.[6,7]

AETIOLOGY/ RISK FACTORS Most people with asthma are atopic. Exposure to certain stimuli initiates inflammation and structural changes in airways causing airway hyperresponsiveness and variable airflow obstruction, which in turn cause most asthma symptoms. There are a large number of such stimuli; the more important include environmental allergens, occupational sensitising agents, and respiratory viral infections.[8,9]

PROGNOSIS **Chronic asthma:** In people with mild asthma, prognosis is good and progression to severe disease is rare. However, as a group, people with asthma lose lung function faster than those without asthma, although less quickly than people without asthma who smoke.[10] People with chronic asthma can improve with treatment. However, some people (possibly up to 5%) have severe disease that responds poorly to treatment. These people are most at risk of morbidity and death from asthma. **Acute asthma:** About 10–20% of people presenting to the emergency department with asthma are admitted to hospital. Of these, fewer than 10% receive mechanical ventilation.[11,12] Those who are ventilated are at 19-fold increased risk of ventilation for a subsequent episode.[13] It is unusual for people to die unless they have suffered respiratory arrest before reaching hospital.[14] One prospective study of 939 people discharged from emergency care found that 17% (95% CI 14% to 20%) relapsed by 2 weeks.[15]

AIMS OF INTERVENTION To minimise or eliminate symptoms; to maximise lung function; to prevent exacerbations; to minimise the need for medication; to minimise adverse effects of treatment; and to provide enough information and support to facilitate self management of asthma.

OUTCOMES Symptoms (daytime and nocturnal); lung function, in terms of peak expiratory flow rate and forced expiratory volume in 1 second(G); need for rescue medication such as inhaled β_2 agonists; variability of flow rates; activities of daily living; adverse effects of treatment.

METHODS *Clinical Evidence* search and appraisal May 2003.

QUESTION **What are effects of treatments for chronic asthma?**

OPTION **SHORT ACTING INHALED β_2 AGONISTS AS NEEDED IN ADULTS WITH MILD OR MODERATE ASTHMA**

One systematic review and one subsequent RCT found no significant difference between regular and as needed short acting inhaled β_2 agonists for clinically important outcomes.

Benefits: We found one systematic review (search date not reported, 22 crossover RCTs, 8 parallel group RCTs)[16] and one subsequent RCT[17] comparing regular with as needed β_2 agonists. Results from crossover RCTs and parallel group RCTs were analysed separately. Only results from crossover RCTs were suitable for pooling. Most of the included studies did not allow the use of concurrent inhaled corticosteroids. The review found no significant difference between regular and as needed use in morning peak expiratory flow rate (PEFR)Ⓖ (5 crossover RCTs, 437 adults: WMD +2.1 L/minute, 95% CI –9.5 L/minute to +13.6 L/minute). Regular β_2 agonists significantly increased evening PEFR compared with as needed β_2 agonists (6 crossover RCTs, 874 adults: WMD 13.1 L/minute, 95% CI 1.9 L/minute to 24.3 L/minute). As needed β_2 agonists significantly increased diurnal variationⒼ of PEFR compared with regular use (2 crossover RCTs, 170 adults: 4.4%, 95% CI 4.3% to 4.5%) and pre-bronchodilator forced expiratory volume in 1 secondⒼ obtained at clinic visits (303 people: WMD 157 mL, 95% CI 123 mL to 192 mL). Use of rescue bronchodilator was measured in most of the RCTs that used a short acting β_2 agonist as a rescue agent. Results for an average 24 hour period showed that, when bronchodilators were given regularly, significantly less relief bronchodilator was used (2 crossover RCTs, 45 adults: WMD –0.68 puffs/day, 95% CI –1.30 puffs/day to –0.07 puffs/day). Two crossover RCTs (174 adults) identified by the review measured exacerbation rates.[16] They found no significant difference between regular and as needed use of β_2 agonists (SMD +0.10, 95% CI –0.11 to +0.31). One parallel group RCT (117 adults) identified by the review found that as needed use significantly improved symptom control over a 24 hour period compared with regular use (WMD 0.120 units, 95% CI 0.001 units to 0.239 units). No significant differences were found in quality of life.[16] The subsequent RCT (983 people with asthma in a general practice setting, 90% using regular inhaled corticosteroids) compared as needed versus regular salbutamolⒼ (400 μg 4 times daily).[17] It found no significant difference between regular and as needed salbutamol in the rate of exacerbations over 1 year (RR 0.96, 95% CI 0.80 to 1.15) or in morning PEFR (see comment below). Evening PEFR was significantly higher with regular salbutamol (WMD 10.7 L/minute, 95% CI 6.7 L/minute to 14.0 L/minute) and diurnal variation of PEFR was also higher (WMD 3.3%, 95% CI 2.5% to 4.1%).[17]

Harms: The systematic review did not find any significant worsening of airways function after stopping regular treatment with β_2 agonists, and concluded that the small increase in lower airways reactivity with regular treatment was unlikely to be of any clinical importance.[16] Non-experimental studies found an association between increased asthma mortality and overuse of short acting inhaled β_2 agonists.[18–23] However, results of these non-randomised studies should be interpreted with caution because of the risk of confounding by factors other than treatment. Other RCTs found that regular use of inhaled β_2 agonists was associated with transient rebound deterioration in airway hyperresponsiveness after stopping the medication[24] and increased allergen induced bronchoconstriction.[25] Tremor was commonly reported, but tolerance developed with more frequent use.[26]

Comment: In the subsequent RCT, 33% (323/983) of people randomised did not complete the RCT, reducing the power of the RCT to detect a significant difference between regular and as needed salbutamol.[17]

OPTION LOW DOSE INHALED CORTICOSTEROIDS IN PEOPLE WITH MILD, PERSISTENT ASTHMA

Systematic reviews and RCTs have found that, in people with mild, persistent asthma, low doses of inhaled corticosteroids improve symptoms and lung function compared with placebo or regular inhaled β_2 agonists.

Benefits: **Versus placebo:** We found one systematic review (search date 1999, 6 RCTs, 393 people)[27] and six subsequent RCTs (5 in 1026 adults and adolescents, 1 in 7241 people aged 5–66 years)[28–33] of budesonide. We found one systematic review (search date 1999, 9 RCTs, 1800 people)[34] and one subsequent RCT (304 people aged ≥ 12 years)[35] of fluticasone. We found one systematic review (search date 1999, 6 RCTs, 492 people) of beclometasone (beclomethasone).[36] We found five additional RCTs (2187 adults and adolescents with mild, persistent asthma using the US classification; see table 1, p 1917) of low doses of triamcinolone,[37–40] flunisolide,[41] or mometasone.[42] The systematic reviews and RCTs all found that low dose inhaled corticosteroids significantly improved lung function and symptoms, and reduced the need for short acting bronchodilators compared with placebo. The largest systematic review,[34] which compared fluticasone 100 μg daily or more versus placebo, found that fluticasone significantly improved forced expiratory volume in 1 second, morning peak expiratory flow rate (PEFR)Ⓖ, use of inhaled β_2 agonists, and the proportion of people who withdrew because of lack of efficiency compared with placebo over 4–12 weeks (forced expiratory volume in 1 second: WMD 0.41 L, 95% CI 0.35 L to 0.47 L; morning PEFR: WMD 30 L/minute, 95% CI 25 L/minute to 35 L/minute; use of inhaled β_2 agonists: WMD 1.36 puffs/day, 95% CI 1.0 puff/day to 1.7 puffs/day; withdrawal because of lack of efficiency: RR 0.32, 95% CI 0.25 to 0.40).[34] The largest subsequent RCT (7241 children and adults aged 5–66 years with mild asthma, no previous steroids) found that budesonide (400 μg once daily for adults and 200 μg once daily for children aged < 11 years) significantly reduced the risk of a severe asthma related event compared with placebo over a period of about 2.4 years (severe asthma related event defined as needing admission or emergency treatment or death owing to asthma: HR 0.56, 95% CI 0.45 to 0.71).[33] **Versus β_2 agonists:** We found one systematic review (search date not reported; 5 RCTs; 3 comparing inhaled corticosteroids *v* placebo; 2 comparing inhaled corticosteroids *v* β_2 agonists; 141 adults with mild, persistent asthma).[43] The review found that regular inhaled corticosteroids (≤ 2 drugs) significantly improved lung function compared with regular β_2 agonists or placebo (overall weighted effect size for PEFR 0.59, 95% CI 0.32 to 0.84).

Harms: We found one systematic review (search date 2001, 2 RCTs) that examined the effects of inhaled corticosteroids on fracture rate.[44] It found no significant difference between conventional doses of inhaled corticosteroids versus placebo for vertebral fracture rates (OR 1.87, 95% CI 0.50 to 7.03). The second review (search date 1998) assessed the harms of inhaled corticosteroids and found that systemic adverse effects increased with dose.[45] It found that, although posterior subcapsular cataracts occurred more frequently in people taking oral corticosteroids, most studies in adults provided no evidence that inhaled corticosteroids increase the risk once the confounding effect of oral corticosteroid use is removed. The review found no significant effect of inhaled low dose corticosteroids on bruising or skin thickness. The systematic review of fluticasone found that fluticasone significantly increased oral candidiasis compared with placebo (13/653 [2%] with fluticasone *v* 3/645 [0.5%] with placebo; RR 3.45, 95% CI 1.29 to 9.26).[34] The largest subsequent RCT (7241 adults and children) found similar rates of adverse events with budesonide and placebo in adults after about 2.4 years.[33] It found that budesonide significantly restricted growth after 2.4 years compared with placebo in children aged 5–15 years (difference in height increase with budesonide *v* placebo: –0.43 cm/year, 95% CI –0.54 cm/year to –0.32 cm/year).[33]

Comment: Two RCTs have found that inhaled corticosteroids delivered using chlorofluorocarbon free propellants such as hydrofluoroalkane are effective at low doses for people with mild, persistent asthma, but dose equivalence varies with each delivery system.[40,41] The dose of inhaled corticosteroid may need to be adjusted if a chlorofluorocarbon free propellant is used.

OPTION ADDING LONG ACTING INHALED β_2 AGONISTS IN PEOPLE WITH MILD, PERSISTENT ASTHMA THAT IS POORLY CONTROLLED BY INHALED CORTICOSTEROIDS

RCTs have found that, in people with asthma that is poorly controlled with inhaled corticosteroids, adding regular long acting inhaled β_2 agonists improves symptoms and lung function compared with placebo or a leukotriene antagonist. One systematic review and three additional RCTs have found that adding regular doses of long acting inhaled β_2 agonists improves lung function and symptoms, and reduces rescue medication compared with increasing the dose of inhaled corticosteroids. However, one further RCT found that increasing inhaled corticosteroid dose reduced exacerbations compared with adding long acting inhaled β_2 agonists. We found insufficient evidence about effects of adding long acting inhaled β_2 agonists on mortality.

Benefits: **Versus placebo:** We found no systematic review. We found three RCTs (1400 people with moderate, persistent asthma, uncontrolled by inhaled corticosteroids 250–2000 µg daily beclometasone diproprionate or equivalent) comparing regular long acting inhaled β_2 agonists versus placebo.[46–48] The RCTs found that twice daily salmeterol or formoterol (eformoterol) improved quality of life scores, peak expiratory flow rate (PEFR), and forced expiratory volume in 1 second (FEV1) and reduced night wakening compared with placebo. In the largest RCT,[48] salmeterol significantly improved the adjusted mean PEFR and significantly increased the proportion of people who did not awaken at night (PEFR: 398 L/minute with salmeterol *v* 386 L/minute with placebo; $P < 0.001$; no night wakening: 74% with salmeterol *v* 68% with placebo; $P < 0.05$). Exacerbation rates were not significantly different between the two groups in any of the RCTs (AR for severe exacerbations in the largest RCT:[48] 20.8% with salmeterol *v* 20.9% with placebo).

Versus increased use of inhaled corticosteroids: We found one systematic review (search date 1999, 9 double blind RCTs, 3685 people with symptomatic asthma on their current dose of inhaled steroids, duration 3–6 months)[49] and three additional RCTs.[50–52] The review compared adding salmeterol with increased use of inhaled corticosteroids (at least double the usual dose). It found that morning PEFR was significantly higher with salmeterol (3 months: WMD in PEFR 22 L/minute, 95% CI 15 L/minute to 30 L/minute; $P < 0.001$; 6 months: WMD 28 L/minute, 95% CI 19 L/minute to 36 L/minute). Salmeterol significantly increased days and nights without symptoms (WMD at 6 months: days: 15 days, 95% CI 12 days to 18 days; nights: 5 nights, 95% CI 3 nights to 7 nights). Salmeterol also significantly reduced the need for rescue medication. No increase in asthma exacerbations of any severity was found in the salmeterol group.[49] The first additional RCT (852 people taking low to moderate dose inhaled corticosteroids) compared adding formoterol, increasing the dose of inhaled corticosteroids, and increasing the dose of corticosteroids plus adding formoterol.[50] It found that increased dose of corticosteroids significantly reduced severe exacerbations compared with adding formoterol at 1 year (AR 46% with increased corticosteroid *v* 67% with added formoterol; P = 0.03). The second additional RCT (454 people with symptomatic asthma on their current dose of inhaled steroids) compared adding salmeterol 42 μg plus fluticasone 88 μg twice daily versus adding fluticasone 220 μg twice daily.[51] It found that salmeterol plus lower dose fluticasone improved lung function, reduced the use of rescue β_2 agonists, and increased the proportion of symptom free days compared with higher dose fluticasone alone. The third additional RCT (663 symptomatic people aged > 12 years taking low to moderate doses of inhaled corticosteroids) compared budesonide 400 μg plus placebo twice daily versus budesonide 400 μg plus formoterol 9 μg twice daily.[52] It found that adding formoterol significantly improved morning and evening PEFR and improved symptoms at 6 months compared with placebo (morning PEFR difference: 19.0 L/minute, 95% CI 12.3 L/minute to 25.6 L/minute; evening PEFR difference: 15.7 L/minute, 95% CI 9.4 L/minute to 22.1 L/minute; P < 0.001; change in symptom score, on a scale from –2 [improvement] to +2 [worsening]: –0.16 with formoterol *v* +0.01 with placebo; P < 0.001). It found no difference between formoterol and placebo in the proportion of people with a clinically important improvement in quality of life (Mini Asthma Quality of Life questionnaire score improved > 0.5 points: 51% with formoterol *v* 47% with placebo, P value not reported). **Versus addition of leukotriene antagonists:** We found four RCTs.[53–56] The first RCT (948 adults with symptomatic asthma on their current dose of inhaled steroids) compared adding salmeterol 50 μg twice daily versus adding montelukast 10 mg daily.[53] It found that salmeterol significantly increased the proportion of symptom free days, improved lung function, and reduced the need for rescue medication and night time awakenings compared with montelukast (symptom free days: 24% with salmeterol *v* 16% with montelukast; difference 8%). It found no significant difference in the proportion of people with asthma exacerbations (26/476 [6%] with salmeterol *v* 23/472 [5%] with montelukast; RR 1.12, 95% CI 0.65 to 1.93) over 12 weeks. The second small RCT (65 people with moderate, persistent asthma all using moderate or high dose inhaled steroid) compared three treatments: adding long acting β agonist formoterol 9 μg twice daily; adding leukotriene antagonist zafirlukast 20 mg twice daily; and adding a sustained release theophylline.[54] Additional short acting β agonists were allowed. It found no significant difference between adding formoterol and adding zafirlukast for lung function at 3 months (FEV_1 as % of predicted at 3 months: 89.5% with added formoterol *v* 87.3% with added zafirlukast; P > 0.05). However, the study may have lacked power to detect clinically important differences. The third RCT (429 people poorly controlled on inhaled corticosteroids) found no significant difference between adding salmeterol 43 μg twice daily through a metered dose inhaler and adding zafirlukast 20 mg twice daily in FEV_1 at 4 weeks (change from baseline in FEV_1: 0.26 L with salmeterol *v* 0.23 L with zafirlukast).[55] However, it found that salmeterol significantly improved symptom scores and reduced night time wakening compared with zafirlukast at 4 weeks (decrease in symptom scores: 35% with salmeterol *v* 21% with zafirlukast; reduction in nocturnal awakenings: 45% with salmeterol *v* 25% with zafirlukast). The fourth RCT (725 adults poorly controlled on their current dose of inhaled corticosteroids) found that adding a fixed salmeterol 50 μg plus fluticasone 100 μg combination significantly increased morning PEFR, FEV_1, and the chance of a symptom free day or night at 12 weeks compared with fluticasone 100 μg twice daily plus montelukast 10 mg once daily (morning PEFR, mean difference: 15 L/minute, 95% CI 11 L/minute to 20 L/minute; mean difference in FEV_1: 0.11 L, 95% CI 0.06 L to 0.16 L; symptom free day: OR 1.32, 95% CI 1.05 to 1.65; symptom free night: OR 1.28, 95% CI 1.02 to 1.61).[56]

Harms: Several studies have found that people taking regular doses of long acting inhaled β_2 agonists develop tolerance to bronchodilatory effects[57–59] and may develop tremor. Regular use of long acting inhaled β_2 agonists has not been linked to deterioration in asthma control.[48–50]

Comment: We found no RCTs or other studies with sufficient power to assess the effect of regular use of long acting inhaled β_2 agonists on mortality.[60]

OPTION ADDING LEUKOTRIENE ANTAGONISTS ALONE IN PEOPLE WITH MILD TO MODERATE, PERSISTENT ASTHMA

RCTs in people taking β_2 agonists alone have found that leukotriene antagonists reduce asthma symptoms and β_2 agonist use compared with placebo. One systematic review and three out of nine subsequent RCTs have found that adding leukotriene antagonists increases exacerbations, reduces lung function, and are less effective for symptom control compared with inhaled corticosteroids. The other six RCTs found no significant difference between adding leukotriene antagonists and adding corticosteroids in asthma control or lung function. Two RCTs have found that an inhaled corticosteroid plus a long acting β_2 agonist improved symptoms, lung function, and exacerbations compared with a leukotriene antagonist alone at 12 weeks.

Benefits: **Versus placebo:** We found no systematic review. We found five RCTs (1400 adults with asthma taking β_2 agonists alone), which compared adding leukotriene antagonists versus adding placebo for 6–13 weeks.[61–65] The first three RCTs all found that the oral leukotriene antagonist zafirlukast 20 mg twice daily significantly reduced daytime and night time asthma symptoms and β_2 agonist use compared with placebo.[61–63] The first and largest of these RCTs (762 people) found that zafirlukast significantly reduced daytime symptoms, night time awakenings, and β agonist use compared with placebo (daytime symptom score: 8.05 with zafirlukast *v* 9.45 with placebo; $P < 0.01$; night time awakenings: 2.05/week with zafirlukast *v* 2.52/week with placebo; $P < 0.05$; β_2 agonist use: 3.1 puffs/day with zafirlukast *v* 3.0 puffs/day with placebo; $P < 0.01$).[61] Morning forced expiratory volume in 1 second (FEV_1) was significantly increased in people taking zafirlukast (morning FEV_1 improvement: by 7% with zafirlukast *v* 3% with placebo; $P < 0.01$). The fourth and fifth RCTs (730 people[64] and 782 people[65] aged > 15 years taking as needed short acting β_2 agonists alone) compared three treatments: oral montelukast 10 mg once daily, inhaled beclomethasone, and placebo. Both RCTs found that oral montelukast significantly improved asthma control compared with placebo at 6 weeks (% days with < 2 puffs of salbutamol**G**, no nocturnal wakening, and no asthma attack; fourth RCT:[64] 50.7% with montelukast *v* 40% with placebo; $P < 0.05$; fifth RCT:[65] 41.4% with montelukast *v* 26.8% with placebo; $P < 0.001$). **Versus inhaled corticosteroids:** We found one systematic review (search date 2002, 12 RCTs in adults, 2 RCTs in children, FEV_1 > 50% predicted)[66] and nine subsequent RCTs.[64,65,67–73] The review compared leukotriene antagonists (montelukast, pranlukast, zafirlukast) versus inhaled corticosteroids (beclomethasone, fluticasone) for 4–37 weeks.[66] It found that leukotriene antagonists increased risk of asthma exacerbations requiring systemic steroids compared with corticosteroids (all leukotriene antagonists: 11 RCTs; significant heterogeneity among trials; RR 1.61, 95% CI 1.15 to 2.25). The review found no significant difference between leukotriene antagonists and inhaled corticosteroids for hospital admission rates for acute asthma (9 RCTs; RR 1.73, 95% CI 0.64 to 4.73). It also found that leukotriene antagonists reduced symptom free days compared with inhaled corticosteroids at 6 weeks (3 RCTs; WMD 9%, 95% CI 5% to 13%).[66] The first subsequent RCT (533 adults with asthma who were symptomatic on β_2 agonists alone) compared fluticasone versus montelukast for 24 weeks.[67] The second subsequent RCT (294 adults and children > 11 years of age previously treated with β_2 agonists alone) compared fluticasone 88 µg twice daily versus zafirlukast 20 µg twice daily.[68] Both RCTs found no significant difference between leukotriene antagonists and inhaled corticosteroids groups for symptom scores. The third subsequent RCT (522 non-smokers with persistent asthma) found that fluticasone propionate 88 µg twice daily increased lung function and quality of life and decreased symptoms compared with oral montelukast 10 mg daily at 24 weeks (mean improvement in FEV_1: 22% with fluticasone *v* 14% with montelukast; $P < 0.001$; mean improvement in asthma symptom score: 0.91 with fluticasone *v* 0.57 with montelukast; $P < 0.001$; mean increase in symptom free days: 34% with fluticasone *v* 20% with montelukast; $P < 0.001$; mean improvement in asthma quality of life questionnaire score: 1.3 with fluticasone *v* 1.0 with montelukast; $P < 0.001$).[69] The fourth subsequent RCT (440 people aged ≥ 12 years, previously treated with inhaled corticosteroids and short acting β agonists, FEV_1 60–80% of predicted) found that inhaled fluticasone 88 µg twice daily increased lung function and symptom free days at 6 weeks compared with zafirlukast 20 mg twice daily (mean difference in morning FEV_1: 0.16 L, 95% CI 0.08 L to 0.24 L; increase in symptom free days 14%, 95% CI 7% to 21%).[70] The fifth subsequent RCT (45 non-smokers with mild asthma) compared three treatments: budesonide 400 µg twice daily, montelukast 10 mg daily, and budesonide plus montelukast (at the same doses).[71] It found no significant difference between budesonide and montelukast alone for lung function at 16 weeks (increase in FEV_1: 2.1% with budesonide *v* 4.2 with montelukast; increase in forced vital capacity 3.1% with budesonide *v* 5.2% with montelukast; P values not reported). The sixth subsequent RCT (730 adults, aged 15–65 years, baseline FEV_1 50% to 85% of predicted, taking short acting β_2 agonist as needed) compared three treatments: montelukast 10 mg once daily, inhaled beclomethasone 200 µg twice daily, and placebo.[64] It found that beclomethasone significantly improved asthma control compared with montelukast at 6 weeks (% days with < 2 puffs of salbutamol, no nocturnal wakening, and no asthma attack: 50.7% with montelukast *v* 57.9% with beclomethasone; $P < 0.05$). The seventh additional RCT (51 non-smokers, mean age 26 years, baseline FEV_1 94–99% of predicted across treatment groups, taking short acting β_2 agonist as needed) compared four treatments: montelukast 10 mg daily, budesonide 400 µg twice daily, montelukast 10 mg plus budesonide 400 µg twice daily, and budesonide 800 µg twice daily.[72] It found no significant difference between montelukast alone and either dose of budesonide in FEV_1 at 12 weeks (results as % of predicted FEV_1 for baseline to post-treatment: 94.8% to 96.3% with montelukast *v* 99.9% to 100.4% with budesonide 400 µg *v* 99.2% to 98.9% with budesonide 800 µg; P values not reported). The eighth additional RCT (40 adults, mean age 25 years, baseline FEV_1 94% of predicted) compared montelukast 10 mg daily versus budesonide 400 mg twice daily.[73] It found no significant difference between montelukast and budesonide in FEV_1 at 16 weeks (% of predicted FEV_1 for baseline to post-treatment: 95.2% to 96.0% with montelukast *v* 94.7% to 96.7% with budesonide; P value not reported). The ninth additional RCT (782 adults, mean age 33 years, baseline FEV_1 66% of predicted, mean weekly short acting β_2 agonist use > 2 puffs/day) compared three treatments: montelukast 10 mg daily, beclomethasone

200 µg twice daily, and placebo.[65] It found no significant difference between montelukast and beclomethasone in asthma control (% days with < 2 puffs of salbutamol, no nocturnal wakening, and no asthma attack: 41.4% with montelukast *v* 41.1% with beclomethasone; P = 0.93). **Versus inhaled corticosteroids plus long acting β_2 agonists:** We found no systematic review. We found two RCTs.[74,75] The first RCT (423 adults with symptomatic asthma taking short acting β_2 agonists) compared montelukast 20 mg once daily versus fluticasone 100 µg plus salmeterol 50 µg twice daily.[74] It found that adding fluticasone plus salmeterol significantly increased symptom free days and reduced exacerbations compared with adding montelukast alone at 12 weeks (increase in symptom free days from baseline: 22% with montelukast *v* 49% with fluticasone plus salmeterol; WMD 27%, 95% CI 20% to 35%; exacerbations: 11 with montelukast *v* 0 with fluticasone plus salmeterol; P < 0.001). The second RCT (432 people aged ≥ 15 years with persistent asthma, symptomatic on short acting β agonists) found that fluticasone 100 µg twice daily plus salmeterol 50 µg twice daily significantly increased lung function and reduced symptoms compared with oral montelukast 10 mg once daily at 12 weeks (increase in FEV_1: 27% with fluticasone plus salmeterol *v* 13% with montelukast; P < 0.001; increase in symptom free days: 40% with fluticasone plus salmeterol *v* 27% with montelukast; P < 0.017).[75]

Harms: **Versus placebo:** In the RCT comparing zafirlukast versus placebo, the incidence of adverse effects (predominantly pharyngitis and headache) was similar in both groups (350/514 [68%] with zafirlukast *v* 160/248 [65%] with placebo).[62] **Versus inhaled corticosteroids:** The systematic review found that leukotriene antagonists significantly increased the risk of "withdrawals for any cause" but there was no significant difference between treatments in withdrawal rates owing to adverse effects (12 RCTs; RR 1.2, 95% CI 0.9 to 1.7).[66] One RCT found no significant difference between fluticasone and montelukast in adverse event rate.[69] One RCT found no significant difference between fluticasone and zafirlukast in adverse event rate (7% with fluticasone *v* 4% with zafirlukast; P = 0.14).[70] It found that the most common adverse events were headache (2% for both fluticasone and zafirlukast), nausea (1% for fluticasone), and hoarseness (1% for fluticasone). The sixth RCT found similar adverse effects between montelukast and beclomethasone (headache: 10% with montelukast *v* 11% with beclomethasone; upper respiratory infection: 7% with montelukast *v* 10% with beclomethasone; P value not reported).[64] The seventh and eighth RCTs found similar adverse effect rates between montelukast and budesonide.[72,73] The ninth RCT found no difference between montelukast and beclomethasone in upper respiratory infection, headache, or sinusitis (no data reported).[65]

Comment: One systematic review (search date 2000) identified 22 cases of the Churg–Strauss Syndrome associated with antileukotriene treatment, but the total number of people exposed was not reported.[76]

OPTION ADDING LEUKOTRIENE ANTAGONISTS PLUS INHALED CORTICOSTEROIDS IN PEOPLE WITH MILD TO MODERATE, PERSISTENT ASTHMA

One systematic review in people taking inhaled corticosteroids found no significant difference between leukotriene antagonists and placebo for exacerbation rates at 4–16 weeks. However, one subsequent RCT in people taking a stable dose of budesonide found that adding montelukast increased asthma free days and decreased nocturnal waking compared with placebo at

16 weeks. One RCT in people taking inhaled corticosteroids found no significant difference between adding montelukast and doubling budesonide in peak expiratory flow rate, daytime symptoms, nocturnal wakening, days with asthma exacerbations, and quality of life.

Benefits: **Versus placebo in people taking inhaled corticosteroids:** We found one systematic review (search date 2001, 12 RCTs in adults, 1 RCT in children with symptomatic asthma on their current dose of inhaled steroids)[77] and one subsequent RCT.[78] The systematic review found no significant different between licensed doses of leukotriene antagonists (montelukast 5 or 10 mg/day, pranlukast 450 mg/day, zafirlukast 80 mg/day) and placebo for exacerbations requiring systemic steroids at 4–16 weeks (2 RCTs: 20/466 [4%] with leukotriene antagonists *v* 33/468 [7%] with placebo; RR 0.61, 95% CI 0.36 to 1.05).[77] The subsequent RCT (639 non-smokers aged 18–70 years, on stable dose of budesonide 400–1600 μg daily or equivalent, baseline forced expiratory volume in 1 second [FEV_1**G**] 81% of predicted) compared adding montelukast 10 mg once daily versus placebo for 16 weeks.[78] It found that montelukast significantly increased asthma free days and decreased nocturnal waking compared with placebo (asthma free days: 66.1% with montelukast *v* 42.3% with placebo; difference 23.8%, 95% CI 10.9% to 41.2%; difference in decrease in nocturnal wakening: 6.6%, 95% CI 1.9% to 13.7%). It found no significant difference between montelukast and placebo in daytime asthma symptoms or change in FEV_1 (difference in symptom score, on a scale from 0 [least severe] to 24 [most severe]: –0.09, 95% CI –0.19 to +0.01; difference in change in morning FEV_1: +0.14%, 95% CI –2.47% to +2.75%). **Versus increasing inhaled steroids:** We found one RCT (889 non-smokers, aged 15–75 years, poorly controlled with budesonide 800 μg daily, baseline FEV_1 69% predicted), which compared adding montelukast 10 mg daily versus doubling the dose of budesonide to 1600 μg daily for 12 weeks.[79] It found no significant difference between adding montelukast and doubled budesonide dose in peak expiratory flow rate**G**, daytime symptoms, nocturnal waking, days with asthma exacerbations, and quality of life (mean increase peak expiratory flow rate: 33.5 L/minute with montelukast *v* 30.1 L/minute with doubled budesonide; difference +3.4 L/minute, 95% CI –12.9 L/minute to +4.8 L/minute; change in daytime symptom score, on a scale from 0 [least severe] to 24 [most severe]: –0.34 with montelukast *v* –0.35 with budesonide; P = 0.91; change in number of nights with nocturnal waking: 12.3% to 2.3% with montelukast *v* 13.8% to 3.9% with budesonide; P = 0.35; median days with exacerbations: 6.7% with montelukast *v* 6.3% with budesonide; P = 0.78; AR for increase in quality of life by ≥ 0.5 points: about 43% with montelukast *v* about 40% with budesonide; P value not reported). **Versus long acting β_2 agonist in people taking inhaled corticosteroids:** See benefits of addition of long acting inhaled β_2 agonists in people with mild, persistent asthma that is poorly controlled by inhaled corticosteroids, p 1897.

Harms: **Versus placebo in people taking inhaled corticosteroids:** The systematic review found that leukotriene antagonists (given at a higher than licensed dose) significantly increased the risk of liver enzyme elevation compared with placebo (13/280 [5%] with leukotriene antagonists *v* 2/276 [0.7%] with placebo; RR 5.36, 95% CI 1.40 to 20.40).[77] The first subsequent RCT found similar adverse effects between montelukast 10 mg once daily and placebo.[78] The most common adverse effects were influenza (11% with both treatments), headache (9% with montelukast *v* 11% with placebo), upper respiratory tract infection (5% with montelukast *v* 7% with placebo), and worsening asthma (7% with montelukast *v* 5% with placebo). **Versus increasing**

inhaled steroids: The RCT comparing added montelukast versus doubled dose of budesonide found no significant difference between treatments in adverse effects at 12 weeks.[79] It found that the most common adverse effects were upper respiratory infection, worsening asthma, and headache (no data reported).

Comment: None.

OPTION THEOPHYLLINE IN PEOPLE WITH MILD TO MODERATE, PERSISTENT ASTHMA POORLY CONTROLLED BY INHALED CORTICOSTEROIDS

Rodolfo Dennis and Ivan Solarte

One RCT has found that adding theophylline improves peak expiratory flow rate compared with continuing low dose corticosteroids plus placebo after 6 months in people with mild to moderate, persistent asthma that was poorly controlled with inhaled corticosteroids alone. One small RCT found no significant difference in lung function or symptoms between theophylline and formoterol (a long acting β agonist) or between theophylline and zafirlukast (a leukotriene antagonist) after 3 months.

Benefits: **Versus placebo:** We found one RCT (155 people with persistent asthma that was poorly controlled with inhaled corticosteroids) which compared three treatments: continuing low dose inhaled corticosteroids 200 μg twice daily plus placebo, continuing low dose inhaled corticosteroids 200 μg twice daily plus slow release theophylline 200 mg twice daily, and high dose inhaled corticosteroids (500 μg twice daily).[80] It found that continuing low dose corticosteroids plus theophylline improved morning and evening peak expiratory flow rate (PEFR) Ⓖ compared with continuing low dose corticosteroids plus placebo after 6 months (mean change in morning PEFR: +4.4 L/minute with corticosteroids plus placebo *v* +21.8 L/minute with corticosteroids plus theophylline; P value not reported; mean change in evening PEFR: 1.9 L/minute with corticosteroids plus placebo *v* 22.5 L/minute with corticosteroids plus theophylline; P value not reported). **Versus leukotriene antagonists:** We found one RCT (64 people with moderate, persistent asthma not well controlled using budesonide daily doses > 800 μg), which compared adding theophylline, zafirlukast, or inhaled formoterol.[54] It found no significant difference between theophylline and zafirlukast in lung function at 3 months (mean improvement in force expiratory volume in 1 second [FEV_1] [% predicted]: 20.7% with adding zafirlukast *v* 21.4% with adding theophylline; P value not reported). It found no significant difference between theophylline and zafirlukast in decrease in daily PEFR variability, daytime or night time asthma symptoms, or in mean number of rescue inhalations after 3 months. The RCT did not present results for asthma exacerbations. **Versus long acting β_2 agonists:** We found one RCT (64 people with moderate, persistent asthma that was poorly controlled with inhaled budesonide > 800 μg/day), which compared three added treatments: theophylline, zafirlukast, and inhaled formoterol.[54] It found no significant difference between theophylline and formoterol in improvement in FEV_1, decrease in daily PEFR variability, daytime or night time asthma symptoms, or in mean number or rescue medications after 3 months (mean improvement in % predicted FEV_1: +21.4% with theophylline *v* +22.9% with formoterol; P > 0.05, CI not reported). No asthma exacerbations in the study period were reported.

Harms: **Versus placebo:** The RCT found no significant differences between low dose steroids, low dose steroids plus theophylline, and high dose inhaled steroids in any common self reported adverse effect (dyspepsia, nausea, dry mouth, headache, coughing, bronchitis, coryza, pharyngitis; $P > 0.05$ for all between group comparisons).[80] **Versus leukotriene antagonists or long acting β_2 agonists:** In the RCT,[54] adverse events, most commonly headache and dyspepsia, were more common with leukotriene than with theophylline (31% with leukotriene antagonists *v* 20% with theophylline, P value not reported), although event rates were the same for theophylline and long acting β_2 agonists (20%). There were no withdrawals because of adverse events in any group.[54]

Comment: The search performed also found two systematic reviews comparing theophylline with long acting β_2 agonists. These reviews included RCTs in people where inhaled steroid use was not required, not well standardised, or not optimally titrated before study randomisation. We, therefore, excluded these reviews. We identified one study comparing oral theophylline versus inhaled formoterol and this will be considered for inclusion when it is translated.[81]

QUESTION What are the effects of treatments for acute asthma?

J Mark FitzGerald

OPTION SPACER DEVICES/HOLDING CHAMBERS FOR DELIVERING β_2 AGONISTS IN ACUTE ASTHMA

One systematic review found no significant difference in forced expiratory volume in 1 second, peak expiratory flow rate, rates of hospital admission, or time spent in the emergency department between nebuliser and spacer devices for delivering β_2 agonists in people with acute but not life threatening asthma.

Benefits: We found one systematic review (search date 1999, 13 RCTs, non-hospitalised adults and children with acute asthma) comparing holding chambers plus metered dose inhalers with nebulisers for delivering β_2 agonists.[82] Results in adults and children were analysed separately (see asthma and other wheezing disorders of childhood, p 239). In adults, there was no significant difference in rates of hospital admission, length of time spent in the emergency department, or in peak expiratory flow rate and forced expiratory volume in 1 second (FEV_1) (hospital admission: OR 1.12, 95% CI 0.45 to 2.76: time in the emergency department: WMD +0.02 hours, 95% CI –0.40 hours to +0.44 hours). There was still no significant difference when the three RCTs involving the most severely affected people ($FEV_1 < 30\%$ predicted) were included (WMD for FEV_1 holding chamber *v* nebuliser –1.5% predicted, 95% CI –8.3% to +5.3%). Symptoms were measured on different scales and findings could not be combined.

Harms: The review found no significant difference in heart rates between holding chambers and nebulisers (WMD with holding chamber *v* nebuliser +1.6% of baseline, 95% CI –2.4% of baseline to +5.5% of baseline).[82]

Comment: The review found no evidence of publication bias.[82] To overcome possible dose confounding, the review was confined to studies that used multiple treatment doses titrated against the individuals' responses. As studies excluded people with life threatening asthma❻, results may not generalise to such people.

OPTION SYSTEMIC CORTICOSTEROIDS FOR ACUTE ASTHMA

Two systematic reviews and one subsequent RCT have found that early treatment with systemic corticosteroids reduce admission and relapse rates compared with placebo in people with acute asthma. One systematic review and one small subsequent RCT found no significant difference between oral and inhaled steroids after emergency department discharge in relapse rates at 7–10 days in adults with acute asthma.

Benefits: **Versus placebo:** We found two systematic reviews[83,84] and one subsequent RCT.[85] The first review (search date 1991, 5 RCTs, 422 people) found that early use of systemic corticosteroids (oral, iv, or im) significantly reduced hospital admissions compared with placebo in the emergency department (OR 0.47, 95% CI 0.27 to 0.79; no significant heterogeneity among RCTs; P = 0.72).[83] The second review (search date 2001, 7 RCTs, about 320 people) compared systematic steroids (im and oral) versus placebo after discharge from the emergency department.[84] It found that systemic corticosteroids significantly reduced relapse at 7–10 days and hospital readmissions within 7 days compared with placebo (relapse rates 5 RCTs, 345 people: RR 0.35, 95% CI 0.17 to 0.73; NNT 13, 95% CI 7 to 91; hospital readmissions 4 RCTs, 210 people: RR 0.32, 95% CI 0.11 to 0.94; NNT 16, 95% CI 7 to 125; no significant heterogeneity was found). Corticosteroids significantly reduced the use of β_2 agonists (WMD –3.3 puffs/day, 95% CI –5.5 puffs/day to –1.0 puff/day). The review found no clear difference between intramuscular and oral corticosteroids.[84] The subsequent RCT (259 adults and children, all given nebulised salbutamol**G** for 5–20 minutes 1–3 times) compared single dose oral prednisolone (30 mg if aged < 5 years or 60 mg if > 5 years) versus placebo given in the emergency room or outpatient department.[85] It found that oral prednisolone significantly reduced hospital admission rate compared with placebo (37/140 [26%] with prednisolone *v* 50/119 [42%] with placebo; P < 0.01). **Versus inhaled steroids:** We found two systematic reviews[86,87] and one small subsequent RCT.[88] The first review (search date 2000) found four RCTs in children but no RCTs in adults (see asthma and other wheezing disorders of childhood, p 239).[86] The second review (search date 2001, 4 RCTs, 772 adults and 22 children) compared oral corticosteroids (prednisone) versus high dose inhaled corticosteroids (≥ 2 mg daily beclomethasone dipropionate or equivalent) in people with acute asthma after emergency department discharge.[87] It found no significant difference between oral and inhaled steroids for relapse rate at 7–10 days (OR relapse 1.00, 95% CI 0.66 to 1.52; no significant heterogeneity among trials; P = 0.88). We found one small subsequent RCT (40 adults aged 18–55 years with asthma exacerbation requiring hospital admission, peak expiratory flow rate**G** < 50% of predicted while in emergency department).[88] Treatment for the first 48 hours was with regular nebulised and then inhaled salbutamol plus methylprednisolone 40 mg intravenously every 6 hours for eight doses. Then people were randomised to inhaled flunisolide (8 puffs twice daily, 250 μg/puff) or oral prednisone 40 mg daily for 7 days. It found no significant difference between inhaled and oral steroids in force expiratory volume in 1 second or symptoms (change in force expiratory volume in 1 second**G**, baseline to 7 days: 1.6 L to 1.3 L with inhaled *v* 1.6 L to 2.3 L with oral steroids; P = 0.33; change in symptoms scores [no details of scoring system reported]: 1.4 to 0.7 with inhaled *v* 1.3 to 0.4 with oral steroids; P = 0.39).

Harms: Systemic corticosteroids can cause the same adverse effects in asthma as in other diseases, even when given for a short time (see asthma and other wheezing disorders of childhood, p 239).

Comment: One RCT (413 adults presenting to general practitioners with acute asthma) found no difference in rates of treatment failure with a short course of oral corticosteroids versus a high dose of inhaled fluticasone.[89] **Stopping treatment:** We found no systematic review but found 1 RCT (35 people admitted to hospital with acute asthma who received 40 mg prednisone for 10 days).[90] It found no significant difference in morning peak expiratory flow rate between tapering of prednisone over 1 week and abrupt stopping (mean increase in peak expiratory flow rate: 45 L/minute with tapering *v* 43 L/minute with abrupt stopping; P = 0.82).[90] **Optimal dose and duration of treatment:** We found no systematic review. One RCT (20 people) compared 1 week with 2 weeks of oral prednisone after a 3 day course of intravenous methylprednisolone and found no difference in peak expiratory flow rate and relapse rates.[91] A second RCT (47 people, 41 analysed) compared 5 versus 10 days of oral prednisolone in people who had been hospitalised with acute asthma.[92] It found no significant difference in lung function. All three RCTs may have been too small to detect a clinically important difference. The optimal duration of treatment is likely to depend on the individual, the severity of the exacerbation, and use of concomitant medications.

OPTION INHALED CORTICOSTEROIDS FOR ACUTE ASTHMA

One systematic review has found that inhaled corticosteroids given in the emergency department reduces hospital admission rates in adults compared with placebo. One systematic review and one subsequent RCT found no significant difference in relapse rates following emergency room discharge between oral and inhaled steroids at 7–10 days. One systematic review found no significant difference in relapse rates between inhaled plus oral corticosteroids and oral corticosteroids alone up to 24 days.

Benefits: **Versus placebo:** We found one systematic review (search date 2001, 3 RCTs, 188 adults).[93] It found that inhaled corticosteroids given in the emergency department significantly reduced admission rates compared with placebo in people with acute asthma (OR 0.38, 95% 0.18 to 0.79). **Versus systemic steroids:** See benefits of systemic corticosteroids, p 1905. **Plus oral corticosteroids versus oral corticosteroids alone:** We found one systematic review (search date 1999, 3 RCTs, 909 adults).[94] It found no significant difference between inhaled plus oral corticosteroids and oral corticosteroids alone in relapse rates at day 7–10 or day 20–24 (day 7–10: OR 0.72, 95% CI 0.48 to 1.10; day 20–24: OR 0.68, 95% CI, 0.46 to 1.02).[94]

Harms: The reviews found no significant differences in adverse effects between the groups, but one review commented that most of the RCTs identified gave little information on adverse effects apart from reporting that they were "rare".[94] See also harms of inhaled corticosteroids under asthma and other wheezing disorders of childhood, p 239.

Comment: None.

OPTION CONTINUOUS NEBULISED SHORT ACTING β_2 AGONISTS FOR ACUTE ASTHMA

One systematic review and one subsequent RCT found no significant difference in admission rates between continuous and intermittent nebulised short acting β_2 agonists for hospital admission rates in adults. The subsequent RCT also found no significant difference between continuous and intermittent nebulised short acting β_2 agonists in lung function.

Benefits: We found one systematic review (search date 2001, 6 RCTs, 393 adults)[95] and one additional RCT.[96] The review found no significant difference in admission rate between 1 hour of continuous and 2 hours of intermittent nebulised salbutamol**G** (2.5–16 mg in first hour) after 1–3 hours (2 RCTs, 80 adults, hospital admission rate: RR 0.68, 95% CI 0.33 to 1.38).[95] The included RCTs also used systemic steroids. The subsequent RCT similarly found no significant difference in lung function or rate of hospital admission between continuous and intermittent nebulised salbutamol.[96]

Harms: Commonly reported mild adverse effects associated with frequent dosing include tachycardia, tremor, and headache. Metabolic abnormalities are less common and include hypokalaemia. One RCT included in the review found the highest rate of adverse effects with high dose intermittent treatment. The most common adverse effect was tremor (24% with intermittent high dose *v* 20% with continuous high dose *v* 9% with hourly standard dose *v* 3% with continuous standard dose).[97]

Comment: We found one RCT (46 adults in hospital), which addressed the slightly different, but related, question of regular nebulised salbutamol (5 mg every 4 hours) versus on demand salbutamol 2.5–5 mg.[98] It found that on demand dosage significantly reduced hospital stay, the proportion of nebulisations and palpitations (hospital stay: 3.7 days with on demand salbutamol *v* 4.7 days with regular salbutamol); proportion of nebulisations: geometric mean 7.0 with on demand salbutamol *v* 14 with regular salbutamol, P = 0.003; palpitations: P = 0.05).

OPTION INTRAVENOUS SHORT ACTING β_2 AGONISTS FOR ACUTE ASTHMA

One systematic review found that intravenous delivery of short acting β_2 agonists was no more effective than nebulised delivery in improving peak expiratory flow rate at 60 minutes.

Benefits: We found one systematic review (search date not reported, 6 RCTs, 337 people) comparing intravenous with inhaled short acting β_2 agonists.[99] Five of the RCTs used nebulised delivery of inhaled β_2 agonists, and one used intermittent positive pressure breathing. It found that intravenous β_2 agonists lowered peak expiratory flow rate**G** at 60 minutes compared with inhaled, but the difference was not significant (WMD +24.7 L/minute, 95% CI –2.9 L/minute to +52 L/minute). It found no significant difference in heart rate at 60 minutes between intravenous and inhaled β_2 agonists (WMD +4.5 beats/minute, 95% CI –4.9 beats/minute to +14 beats/minute).

Harms: The systematic review found that intravenous β_2 agonists significantly reduced the proportion of people with autonomic adverse effects (including palpitations, tachycardia, hypertension, tremor, headache, nausea, and vomiting) compared with inhaled β_2 agonists (53/153 [35%] with intravenous *v* 76/144 [53%] with inhaled; OR 0.38, 95% CI 0.22 to 0.65).[99] However the review found significant heterogeneity between the studies for this analysis, so the harms findings should be interpreted with caution.

Comment: One systematic review (search date 2000, 15 RCTs) compared intravenous β_2 agonists with inhaled β_2 agonists or aminophylline but did not compare intravenous with inhaled β_2 agonists alone.[100] It found no significant difference between treatments in peak expiratory flow rate at 6 hours (7 RCTs, WMD: –3.4, 95% CI –21.6 to +14.7).[100]

OPTION **IPRATROPIUM BROMIDE ADDED TO β_2 AGONISTS IN ACUTE ASTHMA**

Two systematic reviews and one subsequent RCT have found that ipratropium bromide plus salbutamol improves lung function compared with salbutamol alone and is likely to reduce hospital admission in people with severe acute asthma.

Benefits: We found two systematic reviews[101,102] and one subsequent RCT.[103] The first systematic review (search date 1999, 10 RCTs, 1483 people) found that inhaled ipratropium plus salbutamol**G** significantly reduced hospital admissions compared with salbutamol alone (5 RCTs, 1186 people; OR 0.62, 95% CI 0.44 to 0.88; NNT 18, 95% CI 11 to 77).[101] Meta-analysis of the four RCTs that evaluated people with severe airflow obstruction (forced expiratory volume in 1 second [FEV_1] < 35%) found that additional treatment with ipratropium significantly improved FEV_1 over 90 minutes (effect size: 0.38, 95% CI 0.05 to 0.67). The second systematic review (search date 1997, 10 RCTs, including 8 identified by the later reviews, 1377 people) found that adding ipratropium bromide improved lung function compared with adding salbutamol alone. It also found no significant difference in hospital admissions, when assessing the same three RCTs.[102] The subsequent RCT (180 people with acute asthma, mean FEV_1 < 50%) compared salbutamol plus placebo versus salbutamol plus ipratropium.[103] It found that adding ipratropium significantly improved peak expiratory flow rate**G** (difference in improvement with ipratropium *v* placebo: 21%, 95% CI 3% to 38%) and FEV_1 (difference in improvement with ipratropium *v* placebo: 48%, 95% CI 20% to 76%). People taking ipratropium were significantly less likely to require hospital admission at the end of the 3 hour trial period (20% with ipratropium *v* 39% with placebo; P = 0.01).

Harms: The reviews[101,102] and the subsequent RCT[103] found no significant difference in adverse effects with the addition of ipratropium to salbutamol versus salbutamol alone.

Comment: The authors of the second systematic review stated that only three RCTs reported data in sufficient detail to be included in the analysis of hospital admission rates.[102]

OPTION **OXYGEN SUPPLEMENTATION FOR ACUTE ASTHMA**

We found no systematic review or RCTs of oxygen in acute asthma. However, consensus opinion and pathophysiology suggest that its role is vital in acute asthma. One systematic review found no significant difference between helium–oxygen mixture and air or oxygen in pulmonary function tests at 60 minutes for adults and children.

Benefits: **Oxygen alone:** We found no systematic review or RCTs. **Plus helium versus air or oxygen:** We found one systematic review (search date 2002, 8 RCTs, adults and children aged 16 months to 55 years with acute asthma) that compared any mixture of helium plus oxygen (heliox) versus air/oxygen mixtures.[104] Co-interventions included nebulised bronchodilators with and without steroids. It found no significant difference between helium plus oxygen and air/oxygen in peak expiratory flow rate**G** within the first hour (overall WMD, 4 RCTs, 278 people: +3%, 95% CI −2% to +8%). It found no significant difference in peak expiratory flow rate between helium plus oxygen and air/oxygen whether or not nebulised salbutamol**G** was used (WMD, 2 RCTs using nebulised salbutamol, 244 people: –0.03, 95% CI –6.43 to +6.37; WMD in 2 RCTs not using nebulised salbutamol, 34 people: +7.36, 95% CI –1.18 to +15.90). It found that helium plus oxygen slightly improved dyspnoea compared with air/oxygen (WMD in Dyspnoea Index, 2 RCTs, 34 people: 0.60, 95% CI 0.04 to 1.16).

Harms: We found no evidence of adverse effects associated with oxygen alone. **Plus helium versus air or oxygen:** The systematic review (search date 2000) did not report harms.[104] One RCT identified by the review found that one person became hypoxic with 70 : 30 helium : oxygen mixture and another RCT found one person with dizziness with helium.[104]

Comment: The most severe stages of acute asthma are respiratory failure, cardiopulmonary arrest, and death.[12,13] Studies of near fatal asthma suggest that hypoxia rather than arrhythmia account for asthma deaths. It seems reasonable that supplemental oxygen should continue to form a critical part of management even though we found no RCTs providing direct evidence for this. Peak flow readings vary depending on the viscosity of the gas being delivered (helium is less dense than oxygen so non-standardised measures of peak flow will increase relative to air, even if the mixture has no effect on airway narrowing). It was not clear in all RCTs whether peak flow readings were standardised for air and for helium–oxygen mixtures. Evidence for routine use of heliox as a therapeutic option in its own right is currently lacking.

OPTION MAGNESIUM SULPHATE FOR ACUTE ASTHMA

We found limited evidence from one systematic review and two subsequent RCTs that intravenous magnesium improved lung function compared with placebo in people with severe acute asthma. One systematic review and three subsequent RCTs found no significant difference between intravenous magnesium sulphate and placebo for hospital admission rates.

Benefits: **Intravenous magnesium sulphate:** We found one systematic review (search date 1998, 5 RCTs in adults, 2 RCTs in children, 665 people)[105] and three subsequent RCTs.[106–108] The review found no significant difference between intravenous magnesium sulphate and placebo in hospital admission rates (OR 0.31, 95% CI 0.09 to 1.02; significant heterogeneity among trials). Prespecified subgroup analysis of adults with more severe airflow obstruction (5 RCTs, sample size not given; forced expiratory volume in 1 second [FEV_1] < 30% at presentation, failure to respond to initial treatment, or failure to improve beyond 60% in FEV_1 after 1 hour) found magnesium sulphate significantly improved peak expiratory flow rate**G** and reduced rates of hospital admission compared with placebo (hospital admission rates: OR 0.10, 95% CI 0.04 to 0.27, no significant heterogeneity; P > 0.1).[105] The first subsequent RCT (33 evaluable people) found no significant difference in hospital admissions between intravenous magnesium sulphate and placebo (18% with magnesium sulphate *v* 25% with placebo; RR 0.71, 95% CI 0.19 to 2.67).[106] The second subsequent RCT (42 people with acute asthma receiving inhaled bronchodilators and iv corticosteroids) found that intravenous magnesium sulphate significantly improved peak expiratory flow rate (PEFR) at 60 minutes compared with placebo. However, it did not reduce the proportion of people admitted to hospital (PEFR: 174 L/minute with placebo *v* 212 L/minute with magnesium sulphate; P = 0.04; hospital admission: 5/18 [28%] with magnesium sulphate *v* 5/24 [21%] with placebo; RR 1.33, 95% CI 0.45 to 3.92).[107] The third subsequent RCT (248 adults, FEV_1 ≤ 30% predicted, all previously treated with methylprednisolone and nebulised salbutamol**G**) found that intravenous magnesium sulphate (2 g iv given in the emergency department) significantly improved lung function at

4 hours (mean difference in FEV_1: 4.7% predicted, 95% CI 0.3% to 9.3%; P = 0.045). However, it found no significant difference in hospital admission rates compared with placebo; hospital admission rates (39/122 [32%] with magnesium sulphate v 41/126 [32%] with placebo; P value not reported).[108] **Nebulised magnesium sulphate:** We found one RCT (35 people) that compared salbutamol plus 0.9% sodium chloride with salbutamol plus magnesium sulphate through a nebuliser.[109] It found that magnesium sulphate significantly increased PEFR compared with 0.9% sodium chloride (increase in PEFR after 10 minutes: 61% with magnesium sulphate v 31% with sodium chloride; difference 30%, 95% CI 3% to 56%; P = 0.03).

Harms: The RCTs did not specifically address harms.

Comment: Further studies are needed to clarify the role of intravenous magnesium sulphate in acute asthma. Two of the studies involved treatment with aminophylline and one with ipratropium, both of which have been found to affect hospital admission rates without affecting the degree of airflow obstruction.[110] The subgroup analysis in the systematic review and larger RCTs involved intergroup and intragroup analyses specified before the trial was conducted, and so provides reasonably strong evidence of an effect.

OPTION MECHANICAL VENTILATION FOR SEVERE ACUTE ASTHMA

We found no RCTs comparing mechanical ventilation with or without inhaled β_2 agonists versus no mechanical ventilation in people with severe acute asthma. Evidence from cohort studies support its use, although ventilation is associated with a high level of morbidity.

Benefits: **Versus no ventilation:** We found no systematic review or RCTs. **Plus inhaled β agonists versus mechanical ventilation:** We found one systematic review (search date 2001) that evaluated the role of inhaled β agonists for asthma in mechanically ventilated people.[111] It found no RCTs.

Harms: Mechanical ventilation is associated with hypotension, barotrauma, infection, and myopathy, especially when prolonged paralysis is required with muscle relaxants and systemic corticosteroids.[112] Adverse effects reported in one retrospective study of 88 episodes of mechanical ventilation were hypotension (20%), pulmonary barotrauma (14%), and arrhythmia (10%).[113]

Comment: Experience suggests that mechanical ventilation is a life saving intervention needed by a small minority of people with severe acute asthma. Cohort studies[114,115] and one case series[116] found fewer deaths with controlled hypoventilation compared with ventilation in which carbon dioxide levels were normalised (for which historical cohorts and case series have reported mortality of 7.5–23.0%).[113,117–119] Non-invasive ventilation has been used in people with acute exacerbations of chronic obstructive lung disease,[120] but requires prospective validation in people with acute asthma. Future research should also focus on delivery of bronchodilators, optimal use of muscle relaxants, and dose of corticosteroids.

OPTION SPECIALIST VERSUS GENERALIST CARE FOR ACUTE ASTHMA

One systematic review found limited evidence that specialist care improved outcomes in people with acute asthma compared with generalist care.

Benefits: We found one systematic review (search date 1995, 2 RCTs in adults and 2 RCTs in children, 10 observational studies).[121] It found limited evidence that specialist care improved outcomes compared with generalist care and that shared care**G** is as effective as usual outpatient care.[121] The first RCT of adults in the review (801 people attending a UK outpatient clinic) excluded people with severe asthma.[121] It found no significant difference between integrated care and regular outpatient care for most outcomes at 12 months (use of medication, primary care consultation, hospital admissions, restrictions on normal activity, psychological morbidity, patient satisfaction). The second RCT (245 adults admitted to emergency departments in the USA) found a significant reduction in emergency room visits at 2 weeks when educational information was provided by a nurses who themselves had asthma compared with nurses who did not have asthma.[121]

Harms: The review did not report on harms of specialist compared with generalist care.[121]

Comment: Many of the RCTs and observational studies in the systematic review were small.[121] One non-systematic review of RCTs and observational studies found that "expert based" care improved outcomes compared with general care.[122] One quasi-randomised trial (based on day of attendance) identified by the non-systematic review referred people from the emergency department either to specialist care or routine general medical follow up.[123] It found that people receiving specialist care were significantly less likely to wake at night (OR 0.24, 95% CI 0.11 to 0.52), suffer relapse requiring emergency admission by 6 months (for 1 admission RR 0.56, 95% CI 0.34 to 0.95; for 2 admissions RR 0.30, 95% CI 0.16 to 0.60), or suffer multiple relapses. They were more likely to use inhaled corticosteroids (OR 3.6, 95% CI 1.9 to 6.6) and sodium cromoglycate (RR 2.2, 95% CI 1.9 to 2.5).

OPTION EDUCATION ABOUT ACUTE ASTHMA

One systematic review and one subsequent RCT provided evidence that education to facilitate self management of asthma in adults reduced hospital admission, unscheduled visits to the doctor, and days off work compared with usual care. One subsequent RCT provided insufficient evidence about effects of asthma education on quality of life or social functioning at 6 months.

Benefits: We found one systematic review (search date 2002, 36 RCTs, 6090 people)[124] and two subsequent RCTs.[125,126] The included studies compared the following types of self management with usual care: optimal self management (including a written action plan for self management of medications for exacerbations), plus self monitoring plus regular medical review; self monitoring plus regular review; self monitoring only; regular review only; and written action plan but not optimal self management. Included studies recruited people from hospital, emergency room, outpatient clinic, general practice, and the community. It found that self management education reduced hospital admissions, emergency room visits, unscheduled visits to the doctor, days off work or school, nocturnal asthma, and quality of life (hospital admissions: RR 0.64, 95% CI 0.50 to 0.82; emergency room visits: RR 0.82, 95% CI 0.73 to 0.94; unscheduled visits to the doctor: RR 0.68, 95% CI 0.56 to 0.81; days off work or school: RR 0.79, 95% CI 0.67 to 0.93; nocturnal asthma: RR 0.67, 95% CI 0.56 to 0.79; quality of life: SMD 0.29, 95% CI 0.11 to 0.47). It found that optimal self management that included a written plan significantly reduced hospital admissions (9 RCTs; RR 0.58, 95% CI 0.43 to 0.77). It found no significant difference between self management and usual care in lung function (forced expiratory volume in 1 second**G**, 7 RCTs: SMD +0.097, 95% CI −0.024

to +0.217). The first subsequent RCT (131 adults admitted to hospital with asthma).[125] It found no significant difference between an education programme (3 group sessions focused on improving self management skills) and waiting list control on 12 out of 13 scales of health and social functioning at 6 months (115 people included in analysis; scales used were SF-36 and the Asthma Quality of Life Questionnaire). The second subsequent RCT (280 adults admitted to hospital with acute asthma) compared two 30 minute education sessions plus a written action plan versus standard care.[126] It found that the educational intervention significantly reduced daytime wheeze and night disturbance 1 month after discharge (no daytime wheeze: OR 2.6, 95% CI 1.5 to 5.3; no night time disturbance: OR 2.0, 95% CI 1.2 to 3.5). However, it found no significant difference in activity limitation (no activity limitation; OR 1.5, 95% CI 0.9 to 2.7). It found that the educational intervention decreased hospital admissions at 12 months compared with usual care, but the difference was not statistically significant (admission: 17% with self management *v* 27% with usual care; OR 0.5, 95% CI 0.3 to 1.0).

Harms: The systematic review[124] and subsequent RCTs[125,126] gave no information on adverse effects.

Comment: The weight of evidence from other published RCTs and systematic overviews supports the role of asthma education among people with asthma.

GLOSSARY

Diurnal variation A characteristic of people with asthma is increased variation in peak flow rates and forced expiratory volume in 1 second during the day. The diurnal variation is sometimes expressed as the difference between maximum and minimum values expressed as a fraction of the maximum value.

Forced expiratory volume in 1 second The volume breathed out in the first second of forceful blowing into a spirometer, measured in litres.

Life threatening asthma An attack of such severity that the person usually requires management in the emergency department. Some people require endotracheal intubation and, usually in the initial stages of resuscitation, cannot inhale bronchodilator treatment.

Peak expiratory flow rate The maximum rate that gas is expired from the lungs when blowing into a peak flow meter or a spirometer. It is measured at an instant, but the units are expressed as litres a minute.

Salbutamol A short acting β_2 agonist known as albuterol in the USA.

Shared care Involves sharing care between outpatient specialist and general practitioner.

REFERENCES

1. National Heart, Blood and Lung Institute. National Asthma Education and Prevention Program. Expert Panel Report 2. Guidelines for the Diagnosis and Management of Asthma. NIH Publication No. 97–4051;July 1997:20.
2. British Thoracic Society Guidelines. *Thorax* 1997;52:S1–S2.
3. Kaur B, Anderson HR, Austin J, et al. Prevalence of asthma symptoms, diagnosis, and treatment in 12–14 year old children across Great Britain (international study of asthma and allergies in childhood, ISAAC UK). *BMJ* 1998;316:118–124.
4. Woolcock AJ, Peat JK. Evidence for an increase in asthma world-wide. *Ciba Found Symp* 1997;206:122–134.
5. Holgate ST. The epidemic of allergy and asthma. *Nature* 1999;402:B2–B4.
6. The International Study of Asthma and Allergies in Childhood (ISAAC) Steering Committee. Worldwide variation in prevalence of symptoms of asthma, allergic rhinoconjunctivitis, and atopic eczema: ISAAC. *Lancet* 1998;351:1225–1232.
7. Burney P, Chinn DJ, Luczynska C, et al. Variations in the prevalence of respiratory symptoms, self-reported asthma attacks, and use of asthma medication in the European Community Respiratory Health Survey. *Eur Respir J* 1996;9:687–695.
8. Duff AL, Platts-Mills TA. Allergens and asthma. *Pediatr Clin North Am* 1992;39:1277–1291.
9. Chan-Yeung M, Malo JL. Occupational asthma. *N Engl J Med* 1995;333:107–112.
10. Lange P, Parner J, Vestbo J, et al. A 15-year follow-up study of ventilatory function in adults with asthma. *N Engl J Med* 1998;339:1194–1200.
11. FitzGerald JM, Grunfeld A. Acute life-threatening asthma. In: FitzGerald JM, Ernst PP, Boulet LP, et al, eds. *Evidence based asthma management*. Decker: Hamilton, Ontario, 2000:233–244.
12. Nahum A, Tuxen DT. Management of asthma in the intensive care unit. In: FitzGerald JM, Ernst PP, Boulet LP, et al, eds. *Evidence based asthma management*. Decker: Hamilton, Ontario, 2000:245–261.

13. Turner MT, Noertjojo K, Vedal S, et al. Risk factors for near-fatal asthma: a case control study in patients hospitalised with acute asthma. *Am J Respir Crit Care Med* 1998;157:1804–1809.
14. Molfino NA, Nannimi A, Martelli AN, et al. Respiratory arrest in near fatal asthma. *N Engl J Med* 1991;324:285–288.
15. Emmerman CL, Woodruff PG, Cydulka RK, et al. Prospective multi-center study of relapse following treatment for acute asthma among adults presenting to the emergency department. *Chest* 1999;115:919–927.
16. Walters EH, Walters J. Inhaled short acting β_2 agonist use in asthma: regular versus as needed treatment. In: The Cochrane Library, Issue 4, 2001. Oxford: Update Software. Search date not stated; primary sources Cochrane Airways Group Asthma and Wheeze RCT register.
17. Dennis SM, Sharp SJ, Vickers MR, et al. Regular inhaled salbutamol and asthma control: the TRUST randomised trial. *Lancet* 2000;355:1675–1679.
18. Spitzer WO, Suissa S, Ernst P, et al. The use of β-agonists and the risk of death and near death from asthma. *N Engl J Med* 1992;326:501–506.
19. Crane J, Pearce N, Flatt A, et al. Prescribed fenoterol and death from asthma in New Zealand, 1981–1983: case-control study. *Lancet* 1989;1:917–922.
20. Pearce N, Grainger J, Atkinson M, et al. Case-control study of prescribed fenoterol and death from asthma in New Zealand, 1977–81. *Thorax* 1990;45:170–175.
21. Grainger J, Woodman K, Pearce N, et al. Prescribed fenoterol and death from asthma in New Zealand, 1981–7: a further case-control study. *Thorax* 1991;46:105–111.
22. Suissa S, Ernst P, Boivin JF, et al. A cohort analysis of excess mortality in asthma and the use of inhaled beta-agonists. *Am J Respir Crit Care Med* 1994;149:604–610.
23. Abramson MJ, Bailey MJ, Couper FJ, et al. Are asthma medications and management related to deaths from asthma? *Am J Respir Crit Care Med* 2001;163:12–18.
24. Kerrebijn KF, van Essen-Zandvliet EE, Neijens HJ. Effect of long-term treatment with inhaled corticosteroids and β-agonists on the bronchial responsiveness in children with asthma. *J Allergy Clin Immunol* 1987;79:653–659.
25. Cockcroft DW, McParland CP, Britto SA, et al. Regular inhaled salbutamol and airway responsiveness to allergen. *Lancet* 1993;342:833–837.
26. Ahrens RC. Skeletal muscle tremor and the influence of adrenergic drugs. *J Asthma* 1990;27:11–20.
27. Adams N, Bestall J, Jones PW. Budesonide for chronic asthma in children and adults (Cochrane Review). In: The Cochrane Library, Issue 4, 2001. Oxford: Update Software. Search date 1999; primary sources The Cochrane Airways Group Trial Register, reference lists of articles, contact with trialists and hand searches of abstracts of major respiratory society meetings (1997–1999).
28. Kemp J, Wanderer AA, Ramsdell J, et al. Rapid onset of control with budesonide Turbuhaler in patients with mild-to-moderate asthma. *Ann Allergy Asthma Immunol* 1999;82:463–471.
29. McFadden ER, Casale TB, Edwards TB, et al. Administration of budesonide once daily by means of Turbuhaler to subjects with stable asthma. *J Allergy Clin Immunol* 1999;104:46–52.
30. Miyamoto T, Takahashi T, Nakajima S, et al. A double-blind, placebo-controlled dose–response study with budesonide Turbuhaler in Japanese asthma patients. Japanese Pulmicort Turbuhaler study group. *Respirology* 2000;5:247–256.
31. Banov CH, Howland III WC, Lumry WR. Once-daily budesonide via Turbuhaler improves symptoms in adults with persistent asthma. *Ann Allergy Asthma Immunol* 2001;86:627–632.
32. O'Byrne PM, Barnes PJ, Rodriguez-Roisin R, et al. Low dose inhaled budesonide and formoterol in mild persistent asthma: the OPTIMA randomized trial. *J Respir Crit Care Med* 2001;164:1392–1397.
33. Pauwels RA, Pedersen S, Busse WW, et al. Early intervention with budesonide in mild persistent asthma: a randomised, double-blind trial. *Lancet* 2003;361:1071–1076.
34. Adams N, Bestall J, Jones PW. Inhaled fluticasone proprionate for chronic asthma. In: The Cochrane Library, Issue 4, 2001. Oxford: Update Software. Search date 1999; primary sources The Cochrane Airways Group Trial Register, reference lists of articles, contact with trialists, and abstracts of major respiratory society meetings (1997–1999).
35. Wolfe JD, Selner JC, Mendelson LM, et al. Effectiveness of fluticasone propionate in patients with moderate asthma: a dose-ranging study. *Clin Ther* 1996;18:635–646.
36. Adams NP, Bestall JB, Jones PW. Inhaled beclomethasone versus placebo for chronic asthma (Cochrane Review). In: The Cochrane Library, Issue 4, 2001. Oxford: Update Software. Search date 1999; primary sources Cochrane Airways Group Trial Register, hand searches of journals and conference proceedings, and contact with pharmaceutical companies.
37. Bronsky E, Korenblat P, Harris AG, et al. Comparative clinical study of inhaled beclomethasone dipropionate and triamcinolone acetonide in persistent asthma. *Ann Allergy* 1998;80:295–302.
38. Bernstein DI, Cohen R, Ginchansky E, et al. A multicenter, placebo-controlled study of twice daily triamcinolone acetonide (800 μg per day) for the treatment of patients with mild-to-moderate asthma. *J Allergy Clin Immunol* 1998;101:433–438.
39. Ramsdell JW, Fish L, Graft D, et al. A controlled trial of twice daily triamcinolone oral inhaler in patients with mild-to-moderate asthma. *Ann Allergy* 1998;80:385–390.
40. Welch, M Bernstein D. A controlled trial of chlorofluorocarbon-free triamcinolone acetonide inhalation aerosol in the treatment of adult patients with persistent asthma. *Chest* 1999;116:1304–1312.
41. Corren J, Nelson H, Greos LS, et al. Effective control of asthma with hydrofluoroalkane flunisolide delivered as an extrafine aerosol in asthma patients. *Ann Allergy Asthma Immunol* 2001;87:405–411.
42. Nathan RA, Nayak AS, Grant DF, et al. Mometasone furoate; efficacy and safety in moderate asthma compared to beclomethasone dipropionate. *Ann Allergy Asthma Immunol* 2001;86:203–210.
43. Hatoum HT, Schumock GT, Kendzierski DL. Meta-analysis of controlled trials of drug therapy in mild chronic asthma: the role of inhaled corticosteroids. *Ann Pharmacother* 1994;28:1285–1289. Search date not reported; primary source Medline.
44. Jones A, Fay JK, Burr M, et al. Inhaled corticosteroid effects on bone metabolism in asthma and mild chronic obstructive pulmonary disease (Cochrane Review). In Cochrane Library, Issue 4, 2002. Oxford: Update Software. Search date 2001; primary sources Medline, Embase, Cinahl, Bids, Cochrane Controlled Trials Register, Cochrane Airways Group trials register, electronic bibliographies of included studies, and contact with pharmaceutical companies.
45. Lipworth BJ. Systemic adverse effects of inhaled corticosteroid therapy; a systematic review and meta-analysis. *Arch Intern Med* 1999;159:941–955. Search date 1998; primary sources Medline, Embase, BIDS, and hand searches of bibliographies of retrieved articles and abstracts of respiratory and allergy based journals.
46. Kemp JP, Cook DA, Incaudo GA, et al. Salmeterol improves quality of life in patients with asthma requiring inhaled corticosteroids. *J Allergy Clin Immunol* 1998;101:188–195.
47. FitzGerald JM, Chapman KR, Della Cioppa G, et al. Sustained bronchoprotection, bronchodilatation, and symptom control during regular formoterol use in asthma of moderate or greater severity. *J Allergy Clin Immunol* 1999;103:427–435.

48. D'Urzo AD, Chapman KR, Cartier A, et al. Effectiveness and safety of salmeterol in nonspecialist practice settings. *Chest* 2001;119:714–719.
49. Shrewsbury S, Pyke S, Britton M. Meta-analysis of increased dose of inhaled steroid or addition of salmeterol in symptomatic asthma (MIASMA). *BMJ* 2000;320:1368–1373. Search date 1999; primary sources Medline, Embase, and GlaxoSmithKline databases.
50. Pauwels RA, Lofdahl CG, Postma DS, et al. Effect of inhaled formoterol and budesonide on exacerbations of asthma. *N Engl J Med* 1997;337:1405–1411.
51. Baraniuk JM. Fluticasone alone or in combination with salmeterol vs triamcinolone in asthma. *Chest* 1999;116:625–632.
52. Price D, Dutchman D, Mawson A, et al. Early asthma control and maintenance with eformoterol following reduction of inhaled corticosteroid dose. *Thorax* 2002;57:791–798.
53. Fish JE, Israel E, Murray JJ, et al. Salmeterol powder provides significantly better benefit than montelukast in asthmatic patients receiving concomitant inhaled corticosteroid therapy. *Chest* 2001;120:423–430.
54. Yurdakul AS, Calisir HC, Tunctan B, et al. Comparison of second controller medications in addition to inhaled corticosteroid in patients with moderate asthma. *Respir Med* 2002;96:322–329.
55. Chervinsky P, Nelson HS, Bernstein DI, et al. Comparison of mometasone furoate administered by metered dose inhaler with beclomethasone dipropionate. *Int J Clin Pract* 2002;56:419–425.
56. Ringdal N, Eliraz A, Pruzinec R, et al. The salmeterol/fluticasone combination is more effective than fluticasone plus oral montelukast in asthma. *Respir Med* 2003;97:234–241.
57. Cheung D, Timmers MC, Zwinderman AH, et al. Long-term effects of a long-acting β_2-adrenoceptor agonist, salmeterol, on airway hyperresponsiveness in patients with mild asthma. *N Engl J Med* 1992;327:1198–1203.
58. O'Connor BJ. Aikman SL, Barnes PJ. Tolerance to the nonbronchodilating effects of inhaled β_2-agonists in asthma. *N Engl J Med* 1992;327:1204–1208.
59. Nelson JA, Strauss L, Skowronski M, et al. Effect of long-term salmeterol treatment on exercise-induced asthma. *N Engl J Med* 1998;339:141–146.
60. Castle W, Fuller R, Hall J, et al. Serevent nationwide surveillance study: comparison of salmeterol with salbutamol in asthmatic patients who require regular bronchodilator treatment. *BMJ* 1993;306:1034–1037.
61. Fish JE, Kemp JP, Lockey RF, et al. Zafirlukast for symptomatic mild-to-moderate asthma: a 13-week multicenter study. *Clin Ther* 1997;19:675–690.
62. Suissa S, Dennis R, Ernst P, et al. Effectiveness of the leukotriene receptor antagonist zafirlukast for mild-to-moderate asthma. A randomized, double-blind, placebo-controlled trial. *Ann Intern Med* 1997;126:177–183.
63. Nathan RA, Bernstein JA, Bielory L, et al. Zafirlukast improves asthma symptoms and quality of life in patients with moderate reversible airflow obstruction. *Allergy Clin Immunol* 1998;102:935–942.
64. Baumgartner RA, Martinez G, Edelman JM, et al. Distribution of therapeutic response in asthma control between oral montelukast and inhaled beclomethasone. *Eur Respir J* 2003;21:123–128.
65. Israel E, Chervinsky PS, Friedman B, et al. Effects of montelukast and beclomethasone on airway function and asthma control. *J Allergy Clin Immunol* 2002;110:847–854.
66. Ducharme FM, Hicks GC. Anti-leukotriene agents compared to inhaled corticosteroids in the management of recurrent and/or chronic asthma. In: The Cochrane Library, Issue 3, 2002. Oxford: Update Software. Search date 2002; primary sources Medline, Embase, and Cinahl.
67. Busse W, Raphael G, Galant S, et al. Low dose fluticasone propionate compared to montelukast for first-line treatment of persistent asthma: a randomized clinical trial. *J Allergy Clin Immunol* 2001;107:461–468.
68. Nathan RA, Bleecker ER, Kalberg C. A comparison of short-term treatment with inhaled fluticasone propionate and zafirlukast for patients with persistent asthma. *Am J Med* 2001;111:195–202.
69. Meltzer EO, Lockey RF, Friedman BF, et al. Efficacy and safety of low-dose fluticasone propionate compared with montelukast for maintenance treatment of persistent asthma. *Mayo Clin Proc* 2002;77:437–445.
70. Brabson JH, Clifford D, Kerwin E, et al. Efficacy and safety of low-dose fluticasone propionate compared with zafirlukast in patients with persistent asthma. *Am J Med* 2002;113:15–21.
71. Riccioni G, Ballone E, D'Orazio N, et al. Effectiveness of montelukast versus budesonide on quality of life and bronchial reactivity in subjects with mild-persistent asthma. *Int J Immunopathol Pharmacol* 2002;15:149–155.
72. Riccioni G, Vecchia RD, D'Orazio N, et al. Comparison of montelukast and budesonide on bronchial reactivity in subjects with mild-moderate persistent asthma. *Pulm Pharmacol Ther* 2003;16:111–114.
73. Riccioni G, D'Orazio N, Di Ilio C, et al. Effectiveness and safety of montelukast versus budesonide at various doses on bronchial reactivity in subjects with mild persistent asthma. *Clin Ter* 2002;153:317–321. [In Italian]
74. Calhoun WJ, Nelson HS, Nathan RA, et al. Comparison of fluticasone propionate–salmeterol combination therapy and montelukast in patients who are symptomatic on short-acting β_2 agonists alone. *Am J Respir Crit Care Med* 2001;164:759–763.
75. Pearlman DS, White MV, Lieberman AK, et al. Fluticasone propionate/salmeterol combination compared with montelukast for the treatment of persistent asthma. *Ann Allergy Asthma Immunol* 2002;88:227–235.
76. Jamaleddine G, Diab K, Tabbarah Z, et al. Leukotriene antagonists and the Churg-Strauss syndrome. *Semin Arthritis Rheum* 2002;31:218–227. Search date 2000; primary source Medline.
77. Ducharme F. Addition of anti-leukotriene agents to inhaled corticosteroids for chronic asthma. In: The Cochrane Library. Issue 3, 2002. Oxford: Update Software. Search date 2001; primary sources Medline, Embase, Cinahl, reference lists of review articles and trials, contact with international headquarters of anti-leukotriene manufacturers, and ATS meeting abstracts (1998–2000).
78. Vaquerizo MJ, Casan P, Castillo J, et al. Effect of montelukast added to inhaled budesonide on control of mild to moderate asthma. *Thorax* 2003;58:204–211. [Erratum in: *Thorax* 2003;58:370]
79. Price DB, Hernandez D, Magyar P, et al. Randomised controlled trial of montelukast plus inhaled budesonide versus double dose inhaled budesonide in adult patients with asthma. *Thorax* 2003;58:211–216.
80. Lim S, Jatakanon A, Gordon D, et al. Comparison of high dose inhaled steroids, low dose inhaled steroids plus low dose theophylline, and low dose inhaled steroids alone in chronic asthma in general practice. *Thorax* 2000;55:837–841.
81. Malolepszy J. Efficacy and tolerability of oral theophylline slow release versus inhalative formoterol in moderate asthma poorly controlled on low dose steroids. *Atemw Lungenkrkh* 2002;28:78–87. [In German]
82. Cates C. Holding chambers versus nebulisers for β agonist treatment of acute asthma. In: The Cochrane Library, Issue 3, 2002. Oxford: Update Software. Search date 1999; primary sources Cochrane Airways Review Group Register of Trials, Cochrane Controlled Trials Register, bibliographies of all included papers, and authors of included studies.
83. Rowe BH, Keller JL, Oxman AD. Effectiveness of steroid therapy in acute exacerbations of asthma: a meta-analysis. *Am J Emerg Med* 1992;10:301–310.

Search date 1991; primary sources Medline, Science Citation Index, review articles, textbooks, experts, and primary authors.
84. Rowe BH, Spooner CH, Duchrame FM, et al. Corticosteroids for preventing relapse following acute exacerbations of asthma. In: The Cochrane Library, Issue 3, 2002. Oxford: Update Software. Search date 2001; primary sources Cochrane Airways Review Group Register of Trials, Asthma, and Wheeze RCT Register.
85. Mahakalkar SM, Tibdewal S, Khobragade BP. Effect of a single dose of prednisolone on hospitalization in patients of acute bronchial asthma. *Ind J Med Sci* 2000;54:384–387.
86. Edmonds ML, Camargo CA Jr, Pollack CV, et al. Early use of inhaled corticosteroids in the emergency department treatment of acute asthma. In: The Cochrane Library, Issue 3, 2002. Search date 2000; primary sources The Cochrane Airways Review Group Register of Trials, hand searches of reference lists and conference abstracts, and contact with experts and pharmaceutical companies.
87. Edmonds ML, Camargo CA, Brenner BE, et al. Replacement of oral corticosteroids with inhaled corticosteroids in the treatment of acute asthma following emergency department discharge: a meta-analysis. *Chest* 2002;121:1798–1805. Search date 2001; primary sources Embase, Medline, Cinahl, hand searches of 20 respiratory journals and abstracts of meetings, Central, and reference lists, and contact with authors and pharmaceutical companies.
88. Lee-Wong M, Dayrit FM, Kohli AR, Acquah S, Mayo PH. Comparison of high-dose inhaled flunisolide to systemic corticosteroids in severe adult asthma. *Chest* 2002;122:1208–1213.
89. Levy ML, Stevenson C, Maslen T. Comparison of a short course of oral prednisone and fluticasone propionate in the treatment of adults with acute exacerbations of asthma in primary care. *Thorax* 1996;51:1087–1092.
90. O'Driscoll BR, Kalra S, Wilson M, et al. Double-blind trial of steroid tapering in acute asthma. *Lancet* 1993;341:324–327.
91. Hasegawa T, Ishihara K, Takakura S, et al. Duration of systemic corticosteroids in the treatment of asthma exacerbation: a randomized study. *Intern Med* 2000;39:794–797.
92. Jones AM, Munavvar M, Vail A, et al. Prospective, placebo-controlled trial of 5 versus 10 days of oral prednisolone in acute adult asthma. *Respir Med* 2002;96:950–954.
93. Edmonds ML, Camargo CA, Pollack CV, et al. The effectiveness of inhaled corticosteroids in the emergency department treatment of acute asthma: a meta-analysis. *Ann Emerg Med* 2002;40:145–154. Search date 2001; primary sources Embase, Medline, Cinahl, hand searches of 20 respiratory journals and abstracts of meetings, Central, and reference lists, and contact with authors and pharmaceutical companies.
94. Edmonds ML, Camargo CA Jr, Saunders LD, et al. Inhaled steroids in acute asthma following emergency department discharge. The Cochrane Library, Issue 3, 2002. Oxford Software. Search date 1999; primary sources Cochrane Upper Airways Group register of controlled trials, hand searches of bibliographies, 20 respiratory journals, and conference proceedings, and contact with authors of articles retrieved and pharmaceutical companies.
95. Rodrigo GJ, Rodrigo C. Continuous versus intermittent β agonists in the treatment of acute asthma. A systematic review with meta-analysis. *Chest* 2002;122:160–165. Search date 2001; primary sources Medline, Embase, Cinahl, Cochrane Controlled Trials Register, and bibliographies of trials and reviews.
96. Khine H, Fuchs SM, Saville AL. Continuous vs intermittent nebulized albuterol for emergency management of asthma. *Acad Emerg Med* 1969;3:1019–1024.
97. Shrestha M, Bidadi K, Gourlay S, et al. Continuous vs intermittent albuterol, at high and low doses, in the treatment of severe acute asthma in adults. *Chest* 1996;110:42–47.
98. Bradding P, Rushby I, Scullion J, et al. As required versus regular nebulized salbutamol for the treatment of acute severe asthma. *Eur Respir J* 1999;13:290–294.
99. Travers A, Jones AP, Kelly K, et al. Intravenous β_2-agonists for acute asthma in the emergency department. The Cochrane Library, Issue 3, 2002. Oxford Software. Search date not reported; primary sources Cochrane Airways Group Register, hand searches of 20 respiratory journals and bibliographies from included studies, and contact with authors and experts to identify eligible studies.
100. Travers AH, Rowe BH, Barker S, et al. The effectiveness of IV beta-agonists in treating patients with acute asthma in the emergency department: a meta-analysis. *Chest* 2002;122:1200–1207. Search date 2000; primary sources Medline, Embase, Cinahl, Cochrane Controlled Trials Register, Cochrane Airways Group wheeze and asthma specialised register, and hand searches of reference lists of relevant papers and personal contact with authors, pharmaceutical producers and asthma researchers.
101. Rodrigo G, Rodrigo C, Burschtin O. Ipratropium bromide in acute adult severe asthma: a meta-analysis of randomized controlled trials. *Am J Med* 1999;107:363–370. Search date 1999; primary sources Medline, Current Contents, Science Citation Index, review articles, experts, pharmaceutical companies, Medical Editor's Trial Amnesty Register, and hand searches of references.
102. Stoodley RG, Aaron SD, Dales RE. The role of ipratropium bromide in the emergency management of acute asthma exacerbation: a metaanalysis of randomized clinical trials. *Ann Emerg Med* 1999;34:8–18. Search date 1997; primary sources Medline, Embase, Cinahl, Biological Abstracts, Cochrane Library, and Current Contents.
103. Rodrigo GJ, Rodrigo C. First-line therapy for adult patients with acute asthma receiving multiple dose protocol of ipratropium bromide plus albuterol in the emergency department. *Am J Respir Crit Care Med* 2000;161:1862–1868.
104. Ho, AM, Lee A, Karmakar MK, et al. Heliox vs air-oxygen mixtures for the treatment of patients with acute asthma: a systematic overview. *Chest* 2003;123:882–890. Search date 2002; primary sources Medline, Embase, Cochrane Controlled Trials Register, and hand searches of reference lists of relevant articles.
105. Rowe BH, Bretzlaff JA, Bourdon C, et al. Magnesium sulfate for treating exacerbations of acute asthma in the emergency department. In: The Cochrane Library, Issue 3, 2002. Oxford: Update Software. Search date 1998; primary sources Cochrane Airways Review Group Register of Trials, review articles, textbooks, experts, primary authors of included studies, and hand searches of references.
106. Boonyavoroakul C, Thakkinstian A, Charoenpan P. Intravenous magnesium sulfate in acute severe asthma. *Respirology* 2000;5:221–225.
107. Porter RS, Nester S, Braitman LE, et al. Intravenous magnesium is ineffective in adult asthma: a randomised trial. *Eur J Emerg Med* 2001;8:9–15.
108. Silverman RA, Osborn H, Runge J, et al. IV magnesium sulphate in the treatment of acute severe asthma: a multi centre randomized controlled trial. *Chest* 2002;122:489–497.
109. Nannini LJ, Pendino JC, Corna RA, et al. Magnesium sulfate as a vehicle for nebulized salbutamol in acute asthma. *Am J Med* 2000;108:193–197.
110. FitzGerald JM. Commentary: intravenous magnesium in acute asthma. *Evid Based Med* 1999;4:138.

111. Jones A, Rowe B, Peters J, et al. Inhaled beta-agonists for asthma in mechanically ventilated patients. *Cochrane Database Syst Rev* 2000;2:CD 001493. Search date 2001; primary sources Cochrane Airways Group Asthma and Wheeze RCT register, reference lists from identified reports and reviews, and contact with colleagues, collaborators, and trialists.
112. Behbehani NA, Al-Mane FD, Yachkova Y, et al. Myopathy following mechanical ventilation for acute severe asthma: the role of muscle relaxants and corticosteroids. *Chest* 1999;115:1627–1631.
113. Williams TJ, Tuxen DV, Sceinkestel CD, et al. Risk factors for morbidity in mechanically ventilated patients with acute severe asthma. *Am Rev Respir Dis* 1992;146:607–615.
114. Darioli R, Perret C. Mechanical controlled hypoventilation in status asthmaticus. *Am Rev Respir Dis* 1984;129:385–387.
115. Menitove SM, Godring RM. Combined ventilator and bicarbonate strategy in the management of status asthmaticus. *Am J Med* 1983;74:898–901.
116. Higgins B, Greening AP, Crompton GK. Assisted ventilation in severe acute asthma. *Thorax* 1986;41:464–467.
117. Lam KN, Mow BM, Chew LS. The profile of ICU admissions for acute severe asthma in a general hospital. *Singapore Med J* 1992;33:460–462.
118. Mansel JK, Stogner SW, Petrini MF, et al. Mechanical ventilation in patients with acute severe asthma. *Am J Med* 1990;89:42–48.
119. Lim TK. Status asthmaticus in a medical intensive care unit. *Singapore Med J* 1989;30:334–338.
120. Keenan SP, Brake D. An evidence based approach to non invasive ventilation in acute respiratory failure. *Crit Care Clin* 1998;14:359–372.
121. Eastwood AJ, Sheldon TA. Organisation of asthma care: what difference does it make? A systematic review of the literature. *Quality Health Care* 1996;5:134–143. Search date 1995; primary sources Medline, Cinahl, HELMIS, Manchester Primary and Secondary Care Interface, Health Planning and Administration, DHSS databases, hand searches of references, and contact with experts.
122. Bartter T, Pratter MR. Asthma: better outcome at a lower cost? The role of the expert in the care system. *Chest* 1996;110:1589–1596.
123. Zeiger RS, Heller S, Mellon MH, et al. Facilitated referral to asthma specialist reduces relapses in asthma emergency room visits. *J Allergy Clin Immunol* 1991;87:1160–1168.
124. Gibson PG, Powel, Coughlan J, et al. Self-management education and regular practitioner review for adults with asthma. The Cochrane Library Issue 2, 2003. Search date 2002; primary sources Cochrane Airways Group Register of Trials, and hand searches of references.
125. Pereger TV, Sudre P, Muntner P, et al. Effect of patient education on self management skills and health status in patients with: a randomized controlled trial. *Am J Med* 2002;113:7–14.
126. Osman LM, Calder C, Godden DJ, et al. A randomised trial of self-management planning for adult patients admitted to hospital with acute asthma. *Thorax* 2002;57:869–874.

Rodolfo Dennis
Professor of Medicine, Pontificia Universidad Javeriana
Head, Departments of Medicine and Research, Fundacion Cardioinfantil – Instituto de Cardiologia
Bogota
Colombia

Ivan Solarte
Professor of Medicine, Pontificia Universidad Javeriana
Head, Respiratory Unit, Hospital San Ignacio
Bogota
Colombia

J Mark FitzGerald
Respiratory Physician and Director of Center for Clinical Epidemiology and Evaluation
Vancouver General Hospital
Vancouver
Canada

Competing interests: MF has received honoraria for lectures and research funds from GlaxoSmithKline, Merck, AstraZeneca, Novartis, Boehringer Ingelheim, Byk Canada, Schering Canada, and 3M. RJD and IS none declared. *We would like to acknowledge the previous contributors of this chapter, including Chris Cates, Paul O'Byrne, and Bazian Ltd.*

TABLE 1 **Classification of severity for chronic asthma (see text, p 1894).**

In the USA[1]

Asthma is classified by symptoms of severity. Using this system, even people with mild, intermittent asthma can develop severe exacerbations if exposed to appropriate stimuli.

Mild intermittent asthma	Symptoms less than weekly with normal or near normal lung function.
Mild persistent asthma	Symptoms more than weekly but less than daily with normal or near normal lung function.
Moderate persistent asthma	Daily symptoms with mild to moderate variable airflow obstruction.
Severe asthma	Daily symptoms and frequent night symptoms, and moderate to severe variable airflow obstruction.

In the UK[2]

Chronic asthma in ambulatory settings is graded according to the amount of medication required to keep symptoms controlled. People are classified according to whether, for symptom control, they need:

Step 1	Occasional β agonists for symptomatic relief.
Step 2	In addition, regular, inhaled anti-inflammatory agents (such as inhaled corticosteroids, cromoglycate, or nedocromil).
Step 3	In addition, high dose inhaled corticosteroids or low dose inhaled steroids plus long acting inhaled β_2 bronchodilator.
Step 4	In addition, high dose inhaled corticosteroids plus regular bronchodilators.
Step 5	In addition, regular oral corticosteroids.

Bronchiectasis

Search date June 2004

Nick ten Hacken, Huib Kerstjens, and Dirkje Postma

QUESTIONS

INTERVENTIONS

Key Messages

- **Exercise or physical training** One systematic review found that inspiratory muscle training improved quality of life and exercise endurance compared with no intervention or sham training in people with non-cystic fibrosis bronchiectasis.
- **Inhaled steroids** One systematic review found insufficient evidence from two small RCTs to compare inhaled steroids versus placebo in people with bronchiectasis not due to a specific congenital disease.
- **Long acting β_2 agonists** One systematic review identified no RCTs comparing long acting β_2 agonists versus placebo or other treatments in people with non-cystic fibrosis bronchiectasis.
- **Mucolytics (bromhexine or deoxyribonuclease)** One systematic review found insufficient evidence from three RCTs to compare the effects of bromhexine or recombinant human deoxyribonuclease versus placebo in people with non-cystic fibrosis bronchiectasis.
- **Oral steroids** One systematic review found no RCTs comparing steroids versus placebo, no treatment, or any other pharmacological or non-pharmacological treatment in people with non-cystic fibrosis bronchiectasis.

Clin Evid 2005;13:1918–1922.

DEFINITION Bronchiectasis is defined as irreversible widening of medium sized airways (bronchi) in the lung. It is characterised by inflammation, destruction of bronchial walls, and chronic bacterial infection. The condition may be limited to a single lobe or lung segment, or it may affect one or both lungs more diffusely. Clinically, the condition manifests as chronic cough and chronic overproduction of sputum (up to about 500 mL daily), which is often purulent.[1] People with severe bronchiectasis may have life threatening haemoptysis and may develop features of chronic obstructive airways disease, such as wheezing, chronic respiratory failure, pulmonary hypertension, and right sided heart failure.

INCIDENCE/ PREVALENCE We found few reliable data. Incidence has declined over the past 50 years and prevalence is low in higher income countries. Prevalence is much higher in poorer countries and is a major cause of morbidity and mortality.

AETIOLOGY/ RISK FACTORS Bronchiectasis is most commonly a long term complication of previous lower respiratory infections such as measles pneumonitis, pertussis, and tuberculosis. Foreign body inhalation and allergic, autoimmune, and chemical lung damage also predispose to the condition.[2] Underlying congenital disorders such as cystic fibrosis, cilial dysmotility syndromes, α_1 antitrypsin deficiency, and congenital immunodeficiencies may also predispose to bronchiectasis and may be of greater aetiological importance than respiratory infection in higher income countries. Cystic fibrosis is the most common congenital cause.

PROGNOSIS Bronchiectasis is a chronic condition with frequent relapses of varying severity. Long term prognosis is variable. Data on morbidity and mortality are sparse.[3] Bronchiectasis frequently coexists with other respiratory disease, making it difficult to distinguish prognosis for bronchiectasis alone.

AIMS OF INTERVENTION To alleviate symptoms; to reduce morbidity and mortality.

OUTCOMES **Primary outcomes:** Quality of life, admission to hospital, days off work, exacerbation and infection rates, haemoptysis, respiratory failure, mortality, and adverse effects of treatment. **Secondary outcomes:** Sputum volume and lung function indices. We reported secondary outcomes only if trials did not include primary outcomes.

METHODS *Clinical Evidence* search and appraisal June 2004.

QUESTION What are the effects of treatments in people with bronchiectasis but without cystic fibrosis?

OPTION EXERCISE OR PHYSICAL TRAINING

One systematic review found that inspiratory muscle training improved quality of life and exercise endurance compared with no intervention or with sham training in people with non-cystic fibrosis bronchiectasis.

Benefits: We found one systematic review (search date not reported, 2 RCTs published in abstract form only, 43 people with non-cystic fibrosis bronchiectasis).[4] We found no subsequent RCTs. Both RCTs compared inspiratory muscle training (IMT**G**) versus either no intervention or sham IMT for 8 weeks. The review found that IMT significantly improved exercise endurance and quality of life compared with control (endurance [method of assessment not described]: WMD 264 m, 95% CI 16.4 m to 512 m; quality of life [measured on CRQ scale**G**]: WMD 12.4, 95% CI 2.38 to 22.48). The review found no RCTs examining other clinical outcomes.

Harms: The two RCTs did not report anything about adverse effects.[4]

Comment: None.

OPTION MUCOLYTICS (BROMHEXINE AND DEOXYRIBONUCLEASE)

One systematic review found insufficient evidence from three RCTs to compare the effects of bromhexine or recombinant human deoxyribonuclease versus placebo in people with non-cystic fibrosis bronchiectasis.

Benefits: We found one systematic review in people with non-cystic fibrosis bronchiectasis (search date 2003, 3 double blind RCTs, total number of people not reported).[5] **Bromhexine:** The review identified one RCT (45 people with acute exacerbation of bronchiectasis [defined as morning cough and > 20 mL sputum]) comparing bromhexine (30 mg 3 times daily) versus placebo. It found that bromhexine significantly reduced sputum volume compared with placebo after about 2 weeks (WMD –21.5%, 95% CI –38.9% to –4.1%). The review found that bromhexine also improved some symptom scores compared with placebo, although the clinical importance of these score changes is uncertain (see comment below). **Recombinant human deoxyribonuclease (rhDNase):** The review identified two RCTs comparing rhDNase aerosol versus placebo. The first RCT (number of people not reported) found no significant difference between rhDNase (2.5 mg in 2.5 mL, once or twice daily) and placebo in lung function or infection rates (time to outcome not stated; infection rates reported for once daily dose: 4/21 [19%] with placebo *v* 0/21 [0%] with rhDNase; P > 0.1; no further numerical data reported). The second RCT also found similar exacerbation rates between rhDNase (twice daily for 24 weeks) and placebo (AR for exacerbation in 168 days: 0.66 with rhDNase *v* 0.56 with placebo; RR 1.17; CI not reported).

Harms: **Bromhexine:** The review did not report on harms.[5] **Recombinant human deoxyribonuclease:** In one included RCT, more people had influenza type symptoms with rhDNase (5 mg daily) than with placebo (4 people with rhDNase *v* 0 with placebo).[5] Other adverse effects were not specifically reported.

Comment: One included RCT found that bromhexine significantly improved symptom scores compared with placebo for "difficulty with expectoration", "cough", and "quality of sputum" after about 2 weeks.[5] The clinical importance of effects on these scores are uncertain.

OPTION INHALED STEROIDS

One systematic review found insufficient evidence from two small RCTs about the effects of inhaled steroids compared with placebo in people with bronchiectasis not due to a congenital disease.

Benefits: We found one systematic review (search date 2001, 2 double blind RCTs, 54 people with bronchiectasis not due to congenital disease or focal airway obstruction).[6] The included RCTs compared inhaled steroids (beclomethasone 1500 μg daily or fluticasone 1000 μg daily) versus placebo. The review found no significant difference between inhaled steroids and placebo in symptom scores (75 mm visual analogue scale for steroids *v* placebo: mean improvement in cough score +5 mm, 95% CI –28 to +38 mm; mean improvement in dyspnoea score +4 mm, 95% CI –33 to +41 mm), lung function indices (improvement in forced expiratory volume in 1 second: +0.4 L/minute, 95% CI –2.2 L/minute to +1.0 L/minute; improvement in forced vital capacity: +0.6 L, 95% CI –0.1 to +1.3 L), or sputum volume (reduction in sputum volume: +0.2 mL daily, 95% CI –0.4 mL daily to +0.7 mL daily) after 4–6 weeks. The review reported that the RCTs lacked power to detect clinically important effects.

Harms: The review gave no information on harms.[6]

Comment: None.

OPTION ORAL STEROIDS

One systematic review found no RCTs comparing steroids versus placebo, no treatment, or any other pharmacological or non-pharmacological treatment in people with non-cystic fibrosis bronchiectasis.

Benefits: We found one systematic review (search date 2002), which identified no RCTs in people with bronchiectasis without cystic fibrosis.[7] We found no subsequent RCTs.

Harms: We found no RCTs.

Comment: None.

OPTION LONG ACTING β_2 AGONISTS

One systematic review identified no RCTs comparing long acting β_2 agonists versus placebo or other treatments in people with non-cystic fibrosis bronchiectasis.

Benefits: We found one systematic review (search date 2002), which identified no RCTs in people with bronchiectasis without cystic fibrosis.[8] We found no subsequent RCTs.

Harms: We found no RCTs.

Comment: None.

GLOSSARY

Inspiratory muscle training (IMT) People are required to breathe through inspiratory orifices of progressively decreasing diameter, with the goal of increasing the load on the respiratory muscles. Another way is to use a threshold loading device that permits inspiration to commence only after a certain threshold mouth pressure is reached. The threshold pressure can be set by means of a weighted plunger. In most programmes, subjects have to train 30 minutes a day, for 5 days a week.

Chronic Respiratory (Disease) Questionnaire (CRQ) A 20 item questionnaire dealing with dimensions of dyspnoea, fatigue, patients' sense of control over disease (mastery), and emotional dysfunction. A trained interviewer needs 20 minutes to complete it. Answers are scored on a seven point scale ranging from 1, which indicates maximum impairment, to 7, which indicates no impairment.

REFERENCES

1. Nicotra MB, Riveera M, Dale AM, et al. Clinical, pathophysiologic, and microbiologic characterization of bronchiectasis in an aging cohort. *Chest* 1995;108:955–961.
2. Mysliwiec V, Pina JS. Bronchiectasis: the 'other' obstructive lung disease. *Postgrad Med* 1999;106:123–131.
3. Keistinen T, Saynajakangas O, Tuuponen T, et al. Bronchiectasis: an orphan disease with a poorly-understood prognosis. *Eur Respir J* 1997;10:2784–2787.
4. Bradley J, Moran F, Greenstone M. Physical training for bronchiectasis (Cochrane Review). In: The Cochrane Library. Issue 3, 2003. Oxford: Update Software. Search date not reported; primary sources Cochrane Airways Group Trials register, Cochrane Clinical Register of Controlled Trials, hand searching of references, and contact with experts.
5. Crockett AJ, Cranston JM, Latimer KM, et al. Mucolytics for bronchiectasis (Cochrane Review). In: The Cochrane Library, Issue 3, 2003. Oxford, Update Software. Search date 2001; primary sources Cochrane Airways Group register, contact with pharmaceutical manufacturers, contact with experts, and hand searching of references.
6. Kolbe J, Wells A, Ram FSF. Inhaled steroids for bronchiectasis (Cochrane Review). In: The Cochrane Library, Issue 3, 2003. Oxford, Update Software. Search date 2001; primary sources Cochrane Airways Group register, contact with pharmaceutical manufacturers, contact with experts, and hand searching of references.

7. Lasserson T, Holt K, Greenstone M. Oral steroids for bronchiectasis (stable and acute exacerbations) (Cochrane Review). In: The Cochrane Library, Issue 3, 2003. Oxford, Update Software. Search date 2002; primary sources Cochrane Controlled Trials Register, Medline, Embase, and hand searching of references.

8. Sheikh A, Nolan D, Greenstone M. Long-acting beta-2-agonists for bronchiectasis (Cochrane Review). In: The Cochrane Library, Issue 3, 2003. Oxford: Update Software. Search date 2002; primary sources Cochrane Controlled Trials Register, Medline, Embase, hand searching of references.

Nick ten Hacken
Pulmonary physician
Pulmonary Department
University Hospital Groningen
Groningen
The Netherlands

Huib Kerstjens
Professor of Pulmonary Medicine
Pulmonary Department
University Hospital Groningen
Groningen
The Netherlands

Dirkje Postma
Professor of Pulmonary Medicine
Pulmonary Department
University Hospital Groningen
Groningen
The Netherlands

Competing interests: None declared.

Chronic obstructive pulmonary disease

Search date February 2004

Huib Kerstjens, Dirkje Postma, and Nick ten Hacken

QUESTIONS

INTERVENTIONS

†Extrapolated from studies of different types of pulmonary disease, including chronic obstructive pulmonary disease

See glossary Ⓖ

Key Messages

- We found no evidence about effects of most interventions on progression of chronic obstructive pulmonary disease (measured by decline in lung function).

Drug treatments

- **Inhaled anticholinergics (improve exacerbation rate, symptoms, and FEV_1 compared with placebo)** RCTs found that inhaled anticholinergics improved forced expiratory volume in 1 second (FEV1), exercise capacity, and symptoms compared with placebo. One large RCT found that adding ipratropium to a smoking cessation programme had no significant impact compared with the smoking cessation programme alone on decline in FEV_1 over 5 years. RCTs found that inhaled tiotropium (a long acting anticholinergic drug) reduced exacerbation rates compared with placebo or ipratropium.

- **Inhaled anticholinergics plus β_2 agonists (improve FEV_1 compared with either drug alone)** RCTs found that combining a long or short acting β_2 agonist with an anticholinergic drug for 2–12 weeks modestly improved FEV_1 compared with either drug alone. One RCT found that, when combined with an anticholinergic drug, a long acting β_2 agonist improved FEV_1 and peak expiratory flow rate more than a short acting β_2 agonist. We found no RCTs of long term treatment comparing anticholinergics plus β_2 agonists with placebo.
- **Inhaled corticosteroids plus long acting β_2 agonists (improve exacerbation rate, symptoms, quality of life, FEV_1 compared with placebo)** RCTs found that the combination of an inhaled corticosteroid plus a long acting β_2 agonist reduced exacerbation rates and improved lung function, symptoms, and health related quality of life compared with placebo. In general, the combination was more effective than inhaled corticosteroid alone or long acting β_2 agonist alone, although this difference was not significant for all outcomes.
- **Inhaled β_2 agonists (improve FEV_1 compared with placebo)** RCTs found that treatment with inhaled β_2 agonists for 1 week to 12 months improved FEV_1 compared with placebo. RCTs provided insufficient direct evidence about effects of short or long acting β_2 agonists on quality of life or symptoms. RCTs provided insufficient evidence about effects of long acting inhaled β_2 agonists on exacerbation rates.
- **Inhaled anticholinergics compared with β_2 agonists (improve FEV_1 compared with β_2 agonists in long term)** RCTs found inconsistent evidence about the effects of short acting inhaled anticholinergics compared with long acting β_2 agonists for up to 3 months. Two RCTs found that 6 months of a long acting inhaled anticholinergic improved FEV_1 compared with a long acting inhaled β_2 agonist. One RCT found no significant difference between a long acting inhaled anticholinergic and a long acting inhaled β_2 agonist in quality of life or exacerbation rates at 6 months.
- **Long term domiciliary oxygen (beneficial in people with severe hypoxaemia)** One RCT in people with severe daytime hypoxaemia found that domiciliary oxygen improved survival compared with no domiciliary oxygen. A second RCT in people with severe hypoxaemia found that continuous oxygen reduced mortality compared with nocturnal oxygen. Three RCTs in people with milder hypoxaemia or with nocturnal hypoxaemia only, found no significant difference in mortality between long term domiciliary oxygen and no oxygen.
- **Mucolytics (improve exacerbation rates)**† Two systematic reviews found limited evidence that mucolytics for 3–24 months reduced the frequency and duration of exacerbations compared with placebo.
- **Inhaled corticosteroids (improve exacerbation rates, but may have long term harms)** RCTs found no significant difference between inhaled corticosteroids and placebo in lung function (FEV_1) over 10 days to 10 weeks. One systematic review and one subsequent RCT found no significant difference in decline in FEV_1 between inhaled corticosteroids and placebo after 24 months. However, a second systematic review that examined effects of high dose inhaled corticosteroids and four subsequent RCTs found that inhaled corticosteroids slightly reduced the decline in FEV_1 compared with placebo after 12–24 months. One systematic review and one subsequent RCT found that long term inhaled steroids reduced the frequency of exacerbations compared with placebo. Two subsequent RCTs found no significant difference in exacerbation rates. Long term inhaled steroids may predispose to adverse effects, including skin bruising, and oral candidiasis.
- **Theophyllines** One systematic review found that theophyllines slightly improved FEV_1 compared with placebo after 3 months. One large RCT found that theophyllines improved FEV_1 compared with placebo after 12 months' treatment. The usefulness of these drugs is limited by adverse effects and the need for frequent monitoring of blood concentrations.

- **Deoxyribonuclease** We found no RCTs comparing the long term effects of deoxyribonuclease versus placebo.
- **Prophylactic antibiotics** One systematic review found limited evidence of a small reduction in exacerbation rates and days with disability with prophylactic antibiotics. These benefits probably do not outweigh the harms of antibiotics, especially the development of antibiotic resistance. All the identified RCTs were conducted more than 30 years ago, and the results are unlikely to apply to current practice.
- **α_1 Antitrypsin** One RCT in people with α_1 antitrypsin deficiency and moderate emphysema found no significant difference between α_1 antitrypsin infusion and placebo in the decline in FEV_1 after 1 year.
- **Oral corticosteroids (evidence of harm but no evidence of long term benefits)** We found no RCTs on long term benefits. One systematic review found that treatment with oral corticosteroids for 2–4 weeks improved FEV_1 compared with placebo. Long term systemic corticosteroids are associated with serious adverse effects, including osteoporosis and diabetes.
- **Oral versus inhaled corticosteroids (evidence of harm but no evidence of long term benefits)** Two RCTs provided insufficient evidence about effects of oral compared with inhaled corticosteroids over 2 weeks. We found no RCTs of long term treatment with oral compared with inhaled corticosteroids. Long term oral corticosteroids are associated with serious adverse effects, including osteoporosis and diabetes.

Smoking cessation

- **Psychosocial plus pharmacological interventions** One large RCT in people with mild chronic obstructive pulmonary disease found that nicotine gum plus a psychosocial smoking cessation and abstinence maintenance programme (with or without ipratropium) slowed the decline of FEV_1, and reduced respiratory symptoms and lower respiratory illnesses, but increased weight gain compared with usual care (without psychosocial intervention). The RCT found no significant difference between treatments in all cause mortality at 5 years.
- **Pharmacological interventions alone** One systematic review found no RCTs in people with chronic obstructive pulmonary disease.
- **Psychosocial interventions alone** We found no systematic review or RCTs in people with chronic obstructive pulmonary disease.

†Extrapolated from studies of different types of pulmonary disease, including chronic obstructive pulmonary disease

DEFINITION Chronic obstructive pulmonary disease (COPD) is a disease state characterised by airflow limitation that is not fully reversible. The airflow limitation is usually both progressive and associated with an abnormal inflammatory response of the lungs to noxious particles or gases.[1] Classically, it has been thought to be a combination of emphysema and chronic bronchitis, although only one of these may be present in some people with COPD. Emphysema is abnormal permanent enlargement of the air spaces distal to the terminal bronchioles, accompanied by destruction of their walls and without obvious fibrosis. Chronic bronchitis is chronic cough or mucus production for at least 3 months in at least 2 successive years when other causes of chronic cough have been excluded.[2]

INCIDENCE/ PREVALENCE COPD mainly affects middle aged and elderly people. In 1998, the World Health Organization estimated that COPD was the fifth most common cause of death worldwide, responsible for 4.2% of all mortality (estimated 2 249 000 deaths in 1998)[3] and morbidity is increasing. Estimated prevalence in the USA rose by 41% between 1982 and 1994 and age adjusted death rates rose by 71% between 1966 and 1985. All cause age adjusted mortality declined over the same period by 22% and mortality from cardiovascular diseases by 45%.[2] In the UK, physician diagnosed prevalence was 2% in men and 1% in women between 1990 and 1997.[4]

AETIOLOGY/ RISK FACTORS COPD is largely preventable. The main cause in developed countries is exposure to tobacco smoke. The disease is rare in lifelong non-smokers (estimated prevalence 5% in 3 large representative US surveys of non-smokers from 1971–1984), in whom "passive" exposure to environmental tobacco smoke has been proposed as a cause.[5,6] Other proposed causes include bronchial hyperresponsiveness, indoor and outdoor air pollution, and allergy.[7–9]

PROGNOSIS Airway obstruction is usually progressive in those who continue to smoke, resulting in early disability and shortened survival. Smoking cessation reverts the rate of decline in lung function to that of non-smokers.[10] Many people will need medication for the rest of their lives, with increased doses and additional drugs during exacerbations.

AIMS OF INTERVENTION To alleviate symptoms; to prevent exacerbations; to preserve optimal lung function; and to improve activities of daily living, quality of life, and survival.[11]

OUTCOMES Short and long term changes in lung function, including changes in forced expiratory volume in 1 second (FEV_1 Ⓖ); exercise tolerance; peak expiratory flow rate Ⓖ; frequency, severity, and duration of exacerbations; symptom scores for dyspnoea; quality of life; and survival. Symptom and quality of life scores include the St George's Respiratory Questionnaire, which is rated on a scale from 0 to 100 (a 4 point change is considered clinically important); the Transitional Dyspnoea Index, which is rated from −9 to +9 (a 1 point change is considered clinically important), and the Chronic Respiratory Disease Questionnaire (CRDQ), which is rated from 1 to 7 (a 0.5 point change is considered clinically important).

METHODS *Clinical Evidence* search and appraisal February 2004. This review deals only with treatment of stable COPD and not with treatment of acute exacerbations. We were interested in the maintenance treatment of stable COPD; therefore, we did not include single dose or single day cumulative dose–response trials. In this review, short term treatment is defined as less than 6 months and long term as 6 months or over. There is consensus that 6 months is the absolute minimum duration of treatment required to assess effects on decline in lung function. Where RCTs were found, no systematic search for observational studies was performed.

QUESTION What are the effects of maintenance drug treatment in stable chronic obstructive pulmonary disorder?

OPTION INHALED ANTICHOLINERGICS

RCTs found that inhaled anticholinergics improved forced expiratory volume in 1 second (FEV_1), exercise capacity, and symptoms compared with placebo. One large RCT found that adding ipratropium to a smoking cessation programme had no significant impact compared with the smoking cessation programme alone on decline in FEV_1 over 5 years. RCTs found that inhaled tiotropium (a long acting anticholinergic drug) reduced exacerbation rates compared with placebo or ipratropium.

Benefits: **Short term short acting anticholinergics:** We found no systematic review that assessed effects on lung function. We found many small placebo controlled RCTs.[12–15] Most found a significant effect in favour of ipratropium, and the remainder found no significant difference between treatments. We found four larger RCTs comparing ipratropium versus placebo[16–19] and one systematic review comparing any anticholinergic drug versus placebo.[20] The first two of these RCTs (276 people[16] and 405 people[17]) compared ipratropium (36 μg 4 times daily) versus placebo and salmeterol for 12 weeks. In both RCTs, ipratropium significantly improved baseline forced expiratory volume in 1 second (FEV_1 Ⓖ) compared with placebo (results presented graphically). The third RCT (780 people) compared ipratropium (40 μg 4 times daily) versus placebo and versus formoterol (formoterol) for 12 weeks.[18] It found that ipratropium significantly improved FEV_1 compared with placebo (improvement in average FEV_1 over 12 hours after medication 137 mL, 95% CI 88 mL to 186 mL). It found no significant difference in morning premedication peak expiratory flow rate Ⓖ, symptoms, quality of life scores, or need for rescue bronchodilators. The fourth RCT (183 people with moderate to severe chronic obstructive pulmonary disease [COPD], mean FEV_1 40% predicted, mean age 64 years) compared three treatments: ipratropium (80 μg 3 times daily), formoterol (18 μg twice daily), and placebo.[19] It found no significant difference between ipratropium and placebo in shuttle walking distance at 12 weeks (mean increase from baseline: 15.3 m with ipratropium v 6.1 m with placebo; P value not reported, baseline mean distance 325 m). The systematic review (search date 1999) assessed changes in exercise capacity with anticholinergic drugs versus placebo.[20] Meta-analysis was not performed because of heterogeneity in design and outcomes among studies. Sixteen of the 17 RCTs found that anticholinergic drugs improved exercise capacity compared with placebo. **Short term long acting anticholinergics:** We found three RCTs comparing the effects on lung function of tiotropium (a long acting anticholinergic, 18 μg/day) versus placebo or versus ipratropium.[21–23] The first RCT (169 people) compared tiotropium versus placebo for 4 weeks. It found that tiotropium significantly improved FEV_1 during the first 6 hours after treatment compared with placebo and significantly increased trough FEV_1 24 hours after the last dose (mean improvement in post-dose FEV_1: +0.13 L with tiotropium v −0.02 L with placebo; $P < 0.05$; mean trough FEV_1: +0.07 L with tiotropium v −0.03 L with placebo; $P < 0.05$).[21] The second RCT (478 people) compared tiotropium versus placebo for 92 days. It found that tiotropium significantly improved FEV_1 during the first 3 hours after treatment ($P < 0.001$), increased the peak response (CI not reported; $P < 0.001$; results presented graphically), and improved symptoms ($P < 0.01$).[22] The third RCT (288 people, average age 65 years) compared tiotropium (18 μg/day) versus ipratropium (40 μg 4 times daily) for 13 weeks.[23] It found that tiotropium significantly increased post-dose FEV_1 and significantly increased mean trough FEV_1 compared with ipratropium (mean FEV_1 6 hours after treatment on first day: 0.24 L with tiotropium v 0.18 L with ipratropium; difference 0.06 L, 95% CI 0.02 L to 0.09 L; trough FEV_1: 0.15 L with tiotropium v 0.01 L with ipratropium; difference 0.13 L, 95% CI 0.09 L to 0.18 L). **Long term treatment with ipratropium or tiotropium:** We found five RCTs (4 publications).[10,24–26] The first RCT (5887 smokers aged 35–60 years with spirometric signs of early COPD; FEV_1 75% predicted) compared three interventions over a 5 year period: an intensive 12 session smoking cessation programme combining behaviour modification and use of nicotine gum; the same smoking intervention programme plus ipratropium three times daily; or usual care.[10] Although decline in FEV_1 was significantly slower in people in both smoking cessation groups compared with usual care, adding ipratropium had no significant effect (5 year mean cumulative decline in FEV_1 before bronchodilator: usual care 249 mL, 95% CI 236 mL to 262 mL; smoking programme plus ipratropium 188 mL, 95% CI 175 mL to 200 mL; smoking programme plus placebo 172 mL, 95% CI 159 mL to 185 mL). The second RCT (921 people) compared tiotropium 18 μg daily versus placebo for 1 year.[24] It found that tiotropium significantly improved mean trough FEV_1 compared with placebo 3 and 24 hours after dosing (mean improvement compared with placebo at 3 hours: 140–220 mL; P value not reported; at 24 hours: 120–150 mL; $P < 0.01$). It also found that tiotropium significantly reduced exacerbations and hospital admissions compared with placebo (exacerbations per patient year: 0.76 with tiotropium v 0.95 with placebo; $P < 0.05$; admission to hospital for COPD exacerbation: 5.5% with tiotropium v 9.4% with placebo; $P < 0.05$).[24] The third RCT found that 1 year of tiotropium 18 μg daily significantly improved trough FEV_1 and health related quality of life and reduced exacerbations compared with ipratropium (40 μg 4 times daily) at 1 year (improvement in FEV_1 with tiotropium v ipratropium: 150 mL; $P < 0.001$; quality of life: AR for 4 unit improvement in the St George's Respiratory Questionnaire 52% with tiotropium v 35% with ipratropium; $P = 0.001$; exacerbations in 1 year: 0.73 with tiotropium v 0.96 with ipratropium per patient year; $P = 0.006$).[25] It found no significant difference between tiotropium and ipratropium in admissions for COPD exacerbation at 1 year (7.3% with tiotropium *v* 11.7% with ipratropium; P = 0.11).[25] The fourth and fifth RCTs were combined in a single report (total of 1207 people, mean age 64 years, mean baseline FEV_1 from 1.07 L to 1.12 L across treatment groups) that compared three treatments over 6 months: tiotropium 18 µg once daily, salmeterol 50 µg twice daily, and placebo.[26] The RCTs found that tiotropium significantly increased pre-dose FEV_1 and quality of life and reduced exacerbations compared with placebo. They found no significant difference between treatments in hospitalisations for exacerbations (increase in FEV_1 compared with placebo: 0.12 L with tiotropium; P < 0.01; improvement in St George's Respiratory Questionnaire: 4.2 with tiotropium *v* 1.5 with placebo; P < 0.05; exacerbations per person per year: 1.07 with tiotropium *v* 1.49 with placebo; P < 0.05; hospitalisations per person per year: 0.15 with tiotropium *v* 0.10 with placebo; P value not reported).

Harms: **Short term short acting anticholinergics:** One RCT comparing ipratropium found similar rates of adverse events with ipratropium and placebo.[19] **Long term treatment with ipratropium or tiotropium:** The first RCT of long term treatment found no significant difference between ipratropium and placebo in serious adverse events (cardiac symptoms, hypertension, skin rashes, and urinary retention: 1.2% with ipratropium *v* 0.8% with placebo), and dry mouth was the most common mild adverse effect.[10] The long term RCT comparing tiotropium versus placebo found similar rates of adverse effects, except for dry mouth (16.0% with tiotropium *v* 2.7% with placebo; P < 0.05).[24] One RCT found dry mouth was significantly more common with tiotropium compared with ipratropium (12.1% with tiotropium *v* 6.1% with ipratropium; P < 0.05).[25] The report of two RCTs found that tiotropium significantly increased dryness of the mouth compared with placebo (8.2% with tiotropium *v* 2.3% with placebo; P value not reported).[27]

Comment: RCTs of long term treatment found no evidence that people developed tachyphylaxis in response to the bronchodilating effect of ipratropium or tiotropium over a 1–5 year period.[10,24]

OPTION INHALED β_2 AGONISTS

RCTs found that treatment with inhaled β_2 agonists for 1 week to 12 months improved FEV_1 compared with placebo. RCTs provided insufficient direct evidence about effects of short or long acting β_2 agonists on quality of life or symptoms. RCTs provided insufficient evidence about effects of long acting inhaled β_2 agonists on exacerbation rates.

Benefits: **Short term treatment with short acting β_2 agonists:** We found one systematic review (search date 2002, 9 crossover RCTs, 264 people with stable chronic obstructive pulmonary disease [COPD]) comparing short acting β_2 agonists versus placebo for at least 1 week.[28] It found that β_2 agonists delivered by metered dose inhaler slightly but significantly increased forced expiratory volume in 1 second (FEV_1 Ⓖ) compared with placebo (WMD 0.14 L, 95% CI 0.04 L to 0.25 L), and significantly improved daily breathlessness score (results reported as SMD; P < 0.001). There was no significant difference between treatments in exercise tolerance (4 RCTs; SMD +0.18, 95% CI –0.11 to +0.47), although the trials were small and the results were heterogeneous. **Short term treatment with long acting β_2 agonists:** We found one systematic review (search date 2001, 8 RCTs of salmeterol, duration 4–16 weeks, 979 people)[29] and five subsequent RCTs.[17–19,30,31] The review found no significant difference between salmeterol and placebo in FEV_1 (4 RCTs, 717 people; SMD +0.14 L,

95% CI –0.16 L to +0.44 L; see comment below).[29] Other outcomes could not be pooled. The first subsequent RCT (478 people) found that salmeterol 42 μg twice daily significantly increased FEV_1 throughout the 12 week study period compared with placebo (results presented graphically).[17] The second subsequent RCT (780 people) compared four treatments: formoterol 12 μg twice daily, formoterol 24 μg twice daily, ipratropium, and placebo for 12 weeks.[18] It found that both doses of formoterol significantly improved FEV_1 compared with placebo (improvement in average FEV_1 over 12 hours after medication with 12 μg formoterol *v* placebo: 223 mL, 95% CI 174 mL to 273 mL; 24 μg formoterol *v* placebo: 194 mL, 95% CI 145 mL to 243 mL). It also found that 12 or 24 μg formoterol significantly improved quality of life compared with placebo (improvement in total score on St George's Respiratory Questionnaire with 12 μg formoterol *v* placebo: 5; P < 0.001; with 24 μg formoterol *v* placebo: about 3–4, difference presented graphically; P = 0.009). The third subsequent RCT (692 people) compared formoterol (4.5, 9, or 18 μg twice daily) versus placebo for 12 weeks.[30] It found that all doses of formoterol significantly increased FEV_1 compared with placebo (results presented graphically). There was no dose–response effect for FEV_1. The RCT found that the two higher doses of formoterol significantly increased symptom free days compared with placebo (percentage increase in symptom free days compared with placebo +1.4%, 95% CI –2.7% to +5.4% with 4.5 μg formoterol; 4.7%, 95% CI 0.6% to 8.8% with 9 μg formoterol; and 5.7%, 95% CI 1.6% to 9.7% with 18 μg formoterol).[30] The fourth subsequent RCT (34 people, crossover design) compared the effects of three interventions on exercise capacity: formoterol (4.5, 9, or 18 μg twice daily), ipratropium (80 μg 3 times daily), or placebo for 1 week.[31] It found that formoterol or ipratropium slightly but significantly increased time to exhaustion compared with placebo (10.94 minutes with 4.5 μg formoterol; P < 0.0001; 10.78 minutes with 9 μg formoterol; P < 0.01; 10.59 minutes with 18 μg formoterol; P < 0.05; 10.98 minutes with ipratropium; P < 0.0001; 10.20 minutes with placebo).[31] The fifth subsequent RCT (183 people with moderate to severe COPD) compared three treatments: formoterol 18 μg twice daily, ipratropium, and placebo.[19] It found no significant difference between formoterol and placebo in the shuttle walking test after 12 weeks' treatment (increase from baseline: 20.4 m with formoterol *v* 6.0 m with placebo; P value not reported, baseline mean distance 325 m). **Long term treatment with β_2 agonists:** We found no systematic review of long term treatment with short or long acting β_2 agonists versus placebo. We found eight RCTs (7 publications).[26,32–37] The first RCT (623 people) compared salmeterol 50 μg twice daily, tiotropium and placebo for 6 months.[32] It found that salmeterol significantly improved mean pre-dose morning FEV_1 and average FEV_1 (0–12 hours after dose) compared with placebo (mean improvement in mean pre-dose morning FEV_1 85 mL; P < 0.0001; mean improvement in average FEV_1 138 mL; P < 0.0001). However, the RCT found no significant improvement in symptom score (transition dyspnoea index) or health related quality of life score (St George's Respiratory Questionnaire) compared with placebo. A second article combined results from two RCTs (1207 people) that compared salmeterol 50 μg twice daily, tiotropium 18 μg once daily, and placebo over 24 weeks.[26] It found that salmeterol significantly improved pre-dose FEV_1 compared with placebo (difference: 90 mL; P < 0.01). It found no significant difference between treatments in exacerbation rate or quality of life (exacerbations: 1.23 per person per year with salmeterol *v* 1.49 per person per year with placebo; P value not reported; improvement in St George's Respiratory Questionnaire: 2.8 with salmeterol *v* 1.5 with placebo; P value not reported). The fourth and fifth RCTs compared the same four treatments twice daily: salmeterol 50 μg alone, salmeterol plus fluticasone 500 μg, fluticasone alone, and placebo.[33,34] The fourth RCT (691 people) found that salmeterol significantly increased pre-dose and post-dose FEV_1 compared with placebo at 24 weeks (pre-dose increase: 92 mL; $P < 0.05$; post-dose increase: 191 mL; $P < 0.01$).[33] It found no significant difference between salmeterol and placebo in dyspnoea or quality of life (difference in Transitional Dyspnoea Index: 0.5; Chronic Respiratory Disease Questionnaire score: 3.8; P value not reported). The fifth RCT (1465 people) found that salmeterol significantly improved pre-dose FEV_1 and significantly reduced the exacerbation rate at 1 year compared with placebo (FEV_1: 1323 mL with salmeterol *v* 1264 mL with placebo; $P < 0.0001$; exacerbation rate: 1.04 per person per year with salmeterol *v* 1.30 per person per year with placebo; $P = 0.0003$).[34] It found no significant difference between treatments in quality of life (St George's Respiratory Questionnaire score: 45.2 with salmeterol *v* 46.3 with placebo; P value not reported). The sixth RCT (723 people) compared salmeterol 50 μg, fluticasone 250 μg, salmeterol plus fluticasone, and placebo for 24 weeks.[36] It found that salmeterol significantly increased 2 hour post-dose FEV_1 and significantly improved Transitional Dyspnoea Index compared with placebo at 24 weeks. It found no significant difference in health related quality of life (FEV_1: increase 140 mL; $P < 0.001$; Transitional Dyspnoea Index: difference 0.7; $P < 0.05$; Chronic Respiratory Disease Questionnaire score: difference 2.0; $P > 0.05$). The seventh RCT (812 people, FEV_1 36% predicted) compared four treatments twice daily for 1 year: formoterol 12 μg alone, formoterol plus budesonide, budesonide alone, and placebo.[35] It found that formoterol significantly increased post-dose FEV_1 compared with placebo. It found no significant difference in severe exacerbations (increase in FEV_1: 14%, 95% CI 10% to 18%; reduction in exacerbations: 25%, 95% CI –26% to +23%). The eighth RCT (1022 people) compared four inhaled treatments twice daily for 1 year: formoterol 9 μg, budesonide 320 μg plus formoterol 9 μg, budesonide alone 400 μg, and placebo.[37] It found that formoterol significantly improved FEV_1 compared with placebo after 1 year. It found no significant difference in exacerbation rates (FEV_1: increase 85 mL; $P < 0.001$; exacerbations: 1.85 per person per year with formoterol *v* 1.80 per person per year with placebo; difference 0.05 per person per year; $P = 0.828$).

Harms: In people with asthma, β_2 agonists have been linked to increased risk of death, worsened control of asthma, and deterioration in lung function.[38] One crossover RCT (53 people with COPD, $FEV_1 < 70\%$ predicted) compared regular versus as needed treatment with the short acting inhaled β_2 agonist salbutamol for 3 months.[39] It found that regular salbutamol doubled the total daily amount of salbutamol used compared with as needed (13 puffs/day [of which 8 puffs were the allocated regular dose] with regular *v* 6 puffs/day with as needed treatment; significance not reported), with no significant difference in symptoms or lung function. The most common immediate adverse effect is tremor, which is usually worse in the first few days of treatment. High doses of β_2 agonists can reduce plasma potassium, cause dysrhythmia, and reduce arterial oxygen tension.[40] The risk of adverse events may be higher in people with pre-existing cardiac arrhythmias and hypoxaemia.[41] The RCTs comparing salmeterol or formoterol with placebo found no significant increase in adverse effects.[16,17,19,26,33–37]

Comment: It is widely recognised that improvement in symptoms with bronchodilators may not be reflected by a change in FEV_1. Although the systematic review on long acting β_2 agonists showed no significant improvement in FEV_1,[29] two of the four included RCTs (412 people and 97 people) found significant effects, as did the three large subsequent RCTs. Additionally, the generalisability of the systematic review may be limited because RCTs were selected only if they excluded people with 15% or more airflow reversibility to a short acting β_2 agonist, whereas long term studies have found that up to two thirds of people with COPD have at least 15% reversibility with β_2 agonists.[2,42]

OPTION INHALED ANTICHOLINERGICS PLUS β_2 AGONISTS

RCTs found that combining a long or short acting β_2 agonist with an anticholinergic drug for 2–12 weeks modestly improved FEV_1 compared with either drug alone. One RCT found that, when combined with an anticholinergic drug, a long acting β_2 agonist improved FEV_1 and peak expiratory flow rate more than a short acting β_2 agonist. We found no RCTs of long term treatment comparing anticholinergics plus β_2 agonists with placebo.

Benefits: We found no systematic review. **Short term treatment with anticholinergics plus short acting inhaled β_2 agonists:** We found six RCTs (705, 195, 652, 863, and 357 people with stable chronic obstructive pulmonary disease; 1 report combined the results from 2 RCTs) comparing the addition of ipratropium versus no additional ipratropium in people using standard dose short acting inhaled β_2 agonists for 2 weeks to 3 months.[43–47] All found significant improvements in forced expiratory volume in 1 second (FEV_1 Ⓖ) of about 25% with the combination compared with either drug alone. **Short term treatment with anticholinergics plus long acting inhaled β_2 agonists:** One RCT (94 people) compared the long acting β_2 agonist salmeterol (50 μg twice daily) plus ipratropium (40 μg 4 times daily) versus salmeterol alone (50 μg twice daily) for 12 weeks.[48] It found that the combination significantly improved FEV_1 compared with the β_2 agonist alone (mean improvement as a percentage of predicted FEV_1: 8% with combination *v* 5% with β_2 agonist alone, CI not reported; $P < 0.01$), and evening but not morning peak expiratory flow rateⒼ. It found no significant difference in daytime or night time symptoms.[49] **Short term treatment with anticholinergics plus long acting β_2 agonists versus anticholinergics plus short acting β_2 agonists:** One crossover RCT (172 people) compared ipratropium (40 μg 4 times daily) plus formoterol (12 μg twice daily) versus ipratropium (40 μg 4 times daily) plus salbutamol (200 μg 4 times daily).[50] It found that formoterol plus ipratropium significantly improved FEV_1 and peak expiratory flow rate from baseline after 3 weeks of treatment compared with salbutamol plus ipratropium (improvement in mean morning peak expiratory flow rate from baseline over the previous 7 days with formoterol: 12 L/minute, 95% CI 6 L/minute to 19 L/minute; improvement in pre-medication FEV_1 from baseline: 116 mL, 95% CI 83 mL to 150 mL). **Long term treatment with anticholinergics plus inhaled β_2 agonists:** We found no RCTs of long term treatment with anticholinergics plus β_2 agonists compared with placebo.

Harms: The RCTs found no significant differences in adverse effects between treatments.[43–50]

Comment: None.

OPTION INHALED ANTICHOLINERGICS VERSUS β_2 AGONISTS

RCTs found inconsistent evidence about the effects of short acting inhaled anticholinergics compared with long acting β_2 agonists for up to 3 months. Two RCTs found that 6 months of a long acting inhaled anticholinergic

improved FEV_1 compared with a long acting inhaled β_2 agonist. One RCT found no significant difference between a long acting inhaled anticholinergic and a long acting inhaled β_2 agonist in quality of life or exacerbation rates at 6 months.

Benefits: We found no systematic review. **Short term treatment:** We found one non-systematic review (7 RCTs, 1445 people)[51] and three subsequent RCTs[16–18] comparing ipratropium versus different short acting β_2 agonists for 90 days. The review found that ipratropium significantly improved mean forced expiratory volume in 1 second (FEV_1ⓖ) compared with β_2 agonists (28 mL increase with ipratropium *v* 1 mL decrease with β_2 agonist, CI not reported; $P < 0.05$). The first two subsequent RCTs compared ipratropium (36 μg 4 times daily) versus salmeterol (42 μg twice daily).[16,17] The first RCT (411 people) found that salmeterol significantly improved average FEV_1 at 4 and 8 weeks compared with ipratropium (CI not reported; $P < 0.005$), but not immediately after treatment or at 12 weeks.[16] The second RCT (405 people) found no significant difference in FEV_1 between treatments at any time.[17] The third RCT (780 people) compared four treatments: ipratropium, formoterol 12 μg twice daily, formoterol 24 μg twice daily, or placebo for 12 weeks.[18] It found that both doses of formoterol significantly improved FEV_1 compared with ipratropium (improvement in average FEV_1 over 12 hours after medication with 12 μg formoterol *v* with ipratropium: 86 mL, 95% CI 37 mL to 136 mL; with 24 μg formoterol *v* ipratropium: 57 mL, 95% CI 7 mL to 106 mL). Lower dose, but not higher dose, formoterol improved quality of life scores compared with ipratropium (improvement in total score on St George's Respiratory Questionnaire with 12 μg formoterol 3.79; $P < 0.001$; with 24 μg formoterol about 2, difference presented graphically; $P = 0.102$). **Long term treatment:** We found no systematic review comparing long term treatment with anticholinergics versus β_2 agonists. We found two RCTs comparing the same three treatments over 6 months: tiotropium 18 μg daily, salmeterol 50 μg twice daily, or placebo for 6 months.[26,32] The first RCT (total of 623 people) found that tiotropium significantly improved mean pre-dose morning FEV_1, average FEV_1, and health related quality of life compared with salmeterol (improvement in mean pre-dose morning FEV_1 140 mL with tiotropium *v* 90 mL with salmeterol; $P < 0.01$; average FEV_1 [0–12 hours after the dose] 80 mL greater with tiotropium; $P < 0.001$; AR for 4 unit improvement in health related quality of life [St George's Respiratory questionnaire] 51% with tiotropium *v* 40% with salmeterol; $P < 0.05$).[32] The second RCT (1207 people, half of whom were included in the first RCT[32]) found that tiotropium led to a small but significant increase in pre-dose FEV_1 compared with salmeterol (increase in pre-dose FEV_1: 120 mL with tiotropium *v* 90 mL with salmeterol; $P < 0.05$).[25] Over a period of 6 months, the improvements in FEV_1 were maintained with tiotropium but not completely maintained with salmeterol (exact data not reported). The study found no significant difference between the two active treatments in exacerbation rates, hospitalisations, or quality of life (exacerbations: 1.07 per person per year with tiotropium *v* 1.23 with salmeterol; $P = 0.22$; hospitalisation: 0.43 per person per year with tiotropium *v* 0.65 with salmeterol; increase in St George's Respiratory Questionnaire: 4.2 with tiotropium *v* 2.8 with salmeterol; P value not reported).

Harms: Adverse effects such as tremor and dysrhythmia associated with β_2 agonists seem to be more frequent than the adverse effects associated with anticholinergics, although the review provided no evidence for this.[51] The RCTs comparing salmeterol with ipratropium found no significant difference in the frequency of adverse effects.[16,17] In the first

RCT of long term treatment, dry mouth was more frequent with tiotropium than with salmeterol or placebo (experienced by 10% with tiotropium, no further data reported).[32] The second RCT of long term treatment also found that tiotropium significantly increased dryness of the mouth compared with salmeterol (8.2% with tiotropium *v* 1.7% with salmeterol; P value not reported).[26] It found no significant difference between the treatments in other adverse effects.

Comment: It has been suggested that older people experience a greater bronchodilator response with anticholinergic drugs than with β_2 agonists, but we found no evidence for this.

OPTION THEOPHYLLINES

One systematic review found that theophyllines slightly improved FEV_1 compared with placebo after 3 months. One large RCT found that theophyllines improved FEV_1 compared with placebo after 12 months' treatment. The usefulness of these drugs is limited by adverse effects and the need for frequent monitoring of blood concentrations.

Benefits: **Short term treatment:** We found one systematic review (search date 2002, 20 small RCTs, 442 people) comparing theophyllines versus placebo for 1 week to 3 months.[52] It found that theophyllines slightly but significantly improved forced expiratory volume in 1 second (FEV_1Ⓖ) compared with placebo (WMD 100 mL, 95% CI 40 mL to 160 mL). It found no significant difference in maximum walking distance (results presented as SMD).[52] **Long term treatment:** We found one RCT (854 people) comparing four treatments: open label theophylline, double blinded formoterol 12 μg twice daily, formoterol 24 μg twice daily, or placebo for 12 months.[53] It found that theophylline significantly improved FEV_1 compared with placebo (mean difference in FEV_1 with theophylline *v* placebo +120 mL, CI not reported; $P < 0.001$).

Harms: The RCTs identified by the review did not report adverse effects.[54] The therapeutic range for theophyllines is small, with blood concentrations of 10–15 mg/L required for optimal effects. Well documented adverse effects include nausea, diarrhoea, headache, irritability, seizures, and cardiac arrhythmias. These may occur within the therapeutic range.[55] One RCT found that people receiving theophylline were twice as likely to discontinue treatment compared with those taking placebo ($P < 0.002$).[53] Nausea was the most frequent adverse effect.

Comment: None.

OPTION ORAL CORTICOSTEROIDS

We found no RCTs on long term benefits. One systematic review found that treatment with oral corticosteroids for 2–4 weeks improved FEV_1 compared with placebo. Long term systemic corticosteroids are associated with serious adverse effects, including osteoporosis and diabetes.

Benefits: **Short term treatment:** We found one systematic review (search date 1989, 10 RCTs, 445 people), which compared oral corticosteroids versus placebo in people with stable chronic obstructive pulmonary disease.[56] Treatment usually lasted 2–4 weeks. It found that oral corticosteroids significantly increased the proportion of people with a 20% or greater improvement in baseline forced expiratory volume in 1 secondⒼ compared with placebo (WMD 10%, 95% CI 2% to 18%). When five RCTs not meeting all quality criteria were included in the analysis, the difference in effect size was 11% (95% CI 4% to 18%). **Long term treatment:** We found no long term RCTs examining the effects of oral steroids on decline in lung function.

Harms: Many reviews have described the considerable harms of systemic corticosteroids, including osteoporosis and induction of diabetes.[57]

Comment: None.

OPTION INHALED CORTICOSTEROIDS

RCTs found no significant difference between inhaled corticosteroids and placebo in lung function (FEV_1) over 10 days to 10 weeks. One systematic review and one subsequent RCT found no significant difference in decline in FEV_1 between inhaled corticosteroids and placebo after 24 months. However, a second systematic review that examined effects of high dose inhaled corticosteroids and four subsequent RCTs found that inhaled corticosteroids slightly reduced the decline in FEV_1 compared with placebo after 12–24 months. One systematic review and one subsequent RCT found that long term inhaled steroids reduced the frequency of exacerbations compared with placebo. Two subsequent RCTs found no significant difference in exacerbation rates. Long term inhaled steroids may predispose to adverse effects, including skin bruising, and oral candidiasis.

Benefits: **Short term treatment:** We found no systematic review. We found one non-systematic review that identified 10 RCTs of less than 6 months' duration.[58] Nine short term trials (10 days to 10 weeks, 10–127 people) found no significant difference between inhaled steroids and placebo in improvement in lung function forced expiratory volume in 1 second (FEV_1Ⓖ). **Long term treatment:** We found three systematic reviews, each of which examined different questions.[59–61] The first systematic review (search date 2002, 6 RCTs with follow up ≥24 months, 3571 people) compared effects of any dose of inhaled corticosteroids versus placebo on FEV_1.[59] It found no significant difference between inhaled corticosteroids and placebo in the rate of decline of FEV_1 (reduction in annual decline in FEV_1 for corticosteroid *v* placebo: +5 mL, 95% CI –1.2 mL to +11.2 mL). The second systematic review (search date 2003, 4 RCTs, all of which were included in the previous systematic review,[59] 2416 people) compared effects of high dose inhaled corticosteroids versus placebo on FEV_1.[60] It found that high dose inhaled corticosteroids significantly reduced decline in lung function compared with placebo after 24 months (reduction in annual decline in FEV_1 with high dose inhaled corticosteroids *v* placebo: 9.9 mL, 95% CI 2.3 mL to 17.5 mL). The third systematic review (search 2001, 9 RCTs of at least 6 months' duration, 3976 people) examined exacerbation rates.[61] It found that inhaled corticosteroids significantly reduced exacerbations compared with placebo (RR 0.70, 95% CI 0.58 to 0.84).[61] We found five subsequent RCTs, which compared four treatments: combination treatment with inhaled corticosteroids plus long acting β_2 agonist, inhaled steroids alone, inhaled β_2 agonists alone, and placebo.[33–37] The first subsequent RCT (691 people) found that 500 μg fluticasone significantly improved FEV_1 and dyspnoea compared with placebo at 6 months (difference between fluticasone and placebo in FEV_1: 105 mL; $P < 0.05$; difference in Transitional Dyspnoea Index: 1.0; $P < 0.05$).[33] The second subsequent RCT (1465 people) found that fluticasone significantly improved pre-dose FEV_1 and exacerbation rates compared with placebo at 1 year (FEV_1: 1302 mL with fluticasone *v* 1264 mL with placebo; $P < 0.0001$; exacerbation, mean per person per year: 1.05 with fluticasone *v* 1.30 with placebo; $P = 0.003$).[34] It found no significant difference between fluticasone and placebo in quality of life or symptoms (St George's Respiratory Questionnaire: 45.5 with fluticasone *v* 46.3 with placebo; P value not reported). The third subsequent RCT (812 people) found that budesonide 400 μg twice daily significantly increased FEV_1 compared with placebo at 1 year (difference: 5%, 95% CI 2% to 9%).[35] It found no significant difference between budesonide and placebo in exacerbation rate or quality of life (reduction in exacerbations: +15%, 95% CI −10.3% to +34.1%; change in St George's Respiratory Questionnaire: −1.9 with budesonide *v* −0.03 with placebo). The fourth subsequent RCT (1022 people) found no significant difference between budesonide and placebo in time to first exacerbation or decline in FEV_1 at 1 year (median time to first exacerbation: 178 days with budesonide *v* 96 days with placebo; $P = 0.80$; decline in FEV_1 at 1 year: results presented graphically; $P = 0.145$ for difference; CI not reported). However, it found that budesonide significantly improved health related quality of life compared with placebo at 1 year (mean change in St George's Respiratory Questionnaire score from baseline: about 0 with budesonide *v* about −3 with placebo; $P < 0.05$; CI not reported).[37] The fifth subsequent RCT (723 people) found that fluticasone increased post-dose FEV_1 and health related quality of life compared with placebo after 24 weeks (increase in FEV_1 from baseline: 147 mL with fluticasone *v* 58 mL with placebo; $P < 0.048$; improvement in Chronic Respiratory Disease Questionnaire score from baseline: 10.4 with fluticasone *v* 5.0 with placebo; $P = 0.002$; CI not reported).[36] However, it found no significant difference in symptoms at 24 weeks (mean Transitional Dyspnoea Index score: 1.7 with fluticasone *v* 1.0 with placebo; $P = 0.057$).

Harms: **Short term treatment:** The non-systematic review did not report on harms.[58] **Long term treatment:** The first and second reviews did not report on harms.[59,60] The third review found that inhaled corticosteroids significantly increased risks of oropharyngeal candidiasis and skin bruising compared with placebo (candidiasis: RR 2.1, 95% CI 1.5 to 3.1; skin bruising RR 2.1, 95% CI 1.6 to 2.8).[61] The largest RCT identified by the review found that triamcinolone significantly reduced bone mineral density of the lumbar spine ($P = 0.007$) and femur ($P = 0.001$) compared with placebo.[62] The first subsequent RCT found that fluticasone increased oropharyngeal candidiasis compared with placebo but found that other adverse effects were similar between treatments (candidiasis: 10% with fluticasone *v* < 1% with placebo; P value not reported).[33] The second subsequent RCT found that fluticasone increased oropharyngeal candidiasis compared with placebo but found that other adverse effects were similar between treatments (candidiasis: 7% with fluticasone *v* 2% with placebo; P value not reported).[34] The third subsequent RCT found no significant difference between budesonide 400 μg twice daily and placebo in adverse effects.[35] The fourth RCT reported that adverse event rates were similar among all treatment groups (P values not reported),[37] and the fifth RCT reported that serious adverse event rates and rates of adverse events leading to withdrawal of treatment were similar among all treatment groups (serious adverse event rate about 5% in all groups; rate of adverse events leading to withdrawal about 5% in all groups; P values not reported).[36]

Comment: The studies of inhaled corticosteroids have been performed in people with moderate to severe disease (FEV_1 Ⓖ < 50% predicted) and hence apply to that population. The Global Initiative on Obstructive Pulmonary Disease has therefore advocated the use of inhaled corticosteroids only in people with an FEV_1 less than 50% predicted and frequent exacerbations (at least 3 exacerbations in the last 3 years).[1]

OPTION ORAL VERSUS INHALED STEROIDS

Two RCTs provided insufficient evidence about effects of oral compared with inhaled corticosteroids over 2 weeks. We found no RCTs of long term treatment with oral compared with inhaled corticosteroids. Long term oral corticosteroids are associated with serious adverse effects, including osteoporosis and diabetes.

Benefits: We found no systematic review. **Short term treatment:** We found two RCTs comparing oral prednisolone versus inhaled beclometasone (beclomethasone) (12 and 107 people).[63,64] Both were double blind, placebo controlled crossover trials, with treatment periods of 2 weeks. The results of these trials should be interpreted with caution because treatment effects may persist after crossover. The first small RCT found no significant difference in response rate between treatments.[63] The other RCT found greater benefit with oral steroids compared with inhaled steroids (39/107 [36%] with oral steroids v 26/107 [24%] with inhaled steroids, CI not reported; $P < 0.05$).[64] **Long term treatment:** We found no RCTs.

Harms: The RCTs did not report on adverse effects.[63,64] Many reviews have described the considerable harms of systemic corticosteroids, including osteoporosis and induction of diabetes.[57]

Comment: We found one RCT (83 people) that recruited only people known to be responsive to oral steroids, and did not report severity of chronic obstructive pulmonary disease.[65] It found that forced expiratory volume in 1 second (FEV_1 Ⓖ) rose from 650 mL to 1000 mL with prednisolone compared with 630 mL to 800 mL with beclometasone (CI not reported; $P < 0.01$). However, these results may be biased by the selection criteria used in the study. The other two RCTs included people with chronic obstructive pulmonary disease of more than 5 years' duration and FEV_1 less than 70% predicted.[63,64] All trials excluded people with evidence of reversible airflow obstruction.

OPTION INHALED CORTICOSTEROIDS PLUS LONG ACTING β_2 AGONISTS

RCTs found that the combination of an inhaled corticosteroid plus a long acting β_2 agonist reduced exacerbation rates and improved lung function, symptoms, and health related quality of life compared with placebo. In general, the combination was more effective than inhaled corticosteroid alone or long acting β_2 agonist alone, although this difference was not significant for all outcomes.

Benefits: We found five RCTs comparing four treatments: inhaled corticosteroid alone; an inhaled long acting β_2 agonist alone; an inhaled corticosteroid plus a long acting β_2 agonist (combined in 1 inhaler) and placebo.[33–37] The first RCT (691 people, mean age 64 years, current or former smokers, mean forced expiratory volume in 1 second (FEV_1 Ⓖ) 40% predicted) compared a combination of fluticasone 500 µg plus salmeterol 50 µg twice daily versus both components separately versus placebo for 24 weeks.[33] It found that combination treatment significantly improved pre-dose FEV_1 compared with placebo, salmeterol alone, and fluticasone alone, and significantly improved post-dose FEV_1 compared with placebo and fluticasone (difference for combination minus other treatment; pre-dose FEV_1: 159 mL v placebo; 67 mL v salmeterol; 54 mL v fluticasone, all $P < 0.05$; post-dose FEV_1: 231 mL v placebo; 129 mL v fluticasone, both $P < 0.05$; 40 mL v salmeterol, $P > 0.05$). It found that the combination significantly improved dyspnoea compared with placebo, salmeterol alone, and fluticasone alone

(Transition Dyspnoea Index: difference for combination *v* other treatment: 1.7 *v* placebo; 1.2 *v* salmeterol; 0.7 *v* fluticasone, all $P < 0.05$). It found that the combination significantly improved quality of life compared with placebo and fluticasone alone but there was no significant difference between the combination and salmeterol alone (Chronic Respiratory Disease Questionnaire: difference for combination *v* other treatment: 5.3 *v* placebo; 4.8 *v* fluticasone, both $P < 0.05$; 1.6 *v* salmeterol, P value not reported). The second RCT (1465 people, current or former smokers, mean FEV_1 1245–1308 mL at baseline in the treatment groups) compared the same four treatments (salmeterol, fluticasone, salmeterol plus fluticasone, and placebo) for 1 year.[34] It found that the combination significantly improved pre-dose and 2 hour post-dose FEV_1 compared with placebo, fluticasone alone, and salmeterol alone (difference for combination *v* other treatment, pre-dose FEV_1: 133 mL, 95% CI 105 to 161 mL *v* placebo; 73 mL, 95% CI 46 mL to 101 mL *v* salmeterol; 95 mL, 95% CI 67 mL to 122 mL *v* fluticasone; post-dose FEV_1 difference: 155 mL, 95% CI 106 mL to 204 mL *v* placebo; 68 mL, 95% CI 20 mL to 117 mL *v* salmeterol; 94 mL, 95% CI 46 mL to 142 mL *v* fluticasone). It found that the combination, salmeterol alone, and fluticasone alone significantly reduced the exacerbation rate compared with placebo. However, there was no significant difference in exacerbation rate between the combination and either salmeterol alone alone or fluticasone alone (exacerbation rate per person per year: 1.30 with placebo; 1.04 with salmeterol alone, 1.05 with fluticasone alone, 0.97 with combination; $P < 0.0001$ for combination *v* placebo). It found that combination treatment significantly improved quality of life compared with placebo and fluticasone but there was no significant difference between the combination and salmeterol alone (St George's Respiratory Questionnaire: 46.3 with placebo *v* 45.2 with salmeterol *v* 45.5 with fluticasone *v* 44.1 with combination; difference between combination and other treatment: −2.2, 95% CI −3.3 to −1.0 *v* placebo; −1.1, 95% CI −2.2 to +0.1 *v* salmeterol; −1.4, 95% CI −2.5 to −0.2 *v* fluticasone). The third RCT (812 people, mean age 64 years, current or former smokers, mean FEV_1 0.96–1.01 L) compared four treatments twice daily over 1 year: budesonide 320 µg plus formoterol 9 µg twice daily; budesonide 200 µg alone; formoterol 4.5 µg alone; and placebo for 1 year.[35] It found that the combination significantly improved post-dose FEV_1 compared with placebo and budesonide alone but there was no significant difference between combination treatment and formoterol alone (improvement in post-dose FEV_1 for combination *v* placebo: 15%, 95% CI 11% to 19%; combination *v* budesonide: 9.0%, 95% CI 5.4% to 13.0%; combination *v* formoterol: +1.0%, 95% CI −2.2% to +4.9%). It found that combination treatment significantly improved symptoms compared with placebo and budesonide alone but there was no significant difference between combination treatment and formoterol alone (difference in symptoms scored from 0 to 16: combination *v* placebo: −0.77, $P < 0.001$; combination *v* budesonide: −0.70, $P < 0.001$; combination *v* formoterol: −0.27, $P = 0.13$). It found that combination treatment significantly improved quality of life compared with placebo (St George's Respiratory Questionnaire, reduction from baseline: −0.03 with placebo *v* −3.9 with combination *v* −1.9 with budesonide alone *v* −3.6 with formoterol alone; $P = 0.009$ for combination *v* placebo; P for combination *v* each active treatment alone not reported). The fourth RCT (1022 people) found that the combination of budesonide and formoterol significantly reduced time to first exacerbation, rate of exacerbation needing oral corticosteroids, and decline in FEV_1 at 1 year compared with either treatment alone or with placebo (for combination *v* budesonide alone: HR for first exacerbation: 0.77, 95% CI 0.61 to 0.98; RR for exacerbations needing oral steroids: 0.72, 95% CI 0.54 to 0.95;

decline in FEV_1: results presented graphically, $P < 0.001$ in favour of combination; for combination *v* formoterol alone: HR for first exacerbation: 0.71, 95% CI 0.56 to 0.89; RR for exacerbations needing oral steroids: 0.70, 95% CI 0.52 to 0.92; decline in FEV_1: results presented graphically, $P = 0.002$ in favour of combination; for combination *v* placebo: HR for first exacerbation: 0.72, 95% CI 0.56 to 0.91; RR for exacerbations needing oral steroids: 0.55, 95% CI 0.42 to 0.73; decline in FEV_1: results presented graphically, $P < 0.001$ in favour of combination).[37] The RCT also found that combination treatment significantly improved health related quality of life compared with budesonide alone, formoterol alone, or placebo at 1 year (results presented graphically; $P = 0.001$ for combination *v* budesonide; $P = 0.014$ for combination *v* formoterol; $P < 0.001$ for combination *v* placebo). The fifth RCT (723 people) found that combination treatment with fluticasone and salmeterol significantly improved post-dose FEV_1 compared with fluticasone alone, salmeterol alone, or placebo after 24 weeks (difference in post-dose FEV_1: 214 mL for combination *v* placebo; 124 mL for combination *v* fluticasone; 74 mL for combination *v* salmeterol; $P \leq 0.048$ for all comparisons).[36] It found that combination treatment significantly improved symptoms and health related quality of life compared with placebo, but found no significant difference between combination treatment and fluticasone alone or salmeterol alone for these outcomes (adjusted mean difference in Transitional Dyspnoea Index score: 0.8 for combination *v* placebo, $P \leq 0.048$; 0.1 for combination *v* fluticasone, $P > 0.048$; 0.1 for combination *v* salmeterol, $P > 0.048$; adjusted mean difference in Chronic Respiratory Disease Questionnaire score: 5.2 for combination *v* placebo, $P \leq 0.048$; –0.6 for combination *v* fluticasone, $P > 0.048$; 3.2 for combination *v* salmeterol, $P > 0.048$).

Harms: The first RCT found that combination treatment and fluticasone alone increased candidiasis compared with placebo (7% with combination *v* 10% with fluticasone *v* < 1% with placebo and salmeterol; P value not reported).[33] Other adverse effect rates were similar among treatment groups. The second RCT found a slightly lower rate of candidiasis (6% with combination *v* 6% with fluticasone *v* 1% with placebo and salmeterol; P value not reported).[34] It too found similar rates of other adverse effects among treatment groups. The third RCT found similar rates of adverse effects among treatment groups but did not specifically report candidiasis rate.[35] Two RCTs found no clinically relevant decreases in serum cortisol with fluticasone alone or combination treatment.[34,35] The fourth RCT reported that adverse events rates were similar among all treatment groups (P values not reported),[37] and the fifth RCT reported that serious adverse event rates and rates of adverse events leading to withdrawal of treatment were similar among all treatment groups (serious adverse event rate and rate of adverse events leading to withdrawal about 5% in all groups; P values not reported).[36]

Comment: These studies have been performed mainly in people with moderate to severe disease (FEV_1 Ⓖ < 50%) and hence apply to that population. The Global Initiative on Obstructive Pulmonary Disease has, therefore, advocated inhaled corticosteroids and the combination of inhaled corticosteroids plus long acting β_2 agonists only in people with an FEV_1 less than 50% predicted and frequent exacerbations (i.e. at least 3 in the last 3 years).[1]

OPTION MUCOLYTIC DRUGS

Two systematic reviews found limited evidence that mucolytics for 3–24 months reduced the frequency and duration of exacerbations compared with placebo.

Benefits: **Long term treatment:** We found two systematic reviews.[66,67] However, not all included participants had chronic obstructive pulmonary disease (see comment below). The first systematic review (search date 1999, 23 double blind RCTs, 3 RCTs in people with chronic obstructive pulmonary disease, 20 RCTs in people with chronic bronchitis not defined further; > 6000 people) found that mucolytics for 3–6 months significantly reduced the average number of exacerbations and days of disability compared with placebo (exacerbations, WMD: –0.066 exacerbations/month, 95% CI –0.077 exacerbations/month to –0.054 exacerbations/month) and days of disability (disability, WMD: –0.56 days/month, 95% CI –0.77 days/months to –0.35 days/month).[66] The second systematic review (search date 1995, 9 RCTs, 7 of which were included in the first review[66]) compared *N*-acetylcysteine versus placebo for 3–24 months.[67] It found that *N*-acetylcysteine reduced exacerbations compared with placebo (overall weighted effect size: 1.37, 95% CI 1.25 to 1.50, 235 reduction).

Harms: The first systematic review found no significant difference between mucolytics and placebo in the total number of adverse events.[66] Adverse effects of *N*-acetylcysteine were mainly mild gastrointestinal complaints.

Comment: Results of the reviews should be applied with caution.[66,67] It was unclear how many people included in the reviews had chronic obstructive pulmonary disease. In both reviews, there was significant heterogeneity among the RCTs, and symptom scores could not be pooled.[66,67] The effects of *N*-acetylcysteine are usually not ascribed to its mucolytic properties but rather to its antioxidant properties. The effect of *N*-acetylcysteine in slowing the decline in lung function is being examined in a large European multicentre study.[68]

OPTION PROPHYLACTIC ANTIBIOTICS

One systematic review found limited evidence of a small reduction in exacerbation rates and days with disability with prophylactic antibiotics. These benefits probably do not outweigh the harms of antibiotics, especially the development of antibiotic resistance. All the identified RCTs were conducted more than 30 years ago, and the results are unlikely to apply to current practice.

Benefits: **Short term treatment:** We found no systematic review or RCTs. **Long term treatment:** We found one systematic review (search date not reported, 9 RCTs, 1055 people; see comment below) of prophylactic antibiotics (tetracycline, penicillin, trimethoprim, sulphadimidine, and sulphaphenazole) in people with chronic obstructive pulmonary disease or chronic bronchitis.[69] All trials were performed before 1970. The duration of the RCTs ranged from 3 months to 5 years. It found that antibiotics significantly reduced the risk of any exacerbation during the study compared with placebo (RR 0.91, 95% CI 0.84 to 0.99). It found that antibiotics slightly reduced the number of exacerbations per person per year but the reduction was not statistically significant (WMD: –0.15, 95% CI –0.34 to +0.04). It found that antibiotics significantly reduced the number of days of disability per person per month treated (WMD –0.95, 95% CI –1.89 to –0.01, 22% reduction).

Harms: In general, there was a poor reporting of possible adverse effects in most trials. Nevertheless, the review found that antibiotics slightly increased adverse effects compared with placebo (number of adverse effects; WMD per person per year treated: 0.01, 95% CI 0 to 0.02).[69]

Comment: The results of this review should be interpreted with caution.[69] It was unclear from the descriptions of the original studies how many participants had chronic obstructive pulmonary disease (rather than chronic bronchitis without obstruction). Additionally, the data in the review are over 30 years old, so the pathogens and the pattern of antibiotic sensitivity may have changed, and there is a wider range of antibiotics in use. Most people believe that prophylactic antibiotics do not have a place in routine treatment because of concerns about the development of antibiotic resistance and the possibility of adverse effects.

OPTION DOMICILIARY OXYGEN TREATMENT (LONG TERM)

One RCT in people with severe daytime hypoxaemia found that domiciliary oxygen improved survival compared with no domiciliary oxygen. A second RCT in people with severe hypoxaemia found that continuous oxygen reduced mortality compared with nocturnal oxygen. Three RCTs in people with milder hypoxaemia or with nocturnal hypoxaemia only, found no significant difference in mortality between long term domiciliary oxygen and no oxygen.

Benefits: **Long term treatment:** We found one systematic review (search date 2000, 5 RCTs).[70] The review could not perform a meta-analysis because of differences in trial design and participant selection. The first RCT (87 people), which compared daily oxygen supplementation for at least 15 hours versus no oxygen supplementation in people with severe daytime hypoxaemia (arterial oxygen tension [PaO_2] 5.3–8.0 kPa), found that domiciliary oxygen significantly reduced mortality over 5 years.[71] The second RCT (38 people with arterial desaturation at night) comparing nocturnal domiciliary oxygen versus room air found no significant difference in mortality at 3 years (figures not reported).[72] The third RCT (135 people with moderate hypoxaemia [PaO_2 7.4–8.7 kPa] comparing oxygen with no oxygen found no significant difference in survival at 3 years (HR 0.92, 95% CI 0.57 to 1.47; results presented graphically).[73] The fourth RCT (203 people; $PaO_2 < 7.4$ kPa) compared continuous with nocturnal domiciliary oxygen treatment. Continuous oxygen was associated with a significant reduction in mortality over 24 months (22% with continuous oxygen *v* 41% with nocturnal oxygen; OR 0.45, 95% CI 0.25 to 0.81).[74] The fifth RCT (76 people with moderate daytime hypoxaemia [PaO_2 7.4–9.2 kPa] and significant nocturnal desaturation) comparing 2 years of nocturnal oxygen treatment versus placebo found no significant difference in survival.[75]

Harms: The systematic review did not report adverse effects.

Comment: Only one of the studies was double blinded. Domiciliary oxygen treatment seems to be more effective in people with severe hypoxaemia ($PaO_2 < 8.0$ kPa) than in people with moderate hypoxaemia or those who have arterial desaturation only at night.

OPTION α_1 ANTITRYPSIN

One RCT in people with α_1 antitrypsin deficiency and moderate emphysema found no significant difference between α_1 antitrypsin infusion and placebo in the decline in FEV_1 after 1 year.

Benefits: We found no systematic review. **Short term treatment:** We found no RCTs. **Long term treatment:** We found one RCT (56 people with α_1 antitrypsin deficiency and moderate emphysema, forced expiratory volume in 1 second [FEV_1Ⓖ] 30–80% predicted) comparing α_1 antitrypsin infusions 250 mg/kg versus placebo infusion (albumin) given monthly for at least 3 years. It found no significant difference in the decline in FEV_1 after 1 year (decline in FEV_1: 79 mL with α_1 antitrypsin *v* 59 mL with placebo, CI not reported; P = 0.25).[76]

Harms: The RCT reported no adverse effects in people taking α_1 antitrypsin or placebo.[76]

Comment: We found no clear evidence from observational studies on the effect of α_1 antitrypsin. For example, one cohort study (1048 people either homozygous for α_1 antitrypsin deficiency or with an α_1 antitrypsin concentration ≤ 11 µmol/L, with mean FEV_1**G** 49 ± 30% predicted) compared weekly infusions of α_1 antitrypsin 60 mg/kg versus placebo for 3.5–7.0 years.[77] It found that α_1 antitrypsin significantly reduced mortality after an average of 5 years (RR of death 0.64, 95% CI 0.43 to 0.94). It found no significant difference between treatments in the decline in FEV_1, but in a subgroup of people with a mean FEV_1 of 35–49% predicted, α_1 antitrypsin significantly reduced the decline in FEV_1 (mean difference in FEV_1: 80 mL/year, 95% CI 0.003 mL/year to 500 mL/year, P = 0.03). A second cohort study (295 people homozygous for α_1 antitrypsin deficiency with FEV_1 < 65% predicted) compared 198 people who received weekly infusions of α_1 antitrypsin 60 mg/kg (duration not reported) versus 97 people who had never received α_1 antitrypsin. It found that α_1 antitrypsin significantly reduced the decline in FEV_1 (50 mL/year with α_1 antitrypsin *v* 80 mL/year with no α_1 antitrypsin, CI not reported; P = 0.02).[78]

OPTION DEOXYRIBONUCLEASE

We found no RCTs comparing the long term effects of deoxyribonuclease versus placebo.

Benefits: We found no systematic review or RCTs of deoxyribonuclease (DNase) specifically in people with chronic obstructive pulmonary disease (see comment below).

Harms: We found no RCTs.

Comment: **Short term treatment:** We found one RCT (349 people with bronchiectasis but not necessarily chronic airway obstruction) comparing DNase versus placebo given twice daily for 24 weeks.[79] It found that DNase significantly reduced forced expiratory volume in 1 second (FEV_1**G**) (CI not reported; P ≤ 0.05), but found no significant difference in the frequency of exacerbations over 24 weeks (0.66 in people with DNase *v* 0.56 in people with placebo; RR 1.70, 95% CI 0.85 to 1.65). In people with cystic fibrosis, DNase treatment is used to degrade DNA that increases the viscosity of pulmonary secretions. However, we found no evidence that this mechanism is useful to people with chronic obstructive pulmonary disease and chronic sputum production.

QUESTION What are the effects of smoking cessation interventions in stable chronic obstructive pulmonary disease?

OPTION PSYCHOSOCIAL INTERVENTIONS ALONE

We found no systematic review or RCTs in people with chronic obstructive pulmonary disease.

Benefits: We found no systematic review or RCTs examining the effects of psychosocial interventions such as professional advice or counselling alone on the outcomes of interest in this review (forced expiratory volume in 1 second**G**, peak expiratory flow**G** exacerbations, dyspnoea score, quality of life, or survival) specifically in people with chronic obstructive pulmonary disease (see comment below).

Harms: No RCTs were found that reported harms.

Comment: Despite the extensive literature on smoking cessation, we did not identify useful studies because most studies focused on combinations of interventions; continuous abstinence or point prevalence rates of smoking cessation as single outcome measures; healthy people or mixed populations of healthy people and people with disease.

OPTION PHARMACOLOGICAL INTERVENTIONS ALONE

One systematic review found no RCTs in people with chronic obstructive pulmonary disease.

Benefits: We found one systematic review (search date 2002).[80] It found no RCTs examining the effects of pharmacological smoking cessation interventions alone for the outcomes of interest in this review (forced expiratory volume in 1 second❻), peak expiratory flow, exacerbations, dyspnoea score, quality of life, or survival) specifically in people with chronic obstructive pulmonary disease (COPD; see comment below).

Harms: No studies were found of the harms of pharmacological interventions alone.

Comment: The systematic review[80] identified two RCTs, both of which examined pharmacological treatment plus non-pharmacological interventions (see benefits of psychosocial plus pharmacological interventions, p 1943).[10,81] One systematic review (search date 2001, 157 studies) assessed the clinical effectiveness of bupropion and nicotine replacement therapy for smoking cessation, but did not focus solely on people with COPD.[82,83] It found a low incidence of adverse events with nicotine replacement therapy, irrespective of the type of replacement. The most common adverse effects were localised reactions: skin sensitivity and irritation with patches; throat irritation, nasal irritation, and runny nose with nasal spray; hiccups, burning and smarting sensation in the mouth, sore throat, coughing, dry lips, and mouth ulcers with nicotine sublingual tablets; and hiccups, gastrointestinal disturbances, jaw pain, and orodental problems with nicotine gum. Sleep disturbances and alteration of mood may arise because of nicotine withdrawal. A small number of studies were undertaken in specific subgroups (including smokers with lung disease). Results for individual subgroups were generally non-significant, but their direction was consistent with the overall pooled results. The systematic review did not report results separately in people with COPD. Regarding the safety of bupropion, the review concluded that seizure is the most significant and important potential adverse effect. However, this review did not identify RCTs that reported any seizures. Common adverse events of bupropion are: rash, pruritus, urticaria, irritability, insomnia, dry mouth, headache, and tremor. The adverse effect profile of slow release bupropion seem to be better than that of immediate release bupropion. The results for specific subgroups (including smokers with pulmonary disease) were generally consistent with the overall pooled results, although results in people with COPD were not reported separately.

OPTION PSYCHOSOCIAL PLUS PHARMACOLOGICAL INTERVENTIONS

One large RCT in people with mild chronic obstructive pulmonary disease found that nicotine gum plus a psychosocial smoking cessation and abstinence maintenance programme (with or without ipratropium) slowed the decline of FEV_1, and reduced respiratory symptoms and lower respiratory illnesses, but increased weight gain compared with usual care (without psychosocial intervention). The RCT found no significant difference between treatments in all cause mortality at 5 years.

Benefits: One systematic review (search date 2002[84]) identified two RCTs that examined psychosocial plus pharmacological interventions in people with chronic obstructive pulmonary disease (COPD).[10,81] The first RCT (5887 smokers, age 35–60 years, with spirometric signs of early COPD, mean prebronchodilator forced expiratory volume in 1 second [FEV_1] 2640 mL, mean of 30 cigarettes smoked per day) compared three treatments: smoking cessation intervention plus placebo; smoking cessation intervention plus ipratropium; and usual care.[10] The smoking cessation intervention consisted of an intensive 12 session smoking cessation programme combining behaviour modification and use of nicotine gum (nicotine polacrilex 2 mg) with a continuing 5 year maintenance programme that included monitoring of weight gain and nutritional counselling.[85] The RCT found that the smoking cessation intervention (with or without ipratropium) increased the proportion of sustained quitters at 5 years, with a similar proportion remaining abstinent at 11 years, compared with usual care (22% at 5 years and 21.9% at 11 years with smoking cessation intervention *v* 5% at 5 years and 6% at 11 years with usual care; P value not reported).[86] It found that the smoking cessation intervention (with and without ipratropium) significantly improved FEV_1 compared with usual care after 1 and 5 years and that the smoking intervention plus ipratropium significantly improved FEV_1 compared with the smoking cessation intervention alone at 1 and 5 years (change in FEV_1 at 1 year: –34.3 mL with usual care *v* +11.2 mL with smoking cessation intervention *v* +38.8 mL with intervention plus ipratropium; $P < 0.005$ for each between treatment comparison; at 5 years, completer analysis [around 90% of participants]: –267 mL with usual care *v* –208 mL with smoking cessation intervention *v* –184 mL with intervention plus ipratropium; $P \leq 0.002$ for all comparisons).[10] In further analyses, both treatments using a smoking cessation intervention were combined. After 11 years, smoking intervention reduced the decline in FEV_1 compared with usual care (change from baseline: –502 mL with intervention *v* +587 mL with usual care; $P = 0.001$).[87] Smoking cessation intervention significantly reduced self reported lower respiratory illnesses resulting in physician visits compared with usual care at 5 years (results presented graphically; $P = 0.0008$).[88] The smoking cessation intervention significantly reduced cough, phlegm, wheezing, and dyspnoea compared with usual care at 5 years (by intention to treat analysis, cough for ≥ 3 months/year: 15% with intervention *v* 23% with usual care; phlegm for ≥ 3 months/year: 12% with intervention *v* 20% with usual care; presence of wheezing: 25% with intervention *v* 31% with usual care; presence of dyspnoea: 19% with intervention *v* 24% with usual care, all $P < 0.0001$).[89] There was no significant difference between the three treatments in all cause mortality at 5 years (2.60% with usual care *v* 2.24% with smoking cessation intervention *v* 2.75% with intervention plus ipratropium; $P = 0.58$).[90] The second RCT (404 people with mild or moderate COPD, smoking an average of 28 cigarettes per day, mean age 54 years) compared bupropion plus counselling versus placebo plus counselling for 12 weeks with 6 months' follow up, but only reported abstinence rates and adverse effects.[81] This study did not provide data about effects on FEV_1 changes, peak expiratory flow, exacerbations, dyspnoea score, quality of life, or survival. It found that bupropion (slow release 150 mg twice daily) plus counselling significantly increased continuous abstinence rates from weeks 4 to 26 compared with counselling alone (16% with bupropion plus counselling *v* 9% with counselling alone; $P = 0.05$; see comment below).[81]

Harms: In the first RCT,[10] 31% (about 1216 people) were still using nicotine gum after 1 year. About 25% of these reported at least one adverse effect, but most were minor and transient. The most common adverse effects were: indigestion (5.10% for men and 3.95% for women);

mouth irritation (6.2% for men and 6.5% for women); mouth ulcers (4.4% for men and 5.3% for women); nausea (1.8% for men and 3.8% for women); and hiccups (2.8% for men and 3.8% for women).[91] The smoking intervention increased weight at 1 and 5 years in both men and women compared with usual care, but the statistical significance was not reported (weight gain, 1 year: 2.61 kg with intervention *v* 0.61 kg with usual care for men and 2.63 kg *v* 1.10 kg for women; 5 years: 3.9 kg with intervention *v* 2.60 kg with usual care for men and 4.75 kg *v* 2.84 kg for women).[92] The second RCT found similar rates of discontinuation because of adverse effects between treatment groups (6% with placebo *v* 7% with bupropion). It found higher rates of serious adverse effects with placebo (2.5% with placebo *v* 0.5% with bupropion).[81]

Comment: None.

GLOSSARY

Forced expiratory volume in 1 second (FEV_1) The volume breathed out in the first second of forceful blowing into a spirometer, measured in litres

Peak expiratory flow rate The maximum rate that gas is expired from the lungs when blowing into a peak flow meter or a spirometer; the units are expressed as litres per minute

REFERENCES

1. The Global Initiative for Chronic Obstructive Lung Disease. http://www.goldcopd.com. Last accessed 13 February 2004.
2. American Thoracic Society. Standards for the diagnosis and care of patients with chronic obstructive pulmonary disease: ATS statement. *Am J Respir Crit Care Med* 1995;152(5 pt 2) (suppl):77–120.
3. World Health Report 1999. *"Making a difference"*. http://www.who.int/whr2001/2001/archives/1999/en/pdf/StatisticalAnnex.pdf (last accessed January 2004). p 110 Annex Table 4.
4. Soriano JB, Maier WC, Egger P, et al. Recent trends in physician diagnosed COPD in women and men in the UK. *Thorax* 2000;55:789–794.
5. Whittemore AS, Perlin SA, DiCiccio Y. Chronic obstructive pulmonary disease in lifelong nonsmokers: results from NHANES. *Am J Public Health* 1995;85:702–706.
6. Brunekreef B, Fischer P, Remijn B, et al. Indoor air pollution and its effects on pulmonary function of adult non-smoking women: III. passive smoking and pulmonary function. *Int J Epidemiol* 1985;14:227–230.
7. Rijcken B, Weiss ST. Longitudinal analyses of airway responsiveness and pulmonary function decline. *Am J Respir Crit Care Med* 1996;154(suppl):246–249.
8. Dockery DW, Brunekreef B. Longitudinal studies of air pollution effects on lung function. *Am J Respir Crit Care Med* 1996;154(suppl):250–256.
9. O'Connor GT, Sparrow D, Weiss ST. The role of allergy and non-specific airway hyperresponsiveness in the pathogenesis of chronic obstructive pulmonary disease: state of the art. *Am Rev Respir Dis* 1989;140:225–252.
10. Anthonisen NR, Connett JE, Kiley JP, et al. Effects of smoking intervention and the use of an inhaled anticholinergic bronchodilator on the rate of decline of FEV_1: the lung health study. *JAMA* 1994;272:1497–1505.
11. Siafakas NM, Vermeire P, Pride NB, et al. Optimal assessment and management of chronic obstructive pulmonary disease (COPD): a consensus statement of the European Respiratory Society. *Eur Respir J* 1995;8:1398–1420.
12. Braun SR, McKenzie WN, Copeland W, et al. A comparison of the effect of ipratropium bromide and albuterol in the treatment of chronic obstructive airway disease. *Arch Intern Med* 1989;149:544–547.
13. Higgins BG, Powell RM, Cooper S, et al. Effect of salbutamol and ipratropium bromide on airway calibre and bronchial reactivity in asthma and chronic bronchitis. *Eur Respir J* 1991;4:415–420.
14. Ikeda A, Nishimura K, Koyama H, et al. Bronchodilating effects of combined therapy with clinical dosages of ipratropium bromide and salbutamol for stable COPD: comparison with ipratropium bromide alone. *Chest* 1995;107:401–405.
15. Ikeda A, Nishimura K, Koyama H, et al. Comparative dose–response study of three anticholinergic agents and fenoterol using a metered dose inhaler in patients with chronic obstructive pulmonary disease. *Thorax* 1995;50:62–66.
16. Mahler DA, Donohue JF, Barbee RA, et al. Efficacy of salmeterol xinafoate in the treatment of COPD. *Chest* 1999;115:957–965.
17. Rennard SI, Anderson W, ZuWallack R, et al. Use of a long-acting inhaled β_2-adrenergic agonist, salmeterol xinafoate, in patients with chronic obstructive pulmonary disease. *Am J Respir Crit Care Med* 2001;163:1087–1092.
18. Dahl R, Greefhorst LA, Nowak D, et al. Inhaled formoterol dry powder versus ipratropium bromide in chronic obstructive pulmonary disease. *Am J Respir Crit Care Med* 2001;164:778–784.
19. Wadbo M, Lofdahl CG, Larsson K, et al. Effects of formoterol and ipratropium bromide in COPD: a 3-month placebo-controlled study. *Eur Respir J* 2002;20:1138–1146.
20. Liesker JJW, Wijkstra PJ, ten Hacken NHT, et al. A systematic review of the effects of bronchodilators on exercise capacity in patients with COPD. *Chest* 2002;121:597–608. Search date 1999; primary source Medline.
21. Littner MR, Ilowite JS, Tashkin DP, et al. Long-acting bronchodilation with once-daily dosing of tiotropium (Spiriva) in stable chronic obstructive pulmonary disease. *Am J Respir Crit Care Med* 2000;161:1136–1142.
22. Casaburi R, Briggs DD Jr, Donohue JF, et al. The spirometric efficacy of once-daily dosing with tiotropium in stable COPD: a 13-week multicenter trial. *Chest* 2000;118:1294–1302.
23. van Noord JA, Bantje TA, Eland ME, et al. A randomised controlled comparison of tiotropium and ipratropium in the treatment of chronic obstructive pulmonary disease. The Dutch Tiotropium Study Group. *Thorax* 2000;55:289–294.

24. Casaburi R, Mahler DA, Jones PW, et al. A long-term evaluation of once-daily inhaled tiotropium in chronic obstructive pulmonary disease. *Eur Respir J* 2002;19:217–224.
25. Vincken W, van Noord JA, Greefhorst AP, et al. Improved health outcomes in patients with COPD during 1 yr's treatment with tiotropium. *Eur Respir J* 2002;19:209–216.
26. Brusasco V, Hodder R, Miravitlles M, et al. Health outcomes following treatment for six months with once daily tiotropium compared with twice daily salmeterol in patients with COPD. *Thorax* 2003;58:399–404.
27. Van Schayck CP, Dompeling E, van Herwaarden CLA, et al. Bronchodilator treatment in moderate asthma or chronic bronchitis: continuous or on demand? A randomised controlled study. *BMJ* 1991;303:1426–1431.
28. Sestini P, Renzoni E, Robinson S, et al. Short-acting beta-$_2$ agonists for stable chronic obstructive pulmonary disease. In: The Cochrane Library, Issue 4, 2002. Oxford: Update Software. Search date 2002; primary sources Cochrane Airways Group database, and reference lists of review articles and retrieved studies.
29. Appleton S, Smith B, Veale A, et al. Long-acting beta$_2$-adrenoceptor agonists in stable chronic obstructive airways disease. In: The Cochrane Library, Issue 4, 2002. Oxford: Update Software. Search date 2001; primary sources Cochrane Airways Group Register to October 1998, hand searches of reference lists, and pharmaceutical companies contacted for unpublished studies.
30. Aalbers R, Ayres J, Backer V, et al. Formoterol in patients with chronic obstructive pulmonary disease: a randomized, controlled, 3-month trial. *Eur Respir J* 2002;19:936–943.
31. Liesker JJ, Van De Velde V, Meysman M, et al. Effects of formoterol (Oxis Turbohaler) and ipratropium on exercise capacity in patients with COPD. *Respir Med* 2002;96:559–566.
32. Donohue F, van Noord JA, Bateman ED, et al. A 6-month, placebo-controlled study comparing lung function and health status changes in COPD patients treated with tiotropium or salmeterol. *Chest* 2002;122:47–55.
33. Mahler DA, Wire P, Horstman D, et al. Effectiveness of fluticasone propionate and salmeterol combination delivered via the diskus device in the treatment of chronic obstructive pulmonary disease. *Am J Respir Crit Care Med* 2002;166:1084–1091.
34. Calverley P, Pauwels R, Vestbo J, et al. Combined salmeterol and fluticasone in the treatment of chronic obstructive pulmonary disease: a randomised controlled trial. *Lancet* 2003;361:449–456.
35. Szafranski W, Cukier A, Ramirez A, et al. Efficacy and safety of budesonide/formoterol in the management of chronic obstructive pulmonary disease. *Eur Respir J* 2003;21:74–81
36. Hanania NA, Darken P, Horstman D, et al. The efficacy and safety of fluticasone propionate (250 microg)/salmeterol (50 microg) combined in the Diskus inhaler for the treatment of COPD. *Chest* 2003;124:834–843.
37. Calverley PM, Boonsawat W, Cseke Z, et al. Maintenance therapy with budesonide and formoterol in chronic obstructive pulmonary disease. *Eur Respir J* 2003;22:912–919.
38. O'Byrne PM, Kerstjens HAM. Inhaled β_2-agonists in the treatment of asthma. *N Engl J Med* 1996;335:886–888.
39. Cook D, Guyatt G, Wong E, et al. Regular versus as-needed short-acting inhaled beta-agonist therapy for chronic obstructive pulmonary disease. *Am J Respir Crit Care Med* 2001;163:85–90.
40. Hall IP, Tattersfield AE. Beta-agonists. In: Clark TJH, Godfrey S, Lee TH, eds. *Asthma*. 3rd ed. London: Chapman and Hall Medical, 1992:341–365.
41. Cazzola M, Imperatore F, Salzillo A, et al. Cardiac effects of formoterol and salmeterol in patients suffering from COPD with preexisting cardiac arrhythmias and hypoxaemia. *Chest* 1998;114:411–415.
42. Anthonisen NR, Wright EC, and the IPPB Trial Group. Bronchodilator response in chronic obstructive pulmonary disease. *Am Rev Respir Dis* 1986;133:814–819.
43. Friedman M, Serby C, Menjoge S, et al. Pharmacoeconomic evaluation of a combination of ipratropium plus albuterol compared with ipratropium alone and albuterol alone in COPD. *Chest* 1999;115:635–641.
44. Levin DC, Little KS, Laughlin KR, et al. Addition of anticholinergic solution prolongs bronchodilator effect of beta$_2$ agonists in patients with chronic obstructive pulmonary disease. *Am J Med* 1996;100(1A;suppl):40–48.
45. Combivent Inhalation Solution Study Group. Routine nebulized ipratropium and albuterol together are better than either alone in COPD. *Chest* 1997;112:1514–1521.
46. Gross N, Tashkin D, Miller R, et al. Inhalation by nebulization of albuterol–ipratropium combination (Dey combination) is superior to either agent alone in the treatment of chronic obstructive pulmonary disease. Dey Combination Solution study group. *Respiration* 1998;65:354–362.
47. Campbell S. For COPD a combination of ipratropium bromide and albuterol sulfate is more effective than albuterol base. *Arch Intern Med* 1999;159:156–160.
48. Van Noord JA, de Munck DR, Bantje TA, et al. Long-term treatment of chronic obstructive pulmonary disease with salmeterol and the additive effect of ipratropium. *Eur Respir J* 2000;15:878–885.
49. Rutten van Molken M, Roos B, van Noord JA. An empirical comparison of the St George's Respiratory Questionnaire (SGRQ) and the Chronic Respiratory Disease Questionnaire (CRQ) in a clinical trial setting. *Thorax* 1999;54:995–1003.
50. D'Urzo AD, De Salvo MC, Ramirez-Rivera A, et al. In patients with COPD, treatment with a combination of formoterol and ipratropium is more effective than a combination of salbutamol and ipratropium: a 3-week, randomized, double-blind, within-patient, multicenter study. *Chest* 2001;119:1347–1356.
51. Rennard SI, Serby CW, Ghafouri M, et al. Extended therapy with ipratropium is associated with improved lung function in patients with COPD: a retrospective analysis of data from seven clinical trials. *Chest* 1996;110:62–70.
52. Ram FS, Jones PW, Castro AA, et al. Oral theophylline for chronic obstructive pulmonary disease. (Cochrane Review). In: The Cochrane Library, Issue 3, 2002. Oxford: Update Software. Search date 2002; primary sources: Cochrane Airways Group register and Cochrane Controlled Trials Register, Embase, Lilacs, Medline, Cinahl, contact with experts, and hand searches of bibliographies.
53. Rossi A, Kristufek P, Levine BE, et al. Comparison of the efficacy, tolerability, and safety of formoterol dry powder and oral, slow-release theophylline in the treatment of COPD. *Chest* 2002;121:1058–1069.
54. Calverley PMA. Symptomatic bronchodilator treatment. In: Calverley PMA; Pride N, eds. *Chronic obstructive pulmonary disease*. London: Chapman and Hall, 1995:419–446.
55. Ramsdell J. Use of theophylline in the treatment of COPD. *Chest* 1995;107(suppl):206–209.
56. Callahan CM, Dittus RS, Katz BP. Oral corticosteroid therapy for patients with stable chronic obstructive pulmonary disease: a meta-analysis. *Ann Intern Med* 1991;114:216–223. Search date 1989; primary source Medline.
57. McEvoy CE, Niewoehner DE. Adverse effects of corticosteroid therapy for COPD: a critical review. *Chest* 1997;111:732–743.
58. Postma DS, Kerstjens HAM. Are inhaled glucocorticosteroids effective in chronic obstructive pulmonary disease? *Am J Respir Crit Care Med* 1999;160:66–71.

59. Highland KB, Strange C, Heffner JE. Long-term effects of inhaled corticosteroids on FEV_1 in patients with chronic obstructive pulmonary disease. A meta-analysis. *Ann Intern Med* 2003;138:969–973. Search date 2002. [Erratum in: *Ann Intern Med* 2003;139:873]
60. Sutherland ER, Allmers H, Ayas NT, et al. Inhaled corticosteroids reduce the progression of airflow limitation in chronic obstructive pulmonary disease: a meta-analysis. *Thorax* 2003;58:937–941. Search date 2003.
61. Alsaeedi A, Sin DD, McAlister FA. The effects of inhaled corticosteroids in chronic obstructive pulmonary disease: a systematic review of randomized placebo-controlled trials. *Am J Med* 2002;113:59–65. Search date 2001; primary sources Medline, Embase, Cinahl, Sigle, Cochrane Controlled Trial Register, and study bibliographies.
62. The Lung Health Study Research Group. Effect of inhaled triamcinolone on the decline in pulmonary function in chronic obstructive pulmonary disease. *N Engl J Med* 2000;343:1902–1909.
63. Robertson AS, Gove RI, Wieland GA, et al. A double-blind comparison of oral prednisolone 40 mg/day with inhaled beclomethasone dipropionate 1500 μg/day in patients with adult onset chronic obstructive airways disease. *Eur J Respir Dis* 1986;69(suppl 146):565–569.
64. Weir DC, Gove RI, Robertson AS, et al. Corticosteroid trials in non-asthmatic chronic airflow obstruction: a comparison of oral prednisolone and inhaled beclomethasone dipropionate. *Thorax* 1990;45:112–117.
65. Shim CS, Williams MH. Aerosol beclomethasone in patients with steroid-responsive chronic obstructive pulmonary disease. *Am J Med* 1985;78:655–658.
66. Poole PJ, Black PN. Mucolytic agents for chronic bronchitis or chronic obstructive pulmonary disease. In: The Cochrane Library, Issue 2, 2003. Oxford: Update Software. Search date 1999; primary sources Cochrane Airways Group Register, and hand searches of reference lists.
67. Grandjean EM, Berthet P, Ruffmann R, et al. Efficacy of oral long-term *N*-acetylcysteine in chronic bronchopulmonary disease: a meta-analysis of published double-blind, placebo-controlled clinical trials. *Clin Ther* 2000;22:209–221. Search date 1995; primary sources Medline, hand searches of reference list, and personal contact with two experts.
68. Decramer M, Dekhuijzen PN, Troosters T, et al. The Bronchitis Randomized On NAC Cost-Utility Study (BRONCUS): hypothesis and design. BRONCUS trial Committee. *Eur Respir J* 2001;17:329–336.
69. Staykova T, Black P, Chacko E, et al. Prophylactic antibiotic therapy for chronic bronchitis (Cochrane Review). In The Cochrane Library, Issue 4, 2003. Chichester, UK: John Wiley and Sons, Ltd. Search date not reported; primary sources Cochrane Airways Group Register and hand searches of reference lists and reviews.
70. Crockett AJ, Moss JR, Cranston JM, et al. Domiciliary oxygen in chronic obstructive pulmonary disease. In: The Cochrane Library, Issue 1, 2002. Oxford: Update Software. Search date 2000; primary source Cochrane Airways Group Register.
71. Medical Research Council Working Party. Long term domiciliary oxygen therapy in chronic hypoxic cor pulmonale complicating chronic bronchitis and emphysema. *Lancet* 1981;1:681–686.
72. Fletcher EC, Luckett RA, Goodnight-White S, et al. A double-blind trial of nocturnal supplemental oxygen for sleep desaturation in patients with chronic obstructive pulmonary disease and a daytime PaO_2 above 60 mm Hg. *Am Rev Respir Dis* 1992;145:1070–1076.
73. Gorecka D, Gorzelak K, Sliwinski P, et al. Effect of long-term oxygen therapy on survival in patients with chronic obstructive pulmonary disease with moderate hypoxaemia. *Thorax* 1997;52:674–679.
74. Nocturnal Oxygen Therapy Trial Group. Continuous or nocturnal oxygen therapy in hypoxemic chronic obstructive lung disease: a clinical trial. *Ann Intern Med* 1980;93:391–398.
75. Chaouat A, Weitzenblum E, Kessler R, et al. A randomized trial of nocturnal oxygen therapy in chronic obstructive pulmonary disease patients. *Eur Respir J* 1999;14:1002–1008.
76. Dirksen A, Dijkman JH, Madsen F, et al. A randomized clinical trial of alpha$_1$-antitrypsin augmentation therapy. *Am J Respir Crit Care Med* 1999;160:1468–1472.
77. Anonymous. Survival and FEV_1 decline in individuals with severe deficiency of alpha$_1$-antitrypsin. The Alpha-1-Antitrypsin Deficiency Registry Study Group. *Am J Respir Crit Care Med* 1998;158:49–59.
78. Seersholm N, Wencker M, Banik N, et al. Does alpha$_1$-antitrypsin augmentation therapy slow the annual decline in FEV_1 in patients with severe hereditary alpha$_1$-antitrypsin deficiency? *Eur Respir J* 1997;10:2260–2263. [In German]
79. O'Donnell AE, Barker AF, Ilowite JS, et al. Treatment of idiopathic bronchiectasis with aerosolized recombinant human DNase I. rhDNase Study Group. *Chest* 1998;113:1329–1334.
80. Wagena EJ, Zeegers MPA, van Schayck CP, et al. Benefits and risks of pharmacological smoking cessation therapies in chronic obstructive pulmonary disease. *Drug Safety* 2003;26:381–403. Search date 2002.
81. Tashkin D, Kanner R, Bailey W, et al. Smoking cessation in patients with chronic obstructive pulmonary disease: a double-blind, placebo-controlled, randomised trial. *Lancet* 2001;357:1571–1575.
82. National Institute for Clinical Excellence. Guidance on the use of nicotine replacement therapy (NTR) and bupropion for smoking cessation. Technology Appraisal No 39; issue date March 2002. ISBN: 1-84257-163-X. http://www.nice.org.uk derived from 26 electronic databases and Internet resources. In addition, the bibliographies of retrieved articles and submissions from the manufacturers were searched.
83. National Institute for Clinical Excellence. A rapid and systematic review of the clinical and costs effectiveness of bupropion SR and nicotine replacement therapy (NTR) for smoking cessation. NHS Centre for Reviews & Dissemination, University of York in York (UK), February 2002. Primary sources: 26 electronic databases, Internet resources, bibliographies of retrieved articles, and submissions from the manufacturers were searched.
84. van der Meer RM, Wagena EJ, Ostelo RWJG, et al (Cochrane Review). Smoking cessation for chronic obstructive pulmonary disease. In: The Cochrane Library, Issue 1, 2004. Chichester, UK: John Wiley & Sons, Ltd. Search date 2002; primary sources Medline, Embase; Psychlit, Central, Cochrane Controlled Trials Register, and references.
85. O'Hara P, Grill J, Rigdon M, et al. Design and results of the intervention program for the Lung Health Study. *Prev Med* 1993;22:304–315.
86. Murray RP, Connett JE, Rand RCR, et al. Persistence of the effect of the Lung Health Study (LHS) smoking intervention over eleven years. *Prev Med* 2002;35:314–319.
87. Anthonisen NR, Connett JE, Murray RP for the Lung Health Study Research Group. Smoking and lung function of the lung health study participants after 11 years. *Am J Respir Crit Care Med* 2002;166:675–679.
88. Kanner RE, Anthonisen NR, Connett JE, et al. Lower respiratory illnesses promote FEV_1 decline in current smokers but not ex-smokers with mild chronic obstructive pulmonary disease: results from the lung health study. *Am J Respir Crit Care Med* 2001;164:358–364.
89. Kanner RE, Connett JE, Williams DE, et al. Effects of randomized assignment to a smoking cessation intervention and changes in smoking habits on respiratory symptoms in smokers with early chronic obstructive pulmonary disease: the Lung Health Study. *Am J Med* 1999;106:410–416.

90. Anthonisen NR, Connett JE, Enright PL, et al. Hospitalizations and mortality in the lung health study. *Am J Respir Crit Care Med* 2002;166:333–339.
91. Murray RP, Bailey WC, Daniels K, et al. Safety of nicotine polacrilex gum used by 3,094 participants in the Lung Health Study. Lung Health Study Research Group. *Chest* 1996;109:438–445.
92. O'Hara P, Connett JE, Lee WW, et al. Early and late weight gain smoking cessation in the lung health study. *Am J Epidemiology* 1998;148:821–830.

Huib Kerstjens
Professor of Pulmonary Medicine
University Hospital Groningen
Groningen
The Netherlands

Dirkje Postma
Professor of Pulmonary Medicine
University Hospital Groningen
Groningen
The Netherlands

Nick ten Hacken
Pulmonary Physician
University Hospital Groningen
Groningen
The Netherlands

Competing interests: All three authors have received funding from the following manufacturers: AstraZeneca, the manufacturer of budesonide, terbutaline, formoterol; GlaxoSmithKline, the manufacturer of beclometasone, salbutamol, salmeterol, fluticasone; Boehringer Ingelheim, the manufacturer of fenoterol, ipratropium, tiotropium; and Novartis, the manufacturer of formoterol. DP has also received funding from Zambon, the manufacturer of N-acetylcysteine.

Lung cancer

Search date September 2003

Alan Neville

QUESTIONS

INTERVENTIONS

See glossary G

Key Messages

Non-small cell lung cancer

- **Palliative chemotherapy in stage 4 non-small cell lung cancer** Systematic reviews in people with stage 4 non-small cell lung cancer have found that adding chemotherapy regimens containing cisplatin to best supportive care increases survival at 1 year compared with supportive care alone. Limited evidence from RCTs suggests that adding chemotherapy to best supportive care may improve quality of life compared with best supportive care alone.
- **Thoracic irradiation plus chemotherapy in unresectable stage 3 non-small cell lung cancer (compared with thoracic irradiation alone)** Systematic reviews and two RCTs in people with unresectable stage 3 non-small cell lung cancer have found that adding chemotherapy to irradiation improves survival at 2–5 years compared with irradiation alone. One RCT found no significant difference in median survival between radical radiotherapy plus chemotherapy and radiotherapy alone.

Observational evidence suggests that, in people aged over 70 years with unresectable stage 3 non-small cell lung cancer, chemotherapy plus radiotherapy may reduce quality adjusted survival compared with radiotherapy alone. We found insufficient evidence about effects on quality of life.

- **Hyperfractionated radiation treatment in unresectable stage 3 non-small cell lung cancer** One systematic review found no clear evidence that altered fractionation regimens, accelerated, hyperfractionated, or hyperfractionated split course regimens are any more effective than conventional radiotherapy. One RCT identified by the review has found that continuous, hyperfractionated, accelerated radiotherapy reduces mortality at 2 years compared with conventional radiotherapy in people with stage 3A, 3B, 1, or 2 non-small cell lung cancer.
- **Palliative single drug chemotherapy in stage 4 non-small cell lung cancer (not clearly better than combination chemotherapy)** One systematic review and subsequent RCTs in people with stage 3 and 4 non-small cell lung cancer found inconclusive evidence on the effects of single agent chemotherapy compared with combined chemotherapy. One systematic review and subsequent RCTs provided insufficient evidence to compare first line platinum based version non-platinum based chemotherapy.
- **Preoperative chemotherapy in people with resectable stage 3 non-small cell lung cancer** One systematic review of small, weak RCTs and one subsequent RCT provided inconclusive evidence about the effects of preoperative chemotherapy in people with resectable stage 3 non-small cell lung cancer.
- **Postoperative chemotherapy in people with resected stage 1–3 non-small cell lung cancer** Systematic reviews and subsequent RCTs in people with completely resected stage 1–3 non-small cell lung cancer found no significant difference in survival at 5 years between postoperative cisplatin based chemotherapy and surgery alone with or without concomitant radiotherapy, although subgroup analysis in one RCT suggests that postoperative chemotherapy may increase survival in people with stage 3 disease. One systematic review has found that postoperative alkylating agents increase mortality compared with no postoperative chemotherapy.

Small cell lung cancer

- **Chemotherapy plus thoracic irradiation in limited stage small cell lung cancer** Two systematic reviews in people with limited stage small cell lung cancer have found that adding thoracic irradiation to chemotherapy improves survival at 3 years and improves local control. However, one of these reviews has found that chemotherapy plus thoracic irradiation increases deaths related to treatment.
- **Prophylactic cranial irradiation for people in complete remission from limited or extensive stage small cell lung cancer** One systematic review in people with small cell lung cancer in complete remission has found that prophylactic cranial irradiation improves survival at 3 years and reduces the risk of developing brain metastases compared with no irradiation. While long term cognitive dysfunction after cranial irradiation has been described in non-randomised studies, RCTs have not found a cumulative increase in neuropsychological dysfunction.
- **Dose intensification of chemotherapy** One systematic review found limited evidence that intensifying chemotherapy dose by either increasing the number of chemotherapy cycles, increasing chemotherapy dose, or increasing dose intensity per cycle may modestly improve survival compared with standard chemotherapy. However, additional RCTs have found inconclusive evidence about the effects of dose intensification on survival.
- **Oral etoposide in extensive stage small cell lung cancer** Two RCTs in people with extensive stage small cell lung cancer found that oral etoposide reduced survival compared with combination chemotherapy at 1 year. One RCT, in people with extensive stage small cell lung cancer who had not responded to induction combination chemotherapy, found no significant difference between oral etoposide and no further treatment in mortality at 3 years, although overall mortality was lower in people taking etoposide. RCTs found that etoposide may reduce nausea, alopecia, and numbness in the short term compared with combination chemotherapy. They found no evidence that it offered better quality of life overall.

DEFINITION	Lung cancer (bronchogenic carcinoma) is an epithelial cancer arising from the bronchial surface epithelium or bronchial mucous glands. It is broadly divided into small cell and non-small cell lung cancer. For a description of the stages of lung cancer see table 1, p 1967.
INCIDENCE/ PREVALENCE	Lung cancer is the leading cause of cancer death in both men and women annually, affecting about 100 000 men and 80 000 women in the USA and about 40 000 men and women in the UK. Small cell lung cancer constitutes about 20–25% of all lung cancers, the remainder being non-small cell lung cancers of which adenocarcinoma is now the most prevalent form.[1]
AETIOLOGY/ RISK FACTORS	Smoking remains the major preventable risk factor, accounting for about 80–90% of all cases.[2] Other respiratory tract carcinogens have been identified that may enhance the carcinogenic effects of tobacco smoke, either in the workplace (e.g. asbestos and polycyclic aromatic hydrocarbons) or in the home (e.g. indoor radon).[3]
PROGNOSIS	Lung cancer has an overall 5 year survival rate of 10–12%.[4] At the time of diagnosis, 10–15% of people with lung cancer have localised disease. Of these, half will have died at 5 years despite potentially curative surgery. Over half of people have metastatic disease at the time of diagnosis. People with non-small cell cancer who have surgery have a 5 year survival of 60–80% for stage 1 disease and 25–50% for stage 2 disease.[4] In people with small cell cancer, those with limited stage disease who have combined chemotherapy and mediastinal irradiation have a median survival of 18–24 months, whereas those with extensive stage disease who are given palliative chemotherapy have a median survival of 10–12 months.[4] About 5–10% of people with small cell lung cancer present with central nervous system involvement, and half develop symptomatic brain metastases by 2 years. Of these, only half respond to palliative radiation, and their median survival is less than 3 months.[4]
AIMS OF INTERVENTION	To prolong life; to improve quality of life; and to provide palliation of symptoms, with minimum adverse effects of treatment.
OUTCOMES	Survival; clinical response rates; disease related symptoms; adverse effects of treatment; quality of life. Despite recent progress in the development of valid instruments, measuring quality of life in people with lung cancer remains a serious challenge.[5,6]
METHODS	*Clinical Evidence* search and appraisal September 2003. Unless stated otherwise, we have used the term stage 3 non-small cell lung cancer to refer to both stage 3A and stage 3B (see table 1, p 1967).

QUESTION **What are the effects of treatments for non-small cell lung cancer?**

OPTION **PRE- AND POSTOPERATIVE CHEMOTHERAPY IN PEOPLE WITH RESECTABLE NON-SMALL CELL LUNG CANCER**

One systematic review of small, weak RCTs and one subsequent RCT provide inconclusive evidence about the effects of preoperative chemotherapy in people with resectable stage 3 non-small cell lung cancer. Systematic reviews and subsequent RCTs in people with completely resected stage 1–3 non-small cell lung cancer found no significant difference in survival at 5 years between postoperative cisplatin based chemotherapy and surgery alone with or without concomitant radiotherapy, although subgroup analysis in one RCT suggests that postoperative chemotherapy may increase survival in people with stage 3 disease. One systematic review has found that postoperative alkylating agents increase mortality compared with no postoperative chemotherapy.

Benefits: **Preoperative chemotherapy versus no chemotherapy:** We found one systematic review,[7] one non-systematic review,[8] and one subsequent RCT.[9] The systematic review (search date 1997, 4 RCTs, 204 people with technically resectable stage 3A non-small cell lung cancer) compared preoperative cisplatin based chemotherapy with no chemotherapy.[7] It found that preoperative chemotherapy significantly reduced mortality at 2 years compared with no preoperative chemotherapy (2 fully reported RCTs; AR 34/58 [59%] with preoperative chemotherapy v 54/62 [87%] with no chemotherapy; RR 0.67, 95% CI 0.42 to 0.89; NNT 4, 95% CI 2 to 11). The non-systematic review, which identified the same RCTs, suggested that this evidence is limited because the trials were small, staging was clinical rather than pathological, and treatment groups were not balanced for prognostic factors such as K-Ras mutations.[8] The subsequent RCT (355 people with resectable stages 1 [except T1N0] to 3A non-small cell lung cancer) compared preoperative chemotherapy (2 cycles of ifosfamide plus mitomycin plus cisplatin) versus primary surgery alone.[9] It found no significant difference in survival after 4 years follow up between preoperative chemotherapy and surgery alone in people with any disease stage or in people with stage 3 disease (median survival for any disease stage 37 months, 95% CI 26.7 months to 48.3 months with preoperative chemotherapy v 26.0 months, 95% CI 19.8 months to 33.6 months; P = 0.15; RR for survival in people with stage 3 disease 1.04, 95% CI 0.68 to 1.60; P = 0.85). **Postoperative chemotherapy versus surgery alone:** We found one systematic review[10] and two subsequent RCTs.[11,12] The review (search date 1991, 14 RCTs, 1394 people with resected stage 1–3 non-small cell lung cancer) found no significant difference between postoperative cisplatin based chemotherapy compared with surgery alone in mortality at 5 years (8 RCTs; ARR +5%, 95% CI –1% to +10%; HR 0.87, 95% CI 0.74 to 1.02; P = 0.08).[10] However, it found that postoperative alkylating agents significantly increased mortality compared with surgery alone (5 RCTs; HR 1.15; CI not reported; P = 0.005; ARI of death at 5 years +5%, CI not reported). The first subsequent RCT (70 people, stage 1–3B resected non-small cell lung cancer) compared postoperative chemotherapy (4 cycles of iv cyclophosphamide, vincristine, adriamycin, and lomustine, followed by oral ftorafur) versus no chemotherapy for 1 year.[11] It found no significant difference in survival at 5 years between postoperative chemotherapy and no postoperative chemotherapy (49% with postoperative chemotherapy v 31% with no chemotherapy; P > 0.05, absolute numbers not reported).[11] A subgroup analysis in people with stage 3 non-small cell lung cancer (40 people with stage 3A, 9 with stage 3B) found that postoperative chemotherapy significantly increased survival at 5 years compared with no postoperative chemotherapy (44% with postoperative chemotherapy v 21% with no chemotherapy; P < 0.025, absolute numbers not reported). Results for people with stage 3A and 3B non-small cell lung cancer were not reported separately.[11] The second subsequent RCT (221 people, stage 1–2 resected non-small cell lung cancer) compared uracil plus tegafur for 2 years versus no postoperative chemotherapy.[12] It found no significant difference in 5 year survival or 5 year disease free survival between chemotherapy and no chemotherapy (survival: 79% with postoperative chemotherapy v 75% with no chemotherapy; HR 1.13, 95% CI 0.65 to 1.97; disease free survival: 78% with postoperative chemotherapy v 71% with no chemotherapy; HR 1.37, 95% CI 0.81 to 2.32). **Postoperative chemotherapy plus radiotherapy versus postoperative radiotherapy alone:** We found one systematic review (search date 1991, 7 RCTs, 807 people)[10] and one subsequent RCT.[11] The review found no significant difference in overall survival between adding postoperative chemotherapy to postoperative radiotherapy and postoperative radiotherapy alone (overall survival: HR 0.98; CI not reported, P = 0.76; HR for 6 RCTs that used cisplatin based chemotherapy HR 0.94; CI not reported, P = 0.46; ARR for death at 5 years +2%, 95% CI –3% to +8%).[10] The subsequent RCT (488 people with completely resected stage 2 or 3A non-small cell lung cancer) compared postoperative radiotherapy with or without cisplatin plus etoposide.[13] It found no significant difference between postoperative chemotherapy plus radiotherapy and radiotherapy alone in median survival (37.9 months with postoperative chemotherapy plus radiotherapy v 38.8 months with radiotherapy alone; P = 0.56).

Harms: **Preoperative chemotherapy:** One RCT identified by the review, which compared preoperative chemotherapy versus no chemotherapy, found that chemotherapy was associated with grade III or IV neutropenia (80% of people), nausea and vomiting, diarrhoea, hypomagnesaemia, and alopecia (no further data reported).[7] **Postoperative chemotherapy:** The systematic review of postoperative cisplatin based chemotherapy gave no information on adverse effects.[10] One RCT (269 people) identified by the review, which compared four postoperative courses of cyclophosphamide plus adriamycin plus cisplatin versus no postoperative chemotherapy, found that only 53% of people allocated to postoperative chemotherapy completed all four courses.[14] Mild to severe gastrointestinal toxicity was reported in 88% of people receiving postoperative chemotherapy. A second RCT identified by the review reported similar toxicity.[15] Many adjuvant chemotherapy studies were published before serotonin receptor antagonist antiemetics were available. The second subsequent RCT (221 people) reported grade 3–4 toxicity in 0.9% (1/110) of people and grade 1 or more toxicity in 59.8% (64/110) of people with postoperative uracil plus tegafur.[12]

Comment: The systematic review examining effects of preoperative chemotherapy[7] identified one interim report[16] of an RCT in 27 people, which was unsuitable for inclusion in the meta-analysis. The RCT found that preoperative chemotherapy significantly improved median survival after about 30 months' follow up compared with no preoperative chemotherapy (median survival: 28.7 months with preoperative chemotherapy v 15.6 months with no chemotherapy; P = 0.095).[17] Larger trials of preoperative chemotherapy in people with stage 3A non-small cell lung cancer are needed. Most of the chemotherapy regimens in the postoperative RCTs identified by the reviews are no longer used, and more trials examining newer agents are needed.

OPTION THORACIC IRRADIATION FOR UNRESECTABLE STAGE 3 NON-SMALL CELL LUNG CANCER (COMPARED WITH THORACIC IRRADIATION ALONE)

Systematic reviews and subsequent RCTs in people with unresectable stage 3 non-small cell lung cancer have found that adding chemotherapy to irradiation improves survival at 2–5 years compared with irradiation alone. One RCT found no significant difference in median survival between radical radiotherapy plus chemotherapy and radiotherapy alone. Observational evidence suggests that, in people aged over 70 years with unresectable stage 3 non-small cell lung cancer, chemotherapy plus radiotherapy may reduce quality adjusted survival compared with radiotherapy alone. We found insufficient evidence about effects on quality of life.

Benefits: We found three systematic reviews[10,17,18] and three subsequent RCTs.[19–21] The first review (search date 1991, 22 RCTs, 3033 people with unresected stage 3 non-small cell lung cancer) found that chemotherapy plus thoracic irradiation significantly reduced mortality compared with radiotherapy alone, with an absolute survival benefit of 3% with combined treatment compared with radiotherapy alone at 2 years (mortality: HR 0.90, 95% CI 0.83 to 0.97).[10] The second review (search date 1995, 14 RCTs, including 9 RCTs identified by the first review and 1 RCT excluded from the first review because of poor methodology, 1887 people) found that a cisplatin based regimen plus radiotherapy significantly reduced mortality at 2 years compared with radiotherapy alone (OR 0.7, 95% CI 0.5 to 0.9).[17] The third review (search date 1995, 14 RCTs, including 11 RCTs identified by the first or second review, 2589 people) found that chemotherapy (primarily cisplatin based) plus radiotherapy significantly reduced mortality at 3 years compared with radiotherapy alone (RR 0.83, 95% CI 0.77 to 0.90).[18] The first subsequent RCT (458 people) compared 2 months of cisplatin plus vinblastine followed by standard radiotherapy with either standard or hyperfractionated radiotherapy alone.[19] It found that combined treatment significantly improved 5 year survival compared with radiotherapy alone (AR 8% with combined treatment *v* 5% with standard radiotherapy *v* 6% with hyperfractionated radiotherapy; P = 0.04 for combined *v* either comparison). The second subsequent RCT (446 people) compared radical radiotherapy plus four cycles of mitomycin plus ifosfamide plus cisplatin with radical radiotherapy alone.[20] It found no significant difference in median survival between groups (11.7 months with combined treatment *v* 9.7 months with radiotherapy alone; P = 0.14). The third subsequent RCT (506 people randomised, 460 analysed, stage 3A or 3B) compared radiotherapy (60 Gy) plus neoadjuvant cisplatin plus ifosfamide plus and mitomycin for three 21 day cycles versus radiotherapy alone.[21] It found that chemotherapy increased survival at 2 years, but the statistical significance was not reported (20.0% with adjuvant chemotherapy *v* 7.4% with no adjuvant treatment). We found insufficient evidence about the effects of combining thoracic irradiation with chemotherapy on quality of life.

Harms: The reviews and RCTs gave no information on long term adverse effects of treatment.[10,17–21]

Comment: Radioprotector drugs and three-dimensional conformal radiotherapy are being investigated to reduce the toxicities of combined modality treatment.[22] One meta-analysis (6 prospective phase II or III studies) found that, in people aged over 70 years with unresectable stage 3 non-small cell lung cancer, chemotherapy plus radiotherapy significantly reduced quality adjusted survival compared with radiotherapy alone (10.8 months with chemotherapy plus radiotherapy *v* 13.1 months with standard radiotherapy; P < 0.01).[23]

OPTION HYPERFRACTIONATED RADIATION TREATMENT FOR UNRESECTABLE STAGE 3 NON-SMALL CELL LUNG CANCER

One systematic review found no clear evidence that altered fractionation regimens, accelerated, hyperfractionated, or hyperfractionated split course regimens were more effective than conventional radiotherapy. One RCT identified by the review found that continuous, hyperfractionated, accelerated radiotherapy reduced mortality at 2 years compared with conventional radiotherapy in people with stage 3A, 3B, 1, or 2 non-small cell lung cancer.

Benefits: **Hyperfractionation:** We found one systematic review (search date 2001, 7 RCTs, 1369 people, 4 altered fractionation regimens; accelerated, hyperfractionated, hyperfractionated and split course, and continuous, hyperfractionated, accelerated radiotherapy (CHART**G**).[24] It found that of all the regimens examined, only CHART was clearly more effective than standard regimens. **Accelerated radiotherapy:** The review (search date 2001, 1 RCT, 99 people randomised, 77 people with stage 3 analysed) found no significant difference in survival between accelerated radiotherapy and standard radiotherapy (median survival: 14.4 months with accelerated *v* 13.8 months with standard; HR 0.93, 95% CI 0.67 to 1.28).[24] **Accelerated radiotherapy plus chemotherapy:** The review (search date 2001, 1 RCT, 81 people analysed) found no significant difference in survival between accelerated radiotherapy plus chemotherapy and standard radiotherapy alone (median survival: 15.0 months with accelerated plus chemotherapy *v* 13.8 months with standard; HR 0.99, 95% CI 0.73 to 1.32).[24] **Hyperfractionated radiotherapy:** The review (search date 2001, 3 RCTs, 361 people) identified one large RCT (306 people) and two small RCTs.[24] Overall, the review found no significant difference in survival between hyperfractionated radiotherapy and standard radiotherapy, although results were heterogeneous (HR 0.94, 95% CI 0.80 to 1.09, heterogeneity P = 0.025).[24] The large RCT found no significant difference in survival. One small RCT found that hyperfractionated radiotherapy increased survival. The second small RCT found that hyperfractionated radiotherapy decreased survival. **Hyperfractionated radiotherapy plus chemotherapy:** The review (search date 2001, 1 RCT, 17 people) found no significant difference in survival between hyperfractionated radiotherapy plus chemotherapy and standard radiotherapy alone (median survival: 14.5 months with radiotherapy plus chemotherapy *v* 6.0 months with radiotherapy alone; HR 1.72, 95% CI 0.51 to 5.74).[24] **Split-course hyperfractionated radiotherapy plus chemotherapy:** The review (search date 2001, 2 RCTs, 126 people) found that split-course hyperfractionated radiotherapy plus chemotherapy significantly improved survival compared with standard radiotherapy alone (HR 0.48, 95% CI 0.33 to 0.70).[24] However, there was significant heterogeneity among RCTs. One RCT found no significant difference in survival and the other RCT (considered to be of poor quality because of inadequate reporting) found that combined treatment significantly improved survival. **Continuous hyperfractionated accelerated radiotherapy (CHART):** We found no systematic review or RCTs exclusively in people with stage 3 non-small cell lung cancer. The systematic review (search date 2001, 1 RCT, 563 people with non-small cell lung cancer; 61% with stage 3A or 3B, 39% with stage 1 or 2)[24] found that CHART**G** significantly reduced mortality and improved local tumour control compared with standard radiotherapy at 2 years (mortality: AR 71% with CHART *v* 80% with standard radiotherapy, HR 0.78, 95% CI 0.65 to 0.94; P = 0.008; local tumour control: HR 0.79, 95% CI 0.63 to 0.98; P = 0.03).[22]

Harms: **Accelerated radiotherapy:** The review (search date 2001, 1 RCT, 77 people analysed) found that accelerated radiotherapy significantly increased grade 3 and 4 oesophageal toxicity compared with standard radiotherapy (number for each treatment group: 15 people with accelerated *v* 6 people with standard; P value not reported in review).[24] **Accelerated radiotherapy plus chemotherapy:** The review (search date 2001, 1 RCT, 104 people, 78% of people analysed) found that accelerated radiotherapy plus chemotherapy significantly increased grade 3 and 4 oesophageal toxicity compared with standard radiotherapy (24/51[47%] with accelerated *v* 6/53 [11%] with standard, P value not reported in review).[24] **Hyperfractionated radiotherapy:** The large RCT identified by the systematic review (search date 2001) found three treatment related deaths with hyperfractionated radiotherapy.[24] **CHART:** The systematic review (search date 2001)[24] found information on the adverse effects of CHART in further reports.[22,25] It found that CHART significantly increased pain on swallowing, heartburn (both of which were of brief duration), cough (P = 0.01), shortness of breath (P = 0.03), and dizziness (P = 0.03) compared with conventional radiotherapy over the first 3 months. It found no symptoms with a greater than 20% difference between treatment groups at 1 year.[25] The review found that CHART increased pulmonary fibrosis at 2 years (16% with CHART *v* 4% with standard, P value not reported).[24]

Comment: None.

OPTION PALLIATIVE CHEMOTHERAPY IN STAGE 4 NON-SMALL CELL LUNG CANCER

Systematic reviews in people with stage 4 non-small cell lung cancer have found that adding chemotherapy regimens containing cisplatin to supportive care increases survival at 1 year compared with supportive care alone. Limited evidence from RCTs suggests that chemotherapy plus best supportive care may improve quality of life compared with best supportive care alone. Two systematic reviews and subsequent RCTs in people with advanced non-small cell lung cancer found inconclusive evidence on the effects of single agent chemotherapy compared with combined chemotherapy. One systematic review and additional RCTs provided insufficient evidence to compare first line platinum based versus non-platinum based chemotherapy.

Benefits: **First line chemotherapy versus supportive care:** We found three systematic reviews.[10,26,27] The most recent systematic review (search date 1998, 4 earlier systematic reviews)[26] did not fully describe the four earlier systematic reviews it identified, three of which included the same RCTs. The review did not perform a meta-analysis. The first review that performed a meta-analysis (search date 1991, 11 RCTs, 1190 people with advanced non-small cell lung cancer) compared supportive care plus chemotherapy versus supportive care alone.[10] It found that, in trials from the 1970s, long term alkylating agents plus supportive care did not significantly improve survival compared with supportive care alone (HR 1.26, 95% CI 0.96 to 1.66; P = 0.095). However, cisplatin containing regimens plus supportive care significantly increased survival at 1 year (HR 0.73; P < 0.0001) and increased median survival compared with supportive care alone (5.5 months with cisplatin containing regimens plus supportive care *v* 4 months with supportive care alone). It is not possible to deduce from these RCTs to what extent the observed effects are because of the cisplatin or to all the other drugs in the combinations studied. The second review[26] that performed a meta-analysis (search date not reported, 8 RCTs, 7 of which were included in the first review,[10] 712 people with advanced non-small cell lung cancer) comparing chemotherapy plus best supportive care versus best supportive care alone found that chemotherapy significantly reduced mortality at 6 months (OR 0.44, 95% CI 0.32 to 0.59).[26] The third review[27] identified four RCTs, which compared single agent chemotherapy plus best supportive care versus best supportive care alone, and assessed effects on quality of life.[28–31] Overall, the trials consistently found that chemotherapy plus best supportive care improved quality of life compared with best supportive care alone. The difference between groups was not significant in most trials, but they are likely to have been underpowered to detect a clinically important difference. The first RCT (207 people with stage 3B or 4 non-small cell lung cancer) found that adding vinorelbine to supportive care significantly improved emotional functioning (assessed by European Organization for Research and Treatment of Cancer QLQ-C30 questionnaire P = 0.01, absolute numbers not reported), nausea and vomiting (P = 0.04), pain (P < 0.01), and dyspnoea (P = 0.02) compared with supportive care alone.[28] It found no significant difference between groups in other measures of quality of life, although all scores, except those for diarrhoea, were improved in people taking vinorelbine.[28] The second RCT (300 people with symptomatic locally advanced or metastatic non-small cell lung cancer, Karnofsky performance status❻ 60–90) compared gemcitabine plus best supportive care versus best supportive care alone.[29] It found that people receiving gemcitabine had improved quality of life (assessed by European Organization for Research and Treatment of Cancer QLQ-C30 questionnaire) compared with people receiving best supportive care alone.[29] The RCT did not assess the significance of the difference between groups. The third RCT (157 people with stage 3B or 4 non-small cell lung cancer) found no significant difference in overall quality of life between paclitaxel plus supportive care and supportive care alone (assessed by the Rotterdam symptom checklist; lower scores indicate worse symptoms: –0.019 with paclitaxel *v* –0.017 with supportive care alone; P = 0.242), although scores improved in people taking paclitaxel.[31] The fourth RCT (191 people aged ≥70 years with stage 3B or 4 non-small cell lung cancer) found no significant difference in global health status between adding vinorelbine to supportive care and supportive care alone, although functional scale scores were higher in people taking vinorelbine (global health status assessed by European Organization for Research and Treatment of Cancer QLQ-C30 questionnaire, higher score indicates better function, mean difference in score +4.58, 95% CI –0.26 to +9.43).[28] Toxicity scores were also higher in people receiving vinorelbine compared with supportive care alone, but the difference was not significant. **First line single agent versus combined chemotherapy:** We found two systematic reviews[32,33] and five subsequent RCTs.[34–38] The first systematic review (search date 1995–1996, 25 RCTs, 5156 people with stage 4 non-small cell lung cancer) found no significant difference between platinum analogue or vinorelbine containing combination chemotherapy and platinum analogue or vinorelbine alone in 1 year survival (RR 1.10, 95% CI 0.94 to 1.43).[32] The second systematic review (search date 2002, 3 RCTs) compared the single agent gemcitabine versus combination treatment.[33] The review did not pool results. It found that none of the RCTs found any significant difference between treatments in survival (results from the 3 RCTs for gemcitabine *v* combination: 7.9 months with gemcitabine *v* 6.1 months with combination; P = 0.13; 6.6 months with gemcitabine *v* 7.6 months with combination; P reported as not significant; 8.5 months with gemcitabine *v* 11.1 months with combination; P = 0.65). Two subsequent RCTs compared vinorelbine plus gemcitabine versus monotherapy and found different results.[34,37] The first subsequent RCT (120 people with advanced non-small cell lung cancer aged > 70 years) found that gemcitabine plus vinorelbine significantly improved survival at median 14 months compared with vinorelbine alone (median survival: 29 weeks with combined treatment *v* 18 weeks with single treatment; P < 0.01).[34] The second subsequent RCT (698 people aged 63–86 years with stage 3B or 4 disease) found no significant difference in survival between vinorelbine plus gemcitabine and either vinorelbine alone or gemcitabine alone (median survival: 30 weeks with combination *v* 36 weeks with vinorelbine *v* 28 weeks with gemcitabine; HR 1.17, 95% CI 0.95 to 1.44 for combination *v* vinorelbine; HR 1.06, 95% CI 0.86 to 1.29 for combination *v* gemcitabine).[37] The third subsequent RCT (522 chemotherapy naive people with stage 3 or 4 non-small cell lung cancer) found that gemcitabine plus cisplatin significantly improved survival compared with cisplatin alone (median survival: 9.1 months with combination *v* 7.6 months with cisplatin alone; P = 0.004).[35] The fourth subsequent RCT (415 with histologically or cytologically confirmed stage 3 or 4 non-small cell lung cancer) found that cisplatin plus vinorelbine significantly improved survival compared with cisplatin alone (median survival: 8 months with combination *v* 6 months with cisplatin alone; P = 0.002).[36] The fifth subsequent RCT (398 people with stage 3B or 4 non-small cell lung cancer) compared three treatments: irinotecan alone, cisplatin plus vindesine, and cisplatin plus irinotecan.[38] It found no significant difference in survival between irinotecan alone and irinotecan plus cisplatin (median survival time: 46 weeks with irinotecan alone *v* 45.6 weeks with cisplatin plus vindesine *v* 50 weeks with cisplatin plus irinotecan; 2 year survival: 21.9% with irinotecan alone *v* 18.7% with cisplatin plus vindesine v 19.4% with cisplatin plus irinotecan; P = 0.089 for irinotecan alone v cisplatin plus vindesine). **First line platinum based versus non-platinum based chemotherapy:** We found one systematic review of "new" chemotherapy agents (search date 2001, 4 RCTs)[40] and five additional RCTs[39,41–44] that compared platinum based versus non-platinum treatment. The systematic review identified two RCTs that compared cisplatin plus etoposide versus gemcitabine.[40] Neither RCT found any significant difference in survival (median survival in 1 RCT, 146 people; 7.6 with cisplatin plus etoposide v 6.6 months with gemcitabine; P > 0.9; second RCT, 53 people: 48 weeks with cisplatin plus etoposide v 37 weeks with gemcitabine; P = 0.65).[45,46] The systematic review identified two RCTs that compared vinorelbine alone versus vinorelbine plus cisplatin.[40,47,48] The studies used different doses of vinorelbine (50% dose difference) and found different results for survival. One RCT (231 people) found no significant difference between vinorelbine alone (80 mg/m^2) and vinorelbine plus cisplatin (median survival: 32 weeks with vinorelbine alone v 33 weeks with vinorelbine plus cisplatin; P = 0.48).[47] The other RCT (412 people) found that vinorelbine plus cisplatin significantly increased survival compared with vinorelbine alone (median survival: 31 weeks with vinorelbine alone v 40 weeks with vinorelbine plus cisplatin; P = 0.045).[48] The first additional RCT (441 people with stage 3 or 4 non-small cell lung cancer) compared docetaxel plus cisplatin versus docetaxel plus gemcitabine and found no significant difference in survival at 1 year (86/205 [42%] with docetaxel plus cisplatin v 78/201 [39%] with docetaxel plus gemcitabine; RR 1.08, 95% CI 0.84 to 1.33).[39] The second additionalRCT (509 people with stage 3 or 4 non-small cell lung cancer) comparing paclitaxel plus carboplatin versus paclitaxel plus gemcitabine found no significant difference in median survival (10.4 months with paclitaxel plus carboplatin v 9.8 months with paclitaxel plus gemcitabine; P = 0.32).[41] The third additional RCT (90 people with stage 3 or 4 non-small cell lung cancer) found similar median survival time between paclitaxel plus carboplatin and paclitaxel plus gemcitabine (14.1 months with paclitaxel plus carboplatin v 12.6 months paclitaxel plus gemcitabine; CI not reported).[42] The fourth additional RCT (267 people with stage 3B or 4 non-small cell lung cancer) compared four regimens: paclitaxel plus carboplatin plus gemcitabine, paclitaxel plus carboplatin plus vinorelbine, paclitaxel plus gemcitabine, and gemcitabine plus vinorelbine.[43] It found no significant difference in survival at 1 year among groups (range 38–44%, reported as non-significant, no further data reported), but it is likely to have been too small to detect a clinically important difference among regimens. The fifth additional RCT (284 people with stage 4 non-small cell lung cancer) compared three regimens: cisplatin plus carboplatin plus ifosfamide, cisplatin plus carboplatin plus gemcitabine, and ifosfamide plus gemcitabine.[44] It found no significant difference in median survival among groups, although people taking ifosfamide plus gemcitabine had longer median survival time compared with people taking a cisplatin containing regimen (P = 0.2). The RCT is likely to have been underpowered to detect a clinically important difference among regimens. **Any second line chemotherapy:** We found one systematic review (search date not reported, 34 single agent studies and 24 combination regimen studies, 30 published only as an abstract).[49] The review found that results from studies were conflicting and was unable to draw conclusions because of the heterogeneity of participant selection in the studies, and the different definitions of people considered sensitive or refractory to treatment. **Second line single agent docetaxel:** We found one systematic review (search date 2000, 2 RCTs, 477 people resistant to platinum based combination chemotherapy).[50] Results of the RCTs were not combined because of trial heterogeneity. The first RCT identified by the review found that docetaxel 75 mg/m^2 significantly improved survival at 1 year compared with best supportive care (37% with docetaxel *v* 11% with best supportive care; P = 0.003).[51] The second RCT identified by the review found that docetaxel significantly improved survival at 1 year compared with vinorelbine or ifosfamide (32% with docetaxel *v* 19% with vinorelbine or ifosfamide; P = 0.025).[52]

Harms: Over 50% of people with advanced lung cancer treated with chemotherapy reported alopecia, and gastrointestinal and haematological toxicity.[48] One non-systematic review found greater toxicity in people with Eastern Cooperative Oncology Group (ECOG) scale performance status 3 or 4Ⓖ.[53] Subgroup analysis (64 people with ECOG scale performance status 2) from an RCT comparing four cisplatin based chemotherapy regimens found high rates of haematological and gastrointestinal toxicity and low response rates after 1 year; as a result the enrolment of people with ECOG performance status 2 was discontinued (proportion of people who had any grade 3–4 toxicity: 30–60% of people taking paclitaxel plus cisplatin; 8–67% of people taking gemcitabine plus cisplatin; 12–59% of people taking docetaxel plus cisplatin; 27–33% of people taking paclitaxel plus carboplatin; response rate with any type of chemotherapy 14%, 95% CI 5.6% to 22.6%; median survival 4.1 months, 95% CI 0.2 months to 31.0 months).[54] **First line single agent versus combined chemotherapy:** The second subsequent RCT (698 people) found that vinorelbine plus gemcitabine significantly increased thrombocytopenia and liver toxicity compared with vinorelbine alone and significantly increased neutropenia, vomiting, fatigue, extravasation effects, cardiac toxicity, and constipation compared with gemcitabine alone.[37] The fifth subsequent RCT (398 people with stage 3B or 4 non-small cell lung cancer) found that platinum plus vindesine increased overall major adverse effects compared with irinotecan alone.[38] However, irinotecan significantly increased diarrhoea (grade 3 or 4 nausea or vomiting: 23% with platinum plus vindesine *v* 9% with irinotecan alone; P = 0.001; grade 3 or 4 diarrhoea: 3% with platinum plus vindesine *v* 15% with irinotecan alone; P = 0.008). **First line platinum based versus non-platinum based chemotherapy:** The first additional RCT, which compared docetaxel plus cisplatin with docetaxel plus gemcitabine, found that docetaxel plus cisplatin significantly increased neutropenia (P = 0.01), nausea and vomiting (P = 0.001), and diarrhoea (P = 0.001).[39] The RCTs[41,42] comparing paclitaxel plus carboplatin versus paclitaxel plus gemcitabine found similar levels of haematological toxicity between groups, although one RCT[42] found that paclitaxel plus carboplatin significantly increased grade 3 thrombocytopenia compared with paclitaxel plus gemcitabine. The fourth additional RCT found that gemcitabine plus vinorelbine significantly reduced non-haematological toxicity (neuropathy, alopecia, nausea/emesis, diarrhoea, myalgia/arthralgia) compared with paclitaxel plus carboplatin plus gemcitabine, paclitaxel plus carboplatin plus vinorelbine, or paclitaxel plus gemcitabine (P < 0.05 for gemcitabine plus vinorelbine *v* any other regimen).[43]

Comment: For people with stage 4 non-small cell lung cancer, treatment options consist of either chemotherapy or symptomatic care, including palliative radiation. People with Eastern Cooperative Oncology Group (ECOG) scale performance status 3 or 4 have usually been excluded from RCTs of lung cancer chemotherapy. One non-systematic review has found that carboplatin has comparable response rate to, but a better toxicity profile than, cisplatin in people with stage 4 non-small cell lung cancer.[55] One RCT (408 people with stage 3B or 4 non-small cell lung cancer) comparing carboplatin plus paclitaxel versus vinorelbine plus cisplatin found no significant difference in survival at 1 year (36% with carboplatin plus paclitaxel *v* 38% with vinorelbine plus cisplatin; reported as non-significant). It found that vinorelbine plus cisplatin significantly increased withdrawal owing to toxicity (15% with carboplatin plus paclitaxel *v* 28% with vinorelbine plus cisplatin; P = 0.001).[56] Newer agents such as vinorelbine, gemcitabine, irinotecan, paclitaxel, and docetaxel produce objective responses in more than 20% of people with advanced lung cancer,[55] and combinations of some of these agents may be as effective and may cause less toxicity than platinum based regimens. Measuring quality of life in people with lung cancer remains a serious challenge.[40] In the first subsequent RCT comparing first line single agent versus combined chemotherapy, median survival with vinorelbine alone was much shorter than in the second subsequent RCT (18 weeks[34] *v* 36 weeks[37]). The second subsequent RCT speculates that this may be because either the higher doses of vinorelbine used in the first subsequent RCT may be toxic in the elderly based on phase I evidence or there may have been biases in patient selection. The systematic review comparing second line chemotherapy versus supportive care recommended that RCTs of second line chemotherapy report and analyse details of patient characteristics, response to first line treatment, and interval between last chemotherapy and recurrence.[49]

QUESTION **What are the effects of treatments for small cell lung cancer?**

OPTION **DOSE INTENSIFICATION OF CHEMOTHERAPY VERSUS STANDARD CHEMOTHERAPY**

One systematic review found limited evidence that intensifying chemotherapy dose by increasing the number of chemotherapy cycles, increasing chemotherapy dose, or increasing dose intensity per cycle may modestly improve survival compared with standard chemotherapy. However, additional RCTs have found inconclusive evidence about the effects of dose intensification on survival.

Benefits: We found one systematic review (search date 2001, 20 RCTs, 5490 people, most with extensive stage small cell lung cancer)[57] and three additional RCTs[58–60] assessing dose or dose intensity of chemotherapy. Methods of dose intensification differed among RCTs. The review identified eight RCTs comparing an increased (12–14) with a standard (5–6) number of cycles of chemotherapy; five RCTs comparing higher with lower doses of chemotherapy; four RCTs comparing higher with lower intensity chemotherapy, and three RCTs comparing changes in both dose per cycle and number of cycles of chemotherapy with standard dose chemotherapy for standard number of cycles (see comment below). The review found that the median survival time was higher in people receiving dose intensification compared with standard chemotherapy (9.8 months with dose intensification *v* 11.5 months with standard chemotherapy, significance not reported). The difference in median survival was increased if the two RCTs (of the 3 that altered both the dose per cycle and the total number of cycles of chemotherapy) that reduced the number of treatment cycles were excluded (11.5 months with dose intensification *v* 8.7 months with standard chemotherapy, significance not reported). The first additional RCT (229 people with extensive stage small cell lung cancer) comparing dose intensive (cisplatin plus vincristine plus doxorubicin plus etoposide) with standard chemotherapy (alternating cyclophosphamide, doxorubicin, vincristine plus cisplatin) found no significant difference in progression free survival (median 0.66 years in each group) or overall survival (0.98 with dose intensive *v* 0.91 years with standard chemotherapy, reported as non-significant, no further data reported).[58] The second additional RCT (59 people with limited stage and 74 people with extensive stage small cell lung cancer) found no significant difference between paclitaxel plus cisplatin plus etoposide and cisplatin plus etoposide in survival at 1 year (AR 38.2% with paclitaxel plus cisplatin plus etoposide *v* 37% with cisplatin plus etoposide; P = 0.09).[59] The third additional RCT (233 people with extensive disease) found no significant difference in survival over 2 years with three different schedules of epirubicin, vindesine, and ifosfamide (6 cycles every 3 weeks; 6 accelerated cycles every 2 weeks with granulocyte macrophage colony stimulating factor [GM-CSF] support, and 6 accelerated cycles every 2 weeks with oral co-trimoxazole) (2 year survival 5–6%; P = 0.86).[60]

Harms: The review gave no information on adverse effects.[57] The additional RCTs found that, except in people with widespread extensive stage small cell lung cancer, adverse effects of chemotherapy were of short duration.[50,58,61] However, the first RCT found that dose intensive chemotherapy significantly increased deaths related to toxicity compared with standard chemotherapy (9/110 [8%] with dose intensive *v* 1/109 [1%] with standard chemotherapy; RR 8.9, 95% CI 1.1 to 69.0; NNH 14, 95% CI 7 to 60).[58] The second RCT also found that paclitaxel plus cisplatin plus etoposide significantly increased deaths related to toxicity compared with cisplatin plus etoposide (8/62 [13%] with paclitaxel plus cisplatin plus etoposide *v* 0/71 [0%] with cisplatin plus etoposide; P = 0.001).[58]

Comment: Dose escalation and intensification may modestly improve survival; however, the only review of dose intensification available included four different variations of dose and cycle across 20 studies, making comparisons difficult. More research on alternative approaches to the treatment of small cell lung cancer is needed.

OPTION ADDING THORACIC IRRADIATION TO CHEMOTHERAPY IN LIMITED STAGE SMALL CELL LUNG CANCER

Two systematic reviews in people with limited stage small cell lung cancer have found that adding thoracic irradiation to chemotherapy improves survival at 3 years and local control compared with chemotherapy alone. However, one of these reviews has found that thoracic radiation plus chemotherapy increases death related to treatment compared with chemotherapy alone. One systematic review and six additional RCTs found insufficient evidence on the best timing, dose, and fractionation of radiation.

Benefits: We found two systematic reviews.[62,63] The first review (search date not reported, 13 RCTs, 2573 people with limited stage small cell lung cancer) found that radiation plus chemotherapy significantly increased 3 year survival compared with chemotherapy alone (AR 15% with radiation plus chemotherapy *v* 10% with chemotherapy alone; P = 0.001).[62] The second review (search date not reported, 11 RCTs, 10 of which were included in the first review, 1911 people with limited stage small cell lung cancer) pooled data from nine of the RCTs (1521 people) and found that thoracic radiation plus chemotherapy significantly improved local control compared with chemotherapy alone (50% with radiation plus chemotherapy *v* 25% with chemotherapy alone; ARI of improved local control 25%, 95% CI 17% to 34%).[63] **Timing of radiation:** We found one systematic review (search date 2000, 4 RCTs, 927 people with limited stage small cell lung cancer),[64] one additional RCT,[65] and two subsequent RCTs,[66,67] which compared early with late addition of thoracic radiotherapy to chemotherapy. The review found no significant difference between early and late addition of radiotherapy in 5 year survival (AR 66/455 [14.5%] with early addition v 63/472 [13.2%] with late addition; RR 1.09, 95% CI 0.78 to 1.48).[65] The additional RCT, included in the review but not in the meta-analysis, found that early radiotherapy significantly increased 5 year survival compared with late addition of radiotherapy (30% with early addition v 15% with late addition; P = 0.03).[65] The first subsequent RCT (81 people with limited stage small cell lung cancer) compared early radiotherapy (given with the first cycle of chemotherapy) with late radiotherapy (given with the fourth cycle of chemotherapy).[66] It found no significant difference between early and late radiotherapy in survival after median follow up of 35 months (median 17.5 months with early radiotherapy v 17.0 months with late radiotherapy; P = 0.6). The second subsequent RCT (231 people with limited stage small cell lung cancer receiving 4 cycles of cisplatin plus etoposide) compared early addition of thoracic radiotherapy (with the first cycle of chemotherapy [concurrent]) versus late (after the fourth cycle of chemotherapy [sequential]).[67] It found no significant difference in survival at 2, 3, or 5 years between concurrent and sequential radiotherapy (5 year survival: 24% with concurrent v 18% with sequential; P = 0.097). Adjustments for prognostic factors, performance status**G**, age and stage suggested that overall there was a significantly lower risk of death in people receiving concurrent rather than sequential radiotherapy (HR 0.70, 95% CI 0.52 to 0.94; P = 0.02).[67] **Dose:** One RCT (333 people with limited stage small cell lung cancer) found no significant difference between standard dose radiotherapy (25.0 Gy over 2 weeks) and high dose radiotherapy (37.5 Gy over 3 weeks) in overall survival over 3 years (P = 0.18; results presented graphically).[68] **Fractionation:** We found two RCTs.[69,70] The first RCT (417 people) found that hyperfractionation (twice daily treatment) compared with conventional fractionation (once daily treatment) significantly improved 5 year survival (26% with hyperfractionation v 16% with conventional fractionation; P = 0.04).[69] The second RCT (353 people) comparing once daily irradiation with twice daily irradiation found no significant difference in 3 year survival (34% with 50.4 Gy in 28 fractions daily v 29% with 48.0 Gy in 32 fractions twice daily; P = 0.46).[70]

Harms: The second systematic review found that thoracic radiation plus chemotherapy significantly increased death related to treatment compared with chemotherapy alone (29/884 [3.3%] with radiation plus chemotherapy v 12/841 [1.4%] with chemotherapy alone; OR 2.54, 95% CI 1.90 to 3.18).[63] **Fractionation:** One RCT found that hyperfractionation increased the incidence of oesophagitis compared with conventional fractionation.[69]

Comment: Interest in adding thoracic irradiation to chemotherapy derives from the observation that local recurrence in the chest is a major cause of first treatment failure and carries an extremely poor prognosis. One non-systematic review suggested that chest irradiation reduced local failure rates and increased 3 year survival by 50%.[71] The reasons for this improvement have not been established but may include the early use of radiation plus chemotherapy rather than improvements in either modality alone.[72] The RCTs of early versus late addition of radiotherapy used different methods and do not provide strong evidence.[64–66] The different results may be explained by different rates of early toxicity from treatment and different rates of relapse in the central nervous system.

OPTION PROPHYLACTIC CRANIAL IRRADIATION FOR PEOPLE IN COMPLETE REMISSION FROM SMALL CELL LUNG CANCER

One systematic review in people with small cell lung cancer in complete remission has found that prophylactic cranial irradiation improves survival at 3 years and reduces the risk of developing brain metastases compared with no irradiation. Although long term cognitive dysfunction after cranial irradiation has been described in non-randomised studies, RCTs have not found a cumulative increase in neuropsychological dysfunction.

Benefits: We found one systematic review (search date 2000, 7 RCTs, 987 people with small cell lung cancer in complete remission) comparing cranial radiation with no cranial radiation.[73] Of the people in the RCTs, 12% in the irradiation group and 17% in the no irradiation group had extensive stage small cell lung cancer at presentation. It found that cranial irradiation significantly improved survival and increased disease free survival compared with no cranial irradiation (survival: RR of death at 3 years 0.84, 95% CI 0.73 to 0.97, corresponding to a 5.4% increase in survival; disease free survival: RR of recurrence or death at 3 years 0.75, 95% CI 0.65 to 0.86). The review found that cranial irradiation significantly reduced the cumulative incidence of brain metastases compared with no cranial irradiation (RR 0.46, 95% CI 0.38 to 0.57). Larger doses of radiation significantly reduced brain metastases (P = 0.02), but did not significantly improve survival (P = 0.89).

Harms: Non-randomised studies suggest that prophylactic cranial irradiation may lead to neuropsychological sequelae but the review was unable to assess this because adequate assessments were carried out in only two of the seven RCTs.[73] These two RCTs found no cumulative increase in neuropsychological dysfunction in individuals receiving prophylactic cranial irradiation. These RCTs and other non-randomised studies found that 24–60% of participants may have neuropsychological problems before treatment, and other studies have not accounted for potential confounding factors such as age, tobacco use, paraneoplastic syndromes, and neurotoxic chemotherapy effects.

Comment: The clinical importance of cognitive impairment after prophylactic cranial irradiation remains unclear. Differences in survival benefiting those people receiving prophylactic cranial irradiation are small, reflecting the impact of other events not influenced by prophylactic cranial irradiation, e.g. other metastases or thoracic relapse.[74]

OPTION ORAL ETOPOSIDE IN EXTENSIVE STAGE SMALL CELL LUNG CANCER

Two RCTs in people with extensive stage small cell lung cancer found that oral etoposide reduced survival compared with combination chemotherapy at 1 year. One RCT, in people with extensive stage small cell lung cancer who had not responded to induction combination chemotherapy, found no significant difference between oral etoposide and no further treatment in mortality at 3 years, although overall mortality was lower in people taking etoposide. RCTs found that etoposide may reduce nausea, alopecia, and numbness in the short term compared with combination chemotherapy, but found no evidence that it offered better quality of life overall.

Benefits: We found no systematic review but found three RCTs.[75–77] **Versus combination chemotherapy:** The first RCT (155 people with extensive stage small cell lung cancer) compared oral etoposide 100 mg daily for 5 days with combination chemotherapy.[75] It found that etoposide significantly reduced survival at 1 year compared with combined chemotherapy (9.8% with etoposide *v* 19.3% with combined chemotherapy;

P < 0.05). It found similar median survival rates with etoposide compared with combination chemotherapy (4.8 months with etoposide *v* 5.9 months with combined chemotherapy; CI not reported) and found inconclusive results on quality of life. Acute nausea was significantly worse with combination chemotherapy (P < 0.01), but pain, appetite, general well being, and mood were worse with oral etoposide (P < 0.001). Palliation of lung cancer symptoms was of significantly shorter duration with etoposide than with combination chemotherapy (P < 0.01).[75] The second RCT (339 people with extensive stage small cell lung cancer) comparing oral etoposide with combination chemotherapy found that etoposide significantly reduced survival at mean 21 months (HR 1.35, 95% CI 1.03 to 1.70; P = 0.03; absolute numbers not reported).[76] **Versus no further treatment:** The third RCT (233 people with extensive stage small cell lung cancer and Karnofsky performance status**G** ≥ 50 who had not responded after 4 cycles of intravenous cisplatin, etoposide, and ifosfamide) compared oral etoposide 50 mg/m^2 versus no further treatment for 3 months.[77] It found that oral etoposide significantly increased median progression free survival compared with no treatment (8.2 months with etoposide *v* 6.5 months with no treatment; P = 0.0018). It found no significant difference in overall survival at 3 years, although mortality was lower in people taking etoposide (9.1% with etoposide *v* 1.9% with no treatment; P = 0.0704).

Harms: **Versus combination chemotherapy:** The first RCT found that etoposide significantly reduced nausea in the short term (assessed by daily diary card; P < 0.01) compared with combination chemotherapy.[75] However, it found that combination chemotherapy significantly improved general well-being (assessed by daily diary card; P < 0.01) and overall quality of life (assessed by Rotterdam Symptom Checklist; P < 0.01) compared with etoposide.[75] The second RCT found that etoposide reduced alopecia and numbness compared with combination chemotherapy, but increased haematological adverse effects, particularly anaemia.[76] **Versus no further treatment:** The third RCT found that oral etoposide was associated with alopecia and grade 3–4 toxicities, including myelosuppression (40% of people), anaemia (20%), and granulocytopenia (42%).[77] The RCT gave no comparative information about adverse effects in people receiving no treatment.

Comment: Treatment of extensive stage disease is palliative and, because age has been identified as a prognostic factor in small cell lung cancer, studies have looked at outcomes in elderly people with limited and extensive stage disease and in people of all ages with a poor prognosis. Although small cell lung cancer is relatively sensitive to chemotherapy, extensive stage disease remains incurable. Median survival with treatment is 10–12 months, and as yet has been unaffected by high dose combination chemotherapy. Because of its lower acute toxicity, etoposide may be considered for elderly people with extensive stage disease or people with a poor prognosis.

GLOSSARY

Continuous hyperfractionated accelerated radiotherapy (CHART) Radiotherapy given at a rate of two or more radiation fractions a day (each of smaller dose than conventionally fractionated doses). The number of fractions a week is gradually increased to shorten overall duration of treatment.

Performance status Expression used to describe functional status or wellness of participants in studies of cancer. There are two widely accepted scales: the Eastern Cooperative Oncology Group (ECOG) scale (0 = no symptoms; 1 = symptomatic but no extra time in bed; 2 = in bed less than 50% of the day, no work, can care for self; 3 = in bed more than 50% of day, not bedridden, minimal self care; 4 = completely bedridden), and the Karnofsky Scale of symptoms and disability (from 100% = no symptoms to 0% = dead).

Split-course, hyperfractionated radiotherapy Radiotherapy using two or more fractions daily of smaller than conventional fraction size, where the total dose is split into at least two separate courses with an interruption of 10–14 days.

REFERENCES

1. Travis WD, Travis LB, Devesa SS. Lung cancer. *Cancer* 1995;75(suppl 1):191–202.
2. American Thoracic Society/European Respiratory Society Pre-treatment evaluation of non-small cell lung cancer *Am J Respir Crit Care* 1997;156:320–332.
3. Schottenfeld D. Etiology and Epidemiology of Lung Cancer. In: Pass HI, Mitchell JB, Johnson DH, et al, eds. *Lung cancer, principles and practice*, 2nd ed. Philadelphia: Lippincott Williams and Wilkins, 2000:376–388.
4. Ihde DC, Pass HI, Glatstein E. Lung cancer. In: DeVita VT Jr, Hellman S, Rosenberg SA, eds. *Cancer, principles and practice of oncology*, 5th ed. Philadelphia: Lippincott-Raven, 1997;849–959.
5. Montazeri A, Gillis CR, McEwen J. Quality of life in people with lung cancer: a review of literature from 1970 to 1995. *Chest* 1998;113:467–481.
6. Grilli R, Oxman AD, Julian JA. Chemotherapy for advanced non-small-cell lung cancer: how much benefit is enough? *J Clin Oncol* 1993;11:1866–1872. Search date 1991; primary source Medline.
7. Goss G, Paszat L, Newman T, et al. Use of preoperative chemotherapy with or without postoperative radiotherapy in technically resectable stage IIIA non-small cell lung cancer. *Cancer Prev Control* 1998;2:32–39. Search date 1997; primary sources Medline, hand searches of reference lists, and contact with experts.
8. Ramnath N, Hernandez FJ, Bepler G. Neoadjuvant chemotherapy for non-small-call lung cancer: will the answer be in targeted chemotherapy. *Oncol Spect* 2002:1;27–34.
9. Depierre A, Milleron B, Moro-Sibilot D, et al. Pre-operative chemotherapy followed by surgery compared with primary surgery in resectable Stage I (except T1N0), II and IIIA non-small cell lung cancer. *J Clin Oncol* 2002;20:247–253.
10. Non-Small Cell Lung Cancer Collaborative Group. Chemotherapy for non-small cell lung cancer. In: The Cochrane Library, Issue 4, 2002. Oxford: Update Software. Search date 1991; primary sources Medline; Cancerlit; hand searches of meetings abstracts, bibliographies of books, and specialist journals; consultation of trials registers of National Cancer Institute; UK Coordinating Committee for Cancer Research; the Union Internationale Contre le Cancer; and discussion with trialists.
11. Guangchuan XU, Rong T, Lin P. Adjuvant chemotherapy following radical surgery for non-small-cell lung cancer: a randomized study on 70 patients. *Chin Med J* 2000;113:617–620.
12. Endo C, Saito Y, Iwanami H, et al. A randomized trial of postoperative UFT therapy in p stage I, II non-small cell lung cancer: North-east Japan Study Group for Lung Cancer Surgery. *Lung Cancer* 2003;40:181–186.
13. Keller SM, Adak S, Wagner H, et al. A randomized trial of postoperative adjuvant therapy in patients with completely resected stage II or IIIA non-small-cell lung cancer. *N Engl J Med* 2000:343;1217–1222.
14. Feld R, Rubinstein L, Thomas PA, et al. Adjuvant chemotherapy with cyclophosphamide, doxorubicin, and cisplatin in patients with completely resected stage I non-small-cell lung cancer. *J Natl Cancer Inst* 1993;85:299–306.
15. Niiranen A, Niitamo-Korhonen S, Kouri M, et al. Adjuvant chemotherapy after radical surgery for non-small cell lung cancer: a randomized study. *J Clin Oncol* 1992;10:1927–1932.
16. Pass HI, Pogrebniak HW, Steinberg SM, et al. Randomized trial of neoadjuvant therapy for lung cancer: interim analysis. *Ann Thoracic Surg* 1992;53:992–998.
17. Marino P, Preatoni A. Randomized trials of radiotherapy alone versus combined chemotherapy and radiotherapy in stages IIIa and IIIb non small cell lung cancer. *Cancer* 1995;76:593–601. Search date 1995; primary sources Medline and hand searches of references of review articles and abstracts.
18. Pritchard RS, Anthony SP. Chemotherapy plus radiotherapy compared with radiotherapy alone in the treatment of locally advanced, unresectable, non-small-cell lung cancer. *Ann Intern Med* 1996;125:723–729. Search date 1995; primary sources Medline and hand searches of references of review articles and abstracts.
19. Sause W, Kolesar P, Taylor S, et al. Final results of phase III trial in regionally advanced unresectable non-small cell lung cancer: Radiation Therapy Oncology Group, Eastern Cooperative Oncology Group, and Southwest Oncology Group. *Chest* 2000;117:358–364.
20. Cullen MH, Billingham CM, Woodroffe AD, et al. Mitomycin, ifosfamide, and cisplatin in unresectable non-small cell lung cancer: effects on survival and quality of life. *J Clin Oncol* 1999;17:3188–3194.
21. Sharma S, Sharma R, Bhowmik KT. Sequential chemoradiotherapy versus radiotherapy in the management of locally advanced non-small-cell lung cancer. *Adv Ther* 2003;20:14–19.
22. Saunders M, Dische S, Barrett A, et al. Continuous, hyperfractionated, accelerated radiotherapy (CHART) versus conventional radiotherapy in non-small cell lung cancer: mature data from the randomised multicentre trial. *Radiother Oncol* 1999;52:137–148.
23. Mousas B, Scott C, Sause W, et al. The benefit of treatment intensification is age and histology-dependent in patients with locally advanced non-small cell lung cancer (NSCLC): a quality-adjusted survival analysis of Radiation Therapy Oncology Group (RTOG) chemoradiation studies. *Int J Radiat Oncol Biol Phys* 1999;45:1143–1149.
24. Wake B, Taylor R, Sandercock J. Hyperfractionated/accelerated radiotherapy regimens for the treatment of non-small cell lung cancer. A systematic review of clinical and cost-effectiveness. West Midlands Health Technology Assessment Collaboration (WMHTAC); 2002 (DPHE Report No. 35):65. Search date 2001; primary sources Medline, Embase, Cancerlit, Cochrane Library, reference lists, contact with experts in the field and Internet searches.
25. Bailey AJ, Parmar MKB, Stephens RJ. Patient-reported short-term and long-term physical and psychological symptoms: results of the continuous hyperfractionated accelerated radiotherapy (CHART) randomized trial in non-small cell lung cancer. *J Clin Oncol* 1998;16:3082–3093.
26. Marino P, Pampallona S, Preatoni A, et al. Chemotherapy versus supportive care in advanced non-small cell lung cancer: results of a meta-analysis of the literature. *Chest* 1994;106:861–865. Search date not reported; primary sources Medline and hand searches of references from review articles and abstracts.
27. Sorenson S, Glimelius B, Nygren P, et al. A systematic overview of chemotherapy effects in non-small cell lung cancer. *Acta Oncol*

2001;40:327–339. Search date 1998; primary sources Medline, Cancerlit, PDQ database, and hand searches of reference lists and the grey literature.

28. Elderly Lung Cancer Vinorelbine Study Group. Effects of vinorelbine on quality of life and survival of elderly patients with non-small cell lung cancer. *J Natl Cancer Inst* 1999;91:66–72.
29. Anderson H, Hopwood P, Stephens RJ, et al. Gemcitabine plus best supportive care (BSC) versus BSC in inoperable non-small cell lung cancer in a randomised trial with quality of life as the primary outcome. *Br J Cancer* 2000;83:447–453.
30. Roszkowski K, Pluzanska A, Krzakowski M, et al. A multicenter, randomised phase III study of docetaxel plus best supportive care versus best supportive care in chemo-naive patients with metastatic or non-resectable localised non-small cell lung cancer (NSCLC). *Lung Cancer* 2000;27:145–157.
31. Ranson M, Davidson N, Nicolson M, et al. Randomised trial of paclitaxel plus supportive care versus supportive care for patients with advanced non-small cell lung cancer. *J Natl Cancer Inst* 2000;92:1074–1080.
32. Lilenbaum RC, Langenberg P, Dickersin K. Single agent versus combination chemotherapy in patients with advanced non-small cell lung cancer: a meta-analysis of response, toxicity and survival. *Cancer* 1998;82:116–126. Search dates 1995–1996; primary sources Medline, Embase, hand searches of references, Physician Data Query from the National Cancer Institute, and expert consultation.
33. Ellis P, Mackay JA, Evans WK. Use of gemcitabine in non-small-cell lung cancer. *Curr Oncol* 2003;10:3–26. Search date 2002; primary sources Medline, Cancerlit, Cochrane Library, and proceedings of the American Society of Clinical Oncology.
34. Frasci G, Lorusso V, Panza N, et al. Gemcitabine plus vinorelbine versus vinorelbine alone in elderly patients with advanced non-small cell lung cancer. *J Clin Oncol* 2000;18:2529–2536.
35. Sandler AB, Nemunaitis J, Denham C, et al. Phase III trial of gemcitabine plus cisplatin versus cisplatin alone in patients with locally advanced or metastatic non-small cell lung cancer. *J Clin Oncol* 2000;18:122–130.
36. Wozniak AG, Crowley JJ, Balcerzak SP, et al. Randomised trial comparing cisplatin with cisplatin plus vinorelbine in the treatment of advanced non-small cell lung cancer: a Southwest Oncology Group study. *J Clin Oncol* 1998;16:2459–2465.
37. Gridelli C, Perrone F, Gallo C, et al. Chemotherapy for elderly patients with advanced non-small-cell lung cancer: the Multicentre Italian Lung Cancer in the Elderly Study (MILES) phase III randomized trial. *J Natl Cancer Inst* 2003;95:362–372.
38. Negoro S, Masuda N, Takada Y, et al. Randomized phase III trial of irinotecan combined with cisplatin for advanced non-small-cell lung cancer. *Br J Cancer* 2003;88:335–341.
39. Georgoulias V, Papadakis E, Alexopoulos A, et al. Platinum-based and non-platinum-based chemotherapy in advanced non-small cell lung cancer: a randomised multicentre trial. *Lancet* 2001;357:1478–1484.
40. Meert AP, Berghmans T, Lafitte JJ, et al. What progress have the new agents brought for chemotherapy of advanced non-small-cell lung cancer? *Eur Respir Rev* 2002;12:208–216. Search date 2001; primary sources unspecified electronic databases and personal files.
41. Kosmidis P, Mylonakis N, Nicolaides C, et al. Paclitaxel plus carboplatin versus gemcitabine plus paclitaxel in advanced non-small-cell lung cancer: a phase III randomized trial. *J Clin Oncol* 2002;20:3578–3585.
42. Chen Y-M, Perng R-P, Lee Y-C, et al. Paclitaxel plus carboplatin, compared with paclitaxel plus gemcitabine, shows similar efficacy while more cost-effective: a randomised phase II study of combination chemotherapy against inoperable non-small-cell lung cancer previously untreated. *Ann Oncol* 2002;13:108–115.
43. Greco FA, Gray JR, Thompson DS, et al. Prospective randomized study of four novel chemotherapy regimens in patients with advanced non-small cell lung carcinoma. *Cancer* 2002;95:1279–1285.
44. Sculier JP, Lafitte JJ, Lecomte J, et al. A three-arm phase III randomised trial comparing combinations of platinum derivatives, ifosfamide and/or gemcitabine in stage IV non-small-cell lung cancer. *Ann Oncol* 2002;13:874–882.
45. Manegold C, Bergman B, Chemaissani A, et al. Single-agent gemcitabine versus cisplatin-etoposide: early results of a randomised phase II study in locally advanced or metastatic non-small-cell lung cancer. *Ann Oncol* 1997;8:525–529.
46. Perng RP, Chen YM, Ming-Liu J, et al. Gemcitabine versus the combination of cisplatin and etoposide in patients with inoperable non-small-cell lung cancer in a phase II randomized study. *J Clin Oncol* 1997;15:2097–2102.
47. Depierre A, Chastang C, Quoix E, et al. Vinorelbine versus vinorelbine plus cisplatin in advanced non-small cell lung cancer: a randomized trial. *Ann Oncol* 1994;5:37–42.
48. Le Chevalier T, Brisgand D, Douillard JY, et al. Randomized study of vinorelbine and cisplatin versus vindesine and cisplatin versus vinorelbine alone in advanced non-small-cell lung cancer: results of a European multicenter trial including 612 patients. *J Clin Oncol* 1994;12:360–367.
49. Huisman C, Smit EF, Postmus PE. Second-line chemotherapy in relapsing or refractory non-small cell lung cancer: a review. *J Clin Oncol* 2000;18:3722–3730. Search date not reported; primary sources Medline and hand searches of the past five conference abstracts of the American Society of Clinical Oncology, European Cancer Conference, and the European Society of Medical Oncology.
50. Logan D, Laurie S, Markman BR, et al. The role of single-agent docetaxel as second-line treatment for advanced non-small cell lung cancer. *Curr Oncol* 2001;8:50–58. Search date 2000; primary sources Medline, Cancerlit, Cochrane Library, and hand search of reference lists of relevant articles.
51. Shepherd FA, Dancey J, Ramlau, et al. Prospective randomized trial of docetaxel versus best supportive care in patients with non-small-cell lung cancer previously treated with platinum-based chemotherapy. *J Clin Oncol* 2000;18:2095–2103.
52. Fossella FV, DeVore R, Kerr RN. Randomized phase III trial of docetaxel versus vinorelbine or ifosfamide in patients with advanced non-small cell lung cancer previously treated with platinum-containing regimens. *J Clin Oncol* 2000;18:2354–2362.
53. Bunn PA Jr, Kelly K. New chemotherapeutic agents prolong survival and improve quality of life in non-small cell lung cancer: a review of literature and future directions. *Clin Cancer Res* 1998;4:1087–1100.
54. Sweeney CJ, Zhu J, Sandler AB, et al. Outcome of patients with a performance status of 2 in Eastern Cooperative Oncology Group Study E1594. A Phase III trial in patients with metastatic non-small cell lung carcinoma. *Cancer* 2001;92:2639–2647.
55. Bunn PA Jr. Review of therapeutic trials of carboplatin in lung cancer. *Semin Oncol* 1989;16(S5):27–33.
56. Kelly K, Crowley J, Bunn PA, et al. Randomised phase III trial of paclitaxel plus carboplatin versus vinorelbine plus cisplatin in the treatment of patients with advanced non-small-cell lung cancer: a Southwest Oncology Group trial. *J Clin Oncol* 2001;19:3210–3218.
57. Tjan-Heijnen VCG, Wagener DJT, Postmus PE. An analysis of chemotherapy dose and dose-intensity in small-cell lung cancer: lessons to be drawn. *Ann Oncol* 2002;13:1519–1530. Search date 2001, primary sources Medline 1980–2001 and hand searches of reference lists of relevant articles.

58. Murray N, Livingston RB, Shepherd FA, et al. Randomised study of CODE versus alternating CAV/EP for extensive-stage small-cell lung cancer: an intergroup study of the National Cancer Institute of Canada clinical trials group and the Southwest Oncology Group. *J Clin Oncol* 1999;17:2300–2308.
59. Mavroudis D, Papadakis E, Veslemes M, et al. A multicenter randomized clinical trial comparing paclitaxel-cisplatin-etoposide versus cisplatin-etoposide as first-line treatment in patients with small-cell lung cancer. *Ann Oncol* 2001;12:463–470.
60. Sculier JP, Paessmans M, Reconte J, et al. A three-arm Phase III randomized trial assessing in patients with extensive disease small cell lung cancer, accelerated chemotherapy with support of hematological growth factor or oral antibiotics. *Br J Cancer* 2001;85:1444–1451.
61. Noda K, Nishikaa Y, Kawahara M, et al. Irinotecan plus cisplatin compared with etoposide plus cisplatin for extensive small cell lung cancer. *N Engl J Med* 2002;346:85–91.
62. Pignon JP, Arriagada R, Ihde DC, et al. A meta-analysis of thoracic radiotherapy for small-cell lung cancer. *N Engl J Med* 1992;327:1618–1624. Search date not reported; primary sources Medline and hand search of proceedings of key oncology meetings.
63. Warde P, Payne D. Does thoracic irradiation improve survival and local control in limited-stage small cell carcinoma of the lung? A meta-analysis. *J Clin Oncol* 1992;10:890–895. Search date not reported; primary sources Medline and Cancerline.
64. Okawara G, Gagliardi A, Evans WK, et al. The role of thoracic radiotherapy as an adjunct to standard chemotherapy in limited-stage small-cell lung cancer. *Curr Oncol* 2000;7:162–172. Search date 2000; primary sources Medline, Cochrane Library, Physician Data Query File, Cancerlit, and hand searches of conference proceedings.
65. Jeremic B, Shibamoto Y, Acimovic L, et al. Initial versus delayed accelerated hyperfractionated radiation therapy and concurrent chemotherapy in limited small-cell lung cancer. A randomised study. *J Clin Oncol* 1997;15:893–900.
66. Skarlos DV, Samantas E, Briassoulis E, et al. Randomized comparison of early versus late hyperfractionated thoracic irradiation concurrently with chemotherapy in limited disease small-cell lung cancer: A randomized phase II study of the Hellenic Cooperative Oncology Group (HeCOG). *Ann Oncol* 2001;12:1231–1238.
67. Takada M, Fukuoka M, Kawahara M, et al. Phase III study of concurrent versus sequential thoracic radiotherapy in combination with cisplatin and etoposide for limited-stage small-cell lung cancer: results of the Japan Clinical Oncology Group study 9104. *J Clin Oncol* 2002;20:3054–3060.
68. Coy P, Hodson I, Payne DG, et al. The effect of dose of thoracic irradiation on recurrence in patients with limited stage small cell lung cancer. Initial results of a Canadian multicentre randomized trial. *Int J Radiat Oncol Biol Phys* 1988;14:219–226.
69. Turrisi AT, Kim K, Blum R, et al. Twice-daily compared with once-daily thoracic radiotherapy in limited small-cell lung cancer treated concurrently with cisplatin and etoposide. *N Engl J Med* 1999;340:265–271.
70. Bonner JA, Sloan JA, Shanahan TG, et al. Phase III comparison of twice-daily split-course irradiation versus once-daily irradiation for patients with limited stage small-cell lung carcinoma. *J Clin Oncol* 1999;17:2681–2691.
71. Kumar P. The role of radiotherapy in the management of limited-stage small cell lung cancer: past, present, and future. *Chest* 1997;112(suppl):259–265.
72. Murray N, Coy P, Pater JL, et al. Importance of timing for thoracic irradiation in the combined modality treatment of limited-stage small-cell lung cancer. *J Clin Oncol* 1993;11:336–344.
73. Prophylactic Cranial Irradiation Overview Collaborative Group. Cranial irradiation for preventing brain metastasis of small cell lung cancer in patients in complete remission. In: The Cochrane Library, Issue 4, 2002. Oxford: Update Software. Search date 2000; primary sources Medline, Cancerlit, Excerpta Medica, Biosis, hand searches of meeting proceedings, the Physician Data Query clinical trial registry, and personal contact with investigators and experts.
74. Arriagada R, Le Chevalier T, Riviere A. Patterns of failure after prophylactic cranial irradiation in small-cell lung cancer: analysis of 505 randomized patients. *Ann Oncol* 2002;13:748–754.
75. Souhami RL, Spiro SG, Rudd RM, et al. Five day oral etoposide treatment for advanced small cell lung cancer: randomized comparison with intravenous chemotherapy. *J Natl Cancer Inst* 1997;89:577–580.
76. Medical Research Council Lung Cancer Working Party. Comparison of oral etoposide and standard intravenous multidrug chemotherapy for small-cell lung cancer: a stopped multicentre randomised trial. *Lancet* 1996;348:563–566.
77. Hanna NH, Sandler AB, Loehrer PJ, et al. Maintenance daily oral etoposide versus no further therapy following induction chemotherapy with etoposide plus ifosfamide plus cisplatin in extensive small-cell lung cancer: a Hoosier Oncology Group randomized study. *Ann Oncol* 2002; 13:95–102.

Alan Neville
Professor
McMaster University
Hamilton
Canada

Competing interests: None declared.

TABLE 1 **Staging lung cancer** (see text, p 1950).

Non-small cell lung cancer

Stage	Definition*	5 year survival (%)
1	T1–T2, N0, M0	55–75
2	T1–T2, N1, M0	25–50
3A	T3, N0–N1, M0 or T1–T3, N2, M0	20–40
3B	T4, any N, M0 or any T, N3, M0	≤5
4	Any M1	≤5

Small cell lung cancer

Stage	Definition	Median survival
Limited stage disease	Tumour confined to one side of the chest, supraclavicular lymph nodes, or both	18–24 months†
Extensive stage disease	Defined as anything beyond limited stage	10–12 months‡

*M, metastases; N, nodes; T, tumour. †With combined chemotherapy and mediastinal irradiation. ‡With palliative chemotherapy.

Bacterial vaginosis

Search date March 2004

M Riduan Joesoef and George Schmid

QUESTIONS

INTERVENTIONS

To be covered in future updates

Recurrent bacterial vaginosis

Key Messages

- Bacterial vaginosis may resolve spontaneously.

Treating non-pregnant women

- **Antibacterial treatment with metronidazole or clindamycin (short term benefit)** One systematic review found that more women having antibacterial treatment (intravaginal clindamycin cream or intravaginal metronidazole gel) achieved cure than women using placebo. One systematic review found no significant difference in cure rates or adverse effects at 5–10 days or 4 weeks between intravaginal clindamycin and oral metronidazole. However, comparison of results across RCTs found that yeast vulvovaginitis may be less common with intravaginal clindamycin than with oral metronidazole. Intravaginal clindamycin has been associated, rarely, with mild to severe colitis and vaginal candidiasis in non-pregnant women. Another systematic review found that a 7 day course of twice daily oral metronidazole increased cure rates compared with a single 2 g dose; it gave no information on adverse effects. Limited evidence from RCTs found no significant difference in cure rates between oral clindamycin and oral metronidazole, and found that both treatments were associated with nausea and metallic taste. One RCT found no significant difference in cure rates at 35 days between 3 day treatment with intravaginal clindamycin ovules and 7 day treatment with intravaginal clindamycin cream. It found that the proportion of people who had adverse effects was similar in both groups, but ovules were associated with a higher incidence of vaginal pain and headache, and cream with a higher incidence of flu syndrome. Another RCT found no significant difference in cure rates or adverse effects between once and twice daily dosing with intravaginal metronidazole gel. We found no evidence on long term outcomes. One small RCT suggested that more than 50% of women had recurrent bacterial vaginosis 2 months after antibacterial treatment.

Treatment in pregnancy

- **Antibacterial treatment (except intravaginal clindamycin) in pregnant women who have had a previous preterm birth** One systematic review found that antibiotics reduced the risk of low birth weight in women with bacterial vaginosis who had a previous preterm delivery, although results for preterm delivery varied widely between trials. One subsequent RCT found that oral clindamycin given early in the second trimester reduced miscarriages or preterm deliveries compared with placebo in women with previous late miscarriage or preterm delivery.
- **Antibacterial treatment in low risk pregnancy** One systematic review in general populations of pregnant women found no significant difference between antibiotics (oral or vaginal) and placebo or no treatment in the risk of preterm delivery, low birth weight, neonatal sepsis, or perinatal death. However, subsequent RCTs in women with bacterial vaginosis or abnormal genital tract flora (may or may not have included bacterial vaginosis) found that oral or intravaginal clindamycin given early in the second trimester reduced miscarriages or preterm deliveries compared with placebo.
- **Intravaginal clindamycin cream** In studies that assessed women regardless of previous preterm delivery, three RCTs found a non-significant increase in preterm birth and low birth weight in women with bacterial vaginosis treated with clindamycin cream compared with placebo. However, one subsequent RCT found limited evidence in women with abnormal genital tract flora (may or may not have included bacterial vaginosis) that intravaginal clindamycin cream given early in the second trimester reduced preterm birth compared with placebo.

Treating partners

- **Treating a woman's male sexual partner with metronidazole or clindamycin (did not reduce the woman's risk of recurrence)** One systematic review found that in women receiving antibacterial agents, and who have one steady male sexual partner, treating the partner with an oral antibacterial agent did not reduce the woman's risk of recurrence.

Treatment before gynaecological procedures

- **Oral or intravaginal antibacterial treatment before surgical abortion** Three RCTs found a lower rate of post operative pelvic inflammatory disease with oral or intravaginal antibacterial treatment compared with placebo given to women with bacterial vaginosis who were about to have surgical abortion, but the difference was significant only in the largest RCT. The RCTs gave no information on adverse effects. In RCTs in non-pregnant women with bacterial vaginosis, intravaginal clindamycin was associated, rarely, with mild to severe colitis and vaginal candidiasis. Oral metronidazole was associated with nausea and metallic taste.
- **Antibacterial treatment before gynaecological procedures other than abortion** We found no RCTs on the effects of antibacterial treatment in women with bacterial vaginosis about to have gynaecological procedures other than abortion.

DEFINITION Bacterial vaginosis is a microbial disease characterised by a change in the bacterial flora of the vagina from mainly *Lactobacillus* species to high concentrations of anaerobic bacteria. The condition is asymptomatic in 50% of infected women. Women with symptoms have an excessive white to grey, or malodorous vaginal discharge, or both; the odour may be particularly noticeable during sexual intercourse. Commonly practiced clinical diagnosis requires three out of four features: the presence of clue cells on microscopy; a homogenous discharge adherent to the vaginal walls; pH of vaginal fluid greater than 4.5; and a "fishy" amine odour of the vaginal discharge before or after addition of 10% potassium hydroxide. Some experts prefer other methods of diagnosis, (e.g. Gram stain of vaginal secretions), particularly in a research setting. Gram stain using Nugent's criteria[1] categorise the flora of vagina into three categories – normal, intermediate, and flora consistent with bacterial vaginosis. Abnormal vaginal flora includes intermediate flora and bacterial vaginosis.

INCIDENCE/ PREVALENCE Bacterial vaginosis is the most common infectious cause of vaginitis, being about twice as common as candidiasis.[2] Prevalences of 10–61% have been reported among unselected women from a range of settings.[3] Data on incidence are limited but one study found that, over a 2 year period, 50% of women using an intrauterine contraceptive device had at least one episode, as did 20% of women using oral contraceptives.[4] Bacterial vaginosis is particularly prevalent among lesbians.[5]

AETIOLOGY/ RISK FACTORS The cause of bacterial vaginosis is not fully understood. Risk factors include new or multiple sexual partners[2,4,6] and early age of sexual intercourse,[7] but no causative microorganism has been shown to be transmitted between partners. Use of an intrauterine contraceptive device[4] and douching[6] have also been reported as risk factors. Infection seems to be most common around the time of menstruation.[8]

PROGNOSIS The course of bacterial vaginosis varies and is poorly understood. Without treatment, symptoms may persist or resolve in both pregnant and non-pregnant women. Recurrence after treatment occurs in about a third of women. A history of bacterial vaginosis is associated with increased rates of complications in pregnancy: low birth weight;[7] preterm birth (pooled OR from 10 cohort studies: 1.8, 95% CI 1.5 to 2.6);[9] preterm labour; premature rupture of membranes;[7] late miscarriage; chorioamnionitis;[10] endometritis after normal delivery (8.2% v 1.5%; OR 5.6, 95% CI 1.8 to 17.2);[11] endometritis after caesarean section (55% v 17%; OR 5.8, 95% CI 3.0 to 10.9);[12] and surgery to the genital tract.[13,14] Women who have had a previous preterm delivery are especially at risk of complications in pregnancy, with a sevenfold increased risk of preterm birth (24/428 [5.6%] in all women v 10/24 [41.7%] in women with a previous preterm birth).[15] Bacterial vaginosis can also increase the risk of HIV acquisition and transmission.[16]

AIMS OF INTERVENTION To alleviate symptoms and to prevent complications relating to childbirth, termination of pregnancy, and gynaecological surgery, with minimal adverse effects; to reduce adverse neonatal outcomes.

OUTCOMES Preterm delivery; other complications in pregnancy; puerperal and neonatal morbidity and mortality; clinical or microbiological cure rates, usually at 1–2 weeks or 4 weeks after completing treatment; recurrence rates.

METHODS *Clinical Evidence* search and appraisal March 2004. In addition, the authors used information obtained from drug manufacturers.

QUESTION **What are the effects of different antibacterial regimens in non-pregnant women with symptomatic bacterial vaginosis on cure rates and symptom relief?**

OPTION **ANTIBACTERIAL TREATMENT**

One systematic review found that more women having antibacterial treatment (intravaginal clindamycin cream or intravaginal metronidazole gel) achieved cure than women using placebo. One systematic review found no significant difference in cure rates or adverse effects at 5–10 days or 4 weeks between intravaginal clindamycin and oral metronidazole. However, comparison of results across RCTs found that yeast vulvovaginitis may be less common with intravaginal clindamycin than with oral metronidazole. Intravaginal clindamycin has been associated, rarely, with mild to severe colitis and vaginal candidiasis in non-pregnant women. Another systematic review found that a 7 day course of twice daily oral metronidazole increased cure rates compared with a single 2 g dose; it gave no information on adverse effects. Limited evidence from RCTs found no significant difference in cure rates between oral clindamycin and oral metronidazole, and found that both treatments were associated with nausea and metallic taste. One RCT found no significant difference in cure

rates at 35 days between 3 day treatment with intravaginal clindamycin ovules and 7 day treatment with intravaginal clindamycin cream. It found that the proportion of people who had adverse effects was similar in both groups, but ovules were associated with a higher incidence of vaginal pain and headache, and cream with a higher incidence of flu syndrome. Another RCT found no significant difference in cure rates or adverse effects between once and twice daily dosing with intravaginal metronidazole gel. We found no evidence on long term outcomes. One small RCT suggested that more than 50% of women had recurrent bacterial vaginosis 2 months after antibacterial treatment.

Benefits: **Intravaginal antibacterial treatment versus placebo:** We found one systematic review (search date 1996, 4 RCTs, 406 women) comparing antibacterial treatment versus placebo.[17] It found that more women using intravaginal clindamycin cream and intravaginal metronidazole gel achieved cure than women using placebo (cumulative cure rates: 82% with intravaginal clindamycin cream *v* 35% with placebo at 25–39 days after completion of treatment; 2 RCTs, P value and CI not reported; 71% with intravaginal metronidazole gel *v* 50% with placebo at 28–32 days after completion of treatment; 2 RCTs, P value not reported). The relatively high cumulative cure rates with placebo treatment suggest that bacterial vaginosis often resolved spontaneously without treatment.[17] **Oral antibacterial treatment versus placebo:** We found no RCTs. **Intravaginal versus oral antibacterial treatment:** We found one systematic review (search date 1996, 5 RCTs, 741 women)[17] and one subsequent RCT[18] comparing intravaginal versus oral formulations of metronidazole and clindamycin. Three RCTs were conducted in symptomatic non-pregnant women and two were conducted in symptomatic and asymptomatic non-pregnant women.[17] The review found no significant difference in cumulative cure rates 5–10 days after completing treatment (85% with clindamycin vaginal cream 5 g at bedtime for 7 days *v* 81% with metronidazole vaginal gel 5 g twice daily for 5 days *v* 86% with oral metronidazole 500 mg twice daily for 7 days ; P values and CI not reported). Four weeks after completing treatment, the cumulative cure rates were 82% for clindamycin vaginal cream, 71% for metronidazole vaginal gel, and 78% for oral metronidazole (P values not reported). The subsequent RCT (399 women) comparing intravaginal clindamycin cream versus oral metronidazole also found no significant difference in cure rates (68% with clindamycin cream *v* 67% with oral metronidazole; $P = 0.81$).[18] However, a large number of women (166/399 [42%]) were not included in the efficacy analysis making interpretation of the results difficult (results reported on 233 women, many exclusions for different reasons). **Different oral antibacterial regimens:** We found one systematic review (search date 1993[19] updated in 1996[17]), which identified four RCTs comparing oral metronidazole 500 mg twice daily for 7 days versus a single 2 g dose of metronidazole.[17] We also found two additional RCTs comparing metronidazole 500 mg twice daily for 7 days versus clindamycin 300 mg twice daily for 7 days.[20,21] The systematic review found significantly higher cumulative cure rates with 7 day metronidazole than with single dose metronidazole at 3–4 weeks after completing treatment (82% with 7 days of metronidazole *v* 62% with single dose metronidazole; $P < 0.05$).[19] This conclusion remained the same when the review was updated.[17] The first additional RCT (143 symptomatic non-pregnant women) found no significant difference in cure rates within 7–10 days of starting treatment (women cured: 46/49 [94%] with clindamycin *v* 48/50 [96%] with metronidazole; RR 0.98, 95% CI 0.89 to 1.07).[20] A quarter of women were lost to follow up. The second RCT (96 non-pregnant women) found no significant difference in cure rates between clindamycin and metronidazole (39/41 [95%] with clindamycin *v* 41/44 [93%] with metronidazole; ARI 2%; RR 1.00, 95% CI 0.92 to 1.14).[21]

Different intravaginal antibacterial regimens: We found no systematic review but found two RCTs.[22,23] The first RCT (514 women) found no significant difference in cure rates between once daily and twice daily dosing of intravaginal metronidazole gel (118/207 [57%] with once daily gel *v* 129/209 [62%] with twice daily gel; RR 0.92, 95% CI 0.79 to 1.08).[22] The second RCT (662 women) compared 3 day treatment with intravaginal clindamycin ovules versus 7 day treatment with intravaginal clindamycin cream.[23] It found no significant difference in cure rates at 35 day assessment (134/238 [56%] with 3 day ovules *v* 113/224 [50%] with 7 day cream; ARI 6%; RR 1.10, 95% CI 0.94 to 1.30).

Harms: **Intravaginal antibacterial treatment versus placebo:** The review gave no information on adverse effects.[17] **Oral antibacterial treatment versus placebo:** We found no RCTs. **Intravaginal versus oral antibacterial treatment:** The RCT found no significant difference in the frequency of adverse effects between intravaginal clindamycin and oral metronidazole (10.3% with intravaginal clindamycin *v* 16.3% with oral metronidazole; P = 0.104).[18] Taste perversion (0% with intravaginal clindamycin *v* 3.1% with oral metronidazole ; P value not reported) and nausea (1.0% with intravaginal clindamycin *v* 5.6% with oral metronidazole; P value not reported) accounted for most of the difference between the two treatment groups. Rates of vaginal candidiasis were similar between the two treatment groups (3.1% with oral metronidazole *v* 3.4% with intravaginal clindamycin; P value not reported). Comparison of results across RCTs found that yeast vulvovaginitis might be less common with intravaginal metronidazole than with oral metronidazole (4% for intravaginal[24] *v* 8–22% for oral[25]). Intravaginal clindamycin has been associated, rarely, with mild to severe colitis[26] and vaginal candidiasis[27] (vaginal candidiasis with 7 day treatment: 13.3% in pregnant women *v* 10.4% in non-pregnant women). **Different oral antibacterial regimens:** The review gave no information on adverse effects of 7 day or single dose oral metronidazole.[17] The first RCT comparing oral clindamycin versus oral metronidazole reported nausea (7/49 [14%] with oral clindamycin *v* 10/50 [20%] with oral metronidazole; significance not reported) and metallic taste (0/49 [0%] with oral clindamycin *v* 3/50 [6%] with oral metronidazole; significance not reported).[20] **Different intravaginal antibacterial regimens:** The first RCT found no significant difference in the proportion of people who had adverse effects between once and twice daily intravaginal metronidazole gel (38% with once daily *v* 39% with twice daily; reported as non-significant, CI not reported).[22] Once or twice daily intravaginal metronidazole was associated with gastrointestinal symptoms in 7% of people in each group, vulvovaginal candidiasis in 7%, and symptoms of vaginal discharge in 11%.[22] The second RCT found that the proportion of people experiencing adverse effects was similar between 3 day clindamycin ovules and 7 day clindamycin cream, except for vaginal pain (3.4% with 3 day ovules *v* 0.9% with 7 day cream; P value not reported), flu syndrome (0.9% with 3 day ovules *v* 2.7% with 7 day cream; P value not reported), and headache (6.4% with 3 day ovules *v* 3.6% with 7 day cream; P value not reported).[23] Most adverse effects were rated "mild to moderate" intensity (proportion of mild to moderate adverse effects: 177/186 [95%] with 3 day ovules *v* 149/171 [87%] with 7 day cream; proportion with severe adverse effects: 9/186 [5%] with 3 day ovules *v* 19/171 [11%] with 7 day cream; P value not reported).

Comment: Intravaginal administration reduces systemic absorption and systemic adverse effects. Some women may prefer oral medication because it is more convenient. Most of the RCTs followed women for a short period of time (about 4 weeks), therefore it is not possible to fully evaluate long term adverse effects and recurrence rates. **Recurrence:** We found one

RCT (61 women, 19 withdrew) that followed up women who had been treated for bacterial vaginosis with either clindamycin vaginal cream or oral metronidazole.[28] It found that more than 50% of women in both groups had recurrent bacterial vaginosis 2 months after treatment (exact figures and statistical analysis not reported).

QUESTION **What are the effects of antibacterial treatments in pregnant women to reduce adverse outcomes of pregnancy and prevent neonatal complications?**

OPTION **ANTIBACTERIAL TREATMENTS FOR PREGNANT WOMEN TO REDUCE ADVERSE OUTCOMES OF PREGNANCY AND NEONATAL COMPLICATIONS**

One systematic review in general populations of pregnant women with bacterial vaginosis found no significant difference between antibiotics (oral or vaginal) and placebo in the risk of preterm delivery, low birth weight, neonatal sepsis, or perinatal death. However, in women with bacterial vaginosis who had experienced a previous preterm delivery, antibiotics reduced the risk of low birth weight. Results for preterm delivery in this population varied widely among trials. One subsequent RCT found that oral clindamycin given early in the second trimester reduced miscarriages or preterm deliveries compared with placebo, both among all women and in women with previous late miscarriage or preterm delivery. In RCTs that assessed women regardless of previous preterm delivery, three RCTs found a non-significant increase in preterm birth and low birth weight in women with bacterial vaginosis treated with intravaginal clindamycin cream compared with placebo. However, one subsequent RCT found limited evidence in women with abnormal genital tract flora (may or may not have included bacterial vaginosis) that intravaginal clindamycin cream given early in the second trimester reduced preterm birth compared with placebo.

Benefits: We found one systematic review (search date 2002, 10 RCTs, 4249 women) comparing antibacterial treatment versus placebo,[29] and two subsequent RCTs.[30,31] **In all pregnant women, regardless of risk:** The review performed separate analyses of any antibiotic, oral antibiotics, or intravaginal antibiotics versus placebo or no treatment; none found a significant difference in outcomes between antibacterial treatment and placebo or no treatment.[29] Overall, the review found no significant difference between any antibiotic and placebo or no treatment in the risk of preterm delivery, low birth weight, perinatal death, or neonatal sepsis in the general population of pregnant women with bacterial vaginosis (preterm delivery < 37 weeks' gestation, 8 RCTs, 4062 women: OR 0.93, 95% CI 0.78 to 1.12; low birth weight, 4 RCTs, 3131 women: OR 0.97, 95% CI 0.76 to 1.23; perinatal death, 2 RCTs, 749 women: OR 2.26, 95% CI 0.68 to 7.46; neonatal sepsis, 2 RCTs, 428 women: 0.95, 95% CI 0.06 to 15.32).[29] Similarly, it found no significant difference in these outcomes between oral antibiotics and placebo or no treatment (preterm delivery < 37 weeks' gestation, 5 RCTs, 2996 women: OR 0.88, 95% CI 0.72 to 1.09; low birth weight, 3 RCTs, 2459 women: OR 0.90, 95% CI 0.69 to 1.17; perinatal death, 2 RCTs, 739 women: OR 2.03, 95% CI 0.67 to 6.13; neonatal sepsis, 1 RCT, 406 women: OR 0.95, 95% CI 0.06 to 15.28). It also found no significant difference in these outcomes between intravaginal antibiotics and placebo or no treatment (preterm delivery < 37 weeks' gestation, 2 RCTs, 1056 women: OR 1.16, 95% CI 0.78 to 1.72; low birth weight, 1 RCT, 672 women: OR 1.35, 95% CI 0.77 to 2.36; perinatal death, no RCTs: OR and CI not estimable; neonatal sepsis, 1 RCT, 22 women: OR 1.01, 95% CI 0.33 to 3.06).[28] The first subsequent RCT (485 asymptomatic women with bacterial vaginosis) found that oral clindamycin given early in the second trimester significantly reduced the rate of miscarriage or preterm delivery compared with placebo (13/244 [5.3%] with clindamycin v 38/241 [15.8%] with placebo; ARR 10.4%, 95% CI 5.0% to 15.8%).[30] The second subsequent RCT (409 asymptomatic women with abnormal vaginal flora) found that 3 day treatment with intravaginal clindamycin cream at or before 20 weeks of gestation significantly decreased the rate of preterm birth compared with placebo (8/208 [4%] with intravaginal clindamycin v 19/201 [10%] with placebo; OR 0.38, 95% CI 0.16 to 0.90).[31] **In women with previous preterm birth:** The review found that, in women who had a previous preterm birth, antibiotics significantly reduced the risk of low birth weight compared with placebo (2 RCTs of 114 women: OR 0.31, 95% CI 0.13 to 0.75).[29] However, antibiotics did not significantly reduce the risk of preterm delivery or perinatal death (preterm delivery < 37 weeks' gestation, 5 RCTs, 622 women: OR 0.83, 95% CI 0.59 to 1.17; perinatal death, 2 RCTs, 155 women: OR 3.64, 95% CI 0.86 to 15.45), although results for preterm delivery varied widely among RCTs (see comment below). Subgroup analysis in the first subsequent RCT of women who had previous late miscarriage or preterm delivery found that fewer women taking oral clindamycin than placebo had late miscarriage and preterm delivery (miscarriage or preterm delivery: 7/36 [19%] with clindamycin v 16/38 [42%] with placebo; RR and CI not reported).[30] The second RCT did not analyze the results according to whether the women were at high risk (previous preterm birth).[31]

Harms: **General adverse effects:** Overall, the systematic review found that adverse effects of antibiotics were uncommon (although not all of the included RCTs gave information on adverse effects).[29] It found no significant difference between any antibiotic and placebo or no treatment in the risk of adverse effects (adverse effects sufficient to stop treatment, 2 RCTs, 965 women: OR 1.31, 95% CI 0.68 to 2.49; adverse effects not sufficient to stop treatment, 3 RCTs, 1340 women: OR 1.33, 95% CI 0.73 to 2.45). However, one large RCT (1953 women) included in the review found significantly more adverse effects with oral metronidazole compared with placebo, particularly gastrointestinal symptoms (20.0% with metronidazole v 7.5% with placebo; CI not reported).[32] The first subsequent RCT found no significant difference in the proportion of women who had adverse effects, including gastrointestinal upset, nausea, vomiting, vulvovaginal candidiasis, and headache between intravaginal clindamycin and placebo (17/239 [7%] with intravaginal clindamycin v 8/239 [3%] with placebo; P = 0.10).[30] The second subsequent RCT gave no information on adverse effects.[31] **Adverse outcomes of pregnancy and neonatal complications:** Three included RCTs found a non-significant increase in preterm birth in all risk women with bacterial vaginosis who used intravaginal clindamycin cream compared with placebo (first RCT, 271 women: 9/60 [15%] with clindamycin cream v 5/69 [7.2%] with placebo; reported as non-significant, RR and CI not reported; second RCT, 681 women: 51/340 [15.0%] with clindamycin cream v 46/341 [13.5%] with placebo; OR 1.1, 95% CI 0.7 to 1.7; third RCT, 375 women: 9/187 [5%] with clindamycin cream v 7/188 [4%] with placebo; OR 1.3, 95% CI 0.5 to 3.5).[33–35] Two included RCTs found that more women with bacterial vaginosis using intravaginal clindamycin had babies with low birth weight than women using placebo, although the difference was not significant (first RCT, 271 women: 8/59 [13.6%] with clindamycin cream v 3/69 [4.4%] with placebo; second RCT, 681 women: 30/334 [9.0%] with clindamycin cream v 23/338 [6.8%] with placebo; OR 1.3, 95% CI 0.8 to 2.4, reported as non-significant, RR not reported).[34]

Comment: The average quality of the RCTs in the systematic review was good.[29] All trials reported loss to follow up between 1–17% for the various treatment groups. In addition to an increased risk of preterm birth and low birth weight with intravaginal clindamycin treatment, one included RCT found an alteration of normal vaginal flora to flora consistent with bacterial vaginosis among women at high risk of preterm birth who were treated with clindamycin cream. This alteration was reported as significant.[36] The review found two different clusters of results for oral treatment of bacterial vaginosis among high risk women. Different effects may be because of differences in dose and type of treatment regimen or in the timing of treatment.[29] **Differences in oral treatment regimens:** Three RCTs included in the review[29] found that antibiotics reduced preterm birth, of which two[37,38] used the US Centers for Disease Control and Prevention recommended treatment of bacterial vaginosis in pregnancy (oral metronidazole 250 mg 3 times daily for 7 days). The other[15] used a lower dose of oral metronidazole (400 mg twice daily for 2 days), but found a reduction in preterm birth in a small subgroup analysis (17 women in each group). One included RCT, which found no reduction in preterm birth, also used a lower dose of oral metronidazole (2 g single dose, repeated 48 hours later).[32] The subsequent RCT, which also found a benefit from treatment, used oral clindamycin, which has broader activity compared with metronidazole against bacterial vaginosis organisms (especially *Mobiluncus* species). **Differences in timing of treatment:** Differences in timing of treatment (early *v* late gestational age) may also have contributed to different results among RCTs. The two included RCTs[32,39] that found no reduction in preterm birth initiated antibiotic treatment at about 24 weeks of gestation, but the subsequent RCT, which found a reduction in preterm birth, initiated antibiotic treatment earlier in the pregnancy (at about 16 weeks).[30] Another subsequent RCT found a reduction of preterm birth with intravaginal clindamycin treatment, initiated at or before 20 weeks of gestation.[31] However, the treatment was given for vaginal flora which included disturbances of intermediate abnormality as well as of severe abnormality. Unlike severely disturbed flora, intermediate flora is not considered altered sufficiently enough to be a microbiological diagnosis for bacterial vaginosis.[1] To a lesser degree, differences in study population (symptomatic *v* asymptomatic) and diagnosis of bacterial vaginosis (clinical *v* Gram stain diagnosis) may also have contributed to the differing results. **Diagnostic criteria and screening:** Bacterial vaginosis is a condition of altered vaginal flora. There is a continuum of degrees of alteration of vaginal flora that women may have, and bacterial vaginosis may be defined differently according to the diagnostic criteria being used. Given this uncertainty, screening for bacterial vaginosis may result in the treatment of some women who do not have bacterial vaginosis. Thus, it is important to evaluate the harms of treatment among women who have equivocal bacterial vaginosis. Subgroup analyses of RCTs suggest that likely harms of antibiotics in this group include an increase in preterm birth and low birth weight.[37,40]

QUESTION Does treating male partners prevent recurrence?

OPTION TREATMENTS FOR PARTNERS TO PREVENT RECURRENCE

One systematic review found that in women receiving antibacterial agents, and who have one steady male sexual partner, treating the partner with an oral antibacterial agent did not reduce the woman's risk of recurrence.

Benefits: We found one systematic review (search date not reported, 6 RCTs) evaluating the effect of treating male sexual partners of women with bacterial vaginosis on recurrence rates.[41] All RCTs identified by the review found that treating a sexual partner with metronidazole or clindamycin had no effect on recurrence rates in women with bacterial vaginosis receiving the same treatment (significance assessments not reported in the review). The RCTs identified by the review assessed a variety of treatment regimens and populations but excluded women who were pregnant or who had coexistent vaginal infections. The systematic review did not attempt to test for heterogeneity between RCTs or to pool the results.

Harms: The review found that treatment of male partners carries few physiological adverse effects. However, the authors suggested that emotional adverse effects may arise from implying that bacterial vaginosis is a sexually transmitted disease.[41] Adverse effects of metronidazole and clindamycin (oral or intravaginal) are reported elsewhere in this topic (see harms of antibacterial treatments, p 1972).

Comment: The lack of evidence of effectiveness of both metronidazole and clindamycin suggests that anaerobes are unlikely to be the sole pathogenic agents linking bacterial vaginosis with sexual intercourse.

QUESTION **What are the effects of treatment before gynaecological procedures?**

OPTION **ANTIBACTERIAL TREATMENT BEFORE GYNAECOLOGICAL PROCEDURES**

Three RCTs found a lower rate of postoperative pelvic inflammatory disease with oral or intravaginal antibacterial treatment compared with placebo given to women with bacterial vaginosis who were about to have surgical abortion, but the difference was significant only in the largest RCT. The RCTs gave no information on adverse effects. In RCTs in non-pregnant women with bacterial vaginosis, intravaginal clindamycin was associated, rarely, with mild to severe colitis and vaginal candidiasis. Oral metronidazole was associated with nausea and metallic taste. We found no RCTs on the effects of antibacterial treatment in women with bacterial vaginosis about to have gynaecological procedures other than abortion.

Benefits: We found no systematic review. **Before surgical abortion:** We found three RCTs.[13,40,41] The first RCT (174 women with bacterial vaginosis) compared oral metronidazole 500 mg 3 times daily for 10 days versus placebo in women about to have surgical abortion.[13] Fewer women taking oral metronidazole developed pelvic inflammatory disease than those taking placebo, although the difference did not reach significance (3/84 [4%] with metronidazole *v* 11/90 [12%] with placebo; RR 0.29, 95% CI 0.08 to 1.01). The second RCT (1655 women) compared intravaginal clindamycin cream versus placebo in women about to have surgical abortion.[42] It found that significantly fewer women treated with intravaginal clindamycin had an infection after abortion (3/181 [1.7%] with clindamycin *v* 12/181 [6.6%] with placebo; RR: 0.24, 95% CI 0.07 to 0.86). The third RCT compared a single dose metronidazole suppository 2 mg versus placebo.[43] It found that fewer women using metronidazole suppository had postoperative upper genital tract infection, although the difference was not signficant (12/142 [8%] with metronidazole *v* 21/131 [16%] with placebo; RR 0.52, 95% CI 0.27 to 1.02). The broad confidence interval suggests that the RCT was underpowered to rule out clinically important differences. **Before gynaecological surgery:** Cohort studies suggest that bacterial vaginosis is associated with an increased risk of endometritis after caesarean section and vaginal cuff cellulitis after abdominal hysterectomy,[12,14] but we found no RCTs of antibacterial treatment in women before such surgery. **Before insertion of an intrauterine contraceptive device:** Observational evidence suggests that bacterial vaginosis is associated with pelvic inflammatory disease (see pelvic inflammatory disease, p 2031) in women using intrauterine contraceptive devices,[4] but we found no RCTs of antibacterial treatment in women with bacterial vaginosis before insertion of these devices.

Harms: The RCTs gave no information on adverse effects.[13,42,43] Adverse effects of metronidazole and clindamycin (oral or intravaginal) are reported elsewhere in this topic. (see harms of antibacterial treatments in non-pregnant women, p 1972).

Comment: Despite the non-significant findings of infections after abortion and operations,[13,43] the trend in all trials was toward reduced infections among women receiving antibiotics. These trend need to be confirmed in trials with sufficient sample size to reach a conclusion.

Substantive changes

Antibacterial treatments for pregnant women One RCT added;[31] categorisation unchanged.

REFERENCES

1. Nugent RP, Krohn MA, Hillier SL. Reliability of diagnosing bacterial vaginosis is improved by a standardized method of Gram stain interpretation. *J Clin Microbiol* 1991;29:297–301.
2. Barbone F, Austin H, Louv WC, et al. A follow-up study of methods of contraception, sexual activity, and rates of trichomoniasis, candidiasis, and bacterial vaginosis. *Am J Obstet Gynecol* 1990;163:510–514.
3. Mead PB. Epidemiology of bacterial vaginosis. *Am J Obstet Gynecol* 1993;169:446–449.
4. Avonts D, Sercu M, Heyerick P, et al. Incidence of uncomplicated genital infections in women using oral contraception or an intrauterine device: a prospective study. *Sex Transm Dis* 1990;17:23–29.
5. Berger BJ, Kolton S, Zenilman JM, et al. Bacterial vaginosis in lesbians: a sexually transmitted disease. *Clin Infect Dis* 1995;21:1402–1405.
6. Hawes SE, Hillier SL, Benedetti J, et al. Hydrogen peroxide-producing lactobacilli and acquisition of vaginal infections. *J Infect Dis* 1996;174:1058–1063.
7. Hillier SL, Nugent RP, Eschenbach DA, et al. Association between bacterial vaginosis and preterm delivery of a low-birth-weight infant. *N Engl J Med* 1995;333:1737–1742.
8. Schwebke JR, Morgan SC, Weiss HL. The use of sequential self-obtained vaginal smears for detecting changes in the vaginal flora. *Sex Transm Dis* 1997;24:236–239.
9. Flynn CA, Helwig AL, Meurer LN. Bacterial vaginosis in pregnancy and the risk of prematurity: a meta-analysis. *J Fam Pract* 1999;48:885–892.
10. Hillier SL, Martius J, Krohn MA, et al. Case-control study of chorioamnionic infection and chorioamnionitis in prematurity. *N Engl J Med* 1988;319:972–975.
11. Newton ER, Prihoda TJ, Gibbs RS. A clinical and microbiologic analysis of risk factors for puerperal endometritis. *Obstet Gynecol* 1990;75:402–406.
12. Watts D, Krohn M, Hillier S, et al. Bacterial vaginosis as a risk factor for postcesarean endometritis. *Obstet Gynecol* 1990;75:52–58.
13. Larsson PG, Platz-Christensen JJ, Dalaker K, et al. Treatment with 2% clindamycin vaginal cream prior to first trimester surgical abortion to reduce signs of postoperative infection: a prospective, double-blinded, placebo-controlled, multicenter study. *Acta Obstet Gynecol Scand* 2000;79:390–396.
14. Soper DE, Bump RC, Hurt WG. Bacterial vaginosis and trichomoniasis vaginitis are risk factors for cuff cellulitis after abdominal hysterectomy. *Am J Obstet Gynecol* 1990;163:1016–1021.
15. McDonald HM, O'Loughlin JA, Vigneswaran R, et al. Impact of metronidazole therapy on preterm birth in women with bacterial vaginosis flora (*Gardnerella vaginalis*): a randomised, placebo controlled trial. *Br J Obstet Gynaecol* 1997;104:1391–1397.
16. Schmid G, Markowitz L, Joesoef R, et al. Bacterial vaginosis and HIV infection [editorial]. *Sex Transm Infect* 2000;76:3–4.
17. Joesoef MR, Schmid GP. Bacterial vaginosis: review of treatment options and potential clinical indications for therapy. *Clin Infect Dis* 1999;28(suppl 1):S57–S65. Search date 1996; primary sources Medline, hand searches of text books about sexually transmitted diseases and meeting abstracts, and contact with drug manufacturers.
18. Paavonen J, Mangioni C, Martin MA, et al. Vaginal clindamycin and oral metronidazole for bacterial vaginosis: a randomized trial. *Obstet Gynecol* 2000;96:256–260.
19. Joesoef MR, Schmid GP. Bacterial vaginosis: review of treatment options and potential clinical indications for therapy. *Clin Infect Dis* 1995;20(suppl 1):S72–S79. Search date 1993; primary sources Medline, hand searches of text books about sexually transmitted diseases and meeting abstracts, and contact with drug manufacturers.
20. Greaves WL, Chungafung J, Morris B, et al. Clindamycin versus metronidazole in the treatment of bacterial vaginosis. *Obstet Gynecol* 1988;72:799–802.
21. Aubert JM, Oliete S, Leira J. Treatment of bacterial vaginosis: clindamycin versus metronidazol. *Prog Obst Gin* 1994;37:287–292.
22. Livengood CH, Soper DE, Sheehan KL, et al. Comparison of once daily and twice daily dosing of 0.75% metronidazole gel in the treatment of bacterial vaginosis. *Sex Transm Dis* 1999;26:137–142.
23. Sobel J, Peipert JF, McGregor JA, et al. Efficacy of clindamycin vaginal ovule (3-day treatment) versus clindamycin vaginal cream (7-day treatment) in bacterial vaginosis. *Infect Dis Obstet Gynecol* 2001;9:9–15.
24. Hillier SL, Lipinski C, Briselden AM, et al. Efficacy of intravaginal 0.75% metronidazole gel for the treatment of bacterial vaginosis. *Obstet Gynecol* 1993;81:963–967.
25. Schmitt C, Sobel JD, Meriwether C. Bacterial vaginosis: treatment with clindamycin cream versus oral metronidazole. *Obstet Gynecol* 1992;79:1020–1023.
26. Trexler MF, Fraser TG, Jones MP. Fulminant pseudomembranous colitis caused by clindamycin phosphate vaginal cream. *Am J Gastroenterol* 1997;92:2112–2113.

27. CLEOCIN Clindamycin phosphate vaginal cream (product information). *Physicians' desk reference*, 56 Edition. Kalamazoo, MI: Pharmacia & UpJohn Company, 2002, 2788–2789.
28. Sobel JD, Schmitt C, Meriwether C. Long-term follow-up of patients with bacterial vaginosis treated with oral metronidazole and topical clindamycin. *J Infect Dis* 1993;167:783–784.
29. McDonald H, Brocklehurst P, Parsons J, et al. Antibiotics for treating bacterial vaginosis in pregnancy. In: The Cochrane Library, Issue 1, 2004. Chichester, UK: John Wiley & Sons Ltd. Search date 2002; primary sources Cochrane Pregnancy and Childbirth Group trials register.
30. Ugwumadu A, Manyonda I, Reid F, et al. Effect of early oral clindamycin on late miscarriage and preterm delivery in asymptomatic women with abnormal vaginal flora and bacterial vaginosis: a randomised controlled trial. *Lancet* 2003;361:983–988.
31. Lamont RF, Duncan SL, Mandal D, et al. Intravaginal clindamycin to reduce preterm birth in women with abnormal genital tract flora. *Obstet Gynecol* 2003;101:516–522.
32. Carey JC, Klebanoff MA, Hauth JC, et al. Metronidazole to prevent preterm delivery in pregnant women with asymptomatic bacterial vaginosis. *N Engl J Med* 2000;342:534–540.
33. McGregor JA, French JI, Jones W, et al. Bacterial vaginosis is associated with prematurity and vaginal fluid mucinase and sialidase: results of a controlled trial of topical clindamycin cream. *Am J Obstet Gynecol* 1994;170:1048–1059.
34. Joesoef MR, Hillier SL, Wiknjosastro G, et al. Intravaginal clindamycin treatment for bacterial vaginosis: effect on preterm delivery and low birth weight. *Am J Obstet Gynecol* 1995;173:1527–1531.
35. Kekki M, Kurki T, Pelkonen J, et al. Vaginal clindamycin in preventing preterm birth and peripartal infections in asymptomatic women with bacterial vaginosis: a randomized, controlled trial. *Obstet Gynecol* 2001;97:643–648.
36. Vermeulen GM, van Swet AA, Bruinse HW. Changes in the vaginal flora after two percent clindamycin vaginal cream in women at high risk of spontaneous preterm birth. *Br J Obstet Gynaecol* 2001;108:697–700.
37. Hauth JC, Goldenberg RL, Andrews WW, et al. Reduced incidence of preterm delivery with metronidazole and erythromycin in women with bacterial vaginosis. *N Engl J Med* 1995;333:1732–1736.
38. Morales WJ, Schorr S, Albritton J. Effect of metronidazole in patients with preterm birth in preceding pregnancy and bacterial vaginosis: a placebo-controlled, double-blind study. *Am J Obstet Gynecol* 1994;171:345–349.
39. Odendaal HJ, Popov I, Schoeman J, et al. Preterm labour: is bacterial vaginosis involved? *S Afr Med J* 2002;92:231–234.
40. Vermeulen GM, Bruinse HW. Prophylactic administration of clindamycin 2% vaginal cream to reduce the incidence of spontaneous preterm birth in women with an increased recurrence risk: a randomized placebo-controlled double-blind trial. *Br J Obstet Gynaecol* 1999;106:652–657.
41. Hamrick M, Chambliss ML. Bacterial vaginosis and treatment of sexual partners. *Arch Fam Med* 2000;9:647–648. Search date not reported; primary sources Medline and the Cochrane Library.
42. Larsson PG, Platz-Christensen JJ, Thejls H, et al. Incidence of pelvic inflammatory disease after first-trimester legal abortion in women with bacterial vaginosis after treatment with metronidazole: a double-blind, randomized study. *Am J Obstet Gynecol* 1992;166:100–103.
43. Crowley T, Low N, Turner A, et al. Antibiotic prophylaxis to prevent post-abortal upper genital tract infection in women with bacterial vaginosis: randomised controlled trial. *BJOG* 2001;108:396–402.

M Riduan Joesoef
Medical Epidemiologist
National Center for HIV STD and TB Prevention
Atlanta
USA

George Schmid
Medical Epidemiologist
Department of HIV/AIDS
World Health Organization
Geneva
Switzerland

Competing interests: None declared.

Chlamydia (uncomplicated, genital)

Search date March 2004

Nicola Low

QUESTIONS

INTERVENTIONS

Key Messages

- Short term microbiological cure is the outcome used in most RCTs, but this may not mean eradication of *Chlamydia trachomatis*. Long term cure rates have not been studied extensively because of high default rates and difficulty in distinguishing persistent infection from reinfection due to re-exposure.

In men and non-pregnant women

- **Azithromycin (single dose)** A systematic review of 12 blinded and unblinded RCTs found no significant difference in microbiological cure of *C trachomatis* between a single dose of azithromycin and a 7 day course of doxycycline. Rates of adverse effects were similar.
- **Doxycycline, tetracycline (multiple dose regimens)** Small RCTs with short term follow up and high withdrawal rates found that multiple dose regimens of tetracyclines (doxycycline, tetracycline) achieve microbiological cure in at least 95% of people with genital chlamydia. A systematic review of 12 blinded and unblinded RCTs found no significant difference in microbiological cure of *C trachomatis* between a 7 day course of doxycycline and a single dose of azithromycin. Rates of adverse effects were similar. Meta-analysis of two RCTs found that doxycycline reduced microbiological failure compared with ciprofloxacin.

- **Erythromycin (multiple dose regimens)** Three small RCTs found that erythromycin achieved microbiological cure in 77–100% of people, with the highest cure rate with a 2 g rather than a 1 g daily dose.
- **Amoxicillin, ampicillin, clarithromycin, lymecycline, minocycline, ofloxacin, pivampicillin, rifampicin, roxithromycin, sparfloxacin, trovafloxacin (multiple dose regimens)** We found limited evidence on the effects of these regimens.
- **Ciprofloxacin (multiple dose regimens)** Two RCTs found that ciprofloxacin cured 63–92% of people. Meta-analysis of these two RCTs found that ciprofloxacin increased microbiological failure compared with doxycycline.

In pregnant women

- **Azithromycin (single dose)** One systematic review found that a single dose of azithromycin increased microbiological cure and decreased the risk of an adverse effect, sufficient to stop treatment, compared with a 7 day course of erythromycin. Two subsequent unblinded RCTs found no significant difference in cure rate between single dose azithromycin and multiple dose amoxicillin.
- **Erythromycin, amoxicillin (multiple dose regimens)** One small RCT identified in a systematic review found that erythromycin versus placebo increased microbiological cure. The review found that a 7 day course of erythromycin reduced microbiological cure and increased the risk of an adverse event sufficient to stop treatment, compared with a single dose of azithromycin. Two subsequent unblinded RCTs found no significant difference in cure rates between multiple dose amoxicillin and single dose azithromycin. Other RCTs in the review found high cure rates with erythromycin and amoxicillin and no significant difference in microbiological cure between the two drugs.
- **Clindamycin (multiple dose regimens)** One small RCT found no significant difference in cure rates between clindamycin and erythromycin.

DEFINITION Genital chlamydia is a sexually transmitted infection of the urethra in men, and of the endocervix or urethra (or both) in women. It is defined as **uncomplicated** if it has not ascended to the upper genital tract. Infection in women is asymptomatic in up to 80% of cases, but may cause non-specific symptoms, including vaginal discharge and intermenstrual bleeding. Infection in men causes urethral discharge and urethral irritation or dysuria, but may also be asymptomatic in up to half of cases.[1] **Complicated** chlamydial infection includes spread to the upper genital tract (causing pelvic inflammatory disease in women [see pelvic inflammatory disease, p 2031] and epididymo-orchitis in men) and extragenital sites, such as the eye. Interventions for complicated chlamydial infection are not included in this chapter.

INCIDENCE/ PREVALENCE Genital chlamydia is the most commonly reported bacterial sexually transmitted infection in developed countries[1] and reported rates increased by around 20% in the UK and USA between 2000 and 2002.[2,3] In women, infection occurs most commonly between the ages of 16 and 19 years. In this age group, about 1300/100 000 new infections are reported each year in the UK,[2] compared with 1900/100 000 in Sweden,[4] and 2536 per 100 000 in the USA.[3] The peak age group for men is 20–24 years, with about 965/100 000 new infections per year in the UK and USA and 1200/100 000 in Sweden.[2–4] Rates decline markedly with increasing age. Reported rates are highly dependent on the level of testing. The population prevalence of uncomplicated genital chlamydia in 18–44 year olds in the UK in 1999 was 2.2% (95% CI 1.5% to 3.2%) in men and 1.5% (95% CI 1.1% to 2.1%) in women.[5]

AETIOLOGY/ RISK FACTORS Infection is caused by the bacterium *C trachomatis* serotypes D–K. It is transmitted primarily through sexual intercourse, but also perinatally and through direct or indirect oculogenital contact.[1]

PROGNOSIS In women, untreated chlamydial infection that ascends to the upper genital tract causes pelvic inflammatory disease (see pelvic inflammatory disease, p 2031) in an estimated 30–40% of cases.[6] Tubal infertility has been found to occur in about 11% of women after a single episode of pelvic inflammatory disease, and the risk of ectopic pregnancy is increased six- to sevenfold.[7] Ascending infection in men causes epididymitis, but evidence that this causes male infertility is limited.[8] Maternal to infant transmission can lead to neonatal conjunctivitis and pneumonitis in 30–40% of cases.[1] Chlamydia may coexist with other genital infections and may facilitate transmission and acquisition of HIV infection.[1] Untreated chlamydial infection persists in most women for at least 60 days and for a shorter period in men.[9] Spontaneous remission also occurs at an estimated rate of 5% per month.[10]

AIMS OF INTERVENTION To eradicate *C trachomatis*; to prevent the development of upper genital tract infection; to prevent further sexual transmission; and to prevent perinatal transmission, with minimal adverse effects of treatment.

OUTCOMES The primary outcome is short term microbiological cure rate (calculated as the percentage of people attending a follow up visit at least 1 week after the end of antibiotic treatment who had a negative test for *C trachomatis*). This may not mean eradication of *C trachomatis* because of the prolonged life cycle of the organism. Long term cure rates have not been studied extensively because of high default rates and difficulty in distinguishing persistent infection from reinfection. However, studies have found no persistent infection up to 20 weeks after successful antibiotic treatment.[9] Other outcomes include adverse effects of treatment, including effects on the fetus and incidence of pelvic inflammatory disease and infertility. We present cure rates for pregnant women separately from those for men and non-pregnant women because two important drug groups, tetracyclines and quinolones, are contraindicated in pregnancy.

METHODS *Clinical Evidence* search and appraisal March 2004. All relevant systematic reviews and masked clinical RCTs were included. RCTs of treatment for genital chlamydia usually compare a new antibiotic versus an existing regimen because placebo controlled RCTs would be considered unethical. Single trials usually have insufficient statistical power to establish equivalence but meta-analysis is often inappropriate because of differences in the antibiotics used. Therefore, where appropriate, we present the absolute cure rates for individual antibiotics, combining results across trials. We present the range of cure rates (with exact binomial CIs) or, if there was no evidence of statistical heterogeneity between RCTs, the summary cure rate (95% CIs) weighted by the standard error. Summary rates do not include cure rates of 100% because the standard error cannot be computed if there are no treatment failures. In one instance (ciprofloxacin), two RCTs compared the same regimen with no evidence of statistical heterogeneity and we used a fixed effects meta-analysis to calculate the summary odds ratio with 95% confidence intervals. Trial quality was assessed in terms of randomisation, blinding, and numbers of withdrawals from analysis.[11] RCTs with methodological limitations have been included but relevant problems are mentioned in the text. **Categorising interventions:** We considered a regimen beneficial if the summary cure rate from two or more RCTs was 95% or greater, as previously suggested,[12] and if the lower confidence limit was also above 90%. We found insufficient data to differentiate reinfections from persistent infections. We considered regimens to be likely (or unlikely) to be beneficial on the basis of positive (or negative) results from two or more RCTs, and of unknown effectiveness if there was only one RCT or if results were conflicting.

QUESTION **What are the effects of antibiotic treatment in men and non-pregnant women with uncomplicated genital chlamydial infection?**

OPTION **SINGLE DOSE ANTIBIOTICS**

A systematic review of 12 blinded and unblinded RCTs found no significant difference in microbiological cure of *C trachomatis* between a single dose of azithromycin and a 7 day course of doxycycline. Rates of adverse effects were similar.

Benefits: **Versus placebo:** We found no systematic review and no RCTs. **Versus other single dose antibiotics:** We found no systematic review and no RCTs. **Versus multiple dose antibiotics:** We found one systematic review (search date 2001, 12 blinded and unblinded RCTs, 1543 people) comparing azithromycin (1 g as a single dose) versus doxycycline (100 mg twice daily for 7 days).[13] It found no significant difference in microbiological cure of *C trachomatis* (cure rates for single dose azithromycin ranging from 81–100%, for multiple dose doxycycline from 92–100%; pooled efficacy difference for microbiological cure with azithromycin versus doxycycline +0.008, 95% CI –0.007 to +0.022; P = 0.296).

Harms: Short term adverse effects of both azithromycin and doxycycline were reported to be mild and similar.[13]

Comment: When taken as a directly observed treatment, azithromycin has the advantage over multiple dose antibiotics that adherence to therapy can be guaranteed.

OPTION MULTIPLE DOSE ANTIBIOTICS

Small RCTs with short term follow up and high withdrawal rates found that multiple dose regimens of tetracyclines (doxycycline, tetracycline) achieve microbiological cure in at least 95% of people with genital chlamydia. A systematic review of 12 blinded and unblinded RCTs found no significant difference in microbiological cure of *C trachomatis* between a 7 day course of doxycycline and a single dose of azithromycin. Rates of adverse effects were similar. Three small RCTs found that erythromycin achieved microbiological cure in 77–100% of people, with the highest cure rate with a 2 g rather than a 1 g daily dose. Two RCTs found that ciprofloxacin cured 63–92% of people. Meta-analysis of these two RCTs found that ciprofloxacin increased microbiological failure compared with doxycycline. We found limited evidence on the effectiveness of other macrolides, quinolones, and penicillins. The RCTs had short term follow up and high withdrawal rates.

Benefits: **Versus placebo:** We found one small RCT that found trimethoprim–sulfadiazine to be superior to placebo (see comment below).[14] **Versus single dose antibiotics**: See single dose antibiotics in men and non-pregnant women, p 1981. **Versus each other:** We found no systematic review comparing multiple dose antibiotics versus each other. We found 22 RCTs reported to be double blind or with blinded outcome assessment comparing 19 different multiple dose antibiotic regimens. Four RCTs included comparison with single dose azithromycin but only the data on multiple dose antibiotics are presented in this section (see table A on web extra).[15–35] Results were similar in men and women and in populations with proven and presumed infection, so data were combined. **Doxycycline:** We found 11 RCTs (1434 men and women, comparing doxycycline versus another antibiotic).[15–17,19–26] The cure rate was 100% in six and the weighted average 98% (95% CI 96% to 99%) in the other five. We found no RCTs comparing different regimens for doxycycline, but the most frequent schedule (in 6 RCTs) was 100 mg twice daily for 7 days. **Tetracycline:** The summary cure rate in four RCTs (201 men and women) comparing tetracycline hydrochloride (500 mg 4 times daily for 7 days) versus another antibiotic was 97% (95% CI 94% to 99%).[27] **Erythromycin:** Cure rates with erythromycin stearate 1 g daily for 7 days (3 RCTs, 191 people) ranged from 77–95%,[33–35] and with erythromycin 2 g daily for 7 days (2 RCTs, 40 people) from 94–100%.[32,35] **Ciprofloxacin:** In two RCTs (190 men and women) the cure rate for ciprofloxacin ranged from 63–92%.[23,24] Meta-analysis by *Clinical Evidence* found that failure of microbiological cure was significantly more frequent with ciprofloxacin than with doxycycline (OR 5.0, 95% CI 1.2 to 10.0). **Other antibiotics (including macrolides, quinolones, and penicillins):** Ofloxacin, sparfloxacin, trovafloxacin, minocycline, lymecycline, clarithromycin, ampicillin, pivampicillin, rifampicin, and roxithromycin were studied in single RCTs (see table A on web extra). No RCT measured the effect of antibiotics on pelvic inflammatory disease or infertility.

Harms: Reported adverse effects varied widely between RCTs but were mostly gastrointestinal (see table A on web extra). Adverse effects, severe enough to stop treatment, were infrequent. Photosensitivity, which is particularly associated with tetracyclines, was also reported to occur with sparfloxacin (3/231 [1.3%] photosensitive with sparfloxacin *v* 1/230 [0.4%] with doxycycline).[22]

Comment: **Versus placebo:** The single placebo controlled trial was conducted in 1978, when the value of treating non-gonococcal urethritis was disputed.[14] This trial was halted because of the high incidence of complications in the placebo group. **Versus each other:** Most RCTs were conducted in sexually transmitted diseases clinics, where follow up is difficult; in 7/14 RCTs with available data, more than 15% of randomised participants were not included in the analysis.[14,18,25,32–35] Most RCTs were small (3 had fewer than 40 people with chlamydia)[19,27,32] and many antibiotic regimens were compared, so it is difficult to draw conclusions about relative efficacy. Only five RCTs reported that sexual partners of participants were offered treatment. Amoxicillin and ampicillin have not been adequately assessed in the treatment of genital chlamydia infection (see table A on web extra) because *in vitro* studies suggest that amoxicillin does not eradicate *C trachomatis*,[36] raising the concern that infection may persist and recrudesce *in vivo*. A similar effect is presumed for ampicillin.

QUESTION **What are the effects of antibiotic treatment for pregnant women with uncomplicated genital chlamydial infection?**

OPTION **SINGLE DOSE ANTIBIOTICS**

One systematic review found that a single dose of azithromycin increased microbiological cure and decreased the risk of an adverse effect, sufficient to stop treatment, compared with a 7 day course of erythromycin. Two subsequent unblinded RCTs found no significant difference in cure rates between single dose azithromycin and multiple dose amoxicillin.

Benefits: **Versus placebo:** We found no systematic reviews and no RCTs. **Versus other single dose antibiotics:** We found no systematic reviews and no RCTs. **Versus multiple dose antibiotics:** We found one systematic review (search date 1998, 4 non-blinded RCTs, 290 pregnant women),[37] and two subsequent RCTs.[38,39] The review compared a single dose of azithromycin 1 g versus erythromycin 500 mg 4 times daily for 7 days.[37] At first follow up visit 2–3 weeks after treatment, failure of microbiological cure was significantly less frequent with azithromycin than with erythromycin (failure to cure 11/145 [8%] with azithromycin *v* 27/145 [19%] with erythromycin; RR 0.42, 95% CI 0.22 to 0.80). There was no significant difference in the rate of premature delivery in one RCT (OR 0.75, 95% CI 0.28 to 2.04). The two subsequent unblinded RCTs both compared a single dose of azithromycin 1 g versus 7 days of amoxicillin 500 mg.[38,39] The first RCT (39 women) found no significant difference in microbiological cure rate (failure to cure: 1/19 [5.2%] with azithromycin *v* 3/15 [20%] with amoxicillin; OR 0.26, 95% CI 0.005 to 3.79).[38] The second RCT (110 women) found no significant difference in the combined outcome of negative microbiological test and completion of all medication (32/55 [58%] with amoxicillin *v* 35/55 [63%] with azithromycin; RR 0.9, 95% CI 0.7 to 1.2).[39]

Harms: The systematic review found that azithromycin decreased the risk of an adverse effect, sufficient to stop treatment, compared with erythromycin (4/254 [1.6%] with azithromycin *v* 40/249 [16.6%] with erythromycin; RR 0.11, 95% CI 0.04 to 0.28).[36] Fetal anomaly (not further specified) was reported in one infant in each group. The first subsequent RCT found that a non-significantly greater proportion of women reported adverse events with azithromycin compared with amoxicillin (10/19 [52.6%] with azithromycin *v* 5/17 [29.4%] with amoxicillin; RR 1.8, 95% CI 0.8 to 4.2).[38] Similarly, the second subsequent RCT found non-significantly more adverse effects with azithromycin compared with amoxicillin (6/55 [10.9%] with azithromycin *v* 3/55 [5.5%] with amoxicillin; RR 0.5, 95% CI 0.1 to 1.9).[39] We found little good evidence on the effects of azithromycin on pregnancy outcomes.

Comment: Erythromycin is more likely than azithromycin to be discontinued because of its gastrointestinal side effects. Furthermore, azithromycin as a single dose antibiotic is suitable for directly observed treatment where compliance can be guaranteed. However, azithromycin is not yet licensed for use in pregnancy.

OPTION MULTIPLE DOSE ANTIBIOTICS

One small RCT identified in a systematic review found that erythromycin or clindamycin increased microbiological cure compared with placebo. The review found that a 7 day course of erythromycin reduced microbiological cure and increased the risk of an adverse event sufficient to stop treatment, compared with a single dose of azithromycin. Two subsequent unblinded RCTs found no significant difference in cure rates between multiple dose amoxicillin and single dose azithromycin. Other RCTs in the review found no significant difference between erythromycin and amoxicillin in microbiological cure rate, and high cure rates with both drugs. One small RCT in the review found no significant difference in cure rates between clindamycin and erythromycin.

Benefits: **Versus placebo:** We found one systematic review (search date 1998, 1 RCT, 135 women).[37] It found that treatment with erythromycin or clindamycin was more effective than placebo (OR for failure of cure 0.06, 95% CI 0.03 to 0.12). No other information was reported. **Versus single dose antibiotics:** See benefits of single dose antibiotics in pregnant women with uncomplicated genital chlamydia infection, p 1981. **Versus each other:** We found one systematic review (search date 1998, 11 blinded and unblinded RCTs, 1449 people).[37] The review found three RCTs comparing microbiological cure rates between amoxicillin 1.5 g daily for 7 days and erythromycin 2 g daily for 7 days. The RCTs found high rates of microbiological cure with both drugs and a non-significantly higher rate of microbiological cure with amoxicillin than with erythromycin (182/199 [91%] with amoxicillin *v* 163/191 [85%] with erythromycin; RR for failure of cure with amoxicillin compared with erythromycin 0.59, 95% CI 0.34 to 1.03). The review found one small RCT, which found no significant difference in cure rates between clindamycin and erythromycin (cure rate 38/41 [93%] *v* 31/37 [84%]; RR for failure of cure 0.45, 95% CI 0.12 to 1.7).[37]

Harms: Rates of adverse effects were similar for clindamycin and erythromycin, but adverse effects, sufficient to stop treatment, were less frequent with amoxicillin than with erythromycin (OR 0.16, 95% CI 0.09 to 0.30).[37] None of the RCTs gave information on adverse clinical outcomes in the offspring.

Comment: Out of three RCTs conducted between 1982 and 1997, which compared the effects of antibiotic therapy versus placebo, only one reported cure rates in women.[37]

REFERENCES

1. Holmes KK, Sparling PF, M rdh PA, et al, eds. *Sexually transmitted diseases*. 3rd ed. New York: McGraw Hill Inc, 1999.
2. Health Protection Agency. Chlamydia (*Chlamydia trachomatis*). http://www.hpa.org.uk/infections/topics_az/hiv_and_sti/sti-chlamydia/chlamydia.htm (last accessed 19 July 2004).
3. Centers for Disease Control and Prevention. Sexually Transmitted Disease Surveillance, 2001. Atlanta, GA: U.S. Department of Health and Human Services, September 2002.
4. Communicable Diseases in Sweden 2000. The Annual Report of the Department of Epidemiology. 2000, Stockholm, Swedish Institute for Infectious Disease Control.
5. Fenton K, Korovessis C, Johnson AM, et al. Sexual behaviour in Britain: sexually transmitted infections and prevalent *Chlamydia trachomatis* infection. *Lancet* 2001;358:1851–1854.
6. Cates W Jr, Rolfs RT Jr, Aral SO. Sexually transmitted diseases, pelvic inflammatory disease, and infertility: an epidemiologic update. *Epidemiol Rev* 1990;12:199–220.
7. Weström L, Bengtsson LP, M rdh PA. Incidence, trends, and risks of ectopic pregnancy in a population of women. *BMJ* 1981;282:15–18.
8. Ness RB, Markovic N, Carlson CL, et al. Do men become infertile after having sexually transmitted urethritis? An epidemiologic examination [review]. *Fertil Steril* 1997;68:205–213.
9. Golden MR, Schillinger JA, Markowitz L, et al. Duration of untreated genital infections with *Chlamydia trachomatis*: a review of the literature. *Sex Transm Dis 2000;27:329–337.*
10. Morré SA, van den Brule AJC, Rozendaal L, et al. The natural course of asymptomatic *Chlamydia trachomatis* infections: 45% clearance and no development of clinical PID after one-year follow up. *Int J STD AIDS* 2002;13(Suppl 2):12–18.
11. Chalmers I, Adams M, Dickersin K, et al. A cohort study of summary reports of controlled trials. *JAMA* 1990;263:1401–1405.
12. Clinical Effectiveness Group. National guideline for the management of *Chlamydia trachomatis* genital tract infection. *Sex Transm Infect* 1999;75(Suppl 1):4–8
13. Lau C-Y, Qureshi AK. Azithromycin versus doxycycline for genital chlamydial infections: A meta-analysis of randomised clinical trials. *Sex Transm Dis* 2002;29:497–502. Search date 2001; primary sources Medline, HealthSTAR, Ovid, Best Evidence, Cochrane Database of Abstracts and Reviews of Effectiveness.
14. Paavonen J, Kousa M, Saikku P, et al. Treatment of nongonococcal urethritis with trimethoprim-sulphadiazine and with placebo. A double-blind partner-controlled study. *Br J Venereal Dis* 1980;56:101–104.
15. Nilsen A, Halsos A, Johansen A, et al. A double blind study of single dose azithromycin and doxycycline in the treatment of chlamydial urethritis in males. *Genitourin Med* 1992;68:325–327.
16. Steingrímsson Ó, Ólafsson JH, Thórarinsson H, et al. Single dose azithromycin treatment of gonorrhea and infections caused by *C trachomatis* and *U urealyticum* in men. *Sex Transm Dis* 1994;21:43–46.
17. Stamm WE, Hicks CB, Martin DH, et al. Azithromycin for empirical treatment of the nongonococcal urethritis syndrome in men. A randomized double-blind study. *JAMA* 1995;274:545–549.
18. Brihmer C, M rdh PA, Kallings I, et al. Efficacy and safety of azithromycin versus lymecycline in the treatment of genital chlamydial infections in women. *Scand J Infect Dis* 1996;28:451–454.
19. Stein GE, Mummaw NL, Havlichek DH. A preliminary study of clarithromycin versus doxycycline in the treatment of nongonococcal urethritis and mucopurulent cervicitis. *Pharmacotherapy* 1995;15:727–731.
20. Romanowski B, Talbot H, Stadnyk M, et al. Minocycline compared with doxycycline in the treatment of nongonococcal urethritis and mucopurulent cervicitis. *Ann Intern Med* 1993;119:16–22.
21. Boslego JW, Hicks CB, Greenup R, et al. A prospective randomized trial of ofloxacin vs. doxycycline in the treatment of uncomplicated male urethritis. *Sex Transm Dis* 1988;15:186–191.
22. Phillips I, Dimian C, Barlow D, et al. A comparative study of two different regimens of sparfloxacin versus doxycycline in the treatment of non-gonococcal urethritis in men. *J Antimicrob Chemother* 1996;37(suppl A):123–134.
23. Hooton TM, Rogers ME, Medina TG, et al. Ciprofloxacin compared with doxycycline for nongonococcal urethritis. Ineffectiveness against *Chlamydia trachomatis* due to relapsing infection. *JAMA* 1990;264:1418–1421.
24. Jeskanen L, Karppinen L, Ingervo L, et al. Ciprofloxacin versus doxycycline in the treatment of uncomplicated urogenital *Chlamydia trachomatis* infections. A double-blind comparative study. *Scand J Infect Dis Suppl* 1989;60:62–65.
25. McCormack WM, Dalu ZA, Martin DH, et al. Double-blind comparison of trovafloxacin and doxycycline in the treatment of uncomplicated Chlamydial urethritis and cervicitis. Trovafloxacin Chlamydial Urethritis/Cervicitis Study Group. *Sex Transm Dis* 1999;26:531–536.
26. Lassus AB, Virrankoski T, Reitamo SJ, et al. Pivampicillin versus doxycycline in the treatment of chlamydial urethritis in men. *Sex Transm Dis* 1990;17:20–22.
27. Lassus A, Juvakoski T, Kanerva L. Comparison between rifampicin and tetracycline in the treatment of nongonococcal urethritis in males with special reference to *Chlamydia trachomatis*. *Eur J Sex Transm Dis* 1984;2:15–17.
28. Lassus A, Allgulander C, Juvakoski T. Efficacy of rosaramicin and tetracycline in chlamydia-positive and -negative nongonococcal urethritis. *Eur J Sex Transm Dis* 1982;1:29–31.
29. Juvakoski T, Allgulander C, Lassus A. Rosaramicin and tetracycline treatment in *Chlamydia trachomatis*-positive and -negative nongonococcal urethritis. *Sex Transm Dis* 1981;8:12–15.
30. Brunham RC, Kuo CC, Stevens CE, et al. Therapy of cervical chlamydial infection. *Ann Intern Med* 1982;97:216–219.
31. Batteiger BE, Zwickl BE, French ML, et al. Women at risk for gonorrhea: comparison of rosaramicin and ampicillin plus probenecid in the eradication of *Neisseria gonorrhoeae*, *Chlamydia trachomatis* and genital mycoplasmas. *Sex Transm Dis* 1985;12:1–4.
32. Robson HG, Shah PP, Lalonde RG, et al. Comparison of rosaramicin and erythromycin stearate for treatment of cervical infection with *Chlamydia trachomatis*. *Sex Transm Dis* 1983;10:130–134.
33. Worm AM, Hoff G, Kroon S, et al. Roxithromycin compared with erythromycin against genitourinary chlamydial infections. *Genitourin Med* 1989;65:35–38.
34. Worm AM, Avnstorp C, Petersen CS. Erythromycin against *Chlamydia trachomatis* infections. A double blind study comparing 4- and 7-day treatment in men and women. *Dan Med Bull* 1985;32:269–271.
35. Linnemann CCJ, Heaton CL, Ritchey M. Treatment of *Chlamydia trachomatis* infections: comparison of 1- and 2-g doses of erythromycin daily for seven days. *Sex Transm Dis* 1987;14:102–106.
36. Kuo CC, Wang SP, Grayston JT. Antimicrobial activity of several antibiotics and a sulfonamide against *Chlamydia trachomatis* organisms in cell culture. *Antimicrob Agents Chemother* 1977;12:80–83.

37. Brocklehurst P, Rooney G. Interventions for treating genital *Chlamydia trachomatis* infection in pregnancy. In: The Cochrane Library, Issue 3, 2002. Oxford: Update Software. Search date 1998; primary sources Cochrane Pregnancy and Childbirth Review Group Specialised Register of Controlled Trials, and Cochrane Controlled Trials Register.
38. Jacobson GF, Autry AM, Kirby RS, et al. A randomized controlled trial comparing amoxicillin and azithromycin for the treatment of *Chlamydia trachomatis* in pregnancy. *Am J Obstet Gynecol* 2001;184:1352–1356.
39. Kacmar J, Cheh E, Montagno A, et al. A randomized trial of azithromycin versus amoxicillin for the treatment of *Chlamydia trachomatis* in pregnancy. *Infect Dis Obstet Gynecol* 2001;9:197–202.

Nicola Low
Department of Social Medicine University of Bristol
Bristol
UK

Competing interests: None declared.
We would like to acknowledge the previous contributors of this chapter, including Frances Cowan.

Genital herpes

Search date March 2004

Eva Jungmann

QUESTIONS

INTERVENTIONS

PREVENTING SEXUAL TRANSMISSION

Likely to be beneficial

Antiviral treatment of infected sexual partner (reduced transmission to uninfected partner) 1992

Male condom use to prevent sexual transmission from infected men to uninfected sexual partners* . . .1991

Unknown effectiveness

Female condoms 1991

Male condom use to prevent sexual transmission from infected women to uninfected men 1991

Vaccines other than recombinant glycoprotein vaccines 1990

Unlikely to be beneficial

Recombinant glycoprotein vaccines (gB2 and gD2) in people at high risk of infection (unless known to be HSV-1 and HSV-2 negative before vaccination). 1990

PREVENTING TRANSMISSION FROM MOTHER TO NEONATE

Unknown effectiveness

Caesarean delivery in women with genital lesions at term 1993

Oral antiviral maintenance treatment in late pregnancy (36 or more weeks of gestation) in women with a history of genital herpes . . .1992

Serological screening and counselling in late pregnancy 1993

TREATING FIRST EPISODE

Beneficial

Oral antiviral treatment in first episodes of genital herpes. . .1994

Unknown effectiveness

Different types of oral antiviral treatment for first episodes of genital herpes 1995

REDUCING RECURRENCE

Beneficial

Oral antiviral maintenance treatment in people with high rates of recurrence 1996

Oral antiviral treatment taken at the start of recurrence 1995

Unknown effectiveness

Psychotherapy to reduce recurrence 1998

TREATING PEOPLE WITH HIV

Likely to be beneficial

Oral antiviral maintenance treatment for preventing recurrence of genital herpes in people with HIV . . .1999

Unknown effectiveness

Oral antiviral treatment for an acute recurrent episode of genital herpes in people with HIV 1998

Oral antiviral treatment for first episode genital herpes in people with HIV 1998

*Categorisation based on observational or non-randomised evidence in the context of practical and ethical problems of performing RCTs.

See glossary

Key Messages

Preventing sexual transmission

- **Antiviral treatment of infected sexual partner (reduced transmission to uninfected partner)** One RCT found that daily use of valaciclovir reduced the risk of transmission of herpes simplex virus-2 to a previously uninfected sexual partner compared with placebo.
- **Male condom use to prevent sexual transmission from infected men to uninfected sexual partners*** One prospective cohort study found limited evidence that condom use by men infected with genital herpes reduced transmission of herpes simplex virus-2 to their uninfected sexual partners.
- **Female condoms** We found no systematic review or RCTs on the effects of female condoms to prevent sexual transmission.
- **Male condom use to prevent sexual transmission from infected women to uninfected men** Subgroup analysis of one prospective cohort study found no significant difference between male condom use and no male condom use in transmission of herpes simplex virus-2 to uninfected men from their infected female partners.
- **Vaccines other than recombinant glycoprotein vaccines** We found no systematic review or RCTs.
- **Recombinant glycoprotein vaccines (gB2 and gD2) in people at high risk of infection (unless known to be HSV-1 and HSV-2 negative before vaccination)** One RCT found no significant difference between recombinant glycoprotein vaccine (gB2 plus gD2) and placebo in preventing genital herpes simplex virus-2 infection in people at high risk of infection. Subgroup analysis in a second RCT found that recombinant herpes simplex virus-2 glycoprotein-D-adjuvant vaccine reduced the risk of genital herpes infection compared with placebo in women who had been seronegative for herpes simplex virus-1 and herpes simplex virus-2 at baseline and who had regular sexual partners with clinically confirmed genital herpes. Subgroup analyses also found no significant difference between the vaccine and placebo in infection rate for men or in women who had been seropositive for herpes simplex virus-1 and who had regular sexual partners with genital herpes.

Preventing transmission from mother to neonate

- **Caesarean delivery in women with genital lesions at term** We found no systematic review or RCTs on the effects of caesarean delivery on mother to baby transmission of genital herpes in mothers with genital lesions at term. The procedure carries the risk of increased maternal morbidity and mortality.
- **Oral antiviral maintenance treatment in late pregnancy (36 or more weeks of gestation) in women with a history of genital herpes** One systematic review provided insufficient evidence to assess the effects of oral antiviral agents during pregnancy on transmission of infection to neonates. The review found that aciclovir reduced the recurrence of infection at term in women with first or recurrent episodes of genital herpes simplex virus during pregnancy, and reduced the need for caesarean delivery because of genital herpes.
- **Serological screening and counselling in late pregnancy** We found no systematic review or RCTs on the effects of either serological screening or counselling to prevent maternal infection in late pregnancy.

Treating first episode

- **Oral antiviral treatment in first episodes of genital herpes** Three RCTs found that oral aciclovir treatment decreased the duration of lesions, symptoms, and viral shedding compared with placebo.
- **Different types of oral antiviral treatment for first episodes of genital herpes** One RCT found no difference in clinical outcomes between oral aciclovir and valaciclovir.

Reducing recurrence

- **Oral antiviral maintenance treatment in people with high rates of recurrence** RCTs found that daily maintenance treatment with oral antiviral agents (valaciclovir, aciclovir or famciclovir) reduced the frequency of recurrences, and that oral aciclovir and oral valaciclovir improved quality of life compared with placebo.
- **Oral antiviral treatment taken at the start of recurrence** One systematic review, one non-systematic review, and one RCT found that oral antiviral treatment (aciclovir, famciclovir or valaciclovir) taken at the start of recurrence reduced the duration of lesions and viral shedding and increased the rate of aborted recurrences compared with placebo, in people with recurrent genital herpes. RCTs found that aciclovir, famciclovir, and valaciclovir were similarly effective in reducing symptom duration, lesion healing time, and viral shedding compared with placebo. Two RCTs found no difference between valaciclovir taken for 3 days or 5 days.
- **Psychotherapy to reduce recurrence** One systematic review of poor quality studies provided insufficient evidence about the effects of psychosocial interventions to prevent recurrence of genital herpes.

Treating people with HIV

- **Oral antiviral maintenance treatment for preventing recurrence of genital herpes in people with HIV** One RCT found that valaciclovir was more effective than placebo in preventing herpes simplex virus infection. One RCT found no significant difference between valaciclovir and aciclovir in preventing recurrent herpes simplex virus infections over 48 weeks.
- **Oral antiviral treatment for an acute recurrent episode of genital herpes in people with HIV** Two RCTs found no significant differences in duration of lesions and symptoms between famciclovir or valaciclovir or aciclovir.
- **Oral antiviral treatment for first episode genital herpes in people with HIV** We found no RCTs on the treatment of first episode genital herpes in people with HIV.

DEFINITION Genital herpes is an infection with herpes simplex virus type 1 (HSV-1) or type 2 (HSV-2). The typical clinical features include painful shallow anogenital ulceration. Herpes simplex virus infections can be confirmed on the basis of virological and serological findings. Types of infection include **first episode primary infection**, which is defined as herpes simplex virus confirmed in a person without prior findings of HSV-1 or HSV-2 antibodies; **first episode non-primary infection**, which is HSV-2 confirmed in a person with prior findings of HSV-1 antibodies or vice versa; **first recognised recurrence**, which is HSV-1 (or HSV-2) confirmed in a person with prior findings of HSV-1 (or HSV-2) antibodies; and **recurrent genital herpes**, which is caused by reactivation of latent herpes simplex virus. HSV-1 can also cause gingivostomatitis and orolabial ulcers; HSV-2 can also cause other types of herpes infections, such as ocular herpes; and both virus types can cause infection of the central nervous system (e.g. encephalitis).

INCIDENCE/ PREVALENCE Genital herpes infections are among the most common sexually transmitted diseases. Seroprevalence studies showed that 22% of adults in the USA had HSV-2 antibodies.[1] A UK study found that 23% of adults attending sexual medicine clinics and 7.6% of blood donors in London had antibodies to HSV-2.[2] Seroprevalence of HSV-2 increased by 30.0% (95% CI 15.8% to 45.8%) between the periods 1976–1980 and 1988–1994.[1] However, it should be noted that although antibody levels prove the existence of present or past infections, they do not differentiate between possible manifestations of HSV-2 infections (e.g. genital/ocular). Thus, the figures have to be treated with caution when applied to genital herpes only.

AETIOLOGY/ RISK FACTORS Both HSV-1 and HSV-2 can cause a first episode of genital infection, but HSV-2 is more likely to cause recurrent disease.[3] Most people with HSV-2 infection have only mild symptoms and remain unaware that they have genital herpes. However, these people can still pass on the infection to sexual partners and newborns.[4,5]

PROGNOSIS Sequelae of herpes simplex virus infection include neonatal herpes simplex virus infection, opportunistic infection in immunocompromised people, recurrent genital ulceration, and psychosocial morbidity. HSV-2 infection is associated with an increased risk of HIV transmission and acquisition.[6] The most common neurological complications are aseptic meningitis (reported in about 25% of women during primary infection) and urinary retention (reported in up to 15% of women during primary infection).[5] The absolute risk of neonatal infection is high (41%, 95% CI 26% to 56%) in babies born to women who acquire infection near the time of labour and low (< 3%) in women with established infection, even in those who have a recurrence at term.[7,8] About 15% of neonatal infections result from postnatal transmission from oral lesions of relatives or hospital personnel.[5]

AIMS OF INTERVENTION To prevent transmission; to reduce the morbidity of the first episode; to reduce the risk of recurrent disease after a first episode, with minimal adverse effects of treatment.

OUTCOMES Rates of transmission (shown either clinically, virologically, or serologically, depending on the study); seroconversion, severity, and duration of symptoms; healing time; duration of viral shedding (intermediate outcome reflecting the risk of transmitting the infection, although a direct link between the duration of viral shedding and risk of transmission has not been found); recurrence rates; psychosocial morbidity; adverse effects of treatment.

METHODS *Clinical Evidence* search and appraisal March 2004. We also included preliminary results of clinical trials published in the abstracts of the Interscience Conference on Antimicrobial Agents and Chemotherapy and International Society for STD Research.

QUESTION What are the effects of interventions to prevent sexual transmission of herpes simplex virus?

OPTION VACCINATION

One RCT found no significant difference between recombinant glycoprotein vaccine (gB2 plus gD2) and placebo in preventing genital herpes simplex virus-2 infection in people at high risk of infection. Subgroup analysis in a second RCT found that recombinant herpes simplex virus-2 glycoprotein-D-adjuvant vaccine reduced the risk of genital herpes infection compared with placebo in women who had been seronegative for herpes simplex virus-1 and herpes simplex virus-2 at baseline and who had regular sexual partners with clinically confirmed genital herpes. Subgroup analyses also found no significant difference between the vaccine and placebo in infection rate for men or in women who had been seropositive for herpes simplex virus-1 and who had regular sexual partners with genital herpes. We found no systematic review or RCTs on other types of vaccination.

Benefits: **Recombinant glycoprotein vaccines versus placebo:** We found no systematic review. We found two RCTs.[9,10] The first RCT (2393 people seronegative for herpes simplex virus type 2 [HSV-2] and HIV at high risk of exposure to genital herpes) compared recombinant glycoprotein vaccine (gB2 plus gD2) versus placebo.[9] It found no significant difference in the proportion of people with herpes simplex virus infection or positive genital herpes simplex virus culture (4.2 cases per 100 person years with glycoprotein vaccine *v* 4.6 cases per 100 person years with placebo; P = 0.58). Similarly, it found no significant difference in the duration of initial genital herpes (7.1 days with glycoprotein vaccine *v* 6.5 days with placebo; P = 0.45) or in the frequency of subsequent recurrences in people who acquired genital HSV-2 infection (rate of recurring lesions: 13/24 [54%] with glycoprotein vaccine *v* 21/33 [64%]

with placebo; P = 0.47). The second RCT (2 studies; 847 HSV-1 and HSV-2 seronegative people in study 1 and 1867 HSV-2 seronegative people in study 2 but at risk from a regular sexual partner with clinically confirmed genital herpes) compared recombinant HSV-2 glycoprotein-D-adjuvant vaccine versus placebo.[10] Both study arms found that recombinant HSV-2 glycoprotein vaccine reduced the risk of genital herpes compared with placebo in women who were previously uninfected with HSV-1 and HSV-2 (infection defined clinically or by virological or serological investigation; RR for infection 0.27, 95% CI 0.09 to 0.81 in study 1; 0.26, 95% CI 0.07 to 0.91 in study 2). However, no significant effect was found in women who were infected with HSV-1 at baseline or in men (in women with HSV-1: RR for infection 2.06, 95% CI 0.51 to 8.03; in men: RR 1.11, 95% CI 0.47 to 2.61 in study 1; RR 1.10, 95% CI 0.53 to 2.27 in study 2).[10] **Other types of vaccine:** We found no systematic review or RCTs on other types of vaccine.

Harms: The first RCT reported the vaccine to be safe and well tolerated, with frequencies of local and systemic reactions similar to those stated in the literature.[9] In the second RCT, the frequency of soreness at the injection site severe enough to prevent people from engaging in normal actions was higher with vaccine (5%) than with placebo (study 1: 3% and study 2: 1%; P value not reported).[10] The study found no major differences between the two groups in the frequency and type of reported symptoms or withdrawal rates (no statistical values reported).

Comment: Glycoprotein vaccines differ not only in the choice of recombinant herpes simplex virus molecules but also in the use of adjuvants (i.e. substances used to stabilise vaccine components). The use of different adjuvants may explain the inconsistent efficacy results of otherwise similar glycoprotein vaccines.

OPTION CONDOMS

One prospective cohort study found limited evidence that condom use by men infected with genital herpes reduced transmission of herpes simplex virus-2 to uninfected sexual partners. However, subgroup analysis of the cohort study found no significant difference between male condom use and no male condom use in transmission of herpes simplex virus-2 to uninfected men from their infected female partners. We found no systematic review or RCTs on the effects of female condoms to prevent sexual transmission.

Benefits: **Male condom use to prevent sexual transmission from infected men to uninfected sexual partners:** We found no systematic review or RCTs. In one prospective cohort study (528 couples [98% heterosexual] serodiscordant(G) for herpes simplex virus type 2 (HSV-2) infection and followed for 18 months) men infected with genital herpes who used condoms in more than 25% of sexual acts were at lower risk of infecting their sexual partners with HSV-2 (adjusted HR 0.09, 95% CI 0.01 to 0.67).[11] **Male condom use to prevent transmission from infected women to uninfected men:** Subgroup analysis of the prospective cohort study (see above) found no significant difference between male condom use and no male condom use in HSV-2 transmission from infected female partners to uninfected male partners (adjusted HR 2.02, 95% CI 0.32 to 12.50).[11] **Female condoms:** We found no systematic review or RCTs on the effects of female condoms to prevent sexual transmission.

Harms: The study gave no information on adverse effects.[11]

Comment: Only 61% of couples ever used condoms during the study and only 8% used them consistently.[11] Controlled trials of condoms for preventing of HSV-2 transmission are impractical. Even with routine counselling, many couples do not regularly use condoms. Trials of different methods of advising people to use condoms or providing condoms could be performed.

OPTION ANTIVIRAL TREATMENT TO PREVENT SEXUAL TRANSMISSION

One RCT found that daily use of valaciclovir reduced the risk of transmission of herpes simplex virus-2 to a previously uninfected sexual partner compared with placebo.

Benefits: We found no systematic review. We found one RCT (1484 serodiscordant couples**G**).[12] It found that valaciclovir (500 mg once daily, taken by the infected partner) significantly reduced the risk of herpes simplex virus type 2 (HSV-2) transmission compared with placebo after 8 months of treatment (overall risk of sexual transmission: 14/743 [1.9%] with valaciclovir *v* 27/741 [3.6%] with placebo; HR 0.52, 95% CI 0.27 to 0.99; risk of symptomatic HSV-2: 0.5% with valaciclovir *v* 2.2% with placebo; HR: 0.24, 95% CI 0.08 to 0.75).[12] Subgroup analyses found that risks were increased if the uninfected partner was female and the duration of the genital HSV-2 infection in the source partner was less than 2 years (HR for female acquisition: 3.30, 95% CI 1.31 to 8.28; HR for transmission from source partner with shorter duration of genital herpes: 2.89, 95% CI 1.12 to 7.49).

Harms: See individual antiviral drugs (see harms of daily maintenance antiviral treatment, p 1997).

Comment: RCTs have shown that daily antiviral treatment decreases the frequency of clinical and subclinical viral shedding (see antiviral treatment at the start of recurrence and outcomes section, p 1995).

QUESTION What are the effects of interventions to prevent transmission of herpes simplex virus from mother to neonate?

OPTION ANTIVIRAL TREATMENT IN LATE PREGNANCY

One systematic review provided insufficient evidence to assess the effects of oral antiviral agents during pregnancy on transmission of infection to neonates. The review found that aciclovir reduced the recurrence of infection at term in women with first or recurrent episodes of genital herpes simplex virus during pregnancy, and reduced the need for caesarean delivery because of genital herpes.

Benefits: **Rates of neonatal herpes:** We found one systematic review (search date 2003, 5 RCTs, 799 women), which reported no cases of neonatal herpes simplex virus in either the intervention or control groups.[13] **Rate of recurrent genital herpes at term:** We found one systematic review in women with first or recurrent episodes of genital herpes simplex during pregnancy (search date 2003, 5 RCTs, 799 pregnant women at 36 weeks' gestation), which found that aciclovir (800 or 1200 mg/day) significantly reduced herpes simplex virus recurrence at delivery compared with placebo (OR 0.25, 95% CI 0.15 to 0.40; see comment below).[13] **Rate of caesarean delivery for genital herpes:** The review found that aciclovir (800 or 1200 mg/day) significantly reduced the rate of caesarean delivery compared with placebo (AR: 17/424 [4.0%] with aciclovir *v* 85/375 [22.6%] with placebo; OR 0.30, 95% CI 0.13 to 0.67; see comment below).[13]

Harms: The systematic review gave no information on adverse effects.[13] Two RCTs identified by the review found no short term adverse effects in any neonates exposed to aciclovir prenatally or in neonates treated prophylactically with aciclovir after delivery.[14,15] One RCT found no difference in neonatal outcome between the maternal treatment and control groups.[16] However, the studies were underpowered to detect rare adverse events, such as an increase in aciclovir related obstructive uropathy in the newborns. One RCT identified by the review found no evidence of haematological or biochemical toxicity with acyclovir and no difference in adverse effects between maternal treatment and control groups.[17]

Comment: The trials in the review were heterogeneous in terms of the dose and duration of aciclovir and the populations enrolled.[14,17] The studies were underpowered to detect rare effects, such as an increase in asymptomatic viral shedding or neonatal infection. The indication for caesarean delivery for maternal herpes simplex infection was mainly based on clinical diagnosis (presence of prodromal symptoms or genital lesions suspicious for genital herpes) at term. However, in one of the RCTs in the review, delivery by elective caesarean section was performed if a woman experienced a herpes recurrence later than 38 weeks of gestation.[17] In another RCT identified by the review, one woman had a caesarean delivery for genital herpes without a clinical recurrence at term and two women with genital lesions delivered vaginally.[15] In one RCT identified by the review, three women in the placebo group and one woman in the aciclovir group did not have a caesarean delivery because their lesions were distant from the birth canal.[16]

OPTION SEROLOGICAL SCREENING AND COUNSELLING TO PREVENT ACQUISITION OF HERPES SIMPLEX VIRUS DURING LATE PREGNANCY

We found no systematic review or RCTs on the effects of either serological screening or counselling to prevent maternal infection in late pregnancy.

Benefits: We found no systematic review or RCTs that assessed either serological screening with type specific assays to identify women at risk for acquisition of herpes simplex virus infection in late pregnancy, or counselling to avoid genital–genital and oral–genital contact in late pregnancy.

Harms: We found no RCTs.

Comment: None.

OPTION CAESAREAN DELIVERY TO PREVENT NEONATAL HERPES

We found no systematic review or RCTs on the effects of caesarean delivery on mother to baby transmission of genital herpes in mothers with genital lesions at term. The procedure carries the risk of increased maternal morbidity and mortality.

Benefits: We found no systematic review or RCTs that assessed the effects of caesarean delivery on the risk of mother to child transmission of herpes simplex virus.

Harms: Caesarean delivery is associated with significant maternal morbidity (28.5% of women having caesarean section) and mortality (excess maternal mortality 15/100 000 deliveries). A study pooling data from different studies estimated that, for every two neonatal deaths from herpes simplex virus, a policy of caesarean delivery might cause one maternal death.[18]

Comment: The available evidence suggests that efforts to prevent neonatal herpes simplex virus infection should focus on preventing infection in late pregnancy. The absolute risk of neonatal infection is high (AR 41%, 95% CI 26% to 56%) in babies born to women who acquire infection near the time of labour and low (AR < 3%) in women with established infection, even in those who have recurrence at term.[7,8] Most women who acquire infection toward the end of pregnancy are undiagnosed, and most cases of neonatal herpes simplex virus infection are acquired from women without a history of genital herpes. Case studies indicate that the transmission of herpes simplex virus type 2 can occur, despite caesarean delivery.[16] Countries vary in their approach to obstetric management of women with recurrent genital herpes at term. In the USA and the UK, these women are advised to have a caesarean delivery, with its attendant risks to the mother. In the Netherlands, women with recurrent genital herpes at delivery have been allowed vaginal birth since 1987. This policy has not resulted in an increase in neonatal herpes (26 cases from 1981–1986 and 19 cases from 1987–1991).[8]

QUESTION What are the effects of antiviral treatment in people with a first episode of genital herpes?

OPTION ORAL ANTIVIRAL TREATMENT VERSUS PLACEBO

Three RCTs found that oral aciclovir treatment decreased the duration of lesions, symptoms, and viral shedding compared with placebo.

Benefits: **Oral aciclovir versus placebo:** We found no systematic review. We found three RCTs.[19–21] The largest RCT (180 people, 119 of whom had a first episode of genital herpes) compared aciclovir (200 mg 5 times daily for 10 days) versus placebo.[20] Analysis in people with a first episode of genital herpes (119 people) found that aciclovir significantly decreased the time to complete healing of lesions, reduced the formation of new lesions, and the duration of pain and viral shedding compared with placebo (time to complete healing: 12 days with aciclovir *v* 14 days with placebo; P = 0.005; formation of new lesions: 18% with aciclovir *v* 62% with placebo; P = 0.001; median duration of pain: 5 days with aciclovir *v* 7 days with placebo; P = 0.05; median duration of viral shedding: 2 days with aciclovir *v* 9 days with placebo; P < 0.001).[20] The second RCT (31 people with first episode genital herpes) compared aciclovir (200 mg 5 times daily for 5 days) versus placebo.[19] It found that aciclovir significantly reduced the duration of viral shedding, time to healing, and duration of pain (median duration of viral shedding: 1 day with aciclovir *v* 13 days with placebo; P < 0.01; median time to healing: 6 days with aciclovir *v* 11 days with placebo; P = 0.06; median duration of pain: 4 days with aciclovir *v* 8 days with placebo; P < 0.05).[19] The third RCT (48 people, 31 women, 17 men) compared aciclovir (200 mg 5 times daily for 10 days). It found that aciclovir significantly reduced the duration of viral shedding and time to crusting (women: mean duration of viral shedding: 4.9 days with aciclovir *v* 17.7 days with placebo; P = 0.001; men: mean duration of viral shedding: 6 days with aciclovir *v* 15 days with placebo; P = 0.02; women: mean time to crusting: 8.8 days with aciclovir *v* 15.0 days with placebo; P = 0.01; men: mean time to crusting: 5 days with aciclovir *v* 15 days with placebo; P = 0.01).[21]

Harms: Adverse effects were rare and similar in the placebo and treatment group.[19,21]

Comment: No precise estimates of effectiveness were available owing to small numbers. The largest RCT excluded 30/180 [17%] people before analysis: 10 people for not completing the study protocol, 12 because of suspected past infection, and eight because herpes simplex virus was not isolated.[20]

OPTION DIFFERENT TYPES OF ORAL ANTIVIRAL TREATMENT

One RCT found no difference in clinical outcomes between oral aciclovir and valaciclovir.

Benefits: **Valaciclovir versus aciclovir:** We found no systematic review. We found one RCT (643 people), which compared oral valaciclovir (100 mg twice daily for 10 days) versus oral aciclovir (200 mg 5 times daily for 10 days).[22] It found no significant difference between treatments in duration of viral shedding, healing time, and duration of symptoms (HR for duration of viral shedding: 1.00, 95% CI 0.84 to 1.18; HR for healing time: 1.08, 95% CI 0.92 to 1.27; HR for duration of symptoms: 1.02, 95% CI 0.85 to 1.22).[22]

Harms: Headache occurred in 11.5% and nausea in 5.9% of patients treated with aciclovir. There was no difference in adverse events between the aciclovir and valaciclovir group (percentages not given for the valaciclovir group).[22]

Comment: None.

QUESTION What are the effects of interventions to reduce the impact of recurrence?

OPTION ORAL ANTIVIRAL TREATMENT TAKEN AT THE START OF RECURRENCE

One systematic review, one non-systematic review, and one RCT found that oral antiviral treatment (aciclovir, famciclovir or valaciclovir) taken at the start of recurrence reduced the duration of lesions and viral shedding and increased the rate of aborted recurrences compared with placebo, in people with recurrent genital herpes. RCTs found that aciclovir, famciclovir, and valaciclovir were similarly effective in reducing symptom duration, lesion healing time, and viral shedding compared with placebo. Two RCTs found no difference between valaciclovir taken for 3 days or 5 days.

Benefits: **Aciclovir versus placebo:** We found no systematic review. We found one non-systematic review (number of RCTs not reported, 650 people)[23] and one subsequent RCT.[24] The RCTs in the review compared oral aciclovir started at the first sign of recurrence (200 mg 5 times daily or 800 mg twice daily, for 5 days) versus placebo. The review found that aciclovir reduced the period of viral shedding and duration of lesions compared with placebo (duration of viral shedding: 1 day with aciclovir *v* 2 days with placebo; duration of lesions: 5 days with aciclovir *v* 6 days with placebo).[23] The subsequent RCT (131 people with ≥ 3 recurrences in the previous 12 months, observed for ≥ 1 recurrence) found that aciclovir (800 mg 3 times daily for 2 days) significantly reduced the duration of lesions, episodes, and viral shedding compared with placebo (median duration of lesions: 4 days with aciclovir *v* 6 days with placebo; P = 0.001; median duration of episodes: 4 days with aciclovir *v* 6 days with placebo; P < 0.001; median duration of viral shedding: 25.0 hours with aciclovir *v* 58.5 hours with placebo; P = 0.04).[24] **Famciclovir versus placebo:** We found one systematic review (search date not reported; 1 RCT, 467 people).[25] The included RCT found that oral famciclovir (125–500 mg twice daily for 5 days) significantly reduced the duration of lesions and viral shedding compared with placebo (median duration of lesions: 5 days with famciclovir *v* 4 days with placebo; P value not reported; duration of viral shedding: 3 days with famciclovir *v* 2 days with placebo; P value not reported).[25] **Valaciclovir versus placebo:** We found one systematic review (search date not reported, 1 RCT, 987 people).[25] The RCT identified by the review compared oral valaciclovir (500 or 1000 mg twice daily for 5 days) versus placebo. The RCT found that self initiated oral valaciclovir decreased episode duration and viral shedding and increased the rate of aborted recurrences compared with placebo (median episode duration: 4 days with valaciclovir *v* 6 days with placebo; HR 1.9, 95% CI 1.6 to 2.3; median duration of viral shedding: 2 days with valaciclovir *v* 4 days with placebo; HR 2.9, 95% CI 2.1 to 3.9; aborted recurrences: 31% with valaciclovir *v* 21% with placebo; RR 1.5, 95% CI 1.1 to 1.9).[25] **Famciclovir versus aciclovir:** We found one RCT (204 people), which found no significant difference in time to healing between oral famciclovir and aciclovir (mean lesion healing time: 5.1 days with famciclovir *v* 5.4 days with acyclovir; mean difference +0.3 days, 95% CI –0.3 days to +0.8 days).[26] **Valaciclovir versus aciclovir:** We found one systematic review (search date not reported, 1 RCT, 739 people).[25] The included RCT compared oral valaciclovir (500 mg twice daily for 5 days) versus aciclovir (200 mg 5 times a day for 5 days). It found no significant difference in healing time, symptom duration, or viral shedding between the two antiviral agents (HR for healing time: valaciclovir *v* aciclovir: 0.96, 95% CI 0.80 to 1.14; HR for symptom duration: 0.93, 95% CI 0.79 to 1.08; HR for viral shedding: 0.98, 95% CI 0.75 to 1.27).[25] **Valaciclovir 3 days versus 5 days:** We found two RCTs. The first RCT (531 people with ≥6 recurrences of genital herpes a year) found no difference between 3 or 5 days of treatment with valaciclovir (500 mg twice daily) in episode duration or aborted recurrences (median number of days: 4.7 with 3 days of valaciclovir *v* 4.6 with 5 days of valaciclovir; aborted recurrences: 27% with 3 days of valaciclovir *v* 21% with 5 days of valaciclovir).[27] People initiating treatment within 6 hours of first symptoms or signs were more likely to have an aborted episode than those starting treatment after 6 hours (OR 1.93, 95% CI 1.28 to 2.9).[27] The second RCT (800 people with ≥4 outbreaks of genital herpes a year) found no difference between 3 or 5 days of treatment with valaciclovir (500 mg twice daily) in lesion healing time, or aborted lesions (median lesion healing time: 4.4 days with 3 days of valaciclovir *v* 4.7 days with 5 days of valaciclovir; HR 0.95, 95% CI 0.81 to 1.13; aborted lesions: 25.4% with 3 days of valaciclovir *v* 26.6% with 5 days of valaciclovir; RR 1.04, 95% CI 0.83 to 1.32).[28]

Harms: Adverse effects (mostly headache and nausea) were rare, and the frequency was similar for aciclovir, valaciclovir, famciclovir, and placebo (figures not reported in the review).[25]

Comment: The benefit was found to be greater if the person with recurrent herpes initiated treatment at the first symptom or sign of a recurrence.[27,29]

OPTION DAILY ORAL ANTIVIRAL TREATMENT

RCTs found that daily maintenance treatment with oral antiviral agents (valaciclovir, aciclovir or famciclovir) reduced the frequency of recurrences, and that oral aciclovir and oral valaciclovir improved quality of life compared with placebo.

Benefits: **Valaciclovir versus placebo:** We found one systematic review (search date not reported, 2 RCTs, 1861 people), which compared valaciclovir versus placebo for frequently recurring genital herpes.[25] We found one

additional RCT (1479 people), which compared the effect of oral valaciclovir (once and twice daily) with placebo on a genital herpes quality of life scale.[30] The first RCT identified by the review (382 people) found that valaciclovir (500 mg once daily for 16 weeks) significantly increased the time to recurrence compared with placebo (HR 0.10, 95% CI 0.11 to 0.21).[25] The second RCT identified by the review (1479 people) compared valaciclovir (250 mg 4 times daily, 250 mg twice daily, 500 mg 4 times daily, 1000 mg 4 times daily) or aciclovir (400 mg twice daily) with placebo at 1 year. It found a dose–response effect across the valaciclovir regimen on freedom from recurrence compared with placebo (freedom from recurrence: 48–50% with valaciclovir 1000 mg 4 times daily *v* 40% with valaciclovir 500 mg 4 times daily *v* 22% with valaciclovir 250 mg 4 times daily *v* 5% with placebo).[25] The additional RCT found that valaciclovir treatment (once or twice daily) significantly improved health-related quality of life compared with placebo after 3 months ($P < 0.05$).[30,31] **Famciclovir versus placebo:** We found one systematic review (search date not reported, 2 RCTs, 830 people).[25] The first RCT (455 people) identified by the review compared famciclovir (250 mg twice daily, 125 mg 3 times daily, or 250 mg 3 times daily for 1 year) versus placebo. It found that famciclovir significantly increased median time to first recurrence compared with placebo (11 months with famciclovir 250 mg twice daily *v* 10 months with famciclovir 250 mg 3 times daily *v* 8 months with famciclovir 125 mg 3 times daily *v* 1.5 months with placebo).[25] The second RCT identified by the review (375 women) found that famciclovir (125 mg twice or 4 times daily, 250 mg twice or 4 times daily, or 500 mg 4 times daily, for 4 months) significantly increased the proportion of people who had no recurrences compared with placebo (freedom from recurrence: 78% with 250 mg twice daily *v* 42% with placebo).[25] It also found that 250 mg twice daily was the most effective dosage of famciclovir for reducing recurrence.[25] **Aciclovir versus placebo:** We found one non-systematic review (2 RCTs, 107 people) and four subsequent RCTs.[23,30,32–34] The first RCT identified by the non-systematic review (32 people) found that aciclovir 800 mg daily reduced recurrence compared with placebo at 2 years (freedom from recurrence: 5/18 [28%] with aciclovir *v* 0/14 [0%] with placebo; ARR 28%, 95% CI 1% to 51%).[23] The second RCT identified by the non-systematic review (75 people) found that aciclovir (400 mg twice daily) reduced recurrence compared with placebo at 1 year (freedom from recurrence: 21/48 [44%] with aciclovir *v* 0/28 [0%] with placebo; ARR 44%, 95% CI 26% to 56%).[23] The first subsequent RCT (1479 people) found that aciclovir (400 mg twice daily) reduced recurrence compared with placebo at 1 year (freedom from recurrence: 48–50% with aciclovir *v* 5% with placebo).[32] The second RCT (1146 people) also found that aciclovir (400 mg twice daily) reduced recurrence compared with placebo at 1 year (recurrence rate: 1.7% with aciclovir *v* 12.5% with placebo; $P < 0.0001$). Of 210 adults in the trial who completed 5 years of continuous treatment with aciclovir (400 mg twice daily), 53–70% were free of recurrence each year.[33] The third RCT (34 women with recently acquired genital herpes simplex virus type 2 infection) found that aciclovir (400 mg twice daily for 70 days) reduced viral shedding compared with placebo. It also found that, compared with placebo, aciclovir reduced viral shedding by 95% on days with reported lesions and by 94% on days without lesions.[34] The fourth RCT (1479 people) compared the effect of oral aciclovir (once and twice daily) versus placebo on a genital herpes quality of life scale.[30,31] It found that daily aciclovir treatment significantly improved health related quality of life compared with placebo after 3 months ($P < 0.05$).[30]

Harms: Daily treatments with aciclovir, famciclovir, and valaciclovir were well tolerated.[35] People taking aciclovir were followed for up to 7 years, and those taking famciclovir and valaciclovir for up to 1 year. Nausea and

headache were infrequent, and participants rarely discontinued treatment because of adverse effects. We found no studies evaluating whether daily maintenance treatment increases high risk sexual behaviour. We found no evidence that daily treatment with aciclovir results in emergence of aciclovir resistant herpes simplex virus during or after stopping treatment in healthy adults.[35]

Comment: None.

OPTION PSYCHOTHERAPY

One systematic review of poor quality studies provided insufficient evidence about the effects of psychosocial interventions to prevent recurrence of genital herpes.

Benefits: We found one systematic review (search date 1991), which identified six poor quality studies of psychotherapeutic interventions in 69 people (4 studies had < 10 participants).[36] Interventions varied from hypnotherapy and progressive muscle relaxation to cognitive therapy and multifaceted intervention. The largest RCT (31 people with > 4 recurrences a year) compared psychosocial intervention versus social support or waiting list. People receiving psychosocial intervention had significantly lower recurrence rates compared with pretreatment frequency, social support, or waiting list (recurrences per year: 6 with psychosocial intervention *v* 11 (in total) with pretreatment, social support, and waiting list; $P < 0.001$).[37] However, small numbers of people, inadequate controls, and subjective and retrospective assessment of recurrence frequency at baseline limit the usefulness of these studies.[36]

Harms: The review[36] and the RCT[37] gave no information on adverse effects.

Comment: Controlled studies that include prospective clinical evaluation of disease activity are needed.

QUESTION **What are the effects of treatments in people with genital herpes and HIV?**

OPTION ORAL ANTIVIRAL TREATMENT FOR FIRST EPISODE GENITAL HERPES IN PEOPLE WITH HIV

We found no RCTs on the treatment of first episode genital herpes in people with HIV.

Benefits: We found no systematic review and no RCTs examining effects of treatments for first episode genital herpes in people with HIV.

Harms: We found no RCTs.

Comment: None.

OPTION ORAL ANTIVIRAL TREATMENT FOR AN ACUTE RECURRENT EPISODE OF GENITAL HERPES IN PEOPLE WITH HIV

Two RCTs found no significant differences in duration of lesions and symptoms between famciclovir or valaciclovir or aciclovir.

Benefits: **Oral antivirals versus placebo:** We found no systematic review or RCTs. **Famciclovir versus aciclovir:** We found one RCT (193 people on stable antiretroviral treatment), which compared famciclovir (500 mg twice daily) versus aciclovir (400 mg 5 times daily) for 1 week.[38] It found no significant difference between treatments in time to healing, duration

of viral shedding, or time to loss of symptoms (median time to healing: 7 days with both treatments; HR 1.01, 95% CI 0.79 to 1.29; median duration of viral shedding: 2 days for both treatments; HR 0.93, 95% CI 0.68 to 1.27; median time to loss of symptoms: 4 days with both treatments; HR 0.99, 95% CI 0.75 to 1.30). It also found no significant difference between the two treatments in the risk of developing new lesions during treatment (16.7% with famciclovir *v* 13.3% with aciclovir; ARI +3.4%, 95% CI –4.8 to +11.5).[38] **Valaciclovir versus aciclovir:** We found one RCT (467 people), which compared valaciclovir (1000 mg twice daily) versus aciclovir (200 mg 5 times daily) for 5 days.[39] It found no significant difference between treatments in time to lesion healing or episode duration (HR for lesion healing: 0.98, 95% CI 0.79 to 1.22; HR for episode duration: 0.93, 95% CI 0.75 to 1.14).[39]

Harms: **Famciclovir versus aciclovir:** The RCT reported that adverse effects, mostly headache, nausea, diarrhoea, and abdominal pain were experienced by more than 5% of people taking either famciclovir or aciclovir (headache: 16.7% with famciclovir *v* 15.4% with aciclovir; nausea: 10.7% with famciclovir *v* 12.6% with aciclovir; diarrhoea: 6.7% with famciclovir *v* 10.5% with aciclovir; abdominal pain: 3.3% with famciclovir *v* 5.6% with aciclovir). There were no reports of either haemolytic uraemic syndrome or thrombotic thrombocytopenic purpura.[38] **Valaciclovir versus aciclovir:** The RCT reported that adverse effects, mostly headache, nausea, and diarrhoea, were experienced by fewer than 10% of people taking either valaciclovir or aciclovir.[39]

Comment: Although we found no placebo controlled RCTs in people with HIV, consensus regards antiviral treatment as effective for treating recurrences in people with HIV, based on evidence in people without immunocompromise (see oral antiviral treatment taken at the start of recurrence, p 1995) and in immunocompromised people without HIV. One prospective study found an increased rate of herpes simplex virus shedding in people infected with HIV.[40] HIV has also been detected in genital herpes lesions, suggesting that herpes simplex virus infection may increase the risk of sexual transmission of HIV.[41]

OPTION **DAILY ORAL ANTIVIRAL TREATMENT FOR PREVENTING RECURRENCE OF GENITAL HERPES IN PEOPLE WITH HIV**

One RCT found that valaciclovir was more effective than placebo in preventing herpes simplex virus infection. One RCT found no significant difference between valaciclovir and aciclovir in preventing recurrent herpes simplex virus infections over 48 weeks.

Benefits: **Valaciclovir versus placebo:** We found one RCT (239 people with HIV and a history of recurrent herpes simplex virus).[42] The RCT found that valaciclovir (500 mg twice daily) significantly reduced recurrence and increased the median time to first recurrence compared with placebo at 6 months (AR for freedom from recurrence: 65% with valaciclovir *v* 26% with placebo; RR 2.5, 95% CI 1.8 to 3.5; median days to recurrence: > 180 days with valaciclovir *v* 59 days with placebo; HR 16.7, 95% CI 7.3 to 33.3).[42] **Valaciclovir versus aciclovir:** We found one RCT (1062 people), which compared three treatments: valaciclovir (500 mg twice daily), valaciclovir (1000 mg once daily), and aciclovir (400 mg twice daily) for 48 weeks.[39] It found no significant difference between either dose of valaciclovir and aciclovir in time to recurrence (HR for valaciclovir [500 mg twice daily] *v* aciclovir: 0.73, 95% CI 0.50 to 1.06; HR for valaciclovir [1000 mg once daily] *v* aciclovir: 1.31, 95% CI 0.94 to 1.82).[39]

Harms: **Valaciclovir versus aciclovir:** The RCT found that the rate of withdrawal because of adverse effects was similar with aciclovir and valaciclovir (AR adverse effects leading to withdrawal, including nausea and headache: 11% with valaciclovir *v* 9% with aciclovir).[39] **Valaciclovir versus placebo:** The RCT found that valaciclovir increased the risk of headache, fatigue, influenza, nasopharyngitis, and rash compared with placebo, although rates of diarrhoea and nausea were similar between treatments (headache: 13% with valaciclovir *v* 8% with placebo; fatigue: 8% with valaciclovir *v* 5% with placebo; influenza: 8% with valaciclovir *v* 3% with placebo; nasopharyngitis: 8% with valaciclovir *v* 2% with placebo; rash: 8% with valaciclovir *v* 1% with placebo; diarrhoea: 12% with valaciclovir and placebo; nausea: 8% with valaciclovir and placebo).[42] The RCT gave no information on adverse effects in people taking valaciclovir beyond 6 months.

Comment: Valaciclovir significantly reduced the rate of recurrences of genital herpes. However, 35% of people being treated had a recurrence within 6 months.[42] One RCT found that recurrence was more likely with 1000 mg valaciclovir taken once daily than with 500 mg valaciclovir taken twice daily (HR 1.80, 95% CI 1.26 to 2.57; people remaining recurrence free at 48 weeks: 71% with 1000 mg once daily *v* 82% with 500 mg twice daily; $P < 0.05$).[39]

GLOSSARY

Serodiscordant couple A couple in which one partner is infected with herpes simplex virus and the other is not infected.

REFERENCES

1. Fleming DT, McQuillan GM, Johnson RE, et al. Herpes simplex virus type 2 in the United States, 1976 to 1994. *N Engl J Med* 1997;337:1105–1111.
2. Cowan FM, Johnson AM, Ashley R, et al. Antibody to herpes simplex virus type 2 as serological marker of sexual lifestyle in populations. *BMJ* 1994;309:1325–1329.
3. Benedetti J, Corey L, Ashley R. Recurrence rates in genital herpes after symptomatic first-episode infection. *Ann Intern Med* 1994;121:847–854.
4. Mertz GJ, Schmidt O, Jourden JL, et al. Frequency of acquisition of first-episode genital infection with herpes simplex virus from symptomatic and asymptomatic source contacts. *Sex Transm Dis* 1985;12:33–39.
5. Whitley RJ, Kimberlin DW, Roizman B. Herpes simplex viruses. *Clin Infect Dis* 1998;26:541–553.
6. Wald A, Link K. Risk of HIV infection in HSV-2 seropositive persons: a meta-analysis. *J Infect Dis* 2002;185:45–52.
7. Brown ZA, Selke SA, Zeh J, et al. Acquisition of herpes simplex virus during pregnancy. *N Engl J Med* 1997;337:509–515.
8. Smith J, Cowan FM, Munday P. The management of herpes simplex virus infection in pregnancy. *Br J Obstet Gynaecol* 1998;105:255–268. Search date 1996; primary source Medline.
9. Corey L, Langenberg AG, Ashley R, et al. Recombinant glycoprotein vaccine for the prevention of genital HSV-2 infection: two randomised controlled trials. *JAMA* 1999;282:331–340.
10. Stanberry LR, Sprunace SL, Cunningham AL, et al. Glycoprotein-D-adjuvant vaccine to prevent genital herpes. *N Engl J Med* 2002;347:1652–1661.
11. Wald A, Langenberg A, Link K, et al. Effect of condoms on reducing the transmission of herpes simples virus type 2 from men to women. *JAMA* 2001;285:3100–3106.
12. Corey L, Wald A, Patel R, et al. Once-daily valaciclovir to reduce the risk of transmission of genital herpes. *N Engl J Med* 2004;350:11–20.
13. Sheffield JS, Hollier LM, Hill JB, et al. Aciclovir prophylaxis to prevent herpes simplex virus recurrence at delivery: a systematic review. *Obstet Gynecol* 2003;102:1396–1403. Search date 2003.
14. Scott LL, Sanchez PJ, Jackson GL, et al. Acyclovir suppression to prevent Cesarean delivery after first-episode genital herpes. *Obstet Gynecol* 1996;87:69–73.
15. Scott LL, Hollier LM, McIntire D, et al. Acyclovir suppression to prevent recurrent genital herpes at delivery. *Inf Dis Obstet Gynecol* 2002;10:71–77.
16. Watts DH, Brown ZA, Money D, et al. A double-blind, randomized, placebo-controlled trial of aciclovir in late pregnancy for the reduction of herpes simplex virus shedding and cesarean delivery. *Am J Obstet Gynecol* 2003;188:836–843.
17. Brocklehurst P, Kinghorn G, Carney O, et al. A randomised placebo controlled trial of suppressive acyclovir in late pregnancy in women with recurrent genital herpes infection. *Br J Obstet Gynaecol* 1998;105:275–280.
18. Randolph A, Washington A, Prober C. Cesarean delivery for women presenting with genital herpes lesions. *JAMA* 1993;270:77–82.
19. Nilsen AE, Aasen T, Halsos AM, et al. Efficacy of oral acyclovir in treatment of initial and recurrent genital herpes. *Lancet* 1982;2:571–573.
20. Mertz G, Critchlow C, Benedetti J, et al. Double-blind placebo-controlled trial of oral acyclovir in the first episode genital herpes simplex virus infection. *JAMA* 1984;252:1147–1151.
21. Bryson YJ, Dillon M, Lovett M, et al. Treatment of first episodes of genital herpes simplex virus infections with oral acyclovir: a randomized double-blind controlled trial in normal subjects. *N Engl J Med* 1983;308:916–921.
22. Fife KH, Barbarash RA, Rudolph T, et al. Valaciclovir versus acyclovir in the treatment of first-episode genital herpes infection: results of an international, multicenter, double-blind randomized clinical trial. *Sex Transm Dis* 1997;24:481–486.
23. Stone K, Whittington W. Treatment of genital herpes. *Rev Infect Dis* 1990;12(Suppl 6):610–619.
24. Wald A, Carrell D, Remington M, et al. Two-day regimen of acyclovir for treatment of recurrent genital herpes simplex virus type 2 infection. *Clin Infect Dis* 2002;34:944–948.
25. Wald A. New therapies and prevention strategies for genital herpes. *Clin Infect Dis* 1999;28:S4–S13. Search date not reported; primary source Medline.
26. Chosidow O, Drouault Y, Leconte-Veyriac F, et al. Famciclovir versus aciclovir in immunocompetent

patients with recurrent genital herpes infections: a parallel-groups, randomised, double-blind clinical trial. *Br J Dermatol* 2001;144:818–824.
27. Strand A, Patel R, Wulf H C, et al. Aborted genital herpes simplex virus lesions: findings from a randomised controlled trial with valaciclovir. *Sex Transm Infect* 2002;78:435–439.
28. Leone PA, Trottier S, Miller JM. Valaciclovir for episodic treatment of genital herpes: a shorter 3-day treatment course compared with 5-day treatment. *Clin Infect Dis* 2002;34:958–962.
29. Reichman RC, Badger GJ, Mertz GJ, et al. Treatment of recurrent genital herpes simplex infections with oral acyclovir: a controlled trial. *JAMA* 1984;251:2103–2107.
30. Patel R, Tyring S, Strand A, et al. Impact of suppressive antiviral therapy on the health related quality of life of patients with recurrent genital herpes infection. *Sex Transm Infect* 1999;75:398–402.
31. Doward LC, McKenna SP, Kohlmann T, et al. The international development of the RGHQoL: a quality of life measure for recurrent genital herpes. *Qual Life Res* 1998;7:143–153.
32. Reitano M, Tyring S, Lang W, et al. Valaciclovir for the suppression of recurrent genital herpes simplex virus infection: a large-scale dose range finding study. *J Infect Dis* 1998;178:603–610.
33. Goldberg L, Kaufman R, Kurtz T, et al. Continuous five-year treatment of patients with frequently recurring genital herpes simplex virus infection with acyclovir. *J Med Virol* 1993(Suppl 1);45–50.
34. Wald A, Zeh J, Barnum G, et al. Suppression of subclinical shedding of herpes simplex virus type 2 with acyclovir. *Ann Intern Med* 1996;124:8–15.
35. Fife KH, Crumpacker CS, Mertz GJ. Recurrence and resistance patterns of herpes simplex virus following stop of ≥ 6 years of chronic suppression with acyclovir. *J Infect Dis* 1994;169:1338–1341.
36. Longo D, Koehn K. Psychosocial factors and recurrent genital herpes: a review of prediction and psychiatric treatment studies. *Int J Psychiatry Med* 1993;23:99–117. Search date 1991; primary sources Psychological Abstracts, Medline, and hand searches of reference lists.
37. Longo DJ, Clum GA, Yaeger NJ. Psychosocial treatment for recurrent genital herpes. *J Consult Clin Psychol* 1988;56:61–66.
38. Romanowski B, Aoki FY, Martel AY, et al. Efficacy and safety of famciclovir for treating mucocutaneous herpes simplex infection in HIV-infected individuals. Collaborative Famciclovir HIV Study Group. *AIDS* 2000;14:1211–1217.
39. Conant MA, Schacker TW, Murphy RL, et al. International Valaciclovir HSV Study Group. Valaciclovir versus aciclovir for herpes simplex virus infection in HIV-infected individuals: two randomized trials. *Int J STD AIDS* 2002;13:12–21.
40. Schacker T, Zeh J, Hu HL, et al. Frequency of symptomatic and asymptomatic HSV-2 reactivations among HIV-infected men. *J Infect Dis* 1998;178:1616–1622.
41. Schacker T, Ryncarz A, Goddard J, et al. Frequent recovery of HIV from genital herpes simplex virus lesions in HIV infected persons. *JAMA* 1998;280:61–66.
42. DeJesus E, Wald A, Warren T, et al. Valaciclovir for the suppression of recurrent genital herpes in human immunodeficiency virus-infected subjects. *J Infect Dis* 2003;188:1009–1016. [Erratum in: *J Infect Dis* 2003;188:1404]

Eva Jungmann
Camden PCT
London
UK

Competing interests: None declared.

We would like to acknowledge the previous contributors of this chapter, including Anna Wald.

Genital warts

Search date March 2004

Henry W Buck, Jr

QUESTIONS

INTERVENTIONS

To be covered in future updates

Ablative therapy plus imiquimod
Cryotherapy plus interferon
Education
Laser surgery plus interferon
Lifestyle changes
Vaccines

*No placebo controlled RCTs found; categorisation based on consensus opinion.

See glossary

Key Messages

Treatments

- **Cryotherapy (as effective in clearing warts as trichloroacetic acid and more effective than podophyllin)** We found no RCTs comparing cryotherapy versus placebo or no treatment. Two RCTs found no significant difference between cryotherapy and trichloroacetic acid in clearance of warts after 6–10 weeks' treatment. One of the RCTs found no significant difference in recurrence of warts 2 months after the end of treatment. One RCT found limited evidence that cryotherapy was less effective for clearance than electrosurgery after 6 weeks' treatment. However, follow up of the people with successful wart clearance revealed no significant difference in the proportion of people who had warts at 3–5 months. Another RCT found no significant difference in wart clearance at 3 months between cryotherapy and electrosurgery. One RCT found that cryotherapy increased clearance after 6 weeks' treatment compared with podophyllin, and follow up of the people with successful wart clearance found that fewer people receiving cryotherapy had warts at 3–5 months.

- **Electrosurgery (at least as effective as cryotherapy and more effective than podophyllin in clearing warts)** One RCT found that electrosurgery increased clearance of warts at 6 months compared with no treatment. One RCT found that electrosurgery increased clearance of warts at 6 months compared with systemic interferon but the increase was not significant. One RCT found that electrosurgery improved clearance after 6 weeks' treatment compared with cryotherapy. However, follow up of the people with successful wart clearance revealed no significant difference in the proportion of people who had warts at 3–5 months after treatment. It also found that electrosurgery improved clearance after 6 weeks' treatment compared with podophyllin, and follow up of the people with successful wart clearance revealed that the difference was maintained at 3–5 months after treatment. Another RCT found no significant difference in wart clearance at 3 months between electrosurgery and cryotherapy.
- **Imiquimod in people without HIV** One systematic review and one subsequent RCT found that 5% or 1% imiquimod cream increased wart clearance and reduced recurrence compared with placebo in people without HIV. One RCT in women without HIV found that twice daily doses of imiquimod 5% did not increase wart clearance over 20 weeks compared with once daily or three times weekly doses, but found that it increased skin erythema. One RCT in people without HIV found that imiquimod 5% increased moderate to severe erythema, erosion, excoriation, oedema, and scabbing compared with imiquimod 1% or placebo.
- **Interferon, topical** Three RCTs found that topical interferon increased wart clearance at 4 weeks after treatment compared with placebo. One of the RCTs also found that topical interferon increased wart clearance at 4 weeks after treatment compared with podophyllotoxin.
- **Laser surgery (as effective as surgical excision in clearing warts)** We found no RCTs comparing laser surgery versus no treatment. One RCT found no significant difference in wart clearance or recurrence rates over 36 weeks between laser and surgical excision.
- **Podophyllin (as effective as podophyllotoxin or surgical excision in clearing warts but less effective than cryotherapy and electrosurgery; less effective than surgical excision in preventing recurrence)*** We found no RCTs comparing podophyllin versus placebo, but there is consensus that podophyllin is effective for clearing genital warts. Six RCTs provided no consistent evidence of a difference between podophyllotoxin and podophyllin in wart clearance or recurrence. RCTs found no significant difference between surgical (scissor) excision and podophyllin in wart clearance. However, they found that surgical excision was more effective than podophyllin in preventing recurrence at 6–12 months. One RCT found that podophyllin was less effective than cryotherapy or electrosurgery in clearing warts at 6 weeks, and follow up of the people with successful wart clearance revealed that more people receiving podophyllin had warts at 3–5 months. One RCT found no significant difference in wart clearance at 3 months between podophyllin plus trichloroacetic acid and podophyllin alone. One RCT found that podophyllin was more effective than systemic interferon in clearing warts at 3 months.
- **Podophyllotoxin** RCTs found that podophyllotoxin increased wart clearance within 16 weeks compared with placebo. Six RCTs provided no consistent evidence of a difference between podophyllotoxin and podophyllin in wart clearance or recurrence. One RCT found that podophyllotoxin was less effective than topical interferon in clearing warts at 4 weeks.
- **Surgical excision (as effective as laser surgery or podophyllin in clearing warts; more effective than podophyllin in preventing recurrence)** We found no RCTs comparing surgical excision versus no treatment. RCTs found no significant difference between surgical (scissor) excision and laser surgery or podophyllin in wart clearance. However, they found that surgical excision was more effective than podophyllin in preventing recurrence at 6–12 months.

Genital warts

- **Bi- and trichloroacetic acid (as effective as cryotherapy in clearing warts)** We found no RCTs comparing bi- and trichloroacetic acid versus placebo. Two RCTs found no significant difference between trichloroacetic acid and cryotherapy in clearance of warts after 6–10 weeks' treatment, and one of the RCTs found no significant difference in recurrence of warts 2 months after the end of treatment. One RCT found no significant difference in wart clearance at 3 months between trichloroacetic acid plus podophyllin and podophyllin alone.
- **Imiquimod in people with HIV** One RCT in people with HIV found no significant difference in wart clearance over 16 weeks between imiquimod cream and placebo. One RCT in people without HIV found that imiquimod 5% increased moderate to severe erythema, erosion, excoriation, oedema, and scabbing compared with imiquimod 1% or placebo.
- **Interferon, systemic** We found five RCTs comparing different formulations of systemic interferon versus placebo or no treatment. Two of the RCTs found that systemic interferon improved wart clearance compared with placebo or no treatment, whereas three of the RCTs found no significant difference between interferon and placebo in complete or partial wart clearance. Systemic interferon was associated with important adverse effects, including anaphylaxis, blood disorders, flu-like symptoms, headache, fatigue, myalgia, fever, and weight loss. One RCT found no significant difference in wart clearance at 6 months between electrosurgery and systemic interferon. One RCT found that systemic interferon was less effective than podophyllin in clearing warts at 3 months.

Preventing transmission

- **Condoms** Observational studies provided insufficient evidence to assess the effects of condom use on transmission of human papillomavirus. Penetrative intercourse is not required for spread because this can occur with external genital–genital or hand–genital touching. One case control and one cross-sectional study suggested that people who always used condoms were less likely to have genital warts than people who never or occasionally used them.

DEFINITION	External genital warts are benign epidermal growths on the external perigenital and perianal regions. There are four morphological types: condylomatous, keratotic, papular, and flat warts.
INCIDENCE/ PREVALENCE	In 1996, external and internal genital warts accounted for more than 180 000 initial visits to private physicians' offices in the USA, which is about 60 000 fewer than were reported for 1995.[1] In the USA, 1% of sexually active men and women aged 18–49 years are estimated to have external genital warts.[2] It is believed that external and cervical lesions caused by the human papillomavirus (HPV) are the most prevalent sexually transmitted disease among persons 18–25 years of age. In the USA, 50–60% of women aged 18–25 years test positive for HPV DNA, but no more than 10–15% ever have genital warts.[3]
AETIOLOGY/ RISK FACTORS	External genital warts are caused by HPV and are sexually transmitted. They are more common in people with impaired immune function.[3] Although more than 100 types of HPV have been identified, most external genital warts in immunocompetent people are caused by HPV types 6 and 11.[4,5]
PROGNOSIS	The ability to clear and remain free of external genital warts is a function of cellular immunity.[6] In immunocompetent people, the prognosis in terms of clearance and avoiding recurrence is good,[7] but people with impaired cellular immunity (e.g. people with HIV and AIDS) have great difficulty in achieving and maintaining wart clearance.[3] Without treatment, external genital warts may remain unchanged, may increase in size or number, or may resolve completely. Clinical trials have found that recurrences may occur and may necessitate repeated treatment. External genital warts rarely, if ever, progress to cancer.[8] Juvenile laryngeal papillomatosis, a rare and sometimes life threatening condition, occurs in children of women with a history of genital warts. Its rarity makes it difficult to design studies that can evaluate whether treatment in pregnant women alters the risk.[9,10]
AIMS OF INTERVENTION	To eliminate warts from the external genitalia; to prevent recurrence; and to avoid sequelae, with minimal adverse effects.

OUTCOMES Wart clearance, generally accepted as complete eradication of warts from the treated area, rather than elimination of HPV; recurrence; sequelae; adverse effects of treatment; quality of life; transmission.

METHODS *Clinical Evidence* search and appraisal March 2004.

QUESTION **What are the effects of treatments for external genital warts?**

OPTION **BI- AND TRICHLOROACETIC ACID**

We found no RCTs comparing bi- and trichloroacetic acid versus placebo. Two RCTs found no significant difference between trichloroacetic acid and cryotherapy in clearance of warts after 6–10 weeks' treatment, and one of the RCTs found no significant difference in recurrence of warts 2 months after the end of treatment. One RCT found no significant difference in wart clearance at 3 months between trichloroacetic acid plus podophyllin and podophyllin alone.

Benefits: We found no systematic review. **Versus placebo:** We found no RCTs. **Versus cryotherapy:** Two RCTs found no significant difference between trichloroacetic acid and cryotherapy in wart clearance after 6 or 10 weeks of treatment (6 weeks, 1 RCT,[11] 86 people; 21/33 [64%] with trichloroacetic acid *v* 37/53 [70%] with cryotherapy; RR 0.91, 95% CI 0.67 to 1.25; 10 weeks, 1 RCT,[12] 130 men: 43/49 [89%] with trichloroacetic acid *v* 46/57 [81%] with cryotherapy; RR 1.08, 95% CI 0.92 to 2.82). One of the RCTs found no significant difference in recurrence at 2 months after the end of 10 weeks of treatment (14/39 [36%] with trichloroacetic acid *v* 15/38 [40%] with cryotherapy; RR 0.91, 95% CI 0.51 to 1.61).[12] **Plus podophyllin versus podophyllin alone:** One RCT (73 people) found no significant difference in wart clearance at 3 months between trichloroacetic acid plus podophyllin and podophyllin alone (10/35 [28%] with trichloroacetic acid plus podophyllin *v* 9/38 [24%] with podophyllin alone; P value reported as non-significant, CI not reported).[13] **Versus other treatments:** We found no RCTs.

Harms: Safety during pregnancy is unknown. **Versus placebo:** We found no RCTs. **Versus cryotherapy:** The first RCT gave no information on adverse effects.[11] The second RCT found no significant difference in discomfort, ulceration, and scabbing between cryotherapy and trichloroacetic acid (29/57 [51%] with trichloroacetic acid *v* 19/43 [44%] with cryotherapy; reported as non-significant, CI not reported).[12] **Plus podophyllin versus podophyllin alone:** The RCT found that trichloroacetic acid plus podophyllin was associated with ulceration at site of treatment in three people and soreness in two people.[13] It found no adverse effects in people taking podophyllin alone.

Comment: Small numbers of people and inadequate study designs make it difficult to evaluate effectiveness. In pregnant women, only case series are available; 31/32 (97%) pregnant women treated with trichloroacetic acid had wart clearance, and 2/31 (6%) had recurrence.[14]

OPTION **CRYOTHERAPY**

We found no RCTs comparing cryotherapy versus placebo or no treatment. Two RCTs found no significant difference between cryotherapy and trichloroacetic acid in clearance of warts after 6–10 weeks' treatment. One of the RCTs found no significant difference in recurrence of warts 2 months after the end of treatment. One RCT found limited evidence that cryotherapy was less effective for clearance than electrosurgery after 6 weeks' treatment. However, follow up of the people with successful wart clearance revealed no significant

difference in the proportion of people who had warts at 3–5 months. Another RCT found no significant difference in wart clearance at 3 months between cryotherapy and electrosurgery. One RCT found that cryotherapy increased clearance after 6 weeks' treatment compared with podophyllin, and follow up of the people with successful wart clearance found that fewer people receiving cryotherapy had warts at 3–5 months.

Benefits: We found no systematic review. **Versus placebo:** We found no RCTs comparing cryotherapy versus placebo or no treatment. **Versus bi- and trichloroacetic acid:** See benefits of bi- and trichloroacetic acid, p 2005. **Versus electrosurgery:** We found two RCTs.[15,16] The first RCT (450 people) compared three interventions: cryotherapy, electrosurgery**G**, and podophyllin (see comment below).[15] It found that cryotherapy was significantly less effective in clearing warts after 6 weeks' treatment than electrosurgery (68/86 [79%] with cryotherapy *v* 83/88 [94%] with electrosurgery; P = 0.003). The RCT followed up people who had successful wart clearance after 6 weeks' treatment (177 people), and found no significant difference in the proportion of people who had warts at 3–5 months after treatment (9/42 [21%] with cryotherapy *v* 10/46 [22%] with electrosurgery; P = 0.09). The second RCT (42 people) compared cryotherapy versus electrosurgery given at 2 weekly intervals as necessary until warts were completely cleared.[16] It found no significant difference in wart clearance at 3 months' follow up between cryotherapy and electrosurgery (10/18 [56%] with cryotherapy *v* 10/24 [42%] with electrosurgery; RR 1.33, 95% CI 0.71 to 2.50). **Versus podophyllin:** We found one RCT (450 people) that compared three interventions: cryotherapy, electrosurgery, and podophyllin (see comment below).[15] It found that cryotherapy significantly increased wart clearance after 6 weeks' treatment compared with podophyllin (68/86 [79%] with cryotherapy *v* 26/63 [41%] with podophyllin; P < 0.0001). The RCT followed up people who had successful wart clearance after 6 weeks' treatment (177 people) and found that cryotherapy significantly reduced the proportion of people who had warts at 3–5 months after treatment compared with podophyllin (9/42 [22%] with cryotherapy *v* 7/16 [44%] with podophyllin; P < 0.0001).[15] **Versus other treatments:** We found no RCTs.

Harms: **Versus placebo:** We found no RCTs. One case series of 34 pregnant women who received three or fewer treatments of cryotherapy found no subsequent infection or premature rupture of membranes.[17] **Versus bi- and trichloroacetic acid:** See harms of bi- and trichloroacetic acid, p 2005. **Versus electrosurgery or podophyllin:** One RCT reported local infection in 1/86 (1%) people receiving cryotherapy compared with 0/149 (0%) people receiving electrosurgery**G** or podophyllin.[15]

Comment: The results of the RCT comparing cryotherapy versus electrosurgery**G** or podophyllin should be interpreted with caution because no intention to treat analysis was performed and 213/450 (47%) of people withdrew from the trial.[15]

OPTION ELECTROSURGERY

One RCT found that electrosurgery increased clearance of warts at 6 months compared with no treatment. One RCT found that electrosurgery increased clearance of warts at 6 months compared with systemic interferon but the increase was not significant. One RCT found that electrosurgery improved clearance after 6 weeks' treatment compared with cryotherapy. However, follow up of the people with successful wart clearance revealed no significant difference in the proportion of people who had warts at 3–5 months after treatment. It also found that electrosurgery improved clearance after 6 weeks' treatment compared with podophyllin, and follow up of the people with

successful wart clearance revealed that the difference was maintained at 3–5 months after treatment. Another RCT found no significant difference in wart clearance at 3 months between electrosurgery and cryotherapy.

Benefits: We found no systematic review. **Versus no treatment or sham treatment:** We found one RCT (203 women) that compared four treatments: electrosurgery**G** (diathermy); intramuscular or subcutaneous recombinant interferon alpha-2 b; and no treatment.[18] It found that diathermy significantly increased clearance of warts at 6 months after treatment compared with no treatment (82% with diathermy *v* 8% with no treatment; P < 0.001). **Versus cryotherapy:** See benefits of cryotherapy, p 2006. **Versus interferon, systemic:** The RCT (203 women) that compared four treatments found that electrosurgery increased clearance of warts at 6 months compared with interferon but the increase was not significant (35% with diathermy *v* 20% for intramuscular or subcutaneous interferon; P reported as not significant) (see table A on web extra).[18–23] **Versus podophyllin:** We found one RCT (450 people) that compared three interventions: electrosurgery, podophyllin resin, and cryotherapy (see comment below).[15] It found that electrosurgery significantly increased wart clearance after 6 weeks' treatment compared with podophyllin (83/88 [94%] with electrosurgery *v* 26/63 [41%] with podophyllin; P < 0.05). The RCT followed up people who had successful wart clearance after 6 weeks' treatment (177 people), and found that electrosurgery significantly increased the proportion of people who had no warts at 3–5 months (10/46 [22%] with electrosurgery *v* 7/16 [44%] with podophyllin; P < 0.0001). **Versus other treatments:** We found no RCTs.

Harms: **Versus no treatment:** One RCT (203 women) found that the most common adverse effect after electrosurgery**G** was slow cicatrisation, present in 9/51(18%) people and lasting from 30–50 days.[18] Other adverse effects after diathermy included moderate local oedema and pain (17/51 [17%]) and dyspareunia (2/51 [4%]), which lasted from 1–8 weeks (median 2 weeks). **Versus cryotherapy:** See harms of cryotherapy, p 2006. **Versus interferon, systemic:** The RCT comparing diathermy versus interferon did not compare adverse effects between groups (see table A on web extra).[18] See also harms of interferon, systemic, p 2009. **Versus podophyllin:** In the first RCT pain and local irritation were reported in 17% of treated people given electrosurgery.[15]

Comment: **Versus podophyllin:** The results of the RCT should be interpreted with caution because no intention to treat analysis was performed and 213/450 (47%) of people withdrew from the trial.[15]

OPTION IMIQUIMOD

One systematic review and one subsequent RCT found that 5% or 1% imiquimod cream increased wart clearance and reduced recurrence compared with placebo in people without HIV. One RCT in people with HIV identified by the review found no significant difference in wart clearance over 16 weeks between imiquimod cream and placebo. One RCT in people without HIV identified by the review found that imiquimod 5% increased moderate to severe erythema, erosion, excoriation, oedema, and scabbing compared with imiquimod 1% or placebo. One RCT in women without HIV found that twice daily doses of imiquimod 5% did not increase wart clearance over 20 weeks compared with once daily or three times weekly doses, but found that it increased skin erythema.

Benefits: **Versus placebo:** We found one systematic review (search date 2000, 5 RCTs in 588 people with genital warts without HIV infection, 1 RCT in 100 people with HIV)[24] and one subsequent RCT.[25] The review found that, in people without HIV, imiquimod cream (1–5%) significantly increased clearance rates over 16 weeks compared with placebo (5 RCTs; AR for clearance 51% with imiquimod v 6% with placebo; RR 8.3, 95% CI 5.2 to 13.0; NNT 3, 95% CI 2 to 3).[24] The subsequent RCT (60 men without HIV) found similar results (AR for clearance at 4 weeks 70% with imiquimod v 10% with placebo; P = 0.0001).[25] The review found that, in people without HIV, imiquimod 1% or 5% significantly increased the proportion of people with no recurrence at 10–16 weeks after treatment compared with placebo (AR of no recurrence after clearance 37% with imiquimod 5% v 28% with imiquimod 1% v 4–5% with placebo; RR for imiquimod 5% v placebo 9.0, 95% CI 4.9 to 17.0; NNT 3, 95% CI 3 to 4; RR for imiquimod 1% v placebo 2.9, 95% CI 1.5 to 5.9; NNT 10, 95% CI 3 to 91).[24] One RCT (100 people with HIV) included in the review found no significant difference in clearance at 16 weeks between imiquimod cream 5% and placebo (11% with imiquimod v 6% with placebo; P = 0.48).[24] **Different doses of imiquimod:** We found one open label RCT (90 women without HIV) comparing topical imiquimod 5% given either twice daily, once daily, or three times weekly.[26] It found no significant difference among groups in clearance rates over 20 weeks (63% with twice daily v 72% with once daily v 62% with 3 times weekly; P > 0.3). **Versus other treatments:** We found no RCTs.

Harms: **Versus placebo:** The systematic review found no significant difference between imiquimod and placebo in withdrawal from treatment because of adverse effects (4 RCTs; AR 1.8% with imiquimod v 0% with placebo; RR 1.7, 95% CI 0.4 to 9.9).[24] The largest included RCT found that moderate to severe erythema, erosion, excoriation, oedema, and scabbing were more common with imiquimod 5% than with imiquimod 1% or placebo (erythema: 40% v 4% v 3%; erosion: 10% v 1% v 2%; excoriation: 7% v 0% v 0%; oedema: 2% v 0% v 0%; scabbing: 5% v 2% v 0%: no further data reported). The subsequent RCT found that 18% of people taking imiquimod had mild erythema, erosion, or oedema.[25] **Different doses of imiquimod:** The RCT found that imiquimod twice daily significantly increased the proportion of people with severe erythema compared with imiquimod once daily or three times weekly (25% with twice daily v 10% with once daily v 4% with 3 times weekly; P = 0.01).[26]

Comment: A secondary analysis of one of the RCTs identified by the review[24] (209 people without HIV) found that imiquimod significantly increased wart clearance compared with placebo regardless of gender, initial wart size, duration of current outbreak of warts, previous wart treatment, and tobacco use of participants.[27]

OPTION INTERFERON, SYSTEMIC

We found five RCTs comparing different formulations of systemic interferon versus placebo or no treatment. Two of the RCTs found that systemic interferon improved wart clearance compared with placebo or no treatment, whereas three of the RCTs found no significant difference between interferon and placebo in complete or partial wart clearance. Systemic interferon was associated with important adverse effects, including anaphylaxis, blood disorders, flu-like symptoms, headache, fatigue, myalgia, fever, and weight loss. One RCT found no significant difference in wart clearance at 6 months between electrosurgery and systemic interferon. One RCT found that systemic interferon was less effective than podophyllin in clearing warts at 3 months.

Benefits: We found no systematic review. **Versus placebo or no treatment:** We found five RCTs that compared different formulations of systemic interferon versus placebo or no treatment (see table A on web extra).

Two RCTs found that interferon significantly increased wart clearance compared with placebo or no treatment.[18,21] Three RCTs found no significant difference between interferon and placebo in complete or partial (at least 75% reduction in lesion area) wart clearance.[19,20,22] **Versus electrosurgery:** See benefits of electrosurgery, p 2007. **Versus podophyllin:** See benefits of podophyllin, p 2012. **Versus each other:** Three RCTs compared different interferon preparations versus each other and found no consistent differences between preparations (see table A on web extra).[18,19,22] **Plus ablation versus ablation alone:** One RCT (250 people) found no significant difference between interferon plus ablation (diathermy, electric cautery, diathermic loop or laser) and ablation alone in lasting response at 38 weeks (see table A on web extra).[23]

Harms: **Versus placebo:** Two RCTs reported that adverse effects were more common with interferon than with placebo.[19,22] However, the significance of this difference was not always reported (see table A on web extra).[19] Two RCTs found similar incidences of adverse effects in the interferon and placebo groups,[20,21] and one RCT did not report on adverse effects in the placebo group.[18] The most common adverse effect with interferon was flu-like symptoms, which occurred in between 2%[21] and 100%[18] of participants (see table A on web extra). Other adverse effects commonly observed with interferon included headache, fatigue, malaise, myalgia, fever, neuropsychiatric symptoms (drowsiness, lethargy, confusion), and weight loss, which occurred in 5.9–96% of participants. Anaphylactic reaction occurred in 2% of people receiving intramuscular interferon in one RCT;[18] another RCT reported leukopaenia in 6% of people, thrombocytopaenia in 4% of people, and raised liver enzymes in 7.7% of people.[20] One open label dose response study also found raised liver enzymes with intramuscular interferon gamma.[28] **Versus electrosurgery:** See harms of electrosurgery, p 2007. **Versus each other:** Three RCTs compared different interferon preparations versus each other (see table A on web extra).[18,19,22] One RCT found that subcutaneous interferon significantly increased neuropsychiatric problems (drowsiness, lethargy, or confusion) and headache compared with intramuscular interferon (see table A on web extra).[18] One RCT found that a higher dose (9 MIU) of interferon significantly increased flu-like symptoms compared with a lower dose (3 MIU) of interferon (see table A on web extra).[19] One RCT compared three different preparations of interferon versus placebo but did not compare harms of the interferon regimens.[22] **Plus ablation versus ablation alone:** One RCT found that interferon plus ablation increased adverse effects compared with ablation alone, but the statistical significance of this was not reported (see table A on web extra).[23]

Comment: None.

OPTION INTERFERON, TOPICAL

Three RCTs found that topical interferon increased wart clearance at 4 weeks after treatment compared with placebo. One of the RCTs also found that topical interferon increased wart clearance at 4 weeks after treatment compared with podophyllotoxin.

Benefits: We found no systematic review. **Versus placebo:** We found three RCTs (223 people).[29–31] The RCTs found that interferon significantly increased complete wart clearance 4 weeks after treatment compared with placebo (6% with interferon *v* 3% with placebo, CI not reported;[29] 73% with interferon *v* 10% with placebo, $P < 0.0001$;[30] 90% with interferon *v* 20% with placebo, CI not reported[31]). About a third of people in each group in the first RCT had cleared their warts by 16 weeks.[29] Recurrence rates were not evaluated. **Versus podophyllotoxin:** One of the RCTs also compared topical interferon versus podophyllotoxin.[31] It found that topical interferon significantly increased wart clearance at 4 weeks after treatment compared with podophyllotoxin (18/20 [90%] with topical interferon v 12/20 [60%] with podophyllotoxin; P = 0.0285).[31] **Versus other treatments:** We found no RCTs.

Harms: **Versus placebo:** One RCT reported local burning and itching in 39% of people using topical interferon.[29] **Versus podophyllotoxin:** One RCT reported fever, headache, and itching in 18% of people using topical interferon.[31]

Comment: Differences in the clearance rates in the RCTs may be attributable to the preparations used; one preparation was incorporated into a methylcellulose aqueous base[29] and the other two were instilled into a cream base.[30,31]

OPTION SURGICAL EXCISION

We found no RCTs comparing surgical excision versus no treatment. RCTs found no significant difference between surgical (scissor) excision and laser surgery or podophyllin in wart clearance. However, they found that surgical excision was more effective than podophyllin in preventing recurrence at 6–12 months.

Benefits: We found no systematic review. **Versus no treatment:** We found no RCTs comparing surgical excision versus no treatment. **Versus laser surgery:** We found one RCT comparing surgical excision versus carbon dioxide laser.[32] It found no significant difference in clearance between laser and surgical excision (RR 1.2, 95% CI 0.6 to 2.4) and found no significant difference in recurrence rates between the two treatments. **Versus podophyllin:** We found two RCTs (97 people).[33,34] They found no significant difference between surgical excision and podophyllin in wart clearance (16/18 [89%] with surgical excision v 15/19 [79%] with podophyllin; RR 1.13, 95% CI 0.85 to 1.50;[33] 28/30 [93%] with surgical excision v 23/30 [77%]; P = 0.20[34]). However, they found that surgical excision significantly reduced recurrence rates over 6–12 months compared with podophyllin (19% with surgical excision v 60% with podophyllin; P = 0.05;[33] 29% with excision v 65% with podophyllin; P < 0.01[34]). **Versus other treatments:** We found no RCTs.

Harms: All surgically treated people experienced pain.[33,34] **Versus laser surgery:** The RCT found no significant difference in scar formation between surgical excision and laser surgery, although fewer people having surgical excision developed scars (9% had scars with surgical excision v 28% with laser surgery; P > 0.2).[32] Postoperative pain was reported equally in both groups. **Versus podophyllin:** Both RCTs found that more people receiving surgical excision had pain than people receiving podophyllin (11/18 [61%] with excision v 5/19 [26%] with podophyllin;[33] 25/30 [83%] with excision v 7/30 [23%] with podophyllin[34]). The second RCT also found that more people receiving surgical excision had bleeding than people receiving podophyllin (13/30 [43%] with excision v 11/30 [37%] with podophyllin).[34] The RCTs did not assess the significance of the differences between groups.[33,34]

Comment: None.

OPTION LASER SURGERY

We found no RCTs comparing laser surgery versus no treatment. One RCT found no significant difference in wart clearance or recurrence rates over 36 weeks between laser and surgical excision.

Benefits: We found no systematic review. **Versus no treatment:** We found no RCTs comparing laser surgery versus no treatment. **Versus surgical excision:** See benefits of surgical excision, p 2010. **Versus other treatments:** We found no RCTs.

Harms: **Versus surgical excision:** See harms of surgical excision, p 2010.

Comment: We found two case series of laser surgery, which included 47 pregnant women.[14,35] These reported premature rupture of membranes (2/32 [6%] women), prolonged rupture of membranes (1/32 [3%]), the need for postoperative suprapubic catheterisation (7/32 [22%]), pyelonephritis (1/32 [3%]), prolonged healing time (1/52 [2%]), and rectal perforation with secondary abscess (1/52 [2%]).

OPTION PODOPHYLLOTOXIN

RCTs found that podophyllotoxin increased wart clearance within 16 weeks compared with placebo. Six RCTs provided no consistent evidence of a difference between podophyllotoxin and podophyllin in wart clearance or recurrence. One RCT found that podophyllotoxin was less effective than topical interferon in clearing warts at 4 weeks.

Benefits: We found no systematic review. **Versus placebo:** We found eight RCTs (1035 people) comparing podophyllotoxin versus placebo.[31,36–42] All found that, within 16 weeks of treatment, podophyllotoxin was more effective for clearance than placebo (RR values of clearance *v* placebo ranged between 2.0, 95% CI 0.9 to 4.3 and 48.0, 95% CI 3.0 to 773.0). RCTs of 0.5% cream or solution found recurrence rates ranging from 4%[42] to 33%.[37] One RCT (57 people) of 0.5% podophyllotoxin solution as prophylaxis against recurrence of external genital warts (initially treated in an open label study) found fewer recurrences among people taking placebo.[43] **Versus interferon, topical:** See benefits of interferon, topical, p 2009. **Versus podophyllin:** We found six RCTs comparing podophyllotoxin versus podophyllin.[44–49] Five RCTs found no significant difference in wart clearance (RR values for podophyllin *v* podophyllotoxin ranging between 0.7, 95% CI 0.4 to 1.1[45] and 1.7, 95% CI 0.9 to 3.2).[47] One of these RCTs used a 2% solution in a limited study of self treatment for penile warts and found no significant difference in clearance between podophyllotoxin and podophyllin (RR for podophyllin *v* podophyllotoxin 0.6, 95% CI 0.3 to 1.3).[48] The sixth RCT (358 immunocompetent men and women with genital warts for ≤ 3 months, 276 [78%] completed) compared podophyllotoxin (self treatment with 0.5% solution or 0.15% cream twice daily for 3 days with 4 days off) versus podophyllin (25% applied twice weekly at a clinic).[49] Both treatments were given until warts were cleared, up to a maximum of 4 weeks. The RCT found that podophyllotoxin solution, but not podophyllotoxin cream, significantly increased complete remission of warts at 4 weeks compared with podophyllin (intention to treat analysis: OR 1.92, 95% CI 1.13 to 3.27 for solution; OR 1.17, 95 % CI 0.69 to 2.00 for cream). It found no significant difference between treatments in recurrence of warts at 12 weeks among those with initial clearance (74 people analysed: 15/33 [45%] with podophyllotoxin solution *v* 12/22 [55%] with cream *v* 5/19 [26%] with podophyllin, P reported as not significant). High drop–out rates and the potential for selection bias among returning people limits the reliability of these results.

Harms: Cohort studies have reported rare cases of balanoposthitis.[50,51] Safety during pregnancy is unknown. **Versus placebo:** Local inflammation or irritation, erosion, burning, pain, and itching are reported in most trials. Dyspareunia, bleeding, scarring, and insomnia are reported rarely.[36] **Versus interferon, topical:** See harms of interferon, topical, p 2010.

Versus podophyllin: One large RCT reported burning and inflammation in 75% and bleeding in 25% of people treated with podophyllotoxin.[39] Eight RCTs reported pain, erythema, irritation, and tenderness in 3–17% of people treated with podophyllin.[15,33,34,44,45,47,52] Skin burns (1–3%),[33] bleeding (4%),[34] and erosion or ulcerations (1%[45] to 11%[17]) were also reported. Faecal incontinence (4%)[34] and preputial tightening (1%)[44] were reported rarely. One RCT found that podophyllotoxin solution increased local adverse effects and ulceration compared with podophyllotoxin cream and podophyllin (local effects: 33% with solution v 24% with cream v 17% with podophyllin; ulceration: 18% with solution v 12% with cream v 10% with podophyllin; P values not reported).[49]

Comment: RCTs examined the efficacy of podophyllotoxin solutions more often than cream preparations, but cream or gel preparations may be easier to apply than solutions. This and other differences may cause variable efficacy. Podophyllotoxin does not contain the mutagenic flavonoid compounds quercetin and kaempherol, which are contained in podophyllin resin preparations.[53]

OPTION PODOPHYLLIN

We found no RCTs comparing podophyllin versus placebo, but there is consensus that podophyllin is effective for clearing genital warts. Six RCTs provided no consistent evidence of a difference between podophyllotoxin and podophyllin in wart clearance or recurrence. RCTs found no significant difference between surgical (scissor) excision and podophyllin in wart clearance. However, they found that surgical excision was more effective than podophyllin in preventing recurrence at 6–12 months. One RCT found that podophyllin was less effective than cryotherapy or electrosurgery in clearing warts at 6 weeks, and follow up of the people with successful wart clearance revealed that more people receiving podophyllin had warts at 3–5 months. One RCT found no significant difference in wart clearance at 3 months between podophyllin plus trichloroacetic acid and podophyllin alone. One RCT found that podophyllin was more effective than systemic interferon in clearing warts at 3 months.

Benefits: We found no systematic review. **Versus placebo:** We found no RCTs. **Different doses of podophyllin:** One RCT (140 men with anogenital warts) found no significant difference in clearance rates at 3 months between podophyllin 10% and podophyllin 25% (AR 22% in both groups).[54] **Versus cryotherapy:** See benefits of cryotherapy, p 2006. **Versus electrosurgery:** See benefits of electrosurgery, p 2007. **Versus interferon, systemic:** See benefits of interferon, systemic, p 2008. **Versus podophyllotoxin:** See benefits of podophyllotoxin, p 2011. **Versus surgical excision:** See benefits of surgical excision, p 2010. **Plus trichloroacetic acid versus podophyllin alone:** See benefits of bi- and trichloroacetic acid, p 2005.

Harms: Safety during pregnancy is unknown. **Different doses of podophyllin:** The RCT stated that podophyllin 10% or 25% was not associated with hypersensity or ulceration.[54] **Versus cryotherapy:** See harms of cryotherapy, p 2006. **Versus electrosurgery:** See harms of electrosurgery, p 2007. **Versus interferon, systemic:** See harms of interferon, systemic, p 2009. **Versus podophyllotoxin:** See harms of podophyllotoxin, p 2011. **Versus surgical excision:** See harms of surgical excision, p 2010. **Plus trichloroacetic acid versus podophyllin alone:** See harms of bi- and trichloroacetic acid, p 2005.

Comment: Podophyllin may contain the mutagenic flavonoid compounds quercetin and kaempherol.[53]

QUESTION What are the effects of interventions to prevent transmission of human papillomavirus or external genital warts?

OPTION CONDOMS

Observational studies provided insufficient evidence to assess the effects of condom use on transmission of human papillomavirus. Penetrative intercourse is not required for spread because this can occur with external genital–genital or hand–genital touching. One case control and one cross-sectional study suggested that people who always used condoms were less likely to have genital warts than people who never or occasionally used them.

Benefits: We found one systematic review (search date 2000, 1 cohort, 2 cross-sectional, 5 case control studies) comparing the effects of condom use versus no or occasional condom use on transmission of subclinical human papillomavirus (HPV) or transmission of external genital warts.[55] The review could not perform a meta-analysis because of heterogeneity of populations in the studies retrieved. The review was unable to draw firm conclusions about the effects of condom use on transmission of HPV but suggested that condom use may reduce the risk of developing external genital warts. It identified six studies (479 women) assessing the effects of condom use on transmission of subclinical HPV, one of which found that condom use reduced the incidence of HPV. One cross-sectional study (182 women sex workers) identified by the review found that women who always used condoms were significantly less likely to have HPV than women who occasionally or never used condoms (OR 0.2, 95% CI 0.1 to 0.6). However, two case control studies and one cohort study (2638 women) found no significant difference between regular condom use and no use in the proportion of women who had HPV. Another two case control studies (1659 women) found that women who always used condoms were significantly more likely to have HPV than women who never used them (OR 3.8, 95% CI 1.2 to 11.6 in the first study; OR 1.5, 95% CI 1.1 to 2.0 in the second study). One cross-sectional study (432 male military recruits) identified by the review found that men who always used condoms were significantly less likely to have genital warts or HPV than men who occasionally or never used condoms (OR 0.3, 95% CI 0.2 to 0.5). One case control study (1298 people attending a sexually transmitted disease clinic) also found that people who always used condoms were significantly less likely to have genital warts than people who never used them (adjusted OR for men 0.3, 95% CI 0.2 to 0.4; adjusted OR for women 0.6, 95% CI 0.4 to 0.9).[55]

Harms: The review gave no information on adverse effects.[55]

Comment: Penetrative intercourse is not required for spread because this can occur with external genital–genital or hand–genital touching. It is believed that for transmission the virus must be in the form of a virion, which occurs only in lesions. Viable transmission does not occur with contact with the HPV without a lesion.

GLOSSARY

Electrosurgery Includes any method in which an electrical current is used to transect or vaporise tissue, such as diathermy or electrocautery.

Substantive changes

Interferon, systemic Categorisation changed from Unlikely to be beneficial to Likely to be ineffective or harmful on re-evaluation of the evidence.

Podophyllotoxin One RCT added;[49] categorisation unchanged.

REFERENCES

1. US Department of Health and Human Services, Public Health Service. Division of STD Prevention. *Sexually transmitted disease surveillance*. Atlanta: Centers for Disease Control and Prevention, 1996.
2. Koutsky LA, Galloway DA, Holmes KK. Epidemiology of genital human papillomavirus infection. *Epidemiol Rev* 1988;10:122–163.
3. Khanna N. HAART use in women with HIV and influence on cervical intraepithelial neoplasia: a clinical opinion. *J Low Genital Tract Dis* 2002;6:111–115.
4. Gissmann L, zur Hausen H. Partial characterization of viral DNA from human genital warts (condylomata acuminata). *Int J Cancer* 1980;25:605–609.
5. Gissmann L, Boshart M, Durst M, et al. Presence of human papillomavirus in genital tumors. *J Invest Dermatol* 1984;83(suppl 1):26–28.
6. Stanley MA. Imiquimod and the imidazoquinolones: mechanism of action and therapeutic potential. *Clin Exp Dermatol* 2002;27:571–577.
7. Elfgren K, Jacobs M, Walboomers JM, et al. Rate of human papillomavirus clearance after treatment of cervical intraepithelial neoplasia. *Obstet Gynecol* 2002;100:965–971.
8. IARC Working Group on Evaluation of Carcinogenic Risks to Humans. *IARC monographs on the evaluation of carcinogenic risks to humans: human papillomaviruses*. Lyon, France: World Health Organization, International Agency for Research on Cancer, 1995.
9. Bonnez W, Kashima HK, Leventhal B, et al. Antibody response to human papillomavirus (HPV) type 11 in children with juvenile-onset recurrent respiratory papillomatosis (RRP). *Virology* 1992;188:384–387.
10. Hallden C, Majmudar B. The relationship between juvenile laryngeal papillomatosis and maternal condylomata acuminata. *J Reprod Med* 1986;31:804–807.
11. Abdullah AN, Walzman M, Wade A. Treatment of external genital warts comparing cryotherapy (liquid nitrogen) and trichloroacetic acid. *Sex Transm Dis* 1993;20:344–345.
12. Godley MJ, Bradbeer CS, Gellan M, et al. Cryotherapy compared with trichloroacetic acid in treating genital warts. *Genitourin Med* 1987;63:390–392.
13. Gabriel G, Thin RN. Treatment of anogenital warts. Comparison of trichloroacetic acid and podophyllin versus podophyllin alone. *Br J Venereal Dis* 1983;59:124–126.
14. Schwartz DB, Greenberg MD, Daoud Y, et al. Genital condylomas in pregnancy: use of trichloroacetic acid and laser therapy. *Am J Obstet Gynecol* 1988;158(6 pt 1):1407–1416.
15. Stone KM, Becker TM, Hadgu A, et al. Treatment of external genital warts: a randomised clinical trial comparing podophyllin, cryotherapy, and electrodesiccation. *Genitourin Med* 1990;66:16–19.
16. Simmons PD, Langlet F, Thin RN. Cryotherapy versus electrocautery in the treatment of genital warts. *Br J Venereal Dis* 1981;57:273–274.
17. Bergman A, Bhatia NN, Broen EM. Cryotherapy for treatment of genital condylomata during pregnancy. *J Reprod Med* 1984;29:432–435.
18. Benedetti Panici P, Scambia G, Baiocchi G, et al. Randomized clinical trial comparing systemic interferon with diathermocoagulation in primary multiple and widespread anogenital condyloma. *Obstet Gynecol* 1989;74(3 pt 1):393–397.
19. Condylomata International Collaborative Study Group. Recurrent condylomata acuminata treated with recombinant interferon alfa-2a: a multicenter double-blind placebo-controlled clinical trial. *JAMA* 1991;265:2684–2687.
20. Condylomata International Collaborative Study Group. Recurrent condylomata acuminata treated with recombinant interferon α-2a: a multicenter double-blind placebo-controlled clinical trial. *Acta Derm Venereol* 1993;73:223–226.
21. Olmos L, Vilata J, Rodriguez Pichardo A, et al. Double-blind, randomized clinical trial on the effect of interferon-β in the treatment of condylomata acuminata. *Int J STD AIDS* 1994;5:182–185.
22. Reichman RC, Oakes D, Bonnez W, et al. Treatment of condyloma acuminatum with three different interferon-α preparations administered parenterally: a double-blind, placebo-controlled trial. *J Infect Dis* 1990;162:1270–1276.
23. Armstrong DK, Maw RD, Dinsmore WW, et al. Combined therapy trial with interferon α-2a and ablative therapy in the treatment of anogenital warts. *Genitourin Med* 1996;72:103–107.
24. Moore RA, Edwards JE, Hopwood J, et al. Imiquimod for the treatment of genital warts: a quantitative systematic review. *BMC Infect Dis* 2001;1:3. Search date 2000; primary sources Medline, Cochrane Library, and hand searches of review articles and reference lists.
25. Syed TA, Hadi SM, Qureshi ZA, et al. Treatment of external genital warts in men with imiquimod 2% in cream. A placebo-controlled, double-blind study. *J Infect* 2000;41:148–51.
26. Trofatter KF Jr, Ferenczy A, Fife KH. Increased frequency of dosing of imiquimod 5% cream in the treatment of external genital warts in women. *Int J Gynaecol Obstet* 2002;76:191–193.
27. Sauder DN, Skinner RB, Fox TL, et al. Topical imiquimod 5% cream as an effective treatment for external genital and perianal warts in different patient populations. *Sex Transm Dis* 2003;30:124–128.
28. Kirby PK, Kiviat N, Beckman A, et al. Tolerance and efficacy of recombinant human interferon γ in the treatment of refractory genital warts. *Am J Med* 1988;85:183–188.
29. Keay S, Teng N, Eisenberg M, et al. Topical interferon for treating condyloma acuminata in women. *J Infect Dis* 1988;158:934–939.
30. Syed TA, Ahmadpour OA. Human leukocyte derived interferon-α in a hydrophilic gel for the treatment of intravaginal warts in women: a placebo-controlled, double-blind study. *Int J STD AIDS* 1998;9:769–772.
31. Syed TA, Khayyami M, Kriz D, et al. Management of genital warts in women with human leukocyte interferon-α vs podophyllotoxin in cream: a placebo-controlled, double-blind, comparative study. *J Mol Med* 1995;73:255–258.
32. Duus BR, Philipsen T, Christensen JD, et al. Refractory condylomata acuminata: a controlled clinical trial of carbon dioxide laser versus conventional surgical treatment. *Genitourin Med* 1985;61:59–61.
33. Khawaja HT. Podophyllin versus scissor excision in the treatment of perianal condylomata acuminata: a prospective study. *Br J Surg* 1989;76:1067–1068.
34. Jensen SL. Comparison of podophyllin application with simple surgical excision in clearance and recurrence of perianal condylomata acuminata. *Lancet* 1985;2:1146–1148.
35. Kryger-Baggesen N, Falck Larsen J, Hjortkjaer Pedersen P. CO_2 laser treatment of condylomata acuminata. *Acta Obstet Gynecol Scand* 1984;63:341–343.
36. Greenberg MD, Rutledge LH, Reid R, et al. A double-blind, randomized trial of 0.5% podofilox and placebo for the treatment of genital warts in women. *Obstet Gynecol* 1991;77:735–739.
37. Beutner KR, Conant MA, Friedman-Kien AE, et al. Patient-applied podofilox for treatment of genital warts. *Lancet* 1989;i:831–834.
38. Kirby P, Dunne King D, Corey L. Double-blind randomized clinical trial of self-administered podofilox solution versus vehicle in the treatment of genital warts. *Am J Med* 1990;88:465–469.
39. Tyring S, Edwards L, Cherry LK, et al. Safety and efficacy of 0.5% podofilox gel in the treatment of anogenital warts. *Arch Dermatol* 1998;134:33–38.
40. Von Krogh G, Hellberg D. Self-treatment using a 0.5% podophyllotoxin cream of external genital

condylomata acuminata in women. A placebo-controlled, double-blind study. *Sex Transm Dis* 1992;19:170–174.
41. Von Krogh G, Szpak E, Andersson M, et al. Self-treatment using 0.25%–0.50% podophyllotoxin-ethanol solutions against penile condylomata acuminata: a placebo-controlled comparative study. *Genitourin Med* 1994;70:105–109.
42. Syed TA, Lundin S, Ahmad SA. Topical 0.3% and 0.5% podophyllotoxin cream for self-treatment of condylomata acuminata in women: a placebo-controlled, double-blind study. *Dermatology* 1994;189:142–145.
43. Bonnez W, Elswick RK Jr, Bailey-Farchione A, et al. Efficacy and safety of 0.5% podofilox solution in the treatment and suppression of anogenital warts. *Am J Med* 1994;96:420–425.
44. Edwards A, Atma-Ram A, Thin RN. Podophyllotoxin 0.5% *v* podophyllin 20% to treat penile warts. *Genitourin Med* 1988;64:263–265.
45. Hellberg D, Svarrer T, Nilsson S, et al. Self-treatment of female external genital warts with 0.5% podophyllotoxin cream (Condyline) vs weekly applications of 20% podophyllin solution. *Int J STD AIDS* 1995;6:257–261.
46. Kinghorn GR, McMillan A, Mulcahy F, et al. An open, comparative, study of the efficacy of 0.5% podophyllotoxin lotion and 25% podophyllotoxin solution in the treatment of condylomata acuminata in males and females. *Int J STD AIDS* 1993;4:194–199.
47. Lassus A, Haukka K, Forsstrom S. Podophyllotoxin for treatment of genital warts in males: a comparison with conventional podophyllin therapy. *Eur J Sex Transm Dis* 1984;2:31–33.
48. White, DJ, Billingham C, Chapman S, et al. Podophyllin 0.5% or 2.0% *v* podophyllotoxin 0.5% for self treatment of penile warts: a double blind randomised study. *Genitourin Med* 1997;73:184–187.
49. Lacey JN, Goodall RL, Tennvail GR, et al., for the Perstorp Pharma Genital Warts Clinical Trial Group. Randomised controlled trial and economic evaluation of podophyllotoxin solution, podophyllotoxin cream, and podophyllin in the treatment of genital warts. *Sex Transm Infect* 2003;79:270–275.
50. Von Krogh G. Topical self-treatment of penile warts with 0.5% podophyllotoxin in ethanol for four or five days. *Sex Transm Dis* 1987;14:135–140.
51. Von Krogh G. Penile condylomata acuminata: an experimental model for evaluation of topical self-treatment with 0.5–1.0% ethanolic preparations of podophyllotoxin for three days. *Sex Transm Dis* 1981;8:179–186.
52. Condylomata International Collaborative Study Group. A comparison of interferon alfa-2a and podophyllin in the treatment of primary condylomata acuminata. *Genitourin Med* 1991;67:394–399.
53. Petersen CS, Weismann K. Quercetin and kaempherol: an argument against the use of podophyllin? *Genitourin Med* 1995;71:92–93.
54. Simmons PD. Podophyllin 10% and 25% in the treatment of ano-genital warts: a comparative double-blind study. *Br J Venereal Dis* 1981;57:208–209.
55. Manhart LE, Koutsky LA. Do condoms prevent genital HPV infection, external genital warts, or cervical neoplasia? A meta-analysis. *Sex Transm Dis* 2002;29:725–735. Search date 2000; primary sources Medline 1980 to date, hand searches of reference lists, and contact with experts in the field.

Henry Buck, Jr
Courtesy Professor
Health Sports & Exercise Science
Lecturer in Pharmacy
University of Kansas
Lawrence & Kansas City
USA

Competing interests: HWB has been a consultant to 3M Pharmaceuticals and has received research funding from Merck and Co.*We would like to acknowledge the previous contributors of this chapter, including Karl Beutner and DJ Wiley.*

Gonorrhoea

Search date July 2004

John Moran

QUESTIONS

INTERVENTIONS

*Based on comparisons of results across arms of different trials.

†Based on non-RCT evidence and consensus.

See glossary Ⓖ

Key Messages

Treatment

- **Single dose antibiotic regimens*** One systematic review found limited evidence that single dose regimens (ceftriaxone, ciprofloxacin, gatifloxacin, spectinomycin, azithromycin, ofloxacin, cefixime) achieve cure rates of 95% or higher in urogenital or rectal infection. Cure rates were lower (about 80%) for pharyngeal infection. Resistance to penicillins, tetracyclines, and sulphonamides is now widespread, and resistance to fluoroquinolones has become common in some geographic areas.

Treatment in pregnancy

- **Single dose antibiotic regimens** One systematic review found that antibiotic treatment (amoxicillin plus probenecid, spectinomycin, ceftriaxone, cefixime) was effective for curing gonorrhoea in pregnant women. We found no reports of serious adverse effects.

Disseminated gonorrhoea

- **Multidose antibiotic regimens†** We found no RCTs assessing treatments for disseminated gonococcal infection, but there is consensus that multidose regimens using injectable cephalosporins or quinolones (except where quinolone-resistant *Neisseria gonorrhoeae* have been reported) are the most effective treatments. We found no reports of treatment failures with these regimens.

Treatment: gonorrhoea and chlamydia

- **Dual antibiotic treatment** Dual treatment with an antimicrobial effective against gonorrhoea and chlamydia infections is based on theory and expert opinion rather than on evidence from RCTs. The balance between benefits and harms will vary with the prevalence of co-infection in each population.

Clin Evid 2005;13:2016–2023.

DEFINITION Gonorrhoea is caused by infection with *Neisseria gonorrhoeae*. In men, uncomplicated urethritis is the most common manifestation, with dysuria and urethral discharge. Less typically, signs and symptoms are mild and indistinguishable from those of chlamydial urethritis. In women, the most common site of infection is the uterine cervix where infection results in symptoms such as vaginal discharge, lower abdominal discomfort, and dyspareunia in only half of cases. Co-infection with *Chlamydia trachomatis* is reported in 20–40% of people.[1–3]

INCIDENCE/ PREVALENCE Between 1975 and 1997, the reported incidence of gonorrhoea in the USA fell by 74%, reaching a nadir of 122/100 000 people. Since 1997, 125–133 cases have been reported per 100 000 people each year.[4] Rates are highest in younger people. In 2002, the incidence was highest in women aged 15–19 years (676/100 000) and men aged 20–24 years (538/100 000). In England, Wales, and Northern Ireland, diagnoses of gonorrhoea have increased from 1994 to 2002 reaching 296/100 000 for 20–24 year old men and 214/100 000 for 16–19 year old women in 2002.[5] Rates in 2004 were similar to those in 2003.

AETIOLOGY/ RISK FACTORS Most infections result from penile–vaginal, penile–rectal, or penile–pharyngeal contact. An important minority of infections are transmitted from mother to child during birth, which can cause a sight-threatening purulent conjunctivitis (ophthalmia neonatorum). Less common are ocular infections in older children and adults as a result of sexual exposure, poor hygiene, or the medicinal use of urine.

PROGNOSIS The natural history of untreated gonococcal infection is spontaneous resolution and microbiological clearance after weeks or months of unpleasant symptoms.[6] During this time, there is a substantial likelihood of transmission to others and of complications developing in the infected individual.[6] In many women, the lack of readily discernible signs or symptoms of cervicitis means that infections go unrecognised and untreated. An unknown proportion of untreated infections causes local complications, including lymphangitis, periurethral abscess, bartholinitis, and urethral stricture; epididymitis in men; and in women involvement of the uterus, fallopian tubes, or ovaries causing pelvic inflammatory disease (see pelvic inflammatory disease, p 2031). One review found *N gonorrhoeae* was cultured from 8–32% of women with acute pelvic inflammatory disease in 11 European studies and from 27–80% of women in eight US studies.[7] The proportion of *N gonorrhoeae* infections in women that lead to pelvic inflammatory disease has not been well studied. However, one study of 26 women exposed to men with gonorrhoea found that 19 women were culture positive and of these, five women had pelvic inflammatory disease and another four had uterine adnexal tenderness.[8] Pelvic inflammatory disease may lead to infertility (see pelvic inflammatory disease, p 2031). In some people, localised gonococcal infection may disseminate. A US study estimated the risk of dissemination to be 0.6–1.1% among women, whereas a European study estimated it to be 2.3–3.0%.[9,10] The same European study found a lower risk in men, estimated to be 0.4–0.7%.[10] When gonococci disseminate, they cause petechial or pustular skin lesions; asymmetrical arthropathies, tenosynovitis, or septic arthritis; and rarely, meningitis or endocarditis.

AIMS OF INTERVENTION To relieve symptoms; avoid complications; and prevent further transmission, with minimal adverse effects of treatment.

OUTCOMES Microbiological cure rates (number of infected people or infected sites culture negative 1–14 days after treatment, divided by number of infected people or infected sites cultured 1–14 days after treatment).

METHODS *Clinical Evidence* search and appraisal July 2004. Additional Pubmed search conducted by author in October 2004. Key words: gonorrhoea and *N gonorrhoeae* infections, plus a search of references of key articles and books. Studies were excluded if they defined possible treatment failures as "reinfections", if they did not use end points based on microbiological cure, or if they were based on drug regimens unlikely to be of general use (e.g. those using antibiotic regimens that are toxic or to which resistance is now widespread).[11] The authors have not searched for, or included, papers published before 1981 as the susceptibility of *N gonorrhoea* changes over time. The results of particularly old clinical trials may be misleading because of intervening changes in susceptibility.

QUESTION What are the effects of treatments for uncomplicated infections in men and non-pregnant women?

OPTION SINGLE DOSE ANTIBIOTIC REGIMENS

One systematic review found limited evidence that single dose regimens (ceftriaxone, ciprofloxacin, gatifloxacin, spectinomycin, azithromycin, ofloxacin, cefixime) achieve cure rates of 95% or higher in urogenital or rectal infection. Cure rates were lower (about 80%) for pharyngeal infection. Resistance to penicillins, tetracyclines, and sulphonamides is now widespread, and resistance to fluoroquinolones has become common in some geographic areas.

Benefits: **Uncomplicated urogenital, rectal, and pharyngeal infections:** We found one systematic review (search date 1993).[11] The results were updated to 2004 by the author of the review using the original methods (see table 1, p 2022) [10–13] (Moran JS, personal communication, 2004). The original review identified studies (both RCTs and other clinical trials) published from 1981–1993 that used a single dose regimen based on an antimicrobial other than a β-lactamase sensitive penicillin or a tetracycline (ceftriaxane, ciprofloracine, gatifloxacin, spectrinomycin, aithromycin, ofloxacin, cefixime).[11] The search retrieved studies with a total of 24 383 evaluable people. Combining results across arms of trials, 97% were cured on the basis of culture results. Sites of infection, when specified, included the cervix, urethra, rectum, and pharynx. Comparison of cure rates by site of infection found that cure rates were over 95% for all sites except the pharynx, for which they were about 80% (see table 1, p 2022).[14] **Eye infections:** We found no systematic review or RCTs (see comment below).

Harms: Single dose regimens using fluoroquinolones, third generation and extended spectrum cephalosporins, or spectinomycin are generally safe and well tolerated. The most important adverse effects are rare hypersensitivity reactions. Minor adverse effects are most troublesome for the cefixime 800 mg regimen[15,16] and the azithromycin 2 g regimen;[17] both cause frequent gastrointestinal upset. All the other effective doses are associated with a low incidence of adverse outcomes. One large observational cohort study of azithromycin, cefixime, ciprofloxacin, and ofloxacin "in everyday use" found few serious adverse effects.[18] Quinolones may cause arthropathy in animals. One systematic review of harms (search date 2000) found no irreversible fluoroquinolone induced cartilage pathology after 0.3–10.0 months of follow up in 201 adolescents treated for between 7 and 270 days.[19]

Comment: There is good agreement between assessments of antigonococcal activity of antimicrobials *in vitro* and their efficacy in clinical trials. A large number of people were evaluated in a range of settings, suggesting that the results can be generalised. However, comparative results from different settings were not reported. Single dose regimens may make adherence more likely. The ceftriaxone and spectinomycin regimens require intramuscular injection. Resistance is now widespread for all penicillins, sulphonamides, and tetracyclines, and is becoming common for fluoroquinolones in many parts of the world.[5,20–22] Resistance to third generation and extended spectrum cephalosporins or spectinomycin is rarely reported (see table 2, p 2023).[20–25] **Eye infections:** We found two small cohort studies of single dose ceftriaxone for gonococcal eye infections.[26,27] In the first study (12 adults with conjunctivitis), all people responded well to a single 1 g dose of ceftriaxone.[26] In the second study (21 neonates with gonococcal ophthalmia), eye swabs from all neonates were negative 24 hours after a single intramuscular 62.5 mg dose of ceftriaxone.[27]

GLOSSARY

Dual treatment The routine treatment of people with gonorrhoea with an antimicrobial regimen effective against genital *Chlamydia trachomatis* infection in addition to a regimen effective against gonorrhoea (sometimes called dual therapy or co-treatment).

REFERENCES

1. Centers for Disease Control and Prevention. Sexually transmitted diseases treatment guidelines 2002. *MMWR Morb Mortal Wkly Rep* 2002;51:36–42.
2. Creighton S, Tenant-Flowers M, Taylor CB, et al. Co-infection with gonorrhoea and chlamydia: how much is there and what does it mean? *Int J STD AIDS* 2003;14:109–113.
3. Lyss SB, Kamb ML, Peterman TA, et al. *Chlamydia trachomatis* among patients infected with and treated for *Neisseria gonorrhoeae* in sexually transmitted disease clinics in the United States. *Ann Intern Med* 2003;139:178–185.
4. Division of STD Prevention, Centers for Disease Control and Prevention. *Sexually transmitted disease surveillance, 2002*. Atlanta, Georgia: US Department of Health and Human Services, Centers for Disease Control and Prevention, September 2003. http://www.cdc.gov/std/stats (last accessed 10 October 2004).
5. Health Protection Agency. Epidemiological Data — Gonorrhoea. http://www.hpa.org.uk/infections/topics_az/hiv_and_sti/sti-gonorrhoea/epidemiology/epidemiology.htm (last accessed 10 October 2004).
6. Hook EW, Handsfield HH. Gonococcal infections in the adult. In: Holmes KK, Mardh PA, Sparling PF, et al, eds. *Sexually transmitted diseases*. 3rd ed. New York: McGraw-Hill, 1999.
7. Cates WC Jr, Rolfs RT, Aral SG. Sexually transmitted diseases, pelvic inflammatory disease, and infertility: an epidemiologic update. *Epidemiol Rev* 1990;12:199–220.
8. Platt R, Rice PA, McCormack WM. Risk of acquiring gonorrhoea and prevalence of abnormal adnexal findings among women recently exposed to gonorrhoea. *JAMA* 1983;250:3205–3209.
9. Holmes KK, Wiesner PJ, Pedersen AHB. The gonococcal arthritis-dermatitis syndrome. *Ann Intern Med* 1971;75:470–471.
10. Barr J, Danielsson D. Septic gonococcal dermatitis. *BMJ* 1971;1:482–485.
11. Moran JS, Levine WC. Drugs of choice for the treatment of uncomplicated gonococcal infections. *Clin Infect Dis* 1995;20(suppl 1):47–65. Search date range 1981–1993; primary sources Medline, reference lists from retrieved articles, abstracts from the annual Interscience Conference on Antimicrobial Agents and Chemotherapy, and meetings of the International Society for Sexually Transmitted Disease Research.
12. Aplasca De Los Reyes MR, Pato-Mesola V, Klausner JD, et al. A randomized trial of ciprofloxacin versus cefixime for treatment of gonorrhea after rapid emergence of gonococcal ciprofloxacin resistance in the Philippines. *Clin Infect Dis* 2001;32:1313–1318.
13. Rahman M, Alam A, Nessa K, et al. Treatment failure with the use of ciprofloxacin for gonorrhea correlates with the prevalence of fluoroquinolone-resistant *Neisseria gonorrhoeae* strains in Bangladesh. *Clin Infect Dis* 2001;32:884–889.
14. Moran JS. Treating uncomplicated *Neisseria gonorrhoeae* infections: is the anatomic site of infection important? *Sex Transm Dis* 1995;22:39–47.
15. Handsfield HH, McCormack WM, Hook EW III, et al. The Gonorrhea Treatment Study Group. A comparison of single-dose cefixime with ceftriaxone as treatment for uncomplicated gonorrhea. *N Engl J Med* 1991;325:1337–1341.
16. Megran DW, LeFebvre K, Willets V, et al. Single-dose oral cefixime versus amoxicillin plus probenecid for the treatment of uncomplicated gonorrhea in men. *Antimicrob Agents Chemother* 1990;34:355–357.
17. Handsfield HH, Dalu ZA, Martin DH, et al. Azithromycin Gonorrhea Study Group. Multicenter trial of single-dose azithromycin vs. ceftriaxone in the treatment of uncomplicated gonorrhea. *Sex Transm Dis* 1994;21:107–111.
18. Wilton LV, Pearce GL, Mann RD. A comparison of ciprofloxacin, norfloxacin, ofloxacin, azithromycin and cefixime examined by observational cohort studies. *Br J Clin Pharmacol* 1996;41:277–284.
19. Burstein GR, Berman SM, Blumer JL, et al. Ciprofloxacin for the treatment of uncomplicated gonorrhea infection in adolescents: does the benefit outweigh the risk? *Clin Infect Dis* 2002;35(suppl 2):191–199. Search date 2000; primary sources Medline, and citation lists.
20. The WHO Western Pacific Region Gonococcal Antimicrobial Surveillance Programme. Surveillance of antibiotic resistance in *Neisseria gonorrhoeae* in the WHO Western Pacific Region, 2002. *Commun Dis Intell* 2003;26:488–491.
21. Ye S, Su X, Wang Q, et al. Surveillance of antibiotic resistance of *Neisseria gonorrhoeae* isolates in China, 1993–1998. *Sex Transm Dis* 2002;29:242–245.
22. Centers for Disease Control and Prevention: gonococcal isolate surveillance project annual report, 2002. In: *2002 Gonococcal Isolate Surveillance Project (GISP) supplement*. Atlanta, Georgia: US Department of Health and Human Services, October 2003. http://www.cdc.gov/std/GISP2001/ (last accessed 10 October 2004).
23. Dan M, Poch F, Sheinberg B. High prevalence of high-level ciprofloxacin resistance in *Neisseria gonorrhoeae* in Tel Aviv, Israel: correlation with response to therapy. *Antimicrob Agents Chemother* 2002;46:1671–1673.
24. Fenton KA, Ison C, Johnson AP, et al. Ciprofloxacin resistance in *Neisseria gonorrhoeae* in England and Wales in 2002. *Lancet* 2003;361:1867–1869.
25. Fiorito S, Galarza P, Pagano I, et al. Emergence of high level ciprofloxacin resistant *Neisseria gonorrhoeae* strain in Buenos Aires, Argentina. *Sex Transm Infect* 2001;77:77.
26. Haimovici R, Roussel TJ. Treatment of gonococcal conjunctivitis with single-dose intramuscular ceftriaxone. *Am J Ophthalmol* 1989;107:511–514.
27. Hoosen AA, Kharsany AB, Ison CA. Single low-dose ceftriaxone for the treatment of gonococcal ophthalmia: implications for the national programme for the syndromic management of sexually transmitted diseases. *S Afr Med J* 2002;92:238–240.
28. Brocklehurst P. Antibiotics for gonorrhoea in pregnancy. In: The Cochrane Library, Issue 2, 2004. Chichester, UK: John Wiley & Sons, Ltd. Search date 2001; primary sources Cochrane Pregnancy and Childbirth Group Register, and The Cochrane Controlled Trials Register.
29. Cavenee M, Farris J, Spalding T. Treatment of gonorrhea in pregnancy. *Obset Gynaecol* 1993;81:33–38.
30. Ramus RM, Sheffield JS, Mayfield JA, et al. A randomized trial that compared oral cefixime and intramuscular ceftriaxone for the treatment of gonorrhea in pregnancy. *Am J Obstet Gynecol* 2001;185:629–632.
31. Loebstein R, Addis A, Ho E, et al. Pregnancy outcome following gestational exposure to fluoroquinolones: a multicenter prospective controlled study. *Antimicrob Agents Chemother* 1998;42:1336–1339.

John Moran
Medical Epidemiologist
Centers for Disease Control and Prevention, Atlanta, USA
Competing interests: None declared.

TABLE 1 Effectiveness of selected single dose regimens in published clinical trials[10] and updated to 2004 (see text, p 2018).

	Pharyngeal infections	Urogenital and rectal infections
Drug and dose	% cured (95% CI)	% cured (95% CI)
Ceftriaxone 250 mg	98.9 (94.0 to 100)	99.2 (98.8 to 99.5)
Ciprofloxacin 500 mg*	97.2 (85.5 to 99.9)	99.8 (98.7 to 100)
Ciprofloxacin 250 mg	81.5 (81.8 to 95.2)	98.7 (98.0 to 99.4)
Ceftriaxone 125 mg	94.1 (85.6 to 98.4)	98.9 (97.9 to 99.8)
Gatifloxacin 600 mg	100 (82.3 to 100)	99.6 (97.7 to 100)
Spectinomycin 2 g	51.8 (38.7 to 64.9)	98.2 (97.6 to 99.9)
Azithromycin 2 g	100 (82.3 to 100)	99.2 (97.2 to 99.9)
Ofloxacin 400 mg	88.7 (68.8 to 97.8)	98.6 (97.8 to 99.4)
Gatifloxacin 400 mg	100 (63.1 to 100)	99.2 (97.1 to 99.9)
Cefixime 800 mg	80.0 (51.9 to 95.7)	98.4 (95.9 to 99.6)
Cefixime 400 mg	92.3 (74.9 to 99.1)	97.4 (95.9 to 98.6)
Cefuroxime axetil 1 g	56.9 (43.3 to 70.5)	96.2 (94.8 to 97.5)
Cepodoxime proxetil 200 mg	78.9 (54.5 to 94.0)	96.5 (94.3 to 98.5)

*Excludes two published clinical trials among people known to be at high risk of harbouring fluoroquinolone resistant strains; ciprofloxacin 500 mg cured only 48/72 (67%) of cervical infections in one trial [12] and 41/66 (62%) in the other.[13]

TABLE 2 **Reported resistance of *N gonorrhoeae* to antimicrobials (see text, p 2018).**

Drug	Resistance
Sulphonamides	Widespread
Penicillins	Widespread
Tetracyclines	Widespread
Third generation cephalosporins (e.g. ceftriaxone, cefixime)	One report from China[21]
Spectinomycin	Rare
Quinolones	Asia: becoming very common, especially in the Far East (e.g. 80% in China, 64% in Japan, 54% in the Philippines);[20] there are few data from the Middle East, but a high prevalence of resistance (61%) has been reported in Israel.[23]
	USA: in 2002, resistance to ciprofloxacin was reported in 2.2% of 5367 isolates. In the five states bordering the Pacific Ocean, 8.3% of isolates were resistant. In the remaining states, 0.2% were resistant.[22]
	UK: among 2204 gonorrhoeae isolates from England and Wales tested in 2002, 9.8% were fluoroquinolone resistant.[24]
	Australia and New Zealand; 13% and 10%, respectively.[20]
	South America: one fluoroquinolone resistant isolate reported.[25]

Partner notification

Search date July 2003

Catherine Mathews, Nicol Coetzee, Merrick Zwarenstein, and Sally Guttmacher

QUESTIONS

INTERVENTIONS

Key Messages

- We found no good evidence on the effects of partner notification on relationships between patients and partners and, in particular, on the rate of violence, abuse, and abandonment of patient or partner. Also, we found no studies comparing the effects of an intervention across different groups, such as people with different diseases or combinations of diseases, or people from different settings.
- **Contract referral (as effective as provider referral in people with syphilis)** One systematic review of one large RCT comparing different partner notification strategies in people with syphilis found no significant difference in the proportion of partners notified between provider referral and contract referral, when people receiving the contract referral option were given 2 days to notify their partners.
- **Offering a choice between provider and patient referral (v patient referral) in people with HIV** One systematic review of one RCT comparing different partner notification strategies found that, in people with HIV, offering a choice between provider referral (where the identity of the index patient was not revealed) and patient referral improved notification rates compared with offering patient referral alone.
- **Provider referral or contract referral (v patient referral) in people with gonorrhoea or non-gonococcal urethritis (mainly chlamydia)** One systematic review has found that, for people with gonorrhoea, contract versus patient referral increased the rate of partners presenting for treatment. For people with non-gonococcal urethritis, one systematic review found that provider versus patient referral increased the proportion of partners notified and of positive partners detected per patient.
- **Adding telephone reminders and contact cards to patient referral; educational videos; information pamphlets; patient referral by different types of healthcare professionals; patient referral in HIV** We found insufficient evidence about the effects of these interventions in improving partner notification.

Clin Evid 2005;13:2024–2030.

DEFINITION Partner notification is a process whereby the sexual partners of people with a diagnosis of sexually transmitted infection are informed of their exposure to infection. The main methods are patient referral, provider referral, contract referral, and outreach assistance**G**.

INCIDENCE/ PREVALENCE A large proportion of people with sexually transmitted infections will have neither symptoms nor signs of infection. For example, 22–68% of men with gonorrhoea who were identified through partner notification were asymptomatic.[1] Partner notification is one of the two strategies to reach such individuals, the other strategy being screening. Managing infection in people with more than one current sexual partner is likely to have the greatest impact on the spread of sexually transmitted infections.[2]

PROGNOSIS We found no studies showing that partner notification results in a health benefit, either to the partner or to future partners of infected people. Obtaining such evidence would be technically and ethically difficult. One RCT in asymptomatic women compared identifying, testing, and treating women at increased risk for cervical chlamydial infection versus usual care. It found these reduced incidence of pelvic inflammatory disease (RR 0.44, 95% CI 0.20 to 0.90).[3] This evidence suggests that partner notification, which also aims to identify and treat people who are largely unaware of infection, would provide a direct health benefit to partners who are infected.

AIMS OF INTERVENTION To prevent complications of infection in the partner; to prevent transmission to others; to prevent reinfection; and to identify social networks of people practising risky sexual behaviours.

OUTCOMES Partners identified; partners notified; partners presenting for care; partners testing positive; partners treated; rates of reinfection in the patient; incidence of sexually transmitted diseases in the population; harms to patient or partner, such as domestic violence and abuse; ethical outcomes (patient autonomy *v* beneficence). The main outcome presented in each option is the ratio of the number of partners notified to the number of index patients.

METHODS *Clinical Evidence* search and appraisal July 2003. We included RCTs comparing at least two alternative partner notification strategies. The outcome used in this summary was the absolute difference between the ratio of partners identified, notified, presenting for care, testing positive, or treated per index case. Assuming a Poisson distribution for the outcomes, the 95% confidence intervals were calculated using the normal approximation to the Poisson distribution. We excluded studies that did not allow us to extract data on people with specific sexually transmitted diseases, rather than on one of a range of sexually transmitted diseases.

QUESTION **What are the effects of different partner notification strategies in different groups of people?**

OPTION **IN PEOPLE WITH HIV INFECTION**

One systematic review of one RCT found that, for people with HIV infection, offering index patients a choice between provider referral (where the identity of the index patient is not revealed to the partner) and patient referral resulted in more partners being notified than offering patient referral alone. The systematic review found no good evidence on the effects of these strategies on relationships between patients and partners and, in particular, on the rate of violence, abuse, and abandonment of patient or partner.

Benefits: We found one systematic review (search date 2001, 1 RCT, 162 people who tested positive for HIV).[4] **Offering a choice between provider and patient referral versus patient referral:** The RCT (162 people who tested positive for HIV) compared offering a choice between provider referral and patient referral versus patient referral**G**. It was conducted at three public health departments in North Carolina, USA. Of those approached, the 46% who agreed to participate in the study were mostly men (69%), of whom most were homosexual or bisexual

(76%). The choice between provider referral and patient referral significantly increased the likelihood that partners would be notified (rate of number of partners notified to number of index patients 78/39 [2.00] for the group with choice *v* 10/35 [0.29] for the patient referral group; rate increase 1.71, 95% CI 1.35 to 2.07). Thus, for every person offered provider referral compared with using patient referral there will be more than one additional partner notified (see figure A on web extra). **Contract referral:** We found no RCTs assessing contract referral**G** in people with HIV infection. **Outreach assistance:** The systematic review found one RCT, comparing patient referral versus outreach assistance**G** in people with HIV who were injecting drug users, the findings of which have yet to be reported fully.[4,5]

Harms: People's reluctance to disclose their HIV status to partners (see comment below) suggests expectation of harms from doing so. These and other potential harms are poorly understood. The systematic review found no good evidence on the effects of these strategies on relationships between patients and partners and, in particular, on the rate of violence, abuse, and abandonment of patient or partner.

Comment: The number of partners notified is an intermediate outcome. The number of infections in partners that are prevented or treated has not been assessed. Thus, the true benefits and harms of HIV partner notification are unknown. **Rates of disclosure:** One descriptive study (276 people attending for initial primary care for HIV infection in the USA) found that 40% of the respondents had not disclosed their HIV status to all partners over the preceding 6 months.[6] Individuals with more than one partner were significantly less likely to disclose to all partners. Only 42% of the non-disclosers reported that they used condoms all the time, which indicates that many partners were at risk of HIV infection. Another descriptive study conducted in the USA found that, even after repeated individual counselling of people with HIV infection and a 6 month opportunity to disclose HIV status, 30% had not informed any of their past partners and 29% had not informed any of their present partners.[7] **Patient preferences:** The RCT (162 people) comparing offering people a choice between provider and patient referral versus patient referral alone found that, in the group with the choice, most partners (90%) were notified by the provider and only eight people by the index patient.[4] The RCT comparing patient referral versus outreach assistance[5] found, among people allocated to a choice, 82% chose to have the outreach team notify at least one partner, and the team was asked to notify 71% of all partners named by this group. One group in the USA attempted to compare contract referral with provider referral, but cross over between comparison groups made this impossible.[8] The results were therefore analysed as a series without comparison groups, where all patients were assigned to provider referral. The study included 1070 people, who reported having had 8633 partners in the past year. Of these partners, 1035 were successfully located, of whom 248 had previously tested positive for HIV, 560 were tested by the disease intervention specialist, 69 refused testing, and 158 were located by record search only. Of the 560 partners tested, 122 tested positive.

OPTION IN PEOPLE WITH GONORRHOEA OR CHLAMYDIA

One systematic review has found that, for people with gonorrhoea, contract versus patient referral increases the rate of partners presenting for treatment. One RCT also found that contract referral increased the rate of positive partners detected compared with patient referral. For people with non-gonococcal urethritis, one RCT found that provider versus patient referral increased the proportion of partners notified and of positive partners detected

per patient. The systematic review found no good evidence on the effects of these strategies on relationships between patients and partners and, in particular, on the rate of violence, abuse, and abandonment of patient or partner.

Benefits: We found one systematic review (search date 2001, 2 RCTs of partner notification in people with gonorrhoea and 1 RCT in people with non-gonococcal urethritis).[4] **Gonorrhoea:** The two RCTs (2085 people with gonorrhoea) compared patient referral with contract referral**G**. The first RCT (1898 people) found that contract referral significantly increased the number of partners assessed per index patient (392/632 [0.62 partners per index patient] with contract referral *v* 469/1266 [0.37] with patient referral; rate difference 0.25 partners per index patient, 95% CI 0.18 to 0.32). Positive gonorrhoea culture was significantly more likely in the contract referral group than in the patient referral group (233/632 [0.37 positive partners per index patient] with contract referral *v* 315/1266 [0.25] with patient referral; rate difference 0.12, 95% CI 0.06 to 0.18).[4] The second RCT (187 index patients) found contract referral was associated with a non-significantly higher proportion of partners assessed per index patient (119/94 [1.27] with contract referral *v* 107/93 [1.15] in the patient referral group; rate difference +0.12, 95% CI –0.2 to +0.44), and found no significant difference in the number of partners with positive gonorrhoea cultures per index patient.[4] (See figure B on web extra.) **Chlamydia:** One RCT (678 people with non-gonococcal urethritis) compared patient referral with provider referral**G**. It found that provider referral significantly increased the proportion of partners assessed per patient (159/221 [0.72] with provider referral *v* 91/457 [0.20] with patient referral; rate difference 0.52, 95% CI 0.40 to 0.64). In this study, provider referral also significantly increased the proportion of partners with positive culture per index patient (20/221 [0.09] with provider referral *v* 14/457 [0.03] with patient referral; rate difference 0.06, 95% CI 0.02 to 0.10). Provider referral would have to be offered to two index patients with non-gonococcal urethritis for one additional partner to be assessed, and to 17 index patients to identify one additional partner with a positive culture. These findings are likely to over estimate the difference, as partners referred by index patients may have been assessed elsewhere.[4] (See figure C on web extra).

Harms: These are poorly understood. The systematic review found no good evidence on the effects of these strategies on relationships between patients and partners and, in particular, on the rate of violence, abuse, and abandonment of patient or partner.

Comment: One cohort study (265 urban, adolescent girls attending a clinic in Alabama, USA) found that, given the choice, people with gonorrhoea or chlamydia are about as likely to choose provider referral as patient referral.[9] Non-gonococcal urethritis is an old term used when gonorrhoea has been excluded but a positive diagnosis not made. The most common causative agent would be chlamydia.

OPTION IN PEOPLE WITH SYPHILIS

One systematic review of one large RCT found no significant difference between provider referral versus contract referral, when people receiving the contract referral option were given only 2 days in which to notify their partners. We found no RCTs assessing patient referral. The systematic review found no good evidence on the effects of these strategies on relationships between patients and partners and, in particular, on the rate of violence, abuse, and abandonment of patient or partner.

Partner notification

Benefits: We found one systematic review (search date 2001, 1 RCT, 1966 people diagnosed with syphilis in 3 US states).[4] It compared the proportion of partners per patient who were located, tested, tested positive, and treated, using three types of referral process: contract referral**G** (patients were given 2 days to notify partners themselves, before disease intervention specialists would notify them); provider referral**G** (immediate notification by an intervention specialist); and provider referral with the option of a blood test (immediate notification by an intervention specialist who had the option of performing a blood test if he or she thought that the partner would not seek medical attention despite being notified of exposure). There were no significant differences between the three groups: 1.2, 1.1, and 1.1 partners per patient were located; 0.92, 0.87, and 0.86 were tested; and 0.67, 0.61, and 0.62 were treated (CI not provided).[4]

Harms: These are poorly understood. The systematic review found no good evidence on the effects of these strategies on relationships between patients and partners and, in particular, on the rate of violence, abuse, and abandonment of patient or partner.

Comment: In the RCT, the investigators had no way of determining whether disease intervention specialists began actively seeking partners in the contract referral group before waiting 2 days, and they found some evidence of this.[4] Furthermore, the investigators speculated that people may have been allocated to groups not according to the randomisation schedule. These problems may compromise the validity of the study. The use of disease intervention specialists is an approach that may not be generalisable to other settings.

QUESTION What can be done to improve the effectiveness of patient referral?

OPTION COUNSELLING PLUS CONTACT REFERRAL CARDS AND TELEPHONE FOLLOW UP COMPARED WITH COUNSELLING ALONE

One systematic review found one small RCT, which found no significant difference between counselling plus contact referral cards and telephone follow up versus counselling alone.

Benefits: We found one systematic review (search date 2001, 1 RCT).[4] One RCT (38 students from a university clinic in the USA) compared the use of counselling plus contact referral cards and telephone follow up of the index patient with counselling alone. It found no difference between the strategies in the rate of partners presenting for care. The trial also assessed adding a US$3 incentive to the referral card. Charges for clinic visits for patients and partners would be waived after successful recruitment of partners for treatment. This had no effect on the number of partners presenting for care.[4]

Harms: None reported.

Comment: None.

OPTION DIFFERENT HEALTH PROFESSIONALS

One systematic review found one RCT, which found no difference in the effects of patient referral by different healthcare professionals.

Benefits: We found one systematic review (search date 2001, 1 RCT).[4] One RCT (678 index patients) found that there was no difference between patient referral**G** using nurses who did not ask for partners' names and gave referral letters, and disease intervention specialists who took partners' names but no contact details, in terms of the number of partners with positive cultures who were identified (rate difference 0, 95% CI –0.03 to +0.03).[4]

Harms: None reported.

Comment: None.

OPTION INFORMATION PAMPHLETS

One RCT found insufficient evidence on information pamphlets compared with routine counselling.

Benefits: We found one systematic review (search date 2001, 1 unpublished RCT).[4] The unpublished RCT (1898 index patients), conducted in the USA, investigated the use of information pamphlets compared with a routine counselling interview alone. Providing patients with information pamphlets was as effective as the interview alone (rate difference 0, 95% CI –0.07 to +0.07). The two strategies were also equally effective in terms of the number of partners identified with a positive culture per index patient. However, the RCT combined two interventions: different health professionals and asking for partners' names, either of which may have affected the results.[4]

Harms: None reported.

Comment: None.

OPTION EDUCATIONAL VIDEOS

One RCT found no significant difference between educational videos versus standard care, but the outcome reported was potentially inappropriate.

Benefits: We found one systematic review (search date 2001, 1 RCT).[4] The RCT (902 people in the USA) compared a video taped story promoting partner notification versus standard care. No differences in the number of partners assessed were reported (figures not provided).[4] The RCT counted returned contract cards as the main outcome, which has not been shown to be a sensitive enough surrogate indicator for partners presenting for assessment.[10]

Harms: None reported.

Comment: None.

GLOSSARY

Contract referral Also known as conditional referral. Index patients are encouraged to inform their partners, with the understanding that health service personnel will notify those partners who do not visit the health service within a contracted time period.

Outreach assistance At the request of patients, partners are notified by members of an outreach team indigenous to the community, who do not disclose the name of the patient to the partners.

Patient referral Health service personnel encourage index patients to inform partners directly of their possible exposure to sexually transmitted infections.

Provider referral Third parties (usually health service personnel) notify partners identified by index patients, without disclosing the name of the patient to the partners.

REFERENCES

1. Holmes KK, Mardh PA, Sparling PF, et al, eds. *Sexually transmitted diseases*, 2nd ed. New York: McGraw-Hill, 1990:1083.
2. Fenton KA, Peterman TA. HIV partner notification: taking a new look. *AIDS* 1997;11:1535–1546.
3. Scholes D, Stergachis A, Heidrich FE, et al. Prevention of pelvic inflammatory disease by screening for cervical chlamydial infection. *N Engl J Med* 1996;21:1399–1401.
4. Mathews C, Coetzee N, Zwarenstein M, et al. Strategies for partner notification for sexually transmitted diseases. Cochrane Library, Issue 3, 2002. Search date 2001; primary sources Medline, Embase, Psychological Abstracts, Sociological Abstracts, Cochrane Controlled Trials Register, hand searches of the proceedings of International AIDS Conferences and the International Society for STD Research meetings, and personal contact with key experts.
5. Levy JA, Fox SE. The outreach-assisted model of partner notification with IDUs. *Public Health Rep* 1998;113(suppl 1):160–169.
6. Stein MD, Freedberg KA, Sullivan LM, et al. Sexual ethics: disclosure of HIV-positive status to partners. *Arch Intern Med* 1998;158:253–257.
7. Perry SW, Card CAL, Moffatt M, et al. Self-disclosure of HIV infection to sexual partners after repeated counseling. *AIDS Educ Prev* 1994;6:403–411.
8. Toomey KE, Peterman TA, Dicker LW, et al. Human immunodeficiency virus partner notification. *Sex Transm Dis* 1998;25:310–316.
9. Oh MK, Boker JR, Genuardi FJ, et al. Sexual contact tracing in adolescent chlamydial and gonococcal cervicitis cases. *J Adolesc Health* 1996;18:4–9.
10. Potterat JJ, Rothenberg R. The case-finding effectiveness of self-referral system for gonorrhea: a preliminary report. *Am J Public Health* 1977;67:174–176.

Catherine Mathews
Senior Scientist
Health Systems Unit South African Medical Research Council University of Cape Town
Cape Town
South Africa

Nicol Coetzee
Director of Public Health
East Staffordshire Primary Care Trust
Burton on Trent
UK

Merrick Zwarenstein
Director, Health Systems Research Unit
Medical Research Council
Tygerberg
South Africa

Sally Guttmacher
Department of Health Studies New York University
New York
USA

Competing interests: None declared.

Pelvic inflammatory disease

Search date April 2004

Jonathan Ross

QUESTIONS

INTERVENTIONS

Key Messages

Treatment: empirical versus post culture

- **Empirical antibiotic treatment versus treatment guided by test results** We found no RCTs comparing empirical antibiotic treatment (before receiving results of microbiological tests) versus treatment that is guided by test result in women with suspected pelvic inflammatory disease.

Treatment: which antibiotic?

- **Antibiotics (for symptoms and microbiological clearance in women with confirmed pelvic inflammatory disease)** There is consensus that antibiotic treatment is more effective than no treatment for women with confirmed pelvic inflammatory disease. One systematic review of observational studies and RCTs found that several different antibiotic regimens (including parenteral clindamycin plus parenteral aminoglycoside; parenteral cephalosporin with or without probenecid plus oral doxycycline; and oral ofloxacin) were similarly effective in relieving the symptoms of pelvic inflammatory disease, and achieve high rates of clinical and microbiological cure.
- **Oral antibiotics (versus parenteral antibiotics)** Two RCTs found no significant difference between oral ofloxacin and parenteral cefoxitin plus doxycycline.

Pelvic inflammatory disease

- **Outpatient (versus inpatient) antibiotic treatment** One RCT found no significant difference between outpatient treatment with intramuscular cefoxitin plus probenecid plus oral doxycycline and inpatient treatment with parenteral antibiotics in recurrence of pelvic inflammatory disease, infertility, or ectopic pregnancy at 35 months.
- **Different durations of antibiotic treatment** We found no good evidence on the optimal duration of treatment.

Antibiotic prophylaxis before IHD

- **Routine antibiotic prophylaxis before intrauterine device insertion in women at high risk** We found no good evidence about antibiotic prophylaxis before intrauterine device insertion in women at high risk of pelvic inflammatory disease.
- **Routine antibiotic prophylaxis before intrauterine device insertion in women at low risk** One systematic review found no significant difference in the incidence of pelvic inflammatory disease between routine prophylaxis with doxycycline and placebo before intrauterine contraceptive device insertion in women at low risk of pelvic inflammatory disease.

DEFINITION Pelvic inflammatory disease (PID) is inflammation and infection of the upper genital tract in women, typically involving the fallopian tubes, ovaries, and surrounding structures.

INCIDENCE/PREVALENCE The exact incidence of pelvic inflammatory disease (PID) is unknown because the disease cannot be diagnosed reliably from clinical symptoms and signs.[1–3] Direct visualisation of the fallopian tubes by laparoscopy is the best single diagnostic test, but it is invasive and not used routinely in clinical practice. PID is the most common gynaecological reason for admission to hospital in the USA, accounting for 49/10 000 recorded hospital discharges. A diagnosis of PID is made in 1/62 (1.6%) women aged 16–45 years attending their primary care physician in England and Wales.[4] However, because most PID is asymptomatic, this figure underestimates the true prevalence.[1,5] A crude marker of PID in developing countries can be obtained from reported hospital admission rates, where it accounts for 17–40% of gynaecological admissions in sub-Saharan Africa, 15–37% in Southeast Asia, and 3–10% in India.[6]

AETIOLOGY/RISK FACTORS Factors associated with pelvic inflammatory disease (PID) mirror those for sexually transmitted infections: young age, reduced socioeconomic circumstances, lower educational attainment, and recent new sexual partner.[2,7,8] Infection ascends from the cervix, and initial epithelial damage caused by bacteria (especially *Chlamydia trachomatis* and *Neisseria gonorrhoeae*) allows the opportunistic entry of other organisms. Many different microbes, including *Mycoplasma hominis* and anaerobes, may be isolated from the upper genital tract.[9] The spread of infection to the upper genital tract may be increased by instrumentation of the cervix, but reduced by the barrier method, levonorgestrel implants, and oral contraceptives compared with other forms of contraception.[10–14]

PROGNOSIS Pelvic inflammatory disease (PID) has a high morbidity; about 20% of affected women become infertile, 20% develop chronic pelvic pain, and 10% of those who conceive have an ectopic pregnancy.[2] Uncontrolled observations suggest that clinical symptoms and signs resolve in a significant proportion of untreated women.[15] Repeated episodes of PID are associated with a four to six times increase in the risk of permanent tubal damage.[16] One case control study (76 cases and 367 controls) found that delaying treatment by even a few days is associated with impaired fertility (OR 2.6, 95% CI 1.2 to 5.9).[17]

AIMS OF INTERVENTION To alleviate the pain and systemic malaise associated with infection; to achieve microbiological cure; to prevent development of permanent tubal damage with associated sequelae, such as chronic pelvic pain, ectopic pregnancy, and infertility; and to prevent the spread of infection to others with minimal adverse effects.

OUTCOMES Incidence and severity of acute symptoms and signs; microbiological cure of the upper genital tract; incidence of chronic pelvic pain, ectopic pregnancy, and infertility; rate of transmission to others; adverse effects of treatment.

METHODS *Clinical Evidence* search and appraisal April 2004.

QUESTION What are the effects of empirical treatment compared with treatment delayed until the results of microbiological investigations are known?

OPTION EMPIRICAL ANTIBIOTIC TREATMENT

We found no RCTs comparing empirical antibiotic treatment (before receiving results of microbiological tests) versus treatment that is guided by test result in women with suspected pelvic inflammatory disease.

Benefits: We found no systematic review or RCTs comparing empirical versus delayed treatment.

Harms: We found no reliable evidence on harms.

Comment: Because there are no reliable clinical diagnostic criteria for pelvic inflammatory disease, early empirical treatment is common.[3] The positive predictive value of a clinical diagnosis is 65–90% compared with laparoscopy.[1–3] The absence of infection from the lower genital tract, where samples are usually taken, does not exclude pelvic inflammatory disease[2] and so may not influence the decision to treat. One case control study (76 cases and 367 controls) found that delaying treatment by 3 or more days is associated with impaired fertility (OR 2.6, 95% CI 1.2 to 5.9).[17]

QUESTION How do different antimicrobial regimens compare?

OPTION DIFFERENT ANTIMICROBIAL REGIMENS

There is consensus that antibiotic treatment is more effective than no treatment for women with confirmed pelvic inflammatory disease (PID). One systematic review of observational studies and RCTs has found that several different antibiotic regimens (including parenteral clindamycin plus parenteral aminoglycoside; parenteral cephalosporin with or without probenecid plus oral doxycycline; and oral ofloxacin) were similarly effective in relieving the symptoms of PID, and achieve high rates of clinical and microbiological cure. We found no good evidence on the optimal duration of treatment. Two RCTs found no significant difference between oral ofloxacin versus parenteral cefoxitin and doxycycline. One RCT found no significant difference between outpatient treatment with intramuscular cefoxitin plus probenecid plus oral doxycycline and inpatient treatment with parenteral antibiotics in recurrence of pelvic inflammatory disease, infertility, or ectopic pregnancy at 35 months.

Benefits: We found one systematic review (search date 1992, 21 studies),[18] aspects of which were subsequently updated (search date 1997, 26 studies, 1925 women).[19] The earlier version of the review examined all antimicrobial regimens whereas the updated focused on anti-anaerobic treatment. The review evaluated 16 different antimicrobial regimens. The identified studies included case series, and it is not possible to ascertain how many studies were RCTs from the aggregated data published. Inclusion criteria were a diagnosis of pelvic inflammatory disease (PID; clinical, microbiological, laparoscopic, or by endometrial biopsy) and microbiological testing for *C trachomatis* and *N gonorrhoeae*. The review found that antibiotics were effective in relieving the symptoms associated with PID, with clinical and microbiological cure rates of 88–100% (see table 1, p 2037). The only regimen that seemed to perform less well was oral metronidazole plus doxycycline (see table 1, p 2037). However, the studies were of low power and apparent differences in efficacy may have been confounded by differences in disease severity among studies. **Duration of treatment:** We found no RCTs examining the optimal duration of treatment. The duration of treatment were not addressed in the systematic review, although the most common treatment period was 14 days.[19] **Oral versus parenteral treatment:** The review did not analyze outcomes by the oral or parenteral route of administration. Most regimens started with parenteral treatment and continued with oral treatment at different points. Two subsequent RCTs (249 and 72 women) compared oral ofloxacin versus parenteral cefoxitin and doxycycline.[20,21] The RCTs found no significant difference in cure rates between groups (first RCT: RR 1.03, 95% CI 0.97 to 1.10; second RCT: RR 0.97, 95% CI 0.88 to 1.07).[20,21] **Outpatient versus inpatient treatment:** We found one RCT (831 women with mild to moderate PID) published after the review, which compared a single intramuscular dose of cefoxitin with oral probenecid followed by oral doxycycline given to outpatients versus inpatient admission for parenteral antibiotics.[22] It found no significant difference between outpatient and inpatient treatment in tenderness, gonorrhoeal or chlamydial infection, or endometritis at 30 days (tenderness: 20.6% with outpatient treatment *v* 18.4% with inpatient treatment; P = 0.50; gonorrhoeal infection: 3.9% with outpatient treatment *v* 2.4% with inpatient treatment; P = 0.44; chlamydial infection: 2.7% with outpatient treatment *v* 3.6% with inpatient treatment; P = 0.52; endometritis: 45.9% with outpatient treatment *v* 37.6% with inpatient treatment; P = 0.09). At 35 months (mean follow up), the RCT found no significant difference between outpatient and inpatient treatment in PID recurrence, chronic pelvic pain, infertility, or ectopic pregnancy (recurrence: 12.4% with outpatient treatment *v* 16.6% with inpatient treatment; P = 0.11; chronic pelvic pain: 33.7% with outpatient treatment *v* 29.8% with inpatient treatment; P = 0.27; infertility: 18.4% with outpatient treatment *v* 17.9% with inpatient treatment; P = 0.85; ectopic pregnancy: 1.0% with outpatient treatment *v* 0.3% with inpatient treatment; P = 0.37).[22]

Harms: The harms associated with treatment were not specifically addressed by the systematic review.[18,19] In two RCTs reporting adverse effects, withdrawal from treatment was uncommon (2/20 (10%) for doxycycline/metronidazole *v* 0/20 (0%) for pefloxacin/metronidazole *v* 0/16 (0%) for ciprofloxacin; reason for withdrawal not reported).[23,24] The RCT comparing outpatient treatment versus inpatient treatment found no significant difference between treatments in adverse drug reactions (1.7% with outpatient treatment *v* 1.5% with inpatient treatment; event type not reported).[22]

Comment: We found no RCTs comparing antibiotics versus placebo or no treatment. However, such trials would be considered unethical because there is strong consensus that antibiotic treatments are more effective than no treatment in women with PID. We found little evidence about treatment of PID of differing severity, the effect of ethnicity, or the effects of tracing sexual contacts (see partner notification, p 2024). The risks of tubal occlusion and subsequent infertility relate to the severity of PID before starting treatment,[25] and clinical improvement may not translate into preserved fertility.[26,27] The inclusion of observational studies in the systematic review without a sensitivity analysis may compromise the validity of the conclusions. In the review, reliable comparison of different drugs may be confounded by possible differences in disease severity among the included studies.

QUESTION What are the effects of routine antibiotic prophylaxis to prevent pelvic inflammatory disease before intrauterine contraceptive device insertion?

OPTION ROUTINE ANTIBIOTIC PROPHYLAXIS BEFORE INTRAUTERINE CONTRACEPTIVE DEVICE INSERTION

One systematic review found no significant difference in the incidence of pelvic inflammatory disease between routine prophylaxis with doxycycline and placebo before intrauterine contraceptive device insertion in women at low risk of pelvic inflammatory disease. We found no good evidence on the effects in women likely to be at high risk of pelvic inflammatory disease.

Benefits: We found one systematic review (search date 2002, 4 RCTs, 3598 women requesting intrauterine device insertion).[28] The RCTs compared a single dose of doxycycline 200 mg versus placebo 1 hour before intrauterine device insertion. The review found no significant difference in the incidence of pelvic inflammatory disease (PID; doxycycline *v* placebo OR 0.89, 95% CI 0.53 to 1.51). The rate of PID in all women was low (0.5–1.6%), whether or not they received antibiotics, suggesting that this was a low risk group. We found no RCTs on the effects of routine antibiotic prophylaxis in women at high risk of PID.

Harms: The harms associated with treatment were not specifically addressed by the systematic review.[28] Nausea and vomiting has been reported with 17–28% of healthy volunteers on doxycycline, depending on the formulation given.[29] See harms of antimicrobial regimens, p 2034.

Comment: In the populations included in the systematic review, the risk of PID after intrauterine device insertion was low.[28] The occurrence of PID in this group usually reflects the introduction of infection into the uterus during intrauterine device insertion and therefore will vary with the prevalence of sexually transmitted infections in the population. The confidence intervals of results were wide, suggesting that the study may have lacked power to detect a clinically important difference.

REFERENCES

1. Morcos R, Frost N, Hnat M, et al. Laparoscopic versus clinical diagnosis of acute pelvic inflammatory disease. *J Reprod Med* 1993;38:53–56.
2. Metters JS, Catchpole M, Smith C, et al. *Chlamydia trachomatis: summary and conclusions of CMO's expert advisory group*. London: Department of Health, 1998.
3. Centers for Disease Control. 2002 guidelines for treatment of sexually transmitted diseases. Bethesda, Maryland: CDC, 1998, 2002. http://www.cdc.gov/std/treatment/TOC2002TG.htm (last accessed 15 February 2005).
4. Simms I, Rogers P, Charlett A. The rate of diagnosis and demography of pelvic inflammatory disease in general practice: England and Wales. *Int J STD AIDs* 1999;10:448–455.
5. Velebil P, Wingo PA, Xia Z, et al. Rate of hospitalization for gynecologic disorders among reproductive-age women in the United States. *Obstet Gynecol* 1995;86:764–769.
6. Kani J, Adler MW. Epidemiology of pelvic inflammatory disease. In: Berger GS, Westrom L, eds. *Inflammatory disease*. New York: Raven Press, 1992.
7. Simms I, Catchpole M, Brugha R, et al. Epidemiology of genital chlamydia trachomatis in England and Wales. *Genitourin Med* 1997;73:122–126.
8. Grodstein F, Rothman KJ. Epidemiology of pelvic inflammatory disease. *Epidemiology* 1994;5:234–242.
9. Bevan CD, Johal BJ, Mumtaz G, et al. Clinical, laparoscopic and microbiological findings in acute salpingitis: report on a United Kingdom cohort. *Br J Obstet Gynaecol* 1995;102:407–414.
10. Wolner-Hanssen P, Eschenbach DA, Paavonen J, et al. Association between vaginal douching and acute pelvic inflammatory disease. *JAMA* 1990;263:1936–1941.
11. Jacobson L, Westrom L. Objectivized diagnosis of acute pelvic inflammatory disease. Diagnostic and prognostic value of routine laparoscopy. *Am J Obstet Gynecol* 1969;105:1088–1098.
12. Kelaghan J, Rubin GL, Ory HW, et al. Barrier-method contraceptives and pelvic inflammatory disease. *JAMA* 1982;248:184–187.
13. Wolner-Hanssen P, Eschenbach DA, Paavonen J, et al. Decreased risk of symptomatic chlamydial pelvic inflammatory disease associated with oral contraceptive use. *JAMA* 1990;263:54–59.
14. Sivin I. Risks and benefits, advantages and disadvantages of levonorgestrel-releasing contraceptive implants. *Drug Saf* 2003;26:303–335.
15. Curtis AH. Bacteriology and pathology of fallopian tubes removed at operation. *Surg Gynecol Obstet* 1921;33:621.
16. Hillis SD, Owens LM, Marchbanks PA, et al. Recurrent chlamydial infections increase the risks of hospitalization for ectopic pregnancy and pelvic inflammatory disease. *Am J Obstet Gynecol* 1997;176:103–107.

17. Hillis SD, Joesoef R, Marchbanks PA, et al. Delayed care of pelvic inflammatory disease as a risk factor for impaired fertility. *Am J Obstet Gynecol* 1993;168:1503–1509.
18. Walker CK, Kahn JG, Washington AE, et al. Pelvic inflammatory disease: metaanalysis of antimicrobial regimen efficacy. *J Infect Dis* 1993;168:969–978. Search date 1992; primary sources Medline, and bibliographies from reviews, textbooks, and references.
19. Walker CK, Workowski KA, Washington AE, et al. Anaerobes in pelvic inflammatory disease: implications for the Centers for Disease Control and Prevention's guidelines for treatment of sexually transmitted diseases. *Clin Infect Dis* 1999;28(suppl):29–36. Search date 1997; primary sources Medline, and bibliographies from reviews, textbooks, and references.
20. Martens MG, Gordon S, Yarborough DR, et al. Multicenter randomized trial of ofloxacin versus cefoxitin and doxycycline in outpatient treatment of pelvic inflammatory disease. Ambulatory PID Research Group. *South Med J* 1993;86:604–610.
21. Wendel GD, Cox SM, Bawdon RE, et al. A randomized trial of ofloxacin versus cefoxitin and doxycycline in the outpatient treatment of acute salpingitis. *Am J Obstet Gynecol* 1991;164:1390–1396.
22. Ness RB, Soper DE, Holley RL, et al. Effectiveness of inpatient and outpatient treatment strategies for women with pelvic inflammatory disease: results from the Pelvic Inflammatory Disease Evaluation and Clinical Health (PEACH) Randomized Trial. *Am J Obstet Gynecol* 2002;186:929–937.
23. Witte EH, Peters AA, Smit IB, et al. A comparison of pefloxacin/metronidazole and doxycycline/metronidazole in the treatment of laparoscopically confirmed acute pelvic inflammatory disease. *Eur J Obstet Gynecol Reprod Biol* 1993;50:153–158.
24. Heinonen PK, Teisala K, Miettinen A, et al. A comparison of ciprofloxacin with doxycycline plus metronidazole in the treatment of acute pelvic inflammatory disease. *Scand J Infect Dis* 1989;60(suppl):66–73.
25. Soper DE, Brockwell NJ, Dalton HP. Microbial etiology of urban emergency department acute salpingitis: treatment with ofloxacin. *Am J Obstet Gynecol* 1992;167:653–660.
26. Buchan H, Vessey M, Goldacre M, et al. Morbidity following pelvic inflammatory disease. *Br J Obstet Gynaecol* 1993;100:558–562.
27. Brunham RC, Binns B, Guijon F, et al. Etiology and outcome of acute pelvic inflammatory disease. *J Infect Dis* 1988;158:510–517.
28. Grimes DA, Schulz KF. Antibiotic prophylaxis for intrauterine contraceptive device insertion. In: The Cochrane Library, Issue 4, 2002. Oxford: Update Software. Search date 2000; primary sources Medline, Popline, Embase, lists of references, and contacted experts in the field.
29. Story MJ, McCloud PI, Boehm G. Doxycycline tolerance study. Incidence of nausea after doxycycline administration to healthy volunteers: a comparison of 2 formulations (Doryx' vs Vibramycin'). *Eur J Clin Pharmacol* 1991;40:419–421.

Jonathan Ross
Honorary Senior Lecturer
University of Birmingham
Birmingham
UK

Competing interests: Jonthan D C Ross recieved payments as a consultant for Bayer Healthcare including fees for organising Symposia.

TABLE 1 **Cure rates for the antibiotic treatment of acute pelvic inflammatory disease: aggregated data from a systematic review of RCTs and case series (see text, p 2033).[18,19]**

Drug regimen	Number of studies	Number of women	Cure rate (%) clinical	Microbiological*
Inpatient treatment (initially parenteral switching to oral)				
Clindamycin + aminoglycoside	11	470	91	97
Cefoxitin + doxycycline	8	427	91	98
Cefotetan + doxycycline	3	174	95	100
Ceftizoxime + tetracycline	1	18	88	100
Cefotaxime + tetracycline	1	19	94	100
Ciprofloxacin	4	90	94	96
Ofloxacin	1	36	100	97
Sulbactam/ampicillin + doxycycline	1	37	95	100
Co-amoxiclav	1	32	93	–
Metronidazole + doxycycline	2	36	75	71
Outpatient treatment (oral unless indicated otherwise)				
Cefoxitin (im) + probenecid + doxycycline	3	219	89	93
Ofloxacin	2	165	95	100
Co-amoxiclav	1	35	100	100
Sulbactam/ampicillin	1	36	70	70
Ceftriaxone (im) + doxycycline	1	64	95	100
Ciprofloxacin + clindamycin	1	67	97	94

**N gonorrhoeae*, *C trachomatis*, or both, when detected in lower genital tract; im, intramuscular.

Acne vulgaris

Search date April 2004

Sarah Purdy

QUESTIONS

INTERVENTIONS

Key Messages

Topical treatments

- **Benzoyl peroxide** One systematic review identified four RCTs, primarily in people with moderate acne, which found that topical benzoyl peroxide reduced either total lesion count or the number of inflammatory and non-inflammatory lesions at 4, 11, or 12 weeks compared with vehicle; these results were supported by more limited evidence from a fifth RCT with weak methods of analysis. None of the RCTs assessed patient perception of improvement. One of the RCTs found that benzoyl peroxide increased the proportion of people who had adverse effects, including dryness, scaling, burning, tingling, and redness, compared with vehicle. Another RCT found that more people using benzoyl peroxide had peeling compared with people using vehicle. A third RCT found similar rates of local adverse effects between benzoyl peroxide and vehicle.
- **Clindamycin (reduced the number of inflammatory lesions)** RCTs in people with mild, moderate, or severe acne identified by a systematic review found that topical clindamycin reduced the number of inflammatory lesions compared with placebo or vehicle. However, it found inconclusive evidence about the effects of clindamycin on non-inflammatory lesions. Three RCTs found that clindamycin increased the proportion of people who perceived that their acne was "markedly improved" or "improved"; in two of these RCTs the difference between groups was significant. The RCTs gave little information on adverse effects.

- **Erythromycin (reduced the number of inflammatory lesions)** RCTs in people with mild, moderate, or severe acne identified by a systematic review found that topical erythromycin reduced the number of inflammatory lesions at 12 weeks compared with vehicle. One RCT found that a similar proportion of people using erythromycin compared with vehicle perceived that their acne had improved from baseline at 12 weeks; the other RCTs did not assess patient perception of improvement. The RCTs found no significant difference in adverse effects between erythromycin and vehicle.
- **Tretinoin** Four large RCTs, primarily in people with mild to moderate acne, identified by a systematic review found that topical tretinoin reduced the number of inflammatory and non-inflammatory lesions at 8–12 weeks compared with vehicle but increased erythema, peeling, burning, and pruritus. One RCT found that more people taking tretinoin compared with vehicle perceived that their acne had improved; the other RCTs did not assess patient perception of improvement. In the absence of data regarding the risk of birth defects, it is recommended that topical retinoids are not used in pregnancy or by women of childbearing age who are not taking adequate contraceptive precautions.
- **Adapalene** One large RCT in people with moderate acne found that topical adapalene reduced the number of non-inflammatory and inflammatory lesions at 12 weeks compared with vehicle. It found similar quality of life scores in people using adapalene or vehicle. It found that adapalene increased erythema, dryness, scaling, stinging/burning, and pruritus at 2 weeks compared with vehicle, but found no significant difference between groups in these outcomes at 12 weeks. In the absence of data regarding the risk of birth defects, it is recommended that topical retinoids are not used in pregnancy or by women of childbearing age who are not taking adequate contraceptive precautions.
- **Azelaic acid** Two RCTs, primarily in people with moderate acne, identified by a systematic review found limited evidence that topical azelaic acid reduced the number of inflammatory and non-inflammatory lesions after 8–12 weeks compared with placebo or vehicle. Neither of the RCTs assessed patient perception of improvement. The RCTs, and controlled and uncontrolled studies, found that azelaic acid was associated with itching, stinging, burning, and erythema.
- **Erythromycin plus zinc** Two RCTs identified by a systematic review found that topical erythromycin plus zinc reduced acne severity compared with placebo. One RCT found that topical erythromycin plus zinc reduced both inflammatory and non-inflammatory lesions; the other found that it reduced papules but not pustules. Neither RCT assessed patient perception of improvement. The RCTs give little information on adverse effects.
- **Isotretinoin** Two RCTs in people with mild to moderate acne identified by a systematic review found that topical isotretinoin reduced the number of inflammatory and non-inflammatory lesions compared with placebo. These results were supported by more limited evidence from two other RCTs with weak methods of analysis. One of the RCTs found limited evidence from within group comparisons from baseline that a similar proportion of people using isotretinoin compared with vehicle perceived that their acne had improved from baseline at 12 weeks; the other RCTs did not assess patient perception of improvement. The RCTs found that topical isotretinoin was associated with severe erythema, dryness, soreness, and burning. In the absence of data regarding the risk of birth defects, it is recommended that topical retinoids are not used in pregnancy or by women of childbearing age who are not taking adequate contraceptive precautions.
- **Tetracycline** Three RCTs in people with moderate to severe acne identified by a systematic review found that topical tetracycline reduced acne severity at 12–16 weeks compared with placebo. This was supported by more limited evidence from a fourth RCT with weak methods of analysis. One of the RCTs found that a similar proportion of people taking topical tetracycline compared with placebo "considered that their condition was better than before treatment", the other RCTs did not assess participant perception of improvement. Three of the RCTs found that topical tetracycline was associated with skin discolouration.

- **Meclocycline** We found no RCTs comparing topical meclocycline versus vehicle in people with acne vulgaris. One large multicentre non-randomised controlled trial found that meclocycline reduced the number of inflammatory lesions at 11 weeks compared with vehicle but did not reduce comedones. The trial did not assess patient perception of improvement. It found that meclocycline was associated with follicular staining.

Oral treatments

- **Erythromycin** One systematic review identified no RCTs comparing oral erythromycin versus placebo in people with acne vulgaris. One RCT found that both oral erythromycin and oral doxycycline reduced the number of papules and pustules after 6 weeks with no significant difference between groups. The RCT did not assess patient perception of improvement. Two RCTs in people with mild, moderate, or severe acne found that both erythromycin and oral tetracycline improved acne but found no significant difference in the number of lesions or total inflammation scores between the drugs at 3–6 months. A third RCT did not compare oral erythromycin versus oral tetracycline directly but found that fewer people within the group taking erythromycin had a "good" or "very good" response as assessed by their physician than people within the group taking tetracycline although high proportions in both groups responded well. One of the RCTs found no significant difference between oral erythromycin and oral tetracycline in the proportion of people who perceived that their acne had improved; the other RCTs did not assess patient perception of improvement.
- **Doxycycline** One RCT identified by a systematic review provided insufficient evidence to assess oral doxycycline compared with placebo in people with acne vulgaris. One subsequent RCT found that doxycycline reduced inflammatory lesions and comedones after 6 months compared with placebo. It found no significant difference in patient perception of improvement. One systematic review found no significant difference in inflammatory lesions, total lesion count, overall efficacy, or patient perception of improvement between oral doxycycline and oral minocycline. One RCT found that both oral doxycycline and oral erythromycin reduced the number of papules and pustules after 6 weeks with no significant difference between groups and another small RCT found no significant difference in mean lesion count at 8 weeks between oral doxycycline and oral oxytetracycline. The RCTs did not assess patient perception of improvement. Tetracyclines may harm bones and teeth and should not be taken by pregnant or breastfeeding women. They may cause contraceptive failure during the initial weeks of treatment.
- **Lymecycline** One systematic review identified no RCTs comparing oral lymecycline versus placebo in people with acne vulgaris. One RCT in people with moderate to severe acne identified by another systematic review found no significant difference between oral lymecycline and oral minocycline in inflammatory or non-inflammatory lesions or patient perception of improvement at 12 weeks. Tetracyclines may harm bones and teeth and should not be taken by pregnant or breastfeeding women. They may cause contraceptive failure during the initial weeks of treatment.
- **Minocycline** Two RCTs identified by a systematic review provided insufficient evidence to compare oral minocycline versus placebo or oral oxytetracycline. The review found no significant difference in inflammatory lesions, non-inflammatory lesions, total lesion count, overall efficacy, or patient perception of improvement between oral minocycline and oral doxycycline, lymecycline, or tetracycline. Two systematic reviews of one case control study and case reports suggested that oral minocycline was associated with an increased risk of developing the rare but serious condition systemic lupus erythematosus and one review of case reports suggested that it may increase the risk of developing severe hepatic dysfunction. The evidence about adverse effects should be interpreted with caution because of wide variation between studies in numbers of reported adverse events. Tetracyclines may harm bones and teeth and should not be taken by pregnant or breastfeeding women. They may cause contraceptive failure during the initial weeks of treatment.

- **Oxytetracycline** One systematic review identified no RCTs comparing oral oxytetracycline versus placebo in people with acne vulgaris. One small RCT found no significant difference in mean lesion count at 8 weeks between oral doxycycline and oral oxytetracycline. The RCT did not assess patient perception of improvement. Another RCT identified by a systematic review provided insufficient evidence to compare oral oxytetracycline versus oral minocycline. Tetracyclines may harm bones and teeth and should not be taken by pregnant or breastfeeding women. They may cause contraceptive failure during the initial weeks of treatment.
- **Tetracycline** Four RCTs identified by a systematic review found that oral tetracycline reduced acne severity compared with placebo; these results were supported by more limited evidence from two further RCTs with weak methods of analysis. A seventh RCT identified by the review found no significant difference in the number of inflammatory lesions between oral tetracycline and placebo, but may have lacked power to detect a clinically important difference. One of the RCTs found that oral tetracycline increased the proportion of people who perceived that their acne was "markedly improved" or "improved" compared with vehicle; this was supported by weaker evidence from an RCT that compared changes from baseline within groups. RCTs in people with mild, moderate, or severe acne identified by systematic reviews found no significant difference in acne severity between oral tetracycline and oral erythromycin or oral minocycline and that all reduced acne severity. One of the RCTs found no significant difference between oral tetracycline and oral erythromycin in the proportion of people who perceived that their acne had improved; the other RCTs did not assess patient perception of improvement. The RCTs and controlled trials identified by the reviews found few adverse effects associated with oral tetracycline. Tetracyclines may harm bones and teeth and should not be taken by pregnant or breastfeeding women. They may cause contraceptive failure during the initial weeks of treatment.

DEFINITION Acne vulgaris is a common inflammatory pilosebaceous disease characterised by comedones, papules, pustules, inflamed nodules, superficial pus filled cysts, and (in extreme cases) canalising and deep, inflamed, sometimes purulent sacs.[1] Lesions are most common on the face, but the neck, chest, upper back, and shoulders may also be affected. Acne can cause scarring and considerable psychological distress.[2] It is classified as mild, moderate, or severe.[1] Mild acne is defined as non-inflammatory lesions (comedones), a few inflammatory (papulopustular) lesions, or both. Moderate acne is defined as more inflammatory lesions, occasional nodules, or both, and mild scarring. Severe acne is defined as widespread inflammatory lesions; nodules, or both, and scarring; moderate acne which has not settled with 6 months of treatment; or acne of any "severity" with serious psychological upset. This review excludes acne rosacea, acne secondary to industrial occupations, and treatment of acne in people under 13 years of age.

INCIDENCE/ PREVALENCE Acne is the most common skin disease of adolescence, affecting over 80% of teenagers (aged 13–18 years) at some point.[3] Estimates of prevalence vary depending on study populations and the method of assessment used. Prevalence of acne in a community sample of 14–16 year olds in the UK has been recorded as 50%.[4] In a sample of adolescents from schools in New Zealand, acne was present in 91% of males and 79% of females.[5] It has been estimated that up to 30% of teenagers have acne of sufficient severity to require medical treatment.[6] Acne was the presenting complaint in 3.1% of people aged 13–25 years attending primary care in a UK population.[7] Overall incidence is similar in both men and women and peaks at 17 years of age.[6] The number of adults with acne, including people over 25 years, is increasing; the reasons for this increase are uncertain.[8]

AETIOLOGY/ RISK FACTORS The exact cause of acne is unknown. Four factors contribute to the development of acne: increased sebum secretion rate, abnormal follicular differentiation causing obstruction of the pilosebaceous duct, bacteriology of the pilosebaceous duct, and inflammation.[9] The anaerobic bacterium *Proprionibacterium acnes* plays an important role in the pathogenesis of acne. Androgen secretion is the major trigger for adolescent acne.[10]

PROGNOSIS In the absence of treatment, acne persists in most sufferers for an average of 8–12 years.[11]

AIMS OF INTERVENTION To reduce the number of non-inflammatory and inflammatory lesions and scarring; with minimal adverse effects of treatment.

OUTCOMES Number of non-inflammatory lesions (comedones); number of inflammatory lesions (papules, pustules, and nodules); severity scores and scales; patient perception of improvement; quality of life; psychological distress; adverse effects of treatment. The severity scores and scales used in this review include: Leeds Acne Grading Technique, which involves counting and categorising lesions into inflammatory and non-inflammatory;[12] Cook's acne grading scale method, which uses photographs to document severity of acne and grades severity from 0 (least severe) to 8 (most severe);[13] and the Pillsbury Scale, which classifies acne from 1 (mildest) to 4 (severe).[14]

METHODS *Clinical Evidence* search and appraisal April 2004. The review by Lehmann et al[15] included both randomised and non-randomised controlled trials and did not state in all cases whether or not trials were randomised. We have focused on reporting results for RCTs only and, where necessary, have analyzed original papers to ascertain whether trials were randomised. None of the reviews we identified were able to perform a meta-analysis because of heterogeneity among the trials identified. We have described the results of each RCT identified by the reviews, and, where we found numerous RCTs on an intervention, we have tabulated results. We compared all listed oral treatments versus each other and included all RCTs of sufficient quality that we retrieved.

QUESTION What are the effects of topical treatments in people with acne vulgaris? New

OPTION AZELAIC ACID (TOPICAL) New

Two RCTs, primarily in people with moderate acne, identified by a systematic review found limited evidence that topical azelaic acid reduced the number of inflammatory and non-inflammatory lesions after 8–12 weeks compared with placebo or vehicle. Neither of the RCTs assessed patient perception of improvement. The RCTs, and controlled and uncontrolled studies, found that azelaic acid was associated with itching, stinging, burning, and erythema.

Benefits: **Versus placebo or vehicle:** We found one systematic review[15] (search date 1999, 2 RCTs,[16,17] 132 people with acne) comparing topical azelaic acid 20% versus placebo or vehicle. The first RCT (92 people with moderate acne) found that, compared with vehicle, azelaic acid significantly reduced the number of comedones (percentage reduction: 56% with azelaic acid *v* 0% with vehicle; $P = 0.05$ [reported as significant]), the number of inflammatory lesions (percentage reduction: 72% with azelaic acid *v* 47% with vehicle; $P = 0.05$ [reported as significant]). It also found that azelaic acid significantly increased the proportion of people who had physician rating of response to treatment of "excellent" or "good" compared with vehicle (reduction in total lesion count by 75–100% rated as "excellent", 50–75% as "good", 25–50% as "moderate": 28/43 [64%] rated as "excellent/good" with azelaic acid *v* 18/49 [36%] with vehicle; $P = 0.05$ [reported as significant]) after 12 weeks of treatment.[17] These results should be treated with caution because the RCT did not perform an intention to treat analysis and 13% of people did not complete the trial.[17] The RCT did not assess patient perception of improvement. The second RCT (40 people, severity of acne unclear) found that, compared with placebo, azelaic acid significantly reduced the number of inflammatory lesions (percentage reduction: 50% with azelaic acid *v* 12% with placebo; $P = 0.001$) and the number of non-inflammatory lesions (50% with azelaic acid *v* 25% with placebo; $P = 0.027$) after 8 weeks' treatment.[16] These results should be treated with caution as it is unclear whether people taking azelaic acid and placebo had comparable duration and severity of acne.[16] The RCT did not assess patient perception of improvement.

Harms: **Versus placebo or vehicle:** The first RCT found that a higher proportion of people using azelaic acid than vehicle had burning (4/43 [9%] with azelaic acid *v* 1/49 [2%] with vehicle), itching (2/43 [5%] with azelaic acid *v* 0/49 [0%] with vehicle), and erythema (2/43 [5%] with azelaic acid *v* 1/49 [2%] with vehicle; P values not reported for any outcome).[17] The second RCT found that two people taking azelaic acid had itching and stinging compared with one person taking placebo.[16] One non-systematic review of RCTs and uncontrolled studies found that 0–5% of people taking azelaic acid had scaling, 5–23% had burning, and 13–29% had itching.[18]

Comment: None.

OPTION **BENZOYL PEROXIDE (TOPICAL)** New

One systematic review identified four RCTs, primarily in people with moderate acne, which found that topical benzoyl peroxide reduced either total lesion count or the number of inflammatory and non-inflammatory lesions at 4, 11, or 12 weeks compared with vehicle; these results were supported by more limited evidence from a fifth RCT with weak methods of analysis. None of the RCTs assessed patient perception of improvement. One of the RCTs found that benzoyl peroxide increased the proportion of people who had adverse effects, including dryness, scaling, burning, tingling, and redness, compared with vehicle. Another RCT found that more people using benzoyl peroxide had peeling compared with people using vehicle. A third RCT found similar rates of local adverse effects between benzoyl peroxide and vehicle.

Benefits: **Versus vehicle:** We found one systematic review[15] (search date 1999, 5 RCTs,[19–23] 875 people with mild to moderate acne) comparing topical benzoyl peroxide acid versus vehicle (see table A on web extra). The review did not perform a meta-analysis because of heterogeneity among the trials in methods of outcome assessment. Four RCTs, primarily in people with moderate acne, identified by a systematic review, found that topical benzoyl peroxide significantly reduced either total lesion count or the number of inflammatory and non-inflammatory lesions at 4, 11, or 12 weeks compared with vehicle.[19,20,22,23] A fifth RCT found more limited evidence from within group comparisons that benzoyl peroxide reduced total lesion count and the number of inflammatory and non-inflammatory lesions from baseline at 12 weeks.[21] None of the RCTs assessed patient perception of improvement.

Harms: **Versus vehicle:** One of the RCTs found that benzoyl peroxide significantly increased the proportion of people who had adverse effects, including dryness, scaling, burning, tingling, and redness, compared with vehicle[21] and another RCT found that more people using benzoyl peroxide had peeling compared with people using vehicle.[20] One RCT found that benzoyl peroxide was associated with erythema, dryness, soreness, and burning[22] and another that benzoyl peroxide and vehicle were associated with similar rates of local adverse effects.[23] The other RCT gave no information about adverse effects.[19]

Comment: None.

OPTION **ADAPALENE (TOPICAL)** New

One large RCT in people with moderate acne found that topical adapalene reduced the number of non-inflammatory and inflammatory lesions at 12 weeks compared with vehicle. It found similar quality of life scores in people using adapalene or vehicle. It found that adapalene increased erythema, dryness, scaling, stinging/burning, and pruritus at 2 weeks compared with vehicle, but found no significant difference between groups in

these outcomes at 12 weeks. In the absence of data regarding the risk of birth defects, it is recommended that topical retinoids are not used in pregnancy or by women of childbearing age who are not taking adequate contraceptive precautions.

Benefits: **Versus placebo or vehicle:** We found one systematic review (search date 1999), which identified no RCTs comparing adapalene versus placebo or vehicle.[15] One subsequent RCT (327 people with moderate acne) compared adapalene 0.1% daily versus vehicle.[24] It found that adapalene significantly reduced total lesion count at 12 weeks compared with vehicle (mean percentage reduction: 40% with adapalene *v* 20% with vehicle; $P < 0.01$). It also found that, compared with vehicle, adapalene significantly reduced the number of non-inflammatory lesions (mean percentage reduction: 38% with adapalene *v* 20% with vehicle; $P < 0.01$) and the number of inflammatory lesions (mean percentage reduction: 35% with adapalene *v* 19% with vehicle; $P < 0.01$). The RCT assessed quality of life at 12 weeks by a patient questionnaire that evaluated self perception, social and emotional status, and acne symptoms and found similar scores in both groups (no further data reported).

Harms: **Versus vehicle:** The RCT found that adapalene significantly increased erythema, dryness, scaling, stinging/burning and pruritus compared with vehicle ($P < 0.01$), with the highest incidence at 2 weeks. By 12 weeks of follow up, it found no significant difference in adverse effects between the groups. Two people taking adapalene group withdrew, one because of adverse effects. **Birth defects:** We found no RCTs assessing the risk of birth defects in women using topical retinoids. One non-systematic review found that oral retinoids were teratogenic in case reports and case series in humans and experimental studies in animals.[25] In the absence of data regarding the risk of birth defects, it is recommended that topical retinoids are not used in pregnancy or by women of childbearing age who are not taking adequate contraceptive precautions.[6]

Comment: None.

OPTION ISOTRETINOIN (TOPICAL) New

Two RCTs in people with mild to moderate acne identified by a systematic review found that topical isotretinoin reduced the number of inflammatory and non-inflammatory lesions compared with placebo. These results were supported by more limited evidence from two other RCTs with weak methods of analysis. One of the RCTs found limited evidence from within group comparisons from baseline that a similar proportion of people using isotretinoin compared with vehicle perceived that their acne had improved from baseline at 12 weeks; the other RCTs did not assess patient perception of improvement. The RCTs found that topical isotretinoin was associated with severe erythema, dryness, soreness, and burning. In the absence of data regarding the risk of birth defects, it is recommended that topical retinoids are not used in pregnancy or by women of childbearing age who are not taking adequate contraceptive precautions.

Benefits: **Versus vehicle:** We found one systematic review[15] (search date 1999, 3 RCTs,[22,26,27] 472 people with mild to moderate acne) and one subsequent RCT (160 people with mild to moderate acne)[28] comparing isotretinoin versus vehicle. The review did not perform a meta-analysis because of heterogeneity among the trials in methods of outcome assessment.[15] Two RCTs found that isotretinoin 0.05% significantly reduced the number of inflammatory and non-inflammatory lesions and severity scores compared with vehicle; the other two RCTs did not compare isotretinoin versus vehicle directly, assessing only changes from baseline within each group. The first RCT identified by the review (313 people with moderate acne) compared isotretinoin versus vehicle.[26] It found that isotretinoin significantly reduced the number of inflammatory lesions (mean percentage reduction: 55% with isotretinoin *v* 25% with vehicle), the number of non-inflammatory lesions (46% with isotretinoin *v* 14% with vehicle), and severity scores (measured by Cook's acne grading scale method: 40% with isotretinoin *v* 20% with vehicle; reported as significant for all outcomes, CI not reported).[26] The RCT did not assess patient perception of improvement. The second RCT identified by the review (77 people with mild to moderate acne) compared three interventions: isotretinoin, benzoyl peroxide, and vehicle.[22] It also found that, at 12 weeks, isotretinoin significantly reduced the number of inflammatory lesions (mean percentage reduction: –33% with isotretinoin *v* +9 with vehicle; $P = 0.01$), the number of non-inflammatory lesions (–47% with isotretinoin *v* +6% with vehicle; $P = 0.01$), and severity scores compared with vehicle (Leeds score where 0 = no acne and 10 = severest acne: 0 with isotretinoin *v* 1 with vehicle; $P < 0.05$).[22] The RCT did not assess patient perception of improvement. The third RCT identified by the review (82 people with mild to moderate acne) did not assess the effects of isotretinoin on the number of inflammatory or non-inflammatory lesions.[27] It assessed effects on comedones and papules but did not compare isotretinoin versus vehicle directly, rather it assessed within group differences from baseline in each group. It found that isotretinoin 0.05% or 0.1% significantly reduced the number of comedones or papules from baseline at 12 weeks (mean change in comedones from baseline with isotretinoin 0.05%: –9.6; $P < 0.01$; mean change in papules: –7.6; $P < 0.01$).[27] The RCT did not assess patient perception of improvement. The subsequent RCT (160 people with mild to moderate acne) compared four interventions: isotretinoin 0.05% alone, erythromycin 2% alone, isotretinoin plus erythromycin, and vehicle for 12 weeks' treatment.[28] The RCT did not report direct comparisons of isotretinoin alone versus vehicle; it reported changes from baseline within the isotretinoin alone and the vehicle groups. It found limited evidence that isotretinoin significantly reduced total lesion count from baseline at 12 weeks whereas vehicle did not (mean percentage reduction: –21.52%, 95% CI –32.44% to –10.60% with isotretinoin *v* –10.82%, 95% CI –24.29% to +2.65% with vehicle). It also found that isotretinoin significantly reduced the number of non-inflammatory lesions (mean reduction in lesion count: –18.49, 95% CI –35.5 to –1.63 with isotretinoin *v* –7.07, 95% CI –28.31 to +14.16 with vehicle), and inflammatory lesions from baseline whereas vehicle did not (mean reduction in lesion count: –15.66, 95% CI –27.71 to –3.62 with isotretinoin *v* –9.58, 95% CI –24.51 to +5.36 with vehicle).[28] The RCT found that a similar proportion of people using isotretinoin compared with vehicle perceived that their acne had improved from baseline at 12 weeks (66% with isotretinoin *v* 53% with vehicle; P value not reported).

Harms: **Versus vehicle:** The first RCT found that more people using isotretinoin had peeling or erythema than people using vehicle cream (peeling: 71% with isotretinoin *v* 51% with vehicle; erythema: 76% with isotretinoin *v* 62% with vehicle).[26] The second RCT found that isotretinoin was associated with severe erythema (2 people), dryness (3 people), redness (10 people), soreness (4 people), and burning (4 people). One person taking isotretinoin withdrew because of erythema.[22] The third RCT found that isotretinoin significantly increased erythema at 12 weeks compared with vehicle ($P < 0.01$, no further data reported).[27] The subsequent RCT found no significant difference among treatments in "overall tolerance" over 12 weeks (reported as non-significant, P value not reported).[28] The RCT is likely to have been underpowered to detect a clinically important difference in adverse effects among treatments. **Birth defects:** In the absence of data regarding the risk of birth defects, it is recommended that topical retinoids are not used in pregnancy or by women of childbearing age who are not taking adequate contraceptive precautions.[6]

Comment: None.

OPTION TRETINOIN (TOPICAL) New

Four large RCTs, primarily in people with mild to moderate acne, identified by a systematic review found that topical tretinoin reduced the number of inflammatory and non-inflammatory lesions at 8–12 weeks compared with vehicle but increased erythema, peeling, burning, and pruritus. One RCT found that more people taking tretinoin compared with vehicle perceived that their acne had improved; the other RCTs did not assess patient perception of improvement. In the absence of data regarding the risk of birth defects, it is recommended that topical retinoids are not used in pregnancy or by women of childbearing age who are not taking adequate contraceptive precautions.

Benefits: **Versus vehicle:** We found one systematic review[15] (search date 1999, 5 RCTs,[29–33] 802 people with mild to moderate acne, 257 people with moderate to severe acne) comparing topical tretinoin 0.05% or 0.02% versus vehicle twice daily for 8–12 weeks (see table B on web extra). The review did not perform a meta-analysis because of heterogeneity among the RCTs in methods of outcome assessment.[15] Two of the RCTs had weak methods of assessing outcomes.[29,31] Four RCTs found that topical tretinoin significantly reduced the number of inflammatory and non-inflammatory lesions at 8–12 weeks compared with vehicle,[29,30,32,33] the fifth RCT did not assess the differences in outcomes between groups or the significance of the difference in changes from baseline within groups.[31] One RCT found that more people taking tretinoin compared with vehicle perceived that their acne had improved (significance of difference between groups not assessed);[31] the other RCTs did not assess patient perception of improvement.

Harms: **Versus vehicle:** The RCTs found that topical tretinoin 0.02%, 0.025%, or 0.05% significantly increased erythema, peeling, burning, and pruritus compared with vehicle (see table B on web extra). **Birth defects:** In the absence of data regarding the risk of birth defects, it is recommended that topical retinoids are not used in pregnancy or by women of childbearing age who are not taking adequate contraceptive precautions.[6]

Comment: None.

OPTION CLINDAMYCIN (TOPICAL) New

RCTs in people with mild, moderate, or severe acne identified by a systematic review found that topical clindamycin reduced the number of inflammatory lesions compared with placebo or vehicle. However, it found inconclusive evidence about the effects of clindamycin on non-inflammatory lesions. Three RCTs found that clindamycin increased the proportion of people who perceived that their acne was "markedly improved" or "improved"; in two of these RCTs the difference between groups was significant. The RCTs gave little information on adverse effects.

Benefits: **Versus placebo or vehicle:** We found one systematic review[15] (search date 1999, 7 RCTs,[20,34–39] 1502 people with mild, moderate, or severe acne), which compared topical clindamycin (phosphate or hydrochloride) one to four times daily versus placebo or vehicle for 8–12 weeks (see table C on web extra).[15] The review did not perform a meta-analysis because of heterogeneity among the trials in comparisons and outcomes assessed. Three RCTs found inconclusive evidence about the effects of clindamycin compared with placebo on non-inflammatory lesions;[20,36,39] the other RCTs did not assess non-inflammatory lesions. Four RCTs found that clindamycin significantly reduced the number of inflammatory lesions compared with placebo, [20,35,37,38] and a fifth found no significant difference in the number of inflammatory lesions.[36] A sixth RCT found that clindamycin significantly reduced the number of pustules, but not papules.[39] The seventh RCT did not compare clindamycin versus placebo directly, although within group comparisons found that clindamycin significantly reduced the number of inflammatory lesions from baseline.[34] Three RCTs found that clindamycin increased the proportion of people who perceived that their acne was "markedly improved" or "improved", in two of these RCTs the difference between groups was significant.[34,37,38]

Harms: **Versus placebo or vehicle:** Five of the RCTs identified by the review found that clindamycin was associated with diarrhoea and burning in a small proportion of people (see table C on web extra).[34,35,37–39] The fifth RCT found no significant difference in adverse effects between clindamycin and placebo.[20] The seventh RCT gave no information on adverse effects.[36]

Comment: Studies of development of bacterial resistance to antibiotics suggest that topical application of antibiotics in acne may result in antibiotic resistance in *Proprionibacterium acnes*.[6,40]

OPTION ERYTHROMYCIN (TOPICAL) New

RCTs in people with mild, moderate, or severe acne identified by a systematic review found that topical erythromycin reduced the number of inflammatory lesions at 12 weeks compared with vehicle. One RCT found that a similar proportion of people using erythromycin compared with vehicle perceived that their acne had improved from baseline at 12 weeks; the other RCTs did not assess patient perception of improvement. The RCTs found no significant difference in adverse effects between erythromycin and vehicle.

Benefits: **Versus placebo:** We found one systematic review[15] (search date 1999, 8 RCTs,[28,41–47] 347 people with mild to moderate acne, 555 people with moderate to severe acne) that compared topical erythromycin 1–2% versus vehicle for 4–12 weeks (see table D on web extra). The review did not perform a meta-analysis because of heterogeneity among the trials in outcomes assessed. Five RCTs found that erythromycin significantly reduced the number of inflammatory lesions at 12 weeks compared with vehicle.[41–45] The sixth RCT found that more people taking erythromycin had a reduction in the number of inflammatory lesions at 4–8 weeks than people taking placebo, but did not assess the significance of the difference between groups.[46] The seventh RCT found no significant difference in the proportion of people who had greater than 50% reduction in the number of inflammatory lesions at 12 weeks.[47] The eighth RCT did not report direct comparisons of erythromycin alone versus placebo; it reported changes from baseline within the erythromycin and the placebo groups.[28] Few of the RCTs assessed effects on non-inflammatory lesions. One RCT found that a similar proportion of people using erythromycin compared with vehicle perceived that their acne had improved from baseline at 12 weeks;[28] the other RCTs did not assess patient perception of improvement.

Harms: **Versus placebo:** The RCTs identified by the review found no significant difference in adverse effects between topical erythromycin and placebo or vehicle (see table D on web extra).[15]

Comment: Studies of development of bacterial resistance to antibiotics suggest that topical application of antibiotics in acne may result in antibiotic resistance in *Proprionibacterium acnes*.[6,40]

OPTION ERYTHROMYCIN PLUS ZINC (TOPICAL) New

Two RCTs identified by a systematic review found that topical erythromycin plus zinc reduced acne severity compared with placebo. One RCT found that topical erythromycin plus zinc reduced both inflammatory and non-inflammatory lesions; the other found that it reduced papules but not pustules. Neither RCT assessed patient perception of improvement. The RCTs give little information on adverse effects.

Benefits: **Versus placebo:** We found one systematic review[15] (search date 1999, 2 RCTs,[48,49] 222 people with mild, moderate, or severe acne) that compared topical erythromycin 4% plus zinc acetate 1.2% versus placebo. The review did not perform a meta-analysis because of heterogeneity among the trials in outcomes assessed.[15] The first RCT (149 men, severity of acne unclear) compared four interventions: erythromycin 4% plus zinc acetate 1.2% gel twice daily plus oral placebo, erythromycin 4% plus zinc octoate 1.2% liquid twice daily plus oral placebo, oral tetracycline 250 mg twice daily plus topical vehicle, and topical vehicle plus oral placebo for 10 weeks.[48] It found that erythromycin plus zinc (liquid or gel) significantly reduced overall acne severity at 10 weeks compared with topical vehicle plus oral placebo (reduction in severity measured by Cook's acne grading scale: 46% with topical erythromycin plus zinc liquid *v* 7% with topical vehicle plus oral placebo; $P < 0.001$; reduction in severity: 33% with topical erythromycin plus zinc gel *v* 7% with topical vehicle plus oral placebo; $P < 0.01$). It also found that erythromycin plus zinc significantly reduced papules compared with placebo (reduction in papules measured by Cook's acne grading scale: 58% with topical erythromycin plus zinc liquid *v* 25% with topical vehicle plus oral placebo; $P < 0.001$; reduction in papules: 45% with topical erythromycin plus zinc gel *v* 25% with topical vehicle plus oral placebo; $P < 0.05$). It found no significant difference in pustules between treatments (reported as non-significant, no further data reported).[48] The RCT did not assess patient perception of improvement. The second RCT (73 women with Cook's acne grade ≥ 3) compared topical erythromycin 4% plus zinc acetate 1.2% twice daily versus vehicle.[49] It found that topical erythromycin plus zinc acetate significantly reduced both non-inflammatory and inflammatory lesions at 12 weeks compared with vehicle (reduction in non-inflammatory lesions: 61% with topical erythromycin plus zinc acetate *v* 48% with vehicle; $P < 0.01$; reduction in inflammatory lesions: 73% with topical erythromycin plus zinc acetate *v* 46% with vehicle; $P < 0.01$).[49] The RCT did not assess patient perception of improvement.

Harms: **Versus placebo:** One person in the first RCT withdrew from the trial because of irritation with topical erythromycin plus zinc acetate liquid plus oral placebo.[48] The second RCT reported that no-one withdrew from the trial because of irritation or other adverse effects of treatment; it gave no further information on adverse effects.[49]

Comment: Studies of development of bacterial resistance to antibiotics suggest that topical application of antibiotics in acne may result in antibiotic resistance in *Proprionibacterium acnes*.[6,40]

OPTION MECLOCYCLINE (TOPICAL) New

We found no RCTs comparing topical meclocycline versus vehicle in people with acne vulgaris. One large multicentre non-randomised controlled trial found that meclocycline reduced the number of inflammatory lesions at 11 weeks compared with vehicle but did not reduce comedones. The trial did not assess patient perception of improvement. It found that meclocycline was associated with follicular staining.

Benefits: **Versus placebo:** We found one systematic review (search date 1999), which identified no RCTs.[15] The systematic review identified a multicentre non-randomised controlled trial (351 people with mild, moderate, or severe acne) that compared topical meclocycline one or twice daily versus vehicle.[50] It found that meclocycline 1% twice daily significantly reduced the number of inflammatory lesions at 11 weeks compared with vehicle (131 people: reduction: 57% with meclocycline *v* 22% with vehicle; $P < 0.001$). It found a similar number of comedones at 11 weeks with meclocycline compared with vehicle (mean: 59.3 with meclocycline *v* 66.3 with vehicle; P value not reported). The trial did not assess patient perception of improvement.

Harms: **Versus placebo:** We found no RCTs. The controlled trial found that meclocycline was associated with follicular staining in about 16% of people.[50]

Comment: The only trial identified was not randomised.[50] Studies of development of bacterial resistance to antibiotics suggest that topical application of antibiotics in acne may result in antibiotic resistance in *Proprionibacterium acnes*.[6,40]

OPTION TETRACYCLINE (TOPICAL) New

Three RCTs in people with moderate to severe acne identified by a systematic review found that topical tetracycline reduced acne severity at 12–16 weeks compared with placebo. This was supported by more limited evidence from a fourth RCT with weak methods of analysis. One of the RCTs found that a similar proportion of people taking topical tetracycline compared with placebo "considered that their condition was better than before treatment", the other RCTs did not assess participant perception of improvement. Three of the RCTs found that topical tetracycline was associated with skin discolouration.

Benefits: **Versus placebo:** We found one systematic review[15] (search date 1999, 4 RCTs, 355 people with moderate to severe acne). The review did not perform a meta-analysis because of heterogeneity among the trials in outcomes assessed. The first RCT (75 people) identified by the review compared three interventions: topical tetracycline 0.5% plus oral placebo, oral tetracycline 250 mg twice daily plus topical placebo, and topical plus oral placebo for 13 weeks.[51] It found that topical tetracycline significantly reduced acne severity at 12 weeks compared with placebo (mean reduction in severity measured by Cook's acne grading scale: 1.43 with topical tetracycline *v* 0.62 with placebo; $P < 0.05$). The results of the RCT should be interpreted with caution because it did not perform an intention to treat analysis of results and 11/75 [15%] people withdrew from the trial.[51] The RCT did not assess patient perception of improvement. The second RCT (60 male adolescents) identified by the review also compared three interventions: topical tetracycline plus oral placebo, topical vehicle plus oral tetracycline, and topical vehicle plus oral placebo.[52] It found that more people taking topical or oral tetracycline had reduced acne severity compared with people taking placebo (improvement of ≥1 on a scale from 0 [least improvement] to 8 [most improvement]: 12/18 [67%] with topical tetracycline *v* 14/19 [74%] with oral tetracycline *v* 6/17 [35%] with placebo). The RCT did not assess the significance of the difference among groups and did not assess patient perception of improvement.[52] The third RCT (135 people aged 18–25 with mild to moderate acne, Cook's acne grades 0–8) identified by the review compared three interventions: topical tetracycline 0.22% plus oral placebo, oral tetracycline plus topical vehicle, and topical vehicle plus oral placebo for 12 weeks.[53] It found that topical tetracycline significantly reduced acne severity at 7, 10, and 12 weeks compared with placebo ($P < 0.05$; absolute results presented graphically). The RCT did not assess patient perception of improvement.[53] The fourth RCT (85 people with mild to moderate acne) compared topical tetracycline 2.2% versus placebo for 16 weeks. All participants took oral tetracycline for 8 weeks before beginning treatment with topical tetracycline or placebo. The RCT found that topical tetracycline significantly increased the proportion of people who had improved acne at 16 weeks (proportion with improvement measured on a scale from 0 to 8: 29/31 [94%] with topical tetracycline *v* 13/23 [57%] with placebo; $P = 0.035$). The RCT found that a similar proportion of people taking topical tetracycline compared with placebo "considered that their condition was better than before treatment" (25/31 [81%] with topical tetracycline *v* 18/24 [75%] with placebo; P value not reported). It is unclear how the authors dichotomised results to calculate the proportion of people who had improved acne severity.[54]

Harms: **Versus placebo:** Three RCTs found that some people using topical tetracycline had skin discolouration.[51,53,54] In one RCT the difference between groups was significant (proportion with skin discolouration: 17/43 [40%] with tetracycline *v* 4/42 [10%] with placebo; $P < 0.005$).[54] One RCT gave no information on adverse effects.[52]

Comment: Studies of development of bacterial resistance to antibiotics suggest that topical application of antibiotics in acne may result in antibiotic resistance in *Proprionibacterium acnes*.[6,40]

QUESTION What are the effects of oral treatments in people with acne vulgaris? New

OPTION DOXYCYCLINE (ORAL) New

One RCT identified by a systematic review provided insufficient evidence to assess oral doxycycline compared with placebo in people with acne vulgaris. One subsequent RCT found that doxycycline reduced inflammatory lesions and comedones after 6 months compared with placebo. It found no significant difference in patient perception of improvement. One systematic review found no significant difference in inflammatory lesions, total lesion count, overall efficacy, or patient perception of improvement between oral doxycycline and oral minocycline. One RCT found that both oral doxycycline and oral erythromycin reduced the number of papules and pustules after 6 weeks with no significant difference between groups and another small RCT found no significant difference in mean lesion count at 8 weeks between oral doxycycline and oral oxytetracycline. The RCTs did not assess patient perception of improvement. Tetracyclines may harm bones and teeth and should not be taken by pregnant or breastfeeding women. They may cause contraceptive failure during the initial weeks of treatment.

Benefits: **Versus placebo:** We found one systematic review[15] and one subsequent RCT.[55] The review (search date 1999)[15] identified one crossover RCT (62 people with mild acne) that compared oral doxycycline 100 mg daily versus placebo for 8 weeks.[56] The RCT did not report direct comparisons of oral doxycycline versus placebo; it reported changes from baseline within the doxycycline and the placebo groups. Comparing changes from baseline within the oral doxycycline group, it found that oral doxycycline significantly reduced the number of inflammatory lesions from baseline at 4 weeks before crossover whereas placebo did not (percentage reduction from baseline: –36% with doxycycline; P = 0.001; +12% with placebo; reported as non-significant, P value not reported). It found no significant difference in the number of comedones and cysts from baseline within the doxycycline group. The RCT had major losses to follow up (no further data reported). It did not assess patient perception of improvement. The subsequent RCT (51 people with moderate acne) compared doxycycline 20 mg twice daily versus placebo.[55] It found that doxycycline significantly reduced inflammatory lesions and comedones after 6 months compared with placebo (reduction in inflammatory lesions: –50% with doxycycline *v* –30% with placebo; P = 0.04; reduction in comedones: –54% with doxycycline *v* –11% with placebo; P < 0.01). It also found that doxycycline significantly improved clinician's global assessment scores at 6 months compared with placebo (measured by a scale from 1 to 7 where 1 = clear or almost clear skin: 4.4 with doxycycline *v* 5.1 with placebo; P = 0.03).[55] It found no significant difference in patient perception of improvement at 6 months between doxycycline and placebo (global assessment scores measured on same scale as above: 4.8 with doxycycline *v* 5.3 with placebo; reported as non-significant, P value not reported). **Versus oral erythromycin:** We found one RCT (56 people with moderate acne) comparing oral doxycycline 100 mg daily for 2 weeks then on alternate days for 4 weeks versus oral erythromycin 500 mg twice daily for 2 weeks then 250 mg twice daily for 4 weeks.[57] Before treatment, people taking doxycycline had a mean of 38 inflammatory lesions and people taking erythromycin had a mean of 46 inflammatory lesions. It found no significant difference between doxycycline and erythromycin in the number of papules and pustules after 6 weeks (mean number per person: 16 with doxycycline *v* 15 with erythromycin; P > 0.1). The RCT did not assess patient perception of improvement. **Versus oral minocycline:** See benefits of oral minocycline, p 2054. **Versus oral oxytetracycline:** We found no systematic review but found one double blind crossover RCT (28 people with moderate to severe acne) comparing oral doxycycline 100 mg daily for 8 weeks versus oral oxytetracycline 250 mg three times daily for 4 weeks then once daily for 4 weeks.[58] It found no significant difference in mean number of lesions at 8 weeks before crossover between oral doxycycline and oxytetracycline (mean number per person: 62 with doxycycline *v* 32 with oxytetracycline; reported as non-significant, P value not reported). The RCT did not assess patient perception of improvement.

Harms: Tetracyclines may harm bones and teeth and should not be taken by pregnant or breastfeeding women.[59,60] They may cause contraceptive failure during the initial weeks of treatment. **Versus placebo:** The RCT identified by the review found no adverse effects in people taking doxycycline or placebo but may have been underpowered to detect adverse effects. **Versus oral erythromycin:** We found one RCT (56 people) comparing doxycycline with erythromycin, which reported that no withdrawals took place because of adverse effects after 6 weeks with either treatment.[57] **Versus minocycline:** See harms of oral minocycline, p 2055. **Versus oral oxytetracycline:** The RCT reported that there were no "significant adverse effects".[60]

Comment: See comment of oral minocycline, p 2055.

OPTION **ERYTHROMYCIN (ORAL)** New

One systematic review identified no RCTs comparing oral erythromycin versus placebo in people with acne vulgaris. One RCT found that both oral erythromycin and oral doxycycline reduced the number of papules and pustules after 6 weeks with no significant difference between groups. The RCT did not assess patient perception of improvement. Two RCTs in people with mild, moderate, or severe acne found that both erythromycin and oral tetracycline improved acne but found no significant difference in the number of lesions or total inflammation scores between the drugs at 3–6 months. A third RCT did not compare oral erythromycin versus oral tetracycline directly but found that fewer people within the group taking erythromycin had a "good" or "very good" response as assessed by their physician than people within the group taking tetracycline although high proportions in both groups responded well. One of the RCTs found no significant difference between oral erythromycin and oral tetracycline in the proportion of people who perceived that their acne had improved; the other RCTs did not assess patient perception of improvement.

Benefits: **Versus placebo:** We found one systematic review (search date 1999), which identified no RCTs comparing oral erythromycin versus placebo.[15] We found no subsequent RCTs. **Versus oral doxycycline:** See benefits of oral doxycycline, p 2050. **Versus oral tetracycline:** The review[15] identified three RCTs[61–63] (300 people) comparing oral erythromycin versus oral tetracycline in people with mild, moderate, or severe acne. Two RCTs found no significant difference in number of lesions or total inflammation scores between oral erythromycin and oral tetracycline at 3–6 months,[61,62] the third RCT did not directly compare the two treatments.[63] One RCT found no significant difference between erythromycin and tetracycline in the proportion of people who perceived that their acne had improved.[62] The first RCT (60 people with moderate/severe acne) found no significant difference in cure or total inflammation scores between erythromycin 200–400 mg daily and tetracycline 250–400 mg daily for 6 months (proportion symptom free: 9/21 [43%] with erythromycin *v* 7/21 [33%] with tetracycline; inflammation score on face 1 in groups; reported as non-significant, P value not reported).[61] The RCT did not assess patient perception of improvement. The second RCT (200 people with moderate to severe acne) compared erythromycin 333 mg three times daily for 4 weeks, then once daily for 8 weeks versus tetracycline 500 mg twice daily for 4 weeks then once daily for 8 weeks.[62] It found no significant difference between erythromycin and tetracycline in the number of pustules, papules, open comedones, or closed comedones at 12 weeks (percentage change, pustules: –73% with erythromycin *v* –65% with tetracycline; papules: –60% with erythromycin *v* –62% with tetracycline; open comedones: –26% with erythromycin *v* –31% with tetracycline; closed comedones: –17% with erythromycin *v* –36% with tetracycline; P value reported as non-significant for all outcomes, CI not reported). It also found no significant difference between erythromycin and tetracycline in the proportion of people who perceived their acne had improved (proportion who reported acne as "markedly improved" or "improved": 77% with erythromycin *v* 89% with tetracycline; P value reported as non-significant/not not reported, P value not reported). The third RCT (40 people with mild, moderate, or severe acne) compared erythromycin 250 mg twice daily versus tetracycline 250 mg twice daily for 16 weeks.[63] It did not compare the two treatments directly but found that fewer people within the group taking erythromycin had a "good" or "very good" response as assessed by their physician than people within the group taking tetracycline (65% with erythromycin *v* 90% with tetracycline). It did not assess patient perception of improvement.

Harms: **Versus placebo:** We found no RCTs. **Versus oral doxycycline:** The RCT reported no withdrawals because of adverse effects, but gave no further information.[57] **Versus oral tetracycline:** The RCTs found that oral erythromycin and oral tetracycline were associated with similar rates of adverse effects, most of which were gastrointestinal. In the first RCT, one person in each treatment group discontinued treatment because of diarrhoea in first week and 14% of people in the trial had adverse effects, most of which were gastrointestinal.[61] In the second RCT, 12 people taking erythromycin and seven taking tetracycline had adverse effects, again mostly gastrointestinal.[62] One person taking oral tetracycline developed a pseudotumour cerebri but later recovered.[62] In the third RCT, one person taking erythromycin had nausea and vomiting and one person taking tetracycline had mild diarrhoea, one had nausea, and one had pruritus.[63]

Comment: See comment of oral minocycline, p 2055 for data on antibiotic resistance.

OPTION LYMECYCLINE (ORAL) New

One systematic review identified no RCTs comparing oral lymecycline versus placebo in people with acne vulgaris. One RCT in people with moderate to severe acne identified by another systematic review found no significant difference between oral lymecycline and oral minocycline in inflammatory or non-inflammatory lesions or patient perception of improvement at 12 weeks. Tetracyclines may harm bones and teeth and should not be taken by pregnant or breastfeeding women. They may cause contraceptive failure during the initial weeks of treatment.

Benefits: **Versus placebo:** We found one systematic review (search date 1999), which identified no RCTs comparing oral lymecycline versus placebo.[15] We found no subsequent RCTs. **Versus oral minocycline:** See benefits of oral minocycline, p 2054.

Harms: Tetracyclines may harm bones and teeth and should not be taken by pregnant or breastfeeding women.[59,60] They may cause contraceptive failure during the initial weeks of treatment. **Versus oral minocycline:** See harms of oral minocycline, p 2055.

Comment: See comment of oral minocycline, p 2055.

OPTION MINOCYCLINE (ORAL) New

Two RCTs identified by a systematic review provided insufficient evidence to compare oral minocycline versus placebo or oral oxytetracycline. The review found no significant difference in inflammatory lesions, non-inflammatory lesions, total lesion count, overall efficacy, or patient perception of improvement between oral minocycline and oral doxycycline, lymecycline, or tetracycline. Two systematic reviews of one case control study and case reports suggested that oral minocycline was associated with an increased risk of developing the rare but serious condition systemic lupus erythematosus and one review of case reports suggested that it may increase the risk of developing severe hepatic dysfunction. The evidence about adverse effects should be interpreted with caution because of wide variation between studies in numbers of reported adverse events. Tetracyclines may harm bones and teeth and should not be taken by pregnant or breastfeeding women. They may cause contraceptive failure during the initial weeks of treatment.

Benefits: **Versus placebo:** We found one systematic review (search date 2002, 1 crossover RCT, 43 people), comparing oral minocycline versus placebo for 10 weeks.[64] The RCT did not compare minocycline versus placebo directly, rather it assessed within group differences from baseline in each group. It found that minocycline significantly reduced total lesion score from baseline ($P < 0.05$) whereas placebo did not (no further data reported). It found no significant change in patient perception of overall efficacy of minocycline compared with baseline (measured on a 10 cm visual analogue scale: WMD –1.25, 95% CI –7.22 to +4.72). The RCT was of insufficient length to assess effects of minocycline and there was no washout period before crossover so the review could not report results after crossover.[64] **Versus oral doxycycline:** We found one systematic review (search date 2002, 5 RCTs, 419 people with mild to moderate or inflammatory acne) comparing oral minocycline versus oral doxycycline.[64] The review did not perform a meta-analysis because of heterogeneity among the trials in methods, outcomes assessed, and drug doses. All of the RCTs found no significant difference in outcomes between minocycline and doxycycline. Outcomes assessed included proportion of people with 50% or greater reduction in inflammatory lesions, total lesion count, patient perception of improvement, and overall efficacy. The review found problems with the methods of all of the RCTs: three were open label and the two double blind RCTs reported insufficient information to allow calculation of effect sizes. **Versus oral lymecycline:** We found one systematic review (search date 2002, 1 multicentre RCT, 144 people with ≥20 inflammatory lesions on the face) comparing oral minocycline versus oral lymecycline.[64] It found no significant difference between minocycline and lymecycline in the proportion of people with 50% or greater reduction in inflammatory or non-inflammatory lesions at 12 weeks (inflammatory lesions: 46/73 [63%] with minocycline *v* 41/71 [58%] with lymecycline; RR 1.09, 95% CI 0.84 to 1.42; non-inflammatory lesions: 22/73 [30%] with minocycline *v* 33/71 [46%] with lymecycline; RR 0.65, 95% CI 0.42 to 1.00). The RCT also found no significant difference between minocycline and lymecycline in the proportion of people who perceived that there had been "overall improvement" in their acne (59/71 [83%] with minocycline *v* 55/65 [85%] with lymecycline; RR 0.98, 95% CI 0.91 to 1.24). **Versus oral oxytetracycline:** We found one systematic review (search date 2002, 1 open label RCT, 237 people with ≥grade 4 Cook's acne grade), comparing oral minocycline versus oral oxytetracycline.[64] The RCT found that minocycline significantly increased the proportion of people whose acne had improved by at least two grades on the Cook's acne grading severity scale over 12–24 weeks' treatment compared with oxytetracycline (completer analysis: 90/104 [86%] with minocycline *v* 64/90 [71%] with lymecycline; RR 1.22, 95% CI 1.05 to 1.42). The results of the RCT should be interpreted with caution as they are not analyzed by intention to treat and 43 people were excluded from the analysis. The clinical relevance of the results is also unclear as the RCT did not state acne grades after treatment. The RCT did not assess patient perception of improvement. **Versus oral tetracycline:** We found one systematic review (search date 2002, 6 RCTs, 693 people with moderate to severe acne) comparing oral minocycline versus oral tetracycline.[64] The review did not perform a meta-analysis because of heterogeneity among the trials in outcomes assessed. Five RCTs identified by the review found no significant difference between minocycline and tetracycline in overall acne severity assessed on a variety of scales, including Samuelson Lesion and Pillsbury Scale. Two RCTs identified by the review found no significant difference in the proportion of people who felt that there was overall improvement in their acne or felt that their response was "satisfactory" between oral minocycline and oral tetracycline; the other RCTs did not assess patient perception of improvement. One open label RCT identified by the review reported a difference in outcomes between minocycline and tetracycline but had serious methodological flaws, sufficient to question the validity of the result.

Harms: We found three systematic reviews assessing adverse effects of minocycline.[64–66] The first review (search date 2002) identified 21 studies assessing adverse effects of minocycline.[64] It found that 137/1230 (11%) of people had an adverse reaction attributed to minocycline, 36/1230 (3%) of whom withdrew because of adverse effects. It also found that 17/700 (2.4%) people taking minocycline had abnormal pigmentation.[64] One prospective cohort study identified by the review (700 people) assessed adverse effects in people taking minocycline 100–200 mg daily for a mean 10.5 months.[67] It found that adverse effects were reported in 13.6% of people. They included vestibular disturbance, candida infection, gastrointestinal disturbance, cutaneous symptoms (pigmentation, pruritus, photosensitive rash, and urticaria), and benign intracranial hypertension. Tetracyclines may harm bones and teeth and should not be taken by pregnant or breastfeeding women.[59,60] They may cause contraceptive failure during the initial weeks of treatment. **Systemic lupus erythematosus:** We found two systematic reviews.[64,65] The first review[64] identified one case control study[68] (27 688 people aged 15–19 years with acne) assessing the risk of systemic lupus erythematosus (SLE) in people taking tetracyclines compared with matched controls. The case control study found that 29 people (27 women) taking tetracyclines had SLE like syndrome. It found that current minocycline use significantly increased the risk of developing SLE (AR 52.8 cases per 100 000 prescriptions; RR 8.5, 95% CI 2.1 to 35). It found no significant difference in the risk of developing SLE with tetracyclines other than minocycline, although use of tetracyclines was associated with an increased risk (RR 1.7, 95% CI 0.4 to 8.1). Women had a significantly higher risk of developing SLE compared with men (RR 14, 95% CI 1.8 to 111). Cumulative minocycline dose and prolonged exposure (> 100 days) to minocycline may also be risk factors but no quantitative data were reported. The second review (search date 1999) identified 57 case reports of SLE in people taking minocycline.[65] It suggested that minocycline may induce SLE, but did not quantify its conclusions. **Liver damage:** We found one systematic review (search date 1998) of case reports and case series, which found 65 cases of liver damage in people taking minocycline.[66] The review did not quantify the increased risk in people taking minocycline. It suggested that minocycline was associated with severe hepatic dysfunction including hypersensitivity within a few weeks of taking minocycline (16 cases), autoimmune hepatitis within 1 year or more of taking minocycline (29 cases), or unspecified hepatitis (20 cases).

Comment: Evidence about adverse effects should be interpreted with caution because of wide variation between studies in numbers of reported adverse events. The prevalence of SLE in the general population is 30/100 000 in white people, rising to 200/100 000 in Afro Caribbean people.[69] There is increasing *Proprionibacterium acnes* resistance to systemic antibiotics. One systematic review (search date 1998, 12 studies) found an increase in the prevalence of *Proprionibacterium acnes* resistance from 20% in 1978 to 62% in 1996.[70] Resistance to systemic antibiotics varied but was most commonly reported in people taking erythromycin, clindamycin, tetracycline, doxycycline, and trimethoprim. Resistance to minocycline was rare.

OPTION OXYTETRACYCLINE (ORAL) New

One systematic review identified no RCTs comparing oral oxytetracycline versus placebo in people with acne vulgaris. One small RCT found no significant difference in mean lesion count at 8 weeks between oral doxycycline and oral oxytetracycline. The RCT did not assess patient perception of improvement. Another RCT identified by a systematic review provided insufficient evidence to compare oral oxytetracycline versus oral minocycline. Tetracyclines may harm bones and teeth and should not be taken by pregnant or breastfeeding women. They may cause contraceptive failure during the initial weeks of treatment.

Benefits: **Versus placebo:** We found one systematic review (search date 1999) which identified no RCTs comparing oral oxytetracycline versus placebo.[11] We found no subsequent RCTs. **Versus oral minocycline:** See benefits of oral minocycline, p 2054. **Versus oral doxycycline:** See benefits of oral doxycycline, p 2050.

Harms: Tetracyclines may harm bones and teeth and should not be taken by pregnant or breastfeeding women.[59,60] They may cause contraceptive failure during the initial weeks of treatment. **Versus oral minocycline:** See harms of oral minocycline, p 2055. **Versus oral doxycycline:** See harms of oral doxycycline, p 2051.

Comment: See comment of oral minocycline, p 2055.

OPTION TETRACYCLINE (ORAL) New

Four RCTs identified by a systematic review found that oral tetracycline reduced acne severity compared with placebo; these results were supported by more limited evidence from two further RCTs with weak methods of analysis. A seventh RCT identified by the review found no significant difference in the number of inflammatory lesions between oral tetracycline and placebo, but may have lacked power to detect a clinically important difference. One of the RCTs found that oral tetracycline increased the proportion of people who perceived that their acne was "markedly improved" or "improved" compared with vehicle; this was supported by weaker evidence from an RCT that compared changes from baseline within groups. RCTs in people with mild, moderate, or severe acne identified by systematic reviews found no significant difference in acne severity between oral tetracycline and oral erythromycin or oral minocycline and that all reduced acne severity. One of the RCTs found no significant difference between oral tetracycline and oral erythromycin in the proportion of people who perceived that their acne had improved; the other RCTs did not assess patient perception of improvement. The RCTs and controlled trials identified by the reviews found few adverse effects associated with oral tetracycline. Tetracyclines may harm bones and teeth and should not be taken by pregnant or breastfeeding women. They may cause contraceptive failure during the initial weeks of treatment.

Benefits: **Versus placebo:** We found one systematic review (search date 1999, 7 RCTs, 864 people with mild, moderate, or severe acne) that compared oral tetracycline 250 mg twice daily versus placebo (see table E on web extra).[15] The review did not perform a meta-analysis because of heterogeneity among the trials in outcomes assessed. Four RCTs found that oral tetracycline significantly reduced acne severity compared with placebo.[37,51,53,71] One of these RCTs also found that oral tetracycline significantly increased the proportion of people who perceived that their acne was "markedly improved" or "improved" compared with placebo.[37] A fifth RCT compared three interventions: topical tetracycline plus oral placebo, topical vehicle plus oral tetracycline, and topical vehicle plus oral placebo.[52] It found that more people taking oral or topical tetracycline had improved acne compared with people taking placebo but did not assess the significance of the difference among groups. A sixth small RCT, which compared four interventions, found no significant difference in the number of inflammatory lesions between oral tetracycline and placebo, but may have lacked power to detect a clinically important difference among groups.[72] The seventh RCT did not compare tetracycline versus placebo directly, although within group comparisons found that tetracycline significantly reduced the number of inflammatory lesions from baseline and increased the proportion of people who perceived that their acne was "markedly improved" or "improved".[34] **Versus oral erythromycin:** See benefits of oral erythromycin, p 2052. **Versus oral minocycline:** See benefits of oral minocycline, p 2054.

Harms: Tetracyclines may harm bones and teeth and should not be taken by pregnant or breastfeeding women.[59,60] They may cause contraceptive failure during the initial weeks of treatment. **Versus placebo:** The review identified five RCTs that assessed adverse effects and found that 15/579 [3%] people taking tetracycline had adverse effects.[15] **Versus oral minocycline:** See harms of oral minocycline, p 2055.

Comment: See comment of oral minocycline, p 2055.

REFERENCES

1. Healy E, Simpson N. Acne vulgaris. *BMJ* 1994;308:831–833.
2. Mallon E, Newton JN, Klassen A, et al. The quality of life in acne: a comparison with general medical conditions using generic questionnaires. *Br J Dermatol* 1999;140:672–676.
3. Chu TC. Acne and other facial eruptions. *Medicine* 1997;25:30–33.
4. Smithard A, Glazebrook C, Williams HC. Acne prevalence, knowledge about acne and psychological morbidity in mid-adolescence: a community-based study. *Br J Dermatol* 2001;145:274–279.
5. Pearl A, Arroll B, Lello J, et al. The impact of acne: a study of adolescents' attitudes, perception and knowledge. *N Z Med J* 1998;111:269–271.
6. Garner S. Acne vulgaris. In: Williams H. *Evidence-based dermatology*. London: BMJ, 2003.
7. Purdy S, Langston J, Tait L. Presentation and management of acne in primary care: a retrospective cohort study. *Br J Gen Pract* 2003;53:525–529.
8. Cunliffe WJ. Management of adult acne and acne variants. *J Cutan Med Surg* 1998;2(suppl 3):7–13.
9. Brown SK, Shalita AR. Acne vulgaris. *Lancet* 1998:351:1871–1876.
10. Webster GF. Acne vulgaris: state of the science. *Arch Dermatol* 1999;135:1101–1102.
11. Cunliffe WJ. Doctors should not change the way they prescribe for acne. *BMJ* 1996;312:1101.
12. Burke BM, Cunliffe WJ. The assessment of acne vulgaris – the Leeds technique. *Br J Dermatol* 1984;111:83–92.
13. Cook CH, Centner RL, Michaels SE. An acne grading method using photographic standards. *Arch Dermatol* 1979;115:571–575.
14. Pillsbury DM, Shelley WB, Kligman AM. *A manual of cutaneous medicine 1961*. Philadelphia, Saunders.
15. Lehmann HP, Andrews JS, Robinson KA, et al. Management of acne (Evidence Report/Technology Assessment No 17). Agency for Healthcare Research and Quality Publication No 01-E019. Rockville, MD. Agency for Healthcare Research and Quality, 2001. Search date 1999, primary sources Central, Pubmed, Medline, Healthstar, Psychinfo, Cinahl, hand searches, inclusion criteria: management of acne, English language, human data, prospective controlled, randomised/quasi-randomised allocation.
16. Cunliffe WJ, Holland KT. Clinical and laboratory studies on treatment with 20% azelaic acid cream for acne. *Acta Derm Venereol Suppl (Stockh)* 1989;143:31–34.
17. Katsambus A, Graupe K, Stratigos J. Clinical studies of 20% azelaic acid cream in the treatment of acne vulgaris. Comparison with vehicle and topical tretinoin. *Acta Derm Venereol Suppl (Stockh)* 1989;143:35–39.
18. Graupe K, Cunliffe WJ, Gollnick HP, et al. Efficacy and safety of topical azelaic acid (20% cream): an overview of results from European clinical trials and experimental reports. *Cutis* 1996;57(Suppl 1):20–35.
19. Ede M. A double-blind comparative study of benzoyl peroxide, benzoyl peroxide–chlorhydroxyquinolone, benzoyl peroxide–chlorhydroxyquinolone–hydrocortisone, and placebo lotions in acne. *Curr Ther Res Clin Exp* 1973;15:624–629.
20. Lookingbill DP, Chalker DK, Lindholm JS, et al. Treatment of acne with a combination clindamycin/benzoyl peroxide gel compared with clindamycin gel, benzoyl peroxide gel and vehicle gel: combined results of two double-blind investigations. *J Am Acad Dermatol* 1997;37:590–595.
21. Hunt MJ, Barnetson RS. A comparative study of gluconolactone versus benzoyl peroxide in the treatment of acne. *Australas J Dermatol* 1992;33:131–134.
22. Hughes BR, Norris JF, Cunliffe WJ. A double-blind evaluation of topical isotretinoin 0.05%, benzoyl peroxide gel 5% and placebo in patients with acne. *Clin Exp Dermatol* 1992;17:165–168.
23. Smith EB, Padilla RS, McCabe JM, et al. Benzoyl peroxide lotion (20 percent) in acne. *Cutis* 1980;25:90–92.
24. Lucky A, Jorizzo JL, Rodriguez D, et al. Efficacy and tolerance of adapalene cream 0.1% compared with its cream vehicle for the treatment of acne vulgaris. *Cutis* 2001;68:34–40.
25. Pinnock CB, Alderman CP. The potential for teratogenicity of vitamin A and its congeners. *Med J Australia* 1992;157:805–809.
26. Chalker DK, Lesher JL Jr, Smith JG Jr, et al. Efficacy of topical isotretinoin 0.05% gel in acne vulgaris: results of a multicenter, double-blind investigation. *J Am Acad Dermatol* 1987;17:251–254.
27. Langner A, Boorman GC, Stapor V, et al. Isotretinoin cream 0.05% and 0.1% in the treatment of acne vulgaris. *J Dermatol Treat* 1994;5:177–180.
28. Glass D, Boorman GC, Stables GI, et al. A placebo-controlled clinical trial to compare a gel containing a combination of isotretinoin (0.05%) and erythromycin (2%) with gels containing isotretinoin

(0.05%) or erythromycin (2%) alone in the topical treatment of acne vulgaris. *Dermatology* 1999;199:242–247.
29. Christiansen JV, Gadborg E, Ludvigsen K, et al. Topical tretinoin, vitamin A acid (Airol) in acne vulgaris: a controlled clinical trial. *Dermatologica* 1974;148:82–89.
30. Christiansen J, Holm P, Reymann F. The retinoic acid derivative Ro 11–1430 in acne vulgaris: a controlled multicenter trial against retinoic acid. *Dermatologica* 1977;154:219–227.
31. Krishnan G. Comparison of two concentrations of tretinoin solution in the topical treatment of acne vulgaris. *Practitioner* 1976;216:106–109.
32. Lucky AW, Cullen SI, Jarratt MT, et al. Comparative efficacy and safety of two 0.025% tretinoin gels: results from a multicenter double-blind, parallel study. *J Am Acad Dermatol* 1998;38:S17–S23.
33. Lucky AW, Cullen SI, Funicella T, et al. Double-blind, vehicle-controlled, multicenter comparison of two 0.025% tretinoin creams in patients with acne vulgaris. *J Am Acad Dermatol* 1998;38:S24–S30.
34. Braathen LR. Topical clindamycin versus oral tetracycline and placebo in acne vulgaris. *Scand J Infect Dis Suppl* 1984;43:71–75.
35. Ellis CN, Gammon WR, Stone DZ, et al. A comparison of Cleocin T Solution, Cleocin T Gel, and placebo in the treatment of acne vulgaris. *Cutis* 1988;42:245–247.
36. Lucchina LC, Kollias N, Gillies R, et al. Fluorescence photography in the evaluation of acne. *J Am Acad Dermatol* 1996;35:58–63.
37. Gratton D, Raymond GP, Guertin-Larochelle S, et al. Topical clindamycin versus systemic tetracycline in the treatment of acne. Results of a multiclinic trial. *J Am Acad Dermatol* 1982;7:50–53.
38. Becker LE, Bergstresser PR, Whiting DA, et al. Topical clindamycin therapy for acne vulgaris. A cooperative clinical study. *Arch Dermatol* 1981;117:482–485.
39. Kuhlman DS, Callen JP. A comparison of clindamycin phosphate 1 percent topical lotion and placebo in the treatment of acne vulgaris. *Cutis* 1986;38:203–206.
40. Noble WC, Naidoo J. Evolution of antibiotic resistance in *Staphylococcus aureus*: the role of the skin. *Br J Dermatol* 1978;98:481–489.
41. Lesher JL Jr, Chalker DK, Smith JG Jr, et al. An evaluation of a 2% erythromycin ointment in the topical therapy of acne vulgaris. *J Am Acad Dermatol* 1985;12:526–531.
42. Pochi PE, Bagatell FK, Ellis CN, et al. Erythromycin 2% gel in the treatment of acne vulgaris. *Cutis* 1988;41:132–136.
43. Jones EL, Crumley AF. Topical erythromycin vs blank vehicle in a multiclinic acne study. *Arch Dermatol* 1981;117:551–553.
44. Dobson RL, Belknap BS. Topical erythromycin solution in acne. Results of a multiclinic trial. *J Am Acad Dermatol* 1980;3:478–482.
45. Rivkin L, Rapaport M. Clinical evaluation of a new erythromycin solution for acne vulgaris. *Cutis* 1980;25:552–555.
46. Hellgren L, Vincent J. Topical erythromycin for acne vulgaris. *Dermatologica* 1980;161:409–414.
47. Prince RA, Busch DA, Hepler CD, et al. Clinical trial of topical erythromycin in inflammatory acne. *Drug Intell Clin Pharm* 1981;15:372–376.
48. Feucht CL, Allen BS, Chalker DK, et al. Topical erythromycin with zinc in acne. A double-blind controlled study. *J Am Acad Dermatol* 1980;3:483–491.
49. Schachner L, Eaglestein W, Kittles C, et al. Topical erythromycin and zinc therapy for acne. *J Am Acad Dermatol* 1990;22:253–260.
50. Knutson DD, Swinyer LJ, Smoot WH. Meclocycline sulfosalicylate. Topical antibiotic agent for the treatment of acne vulgaris. *Cutis* 1981;27:203–204, 208–210.
51. Blaney DJ, Cook CH. Topical use of tetracycline in the treatment of acne: a double-blind study comparing topical and oral tetracycline therapy and placebo. *Arch Dermatol* 1976;112:971–973.
52. Anderson RL, Cook CH, Smith DE. The effect of oral and topical tetracycline on acne severity and on surface lipid composition. *J Invest Dermatol* 1976;66:172–177.
53. Smith JG Jr, Chalker DK, Wehr RF. The effectiveness of topical and oral tetracycline for acne. *South Med J* 1976;69:695–697.
54. Burton J. A placebo-controlled study to evaluate the efficacy of topical tetracycline and oral tetracycline in the treatment of mild to moderate acne. Dermatology Research Group. *J Int Med Res* 1990;18:94–103.
55. Skidmore, R, Kovach R, Walker C, et al. Effects of subantimicrobial-dose doxycycline in the treatment of moderate acne. *Arch Dermatol* 2003;139:459–464.
56. Plewig G, Petrozzi JW, Berendes U. A double-blind study of doxycycline in acne vulgaris. *Arch Dermatol* 1970;101:435–438.
57. Bleeker J, Hellgren L, Vincent J. Effect of systemic erythromycin stearate on the inflammatory lesions and skin surface fatty acids in acne vulgaris. *Dermatologica* 1981;162:342–349.
58. Juhlin L, Liden S. A quantitative evaluation of the effect of oxytetracycline and doxycycline in acne vulgaris. *Br J Dermatol* 1969;81:154–158.
59. The National Prescribing Centre. The treatment of acne vulgaris: an update. *MeReC Bulletin* 1999;10:29–32.
60. Sanchez AR, Rogers RS, Sheridan PJ. Tetracycline and other tetracycline-derivative staining of the teeth and oral cavity. *Int J Dermatol* 2004;43:709–715.
61. Brandt H, Attila P, Ahokas T, et al. Erythromycin acistrate – an alternative treatment for acne. *J Dermatol Treat* 1994;5:3–5.
62. Gammon WR, Meyer C, Lantis S, et al. Comparative efficacy of oral erythromycin versus oral tetracycline in the treatment of acne vulgaris. A double-blind study. *J Am Acad Dermatol* 1986;14:183–186.
63. Al-Mishari MA. Clinical and bacteriological evaluation of tetracycline and erythromycin in acne vulgaris. *Clin Ther* 1987;9:273–280.
64. Garner SE, Eady EA, Popescu C, et al. Minocycline for acne vulgaris: efficacy and safety. (Cochrane Review). In: The Cochrane Library, Issue 2, 2003. Oxford: Update Software. Search date 2002, primary sources Medline, Embase, Biosis, Biological abstracts, International Pharmaceutical Abstracts, Cochrane Skin Group's Trial Register, Theses Online, Bids, hand searches, inclusion criteria: RCTs comparing minocycline with active/placebo in acne.
65. Schlienger RG, Bircher AJ, Meier CR. Minocycline-induced lupus. A systematic review. *Dermatology* 2000;200:223–231. Search date 1999, primary sources Medline, Embase, hand searches, inclusion criteria: participants to have developed minocycline induced systemic lupus erythematosus.
66. Lawrenson RA, Seaman HE, Sundstrom A, et al. Liver damage associated with minocycline use in acne: a systematic review of the published literature and pharmacovigilance data. *Drug Saf* 2000;23:333–349. Search date 1998, primary sources Medline, Cinahl, The Cochrane Library, Embase, Current Contents, Toxline, Bids, hand searches, pharmaceutical and WHO adverse events databases, inclusion criteria: participants to have developed liver damage from taking minocycline for acne.
67. Goulden V, Glass D, Cunliffe WJ. Safety of long-term high-dose minocycline in the treatment of acne. *Br J Dermatol* 1996;134:693–695.
68. Sturkenboom MC, Meier CR, Jick H, et al. Minocycline and lupuslike syndrome in acne patients. *Arch Intern Med* 1999;159:493–497.
69. Heslett C, Chilvers ER, Boon NA, et al. *Davidsons principals and practices of medicine*. 2002, Churchill Livingstone, London.

70. Cooper AJ. Systematic review of *Propionibacterium acnes* resistance to systemic antibiotics. *Med J Aust* 1998;169:259–261. Search date 1998, primary sources Medline, Embase, hand searches, inclusion criteria: English language, *Proprionibacterium acnes* resistance patterns.
71. Lane P, Williamson DM. Treatment of acne vulgaris with tetracycline hydrochloride: a double-blind trial with 51 patients. *BMJ* 1969;2:76–79.
72. Wong RC, Kang S, Heezen JL, et al. Oral ibuprofen and tetracycline for the treatment of acne vulgaris. *J Am Acad Dermatol* 1984;11:1076–1081.

Sarah Purdy
Honorary Clinical Senior Lecturer in Primary Health Care
University of Newcastle
Newcastle upon Tyne
UK

Competing interests: None declared.

Athlete's foot

Search date December 2003

Fay Crawford

QUESTIONS

INTERVENTIONS

Key Messages

- **Topical allylamines** One systematic review and four subsequent RCTs have found that allylamines are more effective than placebo for curing fungal skin infections. The review found insufficient evidence comparing different allylamines versus one another. It found that topical allylamines increased cure rates at 3–12 weeks compared with azoles. We found no evidence on recurrence rates after clinical cure.
- **Topical azoles** One systematic review has found that azole creams administered for 4–6 weeks increase cure rates compared with placebo. We found no RCTs evaluating differences between individual azoles. It found that topical azoles were less effective than topical allylamines in increasing cure rates at 3–12 weeks. We found no evidence on recurrence rates after clinical cure.
- **Improved foot hygiene, including socks, and hosiery** We found no systematic review or RCTs on the effects of foot hygiene and hosiery in the treatment of athlete's foot.

DEFINITION Athlete's foot is a cutaneous fungal infection caused by dermatophyte infection. It is characterised by itching, flaking, and fissuring of the skin. It may manifest in three ways: the skin between the toes may appear mascerated (white) and soggy; the soles of the feet may become dry and scaly; and the skin all over the foot may become red, and vesicular eruptions may appear.[1] It is conventional in dermatology to refer to fungal skin infections as superficial in order to distinguish them from systemic fungal infections.

INCIDENCE/ PREVALENCE Epidemiological studies have produced various estimates of the prevalence of athlete's foot. Studies are usually conducted in populations of people who attend dermatology clinics, sports centres or swimming pools, or who are in the military. UK estimates suggest that athlete's foot is present in about 15% of the general population.[2] Studies conducted in dermatology clinics in Italy[3] and China (1014 people)[4] found prevalences of 25% and 27%, respectively. A population based study conducted in Israel found the prevalence among children to be 30%.[5]

AETIOLOGY/ RISK FACTORS Swimming pool users and industrial workers may be at increased risk of fungal foot infection. However, one survey identified fungal foot infection in only 9% of swimmers, with the highest prevalence (20%) being in men aged 16 years and older.[2]

PROGNOSIS Fungal infections of the foot are not life threatening in people with normal immune status, but in some people they cause persistent itching and, ultimately, fissuring. Other patients are apparently unaware of persistent infection. The infection can spread to other parts of the body and to other individuals.

AIMS OF INTERVENTION To control symptoms and prevent recurrence, with minimal adverse effects.

OUTCOMES Rates of fungal eradication, shown by negative microscopy and culture, and resolution of clinical signs and symptoms at follow up. We have chosen mycological cure as a primary outcome. Clinical cure is not coherently reported in superficial mycology trials.[6] Like many other diagnostic tests, microscopy and culture are not absolutely accurate. There are several reasons why fungal infections can be missed in laboratory tests.[7] Microscopy and culture are the most frequently used outcomes in athlete's foot research to establish the effect of an intervention.

METHODS *Clinical Evidence* search and appraisal December 2003. We initially searched Medline, Embase, and the Cochrane Controlled Trials Register to May 2003 for systematic reviews and subsequent RCTs (all languages). Studies were excluded if foot specific data could not be extracted. We excluded studies that did not use microscopy and culture (skin infections) or culture (nail infections) for diagnosis and as an outcome measure.

QUESTION What are the effects of topical treatments for athlete's foot?

OPTION TOPICAL ALLYLAMINES (NAFTIFINE, TERBINAFINE)

One systematic review and four subsequent RCTs have found that allylamines are more effective than placebo for curing fungal skin infections. The review found insufficient evidence comparing different allylamines versus one another. It found that topical allylamines increased cure rates at 3–12 weeks compared with topical azoles. We found no evidence on recurrence rates after clinical cure.

Benefits: **Versus placebo:** We found one systematic review (search date 1997),[8,9] and four subsequent RCTs.[10–13] The systematic review (12 RCTs, 1433 people with fungal infections of the foot) found that topical allylamines for 1–4 weeks significantly increased the cure rate, as assessed by culture or microscopy after 6–8 weeks, compared with placebo (at 6 weeks: 532/724 [73%] with allylamines *v* 139/709 [20%] with placebo; RR 3.7, 95% CI 3.2 to 4.4).[8,9] The first subsequent RCT (70 people with interdigital tinea pedis and positive fungal culture) found increased cure rates at 7 weeks after 7 days of treatment with 1% terbinafine cream compared with placebo (mycological cure: 91% with terbinafine *v* 37% with placebo; CI not reported; $P < 0.001$).[10] The second subsequent RCT (60 people with moccasin type tinea pedis**G**) compared three interventions: 1% terbinafine cream, 1% butenafine (a benzylamine derivative) cream, and placebo.[11] People receiving butenafine applied the cream for 1 week, whereas terbinafine and placebo were applied for 2 weeks. The RCT found higher cure rates after 2 weeks with butenafine or terbinafine than with placebo (18/20 [90%] with butenafine *v* 16/20 [80%] with terbinafine *v* 2/20 [10%] with placebo; active treatment *v* placebo P < 0.001). The third subsequent RCT (153 people with interdigital tinea pedis) found significantly higher cure rates with a 1% solution of terbinafine than with placebo after 8 weeks (35/54 [65%] with terbinafine *v* 1/23 [4%] with placebo; RR 14.9, 95% CI 2.2 to 102.3; NNT 2, 95% CI 1.3 to 2.2; figures calculated from graph data).[12] The fourth subsequent RCT (70 people with interdigital tinea pedis) compared 1% terbinafine emulsion gel applied for 7 days versus placebo.[13] It found significantly higher cure rates with 1% terbinafine gel than with placebo at 8 weeks (25/31 [80%] with terbinafine *v* 7/21 [33%] with placebo; RR 2.14, 95% CI 1.3 to 4.5; NNT 3, 95% CI 2 to 5). **Different allylamines:** The systematic review identified one small RCT (60 people), which found no significant difference in cure rates between naftifine and terbinafine (75% with naftifine *v* 81% with terbinafine; ARR +5%, 95% CI –17% to +21%).[8,9] **Versus topical azoles:** See benefits of topical azoles, p 2062.

Harms: None were reported in the systematic review.[8,9] The first subsequent RCT comparing terbinafine versus placebo reported six adverse events, three in the placebo group and three in the terbinafine group.[10] The second RCT did not describe adverse effects.[11] The third RCT found that adverse effects did not significantly differ between terbinafine and placebo (adverse effects: 16/105 [15%] with terbinafine *v* 5/48 [10%] with placebo; RR 1.46, 95% CI 0.57 to 3.76).[12] The nature of these adverse effects was not described in those reports. The fourth subsequent RCT comparing terbinafine versus placebo concluded that both were well tolerated, but some mild to moderate skin reactions and rashes were reported.[13]

Comment: We found no evidence on recurrence rates after clinical cure. One of the subsequent RCTs included multiple comparisons between groups.[11] No apparent adjustment for multiple comparisons was made to reduce the risk of false positive findings.

OPTION TOPICAL AZOLES (CLOTRIMAZOLE, MICONAZOLE NITRATE, TIOCONAZOLE, SULCONAZOLE NITRATE, BIFONAZOLE, ECONAZOLE NITRATE)

One systematic review has found that azole creams administered for 4–6 weeks increase cure rates compared with placebo. We found no RCTs evaluating differences between individual azoles. It found that topical azoles were less effective than topical allylamines in increasing cure rates at 3–12 weeks. We found no evidence on recurrence rates after clinical cure.

Benefits: We found one systematic review (search date 1997).[8,9] **Versus placebo:** The review identified 17 RCTs (1259 people with fungal skin infections of the foot).[8,9] Interventions lasted for 4–6 weeks. The review found that treatment with azoles resulted in a significant increase in cure rate, as determined by culture or microscopy, compared with placebo after 6–10 weeks (cure: 538/664 [81%] with azoles *v* 233/595 [39%] with placebo; RR 2.1, 95% CI 1.85 to 2.3). **Different azoles:** The review found no significant difference between individual azoles administered for 3–4 weeks.[8,9] **Versus topical allylamines:** The review identified 12 RCTs (1487 people with fungal infections of the foot).[8,9] We found two additional RCTs.[14,15] The review compared 1–6 weeks' treatment with topical allylamines versus at least 4 weeks' treatment with topical azoles.[8,9] It found that topical allylamines significantly increased cure rates at 3–12 weeks compared with topical azoles (627/773 [81%] with topical allylamines *v* 490/714 [69%] with topical azoles; RR 2.6, 95% CI 2.3 to 2.9). No significant difference was found in cure rates between a 1 week course of allylamine and a 4 week course of azole (411/464 [85%] with 1 week of allylamine *v* 377/448 [84%] with 4 weeks of azole; RR 1.0, 95% CI 0.99 to 1.10).[8,9] The first additional RCT (429 people with interdigital athlete's foot) found no significant difference in cure rates after 8 weeks with twice daily application of 1% terbinafine solution followed by 3 weeks of placebo compared with 4 weeks of 1% clotrimazole solution (73% with terbinafine *v* 72% with clotrimazole; ARR +1%, 95% CI –5% to +8%).[14] The second additional RCT (48 people) also found no significant difference in number of treatment failures after 10 weeks between 1 week of treatment with 1% terbinafine cream and 4 weeks of treatment with 2% clotrimazole cream (ARR +2%, 95% CI –33% to +28%).[15]

Harms: The second additional RCT found similar adverse events with 1% terbinafine solution and 1% clotrimazole solution.[15] About 5% of the people experienced mild to moderate local skin reactions, such as itching, erythema, or scaling.

Comment: We found no evidence on recurrence rates after clinical cure. Wide confidence intervals and variations in follow up make it difficult to establish clinical equivalence between different azoles.[8,9]

OPTION SOCKS, STOCKINGS, FOOT HYGIENE

We found no systematic review or RCTs on the effects of foot hygiene and hosiery in the treatment of athlete's foot.

Benefits: We found no systematic review or RCTs.

Harms: We found no RCTs.

Comment: Evidence from the placebo arms of RCTs suggests that improved foot hygiene can achieve mycological cure in some patients.[16]

GLOSSARY

Moccasin type tinea pedis A skin fungal infection causing the entire sole of the foot to appear dry and scaly.

REFERENCES

1. Springett K, Merriman L. Assessment of the skin and its appendages. In: Merriman L, Tollafield D, eds. *The assessment of the lower limb*. New York: Churchill Livingstone, 1995:191–225.
2. Gentles JC, Evans EGV. Foot infections in swimming baths. *BMJ* 1973;3:260–262.
3. Aste N, Pau M, Aste N, et al. Tinea pedis observed in Cagliari, Italy, between 1996 and 2000. *Mycoses* 2003;46:38–41.
4. Cheng S, Chong L. A prospective epidemiological study on tinea pedis and onychomycosis in Hong Kong. *Chin Med J (Engl)* 2002;115:860–865.
5. Leibovici V, Evron R, Dunchin M, et al. Population-based epidemiologic study of tinea pedis in Israeli children. *Pediatr Infect Dis J* 2002;21:851–854.
6. Crawford F, Young P, Godfrey C, et al. Oral treatments for toenail onychomycosis. *Arch Dermatol* 2002;138:811–815.
7. Daniel CR, Elewski BE. The diagnosis of nail fungus infection revisited. *Arch Dermatol* 2000; 136:1162–1164.
8. Crawford F, Hart R, Bell-Syer S, et al. Topical treatments for fungal infections of the skin and nails of the foot. In: The Cochrane Library, Issue 3, 2001. Oxford: Update Software. Search date 1997; primary sources Medline, Embase, Cinahl, Cochrane Controlled Trials Register, Science Citation Index, Biosis, CAB-Health, Healthstar, DARE, the NHS Economic Evaluation Database, Econlit, hand searched references and key journals, and pharmaceutical companies contacted.
9. Hart R, Bell-Syer EM, Crawford F, et al. Systematic review of topical treatments for fungal infections of the skin and nails of the feet. *BMJ* 1999;319:79–82. Search date 1997; primary sources Medline, Embase, Cinahl, Cochrane Controlled Trials Register, Science Citation Index, Biosis, CAB-Health, Healthstar, DARE, the NHS Economic Evaluation Database, Econlit, hand searched references and key journals, and pharmaceutical companies contacted.
10. Korting HC, Tietz HJ, Brautigam M. One week terbinafine 1% cream (Lamisil) once daily is effective in the treatment of interdigital tinea pedis: a vehicle controlled study. LAS-INT-06 Study Group. *Med Mycol* 2000;39:335–340.

11. Syed TA, Hadi SM, Quereshi ZA, et al. Butenafine 1% versus terbinafine 1% in cream for the treatment of tinea pedis. A placebo controlled double-blind comparative study. *Clin Drug Invest* 2000;19:393–397.
12. Lebwohl M, Elewski B, Eisen D, et al. Efficacy and safety of terbinafine 1% solution in the treatment of interdigital tinea pedis and tinea corporis or tinea cruris. *Cutis* 2001;67:261–266.
13. Hollmen KA, Kinnunen T, Kiilstala U, et al. Efficacy and tolerability of terbinafine 1% emulsion gel in patients with tinea pedis [letter]. *Eur Acad Dermatol Venereol* 2002;16:87.
14. Schopf R, Hettler O, Brautigam M, et al. Efficacy and tolerability of terbinafine 1% topical solution used for 1 week compared with 4 weeks clotrimazole 1% topical solution in the treatment of interdigital tinea pedis: a randomised controlled clinical trial. *Mycoses* 1999;42:415–420.
15. Leenutaphong V, Tangwiwat S, Muanprasat C, et al. Double-blind study of the efficacy of 1 week topical terbinafine cream compared to 4 weeks miconazole cream in patients with tinea pedis. *J Med Assoc Thai* 1999;82:1006–1009.
16. Crawford F. Athletes foot. In: Williams H, Bigby M, Diepgen T, eds. *Evidence based dermatology*. London: BMJ Publishing Group, 2003.

Fay Crawford
Senior Research Fellow
University of Dundee
Dundee
UK

Competing interests: None declared.

Cellulitis and erysipelas

Search date May 2004

Andrew Morris

QUESTIONS

INTERVENTIONS

Key Messages

- **Antibiotics** We found no RCTs comparing antibiotics versus placebo. RCTs comparing different antibiotic regimens found clinical cure in 50–100% of people.
- **Comparative effects of different antibiotic regimens** RCTs provided insufficient information on differences between regimens. However, most of the RCTs included only a small number of people with cellulitis or erysipelas, and were designed to test equivalence rather than to detect a clinically significant difference in cure rates between antibiotics.
- **Oral versus intravenous antibiotics** We found no satisfactory RCTs comparing oral antibiotics versus intravenous antibiotics.
- **Short versus long courses of antibiotics** We found no RCTs comparing different durations of antibiotics.
- **Treatment of predisposing factors to prevent recurrence** We found no RCTs or observational studies on the effects of treating predisposing factors for recurrence of cellulitis or erysipelas.

Cellulitis and erysipelas

DEFINITION **Cellulitis** is a spreading bacterial infection of the dermis and subcutaneous tissues. It causes local signs of inflammation such as warmth, erythema, pain, lymphangitis, and frequently systemic upset with fever and raised white blood cell count. **Erysipelas** is a form of cellulitis and is characterised by pronounced superficial inflammation. The lower limbs are by far the most common sites, but any area can be affected. The term erysipelas is commonly used when the face is affected.

INCIDENCE/ PREVALENCE We found no specific data on the incidence of cellulitis, but cellulitis and abscess infections were responsible for 158 consultations per 10 000 person years in the UK in 1991.[1] In 1985 in the UK, skin and subcutaneous tissue infections resulted in 29 820 hospital admissions and a mean occupancy of 664 hospital beds each day.[2]

AETIOLOGY/ RISK FACTORS The most common infective organisms for cellulitis and erysipelas in adults are streptococci (particularly *Streptococcus pyogenes*) and *Staphylococcus aureus*.[3] In children, *Haemophilus influenzae* was a frequent cause prior to the introduction of the HiB vaccination. Several risk factors for cellulitis and erysipelas have been identified in a case control study (167 cases and 294 controls): lymphoedema (OR 71.2, 95% CI 5.6 to 908.0), leg ulcer (OR 62.5, 95% CI 7.0 to 556.0), toe web intertrigo (OR 13.9, 95% CI 7.2 to 27.0), and traumatic wounds (OR 10.7, 95% CI 4.8 to 23.8).[4]

PROGNOSIS Cellulitis can spread through the bloodstream and lymphatic system. A retrospective case study of people admitted to hospital with cellulitis found that systemic symptoms such as fever and raised white blood cell count were present in up to 42% of cases at presentation.[5] Lymphatic involvement can lead to obstruction and damage of the lymphatic system that predisposes to recurrent cellulitis. Recurrence can occur rapidly or after months or years. One study found that 29% of people with erysipelas had a recurrent episode within 3 years.[6] Local necrosis and abscess formation can also occur. It is not known whether the prognosis of erysipelas differs from that of cellulitis. We found no evidence about factors that predict recurrence, or a better or worse outcome. We found no good evidence on the prognosis of untreated cellulitis.

AIMS OF INTERVENTION To reduce the severity and duration of infection; to relieve pain and systemic symptoms; to restore the skin to its premorbid state; to prevent recurrence; to minimise adverse effects of treatment.

OUTCOMES Duration and severity of symptoms (pain, swelling, erythema, and fever); clinical cure (defined as the absence of pain, swelling, and erythema); recurrence; adverse effects of treatment. We found no standard scales of severity in cellulitis or erysipelas.

METHODS *Clinical Evidence* search and appraisal May 2004, including a search for observational studies.

QUESTION What are the effects of treatments?

OPTION ANTIBIOTICS

We found no RCTs comparing antibiotics versus placebo or different durations of treatment, and no satisfactory RCTs comparing oral versus intravenous antibiotics. RCTs comparing different antibiotic regimens found clinical cure in 50–100% of people but provided insufficient information on differences between regimens. However, most of the RCTs included only a small number of people with cellulitis or erysipelas, and were designed to test equivalence rather than to detect a clinically significant difference in cure rates between antibiotics.

Benefits: We found no systematic review. **Versus placebo:** We found no RCTs. **Oral versus intravenous antibiotics:** We found no satisfactory RCTs (see comment below). **Different antibiotic regimens:** We found nine RCTs comparing different antibiotic regimens in people with various skin infections (see table 1, p 2069).[7–15] Two of the RCTs were conducted solely in people with moderate to severe cellulitis;[7,8] one RCT was conducted solely in people with erysipelas;[9] and the other six RCTs were conducted in people with a range of skin infections and provided subgroup analysis of people with cellulitis or erysipelas.[10–15] Eight of the RCTs and the subgroup analyses found no significant difference between different antibiotics in clinical cure after 4–30 days.[7,9–15] However, most of the RCTs included only small numbers of people with cellulitis or erysipelas and were designed to test equivalence rather than to detect a clinically significant difference in cure rates between antibiotics. One of the RCTs conducted solely in people with cellulitis (58 people with moderate to severe cellulitis) found that intravenous ceftriaxone significantly increased clinical cure after 4–6 days compared with intravenous flucloxacillin. The results of this study should be treated with caution since only 45 people (78%) completed the study, and it would not appear that an intention to treat analysis was performed.[7] **Short versus long courses of antibiotics:** We found no RCTs comparing different durations of antibiotics.

Harms: **Oral versus intravenous antibiotics:** In a quasi-randomised trial (73 people with erysipelas, see comment below) comparing oral versus intravenous penicillin, adverse events occurred in 15 people taking oral penicillin (rash 4, diarrhoea 7, abscess 4) and in 10 people taking intravenous penicillin (rash 2, diarrhoea 4, cannula phlebitis 4).[16] The RCT comparing flucloxacillin versus ceftriaxone (58 people with moderate to severe cellulitis) found no significant difference in the proportion of people experiencing adverse effects including diarrhoea, nausea and vomiting, abdominal pain, and vaginal candidiasis (6/22 [27%] with flucloxacillin *v* 3/22 [14%] with ceftriaxone; RR 2.00, 95% CI 0.57 to 7.00).[7] **Different antibiotic regimens:** The RCTs found no evidence of a difference in rates of adverse events with different antibiotic regimens. The RCT comparing cefazolin plus probenecid versus ceftriaxone plus placebo (134 people with moderate to severe cellulitis) found no significant difference in the proportion of people who experienced adverse effects, including nausea and vomiting, diarrhoea, headache, and dizziness (14/67 [21%] with cefazolin plus probenecid *v* 7/67 [10%] with ceftriaxone plus placebo; RR 2.00, 95% CI 0.86 to 4.64).[8] The RCT comparing penicillin versus roxithromycin (69 people with erysipelas) found no significant difference in the proportion of people experiencing drug related rashes (2/38 [5%] with penicillin *v* 0/31 [0%] people with roxithromycin).[9] The RCTs comparing different antibiotics in a variety of skin infections gave no discrete information about adverse effects in people with cellulitis.[10–15]

Comment: **Oral versus intravenous antibiotics:** One small quasi-randomised trial (73 people with erysipelas in hospital with a body temperature > 38.5 °C but excluding patients with clinical signs of septicaemia; alternate allocation design) comparing oral versus intravenous penicillin found no significant difference in clinical efficacy, which was assessed by indirect measures such as temperature fall, length of hospital stay, and absence from work.[16] No results were provided on relapse rates.

OPTION **TREATMENT OF PREDISPOSING FACTORS TO PREVENT RECURRENCE**

We found no RCTs or observational studies on the effects of treatment of predisposing factors for recurrence of cellulitis or erysipelas.

Benefits: We found no systematic review, RCTs, or observational studies.

Harms: We found no systematic review, RCTs, or observational studies.

Comment: Although there is a consensus that successful treatment of predisposing factors, such as lymphoedema, leg ulcers, toe web intertrigo and traumatic wounds, reduces the risk of developing cellulitis or erysipelas (see aetiology, p 2066), we found no RCTs or observational studies to support or refute this.

REFERENCES

1. Office of Population Censuses and Surveys. *Morbidity statistics from general practice*. Fourth National Study. London: HMSO (series MB5), 1992, 272.
2. Department of Health, Department of Health and Social Security. *Hospital in-patient enquiry*. London: HMSO (series MB4), 1985, 16, 28.
3. Bernard P, Bedane C, Mounier M, et al. Streptococcal cause of erysipelas and cellulitis in adults. *Arch Dermatol* 1989;125:779–782.
4. Dupuy A, Benchikhi H, Roujeau J-C, et al. Risk factors for erysipelas of the leg (cellulitis): case-control study. *BMJ* 1999;318:1591–1594.
5. Aly AA, Roberts NM, Seipol K, et al. Case survey of management of cellulitis in a tertiary teaching hospital. *Med J Aust* 1996;165:553–556.
6. Jorup-Ronstrom C, Britton S. Recurrent erysipelas: predisposing factors and costs, of prophylaxis. *Infection* 1987;15:105–106.
7. Vinen J, Hudson B, Chan B, et al. A randomized comparative study of once-daily ceftriaxone and 6-hourly flucioxacilin in the treatment of moderate to severe cellulitis. Clinical efficacy, safety and pharmacoeconomic implications. *Clin Drug Invest* 1996;12:221–225.
8. Grayson ML, McDonald M, Gibson K, et al. Once-daily intravenous cefazolin plus oral probenecid is equivalent to once-daily ceftriaxone plus oral placebo for the treatment of moderate-to-severe cellulitis in adults. *Clin Infect Dis* 2002;34:1440–1448.
9. Bernard P, Plantin P, Roger H, et al. Roxithromycin versus penicillin in the treatment of erysipelas in adults: a comparative study. *Br J Dermatol* 1992;127:155–159.
10. Daniel R, Austad J, Debersaques J, et al. Azithromycin, erythromycin and cloxacillin in the treatment of infections of skin and associated soft tissues. *J Int Med Res* 1991;19:433–445.
11. Kiani R. Double-blind, double-dummy comparison of azithromycin and cephalexin in the treatment of skin and skin structure infections. *Eur J Clin Microbiol Infect Dis* 1991;10:880–884.
12. Tack KJ, Littlejohn TW, Mailloux G, et al. Cefdinir versus cephalexin for the treatment of skin and skin-structure infections. *Clin Ther* 1998;20:244–255.
13. Tassler H. Comparative efficacy and safety of oral fleroxacin and amoxicillin/clavulanate potassium in skin and soft tissue infections. *Am J Med* 1993;94:159S–165S.
14. Parish LC, Jungkind DL. Systemic anti-microbial therapy for skin and skin structure infections: comparison of fleroxacin and ceftazidime. *Am J Med* 1993;94:166S–173S.
15. Chan JC. Ampicillin-sulbactam versus cefazolin or cefoxitin in the treatment of skin and skin-structure infections of bacterial etiology. *Adv Ther* 1995;12:139–146.
16. Jorup-Ronstrom C, Britton A, Gavlevik K, et al. The course, costs and complications of oral versus intravenous penicillin therapy of erysipelas. *Infection* 1984;12:390–394.

Andrew Morris
Specialist Registrar in Dermatology
University Hospital of Wales, Cardiff, UK

Competing interests: None declared.

TABLE 1 **Different antibiotic regimens: results of comparative RCTs** **(see text, p 2066).**

Ref	Regimen	Participants	Clinical cure (significance)
7	iv ceftriaxone 1 g od for 7 days *v* iv flucloxacillin 1 g qds for a mean of 9 days	58 people with cellulitis	21/23 (92%) *v* 14/22 (64%) after 4–6 days (RR 1.43, 95% CI 1.02 to 2.02; NNT 4, 95% CI 2 to 17)
8	iv cefazolin 2 g od plus oral probenecid 1 g od *v* ceftriaxone 1 g od plus placebo for median 6–7 days	132 people with cellulitis	51/67 (76%) *v* 55/67 (82%) after 6–7 days (RR 0.93, 95% CI 0.78 to 1.10)
9	iv penicillin 2.5 MU 8 times daily followed by 6 MU orally od for mean 13 days *v* oral roxithromycin 150 mg bd for mean 13 days	69 people with erysipelas	29/38 (76%) *v* 26/31 (84%) after 30 days (RR 0.91, 95% CI 0.72 to 1.15)
10	Oral azithromycin total dose 1.5 g over 5 days *v* oral erythromycin 500 mg qds for 7 days	Subgroup analysis in 128 people with cellulitis	52/72 (72%) *v* 37/50 (74%) after 4–11 days (RR 0.97, 95% CI 0.78 to 1.21)
10	Oral azithromycin total dose 1.5 g over 5 days *v* oral cloxacillin 500 mg qds for 7 days	Subgroup analysis in 62 people with cellulitis	27/41 (66%) *v* 11/21 (52%) after 4–9 days (RR 1.26, 95% CI 0.79 to 2.00)
11	Oral azithromycin total dose 750 mg over 5 days *v* cefalexin 500 mg bd for 10 days	Subgroup analysis in 95 people with suspected cellulitis, 47 of whom had microbiologically proven cellulitis	12/24 (50%) *v* 14/23 (61%) after 11 days (RR 0.82, 95% CI 0.49 to 1.38)
12	Cefdinir 300 mg bd for 10 days *v* cefalexin 500 mg qds for 10 days	Subgroup analysis in 78 people with suspected cellulitis, 34 of whom had microbiologically proven cellulitis	In the 34 people with microbiologically proven cellulitis: 13/17 (76%) *v* 14/17 (82%) after 7–16 days (RR 0.93, 95% CI 0.66 to 1.31)
13	Oral amoxicillin/clavulanate potassium 125–500 mg tds *v* oral fleroxacin 400 mg od	Subgroup analysis in 11 people with cellulitis or erysipelas	7/7 (100%) *v* 4/4 (100%) after 3–9 days
14	iv fleroxacin 400 mg od *v* iv ceftazidime 0.52 g bd/tds	Subgroup analysis in 39 people with cellulitis	26/27 (96%) *v* 9/12 (75%) after 21 days (RR 1.28, 95% CI 0.92 to 1.78)
15	iv ampicillin/sulbactam 0.5–1 g qds *v* iv cefazolin 500 mg qds for 6–7 days	Subgroup analysis in 20 people with cellulitis	8/8 (100%) *v* 9/12 (75%) after 10 days

bd, twice daily; iv, intravenous; od, once daily; qds, four times daily; ref, reference; tds, three times daily.

Chronic plaque psoriasis

Search date June 2004

Luigi Naldi and Berthold Rzany

QUESTIONS

INTERVENTIONS

*Based on consensus.

See glossary G

Key Messages

- RCTs provided insufficient evidence on the effects of non-drug treatments for chronic plaque psoriasis.

Non-drug treatments

- **Acupuncture** One RCT provided insufficient evidence on the effects of acupuncture for chronic plaque psoriasis.
- **Balneotherapy** RCTs provided insufficient evidence on the effects of balneotherapy for chronic plaque psoriasis.
- **Fish oil supplementation** RCTs provided insufficient evidence on the effects of fish oil supplementation for chronic plaque psoriasis.

- **Heliotherapy** One RCT provided insufficient evidence on the effects of heliotherapy for chronic plaque psoriasis.
- **Psychotherapy** One RCT provided insufficient evidence on the effects of psychotherapy for chronic plaque psoriasis.
- **Sunbeds** One RCT provided insufficient evidence on the effects of sunbeds for chronic plaque psoriasis.

Topical treatments

- **Vitamin D derivatives** One systematic review found that topical vitamin D derivatives improved plaque psoriasis compared with placebo. Systematic reviews found no significant difference in effectiveness between topical vitamin D derivatives and "potent" topical steroids, but found that calcipotriol caused more perilesional and lesional irritation. One systematic review and one subsequent RCT found that topical vitamin D derivatives improved psoriasis at 4–12 weeks compared with dithranol, and caused fewer adverse effects. One systematic review found that calcipotriol improved psoriasis compared with coal tar, alone or in combination with allantoin and hydrocortisone. RCTs found that combination treatment with vitamin D derivatives plus "potent" topical steroids improved psoriasis compared with either treatment alone or with placebo. In the short term, the combination of vitamin D derivates plus topical steroids decreased irritation compared with monotherapy. RCTs provided insufficient evidence to assess other combination treatments containing topical vitamin D derivatives.
- **Dithranol** One systematic review of small RCTs found that dithranol improved chronic plaque psoriasis after 4–8 weeks compared with placebo. One systematic review of small RCTs found no significant difference between conventional and short contact dithranol treatment, but the RCTs may have lacked power to detect clinically relevant differences. One systematic review and one subsequent RCT found that dithranol was less effective than topical vitamin D derivatives and caused more adverse effects.
- **Topical retinoids (tazarotene)** RCTs found that tazarotene improved chronic plaque psoriasis in the short term compared with placebo. One RCT found no significant difference between tazarotene and fluocinonide in the reduction of lesion severity at 12 weeks. Three RCTs found that adding topical steroids to tazarotene treatment improved response rate compared with tazarotene treatment alone. One RCT found that combined topical steroid and tazarotene treatment increased the proportion of people with marked improvement compared with calcipotriol.
- **Topical steroids** One systematic review found that topical steroids, especially "potent" and "very potent" ones, improved psoriasis in the short term compared with placebo. Systematic reviews found no significant difference in effectiveness between "potent" topical steroids and vitamin D derivatives, but found that vitamin D derivatives caused more perilesional and lesional irritation. One RCT found no significant difference between fluocinomide and tazarotene in the reduction of lesion severity at 12 weeks. Topical steroids may cause striae and atrophy, which increase with potency and use of occlusive dressings. Continuous use may lead to adrenocortical suppression, and case reports suggest that severe flares of the disease may occur on withdrawal.
- **Emollients and keratolytics** RCTs provided insufficient evidence on the effects of emollients and keratolytics.
- **Tars** One small RCT identified by a systematic review provided insufficient evidence on the effects of coal tar compared with placebo. Small RCTs found conflicting results on the effects of tars in combination with ultraviolet B exposure or dithranol. One systematic review found that coal tar, alone or in combination with allantoin and hydrocortisone, was less effective than topical vitamin D derivatives (calcipotriol).

UV light

- **Psoralen plus ultraviolet A*** We found no systematic review or RCTs that compared psoriasis clearance with psoralen plus ultraviolet A versus no treatment. However, there is consensus that psoralen plus ultraviolet A is effective for clearance of psoriasis. One RCT found that psoralen plus ultraviolet A was more effective than the Ingram regimen in clearing psoriasis. One systematic review found that higher doses of psoralen improved psoriasis clearance more than lower doses of psoralen. One large RCT found that maintenance treatment with psoralen plus ultraviolet A reduced relapse compared with no maintenance treatment. Long term adverse effects of psoralen plus ultraviolet A treatment include photoaging and skin cancer (mainly squamous cell carcinoma).

- **Ingram regimen*** We found no RCTs comparing the Ingram regimen with placebo or no treatment. However, there is consensus that the Ingram regimen is likely to be beneficial for the clearance of psoriasis. One RCT found that the Ingram regimen was less effective than psoralen plus ultraviolet A in clearing psoriasis.
- **Ultraviolet B*** We found no RCTs comparing ultraviolet B with placebo or no treatment. However, there is consensus that ultraviolet B is effective in people with plaque psoriasis. RCTs provided insufficient evidence on the effects of ultraviolet B compared with other treatments, or on the effects of narrow band compared with broad band ultraviolet B for either clearance or maintenance treatment. One RCT found limited evidence that ultraviolet B given three times weekly cleared psoriasis faster than twice weekly treatment.
- **Goeckerman treatment** We found no good evidence on the effects of the Goeckerman treatment.

Systemic treatments

- **Etanercept** Two RCTs found that etanercept increased the proportion of responders at 12–24 weeks compared with placebo. One of the RCTs found that quality of life improved more with etanercept than with placebo at 12 weeks. Etanercept is a relatively new drug for the treatment of psoriasis, and there is limited evidence regarding the possibility of long term or rare adverse events.
- **Cyclosporin** One systematic review found that cyclosporin improved clearance compared with placebo. One RCT found no significant difference between cyclosporin and methotrexate in complete or partial remission, or in duration of remission. Two RCTs found that cyclosporin was more effective than etretinate for reducing psoriasis severity. Two RCTs found that a cyclosporin dose of 5.0 mg/kg daily increased response compared with a cyclosporin dose of 2.5 mg/kg daily. Any advantage of doses greater than 5.0 mg/kg daily may be offset by an increase in dose related adverse effects, particularly increased renal toxicity. The review found that a cyclosporin dose of 3.0 mg/kg daily was more effective than lower doses or than placebo for maintenance.
- **Fumaric acid derivatives** One systematic review of four small RCTs found limited evidence that oral fumaric acid esters improved chronic plaque psoriasis after 16 weeks compared with placebo. However, acute adverse effects were common and included flushing and gastrointestinal symptoms. We found no RCTs on the effects of fumaric acid derivatives as maintenance treatment.
- **Methotrexate*** One small RCT provided insufficient evidence about effects of methotrexate compared with placebo. However, there is consensus that methotrexate is effective for the treatment of psoriasis. One RCT found no significant difference between methotrexate and cyclosporin in complete or partial remission, or in duration of remission of psoriasis. Methotrexate can induce acute myelosuppression. Long term methotrexate carries the risk of hepatic fibrosis and cirrhosis, which is related to the dose regimen employed.
- **Oral retinoids (etretinate, acitretin)** One systematic review found limited evidence that oral retinoids improved clearance compared with placebo in people with chronic plaque psoriasis. RCTs provided insufficient evidence on the effects of oral retinoids as maintenance treatment. Adverse effects led to discontinuation of oral retinoid treatment in 10–20% of people. Teratogenicity renders oral retinoids less acceptable. Etretinate is no longer available in many countries.
- **Tacrolimus** One RCT found limited evidence that tacrolimus improved psoriasis compared with placebo. The adverse effects of tacrolimus are reported to be similar to those of cyclosporin.

- **Anti-CD4 monoclonal antibodies** Two small RCTs provided insufficient evidence on the effects of anti-CD4 monoclonal antibodies.
- **Infliximab** One RCT found that infliximab improved response rates at 10 weeks compared with placebo. Infliximab is a relatively new drug for the treatment of psoriasis, and there is limited evidence regarding the possibility of long term or rare adverse events.

DEFINITION Chronic plaque psoriasis, or psoriasis vulgaris, is a chronic inflammatory skin disease that is characterised by well demarcated erythematous scaly patches on the extensor surfaces of the body and scalp. The lesions may itch, sting, and occasionally bleed. Dystrophic nail changes are found in more than a third of people with chronic plaque psoriasis, and psoriatic arthropathy occurs in 1–3%. The condition waxes and wanes, with wide variations in course and severity among individuals. Other varieties of psoriasis include guttate, inverse, pustular, and erythrodermic psoriasis. This review deals with treatments for chronic plaque psoriasis.

INCIDENCE/ PREVALENCE Psoriasis affects 1–2% of the general population. It is believed to be less frequent in people from Africa and Asia, but we found no reliable epidemiological data.[1]

AETIOLOGY/ RISK FACTORS About a third of people with psoriasis have a family history of psoriasis, but physical trauma, acute infection, and some medications (e.g. lithium salts and β blockers) are believed to trigger the condition. A few observational studies have linked the onset or relapse of psoriasis with stressful life events and personal habits, including cigarette smoking and, less consistently, alcohol consumption. Others have found an association of psoriasis with body mass index Ⓖ and an inverse association with intake of fruit and vegetables.

PROGNOSIS We found no long term prognostic studies. With the exceptions of erythrodermic and acute generalised pustular psoriasis (severe conditions which affect < 1% of people with psoriasis and require intensive hospital care), psoriasis is not known to affect mortality. Psoriasis may substantially affect quality of life, by influencing a negative body image and self image, and limiting daily activities, social contacts, and work. More severe psoriasis is associated with lower levels of quality of life than milder psoriasis.[2] At present, there is no cure for psoriasis.

AIMS OF INTERVENTION To achieve short term suppression of symptoms and long term modulation of disease severity; to improve quality of life, with minimal adverse effects of treatment.

OUTCOMES Clearance or improvement of lesions over time; use of routine treatments; duration of remission; patient satisfaction and autonomy; disease related quality of life; adverse effects of treatment. We found no documented evidence that clinical activity scores, such as the Psoriasis Area and Severity Index (PASI Ⓖ) score, are reliable proxies for these outcomes. Some studies attempt to overcome these limitations by converting PASI score into categories of response deemed to be clinically important – for example, at least a 75% reduction in score from baseline (PASI 75) or at least 90% reduction in score from baseline (PASI 90). Many clinical studies provide no explicit criteria for severity.[3] The effects of placebo treatment have been found to vary across studies in an unpredictable way.[4] Improvements with standardisation of study designs, entry criteria, and outcome measures are needed.

METHODS *Clinical Evidence* search and appraisal June 2004. The authors identified supplementary references through additional electronic literature searches, contact with other experts in the field, and hand searches of several dermatological and medical journals for the years 1976–2004 as a project of the European Dermatoepidemiology Network. The journals searched were the *Journal of Investigative Dermatology*, *British Journal of Dermatology*, *Dermatology*, *Acta Dermo-Venereologica*, *Archives of Dermatology*, *Journal of the American Academy of Dermatology*, *Annales de Dermatologie et de Vénéréologie*, *Giornale Italiano di Dermatologia e Venereologia*, *Hautarzt*, *British Medical Journal*, *Lancet*, *Journal of the American Medical Association*, and *New England Journal of Medicine*.

QUESTION What are the effects of non-drug treatments?

OPTION ACUPUNCTURE

One RCT provided insufficient evidence on the effects of acupuncture for chronic plaque psoriasis.

Benefits: We found one RCT (56 people) comparing classic acupuncture versus sham (placebo) acupuncture.[17] After 3 months, it found no significant difference in the reduction of mean PASI score between the two groups (mean reduction in PASI score 1.3 with classic acupuncture *v* 2.3 with sham acupuncture, $P > 0.05$).[17]

Harms: We found no good evidence on harms.

Comment: Because several trigger and perpetuating factors for psoriasis have been recognised, including physical trauma, acute infections, smoking, diet, and stress, disease severity might be modulated by non-drug treatments. However, we found no good evidence on the effects of non-drug treatments.

OPTION BALNEOTHERAPY

RCTs provided insufficient evidence on the effects of balneotherapy for chronic plaque psoriasis.

Benefits: We found one systematic review (search date 1999)[14] and two additional RCTs of salt water baths.[15,16] The systematic review identified five small RCTs comparing phototherapy plus salt water versus tap water baths. The included RCTs found conflicting results and the review did not report any summary effect estimate. The first additional RCT (71 people) found no significant difference between saline spa water plus phototherapy and phototherapy alone at 21 days, although phototherapy with or without spa water significantly improved symptoms compared with spa water alone (improvement in PASI score: 64% with combination treatment *v* 55% with phototherapy alone *v* 29% with spa water alone; $P < 0.001$ for combination or phototherapy *v* spa water alone).[15] The second, and weaker, additional RCT (50 people) found clinical improvement in more people with a thermal bath (bicarbonate, calcium, and magnesium rich water) than with a tap water bath (64% with thermal bath *v* 11% with tap water bath).[16]

Harms: We found no good evidence on harms.

Comment: Because several trigger and perpetuating factors for psoriasis have been recognised, including physical trauma, acute infections, smoking, diet, and stress, disease severity might be modulated by non-drug treatments. However, we found no good evidence on the effects of non-drug treatments.

OPTION FISH OIL SUPPLEMENTATION

RCTs provided insufficient evidence on the effects of fish oil supplementation for chronic plaque psoriasis.

Benefits: We found six RCTs, which reported inconclusive results (see table 1, p 2096).[8–13]

Harms: We found no good evidence on harms.

Comment: Because several trigger and perpetuating factors for psoriasis have been recognised, including physical trauma, acute infections, smoking, diet, and stress, disease severity might be modulated by non-drug treatments. However, we found no good evidence on the effects of non-drug treatments.

OPTION HELIOTHERAPY

One RCT provided insufficient evidence on the effects of heliotherapy for chronic plaque psoriasis.

Benefits: We found one crossover RCT (95 people), which compared 4 weeks of supervised heliotherapy versus no intervention.[5] Pre-crossover results found that heliotherapy significantly improved psoriasis compared with no intervention at 1 year (Psoriasis Area and Severity Index [PASI**G**] score, taking into consideration scaling, infiltration, and area: 4.2 with heliotherapy *v* 6.2 with no intervention).

Harms: We found no good evidence on harms.

Comment: Because several trigger and perpetuating factors for psoriasis have been recognised, including physical trauma, acute infections, smoking, diet, and stress, disease severity might be modulated by non-drug treatments. However, we found no good evidence on the effects of non-drug treatments.

OPTION PSYCHOTHERAPY

One RCT provided insufficient evidence on the effects of psychotherapy for chronic plaque psoriasis.

Benefits: We found one small RCT, which did not meet *Clinical Evidence* inclusion criteria because of methodological weaknesses.[7]

Harms: We found no good evidence on harms.

Comment: Because several trigger and perpetuating factors for psoriasis have been recognised, including physical trauma, acute infections, smoking, diet, and stress, disease severity might be modulated by non-drug treatments. However, we found no good evidence on the effects of non-drug treatments.

OPTION SUNBEDS

One RCT provided insufficient evidence on the effects of sunbeds for chronic plaque psoriasis.

Benefits: We found one small RCT (38 people with chronic stable plaque psoriasis) comparing ultraviolet A sunbed treatment versus placebo (visible light).[6] In each person, one side of the body was exposed to ultraviolet A light and the other to placebo. The trial found a small improvement in the modified PASI score (median PASI score 3.9 with ultraviolet A *v* 4.2 with placebo; CI not reported; P = 0.04).

Harms: Exposure to ultraviolet light has been associated with adverse effects (see harms of ultraviolet B, p 2082 and harms of psoralen plus ultraviolet A, p 2083).

Comment: Because several trigger and perpetuating factors for psoriasis have been recognised, including physical trauma, acute infections, smoking, diet, and stress, disease severity might be modulated by non-drug treatments. However, we found no good evidence on the effects of non-drug treatments.

QUESTION **What are the effects of topical drug treatments?**

OPTION **EMOLLIENTS AND KERATOLYTICS**

RCTs provided insufficient evidence on the effects of emollients and keratolytics.

Benefits: **Emollients:** We found one small RCT (43 people).[18] It found that emollients temporarily improved psoriasis when they were combined with ultraviolet B radiation. **Keratolytics:** We found one systematic review (search date 1999), which identified one small RCT comparing salicylic acid with placebo.[19] The RCT found no significant difference between treatments after 3 weeks (SMD −0.80, 95% CI −1.71 to +0.11).

Harms: Local irritation and contact dermatitis have been reported with emollients and keratolytics.

Comment: Emollients and keratolytics are usually used as adjuncts to other treatments.

OPTION **TARS**

One small RCT identified by a systematic review provided insufficient evidence on the effects of coal tar compared with placebo. Small RCTs found conflicting results on the effects of tars in combination with ultraviolet B exposure or dithranol. One systematic review found that coal tar, alone or in combination with allantoin and hydrocortisone, was less effective than topical vitamin D derivatives (calcipotriol).

Benefits: **Versus placebo:** We found one systematic review (search date 1999, 1 RCT, 18 people).[19] The RCT found no significant difference between coal tar and placebo after 4 weeks (SMD −0.48, 95% CI −1.14 to +0.19).[19] **Coal tar plus fatty acids versus coal tar alone:** We found one small RCT (20 people; one treatment applied to the right side of the body and the other treatment to the left, the sides determined randomly).[20] After 8 weeks, it found no significant difference in a summed score for erythema, desquamation, and infiltration, between coal tar plus esterified essential fatty acids and coal tar alone (mean improvement in the score: 53.9% with combination treatment *v* 56.1% with coal tar alone; P = 0.52). **Goeckerman treatment:** See benefits of combination regimens, p 2084. **Ingram regimen:** See benefits of combination regimens, p 2084. **Plus ultraviolet B or dithranol:** We found four small RCTs, which found conflicting results about the effects of coal tar when combined with either ultraviolet B exposure[21–23] or dithranol.[24] **Versus vitamin D derivatives:** See benefits of vitamin D derivatives, p 2078.

Harms: Smell, staining, and burning are the main adverse effects of coal tar. **Goeckerman treatment:** See harms of combination regimens, p 2084. **Ingram regimen:** See harms of combination regimens, p 2084. **Versus vitamin D derivatives:** See harms of vitamin D derivatives, p 2080.

Comment: The RCTs were probably too small to detect a clinically important difference.[19,20]

OPTION **DITHRANOL**

One systematic review of small RCTs found that dithranol improved chronic plaque psoriasis after 4–8 weeks compared with placebo. One systematic review of small RCTs found no significant difference between conventional and

short contact dithranol treatment, but the RCTs may have lacked power to detect clinically relevant differences. One systematic review and one subsequent RCT found that dithranol was less effective than topical vitamin D derivatives and caused more adverse effects.

Benefits: **Versus placebo:** We found one systematic review of topical preparations for the treatment of psoriasis (search date 1999, 3 small RCTs).[19] It found that dithranol significantly improved psoriasis at 4–8 weeks compared with placebo (SMD –1.04, 95% CI –1.65 to –0.42; see comment). **Conventional versus short contact treatment:** One systematic review of published studies (search date 1989, 22 small RCTs) compared conventional dithranol treatment versus dithranol short contact treatment (shorter contact time at higher concentrations).[25] It found no significant differences, but the trials were too small to detect clinically important differences (data not reported in the review). **Versus vitamin D derivatives:** See benefits of vitamin D derivatives, p 2078. **Ingram regimen:** See benefits of combination regimens, p 2084.

Harms: Smell, staining, and burning are the main adverse effects of dithranol. **Ingram regimen:** See harms of combination regimens, p 2084. **Versus vitamin D derivatives:** See harms of vitamin D derivatives, p 2080.

Comment: **Versus placebo:** The review performed the meta-analysis using data for the Total Severity Score**G**, the Psoriasis Area and Severity Index score, and the Investigator Assessment of Global Improvement**G** from the included RCTs.[19] **Conventional versus short contact treatment:** Few trials examined participant satisfaction, so it remains unclear whether short contact treatment is easier and more convenient for people at home compared with conventional dithranol treatment.

OPTION TOPICAL STEROIDS

One systematic review found that topical steroids, especially "potent" and "very potent" ones, improved psoriasis in the short term compared with placebo. Systematic reviews found no significant difference in effectiveness between "potent" topical steroids and vitamin D derivatives, but found that vitamin D derivatives caused more perilesional and lesional irritation. One RCT found no significant difference between fluocinomide and tazarotene in the reduction of lesion severity at 12 weeks. Topical steroids may cause striae and atrophy, which increase with potency and use of occlusive dressings. Continuous use may lead to adrenocortical suppression, and case reports suggest that severe flares of the disease may occur on withdrawal.

Benefits: We found one systematic review of topical steroid preparations for the treatment of psoriasis (search date 1999, 12 RCTs, 1686 people)[19] and 12 additional RCTs. **Clearance:** The review found that "potent" and "very potent" topical steroids significantly improved psoriasis compared with placebo (standardised mean difference: "potent" steroids –0.84, 95% CI –0.99 to –0.68; "very potent" steroids –1.51, 95% CI –1.76 to –1.25; see comment).[19] The study duration was usually no longer than 4 weeks. **Maintenance:** One RCT (90 people with 1 target area cleared or nearly cleared of psoriasis by betamethasone dipropionate) found better control at 6 months with topical steroids applied once a week than with placebo (AR for maintenance of clearance in the target area 60% with steroids *v* 20% with placebo; see comment).[26] **Plus occlusive dressings:** Twelve small RCTs, mostly using people as their own controls, found that occlusive polyethylene or hydrocolloid dressings enhanced the clinical activity of topical steroids. **Versus vitamin D derivatives:** See benefits of vitamin D derivatives, p 2078. **Versus topical retinoids:** See benefits of topical retinoids, p 2080.

Harms: Topical steroids can cause striae and atrophy, which increase with clinical potency and use of occlusive dressings. Continuous use may lead to adrenocortical suppression,[27] and case reports suggest that severe flares of the disease may occur on withdrawal. Diminishing clinical response with repeated use (tachyphylaxis) has been described, but we found no estimates of its frequency. **Versus vitamin D derivatives:** See harms of vitamin D derivatives, p 2080.

Comment: **Clearance:** The review performed the meta-analysis using data for the Total Severity Score**G**, the Psoriasis Area and Severity Index score**G**, and the Investigator Assessment of Global Improvement**G**.[19] **Maintenance:** The RCT assessed the effects of treatment on lesions rather than on people.[26]

OPTION VITAMIN D DERIVATIVES

One systematic review found that topical vitamin D derivatives improved plaque psoriasis compared with placebo. Systematic reviews found no significant difference in effectiveness between topical vitamin D derivatives and "potent" topical steroids, but found that calcipotriol caused more perilesional and lesional irritation. One systematic review and one subsequent RCT found that topical vitamin D derivatives improved psoriasis at 4–12 weeks compared with dithranol, and caused fewer adverse effects. One systematic review found that calcipotriol improved psoriasis compared with coal tar, alone or in combination with allantoin and hydrocortisone. RCTs found that combination treatment with vitamin D derivatives plus "potent" topical steroids improved psoriasis compared with either treatment alone or with placebo. In the short term, the combination of vitamin D derivates plus topical steroids decreased irritation compared with monotherapy. RCTs provided insufficient evidence to assess other combination treatments containing topical vitamin D derivatives.

Benefits: **Versus placebo:** We found one systematic review (search date 1999, 14 RCTs, 1537 people).[19] It found that both calcipotriol and tacalcitol were significantly more effective than placebo at 3–8 weeks (calcipotriol, 10 RCTs, standardised WMD –0.74, 95% CI–0.55 to –0.93; tacalcitol, 4 RCTs, standardised WMD –0.89, 95% CI –0.59 to –1.18; WMD based on Total Severity Score**G**, Psoriasis Area and Severity Index (PASI), and Investigator Assessment of Global Improvement**G**).[19] However, the clinical importance of these results is unclear. **Versus each other:** We found six RCTs comparing calcipotriol versus other vitamin D derivatives. One of these RCTs (287 people) found that after 8 weeks, calcipotriol twice daily was more effective than tacalcitol once daily in reducing the severity of pruritus, erythema, infiltration, and scaling (mean reduction in a severity score assessing pruritus, erythema, infiltration, and scaling, on a scale from 0 [least severe] to 16 [most severe]: 4.03 with tacalcitol *v* 5.05 with calcipotriol; $P = 0.0003$).[28] A second RCT (144 people) found that maxacalcitol once daily compared favourably with calcipotriol once daily (people reporting large improvement on summed score for erythema, scaling, and induration or clearance after 8 weeks' treatment: 55% with maxacalcitol *v* 46% with calcipotriol).[29] **Versus topical steroids:** We found one systematic review (search date 1999).[19] The review found no significant difference between vitamin D derivatives and "potent" topical corticosteroids (9 RCTs, 1875 people; SMD +0.06, 95% CI –0.12 to +0.24).[19] The review found significant statistical heterogeneity among trials ($P < 0.01$).[19] One review included in the review found no significant difference between calcipotriol and clobetasol propionate (1 RCT; SMD –0.32, 95% CI –0.95 to +0.30). **Versus dithranol:** We found one systematic review (search date 1999)[19], one additional RCT,[30] and one subsequent RCT.[31] The review (4 RCTs of calcipotriol, 1 RCT of tacalcitol, total of 671 people) found that vitamin D derivatives significantly improved psoriasis compared with dithranol short contact therapy at 4–12 weeks (standardised WMD –0.44, 95% CI –0.72 to –0.16).[19] The additional RCT (171 people) not included in the systematic review found that, of people who initially improved on treatment, more stayed in remission with dithranol than with calcipotriol.[30] The subsequent RCT (88 people) found that calcipotriol ointment (80–100 g/week) plus scalp solution (30–50 mL/week) significantly improved psoriasis at 4 weeks compared with dithranol (change in PASI: –57.4% with calcipotriol *v* –36.1% with dithranol; P = 0.004).[31] **Versus coal tar:** We found one systematic review (search date 1999).[19] It found that calcipotriol significantly improved psoriasis compared with either coal tar alone or a combination of coal tar, allantoin, and hydrocortisone at 6–8 weeks (standardised WMD: coal tar alone, 2 RCTs –0.47, 95% CI–0.83 to –0.11; combination, 1 RCT –0.91, 95% CI –1.36 to –0.46). **Combined with other treatments:** We found two systematic reviews[19,32] and six subsequent RCTs[33–38] comparing combinations of calcipotriol with other therapies. The first systematic review (search date 1999, 11 RCTs, 756 people) found significant improvement in PASI score from adding calcipotriol to acitretin, cyclosporin, or psoralen plus ultraviolet A.[32] It found no significant difference in the rate of marked improvement (at 12 weeks for acitretin plus calcipotriol *v* acitretin RR 1.4, 95% CI 1.0 to 1.9; at 6 weeks for cyclosporin plus calcipotriol *v* cyclosporin RR 1.2, 95% CI 0.9 to 1.6; at 12 weeks for psoralen plus ultraviolet A plus calcipotriol *v* psoralen plus ultraviolet A RR 1.2, 95% CI 0.9 to 1.6; at 8 weeks for ultraviolet B plus calcipotriol *v* ultraviolet B RR 1.0, 95% CI 0.8 to 1.1), in cumulative exposure to phototherapy, or in use of systemic treatment.[32] The second systematic review (search date 1999) found that calcipotriol plus "potent" topical steroids significantly improved psoriasis compared with calcipotriol alone (3 RCTs; SMD 0.42, 95% CI 0.12 to 0.72).[19] It found no significant difference between calcipotriol and calcipotriol plus "very potent" topical steroids (2 RCTs; SMD +0.37, 95% CI –0.08 to +0.81). The first subsequent RCT (164 people) found that fewer ultraviolet B treatments were required to achieve clearance with concomitant calcipotriol compared with no concomitant calcipotriol (median number of ultraviolet B treatments: 22 with calcipotriol plus ultraviolet B *v* 25 with ultraviolet B alone; no statistical analysis reported).[38] The second subsequent RCT (1603 people) compared four treatments: calcipotriol plus steroid combination; calcipotriol alone; steroid alone; and placebo.[33] It found that the combination of calcipotriol plus steroid significantly improved psoriasis at 4 weeks compared with either calcipotriol or steroid alone (mean change in PASI**G** score –71.3% with combination *v* – 57.2% with steroid alone *v* –46.1% with calcipotriol alone *v* –22.7% with placebo; difference for combination *v* steroid alone: –14.2%, 95% CI –17.6% to –10.8%).[33] The third subsequent RCT (1043 people) also compared four treatments: calcipotriene plus betamethasone diproprionate, calcipotriene alone, betamethasone diproprionate alone, and placebo (vehicle alone).[36] It found that after 4 weeks of treatment, calcipotriene plus betamethasone significantly improved lesion severity compared with either drug alone or with placebo (AR clearance or marked improvement of lesions: 229/301 [76.1%] with calcipotriene plus betamethasone *v* 103/308 [33.4%] with calcipotriene *v* 174/312 [55.8%] with betamethasone *v* 8/107 [7.5%] with placebo; OR combination *v* calcipotriene alone 0.14, 95% CI 0.10 to 0.20; OR combination *v* betamethasone alone 0.37, 95% CI 0.26 to 0.53; OR combination *v* placebo 0.02, 95% CI 0.01 to 0.04; analysis not by intention to treat). The fourth subsequent RCT (46 people) compared the combination of calcipotriol plus short contact dithranol versus dithranol alone.[34] It found that combined treatment significantly improved psoriasis at

6 weeks compared with dithranol alone (PASI: 0 with combination *v* 1.21 with dithranol alone; P = 0.0001).[34] The fifth subsequent RCT (143 people) found that the combination of calcipotriol plus oral fumaric acid significantly improved psoriasis at 13 weeks compared with fumaric acid alone (difference between treatments –24.2%, 95% CI –34.2% to –14.2%).[35] **Maintenance:** We found one RCT (97 people), which compared maintenance treatment with calcipotriol versus placebo in people who had stopped taking methotrexate after at least 6 months' treatment, and whose psoriasis had been stable for at least 3 months.[37] Calcipotriol significantly prolonged the time to relapse compared with placebo (relapse defined as doubling of baseline modified psoriasis severity score; median time to relapse 113 days with calcipotriol *v* 35 days with placebo; P < 0.001).[37]

Harms: One systematic review (search date 1999) found that calcipotriol monotherapy caused more lesional or perilesional irritation than "potent" topical steroids (NNH 10, 95% CI 6 to 34).[39] Perilesional irritation from calcipotriol has been reported in as many as 25% of people, the face and skin folds being more susceptible. In the short term, the combination of a topical steroid plus calcipotriene or calcipotriol reduces the incidence of skin irritation.[40,41] Hypercalcaemia and hypercalciuria are dose related adverse effects. One systematic review (4 RCTs, total of 671 people) found that vitamin D derivatives significantly reduced adverse effects compared with dithranol short contact therapy (change: –27%, 95% CI –36% to –17%).[19] One subsequent RCT (88 people) found no significant difference after 4 weeks between calcipotriol ointment (80–100 g/week) plus scalp solution (30–50 mL/week) and dithranol with respect to several parameters of calcium metabolism at 4 weeks.[31]

Comment: There is a consensus that the dosage of calcipotriol should be limited to 100 g a week.

OPTION TOPICAL RETINOIDS (TAZAROTENE)

RCTs found that tazarotene improved chronic plaque psoriasis in the short term compared with placebo. One RCT found no significant difference between tazarotene and fluocinonide in the reduction of lesion severity at 12 weeks. Three RCTs found that adding topical steroids to tazarotene treatment improved response rate compared with tazarotene treatment alone. One RCT found that combined topical steroid and tazarotene treatment increased the proportion of people with marked improvement compared with calcipotriol.

Benefits: We found one systematic review of topical retinoid preparations for treating psoriasis (search date 1999, 1 RCT[33])[19] and nine additional RCTs (published in 8 papers) (see table 2, p 2097).[42–49] **Versus placebo:** Three RCTs (total of 1672 people) compared tazarotene versus placebo.[42–44] All found that tazarotene improved plaque psoriasis compared with placebo (see table 2, p 2097). **Versus steroids:** One RCT (348 people randomised, 275 evaluated) found that once daily treatment with tazarotene (0.1% or 0.05%) was as effective in reducing lesion severity as treatment with the high potency topical steroid fluocinonide (0.05% twice daily) at 12 weeks (see table 2, p 2097).[48] **Plus steroids:** Three RCTs (total of 1198 people) found that adding topical mid- or high potency steroids to tazarotene treatment increased the response rate compared with tazarotene alone (see table 2, p 2097).[45,47,49] One RCT (120 people) found that once daily treatment with tazarotene 0.1% plus topical mometasone furoate 0.1%

significantly increased the number of people with marked improvement in psoriasis symptoms after 2 weeks compared with twice daily treatment with calcipotriol 0.005%.[46] It found no significant difference between groups in the proportion of people attaining complete or almost complete clearance (see table 2, p 2097).

Harms: The RCTs found that some perilesional irritation was reported in most people. Addition of topical steroids to tazarotene reduced the withdrawal rate and treatment related adverse effects.[47,49]

Comment: Tazarotene is contraindicated in women who are, or intend to become, pregnant because it is potentially teratogenic.

QUESTION **What are the effects of treatments with ultraviolet light?**

OPTION **ULTRAVIOLET B**

We found no RCTs comparing ultraviolet B with placebo or no treatment. However, there is consensus that ultraviolet B is effective in people with plaque psoriasis. RCTs provided insufficient evidence on the effects of ultraviolet B compared with other treatments, or on the effects of narrow band compared with broad band ultraviolet B for either clearance or maintenance treatment. One RCT found limited evidence that ultraviolet B given three times weekly cleared psoriasis faster than twice weekly treatment.

Benefits: **Versus placebo or no treatment:** We found no systematic review or RCTs. **Versus other treatments:** We found one systematic review (search date 1999, 2 small RCTs, 78 people).[50] One of the RCTs found that a significantly greater proportion of people achieved 80% clearance of lesions with ultraviolet B plus acitretin compared with acitretin alone (89% with combined treatment *v* 22% with acitretin alone; ARR 67%, 95% CI 33% to 100%). The other RCT compared three treatments: narrow band ultraviolet B alone, narrow band ultraviolet B plus etretinate, and psoralen plus ultraviolet A (PUVA) plus etretinate. It was too small to draw reliable conclusions. It found no significant difference in response rates between PUVA plus etretinate and narrow band ultraviolet B plus etretinate (100% with PUVA plus etretinate *v* 93% with narrow band ultraviolet B plus etretinate; ARR +7%, 95% CI –6% to +20%). It found that significantly fewer people achieved a satisfactory response with narrow band ultraviolet B alone compared with PUVA plus etretinate (100% with PUVA plus etretinate *v* 80% with narrow band ultraviolet B plus etretinate; ARR 20%, 95% CI 0% to 40%). **Narrow band ultraviolet B versus broad band ultraviolet B on clearance:** We found one systematic review (search date 1999, 3 small crossover RCTs, 146 people) of narrow band ultraviolet B versus broad band ultraviolet B.[50] It was not possible to calculate response rates from the results reported by the RCTs. **Twice versus three times weekly narrow band ultraviolet B:** We found one RCT (113 people).[51] It found no significant difference between twice and three times weekly ultraviolet B in clearance rates but found that twice weekly treatment significantly increased the time to reach clearance compared with three times weekly treatment (clearance: 40/58 [69%] with twice weekly *v* 44/55 [80%] with three times weekly, P = 0.21; mean time to clearance: 88 days with twice weekly *v* 58 days with three times weekly, P < 0.0001).[51] **Ultraviolet B versus PUVA:** We found no systematic review but found two RCTs.[52,53] The first RCT (183 people with moderate to severe psoriasis) found no significant difference in clearance rates between PUVA and ultraviolet B (clearance: 88% with PUVA *v* 80% with ultraviolet B; RR of non-clearance with PUVA *v* broad band ultraviolet B 0.62, 95% CI 0.29 to 1.22).[52] Subgroup analysis found that ultraviolet

B radiation was significantly less effective in people with more than 50% body involvement. The second RCT (100 people) found that more people achieved clearance with PUVA compared with narrow band ultraviolet B (clearance: 84% with PUVA *v* 63% with ultraviolet B).[53] **Maintenance:** We found no systematic review but found one RCT.[54] The RCT (104 people with initial clearance of symptoms) found that significantly more people were still clear of symptoms after 181 days with weekly ultraviolet B compared with no maintenance treatment (> 50% with ultraviolet B *v* 28% with no ultraviolet B; RR relapse 0.67, 95% CI 0.41 to 0.92).[54]

Harms: Ultraviolet B radiation may increase photoaging and risk of skin cancer. One systematic review (search date 1996) estimated that the excess annual risk of non-melanoma skin cancer associated with ultraviolet B radiation was likely to be less than 2%.[55]

Comment: We found insufficient evidence from RCTs on the effects of ultraviolet B. However, consensus regards the treatment as effective.

OPTION PSORALEN PLUS ULTRAVIOLET A

We found no systematic review or RCTs that compared psoriasis clearance with psoralen plus ultraviolet A versus no treatment. However, there is consensus that psoralen plus ultraviolet A is effective for clearance of psoriasis. One RCT found that psoralen plus ultraviolet A was more effective than the Ingram regimen in clearing psoriasis. One systematic review found that higher doses of psoralen improved psoriasis clearance more than lower doses of psoralen. One large RCT found that maintenance treatment with psoralen plus ultraviolet A reduced relapse compared with no maintenance treatment. Long term adverse effects of psoralen plus ultraviolet A treatment include photoaging and skin cancer (mainly squamous cell carcinoma).

Benefits: We found one systematic review of phototherapy and photochemotherapy (search date 1999, 51 RCTs).[50] The results could not be pooled because of trial heterogeneity. **Psoralen plus ultraviolet A (PUVA) versus no treatment:** The systematic review found no RCTs (see comment).[50] **Comparison of different doses of psoralen:** The systematic review (2 RCTs, 167 people) found that higher dose psoralen significantly increased success (major improvement or full remission) compared with lower dose psoralen (ARR 72%, 95% CI 54% to 90%; NNT 2).[50] The first RCT included in the systematic review compared 40 mg with 10 mg of 8-methoxypsoralen. The second RCT included in the systematic review compared 1.2 mg/kg 5-methoxypsoralen with 0.6 mg/kg 5-methoxypsoralen. Both RCTs also found that using a higher dose of psoralen reduced the mean cumulative ultraviolet A dose required to achieve success (first RCT: 54 J/cm^2 with 40 mg 8-methoxypsoralen *v* 77 J/cm^2 with 10 mg 8-methoxypsoralen; second RCT: 53 J/cm^2 with 1.2 mg/kg 5-methoxypsoralen *v* 132 J/cm^2 with 0.6 mg/kg 5-methoxypsoralen). **Comparison of different oral psoralens:** The systematic review included two RCTs that compared different oral psoralens.[56] One RCT (169 people) found no significant difference between 5-methoxypsoralen 1.2 mg/kg and 8-methoxypsoralen 0.6 mg/kg in the mean cumulative ultraviolet A dose needed for clearance (53 J/cm^2 with 5-methoxypsoralen *v* 45 J/cm^2 with 8-methoxypsoralen). The other RCT (38 people) found that people treated with 8-methoxypsoralen 0.6 mg/kg required a lower mean cumulative ultraviolet A dose to achieve success than those treated with 1.2 mg/kg 5-methoxypsoralen (155 J/cm^2 with 8-methoxypsoralen *v* 187 J/cm^2 with 5-methoxypsoralen; CI not reported; $P < 0.05$). **Comparison of different topical psoralens:** The systematic review included one RCT (38 people), which found no significant difference between 5-methoxypsoralen and 8-methoxypsoralen in the mean total dose of ultraviolet A required for clearance (56.8 J/cm^2 with 5-methoxypsoralen *v* 59.1 J/cm^2 with 8-methoxypsoralen).[50] **Comparison of different oral psoralen formulations:** The systematic review included one RCT (47 people), which found no significant difference between liquid and crystalline forms of oral 8-methoxypsoralen in the proportion of people with marked improvement or clearance of psoriasis (liquid *v* crystalline: ARI +25%, 95% CI −1% to +51%; mean ultraviolet A dose to achieve clearance 68.7 J/cm^2 with liquid psoralen *v* 80.8 J/cm^2 with crystalline psoralen).[50] **Comparison of oral versus bath psoralen formulations:** The systematic review found two RCTs (137 people), which found no significant difference in the success rate (major improvement or clearance), but found significantly greater mean cumulative ultraviolet A dose for clearance with oral compared with topical psoralens (in the first RCT: 14.5 J/cm^2 with bath 8-methoxypsoralen *v* 60.1 J/cm^2 with oral 8-methoxypsoralen; in the other RCT: 23.5 J/cm^2 with bath 8-methoxypsoralen *v* 131.1 J/cm^2 with oral 8-methoxypsoralen).[50] **Comparison of dose setting strategies:** The systematic review included two RCTs (157 people), which compared the routine use of the minimal phototoxic dose of ultraviolet A at each treatment versus a strategy of setting the ultraviolet A dose according to skin type**G**.[50] Neither study found any significant difference for success rate (clearance). One RCT found that the minimal phototoxic dose strategy**G** had a significantly higher median cumulative ultraviolet A dose for clearance (62.9 J/cm^2 with the minimal phototoxic dose *v* 39.5 J/cm^2 with the dose set on the basis of skin type). The second RCT found similar differences, but they were not significant. **Versus other psoralen based phototherapies:** The systematic review included five RCTs (285 people).[50] The largest RCT (100 people) found no significant difference between PUVA twice weekly and psoralen plus narrow band ultraviolet B twice weekly (ARR for clearance +12%, 95% CI −4% to +28%). **Versus ultraviolet B:** See benefits of ultraviolet B, p 2081. **Versus the Ingram regimen:** See benefits of combination regimens, p 2084. **Versus other treatments:** The systematic review included 25 RCTs (1268 people), which compared different combinations of ultraviolet radiation with systemic or topical treatments, including dithranol, tar, vitamin D_3 analogues, steroids, and fish oil.[50] The RCTs were mostly small and underpowered to detect clinically important differences. The largest of the RCTs (224 people) found that PUVA cleared psoriasis slightly more often than did dithranol (ARR 9%, 95% CI 0% to 18%). **Maintenance:** One large RCT (1005 people whose psoriasis had been cleared by PUVA) found that maintenance treatment with PUVA versus no maintenance treatment reduced relapse at 18 months compared with no maintenance (AR of flares 27% with treatment once a week *v* 34% with treatment once every 3 weeks *v* 62% with no treatment; RR for relapse with once weekly treatment *v* no treatment 0.44, 95% CI 0.32 to 0.56).[57]

Harms: The best evidence on chronic toxicity comes from an ongoing study of more than 1300 people who first received PUVA treatment in 1975.[58] The study found a dose dependent increased risk of squamous cell carcinoma, basal cell carcinoma, and possibly malignant melanoma compared with the risk in the general population. A systematic review (search date 1998) of eight additional studies has confirmed the findings concerning non-melanoma skin cancer.[56] Premature photoaging is another expected adverse effect. After less than 15 years, about a quarter of people exposed to 300 or more treatments of PUVA had at least one squamous cell carcinoma of the skin, with particularly high risk in people with skin types**G** I and II. In people who wear ultraviolet A opaque glasses for 24 hours after psoralen ingestion, the risk of cataract development seems negligible. A combined analysis of two cohort studies (944 people treated with bath PUVA) excluded a three-fold excess risk of squamous cell carcinoma after a mean follow up of 14.7 years, suggesting that bath PUVA is possibly safer than conventional PUVA.[59]

Comment: There is consensus that psoralen plus ultraviolet A is effective for clearance of psoriasis. People receiving PUVA need close monitoring for acute toxicity and long term cutaneous carcinogenic effects.

OPTION COMBINATION REGIMENS

We found no RCTs comparing the Ingram regimen with placebo or no treatment. However, there is consensus that the Ingram regimen is likely to be beneficial for the clearance of psoriasis. One RCT found that the Ingram regimen was less effective than psoralen plus ultraviolet A in clearing psoriasis. We found no good evidence on effectiveness of the Goeckerman treatment.

Benefits: We found one systematic review (search date 1999) of calcipotriol plus phototherapy (see benefits of vitamin D derivatives, p 2078),[32] and one systematic review (search date 1999) examining treatment for severe psoriasis,[50] which compared different combinations of ultraviolet radiation compared with systemic or topical treatments, including dithranol, tar, vitamin D derivatives, steroids, and fish oil (see benefits of psoralen plus ultraviolet A, p 2082). **Ingram regimen:** We found no RCTs comparing the Ingram regimen**Ⓖ** with placebo or no treatment (see comment). One RCT (224 people) compared an inpatient Ingram regimen (dithranol concentration 0.01–1.0%) with psoralen plus ultraviolet A (PUVA).[60] It found that PUVA significantly increased clearance rates compared with the Ingram regimen (clearance rate: 91% with PUVA *v* 82% with the Ingram regimen; ARI for clearance 9%, 95% CI 1% to 17%). **Dithranol plus ultraviolet B:** Five small RCTs (the largest involving 53 people) identified by the systematic review[50] found conflicting results on the added efficacy of dithranol when combined with ultraviolet B exposure. However, the trials were too small to detect a clinically important difference. **Goeckerman treatment:Ⓖ** We found no good evidence on the effects of the Goeckerman treatment. **Calcipotriol plus ultraviolet B or PUVA:** We found one systematic review (search date 1999;)[32] and one additional RCT.[38] The review found no significant difference in the rate of marked improvement between PUVA or ultraviolet B plus calcipotriol and either PUVA or ultraviolet B alone (at 12 weeks for PUVA plus calcipotriol *v* PUVA: RR 1.2, 95% CI 0.9 to 1.6; at 8 weeks for ultraviolet B plus calcipotriol *v* ultraviolet B: RR 1.0, 95% CI 0.8 to 1.1), in cumulative exposure to phototherapy, or in use of systemic treatment.[32] The subsequent RCT (164 people) found that fewer ultraviolet B treatments were required to achieve clearance with calcipotriol plus ultraviolet B compared with ultraviolet B alone (median number of ultraviolet B treatments: 22 with calcipotriol plus ultraviolet B *v* 25 with ultraviolet B alone; no statistical analysis reported).[38]

Harms: Adverse effects vary with the treatments being combined. Local irritation often occurs.

Comment: There is consensus that the Ingram regimen is likely to be beneficial for clearing psoriasis.

QUESTION **What are the effects of systemic drug treatments?**

OPTION **ORAL RETINOIDS (ETRETINATE, ACITRETIN)**

One systematic review found limited evidence that oral retinoids improved clearance compared with placebo in people with chronic plaque psoriasis. RCTs provided insufficient evidence on the effects of oral retinoids as maintenance treatment. Adverse effects led to discontinuation of oral retinoid treatment in 10–20% of people. Teratogenicity renders oral retinoids less acceptable. Etretinate is no longer available in many countries.

Benefits: We found one systematic review of people with severe psoriasis (search date 1999, 32 RCTs; 13 of etretinate, 11 of acitretin, 8 of acitretin *v* etretinate),[50] one systematic review (search date 2000) of people with psoriatic arthropathy,[61] and one (search date 1999) on the combination of acitretin with calcipotriol.[32] The main outcome was treatment success, as indicated by a specific decrease in Psoriasis Area and Severity Index (PASIⒼ) score or the extent of body surface area involved, or by a global improvement. Heterogeneity among trials often prevented pooling of data. **Versus placebo:** The review found 11 RCTs (455 people).[50] Three RCTs allowed concomitant topical steroids. Heterogeneity prevented pooling. Overall, the review found limited evidence that oral retinoids improved symptoms (marked improvement or complete remission) compared with placebo. Three RCTs found that etretinate 1 mg/kg significantly increased response rate compared with placebo (the largest of these RCTs found almost or complete clearance in 35% with etretinate *v* 5% with placebo; ARR 30%, 95% CI 7% to 53%). However, one RCT found no significant difference in clearance rates between etretinate 50 mg and placebo (complete remission: 17% with etretinate *v* 6% with placebo; ARR +11%, 95% CI –2% to +24%). Results were extractable for only two of the RCTs comparing acitretin with placebo. One RCT (38 people) was underpowered and detected no differences between acitretin and placebo. The other RCT (80 people) found no significant difference in the proportion of people achieving 75% or greater decrease in PASI or a PASI score of less than 8 between acitretin 10 mg and placebo (40% with acitretin *v* 25% with placebo; ARI +15%, 95% CI –14% to +44%). However, higher doses of acitretin (25 mg or 50 mg) significantly increased the proportion of people who achieved 75% or greater decrease in PASI or a PASI score of less than 8 compared with placebo (60% with 25 mg acitretin *v* 25% with placebo, ARI 35%, 95% CI 6% to 64%; 70% with 50 mg acitretin *v* 25% with placebo, ARI 45%, 95% CI 17% to 73%). **Acitretin versus etretinate:** The review identified six RCTs (598 people), which found no significant difference between acitretin and etretinate in the proportion of people achieving a marked improvement (≥ 75% decrease in PASI or Psoriasis Severity Index [a modified PASI], or a marked or total clearance for the largest study; 74% of people achieved clearance with 40 mg acitretin *v* 76% with 40 mg etretinate; ARR +2%, 95% CI –17% to +13%).[50] **Etretinate versus cyclosporin:** The review found two RCTs (286 people).[50] The results could not be pooled. The RCT using the higher dose of etretinate (0.7 mg/kg) found that significantly fewer people treated with etretinate than with cyclosporin 5 mg/kg achieved a marked response (≥ 75% decrease in PASI, 97% of people with cyclosporin *v* 73% with etretinate; ARR 24%, 95% CI 9% to 39%). **Retinoid plus psoralen plus ultraviolet A (PUVA) versus PUVA alone:** The review identified six RCTs (305 people).[50] The results could not be pooled. One RCT (30 people) found that retinoid plus PUVA significantly increased clearance rates compared with PUVA alone (93% with etretinate 0.75 mg/kg plus PUVA *v* 60% with PUVA plus placebo; ARR 33%, 95%

CI 5% to 61%). The remaining studies did not report a significant difference between groups. **Retinoid plus PUVA versus retinoid alone:** We found no RCTs. **Retinoid plus ultraviolet B (broad band or narrow band) versus ultraviolet B alone or retinoid alone:** The review included four RCTs (245 people).[50] The results could not be pooled. In each RCT, the combined treatment was superior to ultraviolet B alone. The largest RCT (82 people) found that acitretin 3 mg daily plus ultraviolet B significantly improved psoriasis compared with ultraviolet B alone (≥ 75% decrease in PASI: 57% of people with combination *v* 23% people with ultraviolet B alone; ARR 34%, 95% CI 14% to 54%). One small RCT (18 people) found that acitretin plus ultraviolet B significantly improved clearance rates compared with acitretin alone (achieved ≥80% clearance: 89% with combination *v* 22% with acitretin alone; ARR 67%, 95% CI 33% to 100%). **Retinoid combination with other treatments:** The systematic review included four RCTs (511 people), which found that a retinoid plus topical steroid was superior to the single treatments in improving subjective end points.[50] Another systematic review (search date 1999) found insufficient evidence on the combination of acitretin with calcipotriol (see benefits of vitamin D derivatives, p 2078).[32] **Maintenance:** One systematic review included two RCTs.[50] One of the RCTs (36 people achieving clearance with PUVA plus etretinate) found that low dose etretinate (half of the maximum dose tolerated) significantly reduced relapse rates over 1 year compared with placebo (44% with etretinate *v* 85% with placebo; ARR 41%, 95% CI 12% to 70%). The second RCT found no significant difference between three dosages of acitretin (10 *v* 25 *v* 50 mg daily) and placebo for 6 months.

Harms: Adverse effects led to discontinuation of oral retinoid treatment in 10–20% of people.[50] Most people experience mucocutaneous adverse effects, such as dry skin, cheilitis, and conjunctivitis. Mucocutaneous effects were generally mild. Increased serum cholesterol and triglyceride concentrations occurred in about half of the people. Low grade hepatotoxicity was observed in about 1% of people treated with etretinate.[62] Two people treated with liarozole were withdrawn because of liver enzyme abnormalities. Occasionally, acute hepatitis occurred as a purported idiosyncratic hypersensitivity reaction. Radiographic evidence of extraspinal tendon and ligament calcifications has been documented. In one cohort study, a quarter of 956 people treated with etretinate attributed a joint problem or its worsening to the drug.[62] Etretinate is a known teratogen and may be detected in the plasma for 2–3 years after treatment stops. Acitretin can undergo esterification to etretinate.

Comment: Women of childbearing age are given effective contraception for 1 month before starting etretinate and acitretin, throughout treatment, and after stopping treatment for at least 3 years because it is potentially teratogenic. Etretinate is no longer available in many countries.

OPTION METHOTREXATE

One small RCT provided insufficient evidence about effects of methotrexate compared with placebo. However, there is consensus that methotrexate is effective for the treatment of psoriasis. One RCT found no significant difference between methotrexate and cyclosporin in complete or partial remission, or in duration of remission of psoriasis. Methotrexate can induce acute myelosuppression. Long term methotrexate carries the risk of hepatic fibrosis and cirrhosis, which is related to the dose regimen employed.

Benefits: **Versus placebo:** We found one systematic review (search date 2000).[61] It identified one small RCT (37 people with psoriatic arthritis), which found that methotrexate significantly reduced the surface area of psoriasis after 12 weeks compared with placebo (CI not reported; P = 0.04).[63] **Versus cyclosporin:** We found one single blinded RCT (88 people) which compared oral methotrexate (up to 22.5 mg per week) versus cyclosporin (up to 5 mg/kg per day). It found no significant difference between methotrexate and cyclosporin in complete (at least 90% reduction in Psoriasis Area and Severity Index**G** score) or partial (at least 75% reduction in Psoriasis Area and Severity Index score) remission after 16 weeks' treatment (AR for complete remission: 17/43 [40%] with methotrexate *v* 14/42 [33%] with cyclosporin, P = 0.55; AR for partial remission: 26/43 [60%] with methotrexate *v* 30/42 [71%] with cyclosporin, P = 0.29).[64] It found no significant difference in the duration of either complete or partial remission between groups after treatment was stopped (duration of complete remission P = 0.34; duration of partial remission P = 0.43).

Harms: In one uncontrolled case series, treatment was stopped in 33/113 (29%) people because of adverse effects.[58] The most serious acute reaction, particularly in elderly people, is dose related myelosuppression. In the long term, major adverse events included liver fibrosis and pulmonary toxicity. One systematic review (search date not reported) found that about 28% (95% CI 24% to 32%) of people taking long term methotrexate for psoriasis and rheumatoid arthritis developed liver fibrosis of histological grade I or higher on liver biopsy, whereas 5% developed advanced liver disease (histological grade IIIB or IV).[65] The risk was dose related and was higher with increased alcohol consumption. A limitation of the systematic review was the lack of untreated control groups. Pulmonary disease associated with methotrexate has been described as an acute or chronic interstitial pneumonitis.[66] Adverse pulmonary effects of treatment are considered much rarer in psoriasis than in rheumatoid arthritis, but we found no published evidence to support this claim. Several drug interactions that increase methotrexate toxicity have been described (e.g. with sulphonamides). Methotrexate seems to double the risk of developing squamous cell carcinoma in people exposed to psoralen plus ultraviolet A and may be an independent risk factor for this cancer in people with psoriatic arthritis.[58] A higher risk of lymphoproliferative diseases in long term users has been suggested by a few case reports. On the basis of data from a large case series (248 people), the cumulative incidence of lymphoma is not expected to be much higher than 1%.[67] **Versus cyclosporin:** The RCT reported that 12 people (29%) receiving methotrexate and one person receiving cyclosporin (2%) discontinued treatment because of reversible elevated liver enzyme levels (significance not reported).[64] Significantly more people in the methotrexate group reported nausea, while significantly more people in the cyclosporin group reported headaches, muscle ache, and paresthesias in the fingertips and toes (nausea: 19/43 [44%] with methotrexate *v* 4/42 [10%] with cyclosporin, P < 0.001; headaches: 7/43 [16%] with methotrexate *v* 18/42 [43%] with cyclosporin, P = 0.009; muscle ache: 3/43 [7%] with methotrexate *v* 12/42 [29%] with cyclosporin, P = 0.007; paresthesias: 1/43 [2%] with methotrexate *v* 14/42 [33%] with cyclosporin, P < 0.001).

Comment: There is consensus that methotrexate is effective for the treatment of psoriasis. People using methotrexate are closely monitored for liver toxicity[50] and are advised to limit their consumption of alcohol. The most reliable test of liver damage remains needle biopsy of the liver. It is rare for life threatening liver disease to develop with the first 1.0–1.5 g of methotrexate. In one uncontrolled case series (113 people with severe psoriasis), maintenance treatment with low dose methotrexate (weekly dose not exceeding 15 mg) provided satisfactory control of skin lesions in 81% of people (mean treatment duration 8 years).[68] When treatment was stopped, 45% of people experienced a full relapse within 6 months.

OPTION CYCLOSPORIN

One systematic review found that cyclosporin improved clearance compared with placebo. One RCT found no significant difference between cyclosporin and methotrexate in complete or partial remission, or in duration of remission. Two RCTs found that cyclosporin was more effective than etretinate for reducing psoriasis severity. Two RCTs found that a cyclosporin dose of 5.0 mg/kg daily increased response compared with a cyclosporin dose of 2.5 mg/kg daily. Any advantage of doses greater than 5.0 mg/kg daily may be offset by an increase in dose related adverse effects, particularly increased renal toxicity. The review found that a cyclosporin dose of 3.0 mg/kg daily was more effective than lower doses or than placebo for maintenance.

Benefits: We found one systematic review (search date 1999, 18 RCTs; 13 on induction of remission, 5 on maintenance of remission).[50] Success was defined mostly as reduction in Psoriasis Area and Severity Index (PASI**G**) score or clinical criteria such as "clearance". Dosages of cyclosporin ranged from 1.25–14 mg/kg daily. Duration of treatment ranged from 4–12 weeks. The data could not be pooled. **Cyclosporin versus placebo for clearance:** The review included six RCTs (289 people).[50] It found that cyclosporin significantly increased treatment success compared with placebo (ARI for success 38%, 95% CI 32% to 44%). However, there was heterogeneity, potentially due to differing definitions of "success" (at least 50% decrease in PASI, at least 75% decrease in PASI, PASI < 8, or clinically "clear or almost clear") and differing doses of cyclosporin used in the RCTs. The largest RCT included in the review reported that cyclosporin was significantly more effective than placebo at 10 weeks (ARI for a ≥ 75% reduction of PASI 22%, 95% CI 7% to 37%). **Cyclosporin versus etretinate for clearance:** The review included two RCTs (286 people).[50] The review found that cyclosporin 2.5 mg/kg daily significantly increased rates of achieving a greater than 70% decrease in PASI compared with etretinate 0.5 mg/kg daily (62% with cyclosporin *v* 16% with etretinate; ARI 46%, CI 34% to 58%). Cyclosporin 5 mg/kg daily was more effective than 0.75 mg/kg daily etretinate (97% with cyclosporin *v* 73% with etretinate; ARI 24%, CI 9% to 39%). **Cyclosporin versus methotrexate:** See benefits of methotrexate versus cyclosporin, p 2086. **Comparison of different cyclosporin doses:** The review identified two non-blinded RCTs (468 people) comparing different dosages of cyclosporin.[50] Both RCTs found that cyclosporin 5 mg/kg daily increased the proportion of people achieving a 75% decrease in PASI compared with cyclosporin 2.5 mg/kg daily (first RCT: ARI 19%, 95% CI 4% to 34%; second RCT: ARI 41%, 95% CI 31% to 51%). **Cyclosporin plus calcipotriol versus cyclosporin:** The review identified one RCT (69 people), but the proportions of people responding to each treatment were not extractable. **Comparison of cyclosporin formulations:** The review identified two RCTs (345 people, 12 weeks, 1 with a crossover design). They found no significant difference in the proportion of people achieving a marked response (≥ 75% decrease in PASI) between conventional oil based cyclosporin formulation and the microemulsion preconcentrate formulation (the larger, parallel group RCT results: 78% of people treated with oil based formulation *v* 80% with microemulsion; ARI +2%, 95% CI −7% to +11%). **Maintenance:** The review included five RCTs of treatment to maintain remission.[50] Two RCTs compared two doses of cyclosporin (1.5 mg/kg or 3.0 mg/kg daily) versus placebo.[69,70] Both RCTs found that 3.0 mg/kg daily cyclosporin was better than placebo for maintaining remission (first RCT: AR for "good response" after 24 weeks [defined as < 50% of baseline body surface area affected]; 58% with cyclosporin 3 mg/kg daily *v* 0% with cyclosporin 1.5 mg/kg daily *v* 16% with placebo; no further data reported in review;[69] second RCT: AR for "positive response" after 16 weeks [defined as increase of no more than 2 points on a 7 point severity scale where 1 = complete clearance and 7 = most severe]; 57% with cyclosporin 3 mg/kg daily *v* 21% with cyclosporin 1.5 mg/kg daily *v* 5% with placebo; no further data reported in review[70]). The third RCT compared two different cyclosporin formulations and found no significant difference in response after 24 weeks between an oil based and microemulsion preconcentrate formulation.[71] The fourth RCT (400 people) found that tapering off the cyclosporin dose increased time to relapse compared with abrupt stopping of cyclosporin (time to relapse 113 days with tapered cyclosporin *v* 109 days with abrupt stopping; P = 0.038).[72] The final RCT (37 people) found that, over the 36 months of treatment, continuous cyclosporin was more effective for maintaining remission than intermittent cyclosporin (remission maintained for 69% of the treatment period with continuous cyclosporin *v* 32% with intermittent treatment; P value not reported).[73]

Harms: Cyclosporin is associated with dose related hypertension (diastolic blood pressure > 90 mm Hg over 12 weeks: 4/36 [11%] with 1.25 mg/kg daily *v* 25/121 [21%] with 2.5 mg/kg daily *v* 16/60 [26%] with 5 mg/kg daily) and renal impairment (creatinine ≥ 130% of baseline value: 1% with 1.25 mg/kg daily *v* 5% with 2.5 mg/kg daily *v* 13% with 5 mg/kg daily).[50] The incidence of these adverse events increases over time. In a case series follow up study of 122 consecutive people treated continuously with cyclosporin for 3–76 months at a dose not exceeding 5 mg/kg daily, 104 people discontinued treatment.[74] The mean percentage of people who discontinued treatment because of adverse effects (mostly renal dysfunction and hypertension) rose from 14% at 12 months to 41% at 48 months. One RCT (400 people) found that intermittent treatment with a microemulsion formulation for 1 year (with maximum treatment periods of 12 weeks as 1–4 courses) was well tolerated and produced no clinically significant change in blood pressure or creatinine concentration.[50] With this regimen, only 10 (2.5%) people withdrew because of adverse events. Long term follow up studies are needed to confirm this finding.

Comment: None.

OPTION IMMUNOSUPPRESSIVE DRUGS OTHER THAN METHOTREXATE AND CYCLOSPORIN

One RCT found limited evidence that tacrolimus improved psoriasis compared with placebo. The adverse effects of tacrolimus are reported to be similar to those of cyclosporin. Two small RCTs provided insufficient evidence about the effects of anti-CD4 monoclonal antibodies.

Benefits: **Tacrolimus:** We found no systematic review. We found one RCT (50 people), which found that oral tacrolimus significantly increased response rates at 9 weeks compared with placebo (≥ 70% reduction in Psoriasis Area and Severity Index (PASI**G**) score after treatment: 63% with tacrolimus *v* 25% with placebo; RR 0.62; CI not reported).[75] **Anti-CD4 monoclonal antibodies:** We found no systematic review. We found two small RCTs.[76,77] The first RCT (28 people with moderate to severe psoriasis) compared an anti-CD4 monoclonal antibody (OKTcdr4a) at low dose (225 mg) versus high dose (750 mg) versus placebo.[76] It found no significant difference between treatments (mean decrease in the PASI score at 15 days: 4% with low dose OKTcdr4a *v* 17% with high dose OKTcdr4a *v* 11% with placebo; P reported as not significant). The second RCT (85 people with moderate to severe psoriasis) compared subcutaneous human anti-CD4 monoclonal antibody at doses of 20, 80, 160, or 280 mg once weekly for 4 weeks versus placebo.[77] There was no significant difference in PASI score improvement between any of the antibody groups and placebo at 7 weeks (mean PASI reduction: 24% with 280 mg antibody *v* 16% with 160 mg antibody *v* 14% with 80 mg antibody *v* 12% with 20 mg antibody *v* 8% with placebo; P reported as not significant for all placebo comparisons).

Harms: **Tacrolimus:** Most of the evidence concerning the safety of tacrolimus comes from studies in people who have received transplants. Despite major differences in their chemical structure, tacrolimus and cyclosporin seem to have a notably similar profile of adverse effects.[78] **Anti-CD4 monoclonal antibodies:** The first RCT reported that only mild adverse effects occurred, mostly during infusion (adverse events: 5 with placebo *v* 2 with low dose antibody *v* 9 with high dose antibody; significance not stated).[76] The second RCT reported one serious treatment related adverse effect, an allergy-like rash after infusion in the 160 mg anti-CD4 antibody group.[77] Influenza-like illness occurred more frequently with high dose (160–280 mg) antibody than low dose (20–80 mg) antibody or placebo (8/33 [24%] with high dose antibody *v* 2/35 [6%] with low dose antibody *v* 2/17 [12%] with placebo; significance not stated). A dose dependent decrease in total lymphocyte count was seen with anti-CD4 antibody and was parallel to a dose dependent decrease in CD4+ T cells.[77]

Comment: The benefit and risk profile of these drugs in psoriasis is still poorly defined.

OPTION CYTOKINE BLOCKING AGENTS

Two RCTs found that etanercept increased the proportion of responders at 12–24 weeks compared with placebo. One of the RCTs found that quality of life improved more with etanercept than with placebo at 12 weeks. One small RCT found that infliximab improved response rates at 10 weeks compared with placebo. Etanercept and infliximab are relatively new drugs for the treatment of psoriasis, and there is limited evidence regarding the possibility of long term or rare adverse events.

Benefits: **Etanercept:** We found no systematic review. We found two RCTs.[79,80] The first RCT (112 people with plaque psoriasis involving at least 10% of body surface area) compared subcutaneous etanercept (25 mg twice a week) for 24 weeks versus placebo.[79] Etanercept significantly increased the proportion of people with at least 75% improvement in Psoriasis Area and Severity Index (PASI❻) score compared with placebo at 24 weeks (32/57 [56%] with etanercept *v* 3/55 [5%] with placebo; $P < 0.001$). The second RCT (672 people) compared subcutaneous etanercept at three different dosages (low: 25 mg once weekly; medium: 25 mg twice weekly; or high: 50 mg twice weekly) with placebo for 12 weeks.[50] All three etanercept doses significantly increased the proportion of people with at least a 75% improvement in PASI score compared with placebo at 12 weeks (49% with high dose etanercept *v* 34% with medium dose etanercept *v* 14% with low dose etanercept *v* 4% with placebo; $P < 0.001$ for comparison of each dose of etanercept *v* placebo).[80] Quality of life improved significantly more in the etanercept groups than in the placebo group by week 12 (measured using the Dermatology Life Quality Index❻; mean score improvement: 61.0% with high dose etanercept *v* 50.8% with medium dose etanercept *v* 47.2% with low dose etanercept *v* 10.9% with placebo; $P < 0.001$ for comparison of each dose of etanercept *v* placebo). **Infliximab:** We found no systematic review. We found one RCT (33 people with severe psoriasis), which compared weekly intravenous infliximab 5 mg/kg versus infliximab 10 mg/kg and with placebo.[81] It found that both doses of infliximab significantly increased response rates at 10 weeks compared with placebo (Physician's Global Assessment**G** rating of good, excellent, or clear: 91% with infliximab 10 mg/kg *v* 82% with infliximab 5 mg/kg *v* 18% with placebo; ARI for 10 mg/kg 73%, 95% CI 30% to 94%; ARI for 5 mg/kg 64%, 95% CI 20% to 89%).

Harms: Most of the evidence on the safety of etanercept and infliximab is from studies in people with rheumatoid arthritis or Crohn's disease. Cutaneous reactions to etanercept have been reported with a frequency of up to 5%, including reactions at the injection site and urticarial manifestations.[82] Upper respiratory tract infections have been reported with both etanercept and infliximab. A few cases of lupus-like syndrome and severe infections have been reported with infliximab treatment.[83] **Etanercept:** The first RCT reported a similar frequency and rate of occurrence of adverse effects with etanercept and placebo.[79] Peripheral oedema was significantly less common with etanercept than with placebo (0.04 events per person-year with etanercept *v* 0.41 events per person-year with placebo; $P < 0.05$). Mild injection site reactions were more common with etanercept than with placebo (9% with etanercept *v* 0% with placebo; significance not stated). The second RCT also reported a similar frequency of adverse events in placebo and etanercept groups.[80] Injection site reactions were more frequent with etanercept than with placebo (injection site reaction: 13% with high dose etanercept *v* 17% with medium dose etanercept *v* 11% with low dose etanercept *v* 7% with placebo; significance not stated). **Infliximab:** The RCT found that headache was more common with infliximab 10 mg/kg than with infliximab 5 mg/kg or placebo (7/11 [64%] with infliximab 10 mg/kg *v* 1/11 [9%] with infliximab 5 mg/kg *v* 2/11 [18%] with placebo; significance not stated).[81]

Comment: Etanercept is a recombinant molecule comprising the human tumour necrosis factor-α p75 receptor fused to the Fc portion of the human immunoglobulin G1 molecule. Infliximab is a human-mouse monoclonal antibody that binds to and inhibits the activity of tumour necrosis factor-α. The evidence on the effects of cytokine blocking agents in people with plaque psoriasis is still limited. Further comparative studies are needed to predict precisely how these drugs will fit into current psoriasis management.

OPTION FUMARIC ACID DERIVATIVES

One systematic review of four small RCTs found limited evidence that oral fumaric acid esters improved chronic plaque psoriasis after 16 weeks compared with placebo. However, acute adverse effects were common and included flushing and gastrointestinal symptoms. We found no RCTs on the effects of fumaric acid derivatives as maintenance treatment.

Benefits: We found one systematic review (search date 1999, 4 placebo controlled RCTs, 203 people).[50] Two of the RCTs (123 people) compared a mixture of dimethylfumaric and monoethylfumaric acid esters versus placebo. Pooled analysis found that this mixture of fumaric acid derivatives significantly reduced severity compared with placebo at 16 weeks (pooled ARR for ≥ 70% reduction in Psoriasis Area and Severity Index [PASI**G**] score 0.47, 95% CI 0.33 to 0.61).[50] The remaining RCTs in the review were reported in a single article[84] and compared either monoethylfumaric acid ester or dimethylfumaric acid ester versus placebo. The first of these RCTs found that dimethylfumaric acid ester alone significantly improved severity compared with placebo at 16 weeks (AR for ≥ 50% reduction in PASI 27% with dimethylfumaric acid alone *v* 0% with placebo; ARR 27%, 95% CI 6% to 45%).[84]

However, the other RCT found no significant difference in severity between monoethylfumaric acid ester and placebo at 16 weeks (ARR ≥ 50% improvement in PASI score –5%, 95% CI –22% to +12%).[84] We found no RCTs examining the use of fumaric acid as a maintenance treatment.

Harms: All large RCTs on fumaric acid esters found high withdrawal rates; 39% in the drug group of one RCT terminated the treatment prematurely, mostly because of gastrointestinal adverse effects.[50] Acute adverse effects, including flushing and gastrointestinal symptoms, were reported in up to 75% of people. In one RCT (50 people) of fumaric acid esters versus placebo for 16 weeks, diarrhoea was reported 27 times, stomach ache or stomach cramps 35 times, flushing 21 times, and skin burning twice.[50] Another open study (101 people) reported adverse effects in 69% of people (mainly gastrointestinal [56%] and flushing [31%]).[50] Eosinophilia was often reported. There have been case reports of renal failure, but one recent systematic review found no evidence of significant renal impairment.[50]

Comment: Additional evidence is needed on predictive factors for treatment failure, safety, and long term efficacy.

GLOSSARY

Body mass index A measure of obesity, defined as the weight (in kg) divided by the square of the height (in metres).

Dermatology Life Quality Index Validated 10 item questionnaire for assessing quality or life in people with various skin conditions, including psoriasis. Overall score ranges from 0 to 30, with a higher score indicating a lower quality of life.

Goeckerman treatment A daily application of coal tar followed by ultraviolet B irradiation.

Ingram regimen A daily coal tar bath, ultraviolet B irradiation, and dithranol.

Investigator assessment of global improvement A measure of overall change in lesion severity from baseline, scored on a 6 or 7 point scale, where the lowest score indicates worsening and the highest score indicates clearing of lesions. May also be referred to as the Physician's Global Assessment

Psoriasis Area and Severity Index (PASI) score Composite score grading severity of psoriasis in four body regions according to erythema, scaling, thickness, and the total area of skin affected. Severity of each of erythema, scaling, and thickness is graded from 0–4, and extension in each body region is graded from 1–6). The final composite score ranges from 0–72, with a higher score indicating a greater severity of psoriasis.

Physician's Global Assessment See Investigator assessment of global improvement above.

Skin types A clinical classification of an individual's burning and tanning tendencies. Usually ranges from skin phototype I (which always burns and never tans) to skin phototype VI (marked constitutive pigmentation).

Skin type regimen and minimal phototoxic dose regimen The four parameters of psoralen plus ultraviolet A are the dose of psoralen, the frequency of treatment, the initial dose of ultraviolet A, and the incremental ultraviolet A dose. The initial and incremental ultraviolet A doses are described by at least two regimens. In the minimal phototoxic dose regimen, the initial ultraviolet A dose is a fraction of the minimal phototoxic dose. Weekly increments in dose occur until the maximum dose is reached. In the skin type regimen, the initial dose is based on skin phototype. Weekly dose increments are decreased if erythema develops.

Total severity score Assesses signs (redness, scaling, thickness) and symptoms (itching) of psoriasis on 3- or 4-point scales. The scores for all signs and symptom are summed to obtain the total severity score, which typically ranges from 0–12, where a higher score indicates greater severity.

Substantive changes

Vitamin D derivatives Two RCTs and one review added;[36,37,41] benefits and harms data enhanced.

Combination regimens Ingram regimen re-categorised from Beneficial to Likely to be beneficial based on re-evaluation of the evidence.

Methotrexate One RCT added;[64] benefits and harms data enhanced.

Immunosuppressive drugs other than methotrexate and cyclosporin One RCT on anti-CD4 monoclonal antibodies added;[77] benefits and harms data enhanced.

Cytokine blocking agents Two RCTs on etanercept added;[79,80] benefits and harms data enhanced and categorisation of etanercept changed from Unknown effectiveness to Likely to be beneficial.

REFERENCES

1. Naldi L. Psoriasis. In: Williams HC, Strachan DP, eds. *The challenge of dermato-epidemiology*. Boca Raton: CRC Press, 1997;175–190.
2. De Korte J, Sprangers MAG, Mombers FMC, et al. Quality of life in patients with psoriasis: a systematic literature review. *J Invest Dermatol Symp Proc* 2004; 9:140–147.
3. Petersen LI, Kristensen JK. Selection of patients for psoriasis clinical trials: a survey of the recent dermatological literature. *J Dermatol Treat* 1992;3:171–176.
4. Spuls PI, Witkamp L, Bossuyt PM, et al. The course of chronic plaque-type psoriasis in placebo groups of randomized controlled studies. *Arch Dermatol* 2004;140:338–344.
5. Snellman E, Aromaa A, Jansen CT, et al. Supervised four-week heliotherapy alleviates the long-term course of psoriasis. *Acta Derm Venereol* 1993;73:388–392.
6. Turner RJ, Walshaw D, Diffey BL, et al. A controlled study of ultraviolet A sunbed treatment of psoriasis. *Br J Dermatol* 2000;143:957–963.
7. Zachariae R, Oster H, Bjerring P, et al. Effects of psychologic intervention on psoriasis: a preliminary report. *J Am Acad Dermatol* 1996;34:1008–1015.
8. Mayser P, Mrowietz U, Arenberger P, et al. Omega-3 fatty acid-based lipid infusion in patients with chronic plaque psoriasis: results of a double blind, randomised, placebo-controlled, multicenter trial. *J Am Acad Dermatol* 1998;38:539–547.
9. Veale DJ, Torley HI, Richards IM, et al. A double-blind placebo controlled trial of Efamol Marine on skin and joint symptoms of psoriatic arthritis. *Br J Rheumatol* 1994;33:954–958.
10. Soyland E, Funk J, Rajka G, et al. Effect of dietary supplementation with very-long-chain n-3 fatty acids in patients with psoriasis. *N Engl J Med* 1993;328:1812–1816.
11. Gupta AK, Ellis CN, Goldfarb MT, et al. The role of fish oil in psoriasis. A randomised, double-blind, placebo-controlled study to evaluate the effect of fish oil and topical steroid therapy in psoriasis. *Int J Dermatol* 1990;29:591–595.
12. Gupta AK, Ellis CN, Tellner DC, et al. Double-blind, placebo-controlled study to evaluate the efficacy of fish oil and low dose UVB in the treatment of psoriasis. *Br J Dermatol* 1989;120:801–807.
13. Bjorneboe A, Smith AK, Bjorneboe GE, et al. Effect of dietary supplementation with n-3 fatty acids on clinical manifestations of psoriasis. *Br J Dermatol* 1988;118:77–83.
14. Gambichler T, Kreuter JA, Altmeyer P, et al. Meta-analysis of the efficacy of balneotherapy. *Aktuelle Dermatologie* 2000;26:402–406. Search date 1999; primary sources Medline and Embase/Excerpta Medica.
15. Leaute-Labreze C, Saillour F, Chene G, et al. Saline spa water or combined water and UVB for psoriasis vs conventional UVB: lessons from the Salies de Bearn randomized study. *Arch Dermatol* 2001;137:1035–1039.
16. Zumiani G, Zanoni M, Agostini G. Evaluation of the efficacy of Comano thermal baths water versus tap water in the treatment of psoriasis. *G Ital Dermatol Venereol* 2000;135:259–263.
17. Jerner B, Skogh M, Vahlquist A. A controlled trial of acupuncture in psoriasis: no convincing effect. *Acta Derm Venereol* 1997;77:154–156.
18. Berne B, Blom I, Spangberg S. Enhanced response of psoriasis to UVB therapy after pretreatment with a lubricating base. *Acta Derm Venereol* 1990;70:474–477.
19. Mason J, Mason AR, Cork MJ. Topical preparations for the treatment of psoriasis: a systematic review. *Br J Dermatol* 2002;146:351–364. Search date 1999; primary sources Medline, Embase, Biosis, Healthstar, SIGLE, IHTA, Cochrane Controlled Trials Register, Conference Papers Index, Derwent Drug File, Dissertation Abstracts, Pascal, International Pharmaceutical Abstracts, Science Citation Index, hand searches of reference lists of trial reports and recent reviews, and personal contact with authors and companies.
20. Smith CH, Jackson K, Chinn S, et al. A double-blind randomized controlled clinical trial to assess the efficacy of a new coal tar preparation (Exorex) in the treatment of chronic, plaque type psoriasis. *Clin Exp Dermatol* 2000;25:580–583.
21. Stern RS, Gange RW, Parrish JA, et al. Contribution of topical tar oil to ultraviolet B phototherapy for psoriasis. *J Am Acad Dermatol* 1986;14:742–747.
22. Menkes A, Stern RS, Arndt KA. Psoriasis treatment with suberythemogenic ultraviolet B radiation and a coal tar extract. *J Am Acad Dermatol* 1985;12:21–25.
23. Eells LD, Wolff JM, Garloff J, et al. Comparison of suberythemogenic and maximally aggressive ultraviolet B therapy for psoriasis. *J Am Acad Dermatol* 1984;11:105–110.
24. Duhra P, Ryatt KS. Lack of additive effect of coal tar combined with dithranol for psoriasis. *Clin Exp Dermatol* 1988;13:72–73
25. Naldi L, Carrel CF, Parazzini F, et al. Development of anthralin short-contact therapy in psoriasis: survey of published clinical trials. *Int J Dermatol* 1992;31:126–130. Search date 1989; primary sources Medline, Index Medicus, and Excerpta Medica.
26. Katz HI, Prawer SE, Medansky RS, et al. Intermittent corticosteroid treatment of psoriasis: a double-blind multicenter trial of augmented betamethasone dipropionate ointment in a pulse dose treatment regimen. *Dermatologica* 1991;183:269–274.
27. Wilson L, Williams DI, Marsh SD. Plasma corticosteroid levels in outpatients treated with topical steroids. *Br J Dermatol* 1973;88:373–380.
28. Veien NK, Bjerke JR, Rossmann-Ringdahl I, et al. Once daily treatment of psoriasis with tacalcitol compared with twice daily treatment with calcipotriol: a double-blind trial. *Br J Dermatol* 1997;137:581–586.
29. Barker JN, Ashton RE, Marks R, et al. Topical maxacalcitol for the treatment of psoriasis vulgaris: a placebo controlled, double-blind, dose-finding study with active comparator. *Br J Dermatol* 1999;141:274–278.
30. Christensen OB, Mork NJ, Ashton R, et al. Comparison of a treatment phase and a follow-up phase of short contact dithranol and calcipotriol in outpatients with chronic plaque psoriasis. *J Dermatol Treat* 1999;10:261–265.
31. van der Kerkhof PC, Green C, Hamberg KJ, et al. Safety and efficacy of combined high-dose treatment with calcipotriol ointment and solution in patients with psoriasis. *Dermatology* 2002;204:214–221.
32. Ashcroft DM, Li Wan Po A, Williams HC, et al. Combination regimens of topical calcipotriene in

chronic plaque psoriasis: systematic review of efficacy and tolerability. *Arch Dermatol* 2000;136:1536–1543. Search date 1999; primary sources Medline and Embase.
33. Kaufmann R, Bibby AJ, Bissonnette R, et al. A new calcipotriol/betamethasone dipropionate formulation (Daivobet) is an effective once-daily treatment for psoriasis vulgaris. *Dermatology* 2002;205:389–393.
34. Monastirilj A, Georgiou S, Pasmatzi E, et al. Calcipotriol plus short-contact dithranol: a novel topical combination therapy for chronic plaque psoriasis. *Skin Pharmacol Appl Skin Physiol* 2002;15:246–251.
35. Gollinck H, Altmeyer P, Kaufmann R, et al. Topical calcipotriol plus oral fumaric acid is more effective and faster acting than oral fumaric acid monotherapy in the treatment of severe chronic plaque psoriasis vulgaris. *Dermatology* 2002;205:46–53.
36. Papp K, Guenther L, Boyden B, et al. Early onset of action and efficacy of a combination of calcipotriene and betametasone diproprionate in the treatment of psoriasis. *J Am Acad Dermatol* 2003;48:48–54.
37. de Jong EM, Mork NJ, Seijger MM, et al. The combination of calcipotriol and methotrexate compared with methotrexate and vehicle in psoriasis: results of a multicentre placebo-controlled randomized trial. *Br J Dermatol* 2003;148:318–325.
38. Ramsay CA, Schwartz BE, Lowson D, et al. Calcipotriol cream combined with twice weekly broad-band UVB phototherapy: a safe, effective and UVB-sparing antipsoriatic combination treatment. *Dermatology* 2000;200:17–24.
39. Ashcroft DM, Li Wan Po A, Williams HC, et al. Systematic review of comparative efficacy and tolerability of calcipotriol in treating chronic plaque psoriasis. *BMJ* 2000;320:963–967. Search date 1999; primary sources Medline, Embase, Cochrane Controlled Trials Register, Bids, hand searches of reference lists, and contact with manufacturer of calcipotriol.
40. Kragballe K, Barnes L, Hamberg K, et al. Calcipotriol cream with or without concurrent topical corticosteroid in psoriasis. Tolerability and efficacy. *Br J Dermatol* 1998;139:649–654.
41. Bruner CR, Feldman SR, Ventrapragada M, et al. A systematic review of adverse effects associated with topical treatments for psoriasis. *Dermatol Online J* 2003;9:2.
42. Weinstein GD, Koo JY, Krueger GG, et al. Tazarotene cream in the treatment of psoriasis: two multicenter, double-blind, randomized, vehicle-controlled studies of the safety and efficacy of tazarotene creams 0.05% and 0.1% applied once daily for 12 weeks. *J Am Acad Dermatol* 2003;48:760–767.
43. Krueger GG, Drake LA, Elias PM, et al. The safety and efficacy of tazarotene gel, a topical acetylenic retinoid, in the treatment of psoriasis. *Arch Dermatol* 1998;134:57–60.
44. Weinstein GD, Krueger GG, Lowe NJ, et al. Tazarotene gel, a new retinoid, for topical therapy of psoriasis: vehicle-controlled study of safety, efficacy, and duration of therapeutic effect. *J Am Acad Dermatol* 1997;37:85–92.
45. Green L, Sadoff W. A clinical evaluation of tazarotene 0.1% gel, with and without a high- or mid-high-potency corticosteroid, in patients with stable plaque psoriasis. *J Cutan Med Surg* 2002;6:95–102.
46. Guenther LC, Poulin YP, Pariser DM. A comparison of tazarotene 0.1% gel once daily plus mometasone furoate 0.1% cream once daily versus calcipotriene 0.005% ointment twice daily in the treatment of plaque psoriasis. *Clin Ther* 2000;22:1225–1238.
47. Gollnick H, Menter A. Combination therapy with tazarotene plus a topical corticosteroid for the treatment of plaque psoriasis. *Br J Dermatol* 1999;140(suppl):18–23.
48. Lebwohl M, Ast E, Callen JP, et al. Once-daily tazarotene gel versus twice-daily fluocinonide cream in the treatment of plaque psoriasis. *J Am Acad Dermatol* 1998;38:705–711.
49. Lebwohl MG, Breneman DL, Goffe BS, et al. Tazarotene 0.1% gel plus corticosteroid cream in the treatment of plaque psoriasis. *J Am Acad Dermatol* 1998;39:590–596.
50. Griffiths CEM, Clark CM, Chalmers RJG, et al. A systematic review of treatments for severe psoriasis. *Health Technol Assess* 2000;4:1–125. Search date 1999; primary sources Medline, Embase, and Cochrane Register of RCTs.
51. Cameron H, Dawe RS, Yule S, et al. A randomized, observer-blinded trial of twice vs. three times weekly narrowband ultraviolet B phototherapy for chronic plaque psoriasis. *Br J Dermatol* 2002;147:973–978.
52. Boer J, Hermans J, Schothorst AA, et al. Comparison of phototherapy (UVB) and photochemotherapy (PUVA) for clearing and maintenance therapy of psoriasis. *Arch Dermatol* 1984;120:52–57.
53. Gorden PM, Diffey BL, Mathews JN, et al. A randomised comparison of narrow-band TL-01 phototherapy for psoriasis. *J Am Acad Dermatol* 1999;41:728–732.
54. Stern RS, Armstrong RB, Anderson TF, et al. Effect of continued ultraviolet B phototherapy on the duration of remission of psoriasis. A randomized study. *J Am Acad Dermatol* 1986;15:546–552.
55. Pieternel CM, Pasker-de-Jong M, Wielink G, et al. Treatment with UV-B for psoriasis and nonmelanoma skin cancer. A systematic review of the literature. *Arch Dermatol* 1999;135:834–840. Search date 1996; primary sources Medline, Biosis, and Online Contents.
56. Stern RS, Lunder EJ. Risk of squamous cell carcinoma and methoxsalen (psoralen) and UV-A radiation (PUVA). A meta-analysis. *Arch Dermatol* 1998;134:1582–1585. Search date 1998; primary sources Medline, Healthstar, Aidsline, and Cancerlit.
57. Melski JW, Tanenbaum L, Parrish JA, et al. Oral methoxsalen photochemotherapy for the treatment of psoriasis. A cooperative clinical trial. *J Invest Dermatol* 1977;68:328–335.
58. Stern RS, Laird N. The carcinogenic risk of treatments for severe psoriasis. Photochemotherapy follow-up study. *Cancer* 1994;73:2759–2764.
59. Hannuksela-Svahn A, Sigurgeirsson B, Pukkala E, et al. Trioxsalen bath PUVA did not increase the risk of squamous cell skin carcinoma and cutaneous malignant melanoma in a joint analysis of 944 Swedish and Finnish patients with psoriasis. *Br J Dermatol* 1999;141:497–501.
60. Rogers S, Marks J, Shuster S, et al. Comparison of photochemotherapy and dithranol in the treatment of chronic plaque psoriasis. *Lancet* 1979;i:455–458.
61. Jones G, Crotty M, Brooks P. Interventions for treating psoriatic arthritis. An overview of therapy and toxicity. In: The Cochrane Library, Issue 3, 2001. Oxford: Update Software. Search date 2000; primary sources Medline, Excerpta Medica, and Cochrane Clinical Trials Register.
62. Stern RS, Fitzgerald E, Ellis CN, et al. The safety of etretinate as long-term therapy for psoriasis. Results of the etretinate follow-up study. *J Am Acad Dermatol* 1995;33:44–52.
63. Wilkens RF, Williams HJ, Ward JR, et al. Randomized, double-blind, placebo controlled trial of low-dose pulse methotrexate in psoriatic arthritis. *Arthritis Rheum* 1984;27:376–381.
64. Heydendael VM, Spuls PI, Opmeer BC et al. Methotrexate versus cyclosporine in moderate-to-severe chronic plaque psoriasis. *N Engl J Med* 349:658–665.
65. Whiting-O'Keefe QE, Fye KH, Sack KD. Methotrexate and histologic hepatic abnormalities. *Am J Med* 1991;90:711–716. Search date and primary sources not reported.
66. Cottin V, Tebib J, Souquet PJ, et al. Pulmonary function in patients receiving long-term low-dose methotrexate. *Chest* 1996;109:933–938.
67. Nyfors A, Jensen H. Frequency of malignant neoplasms in 248 long-term methotrexate-treated psoriatics. A preliminary study. *Dermatologica* 1983;167:260–261.

68. Van Dooren-Greebe RJ, Kuijpers AL, Mulder J, et al. Methotrexate revisited: effects of long-term treatment of psoriasis. *Br J Dermatol* 1994;130:204–210.
69. Shupack J, Abel E, Bauer E, et al. Cyclosporine as maintenance therapy in patients with severe psoriasis. *J Am Acad Dermatol* 1997;36:423–432.
70. Ellis CN, Fradin MS, Hamilton TA, et al. Duration of remission during maintenance cyclosporine therapy for psoriasis. Relationship to maintenance dose and degree of improvement during initial therapy. *Arch Dermatol* 1995;131:791–795.
71. Zachariae H, Abrams B, Bleehen SS, et al. Conversion of psoriasis patients from the conventional formulation of cyclosporin A to a new microemulsion formulation: a randomized, open, multicentre assessment of safety and tolerability. *Dermatology* 1998;196:231–236.
72. Ho VC, Griffiths CE, Albrecht G, et al. Intermittent short courses of cyclosporin (Neoral(R)) for psoriasis unresponsive to topical therapy: a 1-year multicentre, randomized study. *Br J Dermatol* 1999;141:283–291.
73. Ozawa A, Sugai J, Ohkido M, et al. Cyclosporin in psoriasis: continuous monotherapy versus intermittent long-term therapy. *Eur J Dermatol* 1999;9:218–223.
74. Grossman RM, Chevret S, Abi-Rached J, et al. Long-term safety of cyclosporin in the treatment of psoriasis. *Arch Dermatol* 1996;132:623–629.
75. The European FK 506 Multicentre Psoriasis Study Group. Systemic tacrolimus (FK 506) is effective for the treatment of psoriasis in a double-blind, placebo-controlled study. *Arch Dermatol* 1996;132:419–423.
76. Gottlieb AB, Lebwohl M, Shirin S, et al. Anti-CD4 monoclonal antibody treatment of moderate to severe psoriasis vulgaris: results of a pilot, multicenter, multiple-dose, placebo-controlled study. *J Am Acad Dermatol* 2000;43:595–604.
77. Skov L, Kragballe K, Zachariae C, et al. HuMax-CD4: a fully human monoclonal anti-CD4 antibody for the treatment of psoriasis vulgaris. *Arch Dermatol* 2003;139:1433–1439.
78. Mihatsch MJ, Kyo M, Morozumi K, et al. The side-effects of cyclosporin A and tacrolimus. *Clin Nephrol* 1998;49:356–363.
79. Gottlieb AB, Matheson RT, Lowe N, et al. A randomized trial of etanercept as monotherapy for psoriasis. *Arch Dermatol* 2003;139:1627–1632.
80. Leonardi CL, Powers JL, Matheson RT, et al. Etanercept as monotherapy in patients with psoriasis. *N Engl J Med* 2003;349:2014–2022.
81. Chaudhari U, Romano P, Mulcahy LD, et al. Efficacy and safety of infliximab monotherapy for plaque-type psoriasis: a randomised trial. *Lancet* 2001;357:1842–1847.
82. Skytta E, Pohjankoski H, Savolainen A. Etanercept and urticaria in patients with juvenile idiopathic arthritis. *Clin Exp Rheumatol* 2000;18:533–534.
83. Kalden JR. How do the biologics fit into the current DMARD armamentarium? *J Rheumatol* 2001;28(suppl 62):27–35.
84. Nieboer C, de Hoop D, van Loenen AC, et al. Systemic therapy with fumaric acid derivates: new possibilities in the treatment of psoriasis. *J Am Acad Dermatol* 1989;20:601–608.

Luigi Naldi
Dermatologist
Ospedali Riuniti Bergamo, Bergamo, Italy

Berthold Rzany
Dermatologist
Klinik für Dermatologie Universittsklinikum Mannheim, Mannheim, Germany

Competing interests: The research activities of the Italian Group for Epidemiologic Research in Dermatology, which is coordinated by one of the authors (LN), have been supported by grants from GlaxoWellcome, Roche, Novartis, Schering, and Schering-Plough. BR has received grant/research support from Fumedica GmbH, Serono, Leo Pharma, Schering, and Biogen.

TABLE 1 RCTs of fish oil supplementation (see text, p 2074).

Ref	Intervention	Control regimen	Number of people	Outcome measure	Duration	Results (intervention *v* control)
8	Infusion of omega-3 fatty acid	Placebo (conventional omega-6)	83	Decrease in PASI by at least 50% from baseline	14 days	16/43 (37%) *v* 9/40 (23%) OR 0.4 (95% CI 0.1 to 1.2)
9	Evening primrose oil + fish oil capsule	Placebo (empty capsule)	38	Skin and joint disease activity	12 months	No difference in disease activity
10	Fish oil capsule	Placebo (corn oil)	145	PASI and total subjective score	4 months	No difference in disease activity
11	Fish oil capsule + topical steroid	Placebo (olive oil) + topical steroid	25	Rate of relapse on withdrawal of topical steroids	9 weeks	No difference in relapse
12	Fish oil capsule + UVB	Placebo (olive oil) + UVB	18	Total body surface area of psoriasis	19 weeks	Significantly greater improvement on fish oil
13	Fish oil	Olive oil	41	Clinical activity	8 weeks	No difference in disease activity

PASI, Psoriasis Area and Severity Index; Ref, reference; UVB, ultraviolet B.

TABLE 2 **RCTs of topical tazarotene alone or in combination (see text, p 2080).**

Ref	Study design	Intervention and control regimens	Number of people	Outcome measure	Duration	Results (intervention *v* control)
42	Parallel group	Tazarotene 0.05% or 0.1% once daily v placebo	1303	Global response, reduction in plaque elevation and scaling	12 weeks	Significantly more effective than vehicle
43 (study A)	Within-participant control: 2 bilateral target plaques	Tazarotene 0.05% or 0.1% twice daily v placebo	45	Treatment success (defined as > 75% improvement from baseline); plaque elevation, scaling, and erythema	6 weeks	Treatment success: 45% with 0.05% tazarotene gel v 13% with placebo after 6 weeks ($P < 0.05$)
43 (study B)	Within-participant control: 2 bilateral target plaques	Tazarotene 0.05% or 0.1% once or twice daily	108	Treatment success (defined as > 75% improvement from baseline); plaque elevation, scaling, and erythema	8 weeks	ARs ranged from 48% to 63% depending on the various tazarotene treatment regimens after 8 weeks of treatment. Between group differences not reported
44	Parallel group	Tazarotene 0.05% or 0.1% v placebo	324 (318 evaluable)	Plaque elevation, scaling, and erythema; percentage treatment success (> 50% improvement) time to initial success	12 weeks	Clinical response was judged to be good, excellent, or completely cleared in 60% of those on tazarotene (0.1%) v 30% of those on placebo (RRR for tazarotene 0.1% v placebo 43%, 95% CI 30% to 60%).
45	Parallel group	Tazarotene 0.1% + high or mid-potency steroid v tazarotene alone	200	Global improvement	12 weeks	Better improvement with tazarotene + mid-potency steroid. No further data reported

TABLE 2 continued

Ref	Study design	Intervention and control regimens	Number of people	Outcome measure	Duration	Results (intervention *v* control)
46	Parallel group	Tazarotene 0.1% + mometasone furoate once daily v calcipotriol twice daily	120 (106 evaluable)	Marked improvement (> 75% global improvement) or clearance (> 90%)	8 weeks	45% marked improvement on tazarotene v 26% on calcipotriol ($P < 0.05$). No significant difference for clearance
47 (study 1)	Within-participant control: 2 bilateral target plaques	Tazarotene + high-potency steroid v tazarotene + mid-potency steroid v tazarotene + placebo	300	Plaque improvement	12 weeks	91% and 95% of plaques improved on the combination regimen v 80% on tazarotene alone; $P < 0.05$
47 (study 2)	Within-participant control: 2 bilateral target plaques	Tazarotene + high-potency steroid each day v tazarotene alternating with a mid-potency corticosteroid or placebo	398	Plaque improvement	12 weeks	75% with tazarotene + high-potency steroid v 55% tazarotene alternating with a mid-potency corticosteroid v 54% with placebo ($P < 0.05$)
48	Parallel group	Once daily tazarotene 0.05% or 0.1% v twice daily fluocinonide	348 (275 evaluable)	Scaling, erythema, elevation	12 weeks	No significant difference at 12 weeks
49	Parallel group	Tazarotene 0.1% with placebo, or with a low, mid-, or high potency steroid	300	Scaling, erythema and overall lesional severity	12 weeks	Higher response rates with combination regimens compared with tazarotene alone

Ref, reference.

Head lice

Search date October 2003

Ian Burgess

QUESTIONS

INTERVENTIONS

See glossary G

Key Messages

- **Insecticide based pharmaceutical products** Two RCTs identified by a systematic review found that permethrin and malathion both increased lice eradication rates compared with placebo. Limited evidence from an earlier systematic review suggested that permethrin increased eradication rates compared with lindane. We found inconclusive evidence from three RCTs about the comparative efficacy of insecticides and combing. One RCT found no significant difference between a herbal product and insecticide.
- **Herbal and essential oils** We found no RCTs that compared herbal treatment with placebo. One RCT found no significant difference in eradication rates between a herbal product (mixture of coconut, anise, and ylang ylang) and insecticide (permethrin, malathion, and piperonyl butoxide). However, results may not generalise to different concentrations of these components or to different herbal preparations.
- **Mechanical removal of lice or viable eggs by combing** We found inconclusive evidence from three RCTs about effects of combing instead of or in addition to insecticides.
- **Repellents** We found insufficient evidence on the effects of these interventions.

Head lice

DEFINITION Head lice are obligate ectoparasites of socially active humans. They infest the scalp and attach their eggs to the hair shafts. Itching, resulting from multiple bites, is not diagnostic but may increase the index of suspicion. Eggs glued to hairs, whether hatched (nits) or unhatched, are not proof of active infection, because eggs may retain a viable appearance for weeks after death. A conclusive diagnosis can only be made by finding live lice.

INCIDENCE/ PREVALENCE We found no studies on incidence and no recent published prevalence results from any developed country. Anecdotal reports suggest that prevalence has increased in the past few years in most communities in the UK and USA.

AETIOLOGY/ RISK FACTORS Observational studies indicate that infections occur most frequently in school children, although there is no proof of a link with school attendance.[1,2] We found no evidence that lice prefer clean hair to dirty hair.

PROGNOSIS The infection is almost harmless. Sensitisation reactions to louse saliva and faeces may result in localised irritation and erythema. Secondary infection of scratches may occur. Lice have been identified as primary mechanical vectors of scalp pyoderma(G) caused by streptococci and staphylococci usually found on the skin.[3]

AIMS OF INTERVENTION To eliminate infestation by killing or removing all head lice and their eggs.

OUTCOMES Treatment success is given as the percentage of people completely cleared of head lice. There are no standard criteria for judging treatment success. Trials used different methods and, in many cases, the method was not stated. Few studies were pragmatic(G).

METHODS *Clinical Evidence* search and appraisal October 2003. The initial search was performed by the Cochrane Infectious Diseases Group at the Liverpool School of Tropical Medicine for a systematic review compiled in July 1998.[4]

QUESTION What are the effects of treatments for head lice?

OPTION INSECTICIDE BASED PHARMACEUTICAL PRODUCTS

Two RCTs identified by a systematic review found that permethrin and malathion both increased lice eradication rates compared with placebo. Limited evidence from an earlier systematic review suggested that permethrin increased eradication rates compared with lindane. We found inconclusive evidence from three RCTs about the comparative efficacy of insecticides and combing. One RCT found no significant difference between a herbal product and insecticide.

Benefits: We found two systematic reviews.[4,5] The first systematic review (search date 1995, 7 RCTs, 1808 people) assessed 11 insecticide products, including lindane, carbaryl, malathion, permethrin, and other pyrethroids in various vehicles.[5] A more recent systematic review (search date 2001, 2 RCTs, 345 children and adults) set stricter criteria for RCTs,[4] and excluded studies on which the earlier review was based.[5] **Versus placebo:** The second systematic review identified one RCT (63 people) comparing permethrin with placebo.[4] It found that permethrin (1% cream rinse) significantly increased eradication rates compared with placebo after 7 and 14 days (7 days: 29/29 [100%] with permethrin *v* 3/34 [9%] with placebo; OR 36, 95% CI 14 to 97; 14 days: 28/29 [97%] with permethrin *v* 2/24 [8%] with placebo; OR 36, 95% CI 13 to 96). The second systematic review also identified one RCT (115 people) comparing malathion (0.5% alcoholic lotion) with placebo.[4] It found that malathion significantly increased eradication rates after 1 week compared with placebo (62/65 [95%] with malathion *v* 21/47 [45%] with placebo; RR 2.1, 95% CI 1.5 to 2.9; NNT 2, 95% CI 1 to 3). **Versus each other:** The first systematic review (7 RCTs, 726 people, search date 1995) found that permethrin (1% cream rinse) significantly increased eradication rates compared with lindane after 14 days (1% shampoo) (lindane *v* permethrin; 2 RCTs; OR for not clearing head lice 15.2, 95% CI 8.0 to 28.8).[5] **Versus mechanical removal of lice:** See mechanical removal of lice or viable eggs by combing, p 2101. **Versus herbal oils:** See herbal and essential oils, p 2102.

Harms: Only minor adverse effects have been reported for most insecticides. The exception is lindane, where there are extensive reports of CNS effects related to overdosing (treatment of scabies) and absorption (treatment of head lice). Transdermal passage of lindane occurs during treatment of head lice,[6] but we found no reports of adverse effects in this setting.

Comment: A number of studies were rejected by reviewers as they followed up participants for only 6 days, which is inadequate as the eggs take 7 days to hatch. Most investigators agree that a final examination after 14 days is necessary to determine cure. Three trials included in the more recent systematic review were conducted in developing countries where insecticide treatments were not regularly available.[4] This may have resulted in greater efficacy, because the insects may have had no previous exposure to the therapeutic agent. Studies *in vitro* suggest that other components of products (e.g. terpenoids and solvents) may be more effective pediculicides❻ than the insecticide itself.[7] Resistance to one or more insecticides is now common.[8–10] One RCT (193 people) investigating resistance compared malathion (0.5% lotion with terpenoids) with phenothrin (0.3% lotion) in a community where lice were identified *in vitro* as being tolerant of phenothrin.[11] After 1 day, malathion increased lice eradication rates compared with phenothrin (louse free: 87/95 [92%] with malathion *v* 39/98 [40%] with phenothrin; RR 2.3, 95% CI 1.7 to 2.9) and this difference had increased by day 7 (90/95 [95%] with malathion *v* 38/98 [39%] with phenothrin; RR 2.4, 95% CI 1.8 to 3.2). However, some children not free from lice on day 1 had become louse free by day 7 in both groups, suggesting that some parental intervention had influenced the results. This study suggests that resistance to pyrethroid insecticide may have influenced about 60% of the treatments.

OPTION MECHANICAL REMOVAL OF LICE OR VIABLE EGGS BY COMBING

We found inconclusive evidence from three RCTs about effects of combing instead of or in addition to insecticides.

Benefits: We found no systematic review. **Combing versus insecticide:** We found two RCTs that compared combing with an insecticide treatment.[12,13] The first RCT (72 people) compared "bug busting" (wet combing with conditioner) versus two applications of 0.5% malathion 7 days apart.[12] It found that malathion significantly improved lice eradication rates compared with "bug busting" after 14 days (12/32 [38%] with "bug busting" *v* 31/40 [78%] with malathion; RR for "bug busting" *v* malathion 0.48, 95% CI 0.30 to 0.78; NNT 3, 95% CI 2 to 5).[12] The second RCT (30 people) compared "bug busting" versus two weekly applications of phenothrin lotion (concentration not specified) plus combing. It found that "bug busting" significantly increased eradication of head lice after 14 days compared with phenothrin (eradication rates: 8/15 [53%] with "bug busting" *v* 2/15 [13%] with phenothrin group; RR 4.0, 95% CI 1.0 to 15.8; NNT 3, 95% CI 2 to 17).[13] **Combing plus insecticide:** We found one RCT (95 adults and children), which compared combing with a metal louse/nit comb plus 1% permethrin cream rinse with permethrin cream rinse alone.[14] In both groups permethrin was applied by a community practitioner and if lice were found after 7 days a further application of permethrin, or permethrin plus combing, was given. It found no significant difference in eradication rates with adjuvant combing compared with permethrin alone at 2, 8, and 15 days (louse free rates, at day 2: 49/59 [83%] with no combing v 24/33 [73%] with combing; RR 1.14, 95% CI 0.90 to 1.50; at day 8 before repeat treatment: 27/59 [46%] with no combing v 11/33 [33%] with combing; RR 0.92, 95% CI 0.60 to 1.40; at day 15: 47/60 [78%] with no combing v 24/33 [73%] with combing; RR 1.08, 95% CI 0.80 to 1.40). We found three RCTs comparing different pediculicides in combination with nit combing, but none included a non-combing or non-insecticide control group.[15–17]

Harms: Apart from discomfort, we found no evidence of harms from combing. Wet combing with conditioner may cause adverse reactions, which have been observed during normal cosmetic use.[18–22]

Comment: The first RCT looking at "bug busting" was designed be a pragmatic RCT**G** with results that are applicable to normal practice.[12] In the second RCT interventions were applied by trained nurses. "Bug busting" involved the use of different graded combs and specific hair conditioner, while people in the phenothrin group used a single head lice comb and unspecified hair conditioners. The follow up strategy for the combing group differed from that offered to the lotion group.[13] This difference may introduce bias and confounding. One observational study compared two groups of children with louse eggs but no lice at initial assessment.[23] These children were followed to see if they developed active infestation over a period of 14 days. More children with five or more eggs within 6 mm of the scalp developed infestations compared with those with fewer than five eggs (infestation rates: 7/22 [32%] with ≥5 eggs v 2/28 [7%] with < 5 eggs; RR 4.45, 95% CI 1.02 to 19.30). The authors concluded that adequate follow up examinations are more likely to be productive than nit removal to prevent reinfestation.

OPTION HERBAL AND ESSENTIAL OILS

We found no RCTs that compared herbal products with placebo. One RCT found no significant difference in eradication rates between a herbal product (coconut, anise, and ylang ylang) and insecticide (permethrin and malathion, synergised with piperonyl butoxide). However, results may not generalise to different concentrations of these components or to different herbal preparations.

Benefits: We found no systematic review. **Versus placebo:** We found no RCTs that compared herbal products with placebo. We found one RCT (143 children) that compared a spray based on herbal oils (coconut, anise, and ylang ylang; concentrations unspecified) versus an insecticide spray (0.5% permethrin and 0.25% malathion, synergised with 2% piperonyl butoxide).[24] The herbal spray was used three times at 5 day intervals and the insecticide twice with 10 days between applications. It found no significant difference in eradication rates between the herbal product and insecticide (60/70 [86%] with herbal product v 59/73 [81%] with insecticide).

Harms: The RCT found no clinically detectable adverse effects with either herbal oils (a mixture of coconut, anise, and ylang ylang) or insecticide spray (permethrin and malathion, synergised with piperonyl butoxide).[24] A potential for toxic effects has been recognised for several essential oils.[25]

Comment: Results may not generalise to different concentrations of these herbal ingredients or to other herbal products.

OPTION **REPELLENTS**

We found no systematic review, RCTs, or cohort studies on the effects of chemicals (such as piperonal) used as repellents.

Benefits: We found no systematic review, RCTs, or cohort studies evaluating repellents.

Harms: We found no evidence of harms.

Comment: None.

GLOSSARY

Pediculicide Any compound or material (possibly a pesticide) that kills lice. This term is used specifically in place of "insecticide" as not all pediculicides are recognised pesticides. A pediculicide is distinct from an "ovicide", which kills louse eggs, although one substance may fulfil both functions.

Pragmatic RCT An RCT designed to provide results that are directly applicable to normal practice (compared with explanatory trials that are intended to clarify efficacy under ideal conditions). Pragmatic RCTs recruit a population that is representative of those who are normally treated, allow normal compliance with instructions (by avoiding incentives and by using oral instructions with advice to follow manufacturers' instructions), and analyse results by "intention to treat" rather than by "on treatment" methods.

Scalp pyoderma Scalp pyoderma involves impetigo-like bacterial infections that result from scratching. In most cases they are due to streptococci with some staphylococcal involvement. Scalp pyoderma of this type is closely associated with long term louse infestation.

REFERENCES

1. Burgess IF. Human lice and their management. *Adv Parasitol* 1995;36:271–342.
2. Gratz NG. *Human lice. Their prevalence, control and resistance to insecticides*. Geneva: World Health Organization, 1997.
3. Taplin D, Meinking TL. Infestations. In: Schachner LA, Hansen RC, eds. *Pediatric dermatology*, Vol 2. New York: Churchill Livingstone, 1988:1465–1493.
4. Dodd CS. Interventions for treating head lice (Cochrane Review). In: The Cochrane Library, Issue 4, 2003. Oxford: Update Software. Search date 2001; primary sources Cochrane Infectious Diseases Group Trials Register, Cochrane Controlled Trials Register, Medline, Embase, Science Citation Index, Biosis, Toxline, hand searches of reference lists from relevant articles, and personal contact with pharmaceutical companies and UK and US Regulatory Authorities.
5. Vander Stichele RH, Dezeure EM, Bogaert MG. Systematic review of clinical efficacy of topical treatments for head lice. *BMJ* 1995;311:604–608. Search date 1995; primary sources Medline, International Pharmaceutical Abstracts, and Science Citation Index.
6. Ginsburg CM, Lowry W. Absorption of gamma benzene hexachloride following application of Kwell shampoo. *Pediatr Dermatol* 1983;1:74–76.
7. Burgess I. Malathion lotions for head lice: a less reliable treatment than commonly believed. *Pharm J* 1991;247:630–632.
8. Burgess IF, Brown CM, Peock S, et al. Head lice resistant to pyrethroid insecticides in Britain [letter]. *BMJ* 1995;311:752.
9. Pollack RJ, Kiszewski A, Armstrong P, et al. Differential permethrin susceptibility of head lice sampled in the United States and Borneo. *Arch Pediatr Adolesc Med* 1999;153:969–973.
10. Lee SH, Yoon KS, Williamson M, et al. Molecular analyses of *kdr*-like resistance in permethrin-resistant strains of head lice, *Pediculus capitis*. *Pestic Biochem Physiol* 2000;66:130–143.
11. Chosidow O, Chastang C, Brue C, et al. Controlled study of malathion and *d*-phenothrin lotions for *Pediculus humanus* var *capitis*-infested schoolchildren. *Lancet* 1994;334:1724–1727.
12. Roberts RJ, Casey D, Morgan DA, et al. Comparison of wet combing with malathion for treatment of head lice in the UK: a pragmatic randomised controlled trial. *Lancet* 2000;356:540–544.
13. Plastow L, Luthra M, Powell R, et al. Head lice infestation: bug busting vs. traditional treatment. *J Clin Nurs* 2001;10:775–783.
14. Meinking TL, Clineschmidt CM, Chen C, et al. An observer-blinded study of 1% permethrin creme rinse with and without adjunctive combing in patients with head lice. *J Pediatr* 2002;141:665–670.
15. Bainbridge CV, Klein GI, Neibart SI, et al. Comparative study of the clinical effectiveness of a pyrethrin-based pediculicide with combing versus a permethrin-based pediculicide with combing. *Clin Pediatr (Phila)* 1998;37:17–22.
16. Clore ER, Longyear LA. A comparative study of seven pediculicides and their packaged nit combs. *J Pediatr Health Care* 1993;7:55–60.
17. Hipolito RB, Mallorca FG, Zuniga-Macaraig ZO, et al. Head lice infestation: single drug versus combination therapy with one percent permethrin and trimethoprim/sulfamethoxazole. *Pediatrics* 2001;107:E30.
18. Korting JC, Pursch EM, Enders F, et al. Allergic contact dermatitis to cocamidopropyl betaine in shampoo. *J Am Acad Dermatol* 1992;27:1013–1015.
19. Niinimaki A, Niinimaki M, Makinen-Kiljunen S, et al. Contact urticaria from protein hydrolysates in hair conditioners. *Allergy* 1998;53:1070–1082.
20. Schalock PC, Storrs FJ, Morrison L. Contact urticaria from panthenol in hair conditioner. *Contact Dermatitis* 2000;43:223.

21. Pasche-Koo F, Claeys M, Hauser C. Contact urticaria with systemic symptoms caused by bovine collagen in hair conditioner. *Am J Contact Dermatol* 1996;7:56–57.
22. Stadtmauer G, Chandler M. Hair conditioner causes angioedema. *Ann Allergy Asthma Immunol* 1997;78:602.
23. Williams LK, Reichert A, MacKenzie WR, et al. Lice, nits, and school policy. *Pediatrics* 2001;107:1011–1015.
24. Mumcuoglu KY, Miller J, Zamir C, et al. The *in vivo* pediculicidal efficacy of a natural remedy. *Isr Med Assoc J* 2002;4:790–793.
25. Veal L. The potential effectiveness of essential oils as a treatment for headlice, *Pediculus humanus capitis*. *Complement Ther Nurs Midwifery* 1996;2:97–101.

Ian Burgess
Director
Insect Research & Development Limited
Cambridge
UK

Competing interests: IB has been a consultant to various makers of pharmaceutical products, alternative therapies, and combs for treating louse infestations.

Herpes labialis

Search date April 2004

Graham Worrall

QUESTIONS

INTERVENTIONS

Key Messages

Prevention

- **Oral antiviral agents (aciclovir)** Six RCTs found limited evidence suggesting that prophylactic oral antiviral agents may reduce the frequency and severity of attacks compared with placebo, but the optimal timing and duration of treatment is uncertain.
- **Sunscreen** Two small crossover RCTs found limited evidence that ultraviolet sunscreen may reduce herpes recurrence compared with placebo.
- **Topical antiviral agents** We found no RCTs on the effects of topical antiviral agents used as prophylaxis.

Treatment for first attack

- **Oral antiviral agents (aciclovir)** One small RCT in children found that oral aciclovir reduced the mean duration of pain compared with placebo. Another small RCT in children found that oral aciclovir reduced the median time to healing compared with placebo.
- **Topical antiviral agents** We found no RCTs on the effects of topical antiviral agents.

Treatment for recurrent attack

- **Oral antiviral agents (aciclovir and valaciclovir)** Four RCTs found that oral aciclovir and valaciclovir (if taken early in the attack) marginally reduced the duration of symptoms and pain compared with placebo. Two large RCTs found no significant difference between a 1 day and a 2 day course of valaciclovir and found that a higher proportion of people experienced headaches with valaciclovir compared with placebo.
- **Topical antiviral agents (aciclovir and penciclovir)** Twelve RCTs found limited evidence that topical penciclovir or aciclovir reduced the duration of pain and symptoms compared with placebo, but found stronger evidence that healing time is reduced.

- **Topical anaesthetic agents** One small RCT found limited evidence that topical tetracaine reduced the mean time to scab loss and increased the proportion of people who subjectively rated the treatment as effective compared with placebo. However, the clinical importance of these results is unclear.
- **Zinc oxide cream** One small RCT found limited evidence that zinc oxide cream reduced time to healing compared with placebo, but found that it increased the risk of skin irritation.

DEFINITION	Herpes labialis is a mild self limiting infection with herpes simplex virus type 1. It causes pain and blistering on the lips and perioral area (cold sores); fever and constitutional symptoms are rare. Most people have no warning of an attack, but some experience a recognisable prodrome.
INCIDENCE/ PREVALENCE	Herpes labialis accounts for about 1% of primary care consultations in the UK each year; 20–40% of people have experienced cold sores at some time.[1]
AETIOLOGY/ RISK FACTORS	Herpes labialis is caused by herpes simplex virus type 1. After the primary infection, which usually occurs in childhood, the virus is thought to remain latent in the trigeminal ganglion.[2] A variety of factors, including exposure to bright sunlight, fatigue, or psychological stress, can precipitate a recurrence.
PROGNOSIS	In most people, herpes labialis is a mild, self limiting illness. Recurrences are usually shorter and less severe than the initial attack. Healing is usually complete in 7–10 days without scarring.[3] Rates of reactivation are unknown. Herpes labialis can cause serious illness in immunocompromised people.
AIMS OF INTERVENTION	To reduce the frequency and severity of recurrent attacks; to speed healing of lesions; to reduce pain, with minimal adverse effects.
OUTCOMES	Severity of symptoms; duration of symptoms; time to crusting of lesions; time to healing; rate of recurrence; adverse effects of treatment.
METHODS	*Clinical Evidence* search and appraisal April 2004.

QUESTION **What are the effects of interventions aimed at preventing attacks?**

OPTION **ORAL/TOPICAL ANTIVIRAL AGENTS**

Six RCTs found limited evidence suggesting that prophylactic oral antiviral agents may reduce the frequency and severity of attacks compared with placebo, but the optimal timing and duration of treatment is uncertain. We found no RCTs on the effects of topical antiviral agents used as prophylaxis.

Benefits: We found no systematic review. **Topical antiviral agents:** We found no good quality RCTs. **Oral antiviral agents:** We found four RCTs[4–7] and one pooled analysis of two further RCTs.[8] The first RCT (147 American skiers with a history of herpes labialis precipitated by ultraviolet light) found that prophylactic oral aciclovir (400 mg twice daily, beginning 12 hours before ultraviolet exposure) reduced frequency of attacks and duration of symptoms compared with placebo ($P < 0.05$).[4] The second RCT (239 Canadian skiers with a history of recurrent herpes labialis) found no significant difference in lesion occurrence between those who took aciclovir (800 mg twice daily, starting on the day before exposure to ultraviolet light for a minimum of 3 days to a maximum of 7 days) and those who took placebo (21/93 [23%] with aciclovir *v* 21/102 [21%] with placebo; $P = 0.92$).[5] The third RCT (20 people with recurrent herpes labialis) found that aciclovir (400 mg twice daily for 4 months) led to 53% fewer clinical recurrences than placebo ($P = 0.05$).[6] The fourth RCT (248 adults with a history of sun-induced recurrent herpes labialis) compared three different dosages of famciclovir (125 mg, 250 mg, and 500 mg) versus placebo.[7] Treatment was given three times daily for 5 days, beginning 48 hours after exposure to artificial ultraviolet light. The RCT found no significant difference in the number of lesions among the four groups (number of lesions: reported as non-significant; P value not reported). However, it found that increasing the dose of famciclovir significantly reduced the size and duration of lesions, in a dose–response relation. Compared with placebo, the 500 mg dose, but not the other doses, significantly reduced the mean size of lesions and reduced the mean time to healing by 2 days (mean size of lesions: $P = 0.04$; mean time to healing: $P = 0.01$; absolute healing times not reported). The pooled analysis of two further RCTs (98 adults with a history of four or more attacks in the previous year) found that oral valaciclovir 500 mg daily significantly decreased the chance of recurrence within 4 months, and significantly increased the time to recurrence compared with placebo (no recurrence within 4 months: 62% with oral valaciclovir *v* 40% with placebo; $P = 0.041$; mean time to recurrence: 13.1 weeks with oral valaciclovir *v* 9.6 weeks with placebo; $P = 0.016$).[8]

Harms: See harms under the effects of antiviral treatments for the first attack, p 2108.

Comment: All participants in the second RCT were allowed to use paracetamol (acetaminophen) and encouraged to use sunscreen.[5]

OPTION SUNSCREEN

Two small crossover RCTs found limited evidence that ultraviolet sunscreen may reduce herpes recurrence compared with placebo.

Benefits: We found no systematic review. We found two small, crossover RCTs.[9,10] The first RCT (38 people with a history of recurrent herpes) found that sunscreen significantly reduced recurrence at 6 days compared with placebo (recurrence 0/35 [0%] with sunscreen *v* 27/38 [71%] with placebo; $P < 0.001$).[9] The second RCT (19 people exposed to a pre-established dose of ultraviolet light in a laboratory) found that sunscreen significantly reduced recurrence at 6 days compared with placebo (11/19 [58%] with placebo *v* 1/19 [5%] with sunscreen; $P < 0.01$; see comment below).[10]

Harms: The RCTs gave no information on adverse effects of treatment with sunscreen.

Comment: The conclusions from the RCTs should be considered with care.[9,10] Crossover studies have important limitations, and the second RCT was conducted under artificial conditions.[10]

QUESTION What are the effects of antiviral treatments for the first attack of herpes labialis?

OPTION ORAL/TOPICAL ANTIVIRAL AGENTS

We found no RCTs on the effects of topical antiviral agents. One small RCT in children found that oral aciclovir reduced the mean duration of pain compared with placebo. Another small RCT in children found that oral aciclovir reduced the median time to healing compared with placebo.

Benefits: We found no systematic review. **Topical antiviral agents:** We found no RCTs. **Oral antiviral agents:** We found two small RCTs in children.[11,12] One double blind RCT (20 children of mean age 2 years with herpetic stomatitis-gingivitis of less than 4 days' duration) found that oral aciclovir (200 mg five times daily) reduced mean duration of pain (4.3 days with aciclovir *v* 5.0 days with placebo, $P = 0.05$).[11] The second RCT (72 children aged 1–6 years with herpes simplex gingivostomatitis of less than 3 days' duration) found that oral aciclovir (15 mg/kg five times daily for 7 days) significantly reduced the median time to healing compared with placebo (4 days with aciclovir *v* 10 days with placebo; median difference 6 days, 95% CI 4 days to 8 days).[12] We found no RCTs in adults.

Harms: Trials have found that topical aciclovir is associated with rash, pruritus, and irritation in some people, but no more frequently than placebo.[13–15] Oral aciclovir is excreted in breast milk. Aciclovir has been used to treat pregnant women with genital herpes, and one systematic review (search date 1996, three RCTs) found no evidence of adverse effects in women or newborn children (see antiviral treatment for genital herpes during pregnancy, p 1987).[15] However, evidence is limited and clinically important adverse effects cannot be ruled out.

Comment: Research in this area is difficult because people may not consult clinicians until they have experienced several attacks of herpes labialis.

QUESTION What are the effects of treatments for recurrent attacks?

OPTION ORAL/TOPICAL ANTIVIRAL AGENTS

Twelve RCTs found limited evidence that topical penciclovir or aciclovir reduced the duration of pain and symptoms compared with placebo, but found stronger evidence that topical penciclovir and aciclovir reduced healing time. Four RCTs found that oral aciclovir and valaciclovir (if taken early in the attack) marginally reduced the duration of symptoms and pain compared with placebo. Two large RCTs found no significant difference between a 1 day and a 2 day course of valaciclovir, and found that a higher proportion of people experienced headaches with valaciclovir compared with placebo.

Benefits: We found no systematic review. **Topical antiviral agents:** We found twelve RCTs (published in eleven papers) (see table 1, p 2112). Seven RCTs found that aciclovir reduced healing time compared with placebo. In six of the RCTS, the reduction was significant, but the absolute benefit was small. One RCT found no significant difference in healing time between aciclovir and placebo. Two RCTs found that penciclovir significantly reduced healing time. Five RCTs found more limited evidence that aciclovir or penciclovir significantly reduced duration of pain. **Oral antiviral agents:** We found four RCTs (published in three papers).[25–27] The first RCT (174 adults with recurrent herpes labialis) found that oral aciclovir (400 mg 5 times daily for 5 days) taken early in the attack (when the person first experienced tingling) significantly reduced the duration of symptoms compared with placebo (8.1 days with oral aciclovir *v* 12.5 days with placebo; $P = 0.02$).[25] The second RCT (149 people) compared oral aciclovir taken within 12 hours of the onset of the first episode with placebo.[26] It found no significant difference in healing time or duration of pain between oral aciclovir and placebo (mean healing time: 7.78 days with aciclovir *v* 8.64 days with placebo; P value not reported; mean duration of pain: 1.31 days with aciclovir *v* 1.35 days with placebo; P value not reported). The third and fourth RCTs (presented in one paper) compared oral valaciclovir for 1 day (2 g twice daily), oral valaciclovir for 2 days (2 g twice daily for the first day followed by 1 g twice daily for the second day), and placebo in people aged at least 12 years with recurrent herpes labialis.[27] The third RCT (902 people) found that both oral valaciclovir regimens significantly reduced the median duration of episode compared with placebo (4.0 days with 1 day course valaciclovir *v* 4.5 days with 2 day course valaciclovir *v* 5.0 days with placebo; $P < 0.001$ for 1 day course valaciclovir *v* placebo; $P = 0.009$ for 2 day course valaciclovir *v* placebo). The fourth RCT (954 people) found that both oral valaciclovir regimens significantly reduced the median duration of episode compared with placebo (5.0 days with 1 day course valaciclovir *v* 5.0 days with 2 day course valaciclovir *v* 5.5 days with placebo; $P < 0.001$ for 1 day course of valaciclovir *v* placebo; $P < 0.001$ for 2 day course of valaciclovir *v* placebo). Neither RCT found a significant difference between 1 day course valaciclovir and 2 day course valaciclovir (P values not reported).

Harms: **Oral antiviral agents:** The large third and fourth RCTs found similar numbers of adverse events for the 1 and 2 day valaciclovir regimens and placebo.[27] However, headache was more common with valaciclovir than with placebo (third RCT: 9% with 1 day course valaciclovir *v* 9% with 2 day course valaciclovir *v* 4% with placebo; P values not reported; fourth RCT: 10% with 1 day course valaciclovir *v* 9% with 2 day course valaciclovir *v* 5% with placebo; P values not reported).[27] The other most common adverse events found were nausea (third RCT: 4% with 1 day valaciclovir *v* 5% with 2 day valaciclovir *v* 4% with placebo; P values not reported; fourth RCT: 4% with 1 day valaciclovir *v* 4% with 2 day valaciclovir *v* 5% with placebo; P values not reported) and diarrhoea (third RCT: 4% with 1 day valaciclovir *v* 3% with 2 day valaciclovir *v* 3% with placebo; P values not reported; fourth RCT: 2% with 1 day valaciclovir *v* 1% with 2 day valaciclovir *v* 3% with placebo; P values not reported). A small number of cases of dyspepsia, dry mouth, and flatulence were reported in all three treatment groups. See harms under the effects of antiviral treatment for the first attack, p 2108.

Comment: We found no RCTs comparing early versus delayed intervention, so no firm conclusions about timing of treatment can be drawn. **Topical antiviral agents:** Fifteen people in the second RCT later took part in a crossover study in which they received two forms of topical aciclovir (in random order) separated by a washout period of at least 1 month.[24] The study found that aciclovir in liposomes significantly reduced the time to crusting of lesions compared with aciclovir cream (1.8 *v* 3.5 days; $P = 0.023$). In the second RCT, too few people experienced pain to enable statistical analysis of the impact of the treatments on discomfort. One RCT was conducted under artificial conditions.[22] A number of the smaller trials that compared topical antiviral agents versus placebo found no significant effect of treatment (see table 1, p 2112). However, these studies may have lacked power to detect clinically important differences.

OPTION TOPICAL ANAESTHETIC AGENTS

One small RCT found limited evidence that topical tetracaine reduced the mean time to scab loss and increased the proportion of people who subjectively rated the treatment as effective compared with placebo. However, the clinical importance of these results is unclear.

Benefits: We found no systematic review. One double blind RCT (72 people) found that 1.8% tetracaine (amethocaine) cream, applied six times daily until scab loss occurred, significantly reduced mean time to scab loss compared with placebo (5.1 days with tetracaine *v* 7.2 days with placebo; $P = 0.002$).[28] It also found that tetracaine cream significantly increased a subjective treatment benefit index (participants rated the benefits of their treatment daily on a scale of 1 to 10; 1 = no benefit at all, 10 = very effective treatment) compared with placebo (7.3 with tetracaine *v* 5.9 with placebo; $P = 0.036$). However, the clinical importance of these results is unclear.

Harms: The RCT found no adverse effects as a result of treatment with 1.8% tetracaine (amethocaine) cream.

Comment: None.

OPTION ZINC OXIDE CREAM

One small RCT found limited evidence that zinc oxide cream reduced time to healing compared with placebo, but increased the risk of skin irritation.

Benefits: One double blind RCT (46 people) found that zinc oxide/glycine (applied twice hourly during waking hours as soon as possible after the onset of an attack) significantly reduced time to healing compared with placebo (5.0 days with cream *v* 6.5 days with placebo; P = 0.018).[29]

Harms: The RCT found adverse effects consisting of transient mild to moderate sensations of burning (7 [22%] people with zinc *v* 2 [7%] with placebo), itching (3 [9%] people with zinc *v* 1 [4%] with placebo), stinging (1 [3%] person with zinc *v* 1 [4%] with placebo), and tingling (1 [3%] person with zinc *v* 0 [0%] with placebo).[29] The RCT reported that all adverse effects resolved spontaneously. One person discontinued the active medication because of burning. One person discontinued the placebo because of lack of improvement.

Comment: See comment under antiviral agents for recurrent attacks, p 2109.

REFERENCES

1. Hodgkin K. *Towards earlier diagnosis: a guide to general practice*. Edinburgh: Churchill Livingstone, 1973.
2. Baringer SR, Swoveland P. Recovery of herpes simplex virus from human trigeminal ganglions. *N Engl J Med* 1973;288:648–650.
3. Bader C, Crumpacker CS, Schnipner LE, et al. The natural history of recurrent facial-oral infections with the herpes simplex virus. *J Infect Dis* 1978;138:897–905.
4. Spruance SL, Hammil ML, Hoge WS, et al. Acyclovir prevents reactivation of herpes labialis in skiers. *JAMA* 1988;260:1597–1599.
5. Raborn GW, Martel AY, Grace MG, et al. Oral acyclovir in prevention of herpes labialis: a randomized, double-blind, placebo controlled trial. *Oral Surg Oral Med Oral Pathol Oral Radiol Endod* 1998;85:55–59.
6. Rooney JF, Strauss SE, Mannix ML, et al. Oral acyclovir to suppress frequently recurrent herpes labialis: a double-blind, placebo controlled trial. *Ann Intern Med* 1993;118:268–272.
7. Spruance SL, Rowe NH, Raborn GW, et al. Peroral famciclovir in the treatment of experimental ultraviolet radiation-induced herpes simplex labialis: a double-blind, dose-ranging, placebo-controlled, multicenter trial. *J Infect Dis* 1999;179:303–310.
8. Baker D, Eisen D. Valacyclovir for prevention of recurrent herpes labialis: 2 double-blind, placebo-controlled studies. *Cutis* 2003;239–242.
9. Rooney JF, Bryson Y, Mannix ML, et al. Prevention of ultraviolet-light-induced herpes labialis by sunscreen. *Lancet* 1991;338:1419–1421.
10. Duteil L, Queille-Roussel C, Loesche C, et al. Assessment of the effect of a sunblock stick in the prevention of solar-simulating ultraviolet light-induced herpes labialis. *J Dermatol Treat* 1998;9:11–14.
11. Ducoulombier H, Cousin J, DeWilde A, et al. Herpetic stomatis-gingivitis in children: controlled trial of acyclovir versus placebo. *Ann Pediatr* 1988;35:212–216. [in French].
12. Amir J, Harel L, Smetana Z, et al. Treatment of herpes simplex gingivostomatitis with aciclovir in children: a randomised double blind placebo controlled trial. *BMJ* 1997;314:1800–1803.
13. Raborn GW, Martel WT, Grace M, et al. Herpes labialis treatment with acyclovir modified aqueous cream: a double-blind randomized trial. *Oral Surg Oral Med Oral Pathol* 1989;67:676–679.
14. Fiddian AP, Ivanyi L. Topical acyclovir in the management of recurrent herpes labialis. *Br J Dermatol* 1983;109:321–326.
15. Smith J, Cowan FM, Munday P. The management of herpes simplex virus infection in pregnancy. *Br J Obstet Gynaecol* 1998;105:255–268. Search date 1996; primary sources Medline and hand searched references.
16. Van Vloten WA, Swart RNJ, Pot F. Topical acyclovir therapy in patients with recurrent orofacial herpes simplex infections. *J Antimicrob Chemother* 1983;12(suppl B):89–93.
17. Spruance SL, Schnipper LE, Overall JC, et al. Treatment of herpes simplex labialis with topical acyclovir in polyethylene glycol. *J Infect Dis* 1982;146:85–90.
18. Spruance SL, Rea TL, Thoming C, et al. Penciclovir cream for the treatment of herpes simplex labialis. *JAMA* 1997;277:1374–1379.
19. Raborn GW, McGraw WT, Grace MG, et al. Herpes labialis treatment with acyclovir 5 per cent ointment. *Sci J* 1989;55:135–137.
20. Shaw M, King M, Best JM, et al. Failure of acyclovir ointment in treatment of recurrent herpes labialis. *BMJ* 1985;291:7–9.
21. Boon R, Goodman JJ, Martinez J, et al. Penciclovir cream for the treatment of sunlight-induced herpes simplex labialis: a randomized, double-blind, placebo-controlled trial. Penciclovir Cream Herpes Labialis Study Group. *Clin Ther* 2000;22:76–90.
22. Evans TG, Bernstein DI, Raborn GW, et al. Double-blind, randomized, placebo-controlled study of topical 5% acyclovir-1% hydrocortisone cream (ME-609) for treatment of UV radiation-induced herpes labialis. *Antimicrob Agents Chemother* 2002;46:1870–1874.
23. Spruance SL, Nett R, Marbury T, et al. Acyclovir cream for treatment of herpes simplex labialis: results of two randomized, double-blind, vehicle-controlled, multicenter clinical trials. *Antimicrob Agents Chemother* 2002;46:2238–2243.
24. Horwitz E, Pisanty S, Czerninski R, et al. A clinical evaluation of a novel liposomal carrier for acyclovir in the topical treatment of recurrent herpes labialis. *Oral Surg Oral Med Oral Pathol Oral Radiol Endod* 1999;87:700–705.
25. Spruance SL, Stewart JC, Rowe NH, et al. Treatment of recurrent herpes simplex labialis with oral acyclovir. *J Infect Dis* 1990;161:185–190.

26. Raborn WG, McGraw WT, Grace M, et al. Oral acyclovir and herpes labialis: a randomized, double-blind, placebo-controlled study. *J Am Dental Assoc* 1987;115:38–42.
27. Spruance SL, Jones TM, Blatte MM, et al. High-does, short-duration, early valacyclovir therapy for episodic treatment of cold sores: results of two randomized, placebo-controlled, multicenter studies. *Antimicrobial Agents Chemother* 2003;47:1072–1080.
28. Kaminester LH, Pariser RJ, Pariser DM, et al. A double-blind, placebo-controlled study of topical tetracaine in the treatment of herpes labialis. *J Am Acad Dermatol* 1999;41:996–1001.
29. Godfrey H, Godfrey N, Godfrey J, et al. A randomized clinical trial on the treatment of oral herpes with topical zinc oxide/glycine. *Altern Ther Health Med* 2001;7:49–56.

Graham Worrall
Professor of Family Medicine, Director,
Centre for Rural Health Studies
Memorial University of Newfoundland
Newfoundland
Canada

Competing interests: None declared.

We would like to acknowledge the previous contributors of this chapter, including Bazian Ltd.

TABLE 1 **Efficacy of topical antiviral agents for treating recurrent attacks of herpes labialis (see text, p 2108).**

Ref	Number of people	Interventions	Efficacy findings
Duration of pain			
13	61	Aciclovir *v* placebo	Mean duration of pain: 1.2 days with aciclovir *v* 1.1 days with placebo; P value not reported
16	30	Aciclovir *v* placebo	Mean duration of pain: 1.7 days with aciclovir *v* 2.3 days with placebo; $P = 0.53$
17	208	Aciclovir *v* placebo	Mean duration of pain: 1.9 days with aciclovir *v* 2.1 days with placebo; $P = 0.30$
18	2209	Penciclovir (twice daily for 4 days) *v* placebo	Median duration of pain: 3.5 days with penciclovir cream *v* 4.1 days with control cream; $P < 0.001$
19	80	Aciclovir *v* placebo	Mean duration of pain: 1.08 days with aciclovir *v* 1.04 with placebo; P value not reported
Healing time			
14	13 (crossover design)	Aciclovir *v* placebo	Mean healing time: 7 days with acyclovir *v* 8 days with placebo; $P < 0.05$
16	30	Aciclovir *v* placebo	Mean healing time: 5.7 days with aciclovir *v* 8.3 days with placebo; $P = 0.022$
20	45	Aciclovir *v* placebo	Mean healing time: 10 days with aciclovir *v* 13 days with placebo; P value not reported
17	208	Aciclovir *v* placebo	Mean healing time: 7.2 days with aciclovir *v* 7.2 days with placebo; $P = 0.67$
18	2209	Penciclovir (twice daily for 4 days) *v* placebo	Median healing time: 4.8 days with penciclovir cream *v* 5.5 days with control cream; $P < 0.001$
19	80	Aciclovir *v* placebo	Mean healing time: 8.9 days with aciclovir *v* 7.9 with placebo; P value not reported
21	534	1% penciclovir cream *v* placebo	Mean healing time of lesions: 7.6 days with penciclovir *v* 8.8 days with placebo; $P < 0.01$
22	380	Aciclovir cream *v* placebo	Mean healing time: 9.0 days with aciclovir *v* 10.1 days with placebo; $P = 0.04$
23	670	Aciclovir *v* placebo	Mean healing time: 4.3 days with aciclovir *v* 4.8 with placebo; $P = 0.010$
23	673	Aciclovir *v* placebo	Mean healing time: 4.6 days with aciclovir *v* 5.2 days with placebo; $P = 0.007$
Time to crusting			
24	31	5% aciclovir cream *v* 5% aciclovir in a liposomal vehicle *v* a drug free vehicle	Mean time to crusting: 1.6 days for aciclovir in liposomes *v* 4.8 days for control; $P < 0.05$); 4.3 days for aciclovir cream *v* 4.8 days for control; P value not stated

Ref, reference.

Malignant melanoma (non-metastatic)

Search date October 2003

Philip Savage, Thomas Crosby, and Malcolm Mason

QUESTIONS

INTERVENTIONS

See glossary G

Key Messages

Preventive interventions

- **Sunscreens** We found no RCTs on the preventive effects of sunscreens. Systematic reviews of case control studies found inconclusive evidence about the effects of sunscreen in preventing malignant melanoma.

Optimum excision margin

- **Wide excision (no better than narrower excision** in people with tumours of < 2 mm Breslow thickness)**)** One systematic review and one subsequent RCT found no significant difference in overall survival over 4–10 years between more radical local surgery (4–5 cm excision margins) and less radical surgery (1–2 cm excision margins). The RCTs also found no significant difference in local recurrence rates between wider and narrower excision margins. One of the RCTs found that wider excision increased the need for skin grafting and the duration of hospital stay compared with narrower excision. Only 8.9% of people in the RCTs had tumours had tumours of > 2 mm thickness, therefore we were unable to draw conclusions about optimum excision margin in these people.

Sentinel lymph node biopsy

- **Sentinel lymph node biopsy** We found no RCTs of sentinel lymph node biopsy that assessed survival in people with malignant melanoma.

Elective lymph node dissection

- **Elective lymph node dissection** One systematic review found no significant difference in survival at 5 years between elective lymph node dissection and delayed or no lymph node dissection in people with malignant melanoma without clinically detectable lymph node metastases.

Adjuvant treatment

- **High dose adjuvant alfa interferon** Two RCTs have found that high dose alfa interferon extends the time to relapse at median follow up of 6.9 years compared with no adjuvant treatment. One of them also found that high dose alfa interferon may improve overall survival. However, a third RCT found no significant difference in relapse rates or overall survival between high dose interferon and no adjuvant treatment. One RCT found that high dose alfa interferon improved both relapse free and overall survival compared with ganglioside GM2 vaccine. Toxicity (myelosuppression, hepatotoxicity, and neurotoxicity) and withdrawal rates were high; in one RCT, toxicity occurred in 15–28% of people.
- **Adjuvant vaccines in people with malignant melanoma** Four RCTs found no significant difference in survival between adjuvant vaccines and surgery alone or surgery plus placebo vaccine in people with malignant melanoma. A different vaccine preparation was used in each RCT, making the results difficult to generalise.
- **Low dose adjuvant alfa interferon** RCTs found inconsistent evidence on the effects of low dose alfa interferon compared with no adjuvant treatment on relapse free and overall survival. In one RCT, toxicity occurred in 10% of people.
- **Surveillance for early treatment of recurrence** We found no RCTs of surveillance for early treatment of recurrent melanoma.

DEFINITION	Cutaneous malignant melanoma is a tumour derived from melanocytes in the basal layer of the epidermis. After undergoing malignant transformation, the tumour becomes invasive by penetrating into and beyond the dermis.
INCIDENCE/ PREVALENCE	Incidence in developed countries has increased by 50% in the past 20 years. Incidence varies in different populations (see table 1, p 2123) and is about 10-fold higher in white than in non-white populations. Despite the rise in incidence, death rates have flattened and even fallen in some populations (e.g. in women and young men in Australia).[1,2] During the same period there has been a sixfold increase in the incidence of melanoma *in situ*, suggesting earlier detection.
AETIOLOGY/ RISK FACTORS	The number of common, atypical, and dysplastic naevi on a person's body correlates closely with the risk of developing malignant melanoma. A genetic predisposition probably accounts for 5–10% of all cases. Although the risk of developing malignant melanoma is higher in fair skinned populations living close to the equator, the relationship between sun exposure, sunscreen use, and skin type and risk is not clear. Exposure to excessive sunlight and severe sunburn in childhood are associated with an increased risk of developing malignant melanoma in adult life. However, people do not necessarily develop tumours at sites of maximum exposure to the sun.
PROGNOSIS	The prognosis of early malignant melanoma (stages I–III) (see table 2, p 2123) relates to the depth of invasion of the primary lesion, the presence of ulceration, and involvement of the regional lymph nodes, with the prognosis worsening with the number of nodes involved.[3] A person with a thin lesion (Breslow thickness Ⓖ < 0.75 mm) and without lymph node involvement has a 3% risk of developing metastases and a 95% chance of surviving 5 years.[4] If regional lymph nodes are macroscopically involved, then there is a 20–50% chance of surviving 5 years. Most studies have shown a better prognosis in women and in people with lesions on the extremities than in those with lesions on the trunk.
AIMS OF INTERVENTION	To prevent melanoma; to detect melanoma earlier; to minimise extent of surgical treatment while still achieving cure of local disease; to optimise quality of life; and to eradicate occult micrometastatic disease, with minimum adverse effects.
OUTCOMES	**Prevention:** Incidence of malignant melanoma; mortality from malignant melanoma; rates and severity of sunburn (proxy measure). **Primary excision:** Local recurrence; overall survival; requirement for skin grafting; adverse effects of treatment. **Lymph node dissection and adjuvant treatment:** Overall survival; disease free survival; quality of life; adverse effects of treatment.

METHODS *Clinical Evidence* search and appraisal October 2003, and hand searches of reference lists of all review articles found and of the main oncological and dermatological textbooks performed by the authors in 1998.

QUESTION **What are the effects of interventions to prevent malignant melanoma?**

OPTION **SUNSCREENS**

We found no RCTs on the preventive effects of sunscreens. Systematic reviews of case control studies found inconclusive evidence about the effects of sunscreen use in preventing malignant melanoma.

Benefits: We found no RCTs assessing the effects of sunscreens in preventing malignant melanoma (see comment below). One RCT (588 people) found that a sunscreen significantly reduced the incidence or progression of solar keratosis compared with placebo (RR 0.62, 95% CI 0.54 to 0.71).[5]

Harms: We found no RCTs (see comment below). One RCT (87 people) found that people who used a sunscreen with a high sun protection factor (SPF 30) spent more hours in the sun over 3 weeks than people who used sunscreen with a lower sun protection factor (SPF 10), although the difference was not significant (mean cumulative exposure 72.6 hours with SPF 30 *v* 58.2 hours with SPF 10; $P < 0.11$).[6]

Comment: We found three systematic reviews of case control studies.[7–9] The first review (search date not reported, 8 case control studies) found conflicting results.[7] Two case control studies (522 people with malignant melanoma, 1039 controls) identified by the review found that people who "regularly" used sunscreen were less likely to develop melanoma than were people who "never" used sunscreen, but three case control studies (831 people with melanoma, 1550 controls) that adjusted for confounding factors (such as fair skin pigmentation, tendency to sunburn, and participation in water sports) found no association between sunscreen use and the development of melanoma. Three case control studies (1389 people with melanoma, 1991 controls) identified by the review found that regular use of sunscreen may be associated with an increased risk of developing melanoma compared with no use.[7] Another three case control studies found no significant difference between sunscreen use and no use in the risk of developing melanoma.[7] The second review (search date 1999, 11 case control studies, including the 8 studies identified by the first review and 2 excluded from the first review because of methodological problems, 3681 cases, 5386 controls) found no significant difference in the risk of developing melanoma between people who "regularly", "often", or "always" used sunscreen and people who "never" used sunscreen (RR 1.11, 95% CI 0.37 to 3.32).[8] However, the review suggested that the results should be treated with caution because there was significant heterogeneity among the case control studies, and eight of the 11 studies found that sunscreen use significantly increased the risk of melanoma compared with no sunscreen use.[8] The third systematic review (17 case control studies, including all of the studies identified by the previous reviews) was only published as a brief communication.[9] The brief communication stated that the review could not draw firm conclusions about the effects of sunscreen in preventing melanoma because of the heterogeneity of the studies identified.[9] Case control studies all have potential biases and confounding factors.[5] Although we found no prospective evidence, it would seem reasonable to take sensible precautions to avoid excessive exposure to sunlight, particularly in children and fair skinned individuals. A possible mechanism for the observed association between regular use of sunscreen and increased risk of developing melanoma may be that, because some sunscreens protect predominantly against ultraviolet B (which induces sunburn), people may spend more time exposed to higher doses of ultraviolet A.[6] Consensus suggests that sunscreens may have a role if used appropriately (SPF ≥ 15 and a star rating for ultraviolet A protection of 3–4), rather than being used to prolong the time spent in direct sunlight.

QUESTION **Is there an optimal margin for primary excision of melanoma of different Breslow thicknesses?**

OPTION **WIDE EXCISION VERSUS NARROWER EXCISION**

One systematic review and one subsequent RCT, primarily in people with primary tumours of less than 2 mm Breslow thickness, found no significant difference in overall survival over 4–10 years between more radical local surgery (4–5 cm excision margins) and less radical surgery (1–2 cm excision margins). The RCTs also found no significant difference in local recurrence rates between wider and narrower excision margins. One of the RCTs found that wider excision increased the need for skin grafting and the duration of hospital stay compared with narrower excision. Only 8.9% of people in the RCTs had tumours had tumours of > 2 mm thickness, therefore we were unable to draw conclusions about optimum excision margin in these people.

Benefits: We found one systematic review[10] and one subsequent RCT.[11] The review (search date 2001, 4 RCTs, 2406 people with stage I and II melanoma [see comment below]) found no significant difference in overall survival at 5 years between narrower (1–2 cm) and wider (4–5 cm) excision margins (4 RCTs: 732/867 [84%] with narrower *v* 796/911 [87%] with wider; OR 0.79, 95% CI 0.61 to 1.04).[10] Three of the RCTs identified by the review were in people with primary tumours of less than 2 mm Breslow thickness**G**; only 8.9% of people in the review had tumours of > 2 mm thickness. The subsequent RCT (337 people with melanoma < 2.1 mm thickness) found no significant difference in progression free or overall survival at 10 years between 2 cm and 5 cm excision margins (progression free survival 85% with 2 cm *v* 83% with 5 cm; P = 0.56; overall survival 87% with 2 cm *v* 86% with 5 cm; P = 0.56). The review[10] identified four RCTs[12–15] that assessed local recurrence, but it could not perform a meta-analysis for this outcome because of different durations of follow up among the trials (see table 3, p 2124). The subsequent RCT also assessed local recurrence (see table 3, p 2124).[11] The RCTs all found similar local recurrence rates and rates of distant metastases between wider and narrower excision margins; not all of the RCTs assessed the significance of the difference between groups.

Harms: One RCT (486 people) included in the review found that wider versus narrower excision margins significantly increased skin grafting (46% with wider *v* 11% with narrower margins; P < 0.001), and inpatient stay (mean 7.0 with wider *v* 5.2 days with narrower margins; P = 0.001).[10] One of the RCTs (612 people) found that narrow (1 cm) margin excision was associated with three local recurrences compared with wide margin excision, all in people with tumours 1–2 mm thick.[12] Local cure was achieved in two people with further surgery. Although not measured in the RCTs, there is potential for psychological and physical morbidity associated with further surgery after local recurrence.

Comment: We found one further RCT published only in abstract form that suggests that reducing the excision margin (from 3 cm to 1 cm) in people with > 2 mm primary melanoma may be associated with increased risk of relapse and mortality (Savage P, personal communication, 2003). For current recommended excision margins see table 4, p 2125.[16,17]

QUESTION **What are the effects of sentinel lymph node biopsy in people with clinically uninvolved lymph nodes?**

OPTION **SENTINEL LYMPH NODE BIOPSY**

We found no RCTs of sentinel lymph node biopsy that assessed survival in people with malignant melanoma.

Benefits: We found no systematic review or RCTs that assessed survival (see comment below).

Harms: We found no RCTs.

Comment: Sentinel lymph node biopsy**G** is currently being evaluated in clinical trials.[18,19]

QUESTION **What are the effects of elective lymph node dissection in people with clinically uninvolved lymph nodes?**

OPTION **ELECTIVE LYMPH NODE DISSECTION**

One systematic review found no significant difference in survival at 5 years between elective lymph node dissection and delayed or no lymph node dissection in people with malignant melanoma without clinically detectable lymph node metastases.

Benefits: We found one systematic review (4 RCTs, 1704 people with stage I and II melanoma with no clinical evidence of lymph node metastases [see comment below]) comparing elective lymph node dissection versus surgery deferred until the time of clinical recurrence.[20] It found no significant difference in mortality at 5 years between elective lymph node dissection and delayed or no lymph node dissection (3 RCTs: 197/768 [26%] with elective dissection *v* 219/765 [29%] with delayed or no dissection; OR 0.86, 95% CI 0.68 to 1.09; see comment below). Retrospective subgroup analyses in the RCTs found non-significant trends in favour of elective lymph node dissection in certain groups of people (those with intermediate thickness tumours, especially those < 60 years of age), but such analyses are subject to bias.[21–24]

Harms: The systematic review gave no information on adverse effects.[20] One retrospective case series found that lymph node dissection was associated with temporary seroma (17%), wound infection (9%), wound necrosis (3%), and lymphoedema (20%).[25]

Comment: In about 20% of people who do not have clinically apparent lymph node involvement, the lymph nodes will contain occult micrometastases. None of the RCTs provided data on morbidity and quality of life in people undergoing lymph node dissection.

QUESTION **What are the effects of adjuvant treatment?**

OPTION **ALFA INTERFERON**

Two RCTs have found that high dose alfa interferon extends the time to relapse at median follow up of 6.9 years compared with no adjuvant treatment. One of them also found that high dose alfa interferon may improve overall survival. However, the other RCT found no significant difference in relapse rates or overall survival between high dose interferon and no adjuvant treatment. One RCT found that high dose alfa interferon improved both

relapse free and overall survival compared with ganglioside GM2 vaccine. RCTs found inconsistent evidence on the effects of low dose alfa interferon compared with no adjuvant treatment on relapse free and overall survival. Toxicity (myelosuppression, hepatotoxicity, and neurotoxicity) and withdrawal rates were high in people taking high dose alfa interferon; in one RCT, toxicity occurred in 15–28% of people. In one RCT, toxicity occurred in 10% of people taking low dose alfa interferon.

Benefits: We found two systematic reviews (search date 2001[26], 8 RCTs,[27–34] 3178 people; search date not reported[35]; 12 RCTs including all 8 RCTs identified by the first review, 6086 people) comparing high or low dose interferon alfa versus no adjuvant treatment, and one RCT comparing high dose interferon versus ganglioside GM2 vaccine.[36] The first review did not perform a meta-analysis because of clinical heterogeneity among the trials, differences in dose and duration of interferon treatment, and stage of disease of participants.[26] The second review found no statistical heterogeneity among the RCTs and performed a meta-analysis of RCTs assessing both high and low dose alfa interferon.[35] **High or low dose versus no adjuvant treatment (observation):** The second review found that alfa interferon (high or low dose) significantly increased recurrence free survival compared with observation (recurrence: 1584/3144 [50%] with interferon *v* 1166/2037 [57%] with observation; HR 0.83, 95% CI 0.77 to 0.90). It found no significant difference in overall survival between alfa interferon and observation, although mortality was lower in people taking alfa interferon (mortality: 1150/3075 [37%] with interferon *v* 848/2007 [42%] with observation; HR 0.93, 95% CI 0.85 to 1.02). It found that higher doses of alfa interferon significantly increased relapse free survival compared with lower doses (P = 0.02), but found no significant difference in overall survival between higher and lower doses (P = 0.8; absolute numbers not reported for either outcome).[35] **High dose versus no adjuvant treatment (observation):** The reviews[26,35] identified three RCTs.[27–29] The first RCT (280 people with resectable stage IIB [primary lesions > 4 mm] or stage III melanoma) compared high dose alfa interferon (20 MU/m^2/day iv for 1 month, followed by 10 MU/m^2 sc 3 times/week for 11 months) versus observation.[27] At a median follow up of 6.9 years, it found that alfa interferon significantly improved disease free survival (median 1.7 *v* 1.0 years; P = 0.023) and overall survival (median 3.8 *v* 2.8 years; P = 0.0237) compared with observation.[27] Retrospective subgroup analysis found prolonged quality of life adjusted survival in people receiving alfa interferon.[37] The clinical importance of this gain varied with the values assigned by people in the trial for the impact of treatment related toxicity and the impact of time with relapsed disease. The second RCT (262 people with completely resected stage I and II melanoma, primary tumours > 0.7 mm, lymph node negative) compared high dose interferon (20 MU/m^2 im 3 times/week for 12 weeks) versus observation and found no significant difference in disease free survival (mean 2.4 years with alfa interferon *v* 2.0 years with observation; P = 0.19) or overall survival (median 6.6 years with alfa interferon *v* 5.0 years with observation; P = 0.40).[29] The third RCT (642 people with stage II or III primary or recurrent nodal involvement) compared three interventions: high dose alfa interferon (20 MU/m^2/day iv 5 days/week for 1 month, followed by 10 MU/m^2 sc 3 times/week for 11 months); low dose alfa interferon (3 MU/m^2/day sc 3 times/week for 2 years); or observation.[28] It found that high dose interferon marginally but significantly improved relapse free survival over 5 years compared with observation (HR 1.28, 95% CI 1.00 to 1.65), but found no significant difference in overall survival (HR 1.0, 95% CI 0.75 to 1.33). **High dose versus ganglioside GM2 vaccine:** The reviews[26,35] identified one RCT[36] (880 people with resected stage IIB and III melanoma) comparing high dose interferon (20 MU/m^2 iv 5 times/week for 4 weeks

plus 10 MU/m^2 sc 3 times/week for 48 weeks) versus ganglioside GM2 vaccine. It found that, compared with ganglioside vaccine, alfa interferon significantly improved both relapse free survival (98/385 [25%] with alfa interferon *v* 151/389 [39%] with ganglioside; HR 1.47, 95% CI 1.14 to 1.90) and overall survival (52/385 [14%] *v* 81/389 [21%]; HR 1.52, 95% CI 1.07 to 2.15) over a median follow up of 16 months.
Low dose versus no adjuvant treatment: The reviews identified seven RCTs.[28,30–34,38] Three of the RCTs identified by the reviews were in people with stage II melanoma (primary tumours > 1.5 mm and lymph node negative).[30,31,33] The first RCT (489 people with stage II melanoma) comparing low dose alfa interferon (3 MU sc 3 times/week for 18 months) versus no adjuvant treatment found that alfa interferon significantly increased relapse free survival over a median 5 years (HR 0.75, 95% CI 0.57 to 0.98; P = 0.035).[30] It found that overall survival rates after a median 5 years were higher with alfa interferon than with no adjuvant treatment, but the difference did not quite reach significance (HR 0.72, 95% CI 0.51 to 1.00; P = 0.059). The second RCT (311 people with stage II melanoma) compared low dose alfa interferon (3 MU/day sc for 3 weeks and 3 times/week for 12 months) versus no adjuvant treatment after excision of the primary tumour.[31] At 41 months' follow up it found that alfa interferon significantly prolonged relapse free survival compared with no adjuvant treatment (P = 0.02). It found no significant difference in overall survival over 41 months between alfa interferon and no adjuvant treatment, but it may have been too small to exclude a clinically important difference (17/154 [11%] with alfa interferon *v* 21/157 [13%] with no adjuvant treatment; RR 0.82, 95% CI 0.45 to 1.50). The third RCT (654 people with stage II melanoma), published only in abstract form, found no significant difference in relapse free survival (P = 0.2) or overall survival (P = 1.0) at 4 years between low dose interferon (3 MU 3 times/week for 2 years or until recurrence) and observation.[33] The fourth RCT (96 people with stage II or III melanoma, primary tumours ≥ 3 mm Breslow thickness**G**, or evidence of regional node involvement) found no significant difference in relapse free survival or overall survival at a median follow up of 6 years between interferon (3 MU sc 3 times/week for 6 months) and observation, but it may have lacked power to exclude a clinically important difference.[34] The fifth RCT (424 people with stage III melanoma, lymph node metastases) compared low dose interferon (3 MU sc 3 times/week for 3 years) versus no adjuvant treatment.[32] It found no significant difference between low dose interferon and no adjuvant treatment in relapse free survival (28.4% with interferon *v* 27.5% with no adjuvant treatment; P = 0.50) or overall survival at 5 years (37% with interferon *v* 37% with no adjuvant treatment; P = 0.72). The sixth RCT (830 people with stage II or III melanoma, primary tumours > 3 mm or lymph node involvement), published only as an abstract, compared low dose gamma or alfa interferon versus no adjuvant treatment for 12 months and found no significant difference in disease free survival (RR alfa interferon *v* no treatment 0.9, 95% CI 0.75 to 1.18; absolute numbers not provided) or overall survival at 6 years (reported as non-significant; no further data provided).[38] The seven RCTs (642 people with stage II or III primary or recurrent nodal involvement) compared three interventions: high dose alfa interferon (20 MU/m^2/day iv 5 days/week for 1 month, followed by 10 MU/m^2 sc 3 times/week for 11 months); low dose alfa interferon (3 MU/m^2/day sc 3 times/week for 2 years); or observation.[28] It found no significant difference between low dose interferon and observation in relapse free survival (HR 1.19, 95% CI 0.93 to 1.53) or overall survival (HR 1.04, 95% CI 0.78 to 1.38) over 5 years.[28]

Harms: Interferons commonly cause malaise, fevers, and flu-like symptoms. **High dose versus no adjuvant treatment (observation):** In the first RCT identified by the reviews, high dose alfa interferon caused severe (> grade 3) myelosuppression in 24% of people, hepatotoxicity in 15% (including 2 deaths), and neurotoxicity in 28%. At 11 months, only 25% of participants were receiving more than 80% of the planned dose.[27] **Low dose versus no adjuvant treatment:** In the first RCT identified by the reviews, 10% of people taking low dose interferon developed toxicity.[30] The fifth RCT identified by the reviews found that 162/225 (72%) taking low dose alfa interferon developed World Health Organization (WHO) grade 1 toxicity,[39] 54/225 (24%) WHO grade 2 toxicity, and 9/225 (4%) no toxicity.[32]

Comment: RCTs investigating sustained release pegylated alfa interferon are underway (Savage P, personal communication, 2003).

OPTION VACCINES

Four RCTs found no significant difference in survival between adjuvant vaccines and surgery alone or surgery plus placebo vaccine in people with malignant melanoma. A different vaccine preparation was used in each RCT, making the results difficult to generalise.

Benefits: Four RCTs found no significant difference in survival between adjuvant vaccines and surgery alone or surgery plus placebo vaccine.[40–43] The first RCT (700 people with stage IIB or III primary or recurrent nodal involvement) compared adjuvant vaccine (prepared from vaccinia melanoma cell lysates) versus surgery alone.[40] It found no significant difference between adjuvant vaccine and surgery alone in relapse free survival (51% with adjuvant treatment *v* 47% with no surgery) or overall survival (60% with adjuvant treatment *v* 55% with no surgery; reported as non-significant, CI not reported) at 5 years or 10 years. The second RCT (689 people with completely resected stage II melanoma, primary tumour 1.5–4 mm Breslow thickness**G**) found no significant difference in relapse free survival at 5 years between adjuvant vaccine (allogeneic melanoma cell lysate) and surgery alone (66% with vaccine *v* 62% with surgery alone; P = 0.17).[41] The third RCT (217 people with resected stage III melanoma) compared adjuvant vaccinia melanoma oncosylate versus placebo vaccine (vaccinia virus).[42] Over 5 years, it found no significant difference between adjuvant melanoma vaccine and placebo vaccine in disease free survival (P = 0.61) or overall survival (P = 0.79, absolute results presented graphically). The fourth RCT (38 people with resected stage III melanoma) compared polyvalent melanoma vaccine versus placebo vaccine (human albumin).[43] It found that melanoma vaccine significantly increased time to recurrence compared with placebo vaccine (1.6 years with vaccine *v* 0.6 years with placebo vaccine; P = 0.03), but found no significant difference in overall survival at 3 years (53% with vaccine *v* 33% with placebo vaccine; reported as non-significant, CI not reported).

Harms: The first RCT found that melanoma vaccine was associated with erythema and ulceration at the injection site (47% of people), malaise (35%), and fever (20%).[40] The second RCT found that most people receiving melanoma vaccine had mild to moderate adverse effects and that 26 (9%) of people had severe adverse effects, including malaise, fatigue, visual complaints, fever, diarrhoea, thrombocytopenia, or skin rash.[41] The third RCT found that both melanoma vaccine and placebo vaccine were associated with erythema, swelling, and tenderness at the injection site, headache, nausea, and fever.[42] The fourth RCT found that both vaccine and placebo vaccine were associated with skin reactions but found no other adverse effects.[43]

Comment: A different vaccine preparation was used in each RCT, making the results difficult to generalise.[40–43] More RCTs of vaccines and other active specific immunostimulants are needed.

OPTION **SURVEILLANCE FOR EARLY TREATMENT OF RECURRENT MELANOMA**

We found no RCTs of surveillance for early treatment of recurrent melanoma.

Benefits: We found no systematic review or RCTs (see comment below).

Harms: We found no RCTs.

Comment: Retrospective studies found that people presented with symptomatic recurrent malignant melanoma regardless of whether they were taking part in an intensive follow up programme.[44] Thinner lesions (< 0.75 mm) may require longer surveillance because recurrence peaks at 5–10 years.[45]

GLOSSARY

Breslow thickness The vertical depth (in mm) to which the tumour has penetrated.

Sentinel lymph node biopsy An alternative to elective lymph node dissection. It involves using a dye or radioactive tracer to identify which nodes are draining the primary lesion. Excision biopsy is then used to determine whether the node is involved with metastatic disease, prior to considering a full lymph node dissection.

REFERENCES

1. International Agency for Research on Cancer. *Globocan 2000: cancer incidence, mortality and prevalence worldwide, version 1.0. IARC CancerBase No. 5*. Lyon: IARC Press, 2001.
2. Giles GG, Armstrong BK, Burton RC, et al. Has mortality from melanoma stopped rising in Australia? Analysis of trends between 1931 and 1994. *BMJ* 1996;312:1121–1125.
3. Balch CM, Buzaid AC, Soong SJ, et al. Final version of the American Joint Committee on Cancer staging system for cutaneous melanoma. *J Clin Oncol* 2001;19:3635–3648.
4. Balch CM, Smalley RV, Bartolucci AA, et al. A randomised prospective clinical trial of adjuvant *C. parvum* immunotherapy in 260 patients with clinically localized melanoma (stage I): prognostic factor analysis and preliminary results of immunotherapy. *Cancer* 1982;49:1079–1084.
5. Thompson SC, Jolley D, Marks R. Reduction of solar keratoses by regular sunscreen use. *N Engl J Med* 1993;329:1147–1151.
6. Autier P, Dore JF, Negrier S, et al. Sunscreen use and duration of sun exposure: a double-blind, randomized trial. *J Natl Cancer Inst* 1999;91:1304–1309.
7. Bastuji-Garin S, Diepgen TL. Cutaneous malignant melanoma, sun exposure, and sunscreen use: epidemiological evidence. *Br J Dermatol* 2002;146:24–30. Search date and primary sources not reported.
8. Huncharek M, Kupelnick B. Use of topical sunscreens and the risk of malignant melanoma: a meta-analysis of 9067 patients from 11 case-control studies. *Am J Public Health* 2002;92:1173–1177. Search date 1999, primary sources Medline, Cancerlit, Current Contents, and hand searches of bibliographies of published reports, review articles, and textbooks.
9. Gefeller O, Pfahlberg A. Sunscreen use and melanoma: a case of evidence-based prevention? *Photodermatol Photoimmunol Photomed* 2002;18:153–156.
10. Lens MB, Dawes M, Goodacre T, et al. Excision margins in the treatment of primary cutaneous melanoma: a systematic review of randomized controlled trials comparing narrow vs wide excision. *Arch Surg* 2002;137:1101–1105.
11. Khayat D, Rixe O, Martin G, et al. Surgical margins in cutaneous melanoma (2 cm versus 5 cm for lesions measuring less than 2.1-mm thick): long-term results of a large European multicentric phase III study. *Cancer* 2003;97:1941–1946.
12. Veronesi U, Cascinelli N, Adamus J, et al. Thin stage I primary cutaneous malignant melanoma: comparison of excision with margins of 1 or 3 cm. *N Engl J Med* 1988;318:1159–1162.
13. Balch CM, Urist MM, Karakousis CP, et al. Efficacy of 2 cm surgical margins for intermediate-thickness melanomas (1 to 4 mm): results of a multi-institutional randomized surgical trial. *Ann Surg* 1993;218:262–267.
14. Cohn-Cedermark G, Rutqvist LE, Andersson R, et al. Long term results of a randomized study by the Swedish melanoma study group on 2- versus 5 cm resection margins for patients with cutaneous melanoma with a tumour thickness of 0.8–2.0 mm. *Cancer* 2000;89:1495–1501.
15. Banzet P, Thomas A, Vuillemin E, et al. Wide versus narrow surgical excision in thin (< 2thinmm) stage I primary cutaneous melanoma: long term results of a French multicentric prospective randomized trial on 319 patients [abstract]. *Proc Am Soc Clin Oncol* 1993;12:1320.
16. American Academy of Dermatology Association. Practice management: guidelines of care for primary cutaneous melanoma. American Academy of Dermatology Association, 2001. http://www.aadassociation.org/Guidelines/CutaneousMel.html (last accessed 2 April 2004).
17. European Society for Medical Oncology Guidelines Task Force. Minimal clinical recommendations for diagnosis, treatment and follow-up of cutaneous malignant melanoma. Lugano, Switzerland: European Society for Medical Oncology Guidelines Task Force, 2002. http://www.esmo.org/reference/referenceGuidelines/pdf/ESMO_17_cutaneous_malignant_melanoma.pdf (last accessed 2 April 2004).
18. Morton DL, Thompson JF, Essner R, et al. Validation of the accuracy of intraoperative lymphatic mapping and sentinel lymphadenectomy for early-stage melanoma: a multicenter trial. Multicenter Selective Lymphadenectomy Trial Group. *Ann Surg* 1999;230:453–463.

19. McMasters KM. The Sunbelt Melanoma Trial. *Ann Surg Oncol* 2001;8:41S–43S.
20. Lens MB, Dawes M, Goodacre T, et al. Elective lymph node dissection in patients with melanoma: systematic review and meta-analysis of randomised controlled trials. *Arch Surg* 2002;137:458–461.
21. Balch CM, Soong SJ, Bartolucci AA, et al. Efficacy of an elective regional lymph node dissection of 1–4 mm thick melanomas for patients 60 years of age and younger. *Ann Surg* 1996;224:255–263.
22. Cascinelli N, Morabito A, Santinami M, et al. Immediate or delayed dissection of regional nodes in patients with melanoma of the trunk: a randomised trial. WHO Melanoma Programme. *Lancet* 1998;351:793–796.
23. Sim FH, Taylor WF, Ivins JC, et al. A prospective randomized study of the efficacy of routine elective lymphadenectomy in management of malignant melanoma: preliminary results. *Cancer* 1978;41:948–956.
24. Veronesi U, Adamus J, Bandiera DC, et al. Inefficacy of immediate node dissection in stage I melanoma of the limbs. *N Engl J Med* 1977;297:627–630.
25. Baas PC, Schraffordt KH, Koops H, et al. Groin dissection in the treatment of lower-extremity melanoma: short-term and long-term morbidity. *Arch Surg* 1992;127:281–286.
26. Lens MB, Dawes M. Interferon alfa therapy for malignant melanoma: a systematic review of randomised controlled trials. *J Clin Oncol* 2002;20:1818–1825.
27. Kirkwood JM, Strawderman MH, Erstoff MS, et al. Interferon alfa-2_b adjuvant therapy of high-risk resected cutaneous melanoma: the Eastern Cooperative Oncology Group trial EST 1684. *J Clin Oncol* 1996;14:7–17.
28. Kirkwood JM, Ibrahim JG, Sondak VK. High- and low-dose interferon alfa-2_b in high risk melanoma: first analysis of intergroup trial E1690/S9111/C9190. *J Clin Oncol* 2000;18:2444–2458.
29. Creagan ET, Dalton RJ, Ahmann DL. Randomized, surgical adjuvant clinical trial of recombinant interferon alfa-2_b in selected patients with malignant melanoma. *J Clin Oncol* 1995;13:2776–2783.
30. Grob JJ, Dreno B, de la Salmoniere P, et al. Randomised trial of interferon alpha-2_a as adjuvant therapy in resected primary melanoma thicker than 1.5 mm without clinically detectable node metastases. French cooperative group on melanoma. *Lancet* 1998;351:1905–1910.
31. Pehamberger H, Peter Soyer H, Steiner A, et al. Adjuvant interferon alfa-2_a treatment in resected primary stage II cutaneous melanoma. *J Clin Oncol* 1998;16:1425–1429.
32. Cascinelli N, Belli F, Mackie RM, et al. Effect of long-term therapy with interferon alpha-2a in patients with regional node metastases from cutaneous melanoma: a randomised trial. *Lancet* 2001;358:866–869.
33. Hancock BW, Wheatley K, Harrison G, et al. Aim high adjuvant interferon in melanoma (high risk), a United Kingdom Co-ordinating Committee on Cancer Research (UKCCCR) randomised study of observation versus adjuvant low dose extended duration interferon alfa 2_a in high risk resected malignant melanoma. *Proc Am Soc Clin Oncol* 2001;20:1393.
34. Cameron DA, Cornbleet MC, Mackie RM, et al. Adjuvant interferon alpha 2b in high risk melanoma — the Scottish study. *Br J Cancer* 2001;84:1146–1149.
35. Wheatley K, Ives N, Hancock B, et al. Does adjuvant interferon-alpha for high-risk melanoma provide a worthwhile benefit? A meta-analysis of the randomised trials. *Cancer Treat Rev* 2003;29:241–252. Search date not reported; primary sources medical databases such as Medline, protocol databases such as PDQ, and hand searches of oncology journals and meeting proceedings.
36. Kirkwood JM, Ibrahim JG, Sosman JA, et al. High-dose interferon alfa2_b significantly prolongs relapse-free and overall survival compared with GM2-KLH/QS-21 vaccine in patients with resected stage IIB–III melanoma: results of the intergroup trial E1694/S9512/C509801. *J Clin Oncol* 2001;19:2370–2380.
37. Cole BF, Gelber RD, Kirkwood JM, et al. Quality-of-life-adjusted survival analysis of high-risk resected cutaneous melanoma: the Eastern Cooperative Oncology Group study. *J Clin Oncol* 1996;14:2666–2673.
38. Kleeberg UR, Brocker EB, Lejeune F. Adjuvant trial in melanoma patients comparing rIFN-alfa to rIFN-gamma to Iscador to a control group after curative resection high risk primary (> 3 mm) or regional lymph node metastasis (EORTC 18871). *Eur J Cancer* 1999;35:S82.
39. Miller AB, Hoogstraten B, Staquet M, et al. Reporting results of cancer treatment. *Cancer* 1981;47:207–214.
40. Hersey P, Coates AS, McCarthy WH, et al. Adjuvant immunotherapy of patients with high-risk melanoma using vaccinia viral lysates of melanoma: results of a randomized trial. *J Clin Oncol* 2002;20:4181–4190.
41. Sondak VK, Liu PY, Tuthill RJ, et al. Adjuvant immunotherapy of resected, intermediate-thickness, node-negative melanoma with an allogeneic tumor vaccine: overall results of a randomized trial of the Southwest Oncology Group. *J Clin Oncol* 2002;20:2058–2066.
42. Wallack MK, Sivanandham M, Balch CM, et al. Surgical adjuvant active specific immunotherapy for patients with stage III melanoma: the final analysis of data from a phase III, randomized, double-blind, multicenter vaccinia melanoma oncolysate trial. *J Am Coll Surg* 1998;187:69–77.
43. Bystryn JC, Zeleniuch-Jacquotte A, Oratz R, et al. Double-blind trial of a polyvalent, shed-antigen, melanoma vaccine. *Clin Cancer Res* 2001;7:1882–1887.
44. Shumate CR, Urist MM, Maddox WA. Melanoma recurrence surveillance: patient or physician based? *Ann Surg* 1995;221:566–569.
45. Rogers GS, Kopf AW, Rigel DS, et al. Hazard-rate analysis in stage I malignant melanoma. *Arch Dermatol* 1986;122:999–1002.

Thomas Crosby
Consultant Clinical Oncologist

Malcolm Mason
Professor of Clinical Oncology

Philip Savage
Consultant in Medical Oncology
Velindre Hospital
Cardiff
UK

Competing interests: None declared.

TABLE 1 Melanoma incidence and mortality in different populations (see text, p 2114).[1]

	New cases/year	ASR/100 000	Deaths/year	ASR/100 000
World	132 602	2.4	37 047	0.75
Australia	8706	40.51	950	4.8
China	2418	0.22	1390	0.13
India	2187	0.34	1274	0.17
UK	5773	6.14	1564	1.81
USA	40 646	13.27	7791	2.74

Reproduced with permission of IARCPress. GLOBOCAN 2000: Cancer Incidence, Mentality and Prevalence Worldwide, Version 1.0 IARC CancerBase No. 5. Lyon IARCPress, 2000 (http://www.iarc.fr)

TABLE 2 Stage of malignant melanoma and 5 year survival (see text, p 2114).[3]

Stage	Description	5 year survival (%)
IA	Primary tumour < 1 mm no ulceration	95
IB	Primary tumour < 1 mm with ulceration or 1–2 mm with no ulceration	90
IIA	Primary tumour 1–2 mm with ulceration or 2–4 mm with no ulceration	78
IIB	Primary tumour 2–4 mm with ulceration or >4 mm with no ulceration	63–67
IIC	Primary tumour >4 mm with ulceration	45
IIIA	Microscopic nodal involvement	63–70
IIIB/C	Macroscopic nodal involvement	46–59
IV	Distant metastases	6.7–18.8

Reprinted with permission from the American Society of Clinical Oncology. Balch CM, Buzaid AC, Soong SJ et al. final version of the American Joint Committee of Cancer staging system for cutaneous melanoma. [Review][83 refs] Journal of Clinical Oncology. 19(16): 3635–48, 2001 Aug 15.

TABLE 3 RCTs for assessing radical versus less radical local surgery for malignant melanoma (see text, p 2116).[12–15]

Ref	Randomisation	Excision margin	Population	Relapse rates	Overall survival
11	Method not described	(a) 2 cm margin (b) 5 cm margin	Multicentre RCT, 327 people in Europe with lesions < 2.1 mm, followed for a median 5 years	Recurrence: 22/161 (14%) with 2 cm margin *v* 33/165 (20%) with 5 cm; P value not reported Distant metastases: 4/161 (2.5%) *v* 10/165 (6%); P value not reported	Overall survival at 10 years: 87% with 2 cm margin *v* 86% with 5 cm Margin; P = 0.56
12	Sealed envelopes, stratified blocks according to centre and previous treatment	(a) 1 cm margin (b) 3 cm margin	International multicentre RCT, 612 people with lesions < 2 mm thick	Local recurrence: 3/321 (1%) with 1 mm margin *v* 0/272 (0%) with 3 mm margin; P value not reported Regional node metastases as first relapse: 14/305 (5%) with 1 mm margin *v* 20/307 (7%) with 3 mm margin; P value not reported Distant metastases: 7/321 (2%) with 1 mm margin *v* 8/272 (3%) with 3 mm margin; P value not reported	4 year actuarial survival rate: 96.8% (305 people) with 1 cm margin *v* 96.0 (307 people) with 3 cm margin; P = 0.66
13	Method not described	(a) 2 cm margin (b) 2 cm margin plus elective node dissection (c) 4 cm margin (d) 4 cm margin plus elective node dissection	Multicentre RCT, 486 people in USA with 1–4 mm thickness lesion and no evidence of metastatic melanoma	Local recurrence at median follow up of 72 months: 2/242 (0.8%) with 2 cm margin *v* 4/244 (1.7%) with 4 cm margin; P = NS A subgroup of all these people had elective node dissection as a co-intervention Distant metastates: 2.5% *v* 2.1%; P = NS	Overall 5 year survival: 79.5% with 2 cm margin *v* 83.7% with 4 cm margin; P = NS
14	Telephone allocation using randomisation lists	(a) 2 cm margin (b) 5 cm margin	Multicentre RCT, 989 people in Sweden, with lesions 0.8–2.0 mm, followed for a median time of 11 years for survival, and 8 years for recurrence	Local recurrence: 1/476 (0.2%) with 2 cm margin *v* 4/513 (1%) with 5 cm margin; P value not reported Distant metastases: 24/479 (5%) with 2 cm margin *v* 34/513 (7%) with 5 cm margin; HR 0.76, 95% CI 0.45 to 1.28; P = 0.29	Overall survival at a median of 8 year follow up: 117/476 (25%) with 2 cm margin: 134/513 (26%) with 5 cm margin; HR 0.96, 95% CI 0.75 to 1.24; P = 0.77
15	Method not described	(a) 2 cm margin (b) 5 cm margin	Multicentre RCT, 319 people in Europe, with lesions < 2 mm, followed for a median 50 months	Recurrence: 14/153 (9%) with 2 cm margin *v* 21/166 (13%) with 5 cm margin; P = 0.31 Distant metastases: not reported	Overall 5 year survival: 93% with 2 cm margin *v* 90% with 5 cm margin; P = 0.57

NS, not significant; Ref, reference.

TABLE 4 **Recommended clinical excision margins.**[16,17]

Tumour thickness	Clinical excision margins
in situ	0.5 cm
mm	1 cm
>2 mm	2 cm

Reprinted from Sober AJ, Chuang TY, Duvic M. Guidelines of care for primary cutaneous melanoma. *J Am Acad Deratol* 2001;45:597–586. © 2001, with permission from the American Academy of Dermatology.

Scabies

Search date January 2003

Godfrey Walker and Paul Johnstone

QUESTIONS

INTERVENTIONS

See glossary

Key Messages

- **Permethrin** One systematic review has found that permethrin increases clinical and parasitic cure after 28 days compared with crotamiton. The systematic review found conflicting results with permethrin versus lindane. One subsequent RCT found limited evidence that permethrin increased clinical cure at 14 days compared with ivermectin.
- **Crotamiton** One systematic review found that crotamiton was less successful in terms of clinical and parasitic cure after 28 days compared with permethrin. One systematic review identified one RCT that found no significant difference between crotamiton and lindane in clinical cure rates at 28 days.
- **Oral ivermectin** One systematic review identified one RCT that found that ivermectin increased clinical cure rates after 7 days compared with placebo. Another small RCT identified by the review found no significant difference between ivermectin and benzyl benzoate in clinical cure rates at 30 days. One subsequent RCT found that, compared with benzyl benzoate, ivermectin increased clinical cure rates at 30 days. One systematic review identified one small RCT that found no significant difference between ivermectin and lindane in cure rates at 15 days. One subsequent RCT found no significant difference between ivermectin and lindane in failed clinical cure rates at 2 weeks, but it found that ivermectin decreased failed clinical cure rates at 4 weeks. One RCT found limited evidence that ivermectin reduced clinical cure rates at 14 days compared with permethrin. Experience suggests oral ivermectin is safe in younger adults being treated for onchocerciasis, but no such experience exists for children, and there have been reports of increased risk of death in elderly people.
- **Lindane** One systematic review identified one RCT that found no significant difference between lindane and crotamiton in clinical cure rates at 28 days. The systematic review found conflicting results between lindane and permethrin after 28 days. Another small RCT identified by the review found no significant difference between lindane and ivermectin in cure rates at 15 days. One subsequent RCT found no significant difference between lindane and ivermectin in failed clinical cure rates at 2 weeks, but it found a higher proportion of people with failed clinical cure with lindane compared with ivermectin at 4 weeks. We found reports of rare, serious adverse effects such as convulsions.

Clin Evid 2005;13:2126–2132.

- **Benzyl benzoate** One systematic review identified one small RCT that found no significant difference between benzyl benzoate and ivermectin in clinical cure rates at 30 days. One subsequent RCT found that benzyl benzoate reduced clinical cure at 30 days compared with ivermectin. One systematic review identified one RCT that found no significant difference between benzyl benzoate and sulphur ointment in clinical cure at 8 or 14 days.
- **Malathion** One systematic review found no RCTs on the effects of malathion. Case series have reported cure rates in scabies of over 80%.
- **Sulphur compounds** One systematic review identified one RCT that found no significant difference between sulphur ointment and benzyl benzoate in clinical cure at 8 or 14 days.

DEFINITION Scabies is an infestation of the skin by the mite *Sarcoptes scabiei*.[1] Typical sites of infestation are skin folds and flexor surfaces. In adults, the most common sites are between the fingers and on the wrists, although infection may manifest in elderly people as a diffuse truncal eruption. In infants and children, the face, scalp, palms, and soles are also often affected.

INCIDENCE/ PREVALENCE Scabies is a common public health problem with an estimated prevalence of 300 million cases worldwide, mostly affecting people in developing countries, where prevalence can exceed 50%.[2] In industrialised countries it is most common in institutionalised communities. Case studies suggest that epidemic cycles occur every 7–15 years and that these partly reflect the population's immune status.

AETIOLOGY/ RISK FACTORS Scabies is particularly common where there is social disruption, overcrowding with close body contact, and limited access to water.[3] Young children, immobilised elderly people, people with HIV/AIDS, and other medically and immunologically compromised people are predisposed to infestation and have particularly high mite counts.[4]

PROGNOSIS Scabies is not life threatening, but the severe, persistent itch and secondary infections may be debilitating. Occasionally, crusted scabies develops. This form of the disease is resistant to routine treatment and can be a source of continued reinfestation and spread to others. A search conducted by the author found no reports of spontaneous remission.

AIMS OF INTERVENTION To eliminate the scabies mites and ova from the skin; to cure pruritus (itching); to prevent reinfestation; to prevent spread to other people.

OUTCOMES **Clinical cure:** Number of visible burrows and papular and vesicular eruptions; pruritus. **Parasitic cure:** Presence of mites, ova, or faecal pellets in skin scrapings under a magnifying lens or microscope. Outcomes should be assessed 28–30 days after the start of treatment, which is the time it takes for lesions to heal and for any eggs and mites to reach maturity if treatment fails.

METHODS *Clinical Evidence* search and appraisal January 2003.

QUESTION What are the effects of topical treatments?

OPTION PERMETHRIN

One systematic review has found that permethrin increases clinical and parasitic cure after 28 days compared with crotamiton. The systematic review found conflicting results between permethrin and lindane. One subsequent RCT found limited evidence that permethrin increased clinical cure at 14 days compared with ivermectin.

Benefits: We found no RCTs that compared permethrin versus placebo. We found one systematic review (search date 1999, 6 RCTs)[5] and one subsequent RCT[6] comparing permethrin versus other topical and oral agents. **Versus crotamiton:** The review (2 RCTs, 194 people) found that permethrin compared with crotamiton significantly increased clinical cure rates after 28 days (2 RCTs; OR for failed clinical cure with permethrin *v* crotamiton 0.21, 95% CI 0.10 to 0.47) and significantly increased parasitic cure after 28 days (1 RCT; 94 people; OR for failed parasitic cure with permethrin *v* crotamiton 0.21, 95% CI 0.08 to

0.53).[5] It found no significant difference between permethrin and crotamiton in self reported pruritus (1 RCT: OR for itch persistence with permethrin *v* with crotamiton 0.38, 95% CI 0.12 to 1.19). **Versus lindane:** The systematic review identified four RCTs that compared permethrin with lindane.[5] Overall, the review found that permethrin appeared to be more effective than lindane in clinical cure after 28 days. However, it found significant trial heterogeneity ($P < 0.005$). Two RCTs (100 people; 52 people) included in the review found that permethrin compared with lindane significantly reduced clinical failure (OR for failed clinical cure of permethrin *v* lindane 0.14, 95% CI 0.05 to 0.43; and 0.19, 95% CI 0.05 to 0.70) whereas two RCTs (99 people; 467 people), including the largest RCT, found no significant difference between permethrin and lindane (OR for failed clinical cure of permethrin *v* lindane 0.8, 95% CI 0.21 to 3.14; and 0.93, 95% CI 0.60 to 1.42).[5] **Versus oral ivermectin:** We found one subsequent RCT that compared topical permethrin versus oral ivermectin.[6] The RCT (85 people attending an outpatient clinic in India) assessed clinical cure at 14 days, and if not assessed as completely cured at that time the same treatment was repeated. It found that permethrin significantly decreased failed clinical cure rate at 14 days compared with ivermectin (OR for failed clinical cure of permethrin *v* ivermectin 0.12, 95% CI 0.04 to 0.39).

Harms: One RCT identified by the review reported five people with adverse effects: two in the permethrin group (rash and possible diarrhoea) and three in the lindane group (pruritic rash, papules, and diarrhoea).[7] During 1990–1995, six adverse events were reported per 100 000 units distributed in the USA (1 central nervous system adverse effect reported per 500 000 units of permethrin distributed).[8] Resistance to permethrin seems to be rare[8] (see harms of lindane, p 2129).

Comment: None.

OPTION LINDANE

One systematic review identified one RCT that found no significant difference between lindane and crotamiton in clinical cure rates at 28 days. The systematic review found conflicting results with lindane compared with permethrin after 28 days. Another small RCT identified by the review found no significant difference between lindane and ivermectin in cure rates at 15 days. One subsequent RCT found no significant difference between lindane and ivermectin in failed clinical cure rates at 2 weeks, but found a higher proportion of people with failed clinical cure with lindane than with ivermectin at 4 weeks. We found reports of rare, serious adverse effects such as convulsions.

Benefits: We found no RCTs comparing lindane versus placebo. We found one systematic review (search date 1999, 6 RCTs)[5] comparing lindane versus other topical and oral agents, and one subsequent RCT comparing lindane versus ivermectin.[9] **Versus crotamiton:** One RCT (100 adults and children) identified by the review found no significant difference in clinical cure rates at 28 days (OR for failed clinical cure with crotamiton *v* lindane 0.41, 95% CI 0.15 to 1.10).[5] However, confidence intervals are broad and a clinically important difference cannot be ruled out. **Versus permethrin:** See benefits of permethrin, p 2127. **Versus oral ivermectin:** One RCT[10] (53 adults referred to hospital with scabies) identified by the review found no significant difference between lindane and ivermectin in clinical cure rates at 15 days (failed clinical cure 14/27 [52%] with lindane *v* 12/26 [46%] with oral ivermectin; RR 0.89, 95% CI 0.51 to 1.55).[5] One subsequent RCT compared topical lindane versus ivermectin.[9] It found no significant difference in failed clinical cure rates between lindane and ivermectin at 2 weeks (failed clinical cure rate 70/100 [70%] with ivermectin *v* 81/100 [81%] with lindane; RR 0.86, 95% CI 0.74 to 1.01) but it found that ivermectin significantly increased clinical cure rates at 4 weeks compared with lindane (failed clinical cure rate 43/100 [43%] with ivermectin *v* 64/100 [64%] with lindane; RR 0.67, 95% CI 0.51 to 0.88).

Harms: One RCT identified by the review reported five people with adverse effects: two in the permethrin group (rash and possible diarrhoea) and three in the lindane group (pruritic rash, papules, and diarrhoea).[7] One RCT identified by the review reported that six people taking lindane had headaches, and one person each had headache, hypotension, abdominal pain, and vomiting in the ivermectin group.[10] Case reports have reported rare severe adverse effects (e.g. convulsions, other long term neurological complications, and aplastic anaemia) particularly when lindane was applied to people with extensive skin diseases and to children.[11–13] Figures from the World Health Organization Collaborating Centre for International Drug Monitoring covering summary reports from 47 countries suggest that lindane is more toxic than other preparations (see comment below).[14] Five convulsions were reported in people on benzyl benzoate, two in people on crotamiton, 48 in people on lindane, two in people on malathion, and 19 in people on permethrin. Deaths reported on benzyl benzoate were none, crotamiton one, lindane four, malathion none, and permethrin five.[14] Resistance to lindane has been reported in many countries.[15]

Comment: Lindane was withdrawn from the market in the UK in 1995 because of concern about possible adverse effects. The evidence linking lindane with convulsions is suggestive but not conclusive.[11–14] It is difficult to draw firm conclusions on the relative occurrence of severe adverse effects of different preparations reported to the World Health Organization Collaborating Centre for International Drug Monitoring because of incomplete information on incidence in relation to use; however, lindane and permethrin appear possibly to be more likely to be related to rare severe adverse effects. Safety results from trials and observational studies need to be summarised, particularly regarding additional risks in infants and pregnant women.

OPTION CROTAMITON

One systematic review found that crotamiton was less successful in terms of clinical and parasitic cure after 28 days compared with permethrin. One systematic review identified one RCT that found no significant difference between crotamiton and lindane in clinical cure rates at 28 days.

Benefits: We found no RCTs comparing crotamiton versus placebo. We found one systematic review (search date 1999, 3 RCTs) comparing crotamiton versus other topical agents.[5] **Crotamiton versus permethrin:** See benefits of permethrin, p 2127. **Crotamiton versus lindane:** See benefits of lindane, p 2128.

Harms: The RCTs reported no serious adverse effects[5] (see harms of lindane, p 2129).

Comment: None.

OPTION MALATHION

One systematic review found no RCTs on the effects of malathion. Case series have reported cure rates in scabies of over 80%.

Benefits: We found one systematic review (search date 1999) that identified no RCTs.[5]

Harms: We found no RCTs (see harms of lindane, p 2129).

Comment: Case series suggest that malathion is effective in curing infestation with scabies, with a cure rate of over 80% of people at 4 weeks.[16–18] The safety results from trials and observational studies need to be systematically reviewed, particularly with regard to additional risks in infants and pregnant women.

OPTION BENZYL BENZOATE

One systematic review identified one small RCT that found no significant difference between benzyl benzoate and ivermectin in clinical cure rates at 30 days. One subsequent RCT found that benzyl benzoate reduced clinical cure at 30 days compared with ivermectin. One systematic review identified one RCT that found no significant difference between benzyl benzoate and sulphur ointment in clinical cure at 8 or 14 days.

Benefits: We found no RCTs comparing benzyl benzoate versus placebo. We found one systematic review (search date 1999, 2 RCTs, 202 people) comparing benzyl benzoate versus other agents[5] and one subsequent RCT comparing ivermectin and benzyl benzoate.[19] **Versus oral ivermectin:** The systematic review identified one RCT[20] and we found one subsequent RCT[19] (see benefits of oral ivermectin, p 2131). **Versus sulphur ointment:** One RCT identified by the review compared benzyl benzoate versus sulphur ointment (158 adults and children identified in a house to house survey of a semi-urban area of India).[21] It found no significant difference in the number of people with apparently cured lesions by 8 days (AR 68/89 [76%] with benzyl benzoate *v* 45/69 [65%] with sulphur ointment; RR 1.17, 95% CI 0.95 to 1.33) or by 14 days (AR 81/89 [91%] with benzyl benzoate *v* 67/69 [97%] with sulphur ointment; RR 0.94, 95% CI 0.86 to 1.01).

Harms: Both RCTs comparing benzyl benzoate versus oral ivermectin found that about a quarter of people treated with benzyl benzoate reported a transient increase in pruritus and dermatitis.[19,20] See harms of lindane, p 2129.

Comment: Non-randomised trials suggest benzyl benzoate has variable effectiveness (as low as 50%).[22,23] The low cure rate may be related to the concentration of the preparation and resistance of the mite to benzyl benzoate.

OPTION SULPHUR COMPOUNDS

One systematic review identified one RCT that found no significant difference between sulphur ointment and benzyl benzoate in clinical cure at 8 or 14 days.

Benefits: We found no RCTs comparing sulphur compounds versus placebo. **Versus benzyl benzoate:** We found one RCT (see benefits of benzyl benzoate, p 2130).[21]

Harms: Use of sulphur has been associated with increased local irritation in about a quarter of cases.[13]

Comment: None.

QUESTION What are the effects of systemic treatments?

OPTION ORAL IVERMECTIN

One systematic review identified one RCT that found that ivermectin increased clinical cure rates after 7 days compared with placebo. Another small RCT identified by the review found no significant difference between ivermectin and benzyl benzoate in clinical cure rates at 30 days. One subsequent RCT found that ivermectin increased clinical cure rates at 30 days compared with benzyl benzoate. One systematic review identified one small RCT that found no significant difference between ivermectin and lindane in cure rates at 15 days. One subsequent RCT found no significant difference between ivermectin and lindane in failed clinical cure rates at 2 weeks, but found that ivermectin increased clinical cure rates at 4 weeks. One RCT found limited evidence that ivermectin reduced clinical cure at 14 days compared with permethrin. Experience suggests that oral ivermectin is safe in younger adults being treated for onchocerciasis, but no such experience exists for children and there have been reports of increased risk of death in elderly people.

Benefits: We found one systematic review (search date 1999, 3 RCTs)[5] and three subsequent RCTs[6,9,19] comparing oral ivermectin versus placebo or other agents. **Versus placebo:** One RCT (55 young adults and children aged > 5 years) identified by the review found that oral ivermectin significantly increased clinical cure rates after 7 days compared with placebo (23/29 [79%] with oral ivermectin *v* 4/26 [15%] with placebo; RR 5.2, 95% CI 2.1 to 12.9; NNT 2, 95% CI 1 to 3).[5] **Versus benzyl benzoate:** One small RCT (44 adults and children) identified by the review found no significant difference in clinical cure rates at 30 days (16/23 [70%] with oral ivermectin *v* 10/21 [48%] with benzyl benzoate; RR 1.5, 95% CI 0.9 to 2.5).[20] One subsequent small RCT (58 adults and children) found that oral ivermectin significantly increased clinical cure rates at 30 days compared with benzyl benzoate (27/29 [93%] with oral ivermectin *v* 14/29 [48%] with benzyl benzoate; RR 1.9, 95% CI 1.3 to 2.8).[19] **Versus lindane:** See benefits of lindane, p 2128. **Versus permethrin:** See benefits of permethrin, p 2127.

Harms: One RCT identified by the review reported that six people had headaches in the lindane group (out of 27 people), and one person each had headache, hypotension, abdominal pain, and vomiting in the ivermectin group (out of 26 people).[10] One RCT reported no adverse effects for oral ivermectin, whereas 7/29 (24%) people taking benzyl benzoate had a mild to moderate increase in skin irritation by day 2 of treatment.[19] One RCT comparing ivermectin versus lindane reported one headache in the ivermectin group.[9] Oral ivermectin has been used widely in adults with onchocerciasis, and even with repeated doses serious adverse effects have been rare.[24,25] Summary reports to the World Health Organization Collaborating Centre for International Drug Monitoring from five countries indicate that it is associated with rare severe side effects, including three convulsions and eight deaths.[26] We found no good evidence about its safety in children. An increased risk of death has been reported among elderly people taking oral ivermectin for scabies in a long term care facility.[27] It is not clear whether this was caused by oral ivermectin, interactions with other scabicides (including lindane and permethrin), or other treatments such as psychoactive drugs. Other studies reported no such complications from its use in elderly people.[28]

Comment: Case series suggest that oral ivermectin may be effective when included in the treatment of hyperkeratotic crusted scabies (also known as Norwegian scabies)[29–31] and in people with concomitant HIV disease.[4] The RCT comparing oral ivermectin versus placebo assessed outcomes 7 days after the intervention was administered, which may be an insufficient time in which to achieve cure.[5]

REFERENCES

1. Meinking TL, Taplin D. Infestations. In: Schachner LA, Hansen RC, eds. *Pediatric dermatology*. New York: Churchill Livingston, 1995.
2. Stein DH. Scabies and pediculosis. *Curr Opin Pediatr* 1991;3:660–666.
3. Green M. Epidemiology of scabies. *Epidemiol Rev* 1989;11:126–150.
4. Meinking TL, Taplin D, Hermida JL, et al. The treatment of scabies with ivermectin. *N Engl J Med* 1995;333:26–30.
5. Walker GJA, Johnstone PW. Interventions for treating scabies. In: The Cochrane Library, Issue 4, 2002. Oxford: Update Software. Search date 1999; primary sources Medline, Embase, records of military trials from UK, USA, and Russia, and specialist register of the Cochrane Diseases Group.
6. Usha V, Gopalakrishnan Nair TV. A comparative study of oral ivermectin and topical permethrin cream in the treatment of scabies. *J Am Acad Dermatol* 2000;42:236–240.
7. Schultz MW, Gomez M, Hansen RC, et al. Comparative study of 5% permethrin cream and 1% lindane lotion for the treatment of scabies. *Arch Dermatol* 1990;126:167–170.
8. Meinking TL, Taplin D. Safety of permethrin vs lindane for the treatment of scabies. *Arch Dermatol* 1996;132:959–962.
9. Madan V, Jaskiran K, Gupta U, et al. Oral ivermectin in scabies patients: a comparison with 1% topical lindane lotion. *J Dermatol* 2001;28:481–484.
10. Chouela EN, Abeldano AM, Pellerano O, et al. Equivalent therapeutic efficacy and safety of ivermectin and lindane in the treatment of human scabies. *Arch Dermatol* 1999;135:651–655.
11. Hall RC, Hall RC. Long-term psychological and neurological complications of lindane poisoning. *Psychosomatics* 1999;40:513–517.
12. Nordt SP, Chew G. Acute lindane poisoning in three children. *J Emerg Med* 2000;18:51–53.
13. Elgart ML. A risk benefit assessment of agents used in the treatment of scabies. *Drug Saf* 1996;14386–393.
14. WHO Collaborating Centre for International Drug Monitoring. Reported adverse reactions to ectoparasiticodes, including scabicides, insecticides and repellents. Uppsala, Sweden, 2002. The WHO Collaborating Centre receives summary clinical reports from National Centres in countries participating in a collaborative programme. The information is not homogenous at least with respect to origin or likelihood that the pharmaceutical product caused the adverse reaction. The information does not represent the opinion of the World Health Organization.
15. Brown S, Belcher J, Brady W. Treatment of ectoparasitic infections: review of the English-language literature. *Clin Infect Dis* 1995;20(suppl 1):104–109.
16. Hanna NF, Clay JC, Harris JRW. *Sarcoptes scabiei* infestation treated with malathion liquid. *Br J Vener Dis* 1978;54:354.
17. Thianprasit M, Schuetzenberger R. Prioderm lotion in the treatment of scabies. *Southeast Asian J Trop Med Public Health* 1984;15:119–120.
18. Burgess I, Robinson RJF, Robinson J, et al. Aqueous malathion 0.5% as a scabicide: clinical trial. *BMJ* 1986;292:1172.
19. Nnoruka EN, Agu CE. Successful treatment of scabies with oral ivermectin in Nigeria. *Trop Doct* 2001;31:15–18.
20. Glaziou P, Cartel JL, Alzieu P, et al. Comparison of ivermectin and benzyl benzoate for treatment of scabies. *Trop Med Parasitol* 1993;44:331–332.
21. Gulati PV, Singh KP. A family based study on the treatment of scabies with benzyl benzoate and sulphur ointment. *Indian J Dermatol Venereol Lepr* 1978;44:269–273.
22. Kaur GA, Nadeswary K. Field trials on the management of scabies in Jengka Triangle, Pahang. *Med J Malaysia* 1980;35:14–21.
23. Haustein UF, Hlawa B. Treatment of scabies with permethrin versus lindane and benzyl benzoate. *Acta Derm Venereol* 1989;69:348–351.
24. Pacque M, Munoz B, Greene BM, et al. Safety of and compliance with community-based ivermectin therapy. *Lancet* 1990;335:1377–1380.
25. De Sole G, Remme J, Awadzi K, et al. Adverse reactions after large-scale treatment of onchocerciasis with ivermectin: combined results from eight community trials. *Bull World Health Organ* 1989;67:707–719.
26. WHO Collaborating Centre for International Drug Monitoring. Reported adverse reactions to ivermectin. Uppsala, Sweden, 2002. The WHO Collaborating Centre receives summary clinical reports from National Centres in countries participating in a collaborative programme. The information is not homogenous at least with respect to origin or likelihood that the pharmaceutical product caused the adverse reaction. The information does not represent the opinion of the World Health Organization.
27. Barkwell R, Shields S. Deaths associated with ivermectin treatment of scabies. *Lancet* 1997;349:1144–1145.
28. Diazgranados JA, Costa JL. Deaths after ivermectin treatment. *Lancet* 1997;349:1698.
29. Sullivan JR, Watt G, Barker B. Successful use of ivermectin in the treatment of endemic scabies in a nursing home. *Australas J Dermatol* 1997;38:137–140.
30. Aubin F, Humbert P. Ivermectin for crusted (Norwegian) scabies. *N Engl J Med* 1995;332:612.
31. Haas N, Henz BM, Ohlendorf D. Is single oral dose of ivermectin sufficient in crusted scabies? *Int J Dermatol* 2001;40:599.

Godfrey Walker
Specialist in Reproductive Health
UNFPA Country Technical Services Team for Eastern Europe and Central Asia
Bratislava, Slovak Republic

Paul Johnstone
Director of Public Health, Visiting Professor in Public Health
University of Teesside, Middlesbrough, UK

Competing interests: None declared.

Seborrhoeic dermatitis

November 2003

Bruce C. Gee

QUESTIONS

INTERVENTIONS

*Based on consensus opinion.

See glossary G

Key Messages

Treatments for seborrhoeic dermatitis of the scalp in adults

- **Ketoconazole** Five RCTs found that ketoconazole 2% shampoo improved scalp symptoms (including scaling, itching, redness, and dandruff) compared with placebo over 4 weeks.
- **Selenium suphide** One RCT found that selenium sulphide shampoo reduced dandruff compared with placebo.
- **Tar shampoo** One RCT found that tar shampoo was more effective at reducing scalp dandruff and redness than placebo.
- **Bifonazole** One small RCT found that bifonazole shampoo improved scalp symptoms compared with placebo.
- **Topical steroids** We found no RCTs comparing topical steroids (hydrocortisone, betamethasone valerate, clobetasone butyrate, mometasone furate, or clobetasol propionate) versus placebo. There is consensus that topical steroids are effective in treating seborrhoeic dermatitis of the scalp in adults.
- **Emollients; terbinafine** We found no RCTs comparing these interventions versus placebo in adults with seborrhoeic dermatitis of the scalp.

Treatments for seborrhoeic dermatitis of the face and body

- **Bifonazole** One RCT found that bifonazole improved symptoms compared with placebo after 4 weeks.
- **Ketoconazole** Two small RCTs found that ketoconazole 2% cream improved symptoms (erythema, scaling, papules, and pruritus) compared with placebo after 4 weeks.

- **Topical steroids (short term episodic treatment)** We found RCTs comparing topical steroids (hydrocortisone, betamethasone valerate, clobetasone butyrate, mometasone furate, or clobetasol propionate) versus placebo. There is consensus that short courses of topical steroids used episodically are effective in treating seborrhoeic dermatitis of the face and body in adults.
- **Emollients; lithium succinate; selenium sulphide; terbinafine** We found no RCTs of sufficient quality comparing these interventions versus placebo in adults with seborrhoeic dermatitis of the face and body.

DEFINITION Seborrhoeic dermatitis occurs in areas of the skin with a rich supply of sebaceous glands and manifests as red, sharply marginated lesions with greasy looking scales. On the face it mainly affects the medial aspect of the eyebrows, the area between the eyebrows, and the nasolabial folds. It also affects skin on the chest (commonly presternal) and the flexures. On the scalp it manifests as dry, flaking desquamation (dandruff) or yellow, greasy scaling with erythema. Dandruff is a lay term commonly used in the context of mild seborrhoeic dermatitis of the scalp. However, any scalp condition that produces scales could be labelled dandruff. Common differential diagnoses for seborrhoeic dermatitis of the scalp are psoriasis, eczema (see atopic eczema, [Web only]), and tinea capitis (see table 1, p 2139).

INCIDENCE/ PREVALENCE Seborrhoeic dermatitis is estimated to affect around 1–3% of the general population.[1] However, this is likely to be an underestimate because people do not tend to seek medical advice for mild dandruff.

AETIOLOGY/ RISK FACTORS *Malassezia* (*Pityrosporum*) *ovale* is considered to be the causative organism of seborrhoeic dermatitis and is responsible for producing an inflammatory reaction involving T cells and complement. Conditions that have been reported to predispose to seborrhoeic dermatitis include HIV,[2] neurological conditions such as Parkinson's disease, neuronal damage such as facial nerve palsy,[3] spinal injury,[4] ischaemic heart disease,[5] and alcoholic pancreatitis.[6] In this chapter we deal with treatment in immunocompetent adults who have no known predisposing conditions.

PROGNOSIS Seborrhoeic dermatitis is a chronic condition that tends to flare and remit spontaneously, and is prone to recurrence after treatment.[1,7]

AIMS OF INTERVENTION To reduce the symptoms and signs of seborrhoeic dermatitis with minimal adverse effects. Most therapeutic options aim to reduce colonisation with *Malassezia* (*Pityrosporum*) *ovale* and reduce inflammation, although they tend to palliate rather than cure.

OUTCOMES Severity of symptoms, including itching, scale, and erythema; adverse effects of treatment.

METHODS *Clinical Evidence* search and appraisal November 2003. Most authors have used the term "dandruff" to mean seborrhoeic dermatitis. If there was any doubt in the diagnosis then the study was excluded.

QUESTION What are the effects of topical treatments for seborrhoeic dermatitis of the scalp in adults?

OPTION TOPICAL STEROIDS

We found no RCTs comparing topical steroids (hydrocortisone, betamethasone valerate, clobetasone butyrate, mometasone furate, or clobetasol propionate) versus placebo. There is consensus that topical steroids are effective in treating seborrhoeic dermatitis of the scalp in adults.

Benefits: We found no systematic reviews or RCTs.

Harms: We found no RCTs.

Comment: Although no systematic reviews or RCTs were identified, there is consensus that topical steroids are effective in treating seborrhoeic dermatitis of the scalp in adults. Betamethasone valerate scalp application in a lotion or mousse are routinely used in practice by dermatologists.

OPTION **EMOLLIENTS**

We found no RCTs comparing emollients versus placebo in adults with seborrhoeic dermatitis of the scalp.

Benefits: We found no systematic review or RCTs.

Harms: We found no RCTs.

Comment: None.

OPTION **ANTIFUNGAL SCALP PREPARATIONS**

Five RCTs found that ketoconazole 2% shampoo improved scalp symptoms (including scaling, itching, redness, and dandruff) compared with placebo over 4 weeks. One small RCT found that bifonazole shampoo improved scalp symptoms compared with placebo. One RCT found that selenium sulphide shampoo reduced dandruff compared with placebo. We found no RCTs comparing terbinafine versus placebo in adults with seborrhoeic dermatitis of the scalp.

Benefits: We found no systematic reviews. **Ketoconazole shampoo:** We found five RCTs ranging in size from 20 to 246 participants.[8–12] All found improvements in symptoms with ketoconazole 2% shampoo after 4 weeks (see table 2, p 2140). **Bifonazole shampoo:** We found one RCT (51 people with seborrhoea or seborrhoeic dermatitis of the scalp) that compared bifonazole (1%) shampoo versus placebo.[13] It found that bifonazole (1%) shampoo significantly improved scalp symptoms (severity of scaling, pruritus, and overall severity graded by a clinician on a 3-point scale from 0 = none to 3 = severe) compared with placebo after 6 weeks (scaling, P = 0.01; pruritus, P = 0.008; overall severity, P = 0.012). **Selenium sulphide shampoo:** We found one RCT (246 people with moderate to severe dandruff) that compared three treatments: selenium sulphide 2.5% shampoo; ketoconazole 2% shampoo; and placebo.[11] It found significantly greater reductions in mean adherent dandruff scores (determined by visual examination of six scalp areas, in which 0 = none and 9–10 = severe/heavy) with selenium sulphide shampoo compared with placebo over 29 days (% reduction in adherent dandruff scores from baseline: 66.7% with selenium sulphide *v* 44.5% with placebo; P value not reported). It also found that significantly more people responded to treatment (global improvement of completely cleared, excellent, or good) with selenium sulphide shampoo than with placebo at 29 days (AR for responding to treatment: 54.7% with selenium sulphide *v* 28.6% with placebo; P = 0.004). **Terbinafine:** We found no RCTs (see comment below).

Harms: **Ketoconazole shampoo:** Four of the five RCTs reported that there were no adverse effects of treatment.[8–11] The fifth RCT reported one instance of scalp tenderness that was probably related to ketoconazole treatment.[12] **Bifonazole shampoo:** The RCT reported no major side effects.[13] **Selenium sulphide shampoo:** The RCT (246 people) reported infrequent adverse events with selenium sulphide shampoo, including pruritus or burning sensation of the scalp (3 people), eruption near the hair line (1 person), psoriasis (1 person), lightening/bleaching of hair colour (2 people), orange staining of the scalp (1 person), and a chemical taste during shampooing (1 person).[11]

Comment: **Ketoconazole shampoo:** We found four additional placebo controlled RCTs in non-English languages, which are awaiting translation. **Terbinafine:** Terbinafine is not manufactured as a scalp preparation in the UK and is not known to be available worldwide.

OPTION TAR SHAMPOO

One RCT found that tar shampoo was more effective at reducing scalp dandruff and redness than placebo.

Benefits: We found no systematic reviews. **Versus placebo:** We found one RCT (111 people with seborrhoeic dermatitis or dandruff) that compared tar shampoo (4% coal tar) versus placebo.[12] It found that, compared with placebo, tar shampoo significantly improved both dandruff (dandruff score, assessed by a technician by multiplying size of affected area by severity; size of affected area scored from 0 = 10% to 4 = >70%; severity scored from 1 = small flakes resembling a white powder to 5 = flakes adhering to the scalp as white or yellow plates) and redness (graded by a clinician on a 5-point scale from 0 = none to 4 = very severe) after 29 days (mean reduction in dandruff score from baseline: 31 with tar shampoo *v* 19 with placebo; $P < 0.01$; mean difference in redness from baseline: 1.2 with tar shampoo *v* 0.6 with placebo; $P < 0.05$). There was no significant difference in scaling or area of seborrhoeic dermatitis after 29 days between tar shampoo and placebo.

Harms: The RCT reported no major adverse events.[12]

Comment: None.

QUESTION What are the effects of topical treatments for seborrhoeic dermatitis of the face and body in adults?

OPTION TOPICAL STEROIDS

We found no RCTs comparing topical steroids (hydrocortisone, betamethasone valerate, clobetasone butyrate, mometasone furate, and clobetasol propionate) versus placebo. There is consensus that short courses of topical steroids used episodically are effective in treating seborrhoeic dermatitis of the face and body in adults.

Benefits: We found no systematic review or RCTs.

Harms: We found no RCTs.

Comment: Although we found no RCTs of topical steroids in adults with seborrhoeic dermatitis of the face or body, consensus regards their use as effective. It is current practice to use short courses of topical steroids episodically in seborrhoeic dermatitis. Affected areas of the body are treated with short courses of potent topical steroids (betamethasone valerate [0.1%], mometasone furoate [0.1%]), while the face is treated with short courses of moderate (clobetasone butyrate [0.05%]) or low potency (hydrocortisone [1%]) steroids.

OPTION EMOLLIENTS

We found no RCTs of emollients in adults with seborrhoeic dermatitis of the face and body.

Benefits: We found no systematic reviews or RCTs.

Harms: We found no RCTs.

Comment: None.

OPTION ANTIFUNGALS

Two small RCTs found that ketoconazole 2% cream improved symptoms (erythema, scaling, papules, and pruritus) compared with placebo after 4 weeks. One RCT found that bifonazole improved symptoms compared with placebo after 4 weeks. We found no RCTs comparing terbinafine or selenium sulphide versus placebo in adults with seborrhoeic dermatitis of the face and body.

Benefits: We found no systematic reviews. **Ketoconazole:** We found two RCTs that compared ketoconazole 2% cream versus placebo.[8,14] The first RCT (37 people with seborrhoeic dermatitis) found that ketoconazole 2% cream improved symptoms (according to a composite clinical score in which 8 sites were graded for erythema, scaling, papules, and pruritus; range not given) compared with placebo after 4 weeks (reduction in approximate mean sum of symptom scores from baseline [see comment below]: 19 with ketoconazole cream *v* 13 with placebo; P value not reported).[14] The second RCT (20 people with seborrhoeic dermatitis of the face, with or without seborrhoeic dermatitis of the scalp, chest or back; see comment below) compared ketoconazole 2% cream plus ketoconazole 2% shampoo versus placebo. It found that ketoconazole 2% cream improved facial symptoms (severity of symptoms graded on a 4-point scale from 0 = none to 3 = severe) compared with placebo after 4 weeks (AR for improving by at least one symptom grade from baseline: 90% [9/10] with ketoconazole *v* 0% [0/10] improving with placebo; P value not reported).[8] **Bifonazole:** We found one RCT (100 people with seborrhoeic dermatitis of the face) that compared bifonazole (1%) cream versus placebo.[15] It found that significantly more people responded to treatment (global improvement graded on a 4-point scale from 0 = no improvement or worsening to 3 = healing) with bifonazole compared with placebo at 4 weeks (AR for healing: 16/37 [43%] with bifonazole *v* 10/43 [23%] with placebo; AR for improvement: 20/37 [54%] with bifonazole *v* 26/43 [61%] with placebo; AR for treatment failure: 1/37 [3%] with bifonazole *v* 7/43 [16%] with placebo; overall P value 0.044; P values for individual outcomes not reported). **Selenium sulphide:** We found no RCTs. **Terbinafine:** We found no RCTs.

Harms: **Ketoconazole:** Both RCTs reported that there were no adverse effects of treatment.[8,14] **Bifonazole:** The RCT reported more minor adverse effects of treatment (including itch, burning, tightness, erythema, papules, and scaling) with bifonazole than with placebo (5/50 [10%] with bifonazole *v* 2/50 [4%] with placebo; P value not reported).[15]

Comment: **Ketoconazole:** Approximate mean scores were extracted from graphs because data were not tabulated.[14] Of the 20 people with seborrhoeic dermatitis of the face, 16 (80%) also had seborrhoeic dermatitis of the scalp, seven (35%) had chest involvement and five (25%) had back involvement.[8]

OPTION LITHIUM SUCCINATE

We found no RCTs of sufficient quality topical lithium succinate in adults with seborrhoeic dermatitis of the face and body.

Benefits: We found no systematic reviews or RCTs of sufficient quality (see comment below).

Harms: We found no systematic reviews or RCTs of sufficient quality (see comment below).

Comment: We found one crossover RCT (30 people with seborrhoeic dermatitis of the face and/or the trunk) that compared lithium succinate 8% cream versus placebo.[16] It found that lithium succinate significantly improved symptoms (graded on a 100-mm scale on severity of redness, scaling, greasiness, and overall clinical impression of the condition) compared with placebo (results not pre-crossover). However, these results should be interpretted with caution because of the potential for persistence of effects after crossover. The RCT also had a high withdrawal rate (37%) and it is not clear whether the analyses were conducted on an intention to treat basis. Withdrawals were due to non-compliance (2 people with lithium succinate, 3 with placebo), local stinging sensation and erythema (1 person with lithium succinate, 2 with placebo), worsening of acne vulgaris (1 person with lithium succinate, 1 with placebo), or resolution of lesions (1 person, group not reported).

REFERENCES

1. Gupta AK, Bluhm R, Cooper EA. Seborrhoeic dermatitis. *Dermatol Clin* 2003;21:401–412.
2. Berger RS. Cutaneous manifestations of early human immunodeficiency virus exposure. *J Am Acad Dermatol* 1988;19:298–303.
3. Bettley FR, Marten RH. Unilateral seborrhoeic dermatitis following a nerve lesion. *Arch Dermatol* 1956;73:110–115.
4. Wilson CL, Walshe M. Incidence of seborrhoeic dermatitis in spinal injury patients. *Br J Dermatol* 1988;119(suppl 33):48
5. Tager A. Seborrhoeic dermatitis in acute cardiac disease. *Br J Dermatol* 1964;76:367–369.
6. Barba A, Piubello W, Vantini I, et al. Skin lesions in chronic alcoholic pancreatitis. *Dermatologica* 1982;164:322–326.
7. Rook et al. *Textbook of Dermatology*, 6th ed. Blackwell and Synergy: 639–643.
8. Green CA, Farr PM, Shuster S. Treatment of seborrhoeic dermatitis with ketoconazole: II. Response of seborrhoeic dermatitis of the face, scalp and trunk to topical ketoconazole. *Br J Dermatol* 1987;116:217–221.
9. Carr MM, Pryce DM, Ive FA. Treatment of seborrhoeic dermatitis with ketoconazole: I. Response of seborrhoeic dermatitis of the scalp to topical ketoconazole. *Br J Dermatol* 1987;116:213–216.
10. Berger R, Mills OH. Double blind placebo-controlled trial of ketoconazole 2% shampoo in the treatment of moderate to severe dandruff. *Adv Ther* 1990;7:247–255.
11. Danby FW, Maddin WS, Margesson LJ. A randomised, double-blind, placebo-controlled trial of ketoconazole 2% shampoo versus selenium sulfide 2.5% shampoo in the treatment of moderate to severe dandruff. *J Am Acad Dermatol* 1993;29:1008–1012.
12. Davies DB, Boorman GC, Shuttleworth D. Comparative efficacy of shampoos containing coal tar (4.0% w/w; Tarmed™), coal tar (4.0% w/w) plus ciclopirox olamine (1.0% w/w; Tarmed™ AF) and ketoconazole (2.0% w/w; Nizoral®) for the treatment of dandruff/seborrhoeic dermatitis. *J Dermatol Treat* 1999;10:177–183.
13. Segal R, David A, Ingber R, Lurie R, Sandbank M. Treatment with bifonazole shampoo for seborrhoea and seborrhoeic dermatitis: a randomised, double blind study. *Acta Derm Venereol (Stockh)* 1992;72:454–455.
14. Skinner RB, Noah PW, Taylor RM, et al. Double-blind treatment of seborrheic dermatitis cream with 2% ketoconazole cream. *J Am Acad Dermatol* 1985;12:852–856.
15. Zienicke H, Korting HC, Braun-Falco O, et al. Comparative efficacy and safety of bifonazole 1% cream and the corresponding base preparation in the treatment of seborrhoeic dermatitis. *Mycoses* 1993;36:325–331.
16. Cuelenaere C, De Bersaques J, Kint A. Use of topical lithium succinate in the treatment of seborrhoeic dermatitis. *Dermatology* 1992;184:194–197.

Bruce C. Gee
Consultant Dermatologist
Warwick Hospital
Warwick
UK

Competing interests: None declared.

TABLE 1 **Differential diagnoses for seborrhoeic dermatitis of the scalp (see text, p 2134).**

Diagnosis	Distinguishing features
Psoriasis	Prominent erythema Tendency for hair line involvement More prominent silver scale Presence of psoriasis elsewhere (skin, nails, joints)
Eczema (atopic and contact dermatitis)	Atopic dermatitis: • General skin examination • History Contact dermatitis: • Distribution of eczema • History
Tinea capitis	Microscopy Fungal culture of scalp scrapings

TABLE 2 **RCTs comparing ketoconazole shampoo versus placebo for seborrhoeic dermatitis of the scalp (see antifungal scalp preparations, p 2135).[8–12]**

Trial details	Ref	Participants	Outcome
Ketoconazole (2% shampoo plus 2% cream) *v* placebo	8	20 people with seborrhoeic dermatitis of the face: 80% had seborrhoeic dermatitis of the scalp, 35% had chest involvement, and 25% had back involvement	Clinician rated scalp scaling (0 = none to 3 = severe): • AR for improvement in scaling at 4 weeks: 86% (6/7) with ketoconazole *v* 0% (0/9) with placebo (P value not reported) Participant rated scalp scaling (100–mm VAS from 0 = none to 100 = severe): • Scalp scaling improved significantly more at 4 weeks with ketoconazole than with placebo (scores shown graphically; P < 0.05)
Crossover RCT comparing ketoconazole 2% shampoo *v* placebo (shampoo base without ketoconazole)	9	20 people (16 male, 4 female) with either dandruff or seborrhoeic dermatitis (no distinction made between these; proportion with seborrhoeic dermatitis not reported)	Participant rated scalp itching and scaling (100–mm VAS from 0 = none to 100 = 'worst ever'): • Approximate median change in itch score at 4 weeks: –20 with ketoconazole *v* +8 with placebo (P value not reported) Approximate median change in scale score at 4 weeks: • –20 with ketoconazole *v* +15 with placebo (P value not reported) (Median scores pre–crossover approximated from graphs)
Ketoconazole 2% shampoo *v* placebo (shampoo base without ketoconazole)	10	53 people with moderate to severe dandruff, 28 [52.8%] of whom had seborrhoeic dermatitis	Adherent dandruff score (six scalp areas assessed; 0 = no scaling to 10 = extremely severe scaling): • Mean change in score at day 15: –12 with ketoconazole *v* –7 with placebo (P < 0.05) • Mean change in score at day 29: –19 with ketoconazole *v* –13 with placebo (P < 0.05) Response to treatment (global evaluation of completely cleared, excellent, or good): • AR for responding to treatment at day 29: 78.6% (22/28) with ketoconazole *v* 37.5% (9/24) with placebo (P = 0.004)
Ketoconazole 2% shampoo *v* selenium sulphide 2.5% shampoo *v* placebo	11	246 people with moderate to severe dandruff	Adherent dandruff score (six scalp areas assessed; 0 = none and 9–10 = severe/heavy): • % Reduction in mean score from baseline at 29 days: 73.0% with ketoconazole *v* 44.5% with placebo (P value not reported) Response to treatment (global evaluation of completely cleared, excellent, or good): • AR for responding to treatment at day 29: 64.9% with ketoconazole *v* 28.6% with placebo (P < 0.001)

TABLE 2 continued

Trial details	Ref	Participants	Outcome
Ketoconazole 2% shampoo *v* coal tar 4.0% plus ciclopirox olamine 1% shampoo *v* placebo	12	163 people with seborrhoeic dermatitis or dandruff	Clinician rated scaling and redness (0 = none to 4 = very severe): • Mean reduction in scale score at 29 days: 1.2 with ketoconazole *v* 0.3 with placebo ($P < 0.01$) • Mean reduction in redness score at 29 days: 1.3 with ketoconazole *v* 0.5 with placebo ($P < 0.001$) Area of scalp affected by seborrhoeic dermatitis: • No significant difference between ketoconazole and placebo at 29 days (area and P value not reported).

VAS = visual–analogue scale.

Squamous cell carcinoma of the skin (non-metastatic)

Search date January 2004

Adèle Green and Robin Marks

QUESTIONS

INTERVENTIONS

See glossary G

Key Messages

Prevention

- **Sunscreens in prevention of squamous cell carcinoma (daily compared with discretionary use)** One RCT in adults in a subtropical community in Queensland, Australia found that daily compared with discretionary use of sunscreen on the head, neck, arms, and hands reduced the incidence of squamous cell carcinoma after 4.5 years.
- **Sunscreens to prevent development of new solar keratoses (compared with placebo or daily compared with discretionary use)** One RCT in people aged over 40 years living in Victoria, Australia who had previous solar keratoses (a risk factor for squamous cell carcinoma) found that daily sunscreen reduced the incidence of new solar keratoses after 7 months compared with placebo. One RCT in adults in a subtropical community in Queensland, Australia found that daily compared with discretionary use of sunscreen reduced the increase of solar keratoses over the whole body after 2.5 years.

Treatment

- **Micrographically controlled surgery (compared with standard surgical excision)** We found no RCTs or observational studies of sufficient quality comparing the effects of micrographically controlled surgery versus standard primary surgical excision on local recurrence rates.
- **Optimal primary excision margin** We found no RCTs or observational studies of sufficient quality relating size of primary excision margin to local recurrence rate.
- **Radiotherapy after surgery (compared with surgery alone)** We found no RCTs or observational studies of sufficient quality comparing the effects of radiotherapy after surgery versus surgery alone on local recurrence rates.

Clin Evid 2005;13:2142–2147.

DEFINITION Cutaneous squamous cell carcinoma is a malignant tumour of keratinocytes arising in the epidermis, showing histological evidence of dermal invasion.

INCIDENCE/ PREVALENCE Incidence rates are often derived from surveys because few cancer registries routinely collect notifications of squamous cell carcinoma of the skin. Incidence rates on exposed skin vary markedly around the world according to skin colour and latitude, and range from negligible rates in black populations and white populations living at high latitudes to rates of about 1/100 in white residents of tropical Australia.[1]

AETIOLOGY/ RISK FACTORS People with fair skin colour who sunburn easily without tanning, people with xeroderma pigmentosum Ⓖ,[2–4] and those who are immunosuppressed[5] are susceptible to squamous cell carcinoma. The strongest environmental risk factor for squamous cell carcinoma is chronic sun exposure. Cohort and case control studies have found that the risk of squamous cell carcinoma is three times greater in people with fair skin colour, a propensity to burn on initial exposure to sunlight, or a history of multiple sunburns. Clinical signs of chronic skin damage, especially solar keratoses, are also risk factors for cutaneous squamous cell carcinoma.[3,4] In people with multiple solar keratoses (> 15), the risk of squamous cell carcinoma is 10–15 times greater than in people with no solar keratoses.[3,4]

PROGNOSIS Prognosis is related to the location and size of tumour, histological pattern, depth of invasion, perineural involvement, and immunosuppression.[6,7] A worldwide review of 95 case series, each consisting of at least 20 people, found that the overall metastasis rate for squamous cell carcinoma on the ear was 11% and on the lip 14%, compared with an average for all sites of 5%.[7] A review of 71 case series found that lesions less than 2 cm in diameter have less than half the local recurrence rate compared with lesions greater than 2 cm (7% *v* 15%), and less than a third of the rate of metastasis (9% *v* 30%).[7]

AIMS OF INTERVENTION To prevent the occurrence of squamous cell carcinoma; to achieve cure by eradicating local disease including microinvasive disease; to reduce mortality.

OUTCOMES **Prevention:** Incidence of cutaneous squamous cell carcinoma; mortality from squamous cell carcinoma. **Primary excision:** Local recurrence; survival; cosmetic outcome. **Radiotherapy after surgery:** Local recurrence; regional recurrence; survival.

METHODS *Clinical Evidence* search and appraisal January 2004, including a search for observational studies. The authors performed a supplementary search in December 2002 of reference lists of all identified review articles and relevant sections of dermatology textbooks.

QUESTION Does the use of sunscreen help to prevent cutaneous squamous cell carcinoma?

Adèle Green

OPTION SUNSCREEN

One RCT in people aged over 40 years living in Australia who had previous solar keratoses (a risk factor for squamous cell carcinoma) found that daily sunscreen reduced the incidence of new solar keratoses after 7 months compared with placebo. One RCT in adults in a subtropical community in Queensland, Australia found that daily compared with discretionary use of sunscreen on the head, neck, arms, and hands reduced the incidence of squamous cell carcinoma after 4.5 years. The RCT found that daily compared with discretionary use of sunscreen reduced the increase of solar keratoses over the whole body after 2.5 years.

Benefits: We found no systematic review. **Versus placebo:** One RCT (588 people with previous solar keratoses, aged > 40 years, living in Victoria, Australia) found that, compared with placebo, daily use of sunscreen significantly reduced the risk of new solar keratoses over 7 months (mean number of new lesions per person: 1.6 with sunscreen *v* 2.3 with placebo; RR 0.62, 95% CI 0.54 to 0.71), and significantly increased lesion remission (OR 1.5, 95% CI 1.3 to 1.8).[8] **Daily versus**

discretionary use: One RCT (1621 adults in a subtropical community in Queensland, Australia) compared daily sunscreen (sun protection factor 15+) versus sunscreen at their usual discretionary rate.[9] People allocated to daily sunscreen were told to apply it to the head, neck, arms, and hands every morning and to reapply it after heavy sweating, bathing, or long sun exposure. They were reminded of this advice every 3 months by research staff when sunscreen supplies were replenished. The RCT found that daily sunscreen significantly reduced the incidence of squamous cell carcinoma tumours after 4.5 years compared with discretionary sunscreen (22 people with 28 new squamous cell carcinomas with daily sunscreen *v* 25 people with 46 new squamous cell carcinomas with discretionary sunscreen use; RR 0.61, 95% CI 0.46 to 0.81). Subgroup analysis found no significant difference between people with a history of skin cancer and those without.[9] However, confidence intervals were wide, suggesting that the subgroup analysis may have lacked sufficient power to rule out a clinically important difference. A subsequent report of this RCT compared the effects of the daily use of sunscreen versus discretionary use on the development of solar keratoses.[10] The RCT found that daily sunscreen significantly reduced the increase of solar keratoses over the whole body in the first 2.5 years compared with discretionary use (increase in solar keratoses: 20% with daily sunscreen *v* 57% with discretionary use; adjusted ratio 76%, $P < 0.05$; regression analysis, see comment below). It found that the rate of increase in solar keratoses was lower with daily compared with discretionary sunscreen use over the next 2 years, but the difference between groups did not reach significance (adjusted ratio 95%, $P > 0.05$; regression analysis, see comment below).[10]

Harms: Daily sunscreen caused contact allergy in a small proportion of users (< 10%)[8,11] and skin irritation in a variable proportion of users (2–15%).[8,9,11] In the placebo controlled RCT, no people tested were allergic to the active ingredients of sunscreen, but irritant reactions both to active sunscreen and the control base cream were observed.[8,11] The RCT of regular versus discretionary use found that daily sunscreen use was not associated with greater sun exposure, including recreational exposure.[9] However, another RCT assessing sun exposure times among young adults who used sunscreen while intentionally exposing themselves to the sun ("sunbathing") found that a sun protection factor 30 sunscreen compared with a sun protection factor 10 sunscreen was associated with significantly longer exposure times.[12]

Comment: In a long term prevention trial with skin cancer as the outcome, placebo sunscreen may be regarded as unethical. It would also be difficult to mask treatment allocation. In the RCT comparing daily versus discretionary sunscreen use in the development of solar keratoses, outcome measures were adjusted for confounding factors including sex, age, beta carotene use, eye and hair colour, skin reaction to acute sun exposure, lifetime occupational sun exposure, smoking, and history of skin cancer.[10]

QUESTION **What is the optimal margin for primary excision of cutaneous squamous cell carcinoma?**

Robin Marks

OPTION **OPTIMAL PRIMARY EXCISION MARGIN**

We found no RCTs or observational studies of sufficient quality relating size of primary excision margin to local recurrence rate.

Benefits: We found no systematic review or RCTs assessing different excision margins at any sites measuring local recurrence (see comment below).

Harms: We found no RCTs. As with all kinds of surgery, there is a potential for tissue destruction and scarring — particularly of vital structures such as eyelids, lip margins, and motor and sensory nerves.

Comment: One case series using micrographically controlled surgery**G** assessed excision margins in relation to histological extension of the tumour and found a 95% clearance rate of squamous cell carcinomas less than 2 cm in diameter with a margin of 4 mm of normal skin, and a 96% clearance rate of tumours greater than 2 cm with a margin of 6 mm.[13] The sites of scalp, ears, eyelid, nose, and lip were found to have more deeply invasive tumours. Another study reported on 37 tumours that had a 4 mm margin of clinically normal skin removed at the time of primary excision. It was estimated that this margin would result in complete excision of 97% of squamous cell carcinomas suitable for excision in an outpatient facility.[14] Numerous case series suggest that primary excision of cutaneous squamous cell carcinoma has a likelihood of local recurrence varying from 5–20% depending on tumour size, site, histopathological differentiation, perineural involvement**G**, and depth of invasion.[7,15–20]

QUESTION **Does micrographically controlled surgery result in lower rates of local recurrence than standard primary excision?**

Robin Marks

OPTION **MICROGRAPHICALLY CONTROLLED SURGERY VERSUS PRIMARY EXCISION**

We found no RCTs or observational studies of sufficient quality comparing the effects of micrographically controlled (Mohs') surgery versus standard primary surgical excision on local recurrence rates.

Benefits: We found no systematic review or RCTs (see comment below).

Harms: Although we found no RCTs, it is thought that with all kinds of surgery there is potential for tissue destruction and scarring particularly of vital structures such as eyelids, lip margins, and motor and sensory nerves. However, Mohs' microscopic surgery**G** is considered more tissue sparing because of its specificity in determining the amount of normal surrounding tissue removed.

Comment: A review of case series since 1940 suggested a local recurrence rate of 3% after Mohs' surgery compared with 8% after primary excision of cutaneous squamous cell carcinoma. However, the evidence must be treated with caution because of differing study quality, the long time period covered, and potential differences between people treated with Mohs' surgery and those treated with non-Mohs' surgery.[7] A site specific comparison found lower 5 year local recurrence rates after Mohs' surgery than after primary excision for squamous cell carcinoma of the lip (2% with Mohs' *v* 16% with primary excision) and of the ear (5% with Mohs' *v* 19% with primary excision).[7]

QUESTION **Does radiotherapy after surgery effect local recurrence of cutaneous squamous cell carcinoma?**

Adèle Green

OPTION **RADIOTHERAPY AFTER SURGERY**

We found no RCTs or observational studies of sufficient quality comparing the effects of radiotherapy after surgery versus surgery alone on local recurrence rates.

Benefits: We found no systematic review or RCTs (see comment below).

Harms: Although not measured, there is the potential for long term scar deterioration with postradiation depigmentation and gradual development of chronic radiodermatitis❻, including telangiectasiae❻, thinning of the skin, and hyperkeratosis❻.

Comment: In rare instances, squamous cell carcinomas cannot be excised completely and these have recurrence rates of over 50%.[21,22] Case series of inadequately excised squamous cell carcinomas, especially those with microscopic perineural invasion❻ found at the time of curative surgery, have reported recurrence rates of 20–25% after 5 years when surgery was followed by radiotherapy.[23,24] Ability to detect advanced perineural invasion can be enhanced by computerised tomography or magnetic resonance imaging.[25]

GLOSSARY

Hyperkeratosis Increased scaling on the surface of the skin.

Micrographically controlled surgery Does not use standard excision margins as the basis for achieving tumour clearance. The visible tumour and a thin margin of apparently normal skin are removed, mapped, and examined microscopically using a specialised sectioning technique at the time of surgery, and the surgery continues until there is microscopic confirmation of complete tumour clearance, at which stage the wound is closed.[26]

Perineural invasion Tumour invasion along (not in) a nerve.

Radiodermatitis Chronic non-malignant changes in the skin due to excessive radiation.

Telangiectasiae Permanently dilated small blood vessels in the skin.

Xeroderma pigmentosum An inherited disorder with defective repair of DNA damage caused by ultraviolet radiation, resulting in sun related skin cancers of all types at an early age.

REFERENCES

1. Buettner PG, Raasch BA. Incidence rates of skin cancer in Townsville, Australia. *Int J Cancer* 1998;78:587–593.
2. Green A, Battistutta D, Hart V, et al, the Nambour Study Group. Skin cancer in a subtropical Australian population: incidence and lack of association with occupation. *Am J Epidemiol* 1996;144:1034–1040.
3. English DR, Armstrong BK, Kricker A, et al. Demographic characteristics, pigmentary and cutaneous risk factors for squamous cell carcinoma: a case-control study. *Int J Cancer* 1998;76:628–634.
4. Kraemer KH, Lee MM, Andrews AD, et al. The role of sunlight and DNA repair in melanoma and nonmelanoma skin cancer. The xeroderma pigmentosum paradigm. *Arch Dermatol* 1994;130:1018–1021.
5. Bouwes Bavinck JN, Claas FH, Hardie DR, et al. The risk of skin cancer in renal transplant recipients in Queensland, Australia: a follow-up study. *Transplantation* 1996;15:715–721.
6. Johnson TM, Rowe DE, Nelson BR, et al. Squamous cell carcinoma of the skin (excluding lip and oral mucosa). *J Am Acad Dermatol* 1992;26:467–484.
7. Rowe DE, Carroll RJ, Day CL. Prognostic factors for local recurrence, metastasis, and survival rates in squamous cell carcinoma of the skin, ear, and lip. *J Am Acad Dermatol* 1992;26:976–990.
8. Thompson SC, Jolley D, Marks R. Reduction of solar keratoses by regular sunscreen use. *N Engl J Med* 1993;329:1147–1151.
9. Green A, Williams G, Neale R, et al. Daily sunscreen application and betacarotene supplementation in prevention of basal cell and squamous-cell carcinomas of the skin: a randomised controlled trial. *Lancet* 1999;354:723–729.
10. Darlington S, Williams G, Neale R, et al. A randomized controlled trial to assess sunscreen application and beta carotene supplementation in the prevention of solar keratoses. *Arch Dermatol* 2003;139:451–455.
11. Foley P, Nixon R, Marks R, et al. The frequency of reactions to sunscreens: results of a longitudinal population-based study on the regular use of sunscreens in Australia. *Br J Dermatol* 1993;128:512–518.

12. Autier P, Dore JF, Negrier S, et al. Sunscreen use and duration of sun exposure: a double blind randomised trial. *J Natl Cancer Inst* 1999;15:1304–1309.
13. Brodland DG, Zitelli JA. Surgical margins for excision of primary cutaneous squamous cell carcinoma. *J Am Acad Dermatol* 1992;27:241–248.
14. Thomas DJ, King AR, Peat BG. Excision margins for nonmelanotic skin cancer. *Plast Reconstr Surg* 2003;112:57–63.
15. de Visscher JGAM, Botke G, Schakenradd JACM, et al. A comparison of results after radiotherapy and surgery for stage 1 squamous cell carcinoma of the lower lip. *Head Neck* 1999:526–530.
16. Ashby MA, Smith J, Ainslie J, et al. Treatment of nonmelanoma skin cancer at a large Australian Center. *Cancer* 1989;6:1863–1871.
17. Eroglu A, Berberoglu U, Berreroglu S. Risk factors related to locoregional recurrence in squamous cell carcinoma of the skin. *J Surg Oncol* 1996;61:124–130.
18. McCombe D, MacGill, Ainslie J, et al. Squamous cell carcinoma of the lip: a retrospective review of the Peter MacCallum Cancer Institute experience 1979–88. *Aust NZ J Surg* 2000;70:358–361.
19. Yoon M, Chougule P, Dufresne R, et al. Localised carcinoma of the external ear is an unrecognised aggressive disease with a high propensity for local regional recurrence. *Am J Surg* 1992;164:574–577.
20. Zitsch RP, Park CW, Renner GJ, et al. Outcome analysis for lip carcinoma. *Otolaryngol Head Neck Surg* 1995;113:589–596.
21. Glass RL, Perez-Mesa C. Management of inadequately excised epidermoid carcinoma. *Arch Surg* 1974;108:50–51.
22. Glass RL, Spratt JS, Perez-Mesa C. The fate of inadequately excised epidermoid carcinoma of the skin. *Surg Gynaecol Obstet* 1966;122:245–248.
23. Shimm DS, Wilder RB. Radiation therapy for squamous cell carcinoma of the skin. *Am J Clin Oncol* 1991;14:381–386.
24. McCord MW, Mendenhall WM, Parsons JT, et al. Skin cancer of the head and neck with clinical perineural invasion. *Int J Radiat Oncol Biol Phys* 2000;47:89–93.
25. Williams LS, Mancuso AA, Mendenhall WM. Perineural spread of cutaneous squamous and basal cell carcinoma: CT and MR detection and its impact on patient management and prognosis. *Int J Radiat Oncol Biol Phys* 2001;49:1061–1069.
26. Holmkvist KA, Roenigk RK. Squamous cell carcinoma of the lip treated with Mohs' micrographic surgery: outcome at 5 years. *J Am Acad Dermatol* 1998;38:960–966.

Adèle Green
Professor
Queensland Institute of Medical Research
Brisbane
Australia

Robin Marks
Professor
University of Melbourne
Melbourne
Australia

Competing interests: AG is the co-author of reference numbers 2, 4, 9, 10, as listed in proof. RM has undertaken studies in association with 3M Pharmaceuticals on the value of topically applied imiquimod in the management of actinic (solar) keratoses and basal cell carcinoma.

Warts

Search date September 2003

Michael Bigby, Sam Gibbs, Ian Harvey, and Jane Sterling

QUESTIONS

INTERVENTIONS

Key Messages

Treatments

- **Topical treatments containing salicylic acid** One systematic review has found that simple topical treatments containing salicylic acid increase complete wart clearance, successful treatment, or loss of one or more warts after 6–12 weeks compared with placebo. The review identified two RCTs comparing salicylic acid versus cryotherapy. These found no significant difference in the proportion of people with wart clearance at 3–6 months.
- **Cryotherapy** One systematic review of two small RCTs found no significant difference between cryotherapy and placebo or no treatment in the proportion of people with wart clearance after 2–4 months. However, the RCTs may have been too small to detect a clinically important difference. The review identified two RCTs that found no significant difference between cryotherapy and salicylic acid in the proportion of people with wart clearance at 3–6 months. The review found that aggressive cryotherapy increased the proportion of people with wart clearance after 1–3 months compared with gentle cryotherapy.
- **Contact immunotherapy (dinitrochlorobenzene)** One systematic review found that contact immunotherapy using dinitrochlorobenzene increased wart clearance compared with placebo.
- **Carbon dioxide laser** One systematic review identified no RCTs on the effects of carbon dioxide laser.
- **Cimetidine** Three small RCTs provided insufficient evidence to compare cimetidine versus placebo, and one small RCT provided insufficient evidence to compare cimetidine versus local treatments. One small RCT found that cimetidine plus levamisole increased wart clearance at 12 weeks compared with cimetidine alone.
- **Distant healing** One RCT provided insufficient evidence to compare distant healing versus no treatment.

- **Hypnotic suggestion** We found no RCTs on the effects of hypnotic suggestion in the clearance of warts.
- **Inosine pranobex** One RCT provided insufficient evidence about the effects of inosine pranobex on wart clearance.
- **Intralesional bleomycin** RCTs found conflicting evidence on the effects of intralesional bleomycin. Two RCTs found that intralesional bleomycin increased the number of warts cured after 6 weeks compared with placebo. One RCT found no significant difference between bleomycin and placebo in the proportion of people with wart clearance after 30 days, and another RCT found weak evidence that bleomycin cured fewer warts than placebo after 3 months. A fifth RCT found no significant difference between different concentrations of bleomycin in the proportion of warts cured after 3 months.
- **Levamisole** Two RCTs and one CCT provided insufficient evidence on the effects of levamisole compared with placebo on the clearance of warts. One RCT found that levamisole plus cimetidine increased wart clearance at 12 weeks compared with cimetidine alone.
- **Photodynamic treatment** RCTs provided insufficient evidence on the effects of photodynamic treatment on wart clearance.
- **Pulsed dye laser** One RCT provided insufficient evidence on the effects of pulsed dye laser.
- **Surgical procedures** One systematic review identified no RCTs on the effects of surgical procedures on wart clearance.
- **Systemic interferon α** We found no RCTs of sufficient quality on the effects of systemic interferon α.
- **Homeopathy** Two RCTs found no significant difference between homeopathy and placebo in the proportion of people with wart clearance after 8–18 weeks.

DEFINITION Non-genital warts (verrucas) are an extremely common, benign, and usually self limiting skin disease. Infection of epidermal cells with the human papillomavirus results in cell proliferation and a thickened, warty papule on the skin. Any area of skin can be infected, but the most common sites involved are the hands and feet. Genital warts are not covered in this review (see chapter on genital warts, p 2002).

INCIDENCE/PREVALENCE There are few reliable, population based data on the incidence and prevalence of non-genital warts. Prevalence probably varies widely between different age groups, populations, and periods of time. Two large population based studies found prevalence rates of 0.84% in the USA[1] and 12.9% in Russia.[2] Prevalence is highest in children and young adults, and two studies in school populations have shown prevalence rates of 12% in 4–6 year olds in the UK[3] and 24% in 16–18 year olds in Australia.[4]

AETIOLOGY/RISK FACTORS Warts are caused by human papillomavirus, of which there are over 70 different types. They are most common at sites of trauma, such as the hands and feet, and probably result from inoculation of virus into minimally damaged areas of epithelium. Warts on the feet can be acquired from walking barefoot in communal areas where other people walk barefoot. One observational study (146 adolescents) found that the prevalence of warts on the feet was 27% in those that used a communal shower room compared with 1.3% in those that used the locker room.[5] Warts on the hand are also an occupational risk for butchers and meat handlers. One cross-sectional survey (1086 people) found that the prevalence of warts on the hand was 33% in abattoir workers, 34% in retail butchers, 20% in engineering fitters, and 15% in office workers.[6] Immunosuppression is another important risk factor. One observational study in immunosuppressed renal transplant recipients found that at 5 years or longer after transplantation 90% had warts.[7]

PROGNOSIS Non-genital warts in immunocompetent people are harmless and usually resolve spontaneously as a result of natural immunity within months or years. The rate of resolution is highly variable and probably depends on several factors, including host immunity, age, human papillomavirus type, and site of infection. One cohort study (1000 children in long stay accommodation) found that two thirds of warts resolved without treatment within a 2 year period.[8] One systematic review (search date 2000, 17 RCTs) comparing local treatments versus placebo found that about 30% of people using placebo (range 0–73%) had no warts after about 10 weeks (range 4–24 weeks).[9]

AIMS OF INTERVENTION	To eliminate warts, with minimal adverse effects.
OUTCOMES	Wart clearance (generally accepted as complete eradication of warts from the treated area); adverse effects of treatment; recurrence.
METHODS	*Clinical Evidence* search and appraisal September 2003 and hand searches by the contributors. We have reported wart clearance where possible. However, some RCTs reported outcomes such as number of warts cured or loss of single warts. Where RCTs have reported outcomes other than wart clearance this has been highlighted in the text.

QUESTION What are the effects of treatments?

OPTION INTRALESIONAL BLEOMYCIN

Sam Gibbs, Ian Harvey, and Jane Sterling

RCTs found conflicting evidence on the effects of intralesional bleomycin. Two RCTs found that intralesional bleomycin increased the number of warts cured after 6 weeks compared with placebo. One RCT found no significant difference between bleomycin and placebo in the proportion of people with wart clearance after 30 days, and another RCT found weak evidence that bleomycin cured fewer warts than placebo after 3 months. A fifth RCT found no significant difference between different concentrations of bleomycin in the proportion of warts cured after 3 months.

Benefits: We found one systematic review (search date 2000, 5 RCTs, 159 people).[9] The review did not perform a meta-analysis because of trial heterogeneity. **Versus placebo:** Four RCTs (133 people) identified by the review compared intralesional bleomycin versus placebo.[10–13] The first RCT (24 adults with warts unsuccessfully treated for > 3 months) compared bleomycin 0.1% versus saline placebo.[10] Matched pairs of warts on the left and right side of the body were injected with bleomycin or saline. It found that bleomycin significantly increased the proportion of people with a more favourable response (not defined) after 6 weeks compared with placebo (21/24 [88%] with bleomycin *v* 3/24 [13%] with placebo; P < 0.001) and increased the number of warts cured after 6 weeks (34/59 [58%] with bleomycin *v* 6/59 [10%] with placebo; P < 0.001).[10] The second small RCT (16 people) found that bleomycin 0.1% significantly increased the number of warts cured at 6 weeks compared with placebo (31/38 [82%] with bleomycin *v* 16/46 [34%] with placebo; P < 0.001; see comment below).[11] The third RCT (62 adults) compared four groups: bleomycin 0.1% in saline, bleomycin 0.1% in oil, saline placebo, and sesame oil placebo.[12] It found no significant difference between individual groups (P value not reported) but combined results for bleomycin compared with combined results for placebo found significantly fewer warts cured with bleomycin after 3 months (4/22 [18%] with bleomycin in saline *v* 5/22 [23%] with bleomycin in oil *v* 8/19 [42%] with saline placebo *v* 5/11 [46%] with sesame oil placebo; P = 0.018; see comment below). The fourth RCT (31 people), which compared 0.1% bleomycin versus placebo, found no significant difference in the proportion of people with wart clearance after 30 days (15/16 [94%] with bleomycin *v* 11/15 [73%] with placebo; RR 1.28, 95% CI 0.92 to 1.78).[13] **Different concentrations of bleomycin:** The fifth RCT (26 adults) found no significant difference between bleomycin 0.25, 0.5, and 1.0% in the proportion of warts cured after 3 months (11/15 [73%] with 0.25% *v* 26/30 [86%] with 0.5% *v* 25/34 [74%] with 1.0%; P > 0.05; see comment below).[14]

Harms: **Versus placebo:** In the first RCT, one person withdrew because of pain during injection and one withdrew because of pain after injection.[10] The third RCT reported dullness, pain, swelling, or bleeding in 19/62 (31%) of all participants but did not specify which treatment they received.[12] The other RCTs found that pain was experienced by most people (no further data reported).[11,14] In two of the RCTs, local anaesthetic was used routinely before the injection of bleomycin.[11,13] **Different concentrations of bleomycin:** The RCT comparing different concentrations of bleomycin reported pain at the injection site in most people, irrespective of dose (no further data reported).[14]

Comment: The results of two of the RCTs should be interpreted with caution as they randomised people but analysed number of warts cured rather than proportion of people cured.[11,12] In the RCT comparing different concentrations of bleomycin, the disparity in the number of warts assessed in each group could be explained by the exclusion of warts that spontaneously regressed from the analysis, and by a high withdrawal rate in people receiving bleomycin 0.25%.[14]

OPTION CARBON DIOXIDE LASER

Sam Gibbs, Ian Harvey, and Jane Sterling

One systematic review identified no RCTs on the effects of carbon dioxide laser.

Benefits: One systematic review (search date 2000) identified no RCTs.[9]

Harms: We found no RCTs.

Comment: None.

OPTION CIMETIDINE

Michael Bigby

Three small RCTs provided insufficient evidence to compare cimetidine versus placebo, and one small RCT provided insufficient evidence to compare cimetidine versus local treatments. One small RCT found that cimetidine plus levamisole increased wart clearance at 12 weeks compared with cimetidine alone.

Benefits: We found no systematic review. **Versus placebo:** We found three small RCTs.[15–17] The first RCT (39 people aged > 15 years), which compared cimetidine 2400 mg daily versus placebo, found no significant difference in the proportion of people with wart clearance after 12 weeks (5/19 [26%] with cimetidine *v* 1/20 [5%] with placebo; RR 3.14, 95% CI 0.75 to 5.66).[15] The second RCT (54 people), which compared cimetidine (400 mg 3 times daily) versus placebo, found no significant difference in the proportion of people with wart clearance after 12 weeks (10/36 [27%] with cimetidine *v* 4/18 [22%] with placebo; RR 1.3, 95% CI 0.5 to 3.4).[16] The third RCT (70 women and children), which compared cimetidine 25–40 mg/kg versus placebo, found no significant difference in the proportion of people with wart clearance after 3 months (9/35 [26%] with cimetidine *v* 8/35 [23%] with placebo; RR 1.1, 95% CI 0.5 to 2.6).[17] **Versus local treatments:** One small RCT (13 people) compared cimetidine 30–40 mg/kg versus topical treatment (cryotherapy**G**, salicylic acid, and other [not specified]).[18] It found no significant difference between cimetidine and topical treatments in the proportion of people with wart clearance after 8 weeks (2/6 [33%] with cimetidine *v* 3/7 [42%] with topical treatments; RR 0.78, 95% CI 0.19 to 3.21). **Cimetidine plus levamisole:** See benefits of levamisole, p 2156.

Harms: **Versus placebo:** Two of the RCTs, which compared cimetidine versus placebo, found no adverse effects associated with cimetidine.[16,17] The third RCT found no significant difference between cimetidine and placebo in the proportion of people with gastrointestinal symptoms, fatigue, dyspnoea, or hair thinning (5/19 [26%] with cimetidine *v* 5/21 [24%] with placebo).[15] **Versus local treatments:** In the RCT comparing cimetidine with local treatments, 1/6 [17%] people taking cimetidine developed watery, green diarrhoea, and 1/6 [17%] had a rash and abdominal pain.[18] **Cimetidine plus levamisole:** See harms of levamisole, p 2156.

Comment: The RCTs may have been too small to exclude a clinically important difference between treatments.[15–18]

OPTION CRYOTHERAPY

Sam Gibbs, Ian Harvey, and Jane Sterling

One systematic review of two small RCTs found no significant difference between cryotherapy and placebo or no treatment in the proportion of people with wart clearance after 2–4 months. However, the RCTs may have been too small to detect a clinically important difference. The review identified two RCTs that found no significant difference between cryotherapy and salicylic acid in the proportion of people with wart clearance at 3–6 months. The review found that aggressive cryotherapy increased the proportion of people with wart clearance after 1–3 months compared with gentle cryotherapy.

Benefits: We found one systematic review (search date 2000, 13 RCTs, 1389 people).[9] **Versus placebo or no treatment:** The review found no significant difference between cryotherapy**Ⓖ** and topical placebo cream or no treatment in the proportion of people with wart clearance at 2–4 months (2 RCTs, 69 people: 11/31 [35%] with cryotherapy *v* 13/38 [34%] with placebo or no treatment; RR 0.95, 95% CI 0.49 to 1.84).[9] **Versus photodynamic treatment:** One RCT identified by the review (28 adults receiving topical salicylic acid) compared cryotherapy versus four different types of photodynamic treatment**Ⓖ** (3 episodes of white light photodynamic treatment, 1 episode of white light photodynamic treatment, 3 episodes of red light photodynamic treatment, and 3 episodes of blue light photodynamic treatment).[19] It found that cryotherapy reduced the number of warts significantly less than white light or red light photodynamic treatment after 4–6 weeks (20% with cryotherapy *v* 73% with white photodynamic treatment 3 times [$P < 0.01$] *v* 71% with white photodynamic treatment once [P value not reported] *v* 42% with red light photodynamic treatment 3 times [$P = 0.03$]). **Versus salicylic acid:** The review found no significant difference between cryotherapy and salicylic acid in the proportion of people with wart clearance at 3–6 months (2 RCTs, 320 people: 107/165 [65%] with cryotherapy *v* 96/155 [62%] with salicylic acid; RR 1.04, 95% CI 0.88 to 1.22).[9] **Aggressive versus gentle cryotherapy (defined by length of freeze):** Four RCTs (592 adults) identified by the review found that aggressive compared with gentle cryotherapy significantly increased the proportion of people with wart clearance after 1–3 months (159/304 [52%] with aggressive cryotherapy *v* 89/288 [31%] with gentle cryotherapy; RR 1.68, 95% CI 1.37 to 2.06; NNT 5, 95% CI 4 to 7).[9] Definitions of aggressive and gentle differed and some RCTs included warts that were resistant to treatment and others did not. **Interval between freezes:** Three RCTs (313 people) identified by the review found no significant difference between cryotherapy at 2, 3, or 4 weekly intervals in wart clearance at the end of the trial (not specified).[9] **Number of freezes:** One RCT (115 people not cured after 3 months of 3 weekly cryotherapy) identified by the review found no significant difference between no further treatment and prolonging cryotherapy for a further 3 months in the proportion of people with wart clearance (after a total of 6 months: 43% with no further treatment *v* 38% with prolonged cryotherapy; no further data reported to calculate RR).[9]

Harms: **Versus placebo or no treatment:** The review did not report on harms. **Versus photodynamic treatment:** In the RCT comparing cryotherapy versus photodynamic treatment, one person receiving cryotherapy withdrew because of pain.[19] Photodynamic treatment was associated with burning and itching during the first few minutes of treatment and mild discomfort throughout treatment in all people receiving it. **Versus salicylic acid:** The review did not report on harms. **Aggressive versus gentle cryotherapy:** One RCT identified by the review found that aggressive compared with gentle cryotherapy significantly increased pain or blistering (64/100 [64%] with aggressive cryotherapy *v* 44/100 [44%] with gentle cryotherapy; RR 1.44, 95% CI 1.14 to 1.75; NNH 5, 95% CI 3 to 16).[20] Five people withdrew from the aggressive group and one from the gentle group because of pain and blistering. **Interval between freezes:** One RCT identified by the review found that cryotherapy at 1 weekly intervals was associated with pain, blistering, or both in 29% of people; at 2 weekly intervals in 7%; and at 3 weekly intervals in 0% (no further data reported).[21] **Number of freezes:** The review did not report on harms.

Comment: The evidence from available RCTs about cryotherapy is both limited and contradictory. Heterogeneity of study design, methodology, and the populations included make it extremely difficult to draw firm conclusions.[9] For instance, some RCTs identified by the review included all types of warts on the hands and feet in all age groups, whereas others were more selective and simply looked at hand warts, or excluded certain groups such as mosaic plantar warts or warts that were resistant to treatment. Of particular note is the likelihood that wart clinic populations used for these studies might have had different characteristics in different periods of time. For instance, hospital based studies carried out in the 1970s in the UK would have included a higher proportion of people with warts that had never been treated before, which have a greater chance of cure, spontaneous resolution, or both. In the 1980s and 1990s more people with warts were being treated in primary care; consequently, the people included in hospital based RCTs were more likely to have warts that were resistant to treatment, with correspondingly lower cure rates.

OPTION DISTANT HEALING

Michael Bigby

One RCT provided insufficient evidence to compare distant healing versus no treatment.

Benefits: We found no systematic review. One double blind RCT (84 people) compared distant healing**G** (see comment below) versus no treatment.[22] Wart clearance was not reported. It found no significant difference between distant healing and no treatment in proportion of warts at 6 weeks (increase of 0.2 warts with distant healing *v* decrease of 1.1 warts with no treatment; P = 0.25) or in mean change in size of three representative warts.

Harms: The RCT gave no information on adverse effects.[22]

Comment: In the RCT 10 experienced healers located within 150 miles of the area in which participants lived performed distant healing for 6 weeks.[22]

OPTION HOMEOPATHY

Michael Bigby

Two RCTs found no significant difference between homeopathy and placebo in the proportion of people with wart clearance after 8–18 weeks.

Benefits: We found no systematic review but found two RCTs comparing homeopathy versus placebo.[23,24] The first RCT (174 people), which compared homeopathy (Thuya 30CH, antimony crudum 7CH, nitricium acidum 7CH for 6 weeks) versus placebo found no significant difference between groups in the proportion of people with wart clearance after 18 weeks (16/80 [20%] with homeopathy *v* 20/82 [24%] with placebo; ARR +4%, 95% CI –8% to +17%).[23] The second RCT (67 people) found no significant difference between homeopathy (individually selected regimen) and placebo in the proportion of people with wart clearance after 8 weeks (5/34 [15%] with homeopathy *v* 1/33 [3%] with placebo; RR 4.85, 95% CI 0.60 to 39.35).[24]

Harms: The first RCT found no significant difference between homeopathy and placebo in the proportion of people with stomach ache, loose stools, fatigue, and acne (2/86 [2%] with homeopathy *v* 4/88 [5%] with placebo; RR 0.51, 95% CI 0.10 to 2.72).[23] The second RCT gave no information on adverse effects.[24]

Comment: Performing RCTs of homeopathic treatment is difficult because a major principle of homeopathy is to individualise treatment to the overall condition of the person. One RCT overcame this difficulty by allowing practitioners to evaluate all people before randomisation and select homeopathic regimens appropriate to each of their overall conditions.[24] People were then randomised to their individually selected regimen (10 different regimens were used) or to placebo.

OPTION HYPNOTIC SUGGESTION

Michael Bigby

We found no RCTs on the effects of hypnotic suggestion in the clearance of warts.

Benefits: We found no systematic review or RCTs that assessed the effects of hypnotic suggestion on complete wart clearance. We found three RCTs that assessed the effects of hypnotic suggestion on the loss of one single wart (see comment below).[25,26]

Harms: The RCTs of loss of one wart gave no information on adverse effects.[25,26]

Comment: **Versus topical salicylic acid, topical placebo, or no treatment:** Three RCTs, two of which were reported in the same article, assessed the effects of hypnotic suggestion on the loss of one wart.[25,26] The first RCT (40 people) compared four treatments: hypnotic suggestion, topical salicylic acid, topical placebo, and no treatment.[25] People were given a 10 minute hypnotic induction procedure involving inter related suggestions for sleep, drowsiness, and entering hypnosis, followed by a 2 minute suggestion of wart regression imagery repeated again after 30 seconds. People were then awakened and instructed to practice their wart regression imagery twice daily for 6 weeks.[25] It found that hypnotic suggestion significantly increased the proportion of people with loss of one wart at 6 weeks compared with salicylic acid, topical placebo, or no treatment (6/10 [60%] with hypnosis *v* 0/10 [0%] with salicylic acid *v* 1/10 [10%] with topical placebo *v* 3/10 [30%] with no treatment; $P < 0.05$). **Versus sham laser or no treatment:** The second RCT (64 people) compared three treatments: hypnotic suggestion, sham laser, and no treatment.[26] It used the same procedure for hypnotic suggestion as the first RCT, except people were given a 5 minute hypnotic induction.[26] The cold laser placebo group in the RCT received two 4 minute treatments with a simulated laser and were told to count their warts daily and assess whether they experienced any sensations in their warts. It found that hypnosis significantly increased the proportion of people with loss of one wart after 6 weeks compared with no treatment (11/22 [50%] with hypnosis *v* 2/17 [12%] with no treatment; $P < 0.01$). It found that a higher proportion of people treated with hypnosis compared with sham treatment lost at least one wart but the difference was not significant (11/22 [50%] with hypnosis *v* 6/24 [25%] with sham treatment; $P = 0.06$). People who lost warts had significantly more warts at baseline than those who did not lose warts ($P < 0.01$).[26] **Versus hypnotic suggestion plus relaxation or no treatment:** The third RCT (76 people) compared four groups: hypnotic suggestion, hypnotic suggestion plus relaxation, suggestion alone, and no treatment.[26] It used the same hypnotic suggestion as the second RCT. The hypnotic suggestion plus relaxation group received a 5 minute relaxation procedure involving interrelated suggestions for relaxation and comfort instead of the induction procedure, and the suggestion alone group received suggestions for wart regression without the hypnotic induction procedure.[26] It found that hypnotic suggestion significantly increased the proportion of people who lost warts after 6 weeks compared with no treatment (4/19 [21%] with hypnotic suggestion *v* 0/19 [0%] with no treatment; $P < 0.05$). However, it found no significant difference between hypnotic suggestion plus relaxation and no treatment (2/19 [11%] with hypnotic suggestion plus relaxation *v* 0/19 [0%] with no treatment; no further data reported).

OPTION CONTACT IMMUNOTHERAPY

Sam Gibbs, Ian Harvey, and Jane Sterling

One systematic review found that contact immunotherapy using dinitrochlorobenzene increased wart clearance compared with placebo.

Benefits: We found one systematic review (search date 2000, 2 RCTs, 80 people).[9] It found that dinitrochlorobenzene 2% solution followed by 1% solution significantly increased the proportion of people with wart clearance at the end of the trial compared with placebo (32/40 [80%] with dinitrochlorobenzene *v* 15/40 [38%] with placebo; RR 1.88, 95% CI 1.27 to 2.79). The end of trial was 4 months in one RCT and unspecified in the other.[9]

Harms: The systematic review gave no information on adverse effects.[9] One of the RCTs identified by the review found that 6/20 (30%) of people developed an inflammatory reaction to dinitrochlorobenzene 2% solution only after the second application, but that all of these people subsequently experienced significant local irritation with or without blistering when they were treated with dinitrochlorobenzene 1% solution.[27] No-one withdrew from the study.

Comment: None.

OPTION INOSINE PRANOBEX

Michael Bigby

One RCT provided insufficient evidence about the effects of inosine pranobex on wart clearance.

Benefits: We found no systematic review. We found one RCT (50 people aged > 12 years receiving topical salicylic acid and cryotherapy**G**), which compared inosine pranobex (1 g 3 times daily for 1 month) versus placebo.[28] It found no significant difference in the proportion of people with wart clearance at 6 months (9/24 [38%] with inosine pranobex *v* 9/26 [35%] with placebo; RR 1.08, 95% 0.52 to 2.27).[28]

Harms: One person taking inosine pranobex developed a sore throat.[28]

Comment: The RCT could have been too small to exclude a clinically important difference between treatments.

OPTION SYSTEMIC INTERFERON α

Michael Bigby

We found no RCTs of sufficient quality on the effects of systemic interferon α.

Benefits: We found no systematic review and no RCTs of sufficient quality.

Harms: We found no RCTs.

Comment: None.

OPTION LEVAMISOLE

Michael Bigby

Two RCTs and one CCT provided insufficient evidence on the effects of levamisole compared with placebo on clearance of warts. One RCT found that levamisole plus cimetidine increased wart clearance at 12 weeks compared with cimetidine alone.

Benefits: We found no systematic review. **Versus placebo:** We found two RCTs[29,30] and one CCT.[31] The first RCT (60 people), which compared levamisole (150 mg 3 times weekly for 10 weeks) versus placebo, found no significant difference between groups in the proportion of people with wart clearance after 3 months (5/29 [17%] with levamisole *v* 6/31 [19%] with placebo; RR 0.89, 95% CI 0.30 to 2.61).[29] The second RCT (32 people), which compared levamisole (2.5 mg/kg twice weekly) versus placebo, found no significant difference between groups in wart clearance after 8 weeks (7/14 [50%] with levamisole *v* 10/18 [55%] with placebo; RR 0.90, 95% CI 0.46 to 1.75).[30] **Levamisole plus cimetidine:** One RCT (48 people) found that levamisole (150 mg twice weekly) plus cimetidine (30 mg/kg daily divided into 3 doses) versus cimetidine alone 30 mg/kg daily significantly increased the proportion of people with wart clearance at 12 weeks (15/24 [62%] with cimetidine plus levamisole *v* 8/24 [33%] with cimetidine alone; RR 1.78, 95% CI 1.01 to 2.49).[32]

Harms: **Versus placebo:** The RCTs and CCT comparing levamisole versus placebo gave no information on adverse effects.[29–31] **Levamisole plus cimetidine:** In the RCT that compared levamisole plus cimetidine versus cimetidine alone, two people taking levamisole plus cimetidine withdrew because of severe nausea.[32] One person taking levamisole plus cimetidine and one person taking cimetidine alone experienced change in taste and constitutional symptoms (fatigue, weakness, and myalgia).[32]

Comment: The RCTs may have been too small to detect a clinically important difference between treatments.[29,30] One CCT (40 people), which compared levamisole (5 mg/kg for 3 days every 2 weeks) versus placebo, found that levamisole significantly increased the proportion of people with wart clearance after 5 months (12/20 [60%] with levamisole *v* 1/20 [5%] with placebo; RR 12.0, 95% CI 1.7 to 83.8).[31] The lack of randomisation in the CCT means that the results should be interpreted with caution.[31]

OPTION PHOTODYNAMIC TREATMENT

Sam Gibbs, Ian Harvey, and Jane Sterling

RCTs provided insufficient evidence on the effects of photodynamic treatment on wart clearance.

Benefits: We found one systematic review (search date 2000, 4 RCTs, 240 people)[9] and one subsequent RCT.[33] **Versus placebo:** The review could not perform a meta-analysis because of trial heterogeneity; one of the RCTs assessed complete wart clearance, the others assessed proportion of warts cured.[9] The first RCT (52 people) in the review compared proflavine photodynamic treatment**Ⓖ** or neutral red photodynamic treatment versus placebo in a left/right hand design.[34] Matched pairs of warts on the left and right hands were treated with photodynamic treatment or placebo. It found no significant difference between proflavine photodynamic treatment and neutral red photodynamic treatment in the proportion of people with wart clearance after 8 weeks (10/27 [37%] with proflavine photodynamic treatment *v* 10/23 [43%] with neutral red photodynamic treatment; RR 0.85, 95% CI 0.43 to 1.68). In all those who responded to treatment, the warts on the placebo treated side also resolved.[34] The second RCT in the review (45 adults with warts unsuccessfully treated for > 3 months), which compared aminolaevulinic acid photodynamic treatment versus placebo photodynamic treatment, found that aminolaevulinic acid photodynamic treatment significantly increased the proportion of warts cured after 18 weeks (64/114 [56%] with aminolaevulinic acid photodynamic treatment *v* 47/113 [42%] with placebo photodynamic treatment; $P < 0.05$).[35] One subsequent RCT (67 people with warts unsuccessfully treated for > 12 months who had received keratolytic ointment under an occlusive dressing for 7 days) compared aminolaevulinic acid photodynamic treatment three times versus placebo photodynamic treatment.[33] It found that aminolaevulinic acid photodynamic treatment compared with placebo significantly increased the number of warts cured after 4 months (48/64 [75%] with aminolaevulinic acid photodynamic treatment *v* 13/57 [23%] with placebo; $P < 0.01$). **Versus cryotherapy:** The review identified one RCT (see benefits of cryotherapy**Ⓖ**, p 2152). **Versus salicylic acid plus creosote:** One RCT (120 people) identified by the review found no significant difference between methylthioninium chloride (methylene blue)/dimethyl sulfoxide (dimethyl sulphoxide) photodynamic treatment and salicylic acid plus creosote in the proportion of people with wart clearance after 8 weeks (5/65 [8%] with methylthioninium chloride/dimethyl sulfoxide *v* 8/55 [15%] with salicylic acid; RR 0.54, 95% CI 0.19 to 1.55).[36]

Harms: **Versus placebo:** One of the RCTs identified by the review found that aminolaevulinic acid photodynamic treatment significantly increased the risk of painful warts (light–unbearable pain) immediately after treatment compared with placebo.[35] Burning and itching continued for up to 48 hours in some people and 3/30 (10%) withdrew because of pain during treatment. The subsequent RCT found that people receiving aminolaevulinic acid photodynamic treatment experienced a burning sensation or slight pain during treatment, and moderate swelling and mild erythema of the treated area 24 hours after treatment.[33] **Versus cryotherapy:** See harms of cryotherapy, p 2153. **Versus salicylic acid plus creosote:** The RCT did not report on harms.

Comment: Unpublished data from the subsequent RCT showed cure rates at 22 months of 45/64 (71%) with photodynamic treatment compared with 13/57 (23%) with placebo and, using patients as the unit of analysis, 26/34 (76%) with photodynamic treatment versus 13/33 (42%) with placebo. Differences in trial methodology makes it difficult to draw conclusions.[9]

OPTION PULSED DYE LASER

Sam Gibbs, Ian Harvey, and Jane Sterling

One RCT provided insufficient evidence on the effects of pulsed dye laser.

Benefits: We found one systematic review (search date 2000, 1 RCT).[9] The RCT (40 people using daily topical salicylic acid, 194 warts) in the review compared pulsed dye laser versus cryotherapy**G** or cantharidin.[37] All treatments were used at monthly intervals up to a maximum of four times. It found no difference between pulsed dye laser and cryotherapy or cantharidin in complete wart clearance at the end of the study (66% with pulsed dye laser *v* 70% with either cryotherapy or cantharidin). Fifteen of the 35 participants were contacted by telephone at an average of 11 months after treatment. It found no significant difference between pulsed dye laser and cryotherapy or cantharidin in the proportion of these people who had recurrence of at least one wart (3/10 [30%] with pulsed dye laser *v* 2/5 [40%] with either cryotherapy or cantharidin; RR 0.75, 95% CI 0.18 to 3.14).[37]

Harms: The RCT found that no significant adverse events occurred in either treatment group.[37]

Comment: None.

OPTION TOPICAL TREATMENTS CONTAINING SALICYLIC ACID

Sam Gibbs, Ian Harvey, and Jane Sterling

One systematic review found that simple topical treatments containing salicylic acid increased complete wart clearance, successful treatment, or loss of one or more warts after 6–12 weeks compared with placebo. The review identified two RCTs comparing salicylic acid versus cryotherapy. These found no significant difference in the proportion of people with wart clearance at 3–6 months.

Benefits: We found one systematic review (search date 2000, 9 RCTs, 816 people) of topical salicylic acid.[9] **Versus placebo or no treatment:** The review (6 RCTs, 376 people) found that salicylic acid compared with placebo significantly increased the proportion of people with either complete wart clearance, successful treatment (not defined), or loss of one or more warts after 6–12 weeks (144/191 [75%] with salicylic acid *v* 89/185 [48%] with placebo; RR 1.55, 95% CI 1.32 to 1.82; NNT 4, 95% CI 3 to 6) (see comment below). **Versus cryotherapy:** The review identified two RCTs (see benefits of cryotherapy**G**, p 2152). **Salicylic acid plus creosote versus photodynamic treatment:** The review identified one RCT (see benefits of photodynamic treatment**G**, p 2157).

Harms: Some of the RCTs identified by the review found that salicylic acid was associated with minor skin irritation.[9]

Comment: Trial heterogeneity and poor quality of the RCTs included in the review mean that the pooled results should be treated with caution.[9] However, sensitivity analysis found that removal of the two RCTs that did not use complete wart clearance did not significantly alter the results.

OPTION SURGICAL PROCEDURES

Sam Gibbs, Ian Harvey, and Jane Sterling

One systematic review identified no RCTs on the effects of surgical procedures on wart clearance.

Benefits: We found one systematic review (search date 2000), which identified no RCTs.[9]

Harms: We found no evidence.

Comment: None.

GLOSSARY

Contact immunotherapy Contact sensitisers such as dinitrochlorobenzene, diphencyprone, and squaric acid dibutyl ester result in allergic dermatitis, which stimulates an immune reaction in close proximity to the wart.

Cryotherapy A destructive treatment based on the targeted freezing of tissue using liquid nitrogen, dimethyl ether propane, or carbon dioxide snow. Liquid nitrogen achieves the lowest temperatures and is now the most commonly used agent.

Distant healing A flow/channelling/projection of energy between healer and participant at a distance.

Photodynamic treatment Combines the application of a photosensitising substance (usually aminolaevulinic acid) to the wart and subsequent irradiation with wavelengths of light that are absorbed by the photosensitising substance and lead to destruction of the target tissue.

REFERENCES

1. Johnson ML, Roberts J. Skin conditions and related need for medical care among persons 1–74 years. *US Department of Health Education and Welfare Publication* 1978;1660:1–26.
2. Beliaeva TL. The population incidence of warts. *Vestn Dermatol Venerol* 1990;2:55–58.
3. Williams HC, Pottier A, Strachan D. The descriptive epidemiology of warts in British schoolchildren. *Br J Dermatol* 1993;128:504–511.
4. Kilkenny M, Merlin K, Young R, et al. The prevalence of common skin conditions in Australian school students: 1. Common, plane and plantar viral warts. *Br J Dermatol* 1998;138:840–845.
5. Johnson LW. Communal showers and the risk of plantar warts. *J Fam Pract* 1995;40:136–138.
6. Keefe M, al-Ghamdi A, Coggon D, et al. Cutaneous warts in butchers. *Br J Dermatol* 1995;132:166–167.
7. Leigh IM, Glover MT. Skin cancer and warts in immunosuppressed renal transplant recipients. *Recent Results Cancer Res* 1995;139:69–86.
8. Massing AM, Epstein WL. Natural history of warts. *Arch Dermatol* 1963;87:303–310.
9. Gibbs S, Harvey I, Sterling J, et al. Local treatments for cutaneous warts: systematic review. *BMJ* 2002;325:461–464 [see comments]. Search date 2000; primary sources Medline, Embase, Cochrane Controlled Trials Register, hand searches of references, and contact with pharmaceutical companies and experts.
10. Bunney MH, Nolan MW, Buxton PK, et al. The treatment of resistant warts with intralesional bleomycin: a controlled clinical trial. *Br J Dermatol* 1984;111:197–207.
11. Rossi E, Soto JH, Battan J, et al. Intralesional bleomycin in verruca vulgaris. Double-blind study. *Dermatol Rev Mex* 1981;25:158–165.
12. Munkvad M, Genner J, Staberg B, et al. Locally injected bleomycin in the treatment of warts. *Dermatologica* 1983;167:86–89.
13. Perez Alfonzo R, Weiss E, Piquero Martin J. Hypertonic saline solution vs intralesional bleomycin in the treatment of common warts. *Dermatol Venez* 1992;30:176–178.
14. Hayes ME, O'Keefe EJ. Reduced dose of bleomycin in the treatment of recalcitrant warts. *J Am Acad Dermatol* 1986;15:1002–1006.
15. Rogers CJ, Gibney MD, Siegfried EC, et al. Cimetidine therapy for recalcitrant warts in adults: is it any better than placebo? *J Am Acad Dermatol* 1999;41:123–127.
16. Karabulut AA, Sahin S, Eksioglu M. Is cimetidine effective for nongenital warts: a double-blind, placebo-controlled study [letter]. *Arch Dermatol* 1997;133:533–534.
17. Yilmaz E, Alpsoy E, Basaran E. Cimetidine therapy for warts: a placebo-controlled, double-blind study. *J Am Acad Dermatol* 1996;34:1005–1007.
18. Bauman C, Francis JS, Vanderhooft S, et al. Cimetidine therapy for multiple viral warts in children [see comments]. *J Am Acad Dermatol* 1996;35:271–272.
19. Stender IM, Lock-Anderson J, Wulf HC. Recalcitrant hand and foot warts successfully treated with photodynamic therapy with topical 5-aminolaevulinic acid: a pilot study. *Clin Exp Dermatol* 1999;24:154–159.
20. Connolly M, Basmi K, O'Connell M, et al. Cryotherapy of viral warts: a sustained 10-s freeze is more effective than the traditional method. *Br J Dermatol* 2001;145:554–557.
21. Bourke JF, Berth-Jones J, Hutchinson PE. Cryotherapy of common viral warts at intervals of 1, 2 and 3 weeks. *Br J Dermatol* 1995;132:433–436.
22. Harkness EF, Abbot NC, Ernst E. A randomized trial of distant healing for skin warts [see comments]. *Am J Med* 2000;108:448–452.
23. Labrecque M, Audet D, Latulippe LG, et al. Homeopathic treatment of plantar warts [see comments]. *CMAJ* 1992;146:1749–1753.
24. Kainz JT, Kozel G, Haidvogl M, et al. Homoeopathic versus placebo therapy of children with warts on the hands: a randomized, double-blind clinical trial [see comments]. *Dermatology* 1996;193:318–320.
25. Spanos NP, Williams V, Gwynn MI. Effects of hypnotic, placebo, and salicylic acid treatments on wart regression. *Psychosom Med* 1990;52:109–114.

26. Spanos NP, Stenstrom RJ, Johnston JC. Hypnosis, placebo, and suggestion in the treatment of warts. *Psychosom Med* 1988;50:245–260.
27. Rosado-Cancino MA, Ruiz-Maldonado R, Tamayo L, et al. Treatment of multiple and stubborn warts in children with 1-chloro-2,4-dinitrobenzene (DNCB) and placebo. *Dermatol Rev Mex* 1989;33:245–252.
28. Benton EC, Nolan MW, Kemmett D, et al. Trial of inosine pranobex in the management of cutaneous viral warts. *J Dermatol Treat* 1991;1:295–297.
29. Morales-Caballero HG, Ruiz MR, Tamayo L. Levamisole in the treatment of warts (double blind study). *Dermatologia* 1978;22:20–25.
30. Saul A, Sanz R, Gomez M. Treatment of multiple viral warts with levamisole. *Int J Dermatol* 1980;19:342–343.
31. Amer M, Tosson Z, Soliman A, et al. Verrucae treated by levamisole. *Int J Dermatol* 1991;30:738–740.
32. Parsad D, Saini R, Negi KS. Comparison of combination of cimetidine and levamisole with cimetidine alone in the treatment of recalcitrant warts. *Australas J Dermatol* 1999;40:93–95.
33. Fabbrocini G, Di Constanzo MP, Riccardo AM, et al. Photodynamic therapy with topical delta-aminolaevulinic acid for the treatment of plantar warts. *J Photochem Photobiol* 2001;61:30–34.
34. Veien NK, Genner J, Brodthagen H, et al. Photodynamic inactivation of *Verrucae vulgares*. II. *Acta Derm Venereol* 1977;57:445–447.
35. Stender IM, Na R, Fogh H, et al. Photodynamic therapy with 5-aminolaevulinic acid or placebo for recalcitrant foot and hand warts: randomised double-blind trial. *Lancet* 2000;355:963–966.
36. Stahl D, Veien NK, Wulf HC. Photodynamic inactivation of virus warts: a controlled clinical trial. *Clin Exp Dermatol* 1979;4:81–85.
37. Robson KJ, Cunningham NM, Kruzan KL. Pulsed dye laser versus conventional therapy for the treatment of warts: a prospective randomized trial. *J Am Acad Dermatol* 2000;43:275–280.

Michael Bigby
Assistant Professor of Dermatology
Harvard Medical School
Boston, Massachusetts
USA

Sam Gibbs
Consultant Dermatologist
Ipswich Hospital NHS Trust
Ipswich
UK

Ian Harvey
Professor of Epidemiology and Public Health
University of East Anglia
Norwich
UK

Jane Sterling
Honorary Consultant Dermatologist
Addenbrooke's NHS Trust
Cambridge
UK

Competing interests: None declared.

Wrinkles

Search date December 2003

Miny Samuel, Rebecca Brooke, and Christopher Griffiths

QUESTIONS

INTERVENTIONS

Key Messages

Prevention

- **Sunscreens; vitamins C or E (topical)** We found no RCTs on the effects of these interventions in preventing wrinkles.

Treatment

- **Tazarotene (improves fine wrinkles)** Two RCTs in people with moderately photodamaged skin found that tazarotene cream improved fine wrinkling compared with placebo at 24 weeks. One RCT found no significant difference between tazarotene and tretinoin cream in fine wrinkling at 24 weeks.
- **Tretinoin (improves fine wrinkles)** RCTs in people with mild to moderate photodamage found that topical tretinoin applied for up to 12 months improved fine wrinkles compared with vehicle cream but the effect on coarse wrinkles differed among studies. Four RCTs in people with moderate to severe photodamage found that topical tretinoin applied for 6 months improved fine and coarse wrinkles on the face compared with vehicle cream. Common short term adverse effects with tretinoin included itching, burning, and erythema. Skin peeling was the most common persistent adverse effect, which was most frequent and severe at 12–16 weeks. One RCT found no significant difference in fine wrinkling between tretinoin and tazarotene cream at 24 weeks.
- **Isotretinoin** In people with mild to severe photodamage, two RCTs found that isotretinoin cream improved fine and coarse wrinkles after 36 weeks compared with vehicle cream. Severe facial irritation occurred in 5–10% of people using isotretinoin.

- **Carbon dioxide laser** We found no RCTs comparing carbon dioxide laser versus placebo or no treatment. Two small RCTs in women with perioral wrinkles found no significant difference between carbon dioxide laser and dermabrasion in improvement in wrinkles at 4–6 months, but a third RCT found that laser was slightly more effective than dermabrasion in improving wrinkles. Adverse effects were commonly reported. Erythema was reported in all three RCTs, two of which found that erythema was more common with laser than with dermabrasion. Small RCTs provided insufficient evidence about carbon dioxide laser compared with chemical peel, or other laser treatments.
- **Dermabrasion** We found no RCTs comparing dermabrasion versus placebo or no treatment. Two small RCTs in women with perioral wrinkles found no significant difference between dermabrasion and carbon dioxide laser in improvement in wrinkles at 4–6 months, but a third RCT found that dermabrasion was slightly less effective than laser in improving wrinkles. Adverse effects were commonly reported. Erythema was reported in all three RCTs, two of which found that erythema was more common with laser than with dermabrasion.
- **Facelift** We found no RCTs on the effects of facelifts in people with wrinkles.
- **Oral natural cartilage polysaccharides** One RCT found no significant difference between an oral preparation of cartilage polysaccharide and placebo in wrinkle appearance at 3 months. Smaller RCTs found that oral cartilage polysaccharide reduced fine, moderate, or severe wrinkles compared with placebo. However, these studies were small and of limited reliability. We found limited evidence that some preparations may be more effective than others.
- **Retinyl esters** We found no systematic review or RCTs of retinyl esters that evaluated clinical outcomes in people with wrinkles.
- **Vitamin C (topical)** One poor quality RCT found limited evidence that an ascorbic acid formulation applied daily to the face for 3 months improved fine and coarse wrinkles compared with a vehicle cream. Stinging and erythema were common but were not analysed by treatment group. We were unable to draw reliable conclusions from this study because of deficiencies in its methodology.
- **Topical natural cartilage polysaccharides** One small RCT found that a topical commercial preparation of natural cartilage polysaccharide reduced the number of fine and coarse wrinkles at 120 days compared with placebo. However, we were unable to draw reliable conclusions from this study.

DEFINITION Wrinkles, also known as rhytides, are visible creases or folds in the skin. Wrinkles less than 1 mm in width and depth are defined as fine wrinkles and those greater than 1 mm as coarse wrinkles. Most RCTs have studied wrinkles on the face, forearms, and hands.

INCIDENCE/ PREVALENCE We found no information on the incidence of wrinkles alone, only on the incidence of skin photodamage Ⓖ, which includes a spectrum of features such as wrinkles, hyperpigmentation, tactile roughness, and telangiectasia. The incidence of skin disorders associated with ultraviolet light increases with age and develops over several decades. One Australian study (1539 people aged 20–55 years living in Queensland) found moderate to severe photodamage in 72% of men and 47% of women under 30 years of age.[1] Severity of photodamage was significantly greater with increasing age, and was independently associated with solar keratoses ($P < 0.01$) and skin cancer ($P < 0.05$). Wrinkling was more common in people with white skin, especially skin phototypes I and II. One study reported that the incidence of photodamage in European and North American populations with Fitzpatrick skin types I, II, and III Ⓖ is about 80–90%.[2] We found few reports of photodamage in black skin (phototypes V and VI).

AETIOLOGY/ RISK FACTORS Wrinkles may be caused by intrinsic factors (for example, aging, hormonal status, and intercurrent diseases) and by extrinsic factors (for example, exposure to ultraviolet radiation and cigarette smoke). These factors contribute to epidermal thinning, loss of elasticity, skin fragility, and creases and lines in the skin. The severity of photodamage varies with skin type, which includes skin colour and the capacity to tan.[3] One review of five observational studies found that facial wrinkles in men and women were more common in smokers than in non-smokers.[4] It also found that the risk of moderate to severe wrinkles in lifelong smokers was more than twice that in current smokers (RR 2.57, 95% CI 1.83 to 3.06). Oestrogen deficiency may contribute to wrinkles in postmenopausal women.[5]

PROGNOSIS Although wrinkles cannot be considered to be a medical illness requiring intervention, concerns about aging may affect quality of life. Such concerns are likely to be influenced by geographical differences, culture, and personal values. In some cases concerns about physical appearance can lead to difficulties with interpersonal interactions, occupational functioning, and self esteem.[6] In societies in which the aging population is growing and a high value is placed on the maintenance of a youthful appearance, there is a growing preference for interventions that ameliorate the visible signs of aging.

AIMS OF INTERVENTION To prevent skin wrinkling; to improve fine and coarse wrinkling in adults; to minimise adverse effects of treatment; to improve quality of life.

OUTCOMES Physician and patient evaluation of improvement in skin texture that reduces the visibility of wrinkles, and adverse effects of treatment. We excluded RCTs based solely on non-clinical outcomes, such as histological assessment, photography, or optical profilometry. Quality of life was not reported in any trial.

METHODS *Clinical Evidence* search and appraisal December 2003. Most RCTs recruited people with moderate to severe photodamage and wrinkles, rather than people with wrinkles alone.

QUESTION What are the effects of interventions to prevent skin wrinkles?

OPTION SUNSCREENS

We found no RCTs on the effects of sunscreens in preventing wrinkles.

Benefits: We found no systematic review or RCTs.

Harms: We found no RCTs.

Comment: We found two non-systematic reviews that reported the effects of sunscreens on the incidence of photodamage and skin cancer but they did not assess the effect of sunscreens in preventing wrinkles.[7,8]

OPTION VITAMINS (TOPICAL)

We found no RCTs on the effects of topical vitamins C or E on wrinkles.

Benefits: We found no systematic review or RCTs.

Harms: We found no RCTs.

Comment: None.

QUESTION What are the effects of treatments for skin wrinkles?

OPTION VITAMIN C OR E (TOPICAL)

One poor quality RCT found limited evidence that an ascorbic acid formulation applied daily to the face for 3 months improved fine and coarse wrinkling compared with a vehicle cream. Stinging and erythema were common but were not quantified according to treatment. We were unable to draw reliable conclusions from this study because of deficiencies in its methodology.

Benefits: We found no systematic review but found one double blind RCT.[9] The RCT (28 people, age 36–72 years, with mild to moderate photodamage❻, split face design) compared topical ascorbic acid (0.5 mL) in a vehicle cream versus the vehicle cream alone applied once daily for 12 weeks.[9] Only 19 people completed the trial. Participants were assigned randomly to treatments to the left and right sides of the face. Improvement was assessed by investigators with reference to pre-treatment photographs, and graded as "much improved", "improved", "no change", or "worse". Analysis, not by intention to treat, found that significantly more people had improvement in fine and coarse wrinkles with ascorbic acid at 12 weeks (fine wrinkles 16/19 [84%] *v* 3/19 [16%]; P = 0.02; coarse wrinkles 13/19 [68%] *v* 6/19 [32%]; P = 0.01). The RCT also found that significantly more participants reported improvement in wrinkles with ascorbic acid than with vehicle cream (proportion of people reporting wrinkles as being "slightly improved", "improved", or "much improved": 16/19 [84%] *v* 3/19 [16%]; RR 5.33, 95% CI 1.85 to 15.34).

Harms: Adverse effects in the RCT, which were not quantified by treatment given, included stinging in 11 people (55%), erythema in five people (24%), and dry skin in one person (0.05%).[9] Symptoms responded to moisturisation and usually resolved within the first 2 months of treatment.

Comment: The RCT is limited by its small sample size and short duration, and by the high withdrawal rate (9/28 [32%]), which compromises the validity of the results.[9]

OPTION TRETINOIN

RCTs in people with mild to moderate photodamage found that topical tretinoin applied for up to 12 months improved fine wrinkles compared with vehicle cream but the effect on coarse wrinkles differed among studies. Four RCTs in people with moderate to severe photodamage found that topical tretinoin applied for 6 months improved fine and coarse wrinkles on the face compared with vehicle cream. Common short term adverse effects with tretinoin included itching, burning, and erythema. Skin peeling was the most common persistent adverse effect, which was most frequent and severe at 12–16 weeks. One RCT found no significant difference between tretinion and tazarotene cream in fine wrinkling at 24 weeks.

Benefits: We found no systematic review. **Versus vehicle cream:** We found 13 double blind, vehicle controlled RCTs (see table A on web extra).[10–21] Seven of the RCTs included people with mild to moderate photodamage with Fitzpatrick skin types I–III**G**.[11–15,17,18] Four of the RCTs (in 3 published articles) included people with moderate to severe photodamage**G**.[19–21] The remaining two RCTs did not define clearly the extent of photodamage.[10,16] The RCTs compared tretinoin (0.1%, 0.05%, 0.02%, 0.01%, 0.025%, and 0.001%) once daily, three times weekly, or once weekly versus a vehicle cream for 12–48 weeks. All of the RCTs that examined higher strength creams (tretinoin 0.1%, 0.05%, and 0.02%) found that tretinoin significantly improved fine wrinkles compared with vehicle cream in people with mild, moderate, or severe photodamage.[10–21] Two of the three RCTs examining lower strength creams (tretinoin 0.01% and 0.001%) in people with mild to moderate photodamage found a significant reduction in fine wrinkles compared with vehicle cream.[15,18] One RCT found no significant difference between lower strength tretinoin cream and vehicle cream.[17] Assessment of improvement in skin texture by the participants and investigators was consistent although the degree of improvement varied. All four RCTs in people with moderate to severe photodamage found that tretinoin cream 0.02% also improved coarse facial wrinkles at 24 weeks (see table A on web extra).[19–21] The effect on coarse wrinkles in people with mild to moderate photodamage was inconsistent.[11–15,17,18] **Versus tazarotene:** See benefits of tazarotene, p 2166.

Harms: The most common adverse effects reported after the application of tretinoin were dry skin/peeling, which were most frequent and severe after 12–16 weeks and tended to be persistent; and itching, burning/stinging, and erythema, which peaked during the first 2 weeks and decreased with time. One RCT found that erythema and scaling occurred in a significantly greater proportion of people using tretinoin 0.1% than in those using tretinoin 0.025% (16/36 [44%] with 0.1% *v* 5/39 [13%] with 0.025%; RR 3.47, 95% CI 1.41 to 8.49).[19] Two RCTs, described in one report, found that more people reported skin irritation for tretinoin cream versus placebo, but that irritation was generally mild and well tolerated (skin irritation 20% with tretinoin *v* 7% with vehicle in 1 RCT, and 38% with tretinoin *v* 11% with vehicle in the other RCT).[20] Signs and symptoms of skin irritation (erythema, peeling, dryness, burning, or stinging) tended to peak during the first 4 weeks of the trial period. We found individual case reports of congenital defects associated with topical tretinoin used during the first trimester of pregnancy.[22,23] We found one observational study that identified 215 case histories of women who used tretinoin cream for acne during the first trimester of pregnancy and compared them with 430 age matched, non-exposed women who delivered infants at the same hospital.[24] It found no significant difference in the incidence of major congenital disorders (1.9% *v* 2.6%; RR 0.7, 95% CI 0.2 to 2.3). **Versus tazarotene:** See harms of tazarotene, p 2167.

Comment: The RCTs were limited by small sample sizes, short duration, and inconsistencies among investigator and participant assessments.[10–21]

OPTION RETINYL ESTERS

We found no RCTs of retinyl esters that evaluated clinical outcomes in people with wrinkles.

Benefits: We found no systematic review or RCTs that evaluated clinical outcomes.

Harms: We found no RCTs.

Comment: None.

OPTION ISOTRETINOIN

In people with mild to severe photodamage, two RCTs found that isotretinoin cream improved fine and coarse wrinkles after 36 weeks compared with vehicle cream. Severe facial irritation occurred in 5–10% of people using isotretinoin.

Benefits: We found no systematic review. We found two double blind RCTs (see table B on web extra).[25,26] The first RCT (776 people in 17 US centres, aged 20–76 years, with mild to moderate facial photodamage Ⓖ) compared once daily application of isotretinoin 0.05% for 12 weeks followed by 0.1% for another 24 weeks versus vehicle cream for 36 weeks.[25] Assessment of photodamage performed by a physician was graded on a 100 mm visual analogue scale (0 = no change from baseline; +50 mm = improvement; and –50 mm = worse). Photographs taken at baseline were compared with photographs taken after 12, 24, and 36 weeks. Only 613 people (79%) remained in the study at 36 weeks and analysis was not by intention to treat. Physician assessment at 36 weeks found that isotretinoin significantly improved overall skin appearance and fine wrinkles compared with vehicle cream (see table B on web extra). Participant assessment found no significant difference between treatments in overall skin appearance, but found that isotretinoin significantly improved fine wrinkles. Pre-treatment and post-treatment photographs were also assessed by five dermatologists; all found that isotretinoin significantly improved fine wrinkles (see table B on web extra). The second RCT (800 people in 20 European centres, mean age 53.5 years, Fitzpatrick skin types I–IV**G** with moderate to severe facial photodamage, mild to severe photodamage of the forearms and hands) compared isotretinoin 0.1% versus vehicle cream for 36 weeks.[26] The methods employed in the trial were the same as those in the first RCT. Physician and participant assessment at 36 weeks found that isotretinoin significantly improved overall appearance, fine and coarse wrinkles of the face, and fine wrinkles of the forearms and hands compared with vehicle cream (see table B on web extra). Panel assessment found similar results but did not assess the significance of the difference between groups.

Harms: The first RCT reported that severe intolerability reactions, which were unspecified, occurred in "less than 5% of people" taking isotretinoin.[25] More people using isotretinoin withdrew from the study because of local irritation (5 with isotretinoin *v* 1 with vehicle). The second RCT found that facial symptoms were more common in people using isotretinoin than in those using vehicle cream (erythema 65% with isotretinoin *v* 26% with vehicle, peeling 54% *v* 8%, burning 64% *v* 16%, and pruritus 45% *v* 13%).[26] Severe facial irritation occurred in 5–10% of people, causing 3.6% of people to discontinue treatment. Irritation usually occurred during the first few weeks of treatment and was alleviated by emollients or brief interruption of treatment.

Comment: None.

OPTION TAZAROTENE

Two RCTs in people with moderately photodamaged skin found that tazarotene cream improved fine wrinkling compared with placebo at 24 weeks. One RCT found no significant difference between tazarotene cream and tretinoin cream in fine wrinkling at 24 weeks.

Benefits: We found no systematic review but found two RCTs.[27,28] The first RCT (349 men and women aged ≥ 18 years with Fitzpatrick skin types I–IV**G**) compared three interventions: tazarotene (0.1%, 0.05%, 0.025%, and 0.01%), placebo cream, and tretinoin (0.05%) applied once daily for 24 weeks.[27] Investigators and participants were not blinded to treatment allocation, but a blinded investigator assessed outcomes. The second RCT (563 men and women aged 18 years or older with Fitzpatrick skin types I–IV, double blind) compared tazarotene 0.1% versus placebo cream applied once daily for 24 weeks.[28] **Versus vehicle cream:** The first RCT found a significant improvement for all concentrations of tazarotene (0.1%, 0.05%, 0.025%, and 0.01%) in fine wrinkling at 24 weeks compared with placebo (proportion of people improved at least 1 grade on a 6 point scale for fine wrinkling, results presented graphically: about 40% for 0.025% tazarotene, about 45% for 0.01% tazarotene, and about 55% for 0.05% and 0.1% tazarotene *v* 18% for placebo; $P < 0.05$).[27] The second RCT found that tazarotene was significantly more effective than placebo in improving both fine and coarse wrinkling after 24 weeks (proportion of people improved at least 1 grade on a 5 point scale for both fine and coarse wrinkling at 24 weeks, results presented graphically: fine wrinkling about 42% with tazarotene *v* about 18% with placebo, $P < 0.001$; coarse wrinkling about 15% with tazarotene 0.1% *v* about 8% with placebo, $P < 0.001$).[28] **Versus tretinoin:** The first RCT found no significant difference in fine wrinkling assessed monthly for 24 weeks between tretinoin and any concentration of tazarotene (proportion of people improved at least 1 grade on a 6 point scale for fine wrinkling at 24 weeks, results presented graphically: about 58% for tretinoin *v* about 40–55% for tazarotene; P value not reported).[27]

Harms: Adverse events were reported by most people in the first RCT (249/349 [71.3%]).[27] Most were considered to be treatment related. The most frequent adverse events were signs and symptoms of local skin irritation, such as mild to moderate desquamation, burning sensation, erythema, pruritus, and dry skin. "Severe" treatment related adverse events were reported by fewer than 3% of people in the 0.1%, 0.05%, and 0.01% tazarotene groups and by 5% in the tretinoin 0.05% group. In the second RCT adverse events were reported mainly during the first 2 weeks of treatment.[28] The main adverse events were desquamation (105/283 [37%] with tazarotene *v* 8/280 [3%] with placebo), erythema (84/283 [30%] with tazarotene *v* 6/280 [2%] with placebo), and burning (82/283 [29%] with tazarotene *v* 1/280 [0.4%] with placebo).

Comment: None.

OPTION TOPICAL NATURAL CARTILAGE POLYSACCHARIDES

One small RCT found that a topical preparation of cartilage polysaccharide reduced fine and coarse wrinkles at 120 days compared with placebo. However, we were unable to draw reliable conclusions from this study.

Benefits: We found no systematic review. **Versus placebo:** We found one double blind RCT (30 women, aged 40–60 years, with moderate to severe facial wrinkles) comparing a topical 1% cartilage polysaccharide twice daily for 120 days on one side of the face versus placebo on the other.[29] It found that active treatment significantly increased the proportion of women with no shallow (< 1 mm), moderate (1 mm), or deep (> 1 mm) wrinkles after 120 days (treatment *v* placebo: no shallow wrinkles 30/30 *v* 0/30; no moderate wrinkles 27/30 *v* 0/30; no deep wrinkles 5/30 *v* 2/30; overall $P < 0.001$). The clinical importance of these results is unclear (see comment below).

Harms: No adverse effects were reported by any of the participants in the RCT.[29]

Comment: The RCT is limited by its small sample size and by potential difficulties with concealment of allocation.[29] Application of creams to each side of the face may result in contamination (one side receiving treatment intended for the other side).

OPTION ORAL NATURAL CARTILAGE POLYSACCHARIDES

One RCT found no significant difference between an oral preparation of cartilage polysaccharide and placebo in wrinkle appearance at 3 months. Smaller RCTs found that oral cartilage polysaccharide reduced fine, moderate, or severe wrinkles compared with placebo. However, these studies were small and of limited reliability. We found limited evidence that some preparations may be more effective than others.

Benefits: We found no systematic review. **Versus placebo:** We found three RCTs.[30–32] The first, a double blind RCT (144 people, aged 35–50 years, with Fitzpatrick skin type II or III and mild to moderate photoaging**G**), compared a commercial preparation of a cartilage polysaccharide (Imedeen® 400 or 200 mg/day) versus placebo for 3 months.[30] It found no significant difference between either dose of active treatment and placebo in face or eye wrinkles at 3 months, as assessed by investigator or subject analyses on a 10 cm visual analogue scale and by assessment of photographs by a dermatologist (reported as non-significant, CI not reported). The second, also a double blind RCT, (30 women, aged 40–60 years, with moderate to severe wrinkles) compared a different commercial oral cartilage polysaccharide preparation (Vivida® 500 mg/day) versus placebo for 90 days.[31] Assessment of wrinkles was measured by the investigator on a three point scale (0 = absent; 1 = moderate; 2 = severe). The RCT found that treatment significantly reduced the proportion of women with moderate or severe wrinkles at 45 days (overall $P < 0.01$) and at 90 days ($P < 0.001$) compared with placebo. The third RCT (30 women, aged 35–60 years, with Fitzpatrick skin types II or III and mild to moderate wrinkles) compared a preparation of 750 mg marine fish cartilage with antioxidant mix (*Ginkgo biloba*, flavonoids, *Centella asiatica*) taken daily versus placebo (soybean oil) for 8 weeks (see comment below).[32] A trained investigator assessed clinical outcome on a 0–9 scale (0 = no signs; 9 = severe signs; based on assessment of dryness, pigmentation, skin tone, and fine superficial wrinkles). It was not clear whether results were directly compared between groups. However, the RCT reported that, at 8 weeks, treatment significantly improved superficial fine wrinkles from baseline whereas placebo did not (results presented graphically: wrinkle score 5.5 at baseline and 4.5 at 8 weeks with treatment; 5.4 at baseline and 5.1 at 8 weeks with placebo). **Versus each other:** We found one double blind RCT (30 women, aged 40–60 years, with moderate to severe wrinkles) comparing two commercial preparations.[33] Participants were given Vivida® 500 mg or Imedeen® 380 mg daily for 90 days. At 90 days, the RCT found that Vivida® significantly increased the proportion of women with no wrinkles (10/15 [66%] *v* 3/15 [20%]) and reduced the proportion of women with severe wrinkles (0/15 [0%] *v* 7/15 [47%]; overall $P < 0.01$) compared with Imedeen®. It found no significant difference in the proportion of women with moderate wrinkles (5/15 [33%] *v* 5/15 [33%]; RR 1.0, 95% CI 0.4 to 2.7).

Harms: **Versus placebo:** The first RCT found no significant difference between Imedeen® and placebo in adverse effects (23/96 [24%] *v* 10/48 [21%]; $P > 0.05$).[30] Acne and seborrhoea were the most common skin related events (24/38 [63%]) and oedema and weight increase were the most frequently reported non-skin related events (18/47 [38%]), but the proportions attributable to active treatment or placebo were not specified. The second RCT reported that "some" people taking Vivida® developed mild pimples during the first 3–4 weeks.[31] The third RCT reported that some people experienced epigastric discomfort (numbers or treatment arm not reported), but no other adverse effects were reported.[32] **Versus each other:** In the RCT, 33% of people using Vivida® had mild facial pimples during the first 3–4 weeks compared with no adverse effects in the Imedeen® group.[33]

Comment: In the RCT of Vivida® versus placebo, the grading of wrinkling is unusual in that wrinkles were graded as severe, moderate, or absent, without a grading of "mild".[31] One might have expected that wrinkles would have reduced from moderate/severe to mild rather than to absent. The RCTs are small, and the possibility of publication bias cannot be excluded. It is not clear whether the RCT of marine fish cartilage with antioxidant was blinded.[32] The available evidence is inadequate to assess accurately the effects of oral cartilage preparations.

OPTION DERMABRASION

We found no RCTs comparing dermabrasion versus placebo or no treatment in people with wrinkles. Two small RCTs in women with perioral wrinkles found no significant difference between dermabrasion and carbon dioxide laser in

improvement in wrinkles at 4–6 months, but a third RCT found that dermabrasion was slightly less effective than laser in improving wrinkles. Adverse effects were commonly reported. Erythema was reported in all three RCTs, two of which found that erythema was more common with laser than with dermabrasion.

Benefits: **Versus placebo/control:** We found no RCTs. **Versus carbon dioxide (CO_2) laser:** We found three RCTs comparing dermabrasion versus a CO_2 laser.[34–36] The first RCT (20 women, 48–76 years old with moderate/severe wrinkles of the upper lip, Fitzpatrick skin types I–III**Ⓖ**) compared dermabrasion with a coarse diamond fraize versus CO_2 laser to the left or right upper lip (see comment below).[34] Upper lip wrinkles were graded as 0 (none) to 5 (severe) by an independent investigator both before treatment and 6 months later. The average pretreatment wrinkle score was 4.3 for the laser side and 4.4 for the dermabrasion side. The RCT found no significant difference in wrinkle score between treatments at 6 months (areas retaining wrinkle score of 4/5: 1/19 [5%] with dermabrasion *v* 2/19 [11%] with laser; P = 0.22). The second RCT (15 women, 46–73 years old with perioral wrinkles, Fitzpatrick skin types I–III) compared dermabrasion versus a CO_2 laser to the left and right sides of the perioral area.[35] The mean pretreatment wrinkle score on both sides of the perioral area was 3.73 (1 = mild; 5 = severe). Investigators and participants were not blinded to treatment allocation, but two independent blinded laboratory assistants familiar with laser resurfacing assessed outcomes. The RCT found no significant difference in mean post-treatment wrinkle score at 4 months, as assessed by the investigator (2.64 with laser *v* 2.79 with dermabrasion; P = 0.35). The third RCT (20 women, 44–74 years old with perioral wrinkles, moderate to severe photodamage**Ⓖ**, Fitzpatrick skin type not specified) compared dermabrasion versus a CO_2 laser to the left or right sides of the perioral area.[36] Photographs of participants assessed by plastic surgeons were graded in terms of improvement in wrinkles (0 = no improvement to 5 = best improvement) at 1 and 6 months after treatment. Investigators and participants were not blinded to treatment allocation, but the panel of plastic surgeons who assessed outcomes were blinded. The RCT found that, compared with dermabrasion, laser significantly improved the wrinkle score at 1 month (2.33 *v* 2.01; P = 0.002) and at 6 months (2.55 *v* 2.22; P = 0.016). The RCT also found that significantly more women reported a greater improvement in wrinkles with laser than with dermabrasion at 6 months (13/20 [65%] *v* 3/20 [15%]; P = 0.001; 4 women reported no difference).[36]

Harms: **Versus carbon dioxide (CO_2) laser:** In the first RCT, 85% of women had erythema on the upper lip, which was similar on sides of the face treated with CO_2 laser and dermabrasion 1 month after treatment.[34] In 10% of people the erythema was worse on the laser treated side, and in 5% it was worse on the dermabraded side. The average duration of erythema was 2.5 months for both treatments. One woman developed a hypertrophic scar on the dermabraded side. Three people developed herpetic lesions several days after treatment, despite valaciclovir prophylaxis. Other complications such as pain, oedema, eczema, and whiteheads resolved either spontaneously or with minimal treatment. The second RCT found that erythema was significantly increased on the laser side compared with the dermabrasion side at 1 month (P = 0.003) but not at 4 months (P = 0.15).[35] The third RCT found that laser significantly increased erythema at 1 month compared with dermabrasion (P < 0.001).[36] Also, significantly more people reported that "post-treatment drainage" was worse with laser than with dermabrasion (10/20 [50%] *v* 2/20 [10%]; P = 0.002).

Comment: The RCTs found inconsistent results, were small, and may not have been powered to detect a significant difference between treatments.[34–36] It is not clear whether the first RCT was blinded.[34] The RCTs varied in their grading of wrinkles, and in participant and investigator assessments. The available evidence is insufficient to define the effects of dermabrasion for wrinkles.

OPTION CARBON DIOXIDE LASER

We found no RCTs comparing carbon dioxide laser versus placebo or no treatment in people with wrinkles. Two small RCTs in women with perioral wrinkles found no significant difference between carbon dioxide laser and dermabrasion in improvement in wrinkles at 4–6 months, but a third RCT found that laser was slightly more effective than dermabrasion in improving wrinkles. Adverse effects were commonly reported. Erythema was reported in all three RCTs, two of which found that erythema was more common with laser than with dermabrasion. Small RCTs provided insufficient evidence about carbon dioxide laser compared with chemical peel, or other laser treatments.

Benefits: We found no systematic review. **Versus placebo/no treatment:** We found no RCTs. **Versus dermabrasion:** See benefits of dermabrasion, p 2169. **Versus chemical peel:** We found two RCTs.[37] The first RCT (20 women, aged 51–71 years, with upper lip wrinkles, Fitzpatrick skin types I–III**G**, double blind) compared a carbon dioxide (CO_2) laser versus a phenol chemical peel.[37] At the start of the RCT, photographs of each participant were graded by an independent investigator in terms of the severity of upper lip wrinkles (0 = none; 5 = severe). Participants were then randomly assigned to receive laser treatment on one side of the upper lip and chemical peel on the other. The RCT found that CO_2 laser was less effective than chemical peel at 6 months (wrinkle score reduced from 4.30 to 1.11 with laser *v* 4.20 to 0.47 with chemical peel; mean difference in post-treatment score 0.54; $P < 0.03$; see comment below). The second RCT (24 men and women, aged 43–73 years, with Fitzpatrick skin types I–III) compared CO_2 laser versus trichloroacetic acid chemical peel applied to opposite sides of the face.[38] Investigators and participants were not blinded to treatment allocation, but an independent blinded investigator assessed outcomes. The RCT found that CO_2 laser was more effective than chemical peel for reducing severity of periorbital wrinkles after 6 months (severity assessed on a 5 point scale [0 = none; 5 = severe]: score improved from 4.00 to 1.75 with laser treatment *v* from 4.13 to 3.29 with chemical peel; $P < 0.001$). **Versus erbium:YAG laser:** We found three RCTs.[39–41] The first RCT (21 women, aged 39–74 years, with upper lip wrinkles, Fitzpatrick skin types I–IV) compared variable pulse erbium:YAG laser**G** versus CO_2 laser to the left or right sides of the upper lip.[39] Photographs and digital images of participants were recorded preoperatively and at intervals up to 2 months after treatment. Investigators and participants were not blinded to treatment allocation, but a blinded panel of plastic surgeons and trained research assistants assessed outcomes. The RCT found that there was a greater overall improvement (which was not defined) in wrinkles with CO_2 laser than with erbium:YAG laser (improvement: 63% *v* 54%; P value not reported). The second RCT (13 people [12 women] aged 30–80 years, with perioral or periorbital wrinkles, Fitzpatrick skin types I–III) compared treatment with one pass pulsed CO_2 laser versus four passes erbium:YAG laser to periorbital or perioral sites or both.[40] Each participant received CO_2 laser on one side of the face and erbium:YAG laser on the other by random allocation. Wrinkles were graded from 0 (absent) to 8 (severe) based on photographs. Investigators and participants were not blinded to treatment allocation, but a blinded panel of physicians familiar with laser resurfacing assessed outcomes. The RCT found no significant difference between treatments for wrinkle improvement (time to outcome not stated; average improvement in wrinkle scores from baseline about 1–2 points in both groups; difference reported as non-significant, P value not reported). However, it may have been too small to exclude a clinically important difference. The third RCT (21 people [19 women] aged 18–90 years, with perioral or periorbital wrinkles, Fitzpatrick skin types I–III) compared variable pulse erbium:YAG laser versus CO_2 laser to the left or right sides of the face by alternate allocation.[41] Photographs of participants were taken preoperatively and at 1 week, 2 weeks, 2 months, and 6 months. Investigators and participants were not blinded to treatment allocation, but a blinded panel of dermatologists also assessed outcomes. The RCT found that CO_2 laser improved wrinkles significantly more than erbium:YAG laser at 6 months (measured by aggregate of investigators', participants', and panel's assessments; $P < 0.03$; further data not reported; see comment below). **Versus CO_2 laser plus variable pulse erbium:YAG laser:** We found one double blind RCT.[42] The RCT (20 people, aged 42–72 years with upper lip wrinkles, Fitzpatrick skin types I–III) compared CO_2 laser versus CO_2 laser plus variable pulse erbium:YAG laser to right or left sides of the upper lip. Photographs recorded before treatment and at intervals after treatment for up to 4 months were graded by investigators, but no details of grading were provided. The RCT found no significant difference in improvement in perioral wrinkles at 4 months (67.5% with laser alone *v* 68.5% with combination; P value not reported).

Harms: **Versus dermabrasion:** See harms of dermabrasion, p 2169.**Versus chemical peel:** The first RCT found that 55% of people had erythema and/or coagulum on the upper lip; in 35% of people this was more severe on the chemical peel side, and in 10% it was more severe on the laser treated side.[37] One person developed an 8 mm hypertrophic scar on the phenol treated side. Herpes simplex infection was reported in three people, which responded to valaciclovir (treatment side not reported). The second RCT found that the erythema lasted for a mean of 4.5 months after laser treatment and 2.5 months after chemical peel.[38] Scarring developed in 13/24 (52%) people with laser treatment and 3/24 (12.5%) with chemical peel. All scars improved or resolved after treatment with topical silicone paste or intralesional steroids. Contact dermatitis to bacitracin–polymyxin B ointment occurred in four participants. This resolved after switching topical therapy to petrolatum and a low potency topical steroid. Hypopigmentation developed in 6/24 (25%) participants in the CO_2 laser treated arm but resolved or improved by the end of the study (no other data given). Whitehead formation was also relatively common during the prolonged healing phase but resolved or improved with tretinoin or manual extraction (no data reported). **Versus erbium:YAG laser:** In the first RCT postoperative erythema occurred with both treatments, but there was no significant difference (P value not reported).[39] Only one person was reported to have mild hyperpigmentation at around 4 weeks after treatment with erbium:YAG laser, which had cleared by 3 months. The second RCT found that postoperative erythema was significantly less frequent with CO_2 laser than with erbium:YAG laser at 2 weeks ($P < 0.04$) but rates were similar at 2 and 6 months.[40] The RCT found no significant difference between treatments for rates of hyperpigmentation. The third RCT found that both treatments were associated with erythema (at 2 weeks AR 67% with erbium:YAG laser *v* 95% with CO_2 laser; at 2 months AR 24% with erbium:YAG laser *v* 62% with CO_2 laser; at 6 months AR for mild erythema 0% with erbium:YAG laser *v* 10% with CO_2 laser).[41] Hypopigmentation (5% with erbium:YAG laser *v* 43% with CO_2 laser; $P < 0.05$) and hyperpigmentation (24% with erbium:YAG laser *v* 29% with CO_2 laser) were seen. Hyperpigmentation resolved spontaneously in all cases within 6 months but hypopigmentation was still visible. **Versus CO_2 laser plus variable pulse erbium:YAG laser:** One RCT reported no significant difference between treatments in erythema or pain (reported as non-significant, absolute results presented graphically).[42]

Comment: The effects of chemical peels and CO_2 lasers are likely to be dependent on the expertise of the dermatological surgeon, and therefore results may not generalise to different populations.[37] The difference in outcomes was not expressed dichotomously, and the clinical importance of the mean "0.54 units" difference in wrinkle score with CO_2 laser compared with chemical peel is difficult to interpret. The available evidence is too weak to define the effects of CO_2 laser on wrinkles.[37] The results of the third RCT comparing CO_2 versus erbium:YAG laser should be interpreted with caution because the participants and investigators were not blinded to treatment allocation.[41]

OPTION FACELIFT

We found no RCTs on the effects of facelifts in people with wrinkles.

Benefits: We found no systematic review and no RCTs.

Harms: We found no RCTs.

Comment: The effectiveness and safety of facelift surgery is likely to depend on the expertise of the surgeon.

GLOSSARY

Erbium:YAG laser An yttrium aluminium garnet laser.

Fitzpatrick skin phototype classification I = always burns easily, never tans; II = always burns easily, tans minimally; III = burns moderately, tans gradually (light brown); IV = burns minimally, always tans well (brown); V = rarely burns, tans profusely (dark brown); VI = never burns, deeply pigmented (black).

Mild/moderate/severe photodamage A spectrum of features including wrinkles, hyperpigmentation, tactile roughness, and telangiectasia. Usually measured on a scale from 0–9 (0 = none; 1–3 = mild; 4–6 = moderate; and 7–9 = severe).

REFERENCES

1. Green AC. Premature ageing of the skin in a Queensland population. *Clin Exp Dermatol* 1991;155:473–478.
2. Maddin S, Lauharanta J, Agache P, et al. Isotretinoin improves the appearance of photodamaged skin: results of a 36-week, multicenter, double-blind, placebo-controlled trial. *J Am Acad Dermatol* 2000;42:56–63.
3. Nagashima H, Hanada K, Hashimoto I. Correlation of skin phototype with facial wrinkle formation. *Photodermatol Photoimmunol Photomed* 1999;15:2–6.
4. Grady D, Ernster V. Does cigarette smoking make you ugly and old? *Am J Epidemiol* 1992;135:839–842.
5. Affinito P, Palomba S, Sorrentino C, et al. Effects of postmenopausal hypoestrogenism on skin collagen. *Maturitas* 1999;15:239–247.
6. Gupta MA, Gupta AK. Photodamaged skin and quality of life: reasons for therapy. *J Dermatol Treat* 1996;7:261–264.
7. Alsarraaf R. Outcomes research in facial plastic surgery: a review and new directions. *Aesthetic Plast Surg* 2000;24:192–197.
8. Boyd AS, Naylor M, Cameron GS, et al. The effects of chronic sunscreen use on the histologic changes of dermatoheliosis. *J Am Acad Dermatol* 1995;33:941–946.
9. Traikovich SS. Use of topical ascorbic acid and its effects on photodamaged skin topography. *Arch Otolaryngol Head Neck Surg* 1999;125:1091–1098.
10. Weiss JS, Ellis CN, Headington JT, et al. Topical tretinoin improves photoaged skin. *JAMA* 1988;259:527–532.
11. Leyden JJ, Grove GL, Grove MJ, et al. Treatment of photodamaged facial skin with topical tretinoin. *J Am Acad Dermatol* 1989;21:638–644.
12. Lever L, Kumar P, Marks R. Topical retinoic acid for treatment of solar damage. *Br J Dermatol* 1990; 122:91–98.
13. Barel AO, Delune M, Clarys P, et al. Treatment of photodamaged facial skin with topical tretinoin: a blinded, vehicle-controlled half-side study. *Nouv Dermatol* 1995;14:585–591.
14. Lowe PM, Woods J, Lewis A, et al. Topical tretinoin improves the appearance of photo damaged skin. *Australas J Dermatol* 1994;35:1–9.
15. Weinstein GD, Nigra TP, Pochi PE, et al. Topical tretinoin for treatment of photodamaged skin. *Arch Dermatol* 1991;127:659–665.
16. Salagnac V, Leonard F, Lacharriere Y, et al. Topical treatment of actinic aging with vitamin A acid at various concentrations. *Rev Fr Gynecol Obstet* 1991;86:458–460.
17. Olsen EA, Katz HI, Levine N, et al. Tretinoin emollient cream: a new therapy for photodamaged skin. *J Am Acad Dermatol* 1992;26:215–224.
18. Andreano J, Bergfeld WF, Medendorp SV. Tretinoin emollient cream 0.01% for the treatment of photoaged skin. *Cleve Clin J Med* 1993;60:49–55.
19. Griffiths CEM, Kang S, Ellis CN, et al. Two concentrations of topical tretinoin (retinoic acid)

cause similar improvement of photoaging but different degrees of irritation. *Arch Dermatol* 1995;131:1037–1044.
20. Nyirady J, Bergfeld W, Ellis C, et al. Tretinoin cream 0.02% for the treatment of photodamaged facial skin: A review of 2 double-blind clinical studies. *Cutis* 2001;68:135–143.
21. Nyirady J, Gisslen H, Lehmann P et al. Safety and efficacy of long-term use of tretinoin cream 0.02% for treatment of photodamage: Review of clinical trials. *Cosmet Dermatol* 2003;3:49–57.
22. Lipson AH, Collins F, Webster WS. Multiple congenital defects associated with maternal use of topical tretinoin. *Lancet* 1993;341:1352–1353.
23. Camera G, Pregliasco P. Ear malformation in baby born to mother using tretinoin cream. *Lancet* 1992;339:687.
24. Jick SS, Terris BZ, Jick H. First trimester topical tretinoin and congenital disorders. *Lancet* 1993;341:1181–1182.
25. Sendagorta E, Lesiewicz J, Armstrong RB. Topical isotretinoin for photodamaged skin. *J Am Acad Dermatol* 1992;27:S15–S18.
26. Maddin S, Lauharanta J, Agache P, et al. Isotretinoin improves the appearance of photodamaged skin: results of a 36-week, multicenter, double blind, placebo-controlled trial. *J Am Acad Dermatol* 2000;42:56–63.
27. Kang S, Leyden JJ, Lowe NJ, et al. Tazarotene cream for the treatment of facial photodamage. *Arch Dermatol* 2001;137:1597–1604.
28. Phillips TJ, Gottlieb AB, Leyden JJ, et al. Efficacy of 0.1% tazarotene cream for the treatment of photodamage. *Arch Dermatol* 2002;138:1486–1493.
29. Lassus A, Eskelinen A, Santalahti J. The effect of Vivida® cream as compared with placebo cream in the treatment of sun-damaged or age-damaged facial skin. *J Int Med Res* 1992;20:381–391.
30. Kieffer ME, Efsen J. Imedeen® in the treatment of photoaged skin: an efficacy and safety trial over 12 months. *J Eur Acad Dermatol Venereol* 1998;11:129–136.
31. Eskelinen A, Santalahti J. Special natural cartilage polysaccharides for the treatment of sun-damaged skin in females. *J Int Med Res* 1992;20:99–105.
32. Distante F, Scalise F, Rona C, et al. Oral fish cartilage polysaccharides in the treatment of photoageing: biophysical findings. *Int J Cosmet Sci* 2002;24:81–87.
33. Eskelinen A, Santalahti J. Natural cartilage polysaccharides for the treatment of sun-damaged skin in females: a double-blind comparison of Vivida® and Imedeen®. *J Int Med Res* 1992; 20:227–233.
34. Gin I, Chew J, Rau KA, et al. Treatment of upper lip wrinkles: a comparison of the 950 μsec dwell time carbon dioxide laser to manual tumescent dermabrasion. *Dermatol Surg* 1999;25:468–474.
35. Holmkvist KA, Rogers GS. Treatment of perioral rhytides. *Arch Dermatol* 2000;136:725–731.
36. Kitzmiller WJ, Visscher M, Page DA, et al. A controlled evaluation of dermabrasion versus CO_2 laser resurfacing for the treatment of perioral wrinkles. *Plast Reconstr Surg* 2000;106:1366–1372.
37. Chew J, Gin I, Rau KA, et al. Treatment of upper lip wrinkles: a comparison of 950 μsec dwell time carbon dioxide laser with unoccluded baker's phenol chemical peel. *Dermatol Surg* 1999; 25:262–266.
38. Reed JT, Joseph AK, Bridenstine JB. Treatment of periorbital wrinkles. *Dermatol Surg* 1997;23:643–648.
39. Newman JB, Lord JL, Ash K, et al. Variable pulse erbium:YAG laser skin resurfacing of perioral rhytides and side-by-side comparison with carbon dioxide laser. *Lasers Surg Med* 2000;26:208–214.
40. Ross EV, Miller C, Meehan K, et al. One-pass CO_2 versus multiple-pass Er:YAG laser resurfacing in the treatment of rhytides: a comparison side-by-side study of pulsed CO_2 and Er:YAG lasers. *Dermatol Surg 2001;27:709–715.*
41. Khatri KA, Ross V, Grevelink LM, et al. Comparison of Erbium:YAG and carbon dioxide lasers in resurfacing of facial rhytides. *Arch Dermatol* 1999;135:391–397.
42. McDaniel DH, Lord J, Ash K, et al. Combined CO_2/Erbium:YAG laser resurfacing of peri-oral rhytides and side-by-side comparison with carbon dioxide laser alone. *Dermatol Surg* 1999;25:285–293.

Miny Samuel
EBM Analyst
NMRC Clinical Trials & Epidemiology Research Unit, Singapore

Rebecca Brooke
Research Fellow
Dermatology Centre, University of Manchester School of Medicine, Manchester, UK

Christopher Griffiths
Professor of Dermatology
University of Manchester, Manchester, UK

Competing interests: MS and RB none declared. CG has been a paid consultant to Johnson & Johnson, the manufacturers of tretinoin; he has also received fees for speaking from Johnson & Johnson.

Insomnia

Search date February 2004

Bazian Ltd

QUESTIONS

INTERVENTIONS

See glossary G

Key Messages

Treatments in older people

- **Cognitive behavioural therapy** One systematic review identified one small RCT, which found that individual or group cognitive behavioural therapy improved sleep quality both immediately after the end of treatment, and at 3 months compared with no treatment, although mean sleep quality scores were consistent with continuing insomnia both with and without treatment.
- **Exercise programmes** One systematic review identified one small RCT. It found that sleep quality improved after a 16 week programme of regular, moderate intensity exercise four times a week compared with no treatment. However, mean sleep quality scores were consistent with persisting insomnia both with and without exercise.
- **Timed exposure to bright light** One systematic review found no RCTs comparing the effects of timed bright light exposure with other treatments or no treatment.

DEFINITION	Insomnia is defined by the US National Institutes of Health as experience of poor quality sleep, with difficulty in initiating or maintaining sleep, waking too early in the morning, or failing to feel refreshed. Chronic insomnia is defined as insomnia occurring for at least three nights a week for 1 month or more.[1] Primary insomnia is defined as chronic insomnia without specific underlying medical or psychiatric disorders such as sleep apnoea, depression, or dementia. This chapter only covers primary insomnia.
INCIDENCE/ PREVALENCE	Across all adult age groups, up to 40% of people have insomnia.[2] However, prevalence increases with age, with estimates ranging from 31–38% in people aged 18–64 years to 45% in people aged 65–79 years.[3]
AETIOLOGY/ RISK FACTORS	The cause of insomnia is uncertain. The risk of primary insomnia increases with age and may be related to changes in circadian rhythms associated with age. Psychological factors and lifestyle changes may exacerbate perceived effects of changes in sleep patterns associated with age, leading to reduced satisfaction with sleep.[4] Other risk factors in all age groups include hyperarousal, chronic stress, and daytime napping.[1,5]
PROGNOSIS	We found few reliable data on long term morbidity and mortality in people with primary insomnia. Primary insomnia is a chronic and relapsing condition.[6] Likely consequences include reduced quality of life and increased risk of accidents owing to daytime sleepiness. People with primary insomnia may be at greater risk of dependence on hypnotic medication, depression, dementia, and falls, and may be more likely to require residential care.[6,7]
AIMS OF INTERVENTION	To improve satisfaction with sleep; to prevent sleepiness and improve functional ability during the daytime.
OUTCOMES	Quality of life; self report of sleep satisfaction; sleep quality scales such as the Pittsburgh Sleep Quality Index (PSQI**G**); performance on attentional task tests; daytime functioning scales such as the Stanford Sleepiness Scale and the Epworth Sleepiness Scale. We excluded measures that record only time or duration of sleep, or wakefulness in the comments, because each of these measures may not directly correlate with symptoms.
METHODS	*Clinical Evidence* search and appraisal February 2004. Only studies examining the effects of treatments in people with chronic primary insomnia were included.

QUESTION What are the effects of non-drug treatments in older people?

OPTION COGNITIVE BEHAVIOURAL THERAPY

One systematic review identified one small RCT, which found that individual or group cognitive behavioural therapy improved sleep quality both immediately after the end of treatment, and at 3 months compared with no treatment, although mean sleep quality scores were consistent with continuing insomnia at 3 months both with and without treatment.

Benefits: We found one systematic review (search date 2002, 6 RCTs, 282 people with primary insomnia, at least 80% of whom were ≥ 60 years old).[8] Only one of the included RCTs (36 people) reported on outcomes relevant to the present review. It found that group or individual cognitive behavioural therapy**G** (consisting of sleep hygiene, stimulus control, sleep restriction, muscle relaxation, and sleep education) significantly improved Pittsburgh Sleep Quality Index**G** scores compared with no treatment, both immediately after treatment and at 3 months (mean scores immediately after treatment: 7.8 with cognitive behavioural therapy *v* 10.6 with no treatment; WMD –2.80, 95% CI –5.44 to –0.16; mean scores at 3 months: 6.20 with cognitive behavioural therapy *v* 10.20 with no treatment; WMD –4.00, 95% CI –6.62 to –1.38).

Harms: The systematic review did not report on harms.[8]

Comment: In the RCT, Pittsburgh Sleep Quality Index was assessed by investigators who were blind to treatment allocation.[8] We found one subsequent RCT (75 adults), in which 45% of participants were older than 55 years.[9] It compared three treatments: cognitive behavioural therapy (sleep education, stimulus control, and restrictions on time spent in bed), relaxation therapy, and a placebo treatment that involved listening to descriptions of neutral activities before going to bed. The trial did not separate results for different age groups. Overall, it found no significant differences among treatments for symptoms (100 point insomnia symptom questionnaire).[9] We found one additional RCT comparing cognitive behavioural therapy against standard care.[10] It appeared to randomise clinics and analyse results by individual patients, making it difficult to interpret the results. The reported results found that cognitive behavioural therapy significantly improved Pittsburgh Sleep Quality at both 3 and 6 months.

OPTION EXERCISE PROGRAMMES

One systematic review identified one small RCT, which found that sleep quality improved after a 16 week programme of regular, moderate intensity exercise four times a week compared with no treatment. However, mean sleep quality scores were consistent with persisting insomnia both with and without exercise.

Benefits: We found one systematic review (search date 2002, 1 RCT, 43 people with primary insomnia, at least 80% of whom were ≥60 years old).[11] The included RCT compared 16 weeks of regular moderate intensity exercise (30–40 minutes of walking or low impact aerobics 4 times a week) with no treatment. It found that, after completion, the exercise programme significantly improved Pittsburgh Sleep Quality Index**G** more than no treatment (mean scores after treatment: 5.4 with exercise therapy *v* 8.8 with no treatment; mean improvement in score for exercise programme *v* no treatment: 3.4, 95% CI 1.9 to 5.4).[11] We found no subsequent RCTs.

Harms: The systematic review did not report on harms.[11]

Comment: None.

OPTION TIMED EXPOSURE TO BRIGHT LIGHT

One systematic review found no RCTs comparing timed bright light exposure with other or no treatment.

Benefits: We found one systematic review that compared the effects of timed bright light exposure with other or no treatment in people aged 60 years and over (search date 2001).[12] It identified no RCTs. We found no RCTs published after the review.

Harms: The review did not report on harms.[12]

Comment: None.

GLOSSARY

Cognitive behavioural therapy The following cognitive behavioural therapies were considered in this review: stimulus control, sleep hygiene education, muscle relaxation, sleep restriction, and cognitive therapy. Stimulus control consists of measures to control the stimuli that affect sleep, such as establishing a standard wake up time, getting out of bed during long periods of wakefulness, and eliminating non-nocturnal sleep. Sleep hygiene education informs people about lifestyle modifications that may impair or enhance sleep, such as avoiding alcohol, heavy meals, and exercise before going to bed, and aims to alter expectations about normal sleep durations. Muscle relaxation involves sequential muscle tensing and relaxing. Sleep restriction reduces the time spent in bed to increase the proportion of time spent asleep while in bed. Cognitive therapy aims to identify and alter beliefs and expectations about sleep and sleep onset (e.g. beliefs about "necessary" sleep duration). Cognitive behavioural therapy may be undertaken on a one-to-one basis (individual therapy) or with a group of people (group therapy).

Pittsburgh Sleep Quality Index (PSQI) A validated 21 point scale (0 = best, 21 = worst) to measure subjective sleep quality. A score above 5 indicates insomnia.

REFERENCES

1. National Heart, Lung and Blood Institute Working Group on Insomnia. Insomnia: assessment and management in primary care. *Am Fam Physician* 1999;59:3029–3038.
2. Liljenberg B, Almqvist M, Hetta J, et al. Age and the prevalence of insomnia in adulthood. *Eur J Psychiatry* 1989;3:5–12.
3. Mellinger GD, Balter MB, Uhlenhuth EH. Insomnia and its treatment. *Arch Gen Psychiatry* 1985;42:225–232.
4. Bliwise DL. Sleep in normal aging and dementia. *Sleep* 1993;16:40–81.
5. National Center on Sleep Disorders Research Working Group. Recognizing problem sleepiness in your patients. *Am Fam Physician* 1999;59:937–944.
6. Reynolds CF, Buysse DJ, Kupfer DJ. Treating insomnia in older adults: taking a long term view. *JAMA* 1999;281:1034–1035.
7. Cricco M, Simonsick EM, Foley DJ. The impact of insomnia on cognitive functioning in older adults. *J Am Geriatr Soc* 2001;49:1185–1189.
8. Montgomery P, Dennis J. Cognitive behavioural interventions for sleep problems in adults aged 60+ (Cochrane Review). In: The Cochrane Library, Issue 1, 2004. Chichester, UK: John Wiley & Sons Ltd. Search date 2002; primary sources Medline, Embase, Cinahl, Psychinfo, The Cochrane Library, National Research Register, hand searches of references and trial reports, and contacts with experts.
9. Edinger JD, Wohlgemuth WK, Radtke RA, et al. Cognitive behavioural therapy for treatment of chronic primary insomnia: a randomized controlled trial. *JAMA* 2002;285:1856–1864.
10. Morgan K, Dixon S, Mathers N et al. Psychological treatment for insomnia in the management of long-term hypnotic use: a pragmatic randomised controlled trial. *Br J of Gen Pract* 2003;53:923–928.
11. Montgomery P, Dennis J. Physical exercise for sleep problems in adults aged 60+ (Cochrane Review). In: The Cochrane Library, Issue 1, 2004. Chichester, UK: John Wiley & Sons Ltd. Search date 2002; primary sources Medline, Embase, Cinahl, Psychinfo, The Cochrane Library, National Research Register, hand searches of references and trial reports, and contacts with experts.
12. Montgomery P, Dennis J. Bright light therapy for sleep problems in adults aged 60+ (Cochrane Review). In: The Cochrane Library, Issue 1, 2004. Chichester, UK: John Wiley & Sons Ltd. Search date 2001; primary sources Medline, Embase, Cinahl, Psychinfo, The Cochrane Library, National Research Register, hand searches of references and trial report, and contacts with experts.

Bazian Ltd
London, UK

Competing interests: None declared.

Jet lag

Search date November 2004

Andrew Herxheimer

QUESTIONS

INTERVENTIONS

*The adverse effects of melatonin have not yet been adequately investigated.

See glossary Ⓖ

Key Messages

Interventions

- **Melatonin*** One systematic review found that melatonin reduced mean jet lag scores on eastward and westward flights compared with placebo. The review found case reports of possible adverse effects, and suggested that people with epilepsy or taking warfarin (or other oral anticoagulants) should not use melatonin without medical supervision. It concluded that the pharmacology and toxicology of melatonin needs systematic study, and routine pharmaceutical quality control of melatonin products is necessary.
- **Hypnotics** Three small RCTs found limited evidence that hypnotics (zopiclone, zolpidem) improved sleep duration or sleep quality or jet lag compared with placebo. Adverse effects reported with hypnotics include headache, dizziness, nausea, confusion, and amnesia. Short term benefits of hypnotics must be considered in the light of potential adverse effects.
- **Lifestyle and environmental adaptations (eating, avoiding alcohol or caffeine, sleeping, daylight exposure, arousal)** We found no RCTs on the effects of eating, avoiding alcohol or caffeine, sleeping, daylight exposure, or arousal. Such RCTs are unlikely to be carried out.

*The adverse effects of melatonin have not yet been adequately investigated.

DEFINITION	Jet lag is a syndrome associated with rapid long haul flights across several time zones, characterised by sleep disturbances, daytime fatigue, reduced performance, gastrointestinal problems, and generalised malaise.[1] As with most syndromes, not all of the components must be present in any one case. It is due to the "body clock" continuing to function in the day–night rhythm of the place of departure. The rhythm adapts gradually under the influence of light and dark, mediated by melatonin secreted by the pineal gland: darkness switches on melatonin secretion, exposure to strong light switches it off.
INCIDENCE/ PREVALENCE	Jet lag affects most air travellers crossing five or more time zones. The incidence and severity of jet lag increases with the number of time zones crossed.
AETIOLOGY/ RISK FACTORS	Someone who has previously experienced jet lag is liable to do so again. Jet lag is worse the more time zones crossed in one flight, or series of flights, within a few days. Westward travel generally causes less disruption than eastward travel as it is easier to lengthen, rather than to shorten, the natural circadian cycle.[2]
PROGNOSIS	Jet lag is worst immediately after travel and gradually resolves over 4–6 days as the person adjusts to the new local time.[2] The more time zones that are crossed, the longer it takes to wear off.
AIMS OF INTERVENTION	To prevent or minimise jet lag, with minimal adverse effects.
OUTCOMES	Subjective jet lag score; sleep duration and quality; daytime alertness.
METHODS	*Clinical Evidence* search and appraisal November 2004. The author added data from the update of his own Cochrane Review. This topic includes studies whose purpose was the prevention of jet lag, in which interventions may have been given before or after travelling. RCTs were included if the authors described the basis of their definition of jet lag, even if not all components of the syndrome were looked for or documented.

QUESTION **What are the effects of interventions to prevent or minimise jet lag?**

OPTION **MELATONIN**

One systematic review found that melatonin reduced mean jet lag scores on eastward and westward flights compared with placebo. One included RCT found no significant difference between zolpidem plus melatonin in alleviating symptoms of jet lag compared with placebo. The review found case reports of possible adverse effects, and suggested that people with epilepsy or taking warfarin (or another oral anticoagulant) should not use melatonin without medical supervision. It concluded that the pharmacology and toxicology of melatonin needs systematic study, and routine pharmaceutical quality control of melatonin products is necessary.

Benefits: **Versus [illegible]** we found one systematic review (search date 2003, 975 people), which compared melatonin versus placebo.[2] Nine RCTs included in the review were in air travellers, and one was in international airline cabin staff (see comment below). In the RCTs, melatonin was given in a varying combination of before the flight, on the day of the flight, and after the flight. The review's primary outcome measure was the subjective rating of jet lag. Four RCTs reported global jet lag scores that could be combined (single scale 0–100 where 0 = no jet lag and 100 = extreme jet lag). The review found that melatonin significantly reduced mean subjective jet lag scores on eastward and westward flights compared with placebo (eastward flights: 4 RCTs, 142 travellers; weighted mean jet lag score 30.9 with melatonin *v* 50.7 with placebo; WMD −19.5, 95% CI −28.1 to −10.9; westward flights: 2 RCTs, 90 travellers; weighted mean jet lag score 22.3 with melatonin *v* 40.6 with placebo; WMD −17.3, 95% CI −27.3 to −7.3).[2] The review reported that melatonin reduced the symptoms of jet lag in eight RCTs, whereas two RCTs found no effect on symptoms between melatonin and placebo (see comment below). **Timing of melatonin:** One RCT included in the review (52 international airline cabin crew completing a 9 day tour of duty) compared melatonin after arrival ("post"), and melatonin before and after arrival ("pre and post") versus placebo. The review reported that "overall recovery" after the flight was no better in the "pre and post" group than with placebo, whereas the "post" group had significantly less jet lag ($P < 0.005$) and sleep disturbance ($P < 0.01$) compared with placebo.[2] However, the review noted that it was difficult to generalise from this finding because the airline staff had complex disordered circadian rhythms due to rapidly repeated flights.[2] **Melatonin plus zolpidem:** See benefits of hypnotics, p 2181.

Harms: The adverse effects of melatonin have not yet been adequately investigated (see comment below). The review noted that most RCTs did not look for adverse effects systematically, and many symptoms were difficult to distinguish from symptoms or manifestations of jet lag itself.[2] One RCT found no significant difference between melatonin and placebo in adverse effects; another found that a disorientating "rocking" feeling was significantly more frequent with melatonin ($P = 0.036$).[2] Hypnotic effects after melatonin occurred in five RCTs, affecting about 10% of people (further details not reported).[2] Other effects included headache or heavy head (2 RCTs); disorientation (1 RCT); ear, nose, and throat problems; nausea; and gastrointestinal problems (absolute numbers not reported; P values not reported).[2] One person had difficulty in swallowing and breathing within 20 minutes of taking melatonin.[2] Symptoms subsided after 45 minutes. They recurred after a further dose of melatonin. The review reported that the adverse events in the trials occurred during treatment and seemed to have been short lived.[2] The review noted that the pharmacology and toxicology of melatonin had not been systematically studied. It found six published and 19 unpublished case reports of possible related adverse effects on the central nervous system (including, confusion, ataxia, headache, and convulsant effects), blood clotting (prothrombin increased or decreased, suspected interaction with warfarin), cardiovascular system (including chest pain and dyspnoea), and skin (fixed drug eruption). Although it noted the difficulty of interpreting such data, it questioned the safety of melatonin in people with epilepsy and in people taking warfarin or other oral anticoagulants. It suggested that people in these groups should not use melatonin without an informed (medical) discussion, and concluded that further investigation was needed.[2] **Melatonin plus zolpidem:** See harms of hypnotics, p 2181.

Comment: The trials reviewed did not state whether travellers we[illegible] or not. Two RCTs found no effect on symptoms with melaton[illegible]vers first of these RCTs, the review noted that there was probably insufficie[illegible] time between inward and outward flights for participants to have fully adjusted to the new time zone. Hence, people may have suffered less jet lag on the return flight than might be expected, making it harder to detect effects. In the second RCT, the data suggested that melatonin may have reduced jet lag after 3 days, but the statistical analysis in the RCT did not test this. One RCT reported details of the source of melatonin; most did not state the pharmaceutical form used.[2] Some melatonin products have been found to contain unidentified impurities.[1] The review concluded that "the pharmacology and toxicology of melatonin needs systematic study, and routine pharmaceutical quality control of melatonin products must be established".[2]

OPTION HYPNOTICS

Three small RCTs found limited evidence that hypnotics (zopiclone, zolpidem) improved sleep duration or sleep quality or jet lag compared with placebo. One of these RCTs found no significant difference between zolpidem plus melatonin in alleviating symptoms of jet lag compared with placebo. Adverse effects reported with hypnotics include headache, dizziness, nausea, confusion, and amnesia. Short term benefits of hypnotics must be considered in the light of potential adverse effects.

Benefits: We found no systematic review but found three RCTs.[3–5] **Versus placebo:** The first RCT (33 people, westward flight crossing 5 time zones; see comment below) compared zopiclone (taken 30 minutes before bedtime on the first 4 nights after the flight) versus placebo.[3] It found no significant difference between zopiclone and placebo in subjective jet lag scores on the first, second, fifth, and sixth days after the flight. The RCT found that zopiclone significantly increased sleep duration on nights two ($P < 0.05$) and three ($P < 0.01$) after the flight compared with placebo. The second RCT (133 people, 25–65 years of age who had travelled overseas at least twice during the past 24 months, eastward flights crossing 5–9 time zones) compared zolpidem (taken immediately before bedtime on the first 3 nights after the flight) versus placebo.[4] It examined sleep disturbance in jet lag. It found that zolpidem significantly reduced the mean number of awakenings on the first two nights after the flight compared with placebo ($P < 0.05$) and significantly improved sleep quality on the first three nights after the flight, measured using a four point rating scale, compared with placebo ($P < 0.05$). **Zolpidem plus melatonin:** The third RCT (137 people, eastward flight crossing 6–9 time zones; see comment below) compared zolpidem alone; melatonin alone; zolpidem plus melatonin; and placebo.[5] Study medication was taken during the flight and at bedtime for 4 consecutive days after the flight. The RCT found that zolpidem alone was significantly more effective in alleviating symptoms of jet lag on the fourth day after the flight than placebo ($P < 0.05$), but the difference between zolpidem plus melatonin and placebo was not significant. It found no significant difference in overall self rated sleep quality during the flight, measured using a five point rating scale, between zolpidem alone and zolpidem plus melatonin, but found that both treatments were more effective than placebo ($P < 0.05$).

Harms: **Versus placebo:** The first RCT did not report on harms.[3] In the second RCT, adverse events included headache (12/68 [17.6%] of people with zolpidem *v* 6/65 [9.2%] with placebo), rhinitis (2/68 [2.9%] *v* 1/65 [1.5%]), diarrhoea (2/68 [2.9%] *v* 1/65 [1.5%]), abnormal dreaming (2/68 [2.9%] *v* 0/65 [0%]), and sinusitis (0/68 [0%] *v* 2/65 [3.1%]).[4] **Zolpidem plus melatonin:** In the third RCT, adverse events were most frequent with zolpidem plus melatonin (see table 1, p 2183) (total adverse events reported: 19 with zolpidem alone *v* 21 with melatonin plus zolpidem *v* 6 with placebo; statistical analysis not reported).[5] The most common adverse events included nausea, vomiting, confusion, dizziness, headache, amnesia, sweating, and dry mouth. One person taking zolpidem plus melatonin was incapacitated by adverse events.

Comment: In the first RCT, subjective jet lag scores were assessed using a 100 mm visual analogue scale: jet lag symptoms were described as feeling tired at unusual times of the day, bad mood, feeling of ill-being, digestive problems, and absence of energy.[3] The third RCT used a 100 mm visual analogue scale to assess the severity of jet lag symptoms and effectiveness of medication.[5] Disruption of sleep is a major component of jet lag, and hypnotics have been used to try to reduce it. The short term benefit seems to be outweighed by the wide range of unpleasant effects, some of them common.

OPTION **LIFESTYLE AND ENVIRONMENTAL ADAPTATIONS (EATING, AVOIDING ALCOHOL OR CAFFEINE, SLEEPING, DAYLIGHT EXPOSURE, AROUSAL)**

We found no RCTs on the effects of eating, avoiding alcohol or caffeine, sleeping, daylight exposure, or arousal. Such RCTs are unlikely to be carried out.

Benefits: We found no systematic review or RCTs looking at the lifestyle and environmental adaptations of eating, avoiding alcohol or caffeine, sleeping, daylight exposure, or arousal (i.e. doing interesting things such as sightseeing or visiting friends; see comment below). We found one RCT that used artificial light exposure (see comment below).

Harms: We found no evidence on harms.

Comment: RCTs on the effects of lifestyle and environmental adaptation are unlikely to be carried out. There is much physiological and anecdotal evidence to support environmental adaptation. Light is the major external environmental cue that pushes the circadian phase towards the light–dark rhythm at the destination. Endogenous melatonin production by the pineal gland is switched on by darkness, normally at dusk, and inhibited by bright light.[2] After a westward flight, it is probably worth staying awake while it is daylight at the destination and trying to sleep when it gets dark; and after an eastward flight, being awake but avoiding bright light in the morning, and being outdoors as much as possible in the afternoon.[1,6] Such behaviour may adjust the body clock and turn on the body's own melatonin secretion at the right time. Other cues may reinforce the effect of light, such as eating modestly at the times that correspond to usual meal times, and taking comfortable exercise.[1] We found one RCT (20 people, age 21–34 years), which compared artificial bright white light via a head mounted light visor versus artificial dim red light for 3 hours on the first two evenings after a westward flight crossing six time zones.[7] Salivary melatonin was measured to detect the onset of evening secretion, and sleep quality and jet lag were rated subjectively. The RCT found that bright light produced a mean delay in salivary melatonin secretion of 1 hour compared with dim light (i.e. put the body clock 1 hour forward). However, the difference in sleep quality or jet lag severity between bright light and dim light was not significant.[7]

REFERENCES

1. Herxheimer A, Waterhouse J. The prevention and treatment of jet lag. *BMJ* 2003;326:296–297.
2. Herxheimer A, Petrie KJ. Melatonin for the prevention and treatment of jet lag. In: The Cochrane Library, Issue 4, 2004. Chichester, UK: John Wiley & Sons, Ltd. Search date 2003; primary sources Cochrane Controlled Trials Register, Medline, Embase, Psychlit, Science Citation Index, hand searches of relevant journals, and contact with authors. A systematic search for harms of melatonin outside randomised trials was also made.
3. Daurat A, Benoit O, Buguet A. Effects of zopiclone on the rest/activity rhythm after a westward flight across five time zones. *Psychopharmacology* 2000;149:241–245.
4. Jamieson AO, Zammit GK, Rosenberg RS, et al. Zolpidem reduces the sleep disturbance of jet lag. *Sleep Med* 2001;2:423–430.
5. Suhner A, Schlagenhauf P, Hofer I, et al. Effectiveness and tolerability of melatonin and zolpidem for the alleviation of jet lag. *Aviat Space Environ Med* 2001;72:638–646.
6. Waterhouse JM, Minors DS, Waterhouse ME, et al. *Keeping in time with your body clock*. Oxford: Oxford University Press, 2002.
7. Boulos Z, Macchi MM, Sturchler MP, et al. Light visor treatment for jet lag after westward travel across six time zones. *Aviat Space Environ Med* 2002;73:953–963.

Andrew Herxheimer
Emeritus Fellow
UK Cochrane Centre
Oxford
UK

Competing interests: None.

TABLE 1 **Adverse events as reported by 137 people in one RCT comparing zolpidem alone, melatonin alone, zolpidem plus melatonin, and placebo.[5] (see text, p 2181).**

Harms	Melatonin (%) (n = 35)	Zolpidem (%) (n = 34)	Melatonin plus zolpidem (%) (n = 29)	Placebo (%) (n = 39)
Number of volunteers reporting adverse events	1 (3%)	6 (18%)	7 (24%)	3 (8%)
Total number of adverse events	2	19	21	6
Most common or relevant adverse events				
Nausea	–	4 (12%)	4 (14%)	1 (3%)
Vomiting	–	2 (6%)	2 (7%)	–
Confusion	–	2 (6%)	4 (14%)	–
Dizziness	–	1 (3%)	2 (7%)	–
Headache	–	1 (3%)	2 (7%)	–
Palpitations	1 (3%)	1 (3%)	–	–
Sweating	–	–	1 (3%)	1 (3%)
Dry mouth	–	1 (3%)	1 (3%)	–
Incapacitation	–	–	1 (3%)	–

– Not found in this treatment group.

Sleep apnoea

Search date August 2003

Michael Hensley and Cheryl Ray

QUESTIONS

INTERVENTIONS

See glossary G

Key Messages

In people with severe obstructive sleep apnoea-hypopnoea syndrome (OSAHS)

- **Nasal continuous positive airway pressure** One systematic review found that nasal continuous positive airway pressure (CPAP) reduced daytime sleepiness compared with placebo, no treatment, or conservative treatment in people with severe OSAHS.
- **Oral appliance** Two small RCTs found that oral appliances that produced anterior advancement of the mandible improved sleep disordered breathing and daytime sleepiness in people with severe OSAHS compared with appliances that did not advance the mandible.
- **Weight loss** One systematic review found no RCTs on the effects of weight loss in people with severe OSAHS.

In people with non-severe OSAHS

- **Nasal continuous positive airway pressure** Two systematic reviews found no significant difference in daytime sleepiness between nasal CPAP and conservative treatment, placebo pill, or sham/subtherapeutic nasal CPAP in people with non-severe OSAHS but found that CPAP improved some measures of cognitive performance, functional outcomes, symptoms, energy and vitality, and depression. One systematic review and one small RCT found that nasal CPAP improved apnoea/hypopnoea index compared with an oral appliance.
- **Oral appliance** Two small RCTs found that an oral appliance that produced mandibular advancement reduced daytime sleepiness and sleep disordered breathing compared with no treatment or a control appliance. One systematic review and one small RCT found that nasal CPAP improved apnoea/hypopnoea index compared with an oral appliance.
- **Weight loss** One systematic review found no RCTs on the effect of weight loss in people with non-severe OSAHS.

DEFINITION Sleep apnoea is the popular term for obstructive sleep apnoea-hypopnoea syndrome (OSAHS). OSAHS is abnormal breathing during sleep that causes recurrent arousals, sleep fragmentation, and nocturnal hypoxaemia. The syndrome includes daytime sleepiness, impaired vigilance and cognitive functioning, and reduced quality of life.[1,2] Apnoea is the absence of airflow at the nose and mouth for at least 10 seconds, and hypopnoea is a major reduction (>50%) in airflow also for at least 10 seconds. Apnoeas may be "central", in which there is cessation of inspiratory effort, or "obstructive", in which inspiratory efforts continue but are ineffective, because of upper airway obstruction. The diagnosis of OSAHS is made when a person with daytime symptoms has significant sleep disordered breathing**G** revealed by polysomnography (study of sleep state, breathing and oxygenation) or by more limited studies. Criteria for the diagnosis of significant sleep disordered breathing have not been rigorously assessed, but they have been set by consensus and convention.[3,4] Diagnostic criteria have variable sensitivity and specificity. For example, an apnoea/hypopnoea index (AHI)**G** of less than five episodes of apnoea or hypopnoea per hour of sleep is considered normal;[5] however, people with upper airway resistance syndrome**G** have an index below five episodes per hour,[6] and many healthy elderly people have an index greater than five episodes per hour.[7] In an effort to obtain an international consensus, new criteria have been proposed and are becoming more widely used.[8] The severity of OSAHS can be classified by the severity of two factors: daytime sleepiness (see table 1, p 2193) and AHI (see table 2, p 2193). Severe OSAHS is defined as severe sleep disordered breathing (AHI >35 episodes per hour) plus symptoms of excessive daytime sleepiness**G** (Epworth Sleepiness Scale >10 or Multiple Sleep Latency Test < 5 minutes — see table 3, p 2194). Central sleep apnoea and sleep associated hypoventilation syndromes are not covered in this chapter.

INCIDENCE/ PREVALENCE The Wisconsin Sleep Cohort Study of over 1000 people (mean age 47 years) in North America found a prevalence of AHI greater than five episodes per hour of 24% in men and 9% in women, and of OSAHS with an index greater than five episodes per hour plus excessive sleepiness of 4% in men and 2% in women.[22] There are international differences in the occurrence of OSAHS, for which obesity is considered to be an important determinant.[23] Ethnic differences in prevalence have also been found after adjustment for other risk factors.[7,23] Little is known about the burden of illness in developing countries.

AETIOLOGY/ RISK FACTORS The site of upper airway obstruction in the OSAHS is around the level of the tongue, soft palate, or epiglottis. Disorders that predispose to either narrowing of the upper airway or reduction in its stability (e.g. obesity, certain craniofacial abnormalities, vocal cord abnormalities, and enlarged tonsils) have been associated with an increased risk of OSAHS. It has been estimated that a 1 kg/m^2 increase in body mass index (3.2 kg for a person 1.8 m tall) leads to a 30% increase (95% CI 13% to 50%) in the relative risk of developing abnormal sleep disordered breathing (AHI ≥ 5 episodes/hour) over a period of 4 years.[23] Other strong associations include increasing age and sex (male to female ratio is 2 : 1). Weaker associations include menopause, family history, smoking, and night time nasal congestion.[23]

PROGNOSIS The long term prognosis of people with untreated severe OSAHS is poor with respect to quality of life, likelihood of motor vehicle accidents, hypertension, and possibly cardiovascular disease and premature mortality.[24] Unfortunately, the prognosis of both treated and untreated OSAHS is unclear.[7] The limitations in the evidence include bias in the selection of participants, short duration of follow up, and variation in the measurement of confounders (e.g. smoking, alcohol use, and other cardiovascular risk factors). Treatment is widespread, making it difficult to find evidence on prognosis for untreated OSAHS. Observational studies support a causal association between OSAHS and systemic hypertension, which increases with the severity of OSAHS (OR 1.21 for non-severe OSAHS to 3.07 for severe OSAHS).[24] OSAHS increases the risk of motor vehicle accidents three- to sevenfold.[24,25] It is associated with increased risk of premature mortality, cardiovascular disease, and impaired neurocognitive functioning.[24]

AIMS OF INTERVENTION To minimise or eliminate symptoms of daytime sleepiness; to improve vigilance and quality of life; to reduce or abolish the increased risk of motor vehicle accidents and cardiovascular events; to enhance compliance with treatment; to minimise adverse effects of treatment.

OUTCOMES **Daytime sleepiness:** Subjective and objective measures such as Epworth Sleepiness Scale, Multiple Sleep Latency Test, and Maintenance of Wakefulness Test.

Quality of life: General measures such as the Medical Outcomes Study 36-item Short Form Health Survey and the General Health Questionnaire; measures of mood such as the Hospital Anxiety and Depression Scale, the Beck Depression Inventory, and the Profile of Mood States; measures of energy and vitality such as the 36-item Short Form SF-36 energy scale, the UWIST Mood Adjective Checklist, and the energy and vitality scale of the Nottingham Health Profile. Disease specific quality of life measures include the Functional Outcomes of Sleep Questionnaire. **Cognitive performance measures:** Steer Clear, Trailmaking Test B, Digit Symbol Substitution, and Paced Auditory Serial Addition-2 Second Timing. **Mortality and morbidity:** For example, road traffic accidents, hypertension, stroke, cardiac failure, and ischaemic heart disease. **Intermediate outcomes:** Measures of the degree of disturbed breathing during sleep, such as the number of apnoeas and hypopnoeas**G** an hour (apnoea/hypopnoea index [AHI]), the frequency of arousals, and the degree of sleep fragmentation. Details of validated outcome measures for daytime sleepiness, quality of life, and cognitive performance are listed in table 3, p 2194.[9–21]

METHODS *Clinical Evidence* search and appraisal August 2003 and ongoing additional hand searches by the author. Different RCTs have used slightly different definitions of OSAHS. Many of the identified studies were crossover RCTs. The results of the crossover trials should be viewed with caution because effects of pre-crossover treatment may persist after crossover.

QUESTION What are the effects of treatment of severe obstructive sleep apnoea-hypopnoea syndrome?

OPTION NASAL CONTINUOUS POSITIVE AIRWAY PRESSURE

One systematic review found that nasal continuous positive airway pressure reduced daytime sleepiness compared with placebo, no treatment, or conservative treatment in people with severe obstructive sleep apnoea-hypopnoea syndrome.

Benefits: **Versus placebo, no treatment, or conservative treatment:** We found one systematic review (search date 2001).[26] The systematic review (12 RCTs in people with mild to severe obstructive sleep apnoea-hypopnoea syndrome [OSAHS], mean apnoea/hypopnoea index**G** 10–64 episodes/hour, mean Epworth Sleepiness Scale 7–16) compared nasal continuous positive airway pressure (CPAP**G**) versus control treatments, including sham CPAP, placebo pill, or conservative treatment (counselling on weight loss, abstinence from alcohol and other sedatives, avoidance of supine position, or the need for adequate sleep). In people with severe OSAHS (≥30 events/hour, Epworth Sleepiness Scale ≥11), it found that CPAP significantly reduced daytime sleepiness compared with control at 4–12 weeks (6 RCTs; 387 people; reduction in Epworth Sleepiness Scale 4.75, 95% CI 2.97 to 6.53).[26]
Versus oral appliances: We found no systematic reviews or RCTs that compared CPAP versus oral appliances in people with severe OSAHS.

Harms: The systematic review did not report on any harmful effects found in the identified RCTs.[26] One previous systematic review (search date 1999) reported a high prevalence of minor adverse effects from nasal CPAP treatment, the most common being dry mouth, nose, and throat (40%).[5] We found one case series (52 consecutive people with severe OSAHS, mean oxygen desaturation index 43/hour), in which the occurrence of nasopharyngeal symptoms was studied systematically before and after nasal CPAP.[27] It found that nasopharyngeal symptoms were common before nasal CPAP in OSAHS (nasal dryness 74%, sneezing 51%, blocked nose 43%, and rhinorrhoea 37%) and increased during nasal CPAP (sneezing 75% and rhinorrhoea 57%), with greater discomfort in the winter. Other adverse effects of nasal CPAP include local effects of the mask on the nasal bridge, mask discomfort, nasal congestion, rhinitis, sore eyes, headache, chest discomfort, and noise disturbance.

Comment: The RCTs included in the review have problems with their methods and with applicability of results.[26] First, severity of sleep disordered breathing (using apnoea/hypopnoea index, etc.) is not a good guide to severity of daytime sleepiness, which is a major symptom.[28] Second, it is not clear whether the sham or subtherapeutic CPAP used in some "placebo" groups are truly inactive treatments. Third, RCT evidence reports short term symptomatic outcomes only, rather than longer term complications such as mortality, motor vehicle accident rate, hypertension, stroke, and ischaemic heart disease. Fourth, several of the RCTs in the reviews were crossover RCTs that did not report results before crossover. Finally, there is evidence of a significant placebo effect for daytime sleepiness, with one RCT finding a significant reduction in Epworth Sleepiness Score with sham CPAP.[29]

OPTION WEIGHT LOSS

One systematic review found no RCTs on the effect of weight loss in people with severe obstructive sleep apnoea-hypopnoea syndrome.

Benefits: We found one systematic review (search date 2000), which identified no RCTs on the effect of weight loss in people with obstructive sleep apnoea-hypopnoea syndrome (OSAHS; see comment below).[30]

Harms: We found no RCTs.

Comment: One review of the effect of body weight in OSAHS found no RCTs but included case series in which weight loss, especially that achieved by surgery, was associated with improvement, mainly in people with severe OSAHS.[31] Large relative improvements in apnoea/hypopnoea index (–72% to –98%) were found after a weight loss of 30–70% of the initial weight.[31] It seems that weight loss has the potential to benefit obese persons with OSAHS. There is consensus that advice about weight reduction is an important component of management. However, weight loss is difficult, and advice may need to be combined with nasal continuous positive airway pressure**G** in people with moderate and severe OSAHS.

OPTION ORAL APPLIANCES

Two small RCTs found that oral appliances that produced anterior advancement of the mandible improved sleep disordered breathing and daytime sleepiness in people with severe OSAHS compared with appliances that did not advance the mandible.

Benefits: **Versus no treatment:** We found no RCTs. **Versus control oral appliances:** We found two RCTs comparing an oral appliance**G** that produced anterior advancement of the mandible (removable mandibular advancement device) versus oral appliances that did not (control intervention).[32,33] The first RCT (24 adults with loud snoring and severe obstructive sleep apnoea-hypopnoea syndrome [OSAHS]) found that mandibular advancement device significantly reduced daytime sleepiness compared with control after 2 weeks (Epworth Sleepiness Scale –3.8 with mandibular advancement device *v* –0.5 with control oral appliance; $P < 0.005$).[32] There was a significant withdrawal rate, with only 10 people in the mandibular advancement group and eight people in the control group providing outcome data after 2 weeks of treatment. The second RCT (85 people, 14 women with mean Epworth Sleepiness Scale of 11, crossover design) found that an active mandibular advancement splint significantly increased sleep latency and improved daytime sleepiness compared with an inactive mandibular advancement splint at 4 weeks (decrease in sleep latency for active v inactive treatment: 1.2 minutes, 95% CI 0.3 minutes to 2.1 minutes; improvement in Epworth Sleepiness Scale for active v inactive treatment: 2 points, 95% CI 1 point to 3 points; proportion of people with normal Epworth Sleepiness score: 82% with active v 62% with inactive, $P < 0.01$).[33] **Versus nasal continuous positive airway pressure:** We found no systematic reviews or RCTs that compared continuous positive airway pressure**G** versus oral appliances in people with severe OSAHS.

Harms: One small case series (22 people with apnoea/hypopnoea index [AHI] > 5) investigated adverse effects with oral appliances over 12–30 months.[34] It found that adverse effects were common (mucosal dryness [86%], tooth discomfort [59%], and hypersalivation [55%]) but did not require discontinuation of treatment. **Versus control oral appliances:** The first RCT did not report on adverse effects.[32]

Comment: Oral appliances are commonly used for snoring. Many studies have been undertaken with a study population of patients with OSAHS ranging from mild to severe, complicating the interpretation of the effects of oral appliances on either severe or non-severe OSAHS separately. We found one systematic review (search date 1994, 304 people with mean AHI in the severe range, but including patients with mild OSAHS, 21 publications, 19 case series), which found that about 70% of people had a 50% or greater reduction in AHI.[35] There is insufficient evidence about long term effectiveness and adverse effects. One RCT (24 people, with AHI ranging from 6 to 47, crossover design), which compared an oral appliance with a small bite opening (4 mm) versus one with a larger opening (14 mm), found no significant difference in sleep disordered breathing**G** or Epworth Sleepiness Scale.[36]

QUESTION What are the effects of treatment for non-severe obstructive sleep apnoea-hypopnoea syndrome?

OPTION NASAL CONTINUOUS POSITIVE AIRWAY PRESSURE

Two systematic reviews found no significant difference in daytime sleepiness between nasal continuous positive airway pressure (CPAP) and conservative treatment, placebo pill, or sham/subtherapeutic nasal CPAP in people with non-severe obstructive sleep apnoea-hypopnoea syndrome but found that CPAP improved some measures of cognitive performance, functional outcomes, symptoms, energy and vitality, and depression. One systematic review and one small RCT found that nasal CPAP improved apnoea/hypopnoea index compared with an oral appliance.

Benefits: **Versus no treatment:** We found no RCTs. **Versus conservative treatment or oral placebo:** We found two systematic reviews.[5,26] The first systematic review (search date 1999, 4 RCTs, 208 people with non-severe obstructive sleep apnoea-hypopnoea syndrome [OSAHS]) compared nasal CPAP**G** versus conservative treatment (sleep hygiene and advice about weight reduction) or oral placebo tablets for at least 4 weeks.[5] It found no significant difference between nasal CPAP and conservative treatment or oral placebo tablets in daytime sleepiness (4 RCTs: mean reduction in Epworth Sleepiness Scale –0.57, 95% CI –1.39 to +0.25; 3 RCTs: Multiple Sleep Latency Test, graphical representation; mean effect about 0, 95% CI about ±0.7). It found no significant difference between nasal CPAP and conservative treatment or oral placebo tablets in two measures of cognitive performance, but found significant improvement in two other measures of cognitive performance (no significant difference in Steer Clear, 2 RCTs, or Digit Symbol Substitution, 2 RCTs; significant improvement in Trailmaking Test B, 3 RCTs: P = 0.003; Paced Auditory Serial Addition-2 Second Timing, 2 RCTs: P < 0.0001; CI not reported). The review found no significant difference between nasal CPAP and oral placebo tablets for quality of life and anxiety measures, but found significant improvement for depression and for energy and vitality (quality of life: 2 RCTs, 36-item Short Form general perception), anxiety measures (2 RCTs, Hospital Anxiety and Depression Scale), depression (2 RCTs, Hospital Anxiety and Depression Scale; 1 RCT, Beck Depression Inventory; combined P = 0.0004); energy and vitality (2 RCTs, 36-item Short Form vitality; 1 RCT, UWIST Mood Adjective Checklist Energetic Arousal Score; combined P = 0.013; 1 RCT, energy/fatigue subscore of MOD; P < 0.05). The three RCTs that reported a symptom score (in-house questionnaires using an analogue scale) showed a significant benefit of appliance over placebo (combined P = 0.006). The second systematic review (search date 2001, 5 RCTs including 4 RCTs also included in the first review, 326 people with non-severe OSAHS, apnoea/hypopnoea index [AHI;Ⓖ < 30, Epworth Sleepiness Scale < 11) found no significant difference in daytime sleepiness between CPAP and control treatment (placebo pill, sham CPAP, or conservative treatment) at 4–10 weeks (difference in Epworth Sleepiness Scale 1.10, 95% CI –0.13 to 2.32).[26] **Versus oral appliances:** See benefits of oral appliances in non-severe OSAHS, p 2190.

Harms: The first systematic review grouped non-severe and severe OSAHS for reporting of adverse effects (see harms of nasal continuous positive airway pressure in severe OSAHS, p 2186).[5] The second systematic review did not report on harms.[26]

Comment: People with non-severe OSAHS find nasal CPAP less acceptable. People with an AHI below 15 episodes per hour have been found to have half the long term use of nasal CPAP compared with people with an AHI greater than 15 episodes per hour.[37] One RCT[38] identified by the second systematic review[26] found that adherence by people with non-severe OSAHS was moderately high (4.8 hours/day). Treatment acceptance was also reasonable (62% of people who finished the trial chose to continue CPAP).

OPTION WEIGHT LOSS

One systematic review found no RCTs on the effect of weight loss in people with non-severe obstructive sleep apnoea-hypopnoea syndrome.

Benefits: We found one systematic review (search date 2000), which found no RCTs on the effect of weight loss in people with obstructive sleep apnoea-hypopnoea syndrome (OSAHS; see comment below).[30]

Harms: We found no RCTs.

Comment: We found one large population based cohort study (690 people with sleep disordered breathingⒼ, including those who did not qualify for a diagnosis of OSAHS) that evaluated sleep disordered breathing at 4 year intervals over 10 years.[39] It found an association between changes in weight and apnoea/hypopnoea index (AHIⒼ; weight gain of 10% was associated with an increase in AHI of 32%, 95% CI 20% to 45%; weight loss of 10% was associated with a decrease in AHI of 26%, 95% CI 18% to 34%).

OPTION **ORAL APPLIANCES**

Two small RCTs found that an oral appliance that produced mandibular advancement reduced daytime sleepiness and sleep disordered breathing compared with no treatment or a control appliance. One systematic review and one small RCT found that nasal continuous positive airway pressure improved apnoea/hypopnoea index compared with an oral appliance.

Benefits: **Versus** no treatment or control oral appliance: We found no systematic reviews. We found two small crossover RCTs that compared an oral appliance**G** versus no appliance or a control appliance, but these did not report results before the crossover.[40,41] The first RCT (24 people, mean apnoea/hypopnoea index [AHI**G**] 26.7 and Epworth Sleepiness Scale [ESS] 11.9) compared two different oral appliances that produced mandibular advancement versus no treatment.[40] It found that both oral appliances significantly reduced daytime sleepiness and sleep disordered breathing after 1 week (ESS: 9.0 with first and second appliance *v* 13.0 with no oral appliance; $P < 0.01$ for each oral appliance *v* control; AHI: 8.7 with first appliance *v* 7.9 with second appliance *v* 22.6 with no oral appliance; $P < 0.05$ for appliance *v* no appliance). It also found that oral appliance significantly reduced interference with daily tasks, snoring frequency and loudness, and improved performance ability and energy level compared with no treatment. The second RCT (28 people with mean AHI 27) compared an active oral appliance versus a control oral appliance, which did not advance the mandible, for 1 week each.[41] It found that the active oral appliance significantly reduced daytime sleepiness and improved AHI (ESS: 3.9 with active *v* 10.1 with control; $P < 0.01$; AHI: 14 with active oral appliance *v* 30 with control oral appliance; $P < 0.001$). **Versus continuous positive airway pressure (CPAP)**: We found one systematic review (search date 2001, 3 RCTs, 60 people)[42] and one small subsequent crossover RCT that compared oral appliances versus CPAP**G**.[43] The systematic review found that nasal CPAP significantly improved AHI compared with oral appliance (3 RCTs; WMD −7.3, 95% CI −10.0 to −4.7).[42] The review only identified one small RCT (38 people) that measured subjective daytime sleepiness, and it found no significant difference between appliance and CPAP (ESS: 5.1 with CPAP *v* 4.7 with control; $P = 0.7$). The review found that significantly more people preferred CPAP than oral appliance (3 RCTs: 35/47 [74%] preferred CPAP *v* 8/47 [17%] preferred appliance; $P = 0.0001$). The subsequent crossover RCT (48 people with a median AHI of 22 episodes/hour and ESS of 14) found that CPAP significantly improved AHI, symptoms (score range 0 = worst to 48 = best), effectiveness rating (10 point Likert scale), functional outcomes, and aspects of quality of life compared with oral appliances after 8 weeks (AHI: 8 with CPAP *v* 15 with oral appliance; ESS: 8 *v* 12; symptoms: 11 v 17; effectiveness rating: 7 *v* 5; Functional Outcomes of Sleep Questionnaire: 14 *v* 13; SF-36 mental component: 52 *v* 48; SF-36 health transition scores: 2.4 *v* 2.9; $P < 0.01$ for all of these outcomes).[43] It found no significant difference between treatments for objective sleepiness, cognitive performance, or preference for treatments.

Harms: The RCTs on oral appliances have generally been too brief to evaluate clinically important adverse effects. The second RCT comparing an oral appliance versus no appliance or a control appliance reported the following adverse effects: excessive salivation (50%), gum irritation (20%), mouth dryness (46%), jaw discomfort (12.5%), and tooth grinding (12.5%).[41] Those adverse effects were described as non-severe to moderate, lasting less than 3 weeks, and not preventing the use of the mandibular advancement splint. See harms of oral appliances in severe obstructive sleep apnoea-hypopnoea syndrome, p 2188.

Comment: Oral appliances are used commonly for people with snoring with or without non-severe sleep apnoea**G**. Although the number and duration of trials are not ideal, there is consensus that oral appliances are effective.[44]

GLOSSARY

Apnoea is absence of airflow at the nose and mouth for at least 10 seconds. It is sometimes defined indirectly in terms of oxygen desaturation index (impact on pulse oximetry saturation is measured as the number of occasions per hour when oxygen saturation falls by ≥ 4%). Apnoeas may be "central", in which there is cessation of inspiratory effort, or "obstructive", in which inspiratory efforts continue but are ineffective because of upper airway obstruction.

Apnoea/hypopnoea index (AHI) The sum of apnoeas and hypopnoeas per hour of sleep. Although the generally accepted cut off point for "normal" is an index of five episodes per hour, there are several definitions of normal, of which at least four are applicable to the situation of sleep disordered breathing: levels that are inside the range found in a "normal" (i.e. healthy) population; levels that are well removed from those found in a target disorder such as obstructive sleep apnoea-hypopnoea syndrome; levels that are not associated with a significant risk of disease and disability; and levels for which there is evidence of a significant benefit of treatment.[4]

Continuous positive airway pressure (CPAP) This involves applying positive pressure from a blower motor to the upper airway through tubing and a soft nasal mask or a facemask. It provides a "pneumatic splint" to the upper airway. Because nasal delivery is the most common in the published literature, we refer to "nasal CPAP".

Excessive daytime sleepiness (EDS) is a condition in which an individual has an overwhelming urge to fall asleep. People with excessive daytime sleepiness feel drowsy and tired, and often nod or doze easily in relaxed or sedentary situations or fall asleep in situations where they need or want to be fully awake and alert. It can interfere with a person's ability to concentrate and perform daily tasks and routines. It can be measured in a sleep laboratory with a Multiple Sleep Latency Test (MSLT) or a Maintenance of Wakefulness Test (MWT), or with questionnaires such as the Epworth Sleepiness Scale (ESS) or Stanford Sleepiness Scale.

Hypopnoea is a major reduction (> 50%) in airflow at the nose and mouth for at least 10 seconds. A smaller reduction in airflow may be accepted as hypopnoea if it is associated with either an arousal or a reduction in oxygen saturation of 4% or more.

Oral appliance The term "oral appliance" is generic for devices that are placed in the mouth in order to change the position of the mandible, tongue, and other structures in the upper airway to reduce snoring or the upper airway obstruction of obstructive sleep apnoea-hypopnoea syndrome. Specific types are referred to as mandibular advancement devices or splints.

Sham/subtherapeutic nasal continuous positive airway pressure This involves the use of the nasal mask and continuous positive airway pressure machine, but with inadequate pressure generated to overcome upper airway obstruction during sleep.

Sleep disordered breathing (SDB) can be described as apnoeas (no airflow for 10 seconds or more) or hypopnoeas (markedly reduced airflow for 10 seconds or more). The choice of 10 seconds is by convention. The usual measure of the degree of SDB is the apnoea/hypopnoea index. Features of SDB include snoring, witnessed episodes of absent breathing (apnoeas), abnormal breathing during sleep, nocturnal hypoxaemia, and abnormal sleep architecture.

Upper airway resistance syndrome Measurement of inspiratory effort by oesophageal pressure shows recurrent episodes of increased inspiratory effort that maintain stable ventilation but are associated with arousals and sleep fragmentation. These episodes are also referred to as respiratory effort related arousal events.[8] More recent techniques of measuring nasal airflow can show changes consistent with upper airway resistance syndrome without the need for an oesophageal pressure catheter.[45]

REFERENCES

1. Gastaut H, Tassarini CA, Duron B. Polygraphic study of the episodic diurnal and nocturnal (hypnic and respiratory) manifestations of the Pickwick syndrome. *Brain Res* 1965;2:167–186.
2. Bassari AG, Guilleminault C. Clinical features and evaluation of obstructive sleep apnea hypopnea syndrome. In: Kryger MH, Roth T, Dement WC, eds. *Principles and practice of sleep medicine*. Philadelphia, PA: WB Saunders, 2000:869–878.
3. Ross SD, Sheinhait IA, Harrison KJ, et al. Systematic review and meta-analysis of the literature regarding the diagnosis of sleep apnea. *Sleep* 2000;23:519–532.
4. Sackett DL, Straus SE, Richardson WS, et al. *Evidence-based medicine. How to practice and teach EBM*. Edinburgh: Churchill Livingstone, 2000:69–70.
5. National Health and Medical Research Council of Australia. *Effectiveness of nasal continuous airway pressure (nCPAP) in obstructive sleep apnoea in adults*. National Health and Medical Research Council of Australia, 2000. http://www.health.gov.uk/nhmrc/publications/pdf/hpr21.pdf (last accessed 4 June 2004). Search date 1999; primary sources Medline, Cochrane Library, some Health Technology Assessment websites, Centre for Reviews and Dissemination website, Veteran Affairs Research website, hand searches of reference lists of review articles, and personal contact with experts.
6. Guilleminault C, Stoohs R, Clerk A, et al. A cause of excessive daytime sleepiness. The upper airway resistance syndrome. *Chest* 1993;104:781–787.
7. Lindberg E, Gislason T. Epidemiology of sleep-related obstructive breathing. *Sleep Med Rev* 2000;4:411–433.
8. American Academy of Sleep Medicine Task Force (Flemons W, Chair). Sleep-related breathing disorders in adults: recommendations for syndrome definition and measurement techniques in clinical research. *Sleep* 1999;22:667–689.
9. Johns MW. A new method for measuring daytime sleepiness: the Epworth Sleepiness Scale. *Sleep* 1991;14:540–545.
10. Carskadon MA, Dement WC, Mitler MM, et al. Guidelines for the Multiple Sleep Latency Test (MSLT): a standard measure of sleepiness. *Sleep* 1986;9:519–524.
11. Poceta JS, Timms RM, Jeong DU, et al. Maintenance of Wakefulness Test in obstructive sleep apnea syndrome. *Chest* 1992;101:893–897.
12. Ware JE and Sherbourne CD. The MOS 36–item short form health survey (SF–36). 1. Conceptual framework and item selection. *Med Care* 1992;30:473–483.
13. NFER website: http://www.nfer-nelson.co.uk/ghq/ghq28.htm
14. Zigmond AS, Snaith RP. The Hospital Anxiety and Depression Scale. *Acta Psychiatr Scand* 1983;67:361–370.
15. Beck AT, Ward CH, Mendelson M, et al. An inventory for measuring depression. *Arch Gen Psychiatry* 1961;4:561–571.
16. McNair D, Lorr M, Droppleman L. *EITS manual for the profile of mood states*. San Diego: Educational and Industrial Test Services, 1971.
17. Matthews G, Jones DM, Chamberlin AG. Refining the measurement of mood: The UWIST Mood Adjective Checklist. *Br J Psychol* 1990;81:17–42.
18. Hunt SM, McEwen J, McKenna SP. Measuring health stats: a new tool for clinicians and epidemiologists. *J R Coll Gen Pract* 1985;35:185–188.
19. Weaver TE, Laizner AM, Evans LK, et al. Instrument to measure functional status outcomes for disorders of excessive sleepiness. *Sleep* 1997;20:835–843.
20. Findley LJ, Fabrizio MJ, Knight H, et al. Driving simulator performance in patients with sleep apnea. *Am Rev Respir Dis* 1989;140:529–530.
21. Weaver TE. Outcome measurement in sleep medicine practice and research. Part 2: assessment of neurobehavioral performance and mood. *Sleep Med Rev* 2001;5:223–236.
22. Young T, Palta M, Dempsey J, et al. The occurrence of sleep-disordered breathing among middle-aged adults. *N Engl J Med* 1993;328:1230–1235.
23. Young TB, Peppard P. Epidemiology of obstructive sleep apnea. In: McNicholas WT, Phillipson EA, eds. *Breathing disorders in sleep*. London, UK: WB Saunders, 2002:31–43.
24. Redline S. Morbidity, mortality and public health burden of sleep apnea. In: McNicholas WT, Phillipson EA, eds. *Breathing disorders in sleep*. London, UK: WB Saunders, 2002:222–235.
25. George CFP. Reduction in motor vehicle collisions following treatment of sleep apnoea with nasal CPAP. *Thorax* 2001;56:508–512.
26. Patel SR, White DP, Malhotra A, Stanchina ML, Ayas NT. Continuous positive airway pressure therapy for treating sleepiness in a diverse population with obstructive sleep apnea: results of a meta–analysis. *Arch Intern Med* 2003;163:565–571.Search date 2001; primary sources Medline, Cochrane database, reference lists and contact with experts.
27. Brander PE, Soirinsuo M, Lohela P. Nasopharyngeal symptoms in patients with obstructive sleep apnea syndrome. *Respiration* 1999;66:128–135.
28. Barbe F, Mayoralas LR, Duran J, et al. Treatment with continuous airway pressure is not effective in patients with sleep apnea but no daytime sleepiness. A randomised, controlled trial. *Ann Intern Med* 2001;134:1015–1023.
29. Jenkinson C, Davies RJO, Mullins R, et al. Comparison of therapeutic and subtherapeutic nasal continuous positive airway pressure for obstructive sleep apnoea: a randomised prospective parallel trial. *Lancet* 1999;353:2100–2105.
30. Shneerson J, Wright J. Lifestyle modification of obstructive sleep apnoea. In: The Cochrane Library, Issue 4, 2002. Oxford: Update Software. Search date 2000; primary sources Cochrane Airways Group Trials Register, Medline, Embase, Cinahl, and hand searches of reference lists of review articles.
31. Barvaux VA, Aubert G, Rodenstein DO. Weight loss as a treatment for obstructive sleep apnoea. *Sleep Med Rev* 2000;4:435–452.
32. Hans MG, Nelson S, Luks VG, et al. Comparison of two dental devices for treatment of obstructive sleep apnea syndrome (OSAS). *Am J Orthod Dentofac Orthop* 1997;111:562–570.
33. Gotsopoulos H, Chen C, Qian J, et al. Oral appliance therapy improves symptoms in obstructive sleep apnea: a randomized, controlled trial. *Am J Respir Crit Care Med* 2002;166:743–748.
34. Fritsch KM, Iselli A, Russi EW, et al. Side effects of mandibular advancement devices for sleep apnea treatment. *Am J Respir Crit Care Med* 2001;164:813–818.
35. Schmidt-Nowra W, Lowe A, Wiegand L, et al. Oral appliance for the treatment of snoring and obstructive sleep apnea: a review. *Sleep* 1995;18:501–510. Search date 1994; primary sources Medline and consultation with experts.
36. Pitsis AJ, Darendeliler MA, Gotsopoulos H, et al. Effect of vertical dimension on efficacy of oral appliance therapy in obstructive sleep apnea. *Am J Respir Crit Care Med* 2002;166:860–864.
37. McArdle N, Dvereux G, Heidarnejad H, et al. Long-term use of CPAP therapy for sleep apnea/hypopnea syndrome. *Am J Respir Crit Care Med* 1999;159:1108–1114.
38. Monasterio C, Vidal S, Duran J, et al. Effectiveness of continuous positive airway pressure in non-severe sleep apnea-hypopnea syndrome. *Am J Respir Crit Care Med* 2001;164:939–943.
39. Peppard PE, Young T, Dempsey J, et al. Longitudinal study of moderate weight change and sleep-disordered breathing. *JAMA* 2000;284:3015–3021.
40. Bloch KE, Iseli A, Zhang JN, et al. A randomized, controlled crossover trial of two oral appliances for sleep apnea treatment. *Am J Respir Crit Care Med* 2000;162:246–251.

41. Mehta A, Qian J, Petocz P, et al. A randomized controlled study of a mandibular advancement splint for obstructive sleep apnea. *Am J Respir Crit Care Med* 2001;163:1457–1461.
42. Wright J, Cates C, White J. Continuous positive airways pressure for obstructive sleep apnoea (Cochrane Review). In: The Cochrane Library, Issue 4, 2003. Chichester, UK: John Wiley & Sons, Ltd. Search date 2001; primary sources Medline, Embase, Cinahl, hand searches of reference lists of identified papers, and personal contact with researchers and clinical experts.
43. Engleman HM, McDonald JP, Graham D, et al. Randomized crossover trial of two treatments for sleep apnea/hypopnea syndrome: continuous positive airway pressure and mandibular repositioning splint. *Am J Respir Crit Care Med* 2002;166:855–859.
44. Ferguson K. Oral appliance therapy for obstructive sleep apnea. Finally evidence you can sink your teeth into (editorial). *Am J Resp Crit Care Med* 2001;163:1294–1295.
45. Ayappa I, Norman RG, Krieger AC, et al. Non-invasive detection of respiratory effort-related arousals (RERAs) by a nasal cannula/pressure transducer system. *Sleep* 2000;23:763–771.

Michael Hensley
Professor of Medicine
University of Newcastle
Newcastle, NSW
Australia

Cheryl Ray
Data Manager
Newcastle Sleep Disorders Centre Royal
Newcastle Hospital
Newcastle, NSW
Australia

Competing interests: None declared.

TABLE 1 Daytime sleepiness (see text, p 2185).

Severity of daytime sleepiness	Activities when unwanted sleepiness or involuntary sleep occurs	Functional effects
Mild	Activities that require little attention (e.g. watching TV, reading)	Only minor impairment of social or occupational function
Moderate	Activities that require some attention (e.g. attending concerts, meetings, or presentations)	Moderate impairment of social or occupational function
Severe	Activities that require more active attention (e.g. eating, during conversation, walking, driving)	Marked impairment in social or occupational function

TABLE 2 Apnoea/hypnoea index (see text, p 2185).

Severity of sleep disordered breathing	AHI (episodes/hour of sleep)
Mild	5–20
Moderate	20–35
Severe	>35

AHI = apnoea/hypnoea index.

TABLE 3 Validated outcome measures (see text, p 2185).[9–21]

Outcome measure (abbreviation)	Description	Scoring
Epworth sleepiness scale (ESS)[9]	Questionnaire developed to measure the general level of sleepiness by the likelihood of falling asleep in eight common situations	The score for each question ranges from 0 (no likelihood of falling asleep) to 3 highly likely to fall asleep). A lower score indicates less daytime sleepiness in the last week. Maximum score 24 Normal < 10 Severe > 16–24
Multiple Sleep Latency test (MSLT)[10]	A daytime sleep laboratory based test in which the patient is asked to try and fall asleep when placed in a quiet dark room for 20 minutes at 2-hourly intervals. Monitoring is by electroencephalography. The time between lights out and sleep onset (sleep latency) is measured in minutes. The mean value of 4–5 test sleeps in the day is calculated. The mean sleep latency is considered an "objective" sleep measure of daytime sleepiness. A reduced score indicates an increase in daytime sleepiness.	Mean adult sleep latency of < 5 minutes is indicative of pathological sleepiness Mild 5–7 minutes Borderline 8–9 minutes Normal ≥ 10 minutes
Maintence of Wakefulness Test (MWT)[11]	Similar to the MSLT, but the patient is asked to stay awake during the 20 minutes in a dark room	Sleep latencies of < 20 minutes are indicative of pathological sleepiness
Quality of life		
Medical Outcomes Survey Short form 36 (SF–36)[12]	A short form health survey that measures generic health related quality of life. The instrument is used widely to evaluate Health Related Quality of Life across various populations It is a 36 item questionnaire comprising eight health concepts : physical functioning; role limitations due to physical health problems; bodily pain; social functioning; general mental health; role limitations due to emotional problems; vitality, energy or fatigue; general health perceptions	Most of the 36 items are scored on a 3–6 point Likert scale. Scaling for different questions includes ranges from excellent to poor; limited a lot to not limited at all; not at all to extremely; and otheres. A higher score reflects a better health related quality of life

TABLE 3 continued

General Health Questionnaire – 28 (GHQ–28)[13]	A self administered screening test, designed to identify short term changes in mental health. The most popular of the GHQ, it has 28 questions, seven in each sub–scale of depression, anxiety, social dysfunction and somatic symptoms	Four subscores as well as a total score are obtained. The higher the score the more severe the condition. A 4 point scoring system ranges from a "better/healthier than normal" option, through a "same as usual" and a "worse/more than usual" to a "much worse/more than usual" option
Hospital Anxiety and Depression scale (HADS)[14]	A 14 item questionnaire designed to identify clinical depression and anxiety. Seven items conceptually assess depression and seven items were derived from psychic manifestations of anxiety neurosis	Overall level of severity of each mood on a 4 point scale (0–3). A score of 8 is clinically significant, a score of 11 or more is highly clinically significant
Beck Depression Inventory (BDI)[15]	A measurement of clinical depression with 21 statements regarding a symptom associated with depression (e.g. appetite, mood, sense of failure)	Scores range from 0, indicating the absence of the particular symptom, to 3 for most severe
Profile of Mood States (POMS)[16]	A self report designed to measure six dimensions of mood, which include: tension–anxiety; depression–dejection; anger–hostility; vigour–activity; fatigue–inertia; and confusion– bewilderment. It consists of 65 short phrases describing feeling and mood, with respondents asked to indicate mood readtions for the "past week including today" or for shorter periods such as "right now"	A five point Likert type scale ranging from 0 for no mood reaction to 5, indicating extreme mood reaction
University of Wales Institute of Science and Technology (UWIST) Mood adaptive checklist (UMACL)[17]	A measurement of mood with four subscales: hedonic tone, anger, tense arousal, and energetic arousal. Except for anger, which only has positively loaded items, each one is made up of a combination of positively loaded and negatively loaded items	The final score is the result of adding the positively loaded answers and subtracting the negatively loaded answers

TABLE 3 continued

Nottingham Health Profile (NHP)[18]	Generic health related quality of life measure made up of 38 items that can be used to produce scores for six domains of health, including: physical mobility (8 items), pain (8 items), social isolation (5 items), emotional reactions (9 items), energy (3 items) and sleep (5 items)	Yes/No answers and domain scores ranging from 0 to 100. Mean score is calculated across all items within each domain. Overall score is the mean across all items. The higher the score the greater the health problem
Functional Outcomes of Sleep Questionnaire (FOSQ)[19]	A sleep specific functional measure designed to evaluate the impact of sleep disorders and excessive sleepiness. Thirty five items represent five subscales: activity level, vigilance, intimacy and sexual relationships, general productivity, and social outcome	Individual scores of each subscale are obtained and summated to produce a global score. The lower the score the greater the dysfunction as a result of sleepiness. Four levels of response: no difficulty, a little, moderate, or extreme plus non–participation. Scored on a 5 point Likert scale
Cognitive performance measures		
SteerClear (SC)[20]	A computer program designed to simulate a long, mundane highway drive and to characterise the decrements in driving ability. The patient is required to avoid obstacles that randomly appear on a two lane highway by pressing a single computer key. Performance on this 30 minute task is reflected by the number of obstacles passed and the number hit	Reducing the number of obstacles hit reflects improved vigilance
Trailmaking B tests (TTB)[21]	A test for broad cognitive performance that uses the connect a dot concept requiring the patient to draw lines from circle to circle to consecutively link numbers and letters in the quickest time possible	Better cognitive performance is indicated by a reduction in score, which reflects the time taken to complete the task
Digit Symbol Substitution (DSS)[21]	Cognitive speed is tested by matching individually presented symbols to their numbers using a reference key	Improved speed of performance is reflected by an increased score
Paced Auditory Serial Addition Task – 2 second timing (PASAT–2)[21]	A test of auditory attention and concentration by evaluating the time taken to add up numbers presented every 2 seconds	An increase in the score indicates improved ability to maintain concentration under distraction

Breast cancer (metastatic)

Search date June 2004

Justin Stebbing and Robert Glassman

QUESTIONS

INTERVENTIONS

Likely to be beneficial

Taxane based combination chemotherapy (may increase response rates compared with non-taxane combination chemotherapy) 2212

Likely to be ineffective or harmful

High dose chemotherapy (no significant difference in overall survival compared with standard chemotherapy and increased adverse effects). 2212

FIRST LINE CHEMO + MONOCLONAL ANTIBODY

Beneficial

Chemotherapy plus monoclonal antibody (trastuzumab) in women with overexpressed *HER2/neu* oncogene 2213

SECOND LINE CHEMOTHERAPY

Likely to be beneficial

Taxane based combination chemotherapy (increases response rate in women with anthracycline resistant disease compared with non-taxane combination chemotherapy) 2214

Unknown effectiveness

Capecitabine for anthracycline resistant disease 2216

Semisynthetic vinca alkaloids for anthracycline resistant disease 2215

TREATING BONE METASTASES

Beneficial

Radiotherapy plus appropriate analgesia* 2217

Likely to be beneficial

Bisphosphonates 2216

TREATING SPINAL CORD METASTASES

Beneficial

Radiotherapy plus high dose steroids in women with spinal cord compression 2218

Radiotherapy* 2218

TREATING CEREBRAL METASTASES

Likely to be beneficial

Radiotherapy* 2218

Unknown effectiveness

Intrathecal chemotherapy. 2219

Radiation sensitisers 2219

Surgical resection 2219

TREATING CHOROIDAL METASTASES

Likely to be beneficial

Radiotherapy* 2219

*Not based on RCT evidence

See glossary Ⓖ

Key Messages

First line hormonal treatment

- **First line hormonal treatment with antioestrogens (tamoxifen) or progestins (no significant difference in survival compared with non-taxane combination chemotherapy so may be preferable in women with oestrogen receptor positive disease)** One systematic review found no significant difference in survival at 12 or 24 months between first line hormonal treatment with tamoxifen or progestins and non-taxane combination chemotherapy. The review suggested that hormonal treatment may be preferable to chemotherapy as first line treatment in women with oestrogen receptor positive disease unless disease is rapidly progressing. It found that response rates were lower with hormonal treatment than with chemotherapy but it was associated with less nausea, vomiting, and alopecia.
- **Selective aromatase inhibitors in postmenopausal women (at least as effective as tamoxifen in delaying disease progression)** Two RCTs found that the aromatase inhibitor anastrozole as first line treatment in metastatic postmenopausal breast cancer was at least as effective as tamoxifen in delaying disease progression and may cause fewer thromboembolic adverse events and vaginal bleeding. One RCT found that the aromatase inhibitor letrozole increased time to disease progression compared with tamoxifen.
- **Tamoxifen in oestrogen receptor positive women** RCTs have found that antioestrogens (primarily tamoxifen) resulted in tumour responses in a substantial proportion of women with metastatic breast cancer. The likelihood of benefit with antioestrogen treatment was greatest in postmenopausal women with oestrogen receptor positive tumours. RCTs found no significant difference in response rates, remission

rates or overall survival between tamoxifen and progestins or ovarian ablation, but tamoxifen was associated with fewer adverse effects. One RCT found that tamoxifen was less effective than medroxyprogesterone in improving bone pain. Two RCTs in women with metastatic postmenopausal breast cancer found that tamoxifen and the aromatase inhibitor anastrozole were similarly effective in delaying disease progression but that tamoxifen may cause more thromboembolic adverse effects and vaginal bleeding. One RCT found that tamoxifen was less effective than the aromatase inhibitor letrozole in increasing time to disease progression.

- **Combined gonadorelin analogues plus tamoxifen in premenopausal women** RCTs in premenopausal women with oestrogen receptor positive metastatic breast cancer found that first line treatment with gonadorelin analogues plus tamoxifen improved response rates, overall survival, and progression free survival compared with gonadorelin analogues alone.
- **Ovarian ablation in premenopausal women (no significant difference in response rates or survival compared with tamoxifen but associated with substantial adverse effects)** One systematic review and one subsequent RCT in premenopausal women found no significant difference in response rate, duration of response, or survival between ovarian ablation (surgery or irradiation) and tamoxifen as first line treatment. Ovarian ablation is associated with substantial adverse effects such as hot flushes and "tumour flare".
- **Progestins (beneficial in women with bone metastases or anorexia compared with tamoxifen; higher doses associated with adverse effects)** RCTs found no significant difference in response rates, remission rates, or survival between medroxyprogesterone and tamoxifen as first line treatment. One non-systematic review found that higher doses of medroxyprogesterone increased nausea, vaginal bleeding, and exacerbations of hypertension. One RCT found that medroxyprogesterone improved bone pain compared with tamoxifen. Observational evidence suggested that progestins may increase appetite, weight gain, and wellbeing. One systematic review found no significant difference in survival at 12 or 24 months between first line hormonal treatment (with progestins or tamoxifen) and non-taxane combination chemotherapy. The review suggested that hormonal treatment may be preferable to chemotherapy as first line treatment in women with oestrogen receptor positive disease unless disease is rapidly progressing. It found that response rates were lower with hormonal treatment than with chemotherapy but it was associated with less nausea, vomiting, and alopecia.

Second line hormonal treatment

- **Selective aromatase inhibitors in postmenopausal women (prolonged survival compared with progestins, as effective in delaying progression as antioestrogens)** RCTs found that, in postmenopausal women with metastatic breast cancer who had relapsed on adjuvant tamoxifen or progressed during first line treatment with tamoxifen, the selective aromatase inhibitors anastrozole, letrozole, and exemestane prolonged survival compared with progestins (megestrol) or non-selective aromatase inhibitors (aminoglutethimide), with fewer adverse effects. Two RCTs found no significant difference between anastrozole and fulvestrant in time to progression. The evidence suggests that selective aromatase inhibitors are most effective in oestrogen receptor positive women.
- **Progestins (less effective in prolonging survival than selective aromatase inhibitors and have more adverse effects)** RCTs found that, in postmenopausal women with metastatic breast cancer who had relapsed on adjuvant tamoxifen or progressed during first line treatment with tamoxifen, progestins were less effective in prolonging survival as second line treatment than selective aromatase inhibitors and were associated with more adverse effects.

First line chemotherapy

- **Anthracycline based non-taxane combination chemotherapy regimens (CAF) containing doxorubicin (increased response rates and survival compared with other regimens)** RCTs found that combination chemotherapy regimens containing an anthracycline, such as doxorubicin (CAF) as first line treatment increased response rates, time to progression, and survival compared with other regimens.

- **Classical non-taxane combination chemotherapy (CMF) (increases response rates and survival compared with modified CMF)** One systematic review found that classical CMF as first line treatment increased response rate and survival compared with modified CMF regimens.
- **Taxane based combination chemotherapy (may increase response rates compared with non-taxane combination chemotherapy)** One systematic review found that taxane based combination chemotherapy as first or second line treatment increased overall survival, time to progression, and overall response compared with non-taxane combination chemotherapy. It found no significant difference in overall survival if the analysis was restricted to RCTs of first line chemotherapy.
- **High dose chemotherapy (no significant difference in overall survival compared with standard chemotherapy and increased adverse effects)** One systematic review found no significant difference in overall survival over 1–5 years between high dose chemotherapy (requiring haematopoietic transplant) and standard dose chemotherapy. It found that high dose chemotherapy increased treatment related morbidity and mortality compared with standard chemotherapy.

First line chemo + monoclonal antibody

- **Chemotherapy plus monoclonal antibody (trastuzumab) in women with overexpressed *HER2/neu* oncogene** One RCT found that, in women whose tumours overexpress the *HER2/neu* oncogene, standard chemotherapy plus the monoclonal antibody trastuzumab as first line treatment increased the time to disease progression, objective response, and overall survival compared with standard chemotherapy alone. The most serious adverse effect observed was cardiac dysfunction in women who received an anthracycline plus trastuzumab.

Second line chemotherapy

- **Taxane based combination chemotherapy (increases response rate in women with anthracycline resistant disease compared with non-taxane combination chemotherapy)** One systematic review has found that taxane based combination chemotherapy as first or second line treatment increased overall survival, time to progression, and overall response compared with non-taxane combination chemotherapy. The difference remained significant if the analysis was limited to women who had previously received anthracyclines. One RCT found no significant difference in progression or overall survival between docetaxel and 5-fluorouracil plus vinorelbine or between paclitaxel and capecitabine given as second line chemotherapy.
- **Capecitabine for anthracycline resistant disease** One RCT found similar response rates and time to disease progression between capecitabine and paclitaxel after anthracycline failure.
- **Semisynthetic vinca alkaloids for anthracycline resistant disease** One RCT found no significant difference in progression or overall survival between 5-fluorouracil plus vinorelbine and docetaxel given as second line chemotherapy. Another RCT found that second line vinorelbine improved survival and reduced progression compared with melphalan. A third RCT found no significant difference in survival or quality of life between vinorelbine plus doxorubicin and doxorubicin alone.

Treating bone metastases

- **Radiotherapy plus appropriate analgesia*** We found no RCTs. We found limited evidence from non-randomised studies that persistent and localised bone pain can be treated successfully in over 80% of women with radiotherapy plus concomitant appropriate analgesia (from non-steroidal anti-inflammatory drugs to morphine and its derivatives) and that cranial nerve compression can be treated successfully with radiotherapy in 50–80% of people. RCTs found no evidence that short courses were less effective for pain relief than long courses of radiotherapy. One RCT found that different fractionation schedules can be used to treat neuropathic bone pain effectively.

- **Bisphosphonates** RCTs in women receiving standard chemotherapy or hormonal treatment for bone metastases secondary to metastatic breast cancer found that bisphosphonates reduced and delayed skeletal complications compared with placebo. They found no significant difference in survival.

Treating spinal cord metastases

- **Radiotherapy plus high dose steroids in women with spinal cord compression** One small RCT in women with spinal cord compression found that adding high dose steroids to radiotherapy improved the chance of walking 6 months after treatment compared with radiotherapy alone.
- **Radiotherapy*** We found no RCTs. Spinal cord compression is an emergency. Retrospective studies suggested that early radiotherapy improved outcomes. However, fewer than 10% of people walked again if severe deterioration of motor function occurred before radiotherapy.

Treating cerebral metastases

- **Radiotherapy*** We found no RCTs. Retrospective studies suggested that whole brain irradiation improved neurological function in some women with brain metastases secondary to breast cancer.
- **Intrathecal chemotherapy** We found no RCTs or observational studies of intrathecal chemotherapy in people with cerebral metastases.
- **Radiation sensitisers** We found no RCTs of radiation sensitisers. One open label case control study found limited evidence that adding intravenous RSR13, a radiation sensitiser, during whole brain radiotherapy may prolong survival.
- **Surgical resection** We found no RCTs. One retrospective cohort study provided insufficient evidence to assess surgical resection in people with cerebral metastases.

Treating choroidal metastases

- **Radiotherapy*** We found no RCTs. Retrospective studies suggested that radiotherapy benefited some women with choroidal metastases.

*Not based on RCT evidence.

DEFINITION Metastatic or advanced breast cancer is the presence of disease at distant sites such as the bone, liver, or lung. It is not treatable by primary surgery and is currently considered incurable. However, young people with good performance status may survive for 15–20 years.[1] Symptoms may include pain from bone metastases, breathlessness from spread to the lung, and nausea or abdominal discomfort from liver involvement.

INCIDENCE/ PREVALENCE Breast cancer is the second most frequent cancer in the world (1.05 million people) and is by far the most common malignant disease in women (22% of all new cancer cases). Worldwide, the ratio of mortality to incidence is about 36%. It ranks fifth as a cause of death from cancer overall (although it is the leading cause of cancer mortality in women — the 370 000 annual deaths represent 13.9% of cancer deaths in women). In the USA, metastatic breast cancer causes 46 000 deaths annually, and in the UK causes 15 000 deaths annually.[2] It is the most prevalent cancer in the world today and there are an estimated 3.9 million women alive who have had breast cancer diagnosed in the past 5 years (compared, for example, with lung cancer, where there are 1.4 million alive). The true prevalence of metastatic disease is high because some women live with the disease for many years. Since 1990, there has been an overall increase in incidence rates of about 1.5% annually.[3]

AETIOLOGY/ RISK FACTORS The risk of metastatic disease relates to known adverse prognostic factors in the original primary tumour. These factors include oestrogen receptor negative disease, primary tumours 3 cm or more in diameter, and axillary node involvement — recurrence occurred within 10 years of adjuvant chemotherapy**G** for early breast cancer**G** in 60–70% of node positive women and 25–30% of node negative women in one large systematic review.[4]

PROGNOSIS Prognosis depends on age, extent of disease, and oestrogen receptor status. There is also evidence that overexpression of the product of the *HER2/neu* oncogene, which occurs in about a third of women with metastatic breast cancer, is associated with a worse prognosis.[5] A short disease free interval**G** (e.g. < 1 year) between surgery for early breast cancer(G) and developing metastases suggests that the recurrent disease is likely to be resistant to adjuvant treatment(G).[6] In women who receive no treatment for metastatic disease, the median survival from diagnosis of metastases is 12 months.[7] The choice of first line treatment(G) (hormonal or chemotherapy(G)) is based on a variety of clinical factors (see table 1, p 2225).[8–11] In many countries, such as the USA, Canada, and some countries in Europe, there is evidence of a decrease in death rates in recent years. This probably reflects improvements in treatment (and therefore improved survival) as well as earlier diagnosis.[2,12]

AIMS OF INTERVENTION To relieve symptoms, prolong life, and improve quality of life, with minimal adverse effects.

OUTCOMES Symptoms; progression free survival(G); overall objective response rate(G); complete response(G); partial response(G); duration of response; disease stabilisation; time to progression of disease (progression defined as $\geq$ 25% increase in lesion size or the appearance of new lesions); quality of life;[13] improvement in performance status (according to validated scales of daily functioning/activity);[14] adverse effects and toxicity of treatment;[15] and overall survival. In people with bone, spinal, cerebral, or choroidal metastases: preservation of function; pain; incidence of fractures; and requirement for radiotherapy or surgery. Response to treatment is a surrogate outcome measure for assessing the effects of treatment on survival or quality of life. The link between clinical and proxy outcomes has not been clearly validated. Women who respond to treatment are more likely to experience improved symptomatic relief, performance status, and survival.[16–18] One recent prospective study (300 women with metastatic breast cancer) found a significant relationship between improvement and objective response for three symptoms, in particular cancer pain, shortness of breath, and abnormal mood.[19] Symptom improvement was greatest in those women who had a complete or partial response.

METHODS *Clinical Evidence* search and appraisal June 2004. Placebo or no treatment controlled trials would be considered unethical in women with metastatic breast cancer. The authors looked for good quality systematic reviews that used the outcome measures listed above. Where they found no good systematic reviews, they included relevant randomised phase III trials using these outcomes. Studies presented only in abstract form were excluded. Response to treatment is often assessed in an unblinded fashion, introducing the possibility of bias. We found few trials of good quality that reported on symptoms or quality of life.

QUESTION What are the effects of first line hormonal treatment?

OPTION ANTIOESTROGENS (TAMOXIFEN)

RCTs found that antioestrogens (primarily tamoxifen) resulted in tumour responses in a substantial proportion of women with metastatic breast cancer. The likelihood of benefit with antioestrogen treatment was greatest in postmenopausal women with oestrogen receptor positive tumours. RCTs found no significant difference in response rates, remission rates or overall survival between tamoxifen and progestins or ovarian ablation, but tamoxifen was associated with fewer adverse effects. One RCT found that tamoxifen was less effective than medroxyprogesterone in improving bone pain. Two RCTs in women with metastatic postmenopausal breast cancer found that tamoxifen and the aromatase inhibitor anastrozole were similarly effective in delaying disease progression but that tamoxifen may cause more thromboembolic adverse effects and vaginal bleeding. One RCT found that tamoxifen was less effective than the aromatase inhibitor letrozole in increasing time to disease progression. One systematic review found no significant difference in survival at 12 or 24 months between first line hormonal treatment with tamoxifen or progestins and non-taxane combination chemotherapy. The review suggested that hormonal treatment may be preferable to chemotherapy as first line

treatment in women with oestrogen receptor positive disease unless disease is rapidly progressing. It found that response rates were lower with hormonal treatment than with chemotherapy but it was associated with less nausea, vomiting, and alopecia.

Benefits: We found no systematic reviews. Non-systematic reviews identified 86 RCTs in 5353 women with metastatic breast cancer unselected for oestrogen receptor status.[8–11] The overall objective response rate**G** to tamoxifen was 34%. Disease stabilisation was achieved in a further 20%, and overall the median duration of response was 12–18 months.[8,9] The likelihood of responding to tamoxifen was highest (60–70%) in postmenopausal women with oestrogen receptor positive disease (see comment below).[10,11] **Versus progestins:** See benefits of progestins as first line hormonal treatment, p 2204. **Versus ovarian ablation in premenopausal women:** See ovarian ablation in premenopausal women, p 2204. **Versus anastrozole in postmenopausal women:** See benefits of selective aromatase inhibitors as first line hormonal treatment in postmenopausal women, p 2205. **Versus letrozole in postmenopausal women:** See benefits of selective aromatase inhibitors as first line hormonal treatment in postmenopausal women, p 2205. **Versus non-taxane combination chemotherapy:** See benefits of non-taxane combination chemotherapy as first line treatment, p 2209.

Harms: **Minor adverse effects:** Tamoxifen is well tolerated in women with metastatic breast cancer; fewer than 3% of women discontinued tamoxifen as a result of toxicity.[20] Reported adverse effects included minor gastrointestinal upset (8%), hot flushes (27%), and menstrual disturbance in premenopausal women (13%).[21] **Tumour flare:** During the first few weeks of treatment, tumour flare**G** occurred in fewer than 5% of women. For those with bone metastases, this may have resulted in increased pain or symptomatic hypercalcaemia. **Relapse:** Most women who initially respond to tamoxifen eventually progress and develop acquired resistance to tamoxifen, although they may still respond to further hormonal treatments**G**.[22]

Comment: An emerging problem is that many women have already received adjuvant tamoxifen for early breast cancer**G** or have developed metastatic disease while still taking tamoxifen, and are thus considered resistant to it. Effective second line treatment**G** hormonal drugs, such as selective aromatase inhibitors, are now used after tamoxifen failure (see selective aromatase inhibitors as second line treatment in postmenopausal women, p 2218), and RCTs have compared selective aromatase inhibitors with tamoxifen as first line treatment**G** (see selective aromatase inhibitors in postmenopausal women, p 2205). New non-steroidal antioestrogens (toremifene, idoxifene, raloxifene) and steroidal antioestrogens (fulvestrant) are more selective than tamoxifen and may have fewer long term adverse effects. RCTs comparing some of these drugs with tamoxifen as first line hormonal treatment in metastatic breast cancer are in progress. So far, one RCT in 658 women has found no evidence of clear clinical superiority of toremifene over tamoxifen.[23]

OPTION PROGESTINS

RCTs found no significant difference in response rates, remission rates, or survival between medroxyprogesterone and tamoxifen as first line treatment. One non-systematic review found that higher doses of medroxyprogesterone increased nausea, vaginal bleeding, and exacerbations of hypertension. One RCT found that medroxyprogesterone improved bone pain compared with tamoxifen. Observational evidence suggested that progestins may increase

appetite, weight gain, and wellbeing. One systematic review found no significant difference in survival at 12 or 24 months between first line hormonal treatment (with progestins or tamoxifen) and non-taxane combination chemotherapy. The review suggested that hormonal treatment may be preferable to chemotherapy as first line treatment in women with oestrogen receptor positive disease unless disease is rapidly progressing. It found that response rates were lower with hormonal treatment than with chemotherapy but it was associated with less nausea, vomiting, and alopecia.

Benefits: **Versus tamoxifen:** We found one systematic review (search date 1991, 7 RCTs, 801 women with metastatic breast cancer)[24] and one subsequent RCT[25] comparing medroxyprogesterone versus tamoxifen. The review found no significant difference in response rates (35–54%), remission rates, or survival between the two groups.[24] The subsequent RCT (166 women) found that medroxyprogesterone increased the rate of response of bone metastases compared with tamoxifen (33% with medroxyprogesterone *v* 13% with tamoxifen; P = 0.01).[25] It found no significant difference in survival. It also found that medroxyprogesterone significantly increased weight gain compared with tamoxifen (mean 17 lb [7.6 kg] with medroxyprogesterone *v* mean 5 lb [2.2 kg] with tamoxifen; P < 0.001). **Versus non-taxane combination chemotherapy:** See benefits of non-taxane based combination chemotherapy as first line treatment, p 2209.

Harms: **Versus tamoxifen:** The systematic review gave no information on adverse effects.[24] The subsequent RCT found that tamoxifen significantly increased nausea and vomiting compared with medroxyprogesterone (P < 0.001).[25] One non-systematic review found that adverse effects associated with medroxyprogesterone were common at higher doses and included nausea (14%), vaginal bleeding (10%), and exacerbation of hypertension. In women with lymphangitis carcinomatosis**G**, progestins**G** may exacerbate symptoms of breathlessness.[26]

Comment: Observational evidence suggested that the benefits of progestins**G** included an analgesic effect (assessed using questionnaires), especially on painful bone metastases,[27] increased appetite, weight gain, and a feeling of wellbeing. In view of the lack of evidence of greater benefit, and the evidence of greater harm, progestins are generally reserved for second or third line hormonal treatment**G** in women with advanced breast cancer who have not responded to tamoxifen.

OPTION OVARIAN ABLATION IN PREMENOPAUSAL WOMEN

One systematic review and one subsequent RCT in premenopausal women found no significant difference in response rate, duration of response, or survival between ovarian ablation (surgery or irradiation) and tamoxifen as first line treatment. Ovarian ablation is associated with substantial adverse effects such as hot flushes and "tumour flare".

Benefits: **Versus tamoxifen:** We found one systematic review (search date not stated, 4 RCTs, 220 premenopausal women)[28] and one subsequent RCT[29] comparing ovarian ablation (carried out by either surgery or irradiation) versus tamoxifen. The review found no significant difference between treatments in response rate, response duration, or survival.[28] The subsequent RCT (39 premenopausal women) comparing initial treatment with ovarian ablation versus tamoxifen found no significant difference in progression, median survival, or mortality (OR for progressive disease**G** 0.71, 95% CI 0.37 to 1.38; median survival 2.46 years with ovarian ablation *v* 2.35 years with tamoxifen; P = 0.98; OR for mortality 1.07, 95% CI 0.55 to 2.06).[29] **Different methods of ovarian ablation:** We found two RCTs comparing gonadorelin analogues🅖 versus surgical ovariectomy or irradiation. They found no significant difference in survival between treatments.[30,31]

Harms: **Versus tamoxifen:** The subsequent RCT found that the adverse effects of tamoxifen included hot flushes and menstrual abnormalities, but these did not result in a reduction of dose.[29] **Different methods of ovarian ablation:** Adverse effects include hot flushes (75% with gonadorelin analogues🅖 *v* 46% with surgical ovariectomy) and "tumour flare"🅖 (16% with gonadorelin analogues v 3% with surgical ovariectomy).[30] In addition, the risks of surgical ovariectomy include those associated with general anaesthesia.

Comment: None.

OPTION COMBINED GONADORELIN ANALOGUES PLUS TAMOXIFEN IN PREMENOPAUSAL WOMEN

RCTs in premenopausal women with oestrogen receptor positive metastatic breast cancer found that first line treatment with gonadorelin analogues plus tamoxifen improved response rates, overall survival, and progression free survival compared with gonadorelin analogues alone.

Benefits: **Versus gonadorelin analogues alone:** We found one non-systematic review (4 RCTs, 506 premenopausal women, primarily with oestrogen receptor positive metastatic breast cancer).[32] It found that combined endocrine treatment with gonadorelin analogues🅖 plus tamoxifen significantly improved both progression free survival🅖 (HR 0.70, 95% CI 0.58 to 0.85; P = 0.0003) and overall survival (HR 0.78, 95% CI 0.63 to 0.96; P = 0.02) compared with a gonadorelin analogue alone.[32] The overall response rate was also significantly higher for combined treatment (OR 0.67, 95% CI 0.46 to 0.96; P = 0.03).

Harms: **Versus gonadorelin analogues alone:** Although the meta-analysis did not analyse differences in tolerability, the largest of the individual trials found that there was no significant difference in expected hormonal adverse effects (hot flushes, vaginal discharge) between the combined treatment and gonadorelin analogues🅖 alone.

Comment: We found that combined endocrine treatment in metastatic breast cancer was more beneficial than single agent treatment. Research to establish whether there is any additional benefit from complete oestrogen deprivation in premenopausal women using ovarian ablation with gonadorelin analogues🅖 combined with aromatase inhibitors🅖 is currently in progress.

OPTION SELECTIVE AROMATASE INHIBITORS IN POSTMENOPAUSAL WOMEN

Two RCTs found that the aromatase inhibitor anastrozole as first line treatment in metastatic postmenopausal breast cancer was at least as effective as tamoxifen in delaying disease progression and may cause fewer thromboembolic adverse events and vaginal bleeding. One RCT found that the aromatase inhibitor letrozole increased time to disease progression compared with tamoxifen.

Benefits: **Anastrozole versus antioestrogens (tamoxifen):** We found two RCTs comparing anastrozole versus tamoxifen.[33,34] The first RCT (668 women) found no significant difference in time to disease progression🅖 (HR 0.99, 95% CI 0.86 to 1.12) or response rate (32.9% with anastrozole *v* 32.6% with tamoxifen; significance not reported).[33] The second

RCT (353 women) found that anastrozole significantly prolonged time to progression (HR for progression, tamoxifen *v* anastrozole 1.44, 95% CI 1.16 to 1.82).[34] Neither trial reported on the effect on survival because of insufficient data, but a survival analysis of data from both RCTs at 2 years found similar survival in both groups (AR for mortality at 2 years: 32% with tamoxifen *v* 31.1% with anastrazole; HR 0.97, lower 95% CI 0.84, upper 95% CI not reported).[35] **Letrozole versus antioestrogens (tamoxifen):** We found one RCT (907 women) comparing letrozole versus tamoxifen, which was described in two publications.[36,37] It found that letrozole significantly increased the time to progression (9.4 months with letrozole *v* 6.0 months with tamoxifen; $P < 0.0001$), time to treatment failure (9.0 months with letrozole *v* 5.7 months with tamoxifen; $P < 0.0001$), and response rates (32% with letrozole *v* 21% with tamoxifen; $P = 0.0002$).[36] It found no significant difference in overall survival (median survival 34 months with letrozole *v* 30 months with tamoxifen; $P = 0.53$; see comment).[36]

Harms: **Anastrozole versus antioestrogens (tamoxifen):** In both trials, anastrozole was associated with reduced thromboembolism and vaginal bleeding compared with tamoxifen (thromboembolic events: 4.8% with anastrozole *v* 7.3% with tamoxifen;[33] vaginal bleeding: 4.1% with anastrozole *v* 8.2% with tamoxifen;[34] significance not reported). **Letrozole versus tamoxifen:** The RCT found that the frequency of adverse events was similar with letrozole and tamoxifen.[36]

Comment: These RCTs[33,34,36,37] have confirmed that the selective third generation aromatase inhibitors**G** are at least as effective as tamoxifen, with a similar, if not better, safety profile. These treatments may, therefore, replace tamoxifen as the first line**G** endocrine treatment of choice for postmenopausal women with oestrogen receptor positive metastatic breast cancer. Results from the letrozole trials suggest an early survival advantage for women treated with letrozole rather than tamoxifen, which was not seen on further follow up owing to the prospective crossover of a large number of participants at progression (51% from the letrozole group and 49% from the tamoxifen group).[36] Subgroup analysis of 562 women with normal *HER2/neu* oncogene expression included in one RCT[38] found that letrozole significantly increased objective response rates and time to progression compared with tamoxifen, but subgroup analysis of 398 women with elevated *HER2/neu* oncogene expression found no significant difference in objective response rates between letrozole and tamoxifen.[36]

QUESTION **What are the effects of second line hormonal treatment in women who have not responded to tamoxifen?**

OPTION **PROGESTINS**

RCTs found that, in postmenopausal women with metastatic breast cancer who had relapsed on adjuvant tamoxifen or progressed during first line treatment with tamoxifen, progestins were less effective in prolonging survival as second line treatment than selective aromatase inhibitors and were associated with more adverse effects.

Benefits: **Versus selective aromatase inhibitors:** See benefits of selective aromatase inhibitors in postmenopausal women, p 2207.

Harms: **Versus selective aromatase inhibitors:** See harms of selective aromatase inhibitors in postmenopausal women, p 2208.

Comment: In women who are not responding to tamoxifen, progestins**G** may have a role in increasing feelings of wellbeing and relieving anorexia.

OPTION SELECTIVE AROMATASE INHIBITORS IN POSTMENOPAUSAL WOMEN

RCTs found that, in postmenopausal women with metastatic breast cancer who had relapsed on adjuvant tamoxifen or progressed during first line treatment with tamoxifen, the selective aromatase inhibitors anastrozole, letrozole, and exemestane prolonged survival compared with progestins (megestrol) or non-selective aromatase inhibitors (aminoglutethimide), with fewer adverse effects. Two RCTs found no significant difference between anastrozole and fulvestrant in time to progression. The evidence suggests that selective aromatase inhibitors are most effective in oestrogen receptor positive women.

Benefits: **Anastrozole versus progestins (megestrol):** A meta-analysis of the two randomised phase III trials comparing anastrozole versus megestrol (764 postmenopausal women with metastatic breast cancer unresponsive to tamoxifen, median age 65 years, 70% oestrogen receptor positive, 30% oestrogen receptor status unknown) found no significant difference in objective response rates (10.3% with anastrozole v 7.9% with megestrol), or in the proportion of women whose disease was stabilised for 6 months (25.1% with anastrozole v 26.1% with megestrol, significance not stated).[39] **Anastrozole versus antioestrogens (fulvestrant):** We found two RCTs comparing anastrozole versus fulvestrant.[40,41] The first RCT (400 postmenopausal women with locally advanced or metastatic breast cancer who had progressed on endocrine treatment) found that fulvestrant increased time to progression🅖 compared with anastrozole, although the difference was not significant (median time to progression: 5.4 months with fulvestrant v 3.4 months with anastrozole; proportion of people who had disease progression over a median 16.8 months: 83.5% with fulvestrant v 86.1% with anastrozole; HR 0.92, 95% CI 0.74 to 1.14).[40] Among 70 women who responded to treatment, fulvestrant increased the duration of response compared with anastrozole (19.0 months with fulvestrant v 10.8 months with anastrozole; P = 0.01). The second RCT (451 postmenopausal women with locally advanced or metastatic breast cancer who had progressed on endocrine treatment) found no significant difference between fulvestrant and anastrozole in time to progression (median time to progression: 5.5 months with fulvestrant v 5.1 months with anastrozole; HR 0.98, 95% CI 0.80 to 1.21).[41] **Exemestane versus progestins (megestrol):** One RCT (769 women) found that exemestane significantly improved median survival time, median duration of treatment success, and time to progression compared with megestrol (median survival time: not reached with exemestane v 123 weeks with megestrol; P = 0.039; median duration of overall success [complete response🅖/partial response🅖 or stable disease ≥24 weeks]: 60.1 weeks with exemestane v 49.1 weeks with megestrol; P = 0.025; time to tumour progression: 20.3 weeks with exemestane v 16.6 weeks with megestrol; P = 0.037).[42] Compared with megestrol, there were similar or greater improvements in pain control, tumour related signs and symptoms, and quality of life with exemestane.[42] **Letrozole versus progestins (megestrol) or non-selective aromatase inhibitors (aminoglutethimide):** We found two large RCTs comparing letrozole 0.5 or 2.5 mg versus megestrol (551 women)[43] and versus aminoglutethimide (555 women).[44] Both RCTs were in postmenopausal women with metastatic breast cancer unresponsive to tamoxifen (median age 64–65 years, 55% oestrogen receptor positive, 45% oestrogen receptor status unknown). The first RCT found that letrozole 2.5 mg significantly increased the response rate, duration of response, and time to treatment failure compared with megestrol ($P < 0.05$ for all outcomes).[43] The second RCT found that letrozole improved overall survival and progression rates compared with aminoglutethimide (overall survival: HR 0.64, 95% CI 0.49 to 0.85; progression: HR 0.72, 95% CI 0.57 to 0.92).[44]

Harms: The selective aromatase inhibitors**G** were generally well tolerated and associated with fewer adverse events than aminoglutethimide or progestins**G**. **Anastrozole:** In the RCTs, anastrozole 1 mg increased minor gastrointestinal disturbance (nausea or change in bowel habit) compared with megestrol (29% with anastrozole *v* 21% with megestrol; $P = 0.005$). However, it reduced weight gain (AR for ≥ 5% weight gain: 13% with anastrozole *v* 34% with megestrol; $P < 0.0001$).[39] The RCTs comparing anastrozole versus fulvestrant found that both treatments were well tolerated.[40,41] The first RCT found that the proportion of women who had hot flushes was similar in both groups (23.5% with fulvestrant *v* 24.9% with anastrozole; CI not reported).[40] The second RCT reported that 1.3% of people stopped anastrozole because of adverse effects compared with 3.2% taking fulvestrant (CI not reported).[41] The incidence of weight gain (1.5% with fulvestrant *v* 1.6% with anastrozole), vaginitis (3.4% with fulvestrant *v* 2.6% with anastrozole), and thromboembolic disease (3.4% with fulvestrant *v* 6.7% with anastrozole) was low in both groups (CI not reported for any outcome).[41] Joint disorders (including arthritis, arthralgia, and arthrosis) were reported by 9.3% of people taking fulvestrant and 13.5% of people taking anastrozole (CI not reported). **Exemestane:** The RCT found that progestin (megestrol) increased adverse events compared with exemestane (45.8% with megestrol *v* 39.1% with exemestane). The most frequently reported adverse events with exemestane were low grade hot flushes (12.6%), nausea (9.2%), and fatigue (7.5%).[42] Both drugs were well tolerated, although grade 3 or 4 weight changes (> 10% weight gain) were more common with megestrol (17.1% with megestrol *v* 7.6% with exemestane; $P = 0.001$). **Letrozole:** The first RCT found that, compared with megestrol, letrozole 2.5 mg significantly reduced the proportion of women who had serious cardiovascular adverse events (10% with letrozole *v* 29% with megestrol; ARR 19%, 95% CI 11% to 27%). It found no significant difference in weight gain, although fewer women taking letrozole had weight gain (≥ 10% weight gain: 6% with letrozole *v* 11% with megestrol; reported as non-significant, CI not reported).[43] The second RCT found that fewer women taking letrozole 2.5 mg had skin rash and serious drug related adverse events compared with women taking aminoglutethimide (skin rash: 3% with letrozole *v* 11% with aminoglutethimide; serious drug related adverse events: 0% with letrozole *v* 3% with aminoglutethimide; CI not reported).[44]

Comment: The evidence indicates greater efficacy and tolerability of anastrozole and letrozole over megestrol acetate or aminoglutethimide, especially in women with oestrogen receptor positive tumours. There is a consensus that they are agents of choice as second line**G** hormonal treatment in postmenopausal women no longer responding to tamoxifen. Exemestane is currently being evaluated in phase III trials.[45] A phase II trial conducted in 2000 evaluated the activity of exemestane in metastatic breast cancer after failure of other non-steroidal aromatase inhibitors**G**.[46] A total of 241 people were enrolled; 56% had received aminoglutethimide, 19% anastrozole, and 17% letrozole. Exemestane produced objective responses in 7% of treated women, including 8% of women after failure of treatment with aminoglutethimide and 5% after failure of other non-steroidal aromatase inhibitors (anastrozole, letrozole, and vorozole), and an overall success rate (complete response plus partial response plus no change for ≥ 24 weeks) of 24%. Women who do not respond to anastrozole or letrozole may respond to exemestane.

QUESTION What are the effects of first line chemotherapy?

OPTION NON-TAXANE COMBINATION CHEMOTHERAPY

We found no RCTs comparing non-taxane combination chemotherapy versus palliative care in women with metastatic breast cancer. Trials comparing one type of chemotherapy versus another found that first line chemotherapy was associated with an objective tumour response in 40–60% of women, with a median response duration of 6–12 months irrespective of menopausal or oestrogen receptor status. A small proportion of women achieve complete remission, which may persist for an extended length of time (see high dose versus standard dose chemotherapy, p 2212). One systematic review found that classical non-taxane combination chemotherapy (CMF) as first line treatment increased response rate and survival compared with modified CMF regimens. RCTs found that combination chemotherapy regimens containing an anthracycline, such as doxorubicin (CAF), as first line treatment increased response rates, time to progression, and survival compared with other regimens. One systematic review found no significant difference in survival at 12 or 24 months between first line non-taxane combination chemotherapy and hormonal treatment with antioestrogens or progestins. The review suggested that hormonal treatment may be preferable to chemotherapy as first line treatment in women with oestrogen receptor positive disease unless disease is rapidly progressing. It found that chemotherapy increased response rates, but also increased nausea, vomiting, and alopecia compared with hormonal treatment. One systematic review found that non-taxane combination chemotherapy as first or second line treatment was less effective than taxane based combination chemotherapy in increasing overall survival, time to progression, and overall response. It found no significant difference in overall survival if the analysis was restricted to RCTs of first line chemotherapy.

Benefits: We found no systematic review and no RCTs comparing first line chemotherapy versus palliative (best supportive) care in women with metastatic breast cancer. We found two systematic reviews (search date 1997,[20] 189 RCTs, 31 510 women; search date not reported,[47] 5 RCTs, 1088 people) and two subsequent RCTs[48,49] evaluating different non-taxane combination chemotherapy regimens; these are discussed further below. **"Classical" versus modified CMF:** In the largest RCT identified by the first review[20] (254 postmenopausal women with metastatic breast cancer who had received no prior chemotherapy), the classical CMF regimen significantly improved survival and response rate compared with a modified version, in which all three drugs were given intravenously every 3 weeks (response rate: 48% with classical CMF *v* 29% with the modified version; P = 0.03; median survival: 17 months with classical CMF *v* 12 months with the modified version; P = 0.016).[50] Another RCT identified by the review[20] (133 women who had received no prior chemotherapy) found that standard dose CMF significantly improved both response rate (30% with standard dose *v* 11% with low dose; P = 0.03) and symptom control compared with low dose CMF.[51] **CAF versus non-anthracycline based regimens:** The second review (5 RCTs, 1088 people) found that CAF regimens increased response rate (HR 0.56, 95% CI 0.43 to 0.73), time to progression (HR 0.69, 95% CI 0.59 to 0.81), and survival (HR 0.78,

95% CI 0.67 to 0.90) compared with non-anthracycline based regimens.[47] However, two of the included RCTs found no evidence of improved survival.[52,53] **Standard versus modified CAF regimens:** Two large multicentre trials identified by the first review[20] comparing CAF (containing doxorubicin) versus FEC**G**, a modified anthracycline based regimen containing epirubicin, found no significant difference in response rates (263 women, response rate 52% with CAF *v* 50% with FEC;[54] 497 women, response rate 56% with CAF *v* 54% with FEC[55]). One subsequent RCT (249 women) comparing standard CAF (containing doxorubicin) versus a modified, better tolerated, anthracycline based regimen containing mitoxantrone (mitozantrone) found that the regimen containing doxorubicin significantly prolonged the time to progression (3.2 months with regimen containing mitoxantrone *v* 5.3 months with regimen containing doxorubicin; P = 0.03) and increased median survival (10.9 months with regimen containing mitoxantrone *v* 15.2 months with regimen containing doxorubicin; P = 0.003).[48] **CAF or modified CAF versus mitoxantrone plus vinorelbine (MV):** One subsequent RCT (281 women) comparing MV versus either CAF or FEC found no significant difference in response rates among treatments (35% with MV *v* 33% with CAF or FEC).[49] Subgroup analysis in women who had received prior adjuvant treatment**G** found that MV significantly improved response rate and progression free survival**G** compared with other treatments (response rate: 33% with MV *v* 13% with CAF or FEC; P = 0.025; progression free survival: 9 months with MV *v* 6 months with CAF or FEC; P = 0.014).[49] **Versus hormonal treatment (antioestrogens or progestins):** We found one systematic review (search date 2002, 10 RCTs, total number of women not reported) comparing chemotherapy alone versus hormonal treatment**G** alone.[56] It found no significant difference in survival at 12 or 24 months (6 RCTs, 112/349 [32%] with chemotherapy *v* 104/330 [31%] with hormonal treatment; HR 1.03, 95% CI 0.74 to 1.43; see comment below).[56] It found that chemotherapy significantly increased response rates compared with hormonal treatment (7 RCTs, 767 women, 131/374 [35%] with chemotherapy *v* 110/393 [28%] with hormonal treatment; RR 1.25, 95% CI 1.01 to 1.54; see comment below). **Versus taxane based combination chemotherapy:** See benefits of taxane based combination chemotherapy as first line treatment, p 2212.

Harms: **Different non-taxane combination chemotherapy regimens:** The toxicity profiles of different combination chemotherapy**G** regimens vary. In RCTs, anthracycline based regimens (CAF**G**) and non-anthracycline based regimens (CMF**G**) are equally associated with haematological toxicity,[53] but CAF is more likely to be associated with alopecia (34% with CAF *v* 22% with CMF) and severe nausea and vomiting (17% with CAF *v* 7% with CMF; P = 0.05). Other studies reported the incidence of greater than grade 3 alopecia (complete hair loss) to be 55–61% with CAF, which was significantly higher than with either mitoxantrone or epirubicin (FEC**G**).[48,55] In one of the trials comparing CAF versus FEC, FEC was associated with fewer episodes of grade 2 or greater neutropenia (10% with FEC *v* 13.1% with CAF), and significantly lower rates of nausea and vomiting (7.8% with FEC *v* 13.3% with CAF; P < 0.01), and no cardiotoxicity (8 women taking CAF discontinued treatment because of cardiac dysfunction compared with none taking FEC).[54] MV was associated with less nausea and vomiting and alopecia than CAF or FEC, although myelosuppression was greater (P = 0.001). **Versus hormonal treatment (antioestrogens or progestins):** The review reported little information on adverse effects.[56] Six RCTs included in the review found that more people receiving chemotherapy had nausea, vomiting, and alopecia than people taking hormonal treatment**G** (CI not reported). **Versus taxane based combination chemotherapy:** See harms of taxane based combination chemotherapy as first line treatment, p 2212.

Comment: Trials comparing one type of chemotherapy versus another found that first line**G** chemotherapy was associated with an objective tumour response in 40–60% of women, with a median response duration of 6–12 months irrespective of menopausal or oestrogen receptor status. A small proportion of women achieve complete remission, which may persist for an extended length of time (see high dose versus standard dose chemotherapy, p 2212). **Versus hormonal treatment (antioestrogens or progestins):** The choice of first line treatment**G** (hormonal or chemotherapy**G**) is based on a variety of clinical factors (see table 1, p 2225).[8–11] The systematic review found significant heterogeneity among the trials analysed for response rates (P = 0.0009).[56] The review suggested that, in women with oestrogen receptor positive disease, hormonal treatment**G** may be recommended except in women with rapidly progressing disease.[56] In one RCT (231 women having first line treatment, 60% oestrogen receptor positive, 40% oestrogen receptor status unknown), women were randomised to receive either chemotherapy (CAF**G**) or chemotherapy plus hormonal treatment (CAF plus tamoxifen and fluoxymesterone). Response rates and time to treatment failure were similar for women who received chemo–hormonal treatment compared with chemotherapy alone (time to treatment failure 13.4 months with chemo–hormonal treatment *v* 10.3 months with chemotherapy; P = 0.087).[57] The effect on time to treatment failure was just significant for women who were oestrogen receptor positive compared with those who were negative (17.4 months for oestrogen receptor positive *v* 10.3 months for oestrogen receptor negative; P = 0.048). Oestrogen receptor status had no effect on overall survival. The choice of a specific drug or regimen is based on which drugs have already been given as adjuvant treatment**G**, together with the likelihood of benefit balanced against a given drug's adverse effects and tolerability profile. Retrospective series in sequential decades (from 1950–1980) have assessed the effect of chemotherapy on the survival of women from the time of diagnosis with metastatic breast cancer. They suggest that the introduction of chemotherapy has improved median survival by about 9 months (from 12 months without treatment to 21 months with treatment).[7,58] This median survival conceals a bimodal distribution of benefit, with the 40–60% of women who respond to treatment achieving survival of 1 year or greater and the non-responders experiencing little or no survival benefit. With the increasing use of adjuvant chemotherapy,[59] more women who develop metastatic disease will have received combination chemotherapy. In the treatment of metastatic breast cancer, better quality of life scores predict better outcome (this is not the case in adjuvant treatment).[60] In one RCT (283 women with metastatic breast cancer) evaluating quality of life as a primary end point, no significant differences were found between women randomised to receive either docetaxel or sequential methotrexate and fluorouracil. This suggests that the choice of treatment should be based on expected clinical effect.[61] This may influence the likelihood of response to further treatment.[61,62] The prevention of nausea and vomiting caused by chemotherapy has been studied in one RCT (619 women).[63] It compared placebo versus dexamethasone versus dexamethasone plus ondansetron after chemotherapy. In people who did not have acute nausea and vomiting with chemotherapy, dexamethasone alone was found to provide adequate protection against delayed nausea and vomiting.[63] **Duration of chemotherapy:** The optimal duration of chemotherapy for metastatic breast cancer is unknown, although a more recent systematic review (search date not stated; 65 publications reporting 97 treatment comparisons) has found that more, rather than fewer, cycles of chemotherapy given at appropriate doses improved survival (ratio of median survivals 1.23, 95% CI 1.01 to 1.49; P = 0.01).[64]

OPTION TAXANE BASED COMBINATION CHEMOTHERAPY

One systematic review found that taxane based combination chemotherapy as first or second line treatment increased overall survival, time to progression, and overall response compared with non-taxane combination chemotherapy. It found no significant difference in overall survival if the analysis was restricted to RCTs of first line chemotherapy.

Benefits: **Versus non-taxane combination chemotherapy:** We found one systematic review (search date 2003, 20 RCTs), which compared taxane based**G** versus non-taxane based combination chemotherapy**G** for first**G** or second line**G** treatment.[65] Twelve RCTs assessed progression free**G** and overall survival. The review found that taxane containing combination chemotherapy as first or second line treatment significantly increased overall survival compared with non-taxane based chemotherapy (AR for mortality: 1397/1947 [72%] with taxane based *v* 1262/1696 [75%] with non-taxane based; HR 0.90, 95% CI 0.84 to 0.97).[65] It found that, compared with non-taxane based combination chemotherapy, taxanes as first or second line treatment significantly increased time to progression**G** (HR 0.87, 95% CI 0.81 to 0.93) and response rates (OR 1.29, 95% CI 1.13 to 1.47). The review found no significant difference in overall survival if the analysis was restricted to RCTs of first line chemotherapy (6 RCTs; HR 0.92, 95% CI 0.84 to 1.02).

Harms: The review found that taxane based combination chemotherapy**G** was associated with more neurotoxicity and alopecia than non-taxane based regimens.[65]

Comment: The review found no significant heterogeneity among the trials included in the analysis of overall survival.[65] However, it found significant heterogeneity among the trials included in the analysis of time to progression**G** and response rates ($P < 0.00001$), probably reflecting the varying efficacy of the comparator regimens used in the trials. When all trials are considered, taxane containing regimens seem to improve overall survival, time to progression, and overall response in women with metastatic breast cancer. The degree of heterogeneity encountered indicates that taxane containing regimens are more effective than some, but not all, non-taxane containing regimens.

OPTION HIGH DOSE VERSUS STANDARD DOSE CHEMOTHERAPY

One systematic review found no significant difference in overall survival over 1–5 years between high dose chemotherapy (requiring haematopoietic transplant) and standard dose chemotherapy. It found that high dose chemotherapy increased treatment related morbidity and mortality compared with standard chemotherapy.

Benefits: We found one systematic review (search date 2002; 5 RCTs of first line**G** high dose chemotherapy**G** plus bone marrow or stem cell transplant; 740 women).[66] It found that high dose chemotherapy significantly increased progression free survival**G** at 1 and 2 years compared with standard dose chemotherapy (at 2 years: RR 1.96, 95%

CI 1.32 to 2.90). It found no significant difference in progression free survival at 3 or 5 years (at 5 years: RR 1.21, 95% CI 0.40 to 3.69). It found no significant difference between high and standard dose chemotherapy in overall survival at 1, 2, 3, or 5 years (at 5 years: RR 1.28, 95% CI 0.72 to 2.27).

Harms: The review found that high dose chemotherapy**G** significantly increased treatment related death compared with standard dose chemotherapy (10/382 [2.6%] with high dose *v* 0/358 [0%] with standard dose; RR 5.70, 95% CI 1.30 to 25.00).[66] It found that high dose chemotherapy significantly increased leucopenia, diarrhoea, cardiotoxicity, thrombocytopenia, and anaemia (leucopenia: RR 1.97, 95% CI 1.58 to 2.45; diarrhoea: RR 22.00, 95% CI 3.05 to 159.00; cardiotoxicity: RR 3.15, 95% CI 1.15 to 8.59; thrombocytopenia: RR 19.50, 95% CI 7.49 to 50.80; anaemia: RR 11.30, 95% CI 4.80 to 26.80).[66]

Comment: Fifteen years' follow up of women with metastatic breast cancer treated with standard dose FAC**G** found that 263/1581 (16.6%) women achieved a complete response**G** and that median time to progression**G** was 2 years; 19% of these women remained free of disease at 5 years.[18] Any long term remissions associated with high dose chemotherapy**G** in metastatic disease must be interpreted in the context of these figures. It remains to be seen if certain women, for example those with a complete response after standard dose chemotherapy, may benefit from subsequent high dose chemotherapy.[67,68]

QUESTION What are the effects of first line chemotherapy in combination with a monoclonal antibody?

OPTION STANDARD CHEMOTHERAPY PLUS TRASTUZUMAB

One RCT found that, in women whose tumours overexpress the *HER2/neu* oncogene, standard chemotherapy plus the monoclonal antibody trastuzumab as first line treatment increased the time to disease progression, objective response, and overall survival compared with standard chemotherapy alone. The most serious adverse effect observed was cardiac dysfunction in women who received an anthracycline plus trastuzumab.

Benefits: **Versus chemotherapy alone:** One RCT (469 women with *HER2/neu* oncogene overexpression) compared standard chemotherapy**G** alone versus standard chemotherapy plus trastuzumab.[69] Women who had not previously received postoperative chemotherapy with an anthracycline were treated with doxorubicin (or epirubicin) and cyclophosphamide with or without trastuzumab. Women who had previously received postoperative anthracycline were treated with paclitaxel with or without trastuzumab. Adding trastuzumab to chemotherapy significantly prolonged the time to disease progression (7.4 months with trastuzumab plus chemotherapy *v* 4.6 months with chemotherapy; $P < 0.001$), increased objective response (50% with trastuzumab plus chemotherapy *v* 32% with chemotherapy; $P < 0.001$), and improved overall survival (25.1 months with trastuzumab plus chemotherapy *v* 20.3 months with chemotherapy alone; $P = 0.046$).[69] We found one subsequent report of this RCT comparing trastuzumab plus chemotherapy versus chemotherapy alone.[70] It reported on quality of life among 400 of the enrolled 469 women and found that trastuzumab plus chemotherapy significantly improved reported global quality of life scores compared with chemotherapy alone (percentage of people with a ≥ 10-point improvement in the European Organisation for Research and Treatment Care Quality of Life Questionnaire score [scale 0–100]: 51% with trastuzumab plus chemotherapy *v* 36% with chemotherapy alone; $P < 0.05$).

Harms: **Versus chemotherapy alone:** Symptomatic or asymptomatic cardiac dysfunction occurred in 27% of women given anthracycline plus cyclophosphamide plus trastuzumab compared with 8% given anthracycline plus cyclophosphamide alone, 13% given paclitaxel plus trastuzumab, and 1% given paclitaxel alone.[69] Symptoms usually improved with standard medical management, although two women died from heart failure (one in the anthracycline plus cyclophosphamide plus trastuzumab group and one in the anthracycline plus cyclophosphamide alone group). About 25% of women had chills, fever, or both during the initial infusion; no episodes of anaphylaxis occurred.

Comment: Trastuzumab based combination treatment was effective at reducing the relative risk of death by 20% at a median follow up of 30 months. Few studies have shown that adding a single agent improves survival to this degree. Cardiac toxicity seems only to be significant in people concurrently receiving an anthracycline. The most appropriate treatment duration in responders is unclear. We found one RCT comparing two different dosing regimens of trastuzumab as first line treatment**G** in 114 women with *HER2/neu* oncogene overexpressing metastatic breast cancer. It found no significant difference between the high dose regimen (8 mg/kg loading dose followed by 4 mg/kg weekly) and low dose regimen (4 mg/kg loading dose followed by 2 mg/kg weekly) for time to progression**G** or time to death (median time to progression: 3.5 months with high dose [95% CI 3.3 months to 5.5 months] *v* 3.8 months with low dose [95% CI 2.4 months to 5.5 months]; median survival: 22.9 months with high dose [95% CI 16.0 months to 37.1 months] *v* 25.8 months with low dose [95% CI 13.3 months to 34.7 months]).[71] Adverse effects included asthenia (23%), fever (22%), nausea (14%), and cardiac dysfunction (2%).

QUESTION What are the effects of second line chemotherapy?

OPTION TAXANE BASED COMBINATION CHEMOTHERAPY

One systematic review has found that taxane based combination chemotherapy as first or second line treatment increased overall survival, time to progression, and overall response compared with non-taxane combination chemotherapy. The difference remained significant if the analysis was limited to women who had previously received anthracyclines. One RCT found no significant difference in progression or overall survival between docetaxel and 5-fluorouracil plus vinorelbine or between paclitaxel and capecitabine given as second line chemotherapy.

Benefits: **Versus non-taxane combination chemotherapy:** We found one systematic review (search date 2003, 20 RCTs), which compared taxane based**G** versus non-taxane based**G** combination chemotherapy**G** for first**G** or second line**G** treatment.[65] Twelve RCTs assessed progression free**G** and overall survival. The review found that taxane containing combination chemotherapy as first or second line treatment significantly increased overall survival compared with non-taxane based chemotherapy (AR for mortality: 1397/1947 [72%] with taxane based *v* 1262/1696 [75%] with non-taxane based; HR 0.90, 95% CI 0.84 to 0.97).[65] It found that this difference remained significant if the analysis was restricted to women who had previously received anthracyclines (5 RCTs, 403/568 [71%] with taxane based *v* 422/555 [76%] with non-taxane based; HR 0.87, 95% CI 0.76 to 0.99). **Versus semisynthetic vinca alkaloids:** One RCT (176 women after anthracycline treatment failure) identified by the review[65] compared docetaxel versus 5-fluorouracil plus vinorelbine.[72] It found no significant difference between treatments in time to progression**G** or overall survival (median time to progression: 5.1 months with docetaxel *v* 6.5 months with 5-fluorouracil plus vinorelbine; P = 0.34; median overall survival: 16.0 months with docetaxel *v* 15.0 months with 5-fluorouracil plus vinorelbine; P value not reported).[72] **Versus capecitabine:** See benefits of capecitabine, p 2216.

Harms: **Versus non-taxane combination chemotherapy:** The review found that taxane based chemotherapyⒼ was associated with more neurotoxicity and alopecia than non-taxane based regimens.[65] **Versus semisynthetic vinca alkaloids:** The RCT found that 5-fluorouracil plus vinorelbine significantly increased severe thrombocytopenia and severe stomatitis compared with docetaxel (severe thrombocytopenia: 10% with 5-fluorouracil plus vinorelbine *v* 1% with docetaxel, P = 0.02; severe stomatitis: 40% with 5-fluorouracil plus vinorelbine *v* 5% with docetaxel, P < 0.0001). Docetaxel significantly increased grade 3/4 neutropenia compared with 5-fluorouracil and vinorelbine (82% with 5-fluorouracil plus vinorelbine *v* 67% with docetaxel, P = 0.02).[72] **Versus capecitabine:** See harms of capecitabine, p 2216.

Comment: The taxanesⒼ, paclitaxel and docetaxel, have an established role as second line treatmentⒼ in metastatic breast cancer, especially in people with disease progression despite a previous anthracycline based regimen, with evidence in some RCTs for a survival advantage over other available options. Trials are in progress to determine the efficacy and tolerability of taxanes in combination with anthracyclines as first line treatmentⒼ, although there are concerns about cardiac toxicity. At present, the indication for docetaxel remains as a single drug for second line treatment, especially in anthracycline resistantⒼ disease, although definitive results on improvement in quality of life are awaited.

OPTION SEMISYNTHETIC VINCA ALKALOIDS

One RCT found no significant difference in progression or overall survival between 5-fluorouracil plus vinorelbine and docetaxel given as second line chemotherapy. Another RCT found that second line vinorelbine improved survival and reduced progression compared with melphalan. A third RCT found no significant difference in survival or quality of life between vinorelbine plus doxorubicin and doxorubicin alone.

Benefits: **Versus non-taxane chemotherapy:** One RCT (183 women with anthracycline resistantⒼ disease) found increased time to progressionⒼ and survival with vinorelbine 30 mg/m^2 weekly compared with intravenous melphalan (median survival 35 weeks with vinorelbine *v* 31 weeks with melphalan; P < 0.001).[73] **Plus non-taxane chemotherapy versus non-taxane chemotherapy alone:** We found one RCT (303 women, firstⒼ or second lineⒼ treatment, no previous vinca alkaloid or anthracycline treatment) comparing doxorubicin plus vinorelbine versus doxorubicin alone. The response rates, quality of life scores, and overall survival were not significantly improved with combined chemotherapyⒼ in this setting.[74] **Versus taxane based combination chemotherapy:** See benefits of taxane based combination chemotherapy, p 2214.

Harms: One RCT comparing vinorelbine versus anthracycline based chemotherapyⒼ (FACⒼ/FECⒼ) as firstⒼ or second lineⒼ treatment found that vinorelbine was associated with considerably lower rates of nausea (8% with vinorelbine *v* 16% with the anthracycline based regimen; P = 0.03) and grade 3 alopecia (7% with vinorelbine *v* 30% with the anthracycline based regimen; P = 0.0001), although haematological toxicity that delayed treatment was more frequent (27% with vinorelbine *v* 17% with the anthracycline based regimen).[75] **Versus taxane based combination chemotherapy:** See harms of taxane based combination chemotherapy, p 2215.

Breast cancer (metastatic)

Comment: One uncontrolled study of vinorelbine found an objective response rate of 31%, with less than 5% grade 3 or 4 toxicities.[76] It seems to have a favourable toxicity profile, but results from phase III trials are awaited. Vinorelbine plus protracted infusional fluorouracil is an active and well tolerated regimen (overall response rate: 61.4%, 95% CI 50.9% to 70.9%), and further trials are underway.[77] One uncontrolled study of vinorelbine plus gemcitabine twice weekly found an objective response rate of 54%.[78]

OPTION CAPECITABINE

One RCT found similar response rates and time to disease progression between capecitabine and paclitaxel after anthracycline failure.

Benefits: **Versus taxane based combination chemotherapy:** We found one systematic review (search date 2000) assessing the oral fluoropyrimidine capecitabine in metastatic breast cancer,[79] which identified one RCT (42 women) comparing capecitabine versus paclitaxel as second**G** or third line treatment after anthracycline failure. It found similar response rates and time to progression**G** between capacitabine and paclitaxel (response: 8/22 [36%] with capecitabine *v* 4/20 [20%] with paclitaxel; time to progression 92 days with capecitabine *v* 95 days with paclitaxel; CI not reported).

Harms: **Versus taxane based combination chemotherapy:** The most commonly reported grade 3/4 toxicities were hand–foot syndrome (13%), diarrhoea (12%), and stomatitis (4%).[79]

Comment: Promising activity has been seen with capecitabine in paclitaxel refractory, heavily pretreated women,[80] and the low toxicity profile, together with evidence of efficacy, all warrant further investigation of this drug as an alternative to more toxic second or third line chemotherapy**G** schedules. It has been suggested that the effectiveness of docetaxel may be increased by the addition of capecitabine,[81] and RCTs are underway.

QUESTION What are the effects of treatments for bone metastases?

OPTION BISPHOSPHONATES

RCTs in women receiving standard chemotherapy or hormonal treatment for bone metastases secondary to metastatic breast cancer found that bisphosphonates reduced and delayed skeletal complications compared with placebo. They found no significant difference in survival.

Benefits: **Plus standard treatment versus standard treatment alone:** We found one systematic review (search date not stated[82]) and one subsequent RCT.[83] The review (13 RCTs, 4395 women with metastatic breast cancer who had bone involvement) compared adding bisphosphonates**G** versus adding placebo to standard treatment (either chemotherapy**G** or hormonal treatment**G**).[82] It found that, compared with placebo, bisphosphonates**G** significantly reduced "skeletal events" (5 RCTs, 416/767 [54%] with bisphosphonates *v* 482/786 [61%] with placebo; RR 0.88, 95% CI 0.81 to 0.96). It found no significant difference in survival (8 RCTs, 594/815 [73%] with bisphosphonates *v* 624/841 [74%] with placebo; RR 0.99, 95% CI 0.93 to 1.04). "Skeletal events" were defined as: new bone metastases, pathological fractures, spinal cord compression, irradiation of or surgery on bone, or the development or progression of bone pain.[82] Four RCTs identified by the review found that bisphosphonates delayed the time to a first "skeletal event" compared with placebo ($P < 0.05$ in all 4 RCTs). One subsequent RCT (466 women) found that, compared with placebo, ibandronate (2 or 6 mg once every 3–4 weeks) reduced new bone events (2.65 events per patient with ibandronate 6 mg *v* 4.24 with ibandronate 2 mg *v* 3.64 events per patient with placebo; $P = 0.032$ for ibandronate 6 mg *v* placebo) and decreased bone pain scores over 2 years' treatment (reported as significant, results presented graphically, CI not reported).[83] **Versus radiotherapy:** We found no RCTs.

Harms: **Plus standard treatment versus standard treatment alone:** RCTs identified by the review suggested that bisphosphonates**G** were well tolerated with no serious adverse events in women treated for up to 2 years.[82] Fever and asymptomatic hypocalcaemia were the most commonly reported adverse effects in women receiving intravenous pamidronate. Mild gastrointestinal toxicity was the most frequently reported adverse effect of oral clodronate. In one RCT identified by the review, gastrointestinal toxicity (nausea and vomiting) was the cause of withdrawal in 25% of women taking oral pamidronate. The subsequent RCT found that three women taking ibandronate had serious adverse effects (asthenia, hydronephrosis, oedema, and bone pain) related to treatment.[83] **Versus radiotherapy:** We found no RCTs.

Comment: Large RCTs are in progress in the adjuvant setting to see whether these agents may delay or prevent the development of bone metastases. The American Society of Clinical Oncology released recent guidelines on the use of bisphosphonates**G**, stating that this treatment reduces the rate of bone complications (although not mortality) in women with lytic bone disease who may or may not also be receiving systemic treatment (chemotherapy**G** or endocrine treatment).[84] It remains unclear exactly when to start or stop treatment, which may affect the costs involved.[85] Although these effects are likely to improve quality of life, this outcome has not been formally evaluated. We found no evidence that bisphosphonates improve survival.

OPTION RADIOTHERAPY

We found no RCTs. We found limited evidence from non-randomised studies that persistent and localised bone pain can be treated successfully in over 80% of women with radiotherapy plus concomitant appropriate analgesia (from non-steroidal anti-inflammatory drugs to morphine and its derivatives) and that cranial nerve compression can be treated successfully with radiotherapy in 50–80% of people. RCTs found no evidence that short courses were less effective for pain relief than long courses of radiotherapy. One RCT found that different fractionation schedules can be used to treat neuropathic bone pain effectively.

Benefits: We found no systematic review and no RCTs comparing radiotherapy versus no treatment or bisphosphonates**G** (see comment below). **Pain control:** Questionnaire studies found that control of pain was successful in over 80% of women who received radiotherapy for bone metastases, with concomitant use of appropriate analgesia according to the World Health Organization ladder (this moves upwards from non-steroidal anti-inflammatory drugs and paracetamol to mild opiates through to morphine and its derivatives).[86] **Cranial nerve compression:** In people with skull base metastases causing cranial nerve involvement, retrospective studies suggest that radiotherapy leads to improvement in 50–80% of women, which is usually maintained.[87] **Different radiotherapy regimens:** We found two RCTs comparing different radiotherapy regimens. These found no significant difference between short courses (8 Gy as a single fraction) and longer courses (e.g. 20 Gy/5 fractions or 30 Gy/10 fractions).[88,89] Studies of accelerated fractionation schedules (e.g. twice daily treatments for 5 days) have failed to show any benefit over conventional regimens in the control of disease secondary to metastatic breast cancer.[90] Published interim results from one RCT (270 women) have found that different fractionation regimens can be used to treat neuropathic bone pain effectively.[91]

Harms: Adverse effects of radiotherapy for bone metastases include nausea and vomiting.[90] Higher dose fractions per day produce more toxic effects.

Comment: Randomised comparisons against no treatment or placebo would be considered unethical in palliative care, and even RCTs comparing one treatment versus another are difficult to undertake because it is reasonable to try many different options in order to make a woman comfortable. Rating of success of end of life care is difficult. Usual outcomes, such as response rates and survival duration, do not apply.[92]

QUESTION What are the effects of treatments for spinal cord metastases?

OPTION RADIOTHERAPY

We found no RCTs. Spinal cord compression is an emergency. Retrospective studies suggested that early radiotherapy improved outcomes. However, fewer than 10% of people walked again if severe deterioration of motor function occurred before radiotherapy. One small RCT in women with spinal cord compression found that adding high dose steroids to radiotherapy improved the chance of walking 6 months after treatment compared with radiotherapy alone.

Benefits: We found no systematic review or RCTs. Retrospective analyses found an improvement with early radiotherapy, but fewer than 10% of people walked again if severe deterioration of motor function occurred before radiotherapy.[93] **Addition of high dose steroids:** One blinded RCT (57 women) evaluated the addition of high dose steroids to radiotherapy. It found that more women were walking 6 months after receiving dexamethasone (96 mg intravenous bolus followed by 96 mg orally for 3 days) compared with those who received no steroids (59% with steroids *v* 33% with no steroids).[94]

Harms: **Addition of high dose steroids:** In the RCT of high dose steroids, significant adverse effects caused withdrawal from treatment in 11% of people.[94] Use of lower doses of glucocorticoids in the control of symptoms from cerebral metastases may result in short term agitation and the longer term development of Cushingoid facies.

Comment: See comment of radiotherapy for bone metastases, p 2218.

QUESTION What are the effects of treatments for cerebral metastases?

OPTION RADIOTHERAPY

We found no RCTs. Retrospective studies suggested that whole brain irradiation improved neurological function in some women with brain metastases secondary to breast cancer.

Benefits: We found no systematic review or RCTs. Retrospective studies suggested that whole brain irradiation produces general improvement in neurological function in 40–70% of women with brain metastases secondary to breast cancer.[95] **Different radiotherapy regimens:** One RCT (544 symptomatic people) that compared two whole brain radiotherapy schedules (30 Gy/10 fractions *v* 12 Gy/2 fractions) found no evidence that the response rate or duration of response in people with multiple brain metastases were improved with higher doses of radiation compared with the lower dose shorter regimen.[90]

Harms: Adverse effects of radiotherapy in the treatment of cerebral metastases include alopecia and somnolence.[90] Higher dose fractions per day produce more toxic effects.

Comment: See comment under radiotherapy for bone metastases, p 2218. There is a consensus that raised intracranial pressure associated with cerebral metastases is best managed by dexamethasone given immediately with anticonvulsants to control seizures if necessary.

OPTION SURGICAL RESECTION

We found no RCTs. One retrospective cohort study provided insufficient evidence to assess surgical resection in people with cerebral metastases.

Benefits: We found no RCTs. One retrospective cohort study nested in one RCT (859 women) found that there may be some beneficial effect on survival with surgical resection in a small subgroup of people (those with Karnofsky Performance Status 70–100, absent or controlled primary tumour, age < 60 years, and cerebral [not other] metastases).[96]

Harms: The cohort study gave no information on harms.[96]

Comment: None.

OPTION INTRATHECAL CHEMOTHERAPY OR RADIATION SENSITISERS

We found no RCTs or observational studies of intrathecal chemotherapy in people with cerebral metastases. We found no RCTs of radiation sensitisers. One open label case control study found limited evidence that adding intravenous RSR13, a radiation sensitiser, during whole brain radiotherapy may prolong survival.

Benefits: **Intrathecal chemotherapy:** We found no RCTs or observational studies of intrathecal chemotherapy**G**. **Radiation sensitisers:** We found no RCTs. One open label case control study (57 women) assessed mortality in women receiving a radiation sensitiser (RSR13) during radiotherapy compared with mortality in a database of women receiving radiotherapy alone. It found that significantly more women receiving RSR13 survived over 2 years than women receiving radiotherapy alone ($P = 0.0267$).[97]

Harms: **Intrathecal chemotherapy:** We found no RCTs or observational studies of sufficient quality of intrathecal chemotherapy**G**. **Radiation sensitisers:** RSR13 requires central line administration during the days when brain radiotherapy is given and seems to be associated with transient hypoxia in a subgroup.

Comment: None.

QUESTION What are the effects of treatments for choroidal metastases?

OPTION RADIOTHERAPY

We found no RCTs. Retrospective studies suggested that radiotherapy benefited some women with choroidal metastases.

Benefits: We found no systematic review and no RCTs. One prospective cohort study (56 people, 62% with breast cancer)[98] and one case series (32 women)[99] suggested that external beam radiotherapy at doses of about 40 Gy prevented functional loss and may increase visual acuity. Retrospective studies suggest that radiotherapy benefits 70% of people.[100]

Harms: People with choroidal metastases who are treated with radiotherapy may lose the sight in that eye. Optic atrophy and proliferative radiation retinopathy are possible late complications.

Comment: See comment of radiotherapy for bone metastases, p 2218. Generally, choroidal metastases occur later than metastases to other organs. Choroidal metastasis is considered a poor prognostic sign; most people die within 6 months of diagnosis. Systemic chemotherapy**G** can induce partial or complete remission of metastatic choroidal breast carcinoma.[101] Recent retrospective studies have shown that krypton red or argon green laser photocoagulation is feasible, easy, rapid, and effective for small choroidal breast carcinoma metastases.[102] Women with deteriorating vision are likely to benefit from emergency assessment and treatment for choroidal metastases.

GLOSSARY

Adjuvant treatment This usually refers to systemic chemotherapy, hormonal treatment, or both, taken after removal of a primary tumour (in this case, surgery for early breast cancer), with the aim of killing any remaining micrometastatic tumour cells and thus preventing recurrence.

Anthracycline resistance This applies to people who have received at least one chemotherapeutic regimen with anthracyclines (doxorubicin or epirubicin) in either an adjuvant setting or for metastatic disease. Primary resistance to an anthracycline is defined as progressive disease during or within 6 months after completion of adjuvant anthracycline. People without any documented tumour response to first line chemotherapy that included anthracyclines for metastatic disease are also classified as having primary resistance. Secondary resistance is defined as disease progression after a documented clinical response to first line chemotherapy with anthracyclines for metastatic disease. Secondary resistance can be divided further into three categories, as follows: (1) absolute resistance, or disease progression during treatment with regimens that contained anthracyclines after a period of response; (2) relative resistance, or disease progression within 6 months after completion of the chemotherapy; and (3) sensitive regrowth, or disease progression more than 6 months after completion of the chemotherapy.[103]

Aromatase inhibitors Drugs that block the conversion of androgens into oestrogens. Aminoglutethimide, anastrozole, and letrozole are non-steroidal aromatase inhibitors. Formestane and exemestane are steroidal aromatase inhibitors. Anastrozole, formestane, exemestane, and letrozole are selective inhibitors of oestrogen synthetase, which is a part of the aromatase enzyme system. Aminoglutethimide also inhibits adrenal steroid production. These drugs cause oestrogen suppression in postmenopausal women.

Bisphosphonates (pamidronate, clodronate) Bone specific palliative drugs that inhibit osteoclast induced bone resorption associated with breast cancer metastases.

Chemotherapy Treatment with cytotoxic drugs (see also non-taxane and taxane based combination chemotherapy regimens below).

Complete response Disappearance of all known lesions on two separate measurements at least 4 weeks apart.

Disease free interval Time between surgery for early breast cancer (see below) and metastatic breast cancer developing.

Early breast cancer Operable disease, restricted to the breast and sometimes to local lymph nodes.

First line treatment Initial treatment for a particular condition that has previously not been treated. For example, first line treatment for metastatic breast cancer may include chemotherapy, hormonal treatment, or both.

Gonadorelin analogues (Also called luteinising hormone releasing hormone [LHRH] agonists.) These are synthetic peptides that occupy the receptors for gonadorelin in the pituitary gland. Continuous administration of gonadorelin agonists may initially increase the release of luteinising hormone, but continuous administration blocks the physiological pulsatile luteinising hormone release, and this causes a fall in oestrogen levels.
Hormonal treatment Includes treatment with antioestrogens such as tamoxifen, aromatase inhibitors, and progestins.
Lymphangitis carcinomatosis dissemination of carcinoma in the lymphoid tissue of the lung.
Non-taxane combination chemotherapy regimens Use of different combinations of cytotoxic drugs: **CAF** Cyclophosphamide (500 mg/m^2 iv), doxorubicin (50 mg/m^2 iv), and fluorouracil (500 mg/m^2 iv) every 3 weeks for up to six cycles of treatment are given, depending on response. **Classical CMF** Cyclophosphamide (100 mg/m^2 orally days 1–14), methotrexate (40 mg/m^2 iv days 1 and 8), and fluorouracil (600 mg/m^2 iv days 1 and 8) every 4 weeks for up to six cycles of treatment are given, depending on response. **FAC** Fluorouracil, doxorubicin, and cyclophosphamide every 3 weeks for up to six cycles of treatment are given, depending on response. **FEC** Fluorouracil, epirubicin, and cyclophosphamide every 3 weeks for up to six cycles of treatment are given, depending on response.
Overall objective response rate The proportion of treated people in whom a complete (see above) or partial response (see below) is observed.
Partial response More than a 50% reduction in the size of lesions.
Progestins (medroxyprogesterone, megestrol) The antitumour effects of progestins may be mediated by a direct action on tumour cells, or an indirect effect on the pituitary–ovarian/adrenal axes.
Progression free survival (or time to progression) Interval between diagnosis of metastatic disease and diagnosis of progression.
Progressive disease More than a 25% increase in the size of lesions, or the appearance of new lesions.
Second line treatment Treatment given after relapse after first line treatment (see above).
Taxane based combination chemotherapy regimens Chemotherapy regimens containing taxanes such as paclitaxel and docetaxel, which are derived from the Pacific yew tree *Taxus brevifolia*.
Tumour flare Diffuse musculoskeletal pain and erythema with increased size of tumour lesions that later regress and which sometimes accompanies initial treatment with drugs such as antioestrogens. It is often accompanied by hypercalcaemia. It does not imply progression.

REFERENCES

1. Hortobagyi GN. Can we cure limited metastatic breast cancer? *J Clin Oncol* 2002;20:620–623.
2. Pisani P, Parkin DM, Ferlay J. Estimates of the worldwide mortality from eighteen major cancers in 1985. Implications for prevention and projections of future burden. *Int J Cancer* 1993;55:891–903.
3. Parkin MD. Global cancer statistics in the year 2000. *Lancet Oncol* 2001;2:533–543.
4. Early Breast Cancer Trialists' Collaborative Group. Polychemotherapy for early breast cancer: an overview of the randomised trials. *Lancet* 1998;352:930–942. Search date 1995; studies were identified using lists prepared by three international cancer research groups, by searching the international Cancer Research Data Bank, meeting abstracts, and references of published trials, and by consulting experts.
5. Slamon DJ, Clark GM, Wong SG, et al. Human breast cancer: correlation of relapse and survival with amplification of the HER-2/neu oncogene. *Science* 1987;235:177–182.
6. Rubens RD, Bajetta E, Bonneterre J, et al. Treatment of relapse of breast cancer after adjuvant systemic therapy. *Eur J Cancer* 1994;30A:106–111.
7. Cold S, Jensen NV, Brincker H, et al. The influence of chemotherapy on survival after recurrence in breast cancer: a population based study of patients treated in the 1950s, 1960s, and 1970s. *Eur J Cancer* 1993;29A:1146–1152.
8. Jackson IM, Litherland S, Wakeling AE. Tamoxifen and other antioestrogens. In: Powels TJ, Smith IE, eds. *Medical management of breast cancer*. London: Martin Dunitz, 1997:51–59.
9. Arafah BM, Pearson OH. Endocrine treatment of advanced breast cancer. In: Jordan VC, ed. *Estrogen/antiestrogen action and breast cancer therapy*. Madison: University of Wisconsin Press, 1986:417–429.
10. McGuire WL. Hormone receptors: their role in predicting prognosis and response to endocrine therapy. *Semin Oncol* 1978;5:428–443.
11. Kuss JT, Muss HB, Hoen H, et al. Tamoxifen as initial endocrine therapy for metastatic breast cancer: long term follow-up of two Piedmont Oncology Association (POA) trials. *Breast Cancer Res Treat* 1997;42:265–274.
12. Olsen O, Gotzsche PC. Cochrane review on screening for breast cancer with mammography. *Lancet* 2001;358:1340–1342.
13. Coates A, Gebski V, Signori D. Prognostic value of quality-of-life scores during chemotherapy for advanced breast cancer. *J Clin Oncol* 1992;10:1833–1838.

14. European Organisation for Research and Treatment of Cancer (EORTC). *A practical guide to EORTC studies*. Brussels: EORTC Data Center, 1996:126.
15. Miller AB, Hoogstraten B, Staquet M, et al. Reporting results of cancer treatment. *Cancer* 1981;47:207–214.
16. Baum M, Priestman T, West RR, et al. A comparison of subjective responses in a trial comparing endocrine with cytotoxic treatment in advanced carcinoma of the breast. In: Mouridsen HT, Palshof T, eds. *Breast cancer — experimental and clinical methods*. London: Pergamon Press, 1980:223–228.
17. Bernhard J, Thurlimann B, Schmitz SF, et al. Defining clinical benefit in postmenopausal patients with breast cancer under second-line endocrine treatment: does quality of life matter? *J Clin Oncol* 1999;17:1672–1679.
18. Greenberg PA, Hortobagyi GN, Smith TL, et al. Long-term follow-up of patients with complete remission following combination chemotherapy for metastatic breast cancer. *J Clin Oncol* 1996;14:2197–2205.
19. Geels P, Eisenhauer E, Bezjak A, et al. Palliative effect of chemotherapy: objective tumor response is associated with symptom improvement in patients with metastatic breast cancer. *J Clin Oncol* 2000;18:2395–2405.
20. Fossati R, Confalonieri C, Torri V, et al. Cytotoxic and hormonal treatment for metastatic breast cancer: a systematic review of published randomised trials involving 31 510 women. *J Clin Oncol* 1998;16:3439–3460. Search date 1997; primary sources Medline, Embase, and hand searches of reference lists from retrieved articles and lists from relevant meetings.
21. Litherland S, Jackson IM. Antioestrogens in the management of hormone-dependent cancer. *Cancer Treat Rev* 1988;15:183–194.
22. Johnston SR. Acquired tamoxifen resistance in human breast cancer — potential mechanisms and clinical implications. *Anticancer Drugs* 1997;8:911–930.
23. Hayes DF, Van Zyl JA, Goedhals L, et al. Randomised comparison of tamoxifen and two separate doses of toremifene in postmenopausal patients with metastatic breast cancer. *J Clin Oncol* 1995;13:2556–2566.
24. Parazzini F, Colli E, Scatigna M, et al. Treatment with tamoxifen and progestins for metastatic breast cancer in postmenopausal women: a quantitative review of published randomised clinical trials. *Oncology* 1993;50:483–489. Search date 1991; primary sources Medline and hand searches of reference lists of articles identified.
25. Muss HB, Case DL, Atkins JN, et al. Tamoxifen versus high-dose oral medroxyprogesterone acetate as initial endocrine therapy for patients with metastatic breast cancer: a Piedmont Oncology Association study. *J Clin Oncol* 1994;12:1630–1638.
26. Pannutti F, Martoni A, Zamagni C, et al. Progestins. In: Powles TJ, Smith IE, eds. *Medical management of breast cancer*. London: Martin Dunitz, 1997:95–107.
27. Pannuti F, Martoni A, Murari G, et al. Analgesic activity of medroxyprogesterone acetate in cancer patients: an anti-inflammatory mediated activity? *Int J Tissue React* 1985;7:505–508.
28. Crump M, Sawka CA, DeBoer G, et al. An individual patient-based meta-analysis of tamoxifen versus ovarian ablation as first-line endocrine therapy for premenopausal women with metastatic breast cancer. *Breast Cancer Res Treat* 1997;44:201–210. Search date not stated; primary sources Medline, Cancerlit, hand searches of bibliographies of related publications, and personal contact with principal investigators of unpublished trials.
29. Sawka CA, Pritchard KI, Shelley W, et al. A randomised crossover trial of tamoxifen versus ovarian ablation for metastatic breast cancer in premenopausal women: a report of the National Cancer Institute of Canada clinical trials group trial MA1. *Breast Cancer Res Treat* 1997;44:211–215.
30. Taylor CW, Green S, Dalton WS, et al. Multicenter randomised clinical trial of goserelin versus surgical ovariectomy in premenopausal patients with receptor-positive metastatic breast cancer: an intergroup study. *J Clin Oncol* 1998;16:994–999.
31. Boccardo F, Rubagotti A, Perotta A, et al. Ovarian ablation versus goserelin with or without tamoxifen in pre-perimenopausal patients with advanced breast cancer: results of a multicentric Italian study. *Ann Oncol* 1994;5:337–342.
32. Klijn JG, Blamey RW, Boccardo F, et al. Combined tamoxifen and luteinising hormone-releasing hormone (LHRH) agonist versus LHRH agonist alone in premenopausal advanced breast cancer: a meta-analysis of four randomised trials. *J Clin Oncol* 2001;19:343–353.
33. Bonneterre J, Thurlimann B, Robertson JFR, et al. Anastrozole versus tamoxifen as first-line therapy for advanced breast cancer in 668 postmenopausal women: results of the tamoxifen or arimidex randomised group efficacy and tolerability study. *J Clin Oncol* 2000;18:3748–3757.
34. Nabholtz JM, Buzdar A, Pollak M, et al. Anastrozole is superior to tamoxifen as first-line therapy for advanced breast cancer in postmenopausal women: results of a North American multicentre randomised trial. *J Clin Oncol* 2000;18:3758–3767.
35. Nabholtz JM, Bonneterre J, Buzdar A, et al. Anastrozole (Arimidex) versus tamoxifen as first-line therapy for advanced breast cancer in postmenopausal women: survival analysis and updated safety results. *Eur J Cancer* 2003;39:1684–1689.
36. Mouridsen H, Gershanovich M, Sun Y, et al. Phase III study of letrozole versus tamoxifen as first-line therapy of advanced breast cancer in postmenopausal women: analysis of survival and update of efficacy from the International Letrozole Breast Cancer Group. *J Clin Oncol* 2003;21:2101–2109.
37. Mouridsen H, Gershanovich M, Sun Y, et al. Superior efficacy of letrozole (Femara) versus tamoxifen as first-line therapy for postmenopausal women with advanced breast cancer: results of a phase III study of the International Letrozole Breast Cancer Group. *J Clin Oncol* 2001:19;2596–2606.
38. Lipton A, Ali SM, Leitzel K, et al. Serum HER-2/neu and response to the aromatase inhibitor letrozole versus tamoxifen. *J Clin Oncol* 2003;21:1967–1972.
39. Buzdar A, Jonat W, Howell A, et al. Anastrozole, a potent and selective aromatase inhibitor, versus megestrol acetate in post-menopausal women with advanced breast cancer: results of overview analysis of two phase III trials. *J Clin Oncol* 1996;14:2000–2011.
40. Osborne CK, Pippen J, Jones SE, et al. Double-blind randomised trial comparing the efficacy and tolerability of fulvestrant versus anastrozole in postmenopausal women with advanced breast cancer progressing on prior endocrine therapy. *J Clin Oncol* 2002;20:3386–3395.
41. Howell A, Robertson JF, Quaresma Albano J, et al. Fulvestrant, formerly ICI 182,780, is as effective as anastrozole in postmenopausal women with advanced breast cancer progressing after prior endocrine treatment. *J Clin Oncol* 2002;20:3396–3403.
42. Kaufman M, Bajetta E, Dirix LY, et al. Exemestane is superior to megestrol acetate after tamoxifen failure in postmenopausal women with advanced breast cancer: results of a phase III randomised double-blind trial. *J Clin Oncol* 2000;18:1399–1411.
43. Dombernowsky P, Smith I, Falkson G, et al. Letrozole, a new oral aromatase inhibitor for advanced breast cancer: double-blind randomised trial showing a dose effect and improved efficacy and tolerability compared with megestrol acetate. *J Clin Oncol* 1998;16:453–461.
44. Gershanovich M, Chaudri HA, Campos D, et al. Letrozole, a new oral aromatase inhibitor: randomised trial comparing 2.5 mg daily, 0.5 mg

daily and aminoglutethimide in postmenopausal women with advanced breast cancer. *Ann Oncol* 1998;9:639–645.

45. Jones S, Vogel C, Arkhipov A, et al. Multicenter phase II trial of exemestane as third-line hormonal therapy of postmenopausal women with metastatic breast cancer. *J Clin Oncol* 1999;17:3418–3425..
46. Lønning PE, Bajetta E, Murray R, et al. Activity of exemestane in metastatic breast cancer after failure of nonsteroidal aromatase inhibitors: a phase II trial. *J Clin Oncol* 2000;18:2234–2244.
47. A'Hern RP, Smith IE, Ebbs SR. Chemotherapy and survival in advanced breast cancer: the inclusion of doxorubicin in Cooper type regimens. *Br J Cancer* 1993;67:801–805. Search date not stated; primary sources Cancerlit and communication with colleagues.
48. Stewart DJ, Evans WK, Shepherd FA, et al. Cyclophosphamide and fluorouracil combined with mitozantrone versus doxorubicin for breast cancer: superiority of doxorubicin. *J Clin Oncol* 1997;15:1897–1905.
49. Namer M, Soler-Michel P, Turpin F. Results of a phase III prospective randomised trial comparing mitoxantrone and vinorelbine in combination with standard FAC/FEC in front-line therapy of metastatic breast cancer. *Eur J Cancer* 2001;37:1132–1140.
50. Engelsman E, Klijn JC, Rubens RD, et al. "Classical" CMF versus a 3-weekly intravenous CMF schedule in postmenopausal patients with advanced breast cancer. *Eur J Cancer* 1991;27:966–970.
51. Tannock IF, Boyd NF, DeBoer G, et al. A randomised trial of two dose levels of cyclophosphamide, methotrexate and fluorouracil chemotherapy for patients with metastatic breast cancer. *J Clin Oncol* 1988;6:1377–1387.
52. Cummings FJ, Gelman R, Horton J. Comparison of CAF versus CMFP in metastatic breast cancer: analysis of prognostic factors. *J Clin Oncol* 1985;3:932–940.
53. Smalley RV, Lefante J, Bartolucci A, et al. A comparison of cyclophosphamide, adriamycin, and 5-fluorouracil (CAF) and cyclophosphamide, methotrexate, 5-fluorouracil, vincristine, and prednisolone (CMFVP) in patients with advanced breast cancer. *Breast Cancer Res Treat* 1983;3:209–220.
54. French Epirubicin Study Group. A prospective randomised phase III trial comparing combination chemotherapy with cyclophosphamide, fluorouracil, and either doxorubicin or epirubicin. *J Clin Oncol* 1988;6:679–688.
55. Italian Multicentre Breast Study with Epirubicin. Randomised phase III study of fluorouracil, doxorubicin, and cyclophosphamide in advanced breast cancer: an Italian multicentre trial. *J Clin Oncol* 1988;6:976–982.
56. Wilcken N, Hornbuckle J, Ghersi D. Chemotherapy alone versus endocrine therapy alone for metastatic breast cancer. In: The Cochrane Library, Issue 3, 2003. Oxford: Update Software. Search date 2002, primary sources Cochrane Breast Cancer Group Specialised Trials Register.
57. Sledge GW, Hu P, Torney D, et al. Comparison of chemotherapy with chemohormonal therapy as first-line therapy for metastatic, hormone sensitive breast cancer. An Eastern Cooperative Oncology Group Study. *J Clin Oncol* 2000;18:262–266.
58. Ross MB, Buzdar AU, Smith TL, et al. Improved survival of patients with metastatic breast cancer receiving combination chemotherapy. *Cancer* 1985;55:341–346.
59. Goldhirsch A, Glick JH, Gelber RD, et al. International consensus panel on the treatment of primary breast cancer. *J Natl Cancer Inst* 1998;90:1601–1608.
60. Coates AS, Hurny C, Peterson HF, et al. Quality of life scores predict outcome in metastatic but not early breast cancer. *J Clin Oncol* 2000;18:3768–3774.
61. Hakamies-Blomquist L, Luoma M, Sjostrom J, et al. Quality of life in patients with metastatic breast cancer receiving either docetaxel or sequential methotrexate and 5-fluorouracil. A multicenter randomised phase III trial by the Scandinavian breast group. *J Clin Oncol* 2000;36:1411–1417.
62. Houston SJ, Richards MA, Bentley AE, et al. The influence of adjuvant chemotherapy on outcome after relapse for patients with breast cancer. *Eur J Cancer* 1993;29A:1513–1518.
63. The Italian Group for Antiemetic Research. Dexamethasone alone or in combination with ondansetron for the prevention of delayed nausea and vomiting induced by chemotherapy. *N Engl J Med* 2000;342:1554–1559.
64. Stockler M, Wilcken NR, Ghersi D, et al. Systematic reviews of chemotherapy and chemotherapy and endocrine therapy in metastatic breast cancer. *Cancer Treat Rev* 2000;26:151–168. Search date not stated; primary source Medline.
65. Ghersi D, Wilcken N, Simes J, et al. Taxane containing regimens for metastatic breast cancer. In: The Cochrane Library, Issue 3, 2003. Oxford: Update Software. Search date 2003, primary sources Cochrane Breast Cancer Group Specialised Trials Register.
66. Farquhar C, Basser R, Hetrick S, et al. High dose chemotherapy and autologous bone marrow or stem cell transplantation versus conventional chemotherapy for women with metastatic breast cancer. In: The Cochrane Library, Issue 3, 2003. Oxford: Update Software. Search date 2002; primary sources Cochrane Breast Cancer Group Specialised Trials register, cooperative research groups' websites, Medline, Embase, Central/CCTR, American Society of Clinical Oncology.
67. Hortobagyi GN, Bodey GP, Buzdar AU, et al. Evaluation of high-dose versus standard FAC chemotherapy for advanced breast cancer in protected environment units: a prospective randomised trial. *J Clin Oncol* 1987;5:354–364.
68. Bastholt L, Dalmark M, Gjedde S, et al. Dose–response relationship of epirubicin in the treatment of postmenopausal patients with metastatic breast cancer: a randomised study of epirubicin at four different dose levels performed by the Danish Breast Cancer Co-operative Group. *J Clin Oncol* 1996;14:1146–1155.
69. Slamon DJ, Leyland-Jones B, Shak S, et al. Use of chemotherapy plus a monoclonal antibody against HER2 for metastatic breast cancer that overexpresses HER2. *N Engl J Med* 2001;344:783–792.
70. Osoba D, Slamon DJ, Burchmore M, et al. Effects on quality of life of combined trastuzumab and chemotherapy in women with metastatic breast cancer. *J Clin Oncol* 2002;20:3106–3113.
71. Vogel CL, Cobleigh MA, Tripathy D, et al. Efficacy and safety of trastuzumab as a single agent in first-line treatment of HER2-overexpressing metastatic breast cancer. *J Clin Oncol* 2002;20:719–726.
72. Bonneterre J, Roche H, Monnier A, et al. Docetaxel vs 5-fluorouracil plus vinorelbine in metastatic breast cancer after anthracycline therapy failure. *Br J Cancer* 2002;87:1210–1215.
73. Jones S, Winer E, Vogel C, et al. Randomised comparison of vinorelbine and melphalan in anthracycline-refractory advanced breast cancer. *J Clin Oncol* 1995;13:2567–2574.
74. Norris B, Pritchard KI, James K, et al. Phase III comparative study of vinorelbine combined with doxorubicin versus doxorubicin alone in disseminated metastatic/recurrent breast cancer: National Cancer Institute of Canada Clinical Trials Group Study MA8. *J Clin Oncol* 2000;18:2385–2394.
75. Namer M, Soler-Michel P, Mefti F, et al. Is the combination FAC/FEC always the best regimen in advanced breast cancer? Utility of mitoxantrone and vinorelbine association as an alternative: results from a randomised trial [abstract]. *Breast Cancer Res Treat* 1997;46:94(A406).
76. Freyer G, Delozier T, Lichinister M, et al. Phase II study of oral vinorelbine in first-line advanced breast cancer chemotherapy. *J Clin Oncol* 2003;21:35–40.
77. Berruti A, Sperone P, Bottini A. Phase II study of vinorelbine with protracted fluorouracil infusion as a

second or third line approach for advanced breast cancer patients previously treated with anthracyclines. *J Clin Oncol* 2000;18:3370–3377.
78. Stathopoulus GP, Rigatos SK, Pergantas N, et al. Phase II trial of biweekly administration of vinorelbine and gemcitabine in pretreated advanced breast cancer. *J Clin Oncol* 2002;20:37–41.
79. Tomiak E, Verma S, Levine M, et al. Use of capecitabine in stage IV breast cancer: an evidence summary. *Curr Oncol* 2000;7:84–90. Search date 2000; primary sources Medline, Cancerlit, Cochrane, Pubmed, US Food and Drug Administration website, Physician Query Database, Clinical Trials Listing service, hand searches of proceedings of the American Society of Clinical Oncology, and contact with Hoffmann-La Roche.
80. Blum JL, Jones SE, Buzdar AU, et al. Multicenter phase II study of capecitabine in paclitaxel-refractory metastatic breast cancer. *J Clin Oncol* 1999;17:485–493.
81. Diasio RB. An evolving role for oral fluoropyrimidine drugs. *J Clin Oncol* 2002;20:894–896.
82. Pavlakis N, Stockler M. Bisphosphonates for breast cancer. In: The Cochrane Library, Issue 3, 2003. Oxford: Update Software. Search date not stated, primary sources Cochrane Breast Cancer Group Specialised Trials Register, Medline, Central/CCTR, Embase, CancerLit, and hand searches from a number of other relevant sources.
83. Body JJ, Diel IJ, Lichinitser MR, et al. Intravenous ibandronate reduces the incidence of skeletal complications in patients with breast cancer and bone metastases. *Ann Oncol* 2003;14:1399–1405.
84. Hillner BE, Ingle JN, Berenson JR, et al. American Society of Clinical Oncology guideline on the role of bisphosphonates in breast cancer: American Society of Oncology Bisphosphonates Expert Panel. *J Clin Oncol* 2000;18:1378–1391.
85. Hillner BE, Weeks JC, Desch CE, et al. Pamidronate in prevention of bone complications in metastatic breast cancer; a cost-effectiveness analysis. *J Clin Oncol* 2000;18:72–79.
86. World Health Organization. *Cancer pain relief*. Geneva: WHO, 1996.
87. Hall SM, Budzar AV, Blumenschein GR. Cranial nerve palsies in metastatic breast cancer due to osseous metastasis without intracranial involvement. *Cancer* 1983;52:180–184.
88. Bone Trial Working Party. 8 Gy single fraction radiotherapy for the treatment of metastatic skeletal pain: randomised comparison with a multifraction schedule over 12 months of patient follow-up. *Radiother Oncol* 1999;52:111–121.
89. Price P, Hoskin PJ, Easton D, et al. Prospective randomised trial of single and multifraction radiotherapy schedules in treatment of painful bony metastases. *Radiother Oncol* 1986;6:247–255.
90. Priestman TJ, Dunn J, Brada M, et al. Final results of the Royal College of Radiologists' trial comparing two different radiotherapy schedules in the treatment of brain metastases. *Clin Oncol* 1996;8:308–315.
91. Roos DE, O'Brien PC, Smith JG, et al. A role for radiotherapy in neuropathic bone pain: preliminary response rates from a prospective trial. *Int J Radiat Oncol Biol Phys* 2000;46:975–981.
92. Bretscher N. Care for dying patients: what is right? *J Clin Oncol* 2000;18:233–234.
93. Rades D, Blach M, Nerreter V, et al. Metastatic spinal cord compression. Influence of time between onset of motor deficits and start of irradiation on therapeutic effect. *Strahlenther Onkol* 1999;175:378–381.
94. Sørensen S, Helweg-Larsen S, Mouridsen H, et al. Effect of high-dose dexamethasone in carcinomatous metastatic spinal cord compression treated with radiotherapy: a randomised trial. *Eur J Cancer* 1994;30A:22–27.
95. Cancer Guidance Subgroup of the Clinical Outcomes Group. *Improving outcomes in breast cancer. The research evidence*. London: NHS Executive, 1996.
96. Diener-West M, Dobbins TW, Phillips TL, et al. Identification of an optimal subgroup for treatment evaluation of patients with brain metastases using RTOG study 7916. *Int J Radiat Oncol Biol Phys* 1989;16:669–673.
97. Shaw E, Scott C, Suh J, et al. RSR13 plus cranial radiation therapy in patients with brain metastases: comparison with the Radiation Therapy Oncology Group Recursive Partitioning Analysis Brain Metastases Database. *J Clin Oncol* 2003;21:2364–2371.
98. Wiegel T, Bottke D, Kreusel KM, et al. External beam radiotherapy of choroidal metastases — final results of a prospective study of the German Cancer Society (ARO 95–08). *Radiother Oncol* 2002;64:13–18.
99. Ratanatharathorn V, Powers WE, Grimm J, et al. Eye metastasis from carcinoma of the breast: radiation treatment and results. *Cancer Treat Rev* 1991;18:261–276.
100. Piccone MR, Maguire AM, Fox KC, et al. Choroidal metastases. Case 1: breast cancer. *J Clin Oncol* 1999;17:3356–3358.
101. Hortobagyi GN. Treatment of breast cancer. *N Engl J Med* 1998;339:974–984.
102. Levinger S, Merin S, Seigal R, et al. Laser therapy in the management of choroidal breast tumor metastases. *Ophthalmic Surg Lasers* 2001;32:294–299.
103. Ando M, Watanabe T, Nagata K, et al. Efficacy of docetaxel 60 mg/m^2 in patients with metastatic breast cancer according to the status of anthracycline resistance. *J Clin Oncol* 2001;19:336–342.

Justin Stebbing
MRC Clinical Training Fellow and Specialist Registrar in Medical Oncology
Chelsea and Westminster Hospital
London
UK

Robert Glassman
Clinical Instructor
Division of Oncology
Weill Medical College
Cornell University
New York
USA

Competing interests: None declared.

We would like to acknowledge the previous contributors of this chapter, including Stephen Johnston.

TABLE 1 **Clinical factors that predict response to hormonal treatment in metastatic breast cancer, based on results of RCTs (see text, p 2201).[8–11]**

Factors predictive of good response to hormonal treatment
Postmenopausal status
Disease limited to soft tissue sites (skin, nodes)
Oestrogen receptor positive tumour
Long disease free interval since primary treatment for early breast cancer (> 18–24 months)
Factors making initial hormonal treatment less appropriate
Symptomatic visceral metastases (e.g. lymphangitis carcinomatosis or progressive liver metastases)
Oestrogen receptor negative tumour
Short disease free interval (12–18 months)
Relapse on adjuvant tamoxifen (unless oestrogen receptor positive tumour and other features predictive of good response)

Breast cancer (non-metastatic)

Search date February 2004

J Michael Dixon, Alan Rodger, and Justin Stebbing

QUESTIONS

INTERVENTIONS

Unlikely to be beneficial
Adding chemotherapy (cyclophosphamide/methotrexate/fluorouracil or anthracycline based regimens) to radiotherapy . . .2250

To be covered in future updates
Intraoperative radiotherapy in early breast cancer

Sentinel node biopsy

Covered elsewhere in *Clinical Evidence*
Breast cancer (metastatic), p 2197

See glossary**G**

Key Messages

Ductal carcinoma in situ

- **Radiotherapy (reduced recurrence)** Two RCTs identified by a systematic review found that radiotherapy after breast conserving surgery for ductal carcinoma *in situ* reduced local recurrence and invasive carcinoma compared with no radiotherapy after 4 and 8 years. However, they found no evidence of an effect on survival. One RCT in women having local excision found no significant difference between tamoxifen plus radiotherapy and radiotherapy alone in total invasive or ductal carcinoma *in situ* events after median follow up of 1 year.
- **Tamoxifen plus radiotherapy (reduced recurrence in women with oestrogen receptor positive tumours)** One RCT found that adjuvant tamoxifen reduced breast cancer events in women who had undergone wide excision and radiotherapy after median follow up of 6 years, although subgroup analysis suggested that benefit may be limited to women with oestrogen receptor positive tumours. It found no evidence of an effect on survival. One RCT in women having local excision found no significant difference between tamoxifen plus radiotherapy and radiotherapy alone in invasive or ductal carcinoma *in situ* events after median follow up of 1 year.

Primary operable breast cancer

- **Adjuvant combination chemotherapy** One systematic review found that adjuvant combination chemotherapy reduced recurrence and improved survival at 10 years compared with no chemotherapy. The benefit seemed to be independent of nodal or menopausal status, although the absolute improvements were greater in women with node positive disease, and probably greater in younger women. Adverse effects of chemotherapy include fatigue, nausea and vomiting, hair loss, bone marrow suppression, neuropathy, and gastrointestinal disturbance. Chemotherapy may impair fertility and ovarian function.
- **Adjuvant tamoxifen (in women with oestrogen receptor positive tumours)** One systematic review found that adjuvant tamoxifen taken for up to 5 years reduced the risk of recurrence and death in women with oestrogen receptor positive tumours irrespective of age, menopausal status, nodal involvement, or the addition of chemotherapy. Five years of treatment was more effective than shorter durations, but available evidence did not find benefit associated with prolongation of treatment beyond 5 years. Tamoxifen slightly increased the risk of endometrial cancer and thrombotic complications, but we found no evidence of an overall adverse effect on non-breast cancer mortality.
- **Anthracycline regimens as adjuvant chemotherapy** One systematic review found that adjuvant regimens containing an anthracycline reduced recurrence, and improved survival compared with a standard multidrug chemotherapy (CMF) regimen at 5 years. Adverse effects of chemotherapy include nausea and vomiting, hair loss, bone marrow suppression, fatigue, and gastrointestinal disturbance. Chemotherapy may impair fertility and ovarian function.
- **Combined chemotherapy plus tamoxifen** One RCT found that adding chemotherapy to tamoxifen improved survival at 5 years in women with lymph node negative, oestrogen receptor positive early breast cancer. It found that adding combined chemotherapy to tamoxifen was associated with increased adverse effects such as nausea, neutropenia, alopecia, thromboembolism, and phlebitis.

Breast cancer (non-metastatic)

- **Less extensive surgery (similar survival to more extensive surgery, and better cosmetic outcome)** Two systematic reviews and long term follow up of included RCTs found that more extensive surgery did not improve outcomes compared with less extensive surgery in women with early invasive breast cancer, providing that all local disease was excised. Cosmetic appearance is worse with more extensive surgery.
- **Ovarian ablation in premenopausal women** One systematic review found that in premenopausal women with early breast cancer, ovarian ablation improved survival compared with no ablation after 15 years follow up.
- **Radiotherapy after breast conserving surgery (reduced local recurrence and had similar survival rates to breast conserving surgery alone)** One systematic review and one subsequent RCT found that adding radiotherapy to breast conserving surgery reduced the risk of local recurrence compared with breast conserving surgery alone. They found no significant difference in survival between breast conserving surgery plus radiotherapy and breast conserving surgery alone. One systematic review and one additional RCT found no significant difference in survival and local recurrence with breast conserving surgery plus radiotherapy compared with mastectomy. One RCT found that radiotherapy (with or without tamoxifen) reduced ipsilateral breast cancer recurrence compared with tamoxifen alone after median follow up of 87 months. It found no significant difference in survival. Radiotherapy may be associated with late adverse effects, which are rare, including pneumonitis, pericarditis, arm oedema, brachial plexopathy, and radionecrotic rib fracture.
- **Radiotherapy after mastectomy in women at high risk of local recurrence** One systematic review found that radiotherapy to the chest wall after mastectomy reduced the risk of local recurrence by about two thirds compared with no postoperative radiotherapy. It found that radiotherapy did not reduce all cause mortality and breast cancer mortality after mastectomy alone or mastectomy plus axillary clearance. However, radiotherapy did reduce all cause mortality and breast cancer mortality after mastectomy plus axillary sampling. Radiotherapy may be associated with late adverse effects, which are rare, including pneumonitis, pericarditis, arm oedema, brachial plexopathy, and radionecrotic rib fracture.
- **Neoadjuvant chemotherapy (reduced mastectomy rates and had similar survival rates to adjuvant chemotherapy)** Five RCTs found no significant difference in survival with neoadjuvant chemotherapy compared with adjuvant chemotherapy. Three RCTs found that neoadjuvant chemotherapy reduced mastectomy rate compared with adjuvant chemotherapy. Adverse effects of chemotherapy include fatigue, nausea and vomiting, hair loss, bone marrow suppression, neuropathy, and gastrointestinal disturbance. Chemotherapy may impair fertility and ovarian function.
- **Total nodal radiotherapy** One systematic review found that postmastectomy radiotherapy, including total nodal irradiation, reduced locoregional recurrence. It found that postmastectomy radiotherapy improved survival in women receiving mastectomy plus axillary sampling, but not in women receiving mastectomy alone or mastectomy plus axillary clearance.
- **Axillary clearance** There is consensus that axillary clearance reduces regional recurrence compared with no axillary management. RCTs found no significant difference in survival at 5–10 years between axillary clearance and axillary sampling (followed by axillary radiotherapy in women found to be node positive) or axillary radiotherapy (regardless of axillary nodal status). One systematic review found that axillary radiotherapy reduced isolated local recurrence compared with axillary clearance, but this difference was not significant. One systematic review of mainly poor quality evidence found that the risk of arm lymphoedema was highest with axillary clearance plus radiotherapy, lower with axillary sampling plus radiotherapy, and lowest with sampling alone.
- **Axillary radiotherapy** One systematic review found that axillary radiotherapy reduced isolated local recurrence compared with axillary clearance, but this difference was not significant. The review found no significant difference in survival at 10

years between axillary radiotherapy and axillary clearance. One systematic review of mainly poor quality evidence found that the risk of arm lymphoedema was highest with axillary clearance plus radiotherapy, lower with axillary sampling plus radiotherapy, and lowest with sampling alone.

- **Axillary sampling** One RCT found no significant difference in survival at 5 years between axillary clearance and axillary sampling (followed by axillary radiotherapy in women found to be node positive). One systematic review of mainly poor quality evidence found that the risk of arm lymphoedema was highest with axillary clearance plus radiotherapy, lower with axillary sampling plus radiotherapy, and lowest with sampling alone.
- **Radiotherapy after mastectomy in women not at high risk of local recurrence** One systematic review found that radiotherapy to the chest wall after mastectomy reduced the risk of local recurrence by about two thirds compared with no postoperative radiotherapy. It found that radiotherapy did not reduce all cause mortality or breast cancer mortality after mastectomy alone or mastectomy plus axillary clearance. However, radiotherapy did reduce all cause mortality and breast cancer mortality after mastectomy plus axillary sampling. Radiotherapy may be associated with late adverse effects, which are rare, including pneumonitis, pericarditis, arm oedema, brachial plexopathy, and radionecrotic rib fracture. There is, therefore, a trade off between absolute benefits and harms in women not at high risk of local recurrence.
- **Different neoadjuvant chemotherapy regimens (insufficient evidence regarding which regimen is most effective)** We found insufficient evidence of any difference between the common neoadjuvant chemotherapy regimens in survival, recurrence, or quality of life.
- **Radiotherapy to the internal mammary chain** One RCT found no significant difference in relapse or survival at 2–3 years between radiotherapy and no radiotherapy to the internal mammary chain. Treatment may increase radiation induced cardiac morbidity.
- **Radiotherapy to the ipsilateral supraclavicular fossa** We found insufficient evidence about the effects of irradiation of the ipsilateral supraclavicular fossa on survival. RCTs have found that radiotherapy to the chest wall and lymph nodes is associated with reduced risk of locoregional recurrence, including supraclavicular fossa nodal recurrence. Morbidity associated with irradiation of the supraclavicular fossa is rare and, where it occurs, is mild and temporary.
- **Enhanced dose regimens of adjuvant combination chemotherapy** RCTs did not find additional survival advantage from enhanced dose regimens of adjuvant combination chemotherapy. Adverse effects of chemotherapy include nausea and vomiting, hair loss, bone marrow suppression, fatigue, and gastrointestinal disturbance. Chemotherapy may impair fertility and ovarian function.
- **Prolonged adjuvant combination chemotherapy (8–12 months *v* 4–6 months)** One systematic review found no additional survival benefit from prolonging adjuvant chemotherapy from 4–6 to 8–12 months. Adverse effects of chemotherapy include nausea and vomiting, hair loss, bone marrow suppression, fatigue, and gastrointestinal disturbance. Chemotherapy may impair fertility and ovarian function.
- **High dose chemotherapy** One systematic review found no significant difference between high dose chemotherapy plus autograft and conventional chemotherapy in 5 year survival for women with early, poor prognosis breast cancer. The review found that high dose chemotherapy plus autograft increased treatment related and non-cancer related deaths compared with conventional chemotherapy.

Locally advanced breast cancer

- **Hormonal treatment plus radiotherapy (improves survival compared with radiotherapy alone)** One RCT found that hormonal treatment (tamoxifen or ovarian ablation) plus radiotherapy delayed locoregional recurrence and improved survival at 8 years in locally advanced breast cancer compared with radiotherapy alone.

- **Radiotherapy** Two small RCTs including women with locally advanced disease (stage III B) found that radiotherapy or surgery as sole local treatments have similar effects on response rates, duration of response, and overall survival for locally advanced breast cancer that is rendered operable by prior chemotherapy. Local skin toxicity (acute and late) after radiotherapy is greater in locally advanced breast cancer than after treatment for less advanced disease, because of the need for a higher radiation dose to skin.
- **Radiotherapy after attempted curative surgery** One RCT found limited evidence that radiotherapy after attempted curative surgery reduced local and regional recurrence compared with no further local treatment, but did not improve time to relapse or overall survival. Local skin toxicity (acute and late) after radiotherapy is greater in locally advanced breast cancer than after treatment for less advanced disease, because of the need for a higher radiation dose to skin.
- **Surgery** Two small RCTs including women with locally advanced disease (stage III B) found that surgery or radiotherapy as sole local treatments have similar effects on response rates, duration of response, and overall survival for locally advanced breast cancer that is rendered operable by prior chemotherapy.
- **Adding chemotherapy (cyclophosphamide/methotrexate/fluorouracil or anthracycline based regimens) to radiotherapy** RCTs found insufficient evidence that radiotherapy plus cytotoxic chemotherapy using cyclophosphamide plus methotrexate plus fluorouracil, or an anthracycline based multidrug regimen improved survival, disease free survival, or long term locoregional control compared with radiotherapy alone in locally advanced breast cancer.

DEFINITION This chapter examines the effects of treatment for non-metastatic, primary breast cancer. **Ductal carcinoma** *in situ* is a non-invasive(G) tumour characterised by the presence of malignant cells in the breast ducts but with no evidence that they breach the basement membrane and invade into periductal connective tissues. **Invasive breast cancer** can be separated into three main groups: early invasive breast cancer(G), locally advanced breast cancer(G), and metastatic breast cancer (see breast cancer (metastatic), p 2197). **Operable breast cancer** is apparently restricted to the breast and sometimes to local lymph nodes and can be removed surgically. Although these women do not have overt metastases at the time of staging, they remain at risk of local recurrence and of metastatic spread. They can be divided into those with tumours greater than 4 cm with multifocal cancers that are usually treated by mastectomy, and those with tumours less than 4 cm with unifocal cancers that can be treated by breast conserving surgery. **Locally advanced breast cancer** is defined according to the TNM staging system(G) of the UICC(G)[1] as stage III B (includes T4 a–d; N2 disease, but absence of metastases). It is a disease presentation with evidence (clinical or histopathological) of skin, or chest wall involvement, or axillary nodes matted together by tumour extension, or a combination of these features. **Metastatic breast cancer** is presented in a separate chapter (see breast cancer (metastatic), p 2197).

INCIDENCE/ PREVALENCE Breast cancer affects 1/10–1/11 women in the UK and causes about 21 000 deaths a year. Prevalence is about five times higher, with over 100 000 women in the UK living with breast cancer at any one time. Of the 15 000 new cases of breast cancer a year in the UK, most will present with primary operable disease.[2]

AETIOLOGY/ RISK FACTORS The risk of breast cancer increases with age, doubling every 10 years up to the menopause. Risk factors include an early age at menarche, older age at menopause, older age at birth of first child, family history, atypical hyperplasia, excess alcohol intake, radiation exposure to developing breast tissue, oral contraceptive use, postmenopausal hormone replacement therapy, and obesity. Risk in different countries varies fivefold. The cause of breast cancer in most women is unknown. About 5% of breast cancers can be attributed to mutations in the genes *BRCA1* and *BRCA2*.[3]

PROGNOSIS **Primary carcinoma** of the breast is potentially curable. The risk of relapse depends on various clinicopathological features, of which axillary node involvement, tumour grade, tumour size, and oestrogen receptor status are the most prognostically important. Of women with operable disease 70% are alive 5 years after diagnosis and treatment (adjuvant treatment(G) is given to most women after surgery). Risk of recurrence is highest during the first 5 years, but the risk remains even 15–20 years after surgery. Those with node positive disease have a 50–60%

chance of recurrence within 5 years, compared with 30–35% for node negative disease. Recurrence at 10 years, according to one large systematic review,[4] is 60–70% compared with 25–30% of node negative women. The prognosis for a disease free survival**G** at 5 years is worse for stage III B (33%) than that for stage III A (71%). Five year overall survival is 44% for stage III B and 84% for stage III A.[5] Poor survival and high rates of local recurrence characterise locally advanced breast cancer**G**.

AIMS OF INTERVENTION To improve survival; to prevent local or regional node recurrence; to obtain prognostic information on the type and extent of tumour and the status of the axillary lymph nodes; to optimise cosmetic results and minimise psychosocial impact; to minimise adverse effects of treatment; and to maximise quality of life.

OUTCOMES Survival; rates of local and regional recurrence; rates of mastectomy after breast conserving treatment; rates of development of metastases; cosmetic outcomes; quality of life; incidence of adverse effects of treatment, including upper limb lymphoedema.

METHODS *Clinical Evidence* search and appraisal February 2004.

QUESTION What are the effects of interventions after breast conserving surgery for ductal carcinoma *in situ*?

OPTION RADIOTHERAPY

Mike Dixon and Alan Rodger

Two RCTs identified by a systematic review found that radiotherapy after breast conserving surgery for ductal carcinoma *in situ* reduced local recurrence and invasive carcinoma compared with no radiotherapy after 4 and 8 years. However, they found no evidence of an effect on survival. One RCT in women having local excision found no significant difference between tamoxifen plus radiotherapy and radiotherapy alone in total invasive or ductal carcinoma *in situ* events after median follow up of 1 year.

Benefits: **Versus no radiotherapy:** We found one systematic review (search date 2001)[6] which found two RCTs[7,8] comparing radiotherapy**G** with no radiotherapy after surgery for ductal carcinoma *in situ* (DCIS). The first RCT identified by the review (814 women) found no significant difference in survival at 8 years with radiotherapy compared with no radiotherapy (survival 95% with radiotherapy *v* 94% with no radiotherapy, reported as not significant).[7] It found significant reductions in risk of local recurrence, recurrent DCIS, and invasive carcinoma with radiotherapy compared with no radiotherapy (local recurrence: 12.1% with radiotherapy *v* 26.8% with no radiotherapy; $P < 0.0005$; risk of recurrent DCIS: 8.2% with radiotherapy *v* 13.4% with no radiotherapy; $P = 0.007$; risk of invasive carcinoma: 3.9% with radiotherapy *v* 13.4% with no radiotherapy; $P < 0.0001$).[7] The second RCT identified by the review (1002 women) found that at 4 years, the proportion of women who were free of local recurrence was significantly greater with surgery plus radiotherapy than with surgery alone (91% with surgery plus radiotherapy *v* 84% with surgery alone; $P = 0.005$; HR 0.62, 95% CI 0.44 to 0.87).[8] More women were free of DCIS recurrence after 4 years with radiotherapy but the difference was not significant (95% with surgery plus radiotherapy *v* 92% with surgery alone; HR 0.65, 95% CI 0.43 to 1.03). Added radiotherapy significantly reduced invasive recurrence (96% with surgery plus radiotherapy *v* 92% with surgery alone; HR 0.60, 95% CI 0.37 to 0.97).[8] There was no significant difference between groups in survival at 4 years (survival rates presented graphically; $P = 0.94$). **Versus radiotherapy plus tamoxifen:** See benefits of tamoxifen plus radiotherapy, p 2232.

Harms: **Versus no radiotherapy:** The second RCT included in the review found an increase in contralateral breast cancer associated with radiotherapy**G** at 4 years (3% with surgery plus radiotherapy *v* 1% with surgery alone; HR 2.57, 95% CI 1.24 to 5.33).[8] **Versus radiotherapy plus tamoxifen:** See harms of tamoxifen plus radiotherapy, p 2233.

Comment: Subgroup analyses may be required to identify groups of women who benefit most from radiotherapy**G** after breast conserving surgery**G**. We found one further large RCT (1694 women), which randomised 912 women to tamoxifen, radiotherapy, both, or none.[9] Of the remaining 782 women, 664 were given the choice between radiotherapy and no radiotherapy, and were further randomised to tamoxifen or no tamoxifen. Similarly, the remaining 118 women were given the choice between tamoxifen and no tamoxifen, and were further randomised to radiotherapy or no radiotherapy. However, the study did not present results comparing radiotherapy alone versus no treatment or versus tamoxifen alone. It found that radiotherapy (with or without tamoxifen) significantly reduced ipsilateral invasive disease (HR 0.45, 95% CI 0.24 to 0.85), ipsilateral DCIS recurrence (HR 0.36, 95% CI 0.19 to 0.66), and all ipsilateral events (HR 0.38, 95% CI 0.25 to 0.59) compared with no radiotherapy (with or without tamoxifen).

OPTION TAMOXIFEN PLUS RADIOTHERAPY

Mike Dixon and Alan Rodger

One RCT found that adjuvant tamoxifen reduced breast cancer events in women who had undergone wide excision and radiotherapy after median follow up of 6 years, although subgroup analysis suggested that benefit may be limited to women with oestrogen receptor positive tumours. It found no evidence of an effect on survival. One RCT in women having local excision found no significant difference between tamoxifen plus radiotherapy and radiotherapy alone in invasive or ductal carcinoma *in situ* events after median follow up of 1 year.

Benefits: We found no systematic review but we found two RCTs.[9,10] **Versus radiotherapy plus placebo:** The first RCT (1804 women with ductal carcinoma *in situ* [DCIS] treated with wide excision and radiotherapy**G** compared adjuvant treatment**G** with tamoxifen 20 mg daily versus placebo for 5 years.[10] At median follow up of 74 months, there were significantly fewer breast cancer events with tamoxifen than with placebo and significantly fewer invasive ipsilateral or contralateral breast cancers (breast cancer events: OR 0.63, 95% CI 0.47 to 0.83; invasive ipsilateral or contralateral breast cancers: OR 0.57, 95% CI 0.38 to 0.85). However, there was no significant difference in overall survival (RR 0.88, 95% CI 0.33 to 2.28). A subsequent subgroup analysis found that only people with oestrogen receptor positive DCIS derive a benefit from tamoxifen.[11] **Versus radiotherapy alone:** The second RCT (1694 women having local excision) compared four treatments in a factorial design: no adjuvant treatment, tamoxifen alone, radiotherapy alone, and tamoxifen plus radiotherapy (see comment of radiotherapy, p 2232).[9] It found no significant difference between tamoxifen plus radiotherapy and radiotherapy alone in ipsilateral invasive disease, ipsilateral DCIS, and invasive or DCIS events after median follow up of 1 year (523 women in comparison; ipsilateral invasive disease: HR 1.25, 95% CI 0.43 to 3.61; ipsilateral DCIS: HR 0.75, 95% CI 0.28 to 2.02; invasive or DCIS: 3% in both groups; HR 0.95, 95% CI 0.51 to 1.77).[9]

Harms: **Versus radiotherapy plus placebo:** The RCT found a higher, but non-significant rate of endometrial cancers associated with tamoxifen (RR 3.4, 95% CI 0.6 to 33.4).[10] **Versus radiotherapy alone:** One RCT did not report results comparing harms of tamoxifen plus radiotherapy**G** versus radiotherapy alone.[9]

Comment: None.

QUESTION **What are the effects of treatments for primary operable breast cancer?**

Mike Dixon, Alan Rodger, and Justin Stebbing

OPTION **NEOADJUVANT CHEMOTHERAPY**

Five RCTs found no significant difference in survival with neoadjuvant chemotherapy compared with adjuvant chemotherapy. Three RCTs found that neoadjuvant chemotherapy reduced mastectomy rate compared with adjuvant chemotherapy. Adverse effects of chemotherapy include fatigue, nausea and vomiting, hair loss, bone marrow suppression, neuropathy, and gastrointestinal disturbance. Chemotherapy may impair fertility and ovarian function.

Benefits: We found no systematic review. **Survival:** We found five RCTs comparing neoadjuvant chemotherapy**G** with adjuvant**G** chemotherapy.[12–16] The first RCT (272 women with tumours > 3 cm in whom mastectomy was indicated) compared preoperative (neoadjuvant) EVMTV (epirubicin, vincristine, mitomycin-C, thiotepa, vindesine) chemotherapy versus mastectomy followed by EVMTV regimen.[12] At an initial median follow up of 34 months, a significant survival difference was reported in favour of neoadjuvant chemotherapy (85% with preoperative EVMTV *v* 95% with mastectomy plus EVMTV; P = 0.04). However, the final analysis at 124 months showed that the survival improvement was no longer significant, with survival of about 55% in both groups.[17] The second RCT (414 women) compared four cycles of FAC**G** chemotherapy given either preoperatively or postoperatively.[13] At 54 months' follow up, the primary (neoadjuvant) chemotherapy group had a better overall survival (86% with preoperative *v* 68% with postoperative; P = 0.039); however, a subsequent analysis at 105 months did not show a long term survival benefit.[18] The third RCT (309 women) compared four cycles of neoadjuvant MM (mitoxantrone [mitozantrone], methotrexate) chemotherapy followed by surgery and four further cycles of MM versus surgery followed by eight cycles of adjuvant MM.[14] At 48 months' follow up, there was no difference in survival between the neoadjuvant and adjuvant groups (84% with neoadjuvant *v* 82% with adjuvant; reported as not significant). The fourth, and largest RCT (NSABP-18), in which 1523 women were randomised to four cycles of AC (adriamycin [doxorubicin], cyclophosphamide) either preoperatively or postoperatively, found identical survival rates (67%) in the two groups at 60 months.[15] The fifth RCT (698 women) compared four cycles of fluorouracil, epirubicin, and cyclophosphamide given either preoperatively or postoperatively.[16] It found no significant difference between preoperative and postoperative chemotherapy in overall survival (82% with preoperative *v* 84% with postoperative; HR 1.16, 95% CI 0.83 to 1.63), progression free survival (65% with preoperative *v* 70% with postoperative; HR 1.15, 95% CI 0.89 to 1.48), or locoregional recurrence at 4 years (21.5% with preoperative *v* 17.8% with postoperative; HR 1.13, 95% CI 0.70 to 1.81). **Mastectomy rates:** We found three RCTs, which compared mastectomy rates with neoadjuvant chemotherapy versus adjuvant chemotherapy.[15,19,20] The first RCT (309 women receiving MM [mitoxantrone, methotrexate] chemotherapy) found that neoadjuvant significantly reduced the mastectomy rate compared with adjuvant chemotherapy (13% with neoadjuvant *v* 28% with adjuvant; $P < 0.005$).[19] The second RCT (1523 women receiving AC [adriamycin [doxorubicin], cyclophosphamide) found that breast conservation rates were lower in the adjuvant arm (60% with adjuvant *v* 67% with neoadjuvant), although this was not significant.[15] The third RCT assessed 272 women at diagnosis in terms of the recommended surgical procedure, and two of three women who were initially advised to have mastectomy were able to have breast conserving surgery**G** after neoadjuvant chemotherapy with FAC.[20]

Harms: We found no evidence that neoadjuvant**G** chemotherapy has a negative impact on survival. None of the RCTs examining effects on mastectomy rates reported a significantly higher local recurrence rate with neoadjuvant chemotherapy compared with adjuvant**G** chemotherapy.[15,19,20] See harms of adjuvant combination chemotherapy, p 2244.

Comment: We found no evidence to support the use of neoadjuvant**G** chemotherapy to improve the chances of survival for operable breast cancers outside the context of an RCT. With an increased number of conservative operations being performed after downstaging by neoadjuvant chemotherapy for large primary tumours, there are theoretical concerns that this may result in an increased rate of local recurrence. Neoadjuvant chemotherapy can lead to a reduction in the requirement for mastectomy and as such an increase in breast conserving surgery**G**. In the three RCTs of women with operable breast cancer receiving breast conserving surgery, this has not been associated with a significant increase in the rate of local recurrence.[15,19,20]

OPTION DIFFERENT NEOADJUVANT CHEMOTHERAPY REGIMENS

We found insufficient evidence of any difference between the common neoadjuvant chemotherapy regimens in survival, recurrence, or quality of life.

Benefits: **Standard versus dose intensified anthracycline based regimens:** We found one RCT (448 women with locally advanced breast cancer) which compared a CEF (cyclophosphamide, epirubicin, fluorouracil) regimen versus a dose intensified ECFi (epirubicin, cyclophosphamide, filgrastim) regimen.[21] It found no significant difference between the regimens in time to progression (recurrence or death) or 5 year survival (median time to progression: 34 months with CEF *v* 33.7 months with ECFi; $P = 0.68$; 5 year survival: 53% with CEF *v* 51% with ECFi; $P = 0.94$). Complete clinical response rates were similar with both regimens (31% with CEF *v* 27% with ECFi; P value and RR not reported). **FAC regimen versus paclitaxel:** We found one RCT (174 women in the USA), which compared conventional FAC**G** versus single agent paclitaxel, and found similar response rates in both groups (79% with FAC *v* 80% with paclitaxel), with no significant difference in survival rates.[22] **Comparison between MPEMi, MPEpiE, and MPEpiV regimens:** We found one RCT (101 women treated with three different combinations: MPEMi [methotrexate, cisplatin, etoposide, mitomycin-C], MPEpiE [methotrexate, cisplatin, epirubicin, etoposide], and MPEpiV [methotrexate, cisplatin, epirubicin, vincristine]. It found that the response rate was 89% in all three groups.[23] **Sequencing of anthracycline based chemotherapy and docetaxel:** We found two RCTs.[24,25] The first RCT (104 women who had achieved complete or partial clinical response to four cycles of CVAP [cyclophosphamide, adriamycin [doxorubicin], vincristine, prednisolone]) compared a further four cycles of CVAP versus four cycles of docetaxel.[24] It found that further treatment with docetaxel significantly improved clinical complete response rate compared with further CVAP (clinical complete response rate: 85% with docetaxel v 64% with CVAP; P = 0.03).[24] In the second RCT (2411 people), all people received four cycles of AC (adriamycin [doxorubicin], cyclophosphamide) and were then randomly allocated to three regimens: surgery alone, four cycles of docetaxel followed by surgery, or surgery followed by four cycles of docetaxel.[25] Preliminary results of this RCT found that, at the time of surgery, preoperative docetaxel improved clinical complete response rate compared with no preoperative docetaxel (65% with docetaxel v 40% with no docetaxel; P < 0.001). Final results, which will also examine effects of postoperative docetaxel, are awaited. **Navelbine based regimens:** We found no fully published RCTs (see comment below). **Comparison between routes of administration:** We found one Japanese study comparing routes of administration.[26] It compared no neoadjuvantⒼ treatment, neoadjuvant intravenous epirubicin, or neoadjuvant intra-arterial epirubicin. Response rates were higher in women receiving intra-arterial epirubicin compared with intravenous epirubicin (68% with intra-arterial epirubicin v 36% with iv epirubicin; P < 0.05); however, this was not associated with a survival benefit.

Harms: **Standard versus dose intensified anthracycline based regimens:** There were similar numbers of serious adverse events requiring hospitalisation in the groups (60 events with CEF v 68 events with ECFi; P value not reported). The dose intensified ECFi regimen increased nausea and vomiting; and induced more grade 3 and 4 anaemia, but fewer febrile neutropenic episodes compared with CEF (AR for nausea: 11.8% with CEF v 22.3% with ECFi; vomiting: 10.9% with CEF v 18.8% with ECFi; anaemia: 16.3% with CEF v 50.9% with ECFi; febrile neutropenia: 14% with CEF v 8.4% with ECFi; no P values reported for comparisons). **FAC versus paclitaxel:** In the RCT comparing FACⒼ versus paclitaxel, rates of septic neutropenia (53% with paclitaxel v 21% with FAC) and granulocyte colony stimulating factor usage (56% with paclitaxel v 25% with FAC) were higher in women taking paclitaxel.[22]

Comment: More work is needed to determine the optimal regimen for neoadjuvantⒼ treatment. We found little evidence in the literature comparing different combinations, but anthracyclineⒼ based combinations probably remain the treatment of choice, with dose intensification not proved to confer additional clinical benefit.[21] Ongoing RCTs are investigating the role of taxane sequencing after anthracycline based treatment (NSABP-27), and anthracycline in combination with fluorouracil infusion. **Navelbine based regimens:** We found one RCT (published as an abstract, 147 women), which compared AC, NM (navelbine, mitoxantrone), and NE (navelbine, epirubicin). Response rates were 65% with AC, 73% with NM, and 86% with NE. The time to outcome was not reported. The trial is ongoing although NM has been stopped because of haematological toxicity.[27]

OPTION LESS EXTENSIVE SURGERY

Two systematic reviews and long term follow up of included RCTs found that more extensive surgery did not improve outcomes compared with less extensive surgery in women with early invasive breast cancer, providing that all local disease was excised. Cosmetic appearance is worse with more extensive surgery.

Benefits: **Comparisons between supraradical, radical, and total mastectomy:** We found one systematic review (search date not reported, 5 RCTs, 2090 women with operable breast cancer) comparing supraradical mastectomyⒼ versus radical mastectomyⒼ (2 RCTs), radical versus total mastectomyⒼ (2 RCTs), and supraradical versus total mastectomy(1 RCT).[28] It found no significant difference in the annual risk of death over a 10 year period (OR for more extensive *v* less extensive surgery 0.98, CI presented graphically; P = 0.7). **Comparisons between radical, total, and simple mastectomy:** The same review included four RCTs comparing either radical versus simple mastectomy**G** (3 RCTs) or total versus simple mastectomy (1 RCT) in 1296 women with operable breast cancer.[28] Meta-analysis found no significant difference in the annual risk of death over a 10 year period (OR for more extensive *v* less extensive surgery 0.98, CI presented graphically; P = 0.8). One included RCT (1079 women) comparing radical mastectomy and total mastectomy with or without axillary radiotherapy**G** has now reported 25 year follow up results.[29] It found no significant difference in survival between total and radical mastectomy, regardless of nodal status (in women with negative nodes: HR for total mastectomy plus radiotherapy *v* radical mastectomy 1.08, 95% CI 0.91 to 1.28; HR for total mastectomy without radiotherapy *v* radical mastectomy 1.03, 95% CI 0.87 to 1.23; in women with positive nodes: HR for total mastectomy plus radiotherapy *v* radical mastectomy 1.06, 95% CI 0.89 to 1.27). **Mastectomy versus breast conservation:** We found two systematic reviews.[28,30] The first review (search date 1995) analysed data on 10 year survival from six RCTs comparing breast conservation with mastectomy.[30] It found no significant difference in the risk of death at 10 years (5 RCTs, 3006 women; OR breast conservation *v* mastectomy 0.91, 95% CI 0.78 to 1.05). Where more than half of node positive women in both mastectomy and breast conservation groups received adjuvant**G** nodal radiotherapy, both groups had similar survival rates. Where fewer than half of node positive women in both groups received adjuvant nodal radiotherapy, survival was better with breast conservation (OR of death: breast conservation *v* with mastectomy 0.69, 95% CI 0.49 to 0.97). The second review (search date not reported, 9 RCTs, 5610 women potentially suitable for breast conserving surgery**G**) compared mastectomy versus breast conservation surgery (with or without radiotherapy; the proportion of women receiving mastectomy who also received radiotherapy was unclear).[28] It found no significant difference in annual risk of death over 10 years between mastectomy and breast conserving surgery either with or without radiotherapy (mastectomy *v* breast conservation alone: 1 RCT, 1432 women, OR 0.97, CI presented graphically; P = 0.4; mastectomy *v* breast conservation plus radiotherapy: 9 RCTs, 4891 women, OR 1.02, CI presented graphically; P = 0.7). It also found no significant difference in overall rates of recurrence or rates of local recurrence between mastectomy and breast conserving surgery plus radiotherapy (6 RCTs, 3107 women; OR for overall recurrence mastectomy *v* breast conservation plus radiotherapy 0.96, 95% CI 0.88 to 1.04; AR for local recurrence: 6.2% with mastectomy *v* 5.9% with breast conservation plus radiotherapy; P value reported as not significant). Three RCTs included in the reviews have now reported 20 year follow up results.[31–33] The first RCT (701 women with breast cancer < 2 cm diameter) found no significant difference between radical mastectomy and quadrantectomy**G** plus radiotherapy for all cause mortality at 20 years (death rate about 42% in both groups; P = 1.0).[31] The second RCT (1851 women) compared lumpectomy**G** alone, lumpectomy plus breast irradiation, and total mastectomy.[32] It found no significant difference between lumpectomy (with or without radiotherapy) and total mastectomy for mortality at 20 years (HR lumpectomy alone *v* mastectomy 1.05, 95% CI 0.90 to 1.23; HR lumpectomy plus radiotherapy *v* mastectomy 0.97, 95% CI 0.77 to 1.06). The third RCT (237 women) found no significant difference between modified radical mastectomy and lumpectomy plus axillary dissection plus radiotherapy in overall survival or in disease free survival**G** at 20 years (AR for overall survival: 58% with mastectomy *v*

54% with lumpectomy; P = 0.67; AR for disease free survival: 67% with mastectomy *v* 63% with lumpectomy; P = 0.64).[33] **Different extents of local excision in breast conservation:** We found no systematic review. We found one RCT (705 women) comparing lumpectomy versus quadrantectomy.[34] There were significantly more local recurrences with lumpectomy than with quadrantectomy (7% with lumpectomy *v* 2% with quadrantectomy), but a major factor associated with local recurrence in the lumpectomy group was incomplete excision (see comment below).[35] We found no RCTs comparing wide local excision (complete excision microscopically) with quadrantectomy.

Harms: More extensive surgery results in a poorer cosmetic result. Between 60–90% of women having breast conservation have an excellent or good cosmetic result (median 83%, 95% CI 67% to 87%).[34,36–44] The single most important factor influencing cosmetic outcome is the volume of tissue excised; the larger the amount of tissue excised the worse the cosmetic result.[34] The RCT of different extents of local excision in breast conservation found that, in a subset of 148 women, there was a significantly higher rate of poor cosmetic outcome with quadrantectomy**G** (RR quadrantectomy *v* lumpectomy**G** 3.1, 95% CI 1.2 to 8.1).[34] Only isolated small studies have shown no correlation between extent of surgical excision and cosmesis.[42]

Comment: The link between completeness of excision and local recurrence after breast conservation has been evaluated in 16 centres.[35] In 13 of these, incomplete excision significantly increased the risk of local recurrence compared with complete excision (RR 1.03, 95% CI 1.03 to 1.05). The three centres not reporting increased rates of local recurrence after incomplete excision gave much higher doses of local radiotherapy**G** (65–72 Gy) to people with involved margins. Two centres also used re-excision, and women with involved margins had only focal margin involvement.

OPTION RADIOTHERAPY AFTER BREAST CONSERVING SURGERY

One systematic review and one subsequent RCT found that adding radiotherapy to breast conserving surgery reduced the risk of local recurrence compared with breast conserving surgery alone. They found no significant difference in survival between breast conserving surgery plus radiotherapy and breast conserving surgery alone. One systematic review and one additional RCT found no significant difference in survival and local recurrence with breast conserving surgery plus radiotherapy compared with mastectomy. One RCT found that radiotherapy (with or without tamoxifen) reduced ipsilateral breast cancer recurrence compared with tamoxifen alone after median follow up of 87 months. It found no significant difference in survival. Radiotherapy may be associated with late adverse effects, which are rare, including pneumonitis, pericarditis, arm oedema, brachial plexopathy, and radionecrotic rib fracture.

Benefits: **Versus breast conserving surgery alone:** We found one systematic review (search date not reported, 10 RCTs)[45] and one subsequent RCT[46] comparing breast conserving surgery**G** plus radiotherapy**G** versus breast conserving surgery alone. Seven RCTs included in the review used megavoltage x rays. The review found that postoperative radiotherapy significantly reduced the annual risk of breast cancer mortality compared with no radiotherapy, but found no significant difference between treatments in the annual risk of all cause mortality (6 RCTs, 4177 women; OR for breast cancer mortality 0.86, CI presented graphically; P = 0.04; OR for all cause mortality 0.94, CI presented graphically; P > 0.1). The review found that postoperative radiotherapy significantly decreased the annual risk of isolated local recurrence compared with no postoperative radiotherapy (6 RCTs, 4177 women; OR 0.32, CI presented graphically; P < 0.00001).[45] Ten year follow up of one RCT included in the review found no significant difference in overall survival, but found that radiotherapy significantly reduced local recurrence rate (overall survival: 82.4% with radiotherapy *v* 76.9% with no radiotherapy; P = 0.33; local recurrence rate: 5.8% with radiotherapy *v* 23.5% with no radiotherapy; P = 0.001).[47] One subsequent RCT (1187 women with stage I–II invasive node negative breast cancer) also found no significant difference in overall survival between adjuvant radiotherapy and no adjuvant radiotherapy, but found that adjuvant radiotherapy significantly reduced ipsilateral breast recurrence compared with no adjuvant radiotherapy at 5 years (overall survival at 5 years: RR 1.16, 95% CI 0.81 to 1.65; ipsilateral breast recurrence at 5 years: AR 14% without radiotherapy *v* 4% with radiotherapy; RR 3.33, 95% CI 2.13 to 5.19).[46] One RCT (381 people) identified by the review was limited to people with "good prognosis disease" (tumour ≤ 2 cm, node negative).[48] It found that radiotherapy significantly reduced local relapse rate compared with breast conserving surgery alone at 5 years (relapse rate 2.3%, 95% CI 1.0% to 4.3% with radiotherapy *v* 18.4%, 95% CI 12.5% to 24.2% with no radiotherapy).[48] Ten year follow up data from this RCT found that radiotherapy significantly reduced local recurrence rates (relapse rate 8.5%, 95% CI 3.9% to 13.1% with radiotherapy *v* 24.0%, 95% CI 17.6% to 30.4% with no radiotherapy).[49] There was no significant difference in overall survival at 10 years (77.5% with radiotherapy *v* 78% with no radiotherapy). **Versus mastectomy:** We found one systematic review (search date not reported, 9 RCTs, 4891 women)[28] and one additional RCT[50] comparing breast radiotherapy after breast conserving surgery versus simple**Ⓖ** or modified radical mastectomy**Ⓖ** in women with invasive breast cancer. The review found no significant difference in annual risk of death over 10 years (OR 1.02, CI presented graphically; P = 0.7), or annual risk of any recurrence or local recurrence (6 RCTs, 3107 women; overall OR for any recurrence: mastectomy *v* breast conservation plus radiotherapy 0.96, 95% CI 0.88 to 1.04; AR for local recurrence: 6.2% with radiotherapy after breast conserving surgery *v* 5.9% with radical mastectomy; P value reported as not significant).[28] Three RCTs included in the review have now reported 20 year follow up results.[31–33] The first RCT (701 women with breast cancer < 2 cm diameter) found no significant difference between radical mastectomy and quadrantectomy**Ⓖ** plus radiotherapy for all cause mortality at 20 years (death rate about 42% in both groups; P = 1.0).[31] The second RCT (1851 women) compared lumpectomy**Ⓖ** alone, lumpectomy plus breast irradiation, and total mastectomy**Ⓖ**.[32] It found no significant difference between lumpectomy plus irradiation and total mastectomy for mortality at 20 years (HR lumpectomy plus irradiation *v* mastectomy 0.97, 95% CI 0.77 to 1.06). The third RCT (237 women) found no significant difference between modified radical mastectomy and lumpectomy plus axillary dissection plus radiotherapy in overall survival or disease free survival**Ⓖ** at 20 years (AR for overall survival: 58% with mastectomy *v* 54% with lumpectomy; P = 0.67; AR for disease free survival: 67% with mastectomy *v* 63% with lumpectomy; P = 0.64).[33] One additional RCT (187 women) found no significant difference in overall or disease free survival between breast conserving surgery plus radiotherapy and modified radical mastectomy at 40 months (overall survival: 94.1% with breast conserving surgery plus radiotherapy *v* 93.7% with mastectomy; disease free survival: 93.9% with breast conserving surgery plus radiotherapy *v* 89.2% with mastectomy; P > 0.05 for both comparisons).[50] The incidence of locoregional recurrence was similar in the two groups (2/76 [2.6%] with breast conserving surgery plus radiotherapy *v* 2/111 [1.8%] with mastectomy; significance not reported). **Versus breast**

conserving surgery plus tamoxifen: We found one RCT (1009 women after lumpectomy for node negative invasive breast cancer ≤ 1 cm), which compared three treatments: radiotherapy (started 2 weeks after surgery, 50 Gy over 5 weeks with or without external beam boost), radiotherapy plus tamoxifen, and tamoxifen alone.[51] It found that radiotherapy (with or without tamoxifen) significantly reduced ipsilateral breast cancer recurrence compared with tamoxifen alone after median follow up of 87 months (23/332 [7%] with radiotherapy alone *v* 9/334 [2.7%] with radiotherapy plus tamoxifen *v* 45/334 [13%] with tamoxifen alone; HR for radiotherapy alone *v* tamoxifen alone 0.51, 95% CI 0.31 to 0.84; P = 0.008; HR for radiotherapy plus tamoxifen *v* tamoxifen alone 0.19, 95% CI 0.09 to 0.39; P < 0.001). It found no significant difference in survival or other events (tumour recurrence, contralateral breast cancer, other second primary breast cancer, or death with no evidence of cancer) between the three treatments (survival: 312/332 [94.0%] with radiotherapy alone *v* 314/334 [94.0%] with tamoxifen alone *v* 312/334 [93.4%] with radiotherapy plus tamoxifen; P = 0.93; events: 61/332 [18.4%] with radiotherapy alone *v* 74/334 [22.2%] with tamoxifen alone *v* 52/334 [15.6%] with radiotherapy plus tamoxifen; P = 0.08).

Harms: **Versus breast conserving surgery alone:** The review found that radiotherapy**Ⓖ** increased the annual rate of non-breast cancer deaths compared with no radiotherapy, this increase was of borderline significance (OR 1.34, CI presented graphically; P = 0.05).[45] The subsequent RCT found similar numbers of non-breast cancer deaths in both groups (20/591 [3.4%] with radiotherapy *v* 18/587 [3.1%] without radiotherapy; P value not reported). **Versus mastectomy:** The review did not report on the harms of breast conserving surgery**Ⓖ** plus radiotherapy compared with mastectomy. However, overall, the review found that adding radiotherapy to mastectomy or breast conserving surgery increased the risk of non-breast cancer death compared with surgery alone (OR 1.24, 95% CI 1.09 to 1.42).[28] **Versus breast conserving surgery plus tamoxifen:** One RCT (1009 women after lumpectomy**Ⓖ** in node negative invasive breast cancer ≤ 1 cm) comparing radiotherapy, radiotherapy plus tamoxifen, and tamoxifen alone found no significant difference between treatments in endometrial cancer or other second primary cancers (endometrial cancer: 1/332 [0.3%] with radiotherapy alone *v* 1/334 [0.3%] with tamoxifen alone *v* 5/334 [1.5%] with radiotherapy plus tamoxifen; P = 0.12; other second primary cancer: 10/332 [3%] with radiotherapy alone *v* 14/334 [4.2%] with tamoxifen alone *v* 15/334 [4.5%] with radiotherapy plus tamoxifen; P = 0.65).[51] **Quality of life:** Two prospective studies of quality of life after breast conserving surgery have been reported and are based on RCTs where participants were randomised to either radiotherapy or no further local treatment after surgery.[52,53] The older study (1984–1989; 837 women)[52] reported that radiotherapy significantly reduced quality of life compared with no radiotherapy at 1 and 2 months (17 item modified Breast Cancer Chemotherapy Questionnaire, higher score indicating better quality of life; mean score change at 1 month: –0.07 with radiotherapy *v* +0.21 without radiotherapy; mean score change at 2 months: –0.05 with radiotherapy *v* +0.30 without radiotherapy; P = 0.0001 for both time points). Radiotherapy significantly increased breast pain at 6 months and breast skin irritation at 3 months (AR for breast pain: 33% with radiotherapy *v* 20% without radiotherapy; P = 0.0002; skin irritation: 28% with radiotherapy *v* 14% without radiotherapy; P = 0.0001). However, there was no significant difference between groups in the risk of breast pain, skin irritation, or upset because of breast appearance at 2 years (AR for breast pain: about 15% for both groups; P reported as not significant; skin irritation: 7% in both groups; P reported as not significant; upset with breast appearance:

4.8% in both groups; P = 0.62).[52] The more recent study (1992–2000),[53] assessed whether breast pain affected quality of life in women who received breast conserving surgery plus tamoxifen plus either radiotherapy or no further treatment. It found no significant difference between groups in pain, physical function, breast symptoms, or global health quality of life at 12 months (measured using the QLQ-C30 and QLQ-BR23 questionnaires; mean scores presented graphically; pain: P = 0.33; physical function: P = 0.76; breast symptoms: P = 0.27; quality of life: P = 0.45).[53] **General adverse effects of adding radiotherapy to breast surgery:** One systematic overview (search date 2001) found limited data on radiotherapy related morbidity and reported that no conclusions could be drawn.[6] A consensus document published in 1998 (mainly of women having breast conserving surgery or mastectomy with variation in radiotherapy techniques, doses, and fractionation) reported two severe adverse effects of radiotherapy, namely acute pneumonitis (0.7–7.0%) and pericarditis (0–0.3%), and the following long term adverse effects: significant arm oedema (1% without axillary dissection), radionecrotic rib fracture (1.1–1.5%), and brachial plexopathy (0–1.8%).[54] The risk and severity of adverse effects increased with volume irradiated, total dose received, dose per fraction, previous surgery (e.g. axillary dissection), and radiotherapy techniques that caused overlap in irradiated tissues. One systematic review (search date not reported)[55] of 10 RCTs found that the excess of non-breast cancer deaths after chest wall radiotherapy was caused by cardiac deaths resulting from the radiotherapy, but recent RCTs with data beyond 10 years did not find an excess of cardiac deaths.[56–58] A more recent systematic review (search date not reported, 40 RCTs in early breast cancer with meta-analysis of 10 and 20 year results) confirms that adding radiotherapy to surgery results in a reduction in local recurrence of two thirds, a reduction in breast cancer mortality, but an increase in other, particularly vascular, mortality.[45] Overall, 20 year survival was 37.1% with radiotherapy compared with 35.9% for controls (P = 0.06). Studies assessing cosmetic results have mainly been retrospective using poorly validated outcomes. The effects of social, psychological, and financial disruptions from attending 5–6 weeks of radiotherapy have not been addressed clearly. There is an extremely low reported incidence of radiation induced malignancy, usually soft tissue sarcomas, in the irradiated breast.

Comment: RCTs comparing breast conserving surgery**G** with and without radiotherapy**G**, as well as retrospective case series, have found that prognostic factors for local recurrence after breast conserving surgery include positive tumour margins, an extensive intraduct component, younger age, lymphovascular invasion, histological grade, and systemic treatment. The only consistent independent risk factor is avoiding radiotherapy. Although there is no published evidence of a difference in survival at 10 years, recent results from the Fifth Early Breast Cancer Trialists' Group meeting suggest a reduction in breast cancer death in women having breast surgery with radiotherapy compared with no radiotherapy (6100 women; 3.9% increase in survival) (Dixon M, personal communication, 2001).One systematic review of radiation effects in breast cancer by the Swedish Council of Technology Assessment in Health Care, which did not carry out meta-analysis, supports the above conclusions for postmastectomy radiotherapy, radiotherapy after breast conserving surgery for ductal carcinoma *in situ*, and for the comparability of breast conserving surgery with radiotherapy and modified radical mastectomy**G** alone for invasive breast cancer for disease free survival**G** and overall survival.[6] It concluded that there are conflicting data about effects of breast conservation surgery plus radiotherapy compared with modified radical mastectomy on local recurrence in people with invasive cancer.

OPTION RADIOTHERAPY AFTER MASTECTOMY

One systematic review found that radiotherapy to the chest wall after mastectomy reduced the risk of local recurrence by about two thirds compared with no postoperative radiotherapy. It found that radiotherapy did not reduce all cause mortality or breast cancer mortality after mastectomy alone or mastectomy plus axillary clearance. However, radiotherapy did reduce all cause mortality and breast cancer mortality after mastectomy plus axillary sampling. Radiotherapy may be associated with late adverse effects, which are rare, including pneumonitis, pericarditis, arm oedema, brachial plexopathy, and radionecrotic rib fracture.

Benefits: We found one systematic review (search date not reported, 34 RCTs, see comment below) comparing mastectomy versus mastectomy followed by radiotherapy**G** to the chest wall.[45] Five RCTs were of mastectomy alone (5397 women), six of mastectomy plus axillary sampling**G** (3901 women), and 23 of mastectomy plus axillary clearance**G** (6700 women). It found that radiotherapy after mastectomy (with or without axillary clearance) did not significantly reduce annual all cause mortality or annual breast cancer mortality (all cause mortality: mastectomy alone OR 0.98; mastectomy plus axillary clearance OR 1.04; breast cancer mortality: mastectomy alone OR 0.95; mastectomy plus axillary clearance OR 0.96; for all comparisons CI presented graphically; $P > 0.1$). However, radiotherapy after mastectomy plus axillary sampling significantly reduced annual all cause mortality and annual breast cancer mortality compared with no postoperative radiotherapy (all cause mortality: OR 0.83, CI presented graphically; $P = 0.00005$; breast cancer mortality: OR 0.82, CI presented graphically; $P = 0.0001$). Postoperative radiotherapy significantly reduced annual isolated local recurrence after mastectomy with or without axillary clearance or axillary sampling (mastectomy alone OR 0.36; mastectomy plus axillary clearance OR 0.37; mastectomy plus axillary sampling OR 0.23; for all comparisons CI presented graphically; $P < 0.00001$). We found no evidence that reduction in relative risk of local recurrence was affected by age, nodal status, receptor status, tumour grade, or tumour size, or that the effect of radiotherapy on mortality varied significantly with extent of surgery, type of radiotherapy (megavoltage or orthovoltage), years the RCTs commenced or completed recruitment, or whether systemic treatment was given.[59]

Harms: See harms of radiotherapy after breast conserving surgery, p 2239. Three RCTs included in the review of total nodal irradiation**G** after mastectomy in high risk disease found no significant increase in cardiac mortality.[56–58,60]

Comment: The RCTs in the large systematic review were heterogeneous, in part because they began when RCT methods were less developed.[45] They varied in randomisation processes, areas irradiated, use of systemic treatment, radiotherapy**G** doses, fractionation, and treatment schedules. We found little good evidence to identify which women should have postmastectomy radiotherapy to prevent local recurrence. One review of retrospective data found that extent of axillary node involvement, larger tumour size, higher histological grade, presence of lymphovascular invasion, and involvement of tumour margins increased the absolute risk of local recurrence or mortality.[59,61–63]

OPTION RADIOTHERAPY TO THE INTERNAL MAMMARY CHAIN

One RCT found no significant difference in relapse or survival at 2–3 years between radiotherapy and no radiotherapy to the internal mammary chain. Treatment may increase radiation induced cardiac morbidity.

Benefits: We found no systematic review. We found one RCT (270 women treated with breast conserving surgery**G** and radiotherapy**G**), which compared internal mammary chain irradiation versus no internal mammary chain irradiation.[64] At median follow up of 2.7 years there was no significant difference in relapse or survival (numbers not reported).

Harms: See harms of radiotherapy after breast conserving surgery, p 2239. Radiotherapy**G** to the internal mammary chain is more likely to affect the heart compared with other types of radiotherapy.[65]

Comment: The risk of internal mammary chain node involvement is related to the location and size of the primary tumour and, most importantly, histopathological axillary nodal status. Up to 30% of women with axillary involvement will also exhibit internal mammary chain nodal metastases. Central or medial breast cancers are more likely to metastasise to the internal mammary chain, as are larger tumours.[66,67] The risk of internal mammary chain recurrence is low, and after modified radical mastectomy**G** alone is 2%.[68] Modern radiotherapy**G** planning and delivery should involve an assessment of the position and depth of the internal mammary chain nodes to be treated (using computerised tomography or ultrasound), and computer assisted placement, arrangement, and determination of dose distribution; these technologies were unavailable at the time of most RCTs included in the reviews.[28,45,55] Recent indirect evidence from RCTs suggests improved survival from nodal irradiation (including radiation to the internal mammary chain) after modified radical mastectomy combined with systemic treatment.[56,57,60] Another RCT of internal mammary chain irradiation has started recently (sponsored by the European Organisation for Research and Treatment of Cancer [EORTC]).

OPTION RADIOTHERAPY TO THE IPSILATERAL SUPRACLAVICULAR FOSSA

We found insufficient evidence about the effects of irradiation of the ipsilateral supraclavicular fossa on survival. RCTs have found that radiotherapy to the chest wall and lymph nodes is associated with reduced risk of locoregional recurrence, including supraclavicular fossa nodal recurrence. Morbidity associated with irradiation of the supraclavicular fossa is rare and, where it occurs, is mild and temporary.

Benefits: We found no systematic review or RCTs on radiotherapy**G** to the ipsilateral supraclavicular fossa. One systematic review (search date not reported) found that postoperative radiotherapy to the chest wall and lymph nodes was associated with reduced locoregional recurrence: see radiotherapy after breast conserving surgery, p 2237; radiotherapy after mastectomy, p 2241; and radiotherapy to internal mammary chain irradiation, p 2242.[45] (RCTs indicate reduced recurrence in the supraclavicular fossa.) One RCT in postmenopausal women at high risk of local recurrence who received tamoxifen after mastectomy found that radiotherapy (chest wall and total nodal irradiation) was associated with lower recurrence in the supraclavicular fossa at median follow up of 123 months (9/689 [1.3%] with radiotherapy *v* 37/686 [5.4%] with no radiotherapy; CI not reported).[60]

Harms: The acute morbidity of irradiation to the supraclavicular fossa is mild and includes temporary upper oesophagitis in nearly all women. The risk of radiation pneumonitis increases with the volume of lung irradiated. Treatment irradiates the lung apex in addition to any lung included in the breast or chest wall fields. Possible late morbidity includes brachial plexopathy but this should not exceed 1.8% if attention is paid to limiting total dose to 50 Gy, the limiting of the dose per fraction to 2 Gy or less, and avoiding field junction overlaps.[54,69] Late apical lung fibrosis is common and usually of no clinical importance. Demyelination of the cervical cord is an extremely rare complication of supraclavicular fossa radiotherapy**G**.

Comment: None.

OPTION TOTAL NODAL RADIOTHERAPY

One systematic review found that postmastectomy radiotherapy, including total nodal irradiation, reduced locoregional recurrence. It found that postmastectomy radiotherapy improved survival in women receiving mastectomy plus axillary sampling, but not in women receiving mastectomy alone or mastectomy plus axillary clearance.

Benefits: We found one systematic review (search date not reported, 34 RCTs of postmastectomy radiotherapy**G**), which included 27 RCTs of total nodal irradiation**G** to the internal mammary chain, supraclavicular fossa, and axilla.[45] It found that postoperative radiotherapy was associated with a significant reduction in locoregional recurrence. However, it found that radiotherapy only improved survival in women receiving mastectomy plus axillary sampling**G**, but not women receiving mastectomy alone or mastectomy plus axillary clearance**G**. See benefits of radiotherapy after mastectomy, p 2241. These results should be interpreted with caution as they include some RCTs that did not give total nodal irradiation**G**.

Harms: See harms of radiotherapy to the internal mammary chain, p 2242, supraclavicular fossa, p 2242, and axilla, p 2239. Three RCTs included in the review found no increase in cardiac mortality because of radiotherapy**G**.[56–58,60]

Comment: None.

OPTION ADJUVANT COMBINATION CHEMOTHERAPY

One systematic review found that adjuvant combination chemotherapy reduced rates of recurrence and improved survival at 10 years compared with no chemotherapy. The benefit seemed to be independent of nodal or menopausal status, although the absolute improvements were greater in those with node positive disease, and probably greater in younger women. The review found no additional survival benefit from prolonging adjuvant chemotherapy from 4–6 to 8–12 months. RCTs did not find additional survival advantage from enhanced dose regimens of combination chemotherapy. The review found that adjuvant regimens containing an anthracycline reduced recurrence, and improved survival compared with a standard multidrug chemotherapy (CMF) regimen at 5 years. Adverse effects of chemotherapy include nausea and vomiting, hair loss, bone marrow suppression, fatigue, and gastrointestinal disturbance. Chemotherapy may impair fertility and ovarian function.

Benefits: **Versus no chemotherapy:** We found one systematic review (search date not reported, 47 RCTs, 18 000 women) comparing prolonged combination chemotherapy**G** versus no chemotherapy.[70] Chemotherapy was associated with significantly lower rates of any kind of recurrence and death from all causes (recurrence: women aged < 50 years, OR 0.65, 95% CI 0.61 to 0.69; women aged 50–69 years, OR 0.80, 95% 0.72 to 0.88; death from all causes: women aged < 50 years, OR 0.73, 95% CI 0.68 to 0.78; women aged 50–69 years, OR 0.89, 95% CI 0.86 to 0.92). Proportional benefits were similar for women with node negative and node positive disease. Ten year survival according to nodal and age group is summarised (see table 1, p 2257). **Duration of treatment:** The same review identified 11 RCTs (6104 women), which compared longer regimens (doubling duration of chemotherapy from between 4–6 months to 8–12 months) with shorter regimens.[70] It found no additional benefit from longer treatment duration. **Different doses:** Several RCTs found no significant improvement from enhanced dose regimens, whereas others found little difference from untreated controls when suboptimal doses were used.[71,72] **Anthracycline regimens versus standard CMF regimen:** The systematic review identified 11 RCTs (5942 women) comparing regimens containing anthracycline**G** (including the drugs adriamycin [doxorubicin] or 4-epidoxorubicin) versus standard CMF**G** regimens.[70] It found a significant reduction in recurrence rates in those on anthracycline regimens (P = 0.006), and a modest but significant improvement in 5 year survival (72% with anthracycline *v* 69% with CMF regimen; P = 0.02).

Harms: **Acute adverse effects:** Adverse effects include fatigue, nausea and vomiting, hair loss, bone marrow suppression, neuropathy, and gastrointestinal disturbance. Prolonged chemotherapy is more likely to be associated with lethargy and haematological toxicity (anaemia and neutropenia), and anthracycline**G** regimens cause complete hair loss. **Long term adverse effects:** Fertility and ovarian function may be permanently affected by chemotherapy, especially in women aged over 40 years, although for some women with hormone dependent cancer, reduced ovarian function may contribute to the benefit of adjuvant**G** treatment. Other potential long term risks include induction of second cancers (especially haematological malignancies, although the risk is low), and cardiac impairment with cumulative anthracycline dosages. Provided the cumulative dose of adriamycin (doxorubicin) does not exceed 300–350 mg/m^2, the risk of congestive heart failure is less than 1%.

Comment: The absolute benefits of these regimens need to be balanced against their toxicity for different women. New and highly active cytotoxic agents such as the taxanes are being examined with anthracyclines**G** either in combination or sequence. Alternating sequences of cytotoxic agents may prove an effective way of circumventing acquired drug resistance and thus enhancing the efficacy of a regimen, such as the Milan regimen**G** of single agent anthracycline followed by standard CMF**G** chemotherapy.[73]

OPTION ADJUVANT TAMOXIFEN

One systematic review found that adjuvant tamoxifen taken for up to 5 years reduced the risk of recurrence and death in women with oestrogen receptor positive tumours irrespective of age, menopausal status, nodal involvement, or the addition of chemotherapy. Five years of treatment was more effective than shorter durations, but available evidence did not find benefit associated with prolongation of treatment beyond 5 years. Tamoxifen slightly increased the risk of endometrial cancer and thrombotic complications, but we found no evidence of an overall adverse effect on non-breast cancer mortality.

Benefits: **Versus placebo:** We found one systematic review (search date not reported, 55 RCTs, 37 000 women), which compared adjuvant**G** tamoxifen with placebo.[74] The review found that taking tamoxifen for a median of 5 years significantly reduced recurrence and mortality compared with placebo (RR for recurrence 0.58; RR for mortality 0.78; CI presented graphically; for both comparisons P < 0.00001). These benefits seemed to be largely irrespective of age, menopausal status, daily tamoxifen dose (generally 20–40 mg), and of whether chemotherapy had been given to both groups. **Oestrogen receptor and lymph node status:** Five years of tamoxifen treatment was associated with a greater reduction in the recurrence rate for women with oestrogen receptor positive rather than negative tumours (RRR 50% with oestrogen receptor positive *v* 6% with oestrogen receptor negative), and with a slightly greater reduction in the absolute risk of 10 year recurrence in women with node positive compared with node negative disease (ARR 15.2% with node positive *v* 14.9% with node negative). Five years of tamoxifen treatment was also associated with a greater absolute improvement in 10 year survival in node positive than node negative women (see table 2, p 2257).[74] **Duration of treatment:** The review found significantly greater reductions in recurrence with increasing duration of adjuvant tamoxifen (RRR 26% with 5 years of tamoxifen use *v* 12% with 1 year of tamoxifen use; $P < 0.0001$).[74] One RCT (3887 women) comparing 2 and 5 years of treatment found similar results.[75] The effects of prolonged treatment beyond 5 years are unclear. In the largest RCT in the systematic review, 1153 women who had completed 5 years of tamoxifen were randomised to either placebo or 5 more years of tamoxifen.[74,76] Disease free survival**G** after 4 years of further follow up was greater for those who switched to placebo rather than continued tamoxifen (86% with continued tamoxifen *v* 92% with placebo; $P = 0.003$), although there was no significant difference in overall survival. Other studies found no detrimental effect or improvement in continuing tamoxifen beyond 5 years.[77] **Versus radiotherapy:** See benefits of tamoxifen plus radiotherapy, p 2231.

Harms: One systematic review found an increased risk of endometrial cancer with tamoxifen (average HR 2.58, 95% CI 2.23 to 2.93).[74] For 5 years of tamoxifen treatment, this resulted in a cumulative risk over 10 years of two deaths per 1000 women (95% CI 0 deaths per 1000 women to 4 deaths per 1000 women). There was no evidence of an increased incidence of other cancers or of non-breast cancer related deaths (i.e. cardiac or vascular), although one extra death per 5000 women years of tamoxifen was attributed to pulmonary embolus. Bone loss was found in premenopausal women (1.4% bone loss a year) but not in postmenopausal women, because of the partial agonist effects of tamoxifen.[78] There were mixed effects on cardiovascular risk, with significant reductions in low density lipoprotein cholesterol associated with a reduced incidence of myocardial infarction in some studies, but an increased risk of thrombosis. Overall, no effect has been found on non-breast cancer mortality (HR 0.99, 95% CI 0.88 to 1.16).[74] **Versus radiotherapy:** See harms of tamoxifen plus radiotherapy, p 2233.

Comment: The risk : benefit ratio may vary between women, with oestrogen receptor negative women deriving little benefit. Even in oestrogen receptor positive women, any benefit on breast cancer could be offset with prolonged treatment (> 5 years), by drug resistance, and by adverse effects on the endometrium. Two multicentre RCTs of tamoxifen duration are in progress (Cancer Research Campaign, personal communication, 2000); however, because of concerns about long term toxicity with tamoxifen (see harms above) and in the absence of further definitive data, current clinical practice has been to recommend tamoxifen for 5 years.[79] For women with completely oestrogen receptor negative disease, the overall benefit of adjuvant**G** tamoxifen needs further research.

OPTION HIGH DOSE CHEMOTHERAPY

One systematic review found no significant difference between high dose chemotherapy plus autograft and conventional chemotherapy in 5 year survival for women with early, poor prognosis breast cancer. The review found that high dose chemotherapy plus autograft increased treatment related and non-cancer related deaths compared with conventional chemotherapy.

Benefits: We found one systematic review (search date 2002, 9 RCTs, 3525 women with early, poor prognosis breast cancer, multiple positive axillary lymph nodes and no distant metastasis) that compared high dose chemotherapy plus bone marrow or peripheral blood stem cell autograft with conventional chemotherapy (see comment below).[80] It found no significant difference between regimens in overall survival at 3 or 5 years (3 years: RR 1.02, 95% CI 0.98 to 1.06; 5 years: RR 0.98, 95% CI 0.93 to 1.05). It found that high dose chemotherapy significantly increased event free survival at 3 years (RR 1.11, 95% CI 1.05 to 1.18). However, there was no significant difference at 5 years (RR 1.00, 95% CI 0.92 to 1.08). It found that high dose chemotherapy significantly reduced quality of life immediately after treatment but found no significant difference between regimens at 1 year (3 RCTs, data not reported in the review).

Harms: The systematic review found that high dose chemotherapy significantly increased treatment related mortality and non-cancer related deaths compared with conventional chemotherapy (treatment related deaths, 5 RCTs: 40/1075 [3.7%] with high dose *v* 0/1087 [0%] with conventional; RR 17.05, 95% CI 4.75 to 61.22; non-cancer related deaths: 48 deaths with high dose *v* 4 deaths with conventional dose, RR 7.74, 95% CI 3.43 to 17.50).[80]

Comment: Most of the RCTs included in the systematic review have only been published as abstracts and reporting of follow up is incomplete.[80] Further results are awaited. Overall survival rates quoted in the review were predominantly based on results to date and showed no differences in overall survival. Quality of life scores were not different between the groups at 1 year but the large excess of non-cancer deaths in the high dose group shows that this intervention is not likely to be beneficial, even in women with poor prognosis primary disease.

OPTION COMBINED CHEMOTHERAPY PLUS TAMOXIFEN

One RCT found that adding chemotherapy to tamoxifen improved survival at 5 years in women with lymph node negative, oestrogen receptor positive early breast cancer. It found that adding combined chemotherapy to tamoxifen was associated with increased adverse effects such as nausea, neutropenia, alopecia, thromboembolism, and phlebitis.

Benefits: We found no systematic review. We found one RCT (2306 women with lymph node negative, oestrogen receptor positive early breast cancer), which compared tamoxifen alone versus tamoxifen plus CMF**G** chemotherapy.[81] It found that adding chemotherapy to tamoxifen caused a further absolute improvement in disease free survival**G** and overall survival (disease free survival at 5 years' follow up: 90% with tamoxifen plus chemotherapy *v* 85% with tamoxifen alone; P = 0.006; overall survival: 97% with tamoxifen plus chemotherapy *v* 94% with tamoxifen alone; P = 0.03).

Harms: Adding CMF**G** chemotherapy to tamoxifen was associated with a greater incidence of grade 3/4 neutropenia (9% with tamoxifen plus chemotherapy *v* 0% with tamoxifen alone), grade 2 or higher nausea

(35% with tamoxifen plus chemotherapy *v* 4% with tamoxifen alone), moderate/severe alopecia (35.6% with tamoxifen plus chemotherapy *v* 0.4% with tamoxifen alone), and thromboembolism/phlebitis (7.5% with tamoxifen plus chemotherapy *v* 2.1% with tamoxifen alone).[81]

Comment: None.

OPTION OVARIAN ABLATION

One systematic review found that in premenopausal women with early breast cancer, ovarian ablation improved survival compared with no ablation after 15 years follow up.

Benefits: We found one systematic review (search date not reported, 12 RCTs with at least 15 years' follow up, 2102 premenopausal women with early breast cancer) comparing ovarian ablation❻ by irradiation or surgery versus no ablation.[82] Significantly more women with ovarian ablation survived (52% with ablation *v* 46% with no ablation; P = 0.001), and survived recurrence free (45% with ablation *v* 39% with no ablation; P = 0.0007). Benefit was independent of nodal status.

Harms: We found no good evidence on long term adverse effects. Concerns exist about late sequelae of ovarian ablation❻, especially effects on bone mineral density and cardiovascular risk. Acute adverse effects are likely to be menopausal symptoms.

Comment: Five of the RCTs compared ovarian ablation❻ plus chemotherapy with chemotherapy alone.[82] In these, the absolute benefit of ablation was smaller than in RCTs of ovarian ablation alone. It may be that cytotoxic chemotherapy itself suppresses ovarian function, making the effect of ablation difficult to detect in combined RCTs. When only premenopausal women were considered in the absence of chemotherapy, there was a 27% improvement in the odds of recurrence free survival. RCTs are underway of reversible oophorectomy using gonadotrophin releasing hormone analogues, which would allow preservation of fertility in younger women with oestrogen receptor positive tumours.

OPTION AXILLARY MANAGEMENT

There is consensus that axillary clearance reduces regional recurrence compared with no axillary management. RCTs found no significant difference in survival at 5–10 years between axillary clearance and axillary node sampling (followed by axillary radiotherapy in women found to be node positive) or axillary radiotherapy (regardless of axillary nodal status). One systematic review found that axillary radiotherapy reduced isolated local recurrence compared with axillary clearance, but this difference was not significant. One systematic review of mainly poor quality evidence found that the risk of arm lymphoedema was highest with axillary clearance plus radiotherapy, lower with axillary sampling plus radiotherapy, and lowest with sampling alone.

Benefits: **Axillary clearance versus axillary sampling:** We found no systematic review but found one RCT (466 women) in women having breast conserving surgery❻.[83] The RCT compared complete axillary clearance❻ (level I, II, and III dissection) versus four node axillary sampling❻ followed by axillary radiotherapy❻ if the nodes were involved. It found that axillary sampling was associated with improved survival compared with axillary clearance❻, but the difference was not significant (overall survival figures presented graphically; P = 0.2; estimated 5 year survival: 88.6% with axillary sampling *v* 82.1% with axillary clearance). Rates of node positivity were similar in both groups. **Axillary**

clearance versus axillary radiotherapy: We found one systematic review (search date not reported, 8 RCTs, 4370 women) comparing axillary clearance (level I, II, and III dissection) versus axillary radiotherapy (regardless of axillary nodal status).[28] It found no significant difference in annual risk of mortality over 10 years or in recurrence (mortality: OR 0.96, CI presented graphically; P = 0.3; recurrence: OR 1.01, CI not reported). Radiotherapy was associated with fewer isolated local recurrences, but this difference did not reach significance (OR 0.85, CI not reported; P = 0.06.[28] **Axillary clearance alone versus axillary clearance plus radiotherapy:** We found no studies assessing the effect of radiotherapy in addition to axillary clearance (level I and II, or level I, II, and III dissection) in regional control of disease.

Harms: **Versus axillary sampling:** Adverse effects of axillary surgery include seroma formation, arm swelling, damage to the intercostobrachial nerve, and shoulder stiffness. We found one RCT comparing the morbidity of different axillary procedures.[83] It compared complete axillary clearance**G** (level I, II, and III dissection) versus four node axillary sampling**G** followed by radiotherapy**G** if the nodes were involved. It found that the rate of arm swelling was higher after clearance than after sampling whether or not women received postoperative radiotherapy (at 3 years, forearm girth was significantly greater with clearance than with sampling alone [P = 0.005] or sampling plus radiotherapy [P = 0.04]). After removal of axillary drains, between 25–50% of women who had had a level I and II, or level I, II, and III axillary dissection developed seromas requiring aspiration. The RCT found that women who received axillary clearance or axillary sampling plus radiotherapy (not to the shoulder joint) had significantly reduced shoulder movement compared with women receiving axillary sampling alone at 6 months (clearance *v* sampling alone; P = 0.003; sampling plus radiotherapy *v* sampling alone: P = 0.004). However, by 3 years, the axillary clearance group had improved and was not significantly different from the sampling alone group (P = 0.1). **Arm lymphoedema:** One Australian systematic review (search date 1996) of lymphoedema prevalence, risks, and management found that, although current information is of poor quality, the combination of axillary dissection (to or beyond level II) and axillary radiotherapy**G** was associated with a risk of lymphoedema of 12–60%, with most studies suggesting that at least a third of women are affected.[84] Studies of axillary sampling followed by irradiation found lower rates (6–32%), and for axillary sampling alone, lower still (0–21%). Studies of dissection beyond level I found rates between 0–42%, with most studies reporting a rate of 20–30% 1 year after operation.[84] In women who receive axillary radiotherapy without axillary surgery, the overall lymphoedema rate is about 8%.

Comment: **Axillary staging:** Both clearance and sampling**G** provide important prognostic information on which decisions on local and systemic treatment can be based. Further RCTs of less invasive and potentially less morbid staging**G** procedures such as sentinel node biopsy are underway. A decision on axillary management should be based on the risk of involvement of axillary nodes (which varies according to tumour size, grade, and the presence of vascular/lymphatic invasion), and potential treatment related morbidity. Two retrospective cohort studies found that level I dissection accurately assessed axillary lymph node status, providing that at least 10 nodes were removed.[85,86] One RCT found that a sample of four nodes provided sufficient information to categorise an axilla as histologically positive or negative.[87] Removal of nodes at level

I and II, or removal of all nodes below the axillary vein (level I, II, and III), accurately stages the axilla.[85,86] RCTs comparing sentinel node biopsy with axillary node clearance and sampling are currently underway, and results of these will be incorporated in future *Clinical Evidence* updates (Dixon M, personal communication, 2000).

QUESTION What are the effects of interventions in locally advanced breast cancer (stage III B)?

Alan Rodger

OPTION LOCAL TREATMENT FOR LOCALLY ADVANCED BREAST CANCER

Two small RCTs including women with locally advanced disease (stage III B) found that radiotherapy or surgery as sole local treatments have similar effects on response rates, duration of response, and overall survival for locally advanced breast cancer that is rendered operable by prior chemotherapy. One RCT found limited evidence that radiotherapy after attempted curative surgery reduced locoregional recurrence compared with no further treatment, but did not improve time to relapse or overall survival. Local skin toxicity (acute and late) after radiotherapy is greater in locally advanced breast cancer than after treatment for less advanced disease, because of the need for a higher radiation dose to skin.

Benefits: We found no systematic review of the role of radiotherapy**G** in locally advanced (stage III B) breast cancer**G**. We found seven RCTs, including women with stage III B, which compared radiotherapy versus no radiotherapy.[57,60,88–92] Other management options varied across these RCTs. Most RCTs were small, but included more than stage III B women. **Postoperative radiotherapy versus no further local treatment after surgery:** We found two RCTs.[88,91] In the first RCT premastectomy and postmastectomy chemo-endocrine treatment were given to all women, and half the women were randomised to postmastectomy radiotherapy to the chest wall and regional lymphatics (45–50 Gy in 5 weeks).[88] However, 43% of the 184 women were excluded and there were more exclusions in the radiotherapy group, and it is impossible to ascertain what percentage of women were stage III B. There were numerous chemotherapy complications, including one death. The RCT found no significant difference in local or distant failures. However, it found that overall crude survival was significantly higher with no radiotherapy compared with radiotherapy (28.7 months with no radiotherapy *v* 21.7 months with radiotherapy; $P < 0.05$). Conclusions cannot be drawn from this RCT. The second RCT of operable locally advanced breast cancer (332 women who were recurrence free after modified radical mastectomy**G** and 6 cycles of chemo-hormone treatment; 38% stage T4 and 14% N2)[90] compared postoperative radiotherapy versus no further treatment. It found no significant difference in time to relapse or median overall survival (time to relapse: 4.7 years with radiotherapy *v* 5.2 years with no further treatment; median overall survival: 8.3 years with radiotherapy *v* 8.1 years with no further treatment). Radiotherapy reduced locoregional sites as first recurrence by 9%. **Postmastectomy radiotherapy in women having systemic treatment after surgery:** Two RCTs of "high risk breast cancer" (including women with stage III B disease) studied postmastectomy radiotherapy in women having systemic treatment after surgery.[57,60] One RCT found that, in a subgroup of 189 postmenopausal women with skin invasion who received postmastectomy radiotherapy plus tamoxifen, 8% developed local recurrence compared with 34% receiving tamoxifen alone (5 year disease free survival**G**: 41% with radiotherapy *v* 37% with tamoxifen; 10 year disease free survival: 23% with radiotherapy *v* 22% with tamoxifen; 5 year survival: 51% with radiotherapy *v* 61% with tamoxifen; 10 year survival: 31% with radiotherapy *v* 27% with tamoxifen). However, the studies used small and retrospective subgroups, making conclusions uncertain. **Surgery alone versus radiotherapy alone:** Two RCTs compared surgery alone with radiotherapy alone as local treatment.[89,90] In one RCT (113 women with stage III breast cancer, 67% stage III B) women were given chemotherapy and 81% became operable; then 87 women were randomised to surgery or radiotherapy.[89] After local treatment, a further 2 years of chemotherapy was given. Both groups had similar duration of disease control (29.2 months with surgery *v* 24.4 months with radiation; P = 0.5), similar overall median survival (39.3 months with surgery *v* 39.0 months with radiation), and similar sites of first relapse. In the other RCT (132 women, 91% stage III B, 9% stage III A) all women received chemotherapy before randomisation to either surgery or radiotherapy.[90] Total response rate was 75% in each group. There was no significant difference in the duration of remission (15 months with surgery *v* 22 months with radiotherapy; P = 0.58). Survival was similar at 4 years (49.1 months with surgery *v* 52 months with radiotherapy). **Low dose radiotherapy versus tamoxifen:** One small RCT (143 women)[92] compared low dose radiotherapy (40 Gy in 15 fractions) versus tamoxifen 20 mg twice daily. Women were given the alternative treatment on relapse. The RCT found no significant difference in response rates (P = 0.34), duration of response (P = 0.76), or survival (P = 0.38).

Harms: The type of harms from radiotherapy**G** for locally advanced breast cancer were similar to those from radiotherapy after mastectomy or breast conserving surgery**G**. However, in stage III B disease with skin involvement (T4 b, c, d), the skin is usually given a higher dose of radiotherapy. In addition, a higher dose (60 Gy) is often given to more of the breast volume. Acute skin toxicity (including moist desquamation) and late skin toxicity (pigmentation and telangiectasia) are also more likely than in women without skin involvement.

Comment: The lack of good quality, large RCTs addressing directly stage III B breast cancer and the role of radiotherapy**G** render it difficult to draw firm conclusions on its value. Such RCTs are small and have varying approaches to management. From the results of two RCTs,[89,90] it can be concluded that in terms of overall response (which includes the response from local treatments such as surgery, radiotherapy, or both, and the effects of any initial systemic treatment), duration of that response, and overall survival, there is no advantage of either surgery alone or radiotherapy alone as sole local treatment over the other. It is more difficult to detail the possible benefits of postoperative radiotherapy in women whose locally advanced breast cancers have been rendered operable by systemic treatment and who have had surgery, usually modified radical mastectomy**G**. It is likely that such postoperative radiotherapy will reduce the risk of local (and regional if nodal areas are irradiated) recurrence. It is not possible to conclude that it will affect survival.

OPTION SYSTEMIC TREATMENT FOR LOCALLY ADVANCED BREAST CANCER

RCTs found insufficient evidence that radiotherapy plus cytotoxic chemotherapy using cyclophosphamide plus methotrexate plus fluorouracil, or an anthracycline based multidrug regimen improved survival, disease free survival, or long term locoregional control compared with radiotherapy alone

in locally advanced breast cancer. One RCT found that hormone treatment (tamoxifen or ovarian ablation) plus radiotherapy delayed locoregional recurrence and improved survival at 8 years in locally advanced breast cancer compared with radiotherapy alone.

Benefits: We found no systematic review. **Radiotherapy versus radiotherapy plus systemic chemotherapy:** We found three RCTs,[93–95] which compared radiotherapy**G** versus radiotherapy plus systemic treatment (hormone treatment, chemotherapy, or both). The first RCT (410 women, most stage III B)[93] compared four treatments in a factorial design: radiotherapy; radiotherapy plus chemotherapy (CMF**G** for 12 cycles); radiotherapy plus hormone treatment (ovarian irradiation for premenopausal women, tamoxifen for postmenopausal women); and radiotherapy plus chemotherapy plus hormone treatment.[93] Adding chemotherapy (P = 0.0002) or hormone treatment (P = 0.0007) to radiotherapy significantly delayed locoregional recurrence, and adding both chemotherapy and hormone treatment had the greatest effect on delaying locoregional recurrence (P = 0.0001). Adding chemotherapy or hormone treatment to radiotherapy reduced locoregional recurrence at 6 years (AR about 60% with radiotherapy alone *v* about 50% with radiotherapy plus chemotherapy or hormonal treatment). The effect of adding chemotherapy or hormone treatment to radiotherapy on distant metastases was similar but less marked. Adding hormone treatment to radiotherapy significantly increased median survival, but adding chemotherapy did not significantly increase survival (median survival: 4.3 years with hormone treatment *v* 3.3 years without hormone treatment, after 8 years HR death 0.75, 95% CI 0.59 to 0.96; median survival: 3.8 years with chemotherapy *v* 3.6 years without chemotherapy, HR 0.84, 95% CI 0.66 to 1.08). The second RCT (118 women with stage III B breast cancer)[94] compared three treatments: radiotherapy; radiotherapy plus chemotherapy (CMF for 12 cycles) plus tamoxifen; and chemotherapy (CMF alternating with adriamycin [doxorubicin] and vincristine [AV]) followed by radiotherapy and further similar chemotherapy plus tamoxifen. The radiotherapy in the third treatment group delivered a lower dose to the skin and a lower total dose than delivered in the other two treatment groups. After a minimum follow up of 14 years, the RCT found no significant difference in survival, disease free survival**G**, or type of first recurrence between groups (figures presented graphically; survival: P = 0.38; disease free survival: P = 0.26; first recurrence: P = 0.4). The third RCT (52 women with T4 breast cancer) compared an anthracycline**G** chemotherapy regimen before radiotherapy versus similar radiotherapy alone.[95] Chemotherapy plus radiotherapy significantly increased initial locoregional control rate compared with radiotherapy alone (complete response: 78.6% with chemotherapy plus radiotherapy *v* 45.8% with radiotherapy alone; P = 0.03). However, the proportion of women free of locoregional spread at death or final follow up was similar (57% with chemotherapy plus radiotherapy *v* 50% with radiotherapy alone). Overall survival and time to distant recurrence were not significantly different between groups. **Adjuvant chemotherapy versus neoadjuvant plus adjuvant chemotherapy:** We found one RCT (101 women with operable T4bN0-2 breast cancer) that compared six cycles of adjuvant CEF (cyclophosphamide, epirubicin, 5-fluorouracil) after surgery (standard or modified radical mastectomy) versus three cycles of neoadjuvant CEF followed by surgery plus three cycles of adjuvant CEF, both groups received chest wall and total nodal radiotherapy.[96] At a median follow up of 25 months there was no significant difference in overall survival or disease free survival (overall survival: 82% with adjuvant *v* 76% with neoadjuvant plus adjuvant chemotherapy; P = 0.42; disease free survival: 76% with adjuvant *v* 61% with neoadjuvant plus adjuvant chemotherapy; P = 0.18). **Multimodal treatment versus hormone treatment:** One RCT (108 women) compared multimodal treatment (preoperative chemotherapy, surgery, radiotherapy, and tamoxifen) with initial hormone treatment plus subsequent salvage treatments upon tumour progression.[97,98] The objective remission after 6 months was higher with multimodal treatment than with tamoxifen alone (31/54 [57%] with multimodal treatment *v* 19/53 [36%] with tamoxifen alone; OR 2.4, 95% CI 1.1 to 5.0).[97] However, at a median follow up of 52 months, there was no significant difference in survival, the development of metastases, the time to metastases, or uncontrolled local disease. Women with oestrogen receptor positive tumours had a higher objective response rate**G** (49% with oestrogen receptor positive *v* 7% with oestrogen recceptor negative; P value not reported), and increased survival (numbers not reported).[98]

Harms: In many RCTs, harms of treatment were not reported (see harms of adjuvant combination chemotherapy, p 2244).

Comment: The lack of large RCTs and the frequent inclusion of less locally advanced disease (T3) with locally advanced breast cancer (defined here as stage III B) make it difficult to draw conclusions. There is, however, no evidence from the studies using CMF**G** chemotherapy or various regimens incorporating anthracyclines**G** that cytotoxic chemotherapy improves survival, disease free survival**G**, or long term locoregional control in stage III B breast cancer.

GLOSSARY

Adjuvant treatment This usually refers to systemic chemotherapy, hormonal treatment, or both, taken by people after removal of a primary tumour (in this case, surgery for early breast cancer), with the aim of killing any remaining micrometastatic tumour cells and thus preventing recurrence.

Anthracyclines Are also known as cytotoxic antibiotics, and are used as adjuvant treatment with radiotherapy. Examples of anthracyclines are aclarubicin, daunorubicin, adriamycin (doxorubicin), epirubicin, and idarubicin.

Axillary clearance Clearance of level I, II, and usually level III axillary lymph nodes. Level I nodes are lateral to the pectoralis minor muscle, level II nodes are under it, and level III nodes are medial to it at the apex of the axilla.

Axillary radiotherapy This usually includes irradiation of the supraclavicular fossa. Irradiation of this area incorporates some underlying lung that increases the risk of radiation pneumonitis. By increasing the volume of the lung irradiated, compared with chest wall or breast radiotherapy alone, the risk of acute pneumonitis is increased.

Axillary sampling Aims to remove the four largest, most easily palpable axillary lymph nodes, for histological examination.

Breast conserving surgery Surgery that consists of lumpectomy (minimal free margins), wide local excision (wider free margins), or segmental or quadrant resection (usually with wide free margins).

CMF (classical) Chemotherapy regimen containing cyclophosphamide, methotrexate, and fluorouracil (5-FU).

Combination chemotherapy Two or more cytotoxic drugs given intravenously every 3–4 weeks for 4–6 months.

Disease free survival Means being alive with no local or distant recurrence or contralateral disease.

Early invasive breast cancer (stage I or II) is M0 with T1 or T2 (tumour diameter ≤ 5 cm, no involvement of skin or chest wall) and N0 or N1 (mobile axillary nodes); or M0 with T3 (tumour diameter > 5 cm, no skin or chest wall involvement), but only N0.

FAC Chemotherapy regimen containing fluorouracil (5-FU), adriamycin (doxorubicin), and cyclophosphamide.

Locally advanced breast cancer Operable locally advanced breast cancer (stage III A) is T3 (tumours > 5 cm) and N1 (non-matted involved axillary nodes). Locally advanced breast cancer (stage III B) is M0 with T4 (skin or chest wall infiltration by tumour), N2 (matted axillary nodes)/N3 (internal mammary node involvement) disease, or both, not classified as non-invasive or early invasive breast cancer. Metastatic breast cancer

(stage IV) is M1 (any supraclavicular fossa node involvement or distant metastases to bone, lung, liver, etc.) with any combination of tumour and node parameters.
Lumpectomy Gross tumour excision.
Milan regimen A sequential regimen of single agent anthracycline followed by CMF.
Modified radical mastectomy Modified radical mastectomy is a total mastectomy with removal of all axillary nodes from level I medial to the pectoralis minor, level II underneath pectoralis minor and up to the apex and including level III nodes medial to pectoralis minor but below the axillary vein up to the first rib. Traditionally a modified radical mastectomy included excision of pectoralis minor, but most surgeons who nowadays perform modified radical mastectomy preserve pectoralis minor.
Neoadjuvant chemotherapy (also known as primary medical treatment.) Involves the use of chemotherapy to treat breast cancer before locoregional treatment (surgery and or radiotherapy) to the breast to downstage large primary cancers that would require mastectomy to improve chances of survival.
Non-invasive breast cancer (stage 0) is Tis (carcinoma *in situ*, intraductal carcinoma, lobular carcinoma *in situ*, or Paget's disease of the nipple with no associated tumour); N0 (no axillary nodal involvement); and M0 (no metastases).
Ovarian ablation Surgical, medical, or radiation induced suppression of ovarian function in premenopausal women.
Overall objective response rate The proportion of treated people in whom a complete response (disappearance of all known lesions on 2 separate measurements at least 4 weeks apart), or partial response (> 50% reduction in the size of lesions) is observed.
Quadrantectomy Tumour excised with ≥ 2 cm of normal surrounding breast tissue and with a segment of breast tissue from the periphery of the breast to the nipple.
Radical mastectomy Removal of breast and pectoralis major and minor muscles and axillary contents.
Radiotherapy Part of initial local and regional treatment. In early stage disease, it may be an adjunct to surgery; in locally advanced disease (T4, N2), it may be the sole locoregional treatment. Radiotherapy may be delivered to the breast or postmastectomy chest wall, as well as to the lymphatic areas of the axilla, supraclavicular fossa, or internal mammary node chain.
Simple mastectomy Removal of the breast tissue, usually in association with an ellipse of skin that includes the nipple and areolar complex. Dissection continues down to but does not usually include the pectoral fascia. It includes removal of the axillary tail of the breast. Lymph nodes are not usually removed other than by additional procedure.
Staging of breast cancer A detailed description by tumour, nodal, and metastatic parameters at a particular time (TNM).[1] These are amalgamated into broader categories called stages (0–IV). Stages can be aggregated into even broader categories (non-invasive, early invasive, and advanced breast cancer).
Supraradical mastectomy Removal of breast, pectoralis major and minor muscles, axillary contents, and internal mammary chain of nodes.
TNM staging system See "staging of breast cancer" above.
Total mastectomy Removal of breast.
Total nodal irradiation Radiotherapy to the regional lymph nodes, including supraclavicular, infraclavicular, axillary nodes, and internal mammary nodes in the upper intercostal spaces.
UICC International Union against Cancer.

REFERENCES

1. UICC International Union Against Cancer. *TNM classification of malignant tumours*, 5th ed. Sobin LH, Wittekind CH, eds. New York: Wiley-Liss, 1997.
2. CRC. Breast Cancer Factsheet. 1996.
3. Easton D, Ford D. Breast and ovarian cancer incidence in BRCA-1 mutation carriers. *Am J Hum Genet* 1995;56:265–271.
4. Carter CL, Allen C, Henson DE. Relation of tumour size, lymph node status and survival in 24 740 breast cancer cases. *Cancer* 1989;63:181–187.
5. Hortobagyi GN, Ames FC, Buzdar AU, et al. Management of stage III primary breast cancer with primary chemotherapy, surgery and radiation therapy. *Cancer* 1988;62:2507–2516.
6. Rutqvist LE, Rose C, Cavallin-Stahl E. A systematic overview of radiation therapy effects in breast cancer. *Acta Oncol* 2003;42:532–545.
7. Fisher B, Dignam J, Wolmark N, et al. Lumpectomy and radiation therapy for the treatment of intraductal breast cancer: findings of the National Surgical Adjuvant Breast and Bowel Project B-17. *J Clin Oncol* 1998;16:441–452.
8. Julien JP, Bijker N, Fentiman IS, et al. Radiotherapy in breast-conserving treatment for ductal carcinoma *in situ*; first results of EORTC randomised Phase III trial 10853. *Lancet* 2000;355:528–533.
9. Houghton J, George WD, Cuzick J, et al. Radiotherapy and tamoxifen in women with completely excised ductal carcinoma in situ of the

breast in the UK, Australia, and New Zealand: randomised controlled trial. *Lancet* 2003;362:95–102.
10. Fisher B, Dignam J, Wolmark N, et al. Tamoxifen in treatment of intraductal breast cancer: National Surgical Adjuvant Breast and Bowel Project B-24 randomised controlled trial. *Lancet* 1999;353:1993–2000.
11. Allred D, Bryant J, Land S, et al. Estrogen receptor expression as a positive marker of the effectiveness of tamoxifen in the treatment of DCIS: findings from NSABP Protocol B-24 [conference abstract]. San Antonio Breast Cancer Symposium, 2002.
12. Mauriac L, Durand M, Avril A, et al. Effects of primary chemotherapy in conservative treatment of breast cancer patients with operable tumours larger than 3 cm: results of a randomised trial in a single centre. *Ann Oncol* 1991;2:347–354.
13. Scholl SM, Fourquet A, Asselain B, et al. Neoadjuvant versus adjuvant chemotherapy in premenopausal patients with tumours considered too large for breast conserving surgery: preliminary results of a randomised trial. *Eur J Cancer* 1994;30A:645–652.
14. Powles TJ, Hickish TF, Makris A, et al. Randomized trial of chemoendocrine therapy started before or after surgery for treatment of primary breast cancer. *J Clin Oncol* 1995;13:547–552.
15. Fisher B, Bryant J, Wolmark N, et al. Effect of preoperative chemotherapy on the outcome of women with operable breast cancer. *J Clin Oncol* 1998;16:2672–2685.
16. Van der Hage JA, van de Velde CJ, Julien JP, et al. Pre-operative chemotherapy in primary operable breast cancer: results from the European Organisation for Research and Treatment of Cancer Trial 10902. *J Clin Oncol* 2001;19:4224–4237.
17. Mauriac L, MacGrogan G, Avril A, et al. Neoadjuvant chemotherapy for operable breast carcinoma larger than 3 cm: a unicentre randomized trial with a 124-month median follow-up. Institut Bergonie Bordeaux Groupe Sein (IBBGS). *Ann Oncol* 1999;10:47–52.
18. Broet P, Scholl S, De la Rochrfordiere A, et al. Short and long term effects on survival in breast cancer patients treated by primary chemotherapy: an updated analysis of a randomised trial. *Breast Cancer Res Treat* 1999;58:151–156.
19. Makris A, Powles TJ, Ashley SE, et al. A reduction in the requirements for mastectomy in a randomized trial of neoadjuvant chemoendocrine therapy in primary breast cancer. *Ann Oncol* 1998;9:1179–1184.
20. Avril A, Faucher A, Bussieres E, et al. Results of 10 years of a randomized trial of neoadjuvant chemotherapy in breast cancers larger than 3 cm. *Chirurgie* 1998;123:247–256. [In French]
21. Therasse P, Mauriac L, Welnicka-Jaskiewicz M, et al. Final results of a randomized phase III trial comparing cyclophosphamide, epirubicin, and fluorouracil with a dose-intensified epirubicin and cyclophosphamide + filgrastim as neoadjuvant treatment in locally advanced breast cancer: an EORTC-NCIC-SAKK multicenter study. *J Clin Oncol* 2003;21:843–850.
22. Buzdar AU, Singletary SE, Theriault RL, et al. Prospective evaluation of paclitaxel versus combination chemotherapy with fluorouracil, doxorubicin, and cyclophosphamide as neoadjuvant therapy in patients with operable breast cancer. *J Clin Oncol* 1999;17:3412–3417.
23. Cocconi G, Bisagni G, Ceci G, et al. Three new active cisplatin-containing combinations in the neoadjuvant treatment of locally advanced and locally recurrent breast carcinoma: a randomized Phase II trial. *Breast Canc Res Treat* 1999;56:125–132.
24. Smith IC, Heys SD, Hutcheon A, et al. Neoadjuvant chemotherapy in breast cancer: significantly enhanced response with docetaxel. *J Clin Oncol* 2002;20:1456–1466.
25. D'Orazio AI, O'Shaughnessy J, Seidman AD. Neoadjuvant docetaxel augments the efficacy of preoperative docetaxel/cyclophosphamide in operable breast cancer: first results of NSABP-27. *Clin Breast Cancer* 2002;2:266–268.
26. Takatsuka Y, Yayoi E, Kobayashi T, et al. Neoadjuvant intra-arterial chemotherapy in locally advanced breast cancer: a prospective randomised study. *Jpn J Clin Oncol* 1994;24:20–25.
27. Webb A, Smith IE, Ahern R. A randomised Phase II trial of pre-operative navelbine/epirubicin (NE) versus navelbine/mitozantrone (NM) versus adriamycin/cyclophosphamide (AC) for early breast cancer. *Eur J Cancer* 2001;37:174.
28. Early Breast Cancer Trialists' Collaborative Group. Fffects of radiotherapy and surgery in early breast cancer: an overview of the randomised trials. *N Engl J Med* 1995;333:1444–1455. Search date not reported; primary sources individual patient data from trials that began before 1985, trials identified from lists from national cancer bodies, the International Cancer Research Data Bank, hand searches of conference proceedings and reference lists, and personal contact with investigators.
29. Fisher B, Jeong JH, Anderson S, et al. Twenty-five year follow-up of a randomized trial comparing radical mastectomy, total mastectomy, and total mastectomy followed by irradiation. *New Engl J Med* 2002;347:567–575.
30. Morris AD, Morris RD, Wilson JF, et al. Breast conserving therapy versus mastectomy in early stage breast cancer: a meta-analysis of 10 year survival. *Cancer J Sci Am* 1997;3:6–12. Search date 1995, primary source Medline.
31. Veronesi U, Cascinelli N, Mariani L, et al. Twenty-year follow-up of a randomised study comparing breast-conserving surgery with radical mastectomy for early breast cancer. *N Engl J Med* 2002;347:1227–1232.
32. Fisher B, Andeson S, Bryant J, et al. Twenty-year follow-up of a randomised trial comparing total mastectomy, lumpectomy and lumpectomy plus irradiation for the treatment of invasive breast cancer. *N Engl J Med* 2002;347:1233–1241.
33. Poggi MM, Danforth DN, Sciuto LC, et al. Eighteen-year results in the treatment of early breast carcinoma with mastectomy versus breast conservation therapy: the National Cancer Institute randomised trial. *Cancer* 2003;98:697–702.
34. Sacchini V, Luini A, Tana S, et al. Quantitative and qualitative cosmetic evaluation after conservative treatment for breast cancer. *Eur J Cancer* 1991;27:1395–1400.
35. Smitt NC, Nowels KW, Zdeblick MJ, et al. The importance of the lumpectomy surgical margin status in long-term results of breast conservation. *Cancer* 1995;76:259–267.
36. Wazer DE, DiPetrillo T, Schmidt-Ullrich R, et al. Factors influencing cosmetic outcome and complication risk after conservative surgery and radiotherapy for early-stage breast carcinoma. *J Clin Oncol* 1992;10:356–363.
37. Abner AL, Recht A, Vicini FA, et al. Cosmetic results after surgery, chemotherapy and radiation therapy for early breast cancer. *Int J Radiat Oncol Biol Phys* 1991;21:331–338.
38. Dewar JA, Benhamou S, Benhamou E, et al. Cosmetic results following lumpectomy axillary dissection and radiotherapy for small breast cancers. *Radiother Oncol* 1988;12:273–280.
39. Rochefordiere A, Abner A, Silver B, et al. Are cosmetic results following conservative surgery and radiation therapy for early breast cancer dependent on technique? *Int J Radiat Oncol Biol Phys* 1992;23:925–931.
40. Sneeuw KA, Aaronson N, Yarnold J, et al. Cosmetic and functional outcomes of breast conserving treatment for early stage breast cancer 1: comparison of patients' ratings, observers' ratings and objective assessments. *Radiother Oncol* 1992;25:153–159.
41. Ash DV, Benson EA, Sainsbury JR, et al. Seven year follow-up on 334 patients treated by breast conserving surgery and short course radical

postoperative radiotherapy: a report of the Yorkshire Breast Cancer Group. *Clin Oncol* 1995;7:93–96.

42. Lindsey I, Serpell JW, Johnson WR, et al. Cosmesis following complete local excision of breast cancer. *Aust N Z J Surg* 1997;67:428–432.
43. Touboul E, Belkacemi Y, Lefranc JP, et al. Early breast cancer: influence of type of boost (electrons vs iridium-192 implant) on local control and cosmesis after conservative surgery and radiation therapy. *Radiother Oncol* 1995;34:105–113.
44. Halyard MY, Grado GL, Schomber PJ, et al. Conservative therapy of breast cancer: the Mayo Clinic experience. *Am J Clin Oncol* 1996;19:445–450.
45. Early Breast Cancer Trialists' Collaborative Group. Favourable and unfavourable effects on long-term survival of radiotherapy for early breast cancer: an overview of the randomised trials. *Lancet* 2000;355:1757–1770. Search date not reported; primary sources individual patient data from trials that began before 1990, trials identified from lists from national cancer bodies, the International Cancer Research Data Bank, hand searches of conference proceedings and reference lists, and personal contact with investigators.
46. Malmstrom P, Holmberg L, Anderson H, et al. Breast conservation surgery, with and without radiotherapy, in women with lymph node-negative breast cancer: a randomised clinical trial in a population with access to public mammography screening. *Eur J Cancer* 2003;39:1690–1697.
47. Veronesi U, Marubini E, Mariani L, et al. Radiotherapy after breast-conserving surgery in small breast carcinoma: long-term results of a randomized trial. *Ann Oncol* 2001;12:997–1003.
48. Liljegren G, Holmberg L, Adami HO, et al, for the Uppsala–cörebro Breast Cancer Study Group. Sector resection with or without postoperative radiotherapy for stage I breast cancer: five year results of a randomised trial. *J Natl Cancer Inst* 1994;86:717–722.
49. Liljegren G, Holmberg J, Bergh, J, et al, and the Uppsala–cörebro Breast Cancer Study Group. 10-year results after sector resection with or without postoperative radiotherapy for stage I breast cancer: a randomized trial. *J Clin Oncol* 1999;17:2326–2333.
50. Lee HD, Yoon DS, Koo JY, et al. Breast conserving therapy in stage I & II breast cancer in Korea. *Breast Cancer Res Treat* 1997;44:193–199.
51. Whelan TJ, Levine M, Julian J, et al. The effects of radiation therapy on quality for life of women with breast carcinoma: results of a randomized trial. *Cancer* 2000;88:2260–2266.
52. Fisher B, Bryant J, Dignam JJ, et al. Tamoxifen, radiation therapy, or both for prevention of ipsilateral breast tumor recurrence after lumpectomy in women with invasive breast cancers of one centimeter or less. *J Clin Oncol* 2002;20:41–49.
53. Rayan G, Dawson LA, Bezjak A, et al. Prospective comparison of breast pain in patients participating in a randomized trial of breast-conserving surgery and tamoxifen with or without radiotherapy. *Int J Radiat Oncol Biol Phys* 2003;55:154–161.
54. Steering Committee on Clinical Practice Guidelines for the Care and Treatment of Breast Cancer. A Canadian consensus document. *Can Med Assoc J* 1998;158(suppl 3):1–84.
55. Cuzick J, Stewart H, Rutqvist L, et al. Cause-specific mortality in long term survivors of breast cancer who participated in trials of radiotherapy. *J Clin Oncol* 1994;12:447–453. Search date not reported; primary source cause specific mortality data from unconfounded randomised trials began before 1975 (trial identification methods not reported).
56. Ragaz J, Jackson SM, Le N, et al. Adjuvant radiotherapy and chemotherapy in node-positive premenopausal women with breast cancer. *N Engl J Med* 1997;337:956–962.
57. Overgaard M, Hansen PS, Overgaard J, et al. Postoperative radiotherapy in high-risk premenopausal women with breast cancer who receive adjuvant chemotherapy. *N Engl J Med* 1997;337:949–955.
58. Hojris I, Overgaard M, Christensen JJ, et al. Morbidity and mortality of ischaemic heart disease in high-risk breast-cancer patients after adjuvant postmastectomy systemic treatment with or without radiotherapy: analysis of DBCG 82b and 82c randomised trials. Radiotherapy Committee of the Danish Breast Cancer Cooperative Group. *Lancet* 1999;354:1425–1430.
59. Ghersi D, Simes J. Draft report of effectiveness of postmastectomy radiotherapy and risk factors for local recurrence in early breast cancer. Report to NHMRC National Breast Cancer Centre, Sydney, 1998.
60. Overgaard M, Jensen MB, Overgaard J, et al. Postoperative radiotherapy in high risk postmenopausal breast cancer patients given adjuvant tamoxifen: Danish Breast Cancer Cooperative Group DBCG 82c randomised trial. *Lancet* 1999;353:1641–1648.
61. O'Rourke S, Gaba MH, Morgan D, et al. Local recurrence after simple mastectomy. *Br J Surg* 1994;81:386–389.
62. Fowble B, Gray R, Gilchrist K, et al. Identification of a subset of patients with breast cancer and histologically positive nodes who may benefit from postoperative radiotherapy. *J Clin Oncol* 1988;6:1107–1117.
63. Houghton J, Baum M, Haybittle JL. Role of radiotherapy following total mastectomy in patients with early breast cancer: the closed trials working party of the CRC breast cancer trials group. *World J Surg* 1994;18:117–122.
64. Kaija H, Maunu P. Tangential breast irradiation with or without internal mammary chain irradiation: results of a randomised trial. *Radiother Oncol* 1995;36:172–176.
65. Gyenes G, Rutqvist LE, Liedberg A, et al. Long-term cardiac morbidity and mortality in a randomized trial of pre- and postoperative radiation therapy versus surgery alone in primary breast cancer. *Radiother Oncol* 1998;48:185–190.
66. Handley R. Carcinoma of the breast. *Ann R Coll Surg Engl* 1975;57:59–66.
67. Veronesi U, Cascinelli NM, Bufalino R, et al. Risk of internal mammary lymph node metastases and its relevance on prognosis in breast cancer patients. *Ann Surg* 1983;198:681–684.
68. Veronesi U, Valagussa P. Inefficacy of internal mammary node dissection in breast cancer surgery. *Cancer* 1981;47:170–175.
69. Bates T, Evans RGB. Report of the Independent Review commissioned by The Royal College of Radiologists into brachial plexus neuropathy following radiotherapy for breast cancer. London: Royal College of Radiologists, 1995.
70. Early Breast Cancer Trialists' Collaborative Group. Polychemotherapy for early breast cancer: an overview of the randomised trials. *Lancet* 1998;352:930–942. Search date not reported; primary sources individual patient data from trials that began before 1990, trials identified from lists from national cancer bodies, the International Cancer Research Data Bank, hand searches of conference proceedings and reference lists, and personal contact with investigators.
71. Fisher B, Anderson S, Wickerham DL, et al. Increased intensification and total dose of cyclophosphamide in a doxorubicin-cyclophosphamide regimen for the treatment of primary breast cancer: findings from national surgical adjuvant breast and bowel project B-22. *J Clin Oncol* 1997;15:1858–1869.
72. Wood WC, Budman DR, Korzun AH. Dose and dose intensity of adjuvant chemotherapy for stage II, node-positive breast carcinoma. *N Engl J Med* 1994;330:1253–1259.
73. Bonadonna G, Zambeti M, Valagussa P. Sequential or alternating doxorubicin and CMF regimens in breast cancer with more than three positive nodes. *JAMA* 1995;273:542–547.

74. Early Breast Cancer Trialists' Collaborative Group. Tamoxifen for early breast cancer: an overview of the randomised trials. *Lancet* 1998;351:1451–1467. Search date not reported; primary sources individual patient data from trials that began before 1990, trials identified from lists from national cancer bodies, the International Cancer Research Data Bank, hand searches of conference proceedings and reference lists, and personal contact with investigators.
75. Swedish Breast Cancer Cooperative Group. Randomised trial of two versus five years of adjuvant tamoxifen for post-menopausal early stage breast cancer. *J Natl Cancer Inst* 1996;88:1543–1549.
76. Fisher B, Dignam J, Bryant J, et al. Five versus more than five years of tamoxifen therapy for breast cancer patients with negative lymph nodes and estrogen receptor-positive tumours. *J Natl Cancer Inst* 1996;88:1529–1542.
77. Stewart HJ, Forrest AP, Everington D, et al. Randomised comparison of 5 years of adjuvant tamoxifen with continuous therapy for operable breast cancer. *Br J Cancer* 1996;74:297–299.
78. Powles TJ, Hickish T, Kanis JA, et al. Effect of tamoxifen on bone mineral density measured by dual-energy x-ray absorptiometry in healthy premenopausal and postmenopausal women. *J Clin Oncol* 1996;14:78–84.
79. Swain SM. Tamoxifen: the long and short of it. *J Natl Cancer Inst* 1996;88:1510–1512.
80. Farquhar C, Basser R, Marjoribanks J, et al. High dose chemotherapy and autologous bone marrow or stem cell transplantation versus conventional chemotherapy for women with early poor prognosis breast cancer. Cochrane Library Issue 2, 2003. Oxford: Update Software. Search date 2002; primary sources Cochrane Breast Cancer Group specialised register, Cochrane Controlled Trials Register, Medline, Embase, Psychinfo, Cinahl, websites of co-operative research groups and American Society of Clinical Oncologists, and reference lists.
81. Fisher B, Dignam J, Wolmark N, et al. Tamoxifen and chemotherapy for lymph node-negative, estrogen receptor-positive breast cancer. *J Natl Cancer Inst* 1997;89:1673–1682.
82. Early Breast Cancer Trialists' Group. Ovarian ablation in early breast cancer: overview of the randomised trials. *Lancet* 1996;348:1189–1196. Search date not reported; primary sources individual patient data from trials that began before 1990, trials identified from lists from national cancer bodies, the International Cancer Research Data Bank, hand searches of conference proceedings and reference lists, and personal contact with investigators.
83. Chetty U, Jack W, Prescott RJ, et al. Management of the axilla in operable breast cancer treated by breast conservation: a randomised controlled trial. *Br J Surg* 2000;87:163–169.
84. Browning C, Redman S, Pillar C, et al. NHMRC National Breast Cancer Centre, Sydney 1998. Lymphoedema: prevalence risk factors and management: a review of research. Search date 1996; primary sources Medline, hand searches of article references, personal contact with key resources of article references, and personal contact with key resources.
85. Axelsson CK, Mouridzsen HT, Zedeler K. Axillary dissection at level I and II lymph nodes is important in breast cancer classification. *Eur J Cancer* 1992;28A:1415–1418.
86. Kiricuta CI, Tausch J. A mathematical model of axillary lymph node involvement based on 1446 complete axillary dissections in patients with breast carcinoma. *Cancer* 1992;69:2496–2501.
87. Steele RJC, Forrest APM, Gibson R, et al. The efficacy of lower axillary sampling in obtaining lymph node status in breast cancer: a controlled randomised trial. *Br J Surg* 1985;72:368–369.
88. Papaioannou A, Lissaios B, Vasilaros S, et al. Pre- and post operative chemoendocrine treatment with or without post-operative radiotherapy for locally advanced breast cancer. *Cancer* 1983;51:1284–1290.
89. Perloff M, Lesnick G J, Korzun A, et al. Combination chemotherapy with mastectomy or radiotherapy for stage III breast carcinoma: a Cancer and Leukaemia Group B Study. *J Clin Oncol* 1988;6:261–269.
90. De Lena M, Varini M, Zucali R, et al. Multimodal treatment for locally advanced breast cancer. Results of chemotherapy–radiotherapy versus chemotherapy–surgery. *Cancer Clin Trials* 1981;4:229–236.
91. Olson JE, Neuberg D, Pandya KJ, et al. The role of radiotherapy in the management of operable locally advanced breast carcinoma: results of a randomised trial by the Eastern Co-operative Oncology Group. *Cancer* 1997;79:1138–1149.
92. Willsher PC, Robertson JF, Armitage NC, et al. Locally advanced breast cancer: long term results of a randomised trial comparing primary treatment with tamoxifen or radiotherapy in post-menopausal women. *Eur J Surg Oncol* 1996;22:34–37.
93. Bartelink H, Rubens RD, Van der Schueren E, et al. Hormonal therapy prolongs survival in irradiated locally advanced breast cancer: a European Organisation for Research and Treatment of Cancer randomised Phase III trial. *J Clin Oncol* 1997;15:207–215.
94. Koning C, Hart G. Long term follow up of a randomised trial on adjuvant chemotherapy and hormonal therapy in locally advanced breast cancer. *Int J Rad Oncol Biol Phys* 1998;41:397–400.
95. Rodger A, Jack WJL, Hardman PDJ, et al. Locally advanced breast cancer: report of a Phase II study and subsequent Phase III trial. *Br J Cancer* 1992;65:761–765.
96. Deo SV, Bhutani M, Shukla NK, et al. Randomized trial comparing neo-adjuvant versus adjuvant chemotherapy in operable locally advanced breast cancer (T4 b N0–2 M0) *J Surg Oncol* 2003;84:192–197.
97. Willsher PC, Robertson JF, Chan SY, et al. Locally advanced breast cancer: early results of a randomised trial of multimodal therapy versus initial hormone therapy. *Eur J Cancer* 1997;33:45–49.
98. Tan SM, Cheung KL, Willsher PC, et al. Locally advanced primary breast cancer: medium term results of a randomised trial of multimodal therapy versus initial hormone therapy. *Eur J Cancer* 2001;37:2331–2338.

J Michael Dixon
Senior Lecturer in Surgery
Western General Hospital
Edinburgh
UK

Justin Stebbing
MRC Clinical Training Fellow
Chelsea and Westminister Hospital
London
UK

Alan Rodger
Professor
Beatson Oncology Centre and
University of Glasgow
Glasgow
UK

Competing interests: None declared.

TABLE 1 Ten year survival with combination chemotherapy versus placebo, according to nodal and age/menopausal status: results of a systematic review of RCTs (see text, p 2243).[70]

	Control (%)	Chemotherapy (%)	Absolute benefit (%)	SD (%)	Significance (two sided)
Age < 50 years					
Node +ve	41.4	53.8	+12.4	2.4	P < 0.0001
Node –ve	71.9	77.6	+5.7	2.1	P = 0.01
Age 50–69 years					
Node +ve	46.3	48.6	+2.3	1.3	P = 0.001
Node –ve	64.8	71.2	+6.4	2.3	P = 0.0025

SD, standard deviation.

TABLE 2 Ten year survival in women treated with tamoxifen for 5 years compared with control treatment (no tamoxifen): results of a systematic review (see text, p 2234).[74]

	Control (%)	Tamoxifen (%)	Absolute benefit (%)	SD (%)	Significance (two sided)
Node +ve	50.5	61.4	+10.9	2.5	P < 0.00001
Node –ve	73.3	78.9	+5.6	1.3	P < 0.00001

SD, standard deviation.

TABLE 3 Staging of breast cancer (the individual terms are explained in the glossary) (see text, p 2252).[1]

	TNM			Stage
Non-invasive	Tis	N0	M0	0
Early invasive	T1–2	N0–1	M0	I, II A or B
	T3	N0	M0	II B
Advanced				
Locally advanced	Tany	N2	M0	III A
	T3	N1–2	M0	III A
	T4	N0–3	M0	III B
	Tany	N3	M0	III B
Metastatic	Tany	Nany	M1	IV

Breast pain

Search date March 2004

Nigel Bundred

QUESTIONS

INTERVENTIONS

Key Messages

Treatments

- **Danazol** One RCT found that danazol reduced cyclical breast pain after 12 months compared with placebo, but increased adverse effects (weight gain, deepening of the voice, menorrhagia, and muscle cramps). It found no significant difference in pain relief between danazol and tamoxifen.
- **Gestrinone** One RCT found that gestrinone reduced breast pain after 3 months compared with placebo, but increased adverse effects (greasy skin, hirsutism, acne, reduction in breast size, headache, and depression).
- **Tamoxifen** Three RCTs found limited evidence that tamoxifen was more effective than placebo at reducing breast pain. The two RCTs which reported on adverse effects found more hot flushes and vaginal discharge with tamoxifen compared with placebo, although differences between groups did not reach significance. One RCT found similar efficacy but fewer adverse effects with a lower dose of 10 mg compared with 20 mg. One RCT found no significant difference in pain relief between tamoxifen and danazol. One meta-analysis of four large breast cancer prevention trials found that tamoxifen used long term was associated with an increased risk of venous thromboembolism. Tamoxifen is not licensed for mastalgia in the UK or USA.
- **Antibiotics** We found no systematic review or RCTs of sufficient quality on the effects of antibiotics.
- **Diet (low fat, high carbohydrate)** One small RCT found limited evidence that advice to follow a low fat, high carbohydrate diet reduced self reported premenstrual breast swelling and breast tenderness at 6 months compared with general dietary advice. However, it found no significant difference between groups in the combined outcome of breast swelling, tenderness, and nodularity on physical examination at 6 months.
- **Diuretics** We found no systematic review or RCTs of sufficient quality on the effects of diuretics.
- **Evening primrose oil** One RCT found no significant difference between evening primrose oil and placebo in frequency of pain at 6 months.

- **Gonadorelin analogues (luteinising hormone releasing hormone analogues)** We found no systematic review or RCTs of sufficient quality on the effects of gonadorelin analogues.
- **Lisuride** One RCT with weak methods found limited evidence that lisuride maleate (a dopamine agonist) reduced breast pain over 2 months compared with placebo.
- **Pyridoxine** We found no systematic review or RCTs of sufficient quality on the effects of pyridoxine.
- **Tibolone** One RCT found no significant difference between tibolone and placebo in breast pain and tenderness at 12 months.
- **Vitamin E** We found no systematic review or RCTs of sufficient quality on the effects of vitamin E.
- **Bromocriptine** One RCT with high withdrawal rates and one small crossover RCT reporting results after crossover found limited evidence that bromocriptine (a dopamine agonist) reduced breast pain compared with placebo. However, both RCTs found a higher incidence of adverse effects with bromocriptine compared with placebo. Adverse events included nausea, dizziness, postural hypotension, and constipation. One of the RCTs found that withdrawals related to adverse effects were more frequent with bromocriptine compared with placebo, although differences between groups did not reach significance. Bromocriptine is now used rarely because of frequent and intolerable adverse effects and the US Food and Drug Administration has withdrawn its licence for this indication.
- **Hormone replacement therapy (oestrogen)** We found no placebo controlled RCTs of hormone replacement therapy for breast pain. Hormone replacement therapy is associated with an increased risk of breast cancer, venous thromboembolism, and gall bladder disease.
- **Progestogens** Two small crossover RCTs found no significant difference between either progesterone cream or medroxyprogesterone acetate tablets and placebo in breast pain.

DEFINITION Breast pain can be differentiated into cyclical mastalgia (worse before a menstrual period) or non-cyclical mastalgia (unrelated to the menstrual cycle).[1,2] Cyclical pain is often bilateral, usually most severe in the upper outer quadrants of the breast, and may be referred to the medial aspect of the upper arm.[1–3] Non-cyclical pain may be caused by true breast pain or chest wall pain located over the costal cartilages.[1,2,4] Specific breast pathology and referred pain unrelated to the breasts are not included in this chapter.

INCIDENCE/ PREVALENCE Up to 70% of women develop breast pain in their lifetime.[1,2] Of 1171 US women attending a gynaecology clinic, 69% suffered regular discomfort, which was judged as severe in 11% of women, and 36% had consulted a doctor about breast pain.[2]

AETIOLOGY/ RISK FACTORS Breast pain is most common in women aged 30–50 years.[1,2]

PROGNOSIS Cyclical breast pain resolves spontaneously within 3 months of onset in 20–30% of women.[5] The pain tends to relapse and remit, and up to 60% of women develop recurrent symptoms 2 years after treatment.[1] Non-cyclical pain responds poorly to treatment but may resolve spontaneously in about 50% of women.[1]

AIMS OF INTERVENTION To reduce breast pain and improve quality of life, with minimal adverse effects.

OUTCOMES Breast pain score based on the number of days of severe (score 2) or moderate (score 1) pain experienced in each menstrual cycle; visual analogue score of breast pain, heaviness, or breast tenderness; questionnaires.

METHODS *Clinical Evidence* search and appraisal March 2004. Overall, the evidence was poor and some studies with weaker methods were included when higher quality evidence was not found, as indicated in the text. Studies were included whatever the definition of breast pain, as indicated in the text.

QUESTION What are the effects of treatments for breast pain?

OPTION DIET (LOW FAT, HIGH CARBOHYDRATE)

One small RCT found limited evidence that advice to follow a low fat, high carbohydrate diet reduced self reported premenstrual breast swelling and breast tenderness at 6 months compared with general dietary advice. However, it found no significant difference between groups in the combined outcome of breast swelling, tenderness, and nodularity on physical examination at 6 months.

Benefits: We found no systematic review. We found one small RCT (21 women attending a clinic in Canada with severe cyclical mastalgia for at least 5 years), which compared instruction to reduce fat content of the diet (to 15% of total calorie intake, while increasing complex carbohydrates to maintain calorie intake) versus general dietary advice (the principles for a healthy diet based on Canada's Food Guide, but not counselled to modify the fat content of their diet) for 6 months.[6] One woman in each group withdrew and was excluded from the analysis. It found that over 6 months, self reported premenstrual breast swelling was significantly reduced in women with low fat, high carbohydrate diet compared with general dietary advice (breast swelling at 6 months: 5/10 [50%] with low fat diet *v* 9/9 [100%] with general diet; NNT 2, 95% CI 2 to 5). It also found that reported premenstrual tenderness was significantly reduced in women receiving low fat dietary advice compared with those receiving general dietary advice at 6 months (6/10 [60%] with low fat diet *v* 9/9 [100%] with general diet; NNT 3, 95% CI 2 to 9). However, it found no significant difference between groups in the combined outcome of breast swelling, tenderness, and nodularity on physical examination at 6 months (6/10 [60%] with low fat diet *v* 2/9 [22%] with general diet; RR 2.7, 95% CI 0.8 to 4.1).[6]

Harms: The RCT reported no adverse effects.[6]

Comment: Diets can be difficult to sustain in the long term.

OPTION EVENING PRIMROSE OIL

One RCT found no significant difference between evening primrose oil and placebo in frequency of pain at 6 months.

Benefits: **Versus placebo:** We found one RCT (112 women with a minimum of 5 days pain each month) comparing four treatments in a factorial design: evening primrose oil plus placebo oil; fish oil plus placebo oil; fish oil plus evening primrose oil, and placebo oil alone.[7] It found no significant difference between evening primrose oil and placebo in frequency or severity of pain at 6 months (decrease in percentage of days with pain from baseline: 12% with evening primrose oil *v* 14% with placebo; P = 0.73; percentage decrease in severity of pain from baseline: 0.06% with evening primrose oil *v* 0.08% with placebo; P = 0.83).

Harms: The RCT found that adverse effects were similar with evening primrose oil and placebo (AR for all adverse effects, about 50% of which were gastric: 14/30 [47%] with evening primrose oil *v* 13/30 [43%] with placebo; P value not reported).[7] Poor quality RCTs found that adverse effects causing treatment discontinuation were similar with evening primrose oil and placebo (3%), and were largely caused by abdominal bloating.[5,8]

Comment: In one RCT, 72 women received evening primrose oil or placebo for 3 months followed by 3 months of evening primrose oil.[8] It reported that pain, tenderness, and lumpiness improved in cyclical but not non-cyclical breast pain. However, the methods of the RCT were poor and included post hoc revision of the inclusion criteria, subgroup analysis, exclusion of withdrawals, and the use of baseline comparisons (with the best response seen in women who were symptomatically worse at baseline). We found one survey of randomised and open studies; however, data were reported as overall summary figures, which makes specific data extraction impossible.[5] In the UK, the Committee for Safety of Medicines has withdrawn the prescription licence from evening primrose oil because of lack of efficacy, but it is still available to purchase without prescription.[9]

OPTION DANAZOL

One RCT found that danazol reduced cyclical breast pain after 12 months compared with placebo, but increased adverse effects (weight gain, deepening of the voice, menorrhagia, and muscle cramps). It found no significant difference in pain relief between danazol and tamoxifen.

Benefits: We found no systematic review. We found one good quality outpatient based RCT in 93 women with severe cyclical mastalgia.[10] **Versus placebo:** The RCT compared three treatments over 6 months: danazol 200 mg daily, tamoxifen 10 mg daily, and placebo. It found that significantly more women achieved greater than 50% pain relief at the end of treatment with danazol compared with placebo (pain relief: 21/32 [66%] with danazol *v* 11/29 [38%] with placebo; RR 1.7, 95% CI 1.0 to 2.9; NNT 4, 95% CI 2 to 29). It found that after 12 months of treatment, the difference between groups remained significant (pain relief after 1 year: 12/32 [38%] with danazol *v* 0/29 [0%] with placebo; NNT 3, 95% CI 2 to 5). **Versus tamoxifen:** The same RCT found no significant difference in pain relief after 6 months of treatment between danazol and tamoxifen (21/32 [66%] with danazol *v* 23/32 [72%] with tamoxifen; RR 0.9, 95% CI 0.7 to 1.3).[10]

Harms: Adverse effects were reported in more women taking danazol than placebo.[10] These included a significant increase in weight gain (10/32 [31%] with danazol *v* 1/29 [3%] with placebo; P = 0.006), and non-significant increases for deepening of the voice (4/32 [13%] with danazol *v* 0/29 [0%] with placebo; P = 0.11), menorrhagia (4/32 [13%] with danazol *v* 0/29 [0%] with placebo; P = 0.11), and muscle cramps (3/32 [9%] with danazol *v* 0/29 [0%] with placebo; P = 0.24).[10]

Comment: Although we found no direct evidence, there is consensus that once a response is achieved, adverse effects can be avoided by reducing the dose of danazol to 100 mg daily and confining treatment to the 2 weeks preceding menstruation.[10,11] Non-hormonal contraception is essential with danazol as danazol has deleterious androgenic effects in the foetus.[12]

OPTION BROMOCRIPTINE

One RCT with high withdrawal rates and one small crossover RCT reporting results after crossover found limited evidence that bromocriptine (a dopamine agonist) reduced breast pain compared with placebo. However, both RCTs found a higher incidence of adverse effects with bromocriptine compared with placebo. Adverse events included nausea, dizziness, postural hypotension, and constipation. One of the RCTs found that withdrawals related to adverse effects were more frequent with bromocriptine compared with placebo,

although differences between groups did not reach significance. Bromocriptine is now used rarely because of frequent and intolerable adverse effects and the US Food and Drug Administration has withdrawn its licence for this indication.

Benefits: We found no systematic review but found two RCTs.[13,14] The first outpatient based, European RCT (272 premenopausal women with diffuse fibrocystic disease of the breast) compared bromocriptine (2.5 mg twice daily) versus placebo.[13] After 3 and 6 months it found that bromocriptine significantly improved symptoms compared with placebo on self assessed visual analogue scoring of breast pain, tenderness, and heaviness (results presented graphically).[13] Results have to be interpreted with care, as overall withdrawal rates were high (see comment below). The second RCT (10 women) used a crossover design, and also found that bromocriptine significantly reduced pain compared with placebo (results after crossover: $P < 0.02$; results before crossover not reported).[14]

Harms: The larger RCT found that adverse effects were significantly more frequent with bromocriptine than with placebo (61/135 [45%] with bromocriptine *v* 41/137 [30%] with placebo; RR 1.5, 95% CI 1.1 to 1.9; NNH 7, 95% CI 4 to 29).[13] It found that withdrawals related to adverse effects were more frequent in women taking bromocriptine, but this difference did not reach significance (15/135 [11%] with bromocriptine *v* 8/137 [6%] with placebo; RR 1.9, 95% CI 0.8 to 4.3). Adverse reactions included nausea (32% with bromocriptine *v* 13% with placebo), dizziness (12% with bromocriptine *v* 7% with placebo), postural hypotension, and constipation.[13] Overall, withdrawal rates were high (see comment below). The second RCT found that nausea and dizziness occurred in 8/10 (80%) women on bromocriptine compared with 0/10 (0%) on placebo.[14] Strokes and death have been reported after use of bromocriptine to inhibit lactation, and the US Food and Drug Administration has withdrawn its licence for this indication.[15]

Comment: Bromocriptine is now used rarely because frequent and intolerable adverse effects at the therapeutic dose outweigh the benefits for this indication. In the larger RCT, analysis was not by intention to treat, and overall withdrawal rates were high (withdrawals: 49/135 [36%] with bromocriptine *v* 36/137 [26%] with placebo; RR 1.4, 95% CI 1.0 to 2.0).[13]

OPTION LISURIDE

One RCT with weak methods found limited evidence that lisuride maleate (a dopamine agonist) reduced breast pain over 2 months compared with placebo.

Benefits: One double blind RCT (60 women with premenstrual breast pain) comparing lisuride maleate 200 μg daily versus placebo over 2 months found significant improvement in visual analogue scores for pain (improved scores in 27/30 [90%] with lisuride maleate *v* 10/30 [33%] with placebo; RR 2.7, 95% CI 1.6 to 4.5; NNT 2, 95% CI 2 to 3) (see comment below).[16]

Harms: During the first month of treatment, nausea was more frequently reported by women taking lisuride maleate; however, the difference was not significant (women reporting nausea: 5/30 [17%] with lisuride maleate *v* 3/30 [10%] with placebo; RR 1.7, 95% CI 0.4 to 6.4).[16]

Comment: Allocation was carried out in blocks of 10 consecutive women. Tablet coding for active treatments and placebo differed, potentially confounding any treatment effect. Response to treatment was defined as a reduction greater than 25% from the baseline score during the first month, or greater than 50% during the second month.[16]

OPTION **HORMONE REPLACEMENT THERAPY (OESTROGEN)**

We found no placebo controlled RCTs of hormone replacement therapy for breast pain. Hormone replacement therapy is associated with an increased risk of breast cancer, venous thromboembolism, and gall bladder disease.

Benefits: We found no systematic review or RCTs examining effects of hormone replacement therapy for treating breast pain.

Harms: See harms of hormone replacement therapy under secondary prevention of ischaemic cardiac events, (Web only).

Comment: One RCT (44 postmenopausal women with or without breast pain) found that hormone replacement therapy (transdermal oestrogen patches 50 μg twice weekly for 3 weeks/month, plus progestogen 5 mg/day for 12 days/month/cycle) significantly increased the risk of developing breast pain compared with tibolone 2.5 mg daily within 1 year (increase in breast pain as assessed by questionnaire: 53% with hormone replacement therapy *v* 5% with tibolone; $P < 0.02$).[17]

OPTION **TIBOLONE**

One RCT found no significant difference between tibolone and placebo in breast pain and tenderness at 12 months.

Benefits: **Versus placebo:** We found no systematic review. We found one RCT (64 women with breast pain secondary to hormone replacement therapy), which compared tibolone versus placebo.[18] It found no significant differences in breast tenderness or breast pain at 12 months (both symptoms measured on a visual analogue scale from 0 [no symptoms] to 10 [greatest severity]); mean breast tenderness score: 7.9 at baseline and 4.1 at 12 months with tibolone *v* 7.4 at baseline and 3.8 at 12 months with placebo; P value not reported; mean mastalgia score: 6.1 at baseline and 2.9 at 12 months with tibolone *v* 5.7 at baseline and 2.7 at 12 months with placebo; P value not reported). **Versus hormone replacement therapy:** We found no RCTs.

Harms: **Versus placebo:** The RCT found that the risk of vaginal bleeding was similar with tibolone and placebo in the first 2 months (6/31 [19%] with tibolone *v* 4/30 [13%] with placebo). The RCT reported that there were no other adverse effects.[18]

Comment: Tibolone is a synthetic steroid reported to have oestrogenic, progestogenic, and weak androgenic properties, which can be used as a form of hormone replacement therapy.[19] See comment in hormone replacement therapy, p 2263.

OPTION **TAMOXIFEN**

Three RCTs found limited evidence that tamoxifen was more effective than placebo at reducing breast pain. The two RCTs which reported on adverse effects found more hot flushes and vaginal discharge with tamoxifen compared with placebo, although differences between groups did not reach significance. One RCT found similar efficacy but fewer adverse effects with a lower dose of 10 mg compared with 20 mg. One RCT found no significant difference in pain relief between tamoxifen and danazol. One meta-analysis of four large breast cancer prevention trials found that tamoxifen used long term was associated with an increased risk of venous thromboembolism. Tamoxifen is not licensed for mastalgia in the UK or USA.

Benefits: We found no systematic review. **Versus placebo:** We found three RCTs.[10,20,21] One double blind RCT (60 premenopausal women with cyclical breast pain) compared tamoxifen 20 mg daily versus placebo.[21] It found that significantly more women experienced pain relief (measured by visual analogue scale over 3 months) with tamoxifen compared with placebo (22/31 [71%] with tamoxifen *v* 11/29 [38%] with placebo; RR 1.9, 95% CI 1.1 to 3.1; NNT 3, 95% CI 2 to 13). The second RCT (93 women) compared tamoxifen, danazol, and placebo.[10] It found that significantly more women with tamoxifen achieved a good outcome (> 50% reduction in mean pain score) at the end of treatment, 6 months later, and 12 months later compared with placebo (pain relief after 6 months of treatment: 23/32 [72%] with tamoxifen *v* 11/29 [38%] with placebo; RR 1.9, 95% CI 1.1 to 3.2; NNT 3, 95% CI 1 to 10). The third RCT (88 women, aged 22–44 years) found that 8 months of tamoxifen increased the proportion of women who achieved complete recovery (outcome not clearly defined) compared with placebo (complete recovery: 40/44 [90%] with tamoxifen *v* 0/44 [0%] with placebo).[20] **Dose response:** One RCT (301 women with cyclical breast pain for > 6 months) compared 10 mg versus 20 mg daily doses of tamoxifen from days 15–25 in the menstrual cycle for 3 months. It found no significant difference in pain relief (127/155 [82%] with 10 mg *v* 107/142 [75%] with 20 mg; RR 1.09, 95% CI 0.96 to 1.18).[22] Another RCT (60 women) compared 10 mg versus 20 mg daily doses of tamoxifen for 3 and 6 months in cyclical and non-cyclical mastalgia.[23] It found that 3 month response rates were similar (pain relief: 12/14 [86%] with 10 mg *v* 14/15 [93%] with 20 mg; RR 0.9, 95% CI 0.4 to 1.1). **Versus danazol:** See benefits of danazol, p 2261.

Harms: The first two RCTs found that hot flushes and vaginal discharge were more common with 20 mg tamoxifen daily than with placebo. However, differences were not significant.[20,21] The first RCT found more hot flushes (8/31 [26%] with tamoxifen *v* 3/29 [10%] with placebo; RR 2.5, 95% CI 0.7 to 8.5) and vaginal discharge (5/31 [16%] with tamoxifen *v* 2/29 [7%] with placebo; ARI 9.2%; RR 2.3, 95% CI 0.5 to 11.0).[21] The second RCT found more hot flushes and vaginal discharge with tamoxifen 20 mg daily compared with placebo (hot flushes: 8/32 [25%] with tamoxifen *v* 3/29 [10%] with placebo; RR 2.4, 95% CI 0.7 to 8.3; vaginal discharge: 5/32 [16%] with tamoxifen *v* 2/29 [7%] with placebo; RR 2.3, 95% CI 0.5 to 10.8).[10] See adverse effects of tamoxifen under treatment of breast cancer, p 2197. The third RCT did not report any significant adverse events.[20] One meta-analysis of the four largest breast cancer prevention trials found that tamoxifen used long term at 20 mg daily was associated with venothromboembolism.[24] **Dose response:** Adverse effects occurred more frequently with the 20 mg dose than with the 10 mg dose between days 15–25 of the menstrual cycle.[22,23] The largest RCT found that adverse effects were reported significantly more frequently with the 20 mg dose than with the 10 mg dose (adverse effects: 94/142 [66%] with 20 mg/day *v* 80/155 [52%] with 10 mg/day; RR 1.28, 95% CI 1.06 to 1.56; NNT 6, 95% CI 3 to 28).[22] Adverse effects were primarily hot flushes (AR 54/142 [38%] with 20 mg/day *v* 33/155 [21%] with the 10 mg/day; RR 1.79, 95% CI 1.24 to 2.58; NNH 6, 95% CI 3 to 16) and gastrointestinal disturbances (AR 54/142 [38%] with 20 mg/day *v* 30/155 [19%] with 10 mg/day; RR 1.97, 95% CI 1.34 to 2.88; NNH 6, 95% CI 4 to 12).

Comment: Tamoxifen is not licensed for mastalgia in the UK or the USA. There is consensus to limit its use to no more than 6 months at a time under expert supervision and with appropriate non-hormonal contraception because of the high incidence of adverse effects. Tamoxifen is contraindicated in pregnancy because of potential teratogenicity.[25]

OPTION GONADORELIN ANALOGUES (LUTEINISING HORMONE RELEASING HORMONE ANALOGUES)

We found no systematic review or RCTs of sufficient quality on the effects of gonadorelin analogues.

Benefits: We found no systematic review or RCTs.

Harms: Adverse effects of goserelin can include hot flushes (90%), headaches (57%), nausea and vomiting (29%), depression and irritability (24%), loss of libido (37%), and amenorrhoea (100%).[26]

Comment: None.

OPTION GESTRINONE

One RCT found that gestrinone reduced breast pain after 3 months compared with placebo, but increased adverse effects (greasy skin, hirsutism, acne, reduction in breast size, headache, and depression).

Benefits: **Versus placebo:** We found no systematic review. We found one double blind, outpatient based RCT (145 premenopausal women with cyclical breast pain) comparing gestrinone (2.4 mg twice weekly) with placebo.[27] It found that gestrinone reduced breast pain significantly more than placebo after 3 months (using visual analogue score where 0 = no pain, 100 = worst pain; mean pain score reduced from 59.5 to 11.0 with gestrinone *v* 58.2 to 36.7 with placebo; $P < 0.0001$).

Harms: **Versus placebo:** The RCT found that adverse effects were significantly more common with gestrinone compared with placebo (at least 1 adverse effect: 41% with gestrinone *v* 14% with placebo; RR 2.96, 95% CI 1.70 to 4.40). Adverse effects included greasy skin (13 with gestrinone *v* 2 with placebo), hirsutism (10 with gestrinone *v* 3 with placebo), acne (9 with gestrinone *v* 2 with placebo), intermenstrual bleeding (7 with gestrinone *v* 0 with placebo), voice change (5 with gestrinone *v* 1 with placebo), reduced libido (5 with gestrinone *v* 3 with placebo), reduction in breast size (3 with gestrinone *v* 0 with placebo), headache (4 with gestrinone *v* 0 with placebo), depression (2 with gestrinone *v* 0 with placebo), and tiredness (2 with gestrinone *v* 0 with placebo).[25]

Comment: Gestrinone is a synthetic steroid, reported to have androgenic, antioestrogenic, and antiprogestogenic properties.[19]

OPTION PROGESTOGENS

Two small crossover RCTs found no significant difference between either progesterone cream or medroxyprogesterone acetate tablets and placebo in breast pain.

Benefits: We found two RCTs.[28,29] The first RCT (crossover, 26 women with cyclical breast pain of at least 6 months' duration) treated all included women with daily 20 mg tablets of medroxyprogesterone acetate for 6 months, followed by a 2 month observation period. Women with persistent symptoms were then randomly allocated to oral medroxyprogesterone acetate (20 mg tablets) or placebo given from day 10–26 of the menstrual cycle, for 3 months and then switched group (crossover) for the remaining 3 months.[28] The RCT found no significant differences in the visual analogue scale for pain at the end of each phase before and after the crossover (data presented graphically). The overall withdrawal rate was 15%.[28] The second RCT (crossover, 80 women with breast pain of at least 2 months' duration) identified women who were able to keep an updated diary with visual analogue scales of pain for 2 months and then randomised them to daily applications of cream with progesterone 1% or placebo, from the 10th day of the cycle to the beginning of the next cycle, for 3 months. The analysis before crossover found no significant difference in pain scores between progesterone and placebo cream (numerical results not reported; see comment below).[29]

Harms: The first RCT found that five women reported adverse effects while on medroxyprogesterone acetate, five while on placebo, and one with both. Symptoms were mostly vague premenstrual symptoms.[28] No further details were reported. The second RCT did not report on harms.[29]

Comment: The second RCT provided insufficient details about the analysis. Withdrawals involved 7/32 (22%) women.[29] Both RCTs have small sample size, significant withdrawals, and a selection phase, which may restrict the generalisibility of the evidence.[28,29]

OPTION OTHER AGENTS

We found no RCTs of the effects of pyridoxine, diuretics, antibiotics, or vitamin E compared with placebo for the treatment of breast pain.

Benefits: We found no systematic review or good quality RCTs on the effects of other agents (pyridoxine, diuretics, antibiotics, or vitamin E) on breast pain.

Harms: We found no RCTs.

Comment: None.

REFERENCES

1. Gateley CA, Mansel RE. Management of the painful and nodular breast. *Br Med Bull* 1991;47:284–294.
2. Ader DN, Shriver CD. Cyclical mastalgia: prevalence and impact in an outpatient breast clinic sample. *J Am Coll Surg* 1997;185:466–470.
3. Harding C, Osundeko O, Tetlow L, et al. Hormonally-regulated proteins in breast secretions are markers of target organ sensitivity. *Br J Cancer* 2000;2:354–360.
4. Maddox PR, Harrison BJ, Mansel RE, et al. Non-cyclical mastalgia: improved classification and treatment. *Br J Surg* 1989;76:901–904.
5. Pye JK, Mansel RE, Hughes LE. Clinical experience of drug treatments for mastalgia. *Lancet* 1985;1:373–377.
6. Boyd NF, McGuire V, Shannon P, et al. Effect of a low-fat high-carbohydrate diet on symptoms of cyclical mastopathy. *Lancet* 1988;2:128–132.
7. Blommers J, de Lange-De Klerk ES, Kuik DJ, et al. Evening primrose oil and fish oil for severe chronic mastalgia: a randomized, double-blind, controlled trial. *Am J Obstet Gynecol* 2002;187:1389–1394.
8. Preece PE, Hanslip JI, Gilbert L, et al. Evening primrose oil (Efamol) for mastalgia. In: Horrobin D, ed. *Clinical uses of essential fatty acids*. Montreal: Eden Press, 1982:147–154.
9. What's new: Epogam and Efamast (gamolenic acid) — withdrawal of marketing authorisations. <extrefLw.mca.gov.uk/whatsnew/epogam.htm> (last accessed 15 September 2004).
10. Kontostolis E, Stefanidis K, Navrozoglou I, et al. Comparison of tamoxifen with danazol for treatment of cyclical mastalgia. *Gynecol Endocrinol* 1997;11:393–397.
11. Maddox PR, Harrison BJ, Mansel RE. Low-dose danazol for mastalgia. *Br J Clin Pract* 1989;68:43–47.
12. Anonymous. Danazol. In: *The ABPI compendium of data sheets and summaries of product characteristics*. London: Datapharm Publications, 1999–2000:1395.
13. Mansel RE, Dogliotti L. European multicentre trial of bromocriptine in cyclical mastalgia. *Lancet* 1990;335:190–193.
14. Blichert-Toft M, Anderson AN, Henrikson OB, et al. Treatment of mastalgia with bromocriptine: a double blind crossover study. *BMJ* 1979;1:237.
15. Arrowsmith-Lowe T. Bromocriptine indications withdrawn. *FDA Med Bull* 1994;24:2.
16. Kaleli S, Aydin Y, Erel CT, et al. Symptomatic treatment of premenstrual mastalgia in premenopausal women with lisuride maleate: a double-blind placebo-controlled randomized study. *Fertil Steril* 2001;75:718–723.
17. Colacurci N, Mele D, De Franciscis P, et al. Effects of tibolone on the breast. *Eur J Obstet Gynecol Reprod Biol* 1998;80:235–238.
18. Palomba S, Di Carlo C, Morelli M, et al. Effect of tibolone on breast symptoms resulting from postmenopausal hormone replacement therapy. *Maturitas* 2003;45:267–273.
19. Parfitt K, ed. *Martindale. The complete drug reference*, 32nd ed. London: Pharmaceutical Press, 1999:1447–1448.
20. Grio R, Cellura A, Geranio R, et al. Clinical efficacy of tamoxifen in the treatment of premenstrual mastodynia. *Minerva Ginecol* 1998;50:101–103.
21. Fentiman IS, Caleffi M, Brame K, et al. Double-blind controlled trial of tamoxifen therapy for mastalgia. *Lancet* 1986;1:287–288.
22. GEMB Group. Tamoxifen therapy for cyclical mastalgia: dose randomised trial. *Breast* 1997;5:212–213.
23. Fentiman IS, Hamed H, Caleffi M, et al. Dosage and duration of tamoxifen treatment for mastalgia: a controlled trial. *Br J Surg* 1988;75:845–846.
24. Cuzick J, Powles T, Veronesi U, et al. Overview of the main outcomes in breast cancer prevention trials. *Lancet* 2003;361:296–300.

25. Anonymous. Nolvadex. In: *The ABPI compendium of data sheets and summaries of product characteristics*. London: Datapharm Publications Ltd, 1999–2000:1799.
26. Hamed H, Caleffi M, Chaudary MA, et al. LHRH analogue for treatment of recurrent and refractory mastalgia. *Ann R Coll Surg Engl* 1990;72:221–224.
27. Peters F. Multicentre study of gestinone in cyclical breast pain. *Lancet* 1992;339:205–208.
28. Maddox PR, Harrison BJ, Horobin JM, et al. A randomised controlled trial of medroxyprogesterone acetate in mastalgia. *Ann R Coll Surg Engl* 1990;72:71–76.
29. McFadyen IJ, Raab GM, Macintyre CC, et al. Progesterone cream for cyclic breast pain. *BMJ* 1989;298:931.

Nigel Bundred
Professor in Surgical Oncology
University of Manchester Department of Surgery
Manchester
UK

Competing interests: The author has received reimbursement by AstraZeneca, the maker of tamoxifen, for attending several conferences and running education programmes. The author has also received support by Searle Pharmacia for attending and speaking at symposia.

Candidiasis (vulvovaginal)

Search date November 2003

Des Spence

QUESTIONS

INTERVENTIONS

See glossary Ⓖ

Key Messages

Acute vulvovaginal candidiasis

- **Intravaginal imidazoles** RCTs found that intravaginal imidazoles (butoconazole, clotrimazole, miconazole, or terconazole) reduced persistent symptoms of vulvovaginal candidiasis after 9–38 days compared with placebo. They found no clear evidence that clinical effects differ among the various intravaginal imidazoles. RCTs found no clear evidence of any difference in persistent symptoms between shorter and longer durations of treatment (1–14 days). RCTs found no significant difference in symptoms between intravaginal imidazoles and oral fluconazole, itraconazole, or ketoconazole. RCTs found that intravaginal imidazoles were associated with less nausea, headache, and abdominal pain but more vulval irritation and vaginal discharge than oral fluconazole or oral ketoconazole. Two RCTs provided insufficient evidence to compare intravaginal imidazoles versus intravaginal nystatin.

Clin Evid 2005;13:2268–2284.

- **Oral fluconazole** We found no RCTs comparing oral fluconazole versus placebo or no treatment. One systematic review found no significant difference in persistent symptoms of vulvovaginal candidiasis over 1–12 weeks between oral fluconazole or oral itraconazole and intravaginal imidazoles, and found that oral fluconazole was associated with more nausea, headache, and abdominal pain but less vulval irritation and vaginal discharge than intravaginal imidazoles. One weak RCT provided insufficient evidence to compare oral fluconazole versus oral itraconazole. One systematic review found no significant difference in persistent symptoms of vulvovaginal candidiasis or in adverse effects between oral fluconazole and oral ketoconazole.
- **Oral itraconazole** One RCT found that oral itraconazole reduced persistent symptoms of vulvovaginal candidiasis at 1 week after treatment compared with placebo. One systematic review found no significant difference in persistent symptoms over 1–12 weeks between oral itraconazole or oral fluconazole and intravaginal imidazoles. One weak RCT provided insufficient evidence to compare oral itraconazole versus oral fluconazole.
- **Intravaginal nystatin** One RCT found that intravaginal nystatin reduced the proportion of women with a poor symptomatic response after 14 days' treatment compared with placebo. Two RCTs provided insufficient evidence to compare intravaginal nystatin versus intravaginal imidazoles. One RCT found that intravaginal nystatin was less effective than boric acid in increasing clinical cure rates at 4 weeks. It gave no information on the adverse effects of intravaginal nystatin compared with intravaginal boric acid. We found no RCTs comparing intravaginal nystatin versus oral fluconazole, itraconazole, or ketoconazole.
- **Douching** We found no RCTs of douching in women with acute vulvovaginal candidiasis. Douching is associated with serious sequelae, including pelvic inflammatory disease, endometritis, and ectopic pregnancy.
- **Garlic** We found no RCTs of garlic in women with acute vulvovaginal candidiasis.
- **Intravaginal boric acid** One RCT found that intravaginal boric acid increased clinical cure rates at 4 weeks compared with intravaginal nystatin. It gave no information on the adverse effects of intravaginal boric acid compared with intravaginal nystatin. Intravaginal boric acid can cause skin irritation.
- **Intravaginal tea tree oil** We found no RCTs of intravaginal tea tree oil in women with acute vulvovaginal candidiasis.
- **Yoghurt containing** ***Lactobacillus acidophilus*** We found no RCTs of lactobacillus yoghurt in women with acute vulvovaginal candidiasis.
- **Oral ketoconazole** We found no RCTs comparing oral ketoconazole versus placebo or no treatment. RCTs found no significant difference between oral ketoconazole and intravaginal imidazoles in persistent symptoms of vulvovaginal candidiasis, and found that oral ketoconazole may cause more nausea, fatigue, and headaches but less vulval irritation. One RCT found no significant difference in persistent symptoms or adverse effects between oral ketoconazole and oral fluconazole. Case reports have associated ketoconazole with a risk of fulminant hepatitis (1/12 000 courses of treatment with oral ketoconazole); there is consensus that the risks may outweigh the benefits in women with vulvovaginal candidiasis.
- **Treating a male sexual partner to resolve symptoms and prevent symptomatic recurrence in women** RCTs found no significant difference between treating and not treating a woman's male sexual partner in the resolution of the woman's symptoms of acute vulvovaginal candidiasis over 1–4 weeks or in the rate of symptomatic recurrence at 4–5 weeks after treatment.

Recurrent vulvovaginal candidiasis

- **Oral itraconazole** One RCT found that monthly prophylaxis with oral itraconazole reduced symptomatic recurrence of vulvovaginal candidiasis over 6 months compared with placebo. One weak, open label RCT provided insufficient evidence to compare twice weekly prophylaxis with oral itraconazole versus intravaginal clotrimazole.

- **Douching** We found no RCTs of douching in women with recurrent vulvovaginal candidiasis. Douching is associated with serious sequelae, including pelvic inflammatory disease, endometritis, ectopic pregnancy, gonorrhoea, and chlamydia.
- **Garlic** We found no RCTs of garlic in women with recurrent vulvovaginal candidiasis.
- **Intravaginal boric acid** We found no RCTs of intravaginal boric acid in women with recurrent vulvovaginal candidiasis.
- **Intravaginal imidazoles** Two RCTs provided insufficient evidence about the effects of regular prophylaxis with intravaginal clotrimazole compared with placebo in preventing symptomatic recurrence of vulvovaginal candidiasis. One RCT found no significant difference in the number of episodes of symptomatic vaginitis over 6 months between monthly prophylaxis with intravaginal clotrimazole and treatment as required, although women who took monthly prophylaxis had fewer episodes. The RCT may have been underpowered to detect a clinically important difference. More women preferred treatment as required. One RCT found insufficient evidence about the effects of regular prophylaxis with intravaginal clotrimazole compared with oral itraconazole.
- **Oral fluconazole** We found no RCTs about the effects of oral fluconazole in preventing symptomatic recurrence of vulvovaginal candidiasis.
- **Intravaginal tea tree oil** We found no RCTs of intravaginal tea tree oil in women with recurrent vulvovaginal candidiasis.
- **Yoghurt containing** *Lactobacillus acidophilus* Two poor quality crossover RCTs identified by a systematic review provided insufficient evidence about the effects of oral lactobacillus yoghurt in women with recurrent vulvovaginal candidiasis. Oral yoghurt may cause gastrointestinal disturbance in people with lactose intolerance. The review identified no RCTs of vaginal lactobacillus yoghurt.
- **Oral ketoconazole** One RCT found that oral ketoconazole, given for 5 days during the menstrual cycle at 400 mg daily or continuously at a lower dose, reduced symptomatic recurrence of vulvovaginal candidiasis over 6 months compared with placebo. This benefit is associated with an increased risk of harms, including rare cases of fulminant hepatitis (1/12 000 courses of treatment with oral ketoconazole); there is consensus that the risks may outweigh the benefits in women with vulvovaginal candidiasis.
- **Treating a male sexual partner to resolve symptoms and prevent symptomatic recurrence in women** One RCT found no significant difference between treating and not treating a woman's male sexual partner in the rate of symptomatic recurrence over 12 months.

DEFINITION **Vulvovaginal candidiasis** is defined as symptomatic vaginitis (inflammation of the vagina), which often involves the vulva, caused by infection with a *Candida* yeast. Predominant symptoms are vulval itching and abnormal vaginal discharge (which may be minimal, a "cheese like" material, or a watery secretion). Differentiation from other forms of vaginitis requires the presence of yeast on microscopy of vaginal fluid. **Recurrent vulvovaginal candidiasis** is commonly defined as four or more symptomatic episodes a year.[1] Studies of asymptomatic women with vaginal colonisation by *Candida* species were excluded.

INCIDENCE/ PREVALENCE Vulvovaginal candidiasis is estimated to be the second most common cause of vaginitis after bacterial vaginosis. Estimates of its incidence are limited and often derived from women who attend hospital clinics. Asymptomatic prevalence has been reported in 10% of women[2] and self-reported history of at least one episode of vulvovaginal candidiasis has been as high as 72%.[3] Recurrent symptoms are common but are caused by candidiasis in only a third of cases.[4]

AETIOLOGY/ RISK FACTORS *Candida albicans* accounts for 85–90% of cases of vulvovaginal candidiasis. Development of symptomatic vulvovaginal candidiasis probably represents increased growth of yeast that previously colonised the vagina without causing symptoms. Risk factors for vulvovaginal candidiasis include pregnancy, diabetes mellitus, and systemic antibiotics. The evidence that different types of contraceptives are risk factors is contradictory. The incidence of vulvovaginal candidiasis rises with initiation of sexual activity, but we found no direct evidence that vulvovaginal candidiasis is sexually transmitted.[5–7]

PROGNOSIS We found few descriptions of the natural history of untreated vulvovaginal candidiasis. Discomfort is the main complication and can include pain while passing urine or during sexual intercourse. Balanitis**G** in male partners of women with vulvovaginal candidiasis can occur, but it is rare.

AIMS OF INTERVENTION To alleviate symptoms with minimal adverse effects from treatment.

OUTCOMES **Acute vulvovaginal candidiasis:** Clinical cure rates, either measured in the short term (5–15 days) or medium term (3–6 weeks) after treatment. The definition of clinical cure varies among RCTs but often includes both complete resolution of symptoms and culture negative for *Candida*. In the option on treating a male sexual partner, we also assessed symptomatic recurrence confirmed by positive culture. **Recurrent vulvovaginal candidiasis:** Symptomatic recurrence confirmed by positive culture.

METHODS *Clinical Evidence* search and appraisal November 2003, and personal contact with the Medical Information Department of Bristol Myers Squibb to retrieve an RCT on nystatin.[8] We included only those RCTs in which most participants were from the target population (for example, to answer the questions for non-pregnant women, we sought RCTs that excluded pregnant women or RCTs in which pregnant women represented < 20% of the participants). We excluded studies of women with HIV infection. Many RCTs excluded women with diabetes mellitus. We included RCTs only if recruitment was restricted to women with both symptoms of vaginal candidiasis and laboratory confirmation of candidal infection.

QUESTION What are the effects of treatments for acute vulvovaginal candidiasis in non-pregnant women?

OPTION INTRAVAGINAL IMIDAZOLES

RCTs found that intravaginal imidazoles (butoconazole, clotrimazole, miconazole, or terconazole) reduced persistent symptoms of vulvovaginal candidiasis after 1–5 weeks compared with placebo. They found no clear evidence that clinical effects differ among the various intravaginal imidazoles. RCTs found no clear evidence of any difference in persistent symptoms between shorter and longer durations of treatment (1–14 days). RCTs found no significant difference in symptoms between intravaginal imidazoles and oral fluconazole, itraconazole, or ketoconazole. RCTs found that intravaginal imidazoles were associated with less nausea, headache, and abdominal pain but more vulval irritation and vaginal discharge than oral fluconazole or oral ketoconazole. Two RCTs provided insufficient evidence to compare intravaginal imidazoles versus intravaginal nystatin.

Benefits: **Versus placebo:** We found one systematic review (search date 1993[9], 3 RCTs[10–12]) and three additional RCTs (see table A on web extra).[13–15] The systematic review did not perform a meta-analysis.[9] Five RCTs found that, compared with placebo, intravaginal imidazoles (butoconazole, clotrimazole, miconazole, or terconazole) significantly reduced persistent symptoms of vaginal candidiasis at 1–5 weeks after treatment.[10–12,14,15] However, only two of these RCTs[14,15] provided results with analysis by intention to treat. The sixth RCT (95 women) found no significant difference in symptoms after 5 weeks between clotrimazole and placebo, but results were not analysed by intention to treat and the follow up rate was very low (62/95 [65%]).[13] **Versus each other:** We found one systematic review (search date 1993,[9] 12 RCTs[10,11,16–25]) and 22 additional RCTs (see table B on web extra).[26–47] Many of the RCTs were too small to exclude clinically important differences in outcomes. The populations selected by each RCT varied considerably in the prevalence of prognostic risk factors (such as diabetes mellitus or a history of recurrent attacks of vulvovaginal candidiasis in the previous year), and a variety of outcomes were assessed. The RCTs provided no clear evidence of any consistent difference in effectiveness between the different imidazoles. **Duration of treatment:** We found one systematic review (search date 1993[9], 14 RCTs[11,16-18,22,48-56]) and seven additional RCTs[57–63] comparing regimens that used the same intravaginal imidazole for different durations (1–14 days). The RCTs found no consistent difference in the proportion of women with persistent symptoms, but they were too small to exclude a clinically important difference. **Versus oral fluconazole or oral itraconazole:** We found one systematic review (search date 2000, 7 RCTs, 1247 women) that found no significant difference between oral fluconazole or oral itraconazole and intravaginal imidazoles (clotrimazole, miconazole, and econazole) in persistent symptoms at 5–15 days (124/627 [20%] with oral fluconazole or itraconazole *v* 121/620 [20%] with intravaginal imidazoles; RR 1.00, 95% CI 0.95 to 1.06) or at 2–12 weeks (74/432 [17%] with oral fluconazole or itraconazole *v* 71/404 [18%] with intravaginal imidazoles; RR 1.04, 95% CI 0.95 to 1.07; see comment below).[65] **Versus oral ketoconazole:** See benefits of oral ketoconazole, p 2274. **Versus intravaginal nystatin:** We found two RCTs.[26,64] The first RCT (70 women) found no significant difference between clotrimazole (100 mg for 14 days) and high strength nystatin vaginal cream (1 million IU, once daily for 7 days) in the proportion of women with persistent symptoms after 4 weeks (2/33 [6%] with nystatin *v* 1/37 [3%] with clotrimazole; OR 2.24, 95% CI 0.23 to 22.40).[26] The second RCT (292 women) compared six interventions: intravaginal clotrimazole, intravaginal econazole, intravaginal miconazole, oral miconazole plus intravaginal nystatin, oral nystatin plus intravaginal nystatin, and intravaginal nystatin alone.[64] It found no significant difference between interventions in symptomatic relapse over 6 months (18/53 [34%] with intravaginal clotrimazole *v* 16/34 [47%] with intravaginal econazole *v* 18/80 [22%] with intravaginal miconazole *v* 6/31 [19%] with oral miconazole plus intravaginal nystatin *v* 14/49 [28%] with oral nystatin plus intravaginal nystatin *v* 26/45 [58%] with intravaginal nystatin alone; reported as non-significant; CI not reported). The RCTs are likely to have been underpowered to detect clinically important differences between treatments.[26,64]

Harms: **Versus placebo:** In the RCTs comparing intravaginal imidazoles versus placebo, most women did not report any adverse effects.[10–15] The most common adverse effect was vulval irritation. Most RCTs did not report frequencies of specific adverse effects in women who took placebo. In one RCT adverse effects were more common in women who took oral placebo than in women who used intravaginal imidazole (9 adverse events, mainly nausea and headache, in 22 women who received oral placebo *v* 1 episode of irritation in 23 women who used intravaginal imidazole).[12] **Versus oral fluconazole or oral itraconazole:** Two large RCTs identified by the review[65] found that oral fluconazole may be associated with increased nausea, headache, and abdominal pain compared with intravaginal imidazoles.[67,68] The first RCT (429 women) found that single dose 150 mg oral fluconazole significantly increased adverse effects over 14 days compared with intravaginal clotrimazole 100 mg daily for 7 days (59/217 [27%] with oral fluconazole *v* 37/212 [17%] with intravaginal clotrimazole; OR 1.75, 95% CI 1.11 to 2.75; NNH 11, 95% CI 6 to 54).[67] The individual events that were more common with oral fluconazole were headache (12% *v* 9%), abdominal pain (7% *v* 3%), and nausea (4% *v* 0%). The second RCT (235 women) found that oral fluconazole significantly increased nausea and other gastrointestinal symptoms compared with intravaginal econazole (9/121 [7%] *v* 2/114 [2%]; OR 3.55, 95% CI 1.06 to 11.90), but intravaginal econazole significantly increased local vulval burning and vaginal discharge (3/121 [2%] with oral fluconazole *v* 25/114 [22%] with intravaginal econazole; OR 0.16, 95% CI 0.07 to 0.35).[68] A third RCT (369 women) identified by the review found very few adverse effects with either oral fluconazole or clotrimazole (8/188 [4%] v 9/181 [5%]).[69] A fourth RCT (double blind, 81 women) identified by the review found no significant difference between oral itraconazole and intravaginal econazole in the proportion of women who had adverse effects (4/40 [10%] with itraconazole v 8/41 [20%] with econazole; OR 0.48, 95% CI 0.14 to 1.61).[70] **Versus intravaginal nystatin:** The first RCT found no adverse effects in women who took intravaginal clotrimazole or intravaginal nystatin.[26] The second RCT gave no information on adverse effects.[64]

Comment: Most RCTs were small and many had weak methods (poorly described randomisation, inadequate concealment and blinding, and definitions of cure based on mycology results rather than symptoms). We excluded all RCTs that defined cure only on the basis of mycology results. Trials in women who obtain intravaginal imidazoles over the counter are needed. **Versus oral fluconazole or oral itraconazole:** The review did not report results in women taking oral fluconazole or oral itraconazole separately.[65]

OPTION ORAL FLUCONAZOLE

We found no RCTs comparing oral fluconazole versus placebo or no treatment. One systematic review found no significant difference in persistent symptoms of vulvovaginal candidiasis over 1–12 weeks between oral fluconazole or oral itraconazole and intravaginal imidazoles, and found that oral fluconazole was associated with more nausea, headache, and abdominal pain but less vulval irritation and vaginal discharge than intravaginal imidazoles. One weak RCT provided insufficient evidence to compare oral fluconazole versus oral itraconazole. One systematic review found no significant difference in persistent symptoms of vulvovaginal candidiasis or in adverse effects between oral fluconazole and oral ketoconazole.

Benefits: **Versus placebo:** We found no systematic review or RCTs. **Versus intravaginal imidazoles:** See benefits of intravaginal imidazoles, p 2271. **Versus oral itraconazole:** We found no systematic review but found one RCT (86 women).[66] The RCT found no significant difference between oral fluconazole 150 mg in a single dose and oral itraconazole 200 mg daily for 3 days in the proportion of women cured at 7 days (13/38 [34%] with fluconazole v 16/32 [50%] with itraconazole; P = 0.18) or at 21 days (18/38 [47%] v 17/32 [53%]; P = 0.63; see comment below). **Versus oral ketoconazole:** See benefits of oral ketoconazole, p 2274. **Versus intravaginal nystatin:** We found no RCTs.

Harms: **Versus intravaginal imidazoles:** See harms of intravaginal imidazoles, p 2272. **Versus oral itraconazole:** The RCT found that oral fluconazole and oral itraconazole were associated with similar rates of adverse effects, including gastrointestinal disturbances, pelvic pain, insomnia, anxiety, and rash.[66] **Versus oral ketoconazole:** See harms of oral ketoconazole, p 2275.

Comment: **Versus intravaginal imidazoles:** See comment of intravaginal imidazoles, p 2273. **Versus oral itraconazole:** In the RCT, women who received oral fluconazole had significantly higher baseline symptom scores than women who received oral itraconazole (9.03 v 7.03; P = 0.003); this makes the results difficult to interpret.[66]

OPTION ORAL ITRACONAZOLE

One RCT found that oral itraconazole reduced persistent symptoms at 1 week after treatment compared with placebo. One systematic review found no significant difference in persistent symptoms over 1–12 weeks between oral itraconazole or oral fluconazole and intravaginal imidazoles. One weak RCT provided insufficient evidence to compare oral itraconazole versus oral fluconazole.

Benefits: **Versus placebo:** We found onc systematic review (search date 2000),[66] which identified one RCT (90 women) that compared three interventions: oral itraconazole, oral clotrimazole, and placebo.[12] The RCT found that oral itraconazole (200 mg/day for 3 days) significantly reduced the proportion of women with persistent symptoms at 1 week after treatment compared with placebo (13/48 [27%] with itraconazole *v* 12/22 [55%] with placebo; $P < 0.05$). **Versus intravaginal imidazoles:** See benefits of intravaginal imidazoles, p 2271. **Versus oral fluconazole:** See benefits of oral fluconazole, p 2273. **Versus oral ketoconazole:** We found no RCTs. **Versus intravaginal nystatin:** We found no RCTs.

Harms: **Versus placebo:** The RCT identified by the review[65] found that itraconazole significantly increased the proportion of women who had adverse effects compared with intravaginal clotrimazole (17/50 [34%] with itraconazole *v* 1/23 [4%] with clotrimazole; OR 4.83, 95% CI 1.55 to 15.1); the adverse effects with increased frequency were nausea (14%), headache (12%), dizziness (6%), and bloating (6%).[12] **Versus intravaginal imidazoles:** See harms of intravaginal imidazoles, p 2272.

Comment: **Versus intravaginal imidazoles:** See comment of intravaginal imidazoles, p 2273.

OPTION ORAL KETOCONAZOLE

We found no RCTs comparing oral ketoconazole versus placebo or no treatment. RCTs found no significant difference between oral ketoconazole and intravaginal imidazoles in persistent symptoms, and found that oral ketoconazole may cause more nausea, fatigue, and headaches but less vulval irritation. One RCT found no significant difference in persistent symptoms or adverse effects between oral ketoconazole and oral fluconazole. Case reports have associated ketoconazole with a risk of fulminant hepatitis (1/12 000 courses of treatment with oral ketoconazole); there is consensus that the risks may outweigh the benefits in women with vulvovaginal candidiasis.

Benefits: **Versus oral placebo:** We found no systematic review or RCTs. **Versus intravaginal imidazoles:** We found one systematic review (search date 1993,[9] 4 RCTs,[71–74] 280 women) and three additional RCTs[75–77] (see table C on web extra). The systematic review concluded that oral treatment is as effective as topical treatment at eliminating *Candida* but did not compare clinical outcomes.[9] Six RCTs found no significant difference in persistent symptoms at 1–4 weeks between oral ketoconazole and intravaginal clotrimazole, miconazole, or tioconazole,[71–76] and one RCT found that significantly more women had persistent symptoms at 4 weeks with oral ketoconazole than with intravaginal isoconazole.[77] **Versus oral itraconazole:** We found no RCTs. **Versus oral fluconazole:** We found one systematic review (search date 1993,[9] 1 RCT,[78] 183 women). The RCT found no significant difference between ketoconazole (400 mg/day for 5 days) and oral fluconazole (1 dose of 150 mg) in the proportion of women with persistent symptoms after

5–16 days (17/72 [24%] with ketoconazole v 17/80 [21%] with fluconazole; OR 1.15, 95% CI 0.53 to 2.45) or after 27–62 days (14/72 [19%] with ketoconazole v 14/76 [18%] with fluconazole; OR 1.07, 95% CI 0.47 to 2.43).[78] **Versus intravaginal nystatin:** We found no RCTs.

Harms: Observational studies have found that asymptomatic elevation in liver enzymes is common in people who take oral ketoconazole, and fulminant hepatitis was observed in about 1/12 000 courses of treatment.[79] **Versus intravaginal imidazoles:** Most of the RCTs gave little information on adverse effects.[71–75,77] In these RCTs, 13 women who took oral ketoconazole had nausea, fatigue, headaches, or abdominal pain, and two women who used intravaginal clotrimazole had vulval irritation or vaginal bleeding. One RCT (151 women) found that more women taking oral ketoconazole had headache (23% v 4%), nausea (22% v 1%), abdominal discomfort (14% v 7%), and fatigue (7% v 2%; CIs not reported) compared with women taking intravaginal clotrimazole.[76] **Versus oral fluconazole:** The RCT (183 women) found that nausea was reported by similar proportions of women who took oral fluconazole and those who took oral ketoconazole (9/92 [10%] with fluconazole v 13/91 [14%] with ketoconazole; CI not reported).[78]

Comment: The possibility of rare but serious hepatitis has led to a consensus that the risks associated with oral ketoconazole may outweigh its benefits in women with vulvovaginal candidiasis.

OPTION INTRAVAGINAL NYSTATIN

One RCT found that intravaginal nystatin reduced the proportion of women with a poor symptomatic response after 14 days' treatment compared with placebo. Two RCTs provided insufficient evidence to compare intravaginal nystatin versus intravaginal imidazoles. One RCT found that intravaginal nystatin was less effective than boric acid in increasing clinical cure rates at 4 weeks. It gave no information on the adverse effects of intravaginal nystatin compared with intravaginal boric acid. We found no RCTs that compared intravaginal nystatin versus oral fluconazole, itraconazole, or ketoconazole.

Benefits: **Versus placebo:** We found no systematic review but found one RCT that compared intravaginal nystatin versus placebo.[8] The RCT (50 women) found that, compared with placebo, intravaginal nystatin (500 000 IU twice daily for 14 days) significantly reduced the proportion of women with a symptomatic response categorised as "poor" (2/25 [8%] with nystatin v 10/25 [40%] with placebo; ARR 32%, 95% CI 8% to 56%; OR 0.18, 95% CI 0.05 to 0.65; NNT 3, 95% CI 2 to 12). **Versus intravaginal imidazoles:** See benefits of intravaginal imidazoles, p 2271. **Versus oral fluconazole, itraconazole, or ketoconazole:** We found no RCTs. **Versus boric acid:** See benefits of boric acid, p 2276.

Harms: **Versus placebo:** The RCT found no reports of adverse effects among 50 women who used intravaginal nystatin.[8]

Comment: None.

OPTION YOGHURT CONTAINING *LACTOBACILLUS ACIDOPHILUS*: ORAL OR VAGINAL

We found no RCTs of lactobacillus yoghurt in women with acute vulvovaginal candidiasis.

Benefits: We found one systematic review (search date 2002), which identified no RCTs.[80]

Harms: The review stated that oral yoghurt may cause gastrointestinal disturbance in people with lactose intolerance.[80]

Comment: None.

OPTION DOUCHING

We found no RCTs of douching in women with recurrent vulvovaginal candidiasis. Douching was associated with serious sequelae, including pelvic inflammatory disease, endometritis, ectopic pregnancy, gonorrhoea, and chlamydia.

Benefits: We found two systematic reviews (search dates 2002), which identified no RCTs.[80,81]

Harms: Case control studies identified by the reviews found that douching is associated with serious sequelae, including pelvic inflammatory disease, endometritis, ectopic pregnancy, gonorrhoea, and chlamydia.[80,81]

Comment: None.

OPTION GARLIC

We found no RCTs of garlic in women with acute vulvovaginal candidiasis.

Benefits: We found one systematic review (search date 2002), which identified no RCTs.[80]

Harms: The review stated that garlic taken orally may cause heartburn, nausea, diarrhoea, flatulence, bloating, and an offensive body odour.[80] Prolonged topical use of garlic can lead to allergic reactions or chemical burns.

Comment: None.

OPTION INTRAVAGINAL TEA TREE OIL

We found no RCTs of intravaginal tea tree oil in women with acute vulvovaginal candidiasis.

Benefits: We found one systematic review (search date 2002), which identified no RCTs.[80]

Harms: The review stated that topical tea tree oil can cause skin irritation and a severe allergic rash.[80] One case report found that topical tea tree oil was associated with systematic hypersensitivity reaction.[82]

Comment: Tea tree oil contains terpinen-4-ol and other terpenes.[80]

OPTION INTRAVAGINAL BORIC ACID

One RCT found that intravaginal boric acid increased clinical cure rates at 4 weeks compared with intravaginal nystatin. It gave no information on the adverse effects of intravaginal boric acid compared with intravaginal nystatin. Intravaginal boric acid can cause skin irritation.

Benefits: We found one systematic review (search date 2002),[80] which identified one RCT (108 women) comparing intravaginal boric acid 600 mg daily versus intravaginal nystatin 100 000 IU daily for 14 days.[83] It found that boric acid significantly increased clinical cure rates at 4 weeks compared with nystatin (36/50 [72%] with boric acid *v* 26/52 [50%] with nystatin; P = 0.02).

Harms: The review stated that intravaginal boric acid can cause skin irritation.[80] The RCT gave no information on adverse effects of boric acid compared with intravaginal nystatin.[83] It stated that it found "no evidence of toxicity" associated with boric acid, but it is too small to exclude clinically important adverse effects. A case series of oral ingestion of boric acid has raised concerns about toxicity because it is associated with vomiting, abdominal pain, diarrhoea, lethargy, headache and dizziness, but serious complications are rare.[84]

Comment: None.

OPTION TREATING A MALE SEXUAL PARTNER

RCTs found no significant difference between treating and not treating a woman's male sexual partner in the resolution of the woman's symptoms of acute vulvovaginal candidiasis over 1–4 weeks or in the rate of symptomatic recurrence at 4–5 weeks after treatment.

Benefits: We found no systematic review but found three RCTs.[85–87] In the first RCT (40 women with acute vulvovaginal candidiasis and their male partners), all of the women received oral itraconazole 100 mg daily for 5 days.[85] Their male partners were randomised to receive oral itraconazole 100 mg daily for 5 days or placebo. The RCT found no significant difference between treating the male partner with oral itraconazole and placebo in the proportion of women with persistent symptoms after 30 days (2/19 [11%] with partners who received itraconazole *v* 4/18 [22%] with partners who received placebo; OR 0.43, 95% CI 0.08 to 2.43). The second RCT (117 women with acute or recurrent vaginal candidiasis and their male partners) treated all of the women with oral ketoconazole 200–600 mg/day for 3 days. Their male partners were randomised to oral ketoconazole 400 mg daily or placebo for 3 days. The RCT found no significant difference in the proportion of women cured 1 week after treatment (48/57 [84%] with partners receiving ketoconazole *v* 53/60 [88%] with partners receiving placebo; OR 0.71, 95% CI 0.25 to 2.02) or in the proportion of initially cured women who relapsed by 4 weeks after treatment (13/48 [27%] with ketoconazole *v* 19/53 [36%] with placebo; OR 0.67, 95% CI 0.29 to 1.54; see comment below). In the third RCT (42 women with acute vulvovaginal candidiasis and their male partners), all the women received topical natamycin for 10 days.[87] Their partners were randomised to receive topical natamycin for 10 days or placebo. The RCT found no significant difference between topical natamycin and placebo in symptoms at 8 days (1/16 [6%] *v* 2/17 [12%]) or in symptomatic relapse at 39 days (6/16 [37%] *v* 6/17 [35%]; reported as non-significant for both outcomes; CI not reported).

Harms: The RCTs gave no information on harms.[85–87]

Comment: The definition of "cured" and "relapsed" in the second RCT is not clear, but it seems to be a combination of improved symptoms and negative cultures.[86] Only a small number of men in the RCT had any penile symptoms, and these were distributed equally between the ketoconazole and placebo groups.

QUESTION What are the effects of treatments for recurrent vulvovaginal candidiasis in non-pregnant women?

OPTION INTRAVAGINAL IMIDAZOLES

Two RCTs provided insufficient evidence about the effects of regular prophylaxis with intravaginal clotrimazole compared with placebo in preventing recurrence of vulvovaginal candidiasis. One RCT found no significant

difference in the number of episodes of symptomatic vaginitis over 6 months between monthly prophylaxis with intravaginal clotrimazole and treatment as required, although women who took monthly prophylaxis had fewer episodes. The RCT may have been underpowered to detect a clinically important difference. More women preferred treatment as required. One RCT found insufficient evidence about the effects of regular prophylaxis with intravaginal clotrimazole versus oral itraconazole.

Benefits: **Versus placebo:** We found one systematic review (search date 1993,[9] 2 RCTs,[88,89] 89 women with recurrent vulvovaginal candidiasis) that compared intravaginal clotrimazole 500 mg monthly versus intravaginal placebo monthly for 6 months. Both RCTs found that intravaginal clotrimazole reduced the proportion of women with symptomatic recurrence over 6 months compared with placebo, although in one RCT the difference was significant (62 women: 30% with clotrimazole *v* 79% with placebo; $P < 0.001$)[88] and in the other RCT it was not (42 women: 53% with clotrimazole *v* 67% with placebo; difference reported as non-significant; CI not reported).[89] **Regular prophylaxis versus as required treatment:** We found one crossover RCT (open label, 23 women with recurrent vaginal candidiasis) that compared regular prophylactic intravaginal clotrimazole 500 mg each month versus intravaginal clotrimazole 500 mg at the onset of symptoms for 12 months.[90] At 12 months after crossover, it found no significant difference between regular clotrimazole and clotrimazole as required in the proportion of women who had symptomatic episodes of vaginitis over 6 months' treatment, although women who took regular clotrimazole had fewer symptomatic episodes (2.2 episodes per woman with regular treatment *v* 3.7 with as needed treatment; $P = 0.05$). The RCT may have been underpowered to detect a clinically important difference. It found that significantly more women preferred treatment as required compared with prophylactic treatment (17/23 [74%] *v* 4/23 [17%]; $P = 0.001$). **Versus oral itraconazole:** See benefits of oral itraconazole, p 2278.

Harms: See harms of intravaginal imidazoles for treatment of acute volvuvaginal candidiasis in non-pregnant women, p 2272.

Comment: None.

OPTION ORAL FLUCONAZOLE

We found no RCTs about the effects of oral fluconazole in preventing recurrent vulvovaginal candidiasis.

Benefits: We found no systematic review or RCTs.

Harms: We found no RCTs.

Comment: None.

OPTION ORAL ITRACONAZOLE

One RCT found that monthly prophylaxis with oral itraconazole reduced symptomatic recurrence of vulvovaginal candidiasis over 6 months compared with placebo. One weak, open label RCT provided insufficient evidence to compare twice weekly prophylaxis with oral itraconazole versus intravaginal clotrimazole.

Benefits: We found no systematic review. **Versus placebo:** One RCT (single blind, 114 women with recurrent vulvovaginal candidiasis) found that oral itraconazole (400 mg monthly) significantly reduced recurrence of symptoms of vulvovaginal candidiasis compared with placebo (recurrence during 6 months' follow up: 20/55 [36%] with itraconazole *v*

34/53 [64%] with placebo; ARR 28%, 95% CI 9% to 47%; OR 0.33, 95% CI 0.16 to 0.71; NNT 4, 95% CI 3 to 11).[91] After discontinuation of oral itraconazole, recurrence rates were similar. **Versus intravaginal imidazoles:** We found one RCT (open label, 44 women) that compared oral itraconazole (200 mg twice weekly) versus intravaginal clotrimazole (200 mg twice weekly) for 6 months.[92] One woman withdrew from itraconazole treatment and five withdrew from clotrimazole treatment. The RCT found that oral itraconazole significantly increased the proportion of women with symptomatic recurrences over 6 months compared with intravaginal clotrimazole (completer analysis: 7/21 [33%] with itraconazole *v* 0/17 [0%] with clotrimazole; P = 0.02; see comment below). **Regular prophylaxis versus as required treatment:** We found no RCTs.

Harms: **Versus placebo:** The RCT gave no information on adverse effects.[91] See harms of oral itraconazole for treatment of acute volvuvaginal candidiasis in non-pregnant women, p 2274. **Versus intravaginal imidazoles:** The RCT found that oral itraconazole significantly increased adverse effects, including nausea, diarrhoea, headache, and dizziness, compared with intravaginal clotrimazole (7/22 [32%] with itraconazole *v* 0/22 [0%] with clotrimazole; P = 0.02).[92]

Comment: **Versus intravaginal imidazoles:** The results of the RCT are difficult to interpret because it was open label, and the unbalanced withdrawal from the RCT could explain the observed difference between groups.[92]

OPTION ORAL KETOCONAZOLE

One RCT found that oral ketoconazole, given during the menstrual cycle at 400 mg daily or continuously at a lower dose, reduced symptomatic recurrence of vulvovaginal candidiasis over 6 months compared with placebo. This benefit is associated with an increased risk of harms, including rare cases of fulminant hepatitis (1/12 000 courses of treatment with oral ketoconazole); there is consensus that the risks may outweigh the benefits in women with vulvovaginal candidiasis.

Benefits: **Versus placebo:** We found one systematic review (search date 1993[9]), which identified one RCT.[93] The RCT (74 women) compared three interventions: intermittent oral ketoconazole (400 mg/day for 5 days of each menstrual cycle), continuous low dose ketoconazole (100 mg/day for 6 months), and placebo over 6 months.[93] It found that intermittent oral ketoconazole significantly reduced symptomatic recurrence over 6 months compared with placebo (6/21 [29%] with intermittent ketoconazole *v* 15/21 [71%] with placebo; OR 0.19, 95% CI 0.06 to 0.62). It also found that continuous low dose oral ketoconazole reduced symptomatic recurrence over 6 months compared with placebo (1/21 [5%] with continuous ketoconazole *v* 15/21 [71%] with placebo; OR 0.06, 95% CI 0.02 to 0.22). **Versus intravaginal imidazoles:** We found no RCTs. **Regular prophylaxis versus as required treatment:** We found no RCTs.

Harms: Ketoconazole is associated with an increased frequency of gastrointestinal adverse effects and case reports of rare fulminant hepatitis. See harms of oral ketoconazole for treatment of acute volvuvaginal candidiasis in non-pregnant women, p 2274.

Comment: The possibility of rare but serious hepatitis has led to a consensus that the risks associated with oral ketoconazole may outweigh its benefits in women with vulvovaginal candidiasis.

OPTION YOGHURT CONTAINING *LACTOBACILLUS ACIDOPHILUS*: ORAL OR VAGINAL

Two poor quality crossover RCTs identified by a systematic review provided insufficient evidence about the effects of a diet containing oral lactobacillus yoghurt in women with recurrent vulvovaginal candidiasis. Oral yoghurt may cause gastrointestinal disturbance in people with lactose intolerance. The review identified no RCTs of vaginal lactobacillus yoghurt.

Benefits: We found one systematic review (search date 2002[80]), which identified two crossover RCTs of oral yoghurt.[94,95] The first RCT (33 women) compared a diet containing 8 ounces oral lactobacillus yoghurt daily versus a diet not containing yoghurt for 6 months.[94] At 1 year follow up, it found that lactobacillus yoghurt 8 ounces daily significantly reduced symptomatic recurrence over 6 months' treatment (mean number of infections: 0.38 with yoghurt *v* 2.54 with no yoghurt; P = 0.001; see comment below). The second RCT (46 women, 18 with recurrent vulvovaginal candidiasis, 20 with bacterial vaginosis, 8 with both infections) compared lactobacillus yogurt 150 mL daily versus pasteurised yoghurt 150 mL daily for 2 months' treatment in a crossover design with a 2 month wash out.[95] The RCT found no significant difference in symptomatic recurrence over 6 months between lactobacillus and pasteurised yoghurt (number of infections over 14 visits: 3 with oral lactobacillus yoghurt *v* 5 with pasteurised; P = 0.67; see comment below). The review identified no RCTs of vaginal lactobacillus yoghurt.

Harms: The review stated that oral yoghurt may cause gastrointestinal disturbance in people with lactose intolerance.[80]

Comment: The results of the first RCT should be treated with caution because it did not provide results before crossover and 20/33 (61%) women did not complete the trial.[94] The second RCT was underpowered to detect a clinically important difference between groups because it did not assess results before crossover and 39/46 (85%) women did not complete the trial.[95]

OPTION DOUCHING

We found no RCTs of douching in women with recurrent vulvovaginal candidiasis. Douching is associated with serious sequelae, including pelvic inflammatory disease, endometritis, ectopic pregnancy, gonorrhoea, and chlamydia.

Benefits: We found two systematic reviews (search dates 2002) which identified no RCTs.[80,81]

Harms: The reviews stated that douching is associated with serious sequelae, including pelvic inflammatory disease, endometritis, ectopic pregnancy, gonorrhoea, and chlamydia.[80,81]

Comment: None.

OPTION GARLIC

We found no RCTs of garlic in women with recurrent vulvovaginal candidiasis.

Benefits: We found one systematic review (search date 2002), which identified no RCTs.[80]

Harms: The review stated that garlic taken orally may cause heartburn, nausea, diarrhoea, flatulence, bloating, and an offensive body odour.[80] Prolonged topical use of garlic can lead to allergic reactions or chemical burns.

Comment: None.

OPTION INTRAVAGINAL TEA TREE OIL

We found no RCTs of intravaginal tea tree oil in women with recurrent vulvovaginal candidiasis.

Benefits: We found one systematic review (search date 2002), which identified no RCTs.[80]

Harms: The review stated that topical tea tree oil can cause skin irritation and a severe allergic rash.[80] One case report found that topical tea tree oil was associated with systematic hypersensitivity reaction.[82]

Comment: Tea tree oil contains terpinen-4-ol and other terpenes.[80]

OPTION INTRAVAGINAL BORIC ACID

We found no RCTs of intravaginal boric acid in women with recurrent vulvovaginal candidiasis.

Benefits: We found one systematic review (search date 2002), which identified no RCTs.[80]

Harms: The review stated that intravaginal boric acid can cause skin irritation.[80] Oral ingestion has raised concerns about toxicity because it is associated with vomiting, abdominal pain, diarrhoea, lethargy, headache and dizziness, but serious complications are rare.[84]

Comment: None.

OPTION TREATING A MALE SEXUAL PARTNER

One RCT found no significant difference between treating and not treating a woman's male sexual partner in the rate of symptomatic recurrence over 12 months.

Benefits: We found one RCT (54 women with a history of 4 episodes of vaginal candidiasis in the past year, and their male partners).[96] All women received ketoconazole 400 mg daily for 7 days. Their partners were then randomised to ketoconazole 200 mg daily for 5 days or no treatment. The RCT did not assess clinical cure rates. It found no significant difference between ketoconazole and no treatment in rates of recurrence at 1 month (8/26 [31%] *v* 9/28 [32%]; P = 0.85), 3 months (17/26 [65%] *v* 17/28 [61%]; P = 0.94), 6 months (17/26 [65%] *v* 20/28 [71%]; P = 0.55), or 12 months (22/26 [85%] *v* 23/28 [82%]; P = 0.55).

Harms: The RCT found that 28% of women taking oral ketoconazole had adverse effects, including nausea, light headedness, and diarrhoea.[96]

Comment: None.

GLOSSARY

Balanitis is inflammation of the glands of the penis. The foreskin is often involved (balanoposthitis).

REFERENCES

1. Sobel JD. Vulvovaginal candidiasis. In: Holmes KK MP-A, Sparling PF, Lemon SM, et al, eds. *Sexually transmitted diseases*. New York: McGraw-Hill, 1999:629–639.
2. de Oliveira JM, Cruz AS, Fonseca AF, et al. Prevalence of *Candida albicans* in vaginal fluid of asymptomatic Portuguese women. *J Reprod Med* 1993;38:41–42.
3. Sobel JD, Faro S, Force RW, et al. Vulvovaginal candidiasis: epidemiologic, diagnostic, and therapeutic considerations. *Am J Obstet Gynecol* 1998;178:203–211.
4. Weissenbacher S, Witkin SS, Tolbert V, et al. Value of *Candida* polymerase chain reaction and vaginal cytokine analysis for the differential diagnosis of women with recurrent vulvovaginitis. *Infect Dis Obstet Gynecol* 2000;8:244–247.
5. Foxman B. The epidemiology of vulvovaginal candidiasis: risk factors. *Am J Public Health* 1990;80:329–331.
6. Geiger AM, Foxman B, Sobel JD. Chronic vulvovaginal candidiasis: characteristics of women with *Candida albicans*, *C glabrata* and no *Candida*. *Genitourin Med* 1995;71:304–307.
7. Geiger AM, Foxman B, Gillespie BW. The epidemiology of vulvovaginal candidiasis among university students. *Am J Public Health* 1995;85:1146–1148.
8. Isaacs JH. Nystatin vaginal cream in monilial vaginitis. *Illinois Med J* 1973;3:240–241.
9. Reef SE, Levine WC, McNeil MM, et al. Treatment options for vulvovaginal candidiasis, 1993. *Clin Infect Dis* 1995;20:S80–S90. Search date 1993; primary sources Medline and hand search of two textbooks.
10. Thomason JL, Gelbart SM, Kellett AV, et al. Terconazole for the treatment of vulvovaginal candidiasis. *J Reprod Med* 1990;35:992–994.
11. Brown D Jr, Henzl MR, LePage ME, et al. Butoconazole vaginal cream in the treatment of vulvovaginal candidiasis: comparison with miconazole nitrate and placebo. *J Reprod Med* 1986;31:1045–1048.
12. Stein GE, Mummaw N. Placebo-controlled trial of itraconazole for treatment of acute vaginal candidiasis. *Antimicrob Agents Chemother* 1993;37:89–92.
13. Bro F. Single-dose 500-mg clotrimazole vaginal tablets compared with placebo in the treatment of *Candida vaginitis*. *J Fam Pract* 1990;31:148–152.
14. Fleury F, Hodgson C. Single-dose treatment of vulvovaginal candidiasis with a new 500mg clotrimazole vaginal tablet. *Adv Ther* 1984;1:349–356.
15. Guess EA, Hodgson C. Single-dose topical treatment of vulvovaginal candidiasis with a new 500mg clotrimazole vaginal tablet. *Adv Ther* 1984;1:137–145.
16. Franklin R. Seven-day clotrimazole therapy for vulvovaginal candidiasis. *South Med J* 1978;71:141–143.
17. Corson SL, Kapikian RR, Nehring R. Terconazole and miconazole cream for treating vulvovaginal candidiasis. *J Reprod Med* 1991;36:561–567.
18. Kjaeldgaard A. Comparison of terconazole and clotrimazole vaginal tablets in the treatment of vulvovaginal candidosis. *Pharmatherapeutica* 1986;4:525–531.
19. Stein GE, Gurwith D, Mummaw N, et al. Single-dose tioconazole compared with 3-day clotrimazole treatment in vulvovaginal candidiasis. *Antimicrob Agents Chemother* 1986;29:969–971.
20. Kaufman RH, Henzl MR, Brown D Jr, et al. Comparison of three-day butoconazole treatment with seven-day miconazole treatment for vulvovaginal candidiasis. *J Reprod Med* 1989;34:479–483.
21. Droegemueller W, Adamson DG, Brown D. Three-day treatment with butoconazole nitrate for vulvovaginal candidiasis. *Obstet Gynecol* 1984;64:530–534.
22. Jacobson JB, Hajman AJ, Wiese J. A new vaginal antifungal agent — butoconazole nitrate. *Acta Obstet Gynecol Scand* 1985;64:241–244.
23. Hajman AJ. Vulvovaginal candidosis: comparison of 3-day treatment with 2% butoconazole nitrate cream and 6-day treatment of 1% clotrimazole cream. *J Int Med Res* 1988;16:367–375.
24. Adamson GD, Brown D Jr, Standard JV, et al. Three-day treatment with butoconazole vaginal suppositories for vulvovaginal candidiasis. *J Reprod Med Obstet Gynecol* 1986;31:131–132.
25. Bradbeer CS, Mayhew SR, Barlow D. Butaconazole and miconazole in treating vaginal candidiasis. *Genitourin Med* 1985;61:270–272.
26. Cassar NL. High-potency nystatin cream in the treatment of vulvovaginal candidiasis. *Curr Ther Res* 1983;34:305–310.
27. Glasser A. Single-dose treatment of vaginal mycoses. Effectiveness of clotrimazole and econazole. *Fortschr Med* 1986;104:259–262.
28. Gastaldi A. Treatment of vaginal candidiasis with fenticonazole and miconazole. *Curr Ther Res Clin Exp* 1985;38:489–493.
29. Gabriel G, Thin RN. Clotrimazole and econazole in the treatment of vaginal candidosis. A single-blind comparison. *Br J Ven Dis* 1983;59:56–58.
30. Amrouni B, Pereiro M, Florez A, et al. A phase III comparative study of the efficacies of flutrimazole versus clotrimazole for the treatment of vulvovaginal candidiasis. *J Mycol Med* 2000;10:62–65.
31. Arendt J. Terconazole versus clotrimazole cream in vulvovaginal candidiasis. *Adv Ther* 1989;6:287–294.
32. Gouveia DC, Jones Da Silva C. Oxiconazole in the treatment of vaginal candidiasis: single dose versus 3-day treatment with econazole. *Pharmatherapeutica* 1984;3:682–685.
33. Brewster E, Preti PM, Ruffmann R, et al. Effect of fenticonazole in vaginal candidiasis: a double-blind clinical trial versus clotrimazole. *J Int Med Res* 1986;14:306–310.
34. Balsdon M-J. Comparison of miconazole-coated tampons with clotrimazole vaginal tablets in the treatment of vaginal candidosis. *Br J Ven Dis* 1981;57:275–278.
35. Bradbeer CS, Thin RN. Comparison of econazole and isoconazole as single dose treatment for vaginal candidosis. *Genitourin Med* 1985;61:396–398.
36. Brown D Jr, Binder CL, Gardner HL, et al. Comparison of econazole and clotrimazole in the treatment of vulvovaginal candidiasis. *Obstet Gynecol* 1980;56:121–123.
37. Brown D, Henzl MR, Kaufman RH, et al. Butoconazole nitrate 2% for vulvovaginal candidiasis. *J Reprod Med* 1999;44:933–938.
38. Cohen L. Single dose treatment of vaginal candidosis: comparison of clotrimazole and isoconazole. *Br J Ven Dis* 1984;60:42–44.
39. Dellenbach P, Thomas J-L, Guerin V, et al. Topical treatment of vaginal candidosis with sertaconazole and econazole sustained-release suppositories. *Int J Gynecol Obstet* 2000;71:S47–S52.
40. Wiest W, Azzollini E, Ruffmann R. Comparison of single administration with an ovule of 600 mg fenticonazole versus a 500 mg clotrimazole vaginal pessary in the treatment of vaginal candidiasis. *J Int Med Res* 1989;17:369–372.
41. Palacio-Hernanz A, Sanz-Sanz F, Rodriquez-Noriega A. Double-blind investigation of R-42470 (terconazole cream 0.4%) and clotrimazole (cream 1%) for the topical treatment of mycotic vaginitis. *Chemioterapia* 1984;3:192–195.
42. Lolis D, Kanellopoulos N, Liappas I, et al. Double-blind evaluation of miconazole tampons, compared with clotrimazole vaginal tablets, in vaginal candidiasis. *Clin Ther* 1981;4:212–216.
43. Studd JW, Dooley MM, Welch CC, et al. Comparative clinical trial of fenticonazole ovule (600 mg) versus clotrimazole vaginal tablet (500 mg) in the treatment of symptomatic vaginal candidiasis. *Curr Med Res Opin* 1989;11:477–484.

44. Herbold H. Comparative studies to the clinical efficacy of two 1-dose-therapies of vaginal candidosis. *Med Welt* 1985;36:255–257.
45. Lappin MA, Brooker DC, Francisco CA, et al. Effect of butoconazole nitrate 2% vaginal cream and miconazole nitrate 2% vaginal cream treatments in patients with vulvovaginal candidiasis. *Infect Dis Obstet Gynecol* 1996;4:323–328
46. Lebherz TB, Goldman L, Wiesmeier E, et al. A comparison of the efficacy of two vaginal creams for vulvovaginal candidiasis, and correlations with the presence of *Candida* species in the perianal area and oral contraceptive use. *Clin Ther* 1983;5:409–416.
47. Stettendorf S, Benijts G, Vignali M, et al. Three-day therapy of vaginal candidiasis with clotrimazole vaginal tablets and econazole ovules: a multicenter comparative study. *Chemotherapy* 1982;28:87–91.
48. Wolfson N, Samuels B, Hodgson C, et al. One-day management of vulvovaginal candidiasis. *J La State Med Soc* 1987;139:27–29.
49. Lebherz T, Guess E, Wolfson N. Efficacy of single- versus multiple-dose clotrimazole therapy in the management of vulvovaginal candidiasis. *Am J Obstet Gynecol* 1985;152:965–968.
50. Fleury F, Hughes D, Floyd R. Therapeutic results obtained in vaginal mycoses after single-dose treatment with 500 mg clotrimazole vaginal tablets. *Am J Obstet Gynecol* 1985;152:968–970.
51. Loendersloot EW, Goormans E, Wiesenhaan PE, et al. Efficacy and tolerability of single-dose versus six-day treatment of candidal vulvovaginitis with vaginal tablets of clotrimazole. *Am J Obstet Gynecol* 1985;152:953–955.
52. Wolfson N, Samuels B, Riley J. A three-day treatment regimen for vulvovaginal candidiasis. *J La State Med Soc* 1982;134:28–31.
53. Oates JK, Davidson F. Treatment of vaginal candidiasis with clotrimazole. *Postgrad Med J* 1974;50:99–102.
54. Lebherz TB, Ford LC, Kleinkopf V. A comparison of a three-day and seven-day clotrimazole regimen for vulvovaginal candidiasis. *Clin Ther* 1981;3:344–348.
55. Robertson WH. Vulvovaginal candidiasis treated with clotrimazole cream in seven days compared with fourteen day treatment with miconazole cream. *Am J Obstet Gynecol* 1978;132:321–323.
56. Pasquale SA, Lawson J, Sargent EC Jr, et al. A dose–response study with Monistat cream. *Obstet Gynecol* 1979;53:250–253.
57. Floyd R, Hodgson C. One-day treatment of vulvovaginal candidiasis with a 500-mg clotrimazole vaginal tablet compared with a three-day regimen of two 100-mg vaginal tablets daily. *Clin Ther* 1986;8:181–186.
58. Hughes D, Kriedman T, Hodgson C. Treatment of vulvovaginal candidiasis with a single 500-mg clotrimazole vaginal tablet compared with two 100-mg tablets daily for three days. *Curr Ther Res Clin Exp* 1986;39:773–777.
59. Mizuno S, Cho N. Clinical evaluation of three-day treatment of vaginal mycosis with clotrimazole vaginal tablets. *J Int Med Res* 1983;11:179–185.
60. Milsom I, Forssman L. Treatment of vaginal candidosis with a single 500-mg clotrimazole pessary. *Br J Ven Dis* 1982;58:124–126.
61. Westphal J. Treatment of *Candida mycoses* of the vulva and vagina with clotrimazole. Comparison of single-dose and six-day therapy. *Fortschr Med* 1988;106:445–448.
62. Upmalis DH, Cone FL, Lamia CA, et al. Single-dose miconazole nitrate vaginal ovule in the treatment of vulvovaginal candidiasis: two single-blind, controlled studies versus miconazole nitrate 100mg cream for 7 days. *J Women's Health Gender-based Medicine* 2000;9:421–429.
63. Wiest W, Ruffmann R. Short-term treatment of vaginal candidiasis with fenticonazole ovules: a three dose schedule comparative trial. *J Int Med Res* 1987;15:319–325.
64. Dennerstein GJ, Langley R. Vulvovaginal candidiasis: treatment and recurrence. *Aust N Z J Obstet Gynaecol* 1982;22:231–233.
65. Watson MC, Grimshaw JM, Bond CM, et al. Oral versus intra-vaginal imidazole and triazole anti-fungal treatment of uncomplicated vulvovaginal candidiasis (thrush). In: The Cochrane Library, Issue 4. Oxford: Update Software, 2001. Search date 2000; primary sources Cochrane Library, Medline, Embase, Cochrane Collaboration Sexually Transmitted Disease Group Specialised Register of Controlled Trials, hand search of reference lists, and UK manufacturers of antifungal drugs.
66. De Punzio C, Garutti P, Mollica M, et al. Fluconazole 150 mg single dose versus itraconazole 200 mg per day for 3 days in the treatment of acute vaginal candidiasis: a double-blind randomized study. *Eur J Obs Gynecol Reprod Biol* 2003;106:193–197.
67. Sobel JD, Brooker D, Stein GE, et al. Single oral dose fluconazole compared with conventional clotrimazole topical therapy of *Candida vaginitis*. *Am J Obstet Gynecol* 1995;172:1263–1268.
68. Osser S, Haglund A, Weström L. Treatment of vaginal candidiasis: a prospective randomized investigator-blind multicenter study comparing topically applied econazole with oral fluconazole. *Acta Obstet Gynecol Scand* 1991;70:73–78.
69. Anonymous. A comparison of single-dose oral fluconazole with 3-day intravaginal clotrimazole in the treatment of vaginal candidiasis. *Br J Obstet Gynaecol* 1989;96:226–232.
70. Timonen H, Hartikainen-Vahtera P, Kivijarvi A, et al. A double-blind comparison of the effectiveness of itraconazole oral capsules with econazole vaginal capsules in the treatment of vaginal candidosis. *Drug Invest* 1992;4:515–520.
71. Puolakka J, Tuimala R. Comparison between oral ketoconazole and topical miconazole in the treatment of vaginal candidiasis. *Acta Obstet Gynecol Scand* 1983;62:575–577.
72. Rohde-Werner H. Topical tioconazole versus systemic ketoconazole treatment of vaginal candidiasis. *J Int Med Res* 1984;12:298–302.
73. Bingham JS. Single blind comparison of ketoconazole 200 mg oral tablets and clotrimazole 100 mg vaginal tablets and 1% cream in treating acute vaginal candidosis. *Br J Ven Dis* 1984;60:175–177.
74. Miller PI, Humphries M, Grassick K. A single-blind comparison of oral and intravaginal treatments in acute and recurrent vaginal candidosis in general practice. *Pharmatherapeutica* 1984;3:582–587.
75. Comninos A, Kapellakis I, Pikouli-Giannopoulou P, et al. Double-blind evaluation of ketoconazole comparatively with clotrimazole in vaginal candidiasis. *Curr Ther Res* 1984;36:100–104.
76. Sobel JD, Schmitt C, Stein G, et al. Initial management of recurrent vulvovaginal candidiasis with oral ketoconazole and topical clotrimazole. *J Reprod Med* 1994;39:517–520.
77. Farkas B, Simon N. Ergebnisse einer Vergleichsstudie mit einem oral und einem lokal zu applizierenden Antimykotikum bei Vaginalmykosen. *Mykosen* 1984;27:554–561.
78. Kutzer E, Oittner R, Leodolter S, et al. A comparison of fluconazole and ketoconazole in the oral treatment of vaginal candidiasis: report of a double-blind multicentre trial. *Eur J Obstet Gynecol Reprod Biol* 1988;29:305–313.
79. Lake-Bakaar G, Scheuer PJ, Sherlock S. Hepatic reactions associated with ketoconazole in the United Kingdom. *BMJ* 1987;294:419–422.
80. Van Kessel K, Assefi N, Marrazzo J, Eckert L. Common complementary and alternative therapies for yeast vaginitis and bacterial vaginosis: a systematic review. *Obstet Gynecol Surv* 2003;58:351–358. Search date 2002; primary sources PubMed, Cochrane Library, Embase, Cinahl, Lilacs, Natural Medicines Comprehensive Databse, Longwood Herbal Taskforce, and Alternative Medicine Alert.
81. Martino JL, Vermund SH. Vaginal douching: evidence for risks or benefits to women's health *Epidemiol Rev*

2002;24:109–124. Search date 2002; primary source Medline, and contact with medical and nursing organisations for policy and education documents and with the US Food and Drug Administration to obtain minutes of a meeting of the Nonprescription Drug Advisory Committee held on April 15 1997.
82. Mozelsio NB, Harris KE, McGrath KG, Grammer LC. Immediate systemic hypersensitivity reaction associated with topical application of Australian tea tree oil. *Allergy Asthma Proc* 2003;24:73–75.
83. Van Slyke K, Michel VP, Rein M. Treatment of vulvovaginal candidiasis with boric acid powder *Am J Obstet Gynecol* 1981;141:145–148.
84. Litovitz TL, Klein-Schwartz W, Oderda GM, Schmitz BF. Clinical manifestations of toxicity in a series of 784 boric acid ingestions. *Am J Emerg Med* 1988;6:209–213.
85. Calderon-Marquez JJ. Itraconazole in the treatment of vaginal candidosis and the effect of treatment of the sexual partner. *Rev Inf Dis* 1987;9:S143–S145.
86. Bisschop MP, Merkus JM, Scheygrond H, et al. Co-treatment of the male partner in vaginal candidosis: a double-blind randomized control study. *Br J Obstet Gynaecol* 1986;93:79–81.
87. Buch A, Skytte Christensen E. Treatment of vaginal candidosis with natamycin and effect of treating the partner at the same time. *Acta Obstet Gynecol Scand* 1982;61:393–396.
88. Roth AC, Milsom I, Forssman L, et al. Intermittent prophylactic treatment of recurrent vaginal candidiasis by postmenstrual application of a 500 mg clotrimazole vaginal tablet. *Genitourin Med* 1990;66:357–360.
89. Sobel JD. Clotrimazole treatment of recurrent and chronic and chronic candida vulvovaginitis. *Obstet Gynecol* 1989;73:330–334.
90. Fong IW. The value of prophylactic (monthly) clotrimazole versus empiric self-treatment in recurrent vaginal candidiasis. *Genitourin Med* 1994;70:124–126.
91. Spinillo A, Colonna L, Piazzi G, et al. Managing recurrent vulvovaginal candidiasis. Intermittent prevention with itraconazole. *J Reprod Med* 1997;42:83–87.
92. Fong IW. The value of chronic suppressive therapy with itraconazole versus clotrimazole in women with recurrent vaginal candidiasis. *Genitourin Med* 1992;68:374–377.
93. Sobel JD. Recurrent vulvovaginal candidiasis. A prospective study of the efficacy of maintenance ketoconazole therapy. *N Engl J Med* 1986;315:1455–1458.
94. Hilton E, Isenberg HD, Alperstein P, et al Ingestion of yoghurt containing *Lactobacillus acidophilus* as prophylaxis for candidal vaginitis. *Ann Intern Med* 1992;116:353–357.
95. Shalev E, Battino S, Weiner E, et al Ingestion of yoghurt containing *Lactobacillus acidophilus* as prophylaxis for recurrent candidal vaginitis and bacterial vaginosis. *Arch Fam Med* 1996;5:593–596.
96. Fong IW. The value of treating the sexual partners of women with recurrent vaginal candidiasis with ketoconazole. *Genitourin Med* 1992;68:174–176.

Des Spence
Dr General Practice
Glasgow University
Glasgow
Scotland

Competing interests: None declared.

We would like to acknowledge the previous contributors of this chapter, including Jeanne Marrazo.

Cervical cancer

Search date June 2003

Sudha Sundar, Amanda Horne and Sean Kehoe

QUESTIONS

INTERVENTIONS

To be covered in future updates

Effects of interventions to manage late stage cervical cancer (stages IIb to IV)

Effects of interventions to manage cervical cancer in pregnancy

Effects of interventions to manage local recurrence of cervical cancer

Effects of interventions to manage metastatic disease

*Based on consensus

See glossary Ⓖ

Key Messages

Early stage cervical cancer

- **Conisation of the cervix for microinvasive carcinoma (stage Ia1)*** We found no systematic review or RCTs of conisation of the cervix versus simple hysterectomy for microinvasive carcinoma (stage Ia1). However, there is consensus that conisation of the cervix is effective for microinvasive carcinoma (stage Ia1), provided that excision margins are clear of cancer or cervical intraepithelial neoplasia. Conisation of the cervix can, unlike hysterectomy, preserve fertility.
- **Radical trachelectomy plus lymphadenectomy (preserved fertility compared with hysterectomy)** We found no systematic review or RCTs comparing radical trachelectomy plus lymphadenectomy versus radical hysterectomy in women with early stage cervical cancer. Radical trachelectomy plus lymphadenectomy can, unlike hysterectomy, preserve fertility.
- **Radiotherapy or surgery*** One RCT found no significant difference in overall survival or disease free survival between radiotherapy and radical hysterectomy plus lymphadenectomy (with or without adjuvant radiotherapy) for early stage cervical cancer. Consensus regards both surgery and radiotherapy as likely to be beneficial.

Bulky early stage cervical cancer

- **Chemoradiotherapy (increased survival compared with radiotherapy alone)** Two RCTs found that chemoradiotherapy improved overall survival and progression free survival compared with radiotherapy, when used either before or after hysterectomy. Combined chemoradiotherapy was associated with more haematological and gastrointestinal toxicity than radiotherapy alone.

- **Neoadjuvant chemotherapy** RCTs found limited evidence that neoadjuvant chemotherapy (before local treatment with surgery, radiotherapy, or both) improved survival and reduced local recurrence compared with local treatment alone.

*Based on consensus.

DEFINITION Cervical cancer is a malignant neoplasm arising from the uterine cervix. Approximately 80% of cervical cancers are of the squamous type; the remainder are adenocarcinomas, adenosquamous carcinomas, and other rare types.[1] Staging of cervical cancer is based on clinical evaluation (FIGO classification (see table 1, p 2291)). Management is determined by tumour bulk and stage. This topic deals with treatments for early stage cancer (defined as FIGO stage Ia1, Ia2, Ib1, and small IIa tumours) and bulky early stage disease (defined as FIGO stage Ib2 and larger IIa tumours).

INCIDENCE/ PREVALENCE Cervical cancer is the second most common cancer in women, with about 450 000 new cases diagnosed worldwide each year.[2] Most (80%) cases occur in less developed countries without an effective screening programme. The incidence of cervical cancer in the UK and Europe has significantly reduced since the introduction of a screening programme for detecting precancerous cervical intraepithelial neoplasia. Cervical cancer incidence fell by 42% between 1988 and 1997 (England and Wales). This fall has been reported to be related to the cervical screening programme.[3] In England and Wales, cervical cancer has an annual incidence of 3200 women, and causes about 1000 deaths each year.[4]

AETIOLOGY/ RISK FACTORS Risk factors for cervical cancer include sexual intercourse at an early age, multiple sexual partners, tobacco smoking, long term oral contraceptive use, low socioeconomic status, immunosuppressive therapy, and micronutrient deficiency. Persistent infection by oncogenic, high risk strains of human papilloma virus is strongly associated with the development of cervical cancer.[5-7] The virus is acquired mainly by sexual intercourse and has a peak prevalence of 20–30% in women aged 20–30 years,[8] although in 80% of cases the infection is transient and resolves within 12–18 months.

PROGNOSIS Overall, 5 year disease free survival is 50–70% for stages Ib2 and IIb, 30–50% for stage III, and 5–15% for stage IV.[1] In people who receive treatment, 5 year survival in stage Ia approaches 100%, falling to 70–85% for stage Ib1 and smaller IIa tumours. Survival in people with more locally advanced tumours is influenced by tumour bulk, the person's age, and coexistent medical conditions. Untreated mortality in locally advanced disease is high.

AIMS OF INTERVENTION To reduce morbidity and mortality; to improve quality of life with minimal adverse effects.

OUTCOMES Overall survival; progression free survival; local recurrence; distant recurrence; quality of life; and adverse effects of treatment. Some treatments — including "fertility preserving treatments" — may affect fertility. We therefore examined the effects of treatment on pregnancy rates and live birth rate. Adverse effects of chemotherapy are usually graded according to severity, using scales such as the Chassagne morbidity scale (grades 0–3), National Cancer Institute Common Toxicity scale (grades 0–4), and the Southwest Oncology Group scale (grades 0–5); unless otherwise stated, grade 0 refers to no adverse effects, and higher scores indicate a greater severity of adverse effects.

METHODS *Clinical Evidence* search and appraisal June 2003. For the bulky early stage disease question, we included RCTs including solely women with stage Ib2 and IIa tumours, as well as studies that comprised women with stage Ib2 and IIa tumours in addition to women with less extensive (lower stage) tumours. We excluded studies that included women with tumours of stage IIb and above, unless they performed prespecified subgroup analyses in women with bulky early stage disease (stage Ib2 or IIa tumours).

QUESTION What are the effects of interventions to manage early stage cervical cancer? New

OPTION CONISATION OF THE CERVIX FOR MICROINVASIVE CARCINOMA (STAGE IA1) New

We found no systematic review or RCTs of conisation of the cervix versus simple hysterectomy for microinvasive carcinoma (stage Ia1). However, there is consensus that conisation of the cervix is effective for microinvasive carcinoma (stage Ia1), provided that excision margins are clear of cancer or cervical intraepithelial neoplasia. Conisation of the cervix can, unlike hysterectomy, preserve fertility.

Benefits: **Versus simple hysterectomy:** We found no systematic review or RCTs of conisation of the cervix(G) versus simple hysterectomy(G) for microinvasive carcinoma (stage Ia1).

Harms: **Versus simple hysterectomy:** We found no systematic review or RCTs.

Comment: Consensus opinion is that conisation is effective for microinvasive carcinoma (stage Ia1), provided that excision margins are clear of cancer or cervical intraepithelial neoplasia, and that there has been an adequate review of histology by a pathologist and multidisciplinary team experienced in dealing with gynaecological cancer. Consensus is based on observational studies, and is consistent with guidelines issued by the NHS cervical screening programme.[9] Conisation of the cervix can, unlike hysterectomy, preserve fertility.

OPTION RADICAL TRACHELECTOMY PLUS LYMPHADENECTOMY New

We found no systematic review or RCTs comparing radical trachelectomy plus lymphadenectomy versus radical hysterectomy in women with early stage cervical cancer. Radical trachelectomy plus lymphadenectomy can, unlike hysterectomy, preserve fertility.

Benefits: **Versus radical hysterectomy:** We found no systematic reviews or RCTs.

Harms: **Versus radical hysterectomy:** We found no systematic reviews or RCTs

Comment: Fertility can be preserved if surgery is restricted to radical trachelectomy(G) and lymphadenectomy(G).[10–14] One retrospective observational study included women with stage Ia2 or Ib tumours of size 2 cm or smaller, and without pelvic lymph node metastasis.[15] Women who had received radical trachelectomy and lymphadenectomy (32 women) were compared with two groups of women who had received radical hysterectomy(G) (one unmatched control group, 556 women and one control group matched for age and tumour characteristics, 30 women). The study found no significant difference in recurrence free survival between groups at 2 years (95% with radical trachelectomy *v* 100% for matched radical hysterectomy controls *v* 97% for unmatched radical hysterectomy controls, P reported as not significant, CI not reported). The conception rate in the radical trachelectomy group was 37% at 1 year.[15] It found that there were significantly more intraoperative complications with radical trachelectomy plus lymphadenectomy than with radical hysterectomy in unmatched controls (AR for complications: 25% with trachelectomy *v* 4% with hysterectomy; $P < 0.05$).[15]

OPTION RADIOTHERAPY VERSUS SURGERY New

One RCT found no significant difference in overall survival or disease free survival between radiotherapy and radical hysterectomy plus lymphadenectomy (with or without adjuvant radiotherapy) for early stage cervical cancer. Consensus regards both surgery and radiotherapy as likely to be beneficial.

Benefits: We found no systematic review. We found one RCT (343 women stage Ib–IIa) comparing radiotherapy versus radical hysterectomy**G** plus lymphadenectomy**G** (see comment).[16] It found no significant difference between radiotherapy and surgery in 5 year survival or disease free survival rates between the two groups (results presented graphically; AR for survival about 83% for both groups; AR for disease free survival approximately 74% for both groups; for both comparisons, P reported as not significant). Recurrence rates were similar in both groups (42/170 [25%] with surgery *v* 44/167 [26%] with radiotherapy; significance not stated).

Harms: Surgery significantly increased the risk of severe adverse effects compared with radiotherapy (grade 2–3 on the Chassagne morbidity scale; 28% with surgery *v* 12% with radiotherapy; $P < 0.0004$).[16] Two women in the surgery group died (one of spontaneous ileal perforation 11 months after adjuvant**G** radiotherapy and one of pulmonary embolism). Pelvic radiotherapy will usually result in ablation of ovarian function. Certain surgical procedures can maintain fertility (See harms of conisation of the cervix, p 2287; see harms of radical trachelectomy plus lymphadenectomy, p 2287).

Comment: The RCT did not report what proportion of women with stage Ib cancer had stage Ib1 and stage Ib2 disease.[16] The radical hysterectomy group in the RCT received a class III abdominal hysterectomy and pelvic lymphadenectomy; women with enlarged para-aortic lymph nodes only received sampling and selective procedures.[16] A large number of women in the surgery group (108/170 [64%]) received postoperative pelvic radiotherapy. The decision to provide adjuvant**G** radiotherapy was taken preoperatively, based on the presence of one or more known risk factors such as UICC surgical stage greater than pT2a (see table 2, p 2292), less than 3 mm of uninvolved cervical stroma, cut-through, or lymph node metastases. The trial excluded people considered medically unfit for surgery. Consensus regards both surgery and radiotherapy as likely to be beneficial.

QUESTION What are the effects of interventions to manage bulky early stage cervical cancer? New

OPTION CHEMORADIOTHERAPY VERSUS RADIOTHERAPY ALONE New

Two RCTs found that chemoradiotherapy improved overall survival and progression free survival compared with radiotherapy, when used either before or after hysterectomy. Combined chemoradiotherapy was associated with more haematological and gastrointestinal toxicity than radiotherapy alone.

Benefits: We found one systematic review (search date 2003),[17,18] which identified two RCTs that compared chemoradiotherapy**G** versus radiotherapy alone in women with bulky early stage cervical carcinoma. The first RCT[19] identified by the review (374 women with stage Ib2 tumours) compared chemoradiotherapy versus radiotherapy, prior to hysterectomy, in all participants. It found that chemoradiotherapy significantly increased progression free survival and overall survival compared with radiotherapy at 3 years (HR for progression 0.51, 95% CI 0.34 to 0.75; HR for mortality 0.54, 95% CI 0.34 to 0.86). The second RCT identified by the review included 268 women who had undergone radical hysterectomy**G** for stage Ia2, Ib, and IIa tumours (tumour diameter 0.2–5.2 cm; see comment).[20] The women had histologically confirmed positive lymph nodes, positive parametrial involvement, or a positive surgical margin. The RCT found that chemoradiotherapy significantly improved progression free survival and overall survival compared with radiotherapy at 4 years (estimated progression free survival: AR 80% with chemoradiotherapy *v* 63% with radiotherapy alone, adjusted HR 2.01, 95% CI not reported, P = 0.003; estimated overall survival: AR 81% with chemoradiotherapy *v* 71% with radiotherapy alone, adjusted HR 1.96, 95% CI not reported, P = 0.007).

Harms: The first RCT[19] found that more women in the chemoradiotherapy group had moderate or severe adverse effects (grade 3 or 4 toxicity according to National Cancer Institute Common Toxicity Criteria; mainly haematological and gastrointestinal toxicity) than in the radiotherapy group (64/183 [35%] *v* 25/186 [13%]; P value not reported).[19] The second RCT[20] found that serious adverse effects (grade 4 Southwest Oncology Group criteria; mainly haematological toxicity) were more common in the chemoradiotherapy group than in the radiotherapy group (21/122 [17%] *v* 4/112 [4%], P value not reported).

Comment: The second RCT did not report what proportion of women had stage Ia2 tumours.[20]

OPTION NEOADJUVANT CHEMOTHERAPY New

RCTs found limited evidence that neoadjuvant chemotherapy (before local treatment with surgery, radiotherapy, or both) improved survival and reduced local recurrence compared with local treatment alone.

Benefits: **Versus local treatment alone:** We found one systematic review[21] (search date not stated) including 1 RCT (see comment). The RCT[22] identified by the review (205 women with stage Ib tumours, 57% stage Ib2) compared neoadjuvant chemotherapy**G** versus no neoadjuvant chemotherapy before local treatment, with surgery plus radiotherapy or radiotherapy alone for unresectable tumours. Prespecified subgroup analysis found that neoadjuvant chemotherapy significantly improved overall survival at 9 years and reduced local recurrence in women with bulky (stage Ib2) tumours (117 women, survival: 80% with neoadjuvant chemotherapy *v* 61% with no neoadjuvant chemotherapy, P < 0.01; local recurrence: 6% with neoadjuvant chemotherapy *v* 23% with no neoadjuvant chemotherapy, P < 0.01).

Harms: **Versus local treatment alone:** The review gave no information on harms.[21] The RCT[22] included in the review reported that in the neoadjuvant chemotherapy group, there were four confirmed cases of peripheral neurotoxicity, one case of renal toxicity with transient tubular failure, and two cases of mild pulmonary toxicity. It did not report on adverse effects in the no neoadjuvant chemotherapy group.

Comment: The review reported that one further trial of neoadjuvant chemotherapy in bulky stage Ib tumours is ongoing. We found one additional RCT (192 women) of neoadjuvant chemotherapy in stages Ib–IIIb cervical cancer.[23] In a post hoc subgroup analysis of women with stages Ib or IIa tumours (126 women, tumour size not stated), it found that neoadjuvant chemotherapy significantly increased disease free survival at 5 years (77.1% with neoadjuvant chemotherapy v 64.3% without neoadjuvant chemotherapy, P < 0.05). Neoadjuvant chemotherapy increased overall survival at 5 years, but this increase was not significant (78.6% with neoadjuvant chemotherapy v 73.2% without neodajuvant chemotherapy, P reported as not significant).

GLOSSARY

Adjuvant Chemotherapy or radiotherapy following definitive treatment (surgery).
Chemoradiotherapy Involves both chemotherapy and radiotherapy given simultaneously for a short duration of time (i.e. completing treatment within 5–6 weeks).
Conisation of the cervix Involves removing the abnormal portion of the cervix using either a diathermy loop or a scalpel.
Simple hysterectomy Surgical removal of the cervix and uterus only.
Lymphadenectomy Surgical removal of lymph nodes.
Neoadjuvant chemotherapy Chemotherapy preceding local or definitive treatment (surgery or radiotherapy).
Radical hysterectomy Surgical removal of the cervix, uterus, vaginal cuff, pelvic lymph nodes, obturator lymph nodes, paracervical tissue, and parametrial tissue.
Radical trachelectomy Surgical removal of the parametrium as well as the cervix.
Trachelectomy Surgical removal of cervix leaving the uterus *in situ*.

REFERENCES

1. Waggoner SE. Cervical cancer. *Lancet* 2003;361:2217–2225.
2. Parkin DM, Whelan SL, Ferlay J et al. *Cancer incidence in five continents, vol 7*. IARC: Lyon, 1997.
3. Quinn M, Babb P, Jones J, et al. Effect of screening on incidence of and mortality from cancer of cervix in England: evaluation based on routinely collected statistics. *BMJ* 1999;318:904–908.
4. London: Office for National Statistics. HMSO, 2001.
5. Walboomers JM, Jacobs MV, Manos MM, et al. Human papillomavirus is a necessary cause of invasive cervical cancer worldwide. *J Pathol* 1999;189:12–19.
6. Ferenczy A, Franco E. Persistent human papillomavirus infection and cervical neoplasia. *Lancet Oncol* 2002;3:11–16.
7. Bosch FX, Manos MM, Munoz N, et al. Prevalence of human papillomavirus in cervical cancer: a worldwide perspective. International biological study on cervical cancer (IBSCC) Study Group. *J Natl Cancer Inst* 1995;87:796–802.
8. Sellors JW, Mahony JB, Kaczorowski J, et al. Prevalence and predictors of human papillomavirus infection in women in Ontario, Canada. Survey of HPV in Ontario Women (SHOW) Group. *Cmaj* 2000;163:503–508.
9. Luesley D, Leeson S, eds. *Colposcopy and programme management. NHS cancer screening programmes 2004*. NHSCP publication No. 20.
10. Dargent D, Franzosi F, Ansquer Y, et al. [Extended trachelectomy relapse: plea for patient involvement in the medical decision]. *Bull Cancer* 2002;89:1027–1030.
11. Dargent D, Martin X, Sacchetoni A, et al. Laparoscopic vaginal radical trachelectomy: a treatment to preserve the fertility of cervical carcinoma patients. *Cancer* 2000;88:1877–1882.
12. Shepherd JH, Mould T, Oram DH. Radical trachelectomy in early stage carcinoma of the cervix: outcome as judged by recurrence and fertility rates. *Bjog* 2001;108:882–885.
13. Roy M, Plante M. Pregnancies after radical vaginal trachelectomy for early-stage cervical cancer. *Am J Obstet Gynecol* 1998;179:1491–1496.
14. Schlaerth JB, Spirtos NM, Schlaerth AC. Radical trachelectomy and pelvic lymphadenectomy with uterine preservation in the treatment of cervical cancer. *Am J Obstet Gynecol* 2003;188:29–34.
15. Covens A, Shaw P, Murphy J, et al. Is radical trachelectomy a safe alternative to radical hysterectomy for patients with stage IA–B carcinoma of the cervix? *Cancer* 1999;86:2273–2279.
16. Landoni F, Maneo A, Colombo A, et al. Randomised study of radical surgery versus radiotherapy for stage Ib–IIa cervical cancer. *Lancet* 1997;350:535–540.
17. Green J, Kirwan J, Tierney J, et al. Concomitant chemotherapy and radiation therapy for cancer of the uterine cervix. *Cochrane Database Syst Rev* 2001;4:CD002225.
18. Green JA, Kirwan JM, Tierney JF, et al. Survival and recurrence after concomitant chemotherapy and radiotherapy for cancer of the uterine cervix: a systematic review and meta-analysis. *Lancet* 2001;358:781–786.
19. Keys HM, Bundy BN, Stehman FB, et al. Cisplatin, radiation, and adjuvant hysterectomy compared with radiation and adjuvant hysterectomy for bulky stage IB cervical carcinoma. *N Engl J Med* 1999;340:1154–1161.
20. Peters WA 3rd, Liu PY, Barrett RJ 2nd, et al. Concurrent chemotherapy and pelvic radiation therapy compared with pelvic radiation therapy alone as adjuvant therapy after radical surgery in high-risk early-stage cancer of the cervix. *J Clin Oncol* 2000;18:1606–1613.
21. Tierney JF, Stewart LA, Parmar MK. Can the published data tell us about the effectiveness of neoadjuvant chemotherapy for locally advanced cancer of the uterine cervix? *Eur J Cancer* 1999;35:406–409.
22. Sardi JE, Giaroli A, Sananes C, et al. Long-term follow-up of the first randomized trial using neoadjuvant chemotherapy in stage Ib squamous carcinoma of the cervix: the final results. *Gynecol Oncol* 1997;67:61–69.
23. Napolitano U, Imperato F, Mossa B, et al. The role of neoadjuvant chemotherapy for squamous cell cervical cancer (Ib-IIIb): a long-term randomized trial. *Eur J Gynaecol Oncol* 2003;24:51–59.
24. Chassagne D, Sismondi P, Horiot JC, et al. *Radiother Oncol* 1993;26:195–202

Cervical cancer

Sudha Sundar
Cheltenham General Hospital
Cheltenham
United Kingdom

Amanda Horne
Churchill Hospital
Oxford
United Kingdom

Sean Kehoe
Nuffield Department of Obstetrics and Gynaecology, John Radcliffe Hospital
Headington
Oxford
UK

Competing interests: None declared.

TABLE 1 **FIGO staging of cervical cancer.**

Stage 0 Carcinoma *in situ*, cervical intraepithelial neoplasia grade III

Stage I The carcinoma is strictly confined to the cervix (extension to the corpus would be disregarded)

Stage Ia Invasive carcinoma which can be diagnosed only by microscopy (all macroscopically visible lesions, even with superficial invasion, are allotted to stage Ib carcinomas)

- Stage Ia1 Measured stromal invasion of not > 3.0 mm in depth and extension of not > 7.0 mm
- Stage Ia2 Measured stromal invasion of > 3.0 mm and not > 5.0 mm, with an extension of not > 7.0 mm

Stage Ib Clinically visible lesions limited to the cervix uteri or preclinical cancers greater than stage Ia

- Stage Ib1 Clinically visible lesions not > 4.0 cm
- Stage Ib2 Clinically visible lesions > 4.0 cm

Stage II Cervical carcinoma invades beyond the uterus but not to the pelvic wall or to the lower third of the vagina

Stage IIa No obvious parametrial involvement.

Stage IIb Obvious parametrial involvement

Stage III The carcinoma has extended to the pelvic wall. On rectal examination, there is no cancer free space between the tumour and the pelvic wall. The tumour involves the lower third of the vagina. All cases with hydronephrosis or non-functioning kidney are included, unless they are known to be due to another cause

*Stage IIIa*Tumour involves lower third of the vagina, with no extension to the pelvic wall

Stage IIIb Extension to the pelvic wall and/or hydronephrosis or non-functioning kidney

Stage IV The carcinoma has extended beyond the true pelvis, or has involved the mucosa of the bladder or rectum (biopsy proven)

Stage IVa Spread of the growth to adjacent organs

Stage IVb Spread to distant organs

TABLE 2 **UICC staging of cervical cancer.**

TNM definitions

The definitions of the primary tumour categories correspond to the FIGO stages.

Primary tumour (T)

TX: Primary tumour cannot be assessed

T0: No evidence of primary tumour

Tis: Carcinoma *in situ*

T1/I: Cervical carcinoma confined to uterus (extension to corpus should be disregarded)

- T1a/IA: Invasive carcinoma diagnosed only by microscopy. All macroscopically visible lesions — even with superficial invasion — are T1b/IB. Stromal invasion with a maximal depth of 5 mm, measured from the base of the epithelium, and a horizontal spread of 7 mm or less. Vascular space involvement, venous or lymphatic, does not affect classification
- T1a1/Ia1: Measured stromal invasion 3 mm or less in depth and 7 mm or less in horizontal spread
- T1a2/IA2: Measured stromal invasion more than 3 mm and not more than 5 mm, with a horizontal spread 7 mm or less
- T1b/IB: Clinically visible lesion confined to the cervix, or microscopic lesion greater than T1a2/IA2
- T1b1/IB1: Clinically visible lesion 4 cm or less in greatest dimension
- T1b2/IB2: Clinically visible lesion more than 4 cm in greatest dimension

T2/II: Cervical carcinoma invades beyond uterus but not to pelvic wall or to the lower third of the vagina

- T2a/IIa: Tumour without parametrial involvement
- T2b/IIb: Tumour with parametrial involvement

T3/III: Tumour extends to the pelvic wall and/or involves the lower third of the vagina, and/or causes hydronephrosis or non-functioning kidney

- T3a/IIIA: Tumour involves lower third of the vagina; no extension to pelvic wall
- T3b/IIIB: Tumour extends to pelvic wall and/or causes hydronephrosis or non-functioning kidney

T4/IVA: Tumour invades mucosa of the bladder or rectum, and/or extends beyond true pelvis (bullous oedema is not sufficient to classify a tumour as T4)

M1/IVB: Distant metastasis

Regional lymph nodes (N)

NX: Regional lymph nodes cannot be assessed

N0: No regional lymph node metastasis

N1: Regional lymph node metastasis

Distant metastasis (M)

MX: Distant metastasis cannot be assessed

M0: No distant metastasis

M1: Distant metastasis

Domestic violence towards women

Search date March 2004

Joanne Klevens and Laura Sadowski

QUESTIONS

INTERVENTIONS

See glossary

Key Messages

- **Advocacy** One RCT and one non-randomised controlled trial found that advocacy reduced reabuse compared with no treatment. The RCT also found an improvement in women's quality of life with advocacy compared with no treatment. One controlled trial in pregnant Hispanic women found no significant difference in rates of reabuse between combined counselling plus mentoring (similar to advocacy) and a resource card, but found that counselling plus mentoring slightly reduced rates of reabuse compared with unlimited counselling.
- **Safety planning** One RCT found that providing telephone sessions on safe behaviour in addition to usual care increased safe behaviour at 6 months compared with usual care alone. We found limited evidence from one non-randomised controlled trial in pregnant women that helping participants to make a safety plan reduced spouse abuse and increased safe behaviour at 12 months.
- **Cognitive behaviour orientated counselling** One controlled trial found that cognitive behaviour orientated therapy improved women's assertiveness and reduced their exposure to abuse compared with baseline levels, whereas non-specific support did not. However, the study did not directly compare effects of interventions.
- **Couple counselling** One non-randomised controlled trial found that both gender specific counselling and couple counselling reduced physical aggression, psychological aggression and depression in wives from baseline levels, but found no significant differences between treatments. One RCT found no significant difference between group and individual couple counselling on reduction in physical violence or on psychological wellbeing.
- **Grief resolution orientated counselling** One controlled trial found that grief resolution orientated counselling improved self esteem and self efficacy from baseline, whereas feminist orientated counselling did not. However, the study did not directly compare effects of interventions.
- **Peer support groups** We found no systematic reviews or controlled trials on the effect of peer support groups.

- **Shelters** We found no reliable controlled trials. One cohort study found a reduced incidence of violence in the weeks following shelter stay for women choosing to use the shelter when they were also engaged in other types of help seeking behaviour compared with women not choosing to stay at the shelter. Women choosing to stay at the shelter who had not sought help elsewhere experienced an increase in violence.
- **Non-specific counselling** Two controlled trials and one comparative cohort study found no effect of counselling compared with no treatment on medical care utilisation rates, reported exposure to violence and threats of violence, or depression, anxiety, and self esteem.

DEFINITION Domestic violence, also called intimate partner violence, is actual or threatened physical or sexual violence, or emotional or psychological abuse (including coercive tactics) by a current or former spouse or dating partner (including same sex partners).[1] Other terms commonly used to describe domestic violence include domestic abuse, spouse abuse, marital violence, and battering.

INCIDENCE/ PREVALENCE Between 10–69% of women participating in population based surveys in 48 countries from around the world reported being physically assaulted by a partner during their lifetime.[2] Rates of assault by a partner are 4.3 times higher among women than men.[3] Nearly 25% of surveyed women in the USA reported being physically and/or sexually assaulted by a current or former partner at some time during their lives, and 1.5% were victimised during the previous 12 months.[3] Rates of violence against pregnant women range from 0.9–20%.[4] Between 11.7–24.5% of women in prenatal clinics[5–8] and 5.5–17% of women in primary or ambulatory care reported being abused by a partner in the past year.[9–12]

AETIOLOGY/ RISK FACTORS A recent systematic review found that physical domestic violence toward women is associated with lower levels of education and unemployment, low family income, marital discord, and with the partner's lower level of occupation, childhood experiences of abuse, witnessing interparental violence, higher levels of anger, depression, heavy or problem drinking, drug use, jealousy, and lack of assertiveness with spouse.[13] A similar review of research on psychological aggression found that the few demographic and psychological variables assessed were either inconsistently associated with psychological domestic violence or were found to be associated with psychological domestic violence in studies with serious methodological limitations.[14]

PROGNOSIS There are few prospective studies documenting the course of domestic violence and its outcomes. Cross sectional surveys suggest that domestic violence persists for at least two thirds of women.[15,16] Among black and Hispanic people, persistence of domestic violence seems to be dependent on initial severity.[17] For all ethnic groups, half of those reporting moderate domestic violence did not report occurrences of domestic violence at the 5 year follow up, but for people of black or Hispanic origin reporting severe domestic violence only a third did not report occurrences of domestic violence at the 5 year follow up. A case control study conducted in middle class working women found that, compared with non-abused women, women abused by their partners during the previous 9 years were significantly more likely to have or report headaches (48% *v* 35%), back pain (40% *v* 25%), sexually transmitted diseases (6% *v* 2%), vaginal bleeding (17% *v* 6%), vaginal infections (30% *v* 21%), pelvic pain (17% *v* 9%), painful intercourse (13% *v* 7%), urinary tract infections (22% *v* 12%), appetite loss (9% *v* 3%), digestive problems (35% *v* 19%), abdominal pain (22% *v* 11%), and facial injuries (8% *v* 1%).[18] After adjusting for age, race, insurance status, and cigarette smoking, a cross sectional survey found that women experiencing psychological abuse are also more likely to report poor physical and mental health, disability preventing work, arthritis, chronic pain, migraine and other frequent headaches, sexually transmitted infections, chronic pelvic pain, stomach ulcers, spastic colon, frequent indigestion, diarrhoea, or constipation (see table 1, p 2302).[19]

AIMS OF INTERVENTION To improve quality of life and psychological and physical wellbeing; to reduce risk of physical and mental illness, injury, or death.

OUTCOMES Self reported rates of domestic violence, mortality, non-fatal injuries, gynaecological and reproductive/obstetrical complications (e.g. chronic pelvic pain, miscarriage, recurrent vaginal infections), chronic disorders that may have a psychosomatic component (e.g. chronic pain, sleep or eating disorders, or hypertension), and psychological conditions (e.g. depression, suicide, substance abuse, anxiety, low self esteem, low self efficacy, or poor assertiveness) associated with intimate partner violence, as well as quality of life, physical and functional status, and adverse effects of treatment. Utilisation of domestic violence services was also considered as an intermediate outcome. Scales frequently used were the Severity of Violence Against Women Scale, Spielberger's 20 item State-Trait Anxiety Inventory, Hudson's Index of Self-esteem, Self-efficacy Scale, Modified Conflict Tactics Scale, Beck Depression Inventory, and Index of Spouse Abuse ScaleⒼ.

METHODS *Clinical Evidence* search and appraisal March 2004. *Clinical Evidence* searched Medline from 1966, Embase from 1980, PsycINFO from 1985, ASSIA from 1987, Cinahl from 1982, MIDIRS from 1990; Cochrane Library 2002 issue 4 and TRIP database; and identified systematic reviews, RCTs, other controlled trials, and observational studies using the following search terms: intimate partner violence, domestic violence, battered women, woman abuse, woman battering, family violence, husband to wife violence, marital violence, battered wives, conjugal violence, spouse abuse, violence against women, and abused women; and prevention, treatment, or intervention. We excluded public education, system level interventions, civil protection orders, screening for domestic violence or protocols focusing on identification of domestic violence victims, as well as interventions targeting only men (e.g. batterer treatment). Couple interventions were included only if women participated regularly in the intervention and reoccurrence of violence or other outcomes among women were measured. Given the paucity of studies, none were excluded because of methodological limitations; however, when high non-participation, attrition, or high rates of loss to follow up were found, these are mentioned in the comment sections.

QUESTION What are the effects of interventions initiated by healthcare professionals, aimed at female victims of domestic violence?

OPTION INDIVIDUAL, COUPLE, OR GROUP COUNSELLING

Two controlled trials and one comparative cohort study found no effect of counselling compared with no treatment on medical care utilisation rates, reported exposure to violence and threats of violence, or depression, state anxiety, and self esteem. One controlled trial found that grief resolution orientated counselling improved self esteem and self efficacy from baseline, whereas feminist orientated counselling did not. However, the study did not directly compare effects of interventions. Similarly, one controlled trial found that cognitive behaviour orientated therapy improved women's assertiveness and reduced exposure to abuse from baseline, whereas non-specific support did not. One RCT and one non-randomised controlled trial reported that gender specific or couple therapy reduced subsequent exposure to violence among couples from baseline, but found no significant differences between these two types of counselling.

Benefits: **Versus no treatment:** We found three systematic reviews (search dates 1997[20] and 2001[21,22]), which between them identified one cohort study[23] and one controlled trial.[24] We found one additional controlled trial.[25] The cohort study (117 women), conducted in Sweden, evaluated an intervention comprising emergency room counsellingⒼ by a social worker and psychiatrist, overnight hospital stay even if not warranted by injuries, counselling after release, and referrals to social and legal services offered to women self identified as battered.[23] Women receiving counselling had similar rates of utilisation of somatic and psychiatric care during the 5 year period after treatment compared with those who declined treatment or withdrew. No numbers or description of types of services were reported. The controlled trial identified by the systematic reviews (290 pregnant Hispanic women) compared three interventions: unlimited counselling, unlimited counselling plus a mentor, or a wallet sized resource card.[24] Clinics were assigned randomly (see comment below). Women in all three groups reported a decrease in levels of violence and threats of violence at follow up 2 months postpartum, which was sustained through follow up at 6, 12, and 18 months. The trial found no significant difference in severity of violence between either type of counselling group and resource card intervention (mean on the Severity of Violence Against Women Scale**G**: 34.7 for counselling plus mentor *v* 39.5 for unlimited counselling only *v* 38.2 for resource card; see note below for explanation of this score). Physical violence and threats of violence scores remained consistently lower at each follow up for the counselling plus mentor group (but not reaching statistical significance), whereas scores for women in the counselling only group were consistently higher than those in the resource card group. The additional controlled trial (33 women in two shelters in South Korea) compared a problem solving/empowerment group intervention versus no intervention.[25] Anxiety proneness scores (measured using Spielberger's 20 item State Trait Anxiety Inventory**G**) decreased significantly in the intervention group compared with the control group (size of change from pre-test to post-test: –11.81 *v* –0.35; $P < 0.01$), but there were no significant differences between groups in current levels of anxiety (–9.88 *v* –9.35; $P = 0.91$), self esteem (measured using Rosenberg's Self-esteem Scale**G**: 1.56 *v* 1.29; $P = 0.84$), or depression (measured using the CES-D**G**: –13.31 *v* –5.76; $P = 0.13$). **Grief resolution orientated counselling versus feminist orientated counselling:** We found one systematic review[22] (search date 2001, 1 quasi-randomised trial, 20 women). In the trial included in the review,[26] women requesting counselling at a battered women's programme were alternately allocated to grief resolution or feminist orientated individual counselling for 8 weeks. Women in both groups improved based on pre–post evaluation with Hudson's Index of Self-esteem**G** and a Self-efficacy Scale**G**. Pre–post score differences were statistically significant only for women in the grief resolution orientated group for both self esteem (66.9 *v* 53.5; $P < 0.01$) and self efficacy (63.3 *v* 74.7; $P < 0.01$), whereas women in the feminist orientated group showed no significant changes between pre- and post-intervention scores (self esteem: 45.7 *v* 39.5; self efficacy: 68.4 *v* 77.7). Differences between treatments were not reported. **Cognitive behaviour orientated counselling:** We found one controlled trial (20 women in Colombia, aged 19–50 years) that compared 20 twice weekly 3 hour sessions of cognitive behavioural treatment versus non-structured support group.[27] Two women in the cognitive behavioural therapy group and four in the non-structured support group reported new episodes of domestic violence after the intervention began. Levels of assertiveness improved significantly in the intervention group (from pre- to post-intervention; $P < 0.05$), whereas in the control group they did not. Differences between treatments were not reported. **Group counselling versus individual couple counselling:** One systematic review (search date 1997) identified one controlled trial (68 couples).[20] It found no difference between group and individual couple intervention in reduction in physical violence or in psychological wellbeing. Withdrawal rates were higher in the group programme. **Gender specific versus couple counselling:** We identified one RCT[28] and one non-randomised controlled trial (124 couples) comparing gender specific counselling versus couple counselling.[29] In the RCT, 49 couples who indicated a desire to remain in their current relationship were randomly assigned to gender specific counselling or couple counselling.[28] There were no differences in victims' reports of subsequent physical violence at 6 month follow up for 26 (62%) of the couples (reports: 8.3% among couple therapy participants *v* 7.1% for gender specific therapy; $P = 0.91$). In the non-randomised controlled trial, volunteer married and intact couples who reported at least two acts of husband to wife physical aggression (75 couples), excluding couples with alcohol dependence, mental disease, and who reported severe injuries, or women who feared their partner, were alternately assigned to couple therapy or gender specific therapy.[29] The past year prevalence of husband to wife physical aggression was reduced from 100% before treatment to 74% after treatment ($P < 0.01$) in both groups, based on the Modified Conflict Tactics Scale❻. With both treatments, there were significant decreases from pre-treatment scores to 1 year follow up in husband to wife psychological aggression (93.37 to 44.79; $P < 0.005$) and mild (19.31 to 8.63; $P < 0.001$) and severe physical aggression (3.34 to 1.71; $P < 0.05$), as well as wives' depression on the Beck Depression Inventory❻ (12.39 to 8.79; $P < 0.005$), with no differences between treatments. Women in couples group therapy reported that physical aggression resulted from content discussed in 2% of the sessions, with no differences between treatments.

Harms: No harms were reported for individual or group counselling. However, a potential harm of any intervention targeting victims of domestic violence is escalation of violence as a result of reprisal. Qualitative assessment of weekly reports did not support the belief that women who received couple counselling were placed in any further danger than those who attended individual therapy.[28]

Comment: It is unclear whether the controlled trial comparing counselling versus no intervention was an RCT because the allocation method was not described.[24] Rotating assignment to groups may have increased the possibility of contamination across groups. In the quasi-randomised trial comparing grief orientated versus feminist orientated counselling, the scoring range was unclear, and the authors did not indicate whether the original 14 point Lickert scale was used.[26] The trial conducted in South Korea, comparing a group problem solving/empowering intervention versus no intervention, had high withdrawal rates (47% in group intervention *v* 43% in the no intervention group).[25] In the second trial comparing gender specific interventions versus couple intervention, two thirds of eligible couples declined to participate.[29] In addition, 67% of the participants withdrew at the start or dropped out during treatment or before follow up.

OPTION ADVOCACY

One RCT and one non-randomised controlled trial found that advocacy reduced reabuse compared with no treatment. The RCT also found an improvement in women's quality of life with advocacy compared with no treatment. One controlled trial in pregnant Hispanic women found no significant difference in rates of reabuse between combined counselling plus mentoring (similar to advocacy) and a resource card, but found that counselling plus mentoring slightly reduced rates of reabuse compared with unlimited counselling.

Benefits: **Versus no treatment:** We found one systematic review[30] (search date 2002, 1 RCT,[31] 278 women) and one additional non-randomised controlled trial.[32] The RCT included in the review allocated 278 battered women leaving shelter stay either to a trainee advocate or to a control group.[31] Advocates worked with participants for about 6.4 hours each week over a 10 week period. Compared with baseline, the RCT found significant reduction in psychological abuse and increased quality of life at 6, 12, 18, and 24 months follow up, but it found no significant change from baseline for depression. The RCT reported no significant differences between groups for psychological abuse or depression, but found that advocacy significantly improved quality of life ($P = 0.01$) and reduced reabuse at 24 months compared with control (reabuse rate: 76% with advocacy *v* 89% with control; $P < 0.01$). The additional non-randomised controlled trial (81 women seeking temporary restraining orders with incomes below the poverty line and access to a telephone, who had no obvious mental disorder, were not already represented by an attorney, or receiving extensive violence related resources) allocated 22 women to law school advocates and 59 to standard court services without an advocate.[32] Women assisted by advocates reported less physical reabuse (5% *v* 25%) and psychological reabuse (10% *v* 47%) compared with women receiving standard court services at 6 months of follow up. **Versus counselling:** We found one systematic review (search date 2001, 1 controlled trial,[24] 290 pregnant Hispanic women).[22] The controlled trial compared unlimited counselling plus a mentor (who might be considered to have acted as an advocate) versus unlimited counselling only versus a resource card.[24] Participants in all three groups reported a reduction in levels of violence and threats of violence at follow up 2 months post partum. Although women receiving unlimited counselling plus mentoring reported less physical violence than women receiving unlimited counselling only (mean on the Severity of Violence Against Women Scale**G** adjusted for entry scores: 34.7 *v* 39.5; $P < 0.05$), neither of these interventions had significantly different results compared with women receiving only a resource card. There were no differences at 6, 12, or 18 month follow up assessments.

Harms: No harms were reported. However, a potential harm for any intervention targeting victims of domestic violence is escalation of violence as a result of reprisal.

Comment: **Versus no treatment:** In the additional controlled trial (81 women below the poverty line), 41% of those approached did not consent to participate.[32] An additional 13% did not appear for their first appointment. Assignment to the intervention group was based on women's acceptance of free legal representation from a law student. The RCT[31] evaluated the effect of advocacy for women exiting shelters, and the controlled trial involving women below the poverty line utilised law school advocates in a legal setting (interventions not available in a healthcare setting).[32] Although referral to an advocate (usually available at community based intimate partner violence services) at any time was considered an intervention to which a healthcare professional could potentially refer a victim; the extent to which the effectiveness of these interventions for women exiting shelter or women seeking restraining orders can be generalised to women in other conditions is unknown.

OPTION SHELTERS

We found no reliable controlled trials. One cohort study found a reduced incidence of violence in the weeks after shelter stay for women choosing to use the shelter when they were also engaged in other types of help seeking behaviour compared with women not choosing to stay at the shelter. Women choosing to stay at the shelter who had not sought help elsewhere experienced an increase in violence.

Benefits: We found one systematic review (search date 1997), which found no reliable studies.[20]

Harms: We found no RCTs (see comment below).

Comment: The systematic review identified one cohort study (243 women) in women who spontaneously went to a shelter**G** and women sent by the prosecutors' offices compared those who voluntarily chose to stay at the shelter compared with those who chose not to stay.[33] Stay ranged from 1–30 days. The study found that women choosing shelter and not seeking any other help were more likely to experience new episodes of violence during the 6 weeks after leaving the shelter compared with those who did not choose to stay at the shelter (OR 1.8; $P = 0.13$, after adjusting for initial risk of violence, days outside the shelter, and attrition). However, women choosing shelters had previously experienced twice as much violence as those not choosing shelters. In women who engaged in at least one other type of help seeking behaviour, shelter use reduced the risk of new violence compared with shelter non-use (OR 0.6; $P < 0.05$), suggesting that shelter stay may only be effective when women use other resources. Conclusions must be drawn carefully from this study because losses to follow up were 36%, and results were based on subgroup analyses.[33] In the study, help seeking behaviour was defined as the number of distinct kinds of help seeking actions taken during the 6 months before the baseline interview and included previous shelter stay, calling the police, trying to get a restraining order, seeking criminal justice prosecution, seeking counselling, and trying to get help from legal aid or a private attorney.[20]

OPTION PEER SUPPORT GROUPS

We found no systematic reviews, RCTs, non-randomised controlled trials, or cohort studies of peer support groups in women experiencing domestic violence.

Benefits: We found no RCTs, non-randomised controlled trials, or cohort studies of peer support groups**G** in women experiencing domestic violence.

Harms: We found no RCTs, non-randomised controlled trials, or cohort studies.

Comment: None.

OPTION SAFETY PLANNING

One RCT found that providing telephone sessions on safe behaviour in addition to usual care increased safe behaviour at 6 months compared with usual care alone. We found limited evidence from one non-randomised controlled trial in pregnant women that helping participants to make a safety plan reduced spouse abuse and increased safe behaviour at 12 months.

Benefits: We found one systematic review (search date 2002, 1 RCT, and 1 non-randomised trial).[30] The RCT (150 English and Spanish speaking women recruited from a family violence unit in an urban District Attorney's office) compared standard services offered by the District Attorney's office versus standard services plus six telephone sessions on safety behaviours.[34] The RCT found that additional sessions on safety behaviours improved safety behaviour compared with standard treatment at 3 and 6 months (safety behaviours were assessed using the Safety Behaviour Checklist of 15 behaviours, adjusted for relevance [e.g. if no firearms in the home, adopting the safety behaviour of removing the firearm was not applicable]; mean increase of two safety behaviours for sessions *v* standard care; effect size 0.91 at 3 months and 0.64 at 6 months). In the non-randomised trial included in the review, 199 pregnant women attending public prenatal clinics who had been physically or sexually assaulted in the past year by their partner were recruited consecutively first into the control group to receive standard prenatal care (67 women) and then into the safety planning group (132 women).[35] Women in the control group received a wallet sized resource card with information on community resources. In the safety planning group, trained nurses helped participants to prepare a safety plan and provided them with information on applying for legal protection orders and filing for criminal charges, as well as community resource phone numbers. This information was provided during three evenly spaced sessions throughout pregnancy and was reinforced with a brochure at the end of each session. After adjusting for entry levels of violence, women in the safety planning group reported less ongoing physical and non-physical abuse on the Index of Spouse Abuse Scale Ⓖ at 12 months (37.6 *v* 56.9; P = 0.007), and fewer threats and instances of actual violence on the Severity of Violence Against Women Scale Ⓖ at 6 months (threats score 27.3 *v* 33.4; actual violence 33.1 *v* 35.9) and 12 months (threats score 27.0 *v* 33.6; actual violence 32.6 *v* 37.1) compared with women in the control group (P = 0.052), although it is unclear to which comparison the statistical test refers to. At 12 months, the safety planning group had used significantly more relevant safety behaviours than women in the control group (P < 0.001).

Harms: None reported. However, a potential harm for any intervention targeting victims of domestic violence is escalation of violence as a result of reprisal. In the RCT, one woman committed suicide after 3 weeks. The study did not report which treatment she was assigned. However, it is not clear that the suicide was related to treatment.[34]

Comment: The RCT recruited participants from a district attorney's office, a setting to which healthcare providers may refer people who have experienced domestic violence.[34] Less than 3% of women refused to participate (4/154). Nearly all women completed the study at 6 months (149/150). The occurrence of intimate partner violence during the trial was not assessed. The intervention ceased at 8 weeks, and a subsequent assessment of effect size showed a decrease between 3–6 months. The authors noted that this may reflect a ceiling effect or a need for reinforcement with additional intervention services. In the non-randomised study, the intervention group was recruited during prenatal care, whereas the comparison group was recruited post partum.[35] The influence of different periods of recruitment on recall of abuse was not explored.

GLOSSARY

Advocacy involves providing information to a client on her legal, medical, and financial options; facilitating her access to and utilisation of community resources such as shelters, counselling, and protection orders; accessing and mobilising her natural support networks; assisting in goal setting and making choices; validating her feelings of being victimised; and providing emotional support.[6]

Beck Depression Inventory in its short version has 13 items. Scores above 4 indicate increasing levels of depression.

CES-D (Centers for Epidemiological Studies Depression) Scale Twenty item 4 point Lickert scale, with scores that range from 0 to 60. Higher scores indicate more symptoms of depression.

Counselling usually involves professional guidance in solving a client's problems. Counselling services tend to focus on providing information rather than the use of psychological techniques. However, counselling, as used in one of the controlled trials referred to above,[25] may also include referral to services and assistance in accessing these services (overlapping with advocacy).

Hudson's Index of Self-esteem Scores vary from 0–100. Higher scores indicate lower self esteem.

Index of Spouse Abuse Scale is a 30 item, self report scale measuring the frequency with which respondents have experienced 11 types of physical abuse and 19 types of non-physical abuse inflicted by a male partner. In scoring the measure, items are weighted differentially based on severity. Scores range from 0–100 on each subscale, with high scores indicating high frequency of severe abuse and low scores indicating relative absence of abuse.

Modified Conflict Tactics Scale (CTS2) has 78 items measuring the frequency (on an 8 point scale from never to more than 20 times) with which partners engage in psychological and physical attacks on each other.

Peer support groups Sometimes facilitated by a professional, peer support groups are hypothesised to help women exposed to domestic violence by reducing social isolation (risk factor for or effect of domestic violence) and providing encouragement and support, for example by allowing women to see that they are not alone in their experience and that there are available alternatives to changing their situation.

Rosenberg's Self-esteem Scale A 10 item scale with a four point response format resulting in a score range of 10 to 40, with higher scores representing higher self steem.

Safety planning helps participants to identify behaviours that might signal increased danger and prepare, ahead of time, codes of communication with family or friends, as well as needed documents, keys, and clothing should a quick exit become necessary.

Self-efficacy Scale Scores on the original 23 item scale vary from 14 to 322, with a mean of 230 ± 39. Higher scores indicate higher self efficacy.[27]

Severity of Violence Against Women Scale Scores on the physical violence component range from 27 to 108, where 27 would equal never being exposed to any of the behaviours and 108 would equal being exposed many times to all of the behaviours in the inventory.

Shelters provide housing, food, and clothing, usually for 30–90 days, to victims and their children under 12 who leave their abuser. Many shelters also offer individual or group therapy or counselling, advocacy, child care, job training, and assistance in finding transitional housing.

Spielberger's 20 item State-Trait Anxiety Inventory Scores range from 20–80, where 20 equals not feeling like that at all (state anxiety) or ever (trait anxiety) and 80 would equal feeling like that very much (state anxiety) or always (trait anxiety).

REFERENCES

1. National Center for Injury Prevention and Control. *Injury fact book 2001–2002*. Atlanta, GA: Centers for Disease Control and Prevention, 2001.
2. Krug EG, Dahlberg LL, Mercy JA, et al. *World report on violence and health*. Geneva: World Health Organization, 2002.
3. Tjaden P, Thoennes N. *Full report of the prevalence, incidence, and consequences of violence against women*. Washington, DC: National Institute of Justice, 2000.
4. Gazmarian JA, Lazorick S, Spitz AM, et al. Prevalence of violence against pregnant women. *JAMA* 1996;275:1915–1920.
5. Savona-Ventura C, Savona-Ventura M, Dregsted-Nielsen S, et al. Domestic abuse in a central Meditarranean pregnant population. *Eur J Obstet Gynecol Reprod Biol* 2001;98:3–8.
6. Purwar MB, Jeyaseelan L, Varhadpande U, et al. Survey of physical abuse during pregnancy GMCH, Nagpur, India. *J Obstet Gynaecol Res* 1999;25:165–171.
7. Lueng WC, Lueng TW, Lam YY, et al. The prevalence of domestic violence against pregnant women in a Chinese community. *Int J Gynaecol Obstet* 1999;66:23–30.
8. Hedin LW, Grimstad H, Moller A, et al. Prevalne of physical and sexual abuse before and during pregnany among Swedish couples. *Acta Obstet Gynecol Scand* 1999;78:310–315.
9. Bauer H, Rodriguez MA, Perez-Stable EJ. Prevalence and determinants of intimate partner abuse among public hospital primary care patients. *J Gen Intern Med* 2000;15:811–817.
10. Richardson J, Coid J, Petruckevitch A, et al. Identifying domestic violence: cross-sectional study in primary care. *BMJ* 2002;324:271–277.
11. McCauley J, Kern DE, Kolodner K, et al. The "battering syndrome": prevalence and clinical characteristics of domestic violence in primary care internal medicine practices. *Ann Intern Med* 1995;123:737–746.
12. Gin NE, Ruker L, Frayne S, et al. Prevalence of domestic violence among patients in three ambulatory care internal medicine clinics. *J Gen Intern Med* 1991;6:317–322.
13. Schumacher JA, Felbau-Kohn S, Smith-Slep AM, et al. Risk factors for male to female physical abuse. *Aggress Violent Behav* 2001;6:281–352.
14. Schumacher JA, Smith-Slep AM, Heyman RE. Risk factors for male-to female psychological abuse. *Aggress Violent Behav* 2001;6:255–268.
15. Gelles RJ. *Intimate violence in families*, 3rd ed. Thousand Oaks, California: Sage, 1997.
16. Rand MR, Saltzman LE. The nature and extent of recurring intimate partner violence against women in the United States. *J Comp Fam Stud* 2003;34:137–149.
17. Caetano R, Schafer J, Fals-Stewart W. Stability and change in intimate partner violence and drinking among white, black, and Hispanic couples over a 5-year interval. *Alcohol Clin Exp Res* 2003;27:292–300.
18. Campbell J, Jones AS, Dienemann J, et al. Intimate partner violence and physical health consequences. *Arch Intern Med* 2002;162:1157–1163.
19. Coker AL, Smith PH, Bethea L, et al. Physical health consequences of physical and psychological intimate partner violence. *Arch Fam Med* 2000;9:451–457.
20. Chalk R, King PA (ed). *Violence in families, assessing prevention and treatment programs*. Washington, DC: National Academy Press, 1998. Search date 1997; primary sources National Criminal Justice Reference Section, National Child Abuse and Neglect Data System, Medline, Legal Resource Index, Criminal Justice Periodical Index, ERIC, Social SciSearch, PsychINFO, Dissertation Abstracts Online, A-V Online, PAIS Online, IAC Business, ARTS, US Political Science Documents, British Education Index, Ageline, Religion Index, Public Opinion Online, National Center on Child Abuse and Neglect Clearinghouse, Family Violence and Sexual Assault Institute, National Clearinghouse for the Defense of Battered Women, National Resource enter on Domestic Violence, Family Violence Prevention Fund.
21. Ramsay J, Richardson J, Carter Y, et al. Should health professionals screen women for domestic violence? Systematic review. *BMJ* 2002;325:314–327. Search date 2001; primary sources Medline, Embase, Cinahl.
22. Centre for Clinical Effectiveness. *Is therapy/counseling/group work more effective than no treatment for women who are victims of domestic violence*? Melbourne: Southern Health/Monash Institute of Public Health, 2001. Search date 2001; primary sources Cochrane Library, Best Evidence, Medline, Cinahl, Current Contents, Premedline, PsychINFO, SocioFile, Journals OVID, National Guideline Clearinghouse, Australasian Medical Index.
23. Bergman B, Brismar B. A 5-year follow-up of 117 battered women. *Am J Public Health* 1991;81:1486–1489.
24. McFarlane J, Soeken K, Wiist W. An evaluation of interventions to decrease intimate partner violence to pregnant women. *Public Health Nurs* 2000;17:443–451.

25. Kim S, Kim J. The effects of group intervention for battered women in Korea. *Arch Psychiatr Nurs* 2001;15:257–264.
26. Mancoske RJ, Standifer D, Cauley C. The effectiveness of brief counseling services for battered women. *Res Soc Work Pract* 1994;4:53–63.
27. Laverde DI. Effects of cognitive-behavioural therapy in controlling wife abuse. *Revista de Analisis del Comportamieno* 1987;3:193–200. [In Spanish]
28. Brannen SJ, Rubin A. Comparing the effectiveness of gender-specific and couples groups in court-mandated spouse abuse treatment program. *Res Soc Work Pract* 1996;6:405–424.
29. O'Leary KD, Heyman RE, Neidig PH. Treatment of wife abuse: a comparison of gender-specific and conjoint approaches. *Behav Ther* 1999;30:475–505.
30. Wathen C, MacMillan H. Interventions for violence against women: scientific review. *JAMA* 2003;289:589–600. Search date 2002; primary sources Medline, PsychINFO, Cinahl, HealthStar, Sociological Abstracts, and hand searches of reference lists from key articles.
31. Sullivan CM, Bybee DI. Reducing violence using community based advocacy for women with abusive partners. *J Consult Clin Psychol* 1999;67:43–53.
32. Bell ME, Goodman LA. Supporting battered women involved with the court system: an evaluation of a law school-based advocacy intervention. *Violence Women* 2001;7:1377–1404.
33. Berk RD, Newton PJ, Berk SF. What a difference a day makes: an empirical study of the impact of shelters for battered women. *J Marriage Fam* 1986;48:481–490.
34. McFarlane J, Malecha A, Gist J, et al. An intervention to increase safety behaviours of abused women: results of a randomised clinical trial. *Nurs Res* 2002;51:347–354.
35. Parker B, McFarlane J, Soeken K, et al. Testing an intervention to prevent further abuse to pregnant women. *Res Nurs Health* 1999;22:59–66.

Joanne Klevens
Epidemiologist
Centers for Disease Control, National Center for Injury Prevention and Control,
Division of Violence Prevention, Atlanta, USA

Laura Sadowski
Co-Director/Associate Professor
Collaborative Research Unit, Cook County Hospital/Department of Internal Medicine,
Rush Medical College, Chicago, USA

Competing interests: None declared.

TABLE 1 **Risks for reported conditions in women experiencing psychological abuse (see text, p 2294).[19]**

Complaint	RR (95% CI)
Poor physical health	1.69 (1.20 to 2.29)
Poor mental health	1.74 (1.07 to 2.73)
Disability preventing work	1.49 (1.06 to 2.14)
Arthritis	1.67 (0.20 to 2.22)
Chronic pain	1.91 (1.49 to 2.36)
Migraine	1.54 (1.16 to 1.93)
Other frequent headaches	1.41 (1.05 to 1.82)
Sexually transmitted infections	1.82 (1.19 to 2.68)
Chronic pelvic pain	1.62 (1.03 to 2.48)
Stomach ulcers	1.72 (1.02 to 2.84)
Spastic colon	3.62 (1.63 to 7.50)
Frequent indigestion, diarrhoea, or constipation	1.30 (1.03 to 1.63)

Dysmenorrhoea

Search date July 2004

Michelle L Proctor and Cynthia M Farquhar

QUESTIONS

INTERVENTIONS

See glossary Ⓖ

Key Messages

Treating dysmenorrhoea

- **Non-steroidal anti-inflammatory drugs (other than aspirin)** Three systematic reviews and five subsequent RCTs found that non-steroidal anti-inflammatory drugs (NSAIDs, including cyclo-oxygenase-2 inhibitors, but excluding niflumic acid) reduced pain compared with placebo. One systematic review found that NSAIDs (excluding cyclo-oxygenase-2 inhibitors) reduced restriction of daily activities, absence from work or school, and the need for additional analgesia compared with placebo. It remains unclear from direct comparisons which NSAIDs have better efficacy or safety. One small RCT identified by one systematic review found no significant difference in pain relief between an NSAID (naproxen) compared with paracetamol. One systematic review found that naproxen was associated with fewer adverse effects than co-proxamol. It also found that mefenamic acid reduced symptoms more than co-proxamol. The harms of NSAIDs including cyclo-oxygenase II inhibitor class, are considered in detail elsewhere in Clinical Evidence (see harms of non-steroidal anti-inflammatory drugs, p 2310) and include gastrointestinal ulceration and haemorrhage for traditional NSAIDs and, for at least some of the COX-2 inhibitors, increased cardiovascular risk. Co-proxamol has been withdrawn in some countries due to evidence that fatal toxicity may occur with a small multiple of the normal therapeutic dose and a proportion of fatalities are caused by inadvertent overdose. Rofecoxib, an NSAID of the COX-2 inhibitor class, has been withdrawn worldwide because of cardiovascular adverse effects.
- **Aspirin, paracetamol, and compound analgesics** One systematic review found that aspirin was more effective than placebo for pain relief. Two systematic reviews found no significant difference between paracetamol compared with placebo, aspirin, or naproxen in pain relief, although some of the RCTs may have been too

small to detect clinically important differences. The first review found limited evidence that co-proxamol reduced pain compared with placebo. One small RCT identified by a systematic review found no significant difference in pain relief between paracetomol and an NSAID (naproxen). One systematic review found that naproxen was associated with fewer adverse effects than co-proxamol. It also found that mefenamic acid reduced symptoms more than co-proxamol.

- **Magnesium** One systematic review found limited evidence from two out of three small RCTs that magnesium reduced pain after 5–6 months compared with placebo. The third RCT found no significant difference between treatments.
- **Thiamine** One systematic review identified one large RCT that found that thiamine reduced pain after 60 days compared with placebo.
- **Toki-shakuyaku-san (herbal remedy)** One systematic review found limited evidence that toki-shakuyaku-san reduced pain after 6 months and reduced the need for additional medication, compared with placebo. We found no RCTs of other herbal remedies.
- **Topical heat (about 39 °C)** One RCT found topical heat treatment to be as effective as ibuprofen and more effective than placebo in reducing pain.
- **Transcutaneous electrical nerve stimulation (high frequency stimulation only; effects of low frequency stimulation remain unclear)** One systematic review found limited evidence from small RCTs that high frequency transcutaneous electrical nerve stimulation reduced pain compared with placebo transcutaneous electrical nerve stimulation but was less effective in achieving pain relief compared with ibuprofen. Small RCTs provided insufficient evidence to assess the effects of low frequency transcutaneous electrical nerve stimulation compared with either placebo tablets, or high frequency or placebo transcutaneous electrical nerve stimulation.
- **Vitamin E** One systematic review identified two RCTs that found that vitamin E reduced pain compared with placebo. A second systematic review identified one RCT that found no difference in pain relief between vitamin E plus ibuprofen compared with ibuprofen alone.
- **Acupuncture** One systematic review of one small RCT provided insufficient evidence to compare clinical effects of acupuncture with placebo or no treatment.
- **Behavioural interventions** Two poor quality RCTs provided insufficient evidence about the effects of behavioural interventions.
- **Combined oral contraceptives** One systematic review and one subsequent RCT provided insufficient evidence about effects of combined oral contraceptives on pain relief compared with placebo.
- **Fish oil** One small crossover RCT identified by a systematic review and one additional RCT provided limited evidence that fish oil (with or without vitamin B_{12}) reduced pain and symptoms after 1–3 months compared with placebo.
- **Herbal remedies (other than toki-shakuyaku-san)** We found no RCTs of other herbal remedies.
- **Surgical interruption of pelvic nerve pathways** One small RCT found limited evidence that laparoscopic uterine nerve ablation increased pain relief compared with diagnostic laparoscopy. A second RCT found that laparoscopic uterine nerve ablation reduced pain at 12 months compared with laparoscopic presacral neurectomy, but no significant difference in pain relief between treatments at 3 months. It also found increased constipation with laparoscopic presacral neurectomy compared with laparoscopic uterine nerve ablation.
- **Vitamin B_{12}** We found no RCTs that compared vitamin B_{12} with placebo. One small RCT provided insufficient evidence for vitamin B_{12} compared with a low fat vegetarian diet. One RCT provided limited evidence that vitamin B_{12} plus fish oil reduced pain and symptoms after 1–3 months compared with placebo.
- **Spinal manipulation** One systematic review found that one good quality RCT found no significant difference between spinal manipulation and placebo manipulation in pain after 1 month. The review found two small poorer quality RCTs which had conflicting results regarding the effectiveness of spinal manipulation versus placebo or no treatment.

DEFINITION Dysmenorrhoea is painful menstrual cramps of uterine origin. It is commonly divided into primary dysmenorrhoea (pain without organic pathology) and secondary dysmenorrhoea (pelvic pain associated with an identifiable pathological condition, such as endometriosis [see endometriosis, p 2326] or ovarian cysts). The initial onset of primary dysmenorrhoea is usually shortly after menarche (6–12 months), when ovulatory cycles are established. Pain duration is commonly 8–72 hours and is usually associated with the onset of menstrual flow. Secondary dysmenorrhoea can also occur at any time after menarche, but may arise as a new symptom during a woman's fourth and fifth decade, after the onset of an underlying causative condition.[1] This chapter deals with both primary and secondary dysmenorrhoea. Endometriosis, which can cause secondary dysmenorrhoea, is covered in a separate chapter (see endometriosis, p 2326).

INCIDENCE/PREVALENCE Variations in the definition of dysmenorrhoea make it difficult to determine prevalence precisely. Studies tend to report on prevalence in adolescent girls, and the type of dysmenorrhoea is not always specified. Adolescent girls tend to have a higher prevalence of primary dysmenorrhoea than older women, as primary dysmenorrhoea can improve with age (see Prognosis). Secondary dysmenorrhoea rates may be lower in adolescents, as onset of causative conditions may not yet have occurred. Therefore, the results from prevalence studies of adolescents may not always be extrapolated to older women, or be accurate estimates of the prevalence of secondary dysmenorrhoea. However, various types of studies have found a consistently high prevalence in women of different ages and nationalities. One systematic review (search date 1996) of the prevalence of chronic pelvic pain, summarising both community and hospital surveys from developed countries, estimated prevalence to be 45–95%.[2] A second systematic review of studies in developing countries (search date 2002) found that 25–50% of adult women and about 75% of adolescents experience pain with menstruation, with 5–20% reporting severe dysmenorrhoea or pain that prevents them from participating in their usual activities.[3] Additional studies of prevalence are summarised in table 1 (see table 1, p 2324).

AETIOLOGY/RISK FACTORS A longitudinal study of a representative sample of women born in 1962 found that the severity of dysmenorrhoea was significantly associated with the duration of menstrual flow (average duration of menstrual flow was 5.0 days for women with no dysmenorrhoea and 5.8 days for women with severe dysmenorrhoea, where severe dysmenorrhoea was defined as pain that did not respond well to analgesics and clearly inhibited daily activity; $P < 0.001$; WMD –0.80, 95% CI –1.36 to –0.24); younger menarche (13.1 years in women without dysmenorrhoea *v* 12.6 years in women with severe dysmenorrhoea; $P < 0.01$; WMD 0.50, 95% CI 0.09 to 0.91); and cigarette smoking (41% of smokers and 26% of non-smokers experienced moderate or severe dysmenorrhoea).[9] There is also some evidence of a dose–response relationship between exposure to environmental tobacco smoke and increased incidence of dysmenorrhoea.[10]

PROGNOSIS Primary dysmenorrhoea is a chronic recurring condition that affects most young women. Studies of the natural history of this condition are sparse. One longitudinal study in Scandinavia found that primary dysmenorrhoea often improves in the third decade of a woman's reproductive life, and is also reduced after childbirth.[9] We found no studies that reliably examined the relationship between the prognosis of secondary dysmenorrhoea and the severity of the underlying pathology, such as endometriosis.

AIMS OF INTERVENTION To relieve pain from dysmenorrhoea, with minimal adverse effects.

OUTCOMES Pain relief, measured either by a visual analogue scale Ⓖ, other pain scales (such as the TOTPAR [TOPAR] score Ⓖ, TOTPAR-8 [TOPAR-8 Ⓖ], or SPID-8 Ⓖ), or as a dichotomous outcome (pain relief achieved yes/no); overall improvement in dysmenorrhoea measured by change in dysmenorrhoeic symptoms either self reported or observed, quality of life scales, or other similar measures such as the Menstrual Distress or Menstrual Symptom Questionnaires; adverse effects of treatment (incidence and type of adverse effects); proportion of women requiring analgesics in addition to their assigned treatment; proportion of women reporting activity restriction or absences from work or school and hours or days of absence as a more selective measure.

METHODS *Clinical Evidence* search and appraisal July 2004.

QUESTION What are the effects of treatments for dysmenorrhoea?

OPTION ACUPUNCTURE

One systematic review of one small RCT provided insufficient evidence to compare clinical effects of acupuncture with placebo or no treatment.

Benefits: We found one systematic review of acupuncture for primary dysmenorrhoea (search date 2001, 1 RCT, 43 women).[11] The RCT identified by the systematic review compared weekly acupuncture (30–40 minutes) for 3 weeks of a menstrual cycle for a total of 3 months (equivalent to three menstrual cycles) with three other treatments: placebo acupuncture❻; monthly medical visits; or no medical visits. Outcomes were assessed after 3 months using non-validated pain scales and symptom questionnaires, and improvement was defined as a reduction in pain by more than half the admission score. It found that acupuncture significantly increased the proportion of women with reduced pain compared with other treatment (10/11 [91%] with acupuncture *v* 4/11 [36%] with placebo acupuncture *v* 1/10 [10%] with monthly medical visits *v* 2/11 [18%] with no medical treatment; $P < 0.05$ for acupuncture *v* all other treatments).

Harms: The RCT identified by the review did not address the harms of acupuncture.[12]

Comment: The scale used to assess outcomes in the RCT identified by the review does not seem to be validated.[11] We found no evidence of statistical adjustment for multiple comparisons (such as Bonferroni's correction) in the published paper.[12] The review identified a second RCT that compared different modalities of acupuncture.[11]

OPTION ASPIRIN, PARACETAMOL, AND COMPOUND ANALGESICS

One systematic review found that aspirin was more effective than placebo for pain relief. Two systematic reviews found no significant difference between paracetamol compared with placebo, aspirin, or naproxen in pain relief, although some of the RCTs may have been too small to detect clinically important differences. The first review found limited evidence that co-proxamol reduced pain compared with placebo. One small RCT identified by a systematic review found no significant difference in pain relief between paracetomol and an NSAID (naproxen). One systematic review found that naproxen was associated with fewer adverse effects than co-proxamol. It also found that mefenamic acid reduced symptoms more than co-proxamol.

Benefits: **Aspirin versus placebo:** We found two systematic reviews.[13,14] The first review (search date 1997, 8 RCTs, 486 women) found that aspirin (650 mg 4 times daily) significantly reduced pain compared with placebo (proportion of women with at least moderate pain relief, 5 RCTs: RR 1.60, 95% CI 1.12 to 2.29; NNT 10, 95% CI 5 to 50). It also found no significant difference between aspirin and placebo in the need for additional medication or restriction of daily activity and absence from work (additional medications, 3 RCTs: RR 0.79, 95% CI 0.58 to 1.08; restriction of activity, 3 RCTs: RR 0.82, 95% CI 0.64 to 1.04; absence from work, 1 RCT: RR 1.28, 95% CI 0.24 to 6.76) (see table 2, p 2325).[13] The second systematic review (search date 2003, 2 RCTs, 143 women) included only double blind RCTs with less than 20% loss to follow up.[14] It found no RCTs for which the results were suitable for quantitative analysis of effects on pain relief. However, it found no significant difference between aspirin and placebo in the need for additional medication (1 RCT, 36 women: RR 0.86, 95% CI 0.46 to

1.60). **Paracetamol versus placebo:** We found one systematic review (search date 1997, 1 RCT, 35 women).[13] It found no significant difference between paracetamol (500 mg 4 times daily) and placebo in pain relief (proportion of women with at least moderate pain relief, 35 women: RR 1.00, 95% CI 0.28 to 3.63).[13] **Co-proxamol versus placebo:** We found one systematic review (search date 1997, 1 RCT, 72 women).[13] It found that co-proxamol**G** significantly increased the proportion of women with at least moderate pain relief compared with placebo (72 women: 650 mg/65 mg 4 times daily; RR 3.72, 95% CI 2.13 to 6.52) (see table 2, p 2325).[13] **Paracetamol versus aspirin:** We found one systematic review (search date 1997, 1 RCT, 35 women).[13] It found no significant difference in pain relief between aspirin (500 mg 4 times daily) and paracetamol (500 mg 4 times daily) (pain measured on 10 cm visual analogue scale**G**: median change from baseline 1.6 cm, 95% CI 0.4 cm to 3.3 cm with paracetamol *v* 1.2 cm, 95% CI 0 cm to 2.7 cm with aspirin). **Aspirin or paracetamol or co-proxamol versus non-steroidal anti-inflammatory drugs:** See benefits of non-steroidal anti-inflammatory drugs, p 2308.

Harms: **Aspirin versus placebo:** The first systematic review found no significant difference in adverse effects between aspirin and placebo (AR for adverse effects 7–17% with aspirin *v* 3–17% with placebo; RR 1.31, 95% CI 0.79 to 2.17).[13] It also found no significant difference in rates of nausea, dizziness, and headache between aspirin and placebo (nausea: RR 1.66, 95% CI 0.59 to 4.67; dizziness: RR 1.29, 95% CI 0.28 to 5.89; headache: RR 0.60, 95% CI 0.18 to 2.04). The second systematic review found no significant difference in adverse effects between aspirin and placebo (AR for adverse effects: 50% with aspirin *v* 33% with placebo; OR 1.93, 95% CI 0.49 to 7.62).[14] It also found no significant difference in rates of gastrointestinal adverse effects and nervous system adverse effects between aspirin and placebo (gastrointestinal adverse effects: OR 1.91, 95% CI 0.39 to 9.26; nervous system adverse effects: OR 3.66, 95% 0.75 to 17.71). **Paracetamol versus placebo:** The systematic review found no difference between paracetamol and placebo in the frequency of adverse effects (any adverse effect for paracetamol *v* placebo: RR 1.00, 95% CI 0.36 to 2.75).[13] **Co-proxamol versus placebo:** The review did not report on adverse effects for this comparison.[13] **Paracetamol versus aspirin:** The review did not report on adverse effects for this comparison.[13] **Aspirin or paracetamol or co-proxamol versus non-steroidal anti-inflammatory drugs:** See harms of non-steroidal anti-inflammatory drugs, p 2310.

Comment: Most RCTs included in the first systematic review were short (usually only 1 menstrual cycle on each treatment), small, and used a crossover design without a washout period.[13] All of the RCTs (except one of co-proxamol**G** *v* naproxen) used double blinding. All of the RCTs used oral administration of treatment in the form of tablets or capsules. Negative RCTs may have been too small to detect clinically important differences.

OPTION NON-STEROIDAL ANTI-INFLAMMATORY DRUGS (OTHER THAN ASPIRIN)

Three systematic reviews and five subsequent RCTs found that non-steroidal anti-inflammatory drugs (NSAIDs, including cyclo-oxygenase-2 inhibitors, but excluding niflumic acid) reduced pain compared with placebo. One systematic review found that NSAIDs (excluding cyclo-oxygenase-2 inhibitors) reduced restriction of daily activities, absence from work or school, and the need for additional analgesia compared with placebo. It remains unclear from direct comparisons which NSAIDs have better efficacy or safety. One small RCT

identified by one systematic review found no significant difference in pain relief between an NSAID (naproxen) compared with paracetamol. One systematic review found that naproxen was associated with fewer adverse effects than co-proxamol. It also found that mefenamic acid reduced symptoms more than co-proxamol. The harms of NSAIDs including cyclo-oxygenase II inhibitor class, are considered in detail elsewhere in Clinical Evidence (see harms of non-steroidal anti-inflammatory drugs, p 2310) and include gastrointestinal ulceration and haemorrhage for traditional NSAIDs and, for at least some of the COX-2 inhibitors, increased cardiovascular risk. Co-proxamol has been withdrawn in some countries due to evidence that fatal toxicity may occur with a small multiple of the normal therapeutic dose and a proportion of fatalities are caused by inadvertent overdose. Rofecoxib, an NSAID of the COX-2 inhibitor class, has been withdrawn worldwide because of cardiovascular adverse effects.

Benefits: **Versus placebo:** We found three systematic reviews and five subsequent RCTs.[14–20] The first systematic review (search date 2003) included only double blind RCTs with less than 20% loss to follow up and examined the effects of any non-steroidal anti-inflammatory drug (NSAID; excluding cyclo-oxygenase-2 [COX-2] selective inhibitors).[14] It found that, with the exception of niflumic acid, each NSAID significantly relieved moderate to severe pain compared with placebo (14 RCTs, 599 women: RR 3.43, 95% CI 2.70 to 4.35).[14] It also found that NSAIDs significantly reduced restriction of daily activities, absence from work or school, and the need for additional analgesia compared with placebo (additional analgesia: 10 RCTs, 667 women, pooled RR 0.57, 95% CI 0.47 to 0.69; restriction of daily activities: 3 RCTs, 216 women, RR 0.65, 95% CI 0.51 to 0.83; absence from school or work: 4 RCTs, 229 women, RR 0.46, 95% CI 0.34 to 0.61; see comment below).[14] The second systematic review (search date not stated) examined the effects of rofecoxib (a COX-2 selective NSAID).[15] It found one RCT (127 women), which compared four treatments: rofecoxib (25 mg/day), rofecoxib (50 mg loading dose then 25 mg/day), naproxen sodium (550 mg every 12 hours), and placebo over four consecutive cycles.[21] It found that both doses of rofecoxib and naproxen provided more pain relief compared with placebo (pain relief measured by combining the total pain relief [TOTPAR] scores at 8 and 12 hours; $P < 0.05$ for all treatments *v* placebo). The third systematic review (search date 2002) assessed the effects of valdecoxib (another COX-2 selective NSAID).[16] It found three RCTs (363 women) which compared valdecoxib, naproxen, and placebo. The review found that valdecoxib (20 mg or 40 mg) and naproxen sodium significantly relieved pain compared with placebo (pain relief measured by TOTPAR scores at 8 and 12 hours; $P < 0.05$ for all treatments *v* placebo).[16] The first subsequent RCT (104 women, crossover design; see comment below) compared ibuprofen arginate (200 mg or 400 mg), ibuprofen (200 mg or 400 mg), and placebo over five menstrual cycles.[17] It found that ibuprofen arginate (200 mg or 400 mg) and ibuprofen (400 mg) significantly relieved pain compared with placebo (TOTPAR scores at 8 and 12 hours, time to pain relief, and time to remedication; $P < 0.05$). The second and third subsequent RCTs (both crossover designs) were meta-analysed together in one paper.[18] One of the RCTs (84 women with moderate to severe primary dysmenorrhoea) compared lumiracoxib (400 mg once daily), rofecoxib (50 mg once daily), and placebo. The other RCT (99 women with moderate to severe primary dysmenorrhoea) compared lumiracoxib (400 mg once daily), naproxen (500 mg twice daily), and placebo. Both studies found that all active treatments (lumiracoxib, naproxen, and rofecoxib) significantly reduced pain compared with placebo up to 12 hours (SPID-8 score from 0 to 8 hours on day 1: active treatments *v* placebo, $P < 0.001$, results presented graphically; pain intensity difference from 2 to 12 hours: active treatments *v* placebo, $P < 0.05$). The fourth subsequent RCT (crossover design; 73 women with moderate to severe primary dysmenorrhoea) compared etoricoxib (120 mg), naproxen sodium (550 mg), and placebo taken at the onset of painful menses.[19] It found that both etoricoxib and naproxen sodium significantly reduced pain compared with placebo over 8 hours (TOPAR-8 score: 20.0 with etoricoxib *v* 21.5 with naproxen sodium *v* 12.6 with placebo, $P < 0.001$ for each active treatment *v* placebo). The fifth subsequent RCT (crossover design; 55 women, 41 of whom had primary dysmenorrhoea) compared rofecoxib (25 mg), rofecoxib (50 mg), naproxen sodium (550 mg), and placebo.[20] It found that all active treatments significantly reduced pain compared with placebo (pain intensity score: active treatments *v* placebo, $P < 0.001$, results presented graphically). **Comparison of NSAIDs:** We found three systematic reviews and five subsequent RCTs.[14–20] The first systematic review identified 26 RCTs that compared different NSAIDs,[14] but only three reported data that were suitable for meta-analysis. These RCTs compared mefenamic acid (500 mg 3 times daily) versus tolfenamic acid (200 mg 3 times daily), diclofenac (50 mg up to 3 times daily as required) versus nimesulide (100 mg up to 3 times daily as required), and naproxen sodium (up to a maximum daily dose of 660 mg) versus ibuprofen (up to a maximum daily dose of 1200 mg). The review found no significant differences in pain relief between treatments (mefenamic acid *v* tolfenamic acid, 1 RCT, 73 women: WMD +0.23, 95% CI –0.64 to +1.10; diclofenac *v* nimesulide, 1 RCT, 304 women: OR 0.69, 95% CI 0.38 to 1.25; ibuprofen *v* naproxen, 1 RCT, 81 women: OR 0.57, 95% CI 0.23 to 1.38). The RCT[21] identified by the second systematic review[15] found no significant difference between rofecoxib (25 mg/day), rofecoxib (50 mg loading dose then 25 mg/day), and naproxen sodium (550 mg every 12 hours) (pain relief measured by combining the TOTPAR scores to 8 hours; mean TOTPAR scores were 17.4, 18.0, and 18.4, respectively, $P > 0.05$). The third systematic review (search date 2002) identified two RCTs (363 women), which compared valdecoxib (another COX-2 selective NSAID) versus naproxen.[16] Two RCTs found that valdecoxib (either 20 mg or 40 mg at onset of pain and again 8–12 hours later if needed) was as effective at reducing pain as naproxen, although no statistical data were reported.[16] The first subsequent RCT (104 women, crossover design; see comment) compared ibuprofen arginate (200 mg or 400 mg), ibuprofen (200 mg or 400 mg), and placebo over five menstrual cycles.[17] It found that ibuprofen arginate (200 mg or 400 mg) significantly relieved pain compared with placebo and that ibuprofen arginate (400 mg) relieved pain significantly faster than ibuprofen (200 mg or 400 mg) (TOTPAR scores at 8 and 12 hours, $P < 0.05$; time to pain relief: 56 minutes with ibuprofen arginate *v* 90 minutes with 200 mg ibuprofen *v* 86 minutes with ibuprofen 400 mg; $P < 0.05$ for both comparisons). The RCT found no significant difference between all active treatments for time to remedication ($P > 0.05$). The second and third subsequent RCTs (total of 183 women with moderate to severe primary dysmenorrhoea; both crossover design) were meta-analysed together in one paper.[18] Both compared three treatments (two different NSAIDs versus placebo; see above). The studies found no significant difference in pain among NSAIDs up to 12 hours (SPID-8: lumiracoxib *v* rofecoxib, $P = 0.988$, lumiracoxib *v* naproxen, $P = 0.159$, results presented graphically; pain intensity difference from 2 to 12 hours: lumiracoxib *v* naproxen and rofecoxib, P reported as non-significant). The fourth subsequent RCT (crossover design, 73 women with moderate to severe primary dysmenorrhoea; see above) found no significant difference in pain between etoricoxib and naproxen over 8 hours (mean TOPAR-8 score: 20.0 units with etoricoxib *v* 21.5 units with naproxen sodium, $P = 0.326$).[19] The fifth subsequent RCT (55 women with primary dysmenorrhoea, 41of whom had primary dysmenorrhoea; see above) found no significant difference between rofecoxib 25 mg or 50 mg and naproxen sodium in pain up to 8 hours. (SPID-8: 21.05 with rofecoxib 50 mg *v* 18.05 with rofecoxib 25 mg *v* 18.10 with naproxen sodium, $P > 0.05$).[20] **Versus aspirin or paracetamol:** We found one systematic review (search date 2003).[14] It identified no RCTs comparing NSAIDs versus aspirin that were suitable for meta-analysis. It found one small RCT that found no significant difference between an NSAID (naproxen) compared with paracetamol in pain relief (68 women, RR for pain relief 2.25, 95% CI 0.81 to 6.19). **Versus co-proxamol:** We found one systematic review (search date 1997, 3 RCTs), which compared NSAIDs versus co-proxamol❻.[13] The first of these RCTs compared mefenamic acid (500 mg 3 times daily) versus co-proxamol (650 mg/65 mg 3 times daily). It found that mefenamic acid significantly reduced dysmenorrhoea related symptoms compared with co-proxamol ($P < 0.01$). Mefenamic acid also reduced the need for additional medication compared with co-proxamol (mean number of tablets of additional medication: 2.6 with mefenamic acid *v* 6.8 with co-proxamol; P value not reported). The RCT found similar rates of absences from work or school between treatments (total days of absence: 10.5 with mefenamic acid *v* 15.25 with co-proxamol; P value not stated). Two RCTs (98 women) identified by the review compared naproxen (275 mg 3 times daily) versus co-proxamol (650 mg/65 mg 3 times daily). Neither RCT found a significant difference in pain severity.[13]

Harms: The harms of NSAIDs including cyclo-oxygenase II inhibitor class, are considered in detail elsewhere in Clinical Evidence (see non-steroidal anti-inflammatory drugs, p 2307) and include gastrointestinal ulceration and haemorrhage for traditional NSAIDs and, for at least some of the COX-2 inhibitors, increased cardiovascular risk. Co-proxamol has been withdrawn in some countries due to evidence that fatal toxicity may occur with a small multiple of the normal therapeutic dose and a proportion of fatalities are caused by inadvertent overdose. Rofecoxib, an NSAID of the COX-2 inhibitor class, has been withdrawn worldwide because of cardiovascular adverse effects. **Versus placebo:** The most commonly reported adverse effects in the RCTs identified by the first review were mild neurological and gastrointestinal symptoms.[14] The review found no significant difference between any particular NSAID and placebo in the frequency of adverse effects. However, pooled results showed that, overall, NSAIDs significantly increased adverse effects compared with placebo (RR 1.29, 95% CI 1.05 to 1.59). The RCT[21] identified by the second review[15] reported minor adverse effects including nausea and dry mouth (4/127 [3%] with placebo *v* 7/127 [6%] with rofecoxib [25 mg followed by 25 mg/day] *v* 13/127 [11%] with rofecoxib [50 mg followed by 25 mg/day] *v* 11/127 [9%] with naproxen sodium [550 mg twice daily for 3 days]; $P < 0.05$ for rofecoxib [50 mg followed by 25 mg/day] *v* placebo).[21] One of the three RCTs (96 women) identified by the third systematic review[16] reported that the incidence of adverse effects was similar between all treatment groups except for headache, which was more common with valdecoxib 20 mg and with placebo than with valdecoxib 40 mg and naproxen sodium 500 mg (AR 15.7% with valdecoxib 20 mg *v* 9.2% with valdecoxib 40 mg *v* 8.2% with naproxen sodium 500 mg *v* 19.6% with placebo; P values not reported). The first subsequent RCT[17] found no significant difference between ibuprofen arginate, ibuprofen, or placebo in the incidence of headache, nausea, and dizziness (P values not reported). No participants discontinued treatment due to adverse effects. The paper reporting the results from the second and third RCTs found similar rates of adverse effects between the active treatments and placebo (first RCT: 21.3% with lumiracoxib *v* 19.5% with rofecoxib *v* 21.5% with placebo, P values not reported; second RCT: 15.7% with lumiracoxib *v* 19.1% with naproxen *v* 25% with placebo, P values not reported).[18] The fourth RCT found similar rates of adverse effects with active treatments and placebo. The most common adverse effects were headache and nausea. No serious adverse experiences were reported (incidence of adverse effects: 12% with etoricoxib *v* 25% with naproxen sodium *v* 15% with placebo, P values not reported; headache: 1.5% with etoricoxib *v* 7.5% with naproxen sodium *v* 4.5% with placebo, P values not reported; nausea: 3% with etoricoxib *v* 3% with naproxen sodium *v* 1.5% with placebo, P values not reported).[19] The fifth RCT reported no serious adverse effects. However, it found that gastrointestinal adverse effects were significantly more common with naproxen sodium than with placebo, although gastrointestinal adverse effects were similar with rofecoxib and placebo (gastrointestinal adverse effects: 63.6% with naproxen sodium *v* 10.9% with placebo, $P < 0.01$; 9.1% with rofecoxib 25 mg *v* 10.9% with placebo, $P > 0.05$; 7.3% with rofecoxib 50 mg *v* 10.9% with placebo, $P > 0.05$).[20] **Comparison of NSAIDs:** The first systematic review[14] found no significant difference in rates of adverse effects between different NSAIDS in any of the RCTs identified (all adverse effects: ibuprofen *v* fenoprofen, 1 RCT, 111 women: OR 1.51, 95% CI 0.72 to 3.18; naproxen *v* other NSAIDs, 2 RCTs, 323 women: OR 1.09, 95% CI 0.54 to 2.22). The RCT[21] identified by the second review[15] reported minor adverse effects including nausea and dry mouth (4/127 [3%] with placebo *v* 7/127 [6%] with rofecoxib [25 mg followed by 25 mg/day] *v* 13/127 [11%] with rofecoxib [50 mg followed by 25 mg/day] *v* 11/127 [9%] with naproxen sodium [550 mg twice daily for 3 days]).[21] The subsequent RCT (described above)[17] found no significant difference between ibuprofen arginate, ibuprofen, or placebo in the incidence of headache, nausea, and dizziness (P values not reported). The paper reporting the results from the second and third RCTs found no significant difference in the incidence of adverse effects between lumiracoxib, rofecoxib, and naproxen (incidence of adverse effects in first RCT: 21.3% with lumiracoxib *v* 19.5% with rofecoxib, P values not reported; incidence of adverse events in second RCT: 15.7% with lumiracoxib *v* 19.1% with naproxen, P values not reported.[18] The fourth RCT found no significant differences in the incidence of clinical adverse effects between etoricoxib and naproxen sodium. The most common adverse effects were headache and nausea. No serious adverse experiences were found (incidence of clinical adverse effects: 12% with etoricoxib *v* 25% with naproxen sodium, P values not reported; headache: 1.5% with etoricoxib *v* 7.5% with naproxen sodium, P values not reported; nausea: 3% with etoricoxib *v* 3% with naproxen sodium, P values not reported).[19] The fifth RCT found no serious adverse effects. However, it did find that gastrointestinal adverse effects with naproxen sodium were significantly higher than with either dose of rofecoxib (gastrointestinal adverse effects: 63.64% with naproxen sodium *v* 9.1% with rofecoxib 25 mg *v* 7.3% with rofecoxib 50 mg, $P < 0.01$).[20] **Versus aspirin or paracetamol:** The first systematic review[14] found no significant difference in adverse effects between aspirin compared with fenoprofen (1 RCT, 61 women: OR 1.46, 95% CI 0.52 to 4.07). It also found no significant difference in gastrointestinal adverse effects or nervous system adverse effects between paracetamol compared with naproxen (1 RCT, 78 women, gastrointestinal effects: OR 1.00, 95% 0.06 to 16.58; nervous system effects: OR 1.54, 95% CI 0.24 to 9.78). The review[14] identified one RCT (67 women; crossover design), which found no significant difference in adverse effects between paracetamol compared with ibuprofen (P value not reported). **Versus co-proxamol:** Co-proxamol was associated with significantly more adverse effects than naproxen (2 RCTs, 98 women; RR 1.94, 95% CI 1.11 to 3.41). (See NSAIDS, p 1525).

Comment: All RCTs identified used oral treatment.[14–20] NSAIDs can be given as suppositories, which seem to have a similar effect on overall pain relief but less effect than oral treatment on spasmodic pain.[22] In the first systematic review[14], only five of the included RCTs clearly described methods of randomisation and allocation concealment. At least half of the studies were co-authored or financially supported by pharmaceutical company associates; it was unclear how the others were funded, with the exception of a single study that reported receipt of a grant from an academic institution. The measurement and reporting of adverse effects by individual RCTs was generally poor, even taking into account the challenge of distinguishing between dysmenorrhoeic symptoms and medication effects. Methods of collecting this information varied: about one third of the studies described the use of prospective self report forms or diaries, but another third assessed adverse effects retrospectively (at follow up appointments) and the others were not specific about their methods. In some cases, the adverse effects recorded were those deemed by the study investigator to be medication related. Few studies provided adverse effect data suitable for meta-analysis and many provided no numerical data at all. Despite the large number of included trials, it is not clear as to which NSAIDs are most effective for dysmenorrhoea. This was because most of the trials were relatively small, they covered a large number of different comparisons, and few of them provided data suitable for meta-analysis (only 14/36 RCTs were included in meta-analyses). Of the 24 additional comparisons of 12 different NSAIDs versus placebo, 19 found that NSAIDs significantly relieved pain (P < 0.05), three found no significant difference (aspirin, diclofenac, and ibuprofen), and two did not report statistical results. The meta-analytical results for assessing restriction of daily activities and the need for additional analgesia[14] included data from one arm of an RCT (85 women; 4 treatment arms) that compared aspirin versus placebo. However, these data are unlikely to affect the applicability of the results. The second systematic review identified one additional crossover trial (63 women) that compared rofecoxib (50 mg loading dose then 25 mg/day), naproxen (550 mg every 12 hours), and placebo as needed. It found no difference in outcomes between rofecoxib and naproxen, but found that rofecoxib significantly reduced pain, as measured by TOPAR scores (P < 0.002) and time to remedication (P < 0.009) compared with placebo.[15] The first subsequent RCT[17] used a crossover design without a washout period and was co-authored by a pharmaceutical company.

OPTION BEHAVIOURAL INTERVENTIONS

Two poor quality RCTs provided insufficient evidence about the effects of behavioural interventions.

Benefits: We found no systematic review. We found two small RCTs on behavioural interventions**G**. One involved relaxation and imagery for women with congestive**G** or spasmodic**G** dysmenorrhoea,[23] and the other involved aerobic exercise for women with primary dysmenorrhoea.[24] **Relaxation treatment:** The first RCT (69 women) compared relaxation treatment plus positive imagery regarding menstruation versus self directed group discussion about menstruation versus waiting list control. The groups were divided into women with congestive or spasmodic dysmenorrhoea using the Menstrual Symptom Questionnaire. It found that, in women with spasmodic or congestive dysmenorrhoea, relaxation treatment significantly improved symptoms compared with waiting list control (P < 0.01). However, it found that only the women with spasmodic dysmenorrhoea experienced significantly less pain with relaxation compared with group discussion or waiting list control (P < 0.001).[23]

Aerobic exercise: The second RCT (36 women) compared a training group that participated in 30 minutes of exercise 3 days a week with a sedentary control group, and found that aerobic exercise significantly lowered Menstrual Distress Questionnaire scores ($P < 0.05$; results presented graphically).[24]

Harms: The RCTs gave no information on adverse effects.

Comment: Both RCTs were small and of poor methodological quality.[23,24] In one RCT, spasmodic dysmenorrhoea(G) was defined as spasms of pain mainly in the abdomen, and congestive dysmenorrhoea(G) was defined as a dull aching pain in the lower abdomen and other areas of the body.[23] However, the classification of dysmenorrhoea into spasmodic and congestive categories is no longer commonly used and has little meaning.[24] The RCT (36 women) that compared aerobic exercise with a sedentary control group analysed results for the 26 women (72%) who completed the trial (11 in the exercise group and 15 in the control group).[24] A systematic review is underway.[25]

OPTION COMBINED ORAL CONTRACEPTIVES

One systematic review and one subsequent RCT provided insufficient evidence about effects of combined oral contraceptives on pain relief compared with placebo.

Benefits: We found one systematic review of combined oral contraceptives for primary dysmenorrhoea (search date 1999, 5 RCTs, 379 women)[26] and one subsequent RCT.[27] The systematic review found no significant difference between medium dose oestrogen (> 35 μg) plus first or second generation progestogens compared with placebo in pain relief at 1–3 months (4 RCTs, 320 women; RR 1.40, 95% CI 0.58 to 3.42). It found that combined oral contraceptives reduced the proportion of women absent from work or school compared with placebo but the difference was of borderline statistical significance (1 RCT; 19/49 [39%] with contraceptives *v* 24/40 [60%] with placebo; RR 0.65, 95% CI 0.42 to 1.00).[26] The subsequent RCT (77 women) compared a low dose combined oral contraceptive containing desogestrel (a third generation progestogen) plus a low dose of ethinyl estradiol versus placebo for four consecutive monthly cycles. It found that the combined oral contraceptive significantly reduced the severity of menstrual cramping compared with placebo (mean reduction of score for cramping on the Menstrual Distress Questionnaire: 1.4 with combined oral contraceptive *v* 0.3 with placebo; $P < 0.01$). The combined oral contraceptive reduced overall menstrual pain compared with placebo but the difference did not reach statistical significance (mean reduction of score on the Menstrual Distress Questionnaire: 13.7 with combined contraceptive *v* 6.2 with placebo; $P = 0.074$). The RCT found no significant difference between the combined oral contraceptive and placebo in the proportion of women absent from work or school.[27]

Harms: The review found no significant difference between combined oral contraceptives and placebo in adverse effects such as nausea, vomiting, depression, and abdominal pain (1 RCT, 89 women: 15/49 [31%] with contraceptives *v* 8/40 [20%] with placebo; RR 1.53, 95% CI 0.72 to 3.24).[26] The results of two RCTs are difficult to interpret and could not be included in the meta-analysis of adverse effects performed by the review because the RCTs randomised menstrual cycles and not women.[28,29] One small RCT (18 women) identified by the review that compared combined oral contraceptives versus placebo found that more women receiving oral contraceptives experienced breakthrough bleeding (2/12 [17%] with contraceptives *v* 0/6 [0%] with placebo).[28]

Another RCT (59 women) identified by the review found that combined oral contraceptives increased weight gain, nausea, and vomiting compared with placebo (no further data reported).[29] The subsequent RCT found no difference between a low dose combined oral contraceptive and placebo in adverse effects such as headache, nausea, abdominal pain, bloating, anxiety, loneliness, weight gain, and acne (no further data reported). The most frequently reported adverse effect was headache (9/38 [24%] with combined contraceptive *v* 3/35 [9%] with placebo; P value not reported). There were no withdrawals due to adverse effects in either treatment group.[27]

Comment: Most of the RCTs identified by the review had weak methods.[26] Because of the small number of included trials and participants, the results of the systematic review are sensitive to the statistical methods of calculation used. One of the RCTs identified by the review could not be included in the meta-analysis because of poor reporting of data.[29] All of the RCTs identified by the review used combined oral contraceptives that are no longer commonly prescribed, so the results may not be applicable to women today, who take different preparations.[26]

OPTION FISH OIL

One small crossover RCT identified by a systematic review and one additional RCT provided limited evidence that fish oil (with or without vitamin B_{12}) reduced pain and symptoms after 1–3 months compared with placebo.

Benefits: **Versus placebo:** We found one systematic review (search date 2000, 1 RCT; crossover design; 42 women)[30] and one additional RCT[31] that compared fish oil versus placebo. The RCT identified by the review compared fish oil capsules with placebo twice daily for 1 month. It found that menstrual symptom scores were significantly lower with fish oil compared with placebo; however, these results should be interpreted with caution (see comment below).[30] Less additional medication (ibuprofen 200 mg) was used in the fish oil group (mean 4.7 tablets with fish oil *v* 10.1 with placebo; P = 0.015). **Plus vitamin B_{12}:** One additional RCT (78 women) compared four interventions: fish oil (0.5–1.0 g 5 times daily); fish oil plus vitamin B_{12}; seal oil (higher in saturated fat than fish oil); and placebo for a minimum of 3 months.[31] It found that pain measured on a visual analogue scale❻ significantly decreased only in the fish oil plus vitamin B_{12} group (pain measured on 10cm visual analogue scale: reduction in mean scores: 0.15cm with fish oil *v* 0.73cm with fish oil plus vitamin B_{12} *v* 0.2cm with seal oil *v* 0.19cm with placebo; P = 0.015 for fish oil plus vitamin B_{12} *v* placebo). However, all three active treatment groups experienced a significant change in the number of other menstrual symptoms and the amount of interference with daily activities (P < 0.05).

Harms: **Versus placebo:** One RCT (42 women) identified by the review found that two women taking fish oils reported nausea and one woman reported acne.[30] No adverse effects were reported in women receiving placebo.

Comment: Both RCTs included women with dysmenorrhoea and no additional health problems.[30,31] This could include women with either primary or secondary dysmenorrhoea. The results from the RCT identified by the review refer to the average of the two groups after the allocated treatments were crossed over, and should be interpreted with caution, as treatment effects may persist after crossover.[30]

OPTION MAGNESIUM

One systematic review found limited evidence from two out of three small RCTs that magnesium reduced pain after 5–6 months compared with placebo. The third RCT found no significant difference between treatments.

Benefits: **Versus placebo:** We found one systematic review (search date 2000, 3 RCTs).[30] The first RCT (50 women) identified by the review compared magnesium aspartate three times daily versus placebo. It found that magnesium aspartate significantly increased the proportion of women without pain after 6 months compared with placebo (21/25 [84%] with magnesium *v* 7/25 [28%] with placebo; RR 3.0, 95% CI 1.6 to 5.8; NNT 2, 95% CI 2 to 3). The second RCT (27 women) identified by the review found no significant difference between magnesium (5 mmol 3 times daily) and placebo in reducing pain, as measured by visual analogue scale**G** pain scores, or in the number of ibuprofen tablets taken after 4 months ($P = 0.07$; no further data reported). The third RCT (21 women) identified by the review found that magnesium (500 mg/day during menses) significantly reduced pain after 5 months compared with placebo ($P < 0.01$).[30]

Harms: One RCT identified by the review found that magnesium significantly increased the proportion of women who experienced intestinal discomfort and other minor adverse effects compared with placebo (5/25 [20%] with magnesium *v* 0/25 [0%] with placebo; NNH 5, 95% CI 2 to 38), although relief of these symptoms occurred when the dose was reduced from three to two tablets daily.[30]

Comment: None.

OPTION THIAMINE

One systematic review identified one large RCT that found that thiamine reduced pain after 60 days compared with placebo.

Benefits: We found one systematic review (search date 2000, 1 RCT).[30] The RCT identified by the review (crossover design; 556 Indian adolescents attending school) compared thiamine 100 mg/day versus placebo for 3 months. It found that thiamine significantly increased the proportion of women with no pain before crossover after 60 days compared with placebo (142/277 [51%] with thiamine *v* 0/279 [0%] with placebo; NNT 2, 95% CI 2 to 3). After completion of the RCT, 87% of all women experienced no pain.[30]

Harms: The review did not report any harms of thiamine.[30]

Comment: None.

OPTION VITAMIN B_{12}

We found no RCTs that compared vitamin B_{12} with placebo. One small RCT provided insufficient evidence for vitamin B_{12} compared with a low fat vegetarian diet. One RCT provided limited evidence that vitamin B_{12} plus fish oil reduced pain and symptoms after 1–3 months compared with placebo.

Benefits: **Versus placebo:** We found no systematic reviews or RCTs. **Versus dietary change:** We found no systematic review. We found one RCT (crossover design; 33 women), which compared a supplement tablet containing vitamin B_{12} (0.02 mg/day) versus advice to follow a low fat vegetarian diet.[32] However, the results were difficult to interpret because no pre-crossover results were reported. **Plus fish oil:** We found one RCT (78 women), which compared four interventions (see benefits of fish oil, p 2314): fish oil (0.5–1.0 g 5 times daily); fish oil plus vitamin B_{12}; seal oil (higher in saturated fat than fish oil); and placebo for a minimum of 3 months.[31] It found that pain measured on a visual analogue scale**G** significantly decreased only in the fish oil plus vitamin B_{12} group (reduction in mean scores: 0.15 with fish oil *v* 0.73 with fish oil plus vitamin B_{12} *v* 0.2 with seal oil *v* 0.19 with placebo; $P = 0.015$ for fish oil plus vitamin B_{12} *v* placebo). However, all three active treatment groups experienced a significant change in the number of other menstrual symptoms and the amount of interference with daily activities ($P < 0.05$).

Harms: The RCT that compared a vitamin B_{12} tablet with advice to follow a low fat vegetarian diet found that stomach upset, slight nausea, burping, and a bad taste in the mouth were reported by eight women across the different treatment groups.[32] No additional information was reported in the trial.

Comment: The RCT that compared vitamin B_{12} with dietary advice may have been too small to detect clinically important differences.[32]

OPTION VITAMIN E

One systematic review identified two RCTs that found that vitamin E reduced pain compared with placebo. A second systematic review identified one RCT that found no difference in pain relief between vitamin E plus ibuprofen compared with ibuprofen alone.

Benefits: **Versus placebo:** We found one systematic review (search date 2002, 2 RCTs).[33] The first RCT identified by the review (100 women aged 16–18 years) compared vitamin E (500 units/day [about 333 mg], from 2 days prior to expected menses until the third day of menses) versus placebo for 2 months. It found that vitamin E significantly reduced pain compared with placebo (median 10 cm visual analogue scale**G** pain scores: 3.5cm with vitamin E *v* 4.3cm with placebo; $P = 0.02$).[34] The second RCT identified by the review (100 women aged 18–21 years) compared vitamin E (500 mg three times daily from 10 days prior to expected menses until the fourth day of menses) versus placebo for 3 months. It found that vitamin E increased pain relief compared with placebo (proportion with improvement in pain: 34/50 [68%] with vitamin E *v* 9/50 [18%] with placebo; P value not reported).[33] **Vitamin E plus ibuprofen versus ibuprofen alone:** We found one systematic review (search date 2000, 1 RCT).[33] The RCT identified by the review (crossover design; 50 women) compared vitamin E (100 mg/day for 20 days before menses) plus ibuprofen (400 mg 3 times daily at the onset of painful menstruation) versus ibuprofen alone (400 mg 3 times daily at the onset of pain). It found no significant difference between vitamin E plus ibuprofen and ibuprofen alone in pain relief (proportion of women experiencing pain relief: 23/26 [88%] with vitamin E plus ibuprofen *v* 17/24 [71%] with ibuprofen; RR 1.25, 95% CI 0.93 to 1.67).[30]

Harms: The RCTs did not report harms.[30,33]

Comment: None.

OPTION HERBAL REMEDIES

One systematic review found limited evidence that toki-shakuyaku-san reduced pain after 6 months and reduced the need for additional medication, compared with placebo. We found no RCTs of other herbal remedies.

Benefits: We found one systematic review (1 RCT, search date 2000, 50 women), which compared herbal and dietary remedies versus placebo.[30] It found that a Japanese herbal remedy (see comment below), toki-shakuyaku-san (2.5 g 3 times daily), significantly reduced pain, as measured by a visual analogue scale❻ after 6 months compared with placebo ($P < 0.005$), and reduced the need for additional medication (diclofenac sodium) ($P < 0.01$; results presented graphically). We found no RCTs of other herbal remedies.

Harms: The RCT gave no information on adverse effects.[30]

Comment: Toki-shakuyaku-san is a mixture of six herbs, including angelica and peony root. The allocation method was not clearly described in the RCT.[30]

OPTION SPINAL MANIPULATION

One systematic review found that one good quality RCT found no significant difference between spinal manipulation and placebo manipulation in pain after 1 month. The review found two small poorer quality RCTs which had conflicting results regarding the effectiveness of spinal manipulation versus placebo or no treatment.

Benefits: We found one systematic review (search date 2000, 3 RCTs that met *Clinical Evidence* inclusion criteria), which compared spinal manipulation versus placebo or no treatment.[35] The review did not perform a meta-analysis because of heterogeneity. The largest RCT (138 women) identified by the review found no difference in pain (as measured by mean change in visual analogue scale pain score) between high velocity, low amplitude manipulation (HVLA❻) compared with placebo manipulation❻ after one menstrual cycle (WMD +2.08, 95% CI –3.20 to +7.36). The second RCT identified by the review (44 women) found that HVLA significantly reduced pain intensity, as measured by a 10 cm visual analogue scale❻ pain score after one treatment and one menstrual cycle, compared with placebo manipulation (WMD –1.41, 95% CI –2.55 to –0.27). The third RCT (26 women) identified by the review compared 3 months of Toftness manipulation❻ versus placebo manipulation. It found that manipulation significantly reduced pain intensity after 6 months compared with placebo, but not at 3 months (WMD at 6 months –1.40, 95% CI –2.21 to –0.59; WMD at 3 months 2.20, 95% CI 1.38 to 3.02).[35]

Harms: One RCT (138 women) identified by the review found no significant difference between HVLA❻ and placebo manipulation❻ in the proportion of women experiencing soreness in the lower back region within 48 hours of the intervention (3/69 [4%] with HVLA *v* 2/69 [3%] with placebo; RR 1.50, 95% CI 0.26 to 8.70).[35] Soreness resolved within 24 hours. No other adverse effects were reported. The other RCTs identified by the review gave no information on adverse effects.

Comment: Two of the three studies included in the review had small sample sizes and methodological weaknesses, such as inadequate allocation concealment, and lack of blinding of outcome assessors. The study receiving the highest methodological score was also the largest study, and was therefore considered to be the most reliable.

OPTION TRANSCUTANEOUS ELECTRICAL NERVE STIMULATION

One systematic review found limited evidence from small RCTs that high frequency transcutaneous electrical nerve stimulation reduced pain compared with placebo transcutaneous electrical nerve stimulation but was less

effective in achieving pain relief compared with ibuprofen. Small RCTs provided insufficient evidence to assess the effects of low frequency transcutaneous electrical nerve stimulation compared with either placebo tablets, or high frequency or placebo transcutaneous electrical nerve stimulation.

Benefits: We found one systematic review including women with primary dysmenorrhoea (search date 2001, 8 RCTs, 172 women).[11] **High frequency transcutaneous electrical nerve stimulation (TENS) versus placebo TENS:** The review found that high frequency TENS**G** significantly increased pain relief compared with placebo TENS, as measured by subjective assessment or by a visual analogue scale**G** (pain relief by subjective assessment, 2 RCTs, 53 women: OR 7.2, 95% CI 3.1 to 16.5; pain relief by visual analogue scale range 0–100 [0 meaning no pain relief and 100 total pain relief], 1 RCT, 18 women: WMD 45.0 scale units, 95% CI 22.5 scale units to 67.5 scale units). The review found no significant difference in the proportion of women needing additional analgesics between high frequency TENS and placebo TENS (1 RCT, 64 women: OR 0.3, 95% CI 0.1 to 1.1). It also found no significant difference in the number of analgesic tablets taken between high frequency TENS and placebo TENS (1 RCT, 24 women, mean number of tablets taken each day: 6.92 with high frequency TENS *v* 6.78 with placebo; WMD +0.1 tablets, 95% CI –2.1 tablets to +2.4 tablets). It found no difference between high frequency TENS and placebo TENS in absence from work or school, as measured by the number of lost hours each menstrual cycle (1 RCT, 24 women: WMD +0.04 hours, 95% CI –0.4 hours to +0.5 hours). **Low frequency TENS versus placebo TENS:** The review found no significant difference in pain relief between low frequency TENS and placebo TENS (pain relief by subjective assessment, 2 RCTs, 29 women: OR 1.3, 95% CI 0.4 to 4.1; pain relief by visual analogue scale 0–100, 1 RCT, 18 women: WMD +24.1 scale units, 95% CI –2.9 scale units to +51.1 scale units). One additional RCT (24 women), which could not be included in the meta-analysis because of the way in which the results were reported, found that pain relief was significantly increased by low frequency TENS compared with placebo TENS ($P < 0.05$). Low frequency TENS reduced the number of additional tablets of analgesic used compared with placebo TENS (1 RCT, 24 women: WMD –3.1 tablets, 95% CI –5.5 tablets to –0.7 tablets). However, there was no difference between the two groups for hours of absence from work or school (1 RCT, 24 women: WMD –0.2 hours, 95% CI –0.6 hours to +0.2 hours). **Low frequency TENS versus placebo tablets:** The review found no difference in pain relief between low frequency TENS and placebo tablets (1 RCT, 21 women: OR 2.9, 95% CI 0.4 to 24.4). One additional RCT (20 women), which could not be included in the meta-analysis found that low frequency TENS increased pain relief compared with placebo tablets ($P < 0.05$). **High frequency TENS versus low frequency TENS:** The review found that high frequency TENS was more effective than low frequency TENS for pain relief measured by subjective assessment (1 RCT, 21 women: OR 3.9, 95% CI 1.1 to 13.0), but not for pain relief measured with a visual analogue scale (1 RCT, 18 women: WMD +21, 95% CI –4.4 to +46). One additional RCT, which that could not be included in the meta-analysis, found that low frequency TENS significantly reduced pain compared with high frequency TENS ($P < 0.05$). The review found that low frequency TENS significantly reduced the number of additional analgesic tablets taken compared with high frequency TENS (WMD 3.2 tablets, 95% CI 0.5 tablets to 5.9 tablets). There was no difference between the two groups in absence from work or school (WMD +0.2 hours, 95% CI –0.2 hours to +0.6 hours). **TENS versus non-steroidal anti-inflammatory drugs:** The review[8] identified two RCTs[36,37], which compared TENS versus non-steroidal anti-inflammatory drugs. The first

RCT (crossoverdesign 32 women) compared high frequency TENS, ibuprofen, and placebo. It found that high frequency TENS was significantly less effective than ibuprofen in achieving pain relief (proportion of women experiencing pain relief: 14/32 [44%] with TENS *v* 24/32 [75%] with ibuprofen; OR 0.26, 95% CI 0.09 to 0.75).[36] The second RCT (unblinded, crossover design; 12 women) found no significant difference between naproxen and high frequency/high intensity TENS in pain relief (data presented in graphical form, and neither OR nor P values reported).[37]

Harms: The adverse effects of muscle vibrations, tightness, headaches, and slight burning or redness after use were experienced by four women on treatment and none on placebo (RR 9.00, 95% CI 0.50 to 160.59).[11] There were no reported adverse effects from low frequency TENS or placebo TENS. The systematic review[11] identified one RCT that compared high frequency TENS with naproxen.[37] It reported an increase in the number of adverse effects experienced by participants with low frequency TENS compared with naproxen (OR 26.7, 95% CI 5.5 to 130.9).[11] Ten women (83%) experienced pain from TENS treatment, whereas there were no reported adverse effects with naproxen. The women who reported pain from TENS stated that they were prepared to accept the short term pain from the treatment in return for relief of dysmenorrhoea.[11,37]

Comment: None.

OPTION TOPICAL HEAT (ABOUT 39 °C)

One RCT found topical heat treatment to be as effective as ibuprofen and more effective than placebo in reducing pain.

Benefits: We found no systematic review. We found one efficacy RCT**G** (84 women with moderate or greater pain in at least four of their last six cycles who experienced pain relief with non-prescription analgesics and had a history consistent with a diagnosis of primary dysmenorrhoea) of topically applied heat, which used a double dummy**G** design with a heated or unheated patch plus oral ibuprofen or placebo.[38] An abdominal patch (heated to 38.9 °C versus unheated) was applied for about 12 hours daily for 2 days from the start of menses. In addition, oral medication (placebo *v* ibuprofen 400 mg) was given three times daily for 2 days. There were four treatment groups: heated patch plus placebo; heated patch plus ibuprofen; unheated patch plus placebo; and unheated patch plus ibuprofen. Pain relief was measured on a scale from 0 to 5; 0 was no relief and 5 complete relief of pain. After 2 days of treatment, significant pain relief compared with the unheated patch plus placebo group (mean pain relief score 1.95) was obtained with the heated patch plus placebo (mean pain relief score 3.27; $P < 0.001$), with the heated patch plus ibuprofen (mean pain relief score 3.55; $P < 0.001$), and with the unheated patch plus ibuprofen (mean pain relief score 3.07; $P = 0.001$). There was no difference in pain relief between the heated patch plus ibuprofen and the unheated patch plus ibuprofen groups ($P = 0.09$). However, the "time to noticeable pain relief" was significantly shorter for the heated patch plus ibuprofen compared with the unheated patch plus ibuprofen group (median 1.50 hours with the heated patch plus ibuprofen *v* 2.79 hours with the unheated patch plus ibuprofen; $P = 0.01$; no further data were provided). Pain intensity was measured on a 101 point numerical scale ranging from 0 (no pain) to 100 (worst possible pain). After 2 days of treatment, all treatment groups had a significant reduction in pain intensity compared with unheated patch plus placebo (mean pain intensity reduction: 40.4 heated patch plus placebo *v* 39.0 unheated patch plus ibuprofen *v* 43.8 heated patch plus ibuprofen *v* 21.9 unheated patch plus placebo; P < 0.003 for individual group comparisons *v* unheated patch plus placebo). There was no significant difference between heated patch plus placebo and unheated patch plus ibuprofen in the reduction in pain intensity at 2 days (P = 0.8).

Harms: The RCT found that women using a heated patch were more likely to report pinkness or redness of the skin than those using an unheated patch at the end of day 2 after 12 continuous hours of use (23/40 [58%] with a heated patch *v* 5/41 [12%] with an unheated patch; OR 9.74, 95% CI 3.16 to 30.04). All women reported normal skin 3–7 days after starting treatment.

Comment: Participants in the RCT included volunteer women. Disease in these women may have a different pattern and response to treatment than disease in women seeking health care.

OPTION SURGICAL INTERRUPTION OF PELVIC NERVE PATHWAYS

One small RCT found limited evidence that laparoscopic uterine nerve ablation increased pain relief compared with diagnostic laparoscopy. A second RCT found that laparoscopic uterine nerve ablation reduced pain at 12 months compared with laparoscopic presacral neurectomy, but no significant difference in pain relief between treatments at 3 months. It also found increased constipation with laparoscopic presacral neurectomy compared with laparoscopic uterine nerve ablation.

Benefits: We found one systematic review (search date 1998, 6 RCTs) of surgical pelvic nerve interruption for primary and secondary dysmenorrhoea.[39] Two of the six RCTs included women with primary dysmenorrhoea. The remainder included women with dysmenorrhoea associated with endometriosis, which is not the focus of this chapter. Meta-analysis was not performed because of RCT heterogeneity. **Versus diagnostic laparoscopy:** One RCT identified by the review (21 women) compared laparoscopic uterine nerve ablation (LUNA**G**) versus diagnostic laparoscopy and found that LUNA significantly increased pain relief at 3 months (OR 15.5, 95% CI 2.9 to 83.0) and at 12 months (OR 10.9, 95% CI 1.5 to 77.0). **LUNA versus laparoscopy presacral neurectomy:** The other RCT (68 women) found no significant difference between LUNA and laparoscopic presacral neurectomy (LPSN**G**) in pain relief at 3 months' follow up (OR 0.7, 95% CI 0.2 to 2.7). However, at 12 months' follow up, the LPSN group had significantly better pain relief scores (OR 0.26, 95% CI 0.10 to 0.71).[39]

Harms: One RCT identified by the review found that LPSN**G** increased constipation compared with LUNA**G** (31/33 [94%] with LPSN *v* 0/35 [0%] with LUNA; RR 0.01, 95% CI 0.00 to 0.24).[39]

Comment: Two larger RCTs of LUNA**G** are underway, and data will be included in an update of the systematic review (Proctor M, personal communication, 2004).[40] We found a second relevant systematic review but have not included this because it includes lower levels of evidence, such as case studies.[41]

GLOSSARY

Behavioural interventions Treatments that attempt modification of thought and beliefs (cognition) about symptoms and pain; modification of behavioural or physiological responses to symptoms, pain; or both.

Co-proxamol Non-proprietary label for a dextropropoxyphene hydrochloride and paracetamol combination. The most common presentation is tablets containing dextropropoxyphene hydrochloride 32.5 mg and paracetamol 325 mg.

Congestive dysmenorrhoea A dull aching pain in the lower abdomen as well as other areas of the body that may begin several days before menstruation and can include other premenstrual symptoms such as irritability.[42]

Double dummy Design pertaining to an RCT in which multiple treatments are compared (usually against a placebo) and the treatments have dissimilar presentations. Each participant will receive either active treatment or placebo for each treatment. Because multiple treatments are being compared (at least two), it allows identification of treatment effects against placebo, as well as the additive effects of treatments.

Efficacy RCT A trial designed to study if an intervention works in ideal conditions (e.g. when people receive treatments exactly as prescribed). In contrast, effectiveness trials evaluate the effects of treatments in "real life" conditions. Analysis in efficacy trials usually involves only the participants who were fully compliant with the therapeutic regimen. The applicability of the results from efficacy trials may be limited because conditions are artificial and hence response may be different in real life situations.

High velocity, low amplitude manipulation (HVLA) A technique of spinal manipulation that uses high velocity, low amplitude thrusts to manipulate vertebral joints. The technique is designed to restore motion to a restricted joint and improve function. The physician positions the person at the barrier of restricted motion and then gives a rapid, accurate thrust in the direction of the restricted barrier to resolve the restriction and improve motion.

Laparoscopic presacral neurectomy (LPSN) Involves the total removal of the presacral nerves lying within the boundaries of the interiliac triangle. This procedure interrupts most of the cervical sensory nerve fibres and is used to diminish uterine pain.

Laparoscopic uterine nerve ablation (LUNA) Involves laparoscopic surgery to transect (usually involves cutting and then electrocauterisation) the uterosacral ligaments at their insertion into the cervix. This procedure interrupts most of the cervical sensory nerve fibres and is used to diminish uterine pain.

Placebo acupuncture Also known as sham acupuncture, this is a commonly used control intervention involving the use of acupuncture needles to stimulate non-acupuncture points in areas outside of Chinese meridians. These points can be identified by a point detector as areas of the skin that do not have skin electrical activity similar to acupuncture points. There is some disagreement over correct needle placement, as placement of a needle in any position may elicit some biological response that can complicate the interpretation of results.

Placebo manipulation Also known as sham manipulation, this is a control intervention. The main principle is to use a non-therapeutic level of torque. There are two common techniques for placebo manipulation. In one, thrust is administered but the posture of the participant is such that the mechanical torque of the manipulation is substantially reduced. In the other, an activator adjusting tool is used; this can make spinal adjustments using spring recoil, whereby the spring is set so that no force is exerted on the spine.

Spasmodic dysmenorrhoea Spasms of acute pain that typically begin on the first day of menstruation.[37]

SPID-8 An outcome measure commonly used in pharmaceutical trials of treatments for pain. The difference in pain intensity from baseline up to 8 hours after dosing is measured. The SPID-8 is the sum of the pain intensity differences of all participants up to 8 hours after dosing. Pain intensity can be measured on any categorical scale, but typically a low score will mean less pain and a high score more pain.

Toftness manipulation A low force technique of chiropractic adjustment that uses a sensometer to detect sites of abnormal electromagnetic radiation, and to determine which sites to adjust. Adjustment is then delivered using a metered, hand held pressure applicator.

TOTPAR (TOPAR) score An outcome measure commonly used in pharmaceutical trials of treatment for pain. The pain relief scores for all participants at various time points after dosing are totalled and a mean calculated. Pain relief can be measured on any categorical scale, but typically a low score will mean less pain relief and a high score more pain relief.

TOTPAR-8 (TOPAR-8) score The same as TOTPAR (see above) but measured up to 8 hours after dosing.

Transcutaneous electrical nerve stimulation (TENS) Electrodes are placed on the skin and different electrical pulse rates and intensities are used to stimulate the area. Low frequency TENS (also referred to as acupuncture-like TENS) usually consists of pulses delivered at 1–4 Hz at high intensity so they evoke visible muscle fibre contractions. High frequency TENS (conventional TENS) usually consists of pulses delivered at 50–120 Hz at a low intensity, so there are no muscle contractions.

Visual analogue scale A commonly used scale in pain assessment. It is a 10 cm horizontal or vertical line with word anchors at each end, such as "no pain" and "pain as bad as it could be". The person is asked to make a mark on the line to represent pain intensity. This mark is converted to distance in either centimetres or millimetres from the "no pain" anchor to give a pain score that can range from 0-10 cm or 0–100 mm.

Substantive changes

Non-steroidal anti-inflammatory drugs (other than aspirin) Three papers, reporting four RCTs, added.[18–20] Benefits and harms data enhanced and categorisation unchanged.

REFERENCES

1. Fraser I. Prostaglandins, prostaglandin inhibitors and their roles in gynaecological disorders. *Bailliere's Clinical Obstet Gynaecol* 1992;6:829–857.
2. Zondervan KT, Yudkin PL, Vessey MP, et al. The prevalence of chronic pelvic pain in the United Kingdom: a systematic review. *Br J Obstet Gynaecol* 1998;105:93–99. Search date 1996; primary sources Medline, Embase, and Psychlit.
3. Harlow SD, Campbell OM. Epidemiology of menstrual disorders in developing countries: a systematic review. *BJOG* 2004;111:6–16.
4. Harlow SD, Park M. A longitudinal study of risk factors for the occurrence, duration and severity of menstrual cramps in a cohort of college women. *Br J Obstet Gynaecol* 1996;103:1134–1142.
5. Campbell MA, McGrath PJ. Use of medication by adolescents for the management of menstrual discomfort. *Arch Pediatr Adolesc Med* 1997;151:905–913.
6. Robinson JC, Plichta S, Weisman CS, et al. Dysmenorrhoea and the use of oral contraceptives in adolescent women attending a family planning clinic. *Am J Obstet Gynecol* 1992;166:578–583.
7. Andersch B, Milsom I. An epidemiologic study of young women with dysmenorrhea. *Am J Obstet Gynecol* 1982;144:655–660.
8. Klein JR, Litt IF. Epidemiology of adolescent dysmenorrhea. *Pediatrics* 1981;68:661–664.
9. Sundell G, Milsom I, Andersch B. Factors influencing the prevalence and severity of dysmenorrhoea in young women. *Br J Obstet Gynaecol* 1990;97:588–594.
10. Chen C, Cho SI, Damokosh AI, et al. Prospective study of exposure to environmental tobacco smoke and dysmenorrhea. *Environ Health Perspect* 2000;108:1019–1022.
11. Proctor ML, Smith CA, Farquhar CM, et al. Transcutaneous electrical nerve stimulation and acupuncture for primary dysmenorrhoea. In: The Cochrane Library, Issue 1, 2004. Oxford: Update Software. Search date 2001; primary sources Cochrane Controlled Trials Register, Medline, Embase, Cinahl, Bio extracts, Psychlit, SportDiscus, Cochrane Complementary Medicine Field's Register of Controlled Trials (CISCOM), and hand searches of citation lists.
12. Helms JM. Acupuncture for the management of primary dysmenorrhea. *Obstet Gynecol* 1987;69:51–56.
13. Zhang WY, Li Wan Po A. Efficacy of minor analgesics in primary dysmenorrhoea: a systematic review. *Br J Obstet Gynaecol* 1998;105:780–789. Search date 1997; primary sources Medline, Embase, and Science Citation Index.
14. Marjoribanks J, Proctor ML, Farquhar C. Nonsteroidal anti-inflammatory drugs for primary dysmenorrhoea. In: The Cochrane Library, Issue 1, 2004. Chichester, UK: John Wiley & Sons, Ltd. Search date 2003; primary sources Cochrane Menstrual Disorders and Subfertility Group Trials Register, Cochrane Controlled Trials Register, Medline, Embase, National Research Register, and hand searches of citation lists and conference proceedings.
15. Weaver AL. Rofecoxib: clinical pharmacology and clinical experience. *Clin Ther* 2001;23:1323–1338. Search date not stated; primary sources Medline, Embase, relevant web sites, and hand searches of proceedings of relevant scientific meetings.
16. Chavez ML, DeKorte CJ. Valdecoxib: a review. *Clin Ther* 2003:25;817–851. Search date 2002; PubMed, Medline, International Pharmaceutical Abstracts, and hand searches of citation lists.
17. Mehlisch DR, Ardia A, Pallotta T. Analgesia with ibuprofen arginate versus conventional ibuprofen for patients with dysmenorrhea: a crossover trial. *Curr Ther Res* 2003:64;327–337.
18. Bitner M, Kattenhorn J, Hatfield C, et al. Efficacy and tolerability of lumiracoxib in the treatment of primary dysmenorrhoea. *Int J Clin Pract* 2004;58:340–345.
19. Malmstrom K, Kotey P, Cichanowitz N, et al. Analgesic efficacy of etoricoxib in primary dysmenorrhea: results of a randomized, controlled trial. *Gynecol Obstet Invest* 2003;56:65–69.
20. Sahin I, Saracoglu F, Kurban Y, et al. Dysmenorrhea treatment with a single daily dose of rofecoxib. *Int J Gynaecol Obstet* 2003;83:285–291.
21. Morrison BW, Daniels SE, Kotey P, et al. Rofecoxib, a specific cyclooxygenase-2 inhibitor, in primary dysmenorrhea: a randomized controlled trial. *Obstet Gynecol* 1999;94:504–508.
22. Ylikorkala O, Puolakka J, Kauppila A. Comparison between naproxen tablets and suppositories in primary dysmenorrhea. *Prostaglandins* 1980;20:463–468.
23. Chesney MA, Tasto DL. The effectiveness of behavior modification with spasmodic and congestive dysmenorrhea. *Behav Res Ther* 1975;13:245–253.
24. Israel RG, Sutton M, O'Brien KF. Effects of aerobic training on primary dysmenorrhea symptomatology in college females. *J Am Coll Health* 1985;33:241–244.
25. Proctor ML, Murphy PA, Pattison HM, et al. Behavioural interventions for primary and secondary dysmenorrhoea (Protocol for a Cochrane Review). In: The Cochrane Library, Issue 1, 2004. Oxford: Update Software.
26. Proctor ML, Roberts H, Farquhar C. Combined oral contraceptives for primary dysmenorrhoea. In: The Cochrane Library, Issue 1, 2004. Oxford, Update Software. Search date 1999; primary sources Medline, Embase, Cinahl, Cochrane Controlled Trials Register, and hand searches of citation lists.
27. Hendrix SL, Alexander NJ. Primary dysmenorrhea treatment with a desogestrel-containing low-dose oral contraceptive. *Contraception* 2002:66;393–399.

28. Nakano R, Takemura H. Treatment of function dysmenorrhoea: a double-blind study. *Acta Obstet Gynaecol Jpn* 1971;18:41–44.
29. Matthews AE, Clarke JE. Double-blind trial of a sequential oral contraceptive (Sequens) in the treatment of dysmenorrhoea. *J Obstet Gynaecol Br Commonw* 1968;75:1117–1122.
30. Proctor ML, Murphy PA. Herbal and dietary therapies for primary and secondary dysmenorrhoea. In: The Cochrane Library, Issue 4, 2003. Oxford: Update Software. Search date 2000; primary sources Medline, Embase, Cinahl, Psychlit, Bioabstracts, Cochrane Controlled Trials Register, and hand searches of citation lists.
31. Deutch B, Jorgensen EB, Hansen JC. Menstrual discomfort in Danish women reduced by dietary supplements of omega-3 PUFA and B12 (fish oil or seal oil capsules). *Nutr Res* 2000;20:621–631.
32. Barnard ND, Scialli AR, Hurlock D, et al. Diet and sex-hormone binding globulin, dysmenorrhea, and premenstrual symptoms. *Obstet Gynecol* 2000;95:245–250.
33. Fugh-Berman A, Kronenberg F. Complementary and alternative medicine (CAM) in reproductive-age women: a review of randomized controlled trials. *Reprod Toxicol* 2003:17;137–152. Search date 2002; primary sources Medline, Alternative and Complementary Database, and hand searches of citation lists.
34. Ziaei S, Faghihzadeh S, Sohrabvand F, et al. A randomised placebo-controlled trial to determine the effect of vitamin E in treatment of primary dysmenorrhoea. *BJOG* 2001;108:1181–1183.
35. Proctor ML, Hing W, Johnson TC, et al. Spinal manipulation for primary and secondary dysmenorrhoea. In: The Cochrane Library, Issue 4, 2003. Oxford: Update Software. Search date 2000; primary sources Medline, Embase, Cinahl, Psychlit, Bioabstracts, SportDiscus, Cochrane Controlled Trials Register, and hand searches of citation lists.
36. Dawood MY, Ramos J. Transcutaneous electrical nerve stimulation (TENS) for the treatment of primary dysmenorrhea: a randomized crossover comparison with placebo TENS and ibuprofen. *Obstet Gynecol* 1990;75:656–660.
37. Hedner N, Milsom I, Eliasson T, et al. TENS is effective in painful menstruation. *Lakartidningen* 1996;93:1219–1222. [In Swedish]
38. Akin MD, Weingand KW, Hengehold DA, et al. Continuous low-level topical heat in the treatment of dysmenorrhea. *Obstet Gynecol* 2001;97:343–349.
39. Proctor ML, Farquhar CM, Sinclair OJ, et al. Surgical interruption of pelvic nerve pathways for primary and secondary dysmenorrhoea. In: The Cochrane Library, Issue 4, 2003. Oxford: Update Software. Search date 1999; primary sources Medline, Embase, Cochrane Controlled Trials Register, and hand searches of citation lists and conference proceedings.
40. Birmingham Women's Health Care NHS Trust. An RCT to assess the efficacy of laparoscopic uterosacral nerve ablation (LUNA) in the treatment of chronic pelvic pain. *The National Research Register* 2002;4:N0047063419. http://www.update-software.com/national/provUpdate.htm (last accessed 8 July 2003).
41. Khan KS, Khan SF, Nwosu CR, et al. Laparoscopic uterosacral nerve ablation in chronic pelvic pain: an overview. *Gynaecol Endosc* 1999;8:257–265. Search date 1997; primary sources Medline, Embase, and Science Citation Index.
42. Rosenwaks Z, Jones GS, Henzl MR, et al. Naproxen sodium, aspirin, and placebo in primary dysmenorrhoea. Reduction of pain and blood levels of prostaglandin-F2-alpha metabolite. *Am J Obstet Gynecol* 1981:140;592–598.

Michelle L Proctor
Cochrane Review Group Co-ordinator
Cochrane Menstrual Disorders and Subfertility Group
Department of Obstetrics and Gynaecology
University of Auckland
Auckland
New Zealand

Cynthia M Farquhar
School of Medicine
University of Auckland
Auckland
New Zealand

Competing interests: None declared.

TABLE 1 Prevalence of dysmenorrhoea: results of community and hospital surveys (see text, p 2305).[4–8]

Study population	Population size	Location	Year	Prevalence
College students aged 17–19 years[4]	165	USA	1996	72% (13% severe)
High school students aged 14–21 years[5]	291	Canada	1997	93% (5% severe)
Adolescents attending an inner city family planning clinic[6]	308	USA	1992	80% (18% severe)
Women from an urban population aged 19 years[7]	596	Sweden	1982	73% (15% severe)
Adolescents aged 12–17 years[8]	2699	USA	1981	60% (14% severe)

TABLE 2 **Effects of aspirin, paracetamol, and compound analgesics for dysmenorrhoea: results of two systematic reviews (see text, p 2306).[13,14]**

Comparison	Usual dosage	Number of RCTs	Number of women	Pain relief	Adverse effects	Conclusion
Aspirin *v* placebo	650 mg four times daily	8	486	RR 1.60 (95% CI 1.12 to 2.29)	No significant difference (7–17% *v* 3–17% on placebo; RR 1.3, 95% CI 0.79 to 2.17)	Aspirin more effective than placebo (NNT 10, 95% CI 5 to 50)
Aspirin *v* paracetamol	650 mg *v* 500 mg four times daily	1	35	Median pain relief: paracetamol 1.6 (95% CI 0.4 to 3.3); aspirin 1.2 (95% CI 0 to 2.7)	NA	No significant difference
Aspirin *v* naproxen	650 mg *v* 275 mg four times daily	1	32	RR 2.29 (95% CI 1.09 to 4.79)	NA	Naproxen more effective than aspirin
Aspirin *v* ibuprofen	650 mg *v* 400 mg four times daily	1	56	RR 1.9 (95% CI 1.13 to 2.78)	NA	Ibuprofen more effective than placebo
Paracetamol *v* placebo	500 mg four times daily	1	35	RR 1.00 (95% CI 0.28 to 3.63)	No significant difference (RR 1.00, 95% CI 0.36 to 2.75)	No significant difference
Paracetamol *v* ibuprofen	1000 mg *v* 400 mg three times daily	1	67	RR 0.86 (95% CI 0.68 to 1.10)	NA	No significant difference
Co-proxamol *v* placebo	650 mg/65 mg four times daily	1	72	RR 3.72 (95% CI 2.13 to 6.52)	NA	Co-proxamol more effective than placebo
Co-proxamol *v* naproxen	650 mg/65 mg *v* 275 mg three times daily	2	98	$P > 0.05$ (no other data could be obtained from the report)	More frequent on co-proxamol (23–58% *v* 15–25% on naproxen; RR 1.94, 95% CI 1.11 to 3.41)	No significant difference
Co-proxamol *v* mefenamic acid	650 mg/65 mg *v* 500 mg three times daily	1	30	$P < 0.01$ (no other evidence can be obtained from the trial)	NA	Mefenamic acid more effective than co-proxamol

NA, not available.

Endometriosis

Search date March 2004

Neil Johnson and Cynthia Farquhar

QUESTIONS

INTERVENTIONS

See glossary Ⓖ

Key Messages

- We found no RCTs comparing medical with surgical treatments.

Hormones at diagnosis

- **Combined oral contraceptives or medroxyprogesterone** RCTs found that hormonal treatments at diagnosis (combined oral contraceptives, danazol, gestrinone, gonadorelin analogues, or medroxyprogesterone acetate) reduced pain attributed to endometriosis over 3–6 months of treatment, and were all similarly effective. One small RCT identified by a systematic review found that low dose combined oral contraceptive reduced dysmenorrhoea compared with goserelin during 6 months of treatment, but all women improved 6 months after stopping treatment. One additional, larger RCT found no significant difference in relief of menstrual or non-menstrual pain between combined oral contraceptives and combined oral contraceptives plus gonadorelin analogues. Adverse effects of hormonal treatments are common. One RCT found that combined oral contraceptives reduced hot flushes, insomnia, and vaginal dryness compared with gonadorelin analogues.

- **Danazol, gestrinone, or gonadorelin analogues** RCTs found that hormonal treatments at diagnosis (combined oral contraceptives, danazol, gestrinone, gonadorelin analogues, or medroxyprogesterone acetate) reduced pain attributed to endometriosis over 3–6 months of treatment, and were all similarly effective. One small RCT identified by a systematic review found that low dose combined oral contraceptive reduced dysmenorrhoea compared with goserelin during 6 months of treatment, but all women improved 6 months after stopping treatment. One additional, larger RCT found no significant difference in relief of menstrual or non-menstrual pain between combined oral contraceptives and combined oral contraceptives plus gonadorelin analogues. Adverse effects of hormonal treatments are common, and include hot flushes and bone loss with gonadorelin analogues or gestrinone and androgenic adverse effects with danazol. One RCT found that combined oral contraceptives reduced hot flushes, insomnia, and vaginal dryness compared with gonadorelin analogues.
- **Dydrogesterone** One small RCT provided insufficient evidence to compare dydrogesterone with placebo.

Preoperative hormones

- **Hormonal treatment before surgery** Two RCTs provided insufficient evidence on the effects of hormonal treatment before surgery in women with pain attributed to endometriosis.

Surgery

- **Combined laparoscopic ablation of endometrial deposits and uterine nerve** One RCT found limited evidence that laparoscopic ablation of endometrial deposits plus laparoscopic uterine nerve ablation reduced pain at 6 months compared with diagnostic laparoscopy, and that pain reduction persisted for up to 5 years in more than 50% of the women. Two small RCTs identified by a systematic review and one larger subsequent RCT found no significant difference between laparoscopic ablation of endometrial deposits plus laparoscopic uterine nerve ablation and laparoscopic ablation alone in rates of recurrent dysmenorrhoea at 6 months to 3 years. The subsequent RCT found no significant difference between treatments in treatment satisfaction at 1 year. However, the RCTs may have been too small to detect clinically important differences.
- **Laparoscopic ablation of endometrial deposits alone** We found no RCTs comparing laparoscopic ablation of endometrial deposits alone in women with pain attributed to endometriosis. Two small RCTs identified by a systematic review and one larger subsequent RCT found no significant difference between laparoscopic ablation alone and laparoscopic ablation of endometrial deposits plus laparoscopic uterine nerve ablation alone in rates of recurrent dysmenorrhoea at 6 months to 3 years. The subsequent RCT found no significant difference between treatments in treatment satisfaction at 1 year. However, the RCTs may have been too small to detect clinically important differences. We found no RCTs comparing laser versus diathermy ablation of endometrial deposits.
- **Laparoscopic uterine nerve ablation alone** We found no RCTs evaluating laparoscopic uterine nerve ablation alone in women with pain attributed to endometriosis.

Hormones post conservative surgery

- **Hormonal treatment after conservative surgery** RCTs found that, compared with placebo or expectant management, 6 months of hormonal treatment with danazol or gonadorelin analogues after surgery reduced pain and delayed the recurrence of pain at 12 and 24 months. Treatment for 3 months with danazol or gonadorelin analogues or treatment with combined oral contraceptives for 6 months did not seem to be effective. One RCT found that cyproterone acetate and combined oral contraceptives were similarly effective in women with modest and severe pain. One small RCT found that a levonorgestrel releasing intrauterine device inserted after surgery reduced dysmenorrhoea compared with surgery alone at 1 year. Adverse effects of hormonal treatment are common and include hot flushes and bone loss with gonadorelin analogues and androgenic adverse effects with danazol.

Hormones post oophorectomy

- **Hormonal treatment after oophorectomy** One RCT in women who previously had an oophorectomy found insufficient evidence on the effects of hormone replacement therapy in recurrence of endometriosis compared with no treatment.

Treating ovarian endometrioma

- **Laparoscopic cystectomy for ovarian endometrioma (reduces pain compared to drainage)** One RCT found that laparoscopic cystectomy reduced pain caused by ovarian endometrioma at 2 years compared with laparoscopic drainage. Complication rates were similar.

DEFINITION Endometriosis is characterised by ectopic endometrial tissue, which can cause dysmenorrhoea, dyspareunia, non-cyclical pelvic pain, and subfertility. Diagnosis is made by laparoscopy. Most endometrial deposits are found in the pelvis (ovaries, peritoneum, uterosacral ligaments, pouch of Douglas, and rectovaginal septum). Extrapelvic deposits, including those in the umbilicus and diaphragm, are rare. Severity of endometriosis(G) is defined by the American Fertility Society: this review uses the terms mild (stage I and II), moderate (stage III), and severe (stage IV).[1] Endometriomas are cysts of endometriosis within the ovary. This review assesses dysmenorrhoea, dyspareunia, and non-cyclical pelvic pain associated with endometriosis. For subfertility associated with endometriosis see infertility and subfertility, p 2365.

INCIDENCE/ PREVALENCE In asymptomatic women, the prevalence of endometriosis is 2–22%.[2-5] Variations in estimates of prevalence are thought to be mostly due to differences in diagnostic thresholds and criteria between studies, and in variations in childbearing age between populations, rather than underlying genetic differences. In women with dysmenorrhoea, the incidence of endometriosis is 40–60%, and in women with subfertility is 20–30%.[3,6,7] The severity of symptoms and the probability of diagnosis increase with age.[8] Incidence peaks at about 40 years of age.[9] Symptoms and laparoscopic appearance do not always correlate.[10]

AETIOLOGY/ RISK FACTORS The cause of endometriosis is unknown. Risk factors include early menarche and late menopause. Embryonic cells may give rise to deposits in the umbilicus, whereas retrograde menstruation may deposit endometrial cells in the diaphragm.[11,12] Use of oral contraceptives reduces the risk of endometriosis, and this protective effect persists for up to 1 year after their discontinuation.[9]

PROGNOSIS We found two RCTs in which laparoscopy was repeated after treatment in women given placebo.[13,14] Over 6–12 months, endometrial deposits resolved spontaneously in up to a third of women, deteriorated in nearly half, and were unchanged in the remainder.

AIMS OF INTERVENTION To relieve pain (dysmenorrhoea, dyspareunia, and other pelvic pain), with minimal adverse effects.

OUTCOMES American Fertility Society scores for size and number of deposits;[1] recurrence rates; time between stopping treatment and recurrence; rate of adverse effects of treatment. **In women with pain:** Relief of pain, assessed by a visual analogue scale ranging from 0 to 10, and subjective improvement. **In women having surgery:** Ease of surgical intervention (rated by the surgeon as easy, average, difficult, or very difficult).[15]

METHODS *Clinical Evidence* search and appraisal March 2004. The authors also sought RCTs by electronic searching of databases, hand searches of 30 key journals, searches of reference lists of other RCTs, and identifying unpublished studies from abstracts, proceedings, and pharmaceutical companies. The authors' most recent search was completed in May 2004. They used the search strategy and database of the Cochrane Menstrual Disorders and Subfertility Group, updated on a monthly basis, to identify RCTs on Medline and Embase. They included RCTs that used adequate diagnostic criteria for inclusion of participants (endometriosis diagnosed either by laparoscopy or laparotomy in association with dysmenorrhoea, dyspareunia, other pelvic pain, or infertility) and that assessed clinical outcomes (see outcomes above). Trials comparing different hormonal treatments of the same class were not assessed.

QUESTION What are the effects of hormonal treatments given at diagnosis?

OPTION HORMONAL TREATMENTS AT DIAGNOSIS

RCTs found that hormonal treatments at diagnosis (combined oral contraceptives, danazol, gestrinone, gonadorelin analogues, or medroxyprogesterone acetate) reduced pain attributed to endometriosis over 3–6 months of treatment, and were all similarly effective. One small RCT provided insufficient evidence to compare dydrogesterone with placebo. One small RCT identified by a systematic review found that low dose combined oral contraceptive reduced dysmenorrhoea compared with goserelin during 6 months of treatment, but all women improved 6 months after stopping treatment. One additional, larger RCT found no significant difference in relief of menstrual or non-menstrual pain between combined oral contraceptives and combined oral contraceptives followed by gonadorelin analogues. Adverse effects of hormonal treatments are common, and include hot flushes and bone loss with gonadorelin analogues or gestrinone and androgenic adverse effects with danazol. One RCT found that combined oral contraceptives reduced hot flushes, insomnia, and vaginal dryness compared with gonadorelin analogues.

Benefits: We found four systematic reviews (search dates 1998,[16] 2000,[17] 2001,[18] and 2003[19]) of 6 months of continuous ovulation suppression (using combined oral contraceptives, danazol, gestrinone, gonadorelin analogues, or medroxyprogesterone acetate). The reviews found that all treatments were similarly effective in reducing severe and moderate**G** pain at 6 months. **Versus placebo or no treatment:** Three RCTs (155 women) identified by the reviews[16–18] found that danazol, gonadorelin analogues, and medroxyprogesterone acetate all significantly reduced pain at 3–6 months compared with placebo (see table 1, p 2339). One RCT (22 women) identified by the second review[17] found no significant difference between dydrogesterone and placebo in the proportion of women who had pain relief, but it may have been underpowered to detect a clinically important difference. Additional placebo-controlled RCTs found that, in women who received 12 months of leuprolide (a gonadorelin agonist) or norethisterone (a progestogen) with or without oestrogen, pain relief was maintained for the duration of treatment and up to 8 months after treatment was stopped.[20,21] **Combined oral contraceptives versus gonadorelin analogues:** The fourth review[19] (1 RCT,[22] 57 women with laparoscopically diagnosed endometriosis and moderate or severe**G** pain) found that cyclic low dose monophasic combined oral contraceptive was significantly more effective for relief of dysmenorrhoea than goserelin (3.6 mg subcutaneous depot formulation monthly for 6 months of treatment; 21/24 [88%] with combined oral contraceptive *v* 0/25 [0%] with goserelin; OR 33.1, 95% CI 10.8 to 101.0).[19] After 6 months of follow up without treatment, all women improved (24/24 [100%] with combined oral contraceptive *v* 25/25 [100%] with goserelin). The review found no significant difference between combined cyclic low dose monophasic oral contraceptives and goserelin in the relief of dyspareunia or non-menstrual pain at the end of 6 months of treatment (OR 0.93, 95% CI 0.25 to 3.53).[19] One additional RCT (102 women) compared combined oral contraceptive for 12 months versus combined oral contraceptive for 4 months followed by gonadorelin analogues for 8 months.[23] It found no difference in the proportion of women with pain (either menstrual or non-menstrual) at 12 months (menstrual pain: 14/47 [29.8%] with combined oral contraceptive *v* 16/55 [29.1%] with combined oral contraceptive followed by gonadorelin analogues; non-menstrual pain: 15/47 [31.9%] with combined oral contraceptive *v* 17/55 [30.9%] with combined oral contraceptive followed by gonadorelin analogues; reported as non-significant, CI not reported). **Danazol versus gestrinone:** The second review identified one RCT (269 women) comparing danazol 200 mg daily versus gestrinone 2.5 mg twice weekly.[24] It found no significant difference in dysmenorrhoea over 6 months of treatment between danazol and gestrinone (reported as non-significant, results presented graphically), although both groups significantly improved from baseline ($P < 0.001$). **Danazol versus gonadorelin analogues:** The first systematic review identified 15 RCTs (1299 women) comparing gonadorelin analogues versus danazol.[16] After 6 months of treatment, the review found no significant difference in menstrual pain (5 RCTs, 386 women; RR 1.09, 95% CI 0.99 to 1.20), dyspareunia (6 RCTs, 476 women; RR 0.98, 95% CI 0.93 to 1.02), or resolution of endometrial deposits (3 RCTs, 426 women; RR 0.84, 95% CI 0.56 to 1.26).[16] **Gestrinone versus gonadorelin analogues:** One RCT identified by the second systematic review[17] found that both gestrinone and gonadorelin analogues significantly reduced all types of pain from baseline over 3 months. It found that gestrinone modestly, but significantly, reduced dyspareunia after 6 months' treatment compared with gonadorelin analogues (measured by a visual analogue scale: WMD –1.16, 95% CI –2.08 to –0.24), but gonadorelin analogues significantly reduced dysmenorrhoea (WMD 0.82, 95% CI 0.15 to 1.49). It found no significant difference in non-menstrual pain between gestrinone and gonadorelin analogues (WMD –0.41, 95% CI –1.76 to +0.94). **Medroxyprogesterone acetate versus combined oral contraceptives plus danazol:** One RCT (80 women) identified by the second review[17] compared medroxyprogesterone acetate (150 mg every 3 months) versus combined oral contraceptive plus danazol 50 mg daily. It found that medroxyprogesterone acetate was more effective at reducing dysmenorrhoea, but not dyspareunia or non-menstrual pain (CI not reported). **Medroxyprogesterone acetate versus gonadorelin analogues:** We found one RCT (double blind; 48 women with endometriosis treated for 6 months and followed for 1 year after allocation) that compared medroxyprogesterone versus gonadorelin analogues.[25] It found that both treatments significantly improved symptoms attributable to endometriosis, sleep disturbances, and anxiety–depression scores from baseline measurements ($P < 0.05$ for all outcomes). It found no significant difference between treatments (reported as non-significant, CI not reported).

Harms: **Versus placebo or no treatment:** One review found that gonadorelin analogues significantly increased hot flushes and headaches compared with placebo (hot flushes: about 80% with gonadorelin analogues *v* 30% with placebo; RR 2.7, 95% CI 1.5 to 4.8; headaches: 33% gonadorelin analogues *v* 10% with placebo; RR 3.6, 95% CI 1.1 to 11.5).[16] Gonadorelin analogues are associated with hypo-oestrogenic symptoms, such as hot flushes and vaginal dryness. RCTs have found that adding oestrogen, progestogens, or tibolone significantly relieves hot flushes caused by gonadorelin analogues (reducing symptom scores by ≥ 50%).[20,21,26–28] One RCT found that danazol 100 mg daily after surgery increased adverse effects after 6 months compared with no treatment (spotting: 12% with danazol *v* 7% with no treatment; bloating: 16% with danazol *v* 9% with no treatment; headache: 21% with danazol *v* 13% with no treatment; weight gain: 22% with danazol *v* 14% with no treatment) (see hormonal treatment after surgery, p 2334).[29] **Combined oral contraceptives versus gonadorelin analogues:** The fourth review found that goserelin significantly increased hot flushes, insomnia, and vaginal dryness compared with combined oral contraceptives (hot flushes, 1 RCT: 1/28 [4%] with combined oral contraceptives *v* 24/29 [83%] with goserelin; OR 0.04, 95% CI 0.02 to 0.12; insomnia, 1 RCT: 0/28 [0%] with combined oral contraceptives *v* 7/29 [24%] with goserelin; OR 0.11, 95% CI 0.02 to 0.53; vaginal dryness: 0/28 [0%] with combined oral contraceptives *v* 5/29 [17%] with goserelin; OR 0.12, 95% CI 0.02 to 0.74).[19] **Danazol versus gestrinone:** The second review found that gestrinone significantly increased greasy skin and hirsutism compared with danazol (greasy skin, 2 RCTs: 69/149 [46%] with gestrinone *v* 37/153 [24%] with danazol; OR 2.68, 95% CI 1.67 to 4.31; hirsutism, 2 RCTs: 68/149 [46%] with gestrinone *v* 38/153 [25%] with danazol; OR 2.63, 95% CI 1.62 to 4.28).[17] However, it found that gestrinone significantly reduced muscle cramps, hunger, and breast size reduction compared with danazol (muscle cramps, 2 RCTs: 48/149 [32%] with gestrinone *v* 75/153 [49%] with danazol; OR 0.49, 95% CI 0.31 to 0.78; hunger, 1 RCT: 69/130 [53%] with gestrinone *v* 88/134 [66%] with danazol; OR 0.59, 95% CI 0.36 to 0.97; reduction in breast size, 2 RCTs: 54/149 [36%] with gestrinone *v* 73/153 [48%] with danazol; OR 0.62, 95% CI 0.39 to 0.98).[17] **Gestrinone versus gonadorelin analogues:** One RCT identified by the second systematic review found that gestrinone significantly reduced hot flushes compared with gonadorelin analogues (8/27 [30%] with gestrinone *v* 19/28 [68%] with gonadorelin analogues; OR 0.22, 95% CI 0.08 to 0.64).[17] **Medroxyprogesterone versus combined oral contraceptives plus danazol:** One RCT (80 women) found that medroxyprogesterone significantly increased bloating and spotting compared with combined oral contraceptives plus danazol (bloating: OR 4.04, 95% CI 1.68 to 9.70; spotting: OR 16.3, 95% CI 6.8 to 39.2).[17] One small RCT (28 women with previous laparoscopic surgery) found that medroxyprogesterone acetate increased amenorrhoea, breakthrough bleeding, bloating, and weight gain compared with combined oral contraceptives plus danazol (amenorrhoea: 20% with medroxyprogesterone acetate *v* 0% with combined oral contraceptives plus danazol; breakthrough bleeding: 15% with medroxyprogesterone acetate *v* 0% with combined oral contraceptives plus danazol; bloating: 63% with medroxyprogesterone acetate *v* 28% with combined oral contraceptives plus danazol; weight gain: 53% with medroxyprogesterone acetate *v* 30% with combined oral contraceptives plus danazol).[29] **Medroxyprogesterone acetate versus gonadorelin analogues:** The RCT gave no information on adverse effects.[25]

Comment: The RCTs were mainly small with no long term follow up. The RCT addressing quality of life had high withdrawal rates (18/48 [38%]).[25] One RCT suggested that bone loss associated with prolonged use of gonadorelin analogue (12 months) may be prevented by using norethisterone with or without oestrogen.[21]

QUESTION What are the effects of hormonal treatments before surgery?

OPTION PREOPERATIVE HORMONAL TREATMENT

Two RCTs provided insufficient evidence on the effects of hormonal treatment before surgery in women with pain attributed to endometriosis.

Benefits: We found no systematic review but found two RCTs comparing treatment with a gonadorelin analogue before surgery versus no preoperative hormonal treatment.[15,30] The first RCT (75 women with moderate or severe**Ⓖ** endometriosis) compared 6 months of nafarelin before surgery versus surgery followed by 6 months of nafarelin.[15] It found that 6 months of nafarelin 200 μg before surgery significantly reduced symptom scores compared with 6 months of nafarelin after surgery (mean American Fertility Society score: 0 with nafarelin before surgery *v* 6 with nafarelin after surgery; P = 0.007).[15] It found no significant difference in ease of surgery as assessed by the surgeon (proportion of women judged easy to treat: 14/25 [56%] with nafarelin before surgery v 10/28 [36%] with no treatment before surgery; RR 1.60, 95% CI 0.86 to 2.90).[15] The second RCT (48 women with moderate or severe**G** endometriosis) compared 3 months goserelin treatment before surgery with no pre-operative hormonal treatment, and found similar symptoms in both groups at 6 months after surgery.[30] It also found no significant difference in the proportion of women whose surgery was rated as "moderately" or "very" difficult (14/20 [70%] with goserelin before surgery v 20/27 [74%] with no treatment before surgery; RR 0.94, 95% CI 0.60 to 1.50).

Harms: The first RCT found that nafarelin was associated with hot flushes (96% with nafarelin before surgery v 92% with nafarelin after surgery), vaginal dryness (43% with nafarelin before surgery v 32% with nafarelin after surgery), and decreased libido (36% with nafarelin before surgery v 36% with nafarelin after surgery).[15] In the second RCT, adverse events were also reported frequently both in women receiving gonadorelin analogues before surgery and in women receiving no treatment (AR for at least 1 adverse event: 18/21 [86%] with gonadorelin analogue v 21/27 [78%] with no treatment; RR 1.1, 95% CI 0.8 to 1.4).[30] The most frequently reported adverse effects were hot flushes and headaches, and these happened only in women receiving gonadorelin analogue (hot flushes 13/21 [62%], headaches 6/21 [29%]). See also harms of hormonal treatments, p 2329.

Comment: The second RCT may have been too small to exclude a clinically important effect.[30]

QUESTION What are the effects of surgical treatments?

OPTION LAPAROSCOPIC ABLATION OF ENDOMETRIAL DEPOSITS

We found no RCTs evaluating laparoscopic ablation of endometrial deposits alone. One RCT found limited evidence that ablation of deposits plus laparoscopic uterine nerve ablation reduced pain at 6 months compared with diagnostic laparoscopy, and that pain reduction persisted for up to 5 years in more than half of the women. Two small RCTs identified by a systematic review and one larger subsequent RCT found no significant difference between laparoscopic ablation of endometrial deposits plus laparoscopic uterine nerve ablation and laparoscopic ablation alone in rates of recurrent dysmenorrhoea at 6 months to 3 years. The subsequent RCT found no significant difference between treatments in overall treatment satisfaction at 1 year. However, the RCTs may have been too small to detect clinically important differences. We found no RCTs comparing laser versus diathermy ablation.

Benefits: **Laparoscopic ablation alone versus diagnostic laparoscopy or no treatment:** We found no RCTs comparing laparoscopic ablation alone versus diagnostic laparoscopy or no treatment in women with pain attributed to endometriosis. **Laparoscopic ablation plus laparoscopic uterine nerve ablation (LUNA) versus diagnostic laparoscopy:** We found one systematic review (search date 1999), which identified one RCT (63 women with mild to moderate endometriosis**G**) comparing laparoscopic ablation of deposits**G** plus LUNA**G** versus diagnostic laparoscopy.[31–33] The RCT found that ablation plus LUNA significantly reduced pain at 6 months (median decrease in pain score on a 10 cm visual analogue scale: 2.85cm with ablation v 0.05cm with diagnostic laparoscopy; P = 0.01).[31] Follow up of the RCT suggested that 90% of the women who responded continued to have pain improvement at 1 year,[32] and 55% at 5 years.[33] **Laparoscopic ablation plus LUNA versus laparoscopic ablation alone:** We found one systematic review[34] and one subsequent RCT[35] of laparoscopic ablation of endometrial deposits**G** plus LUNA. The review (search date 1998) identified two RCTs (132 women with mild to severe endometriosis**G**; age range 18–40 years) comparing laparoscopic ablation plus LUNA versus laparoscopic ablation alone.[34] The RCTs found no clinically important difference in pain relief at 6–9 months after laparoscopic ablation plus LUNA and laparoscopic ablation alone (pain measured by a visual analogue scale; P = 0.12 in one RCT, CI not reported in the other). The largest RCT (81 women) identified by the review found that satisfaction with treatment was high in both groups (68% with laparoscopic ablation plus LUNA *v* 73% laparoscopic ablation alone). The subsequent RCT (180 women with stage I–IV endometriosis, 156 analyzed at 1 year, 116 analyzed at 3 years) found no significant difference in recurrence of dysmenorrhoea between laparoscopic surgery plus LUNA and laparoscopic ablation alone at 1 or 3 years (1 year: 23/78 [29%] with laparoscopic ablation plus LUNA *v* 21/78 [27%] with laparoscopic ablation alone; P = 0.86; 3 years: 21/59 [36%] with laparoscopic ablation plus LUNA *v* 18/57 [32%] with laparoscopic ablation alone, P = 0.79).[35] It found no significant difference between treatments in satisfaction with treatment rates at 1 year (satisfied or very satisfied: 55/90 [61%] with laparoscopic ablation plus LUNA *v* 59/90 [65%] with laparoscopic ablation alone; P = 0.76). **Laser versus diathermy ablation:** We found no RCTs.

Harms: **Laparoscopic ablation plus LUNA versus diagnostic laparoscopy:** The RCT identified by the first review reported that no adverse effects were observed.[31] **Laparoscopic ablation plus LUNA versus laparoscopic ablation alone:** The RCTs identified by the second review gave no information on adverse effects.[34] The subsequent RCT found no adverse effects (specifically changes in bladder or intestinal function) attributable to LUNA**G**.[35] Potential harms of laparoscopic ablation include adhesions, reduced fertility, and damage to other pelvic structures.

Comment: The RCTs included in the review may have been underpowered to exclude a clinically important difference in outcomes.[34] Further trials are needed. An RCT of LUNA**G** is underway in Auckland, New Zealand. One hundred and ten women were randomised and 12 months of follow up data were due by the end of 2003 (Farquhar C, personal communication, 2003).

OPTION LAPAROSCOPIC UTERINE NERVE ABLATION (LUNA)

We found no RCTs evaluating laparoscopic uterine nerve ablation alone. One RCT found limited evidence that laparoscopic uterine nerve ablation plus laparoscopic ablation of endometrial deposits reduced pain at 6 months compared with diagnostic laparoscopy, and that pain reduction persisted for up to 5 years in more than half of the women. Two small RCTs identified by a systematic review and one larger subsequent RCT found no significant difference between laparoscopic ablation of endometrial deposits plus laparoscopic uterine nerve ablation and laparoscopic ablation alone in rates of recurrent dysmenorrhoea at 6 months to 3 years. The subsequent RCT found no significant difference between treatments in overall treatment satisfaction at 1 year. The RCTs may have been too small to detect a clinically important difference.

Benefits: We found no RCTs evaluating laparoscopic uterine nerve ablation**G** alone in women with pain attributed to endometriosis. **Plus laparoscopic ablation of endometrial deposits:** See benefits of laparoscopic ablation of endometrial deposits, p 2333.

Harms: Potential harms of laparoscopic uterine nerve ablationⒼ include denervation of pelvic structures and uterine prolapse (see harms of laparoscopic ablation of endometrial deposits, p 2334).

Comment: None.

QUESTION What are the effects of hormonal treatment after conservative surgery?

OPTION HORMONAL TREATMENT AFTER CONSERVATIVE SURGERY

RCTs found that, compared with placebo or expectant management, 6 months of hormonal treatment with danazol or gonadorelin analogues after surgery reduced pain and delayed the recurrence of pain at 12 and 24 months. Treatment for 3 months with danazol or gonadorelin analogues or treatment with combined oral contraceptives for 6 months did not seem to be effective. One RCT found that cyproterone acetate and combined oral contraceptives were similarly effective in women with modest and severe pain. One small RCT found that a levonorgestrel releasing intrauterine device inserted after surgery reduced dysmenorrhoea compared with surgery alone at 1 year. Adverse effects of hormonal treatment are common and include hot flushes and bone loss with gonadorelin analogues and androgenic adverse effects with danazol.

Benefits: We found no systematic review. We found nine RCTs.[29,36–43] Four RCTs found that 6 months of treatment with danazol, medroxyprogesterone acetate, or gonadorelin analogues after laparoscopic conservative surgeryⒼ significantly reduced pain over 1–2 years compared with placebo or expectant management. However, three RCTs found no significant difference in pain relief if treatment was given for 3 months. One RCT found no significant difference between 6 months of treatment with a monophasic combined oral contraceptive and placebo in pain at 22 months. One small RCT found that a levonorgestrel releasing intrauterine device inserted after surgery significantly reduced dysmenorrhoea compared with surgery alone at 1 year.[43] **Combined oral contraceptive versus placebo for 6 months:** One RCT (70 women who had had laparoscopic conservative surgeryⒼ) comparing combined oral contraceptives after surgery versus placebo for 6 months found no significant difference in recurrence of endometriosis (mean follow up 22 months; recurrences: 2/33 [6%] with oral contraceptives *v* 1/35 [3%] with no treatment; RR 2.1, 95% CI 0.2 to 22.3).[41] The RCT may have been underpowered to detect a clinically important difference. **Danazol versus placebo or versus expectant management for 6 months:** We found two RCTs.[29,38] The first RCT (28 women with moderateⒼ endometriosis who had had conservative surgery followed by monthly injections of decapeptyl for 6 months) compared danazol 100 mg daily for 6 months versus expectant management.[29] It found that danazol significantly reduced pain at both 12 months ($P < 0.01$) and 24 months ($P < 0.05$). Overall, recurrence at 24 months was 44% with danazol compared with 67% with expectant management ($P < 0.05$). The second RCT (60 women with mild to severeⒼ endometriosis who had had conservative surgery) compared three interventions: danazol 600 mg daily, medroxyprogesterone 100 mg daily, or placebo for 180 days after surgery. It found that danazol significantly reduced pain compared with placebo at 6 months (absolute results presented graphically; $P < 0.05$).[38] **Danazol versus placebo for 3 months:** One RCT (77 women with moderate to severe endometriosis who had had laparoscopic conservative surgery) compared danazol 600 mg daily after surgery versus placebo for 3 months.[37] It found no significant difference in pain relief 6 months after finishing treatment (moderate to severe pain: 7/31 [23%] with danazol v 9/29 [31%] with placebo; RR 0.73, 95% CI 0.31 to 1.70). **Gonadorelin (gonadotrophin releasing hormone) analogues versus placebo or expectant management for 6 months:** We found two RCTs.[39,40] The first RCT (109 women with mild to moderate symptomatic endometriosis who had had laparoscopic conservative surgery) found that nafarelin 200 μg twice daily after surgery significantly reduced pain after 6 months of treatment compared with placebo ($P = 0.001$).[39] The second RCT (269 women with mild to moderate symptomatic endometriosis who had had laparoscopic conservative surgery) compared 6 months of open label allocation of 3.6 mg of subcutaneous goserelin versus expectant management with 2 years of follow up.[40] It found that goserelin significantly reduced pain scores over 2 years ($P = 0.008$) and delayed the recurrence of pain by more than 12 months.[40] **Gonadorelin analogues versus placebo or expectant management for 3 months:** We found two RCTs.[36,42] The first RCT (75 women with mild to moderate endometriosis who had had laparotomy) compared nafarelin after surgery versus placebo for 3 months.[36] It found no significant difference in pain at 12 months (assessed by a visual analogue scale: 7.0 with nafarelin v 6.9 with placebo; reported as non-significant, CI not reported).[36] The second RCT (89 women with moderate to severe endometriosis who had had laparoscopic conservative surgery) compared monthly intramuscular leuprolide acetate depot injections after surgery for 3 months versus expectant management with 36 months of follow up.[42] It found no significant difference in pain (moderate to severe pain recurrence during follow up: 10/44 [23%] with leuprolide acetate v 11/45 [24%] with expectant management; cumulative pain recurrence rates at 18 months: 23% with leuprolide acetate v 29% with expectant management; log rank test not significant). **Medroxyprogesterone acetate versus placebo for 6 months:** We found one RCT (60 women with mild to severe endometriosis who had had conservative surgery) comparing three interventions: medroxyprogesterone 100 mg daily, danazol 600 mg daily, or placebo for 180 days after surgery. It found that medroxyprogesterone significantly reduced pain compared with placebo at 6 months (absolute results presented graphically; $P < 0.05$).[38] **Cyproterone acetate versus combined oral contraceptive:** One RCT (open label, 90 women with recurrent pelvic pain of more than 6 months of duration after complete surgical eradication of endometriosis) compared low dose continuous cyproterone acetate after surgery versus a continuous monophasic combined oral contraceptive.[44] It found that both treatments were similarly effective in women with modest and severe pain. It found no significant difference between treatments in the proportion of women who were satisfied with treatment (33/45 [73%] with cyproterone acetate v 30/45 [67%] with oral contraceptive; RR 1.1, 95% CI 0.8 to 1.4). **Levonorgestrel intrauterine systems:** We found one small RCT (40 women who had conservative laparoscopic surgery).[43] After 1 year of follow up, it found that a levonorgestrel intrauterine device (Lng-IUD) inserted after surgery significantly reduced moderate or severe dysmenorrhoea compared with surgery alone (dysmenorrhoea assessed on 0–100 mm visual analogue scale [0 = no pain, 100 = most severe pain]; AR for score > 51: 2/20 [10%] with Lng-IUD v 9/20 [45%] with no Lng-IUD; $P = 0.03$). It found no significant difference between treatments in the proportion of women who were satisfied with treatment after 1 year (15/20 [75%] with Lng-IUD v 10/20 [50%] with with no Lng-IUD; P value not reported). The RCT may have been too small to detect a clinically important difference in satisfaction.

Harms: See harms of hormonal treatments, p 2329. **Levonorgestrel intrauterine systems:** The RCT comparing Lng-IUD versus no Lng-IUD reported adverse effects in eight women who had a Lng-IUD inserted.

The Lng-IUD was removed in one woman because the system became displaced.[43] Adverse effects among women with Lng-IUD included bloating (6/20 [30%]), weight gain (6/20 [30%]), headache (3/20 [15%]), seborrhoea and acne (2/20 [10%]), breast tenderness (1/20 [5%]), decreased libido (1/20 [5%]), and pelvic pain (1/20 [5%]). The study did not report on adverse effects in the control group.

Comment: The RCTs were mainly small with no long term follow up.

QUESTION **What are the effects of hormonal treatment after oophorectomy (with or without hysterectomy)?**

OPTION **HORMONAL TREATMENT AFTER OOPHORECTOMY**

One RCT in women who previously had an oophorectomy found insufficient evidence on the effects of hormone replacement therapy in recurrence of endometriosis compared with no treatment.

Benefits: We found no systematic review. We found one RCT (172 women who previously had bilateral salpingo-oophorectomy, 91.8% of whom had total abdominal hysterectomy**G**) comparing hormone replacement therapy (HRT; 115 women) versus no treatment (57 women).[45] HRT consisted of two, weekly 1.5 mg oestradiol patches and 200 mg daily of micronised progesterone given orally during 14 days followed by a 16 day interval free of treatment. HRT was started 4 weeks after the salpingo-oophorectomy. It found no significant difference in recurrence rates at a mean of 45 months (4/115 [3.5%] with HRT *v* 0/57 [0%] with no HRT; ARI +3.5%, 95% CI –3.2% to +8.6%). The risk factors for recurrence were women who had endometriotic peritoneal involvement > 3 cm (2.4% with HRT *v* 0.3% with no HRT) and incomplete hysterectomy (22.2% with HRT *v* 1.9% with no HRT).

Harms: The RCT found that surgical re-interventions were more frequent with HRT but this difference was not significant (2.6% with HRT *v* 0% with no HRT; OR 4.5, 95% CI 0.4 to 60.0).[45]

Comment: The RCT had insufficient power to exclude clinically important differences.[45]

QUESTION **What are the effects of treatments for ovarian endometrioma?**

OPTION **LAPAROSCOPIC CYSTECTOMY**

One RCT found that laparoscopic cystectomy reduced pain caused by ovarian endometrioma at 2 years compared with laparoscopic drainage. Complication rates were similar.

Benefits: **In women with pain attributed to endometrioma:** We found no systematic review. We found one RCT (64 women) comparing laparoscopic cystectomy**G** versus laparoscopic drainage**G** and coagulation.[46] It found that cystectomy significantly reduced the recurrence of pain at 2 years (OR 0.2, 95% CI 0.1 to 0.8) and increased the pain free interval after operation compared with drainage (median interval: 19.0 months with cystectomy *v* 9.5 months with drainage; $P < 0.05$).[46]

Harms: The RCT reported no intraoperative or postoperative complications in either group.[46]

Comment: None.

GLOSSARY

Conservative surgery Surgery to conserve the pelvic organs.

Laparoscopic ablation of endometrial deposits A surgical procedure where a long tube with a fibre-optic telescope (the laparoscope) is inserted into a woman's abdomen to ablate (destroy) the endometrial deposits around the ovaries and uterus in order to relieve pain.

Laparoscopic cystectomy During laparoscopy the cyst wall of the endometrioma is excised or stripped.

Laparoscopic drainage During laparoscopy the endometrioma contents are drained out.

Laparoscopic uterine nerve ablation (LUNA) The cutting of nerves in the uterus to stop chronic pain. This is carried out laparoscopically through a small incision in the abdomen so the outside surface of the uterus and uterine nerves can be seen.

Severity of endometriosis Determination of the stage or degree of endometrial involvement is based on the American Fertility Society Scale of weighted point scale of estimations, evaluating the degree of involvement of the peritoneum, ovaries, and fallopian tubes.[1] According to the allocated score, endometriosis is categorised as: **Mild (stage I and II)** American Fertility Society score of 1–15 points **Moderate (stage III)** American Fertility Society score of 16–40 points. **Severe (stage IV)** American Fertility Society score of > 40 points.

Total abdominal hysterectomy Open operation through the abdominal wall to remove the uterus. In some situations, this is performed in conjunction with a bilateral salpingo-oophorectomy, the removal of both ovaries and fallopian tubes.

Substantive changes

Laparoscopic deposit ablation One RCT added.[35] Categorisation unchanged.

Hormonal treatments after conservative surgery One RCT added.[43] Categorisation unchanged.

REFERENCES

1. American Fertility Society. Revised American Fertility Society (RAFS) classification of endometriosis. *Fertil Steril* 1985;43:351–352.
2. Mahmood TA, Templeton A. Prevalence and genesis of endometriosis. *Hum Reprod* 1991;6:544–549.
3. Gruppo Italiano per lo studio dell'endometriosi. Prevalence and anatomical distribution of endometriosis in women with selected gynaecological conditions: results from a multicentric Italian study. *Hum Reprod* 1994;9:1158–1162.
4. Moen MH, Schei B. Epidemiology of endometriosis in a Norwegian County. *Acta Obstet Gynecol Scand* 1997;76:559–562.
5. Eskenazi B, Warner ML. Epidemiology of endometriosis. *Obstet Gynecol Clin North Am* 1997;24:235–258.
6. Ajossa S, Mais V, Guerriero S, et al. The prevalence of endometriosis in premenopausal women undergoing gynecological surgery. *Clin Exp Obstet Gynecol* 1994;21:195–197.
7. Waller KG, Lindsay P, Curtis P, et al. The prevalence of endometriosis in women with infertile partners. *Eur J Obstet Gynecol Reprod Biol* 1993;48:135–139.
8. Berube S, Marcoux S, Maheux R. Characteristics related to the prevalence of minimal or mild endometriosis in infertile women. Canadian Collaborative Group on Endometriosis. *Epidemiology* 1998;9:504–510.
9. Vessey MP, Villard-Mackintosh L, Painter R. Epidemiology of endometriosis in women attending family planning clinics. *BMJ* 1993;306:182–184.
10. Vercellini P, Trespidi L, De Giorgi O, et al. Endometriosis and pelvic pain: relation to disease stage and localization. *Fertil Steril* 1996;65:299–304.
11. Rock JA, Markham SM. Pathogenesis of endometriosis. *Lancet* 1992;340:1264–1267.
12. McLaren J, Prentice A. New aspects of pathogenesis of endometriosis. *Curr Obstet Gynaecol* 1996;6:85–91.
13. Cooke ID, Thomas EJ. The medical treatment of mild endometriosis. *Acta Obstet Gynecol Scand Suppl* 1989;150:27–30.
14. Harrison RF, Barry-Kinsella C. Efficacy of medroxyprogesterone treatment in infertile women with endometriosis: a prospective, randomized, placebo-controlled study. *Fertil Steril* 2000;74:24–30.
15. Audebert A, Descampes P, Marret H, et al. Pre or post operative medical treatment with nafarelin in Stage III–IV endometriosis: a French multicentred study. *Eur J Obstet Gynecol Reprod Biol* 1998;79:145–148.
16. Prentice A, Deary AJ, Goldbeck-Wood S, et al. Gonadotrophin releasing hormone analogues for pain associated with endometriosis. In: The Cochrane Library, Issue 2, 2001. Oxford: Update Software. Search date 1998; primary sources Medline, Embase, Cochrane Controlled Trials Register, and unpublished trials by UK distributors of gonadotrophin releasing hormone analogues.
17. Prentice A, Deary AJ, Bland E. Progestagens and antiprogestagens for pain associated with endometriosis. In: The Cochrane Library, Issue 1, 2004. Chichester, UK: John Wiley & Sons Ltd. Update Software. Search date 2000; primary sources Medline, Embase, and Cochrane Controlled Trials Register.
18. Selak V, Farquhar C, Prentice A, et al. Danazol for pelvic pain associated with endometriosis. In: The Cochrane Library, Issue 1, 2004. Chichester: John Wiley & Sons Ltd. Update Software. Search date 2003; primary sources Medline, Embase, Cochrane Controlled Trials Register, and hand searches of journals and conference proceedings.

19. Moore J, Kennedy S, Prentice A. Modern combined oral contraceptives for pain associated with endometriosis. In: The Cochrane Library, Issue 1, 2004. Chichester, UK: John Wiley & Sons Ltd. Update Software. Search date 2003; primary sources Medline, Embase, and Cochrane Controlled Trials Register.
20. Hornstein MD, Surrey ES, Weisberg GW, et al. Leuprolide acetate depot and hormonal add-back in endometriosis: a 12-month study. Lupron Add-Back Study Group. *Obstet Gynecol* 1998; 91:16–24.
21. Surrey ES, Hornstein MD. Prolonged GnRH agonist and add-back therapy for symptomatic endometriosis: long-term follow-up. *Obstet Gynecol* 2002;99:709–719.
22. Vercellini P, Trespidi L, Colombo A, et al. A gonadotropin-releasing hormone agonist versus a low-dose oral contraceptive for pelvic pain associated with endometriosis. *Fertil Steril* 1993;60:75–79.
23. Parazzini F, Di Cintio E, Chatenoud L, et al. Estroprogestin vs. gonadotrophin agonists plus estroprogestin in the treatment of endometriosis-related pelvic pain: a randomized trial. *Eur J Obstet Gynecol Reprod Biol* 2000;88:11–14.
24. Bromham DR, Bookere MW, Rose GR, et al. Updating the clinical experience in endometriosis — the European perspective. *Br J Obstet Gynaecol* 1995;102(suppl):12–16.
25. Bergqvist A, Theorell T. Changes in quality of life after hormonal treatment of endometriosis. *Acta Obstet Gynecol Scand* 2001;80:628–637.
26. Compston JE, Yamaguchi K, Croucher PI, et al. The effects of gonadotrophin-releasing hormone agonists on iliac crest cancellous bone structure in women with endometriosis. *Bone* 1995;16:261–267.
27. Gregoriou O, Konidaris S, Vitoratos N, et al. Gonadotropin-releasing hormone analogue plus hormone replacement therapy for the treatment of endometriosis: a randomized controlled trial. *Int J Fertil Womens Med* 1997;42:406–411.
28. Taskin O, Yalcinoglu AI, Kucuk S. Effectiveness of tibolone on hypoestrogenic symptoms induced by goserelin treatment in patients with endometriosis. *Fertil Steril* 1997;67:40–45.
29. Morgante G. Low-dose danazol after combined surgical and medical therapy reduces the incidence of pelvic pain in women with moderate and severe endometriosis. *Hum Reprod* 1999;14:2371–2374.
30. Shaw R, Garry R, McMillan L, et al. A prospective randomized open study comparing goserelin (Zoladex) plus surgery and surgery alone in the management of ovarian endometriomas. *Gynaecol Endosc* 2001;10:151–157.
31. Jacobson TZ, Barlow DH, Garry R, et al. Laparoscopic surgery for pelvic pain associated with endometriosis. In: The Cochrane Library, Issue 1, 2004. Chichester, UK: John Wiley & Sons Ltd. Update Software. Search date 2001; primary sources Medline, Embase, The Cochrane Menstrual Disorders and Subfertility Group's Specialised Register of controlled trials, and the National Research Register.
32. Sutton CJG, Ewen SP, Whitelaw N, et al. A prospective, randomised, double-blind, controlled trial of laser laparoscopy in the treatment of pelvic pain associated with minimal, mild and moderate endometriosis. *Fertil Steril* 1994;62:696–700.
33. Sutton CJG, Pooley AS, Ewen SP. Follow-up report on a randomised, controlled trial of laser laparoscopy in the treatment of pelvic pain associated with minimal to moderate endometriosis. *Fertil Steril* 1997;68:170–174.
34. Proctor M, Farquhar CM, Sinclair O, et al. Surgical interruption of pelvic nerve pathways for primary and secondary dysmenorrhoea. In: The Cochrane Library, Issue 1, 2004. Chichester, UK: John Wiley & Sons Ltd. Update Software. Search date 1998; primary sources Medline, Embase, Cochrane Controlled Trials Register, and hand searches of journals, conference proceedings, and references.
35. Vercellini P, Aimi G, Busacca, M, et al. Laparoscopic uterosacral ligament resection for dysmenorrhea associated with endometriosis: results of a randomized, controlled trial. *Fertil Steril* 2003;80:310–319.
36. Parazzini F, Fedele L, Busacca M, et al. Postsurgical medical treatment of advanced endometriosis: results of a randomized clinical trial. *Am J Obstet Gynecol* 1994;171:1205–1207.
37. Bianchi S, Busacca M, Agnoli B, et al. Effects of 3 month therapy with danazol after laparoscopic surgery for stage III/IV endometriosis: a randomized study. *Hum Reprod* 1999;14:1335–1337.
38. Telimaa S, Ronnberg L, Kauppila A. Placebo-controlled comparison of danazol and high-dose medroxyprogesterone acetate in the treatment of endometriosis after conservative surgery. *Gynecol Endocrinol* 1987;1:363–371.
39. Hornstein MD, Hemmings R, Yuzpe AA, et al. Use of nafarelin versus placebo after reductive laparoscopic surgery for endometriosis. *Fertil Steril* 1997;68:860–864.
40. Vercellini P, Crosignani PG, Fadini R, et al. A gonadotrophin-releasing hormone agonist compared with expectant management after conservative surgery for symptomatic endometriosis. *Br J Obstet Gynaecol* 1999;106:672–677.
41. Muzii L, Marana R, Caruana P, et al. Postoperative administration of monophasic combined oral contraceptives after laparoscopic treatment of ovarian endometriosis: a prospective, randomized trial. *Am J Obstet Gynecol* 2000;183:588–592.
42. Busacca M, Somigliana E, Bianchi S, et al. Post-operative GnRH analogue treatment after conservative surgery for symptomatic endometriosis stage III–IV: a randomized controlled trial. *Hum Reprod* 2001;16:2399–2402.
43. Vercellini P, Frontino G, de Giorgi O, et al. Comparison levonorgestrel-releasing intrauterine device versus expectant management after conservative surgery for symptomatic endometriosis: a pilot study. *Fertil Steril* 2003;80:305–309.
44. Vercellini P, De Giorgi O, Mosconi P, et al. Cyproterone acetate versus a continuous monophasic oral contraceptive in the treatment of recurrent pelvic pain after conservative surgery for symptomatic endometriosis. *Fertil Steril* 2002;77:52–61.
45. Matorras R, Elorriaga MA, Pijoan JI, et al. Recurrence of endometriosis in women with bilateral adnexectomy (with or without total hysterectomy) who received hormone replacement therapy. *Fertil Steril* 2002;77:303–308.
46. Beretta P, Franchi M, Ghezzi F, et al. Randomised clinical trial of two laparoscopic treatments of endometriomas: cystectomy versus drainage and coagulation. *Fertil Steril* 1998;709:1176–1180.

Neil Johnson
Senior lecturer in Obstetrics and Gynaecology
University of Auckland, Auckland, New Zealand

Cynthia Farquhar
Professor School of Medicine
University of Auckland, Auckland, New Zealand

Competing interests: None declared.

TABLE 1 RCTs comparing hormonal treatment at diagnosis versus placebo.

Ref	Comparison	Number of RCTs	Number of Women	Outcome	Results (95% CI)
16	Gonadorelin analogues *v* placebo	1	63	Symptoms at 3 months	Mean change in dysmenorrhoea: –2.3 with gonadorelin analogues *v* –0.3 with placebo Mean change in pelvic pain: –1.2 with gonadorelin analogues *v* –0.2 with placebo Mean change in dyspareunia: –0.2 with gonadorelin analogues *v* + 0.1 with placebo
17	Dydrogesterone *v* placebo	1	22	Proportion of women with pain relief at 6 months	4/11 (36%) with dydrogesterone *v* 5/11 (45%) with placebo; RR 0.80 (0.29 to 2.21)
17	Medroxyprogesterone acetate 100 mg daily *v* placebo	1	33	Symptoms at 6 months	WMD–5.20 (–6.80 to –3.60)
18	Danazol *v* placebo	1	59	Pain relief at 6 months	WMD –5.70 (–7.51 to –3.89)

Ref, reference.

Fibroids (uterine myomatosis, leiomyomas)

Search date December 2003

Anne Lethaby and Beverley Vollenhoven

QUESTIONS

INTERVENTIONS

Covered elsewhere in *Clinical Evidence*
Menorrhagia (many women with fibroids experience symptoms of heavy menstrual bleeding) (see menorrhagia, p 2407)

*Based on consensus. RCTs unlikely to be conducted.

See glossary

Key Messages

Medical treatment alone

- **Gonadorelin analogues (GnRHa) plus progestogen (no significant difference in heavy bleeding compared with GnRHa alone, but adding progestogen reduces vasomotor symptoms and hot flushes associated with GnRHa)** One small RCT found no significant difference between leuprorelin (leuprolide) acetate plus progestogen and leuprorelin acetate alone in the proportion of women who had heavy bleeding at 12 months. One small RCT found that GnRHa plus medroxyprogesterone acetate significantly reduced vasomotor symptoms over 12 months compared with GnRHa alone. One small RCT found that leuprorelin acetate plus progestogen significantly reduced the proportion of women with hot flushes over 24 weeks compared with leuprorelin acetate alone.
- **Gonadorelin analogues plus tibolone (no significant difference in fibroid symptoms compared with GnRHa alone, but adding tibolone reduces hot flushes and prevents loss in bone mineral density associated with GnRHa)** Two small RCTs found no significant difference between GnRHa alone and GnRHa plus tibolone in fibroid related symptoms or uterine and fibroid size. They found that adding tibolone reduced hot flushes, vaginal dryness, and night sweats and prevented loss in bone mineral density.
- **Gonadorelin analogues alone** RCTs found that GnRHa reduced fibroid related symptoms compared with placebo, but were associated with important adverse effects. Two RCTs found that GnRHa increased amenorrhoea compared with placebo after about 3 months. One RCT provided insufficient evidence to compare nafarelin versus buserelin. One RCT found that higher doses of nafarelin increased amenorrhoea at 16 weeks compared with lower doses. Two RCTs found that nafarelin reduced bone density from baseline after 16 weeks' treatment compared with placebo, but that bone density returned to pretreatment levels 6 months after treatment was stopped. Two RCTs found that hot flushes were more common with nafarelin than with placebo or buserelin. One RCT found that hot flushes and sweating were more common with goserelin than placebo.
- **Gonadorelin analogues plus combined oestrogen–progestogen (insufficient evidence on effects compared with GnRHa plus progestogen)** One small RCT provided insufficient evidence to compare GnRHa plus combined oestrogen–progestogen hormone replacement therapy versus GnRHa plus progestogen hormone replacement therapy.
- **Gonadorelin analogues plus raloxifene (insufficient evidence on effects compared with GnRHa alone)** One RCT found that adding raloxifene to GnRHa reduced fibroid size compared with GnRHa alone. It found no significant difference in fibroid related symptoms or hot flushes.
- **Non-steroidal anti-inflammatory drugs** Two small RCTs provided insufficient evidence to assess non-steroidal anti-inflammatory drugs in women with fibroids.
- **Gestrinone; levonorgestrel intrauterine system; mifepristone** We found no RCTs on the effects of these interventions.

Preoperative medical treatment

- **Gonadorelin analogues** One systematic review found that GnRHa for at least 3 months before fibroid surgery improved preoperative haemoglobin concentration and haematocrit, and reduced uterine and pelvic symptoms compared with placebo or no pretreatment. Preoperative gonadorelin also reduced the rate of vertical incisions during laparotomy. Women having hysterectomy were more likely to have a vaginal rather than an abdominal procedure after GnRHa pretreatment compared with placebo or no pretreatment. Preoperative goserelin reduced intra-operative blood loss although the difference was small and the clinical importance is uncertain. One subsequent RCT found no significant difference between preoperative triptorelin and immediate surgery in intra-operative blood loss. One small RCT found that GnRHa combined with endometrial resection reduced the need for further treatment (either medical or surgical) over 1 year compared with GnRHa alone. However, preoperative GnRHa is associated with adverse hypo-oestrogenic effects, such as hot flushes, vaginal symptoms, and sweating, and women receiving GnRHa were more likely to withdraw from treatment because of adverse effects.

Surgical treatments

- **Laparoscopic myomectomy (maintains fertility compared to hysterectomy; reduces recovery time and postoperative pain compared with abdominal myomectomy)** Two RCTs found limited evidence that laparosopic myomectomy reduced postoperative pain, fever, and recovery time compared to abdominal myomectomy. We found no RCTs comparing laparoscopic myomectomy versus total abdominal, vaginal, or laparoscopic hysterectomy, but the main benefit of myomectomy compared with hysterectomy is that it maintains fertility.
- **Laparoscopically assisted vaginal hysterectomy (reduces recovery time and postoperative pain compared with total abdominal hysterectomy, but increases operating time and blood loss compared with total vaginal hysterectomy)** Two RCTs found that women having laparoscopically assisted vaginal hysterectomy had shorter recovery times and less postoperative pain compared with women having total abdominal hysterectomy. One RCT found that women having laparoscopically assisted vaginal hysterectomy had longer operating time and more blood loss than women having total vaginal hysterectomy.
- **Total abdominal hysterectomy (reduces fibroid related symptoms compared with no treatment)*** We found no RCTs comparing total abdominal hysterectomy versus no treatment or sham surgery. An RCT is unlikely to be conducted. There is consensus that total abdominal hysterectomy is superior to no treatment in reducing fibroid related symptoms. RCTs found that women having total abdominal hysterectomy had longer surgery, more blood loss, pain and fever, longer hospital stay, later return to work, and less satisfaction than women having total vaginal hysterectomy. Two RCTs found that women having total abdominal hysterectomy had longer recovery times and more postoperative pain but shorter operating times and less blood loss than women having laparoscopically assisted vaginal hysterectomy. One RCT found that women having total abdominal hysterectomy had more postoperative fever, longer hospital stay, and recovery times than women having total laparoscopic hysterectomy.
- **Total laparoscopic hysterectomy (reduces postoperative fever, hospital stay, and recovery time compared with total abdominal hysterectomy)** One RCT found that women having total laparoscopic hysterectomy had less postoperative fever, shorter hospital stay, and shorter recovery times compared with women having total abdominal hysterectomy.
- **Total vaginal hysterectomy (reduces operation time, blood loss, pain, fever, and hospital stay compared with total abdominal hysterectomy and increases satisfaction with operation)** Two RCTs found that women having total vaginal hysterectomy had shorter operation time, less blood loss, pain and fever, shorter hospital stay, earlier return to work, and greater satisfaction than women having total abdominal hysterectomy. One RCT found that women having total vaginal hysterectomy had shorter operation times and less blood loss than women having laparoscopically assisted vaginal hysterectomy.
- **Thermal balloon ablation** We found no RCTs comparing thermal balloon ablation versus non-surgical treatment or hysterectomy. One RCT compared thermal balloon ablation versus rollerball endometrial ablation in women with fibroids smaller than the average size of a 12 week pregnancy, all of whom had been pretreated with

gonadorelin analogues. It found no significant difference between thermal balloon and rollerball ablation in amenorrhoea rates, pictorial bleeding assessment chart score, haemoglobin, or hysterectomy rates at 12 months. It found that thermal balloon ablation reduced operation time and intraoperative complication rate compared with rollerball ablation. About one third of women reported being "not very satisfied" with either operation.

*Based on consensus. RCTs unlikely to be conducted.

DEFINITION Fibroids (uterine leiomyomas) are benign tumours of the smooth muscle cells of the uterus. Women with fibroids can be asymptomatic or may present with menorrhagia (30%), pelvic pain with or without dysmenorrhoea or pressure symptoms (34%), infertility (27%), and recurrent pregnancy loss (3%).[1] Much of the data describing the relationship between the presence of fibroids and symptoms are based on uncontrolled studies that have assessed the effect of myomectomy**G** on the presenting symptoms.[2] The prevalence of fibroids in infertile women can be as high as 13%, but no direct causal relationship between fibroids and infertility has been established.[3]

INCIDENCE/PREVALENCE The reported incidence of fibroids varies from 5.4–77.0% depending on the method of diagnosis (the gold standard is histological evidence). A random sample of 335 Swedish women aged 25–40 years was reported to have an incidence of fibroids of 5.4% (95% CI 3.0% to 7.8%) based on transvaginal ultrasound examination.[4] The prevalence of these tumours increased with age (age 25–32 years: 3.3%, 95% CI 0.7% to 6.0%; 33–40 years: 7.8%, 95% CI 3.6% to 12.0%).[4] Another large case control study found that the rate of fibroids was higher in women aged less than 50 years; it found a rate of pathologically confirmed fibroids of 4.24/1000 woman years in women aged 50 years or more compared with 6.20/1000 in women aged 45–50 years, 4.63/1000 in women aged 40–45 years, 2.67/1000 in women aged 35–40 years, 0.96/1000 in women aged 30–35 years and 0.31/1000 in women aged 25–30 years.[5] Based on postmortem examination, 50% of women were found to have these tumours.[6] Gross serial sectioning at 2 mm intervals of 100 consecutive hysterectomy specimens revealed the presence of fibroids in 50/68 [73%] premenopausal women and 27/32 [84%] postmenopausal women. These women were having hysterectomies for reasons other than fibroids.[7] The incidence of fibroids in black women is three times greater than that in white women, based on ultrasound or hysterectomy diagnosis.[8] Submucosal fibroids have been diagnosed in 6–34% of women having a hysteroscopy for abnormal bleeding, and in 2–7% of women having infertility investigations.[9]

AETIOLOGY/RISK FACTORS The cause of fibroids is unknown. It is known that each fibroid is of monoclonal origin and arises independently.[10,11] Factors thought to be involved include the sex steroid hormones oestrogen and progesterone as well as the insulin-like growth factors, epidermal growth factor and transforming growth factor. Risk factors for fibroid growth include nulliparity and obesity. There is a risk reduction to a fifth with five term pregnancies, compared with nulliparous women ($P < 0.001$).[5] Obesity increases the risk of fibroid development by 21% with each 10 kg weight gain ($P = 0.008$).[5] The combined oral contraceptive pill also reduces the risk of fibroids with increasing duration of use (women who have taken oral contraceptives for 4–6 years compared with women who have never taken oral contraceptives: OR 0.8, 95% CI 0.5 to 1.2; women who have taken oral contraceptives for ≥ 7 years compared with women who have never taken oral contraceptives: OR 0.5, 95% CI 0.3 to 0.9).[12] Women who have had injections containing 150 mg depot medroxyprogesterone acetate also have a reduced incidence compared with women who have never had injections of this drug (OR 0.44, 95% CI 0.36 to 0.55).[13]

PROGNOSIS There are few data on the long term untreated prognosis of these tumours, particularly in women who are asymptomatic at diagnosis. One small case control study reported that in a group of 106 women treated with observation alone over 1 year there was no significant change in symptoms and quality of life over that time.[14] Fibroids tend to shrink or fibrose after the menopause.[5]

AIMS OF INTERVENTION To reduce menstrual bleeding; prevent or correct iron deficiency anaemia; reduce pressure symptoms; reduce pelvic pain; and induce a change in fertility status, with minimal adverse effects.

OUTCOMES Menstrual blood flow (assessed objectively [mL/cycle] or subjectively); haemoglobin and haematocrit concentration; pelvic pain, pressure, or both (measured by a validated scale or subjective report); reduction in fibroid and uterine volume;

pregnancy rate; quality of life. Some of the outcomes relate to surgery: ease of surgery as assessed by the surgeon, complication rates during and after surgery; blood loss during surgery; duration of surgery; length of hospital stay; rate of blood transfusions; probability of transverse versus vertical incisions during surgery; probability of vaginal versus abdominal hysterectomy; recurrence rate; patient satisfaction rate.

METHODS *Clinical Evidence* search and appraisal December 2003.

QUESTION What are the effects of medical treatment alone?

OPTION GONADORELIN ANALOGUES ALONE

RCTs found that gonadorelin analogues (GnRHa) reduced fibroid related symptoms compared with placebo, but were associated with important adverse effects. Two RCTs found that GnRHa increased amenorrhoea after about 3 months compared with placebo. One RCT provided insufficient evidence to compare nafarelin versus buserelin. One RCT found that higher doses of nafarelin increased amenorrhoea at 16 weeks compared with lower doses. Two RCTs found that nafarelin reduced bone density from baseline after 16 weeks' treatment compared with placebo, but that bone density returned to pretreatment levels 6 months after treatment was stopped. Two RCTs found that hot flushes were more common with nafarelin than with placebo or buserelin. One RCT found that adverse effects, mainly hot flushes and sweating, were more common with goserelin than placebo.

Benefits: **Versus placebo:** We found one systematic review of nafarelin (search date 1997, 1 RCT, 101 women).[15] The RCT identified by the review found that intranasal nafarelin (200 μg twice daily) significantly increased the proportion of women with amenorrhoea at 3 months compared with placebo (33/64 [51%] women amenorrhoeic with nafarelin *v* 3/37 [8%] with placebo, $P \leq 0.05$).[15] We found one subsequent RCT (307 women awaiting surgery for fibroids), which compared three treatments: goserelin; fulvestrant and placebo. It found that goserelin (3.6 mg every 4 weeks) increased amenorrhoea compared with placebo at 13 weeks (AR of amenorrhoea: 0.18% at baseline to 92.5% at with goserelin *v* no change from baseline with placebo; P value not reported).[16] **Versus each other:** We found one systematic review (search date 1997) that identified one RCT (211 women enrolled) comparing intranasal nafarelin (200 μg twice daily) versus intranasal buserelin (300 μg 3 times daily).[15] The RCT found that nafarelin significantly increased haemoglobin at 16 weeks compared with buserelin (haemoglobin 12.8 g/dL with nafarelin *v* 12.3 g/dL with buserelin; $P = 0.03$). However, the RCT did not describe the clinical importance of this difference. **Different doses:** We found one systematic review (search date 1997) that identified one RCT (257 women) comparing different doses of nafarelin (50, 100, 200, and 400 μg twice daily).[15] The RCT found that higher doses of nafarelin significantly increased the proportion of women who were amenorrhoeic at 16 weeks compared with lower doses (women amenorrhoeic 41/59 [69.5%] with 50 μg *v* 46/54 [85.2%] with 100 μg *v* 40/48 [83.3%] with 200 μg *v* 52/57 [91.2%] with 400 μg; $P = 0.0053$ for dose-response effect). **Different modes of administration:** We found no systematic review and no RCTs that measured clinical outcomes (see comment below). **Versus gonadorelin analogues (GnRHa) plus hormonal treatment:** See benefits of GnRHa plus hormone replacement therapy, p 2346.

Harms: **Versus placebo:** The systematic review identified two RCTs, which found that intranasal nafarelin (200 μg twice daily) reduced bone density by 2.5% from baseline after 16 weeks' treatment compared with placebo.[15] Six months after treatment was withdrawn, bone density had increased to values that were not significantly different from baseline. Many women reported hot flushes during nafarelin treatment (rates ranged from 39% to 100% across 5 RCTs in the review). One RCT found that nafarelin significantly increased the proportion of women who had hot flushes compared with placebo (61% with nafarelin *v* 36% with placebo; P = 0.02).[15] One RCT found that adverse effects, mainly hot flushes and sweating, were more common with goserelin than placebo (63.3% with goserelin *v* 28.3% with placebo, P value not reported).[16] **Versus each other:** The RCT identified by the review found that nafarelin significantly increased the proportion of women who had hot flushes compared with buserelin (38.5% with nafarelin *v* 23.4% with buserelin; P = 0.025), but few women discontinued treatment (data not reported).[15] **Versus GnRHa plus hormonal treatment:** See harms of GnRHa plus hormone replacement, p 2347.

Comment: The RCTs did not assess effects on pregnancy rates. GnRHa control bleeding, reduce some fibroid related symptoms, and reduce fibroid and uterine size. However, they may cause menopausal symptoms and bone loss, which make them unacceptable for long term use. **Versus placebo:** We found four additional RCTs (154 women) comparing GnRHa versus placebo.[17–20] All had important methodological weaknesses. The first RCT (13 participating centres, 128 women, 24 weeks' treatment) had high withdrawal rates, precluding reliable comparison of the benefits of treatments.[17] It found that leuprorelin was associated with vasomotor flushes, vaginitis, arthralgia/myalgia, asthenia, peripheral oedema, insomnia, nausea, and nervousness compared with placebo (see table 1, p 2359).[17] It found no significant difference between nafarelin and placebo in the risk of developing emotional lability/nervousness, depression, headaches, or decreased libido, although sample size may have been insufficient to rule out clinically important differences for these outcomes (see table 1, p 2359).[17] The second RCT (38 premenopausal women) did not assess clinical outcomes.[18] The other two RCTs were too small to yield reliable results (12 women[19] and 15 women[20]). Two of these RCTs found that fibroids returned to their previous size after stopping treatment.[17,18] **Versus each other:** We found two additional small RCTs.[21,22] The first RCT (67 women) compared buserelin (1.8 mg every 4 weeks) versus leuprorelin (1.88 mg every 4 weeks) by subcutaneous injection.[21] The second RCT (27 women) compared triptorelin standard dose treatment plus three different types of dosage regimen.[22] Neither of the RCTs compared clinical outcomes among treatment groups. **Different doses:** Two RCTs (77 women) compared two different doses of leuprorelin (leuprolide) acetate (1.88 mg *v* 3.75 mg every 4 weeks for 24 weeks).[23,24] Neither of the RCTs compared clinical outcomes among treatment groups, but one RCT reported that all women experienced partial or complete relief from symptoms throughout their treatment.[23] **Different modes of administration:** We found three RCTs (96 women) comparing intranasal versus subcutaneous GnRHa, none of which reported quantitative results for clinical outcomes.[25–27] One RCT reported that all women had a subjective improvement in menstrual symptoms after 6 months' treatment, especially menorrhagia and dysmenorrhoea, but no figures were reported.[25] The RCTs found no differences in uterine and fibroid shrinkage depending on how GnRHa treatment was given.[25–27]

OPTION GONADORELIN ANALOGUES PLUS HORMONE REPLACEMENT

One small RCT found no significant difference between leuprorelin (leuprolide) acetate plus progestogen and leuprorelin acetate alone in the proportion of women who had heavy bleeding at 12 months. One small RCT found that GnRHa plus medroxyprogesterone acetate significantly reduced vasomotor symptoms over 12 months compared with GnRHa alone. One small RCT found

that leuprorelin acetate plus progestogen significantly reduced the proportion of women with hot flushes over 24 weeks compared with leuprorelin acetate alone. Two small RCTs found no significant difference between gonadorelin analogues alone and gonadorelin analogues plus tibolone in fibroid related symptoms or uterine and fibroid size. They found that adding tibolone reduced hot flushes, vaginal dryness, and night sweats, and prevented loss in bone mineral density. One small RCT provided insufficient evidence to compare gonadorelin analogues plus combined oestrogen–progestogen hormone replacement therapy versus gonadorelin analogues plus progestogen only hormone replacement therapy. Another RCT found that adding raloxifene to gonadorelin analogues reduced fibroid size compared with gonadorelin analogues alone. It found no significant difference in fibroid related symptoms or hot flushes.

Benefits: **Gonadorelin analogue (GnRHa) plus progestogen versus GnRHa alone:** We found no systematic review but found one RCT (41 women).[28] It found no significant difference between leuprorelin (leuprolide) acetate plus progestogen and leuprorelin acetate plus placebo in heavy bleeding at 12 months (proportion of women with bleeding for ≤ 7 days/month or self reported improvement in bleeding assessed by menstrual calendar: 8/21 [38%] with added progestogen *v* 11/20 [55%] with added placebo; RR 0.69, 95% CI 0.35 to 1.36). We found two RCTs that did not assess effects on fibroid related symptoms but studied whether adding progestogen to GnRHa reduced the harms associated with giving GnRHa alone.[29,30] The first RCT (24 women) assessing harms found that GnRHa plus medroxyprogesterone acetate significantly reduced vasomotor symptoms over 12 months compared with GnRHa alone ($P < 0.05$; absolute numbers not reported).[29] The second RCT (16 women) found that leuprorelin acetate plus progestogen hormone replacement significantly reduced the proportion of women with hot flushes over 24 weeks compared with leuprorelin acetate alone (1/9 [11%] with leuprorelin acetate plus progestogen *v* 6/7 [86%] with leuprorelin acetate alone; RR 0.13, 95% CI 0.02 to 0.84).[30] **GnRHa plus tibolone versus GnRHa alone:** We found two RCTs.[31,32] Both RCTs found no significant difference in symptoms at 6 months between adding tibolone to GnRHa and GnRHa alone. They found that fewer women taking tibolone had hot flushes. The first RCT (50 women) found no significant difference between GnRHa plus tibolone and GnRHa plus placebo in uterine and fibroid size or fibroid related symptoms at 6 months (mean uterine volume 415 cm^3 with added tibolone *v* 386 cm^3 with added placebo; mean fibroid volume 139 cm^3 with added tibolone *v* 133 cm^3 with added placebo; symptom intensity on a visual analogue scale from 0–10: 3.3 with added tibolone *v* 3.5 with added placebo for pelvic pressure; 2.0 with added tibolone *v* 2.5 with added placebo for pelvic pain; 3.0 in both groups for urinary frequency; P value for all comparisons reported as non-significant).[31] It found that, after 6 months' treatment, GnRHa plus tibolone significantly reduced the mean number of hot flushes each day compared with GnRHa alone (1.5 with added tibolone *v* 4.6 with added placebo; $P < 0.01$; data presented graphically).[31] The RCT also found that the significant reduction in bone mineral density after 6 months' treatment with gonadorelin alone was prevented with the concurrent administration of tibolone (mean difference $P < 0.01$).[31] The risk of fractures was not assessed. The second RCT (20 women) comparing GnRHa (triptoreline) plus tibolone versus GnRHa alone also found no significant difference in fibroid volume at 6 months (reduction in volume 64% with GnRHa plus tibolone *v* 60% with GnRHa alone; reported as non-significant, CI not reported).[32] The RCT is likely to have been too small to detect a clinically important difference. It found that fewer women taking tibolone plus GnRHa had hot flushes (30% with GnRHa plus tibolone *v* 80% with GnRHa alone), vaginal dryness (20% with GnRHa plus tibolone v 50% with GnRHa alone), and night sweats (20% with GnRHa plus tibolone v 30% with GnRHa alone) compared with women taking GnRHa alone.[32] The RCT did not assess the significance of the difference between groups. **GnRHa plus progestogen versus GnRHa plus combined oestrogen–progestogen:** We found one RCT (51 women) that compared GnRHa plus progestogen hormone replacement versus GnRHa plus combined oestrogen–progestogen hormone replacement over a 2 year period.[33] After 3 months of leuprorelin treatment, it found a decrease in the mean uterine volume in both groups compared with baseline estimates (416 cm^3 with oestrogen–progestogen v 440 cm^3 with progestogen alone; CI of the difference not reported). After 21 months of treatment, the mean uterine volume was reduced only in women taking oestrogen–progestogen hormone replacement (414 cm^3 with oestrogen–progestogen v 647 cm^3 with progestogen alone; CI not reported). Most women experienced a reduction in fibroid related symptoms (comparison of results between groups not reported). Menorrhagia improved or resolved in 85%, pelvic pressure in 63%, and pelvic pain in 100% of women. **GnRHa plus raloxifene versus GnRHa alone:** We found one RCT (100 women) that compared adding raloxifene to GnRHa versus GnRHa alone for 6 months.[34] It found that both treatments were associated with a reduction in both uterine and fibroid size from baseline, and found that raloxifene plus GnRHa caused a significantly greater reduction in fibroid size at 6 months compared with GnRHa alone (reduction 7% with raloxifene plus GnRHa v 4% with GnRHa alone, absolute data read from graph, $P < 0.05$). It found no significant difference between groups in fibroid related symptoms (menorrhagia or constipation: no women in either group; pelvic pressure: 6.7% with raloxifene plus GnRHa v 6.5% with GnRHa alone; pelvic pain: 4.4% with raloxifene plus GnRHa v 6.5% with GnRHa alone; urinary frequency: 6.7% with raloxifene plus GnRHa v 4.3% with GnRHa alone; reported as non-significant, CI not reported).[34]

Harms: See harms of hormone replacement therapy under menopausal symptoms topic, p 2392. **GnRHa plus progestogen versus GnRHa alone:** The first RCT gave no information on adverse effects.[28] **GnRHa plus tibolone versus GnRHa alone:** See also GnRHa without hormonal replacement therapy, p 2344. **GnRHa plus raloxifene versus GnRHa alone:** The RCT found that both GnRHa alone and raloxifene plus GnRHa significantly increased the mean number of hot flushes a day after 15 days' treatment (mean 3–6 flushes a day; $P < 0.05$). However, it found no significant difference between groups (reported as non-significant, CI not reported).

Comment: Most of the RCTs were small. There is insufficient evidence to determine the optimum hormone replacement regimen that minimises the adverse effects of GnRHa. The RCTs did not assess effects on pregnancy rates.

OPTION NON-STEROIDAL ANTI-INFLAMMATORY DRUGS

Two small RCTs provided insufficient evidence to assess non-steroidal anti-inflammatory drugs in women with fibroids.

Benefits: We found two small RCTs, which assessed the effects of non-steroidal anti-inflammatory drugs (ibuprofen and naproxen) on heavy menstrual bleeding in women with fibroids.[35,36] The first RCT (25 women with menorrhagia; 11 with fibroids) found no significant difference in menstrual blood loss over 4 months between naproxen and placebo in women with fibroids (total menstrual blood loss over 4 cycles 221 mL with placebo v 196 mL with naproxen; P value not reported).[35] The second RCT (24 women; 10 with fibroids) also found no significant difference in menstrual blood loss over 2 months between ibuprofen 600–1200 mg/day and placebo (34 women: total menstrual blood loss over 2 cycles about 130 mL in all groups; P value not reported).[36] Both RCTs may have been underpowered to assess a clinically important difference in outcomes.[35,36]

Harms: See harms under non-steroidal anti-inflammatory drugs, p 1525.

Comment: The RCTs did not assess effects on pregnancy rates.

OPTION GESTRINONE

We found no RCTs about the effects of gestrinone on fibroid related symptoms. Androgenic adverse effects limit its use.

Benefits: We found no systematic review and no RCTs that assessed clinical outcomes (see comment below).

Harms: Two uncontrolled trials found that gestrinone was associated with seborrhoea and acne, which increased with duration of treatment.[37,38] One RCT found that after 1 year of treatment, seborrhoea affected 71–93% of women, and acne was reported by 31–63% of women after 2 years of treatment. Myalgia and arthralgia, mild hirsutism, and hoarseness were also reported. Body weight also increased after 2 years of treatment, from a mean of 57.4 kg to 60.9 kg. These changes reversed when treatment was discontinued.

Comment: We found two uncontrolled trials (197 women) that assessed the mode of administration of gestrinone in reducing uterine volume.[37,38] The effects of gestrinone were assessed as comparisons with baseline values. After 3 months of treatment in one trial, 76–86% of women reported amenorrhoea. Pelvic pain was resolved in 76–98% of women.[37] Haemoglobin increased from a mean of 12.38 g/dL to 13.26 g/dL and haematocrit increased from 36.9% to 38.4%.[37] The trials did not assess effects on pregnancy rates.

OPTION MIFEPRISTONE

We found no RCTs of mifepristone in women with fibroids.

Benefits: We found no systematic review or RCTs.

Harms: Mild atypical hot flushes were reported in 28–40% of women in one observational study.[39]

Comment: None.

OPTION LEVONORGESTREL INTRAUTERINE SYSTEM

We found no RCTs of the levonorgestrel intrauterine system in women with fibroids.

Benefits: **Versus no treatment:** One systematic review (search date 2000) identified no RCTs.[40] We found no additional RCTs.

Harms: We found no RCTs.

Comment: None.

QUESTION In women scheduled for fibroid surgery, what are the effects of preoperative medical treatments?

OPTION GONADORELIN ANALOGUES

One systematic review found that gonadorelin analogues for at least 3 months before fibroid surgery improved preoperative haemoglobin concentration and haematocrit, and reduced uterine and pelvic symptoms compared with placebo or no pretreatment. Preoperative gonadorelin also reduced the rate of vertical incisions during laparotomy. Women having hysterectomy were more likely to have a vaginal rather than an abdominal procedure after gonadorelin analogue pretreatment compared with placebo or no pretreatment. Preoperative goserelin reduced intra-operative blood loss although the difference was small and the clinical importance is uncertain. One subsequent RCT found no significant difference between preoperative triptorelin and immediate surgery in intra-operative blood loss. One small RCT found that gonadorelin analogues combined with endometrial resection reduced the need for further treatment (either medical or surgical) over 1 year compared with gonadorelin analogues alone. However, preoperative GnRHa is associated with adverse hypo-oestrogenic effects, such as hot flushes, vaginal symptoms, and sweating, and women receiving GnRHa were more likely to withdraw from treatment because of adverse effects.

Benefits: **Versus placebo or no preoperative treatment:** We found one systematic review (search date 2000, 21 RCTs, 1886 women)[41] and one subsequent RCT.[42] The systematic review assessed gonadorelin analogue (GnRHa) pretreatment (given at least 3 months before surgery) compared with placebo or no treatment, in separate categories: before, during, and after myomectomy**G** or hysterectomy. The review found that, compared with placebo or no treatment, pretreatment with GnRHa significantly improved preoperative haemoglobin concentration (9 RCTs, 541 women: WMD 0.98 g/dL, 95% CI 0.74 g/dL to 1.22 g/dL) and haematocrit (4 RCTs, 138 women: WMD 3.14%, 95% CI 1.78% to 4.51%). It also found that GnRHa significantly improved preoperative pelvic symptoms when measured on a symptom scale (pelvic symptom score**G**: 3 RCTs, 372 women: WMD –2.12, 95% CI –2.38 to –1.87). It found that significantly fewer women receiving GnRHa pretreatment had no improvement in pelvic symptoms compared with women receiving no pretreatment (1 RCT: OR 0.38, 95% CI 0.22 to 0.60). It found that pretreatment with GnRHa significantly reduced intraoperative blood loss (estimated by measuring the weight of swabs and the volume of blood collected in receptacles) compared with placebo or no treatment (8 RCTs, 263 women: WMD 67 mL, 95% CI 44 mL to 91 mL during myomectomy; 6 RCTs, 419 women: WMD 58 mL, 95% CI 40 mL to 76 mL during hysterectomy), although these differences may not be clinically important. The review also found that GnRHa significantly reduced the duration of operation in women having hysterectomy (8 RCTs, 748 women: WMD 5.2 minutes, 95% CI 1.8 minutes to 8.6 minutes) and reduced hospital stay compared with placebo or no treatment (4 RCTs, 392 women: WMD 1.0 day, 95% CI 0.9 days to 1.2 days). GnRHa pretreatment significantly reduced vertical incision rate in women having laparotomy compared with placebo or no treatment (myomectomy; 1 RCT, 28 women: OR 0.11, 95% CI 0.02 to 0.75; hysterectomy; 4 RCTs, 529 women: OR 0.36, 95% CI 0.23 to 0.55). There was also a suggestion that hysterectomy was subjectively graded by the surgeons as "not as difficult" in the pretreated women (2 RCTs: OR 0.73, 95% CI 0.25 to 0.97). A significantly higher proportion of these women also converted to a vaginal procedure (3 RCTs: OR 4.7, 95% CI 3.0 to 7.5). The review found that pretreated compared with non-pretreated women maintained marginally but significantly higher postoperative blood counts (postoperative haemoglobin: 3 RCTs, 240 women: WMD 0.8 g/dL, 95% CI 0.5 g/dL to 1.1 g/dL) for both types of surgery and higher haematocrit levels after hysterectomy (2 RCTs, 173 women: WMD 1.8%, 95% CI 1.1% to 2.4%), although the clinical significance of these results is unclear. One small RCT (60 women, 18 infertile, 6 with recurrent abortion) identified by the review[41] assessed pregnancy rate in infertile women who had had myomectomy for fibroids at a mean follow up of 13 months.[44] Pregnancy rate was higher for pretreated versus non-pretreated women, although the difference was not significant (AR 7/11 [64%] for pretreated *v* 6/13 [46%] for non-pretreated; RR 1.4, 95% CI 0.7 to 2.9). The RCT may have been too small to detect a clinically important difference. The subsequent RCT (100 women) comparing 2 months of pretreatment with triptorelin with immediate surgery (myomectomy) found no significant difference in blood loss during surgery between the two groups (mean blood loss 265 ml in the pretreated group *v* 296 ml in the immediate surgery group, WMD –31 ml, 95% CI –108 to 46 ml).[42] **Surgery plus GnRHa versus GnRHa alone:** We found one RCT (25 women) comparing goserelin acetate plus endometrial resectionⒼ versus goserelin acetate alone.[45] It found that, compared with goserelin acetate alone, combined treatment reduced the proportion of women who required further treatment (either medical or surgical) over 1 year (17% with combined treatment *v* 69% with goserelin acetate alone; RR 4.3, 95% CI 1.1 to 15.4).

Harms: **Versus placebo or no preoperative treatment:** The review found that women pretreated with GnRHa versus placebo or no treatment were significantly more likely to experience hypo-oestrogenic symptoms, such as hot flushes (534 women: OR 6.5, 95% CI 4.6 to 9.2), change in breast size (261 women: OR 7.7, 95% CI 2.4 to 24.9), and vaginal symptoms (534 women: OR 4.0, 95% CI 2.1 to 7.6).[41] Women receiving GnRHa were also more likely to withdraw from treatment because of adverse effects (4 RCTs, 628 women: OR 2.5, 95% CI 1.0 to 5.9). The systematic review identified two small RCTs that evaluated long term follow up in women receiving pretreatment with GnRHa before myomectomy. In one of these, all 24 women were checked for fibroid recurrence at 6 months and 63% of the pretreated group had a recurrence of their fibroids compared with 13% of the control group. Fibroid recurrence 2–3 years after surgery was over 50% in the 18 women from the second RCT, but no significant difference was found between pretreated and non-pretreated women. No other adverse effects were assessed. One subsequent RCT also found that GnRH pretreatment increased fibroid recurrence compared with no pretreatment at 6 months, although this difference was not significant (OR 4.10, 95% CI 0.44 to 38.25).[42] **Surgery plus GnRHa versus GnRHa alone:** The RCT gave no information on harms.[45]

Comment: Only one of the RCTs[44] assessed effects on pregnancy rates. One RCT was not included in the systematic review because the outcome of avoiding scheduled hysterectomy was assessed in the GnRHa group only.[43]

QUESTION What are the effects of surgical treatments?

OPTION TOTAL ABDOMINAL HYSTERECTOMY

We found no RCTs comparing total abdominal hysterectomy versus no treatment or sham surgery. An RCT is unlikely to be conducted. There is consensus that abdominal hysterectomy is superior to no treatment in improving fibroid related symptoms. RCTs found that women having total

abdominal hysterectomy had longer surgery, more blood loss, pain and fever, longer hospital stay, later return to work, and less satisfaction than women having total vaginal hysterectomy. Two RCTs found that women having total abdominal hysterectomy had longer recovery times and more postoperative pain but shorter operating times and less blood loss than women having laparoscopically assisted vaginal hysterectomy. One RCT found that women having total abdominal hysterectomy had more postoperative fever, longer hospital stay, and recovery times than women having total laparoscopic hysterectomy.

Benefits: We found no systematic review. We found no RCTs comparing total abdominal hysterectomy**G** versus no intervention or sham surgery (see comment below). **Versus total vaginal hysterectomy G:** See benefits of total vaginal hysterectomy, p 2351. **Versus laparoscopically assisted vaginal hysterectomy G:** See benefits of laparoscopically assisted vaginal hysterectomy, p 2352. **Versus laparoscopic myomectomy:** See benefits of laparoscopic myomectomy, p 2354.

Harms: **Versus total vaginal hysterectomy:** See harms of total vaginal hysterectomy, p 2352. **Versus laparoscopically assisted vaginal hysterectomy:** See harms of laparoscopically assisted vaginal hysterectomy, p 2353. **Versus laparoscopic myomectomy:** See harms of laparoscopic myomectomy, p 2355.

Comment: There is consensus that abdominal hysterectomy is superior to no treatment in improving fibroid related symptoms. An RCT is unlikely to be conducted. Other RCTs have compared different types of hysterectomy in various groups of women but results from these RCTs are not generalisable to women with fibroids.

OPTION TOTAL VAGINAL HYSTERECTOMY

Two RCTs found that women having total vaginal hysterectomy had shorter operation times, less blood loss, pain and fever, shorter hospital stay, earlier return to work, and greater satisfaction than women having total abdominal hysterectomy. One RCT found that women having total vaginal hysterectomy had shorter operation times and less blood loss than women having laparoscopically assisted vaginal hysterectomy.

Benefits: We found no systematic review. We found no RCTs comparing total vaginal hysterectomy**G** versus no intervention or sham surgery. **Versus total abdominal hysterectomy:** We found no systematic review. We found two RCTs (179 women) comparing total vaginal hysterectomy versus total abdominal hysterectomy.[47,48] Both RCTs found that vaginal hysterectomy improved intraoperative and postoperative outcomes compared with abdominal hysterectomy. The first RCT (90 women) compared three interventions: total vaginal hysterectomy, total abdominal hysterectomy, and laparoscopically assisted vaginal hysterectomy (LAVH)**G**.[47] The women in each group did not differ significantly in age, weight, or other relevant demographic characteristics. The RCT found that, compared with either total abdominal hysterectomy or LAVH, total vaginal hysterectomy significantly reduced intraoperative blood loss (215 mL with vaginal hysterectomy *v* 293 mL with abdominal hysterectomy *v* 343 mL with LAVH; $P = 0.04$). It found that, compared with total abdominal hysterectomy, both total vaginal hysterectomy and LAVH significantly reduced postoperative pain scores at 24 hours (measured on a scale from 0–10; 3 with vaginal hysterectomy *v* 6 with abdominal hysterectomy *v* 4 with LAVH; $P < 0.001$), and the number of days of postoperative antibiotic use (1.3 days with vaginal hysterectomy *v* 1.7 days with abdominal hysterectomy *v* 1.3 days with LAVH; $P < 0.001$). It also found that both total vaginal hysterectomy and LAVH significantly reduced the time to return to work (mean: 29 days with vaginal hysterectomy *v* 41 with abdominal hysterectomy *v* 30 with LAVH; $P < 0.001$), reduced the proportion of women with febrile morbidity (13% with vaginal hysterectomy *v* 27% with total abdominal hysterectomy *v* 3% with LAVH; $P < 0.05$), and reduced mean hospital stay (4.7 days with vaginal hysterectomy *v* 5.0 days with abdominal hysterectomy *v* 4.7 days with LAVH; $P = 0.003$). The second RCT found that, compared with total abdominal hysterectomy, total vaginal hysterectomy significantly reduced the duration of operation (86 minutes with vaginal hysterectomy *v* 102 minutes with abdominal hysterectomy; $P < 0.001$), reduced the proportion of women with postoperative fever (17% with vaginal hysterectomy *v* 30% with abdominal hysterectomy; $P < 0.05$), and reduced the proportion of women who needed postoperative analgesics (66% with vaginal hysterectomy *v* 86.4% with abdominal hysterectomy; $P < 0.05$).[48] It found that total vaginal hysterectomy significantly reduced hospital stay compared with abdominal hysterectomy (3.4 days with vaginal hysterectomy *v* 4.3 days with abdominal hysterectomy; $P < 0.001$). More women having vaginal hysterectomy rated treatment as "good" or "very good" (83% with vaginal hysterectomy *v* 32% with total hysterectomy, P value not reported). **Versus laparoscopically assisted vaginal hysterectomy:** See benefits of laparoscopically assisted vaginal hysterectomy, p 2352.

Harms: The RCTs found no major complications associated with total vaginal hysterectomy.[47,48]

Comment: Other RCTs have compared different types of hysterectomy in various groups of women but results from these RCTs are not generalisable to women with fibroids. The RCTs did not assess effects on pregnancy rates.

OPTION LAPAROSCOPICALLY ASSISTED VAGINAL HYSTERECTOMY

Two RCTs found that women having laparoscopically assisted vaginal hysterectomy had shorter recovery times and less postoperative pain but longer operating time and more blood loss than women having total abdominal hysterectomy. One RCT found that women having laparoscopically assisted vaginal hysterectomy had longer operating time and more blood loss than women having total vaginal hysterectomy.

Benefits: We found no systematic review. We found no RCTs comparing laparoscopically assisted vaginal hysterectomy (LAVH)Ⓖ versus no intervention or sham surgery. **Versus total abdominal hysterectomy or total vaginal hysterectomy:** We found two RCTs in women with symptomatic fibroids scheduled for hysterectomy comparing the effects of LAVH versus total abdominal hysterectomy (TAH) on operating time, blood loss, complications (not clearly specified), febrile morbidity, postoperative analgesic requirement, and hospital stay.[46,47] Both RCTs found that LAVH improved intraoperative and postoperative outcomes compared with abdominal hysterectomy. The first RCT (62 women) found that LAVH significantly reduced hospital stay and analgesic use compared with TAH (mean hospital stay 3.8 days with LAVH *v* 5.8 days with TAH; $P < 0.001$; analgesic use for > 24 hours postoperatively 23% with LAVH *v* 77% with TAH; CI not reported).[46] Post hoc subgroup analyses found limited evidence that relative effects of LAVH and TAH depended on uterine weight (see comment below).[46] The second RCT (90 women) compared three interventions: LAVH, total vaginal hysterectomy, and TAH.[47] There was no significant difference in age, weight, or other relevant demographic characteristics among groups. The RCT found that, compared with either LAVH or TAH, total vaginal hysterectomy significantly reduced intraoperative blood loss (343 mL with LAVH *v* 215 mL with vaginal hysterectomy *v* 293 mL with TAH; P = 0.04). It found that, compared with TAH, both LAVH and total vaginal hysterectomy significantly reduced postoperative pain scores at 24 hours (measured on a scale from 0–10; 4 with LAVH *v* 3 with total vaginal hysterectomy *v* 6 with TAH; P < 0.001), and the number of days of postoperative antibiotic use (1.3 days with LAVH *v* 1.3 days with total vaginal hysterectomy *v* 1.7 days with TAH; P < 0.001). It also found that both LAVH and total vaginal hysterectomy significantly reduced the time to return to work (mean 30 days with LAVH *v* 29 days with vaginal hysterectomy *v* 41 days with TAH; P < 0.001), reduced the proportion of women with febrile morbidity (3% with LAVH *v* 13% with total vaginal hysterectomy *v* 27% with TAH; P < 0.05), and reduced mean hospital stay (4.7 days with LAVH *v* 4.7 days with vaginal hysterectomy *v* 5.0 days with TAH; P = 0.003). The second RCT found no significant difference in postoperative pain, time to return to work, or febrile morbidity between LAVH and vaginal hysterectomy.[47]

Harms: **Versus total abdominal hysterectomy:** The first RCT found that LAVH significantly increased operating time (in women who did not have a second operation [oophorectomy and/or adhesiolysis]) compared with TAH (mean operating time 135 minutes with LAVH *v* 120 minutes with TAH; P = 0.001).[46] The second RCT also found that LAVH significantly increased mean operating time (without second procedure) and blood loss compared with TAH (mean 109 minutes with LAVH *v* 98 minutes with TAH; P < 0.001; mean blood loss 343 mL with LAVH *v* 293 mL with TAH; P = 0.04).[47] No major complications were reported in either RCT, although there was insufficient information to determine which complications were addressed.

Comment: The RCTs did not assess effects on pregnancy rates. **In women with uterus estimated to weigh 500 g or less:** Subgroup analysis of the first RCT in 41 women with uterus estimated to weigh 500 g or less in the preoperative assessment found that LAVH and TAH required comparable operating times (130 minutes on average with LAVH *v* 120 minutes with TAH).[46] Women in the LAVH group had less postoperative pain and shorter recovery compared with the TAH group. Sonograms were used to estimate uterine weight. Analgesia requirement was reduced with LAVH (1/20 [5%] with LAVH *v* 6/11 [55%] with TAH; RR 0.09, 95% CI 0.01 to 0.67; NNT 2, 95% CI 1 to 6). Hospital stay was also reduced with LAVH (3.8 days, 95% CI 3.2 days to 4.0 days with LAVH *v* 5.8 days, 95% CI 5.0 days to 6.4 days with TAH; P < 0.0001). **In women with uterus estimated to weigh more than 500 g:** Subgroup analysis of the RCT in 21 women with uteri weighing more than 500 g found that LAVH was associated with a shorter recovery but a longer operating time compared with TAH.[46] About 27% of women randomised to LAVH converted to laparotomy. Mean operating time was increased with LAVH (150 minutes, 95% CI 125 minutes to 173 minutes with LAVH *v* 108 minutes, 95% CI 83 minutes to 120 minutes with TAH; P = 0.002). Mean hospital stay was reduced with LAVH (4.0 days, 95% CI 3.9 days to 5.8 days with LAVH *v* 6.0 days, 95% CI 5.8 days to 6.0 days with TAH). **Extrapolating results of hysterectomy for other disorders to women with fibroids:** Other RCTs have compared different types of hysterectomy in other groups of women but results from these RCTs are not generalisable to women with fibroids.

OPTION TOTAL LAPAROSCOPIC HYSTERECTOMY

One RCT found that women having total laparoscopic hysterectomy had less postoperative fever, shorter hospital stay, and shorter recovery times compared with women having total abdominal hysterectomy.

Benefits: We found no systematic review. We found no RCTs comparing total laparoscopic hysterectomy**G** versus no intervention or sham surgery. **Versus total abdominal hysterectomy:** We found no systematic review but found one RCT (122 women with an enlarged uterus [equivalent to > 14 weeks' gestation] because of fibroids) comparing total laparoscopic hysterectomy versus total abdominal hysterectomy.[49] It found that, compared with total abdominal hysterectomy, total laparoscopic hysterectomy significantly reduced the proportion of women who had postoperative fever (13% with total laparoscopic hysterectomy *v* 29% with total abdominal hysterectomy; $P < 0.05$), and reduced duration of hospital stay (mean 76.4 hours with total laparoscopic hysterectomy *v* 121.8 hours with total abdominal hysterectomy) and recovery times (mean 22 days with total laparoscopic hysterectomy *v* 36 days with total abdominal hysterectomy; $P < 0.001$ for both outcomes).

Harms: The RCT reported that one woman randomised to total laparoscopic hysterectomy converted to abdominal hysterectomy because of incidental bowel injury.[49] It found no other major complications associated with laparoscopic or abdominal hysterectomy.

Comment: Women were only included in the RCT if they had an enlarged uterus.[49] This would usually be a contraindication to total laparoscopic hysterectomy. The RCT did not assess effects on pregnancy rates.[49] Other RCTs have compared different types of hysterectomy in various groups of women but results from these RCTs are not generalisable to women with fibroids.

OPTION LAPAROSCOPIC MYOMECTOMY

Two RCTs found limited evidence that laparosopic myomectomy reduced postoperative pain, fever, and recovery time compared to abdominal myomectomy. We found no RCTs comparing laparoscopic myomectomy versus total abdominal, vaginal, or laparoscopic hysterectomy, but the the main benefit of myomectomy over hysterectomy is that it maintains fertility.

Benefits: We found no systematic review. **Versus no intervention or sham surgery:** We found no RCTs. **Versus abdominal myomectomy:** We found two RCTs comparing laparoscopic versus abdominal myomectomy**G**.[50,51] The first RCT (40 women with < 5 myomas and the size of the largest myoma < 7 cm) found no differences in length of surgery, blood loss, or postoperative complications (fever). Women having laparoscopic myomectomy reported a lower intensity of postoperative pain (unlabelled scale), required less analgesia, and had a shorter recovery time than women having abdominal myomectomy by laparotomy. Two days after surgery, a significantly smaller proportion of women required analgesia with laparoscopic myomectomy versus abdominal myomectomy (analgesia free women: 17/20 [85%] with laparoscopy *v* 3/20 [15%] with abdominal; RR 5.7, 95% CI 2.0 to 16.4; NNT 2, 95% CI 1 to 3), and by day 15 more women were fully recovered after laparoscopic myomectomy (18/20 [90%] with laparoscopy *v* 1/20 [5%] with abdominal; RR 18.0, 95% CI 2.7 to 122.0; NNT 2, 95% CI 1 to 2). The second RCT (131 women with at least 1 myoma ≥ 5 cm) found similar length of surgery with laparoscopic and abdominal myomectomy.[51] However, it found a significantly greater drop in haemoglobin with abdominal than with laparoscopy (1.33 g/dL with laparoscopy *v* 2.17 g/dL with abdominal; $P < 0.001$). Women who had laparoscopic myomectomy were marginally but significantly less likely to experience postoperative fever than women who had abdominal myomectomy (8/66 [12%] with laparoscopy v 17/65 [26%] with abdominal; RR 0.46, 95% CI 0.22 to 1.00; NNT 9, 95% CI 4 to 116) and were more likely to have a shorter hospital stay (75.6 hours with laparoscopy v 142.8 hours with abdominal; CI not reported; $P < 0.001$). It found no significant difference in pregnancy rate after surgery between laparoscopic and abdominal myomectomy (53.6% with laparoscopy v 55.9% with abdominal; reported as non-significant, CI not reported). **Versus total abdominal, vaginal, or laparoscopic hysterectomy:** We found no RCTs (see comment).

Harms: No major complications were reported in the two RCTs.[50,51] The second RCT found that more people having abdominal compared with laparoscopic myomectomy had transfusions (transfusion risk: 3/65 [5%] with abdominal v 0/66 [0%] with laparoscopy; CI not reported).[51]

Comment: We found no RCTs comparing laparoscopic myomectomy versus hysterectomy, the main benefit of myomectomy compared with hysterectomy is that it maintains fertility.

OPTION THERMAL BALLOON ABLATION

We found no RCTs comparing thermal balloon ablation versus non-surgical treatment or versus hysterectomy. One RCT compared thermal balloon ablation versus rollerball endometrial ablation in women with fibroids smaller than the average size of a 12 week pregnancy, all of whom had been pretreated with gonadorelin analogues. It found no significant difference between thermal balloon and rollerball ablation in amenorrhoea rates, pictorial bleeding assessment chart score, haemoglobin, or hysterectomy rates at 12 months. It found that thermal balloon ablation reduced operation time and intraoperative complication rate compared with rollerball ablation. About one third of women reported being "not very satisfied" with either operation.

Benefits: **Versus other surgical treatment:** We found no RCTs comparing thermal balloon ablation**G** versus hysterectomy. We found one RCT (96 women with fibroids smaller than the average size of a 12 week pregnancy who had received 2 months of preoperative treatment with gonadorelin analogues) that compared thermal balloon ablation versus rollerball endometrial ablation**G**.[52] Thermal balloon ablation was performed by staff surgeons or supervised residents under local intracervical and paracervical anaesthesia with intravenous sedation. Rollerball ablation was performed under general anaesthesia by experienced surgeons. The RCT found no significant difference between thermal balloon ablation compared with rollerball endometrial ablation in hysterectomy rates, amenorrhoea rates, pictorial bleeding assessment chart score**G**, or haemoglobin at 12 months (women having hysterectomy: 4/45 [9%] with thermal balloon v 4/48 [8%] with rollerball; amenorrhoea: 5 women with thermal balloon v 8 women with rollerball; mean decrease in pictorial bleeding assessment chart score: 343 with thermal balloon v 345 with rollerball; mean increase in haemoglobin: 2.7 g/dL with thermal balloon v 3.0 g/dL with rollerball; P values reported as non-significant for all comparisons; CI not reported). Operating time was significantly shorter in the thermal balloon group compared with the rollerball group (11.5 minutes with thermal balloon v 37.3 minutes with rollerball, $P < 0.0001$). About a third of women in both groups reported that they were "not very satisfied" with their operation (33% with thermal balloon v 39% with rollerball).[52]

Harms: The RCT found that a significantly higher proportion of women had intraoperative complications with rollerball ablation than with thermal balloon ablation (5/45 [11%] with rollerball v 0/48 [0%] with thermal balloon, $P < 0.05$; 2 women had fluid overload, 2 had major bleeding, and 1 had injury to the cervix).[52] It found no significant difference between rollerball ablation and thermal balloon ablation in postoperative complications (3 women in each group) or postoperative pain score at 12 hours.

Comment: The RCT did not assess effects on pregnancy rates.

GLOSSARY

Endometrial resection Destruction of the endometrium using a cutting tool.

Myomectomy Removal of fibroids from the uterus. The mode of removal may be abdominal, laparoscopic, or hysteroscopic.

Pelvic symptom score scale An ordinal scale that adds the results of pelvic pain and pelvic pressure. Each symptom is evaluated in a scale ranging of 0–3, where 0 means absence of pain, and increasing numbers represent mild, moderate, and severe pain. Because both results are added, absence of symptoms is represented by 0 and severe pain and pelvic pressure by 6. We found no data on validation of the scale. However, it is commonly used in studies evaluating pelvic pain.

Pictorial bleeding assessment chart (PBAC) Used to measure menstrual bleeding. Validation studies indicate that a PBAC score of 100–185 is suggestive of menorrhagia (heavy menstrual bleeding) which is objectively defined by the alkaline haematin test as a menstrual blood loss greater than 80 mL.

Rollerball endometrial ablation Destruction of the endometrium using electrical coagulation with a rollerball electrode applied through the cervical os.

Thermal balloon ablation Destruction of the endometrium using pressure from a balloon catheter inserted through the cervical os and then filled with fluid to a pressure of 160–180 mm Hg and heated to about 87 °C.

Total hysterectomy Removal of the uterus. The mode of removal may be through the abdominal wall (total abdominal hysterectomy), through the vagina (total vaginal hysterectomy), partially through the vagina and partially morcellated and removed by laparoscopic incision (laparoscopically assisted vaginal hysterectomy), or entirely by laparoscopic excision (total laparoscopic hysterectomy). In some situations, total abdominal hysterectomy is performed in conjunction with a bilateral salpingo-oophorectomy, the removal of both ovaries and fallopian tubes.

REFERENCES

1. Buttram VC, Reiter RC. Uterine leiomyomata: etiology, symptomatology and management. *Fertil Steril* 1981;6:433–445.
2. Lumsden MA, Wallace EM. Clinical presentation of uterine fibroids. *Baillieres Clin Obstet Gynaecol* 1998;12:177–195.
3. Valle RF. Hysteroscopy in the evaluation of female infertility. *Am J Obstet Gynecol* 1980;137:425–431.
4. Borgfeldt C, Andolf E. Transvaginal ultrasonographic findings in the uterus and the endometrium: low prevalence of leiomyoma in a random sample of women age 25–40 years. *Acta Obstet Gynecol Scand* 2000;79:202–207.
5. Ross RK, Pike MC, Vessey MP, et al. Risk factors for uterine fibroids: reduced risk associated with oral contraceptives. *BMJ* 1986;293:359–363.
6. Thompson JD, Rock JA, eds. *Te Linde's operative gynecology*, 7th edition. 1992, JB Lippincott Company: London, Hagerstrom.
7. Cramer SF, Patel A. The frequency of uterine leiomyomas. *Am J Clin Pathol* 1990;90:435–438.
8. Schwartz SM, Marshall LM, Baird DD. Epidemiologic contributions to understanding the etiology of uterine leiomyomata. *Environ Health Perspect* 2000;108:821–827.
9. Farquhar C, Arroll B, Ekeroma A, et al. An evidence-based guideline for the management of uterine fibroids. *Aust N Z J Obstet Gynaecol* 2001;41:125–140.
10. Townsend DE, Sparkes RS, Baluda MC, et al. Unicellular histogenesis of uterine leiomyomas as determined by electrophoresis of glucose-6-phosphate dehydrogenase. *Am J Obstet Gynecol* 1970;107:1168–1174.
11. Hashimoto K, Azuma C, Kamiura S, et al. Clonal determination of uterine leiomyomas by analyzing differential inactivation of the X-chromosome-linked phosphoglycerokinase gene. *Gynecol Obstet Invest* 1995;40:204–208.
12. Chiaffarino F, Parazzini F, La Vecchia C, et al. Use of oral contraceptives and uterine fibroids: results from a case-control study. *Br J Obstet Gynaecol* 1999;106:857–860.
13. Lumbiganon P, Rugpao S, Phandhu-Fung S, et al. Protective effect of depot-medroxyprogesterone acetate on surgically treated uterine leiomyomas: a multicentre-case control study. *Br J Obstet Gynaecol* 1995;103:909–914.
14. Carlson KJ, Miller BA, Fowler FJ Jr. The Maine Women's Health Study: II. Outcomes of nonsurgical management of leiomyomas, abnormal bleeding, and chronic pelvic pain. *Obstet Gynecol* 1994;83:566–572.
15. Minaguchi H, Wong JM, Snabes MC. Clinical use of nafarelin in the treatment of leiomyomas. A review of the literature. *J Reprod Med* 2000;45:481–489. Search date 1997; primary sources Medline, Refline, bibliographies, relevant journals, and abstracts from conferences and other meetings.
16. Donnez J, Vivancos BH, Kudela M, et al. A randomized, placebo-controlled, dose-ranging trial comparing fulvestrant with goserelin in

premenopausal patients with uterine fibroids awaiting hysterectomy. *Fertil Steril* 2003;79:1380–1389.
17. Friedman AJ, Hoffman DI, Comite F, et al. Treatment of leiomyomata uteri with leuprolide acetate depot: a double-blind, placebo-controlled, multicenter study. *Obstet Gynecol* 1991;77:720–725.
18. Friedman AJ, Harrison-Atlas D, Barbieri RL, et al. A randomized placebo-controlled double-blind study evaluating the efficacy of leuprolide acetate depot in the treatment of uterine leiomyomata. *Fertil Steril* 1989;51:251–254.
19. Schlaff WD, Zerhouni EA, Huth JA, et al. A placebo-controlled trial of a depot gonadotropin-releasing hormone analogue (leuprolide) in the treatment of uterine leiomyomata. *Obstet Gynecol* 1989;74:856–862.
20. Espinos JJ, Marti A, Asins E, et al. Efectos de dos dosis de un analogo de la GnRH (leuprorelina depot) sobre la miomatosis uterina. *Clin Invest Gin Obst* 1993;20:382–387.
21. Takeuchi H, Kobori H, Kikuchi I, et al. A prospective randomised study comparing endocrinological and clinical effects of two types of GnRH agonists in cases of uterine leiomyomas or endometriosis. *J Obstet Gynecol Res* 2000;26:325–331.
22. Broekmans FJ, Hompes PG, Heitbrink MA, et al. Two-step gonadotropin-releasing hormone agonist treatment of uterine leiomyomas: standard-dose therapy followed by reduced-dose therapy. *Am J Obstet Gynecol* 1996;175:1208–1216.
23. Watanabe Y, Nakamura G, Matsuguchi H, et al. Efficacy of a low-dose leuprolide acetate depot in the treatment of uterine leiomyomata in Japanese women. *Fertil Steril* 1992;58:66–71.
24. Watanabe Y, Nakamura G. Effects of two different doses of leuprolide acetate depot on uterine cavity area in patients with uterine leiomyomata. *Fertil Steril* 1995;63:487–490.
25. Vollenhoven BJ, Shekleton P, McDonald J, et al. Clinical predictors for buserelin acetate treatment of uterine fibroids: a prospective study of 40 women. *Fertil Steril* 1990;54:1032–1038.
26. Friedman AJ, Barbieri RL, Benacerraf BR, et al. Treatment of leiomyomata with intranasal or subcutaneous leuprolide, a gonadotropin-releasing hormone agonist. *Fertil Steril* 1987;48:560–564.
27. Costantini S, Anserini P, Valenzano M, et al. Luteinizing hormone-releasing hormone analog therapy of uterine fibroid: analysis of results obtained with buserelin administered intranasally and goserelin administered subcutaneously as a monthly depot. *Eur J Obstet Gynaecol Reprod Biol* 1990;37:63–69.
28. Scialli AR, Jestila KJ. Sustained benefits of leuprolide acetate with or without subsequent medroxyprogesterone acetate in the nonsurgical management of leiomyomata uteri. *Fertil Steril* 1995;64:313–320.
29. Caird LE, West CP, Lumsden MA, et al. Medroxyprogesterone acetate with Zoladex for long-term treatment of fibroids: effects on bone density and patient acceptability. *Hum Reprod* 1997;2:436–440.
30. Friedman AJ, Barbieri RL, Doubilet PM, et al. A randomized double-blind trial of a gonadotropin releasing-hormone agonist (leuprolide) with or without medroxyprogesterone acetate in the treatment of leiomyomata uteri. *Fertil Steril* 1988;49:404–409.
31. Palomba S, Affinito P, Giovanni MD, et al. A clinical trial of the effects of tibolone administered with gonadotropin-releasing hormone analogues for the treatment of uterine leiomyomata. *Fertil Steril* 1998;70:111–118.
32. Gocmen A, Kara IH, Karaca M. The effect of add-back treatment with tibolone on patients with myoma uteri treated with triptorelin. *Clin Exp Obstet Gynecol* 2002:29;222–224.
33. Friedman AJ, Daly M, Juneau-Norcross M, et al. Long-term medical therapy for leiomyomata uteri: a prospective, randomized study of leuprolide acetate depot plus oestrogen-progestin or progestin 'add-back' for 2 years. *Hum Reprod* 1994;9:1618–1625.
34. Palomba S, Russo T, Orio F Jr, et al. Effectiveness of combined GnRH analogue plus raloxifene administration in the treatment of uterine leiomyomas: a prospective, randomized, single-blind, placebo-controlled clinical trial. *Hum Reprod* 2002;17:3213–3219.
35. Ylikorkala O, Pekonen F. Naproxen reduces idiopathic but not fibromyoma-induced menorrhagia. *Obstet Gynecol* 1986;68:10–12.
36. Makarainen L, Ylikorkala O. Primary and myoma-associated menorrhagia: role of prostaglandins and effects of ibuprofen. *Br J Obstet Gynaecol* 1986;93:974–978.
37. Coutinho EM, Goncalves MT. Long-term treatment of leiomyomas with gestrinone. *Fertil Steril* 1989;51:939–946.
38. Coutinho EM, Boulanger GA, Goncalves MT. Regression of uterine leiomyomas after treatment with gestrinone, an antiestrogen, antiprogesterone. *Am J Obstet Gynecol* 1986;155:761–767.
39. Mahajan DK, London SN. Mifepristone (RU486): a review. *Fertil Steril* 1997;68:967–976.
40. Ikomi A, Pepra EF. Efficacy of the levonorgestrel intrauterine system in treating menorrhagia: actualities and ambiguities. *J Fam Plann Reprod Health Care* 2002;28:99–100.
41. Lethaby A, Vollenhoven B, Sowter M, et al. Preoperative GnRH analogue therapy before hysterectomy or myomectomy for uterine fibroids. In: The Cochrane Library, Issue 4, 2000. Oxford: Update Software. Search date 2000; primary sources the Cochrane Menstrual Disorders and Subfertility Group Register of Trials, Medline, Embase, the National Research Register, the National Library of Medicine's Clinical Trials Register, and Current Contents. Published trials were also identified from citation lists of review articles and direct contact with drug companies for unpublished trials. In most cases, the first author of each included trial was contacted for additional information.
42. Vercellini P, Trespidi L, Zaina B, et al. Gonadotropin-releasing hormone agonist treatment before abdominal myomectomy: a controlled trial. *Fertil Steril* 2003;79:1390–1395.
43. Parazzini F, Bortolotti A, Chiantera V, et al. Goserelin acetate to avoid hysterectomy in pre-menopausal women with fibroids requiring surgery. *Eur J Obstet Gynecol Reprod Biol* 1999;87:31–33.
44. Campo S, Garcea N. Laparoscopic myomectomy in premenstrual women with and without preoperative treatment using gonadotrophin-releasing hormone analogues. *Hum Reprod* 1999;14:44–48.
45. Rees M, Chamberlain P, Gillmer M. Management of uterine fibroids with goserelin acetate alone or goserelin acetate plus endometrial resection. *Gynaecol Endosc* 2001;10:33–35.
46. Ferrari MM, Berlanda N, Mezzopane R, et al. Identifying the indications for laparoscopically assisted vaginal hysterectomy: a prospective, randomised comparison with abdominal hysterectomy in patients with symptomatic uterine fibroids. *Br J Obstet Gynaecol* 2000;107:620–625.
47. Hwang JL, Seow KM, Tsai YL, et al. Comparative study of vaginal, laparoscopically assisted vaginal and abdominal hysterectomies for uterine myoma larger than 6 cm in diameter or uterus weighing at least 450 g: a prospective randomized study. *Acta Obstet Gynecol Scand* 2002;81:1132–1138.
48. Benassi L, Rossi T, Kaihura CT, et al. Abdominal or vaginal hysterectomy for enlarged uteri: a randomized clinical trial. *Am J Obstet Gynecol* 2002;187:1561–1565.
49. Seracchioli R, Venturoli S, Vianello F, et al. Total laparoscopic hysterectomy compared with abdominal hysterectomy in the presence of a large uterus. *J Am Assoc Gynecol Laparosc* 2002;9:333–338.
50. Mais V, Ajossa S, Guerriero S, et al. Laparoscopic versus abdominal myomectomy: a prospective, randomized trial to evaluate benefits in early outcome. *Am J Obstet Gynecol* 1996;174:654–658.

51. Seracchioli R, Rossi S, Govoni F, et al. Fertility and obstetric outcome after laparoscopic myomectomy of large myomata: a randomised comparison with abdominal myomectomy. *Hum Reprod* 2000;15:2663–2668.

52. Soysal ME, Soysal SK, Vicdan K. Thermal balloon ablation in myoma-induced menorrhagia under local anesthesia. *Gynecol Obstet Invest* 2001;51:128–133.

Anne Lethaby
Cochrane Menstrual Disorders and Subfertility Group
Auckland
New Zealand

Beverley Vollenhoven
Department of Obstetrics and Gynaecology
Monash University
Clayton, Victoria
Australia

Competing interests: None declared.

TABLE 1 Harms of leuprotelin versus placebo in one RCT (65 women).[17] See text, p 2344.

Harms	Gonadorelin			Placebo				
	Outcome	Population	%	Outcome	Population	%	RR*	95% CI*
Vasomotor flushes	52	63	83%	5	65	8%	10.7	4.6 to 25.1
Vaginitis	11	63	17%	0	65	0%		
Arthralgia/mialgia	9	63	14%	0	65	0%		
Asthenia	10	63	16%	3	65	5%	3.4	0.97 to 996
Peripheral oedema	7	63	11%	1	65	2%	7.2	0.9 to 57
Insomnia	6	63	10%	0	65	0%		
Nausea	6	63	10%	1	65	2%	6.2	0.8 to 50
Emotional ability /nervousness	5	63	8%	1	65	2%	5.2	0.6 to 42.9
Depression	7	63	11%	2	65	3%	3.6	0.8 to 16.7
Headaches	18	63	29%	13	65	20%	1.4	0.8 to 2.7
Decreased libido	2	63	3%	0	65	0%		

*_Clinical Evidence_ recalculation.

Genital prolapse

Search date August 2004

Joseph Loze Onwude

QUESTIONS

INTERVENTIONS

NON-SURGICAL TREATMENTS
Unknown effectiveness

To be covered in future updates
Effects of surgical treatments in women with genital prolapse

Covered elsewhere in *Clinical Evidence*
See urinary stress incontinence, p 2463

*Consensus regards vaginal pessaries as effective

See glossary G

Key Messages

Non-surgical treatments

- **Pelvic floor muscle exercises** We found no RCTs or observational studies of sufficient quality examining the effects of pelvic floor muscle exercises on the symptoms of genital prolapse.
- **Vaginal oestrogen** We found no systematic review or RCTs on the effects of vaginal oestrogen.
- **Vaginal pessaries*** We found no RCTs or observational studies of sufficient quality examining effects of vaginal pessaries on the symptoms of genital prolapse. However, consensus opinion suggests that they are effective for short term relief of genital prolapse prior to surgery, or in the long term if surgery is contraindicated.

  *Consensus regards vaginal pessaries as effective

Clin Evid 2005;13:2360–2364.

DEFINITION Genital prolapse (also known as pelvic organ prolapse) refers to uterine, uterovaginal, or vaginal prolapse. Genital prolapse results from loss of muscle support in the pelvic region. In uterine prolapse the uterus descends into the vaginal canal with the cervix at its leading edge; this may in turn pull down the vagina, in which case it may be referred to as uterovaginal prolapse. In vaginal prolapse one or more regions of the vaginal wall protrude into the vaginal canal. Vaginal prolapse is classified according to the region of the vaginal wall that is affected: a cystocoele involves the anterior upper vaginal wall, urethrocoele the lower anterior vaginal wall, rectocoele the posterior vaginal wall, and enterocoele the upper posterior vaginal wall. After hysterectomy, the apex of the vagina may prolapse as a vault prolapse. This usually pulls down the anterior and posterior walls as well. The two main systems for grading the severity of genital prolapse, the Baden–Walker halfway system[1] and the Pelvic Organ Prolapse Quantification (POPQ) system,[2] are summarised in Table 1, p 2364. Mild genital prolapse may be asymptomatic. Symptoms of genital prolapse are mainly non-specific. Common symptoms include pelvic heaviness, genital bulge, and difficulties during sexual intercourse, such as pain or loss of vaginal sensation. Symptoms that may be more commonly associated with specific forms of prolapse include urinary incontinence, which is associated with cystocoele; incomplete urinary emptying, which is associated with cystocoele or uterine prolapse, or both; and need to apply digital pressure to the perineum or posterior vaginal wall for defaecation, which is associated with rectocoele.[3]

INCIDENCE/ PREVALENCE Prevalence estimates vary widely, depending on the population and the way in which women were recruited into studies. One study conducted in the USA (497 women aged 18–82 years attending a routine general gynaecology clinic) found that 93.6% had some degree of genital prolapse (43.3% POPQ stage 1, 47.7% POPQ stage 2, 2.6% POPQ stage 3, and 0% POPQ stage 4).[4] In that study the incidence of clinically relevant prolapse (POPQ stage 2 or greater) was found to increase with advancing parity: non-parous, 14.6%; one to three births, 48%; and more than three births, 71.2%. One Swedish study (487 women) found that 30.8% of women between the ages of 20 and 59 years had some degree of genital prolapse on clinical assessment.[5] The prevalence of genital prolapse increased with age, from 6.6% in women aged 20–29 years to 55.6% in women aged 50–59 years. Prevalence of genital prolapse was also higher in parous women (44%) than in non-parous women (5.8%). A cross-sectional study (241 perimenopausal women aged 45–55 years seeking to enter a trial of hormone replacement therapy) found that 23% had POPQ stage 1 genital prolapse, 4% had POPQ stage 2 prolapse, and no women had POPQ stage 3 or 4 prolapse.[6] One cross-sectional study conducted in the UK (285 perimenopausal and postmenopausal women attending a menopause clinic with climacteric symptoms) found that 20% had some degree of uterovaginal or vault prolapse, 51% some degree of anterior wall vaginal prolapse, and 27% some degree of posterior wall vaginal prolapse.[7] Severe prolapse (equivalent to POPQ stage 3 or 4) was found in 6% of women. One prospective study (412 postmenopausal women aged 50–79 years) found that the baseline prevalence of cystocoele was 24.6% (for grades 1, 2, and 3 the prevalences were 14.4%, 9.5%, and 0.7%, respectively), the baseline prevalence of rectocoele was 12.9% (for grades 1 and 2 the prevalences were 7.8% and 5.1%, respectively), and the baseline prevalence of uterine prolapse was 3.8% (for grades 1 and 2 the prevalences were 3.3% and 0.6%, respectively).[8] Among women who entered the study the annual incidences of cystocoele, rectocoele, and uterine prolapse were 9%, 6%, and 2%, respectively.

AETIOLOGY/ RISK FACTORS One case control study found that the strongest risk factors for severe (POPQ stages 3 or 4) genital prolapse are increasing age (OR 1.12 for each additional year, 95% CI 1.09 to 1.15), increasing weight of largest baby delivered vaginally (OR 1.24 for each additional pound, 95% CI 1.06 to 1.44), previous hysterectomy (OR 2.37, 95% CI 1.16 to 4.86), and previous surgery for genital prolapse (OR 5.09, 95% CI 1.49 to 17.26).[10] The study did not find a significant association between severe genital prolapse and chronic medical conditions such as obesity, hypertension, or chronic obstructive pulmonary disease.

PROGNOSIS We found no reliable information about the natural history of untreated mild genital prolapse (POPQ stages 1 and 2, Baden–Walker grades 1 and 2). We found one prospective study on the progression of genital prolapse in women who were treated or untreated with hormone replacement therapy (oestrogen + progesterone).[8] However, the results were not reported separately by treatment group and therefore they may not apply to untreated women. In addition, the investigators used an examination technique whose reliability, reproducibility, and ability to discriminate between absence of prolapse and mild prolapse was not known. It found that, over 1 year, cystocoeles progressed from grade 1 to grades 2–3 in 9% of cases, regressed from grades 2–3 to grade 0 in 9%, and regressed from grade 1 to grade 0 in 23%. Rectocoeles progressed from grade 1 to grades 2–3 in 1%, but regressed from grades 2–3 to grade 0 in 3%, and from grade 1 to grade 0 in 2%. Uterine prolapse regressed from grade 1 to grade 0 in 48%. The incidence of morbidity associated with genital prolapse is also difficult to estimate. The annual incidence of hospital admission for prolapse in the UK has been estimated at 2.04 per 1000 women under the age of 60 years.[9] Genital prolapse is also a major cause of gynaecological surgery.

AIMS OF INTERVENTION To relieve symptoms; to remove the vaginal mass; to improve urinary incontinence, poor flow, or urinary retention; to alleviate problems with sexual intercourse or emptying the bowel.

OUTCOMES Quality of life scores such as the Prolapse Quality of Life Questionnaire;[11] symptom scores.

METHODS *Clinical Evidence* search and appraisal August 2004. We searched Medline from June 1966 to August 2004 using a McMaster validated search strategy (key words: uterine prolapse, vaginal prolapse, exercise therapy, pelvic floor, pessaries, vagina pessary, estrogens, estrogen therapy, muscle training). We searched Embase 1980 to August 2004, and the Cochrane Library 2004 Issue 2, and some evidence-based medicine web sites. Two independent appraisers critically appraised the results of the search.

QUESTION What are the effects of non-surgical treatments in women with genital prolapse?

OPTION PELVIC FLOOR MUSCLE EXERCISES

We found no RCTs or observational studies of sufficient quality examining the effects of pelvic floor muscle exercises on the symptoms of genital prolapse.

Benefits: We found one systematic review (search date 2003, and 2004 for some sources), which identified no RCTs.[12] We found no RCTs or observational studies of sufficient quality (see comment below).

Harms: We found no RCTs or observational studies of sufficient quality.

Comment: Although pelvic floor muscle exercises**G** appear to be effective in reducing the symptoms of urinary stress incontinence (see benefits of pelvic floor muscle exercises in stress incontinence chapter, p 2463), their usefulness in the treatment of genital prolapse is unproven. We found one RCT in elderly women in Thailand that compared pelvic floor muscle exercises versus no treatment.[13] However, this RCT was excluded because it did not use a standard system for grading prolapse, did not assess the effects of treatments on the symptoms of prolapse or quality of life, and had high loss to follow up (28%).

OPTION VAGINAL PESSARIES

We found no RCTs or observational studies of sufficient quality examining effects of vaginal pessaries on the symptoms of genital prolapse. However, consensus opinion suggests that they are effective for short term relief of genital prolapse prior to surgery, or in the long term if surgery is contraindicated.

Benefits: We found one systematic review (search date 2003, and 2004 for some sources), which identified no RCTs.[14] We found no observational studies of sufficient quality.

Harms: We found one systematic review (search date 2003, and 2004 for some sources), which identified no RCTs.[14] Observational studies have found that vaginal pessaries**G** are associated with minimal morbidity. The most common adverse effects are pelvic pain, vaginal bleeding, vaginal discharge or odour, and unmasking of latent urinary stress incontinence.[15,16] Regular surveillance involving removing the pessary and inspecting the vaginal wall for evidence of erosion is required.

Comment: Consensus opinion suggests that vaginal pessaries**G** are effective as a short term option to relieve symptoms of genital prolapse during the preoperative waiting period, or over the long term if surgical treatment is contraindicated. Women with severe (Baden–Walker grades 3 and 4) prolapse are more likely than women with less severe prolapse (grades 1 and 2) to continue use long term because they are more likely to find them useful and because they must continue to use them long term to alleviate symptoms.[17]

OPTION VAGINAL OESTROGEN

We found no systematic review or RCTs on the effects of vaginal oestrogen.

Benefits: We found no systematic review or RCTs.

Harms: We found no RCTs.

Comment: There is currently no consensus on the efficacy of vaginal oestrogen in women with genital prolapse. Oestrogen deficiency may lead to a weakening of the connective tissue surrounding the uterus and vagina, and an increased risk of prolapse.[18,19] In women with oestrogen deficiency, such as menopausal women, vaginal oestrogen might therefore strengthen the connective tissue or prevent further damage. However, the clinical effectiveness of this treatment is unproven.

GLOSSARY

Pelvic floor muscle exercises Repetitive contraction exercises designed to strengthen the pelvic floor muscles.

Vaginal pessary A small device, usually made of latex or silicon, which is inserted into the vagina to hold the prolapsed uterus or vagina in place. Pessaries vary in shape, with two common types being ring and shelf pessaries.

Valsalva manoeuvre The woman bears down in order to apply pressure to the pelvic floor and elicit maximal protrusion of the prolapse site.

Substantive changes

Pelvic floor muscle exercise One systematic review added;[12] categorisation unchanged.

Vaginal pessaries One systematic review added;[14] categorisation unchanged.

REFERENCES

1. Baden WF, Walker TA, Lindsay HJ. The vaginal profile. *Tex Med J* 1968;64:56–58.
2. Bump RC, Mattiasson A, Bo K, et al. The standardization of terminology of female pelvic floor dysfunction. *Am J Obstet Gynecol* 1996;175:10–17.
3. Eva UF, Gun W, Preben K. Prevalence of urinary and fecal incontinence and symptoms of genital prolapse in women. *Acta Obstet Gynecol Scand* 2003;82:280–286.
4. Swift SE. The distribution of pelvic organ support in a population of female subjects seen for routine gynaecology health care. *Am J Obstet Gynecol* 2000;183:277–285.
5. Samuelsson EU, Victor FTA, Tibbin G, et al. Signs of genital prolapse in a Swedish population of women 20–59 years of age and possible related factors. *Am J Obstet Gynecol* 1999;180:299–305.
6. Bland DR, Earle BB, Vitolins MZ, et al. Use of the Pelvic Organ Prolapse staging system of the International Continence Society, American Urogynecologic Society, and Society of Gynecologic Surgeons in perimenopausal women. *Am J Obstet Gynecol* 1999;181:1324–1327.
7. Versi E, Harvey MA, Cardozo L, et al. Urogenital prolapse and atrophy at menopause: a prevalence study. *Int Urogynecol J* 2001;12:107–110.
8. Handa VL, Garrett E, Hendrix S, et al. Progression and remission of pelvic organ prolapse: a longitudinal study of menopausal women. *Am J Obstet Gynecol* 2004;190:27–32.
9. Mant J, Painter R, Vessey M. Epidemiology of genital prolapse: observations from the Oxford Family Planning Association Study. *Br J Obstet Gynaecol* 1997;104:579–585.
10. Swift SE, Pound T, Dias JK. Case-control study of the etiology of severe pelvic organ prolapse. *Int Urogynecol J* 2001;12:187–192.
11. Digesu GA, Khullar V, Cardoso L, et al. P-QoL: a validated quality of life questionnaire for the symptomatic assessment of women with uterogenital prolapse. *Int Urogynecol J* 2000;11:S25.

12. Hagen S, Stark D, Maher C, Adams E. Conservative management of pelvic organ prolapse in women (Cochrane Review). In: The Cochrane Library, Issue 2, 2004. Chichester, UK: John Wiley & Sons, Ltd. Search date 2003 for most sources and 2004 for the Cochrane Incontinence Group Trials Register; primary sources the Cochrane Incontinence Group Trials Register, Medline, Premedline, Embase, Cinahl, PEDro, the UK National Research Register, Controlled Clinical Trials and Zetoc.
13. Piya-Anant M, Therasakvichya S, Leelaphatanadit C, et al. Integrated health research program for the Thai elderly: prevalence of genital prolapse and effectiveness of pelvic floor exercise to prevent worsening of genital prolapse in elderly women. *J Med Assoc Thai* 2003;86:509–515.
14. Adams E, Thomson A, Maher C, Hagen S. Mechanical devices for pelvic organ prolapse in women (Cochrane Review). In: The Cochrane Library, Issue 2, 2004 Chichester, UK: John Wiley & Sons, Ltd. Search date 2003 for most sources and 2004 for the Cochrane Incontinence Group Trials Register; primary sources the Cochrane Incontinence Group Trials Register, Medline, Premedline, Embase, Cinahl, PEDro, the UK National Research Register, Controlled Clinical Trials and Zetoc.
15. Wu V, Farrell SA, Baskett TF, et al. A simplified protocol for pessary management. *Obstet Gynecol* 1997;90:990–994.
16. Farrell SA. Practical advice for ring pessary fitting and management. *J Obstet Gynaecol Can* 1997;19:625–632.
17. Sulak PJ, Kuehl TJ, Shull BL. Vaginal pessaries and their use in pelvic relaxation. *J Reprod Med* 1993;38:919–923.
18. Makinen J, Soderstrom K, Kiilhoma P, et al. Histological change in the vaginal connective tissue of women with and without uterine prolapse. *Arch Gynecol* 1986;239:17–20.
19. Norton P, Boyd C, Deak S. Abnormal collagen ratios in women with genitourinary prolapse. *Neurourol Urodyn* 1992;11:2–4.

Joseph Loze Onwude
Consultant Gynaecologist and Medical Statistician
Springfield Hospital
Chelmsford
United Kingdom

Competing interests: None declared.

TABLE 1 **Standard grading systems for the severity of genital prolapse (see text, p 2361).**

Baden–Walker halfway system[1]		POPQ system‡[2]	
Grade	**Position of prolapse site***	**Stage**	**Position of prolapse site***
0	No prolapse	0	No prolapse
1	Halfway to hymen	1	> 1 cm above the hymen
2	To hymen	2	≤1 cm proximal or distal to the plane of the hymen
3	Halfway past hymen	3	> 1 cm below the plane of the hymen, but protrudes no further than 2 cm less than the total vaginal length
4	Maximum descent	4	Eversion of the lower genital tract is complete

*Both systems measure the position of the most distal portion of the prolapse site during the Valsalva manoeuvre (See glossary). ‡The Pelvic Organ Prolapse Quantification (POPQ) system is an adaptation of the Baden–Walker halfway system.[2] Since 1996, the POPQ has been internationally recognised as a standard classification system for genital prolapse. The POPQ is more accurate than the Baden–Walker system because it measures the positions of nine sites of the vagina and the perineal body in relation to the hymen, to create a tandem vaginal profile before assigning site specific ordinal stages. The main limitation of the POPQ system is that it is more complex to learn and communicate verbally than the original Baden–Walker system.

Infertility and subfertility

Search date June 2003

Kirsten Duckitt

QUESTIONS

INTERVENTIONS

See interventions in women with pain attributed to endometriosis under endometriosis, p 2326

*No RCT, but strong observational evidence that increases live birth rates

See glossary G

Key Messages

In women with infertility caused by ovulation disorders

- **Clomifene** One systematic review has found that clomifene (clomiphene) increases pregnancy rate compared with placebo in women who ovulate infrequently. Four other studies, including two RCTs, have found no significant difference in ovulation or pregnancy rates between clomifene and tamoxifen. One RCT found that clomifene plus metformin increased pregnancy rates after 6 months' treatment compared with clomifene alone.
- **Gonadotrophins** We found no RCTs comparing gonadotrophins versus placebo or clomifene. One systematic review found that pregnancy rates with human menopausal gonadotrophins or urofollitropin (urofollitrophin, urinary follicle stimulating hormone) ranged from 10–12%. The review found no significant difference in pregnancy rates between treatments. Two RCTs found that pregnancy rates with follitropin (recombinant follicle stimulating hormone) or urofollitropin ranged from 24–27%. It found no significant difference between treatments. The review found that urofollitropin reduced the risk of ovarian hyperstimulation syndrome compared with human menopausal gonadotrophins, although this was confined to women who were not treated with concomitant gonadotrophin releasing hormone analogues. One systematic review and one subsequent RCT found no significant difference in pregnancy rates between gonadotrophins and laparoscopic ovarian drilling but found that gonadotrophins increased rates of multiple pregnancies. Observational evidence suggests that gonadotrophins may be associated with an increased risk of non-invasive ovarian tumours and multiple pregnancies.
- **Cyclofenil** One RCT provided insufficient evidence about the effects of cyclofenil in women with ovulatory disorders.
- **Laparoscopic ovarian drilling** We found no RCTs comparing laparoscopic ovarian drilling versus no treatment. One systematic review and one subsequent small RCT found no significant difference in pregnancy rates between laparoscopic ovarian drilling and gonadotrophins. They found that laparoscopic ovarian drilling reduced rates of multiple pregnancies.
- **Pulsatile gonadotrophin releasing hormone** One systematic review of small, weak RCTs provided insufficient evidence to assess pulsatile gonadotrophin releasing hormone treatment.

In women with tubal infertility

- **In vitro fertilisation** We found no RCTs comparing in vitro fertilisation versus no treatment. RCTs are unlikely to be conducted. Observational evidence in the UK and the USA suggests an average live birth rate of 22–25% per in vitro fertilisation cycle if intracytoplasmic sperm injection is taken into account. One RCT found that immediate compared with delayed in vitro fertilisation increased pregnancy and live birth rates. Three RCTs found no significant difference in numbers of live births between in vitro fertilisation and intracytoplasmic sperm injection. Observational evidence suggests that adverse effects associated with in vitro fertilisation include multiple pregnancies and ovarian hyperstimulation syndrome.
- **Tubal flushing with oil soluble media** One systematic review found that tubal flushing with oil soluble media increased pregnancy rates compared with no intervention. It found that tubal flushing with oil soluble media increased the live birth rate compared with flushing with water soluble media.

- **Tubal surgery before in vitro fertilisation** One systematic review in women with hydrosalpinges undergoing in vitro fertilisation has found that tubal surgery increases pregnancy and live birth rates compared with no treatment or medical treatment. One systematic review found no significant difference in pregnancy rates among different types of tubal surgery. One systematic review found no significant difference in pregnancy rates between tubal surgery plus additional treatments to prevent adhesion formation (steroids, dextran, noxytioline) and tubal surgery alone. Another systematic review provided insufficient evidence to assess postoperative hydrotubation or second look laparoscopy.
- **Selective salpingography plus tubal catheterisation** We found no RCTs on the effects of selective salpingography plus tubal catheterisation.
- **Tubal flushing with water soluble media** One systematic review identified no RCTs comparing tubal flushing with water soluble media versus no intervention. It found that tubal flushing with water soluble media decreased live birth rate compared with flushing with oil soluble media.

In women with infertility associated with endometriosis

- **Intrauterine insemination plus gonadotrophins** One RCT found that intrauterine insemination plus gonadotrophins increased live birth rates compared with no treatment. A second RCT found no significant difference in birth rates between intrauterine insemination plus pituitary down regulation plus gonadotrophins and expectant management, but it is likely to have been underpowered to detect a clinically important difference. A third RCT found that intrauterine insemination plus gonadotrophins increased pregnancy rates after the first treatment cycle compared with intrauterine insemination alone.
- **In vitro fertilisation** We found no RCTs comparing in vitro fertilisation versus no treatment in women with endometriosis related infertility. RCTs are unlikely to be conducted. Observational evidence in the UK and the USA suggests an average live birth rate of 22–25% per in vitro fertilisation cycle if intracytoplasmic sperm injection is taken into account. Observational studies found inconclusive evidence about whether in vitro fertilisation is as effective in women with endometriosis as in women with tubal infertility.
- **Laparoscopic ablation of endometrial deposits** We found no RCTs comparing laparoscopic surgery versus no treatment or versus ovarian suppression. One systematic review has found that laparoscopic resection or ablation of endometrial deposits increases live birth rates and ongoing pregnancy rates compared with diagnostic laparoscopy. Operative complications were not increased with laparoscopic surgery.
- **Drug induced ovarian suppression** One systematic review found no significant difference in pregnancy rates between drugs that induce ovarian suppression and placebo. The review found that ovulation suppression agents (medroxyprogesterone, gestrinone, combined oral contraceptives, and gonadotrophin releasing hormone analogues) cause adverse effects, including weight gain, hot flushes, and osteoporosis, and that danazol may cause dose related weight gain and androgenic effects.

In couples with male factor infertility

- **Intracytoplasmic sperm injection plus in vitro fertilisation** We found no RCTs of intracytoplasmic sperm injection plus in vitro fertilisation that assessed pregnancy and live birth rates. Observational evidence in the UK suggests an average live birth rate of 22% per in vitro fertilisation cycle if intracytoplasmic sperm injection is taken into account.
- **Intrauterine insemination** Two systematic reviews have found that intrauterine insemination increases pregnancy rates per cycle compared with intracervical insemination or timed intercourse.
- **Donor insemination** We found no RCTs on the effects of donor insemination. Observational evidence suggests an average live birth rate of 11%, but it is sometimes unclear whether ovarian stimulation was used in addition to donor insemination.

- **In vitro fertilisation versus gamete intrafallopian transfer** One small RCT provided insufficient evidence to compare in vitro fertilisation versus gamete intrafallopian transfer.

In couples with unexplained infertility

- **Intrauterine insemination plus gonadotrophins** Two systematic reviews and one subsequent RCT have found that intrauterine insemination plus gonadotrophins increases pregnancy rates compared with timed intercourse or intracervical insemination. One systematic review found no significant difference between intrauterine insemination and timed intercourse or intracervical insemination in pregnancy rates. However, it found that adding gonadotrophins to any of the three interventions increased pregnancy rates per cycle. One systematic review and one subsequent RCT have found that fallopian tube sperm perfusion increases pregnancy rates compared with intrauterine insemination. One systematic review found no significant difference in live birth rate between intrauterine insemination with or without ovarian stimulation and in vitro fertilisation.
- **Clomifene** One systematic review found limited evidence that clomifene (clomiphene) increased rates of pregnancy per cycle compared with placebo.
- **Fallopian tube sperm perfusion** One systematic review and one subsequent RCT have found that fallopian tube sperm perfusion increases pregnancy rates compared with intrauterine insemination.
- **Gamete intrafallopian transfer** We found no RCTs comparing gamete intrafallopian transfer versus no treatment. RCTs found conflicting effects on pregnancy rates of gamete intrafallopian transfer versus other treatments (intrauterine insemination, timed intercourse, and in vitro fertilisation).
- **In vitro fertilisation** Observational evidence in the UK and the USA suggests an average live birth rate of 22–25% per in vitro fertilisation cycle. However, one systematic review identified one RCT in couples with unexplained infertility that found no significant difference in pregnancy rates between in vitro fertilisation and expectant management. RCTs included in the review found no significant difference in live birth rate between in vitro fertilisation and either gamete intrafallopian transfer or intrauterine insemination with or without ovarian stimulation.

DEFINITION Normal fertility has been defined as achieving a pregnancy within 2 years by regular sexual intercourse.[1] However, many define infertility as the failure to conceive after 1 year of unprotected intercourse. Infertility can be primary, in couples who have never conceived, or secondary, in couples who have previously conceived. Infertile couples include those who are sterile (who will never achieve a natural pregnancy) and those who are subfertile (who could eventually achieve a natural pregnancy).

INCIDENCE/ PREVALENCE Although there is no evidence of a major change in the prevalence of infertility, many more couples are seeking help than previously. Currently, about 1/7 couples in industrialised countries will seek medical advice for infertility.[2] Rates of primary infertility vary widely between countries, ranging from 10% in Africa to about 6% in North America and Europe.[1] Reported rates of secondary infertility are less reliable.

AETIOLOGY/ RISK FACTORS In the UK, nearly a third of infertility cases are unexplained.[3] The rest are caused by ovulatory failure (27%), low sperm count or quality (19%), tubal damage (14%), endometriosis (5%), and other causes (5%).[3]

PROGNOSIS In developed countries, 80–90% of couples attempting to conceive are successful after 1 year and 95% after 2 years.[3] The chances of becoming pregnant vary with the cause and duration of infertility, the woman's age, the couple's previous pregnancy history, and the availability of different treatment options.[2,4] For the first 2–3 years of unexplained infertility, cumulative conception rates remain high (27–46%) but decrease with increasing age of the woman and duration of infertility.[4] The background rates of spontaneous pregnancy in infertile couples can be calculated from longitudinal studies of infertile couples who have been observed without treatment.[4]

AIMS OF INTERVENTION To achieve the delivery of one healthy baby; to reduce the distress associated with infertility, with minimal adverse effects.

OUTCOMES Live births, miscarriages, multiple pregnancies, incidence of ovarian hyperstimulation syndrome(G), satisfaction with services and treatments, acceptance of childlessness if treatment is unsuccessful, and pregnancy rate. Pregnancy rate is an intermediate outcome, but one that is important in itself to many people. Ovulation is an intermediate outcome. Pregnancies in infertile couples will occur spontaneously without treatment.[4] Effectiveness of treatments for infertility should be assessed on the basis of pregnancy rates over and above the spontaneous pregnancy rates, otherwise the impacts of treatments may be overestimated.

METHODS *Clinical Evidence* search and appraisal June 2003. **Crossover design:** For infertility, RCTs with a crossover design may overestimate the treatment effect because pregnancies occurring in the first half of the trial will remove couples from the second half.[5] Crossover trials were included in some systematic reviews where no or few RCTs using a parallel group design were available. Ideally, only data from the first half of the trial, before crossover, should be used. However, a study that used a computer model to compare the results of crossover and parallel designed trials suggests that any overestimation may be clinically irrelevant.[6]

QUESTION What are the effects of treatments for infertility caused by ovulation disorders?

OPTION CLOMIFENE

One systematic review has found that clomifene (clomiphene) increases pregnancy rate compared with placebo in women who ovulate infrequently. Four other studies, including two RCTs, have found no significant difference in ovulation or pregnancy rates between clomifene and tamoxifen. One RCT found that clomifene plus metformin increased pregnancy rates alone after 6 months' treatment compared with clomifene alone.

Benefits: **Versus placebo:** We found one systematic review (search date not reported, 3 crossover RCTs) that compared clomifene 50–200 mg versus placebo in 217 cycles in women who ovulate infrequently (see table 1, p 2390).[7] It found that clomifene significantly increased pregnancy rates compared with placebo (OR 3.4, 95% CI 1.2 to 9.5). **Versus tamoxifen:** We found no systematic review, but found four studies (2 RCTs, 1 quasi-randomised study, and 1 observational study; 197 anovulatory or infrequently ovulating women; see comment below).[32–35] The first RCT (86 anovulatory women aged < 40 years) compared tamoxifen (maximum 60 mg daily) versus clomifene (maximum 150 mg daily).[33] It found no significant difference in the overall rate of ovulation between tamoxifen and clomifene (50/113 [44%] ovulatory cycles with tamoxifen *v* 41/91 [45%] ovulatory cycles with clomifene; $P > 0.05$; see comment below) or in the number of pregnancies (10/46 [22%] with tamoxifen *v* 6/40 [15%] with clomifene; RR 1.7, 95% CI 0.7 to 4.2). The other studies found similar results.[32,34,35] **Versus other drug combinations:** We found no systematic review but found one RCT (90 infertile women with polycystic ovary syndrome, infrequent menstruation, high insulin levels, and body mass indexes > 28) comparing clomifene (at its lowest effective dose; see comment below) plus metformin (500 mg orally 3 times daily) versus clomifene alone (at its lowest effective dose; see comment below).[36] The RCT found that clomifene plus metformin significantly increased pregnancy rates per person after 6 months' treatment compared with clomifene alone (13/45 [29%] with clomifene plus metformin *v* 4/45 [9%] with clomifene alone; RR 3.3, 95% CI 1.2 to 9.2; NNT 5, 95% CI 3 to 22).

Harms: **Ovarian cancer:** In a cohort study of 3837 infertile women, 11 women were found to have ovarian cancer.[14] In 135 women that were randomly selected as a subcohort from these 3837 women, there was an 11-fold increase in risk of ovarian cancer in women using clomifene for 12 or more cycles (RR 11.1, 95% CI 1.5 to 82.3). The association was present for both gravid and nulligravid women, and for infertile women both with ovulatory disorders and with infertility from other causes. Subsequent cohort[37] and case-control[38–40] studies have found no association between clomifene and ovarian cancer. **Multiple pregnancy:** Multiple pregnancy occurs in 2–13% of women with all causes of infertility taking clomifene compared with a spontaneous multiple pregnancy rate of about 1–2% of women in North American and European populations.[41,42] In a 1 year survey in the UK, 25/44 (57%) triplet pregnancies reported were attributable to clomifene.[43] Clomifene was also implicated in 2/8 sets of quadruplets and quintuplets reported. **Ovarian hyperstimulation syndrome:** Clomifene tends to cause only mild ovarian hyperstimulationⒼ that does not require treatment.

Comment: Clomifene was first introduced in the 1960s and most of the trials testing its efficacy took place in the 1970s before more recent quality standards for RCTs were established. Three of the studies comparing clomifene versus tamoxifen based estimates of pregnancy rates on fewer than 30 pregnancies.[32,33,35] In the first RCT comparing tamoxifen versus clomifene, the different number of treatment cycles between groups could potentially bias the results.[33] In the RCT comparing clomifene plus metformin versus clomifene alone, the dose of clomifene was initially 50 mg daily for 5 days and only increased to 100 mg or 150 mg daily for 5 days if the lower dose was insufficient to enable ovulation to be triggered with human chorionic gonadotrophin.[36] In the cohort study, 5/11 (45%) people with ovarian cancer were diagnosed with borderline epithelial tumours that had low malignant potential, and two with granulosa cell tumours that had different embryological, pathological, and epidemiological features from epithelial tumours.[14] Borderline and malignant tumours pose different risks that are not easy to combine and excluding the two granulosa cell tumours from the number of ovarian cancers found diminishes the increased risk attributed to clomifene treatment.

OPTION CYCLOFENIL

One RCT provided insufficient evidence about the effects of cyclofenil in women with ovulatory disorders.

Benefits: **Versus placebo:** We found one RCT (213 women with either ovulatory disorders or unexplained infertility) comparing three cycles of cyclofenil (800 mg daily) versus placebo from days 4–8 of the ovulatory cycle (see comment below).[44] It found no significant difference in cumulative pregnancy rates (26/114 [23%] with cyclofenil *v* 21/99 [21%] with placebo; RR 1.1, 95% CI 0.7 to 1.8).

Harms: The RCT gave no information on adverse effects.[44]

Comment: Only 123/213 (58%) women in the RCT had ovulatory disorders and the results for these women were not presented separately.[44] The RCT does not, therefore, exclude a possible benefit of cyclofenil.

OPTION GONADOTROPHINS

We found no RCTs comparing gonadotrophins versus placebo or clomifene (clomiphene). One systematic review found that pregnancy rates with human menopausal gonadotrophins or urofollitropin (urofollitrophin, urinary follicle stimulating hormone) ranged from 10–12% and found no significant difference in pregnancy rates between treatments. Two RCTs found that pregnancy rates with follitropin (recombinant follicle stimulating hormone) or urofollitropin

ranged from 24–27% and found no significant difference between treatments. The review found that urofollitropin reduced the risk of ovarian hyperstimulation syndrome compared with human menopausal gonadotrophins, although this was confined to women who were not treated with concomitant gonadotrophin releasing hormone analogues. One systematic review and one subsequent RCT found no significant difference in pregnancy rates between gondaotrophins and laparoscopic ovarian drilling but found that gonadotrophins increased rates of multiple pregnancies. Observational evidence suggests that gonadotrophins may be associated with an increased risk of non-invasive ovarian tumours and multiple pregnancies.

Benefits: **Versus placebo:** We found no RCTs. **Versus clomifene:** We found no RCTs. **Human menopausal gonadotrophins versus urofollitropin:** We found one systematic review (search date not reported, 14 RCTs, 388 women with subfertility associated with polycystic ovary syndrome) that compared human menopausal gonadotrophins versus urofollitropin.[15] It found no significant difference in pregnancy rates (19/183 [10%] with human menopausal gonadotrophins *v* 26/213 [12%] with urofollitropin; OR 0.8, 95 % CI 0.4 to 1.5) (see table 1, p 2390). **Follitropin versus urofollitropin:** We found no systematic review, but found two RCTs comparing urofollitropin versus follitropin.[16,45] The first RCT (172 women with clomifene resistant, normogonadotrophic anovulation) found no significant difference between follitropin and urofollitropin in cumulative ovulation rates (95% with follitropin *v* 96% with urofollitropin), cumulative pregnancy rates (27% with follitropin *v* 24% with urofollitropin), or miscarriage rates (31% with follitropin *v* 32% with urofollitropin).[16] The second RCT (51 women with clomifene resistant, normogonadotrophic anovulation) found similar results, although a much lower total dose and shorter duration of follitropin was used to achieve ovulation.[45] **Versus laparoscopic ovarian drilling**Ⓖ: See benefits of laparoscopic ovarian drilling, p 2372.

Harms: **Ovarian cancer:** One case control study (200 women with ovarian cancer and 408 area matched controls) found that women with non-invasive ovarian tumours were more than three times more likely to have been exposed to an ovulation induction agent (adjusted OR 3.5, 95% CI 1.2 to 10.1), particularly to human menopausal gonadotrophins (adjusted OR 9.4, 95% CI 1.7 to 52.1).[40] Women with invasive ovarian tumours were no more likely to have been exposed to any ovulation induction agents. **Multiple pregnancy:** One case series found that multiple pregnancy occurred in 29% of women with polycystic ovary syndrome when conventional regimens of gonadotrophins were used to induce ovulation.[17] The first RCT comparing urofollitropin versus follitropin found no significant difference in the risk of multiple pregnancy, although the low event rates found with either treatment limit the usefulness of the result.[17] **Ovarian hyperstimulation:** The systematic review (search date not reported, 7 RCTs) found that urofollitropin significantly reduced the risk of ovarian hyperstimulation compared with human menopausal gonadotrophins (OR 0.3, 95% CI 0.2 to 0.7).[15] However, this effect was only present where no concomitant gonadotrophin releasing hormone analogue was used (5 RCTs; OR 0.2, 95% CI 0.1 to 0.5). The review found that concomitant use of a gonadotrophin releasing hormone analogue increased the risk of ovarian hyperstimulation (2 RCTs; OR 3.2, 95% CI 1.5 to 6.7).[15] The first RCT comparing urofollitropin versus follitropin found no significant difference in the risk of ovarian hyperstimulation syndromeⒼ, although the low event rates found with either treatment limit the usefulness of the result.[16]

Comment: Despite not being placebo controlled, trials in the review of gonadotrophins often included women who were not ovulating and, therefore, provide some evidence that treatment is effective.[15] Follitropin is not derived from human tissues.

OPTION LAPAROSCOPIC OVARIAN DRILLING

We found no RCTs comparing laparoscopic ovarian drilling versus no treatment. One systematic review and one subsequent small RCT found no significant difference in pregnancy rate between laparoscopic ovarian drilling and gonadotrophins. It found that laparoscopic ovarian drilling reduced rates of multiple pregnancies.

Benefits: **Versus no treatment:** We found no RCTs. **Versus gonadotrophins:** We found one systematic review (search date 2001, 4 RCTs, 303 women with anovulatory clomifene [clomiphene] resistant polycystic ovary syndrome)[18] (see table 1, p 2390) and one subsequent RCT (see comment below) comparing laparoscopic ovarian drilling**G** versus gonadotrophins.[19] The review found no significant difference between laparoscopic ovarian drilling and gonadotrophins in pregnancy rates after 6–12 months' follow up (81/127 [64%] with laparoscopic ovarian drilling *v* 72/126 [57%] with gonadotrophins; OR 1.42, 95% CI 0.84 to 2.42).[18] The subsequent RCT (18 women with polycystic ovary syndrome who had failed to ovulate after treatment with clomifene or purified follicle stimulating hormone) compared laparoscopic ovarian drilling versus a gonadotrophin releasing hormone analogue plus a combined oral contraceptive.[19] All the women also received three cycles of follitropin plus intrauterine insemination. The RCT found no significant difference in the number of pregnancies or live births after 6 months' treatment (pregnancies: 5/10 [50%] with laparoscopic ovarian drilling *v* 5/8 [63%] with gonadotrophin releasing hormone analogue plus combined oral contraceptive; RR 0.8, 95% CI 0.4 to 1.8; live births: 5/10 [50%] with laparoscopic ovarian drilling *v* 4/8 [50%] with gonadotrophin releasing hormone analogue plus combined oral contraceptive; RR 1.00, 95% CI 0.34 to 2.93).

Harms: **Versus gonadotrophins:** The systematic review found that laparoscopic ovarian drilling significantly reduced rates of multiple pregnancies compared with gonadotrophins (OR 0.16, 95% CI 0.03 to 0.98).[18] Adverse effects associated with laparoscopic ovarian drilling include the risks of general anaesthesia, postoperative adhesion formation,[46] and pelvic infection.[47] We found no evidence to support the suggestion that laparoscopic drilling increases the long term risk of premature ovarian failure. Laparoscopic drilling is thought not to increase the risk of multiple pregnancy as it usually induces spontaneous ovulation, in contrast to the multifollicular ovulation that may be induced by the use of gonadotrophins.

Comment: The trials of laparoscopic ovarian drilling included women who were not ovulating and, therefore, provide some evidence that treatment is effective despite the lack of placebo controls.[18,19]

OPTION PULSATILE GONADOTROPHIN RELEASING HORMONE

One systematic review of small, weak RCTs provided insufficient evidence to assess pulsatile gonadotrophin releasing hormone treatment.

Benefits: We found one systematic review (search date not reported, 3 RCTs, 29 women with subfertility and clomifene [clomiphene] resistant polycystic ovary syndrome) that compared pulsatile gonadotrophin releasing hormone (GnRH) versus other treatments to induce ovulation.[48] The RCTs included in the review assessed three different comparisons: pulsatile GnRH plus follicle stimulating hormone versus pulsatile GnRH alone; pulsatile GnRH plus 3 weeks' pretreatment with GnRH versus pulsatile GnRH alone; and pulsatile GnRH versus human menopausal gonadotrophins. The RCTs were also small (each reporting 1–4 pregnancies) and of short duration (1–3 cycles), and therefore provided insufficient evidence to assess pulsatile GnRH in women with polycystic ovary syndrome.

Harms: One retrospective analysis (229 cycles in 71 women) compared pulsatile GnRH versus gonadotrophins alone and found no significant difference in multiple pregnancy rates after six cycles.[49] However, 75% of the multiple pregnancies in the gonadotrophin group were triplets or higher order multiple pregnancies, whereas all multiple pregnancies in the GnRH group were twins.

Comment: Pulsatile GnRH is used in women with anovulation caused by low serum gonadotrophins and oestrogen concentrations (hypogonadotropic hypogonadism). Hypogonadotropic hypogonadism is a well defined condition and so evidence from case series should be generalisable to most affected women. Case series (256 anovulatory women with hypogonadotropic hypogonadism undergoing 1043 treatment cycles) found cumulative pregnancy rates of 59–73% at 6 months and 81–92% at 12 months.[50–53] Only one series reported the live birth rate; this was 65% after 12 treatment cycles.[53]

QUESTION What are the effects of treatments for tubal infertility?

OPTION SELECTIVE SALPINGOGRAPHY PLUS TUBAL CATHETERISATION

We found no RCTs on the effects of selective salpingography plus tubal catheterisation in women with tubal infertility.

Benefits: We found no systematic review or RCTs.

Harms: Observational studies found that ectopic pregnancy occurred in 3–9% of women undergoing selective salpingography and tubal catheterisation and that tubal perforation, which does not seem to be clinically important, occurred in 2%.[52,54]

Comment: One systematic review (search date not reported) combined data from 10 cohort and other observational studies of selective salpingography and tubal cannulation (482 women), and four observational studies of hysteroscopic cannulation for proximal tubal blockage (133 women).[52] It found that hysteroscopy was associated with a higher pregnancy rate compared with selective salpingography and tubal catheterisation (pregnancies exceeding 20 weeks' gestation: 65/133 [49%] with hysteroscopy *v* 103/482 [21%] with salpingography). None of the observational studies included an untreated group, so it is not possible to estimate the treatment related pregnancy rate over and above the spontaneous pregnancy rate. Tubal patency and pregnancy without treatment have been reported in women diagnosed with bilateral proximal tube obstruction.[55]

OPTION TUBAL FLUSHING

One systematic review identified no RCTs comparing tubal flushing with water soluble media versus no intervention. It found that tubal flushing with oil soluble media increased pregnancy rates compared with no intervention. It also found that tubal flushing with oil soluble media increased the live birth rate compared with flushing with water soluble media.

Benefits: We found no RCTs reporting solely on women with tubal infertility. We found one systematic review (search date 2001, 8 RCTs, 1706 women) that evaluated flushing of the woman's fallopian tubes with oil or water soluble media in couples with infertility.[56] **Versus no intervention:** The review found no RCTs comparing tubal flushing with water soluble media versus no intervention.[56] It found that tubal flushing with oil soluble media significantly increased the chance of pregnancy compared with no intervention (2 RCTs; 224 women; OR 3.57, 95% CI 1.76 to 7.23). **Oil soluble versus water soluble media:** The review found no significant difference in pregnancy rates between tubal flushing with oil soluble versus water soluble media.[56] However, oil soluble media significantly increased live birth rates (live birth: 2 RCTs; 951 women; OR 1.49, 95% CI 1.05 to 2.11; pregnancy: 5 RCTs; 1241 women; OR 1.23, 95% CI 0.95 to 1.60).

Harms: **Versus no intervention:** The RCTs included in the review gave no information on miscarriage, ectopic pregnancy, procedural pain, or short or long term procedural complications.[56] **Oil soluble versus water soluble media:** The systematic review found that oil soluble media reduced procedural pain and procedural complications compared with water soluble media (pain: 2 RCTs; 834 women; OR 0.40, 95% CI 0.28 to 0.57; procedural complications: 4 RCTs; 1357 women; OR 0.22, 95% CI 0.14 to 0.34).[56] It found no significant difference in miscarriage or ectopic pregnancy (miscarriage per pregnancy: 1 RCT; 158 women; OR 0.82, 95% CI 0.41 to 1.64; ectopic pregnancy: 2 RCTs; 562 women; OR 0.49, 95% CI 0.10 to 2.42).

Comment: RCTs comparing oil soluble versus water soluble media were statistically heterogeneous.[56] The RCTs were not solely in women with tubal infertility and so may also be relevant to couples with unexplained infertility. One RCT included in the review only included women with unexplained infertility or mild endometriosis.[57]

OPTION TUBAL SURGERY

One systematic review in women with hydrosalpinges undergoing in vitro fertilisation has found that tubal surgery increases pregnancy and live birth rates compared with no treatment or medical treatment. One systematic review found no significant difference in pregnancy rates among different types of tubal surgery. One systematic review found no significant difference in pregnancy rates between tubal surgery plus additional treatments to prevent adhesion formation (steroids, dextran, noxytioline) and tubal surgery alone. Another systematic review provided insufficient evidence to assess postoperative hydrotubation or second look laparoscopy.

Benefits: **Versus no treatment or medical treatment:** We found one systematic review (search date 2000, 3 RCTs, 295 women with hydrosalpinges undergoing in vitro fertilisation [IVF]; see comment below), which found that tubal surgery significantly increased pregnancy rates compared with no treatment or medical treatment (OR 1.75, 95% CI 1.07 to 2.86) and the live birth rate (OR 2.13, 95% CI 1.24 to 3.65; see comment below).[58] **Different types of tubal surgery versus each other:** We found one systematic review (search date not reported, 8 RCTs, 557 women).[59] Two RCTs (130 women) identified by the review found no significant difference in pregnancy rates between CO_2 laser adhesiolysis**G** and diathermy adhesiolysis (1 RCT; 16/30 [53%] with laser *v* 17/33 [52%] with diathermy; RR 1.04, 95% CI 0.65 to 1.67) or between CO_2 laser salpingostomy and diathermy salpingostomy (1 RCT; 26/75 [35%] with laser *v* 16/60 [27%] with diathermy; RR 1.30, 95% CI 0.77 to 2.19).[59] A third RCT (72 women) identified by the first review found no significant difference in pregnancies after 2 years between the use of an operating microscope and the use of magnifying lenses (loupes) during microsurgical reversal of sterilisations (26/36 [72%] with microscope *v* 28/36 [78%] with loupes; OR 0.75, 95% CI 0.26 to 2.15).[59] **Adding postoperative treatments to tubal surgery:** We found two systematic reviews (search date not reported, 10 RCTs, 1086 women;[60] search date not reported, 5 RCTs, 588 women[61]). The first review compared tubal surgery plus additional treatments to prevent adhesion formation (steroids, dextran, and noxytioline) versus tubal surgery alone.[60] It found no significant difference in pregnancy rates between tubal surgery plus steroids (systemic or intraperitoneal) and no steroids (4 RCTs; OR 1.10, 95% CI 0.74 to 1.64), tubal surgery plus dextran (intraperitoneal) and no dextran (3 RCTs; OR 0.65, 95% CI 0.37 to 1.14), or tubal surgery plus noxytioline (intraperitoneal) and no noxytioline (1 RCT; OR 0.67, 95% CI 0.30 to 1.47). The second review compared early postoperative hydrotubation**Ⓖ** or second look laparoscopy**Ⓖ** plus adhesiolysis after tubal surgery versus control (late postoperative hydrotubation, postoperative irrigation with antibiotics plus late postoperative hydrotubation, no postoperative hydrotubation, or no second look laparoscopy).[61] It found that all the RCTs were either poor quality or underpowered. It found insufficient evidence to support the routine practice of hydrotubation (1 RCT; OR 1.12, 95% CI 0.57 to 2.21) or second look laparoscopy (2 RCTs; OR 0.96 95% CI 0.44 to 2.07) after tubal surgery. **Versus IVF:** We found no RCTs (see comment below).

Harms: **Versus no treatment or medical treatment:** The review found no significant difference between tubal surgery and no treatment or medical treatment in the rate of ectopic pregnancy (OR 0.42, 95% CI 0.08 to 2.14), miscarriage per pregnancy (OR 0.49, 95% CI 0.16 to 1.52), or treatment related complications (OR 5.80, 95% CI 0.35 to 96.79).[58] Tubal surgery involves general anaesthesia and admission to hospital. There is a risk of ectopic pregnancy caused by pre-existing tubal damage; retrospective studies have reported rates of 7–9% with tubal surgery, compared with 1–3% with IVF.[9,10] IVF carries the risk of multiple pregnancy and ovarian hyperstimulation syndrome**Ⓖ** (see harms of IVF under treatments for tubal infertility, p 2376).

Comment: Success rates with tubal surgery depend on the severity and site of disease. The best figures from surgery in women with distal tubal occlusion are live birth rates of 20–30%, with rates of 40–60% reported for the less common proximal occlusion (see table 1, p 2390).[20–24] Success rates with reversal of female sterilisation vary depending on the method used for sterilisation, with live birth rates of 50–90%.[25] **Versus no treatment or medical treatment:** In the systematic review comparing tubal surgery versus non-surgical treatment, although a variety of different surgical techniques were used, laparoscopic unilateral or bilateral salpingectomy were the most common (numerical data not reported).[58] **Different types of tubal surgery versus each other:** Of the eight RCTs included in the review, five used outdated surgical techniques, were small, and had problems relating to methods of randomisation.[59] These data precede recent improvements in case selection and laparoscopic training. One additional systematic review (search date not reported, 7 observational studies, 279 women with proximal tubal blockage) compared microsurgery**Ⓖ** (275 women) versus macrosurgery**Ⓖ** (104 women).[52] It found that microsurgery significantly increased pregnancy rates compared with macrosurgery (RR 2.2, 95% CI 1.5 to 3.2). **Versus IVF:** Fertility rates from case series of tubal surgery and from large databases of couples undergoing IVF suggest that tubal surgery is as effective as IVF in women with filmy adhesions, mild distal tubal occlusion, or proximal obstruction.[20,62–66] If successful, tubal surgery allows women to have more pregnancies without further medical intervention and without the risks associated with IVF.[67]

OPTION IN VITRO FERTILISATION

We found no RCTs comparing in vitro fertilisation versus no treatment. RCTs are unlikely to be conducted. Observational evidence in the UK and the USA suggests an average live birth rate of 22–25% per in vitro fertilisation cycle if intracytoplasmic sperm injection is taken into account. One RCT found that immediate compared with delayed in vitro fertilisation increased pregnancy and live birth rates. Three RCTs found no significant difference in numbers of live births between in vitro fertilisation and intracytoplasmic sperm injection. Observational evidence suggests that adverse effects associated with in vitro fertilisation include multiple pregnancies and ovarian hyperstimulation syndrome.

Benefits: We found no systematic review. **In vitro fertilisation (IVF) versus no treatment:** We found no RCTs. **Immediate versus delayed IVF:** We found one RCT (399 couples with any cause of infertility; the couples who received delayed IVF acted as untreated controls for at least 6 months), which found that immediate IVF**G** compared with delayed IVF**G** significantly increased the pregnancy rate (33/190 [17%] with immediate IVF *v* 13/163 [8%] with delayed IVF; RR 2.18, 95% CI 1.19 to 4.0), and significantly increased the numbers of live births (22/190 [12%] with immediate IVF *v* 8/163 [5%] with delayed IVF; RR 2.36, 95% CI 1.08 to 5.16).[68] **Versus tubal surgery:** See benefits of tubal surgery, p 2374. **Plus intracytoplasmic sperm injection (ICSI):** We found one systematic review (search date 2002, 1 RCT, 415 couples) that found no significant difference in pregnancy rates between IVF plus ICSI and IVF alone in couples with non-male subfertility (70/213 [33%] with IVF alone *v* 51/202 [25%] with IVF plus ICSI; OR 1.4 95% CI 0.95 to 2.2).[69]

Harms: **Multiple pregnancy:** One RCT did not report on multiple pregnancy rates,[70] and the other RCTs were underpowered to detect clinically important differences in multiple pregnancy rates between treatments.[68,71,72] However, of the 6309 live births after IVF in the UK in 2000–2001, 27% were multiple, including 109 (2%) triplets.[8] In the UK, the number of embryos that can be replaced is restricted to two (see table 1, p 2390).[8] In the USA, where there are no such restrictions, 15 367 live births included 38% multiple births, 6% of which were triplets and above.[11] **Ovarian hyperstimulation syndrome:** The RCT comparing IVF versus ICSI found that ovarian hyperstimulation occurred in seven (4%) IVF cycles and nine (5%) ICSI cycles.[71] The other RCTs gave no information about rates of ovarian hyperstimulation syndrome**G**.[68,70,72] One non-systematic review suggests that severe ovarian hyperstimulation syndrome occurs in 0.5–2.0% of all IVF cycles.[12] **Obstetric outcome:** We found one systematic review (search date 1998, 42 high quality observational studies) that compared obstetric outcome in mothers receiving IVF versus either a population based control group or a selected control group matched for different variables.[73] It found that children born after IVF had a considerably higher risk of being born preterm and with a lower birth weight than children conceived naturally, although this was likely to be because of the high incidence of multiple births and maternal characteristics such as nulliparity, increased age, previous infertility, and obstetric history (absolute numbers not reported). There was no evidence of an increased overall incidence of congenital malformations in children born after conventional IVF or after embryo cryopreservation.

Comment: The success of IVF is influenced by a woman's age, duration of infertility, and previous pregnancy history.[2] Pregnancy rates are highest between the ages of 25 and 35 years and decline steeply after 35 years . Similar clinics, which describe the same methods, report different success rates for IVF.[2] In the UK Human Fertilisation and Embryology Authority database, the average live birth rate per IVF cycle over 2000–2001 was 22% if ICSI cycles were taken into account (see table 1, p 2390).[8] The equivalent average figure in the USA is 25%, but again results vary among centres.[11,74] In the UK, larger centres (≥ 200 cycles a year) report slightly higher live birth rates than smaller centres (20% per cycle started compared with 16%).[75] Such a difference has not been reported consistently in the USA.

QUESTION What are the effects of treatment for infertility associated with endometriosis?

OPTION DRUG INDUCED OVARIAN SUPPRESSION

One systematic review found no significant difference in pregnancy rates between drugs that induce ovarian suppression and placebo. The review found that ovulation suppression agents (medroxyprogesterone, gestrinone, combined oral contraceptives, and gonadotrophin releasing hormone analogues) cause adverse effects, including weight gain, hot flushes, and osteoporosis, and that danazol may cause dose related weight gain and androgenic effects.

Benefits: We found one systematic review (search date not reported, 13 RCTs).[76] **Versus placebo:** The review identified five RCTs (244 women with visually diagnosed endometriosis who had been attempting conception for < 12 months) comparing ovulation suppression agents (medroxyprogesterone, gestrinone, combined oral contraceptives, and gonadotrophin releasing hormone analogues) versus placebo. It found no significant difference in pregnancy rates between ovulation suppression agents and placebo (OR 0.8, 95% CI 0.5 to 1.4).[76] **Versus danazol:** The review identified eight RCTs (658 women with visually diagnosed endometriosis who had been attempting conception for < 12 months).[76] It found no significant difference in pregnancy rates between ovulation suppression agents and danazol (OR 1.2, 95% CI 0.9 to 1.7).[76] **Versus surgery:** See benefits of laparoscopic ablation of endometrial depositis, p 2379.

Harms: The review found that ovulation suppression agents caused adverse effects that included weight gain, hot flushes, and osteoporosis.[76] Adverse effects of danazol were dose related and included an average weight gain of 2–4 kg with 3 months' treatment; androgenic effects such as acne, seborrhoea, hirsutism, voice changes; and general complaints, including irritability, musculoskeletal pains, and tiredness. Hot flushes and breast atrophy were sometimes observed. One RCT (40 women with menorrhagia) comparing danazol versus mefenamic acid found that most of these adverse effects were reversible on stopping treatment.[77]

Comment: In the review, three of the RCTs used a combination of clomifene (clomiphene) plus ovarian suppression agents.[76] Treatment using ovulation suppression could waste valuable time for women who are trying to get pregnant, as the opportunity for spontaneous conceptions is lost during treatment.

OPTION INTRAUTERINE INSEMINATION PLUS GONADOTROPHINS

One RCT found that intrauterine insemination plus gonadotrophins increased live birth rates compared with no treatment. A second RCT found no significant difference in birth rates between intrauterine insemination plus pituitary down regulation plus gonadotrophins and expectant management,

but it is likely to have been underpowered to detect a clinically important difference. A third RCT found that intrauterine insemination plus gonadotrophins increased pregnancy rates after the first treatment cycle compared with intrauterine insemination alone.

Benefits: We found no systematic review but found three RCTs.[78–80] The first RCT (103 couples with infertility associated with minimal or mild endometriosis) compared intrauterine insemination plus gonadotrophins (53 couples, 127 cycles) versus no treatment (50 couples, 184 cycles).[78] It found that intrauterine insemination plus follicle stimulating hormone (FSH) significantly increased live birth rates compared with no treatment (14/53 [26%] with intrauterine insemination plus FSH *v* 4/50 [8%] with no treatment; RR 3.3, 95% CI 1.2 to 9.4; NNT 6, 95% CI 3 to 28).[78] The second RCT (49 women with minimal or mild endometriosis) compared three cycles of pituitary down regulation plus gonadotrophins plus intrauterine insemination versus 6 months of expectant management.[79] It found no significant difference in birth rates (7/24 [29%] with intrauterine insemination plus pituitary down regulation plus gonadotrophins *v* 5/25 [20%] with expectant management; RR 1.5, 95% CI 0.5 to 4.0). The RCT is likely to have been underpowered to detect a clinically important difference in pregnancy rates between the two groups. The third RCT (119 couples with primary pelvic or cervical factor infertility for a mean of 3.7 years, 57 couples with infertility associated with endometriosis) compared alternate cycles of gonadotrophins plus intrauterine insemination versus intrauterine insemination alone.[80] It found that gonadotrophins plus intrauterine insemination significantly increased the pregnancy rate after the first treatment cycle compared with intrauterine insemination alone (11/58 [19%] with gonadotrophins plus intrauterine insemination *v* 0/61 [0%] with intrauterine insemination alone; NNT 5, 95% CI 4 to 14). The 119 couples were subsequently followed up longitudinally and it was found that, in the 57 couples with a diagnosis of endometriosis, gonadotrophins plus intrauterine insemination significantly increased the probability of pregnancy over a total of 127 cycles compared with intrauterine insemination alone (RR 5.1, 95% CI 1.1 to 22.5).[80]

Harms: No cases of severe ovarian hyperstimulation or hospital admission were reported in the first or third RCTs.[78,80] In the second RCT, one severe case (1/24 [4%]), one moderate case (1/24 [4%]), and three mild cases (3/24 [13%]) of ovarian hyperstimulation syndrome**G** were reported.[79]

Comment: We found one systematic review (search date 2002, 3 RCTs, 386 women) that compared single versus double inseminations in stimulated cycles of intrauterine insemination.[81] Although live birth rates per couple could not be estimated, the pregnancy rates per couple were not significantly increased by performing an additional insemination (OR 1.45, 95% CI 0.78 to 2.68). One small crossover RCT assessed the timing of insemination in clomifene (clomiphene) stimulated cycles.[82] It found similar pregnancy rates per cycle whether insemination was timed with a urinary luteinising hormone kit or whether ultrasound monitoring with human chorionic gonadotrophin induction of ovulation was used.

OPTION LAPAROSCOPIC ABLATION OF ENDOMETRIAL DEPOSITS

We found no RCTs comparing laparoscopic surgery versus no treatment or versus ovarian suppression. One systematic review has found that laparoscopic ablation or resection of endometrial deposits increases live births and ongoing pregnancy rates compared with diagnostic laparoscopy. Operative complications were not increased with laparoscopic surgery.

Benefits: **Versus no treatment or ovarian suppression:** We found no RCTs (see comment below). **Laparoscopic surgery versus diagnostic laparoscopy:** We found one systematic review (search date 2000–2001, 2 RCTs, 437 women) comparing laparoscopic surgery (ablation or resection of endometrial deposits) versus diagnostic laparoscopy.[26] It found that laparoscopic surgery significantly increased the proportion of women who had a live birth or pregnancy continuing beyond 20 weeks compared with diagnostic laparoscopy (60/223 [27%] with laparoscopic surgery *v* 39/214 [18%] with diagnostic laparoscopy; OR 1.65, 95% CI 1.05 to 2.60) (see table 1, p 2390). See also laparoscopic ablation of endometrial deposits under endometriosis, p 2326.

Harms: The review found no significant difference in the proportion of women who had intraoperative complications between laparoscopic surgery and diagnostic laparoscopy (3/172 [1.7%] with laparoscopic surgery *v* 1/169 [0.6%] with diagnostic laparoscopy; OR 2.69, 95% CI 0.38 to 19.30).[26] One multicentre series of 29 966 diagnostic and operative gynaecological laparoscopies found a mortality of 3.3/100 000 laparoscopies and a complication rate of 3.2/1000 laparoscopies.[27]

Comment: The risks and morbidity of surgery under general anaesthesia and of postoperative adhesion formation need to be balanced against the adverse effects of treatments involving ovarian suppression or stimulation. In the larger RCT comparing laparoscopic surgery versus diagnostic laparoscopy, 48/341 (14%) women who received laparoscopic surgery for their endometriosis also had periadnexal adhesions treated, which may have affected their fertility.[26] We found one systematic review (search date not reported)[83] and one non-systematic review,[84] which together identified 21 cohort studies and one quasi-randomised trial in a total of 3879 women with all stages of endometriosis. Interventions were laparoscopic or open surgery versus medical treatment or no treatment. The non-systematic review combined data from all 21 studies and found that surgery significantly increased pregnancy rates compared with medical treatment or no treatment (RR 1.4, 95% CI 1.3 to 1.5).[84] It found no significant difference in pregnancy rates between laparoscopic and open surgery (RR 0.9, 95% CI 0.8 to 1.0). It found that, in women with mild or minimal endometriosis, laparoscopic surgery significantly increased pregnancy rates compared with danazol or no treatment (OR 2.7, 95% CI 2.1 to 3.5; absolute results presented graphically).

OPTION IN VITRO FERTILISATION

We found no RCTs comparing in vitro fertilisation versus no treatment in women with endometriosis related infertility. RCTs are unlikely to be conducted. Observational evidence in the UK and the USA suggests an average live birth rate of 22–25% per in vitro fertilisation cycle if intracytoplasmic sperm injection is taken into account. Observational studies found inconclusive evidence about whether in vitro fertilisation is as effective in women with endometriosis as in women with tubal infertility.

Benefits: We found no systematic review or RCTs (see comment below).

Harms: See harms of in vitro fertilisation under treatments for tubal infertility, p 2376.

Comment: In the UK Human Fertilisation and Embryology Authority database, the live average birth rate per in vitro fertilisation cycle over 2000–2001 was 22% if intracytoplasmic sperm injection cycles were taken into account.[8] We found one systematic review[85] and two retrospective cohort studies[86,87] that examined the effects of endometriosis compared with other causes of infertility, or the effects of severity of endometriosis, on in vitro fertilisation outcome. The cohort studies found no significant difference in pregnancy rates among groups.[86,87] The systematic review (search date 1999, 22 non-randomised studies) found that women with endometriosis were less likely to become pregnant than women with infertility because of blocked or damaged tubes (pregnancy assessed by human chorionic gonadotrophin levels; adjusted OR 0.56, 95% CI 0.44 to 0.70).[85] There is a need for properly controlled prospective randomised studies that present fertility rates with in vitro fertilisation in different stages of endometriosis using a validated classification system. Comparisons with assisted reproductive techniques are also required.

QUESTION **What are the effects of treatments for male factor infertility?**

OPTION **INTRAUTERINE INSEMINATION**

Two systematic reviews have found that intrauterine insemination increases pregnancy rates per cycle compared with intracervical insemination or timed intercourse.

Benefits: We found two systematic reviews (search date not reported[28] and search date 1996–1997[88]). The first review (10 RCTs, 2082 treatment cycles in couples with male infertility) compared intrauterine insemination with or without gonadotrophins versus intracervical insemination or timed intercourse.[28] It found that intrauterine insemination significantly increased the pregnancy rate per cycle compared with other treatments (6.5% with intrauterine insemination *v* 3.1% with intracervical insemination or timed intercourse; OR for intrauterine insemination *v* either intracervical insemination or timed intercourse 2.2, 95% CI 1.4 to 3.4) (see table 1, p 2390).[28] The second review (17 RCTs including 8 RCTs identified by the first review, 3662 completed treatment cycles in couples with male subfertility) found that, compared with timed intercourse, intrauterine insemination with or without ovarian stimulation significantly increased conception rates both in natural cycles (OR 2.4, 95% CI 1.5 to 3.8) and in controlled cycles (OR 2.1, 95% CI 1.3 to 3.5).[88] The review found that intrauterine insemination in controlled cycles also significantly increased the probability of conception compared with timed intercourse in natural cycles (OR 6.2, 95% CI 2.4 to 16.5). It found no significant difference in conception rates between intrauterine insemination in controlled cycles and intrauterine insemination in natural cycles (OR 1.8, 95% CI 1.0 to 3.3).[88]

Harms: Apart from the risks of ovarian hyperstimulation syndrome Ⓖ and multiple pregnancy associated with ovarian stimulation, intrauterine insemination may increase the likelihood of infection and may cause discomfort. However, data from RCTs are scarce.

Comment: The evidence from RCTs for timing and the optimum number of inseminations per cycle is inconclusive (see comments on intrauterine insemination under treatments for infertility associated with endometriosis, p 2378).

OPTION **INTRACYTOPLASMIC SPERM INJECTION PLUS IN VITRO FERTILISATION**

We found no RCTs of intracytoplasmic sperm injection plus in vitro fertilisation that assessed pregnancy and live birth rates. Observational evidence in the UK suggests an average live birth rate of 22% per in vitro fertilisation cycle if intracytoplasmic sperm injection is taken into account.

Benefits: **Versus in vitro fertilisation alone:** We found no RCTs of intracytoplasmic sperm injection (ICSI) plus in vitro fertilisation that assessed pregnancy and live birth rates (see comment below).

Harms: Observational studies have found conflicting reports of congenital abnormalities[89,90] and sex chromosomal abnormalities in children born after ICSI (see comment below).[91,92] One systematic review (search date 2001, 30 observational studies) concluded that although there was a small increased risk of major birth defects in children born after ICSI, this increase was not significant and no particular type of malformation was increased.[93] It could not clarify whether ICSI increased the occurrence of chromosomal abnormalities in the offspring of infertile couples with normal karyotypes.

Comment: The data on congenital and chromosome abnormalities with ICSI are constantly being revised as experience increases. Many couples have a strong preference for a child that is genetically related to both partners.[94] In the UK Human Fertilisation and Embryology Authority database, the average live birth rate per in vitro fertilisation cycle over 2000–2001 was 22% if ICSI cycles were taken into account (see table 1, p 2390).[8]

OPTION IN VITRO FERTILISATION VERSUS GAMETE INTRAFALLOPIAN TRANSFER

One small RCT provided insufficient evidence to compare in vitro fertilisation versus gamete intrafallopian transfer.

Benefits: We found no systematic review. We found one RCT (13 couples with male infertility), which found no significant difference between in vitro fertilisation and gamete intrafallopian transfer in pregnancy rates over 1 year (2/7 [29%] with in vitro fertilisation *v* 2/6 [33%] with gamete intrafallopian transfer; RR 1.20, 95% CI 0.23 to 5.95).[95]

Harms: See harms of in vitro fertilisation under treatments for tubal infertility, p 2376.

Comment: Data from large databases suggest the live birth rate per cycle of gamete intrafallopian transfer in women with infertility other than tubal infertility is 23% and the risk of ectopic pregnancy 5% (see table 1, p 2390).[13]

OPTION DONOR INSEMINATION

We found no RCTs on the effects of donor insemination. Observational evidence suggests an average live birth rate of 11%, but it is sometimes unclear whether ovarian stimulation was used in addition to donor insemination.

Benefits: **Versus no treatment:** We found no systematic review or RCTs in couples with male infertility that compared donor insemination versus no treatment or other interventions (see comment below).

Harms: We found no RCTs.

Comment: One systematic review (search date 1996, 12 RCTs, 2215 treatment cycles) found limited evidence that intrauterine compared with intracervical insemination of frozen donor sperm increased pregnancy rates.[96] The review included RCTs that were poor in their methodology, contained several different treatment variations making direct comparisons difficult, and included a mixture of women with and without fertility problems. Data are available from large databases, but it is sometimes unclear whether ovarian stimulation was used in addition to donor insemination. The average live birth rate per cycle in the UK Human

Fertilisation and Embryology Authority database in 2000–2001 was 11% with donor insemination (see table 1, p 2390).[8] Similar rates are reported from the French donor insemination database (23 700 women over 4 years), with a mean pregnancy rate of 10% per cycle, and the Sheffield database (UK, 343 women, 980 treatment cycles), with an 11% overall live birth rate.[29,30] Comparisons of donor insemination versus no treatment or other interventions may be inappropriate as, for many couples, donor insemination is not an acceptable option. RCTs have tended to concentrate on comparisons between different techniques of donor insemination.

QUESTION What are the effects of treatments for unexplained infertility?

OPTION CLOMIFENE

One systematic review found limited evidence that clomifene (clomiphene) increased rates of pregnancy per cycle compared with placebo.

Benefits: We found one systematic review (search date 2000, 5 RCTs, 4 using crossover designs; 458 cycles in women with unexplained infertility), which found that clomifene significantly increased pregnancy rates per cycle compared with placebo (OR 2.5, 95% CI 1.4 to 4.6; see comment below).[97] When only cycles before crossover were analysed (which was only possible with the data from 3 of the RCTs), the positive effect increased (OR 5.0, 95% CI 1.8 to 14.3).

Harms: See harms of clomifene under treatments for infertility caused by ovulation disorders, p 2369.

Comment: The systematic review[97] excluded one RCT[98] because of the risk of selection bias with a pseudo-random allocation method based on odd or even chart numbers. The other RCTs identified by the review were generally poor and it is possible that if one further medium sized RCT was performed, the direction of the overall effect found with meta-analysis could change again.[97] The review highlighted important differences between the trials: two RCTs included women with surgically treated endometriosis, one included only couples with primary infertility, and one included couples with a short duration of infertility (median of 28 months). Three of the RCTs included co-intervention with intrauterine insemination or cervicovaginal insemination. The RCTs also differed in their design (4 were crossover trials) and in the quality of randomisation (only 1 used properly concealed randomisation). The authors of the review commented that, as the baseline cycle fecundity of the women included in these trials would only be about 1–2%, even with clomifene their cycle fecundity would be unlikely to exceed 5%.[97]

OPTION INTRAUTERINE INSEMINATION PLUS GONADOTROPHINS

Two systematic reviews and one subsequent RCT have found that intrauterine insemination plus gonadotrophins increases pregnancy rates compared with timed intercourse or intracervical insemination. One systematic review found no significant difference between intrauterine insemination and timed intercourse or intracervical insemination in pregnancy rates. It found that adding ovarian stimulation to any of the three interventions increased pregnancy rates per cycle. One systematic review and one subsequent RCT have found that fallopian tube sperm perfusion increases pregnancy rates compared with intrauterine insemination. One systematic review found no significant difference in live birth rate between intrauterine insemination with or without ovarian stimulation and in vitro fertilisation.

Benefits: **Versus timed intercourse or intracervical insemination:** We found three systematic reviews,[28,31,99] which between them identified 12 RCTs and we found one subsequent RCT,[100] in couples with unexplained infertility. The first review (search date not reported, 8 RCTs, number of treatment cycles not reported) compared intrauterine insemination plus gonadotrophins versus timed intercourse plus gonadotrophins.[99] It found that intrauterine insemination plus ovarian stimulation significantly increased pregnancy rates (OR 2.4, 95% CI 1.4 to 3.9). The second review (search date 1997, 7 RCTs including 6 RCTs identified by the first review, 980 treatment cycles) compared intrauterine insemination plus ovarian stimulation with gonadotrophins versus timed intercourse plus ovarian stimulation with gonadotrophins.[31] It found that intrauterine insemination plus ovarian stimulation significantly increased the pregnancy rate per cycle (110/549 [20%] with intrauterine insemination plus ovarian stimulation *v* 49/431 [11%] with timed intercourse plus ovarian stimulation; RR 0.20, 95% CI 0.08 to 0.31). The third systematic review (search date not reported, 7 RCTs, including 4 RCTs identified by the first or second reviews, 934 treatment cycles) compared intrauterine insemination versus timed intercourse or intracervical insemination.[28] Four RCTs used gonadotrophins, two used clomifene (clomiphene), and three used no ovarian stimulation. The review found no significant difference between intrauterine insemination and intracervical insemination or timed intercourse in pregnancy rates (OR 1.5, 95% CI 1.0 to 2.2). The review also found that the addition of ovarian stimulation with gonadotrophins to any of the three interventions significantly increased the overall pregnancy rates (45/249 [18%] with intrauterine insemination or favourable timed intracervical insemination or timed intercourse plus gonadotrophin stimulation *v* 9/108 [8%] with intrauterine insemination or favourable timed intracervical insemination or timed intercourse alone; RR 2.17, 95% CI 1.10 to 4.28; NNT 11, 95% CI 7 to 58).[28] The subsequent RCT (932 couples) compared intracervical insemination alone, intrauterine insemination alone, intracervical insemination plus ovarian stimulation, and intrauterine insemination plus ovarian stimulation for four cycles or until pregnancy was achieved.[100] It found that intrauterine insemination plus ovarian stimulation versus intracervical insemination alone significantly increased the chance of becoming pregnant (OR 3.2, 95% CI 2.0 to 5.3). The RCT also found pregnancy rates of 14/233 (6%) with intracervical insemination, 35/234 (15%) with intrauterine insemination, 26/234 (11%) with ovarian stimulation plus intracervical insemination, and 54/231 (23%) with ovarian stimulation plus intrauterine insemination.[100] **Versus intrauterine insemination alone:** We found one RCT (932 couples), which found that intrauterine insemination plus ovarian stimulation versus intrauterine insemination alone significantly increased the chance of becoming pregnant (OR 1.7, 95% CI 1.2 to 2.6).[100] **Versus fallopian tube sperm perfusion:** See benefits of fallopian tube sperm perfusionⒼ, p 2384. **Versus gamete intrafallopian transfer:** See benefits of gamete intrafallopian transfer, p 2384. **Versus in vitro fertilisation:** See in vitro fertilisation for unexplained infertility, p 2385.

Harms: Apart from the risks of ovarian hyperstimulation syndromeⒼ and multiple pregnancy, intrauterine insemination may increase the likelihood of infection and may be associated with some discomfort. However, data from RCTs are scarce. **Versus in vitro fertilisation:** See in vitro fertilisation for unexplained infertility, p 2385. **Different gonadotrophins:** One RCT (97 couples with unexplained infertility) compared intrauterine insemination plus low dose, step up follicle stimulating hormone (FSH) versus intrauterine insemination plus a conventional FSH regimen.[101] It found no significant difference in pregnancy rates (7/49 [14%] with low dose FSH plus intrauterine insemination *v* 7/48 [15%] with conventional

FSH plus intrauterine insemination; RR 0.98, 95% CI 0.37 to 2.58). Low dose FSH versus conventional FSH significantly reduced the proportion of women with ovarian hyperstimulation syndrome (4/49 [8%] with low dose FSH v 13/48 [27%] with conventional FSH; RR 0.30, 95% CI 0.11 to 0.86; NNT 6, 95% 3 to 28), and ovarian hyperstimulation syndrome requiring hospital admission (0% with low dose FSH v 16.7% with conventional FSH). However, the low dose regimen did not completely prevent multiple pregnancies.

Comment: Only three of the RCTs were common to all three systematic reviews. One of the reviews scored the included studies for validity.[31] They scored from 49–70% when 100% was taken as the ideal study. The evidence from RCTs for timing and the optimum number of inseminations per cycle is inconclusive (see comments on intrauterine insemination under treatments for infertility associated with endometriosis, p 2378).

OPTION FALLOPIAN TUBE SPERM PERFUSION

One systematic review and one subsequent RCT have found that fallopian tube sperm perfusion increases pregnancy rates compared with intrauterine insemination.

Benefits: **Versus intrauterine insemination:** We found one non-systematic review (search date not reported, 5 RCTs in couples with unexplained infertility)[102] and one subsequent RCT that compared fallopian tube sperm perfusion**G** versus intrauterine insemination.[103] All five RCTs in the review used gonadotrophins or gonadotrophins plus clomifene (clomiphene), and in total 293 cycles of intrauterine insemination and 317 cycles of fallopian tube sperm perfusion were assessed.[102] The review found that fallopian tube sperm perfusion significantly increased pregnancy rate per cycle compared with intrauterine insemination (70/317 [22%] with fallopian tube sperm perfusion v 38/293 [13%] with intrauterine insemination; RR 1.70, 95% CI 1.19 to 2.44; NNT 11, 95% CI 7 to 33). The subsequent RCT (132 cycles in 65 couples) also found that, compared with intrauterine insemination, fallopian tube sperm perfusion significantly increased pregnancy rates per cycle (16/66 [24%] with fallopian tube sperm perfusion v 6/66 [9%] with intrauterine insemination; RR 2.67, 95% CI 1.11 to 6.40; NNT 7, 95% CI 4 to 38) and pregnancy rates per person after a maximum of three treatment cycles (16/33 [48%] with fallopian tube sperm perfusion v 6/32 [19%] with intrauterine insemination; RR 2.59, 95% CI 1.16 to 5.77; NNT 4, 95% CI 2 to 9).[103]

Harms: See harms of intrauterine insemination, p 2383. The non-systematic review did not report on harms.[102] The subsequent RCT reported that complications, including cervical bleeding, vasovagal episodes, uterine cramping, or pelvic infections, were not reported with either treatment.[103]

Comment: None.

OPTION GAMETE INTRAFALLOPIAN TRANSFER

We found no RCTs comparing gamete intrafallopian transfer versus no treatment. RCTs found conflicting results with gamete intrafallopian transfer versus other treatments (intrauterine insemination, timed intercourse, and in vitro fertilisation in pregnancy rates).

Benefits: **Versus no treatment:** We found no systematic review or RCTs. **Versus intrauterine insemination or timed intercourse:** We found no systematic review. We found three RCTs (283 couples with unexplained infertility).[104–106] The first RCT (50 couples) compared gamete intrafallopian transfer (GIFT) versus ovarian stimulation plus either timed intercourse or timed cervical donor insemination and found no significant difference in pregnancy rates (2/24 [8%] with GIFT cycles *v* 2/15 [13%] with ovarian stimulation plus either timed intercourse or timed cervical donor insemination; RR 0.63, 95% CI 0.10 to 3.98).[104] Of the other two RCTs, one (174 couples) found that GIFT increased pregnancy rates compared with ovarian stimulation with or without intrauterine insemination, and the other (59 couples) found no significant difference in pregnancy rates.[105,106] **Versus in vitro fertilisation:** See benefits of in vitro fertilisation for the treatment of unexplained infertility, p 2385.

Harms: Potential harms include the risks attributable to general anaesthesia and laparoscopy. One of the RCTs found that multiple pregnancy rates varied with the number of oocytes transferred.[106]

Comment: One prospective cohort study (99 treatment cycles, 53 couples) found that GIFT versus no treatment increased numbers of pregnancies.[107] GIFT, unlike in vitro fertilisation, gives no diagnostic information regarding fertilisation, and involves a laparoscopy and general anaesthetic, both of which are usually avoided with in vitro fertilisation. Observational data suggest that success rates decrease with increasing age.[108,109]

OPTION IN VITRO FERTILISATION

Observational evidence in the UK and the USA suggests an average live birth rate of 22–25% per in vitro fertilisation cycle. However, one systematic review identified one RCT in couples with unexplained infertility that found no significant difference in pregnancy rates between in vitro fertilisation and expectant management. RCTs included in the review found no significant difference in live birth rate between in vitro fertilisation and either gamete intrafallopian transfer or intrauterine insemination with or without ovarian stimulation.

Benefits: We found one systematic review (search date 2001, 5 RCTs, 353 women).[110] **Versus expectant management:** The review found no significant difference between in vitro fertilisation (IVF) and expectant management in pregnancy rates (1 RCT; 35 women; OR 0.30, 95% CI 0.02 to 3.67).[110] **Versus intrauterine insemination:** Three included RCTs found no significant difference in live birth rate between IVF and intrauterine insemination with or without ovarian stimulation (without ovarian stimulation: 1 RCT, 113 women; OR for live birth 1.96, 95% CI 0.88 to 4.36; with ovarian stimulation: 1 RCT, 118 women; OR 1.15, 95% CI 0.55 to 2.42).[110] **Versus gamete intrafallopian transfer:** One included RCT (69 women) found no significant difference between IVF and gamete intrafallopian transfer in live birth rate (OR 2.57, 95% CI 0.93 to 7.08).[110]

Harms: **Versus intrauterine insemination:** In one RCT (113 women) comparing intrauterine insemination versus IVF identified by the review, multiple pregnancy rates were 4% with intrauterine insemination in natural cycles, 29% with intrauterine insemination in stimulated cycles, and 21% with IVF (see harms of gonadotrophins, p 2371).[110] Mild ovarian hyperstimulation syndrome G occurred in two women in the stimulated intrauterine insemination group, and severe ovarian hyperstimulation syndrome occurred in three women in the IVF group. See also harms of in vitro fertilisation under treatments for tubal infertility, p 2376.

Comment: The RCTs included in the systematic review may have lacked power to detect clinically important differences between treatments.[110]

Infertility and subfertility

GLOSSARY

Adhesiolysis Division of adhesions, which are bands of scar tissue that form after infection or surgery.

Delayed in vitro fertilisation In vitro fertilisation treatment after 6 months of being assessed in an infertility clinic after at least 12 months of infertility.

Fallopian tube sperm perfusion Fallopian tube sperm perfusion is based on a pressure injection of 4 mL sperm suspension with an attempt to seal the cervix to prevent semen reflux. It attempts to ensure a sperm flushing of the fallopian tubes and an overflowing of the inseminate into the pouch of Douglas.

Hydrotubation Flushing of the fallopian tubes through the cervix and uterine cavity to remove surgical debris and reduce the incidence of tubal reocclusion.

Immediate in vitro fertilisation In vitro fertilisation treatment within 6 months of being assessed in an infertility clinic after at least 12 months of infertility.

Laparoscopic ovarian drilling Ovarian drilling can be performed laparoscopically by either cautery or laser vapourisation (using CO_2, argon, or Nd:YAG lasers), which are used to create multiple perforations (about 10 holes per ovary) of the ovarian surface and stroma (inner area of the ovary). This is thought to cause ovulation by restoring the intra-ovarian hormonal environment to normal, which in turn beneficially affects the hypothalamic–pituitary–ovarian axis.

Macrosurgery Surgery without dedicated optical magnification.

Microsurgery Surgery involving optical magnification to allow the use of much finer instruments and suture material in addition to a non-touch technique, with the aim of minimising tissue handling and damage.

Ovarian hyperstimulation syndrome Can occur in mild, moderate, and severe forms. Mild ovarian hyperstimulation syndrome is characterised by fluid accumulation, as shown by weight gain, abdominal distension, and discomfort. Moderate ovarian hyperstimulation syndrome is associated with nausea and vomiting, ovarian enlargement, abdominal distension, discomfort, and dyspnoea. Severe ovarian hyperstimulation syndrome is a life threatening condition, in which there is contraction of the intravascular volume, tense ascites, pleural and pericardial effusions, severe haemoconcentration, and the development of hepatorenal failure. Deaths have occurred, caused usually by cerebrovascular thrombosis, renal failure, or cardiac tamponade.

Second look laparoscopy Laparoscopy performed some time after tubal surgery (either open or laparoscopic) with the aim of dividing adhesions relating to the initial procedure.

REFERENCES

1. European Society for Human Reproduction and Embryology. Guidelines to the prevalence, diagnosis, treatment and management of infertility, 1996. *Hum Reprod* 1996;11:1775–1807.
2. Templeton A, Morris JK. IVF – factors affecting outcome. In: Templeton A, Cooke ID, O'Brien PMS, eds. *35th RCOG study group evidence-based fertility treatment*. London: RCOG Press, 1998:265–273.
3. Effective Health Care. The management of subfertility. *Effective Health Care Bulletin* 1992;3:13. Search date and primary sources not reported.
4. Collins JA, Burrows EA, Willan AR. The prognosis for live birth among untreated infertile couples. *Fertil Steril* 1995;64:22–28.
5. Khan KS, Daya S, Collins JA, et al. Empirical evidence of bias in infertility research: overestimation of treatment effect in crossover trials using pregnancy as the outcome measure. *Fertil Steril* 1996;65:939–945.
6. Cohlen BJ, Te Velde ER, Looman CW, et al. Crossover or parallel design in infertility trials? The discussion continues. *Fertil Steril* 1998;70:40–45.
7. Hughes E, Collins J, Vandekerckhove P. Clomiphene citrate for ovulation induction in women with oligo-amenorrhoea. In: The Cochrane Library, Issue 2, 2003. Oxford: Update Software. Search date not reported; primary source Cochrane Subfertility Group Register of Controlled Trials.
8. Human Fertilisation and Embryology Authority. www.hfea.gov.uk (last accessed 21 January 2004).
9. Holst N, Maltau JM, Forsdahl F. Handling of tubal infertility after introduction of in vitro fertilization: changes and consequences. *Fertil Steril* 1991;55:140–143.
10. Vilos GA, Verhoest CR, Martin JS. Economic evaluation of in vitro fertilization-embryo transfer and neosalpingostomy for bilateral tubal obstruction. *J Soc Obstet Gynecol Can* 1998;20:139–147.
11. Centers for Disease Control and Prevention. US Department of Health and Human Services, 1998. Assisted Reproductive Technology Success Rates. National Summary and Clinic Reports. December 2000.
12. Brinsden PR, Wada I, Tan SL, et al. Diagnosis, prevention and management of ovarian hyperstimulation syndrome. *Br J Obstet Gynaecol* 1995;102:767–772.
13. Meirow D, Schenker JG. Appraisal of GIFT. *Eur J Obstet Gynecol Reprod* 1995;58:59–65.
14. Rossing MA, Daling JR, Weiss NS, et al. Ovarian tumours in a cohort of infertile women. *N Engl J Med* 1994;331:771–776.
15. Nugent D, Vandekerckhove P, Hughes E, et al. Gonadotrophin therapy for ovulation induction in subfertility associated with polycystic ovarian syndrome. In: The Cochrane Library, Issue 2, 2003. Oxford: Update Software. Search date not reported; primary sources Cochrane Menstrual Disorders and Subfertility Group Specialised Trials Register, Medline, and bibliographies of identified studies.

16. Coelingh-Bennink HJ, Fauser BC, Out HJ. Recombinant follicle-stimulating hormone (FSH; Puregon) is more efficient than urinary follicle stimulating hormone (Metrodin) in women with clomiphene-resistant, normogonadotrophic, chronic anovulation: a prospective, multicenter, assessor-blind, randomized, clinical trial. European Puregon collaborative anovulation study group. *Fertil Steril* 1998;69:19–25.
17. Wang CF, Gemzell C. The use of human gonadotrophins for the induction of ovulation in women with polycystic ovarian disease. *Fertil Steril* 1980;33:479–486.
18. Farquhar C, Vandekerckhove P, Arnot M, et al. Laparoscopic "drilling" by diathermy or laser for ovulation induction in anovulatory polycystic ovary syndrome. In: The Cochrane Library, Issue 2, 2003. Oxford: Update Software. Search date 2001; primary source Cochrane Menstrual Disorders and Subfertility Group Specialised Trials Register.
19. Muenstermann U, Kleinstein J. Long-term GnRH analogue treatment is equivalent to laparoscopic laser diathermy in polycystic ovarian syndrome patients with severe ovarian dysfunction. *Hum Reprod* 2000;15:2526–2530.
20. Winston RM, Margara RA. Microsurgical salpingostomy is not an obsolete procedure. *Br J Obstet Gynaecol* 1991;98:637–642.
21. Singhal V, Li TC, Cooke ID. An analysis of factors influencing the outcome of 232 consecutive tubal microsurgery cases. *Br J Obstet Gynaecol* 1991;98:628–636.
22. Marana R, Quagliarello J. Distal tubal occlusion: microsurgery versus in vitro fertilization: a review. *Int J Fertil* 1988;33:107–115.
23. Marana R, Quagliarello J. Proximal tubal occlusion: microsurgery versus IVF – a review. *Int J Fertil* 1988;33:338–340.
24. Patton PE, Williams TJ, Coulam CB. Results of microsurgical reconstruction in patients with combined proximal and distal occlusion: double obstruction. *Fertil Steril* 1987;47:670–674.
25. Wahab M, Li TC, Cooke ID. Reversal of sterilization versus IVF. *J Obstet Gynaecol* 1997;17:180–185.
26. Jacobson TZ, Barlow DH, Koninckx PR, et al. Laparoscopic surgery for subfertility associated with endometriosis. In: The Cochrane Library, Issue 2, 2003. Oxford: Update Software. Search date 2000–2001; primary sources Cochrane Menstrual Disorders and Subfertility Group Specialised Trials Register, the Cochrane Controlled Trials Register, Medline, Embase, and the National Research Register.
27. Chapron C, Querleu D, Bruhat M, et al. Surgical complications of diagnostic and operative gynaecological laparoscopy: a series of 29 966 cases. *Hum Reprod* 1998;13:867–872.
28. Ford WCL, Mathur RS, Hull MGR. Intrauterine insemination: is it an effective treatment for male factor infertility? *Balliere Clin Obstet Gynecol* 1997;11:691–710. Search date not reported; primary sources Medline, Bids, and manual scanning of leading reproductive journals.
29. Le Lannou D, Lansac J. Artificial procreation with frozen donor sperm: the French experience of CECOS. In: Barratt CLR, Cooke ID, eds. *Donor insemination*. Cambridge: Cambridge University Press, 1993;152–169.
30. Cooke ID. Donor insemination — timing and insemination method. In: Templeton A, Cooke ID, O'Brien PMS, eds. *35th RCOG Study Group evidence-based fertility treatment*. London: RCOG Press, 1998.
31. Zeyneloglu HB, Arici A, Olive DL, et al. Comparison of intrauterine insemination with timed intercourse in superovulated cycles with gonadotrophins: a meta-analysis. *Fertil Steril* 1998;69:486–491. Search date 1997; primary sources Medline, and hand searches of bibliographies of relevant publications and review articles.
32. Buvat J, Buvat-Herbaut M, Marcolin G, et al. Antiestrogens as treatment of female and male infertilities. *Horm Res* 1987;28:219–229.
33. Boostanfar R, Jain JK, Mishell DR Jr, et al. A prospective randomized trial comparing clomiphene citrate with tamoxifen citrate for ovulation induction. *Fertil Steril* 2001;75:1024–1026.
34. Messinis IE, Nillius SJ. Comparison between tamoxifen and clomiphene for induction of ovulation. *Acta Obstet Gynecol Scand* 1982;61:377–379.
35. Gerhard I, Runnebaum B. Comparison between tamoxifen and clomiphene therapy in women with anovulation. *Arch Gynecol* 1979;227:279–288.
36. El Biely MM, Habba M. The use of metformin to augment the induction of ovulation in obese infertile patients with polycystic ovary syndrome. *Middle East Fertil Soc J* 2001;6:43–49.
37. Venn A, Watson L, Lumley J, et al. Breast and ovarian cancer incidence after infertility and IVF. *Lancet* 1995;346:995–1000.
38. Parazzini F, Negri E, La Vecchia C, et al. Treatment for infertility and risk of invasive epithelial ovarian cancer. *Hum Reprod* 1997;12:2159–2161.
39. Mosgaard BJ, Lidegaard O, Kjaer SK, et al. Infertility, fertility drugs, and invasive ovarian cancer: a case-control study. *Fertil Steril* 1997;67:1005–1012.
40. Shushan A, Paltiel O, Iscovich J, et al. Human menopausal gonadotrophin and the risk of epithelial ovarian cancer. *Fertil Steril* 1996;65:13–18.
41. Dunn A, Macfarlane A. Recent trends in the incidence of multiple births and associated mortality in England and Wales. *Arch Dis Child Fetal Neonatal Ed* 1996;75:F10–F19.
42. State-specific variation in rates of twin births — United States, 1992–1994. *MMWR Morb Mortal Wkly Rep* 1997;46:121–125.
43. Levene MI, Wild J, Steer P. Higher multiple births and the modern management of infertility in Britain. British Association of Perinatal Medicine. *Br J Obstet Gynecol* 1992;99:607–613.
44. Cabau A, Krulik DR. Stérilités de cause hormonale et stérilitées inexpliquées. Traitement par le cyclofenil. Etude controlée à double insu. *J Gynécol Obstet Biol Reprod* 1990;19:96–101.
45. Yarali H, Bukulmez O, Gurgan T. Urinary follicle stimulating hormone (FSH) versus recombinant FSH in clomiphene citrate resistant normogonadotropic, chronic anovulation: a prospective randomised study. *Fertil Steril* 1999;72:276–281.
46. Greenblatt E, Casper R. Adhesion formation after laparoscopic ovarian cautery for polycystic ovarian syndrome: lack of correlation with pregnancy rates. *Fertil Steril* 1993;60:766–770.
47. Deans A, Wayne C, Toplis P. Pelvic infection: a complication of laparoscopic ovarian drilling. *Gynaecol Endoscopy* 1997;6:301–303.
48. Bayram N, Van Wely M, Vandekerckhove P, et al. Pulsatile luteinising hormone releasing hormone for ovulation induction in subfertility associated with polycystic ovary syndrome. In: The Cochrane Library, Issue 2, 2003. Oxford: Update Software. Search date not reported; primary sources Cochrane Menstrual Disorders and Subfertility Group Specialised Trials Register and hand searches of reference lists of included trials.
49. Martin KA, Hall JE, Adams JM, et al. Comparison of exogenous gonadotropins and pulsatile gonadotropin-releasing hormone for induction of ovulation in hypogonadotropic amenorrhea. *J Clin Endocrinol Metab* 1993;77:125–129.
50. Braat DD, Schoemaker R, Schoemaker J. Life table analysis of fecundity in intravenously gonadotropin-releasing hormone-treated patients with normogonadotropic and hypogonadotropic amenorrhea. *Fertil Steril* 1991;55:266–271.
51. Filicori M, Flamigni C, Dellai P, et al. Treatment of anovulation with pulsatile gonadotropin-releasing hormone: prognostic factors and clinical results in 600 cycles. *J Clin Endocrinol Metab* 1994;79:1215–1220.
52. Honore GM, Holden AE, Schenken RS. Pathophysiology and management of proximal tubal blockage. *Fertil Steril* 1999;71:785–795. Search date not reported; primary sources Medline and Science Citation Index.

53. Balen AH, Braat DD, West C, et al. Cumulative conception and live birth rates after the treatment of anovulatory infertility: safety and efficacy of ovulation induction in 200 patients. *Hum Reprod* 1994;9:1563–1570.
54. Thurmond AS. Pregnancies after selective salpingography and tubal recanalization. *Radiology* 1994;190:11–13.
55. Marana R. Proximal tubal obstruction: are we overdiagnosing and overtreating? *Gynaecol Endoscopy* 1992;1:99–101.
56. Johnson N, Vandekerckhove P, Watson A, et al. Tubal flushing for subfertility. In: The Cochrane Library, Issue 2, 2003. Oxford: Update Software. Search date 2001; primary sources Cochrane Menstrual Disorders and Subfertility Group Specialised Trials Register, Medline; Embase; Biological Abstracts; the National Research Register; the Clinical Trials Register; search of citation lists of included trials, eligible studies, and relevant review articles; contact with authors of trials eligible for inclusion; and search of abstract booklets from scientific meetings.
57. Nugent D, Watson AJ, Killick SR, et al. A randomized controlled trial of tubal flushing with lipiodol for unexplained infertility. *Fertil Steril* 2002;77:173–175.
58. Johnson NP, Mak W, Sowter MC. Surgical treatment for tubal disease in women due to undergo in vitro fertilisation. In: The Cochrane Library, Issue 2, 2003. Oxford: Update Software. Search date 2000; primary sources Cochrane Menstrual Disorders and Subfertility Group Specialised Trials Register, Medline, Embase, Psychlit, Current Contents, Biological Abstracts, Social Sciences Index, and the National Research Register.
59. Watson A, Vandekerckhove P, Lilford R. Techniques for pelvic surgery in subfertility. In: The Cochrane Library, Issue 2, 2003. Oxford: Update Software. Search date not reported; primary source Cochrane Menstrual Disorders and Subfertility Group Specialised Trials Register.
60. Watson A, Vandekerckhove P, Lilford R. Liquid and fluid agents for preventing adhesions after surgery for subfertility. In: The Cochrane Library, Issue 2, 2003. Oxford: Update Software. Search date not reported; primary source Cochrane Menstrual Disorders and Subfertility Group Specialised Trials Register.
61. Johnson NP, Watson A. Postoperative procedures for improving fertility following pelvic reproductive surgery. In: The Cochrane Library, Issue 2, 2003. Oxford: Update Software. Search date not reported; primary source Cochrane Menstrual Disorders and Subfertility Group Specialised Trials Register.
62. Filippini F, Darai E, Benifla JL, et al. Distal tubal surgery: a critical review of 104 laparoscopic distal tuboplasties. *J Gynecol Obstet Biol Reprod* 1996;25:471–478. [In French].
63. Donnez J, Casanas-Roux F. Prognostic factors of fimbrial microsurgery. *Fertil Steril* 1986;46:200–204.
64. Tomazevic T, Ribic-Pucelj M, Omahen A, et al. Microsurgery and in vitro fertilization and embryo transfer for infertility resulting from pathological proximal tubal blockage. *Hum Reprod* 1996;11:2613–2617.
65. Wu CH, Gocial B. A pelvic scoring system for infertility surgery. *Int J Fertil* 1988;33:341–346.
66. Oelsner G, Sivan E, Goldenberg M, et al. Should lysis of adhesions be performed when in vitro fertilization and embryo transfer are available? *Hum Reprod* 1994;9:2339–2341.
67. Gillett WR, Clarke RH, Herbison GP. First and subsequent pregnancies after tubal surgery: evaluation of the fertility index. *Fertil Steril* 1998;68:1033–1042.
68. Jarrell J, Labelle R, Goeree R, et al. In vitro fertilization and embryo transfer: a randomized controlled trial. *Online J Curr Clin Trials* 1993;2:Doc 73.
69. van Rumste MME, Evers JLH, Farquhar CM. Intra-cytoplasmic sperm injection versus conventional techniques for oocyte insemination during in vitro fertilisation in patients with non-male subfertility. In: The Cochrane Library, Issue 2, 2003. Oxford: Update Software. Search date 2002; primary sources Cochrane Menstrual Disorders and Subfertility Group Specialised Trials Register, the Cochrane Controlled Trials Register, and Pubmed.
70. Bukulmez O, Yarali H, Yucel A, et al. Intracytoplasmic sperm injection versus in vitro fertilization for patients with a tubal factor as their sole cause of infertility: a prospective, randomized trial. *Fertil Steril* 2000;73:38–42.
71. Bhattacharya S, Hamilton MP, Shaaban M, et al. Conventional in-vitro fertilisation versus intracytoplasmic sperm injection for the treatment of non-male-factor infertility: a randomised controlled trial. *Lancet* 2001;357:2075–2079.
72. Poehl M, Holagschwandtner M, Bichler K, et al. IVF-patients with nonmale factor "to ICSI" or "not to ICSI" that is the question? *J Assist Reprod Genet* 2001;18:205–208.
73. Wennerholm U, Bergh C. Obstetric outcome and follow-up of children born after in vitro fertilization (IVF). *Hum Fertil* 2000;3:52–64. Search date 1998; primary source Medline.
74. Chapko KM, Weaver MR, Chapko MK, et al. Stability of in vitro fertilization-embryo transfer success rates from the 1989, 1990, and 1991 clinic-specific outcome assessments. *Fertil Steril* 1995;64:757–763. Search date not reported; primary source Medline.
75. Human Fertilisation and Embryology Authority. *The patients' guide to IVF clinics*. London: HFEA, 2000.
76. Hughes E, Fedorkow D, Collins J, et al. Ovulation suppression for endometriosis. In: The Cochrane Library, Issue 2, 2003. Oxford: Update Software. Search date not reported; primary source Cochrane Subfertility Group Register of Controlled Trials.
77. Dockeray CJ, Sheppard BL, Bonnar J. Comparison between mefenamic acid and danazol in the treatment of established menorrhagia. *Br J Obstet Gynaecol* 1989;96:840–844.
78. Tummon IS, Asher LJ, Martin JSB, et al. Randomized controlled trial of superovulation and insemination for infertility associated with minimal or mild endometriosis. *Fertil Steril* 1997;68:8–12.
79. Fedele L, Bianchi S, Marchini M, et al. Superovulation with human menopausal gonadotrophins in the treatment of infertility associated with endometriosis: a controlled randomised study. *Fertil Steril* 1992;58:28–31.
80. Nulsen JC, Walsh S, Dumez S. A randomised and longitudinal study of human menopausal gonadotrophin with intrauterine insemination in the treatment of infertility. *Obstet Gynaecol* 1993;82:780–786.
81. Cantineau AEP, Heineman MJ, Cohlen BJ. Single versus double intrauterine insemination (IUI) in stimulated cycles for subfertile couples. In: The Cochrane Library, Issue 2, 2003. Oxford: Update Software. Search date July 2002; primary sources Cochrane Menstrual Disorders and Subfertility Group Specialised Trials Register, the Cochrane Controlled Trials Register, Medline, Embase, Science Direct Database, Confsci, and Pascal.
82. Zreik TG, Garcia-Velasco JA, Habboosh MS, et al. Prospective, randomized, crossover study to evaluate the benefit of human chorionic gonadotrophin-timed versus urinary luteinising hormone-timed intrauterine inseminations in clomiphene citrate-stimulated treatment cycles. *Fertil Steril* 1998;71:1070–1074.
83. Hughes EG, Fedorkow DM, Collins J. A quantitative overview of controlled trials in endometriosis-associated infertility. *Fertil Steril* 1993;59:963–970. Search date not reported; primary sources Medline, Science Citation Index, abstracts from scientific meetings, and hand searches of relevant trials and personal contacts.
84. Adamson GD, Pasta DJ. Surgical treatment of endometriosis-associated infertility: meta-analysis compared with survival analysis. *Am J Obstet Gynecol* 1994;171:1488–1504.
85. Barnhart K, Dunsmoor-Su R, Coutifaris, C. Effect of endometriosis on in vitro fertilization. *Fertil Steril*

2002;77:1148–1155. Search date 1999; primary sources Medline and hand searches of references.
86. Geber S, Paraschos T, Atkinson G, et al. Results of IVF in patients with endometriosis: the severity of the disease does not affect outcome or the incidence of miscarriage. *Hum Reprod* 1995;10:1507–1511.
87. Olivennes F, Feldberg D, Liu H-C, et al. Endometriosis: a stage by stage analysis — the role of in vitro fertilization. *Fertil Steril* 1995;64:392–398.
88. Cohlen BJ, Vandekerckhove P, Te Velde ER, et al. Timed intercourse versus intra-uterine insemination with or without ovarian hyperstimulation for subfertility in men. In: The Cochrane Library, Issue 2, 2003. Oxford: Update Software. Search date 1996–1997; primary sources Medline, Embase, DDFU, Biosis, Scisearch, hand searches, and conference abstracts.
89. Kurinczuk J, Bower C. Birth defects in infants conceived by intracytoplasmic sperm injection: an alternative interpretation. *BMJ* 1997;315:1260–1265.
90. Bonduelle M, Legein J, Buyesse A, et al. Prospective follow up study of 423 children born after intracytoplasmic sperm injection. *Hum Reprod* 1996;11:1558–1564.
91. Bonduelle M, Legein J, Derde M, et al. Comparative follow-up study of 130 children born after ICSI and 130 children born after IVF. *Hum Reprod* 1995;10:3327–3331.
92. Velde E, Van Baar A, Van Kooije R. Concerns about assisted reproduction. *Lancet* 1998;351:1524–1525.
93. Tanbo T, Bakketeig LS, Jacobsen G, et al. SMM Report 3/2002: children born from intracytoplasmic sperm injection – systematic review. The Norwegian Centre for Health Technology Assessment: SINTEF Unimed. Search date 2001; primary sources Medline, Embase, Cochrane Controlled Clinical Database Register (CCTR), INAHTA database, and Cochrane Database of Systematic Reviews (CDSR).
94. De Wert G. Ethics of intracytoplasmic sperm injection: proceed with care. *Hum Reprod* 1998;13(suppl 1):219–227.
95. Leeton J, Healy D, Rogers P. A controlled study between the use gamete intrafallopian transfer (GIFT) and in vitro fertilization and embryo transfer in the management of idiopathic and male infertility. *Fertil Steril* 1987;48:605–607.
96. O'Brien P, Vandekerckhove P. Intra-uterine versus cervical insemination of donor sperm for subfertility. In: The Cochrane Library, Issue 2, 2003. Oxford: Update Software. Search date 1996; primary source Cochrane Menstrual Disorders and Subfertility Group Specialised Trials Register.
97. Hughes E, Collins J, Vandekerckhove P. Clomiphene citrate for unexplained subfertility in women. In: The Cochrane Library, Issue 2, 2003. Oxford: Update Software. Search date 2000; primary sources Cochrane Menstrual Disorders and Subfertility Group Specialised Trials Register, Medline, Embase, and Cinahl.
98. Fujii S, Fukui A, Fukushi Y, et al. The effects of clomiphene citrate on normally ovulatory women. *Fertil Steril* 1997;68:997–999.
99. Hughes EG. The effectiveness of ovulation induction and intrauterine insemination in the treatment of persistent infertility: a meta-analysis. *Hum Reprod* 1997;12:1865–1872. Search date not reported; primary source Cochrane Menstrual Disorders and Subfertility Group Specialised Trials Register.
100. Guzick DS, Carson SA, Coutifaris C, et al. Efficacy of superovulation and intrauterine insemination in the treatment of infertility. National Cooperative Reproductive Medicine Network. *N Engl J Med* 1999;340:177–183.
101. Sengoku K, Tamate K, Takaoka Y, et al. The clinical efficacy of low-dose step-up follicle stimulating hormone administration for treatment of unexplained infertility. *Hum Reprod* 1999;14:349–353.
102. Trout SW, Kemmann E. Fallopian sperm perfusion versus intrauterine insemination: a randomized controlled trial and meta-analysis of the literature. *Fertil Steril* 1999;71:881–885. Search date not reported; primary source Medline.
103. Ricci G, Nucera G, Pozzobon C, et al. A simple method for fallopian tube sperm perfusion using a blocking device in the treatment of unexplained infertility. *Fertil Steril* 2001;76:1242–1248.
104. Hogerzeil HV, Spiekerman JCM, De Vries JWA, et al. A randomized trial between GIFT and ovarian stimulation for the treatment of unexplained infertility and failed artificial insemination by donor. *Hum Reprod* 1992;7:1235–1239.
105. Murdoch AP, Harris M, Mahroo M, et al. Gamete intrafallopian transfer (GIFT) compared with intrauterine insemination in the treatment of unexplained infertility. *Br J Obstet Gynaecol* 1991;98:1107–1111.
106. Wessels PHX, Cronje HS, Oosthuizen AP, et al. Cost-effectiveness of gamete intrafallopian transfer in comparison with induction of ovulation with gonadotrophins in the treatment of female infertility: a clinical trial. *Fertil Steril* 1992;57:163–167.
107. Murdoch AP, Harris M, Mahroo M, et al. Is GIFT (gamete intrafallopian transfer) the best treatment for unexplained infertility? *Br J Obstet Gynaecol* 1991;98:643–647.
108. Rombauts L, Dear M, Breheny S, et al. Cumulative pregnancy rates and live birth rates after gamete intra-fallopian transfer. *Hum Reprod* 1997;12:1338–1342.
109. Society for Assisted Reproductive Technology and the American Society for Reproductive Medicine. Assisted reproductive technology in the United States and Canada: 1995 results generated from the American Society for Reproductive Medicine/Society for Assisted Reproductive Technology Registry. *Fertil Steril* 1998;69:389–398.
110. Pandian Z, Bhattacharya S, Nikolaou D, et al. In vitro fertilisation for unexplained subfertility. In: The Cochrane Library, Issue 2, 2003. Oxford: Update Software. Search date 2001; primary sources Cochrane Menstrual Disorders and Subfertility Group Specialised Trials Register, the Cochrane Controlled Trials Register, Medline, Embase, reference lists of articles, hand searches of relevant conference proceedings, and contact with researchers in the field.

Kirsten Duckitt
Consultant Obstetrician and Gynaecologist
John Radcliffe Hospital
Oxford
UK

Competing interests: None declared.

TABLE 1 Success rates of treatments for infertility: evidence from RCTs and observational studies.

Treatment	Live birth rates	Pregnancy rates	Adverse effects
All causes of infertility			
IVF (per treated cycle)	UK 22%[8]; USA 20%[2]		Ectopic pregnancy 1–3%[9,10]; MB 27%[8]; Severe OHSS 0.5–2.0%[11,12]
GIFT (per cycle) (not including tubal infertility)	23%[13]		Ectopic pregnancy 5%
Infertility caused by ovulation disorders			
Clomifene in amenorrhoeic women (after 2–4 cycles of treatment)		Ovulation rate 61%; pregnancy rate 14%[7]	Risk of ovarian cancer unproved. MP 2–13%, mostly twins[14] OHSS infrequent and mild
Gonadotrophins in women with clomifene resistant PCOS (per cycle)		Human menopausal gonadotrophin 10%;[15] urofollitropin/follitropin 12–27%[15,16]	Risk of ovarian cancer unproved. MP 29%[17]
Laparoscopic drilling in women with clomifene resistant PCOS (per cycle) (cumulative rate 6–12 months after treatment)		50–57%[18,19]	Risks of laparoscopy, general anaesthesia, adhesions, and pelvic infection. Risk of premature ovarian failure unproved
Tubal infertility			
Tubal surgery for distal occlusion (cumulative rate 2 years after surgery)	20–30%[20–22]		Risks of general anaesthesia. Ectopic pregnancy 7–9%[9,10]
Tubal surgery for proximal occlusion (cumulative rate)	40–60%[23,24]		
Reversal of female sterilisation (cumulative live birth rate 1–2 years after surgery)	50–90% depending on method used for sterilisation[25]		

TABLE 1 continued

Treatment	Live birth rates	Pregnancy rates	Adverse effects
Infertility associated with endometriosis			
Surgery (per cycle)	27%[26]		Risks of surgery and general anaesthesia. Mortality 3.33/100 000; complication rate 3.2/1000[27]
Male infertility			
IUI ± gonadotrophins (per cycle)		6.5%[28]	
ICSI plus IVF (per cycle)	22%[8]		
Donor insemination (per cycle)	10–11%[8,29,30]		No adverse effects if no ovarian stimulation is given, but child is not male partner's genetic offspring
Unexplained infertility			
IUI ± gonadotrophins (per cycle)		9–12% without stimulation; 19–20% with stimulation[28,31]	

FSH, follicle stimulating hormone; GIFT, gamete intrafallopian transfer; ICSI, intracytoplasmic sperm injection; IUI, intrauterine insemination; IVF, in vitro fertilisation; MB, multiple birth; MP, multiple pregnancy; OHSS, ovarian hyperstimulation syndrome; PCOS, polycystic ovary syndrome.

Menopausal symptoms

Search date March 2004

Edward Morris and Janice Rymer

QUESTIONS

INTERVENTIONS

See glossary G

Key Messages

Medical treatments

- **Progestogens alone** Five RCTs found that progestogens alone reduced vasomotor symptoms compared with placebo and one RCT found no significant difference in vasomotor symptoms between progestogens and placebo. One RCT found no significant difference in vasomotor symptoms between progesterone alone and oestrogen alone. We found no RCTs examining effects of progestogens alone on urogenital symptoms. One RCT found no significant difference in psychological symptoms or quality of life between progesterone and placebo.
- **Tibolone** Two RCTs found that tibolone improved vasomotor symptoms compared with placebo. One RCT found that tibolone improved sexual function compared with placebo. Two RCTs provided limited evidence that tibolone was not as effective for reducing vasomotor symptoms as oestrogen plus progestogen. Two RCTs found that tibolone improved sexual function compared with oestrogen plus progestogen. We found no RCTs assessing psychological symptoms or quality of life.
- **Oestrogens alone (improved menopausal symptoms but increased risk of breast cancer, endometrial cancer, stroke, and venous thromboembolism after long term use)** Systematic reviews and subsequent RCTs found that oestrogen improved vasomotor symptoms, urogenital symptoms, psychological symptoms, and quality of life in the short term compared with placebo. However, important adverse effects of oestrogen include increased risk of breast cancer, endometrial cancer, stroke, and venous thromboembolic disease. Adding progestogen reduces the risk of endometrial hyperplasia.
- **Oestrogens plus progestogens (improved menopausal symptoms but increased risk of breast cancer, stroke, and venous thromboembolism after long term use)** One systematic review and subsequent RCTs found that oestrogen plus progestogens improved vasomotor symptoms, urogenital symptoms, and psychological symptoms in the short term compared with placebo. However, important adverse effects include increased risk of breast cancer, stroke, and venous thromboembolic disease. Two RCTs provided limited evidence that oestrogen plus progestogen reduced vasomotor symptoms compared with tibolone, but that tibolone improved sexual function compared with oestrogen plus progestogen.

Clin Evid 2005;13:2392–2406.

- **Antidepressants** We found no RCTs on the effects of antidepressants on menopausal symptoms.
- **Clonidine** One small RCT found that transdermal clonidine reduced the number and intensity of hot flushes after 8 weeks compared with placebo. However, we were unable to draw reliable conclusions from this study. We found no RCTs that assessed the effects of clonidine on sexual function, psychological symptoms, or quality of life.
- **Phyto-oestrogens** Nine RCTs provided no consistent evidence that phyto-oestrogens reduced vasomotor or other menopausal symptoms compared with placebo. We found no RCTs that assessed quality of life.
- **Testosterone** Small RCTs provided no consistent evidence about the effects of testosterone plus oestrogens on vasomotor symptoms or sexual function compared with oestrogen alone or placebo. We found no RCTs that assessed psychological symptoms or quality of life.

DEFINITION Menopause is defined as the end of the last menstrual period. A woman is deemed to be postmenopausal 1 year after her last period. For practical purposes, most women are diagnosed as menopausal after 1 year of amenorrhoea. Menopausal symptoms often begin in the perimenopausal years. The complex of menopausal symptomatology includes vasomotor symptoms (hot flushes), sleeplessness, mood changes, reduction in energy levels, loss of libido, vaginal dryness, and urinary symptoms.

INCIDENCE/ PREVALENCE In the UK, the mean age for the start of the menopause is 50 years and 9 months. The median onset of the perimenopause is 45.5–47.5 years. One Scottish survey (6096 women aged 45–54 years) found that 84% of women had experienced at least one of the classic menopausal symptoms, with 45% finding one or more symptoms to be a problem.[1]

AETIOLOGY/ RISK FACTORS Urogenital symptoms of menopause are caused by decreased oestrogen concentrations, but the cause of vasomotor symptoms and psychological effects is complex and remains unclear.

PROGNOSIS Menopause is a physiological event. Timing of the natural menopause in healthy women may be determined genetically. Although endocrine changes are permanent, menopausal symptoms such as hot flushes, which are experienced by about 70% of women, usually resolve with time.[2] Some symptoms, however, such as genital atrophy, may remain the same or worsen.

AIMS OF INTERVENTION To reduce or prevent menopausal symptoms; and to improve quality of life, with minimum adverse effects.

OUTCOMES Frequency and severity of vasomotor, urogenital, and psychological symptoms; quality of life.

METHODS *Clinical Evidence* search and appraisal March 2004. Many of the RCTs included were crossover trials, which may have important limitations because treatment effects may persist after crossover, confounding the results for each treatment. Where results are reported only for comparisons with pretreatment values, they have been omitted because these comparisons may be influenced in many (often unquantifiable) ways by factors other than treatment effect.

QUESTION What are the effects of medical treatments?

OPTION OESTROGENS ALONE

Systematic reviews and subsequent RCTs found that oestrogen improved vasomotor symptoms, urogenital symptoms, psychological symptoms, and quality of life in the short term compared with placebo. However, important adverse effects of oestrogen include increased risk of breast cancer, endometrial cancer, stroke, and venous thromboembolic disease. Adding progestogen reduces the risk of endometrial hyperplasia.

Benefits: **Vasomotor symptoms:** We found one systematic review[3] and four subsequent RCTs.[4–7] The systematic review (search date 2000, 21 RCTs, 2511 women) found that oestrogen only hormone replacement therapy (HRT) significantly reduced the frequency of hot flushes compared with placebo (6 RCTs, 371 women; RR of a hot flush in 1 week: 0.23, 95% CI 0.12 to 0.42; WMD –15.7, 95% CI –20.0 to –11.5 flushes/week).[3] It also found that oestrogen only HRT significantly reduced the number of women with hot flushes at the end of the study compared with placebo (8 RCTs, 1240 women; 139/906 [15%] with oestrogen *v* 158/334 [47%] with placebo; RR 0.37, 95% CI 0.30 to 0.45; NNT 4, 95% CI 3 to 4). There was a wide variation in the frequency of hot flushes in both placebo and treatment groups among the RCTs (range of means for each RCT 0.9–13.8 flushes/week with oestrogen *v* 12.6–33.5 with placebo). The first subsequent RCT (2673 women entered, 2152 analysed) compared eight combinations of different doses of oral conjugated equine oestrogen (0.625 mg, 0.45 mg, and 0.3 mg) either alone or plus different doses of medroxyprogesterone acetate (2.5 mg or 1.5 mg) versus placebo.[4] It found that daily doses of 0.3 mg, 0.45 mg, or 0.625 mg conjugated equine oestrogens alone significantly reduced vasomotor symptoms from weeks 3–12, as assessed using diary cards to record number and severity of hot flushes, compared with placebo ($P < 0.05$). It found that 0.625 mg conjugated oestrogen alone significantly reduced the number of hot flushes by week 3 compared with 0.45 mg and 0.3 mg oestrogen dosages (data presented graphically). The second subsequent RCT (165 women) compared two doses of intranasal estradiol (oestradiol, 150 or 300 μg/day) versus placebo over 12 weeks.[5] Symptoms were assessed with diaries and the Kupperman Index**G**. It found that both doses of oestrogen reduced moderate to severe symptoms at 12 weeks compared with placebo (mean reduction from baseline in number of moderate to severe vasomotor symptoms per day: 9.39 with 300 μg estradiol *v* 7.86 with 150 μg estradiol *v* 5.22 with placebo; $P = 0.002$ for high dose *v* placebo and $P < 0.001$ for low dose *v* placebo). The third subsequent RCT (333 women) compared a vaginal ring releasing either 50 or 100 μg estradiol daily versus a placebo vaginal ring for 12 weeks.[7] It found that both doses of estradiol significantly reduced moderate to severe hot flushes and scores on the Greene Climacteric Scale**G** compared with placebo after 12 weeks of treatment (hot flushes/week measured using 4-point scale in daily dairy: 15.5 with 50 μg estradiol *v* 8.3 with 100 μg estradiol *v* 42.2 with placebo; $P < 0.05$; reduction in Greene Climacteric Scale [score range 0–63]: 10.52 with 50 μg estradiol *v* 10.72 with 100 μg estradiol *v* 5.95 with placebo; $P < 0.002$). The fourth subsequent RCT (43 menopausal women) compared oral oestrogen alone versus progestin (150 mg depot medroxyprogesterone for 25 days/month).[6] It found a similar reduction in vasomotor symptoms between treatments at 3 months (P value not reported). **Urogenital system:** We found one systematic review (search date 1998, 6 RCTs, 334 people[8]) and four subsequent RCTs.[5,7,9,10] The systematic review found a significant reduction in the incidence of urinary tract infection with oral or vaginal oestrogen HRT compared with placebo or no treatment (OR for infection; no HRT *v* HRT: 2.51, 95% CI 1.48 to 4.25).[8] Vaginal oestrogens significantly reduced the risk of urinary tract infections compared with oral oestrogens ($P < 0.008$). The first subsequent RCT (145 women) found that low dose estradiol reduced vaginal dryness at weeks 9–12 compared with placebo (86% of days free from vaginal dryness with 1 mg estradiol *v* 76% with 0.5 mg estradiol *v* 74% with placebo), but significance was not tested.[9] The second RCT (multicentre, 84 women treated for 24 weeks, 20% withdrawals) found that an estradiol ring significantly increased relief from dyspareunia compared with placebo (freedom from dyspareunia: 90% with estradiol ring *v* 45% with placebo; $P = 0.028$).[10] The third RCT (165 women) compared the effects of two doses of intranasal estradiol (150 or 300 μg/day) versus placebo on dyspareunia and "urinary troubles" (measured on a visual analogue scales).[5] It found that the 150 µg dose significantly reduced symptoms compared with placebo at 12 weeks ($P < 0.001$), and that the 300 µg dose significantly reduced urogenital symptoms compared with placebo at 4 weeks ($P = 0.014$). The fourth subsequent RCT (333 women) compared vaginal rings releasing either 50 or 100 µg estradiol daily versus placebo for 12 weeks.[7] It found no significant difference between estradiol and placebo for symptoms of vaginal dryness, vaginal itching, urinary frequency, or urinary leakage (reduction in symptoms assessed using 4-point scale scored from none to severe; vaginal dryness: 0.9 with 50µg estradiol *v* 1.3 with 100µg estradiol *v* 0.8 with placebo; vaginal itching: 0.5 with 50µg estradiol *v* 0.4 with 100µg estradiol *v* 0.8 with placebo; urinary frequency: 0.8 with 50µg estradiol *v* 1.0 with 100µg estradiol *v* 0.7 with placebo; urinary leakage: 0.6 with 50µg estradiol *v* 0.5 with 100µg estradiol *v* 0.4 with placebo; P values not reported). It found that estradiol 100 µg daily significantly reduced dyspareunia compared with placebo (score range 0–4; mean score reduction: 1.2 with 50 µg estradiol *v* 1.3 with 100 µg estradiol *v* 0.8 with placebo; $P \leq 0.05$). **Psychological, cognitive, and sleep symptoms:** We found one systematic review on the effect of HRT on menopausal depressed mood (search date 1995, 14 RCTs including several crossover RCTs, 12 cohort studies; duration of treatment ranged from 1 month to 2 years)[11] and one systematic review of the effects of oestrogen on cognitive function in postmenopausal women (search date 1996, 10 controlled trials, and 9 observational studies).[12] We found no RCTs of oestrogen treatment in women with clinically proven depression. The first review found that oestrogen significantly reduced depressed mood (measured using different scales) compared with placebo or no treatment ($P < 0.0001$).[11] The second review found that studies were too weak to allow reliable conclusions to be drawn.[12] **Quality of life:** We found no systematic review. We found one RCT of transdermal estradiol versus placebo[13]and one RCT of oral estradiol versus placebo.[14] The first RCT (242 postmenopausal women) found that estradiol transdermal patches (50 µg/24 hours) significantly improved quality of life ($P = 0.0003$) and wellbeing ($P = 0.003$) over 12 weeks compared with placebo patches.[13] The second RCT (82 women aged 40–60 years) found that oral estradiol significantly improved quality of life scores compared with placebo (assessed using the Kupperman Index [$P = 0.0015$], 3-Factor Green Index [$P = 0.0037$; $P = 0.0026$; $P = 0.0003$], and the Beck Depression Inventory [$P = 0.0242$]).[14]

Harms: Women often report an increase in weight when starting oestrogen, but we found no evidence from RCTs that oestrogen causes significant weight gain in the long term. One systematic review (search date 1998; 22 RCTs) found no effect of oestrogen alone on body weight.[15] The most important long term adverse effects with oestrogens are increased risk of venous thromboembolic disease (see hormone replacement therapy under secondary prevention of ischaemic cardiac events, [web only]), endometrial cancer, and breast cancer.[15–18] One systematic review (search date not reported; 51 RCTs, > 160 000 women) found that HRT (oestrogen alone or oestrogen plus progesterone) increased the relative risk of breast cancer by 2.3% (95% CI 1.1% to 3.6%) each year.[19] Five or more years after HRT was stopped, there was no significant excess of breast cancer. One systematic review (search date not reported, 18 RCTs, 5247 women) of the effects of HRT found significantly increased risks of endometrial hyperplasia in women taking unopposed oestrogen (RR 8.14, 95% CI 1.05 to 63.1 for 6 months of treatment; RR 37.0, 95% CI 9.3 to 147 for 36 months of treatment).[18] It found significant reductions in the incidence of endometrial hyperplasia when women were given progestogens either cyclically or continuously, with continuous combined HRT having the greatest effect at 36 months (RR 0.17,

95% CI 0.02 to 1.26). Meta-analysis of four large RCTs (> 20 000 women) found that long term combined HRT or oestrogen only HRT significantly increased the risk of developing breast cancer (RR 1.27, 95% CI 1.03 to 1.56) and pulmonary embolism (RR 2.16, 95% CI 1.47 to 3.18) compared with placebo, but decreased the risk of colorectal cancer (RR 0.64, 95% CI 0.45 to 0.92) and fractured neck of femur (RR 0.72, 95% CI 0.52 to 0.98) (see harms of hormone replacement therapy in fracture prevention in postmenopausal women, p 1419).[20] The meta-analysis found no significant difference between combined HRT and placebo in risk of endometrial cancer (RR 0.76, 95% CI 0.45 to 1.31) or coronary heart disease (slight increase but not significant; RR 1.11, 95% CI 0.96 to 1.30).[20] The RCT comparing estradiol releasing vaginal rings versus placebo found no difference in adverse effects between treatments apart from "events expected to occur during oestrogen replacement therapy" (no details reported).[7]

Comment: Based on the evidence of important adverse effects, there has been a change in prescribing attitude toward HRT. Before starting HRT, it is now considered important for prescribers to discuss with women the excess risks associated with HRT. Based on the evidence presented under harms above, it remains important that women with an intact uterus who are prescribed any form of oestrogen take either continuous or cyclic progestogens. Applicability of the large RCT may be limited because the average age of women enrolled in the study (63.3 years) is much older than that of women who typically start HRT.[21] A parallel study of the effects of oestrogen alone in women who have had a hysterectomy continues.

OPTION OESTROGENS PLUS PROGESTOGENS

One systematic review and subsequent RCTs found that oestrogen plus progestogens improved vasomotor symptoms, urogenital symptoms, and psychological symptoms in the short term compared with placebo. However, important adverse effects include increased risk of breast cancer, stroke, and venous thromboembolic disease. Two RCTs provided limited evidence that oestrogen plus progestogen reduced vasomotor symptoms compared with tibolone, but that tibolone improved sexual function compared with oestrogen plus progestogen.

Benefits: **Vasomotor symptoms:** We found two RCTs comparing oestrogens plus progestogens versus tibolone (see benefits of tibolone, p 2399).[22,23] We found one systematic review[3] and one subsequent RCT comparing oestrogens plus progestogens versus oestrogen alone.[4] The systematic review (search date 2000, 21 RCTs, 2511 women, follow up for 3–36 months) included comparisons of progesterone plus oestrogen hormone replacement therapy (HRT) versus placebo.[3] It found that progesterone plus oestrogen significantly reduced hot flushes compared with placebo (OR 0.1, 95% CI 0.06 to 0.19).[3] The subsequent RCT (2673 women entered, 2152 analysed) compared eight combinations of different doses of oral conjugated equine oestrogen (0.625 mg, 0.45 mg, and 0.3 mg) either alone or plus different doses of medroxyprogesterone acetate (2.5 mg or 1.5 mg) versus placebo.[4] It found that daily doses of 0.3 mg, 0.45 mg, or 0.625 mg conjugated equine oestrogens plus medroxyprogesterone acetate (2.5 mg/day) significantly reduced vasomotor symptoms from weeks 3–12 compared with placebo ($P < 0.05$). There was no significant difference in the number or severity of hot flushes between different doses of medroxyprogesterone acetate. **Urogenital system:** We found one RCT (136 women).[24] It found that low dose transdermal oestrogen (25 µg/day) plus norethisterone acetate significantly reduced vaginal dryness and dyspareunia over 6 months compared with placebo ($P < 0.001$). **Psychological,**

cognitive, and sleep symptoms: We found one large RCT.[25,21] The RCT (16 608 postmenopausal women with an intact uterus aged 50–79 years) compared conjugated equine oestrogens (0.625 mg/day) plus medroxyprogesterone acetate (2.5 mg/day) versus placebo.[21] It found that oestrogen plus progestin did not significantly improve mental health or depressive symptoms (assessed using the RAND 36-Item Health Survey) compared with placebo after 1 year (range in mean change of scores from baseline: –0.1 to +0.6 with oestrogen plus progestin *v* –0.1 to +0.7 with placebo; P value ranged from 0.40–0.81). However, it did find significant improvements in sleep disturbance (mean change of scores from baseline: 0.5 with oestrogen plus progestin *v* 0.1 with placebo; $P < 0.001$), although the generalisability of these results may be limited (see comment below).[25] **Quality of life:** We found two RCTs.[21,26] The first large RCT (16 608 postmenopausal women with an intact uterus aged 50–79 years of age) compared conjugated equine oestrogens (0.625 mg/day) plus medroxyprogesterone acetate (2.5 mg/day) versus placebo.[21] It found that oestrogen plus progestin did not significantly improve general health, social functioning, vitality, or sexual satisfaction (assessed using the RAND 36-Item Health Survey) compared with placebo after 1 year (range in mean change in quality of life scores from baseline: –1.9 to +0.2 with oestrogen plus progestin *v* –2.3 to 0 with placebo; P value ranged from 0.08–0.76). However, it did find significant improvements in physical functioning and bodily pain ($P < 0.001$ for both outcomes), although the generalisability of these results may be limited (see comment below).[25] The second RCT (74 women with an intact uterus and ovaries, 2–7 years after menopause) found that quality of life was similarly improved with either oral conjugated equine oestrogen (0.625 mg/day for four 4 week cycles) plus medroxyprogesterone acetate (10 mg for the last 12 days of each cycle) or with continuous transdermal estradiol-17β (50 μg twice weekly for four 4 week cycles) plus medroxyprogesterone acetate (10 mg for the last 12 days of each cycle).[26]

Harms: One systematic review (search date not reported; 18 RCTs, 5247 women) found significant reductions in the incidence of endometrial hyperplasia when women receiving oestrogen were given progestogens either cyclically or continuously, with continuous combined HRT having the greatest effect at 36 months (RR for continuous combined HRT *v* oestrogen only HRT 0.17, 95% CI 0.02 to 1.26).[18] A meta-analysis of four large RCTs found no significant difference between combined HRT and placebo in risk of endometrial cancer (RR 0.76, 95% CI 0.45 to 1.31) or coronary heart disease (slight increase but not significant; RR 1.11, 95% CI 0.96 to 1.30).[20] The large RCT[21] (described under benefits above) found similar results (HR for coronary heart disease: 1.29, 95% CI 1.02 to 1.63; HR for pulmonary embolus: 2.13, 95% CI 1.39 to 3.25). Although the intended duration of the large RCT study was 8.5 years, it was stopped after a mean follow up of 5.2 years because of a significant increase in risks associated with treatment compared with placebo.[21] Further analysis of the RCT found that combined oestrogen plus progesterone increased the risk of breast cancer and, in women who developed breast cancer, it increased the size of tumours and the risk of tumour spread compared with placebo (size: 1.7 cm with treatment *v* 1.5 cm with placebo; $P = 0.04$; spread: 25.4% with treatment *v* 16% with placebo; $P = 0.04$) (see table 1, p 2405).[27] Analyses found no significant difference between treatments in the risk of gynaecological tumours (see table 1, p 2405),[28] and found that treatment increased risk of stroke, regardless of age, race, or risk group.[29] Two RCTs also assessed the harms of oestrogen plus progestogens.[30,31] The first RCT (321 women who had undergone hysterectomy and were already taking conjugated oestrogen) compared continuous progestogen (norgestrel) versus placebo.[30] It found no difference in adverse effects of treatments (including weight gain and bloating). The second RCT (875 women) compared various oestrogen/progestogen combinations over 3 years.[31] It found that addition of progestogen to oestrogen therapy increased breast discomfort compared with oestrogen alone (OR 1.92, 95% CI 1.16 to 3.09). Neither RCT found evidence of an effect on cardiovascular events. Adding oestrogen to progestogen is associated with an increased risk of breast cancer, stroke, and venous thromboembolic disease compared with progestogen alone (see harms of oestrogen, p 2395).[20,21]

Comment: Applicability of the large RCT[21] may be limited because the average age of women enrolled in the study (63.3 years) is much older than that of women who typically start HRT. Based on the evidence for harms associated with oestrogen (see harms of oestrogens alone, p 2395), it remains important that women with an intact uterus who are prescribed any form of oestrogen take either continuous or cyclical progestogens.

OPTION PROGESTOGENS ALONE

Five RCTs found that progestogens alone reduced vasomotor symptoms compared with placebo and one RCT found no significant difference in vasomotor symptoms between progestogens and placebo. One RCT found no significant difference in vasomotor symptoms between progesterone alone and oestrogen alone. We found no RCTs examining effects of progestogens alone on urogenital symptoms. One RCT found no significant difference in psychological symptoms or quality of life between progesterone and placebo.

Benefits: **Vasomotor symptoms:** We found no systematic review. We found three RCTs of oral progestogens versus placebo,[32–34] two RCTs of transdermal progesterone versus placebo,[35,36] and one RCT of oral progestogens versus oral oestrogen.[6] The three RCTs comparing oral progestogens alone versus placebo (all ≤ 24 weeks in duration) found that progestogens significantly reduced vasomotor symptoms (see table 2, p 2406).[32–34] The two RCTs comparing transdermal progesterone alone versus placebo found different results.[35,36] The first RCT found that progesterone significantly reduced vasomotor symptoms (see table 2, p 2406).[35] The second RCT found no significant difference in vasomotor symptoms (assessed using the Greene Climacteric Scale**G**) between treatments (see table 2, p 2406).[36] The remaining RCT (43 menopausal women) compared oral progesterone versus oral oestrogen alone.[6] It found a similar reduction in vasomotor symptoms between treatments at 3 months (no decrease in vasomotor symptoms in 18% of women in each group; P value not reported). **Urogenital system:** We found no RCTs evaluating the effects of progestogens alone on urinary incontinence, the lower genital tract, or libido. **Psychological symptoms:** We found one RCT (see table 2, p 2406).[36] It found no significant difference in depression or anxiety symptoms between transdermal progesterone and placebo after 12 weeks (anxiety: $P = 0.10$; depression: $P = 0.56$). **Quality of life:** We found one RCT (see table 1, p 2405),[36] which found no significant difference between transdermal progesterone and placebo for each of four quality of life domains (vasomotor, physical, psychosocial, sex-related; P value ranged from 0.28–0.94).

Harms: The RCTs did not report any harms.[32–36] See also harms of oral progestogen in the chapters on menorrhagia, p 2407.

Comment: Progestogens are seldom given alone, which makes it difficult to isolate their effects. When given without oestrogen, doses of progestogens were high, the lowest dose being 20 mg medroxyprogesterone acetate daily. We found one further RCT, which compared depomedroxyprogesterone acetate versus placebo, but the disparity in size between the experimental and control groups (57 *v* 12 women) and lack of detail on randomisation strategies make the results difficult to interpret.[37] Three of the placebo controlled RCTs had crossover comparisons, which make conclusions difficult to draw.[32–34]

OPTION TIBOLONE

Two RCTs found that tibolone improved vasomotor symptoms compared with placebo. One RCT found that tibolone improved sexual function compared with placebo. Two RCTs provided limited evidence that tibolone was not as effective for reducing vasomotor symptoms as oestrogen plus progestogen. Two RCTs found that tibolone improved sexual function compared with oestrogen plus progestogen. We found no RCTs assessing psychological symptoms or quality of life.

Benefits: We found no systematic review. **Vasomotor symptoms:** We found two RCTs comparing tibolone versus placebo,[38,39] and two RCTs comparing tibolone versus oestrogen/progestogen combinations.[22,23] The first RCT (82 women with menopausal symptoms) found that tibolone significantly reduced vasomotor symptoms at 16 weeks compared with placebo (39% reduction in mean score; P = 0.001).[38] The second RCT (775 women) compared four different doses of tibolone (0.625, 1.25, 2.5, and 5 mg/day) versus placebo.[39] It found that 1.25 mg, 2.5 mg, and 5 mg tibolone reduced the frequency of hot flushes and sweating episodes compared with placebo (assessed using symptom diaries, results presented graphically; P < 0.0001). It found no significant difference in frequency of hot flushes and sweating episodes between 0.625 mg tibolone and placebo. The third RCT (437 women with menopausal symptoms) compared combined oestrogen and progestogen versus tibolone.[22] It found that combined oestrogen/progestogen significantly reduced hot flushes over 48 weeks compared with tibolone (P = 0.01). The fourth RCT (235 postmenopausal women) found no significant difference in vasomotor symptoms between combined oestrogen/progestogen and tibolone at 52 weeks (figures not reported).[23] **Urogenital system:** We found three RCTs published in four reports: one comparing tibolone versus placebo, and two comparing tibolone versus oestrogen plus progestogen.[22,40–42] The first RCT (crossover, 38 women) found that tibolone significantly increased sexual fantasies (P < 0.03) and arousability over 3 months compared with placebo (P < 0.01).[42] The second RCT (437 women) found that tibolone significantly improved vaginal dryness from baseline compared with estradiol plus norethisterone after 48 weeks of treatment (assessed using a 5-point scoring system: 2.16 at baseline to 1.33 after treatment with tibolone *v* 2.12 at baseline to 1.27 after treatment with hormone replacement therapy; P < 0.001).[22] The RCT also found that tibolone improved sexual satisfaction as measured using McCoy's Sex Scale Questionnaire compared with estradiol plus norethisterone (P < 0.05).[40] The third RCT (50 women attending a university gynaecology clinic) found that tibolone significantly improved sexual desire and coital frequency as measured using a questionnaire compared with conjugated oestrogen (0.625 mg) plus medroxyprogesterone acetate (2.5 mg) after 12 months (P < 0.05 for both outcomes).[41] We found no RCTs examining the effects on urinary incontinence. **Psychological symptoms:** We found no RCTs. **Quality of life:** We found no RCTs.

Harms: One RCT reported that two women randomised to receive tibolone (at 1.25 mg and 5.0 mg daily doses) discontinued treatment because of vaginal bleeding.[39] One non-randomised controlled trial found that the main adverse effect of tibolone was breakthrough bleeding, which occurred in about 10% of users.[43] We found no good evidence of androgenic adverse effects, such as hair growth and greasiness of the skin. Two RCTs of short term use found a 33% reduction in plasma high density lipoproteins with tibolone,[44,45] although the long term effects on cardiovascular disease are unknown.

Comment: None.

OPTION PHYTO-OESTROGENS

Nine RCTs provided no consistent evidence that phyto-oestrogens reduced vasomotor or other menopausal symptoms compared with placebo. We found no RCTs that assessed quality of life.

Benefits: We found no systematic review. **Vasomotor symptoms:** We found nine placebo controlled RCTs.[46–54] The first RCT (58 postmenopausal women) compared soy flour (which contains phyto-oestrogens) versus wheat flour for 12 weeks.[46] It found no significant difference between soy flour and wheat flour in hot flushes at 12 weeks (reduction in hot flushes: 40% with soy flour *v* 25% with wheat flour; P = 0.82). The second RCT (crossover, 51 women) compared a daily dietary supplement containing no phyto-oestrogens versus a supplement containing 34 mg soy protein.[47] It found that soy protein reduced the severity (P < 0.001) but not the frequency of vasomotor symptoms at 6 weeks. The third RCT (unblinded crossover, 51 women) compared isoflavone 40 mg daily versus placebo.[48] It found no significant difference between isoflavone and placebo in vasomotor symptoms assessed after 12 weeks by flush count (mean hot flush count: 3.72 in 46 women receiving placebo *v* 4.22 in 42 women receiving isoflavone; SMD –0.5, 95% CI –8.9 to +7.9) and Greene Climacteric Scale**G**; mean 7.23 in 42 women with isoflavone *v* 6.93 in 46 women with placebo; SMD –0.3, 95% CI –19.2 to +18.6). The fourth RCT (39 women) found that soy flour significantly reduced mean flushes per week compared with placebo (45% reduction with soy flour *v* 25% with placebo tablets after 12 weeks; P < 0.01), although women taking soy extract had a greater number of vasomotor symptoms at baseline than the placebo group.[49] The fifth RCT (94 women) found no significant difference between soy protein and placebo at 3 months for vasomotor symptoms as assessed using a 4-point subjective rating scale.[50] The sixth RCT (177 women) found that a 50 mg daily dose of an isoflavone extract significantly reduced hot flush severity over 12 weeks compared with placebo (P = 0.01).[51] It found no significant difference between groups in hot flush frequency. The seventh RCT (80 women) found that 100 mg soy isoflavone daily significantly reduced menopausal symptoms compared with placebo (change in Kupperman Index**G** from baseline to 16 weeks: 44.6 at baseline to 24.9 at 16 weeks with isoflavone *v* 40.3 at baseline to 41.6 at 16 weeks with placebo; P < 0.01).[52] The eighth RCT (62 women) found no significant difference in vasomotor symptoms at 6 months between soy isoflavones and placebo (mean number of hot flushes/day at 6 months recorded using daily dairy: 4.6 with isoflavone *v* 4.0 with placebo; P value not reported).[53] The ninth RCT (252 women) found no significant difference after 12 weeks between isoflavone (57 mg/day or 82 mg/day) and placebo in either the number of hot flushes or vasomotor symptoms assessed using the Greene Climacteric Scale (hot flushes/day at 12 weeks: 5.0 with 57 mg isoflavone *v* 5.4 with 82 mg isoflavone *v* 5.1 with placebo; P > 0.2; reduction in Greene vasomotor subscale score: 0.9 with 57 mg isoflavone *v* 1.1 with 82 mg isoflavone *v* 1.2 with placebo; P > 0.36).[54] **Other symptoms:** One RCT (94 women) found no significant difference between soy protein and placebo at 3 months in psychological, musculoskeletal, and genitourinary symptoms, as assessed using a 4-point subjective rating scale.[50] **Quality of life:** We found no RCTs.

Harms: We found no evidence of significant adverse effects.

Comment: Few studies have specifically investigated adverse effects of phytooestrogens. Results of studies are difficult to interpret because phytooestrogen preparations are not standardised. One recent RCT (80 women) compared the effects of 100 mg soy isoflavone daily versus placebo on blood pressure, plasma glucose, serum lipid and lipoprotein concentrations, and endometrial thickness.[52] It found that phytooestrogens reduced serum total cholesterol and low density lipoprotein compared with placebo (P < 0.01).

OPTION CLONIDINE

One small RCT found that transdermal clonidine reduced the number and intensity of hot flushes after 8 weeks compared with placebo. However, we were unable to draw reliable conclusions from this study. We found no RCTs that assessed the effects of clonidine on sexual function, psychological symptoms, or quality of life.

Benefits: We found no systematic review. **Vasomotor symptoms:** One RCT (30 women) found that transdermal clonidine (3.5 cm^2 patch delivering 0.1 mg clonidine/day for 7 days) significantly reduced the proportion of women with hot flushes and increased the proportion of women perceiving a reduction in severity of the hot flushes compared with placebo at 8 weeks (women reporting reduction in number of hot flushes: 12/15 [80%] with clonidine *v* 5/14 [35%] with placebo; RR 2.4, 95% CI 1.1 to 4.7; NNT 3, 95% CI 2 to 12; women reporting reduction in severity of hot flushes: 11/15 [73%] with transdermal clonidine *v* 4/14 [29%] with placebo; RR 2.7, 95% CI 1.09 to 6.6; NNT 3, 95% CI 2 to 5).[55] **Urogenital system:** We found no RCTs. **Psychological symptoms:** We found no RCTs. **Quality of life:** We found no RCTs.

Harms: The RCT found no significant difference in the incidence of adverse effects between clonidine and placebo.[55] The analysed adverse effects included transient local skin reactions (4/15 [27%] with clonidine patch *v* 3/14 [21%] with placebo; RR 1.2, 95% CI 0.34 to 4.6).

Comment: Transdermal patches of clonidine are not widely available. Results may not be generalisable and may not extrapolate to oral clonidine.

OPTION TESTOSTERONE

Small RCTs provided no consistent evidence about the effects of testosterone plus oestrogens on vasomotor symptoms or sexual function compared with oestrogen alone or placebo. We found no RCTs that assessed psychological symptoms or quality of life.

Benefits: We found no systematic review. **Vasomotor symptoms:** We found no RCTs comparing testosterone alone versus placebo. We found two RCTs comparing testosterone/oestrogen combinations versus oestrogen alone.[56,57] The first RCT (93 postmenopausal women) compared oestrogen plus methyltestosterone (1.25 mg/day or 2.5 mg/day) versus oestrogen alone (0.625 mg/day or 1.25 mg/day).[56] It found that adding a small dose of methyltestosterone significantly reduced hot flushes (P = 0.008) and reduced the oestrogen dose required to control menopausal symptoms. The second RCT (40 women) compared estradiol plus testosterone versus estradiol alone.[57] It found no significant difference in vasomotor symptoms after 2 and 6 months of treatment (numbers not reported). **Urogenital system:** We found one RCT (40 women; described above).[57] It found no significant difference between estradiol alone and estradiol plus testosterone in level of self reported sexual enjoyment and desire.[57] The second RCT (crossover, 53 surgically menopausal women; see comment below) compared four treatments: oestrogen alone, testosterone plus oestrogen, testosterone alone, and placebo.[58] It found that testosterone with or without oestrogen significantly increased sexual desire ($P < 0.01$), sexual arousal ($P < 0.01$), and number of sexual fantasies ($P < 0.01$) compared with placebo or oestrogen alone during the treatment months. **Psychological symptoms:** We found no RCTs. **Quality of life:** We found no RCTs.

Harms: We found no evidence from RCTs or other controlled studies on the incidence of androgenic adverse effects with testosterone in women with menopausal symptoms.

Comment: The crossover RCT addressing urogenital symptoms did not provide an analysis before crossover.[58] Results are therefore likely to be confounded by carry over effects of treatments.

OPTION ANTIDEPRESSANTS

We found no RCTs on the effects of antidepressants on menopausal symptoms.

Benefits: We found no systematic review or RCTs on the effects of antidepressants on menopausal symptoms or quality of life in menopausal women.

Harms: We found no evidence on adverse effects in postmenopausal women. Antidepressants as a group can cause many central nervous system adverse effects, including sedation and agitation, as well as urinary and vision problems, liver dysfunction, and cardiac dysrhythmias (see antidepressants under depressive disorders, p 1238).

Comment: None.

GLOSSARY

Greene Climacteric Scale A numerical index that scores 21 menopausal symptoms in three domains: psychological, somatic, and vasomotor. Each symptom is rated from 0–3 where 0 = no symptoms and 3 = extreme symptoms.

Kupperman Index A numerical index that scores 11 menopausal symptoms: hot flushes, paraesthesia, insomnia, nervousness, melancholia, vertigo, weakness, arthralgia or myalgias, headache, palpitations, and formication. Each symptom is rated from 0–3 according to severity and symptoms (where 0 = no symptoms and 3 = most severe) are then weighted and the total sum calculated. The maximum score is 51 points.

REFERENCES

1. Porter M, Penney G, Russell D, et al. A population based survey of women's experience of the menopause. *Br J Obstet Gynaecol* 1996;103:1025–1028.
2. Hagsta TA, Janson PO. The epidemiology of climacteric symptoms. *Acta Obstet Gynecol Scand* 1986;134(suppl):59.
3. MacLennan A, Lester S, Moore V. Oral oestrogen replacement therapy versus placebo for hot flushes. In: The Cochrane Library, Issue 2, 2001. Oxford: Update Software. Search date 2000; primary sources Medline, Embase, Cinahl, and hand searched relevant journals and conference abstracts.
4. Utian WH, Shoupe D, Bachmann G, et al. Relief of vasomotor symptoms and vaginal atrophy with lower doses of conjugated equine estrogens and medroxyprogesterone acetate. *Fertil Steril* 2001;75:1065–1079.
5. Rozenbaum H, Chevallier O, Moyal M, et al. Efficacy and tolerability of pulsed estrogen therapy: a 12-week double-blind placebo-controlled study in highly symptomatic postmenopausal women. *Climacteric* 2002;5:249–258.
6. Lobo RA, McCormick W, Singer F, et al. DMPA compared with conjugated oestrogens for the treatment of postmenopausal women. *Obstet Gynecol* 1984;63:1–5.
7. Speroff L. Efficacy and tolerability of a novel estradiol vaginal ring for relief of menopausal symptoms. *Obstet Gynecol* 2003;102:823–834.

8. Cardozo L, Lose G, McClish D, et al. A systematic review of estrogens for recurrent urinary tract infections: third report of the hormones and urogenital therapy (HUT) committee. *Int Urogynecol J Pelvic Floor Dysfunct* 2001;12:15–20. Search date 1998; primary sources Excerpta Medica, Medline, Science Citation Index, and hand-searching relevant journals.
9. Notelovitz M, Mattox JH. Suppression of vasomotor and vulvovaginal symptoms with continuous oral 17β-estradiol. *Menopause* 2000;7:310–317.
10. Casper F, Petri E. Local treatment of urogenital atrophy with an estradiol-releasing vaginal ring: a comparative and a placebo-controlled multicenter study. Vaginal Ring Study Group. *Int Urogynecol J Pelvic Floor Dysfunct* 1999;10:171–176.
11. Zweifel JE, O'Brien WH. A meta-analysis of the effect of HRT upon depressed mood. *Psychoneuroendocrinology* 1997;22:189–212. Search date 1995; primary sources Psychological Abstracts, Medline, and hand searches of Dissertation Abstracts International.
12. Haskell SG, Richardson ED, Horwitz RI. The effect of ORT on cognitive function in women: a critical review of the literature. *J Clin Epidemiol* 1997;50:1249–1264. Search date 1996; primary sources Medline, and hand searched reference lists.
13. Wiklund I, Karlberg J, Mattsson L. Quality of life of postmenopausal women on a regimen of transdermal estradiol therapy: a double-blind placebo-controlled study. *Am J Obstet Gynecol* 1993;168:824–830.
14. Derman RJ, Dawood MY, Stone S. Quality of life during sequential hormone replacement therapy — a placebo-controlled study. *Int J Fertil Menopausal Stud* 1995;40:73–78.
15. Norman RJ, Flight IHK, Rees MCP. Oestrogen and progestogen hormone replacement therapy for peri-menopausal and post-menopausal women: weight and body fat distribution. In: The Cochrane Library, Issue 2, 2001. Search date 1998; primary sources Medline, Embase, Current Contents, Biological Abstracts, Cinahl, citation lists, and contact with authors of eligible trials retrieved.
16. Grady D, Sawaya G. Postmenopausal hormone therapy increases risk of deep vein thrombosis and pulmonary embolism. *Am J Med* 1998;105:41–43.
17. Barrett-Connor E. Fortnightly review: hormone replacement therapy. *BMJ* 1998;317:457–461.
18. Lethaby A, Farquhar C, Sarkis A, et al. Hormone replacement therapy in postmenopausal women: endometrial hyperplasia and irregular bleeding. In: The Cochrane Library, Issue 1, 2004. Oxford: Update Software. Search date not reported; primary sources Cochrane Menstrual Disorders and Subfertility Group Trials Register, Medline, Embase, Current Contents, Biological Abstracts, Social Sciences Index, Psychlit, Cinahl, hand searched citation lists, and contact with drug companies and trials authors.
19. Collaborative Group on Hormonal Factors in Breast Cancer. Breast cancer and hormone replacement therapy: collaborative reanalysis of data from 51 epidemiological studies of 52 705 women with breast cancer and 108 411 women without breast cancer. *Lancet* 1997;350:1047–1059. Search date and primary sources not reported; the authors collected epidemiological data on 52 705 women with breast cancer and 108 411 women without breast cancer from 51 studies identified from literature searches, review articles, and discussions with colleagues.
20. Beral V, Banks E, Reeves G. Evidence from randomized trials on the long-term effects of hormone replacement therapy. *Lancet* 2002;360:942–944.
21. Writing Group for the Women's Health Initiative Investigators. Risks and benefits of estrogen plus progestin in healthy postmenopausal women: principal results from the Women's Health Initiative randomized controlled trial. *JAMA* 2002;288:321–333.
22. Hammar M, Christau S, Nathorst-Boos J, et al. A double-blind, randomised trial comparing the effects of tibolone and continuous combined hormone replacement therapy in postmenopausal women with menopausal symptoms. *Br J Obstet Gynaecol* 1998;105:904–911.
23. Al Azzawi F, Wahab M, Habiba M, et al. Continuous combined hormone replacement therapy compared with tibolone. *Obstet Gynecol* 1999;93:258–264.
24. Mattsson LA. Clinical experience with continuous combined transdermal hormone replacement therapy. *J Menopause* 1999;6:25–29.
25. Hays J, Ockene JK., Brunner RL, et al. Effects of estrogen plus progestin on health-related quality of life. *N Engl J Med* 2003;348:1839–1854.
26. Hilditch JR, Lewis J, Ross AH, et al. A comparison of the effects of oral conjugated equine estrogen and transdermal estradiol-17 β combined with an oral progestin on quality of life in postmenopausal women. *Maturitas* 1996;24:177–184.
27. Chlebowski RT, Hendrix SL, Langer RD, et al. Influence of estrogen plus progestin on breast cancer and mammography in healthy postmenopausal women: the Women's Health Initiative Randomized Trial. *JAMA* 2003;289:3243–3253.
28. Anderson GL, Judd HL, Kaunitz AM, et al. Effects of estrogen plus progestin on gynecologic cancers and associated diagnostic procedures: the Women's Health Initiative Randomized Trial. *JAMA* 2003;290:1739–1748.
29. Wassertheil-Smoller S, Hendrix SL, Limacher M, et al. Effect of estrogen plus progestin on stroke in postmenopausal women: the Women's Health Initiative: a randomized trial. *JAMA* 2003;289:2673–2684.
30. Medical Research Council's General Practice Research Framework. Randomised comparison of oestrogen versus oestrogen plus progesterone hormone replacement therapy in women with hysterectomy. *BMJ* 1996;312:473–478.
31. Greendale GA, Reboussin BA, Hogan P, et al. Symptom relief and side effects of postmenopausal hormones: results from the postmenopausal estrogen/progestin interventions trial. *Obstet Gynecol* 1998;92:982–988.
32. Loprinzi CL, Michalak JC, Quella SK, et al. Megestrol acetate for the prevention of hot flashes. *N Engl J Med* 1994;331:347–352.
33. Aslaksen K, Frankendal B. Effect of oral MPA on menopausal symptoms on patients with endometrial carcinoma. *Acta Obstet Gynecol Scand* 1982;61:423–428.
34. Schiff I, Tulchinsky D, Cramer D, et al. Oral medroxyprogesterone in the treatment of postmenopausal symptoms. *JAMA* 1980;244:1443–1445.
35. Leonetti HB, Longo S, Anasti JN. Transdermal progesterone cream for vasomotor symptoms and postmenopausal bone loss. *Obstet Gynecol* 1999;94:225–228.
36. Wren BG, Champion SM, Willetts K, et al. Transdermal progesterone and its effect on vasomotor symptoms, blood lipid levels, bone metabolic markers, moods, and quality of life for postmenopausal women. *Menopause* 2003;10:13–18.
37. Bjorn I, Bixo M, Noid KS, et al. Negative mood changes during hormone replacement therapy: a comparison between two progestogens. *Am J Obstet Gynecol* 2000;183:1419–1426.
38. Kicovic PM, Cortes-Prieto J, Luisi M, et al. Placebo-controlled cross-over study of effects of Org OD14 in menopausal women. *Reproduction* 1982;6:81–91.
39. Landgren MB, Bennink HJ, Helmond FA, et al. Dose-response analysis of effects of tibolone on climacteric symptoms. *BJOG* 2002;109:1109–1114.
40. Nathorst-Boos J, Hammar M. Effect on sexual life — a comparison between tibolone and a continuous estradiol-norethisterone acetate regimen. *Maturitas* 1997;26:15–20.
41. Kokcu A, Cetinkaya MB, Yanik F, et al. The comparison of effects of tibolone and conjugated

estrogen- medroxyprogesterone acetate therapy on sexual performance in postmenopausal women. *Maturitas* 2000;36:75–80.
42. Laan E, Van Lunsen RHW, Everaerd W. The effects of tibolone on vaginal blood flow, sexual desire and arousability in postmenopausal women. *Climacteric* 2001;4:28–41.
43. Morris EP, Wilson POG, Robinson J, et al. Long term effects of tibolone on the genital tract in postmenopausal women. *Br J Obstet Gynaecol* 1999;106:954–959.
44. Benedek-Jaszmann LJ. Long-term placebo-controlled efficacy and safety study of Org OD14 in climacteric women. *Maturitas* 1987;1:25–33.
45. Walker ID, Davidson JF, Richards A, et al. The effect of the synthetic steroid Org OD14 on fibrinolysis and blood lipids in postmenopausal women. *Thromb Haemost* 1985;53:303–305.
46. Murkies AL, Lombard C, Stauss BJ, et al. Dietary flour supplementation decreases postmenopausal hot flushes: effect of soy and wheat. *Maturitas* 1995;21:189–195.
47. Washburn S, Burke GL, Morgan T, et al. Effect of soy protein supplementation on serum lipoproteins, blood pressure, and menopausal symptoms in perimenopausal women. *Menopause* 1999;6:7–13.
48. Baber RJ, Templeman C, Morton T, et al. Randomized placebo-controlled trial of an isoflavone supplement and menopausal symptoms in women. *Climacteric* 1999;2:85–92.
49. Scambia G, Mango D, Signorile PG, et al. Clinical effects of a standardized soy extract in postmenopausal women: a pilot study. *Menopause* 2000;7:105–111.
50. Kotsopoulos D, Dalais FS, Liang Y-L, et al. The effects of soy protein containing phytoestrogens on menopausal symptoms in postmenopausal women. *Climacteric* 2000;3:161–167.
51. Upmalis DH, Lobo R, Bradley L, et al. Vasomotor symptom relief by soy isoflavone extract tablets in postmenopausal women: a multicenter, double-blind, randomized, placebo-controlled study. *Menopause* 2000;7:236–242.
52. Han KK, Soares JM Jr, Haidar MA, et al. Benefits of soy isoflavone therapeutic regimen on menopausal symptoms. *Obstet Gynecol* 2002;99:389–394.
53. Penotti M, Fabio E, Modena AB, et al. Effect of soy-derived isoflavones on hot flushes, endometrial thickness, and the pulsatility index of the uterine and cerebral arteries. *Fertil Steril* 2003;79:1112–1117.
54. Tice JA, Ettinger B, Ensrud K, et al. Phytoestrogen supplements for the treatment of hot flashes: the Isoflavone Clover Extract (ICE) Study: a randomized controlled trial. *JAMA* 2003;290:207–214.
55. Nagamani M, Kelver ME, Smith ER. Treatment of menopausal hot flashes with transdermal administration of clonidine. *Am J Obstet Gynecol* 1987;156:561–565.
56. Simon J, Klaiber E, Wiita B, et al. Differential effects of estrogen-androgen and estrogen-only therapy on vasomotor symptoms, gonadotropin secretion, and endogenous androgen bioavailability in postmenopausal women. *Menopause* 1999;6:138–146.
57. Dow MG, Hart DM, Forrest CA. Hormonal treatments of sexual unresponsiveness in postmenopausal women: a comparative study. *Br J Obstet Gynaecol* 1983;90:361–366.
58. Sherwin BB, Gelfand MM, Brender W. Androgen enhances sexual motivation in females: a prospective crossover study of sex steroid administration in the surgical menopause. *Psychosom Med* 1985;47:339–351.

Edward Morris
Consultant in Obstetrics and Gynaecology
Norfolk and Norwich University Hospital
Norwich
UK

Janice Rymer
Senior Lecturer/Consultant in Obstetrics and Gynaecology
Guy's, King's and St Thomas' Medical School
London
UK

Competing interests: EM has been sponsored to attend conferences and has received speakers' fees from Eli Lilly, Organon, Novo Nordisk, Astra Zeneca, and Pharmacia; JR has been sponsored to attend conferences by Organan, Solvay Healthcare Ltd, Wyeth, Novo Nordish, Janssen-Cilag, and Servier. JR has also received research funding from Organon and Novo Nordish, and consultancy fees from Organon, Wyeth, Janssen-Cilag, and Pfizer.

TABLE 1 **Harms of oestrogen: summary data regarding stroke, breast, ovarian, and endometrial cancer incidence from the Women's Health Initiative Trial (see text, p 2397).**

Trial	Total participants	Comparison	Duration	Outcome	Difference	Effect
Loprinzi[32]	163	Oral medroxyprogesterone acetate 200 mg twice daily versus placebo (crossover)	9 weeks	50% reduction in daily hot flush frequency at 4 weeks (pre-crossover)	34/48 (71%) with medroxyprogesterone acetate *v* 12/49 (24%) with placebo	RR 2.9, 95% CI 1.71 to 4.89; NNT 3, 95% CI 2 to 4
Aslaksen[33]	21	Oral medroxyprogesterone acetate 100 mg twice daily versus placebo (crossover)	24 weeks	Free from hot flushes at end of study	18/21 (86%) with medroxyprogesterone acetate *v* 7/21 (33%) with placebo	RR for no flush 2.6, 95% CI 1.37 to 4.83; NNT 2, 95 % CI 2 to 3
				Free from sweating	18/21 (86%) with medroxyprogesterone acetate *v* 3/21 (14%) with placebo	RR for no sweating 6.0, 95% CI 2.1 to 17.4; NNT 2, 95% CI 1 to 2
Schiff[34]	27	Oral medroxyprogesterone acetate 20 mg daily versus placebo (crossover)	24 weeks	% reduction in hot flushes at 12 week crossover to alternative treatment	74% with medroxyprogesterone acetate *v* 26% with placebo	$P < 0.05$
Leonetti[35]	102	Transdermal progesterone cream 20 mg versus placebo	1 year	Improvement or resolution of vasomotor symptoms as determined by review of weekly symptom diaries	25/30 (83%) with transdermal progesterone *v* 26/47 (55%) with placebo	RR 1.5, 95% CI 1.1 to 2.0; NNT 4, 95% CI 2 to 9
Wren[36]	80	Transdermal progesterone cream 32 mg daily versus placebo	12 weeks	Greene Climacteric Scale and the Menopause Quality of Life Questionnaire	Median change in Greene Climacteric Scale (vasomotor symptoms) from baseline –1.0 with progesterone *v* 0 with placebo	$P = 0.07$

TABLE 2 Placebo controlled RCTs evaluating the effect of progestogens on vasomotor symptoms (see text, p 2398).

Event type		Cumulative absolute risk with oestrogen/progesterone	Cumulative absolute risk with placebo	Hazard ratio (95% CI)
Breast cancer[27]	Total cancers	245/8506 [2.9%]	185/8102 [2.3%]	1.24 (1.02 to 1.50)
	Invasive cancers	199/8506 [2.3%]	150/8102 [1.9%]	1.24 (1.01 to 1.54)
	In *situ cancers*	47/8506 [0.6%]	37/8102 [0.5%]	1.18 (0.77 to 1.82)
Ovarian cancer[28]	Total cancers	20/8506 [0.2%]	12/8102 [0.1%]	1.58 (0.77 to 3.24)
Endometrial cancer[28]	Total cancers	27/8506 [0.3%]	31/8102 [0.4%]	0.81 (0.48 to 1.36)
Stroke[29]	Total strokes	151/8506 [1.8%]	107/8102 [1.3%]	1.31 (1.02 to 1.68)
	Ischaemic stroke	125/8506 [1.5%]	81/8102 [1.0%]	1.44 (1.09 to 1.90)
	Haemorrhagic stroke	18/8506 [0.2%]	20/8102 [0.2%]	0.82 (0.43 to 1.56)

Menorrhagia

Search date October 2003

Kirsten Duckitt and Keri McCully

QUESTIONS

INTERVENTIONS

Beneficial

Gonadorelin analogues for endometrial thinning before endometrial destruction 2423
Hysterectomy (reduces menstrual blood loss compared with intrauterine progestogens or endometrial destruction; also reduces need for further surgery compared with endometrial destruction) 2419
Non-steroidal anti-inflammatory drugs. 2410
Tranexamic acid 2411

Likely to be beneficial

Hysteroscopic endometrial destruction (increases amenorrhoea compared with non-hysteroscopic destruction) 2420

Trade off between benefits and harms

Danazol. 2413
Endometrial destruction (reduces menstrual blood loss compared with medical treatment) 2420

Unknown effectiveness

Combined oral contraceptives . .2414
Danazol for endometrial thinning before endometrial destruction 2424
Dilatation and curettage 2418
Etamsylate. 2413
Gonadorelin analogues. 2418
Intrauterine progestogens. 2416
Myomectomy 2422
Oral progestogens for endometrial thinning before endometrial destruction 2424

Unlikely to be beneficial

Oral progestogens (longer cycle). 2415

Likely to be ineffective or harmful

Oral progestogens in luteal phase only. 2415

See glossary G

Key Messages

Treatments

- **Gonadorelin analogues for endometrial thinning before endometrial destruction** One systematic review found that preoperative gonadorelin analogues reduced postoperative moderate or heavy periods at 6–12 months after surgery and increased amenorrhoea at 24 months after surgery compared with placebo or no preoperative treatment. It found no significant difference between gonadorelin analogues and danazol in postoperative amenorrhoea at 12 months.
- **Hysterectomy (reduces menstrual blood loss compared with intrauterine progestogens or endometrial destruction; also reduces need for further surgery compared with endometrial destruction)** One systematic review found that surgery (hysterectomy or endometrial destruction) reduced menstrual blood loss over 1 year compared with intrauterine progestogens but that hysterectomy was associated with more serious adverse effects than progestogens. Two systematic

reviews found that hysterectomy reduced menstrual blood loss and the number of women requiring further operations, and increased participant satisfaction compared with endometrial destruction. Five small RCTs found no evidence of a difference in effectiveness between different types of hysterectomy, although operating and recovery times differed. One large cohort study reported major or minor complications in about a third of women undergoing hysterectomy.

- **Non-steroidal anti-inflammatory drugs** One systematic review found that non-steroidal anti-inflammatory drugs reduced menstrual blood loss compared with placebo. Systematic reviews found no significant difference in menstrual blood loss between mefenamic acid and naproxen, or between non-steroidal anti-inflammatory drugs and oral progestogens given in the luteal phase, but the comparisons may have lacked power to exclude clinically important differences between treatments. Systematic reviews found that mefenamic acid was less effective than tranexamic acid or danazol in reducing menstrual blood loss, but caused fewer adverse effects than danazol. RCTs identified by several systematic reviews provided insufficient evidence to compare non-steroidal anti-inflammatory drugs versus etamsylate, combined oral contraceptives, or intrauterine progestogens. We found no RCTs comparing non-steroidal anti-inflammatory drugs versus gonadorelin analogues. One RCT identified by a systematic review found that medical treatment, including non-steroidal anti-inflammatory drugs, was less effective than endometrial resection in reducing menstrual blood loss at 4 months and 2 years, and increased the proportion of women who had adverse effects over 4 months.
- **Tranexamic acid** Systematic reviews found that tranexamic acid reduced menstrual blood loss compared with placebo, mefenamic acid, flurbiprofen, diclofenac, etamsylate (ethamsylate), or oral progestogens. We found no RCTs comparing tranexamic acid versus danazol, combined oral contraceptives, or gonadorelin analogues. RCTs identified by several systematic reviews provided insufficient evidence to compare tranexamic acid versus intrauterine progestogens. One RCT identified by a systematic review found that medical treatment, including tranexamic acid, was less effective than endometrial resection in reducing menstrual blood loss at 4 months and 2 years, and increased the proportion of women who had adverse effects over 4 months. Adverse effects of tranexamic acid include leg cramps and nausea, which occur in about a third of women using this drug. One long term population based observational study found no evidence that tranexamic acid increased the risk of thromboembolism.
- **Hysteroscopic endometrial destruction (increases amenorrhoea compared with non-hysteroscopic destruction)** One systematic review and three subsequent RCTs found that hysteroscopic methods of endometrial destruction increased amenorrhoea at 12 months compared with non-hysteroscopic methods. We found no consistent evidence of a difference in amenorrhoea or satisfaction rates among different types of hysteroscopic procedure. RCTs found that complications, such as infection, haemorrhage, and uterine perforation, occurred in up to 15% of women undergoing endometrial destruction.
- **Danazol** Systematic reviews found that danazol reduced blood loss compared with placebo, mefenamic acid, naproxen, or luteal phase oral progestogens but found that danazol increased adverse effects compared with either non-steroidal anti-inflammatory drugs or oral progestogens. RCTs identified by several systematic reviews provided insufficient evidence to compare danazol versus combined oral contraceptives or intrauterine progestogens. We found no RCTs comparing danazol versus tranexamic acid or gonadorelin analogues. One RCT identified by a systematic review found that medical treatment, including danazol, was less effective than endometrial resection in reducing menstrual blood loss at 4 months and 2 years, and increased the proportion of women who had adverse effects over 4 months.
- **Endometrial destruction (reduces menstrual blood loss compared with medical treatment)** One systematic review found that surgery (hysterectomy or endometrial destruction) reduced menstrual blood loss over 1 year compared with intrauterine progestogens. One RCT identified by a systematic review found that endometrial resection reduced blood loss at 4 months and 2 years compared with

medical treatment, and reduced the proportion of women who had adverse effects over 4 months. Two systematic reviews found that endometrial destruction increased menstrual blood loss and the need for further operations and reduced participant satisfaction compared with hysterectomy. RCTs found that complications, such as infection, haemorrhage, and uterine perforation, occurred in up to 15% of women undergoing endometrial destruction.

- **Combined oral contraceptives** One RCT identified by three systematic reviews provided insufficient evidence to compare oral contraceptives versus other drugs. Another RCT identified by a systematic review found that medical treatment, including oral contraceptives, was less effective than endometrial resection in reducing menstrual blood loss at 4 months and 2 years, and increased the proportion of women who had adverse effects over 4 months.
- **Danazol for endometrial thinning before endometrial destruction** Two small RCTs identified by a systematic review and one subsequent RCT provided insufficient evidence to compare preoperative danazol versus placebo or no preoperative treatment. One systematic review found no significant difference between danazol and gonadorelin analogues in postoperative amenorrhoea at 12 months. Two RCTs identified by a systematic review provided insufficient evidence to compare danazol versus other medical treatments.
- **Etamsylate** One systematic review provided insufficient evidence to compare etamsylate (ethamsylate) versus placebo or mefenamic acid. Two systematic reviews found that etamsylate was less effective than tranexamic acid in reducing menstrual blood loss. We found no RCTs comparing etamsylate versus danazol, combined oral contraceptives, oral progestogens, intrauterine progestogens, or gonadorelin analogues.
- **Intrauterine progestogens** We found no RCTs comparing intrauterine progestogens versus placebo. RCTs identified by several systematic reviews provided insufficient evidence to compare intrauterine progestogens versus other drugs. RCTs identified by two systematic reviews provided insufficient evidence to compare intrauterine versus oral progestogens. One systematic review found that intrauterine progestogens were less effective than hysterectomy or endometrial destruction in reducing menstrual blood loss over 1 year, but caused fewer serious adverse effects than hysterectomy.
- **Oral progestogens for endometrial thinning before endometrial destruction** RCTs provided insufficient evidence about the effects of preoperative progestogens compared with placebo, no preoperative treatment, or other medical treatments.
- **Dilatation and curettage; gonadorelin analogues; myomectomy** We found no RCTs on the effects of these interventions.
- **Oral progestogens (longer cycle)** We found no RCTs comparing oral progestogens versus placebo. One RCT identified by a systematic review found no significant difference in menstrual blood loss between a longer treatment cycle of oral progestogen and a levonorgestrel releasing intrauterine device.
- **Oral progestogens in luteal phase only** We found no RCTs comparing oral progestogens versus placebo. One systematic review found no significant difference in menstrual blood loss between oral progestogens given in the luteal phase and non-steroidal anti-inflammatory drugs, but the comparison may have lacked power to exclude clinically important differences between treatments. One systematic review found that luteal phase oral progestogens were less effective in reducing mean menstrual blood loss than tranexamic acid or danazol. RCTs identified by two systematic reviews provided insufficient evidence to compare oral versus intrauterine progestogens. One RCT identified by a systematic review found that medical treatment, including oral progestogens, was less effective than endometrial resection in reducing menstrual blood loss at 4 months and 2 years, and increased the proportion of women who had adverse effects over 4 months.

DEFINITION Menorrhagia is defined as heavy but regular menstrual bleeding. Idiopathic ovulatory menorrhagia is regular heavy bleeding in the absence of recognisable pelvic pathology or a general bleeding disorder. Objective menorrhagia is taken to be a total menstrual blood loss of 80 mL or more in each menstruation.[1] Subjectively, menorrhagia may be defined as a complaint of regular excessive menstrual blood loss occurring over several consecutive cycles in a woman of reproductive years.

INCIDENCE/ PREVALENCE In the UK, 5% of women (aged 30–49 years) consult their general practitioner each year with menorrhagia.[2] In New Zealand, 2–4% of primary care consultations by premenopausal women are for menstrual problems.[3]

AETIOLOGY/ RISK FACTORS Idiopathic ovulatory menorrhagia is thought to be caused by disordered prostaglandin production within the endometrium.[4] Prostaglandins may also be implicated in menorrhagia associated with uterine fibroids, adenomyosis, or the presence of an intrauterine device. Fibroids have been reported in 10% of women with menorrhagia (80–100 mL/cycle) and 40% of those with severe menorrhagia (≥ 200 mL/cycle).[5]

PROGNOSIS Menorrhagia limits normal activities and causes iron deficiency anaemia in two thirds of women proved to have objective menorrhagia.[1,6,7] One in five of all women in the UK and one in three women in the USA have a hysterectomy before the age of 60 years; menorrhagia is the main presenting problem in at least 50% of these women.[8–10] About 50% of the women who have a hysterectomy for menorrhagia are found to have a normal uterus.[11]

AIMS OF INTERVENTION To reduce menstrual bleeding; improve quality of life; and prevent or correct iron deficiency anaemia, with minimum adverse effects. Women may regard amenorrhea as a benefit or a harm of treatment depending on their perspective.

OUTCOMES Menstrual blood flow (assessed objectively [mL/cycle] or subjectively); haemoglobin concentration; quality of life; patient satisfaction; incidence of adverse drug effects; and incidence of postoperative complications. Whether a particular percentage reduction in menstrual blood loss is considered clinically important will depend on pretreatment menstrual loss and the individual woman's perception of acceptable menstrual loss.

METHODS *Clinical Evidence* search and appraisal October 2003. The author also hand searched reference lists of non-systematic reviews and studies obtained from the initial search, and recent issues of key journals. We found several systematic reviews that assessed the same RCTs in relation to different treatment options. When presenting comparative data regarding an option, we have reported the data from the review that presented the most data on that option.

QUESTION What are the effects of medical treatments?

OPTION NON-STEROIDAL ANTI-INFLAMMATORY DRUGS

One systematic review found that non-steroidal anti-inflammatory drugs reduced menstrual blood loss compared with placebo. Systematic reviews found no significant difference in menstrual blood loss between mefenamic acid and naproxen, or between non-steroidal anti-inflammatory drugs and oral progestogens given in the luteal phase, but the comparisons may have lacked power to exclude clinically important differences between treatments. Systematic reviews found that mefenamic acid was less effective than tranexamic acid or danazol in reducing menstrual blood loss, but caused fewer adverse effects than danazol. RCTs identified by several systematic reviews provided insufficient evidence to compare non-steroidal anti-inflammatory drugs versus etamsylate, combined oral contraceptives, or intrauterine progestogens. We found no RCTs comparing non-steroidal anti-inflammatory drugs versus gonadorelin analogues. One RCT identified by a systematic review found that medical treatment, including non-steroidal anti-inflammatory drugs, was less effective than endometrial resection in reducing menstrual blood loss at 4 months and 2 years, and increased the proportion of women who had adverse effects over 4 months.

Benefits: **Versus placebo:** We found one systematic review (search date 1996, 12 RCTs, 313 women) comparing non-steroidal anti-inflammatory drugs (NSAIDs; mefenamic acid, naproxen, mefenamic acid, ibuprofen, and diclofenac) versus placebo.[3] Treatment was taken only during menstruation and doses varied depending on the drug used. The review found that NSAIDs significantly reduced mean menstrual blood loss compared with placebo (WMD for blood loss for all NSAIDs *v* placebo –35 mL, 95% CI –43 mL to –27 mL). **Versus each other:** We found one systematic review (search date 2001, 2 RCTs, 61 women), which found no significant difference in menstrual blood loss between mefenamic acid and naproxen (WMD for blood loss +21.0 mL, 95% CI –5.9 mL to +47.9 mL; see comment below).[12] **Versus tranexamic acid:** See benefits of tranexamic acid, p 2411. **Versus etamsylate:** See benefits of etamsylate, p 2413. **Versus danazol:** We found two systematic reviews (search dates 2001), both of which identified the same three RCTs (79 women).[12,13] The first review found that NSAIDs were significantly less effective than danazol in reducing menstrual blood loss (WMD for blood loss 45.1 mL, 95% CI 18.7 mL to 71.4 mL; see comment below).[12] **Versus combined oral contraceptives:** See benefits of combined oral contraceptives, p 2414. **Versus oral progestogens:** We found one systematic review (search date 2001, 2 RCTs, 48 women), which found no significant difference in menstrual blood loss between NSAIDs and oral progestogens given in the luteal phase (WMD for blood loss –23.0 mL, 95% CI –46.6 mL to +0.625 mL).[12] **Versus intrauterine progestogens:** See benefits of intrauterine progestogens, p 2416. **Versus gonadorelin analogues:** We found no RCTs.

Harms: The reviews found that commonly reported adverse effects included headaches and gastrointestinal disturbances such as indigestion, nausea, vomiting, and diarrhoea.[3,12] These occurred in at least 50% of women taking NSAIDs in the RCTs that reported data on adverse effects, but similar levels of adverse effects were found in placebo cycles (see non-steroidal anti-inflammatory drugs, p 1525).

Comment: The comparisons of NSAIDs versus other drugs may have lacked power to exclude clinically important differences between treatments.[12] NSAIDs have the additional benefit of relieving dysmenorrhoea (see dysmenorrhoea, p 2303). Both reviews comparing NSAIDs versus danazol found that NSAIDs were less effective than danazol in reducing blood loss but the second review[13] did not perform a meta-analysis for this comparison.

OPTION TRANEXAMIC ACID

Systematic reviews found that tranexamic acid reduced menstrual blood loss compared with placebo, mefenamic acid, flurbiprofen, diclofenac, etamsylate (ethamsylate), or oral progestogens. We found no RCTs comparing tranexamic acid versus danazol, combined oral contraceptives, or gonadorelin analogues. RCTs identified by several systematic reviews provided insufficient evidence to compare tranexamic acid versus intrauterine progestogens. One RCT identified by a systematic review found that medical treatment, including tranexamic acid, was less effective than endometrial resection in reducing menstrual blood loss at 4 months and 2 years, and increased the proportion of women who had adverse effects over 4 months. Adverse effects of tranexamic acid include leg cramps and nausea, which occur in about a third of women using the drug. One long term population based observational study found no evidence that tranexamic acid increased the risk of thromboembolism.

Benefits: **Versus placebo:** We found two systematic reviews.[3,14] The first review (search date 1996, 5 RCTs, 153 women) found that tranexamic acid (250–500 mg 4 times daily during menstruation) significantly reduced mean menstrual blood loss compared with placebo (WMD –52 mL; other results and significance presented graphically).[3] Few RCTs in the review measured patient satisfaction. The second review (search date 1997, 7 RCTs) identified two RCTs that compared tranexamic acid (1 g 4 times daily) or a prodrug of tranexamic acid (Kabi 2161; 1.2 g twice daily) versus placebo.[14] It found that either active drug significantly reduced mean menstrual blood loss compared with placebo (WMD −94 mL, 95% CI −151 mL to −37 mL). One of the RCTs identified by the second review found limited evidence from indirect comparisons that tranexamic acid significantly reduced limitations in social activities compared with placebo (proportion of women who reported reduced limitation in social activities when taking tranexamic acid compared with when taking placebo: 67%, reported as significant, CI not reported) and increased the proportion of women with improved sex life (proportion reporting improved sex life when taking tranexamic acid compared with when taking placebo: 46% with tranexamic acid, P = 0.029).[15] **Versus non-steroidal anti-inflammatory drugs:** We found three systematic reviews (search date 1997,[14] search date 1996,[3] search date not reported[16]). Two of the reviews[3,14] identified the same RCT (49 women) comparing tranexamic acid versus mefenamic acid. The RCT found that tranexamic acid significantly reduced mean menstrual blood loss compared with mefenamic acid (WMD −73 mL, 95% CI −123 mL to −23 mL).[14] The second review[3] identified two further RCTs comparing tranexamic acid versus flurbiprofen (15 women) or diclofenac (19 women).[3] Both RCTs found that tranexamic acid improved outcomes compared with flubiprofen or diclofenac. The third review[16] identified one RCT[19] (81 women) comparing three interventions: tranexamic acid, mefenamic acid, and etamsylate(see comment below).[16] The RCT found that tranexamic acid significantly reduced mean menstrual blood loss compared with mefenamic acid WMD −56 mL, 95% CI −90 mL to −2 mL). **Versus etamsylate:** We found two systematic reviews (search date 1996,[3] search date not reported[16] that identified the same RCT (81 women).[19] The RCT compared three interventions: tranexamic acid, etamsylate, and mefenamic acid (see comment below). It found that tranexamic acid significantly reduced mean menstrual blood loss compared with etamsylate (WMD −97 mL, 95% CI −140 mL to −54 mL).[19] **Versus danazol:** We found no RCTs. **Versus combined oral contraceptives:** We found no RCTs. **Versus oral progestogens:** We found three systematic reviews (search date 1996,[3] search date 1997,[14] search date not reported[17]). All of the reviews identified the same single RCT[15] (46 women). The RCT did not directly compare the difference in menstrual blood loss between groups.[15] One of the reviews performed an analysis directly comparing tranexamic acid versus norethisterone.[14] It found that tranexamic acid significantly reduced mean menstrual blood loss compared with norethisterone (WMD −111 mL, 95% CI −179 mL to −44 mL).[14] **Versus intrauterine progestogens:** See benefits of intrauterine progestogens, p 2416. **Versus gonadorelin analogues:** We found no RCTs. **Versus endometrial destruction:** See benefits of endometrial destruction, p 2420.

Harms: Nausea and leg cramps occur in a third of women taking tranexamic acid. Isolated case reports have suggested a risk of thromboembolism associated with tranexamic acid, but a large population based study conducted over 19 years found no evidence that this was higher than expected in the normal population.[18] **Versus placebo or other drugs:** One systematic review (search date 1997) found no increase in gastrointestinal adverse effects compared with either placebo or other drugs.[14] **Versus endometrial destruction:** See harms of endometrial destruction, p 2421.

Comment: Unlike non-steroidal anti-inflammatory drugs, tranexamic acid has no effect on dysmenorrhoea. The RCT comparing tranexamic acid, etamsylate, and mefenamic acid reported that 27% of women had withdrawn from the study before its completion, and made no adjustment for the multiple treatment comparisons involved.[19]

OPTION ETAMSYLATE

One systematic review provided insufficient evidence to compare etamsylate (ethamsylate) versus placebo or mefenamic acid. Two systematic reviews found that etamsylate was less effective than tranexamic acid in reducing menstrual blood loss. We found no RCTs comparing etamsylate versus danazol, combined oral contraceptives, oral progestogens, intrauterine progestogens, or gonadorelin analogues.

Benefits: We found one systematic review (search date not reported, 4 RCTs) of etamsylate.[16] The results were presented as a comparison versus baseline rather than direct comparisons of etamsylate versus placebo or other drugs. The review found that etamsylate achieved an overall reduction in menstrual blood loss compared with baseline of 13% (95% CI 11% to 15%), which may not be clinically important.[16] **Versus non-steroidal anti-inflammatory drugs:** The review[16] identified one RCT (double blind, 81 women; see comment below) that compared three treatments: etamsylate, tranexamic acid, and mefenamic acid.[19] The RCT found that etamsylate was significantly less effective in reducing mean menstrual blood loss compared with mefanamic acid (WMD –51 mL, 95% CI –96 mL to –6 mL). **Versus tranexamic acid:** See benefits of tranexamic acid, p 2411. **Versus other drugs:** We found no RCTs.

Harms: The review found no significant difference in the rate of adverse effects (nausea, headaches, and dizziness) between different drug regimens, and these adverse effects seldom caused women to withdraw from studies.[16]

Comment: The RCT comparing tranexamic acid, etamsylate, and mefenamic acid reported that 27% of women had withdrawn from the study before its completion, and made no adjustment for the multiple treatment comparisons involved.[19]

OPTION DANAZOL

Systematic reviews found that danazol reduced blood loss compared with placebo, mefenamic acid, naproxen, or luteal phase oral progestogens but found that danazol increased adverse effects compared with either non-steroidal anti-inflammatory drugs or oral progestogens. RCTs identified by several systematic reviews provided insufficient evidence to compare danazol versus combined oral contraceptives or intrauterine progestogens. We found no RCTs comparing danazol versus tranexamic acid or gonadorelin analogues. One RCT identified by a systematic review found that medical treatment, including danazol, was less effective than endometrial resection in reducing menstrual blood loss at 4 months and 2 years, and increased the proportion of women who had adverse effects over 4 months.

Benefits: **Versus placebo:** We found two systematic reviews (search date 2001,[13] 1 RCT, 66 women; search date 1996[13], 3 RCTs, 127 women) comparing danazol versus placebo. The RCT identified by the first review did not directly compare danazol versus placebo; it reported blood loss scores within each group before and after treatment. It found that danazol significantly improved blood loss scores from baseline whereas placebo had no significant effect at 3 months.[13] However, it is unclear how this result was calculated as blood loss scores and significance assessments were not reported. The second review found that danazol (200 mg/day continuously for 2–3 months) significantly reduced mean menstrual blood loss compared with placebo (WMD −108 mL; CI presented graphically; see comment below).[3] **Versus non-steroidal anti-inflammatory drugs (NSAIDs):** See benefits of NSAIDs, p 2410. **Versus tranexamic acid:** We found no RCTs. **Versus etamsylate:** We found no RCTs. **Versus combined oral contraceptives:** See benefits of combined oral contraceptives, p 2414. **Versus oral progestogens:** See benefits of oral progestogens, p 2415. **Versus intrauterine progestogens:** See benefits of intrauterine progestogens, p 2416. **Different regimens:** We found one systematic review (search date 2001), which included two small RCTs comparing different danazol regimens: standard dose danazol (200 mg/day), lower dose danazol (100 mg/day), and a reducing dose regimen.[13] It found no significant difference in blood loss (WMD for mean menstrual blood loss +33.5 mL, 95% CI −32.4 mL to +99.4 mL), frequency of adverse events (OR for number of women reporting adverse events 1.13, 95% CI 0.14 to 9.07), or duration of menstruation (WMD for duration of menstruation +1.3 days, 95% CI −0.76 days to +3.36 days) when a dose of 200 mg daily was compared with a reducing dose regimen. **Versus endometrial destruction:** See benefits of endometrial destruction, p 2420.

Harms: **Versus placebo:** RCTs included in the first review reported that danazol may be associated with weight gain; androgenic effects such as acne, seborrhoea, hirsutism, and voice changes; and general complaints including irritability, musculoskeletal pains, and tiredness.[13] Hot flushes and breast atrophy can sometimes occur. Most of these adverse effects are reversible on cessation of treatment (see harms of hormonal treatments under endometriosis, p 2326, and harms of danazol under breast pain, p 2258). Women using danazol may be advised to use barrier methods of contraception because of potential virilisation of the fetus if pregnancy occurs during treatment with this drug. **Versus NSAIDs:** One RCT (40 women) identified by the first review found that adverse effects, including musculoskeletal pains, dizziness, flushes, acne, behavioural changes, tiredness, and hirsutism, were significantly more frequent with danazol than with mefenamic acid (OR 7.0, 95% CI 1.7 to 28.2).[13] However, the RCT found no significant difference in adherence to treatment (OR 1.11, 95% CI 0.32 to 3.90). **Versus oral progestogens:** See harms of oral progestogens, p 2416. **Versus endometrial destruction:** See harms of endometrial destruction, p 2421.

Comment: **Versus placebo:** The second systematic review comparing danazol versus placebo had less rigorous inclusion criteria and included two RCTs that were excluded in the first review.[3]

OPTION COMBINED ORAL CONTRACEPTIVES

One RCT identified by three systematic reviews provided insufficient evidence to compare oral contraceptives versus other drugs. Another RCT identified by a systematic review found that medical treatment, including oral contraceptives, was less effective than endometrial resection in reducing menstrual blood loss at 4 months and 2 years, and increased the proportion of women who had adverse effects over 4 months.

Benefits: **Versus placebo:** We found no RCTs. **Versus non-steroidal anti-inflammatory drugs or danazol:** We found three systematic reviews (search dates 2001,[12,13] search date 1997[20]), all of which identified the same small RCT (38 women) comparing four interventions: a combined oral contraceptive, mefenamic acid, naproxen, or danazol (doses not reported). It found no significant difference between any of the treatments but was too small to rule out a clinically important difference (WMD for oral contraceptive *v* mefenamic acid: −17.5 mL, 95% CI −22.5 mL to +47.5 mL, WMD for oral contraceptive *v* naproxen: +8.37, 95% CI −27.3 to +44.0, WMD for oral contraceptive *v* danazol: +19.3, 95% CI −24.47 to +63.01). **Versus other drugs:** We found no RCTs. **Versus endometrial destruction:** See benefits of endometrial destruction, p 2420.

Harms: Minor adverse effects are common and include nausea, headache, breast tenderness, changes in body weight, hypertension, changes in libido, and depression. **Versus endometrial destruction:** See harms of endometrial destruction, p 2421.

Comment: One non-randomised controlled trial (164 women) found that a 50 mg oral contraceptive pill led to a 53% reduction in menstrual blood loss from baseline.[21] Two longitudinal case control studies found that women taking the contraceptive pill were less likely than those not taking the pill to experience heavy menstrual bleeding or anaemia.[22,23]

OPTION ORAL PROGESTOGENS

We found no RCTs comparing oral progestogens versus placebo. One systematic review found no significant difference in menstrual blood loss between oral progestogens given in the luteal phase and non-steroidal anti-inflammatory drugs, but the comparison may have lacked power to exclude clinically important differences between treatments. One systematic review found that luteal phase oral progestogens were less effective in reducing mean menstrual blood loss than tranexamic acid or danazol. RCTs identified by two systematic reviews provided insufficient evidence to compare oral versus intrauterine progestogens. One RCT identified by a systematic review found no significant difference in menstrual blood loss between a longer treatment cycle of oral progestogen and a levonorgestrel releasing intrauterine device. Another RCT identified by a systematic review found that medical treatment, including oral progestogens, was less effective than endometrial resection in reducing menstrual blood loss at 4 months and 2 years, and increased the proportion of women who had adverse effects over 4 months.

Benefits: **Versus placebo:** We found no RCTs. **Versus non-steroidal anti-inflammatory drugs:** See benefits of non-steroidal anti-inflammatory drugs, p 2410. **Versus tranexamic acid:** See benefits of tranexamic acid, p 2411. **Versus etamsylate:** We found no RCTs. **Versus danazol:** We found one systematic review (search date not reported; 2 RCTs, 51 women), which found that oral progestogens were significantly less effective in reducing menstrual blood loss than danazol (WMD −56 mL, 95% CI −96 mL to −15 mL).[17] The review also found that luteal phase oral progestogens significantly increased the proportion of women who reported a greater self assessed menstrual blood loss after treatment compared with danazol (2 RCTs: 19/28 [68%] with luteal phase progestogens *v* 8/26 [31%] with danazol; RR 2.2, 95% CI 1.2 to 4.1; NNH 2, 95% CI 1 to 9). **Versus combined oral contraceptives:** We found no RCTs. **Versus intrauterine progestogens:** See benefits of intrauterine progestogens, p 2416. **Longer treatment cycle:** We found one systematic review (search date not reported).[17] One RCT (44 women) identified by the review found no significant difference between a longer regimen of oral progestogen (norethisterone, 21 days/cycle) and a levonorgestrel releasing intrauterine device (IUD) in menstrual blood loss (94 mL with oral norethisterone *v* 104 mL with levonorgestrel IUD, WMD +7.5 mL, 95% CI −21.2 mL to +36.5 mL). **Versus endometrial destruction:** See benefits of endometrial destruction, p 2420.

Harms: The review found that adverse effects (including headache, breast tenderness, premenstrual symptoms, and gastrointestinal disturbances) were reported in a third to a half of the women who received oral progestogens.[17] **Versus danazol:** The review found that oral progestogens were associated with significantly fewer adverse effects than danazol (OR 4.05, 95% CI 1.6 to 10.2).[17] **Longer treatment cycle:** In the RCT that compared longer treatment cycle with oral progestogens versus a levonorgestrel releasing IUD, 56% of women taking oral progestogens did not feel "well" or "very well" and 22% elected to continue treatment with oral progestogens after the 3 months of the study.[17] **Versus endometrial destruction:** See harms of endometrial destruction, p 2421.

Comment: None.

OPTION INTRAUTERINE PROGESTOGENS

We found no RCTs comparing intrauterine progestogens versus placebo. RCTs identified by several systematic reviews provided insufficient evidence to compare intrauterine progestogens versus other drugs. RCTs identified by two systematic reviews provided insufficient evidence to compare intrauterine versus oral progestogens. One systematic review found that intrauterine progestogens were less effective than hysterectomy or endometrial destruction in reducing menstrual blood loss over 1 year, but caused fewer serious adverse effects than hysterectomy.

Benefits: We found no systematic review or RCTs comparing intrauterine progestogens versus placebo. We found three systematic reviews (search date 1999, 5 RCTs;[24] search date 1999, 5 RCTs, including 4 RCTs identified by the first review;[25] search date 2002, 5 RCTs, including 1 RCT identified by the earlier reviews[26]) and one subsequent RCT[27] comparing intrauterine progestogens versus other drugs or versus surgical treatment. **Progesterone releasing intrauterine device (IUD) versus other drugs:** The first systematic review identified one RCT that compared four interventions: a progesterone releasing IUD (65 μg/day), mefenamic acid, danazol, or norethisterone.[24] The RCT did not compare treatments versus each other, but found that all treatments reduced menstrual blood loss compared with baseline values. **Levonorgestrel intrauterine system versus other drugs:** The first two reviews identified three RCTs between them.[24,25] The first RCT (44 women) found no significant difference between a levonorgestrel intrauterine system and norethisterone (15 mg/day, days 5–26 of cycle) in reduction in blood loss (median reduction from baseline 6 mL/cycle with norethisterone *v* 20 mL/cycle with levonorgestrel; reported as non-significant; CI not reported) or in the proportion of women satisfied with treatment (RR 1.43, 95% CI 0.78 to 2.62). The second RCT (35 women) compared three interventions: a levonorgestrel intrauterine system, flurbiprofen, and tranexamic acid (see comment below). It found that a levonorgestrel intrauterine system significantly reduced mean menstrual flow after 12 months compared with both other treatments (mean menstrual blood flow reduction: 96% with levonorgestrel *v* 21% with flurbiprofen, $P < 0.001$; 96% with levonorgestrel *v* 44% with tranexamic acid, $P < 0.01$). The third RCT (56 women scheduled for hysterectomy) compared a levonorgestrel intrauterine system versus continuing on existing medical treatment. Details of medical treatment were not reported. The RCT found that, compared with medical treatment, a levonorgestrel intrauterine system significantly increased the number of women who cancelled their hysterectomy after 6 months of treatment and improved all of the quality of life scores that were assessed (cancelled hysterectomy: 8/28 [64%] with levonorgestrel intrauterine system *v* 4/28 [14%] with medical treatment; RR 4.5, 95% CI 1.7 to 11.6; results of quality of life assessment not reported). **Levonorgestrel intrauterine system versus surgery:** The third systematic review included four RCTs (438 women) comparing the levonorgestrel intrauterine system versus endometrial destruction (2 RCTs), thermal balloon ablation (1 RCT), or hysterectomy (1 RCT).[26] The review did not assess menstrual blood loss in the RCT comparing levonorgestrel intrauterine system versus hysterectomy because menstrual blood loss stopped in all women receiving hysterectomy. The review found that both the levonorgestrel intrauterine system and conservative surgery (endometrial destruction or thermal balloon ablation) significantly reduced pictorial blood loss assessment chart (PBAC)Ⓖ scores from baseline (reported as significant, no further data reported). However, it found that mean reduction in PBAC score from baseline was significantly greater at 1 year in women undergoing conservative surgery compared with the levonorgestrel intrauterine system (3 RCTs: WMD 44.07, 95% CI 33.01 to 55.12). All RCTs comparing a levonorgestrel intrauterine system versus surgery found an increase in haemoglobin from baseline in both groups at 6 months (2 RCTs, CI not reported) and at 1 year (2 RCTs, CI not reported). The three RCTs comparing a levonorgestrel intrauterine system versus conservative surgery found no significant difference in haemoglobin between levonorgestrel uterine system and conservative surgery (reported as non-significant, CI not reported). The RCT comparing a levonorgestrel intrauterine system versus hysterectomy did not assess the significance of the difference between groups. The review found no significant difference in patient satisfaction between a levonorgestrel intrauterine system and conservative surgery (2 RCTs, 59/71 [83%] with surgery *v* 51/70 [73%] with a levonorgestrel intrauterine system; RR 1.14, 95% CI 0.96 to 1.35). The subsequent RCT (50 women) found no significant difference between a levonorgestrel intrauterine system and thermal balloon ablation in reducing blood loss from baseline at 6 month follow up (mean postoperative menstrual score measured on a pictorial chart: 31 with levonorgestrel intrauterine system *v* 61 with thermal balloon ablation; P = 0.689).[27] There was a significantly higher menstrual score before treatment in women treated with thermal balloon ablation compared with women treated with the levonorgestrel intrauterine system (122 with thermal balloon ablation *v* 107 with levonorgestrel intrauterine system; P = 0.025).

Harms: There are concerns that progesterone releasing IUDs increase rates of ectopic pregnancy, although the RCTs identified by the reviews did not report this adverse effect.[24,25] RCTs looking at the contraceptive effect of levonorgestrel intrauterine systems in younger women found that during the first few months of use the total number of bleeding days (including menstrual bleeding, intermenstrual bleeding, and spotting) increased in most women.[28] However, most women bled lightly for only 1 day a month and about 15% were amenorrhoeic after 12 months.[29] **Levonorgestrel intrauterine system versus other drugs:** The first review found that most adverse effects in women using a levonorgestrel intrauterine system were typical of progestogens (bloating, weight gain, breast tenderness).[24] One further trial found that a levonorgestrel intrauterine system significantly increased the proportion of women who were amenorrhoeic after 3 months of treatment compared with norethisterone (32% with a levonorgestrel intrauterine system *v* 0% with norethisterone).[30] The other main adverse effect reported with levonorgestrel intrauterine systems was irregular, although not usually heavy, menstrual bleeding.[24] **Levonorgestrel intrauterine system versus surgery:** The third review found that surgery was significantly less likely to cause adverse effects compared with the levonorgestrel intrauterine system (4 RCTs; OR 0.24, 95%CI 0.11 to 0.49).[26] However, the adverse effects in the RCT that assessed hysterectomy were much more serious than those reported in the levonorgestrel intrauterine system group. Adverse effects in women undergoing hysterectomy included bladder and bowel perforation, vesicovaginal fistula, urinary retention, intestinal obstruction, postoperative bleeding, severe postoperative pain, peritonitis, fever, wound infection, wound rupture, and infected pelvic haematoma. In women using a levonorgestrel intrauterine system, the adverse effects were failure of insertion, intermenstrual bleeding, and hormonal symptoms.

Comment: In the additional RCT (35 women) identified by the second review, the first 20 women were given a levonorgestrel releasing IUD and the following 15 women were randomised in a crossover design to receive either flurbiprofen or tranexamic acid.[25] Long term follow up in women with menorrhagia is required to assess continuation rates, satisfaction, and whether surgical treatment is avoided or just postponed. The trials that considered long term bleeding patterns were mainly in women under 40 years of age. It is not yet known whether these results can be extrapolated to older women with menorrhagia.

OPTION GONADORELIN ANALOGUES

We found no RCTs of gonadorelin analogues in women with menorrhagia.

Benefits: We found no systematic review or RCTs.

Harms: We found no RCTs (see comment below).

Comment: A few small non-randomised studies have looked at gonadorelin analogues in menorrhagia. Others have examined their effects in women with fibroids or on thinning the endometrium before ablation or resection. Adverse effects of gonadorelin analogues are mainly caused by reduced oestrogens. Hormone replacement to counteract hypo-oestrogenism has been tried to reduce hot flushes, with limited success.[31] Bone demineralisation occurs in most women after 6 months of treatment but is reversible after treatment is stopped.[32] Contraception while using these drugs is not guaranteed.[33]

QUESTION What are the effects of surgical treatments?

OPTION DILATATION AND CURETTAGE

We found no RCTs of dilatation and curettage in women with menorrhagia.

Benefits: We found no systematic review or RCTs.

Harms: Observational evidence suggest that dilatation and curettage may cause adverse effects including uterine perforation and cervical laceration, as well as the usual risks of general anaesthesia.[34]

Comment: Dilatation and curettage still plays a role in the investigation of menorrhagia. We found one uncontrolled cohort study (50 women) that measured blood loss before and after dilatation and curettage.[35] It found a reduction in menstrual blood loss immediately after the procedure, but losses returned to previous levels or higher by the second menstrual period.

OPTION HYSTERECTOMY

One systematic review found that surgery (hysterectomy or endometrial destruction) reduced menstrual blood loss over 1 year compared with intrauterine progestogens but that hysterectomy was associated with more serious adverse effects than progestogens. Two systematic reviews found that hysterectomy reduced menstrual blood loss and the number of women requiring further operations, and increased participant satisfaction compared with endometrial destruction. Five small RCTs found no evidence of a difference in effectiveness between different types of hysterectomy, although operating and recovery times differed. One large cohort study reported major or minor complications in about a third of women undergoing hysterectomy.

Benefits: **Versus intrauterine progestogens:** See benefits of intrauterine progestogens, p 2416. **Versus endometrial destruction:** We found two systematic reviews (search date 1996[3] and search date not reported[36]) and one subsequent RCT.[37] Both reviews identified the same five RCTs (708 premenopausal women) comparing hysterectomy versus endometrial destruction (transcervical endometrial resection or laser ablation).[3,36] The reviews found that hysterectomy significantly reduced menstrual blood loss, and significantly increased the proportion of women with a reduction in menstrual blood loss after 12 months (3 RCTs; 220/220 [100%] with hysterectomy *v* 191/220 [87%] with endometrial destruction; NNT 8, 95% CI 6 to 13). However, the reviews reported that the differences in reduction in blood loss between treatments seemed to narrow with longer follow up, possibly because of retreatment in the endometrial ablation group or because of menopause. The reviews also found that women were more satisfied with hysterectomy than with endometrial ablation after 12 months compared with hysterectomy (RR 0.93, 95% CI 0.89 to 0.99) and after 2 years (RR for being "moderately" or "very" satisfied with endometrial ablation *v* hysterectomy: 0.87, 95% CI 0.81 to 0.94).[3,36] Two RCTs included in the reviews found no significant difference between treatments in satisfaction rates after 3 and 4 years. The reviews found that endometrial destruction significantly increased the number of women requiring repeat surgery compared with hysterectomy (after 12 months, 5 RCTs: 1/320 [0.3%] with hysterectomy *v* 54/386 [14%] with endometrial destruction; RR 44.8, 95% CI 6.2 to 321.8; after 4 years, 1 RCT: 1/95 [1%] with hysterectomy *v* 39/102 [38%] with endometrial destruction; RR 36.3, 95% CI 5.1 to 259.2), but found that endometrial destruction significantly reduced the duration of surgery (–23 minutes), duration of hospital stay (–5 days), and time to return to work (–4.5 weeks). The subsequent RCT (181 women) compared laparoscopic supracervical hysterectomy**G** versus transcervical endometrial resection.[37] It found no significant difference in blood loss, discharge home and return to normal activity between hysterectomy and endometrial resection (P value reported as non-significant for all outcomes, no further data reported). It found that hysterectomy significantly increased pain scores at discharge ($P < 0.01$) and duration of surgery compared with endometrial resection (mean 71.5 minutes with hysterectomy *v* 41.7 minutes with endometrial resection; $P < 0.01$). However, at 2 year follow up it found that, compared with hysterectomy, endometrial resection significantly increased bleeding recurrence (0/92 [0%] with hysterectomy *v* 11/89 [12%] with endometrial resection; $P < 0.01$) and need for further surgery (1/92 [1%] after hysterectomy *v* 12/89 [13%] after endometrial resection; $P < 0.01$). There was an improvement in all quality of life scores following surgery in both groups; general health and social function significantly improved with both endometrial resection and hysterectomy ($P < 0.01$), and emotional role and vitality also significantly improved with hysterectomy ($P < 0.01$).[37] **Different**

techniques: We found no systematic review. Five small RCTs (total of 334 women) compared abdominal, vaginal, or laparoscopic hysterectomy.[38–42] They found no evidence of a difference in effectiveness or complication rates. However, operating and recovery times varied.

Harms: **Versus intrauterine progestogens:** See harms of intrauterine progestogens, p 2417. Large population based analyses stratified by age have found that mortality after hysterectomy for non-malignant conditions is about 1/2000 in women aged under 50 years.[43] One large, prospective cohort study of hysterectomy for non-malignant conditions found combined major and minor complication rates (mainly infectious morbidity) of 25% for vaginal hysterectomy and 43% for abdominal hysterectomy.[44] It is possible that the difference seen was attributable to the prevalence and efficacy of prophylactic antibiotic use among the vaginal hysterectomy group. Prophylactic antibiotics are now used more routinely in both groups. **Versus endometrial destruction:** The reviews found that, compared with endometrial destruction, hysterectomy increased the risk of sepsis, blood transfusion, urinary retention, anaemia, pyrexia, vault and wound haematoma, and cautery of hypergranulation before hospital discharge.[3,36] The subsequent RCT found no significant difference in intraoperative and postoperative complications between hysterectomy and endometrial resection (P value reported as non-significant, CI not reported).

Comment: None.

OPTION ENDOMETRIAL DESTRUCTION (RESECTION OR ABLATION)

One systematic review found that surgery (hysterectomy or endometrial destruction) reduced menstrual blood loss over 1 year compared with intrauterine progestogens. One RCT identified by a systematic review found that endometrial resection reduced blood loss at 4 months and 2 years compared with medical treatment, and reduced the proportion of women who had adverse effects over 4 months. Two systematic reviews found that endometrial destruction increased menstrual blood loss and the need for further operations and reduced participant satisfaction compared with hysterectomy. One systematic review and three subsequent RCTs found that hysteroscopic methods of endometrial destruction increased amenorrhoea at 12 months compared with non-hysteroscopic methods. We found no consistent evidence of a difference in amenorrhoea or satisfaction rates among different types of hysteroscopic procedure. RCTs identified by the reviews found that complications, such as infection, haemorrhage, and uterine perforation, occurred in up to 15% of women undergoing endometrial destruction.

Benefits: **Versus intrauterine progestogens:** See benefits of intrauterine progestogens, p 2416. **Versus other drugs:** We found one systematic review (search date 2002, 1 RCT, 187 women) comparing endometrial resection (93 women) versus tranexamic acid (22 women), danazol (15 women), combined oral contraceptives (24 women), oral progestogens (31 women), or hormone replacement therapy plus a non-steroidal anti-inflammatory drug (2 women).[26] It found that surgery significantly reduced blood loss at 4 months and 2 years follow up compared with medical treatment (at 4 months: 77/93 [83%] *v* 29/93 [31%]; RR 2.66, 95% CI 1.94 to 3.64).[26] At 5 years of follow up it found no significant difference in blood loss between groups, but by then 77% of the women randomised to medical treatment had received surgery. **Versus hysterectomy:** See benefits of hysterectomy, p 2419. **Hysteroscopic resection or ablation versus non-hysteroscopic techniques**: We found one systematic review (search date 2001, 5 RCTs, 1106 premenopausal women).[45] Hysteroscopic methods included in the review were laser ablation, rollerball ablation, transcervical endometrial resection❻, and vaporising electrode ablation. Non-hysteroscopic methods included thermal uterine balloon therapy, multielectrode balloon ablation, microwave ablation❻, and heated saline. All methods reduced menstrual blood loss compared with baseline assessment. The review found that hysteroscopic ablation significantly increased amenorrhoea at 12 months compared with non-hysteroscopic ablation (OR 0.76, 95% CI 0.60 to 0.90).[45] The review found no significant difference between hysteroscopic and non-hysteroscopic methods in satisfaction rate (OR 0.74, 95% CI 0.54 to 1.63), inability to work (OR 0.81, 95% CI 0.33 to 2.01), or subsequent requirement for additional surgery (OR 0.83, 95% CI 0.45 to 1.58) after 12 months. **Hysteroscopic techniques versus each other:** We found one systematic review (search date 2001, 3 RCTs, 489 women) and three subsequent RCTs.[46–48] Among hysteroscopic techniques the review found no significant difference in rates of amenorrhoea between laser ablation and transcervical endometrial resection (OR 1.67, 95% CI 0.63 to 1.83). The review also found no significant difference between vaporising electrode ablation and transcervical endometrial resection in amenorrhoea rate (OR 0.95, 95% CI 0.35 to 2.60) or satisfaction rate (OR 1.65, 95% CI 0.26 to 10.35) after 12 months.[45] The first subsequent RCT (120 women, 113 followed up at 5 years) found no significant difference between transcervical endometrial resection and rollerball ablation in reduction in bleeding, hysterectomy rates, or satisfaction at 5 years (median number of days bleeding in 3 months: 18 days with resection *v* 16 days with rollerball ablation; hysterectomy: 8/59 [14%] with resection *v* 10/61 [16%] with rollerball ablation, $P > 0.05$; number of women who would recommend procedure to a friend: 46 with resection *v* 49 with rollerball ablation, the number of women responding to this question was not reported by treatment group, $P > 0.05$).[46] The second subsequent RCT (82 women) found that recurrent bleeding and reoperation rate were higher at 2 years with transcervical endometrial resection increased than with thermal ablation (68 women included in analysis; recurrent bleeding 24.2% with endometrial resection *v* 8.5% with thermal ablation; reoperation 15.1% with endometrial resection *v* 5.7% with thermal ablation).[47] It also found higher satisfaction rates with thermal ablation at 1 and 2 years (2 years: health excellent or good 79.9% with thermal ablation *v* 60.5% with endometrial resection). The third subsequent RCT (265 women) compared NovaSure endometrial ablation❻ versus transcervical endometrial resection plus rollerball ablation.[48] It found similar "success" rates at 12 months between groups (success defined as PBAC score of ≤75: 136/154 [88%] with NovaSure endometrial ablation *v* 67/82 [82%] with rollerball ablation; CI not reported). It also found that a similar proportion of had amenorrhoea (63/154 [41%] with NovaSure endometrial ablation *v* 29/82 [35%] with resection plus rollerball ablation) and were satisfied with the procedure (92.8% with endometrial ablation *v* 93.3% with resection plus rollerball ablation; CI not reported for either outcome). It found that significantly more women receiving resection plus rollerball ablation had dysmenorrhoea at 12 months compared with women receiving NovaSure endometrial ablation ($P = 0.02$).

Harms: Intraoperative complications of endometrial destruction include uterine perforation, haemorrhage, and fluid overload from the distension medium. Immediate postoperative complications include infection, haemorrhage, and, rarely, bowel injury. One large prospective survey of 10 686 women undergoing endometrial destruction in the UK found an immediate complication rate of 4%.[49] Intraoperative emergency procedures were performed in 1%, and two procedure related deaths occurred. **Versus intrauterine progestogens:** See harms of intrauterine progestogens, p 2417. **Versus other drugs:** The RCT found that endometrial resection significantly reduced the proportion of women who had adverse effects at 4 months follow up compared with oral medication (12/93 [13%] with endometrial resection *v* 46/93 [49%] with oral medication; RR 0.26, 95% CI 0.15 to 0.46).[26] **Versus hysterectomy:** See harms of hysterectomy, p 2420. **Hysteroscopic resection or ablation versus non-hysteroscopic techniques:** Complication rates in the RCTs included in the systematic review above ranged from 0% to 15%.[45] Newer non-hysteroscopic methods of endometrial destruction have been evaluated only in small numbers of women and, although complications in the RCTs seem minimal, safety data for routine use are awaited. **Hysteroscopic techniques versus each other:** The first subsequent RCT (120 women) found similar postoperative infection rates at 5 years between transcervical endometrial resection and rollerball ablation (6/59 [10%] infections with resection *v* 9/61 [15%] infections with ablation; CI not reported).[46] Prophylactic antibiotics were given to 48/74 (65%) having resection compared with 35/61 (57%) having ablation. The second subsequent RCT (82 women) found that more women undergoing transcervical endometrial resection had short and long term complications compared with women undergoing thermal ablation (intraoperative complications 5/42 [12%] with endometrial resection *v* 0/40 [0%] with thermal ablation, CI not reported).[47] Intraoperative complications of endometrial resection included open hysterectomy for uterine perforation (2 women).The third subsequent RCT reported adverse events in 23/154 (13%) of women after NovaSure ablation and in 23/82 (25%) after rollerball ablation.[48] The RCT did not assess the significance of the difference between groups.

Comment: **Hysteroscopic resection or ablation versus non-hysteroscopic techniques:** The review found that hysteroscopic ablation significantly increased the duration of procedure compared with non-hysteroscopic ablation and significantly increased the number of times general anaesthesia was required, although equipment failure was more likely with non-hysteroscopic methods (duration of procedure: WMD 8.4 minutes, 95% CI 6.8 minutes to 10.1 minutes; general anaesthesia required: OR 6.8, 95% CI 4.5 to 10.4; equipment failure: OR 4.1, 95% CI 1.1 to 15.0).[45] The review found no significant difference in complication rates between hysteroscopic and non-hysteroscopic methods. Among hysteroscopic techniques the review found that laser ablation significantly increased procedural length compared with transcervical endometrial resection (WMD 9.15 minutes, 95% CI 7.20 minutes to 11.10 minutes), and significantly increased rates of equipment failure (OR 6.0, 95% CI 1.7 to 20.9) and fluid overload (OR 5.2, 95% CI 1.5 to 18.4).[49] The review found that vaporising electrode ablation significantly reduced duration of surgery compared with transcervical endometrial resection (WMD 1.50 minutes, 95% CI 0.35 minutes to 2.65 minutes). The subsequent RCT found that NovaSure endometrial ablation significantly reduced duration of surgery compared with rollerball ablation (mean 4.2 minutes *v* 24.2 minutes; $P < 0.0001$) and reduced time was spent in the recovery room (mean 85 minutes with endometrial ablation *v* 135 minutes with resection plus rollerball ablation; $P < 0.0001$).[48]

OPTION MYOMECTOMY

We found no RCTs of myomectomy in women with menorrhagia.

Benefits: We found no systematic review. **Open versus laparoscopic myomectomy:** We found no RCTs or other studies in women with menorrhagia that measured menstrual blood loss. **Hysteroscopic myomectomy:** We found no RCTs.

Harms: Intraoperative complications for hysteroscopic myomectomy are similar to those with endometrial destructive procedures that use a hysteroscope (see harms of endometrial destruction, p 2421). The main complication of open myomectomy is haemorrhage, making a hysterectomy necessary.

Comment: One uncontrolled study (15 women with menorrhagia, 10 with additional symptoms) reported objective measures of menstrual blood loss after myomectomy.[50] Mean menstrual blood loss, assessed preoperatively and at 3 and 6 months postoperatively, was significantly reduced (261 mL at baseline, 76 mL at 3 months, and 57 mL at 6 months; $P < 0.05$). The study found a significant reduction in pain scores and menstrual duration ($P < 0.001$), despite the fibroids removed measuring only 1–4 cm. RCTs are needed that use objective assessment of menstrual blood loss. This is especially important in the evaluation of surgical procedures because of the greater difficulty in blinding.

QUESTION What are the effects of endometrial thinning before endometrial destruction or surgery in general?

OPTION GONADORELIN ANALOGUES

One systematic review found that preoperative gonadorelin analogues reduced moderate or heavy periods at 6–12 months after surgery and increased amenorrhoea at 24 months after surgery compared with placebo or no preoperative treatment. It found no significant difference between gonadorelin analogues and danazol in postoperative amenorrhoea at 12 months.

Benefits: We found one systematic review (search date 2001, 11 RCTs, 998 women).[51] **Versus placebo or no treatment:** Eight RCTs (618 women) identified by the review compared preoperative gonadorelin analogues versus placebo or no treatment. The review found that gonadorelin analogues significantly increased the rate of postoperative amenorrhoea at 24 months and significantly reduced the risk of continued moderate or heavy periods after 6–12 months (amenorrhoea, 2 RCTs: RR 1.62, 95% CI 1.04 to 2.52; moderate or heavy periods, 4 RCTs: RR 0.74, 95% CI 0.59 to 0.92). The review found no significant difference in patient satisfaction or the likelihood of undergoing further surgery. **Versus danazol:** Three RCTs (340 women) identified by the review compared gonadorelin analogues (goserelin or decapeptyl) versus danazol. The review found no significant difference between gonadorelin analogues and danazol in postoperative amenorrhoea at 12 months (RR 1.18, 95% CI 0.18 to 1.57).[51] **Versus other medical treatments:** One RCT included in the review (40 women) compared four interventions: preoperative gonadorelin analogues, danazol, progestogens, and no treatment. The trial was too small to allow firm conclusions to be drawn.[51]

Harms: **Versus placebo or no treatment:** The review found no significant difference between goserelin and either placebo or no treatment in intraoperative uterine perforations (2/266 [0.8%] with goserelin *v* 1/275 [0.4%] with no treatment/placebo; RR 2.01, 95% CI 0.19 to 22.67).[51] **Versus danazol:** The review found that goserelin significantly increased hot flushes, depression, and vaginal dryness and reduced libido compared with danazol. Oily skin, hirsutism, and weight gain were significantly more common with danazol. The review also found that danazol significantly increased withdrawal due to adverse effects compared with goserelin (11/139 [8%] with danazol *v* 1/566 [0.2%] with goserelin; RR 44.80, 95% CI 5.83 to 344.00).

Comment: **Versus placebo or no treatment:** None of the RCTs included in the review used objective measures of postoperative menstrual blood loss.[51] Rates of withdrawal or loss to follow up were low in all RCTs. One systematic review found that gonadorelin analogues significantly reduced both the duration of surgery and operative difficulty compared with placebo or no treatment (duration of surgery, 3 RCTs: WMD −4.8 minutes, 95% CI −6.5 minutes to −3.0 minutes; difficulty during procedure, 2 RCTs: RR 0.32, 95% CI 0.22 to 0.46).[51] **Versus danazol:** The review found that gonadorelin analogues significantly reduced the duration of surgery compared with danazol (3 RCTs: WMD −3.9 minutes, 95% CI −6.1 minutes to −1.7 minutes). It found no significant difference in operative difficulty between gonadorelin analogues and danazol (RR 0.68, 95% CI 0.31 to 1.51).[51]

OPTION DANAZOL

Two small RCTs identified by a systematic review and one subsequent RCT provided insufficient evidence to compare preoperative danazol versus placebo or no preoperative treatment. One systematic review found no significant difference between danazol and gonadorelin analogues in postoperative amenorrhoea at 12 months. Two RCTs identified by a systematic review provided insufficient evidence to compare danazol versus other medical treatments.

Benefits: We found one systematic review (search date 2001, 3 RCTs, 110 women)[51] and one subsequent RCT.[52] **Versus placebo:** The review identified two small RCTs and we found one subsequent RCT.[51,52] Both RCTs identified by the review found no significant difference in amenorrhoea between preoperative danazol and placebo at 12 and 24 months (1 RCT, 50 women: RR 1.31, 95% CI 0.82 to 2.08; 1 RCT, 20 women: RR 3.00, 95% CI 0.79 to 11.44). The subsequent RCT (132 women) found no significant difference in amenorrhoea between preoperative danazol and placebo at 1 year (129 women analysed; amenorrhoea rate: 49% with danazol *v* 52% with placebo, CI and P values not reported).[52] It found that danazol significantly reduced operating time compared with placebo (25.7 minutes with danazol *v* 33.6 minutes with placebo, $P < 0.001$) **Versus gonadorelin analogues: Versus other medical treatments:** One RCT included in the review (40 women) compared four interventions: preoperative danazol, gonadorelin analogues, progestogens, and no treatment.[51] The trial was too small to allow firm conclusions to be drawn.

Harms: **Versus placebo:** The review and subsequent RCT gave no information on adverse effects.[51,52] **Versus gonadorelin analogues:** See harms of gonadorelin analogues, p 2423.

Comment: None.

OPTION ORAL PROGESTOGENS

Three RCTs identified by a systematic review provided insufficient evidence about the effects of preoperative oral progestogens compared with placebo, no preoperative treatment or other medical treatments.

Benefits: We found one systematic review (search date 2001, 3 RCTs, 110 women).[51] **Versus no treatment:** Two RCTs included in the review (70 women) compared preoperative oral progestogens versus no preoperative treatment. The review found no significant difference between oral progestogens and no preoperative treatment in amenorrhoea at 2 years after endometrial destruction (RR 0.75, 95% CI 0.36 to 1.54).[51] **Versus other medical treatments:** Two RCTs included in the review (140 women) compared four interventions: oral progestogens, gonadorelin analogues, danazol, and no treatment. The trials were too small to allow firm conclusions to be drawn.[51]

Harms: The review gave no information on adverse effects.[51]

Comment: None.

GLOSSARY

Laparoscopic supracervical hysterectomy A laparoscopic procedure where the uterus, but not the cervix, is removed.

Laser ablation A hysteroscopic procedure in which endometrium is destroyed under direct vision by a laser beam.

Microwave endometrial ablation A procedure in which a microwave probe is passed through the cervix into the uterine cavity. When activated it is moved slowly from side to side over the whole surface of the uterine cavity in order to destroy the endometrium.

Multielectrode balloon ablation A procedure in which an inflatable device with electrodes on the outside is inserted into the uterine cavity through the cervix. The electrodes make contact with the endometrium and cause necrosis.

NovaSure endometrial ablation A procedure in which a disposable, conformable bipolar electrode array mounted on an expandable frame desiccates and coagulates endometrial tissue.

Pictorial blood loss assessment chart (PBAC) A semi-quantitative assessment of menstrual blood loss based on women filling in the number and appearances of their sanitary protection and size of blood clots on a pictorial chart. Scores of 100 or more equate to a menstrual blood loss of 80 mL or more.[53]

Rollerball ablation A hysteroscopic procedure in which endometrium is destroyed under direct vision by diathermy applied by a rollerball.

Thermal uterine balloon therapy/thermal ablation A procedure in which a balloon catheter is passed through the cervix into the uterine cavity. The balloon is then filled with fluid, which is heated to about 87 °C, and left for 8 minutes. This causes necrosis of the endometrium.

Transcervical endometrial resection A hysteroscopic procedure in which endometrium is removed under direct vision by using an electrosurgical loop.

REFERENCES

1. Hallberg L, Hogdahl A, Nilsson L, et al. Menstrual blood loss – a population study: variation at different ages and attempts to define normality. *Acta Obstet Gynecol Scand* 1966;45:320–351.
2. Vessey MP, Villard-Mackintosh L, McPherson K, et al. The epidemiology of hysterectomy: findings in a large cohort study. *Br J Obstet Gynaecol* 1992;99:402–407.
3. Working Party of the National Health Committee New Zealand. *Guidelines for the management of heavy menstrual bleeding*. Wellington: Ministry of Health, 1998. (Available from The Ministry of Health, 133 Molesworth Street, PO Box 5013, Wellington, New Zealand.) Search date 1996; primary sources Medline, Embase, Current Contents, Biological Abstracts, Social Sciences Index, Psychlit, and Cinahl.
4. Smith SK, Abel MH, Kelly RW, et al. A role for prostacyclin (PGI_2) in excessive menstrual bleeding. *Lancet* 1981;1:522–524.
5. Rybo G, Leman J, Tibblin R. Epidemiology of menstrual blood loss. In: Baird DT, Michie EA, eds. *Mechanisms of menstrual bleeding*. New York: Raven Press, 1985:181–193.
6. Alexander DA, Naji AA, Pinion SB, et al. Randomised trial comparing hysterectomy with endometrial ablation for dysfunctional uterine bleeding: psychiatric and psychosocial aspects. *BMJ* 1996;312:280–284.
7. Coulter A, Peto V, Jenkinson C. Quality of life and patient satisfaction following treatment for menorrhagia. *Fam Pract* 1994;11:394–401.
8. Coulter A, McPherson K, Vessey M. Do British women undergo too many or too few hysterectomies? *Soc Sci Med* 1988;27:987–994.
9. Pokras R, Hufnagel VG, NCHS. Hysterectomies in the United States, 1965–84. Hyattsville, Maryland: US Department of Health and Human Services, Public Health Service, CDC, 1987; DHHS publication no. (PHS)87–1753. (Vital and health statistics; series 13, no. 92).
10. Coulter A, Kelland J, Long A. The management of menorrhagia. *Effective Health Care Bull* 1995;9:1–14.
11. Clarke A, Black N, Rowe P, et al. Indications for and outcome of total abdominal hysterectomy for benign disease: a prospective cohort study. *Br J Obstet Gynaecol* 1995;102:611–620.

12. Lethaby A, Augood C, Duckitt K. Nonsteroidal anti-inflammatory drugs for heavy menstrual bleeding In: The Cochrane Library, Issue 3, 2003. Oxford: Update Software. Search date 2001; primary sources Cochrane Menstrual Disorders and Subfertility Group trials register, Medline, Embase, Psychlit, Current Contents, Biological Abstracts, Social Sciences Index, Cinahl, reference lists, and drug companies.
13. Beaumont H, Augood C, Duckitt K, et al. Danazol for heavy menstrual bleeding (Cochrane Review). In: The Cochrane Library, Issue 3, 2003. Oxford: Update Software. Search date 2001; primary sources Medline, Embase, Current Contents, Cinahl, National Research Register, Menstrual Disorders and Subfertility Group's Specialised Register, reference lists, and authors contacted.
14. Lethaby A, Farquhar C, Cooke I. Antifibrinolytics for heavy menstrual bleeding (Cochrane review). In: The Cochrane Library, Issue 3, 2003. Oxford: Update Software. Search date 1997; primary sources Cochrane Menstrual Disorders and Subfertility Group trials register, Medline, Embase, and hand searches of reference lists from experts, and drug companies.
15. Preston JT, Cameron IT, Adams EJ, et al. Comparative study of tranexamic acid and norethisterone in the treatment of ovulatory menorrhagia. *Br J Obstet Gynaecol* 1995;102:401–406.
16. Coulter A, Kelland J, Peto V, et al. Treating menorrhagia in primary care. An overview of drug trials and a survey of prescribing practice. *Int J Technol Assess Health Care* 1995;11:456–471. Search date not reported; primary sources Medline and Embase.
17. Lethaby A, Irvine G, Cameron I. Cyclical progestogens for heavy menstrual bleeding (Cochrane review). In: The Cochrane Library, Issue 3, 2003. Oxford: Update Software. Search date not reported; primary sources Cochrane Menstrual Disorders and Subfertility Group trials register, Medline, Embase, Psychlit, Current Contents, Biological Abstracts, Social Sciences Index, Cinahl, and reference lists.
18. Rybo G. Tranexamic acid therapy is effective treatment in heavy menstrual bleeding: clinical update on safety. *Ther Adv* 1991;4:1–8.
19. Bonnar J, Sheppard BL. Treatment of menorrhagia during menstruation: randomised controlled trial of etamsylate, mefenamic acid, and tranexamic acid. *BMJ* 1996;313:579–582.
20. Iyer V, Farquhar C, Jepson R. Oral contraceptive pills for heavy menstrual bleeding. In: The Cochrane Library, Issue 3, 2003. Oxford: Update Software. Search date 1997; primary source Cochrane Register of Controlled Trials.
21. Nilsson L, Rybo G. Treatment of menorrhagia. *Am J Obstet Gynecol* 1971;5:713–720.
22. Ramcharan S, Pellegrin FA, Ray MR, et al. The Walnut Creek contraceptive drug study — a prospective study of the side effects of oral contraceptives. Vol III. An interim report: a comparison of disease occurrence leading to hospitalization or death in users and nonusers of oral contraceptives. *J Reprod Med* 1980;25:345–372.
23. Royal College of General Practitioners. *Oral contraceptives and health*. London: Pitman Medical, 1974.
24. Lethaby AE, Cooke I, Rees M. Progesterone/progestogen intrauterine releasing systems for heavy menstrual bleeding (Cochrane review). In: The Cochrane Library, Issue 3, 2003. Oxford: Update Software. Search date 1999; primary sources Cochrane Menstrual Disorders and Subfertility Group trials register, Medline, Embase, and experts contacted.
25. Stewart A, Cummins C, Gold L, et al. The effectiveness of the levonorgestrel-releasing intrauterine system in menorrhagia: a systematic review. *Br J Obstet Gynaecol* 2001;108:74–86. Search date 1999; primary sources Medline, Cinahl, Embase, Cochrane Library, Best Evidence, BMJ website archive facility, various internet search engines, hand searches of the *J Family Plan* and *The Diplomate*, and personal contact with Schering Health Care Ltd and the Royal College of Obstetricians and Gynaecologists Audit Unit.
26. Marjoribanks J, Lethaby A, Farquhar C. Surgery versus medical therapy for heavy menstrual bleeding (Cochrane Review). In: *The Cochrane Library*, Issue 3, 2003. Oxford: Update Software. Search date 2002, primary sources Cochrane Menstrual Disorders and Subfertility Group Trials Register, Cochrane Controlled Trials Register, Medline, Embase, Current Contents, Biological Abstracts, Psychinfo, Cinahl, hand searches of reference lists of articles, and personal contact with experts in the field.
27. Barrington J, Arunkalaivanan A, Abdel-Fattah M. Comparison between the levonorgestrel intrauterine system and thermal balloon ablation in the treatment of menorrhagia. Eur J Obstet Gynaecol Reprod Biol 2003;108:72–74.
28. Anonymous. Long-acting progestogen-only contraception. *Drug Ther Bull* 1996;34:93–96.
29. Luukkainen T. The levonorgestrel-releasing IUD. *Br J Fam Plann* 1993;19:221–224.
30. Irvine GA, Campbell-Brown MB, Lumsden MA, et al. Randomised comparative study of the levonorgestrel intrauterine system and norethisterone for the treatment of idiopathic menorrhagia. *Br J Obstet Gynaecol* 1998;105:592–598.
31. Thomas EJ, Okuda KJ, Thomas NM. The combination of a depot gonadotrophin releasing hormone agonist and cyclical hormone replacement therapy for dysfunctional uterine bleeding. *Br J Obstet Gynaecol* 1991;98:1155–1159.
32. Eldred JM, Haynes PJ, Thomas EJ. A randomized double blind placebo controlled trial of the effects on bone metabolism of the combination of nafarelin acetate and norethisterone. *Clin Endocrinol* 1992;37:354–359.
33. Pickersgill A, Kingsland CR, Garden AS, et al. Multiple gestation following gonadotrophin releasing hormone therapy for the treatment of minimal endometriosis. *Br J Obstet Gynaecol* 1994;101:260–262.
34. Smith JJ, Schulman H. Current dilatation and curettage practice: a need for revision. *Obstet Gynecol* 1985;65:516–518.
35. Haynes PJ, Hodgson H, Anderson AB, et al. Measurement of menstrual blood loss in patients complaining of menorrhagia. *Br J Obstet Gynaecol* 1977;84:763–768.
36. Lethaby A, Sheppers S, Cooke I, et al. Endometrial resection and ablation versus hysterectomy for heavy menstrual bleeding. In: The Cochrane Library, Issue 3, 2003. Oxford: Update Software. Search date not reported; primary sources Cochrane Menstrual Disorders and Subfertility Group trials register, Medline, Embase, Psychlit, Current Contents, Biological Abstracts, Social Sciences Index, and Cinahl.
37. Zupi E, Zullo F, Marconi D, et al. Hysteroscopic endometrial resection versus laparoscopic supracervical hysterectomy for menorrhagia: A prospective randomized trial. Am J Obstet Gynecol 2003;188:7–12.
38. Phipps JH, John M, Nayak S. Comparison of laparoscopically assisted vaginal hysterectomy and bilateral salpingo-oophorectomy with conventional abdominal hysterectomy and bilateral salpingo-oophorectomy. *Br J Obstet Gynaecol* 1993;100:698–700.
39. Raju KS, Auld BJ. A randomised prospective study of laparoscopic vaginal hysterectomy versus abdominal hysterectomy each with bilateral salpingo-oophorectomy. *Br J Obstet Gynaecol* 1994;101:1068–1071.
40. Richardson RE, Bournas N, Magos AL. Is laparoscopic hysterectomy a waste of time? *Lancet* 1995;345:36–41.
41. Summitt RL Jr, Stovall TG, Lipscomb GH, et al. Randomized comparison of laparoscopy-assisted

vaginal hysterectomy with standard vaginal hysterectomy in an outpatient setting. *Obstet Gynecol* 1992;80:895–901.
42. Langebrekke A, Eraker R, Nesheim B, et al. Abdominal hysterectomy should not be considered as primary method for uterine removal. *Acta Obstet Gynecol Scand* 1996;75:404–407.
43. Carlson KJ. Outcomes of hysterectomy. *Clin Obstet Gynecol* 1997;40:939–946.
44. Dicker RC, Greenspan JR, Strauss LT, et al. Complications of abdominal and vaginal hysterectomy among women of reproductive age in the United States. The Collaborative Review of Sterilization. *Am J Obstet Gynecol* 1982;144:841–848.
45. Lethaby A, Hickey M. Endometrial destruction techniques for heavy menstrual bleeding (Cochrane Review). In: The Cochrane Library, Issue1, 2003. Oxford: Update Software. Search date 2001; primary sources Conchrane Controlled Trials Register, Medline, Embase, Current Contents, Biological Abstracts, Psychlit, Cinahl, Register of Cochrane Menstrual Disorders and Subfertility Group, reference lists of articles, contacted pharmaceutical companies, and experts in the field.
46. Boujida VH, Philipsen T, Pelle J, et al. Five-year follow-up of endometrial ablation: endometrial coagulation versus endometrial resection. *Obstet Gynecol* 2002;99:988–992.
47. Pellicano M, Guida M, Acunzo G, et al. Hysteroscopic transcervical endometrial resection versus thermal destruction for menorrhagia: a prospective randomized trial on satisfaction rate. *Am J Obstet Gynecol* 2002;187:545–550.
48. Cooper J, Gimpelson R, Laberge P, et al. A randomized, multicenter trial of safety and efficacy of the NovaSure system in the treatment of menorrhagia.. J American Association of Gynecologic Laparoscopists 2002;9:418–428.
49. Overton C, Hargreaves J, Maresh M. A national survey of the complications of endometrial destruction for menstrual disorders: the MISTLETOE study. Minimally invasive surgical techniques — laser, endothermal or endoresection. *Br J Obstet Gynaecol* 1997;104:1351–1359.
50. Broadbent JAM, Magos AL. Menstrual blood loss after hysteroscopic myomectomy. *Gynaecol Endoscop* 1995;4:41–44.
51. Sowter MC, Singla AA, Lethaby A. Pre-operative endometrial thinning agents before endometrial destruction for heavy menstrual bleeding (Cochrane review). In: The Cochrane Library, Issue 3, 2003. Oxford: Update Software. Search date 2001; primary sources Cochrane Menstrual Disorders and Subfertility Group trials register, Medline, Embase, Psychlit, Biological Abstracts, Cinahl, reference lists, authors of conference abstracts, Zeneca Pharmaceuticals, and Sanofi Winthrop.
52. Kriplani A, Manchanda R, Nath J, et al. A randomized trial of danazol pretreatment prior to endometrial resection. *Eur J Obstet Gynecol Reprod Biol* 2002;103:68–71.
53. Higham JM, O'Brien PMS, Shaw RW. Assessment of menstrual blood loss using a pictorial chart. *Br J Obstet Gynaecol* 1990;97:734–739.

Kirsten Duckitt
Consultant Obstetrician and Gynaecologist

Keri McCully
Specialist Registrar Obstetrics and Gynaecology
John Radcliffe Hospital
Oxford
UK

Competing interests: None declared.

Ovarian cancer

Search date June 2003

Richmal Oates-Whitehead

QUESTIONS

INTERVENTIONS

See glossary Ⓖ

Key Messages

- We found insufficient evidence on the effects of any treatments on quality of life.

Surgical treatments

- **Primary surgery versus no surgery; primary surgery plus chemotherapy versus chemotherapy alone** We found no RCTs.
- **Routine interval debulking** One RCT found that routine interval debulking, after primary surgery plus chemotherapy, improved overall survival over about 3.5 years compared with chemotherapy alone. A second RCT found that interval debulking had no effect on survival, but it was probably underpowered to detect a clinically important effect.

- **Routine second look surgery** Two RCTs found no evidence that routine second look surgery improved overall survival compared with watchful waiting in women undergoing chemotherapy after primary surgery for advanced ovarian cancer.

Cytotoxic chemotherapy

- **Adding a single platinum agent to a non-platinum combination regimen** One systematic review (4 RCTs, 1024 women) found that adding a platinum agent to a non-platinum combination regimen reduced mortality compared with the non-platinum regimen alone.
- **Adding a taxane (paclitaxel) to a platinum regimen** One systematic review and one additional RCT have found that adding paclitaxel to platinum based chemotherapy significantly improves progression free survival and overall survival after primary surgery for advanced ovarian cancer.
- **Platinum based chemotherapy (at least as effective as non-platinum regimens)** A systematic review and subsequent RCTs have found that platinum based regimens are at least as effective as non-platinum regimens, and that adding a platinum compound to a non-platinum combination regimen improves survival.
- **Single agent platinum regimens (as effective as combination platinum chemotherapy, but with fewer adverse effects and better than single agent non-platinum regimens)** One systematic review and three subsequent RCTs found that single agent platinum based regimens were at least as effective for progression free or overall survival as combination platinum regimens, and had fewer adverse effects. One RCT found that the platinum agent cisplatin improved progression free survival but not overall survival compared with the non-platinum agent thiotepa.
- **Relative efficacy of different platinum agents (cisplatin versus carboplatin) added to a taxane (paclitaxel)** One RCT found no significant difference in progression free or overall survival between adding cisplatin and adding carboplatin to paclitaxel, although it may have lacked power to detect clinically important effects.
- **Relative efficacy of different taxanes (paclitaxel versus docetaxel) added to a platinum agent docetaxel** We found no reliable RCTs comparing the effects of carboplatin plus paclitaxel versus those of carboplatin plus docetaxel.

DEFINITION Ovarian tumours are classified according to the assumed cell type of origin (surface epithelium, stroma, or germ cells). Most malignant ovarian tumours (85–95%) are derived from the epithelium of the ovarian surface, and thus are termed epithelial.[1] These can be further grouped into histological types (serous, mucinous, endometroid, and clear cell). Epithelial ovarian cancer is staged using the FIGO classification (see table A on web extra). This review concerns only advanced epithelial ovarian cancer, which is regarded as FIGO stages II–IV.

INCIDENCE/ PREVALENCE The worldwide annual incidence of ovarian cancer exceeds 140 000.[2] Rates vary between countries. Differences in reproductive patterns, including age of menarche and menopause, gravidity, breast feeding, and use of the oral contraceptive pill, may contribute to this variation. Rates are highest in Scandinavia, northern America, and the UK; and lowest in Africa, India, China, and Japan.[3] In the UK ovarian cancer is the fourth most common malignancy in women and is the leading cause of death from gynaecological cancers, with a lifetime risk of about 2%.[4] In the UK the incidence was 5174 in 1988[5] and 6880 in 1998.[6] The incidence of ovarian cancer appears to be stabilising in some other countries, and in some affluent countries (Finland, Denmark, New Zealand, and the USA) rates are declining.

AETIOLOGY/ RISK FACTORS Risk factors include increasing age, family history of ovarian cancer, low fertility, use of fertility drugs, and low parity.[7–11] Case control studies found that using the combined oral contraceptive pill for more than 5 years was associated with a 40% reduction in the risk of ovarian cancer.[3,7,12,13]

PROGNOSIS More than 80% of women present with advanced disease, and the overall 5 year survival rates are poor (< 30%).[6] For advanced disease the major independent prognostic factors appear to be stage, and residual tumour mass after surgery.

AIMS OF INTERVENTION To prolong survival and reduce disability; to minimise adverse effects of treatment.

OUTCOMES Mortality; disease free survival; disease related symptoms; quality of life; adverse effects of treatment.

METHODS *Clinical Evidence* search and appraisal June 2003. RCTs with greater than 20% withdrawal or with less than 18 months' follow up were excluded.

QUESTION **What are the effects of surgical treatments for ovarian cancer that is advanced at first presentation?**

OPTION **PRIMARY SURGERY**

We found no RCTs in women with advanced ovarian cancer comparing the effects of primary surgery versus those of no surgery, or the effects of primary surgery plus chemotherapy versus those of chemotherapy alone.

Benefits: **Primary surgery alone versus no surgery:** We found one systematic review (search date not reported), which found no RCTs comparing primary debulking**G** surgery versus no surgery.[1] We found no subsequent RCT. **Primary surgery plus chemotherapy versus chemotherapy alone:** We found no systematic review and no RCT.

Harms: We found no RCT.

Comment: None.

OPTION **ROUTINE SECOND LOOK SURGERY**

Two RCTs found no evidence that routine second look surgery improved overall survival compared with watchful waiting in women undergoing chemotherapy after primary surgery for advanced ovarian cancer.

Benefits: **Primary surgery plus chemotherapy with or without second look surgery:** We found two RCTs in women with advanced ovarian cancer.[14,15] The first RCT (102 women in complete remission after primary debulking**G** surgery and first line chemotherapy consisting of cisplatin plus cyclophosphamide or doxorubicin plus cyclophosphamide every 3 weeks for 5 cycles) compared second look surgery**G**, which included visual inspection and biopsy, versus watchful waiting.[14] Complete remission before trial entry was confirmed by clinical and biochemical assessment, computed tomography, and laparoscopy. The RCT found no significant difference between interventions for overall survival after 60 months (AR for survival 65% with second look laparotomy *v* 78% with watchful waiting; CI not reported; P = 0.14). The second RCT (166 women, after primary debulking surgery plus cisplatin every 3 weeks for 5 cycles) compared three groups.[15] One group underwent a second look laparotomy (which included visual inspection, cytology of any free fluid, total hysterectomy, bilateral salpingo-oophorectomy, omentectomy, and multiple biopsies) followed by oral chlorambucil (12 courses of 0.2 mg/kg daily for 14 days). The second group received second look laparotomy plus pelvic irradiation. The third group received chlorambucil without second look surgery. The RCT found no significant difference among groups for overall survival after 46 months (median survival time 21 months, 95% CI 11 months to 31 months with second look laparotomy plus chlorambucil; 15 months, 95% CI 11 months to 19 months with second look laparotomy plus pelvic irradiation; 17 months, 95% CI 8 months to 26 months with chlorambucil without second look surgery).

Harms: The first RCT did not report on harms.[14] The second RCT reported that one woman died of a cerebrovascular accident 10 days after second look laparotomy.[15] Other reported surgical complications were ileus, wound infection, urinary and respiratory tract infection, and anaemia (rates not reported).

Comment: None.

OPTION **ROUTINE INTERVAL DEBULKING**

One RCT found that routine interval debulking, after primary surgery plus chemotherapy, improved overall survival after about 3.5 years compared with no interval debulking. A second RCT found that interval debulking had no effect on survival, although it was probably underpowered to detect a clinically important effect.

Benefits: We found no systematic review but found two RCTs.[16,17] The first RCT (319 women with non-progressive disease after 3 cycles of cisplatin and cyclophosphamide chemotherapy following primary surgery) compared interval debulking❻ plus continued chemotherapy versus continued chemotherapy alone.[16] All women had a residual tumour diameter of more than 1 cm after primary surgery. It found that interval debulking significantly improved progression free and overall survival after a median of 3.5 years (278 women; median progression free survival 18 months with interval debulking *v* 13 months without, P = 0.01; median overall survival 26 months *v* 20 months, P = 0.01; adjusted HR for death for interval debulking *v* no interval debulking 0.77, 95% CI 0.50 to 0.90).[16] The second RCT (79 women with advanced ovarian cancer with residual tumour of at least 2 cm maximal diameter after primary surgery) compared interval debulking plus continued chemotherapy versus continued chemotherapy alone.[17] Chemotherapy consisted of either cisplatin plus cyclophosphamide or cisplatin plus bleomycin plus doxorubicin followed by escalating cyclophosphamide. Of the women allocated to interval debulking, 11 had non-responsive or progressive disease after three cycles of chemotherapy and were excluded from surgery. Interval debulking (which could include hysterectomy, oophorectomy, and omentectomy) was undertaken at a median of 13 weeks after primary surgery. The RCT found no significant difference between interval debulking and no interval debulking for overall survival after median follow up of 48 months, but it may have lacked power to exclude a clinically important effect (intention to treat analysis: median survival 15 months with interval debulking *v* 12 months without; HR 0.71, 95% CI 0.44 to 1.33).

Harms: The second RCT found that, among 26 women who received interval debulking, 11 received a blood transfusion, two developed intestinal fistulae, and one developed a deep vein thrombosis.[17]

Comment: None.

QUESTION **What are the effects of cytotoxic chemotherapy for ovarian cancer that is advanced at first presentation?**

OPTION **PLATINUM BASED REGIMENS**

One systematic review and subsequent RCTs have found that platinum based regimens are at least as effective as non-platinum regimens, and that adding a platinum compound to a non-platinum combination regimen improves survival. The systematic review and three subsequent RCTs found that single agent platinum based regimens were at least as effective for progression free

or overall survival as combination platinum regimens, and had fewer adverse effects. One RCT found that a single platinum agent, cisplatin, improved progression free survival but not overall survival compared with a single non-platinum agent, thiotepa. The review found that adding a platinum agent to a non-platinum combination regiment reduced mortality compared with the non-platinum regimen alone. One RCT found no significant difference in progression free or overall survival between adding cisplatin and adding carboplatin to paclitaxel, although it may have lacked power to detect clinically important effects.

Benefits: We found one systematic review (search date 1998, 37 RCTs)[18] and six subsequent RCTs[19–24] in women with advanced ovarian cancer. **Platinum based combination chemotherapy versus single agent non-platinum based chemotherapy:** The review identified 11 RCTs (1329 women) comparing platinum based combination chemotherapy versus single agent non-platinum chemotherapy.[18] It found no significant difference between treatments for overall survival (9 RCTs, 1704 women; HR 0.93, 95% CI 0.83 to 1.05; P = 0.23; estimated ARR for 2 and 5 year survival with single agent non-platinum versus combination platinum +3%, 95% CI −2% to +7%). **Adding a platinum based compound to a non-platinum single agent regimen:** The systematic review found no significant difference in mortality between a single agent chemotherapy regimen and the same single agent plus a platinum based compound, although results of trials were statistically heterogeneous (5 RCTs, 680 women; HR for death with platinum added to single agent *v* single agent alone 0.93, 95% CI 0.78 to 1.10).[18] **Adding a platinum based compound to a non-platinum combination regimen:** The systematic review found that adding a platinum based compound to a non-platinum combination regimen significantly reduced mortality compared with the same non-platinum regimen alone (4 RCTs, 1024 women; HR 0.85, 95% CI 0.74 to 0.97).[18] The first subsequent RCT (228 women) found similar results.[19] It found that adding cisplatin (50 mg/m^2 every 3–4 weeks) to 12 cycles of doxorubicin plus cyclophosphamide with or without Bacillus Calmette-Guérin significantly improved overall survival compared with same regimen without cisplatin (median survival 17.8 months with cisplatin *v* 9.9 months without cisplatin; P < 0.005). **Platinum based combination regimens versus non-platinum based combination regimens:** The second subsequent RCT (169 women) compared 12 cycles at four weekly intervals of cisplatin (60 mg/m^2/cycle) plus melphalan (1 mg/kg/cycle) versus hexamethylmelamine plus doxorubicin plus cyclophosphamide.[20] It found no significant difference between treatments for overall survival (153 women; median survival 29.6 months with a platinum based regimen *v* 26.4 months with non-platinum based regimen; P value not reported) but the trial may have lacked power to exclude a clinically important difference. The third subsequent RCT (120 women) found no significant difference between hexamethylmelamine plus doxorubicin plus cyclophosphamide versus cisplatin plus doxorubicin plus cyclophosphamide for overall survival after 10 years (median survival 126 months without a platinum based regimen *v* 138 months with a platinum based regimen; P = 0.54).[21] The fourth subsequent RCT (83 women) compared 12 cycles at four weekly intervals of doxorubicin (60 mg/m^2) plus cyclophosphamide (750 mg/m^2) combined with either cisplatin (80 mg/m^2) or vincristine (1.4 mg/m^2).[22] It found that the platinum based regimen increased progression free and overall survival compared with the non-platinum regimen after 5 years (median progression free survival 14 months with platinum based regimen *v* 10 months without the platinum based regimen, P < 0.05; median overall survival 24 months with platinum *v* 15 months without platinum, P < 0.01). The fifth subsequent RCT (186 women) compared hexamethylmelamine plus cyclophosphamide plus methotrexate plus 5-fluorouracil versus a regimen that alternated between cyclophosphamide plus hexamethylmelamine and doxorubicin plus cisplatin.[23] It found that the platinum based regimen significantly improved progression free and overall survival after about 50 months compared with the non-platinum regimen (median progression free survival 19.5 months with platinum *v* 6.8 months without platinum, $P < 0.0001$; median overall survival 30.7 months with platinum *v* 19.6 months without platinum, $P < 0.002$). A follow up study at 10 years found a survival rate of 9% among women who received non-platinum chemotherapy as first line treatment compared with 23% among those treated with the platinum based regimen (P value not reported).[25] **Single platinum based agent versus single non-platinum agent:** The sixth additional RCT (171 women) compared a single platinum based compound (cisplatin, 75 mg/m^2 every 28 days for 6 cycles) versus a single non-platinum compound (thiotepa, 60 mg loading dose im followed by 10 cycles of 30 mg im every 14 days).[24] It found that cisplatin significantly improved progression free survival after a median follow up of 110 months compared with the non-platinum agent, thiotepa (median progression free survival 10.5 months with cisplatin *v* 6.3 months with thiotepa, $P = 0.025$; HR for thiotepa *v* cisplatin 1.64, 95% CI 1.17 to 2.30). Cisplatin did not significantly improve overall survival compared with thiotepa (median overall survival 20 months with cisplatin *v* 14 months with thiotepa, $P = 0.155$; AR for survival at 8 years 10.6% with cisplatin *v* 7.4% with thiotepa, CI and P value not reported). **Combination platinum based chemotherapy versus single agent platinum based chemotherapy:** We found one systematic review (search date 1998, 9 RCTs, 1095 women with advanced ovarian cancer)[18] and three additional RCTs.[26–28] The review found no significant difference between treatments for risk of death (HR 0.91, 95% CI 0.80 to 1.05).[18] Separate analyses of cisplatin and carboplatin containing regimens yielded similar findings (HR of death for single agent *v* combination cisplatin regimens 0.86, 95% CI 0.73 to 1.02; HR of death for single agent *v* combination carboplatin regimens 1.05, 95% CI 0.82 to 1.35). The first additional RCT (multicentre, 1526 women, 36% of women < 55 years old) compared six cycles of cisplatin (50 mg/m^2) plus cyclophosphamide (500 mg/m^2) plus doxorubicin (50 mg/m^2) versus carboplatin alone (3 times weekly for 6 cycles; dose calculated as follows: [glomerular filtration rate 5] + 25mg).[26] After a median follow up of 35 months, the RCT found no significant difference between treatments for progression free survival or overall survival (HR for progression free survival for combined treatment *v* carboplatin alone 0.92, 95% CI 0.81 to 1.04; HR for overall survival 1.00, 95% CI 0.86 to 1.16). The second additional RCT (611 women aged < 75 years) compared cisplatin alone (50 mg/m^2) weekly for nine cycles versus cisplatin (75 mg/m^2) plus cyclophosphamide (750 mg/m^2) three times weekly for six cycles.[27] It found no difference between groups either for 3 year progression free survival or overall survival (3 year progression free survival 33.8% with cisplatin alone *v* 35.1% with combined treatment, CI and P values not reported; 3 year overall survival 44.1% with cisplatin alone *v* 44.6% with combined treatment, CI not reported, $P = 0.96$). The third RCT (176 women) compared cisplatin alone (75 mg/m^2) for six four weekly courses versus cisplatin (50 mg/m^2) plus cyclophosphamide (500 mg/m^2) every 28 days for six courses.[28] It found no significant difference between treatments for progression free survival or overall survival after a median of 10 years (median progression free survival 11.9 months with single *v* 10.0 months with combination, $P = 0.092$; median overall survival 21.5 months with single *v* 19.4 months with combination, $P = 0.1299$). We found one further RCT that was reported as a conference abstract (see comment below). **Comparison of different platinum agents (cisplatin versus**

carboplatin) added to a taxane: We found one RCT (208 women).[29] It compared cisplatin (75 mg/m^2) plus paclitaxel (175 mg/m^2 over 3 hours) versus carboplatin plus the taxane paclitaxel for at least six cycles (dose of carboplatin calculated as follows: [glomerular filtration rate 5] + 25mg). It found no significant difference between treatments for either progression free survival or overall survival after a median of 37 months, although it may have lacked power to detect clinically important effects (median progression free survival 16 months in both groups; HR 1.07, 95% CI 0.78 to 1.48; median overall survival 30 months with paclitaxel plus cisplatin *v* 32 months with paclitaxel plus carboplatin; HR 0.85, 95% CI 0.59 to 1.24).

Harms: The first systematic review did not report adverse effects.[18] One cohort analysis of two RCTs comparing platinum and non-platinum based regimens found that grade 3 nausea and vomiting (see table 1, p 2439), mild renal toxicity, and neurotoxicity were significantly more common with platinum containing regimens than with non-platinum regimens (AR grade 3 nausea and vomiting about 6–10% with platinum based regimens *v* 4% with non-platinum based regimens, P = 0.004; AR any renal toxicity 17–20% with platinum *v* 4% with non-platinum, P value not reported; AR neurotoxicity 1–4% with platinum *v* 0% with non-platinum, P value not reported).[30] **Adding a platinum based compound to a non-platinum combination regimen:** We found one analysis of data from two RCTs (387 women with advanced ovarian cancer) comparing hexamethylmelamine plus cyclophosphamide plus methotrexate plus 5-fluorouracil with or without cisplatin, or with cyclophosphamide plus cisplatin.[31] After a median follow up of 45 months, it found that neurotoxicity was more common and more severe with regimens that included platinum based compounds than with those that did not include platinum (AR for any neurotoxicity 47% with platinum *v* 25% without platinum; AR for grade 2–3 neurotoxicity 25% with platinum *v* 3% without platinum; CI and P values not reported). **Platinum based combination regimens versus non-platinum based combination regimens:** The RCT comparing cisplatin plus melphalan versus hexamethylmelamine plus doxorubicin plus cyclophosphamide found that haematological toxicity was significantly more common with the platinum based regimen (white cells $< 3000/m^3$, $P < 0.0001$; platelets $< 75\,000/m^3$, $P < 0.0001$; anaemia, $P = 0.001$).[20] The RCT comparing doxorubicin plus cyclophosphamide combined with either vincristine or cisplatin reported that platinum increased haematological toxicity (rates not reported).[22] **Single platinum based agent versus single non-platinum agent:** One additional RCT comparing cisplatin versus thiotepa found that 1/85 (1%) women taking cisplatin stopped because of weakness and dizziness.[24] **Single platinum based agent versus combined platinum based chemotherapy:** In the RCT comparing carboplatin alone versus cyclophosphamide plus doxorubicin plus cisplatin, 875 women (57%) were assessed for adverse effects.[26] Leucopenia, hair loss, nausea, and vomiting were more common with combination treatment than with carboplatin alone (AR for leucopenia 36% with combination *v* 10% with carboplatin alone; AR for hair loss 70% with combination *v* 4% with carboplatin alone; AR for nausea and vomiting 20% with combination *v* 9% with carboplatin alone). Thrombocytopenia was more common with carboplatin (AR 6% with combination *v* 16% with carboplatin alone). Renal, cardiac, and neurotoxicity were rare in both groups (1–2% in both groups for each category). **Comparison of different platinum agents (cisplatin versus carboplatin) added to a taxane:** The RCT comparing carboplatin plus the taxane paclitaxel, versus cisplatin plus paclitaxel, found no significant difference between treatments for rates of hair loss, fever, mucositis, diarrhoea, allergic reaction, cardiorespiratory complications, skin reactions, muscle or joint pain, constipation, fever, or renal toxicity.[29]

However, after six cycles of treatment, grade 4 nausea and vomiting (see table 1, p 2439) was more common with cisplatin plus paclitaxel (AR 17% with cisplatin plus paclitaxel *v* 14% with carboplatin plus paclitaxel; P < 0.01). Grade 3–4 thrombocytopenia and grade 4 granulocytopenia (see table 1, p 2439) were more common with carboplatin plus paclitaxel (AR for grade 3–4 thrombocytopenia 6% with carboplatin plus paclitaxel *v* 1% with cisplatin plus paclitaxel, P < 0.01; AR for grade 4 granulocytopenia 40% with carboplatin plus paclitaxel *v* 23% with cisplatin plus paclitaxel, P < 0.01). Two other RCTs reported as conference abstracts reported on harms (see comment below).

Comment: **Single agent platinum versus combined platinum chemotherapy:** We found one RCT (120 women with advanced ovarian cancer) reported as a conference abstract, which compared six cycles of cisplatin plus cyclophosphamide versus three cycles of epirubicin plus ifosfamide followed by four cycles of cisplatin.[32] It found no significant differences between treatments for relapse free survival or overall survival (relapse free survival at 3 years 24% with cisplatin plus cyclophosphamide *v* 41% with epirubicin plus ifosfamide plus cisplatin, CI and P values not reported; median overall survival 141 weeks with cisplatin plus cyclophosphamide *v* 172 weeks with epirubicin plus ifosfamide plus cisplatin, CI and P values not reported). **Comparison of different platinum agents (cisplatin versus carbaplatin) added to a taxane:** We found two additional RCTs that were reported in three conference abstracts. The first RCT (797 women) compared carboplatin plus paclitaxel versus cisplatin plus paclitaxel, and was reported in two conference abstracts.[33,34] It found no significant difference between treatments for either progression free survival or overall survival after a median follow up of 2 years (P > 0.05).[34] A preliminary safety report on 488/797 of the women (61.2%) found that grade 3–4 haematological toxicity (see table 1, p 2439) was more common with the carboplatin regimen, and non-haematological toxicity (other than hair loss) was more common with the cisplatin regimen (ARs not reported).[33] The second RCT compared carboplatin plus paclitaxel versus paclitaxel plus alternating cisplatin and carboplatin in 164 women and was reported in a single conference abstract.[35] It found no significant differences for disease free survival or overall survival (P = 0.4 for both outcomes).

OPTION TAXANES

One systematic review and one additional RCT have found that adding paclitaxel to platinum based chemotherapy significantly improves progression free survival and overall survival after primary surgery for advanced ovarian cancer compared with platinum based chemotherapy alone. We found no reliable RCTs comparing carboplatin plus docetaxel versus carboplatin plus paclitaxel.

Benefits: **Adding a taxane (paclitaxel) to a platinum regimen:** We found one systematic review[36] and one additional RCT[37] in women with advanced ovarian cancer. The systematic review (search date not reported, 4 RCTs, 3754 women) included one published RCT[38] and three unpublished RCTs, all of which have since been published.[39–41] The first RCT (386 women) compared cisplatin (75 mg/m^2) plus cyclophosphamide versus cisplatin (75 mg/m^2) plus paclitaxel (135 mg/m^2).[38] It found that cisplatin plus paclitaxel improved progression free survival and overall survival when compared with cisplatin plus cyclophosphamide (median progression free survival 18 months with cisplatin plus paclitaxel *v* 13 months with cisplatin plus cyclophosphamide, P < 0.001; median overall survival 38 months with cisplatin plus paclitaxel *v* 24 months with cisplatin plus cyclophosphamide, P < 0.001). The second RCT (680 women) compared cisplatin (75 mg/m^2) plus cyclophosphamide versus cisplatin (75 mg/m^2) plus paclitaxel (175 mg/m^2).[39] It found that cisplatin plus paclitaxel significantly improved progression free survival and overall survival compared with cisplatin plus cyclophosphamide (median progression free survival 17 months with cisplatin plus paclitaxel *v* 12 months with cisplatin plus cyclophosphamide, P = 0.001; median survival 35 months with cisplatin plus paclitaxel *v* 25 months with cisplatin plus cyclophosphamide, P = 0.001). The third RCT (614 women) compared three treatments: cisplatin alone (100 mg/m^2), paclitaxel alone (200 mg/m^2), and paclitaxel (135 mg/m^2) followed by cisplatin (75 mg/m^2).[40] It found no significant difference between cisplatin alone versus cisplatin plus paclitaxel for progression free survival or overall survival after a median follow up of 61 months (progression free survival: median 16 months with cisplatin alone *v* 14 months with cisplatin plus paclitaxel; HR 1.06, 95% CI 0.90 to 1.30; overall survival: median 30 months with cisplatin alone *v* 27 months with cisplatin plus paclitaxel; HR 0.99, 95% CI 0.80 to 1.23). The fourth RCT (2074 women) compared three treatments: paclitaxel (175 mg/m^2) plus carboplatin, carboplatin alone, and cyclophosphamide plus doxorubicin plus cisplatin.[41] It found no significant difference in progression free survival or overall survival between paclitaxel plus carboplatin versus carboplatin alone after 24 months (overall free survival: HR 0.98, 95% CI 0.87 to 1.10; progression free survival: HR 0.93, 95% CI 0.84 to 1.04). The additional RCT (45 women) compared cisplatin (75 mg/m^2) plus paclitaxel (175 mg/m^2) versus cisplatin (75 mg/m^2) plus cyclophosphamide (750 mg/m^2).[37] It found that cisplatin plus paclitaxel significantly increased the time to relapse and relapse free survival after 25 months compared with cisplatin plus cyclophosphamide (38 women; median time to relapse 17.5 months with cisplatin plus paclitaxel *v* 9.9 months with cisplatin plus cyclophosphamide, CI and P value not reported; P value for difference in relapse free survival = 0.001, mean values and CI not reported). **Comparison of different agents (cisplatin versus carboplatin) added to a taxane:** See benefits of platinum based regimens, p 2432. **Comparison of different taxanes (paclitaxel versus docetaxel) added to a platinum agent:** We found no RCTs with sufficient follow up for inclusion (see comment below).

Harms: **Adding a taxane (paclitaxel) to a platinum regimen:** The systematic review found that reporting of adverse effects was not consistent among trials.[36] One RCT found that adding paclitaxel to platinum based regimens did not significantly increase haematological toxicity, fever, or anaemia (any haematological toxicity: RR about 1, 95% CI about 0.8 to 1.3; anaemia: RR 1.10, 95% CI 0.57 to 2.13; fever: RR 16.38 in favour of non-paclitaxel regimen, 95% CI 0.83 to 284).[38] In one RCT, compared with the platinum based regimen alone, infection was more common with paclitaxel plus a platinum compound (RR 3.38, 95% CI 2.15 to 5.32) but less common with cyclophosphamide plus doxorubicin plus a platinum compound (RR 0.59, 95% CI 0.40 to 0.86).[41] Nausea and vomiting was reported in 7–18% of women receiving paclitaxel, and hair loss was reported in 68–77% of women receiving paclitaxel. Cardiac toxicity was not reported in the included RCTs. One RCT (614 women) found that adverse effects were significantly more common with paclitaxel or paclitaxel plus cisplatin (neutropenia, $P < 0.008$; hair loss, $P < 0.001$; fever, $P < 0.001$) than with cisplatin alone.[40] Another RCT found that grades 3 and 4 muscle pain (see table 1, p 2439), neurosensory and neuromotor symptoms, and hair loss were more common with cisplatin plus paclitaxel than with cisplatin plus cyclophosphamide (AR muscle pain 6% with cisplatin plus paclitaxel *v* 0% with cisplatin plus cyclophosphamide; neurosensory symptoms 19.6% with cisplatin plus paclitaxel *v* 1% with cisplatin plus cyclophosphamide; neuromotor symptoms 5% with cisplatin plus paclitaxel v 0.6% with cisplatin plus cyclophosphamide; hair loss 51% with cisplatin plus paclitaxel v 21% with cisplatin plus cyclophosphamide; CI and P values not reported).[35] Grade 3 and 4 leucopenia (see table 1, p 2439), anaemia, and thrombocytopenia were less common with cisplatin plus paclitaxel than with cisplatin plus cyclophosphamide (AR, CI, and P values not reported). Febrile neutropenia rates were similar between groups (AR 3% for both groups).

Comment: **Comparison of different taxanes (paclitaxel versus docetaxel) added to a platinum regimen:** We found one ongoing RCT (1077 women from 83 centres), that will compare effects of six cycles of carboplatin (dose calculated as follows: [glomerular filtration rate 5] + 25 mg) combined with either paclitaxel (175 mg/m²) or docetaxel (75 mg/m²).[42]

GLOSSARY

Debulking is removal of a major proportion of the tumour. Initial and primary debulking both refer to surgery performed at first presentation.

Interval debulking is a second operation to remove residual tumour after a specified number of cytotoxic chemotherapy cycles, which is then followed by further chemotherapy.

Routine second look surgery is an operation to assess the response to cytotoxic chemotherapy in women who have already undergone primary surgery.

REFERENCES

1. Allen DG, Heintz AP, Touw FW. A meta-analysis of residual disease and survival in stage III and IV carcinoma of the ovary. *Eur J Gynaecol Oncol* 1995;16:349–356. Search date not reported; primary sources literature search of Silver-Platter 3.1, hand searches, and personal communications.
2. Beral V. *The epidemiology of ovarian cancer.* In: Sharp F, Soutter WP, eds. *Proceedings of the Seventeenth Study Group of the Royal College of Obstetricians and Gynaecologists in conjunction with the Helene Harris Memorial Trust*. London: RCOG, 1987:21–31.
3. Banks E, Beral V, Reeves G. The epidemiology of ovarian cancer: a review. *Int J Gynecol Cancer* 1997;7:425–438.
4. Parkin DM, Laara E, Muir CS. Estimates of the worldwide frequency of sixteen major cancers in 1980. *Int J Cancer* 1988;41:184–197.
5. Blake P, Lambert H, Crawford R. *Cancer of the ovary and fallopian tube.* In: Blake P, Lambert H, Crawford R, eds. *Gynaecological oncology. A guide to clinical management*. Oxford: Oxford University Press, 1998:12–44.
6. Cancer Statistics: Cancer Research Campaign, 2002. http:/www.cancerresearchuk.org/aboutcancer/statistics/incidence. Last accessed 14 January 2004.
7. Whittemore AS, Harris R, Itnyre J. Characteristics relating to ovarian cancer risk: collaborative analysis of 12 US case-control studies. II. Invasive epithelial ovarian cancers in white women. Collaborative Ovarian Cancer Group. *Am J Epidemiol* 1992;136:1184–1203.
8. Yancik R. Ovarian cancer. Age contrasts in incidence, histology, disease stage at diagnosis and mortality. *Cancer* 1993;71:517–523.
9. Adami H-O, Hseih C-C, Lambe M, et al. Parity, age at first childbirth, and risk of ovarian cancer. *Lancet* 1994;344:1250–1254.
10. Rossing MA, Daling JR, Weiss NS, et al. Ovarian tumours in a cohort of infertile women. *N Engl J Med* 1994;331:771–776.
11. Venn A, Watson L, Bruinsma F, et al. Risk of cancer after use of fertility drugs with in-vitro fertilisation. *Lancet* 1999;354:1586–1590.
12. Mant JWF, Vessey MP. *Ovarian and endometrial cancers.* In: Doll R, Fraumeni JF Jr, Muir CS, eds. *Trends in cancer incidence and mortality*. Plainview, NY: Cold Spring Harbor Laboratory Press, 1994:287–307.
13. Booth M, Beral V, Smith P. Risk factors for ovarian cancer: a case-control study. *Br J Cancer* 1989;60:592–598.
14. Nicoletto MO, Tumolo S, Talamini R, et al. Surgical second look in ovarian cancer: a randomized study in patients with laparoscopic complete remission — a Northeastern Oncology Cooperative Group-Ovarian Cancer Cooperative Group Study. *J Clin Oncol* 1997;15:994–999.
15. Luesley D, Lawton F, Blackledge G, et al. Failure of second-look laparotomy to influence survival in epithelial ovarian cancer. *Lancet* 1988;2:599–603.
16. Van der Burg ME, van Lent M, Buyse M, et al. The effect of debulking surgery after induction chemotherapy on the prognosis in advanced epithelial ovarian cancer. Gynecological Cancer Cooperative Group of the European Organization for Research and Treatment of Cancer. *N Engl J Med* 1995;332:629–634.
17. Redman CW, Warwick J, Luesley DM, et al. Intervention debulking surgery in advanced epithelial ovarian cancer. *Br J Obstet Gynaecol* 1994;101:142–146.
18. Advanced Ovarian Cancer Trialists Group. Chemotherapy for advanced ovarian cancer. In: The Cochrane Library, Issue 1, 2002. Oxford: Update Software. Search date 1998; primary sources Medline, Cancerlit, the trial registers produced by the National Cancer Institute (Physicians Data Query) and the United Kingdom Co-ordinating Committee on Cancer Research, hand searches of relevant meeting proceedings, and contact with experts in the field and pharmaceutical companies.
19. Alberts DS, Mason-Liddil N, O'Toole RV, et al. Randomized phase III trial of chemoimmunotherapy in patients with previously untreated stages III and IV suboptimal disease ovarian cancer: a Southwest Oncology Group Study. *Gynecol Oncol* 1989;32:8–15.
20. Edwards CL, Herson J, Gershenson DM, et al. A prospective randomized clinical trial of melphalan and cis-platinum versus hexamethylmelamine, adriamycin, and cyclophosphamide in advanced ovarian cancer. *Gynecol Oncol* 1983;15:261–277.

21. Sessa C, Colombo N, Bolis G, et al. Randomized comparison of hexamethylmelamine, adriamycin, cyclophosphamide (HAC) vs. cisplatin, adriamycin, cyclophosphamide (PAC) in advanced ovarian cancer: long-term results. *Cancer Treat Rev* 1991;18(suppl A):37–46.
22. Krommer CF, Szalai JP. Cyclophosphamide, adriamycin and cisplatin (CAP) versus cyclophosphamide, adriamycin and vincristin (CAV) in the treatment of advanced ovarian cancer: a randomized study. *Ann Oncol* 1992;3:37–39.
23. Neijt JP, Bokkel Huinink WW, van der Burg ME, et al. Randomised trial comparing two combination chemotherapy regimens (Hexa-CAF vs CHAP-5) in advanced ovarian carcinoma. *Lancet* 1984;2:594–600.
24. Dorum A, Kristensen GB, Trope C. A randomised study of cisplatin versus thiotepa as induction chemotherapy in advanced ovarian carcinoma. *Eur J Cancer* 1994;30A:1470–1474.
25. Neijt J, ten Bokkel Huinink W, van der Burg M, et al. Long-term survival in ovarian cancer. Mature data from The Netherlands Joint Study Group for Ovarian Cancer. *Eur J Cancer* 1991;27:1367–1372.
26. The ICON Collaborators. ICON2: randomised trial of single-agent carboplatin against three-drug combination of CAP (cyclophosphamide, doxorubicin, and cisplatin) in women with ovarian cancer. ICON Collaborators. International Collaborative Ovarian Neoplasm Study. *Lancet* 1998;352:1571–1576.
27. Bolis G, Favalli G, Danese S, et al. Weekly cisplatin given for 2 months versus cisplatin plus cyclophosphamide given for 5 months after cytoreductive surgery for advanced ovarian cancer. *J Clin Oncol* 1997;15:1938–1944.
28. Marth C, Trope C, Vergote IB, et al. Ten-year results of a randomised trial comparing cisplatin with cisplatin and cyclophosphamide in advanced, suboptimally debulked ovarian cancer. *Eur J Cancer* 1998;34:1175–1180.
29. Neijt JP, Engelholm SA, Tuxen MK, et al. Exploratory phase III study of paclitaxel and cisplatin versus paclitaxel and carboplatin in advanced ovarian cancer. *J Clin Oncol* 2000;18:3084–3092.
30. US Food and Drug Administration. Center for Drug Evaluation and Research. http://www.fda.gov/cder/cancer/toxicityframe.htm. Last accessed 14 January 2004.
31. van der Hoop RG, van der Burg ME, Bokkel Huinink WW, et al. Incidence of neuropathy in 395 patients with ovarian cancer treated with or without cisplatin. *Cancer* 1990;66:1697–1702.
32. Bella M, Cocconi A, Mambrini A, et al. The concept of a medical debulking in advanced ovarian carcinoma before cisplatin treatment. Final results of a prospective randomized trial [abstract]. *Tumori* 1998;84(suppl 54):A146.
33. Mobus V, Schoder W, Luck HJ, et al. Cisplatin/paclitaxel vs carboplatin/paclitaxel as first-line chemotherapy in ovarian cancer: an AGO study group phase III trial [abstract]. *Ann Oncol* 1998;9:173.
34. Shröeder W, DuBois A, Kuhn W, et al. Treatment of patients with advanced ovarian cancer (FIGO IIB-IV) with cisplatin/paclitaxel or carboplatin/paclitaxel — an interim analysis of the AGO study protocol ovar-3 [abstract 908]. *Eur J Cancer* 1999; 35(suppl 4):S231.
35. Skarlos DV, Aravantinos G, Kosmidis P, et al. Paclitaxel with carboplatin versus paclitaxel with carboplatin alternating with cisplatin as first-line chemotherapy in advanced epithelial ovarian cancer: preliminary results of a Hellenic Cooperative Oncology Group study [abstract]. *Semin Oncol* 1997;24(suppl 15):S15.
36. Lister-Sharp D, McDonagh MS, Khan KS, et al. A rapid and systematic review of the effectiveness and cost-effectiveness of the taxanes used in the treatment of advanced breast and ovarian cancer. *Health Technol Assess* 2000;4:17–115. Search date not reported; primary sources Medline, Embase, Cancerlit, Cochrane Controlled Trials Register, National Research Register, and contact with researchers and review groups.
37. Smith-Sorensen B, Kaern J, Holm R, et al. Therapy effect of either paclitaxel or cyclophosphamide combination treatment in patients with epithelial ovarian cancer and relation to TP53 gene status. *Br J Cancer* 1998;78:375–381.
38. McGuire WP, Hoskins WJ, Brady MF, et al. Cyclophosphamide and cisplatin compared with paclitaxel and cisplatin in patients with stage III and stage IV ovarian cancer. *N Engl J Med* 1996;334:1–6.
39. Piccart MJ, Bertelsen K, James K, et al. Randomized intergroup trial of cisplatin–paclitaxel versus cisplatin–cyclophosphamide in women with advanced epithelial ovarian cancer: three-year results. *J Natl Cancer Inst* 2000;92:699–708.
40. Muggia FM, Braly PS, Brady MF, et al. Phase III randomized study of cisplatin versus paclitaxel versus cisplatin and paclitaxel in patients with suboptimal stage III or IV ovarian cancer: a gynecologic oncology group study. *J Clin Oncol* 2000;18:106–115.
41. International Collaborative Ovarian Neoplasm Group. Paclitaxel plus carboplatin versus standard chemotherapy with either single-agent carboplatin or cyclophosphamide, doxorubicin, and cisplatin in women with ovarian cancer: the ICON3 randomised trial. *Lancet* 2002;360:505–515.
42. Vasey PA. First results of the SCOTROC trial: a phase III comparison of paclitaxel–carboplatin and docetaxel–carboplatin as first line chemotherapy for epithelial ovarian cancer. *Proc ASCO* 2001;84:170–178.

Richmal Oates-Whitehead
Clinical Editor/Editor Cochrane Heart Group
BMJ Knowledge
BMA House
London
UK

Competing interests: None declared.
We would like to acknowledge the previous contributors of this chapter, including Hani Gabra, Charles Redman, and Jennifer Byrom.

TABLE 1 Adverse effects of chemotherapy — Common Toxicity Criteria (see text, p 2434).[28] Published with permission.

Toxicity grade	0	1	2	3	4
Blood and bone marrow					
WBC (10^9/L)	≥ 4.0	3.0–3.9	2.0–2.9	1.0–1.9	< 1.0
Platelets (10^9/L)	WNL	75.0 normal	50.0–74.9	25.0–49.9	< 25.0
Haemoglobin (g/L)	WNL	10.0 normal	8.0–10.0	6.5–7.9	< 6.5
Granulocytes and bands (10^9/L)	≥ 2.0	1.5–1.9	1.0–1.4	0.5–0.9	< 0.5
Lymphocytes (10^9/L)	≥ 2.0	1.5–1.9	1.0–1.4	0.5–0.9	< 0.5
Nausea	None	Able to eat	Oral intake significantly decreased	No significant intake, requiring iv fluids	
Vomiting	None	1 episode in 24 hours over pretreatment	≥ 6 episodes in 24 hours over pretreatment; or need for iv fluids	Requiring parenteral nutrition; or physiological consequences requiring intensive care; haemodynamic collapse	
Muscle pain	None	Mild pain not interfering with function	Moderate pain: pain or analgesics interfering with function, but not interfering with activities of daily living	Severe pain: pain or analgesics severely interfering with activities of daily living	Disabling

iv, intravenous; WBC, white blood cells; WNL, within normal limits.

Polycystic ovary syndrome

Search date October 2003

Hesham Al-Inany

QUESTIONS

INTERVENTIONS

To be covered in future updates

Treatments for insulin resistance in women with polycystic ovary syndrome

Covered elsewhere in *Clinical Evidence*

For interventions in women with infertility attributed to polycystic ovary syndrome, see Infertility and subfertility chapter, p 2365)

See glossary Ⓖ

Key Messages

- **Cyproterone acetate–ethinylestradiol (co-cyprindiol; reduced hirsutism from baseline, no significant difference in hirsutism between cyproterone acetate–ethinylestradiol and other combined oral contraceptives)** We found no RCTs comparing cyproterone acetate–ethinylestradiol versus placebo. One RCT found limited evidence by assessing within group changes from baseline that cyproterone acetate–ethinylestradiol reduced hirsutism and oligomenorrhoea. Two RCTs found that cyproterone acetate–ethinylestradiol and other combined oral contraceptive regimens were effective in reducing hirsutism at 6 months. One of these RCTs also found limited evidence that cyproterone acetate–ethinylestradiol may be less effective than ketoconazole in reducing hirsutism at 6 months. A fourth RCT found that cyproterone acetate–ethinylestradiol was less effective in reducing hirsutism at 6 months than metformin. A fifth RCT found that adding finasteride to cyproterone acetate–ethinylestradiol reduced hirsutism at 6 months compared with cyproterone acetate–ethinylestradiol alone. Cyproterone acetate–ethinylestradiol is associated with an increased risk of venous thromboembolism.
- **Finasteride (may be equally effective in reducing hirsutism compared with flutamide and spironolactone)** Two RCTs found that finasteride reduced hirsutism after 6 months' treatment compared with placebo and three others found more limited evidence that it reduced hirsutism from baseline. Small RCTs, which included women with idiopathic hirsutism, provided insufficient evidence to compare the

relative effectiveness of finasteride, flutamide, and spironolactone. Of the three RCTs that directly compared treatments, two found no significant difference in hirsutism among treatments, and the third found that finasteride was less effective than flutamide in reducing hirsutism at 12 months. Another RCT found that adding finasteride to cyproterone acetate–ethinylestradiol reduced hirsutism at 6 months compared with cyproterone acetate–ethinylestradiol alone. We found no RCTs that assessed effects on oligomenorrhoea.

- **Flutamide (may be equally effective in reducing hirsutism compared with finasteride and spironolactone)** Small RCTs, which included women with idiopathic hirsutism, provided insufficient evidence to compare the relative effectiveness of flutamide, finasteride, and spironolactone. One of the RCTs found that flutamide improved hirsuitism compared with placebo, and three other RCTs found more limited evidence that it improved hirsuitism from baseline. Of the three RCTs that directly compared treatments, two found no significant difference in hirsutism among treatments, and the third found that flutamide was more effective than finasteride in reducing hirsutism at 12 months. We found no RCTs that assessed effects on oligomenorrhoea.
- **Metformin (improved menstrual pattern compared with placebo; reduced hirsutism compared with cyproterone acetate–ethinylestradiol)** One RCT found limited evidence that metformin improved menstrual pattern over 3 months compared with placebo. Another RCT found that adding metformin to a low calorie diet reduced oligomenorrhoea at 6 months compared with placebo, and found more limited evidence by assessing within group changes from baseline that it also reduced hirsutism. A third RCT found that metformin was more effective in reducing hirsutism at 12 months than cyproterone acetate–ethinylestradiol.
- **Spironolactone (may be equally effective in reducing hirsutism compared with finasteride and flutamide)** One systematic review of two small RCTs in women with hirsutism attributed to polycystic ovary syndrome or idiopathic hirsutism found that spironolactone reduced hirsutism at 6 months compared with placebo. One small RCT found limited evidence that spironolactone was less effective in reducing hirsuitism at 6 months than ketoconazole. One small RCT found that spironolactone, finasteride, and flutamide all reduced hirsutism at 6 months compared with placebo, and found no significant difference among groups. This RCT may have been underpowered to detect a clinically important difference among active treatments. We found no RCTs that assessed the effects of spironolactone on oligomenorrhoea.
- **Cyproterone acetate–ethinylestradiol (co-cyprindiol; for reducing oligomenorrhoea)** We found no RCTs comparing cyproterone acetate–ethinylestradiol versus placebo. One RCT found limited evidence by assessing within group changes from baseline that cyproterone acetate–ethinylestradiol reduced oligomenorrhoea.
- **Interventions to achieve weight loss** We found no systematic review or RCTs comparing interventions to achieve weight loss versus no intervention that assessed clinical outcomes in women with polycystic ovary syndrome. One RCT found limited evidence by assessing within group changes from baseline that a high or a low protein diet aimed at achieving weight loss may improve menstrual pattern over 16 weeks.
- **Ketoconazole** One RCT found limited evidence that ketoconazole reduced hirsutism at 6 months compared with cyproterone acetate–ethinylestradiol or spironolactone. We found no RCTs that assessed effects on oligomenorrhoea.
- **Mechanical hair removal** We found no RCTs of the effects of mechanical hair removal in women with hirsutism attributed to polycystic ovary syndrome.

DEFINITION Polycystic ovary syndrome (PCOS; Stein–Leventhal syndrome, sclerocystic ovarian disease) is defined as an accumulation of many incompletely developed follicles in the ovaries due to chronic anovulation with an increase in ovarian androgen production. The diagnosis excludes secondary causes such as androgen producing neoplasm, hyperprolactinaemia, and adult onset congenital adrenal hyperplasia.[1] It is characterized by irregular menstrual cycles, scanty or absent menses, multiple small cysts on the ovaries (polycystic ovaries), mild hirsutism, and infertility. Many women also have insulin resistance, acne, and weight gain.[1] Until recently, there was no overall consensus on the criteria for diagnosing PCOS. In some studies, it has been diagnosed based on the ultrasound findings of polycystic ovaries, rather than on clinical criteria. An international consensus definition of PCOS has now been published, which defines PCOS as the presence of at least 12 follicles measuring 2–9 mm in diameter and/or an ovarian volume in excess of 10 mL.[2]

INCIDENCE/ PREVALENCE PCOS is diagnosed in 4–10% of women attending gynaecology clinics in developed countries,[1,3] but this figure may not reflect the true prevalence because there have been no specific population based studies and the criteria used for diagnosis are varied. Most women present in their thirties.[3]

AETIOLOGY/ RISK FACTORS The aetiology is unknown. Genetic factors may play a part, but the exact mechanisms are unclear. Two studies demonstrated some evidence of familial aggregation of hyperandrogenaemia (with or without oligomenorrhoea) in first degree relatives of women with PCOS.[3,4] In the first study, 22% of sisters of women with PCOS fulfilled diagnostic criteria for PCOS.[3] In the second study, of the 78 mothers and 50 sisters evaluated clinically, 19 (24%) mothers and 16 (32%) sisters had PCOS.[4]

PROGNOSIS There is some evidence that women with PCOS are at increased risk of developing type 2 diabetes and cardiovascular disorders secondary to hyperlipidaemia compared with women who do not have PCOS.[5] Oligomenorrhoeic and amenorrhoeic women are at increased risk of developing endometrial hyperplasia and, later, endometrial carcinoma.[6]

AIMS OF INTERVENTION To reduce hirsutism and restore regular menstrual cycle, with minimal adverse effects.

OUTCOMES **In women with hirsutism:** Objective scales of reduction in hirsutism such as the Ferriman–Gallwey scale, which quantifies the extent of hair growth in nine anatomical sites, scoring 0 (no hair) to 4 (maximal growth), with a maximum score of 36; personal perception of reduction in hirsutism; adverse effects of treatment. **In women with oligomenorrhoea:** menstruation rate; adverse effects of treatment.

METHODS *Clinical Evidence* search and appraisal October 2003. We also searched *WHO Pharmaceuticals Newsletter* 1997–2004 for safety alerts regarding the included drugs.

QUESTION What are the effects of treatments?

OPTION CYPROTERONE ACETATE–ETHINYLESTRADIOL (CO-CYPRINDIOL)

We found no RCTs comparing cyproterone acetate–ethinylestradiol versus placebo. One RCT found limited evidence by assessing within group changes from baseline that cyproterone acetate–ethinylestradiol reduced hirsutism and oligomenorrhoea. Two RCTs found that cyproterone acetate–ethinylestradiol and other combined oral contraceptive regimens were effective in reducing hirsutism at 6 months. One of these RCTs also found limited evidence that cyproterone acetate–ethinylestradiol may be less effective than ketoconazole in reducing hirsutism at 6 months. A fourth RCT found that cyproterone acetate–ethinylestradiol was less effective in reducing hirsutism at 6 months than metformin. A fifth RCT found that adding finasteride to cyproterone acetate–ethinylestradiol reduced hirsutism at 6 months compared with cyproterone acetate–ethinylestradiol alone. Cyproterone acetate–ethinylestradiol is associated with an increased risk of venous thromboembolism.

Benefits: **Versus placebo:** We found no RCTs. **Versus other combined oral contraceptives:** We found one RCT (28 adolescent girls) comparing cyproterone acetate–ethinylestradiol (ethinylestradiol 35 μg plus cyproterone acetate 2 mg daily) versus ethinylestradiol 30 μg plus desogestrel 0.15 mg daily for 21 days followed by a 7 day rest for a period of 12 months.[7] It did not directly compare interventions; rather, it reported changes from baseline within each group. It found that both treatments significantly reduced hirsutism**G** after 6 months' treatment (measured by mean reduction in Ferriman–Gallwey score; $P < 0.05$, absolute results presented graphically). The RCT did not assess effects on oligomenorrhoea**G**. **Versus other combined oral contraceptives, ketoconazole, or spironolactone:** We found one open label RCT (141 women) comparing four interventions: cyproterone acetate–ethinylestradiol (48 women) for 21 days, cyproterone acetate–ethinylestradiol for 21 days plus cyproterone acetate 100 mg daily for the first 10 days of the cycle (65 women), oral spironolactone 100–200 mg daily (12 women), or ketoconazole 400 mg daily (16 women) for 6 months.[8] It found that all four interventions reduced hirsutism at 6 months, but that ketoconazole was significantly more effective than the other three interventions (mean reduction in Ferriman–Gallwey score –34.6 with ketoconazole *v* –18 with cyproterone acetate–ethinylestradiol *v* –20.1 with cyproterone acetate–ethinylestradiol plus cyproterone acetate *v* –12.8 with spironolactone; $P < 0.001$ for ketoconazole *v* all other treatments).[8] It found no significant difference between cyproterone acetate–ethinylestradiol alone and cyproterone acetate–ethinylestradiol plus cyproterone acetate (reported as non-significant, CI not reported). It did not directly compare cyproterone acetate–ethinylestradiol versus spironolactone. The RCT did not assess effects on oligomenorrhoea. **Versus gonadotrophic releasing hormone (GnHR) agonist:** We found one RCT (45 adolescents aged 15–18 years) comparing cyproterone acetate–ethinylestradiol versus triptorelin.[9] The RCT did not directly compare clinical outcomes between groups, rather it reported changes from baseline within groups. It found that both cyproterone acetate–ethinylestradiol and triptorelin significantly reduced hirsutism from baseline after 6 months' treatment (mean percentage reduction in Ferriman–Gallwey score from baseline 4.1% with cyproterone acetate–ethinylestradiol; $P < 0.001$; 3.1% with triptorelin; $P < 0.01$). It also found that all women taking cyproterone acetate–ethinylestradiol had regular menstruation. All taking the GnHR agonist developed amenorrhoea. **Versus metformin:** We found one RCT (52 women with polycystic ovary syndrome [PCOS] with Ferriman–Gallwey score > 8) comparing cyproterone acetate–ethinylestradiol versus metformin 500 mg three times daily for 12 months.[10] It found that cyproterone acetate–ethinylestradiol was significantly less effective than metformin in reducing hirsutism at 12 months (mean percentage reduction –5% with cyproterone acetate–ethinylestradiol *v* –25% with metformin; $P < 0.001$), although both treatments significantly reduced hirsutism from baseline ($P < 0.005$ with cyproterone acetate–ethinylestradiol; $P < 0.0001$ with metformin). The RCT did not assess effects on oligomenorrhoea. **Plus finasteride versus cyproterone acetate–ethinylestradiol alone:** We found one RCT (50 women, 20 with PCOS) comparing cyproterone acetate–ethinylestradiol plus finasteride for 2 weeks per cycle versus acetate–ethinylestradiol alone.[11] It found that, in women with PCOS, cyproterone acetate–ethinylestradiol plus finasteride significantly reduced hirsutism at 3 and 6 months compared with cyproterone acetate–ethinylestradiol alone ($P < 0.05$ at both time points, absolute results presented graphically). The RCT did not assess effects on oligomenorrhoea.

Harms: Cyproterone acetate–ethinylestradiol is associated with an increased risk of venous thromboembolism.[12] The risk may be higher than that with other combined oral contraceptives. **Versus other combined oral contraceptives:** The RCT gave no information on adverse effects.[7] **Versus other combined oral contraceptives, ketoconazole, or spironolactone:** The RCT gave no information on adverse effects.[8] **Versus GnRH agonist:** The RCT reported no adverse effects in women taking cyproterone acetate–ethinylestradiol.[9] It found that three women taking the GnRH agonist developed atrophic vaginitis. **Versus metformin:** The RCT found that significantly more women taking metformin had reduced appetite at 12 months compared with women taking cyproterone acetate–ethinylestradiol (33% with metformin *v* 0% with cyproterone acetate–ethinylestradiol; P = 0.001).[10] **Plus finasteride versus cyproterone acetate–ethinylestradiol alone:** The RCT found that significantly more people taking cyproterone acetate–ethinylestradiol plus finasteride had reduced libido at 3 and 6 months compared with cyproterone acetate–ethinylestradiol alone (at 6 months: 20% *v* 10%; P < 0.05).[11]

Comment: None of the RCTs assessed patient satisfaction or compliance.

OPTION FINASTERIDE

Two RCTs found that finasteride reduced hirsutism after 6 months' treatment compared with placebo and three others found more limited evidence that it reduced hirsutism from baseline. Small RCTs, which included women with idiopathic hirsutism, provided insufficient evidence to compare the relative effectiveness of finasteride, flutamide, and spironolactone. Of the three RCTs that directly compared treatments, two found no significant difference in hirsutism among treatments, and the third found that finasteride was less effective than flutamide in reducing hirsutism at 12 months. Another RCT found that adding finasteride to cyproterone acetate–ethinylestradiol reduced hirsutism at 6 months compared with cyproterone acetate–ethinylestradiol alone. We found no RCTs that assessed effects on oligomenorrhoea.

Benefits: **Versus placebo or other treatments:** We found five RCTs.[13–17] None of the RCTs assessed effects on oligomenorrhoea**G**. The first RCT (24 women, 14 with polycystic ovary syndrome [PCOS]) compared finasteride 5 mg daily versus placebo for 6 months.[13] It found that finasteride significantly reduced hirsutism**G** at 6 months compared with placebo (measured by change in Ferriman–Gallwey score: 6.7 with finasteride *v* 10.6 with placebo; P < 0.01). The second RCT (40 women, 21 of whom had PCOS) compared four interventions: finasteride 5 mg daily, spironolactone 100 mg daily, flutamide 250 mg daily, and placebo for 6 months.[14] It found that finasteride, spironolactone, and flutamide significantly reduced hirsutism at 6 months compared with placebo (measured by mean reduction in Ferriman–Gallwey score, P < 0.01 *v* placebo for all treatments; absolute results presented graphically). It found no significant difference in hirsutism among active groups, although all active treatments reduced hirsutism from baseline (reported as non-significant, CI not reported, absolute results presented graphically). The RCT may have been underpowered to detect a clinically important difference among active treatments. The third RCT (44 women with PCOS) found that both finasteride 5 mg daily and flutamide 250 mg twice daily significantly reduced hirsutism from baseline after 6 months' treatment (P < 0.05 for reduction in Ferriman–Gallwey score in both groups *v* baseline).[15] It found no significant difference in hirsutism between groups (reduction in Ferriman–Gallwey score 25% with finasteride *v* 20% with flutamide; reported as non-significant, CI not reported). The fourth RCT (70 women, 36 with PCOS, 34 with idiopathic hirsutism, mean age 25 years) compared finasteride 5 mg daily versus flutamide 250 mg daily.[17] The RCT did not directly compare finasteride versus flutamide, rather it reported changes from baseline within each group. It found that both finasteride and flutamide significantly reduced hirsutism from baseline at 12 months (percentage reduction in Ferriman–Gallwey score: 41% with finasteride, 71% with flutamide; P < 0.01 *v* placebo in both groups). The fifth RCT (110 women aged

18–29 years, 64 with PCOS) found that, in women with PCOS, finasteride was significantly less effective than flutamide in reducing hirsutism at 12 months, although both treatments reduced hirsutism from baseline (mean Ferriman–Gallwey score 10.9 with finasteride *v* 7.1 with flutamide; $P < 0.01$).[16] **Plus cyproterone acetate–ethinylestradiol:** See benefits of cyproterone acetate–ethinylestradiol, p 2442.

Harms: **Versus placebo or other treatments:** The first RCT found that 3/12 (25%) women taking finasteride had dizziness compared with 1/12 (8%) women taking placebo.[13] The fifth RCT found that 13/55 (24%) women taking finasteride and 37/55 (67%) taking flutamide had dry skin. It also found that 6/55 (11%) women taking finasteride and 9/55 (16%) taking flutamide had decreased libido. Flutamide was associated with gastrointestinal disorders in 7/55 (13%) women. The fifth RCT found that four women taking finasteride had gastric discomfort.[17] It suggested that flutamide may be associated with hepatotoxicity, but risk was lower with flutamide 250 mg daily as given in the trial. The other RCTs gave no information on adverse effects.[14,15] **Plus cyproterone acetate–ethinylestradiol:** See harms of cyproterone acetate–ethinylestradiol, p 2443.

Comment: Although the RCTs included women with idiopathic hirsutism (women with hirsutism who have regular menstrual cycles and normal circulating androgen levels), it is likely that the results are generalisable to women with hirsutism associated with PCOS.

OPTION FLUTAMIDE

Small RCTs, which included women with idiopathic hirsutism, provided insufficient evidence to compare the relative effectiveness of flutamide, finasteride, and spironolactone. One of the RCTs found that flutamide improved hirsuitism compared with placebo, and three other RCTs found more limited evidence that it improved hirsuitism from baseline. Of the three RCTs that directly compared treatments, two found no significant difference in hirsutism among treatments, and the third found that flutamide was more effective than finasteride in reducing hirsutism at 12 months. We found no RCTs that assessed effects on oligomenorrhoea.

Benefits: **Versus placebo:** See benefits of finasteride, p 2444. **Versus finasteride:** See benefits of finasteride, p 2444.

Harms: **Versus placebo:** We found no RCTs. **Versus finasteride:** See harms of finasteride, p 2445.

Comment: None.

OPTION INTERVENTIONS TO ACHIEVE WEIGHT LOSS

We found no systematic review or RCTs comparing interventions to achieve weight loss versus no intervention that assessed clinical outcomes in women with polycystic ovary syndrome. One RCT found limited evidence by assessing changes within group from baseline that a high or a low protein diet aimed at achieving weight loss may improve menstrual pattern over 16 weeks.

Benefits: We found no systematic review or RCTs comparing interventions to achieve weight loss versus no intervention that assessed clinical outcomes (see comment below). We found one RCT (28 women with polycystic ovary syndrome [PCOS]) comparing two diets to achieve weight loss: a high protein (40% carbohydrate, 30% protein) versus a low protein (55% carbohydrate, 15% protein) diet for 16 weeks.[18] The RCT found similar effects with either diet and so did not assess results comparing different diets; rather, it combined results for both diets and assessed changes in both groups from baseline. It found that menstrual pattern improved in 11/25 (44%) women, but found no effect on hirsutism**G** (mean Ferriman–Gallwey score increased from 19.5 to 19.7, P values not reported).

Harms: The RCT gave no information on adverse effects.[18]

Comment: Obesity and hyperinsulinaemia play a key role in the development of PCOS. Weight loss could, therefore, be of help in its management. We found another RCT that assessed adding metformin to a weight loss diet.[19] Unfortunately, it did not assess clinical outcomes of weight loss; for clinical outcomes of adding metformin to weight loss, see benefits of metformin, p 2446. More RCTs assessing interventions to achieve weight loss in women with PCOS are needed.

OPTION KETOCONAZOLE

One RCT found limited evidence that ketoconazole reduced hirsutism at 6 months compared with low dose cyproterone acetate–ethinylestradiol or spironolactone. We found no RCTs that assessed effects on oligomenorrhoea.

Benefits: **Versus placebo:** We found no RCTs. **Versus cyproterone acetate–ethinylestradiol or spironolactone:** See benefits of cyproterone acetate–ethinylestradiol, p 2442.

Harms: **Versus cyproterone acetate–ethinylestradiol or spironolactone:** See harms of cyproterone acetate–ethinylestradiol, p 2443.

Comment: None.

OPTION MECHANICAL HAIR REMOVAL

We found no RCTs of mechanical hair removal in women with hirsutism associated with polycystic ovary syndrome.

Benefits: We found no systematic review or RCTs.

Harms: We found no RCTs.

Comment: Mechanical methods of hair removal searched for by *Clinical Evidence* included epilators, depilatory creams or lotions, waxing, electrolysis, and laser treatment.

OPTION METFORMIN

One RCT found limited evidence that metformin improved menstrual pattern over 3 months compared with placebo. Another RCT found that adding metformin to a low calorie diet reduced oligomenorrhoea at 6 months compared with placebo, and found more limited evidence by assessing within group changes from baseline that it also reduced hirsutism. A third RCT found that metformin was more effective in reducing hirsutism at 12 months than cyproterone acetate–ethinylestradiol.

Benefits: **Versus placebo:** We found two RCTs.[19,20] The first RCT (23 women with polycystic ovary syndrome) comparing metformin 500 mg twice daily versus placebo for 26 weeks.[20] It found that metformin significantly increased the proportion of women whose menstrual pattern was "substantially improved" over 3 months compared with placebo (5/11 [45%] with metformin *v* 0/12 [0%] with placebo; OR 12.88, 95% CI 1.85 to 89.61; see comment below).[20] The RCT did not define "substantial improvement" in menstrual pattern. The second RCT (40 women, 20 with polycystic ovary syndrome, all with body mass index

> 28) compared metformin versus placebo for 6 months.[19] All women were given a low calorie (1200–1400 kcal daily) diet for 1 month prior to metformin treatment. The RCT found that metformin significantly improved menstrual frequency over 6 months compared with placebo (mean 4.7 with metformin *v* 3.5 with placebo; $P < 0.05$). The RCT did not directly compare the effects on hirsutism**G** between metformin and placebo; rather, it assessed changes from baseline within each group. It found that hirsutism was significantly reduced from baseline in women taking metformin (reduction in Ferriman–Gallwey score from mean 14.8 to 12.9; $P < 0.05$), but was not significantly reduced from baseline in women taking placebo (from mean 11.5 to 10.5; P value reported as non-significant, CI not reported). **Versus cyproterone acetate–ethinylestradiol:** See benefits of cyproterone acetate–ethinylestradiol, p 2442.

Harms: **Versus placebo:** The RCT found mild adverse effects, including nausea, diarrhoea, and heartburn, in five women taking metformin and two women taking placebo.[20] **Versus cyproterone acetate–ethinylestradiol:** See harms of cyproterone acetate–ethinylestradiol, p 2443.

Comment: Women taking placebo had a significantly higher body mass index at baseline compared with women taking metformin ($P < 0.05$). Women taking placebo also had higher fasting insulin than women taking metformin (P value reported as non-significant), but similar insulin sensitivity. This may have biased results in favour of metformin.

OPTION SPIRONOLACTONE

One systematic review of two small RCTs in women with hirsutism attributed to polycystic ovary syndrome or idiopathic hirsutism found that spironolactone reduced hirsutism at 6 months compared with placebo. One small RCT found limited evidence that spironolactone was less effective in reducing hirsuitism at 6 months than ketoconazole. One small RCT found that spironolactone, finasteride, and flutamide all reduced hirsutism at 6 months compared with placebo, and found no significant difference among groups. This RCT may have been underpowered to detect a clinically important difference among active treatments. We found no RCTs that assessed the effects of spironolactone on oligomenorrhoea.

Benefits: **Versus placebo:** We found one systematic review (search date not reported, 2 RCTs, 78 women, 21 with polycystic ovary syndrome) comparing spironolactone 100 mg versus placebo for 6 months' treatment.[21] It found that spironolactone significantly reduced hirsutism**G** compared with placebo (women who reported subjective improvement: 12/21 [57%] with spironolactone *v* 3/21 [14%] with placebo; OR 7.18, 95% CI 1.96 to 26.28; WMD in Ferriman–Gallwey score –7.20, 95% CI –10.98 to –3.42).[21] The review did not assess the effects on oligomenorrhoea**G**. **Versus cyproterone acetate–ethinylestradiol or ketoconazole:** See benefits of cyproterone acetate–ethinylestradiol, p 2442. **Versus finasteride or flutamide:** See benefits of finasteride, p 2444.

Harms: **Versus placebo:** In one of the RCTs identified by the review, three women taking spironolactone withdrew from the trial because of menorrhagia.[21] Adverse effects of spironolactone may include polyuria, fatigue, nausea, headache, decreased libido, and sexual dysfunction, but these were not reported by the review.[21] **Versus cyproterone acetate–ethinylestradiol or ketoconazole:** See harms of cyproterone acetate–ethinylestradiol, p 2443. **Versus finasteride:** See harms of finasteride, p 2445.

Polycystic ovary syndrome

Comment: The included trials were small and confidence intervals were wide, so firm conclusions of treatment effectiveness could not be drawn. Although the RCTs included women with idiopathic hirsutism (hirsutism in women with regular, ovulatory menstrual cycles, and normal circulating androgen levels), it is likely that the results are generalisable to women with hirsutism attributed to polycystic ovary syndrome.

GLOSSARY

Hirsutism is the presence of excessive male pattern hair growth in women on the face, chest, linea alba, or lower back. It usually occurs in women with polycystic ovary syndrome, but "idiopathic hirsutism" may occur in women with regular menstrual cycles and normal circulating androgen levels.

Oligomenorrhoea is infrequent or scanty menstruation.

REFERENCES

1. Dunaif A. Insulin resistance and the polycystic ovary syndrome: mechanism and implications for pathogenesis. *Endocr Rev* 1997;18:774–800.
2. The Rotterdam ESHRE/ASRM-sponsored PCOS consensus workshop group. Revised 2003 consensus on diagnostic criteria and long-term health risks related to polycystic ovary syndrome (PCOS). *Hum Reprod* 2004;19:41–47.
3. Legro RS, Driscoll D, Strauss JF 3rd, et al. Evidence for a genetic basis for hyperandrogenemia in polycystic ovary syndrome. *Proc Natl Acad Sci U S A* 1998;95:14956–14960.
4. Kahsar-Miller MD, Nixon C, Boots LR, et al. Prevalence of polycystic ovary syndrome (PCOS) in first-degree relatives of patients with PCOS. *Fertil Steril* 2001;75:53–58.
5. Legro RS, Kunselman AR, Dunaif A. Prevalence and predictors of dyslipidemia in women with polycystic ovary syndrome. *Am J Med* 2001;111:607–613.
6. Hardiman P, Pillay OS, Atiomo W. Polycystic ovary syndrome and endometrial carcinoma. *Lancet* 2003;361:1810–1812.
7. Mastorakos G, Koliopoulos C, Creatsas G. Androgen and lipid profiles in adolescents with polycystic ovary syndrome who were treated with two forms of combined oral contraceptives. *Fertil Steril* 2002;77: 919–927.
8. Gokmen O, Senoz S, Gulekli B, Isik AZ. Comparison of four different treatment regimes in hirsutism related to polycystic ovary syndrome. *Gynecol Endocrinol* 1996;10:249–255.
9. Creatsas G, Hassan E, Deligeoroglou E, et al. Treatment of polycystic ovarian disease during adolescence with ethinylestradiol/cyproterone acetate versus a D-Tr-6-LHRH analog. *Int J Gynaecol Obstet* 1993;42:147–153.
10. Harborne L, Fleming R, Lyall H, et al. Metformin or antiandrogen in the treatment of hirsutism in polycystic ovary syndrome. *J Clin Endocrinol Metab* 2003;88:4116–4123.
11. Tartagni M, Schonauer LM, De Salvia MA, et al. Comparison of Diane 35 and Diane 35 plus finasteride in the treatment of hirsutism. *Fertil Steril* 2000;73:718–723.
12. World Health Organization. WHO Pharmaceuticals Newsletter 2003;3:5.
13. Lakryc EM, Motta ELA, Soares JM Jr, et al. The benefits of finasteride for hirsute women with polycystic ovary syndrome or idiopathic hirsutism. *Gynecol Endocrinol* 2003;17:57–63.
14. Moghetti P, Tosi F, Tosti A, et al. Comparison of spironolactone, flutamide, and finasteride efficacy in the treatment of hirsutism: a randomized, double blind, placebo-controlled trial. *J Clin Endocrinol Metab* 2000;85:89–94.
15. Falsetti L, De Fusco D, Eleftheriou G, et al. Treatment of hirsutism by finasteride and flutamide in women with polycystic ovary syndrome. *Gynecol Endocrinol* 1997;11:251–257.
16. Falsetti L, Gambera A, Legrenzi L, et al. Comparison of finasteride versus flutamide in the treatment of hirsutism. *Eur J Endocrinol* 1999;141:361–367.
17. Muderris II, Bayram F, Guven M. A prospective, randomized trial comparing flutamide (250 mg/d) and finasteride (5 mg/d) in the treatment of hirsutism. *Fertil Steril* 2000;73:984–987.
18. Moran LJ, Noakes M, Clifton PM, et al. Dietary composition in restoring reproductive and metabolic physiology in overweight women with polycystic ovary syndrome. *J Clin Endocrinol Metab* 2003;88:812–819.
19. Pasquali R, Gambineri A, Biscotti D, et al. Effect of long-term treatment with metformin added to hypocaloric diet on body composition, fat distribution, and androgen and insulin levels in abdominally obese women with and without the polycystic ovary syndrome. *J Clin Endocrinol Metab* 2000;85:2767–2774.
20. Moghetti P, Castello R, Negri C, et al. Metformin effects on clinical features, endocrine and metabolic profiles, and insulin sensitivity in polycystic ovary syndrome: a randomized, double-blind, placebo-controlled 6-month trial, followed by open, long-term clinical evaluation. *J Clin Endocrinol Metab* 2000;85:139–146.
21. Farquhar C, Lee O, Toomath R, et al. Spironolactone versus placebo or in combination with steroids for hirsutism and/or acne (Cochrane Review). In: The Cochrane Library, Issue 2, 2003. Oxford: Update Software. Search date not reported, primary sources Medline, Bioabstracts, Psychlit, Cinahl, Social Sciences Index, Dissertation Abstracts, Current Contents, Embase, and hand searches of reference lists of relavant trials and personal contact with drug companies.

Hesham Al-Inany
Cairo University
Cairo
Egypt

Competing interests: None reported.

Pyelonephritis in non-pregnant women

Search date July 2003

Adriana Wechsler

QUESTIONS

INTERVENTIONS

*Categorisation is not based on placebo controlled RCTs. Such studies are likely to be considered unethical.

Key Messages

- **Intravenous antibiotics in women admitted to hospital with uncomplicated infection** We found no RCTs comparing intravenous antibiotics versus no antibiotics. Consensus holds that intravenous antibiotics are effective, and it is unlikely that a placebo controlled RCT would now be performed. One RCT found no significant difference between intravenous ampicillin plus intravenous gentamicin and intravenous co-trimoxazole plus intravenous gentamicin for relief of symptoms and recurrence of bacteriuria at 28 days. We found insufficient evidence to compare clinical effects of different intravenous regimens.
- **Oral antibiotics for women with uncomplicated infection** We found no RCTs comparing oral antibiotics with no antibiotics. However, consensus holds that these drugs are effective, and it is unlikely that such an RCT would now be performed. One systematic review and one subsequent RCT in women with uncomplicated pyelonephritis (none of whom were admitted to hospital) have found no consistent differences between co-amoxiclav, or quinolones (ciprofloxacin, norfloxacin, levofloxacin, or lomefloxacin) in bacteriological or clinical cure rates. However, observational data suggest that broader spectrum antibiotics, such as quinolones, are more effective than narrow spectrum antibiotics such as amoxicillin and trimethoprim–sulphamethoxazole in areas with high prevalence of resistance to these drugs.
- **Relative effectiveness of different oral and antibiotic regimens, inpatient versus outpatient management, intravenous versus oral antibiotics** We found no RCTs in women with acute uncomplicated pyelonephritis.

Pyelonephritis in non-pregnant women

DEFINITION	Acute pyelonephritis, or upper urinary tract infection, is an infection of the kidney characterised by pain when passing urine, fever, flank pain, nausea, and vomiting. White blood cells are almost always present in the urine and occasionally white blood cell casts are also seen on urine microscopy. There is no real consensus on the definitions for grades of severity. However, people with acute pyelonephritis may be divided into those able to take oral antibiotics and without signs of sepsis, who may be managed at home, and those requiring intravenous antibiotics in hospital. There is little difference in the application of treatments between men and non-pregnant women.
INCIDENCE/ PREVALENCE	In the USA, there are 250 000 cases of acute pyelonephritis a year.[1] Worldwide prevalence and incidence are unknown.
AETIOLOGY/ RISK FACTORS	Pyelonephritis is most commonly caused when bacteria in the bladder ascend the ureters and invade the kidneys. In some cases, this may result in bacteria entering and multiplying in the bloodstream. People with structural or functional urinary tract abnormalities are more prone to pyelonephritis that is refractory to oral therapy or complicated by bacteraemia. Repeated urinary tract infections also predispose them to drug resistant organisms.
PROGNOSIS	Complications include urosepsis, renal impairment, and renal abscess. Conditions such as underlying renal disease, diabetes mellitus, and immunosuppression may worsen prognosis, but we found no good long term evidence about rates of sepsis or death among people with such conditions.
AIMS OF INTERVENTION	To reduce the duration and severity of symptoms; to prevent or minimise potential complications, with minimum adverse effects.
OUTCOMES	Urine culture after treatment; signs and symptoms of infection; rates of complications of infection; and adverse effects of treatment.
METHODS	*Clinical Evidence* search and appraisal July 2003. We excluded studies that were primarily in men, pregnant women, and people with complicated pyelonephritis, or prone to pyelonephritis because of indwelling catheters, or anatomical or functional bladder abnormalities. Most studies examined both men and women and we have stated how many women were included when available.

QUESTION What are the effects of treatments for acute pyelonephritis?

OPTION ORAL ANTIBIOTICS FOR WOMEN WITH UNCOMPLICATED INFECTION

We found no RCTs comparing oral antibiotics with no antibiotics. However, consensus holds that these drugs are effective, and it is unlikely that such an RCT would now be performed. One systematic review and one subsequent RCT in women with uncomplicated pyelonephritis (some of whom were admitted to hospital) have found no consistent differences between co-amoxiclav, or a quinolone (ciprofloxacin, norfloxacin, levofloxacin, or lomefloxacin) in bacteriological or clinical cure rates. However, observational data suggest that broader spectrum antibiotics, such as quinolones, are more effective than narrow spectrum antibiotics such as amoxicillin and trimethoprim–sulphamethoxazole in areas with high prevalence of resistance to these drugs.

Benefits: **Versus placebo:** We found no systematic review or RCTs. **Oral antibiotics versus each other:** We found one systematic review (search date 1991, 9 RCTs, 470 men and non-pregnant women) (see table 1, p 2454),[2] and one subsequent RCT[3] comparing different oral antibiotics in acute pyelonephritis. Five RCTs identified by the review were conducted in people outside hospital and four in people admitted to hospital. The studies were conducted in the USA, Europe, and Peru. All RCTs included in the review included more women than men. Most excluded people with complicating factors such as structural abnormalities of the urinary tract, additional diseases, pregnancy, or signs of possible sepsis. All but one of the RCTs in the review found no significant difference between different antibiotics in rates of early cure (negative urine culture within 7–10 days), and six of the RCTs found no significant difference in rates of late cure (negative urine culture 2–4 weeks or more after stopping treatment). However, several of the included RCTs were too small to rule out a clinically important difference between antibiotic regimens. The subsequent RCT (186 people with acute uncomplicated pyelonephritis treated at home) compared oral levofloxacin (250 mg/day for 10 days) versus either oral ciprofloxacin (500 mg twice daily for 10 days) or oral lomefloxacin (400 mg/day for 14 days) and found similar clinical cure rates for all three antibiotics (92% with levofloxacin *v* 88% with ciprofloxacin *v* 80% with lomefloxacin; significance not reported).[3] **Oral versus intravenous antibiotics:** We found no RCTs in women with uncomplicated pyelonephritis.

Harms: The subsequent RCT reported adverse effects in 3/124 (2%) people taking levofloxacin, 6/80 (8%) people taking ciprofloxacin, and 3/55 (5%) people taking lomefloxacin.[3] Gastrointestinal symptoms were common with both ciprofloxacin and levofloxacin, whereas rash was the most common adverse effect with lomefloxacin. One of the 186 people discontinued treatment (lomefloxacin) because of adverse effects.[3]

Comment: The lack of placebo-controlled RCTs may reflect the fact that experimental trials would be considered unethical. **Cure rates:** Calculated cure rates from the systematic review comparing the oral antibiotic regimens are likely to overestimate rates that would be achieved in clinical practice, because many people were excluded from the studies, including those who experienced adverse effects, had growth of resistant bacteria on initial culture, or did not adhere to treatment.[2] **Antibiotic resistance:** Consensus does not recommend ampicillin or amoxicillin (amoxycillin), because of concerns about increasing bacterial resistance. One UK multicentre study (108 people; 87 women) found that *Escherichia coli* was the most prevalent organism (68.5%), followed by *Klebsiella pneumoniae* (6.5%) and *Enterococcus faecalis* (6.5%).[4] It found a high rate of ampicillin resistance (40%). *E coli*, the most common pathogen in pyelonephritis, had low susceptibility to tetracycline, sulphamethoxazole, and trimethoprim, although it had 95% susceptibility to ciprofloxacin and nitrofurantoin.[4] *K pneumoniae*, however, was highly resistant to nitrofurantoin. Susceptibility patterns were not separated out by type of urinary tract infection, making it hard to interpret these results specifically for pyelonephritis. Recent recommendations by the Infectious Disease Society of America and the European Society of Clinical Microbiology and Infectious Disease warn against the empiric use of trimethoprim–sulfamethoxazole in geographical areas where resistance reaches 10–20%.[5] These recommendations are based on two studies, which found that women with acute pyelonephritis caused by organisms that were resistant to trimethoprim–sulphamethoxazole had significantly lower clinical cure rates with trimethoprim–sulphamethoxazole compared with women in whom the causative organism was not resistant (88–92% clinical cure with non-resistant organisms *v* 35–54%, cure with resistant organisms; $P < 0.01$).[6,7]

OPTION — INTRAVENOUS ANTIBIOTICS (AMPICILLIN, CO-TRIMOXAZOLE) IN WOMEN ADMITTED TO HOSPITAL WITH UNCOMPLICATED INFECTION

We found no RCTs comparing intravenous antibiotics versus no antibiotics. Consensus holds that intravenous antibiotics are effective, and it is unlikely that a placebo controlled RCT would now be performed. We found insufficient evidence to compare clinical effects of different intravenous regimens. One RCT found no significant difference between intravenous ampicillin and intravenous co-trimoxazole, both combined with intravenous gentamicin, in terms of relief of symptoms and recurrence of bacteriuria at 28 days.

Benefits: **Versus placebo:** We found no systematic review and no RCTs. **Intravenous antibiotics versus each other:** We found no systematic review. We found one RCT (85 women admitted to hospital for acute uncomplicated pyelonephritis; see comment below), which compared intravenous ampicillin (1 g every 6 hours) versus intravenous co-trimoxazole (160 mg/800 mg twice daily), initiated before culture results were known.[8] Both regimens were combined with intravenous gentamicin and followed by oral treatment with either ampicillin or co-trimoxazole. The RCT found that symptoms of infection resolved in all women who completed the trial, but found no significant difference between ampicillin and co-trimoxazole in the recurrence of bacteria in the urine after 28 days (1/20 [5%] with ampicillin *v* 2/27 [7%] with co-trimoxazole; RR 0.70, 95% CI 0.07 to 6.94). We found no other reliable RCTs comparing treatments that included intravenous quinolones, cephalosporins, broad spectrum β lactams, or co-trimoxazole. **Intravenous plus oral antibiotics versus oral antibiotics alone:** We found one RCT (118 women admitted with acute uncomplicated pyelonephritis), which compared a single dose of intravenous tobramycin (2 mg/kg) plus oral ciprofloxacin (500 mg twice daily for 10 days) versus oral ciprofloxacin plus intravenous placebo (0.9% saline solution).[9] Clinical success or failure was assessed, with failure defined as the persistence of fever or pain after 48 hours of treatment and success, the absence of these. The RCT found no significant difference in rates of clinical success (58/60 [97%] with intravenous tobramycin plus oral ciprofloxacin *v* 54/58 [93%] with oral ciprofloxacin plus placebo; RR 1.04, 95% CI 0.95 to 1.13). **Intravenous versus oral antibiotics:** We found no RCTs in women with uncomplicated pyelonephritis.

Harms: **Intravenous antibiotics versus each other:** The RCT comparing intravenous regimens found no significant difference between treatment adverse effects (10/32 [32%] with ampicillin *v* 13/39 [33%] with co-trimoxazole; RR 0.90, 95% CI 0.48 to 1.85).[9] Common adverse effects with ampicillin include rash, diarrhoea, and vaginitis, and with co-trimoxazole include nausea, vomiting, and vaginitis. **Intravenous plus oral antibiotics versus oral antibiotics alone:** The RCT comparing intravenous tobramycin plus ciprofloxacin versus ciprofloxacin plus placebo reported that "no undesirable side effects were observed".[9] No further details were reported.

Comment: RCTs comparing antibiotics versus placebo would be considered unethical in women with uncomplicated pyelonephritis. The RCT comparing intravenous regimens reported that 47/85 (55%) women completed the trial to the 28 days' follow up assessment; 14/42 (33%) women receiving ampicillin were infected with ampicillin resistant isolates and were withdrawn from the study.[8] There is a consensus view that the choice of empirical antibiotics should take into account the setting, medical history of the patient, Gram stain of the urine, previous infecting organism, and local antibiotic sensitivities. We found two RCTs (258 adults with complicated urinary tract infection or either uncomplicated or complicated pyelonephritis, 58% women and 592 adults, 70% women) comparing intravenous ertapenem with intravenous ceftriaxone.[10,11] Neither RCT found any significant difference between treatments in microbiologic and clinical cure rates, though the first RCT was limited by inclusion of only three quarters of the participants in the final analysis.[11]

OPTION INPATIENT VERSUS OUTPATIENT MANAGEMENT

We found no RCTs comparing inpatient with outpatient management of women with acute uncomplicated pyelonephritis.

Benefits: We found no systematic review and no RCTs.

Harms: We found no RCTs.

Comment: Hospitals might be able to provide closer monitoring and supervision of people with pyelonephritis than can be provided outside hospital. However, we found no RCTs to clarify whether treatment in hospital delivers any benefit in terms of outcomes or whether there is an increased risk of harm from hospital treatment.

REFERENCES

1. Stamm WE, Hooton TM, Johnson JR. Urinary tract infection: from pathogenesis to treatment. *J Infect Dis* 1989;15:400–406.
2. Pinson AG, Philbrick JT, Lindbeck GH, et al. Oral antibiotic therapy for acute pyelonephritis: a methodologic review of the literature. *J Gen Intern Med* 1992;7:544–553. Search date 1991; primary sources Medline and Current Contents.
3. Richard GA, Klimberg IN, Fowler CL, et al. Levofloxacin versus ciprofloxacin versus lomefloxacin in acute pyelonephritis. *Urology* 1998;52:51–55.
4. Farrell DJ, Morrissey I, De Rubeis D, et al. A UK multicentre study of the antimicrobial susceptibility of bacterial pathogens causing urinary tract infection. *J Infect* 2003;46:94–100.
5. Hoiby N, Tvede M. Therapeutic failure with trimethoprim+sulfamethoxazole in uncomplicated acute bacterial cystitis and pyelonephritis in women with resistant bacteria. *Ugeskr Laeger* 2002;164:4672–4673. [In Danish]
6. Talan DA, Stamm WE, Hooton TM, et al. Comparison of ciprofloxacin (7 days) and trimothoprim-sulfamethoxazole (14 days) for acute uncomplicated pyelonephritis in women: a randomized trial. *JAMA* 2000;283:1583–1590.
7. Raz R, Chazan B, Kennes Y, et al. Empiric use of trimthoprim–sulfamethoxazole (TMP–SMX) in the treatment of women with uncomplicated urinary tract infections, in a geographical area with high prevalence of TMP–SMX-resistant uropathogens. *Clin Infect Dis* 2002;34:1165–1169.
8. Johnson JR, Lyons MF, Pearce W, et al. Therapy for women hospitalized with acute pyelonephritis: a randomized trial of ampicillin versus trimethoprim–sulfamethoxazole for 14 days. *J Infect Dis* 1991;163:325–330.
9. Le Conte P, Simon N, Bourrier P, et al. Acute pyelonephritis. Randomized multicentre double-blind study comparing ciprofloxacin with combined ciprofloxacin and tobramycin. *Presse Med* 2001;30:11–15. [In French]
10. Jimenez-Cruz F, Jasovich A, Cajigas J, et al. A prospective, multicenter, randomized, double-blind study comparing ertapenem and ceftriaxone followed by appropriate oral therapy for complicated urinary tract infections in adults. *Urology* 2002;60:16–22.
11. Tomera KM, Burdmann EA, Reyna OG, et al. Ertapenem versus ceftriaxone followed by appropriate oral therapy for treatment of complicated urinary tract infections in adults: results of a prospective, randomized, double-blind multicenter study. *Antimicrob Agents Chemother* 2002;46:2895–2900.

Adriana Wechsler
M.D.
Baylor College of Medicine
Houston, Texas
USA

Competing interests: None declared.

We would like to acknowledge the previous contributors of this chapter, including Lisa Chew, Stephan Finn, Ruth Jepson, Bruce Cooper, and Bazian Ltd.

TABLE 1 Oral antibiotic treatment for acute pyelonephritis: results of RCTs (see text, p 2450).[2]

Oral antibiotic regimens	Total number of people	Early cure* rates %	Late cure* rates %	P value
Amoxicillin 500 mg three times daily for 14 days	16	NA	94	NS
Co-trimoxazole 160 mg/800 mg twice daily for 14 days	12	NA	92	
Norfloxacin 400 mg twice daily for 10 days	14	100	86	NS
Co-trimoxazole 160 mg/800 mg twice daily for 10 days	10	100	90	
Ampicillin 500 mg four times daily for 10 days	8	88	NA	NS
Cefaclor 250 mg twice daily for 10 days	6	67	NA	
Norfloxacin 400 mg twice daily for 7 days or longer	3	67	NA	NS
Co-trimoxazole 160 mg/800 mg twice daily for 7 days or longer	12	92	NA	
Co-amoxiclav 250 mg/125 mg three times daily for 10 days	54	94	85	P = 0.02 for late cure; NS for early cure
Co-trimoxazole 160 mg/800 mg twice daily for 10 days	50	82	64	
Ampicillin 500 mg four times daily for 2 or 6 weeks	17	100	47	P = 0.004 for late cure; NS for early cure
Co-trimoxazole 160 mg/800 mg twice daily for 2 or 6 weeks	22	100	91	
Amoxicillin 2000 mg one time dose then 1000 mg twice daily for 9 days	22	100	100	NS
Amoxicillin 750 mg three times daily for 12 days	23	96	87	
Cefetamet 2000 mg once daily or 1000 mg twice daily for 10–15 days	28	93	79	NS
Cefadroxil 1000 mg twice daily for 10–15 days	22	73	52	
Norfloxacin 400 mg twice daily for 14 days	76	91	82	P < 0.0001 for both early and late cures
Cefadroxil 1000 mg twice daily for 14 days	75	59	44	

*Early cure: negative urine culture within 7–10 days of starting treatment; late cure: negative urine culture 2–4 weeks or more after stopping treatment. NA, not available; NS, not significant. Pinson AG, Philbrick JT, Lindbeck GH, et al. Oral antibiotic therapy for acute pyelonephritis; a methodologic review of the literature. *J Gen Intern Med* 1992;7:544–553. Reprinted by permission of Blackwell Science, Inc.

Recurrent cystitis in non-pregnant women

Search date April 2003

Adriana Wechsler

QUESTIONS

INTERVENTIONS

Key Messages

- **Continuous antibiotic prophylaxis (trimethoprim, co-trimoxazole, nitrofurantoin, cefaclor, or a quinolone)** RCTs have found that continuous antibiotic prophylaxis for 6–12 months with trimethoprim, co-trimoxazole, nitrofurantoin, cefaclor, or a quinolone reduces rates of recurrent cystitis compared with placebo, and have found no consistent difference in recurrence rates among different continuous regimens. One RCT comparing continuous daily antibiotic prophylaxis versus postcoital antibiotic prophylaxis found no significant difference in rates of positive urine culture after 1 year.
- **Postcoital antibiotic prophylaxis (co-trimoxazole, nitrofurantoin, or a quinolone)** RCTs have found that co-trimoxazole, nitrofurantoin, or a quinolone up to 2 hours after sexual intercourse reduces the rates of cystitis compared with placebo. One RCT comparing continuous daily antibiotic prophylaxis versus postcoital antibiotic prophylaxis found no significant difference in rates of positive urine culture after 1 year.
- **Cranberry juice and cranberry products** One systematic review of two weak RCTs provided insufficient evidence to assess cranberry juice and other cranberry products in women with recurrent cystitis.
- **Prophylaxis with methenamine hippurate** One systematic review of weak RCTs provided insufficient evidence to assess methenamine hippurate (hexamine hippurate) in women with recurrent cystitis.
- **Single dose self administered co-trimoxazole** One small RCT that single dose, self administered co-trimoxazole started at the onset of cystitis symptoms was less effective in reducing recurrence rates over 1 year than continuous co-trimoxazole prophylaxis. However, evidence was too limited to draw firm conclusions.

Recurrent cystitis in non-pregnant women

DEFINITION Cystitis is an infection of the lower urinary tract, which causes pain when passing urine, and causes frequency, urgency, haematuria, or suprapubic pain not associated with passing urine. White blood cells and bacteria are almost always present in the urine. The presence of fever, flank pain, nausea, or vomiting suggests pyelonephritis (upper urinary tract infection) (see pyelonephritis in non-pregnant women, p 2449). Recurrent cystitis may be either a reinfection (after successful eradication of infection) or a relapse after inadequate treatment.

INCIDENCE/ PREVALENCE The incidence of cystitis among premenopausal sexually active women is 0.5–0.7 infections per person year,[1] and 20–40% of women will experience cystitis during their lifetime. Of those, 20% will develop recurrence, almost always (90% of cases) because of reinfection rather than relapse. Rates of infection fall during the winter months.[2]

AETIOLOGY/ RISK FACTORS Cystitis is caused by uropathogenic bacteria in the faecal flora that colonise the vaginal and periurethral openings, and ascend the urethra into the bladder. Prior infection, sexual intercourse, and exposure to vaginal spermicide are risk factors for developing cystitis.[3,4]

PROGNOSIS We found little evidence on the long term effects of untreated cystitis. One study found that progression to pyelonephritis was infrequent, and that most cases of cystitis regressed spontaneously, although symptoms sometimes persisted for several months.[5] Women with a baseline rate of more than two infections a year, over many years, are likely to have ongoing recurrent infections.[6]

AIMS OF INTERVENTION To prevent recurrent cystitis in women predisposed to frequent infections, with minimal adverse effects of treatment.

OUTCOMES Rate of infection based on symptoms and urine culture.

METHODS *Clinical Evidence* search and appraisal January 1998 to April 2003. We reviewed all systematic reviews and RCTs comparing different forms of prophylaxis, or comparing prophylaxis versus placebo in non-pregnant women with a history of recurrent cystitis. We excluded studies in populations consisting mainly of men or pregnant women.

QUESTION **Which interventions prevent further recurrence of cystitis in women experiencing at least two infections per year?**

OPTION **CONTINUOUS ANTIBIOTIC PROPHYLAXIS (TRIMETHOPRIM, CO-TRIMOXAZOLE, NITROFURANTOIN, CEFACLOR, OR A QUINOLONE)**

RCTs have found that continuous antibiotic prophylaxis for 6–12 months with trimethoprim, co-trimoxazole, nitrofurantoin, cefaclor, or a quinolone reduces rates of recurrent cystitis compared with placebo, and have found no consistent difference in recurrence rates among different continuous regimens. One RCT comparing postcoital versus continuous daily antibiotic prophylaxis found no significant difference in rates of positive urine culture after 1 year.

Benefits: We found no systematic review. We found eight RCTs (in women with at least 2 episodes of cystitis per year) comparing different regimens for continuous antibiotic prophylaxis lasting 6–12 months (see table 1, p 2461).[7–14] **Versus placebo or no treatment:** Four of the RCTs (225 women) found that active treatment (co-trimoxazole, nitrofurantoin, or a quinolone) significantly reduced rates of cystitis compared with placebo or no treatment.[7–9] **Versus each other:** One RCT (72 women) found that women taking oral nitrofurantoin (100 mg at night) compared with oral trimethoprim (100 mg at night) had significantly fewer episodes of cystitis after 12 months ($P < 0.05$; absolute numbers not reported).[10] Four other RCTs compared different antibiotic regimens versus each other and found no significant difference in numbers of infections among treatments over 6–12 months.[7,11–13] **Versus postcoital prophylaxis:** One RCT (135 women) compared daily oral ciprofloxacin (125 mg) versus postcoital (within 2 hours of sexual intercourse) oral ciprofloxacin (125 mg) (see benefits of postcoital prophylaxis, p 2457). It found no significant difference in the number of positive urine cultures after 1 year (27/239 [11%] positive urine cultures with daily prophylaxis v 32/254 [13%] with postcoital prophylaxis; RR 0.9, 95% CI 0.55 to 1.45).[8]

Harms: Rates of adverse effects in the RCTs ranged from 7–40% for trimethoprim, 0–40% for nitrofurantoin, 5% for cefaclor, 7–21% for norfloxacin, and 13% for ciprofloxacin.[7–9,11–13] The most common adverse effects for all agents were gastrointestinal symptoms, rash, and yeast vaginitis. One cohort study (see comment below) reported no significant adverse effects in women taking trimethoprim, co-trimoxazole, or nitrofurantoin, even when treatment continued for as long as 5 years. The development of bacterial resistance from continuous antibiotic prophylaxis was rare. However, the number of co-trimoxazole resistant infections increased during the latter part of the study.[2]

Comment: Many of the RCTs were not placebo controlled or blinded, and had small study populations. However, most of the reported rates of infection in the RCTs comparing different antibiotic regimens versus each other were much less than 0.6 per person year, suggesting that they were all effective in reducing the rate of infection in people with a history of recurrent cystitis.[7,10–13] These studies were not powered to exclude a clinically important difference between treatments, and adjustments were not made for confounding factors such as frequency of sexual intercourse. We found one cohort study (51 non-pregnant women with a baseline rate of more than 2 urinary tract infections a year over many years), which compared continuous treatment with three different antibiotics (trimethoprim, co-trimoxazole, or nitrofurantoin) for more than 12 months.[2] It found that all were effective in preventing both cystitis and pyelonephritis for over 112 person years.

OPTION POSTCOITAL ANTIBIOTIC PROPHYLAXIS

RCTs have found that co-trimoxazole, nitrofurantoin, or a quinolone up to 2 hours after sexual intercourse reduces the rates of cystitis compared with placebo. One RCT comparing postcoital versus continuous daily antibiotic prophylaxis found no significant difference in rates of cystitis after 1 year.

Benefits: We found no systematic review. **Versus placebo or no treatment:** We found four RCTs (in women with at least 2 episodes of cystitis per year) comparing postcoital (within 2 hours of sexual intercourse) antibiotic regimens versus placebo or no treatment evaluated over 6–14 months.[8,15–17] All four RCTs found that active treatment (co-trimoxazole, nitrofurantoin, or a quinolone) significantly reduced rates of cystitis (see table 2, p 2462). **Versus continuous daily prophylaxis:** See benefits of continuous antibiotic prophylaxis, p 2456.

Harms: Rates of adverse effects were as follows: co-trimoxazole 18%, ciprofloxacin 6%, and nitrofurantoin less than 1%.[8,15–17] The most common adverse effects for all agents were gastrointestinal symptoms, rash, and yeast vaginitis.

Comment: Only one of the studies was placebo controlled and blinded.[15] Adjustments were not made for confounding factors such as frequency of sexual intercourse.

OPTION SINGLE DOSE SELF ADMINISTERED CO-TRIMOXAZOLE

One small RCT found that single dose, self administered co-trimoxazole started at the onset of cystitis symptoms was less effective in reducing recurrence rates over 1 year than continuous co-trimoxazole prophylaxis. However, evidence was too limited to draw firm conclusions.

Recurrent cystitis in non-pregnant women

Benefits: We found no systematic review but found one RCT (38 non-pregnant women with 2 or more culture documented urinary tract infections in the previous 12 months; see comment below).[18] The RCT compared continuous oral co-trimoxazole prophylaxis (40 mg/200 mg) versus single dose, self administered co-trimoxazole (40 mg/200 mg) to be taken at the onset of cystitis symptoms. It found that single dose co-trimoxazole was significantly less effective in reducing the number of episodes of cystitis compared with continuous co-trimaxazole (2.2 infections per person year with treatment at onset of symptoms *v* 0.22 infections per person year with continuous prophylaxis; $P < 0.001$; see comment below).

Harms: The RCT reported a total of eight adverse reactions; five in women taking continuous antibiotic prophylaxis compared with three in women taking single dose treatment (CI not reported).[18] Adverse reactions included mild nausea, abdominal pain, rash, mouth ulcers, and yeast vulvovaginitis.

Comment: The RCT reported that 10/38 (26%) women did not complete the full study protocol, and it is not clear whether analysis of results was by intention to treat.[18] It found that the women were almost always able to diagnose their own episodes of cystitis from symptoms (positive predictive value 92%). The higher rate of cystitis in women using single dose prophylaxis is to be expected because treatment was only administered after the onset of symptoms.

OPTION CRANBERRY JUICE AND CRANBERRY PRODUCTS

One systematic review of two weak RCTs provided insufficient evidence to assess cranberry juice and other cranberry products in women with recurrent cystitis.

Benefits: We found one systematic review (search date 2001, 2 RCTs, 211 women) comparing cranberry juice or other cranberry products versus placebo in the prevention of urinary tract infections (see comment below).[19] The first RCT (19 women with recurrent cystitis) included in the review compared cranberry capsules versus placebo (see comment below). The review reported 21 infections among 10 women who completed the study; six of these infections occurred in women taking cranberry capsules (the number of infections/women in the different groups was not reported; significance testing not possible). The second RCT (192 elderly women) compared cranberry juice versus placebo and found that cranberry juice significantly reduced the rate of infection (defined as ≥ 100 000 organisms/mL of urine plus white blood cells in the urine; OR 0.42, $P = 0.004$; see comment below).

Harms: The review gave no information on adverse effects.[19]

Comment: The RCTs identified by the review were small, with high withdrawal rates (47% in the first RCT and 20% in the second RCT), and the lack of intention to treat analyses in either trial may mean that they overestimated the effectiveness of cranberry juice and products.[19] High withdrawal rates suggest that long term adherence may be difficult to achieve.

OPTION PROPHYLAXIS WITH METHENAMINE HIPPURATE

One systematic review of weak RCTs provided insufficient evidence to assess methenamine hippurate (hexamine hippurate) in women with recurrent cystitis.

Benefits: We found one systematic review (search date 2000, 3 RCTs, 372 women) comparing methenamine hippurate versus placebo or antibiotics.[20] The review concluded that there was insufficient evidence about effects of methenamine hippurate (see comment below).

Harms: We found no reliable RCTs.

Comment: The review found three RCTs comparing methenamine hippurate versus placebo or versus antibiotics in women with recurrent urinary tract infection.[20] All had important problems with their methods, principally that each participant could contribute more than once to assessment of recurrence rate.[21–23] Two of the included RCTs were small (30 and 52 women with recurrent lower urinary tract infection).[21,22] Both found that methenamine hippurate reduced recurrence compared with placebo (monthly recurrence rate 0.03–0.08 episodes per month with methenamine hippurate *v* 0.25–0.34 episodes per month with placebo; CI not reported).[21,22] The largest of the RCTs (290 people [92% women] with recurrent urinary tract infection) also included women with chronic pyelonephritis. It found that methenamine hippurate reduced recurrence of cystitis compared with placebo after 1 year (recurrence was observed on 34% of tests in women receiving methenamine hippurate *v* 63.2% with placebo; CI not reported).[23]

REFERENCES

1. Hooton TM, Scholes D, Hughes JP, et al. A prospective study of risk factors for symptomatic urinary tract infection in young women. *N Engl J Med* 1996;335:468–474.
2. Stamm WE, McKevitt M, Roberts PL, et al. Natural history of recurrent urinary tract infections in women. *Rev Infect Dis* 1991;13:77–84.
3. Fihn SD, Latham RH, Roberts P, et al. Association between diaphragm use and urinary tract infection. *JAMA* 1985;254:240–245.
4. Fihn SD, Boyko EJ, Normand EH, et al. Association between use of spermicide-coated condoms and *Escherichia coli* urinary tract infection in young women. *Am J Epidemiol* 1996;144:512–520.
5. Mabeck CE. Treatment of uncomplicated urinary tract infection in non-pregnant women. *Postgrad Med J* 1972;48:69–75.
6. Stamm WE, Counts GW, McKevitt M, et al. Urinary prophylaxis with trimethoprim and trimethoprim-sulfamethoxazole: efficacy, influence on the natural history of recurrent bacteriuria and cost control. *Rev Infect Dis* 1982;4:450–455.
7. Stamm WE, Counts GW, Wagner KF, et al. Antimicrobial prophylaxis of recurrent urinary tract infections: a double-blind placebo-controlled trial. *Ann Intern Med* 1980;92:770–775.
8. Melekos MD, Asbach HW, Gerharz E, et al. Post-intercourse versus daily ciprofloxacin prophylaxis for recurrent urinary tract infections in premenopausal women. *J Urol* 1997;157:935–939.
9. Nicolle LE, Harding GKM, Thompson M, et al. Prospective, randomized, placebo-controlled trial of norfloxacin for the prophylaxis of recurrent urinary tract infection in women. *Antimicrob Agents Chemother* 1989;33:1032–1035.
10. Brumfitt W, Smith GW, Hamilton-Miller JMT, et al. A clinical comparison between macrodantin and trimethoprim for prophylaxis in women with recurrent urinary infection. *J Antimicrob Chemother* 1985;16:111–120.
11. Raz R, Boger S. Long-term prophylaxis with norfloxacin versus nitrofurantoin in women with recurrent urinary tract infection. *Antimicrob Agents Chemother* 1991;35:1241–1242.
12. Brumfitt W, Hamilton-Miller JMT, Smith GW, et al. Comparative trial of norfloxacin and macrocrystalline nitrofurantoin (Macrodantin) in the prophylaxis of recurrent urinary tract infection in women. *Q J Med* 1991;81:811–820.
13. Brumfitt W, Hamilton-Miller JMT. A comparative trial of low-dose cefaclor and macrocrystalline nitrofurantoin in the prevention of recurrent urinary tract infection. *Infection* 1995;23:98–102.
14. Martorana C, Giberti C, Damonte P: Preventive treatment of recurring cystitis in women. Double-blind randomised study using cinoxacin and placebo. *Minerva Urol Nefrol* 1984;36:43–49.
15. Stapleton A, Latham RH, Johnson C, et al. Postcoital antimicrobial prophylaxis for recurrent urinary tract infection: a randomized, double-blind placebo-controlled trial. *JAMA* 1990;264:703–706.
16. Pfau A, Sacks TG. Effective postcoital quinolone prophylaxis of recurrent urinary tract infection in women. *J Urol* 1994;152:136–138.
17. Pfau A, Sacks T, Englestein D. Recurrent urinary tract infections in premenopausal women: prophylaxis based on an understanding of the pathogenesis. *J Urol* 1983;129:1153–1156.
18. Wong ES, McKevitt M, Running K, et al. Management of recurrent urinary tract infections with patient-administered single-dose therapy. *Ann Intern Med* 1985;102:302–307.
19. Jepson RG, Mihaljevic L, Craig J. Cranberries for preventing urinary tract infections. In: The Cochrane Library, Issue 3, 2002. Oxford: Update Software. Search date 2001; primary sources Cochrane Collaboration Field in Complementary Medicine Registry of randomised trials, Cochrane Controlled Trials Register (CCTR) and CENTRAL, Psychlit, LILACS, Cinahl, Medline, Embase, Biological Abstracts, Current Contents, the Internet, hand searches of reference lists of review articles and relevant trials, conference abstracts from relevant meetings, and personal contact with companies involved with the manufacture of cranberry preparations.
20. Lee B, Bhuta T, Craig J, et al. Methenamine hippurate for preventing urinary tract infections. In: The Cochrane Library, Issue 3, 2002. Oxford: Update Software. Search date 2000; primary sources Cochrane Controlled Trials Register, Medline, Embase, Cinahl, Current Contents, reference lists of review articles, and retrieved trials. The manufacturers of methenamine salts were contacted for unpublished studies, and contact was made with known investigators in the area.
21. Hoivik HO, Gundersen R, Osmundsen K, et al. Prevention of recurrent cystitis in fertile women. A double-blind comparison of hiprex and placebo in general practice. [Norwegian]. *Tidsskr Nor Laegeforen* 1984;104:1150–1152.

22. Gundersen R, Hoivik HO, Osmundsen K. Frequent cystitis in elderly women. A double-blind comparison of hiprex and placebo in general practice. [Norwegian]. *Tidsskr Nor Laegeforen* 1986;106:2048–2049.
23. Kasanen A, Junnila SY, Kaarsalo E, et al. Secondary prevention of recurrent urinary tract infections. Comparison of the effect of placebo, methenamine hippurate, nitrofurantoin and trimethoprim alone. *Scand J Infect Dis* 1982;14:293–296.

Adriana Wechsler
Assistant Professor of Medicine
Baylor College of Medicine
Houston, Texas
USA

Competing interests: None declared.

We would like to acknowledge the previous contributors of this chapter, including Lisa Chew, Bruce Cooper, Stephan Finn, Ruth Jepson, and Bazian Ltd.

TABLE 1 **Continuous antimicrobial prophylactic regimens for recurrent urinary tract infections: results of RCTs (see text, p 2456).**

Study design	Total number of people	Regimen	Duration of prophylaxis (months)	Infections per patient year	P value
Placebo controlled RCT[7]	60	Placebo	6	2.80	< 0.001 (drug treatment *v* placebo)
		Co-trimoxazole (40 mg/200 mg) at bedtime		0.15	
		Nitrofurantoin 100 mg at bedtime		0.14	
		Nitrofurantoin 100 mg at bedtime		0	
No treatment controlled and comparative RCT[8]	135	Without prophylaxis	12	3.62–3.66	< 0.001
		Ciprofloxacin 125 mg postcoital		0.043	
		Ciprofloxacin 125 mg daily		0.031	
Placebo controlled RCT[9]	30	Placebo	12	1.6	< 0.001
		Norfloxacin 200 mg at bedtime		0	
Comparative RCT[10]	72	Trimethoprim 100 mg at bedtime	12	1.00	< 0.05
		Nitrofurantoin 100 mg bedtime		0.17	
Comparative RCT[11]	94	Norfloxacin 200 mg at bedtime	6	0.04	= 0.05
		Nitrofurantoin 50 mg at bedtime		0.60	
Comparative RCT[12]	88	Norfloxacin 200 mg at bedtime	12	0.002	Not reported
		Nitrofurantoin 100 mg at bedtime		0.003	
Comparative RCT[13]	97	Cefaclor 250 mg at bedtime	12	0.006	Not reported
		Nitrofurantoin 50 mg at bedtime		0.006	
Placebo controlled RCT[14]	40	Cinoxacin 500 mg at bedtime	6		< 0.001 Cimoxacin *v* placebo

TABLE 2 Postcoital regimens for recurrent urinary tract infections: results of RCTs (see text, p 2457).

Study design	Total number of people	Regimen	Duration of prophylaxis (months)	Infections per patient year	P value
Placebo controlled RCT[15]	27	Placebo	6	3.6	= 0.0001
		Postcoital co-trimoxazole 40 mg/20 mg		0.3	
Comparative RCT[16]	33	Without prophylaxis	14	6.13	= 0.0000
		Postcoital prophylaxis with either ofloxacin 100 mg, norfloxacin 200 mg, or ciprofloxacin 125 mg		0.02	
Comparative RCT[8]	135	Without prophylaxis	12	3.62–3.66	< 0.0001
		Ciprofloxacin 125 mg daily		0.031	
		Ciprofloxacin 125 mg postcoital		0.043	
Comparative RCT[17]	56	Without prophylaxis	12	4.6	< 0.001
		Postcoital prophylaxis with either			
		Co-trimoxazole 80 mg/400 mg		0	
		Nitrofurantoin 50–100 mg		0.1	

Stress incontinence

Search date December 2003

Joseph Onwude

QUESTIONS

INTERVENTIONS

See glossary G

Key Messages

Non-surgical interventions

- **Oestrogen supplements (short term treatment only; effectiveness of long term treatment is uncertain, and may be associated with increased risk of stroke and endometrial cancer if unopposed, and breast cancer, coronary heart disease, and pulmonary embolism if combined with progestogen)** One systematic review found that short term treatment with oestrogen supplements improved cure or improvement rates compared with placebo. The review found that pelvic floor muscle exercises increased rates of cure or improvement compared with short term treatment with oestrogen supplements. It found no significant difference in rates of cure or improvement between pelvic floor electrical stimulation and short term treatment with oestrogen supplements, but it may have lacked the power to detect a clinically important difference. There are concerns about the safety of long term oestrogen use. One RCT found that combined oral oestrogen and progestogen supplements increased the risk of invasive breast cancer, coronary heart disease, stroke, and pulmonary embolism in postmenopausal women with a uterus at 5 years. One RCT found that oral oestrogen supplements increased the risk of stroke in women without a uterus at 6 years. There is limited evidence that unopposed oestrogen is associated with an increased risk of endometrial cancer in women with a uterus.

- **Pelvic floor electrical stimulation** RCTs found that pelvic floor electrical stimulation reduced symptoms compared with no treatment or sham pelvic floor electrical stimulation. One systematic review found no significant difference in cure or improvement rates at 12 months between pelvic floor electrical stimulation and pelvic floor muscle exercises. It found that pelvic floor electrical stimulation was associated with a small number of cases of vaginal irritation and difficulties in maintaining motivation for treatment. RCTs found no significant difference between pelvic floor electrical stimulation and vaginal cones in self reported cure or improvement rates, or in urinary leakage over 4 weeks to 12 months, but they may have lacked power to detect a clinically important difference. One systematic review found no significant difference in cure or improvement rates between pelvic floor electrical stimulation and oestrogen supplements, but it may have lacked the power to detect a clinically important difference.
- **Pelvic floor muscle exercises** One systematic review found that pelvic floor muscle exercises increased cure or improvement rates and reduced the number of leakages over 3–6 months compared with no treatment or placebo. It found no significant difference in cure or improvement rates at 12 months between pelvic floor muscle exercises and pelvic floor electrical stimulation. It found that pelvic floor muscle exercises reduced the number of leakage episodes at 6 months compared with vaginal cones, but there was no significant difference between treatments in cure or improvement rates at 12 months. One systematic review found that pelvic floor muscle exercises increased cure or improvement rates compared with oestrogen supplements.
- **Vaginal cones** One systematic review found that vaginal cones improved self reported cure or improvement rates compared with control over 6–12 months. It found no significant difference in leakage episodes. RCTs found no significant difference between vaginal cones and pelvic floor muscle exercises in self reported cure or improvement rates over 12 months. It found that vaginal cones were less effective than pelvic floor muscle exercises in reducing the number of leakage episodes over 6 months. RCTs also found no significant difference between vaginal cones and pelvic floor electrical stimulation in self reported cure or improvement rates, or in urinary leakage over 4 weeks to 12 months, but they may have lacked power to detect a clinically important difference. The most common adverse effect associated with vaginal cones was difficulty maintaining motivation for use, but a small number of more serious events such as vaginitis and abdominal pain were reported.

Surgical interventions

- **Laparoscopic colposuspension (similar cure rates to open retropubic colposuspension and tension free vaginal tape)** We found no RCTs comparing laparoscopic colposuspension versus no treatment, sham treatment, non-surgical treatment, anterior vaginal repair, suburethral slings, or needle colposuspension. One systematic review found that open retropubic colposuspension improved objective cure rates at 1 year compared with laparoscopic colposuspension. However, it found no significant difference in objective cure rates at 5 years, or in subjective cure rates at 1 or 5 years. One RCT identified by a review found a higher cure rate with tension free vaginal tape than with laparoscopic colposuspension at 6 months to 2 years, while two subsequent RCTs found no significant difference in cure rate between treatments at 6 weeks to 1 year.

- **Open retropubic colposuspension (higher cure rates than non-surgical treatment, anterior vaginal repair, or needle colposuspension, but more adverse effects than non-surgical treatment)** We found no RCTs comparing open retropubic colposuspension versus no treatment or sham treatment. One systematic review found that open retropubic colposuspension increased cure rates at 1–5 years compared with non-surgical treatment, anterior vaginal repair, or needle colposuspension. Open retropubic colposuspension was associated with more adverse effects than non-surgical treatment, but fewer surgical complications than needle colposuspension. It found that open retropubic colposuspension improved objective cure rates at 1 year compared with laparoscopic colposuspension. However, it found no significant difference in objective cure rates at 5 years, or in subjective cure rates at 1 or 5 years. It found no significant difference in cure rates at 1 year between open retropubic colposuspension and suburethral slings. One systematic review found no significant difference in cure rate between tension free vaginal tape and open retropubic colposuspension at up to 2 years. However, the included trials may have lacked power to exclude a clinically important difference in cure rates. RCTs included in the review found that open retropubic colposuspension was associated with a lower incidence of bladder perforation than tension free vaginal tape, but a higher incidence of postoperative fever.
- **Tension free vaginal tape (similar cure rates to open retropubic colposuspension and laparoscopic colposuspension)** We found no RCTs comparing tension free vaginal tape versus no treatment, sham treatment, non-surgical treatment, anterior vaginal repair, or needle colposuspension. One RCT found no significant difference in cure rates between tension free vaginal tape and suburethral slings at 12 months. One systematic review found no significant difference in cure rate between tension free vaginal tape and open retropubic colposuspension at up to 2 years. However, the included trials may have lacked statistical power to exclude a clinically important difference in cure rates. RCTs included in the review found that tension free vaginal tape was associated with a higher incidence of bladder perforation than open retropubic colposuspension, but a lower incidence of postoperative fever. One RCT identified by a systematic review found a higher cure rate with tension free vaginal tape than with laparoscopic colposuspension at 6–24 months, while two subsequent RCTs found no significant difference in cure rate between groups at 6 weeks to 1 year.
- **Suburethral slings other than tension free vaginal tape (similar cure rates to open retropubic colposuspension and needle colposuspension, but more perioperative complications than needle colposuspension)** We found no RCTs comparing suburethral slings versus no treatment, non-surgical treatment, anterior vaginal repair, or laparoscopic colposuspension. Five RCTs identified by a systematic review found no significant difference in cure rates between suburethral slings and open retropubic colposuspension at up to 6 years, although the studies may have lacked power to detect a clinically important difference. One small RCT identified by the review found no significant difference in cure rates at 1 year between suburethral slings and needle colposuspension, but it may have lacked power to detect a clinically important difference. The RCT found that suburethral slings increased perioperative complications compared with needle colposuspension. One RCT found no significant difference in subjective cure rates between tension free vaginal tape and suburethral slings at 12 months.
- **Anterior vaginal repair (lower cure rates than open retropubic colposuspension)** We found no RCTs comparing anterior vaginal repair (anterior colporrhaphy) versus no treatment, suburethral slings, tension free vaginal tape, or laparoscopic colposuspension. One RCT provided insufficient evidence to compare anterior vaginal repair versus non-surgical treatment. One systematic review found that anterior vaginal repair was less effective than open retropubic colposuspension in increasing cure rates at 12 months or 5 years, and found no significant difference in overall operative complications between the two procedures. It found no significant difference in cure rates at 12 months between anterior vaginal repair and needle colposuspension.

- **Needle colposuspension (lower cure rates and more surgical complications than open retropubic colposuspension)** We found no RCTs comparing needle colposuspension versus no treatment, non-surgical treatment, tension free vaginal tape, or laparoscopic colposuspension. One systematic review found no significant difference in cure rates between needle colposuspension and anterior vaginal repair or suburethral slings, but found that needle colposuspension was associated with fewer perioperative complications than suburethral slings. Another systematic review found that open retropubic colposuspension improved cure rates and was associated with fewer surgical complications than needle colposuspension at 5 years.

DEFINITION Stress incontinence is involuntary leakage on effort or exertion, or on sneezing or coughing.[1] Stress incontinence predominantly affects women, and can cause social and hygiene problems. Typically, there is no anticipatory feeling of needing to pass urine. Physiologically, stress incontinence is defined as intravesical pressure that exceeds urethral pressure in the absence of a detrusor contraction.

INCIDENCE/ PREVALENCE Stress incontinence is a common problem. Prevalence has been estimated at 17–45% of adult women in the setting of a high income country.[2] One cross-sectional study (15 308 women in Norway under the age of 65 years) found that the prevalence of stress incontinence was 4.7% in women who have not borne a child, 6.9% in women who had caesarian deliveries only, and 12.2% in women who had vaginal deliveries only.[3] During 2000–2001, about 10 000 operations on the outlet of the female bladder were carried out in England.[4] About 4000 were open abdominal operations, about 3000 were vaginal, about 1500 were endoscopic, and the rest were categorised as "other".

AETIOLOGY/ RISK FACTORS Aetiological factors include pregnancy, vaginal or caesarean delivery, cigarette smoking, and obesity.[3–7] One cross-sectional study (15 308 women in Norway) found that when compared with women who have not borne a child, the risk of stress incontinence was increased in women who have delivered by caesarean section (age adjusted OR 1.4, 95% CI 1.0 to 2.0) or by vaginal delivery (age adjusted OR 3.0, 95% CI 2.5 to 3.5).[3] The risk of stress incontinence was also increased in women who had a vaginal delivery compared with women who had a caesarean section (adjusted OR 2.4, 95% CI 1.7 to 3.2). One case control study (606 women) found that the risk of genuine stress incontinence was increased in former smokers (adjusted OR 2.20, 95% CI 1.18 to 4.11) and in current smokers (adjusted OR 2.48, 95% CI 1.60 to 3.84).[7] We found no reliable data measuring the risks associated with obesity.

PROGNOSIS We found no reliable data about the natural history of stress incontinence. Untreated stress incontinence is believed to be a persistent, lifelong condition.

AIMS OF INTERVENTION To improve quality of life and social function; to reduce embarrassment; and to reduce frequency and volume of involuntary urine leakage, with minimal adverse effects.

OUTCOMES **Primary outcomes:** quality of life, social functioning, subjective reduction in urine loss, and adverse effects of treatment. **Secondary outcomes:** reduced urine leakage on urodynamic testing, and pad tests(G) for objective demonstration of leakage. **Excluded proxy/surrogate outcomes:** pelvic floor strength, tension, contractility, physiological measures, and perineometry.

METHODS *Clinical Evidence* search and appraisal December 2003. We excluded studies comparing different techniques within a single intervention type (e.g. high intensity *v* low intensity pelvic floor muscle training, or Burch colposuspension *v* Marshall–Marchetti–Krantz urethropexy). We excluded RCTs that reported only within group comparisons. We have included only RCTs that stated that more than half of the participants had stress incontinence. Ideally, studies would include a follow up length of 5–10 years, but most studies reported outcomes of less than 1 year. We have not excluded studies based on length of follow up.

QUESTION What are the effects of non-surgical interventions for women with stress incontinence?

OPTION PELVIC FLOOR MUSCLE EXERCISES

One systematic review found that pelvic floor muscle exercises increased cure or improvement rates and reduced the number of leakages over 3–6 months compared with no treatment or placebo. It found no significant difference in cure or improvement rates at 12 months between pelvic floor muscle exercises and pelvic floor electrical stimulation. It found that pelvic floor muscle exercises reduced the number of leakage episodes at 6 months compared with vaginal cones, but there was no significant difference between treatments in cure or improvement rates at 12 months. One systematic review found that pelvic floor muscle exercises increased cure or improvement rates compared with oestrogen supplements.

Benefits: We found one systematic review (search date 2000).[8] **Versus no treatment:** The review identified seven RCTs (816 women) comparing pelvic floor muscle exercises**G** (PFME) versus no treatment.[8] It found that PFME significantly improved self reported cure rates and self reported cure or improvement rates over 3–6 months compared with no treatment (cure rates: 2 RCTs; 18/108 [17%] with PFME *v* 2/108 [2%] with no treatment; RR 7.25, 95% CI 1.99 to 26.49; cure or improvement rates: 2 RCTs; 62/78 [79%] with PFME *v* 3/86 [3%] with no treatment; RR 23.04, 95% CI 7.56 to 70.22). It also found that PFME significantly reduced the number of daily leakage episodes over 3–6 months (3 RCTs; $P < 0.00001$; pooled absolute numbers not reported, WMD reported graphically). **Versus placebo:** The review identified three RCTs (284 women) comparing PFME versus placebo (sham PFME, sham pelvic floor electrical stimulation [PFES**G**], or placebo tablet).[8] It found that PFME significantly improved self reported cure rates and self reported cure or improvement rates over 3–6 months compared with placebo (cure rates: 2 RCTs; 28/85 [33%] with PFME *v* 8/82 [10%] with placebo; RR 3.12, 95% CI 1.56 to 6.23; cure or improvement rates: 3 RCTs; 85/107 [79%] with PFME *v* 54/107 [50%] with placebo; RR 1.53, 95% CI 1.26 to 1.87). It also found that PFME significantly reduced the number of daily leakage episodes over 3–6 months (1 RCT; mean episodes 0.4 with PFME *v* 1.17 with placebo; $P < 0.0007$). **Versus pelvic floor electrical stimulation (PFES):** The review identified six RCTs (382 women) comparing PFME versus PFES.[8] It found no significant difference in cure rates and self reported cure or improvement rates between PFME and PFES at up to 12 months (cure rates: 4 RCTs; 11/63 [17%] with PFME *v* 4/69 [6%] with PFES; RR 2.94, 95% CI 0.99 to 8.67; cure or improvement rates: 4 RCTs; 47/63 [75%] with PFME *v* 41/69 [60%] with PFES; RR 1.24, 95% CI 0.97 to 1.57). It also found no significant difference in the number of daily leakage episodes over 6 months between PFME and PFES (1 RCT, 57 women, mean daily episodes 0.27 with PFME *v* 0.56 with PFES; $P = 0.06$). The RCT may have been underpowered to detect a clinically important difference. **Versus vaginal cones:** One systematic review (search date 2003) identified seven RCTs (661 women) comparing PFME versus vaginal cones**G**.[9] It found no significant difference in self reported cure rates and self reported cure or improvement rates between PFME and vaginal cones over 12 months (failure to cure: 3 RCTs; 41/63 [65%] with PFME *v* 46/66 [70%] with vaginal cones; RR 0.93, 95% CI 0.72 to 1.16; failure to cure or improve: 4 RCTs; 30/90 [33%] with PFME *v* 35/92 [38%] with vaginal cones; RR 0.87, 95% CI 0.58 to 1.28). It found that PFME significantly reduced the number of daily leakage episodes at 6 months compared with vaginal cones (2 RCTs; $P = 0.008$; pooled absolute numbers not reported, WMD reported graphically). **Versus**

oestrogen supplements: One systematic review (search date 2003, 2 RCTs, 69 women) found that pelvic floor muscle exercises significantly improved objective cure or improvement rates compared with oestrogen supplements at 9 months (21/34 [61.7%] with PFME *v* 3/35 [8.6%] with oestrogen; RR 5.9, 95% CI 2.2 to 16.7).[10]

Harms: **Versus no treatment:** One RCT identified by the review reported that one woman doing pelvic floor muscle exercises felt pain when contracting pelvic muscles, three women had an uncomfortable feeling, and two had difficulty in complying with treatment.[8] **Versus placebo:** One RCT identified by the review found that PFME were associated with significantly less dry mouth than placebo tablets (absolute numbers not reported; P = 0.03).[8] **Versus pelvic floor electrical stimulation:** One RCT identified by the review found that two women receiving pelvic floor electrical stimulation had vaginal irritation, two had urinary tract infection, and two had tingling in the thigh.[8] It found no adverse effects associated with PFME. A second RCT identified by the review also found that two women receiving PFES reported vaginal "smarting", and eight women had difficulties using the stimulator and maintaining motivation for use. **Versus vaginal cones:** Three RCTs identified by the review gave information on adverse events, all of which were in women using vaginal cones.[8] In one RCT (29 women), 14 women (48%) had difficulty in using the cones and maintaining motivation for use, two women (7%) had vaginitis, one woman (3%) had abdominal pain, and one woman (3%) had bleeding. The second RCT (30 women) found that cones produced an unpleasant feeling in five women (17%), three women (10%) said that cones were time consuming, two women (7%) said that cones were difficult to insert when anxious or in a hurry, two women (7%) said that cones interfered with menstruation, and two women (7%) suffered from muscle fatigue. **Versus oestrogen supplements:** The systematic review reported no information on harms.[10]

Comment: None.

OPTION PELVIC FLOOR ELECTRICAL STIMULATION

RCTs found that pelvic floor electrical stimulation reduced symptoms compared with no treatment or sham pelvic floor electrical stimulation. One systematic review found no significant difference in cure or improvement rates at 12 months between pelvic muscle electrical stimulation and pelvic floor muscle exercises. It found that pelvic floor electrical stimulation was associated with a small number of cases of vaginal irritation and difficulties in maintaining motivation for treatment. RCTs found no significant difference between pelvic floor electrical stimulation and vaginal cones in self reported cure or improvement rates, or in urinary leakage over 4 weeks to 12 months, but they may have lacked power to detect a clinically important difference. One systematic review found no significant difference in cure or improvement rates between pelvic floor electrical stimulation and oestrogen supplements, but it may have lacked the power to detect a clinically important difference.

Benefits: **Versus no treatment or sham treatment:** We found one systematic review (search date 1998, 1 RCT),[11] three additional RCTs,[12–14] and two subsequent RCTs.[15,16] The RCT identified by the review (52 women) found that pelvic floor electrical stimulation❻ (PFES) significantly reduced the number of weekly incontinence episodes compared with sham PFES (mean reduction of 4.1 episodes/week with PFES *v* mean increase of 6.9 episodes/week with sham PFES; P = 0.009).[11] The first additional RCT (121 women; 60 [49.5%] with stress incontinence, 28 [23.2%] with urge incontinence❻, and 33 [27.3%] with mixed incontinence) found that PFES significantly increased the proportion of women with self reported improvement in symptoms after 6 weeks compared with sham PFES (35% with PFES *v* 17% with sham PFES; $P = 0.03$; results not analysed by intention to treat; see comment below).[12] The second additional RCT (33 men and women with stress incontinence; see comment below) found that PFES significantly increased the proportion of people with self reported improvement in symptoms and reduced urine loss (measured with the 1 hour pad test**G** over 4 weeks compared with sham PFES; proportion with subjective improvement: 60% with PFES *v* 8% with sham PFES, $P = 0.005$; proportion with reduced urine loss: AR not reported, $P = 0.008$).[13] The third additional RCT (43 women) found that more people receiving PFES reported improvement or cure compared with no treatment (27% with PFES *v* 0% with no treatment; P value not reported).[14] The first subsequent RCT (60 women) found that PFES significantly reduced the frequency and severity of incontinence after 6 weeks compared with no treatment (each symptom scored using the Bristol Urinary Symptoms Questionnaire scoring, 1 [not a problem] to 5 [very serious problem]; mean reduction in frequency score 0.97 with PFES *v* 0 with no treatment; $P < 0.01$; mean reduction in severity score: 1.2 with PFES *v* 0 with no treatment; $P < 0.01$).[15] The second subsequent RCT (27 women) found that PFES significantly reduced scores on the Urogenital Distress Inventory Questionnaire after 8 weeks (score 0–100, greater score indicating worse distress) compared with sham PFES (31% reduction in score with PFES *v* 9% increase in score with sham PFES; $P = 0.01$).[16] **Versus pelvic floor muscle exercises:** See benefits of pelvic floor muscle exercises**G**, p 2467. **Versus vaginal cones:** We found one systematic review (search date 2003, 4 RCTs, 274 women).[9] It found no significant difference between PFES and vaginal cones**G** in self reported cure rates, self reported cure or improvement rates, daily leakage episodes, or grams of daily leakage after treatment over 4 weeks to 12 months (failure to cure: 50/55 [91%] with PFES *v* 47/51 [92%] with vaginal cones; RR 0.99, 95% CI 0.88 to 1.12; failure to improve or cure: 18/61 [30%] with PFES *v* 24/60 [40%] with vaginal cones; RR 0.74, 95% CI 0.45 to 1.22; daily leakage episodes: 1 RCT; 0.57 with PFES *v* 1.17 with vaginal cones; $P = 0.1$; grams of daily leakage after 6 months: 1 RCT; 0.8 with PFES *v* 0.6 with vaginal cones; $P = 0.6$). The review may have lacked the power to detect a clinically important difference in outcomes. **Versus oestrogen supplements:** We found one systematic review (search date 2003, 1 RCT, 49 women).[10] It found no significant difference in objective cure or improvement rate between PFES and oestrogen supplements at 6 weeks (8/25 [32%] with PFES *v* 3/24 [12.5%] with oestrogen; RR 2.56, 95% CI 0.77 to 8.33)[10]. The RCT included in the review may have lacked the power to detect a clinically important difference.

Harms: **Versus no treatment or sham treatment:** The RCTs gave no information on harms.[11–16] **Versus pelvic floor muscle exercises:** See harms of pelvic floor muscle exercises, p 2468. **Versus vaginal cones:** Two women in one of the RCTs included in the review[9] reported vaginitis with vaginal cones, one reported bleeding, and 14 reported difficulty with use.[18] **Versus oestrogen supplements:** The systematic review reported no information on harms.[10]

Comment: **Versus no treatment or sham treatment:** The first additional RCT enrolled 148 women but only 121 completed the study.[12] The RCT did not perform an intention to treat analysis. It found no significant difference in withdrawal rates between pelvic floor electrical stimulation and sham treatment (14% with PFES *v* 21% with sham treatment; $P = 0.27$). The second additional RCT included men, so the findings of this RCT may not be fully generalisable to women with stress incontinence.[13]

OPTION VAGINAL CONES

One systematic review found that vaginal cones improved self reported cure or improvement rates compared with control over 6–12 months. It found no significant difference in leakage episodes. RCTs found no significant difference between vaginal cones and pelvic floor muscle exercises in self reported cure or improvement rates over 12 months. It found that vaginal cones were less effective than pelvic floor muscle exercises in reducing the number of leakage episodes over 6 months. RCTs also found no significant difference between vaginal cones and pelvic floor electrical stimulation in self reported cure or improvement rates, or urinary leakage over 4 weeks to 12 months, but they may have lacked power to detect a clinically important difference. The most common adverse effect associated with vaginal cones was difficulty maintaining motivation for use, but a small number of more serious events such as vaginitis and abdominal pain were reported.

Benefits: **Versus control:** We found one systematic review (search date 2003, 2 RCTs, 252 women) comparing vaginal cones**G** versus control (no treatment or advice to use a continence guard).[9] It found that vaginal cones significantly improved the self reported cure and self reported improvement or cure rates over 6–12 months compared with control (failure to cure: 2 RCTs; 32/48 [67%] with vaginal cones *v* 98/121 [81%] with control; RR 0.74, 95% CI 0.59 to 0.93; failure to improve or cure: 1 RCT; 10/27 [37%] with vaginal cones *v* 29/30 [97%] with no treatment; RR 0.38, 95% CI 0.23 to 0.63). It found no significant difference in the number of daily leakage episodes over 6–12 months between vaginal cones and control (mean daily leakage episodes: 1.17 with vaginal cones *v* 1.07 with control; P = 0.8). **Versus pelvic floor muscle exercises:** See benefits of pelvic floor muscle exercises versus vaginal cones, p 2467. **Versus pelvic floor electrical stimulation:** See benefits of pelvic floor electrical stimulation versus vaginal cones, p 2468. **Versus oestrogen supplements:** We found no systematic reviews or RCTs.

Harms: **Versus control:** The systematic review gave little information on adverse effects.[9] It gave some reasons for withdrawal from RCTs in women using vaginal cones, including motivation problems, unpleasantness, aesthetic dislike, discomfort, bleeding, and vaginal prolapse. **Versus pelvic floor muscle exercises:** See harms of pelvic floor muscle exercises versus vaginal cones, p 2468. **Versus pelvic floor electrical stimulation:** See harms of pelvic floor electrical stimulation versus vaginal cones, p 2469. **Versus oestrogen supplements:** We found no RCTs.

Comment: None.

OPTION OESTROGEN SUPPLEMENTS

One systematic review found that short term treatment with oestrogen supplements improved cure or improvement rates compared with placebo. The review found that pelvic floor muscle exercises increased rates of cure or improvement compared with short term treatment with oestrogen supplements. It found no significant difference in rates of cure or improvement between pelvic floor electrical stimulation and short term treatment with oestrogen supplements, but it may have lacked the power to detect a clinically important difference. There are concerns about the safety of long term oestrogen use. One RCT found that combined oral oestrogen and progestogen supplements increased the risk of invasive breast cancer, coronary heart disease, stroke, and pulmonary embolism in postmenopausal women with a uterus at 5 years. One RCT found that oral

oestrogen supplements increased the risk of strokes in postmenopausal women without a uterus at 6 years. There is limited evidence that unopposed oestrogen is associated with an increased risk of endometrial cancer in women with a uterus.

Benefits: **Versus placebo:** We found one systematic review (search date 2003, 15 RCTs, 718 women), which compared oestrogen supplementation versus placebo (see comment).[10] This review found that, in the short term, oestrogen supplements significantly improved cure or improvement rates compared with placebo at 11 weeks to 9 months (6 RCTs; 46/107 [43%] with oestrogen *v* 29/109 [27%] with placebo; RR 1.62, 95% CI 1.15 to 2.28). **Versus pelvic floor muscle exercises:** See benefits of pelvic floor muscle exercises**G** versus oestrogen supplements, p 2467. **Versus pelvic floor electrical stimulation:** See benefits of pelvic floor electrical stimulation**G** versus oestrogen supplements, p 2468. **Versus vaginal cones:** We found no systematic reviews or RCTs.

Harms: **Versus placebo:** The review found that common adverse effects with oestrogen were vaginal bleeding (AR about 25%) and breast tenderness (AR about 20%).[10] There are concerns about the safety of long term oestrogen use. One RCT (16 608 healthy postmenopausal women with a uterus) found that after an average follow up of 5.2 years, combined oral oestrogen and progestogen increased the risk of invasive breast cancer (HR 1.26, 95% CI 1.00 to 1.59), coronary heart disease (HR 1.29, 95% CI 1.02 to 1.63), stroke (HR 1.41, 95% CI 1.07 to 1.85), and pulmonary embolism (HR 2.13, 95% CI 1.39 to 3.25).[19] Most of these adverse outcomes appeared within 1–2 years, but the increased risk of breast cancer began after 3 years of use. One RCT (10 739 healthy postmenopausal women without a uterus) found that after an average follow up of 6.8 years, oestrogen alone increased the risk of stroke (HR 1.39, 95% CI 1.10 to 1.77), but not of breast cancer (HR 0.77, 95% CI 0.59 to 1.01), coronary heart disease (HR 0.91, 95% CI 0.75 to 1.12), or pulmonary embolism (HR 1.34, 95% CI 0.87 to 2.06).[20] One meta-analysis of observational studies found that unopposed oestrogens were associated with an increased risk of endometrial cancer (RR 2.3, 95% CI 2.1 to 2.5).[21] However, this meta-analysis should be interpreted with caution, as it is based on observational studies only, which may be subject to bias and confounding. It is not clear whether these harms are associated with short term oestrogen therapy. **Versus pelvic floor muscle exercises:** See harms of pelvic floor muscle exercises versus oestrogen supplements, p 2468. **Versus pelvic floor electrical stimulation:** See harms of pelvic floor electrical stimulation versus oestrogen supplements, p 2469. **Versus vaginal cones:** We found no RCTs.

Comment: The systematic review[10] included many small studies with different types of oestrogen, methods of administration, doses, treatment durations, and periods of follow up. The review did not provide information on whether the benefits of oestrogen therapy were sustained after treatment was stopped.

QUESTION **What are the effects of surgical interventions for women with stress incontinence?**

OPTION **ANTERIOR VAGINAL REPAIR (ANTERIOR COLPORRHAPHY)**

We found no RCTs comparing anterior vaginal repair versus no treatment, suburethral slings, tension free vaginal tape, or laparoscopic colposuspension. One RCT provided insufficient evidence to compare anterior vaginal repair versus non-surgical treatment. One systematic review found

that anterior vaginal repair was less effective than open retropubic colposuspension in increasing cure rates at 12 months or at 5 years, and found no significant difference in overall operative complications between the two procedures. It found no significant difference in cure rates at 12 months between anterior vaginal repair and needle colposuspension.

Benefits: We found one systematic review (search date 2003) of anterior vaginal repair❻.[22] **Versus no treatment or sham treatment:** The review identified no RCTs.[22] **Versus non-surgical treatment:** The review identified one RCT (50 women), which compared anterior vaginal repair versus pelvic floor muscle exercises❻. Only 16 women were suitable for anterior vaginal repair (7 received anterior repair and 9 received pelvic floor muscle exercises), so no reliable conclusions could be drawn.[22] **Versus suburethral slings:** The review identified no RCTs.[22] **Versus open retropubic colposuspension:** The review identified eight RCTs (929 women).[22] It found that anterior vaginal repair was significantly less effective than open retropubic colposuspension❻ in increasing cure rates at 12 months or 5 years (failure to cure at 12 months: 82/279 [29%] with anterior repair *v* 50/346 [14%] with open retropubic colposuspension; RR 1.89, 95% CI 1.39 to 2.59; failure to cure at 5 years: 49/128 [38%] with anterior repair *v* 31/145 [21%] with open retropubic colposuspension; RR 2.02, 95% CI 1.36 to 3.01). **Versus laparoscopic colposuspension:** The review identified no RCTs.[22] **Versus needle colposuspension:** The review identified two RCTs (469 women).[22] It found no significant difference between anterior vaginal repair and needle colposuspension❻ in cure rates at 1 year (failure to cure: 33/134 [25%] with anterior vaginal repair *v* 31/132 [23%] with needle colposuspension; RR 1.05, 95% CI 0.69 to 1.59).**Versus tension free vaginal tape:** We found no RCTs.

Harms: **Versus no treatment or sham treatment:** We found no RCTs. **Versus non-surgical treatment:** The RCT identified by the review gave no information on harms.[22] **Versus suburethral slings:** We found no RCTs. **Versus open retropubic colposuspension:** One RCT identified by the review reported more positive urine cultures after anterior vaginal repair than after open retropubic colposuspension. Another RCT identified by the review found one bladder perforation in the open retropubic colposuspension group. A third RCT identified by the review reported more intraoperative complications in women receiving open retropubic colposuspension, but more postoperative pyrexia and bleeding in women receiving anterior vaginal repair. It found no significant difference in overall operative complications between anterior vaginal repair and open retropubic colposuspension (14/73 [19%] *v* 12/91 [13%]; RR 1.57, 95% CI 0.84 to 2.95).[22] **Versus laparoscopic colposuspension:** We found no RCTs. **Versus needle colposuspension:** The systematic review gave no information on adverse effects.[22] An earlier systematic review (search date 1995) found one non-randomised study assessing complications after surgery.[23] The review reported that anterior vaginal repair caused fewer major complications than needle suspension (no further data reported).[23] **Versus tension free vaginal tape:** We found no RCTs.

Comment: None.

OPTION SUBURETHRAL SLINGS OTHER THAN TENSION FREE VAGINAL TAPE

We found no RCTs comparing suburethral slings versus no treatment, non-surgical treatment, anterior vaginal repair, or laparoscopic colposuspension. Five RCTs identified by a systematic review found no significant difference in cure rates at up to 6 years between suburethral slings

and open retropubic colposuspension, although the studies may have lacked power to detect a clinically important difference. One small RCT identified by the review found no significant difference in cure rates at 1 year between suburethral slings and needle colposuspension, but it may have lacked power to detect a clinically important difference. The RCT found that suburethral slings increased perioperative complications compared with needle colposuspension. One RCT found no significant difference in subjective cure rates between tension free vaginal tape and suburethral slings at 12 months.

Benefits: **Versus no treatment, sham treatment, or non-surgical treatment:** We found one systematic review (search date 2003), which identified no RCTs.[24] **Versus anterior vaginal repair:** We found one systematic review (search date 2003), which identified no RCTs.[22] **Versus open retropubic colposuspension:** We found one systematic review (search date 2003, 5 RCTs, 206 women).[24] The systematic review did not perform a meta-analysis for non-tension free vaginal tape (TVT) suburethral sling procedures. None of the RCTs found a significant difference in outcome between non-TVT suburethral sling techniques and open retropubic colposuspension**G**. The first RCT included in the review (30 women) found no significant difference between suburethral slings**G** and open retropubic colposuspension groups in cure rate at 4–6 months' follow up (15/15 [100%] participants cured in both groups; RR and CI not reported). The second RCT included in the review (72 women) found no significant difference between suburethral slings and open retropubic colposuspension in cure rate at up to 2 years (failure to cure: 3/36 [8%] with sling *v* 5/36 [14%] with colposuspension; RR 0.60, 95% CI 0.15 to 2.33). The third RCT included in the review (46 women) found no significant difference between suburethral slings and open retropubic colposuspension in cure rate (failure to cure: 1/17 [6%] with sling *v* 2/17 [12%] with colposuspension; RR 0.50, 95% CI 0.05 to 5.01). The fourth RCT included in the review (22 women) found no significant difference between suburethral slings and open retropubic colposuspension in cure rate at 6 months (failure to cure: 0/11 [0%] with sling *v* 2/9 [22.2%] with colposuspension; reported as non-significant). The review reported the short term results of the fifth RCT (36 women),[24] and long term follow up was reported in a subsequent publication.[25] The RCT found no significant difference between suburethral slings and open retropubic colposuspension in cure rate at 3 months or at 6 years (cure rate at 3 months: 100% with sling *v* 90% with colposuspension, P = 0.49; cure rate at 6 years: 100% with sling *v* 84.6% with colposuspension, P = 0.17). **Versus laparoscopic colposuspension:** We found one systematic review (search date 2003) which found no RCTs.[24] **Versus needle colposuspension:** We found one systematic review (search date 2003, 1 RCT, 20 women).[24] The RCT included in the review found no significant difference in cure rate at 1 year between suburethral slings and needle colposuspension**G** (failure to cure: 1/10 [10%] with suburethral slings *v* 3/10 [30%] with needle colposuspension; RR 0.33, 95% CI 0.04 to 2.69), but it may have lacked power to detect a clinically important difference.[24] **Versus tension free vaginal tape:** See benefits of tension free vaginal tape**G** versus suburethral slings, p 2474.

Harms: **Versus no treatment, sham treatment, or non-surgical treatment:** We found no RCTs. **Versus anterior vaginal repair:** We found no RCTs. An earlier systematic review (search date 1995) identified one retrospective study assessing complications after surgery.[23] It found that significantly more women had perioperative complications, including residual urine, urinary retention, and uterine prolapse with suburethral slings than with anterior vaginal repair**G** ($P < 0.01$).[23] **Versus open retropubic colposuspension:** One RCT included in the review found no significant difference in the incidence of perioperative complications between suburethral slings and open retropubic colposuspension (3/36 [8.3%] with sling *v* 4/36 [11.1%] with colposuspension; RR 0.75, 95% CI 0.18 to 3.11).[24] Another RCT included in the review also found no significant difference in the incidence of perioperative complications between groups (0/17 [0%] with sling *v* 1/19 [5.2%] with colposuspension, difference reported as non-significant). The same study found that long term complications of suburethral slings were partial sling erosion (2 people) and prolonged urinary retention (one person).[25] In a third RCT included in the review, five participants from both groups had late complications (including genital prolapse, detrusor instability, dyspareunia, and suprapubic pain).[24] **Versus laparoscopic colposuspension:** We found no RCTs. **Versus needle colposuspension:** The systematic review found that suburethral slings significantly increased perioperative complications, including pyrexia, blood loss, wound infection, and pulmonary embolus, compared with needle colposuspension (1 RCT; 9/10 [90%] with suburethral slings *v* 2/10 [20%] with needle colposuspension; RR 4.50, 95% CI 1.28 to 15.81).[24] **Versus tension free vaginal tape:** See harms of tension free vaginal tape versus suburethral slings, p 2475.

Comment: None.

OPTION TENSION FREE VAGINAL TAPE

We found no RCTs comparing tension free vaginal tape versus no treatment, sham treatment, non-surgical treatment, anterior vaginal repair, or needle colposuspension. One RCT found no significant difference in subjective cure rates between tension free vaginal tape and suburethral slings at 12 months. One systematic review found no significant difference in cure rate between tension free vaginal tape and open retropubic colposuspension at up to 2 years. However, the included trials may have lacked power to exclude a clinically important difference in cure rates. RCTs included in the review found that tension free vaginal tape was associated with a higher incidence of bladder perforation than open retropubic colposuspension, but a lower incidence of postoperative fever. One RCT identified by a review found a higher cure rate with tension free vaginal tape than with laparoscopic colposuspension at 6 months to 2 years, while two subsequent RCTs found no significant difference in cure rate between groups at 6 weeks to 1 year.

Benefits: **Versus no treatment, sham treatment, or non-surgical treatment:** We found no RCTs. **Versus anterior vaginal repair:** We found no RCTs. **Versus other types of suburethral slings:** We found one systematic review (search date 2002), which found no RCTs,[17] and one subsequent RCT.[29] The RCT (142 women) found no significant difference between other types of suburethral slingsⒼ and tension free vaginal tapeⒼ (TVT) in cure rate at 12 months (AR 85% [58/68] with TVT *v* 89% [66/74] with suburethral slings; P = 0.99].[29] **Versus open retropubic colposuspension:** We found one systematic review (search date 2002, 2 RCTs).[17] The first RCT (344 women) identified by the review [17] found no significant difference between TVT and open retropubic colposuspensionⒼ in cure rates at 6 months (AR for subjective cure: 64.8% [103/159] with TVT *v* 70.9% [90/127] with open retropubic colposuspension; RR 0.91, 95% CI 0.78 to 1.07; AR for objective cure: 82.1% [128/156] *v* 83.2% [109/131]; RR 0.99, 95% CI 0.89 to 1.10; analysis not by intention to treat; see comments). The second RCT (71 women; see comment) identified by the review [17] found no significant difference in cure rate between TVT and open retropubic colposuspension at 24 months (AR 83.3% [30/36] with TVT *v* 86% [30/35] with open retropubic colposuspension; P reported as not significant). It also found that return to normal activities was significantly shorter with TVT than with open retropubic colposuspension (21 days with open retropubic colposuspension *v* 10 days with TVT, P < 0.05). The review identified two further RCTs, which did not assess cure rates.[17] **Versus laparoscopic colposuspension:** We found one systematic review (search date 2002, 1 RCT)[17] and two subsequent RCTs.[27,28] The RCT identified by the review (113 women) found that both groups had 100% subjective cure rate at 3 months' follow up, but that at 6 months to 2 years TVT had a higher subjective cure rate than laparoscopic colposuspension**G**, although this difference was only of borderline significance (AR for subjective cure: 93% [53/57] with TVT *v* 80% [45/56] with laparoscopic colposuspension; RR 1.16, 95% CI 1.00 to 1.34).[17] The first subsequent RCT (128 women) found no significant difference in cure rates between TVT and laparoscopic colposuspension at 6 weeks (AR for objective cure: 92.9% [65/70] with TVT *v* 88.2% [45/51] with laparoscopic colposuspension; P reported as not significant).[27] The second subsequent RCT (46 women) found no significant difference in cure rates between groups at 1 year (AR for subjective cure: 82.6% [19/23] for both TVT and laparoscopic colposuspension; P reported as not significant).[28] **Versus needle colposuspension:** One systematic review (search date 2002) found no RCTs.[17] We found no subsequent RCTs.

Harms: **Versus no treatment, sham treatment, or non-surgical treatment:** We found no RCTs. **Versus anterior vaginal repair:** We found no RCTs. **Versus other types of suburethral slings:** The subsequent RCT[29] found similar rates of minor perioperative complications (mainly urinary retention; 13/68 [19%] with TVT *v* 17/74 [23%] with suburethral slings; P value not reported). **Versus open retropubic colposuspension:** The first RCT identified by the systematic review[17] found that bladder perforation was significantly more common with TVT, while postoperative fever was significantly less common with TVT than with open retropubic colposuspension (AR for bladder perforation: 9% [15/170] with TVT *v* 2% [3/146] with open retropubic colposuspension; RR 4.29, 95% CI 1.27 to 14.54; AR for fever: 1% [1/170] with TVT *v* 5% [7/146] with open retropubic colposuspension; P = 0.03). It found no significant difference between groups in the incidence of postoperative urinary tract infection (UTI) or wound infection (AR for UTI in the first 6 weeks after operation: 22% [38/170] with TVT *v* 32% [46/146] with open retropubic colposuspension, P = 0.07; wound infection: 2% [4/170] *v* 7% [10/146], P = 0.06). The second RCT identified by the review[17] found that bladder perforation and postoperative UTI were more common with TVT, while haematoma was more common with open retropubic colposuspension (AR for bladder perforation: 11% [4/36] with TVT *v* 0% [0/35] with open retropubic colposuspension; UTI: 13.9% [5/36] *v* 5.7% [2/35]; haematoma: 0% [0/36] *v* 5.5% [2/36]; P values not reported). It found no significant difference between groups in the proportion of women with new detrusor overactivity at 6 months (3/36 [16.6%] for TVT *v* 5/35 [14%] for open retropubic colposuspension; RR 1.17, 95% CI 0.39 to 3.48). **Versus laparoscopic colposuspension:** The RCT identified by the review[17] found no significant difference between groups in the incidence of bladder perforation or haematoma (AR bladder perforation: 5% [3/57] with TVT *v* 0% [0/56] with laparoscopic bladder perforation; RR 6.88, 95% CI 0.36 to 130.21; haematoma: 0% [0/57] *v* 4% [2/56]; RR 0.20, 95% CI 0.01 to 4.00). The first subsequent RCT[27] found similar rates of minor operative and 6 week postoperative complications (ARs for most common adverse effects: prolonged urinary retention: 2.9% [2/70] with TVT *v* 3.9% [2/51] with laparoscopic colposuspension; urinary tract infection: 4.3% [3/70] *v* 1.9% [1/51]; urge symptoms: 2.9% [2/70] *v* 0% [0/51]; P values not reported). The second subsequent RCT[28] found similar rates of complications for TVT and laparoscopic colposuspension (5/23 [22%] in both groups; P value not reported). **Versus needle colposuspension:** We found no RCTs.

Comment: TVT has been separated from traditional suburethral sling operations because the operative procedure is substantially different. **Versus open retropubic colposuspension:** The first RCT identified by the review trial was weakened by differential withdrawal from the two groups after randomisation (5 in the TVT group and 23 in open retropubic colposuspension group).[17] At later stages of the trial, the number of women withdrawing was similar in both groups. The reasons for the differential dropout were not reported. In addition, the trial was smaller than planned, so it lacked the statistical power to detect a 10% difference in cure rates between the groups. Participants in the second RCT identified by the review[17] were allocated into groups alternately, rather than by true randomisation.[26]

OPTION OPEN RETROPUBIC COLPOSUSPENSION

We found no RCTs comparing open retropubic colposuspension versus no treatment or sham treatment. One systematic review found that open retropubic colposuspension increased cure rates at 1–5 years compared with non-surgical treatment, anterior vaginal repair, or needle colposuspension. Open retropubic colposuspension was associated with more adverse effects than non-surgical treatment, but fewer surgical complications than needle colposuspension. It found that open retropubic colposuspension improved objective cure rates at 1 year compared with laparoscopic colposuspension. However, it found no significant difference in objective cure rates at 5 years, or in subjective cure rates at 1 or 5 years. It also found no significant difference in cure rates at 1 year between open retropubic colposuspension and suburethral slings. One systematic review found no significant difference in cure rate between tension free vaginal tape and open retropubic colposuspension at up to 2 years. However, the included trials may have lacked power to exclude a clinically important difference in cure rates. RCTs included in the review found that open retropubic colposuspension was associated with a lower incidence of bladder perforation than tension free vaginal tape, but a higher incidence of postoperative fever.

Benefits: **Versus no treatment or sham treatment:** We found one systematic review (search date 2003), which identified no RCTs.[30] **Versus non-surgical treatment:** We found one systematic review (search date 2003, 2 RCTs, 120 women) comparing open retropubic colposuspension**G** versus non-surgical treatments (pelvic floor muscle exercises**G** alone or pelvic floor muscle exercises plus pelvic floor electrical stimulation).[30] It found that open retropubic colposuspension significantly improved self reported and objective cure rates at 1 year compared with non-surgical treatment (self reported failure to cure: 1 RCT; 3/16 [19%] with open retropubic colposuspension *v* 10/13 [77%] with conservative treatments; RR 0.24, 95% CI 0.08 to 0.71; objective failure to cure: 1 RCT; 6/24 [25%] with open retropubic colposuspension *v* 42/44 [95%] with conservative treatments; RR 0.26, 95% CI 0.13 to 0.53). **Versus anterior vaginal repair:** See benefits of anterior vaginal repair**G** versus open retropubic colposuspension, p 2472. **Versus suburethral slings:** See benefits of suburethral slings versus open retropubic colposuspension, p 2473. **Versus laparoscopic colposuspension:** We found one systematic review (search date 2003, 7 RCTs, 599 women).[30] It found no significant difference between open retropubic colposuspension and laparoscopic colposuspension**G** in self reported cure rates at 1 or 5 years (failure to cure at 1 year: 4 RCTs; 13/207 [6%] with open retropubic colposuspension *v* 13/196 [6%] with laparoscopic colposuspension; RR 0.97, 95% CI 0.47 to 2.03; failure to cure at 5 years: 1 RCT; 6/40 [15%] with open retropubic colposuspension *v* 4/33 [12%] with laparoscopic colposuspension; RR 1.24, 95% CI 0.38 to 4.02). It found that open retropubic colposuspension significantly increased objective cure rates at 1 year but found no significant difference in objective cure rates at 5 years (failure to cure at 1 year: 5 RCTs; 30/241 [12%] with open retropubic colposuspension *v* 45/224 [20%] with laparoscopic colposuspension; RR 0.63, 95% CI 0.42 to 0.95; failure to cure at 5 years: 2 RCTs; 10/68 [15%] with open retropubic colposuspension *v* 6/57 [11%] with laparoscopic colposuspension; RR 1.39, 95% 0.54 to 3.60). **Versus needle colposuspension:** We found one systematic review (search date 2003, 7 RCTs, 570 women).[30] It found that open retropubic colposuspension significantly improved self reported and objective cure rates at 5 years compared with needle colposuspension**G** (self reported failure to cure: 6 RCTs; 38/278 [14%] with open retropubic colposuspension *v* 66/291 [23%] with needle colposuspension; RR 0.56, 95% CI 0.39 to 0.81; objective failure to cure: 5 RCTs; 32/248 [13%] with open retropubic colposuspension *v* 57/271 [21%] with needle colposuspension; RR 0.59, 95% CI 0.40 to 0.88).[30] **Versus tension free vaginal tape:** See benefits of tension free vaginal tape**G** versus open retropubic colposuspension, p 2474.

Harms: **Versus anterior vaginal repair:** See harms of anterior vaginal repair versus open retropubic colposuspension, p 2472. **Versus non-surgical treatment:** The review identified one RCT, which gave information on adverse effects.[30] It found that open retropubic colposuspension was associated with more adverse events than non-surgical treatments (pelvic floor muscle exercises alone or pelvic floor muscle exercises plus pelvic floor electrical stimulation). These included retropubic pain (1/16 [6.25%] with open retropubic colposuspension v 0/24 [0%] with non-surgical treatment; CI not reported), detrusor overactivity (1/16 [6.25%] with open retropubic colposuspension v 0/24 [0%] with non-surgical treatment; significance not reported), and persistent dyspareunia with loss of libido (1/16 [6.25%] with open retropubic colposuspension v 0/24 [0%] with non-surgical treatment; CI not reported). **Versus suburethral slings**: See harms of suburethral slings versus open retropubic colposuspension, p 2473. **Versus laparoscopic colposuspension:** We found one systematic review (search date 2003, 7 RCTs, 599 women).[30] It found no significant difference in perioperative complications between open retropubic colposuspension and laparoscopic colposuspension (14/120 [12%] with open retropubic colposuspension v 10/107 [9%] with laparoscopic colposuspension; RR 1.28, 95% CI 0.60 to 2.75). The review gave no information on the nature or severity of perioperative complications. **Versus needle colposuspension:** We found one systematic review (search date 2003, 7 RCTs, 570 women).[30] It found that open retropubic colposuspension significantly reduced the risk of surgical complications compared with needle colposuspension (3 RCTs: 23/77 [30%] with open retropubic colposuspension v 36/75 [48%] with needle colposuspension; RR 0.66, 95% CI 0.46 to 0.94). The review gave no information on the nature or severity of surgical complications.[30] **Versus tension free vaginal tape:** See harms of tension free vaginal tape versus open retropubic colposuspension, p 2475.

Comment: The studies included in the systematic review comparing colposuspension versus needle colposuspension had weak methods.[30]

OPTION LAPAROSCOPIC COLPOSUSPENSION

We found no RCTs comparing laparoscopic colposuspension versus no treatment, non-surgical treatment, anterior vaginal repair, suburethral slings, or needle colposuspension. One systematic review found that open retropubic colposuspension improved objective cure rates at 1 year compared with laparoscopic colposuspension. However, it found no significant difference in objective cure rates at 5 years, or in subjective cure rates at 1 or 5 years.

Stress incontinence

One RCT identified by a review found a higher cure rate with tension free vaginal tape than with laparoscopic colposuspension at 6 months to 2 years, while two subsequent RCTs found no significant difference in cure rate between treatments at 6 weeks to 1 year.

Benefits: **Versus no treatment, sham treatment, or non-surgical treatment:** We found one systematic review (search date 2002) which identified no RCTs.[31] **Versus anterior vaginal repair:** See benefits of anterior vaginal repairⒼ versus laparoscopic colposuspension, p 2472. **Versus suburethral slings:** See benefits of suburethral slingsⒼ versus laparoscopic colposuspension, p 2473. **Versus open retropubic colposuspension:** See benefits of open retropubic colposuspensionⒼ versus laparoscopic colposuspension, p 2476. **Versus needle colposuspension:** We found no RCTs. **Versus tension free vaginal tape:** See benefits of tension free vaginal tapeⒼ versus laparoscopic colposuspension, p 2474.

Harms: **Versus no treatment, sham treatment, surgery, or non-surgical treatments:** We found no RCTs. **Versus anterior vaginal repair:** See harms of anterior vaginal repair versus laparoscopic colposuspension, p 2472. **Versus suburethral slings:** See harms of suburethral sling versus laparoscopic colposuspension, p 2473. **Versus open retropubic colposuspension**: See harms of open retropubic colposuspension versus laparoscopic colposuspension, p 2477. **Versus tension free vaginal tape**: See harms of tension free vaginal tape versus laparoscopic colposuspension, p 2475.

Comment: None.

OPTION NEEDLE COLPOSUSPENSION

We found no RCTs comparing needle colposuspension versus no treatment, non-surgical treatment, tension free vaginal tape, or laparoscopic colposuspension. One systematic review found no significant difference in cure rates between needle colposuspension and anterior vaginal repair or suburethral slings, but found that needle colposuspension was associated with fewer perioperative complications than suburethral slings. Another systematic review found that open retropubic colposuspension improved cure rates and was associated with fewer surgical complications than needle colposuspension at 5 years.

Benefits: **Versus no treatment, sham treatment, or non-surgical treatment:** We found one systematic review (search date 2002), which found no RCTs.[32] **Versus anterior vaginal repair:** See benefits of anterior vaginal repairⒼ versus needle colposuspension, p 2472. **Versus suburethral slings:** See benefits of suburethral slingsⒼ versus needle colposuspension, p 2473. **Versus open retropubic colposuspension:** See benefits of open retropubic colposuspensionⒼ versus needle colposuspension, p 2476. **Versus laparoscopic colposuspension:** See benefits of laparoscopic colposuspensionⒼ versus needle colposuspension, p 2478. **Versus tension free vaginal tape:** See benefits of tension free vaginal tapeⒼ versus needle colposuspension, p 2474.

Harms: **Versus no treatment, sham treatment, or non-surgical treatment:** We found no RCTs. **Versus anterior vaginal repair:** See harms of anterior vaginal repair versus needle colposuspension, p 2472. **Versus suburethral slings:** See harms of suburethral sling versus needle colposuspension, p 2473. **Versus open retropubic colposuspension:** See harms of open retropubic colposuspension versus needle colposuspension, p 2477. **Versus laparoscopic colposuspension:** See harms of laparoscopic colposuspension versus needle colposuspension, p 2478. **Versus tension free vaginal tape:** See harms of tension free vaginal tape versus needle colposuspension, p 2469.

Comment: None.

GLOSSARY

Anterior vaginal repair (anterior colporrhaphy) The vaginal mucosa below the urethra is dissected, ending just in front of the cervix. Sutures are placed in the periurethral tissue and the pubocervical fascia to support and elevate the bladder neck. Excess vaginal tissue is removed and then the dissected area is closed. The operation may be performed under general, regional, or local anaesthetic.

Laparoscopic colposuspension An endoscope is inserted into or through the abdominal wall to view abdominal and pelvic organs. Sutures are inserted into the paravaginal tissues on either side of the bladder neck and then attached to the ileopectineal ligaments on the same side. The operation is performed under general anaesthetic.

Needle colposuspension To support the bladder neck, a needle threads sutures from the vagina to the anterior abdominal fascia through the paraurethral tissue of the bladder neck. The operation is performed under general or regional anaesthetic.

Open retropubic colposuspension Open retropubic colposuspension involves lifting the tissues near the bladder neck and proximal urethra in the area of the pelvis behind the anterior pubic bones through an incision over the lower abdomen. The operation is performed under general or regional anaesthetic.

Pad test After the placement of a preweighed sanitary pad, the woman is asked to exercise. The pad is then reweighed to determine the amount of urine loss.

Pelvic floor electrical stimulation A recurrent electrical pulse is delivered by vaginal probe to stimulate pelvic floor muscle contractions.

Pelvic floor muscle exercises Repetitive contraction exercises designed to strengthen the pelvic floor muscles based on the rationale that a strong, fast pelvic floor muscle contraction will clamp the urethra, thus increasing the intraurethral pressure, preventing leakage during abrupt increases in intra-abdominal pressure.

Suburethral slings Strips of material are tunnelled under the urethra, attached either to the rectus muscle or the ileopectineal ligaments, resulting in a tightening of the sling and increased bladder support every time the woman contracts her rectus muscles. The operation is performed under general or regional anaesthetic.

Tension free Vaginal Tape (TVT) A minimal access surgical sling procedure, in which a tape is passed beneath the urethra, aiming to restore the urethra to its normal position. The TVT is placed with minimal tension, and support is thought to be achieved by causing a tissue reaction with a subsequent collagen scar. The operation is performed under general or regional anaesthetic.

Urge incontinence Urge incontinence is typically caused by a spontaneous or inappropriately provoked involuntary bladder contraction (detrusor instability). Urge incontinence, unlike stress incontinence, is associated with a feeling of needing to void. It can exist alone, or more commonly as mixed urinary incontinence, when it is combined with stress incontinence.

Vaginal cones A women inserts a weighted cone into the vagina. When she can successfully retain that cone while standing, moving around, and coughing, she will move onto the next heaviest cone, and so on.

REFERENCES

1. Abrams P, Cardozo L, Fall M, et al. The standardisation of terminology in lower urinary tract function. *Neurourol Urodyn* 2002;21:167–178.
2. Jolleys JV. Reported prevalence of urinary incontinence in women in a general practice. *BMJ* 1988;296:1300–1302.
3. Rortveit G, Daltveit AK, Hannestad YS, et al; Norwegian EPINCONT Study. Urinary incontinence after vaginal delivery or cesarean section. *N Engl J Med* 2003;348:900–907.
4. Department of Health. Hospital episode statistics; England: financial year 2000–01. http://www.doh.gov.uk/hes/tables/tbcv100a.pdf (last accessed 1 December 2003).
5. Wilson PD, Herbison RM, Herbison GP. Obstetric practice and the prevalence of urinary incontinence three months after delivery. *B J Obstet Gynaecol* 1996;103:154–161.
6. Bump RC, Sugerman HJ, Fantl JA, et al. Obesity and lower urinary tract function in women: effect of surgically induced weight loss. *Am J Obstet Gynecol* 1992;167:392–397.

7. Bump RC, McClish DK. Cigarette smoking and urinary incontinence in women. *Am J Obstet Gynecol* 1992;167:1213–1218.
8. Hay-Smith EJ, Bo K, Berghmans LC, et al. Pelvic floor muscle training for urinary incontinence in women. In: The Cochrane Library, Issue 4, 2003. Chichester: Wiley. Search date 2000; primary sources Medline, Embase, the database of the Dutch National Institute of Allied Health Professions, the database of the Cochrane Rehabilitation and Related Therapies Field, Physiotherapy Index, reference lists of relevant articles, the proceedings of the International Continence Society and contact with investigators in the field.
9. Herbison P, Plevnik S, Mantle J. Weighted vaginal cones for urinary incontinence. In: The Cochrane Library, Issue 4, 2003. Chichester: Wiley. Search date 2003; primary sources Cochrane Incontinence Group Specialised Register, Medline, Cihahl, and reference lists of relevant articles.
10. Moehrer B, Hextall A, Jackson S. Oestrogens for urinary incontinence in women. In: Cochrane Library, Issue 4, 2003. Chichester: Wiley. Search date 2003, primary sources Cochrane Incontinence Group Specialized Register, Medline, Cinahl, CCT, hand searching of journals.
11. Berghmans LCM, Hendriks HJM, Bo K, et al. Conservative treatment of stress urinary incontinence in women: a systematic review of randomized clinical trials. *Br J Urol* 1998;82:181–191. Search date 1998; primary sources Medline, Excerpta Medica, database of the Dutch National Institute of Allied Health Professions, database of the Cochrane Field in Therapies and Rehabilitation, and hand searches of references.
12. Brubaker L, Benson JT, Bent A, et al. Transvaginal electrical stimulation for female urinary incontinence. *Am J Obstet Gynecol* 1997;177:536–540.
13. Yamanishi R, Yasuda K, Sakakibara R, et al. Pelvic floor electrical stimulation in the treatment of stress incontinence: an investigation study and a placebo controlled double-blind trial. *J Urol* 1997;158:2127–2131.
14. Preisinger E, Hofbauer J, Numberger N, et al. Possibilities of physiotherapy for urinary stress incontinence. *Z Phys Med Bain Med Klim* 1990;19:75–79.
15. Sung MS, Choi YH, Back SH, et al. The effect of pelvic floor muscle exercises on genuine stress incontinence among Korean women – focusing on its effects on the quality of life. *Yonsei Med J* 2000;41:237–251.
16. Jeyaseelan SM, Haslam EJ, Winstanley J, et al. An evaluation of a new pattern of electrical stimulation as a treatment for urinary stress incontinence: a randomized, double-blind, controlled trial. *Clinic Rehabil* 2000;14:631–640.
17. Cody J, Wyness L, Wallace S, et al. Systematic review of the clinical effectiveness of tension-free vaginal tape for treatment of urinary stress incontinence. *Health Technol Assess* 2003;7:1–218. Search date 2002, primary sources Medline, Embase, Dane, Cochrane Incontinence Review Group, references lists, conference proceedings, and experts in the area.
18. Bo K, Talseth R, Holme I. Single blind, randomised controlled trial of pelvic floor exercises, electrical stimulation, vaginal cones, and no treatment in management of genuine stress incontinence in women. *BMJ* 1999;318:487–493.
19. WHI Writing Group. Risk and benefits of estrogen plus progestin in healthy postmenopausal women: principal results From the Women's Health Initiative randomized controlled trial. *JAMA* 2002;288:321–333.
20. WHI Steering Committee. Effects of conjugated equine estrogens in postmenopausal women with hysterectomy. *JAMA* 2004;291:1701–1712.
21. Grady D, Gebretsadik T, Kerlikowske K, et al. Hormone replacement therapy and endometrial cancer: a meta-analysis. *Obstet Gynecol* 1995;85:304–313.
22. Glazener CMA, Cooper K. Anterior vaginal repair for urinary incontinence in women. In: The Cochrane Library, Issue 4, 2003. Chichester: Wiley. Search date 2003; primary sources the Medline, Cinahl, CCT, Cochrane Incontinence Trials Register, hand searching of journals, and reference lists of relevant articles.
23. Black NA, Downs SH. The effectiveness of surgery for stress incontinence in women: a systematic review. *B J Urol* 1996;78:497–510. Search date 1995; primary sources Medline, Embase, Science Citation Index, British Library Information Index, and reference lists of relevant articles.
24. Bezerra CA, Bruschini H, Cody DJ. Suburethral sling operations for urinary incontinence in women. In: The Cochrane Library, Issue 4, 2003. Chichester: Wiley. Search date 2003; primary sources the Cochrane Incontinence Group's Trials Register, Medline. Cinahl, CCT, and hand searches of journals.
25. Culligan PJ, Goldberg RP, Sand PK. A randomized controlled trial comparing a modified Burch procedure and a suburethral sling: long-term follow-up. *Int Urogynecol J Pelvic Floor Dysfunct* 2003;14:229–233.
26. Liapis A, Bakas P, Creatsas G. Burch colposuspension and tension-free vaginal tape in the management of stress urinary incontinence in women. *Eur Urol* 2002;41:469–473.
27. Valpas A, Kivela A, Penttinen J, et al. Tension-free vaginal tape and laparoscopic mesh colposuspension in the treatment of stress urinary incontinence: immediate outcome and complications – a randomized clinical trial. *Acta Obstet Gynecol Scand* 2003;82:665–671.
28. stün Y, Engin- stün Y, Güngör M, et al. Tension-free vaginal tape compared with laparoscopic Burch urethropexy. *J Am Assoc Gynecol Laparosc* 2003;10:386–389.
29. Arunkalaivanan AS, Barrington JW. Randomised trial of porcine dermal sling (Pelvicol implant) vs. tension-free vaginal tape (TVT) in the surgical treatment of stress incontinence: a questionnaire-based study. *Int Urogynecol J Pelvic Floor Dysfunct* 2003;14:17–23.
30. Lapitan MC, Cody DJ, Grant AM. Open retropubic colposuspension for urinary incontinence in women. In: The Cochrane Library, Issue 4, 2003. Chichester: Wiley. Search date April 2003; primary sources the Cochrane Incontinence Group Specialised Register, Medline, Cinahl, CCT, and hand searches of journals.
31. Moehrer B, Ellis G, Carey M, et al. Laparoscopic colposuspension for urinary incontinence in women. In: The Cochrane Library, Issue 4, 2003. Chichester: Wiley. Search date April 2002; primary sources the Cochrane Incontinence Group Specialised Register, reference lists of relevant articles, conference proceedings, reviews, and unpublished research.
32. Glazener CMA, Cooper K. Bladder neck needle suspension for urinary incontinence in women. In: The Cochrane Library, Issue 4, 2003. Chichester: Wiley. Search date December 2002; primary sources the Cochrane Incontinence Trials Register, Medlines, Cinahl, CCT, hand searching of journals, and reference lists of relevant articles.

Joseph Onwude
Consultant Gynaecologist and Medical Statistician
Springfield Hospital, Chelmsford, UK

Competing interests: None declared.

The following previous author of this topic would like to be acknowledged: Bazian Ltd.

Bites (mammalian)

Search date November 2003

Iara Marques de Medeiros and Humberto Saconato

QUESTIONS

INTERVENTIONS

PREVENTION OF BITES
Likely to be beneficial
Education 2482

Unknown effectiveness
Education in specific occupational groups 2482

PREVENTION OF COMPLICATIONS
Likely to be beneficial
Antibiotic prophylaxis 2483
Debridement, irrigation, and decontamination* 2484

Unknown effectiveness
Primary wound closure 2484
Tetanus immunisation after mammalian bites 2483

TREATMENT FOR INFECTED BITES
Likely to be beneficial
Antibiotics* 2485

Unknown effectiveness
Comparative effectiveness of different antibiotics. 2485

To be covered in future updates
Prevention of rabies

*No RCT evidence, but there is consensus that treatment is likely to be beneficial

See glossary G

Key Messages

Prevention of bites

- **Education** We found no RCTs of the effect of education programmes on the incidence of mammalian bites. One RCT in school children found that an educational programme increased precautionary behaviour around dogs compared with no education.
- **Education in specific occupational groups** We found no RCTs of education to prevent bites in specific occupational groups.

Prevention of complications

- **Antibiotic prophylaxis** The effects of antibiotic prophylaxis in preventing complications of mammalian bites remain unclear. Limited evidence from one systematic review found that, when all causes and sites of mammalian bite were combined, there was no evidence of a difference in infection rate between antibiotics and placebo. Meta-analysis according to the site of the wound found that antibiotics reduced infections of the hand only. One small RCT in the review found that in people with human bites, antibiotics reduced the rate of infection compared with placebo.
- **Debridement, irrigation, and decontamination** We found no reliable studies assessing debridement, irrigation, decontamination measures, or infiltration of serum into the wound. However, there is consensus that such measures are likely to be beneficial.
- **Primary wound closure** One poor quality RCT comparing primary wound closure with no closure in people with dog bites found no significant difference in the incidence of infection, but the RCT was too small to exclude clinically important effects.

- **Tetanus immunisation after mammalian bites** We found no evidence on the effects of tetanus toxoid or tetanus immunoglobulin in preventing tetanus after human or animal bites.

Treatment for infected bites

- **Antibiotics** We found no RCTs of antibiotics compared with placebo for infected mammalian bites. However, there is consensus that antibiotics are likely to be beneficial.
- **Comparative effectiveness of different antibiotics** One RCT in people with infected and uninfected animal and human bites found no significant difference in failure rate (which was undefined) with penicillin, with or without dicloxacillin, compared with amoxicillin/clavulanic acid.

DEFINITION	Bite wounds are mainly caused by humans, dogs, or cats. They include superficial abrasions (30–43%), lacerations (31–45%), and puncture wounds(G) (13–34%).[1]
INCIDENCE/ PREVALENCE	In areas where rabies is poorly controlled among domestic animals, dogs account for 90% of reported mammalian bites compared with less than 5% in areas where rabies is well controlled. In the USA, an estimated 3.5–4.7 million dog bites occur each year.[2] About 1 in 5 people bitten by a dog seek medical attention, and 1% of those require admission to hospital.[3,4] Between a third and half of all mammalian bites occur in children.[5]
AETIOLOGY/ RISK FACTORS	In over 70% of cases, people are bitten by their own pets or by an animal known to them. Males are more likely to be bitten than females, and are more likely to be bitten by dogs, whereas females are more likely to be bitten by cats.[2] One study found that children under 5 years old were significantly more likely than older children to provoke animals before being bitten.[6] One study of infected dog and cat bites found that the most commonly isolated bacteria was *Pasteurella*, followed by *Streptococci*, *Staphylococci*, *Moraxella*, *Corynebacterium*, and *Neisseria*.[7] Mixed aerobic and anaerobic infection was more common than anaerobic infection alone.
PROGNOSIS	In the USA, dog bites cause about 20 deaths a year.[8] In children, dog bites frequently involve the face, potentially resulting in severe lacerations and scarring.[9] Rabies, a life threatening viral encephalitis, may be contracted as a consequence of being bitten or scratched by a rabid animal. More than 99% of human rabies occurs in developing countries where canine rabies is endemic.[10]
AIMS OF INTERVENTION	To prevent mammalian bites; to prevent or achieve rapid resolution of complications after mammalian bites, with minimal adverse effects.
OUTCOMES	**Prevention of bites:** Incidence of mammalian bites. **Prevention of complications:** Rate of infection after mammalian bites, incidence of tetanus. **Treatment of infected bites:** Cure rate of infection owing to mammalian bites.
METHODS	*Clinical Evidence* search and appraisal November 2003, including a search for observational studies. In addition, the authors searched Web of Science (Science Citation Index to October 2001).

QUESTION What are the effects of interventions to prevent mammalian bites?

OPTION EDUCATION

We found no RCTs of the effect of education programmes on the incidence of mammalian bites. One RCT found that an educational programme compared with no education in school children increased precautionary behaviour around dogs. We found no RCTs of education to prevent bites in specific occupational groups.

Benefits: We found no systematic review. **In the general population:** We found no RCTs on the effect of education programmes on the incidence of mammalian bites. One RCT (346 school children aged 7–8 years in 8 primary schools in Sydney, Australia) cluster randomised schools to either an educational programme or no education.[11] The educational programme consisted of one 30 minute lesson demonstrating behavioural techniques around dogs, such as how to recognise friendly, angry, or frightened dogs; how to approach dogs and owners when wanting to pat a dog; and how to use a precautionary and protective body posture when approached or knocked over by a dog. After 10 days, children were videotaped for 10 minutes while playing in school grounds where a dog was leashed. The trial found that children in schools receiving education were significantly less likely to pat the dog without hesitation and try to excite it (118/149 [79%] *v* 18/197 [9%]; RR 0.16, 95% CI 0.064 to 0.20). **In specific occupational groups:** We found no RCTs.

Harms: The RCT did not report on adverse effects.[11]

Comment: The RCT was brief and reported only the proxy outcome of behaviour modification. The effect of such a programme on the incidence of dog bites in the long term is unclear.

QUESTION What are the effects of interventions to prevent complications from mammalian bites?

OPTION IMMUNISATION AGAINST TETANUS

We found no evidence on the effects of tetanus toxoid or tetanus immunoglobulin in preventing tetanus after human or animal bites.

Benefits: We found no systematic review. **Tetanus toxoid:** We found no RCTs or cohort studies. **Tetanus immunoglobulin:** We found no RCTs or cohort studies.

Harms: We found no evidence.

Comment: None.

OPTION ANTIBIOTIC PROPHYLAXIS

The effects of antibiotic prophylaxis in preventing complications of mammalian bites remain unclear. Limited evidence from one systematic review found that, when all causes and sites of mammalian bite were combined, there was no evidence of a difference in infection rate between antibiotic prophylaxis and placebo. Meta-analysis according to the site of the wound found that antibiotic prophylaxis reduced infections of the hand only. One small RCT in the review found that in people with human bites, antibiotic prophylaxis reduced the rate of infection compared with placebo.

Benefits: We found one systematic review (search date 2001, 7 RCTs and 1 quasi-randomised controlled trial, 522 people bitten by dogs, cats, or humans in the preceding 24 hours) comparing prophylactic antibiotics versus placebo or no treatment.[12] There was significant heterogeneity between trials. The review found no significant difference in infection rate with antibiotic prophylaxis compared with placebo after dog, cat, or human bites (OR 0.49, 95% CI 0.15 to 1.58; timescale not reported). When the results were analysed for each wound site (hands, trunk, arms, or head/neck), antibiotic prophylaxis significantly reduced infections of the hand only (3 RCTs: 2% with antibiotic prophylaxis *v* 28% with control; OR 0.10, 95% CI 0.01 to 0.86; NNT 4, 95% CI 2 to 50). **Animal bites:** The review identified six RCTs of dog bites (463 people) and found no significant difference in infection rate with antibiotic prophylaxis compared with control (10/225 [4%] with antibiotic prophylaxis *v* 13/238 [5%] with control; OR 0.74, 95% CI 0.30 to 1.85). The review identified one small RCT of cat bites (12 people), which found no significant difference in infection rate with antibiotic prophylaxis compared with control (4/6 [67%] with antibiotic prophylaxis *v* 0/5 [0%] with control; $P < 0.06$).[12] **Human bites:** The review included one RCT of human bites (48 people with uncomplicated bites on the hand in the preceding 24 hours) comparing oral cephalosporin versus intravenous cephalosporin plus penicillin versus placebo. All participants received debridement, irrigation, and sterile dressing and remained in hospital for 5 days. It found that antibiotic prophylaxis by either route significantly reduced the proportion of people with wound infection compared with placebo (0/33 [0%] with oral or iv antibiotic prophylaxis *v* 7/15 [47%] with placebo; $P < 0.05$; timescale not reported).[12]

Harms: The review did not report on adverse effects.[12]

Comment: Most of the RCTs were small and gave insufficient information about allocation concealment and randomisation. Some studies were not double blind, and four studies had withdrawal rates greater than 10%.[12] The effects of antibiotic prophylaxis in preventing complications of mammalian bites remain unclear. Only a few studies analysed the effect of antibiotic prophylaxis on specific wound types (lacerations, puncture, or avulsions❻).[12]

OPTION PRIMARY WOUND CLOSURE

One poor quality RCT comparing primary wound closure with no closure in people with dog bites found no significant difference in the incidence of infection, but the RCT was too small to exclude clinically important effects.

Benefits: We found no systematic review. We found one RCT comparing primary wound closure versus no closure (96 people bitten by dogs in the preceding 24 hours).[13] All wounds were debrided and irrigated, and tetanus immunisation was updated, but no antibiotic prophylaxis was given. In uncomplicated lacerations❻, closure was performed by an experienced nurse; in complicated lacerations closure was performed by a specialist physician. The RCT found no difference in the incidence of infection with closed compared with open wounds (7/92 [8%] with closed *v* 6/77 [8%] with open; RR 0.98, 95% CI 0.33 to 2.62; timescale not reported). There were significantly more infections of the hand compared with the rest of the body (69% *v* 31% of body), but there was no difference between closure and non-closure groups in the rate of hand infection (5/9 [56%] with closure *v* 4/9 [44%] with non-closure).

Harms: The RCT did not report on adverse effects.[13]

Comment: Although the RCT found no increased risk of infection with primary wound closure, further RCTs are required to confirm this conclusion, and also to evaluate if wound closure of bites from a rabid animal may increase the risk of rabies.

OPTION DEBRIDEMENT, IRRIGATION, AND DECONTAMINATION

We found no reliable studies assessing debridement, irrigation, decontamination measures, or infiltration of serum into the wound. However, there is consensus that such measures are likely to be beneficial.

Benefits: We found no systematic review, RCTs, or good cohort studies.

Harms: We found no evidence.

Comment: It would be regarded as unethical to conduct an RCT comparing debridement, irrigation, and decontamination versus no treatment. There is consensus that such measures are likely to be beneficial.

QUESTION What are the effects of treatments for infected mammalian bites?

OPTION ANTIBIOTICS

We found no RCTs comparing antibiotics versus placebo for infected mammalian bites; however, there is consensus that they are likely to be beneficial. One RCT in people with infected and uninfected animal and human bites found no significant difference in failure rate (which was undefined) with penicillin, with or without dicloxacillin, compared with amoxicillin/clavulanic acid.

Benefits: We found no systematic review. **Versus placebo:** We found no RCTs. **Comparison of different antibiotics:** We found one RCT (61 people bitten in the preceding 10 days; 48 by animals, 13 by humans) comparing penicillin with or without dicloxacillin versus amoxicillin (amoxycillin)/clavulanic acid.[10] Treatment was given for 5 days in people bitten less than 8 hours previously or in those without clinical infection (34 people), and for 10 days in people bitten more than 8 hours previously or with clinical infection (27 people). All wounds received usual care and were left closed or open at the discretion of the attending physician. The RCT found no significant difference in failure rate (which was undefined) with penicillin/dicloxacillin compared with amoxicillin/clavulanic acid (1/31 [3%] with penicillin/dicloxacillin *v* 3/30 [10%] with amoxicillin/clavulanic acid; RR 0.32, 95% CI 0.03 to 2.54; timescale not reported).

Harms: Adverse effects were significantly more common in people using amoxicillin/clavulanic acid compared with penicillin/dicloxacillin (3/30 [10%] penicillin/dicloxacillin *v* 13/31 [42%] with amoxicillin/clavulanic acid; RR 4.2, 95% CI 1.5 to 7.4; NNH 3, 95% CI 2 to 19). Diarrhoea was the most common adverse event (1/30 [3%] with penicillin/dicloxacillin *v* 9/31 [29%] with amoxicillin/clavulanic acid; RR 8.71, 95% CI 1.34 to 23.3; NNH 4, 95% CI 1 to 79).[10]

Comment: Interpretation of the results of the RCT is difficult as the main outcome measure of "failure rate" was not defined. Also, failure rates were not separated according to whether people had infected or uninfected wounds at inclusion.[10] We found no RCTs comparing antibiotics versus placebo for infected mammalian bites; however, there is consensus that they are likely to be beneficial.

GLOSSARY

Abrasion The scraping or rubbing away of a small area of skin or mucous membrane.
Avulsion A wound resulting from the ripping or tearing away of a part.
Laceration Occurs when the skin, soft tissues, or both are torn by the crushing and shearing forces produced on impact; characterised by ragged, irregular margins, surrounding contusion, marginal abrasion, and tissue bridging in the wound depths.
Puncture A wound caused by perforation of the skin with a sharp point.

REFERENCES

1. Dire DJ. Emergency management of dog and cat bite wounds. *Emerg Med Clin North Am* 1992;10:719–736.
2. Overall KL, Love M. Dog bites to humans — demography, epidemiology, injury and risk. *JAMA* 2001;218:1923–1934.
3. Sacks JJ, Kresnow M, Houston B. Dog bites: how big a problem? *Injury Prev* 1996;2:52–54.
4. Quinlan KP, Sacks JJ. Hospitalizations for dog bite injuries. *JAMA* 1999;281:232–233.
5. Fishbein DB, Bernard KW. Rabies virus. In: *Mandell, Douglas and Bennett's principles and practice of infectious diseases*. 4th ed. Vol 2:1527–1543. New York: Churchill Livingstone.
6. Avner JR, Baker MD. Dog bites in urban children. *Pedriatrics* 1991;88:55–57.
7. Talan DA, Citron DM, Abrahamian FM, et al. Bacteriologic analysis of infected dog and cat bites. Emergency Medicine Animal Bite Infection Study Group. *N Engl J Med* 1999;340:85–92.

8. Sacks JJ, Sattin RW, Bonzo SE. Dog bite-related fatalities from 1979 through 1988. *JAMA* 1989;262:1489–1492.
9. Karlson TA. The incidence of facial injuries from dog bites. *JAMA* 1984;251:3265–3267.
10. Goldstein EJC, Reinhardt JF, Murray PM, et al. Outpatient therapy of bite wounds. Demographic data, bacteriology, and prospective, randomized trial of amoxicillin/clavulanic acid versus penicillin +/− dicloxacillin. *Int J Dermatol* 1987;26:123–127.
11. Chapman S, Cornwall J, Righetti J, et al. Preventing dog bites in children: randomised controlled trial of an educational intervention. *BMJ* 2000;320:1512–1513.
12. Medeiros I, Saconato H. Antibiotic prophylaxis for mammalian bites (Cochrane Review). In: The Cochrane Library, Issue 1, 2003. Oxford: Update Software. Search date 2001; primary sources Medline, Embase, Lilacs, the Cochrane Controlled Trials Register and hand searches of Brazilian Infectious Diseases Meetings (1980–1995).
13. Maimaris C, Quinton DN. Dog-bite lacerations: a controlled trial of primary wound closure. *Arch Emerg Med* 1988;5:156–161.

Iara Marques de Medeiros

Humberto Saconato
Universidade Federal do Rio Grande do Norte
Natal
Brazil

Competing interests: None declared.

Minor thermal burns

Search date December 2003

Jason Wasiak and Heather Cleland

QUESTIONS

INTERVENTIONS

See glossary G

Key Messages

- **Antibiotics** We found no RCTs comparing the use of topical or oral antibiotics versus placebo or no treatment in the management of minor burns. Routine prophylactic use of antibiotics may promote the emergence of resistant organisms in the community.
- **Chorhexidine impregnated paraffin gauze dressing** Two RCTs comparing chlorhexidine impregnated paraffin gauze versus hydrocolloid dressing found no significant difference in time to wound healing but, subjectively, both investigators and patients in one of the RCTs rated the hydrocolloid dressing more favourably. One RCT found that chlorhexidine impregnated paraffin gauze increased time to wound healing and was perceived as more painful compared with polyurethane film.
- **Hydrocolloid dressing** Two RCTs comparing hydrocolloid dressing versus paraffin impregnated gauze dressings found no significant difference in time to wound healing between the two treatment groups but, subjectively, both investigators and patients in one of the RCTs rated the hydrocolloid dressing more favourably. One RCT found no significant difference in time to wound healing, pain, or interference with activities of daily living between hydrocolloid dressing and a combination of chlorhexidine impregnated paraffin gauze dressing plus silver sulfadiazine cream. One RCT found that hydrocolloid dressing reduced time to healing, pain, and limitation of activity compared with silver sulfadiazine dressing. One RCT found that healing time was shorter with hydrocolloid dressing alone compared with hydrocolloid dressing plus silver sulfadiazine cream and found no difference in pathogenic bacteria growth with hydrocolloid dressing alone compared with hydrocolloid dressing plus silver sulfadiazine cream.
- **Paraffin gauze dressing** One RCT found no significant difference in pain or time to wound healing with paraffin gauze compared with polyurethane film.
- **Polyurethrane film** One RCT comparing polyurethane film versus paraffin gauze found no significant difference in pain or the number of days to wound healing. One RCT found that polyurethane film reduced time to wound healing and was perceived as less painful compared with chlorhexidine impregnated paraffin gauze.
- **Silicone coated nylon dressing** One RCT found that silicone coated nylon dressing reduced time to wound healing in children compared with silver sulfadiazine dressing.
- **Silver sulfadiazine cream** One RCT comparing a combination of chlorhexidine impregnated paraffin gauze dressing plus silver sulfadiazine cream versus hydrocolloid dressing found no significant difference in time to wound healing, pain levels, or interference with activities of daily living. One RCT found that silver sulfadiazine dressing increased time to healing, pain, and limitation of activity compared with

hydrocolloid dressing. One RCT found that healing time was longer with hydrocolloid dressing plus silver sulfadiazine cream compared with hydrocolloid dressing alone and found no significant difference in pathogenic bacteria growth between the two groups. One RCT found that silver sulfadiazine dressing increased time to wound healing in children compared with silicone coated nylon dressing.

DEFINITION Minor thermal burns can be defined as being caused by exposure to heat sufficient to cause damage to the epidermis and papillary dermis of the skin. They are characterised by pain and hypersensitivity. The skin appears moist and pink or red and is perfused, as demonstrated by blanching on pressure. This type of injury will blister and heal within 2–3 weeks with minimal scarring if no infection is present.

INCIDENCE/ PREVALENCE The incidence of minor thermal burns is difficult to estimate. Generally, less than 5% of all burn injuries requiring treatment will necessitate admission to hospital.[1] Worldwide estimates surrounding all thermal burn injuries suggest that approximately two million people are burned, up to 80 000 are hospitalised and 6500 die of burn wounds every year.

AETIOLOGY/ RISK FACTORS The pattern of injury varies among different age groups. Males aged 18–25 years appear more susceptible to injury due to a variety of causes — mainly flame, electrical, and, to a lesser extent, chemicals.[2] Many burn injuries in this age group are due to the inappropriate use of flammable agents such as petrol; however, the majority of burns occur in the home. Thermal burns, in particular scalds, are common among the young as well as the elderly. The kitchen is reported to be the most common place of injury for children, as is the bathroom for the elderly. Those with concomitant conditions or complicating factors such as motor or neurological impairment are at greater risk.

PROGNOSIS Superficial thermal burns will heal spontaneously with minimal hypertrophic scarring within 2–3 weeks if the wound remains free of infection.[3] The capacity to heal is also dependent on the health and age of the individual, with the elderly and those with concomitant medical conditions prone to delayed healing. Cooling the burn significantly reduces pain and wound oedema if started within 3 hours of injury. The optimal duration of cooling may vary, but recommended periods of 20–30 minutes with tap water (at a temperature of 5–25 °C) have been suggested.[4] Use of iced water or prolonged periods of cooling can deepen tissue injury, induce hypothermia, and are best avoided. Cleaning solutions and dressings aim to prevent wound infection. The ideal dressing will establish an optimum microenvironment for wound healing. It will maintain the wound temperature and moisture level, permit respiration, allow epithelial migration,[5] and exclude environmental bacteria.

AIMS OF INTERVENTION To promote wound healing; to prevent infection, with minimal adverse effects and discomfort.

OUTCOMES Time to healing; quality of healing with regard to scarring, re-epithelisation, repigmentation, and cosmetic results; prevention of wound infection; quality of life during treatment regimen; pain (during procedures and background); ease of dressing application and removal; patient/investigator preference and satisfaction; number and frequency of dressing change; adverse effects.

METHODS *Clinical Evidence* search and appraisal December 2003.

QUESTION What are the effects of treatments for minor thermal burns?

OPTION ANTIBIOTICS

We found no RCTs comparing the use of topical or oral antibiotics versus placebo or no treatment in the management of superficial burn wounds. Routine prophylactic use of antibiotics may promote the emergence of resistant organisms in the community.

Benefits: We found no systematic reviews or RCTs.

Harms: We found no RCTs.

Comment: We found no evidence to suggest that the routine prophylactic use of topical or oral antibiotics decreases the rate of wound infection or improves clinical outcomes such as time to wound healing of superficial burn wounds. Furthermore, unnecessary and excessive antibiotic use promotes the emergence of resistant organisms in the community for no therapeutic gain in the individual case.[6] Therefore, antibiotics should only be used if signs of infection develop, in order to prevent significant complications such as toxic shock syndrome, especially in children and young adults.[7]

OPTION CHLORHEXIDINE IMPREGNATED PARAFFIN GAUZE DRESSING

Two RCTs comparing chlorhexidine impregnated paraffin gauze versus hydrocolloid dressing found no significant difference in time to wound healing but, subjectively, both investigators and patients in one of the RCTs rated the hydrocolloid dressing more favourably. One RCT found that chlorhexidine impregnated paraffin gauze increased time to wound healing and was perceived as more painful compared with polyurethane film.

Benefits: We found no systematic review but we found three RCTs (see table A on web extra).[8–10] **Versus hydrocolloid dressing:** See benefits of hydrocolloid dressing(G), p 2489. **Versus polyurethane film:** See benefits of polyurethane film(G), p 2492.

Harms: **Versus hydrocolloid dressing:** See harms of hydrocolloid dressing, p 2490. **Versus polyurethane film:** See harms of polyurethane film, p 2492.

Comment: In common with other antibacterial substances, chlorhexidine shows some toxicity to regenerating epithelial cells such as keratinocytes and fibroblasts, although the applicability of these studies to clinical situations remains unclear. Topical antimicrobials seem to be clinically indicated in infected burns and may delay wound healing to a lesser extent than does an uncontrolled infection. However, the toxicity associated with topical antibacterial products makes them relatively contraindicated in wounds that are not infected or heavily contaminated. (See comments under hydrocolloid dressing, p 2491 and polyurethane film, p 2493.)

OPTION HYDROCOLLOID DRESSING

Two RCTs comparing hydrocolloid dressing versus paraffin impregnated gauze dressings found no significant difference in time to wound healing between the two treatment groups but, subjectively, both investigators and patients in one of the RCTs rated the hydrocolloid dressing more favourably. One RCT found no significant difference in time to wound healing, pain, or interference with activities of daily living between hydrocolloid dressing and a combination of chlorhexidine impregnated paraffin gauze dressing plus silver sulfadiazine cream. One RCT found that hydrocolloid dressing reduced time to healing, pain, and limitation of activity compared with silver sulfadiazine dressing. One RCT found that healing time was shorter with hydrocolloid dressing alone compared with hydrocolloid dressing plus silver sulfadiazine cream, and found no difference in pathogenic bacteria growth with hydrocolloid dressing alone compared with hydrocolloid dressing plus silver sulfadiazine cream.

Benefits: We found no systematic review but we found four RCTs (see table A on web extra).[8,9,11,12] **Versus chlorhexidine impregnated paraffin gauze dressing:** We found two RCTs comparing hydrocolloid dressing(G) versus chlorhexidine impregnated paraffin gauze dressing.[8,9] The first RCT (67 people) found no significant difference in time to wound healing (median 12 days in each group, P = 0.89) or background pain (rated using a visual analogue scale, data for mean scores not provided, P = 0.28).[8] After complete wound healing, wound appearance was more frequently rated as "excellent" with hydrocolloid dressing compared with chlorhexidine impregnated paraffin gauze dressing (19/34 [56%] with hydrocolloid dressing *v* 3/28 [11%] with chlorhexidine impregnated paraffin gauze dressing, P < 0.001). Investigators and patients rated the hydrocolloid dressing more highly than the chlorhexidine impregnated paraffin gauze (10 item visual analogue scale, with 0 = useless and 10 = excellent: patients' rating 9.04 with hydrocolloid *v* 6.86 with chlorhexidine impregnated paraffin gauze, P < 0.02; investigators' rating: 9.31 with hydrocolloid *v* 6.9 with chlorhexidine impregnated paraffin gauze, P = 0.005). The second RCT (54 people presenting within 24 hours of injury affecting less than 5% of total body surface area) had three study arms, comparing hydrocolloid dressing, hydrocolloid dressing plus silver sulfadiazine, and chlorhexidine impregnated paraffin gauze dressing.[9] It found no significant difference in time to healing between hydrocolloid dressing and the chlorhexidine impregnated paraffin gauze dressing (10.6 days with hydrocolloid *v* 11.1 days with chlorhexidine impregnated paraffin gauze dressing, P value reported as not significant). **Versus chlorhexidine impregnated paraffin gauze dressing plus silver sulfadiazine cream:** We found one RCT (30 people), which compared hydrocolloid dressing versus chlorhexidine impregnated paraffin gauze plus silver sulfadiazine cream after initial burn cleaning.[11] It found no significant difference in any of the outcomes measured: time to wound healing (11 days in each group, P value not reported), pain levels (median pain score baseline 3/10 with hydrocolloid *v* 2/10 with chlorhexidine impregnated paraffin gauze plus silver sulfadiazine; median pain score at second visit 0/10 with hydrocolloid *v* 1/10 with chlorhexidine impregnated paraffin gauze plus silver sulfadiazine, P values not reported), people reporting interference of daily living (6/15 [40%] in each group), or investigator/patient satisfaction ratings (patients' overall satisfaction rated as "excellent" by 8/15 [57%] with hydrocolloid *v* 11/15 [79%] with chlorhexidine impregnated paraffin gauze plus silver sulfadiazine; investigators' overall evaluation rated as "excellent" by 11/15 [79%] with hydrocolloid *v* 13/15 [87%] with chlorhexidine impregnated paraffin gauze plus silver sulfadiazine; P values not reported). **Versus silver sulfadiazine dressing:** We found one RCT (42 people) comparing hydrocolloid dressing versus silver sulfadiazine dressing after initial burn cleaning.[12] It found that, compared with silver sulfadiazine dressing, hydrocolloid dressing significantly reduced time to wound healing (10.23 days *v* 15.59 days, P < 0.01), pain (results represented graphically, P < 0.01), and limitation of activity (in 2/22 [9%] people with hydrocolloid *v* in 11/20 [55%] people with silver sulfadiazine, P < 0.01). After complete wound healing, wound appearance (P < 0.01), repigmentation (P < 0.01), and overall investigator/patient satisfaction (P < 0.001) were rated as better with hydrocolloid dressing compared with silver sulfadiazine. **Versus hydrocolloid plus silver sulfadiazine cream:** We found one RCT (54 people presenting within 24 hours of injury affecting less than 5% of total body surface area) with three study arms, comparing hydrocolloid dressing, hydrocolloid dressing plus silver sulfadiazine cream, and chlorhexidine impregnated paraffin gauze dressing.[9] It found a shorter mean healing time with hydrocolloid dressing alone compared with hydrocolloid plus silver sulfadiazine cream (10.6 days with hydrocolloid dressing *v* 14.2 days with hydrocolloid plus silver sulfadiazine cream, reported as a significant difference).

Harms: **Versus chlorhexidine impregnated paraffin gauze dressing:** In the first RCT, pain was reported in one person and rash in two people with hydrocolloid dressing.[8] Infection occurred in one person in the hydrocolloid group, and healing was delayed in one person in each treatment group. The RCT found no significant difference in pain associated with dressing changes (rated using a visual analogue scale, data for mean scores not provided, P = 0.96) or the ease of dressing removal (P = 0.49) between the two treatment groups. Dressings were changed more often due to leakage with hydrocolloid compared with chlorhexidine impregnated paraffin gauze dressing (15/94 [15%] with hydrocolloid *v* 3/89 [3%] with chlorhexidine impregnated paraffin gauze dressing, P < 0.02). The second RCT found no significant difference in increase in pathogenic bacterial isolates between hydrocolloid dressing and the chlorhexidine impregnated paraffin gauze dressing (P = 0.12).[9] The number of wound infections was not reported but none of the people in either treatment group required antibiotic treatment. The RCT found significantly fewer dressing changes with hydrocolloid dressing compared with chlorhexidine impregnated paraffin gauze dressing (2.3 with hydrocolloid dressing *v* 4.1 with chlorhexidine impregnated paraffin gauze dressing, P < 0.0001); reasons for dressing changes were not listed. **Versus chlorhexidine impregnated paraffin gauze dressing plus silver sulfadiazine cream:** The RCT reported no wound infections.[11] However, three people who developed cellulitis during treatment were excluded from the RCT. Dressings were changed less frequently with hydrocolloid dressing compared with chlorhexidine impregnated paraffin gauze plus silver sulfadiazine cream (P < 0.02). Although reasons for dressing changes were not given, this result was to be expected, as chlorhexidine impregnated paraffin gauze plus silver sulfadiazine dressings were routinely changed, whereas there was no indication to change hydrocolloid dressings without leakage or suspected infection. The RCT found that application and removal were more frequently rated as "easy" with hydrocolloid dressing compared with chlorhexidine impregnated paraffin gauze plus silver sulfadiazine (P < 0.001). **Versus silver sulfadiazine dressing:** The RCT reported no infections in either group.[12] It found fewer dressing changes with hydrocolloid dressing compared with silver sulfadiazine (mean number of dressing changes 3.55 [range 3.39–3.71] with hydrocolloid dressing *v* 22.2 [range 20.22–24.18] with silver sulfadiazine, P < 0.001). However, this result was to be expected, as silver sulfadiazine dressings were routinely changed, whereas there was no indication to change hydrocolloid dressings without leakage or suspected infection. Dressing application and removal were rated as easier, and dressing comfort as better with hydrocolloid dressing compared with silver sulfadiazine (P < 0.01). **Versus hydrocolloid plus silver sulfadiazine cream:** The RCT found no significant difference in increase in pathogenic bacterial isolates between the groups (P = 0.12).[9] One person in the combination treatment group required antibiotic treatment, presumably for wound infection. The RCT found fewer dressing changes with hydrocolloid dressing compared with hydrocolloid dressing plus silver sulfadiazine cream (2.3 with hydrocolloid dressing *v* 3.9 with hydrocolloid dressing plus silver sulfadiazine cream, P < 0.0001); reasons for dressing changes were not given.

Comment: **Versus chlorhexidine impregnated paraffin gauze dressing:** Neither RCT reported the methods used for randomisation or allocation concealment.[8,9] The first RCT had a high withdrawal rate (31/98 [32%]), which may limit the validity of its results.[8] **Versus chlorhexidine impregnated paraffin gauze dressing plus silver sulfadiazine cream:** The RCT gave insufficient information about the methods used for randomisation and allocation concealment. Furthermore, the RCT was limited by a small sample size and a high withdrawal rate (18/48 [38%]), which may limit the validity of its results.[11] Excluding people with cellulitis compromises the ability of the study to assess infection rates for the dressings used. **Versus silver sulfadiazine dressing:** The RCT had a number of shortcomings, including a small sample size and unspecified methods for randomisation or allocation concealment.[12] The withdrawal rate was 8/50 (16%).

OPTION PARAFFIN GAUZE DRESSINGS

One RCT found no significant difference in pain or time to wound healing with paraffin gauze compared with polyurethane film.

Benefits: We found no systematic review but we found one RCT (see table A on web extra).[13] **Versus polyurethane film:** See benefits of polyurethane film, p 2492.

Harms: See harms of polyurethane film, p 2492.

Comment: See comment under polyurethane film, p 2493.

OPTION POLYURETHANE FILM

One RCT comparing polyurethane film versus paraffin gauze found no significant difference in pain or the number of days to wound healing. One RCT found that polyurethane film reduced time to wound healing and was perceived as less painful compared with chlorhexidine impregnated paraffin gauze.

Benefits: We found no systematic review but found two RCTs (see table A on web extra).[10,13] **Versus paraffin gauze dressing:** The first RCT (55 people) found no significant difference in time to healing between polyurethane film**Ⓖ** and paraffin impregnated gauze, although burn wounds tended to heal faster with paraffin gauze dressing (median days to wound healing: 7 days with paraffin gauze *v* 10 days with polyurethane film, $P > 0.05$).[13] Pain and patient satisfaction ratings were not significantly different between groups (pain: 4 item assessment scale for degrees of no pain, mild, moderate, and severe pain; grouped scores listed, difference reported as not significant; patient satisfaction: people, or, in the case of children, their parents, reporting themselves "satisfied": 27/29 [96%] with polyurethane *v* 20/25 [80%] with paraffin gauze, P value not given but reported as not significant). **Versus chlorhexidine impregnated paraffin gauze:** The second RCT (51 people with small blistered burns) found that mean healing time was significantly shorter with polyurethane film compared with chlorhexidine impregnated paraffin gauze (10 days, 95% CI 5 days to 15 days with polyurethane film *v* 14.08 days, 95% CI 7.08 days to 21.08 days with chlorhexidine impregnated paraffin gauze, $P < 0.04$).[10] Comparative ranking on a "pain" perception diagram (assessing intensity and duration) was lower with polyurethane film compared with chlorhexidine impregnated paraffin gauze ($P < 0.01$). Although the RCT found a significantly higher number of people healed in the polyurethane film group at 10 days after injury (presented graphically, $P < 0.05$), there was no significant difference in wound healing between the two treatment groups at times greater than 10 days after injury (presented graphically, no P value given but reported as not significant).

Harms: **Versus paraffin gauze dressing:** The RCT reported skin reactions such as follicular exanthema and itching in 2/30 people with polyurethane.[13] Wound infection was seen in 3/30 people with polyurethane and 2/25 people with paraffin gauze (P value not reported). No infection required antibiotic treatment. Leakages were observed 43 times in 19/30 (63%) people and new dressings were required 32 times in 15/30 (50%)

people with polyurethane, whereas the dressing was soaked in 7/25 (28%) people with paraffin gauze (P value not reported; see comment below). Review at 3 months after injury showed that more people in the polyurethane film group than in the paraffin gauze group had residual scars (6/29 [21%] with polyurethane *v* 2/25 [8%] with paraffin gauze, difference reported as not significant). **Versus chlorhexidine impregnated paraffin gauze:** The RCT found no significant difference in rate of wound infection between the two treatment groups (1/26 [4%] with polyurethane *v* 2/25 [8%] with chlorhexidine impregnated paraffin gauze, P value not reported). Comparative ranking on a "social inconvenience" perception diagram (assessing embarrassment and difficulty in coping) was lower with polyurethane compared with chlorhexidine impregnated paraffin gauze ($P < 0.01$).[10]

Comment: **Versus paraffin gauze dressing:** The paraffin gauze dressing was routinely changed on day 6, whereas the polyurethane dressing was not touched, unless there was significant leakage, infection, or skin reaction.[13] **Versus chlorhexidine impregnated paraffin gauze:** The RCT was conducted in the early 1980s and gave no information on the methods used for randomisation or concealment strategies.[10]

OPTION SILICONE COATED NYLON

One RCT found that silicone coated nylon dressing reduced time to wound healing in children compared with silver sulfadiazine dressing.

Benefits: We found no systematic review but we found one RCT (see table A on web extra).[14] **Versus silver sulfadiazine dressing:** One RCT (76 children presenting within 24 hours of injury with a previously untreated burn) comparing silicone coated nylon net dressing versus silver sulfadiazine cream covered by gauze dressing.[14] It found that silicone coated nylon resulted in a shorter mean healing time compared with silver sulfadiazine (7.58 days, 95% CI 4.46 days to 10.70 days with silicone coated nylon *v* 11.26 days, 95% CI 5.24 days to 17.28 days with silver sulfadiazine, $P < 0.01$).

Harms: **Versus silver sulfadiazine dressing:** The RCT found no allergies in either treatment group.[14] One reported case of wound infection was reported among the 30 children in the silver sulfadiazine dressing group. The number of dressings was lower with silicone coated nylon net dressing compared with silver sulfadiazine (3.64 [range 2.14–4.14] with silicone coated nylon net dressing *v* 5.13 [range 2.23–8.03] with silver sulfadiazine, $P < 0.05$). As dressings were changed every 2–3 days until complete healing was obtained, this result is not surprising but simply results from the longer healing period with the silver sulfadiazine dressing. The RCT found no fluid collection, haematoma, or secondary displacement in either group. Dressing removal was reported as easy and atraumatic.

Comment: **Versus silver sulfadiazine dressing:** The RCT gave no information on the methods used for randomisation or allocation concealment.[14]

OPTION SILVER SULFADIAZINE CREAM

One RCT found no significant difference in time to wound healing, pain levels, or interference with activities of daily living comparing a combination of chlorhexidine impregnated paraffin gauze dressing plus silver sulfadiazine cream versus hydrocolloid dressing. One RCT found that silver sulfadiazine dressing increased time to healing, pain, and limitation of activity compared with hydrocolloid dressing. One RCT found that healing time was longer with hydrocolloid dressing plus silver sulfadiazine cream compared with

hydrocolloid dressing alone and found no significant difference in pathogenic bacteria growth between the two groups. One RCT found that silver sulfadiazine dressing increased time to wound healing in children compared with silicone coated nylon dressing.

Benefits: We found no systematic review but we found three RCTs (see table A on web extra).[9,12,14] **Versus hydrocolloid dressing:** See benefits of hydrocolloid dressing**G**, p 2489. **Versus silicone coated nylon:** See benefits of silicone coated nylon, p 2493.

Harms: **Versus hydrocolloid dressing:** See harms of hydrocolloid dressing, p 2490. **Versus silicone coated nylon:** See harms of silicone coated nylon, p 2493.

Comment: Silver sulfadiazine cream is well known to be toxic to regenerating epithelial cells and may retard healing of minor burns, which are known to heal by re-epithelialisation.[2] (See comments under hydrocolloid dressing, p 2491 and silicone coated nylon, p 2493.)

GLOSSARY

Hydrocolloid dressings such as Comfeel® and Duoderm® are adhesive, water and gas impermeable membranes, which form a gel when their inner layer comes into contact with exudate and thus help to debride the wound.[5] They provide a seal around the edges of the wound and can protect pressure areas. Furthermore, they may have an antimicrobial effect due to wound acidification.[15] However, difficulties can arise from leakage and subsequently increased risk of wound contamination.

Polyurethane film dressings such as Opsite® or Tegaderm® serve as a barrier to bacteria and water. The dressings can be left in place for several days, but usually leak if exudate builds up, thus increasing the risk of wound contamination.[5]

REFERENCES

1. 1.Brigham PA, McLoughlin E. Burn incidence and medical care use in the United States: estimates, trends and data sources. *J Burn Care Rehabil* 1996;17:95–107.
2. 2.Haertsch PA. Burn injuries. *Australian Doctor* 2003;August:37–44.
3. 3.Deitch EA, Wheelahan TM, RoseMP. Hypertrophic burns scars: analysis of variables. *J Trauma* 1983;3:895.
4. 4.McCormick RA, La Hei ER, Martin HCO. First-aid management of minor burns in children: a prospective study of children presenting to the Children's Hospital at Westmead, Sydney. *Med J Aust* 2003;178:31–33.
5. 5.Hayward PG, Morrsion WA. Current concepts in wound dressings. *Australian Prescriber* 1996;19:11–13.
6. 6.Wise R, Hart T, Cars O, et al. Antimicrobial resistance is a major threat to public health [Editorial]. *BMJ* 1998;317:609–610.
7. 7.Brown AP, Khan K, Sinclair S. Bacterial toxicosis/toxic shock syndrome as a contributor to morbidity in children with burn injuries. *Burns* 2003;29:733–738.
8. 8.Wright A, MacKechnie DW, Paskins JR. Management of partial thickness burns with Granuflex 'E' dressings. *Burns* 1993;19:128–130.
9. 9.Thomas SS, Lawrence, JC, Thomas A. Evaluation of hydrocolloids and topical medication in minor burns. *J Wound Care* 1995;4:218–220.
10. 10.Neal DE, Whalley PC, Flowers MW, et al. The effects of an adherent polyurethane film and conventional absorbent dressing in patients with small partial thickness burns. *Br J Clin Pract* 1981;35:254–257.
11. 11.Afilalo M, Dankoff J, Guttman A, et al. DuoDERM hydroactive dressing versus silver sulphadiazine/Bactigras in the emergency treatment of partial skin thickness burns. *Burns* 1992;18:313–316.
12. 12.Wyatt D, McGowan DN, Najarian, MP. Comparison of a hydrocolloid dressing and silver sulfadiazine cream in the outpatient management of second-degree burns. *J Trauma* 1990;30:857–865.
13. 13.Poulsen TD, Freund KG, Arendrup K, et al. Polyurethane film (Opsite) vs. impregnated gauze (Jelonet) in the treatment of outpatient burns: a prospective, randomized study. *Burns* 1991;17:59–61.
14. 14.Bugmann PH, Taylor S, Gyger D, et al. A silicone-coated nylon dressing reduces healing time in burned paediatric patients in comparison with standard sulfadiazine treatment: a prospective randomized trial. *Burns* 1998;24:609–612.
15. 15.Kaufman T, Eichealanb EH, Angel MF, et al. Topical acidification promotes healing of experimental deep partial thickness burns. *Burns Incl Therm Inj* 1985; 12:84–90.

Jason Wasiak
Therapeutic Guidelines Limited
Melbourne
Australia

Heather Cleland
The Alfred Hospital
Melbourne
Australia

Competing interests: None declared.

Pressure sores

Search date January 2004

Nicky Cullum, E Andrea Nelson, and Jane Nixon

QUESTIONS

INTERVENTIONS

See glossary G

Key Messages

Prevention

- **Foam alternatives (compared with standard foam mattresses)** One systematic review found that foam alternatives to the standard hospital foam mattress reduced the incidence of pressure sores over 10–14 days in people at high risk. One subsequent RCT found no significant difference in pressure sores between a standard mattress and a foam alternative. We found no clear evidence of a "best" foam alternative.
- **Pressure relieving overlays on operating tables** Three RCTs identified by a systematic review found that pressure relieving overlays on operating tables reduced the incidence of pressure sores.
- **Low air loss beds in intensive care (compared with standard beds)** One RCT in people in intensive care found that low air loss beds reduced the risk of new pressure sores compared with standard intensive care beds.
- **Medical sheepskin overlays** One RCT found that medical sheepskin overlays reduced the incidence of pressure sores compared with standard treatment in people aged 60 years or more who underwent orthopaedic surgery.

- **Alternating pressure surfaces** Two RCTs identified by a systematic review and one subsequent RCT found that alternating pressure mattresses reduced pressure sores compared with a standard foam mattress or a constant low pressure mattress, but seven other smaller RCTs identified by the review found no significant difference between alternating pressure devices and constant low pressure mattresses.
- **Different seat cushions** We found insufficient evidence about the effects of different seat cushions in preventing pressure sores.
- **Electric profiling beds** We found insufficient evidence about the effects of electric profiling beds in preventing pressure sores.
- **Low tech constant low pressure supports** We found insufficient evidence about the effects of low tech constant low pressure supports in preventing pressure sores.
- **Repositioning (regular "turning")** One systematic review found insufficient evidence about the effects of repositioning (regular "turning").
- **Topical lotions and dressings** One systematic review found insufficient evidence about the effects topical lotions or dressings.
- **Air filled vinyl boots with foot cradle** One small RCT found that air filled vinyl boots with foot cradles were associated with more rapid development of pressure sores compared with hospital pillows.
- **Low air loss hydrotherapy beds** One RCT found that low air loss hydrotherapy beds increased the risk of developing a pressure sore compared with a range of support surfaces in people with incontinence.

Treatment

- **Air fluidised supports (compared with standard care)** Two RCTs found that air fluidised supports reduced pressure sores after 15 days compared with standard care. One RCT with methodological weaknesses and one very small RCT found no significant difference between air fluidised supports and standard care.
- **Alternating pressure surfaces** We found insufficient evidence on the effects of alternating pressure surfaces in healing pressure sores.
- **Debridement** RCTs provided insufficient evidence to compare effects of different debriding agents on healing.
- **Dressings other than hydrocolloid** Small, methodologically weak RCTs provided insufficient evidence about the effect of dressings other than hydrocolloid.
- **Electrotherapy** Three RCTs found limited evidence that electrotherapy increased healing compared with sham therapy. However, the RCTs were small and of limited quality, and their conclusions are therefore unreliable.
- **Hydrocolloid dressings** We found inconclusive evidence about the effects of hydrocolloid dressings.
- **Low air loss beds** We found insufficient evidence on the effects of low air loss beds in healing pressure sores.
- **Low level laser therapy** We found insufficient evidence from two RCTs about the effects of low level laser therapy on healing.
- **Low tech constant low pressure supports** We found insufficient evidence on the effects of low tech constant low pressure supports in healing pressure sores.
- **Nutritional supplements** RCTs found no significant difference in healing between nutritional supplements and control interventions (low dose or no supplements). However, studies were small and may have lacked power to detect clinically important differences between treatments.
- **Seat cushions** We found insufficient evidence on the effects of seat cushions in healing pressure sores.
- **Surgery** We found no RCTs of surgical treatments for pressure sores.
- **Therapeutic ultrasound** Two RCTs identified by a systematic review found no significant difference in healing between ultrasound and sham ultrasound.
- **Topical negative pressure** We found insufficient evidence from two small RCTs about the effects of topical negative pressure on healing.

■ **Topical phenytoin** One small RCT provided insufficient evidence about the effects of topical phenytoin on healing.

DEFINITION	Pressure sores (also known as pressure ulcers, bed sores, and decubitus ulcers) may present as persistently hyperaemic, blistered, broken, or necrotic skin and may extend to underlying structures, including muscle and bone.
INCIDENCE/ PREVALENCE	Reported prevalence rates range between 4.7–32.1% for hospital populations, between 4.4–33% for community care populations, and between 4.6–20.7% for nursing home populations.[1]
AETIOLOGY/ RISK FACTORS	Pressure sores are caused by unrelieved pressure, shear, or friction. They are most common below the waist and at bony prominences, such as the sacrum, heels, and hips. They occur in all health care settings. Increased age, reduced mobility, impaired nutrition, vascular disease, faecal incontinence, and skin condition at baseline consistently emerge as risk factors.[2,3] However, the relative importance of these and other factors is uncertain.
PROGNOSIS	The presence of pressure sores has been associated with a twofold to fourfold increased risk of death in elderly people and people in intensive care.[4,5] However, pressure sores are a marker for underlying disease severity and other comorbidities rather than an independent predictor of mortality.[4]
AIMS OF INTERVENTION	To prevent pressure sore formation; heal existing pressure sores; and improve quality of life.
OUTCOMES	Incidence and severity of pressure sores; rate of change of area and volume; and time to heal. Interface pressure recorded at various anatomical sites is a surrogate outcome that is sometimes used in studies of preventive interventions but has not yet been linked to clinical outcomes.
METHODS	*Clinical Evidence* search and appraisal January 2004. We reviewed all RCTs that used objective clinical outcome measures. For many trials we could not be sure that the size of pressure sores was distributed evenly between groups at baseline. Unequal distribution of wound size at baseline would have an impact on all measures of wound healing. Ideally, studies of treatment should stratify randomisation by initial wound area and be of sufficient size to ensure even distribution of baseline wound size.

QUESTION What are the effects of preventive interventions?

OPTION PRESSURE RELIEVING SURFACES

One systematic review found that foam alternatives to the standard hospital foam mattress reduced the incidence of pressure sores over 10–14 days in people at high risk. One subsequent RCT found no significant difference in pressure sores between a standard mattress and a foam alternative. We found no clear evidence of a "best" foam alternative. We found insufficient evidence on the effects of electric profiling beds, different seat cushions, and low tech constant low pressure supports. Two RCTs identified by a systematic review and one subsequent RCT found that alternating pressure mattresses reduced pressure sores compared with a standard foam mattress or a constant low pressure mattress, but seven other smaller RCTs identified by the review found no significant difference between alternating pressure devices and constant low pressure mattresses. One RCT in people in intensive care found that low air loss beds reduced the risk of new pressure sores compared with standard intensive care beds. One RCT found that low air loss hydrotherapy beds increased the risk of developing a pressure sore compared with a range of support surfaces in people with incontinence. Three RCTs identified by the systematic review found that pressure relieving overlays on operating tables reduced the incidence of pressure sores. One small RCT found that air filled vinyl boots with foot cradles were associated with more rapid development of pressure sores compared with hospital pillows. One RCT found that medical sheepskin overlays reduced the incidence of pressure sores compared with standard treatment in people aged 60 years or more who underwent orthopaedic surgery.

Benefits: We found one systematic review (search date 2000).[6] **Foam alternatives versus standard hospital mattress:** The systematic review[6] identified four RCTs (850 people), and we found one subsequent RCT (101 people).[7] All five RCTs were undertaken primarily in elderly people in orthopaedic hospital wards. The systematic review found that foam alternatives to the standard hospital mattress significantly reduced the incidence of sores over 10–14 days (RR 0.29, 95% CI 0.19 to 0.43).[6] The subsequent RCT (101 people with acute hip fracture) compared foam mattresses (viscoelastic foam mattress in the emergency room followed by a viscoelastic foam overlay on top of a standard mattress) versus standard mattresses (standard trolley mattress in the emergency room followed by a standard hospital foam mattress).[7] It found no significant difference between mattress types in the incidence of pressure ulcers up to 14 days (12/48 [25%] with foam mattress *v* 17/53 [32%] with standard mattress; P value not reported). **Different foam alternatives:** The systematic review identified five RCTs (795 people) that compared different foam alternatives.[6] One RCT (40 people) found that a foam and fibre replacement that comprised five sections reduced the risk of pressure sores compared with a 4 inch (10 cm) thick dimpled foam (RR for development of pressure sore 0.42, 95% CI 0.18 to 0.96; NNT for 10–21 days' treatment 3, 95% CI 2 to 25). The other RCTs were too small to detect a difference between the foam alternatives. **Electric profiling beds:** We found one RCT (70 people in medical or surgical hospital wards), which compared an electrically operated profiling bed (comprising four sections plus a pressure relieving foam mattress) versus a standard hospital bed with pressure relieving mattress (foam or alternating pressure).[8] It found no significant difference in the incidence of pressure sores up to 10 days (no one who received either intervention developed a sore). The RCT may have been underpowered to detect a clinically important difference. **Different seat cushions:** The systematic review identified two RCTs.[6] The first RCT (53 people) compared slab foam versus bespoke contoured foam cushions, and the other RCT (141 people) compared a gel and foam wheelchair cushion versus a foam cushion. The RCTs found no significant difference in the incidence of pressure sores among different types of cushions after 5 months' use of a slab foam cushion and 3 months of the gel and foam cushion, but they may have been too small to detect a clinically important difference. **Low tech constant low pressure supports:** The systematic review identified seven RCTs (1451 people), which were too small or flawed to draw reliable conclusions.[6] **Alternating pressure surfaces:** The systematic review[6] identified nine RCTs (1242 people) that compared alternating pressure surfaces**G** versus standard foam or constant low pressure supports and we found one subsequent RCT.[9] Most RCTs were too small to rule out a clinically important difference in the prevention of pressure sores. One RCT (327 people) included in the review found that an alternating pressure surface significantly reduced the incidence of pressure sores compared with a standard foam mattress (RR 0.32, 95% CI 0.14 to 0.72; NNT for 10 days' treatment 11, 95% CI 6 to 34). Another RCT (230 people) included in the review found that a range of alternating pressure surfaces significantly reduced the incidence of pressure sores compared with a range of constant low pressure supports after an average of 16 days. The subsequent RCT (108 older hospitalised people confined to bed) compared alternating pressure (both single and double layer air cell) mattresses versus a standard polyester foam mattress.[9] It found that both alternating mattresses significantly reduced pressure sores compared with standard foam mattresses (3.4% with double layer *v* 19.2% with single layer *v* 37.0% with standard; P < 0.01 between all groups). However, this RCT did not undertake intention to treat analysis, and only 68% of randomised patients were included in the analysis. The other smaller RCTs found no significant difference between alternating pressure devices and constant low pressure supports over periods ranging from 8 days to 3 months. **Low air loss beds:** The systematic review identified one RCT (98 people).[6] It found that low air loss beds**G** in intensive care significantly reduced the risk of new pressure sores compared with standard intensive care beds (duration of trial not reported; RR 0.24, 95% CI 0.11 to 0.51; NNT 3, 95% CI 2 to 5). **Low air loss hydrotherapy beds:** The systematic review identified one RCT (98 people with incontinence admitted to acute and long stay hospital wards).[6] It found that low air loss hydrotherapy beds**G** significantly increased the risk of developing a pressure sore compared with a range of support surfaces after 60 days (RR 3.6, 95% CI 6.7 to 11.3). **Pressure relieving overlays on the operating table:** The systematic review identified three RCTs.[6] The first RCT (446 people who had undergone elective major general, gynaecological, or vascular surgery) found that a pressure relieving viscoelastic polymer pad significantly reduced the incidence of postoperative pressure sores compared with a standard table after 8 days (RR 0.52, 95% CI 0.32 to 0.83; NNT for intraoperative use 11, 95% CI 6 to 36). Meta-analysis of results from the two other RCTs (368 people) found that an alternating pressure surface (used during and for 7 days after surgery) significantly reduced the incidence of pressure sores over 7 days compared with a gel pad (used during surgery) plus a standard mattress (used for 7 days after surgery) (RR 0.21, 95% CI 0.06 to 0.70; NNT for 7 days' treatment 16, 95% 9 to 48). Whether the reduced incidence of pressure sores was because of intraoperative or postoperative pressure relief, or both, is unclear.[6] **Air filled vinyl boot with foot cradle:** The systematic review identified one small RCT (52 people), which found that hospital pillows significantly reduced the rate of developing pressure sores compared with a vinyl boot (air filled with a built in foot cradle) (mean time to skin breakdown 10 days *v* 13 days; $P < 0.036$ log rank test).[6] **Medical sheepskin overlays:** The systematic review[6] identified one small, poor quality RCT (36 people) and we found one subsequent RCT[10] of sheepskin overlays compared with standard treatment. The systematic review found no conclusive evidence.[6] The subsequent RCT (297 people aged ≥ 60 years who underwent orthopaedic surgery) found that medical sheepskin overlays plus standard pressure area care significantly reduced the incidence of pressure sores over an unspecified period (14/155 [9.0%] with sheepskin *v* 43/142 [30.3%] with standard care; RR 0.3, 95% CI 0.17 to 0.52).[10]

Harms: The systematic review noted that hypothermia was found in a few people who used low air loss hydrotherapy beds**G**.[6]

Comment: Most RCTs were small and of poor quality, and few performed the same comparison. Alternative foam mattresses comprised foam of varying densities, often within the same mattress, and sometimes were sculptured. **Medical sheepskin overlays:** Although these have been included in this option, it is debatable whether pressure relief is their main mechanism of action.

OPTION REPOSITIONING (REGULAR "TURNING")

One systematic review found insufficient evidence about the effects of repositioning (regular "turning").

Benefits: We found one systematic review (search date 1995, three small RCTs, 56 people [see comment below]), which found no significant difference in the incidence of pressure sores between regular manual repositioning and control treatment.[11] We found no RCTs that evaluated placement of people in different positions.

Harms: The review did not report on harms.[11]

Comment: The RCTs identified by the review were small, of poor quality, and few comparisons were undertaken more than once.[11] In one of the RCTs of regular repositioning identified by the review, 23 people were randomised to repositioning but only 10 people actually were repositioned regularly.[11]

OPTION TOPICAL LOTIONS AND DRESSINGS

One systematic review found insufficient evidence about the effects topical lotions or dressings.

Benefits: **Topical lotions and dressings:** We found one systematic review (search date 2000) that identified two RCTs of topical lotions.[12] The first RCT (319 people), which compared hexachlorophene (hexachlorophane) lotion versus cetrimide lotion, found no significant difference in the incidence of new pressure sores over 3 weeks (OR 0.97, 95% CI 0.46 to 1.65; no raw data reported). These results must be interpreted with caution because they were based on a completer analysis of 167 people. The other RCT (120 people) compared hexachlorophene lotion versus an inert lotion and found no significant difference in the proportion of people with changes in skin condition over 3 weeks.

Harms: The review did not report on harms.[11]

Comment: None.

QUESTION What are the effects of treatments?

OPTION PRESSURE RELIEVING SURFACES

Two RCTs found that air fluidised supports reduced pressure sores after 15 days compared with standard care. One RCT with methodological weaknesses and one very small RCT found no significant difference between air fluidised supports and standard care. We found insufficient evidence on the effects of low tech constant low pressure supports, alternating pressure surfaces, low air loss beds, or seat cushions.

Benefits: We found one systematic review (search date 2000[6]). **Air fluidised supports:** The systematic review identified four RCTs (214 people) that compared air fluidised supports**G** versus standard care.[6] Two RCTs (105 people in hospital) found that air fluidised supports healed more established sores than standard care (alternating pressure mattresses, regular changes of position, sheepskin, gel pads, or limb protectors) after 15 days. The third RCT (97 people being cared for at home) found no significant difference after 36 weeks, although this RCT had a high withdrawal rate. The fourth RCT (12 people) was too small to detect a clinically important difference. **Low tech constant low pressure supports:** The systematic review identified one RCT (120 elderly people with pressure sores in a nursing home) that found no significant difference in rates of pressure sore healing between a layered foam replacement mattress and a water mattress after 4 weeks. **Alternating pressure surfaces:** The systematic review[6] identified three RCTs and we found one subsequent RCT.[13] Two RCTs identified by the review (182 older people with pressure sores in hospital) found no significant differences in rates of pressure sore healing with different alternating pressure mattresses**G** after 4 and 18 weeks.[6] The third RCT in the review (32 older people in hospital and nursing homes) found no significant difference in pressure sore healing between an alternating pressure mattress and standard care after 2 weeks. The subsequent

RCT (158 people with pressure sores) found no significant difference in pressure ulcer progress between an alternating pressure mattress replacement and a static, fluid filled mattress overlay (overall ulcer and worst ulcer progress classified as worse, no change or improved: overall ulcer progress, P = 0.67; worst ulcer progress, P = 0.053).[13] **Low air loss beds:** The systematic review identified two RCTs (133 people), which found no significant difference in healing of pressure sores between low air loss beds**G** and convoluted foam.[6] We found no RCTs that compared low air loss beds versus alternating pressure or air fluidised supports. **Seat cushions:** The systematic review identified one RCT (25 people) that compared seat cushions with dry flotation versus alternating pressure and found no significant difference in healing rates (mean healing time: 44 days with dry flotation *v* 59 days with alternating pressure).[6]

Harms: The systematic review[6] noted that, in one of the RCTs identified,[14] hypothermia was found in a few people who used low air loss hydrotherapy beds**G**. The subsequent RCT did not report on harms.[13]

Comment: People are unable to move in and out of bed independently when they use air fluidised beds**G**, and this limits the type of people for whom they are suitable.

OPTION HYDROCOLLOID DRESSINGS

We found inconclusive evidence about the effects of hydrocolloid dressings.

Benefits: **Versus gauze soaked in saline or hypochlorite:** We found one systematic review (search date 1997, five RCTs; 396 wounds)[15] and one subsequent RCT (32 people)[16] of dressings or topical agents for pressure sores. The review found that hydrocolloid significantly improved healing up to 75 days compared with control (wounds healed: 102/205 [50%] with hydrocolloid dressing *v* 59/191 [31%] with traditional dressings; OR 2.57, 95% CI 1.58 to 4.18).[15] Findings were similar in the subsequent RCT (relative volume of wound at 12 weeks relative to 100% at baseline: 26% with hydrogel *v* 64% with saline; P < 0.02).[16] However, RCTs were small and of poor quality, and the significance of the meta-analysis was sensitive to the method of calculation (see comment below). **Versus other dressings:** The systematic review (search date 1997) identified nine RCTs (713 people) that compared hydrocolloid versus other dressings.[15] The RCTs had weak methods and were too small to draw reliable conclusions.

Harms: We found no reports on harms with these treatments.

Comment: Given the large absolute risks of events in the review, a relative risk would be a preferable outcome measure for results.[17] If the meta-analysis is re-worked using relative risk instead of odds ratio, the result is no longer significant (Cullum N, 2004; personal communication).

OPTION DRESSINGS OTHER THAN HYDROCOLLOID

Small, methodologically weak RCTs provided insufficient evidence about the effect of dressings other than hydrocolloid.

Benefits: We found one systematic review (search date 1997), which found seven RCTs (463 people) that compared dressings other than hydrocolloid.[15] We found five subsequent RCTs.[18–22] The RCTs had weak methods and were too small to draw reliable conclusions.

Harms: We found no good evidence on harms.

Comment: None.

OPTION DEBRIDEMENT

RCTs provided insufficient evidence to compare effects of different debriding agents on healing.

Benefits: We found one systematic review (search date 1998)[23] and five subsequent RCTs.[24–28] The systematic review found no RCTs that compared debridement versus no debridement.[23] It identified 32 RCTs that compared different debriding agents, but the studies were small, included a range of wounds, and few comparisons were undertaken in more than one RCT. The review concluded that there was insufficient evidence to promote the use of any particular debriding agent over another. The subsequent RCTs compared a variety of agents versus each other or versus dressings.[24–28] All but one were small, and together they provided no conclusive evidence about the relative effectiveness of the agents (see table A on web extra).

Harms: We found no good evidence on harms.

Comment: None.

OPTION TOPICAL PHENYTOIN

One small RCT provided insufficient evidence about the effects of topical phenytoin on healing.

Benefits: We found one RCT (48 patients) that compared topical phenytoin suspension (100 mg capsule in 5 mL saline) versus hydrocolloid dressings or antibiotic ointment as a treatment for partial thickness pressure sores.[29] It found that topical phenytoin significantly increased the healing rate compared with hydrocolloid dressings or antibiotic ointment (mean time to healing 35.3 ± 14.3 days with phenytoin *v* 51.8 ± 19.6 days with hydrocolloid *v* 53.8 ± 8.5 days with antibiotic; $P < 0.005$ for both comparisons), but no data that showed baseline equivalence for wound size were presented.

Harms: We found no good evidence on harms.

Comment: None.

OPTION SURGERY

We found no RCTs of surgical treatments for pressure sores.

Benefits: We found no RCTs of surgical treatments for pressure sores.

Harms: We found no good evidence on harms.

Comment: None.

OPTION NUTRITIONAL SUPPLEMENTS

RCTs found no significant difference in healing between nutritional supplements and control interventions (low dose or no supplements). However, studies were small and may have lacked power to detect clinically important differences between treatments.

Benefits: We found one systematic review (search date 2002, 4 RCTs, 134 people with existing pressure ulcers).[30] The review did not pool data. The first RCT (88 people with pressure sores in nursing homes or hospital, some of whom were receiving ultrasound treatment for their pressure sores) found no significant difference in ulcer healing at 84 days between 1000 mg ascorbic acid daily and 20 mg ascorbic acid daily (healing: 17/43 [39.5%] with 1000 mg ascorbic acid *v* 22/45 [48.9%] with control; RR 0.81, 95% CI 0.50 to 1.30). The second RCT (20 people with pressure sores undergoing surgery) found no significant difference in ulcer healing at 4 weeks between ascorbic acid (1000 mg/day for 4 weeks) and placebo (RR of ulcer healing 2, 95% CI 0.68 to 5.85). The third RCT (12 institutionalised people being fed via tube) found no significant difference in ulcer healing at 8 weeks between a very high protein diet and a high protein diet (RR of healing 0.11, 95% CI 0.01 to 1.70). The other RCT (14 people) was a crossover RCT that did not report results before the crossover period and had a high dropout rate.

Harms: The review did not report on harms.[30]

Comment: The studies identified by the review were small and may have lacked power to detect clinically important differences between treatments.

OPTION ELECTROTHERAPY

Three RCTs found limited evidence that electrotherapy increased healing compared with sham therapy. However, the RCTs were small and of limited quality, and their conclusions are therefore unreliable.

Benefits: **Electrotherapy:** We found one systematic review (search date 2000, 3 RCTs).[6] Two of the RCTs (91 pressure sores) were suitable for inclusion in a meta-analysis, which found that electrotherapy**G** significantly increased healing compared with sham therapy after about 3–5 weeks (RR 7.92, 95% CI 2.4 to 26.3). The third RCT included in the review found similar results after 4 weeks (percentage area of pressure sore healed: 49.8% with electrotherapy *v* 23.4% with sham; P = 0.042).[31] These RCTs were small, however, and had important weaknesses in their methods. Results should therefore be interpreted with caution.

Harms: We found no good evidence on harms.

Comment: None.

OPTION THERAPEUTIC ULTRASOUND

Two RCTs identified by a systematic review found no significant difference in healing between ultrasound and sham ultrasound.

Benefits: We found one systematic review (search date 1999, two RCTs comparing therapeutic ultrasound**G** *v* sham ultrasound, 128 people).[32] The review found no significant difference between ultrasound and sham ultrasound (2 RCTs, 128 people: RR 0.97, 95% CI 0.65 to 1.45). One RCT assessed outcomes at 12 weeks the other RCT did not report the timing of outcome assessment.

Harms: We found no good evidence on harms.

Comment: None.

OPTION LOW LEVEL LASER THERAPY

We found insufficient evidence from two RCTs about the effects of low level laser therapy on healing.

Benefits: **Low level laser therapy:** We found one systematic review (search date 1998, 1 RCT, 18 people) of low level laser therapy**G** in pressure sores.[33] It found no evidence of benefit. One subsequent RCT (86 people) similarly found no significant difference between low level laser therapy and standard care in reduction in wound size at 6 weeks (P = 0.23).[34]

Harms: We found no good evidence on harms.

Comment: None.

OPTION **TOPICAL NEGATIVE PRESSURE**

We found insufficient evidence from two small RCTs about the effects of topical negative pressure on healing.

Benefits: We found one systematic review (search date 2000, two small RCTs, one of which included 34 people with pressure sores).[35] The review found no clear evidence of improved healing of pressure sores with topical negative pressure**G** compared with no topical negative pressure.

Harms: We found no good evidence on harms.

Comment: None.

GLOSSARY

Air fluidised supports Membranes that cover a layer of particles that are fluidised by having air forced through them. The airflow can be turned off, which makes the surface solid again, to allow the person to be moved. People find it difficult to get in and out of these beds independently; therefore, they are usually reserved for people who spend most of the day in bed.

Alternating pressure surfaces Mattresses or overlays made of one or two layers of parallel air sacs. Alternate sacs are inflated and deflated, which provides alternating pressure and release for each area of skin.

Dextranomer paste Anhydrous, porous beads 0.1–0.3 mm in diameter. These beads are hydrophilic and absorb and adsorb exudate, wound debris, and bacteria, depending on particle size.

Electrotherapy The application of electrical fields by placing electrodes near a wound. Treatments include pulsed electromagnetic therapy, low intensity direct current, negative polarity and positive polarity electrotherapy, and alternating polarity electrotherapy.

Low air loss beds Mattresses that comprise inflatable upright sacs of semi-permeable fabric. Inflation of the sacs increases the area of contact between the individual and the support surface and reduces the pressure on the skin. People find it difficult to get in and out of these beds independently; therefore, they are usually reserved for people who spend most of the day in bed.

Low air loss hydrotherapy beds A mattress that comprises cushions covered by a permeable, fast drying filter sheet, through which air is circulated. The bed also contains a urine collecting device.

Low level laser therapy Also known as low intensity or low power therapy. It is thought to work by inducing a photochemical response to laser light, which results in biochemical alterations in cells and physiological changes.

Low or high tech constant low pressure supports Mattresses, overlays, and cushions made of high density or contoured foam or filled with fibre, gel, water, beads, or air. They increase the area of contact between the person and the support surface and thus reduce the pressure at the interface. See also air fluidised supports, low air loss beds, and low air loss hydrotherapy beds.

Therapeutic ultrasound The application of ultrasound to a wound with a transducer and water based gel. The power of ultrasound waves used in wound healing is low to avoid heating the tissues.

Topical negative pressure Negative pressure (suction) applied to a wound through an open cell dressing (for example, foam or felt).

Substantive changes

Pressure relieving surfaces (prevention) One RCT added;[9] categorisation of low air loss hydrotherapy beds changed from Unknown effectiveness to Likely to be ineffective or harmful based on re-evaluation of the evidence.

Pressure relieving surfaces (treatment) One RCT added;[13] categorisation unchanged.

Nutritional supplements (treatment) One systematic review added;[30] categorisation unchanged.

Low level laser therapy (treatment) One RCT added;[34] categorisation unchanged.

REFERENCES

1. Kaltenhaler E, Whitfield MD, Walters SJ, et al UK, USA, and Canada: how do their pressure ulcer prevalence and incidence data compare? *J Wound Care* 2001;10:530–535.
2. Reed RL, Hepburn K, Adelson R et al Low serum albumin levels, confusion and faecal incontinence: are these risk factors for pressure ulcers in mobility-impaired hospitalised adults? *Gerontology* 2003;49:255–259.
3. Allman RM. Pressure ulcer prevalence, incidence, risk factors, and impact. *Clin Geriatr Med* 1997;13:421–436.
4. Thomas DR, Goode PS, Tarquine PH, et al. Hospital acquired pressure ulcers and risk of death. *J Am Geriatr Soc* 1996;44:1435–1440.
5. Clough NP. The cost of pressure area management in an intensive care unit. *J Wound Care* 1994;3:33–35.
6. Cullum N, Nelson EA, Flemming K, et al. Systematic reviews of wound care management: (5) beds; (6) compression; (7) laser therapy, therapeutic ultrasound, electrotherapy and electromagnetic therapy. *Health Technol Assess* 2001;5:1–221. Search date 2000; primary sources 19 electronic databases, including Medline, Cinahl, Embase, and Cochrane Controlled Trials Register and hand searches.
7. Gunningberg L, Lindholm C, Carlsson M, et al. Effect of viscoelastic foam mattresses on the development of pressure ulcers in patients with hip fractures. *J Wound Care* 2000;9:455–460.
8. Keogh A, Dealey C. Profiling beds versus standard hospital beds: effects on pressure ulcer incidence outcomes. *J Wound Care* 2001;10:15–19.
9. Sanada H, Sugama J, Matsui Y, et al. Randomised controlled trial to evaluate a new double layer air cell overlay for elderly patients requiring head elevation. *J Tissue Viability* 2003;13:112–121.
10. McGowan S, Montgomery K, Jolley D, et al. The role of sheepskins in preventing pressure ulcers in elderly orthopaedic patients. *Prim Intention* 2000;8:1–8.
11. Cullum N, Deeks JJ, Fletcher AW, et al. Preventing and treating pressure sores. *Qual Health Care* 1995;4:289–297. Search date 1995; primary sources Medline, Cinahl, and hand searching of five journals.
12. O'Meara SM, Cullum NA, Majid M, et al. Systematic review of antimicrobial agents used for chronic wounds. *Br J Surg* 2001;88:4–21. Search date 2000; primary sources 19 electronic databases, including Medline and Cinahl, hand searches, and a panel of experts.
13. Russell L, Reynolds TM, Towns A, Worth W, Greenman A, Turner R. Randomized comparison trial of the RIK and the Nimbus 3 mattresses. *Br J Nurs* 2003;12:254, 256–259.
14. Bennett RG, Baran PJ, DeVone L, et al. Low airloss hydrotherapy versus standard care for incontinent hospitalized patients. *J Am Geriatr Soc* 1998;46:569–576.
15. Bradley M, Cullum N, Nelson EA, et al. Systematic reviews of wound care management: (2). Dressings and topical agents used in the healing of chronic wounds. *Health Technol Assess* 1999;3:1–35. Search date 1997; primary source Medline.
16. Matzen S, Peschardt A, Alsbjø rn B. A new amorphous hydrocolloid for the treatment of pressure sores: a randomised controlled study. *Scand J Plast Reconstr Hand Surg* 1999;33:13–15.
17. Altman DG, Deeks JJ, Sackett DL. Odds ratios should be avoided when events are common. *BMJ* 1998;317:1318.
18. Thomas DR, Goode PS, LaMaster K, et al. Acemann hydrogel dressing versus saline dressing for pressure ulcers. A randomized, controlled trial. *Adv Wound Care* 1998;11:273–276.
19. Rees RS, Robson MC, Smiell JM, et al. Becaplermin gel in the treatment of pressure ulcers: a phase II randomized, double-blind, placebo controlled study. *Wound Repair Regen* 1999;7:141–147.
20. Seaman S, Herbster S, Muglia J, et al. Simplifying modern wound management for nonprofessional caregivers. *Ostomy Wound Manage* 2000;46:18–27.
21. Price P, Bale S, Crook H, et al. The effect of a radiant heat dressing on pressure ulcers. *J Wound Care* 2000;9:201–205.
22. Graumlich JF, Blough LS, McLaughlin RG, et al. Healing pressure ulcers with collagen or hydrocolloid: a randomized, controlled trial. *J Am Geriatr Soc* 2003;51:147–154.
23. Bradley M, Cullum N, Sheldon T. The debridement of chronic wounds: a systematic review. *Health Technol Assess* 1999;3:1–78. Search date 1998; primary sources 19 electronic databases, including Medline and Embase.
24. Ljunberg S. Comparison of dextranomer paste and saline dressings for the management of decubital ulcers. *Clin Ther* 1998;20:737–743.
25. Burgos A, Gimenez J, Moreno E, et al. Cost, efficacy, efficiency and tolerability of collagenase ointment versus hydrocolloid occlusive dressing in the treatment of pressure sores. A comparative, randomised, multicentre study. *Clin Drug Invest* 2000;19:357–365.
26. Müller E, Van Leen MWF, Bergemann R. Economic evaluation of collagenase containing ointment and hydrocolloid dressing in the treatment of pressure ulcers. *Pharmacoeconomics* 2001;19:1209–1216.
27. Alvarez OM, Fernandez OA, Rogers RS, et al. Chemical debridement of pressure ulcers: a prospective randomized comparative trial of collagenase and papain/urea formulations. *Wounds* 2000;12:15–25.
28. Pullen R, Popp R, Volkers P, et al. Prospective randomized double-blind study of the wound-debriding effects of collagenase and fibrinolysin/deoxyribonuclease in pressure ulcers. Age Ageing 2002;31:126–30.
29. Rhodes RS, Heyneman CA, Culbertson VL, et al. Topical phenytoin treatment of stage II decubitus ulcers in the elderly. *Ann Pharmacother* 2001;35:675–681.
30. Langer G, Schloemer G, Knerr A, Kuss O, Behrens J. Nutritional interventions for preventing and treating pressure ulcers (Cochrane Review). In: The Cochrane Library, Issue 2, 2004. Chichester, UK: John Wiley & Sons, Ltd. Search date 2002; primary sources Cochrane Wounds Group Specialised Trials Register, Cochrane Central register of Controlled Trials, PubMed, Cinahl, reference lists, hand searches of conference proceedings and journals, and contact with manufacturers and experts in the field.

31. Gentzkow GD, Pollack SV, Kloth LC, et al. Improved healing of pressure ulcers using dermapulse, a new electrical stimulation device. *Wounds* 1991;3:158–170.

32. Flemming K, Cullum N. Therapeutic ultrasound for pressure sores. In: The Cochrane Library, Issue 4, 2003. Chichester, UK: John Wiley & Sons, Ltd. Search date 1999; primary sources 19 electronic databases, including Medline, Cinahl, Embase, and Cochrane Controlled Trials Register; hand searches; and contact with companies and experts in the field.

33. Lucas C, Stanborough RW, Freeman CL, et al. Efficacy of low level laser therapy on wound healing in human subjects. A systematic review. *Lasers Med Sci* 2000;15:84–93. Search date 1998; primary sources Medline, Embase, and Cinahl.

34. Lucas C, van Gemert MJ, de Haan RJ. Efficacy of low-level laser therapy in the management of stage III decubitus ulcers: a prospective, observer-blinded multicentre randomised clinical trial. *Lasers Med Sci* 2003;18:72–77.

35. Evans D, Land L. Topical negative pressure for treating chronic wounds. In: The Cochrane Library, Issue 4, 2003. Chichester, UK: John Wiley & Sons, Ltd. Search date 2000; primary sources Cochrane Wounds Group Specialised Trials Register, hand searches of reference lists, and contact with relevant companies and a panel of experts.

Nicky Cullum
Department of Health Sciences
University of York
York
UK

E Andrea Nelson
Senior Research Fellow
Centre for Evidence Based Nursing
Department of Health Sciences
University of York
York
UK

Jane Nixon
Deputy Head of Unit
Clinical Trials and Research Unit
University of Leeds
UK

Competing interests: EAN and NC are coinvestigators on a trial for which Beiersdorf provided trial related education. EAN, NC, and JN are coinvestigators on a trial of pressure relieving surfaces for which Huntleigh Healthcare Ltd provided trial related education. JN has been reimbursed for attending conferences and received speakers fees and research funding from Huntleigh Healthcare Ltd.

Venous leg ulcers

Search date July 2004

E Andrea Nelson, Nicky Cullum, and June Jones

QUESTIONS

INTERVENTIONS

See glossary **G**

Key Messages

Treatments

- **Compression bandages and stockings** One systematic review and one additional RCT found that compression bandages or stockings healed more venous leg ulcers than no compression. One systematic review and one subsequent RCT found insufficient evidence to suggest a difference between multilayer elastomeric and non-elastomeric high compression bandages. One systematic review and four subsequent RCTs found no significant difference in healing rates between multilayer elastomeric high compression bandages and short stretch bandages or Unna's boot. One systematic review found that multilayer compression increased ulcer healing compared with single layer bandages. One systematic review and two subsequent RCTs found no significant difference in the proportion of people healed with four layer elastomeric bandages compared with other high compression multilayer bandages. We found insufficient evidence from one small RCT about the effects of compression bandages compared with intermittent pneumatic compression.

Venous leg ulcers

- **Oral pentoxifylline** One systematic review and two subsequent RCTs found that oral pentoxifylline increased the proportion of ulcers healed over 6–12 months compared with placebo.
- **Cultured allogenic bilayer skin replacement** One RCT found that cultured allogenic bilayer skin replacement increased the proportion of ulcers healed after 6 months compared with a non-adherent dressing.
- **Oral flavonoids** Two RCTs found that adding flavonoids to compression increased the proportion of ulcers healed after 2–6 months compared with compression alone.
- **Oral sulodexide** Two RCTs found that sulodexide plus compression increased the proportion of ulcers healed after 2–3 months' treatment compared with compression alone.
- **Peri-ulcer injection of granulocyte-macrophage colony stimulating factor** One RCT found that peri-ulcer injection of granulocyte-macrophage colony stimulating factor increased the proportion of ulcers healed after 13 weeks' treatment compared with placebo.
- **Systemic mesoglycan** One RCT found that systemic mesoglycan plus compression increased the proportion of ulcers healed after 24 weeks' treatment compared with compression alone.
- **Debriding agents** One systematic review of small RCTs provided insufficient evidence about the effects of debriding agents on ulcer healing.
- **Foam, film, hyaluronic acid-derived dressings, or alginate (semi-occlusive) dressings** One systematic review provided insufficient evidence to compare the effects of semi-occlusive dressings (foam, film, hyaluronic acid-derived, or alginate) versus simple low adherent dressings, in the presence of compression. One systematic review and two subsequent RCTs found no significant difference in healing rates between semi-occlusive and occlusive dressings.
- **Intermittent pneumatic compression** One small RCT found insufficient evidence to compare intermittent pneumatic compression with compression bandages or stockings. One RCT found that intermittent pneumatic compression plus compression stockings improved ulcer healing at 3 months compared with compression stockings alone. Two other RCTs found no significant difference in healing at 6 months between intermittent pneumatic compression plus elastic stockings, and Unna's boot, and between intermittent pneumatic compression plus Unna's boot, and Unna's boot alone.
- **Laser treatment (low level)** RCTs provided insufficient evidence about the effects of low level laser on ulcer healing.
- **Oral aspirin** One RCT provided insufficient evidence about the effects of oral aspirin on ulcer healing.
- **Oral rutosides** RCTs provided insufficient evidence about the effects of oral rutosides on ulcer healing.
- **Oral thromboxane α_2 antagonists** One RCT provided insufficient evidence about the effects of oral thromboxane α_2 antagonists on ulcer healing.
- **Oral zinc** RCTs provided insufficient evidence about the effects of oral zinc on ulcer healing.
- **Skin grafting** RCTs provided insufficient evidence about the effects of skin grafting on ulcer healing.
- **Superficial vein surgery** Three RCTs found no evidence of a benefit associated with superficial vein surgery for ulcer healing. One systematic review identified one RCT which compared two forms of surgery. It found no difference between open surgery and endoscopic surgery in healing rates, but it found that higher rates of infection were associated with open surgery.
- **Therapeutic ultrasound** RCTs provided insufficient evidence about the effects of therapeutic ultrasound on ulcer healing.
- **Topical antimicrobial agents** RCTs provided insufficient evidence about the effects of topical antimicrobial agents on ulcer healing.

- **Topical calcitonin gene related peptide plus vasoactive intestinal polypeptide** One RCT provided insufficient evidence about the effects of topical calcitonin gene related peptide plus vasoactive intestinal polypeptide on ulcer healing.
- **Topical mesoglycan** One RCT provided insufficient evidence about the effects of topical mesoglycan on ulcer healing.
- **Topical negative pressure** RCTs provided insufficient evidence about the effects of topical negative pressure on ulcer healing.
- **Topical recombinant keratinocyte growth factor 2** RCTs provided insufficient evidence about the effects of topical recombinant keratinocyte growth factor 2 on ulcer healing.
- **Hydrocolloid (occlusive) dressings in the presence of compression** One systematic review found that, in the presence of compression, hydrocolloid dressings did not heal more venous leg ulcers than simple, low adherent dressings. One systematic review and two subsequent RCTs found no significant difference in healing rates between occlusive and semi-occlusive dressings.
- **Topically applied autologous platelet lysate** One RCT found no significant difference in the proportion of people with healed ulcers after 9 months between topically applied autologous platelet lysate compared with placebo.

Preventing recurrence

- **Compression stockings** RCTs found that compression stockings reduced recurrence at 6 months compared with no compression, but non-compliance with compression is a risk factor for recurrence.
- **Superficial vein surgery** Three RCTs provided evidence that superficial vein surgery with or without compression reduced recurrence compared with compression alone. One RCT identified by a systematic review compared open versus endoscopic surgery and found no recurrences in either group, but higher infection rates with open surgery. Vein surgery has the usual risks of surgery and anaesthesia.
- **Oral rutoside** One RCT identified by a systematic review provided insufficient evidence on the effects of oral rutoside versus placebo on ulcer recurrence.
- **Oral stanozolol** One RCT identified by a systematic review provided insufficient evidence on the effects of oral stanozolol versus placebo on ulcer recurrence.

DEFINITION Definitions of leg ulcers vary, but the following is widely used: loss of skin on the leg or foot that takes more than 6 weeks to heal. Some definitions exclude ulcers confined to the foot, whereas others include ulcers on the whole of the lower limb. This review deals with ulcers of venous origin in people without concurrent diabetes mellitus, arterial insufficiency, or rheumatoid arthritis.

INCIDENCE/ PREVALENCE Between 1.5 and 3.0/1000 people have active leg ulcers. Prevalence increases with age to about 20/1000 in people aged over 80 years.[1]

AETIOLOGY/ RISK FACTORS Leg ulceration is strongly associated with venous disease. However, about a fifth of people with leg ulceration have arterial disease, either alone or in combination with venous problems, which may require specialist referral.[1] Venous ulcers (also known as varicose or stasis ulcers) are caused by venous reflux or obstruction, both of which lead to poor venous return and venous hypertension.

PROGNOSIS People with leg ulcers have a poorer quality of life than age matched controls because of pain, odour, and reduced mobility.[2] In the UK, audits have found wide variation in the types of care (hospital inpatient care, hospital clinics, outpatient clinics, home visits), in the treatments used (topical agents, dressings, bandages, stockings), in healing rates, and in recurrence rates (26–69% in 1 year).[3,4]

AIMS OF INTERVENTION To promote healing; to reduce recurrence; to improve quality of life, with minimal adverse effects.

OUTCOMES Ulcer area; number of ulcers healed; time to complete ulcer healing; number of ulcer free limbs; recurrence rates; number of new ulcer episodes; number of ulcer free weeks or months; number of people who are ulcer free; frequency of dressing/bandage changes; quality of life; adverse effects of treatment.

METHODS *Clinical Evidence* search and appraisal July 2004.

QUESTION What are the effects of treatments?

OPTION COMPRESSION BANDAGES AND STOCKINGS

One systematic review and one additional RCT found that compression bandages or stockings healed more venous leg ulcers than no compression. One systematic review and one subsequent RCT found insufficient evidence to suggest a difference between multilayer elastomeric and non-elastomeric high compression bandages. One systematic review and four subsequent RCTs found no significant difference in healing rates between multilayer elastomeric high compression bandages and short stretch bandages or Unna's boot. One systematic review found that multilayer compression increased ulcer healing compared with single layer bandages. One systematic review and two subsequent RCTs found no significant difference in the proportion of people healed with four layer elastomeric bandages compared with other high compression multilayer bandages. We found insufficient evidence from one small RCT about the effects of compression bandages compared with intermittent pneumatic compression.

Benefits: **Compression bandages and stockings versus no compression:** We found one systematic review[5] and one additional RCT.[6] Overall, the studies found that compression (e.g. multilayer elastomeric high compression bandages❻, short stretch bandages❻, double layer bandages, compression stockings, or Unna's boot❻) healed more venous leg ulcers compared with no compression (dressing alone, non-compressive bandages, usual care). The review (search date 2000, 6 RCTs, 260 people) compared all forms of compression versus no compression.[5] The RCTs included in the review were heterogeneous, using different forms of compression in different settings and populations. Therefore, the results were not pooled. The first RCT (50 people) identified by the review found that compression healed significantly more ulcers compared with no compression (19/27 [70%] with compression *v* 6/23 [26%] with no compression; RR 2.70, 95% CI 1.30 to 5.60). The second RCT (34 people) identified by the review found no significant difference between compression and no compression in healing (9/17 [53%] with compression *v* 7/17 [41%] with no compression; RR 1.29, 95% CI 0.62 to 2.65). The third RCT (69 people) found that compression healed significantly more ulcers compared with no compression (21/30 [70%] with compression *v* 15/39 [38%] with no compression; RR 1.82, 95% CI 1.15 to 2.89). The fourth RCT (36 people) found that compression healed significantly more ulcers compared with no compression (18/19 [95%] with compression *v* 7/17 [41%] with no compression; RR 2.30 95% CI 1.29 to 4.10). The fifth RCT (42 people) found no significant difference between compression and no compression in healing (17/21 [81%] with compression *v* 15/21 [71%] with no compression; RR 1.13 95% CI 0.81 to 1.59). The sixth RCT (36 people) found that compression healed significantly more ulcers compared with no compression (12/18 [67%] with compression *v* 4/18 [22%] with no compression; RR 3.00, 95% CI 1.19 to 7.56). The additional RCT (200 people) found that four layer elastomeric high compression bandaging healed significantly more ulcers over 12 weeks compared with no compression (54% with compression *v* 34% with no compression; $P < 0.001$).[6] **Multilayer elastomeric versus non-elastomeric high compression bandages:** We found one systematic review (search date 2000, 3 RCTs, 273 people)[5] and one subsequent RCT.[7] The review found that elastomeric high compression bandaging significantly increased healing rates compared with non-elastomeric bandaging (77/134 [57%] with elastomeric compression *v* 52/139 [37%] with non-elastomeric compression; RR 1.54, 95% CI 1.19 to

2.00, NNT for variable periods of treatment 5, 95% CI 3 to 12) (see table 1, p 2526). The subsequent RCT (112 people) found no significant difference in healing rates between elastomeric and non-elastomeric layered compression (58% with elastomeric compression *v* 62% with non-elastomeric compression; P = 0.623).[7] **Multilayer elastomeric high compression bandages versus short stretch bandages or Unna's boot:** We found one systematic review (search date 2000, 4 small RCTs, 164 people)[5] and four subsequent RCTs (357 people).[13–16] The review found no significant difference in healing rate between multilayer elastomeric compression bandages and short stretch bandages or Unna's boot (37/83 [44%] with multilayer elastomeric bandages *v* 33/81 [41%] with short stretch bandages or Unna's boot; RR for 1.10, 95% CI 0.78 to 1.55).[5] The first subsequent RCT (116 people) found no significant difference in healing rates between four layer compression bandages and short stretch bandages (33/53 [62%] with compression bandages *v* 43/59 [73%] with short stretch bandages; P = 0.49).[13] The second subsequent RCT (89 people) found that four layer elastomeric multilayer compression bandages significantly increased healing compared with short stretch bandages at 12 weeks (30% with elastomeric multilayer compression bandages *v* 22% with short stretch bandages; HR 2.9, 95% CI 1.1 to 7.5).[14] The third subsequent RCT (156 people) found no significant difference in healing between four layer bandages and cohesive short stretch bandages over 24 weeks (51/74 [69%] with four layer bandages *v* 60/82 [73%] with cohesive short stretch bandages; HR 1.08, 95% CI 0.63 to 1.85).[15] The fourth subsequent RCT (68 people) found no difference in healing with a four layer bandage compared with Unna's boot at 24 weeks (hazard for healing in four layer: 1.62, 95% CI 0.87 to 3.02).[16] The lack of power in these small studies means that a clinically important difference cannot be excluded. **Multilayer elastomeric high compression bandages versus single layer bandage:** We found one systematic review (search date 2000, 4 RCTs, 280 people), which compared multilayer high compression bandages versus a single layer of bandage.[5] It found a significant increase in the proportion of people whose reference ulcer had healed with multilayer compression bandages compared with single layer bandages (82/139 [59%] with multilayer compression bandages *v* 59/141 [42%] with single layer bandages; RR 1.41, 95% CI 1.12 to 1.77; NNT for variable periods of treatment: 6, 95% CI 4 to 18) (see table 1, p 2526). **Multilayer elastomeric high compression regimens versus each other:** We found one systematic review (3 RCTs, 285 people)[5] and two subsequent RCTs.[17,18] The RCTs identified by the review compared the original "Charing Cross" four layer bandages versus other types of four layer compression, and one compared four layer versus three layer compression bandages. The review found no significant difference in the proportion of people healed with four layer elastomeric bandages compared with other high compression multilayer bandages (99/142 [70%] with four layer elastomeric bandages *v* 98/143 [68%] with other high compression multilayer bandages; RR 1.02, 95% CI 0.87 to 1.18).[5] The first subsequent RCT (133 people) found that three layer paste significantly increased healing rates compared with four layer bandages (80% with three layer paste *v* 65% with four layer bandage: P = 0.031), and reduced time to complete ulcer healing (median: 12 weeks with three layer paste *v* 16 weeks with four layer).[17] The second subsequent RCT (149 people) found no significant difference in healing rates between an original Charing Cross four layer bandage and two commercial "kits" making a four layer bandage at 20 weeks (87% with Charing Cross system *v* 84% and 83% with the two commercial kits; P = 0.56).[18] **Versus intermittent pneumatic compression:** See benefits of intermittent pneumatic compression, p 2512.

Harms: Complication rates were rarely reported in RCTs.[5,6,7,13,14,16,18] High levels of compression applied to limbs with insufficient arterial supply, or inexpert application of bandages, can lead to tissue damage and, at worst, amputation.[19] One observational study (194 people) found that four layer compression bandaging for several months was associated with toe ulceration in 12 (6%) people.[20]

Comment: People thought to be suitable for high compression bandages are those with clinical signs of venous disease (ulcer in the gaiter region, from the upper margin of the malleolus to the bulge of the gastrocnemius, staining of the skin around an ulcer, or eczema), no concurrent diabetes mellitus or rheumatoid arthritis, and adequate arterial supply to the foot as determined by ankle/brachial pressure index. The precise ankle/brachial pressure index below which compression is contraindicated is often quoted as 0.8; however, many RCTs used the higher cut off of 0.9.[5] Effectiveness is likely to be influenced by the ability of those applying the bandage to generate safe levels of compression. Bandages may be applied by the person with the leg ulcer, their carer, nurse, or doctor. We found no comparisons of healing rates between specialist and non-specialist application of compression. Training improves bandaging technique among nurses.[21] Bandages containing elastomeric fibres can be applied weekly as they maintain their tension over time. Bandages made of wool, cotton, or both, such as short stretch bandages**G**, may need to be reapplied more frequently as they do not maintain their tension.

OPTION INTERMITTENT PNEUMATIC COMPRESSION

One small RCT found insufficient evidence to compare intermittent pneumatic compression with compression bandages or stockings. One RCT found that intermittent pneumatic compression plus compression stockings improved ulcer healing at 3 months compared with compression stockings alone. Two other RCTs found no significant difference in healing at 6 months between intermittent pneumatic compression plus elastic stockings, and Unna's boot, and between intermittent pneumatic compression plus Unna's boot, and Unna's boot alone.

Benefits: **Versus compression bandages:** We found one systematic review (search date 2001, 1 RCT, 16 people).[22] The RCT identified by the review found no significant difference in the proportion of people with healed ulcers over 2–3 months between intermittent pneumatic compression**G** and compression bandages (0/10 with intermittent pneumatic compression *v* 0/6 with compression bandages), but it was probably too small to exclude a clinically important difference. **Plus compression stockings versus compression stockings or bandages alone:** We found one systematic review (search date 2001, 3 RCTs, 115 people).[22] The review did not perform a meta-analysis because of clinical and methodological heterogeneity among the trials. The first RCT identified by the review (45 people) found that intermittent pneumatic compression plus graduated compression stockings significantly increased the proportion of people with healed ulcers at 3 months compared with graduated compression stockings alone (10/21 [48%] with intermittent pneumatic compression plus graduated compression stockings *v* 1/24 [4%] with graduated compression stockings alone; RR 11.4, 95% CI 1.6 to 82.0). The second RCT (53 people) found no significant difference between intermittent pneumatic compression plus elastic stockings, and Unna's boot**G** in the proportion of people healed at 6 months (20/28 [71%] with intermittent pneumatic compression plus elastic stockings *v* 15/20 [75%] with Unna's boot; RR 0.95, 95% CI 0.67 to 1.34). The third RCT (22 people) found no significant difference in healing at 6 months between intermittent pneumatic compression plus Unna's boot and Unna's boot alone (12/12 [100%] with intermittent pneumatic compression plus Unna's boot *v* 8/10 [80%] with Unna's boot alone; RR 1.25, 95% CI 0.92 to 1.70).[22]

Harms: The RCTs identified by the review gave no information on adverse effects.[22]

Comment: Availability may vary widely in different health care settings. Treatment can be delivered in the home, in outpatient clinics, or in the hospital ward. RCTs have evaluated the use of intermittent pneumatic pressure**G** for 1 hour twice weekly and 3–4 hours daily. Treatment requires resting for 1–4 hours daily, which may reduce quality of life.

OPTION DRESSINGS

One systematic review provided insufficient evidence to compare the effects of semi-occlusive dressings (foam, film, hyaluronic acid-derived or alginate) versus simple low adherent dressings, in the presence of compression. The review found that, in the presence of compression, hydrocolloid dressings did not heal more venous leg ulcers than simple, low adherent dressings. One systematic review and two subsequent RCTs found no significant difference in healing rates between semi-occlusive and occlusive dressings.

Benefits: **Foam, film, hyaluronic acid-derived dressings or alginate (semi-occlusive) dressings versus simple low adherent dressings, in the presence of compression:** We found one systematic review (search date 1997, 5 RCTs)[23] and one subsequent RCT.[24] The review identified five RCTs comparing semi-occlusive dressings (foam, film, alginates) versus simple (traditional) low adherent dressings (such as paraffin-tulle or knitted viscose dressings).[23] The first RCT (71 people) identified by the review compared film versus saline soaked gauze. It found no significant difference between dressings in wound healing (11/36 [31%] with film *v* 8/35 [23%] with gauze; OR 1.48, 95% CI 0.5 to 4.3).[23] The second RCT (11 people, 12 ulcers) compared film versus Unna's boot**G**. It found that film significantly reduced the wound area compared with the simple dressing (mean reduction in wound area: 39% with film *v* 7% with traditional dressing; mean difference 32%, 95% CI 10% to 54%).[23] The third RCT (132 people) identified by the review compared foam versus a knitted viscose dressing. It found no significant difference between dressings in wound healing (31/66 [47%] with foam *v* 23/66 [35%] with knitted viscose; OR 1.67, 95% CI 0.80 to 3.30).[23] The fourth RCT (48 people) compared foam versus a sterile gauze compress. It found that foam significantly reduced the wound area compared with the sterile gauze (mean change in wound area: −66% with foam *v* +78% with sterile gauze; mean difference between treatments: 144%, 95% CI 49% to 239%).[23] The fifth RCT (60 people) compared an alginate dressing versus a knitted viscose dressing. It found no significant difference between dressings in wound healing (26/30 [87%] with alginate *v* 24/30 [80%] with knitted viscose; OR 1.62 95% CI 0.40 to 6.50).[23] However, the RCTs identified by this review may have been too small to detect anything but a very large difference in effectiveness. The subsequent RCT (17 people) compared hyaluronic dressings versus paraffin gauze. It found no significant difference between hyaluronic dressings and paraffin gauze in rates of ulcer healing (2/12 [17%] with hyaluronic dressing *v* 1/12 [8%] with paraffin gauze).[24] However this RCT may have been too small to detect anything but a very large difference in effectiveness. **Hydrocolloid (occlusive) dressings versus simple dressings, in the presence of compression:** We found one systematic review (search date 1997, 9 RCTs).[23] A pooled analysis of seven of the RCTs identified by the review

(714 people) found no significant difference in rates of ulcer healing between hydrocolloid dressings and simple low adherent dressings in the presence of compression (OR 1.45, 95% CI 0.83 to 2.54). **Comparisons between different occlusive or semi-occlusive dressings:** We found one systematic review (search date 1997, 12 small RCTs)[23] and two subsequent RCTs[25,26] comparing different occlusive or semi-occlusive dressings. The review found no significant difference in healing rates between dressings, or insufficient data were reported to calculate their significance.[23] The first subsequent RCT (40 people) compared hydrocolloid (occlusive) versus hydrocellular (semi-occlusive) dressings. It found no significant difference between treatments in healing rates at 8 weeks (8/20 [40%] in both groups; CI not reported).[25] The second subsequent RCT (91 people) compared two hydrocolloid dressings versus a foam dressing. It found no significant difference between treatments in healing rates at 12 weeks (58% and 55% with the two hydrocolloid dressings *v* 59% with foam dressing; CI not reported).[26]

Harms: The review and subsequent RCT gave no information on adverse effects.[23,24] It is unlikely that low adherent primary wound dressings cause harm, although dressings containing iodine may affect thyroid function if used over large surface areas for extended periods.[27] Many people (50–85%) with venous leg ulcers have contact sensitivity to preservatives, perfumes, or dyes.[28] The subsequent RCT reported that no serious adverse effects were observed with any of the treatments.[26]

Comment: Simple primary dressings maintain a moist environment beneath compression bandages by preventing loss of moisture from the wound.[29]

OPTION TOPICAL AGENTS

One systematic review provided insufficient evidence from small, heterogeneous RCTs about the effects of topical agents, such as growth factors, compared with inert comparators. One RCT found that cultured allogenic bilayer skin replacement increased complete ulcer healing at 6 months compared with non-adherent dressings. One RCT found no significant difference in the proportion of people with healed ulcers after 12 weeks' iontophoretic treatment with calcitonin gene related peptide plus vasoactive intestinal polypeptide compared with placebo. One RCT found no significant difference in the proportion of people with healed ulcers after 9 months between topical autologous platelet lysate and placebo. One RCT found no significant difference between topical mesoglycan and a plant based extract. One RCT found no significant difference in ulcer healing after 12 weeks between topical recombinant keratinocyte growth factor 2 and placebo. One RCT found no significant difference in ulcer healing with various doses of human dermal replacement plus compression compared with compression alone after 12 weeks. One systematic review provided insufficient evidence on the effects of topical negative pressure compared with usual care. One systematic review of small RCTs provided insufficient evidence to compare topical antimicrobial agents versus placebo or usual care or debriding agents versus traditional dressing or each other.

Benefits: We found one systematic review which provided insufficient evidence about the effects of topical agents, such as growth factors, compared with inert comparators.[23] The studies were small (9–233 people) and heterogeneous. Therefore, results could not be pooled. **Cultured allogenic bilayer skin replacement versus usual care:** We found one RCT (293 people).[30] It found that a cultured allogenic bilayer skin replacement®, containing both epidermal and dermal components, significantly increased the proportion of ulcers healed completely in 6 months compared with a simple non-adherent dressing (92/146 [63%]

with cultured allogenic bilayer skin replacement v 63/129 [49%] with non-adherent dressing; RR 1.29, 95% CI 1.04 to 1.60; NNT for 6 months' treatment 7, 95% CI 4 to 41) (see table 1, p 2526).[30] **Topical calcitonin gene related peptide plus vasoactive intestinal polypeptide versus placebo:** We found one RCT (66 people) which compared calcitonin (salcatonin) gene related peptide plus vasoactive intestinal polypeptide given by iontophoresis**G** with placebo iontophoresis.[31] It found no significant difference between treatments in the proportion of people with healed ulcers after 12 weeks (11/33 [37%] with calcitonin (salcatonin) gene related peptide plus vasoactive intestinal polypeptide v 6/33 [28%] with placebo; RR 1.83, 95% CI 0.77 to 4.38).[31] However, the RCT may have been too small to exclude a clinically important difference. **Topical mesoglycan versus a plant based extract:** We found one RCT (40 people) which found similar cure rates at 2 months between topically applied mesoglycan, a profibrinolytic agent, and a plant based extract (19/20 [95%] with topical mesoglycan v 16/20 [85%] with plant extract; CI not reported).[32] **Topically applied autologous platelet lysate versus placebo:** We found one RCT (86 people) which found no significant difference in the proportion of people healed at 9 months between topical autologous platelet lysate and placebo (33/42 [78%] with topical autologous platelet lysate v 34/44 [77%] with placebo; RR 1.05, 95% CI 0.80 to 1.30).[33] **Topical recombinant human keratinocyte growth factor 2 versus placebo:** We found one RCT (94 people) which compared topically applied recombinant human keratinocyte growth factor 2 (repifermin 20 or 60 μg/cm^2) versus placebo (beneath compression).[34] It found no significant difference in the rate of complete ulcer healing between human keratinocyte growth factor 2 and placebo after 12 weeks (32% with 20 μg/cm^2 v 38% with 60 μg/cm^2 v 29% with placebo; for all doses of human keratinocyte growth factor 2 v placebo, $P = 0.57$). **Cultured allogenic single layer dermal replacement versus usual care:** We found one RCT (53 people) which compared 12, four or one piece of human dermal replacement plus compression versus compression alone. It found no difference between treatments in the number of ulcers healed at 12 weeks (5/13 [38%] with 12 pieces v 5/13 [38%] with 4 pieces v 1/14 [7%] with 1 piece v 2/13 [15%] with compression alone). However this RCT may have been too small to detect anything but a very large difference in effectiveness.[35] **Topical negative pressure versus usual care:** We found one systematic review (search date 2002, 1 RCT, 24 people) which compared topical negative pressure**G** versus simple dressings.[36] The RCT identified by the review was carried out in people with any type of chronic wound but included some people with venous leg ulcers. However, it may have been too small to detect a clinically important difference in outcomes between topical negative pressure and simple dressings. **Topical antimicrobial agents versus placebo or usual care:** We found one systematic review (search date 1997, 14 RCTs) which compared antimicrobial agents versus either placebo or usual care.[37] The RCTs identified by the review were small (25–153 people), of poor quality, and no firm conclusions could be drawn. **Debriding agents versus usual care or versus each other:** We found one systematic review (search date 1997, 23 RCTs) which compared debriding agents versus traditional dressings.[38] The review did not perform a meta-analysis specifically in people with venous leg ulcers.[38] Six RCTs (277 people) identified by the review compared dextranomer polysaccharide bead dressings with traditional dressings, but only two RCTs reported complete ulcer healing. The incomplete reporting of healing rates and small sample sizes mean we cannot draw any firm conclusions from these trials. Seven RCTs (451 people) identified by the review compared cadexomer iodine versus traditional dressings, but only three RCTs reported complete ulcer healing. The incomplete reporting of healing rates means we cannot draw any firm conclusions from these trials. Two RCTs identified by the review compared enzymatic preparations versus traditional dressings (52 ulcers) and found no evidence of a difference in ulcer healing rates.[38] Four RCTs identified by the review compared debriding agents versus each other; two compared cadexomer iodine versus dextranomer (69 people), one compared cadexomer iodine versus hydrogel (95 people), and one compared dextranomer versus hyaluronic acid (50 people). The RCTs found no significant difference in ulcer healing with different debriding agents, but may have been too small to detect a clinically important difference.[38]

Harms: Preparations containing iodine may affect thyroid function if used over large surface areas for extended periods.[27] Many people (50–85%) with venous leg ulcers have contact sensitivity to preservatives, perfumes, or dyes.[28] **Topical recombinant human keratinocyte growth factor 2:** One RCT (94 people) found no significant difference in adverse effects (leg pain, pruritus, skin ulcer, rash abrasion, reopening of venous ulcer) between repifermin and placebo.[34] However, this study may have lacked power to detect a clinically important difference between groups. **Cultured allogenic dermal replacement versus usual care:** The incidence of adverse events was similar between groups (adverse events: 19 with 12 pieces *v* 15 with 4 pieces *v* 15 with 1 piece *v* 17 with usual care).[35]

Comment: None.

OPTION THERAPEUTIC ULTRASOUND

RCTs provided insufficient evidence about the effects of therapeutic ultrasound on ulcer healing.

Benefits: We found one systematic review (search date 1999, 7 RCTs, 470 people) comparing therapeutic ultrasound**G** with no ultrasound or sham ultrasound for venous leg ulcers.[8] Ultrasound improved ulcer healing in all studies, but a significant difference was found in only four of the seven RCTs, and heterogeneity precluded pooling the seven RCTs.

Harms: Mild and severe erythema, local pain, and small areas of bleeding were reported in RCTs identified by the review.[39,40]

Comment: None.

OPTION SYSTEMIC DRUG TREATMENTS

One systematic review and two subsequent RCTs found that oral pentoxifylline increased ulcer healing over 6–12 months in people receiving compression compared with placebo. Two RCTs found that adding oral flavonoids to compression increased the proportion of ulcers healed after 2–6 months compared with compression alone. One RCT found that peri-ulcer injections of granulocyte-macrophage colony stimulating factor increased complete healing after 13 weeks treatment compared with placebo. Two RCTs found that oral sulodexide plus compression increased the proportion of ulcers healed after 2–3 months' treatment compared with compression alone. One RCT found that systemic mesoglycan plus compression increased the proportion of ulcers healed after 24 weeks treatment compared with compression alone. RCTs found insufficient evidence on the effects of oral thromboxane α_2 antagonists, oral aspirin, oral rutosides, or oral zinc supplements.

Benefits: **Oral pentoxifylline:** We found one systematic review (search date 2001, 9 RCTs, 572 people)[41] and two subsequent RCTs.[9,42] The systematic review compared pentoxifylline (oxpentifylline) 1200 or 2400 mg daily versus placebo or versus other treatments, with or without compression.[41] It found that, in the presence of compression, pentoxifylline significantly increased the proportion of people with healed ulcers over 8–24 weeks compared with placebo (5 RCTs: 155/243 [64%] with pentoxifylline *v* 96/204 [47%] with placebo; RR 1.30, 95% CI 1.10 to 1.54; NNT for 6 months' treatment 6, 95% CI 4 to 14) (see table 1, p 2526). One RCT identified by the review found no significant difference in healing rates at 3 months between pentoxifylline and defibrotide in people receiving compression (11/12 [92%] with pentoxifylline *v* 9/11 [82%] with defibrotide; RR 1.12, 95% CI 0.81 to 1.55).[41] The two subsequent RCTs compared pentoxifylline (400 mg 3 times daily) versus placebo in people receiving compression.[9,42] The first RCT (172 people, 160 analysed) found that pentoxifylline for 6 months significantly increased rates of complete healing compared with placebo (55/82 [67%] with pentoxifylline *v* 24/78 [30.7%] with placebo; $P < 0.02$).[42] The second subsequent RCT (85 people, 80 analyzed) found that pentoxifylline for 12 months significantly increased rates of complete healing compared with placebo (complete healing: 36/41 [88%] with pentoxifylline *v* 17/39 [44%] with placebo; $P < 0.02$).[9] **Oral flavonoids:** We found two RCTs that compared micronised purified flavonoid fraction 1 g daily plus compression versus compression with or without placebo.[11,12] The first RCT (107 people) found no significant difference in cure rates at 2 months between adding flavonoids to compression and adding placebo (14/53 [26%] with flavonoids *v* 6/52 [11%] with placebo; RR 2.29, 95% CI 0.99 to 5.43).[11] It found that flavonoids significantly reduced time to healing of ulcers less than 10 cm^2 compared with placebo ($P = 0.037$). The second RCT (140 people) found that flavonoids plus compression significantly increased cure rates at 6 months compared with compression alone (33/71 [46.5%] with adding flavonoids *v* 19/69 [27.5%] with compression alone; OR 2.3, 95% CI 1.1 to 4.6).[12] **Peri-ulcer injection of granulocyte-macrophage colony stimulating factor:** One RCT (60 people) found that a 4 week course of injections of granulocyte-macrophage colony stimulating factor 200 or 400 μg around the ulcer significantly increased the proportion of people whose ulcers had completely healed after 13 weeks' treatment compared with placebo (23/39 [59%] with granulocyte-macrophage colony stimulating factor *v* 4/21 [19%] with placebo; Combined RR for 200 and 400 μg: 3.21, 95% CI 1.23 to 8.34; NNT for 13 weeks' treatment 2, 95% CI 1 to 7) (see table 1, p 2526).[43] **Oral sulodexide:** We found two RCTs (330 people).[44,45] The first RCT (235 people) found that adding sulodexide to compression significantly increased cure rates at 3 months compared with adding placebo (63/121 [52%] with adding sulodexide *v* 36/114 [32%] with adding placebo; RR 1.65, 95% CI 1.28 to 18.54).[44] The second RCT (140 people) also found that adding sulodexide to compression significantly increased cure rates at 2 months compared with compression alone (30/52 [58%] with adding sulodexide *v* 15/43 [35%] with adding placebo; RR 1.65, 95% CI 1.06 to 2.7) (see table 1, p 2526).[45] **Systemic mesoglycan:** We found one RCT (183 people) comparing systemic mesoglycan (daily im injection for 21 days and then orally for 21 weeks) plus compression versus placebo plus compression.[46] It found that systemic mesoglycan significantly increased the proportion of people with healed ulcers after 24 weeks' treatment compared with placebo (82/92 [89%] with mesoglycan *v* 69/91 [76%] with placebo; RR 1.17, 95% CI 1.03 to 1.35). **Oral thromboxane α_2 antagonists:** We found one RCT (165 people) comparing an oral thromboxane α_2 antagonist versus placebo. It found no significant difference in the proportion of ulcers healed (54% with thromboxane α_2 antagonist *v* 55% with placebo).[47] **Oral zinc:** We found one systematic review (search date 1997, 5 RCTs, 151 people) comparing daily doses of 440–660 mg oral zinc sulphate versus placebo.[48] The review found no evidence of benefit for oral zinc. **Oral aspirin:** We found one small RCT comparing aspirin (300 mg daily, enteric coated) versus placebo.[49] It found that aspirin increased ulcer healing rates compared with placebo (38% with aspirin *v* 0% with placebo), but the RCT had several methodological weaknesses so the result should be treated with caution. **Oral rutosides:** We found one report of two RCTs.[50] The RCTs (total of 119 people) compared two different doses of oral hydroxyethyl rutosides (500 and 1000 mg twice daily) with placebo. The RCTs found no significant difference between either dose of rutosides and placebo in rates of complete ulcer healing at 12 weeks (1 RCT, 55 people, 48 analyzed: 12/23 [52%] with 1 g/day rutoside *v* 7/25 [28%] with placebo; $P = 0.087$; results for the other RCT not reported). The RCTs may have been too small to detect a clinically important difference.

Harms: **Oral pentoxifylline:** The systematic review of oral pentoxifylline found no significant difference in adverse effects between pentoxifylline and placebo, although people taking pentoxifylline had more adverse effects (55/297 [18%] with pentoxifylline *v* 33/252 [13%] with placebo; RR 1.27, 95% CI 0.89 to 1.83).[41] Nearly half of the adverse effects were gastrointestinal (dyspepsia, vomiting, or diarrhoea). **Oral flavonoids:** Adverse effects of flavonoids, such as gastrointestinal disturbance, were reported in 10% of people.[11,12] **Oral rutosides:** One report of two RCTs (119 people) found no significant difference in adverse effects between oral rutosides and placebo (no details reported).[50] However, they may have lacked power to detect a clinically important difference between the groups.

Comment: Sulodexide is not widely available, and daily injections may be unacceptable to some people.

OPTION SUPERFICIAL VEIN SURGERY

Three RCTs found no evidence of a benefit associated with superficial vein surgery for ulcer healing. One systematic review identified one RCT which compared two forms of surgery. It found no difference between open surgery and endoscopic surgery in healing rates, but it found that higher rates of infection were associated with open surgery.

Benefits: **Surgery versus no surgery:** We found no systematic review. **Perforator ligation:** We found one RCT (47 people) which compared perforator ligation**G** versus no surgery or surgery plus skin grafting.[51] All participants were also treated with a compression bandage. The RCT found no significant difference in the number of ulcers healed after 1 year or in the time to complete ulcer healing (reported as $P > 0.05$ for both outcomes; see comment below).[51] The RCT is likely to have been underpowered to detect a clinically important difference among groups. **Minimally invasive surgery:** We found one RCT (45 people), which compared minimally invasive surgery**G** versus compression bandages.[52] People randomised to surgery were treated with a compression bandage before surgery. The RCT found high healing rates in both groups (100% with surgery *v* 96% with compression). It found that surgery significantly reduced time to complete healing compared with compression bandages (median: 31 days with surgery *v* 63 days with compression; $P < 0.005$).[52] **Venous surgery (based on duplex scan):** We found one RCT (341 people), which compared venous surgery (type of surgery based on duplex scan) plus compression versus compression alone.[53] The RCT found no significant difference in healing rates between treatments at 24 weeks (ulcer healing rates: 65% in both arms; HR for healing: 0.84, 95% CI 0.77 to 1.24).[53] **Open perforator surgery versus subfascial endoscopic perforator surgery:** We found one systematic review (search date 2003, 1 RCT, 39 people).[54] The RCT identified by the review found no significant difference between treatments in healing rates at 4 months (17/20 [85%] with subfascial endoscopic perforator surgery**G** *v* 17/19 [89%] with open surgery).[54,55]

Harms: The first RCT found no postoperative complications but may have been too small to detect clinically important adverse effects.[51] Two RCTs gave no information on adverse effects.[52,53] Vein surgery carries the usual risks of surgery and anaesthesia. One RCT (39 people) identified by a systematic review found higher wound infection rates with open surgery compared with subfascial endoscopic perforator surgery**G** (53% with open surgery *v* 0% with subfascial endoscopic perforator surgery; $P < 0.001$).[55] The review reported that deep vein thrombosis occurred in 1%, wound infection in 6%, neuralgia in 7%, and haematoma in 9% of all people with venous ulcers having surgical treatment involving subfascial endoscopic perforator surgery.[54]

Comment: The first RCT did not perform an intention to treat analysis and 7/47 (15%) people withdrew from the trial.[51] The second RCT randomised legs rather than people.[52] Several operative approaches are commonly used, including perforator ligation**G**, saphenous vein stripping, and a combination of both procedures. The RCT comparing open perforator surgery versus subfascial endoscopic surgery (SEPS) found that hospital stay was shorter with SEPS (4 days SEPS *v* 7 days open surgery).[55] Around 25% of people who were offered venous surgery in one study, refused it.[56]

OPTION SKIN GRAFTING

RCTs provided insufficient evidence about the effects of skin grafting on ulcer healing.

Benefits: We found one systematic review (search date 1999, 6 RCTs, 197 people) of skin grafts (autografts or allografts) for venous leg ulcers.[57] In five RCTs, people also received compression bandaging; two of the RCTs (98 people) evaluated split thickness autografts, three RCTs (92 people) evaluated cultured keratinocyte allografts, and one RCT (7 people, 13 ulcers) compared tissue engineered skin (artificial skin) with split thickness skin grafts. The review found insufficient evidence to determine whether skin grafting increased the healing of venous ulcers.[57]

Harms: Taking a skin graft leaves a wound that itself requires management and may cause pain. We found no evidence of harm from tissue engineered skin.[57]

Comment: None.

OPTION LASER (LOW LEVEL)

RCTs provided insufficient evidence about the effects of low level laser on ulcer healing.

Benefits: We found two systematic reviews[58,59] and two subsequent RCTs.[60,61] Two RCTs identified by the first review (search date 1998, 4 RCTs, 139 people)[58] compared low level laser treatment**G** versus sham treatment and found no significant difference in healing rates over 12 weeks (17/44 [39%] with laser treatment *v* 14/44 [32%] with sham treatment; RR 1.21, 95% CI 0.73 to 2.03). The third RCT (30 people) compared three interventions: low level laser treatment, low level laser treatment plus infrared light, and non-coherent, unpolarised red light. It found that significantly more ulcers healed completely after 9 months' treatment in the group receiving a combination of laser plus infrared light compared with non-coherent, unpolarised red light (12/15 [80%] with laser plus infrared light *v* 5/15 [33%] with non-coherent, unpolarised red light; RR 2.40, 95% CI 1.12 to 5.13). The fourth RCT compared laser versus ultraviolet light and found no significant difference in healing over 4 weeks.[58] The second review (search date 1999, 5 RCTs, 148 people)[59] identified but did not fully describe the four RCTs identified by the first review. The review did not perform a meta-analysis. The fifth RCT identified by the review (9 people, 12 venous leg ulcers) compared low level laser treatment versus sham treatment and found limited evidence that ulcer area reduction was greater with laser over 10 weeks (ulcer area remaining unhealed: 25% with laser treatment *v* 85% with sham treatment; CI not reported).[59] The RCT did not assess complete ulcer healing. The first subsequent RCT (15 people) compared low level laser treatment plus phototherapy once weekly for 4 weeks versus sham treatment.[60] It found no significant difference between laser and sham in ulcer area at 12 weeks ($P = 0.14$). The second subsequent RCT (65 people receiving compression and drug treatment) compared three interventions: low level laser, sham laser, and "no additional treatment" (although it is unclear if the "no additional treatment" was established by randomisation).[61] It found no significant difference between treatments in the change in area of ulceration (reduction in area: 4.25 cm^2 [27%] with laser *v* 5.21 cm^2 [39%] with sham laser *v* 2.98 cm^2 [18%] with no treatment; reported as non-significant, P value not reported).

Harms: Eye protection is required when using some types of laser, as the high energy beam may lead to damage of the retina.

Comment: The laser power, wavelength, frequency, duration, and follow up of treatment were different for all of the studies. The subsequent RCTs may have lacked power to detect clinically important differences between laser and sham treatment.

QUESTION What are the effects of interventions to prevent recurrence?

OPTION COMPRESSION BANDAGES AND STOCKINGS

RCTs found that compression stockings reduced recurrence at 6 months compared with no compression, but non-compliance with compression is a risk factor for recurrence.

Benefits: **Versus no compression:** We found one systematic review (search date 2000),[62] which found no RCTs comparing compression stockings versus no compression and one subsequent RCT.[63] The RCT (153 people) found that wearing compression stockings significantly reduced recurrence at 6 months compared with not wearing compression stockings (21% with compression stockings *v* 46% with no compression stockings; RR 0.46, 95% CI 0.28 to 0.76; NNT for 6 months' treatment 2, 95% CI 2 to 5).[63] **Versus other forms of compression:** We found one systematic review (search date 2000, 2 RCTs).[62] The first RCT identified by the review (166 people) compared two brands of UK Class 2 stockings (see comment below) and found no significant difference in recurrence. The second RCT identified by the review (300 people) compared Class 2 and Class 3 stockings (see comment below). With intention to treat analysis, the RCT found no significant reduction in recurrence after 5 years with high compression stockings (UK Class 3) compared with moderate compression stockings (UK Class 2). This analysis may underestimate the effectiveness of the Class 3 stockings because a significant proportion of people changed from Class 3 to Class 2. Both RCTs found that non-compliance with compression stockings was associated with recurrence.

Harms: The application of high compression to limbs with reduced arterial supply may result in ischaemic tissue damage and, at worst, amputation.[41]

Comment: Compression hosiery is classified according to the magnitude of pressure exerted at the ankle; the UK classification states that Class 2 stockings are capable of applying 18–24 mm Hg pressure and Class 3 are capable of applying 25–35 mm Hg pressure at the ankle. Other countries use different classification systems. Stockings reduce venous reflux by locally increasing venous pressure in the legs relative to the rest of the body. This effect only takes place while hosiery is worn. The association between non-compliance with compression and recurrence of venous ulceration provides some indirect evidence of the benefit of compression in prevention. People are advised to wear compression stockings for life and may be at risk of pressure necrosis from their compression stockings if they subsequently develop arterial disease. Regular reassessment of the arterial supply is considered good practice, but we found no evidence about the optimal frequency of assessment. Other measures designed to reduce leg oedema, such as resting with the leg elevated, may be useful.

OPTION SYSTEMIC DRUG TREATMENT

Two RCTs identified by a systematic review provided insufficient evidence on the effects of oral rutoside or oral stanozolol versus placebo on ulcer recurrence.

Benefits: **Oral rutoside:** We found one systematic review (search date 1997, 1 RCT, 139 people).[64] The RCT found no significant difference between rutoside and placebo in recurrence at 18 months (32% with rutoside *v* 34% with placebo; P = 0.93). **Oral stanozolol:** We found one systematic review (search date 1997, 1 RCT, 60 people).[64] The RCT found no significant difference between treatment with stanozolol and placebo for 6 months in ulcer recurrence (length of follow up not reported; recurrence in 7/25 [28%] legs with stanozolol *v* 4/23 [17%] legs with placebo; RR 1.61, 95% CI 0.54 to 4.79).[64]

Harms: The review gave no information on adverse effects.[64] One RCT (31 people with obstructive arm lymphoedema) found that rutoside was associated with headache, flushing, rashes, and mild gastrointestinal disturbances.[65] Stanozolol is an anabolic steroid; adverse effects include acne, hirsutism, amenorrhoea, oedema, headache, dyspepsia, rash, hair loss, depression, jaundice, and changes in liver enzymes.

Comment: None.

OPTION SUPERFICIAL VEIN SURGERY

Three RCTs provided evidence that superficial vein surgery with or without compression reduced recurrence compared with compression alone. One RCT identified by a systematic review compared open versus endoscopic surgery and found no recurrences in either group, but higher infection rates with open surgery. Vein surgery has the usual risks of surgery and anaesthesia.

Benefits: **Surgery plus compression versus compression alone:** We found one systematic review (search date 1997, 1 RCT)[64] and two subsequent RCTs.[52,53] The RCT (30 people) identified by the review compared surgery plus compression stockings versus compression stockings alone for prevention of recurrence (see comment below).[64] It found that surgery plus compression stockings significantly reduced recurrence rates compared with compression stockings alone (5% with surgery plus compression stockings *v* 24% with compression stockings alone; RR 0.21, 95% CI 0.03 to 0.80).[64] The first subsequent RCT (45 people) compared minimally invasive surgery**G** versus compression bandages.[52] People randomised to surgery wore compression stockings immediately after surgery and people randomised to compression wore compression stockings after ulcer healing was achieved. The RCT found that surgery significantly reduced recurrence rates over 3 years compared with compression (2/21 [10%] with surgery *v* 9/24 [38%] with compression bandages; $P < 0.05$).[52] The second subsequent RCT (428 people), which compared superficial vein surgery plus compression versus compression alone, found that after 12 months recurrence rates were significantly lower with surgery plus compression compared with compression alone (12% with surgery plus compression *v* 28% with compression alone; HR –2.76, 95% CI –1.78 to +4.27).[53] **Open versus endoscopic surgery:** We found one systematic review (search date 2003, 1 RCT, 39 people), which compared open surgery versus subfascial endoscopic perforator surgery**G**.[54] The RCT found no recurrences at 12 months in either group (data represented graphically).[55]

Harms: Only one RCT gave information on adverse effects.[55] It found that higher wound infection rates were associated with open surgery compared with subfascial endoscopic perforator surgery**G** (53% with open surgery *v* 0% with subfascial endoscopic perforator surgery; $P < 0.001$).[55] The systematic review found that deep vein thrombosis was reported in 1%, wound infection in 6%, neuralgia in 7%, and haematoma in 9% of all people having surgical treatment involving subfascial endoscopic perforator surgery.[54] Vein surgery has the usual risks of surgery and anaesthesia.

Comment: The results of the small RCT identified by the systematic review, which compared surgery plus compression versus compression alone, should be interpreted with caution because it was poorly controlled.[64] The subsequent small RCT randomised legs rather than people.[52]

GLOSSARY

Cultured allogenic bilayer skin replacement Also called human skin equivalent. This is made of a lower (dermal) layer of bovine collagen containing living human dermal fibroblasts and an upper (epidermal) layer of living human keratinocytes.

Intermittent pneumatic compression External compression applied by inflatable leggings or boots either over, or instead of, compression bandages or stockings. A pump successively inflates and deflates the boots to promote the return of blood from the tissues. Newer systems have separate compartments in the boots so that the foot is inflated before the ankle, which is inflated before the calf.

Iontophoresis The delivery of an ionic substance by application of an electrical current.

Laser treatment (low level) Application of treatment energy (< 10 J/cm^2) using lasers of 50 mW or less.

Minimally invasive surgery Surgery in which small incisions are made in the skin and the use of surgical instruments with cameras or direct viewing via eyepieces allows the surgeon to operate. Often performed under local anaesthetic and as a day case.

Multilayer elastomeric high compression bandages Usually a layer of padding material followed by one to four additional layers of elastomeric bandages.

Perforator ligation involves tying off the blood vessels which link the deep and superficial venous systems. The one way valves in these veins prevent flow from the deep to the superficial system. Malfunctioning perforator vessels may be responsible for increasing venous pressure in the superficial venous system, leading to ulceration.

Subfascial endoscopic perforator surgery (SEPS) is a minimally invasive endoscopic procedure, which eliminates the need for a large incision in the leg. An endoscope is used to directly visualise and tie off incompetent medial calf perforating veins to decrease venous reflux and reduce ambulatory venous pressure.

Short stretch bandages Minimally extensible bandages, usually made of cotton, with few or no elastomeric fibres. They are applied at near full extension to form a semirigid bandage.

Therapeutic ultrasound Application of ultrasound to a wound, using a transducer and a water based gel. Prolonged application can lead to heating of the tissues but, when used in wound healing, the power used is low and the transducer is constantly moved by the therapist, so that the tissue is not significantly heated.

Topical negative pressure Negative pressure (suction) applied to a wound through an open cell dressing (e.g. foam, felt).

Unna's boot An inner layer of zinc oxide impregnated bandage, which hardens as it dries to form a semirigid layer against which the calf muscle can contract. It is usually covered in an elastomeric bandage.

Substantive changes

Compression bandages and stockings Two RCTs added;[15,16] categorisation unchanged.

Dressings Two RCTs added;[24,26] categorisation unchanged.

Topical agents One RCT added;[35] categorisation unchanged.

Superficial vein surgery One systematic review[54] and two RCTs added;[53,55] categorisation of vein surgery for treatment unchanged.

Superficial vein surgery One systematic review[54] and two RCTs added;[53,55] categorisation of vein surgery for prevention of recurrence changed from Unknown effectiveness to Likely to be beneficial.

REFERENCES

1. Callam MJ, Ruckley CV, Harper DR, et al. Chronic ulceration of the leg: extent of the problem and provision of care. *BMJ* 1985;290:1855–1856.
2. Roe B, Cullum N, Hamer C. Patients' perceptions of chronic leg ulceration. In: Cullum N, Roe B, eds. *Leg ulcers: nursing management*. Harrow: Scutari, 1995:125–134.
3. Roe B, Cullum N. The management of leg ulcers: current nursing practice. In: Cullum N, Roe B, eds. *Leg ulcers: nursing management*. Harrow: Scutari, 1995:113–124.
4. Vowden KR, Barker A, Vowden P. Leg ulcer management in a nurse-led, hospital-based clinic. *J Wound Care* 1997;6:233–236.
5. Cullum N, Nelson EA, Fletcher AW, et al. Compression for venous leg ulcers. In: The Cochrane Library, Issue 4, 2003. Chichester, UK: John Wiley & Sons, Ltd. Search date 2000; primary sources 19 electronic databases, hand searches, and personal contacts.
6. O'Brien JF, Grace PA, Perry IJ, et al. Randomized clinical trial and economic analysis of four-layer compression bandaging for venous ulcers. *Br J Surg* 2003;90:794–798.
7. Meyer F, Burnand KG, McGuiness C, et al. Randomized clinical RCT comparing the efficacy of two bandaging regimens in the treatment of venous leg ulcer. *Br J Surg* 2002;89:40–44.
8. Flemming K, Cullum N. Therapeutic ultrasound for venous leg ulcers. In: The Cochrane Library, Issue 3, 2004. Oxford: Update Software. Search date 1999; primary sources Cochrane Wounds Group Specialised register and hand searches of citation lists.
9. De Sanctis MT, Belcaro G, Cesarone MR, et al. Treatment of venous ulcers with pentoxfylline: a 12-month double-blind placebo controlled trial. Microcirculation and healing. *Angiology* 2002;53:S49–S51.
10. Berliner E, Ozbilgin B, Zarin DA. A systematic review of pneumatic compression for treatment of chronic venous insufficiency and venous ulcers. *J Vasc Surg* 2003;37:539–544. Search date 2001; primary source Medline, Embase, Amed, hand searches from reference lists, and suggestions from experts.
11. Guilhou JJ, Dereure O, Marzin L, et al. Efficacy of Daflon 500 mg in venous leg ulcer healing: a double-blind, randomized, controlled versus placebo RCT in 107 patients. *Angiology* 1997;48:77–85.
12. Glinski W, Chodynicka B, Roszkiewicz J, et al. The beneficial augmentative effect of micronised purified flavonoid fraction (MPFF) on the healing of leg ulcers: an open, multicentre, controlled randomised study. *Phlebology* 1999;14:151–157.
13. Partsch H, Damstra RJ, Tazelaar DJ, et al. Multicentre, randomised controlled RCT of four-layer bandaging versus short-stretch bandaging in the treatment of venous leg ulcers. *VASA* 2001;30:108–113.
14. Ukat A, Konig M, Vanscheidt W, et al. Short-stretch versus multilayer compression for venous leg ulcers: a comparison of healing rates. *J Wound Care* 2003;12:139–143.
15. Franks PJ, Moody M, Moffatt CJ, et al. Randomized trial of cohesive short-stretch versus four-layer bandaging in the management of venous ulceration. *Wound Repair Regen* 2004;12:157–162.
16. Polignano R, Bonadeo P, Gasbarro S, et al. A randomised controlled study of four-layer compression versus Unna's Boot for venous ulcers. *J Wound Care* 2004;13:21–24.
17. Meyer FJ, Burnand KG, Lagattolla NRF, et al. More venous leg ulcers are healed by three-layer paste

than by four-layer bandages: a randomised, controlled, prospective study. Proceedings of the First World Wound Healing Congress, 74–75, 2000. Australian Wound Management Association.

18. Vowden KR, Mason A, Wilkinson D, et al. Comparison of the healing rates and complications of three four-layer bandage regimens. *J Wound Care* 2000;9:269–272.
19. Callam MJ, Ruckley CV, Dale JJ, et al. Hazards of compression treatment of the leg: an estimate from Scottish surgeons. *BMJ* 1987;295:1382.
20. Chan CLH, Meyer FJ, Hay RJ, et al. Toe ulceration associated with compression bandaging: observational study. *BMJ* 2001;323:1099.
21. Nelson EA, Ruckley CV, Barbenel J. Improvements in bandaging technique following training. *J Wound Care* 1995;4:181–184.
22. Mani R, Vowden K, Nelson EA. Intermittent pneumatic compression for treating venous leg ulcers. In: The Cochrane Library, Issue 4, 2003. Chichester, UK: John Wiley & Sons, Ltd. Search date 2001; primary sources The Cochrane Wound Group Trials Register and hand searches of journals, relevant conference proceedings and citations within obtained reviews and papers and personal contact with relevant companies.
23. Bradley M, Cullum N, Nelson EA, et al. Dressings and topical agents for healing of chronic wounds: a systematic review. *Health Technol Assess* 1999;3(17 Pt 2):1–35. Search date 1997; primary sources Cochrane Library, Medline, Embase, and Cinahl.
24. Taddeucci P, Pianigiani E, Colletta V, et al. An evaluation of Hyalofill-F plus compression bandaging in the treatment of chronic venous ulcers. *J Wound Care* 2004;13:202–204.
25. Seeley J, Jensen JL, Hutcherson J. A randomised clinical study comparing a hydrocellular dressing to a hydrocolloid dressing in the management of pressure ulcers. *Ostomy Wound Manage* 1999;45:39–47.
26. Charles H, Callicot C, Mathurin D, et al. Randomised, comparative study of three primary dressings for the treatment of venous ulcers. *Br J Community Nurs* 2002;7:48–54.
27. Thomas S. *Wound management and dressings*. London: Pharmaceutical Press, 1990.
28. Cameron J, Wilson C, Powell S, et al. Contact dermatitis in leg ulcer patients. *Ostomy Wound Manage* 1992;38:10–11.
29. Wu P, Nelson EA, Reid WH, et al. Water vapour transmission rates in burns and chronic leg ulcers: influence of wound dressings and comparison with in vitro evaluation. *Biomaterials* 1996;17:1373–1377.
30. Falanga V, Margolis D, Alvarez O, et al. Rapid healing of venous ulcers and lack of clinical rejection with an allogeneic cultured human skin equivalent. Human Skin Equivalent Investigators Group. *Arch Dermatol* 1998;134:293–300.
31. Gherardini G, Gurlek A, Evans GRD, et al. Venous ulcers: improved healing by iontophoretic administration of calcitonin gene-related peptide and vasoactive intestinal polypeptide. *Plast Reconstr Surg* 1998;101:90–93.
32. La Marca G, Pumilia G, Martino A. Effectiveness of mesoglycan topical treatment of leg ulcers in subjects with chronic venous insufficiency. *Minerva Cardioangiol* 1999;47:315–319.
33. Stacey MC, Mata SD, Trengove NJ, et al. Randomised double-blind placebo controlled RCT of autologous platelet lysate in venous ulcer healing. *Eur J Vasc Endovasc Surg* 2000;20:296–301.
34. Robson MC, Phillips TJ, Falanga V, et al. Randomized trial of topically applied repifermin (recombinant human keratinocyte growth factor-2) to accelerate wound healing in venous ulcers. *Wound Repair Regen* 2001;9:347–352.
35. Krishnamoorthy L, Harding K, Griffiths D, et al. The clinical and histological effects of Dermagraft in the healing of chronic venous leg ulcers. *Phlebology* 2003;18:12–22.
36. Evans D, Land L. Topical negative pressure for treating chronic wounds. In: The Cochrane Library, Issue 3, 2004. Chichester, UK: John Wiley & Sons, Ltd. Search date 2002; primary sources Cochrane Wounds Group specialised register, contact with experts and relevant companies, and hand searches.
37. O'Meara S, Cullum N, Majid M, et al. Systematic reviews of wound care management: (3) antimicrobial agents for chronic wounds. *Health Technol Assess* 2000;4:1–237. Search date 1997; primary sources Cochrane Library, Medline, Embase, and Cinahl.
38. Bradley M, Cullum N, Sheldon T. The debridement of chronic wounds: a systematic review. *Health Technol Assess* 1999;3(17 Pt 1):1–78. Search date 1997; primary sources 19 electronic databases (including the Cochrane Wounds Group Specialised Register); hand searches of specialist wound care journals, conference proceedings, and bibliographies of retrieved relevant publications; and personal contact with appropriate companies and an advisory panel of experts.
39. Peschen M, Vanscheidt W. Low frequency ultrasound of chronic venous leg ulcers as part of an out-patient treatment [abstract]. In: Cherry GW, Gottrup F, Lawrence JC, et al. *Fifth European Conference on Advances in Wound Management*. Macmillan, 1996.
40. Weichenthal M, Mohr P, Stegmann W, et al. Low-frequency ultrasound treatment of chronic venous ulcers. *Wound Repair Regen* 1997;5:18–22.
41. Jull AB, Waters J, Arroll B. Oral pentoxifylline for treatment of venous leg ulcers. In: The Cochrane Library, Issue 3, 2004. Chichester, UK: John Wiley & Sons, Ltd. Search date 2001; primary sources Cochrane Peripheral Vascular Diseases and Wounds Group Specialised Registers; hand searches of reference lists, relevant journals, and conference proceedings; and personal contact with manufacturer of pentoxifylline and experts in the field.
42. Belcaro G, Cesarone MR, Nicolaides AN, et al. Treatment of venous ulcers with pentoxifylline: a 6-month randomized double-blind placebo controlled trial. *Angiology* 2002;53:S45–S47.
43. Da Costa RM, Ribeiro Jesus FM, Aniceto C, et al. Randomized, double-blind, placebo-controlled, dose-ranging study of granulocyte-macrophage colony stimulating factor in patients with chronic venous leg ulcers. *Wound Repair Regen* 1999;7:17–25.
44. Coccheri S, Scondotto G, Agnelli G, et al. Randomised, double blind, multicentre, placebo controlled study of sulodexide in the treatment of venous leg ulcers. *Thromb Haemost* 2002;87:947–952.
45. Scondotto G, Aloisi D, Ferrari P, et al. Treatment of venous leg ulcers with sulodexide. *Angiology* 1999;50:883–889.
46. Arosio E, Ferrari G, Santoro F, et al. A placebo-controlled, double blind study of mesoglycan in the treatment of chronic venous ulcers. *Eur J Vasc Endovas Surg* 2001;22:365–372.
47. Lyon RT, Veith FJ, Bolton L, et al. Clinical benchmark for healing of chronic venous ulcers. Venous Ulcer Study Collaborators. *Am J Surg* 1998;176:172–175.
48. Wilkinson EAJ, Hawke CI. Does oral zinc aid the healing of chronic leg ulcers? A systematic literature review. *Arch Dermatol* 1998;134:1556–1560. Search date 1997; primary sources Medline, Embase, Cinahl, Science Citation Index, Biosis, British Diabetic Association Database, Ciscom, Cochrane Controlled Register of Clinical RCTs, Dissertation Abstracts, Royal College of Nursing Database, electronic databases of ongoing research, hand searches of wound care journals and conference proceedings, and contact with manufacturer of zinc sulphate tablets.
49. Layton AM, Ibbotson SH, Davies JA, et al. Randomised RCT of oral aspirin for chronic venous leg ulcers. *Lancet* 1994;344:164–165.
50. Schultz-Ehrenburg U, Müller B. Two multicentre clinical trials of two different dosages of O-β-hydroxyethyl)-rutosides in the treatment of leg ulcers. *Phlebology* 1993;8:29–30.

51. Warburg FE, Danielsen L, Madsen SM, et al. Vein surgery with or without skin grafting versus conservative treatment for leg ulcers. *Acta Dermatol Venereol* 1994;74:307–309.
52. Zamboni P, Cisno C, Marchetti F, et al. Minimally invasive surgical management of primary venous ulcers vs. compression treatment: a randomized clinical trial. *Eur J Vasc Endovasc Surg* 2003;25:313–318.
53. Barwell JR, Davies CE, Deacon J, et al. Comparison of surgery and compression with compression alone in chronic venous ulceration (ESCHAR study): randomised controlled trial. *Lancet* 2004;363:1854–1859.
54. Tenbrook JA Jr, Iafrati MD, O'Donnell TF Jr, et al. Systematic review of outcomes after surgical management of venous disease incorporating subfascial endoscopic perforator surgery. *J Vasc Surg* 2004;39:583–589. Search date 2003, primary sources Medline (restricted to English studies), reference lists of review articles and retrieved studies, and consultation with local experts.
55. Pierik EG, van Urk H, Hop WC, et al. Endoscopic versus open subfascial division of incompetent perforating veins in the treatment of venous leg ulceration: a randomized trial. *J Vasc Surg* 1997;26:1049–1054.
56. Ghauri AS, Nyamekye I, Grabs AJ, et al. Influence of a specialised leg ulcer service and venous surgery on the outcome of venous leg ulcers. *Eur J Vasc Endovasc Surg* 1998;16:238–244.
57. Jones JE, Nelson EA. Skin grafting for venous leg ulcers. In: The Cochrane Library, Issue 3, 2004. Chichester, UK: John Wiley & Sons, Ltd. Search date 1999; primary sources Cochrane Wounds Group specialised register; hand searches of reference lists, relevant journals, and conference proceedings; and personal contact with experts in the field.
58. Flemming K, Cullum N. Laser therapy for venous leg ulcers. In: The Cochrane Library, Issue 3, 2004. Chichester, UK: John Wiley & Sons, Ltd. Search date 1998; primary sources 19 electronic databases and hand searches of journals, conference proceedings, and bibliographies.
59. Schneider WL, Hailey D. Low level laser therapy for wound healing. Alberta Heritage Foundation Report 1999. Search date 1999; primary sources Medline, Healthstar, Embase, Dissertation Abstracts, Current Contents, Cinahl, Cochrane Library, and the Internet.
60. Lagan KM, McKenna T, Witherow A, et al. Low-intensity laser therapy/combined phototherapy in the management of chronic venous ulceration: a placebo-controlled study. *J Clin Laser Med Surg* 2002;20:109–116.
61. Franek A, Krol P, Kucharzewski M. Does low output laser stimulation enhance the healing of crural ulceration? Some critical remarks. *Med Eng Phys* 2002;24:607–615.
62. Cullum N, Nelson EA, Flemming K, et al. Systematic reviews of wound care management: (5) beds; (6) compression; (7) laser therapy, therapeutic ultrasound, electrotherapy and electromagnetic therapy. *Health Technol Assess* 2001;5;1–221. Search date 2000; primary sources Cochrane Wounds Group specialised register, 19 electronic databases (up to December 1999); hand searches of relevant journals, conference proceedings, and bibliographies of retrieved publications; and personal contact with manufacturers and an advisory panel of experts.
63. Vandongen YK, Stacey MC. Graduated compression elastic stockings reduce lipodermatosclerosis and ulcer recurrence. *Phlebology* 2000;15:33–37.
64. Cullum N, Fletcher A, Semlyen A, et al. Compression therapy for venous leg ulcers. *Qual Health Care* 1997;6:226–231. Search date 1997; primary sources 18 databases, including Medline, Embase, Cinahl with no restriction on date, hand searches of relevant journals, conference proceedings, and correspondence with experts to obtain unpublished papers.
65. Taylor HM, Rose KE, Twycross RG. A double-blind clinical RCT of hydroxyethylrutosides in obstructive arm lymphoedema. *Phlebology* 1993;8:22–28.

E Andrea Nelson
Senior Research Fellow
Centre for Evidence Based Nursing
Department of Health Sciences
University of York
York
UK

Nicky Cullum
Professor
Centre for Evidence Based Nursing
Department of Health Sciences
University of York
York
UK

June Jones
Clinical Nurse Specialist
Southport and Formby PCT
Southport
UK

Competing interests: EAN and NC are applicants on a RCT of compression bandages for which Beirsdorf UK Ltd provided RCT related education. EAN, NC and JJ are authors of systematic reviews included in this review. EAN is an author of additional studies referenced in the chapter (references 21 and 22). JJ has been reimbursed for attending symposia by Activia Healthcare.

TABLE 1 **Number needed to treat for healing of leg ulcers (see text,** **p 2511)**

Intervention	NNT (95% CI)
Multilayer elastomeric compression *v* non–elastomeric compression bandages	5 (3 to 12)[5]
Multilayer high compression *v* single layer compression bandages	6 (4 to 18)[5]
Pentoxifylline 400 mg 3 times daily *v* placebo (concurrent use of compression)	6 (4 to 14)[41]
Peri–ulcer injection of GM–CSF (400 μg) *v* placebo	2 (1 to 7)[43]
Cultured allogenic bilayer skin equivalent *v* non–adherent dressing	7 (4 to 41)[30]
Sulodexide plus compression *v* compression alone	4 (3 to 9)[44,45]

Key: GM–CSF, granulocyte–macrophage colony stimulating factor.

Note

When looking up a class of drug, the reader is advised to also look up specific examples of that class of drug where additional entries may be found. The reverse situation also applies. Abbreviations used: CVD, cardiovascular disease; HRT, hormone replacement therapy; IVF, in vitro fertilisation; MI, myocardial infarction; NSAIDs, non-steroidal anti-inflammatory drugs; STD, sexually transmitted disease.

INDEX

Subject index

Subject index

Subject index

Subject index

Subject index

Subject index

Subject index

Subject index

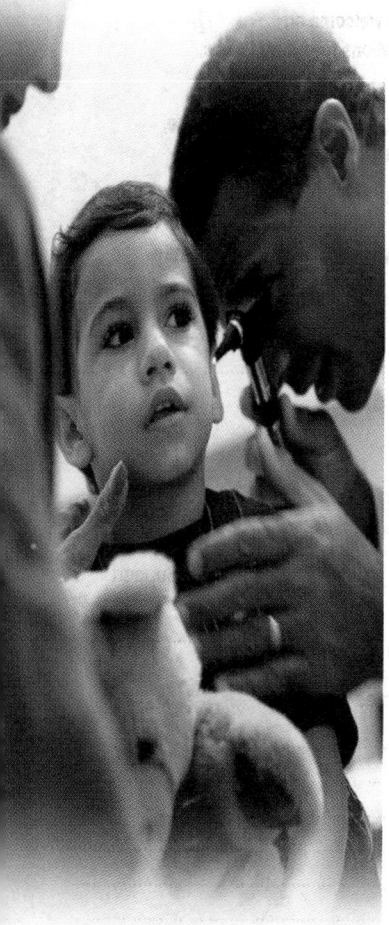

Clinical evidence comments

Clinical Evidence is an evolving resource and we welcome any feedback on the content of this issue and suggestions for future issues.

Please photocopy and complete this form, then return it to us.

For UK and rest of world - Fax: + 44 (0) 20 7383 6242, mail: BMJ Clinical Evidence, BMJ Publishing Group, BMA House, Tavistock Square, London WC1H 9JR, UK

For North and South America - Fax: 1-240-646-7005, mail: BMJ Clinical Evidence, PO Box 512, Annapolis Jct, MD20701-0512, USA

Alternatively, email us at CEfeedback@bmjgroup.com

Name: ....

Address: ....

....

....Email: ....

Position

- ☐ GP/Primary Care Physician
- ☐ Hospital Doctor/ Specialist Physician
- ☐ Pharmacist
- ☐ Resident/Registrar
- ☐ Nurse
- ☐ PAM
- ☐ Manager
- ☐ Press
- ☐ Researcher
- ☐ Administrator
- ☐ Librarian
- ☐ Medical Student
- ☐ Member of Public/ Patient Support Group
- ☐ Other.........................

1. Comments concerning the selection of studies

Section..

Topic ....

Reference ....

Comment..

....

....

2. Suggestions for future issues

....

....

....

3. Other comments/questions

....

....

....

Clinical evidence issue 13